SEVENTH EDITION

BAUM'S TEXTBOOK OF PULMONARY DISEASES

SEVENTH EDITION

BAUM'S TEXTBOOK OF PULMONARY DISEASES

EDITORS

James D. Crapo, MD

Chairman, Department of Medicine
Executive Vice President of Academic Affairs
National Jewish Medical and Research Center
Denver, Colorado

Jeffrey Glassroth, MD

George R. and Elaine Love Professor and Chair
Department of Medicine
University of Wisconsin–Madison
Chair, Department of Medicine
University of Wisconsin Hospitals and Clinics
Madison, Wisconsin

Joel B. Karlinsky, MD, MBA

Professor of Medicine
Department of Pulmonary and Critical Care Medicine
Boston University School of Medicine
Boston, Massachusetts
Director, Pulmonary Outpatient Services
Department of Pulmonary and Critical Care Medicine
VA Boston Healthcare System
West Roxbury, Massachusetts

Talmadge E. King, Jr., MD

The Constance B. Wofsy Distinguished Professor
Department of Medicine
University of California, San Francisco
Chief, Medical Services
Department of Medicine
San Francisco General Hospital
San Francisco, California

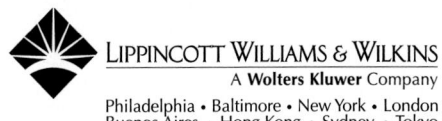

LIPPINCOTT WILLIAMS & WILKINS
A **Wolters Kluwer** Company
Philadelphia • Baltimore • New York • London
Buenos Aires • Hong Kong • Sydney • Tokyo

Acquisitions Editor: Danette Somers
Developmental Editor: Michelle M. LaPlante
Manufacturing Manager: Benjamin Rivera
Production Editor: Timothy Prairie
Cover Designer: Karen Quigley
Compositor: TechBooks
Printer: Maple Press

Printed in United States of America

9 8 7 6 5 4 3 2 1

Library of Congress Cataloging-in-Publication Data

Baum's textbook of pulmonary diseases.—7th ed./editors, James D. Crapo . . . [et al.].
   p. ; cm.
   Rev. ed. of: Textbook of pulmonary diseases. 6th ed. c1998.
   Includes bibliographical references and index.
   ISBN 0-7817-3727-3 (alk. paper)
   1. Lungs—Diseases.   2. Pleura—Diseases.   I. Title: Textbook of pulmonary diseases.
II. Baum, Gerald L.   III. Crapo, James D.
   [DNLM: 1. Lung Diseases. WF 600 B3471 2004]
RC756.T48   2004
616.2′4—dc21   2003047508

To Donald F. Tierney, who introduced me to the challenges of pulmonary medicine and exposed me to the excitement of exploring new frontiers in knowledge.
James D. Crapo, MD

To Gordon Snider and Dixie E. Snider, Jr., two men with the same last name and one student in common and to the late Larry Farer, a mentor and friend.
Jeffrey Glassroth, MD

To my wife and children.
Joel B. Karlinsky, MD, MBA

To my parents, Talmadge and Almetta, for instilling in me the values of hard work and education and to my mother-in-law, Ida Spann, for her love and encouragement.
Talmadge E. King, Jr., MD

CONTENTS

CONTRIBUTING AUTHORS

Muzaffar Ahmad, MD   Professor of Medicine, Department of Pulmonary and Critical Care Medicine, The Cleveland Clinic, Cleveland, Ohio

Vivek N. Ahya, MD   Associate Professor of Medicine, Pulmonary, Allergy, and Critical Care Division, University of Pennsylvania; Associate Medical Director, Lung Transplantation Program, University of Pennsylvania Medical Center, Philadelphia, Pennsylvania

James N. Allen, MD   Associate Professor, Pulmonary and Critical Care Medicine, Ohio State University; Battelle Professor of Pulmonary Therapy, Department of Internal Medicine, Ohio State University Medical Center, Columbus, Ohio

Nicholas R. Anthonisen, MD, PhD   Professor, Department of Medicine, University of Manitoba; Department of Medicine, Respiratory Hospital, Winnipeg, Manitoba, Canada

Veena B. Antony, MD   B. Calvin H. English Professor of Medicine, Department of Medicine Indiana University School of Medicine; Chief, Pulmonary and Critical Care Medicine, Richard L. Roudebush VA Medical Center, Indianapolis, Indiana

Safwan Badr, MD   Professor of Medicine and Biomedical Engineering, Chief, Division of Pulmonary, Critical Care, and Sleep Medicine, Department of Internal Medicine, Wayne State University School of Medicine; Chief, Section of Pulmonary and Critical Care, Harper University Hospital, Detroit, Michigan

Peter J. Barnes, DM, DSc, FRCP   Head, Department of Thoracic Medicine, National Heart and Lung Institute, Imperial College, London, United Kingdom

William S. Beckett, MD, MPH   Professor, Department of Environmental Medicine and Medicine, University of Rochester School of Medicine; Medical Staff, Department of Environmental Medicine and Pulmonary Medicine, Strong Memorial Hospital, Rochester, New York

Jeffrey S. Berman, MD   Professor of Medicine, Pulmonary Center, Boston University School of Medicine; Chief, Department of Pulmonary and Critical Care, Boston VA Healthcare Systems, West Roxbury, Massachusetts

Richard J. Blinkhorn, Jr., MD   Associate Professor, Department of Medicine, Case Western Reserve University; Vice Chairman, Department of Medicine, MetroHealth Medical Center, Cleveland, Ohio

Esteban González Burchard, MD   Assistant Professor of Medicine, Department of Pulmonary and Critical Care Medicine, University of California, San Francisco; Staff Physician, Department of Pulmonary and Critical Care Medicine, San Francisco General Hospital, San Francisco, California

Marco Chilosi, MD   Professor, Department of Pathology, Universitá di Verona, Verona, Italy

James D. Crapo, MD   Chairman, Department of Medicine, Executive Vice President of Academic Affairs, National Jewish Medical and Research Center, Denver, Colorado

Robert O. Crapo, MD   Professor of Medicine, Pulmonary Department, University of Utah; Medical Director, Pulmonary Lab, LDS Hospital, Salt Lake City, Utah

Christopher J. Crnich, MD   Fellow, Department of Infectious Diseases, University of Wisconsin Hospitals and Clinics, Madison, Wisconsin

Scott F. Davies, MD   Professor of Medicine, Department of Pulmonary and Critical Care Medicine, Hennepin County Medical Center, Minneapolis, Minnesota

Stephen L. Demeter, MD   Professor of Medicine, Head, Pulmonary Division, Northeastern Ohio Universities College of Medicine, Rootstown, Ohio

Tushar J. Desai, MD, MPH   Department of Internal Medicine, The Pulmonary Center, Boston Medical Center; Division of Pulmonary and Critical Care Medicine, VA New England Healthcare System, Boston Division, Boston, Massachusetts

Raed A. Dweik, MD   Staff Physician, Department of Pulmonary and Critical Care Medicine, Cleveland Clinic Foundation, Cleveland, Ohio

Jack A. Elias, MD   Chief, Pulmonary and Critical Care Medicine, Yale University School of Medicine, New Haven, Connecticut

Gary R. Epler, MD   Clinical Associate Professor, Department of Medicine, Harvard Medical School; Department of Pulmonary and Critical Care Medicine, Brigham and Women's Hospital, Boston, Massachusetts

Scott K. Epstein, MD   Associate Professor of Medicine, Tufts University School of Medicine; Director, Medical Intensive Care Unit, Department of Pulmonary, Critical Care, and Sleep, Tufts-New England Medical Center, Boston, Massachusetts

John L. Faul, MD   Assistant Professor, Division of Pulmonary and Critical Care Medicine, Stanford University Medical Center, Stanford, California

Michael C. Fiore, MD, MPH   Professor, Department of Medicine, Director, Center for Tobacco Research and Intervention, University of Wisconsin Medical School, Madison, Wisconsin

Andrew P. Fontenot, MD   Assistant Professor, Department of Medicine, University of Colorado Health Sciences Center, Denver, Colorado

Wolfgang Frank, MD   Johanniter-Krankenhaus Treuenbrietzen, Pneumologische Klinik III, Treuenbrietzen, Germany

Suzette Garofano, MD   Clinical Assistant Professor, Department of Medicine, New York University Medical School; Clinical Assistant Attending, Department of Medicine, New York University Medical Center, New York, New York

Jeffrey Glassroth, MD   George R. and Elaine Love Professor and Chair, Department of Medicine, University of Wisconsin-Madison; Chair, Department of Medicine, University of Wisconsin Hospitals and Clinics, Madison, Wisconsin

David R. Graham, MD   Dean of Postgraduate Education, University of Liverpool Medical School, Liverpool, United Kingdom

Colin K. Grissom, MD   Assistant Professor, Division of Pulmonary and Critical Care, Department of Medicine, University of Utah School of Medicine; Critical Care Attending, Division of Pulmonary and Critical Care, Department of Medicine, LDS Hospital, Salt Lake City, Utah

Thomas J. Gross, MD   Associate Professor, Department of Internal Medicine, Roy J. and Lucille A. Carver College of Medicine; Director, Medical Intensive Care Unit, Department of Internal Medicine, University of Iowa Health Care, Iowa City, Iowa

Ronald F. Grossman, MD, FRCPC, FACP, FCCP   Professor, Department of Medicine, University of Toronto, Toronto, Ontario; Chief, Department of Medicine, Credit Valley Hospital, Mississauga, Ontario, Canada

James E. Hansen, MD   Professor, Department of Medicine, University of California, Los Angeles School of Medicine, Los Angeles, California; Professor, Department of Medicine, Harbor-UCLA Medical Center, Torrance, California

John E. Heffner, MD   Professor, Department of Medicine, Medical University of South Carolina; Medical Director, Division of Pulmonary and Critical Care Medicine, Medical University Hospital, Charleston, South Carolina

Tim Higenbottam, MA, MD, DSc, FRCP   Professor of Medicine, Department of Clinical Science (South), University of Sheffield; Honorary Consultant Physician, Department of Respiratory Medicine, Royal Hallamshire Hospital, Sheffield, United Kingdom

Nicholas S. Hill, MD   Professor of Medicine, Pulmonary, Critical Care, and Sleep Division, Tufts University School of Medicine; Chief, Pulmonary, Critical Care, and Sleep Division, Tufts-New England Medical Center, Boston, Massachusetts

Gary W. Hunninghake, MD   Sterba Professor of Medicine, Department of Internal Medicine, Roy J. and Lucille A. Carver College of Medicine and Veterans Administration Medical Center; University of Iowa Hospitals and Clinics and Veterans Administration Medical Center, Iowa City, Iowa

Bruce D. Johnson, PhD   Associate Professor of Medicine, Department of Internal Medicine, Division of Cardiovascular Diseases, Mayo Clinic and Foundation, Rochester, Minnesota

Douglas E. Jorenby, PhD   Associate Professor, Department of Medicine, University of Wisconsin Medical School; Director of Clinical Services, Center for Tobacco Research and Intervention, University of Wisconsin Medical School, Madison, Wisconsin

Joel B. Karlinsky, MD, MBA   Professor of Medicine, Department of Pulmonary and Critical Care Medicine, Boston University School of Medicine, Boston, Massachusetts; Director, Pulmonary Outpatient Services, Department of Pulmonary and Critical Care Medicine, VA Boston Healthcare System, West Roxbury, Massachusetts

Jason Kelley, MD   Professor and Deputy Chairman, Department of Medicine, University of Louisville; Chief of Medicine Service, Louisville Veteran Affairs Hospital, Louisville, Kentucky

Talmadge E. King, Jr., MD   The Constance B. Wofsy Distinguished Professor, Department of Medicine, University of California, San Francisco; Chief, Medical Services, Department of Medicine, San Francisco General Hospital, San Francisco, California

Masanori Kitaichi, MD   Associate Professor, Department of Anatomical Pathology, Kyoto University; Acting Chief, Department of Anatomical Pathology, Kyoto University Hospital, Kyoto, Japan

James R. Klinger, MD   Associate Professor, Department of Medicine, Brown Medical School; Medical Director, Respiratory Care Unit, Department of Pulmonary and Critical Care Medicine, Rhode Island Hospital, Providence, Rhode Island

Robert M. Kotloff, MD   Associate Professor of Medicine, Pulmonary, Allergy, and Critical Care Division, University of Pennsylvania; Chief, Section of Advanced Lung Disease and Lung Transplantation, University of Pennsylvania Medical Center, Philadelphia, Pennsylvania

Monica Kraft, MD   Associate Professor, Department of Medicine, Medical Director, Pulmonary Physiology Unit, National Jewish Medical and Research Center, Denver, Colorado

Robert J. Kruklitis, MD, PhD   Senior Fellow, Pulmonary, Allergy, and Critical Care Division, University of Pennsylvania, Philadelphia, Pennsylvania

Paul A. Kvale, MD   Professor, Department of Medicine, Case Western Reserve University; Senior Staff Physician, Department of Medicine, Henry Ford Health System, Detroit, Michigan

Robert Loddenkemper, MD   Professor, Medical Faculty, Humboldt University; Chief, Department of Pneumology, Zentralklinik Emil von Behring, Lungenklinik Heckeshorn, Berlin, Germany

R. John Looney, MD   Associate Professor, Department of Medicine, University of Rochester School of Medicine; Clinical Director, Allergy, Immunology, and Rheumatology, Department of Medicine, Strong Memorial Hospital, Rochester, New York

David A. Lynch, MD   Professor of Radiology and Medicine, Department of Radiology, University of Colorado Health Sciences Center; Attending Radiologist, Department of Radiology, University of Colorado Hospital, Denver, Colorado

Joseph P. Lynch, III, MD   Professor, Department of Internal Medicine, University of Michigan, Ann Arbor, Michigan

Roberto F. Machado, MD   Senior Fellow, Department of Pulmonary and Critical Care Medicine, Cleveland Clinic Foundation, Cleveland, Ohio

Neil MacIntyre, MD   Professor, Department of Medicine, Duke University; Medical Director, Respiratory Care Services, Duke University Medical Center, Durham, North Carolina

Barry Make, MD   Professor, Department of Medicine, University of Colorado School of Medicine; Director, Emphysema Center, Department of Medicine, National Jewish Medical and Research Center, Denver, Colorado

Atul Malhotra, MD   Instructor, Department of Medicine, Harvard Medical School; Attending Physician, Pulmonary, Critical Care, and Sleep Medicine Division, Brigham and Women's Hospital, Boston, Massachusetts

Jure Manfreda, MD   Associate Professor, Department of Medicine, University of Manitoba, Winnipeg, Manitoba, Canada

Mitchell L. Margolis, MD   Clinical Associate Professor of Medicine, Pulmonary, Allergy and Critical Care Division, University of Pennsylvania; Director, Clinical Pulmonary Medicine, Department of Primary Care and Consultative Medicine, Philadelphia VA Medical Center, Philadelphia, Pennsylvania

John J. Marini, MD   Professor, Department of Medicine, University of Minnesota; Director of Physiological and Translational Research, Department of Pulmonary and Critical Care, Regions Hospital, St. Paul, Minnesota

Fernando D. Martinez, MD   Director, Arizona Respiratory Center, University of Arizona; Swift-McNear Professor of Pediatrics, Department of Pediatrics, Arizona Health Sciences Center, Tucson, Arizona

John W. Martyny, PhD, CIH   Associate Professor, Department of Preventive Medicine, University of Colorado Health Sciences Center; Industrial Hygienist, National Jewish Medical and Research Center, Denver, Colorado

Semil Mehta, MD   Department of Pulmonary and Critical Care Medicine, Office of Clinical Research and Training, Northwestern University Medical School, Chicago, Illinois

Priya Menon, MD   Department of Radiology, University of Colorado Health Sciences Center, Denver, Colorado

W. Keith C. Morgan, MD   Professor Emeritus, Department of Medicine, University of Western Ontario, London, Ontario, Canada

David G. Morris, MD   Assistant Professor of Medicine, Department of Pulmonary and Critical Care Medicine, Yale University; Staff Physician, Department of Pulmonary and Critical Care Medicine, Yale-New Haven Hospital, New Haven, Connecticut

Timothy A. Morris, MD   Associate Professor, Department of Medicine, Division of Pulmonary and Critical Care Medicine, University of California, San Diego Medical Center, San Diego, California

Ali I. Musani, MD   Instructor, Department of Pulmonary and Critical Care Medicine, and Associate Director, Interventional Pulmonology Program, Hospital of the University of Pennsylvania, Philadelphia, Pennsylvania

Sonoko Nagai, MD, PhD   Associate Professor, Department of Respiratory Medicine, Kyoto University; Acting Chief, Department of Respiratory Medicine, Kyoto University Hospital, Kyoto, Japan

Michael S. Niederman, MD   Professor, Department of Medicine, State University of New York at Stony Brook; Chairman, Department of Medicine, Winthrop-University Hospital, Mineola, New York

Catherine B. Niewoehner, MD   Professor, Department of Medicine, University of Minnesota Medical School; Staff Physician, Endocrinology, Department of Medicine, VA Medical Center, Minneapolis, Minnesota

Anthony W. O'Regan, MD   Assistant Professor of Medicine, Pulmonary Center, Boston University School of Medicine; Attending Physician, Department of Pulmonary and Critical Care Medicine, Boston Medical Center, Boston, Massachusetts

Claude A. Piantadosi, MD   Professor, Department of Medicine, Duke University Medical Center, Durham, North Carolina

Venerino Poletti, MD   Clinical Professor, Dipartimento di Malattie Apparato Respiratorio, Scuola di Specialitá, Universitá di Parma, Parma, Italy; Head, Dipartimento di Malattie Apparato Respiratorio e del Torace, Ospedale G.B. Morgagni, Forli, Italy

Udaya B. S. Prakash, MD   Edward W. Scripps Professor of Medicine, Mayo Medical School and Mayo Graduate School of Medicine; Consultant in Pulmonary, Critical Care, and Internal Medicine; Director of Bronchoscopy, Mayo Medical Center and Mayo Clinic, Rochester, Minnesota

Thomas A. Raffin, MD   Colleen and Robert Haas Professor of Medicine and Biomedical Ethics, Co-Director, Stanford University Center for Biomedical Ethics, Stanford University; Chief, Department of Pulmonary and Critical Care Medicine, Stanford University Medical Center, Stanford, California

Ganesh Raghu, MD   Professor, Department of Medicine, University of Washington; Chief, Chest Clinic, Director, Lung Transplant Program, University of Washington Medical Center, Seattle, Washington

Ritesh Rathore, MD   Assistant Professor, Department of Medicine, Boston University; Assistant Professor, Department of Medicine, Roger Williams Hospital, Providence, Rhode Island

Christine Reardon, MD   Assistant Professor, Department of Internal Medicine, Boston University; Associate Director of Medical Intensive Care Unit, Department of Pulmonary and Critical Care Medicine, Boston Medical Center, Boston, Massachusetts

Robert B. Reger, PhD   Retired Research Professor, Physician Assistant Program, Alderson-Broaddus College, Philippi, West Virginia

Cecile S. Rose, MD, MPH   Associate Professor, Department of Medicine, University of Colorado Health Sciences Center; Staff Physician, Department of Medicine, National Jewish Medical and Research Center, Denver, Colorado

Sharon I. S. Rounds, MD   Professor, Departments of Medicine, Pathology, and Laboratory Medicine, Brown Medical School; Chief, Department of Pulmonary and Critical Care, Providence VA Medical Center, Providence, Rhode Island

Lewis J. Rubin, MD   Professor, Department of Medicine, University of California, San Diego, La Jolla, California

Steven A. Sahn, MD   Professor, Department of Medicine, Medical University of South Carolina; Director, Division of Pulmonary and Critical Care Medicine, Medical University Hospital, Charleston, South Carolina

Jean T. Santamauro, MD   Associate Professor, Department of Medicine, Weill Medical College of Cornell University; Associate Attending, Department of Pulmonary Service, Memorial Sloan-Kettering Cancer Center, New York, New York

George A. Sarosi, MD   Professor of Medicine, Indiana University School of Medicine; Chief of Medical Service, Indianapolis VA Medical Center, Indianapolis, Indiana

Robert B. Schoene, MD   Professor, Pulmonary and Critical Care Division, Department of Medicine, University of Washington, Seattle, Washington

Mark Schuyler, MD   Professor, Department of Medicine, University of New Mexico School of Medicine; Department of Medicine, Albuquerque VA Medical Service, Albuquerque, New Mexico

Marvin Schwarz, MD   The James C. Campbell Professor of Pulmonary Medicine, Head, Division of Pulmonary Science and Critical Care Medicine, Department of Medicine, University of Colorado Health Sciences Center, Denver, Colorado

Lewis J. Smith, MD   Professor, Division of Pulmonary and Critical Care Medicine, Department of Medicine, Northwestern University, Chicago, Illinois

Linda S. Snyder, MD Associate Professor, Arizona Respiratory Center, University of Arizona; Associate Professor, Department of Internal Medicine, Arizona Health Sciences Center, Tucson, Arizona

Michael Stanchina, MD Assistant Professor, Department of Medicine, Brown Medical School; Associate Director, Sleep Disorders Center, Department of Medicine, Pulmonary, Critical Care, and Sleep Medicine Division, Rhode Island Hospital, Providence, Rhode Island

Daniel H. Sterman, MD Director, Interventional Pulmonology Program; Clinical Director, Thoracic Oncology Gene Therapy Program; Department of Pulmonary, Allergy, and Critical Care Medicine, University of Pennsylvania, Philadelphia, Pennsylvania

Diane E. Stover, MD Professor, Department of Medicine, Weill Medical College of Cornell University; Chief, Department of Pulmonary Service, Memorial Sloan-Kettering Cancer Center, New York, New York

Gary M. Strauss, MD, MPH Professor, Department of Medicine, Brown University Medical School; Division of Hemotology-Oncology, Rhode Island Hospital, Providence, Rhode Island

Kingman P. Strohl, MD Professor, Department of Medicine, Case Western Reserve University; Director, Center for Sleep Disorders Research, Department of Medicine, Louis Stokes DVA, Medical Center, Cleveland, Ohio

E. Rand Sutherland, MD, MPH Assistant Professor, Department of Medicine, National Jewish Medical and Research Center, Denver, Colorado

Lynn T. Tanoue, MD Associate Professor of Medicine, Department of Pulmonary and Critical Care Medicine, Yale University School of Medicine, New Haven, Connecticut

Victor F. Tapson, MD Associate Professor of Medicine, Division of Pulmonary and Critical Care Medicine, Duke University Medical Center, Durham, North Carolina

Mark J. Utell, MD Professor, Department of Medicine and Environmental Medicine, University of Rochester School of Medicine; Director, Pulmonary/Critical Care and Occupational/Environmental Medicine, Department of Medicine and Environmental Medicine, Strong Memorial Hospital, Rochester, New York

Anil Vachani, MD Senior Fellow, Pulmonary, Allergy, and Critical Care Medicine Division, University of Pennsylvania, Philadelphia, Pennsylvania

Nicholas J. Vander Els, MD Assistant Professor, Department of Medicine, Weill Medical College of Cornell University; Associate Attending, Department of Pulmonary Service, Memorial Sloan-Kettering Cancer Center, New York, New York

Janine R. E. Vintch, MD Assistant Clinical Professor, Department of General Internal Medicine, David Geffen School of Medicine, University of California, Los Angeles; Assistant Clinical Professor, Department of General Internal Medicine, Harbor-UCLA Medical Center, Torrance, California

Idelle M. Weisman, MD Clinical Professor, Departments of Internal Medicine and Pulmonary and Critical Care, University of Texas Health Science Center at San Antonio, San Antonio, Texas; Chief, Department of Clinical Investigations, Director, Human Performance Laboratory, Pulmonary and Critical Care Service, William Beaumont Army Medical Center, El Paso, Texas

Scott T. Weiss, MD, MS Professor, Department of Medicine, Harvard Medical School; Director, Respiratory, Environmental, and Genetic Epidemiology, Department of Medicine, Channing Laboratory, Brigham and Women's Hospital, Boston, Massachusetts

David P. White, MD Associate Professor, Department of Medicine, Harvard Medical School; Director, Sleep Disorders Program, Sleep Medicine Division, Pulmonary and Critical Care Division, Brigham and Women's Hospital, Boston, Massachusetts

Tanya Wiese, DO Staff, Department of Pulmonary and Critical Care Medicine, Jewish Hospital Louisville, Louisville, Kentucky

Laurel A. Wright, MD Assistant Professor, Department of Pulmonary and Critical Care, University of Minnesota, Minneapolis; Department of Pulmonary, Critical Care and Sleep, Park Nicollet Clinic, St. Louis Park, Minnesota

Rosalind J. Wright, MD, MPH Assistant Professor, Department of Medicine, Channing Laboratory, Harvard Medical School; Department of Medicine, Brigham and Women's Hospital, Boston, Massachusetts

James R. Yankaskas, MD Professor, Department of Medicine, University of North Carolina, Chapel Hill, North Carolina

Maurizio Zompatori, MD Professor of Radiology, Department of Clinical Sciences, Section of Radiology, Department of Clinical Sciences, Universitá di Parma, Parma, Italy

PREFACE

Our challenge in revising and editing this seventh edition was to meet the changing demands of a rapidly evolving and expanding medical profession while keeping the focus and the tradition that has made the *Textbook of Pulmonary Diseases* ideal for those interested in the fundamentals and practice of pulmonary medicine. From the beginning, Dr. Gerald L. Baum designed this textbook for the introduction of pulmonary medicine to medical students and residents, while making it sufficiently comprehensive to provide the updates, background, and recommendations needed by the practicing pulmonologist. The first edition of this book, published in 1964, was the first multi-authored text representing a "comprehensive collection of current pulmonary knowledge." Each subsequent edition—the second in 1974, the third in 1983, the fourth in 1989, the fifth in 1994, and the sixth in 1998—has continued that tradition. With Dr. Baum's retirement as the founder and senior editor of this long-established textbook series, we now rename and dedicate the seventh and future editions as *Baum's Textbook of Pulmonary Diseases.*

The seventh edition has been completely rewritten in an attempt to address new diagnostic and therapeutic advances in the field of pulmonary diseases. In preparing this edition, our commitment has been to create a comprehensive collection of current pulmonary knowledge while keeping it sufficiently focused so that it can be read easily and will serve as the optimum desk reference for the practitioner of pulmonary medicine at any level, from medical student to subspecialist. The fifth and sixth editions of this textbook grew to two volumes each. As editors, we felt it important to condense and focus the seventh edition into a single volume to improve its ease of use. This required us to choose topics judiciously in order to address all of the primary elements that represent the core body of knowledge needed for the clinical practice of pulmonary medicine. An outstanding group of 106 authors have each written their chapters with the challenge to be concise, clear, and complete. In addition, each of the book's 70 chapters now includes a critical evaluation of the underlying literature supporting the chapter's primary recommendations as well as simplified evidence-based medicine tables to guide the reader as to the level of scientific scrutiny underlying critical recommendations or conclusions. The highest level of evidence is generally considered to be the prospective randomized clinical trial. However, many critical recommendations are still formed on the basis of different types of evidence including expert opinion and consensus statements, and these are identified as such in the tables.

The goal of the seventh edition, as with each of the prior six editions, is to create a highly readable, concise textbook that is user friendly and hopefully will be at the fingertips of the practitioners of pulmonary medicine who will continue to shape the exciting evolution of this field. The textbook takes advantage of the diverse skills of an outstanding team of authors and their willingness to do a renewed critical review of the scientific literature underlying the current practice of pulmonary medicine.

J.D.C.
J.G.
J.B.K.
T.E.K.

PREFACE TO THE FIRST EDITION

Why another textbook? A few years ago when this work began, I approached the prospective contributors and found that they felt, as I did, that the available compilations and texts were weak in one or another of the major areas in the field of chest diseases. It seemed that by using specialists whose major interests were in these areas and allowing them to be responsible for covering all that they felt belonged in their area, a more complete and current textbook would result. Thus, the authors were assembled with an overall plan to cover the field completely and in a coordinated way with current material being woven into concepts by each author.

The difficulties of such a project are apparent. As part of internal medicine, the study of pulmonary diseases involves a wide variety of disciplines. Anatomy, physiology, immunology, bacteriology, mycology, biochemistry, epidemiology, and pathology, among the basic sciences, must be blended with physical diagnosis, therapeutics, radiology, clinical pathology, physiatry, and psychiatry to present a complete picture of this field of medicine. In addition, emphasis must be placed on the more important problems in public health as they bear on each area. Putting this material into an orderly and readable form is crucial to the value of the book, and providing a complete but selective bibliography is essential to making this a true textbook and not just a review.

In many areas, such as allergic disease and interstitial diseases, extensive background discussions precede the actual clinical presentations. This was done in order to provide sound physiologic basis for the clinical expressions of pathology that direct the activities of the clinician. In addition, embryology of the lung is discussed within the areas of congenital, developmental, and hereditary diseases and in continuity with this material rather than in a remote part of the book where its application would not be directly apparent. For the same reason, details of bronchial and parenchymal anatomy are followed by well-illustrated chapters on emphysema and pulmonary insufficiency.

At the clinical level, the approach to the various infectious diseases is consistent, and it makes use of principles proven reliable in the field of clinical bacteriology as the basis of the approach to viral, rickettsial, and fungal diseases. The mycobacterioses are described in a fresh way which clearly integrates new knowledge of chemotherapy and rehabilitation with established pathogenetic and clinical principles. It is in this historically prime subject in the field of pulmonary diseases that this book offers something that has not been available before. The established treatises dealing with tuberculosis have merely modified and appended the old format to include the subjects of drug therapy, drug resistance, resectional therapy, and rehabilitation based on physical activity early rather than late in the course of treatment. No continuity of approach was projected in such an exposition. By contrast, in this textbook, Drs. Jenkins and Wolinsky have synthesized a discussion that deals with broad principles in light of current information on one hand and provide orderly presentation of details on the other.

Diagnosis is the first subject dealt with in this book, and this is appropriate. Drs. Smith and Kory have developed a unique set of tables at the end of their chapters which should be extremely useful to the student and to the practitioner alike. It is no coincidence that Drs. Amberson, Middleton, and Schwarz have each repeatedly stressed the primacy of accurate diagnosis to many generations of students.

The authors and I have attempted to make this book detailed and current enough to appeal to the sophisticated specialist and clinical researcher and orderly, clearly organized, and well indexed to be of use to the beginning student. Because this book deals with pulmonary diseases primarily, specific discussions of mediastinal diseases other than tumors or gastrointestinal diseases with thoracic manifestations have not been included. Finally, I have written nothing myself, but have devoted my efforts to organization of material and exhortation of the authors.

This textbook is only a beginning, since new work will make much of what is written here obsolete; possibly obsolescence will have set in before publication. Nevertheless, the soundness of the physiologic approach allows for the addition of current knowledge to that discussed here without loss of continuity.

I sincerely hope that this book will, through the authority of the authors' material, stimulate the most important ingredient of any textbook in any field: the curiosity of the student.

G.L.B.
Cincinnati

FOREWORD

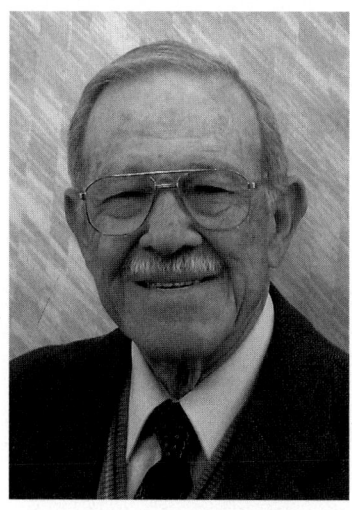

In the summer of 1958, I became Chief of the Pulmonary Section at the Veterans Administration (VA) Hospital in Cincinnati, after having spent two and half years working with Jan Schwarz in mycology. Previously, I had been a resident on the Bellevue Chest Service, with J. Burns Amberson and Julia Jones as my mentors; thus, I felt prepared to run a chest service and assume responsibilities for both patient care and teaching. While I was engaged in the latter, residents and medical students frequently asked me what textbook of pulmonary medicine I would recommend. "Aye, there's the rub," I quoted more than once!

Within a short time, I learned of the remarkable group of colleagues in pulmonary medicine who were working within the network of VA hospitals around the United States. At the first of several VA research meetings that I attended in the autumn of 1958, I encountered firsthand the exciting work of these colleagues in pulmonary medicine. In addition, through contacts at the University of Cincinnati College of Medicine, where I had a teaching appointment, I had many opportunities to learn from a friend who had been a fellow resident with me at the Jewish Hospital in Cincinnati, I. Leonard Bernstein, about the explosion of information in the field of allergy, especially pulmonary allergy. My experience at Bellevue had included contacts with Drs. Andre Cournand and Dickenson Richards, who generated in me a sense of wonder about the burgeoning field of pulmonary physiology.

These experiences, all put together, made quite clear to me the deficiency that existed at that time—the lack of a summary of the current status of pulmonary medicine in textbook form. From my encounters with these colleagues, the "germ of an idea" to produce a new textbook was born.

I was then a youngster, 33 years old, and just beginning to work in the academic world of pulmonary medicine. I had had experience in writing articles for the medical literature but none in producing a book. Despite all these negative factors, the idea of somehow generating a new and better textbook kept biting me. My presumption in entertaining such an idea was all too apparent to me and kept me from moving ahead until a chance encounter with an older and very accomplished medical luminary changed everything.

I had been invited to attend a meeting at Saranac Lake, New York, early in 1959, and I was scheduled to travel on a feeder airline operating a small plane service from LaGuardia Field, in Queens, to upstate New York. Also invited to the meeting was Julius Wilson, Director of the Phipps Institute in Philadelphia, and he was on the same flight. By chance, he and I sat next to each another, and this was the fortuitous encounter that resulted in the creation of the first edition of the *Textbook of Pulmonary Diseases.* In the course of conversation, I happened to mention my crazy idea and also my disclaimer, "Who am I to presume to do such a thing!" He replied that every youngster who ever achieved anything felt the same way starting out, and that if I was convinced that a new textbook was needed, then I should go ahead and produce one.

The form of the book was already clear to me; one or two authors could no longer cover the field in an authoritative way, so a textbook with multiple authors was the obvious choice. As for me, my duties would be solely to edit the book—I did not feel expert enough to presume to write a chapter. Thus, my next task was to assemble a team for the project.

By this time, I had become familiar with some very articulate and productive clinicians and scientists within the VA system. Among them were Hollis Boren in Houston, Ross Kory and Josef Smith at the Milwaukee VA Hospital, Charles Andrews in Kansas City, and Robert Green at the VA facility in Ann Arbor, Michigan. In addition, attendance at a number of national meetings in pulmonary medicine had exposed me to the work of other impressive investigators and provided an opportunity to know them personally. This group included the Bader twins, Mortimer and Richard, Roger Mitchell, Daniel Jenkins (with help from Hollis Boren), and Gustave Laurenzi, in addition to John Rankin, who worked at my medical school alma mater, the

University of Wisconsin, Madison. During my training days with Dr. Jan Schwarz, I had met Donald Louria, who subsequently became an infectious disease specialist at Cornell Medical College. Two physicians had impressed me while I was serving at St. Albans Naval Hospital some years previously, Captain J. A. C. Gray and Joseph Timmes. In my own town of Cincinnati were I. Leonard Bernstein, already mentioned, and Noble Fowler, who was on the cardiology staff of the medical school. Through the Ohio State Chest Physicians Society I met Myron Perlich and Emanuel Wolinsky.

On the basis of my experiences, I created the table of contents of a proposed book with these physicians as authors. Within a short time, I had contacted all of them and persuaded them to write their chapters, and we were ready to go.

One small matter remained— we needed a publisher. I did my homework in the medical library of the VA Hospital, checking the current publications list of the major medical publishers, and I found three very well-known publishing houses with no textbook of pulmonary medicine of any kind. I sent letters to all three with the table of contents I had developed, and all three sent a representative to discuss the terms of publication! Of the three, the most impressive was the ultimate publisher of the first several editions of the book, Little, Brown and Company.

What impressed me was that the representative who visited me was the director of the medical books division of the company, Mr. Fred Belliveau, Jr. He told me that Little, Brown and Company had only recently entered the world of medical publishing, and they were eager to expand their enterprise with major textbooks in important fields of medicine. In addition to all this, Fred Belliveau was a charming and enthusiastic person, and he definitely appeared to be a highly capable publishing executive. A decision was made on the spot, and the book was converted from a nebulous dream to a working potential reality. All that remained was to write it!

The rest of the story, which continued for some 40 years and a total of six editions of the textbook, is objectively mundane, although for me each edition brought its own highly significant experiences. Urging authors to complete their work according to schedule, cajoling them some of the time, threatening them at other times, and working with them in remarkable harmony almost all the time was my fate. I edited the first two editions alone and the next three with Emanuel Wolinsky, and for the last edition, my co-editors were James Crapo, Bartolome Celli, and Joel Karlinsky. At Little, Brown and Company and for the most recent edition at Lippincott, Williams & Wilkins, I had the good fortune to work with highly professional editors. Within that context, I must mention the names of three ladies, Ms. Lin Richter, Ms. Laurie Anello, and Ms. Joyce-Rachel John, all three of whom were responsible for the overall production of one or another edition of the textbook and all of whom were truly a delight to work with. Ms. Richter passed away some years ago, but the other two are alive and well and still smiling.

It's hard for me to believe that this project has come so far. I can still remember that plane ride with Julius Wilson and can only wonder what would have happened had I missed that flight. Happily, I didn't.

Gerald L. Baum, MD
Tel Aviv, Israel

ACKNOWLEDGMENTS

Thanks to my assistant, Peggy Hammond, for overseeing the timing and accuracy of each step in editing this text, and to Kathy and my family for support and allowing me time to do this work.

James D. Crapo, MD

Thanks go to my assistant, Madelyn Alt, for her work on behalf of the book, and my understanding wife and two semi-understanding kids.

Jeffrey Glassroth, MD

I would like to acknowledge my wife and children.

Joel B. Karlinsky, MD, MBA

I wish to acknowledge the unending support of my wife, Mozelle, during the work on this book and other academic efforts. I thank my colleagues and staff for their input and assistance. Finally, I am particularly grateful to my patients for allowing me to participate in their care.

Talmadge E. King, Jr., MD

Imaging of Lung Disease

David A. Lynch · Priya Menon

The purposes of this chapter are to explain the range of imaging modalities available to the pulmonary physician, to describe and illustrate common radiologic signs of lung disease, and to show how imaging can help elucidate some common clinical problems.

CHEST RADIOGRAPHIC TECHNIQUES

The conventional chest radiograph is usually the first imaging procedure performed in a patient with known or suspected chronic obstructive pulmonary disease, and may be the only examination required. Pulmonologists should pay careful attention to the technique used in acquiring chest radiographs. Variation in quality of chest images obtained in outpatient offices may lead to misdiagnoses. Overexposure of the radiograph may simulate emphysema, whereas underexposure may lead to a false diagnosis of interstitial lung disease (ILD). The use of a wide-latitude asymmetric screen-film combination, such as Kodak Insight, and a high-kilovoltage technique (kilovolt peak between 120 and 140), with a fine grid, are strongly recommended (1).

At most medical centers and hospitals, conventional analog chest imaging is being replaced by digital imaging. *Digital image acquisition* allows immediate electronic distribution of images to workstations on patient care floors and outpatient clinics by use of a *picture archiving and communication system* (PACS). Modalities for digital imaging of the thorax include *computed radiography* (CR) and *direct capture radiography* (DR). In CR, the image is obtained on a photostimulable phosphor plate within a cassette, which is then processed through a reader. With DR, the images are directly captured onto a grid of receptors, which generate the image without the need for a processor. Two recent innovations in digital imaging may enhance the ability of chest radiographs to detect abnormalities. *Dual energy imaging* allows "subtraction" of overlying bones to create an image composed almost entirely of soft tissues. *Temporal subtraction* electronically subtracts a previous radiograph from the current image to enhance detection of changes. Temporal subtraction enhances detection of hazy pulmonary opacities and lung nodules. These techniques require further evaluation, but could ultimately rival computed tomography (CT) as cost-effective modalities for screening for lung cancer.

COMPUTED TOMOGRAPHY TECHNIQUES

Spiral (Helical) Computed Tomography

In spiral CT, the x-ray tube is continuously rotated as the patient table passes through the CT aperture, producing a three-dimensional volumetric data set. In spiral CT of the lungs, the images are usually acquired during a single inspiratory breath-hold of 20 to 30 seconds. For patients with significant dyspnea, multiple shorter acquisitions may be required to cover the lung volumes. This type of acquisition allows construction of overlapping images, multiplanar images, and three-dimensional models.

Initial spiral CT models used one set of CT detectors to acquire information from one slice position at a time. The newer technique of *multidetector CT* uses multiple CT detectors to acquire information from multiple levels. Currently available scanners allow slice thicknesses as low as 0.6 mm in the z-axis, and promise three-dimensional or multiplanar reconstructions of excellent quality, with acceptable patient dose and shorter acquisition times. Multidetector CT is of particular value for *CT angiography* of the pulmonary

D. A. Lynch and **P. Menon:** Department of Radiology, University of Colorado Health Sciences Center, Denver, Colorado.

and mediastinal vessels, allowing rapid acquisition of angiographic images of these vessels.

With specialized workstations, thin slices acquired from spiral CT acquisitions can be integrated to create simulated images of the internal surface of the bronchial tree *(virtual bronchoscopy)*. Although virtual bronchoscopy provides images of excellent quality, it contributes little to diagnostic accuracy, because all the information is available on the source images. Its main value is to allow the bronchoscopist to plan interventional procedures, such as transtracheal or transbronchial biopsy of masses, and bronchial stenting.

Contrast administration is not necessary for most chest CT examinations. Intravenous contrast is useful when the pulmonary or mediastinal vessels, or the heart, are being evaluated or when hilar adenopathy is being sought.

High-Resolution Computed Tomography

The technique of high-resolution CT (HRCT) uses thin (1–1.5-mm) sections and a special reconstruction algorithm to maximize detail in the lung parenchyma (Fig. 1.1) (2). Careful attention to technique is required to ensure high-quality images. In particular, technologists must work with the patient to ensure the absence of respiratory motion, which is the most common cause of suboptimal images. Respiratory motion can almost always be prevented by careful communication between technologist and patient. Because atelectasis in the dependent lung can obscure detail, prone HRCT imaging is frequently performed to evaluate the posterior lung, in which the early changes of asbestosis, collagen vascular-related lung disease, and idiopathic interstitial pneumonias may be first seen.

In patients with lung nodules, HRCT is obtained contiguously through the nodule. In patients with suspected diffuse lung disease, HRCT is usually used to sample the lung at 1- to 4-cm intervals. Many radiologists choose to supplement this sampling approach with a contiguous CT acquisition, to identify important focal abnormalities such as nodules, cavities, or consolidation. Multidetector CT can meet both goals by allowing thin section imaging of the entire lung volume, although at the cost of some increase in x-ray exposure. The resultant images can then be reconstructed at appropriate thicknesses to provide both thick-section and thin-section samples from a single acquisition.

Expiratory Computed Tomography

CT imaging during expiration is useful for identification of air trapping (Fig. 1.2) and may accentuate subtle areas of centrilobular emphysema. Because diseases such as hypersensitivity pneumonitis and sarcoidosis are frequently associated with air trapping, expiratory CT should be an integral part of the CT acquisition in patients with known or suspected infiltrative lung disease. The patient is usually asked to expire to residual volume, but the reproducibility of this level of expiration is variable. Expiratory images are usually obtained at several levels in the chest.

Volumetric Computed Tomography

Inspiratory and expiratory spiral CT can be used to calculate total lung capacity (TLC) and residual volume. In a study by Kauczor et al., the volume of the lungs measured on inspiratory helical CT, performed without spirometric control, was approximately 12% less than TLC, but was highly correlated with TLC (3). The volume of the lungs on deep expiration was highly correlated with thoracic gas volume, but correlated less well with residual volume. These findings

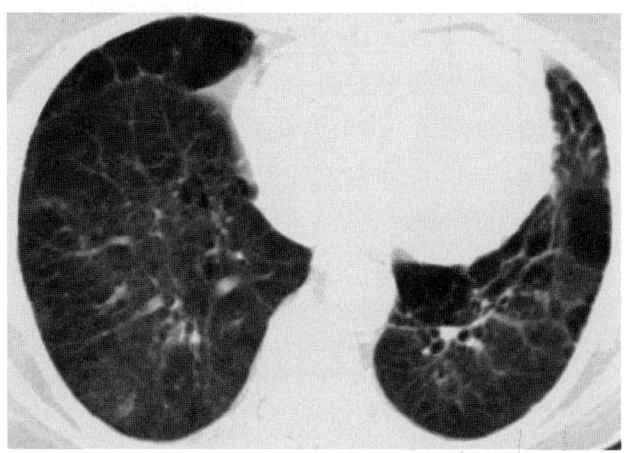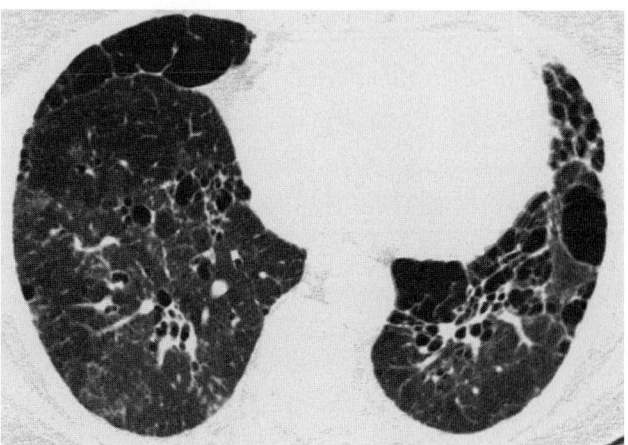

A   B

FIGURE 1.1. Comparison of thick-section computed tomography (CT) and thin-section high-resolution CT (HRCT) in a patient with sarcoidosis. **A:** Thick-section CT shows basal ground-glass abnormality, with some anterior subpleural cysts. **B:** HRCT scan at the same level shows that the ground-glass abnormality is due to fine micronodules. Extensive traction bronchiectasis is also shown much more clearly.

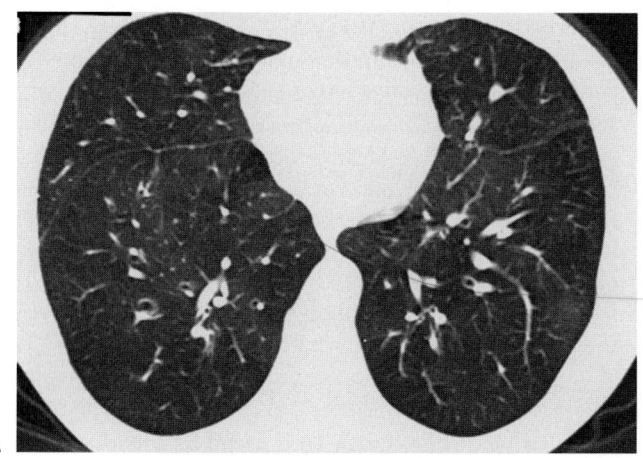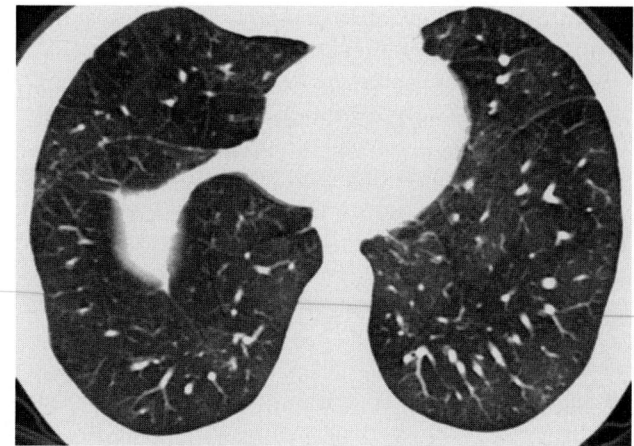

A   B

FIGURE 1.2. Inspiratory and expiratory computed tomography (CT) in a patient with bronchiolitis obliterans. **A:** Inspiratory CT shows mild heterogeneity of lung attenuation and mild cylindric bronchiectasis. **B:** Expiratory CT shows substantial airtrapping, particularly evident anteriorly, where the attenuation of the lung is unchanged from the inspiratory scan.

suggest that the level of inspiration for an inspiratory helical CT is approximately 12% lower than TLC, whereas on an expiratory CT, the level of expiration is closer to functional residual capacity than to residual volume. Similarly, in a study of patients before and after lung volume reduction surgery, the TLC calculated by CT correlated very well with plethysmographic TLC, but calculated residual volume tended to overestimate the plethysmographic residual volume (4). Calculation of lung volumes by CT, although effort dependent, may become part of routine CT evaluation in the future.

Quantitative Computed Tomography

CT attenuation values can be used to quantify the amount of air, soft tissue, and blood in the lung. Spiral CT can be used to calculate lung volumes. For this reason, CT can be used to provide a valid index of the extent of emphysema, air trapping, and lung fibrosis, and is increasingly being used for this purpose in clinical trials (5, 6). The optimal CT acquisition technique for quantification of lung disease remains unresolved. There is a choice between sampling the lungs with high-resolution thin sections at selected intervals and use of spiral CT to acquire a three-dimensional CT data set. The use of a volumetric data set ensures that the lung has been completely sampled, and allows the creation of impressive three-dimensional models and the calculation of lung volumes. However, subtle inhomogeneities of lung density due to emphysema, fibrosis, or air trapping may be lost in the relatively large voxel sizes. A thin-section sampling technique will allow detection of greater lung detail. In the National Emphysema Treatment Trial, both spiral and thin sections are obtained, along with expiratory CT performed at selected intervals, to obtain the most comprehensive data set possible. The results of this study should help determine

which technique provides the best overall measure of the extent of emphysema.

Spirometric standardization of the inspired volume of air can be important in ensuring reproducibility of quantitative CT measurements on lung CT. Several investigators have used spirometric triggering devices, but these are not widely available. If spiral CT is used to acquire volumetric information in a single breath-hold, the lung volumes can be measured directly, obviating the need for spirometric gating (3).

Dynamic Computed Tomography

Dynamic CT refers to any process whereby serial CT images are obtained through an area during a physiologic maneuver or after administration of contrast. Dynamic CT during inspiration and expiration can be used to document air trapping (7, 8). Dynamic contrast-enhanced CT is commonly used to evaluate lung nodules.

NUCLEAR MEDICINE TECHNIQUES

Ventilation Agents

A variety of agents is available for the scintigraphic evaluation of emphysema. They include gases such as ^{133}Xe and ^{81m}Kr, as well as the radioaerosols ^{99m}Tc pentetate (^{99m}Tc-DTPA) and Technegas (Daiichi Radioisotope, Tokyo, Japan) (9). The choice of ventilation agent often depends on availability. Gaseous ^{81m}Kr is the ideal ventilation agent, providing near instant regional ventilatory mapping with ability to perform single photon emission CT (SPECT) imaging. However, ^{81m}Kr must be obtained from a ^{81}Rb generator, which has a clinical lifespan of about one working day. Also, its 13-second half-life means that imaging must be performed during steady state and that washout imaging cannot be performed.

Because of its availability, ^{133}Xe is the most widely used gaseous ventilation agent, with a half-life of 5.1 days. It allows imaging of wash-in, equilibrium, and washout phases. Images taken at equilibrium correspond to regional lung volume. Delayed washout is a sensitive indicator of air trapping. Limitations of ^{133}Xe include the fact that the photon that it emits has relatively low energy, resulting in greater attenuation in the chest wall and lower-resolution images. Also, if dynamic imaging is performed, scanning is limited to one projection only, a disadvantage in ventilation/perfusion imaging for pulmonary embolism. ^{127}Xe has a higher photon energy (203 keV) but has a longer half-life of 36 days and is less widely available.

Modern radioaerosols provide excellent images of ventilation in patients without airway disease (Fig. 1.3), but are deposited in the airways to a variable extent in patients with chronic obstructive pulmonary disease, with resultant nonuniform demonstration of the distal airspaces. The most commonly used aerosol in clinical practice is ^{99m}Tc-DTPA. The clearance of this aerosol has also been used as an index of the severity of ILD; patients with ILD have faster clearance of this agent. However, the value of this washout index is limited by the fact that washout is also increased in cigarette smokers, and the technique is not widely used in clinical practice.

Technegas (Daiichi Radioisotope, Tokyo, Japan), is a ^{99m}Tc-labeled ultrafine carbon particle radioaerosol (9). These particles are small enough to reach the lung periphery but probably do not reach the alveoli, as movement of gas in the smallest airways, beyond the 16th-order division, is largely by molecular diffusion (9). Central airway deposition is less with Technegas than with ^{99m}Tc-DTPA, and Technegas appears to provide an effective measure of ventilation in patients with obstructive lung disease (10).

Perfusion Agents

Perfusion imaging is almost always performed with ^{99m}Tc-labeled human albumin microparticles, the most common of which is macroaggregated human serum albumin (^{99m}Tc-MAA), with a particle size of 10 to 100 microns, allowing these particles to be trapped in pulmonary capillaries. ^{99m}Tc-albumin microspheres have more uniform size (20–45 microns), but are more expensive and less widely available. Usually 200,000 to 400,000 particles are injected intravenously, and about 95% of them are trapped in the lung on the first pass, occluding less than 1 in 1,000 capillaries (11). Distribution within the lungs via microembolization is proportional to regional pulmonary arterial flow. In patients with right-to-left shunts, the agents can bypass the lungs and be trapped in capillaries in brain and kidneys. Images obtained over the kidneys and brain may help diagnose the presence of such a shunt.

Ventilation and Perfusion Imaging

Perfusion imaging with microparticles is an excellent method for identifying perfusion defects due to pulmonary embolism (Fig. 1.3). However, the excellent matching of ventilation and perfusion means that patients with pneumonia or airway obstruction will have perfusion defects that must be distinguished from pulmonary embolism by ventilation imaging. Use of radioaerosols is preferred for this

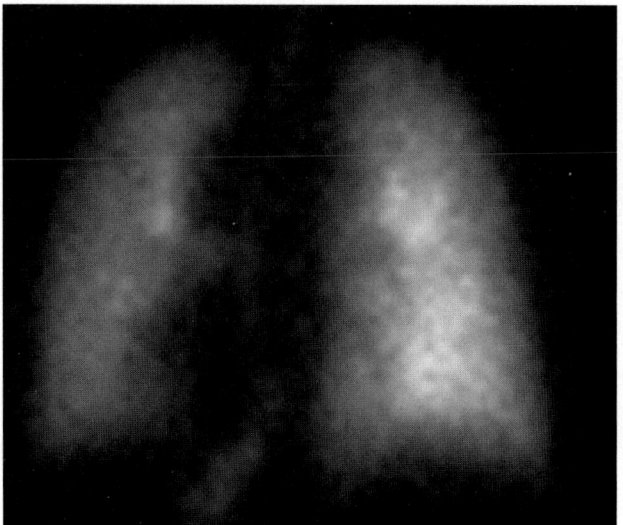
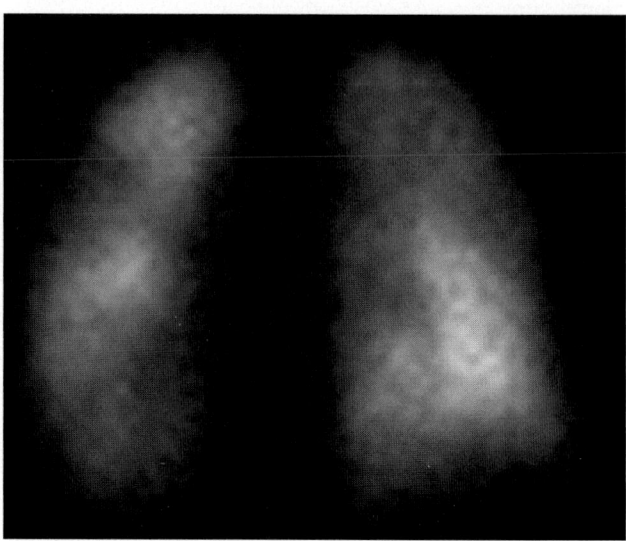

A   B

FIGURE 1.3. Ventilation-perfusion imaging in diagnosis of pulmonary embolism. **A:** Ventilation image, obtained with ^{99m}Tc pentetate aerosol, shows homogenous ventilation on posterior view. **B:** Matched perfusion image shows large (segmental) perfusion defects in the left mid lung, and in the lateral segment of the left lower lobe. There is also decreased perfusion in the right upper lobe. The presence of unmatched segmental abnormalities indicates a high probability for pulmonary embolism.

purpose because matching images of ventilation and perfusion can be obtained in eight projections. Unmatched segmental or large subsegmental perfusion defects are usually (>90%) due to pulmonary embolism. Smaller unmatched defects are less specific and must be regarded as indeterminate or intermediate probability for pulmonary embolism. Small perfusion defects (<25% of a segment) are usually associated with a low (<10%) probability of pulmonary embolism. A normal perfusion scan is associated with a very low probability of pulmonary embolism.

Unilateral absence of perfusion on perfusion scanning is usually not due to pulmonary embolism. Differential diagnosis of this finding includes obstruction of the pulmonary artery or main bronchus by a mass, unilateral small-airway disease (Swyer-James syndrome), and pulmonary artery agenesis.

Positron Emission Tomography

Positron emission tomography (PET) with [18]fluorodeoxyglucose (18-FDG) has revolutionized the evaluation of thoracic malignancy by its ability to depict metabolically active tumor within and outside the thorax. FDG is a glucose analog that is avidly imbibed by metabolically active cells and is phosphorylated into FDG-6-phosphate, which cannot be further metabolized in the glycolytic pathway. It therefore accumulates in metabolically active cells. The positrons emitted simultaneously when the ^{18}F isotope decays can be detected and localized with a coincidence-detecting tomographic camera. Images obtained by PET can be reconstructed in any plane (sagittal, axial, coronal). To precisely localize the abnormality, PET images must be correlated with corresponding axial CT images. *PET-CT fusion scanners* can perform PET and CT almost simultaneously, allowing direct mapping of the site of PET activity to the corresponding axial CT image. However, experienced cross-sectional imagers can usually perform the same correlation without the need for synchronous acquisition of PET and CT. 18-FDG PET is widely used for discriminating between benign and malignant lung nodules and for staging of lung cancer.

The most important role of PET is in staging of established lung cancer. PET may also show increased uptake in the pleura in patients with malignant effusions. In patients with malignant pleural mesothelioma, PET may be useful in showing occult mediastinal nodal metastases (12).

LUNG MAGNETIC RESONANCE IMAGING

There are several theoretical reasons to advocate the use of magnetic resonance imaging (MRI) in the lung. MRI uses nonionizing radiation, can quantify the amount of lung water (13, 14), and can distinguish fibrosis from active inflammation (15–17). However, MRI of the lung has been gravely hampered by the problems of respiratory motion and in-

duced inhomogeneity of the magnetic field within individual voxels. The magnetic inhomogeneity problem arises because the lung is composed of innumerable air–soft tissue interfaces. Magnetic field inhomogeneity is created at each of these interfaces, causing dramatic loss of signal with standard MRI techniques.

The use of inhaled hyperpolarized helium (18, 19) or oxygen (20, 21) as contrast agents to image pulmonary ventilation is the latest technical advance in MRI, currently under evaluation in patients with obstructive lung diseases. The enormous gain in polarization overcomes the loss in signal owing to the low density of the gas in the lungs (22). With helium imaging, normally ventilated lung parenchyma has homogeneous intermediate-to-high signal, whereas patients with chronic obstructive lung disease and emphysema demonstrate severe signal inhomogeneities with patchy or wedge shaped defects (23). Although evaluation has been limited, this technique appears to have great potential in directly visualizing the small, reversible ventilation defects that are characteristic of asthma (24). However, its use is limited by the requirement for specialized equipment, including the helium polarizer and dedicated magnetic resonance coils. Regional ventilation has also been assessed by using oxygen-enhanced MRI. Although molecular oxygen is only weakly paramagnetic, it produces substantial signal changes in the lungs because of their large surface areas. Edelman et al. used inhaled molecular oxygen as a contrast agent, directly depicting transfer of oxygen across the alveolus into the pulmonary vasculature (20). A limitation of this technique may be the requirement for patients to inhale 100% oxygen, which may be dangerous for patients with blunted respiratory drives.

MRI has a limited role in the evaluation of patients with lung cancer and with mediastinal masses. Because of excellence in imaging soft tissues, MRI is useful for identifying the degree of soft tissue invasion by lung cancer and other tumors such as mesothelioma. In particular, MRI is used for evaluation of neurovascular involvement by Pancoast tumor (25) and for the preoperative staging of mesothelioma (26). In the mediastinum, MRI is used to assess the degree of cardiac invasion by paracardiac masses and to characterize mediastinal masses as solid or cystic (Fig. 1.4).

ULTRASOUND

The primary role of ultrasound in the chest is determination of the presence and extent of pleural fluid. When small or loculated pleural effusions are present, ultrasound is recommended to mark the precise location of the fluid, and to determine its depth, before thoracentesis. Ultrasound is also very useful for guiding placement of pigtail catheters and for biopsying peripheral lung lesions. For the pulmonologist, a further role of ultrasound is to make the diagnosis of venous thromboembolic disease, when lower extremity symptoms are present.

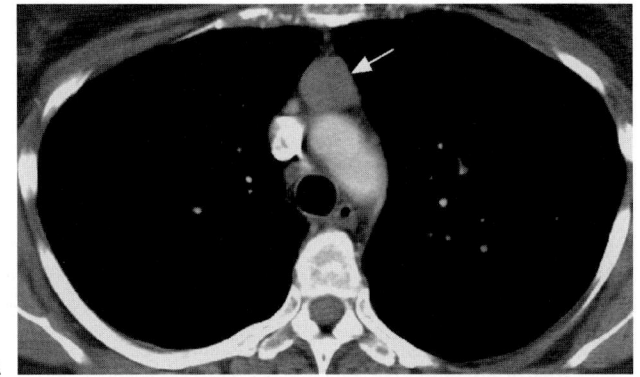

A

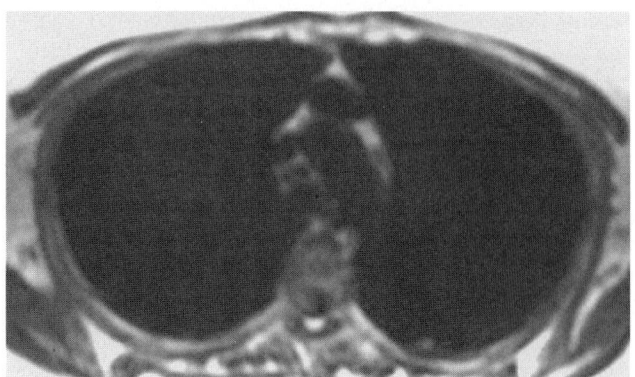

B

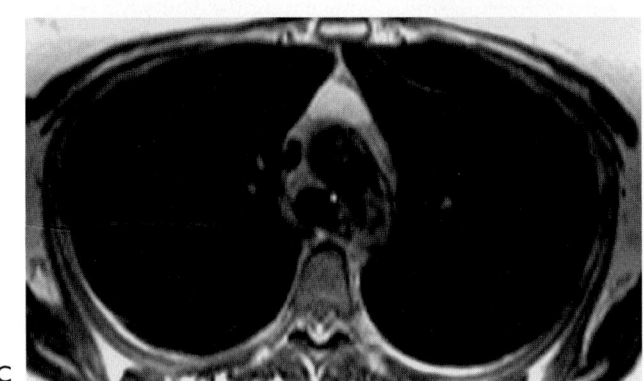

C

FIGURE 1.4. The role of magnetic resonance imaging (MRI) in the evaluation of mediastinal masses. **A:** Computed tomography scan of the chest shows a well-defined low-attenuating lesion in the anterior mediastinum *(arrow)*. The attenuation values of this lesion were not sufficiently low to allow the diagnosis of a simple cyst. **B:** T$_1$-weighted MRI shows that the lesion is of low signal intensity on T$_1$-weighted imaging. **C:** T$_2$-weighted image shows marked increase in signal attenuation, indicating predominantly fluid content. The mass was diagnosed as a thymic cyst, thus avoiding the need for thoracotomy.

INTERVENTIONAL THORACIC RADIOLOGY

The use of imaging to guide thoracic procedures is an important part of the work of the thoracic radiologist. Image-guided small-bore catheter drainage of infected pleural collections (empyema and complicated parapneumonic effusion) is successful in 72% to 88% of cases, and may be facilitated by intrapleural thrombolytic therapy with streptokinase, urokinase, or tissue plasminogen activator. Malignant pleural effusions are also amenable to image-guided palliative drainage, and chemical pleurodesis of malignant effusions via small bore catheters is successful in 70% to 90% of cases (27, 28). Small-bore catheter drainage is highly effective for evacuation of spontaneous or iatrogenic pneumothorax. Image guidance for drainage of fluid collections is usually accomplished by ultrasound. CT-guided drainage is effective only for loculated collections.

Image-guided biopsy of lung or mediastinal lesions is almost always accomplished with CT, but ultrasound can be used in selected peripheral or chest wall lesions. CT-guided biopsy to obtain a cytologic specimen is diagnostic in up to 95% of malignant lesions, but is less accurate for making specific benign diagnoses (29). The use of a biopsy gun to provide a histologic specimen increases the likelihood of a diagnosis of benign disease such as hamartoma (30). Pneumothorax occurs in about 30% of lung biopsies when the needle traverses aerated lung but is self-limiting in most, with only about 20% of pneumothoraces requiring chest

tube drainage (31, 32). The risk of pneumothorax increases with increasing depth of the lesion, and with the presence of obstructive lung disease.

IMAGE-GUIDED THORACIC PROCEDURES	
Summary Statement	**Level of Evidence**
In complex parapneumonic effusions and empyema, image-guided catheter drainage with fibrinolysis is effective in 60%–90% of cases	Retrospective studies
Image-guided biopsy is diagnostic in 80%–90% of malignant lesions, and is less diagnostic in benign lesions	Retrospective studies
Pneumothorax rate for percutaneous biopsy is 20%–30%	Retrospective studies
Chest tube rate is 5%	Retrospective studies

RADIOLOGIC ANATOMY

Understanding of the anatomy of the frontal and lateral chest radiograph is critical for the pulmonologist (Fig. 1.5). On CT, an understanding of bronchial anatomy is particularly important, as CT provides a valuable roadmap for bronchoscopy. The main requirement for understanding CT anatomy is the ability to integrate the axial images in the craniocaudal dimension. Figure 1.6 provides a series of axial CT images that illustrate the anatomy of the lobar and segmental bronchi.

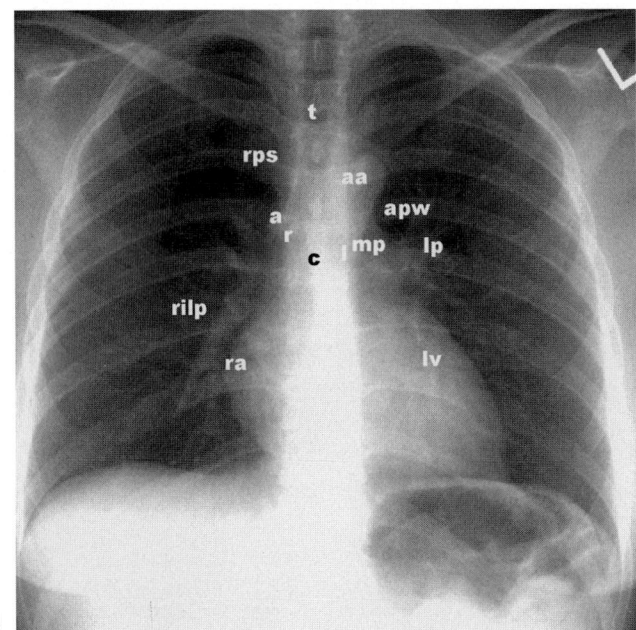

A

FIGURE 1.5. Normal radiologic anatomy. *T,* trachea; *r,* right main bronchus; *l,* left main bronchus; *c,* carina; *a,* azygos vein; *Rps,* right paratracheal stripe; *aa,* aortic arch; *mp,* main pulmonary artery; *apw,* aorto-pulmonary window; *ra,* right atrium; *lv,* left ventricle; *rilp,* right interlobular pulmonary artery; *lp,* left pulmonary artery; *rv,* right ventricle; *la,* left atrium; *bi,* bronchus intermedius. **A:** Frontal radiograph. Note that the left pulmonary artery, which passes over the left main bronchus, is always higher than the right by up to 2 cm. **B:** Lateral radiograph. The *black asterisk* indicates the right posterior ribs, which are slightly magnified relative to the left ribs, and are projected behind the left ribs. **C:** Detail of lateral view of hilum The *white arrow* indicates the thin posterior wall of bronchus intermedius. The *black arrow* indicates the round lucency of the left upper lobe bronchus, passing below the left pulmonary artery. Note that the left pulmonary artery arches above the left main bronchus, whereas the right interlobar pulmonary artery passes in front of the bronchus intermedius.

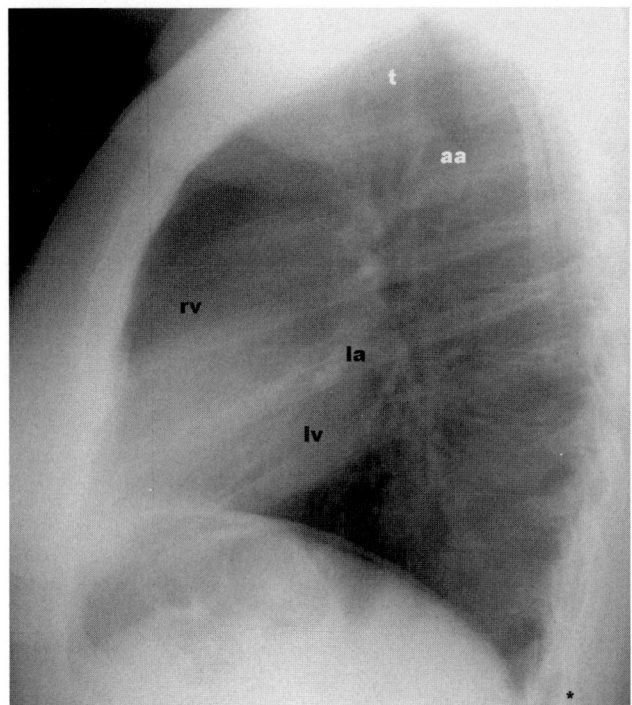

B

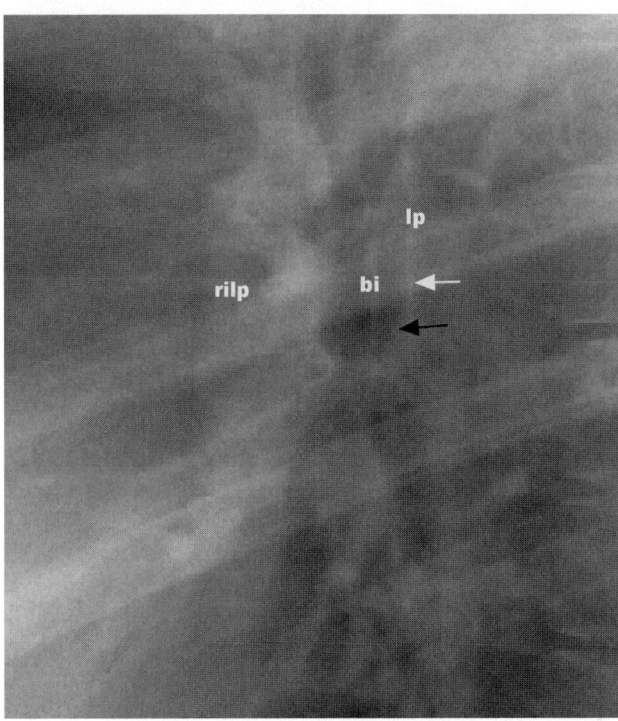

C

An appreciation of normal and abnormal HRCT findings in the lung requires an understanding of the anatomy of the secondary pulmonary lobule, which is a basic anatomic and physiologic unit of mammalian lung (33). In humans, the irregularly polyhedral secondary pulmonary lobule is composed of several acini, each supplied by a terminal bronchiole (Fig. 1.7). The secondary lobules are separated from each other by interlobular septa, which contain branches of the pulmonary veins and lymphatics. The septa are best developed in the peripheral anterior lung and are less well developed posteriorly and in the central lung. Interlobular septa become visible as septal lines on the chest radiograph when they are thickened by interstitial fluid, cellular infiltration, or fibrosis. On HRCT, the interlobular septa may be visible in the normal anterior lung as scattered, thin, nontapering lines that are 1 to 2 cm long, that are perpendicular to the pleura, and that often contact the pleural surface (33).

In the center of the secondary pulmonary lobule are the distal bronchus and its terminal bronchioles with the associated distal pulmonary artery branches. These structures are often called centrilobular or core structures and may

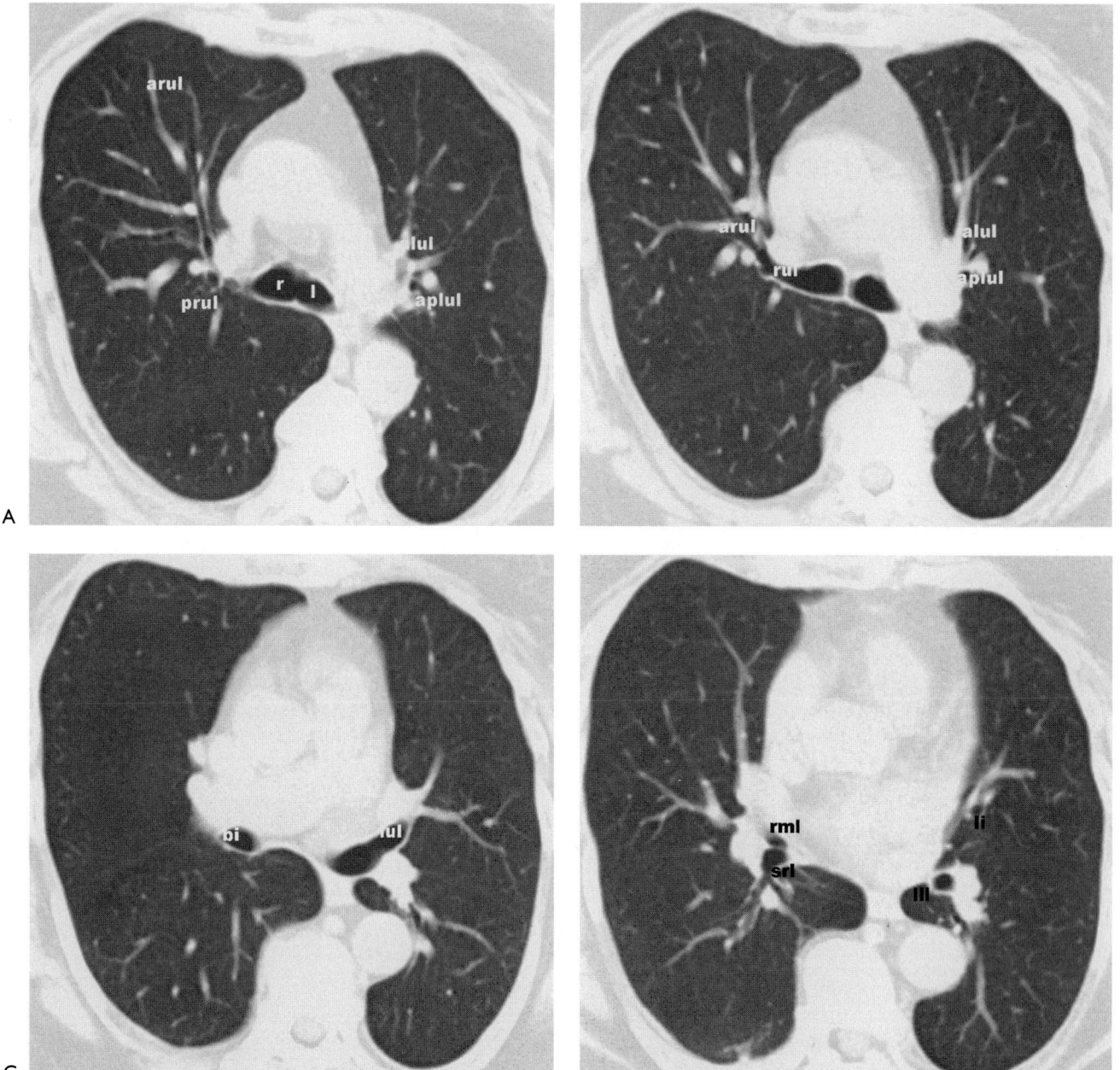

FIGURE 1.6. Computed tomography depictions of segmental bronchial anatomy. *R,* right main bronchus; *l,* left main bronchus; *rul,* right upper lobe bronchus; *bi,* bronchus intermedius; *arul,* anterior segment right upper lobe bronchus; *prul,* posterior segment right upper lobe bronchus; *rml,* right middle lobe bronchus; *mrml,* medial segment right middle lobe bronchus; *lrml,* lateral segment right middle lobe bronchus; *srll,* superior segment right lower lobe bronchus; *mrll,* medial segment right lower lobe bronchus; *arll,* anterior segment right lower lobe bronchus; *lrll,* lateral segment right lower lobe bronchus; *prll,* posterior segment right lower lobe bronchus; *lul,* left upper lobe bronchus; *aplul,* apical posterior segment left upper lobe bronchus; *alul,* anterior segment left upper lobe bronchus; *li,* lingular bronchus; *il,* inferior segment lingular bronchus; *lll,* left lower lobe bronchus; *sllll,* superior segment left lower lobe bronchus; *mlll,* medial subsegment left lower lobe bronchus; *alll,* anterior subsegment left lower lobe bronchus; *llll,* lateral segment left lower lobe bronchus; *plll,* posterior segment left lower lobe bronchus. *(continued)*

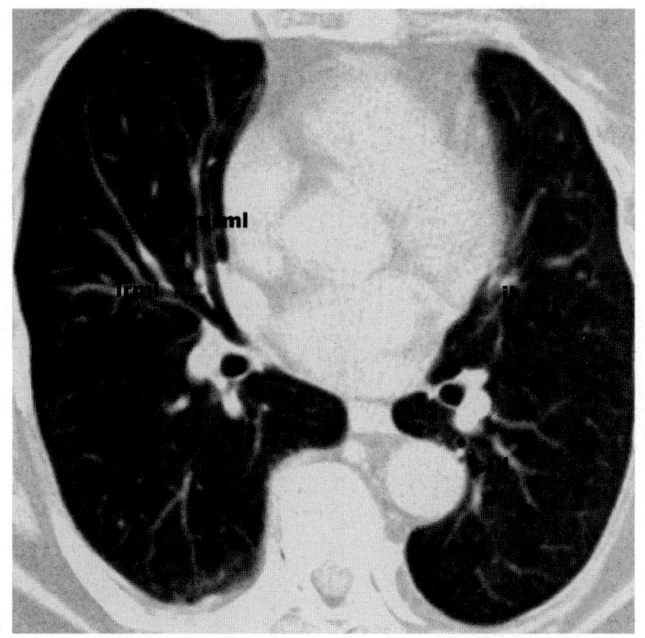

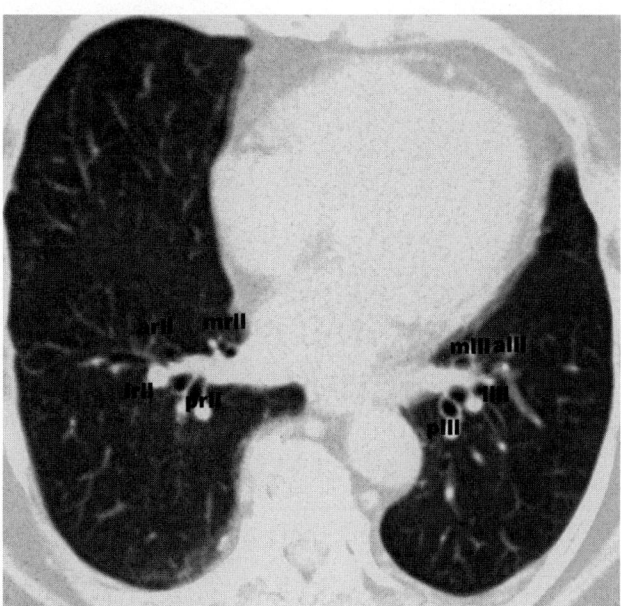

E   F

FIGURE 1.6. (*continued*)

be visible on HRCT as a dot or branching structure 5 to 10 mm deep to the pleural surface. This visualized centrilobular structure represents the distal pulmonary artery branch; its accompanying bronchus is not normally seen.

APPROACH TO CHEST RADIOGRAPHS

A systematic approach to the chest radiograph should incorporate a review of technical adequacy; a systematic survey of the soft tissues, lungs, and mediastinum; and a review of the areas where lesions are most likely to be missed.

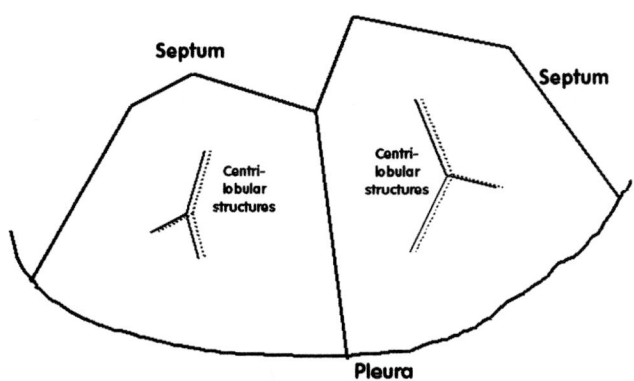

FIGURE 1.7. Schematic diagram of secondary pulmonary lobule. The secondary pulmonary lobule is supplied by the centrilobular pulmonary arteriole and its accompanying bronchiole. It is drained by veins and lymphatics running in the interlobular septa. The septa are best developed by the periphery of the lung.

Technical Adequacy

On an adequately exposed radiograph, the outlines of the vertebral bodies should be visible through the heart, and the pulmonary vasculature should be clearly visible. The degree of rotation of the radiograph can be evaluated by determining whether the thoracic spinous processes are projected midway between the clavicles. Caudal or cranial displacement of the x-ray beam will result in apparent displacement of the clavicles superiorly or inferiorly relative to the posterior ribs. The radiograph should include all parts of the lungs. The peak of the right hemidiaphragm should project over the posterior 10th intercostal space.

On a technically adequate lateral radiograph, the arms should be elevated so that the anterior mediastinum is not obscured. Because lateral images are usually obtained with the left side of the chest closest to the x-ray detection device, the right ribs will be projected slightly behind the left ribs on a well-positioned lateral image and will be more magnified than the left ribs (Fig. 1.5).

Systematic Survey

A systematic survey (Fig. 1.8) of the frontal chest radiograph begins with an overall glance to detect major abnormalities and identify asymmetry of lung density. A detailed search begins at the outside of the image, with a review of the soft tissues and bones of the supraclavicular regions, shoulders, lateral chest wall, and upper abdomen. This should be followed by a sweeping search of the lungs, ribs, and intercostal spaces, comparing right with left. Next, the eye moves along

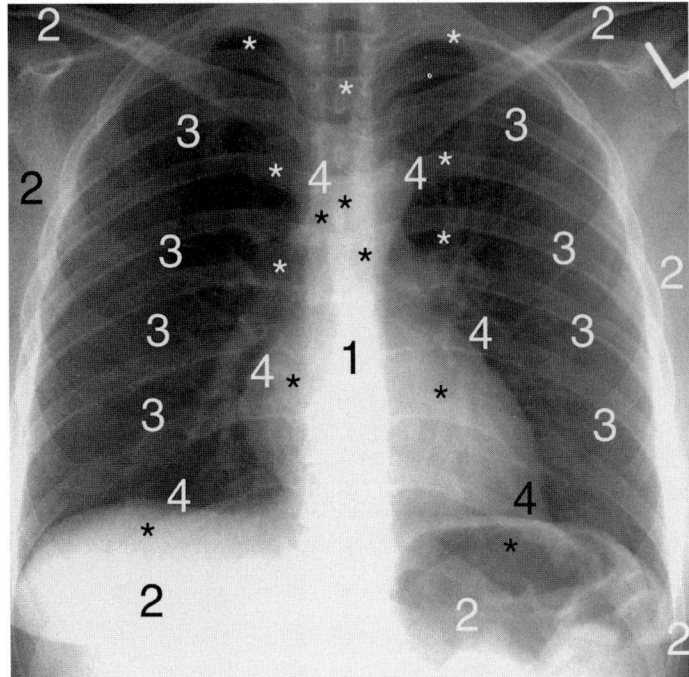

A

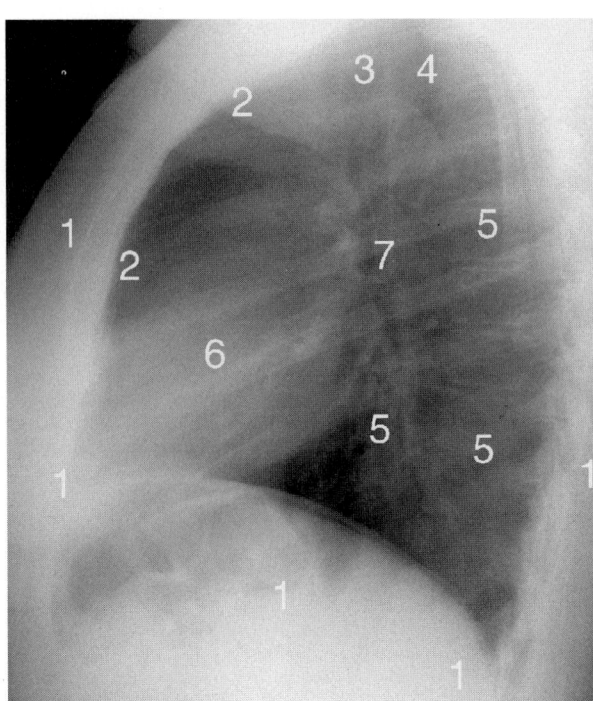

B

FIGURE 1.8. A systematic approach to chest radiographic evaluation. **A:** A typical systematic approach to the chest radiograph begins with an overall evaluation of the image to detect gross abnormalities and asymmetry of density *(1)*. After this, the eyes move around the periphery of the image *(2)*. Next comes a side-to-side sweep of the lungs, using the intercostal spaces as a guide and comparing one side with the other *(3)*. Next comes a review of the mediastinal interfaces and the diaphragm *(4)*. Finally comes a review of the "miss areas" (marked with an *asterisk*): the apices, the hila and suprahilar regions, the right and left retrocardiac regions, and the right and left retrodiaphragmatic regions. **B:** Systematic search pattern for the lateral chest radiograph begins with a review of the periphery of the radiograph *(1)*. Next comes a review of the sternum and the retrosternal region *(2)*. Next is a look at the trachea *(3)* and retrotracheal triangle *(4)*. The eye then moves down along the spine and the area of the lungs behind the heart *(5)*. Next comes the area overlying the heart *(6)*. The final review is reserved for the anatomically complex area of the hila *(7)*.

the right and left borders of the mediastinum and along the right and left hemidiaphragms. Finally, one reviews the areas in which abnormalities are commonly missed: the lung apices, the hila and suprahilar regions, the major airways, the right and left retrocardiac regions, and the right and left retrodiaphragmatic regions. In all of these areas, symmetry of the right and left lungs is probably the most important feature.

On the lateral image, the search begins at the periphery, with a review of the soft tissues and bones of the shoulders, chest wall, and abdomen. Next comes a review of the sternum and retrosternal region, followed by review of the trachea, retrotracheal triangle, the area over the heart, and the area of the lower lobes. The final part of the review covers the anatomically complex pulmonary hila.

RADIOLOGIC SIGNS OF LUNG DISEASE

Terminology

Radiologists are trained to apply a standard terminology to their descriptions of radiologic abnormalities. The Fleischner Society has published helpful glossaries of the descriptors used for chest radiographs (34) and chest CT scans (35). Nonspecific terms such as increased interstitial markings and infiltrate are best avoided. Specificity of radiologic descriptors enhances the ability of radiologists to communicate their findings and generate appropriate differential diagnoses. One of the basic radiologic distinctions is between disorders that increase the attenuation of x-rays by the lung (opacities), and those that decrease x-ray attenuation (lucencies). On radiographs and chest CT scans, opacities will appear whiter than normal lung, whereas lucent lesions will appear blacker.

Identification of radiographic categories of abnormality such as airspace disease, interstitial disease, airway disease, and emphysema must be based on the recognition of appropriate signs, as indicated in Table 1.1. Common signs of lung disease are illustrated on chest radiograph and chest CT in Figures 1.9 through 1.14.

Distribution of Lung Diseases

Many ILDs have a peripheral predominance (Table 1.2). In particular, the characteristic peripheral distribution of idiopathic pulmonary fibrosis (36) and of eosinophilic

TABLE 1.1. PATTERN-BASED ANALYSIS OF CHEST RADIOGRAPHS

Radiographic Findings	Pattern	Common Differential Diagnosis

Poorly defined opacities
Coalescence
Air bronchograms
	Airspace (alveolar) disease	Acute
		  Pneumonia
		  Edema
		  Aspiration
		  Hemorrhage
		Chronic
		  Chronic infection (tuberculosis, fungal)
		  Organizing pneumonia
		  Sarcoidosis (pseudoalveolar)
		  Pulmonary alveolar proteinosis
		  Cellular infiltrations
		  Bronchioloalveolar cell carcinoma
		  Lymphoma
		  Eosinophilic pneumonia
		  Vasculitis
		  Chronic aspiration (especially lipid)

Well-defined nodule	Solitary pulmonary nodule	Granuloma Hamartoma Primary neoplasm Metastasis Pulmonary arteriovenous malformation Mucous plug

Multiple well-defined
  nodules <5 mm
	Nodular disease	Malignancy
		Pneumoconiosis
		  Silicosis
		  Pneumoconiosis of coal workers
		Granulomas
		  Infectious (miliary)
		  Sarcoid
		  Berylliosis
		  Langerhans histiocytosis

Poorly defined nodules		Malignancy
		  Bronchioloalveolar
		  Lymphoma
		  Hemorrhagic metastases
		Granulomas
		  Infection (tuberculosis/fungal)
		  Sarcoid
		  Langerhans histiocytosis
		Infection
		  Viral (varicella, cytomegalovirus)

Reticular lines Honeycombing	Fibrotic disease	Idiopathic pulmonary fibrosis Asbestosis Collagen vascular disease Sarcoidosis Chronic hypersensitivity pneumonitis
Kerley A, B, C lines	Septal thickening	Lung edema Lymphangitic spread Infection (*Pneumocystis carinii* pneumonia, mycoplasma) Drug reaction
Ring shadows Train track Hyperinflation	Airway disease	Bronchitis Asthma Bronchiectasis
Hyperlucency Oligemia Distorted vessels Hyperinflation	Emphysema	Cigarette smoking α_1-antitrypsin deficiency
Cavities	Cavitary disease	Infection Neoplasm Pulmonary infarction Vasculitis

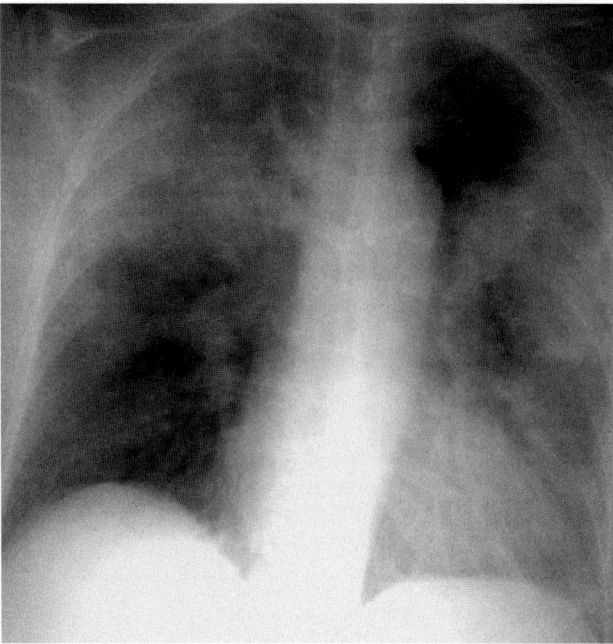

FIGURE 1.9. Lung consolidation. Chest radiograph in a 50-year-old patient with chronic eosinophilic pneumonia shows poorly defined confluent opacity, compatible with lung consolidation.

pneumonia (37) are much better demonstrated on CT than on conventional radiographs. The upper-lobe predominance of the cysts and nodules of pulmonary Langerhans histiocytosis (38, 39) helps to distinguish this entity from the diffuse cysts seen in lymphangiomyomatosis (40).

TABLE 1.2. CRANIOCAUDAL AND AXIAL DISTRIBUTION OF LUNG DISEASES

Peripheral disease	UIP, OP
	Asbestosis
	Collagen vascular disease
	Eosinophilic pneumonia
Central/peribronchovascular disease	Sarcoidosis
	Lymphangitis carcinomatosa
	Lymphoproliferative disorders
	Organizing pneumonia
Upper-lobe predominance	Sarcoidosis
	Pneumoconiosis of coal workers
	Silicosis
	Eosinophilic pneumonia
	Pulmonary histiocytosis X
	Hypersensitivity pneumonitis
Lower-lobe predominance	UIP, NSIP, OP
	Asbestosis
	Collagen vascular disease

UIP, usual interstitial pneumonitis; OP, organizing pneumonia; NSIP, nonspecific interstitial pneumonia.

ABNORMALITIES OF THE SECONDARY PULMONARY LOBULE

A valuable approach to differential diagnosis of ILD on HRCT involves assessment of the distribution of disease in relation to bronchovascular structures, pleura, and the secondary pulmonary lobule (41, 42) (Table 1.3). In patients with inflammation or plugging of small airways, the normally invisible centrilobular structures become visible as nodules or short branching structures. When these

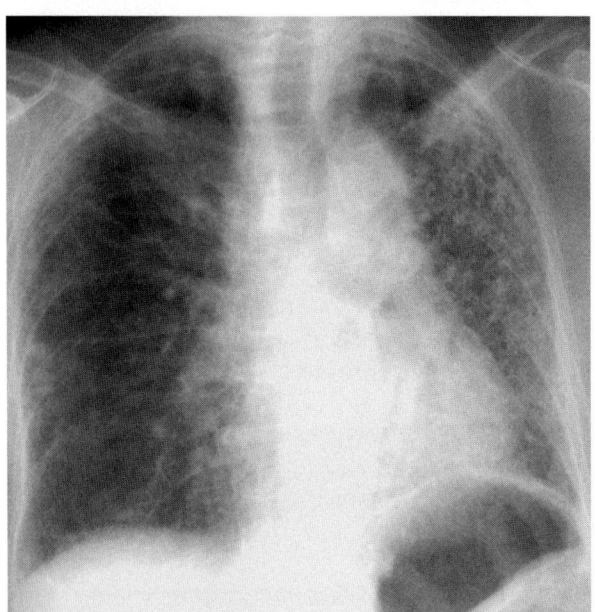

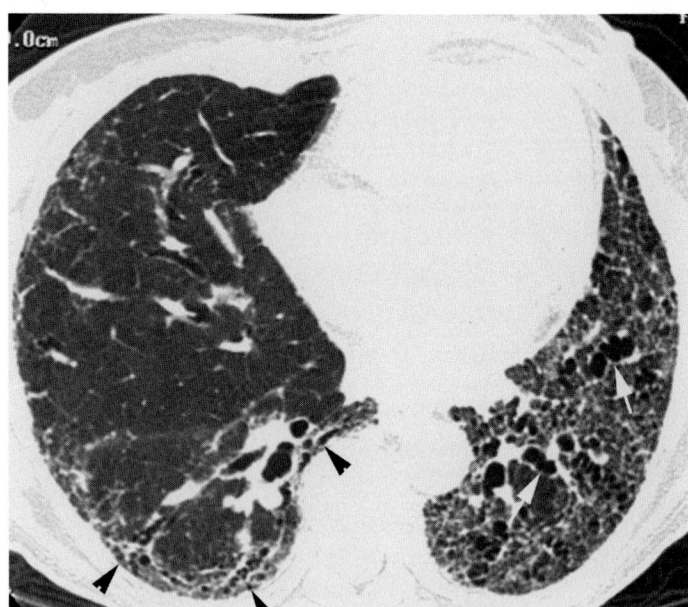

A   B

FIGURE 1.10. A: Reticular and honeycomb pattern in a 73-year-old woman with idiopathic pulmonary fibrosis. Chest radiograph shows asymmetric fine reticular pattern with basal honeycombing. **B:** Computed tomography shows left-sided predominant reticular abnormality with traction bronchiectasis *(white arrows)* and peripheral subpleural rows of honeycomb cysts *(black arrowheads).*

TABLE 1.3. LOBULAR DISTRIBUTION OF INFILTRATIVE LUNG DISEASES ON HIGH-RESOLUTION COMPUTED TOMOGRAPHY

Centrilobular nodules	Pneumoconiosis
	Sarcoidosis
	Hypersensitivity pneumonitis
Centrilobular thickening with tree in bud	Bronchiolitis
Dominant septal thickening	Lymphangitic carcinoma
	Left heart failure
Mixed septal and centrilobular thickening	Sarcoidosis
	Lymphangitic carcinoma
Panlobular increased density	Hypersensitivity pneumonitis
	Drug toxicity
	Desquamative interstitial pneumonitis
Panlobular decreased density	Pulmonary embolism
	Constrictive bronchiolitis
	Panlobular emphysema

branching structures terminate in a nodule, the *tree-in-bud* sign is present (Fig. 1.15A). The tree-in-bud sign is usually due either to small airway inflammation or to disease that spreads by the airways, such as tuberculosis (43). Nodules that are centrilobular without a tree-in-bud appearance are usually due to some form of inhalational disease. Thickening of interlobular septa (Fig. 1.15B) is usually due to edema or infiltration of the lymphatic structures, and is often associated with thickening of the other lymphatic pathways (subpleural and peribronchovascular). Panlobular ground-glass attenuation, often associated with sparing of one or more lobules, commonly represents an active inflammatory process. A limitation of analysis of the secondary pulmonary lobule is that many common ILDs such as idiopathic pulmonary fibrosis, sarcoidosis, and lymphangiomyomatosis are associated with distortion of lobular anatomy (44), so that assessment of the lobular anatomy is not very useful in these individuals.

Computed Tomography Patterns of Lung Disease

A very useful standard terminology for describing the CT findings in parenchymal lung diseases has been published by the Fleischner Society (35). Some of the more important features are listed below and in Table 1.4.

Nodules

Nodules seen on HRCT can be classified according to their size (micronodules or larger nodules), density (ground-glass, soft tissue, or calcific densities), definition (well defined or poorly defined), and distribution. Micronodules measure less than 3 mm in diameter (45). Gruden et al.

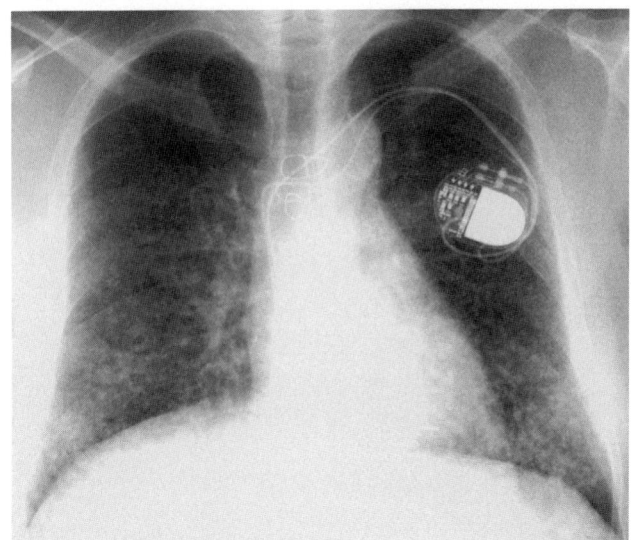

A

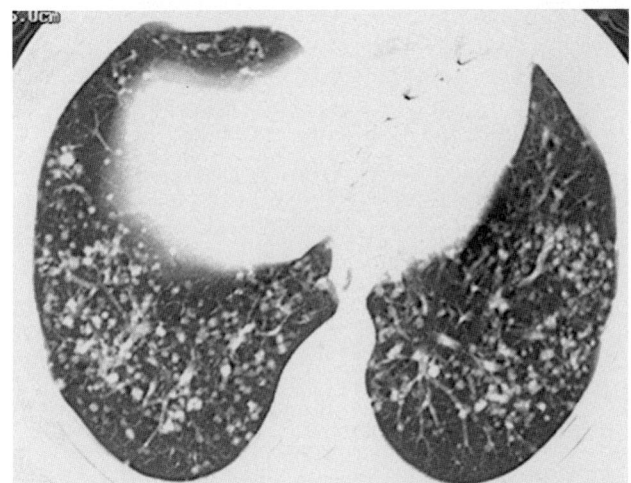

B

FIGURE 1.11. A 60-year-old man with nodular parenchymal pattern on chest radiograph, due to metastases from thyroid carcinoma. **A:** Chest radiograph shows multiple nodules, mainly in the lower lungs, and an automatic implantable cardioverter defibrillator (AICD) is also present. Note that the nodules are of varying sizes. **B:** Computed tomography through the lung bases confirms the presence of multiple nodules of varying sizes.

(46) classified nodules on the basis of their location (random, perilymphatic, centrilobular, or airway-associated). Perilymphatic micronodules are seen in subpleural and septal locations, and are most profuse in subjects with lymphangitic carcinomatosis and sarcoidosis, but may also be seen in pneumoconiosis. Scattered subpleural micronodules may be seen in normal subjects. Centrilobular nodules differ from small airway–associated nodules in that the small-airway nodules are frequently patchy, tend to be related to small branching structures (tree-in-bud phenomenon), and are often associated with patches of airspace opacification.

Nodules of ground-glass density are typically seen in hypersensitivity pneumonitis (Fig. 1.16) but may also be

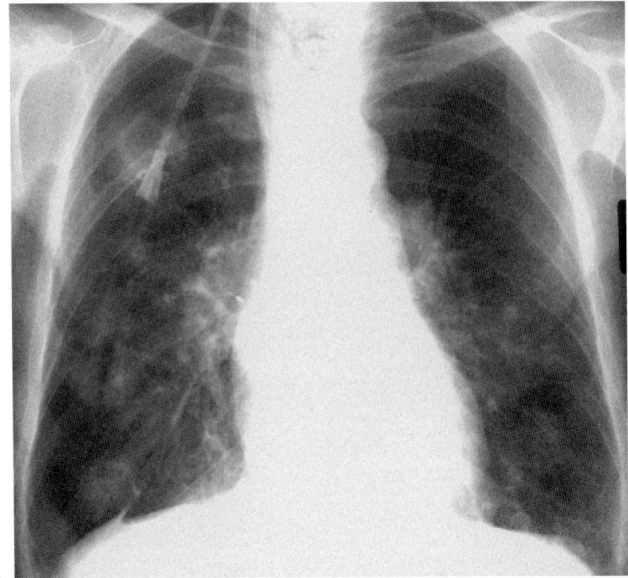

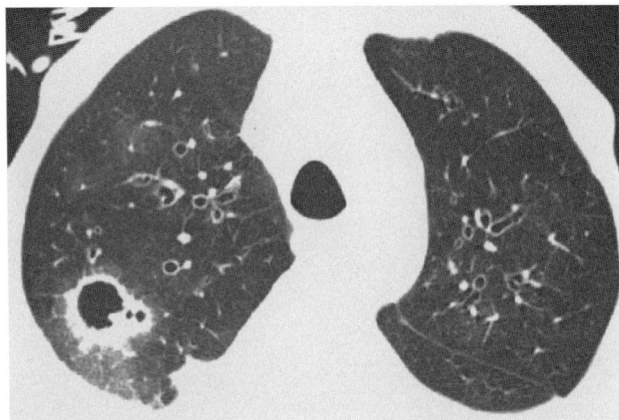

FIGURE 1.12. A 60-year-old allogeneic bone marrow transplant recipient with fever. **A:** Chest radiograph shows a large cavity in the right upper lung, with a further cavitary nodule in the right lower lung. **B:** Computed tomography confirms the presence of a cavity, with an irregular wall, subsequently proven to be caused by *Aspergillus*. The patient has widespread cylindric bronchiectasis due to bronchiolitis obliterans, indicating graft-versus-host disease.

TABLE 1.4. COMPUTED TOMOGRAPHY FEATURES OF COMMON LUNG DISEASES

Nodules	Sarcoidosis
	Pulmonary histiocytosis X
	Hypersensitivity pneumonitis
	Silicosis
	Metastatic cancer
Centrilobular nodules	See Table 1.2
Lines	
Thickened septa	See Table 1.2
Intralobular or reticular	UIP, NSIP
	Asbestosis
	Collagen vascular disease
	Pulmonary alveolar proteinosis
Curvilinear subpleural	Asbestosis
	Congestion in dependent lung
Parenchymal band	Asbestosis
	Scarring from pleural disease
Lung cysts	Distinguish from emphysema
	Pulmonary histiocytosis X
	Lymphangiomyomatosis
	Lymphoid interstitial pneumonitis
Honeycombing	Asbestosis
	UIP
	Collagen vascular disease
	Sarcoidosis
	Hypersensitivity pneumonitis
Parenchymal Opacification	OP
Ground-glass attenuation	Hypersensitivity pneumonitis
	Drug toxicity
	Desquamative interstitial pneumonitis
	Pulmonary alveolar proteinosis
	Sarcoidosis
Consolidation	Organizing pneumonia
	Eosinophilic pneumonia
	Alveolar cell carcinoma
	Lipoid pneumonia
	Pulmonary alveolar proteinosis
Decreased Lung Attenuation	Pulmonary embolism
	Constrictive bronchiolitis
	Panlobular emphysema
Mosaic Pattern	Constrictive bronchiolitis
	Pulmonary thromboembolism
	Diseases causing ground-glass attenuation

UIP, usual interstitial pneumonia; NSIP, nonspecific interstitial pneumonia; OP, organizing pneumonia.

seen in respiratory bronchiolitis. Soft tissue density nodules are seen in patients with granulomatous lung diseases, malignancy, or pneumoconiosis. Calcific nodules are seen in prior granulomatous infection or in pulmonary alveolar microlithiasis.

Lines

A variety of linear densities may be seen on HRCT. Thickened interlobular septa (Fig. 1.15B) are identified because they are perpendicular to the pleura (47) or because they form polygonal structures (48). Reticular lines are probably the commonest type of linear abnormality (Fig. 1.10). These lines are less than 5 mm long, forming a fine lacelike network that usually does not conform to lobular anatomy. They are seen in all types of fibrotic lung conditions, particularly idiopathic pulmonary fibrosis (49), collagen vascular disease, and asbestosis (Fig. 1.17). Reticular lines are also a prominent CT feature in patients with the crazy paving pattern (discussed below) (Fig. 1.18).

Cysts

The cysts of ILD are air-containing lucencies with a well-defined, complete wall (Fig. 1.19). They are usually round but may sometimes be irregular in shape, particularly in Langerhans histiocytosis. They must be distinguished from

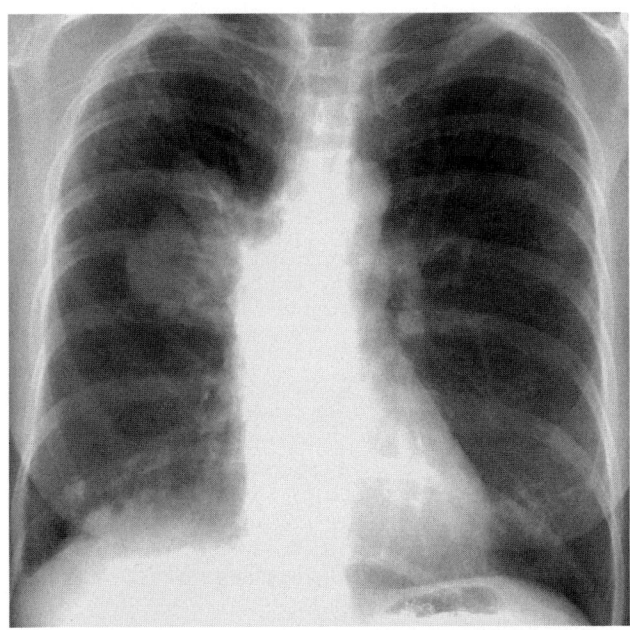

A

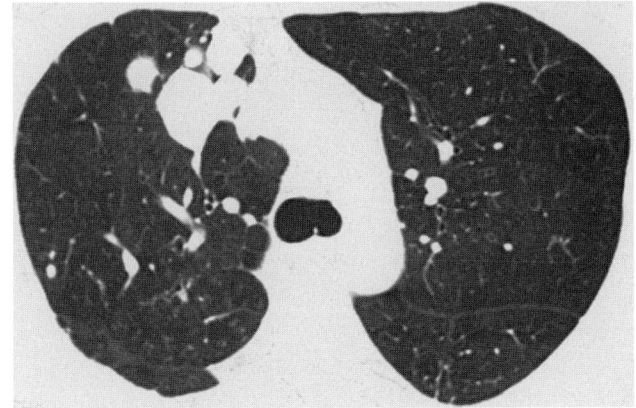

B

FIGURE 1.13. Mucoid impaction in patient with proximal bronchial obstruction. **A:** Chest radiograph shows lobulated, tubular, branching mass extending from the right hilum. **B, C:** Computed tomography confirms the tubular nature of the mass.

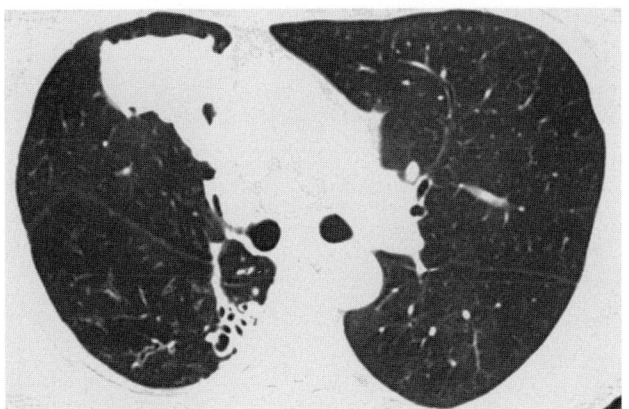

C

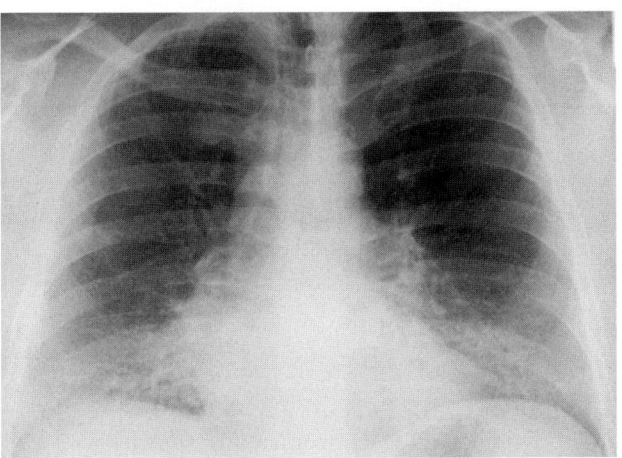

A

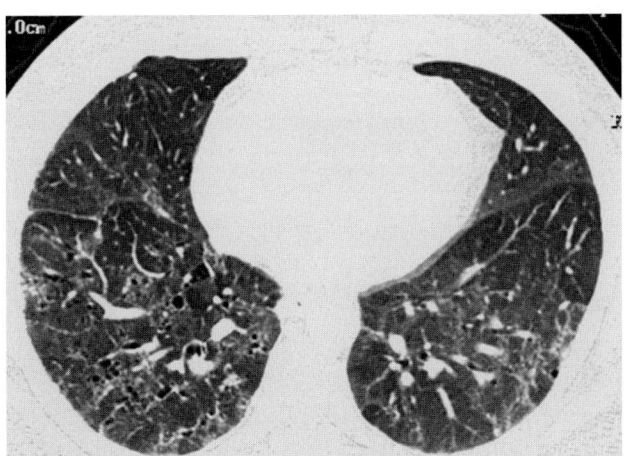

B

FIGURE 1.14. Ground-glass attenuation in a patient with desquamative interstitial pneumonia. **A:** Chest radiograph shows basal ground-glass attenuation. **B:** Computed tomography confirms patchy ground-glass attenuation, with traction bronchiectasis and scattered cysts.

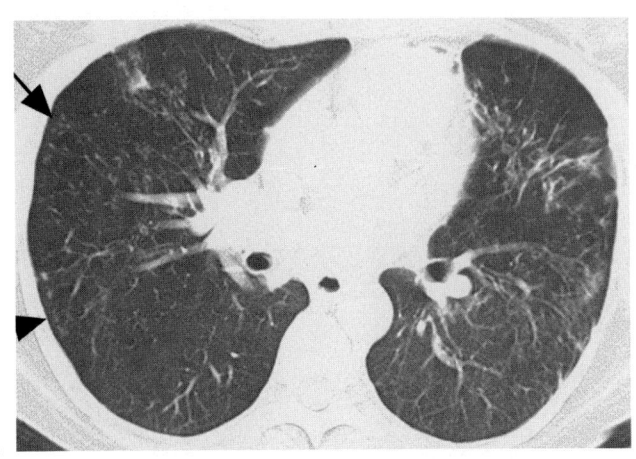
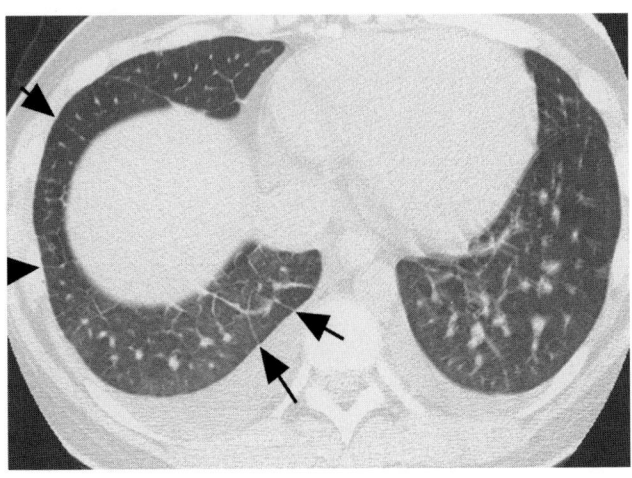

FIGURE 1.15. A: A 22-year-old woman with cystic fibrosis. Computed tomography (CT) shows multiple centrilobular nodules connected to more central branching structures (tree-in-bud sign) *(arrows).* **B:** A 22-year-old woman with postpartum pulmonary edema, scanned to rule out pulmonary embolism. High-resolution CT through the lung bases shows smooth thickening of multiple interlobular septa *(arrows).* The septa outline the typical polygonal structure of the secondary pulmonary lobule.

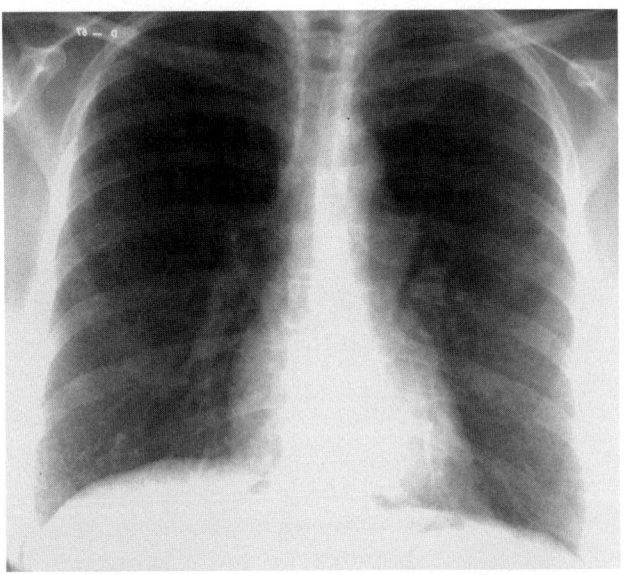
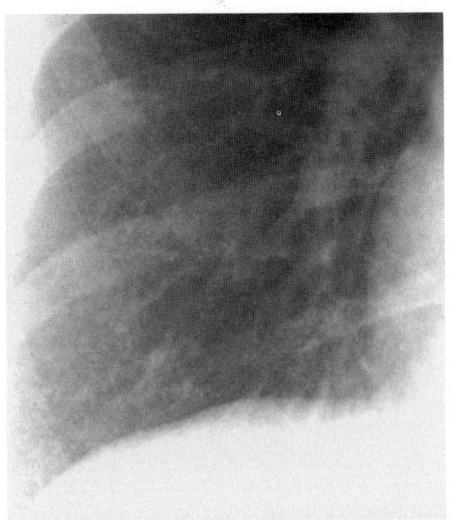
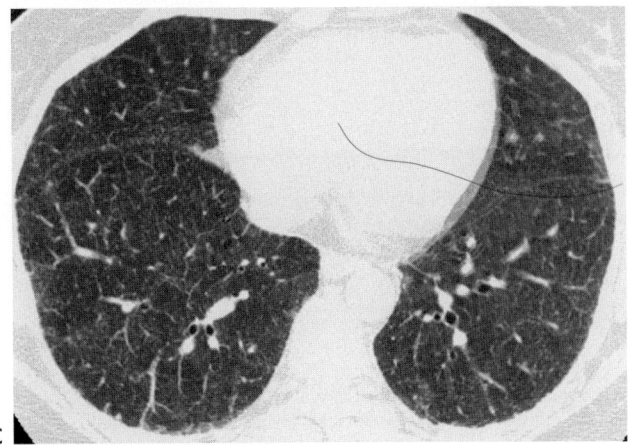

FIGURE 1.16. Micronodular pattern in a patient with hypersensitivity pneumonitis. **A, B:** Posterior-anterior chest radiograph, with detail view, shows fine micronodular pattern. **C:** High-resolution chest computed tomography confirms the presence of a fine micronodular pattern, associated with ground-glass abnormality.

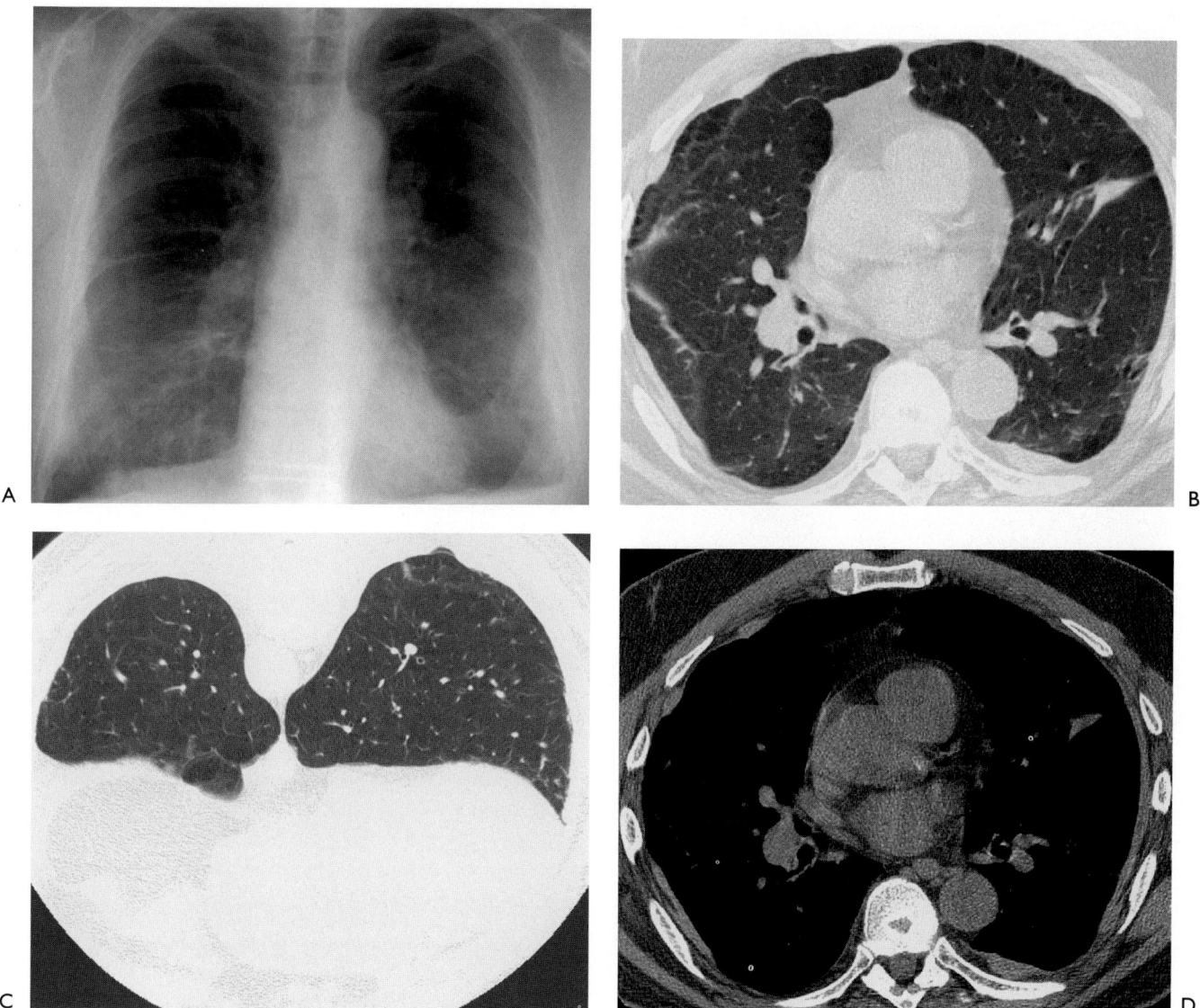

FIGURE 1.17. A 72-year-old man with asbestosis. **A:** Chest radiograph shows bilateral pleural thickening, with blunting of both costophrenic sulci, and lobulated thickening along both lateral chest walls owing to pleural plaques. Coarse parenchymal bandlike opacities are present, but it is difficult to determine whether there is true underlying lung fibrosis because of the extent of pleural disease. **B:** High-resolution computed tomography (HRCT) through the mid lungs shows coarse parenchymal bandlike scarring, **C:** Prone HRCT through the lung bases shows mild peripheral linear abnormality. This was present at multiple levels and bilaterally, and is consistent with early asbestosis. **D:** Soft tissue windows confirm the presence of asbestos related pleural thickening.

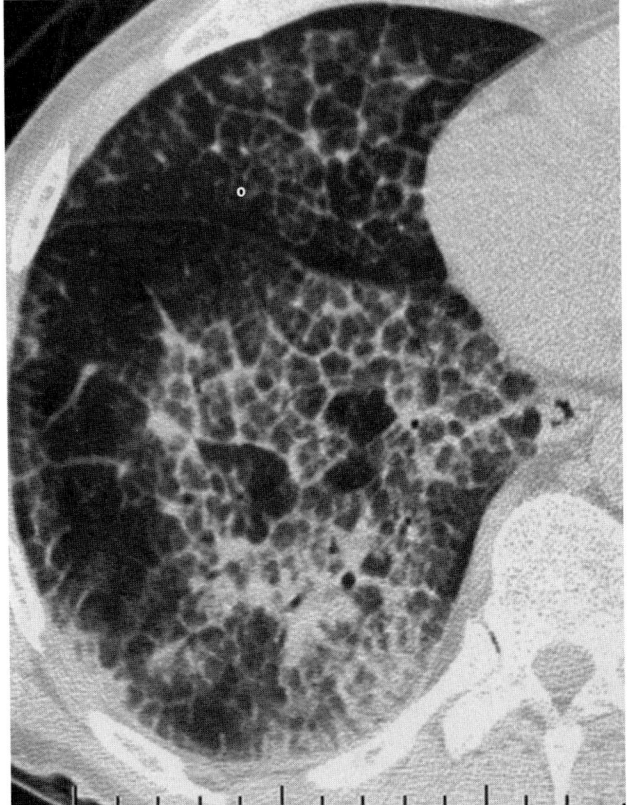

FIGURE 1.18. A 54-year-old man with mild dyspnea on exertion. Computed tomography shows typical crazy paving pattern of alveolar proteinosis. (From Lynch DA, Newell JD, Lee S, eds. *Imaging of diffuse lung disease.* Hamilton, Ontario: BC Decker, 2000, with permission.)

the "moth-eaten" lucencies of centrilobular emphysema, which are usually irregular in outline and do not have a definable wall (Fig. 1.20). Cysts may be distinguished from bronchiectatic bronchi because bronchi are usually accompanied by a smaller pulmonary artery, and cysts

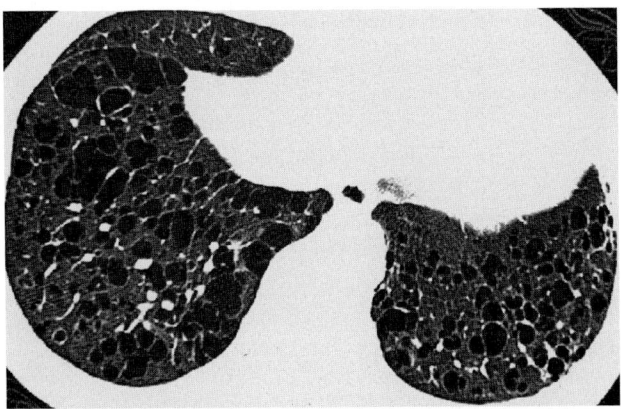

FIGURE 1.19. Multiple pulmonary cysts in a young girl with lymphangiomyomatosis. High-resolution computed tomography through the lung bases shows multiple discrete cysts. All of the cysts have a thin, well-defined wall.

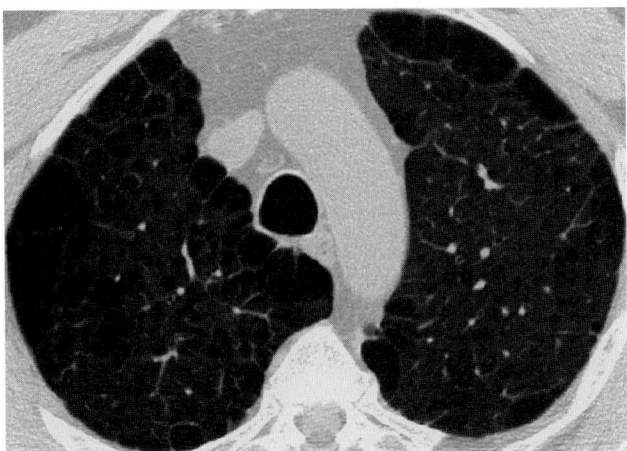

FIGURE 1.20. High-resolution computed tomography scan shows widespread centrilobular emphysema. The small holes within the lung are distinguished from cysts by the lack of a visible wall. The larger subpleural areas of low attenuation represent areas of distal acinar emphysema.

can usually be traced back to the hilum on serial CT sections.

Honeycombing is defined as a cluster or row of cysts (Fig. 1.10). Honeycomb cysts are usually very small (<5 mm in diameter). This CT finding correlates with histologic honeycombing and is found in end-stage lung of any cause (50). Larger honeycomb cysts may sometimes be found in patients with sarcoidosis.

Traction Bronchiectasis/Bronchiolectasis

Traction bronchiectasis and bronchiolectasis (Fig. 1.10) refers to dilatation and distortion of the bronchi and bronchioles in areas of fibrosis, presumed to be due to the forces of increased elastic recoil acting on these structures (51). It is usually associated with a reticular pattern or with ground-glass attenuation and is reliable evidence of lung fibrosis (52).

Consolidation/Ground-Glass Attenuation

The term parenchymal opacification (35, 53) is applied to any homogeneous increase in lung density on chest radiographs or chest CT. When this parenchymal opacification is dense enough to obscure the vessels and other parenchymal structures, it is called *consolidation* (Fig. 1.21). *Ground-glass attenuation* (sometimes called hazy increase in lung density) is defined as an increase in lung density that is not sufficient to obscure vessels (Fig. 1.14). Ground-glass attenuation is commonly, although not always, associated with reversible or potentially reversible lung disease. When consolidation is superimposed on a background of emphysema, it produces the "Swiss cheese pattern" (Fig. 1.21).

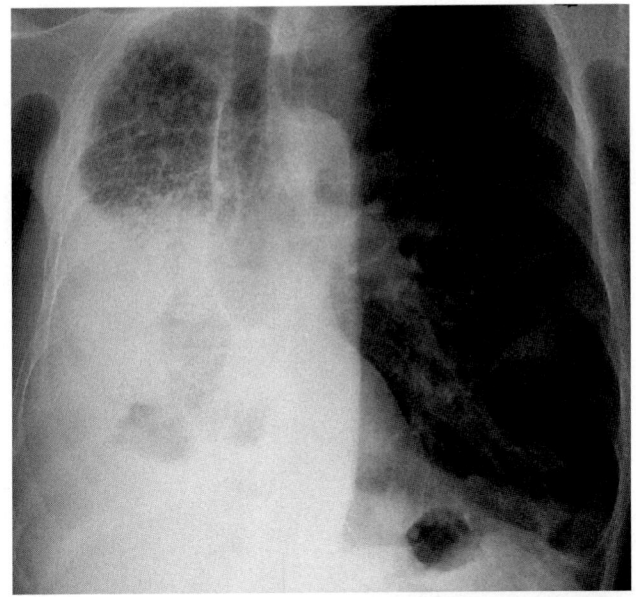

A

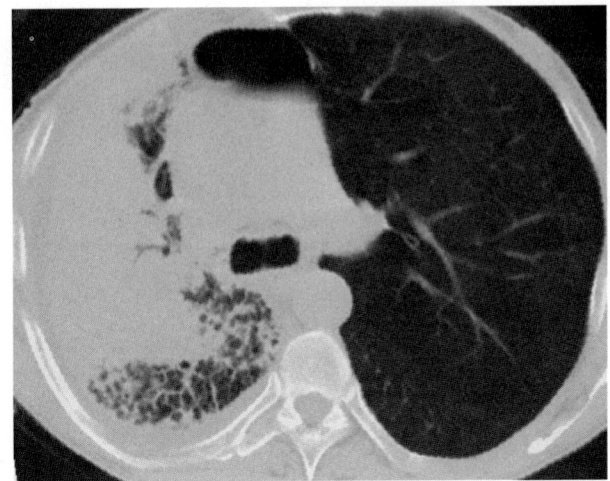

B

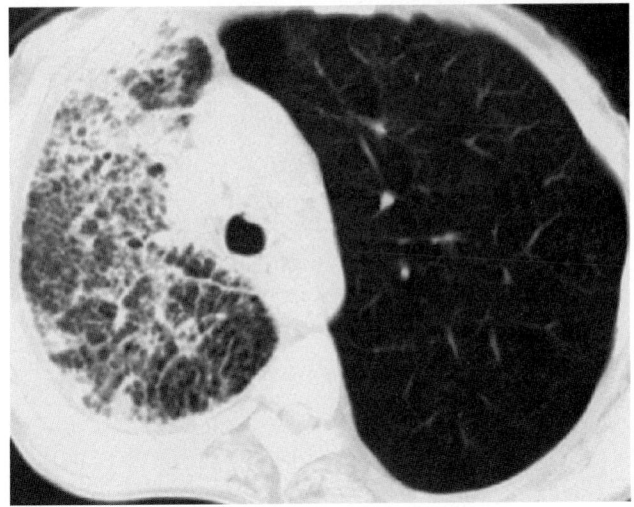

C

FIGURE 1.21. A 70-year-old man with lung consolidation due to bronchioloalveolar carcinoma. **A:** Chest radiograph shows dense consolidation in the right lower lung, with a more reticular pattern in the right upper lung. **B:** Computed tomography (CT) through the lower lung shows consolidation. **C:** CT scan through the upper lung shows that the apparent reticular abnormality is owing to consolidation superimposed on emphysema (Swiss cheese effect).

Decreased Lung Attenuation/Mosaic Pattern

The attenuation (density) of a given area of lung depends on the amount of parenchymal tissue, air, and blood in that area. Therefore, decreased attenuation of the lung may be due to lung destruction (in panlobular emphysema), to decreased blood flow (Fig. 1.22) (in vascular disease such as pulmonary thromboembolism), or to decreased ventilation with air trapping and reflex pulmonary oligemia (in small-airway diseases with constrictive bronchiolitis). Panlobular emphysema differs from vascular lung disease and small-airway disease in that it usually causes a diffuse decrease in lung attenuation (increased blackness), whereas thromboembolic disease and obliterative bronchiolitis are commonly (although not always) more patchy in distribution. Vascular disease can often be distinguished from airway disease by comparing inspiratory and expiratory scans. In airway disease, one will expect to see air trapping on the expiratory scans, resulting in an increase in the number of areas of decreased attenuation. In patients with occlusive vascular disease, the areas of decreased attenuation should not increase on expiration (54).

Because patients with thromboembolic disease and obliterative bronchiolitis commonly have patchy decreases in lung attenuation, they may present with a *mosaic pattern,* with lobules of normal attenuation adjacent to lobules or subsegments of decreased attenuation. A similar mosaic pattern may be caused by parenchymal disease, which causes lobular areas of ground-glass attenuation. With the mosaic pattern, it can be difficult to decide whether the abnormal

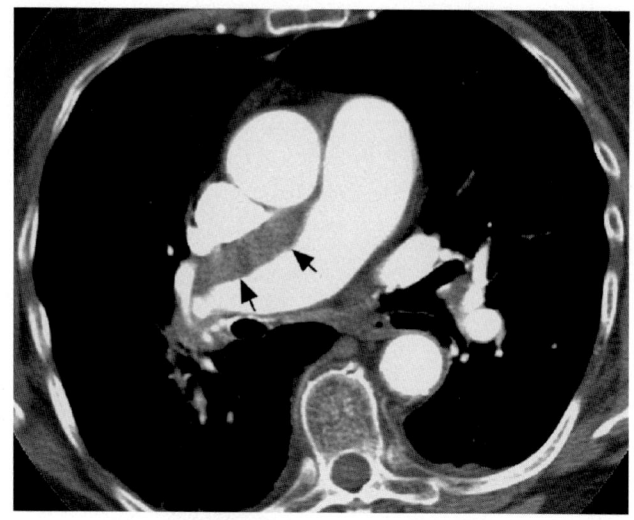

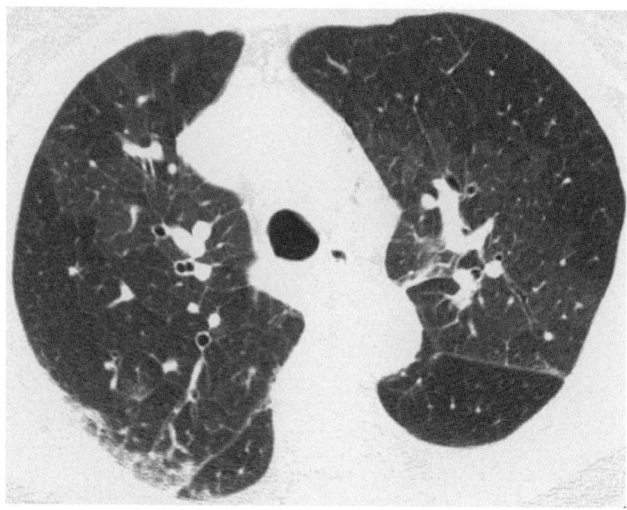

A   B

FIGURE 1.22. Mosaic pattern related to chronic pulmonary thromboembolic disease. **A:** Computed tomography (CT) pulmonary arteriogram shows extensive mural thrombus along the course of the right pulmonary artery *(arrows).* **B:** High-resolution CT shows alternating areas of increased and decreased lung attenuation (mosaic pattern). Note the decreased vessel size in the areas of decreased lung attenuation, indicating that the decreased lung attenuation is caused by decreased blood flow.

areas are those of decreased attenuation or those of increased attenuation. This distinction can be made by observing the pulmonary vessels, which will be reduced in size in areas affected by vascular occlusive disease (Fig. 1.22) or obliterative bronchiolitis, but will be normal in size in patients with parenchymal infiltrative lung diseases (54). One can then use expiratory images to distinguish between airway obstruction and thromboembolic disease (55). Of course, physiologic evaluation will also help to distinguish between vascular disease, airway obstruction, and parenchymal infiltration.

Crazy Paving Pattern

In the crazy paving pattern, thickened intralobular and interlobular lines form a fine geographic network superimposed on a background of ground-glass attenuation (56) (Fig. 1.18). In the correct clinical context, this pattern is strongly suggestive of pulmonary alveolar proteinosis. The pattern can also be seen in patients with other lung diseases, including resolving pneumonia, adult respiratory distress syndrome, lipoid pneumonia, and mucinous bronchioloalveolar carcinoma, but in these conditions, it is usually associated with other types of CT abnormality (57–59).

Signs of Pleural Disease

Pleural effusion. Pleural effusion is usually manifested by rounded blunting of the costophrenic sulci. The posterior costophrenic sulcus, being deeper, usually becomes abnormal before the lateral costophrenic sulcus, so the lateral

chest radiograph is more sensitive than is the frontal radiograph for detecting small effusions. In subpulmonic pleural effusions, pleural fluid accumulates beneath the lung and may be difficult to distinguish from an elevated hemidiaphragm (Fig. 1.23). In other cases, loculation of pleural fluid within a fissure may simulate a parenchymal mass (pseudotumor).

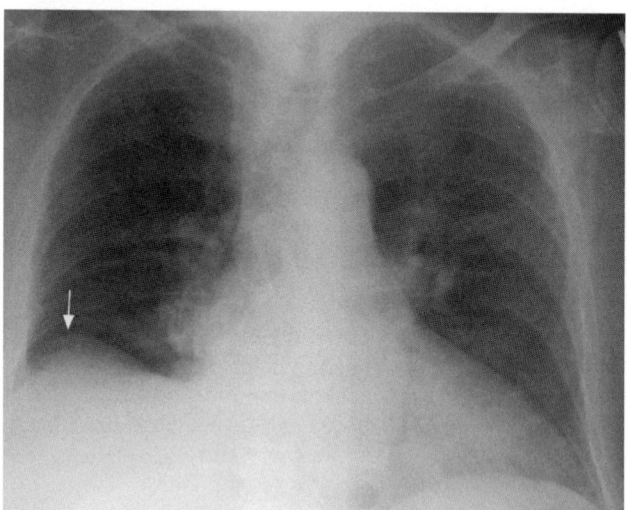

FIGURE 1.23. Subpulmonic pleural effusion. Frontal chest radiograph shows apparent elevation of the right hemidiaphragm. However, the appearance differs from the typical appearance of an elevated hemidiaphragm because the peak of the effusion is more lateral than one would expect for an elevated hemidiaphragm *(arrow).* Second, the vessels of the retrodiaphragmatic lung cannot be visualized, because pleural fluid is filling the posterior costophrenic sulcus. Third, the right lateral costophrenic sulcus is blunted.

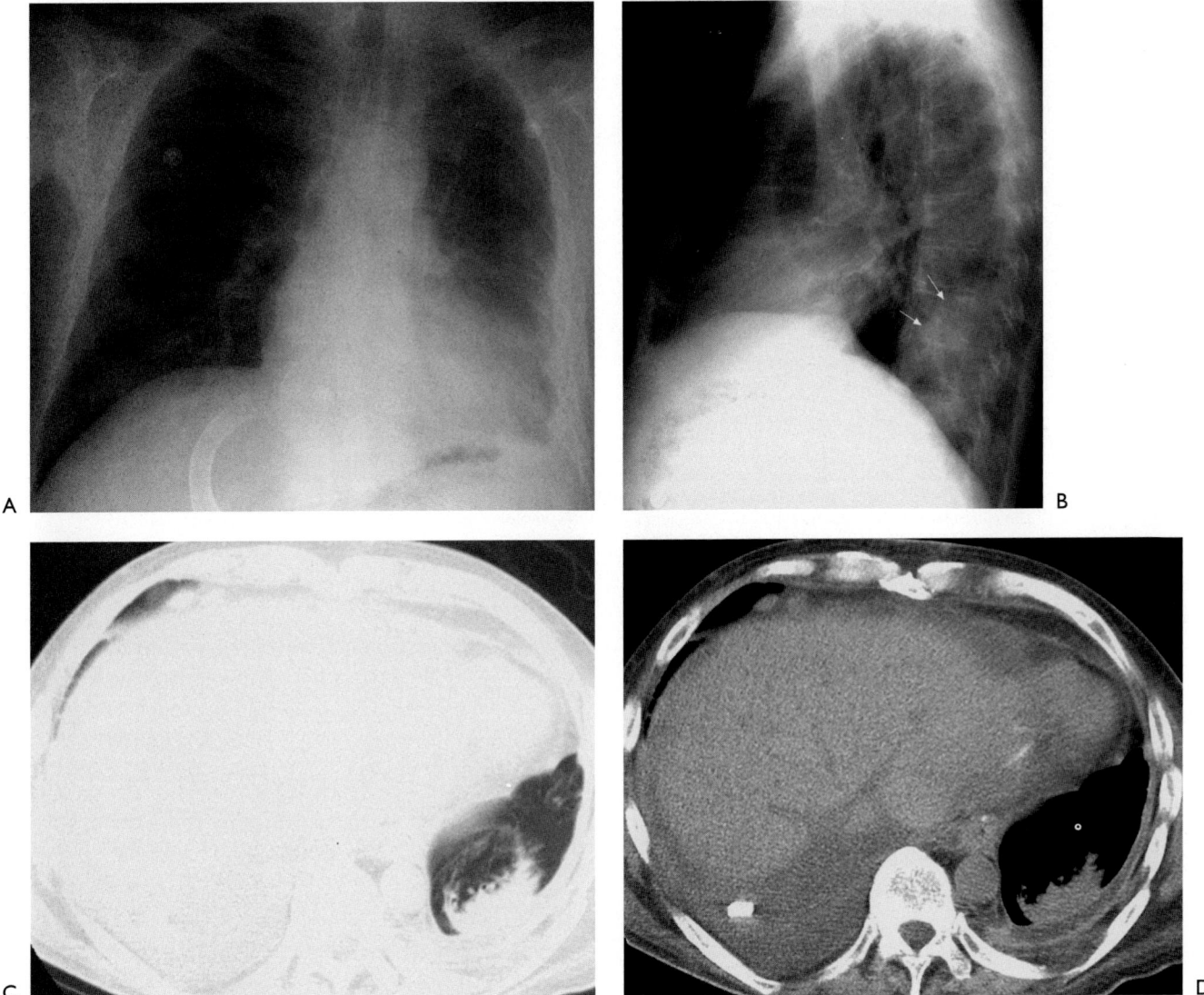

FIGURE 1.24. Pleural thickening with rounded atelectasis. **A, B:** Frontal and lateral chest radiographs show a transjugular intrahepatic portosystemic shunt (TIPS) for chronic portal hypertension. Marked pleural thickening is evident along the left lateral chest wall. The "meniscus" of the pleural thickening is sharper than one would expect with pleural fluid. The lateral view shows a masslike opacity posteriorly *(arrows)*. **C, D:** Computed tomography of the chest shows a masslike opacity. The contiguity of the mass with an area of thickened pleura, the lobar volume loss, and the curving of vessels into the medial and lateral aspects of the mass are all typical of rounded atelectasis.

Pleural thickening. Pleural thickening is usually manifested by straighter lines than is pleural fluid. Pleural thickening is often associated with rounded atelectasis, a masslike opacity associated with significant lobar volume loss (Fig. 1.24).

Pleural plaques. When noncalcified, these are usually best seen in profile along the lateral chest wall (Fig. 1.17).

Pleural/extrapleural sign. Masses that are pleural or extrapleural tend to displace the pleura in a gradual fashion, resulting in an obtuse angle with the chest wall (Fig. 1.25). Conversely, masses that are within the lung parenchyma tend to form acute angles with the adjacent lung. If a pleural or extrapleural mass is present, underlying bone destruction should be carefully sought.

Pneumothorax. The thin white line of the visceral pleura is the salient feature of pneumothorax (Fig. 1.26). This must be differentiated from the interface sometimes seen in patients with skinfolds overlying the lung. If pneumothorax is not seen on an inspiratory radiograph, expiratory images are rarely of additional benefit. In supine patients imaged in the intensive care unit, air will accumulate in the costophrenic sulci, producing the "deep sulcus" sign. Decubitus views may help confirm pneumothorax in patients who cannot sit up.

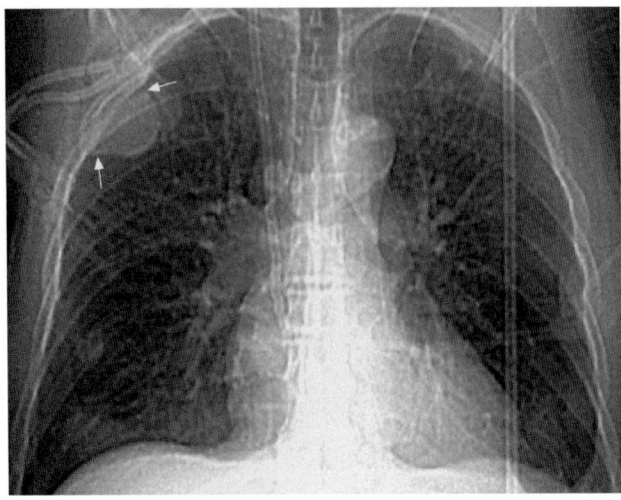
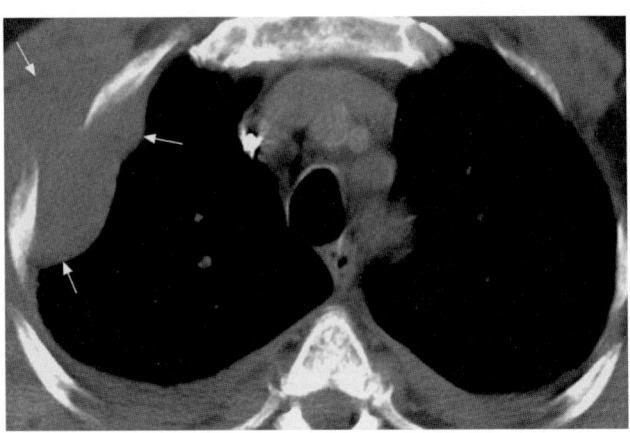

FIGURE 1.25. Extrapleural mass in a 60-year-old man with multiple myeloma. **A:** Scout view from computed tomography (CT) scan shows a pleural-based mass in the right upper chest, which forms obtuse angles with the pleura *(arrows)*. **B:** CT confirms the extrapleural nature of this myeloma deposit, which appears to be invading the chest wall although not destroying the underlying ribs *(arrows)*.

Other Radiologic Signs

Silhouette sign. Radiographic opacities will commonly obscure adjacent structures such as the diaphragm or mediastinum (silhouette sign) (Fig. 1.27). The structures that are obscured allow one to deduce the location of the pulmonary abnormality. For instance, if an opacity in the left lower lung obscures the left hemidiaphragm or descending aorta, the abnormality is probably in the lower lobe, whereas if the opacity obscures the heart border, it is likely to be in the lingula.

Air crescent sign. The air crescent sign occurs when a mass of tissue is present within a cavity. It occurs in patients with angioinvasive pulmonary infection (usually with aspergillus). In a different clinical context, the air crescent sign is found in patients with a mycetoma occurring in a preexisting cavity (Fig. 1.28).

CT halo sign. The CT halo sign refers to the presence of a "halo" of ground-glass attenuation surrounding a central area of consolidation (Fig. 1.29). The halo is usually caused by hemorrhage surrounding a solid nodule. In

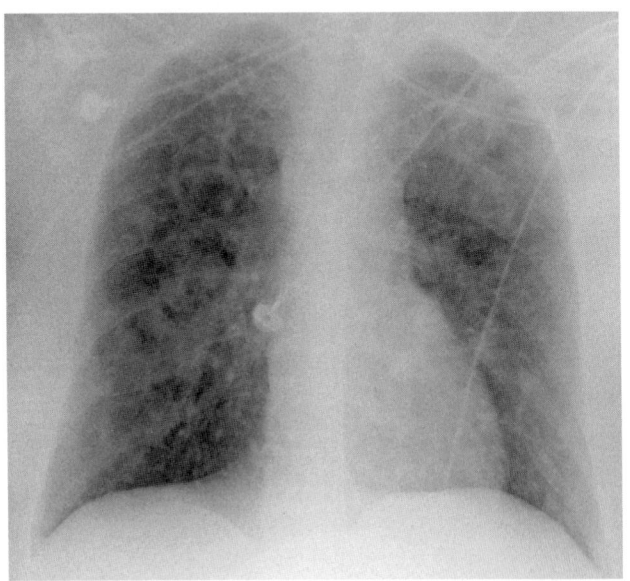
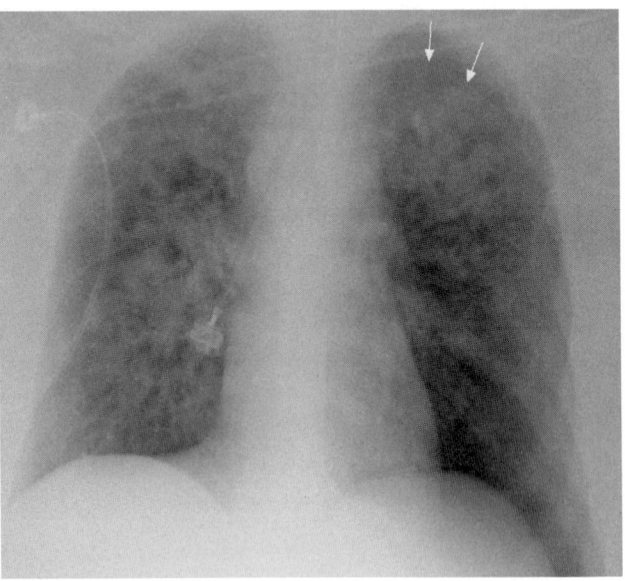

FIGURE 1.26. A 40-year-old man who developed a left pneumothorax while being ventilated for acute respiratory distress syndrome (ARDS). **A:** Baseline chest radiograph shows diffuse parenchymal airspace opacity compatible with ARDS. **B:** A chest radiograph obtained during respiratory deterioration shows a new lucency over the region of left hemidiaphragm (deep anterior sulcus). There is also increased depth of the lateral costophrenic sulcus. The thin white line of pneumothorax is evident superiorly *(arrows)*.

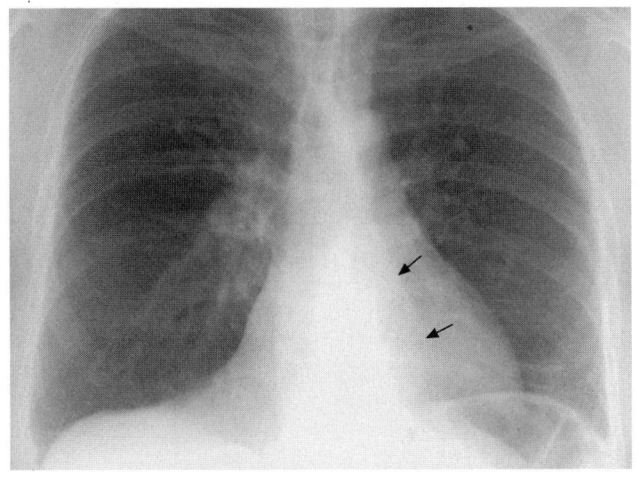
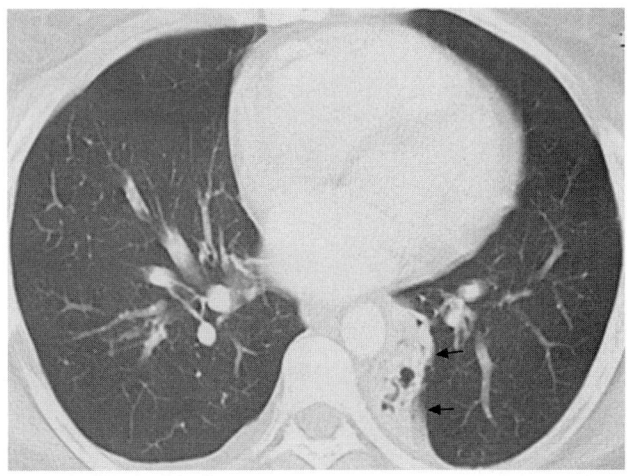

A

B

FIGURE 1.27. Chronic left lower lobe collapse with silhouette sign. **A:** Chest radiograph shows collapse of the left lower lobe *(arrows)*. The outlines of the descending aorta and the medial left hemidiaphragm are obscured. The right pulmonary artery is enlarged because of increased blood flow to the right lung. **B:** Computed tomography scan on the same patient shows the collapsed lower lobe *(arrows)* in contact with the descending aorta.

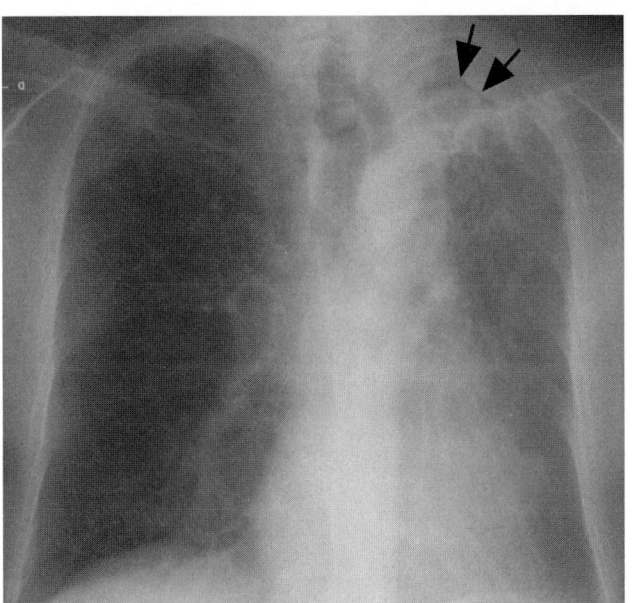

A

immunocompromised patients, it is usually caused by infection by *Aspergillus fumigatus,* although candidiasis or viral infection can cause similar appearances. In other contexts, this finding can be seen in patients with vasculitis or hemorrhagic metastases (60).

SPECIFIC IMAGING ISSUES IN EVALUATION OF LUNG DISEASE

Solitary Pulmonary Nodule

The solitary pulmonary nodule (Fig. 1.30) remains a common cause for referral to pulmonologists. Most commonly, the nodule is identified incidentally on chest radiograph or chest CT. Pulmonary nodules are a growing problem because of the increasing use of chest CT. Depending on the choice of imaging technique and the geographic location, between 25% and 50% of patients screened for lung cancer

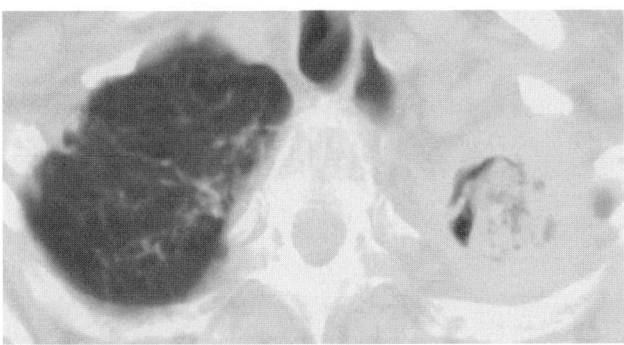

B

FIGURE 1.28. Air crescent sign in a patient with mycetoma. **A:** Chest radiograph shows marked left upper lobe volume loss. A crescent of air is seen within a left apical cavity *(arrows),* indicating the presence of a solid intracavitary mass. There is marked adjacent pleural thickening. **B:** Computed tomography scan in the same patient confirms the presence of an intracavitary mass.

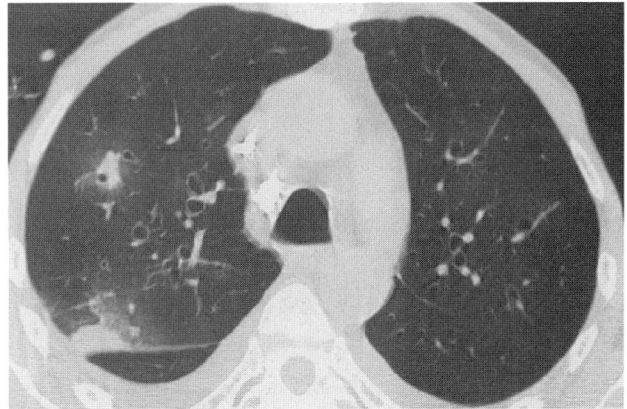

FIGURE 1.29. Computed tomography (CT) halo sign in invasive pulmonary aspergillosis (same patient as in Figure 1.12). CT shows two right upper lobe nodules, with surrounding ground-glass abnormality.

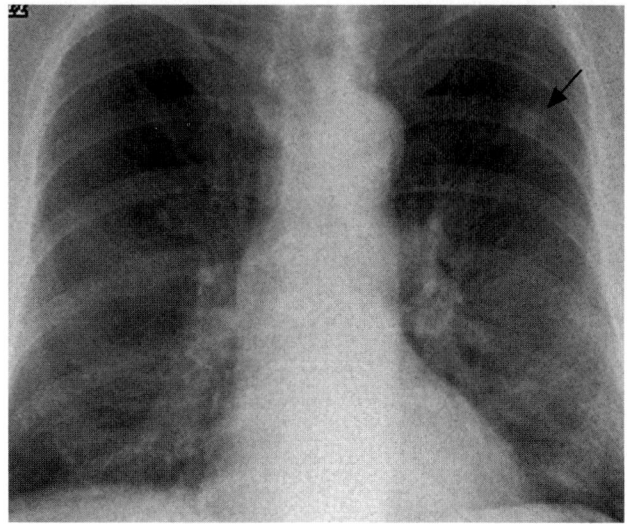
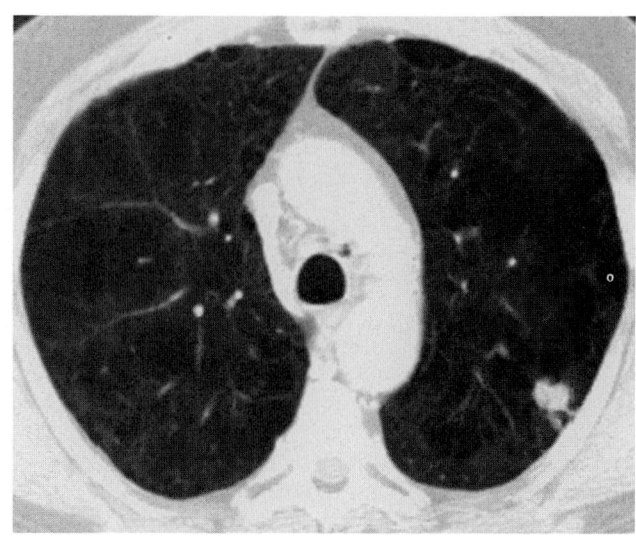

FIGURE 1.30. Solitary pulmonary nodule evaluated by computed tomography (CT). **A:** Chest radiograph shows nodule in the left upper lobe *(arrow)*. **B:** CT shows extensive emphysema and a noncalcified nodule in the posterior-segment, left upper lobe, with a "tail" extending to the pleura. The nodule is noncalcified and was proven to be a non–small cell lung cancer.

will have one or more noncalcified lung nodules detected by CT. These nodules usually measure less than 1 cm.

When a solitary pulmonary nodule is identified or suspected on the chest radiograph, one must first evaluate whether or not the nodule is truly intrathoracic. Pulmonary nodules must be distinguished from extrathoracic abnormalities such as bone islands and nipple shadows. Fluoroscopy can help to determine whether a nodule is in the lung or in the bones. Significant calcification should be suspected if the nodule is equal or greater in opacity to the adjacent rib.

The most important part of the evaluation of the solitary pulmonary nodule is obtaining old radiographs or CT scans. Noncalcified nodules that have been stable in size for 2 years are usually assumed to be benign. However, lung cancers may rarely be seen to grow over an interval longer than 2 years (61). Therefore, chest radiographs should be performed at yearly intervals in any patient with a noncalcified nodule to exclude such slow-growing malignancies.

If prior images are not available, chest HRCT is usually the first line of investigation for pulmonary nodules. HRCT is obtained contiguously through the nodule to determine the presence of calcification or fat, to identify cavitation, and to evaluate the edge characteristics such as spiculation or lobulation. Homogenous calcification almost always indicates benignity (62), but eccentric calcification or small areas of calcification may be seen in lung cancer. The presence of significant amounts of fat almost always indicates a hamartoma (63). In a study by Siegelman et al., 30 (63%) of 47 hamartomas were diagnosed on thin-section CT by the presence of fat and/or calcification (63).

In dynamic nodule CT, images are obtained through the nodule at 1-minute intervals after administration of intravenous iodinated contrast (64). In a multicenter study, a threshold for nodule enhancement of 15 Hounsfield units was shown to have a 98% sensitivity for malignancy, with a specificity of 58% (64). The degree of nodule enhancement appears to be related to the degree of vascularity of the lesion. Dynamic CT can be used for nodules as small as 7 mm, but evaluation of small nodules may be technically compromised by variation in breath-holding.

The sensitivity of FDG PET for malignancy in a solitary pulmonary nodule is approximately 95%, with a specificity of 81%. In a study by Gould and Lillington (65), Bayesian analysis showed that the likelihood ratio for malignancy in a solitary pulmonary nodule with an abnormal FDG PET scan was 7.11 (95% confidence interval, 6.36–7.96), suggesting a high probability for malignancy, and 0.06 (95% confidence interval, 0.05–0.07) when the PET scan was normal, suggesting that PET scanning was a useful test for evaluation of the solitary pulmonary nodule. Similarly, Gambhir (65a) showed that an approach based on PET and CT was the most cost-effective method for evaluation of lung nodules. However, neither of these studies compared PET with dynamic nodule CT. PET scanning is usually restricted to nodules measuring more than 1 cm, and its accuracy for smaller nodules has not been systematically established. The limited specificity of PET is because metabolically active processes such as infection may also show increase in uptake of FDG. A further limitation is that PET scanning is less sensitive for slowly growing malignancies such as bronchioloalveolar carcinoma and carcinoid tumors. An advantage of PET is that it can detect local or distant metastasis.

The new technique of scanning with ^{99m}Tc depreotide, a somatostatin analog, has been shown to have a similar sensitivity and specificity to that of PET (66). The size limitations are similar to those of PET, but depreotide scanning is less expensive because it can be performed by using conventional nuclear scanners. The impact of ^{99m}Tc depreotide on staging of lung cancer has not been established.

The appropriate imaging modality in nodules that remain indeterminate after thin-section CT remains unclear. For nodules measuring more than 7 to 10 mm in diameter, PET, dynamic CT, and ^{99m}Tc depreotide scanning are all acceptable. For smaller nodules, follow-up imaging is usually performed, but the appropriate interval for follow-up has not been established. It is hoped that the National Lung Screening Trial will provide useful information regarding the appropriate follow-up of patients with incidental lung nodules discovered on CT.

SOLITARY PULMONARY NODULE

Summary Statement	Level of Evidence
Stability over 2 y is usually, although not always, indicative of benignity	Expert opinion
Enhancement by <15 Hounsfield units on dynamic computed tomography indicates benignity in 98% of cases	Multicenter prospective study
Normal uptake of ^{18}fluorodeoxyglucose indicates benignity in at least 95% of cases	Retrospective and prospective studies
Normal uptake of ^{99m}Tc depreotide indicates benignity in 96% of cases	Prospective multicenter study
For nodules <7–10 mm, follow-up by computed tomography is usually the most appropriate evaluation method	Expert opinion

Staging of Lung Cancer

The critical issue in staging of lung cancer is to distinguish between resectable and unresectable cancer. CT is an established part of the staging of lung cancer because of its ability to demonstrate the local extent of disease, the presence of enlarged mediastinal lymph nodes, and the presence of metastases to liver, adrenals, or bones. However, 20 years of evaluation have led to an understanding of the limitations and advantages of CT. CT can demonstrate that resection is not possible by showing encasement of mediastinal structures, but it is often difficult to determine whether tumor is truly invading the structure or is merely contiguous with it. With regard to determination of node (N) status, CT relies solely on nodal size in determining the presence or absence of malignancy. The generally accepted upper limit of normal for short-axis nodal diameter is 10 mm. The sensitivity and specificity of this threshold for mediastinal nodal invasion are both between 60% and 70% (67). The lack of sensitivity is because nodal metastases may be present in normal-sized lymph nodes (Fig. 1.31). The lack of specificity is because enlarged lymph nodes may be reactive rather than neoplastic. However, CT has an important role in nodal staging by suggesting a route for biopsy of suspicious nodes.

In general, MRI confers no advantage over CT in staging of patients with lung cancer (68). However, in individual cases, MRI may be valuable in determining the extent of soft tissue or mediastinal invasion. In particular, MRI can be useful in determining the extent of involvement of the brachial plexus, subclavian artery, and vertebral body in patients with Pancoast tumor (25).

In multiple studies, PET has been shown to detect unsuspected nodal or distant metastases in 20% to 30% of cases, with an important impact on choice of treatment strategy and prognosis (69, 70) (Fig. 1.31). A smaller percentage of patients are "down-staged" when PET detects no uptake in areas suspicious for metastasis on CT, such as enlarged mediastinal nodes. The sensitivity of PET for mediastinal metastasis ranges from 67% to 90%, with specificities ranging from 85% to 95% (71–73). A randomized controlled study of 188 patients with lung cancer showed that the addition of PET to the conventional evaluation resulted in a decrease in the rate of futile thoracotomy, from 41% to 21% (74).

STAGING OF LUNG CANCER

Summary Statement	Level of Evidence
MRI adds little to CT in staging of lung cancer, except for chest-wall invasion	Prospective studies
PET upstages 20%–30% of lung cancer compared with CT	Nonrandomized studies
PET reduces the rate of futile thoracotomy in potentially resectable lung cancer	Randomized study

MRI, magnetic resonance imaging; CT, computed tomography; PET, positron emission tomography.

Pulmonary Vascular Disease

Enlargement of the pulmonary arteries on the chest radiograph is a useful but relatively insensitive sign of pulmonary hypertension (75) (Fig. 1.32). The upper limit of normal for the right interlobar pulmonary artery on the chest radiograph is 17 mm, whereas the upper limit of normal of the left pulmonary artery on the lateral view is 20 mm. The size of the right interlobar pulmonary artery increases with age and with the altitude of residence (76). Enlargement of the main pulmonary artery (>30 mm) may be identified on CT, but it remains unclear whether this is any more sensitive or specific than the chest radiographic measurements.

The relative roles of ventilation-perfusion imaging and computed tomographic pulmonary angiography (CTPA) in diagnosis of pulmonary embolism are still undergoing evaluation. CTPA (Fig. 1.33) is more than 95% sensitive for central thrombus, but it is less sensitive for subsegmental emboli. The lower sensitivity in some earlier studies seems to have been due to use of 5-mm collimation, compared to

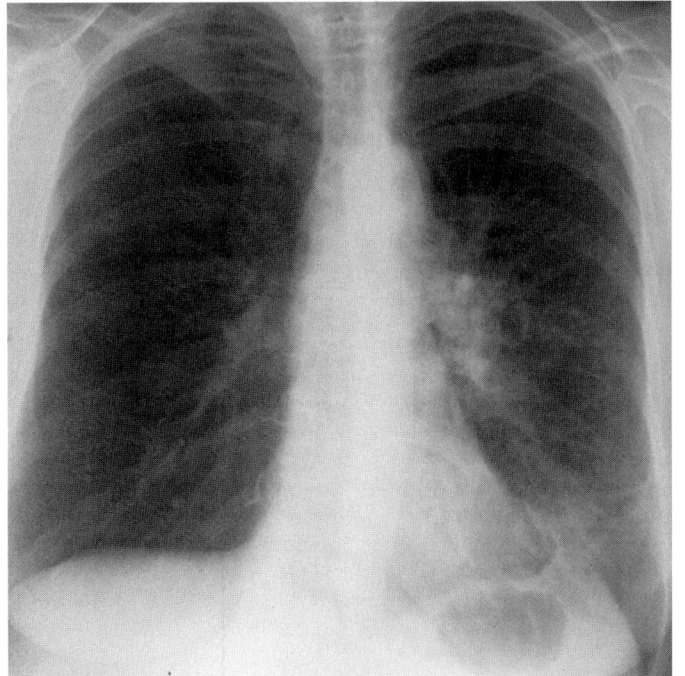

A

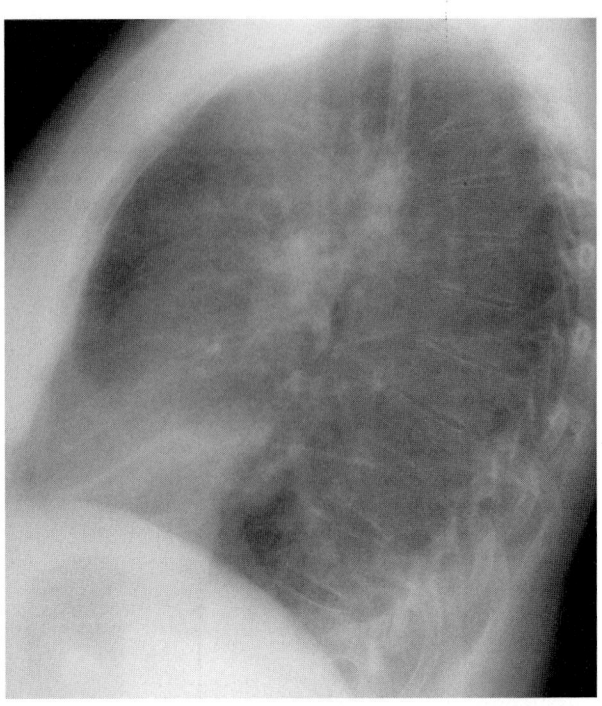

B

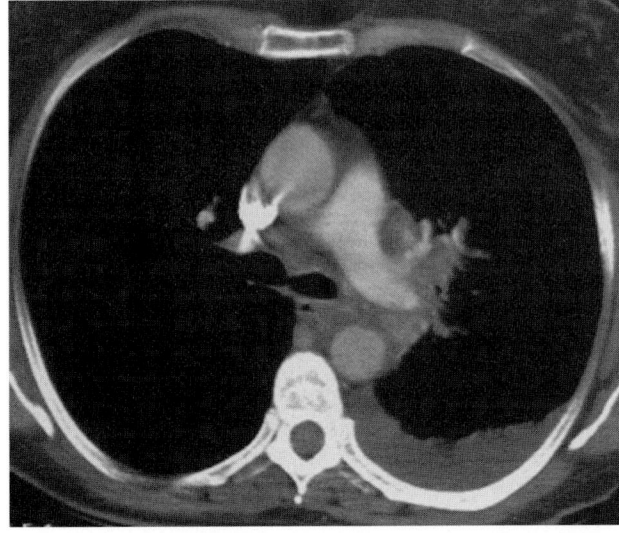

C

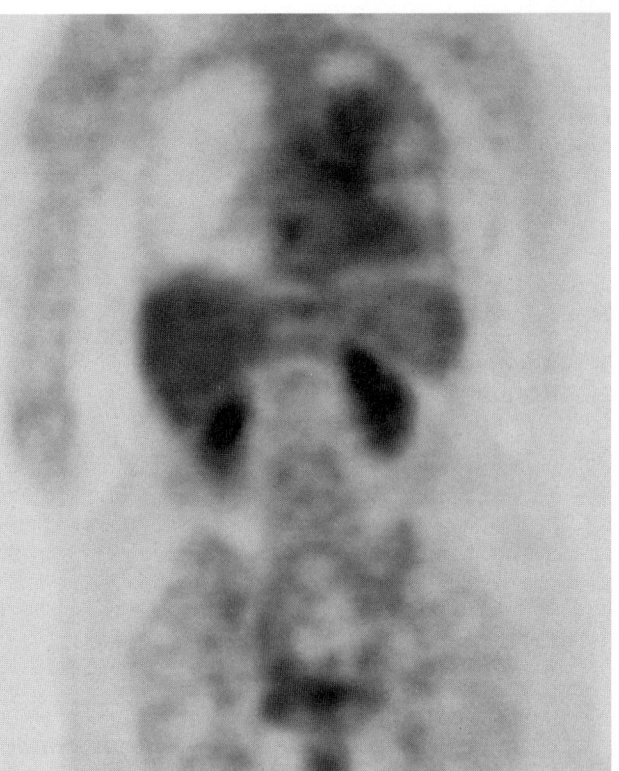

D

FIGURE 1.31. Positron emission tomography (PET) in staging of lung cancer. **A, B:** Chest radiographs in a 64-year-old woman show a left hilar mass. **C:** Computed tomography (CT) confirms a left hilar mass and shows a left effusion. **D:** PET scan confirms marked increased uptake in the left hilar mass. (*continued*)

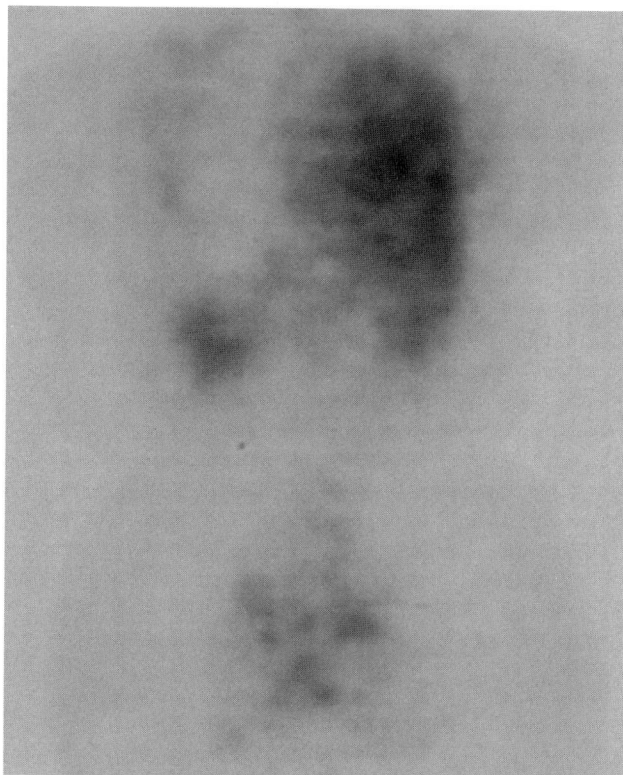

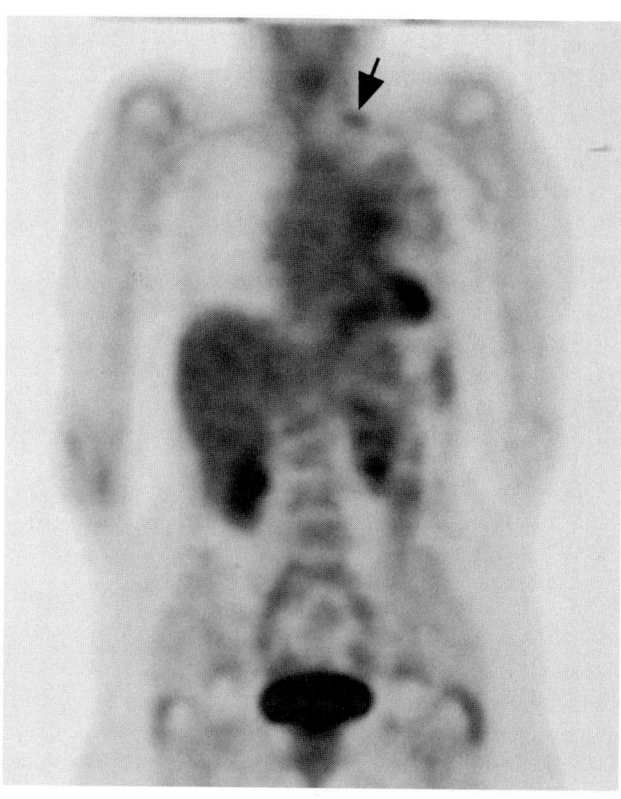

E   F

FIGURE 1.31. *(continued)* **E:** PET also shows diffuse increased uptake in the left pleural space, compatible with malignant pleural effusion. **F:** In addition, a left supraclavicular node is found on PET that was not identified on CT. The staging of this patient was therefore upgraded from T3 N0 MX to T4 N3 MX based on the PET findings.

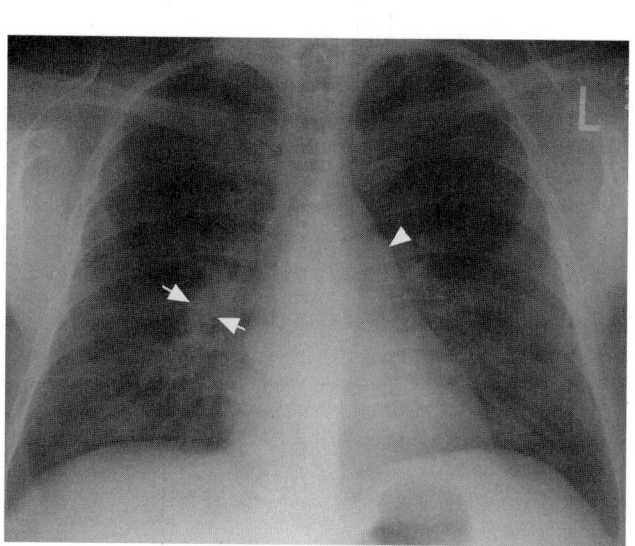

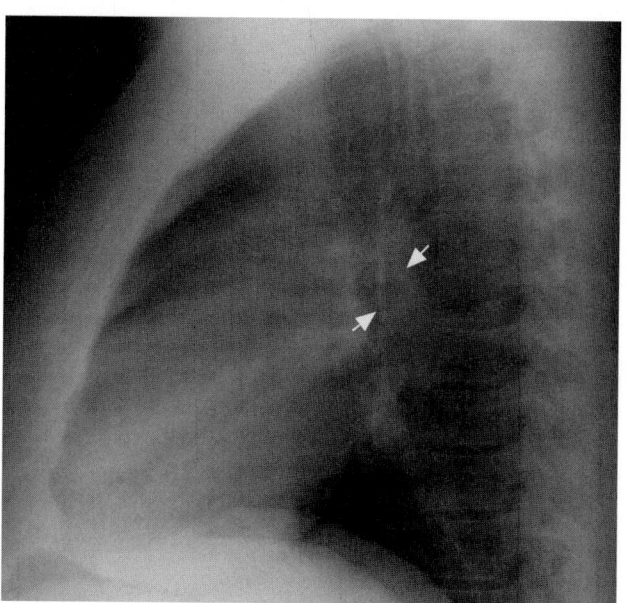

A   B

FIGURE 1.32. A 60-year-old man with pulmonary hypertension due to chronic liver disease. **A:** On the frontal chest radiograph, the main pulmonary artery is enlarged *(arrow)*. The right interlobar pulmonary artery is enlarged, measuring 20 mm. The normal value is 17 mm *(arrows)*. **B:** On the lateral view, the left pulmonary artery is enlarged, measuring 23 mm, compared with a normal value of 20 mm.

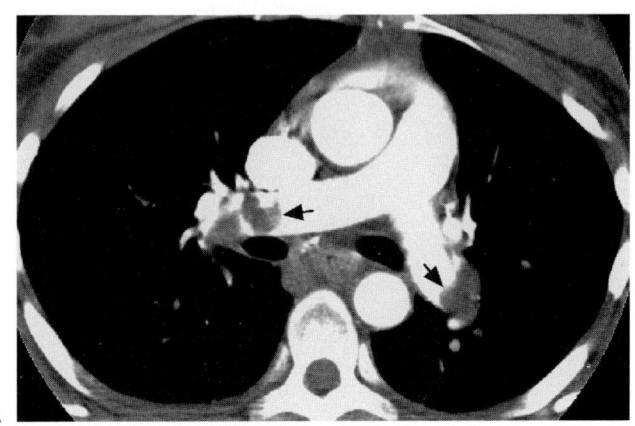
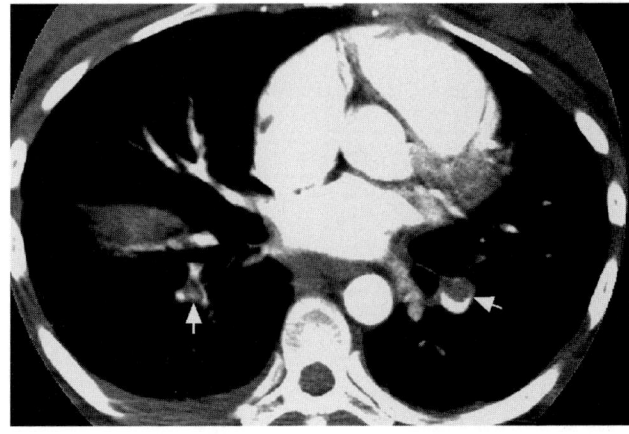

A   B

FIGURE 1.33. Computed tomography (CT) diagnosis of pulmonary thromboembolism. CT angiogram shows intraluminal filling defects in the right and left main pulmonary arteries, in the left lower lobe pulmonary artery, and in a right lower lobe segmental pulmonary artery *(arrows).*

3-mm or finer collimation in more recent studies. Careful attention to technique and knowledge of normal anatomy are critical for optimizing sensitivity. There is also a substantial learning curve for interpretation of CTPA.

Because of the high predictive values of normal or high-probability ventilation perfusion scans, ventilation perfusion imaging remains an excellent test for patients who do not have significant underlying lung disease and who have a normal or near-normal chest radiograph. CT angiography has several important advantages over ventilation-perfusion scintigraphy: the low prevalence of indeterminate scans, the direct visualization of the presence and extent of thrombus, and the ability to identify other causes for the patient's symptoms. The ability to perform CT venography as an "add-on" study is of particular value in those with symptoms of lower extremity thrombus.

Although MRI of ventilation and perfusion shows promise, it currently has no clinical role in evaluation of thromboembolism, except perhaps in the patient with a contraindication to intravenous contrast (77). Figure 1.34 displays an algorithm in current use at our institution for choosing imaging modalities in suspected venous thromboembolism. The PIOPED II study currently in progress should yield an excellent understanding of the relative roles of these two modalities.

CT can be valuable in detection of arteriovenous malformations. Even small arteriovenous malformations may be recognizable by identifying the characteristic feeding artery and draining vein (78) (Fig. 1.35). Administration of intravenous contrast is not necessary.

Evaluation of Diffuse Lung Disease

Detection of Early Interstitial Lung Disease

The chest radiograph is relatively insensitive for detection of diffuse lung disease. Although it is commonly stated that the chest radiograph is normal in 10% to 15% of patients

with diffuse lung disease, the true sensitivity of the chest radiograph is impossible to determine, as it depends on the severity and type of disease present in the population being studied. CT has been shown to be more sensitive than the chest radiograph in many diseases, including asbestosis (79) (Fig. 1.17), silicosis (80), sarcoidosis (81), scleroderma (82, 83), and hypersensitivity pneumonitis (84, 85). In asbestosis, HRCT may detect abnormality before resting pulmonary function tests become abnormal (79, 86). It is also clear that the HRCT scan may be normal despite the presence of biopsy-proven ILD. In a population-based study of subjects with hypersensitivity pneumonitis who had normal resting pulmonary function, the sensitivity of HRCT was 38% (87). Similarly, in a paper by Gamsu (87a), CT scanning was normal or near-normal in five of 25 patients with histologic asbestosis. These studies emphasize the fact that there is a phase in the evolution of any lung disease when the degree of parenchymal infiltration is too slight or too focal to cause a recognizable increase in lung attenuation on CT. Therefore, although CT is substantially more sensitive than is chest radiograph for ILD, normal findings on HRCT cannot be used to exclude ILD. In future, it is possible that computer-based characterization systems might help to detect lung disease in patients with visually normal CT.

Characterization of Interstitial Lung Disease

Several large retrospective studies have compared the diagnostic accuracy of chest CT and chest radiography for diagnosis of specific lung diseases. A study by Mathieson et al. examined the chest radiographs and CT scans of 118 patients with diffuse infiltrative lung diseases (88). For usual interstitial pneumonitis, the first-choice diagnosis was correct in 75% of the cases on chest radiograph and 89% of the cases on CT. For silicosis, the corresponding figures were 63% and 93%; for sarcoidosis, 61% and 77%. For lymphangitic carcinomatosis, the first-choice diagnosis was correct in 56% of cases on the chest radiograph and 85% on CT. In addition,

PE/DVT IMAGING ALGORITHM

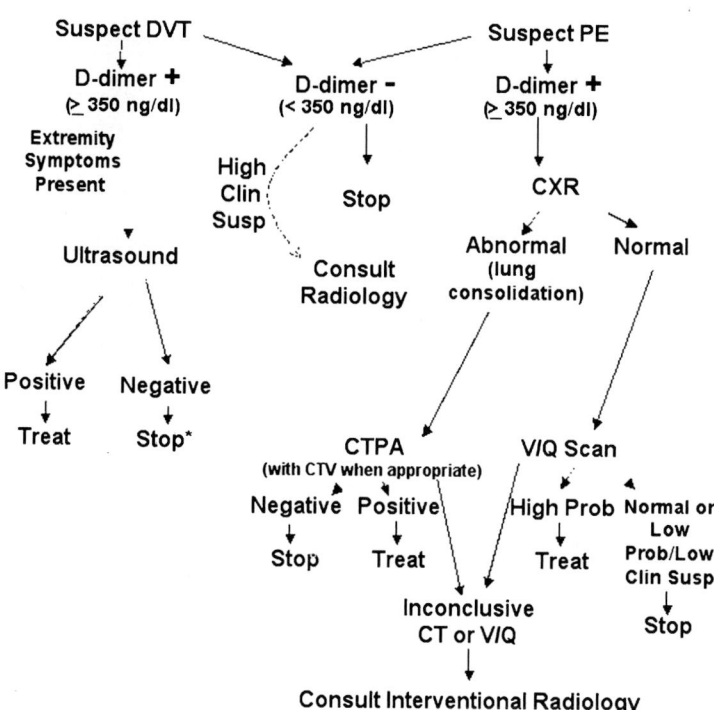

FIGURE 1.34. Algorithm used to choose the appropriate imaging modality for diagnosis of pulmonary thromboembolic disease. PE, pulmonary embolism; DVT, deep venous thrombosis; CXR, chest radiograph; CTPA, computed tomography pulmonary arteriogram; CTV, computed tomography venogram; V/Q, ventilation-perfusion. (From Deb Dyer, M.D., and Phyllis Siracusano, University of Colorado Health Sciences Center, with permission.)

interobserver variation appeared to be less for CT scanning than for chest radiographs. Overall, a correct first-choice diagnosis was made with 57% of radiographs and 76% of CT scans.

One of the defects of these earlier studies was that they may have included patients with well-established disease. In a more recent study of 85 patients who were scanned before surgical lung biopsy, the accuracy of a confident first-choice diagnosis of disease was 90%, but such a confident diagnosis was made in only about 25% of cases (89). This relatively low level of diagnostic confidence was most likely due to

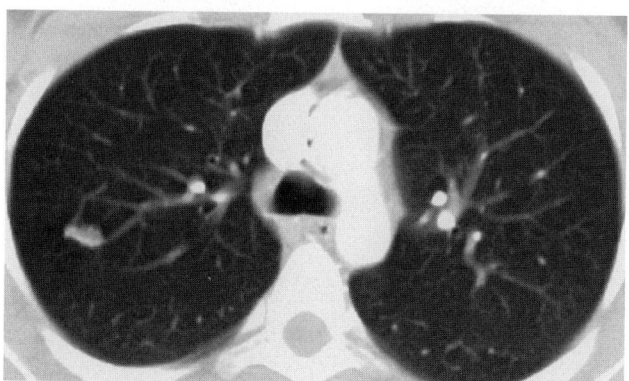

FIGURE 1.35. A 25-year-old woman with pulmonary arteriovenous malformation. Axial computed tomography images show a nodule in the right upper lobe, with feeding and draining vessels, characteristic for pulmonary arterio-venous malformations (AVM).

selection bias (patients in whom confident CT diagnoses could be made would likely not undergo biopsy). However, it is also possible that confident diagnoses are more difficult to make in those with earlier disease.

A prospective, multicenter study of the accuracy of diagnosis of usual interstitial pneumonitis (UIP) found that a confident CT diagnosis of UIP, based on typical features, was correct in 96% of cases (90), consistent with the results of several other studies, indicating that the correctness of a confident first-choice diagnosis of UIP, made by an experienced radiologist, is greater than 90% (89, 91, 92). Univariate and multivariate analysis showed that radiologic features were the primary discriminants between UIP and other causes of diffuse lung disease (93). None of the other classic clinical features of UIP were useful in diagnosis. However, it should be noted that in this study, a confident CT diagnosis of UIP was made in only about 50% of cases. In other cases of histologically confirmed UIP, the CT features were not typical enough to make a confident diagnosis. Similar findings were reported in a study by Raghu et al. (94). Other diseases in which a confident CT diagnosis is highly likely to be correct include lymphangitic carcinoma (48), Langerhans histiocytosis (95), lymphangiomyomatosis (95) (Fig. 1.19), and hypersensitivity pneumonitis with micronodules (96) (Fig. 1.16).

It must be clearly understood that even a confident CT diagnosis should be integrated with the available clinical information. Patients with discrepant findings on clinical evaluation and CT should usually undergo biopsy. Biopsy is also indicated in patients with nonspecific CT findings. HRCT can be valuable for predicting whether transbronchial biopsy would be helpful (in suspected sarcoidosis or lymphangitic carcinoma) and for identifying a suitable site for biopsy by the bronchoscopist or surgeon. When a biopsy is performed, it is important to review the biopsy in conjunction with the CT findings. Discrepancies between the CT pattern and the biopsy findings may be due to sampling of a nonrepresentative part of the lung.

CT CHARACTERIZATION OF INTERSTITIAL LUNG DISEASE	
Summary Statement	**Level of Evidence**
CT is more sensitive than is chest radiograph for lung disease, but a normal CT does not exclude disease	Prospective and retrospective studies
A confident diagnosis of idiopathic pulmonary fibrosis based on CT appearances is correct in >90% of cases	Prospective and retrospective studies

CT, computed tomography.

Evaluation of Hemoptysis

In the evaluation of the patient with hemoptysis, the role of CT is complementary to that of bronchoscopy (97). HRCT will identify conditions that are beyond the reach of the bronchoscope, such as mycetoma or bronchiectasis. CT will also identify most endobronchial lesions (Fig. 1.36) and is of particular value in identifying an extraluminal component of these lesions.

Diagnosis of Bronchiectasis

Though relatively insensitive, the chest radiograph may sometimes detect bronchiectasis, by the recognition of dilated or nontapering bronchi. Moderate or severe bronchiectasis is usually associated with lobar volume loss. The diagnosis of milder bronchiectasis usually requires HRCT scanning.

CT has supplanted bronchography as the gold standard for diagnosing bronchiectasis. To diagnose bronchiectasis, the use of high-resolution thin sections (usually 1 mm) is essential. Based on bronchographic criteria, now adapted for CT, bronchiectasis is classified as cylindric, varicose, or cystic (98). Cylindric bronchiectasis is characterized by uniform bronchial dilation (Fig. 1.37). Varicose bronchiectasis is evident by the presence of beading or irregular outpouchings from the dilated bronchus. Cystic (or saccular) bronchiectasis is diagnosed by the presence of thin-walled cysts measuring 3 to 20 mm (Fig. 1.38). The adjacent pulmonary artery is usually substantially smaller than is the bronchus (signet ring sign). Sometimes a string or cluster of cysts is evident, and some of the cysts may contain air-fluid levels. The morphologic classification of bronchiectasis correlates with physiologic and clinical features (99): Patients with cylindric bronchiectasis usually have predominantly obstructive physiology, whereas those with varicose or cystic bronchiectasis are predominantly restricted. Patients with cystic bronchiectasis are highly likely to have purulent sputum and to grow pseudomonas from their sputum.

When a bronchus is imaged in cross section, the diagnosis of bronchiectasis is made if the internal diameter of the bronchus is significantly greater than that of the adjacent pulmonary artery (broncho-arterial diameter ratio). Bronchial wall thickening is not required for the diagnosis.

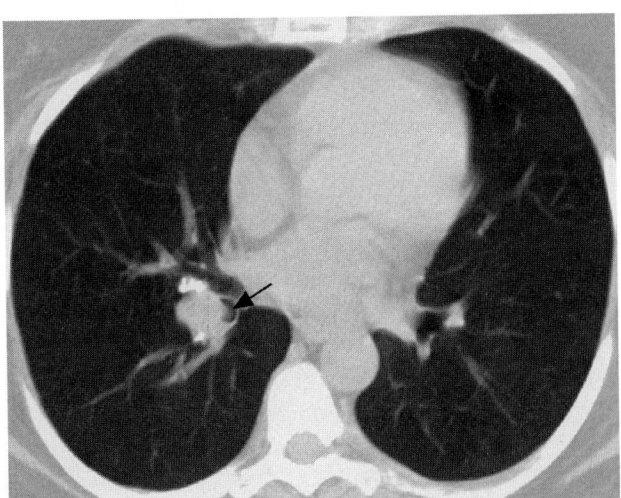

FIGURE 1.36. A 25-year-old woman with hemoptysis. Chest radiograph was normal. Computed tomography scan shows an endobronchial mass in the right lower lobe bronchus *(arrow)*. On bronchoscopy, the patient was diagnosed with carcinoid tumor.

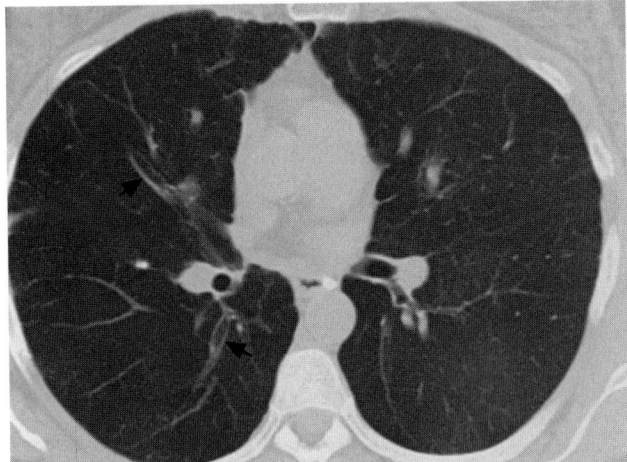

FIGURE 1.37. Computed tomography (CT) diagnosis of bronchiectasis. High-resolution CT shows multiple cylindrically dilated bronchi that are not tapering. The diameter is substantially greater than that of adjacent pulmonary vessels *(arrows)*.

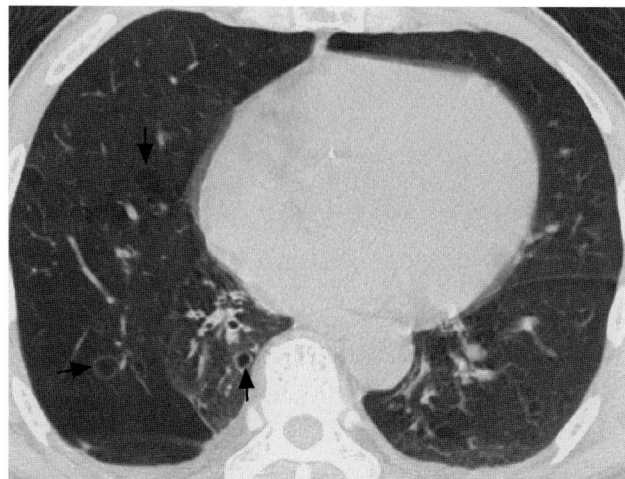

FIGURE 1.38. Cystic bronchiectasis. High-resolution computed tomography through the lower lungs in a 30-year-old patient with postinfectious bronchiectasis and unilateral hyperlucent lung (Swyer-James syndrome) shows multiple cystic dilated bronchi.

Other reliable signs of cylindric bronchiectasis include lack of bronchial tapering and visibility of peripheral bronchi within 1 or 2 cm of the pleura (100). The lung parenchyma supplied by bronchiectatic bronchi is often decreased in attenuation, probably because of associated bronchiolitis with air trapping. In a study by Roberts et al., the extent of air trapping on expiratory CT was closely associated with decreased forced expiratory volume in one second (FEV_1) (101).

In interpreting the broncho-arterial diameter ratio, one must be aware that the sizes of the bronchi and pulmonary arteries are each subject to physiologic variation. Pulmonary arterial vasoconstriction is an important response to hypoxia. For example, patients undergoing CT scans at 1,700 m above sea level have a mean broncho-arterial ratio that is significantly higher than that in patients scanned at sea level (102). Because of these physiologic variations in the broncho-arterial ratio, the CT diagnosis of cylindric bronchiectasis should be reserved for bronchi that are significantly larger than the adjacent pulmonary arteries. The CT diagnosis of mild cylindric bronchiectasis should be supported by other findings such as bronchial wall thickening, lack of bronchial tapering, visibility of dilated peripheral bronchi, or decreased CT attenuation in the lung.

SUMMARY

An awareness of the range of imaging modalities available to the pulmonologist for evaluation of lung disease should help optimize the selection of imaging evaluation in individual patients.

REFERENCES

1. Ravin CE, Chotas HG. Chest radiography. *Radiology* 1997;204:593–600.
2. Mayo J, Webb W, Gould R, et al. High-resolution CT of the lungs: an optimal approach. *Radiology* 1987;163:507–510.
3. Kauczor HU, Heussel CP, Fischer B, et al. Assessment of lung volumes using helical CT at inspiration and expiration: comparison with pulmonary function tests. *AJR Am J Roentgenol* 1998;171:1091–1095.
4. Becker MD, Berkmen YM, Austin JH, et al. Lung volumes before and after lung volume reduction surgery: quantitative CT analysis. *Am J Respir Crit Care Med* 1998;157:1593–1599.
5. Goldin JG, Tashkin DP, Kleerup EC, et al. Effects of HFA- and CFC-beclomethasone dipropionate inhalation on small airways: assessment using functional helical thin-section computed tomography. *J Allergy Clin Immunol* 1999;104:S258–S267.
6. Best A, Lynch A, Bozic C, et al. Quantitative CT indices in IPF: relationship to physiologic Impairment. *Radiology* 2003 (in press).
7. Johnson JL, Kramer SS, Mahboubi S. Air trapping in children: evaluation with dynamic lung densitometry with spiral CT. *Radiology* 1998;206:95–101.
8. Stern EJ, Webb WR, Gamsu G. Dynamic quantitative computed tomography: a predictor of pulmonary function in obstructive lung diseases. *Invest Radiol* 1994;29:564–569.
9. Burch WM, Sullivan PJ, McLaren CJ. Technegas: a new ventilation agent for lung scanning. *Nucl Med Commun* 1986;7:865–871.
10. Satoh K, Nakano S, Tanabe M, et al. A clinical comparison between Technegas SPECT, CT, and pulmonary function tests in patients with emphysema. *Radiat Med* 1997;15:277–282.
11. Mettler F, Guiberteau M. *Essentials of nuclear medicine imaging,* 2nd ed Philadelphia: WB Saunders, 1985.
12. Schneider DB, Clary-Macy C, Challa S, et al. Positron emission tomography with F18-fluorodeoxyglucose in the staging and preoperative evaluation of malignant pleural mesothelioma. *J Thorac Cardiovasc Surg* 2000;120:128–133.
13. Cutillo AG, Morris AH, Ailion DC, et al. Quantitative assessment of pulmonary edema by nuclear magnetic resonance methods. *J Thorac Imaging* 1988;3:51–58.
14. Cutillo AG, Morris AH, Ailion DC, et al. Clinical implications of nuclear magnetic resonance lung research. *Chest* 1989;96:643–652.
15. Glazer HS, Lee JK, Levitt RG, et al. Radiation fibrosis: differentiation from recurrent tumor by MR imaging. *Radiology* 1985;156:721–726.
16. Glazer HS, Levitt RG, Lee JK, et al. Differentiation of radiation fibrosis from recurrent pulmonary neoplasm by magnetic resonance imaging. *AJR Am J Roentgenol* 1984;143:729–730.
17. Vinitski S, Pearson MG, Karlik SJ, et al. Differentiation of parenchymal lung disorders with in vitro proton nuclear magnetic resonance. *Magn Reson Med* 1986;3:120–125.
18. Kauczor HU, Hofmann D, Kreitner KF, et al. Normal and abnormal pulmonary ventilation: visualization at hyperpolarized He-3 MR imaging. *Radiology* 1996;201:564–568.
19. de Lange EE, Mugler JP 3rd, Brookeman JR, et al. Lung air spaces: MR imaging evaluation with hyperpolarized ^{3}He gas. *Radiology* 1999;210:851–857.
20. Edelman RR, Hatabu H, Tadamura E, et al. Noninvasive assessment of regional ventilation in the human lung using oxygen-enhanced magnetic resonance imaging. *Nat Med* 1996;2:1236–1239.
21. Kauczor HU, Kreitner KF. Contrast-enhanced MRI of the lung. *Eur J Radiol* 2000;34:196–207.

22. Johnson GA, Cates G, Chen XJ, et al. Dynamics of magnetization in hyperpolarized gas MRI of the lung. *Magn Reson Med* 1997;38:66–71.

23. Kauczor HU, Ebert M, Kreitner KF, et al. Imaging of the lungs using ³He MRI: preliminary clinical experience in 18 patients with and without lung disease. *J Magn Reson Imaging* 1997;7:538–543.

24. Altes TA, Powers PL, Knight-Scott J, et al. Hyperpolarized ³He MR lung ventilation imaging in asthmatics: preliminary findings. *J Magn Reson Imaging* 2001;13:378–384.

25. Heelan RT, Demas BE, Caravelli JF, et al. Superior sulcus tumors: CT and MR imaging. *Radiology* 1989;170:637–641.

26. Patz EJ, Shaffer K, Piwnica WD, et al. Malignant pleural mesothelioma: value of CT and MR imaging in predicting resectability. *AJR Am J Roentgenol* 1992;159:961–966.

27. Marom EM, Patz EF Jr, Erasmus JJ, et al. Malignant pleural effusions: treatment with small-bore-catheter thoracostomy and talc pleurodesis. *Radiology* 1999;210:277–281.

28. Patz EF Jr, McAdams HP, Erasmus JJ, et al. Sclerotherapy for malignant pleural effusions: a prospective randomized trial of bleomycin vs doxycycline with small-bore catheter drainage. *Chest* 1998;113:1305–1311.

29. Dahlstrom JE, Langdale-Smith GM, James DT. Fine needle aspiration cytology of pulmonary lesions: a reliable diagnostic test. *Pathology* 2001;33:13–16.

30. Laurent F, Latrabe V, Vergier B, et al. CT-guided transthoracic needle biopsy of pulmonary nodules smaller than 20 mm: results with an automated 20-gauge coaxial cutting needle. *Clin Radiol* 2000;55:281–287.

31. Cox JE, Chiles C, McManus CM, et al. Transthoracic needle aspiration biopsy: variables that affect risk of pneumothorax. *Radiology* 1999;212:165–168.

32. Laurent F, Michel P, Latrabe V, et al. Pneumothoraces and chest tube placement after CT-guided transthoracic lung biopsy using a coaxial technique: incidence and risk factors. *AJR Am J Roentgenol* 1999;172:1049–1053.

33. Webb W, Stein M, Finkbeiner W, et al. Normal and diseased isolated lungs: high resolution CT. *Radiology* 1988;166:81–87.

34. Tuddenham WJ. Glossary of terms for thoracic radiology: recommendations of the Nomenclature Committee of the Fleischner Society. *AJR Am J Roentgenol* 1984;143:509–517.

35. Austin J, Muller N, Friedman P, et al. Glossary of terms for CT of the lungs: recommendations of the nomenclature committee of the Fleischner Society. *Radiology* 1996;200:327–331.

36. Staples C, Muller N, Vedal S, et al. Usual interstitial pneumonia: correlation of CT with clinical, functional, and radiographic findings. *Radiology* 1987;162:377–381.

37. Mayo JR, Muller NL, Road J, et al. Chronic eosinophilic pneumonia: CT findings in six cases. *AJR Am J Roentgenol* 1989;153:727–730.

38. Brauner MW, Grenier P, Mouelhi MM, et al. Pulmonary histiocytosis X: evaluation with high-resolution CT. *Radiology* 1989;172:255–258.

39. Moore A, Godwin J, Muller N, et al. Pulmonary histiocytosis X: comparison of radiographic and CT findings. *Radiology* 1989;172:249–254.

40. Aberle DR, Hansell DM, Brown K, et al. Lymphangiomyomatosis: CT, chest radiographic, and functional correlations. *Radiology* 1990;176:381–387.

41. Murata K, Khan A, Herman PG. Pulmonary parenchymal disease: evaluation with high-resolution CT. *Radiology* 1989;170:629–635.

42. Noma S, Khan A, Herman PG, et al. High-resolution computed tomography of the pulmonary parenchyma. *Semin Ultrasound CT MR* 1990;11:365–379.

43. Murata K, Itoh H, Todo G, et al. Centrilobular lesions of the lungs: demonstration by high-resolution CT and pathologic correlation. *Radiology* 1986;161:641–645.

44. Bergin C, Roggli V, Coblentz C, et al. The secondary pulmonary lobule: normal and abnormal CT appearances. *AJR Am J Roentgenol* 1988;151:21–25.

45. Remy-Jardin M, Beuscart R, Sault MC, et al. Subpleural micronodules in diffuse infiltrative lung diseases: evaluation with thin-section CT scans. *Radiology* 1990;177:133–139.

46. Gruden JF, Webb WR, Naidich DP, et al. Multinodular disease: anatomic localization at thin-section CT–multireader evaluation of a simple algorithm. *Radiology* 1999;210:711–720.

47. Aberle DR, Gamsu G, Ray CS, et al. Asbestos-related pleural and parenchymal fibrosis: detection with high-resolution CT. *Radiology* 1988;166:729–734.

48. Stein M, Mayo J, Muller N, et al. Pulmonary lymphangitic spread of carcinoma: appearance on CT scans. *Radiology* 1987;162:371–375.

49. Muller NL, Miller RR, Webb WR, et al. Fibrosing alveolitis: CT-pathologic correlation. *Radiology* 1986;160:585–588.

50. Meziane M, Hruban R, Zerhouni E, et al. High resolution CT of the lung parenchyma with pathologic correlation. *RadioGraphics* 1988;8:27–54.

51. Westcott JL, Cole SR. Traction bronchiectasis in end-stage pulmonary fibrosis. *Radiology* 1986;161:665–669.

52. Remy-Jardin M, Giraud F, Remy J, et al. Importance of ground-glass attenuation in chronic diffuse infiltrative lung disease: pathologic-CT correlation. *Radiology* 1993;189:693–698.

53. Leung A, Miller R, Muller N. Parenchymal opacification in chronic infiltrative lung disease: CT-pathologic correlation. *Radiology* 1993;188:209–214.

54. Stern E, Swensen S, Hartman T, et al. CT mosaic pattern of lung attenuation: distinguishing different causes. *AJR Am J Roentgenol* 1995;165:813–816.

55. Arakawa H, Webb WR, McCowin M, et al. Inhomogeneous lung attenuation at thin-section CT: diagnostic value of expiratory scans. *Radiology* 1998;206:89–94.

56. Godwin J, Muller N, Takasugi J. Pulmonary alveolar proteinosis: CT findings. *Radiology* 1988;169:609–613.

57. Tan RT, Kuzo RS. High-resolution CT findings of mucinous bronchioloalveolar carcinoma: a case of pseudopulmonary alveolar proteinosis. *AJR Am J Roentgenol* 1997;168:99–100.

58. Laurent F, Philippe JC, Vergier B, et al. Exogenous lipoid pneumonia: HRCT, MR, and pathologic findings. *Eur Radiol* 1999;9:1190–1196.

59. Murayama S, Murakami J, Yabuuchi H, et al. "Crazy paving appearance" on high resolution CT in various diseases. *J Comput Assist Tomogr* 1999;23:749–752.

60. Primack SL, Hartman TE, Lee KS, et al. Pulmonary nodules and the CT halo sign. *Radiology* 1994;190:513–515.

61. Yankelevitz DF, Henschke CI. Does 2-year stability imply that pulmonary nodules are benign? *AJR Am J Roentgenol* 1997;168:325–328.

62. Huston J 3rd, Muhm JR. Solitary pulmonary nodules: evaluation with a CT reference phantom. *Radiology* 1989;170:653–656.

63. Siegelman SS, Khouri NF, Scott WW Jr, et al. Pulmonary hamartoma: CT findings. *Radiology* 1986;160:313–317.

64. Swensen SJ, Viggiano RW, Midthun DE, et al. Lung nodule enhancement at CT: multicenter study. *Radiology* 2000;214:73–80.

65. Gould MK, Lillington GA. Strategy and cost in investigating solitary pulmonary nodules. *Thorax* 1998;53[Suppl 2]:S32–S37.

65a. Gambhir SS, Shepherd JE, Shah BD, et al. Analytical decision model for the cost effective management of solitary pulmonary nodules. *J Clin Oncol* 1998;16:2113–2135.

66. Blum J, Handmaker H, Lister-James J, et al. A multicenter trial

with a somatostatin analog ^{99m}Tc depreotide in the evaluation of solitary pulmonary nodules. *Chest* 2000;117:1232–1238.

67. McLoud TC, Bourgouin PM, Greenberg RW, et al. Bronchogenic carcinoma: analysis of staging in the mediastinum with CT by correlative lymph node mapping and sampling. *Radiology* 1992;182:319–323.

68. Webb WR, Gatsonis C, Zerhouni EA, et al. CT and MR imaging in staging non-small cell bronchogenic carcinoma: report of the Radiologic Diagnostic Oncology Group. *Radiology* 1991;178:705–713.

69. MacManus MP, Hicks RJ, Matthews JP, et al. High rate of detection of unsuspected distant metastases by pet in apparent stage III non–small-cell lung cancer: implications for radical radiation therapy. *Int J Radiat Oncol Biol Phys* 2001;50:287–293.

70. Hicks RJ, Kalff V, MacManus MP, et al. ^{18}F-FDG PET provides high-impact and powerful prognostic stratification in staging newly diagnosed non–small cell lung cancer. *J Nucl Med* 2001;42:1596–1604.

71. Poncelet AJ, Lonneux M, Coche E, et al. PET-FDG scan enhances but does not replace preoperative surgical staging in non–small cell lung carcinoma. *Eur J Cardiothorac Surg* 2001;20:468–474;discussion 474–475.

72. Pieterman RM, van Putten JW, Meuzelaar JJ, et al. Preoperative staging of non–small-cell lung cancer with positron-emission tomography. *N Engl J Med* 2000;343:254–261.

73. Fischer BM, Mortensen J, Hojgaard L. Positron emission tomography in the diagnosis and staging of lung cancer: a systematic, quantitative review. *Lancet Oncol* 2001;2:659–666.

74. van Tinteren H, Hoekstra OS, Smit EF, et al. Effectiveness of positron emission tomography in the preoperative assessment of patients with suspected non–small-cell lung cancer: the PLUS multicentre randomised trial. *Lancet* 2002;359:1388–1393.

75. Matthay RA, Schwarz MI, Ellis JH Jr, et al. Pulmonary artery hypertension in chronic obstructive pulmonary disease: determination by chest radiography. *Invest Radiol* 1981;16:95–100.

76. Ghio AJ, Meyer GA, Crapo RO. Association of pulmonary artery size on chest radiograph with residence at elevated altitudes. *J Thorac Imaging* 1996;11:53–57.

77. Sonnet S, Buitrago-Tellez C, Scheffler K, et al. Dynamic time-resolved contrast-enhanced two-dimensional MR projection angiography of the pulmonary circulation: standard technique and clinical applications. *AJR Am J Roentgenol* 2002;179:159–165.

78. Remy J, Remy-Jardin M, Wattinne L, et al. Pulmonary arteriovenous malformations: evaluation with CT of the chest before and after treatment. *Radiology* 1992;182:809–816.

79. Staples CA, Gamsu G, Ray CS, et al. High resolution computed tomography and lung function in asbestos-exposed workers with normal chest radiographs. *Am Rev Respir Dis* 1989;139:1502–1508.

80. Begin R, Ostiguy G, Fillion R, et al. Computed tomography in the early detection of silicosis. *Am Rev Respir Dis* 1991;144:697–705.

81. Bergin C, Bell D, Coblentz C, et al. Sarcoidosis: correlation of pulmonary parenchymal pattern at CT with results of pulmonary function tests. *Radiology* 1989;171:619–624.

82. Harrison NK, Glanville AR, Strickland B, et al. Pulmonary involvement in systemic sclerosis: the detection of early changes by thin section CT scan, bronchoalveolar lavage and [99m]Tc- DTPA clearance. *Respir Med* 1989;83:403–414.

83. Schurawitzki H, Stiglbauer R, Graninger W, et al. Interstitial lung disease in progressive systemic sclerosis: high-resolution CT versus radiography. *Radiology* 1990;176:755–759.

84. Hansell D, Moskovic E. High-resolution computed tomography in extrinsic allergic alveolitis. *Clin Rad* 1991;43:8–12.

85. Silver S, Muller N, Miller R, et al. Hypersensitivity pneumonitis: evaluation with CT. *Radiology* 1989;173:441–445.

86. Aberle DR, Gamsu G, Ray CS. High-resolution CT of benign asbestos-related diseases: clinical and radiographic correlation. *AJR Am J Roentgenol* 1988;151:883–891.

87. Lynch DA, Rose CS, Way D, et al. Hypersensitivity pneumonitis: sensitivity of high-resolution CT in a population-based study. *AJR Am J Roentgenol* 1992;159:469–472.

87a. Gamsu G, Salmon CT, Warnock ML, et al. CT quantification of interstitial fibrosis in patients with asbestosis: a comparison of two methods. *AJR Am J Roentgenol* 1995;16:63–68.

88. Mathieson JR, Mayo JR, Staples CA, et al. Chronic diffuse infiltrative lung disease: comparison of diagnostic accuracy of CT and chest radiography. *Radiology* 1989;171:111–116.

89. Swensen S, Aughenbaugh G, Myers J. Diffuse lung disease: Diagnostic accuracy of CT in patients undergoing surgical biopsy of the lung. *Radiology* 1997;205:229–234.

90. Hunninghake GW, Zimmerman MB, Schwartz DA, et al. Utility of a lung biopsy for the diagnosis of idiopathic pulmonary fibrosis. *Am J Respir Crit Care Med* 2001;164:193–196.

91. Tung KT, Wells AU, Rubens MB, et al. Accuracy of the typical computed tomographic appearances of fibrosing alveolitis. *Thorax* 1993;48:334–338.

92. Lynch D, Newell J, Logan P, et al. Can CT distinguish idiopathic pulmonary fibrosis from hypersensitivity pneumonitis? *AJR Am J Roentgenol* 1995;165:807–811.

93. Hunninghake G, Lynch D, Galvin J, et al. Radiological findings are most strongly associated with a pathological diagnosis of IPF. *Chest* 2003 (in press).

94. Raghu G, Mageto YN, Lockhart D, et al. The accuracy of the clinical diagnosis of new-onset idiopathic pulmonary fibrosis and other interstitial lung disease: a prospective study. *Chest* 1999;116:1168–1174.

95. Bonelli FS, Hartman TE, Swensen SJ, et al. Accuracy of high-resolution CT in diagnosing lung diseases. *AJR Am J Roentgenol* 1998;170:1507–1512.

96. Nishimura K, Izumi T, Kitaichi M, et al. The diagnostic accuracy of high-resolution computed tomography in diffuse infiltrative lung diseases. *Chest* 1993;104:1149–1155.

97. McGuinness G, Beacher JR, Harkin TJ, et al. Hemoptysis: prospective high-resolution CT/bronchoscopic correlation. *Chest* 1994;105:1155–1162.

98. McGuinness G, Naidich D. Bronchiectasis: CT/clinical correlations. *Semin Ultrasound CT MRI* 1995;16:395–419.

99. Lynch DA, Newell J, Hale V, et al. Correlation of CT findings with clinical evaluations in 261 patients with symptomatic bronchiectasis. *AJR Am J Roentgenol* 1999;173:53–58.

100. Kim J, Muller N, Park C, et al. Cylindric bronchiectasis: diagnostic findings on thin-section CT. *AJR Am J Roentgenol* 1997;168:751–754.

101. Roberts HR, Wells AU, Milne DG, et al. Airflow obstruction in bronchiectasis: correlation between computed tomography features and pulmonary function tests. *Thorax* 2000;55:198–204.

102. Kim J, Muller N, Park C, et al. Bronchoarterial ratio on thin section CT: comparison between high altitude and sea level. *J Comput Assist Tomogr* 1997;21:306–311.

Baum's Textbook of Pulmonary Diseases, 7th ed. Edited by James D. Crapo, Jeffrey Glassroth, Joel Karlinsky, and Talmadge E. King, Jr.
Lippincott Williams & Wilkins, Philadelphia © 2004.

2 Pulmonary Function Testing

Robert O. Crapo

Pulmonary function tests provide objective measures of lung function for (a) detecting and quantifying pulmonary impairment in cardiopulmonary diseases; (b) monitoring the evolution of diseases and response to therapy; (c) monitoring the effects of environmental, occupational, and drug exposures associated with lung injury; (d) assessing preoperative risk; and (e) assessing disability and impairment (1). This chapter focuses on the practical pulmonary function tests of most use in day-to-day clinical medicine.

Following the steps in gas exchange from ambient air to cell (Table 2.1) helps put pulmonary function testing in perspective. Respiratory gases move by passive diffusion, which means optimal concentrations of oxygen (O_2) and carbon dioxide (CO_2) in alveolar gas are necessary to transfer them to and from pulmonary capillary blood. The environment for gas transfer is established by alveolar ventilation accomplished with the bellows action of the lung. Many lung function tests (static lung volumes, spirometry, airway resistance, and respiratory muscle function) characterize mechanical aspects of the air pump. The second step, gas transfer from the alveolar air to blood, is traditionally assessed with carbon monoxide (CO) diffusing capacity and arterial blood gas measurements. Diffusing capacity is an indirect test, whereas arterial blood gases provide a more direct assessment of successful O_2 loading and CO_2 removal from blood. The third and fourth steps, assessing gas transport and gas transfer from blood to cells, require evaluation of arterial and mixed venous blood gases, cardiac output, and end-organ function. These aspects of gas transfer are usually the focus in intensive care units; they are not usually assessed in traditional pulmonary function laboratories.

Control of breathing can be assessed by measuring the ventilatory response to progressive hypercarbia or hypoxemia, but these are measurements not commonly used in clinical practice. The final element in practical lung function testing is measuring cardiac and respiratory responses to exercise. Because exercise stresses the entire heart, lung, and blood system, exercise testing provides an opportunity to tease out the factors that lead to dyspnea and impaired exercise capacity. Exercise testing is covered in Chapter 3.

Lung function tests differ from most other medical tests in the level of patient participation required. Test quality depends on how well the patient has been coached to a vigorous effort. In a general population study, in which test quality was carefully controlled, Hankinson and colleagues found about 85% of more than 6,000 spirometry studies met American Thoracic Society (ATS) quality standards (2). In contrast, a study of spirometry performed in 30 primary care practices found ATS criteria were met in only 13.5% (3). Although some patients are unable to perform acceptable tests, training staff to recognize quality tests and providing feedback to the staff on test quality will result in consistently good quality tests. A modest investment of time and effort can bring test quality to acceptable standards in most pulmonary laboratories (4).

STATIC LUNG VOLUMES

The static lung volume subdivisions, illustrated in Figure 2.1, are grouped into volumes and capacities. Volumes, the primary subdivisions, cannot be subdivided. Capacities contain two or more volumes and can, therefore, be subdivided. Total lung capacity (TLC), the volume of air in the lungs at the end of a maximal inspiration, is attained when maximal inspiratory muscle force is counterbalanced by the recoil forces of the lung and chest wall. The maximal volume of air that

R. O. Crapo: Pulmonary Laboratory, LDS Hospital, University of Utah School of Medicine, Salt Lake City, Utah.

TABLE 2.1. GAS EXCHANGE BETWEEN THE ATMOSPHERE AND BODY CELLS: GAS TRANSPORT SYSTEM STEPS

Step	Purpose	Structure(s)	Tests to Characterize Structure or Function
Ventilation	Maintain normal P_{AO_2} and P_{ACO_2}	Air pump (lungs, chest wall, and neuromuscular apparatus)	P_{ACO_2}, spirometry, lung volumes, airway resistance, respiratory muscle strength
Gas transfer (lung)	Transfer of gases between alveolar air and pulmonary capillary blood	Alveolar capillary membrane	Arterial blood gases (P_{aO_2} and P_{aCO_2}, $P_{AO_2} - P_{aO_2}$), oxygen content, carbon monoxide diffusing capacity
Circulation	Delivery of oxygen from the lungs to the peripheral capillaries, and carbon dioxide from the peripheral capillaries to the lungs	Blood pump (heart and blood)	Heart function (e.g., cardiac output, oxygen content, oxygen delivery)
Gas transfer (periphery)	Transfer of gases between systemic capillaries and metabolizing cells	Systemic capillary membranes and metabolizing cells	Difficult to assess. Tests of end-organ function (e.g., central nervous system and renal function) provide regional information and are the best clinical indicators. Lactic acidosis may occur with tissue hypoxemia but is not a definite indicator of its presence.

P_{AO_2}, alveolar partial pressure of oxygen; P_{ACO_2}, alveolar partial pressure of carbon dioxide; P_{aCO_2}, arterial partial pressure of carbon dioxide; $P_{AO_2} - P_{aO_2}$, alveolar-arterial gradient in partial pressure of oxygen.

can be exhaled after a maximal inhalation is vital capacity (VC). VC can be measured with either an inspiratory or an expiratory maneuver and with either an unforced slow exhalation (SVC) or a nearly maximally forced maneuver (FVC). The volume of air remaining in the lungs after a maximal exhalation is residual volume (RV). RV is determined by the balance of the forces tending to reduce lung volume (maximal expiratory muscle force and inward lung recoil) against the force tending to increase lung volume (outward recoil of the chest wall). Tidal volume (V_T) is the volume of air moved with each breath during normal breathing. Functional residual capacity (FRC) is usually defined as the volume of air in the lungs at the end of a quiet relaxed exhalation, although it is sometimes used to indicate the volume of air in the lungs at the end of a tidal breath, whether exhalation is active or passive. Inspiratory capacity (IC) is the maximal volume of air that can be inhaled from FRC. Expiratory reserve vol-

ume (ERV) is the maximal volume of air that can be exhaled from FRC. IC and ERV have little role in diagnostic testing, although ERV is the lung volume most commonly reduced in the morbidly obese (5).

The displaceable lung volumes—those that can be inhaled and exhaled from the mouth—are measured with a spirometer. Two types of spirometer are schematically illustrated and described in Figure 2.2. The parameters measured by a spirometer are VC, V_T, IC, and ERV (Fig. 2.1). The remaining volumes and capacities contain RV and cannot be measured with a spirometer. Plethysmographic, gas dilution, and radiographic techniques each measure one of the capacities containing RV. Once determined, they can be combined with the appropriate displaceable volumes to calculate the remaining lung volumes and capacities. The following descriptions are brief overviews. The tests are all discussed in greater detail in standard texts on lung function (6–8).

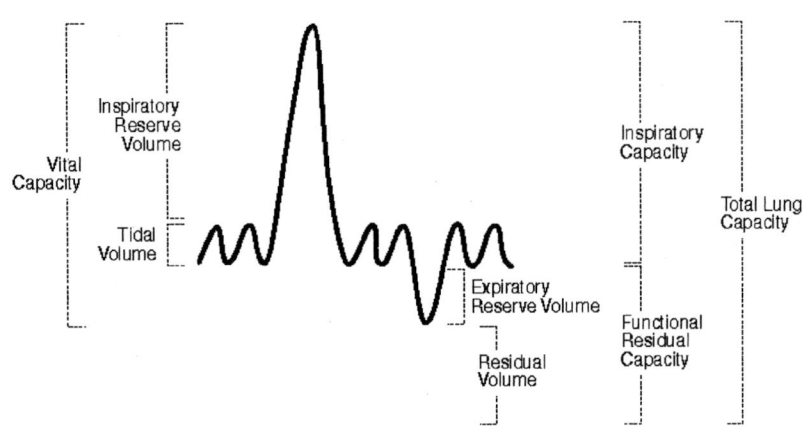

FIGURE 2.1. Lung volumes and capacities. Volumes cannot be subdivided. Capacities contain two or more volumes. (From Aldose MD. Practical aspects of pulmonary function testing. In: Baum GL, Wolinsky E, eds. *Textbook of pulmonary diseases.* Boston: Little, Brown and Company, 1993, with permission.)

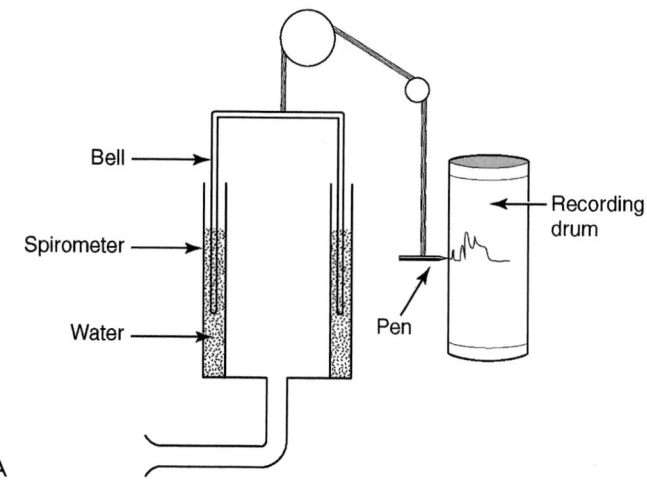

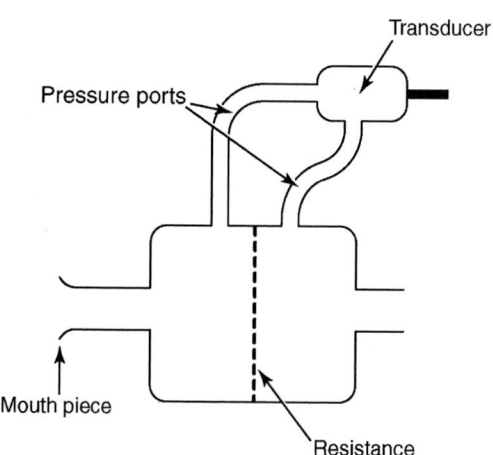

FIGURE 2.2. Two types of spirometers. **A:** Volume-based spirometer that uses water as a seal. Air blown into the spirometer causes the bell to rise, inscribing the height of a cylinder and, therefore, volume. Time is also recorded to allow measurement of volumes as a function of time. As volume is the primary measurement, flows are derived by differentiating the volume–time information. **B:** Flow-based spirometer. Air is blown across a resistor; differential pressures measured across the resistor are related to flow. As flow is the primary measurement, it must be integrated to get volumes. (From Aldose MD. Practical aspects of pulmonary function testing. In: Baum GL, Wolinsky E, eds. *Textbook of pulmonary diseases.* Boston: Little, Brown and Company, 1993, with permission.)

Gas Dilution Techniques

Gas dilution techniques measure the gas volume in the lungs that communicates via the airways. The techniques vary in details but all use a mass balance approach. The most common approach is schematically illustrated in Figure 2.3. The patient breathes from a known volume and concentration of a relatively insoluble and inert tracer gas (e.g., helium). Mixing is allowed to occur for a variable length of time, and the final mixed concentration of tracer gas is measured. A mass balance equation uses the initial volume and tracer gas concentration and the final tracer gas concentration to calculate the volume in the patient's lungs at

the moment tracer gas breathing began. The assumptions that the tracer gas is relatively insoluble and inert and is well mixed in lung air are critical. Use of a relatively soluble gas would result in an overestimation of lung volumes; incomplete gas mixing would cause them to be underestimated. By using the helium rebreathing method, the patient quietly breathes from the test circuit for 4 to 7 minutes, with occasional deep breaths, until gas measurements demonstrate the concentration of helium in the circuit is stable, an indication gas mixing is complete. The long rebreathing time (up to 7 minutes) allows complete mixing of helium in the circuit, but it also means that CO_2 has to be removed from and O_2 added to the circuit for patient safety and comfort.

A gas dilution measurement of TLC (usually reported as alveolar volume, or V_A) accompanies every measurement of the single-breath CO diffusing capacity test. In this test, subjects inhale a VC-sized volume of gas that contains 10% helium, 0.3% CO, and 21% O_2, hold the breath for 10 seconds, and then exhale. An alveolar gas sample is analyzed to get the diluted alveolar helium concentration. The assumption that helium is completely mixed during the 10-second breath-hold is reasonably acceptable in healthy individuals. TLC is only minimally underestimated compared with the multibreath technique in healthy people. In people with airway obstruction, mixing is less complete and becomes less so as obstruction worsens. TLC is progressively underestimated with increasing obstruction, and the single-breath technique has little utility as a technique for measuring TLC in people with airway obstruction (9).

The nitrogen (N_2) washout techniques also use a mass balance approach to estimate TLC. In the multibreath N_2 washout method, the subject begins breathing 100% O_2 at FRC and continues to breathe O_2 until N_2 is displaced from the lungs. The displaced N_2 is measured. FRC is calculated by assuming (a) that the mass of displaced N_2 is equal to the mass of N_2 in the lungs at the beginning of the test, and (b) that the initial concentration of N_2 in the lungs was 80%. N_2 washout techniques also underestimate TLC when airway obstruction is present.

Plethysmography

Plethysmography is used to measure lung volumes and airway resistances. For lung volumes, plethysmography measures the compressible gas volume in the chest by using Boyle's law; i.e., the product of gas volume and pressure is a constant ($V_1 \times P_1 = k$) when temperature is held constant. The test is performed by having the patient sit in a sealed box and gently pant against a closed shutter located at the mouth. During the inspiratory phase of the panting maneuver, the thoracic volume increases, slightly decompressing the volume of air in the lungs while compressing the air in the box. In the expiratory phase, thoracic gas volume decreases slightly, compressing the air in the lungs and decompressing

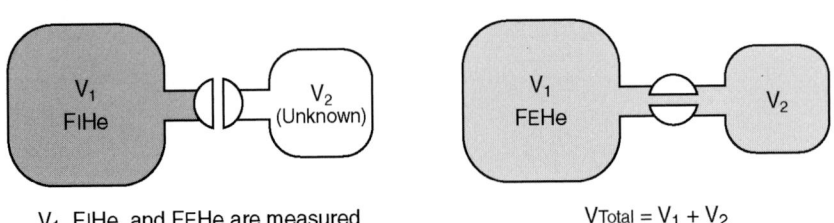

V_1, FIHe, and FEHe are measured   VTotal = V_1 + V_2

$$FIHe \times V_1 = FEHe \times VTotal$$

$$\frac{FIHe}{FEHe} \times V_1 = VTotal$$

$$V_2 = VTotal - V_1$$

FIGURE 2.3. Schematic illustration of the basic theory of gas dilution measurement of lung volume. Air in a subject's lungs is allowed to come into equilibrium with a known mass of a relatively insoluble and inert gas, such as helium (He). Initial volume (V_1) and He concentration (FIHe) are known. The diluted final He concentration (FEHe) is used to calculate the unknown volume (V_2).

box air. By Boyle's law (Equation 1):

$$V_1 \times P_1 = V_2 \times P_2 \qquad (Eq. 1)$$

The initial pressure and volume at FRC (the beginning volume before panting) are P_1 and V_1. Pressure and volume at the end of the inspiratory phase of the pant are P_2 and V_2, which can be rewritten as $[(P_1 + \Delta P) \times (V_1 + \Delta V)]$. P_1 and ΔP are measured at the mouth, assuming that mouth pressure is equal to alveolar pressure, and ΔV is measured by using the change in box pressure. The equation can then be solved for V_1.

Body plethysmography is still considered the gold standard of techniques used to measure static lung volumes. It is sensitive to technical and procedural errors and, like all other lung volume techniques, requires exquisite attention to quality control. For example, the assumption that mouth pressure equals alveolar pressure tends to fail when panting frequency exceeds one pant per second because there is insufficient time for the pressure changes at the mouth to equilibrate with alveolar pressure. This is primarily a problem in patients with airway obstruction, in whom rapid panting causes a significant overestimation of TLC (10).

When plethysmographic and single-breath gas dilution measurements of TLC are made during the same test session, the difference between the two (TLC$_{PL}$ − TLC$_{GAS}$) can be used as an estimate of the poorly ventilated gas volume in the lungs, commonly referred to as trapped gas. The volume of trapped gas increases with airway obstruction.

Radiographic Total Lung Capacity

TLC can also be estimated from standard posteroanterior and lateral chest radiographs. A radiographic TLC measurement starts with a calculation of total intrathoracic gas volume, from which estimated volumes for the mediastinum, heart, blood, and diaphragm are subtracted. Studies show excellent correlation between radiographic TLC and plethysmographic TLC in healthy individuals and in those with

airway obstruction (9). The advantages of this method are that the methodology is simple, requires no special equipment, and takes little time. Chest radiographs are commonly included in evaluations for respiratory diseases and thus are often available. The radiographic method can also be used to re-create a history of TLC. Old chest radiographs are often the only source of lung volume information from a patient's past and can provide evidence of change in a patient whose loss of lung volume would otherwise not have been detectable. This advantage is being compromised by the current trend to destroy radiographs earlier.

Disadvantages of the method are that the radiographic TLC method has not yet been proven accurate in patients with interstitial lung diseases, and test variability is larger than that for other methods (11). Chest structures are magnified slightly on chest radiographs. Published methods usually use a magnification factor based on a target–film distance of 72 in. (183 cm). For other target–film distances, magnification factors will differ. The method has not kept up with the technology, and there are no computation schemes available for digitized chest radiographs.

Pathophysiologic Correlates with Lung Volumes

The three basic patterns of lung volumes illustrated in Figure 2.4 are normal, overinflation (too large), and restriction (too small). In the normal pattern, TLC, VC, and RV fall within a reference range based on healthy people. In young people, RV constitutes about 25% of TLC, and FRC about 40%. As people age, lung recoil decreases, causing a slight shift toward obstruction in the pattern of airflow. With aging, TLC remains essentially unchanged, RV increases, and FRC either increases slightly or does not change. RV increases with aging primarily because the slight shift toward an obstructive pattern makes it impossible for a true expiratory plateau to be reached and RV becomes a dynamic measurement, dependent on expiratory time.

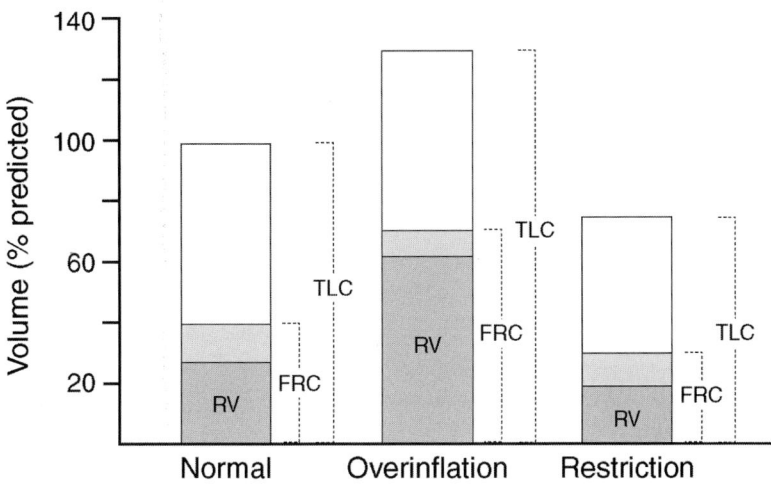

FIGURE 2.4. The three basic lung volume patterns: normal, overinflation (too large), and restriction (too small). TLC, total lung capacity; FRC, functional residual capacity; RV, residual volume. (From Aldose MD. Practical aspects of pulmonary function testing. In: Baum GL, Wolinsky E, eds. *Textbook of pulmonary diseases.* Boston: Little, Brown and Company, 1993, with permission.)

Diseases that alter the elastic properties of either the chest wall or lungs may alter lung volumes. Diseases such as emphysema reduce lung recoil and may cause TLC, FRC, and RV to be increased, even when minimal airflow obstruction is present. In emphysema, airway obstruction commonly accompanies decreased lung recoil, and both contribute to overinflation. Mechanically, airway obstruction impedes exhalation and inspiration begins before exhalation is complete, resulting in overinflation. The process is exacerbated when respiratory rate increases, causing expiratory time to shorten. Asthma is a classic illustration of a disease with overinflation secondary to airflow obstruction. There is also evidence in asthma that inspiratory muscle activity persists throughout expiration, contributing to overinflation (12).

Overinflation is primarily determined by an elevated TLC. Other patterns, such as elevated RV or FRC, suggest the presence of overinflation, but one should be cautious about making an interpretation of overinflation when TLC is within the normal range.

Lung volumes may be reduced (restriction) in any disease process that increases lung recoil (e.g., pulmonary fibrosis), compresses the lungs (pleural effusion), decreases chest wall compliance (kyphoscoliosis, morbid obesity), alters the shape of the chest (kyphoscoliosis), or decreases respiratory muscle function (neuromuscular diseases, diaphragmatic paralysis).

TLC is the primary variable used to determine the presence of restriction. By definition, the presence of restriction is determined by a reduction in TLC. A spirometric pattern of a reduced VC in the absence of airway obstruction has been used to suggest the presence of a reduced TLC (restrictive pattern). Aaron and colleagues found the low VC predicted a low TLC only 58% of the time (13). However, a normal VC predicted a normal TLC 98% of the time. The study may have some ascertainment bias, and the predictive numbers reported by Aaron and colleagues should be interpreted with some caution.

DYNAMIC TESTS OF LUNG FUNCTION

Spirometry

Spirometry, which can include both quiet and forced VC maneuvers, is the most common and useful of the lung function tests. Its clinical utility is accepted, it is the least expensive test to perform, and it should be the test most widely available in doctors' offices, clinics, and hospitals. The FVC test is performed by having a patient inhale to TLC and then make a maximally forced exhalation into a spirometer. Classically, exhaled volume is measured as a function of time. Flow may also be measured and displayed as a function of exhaled volume. The three primary spirometric indices in the forced test are FVC, forced expired volume in 1 second (FEV_1), and the ratio FEV_1/FVC. Other spirometric measures are available, but their clinical utility is less well established. Typical volume–time and flow–volume spirographic displays for a healthy individual are shown in Figure 2.5.

Test quality depends on achieving a maximal inhalation, a nearly maximal effort during the initial few seconds of exhalation, and a reasonable duration of exhalation. A plateau in the volume–time tracing or a minimum expiratory time of 6 seconds indicates a reasonable duration of exhalation. A plateau is rarely reached in individuals with airflow obstruction or in healthy older people who have reduced airflow at low lung volumes because of the normal age-related loss of lung recoil. Because expiratory flow never truly reaches a plateau in these individuals, VC increases and FEV_1/VC falls with increased expiratory time. The volume exhaled in 6 seconds (FEV_6) has been proposed as a surrogate for FVC. Swanney demonstrated that FEV_1/FEV_6 performed the same as FEV_1/FVC in identifying airway obstruction (14).

Syncope may occur, even in healthy subjects, when maximal expiratory force is exerted throughout the entire maneuver. Spirogram quality is not altered if patients are allowed to reduce their expiratory effort after about 2 to 3 seconds and continue to exhale without squeezing hard (15).

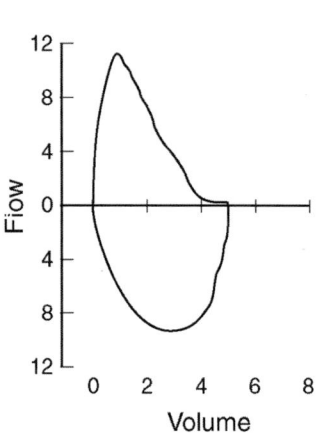
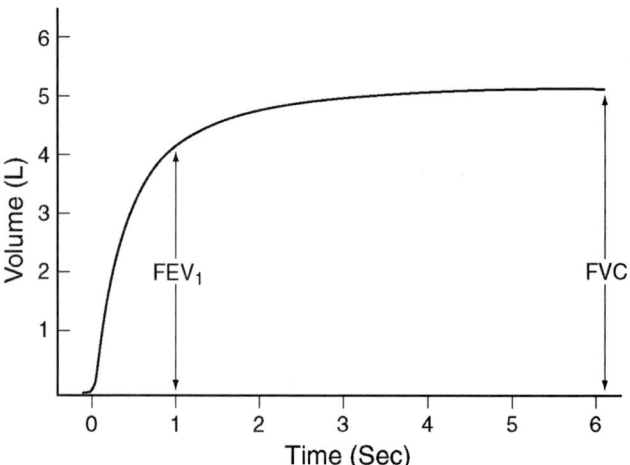

FIGURE 2.5. Spirogram of acceptable quality in a healthy 54-year-old man. In the flow–volume display, markers of good quality include a quick start with a rapid rise in expiratory flow, a well-defined early peak in flow, the absence of a cough or hesitation in the early portion of the spirogram, and an exhalation that exceeds 6 seconds. The slight tail at the end of exhalation and the continued increase in volume even after 6 seconds of exhalation (volume–time tracing) reflect normal age-related changes. FEV_1, forced expiratory volume in 1 second; FVC, forced vital capacity.

Detailed quality standards have been published by the ATS and the European Respiratory Society (ERS) (16, 17). The first step is to use a spirometer demonstrated to meet accuracy and precision standards. Although this may seem flagrantly obvious, a study of more than 50 instruments on the market in the early 1980s found only about half met ATS accuracy standards (18). The problems have largely been corrected. Now, most, but not all, commercially marketed spirometers meet standards, and it would be unwise to choose a spirometer that cannot demonstrate accuracy and precision. Once in use, spirometers need regular quality control checks to assure proper performance. Such checks are especially important after an instrument has been serviced or upgraded.

As instrumentation has improved, the major quality issues are procedural. Test quality includes acceptability criteria for each effort and reproducibility criteria for the series of tests performed. Current standards require at least three acceptable quality spirograms be obtained. Reproducibility criteria are then applied to the acceptable spirograms to ensure the data are representative of the patient. If spirograms of acceptable quality do not meet reproducibility criteria, the patient should be asked to perform the test again. If acceptability and reproducibility criteria are not met in eight tries, the study may be terminated (16). Efforts to improve procedural aspects of spirometry include immediate computerized analysis of each test waveform with feedback to the technician about test quality.

Acceptability and reproducibility criteria are target ideals for test performance. Even suboptimal tests may provide useful information, and patient data should not be discarded solely because acceptability and reproducibility criteria are not met. The best data available should be submitted for interpretation, and the interpretation should deal with the limitations (16). For example, a test with completely inadequate initial effort still may yield an acceptable VC if a reasonable end of test is achieved. Failure to meet acceptability criteria in an individual test occurs for a variety of reasons, including inability or unwillingness of a patient to perform the test, even with vigorous coaching. Failure to meet reproducibility criteria in an individual test may also indicate the presence of hyperreactive airways. Frequent test failures in a laboratory are evidence of quality control problems.

Most quality issues are the responsibility of the laboratory and its director, but clinicians who use pulmonary function tests in their medical practice should be able to recognize good-quality tests, as well as various disease patterns. Spirograms should be analyzed for quality by visually inspecting both flow–volume and volume–time displays. Good-quality spirograms, along with several faulty spirogram patterns, are illustrated in Figures 2.5 through 2.7.

Full spirometry should include both FVC (forced) and SVC (unforced) maneuvers. SVC is often larger than FVC, especially in older people and in those with airway obstruction in whom the forced maneuver effectively causes some air trapping. However, VC will be underestimated if the unforced maneuver is excessively slow. The largest VC found during testing, whether from the forced or the unforced maneuver, should be used to calculate the FEV_1/VC ratio.

When studies meet acceptability and reproducibility standards, the next question is choosing which measurements to use for interpretation. In general, the largest FVC, FEV_1, and peak flow from acceptable tests are used for interpretative purposes; they need not come from the same trial (16). If midflows (e.g., forced expiratory flow [FEF]$_{25\%–75\%}$) or instantaneous flows (e.g., $V_{max50\%}$) are used for interpretation, they should be selected from the single, acceptable-quality spirogram with the largest sum of FVC and FEV_1 (16).

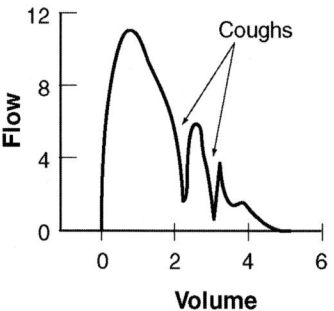

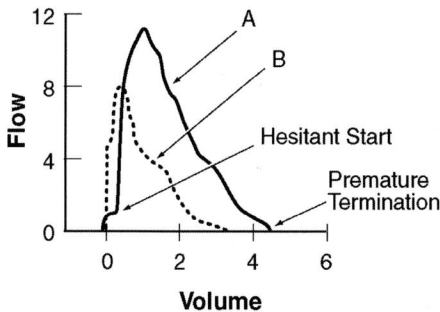

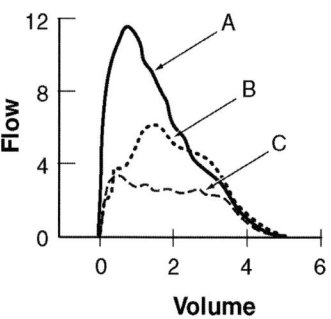

FIGURE 2.6. Several types of faulty spirograms. **Top:** Multiple coughs begin early in exhalation (before I second). Coughs are characterized by sudden falls in flow, followed by quick restoration of flow. Early coughs may cause forced expiratory volume in I second (FEV_1) to be underestimated. **Middle:** A hesitant start (waveform A) could cause FEV_1 to be overestimated, and a premature termination of exhalation would cause forced VC (FVC) to be underestimated. Waveform B, from the same patient, illustrates an inadequate inhalation followed by a good expiratory effort. Alone, the curve would be graded acceptable; it is unacceptable when compared with waveform A. **Bottom:** Nonreproducible tracings. Waveform A is an acceptable tracing. Waveforms B and C show two different but submaximal initial efforts. FEV_1 may be underestimated with the submaximal efforts; FVC may be acceptable in all tracings, depending on the presence of an adequate inhalation and end of test. (From Paul Enright, M.D., University of Arizona, Tucson, Arizona, with permission.)

Average ($FEF_{25\%-75\%}$) and instantaneous flows ($V_{max50\%}$) variables have limited clinical utility. They should be used to assist in decision making when the primary indices (FVC, FEV_1, FEV_1/VC) are close to the lower limits of their normal ranges (19).

Pathophysiologic Correlations with Spirometry

Spirometry is used diagnostically only to classify patients as having one of three patterns: normal, airflow obstruc-

tion, and restriction. Specific diagnoses cannot be made with spirometry alone, and the patterns must be interpreted in light of the clinical questions being asked (19). The interpretation of spirometry is discussed in detail in the section "General Interpretative Guidelines."

Bronchodilator Administration and Testing

In patients with airway obstruction, it is common practice to perform spirometry before and after the administration of an inhaled, fast-acting β_2-selective agonist. The test is performed by obtaining baseline spirometry, administering the bronchodilator medication, waiting a brief period (usually about 15 minutes), and then repeating the spirometry. The test is best performed with a spirometer but can be done with a peak flow meter. An improvement in FEV_1 of 12% and 200 mL is considered an unequivocally positive response (19). There is, however, controversy on how to calculate the percentage of change. The ATS calculates it as percentage of change from the baseline study (16), and the ERS as a percentage of the reference value for FEV_1 (17). An increase in peak flow of 60 L/min is considered a positive response.

A positive response in an appropriate clinical setting should be considered reasonable evidence that the patient will benefit from bronchodilator therapy. The converse, however, is not true. The absence of a bronchodilator response in a single laboratory setting does not predict whether bronchodilator therapy will benefit an individual patient. The laboratory outcome can be affected by several technical issues, including the dose and method of administration of the bronchodilator, the wait time, the quality of the effort, the choice of spirometric parameter used to measure response, the threshold used to define response, and recent prior use of bronchodilator medications (20). In addition, patient response is variable from one day to the next. Finally, the obstructive effect of mucous plugging and mucosal edema might be large enough to mask a smooth muscle response to bronchodilator medication. Patients with chronic obstructive pulmonary disease may improve clinically in response to bronchodilation with little or no change in FEV_1. The improvement is better correlated to a reduction in the degree of overinflation, as reflected in increases in IC and decreases in FRC (21). A several-week trial of regular bronchodilator therapy and consideration of outcome variables other than FEV_1 are often required to assess benefit.

Maximum Voluntary Ventilation

Maximum voluntary ventilation (MVV) is the maximum amount of air a person can exhale while breathing as fast and deep as possible with vigorous coaching. It is measured for 12 to 15 seconds and is expressed as liters per minute at BTPS (body temperature, ambient pressure, and saturated with water vapor) conditions. Test duration is short, because people cannot sustain the MVV maneuver much beyond

A. Mild Airflow Obstruction

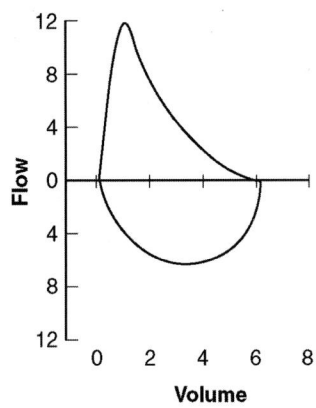
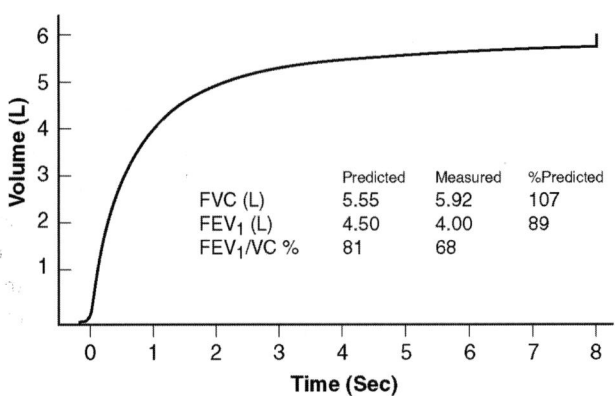

	Predicted	Measured	%Predicted
FVC (L)	5.55	5.92	107
FEV$_1$ (L)	4.50	4.00	89
FEV$_1$/VC %	81	68	

B. Moderate Airflow Obstruction

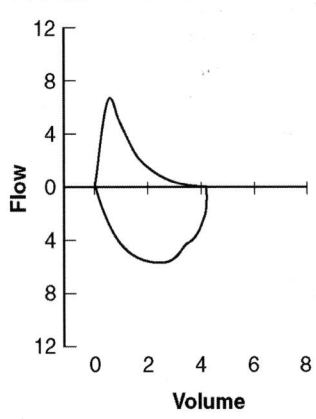
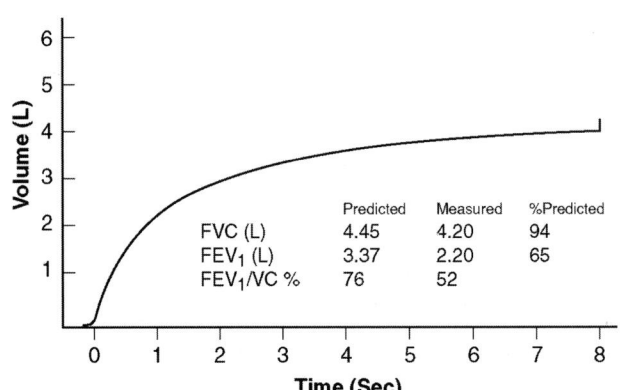

	Predicted	Measured	%Predicted
FVC (L)	4.45	4.20	94
FEV$_1$ (L)	3.37	2.20	65
FEV$_1$/VC %	76	52	

C. Severe Airflow Obstruction

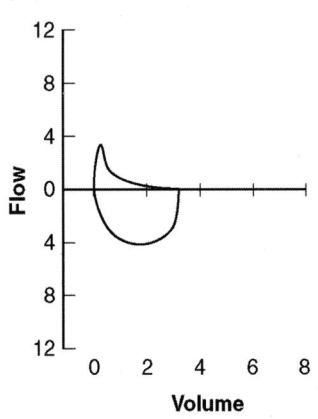
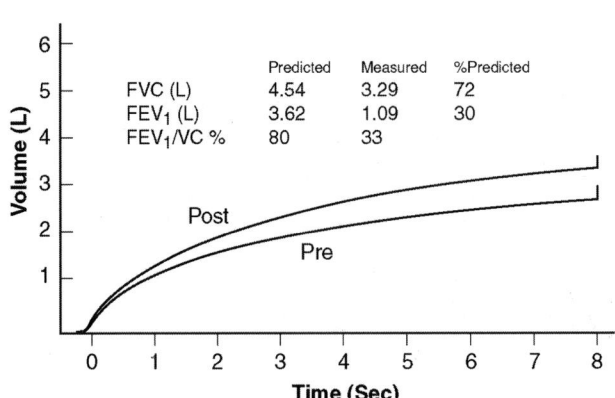

	Predicted	Measured	%Predicted
FVC (L)	4.54	3.29	72
FEV$_1$ (L)	3.62	1.09	30
FEV$_1$/VC %	80	33	

FIGURE 2.7. Typical spirograms for mild **(A)**, moderate **(B)**, and severe **(C)** airway obstruction. Note that with increasing obstruction, the flow–volume tracings show increasing concavity toward the horizontal axis. Prebronchodilator and postbronchodilator tracings **(C, right)** illustrate a good response to administration of an inhaled bronchodilator. FVC, forced vital capacity; FEV$_1$, forced expiratory volume in 1 second; VC, vital capacity; FEV$_1$/VC%, percent of vital capacity exhaled in the first second.

15 seconds. It is often estimated rather than measured, by multiplying the FEV_1 by 35 or the $FEV_{0.75}$ by 40. Ajelabi and colleagues found no difference in MVV with breathing frequencies from 70 to 150 breaths/min (22). However, there is little reason to push patients past 100 breaths/min.

The MVV is a nonspecific test. Reductions in MVV occur in the presence of airway obstruction, chest restriction, neuromuscular diseases, loss of coordination, and diminished cognitive function. It may also be reduced because the subject is unwilling to work maximally during the test (most often elderly patients, those with chronic illness, and those for whom a poor test result promises secondary gain). The clinical utility of MVV is limited because it is so nonspecific. However, the nonspecific nature of the test might also be an advantage in some instances. Reductions in MVV correlate with postoperative risks for respiratory complications and with dyspnea from any cause (23). If measured MVV is significantly below calculated MVV, nonpulmonary factors may be involved in the reduction (24).

The primary use of MVV is to estimate ventilatory reserve in exercise studies. If it is used, it is better measured than estimated. The common practice of using an estimated MVV for this purpose is problematic because the normal between-individual variation in measured MVV is large and because so many variables affect MVV.

Peak Expiratory Flow and Peak Flow Meters

Peak expiratory flow (PEF) is the maximum flow achieved during an FVC maneuver. It occurs very early in the FVC maneuver (usually within the first 0.2 second if the maneuver is well performed). This places the measurement in the most effort-dependent portion of the FVC maneuver. Thus, PEF is significantly more effort-dependent than is FEV_1 and, in my opinion, of less clinical utility. The value of PEF in clinical medicine derives from the availability of small, easily portable, highly reproducible, inexpensive peak flow meters. The meters are acceptably accurate but are less accurate than are good spirometers. Reproducibility is excellent for individual PEF meters, but there is less reproducibility between meters, and there can be marked differences among different PEF meter models. The low cost and reproducibility of PEF meters makes them a practical monitoring device for patients with asthma, especially useful because asthma symptoms and physical findings are imperfect indicators of asthma severity. Monitoring information from PEF meters is of two basic types: (a) trending over days to months, and (b) trending across a day. Increased variability across a day (>20%) indicates airway hyperreactivity and may be an indication of diminished asthma control. At the present time, PEF meters should not be used diagnostically to define normal or abnormal function, because there are no reference values applicable to all PEF meter models.

Peak flow meters can be used to track response to medication, monitor the course of asthma, and quantify the effects of exposures to potential triggers or other environmental factors. National and international guidelines use peak flow data to structure individualized asthma management plans (25). However, the enthusiasm for peak flow meters must be tempered with a note of caution. Their role in the management of asthma is largely based on reasonable suppositions; there is little science to document exactly what the benefits are and who should be using them (26, 27).

Bronchial Reactivity Testing

Airway hyperresponsiveness, an index of the degree of airway narrowing on exposure to provocative stimuli, is one of the primary characteristics of asthma. On average, the airways of asthmatic patients are far more sensitive to provocative stimuli than are those of nonasthmatic subjects. Airway hyperreactivity is suggested by simple tests, such as documenting a response to a bronchodilator or documenting excessive variation in peak flow during a day (most nonasthmatic subjects have a within-day variation in peak flow of <20%). Sometimes specific tests measuring response to provocative stimuli are needed to document the presence of airway hyperresponsiveness.

Two broad categories of stimuli are used to provoke airway narrowing: (a) specific stimuli such as aeroallergens like ragweed antigen or chemicals like toluene diisocyanate, or (b) nonspecific stimuli such as methacholine, histamine, exercise, hyperventilation, or cold dry air. The bronchoconstrictive response will vary with the individual stimulus regardless of category.

Methacholine Challenge Testing

The most common nonspecific bronchoprovocation test uses methacholine, a parasympathomimetic analogue of acetylcholine, as the bronchoconstricting agent (28). Methacholine chloride is prepared in several dilutions and administered as a nebulized aerosol in progressively increasing doses. The test begins with baseline measurements of FEV_1. A second set of measurements may be made after administration of the diluent. Each methacholine dose is followed, after a brief wait, by measurement of FEV_1. The test is terminated if a sustained 20% fall (calculated from the baseline or post diluent value) in FEV_1 is observed within the prescribed dosage schedule (Fig. 2.8). Current ATS recommendations suggest the PC_{20} (the concentration at which the 20% fall in FEV_1 is observed) be used to define the methacholine response (28). As the study is performed in steps, the PC_{20} is calculated either mathematically or graphically from the stepwise changes in FEV_1 (Fig. 2.8). The response is actually a continuum; the lower the PC_{20}, the more reactive the airways. Most asthmatic patients have a PC_{20} of less than or equal to 8 mg/mL. Methacholine challenge testing deals with complex issues and requires rigid standardization to ensure that proper doses of active drug are administered on

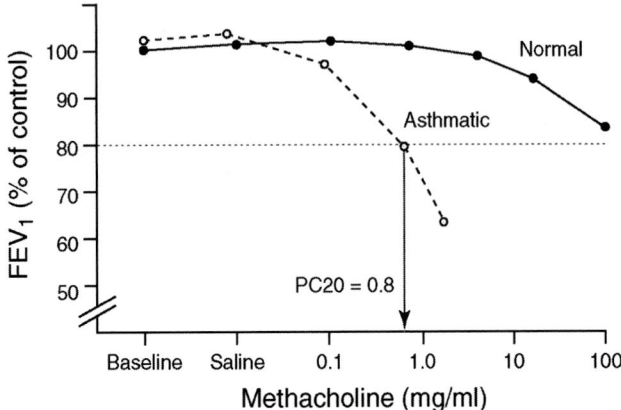

FIGURE 2.8. Graphic display of normal and asthmatic responses to a methacholine challenge test. Forced expiratory volume in 1 second (FEV$_1$) expressed as a percentage of the control (diluent value) is graphed against the methacholine dose. The point at which the fall in FEV$_1$ exceeds 20% is used to calculate the provocative concentration (PC$_{20}$). (From Charles Irvin, Ph.D., Vermont Lung Center and Department of Medicine, University of Vermont, College of Medicine, Burlington, Vermont, with permission.)

a proper schedule, that timing of spirometry relative to the dose is controlled, and that spirometry quality and patient safety are properly addressed. Details of these issues and protocols are published in the ATS standards (28) and elsewhere (29).

Methacholine challenge studies are common in research protocols involving asthma because they allow bronchial hyperreactivity to be quantified and monitored. In most clinical settings, it is not necessary to document or quantify airway hyperreactivity with formal challenge tests. However, when the diagnosis of asthma is uncertain, bronchoprovocation studies may be clinically useful, as in a patient who has normal spirometry results but also has chest symptoms, such as cough or chest tightness, that suggest asthma. A positive methacholine challenge test result in this setting is highly suggestive of asthma. Clinical monitoring of airway hyperreactivity during asthma therapy as a guide to treatment is controversial. Sont and colleagues found improved clinical outcomes and reduced inflammation markers by using airway reactivity (as measured by methacholine challenge) to guide therapy (30). Currently, such monitoring would be indicated only in selected patients under special circumstances.

Though methacholine challenge testing is generally safe, large doses in asthmatic patients can provoke severe attacks. Other reactions to excessive doses include increased salivation, abdominal cramping, diarrhea, and sweating. Atropine is a specific antidote. Contraindications and precautions are well described in standard references (28).

Bronchoprovocation with specific sensitizing agents such as antigens or occupational sensitizers is associated with higher risks, and more caution is warranted. Testing with sensitizing agents should be limited to laboratories specializing in such studies.

Exercise Bronchoprovocation and Eucapnic Voluntary Hyperpnea

Exercise provokes bronchoconstriction in 60% to 90% of asthmatics, but some individuals who experience exercise-induced bronchoconstriction do not have classic asthma (31). The mechanism by which exercise induces bronchoconstriction is related to cooling and drying of the airways (32). The dominant theory is that the rapid breathing associated with exercise causes airway drying, resulting in hyperosmolarity in the surface liquids. The osmotic changes cause fluid to move from the cells, resulting in cell shrinkage (32, 33).

Exercise-induced asthma can be established in several ways: (a) a clear symptoms response to a specific therapy such as a β_2-agonist, and (b) using one of several bronchoprovocation techniques. Provocation techniques include laboratory exercise (28), event specific exercise for symptomatic athletes (34), methacholine, and eucapnic voluntary hyperpnea (34, 35). Eucapnic voluntary hyperpnea appears to be the most sensitive (34). In the eucapnic voluntary hyperpnea test, subjects breathe dry air containing 5% CO_2 at a rate 30 times measured FEV$_1$ for 6 minutes. A 10% fall in FEV$_1$ from baseline is a positive test (34, 35).

DIFFUSION

The most common test of gas transfer across the lungs is the CO diffusing capacity (D$_{LCO}$), also called *transfer factor* (T$_{LCO}$). The test measures the rate of CO transfer from the lungs to the blood. The result is reported in two ways: In North America, D$_{LCO}$ is expressed as milliliters of CO per minute per millimeters of mercury; in Europe, T$_{LCO}$ is expressed as millimoles of CO per minute per kilopascals. CO is the gas of interest because it behaves similarly to O_2, with the advantage that D$_{LCO}$ can be measured and D$_{LO_2}$ cannot. The pathway for the movement of CO or O_2 from alveolus to hemoglobin (Hb) molecule is illustrated in Figure 2.9.

Diffusing capacity can be measured with single-breath, steady-state, and rebreathing techniques. The single-breath technique is the most common, best standardized, and most readily available (17, 36). Most of the available clinical information relating D$_{LCO}$ to disease states is based on the studies using the single-breath technique.

The single-breath test is performed as follows: The patient exhales to RV, a valve is opened, the patient inhales to full VC the test gas, which contains N$_2$, 0.3% CO, an inert insoluble tracer gas (e.g., helium), and 18% to 21% O_2. The patient relaxes into a breath-hold at TLC for 10 seconds and then exhales rapidly. Anatomic and mechanical dead space is flushed out by exhaled air, and an alveolar sample is collected for analysis. The test is safe and easy to perform. Details of the technique and the computations involved are well described in current ATS and ERS standards documents (17, 36).

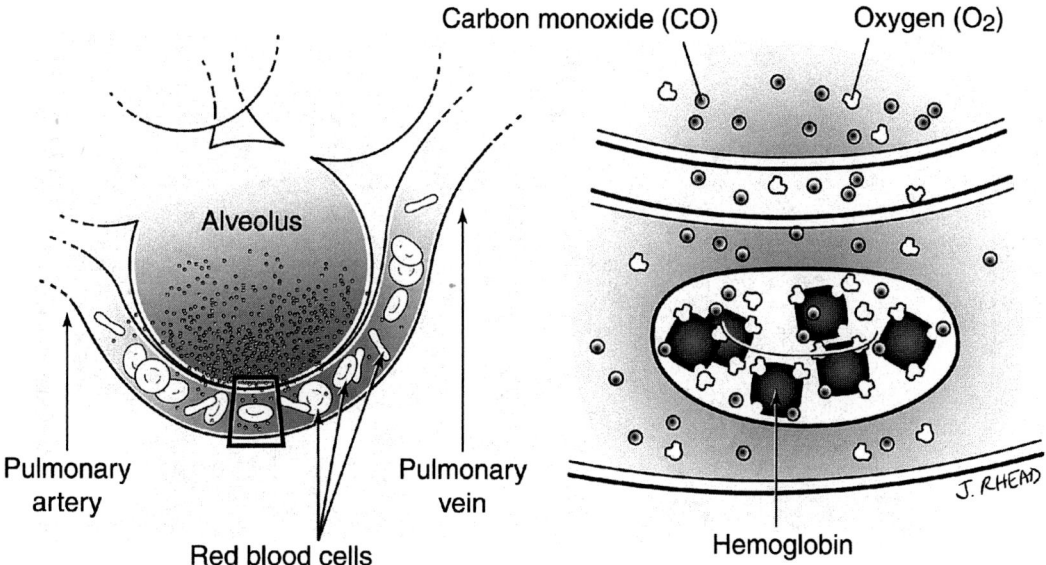

FIGURE 2.9. The diffusion pathway for oxygen (O_2). Pathway lengths in this figure do not reflect true pathway distances. The pathway is identical for carbon monoxide (CO), the gas used in the diffusing capacity test. O_2 and CO move across the alveolar-capillary membrane, traverse a very thin plasma layer, cross the red cell membrane, diffuse within the red cell interior, and chemically react, binding with hemoglobin. O_2 and CO compete for the same binding sites on the hemoglobin molecule (From Crapo RO, Jensen RL, Wanger JS. Single-breath carbon monoxide diffusing capacity. *Clin Chest Med* 2001;22:637–649, with permission.)

Variations in test procedure and computation techniques affect test results. The selection of reference values for D_{LCO} is confounded by large interlaboratory differences in D_{LCO}. In early studies, D_{LCO} measured in the same person in different laboratories could vary by as much as 90% (19, 37). More recent studies demonstrate reduced interlaboratory variability, but variability still seems excessive (38, 39). Thus, reference data must be carefully selected to ensure a laboratory's measured values correspond technically to the measurement techniques used to create the reference values. Without such technical correspondence, interpretative errors will be frequent.

Other issues center on physiologic variables that can influence D_{LCO} in the absence of a lung function abnormality. CO competes with O_2 for Hb binding sites, and the number of sites available influences D_{LCO} (36, 40, 41). Anemia decreases and polycythemia increases D_{LCO}. Interpreting D_{LCO} without knowing the Hb concentration is potentially misleading, especially in settings in which hemoglobin is likely to be altered. In patients being monitored for pulmonary injury while receiving chemotherapy, for example, a fall in D_{LCO} could reflect lung injury, the development of anemia, or both. If carboxyhemoglobin (Hbco) is elevated, as it is in smokers, the Hbco effectively reduces the available binding sites while at the same time creating a small CO backpressure in the plasma. These effects combine to artifactually lower D_{LCO} about 1% for each 1% increase in Hbco (41, 42). The best (although, not the easiest) method of avoiding problems with Hbco is to have patients refrain from smoking overnight before testing. An optimal procedure is to measure

Hb and Hbco along with D_{LCO} and adjust the predicted D_{LCO} accordingly. The small backpressure created by CO has other implications in testing. The CO in the test gas itself will raise Hbco about 0.5% for each trial (43).

Because CO and O_2 compete for the same Hb binding site, changes in O_2 pressure also artifactually alter D_{LCO} (42, 44, 45). For example, as an individual moves from sea level to higher altitudes, the decreased barometric pressure lowers partial pressure of inspired O_2 (P_{IO_2}) and gives the advantage to CO, causing D_{LCO} to increase about 0.35% for each decrease of 1 mmHg in the alveolar partial pressure of O_2 (P_{AO_2}) (44, 45). Using a correction factor in the computation or simulating the fraction of inspired O_2 at sea level (150 mm Hg) by adding O_2 to the test gas mixture will compensate for the effect of altitude (46).

RESPIRATORY MUSCLE STRENGTH

Tests of respiratory muscle strength may be useful when neurogenic and myopathic processes are known or suspected and when diaphragmatic weakness, fatigue, or paralysis is suspected. Severe diaphragmatic weakness can cause dyspnea and tachypnea, and even mild diaphragmatic weakness can contribute to dyspnea from other disease processes.

Routine pulmonary function tests may suggest moderate to severe respiratory muscle dysfunction. In patients with such disorders, VC measured in the supine position may be less (<20%) than it is when the patient is sitting upright. MVV is also commonly reduced in the presence of respiratory muscle dysfunction, but its use is limited because so many other factors affect the test.

Respiratory muscle strength is usually assessed by measurement of maximum inspiratory (PImax) and expiratory (PEmax) pressures at the mouth. These pressures can be easily measured with portable pressure meters in most clinical settings. PImax is usually measured from RV, and PEmax from TLC. The measurements are made against a closed valve; a small, 1-mm fixed air leak is introduced to reduce the effect of using the cheek muscles to generate pressure. Mouth pressures well within a normal range (PImax >80 cm H₂O), along with a decrease of less than 20% in VC measured in the supine position compared with upright VC, can be used to exclude clinically significant respiratory muscle weakness (47).

In patients for whom measurements of PImax and PEmax do not resolve the question being asked, transdiaphragmatic pressures and nerve stimulation tests provide more sophisticated assessment of respiratory muscle function. These tests are more technically demanding and are therefore usually available only in specialty laboratories.

TESTS OF ELASTIC PROPERTIES

These tests are used to characterize the elastic properties of the lung and chest wall. They require the measurement of transmural pressures across the lung (lung elastic recoil pressure, or PLe) and across the chest wall (chest wall elastic recoil pressure, or PTH). Measurement of these transmural pressures requires estimates of pleural pressure (PPL) and alveolar pressure. A small esophageal balloon is inserted into the lower third of the esophagus; esophageal pressure is used to approximate pleural pressure. Mouth pressure under static conditions (no air flow in a relaxed patient with an open glottis) is used to approximate alveolar pressure. Under static conditions, esophageal and mouth pressures are measured at several lung volumes between TLC and RV. Curves relating transmural pressures to lung volume (pressure–volume curves) are calculated separately for the lungs and chest wall and for the respiratory system (lung and chest wall combined). Compliance is calculated as change in lung volume divided by change in pressure ($\Delta V/\Delta P$).

Normal aging and diseases such as pulmonary emphysema, which involve disruption of the alveolar walls, are associated with decreased lung recoil pressures for a given lung volume and, consequently, increased lung compliance. Diseases like pulmonary fibrosis increase lung elastic recoil pressures and reduce lung compliance. Aging and chest wall disorders are associated with decreased chest wall compliance.

Although these tests are critical for clarifying the pathophysiology of lung function in various diseases, their clinical utility in routine patient care has never been proved. Interested readers should consult pulmonary physiology texts for further information.

ARTERIAL BLOOD GASES

The discussion thus far has addressed tests of the mechanical properties of the lung—the bellows action that moves air into and out of the lungs. The mechanical studies, including spirometry, lung volumes, and respiratory muscle testing, characterize the function of the lung but do not provide any estimate of how well the lung is performing its primary function, i.e., transferring O₂ to and CO₂ from the blood. Arterial blood gases provide direct evidence about the adequacy of gas transfer across the lungs.

It is important to understand both what information arterial blood gases provide and what they do not. Arterial blood gases define how well the lung is loading O₂ into and removing CO₂ from blood. However, these are only the first and last steps in the gas transport system (Table 2.1). They do not assess how well O₂ is being delivered to cells or the adequacy of cellular function.

Blood gas technology is advancing rapidly. Blood gas machines are now highly automated. They calibrate and monitor themselves for errors. They wash and rinse themselves and provide numerous alert messages when conditions are not properly controlled. They measure temperature and barometric pressure and compensate for electrode nonlinearity with empirically derived mathematical algorithms. Because they do so much and the technician needs to do so little, laboratory physicians and technicians may become less knowledgeable about the details of blood gas analysis. The increased accuracy of modern blood gas machines partially compensates for this lack of knowledge but exacerbates it at the same time. Noninvasive monitoring of blood gas parameters is also advancing rapidly. Pulse oximeters are widely used, and other techniques for continuously monitoring blood gas parameters are being developed.

Arterial blood gases assess three areas: (a) acid-base status, (b) ventilation status, and (c) oxygenation status. The lungs are an important part of maintaining the body's acid–base balance, excreting approximately 13,000 mEq of CO₂ per day. In contrast, the kidneys excrete 40 to 80 mEq of fixed acid per day (48, 49). The two measured elements relating to acid–base balance are pH and PaCO₂. These two measured values are used to calculate bicarbonate concentration by using the Henderson-Hasselbalch equation. Calculated bicarbonate provides a quick insight into the metabolic component of acid–base derangements.

The adequacy of ventilation is assessed with PaCO₂, according to Equation 2:

$$\text{PaCO}_2 \propto \frac{\dot{V}\text{CO}_2}{\dot{V}\text{A}} \propto \frac{\dot{V}\text{CO}_2}{\dot{V}\text{E} - \dot{V}\text{D}} \qquad \text{(Eq. 2)}$$

where $\dot{V}\text{CO}_2$ is CO₂ production, $\dot{V}\text{A}$ is alveolar ventilation, $\dot{V}\text{E}$ is minute ventilation, and $\dot{V}\text{D}$ is dead-space ventilation.

As Equation 2 illustrates, PaCO₂ is determined by the matching alveolar ventilation ($\dot{V}\text{A}$) to CO₂ production ($\dot{V}\text{CO}_2$). An elevated PaCO₂ indicates hypoventilation; that is, $\dot{V}A$ is inadequate relative to $\dot{V}CO_2$. Inadequate $\dot{V}A$ can occur because $\dot{V}E$ is reduced and/or $\dot{V}D$ is increased. If $PaCO_2$ is low, hyperventilation is present. A normal $PaCO_2$ indicates adequate matching of $\dot{V}A$ to $\dot{V}CO_2$, but it is not the sole determinate of the efficiency of ventilation. Efficiency of ventilation must be interpreted in light of the clinical setting, including breathing parameters and $\dot{V}CO_2$. Problems with $\dot{V}CO_2$ can usually be diagnosed simply by looking for what may be driving the metabolic processes. In the intensive care unit, these include fever and overfeeding with parenteral nutrition. Increases in $\dot{V}CO_2$ are rarely reflected directly into increases in $PaCO_2$ because the ventilatory reserve is so large.

Evaluation of oxygenation parameters includes assessment of the PaO_2 and arterial O_2 content. The PaO_2 provides a valuable—but incomplete—estimate of the adequacy of O_2 loading in the pulmonary capillary blood. It is useful to think of PaO_2 (a pressure) as an intensive rather than a quantitative variable. Although very useful, PaO_2 by itself gives no information about the volume of O_2 contained in the blood (O_2 content). Analyzing both PaO_2 and O_2 content enhances blood gas information.

CO oximeters are available for accurate measurement of Hb concentration, arterial O_2 saturation (SaO_2), carboxyhemoglobin concentration, and methemoglobin concentration. Their availability improves the accuracy of estimations of SaO_2 and simplifies the diagnosis of CO poisoning. Blood gas reports should now routinely include a calculation of arterial O_2 content (CaO_2) using CO-oximeter measurements (Equation 3).

$$CaO_2 = 1.39Hb \times SaO_2 + 0.0031\,PaO_2 \qquad \text{(Eq. 3)}$$

Calculation of the alveolar-to-arterial pressure gradient for O_2, or $PAO_2 - PaO_2$, when the patient is breathing room air can be useful in separating the physiologic causes of hypoxemia. The method of calculating $PAO_2 - PaO_2$ is shown in Equation 4 (48, 50):

$$PAO_2 - PaO_2 = F_1O_2(P_B - 47)$$
$$- PaCO_2\left[F_1O_2 + \frac{1 - F_1O_2}{R}\right] - PaO_2 \qquad \text{(Eq. 4)}$$

where $PAO_2 - PaO_2$ is the alveolar-to-arterial pressure gradient for O_2, F_1O_2 is the inspired O_2 concentration, ($P_B - 47$) is the barometric pressure minus water vapor pressure at $37°C$, and R is the respiratory quotient (usually assumed to be 0.8). For blood gases obtained at sea level with a patient breathing room air, Equation 3 can be reduced for rapid clinical use as follows:

$$P(A - a)O_2 = 150 - 1.2 \times PaCO_2 - PaO_2 \qquad \text{(Eq. 5)}$$

It is clinically useful to categorize the physiologic causes of hypoxemia. Physiologic causes of hypoxemia are summarized in Table 2.2, along with corresponding alveolar-to-arterial gradients when appropriate.

TABLE 2.2. PHYSIOLOGIC CAUSES OF HYPOXEMIA

Cause	$PAO_2 - PaO_2$
Low PAO_2	
Low inspired PO_2 (P_1O_2)	Normal
Low P_B (e.g., high altitude)	Normal
F_1O_2 is low	If inspired PO_2 is incorrectly assumed to be 21%, the alveolar-arterial gradient may be elevated
Hypoventilation (Elevated $PaCO_2$)	Normal
$\dot{V}/\dot{Q}$ mismatching	Elevated
Diffusion impairment	Elevated. Rarely a cause of hypoxemia
Right-to-left shunting	Elevated. Response to oxygen poor with large shunt
Low arterial oxygen content	
Anemia	
Low arterial oxygen saturation	
Presence of other hemoglobin species such as carboxyhemoglobin or methemoglobin	
Shift of oxyhemoglobin curve to right	

$PAO_2 - PaO_2$, alveolar-arterial gradient for oxygen; PaO_2, arterial partial pressure for oxygen; PO_2, partial pressure for oxygen; F_1O_2, fraction of inspired oxygen; $PaCO_2$, arterial partial pressure for carbon dioxide; V/Q, ventilation/perfusion, P_B, barometric pressure.

Noninvasive Measurement of Oxygenation Status

The most common noninvasive measurement of oxygenation status is made by pulse oximetry. Pulse oximeters do not directly measure SaO_2 but relate light absorption across the finger to arterial blood gas data from volunteers in whom arterial blood gases and pulse oximeter light absorption readings have been simultaneously obtained (51–53). One side of a pulse oximeter probe contains two light-emitting diodes, each emitting light at a different wavelength (one at about 660 nm and one at about 940 nm). The other side contains a photocell to measure light intensity after light has passed through a finger or ear lobe. A clever variation of Beer's law (the light absorbed by a solute in a solution is related to the concentration of the solute) is used to estimate SaO_2. Light is absorbed in a pulsatile fashion, increasing with each heartbeat. The assumption is that the increased absorption is owing to arterial blood.

With such a useful and simple tool, it is important to keep its limitations in mind. These include the margin of error, the fact that pulse oximetry does not differentiate between different Hb species, and the effect of substances in the body that may affect light absorption. As a general rule, in the absence of a source of interference, a single isolated measurement of O_2 saturation by pulse oximetry (SpO_2) will be within $\pm 3\%$ to 4% of the saturation directly measured in blood. A pulse oximeter reading of 90% could, therefore,

TABLE 2.3. PULSE OXIMETRY: SOURCES OF ERROR

Source of Error	Direction of Error
Probe slightly beyond fingertip	Low
Low-quality signal	High or low
Vasoconstriction	High or low
Motion artifact	High or low
Venous pulsations (e.g., tricuspid insufficiency)	Low
Ventilator pulse interference	May cause continuous searching for signal
Skin pigment	High in black patients, jaundice, no effect
Nail polish	Low, varies with polish and color
Anemia	Low, inversely related to hemoglobin for Spo$_2$ <80%
Carboxyhemoglobin	High roughly by the percentage of carboxyhemoglobin
Methemoglobin	Low by about half the percentage of methemoglobin
	Essentially no change after Spo$_2$ = 85%
Dye, leukomethylene blue	Low–transient
Dye, indocyanine green	Low–transient
Ambient light	High or low

Spo$_2$; oxygen saturation as measured by pulse oximetry. (Data from refs. 51–53.)

actually be between 87% and 93%. If the device is being used to monitor Spo$_2$ in a single individual, a 2% to 3% change is considered significant (54). Pulse oximetry uses only two wavelengths of light and cannot distinguish either Hbco or methemoglobin. Since pulse oximeters measure Hbco as if it were oxyhemoglobin, Spo$_2$ in a patient with CO poisoning will be falsely high by about the percentage of Hbco (51).

Other conditions that may result in misleading readings include presence of dyes (methylene blue), elevated bilirubin, states of low perfusion, anemia, and presence of strong external light sources, which may interfere with absorbance measurement. On occasion, the assumption that the pulsatile waveform marks arterial blood does not hold. For example, in a patient with tricuspid regurgitation and strong venous pulsations, the pulse oximeter cannot separate arterial from venous pulsations, and an erroneous reading may occur. Sources of interference are summarized in Table 2.3.

REFERENCES VALUES

Background

The first step in interpreting pulmonary function tests is selecting the best possible reference values. The selection is made at the testing site; traditionally that has meant reference values have been selected by laboratory medical directors, but as equipment moves into offices and clinics, individual clinicians will be called on to make the choice. Guide-lines for selecting reference values are widely available. For pulmonary function tests, the ATS and ERS provide access to appropriate reference values (19, 55).

Medical decisions are made after comparing clinical observations with one or more sets of reference data. This is not as simple as defining a normal range. Clinical test results within a normal range may be taken as absence or low risk of disease, an implication that may not be correct. For example, a cholesterol value may fall well within an average range from a general population sample but still indicate increased risk for coronary disease when compared with reference data based on risk assessment. In pulmonary function testing, the assumption may also be incorrect. For example, an individual who starts out with an FEV$_1$ at 110% of the predicted value could suffer a reduction of 25% or more in FEV$_1$ and still have a value within the normal range. The loss—and thus the underlying disease process—would not be detected by routine lung function testing.

Lung function test interpretation is commonly based on comparisons of observed values with reference values based on healthy subjects, comparisons with recognized disease patterns and/or values previously measured in the same patient. Using historical lung function data from the same patient eliminates the between-individual variability that exists in the representative group comparison, so changes as small as 5% can be detected. However, it is not practical to perform baseline studies on every person against the unlikely chance that a pulmonary disease will develop. It is practical to track individual lung function in at-risk populations, such as those in occupations with a known risk for lung injury and patients receiving therapy with a known potential for lung damage.

Selecting and using reference values has been the subject of many expert panels and is well described by Solberg (56) and Grasbeck (57). The general rules, modified slightly for pulmonary applications, are as follows: (a) the reference population must be clearly defined and described; and (b) the patient being examined must resemble the reference study subjects in the biologic factors known to contribute to variability. For lung function, these factors are sex, age, height, weight, ethnic group, past and present health, socioeconomic status, and environmental exposures, including cigarette smoke, air pollution, and occupational exposures (Fig. 2.10). (c) Clinical and reference value measurements should be made with adequately standardized methods and appropriate quality control. Technical variability is reduced when a clinical laboratory makes measurements with the same standardized methods as those used in a reference value study. This last criterion is the basis for the development of equipment and procedural standards published by many different respiratory societies.

Reference data vary depending on the population being sampled, the method of sampling the population, and the methods of analyzing the data. The data may be gathered

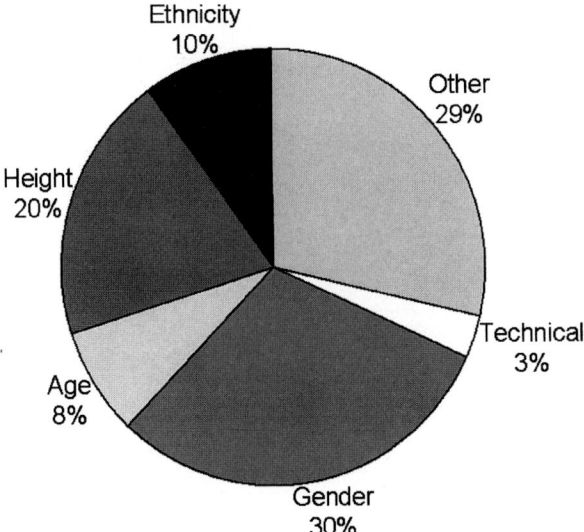

FIGURE 2.10. Schematic illustration of the sources of variability in lung function tests. These sources of variability must be dealt with as part of the performance and interpretation of lung function tests, or else the noise encountered in the testing will overwhelm the signal of interest, which in a clinical setting is usually change in lung function with disease. Note that the 3% technical variability assumes high-quality tests. Substandard tests can cause technical variability to exceed all other sources of variability. (From data in Becklake MR, White N. Sources of variation in spirometric measurements. *Occup Med* 1993;8:241–264.)

from a subset of a population sample in a larger epidemiologic study, or it may come from a study specifically designed as a reference value study. Although the optimal method of sampling a population is random sampling, volunteer samples are less expensive and easier to perform and thus are more frequently used. Sample size is important. In general, lung function reference studies are better if they include at least 10 subjects of each sex for each decade; larger numbers are better. The method of analysis also influences reference ranges. In some pulmonary function reference studies, only linear relationships are considered; in others, complex models are used. The reference data from Hankinson and colleagues are the best available in the United States at this time (2). The data are drawn from a random sample of the U.S. population, including children and adults, and an overrepresentation of two major ethnic minorities (African Americans and Mexican Americans). Equations for both mean values and lower limits of normal are included.

Lower Limits for Reference Ranges (Lower Limits of Normal)

Once reference values have been selected, a reference range defines the limits for comparisons. In pulmonary function testing, three sets of limits are commonly used. The most common is also the least desirable. It defines the normal

range for FEV_1/VC as greater than 70% or greater than 75%, and the normal range for everything else as the predicted value $\pm 20\%$. This method is popular because of its simplicity, but it is statistically incorrect and should be abandoned. The FEV_1/VC ratio falls with aging, so a fixed ratio to define normal is inappropriate. Using $\pm 20\%$ to define a reference range causes false-negative results in younger and taller patients and false-positive tests in shorter and older patients. It causes large numbers of false-positive errors in the interpretation of midflows and instantaneous flow variables, for which statistically appropriate lower limits of normal approach 50% of the predicted value (58).

Two statistically acceptable approaches to lower limits of normal are available. One, based on an assumption that the data distribution is gaussian, uses 95% confidence intervals, usually calculated as 1.645 times the standard error of the estimate in a linear regression equation. The other is based on a calculated lower (or upper) fifth percentile. The percentile calculation is usually based on data expressed as a percentage of the predicted value. Calculation of percentiles avoids the gaussian distribution assumption. Both are probably acceptable for basic pulmonary function tests that involve FVC and FEV_1. The instantaneous and midflow variables are more likely to have skewed distributions; reference ranges defined with percentiles are preferable for these variables (58).

Lower limits of normal are variable and should not be treated as absolute demarcations. Measured values that lie well within or outside the normal range can be interpreted with confidence. Those close to lower or upper limits should be interpreted with caution. In these borderline cases, clinical information is the best guide to categorizing a test result (19).

GENERAL INTERPRETATIVE GUIDELINES

Restricting the Number of Tests Used in an Interpretation

More than 30 parameters can be obtained from spirometry, lung volumes, and diffusing capacity. By chance alone, more than 25% of healthy subjects would have an abnormal result in one or more tests if all 30 were used (59). The chances for a false-positive test decrease when one is selective about the number of results analyzed. For spirometry, the interpretation should focus on three variables: VC, FEV_1, and FEV_1/VC (19). For static lung volumes, the interpretation should focus on TLC; for diffusing capacity, on D$_{LCO}$. The other results reported may help guide decisions in borderline cases, but clinical data are even more helpful.

Dynamic Spirometry

A simple algorithm for interpreting spirometry by using three variables is outlined in Figure 2.11 (19). Obstructive lung

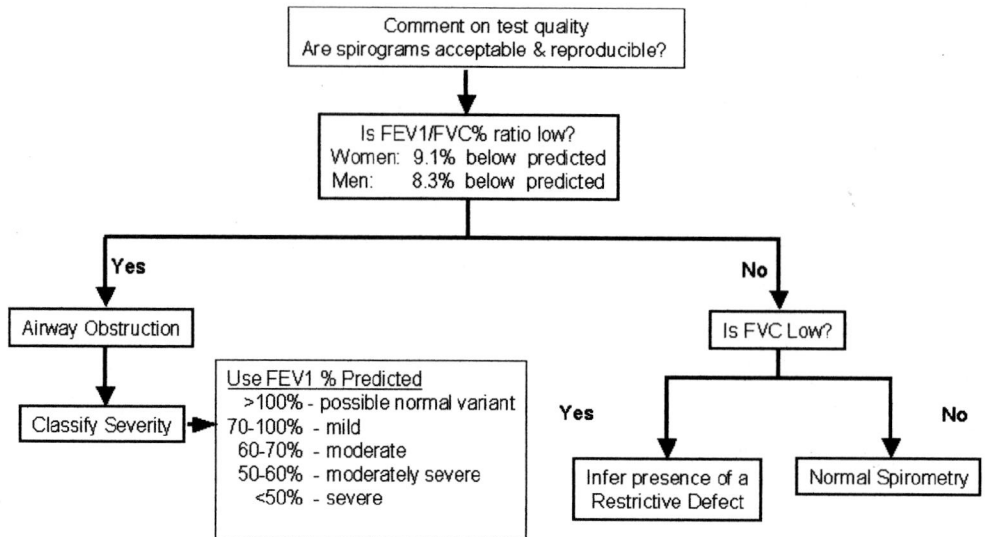

FIGURE 2.11. Simple algorithm for interpretation of spirometry. For simplicity, the severity of restriction based on vital capacity (VC) is not diagrammed. Severity of restriction here would use percentage of predicted VC and use a scale similar to that for obstruction. FEV_1, forced expiratory volume in 1 second; FVC, forced vital capacity. (From information in Becklake MR, Crapo RO. Lung function testing: selection of reference values and interpretative strategies. *Am Rev Respir Dis* 1991;144:1202–1218, with permission.)

diseases are characterized by decreased expiratory flows compared with flows in healthy persons. Early airway obstruction, which begins in the small airways, tends to reduce flows at lower lung volumes. Numerous tests for small-airway disease have been studied. Some, including closing volume, $V_{max50\%}$, and $FEF_{25\%-75\%}$, tend to correlate well with small-airway disease in groups, but there is no convincing evidence they can be effectively used in a clinical setting to diagnose the presence of small-airway disease in a given individual (19). The pattern of reduced airflow at lower lung volumes is also seen as part of normal aging, reflecting the loss of elastic recoil of the lungs with age.

As airway obstruction worsens, airflow is reduced at higher lung volumes. The flow–volume display shows progressively more concavity toward the horizontal axis; the volume–time curve shows a slowly rising volume even after 6 to 10 seconds of exhalation. The primary marker for the presence of airway obstruction is the FEV_1/VC ratio. When airway obstruction has been diagnosed on the basis of FEV_1/VC, severity is classified by using the $FEV_1\%$ (FEV_1 as a percentage of the predicted value) (19) (Fig. 2.11). The characteristic patterns of severe airway obstruction are illustrated in Figure 2.7. All expiratory flows are reduced. With good effort, a well-defined but reduced peak flow is seen, followed by a rapid fall in flow to a very low level.

Central airway obstruction has a characteristic pattern, depending on the location of the obstruction (60) (Fig. 2.12). The sensitivity of this test is low because the classic pattern is not seen until the obstruction is rather advanced. Vigorous patient effort is especially important when central airway obstruction is suspected because submaximal inspiratory and expiratory efforts can produce the same pattern as that of central airway obstruction.

Restrictive patterns in spirometry are commonly characterized by a reduced VC in the absence of airway obstruction (FEV_1/VC is normal). Recent work by Aaron and colleagues suggests reduced VC without airway obstruction predicts low TLC only about half the time (13). Small VCs commonly occur in the presence of obstruction because expiratory time is relatively short. If airway obstruction is present and VC is low, no certain determination of restriction can be made on the basis of spirometry alone. If it is clinically indicated, a measurement of TLC will confirm the presence of a combined obstructive and restrictive pattern. Restriction can also be determined by reviewing the chest radiograph, which will usually have been obtained for other clinical reasons.

Static Lung Volumes

The number of static lung volume variables used for interpretation should be limited to avoid excessive false-positive results. The variables used depend on the question being asked. For example, TLC is the primary variable when restriction is being considered. Statistically based lower limits of normal should be used. Occasionally TLC and VC findings will conflict. If there are no obvious technical problems, TLC should determine the estimation of restriction. The classic pattern of overinflation includes elevations in TLC, FRC, and RV. Increases in FRC and RV may precede increases in TLC, but one should be cautious in using them to diagnose overinflation, because they also increase the risk for a false positive result. The chest radiograph may also show overinflation.

Fixed Upper Airway Obstruction

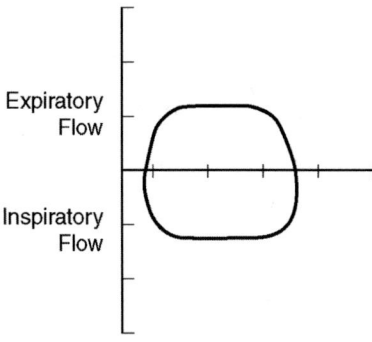

Variable Extrathoracic Obstruction

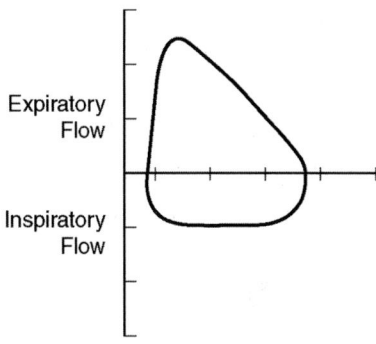

Variable Intrathoracic Obstruction

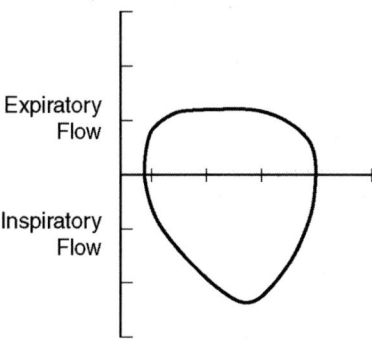

FIGURE 2.12. Central airway obstruction patterns. Three basic forced expiratory flow–volume patterns seen in the presence of at least moderate upper airway obstruction are schematically illustrated. The basic pattern of airflow obstruction in central airways is constant flow over a significant portion of the inhaled and/or exhaled volumes. In fixed central airway obstruction, the pattern does not vary with inspiration or expiration. Variable extrathoracic obstruction is associated with a relatively normal pattern during expiration, as extrathoracic airways widen during exhalation and narrow during inspiration. Conversely, variable intrathoracic obstruction tends to have a more normal pattern during inspiration, as intrathoracic airways tend to widen during inspiration and narrow during expiration. The patterns may also be seen with submaximal effort. The patterns are present to some degree in patients with milder degrees of obstruction but may be more subtle.

Diffusing Capacity

The primary variable used for interpretation is DLCO. A laboratory can usually categorize DLCO only as within or outside the reference range. The one pattern of findings that immediately suggests a clinical diagnosis is the combination of airway obstruction, evidence of overinflation, and a low DLCO (suggesting emphysema) (61). Further interpretation of alterations in DLCO requires knowledge of the clinical question being asked. For example, it is not uncommon to find a reduced DLCO as the only abnormality in a battery of pulmonary function tests. In the absence of other clinical or functional information, an isolated reduction in DLCO does not have clinical significance and need not be pursued further.

Using DL/VA in interpretative schemes is somewhat controversial. It is sometimes simplistically used to normalize DLCO for lung volume, ignoring the fact that DL/VA does not remain constant with lung volume (62). Several interpretative schemes using DL/VA have been proposed (62, 63). Other investigators argue the original DL/VA is useful in interpreting DLCO (64).

Changes in Lung Function Measurements with Time

It is difficult to precisely define a significant change with time. A consistent trend in lung function revealed with multiple measurements will signify significant change more accurately than will two or three measurements. For VC and FEV_1 performed within a few weeks, a 12% change in healthy subjects and 20% change in subjects with obstruction is likely to be significant (19). When there are years between testing, a 15% change (adjusting for age) is probably significant for VC and FEV_1. For DLCO and TLC, within-test and between-test variability are increased, and criteria defining change with time are largely absent. When no trending information is available, I tend to consider changes of more than 10% significant, but I do so with some discomfort, knowing there are no good criteria.

SUMMARY

Pulmonary function tests are useful in detecting and monitoring lung impairments. They are most useful when the practitioner keeps both the question being asked and the limitations of the tests in mind.

REFERENCES

1. Crapo RO. Review article: pulmonary function testing. *N Engl J Med* 1994;331:25–30.
2. Hankinson JL, Odencrantz JR, Fedan KB. Spirometric reference values from a sample of the general U.S. population. *Am J Resp Crit Care Med* 1999;159:179–187.

3. Eaton T, Withy S, Garrett JE, et al. Spirometry in primary care practice: the importance of quality assurance and the impact of spirometry workshops. *Chest* 1999;116:416–423.

4. Malmstrom K, Peszak I, Botton A, et al. Quality assurance of asthma clinical trials. *Control Clin Trials* 2002;23:143–156.

5. Biring MS, Lewis MI, Liu JT, et al. Pulmonary physiologic changes of morbid obesity. *Am J Med Sci* 1999;318:293–297.

6. Hughes JMB, Pride NB, eds. *Lung function tests: physiological principles and clinical applications.* London: WB Saunders, 1999.

7. Cotes JE. *Lung function: assessment and application in medicine,* 5th ed Oxford: Blackwell Science, 1993.

8. Wanger J. *Pulmonary function testing: a practical approach,* 2nd ed Baltimore: Williams and Wilkins, 1996.

9. Ferris BG. Epidemiology standardization project. *Am Rev Respir Dis* 1978;118:1–120.

10. Begin P, Peslin R. Influence of panting frequency on thoracic gas measurements in chronic obstructive pulmonary disease. *Am Rev Respir Dis* 1984;130:121–123.

11. Clausen JL, ed. *Pulmonary function testing: guidelines and controversies. equipment, methods, and normal values.* New York: Academic Press, 1982.

12. Muller N, Bryan AC, Zamel N. Tonic inspiratory muscle activity as a cause of hyperinflation in asthma. *J Appl Phys* 1981;50:279–282.

13. Aaron SD, Dales RE, Cardinal P. How accurate is spirometry at predicting restrictive pulmonary impairment? *Chest* 1999;115:869–873.

14. Swanney MP, Jensen RL, Crichton DA, et al. FEV$_6$ is an acceptable surrogate for FVC in the spirometric diagnosis of airway obstruction and restrictions. *Am J Resp Crit Care Med* 2000;162:917–919.

15. Stoller JK, Basheda S, Laskowski D, et al. Trial of standard versus modified expiration to achieve end-of-test spirometry criteria. *Am Rev Respir Dis* 1993;148:275–280.

16. Standardization of spirometry: 1994 update. *Am J Resp Crit Care Med* 1995;152:1107–1136.

17. Standardized lung function testing: official statement of the European Respiratory Society. *Eur Respir J* 1993;16:1–100.

18. Nelson SB, Gardner RM, Crapo RO, et al. Performance evaluation of contemporary spirometers. *Chest* 1990;97:288–297.

19. Becklake MR, Crapo RO. Lung function testing: selection of reference values and interpretative strategies. *Am J Resp Crit Care Med* 1991;144:1202–1218.

20. Shim C. Response to bronchodilators. *Clin Chest Med* 1989;10:155–164.

21. Hadcroft J, Calverley PM. Alternative methods for assessing bronchodilator reversibility in chronic obstructive pulmonary disease. *Thorax* 2001;56:713–720.

22. Ajelabi A, McGee RV, Petrini MF. Standards for performing the maximum voluntary ventilation (MVV). *Am J Resp Crit Care Med* 2002;165: A497.

23. Launo C, Palermo S, Reillo R, et al. Respiratory function tests and operative risk in thoracic surgery. *Minerva Anestesiol* 1992;58:458–501.

24. Morris AH, Kanner RE, Crapo RO, et al. *Clinical pulmonary function testing: a manual of uniform laboratory procedures,* 2nd ed Salt Lake City, UT: Intermountain Thoracic Society, 1984.

25. National Institutes of Health. Expert panel report 2: guidelines for the diagnosis and management of asthma. Bethesda, MD: National Institutes of Health, National Heart, Lung, and Blood Institute; 1997;97-4051.

26. Adams RJ, Boath K, Homan S, et al. A randomized trial of peak-flow and symptom-based action plans in adults with moderate-to-severe asthma. *Respirology* 2001;6:297–304.

27. Jones KP, Mullee MA, Middleton M, et al. Peak flow–based asthma self-management: a randomised controlled study in general practice. *Thorax* 1995;50:851–857.

28. Crapo RO, Casaburi R, Coates AL, et al. Guidelines for methacholine and exercise challenge testing, 1999. *Am J Resp Crit Care Med* 2000;161:309–329.

29. Rosenthal RR. Approved methodology for methacholine challenge. *Allergy Proc* 1989;10:301–312.

30. Sont SK, Willems LN, Bell EH, et al. Clinical control and histopathologic outcome of asthma when using airway hyperresponsiveness as an additional guide to long-term treatment: the AMPUL Study Group. *Am J Resp Crit Care Med* 1999;159:1045–1051.

31. Anderson SD, Holzer K. Exercise-induced asthma: is it the right diagnosis in athletes? *J Allergy Clin Immunol* 2000;106:419–428.

32. Anderson SD, Daviskas E. The mechanisms of exercise-induced asthma is.... *J Allergy Clin Immunol* 2000;106:453–459.

33. Mihalyka M, Wong J, James AL, et al. The effect on airway function of inspired air conditions after isocapnic hyperventilation with dry air. *J Allergy Clin Immunol* 1988;82:842–848.

34. Eliasson AH, Phillips YY, Rajogopal KR. Sensitivity and specificity of bronchial provocation of testing: an evaluation of four techniques in exercise-induced bronchospasm. *Chest* 1992;102:347–355.

35. Anderson SD, Argyros GJ, Magnussen H, et al. Provocation by eucapnic voluntary hyperpnea to identify exercise induced bronchoconstriction. *Br J Sports Med* 2001;35:344–347.

36. Single-breath carbon monoxide diffusing capacity (transfer factor): recommendations for a standard technique, 1995 update. *Am J Resp Crit Care Med* 1995;152:2185–2198.

37. Johns DP, Rochford PD. Questionnaire based study of interlaboratory variability of the single breath TLCO test: instrumentation, technique, calculation, quality control, and predicted values. *Volume* 1985;5:4–13.

38. Wanger J, Irvin C. Comparability of pulmonary function results from 13 laboratories in a metropolitan area. *Resp Care* 1991;36:1375–1382.

39. Clausen J, Crapo R, Gardner R. Interlaboratory comparisons of pulmonary function testing. *Am Rev Respir Dis* 1984;129: A37.

40. Marrades RM, Diaz O, Roca J, et al. Adjustment of D$_{LCO}$ for hemoglobin concentration. *Am J Resp Crit Care Med* 1997;155:236–241.

41. Mohsenifar Z, Brown HV, Schnitzer B, et al. The effect of abnormal levels of hematocrit on the single breath diffusing capacity. *Lung* 1982;160:325–330.

42. Frey TM, Crapo RO, Jensen RL, et al. Adjustment of D$_{LCO}$ for varying COHb and alveolar Po$_2$ using a theoretical adjustment equation. *Respir Physiol* 1990;81:303–311.

43. Frey TM, Crapo RO, Jensen RL, et al. Diurnal variation of the diffusing capacity of the lung: is it real? *Am Rev Respir Dis* 1987;136:1381–1384.

44. Kanner RE, Crapo RO. The relationship between alveolar oxygen tension and the single-breath carbon monoxide diffusing capacity. *Am Rev Respir Dis* 1986;133:676–678.

45. Crapo RO, Kanner RE, Jensen RL, et al. Variability of the single-breath carbon monoxide transfer factor as a function of inspired oxygen pressure. *Eur Respir J* 1988;1:573–574.

46. Gray G, Zamel N, Crapo RO. Magnitude of the effect of a simulated 3,048-meter altitude on the single breath transfer factor (diffusing capacity). *Clin Respir Physiol* 1986;22:429–431.

47. Polkey MI, Green M, Moxham J. Measurement of respiratory muscle strength. *Thorax* 1995;50:1131–1135.

48. Shapiro BA, Harrison RA, Cane RD, et al. *Clinical application of blood gases,* 4th ed Chicago: Mosby–Year Book, 1989.

49. Malley WJ. *Clinical blood gases.* Philadelphia: WB Saunders, 1990.

50. Forster RE, DuBois AB, Brisco WA, et al. *The lung: physiologic basis of pulmonary function tests,* 3rd ed Chicago: Mosby–Year Book, 1986.

51. Severinghaus JW, Kelleher JF. Recent developments in pulse oximetry. *Anesthesiology* 1992;76:1018–1038.

52. Schnapp LM, Cohen NH. Pulse oximetry: uses and abuses. *Chest* 1990:98:1244–1250.

53. Sinex JE. Review: pulse oximetry: principles and limitations. *Am J Emerg Med* 1999;17:59–67.

54. Reis AL, Farrow JT, Clausen JL. Pulmonary function tests cannot predict exercise-induced hypoxemia in chronic obstructive pulmonary disease. *Chest* 1988;93:454–459.

55. Standardized lung function testing: report of the Working Party. *Bull Eur Physiopathol Respir* 1983;9[Suppl 5]:1–95.

56. Solberg HE, Grasbeck R. Reference values. *Adv Clin Chem,* 989;27:1–79.

57. Grasbeck R. Reverence values, why and how. *Scand J Clin Lab Invest* 1990;201:45–53.

58. Knudson RJ, Lebowitz MD, Holberg CJ, et al. Changes in the normal maximal expiratory flow–volume curve with growth and aging. *Am Rev Respir Dis* 1983;127:725–734.

59. Vedal S, Crapo RO. False-positive rates of multiple pulmonary function tests in healthy subjects. *Bull Eur Physiopathol Respir* 1983;19:263–266.

60. Aboussouan LS, Stoller JK. Diagnosis and management of upper airway obstruction. *Clin Chest Med* 1994;15:35–53.

61. West WW, Nagai A, Hodgkin JE, et al. The National Institutes of Health Intermittent Positive Pressure Breathing Trial—pathology studies, III: the diagnosis of emphysema. *Am Rev Respir Dis* 1987;135:123–129.

62. Chinn DJ, Cotes JE, Flowers R, et al. Transfer factor (diffusing capacity) standardized for alveolar volume: validation, reference values and applications of a new linear model to replace Kco (TL/Va). *Eur Respir J* 1996;9:1269–1277.

63. Johnson DC. Importance of adjusting carbon monoxide diffusing capacity (DLco) and carbon monoxide transfer coefficient (Kco) for alveolar volume. *Respir Med* 2000;94:28–37.

64. Hughes JM, Pride NB. In defense of the carbon monoxide transfer coefficient Kco (TL/Va). *Eur Respir J* 2001;17:168–174.

3

Clinical Exercise Testing

Bruce D. Johnson · Idelle M. Weisman

Exercise testing is playing an increasingly important role in the physiologic assessment and optimal management of patients in different clinical settings, especially those with known or suspected cardiopulmonary disorders. This reflects several factors that include the current emphasis on objective functional physiologic assessment in clinical decision analysis; heightened awareness that resting pulmonary and cardiac function testing cannot reliably predict exercise performance and functional capacity; knowledge that health status assessment (high-related quality of life) better relates to exercise tolerance rather than to resting indices; and exertional symptoms, especially dyspnea and unexplained exercise intolerance, correlate poorly with resting indices and are best evaluated during a structured exercise test. Finally, the increased use of exercise testing in clinical trials highlights the importance of assessing functional capacity in determining the benefits of treatment. Given the prognostic importance of exercise capacity and peak oxygen consumption ($\dot{V}o_2$) in various populations, improvement of exercise tolerance through new medications, surgical interventions, new devices, and evolving rehabilitation programs may also imply improved clinical outcomes.

Various degrees of sophistication can be applied to clinical exercise testing, ranging from those that have low technical requirements and are simple to perform but provide limited physiologic information to those that are more comprehensive in assessing all the components of the exercise response

B. D. Johnson: Department of Internal Medicine, Division of Cardiovascular Diseases, Mayo Clinic and Foundation, Rochester, Minnesota.

I. M. Weisman: Departments of Clinical Investigation and Pulmonary Medicine, William Beaumont Army Medical Center, El Paso, Texas, and Department of Internal Medicine, Pulmonary Critical Care Service, University of Texas Health Science Center at San Antonio, San Antonio, Texas.

The opinions or assertions contained herein are the private views of the authors and are not to be construed as official or as reflecting the views of the Department of the Army or the Department of Defense.

but are more technically demanding and costly (Table 3.1). Clinical exercise tests that are used include stair climbing, 6-minute walk test (6MWT), shuttle walk test, exercise-induced bronchoconstriction (EIB) test, cardiac stress test, and, finally, the most comprehensive cardiopulmonary exercise test (CPET) (Table 3.1). Decision analysis for use of these tests reflects the clinical questions being asked and the available resources. The salient features and recommended use of these clinical exercise tests will be discussed briefly. The main focus of this chapter will be CPET indications, implementation of a clinical exercise test, physiological principles, measurements, and current concepts in exercise limitation and interpretation.

CLINICAL EXERCISE TESTING

Stair Climbing

Functional assessment using stair climbing is simple, technically nondemanding, and cost-effective. Historically, surgeons have used stair climbing for preoperative evaluation and postoperative risk assessment before the availability of more advanced technology and more structured exercise tests. Symptom-limited stair climbing may represent near maximal/maximal exercise intensity, depending on the instructions given to the patient. The energy cost of stair climbing has been evaluated in several studies (1). $\dot{V}o_2$ peak measured during stair climbing correlated well ($r = 0.7$) with number of stairs climbed and was higher, as was the heart rate (HR) response, than that measured during CPET in patients with chronic obstructive pulmonary disease (COPD) (2). Several studies have suggested that stair climbing is useful in identifying patients at increased risk for postoperative complications after upper abdominal surgery (3) and after lung resection surgery (3–6). Inability to climb two flights of stairs may be associated with increased risk of postoperative

TABLE 3.1. CLINICAL EXERCISE TESTS

Test	Technology Required	Intensity	Clinical Question Evaluated	Standardization	Reproducibility
Stair climbing	0	Near max/ maximal	Postoperative risk. Functional capacity.	0	0
6MWT	+	Sub max/ Near max	Functional capacity. Therapeutic effects.	++	++
SWT	++	Maximal	Functional capacity. Therapeutic effects.	+++	++
EIB	+++	Sub maximal	Airway hyperreactivity.	++	++
GXT	+++	Sub maximal	Ischemia. Arrythmias.	+++	+++
CPET	++++	Maximal	$\dot{V}o_2$max-gold standard-functional capacity. Global/individual system function and contribution to exercise limitation. Therapeutic effects. Postoperative risk. Exercise prescription.	++	+++
Constant work	+++/++++	Sub maximal	Therapeutic effects.	+++	+++

6MWT, 6-min walk test; SWT, Shuttle walk test; EIB, exercise-induced bronchospasm; GXT, graded exercise cardiac stress test; CPET, cardiopulmonary exercise test.
Adapted from Zeballos RJ, Weisman IM. Modalities of clinical exercise testing. In: Weisman IM, Zeballos RJ, eds. *Clinical exercise testing: Progress in respiratory research.* Basel: Karger, 2002:30–42, with permission.

complications (3). Comparing data from different stair climbing studies, however, is complicated by the lack of standardization and consensus on many important issues related to methodology, conduct of the test, outcome measures, and practical safety monitoring. Additional studies addressing these issues would be useful.

Six-Minute Walk Test

The 6MWT is a self-paced, simple, and practical test of submaximal functional capacity that measures the maximal distance walked by a subject in 6 minutes while traversing a 30-m indoor corridor (7, 8). Standardized encouragement improves results and reproducibility (9). As with other walk tests (10), the 6MWT provides a global assessment of functional capacity but is unable to provide specific information on each of the different organ systems involved in exercise, including mechanisms of exercise limitation. Consequently, it has limited diagnostic capability especially for (occult) ischemia and combined heart-lung disease. However, 6MWT may be adequate if the clinical question is as follows: does a patient desaturate with exercise, and is the absolute value/magnitude of desaturation not critical and the etiology of exercise limitation not important. Subsequent improvement with titration of supplemental oxygen (O_2) can then be objectively determined by monitoring O_2 saturation as measured by pulse oximetry (SpO_2), HR, dyspnea Borg scale, and the 6-minute walk distance responses. A good correlation of 6-minute walk distance and maximum O_2 consumption ($\dot{V}o_2$max; $r = 0.75$) has been reported in patients with end-stage lung disease (11).

The 6MWT has been used for the following: (a) preoperative and postoperative evaluation of lung transplantation and lung volume reduction surgery (12–14), (b) monitoring response to therapeutic interventions and pulmonary rehabilitation (15–17), and (c) predicting mortality and morbidity in cardiac patients and in patients with pulmonary vascular disease (11, 18–20). Reference equations for 6MWT in normal subjects and an American Thoracic Society statement on 6MWT, which addresses standardization and clinical application issues, have recently been published (7, 21).

The 6MWT and CPET provide complementary albeit different information (7, 22). As such, it is unlikely that a 6MWT would replace CPET in those circumstances in which important information not available from 6MWT results is required for clinical decision making. This is underscored in recent clinical commentary in heart failure patients, which noted that although the 6MWT correlates generally with outcome (20) and is easier to perform, it is "not precise enough" for indications, including measuring important risk stratification determinants ($\dot{V}o_2$max), adjusting exercise prescriptions, and gauging ability to perform physical work (important for impairment/disability evaluation) (23). Finally, an endurance constant work exercise protocol was more sensitive than was conventional 6MWT in detecting the effects of therapeutic interventions (inhaled anticholinergic agents) on exercise performance in patients with COPD (15).

Six-Minute Walk Test on the Treadmill

The 6MWT can be performed on a treadmill and has been proposed when facilities for a standard 6MWT are unavailable. During this test, the patient walks on the treadmill for 6 minutes, continuously self-adjusting the speed of the treadmill in order to set the pace. The advantages of a treadmill 6MWT include the availability of continuous cardiovascular and oximetry monitoring, the ease of supplemental O_2 device carriage, and the avoidance/inconvenience of performing the test outside the laboratory. However, a treadmill 6MWT may undermine the low technical and self-paced basic principles of the standard 6MWT. Furthermore, a treadmill 6MWT may be difficult for the elderly. Importantly, 6MWT and treadmill 6MWT results are not interchangeable, as reported in a recent study in lung disease patients (24). This study compared treadmill 6MWT versus conventional 6MWT, and demonstrated that the distance walked on the treadmill was, not surprisingly, 14% less than hallway walking, reflecting less familiarity with treadmill walking.

Shuttle Walk Test

The shuttle walk test (SWT) measures the maximal distance walked by a subject on a 10-m course while being externally paced by audio signals from a cassette tape (25). This is a progressive test in which minute-by-minute walking speed is increased until the patient achieves exhaustion. In essence, the SWT is a maximal symptom-limited test comparable in intensity to (near) maximal tests performed on the treadmill. As such, the SWT not surprisingly, correlates better with $\dot{V}o_2$max than with the 6MWT (26, 27), although a good correlation with 6MWT has been reported (25). The SWT most probably does not reflect daily activities, as does the 6MWT, which is a submaximal test. Whether SWT has a potential greater risk of medical complications because of the lack of electrocardiogram (ECG) monitoring compared with CPET is unknown. Currently, the SWT is less popular than is the 6MWT, with its main use reported in the United Kingdom. There are only a limited number of studies available in the literature. Additional studies that address safety issues, reference values, and guidelines for the determination of clinical significance are necessary.

Exercise-Induced Bronchoconstriction Test

EIB testing is used to determine the presence of airway hyperreactivity when inhalational challenge testing is not available or the results are indeterminate, especially in individuals with exercise-induced symptoms (28). EIB classically occurs after exercise, peaking at 5 to 10 minutes and usually resolving in another 20 to 30 minutes, often spontaneously (29, 30). EIB, however, can occur during exercise (31). Current knowledge suggests that EIB is owing to airway drying and cooling, resulting from exercise-induced hyperventilation (32). Therefore, controlling factors that affect airway drying and cooling can optimize conditions for eliciting a positive test. Withholding bronchodilators and other inhaled agents and assessing other medications and foods (caffeine containing) before testing may also be of importance (28).

Spirometry (forced vital capacity [FVC] and forced expiratory volume in 1 second [FEV$_1$]) is measured before (baseline) and at 5, 10, 15, and 30 minutes after exercise. A positive test is reflected as a reduction of FEV$_1$ or FVC of 10% to 15% from baseline (33). Short intense bouts of exercise without a warm-up and with ambient relative humidity of approximately 50% and temperature of 25°C are optimal. A widely used protocol involves constant work exercise on the treadmill or on the cycle ergometer for 6 to 8 minutes at an intensity necessary to elicit a HR of approximately 80% of the maximum predicted, so that expired volume ($\dot{V}$E) will increase sufficiently to trigger bronchoconstriction in those with hyperreactive airways (30). Exercise induced bronchoconstriction is observed in 70% to 80% of patients with clinically recognized asthma. Importantly, EIB testing is less sensitive than is inhalational challenge testing with methacholine (28, 34) for the evaluation of airway hyperactivity, especially in young patients with unexplained exertional dyspnea (35).

Cardiac Stress Test or Graded Exercise Test

A cardiac stress test or graded exercise test is the most widely used clinical exercise testing modality in the United States, with extensive literature documenting its efficacy (36, 37). Its major use is in the diagnosis of coronary artery disease (myocardial ischemia) and arrhythmias, and for the assessment of therapeutic interventions, including medications, interventional procedures, and surgery. The test is performed on a treadmill while monitoring ECG and blood pressure responses. The Bruce protocol is the most widely used and consists of five progressive stages, each 3 minutes in duration. Stage I is 1.7 mph and 10% grade; stage II, 2.5 mph and 12% grade; stage III, 3.4 mph and 14% grade; stage IV, 4.2 mph and 16% grade; and stage V, 5.0 mph and 18% grade. The single most reliable indicator of exercise-induced ischemia is ST-segment depression (36, 37). Other ECG abnormalities are also used as supplementary indicators of ischemia. The increment in workload per stage is approximately 50 W, which although good for diagnosing ischemia is too great for most patients with respiratory disease. Importantly, standard cardiac stress tests cannot generally define underlying pathophysiology in patients with exercise intolerance of nonischemic origin. The diagnostic potential of standard exercise testing can be enhanced by the concurrent measurement of respiratory gas exchange during a CPET.

Cardiopulmonary Exercise Test

CPET involves the measurement of O$_2$ uptake ($\dot{V}o_2$), CO$_2$ output ($\dot{V}co_2$), minute ventilation ($\dot{V}$E), and other variables while monitoring a 12-lead ECG, blood pressure, Spo$_2$, and ratings of perceived exertion (Borg scale) during a maximal symptom-limited incremental exercise test on the cycle ergometer or on the treadmill. In some circumstances, a constant work exercise test (based on maximal test results) is performed. Measurement of arterial blood gases provides more detailed information on pulmonary gas exchange. Spirometry and exercise tidal flow volume loops may also be performed to assess the degree of pulmonary constraint.

CPET provides a global assessment of the integrative exercise responses involving the pulmonary, cardiovascular, blood, brain, and skeletal muscle systems, which are not adequately reflected through the measurement of individual organ system function. CPET is unparalleled compared with other exercise testing modalities. This relatively noninvasive, dynamic physiologic overview permits the objective determination of both submaximal and peak exercise responses, providing the physician with relevant information for clinical decision making. CPET is increasingly being used in a wide spectrum of clinical applications for the evaluation of undiagnosed exercise intolerance, exercise-related symptoms, determination of mechanisms of exercise limitation (i.e., heart, lungs, skeletal muscles), objective assessment of therapeutic interventions, and unique, objective determination of functional capacity ($\dot{V}o_2$max) and impairment.

Indications

Indications for comprehensive CPET appear in Table 3.2 (38) and reflect its utility in a wide spectrum of clinical scenarios and potential impact on all phases of clinical decision analysis and diagnosis, disease progression, prognosis, and response to treatment. In practice, CPET is considered when specific questions remain unanswered after evaluation of basic clinical data, including history, physical examination, chest x-ray, pulmonary function tests (PFTs), and resting ECG.

Evaluation of Exercise Intolerance

The use of CPET in patient management is increasing in patients with cardiopulmonary disease because resting pulmonary (FEV_1, diffusing capacity of lung for carbon monoxide [D_{LCO}], arterial blood gases) and cardiac function (ECG, left ventricular ejection fraction) testing cannot reliably predict exercise performance and functional capacity ($\dot{V}o_2$max) in the individual patient (39–52). Furthermore, exertional symptoms correlate poorly with resting cardiopulmonary measurements (48, 50, 53), and although exertional dyspnea is common in patients with cardiopulmonary disease, other symptoms—leg discomfort, chest pain, or fatigue—other than dyspnea are often exercise limiting (47, 53). Interestingly, a patient's health status (health-related quality of life) reveals a stronger correlation with exercise tolerance than with either spirometry or oxygenation (54).

In addition to providing the traditional gold standard objective determination of functional capacity ($\dot{V}o_2$max) and impairment, CPET permits the prioritization/quantification of exercise limiting factors, the definition of underlying pathophysiological mechanisms important for distinguishing between entities (i.e., respiratory versus cardiac etiology when both diseases coexist), the timely detection of early (occult) diseases (ischemia, gas exchange in interstitial lung disease [ILD]) and, an objective measure of performance indices and exertional symptoms for evaluating disease progression and response to treatment. Based on the more thorough assessment that CPET provides, the weight of evidence supports that comprehensive CPET is useful in evaluating exercise intolerance (37, 39, 49, 52, 55–59).

TABLE 3.2. INDICATIONS FOR CARDIOPULMONARY EXERCISE TESTING

Evaluation of exercise intolerance and unexplained exertional dyspnea

- Functional impairment ($\dot{V}o_2$ peak)
- Exercise limitation: determination of factors and pathophysiologic mechanisms
- Assessment of contribution of cardiac and pulmonary etiology in coexisting disease
- Symptoms disproportionate to resting pulmonary and cardiac tests
- Initial resting cardiopulmonary testing is nondiagnostic

Evaluation of patients with cardiovascular disease

- Heart failure
- Selection for cardiac transplantation
- Exercise prescription and monitoring response to cardiac rehabilitation

Evaluation of patients with respiratory diseases

- Assessment of functional impairment
- COPD, ILD, PVD, exercise-induced bronchoconstriction, cystic fibrosis
- Detection of gas exchange abnormalities
- Determination of magnitude of hypoxemia for oxygen prescription
- Evaluation of therapeutic interventions

Specific clinical applications

- Preoperative evaluation: lung resection surgery; lung volume reduction surgery, elderly undergoing major abdominal surgery
- Exercise prescription for pulmonary rehabilitation
- Evaluation for lung, heart-lung transplantation
- Evaluation for impairment or disability
- Health promotion (wellness)

$\dot{V}o_2$, oxygen consumption; COPD, chronic obstructive pulmonary disease; ILD, interstitial lung disease; PVD, pulmonary vascular disease.
Adapted from Weisman IM, Zeballos RJ. Clinical exercise testing. *Clin Chest Med* 2001;22:679–701, with permission.

Evaluation of Unexplained Exertional Dyspnea

For patients with unexplained dyspnea after initial test results are not diagnostic, the weight of evidence suggests that CPET is a useful tool in identifying cardiac and/or pulmonary causes; metabolic myopathy; and it is a useful tool when psychological factors (e.g., hyperventilation, panic, anxiety syndromes) or deconditioning are suspected (37, 39, 60–62). Results from CPET may efficiently direct further diagnostic testing to target the suspected organ system involved. Moreover, a normal CPET would provide reassurance to the patient and limit subsequent testing.

Evaluation of Patients with Cardiovascular Disease

Strong evidence exists to support the use of CPET in the evaluation of exercise capacity and response to therapy in patients with heart failure who are being considered for heart transplantation (37, 63, 64). More recent work has confirmed the prognostic value of CPET in patients with ischemic and dilated cardiomyopathies. In one study, $\dot{V}O_2$max greater than 50% predicted was the most significant predictor of cardiac death in multivariate analysis (57).

Evaluation of Patients with Respiratory Disease

Chronic Obstructive Pulmonary Disease

CPET is clinically useful in the evaluation of patients with COPD: to get an objective determination of exercise capacity ($\dot{V}O_2$ peak) when necessary; to establish exercise limitations (56, 65, 66); and to assess other factors that may be contributing to exercise limitation (occult ischemia), as well as when heart and lung disease coexist (39, 59); when relating symptoms to exercise limitation (47, 67), especially when exertional symptoms are disproportionate to resting PFTs; and when hypoxemia may contribute to exercise limitation and O_2 requirements may be directly quantified (65).

Furthermore, CPET permits the evaluation of therapeutic interventions on exercise capacity, relief of dyspnea, and improvement in exercise tolerance. The efficacy of CPET in monitoring a variety of treatment modalities (e.g., continuous positive airway pressure, bronchodilators, exercise training, lung volume reduction surgery) directed at improving breathing strategy and/or reducing dynamic hyperinflation (resulting in improved breathlessness and exercise capacity) has recently been demonstrated (56, 68–72).

Interstitial Lung Disease

CPET is efficacious in providing for the early detection of subtle pulmonary gas exchange abnormalities that are not revealed by routine testing and an overall assessment of pulmonary gas exchange during exercise, which is important in establishing a timely diagnosis, accurately assessing physiologic severity, and permitting the monitoring of therapeutic interventions (44, 73–77).

Chronic Pulmonary Vascular Disease

In chronic pulmonary vascular disease, $\dot{V}O_2$max provides an index of severity, being lower in patients with high pulmonary vascular resistance and lower cardiac index, as well as being significantly correlated with the amount of functional vascular bed (78, 79). CPET can be safely performed in patients with primary pulmonary hypertension (80). Previous studies have suggested that $\dot{V}O_2$max correlated with results of 6MWT in this patient population (19). Because of significant mortality risk, exercise testing should be approached cautiously, especially in primary pulmonary hypertension. If syncope, arrhythmia, and/or right heart failure are evident, exercise testing should generally be avoided (81). Indications for CPET in the individual patient must reflect careful risk/benefit analysis.

Cystic Fibrosis

Recent work has provided convincing evidence that the measurement of $\dot{V}O_2$ peak is valuable for prognosis and management in patients with cystic fibrosis (82). A more optimized exercise prescription for patients with cystic fibrosis may be achieved by using CPET results and estimates of muscle size (cross-sectional area) (83).

Preoperative Evaluation of Lung Cancer Resection Surgery

Although routine pulmonary function tests (FEV_1, D_{LCO}) have the greatest utility in documenting physiologic operability in low-risk patients, other diagnostic modalities, including CPET and/or split function assessment by quantitative lung scintigraphy, are necessary to more accurately assess moderate- to high-risk patients (59, 84–87). Although which diagnostic modality should be used initially remains controversial, recent work would suggest, however, that CPET and the measurement of $\dot{V}O_2$ peak, especially when expressed as percentage predicted, appears to be particularly useful in predicting postoperative pulmonary complications (84, 88, 89). A $\dot{V}O_2$ peak more than 50% to 60% predicted is associated with higher morbidity and mortality after lung resection (84, 88–90).

Preoperative Evaluation in the Elderly

Recent work has shown that CPET is helpful in objectively assessing the adequacy of cardiovascular reserve and in predicting cardiovascular risk in an elderly population (91).

Lung Volume Reduction Surgery

The potential utility of CPET is highlighted by its emergence as an important tool in the evaluation of emphysema patients being considered for lung volume reduction surgery (LVRS). The range of application of CPET in this patient group includes the determination of cardiopulmonary functional status and assessment of potential operative risk before surgery, the determination of exercise training prescription before and after LVRS, quantification and monitoring of the clinical response to surgery, and definition of the underlying pathophysiologic mechanisms responsible for improvements in exercise performance resulting from LVRS (69, 92–96).

Evaluation for Lung, Heart-Lung Transplantation

With the emergence of lung and heart-lung transplantation for patients with end-stage pulmonary vascular and parenchymal lung disease as a viable therapeutic option, comprehensive CPET is increasingly being used to evaluate these complex patients before and after transplantation. As such, CPET is useful in assessing disease progression before transplantation and in assessing functional capacity, quantitating causes of exercise limitation, and providing exercise prescription for pulmonary rehabilitation before and after transplantation (37, 97, 98). However, there is presently no consensus on how indices of exercise performance may impact the clinical decision-making process for lung transplantation selection. Although a 6MWT distance less than 400 m is used for listing for lung transplantation (12), information from a 6MWT in general may be too imprecise in providing answers to important questions relating to patient management. From a clinical perspective, integrative CPET results in the transplantation arena have reinforced the importance of the multifactorial etiology of exercise limitation and of skeletal muscle dysfunction in patients with chronic lung disease (58, 97–102).

Exercise Prescription for Pulmonary Rehabilitation

Exercise training is a recommended, integral component of comprehensive pulmonary rehabilitation in patients with COPD and other chronic lung diseases (103, 104). CPET provides valuable information before exercise training to determine exercise capacity, lactic acidosis, safety (ischemia, arrhythmias, O_2 desaturation), and training intensity (105, 106) and can be repeated after training to objectively document improvement and to refine training levels. CPET results have documented improvement in exercise tolerance and $\dot{V}O_2$ peak, reduced ventilatory requirements, and improved muscle oxidative capacity (107, 108) resulting from exercise training in COPD. Controversy persists, however, regarding optimal training intensity for COPD (51, 103, 109, 110). Combined strength and endurance training is an effective training strategy (111). CPET and pulmonary rehabilitation are underutilized in patients with ILD (112).

Evaluation of Impairment or Disability

Increasing awareness of the inadequacies of resting cardiopulmonary tests in accurately predicting functional impairment (work capacity) and exercise limitation in patients with respiratory disease has focused attention on the expanded role of CPET in the evaluation of impairment or disability (113–115). CPET complements other clinical and diagnostic modalities and, by directly quantitating work capacity, improves the diagnostic accuracy of impairment/disability evaluation. $\dot{V}O_2$ max is used for defining energy requirements for physical activities (116), which is the cornerstone for impairment evaluation. Although an earlier American Thoracic Society statement concluded that CPET might be helpful only in selected cases of impairment evaluation (117), more recent work has demonstrated its enhanced diagnostic accuracy and impact in clinical decision making in cases ranging

from mild to moderate impairment (118, 119) to those with severe COPD (120).

Implementation of CPET

The goal of CPET is to assess the component and integrative exercise responses during progressive increases in external work involving large muscle groups so that a range of exercise intensities and metabolic stresses can be safely studied in a short time frame. That is roughly 25 minutes from rest through recovery, with actual exercise lasting approximately 8 to 12 minutes (121).

Methodology

Commercially available automated systems process four primary signals—air flow, O_2, CO_2, and HR—that form the basis for the determination of all the measured and derived cardiopulmonary variables (121). The current systems are technically advanced and provide on-line analysis of expired respiratory gas exchange by using either breath-by-breath or modern mixing chamber techniques (122, 123). Both are acceptable for clinical exercise testing (22, 121). The more popular breath-by-breath technique is associated with a high degree of breath-to-breath variability "noise," which can be minimized by 30- to 60-second interval averaging of the data (22, 124). Cardiopulmonary measurements obtained during maximal CPET in both normal subjects and patients are reproducible, provided that calibration and quality assurance procedures are followed (22, 121, 125).

Exercise testing can be performed by using either a cycle ergometer or a treadmill. Traditionally, exercise testing in respiratory patients has used cycle ergometry. However, depending on the reasons for which CPET was requested, a treadmill might be an acceptable or better alternative. For clinical CPET purposes, electronically braked cycle ergometry, which maintains a given work level independent of cycling frequency, offers several advantages to treadmill testing. These include direct quantitation of work rate, less noise (artifact) on ECG, easier-to-collect blood samples during exercise, less expense, and better safety (22, 121). However, the $\dot{V}O_2$ max achieved on a cycle ergometer is usually 5% to 11% less than that achieved on a treadmill. This is likely owing to more local fatigue and less muscle mass involved in exercise, as well as the possibility that patients are pushed beyond usual comfort levels because of the electrically propelled treadmill.

Protocols

There are several symptom-limited protocols that can be used with either cycle ergometry or treadmill (22, 121). These include an incremental protocol in which the work intensity is increased in a square wave fashion, from 5 W every 1 to 3 minutes for debilitated patients to 25 W every 1 to

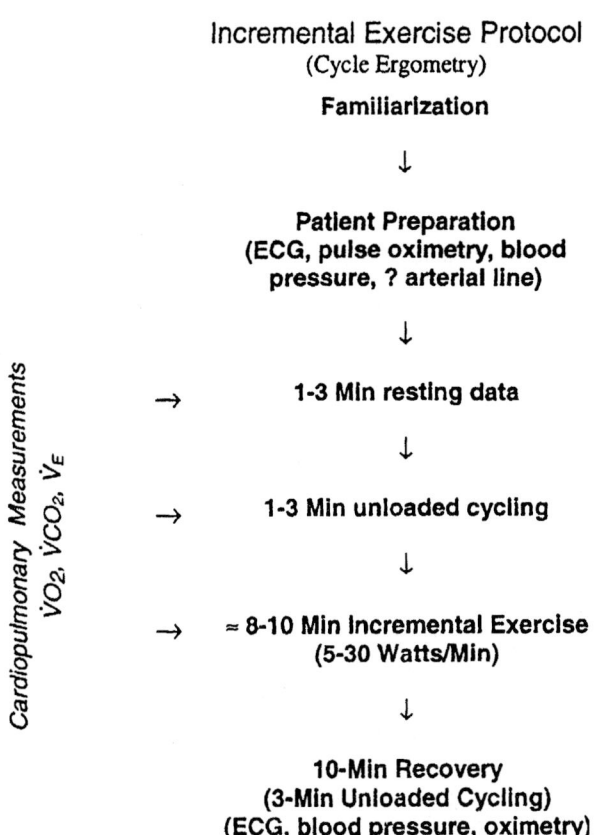

Incremental Exercise Protocol
(Cycle Ergometry)

Familiarization

↓

Patient Preparation
(ECG, pulse oximetry, blood
pressure, ? arterial line)

↓

→ **1-3 Min resting data**

↓

→ **1-3 Min unloaded cycling**

↓

→ **≈ 8-10 Min Incremental Exercise**
(5-30 Watts/Min)

↓

10-Min Recovery
(3-Min Unloaded Cycling)
(ECG, blood pressure, oximetry)

Cardiopulmonary Measurements
$\dot{V}O_2$, $\dot{V}CO_2$, $\dot{V}_E$

FIGURE 3.1. Typical incremental cycle ergometer exercise protocol used for clinical testing. (Adapted from Beck KC, Weisman IM. Methods for cardiopulmonary exercise testing. In: Weisman IM, Zeballos RJ, eds. *Clinical exercise testing: progress in respiratory research.* Basel: Karger, 2002:43–59, with permission.)

3 minutes for mildly diseased or healthy subjects, and the ramp protocol in which the power is increased continuously. Both should be programmed to achieve maximal aerobic capacity in 8 to 12 minutes. The comparability of these protocols for metabolic and cardiopulmonary measurements is well established (52). Subsequently, these results can then be used to establish constant work (steady-state) protocols (see below). A popular protocol for performing a maximal CPET appears in Figure 3.1.

Constant Work

Increasingly, constant work exercise at a standardized work load (based on an initial incremental exercise test) is being used to evaluate the impact of therapeutic interventions, including exercise training, O_2 therapy, and lung volume reduction surgery. Recent work has suggested that Borg dyspnea ratings, measurements of inspiratory capacity (IC, as a reflection of dynamic hyperinflation), and endurance times during submaximal exercise were highly reproducible and sensitive in patients with severe COPD (15, 71). Furthermore, constant work endurance times were more sensitive than was 6MWT in determining therapeutic effectiveness

of pharmacological intervention (15, 71). A constant work protocol is also useful as a possible alternative approach to obtain partial pressure of arterial O_2 (P_{AO_2}), alveolar-arterial difference in partial pressure of O_2 ($P_{AO_2} - P_{aO_2}$), and tidal volume (V_D/V_T) in lieu of arterial line placement during incremental exercise testing (39, 126). A work rate of 70% of the maximum work rate achieved during the incremental exercise test is used for the constant work rate test, which results in $\dot{V}O_2$ peak greater than 90% of the value obtained in the maximal exercise evaluation. Additional validation of this approach is warranted.

Patient Safety

Extensive literature documents that symptom-limited exercise testing is safe, with the risk of medical complications

CARDIOPULMONARY EXERCISE TEST	
Summary Statement	**Level of Evidence**
CPET provides the most comprehensive and insightful evaluation of exercise intolerance and unexplained exertional dyspnea not adequately reflected in resting cardiopulmonary measurements or other exercise tests	Randomized controlled trials, consensus recommendations, and observational studies
$\dot{V}O_2$max provides important risk stratification and prognostic information in patients with heart failure being evaluated for cardiac transplantation	Multiple randomized controlled trials
CPET provides important clinically relevant information ranging from early diagnosis (ILD) to prognosis (CF) and management (COPD) useful in the care of patients with respiratory disease	Moderate quality on the basis of randomized controlled trials and consensus recommendations.
CPET optimizes exercise prescription for pulmonary rehabilitation	Randomized control trials and consensus recommendations
$\dot{V}O_2$max is helpful in predicting postoperative complications after lung resection surgery	Randomized control trials and consensus recommendations
CPET can be useful both before and after lung and heart-lung transplantation, but its role in the selection process requires clarification	Expert opinion
CPET plays an important role in optimally assessing respiratory patients for impairment disability, although the precise role requires additional study	Observational studies and consensus of expert opinion

CPET, cardiopulmonary exercise test; $\dot{V}O_2$max, maximum oxygen consumption; ILD, interstitial lung disease; CF, cystic fibrosis; COPD, chronic obstructive pulmonary disease.

during exercise testing related to the underlying disease and with morbidity for patients in the range of two to five per 100,000 clinical exercise tests (127, 128). Advantages to performing CPET over less-structured exercise include not only the extensive amount of physiological information gained but also safety. Typically, trained personnel (physicians, exercise physiologists, and nurses) perform exercise testing under controlled and stable conditions for temperature and humidity, with emergency equipment and a bed available while carefully monitoring the ECG, blood pressure, symptoms, and O_2 saturation (22, 121, 127, 129, 130). These trained individuals should be knowledgeable with the conduct and risks of testing, contraindications to testing, and the criteria for terminating exercise tests (22, 121).

MEASUREMENTS

Computerized metabolic systems allow an impressive number of variables to be measured or derived during exercise (Table 3.3). The number of variables actually used will vary and be a function of the reasons for exercise testing. A listing of selected measurements and important caveats, including suggested guidelines for interpretation, appears in Table 3.4.

Oxygen Consumption

$\dot{V}O_2$ rises linearly with increases in work rate to a maximal value. The measurement of $\dot{V}O_2$max or $\dot{V}O_2$peak remains the best available index for the assessment of aerobic capacity. $\dot{V}O_2$ peak can be estimated from work rate; however, previous studies have suggested such estimates may not always be reliable (37). $\dot{V}O_2$ peak may be expressed in absolute values (liters per minute), per kilogram body weight (milliliters per kilogram per minute), and as the percentage predicted. The optimal normalization for body mass remains somewhat controversial. In addition to the typical expression in milliliters per kilogram per minute (e.g., American Heart Association and American College of Sports Medicine), others have expressed $\dot{V}O_2$ relative to body mass index (kilogram per squared meter) or fat-free mass (milliliters per kilogram per minute) (131). $\dot{V}O_2$max values have been regarded as most reliable when $\dot{V}O_2$ does not increase (plateau) despite further increases in work rate (132, 133). Such a plateau, however, is not often observed, and the $\dot{V}O_2$max achieved has been called $\dot{V}O_2$peak (134, 135). This implies that if a subject could be pushed harder, there may be a small further increase in the peak value. For practical purposes, however, $\dot{V}O_2$peak is likely quite close to $\dot{V}O_2$max, and thus, they are often used interchangeably.

A reduced $\dot{V}O_2$ peak (defined by the *Fick equation:* $\dot{V}O_2 =$ heart rate × stroke volume × arteriovenous oxygen difference) reflects problems with O_2 delivery (heart, lung, systemic and pulmonary circulation; and blood) and/or peripheral abnormalities (i.e., reduced O_2 utilization and/or muscle dysfunction) (47, 55, 99, 102). A reduced $\dot{V}O_2$ peak may also reflect poor effort. $\dot{V}O_2$ peak is modulated by physical activity and, as such, has been the gold standard for the evaluation of fitness. A number of normative studies have derived predicted equations based on age and sex. A normal $\dot{V}O_2$ peak reflects a normal aerobic power and exercise capacity and suggests that no significant functional abnormality exist. In some subjects, however, even though the $\dot{V}O_2$ peak may be near normal, exercise testing may reveal other abnormalities (e.g., abnormal breathing patterns) (39, 62) that may be of diagnostic value. A reduced $\dot{V}O_2$ peak is usually the starting point in the evaluation of a CPET (39, 52, 123).

Although $\dot{V}O_2$ peak is most commonly reported, it may also be of interest to assess the slope of rise in $\dot{V}O_2$ relative to work ($\Delta\dot{V}O_2/\Delta WR$). In health, this slope is approximately a rise in $\dot{V}O_2$ of 10 mL for every watt increase in work. Clinically, an abnormal slope of this relationship is most often owing to O_2 transport dysfunction (heart failure and pulmonary hypertension); less commonly, O_2 utilization dysfunction may also be associated with a reduced slope (60, 83). Obese individuals may show an increase in $\dot{V}O_2$ for a given external work rate, but the slope of the relationship is usually normal.

TABLE 3.3. CARDIOPULMONARY VARIABLES MEASURED DURING CARDIOPULMONARY EXERCISE TESTING

Work	WR
Metabolic	$\dot{V}O_2$, $\dot{V}CO_2$, RER, AT
Cardiovascular	HR, ECG, BP, O_2 pulse
Ventilatory	$\dot{V}E$, V_T, fb
Pulmonary gas exchange	$\dot{V}E/\dot{V}CO_2$, $\dot{V}E/\dot{V}O_2$, $P_{ET}O_2$, $P_{ET}CO_2$, SpO_2 SaO_2, PaO_2, PAO_2-PaO_2, V_D/V_T
Acid base	pH, $PaCO_2$, HCO_3^-, lactate
Symptoms	Dyspnea, leg fatigue, chest pain

Abnormality of a variable does not necessarily define exercise limitation in that category.
WR, work rate; $\dot{V}O_2$, oxygen consumption; $\dot{V}CO_2$, carbon dioxide production; RER, respiratory exchange ratio; AT, anaerobic threshold; HR, heart rate; ECG, electrocardiogram; BP, blood pressure; $\dot{V}E$, minute ventilation; V_T, tidal volume; fb, breathing frequency; $P_{ET}O_2$, end-tidal partial pressure of oxygen; $P_{ET}CO_2$, end-tidal partial pressure of carbon dioxide; SpO_2, pulse oximetry; SaO_2, arterial oxygen saturation; PaO_2, partial pressure of oxygen in the arterial blood; PAO_2, partial pressure of oxygen in the alveolar air; V_D/V_T, dead space to tidal volume ratio; $PaCO_2$, partial pressure of carbon dioxide in the arterial blood; HCO_3^-, bicarbonate.
Adapted from Zeballos RJ, Weisman IM. Behind the scenes of cardiopulmonary exercise testing. *Clin Chest Med.* 1994;15:193–213, with permission.

Carbon Dioxide Production

Paralleling the changes in $\dot{V}O_2$ with exercise are the changes in the volume of CO_2 expired ($\dot{V}CO_2$). At low levels of exercise, $\dot{V}CO_2$ tends to be slightly less than the uptake of O_2; however, this becomes equimolar in moderate exercise and exceeds O_2 uptake with moderate-to-heavy exercise. The relationship of $\dot{V}CO_2$ to $\dot{V}O_2$ is known as the respiratory exchange ratio. Under steady-state conditions, this ratio may reflect the

TABLE 3.4. SELECTED PEAK CARDIOPULMONARY EXERCISE TESTING MEASUREMENTS

Variables	Measurement caveats	Comments	Suggested Guidelines
$\dot{V}O_2$max or $\dot{V}O_2$peak	Max: when plateau is achieved Peak: $\dot{V}O_2$ at maximum exercise, but no plateau	Global assessment of respiratory, cardiovascular, blood, and muscle function	>84% predicted
Anaerobic threshold (or lactate threshold)	Direct: lactate in arterial blood. Indirect: modified V-slope ($\dot{V}CO_2$ vs. $\dot{V}O_2$) and conventional ($\dot{V}E/\dot{V}O_2$, $\dot{V}E/\dot{V}CO_2$, $P_{ET}O_2$, $P_{ET}CO_2$). No noninvasive method is consistently superior	Estimator of the onset of metabolic acidosis during exercise. Not an effective discriminator among different clinical entities. Appears nonessential for exercise prescription in COPD. 50%–60% $\dot{V}O_2$max in average persons; higher in fit persons	>40% $\dot{V}O_2$max predicted. Wide range of normal: 35%–80%. Clinical validation is required
Heart rate reserve	Predicted HR max: $210 - (age \times 0.65)$ HRR: age-predicted HR max − HR max achieved	Age related variability in HR max predicted. Normal subjects usually have no HRR	HR max >90% age-predicted HRR <15 bpm
O_2 Pulse ($\dot{V}O_2$/HR)	Determined at plateau, when O_2 max extraction and stroke volume have been reached	Reflects stroke volume assuming that O_2 extraction is normal. Its use in COPD/congestive heart failure remains unvalidated.	>80%
$\Delta\dot{V}O_2/\Delta$WR	Measured during incremental cycle ergometry. ($\dot{V}O_2$peak-$\dot{V}O_2$ at min 3 unloaded)/(W/min × duration test − 0.75). Recently, simple linear regression is also being used.	Used as index of O_2 delivery/utilization by the muscle. Could be abnormal in patients with cardiovascular/pulm vascular disease. Normal in patient with pulmonary disease	>8.3 mL/min/W
Ventilatory reserve	MVV − $\dot{V}E$max or $\dot{V}E$max/MVV × 100 (widely used). MVV can be measured directly or calculated ($FEV_1 \times 40$). ExtFVL/MFVL to visualize "limitation"; Quantitate:IC = TLC − EELV, EILV/TLC	Potential ventilation in L that could be increased Percentage of the maximum breathing capacity used No gold standard for its determination	MVV − $\dot{V}E$max: >11 L $\dot{V}E$max/MVV × 100: <75%. Wide normal range: 72 ± 15%
Breathing frequency	Different breathing strategies in COPD and interstitial lung disease. Erratic in malingers. High in psychogenic disorders	Reflects abnormalities in the mechanics of breathing, control of breathing, and/or hypoxemia or psychological disorders.	<60 breaths/min
$\dot{V}E/\dot{V}CO_2$ (at AT)	Measured throughout but reported at AT (or near nadir) when P_aCO_2 is steady, to avoid the effect of hyperventilation acidosis, etc.	Noninvasive measurement of efficiency of ventilation (L of $\dot{V}E$ to eliminate 1L of $\dot{V}CO_2$). Reflects increase in VD/VT and or hyperventilation.	<34
VD/VT	P_aCO_2 should be used in its determination. $P_{ET}CO_2$ produces unreliable results	Reflects efficiency of CO_2 exchange or lung units with proportionally higher VA than Q (increased VD). Normally decreases with increased exercise intensity.	<0.30
P_aO_2	Careful anaerobic collection near maximal and peak exercise for consistency in the results	Ability to exchange O_2 is best assessed by measurement of P_aO_2 and not by pulse oximetry, particularly in suspect cases.	>80 mm Hg
$P_AO_2 - P_aO_2$	Arterial blood should be collected slowly in the middle to end of the respective interval	Evaluates gas transfer. Abnormal high values may reflect V/Q mismatching (shunt type), diffusion limitation, shunt and or reduced P_vO_2	<35 mm Hg

$\dot{V}O_2$max, maximum oxygen consumption; $\dot{V}CO_2$, carbon dioxide production; $\dot{V}E$, minute ventilation; $P_{ET}O_2$, end-tidal partial pressure of oxygen; $P_{ET}CO_2$, end-tidal partial pressure of carbon dioxide; COPD, chronic obstructive pulmonary disease; HR, heart rate; HRR, heart rate reserve; MVV, maximum voluntary ventilation; FEV_1, forced expiratory volume in 1s; MFVL, maximum flow–volume envelope; IC, inspiratory capacity; TLC, total lung capacity; EELV, end expiratory lung volume; AT, anaerobic threshold.
Modified from Weisman IM, Zeballos RJ. Clinical evaluation of unexplained dyspnea. *Cardiologia* 1996;41:621–634, with permission.

fuels being consumed at the muscle (similar to the respiratory quotient). However, with non—steady-state or heavy exercise, this more accurately reflects transient changes in CO_2 stores and exceeds 1.0 when lactate buffering occurs, and when arterial pH falls causing a significant hyperventilation. Anxiety-related hyperventilation will also cause a high $\dot{V}CO_2$ and respiratory exchange ratio. As noted, $\dot{V}CO_2$ is typically assessed in combination with $\dot{V}O_2$ or with minute ventilation ($\dot{V}E$).

Heart Rate

The best index for the evaluation of cardiac function during exercise would be the measurement of cardiac output. However, this is not routinely performed in the clinical exercise laboratory. Because it is well established that increases in cardiac output are initially accomplished by increases in stroke volume and HR, and then at higher work rates almost exclusively by increases in HR (132), the evaluation of HR yields an estimate of the level of cardiac output achieved during exercise. Achievement of age-predicted values for HR typically reflects maximal or near maximal effort and presumably signals attainment of $\dot{V}O_2$max and, in turn, maximal cardiac output.

For interpretive purposes, it is extremely important to remember that there is considerable variability (10 to 20 beats per minute) within an age group when estimates of maximal HR are used. The difference between the age-predicted maximal HR and the maximum HR achieved during exercise is referred to as the HR reserve (HRR). Normally, at maximal exercise, there is little or no HRR. In patients with pulmonary disease, the achievement of peak HR during exercise may vary considerably, depending on the disease severity and medications.

Oxygen Pulse

The O_2 pulse is $\dot{V}O_2$ divided by HR. According to the Fick equation, this is equivalent to the product of stroke volume multiplied by the arterial-mixed venous O_2 difference (a − vDO_2). As such, several factors that affect stroke volume (SV)—including heart disease, deconditioning, ventilatory limitation, and possibly even the hemodynamic consequences of dynamic hyperinflation—as well as factors that affect arterial O_2 concentration (CaO_2) − venous O_2 concentration (CvO_2)—including abnormal O_2 utilization (60), desaturation, anemia, and carboxyhemoglobinemia—may impact the O_2 pulse (39). Recent work in normal subjects suggests that the relationship between stroke volume and O_2 pulse can be defined as follows: $SV = \Delta \dot{V}O_2 / \Delta HR / CaO_2$, or $5\times$ slope of $\Delta \dot{V}O_2 / \Delta HR$. Although valid in normal subjects, this may not be applicable in lung disease, desaturation, and carboxyhemoglobinemia (136). A well-executed comparative study between SV and O_2 pulse would be helpful to ensure the accuracy of this noninvasive estimate in various patient populations.

Ventilation

$\dot{V}E$ (expressed in liters per minute) is typically determined from respiratory rate and V_T. Ventilation includes both alveolar and dead-space ventilation and is most often expressed relative to ventilatory capacity (see section "Ventilatory Reserve") or metabolic demand (see section "Ventilatory Efficiency").

Ventilatory Reserve

This concept is used to determine the degree of mechanical limitation or constraint to breathing during exercise. It is typically expressed as the maximal ventilation achieved during exercise relative to the maximal voluntary ventilation ($\dot{V}E$/MVV) or some estimate of the MVV (e.g., $FEV_1 \times 35$–40) used as an index of ventilatory capacity (52). Ventilatory reserve (VR) is dependent on many factors responsible for altering ventilatory demand, including metabolic demand (fitness), body weight, mode of testing, dead-space ventilation, and neuroregulatory and behavioral considerations. Ventilatory capacity, in turn, is influenced by multiple factors as well, including ventilatory muscle function, genetic endowment, aging, and disease (137). The ventilatory capacity may also vary during exercise, depending on bronchodilation or bronchoconstriction and the regulation of the operational lung volume (where one breathes relative to the constraints imposed by the boundaries of the maximal flow-volume envelope) (see "Limitations to the Use of Classical Ventilation Reserve," below) (138).

A high $\dot{V}E$/MVV ratio is one of the criteria often used to indicate encroachment on the VR and an increasing ventilatory constraint to breathing. A reduced or absent VR, especially when accompanied by other respiratory abnormalities (and an inability to achieve maximal HR), increases the likelihood that respiratory limitation may be a significant contributing factor to exercise limitation.

Limitations to the Use of Classical Ventilation Reserve

Although widely used and practical, MVV may not always be a reliable indicator of the maximal available ventilation (Fig. 3.2) (138) or may not provide adequate insight into abnormalities in breathing strategy. The MVV is typically a 15-second test, and patients will typically produce pulmonary pressures in excess of those produced even during maximal exercise. In addition, as shown in Figure 3.2, patients have a tendency to perform the MVV at higher lung volumes than those achieved during exercise, although allowing full advantage of the higher available maximal expiratory air flows at higher lung volumes. This can increase the work of breathing as inspiratory muscle length decreases, and the elastic load is also increased.

A more comprehensive assessment of the degree of ventilatory constraint can be gained by comparison of the exercise tidal flow–volume loop to the maximal volitional

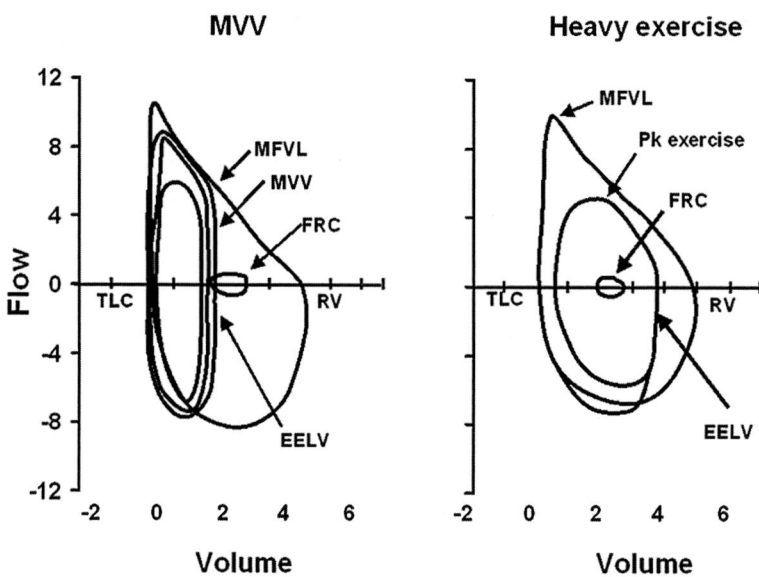

FIGURE 3.2. Comparison of the tidal flow–volume responses during a maximum voluntary ventilation (MVV) maneuver relative to the same subject breathing during maximal exercise. Note differences in breathing strategy, which include significant hyperinflation and expiratory flow limitation during the MVV maneuver. (From Johnson BD, Weisman IM, Zeballos RJ, et al. Emerging concepts in the evaluation of ventilatory limitation during exercise. *Chest* 1999;116:488–503, with permission.)

flow–volume envelopes (MFVLs) (139) (Fig. 3.3). This display of the exercise breathing pattern provides visual insight into the degree of ventilatory constraint and the strategies used to achieve a given level of ventilation relative to that which is available. Quantification of the degree of constraint from the tidal flow and volume responses to exercise relative to the MFVL has been suggested. In addition to a more in-depth assessment of ventilatory constraint during exercise, a more precise assessment of ventilatory capacity can be obtained. This assessment of ventilatory capacity takes into account the V_T, the operational lung volume (EELV), and the constraints imposed by the maximal expiratory flow–volume curve. To account for changes in ventilatory capacity during exercise (i.e., bronchodilation or constriction), comparisons can be made to a MFVL obtained during or immediately after exercise (139). Exercise tidal flow–volume loop analysis

has been applied in several clinical settings (68, 69, 139, 140). Exercise tidal flow–volume loops in a normal young subjects and in fit older subjects appear in Figure 3.4 (138, 139).

Anaerobic Threshold

The anaerobic threshold (AT) is an estimator of the onset of metabolic acidosis caused predominantly by increases in lactic acid during exercise. This was initially termed the lactate threshold, and subsequently, it was determined that noninvasive gas exchange measurements could fairly closely approximate these changes in lactate accumulation. Although the exact mechanism for the rise remains somewhat controversial and may vary depending on disease population, the lactate rise in health most likely reflects accumulative recruitment of obligatory glycolytic fibers. The lactic acid is subsequently

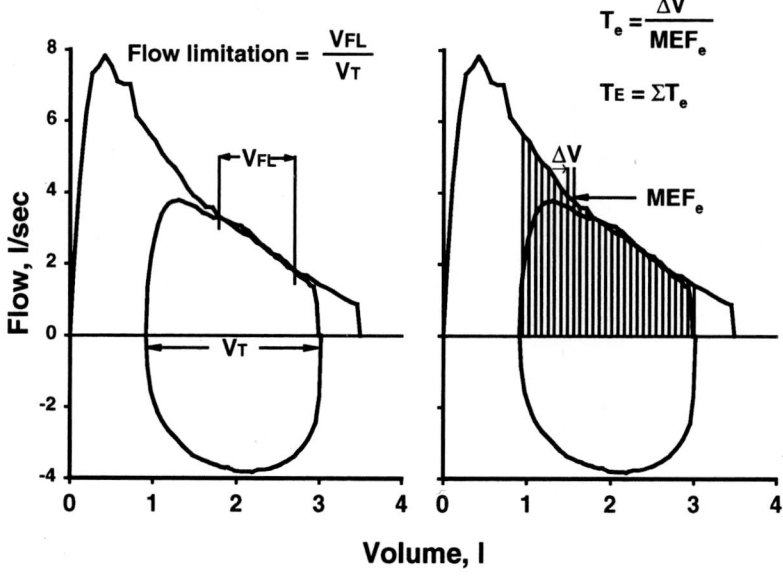

FIGURE 3.3. Flow–volume curve analysis. **Left:** Determination of ventilatory constraint using the flow–volume loop analysis. The tidal exercise loops are plotted within the maximal flow–volume envelope (MFVL) according to a measured end expiratory lung volume. From this plot, the degree of expiratory flow limitation can be assessed by the degree of overlap of the tidal loops with the expiratory boundary of the MFVL. In addition, a rising end expiratory lung volume along with an end inspiratory lung volume that approaches total lung capacity implies expiratory flow limitation and an increasing elastic load. **Right:** Assessment of ventilatory capacity based on the tidal volume achieved during exercise, the shape of the expiratory boundary of the MFVL, and the measured end expiratory lung volume. Integration of small volume segments throughout the tidal breath leads to an estimation of the amount of ventilation truly available for the given breathing pattern. (Modified from Johnson BD, Weisman IM, Zeballos RJ, et al. Emerging concepts in the evaluation of ventilatory limitation during exercise. *Chest* 1999;116:488–503, with permission.)

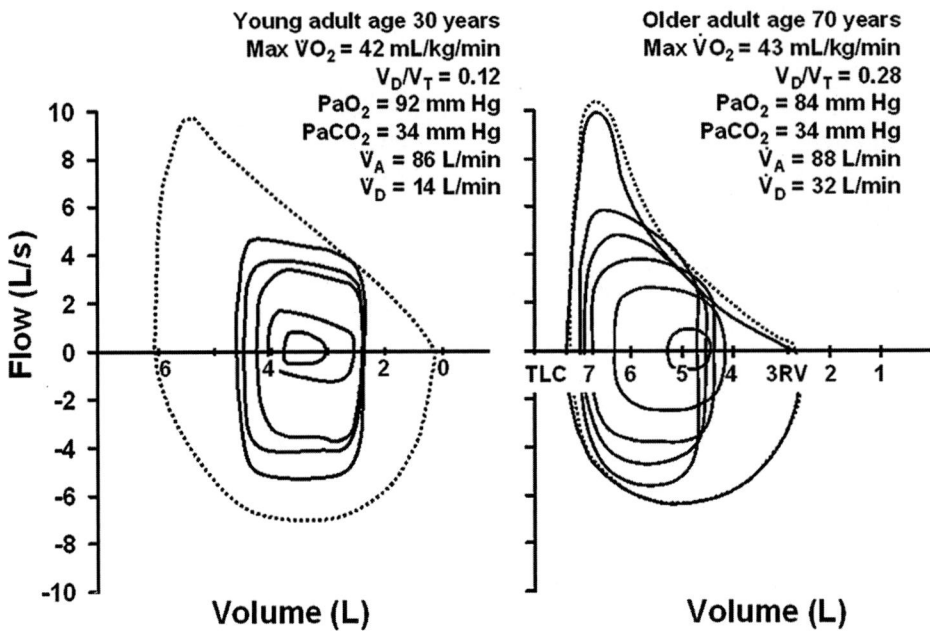

FIGURE 3.4. Flow–volume responses to exercise in younger **(left)** and older **(right)** adults. Subjects were matched for similar peak oxygen consumption per time unit ($\dot{V}o_2$) values. Key differences in the ventilatory response to exercise for young adult are as follows: drop in functional residual capacity (a), encroachment equally on the inspiratory reserve volume (IRV) and expiratory reserve volume (ERV) (b), little or no expiratory flow limitation (c), available inspiratory flow reserve (d), and significant volume reserve (e). Key differences in the ventilatory response to exercise for older adult are as follows: drop in functional residual capacity followed by an increase with flow limitation (a), encroachment mostly on IRV (b), significant expiratory flow limitation (c), minimal inspiratory flow reserve (d), and little reserve to increase either flow or volume at peak exercise (e). It should be noted that the young adults have average levels of fitness, whereas the older adults studied are much fitter than age predicted (maximum oxygen consumption is approximately twice age predicted). (From Johnson BD, Badr MS, Dempsey JA. Impact of the aging pulmonary system on the response to exercise. *Clin Chest Med* 1994;15:229–246, with permission.)

buffered by bicarbonate and the by-product becomes CO_2 production in excess of typical metabolic CO_2 production. This results in a rise in the $\dot{V}co_2$ and a parallel increase in $\dot{V}e$ to maintain iso-pH.

Current knowledge would suggest that the AT may be considered to be affected by factors that impact both O_2 delivery and O_2 utilization processes, pattern of muscle fiber recruitment, and possibly others (141). The AT usually occurs at 50% to 70% $\dot{V}o_2$max in sedentary individuals and is higher in fit individuals (52). There is a wide range of normal predicted values (35%–70%) making its usefulness in clinical decision making somewhat limited (142).

Although there are several ways to determine the AT noninvasively, none appears consistently superior. Currently, the modified V-slope method ($\dot{V}co_2$ versus $\dot{V}o_2$ plot) is most popular (143). The AT, using the ventilatory equivalents method is defined as the lowest (nadir) for $\dot{V}e/\dot{V}o_2$ and partial pressure of end-tidal oxygen ($Peto_2$) before beginning to consistently increase, whereas $\dot{V}e/\dot{V}co_2$ and partial pressure of end-tidal CO_2 ($Petco_2$) remain unchanged, and R is approximately 1.0. An approach that combines the modified V-slope and the ventilatory equivalents method is recommended (124). Blood samples for standard bicarbonate or lactates help avoid false-positive noninvasive AT

determinations that have been reported in COPD (102). The AT determination is helpful as an indicator of level of fitness and as a monitor of the effect of physical training (105). The AT is reduced in a wide spectrum of clinical entities—e.g., heart disease, lung disease, deconditioning, lung and heart transplantation, muscle abnormalities (metabolic myopathy)—and, therefore, may be of limited discriminatory value in interpretative schemes (39).

Ventilatory Efficiency

Ventilatory efficiency is determined by how much ventilation is achieved for a given level of metabolic demand (i.e., $\dot{V}e/\dot{V}co_2$ and or $\dot{V}e/\dot{V}o_2$). Because $\dot{V}e$ is more closely linked to $\dot{V}co_2$, the relationship of $\dot{V}e$ to $\dot{V}co_2$ has typically been reported. In healthy subjects, it typically requires approximately 25 L of ventilation for every 1 L of CO_2 produced. $\dot{V}e/\dot{V}co_2$ and $\dot{V}e/\dot{V}o_2$ are typically similar until near where the AT occurs, and then $\dot{V}e/\dot{V}co_2$ tends to stay constant while $\dot{V}e/\dot{V}o_2$ starts to rise. The degree of ventilation produced is best described in the alveolar air equation, where $\dot{V}e = K \times \dot{V}co_2/Paco_2 \times (1/Vd/Vt)$. Dead-space ventilation and arterial CO_2 levels critically influence the relationship of $\dot{V}e/\dot{V}co_2$. High dead-space ventilation increases the $\dot{V}E/\dot{V}CO_2$ ratio as does hyperventilation (reduced $PaCO_2$ values). An inadequate hyperventilation during exercise (high or rising $PaCO_2$) may result in a low $\dot{V}E/\dot{V}CO_2$, particularly if the VD/VT is normal. Various $\dot{V}E/\dot{V}CO_2$ values have been reported, including the lowest point in an incremental test, at or near the AT, the slope of $\dot{V}E$ relative to $\dot{V}CO_2$ and peak. For most purposes, the $\dot{V}E/\dot{V}CO_2$ nadir occurs near the AT, where it is usually reported because during heavy and maximal exercise, it is more susceptible to variation in the degree of hyperventilation, altered breathing pattern, anxiety, and the degree of acidosis. Under some circumstances, the peak values may be important, as when a relatively sudden increase in $\dot{V}E/\dot{V}CO_2$ with heavier exercise occurs in patients with pulmonary hypertension, likely related to the high pulmonary pressures and the shunting of blood through a patent foramen ovale.

In patients with heart failure, the slope of the $\dot{V}E$ versus $\dot{V}CO_2$ relationship may provide important prognostic information similar to peak $\dot{V}O_2$ measurements (144). Examining the $PETCO_2$, or preferably $PaCO_2$ (if available), is useful in distinguishing between a hyperventilation-induced increase in $\dot{V}E/\dot{V}CO_2$ versus that related to a high dead space (52, 58, 123).

Blood Gases

In the clinical laboratory where more specific gas exchange information is needed, direct arterial blood gas sampling during exercise should be considered. This may be useful in a patient with significant O_2 desaturation (<85%) during a noninvasive CPET or in patients with a markedly elevated $\dot{V}E/\dot{V}CO_2$. It may also be of importance in patients in whom it is difficult to obtain clean noninvasive gas exchange data owing to problems with the mouthpiece or noninvasive estimates of O_2 saturation.

Measurements of PaO_2, $PaCO_2$, combined with ventilatory measurements also allows the assessment of the alveolar-arterial difference in PO_2 ($PAO_2 - PaO_2$) and the physiologic dead space–to-VT ratio (VD/VT) (145). VD/VT determined noninvasively by using $PETCO_2$ can often yield unreliable results (146). Abnormal widening of the $PAO_2 - PaO_2$ with exercise usually reflects $\dot{V}A/\dot{Q}$ mismatching but may also be owing to lung diffusion abnormalities, anatomical shunt, and/or reduced O_2 saturation in mixed venous blood (thereby worsening the $\dot{V}A/\dot{Q}$ mismatching, shunt effect) (147). Failure of VD/VT to decrease normally with exercise is indicative of $\dot{V}A/\dot{Q}$ abnormalities caused by increases in physiologic dead space (wasted ventilation) (52, 58).

Pulse Oximetry

SpO_2 is only an estimation of the arterial O_2 saturation with actual SaO_2 ± 4% of the pulse oximetry readings (148, 149). Each laboratory should validate its pulse oximeter(s) with arterial O_2 saturation. This is important because some pulse oximeters underestimate, and others overestimate true arterial O_2 saturation, especially at SaO_2 less than 88% (150). Caution should be exercised in the use of pulse oximetry in darker skinned subjects, because the inaccuracies reported in white subjects appear to be exaggerated (151). Pulse oximeters cannot be used in patients with high levels of carboxyhemoglobin (Hbco), owing to smoking or CO exposure, as Hbco is not measured independently. Pulse oximeters measure functional SaO_2 and not fractional saturation as do CO oximeters. For example, if a patient has 5% Hbco and 85% SaO_2, the pulse oximeter will read approximately 90% (124). Pulse oximetry may also be misleading in some patients with heart failure and impaired peripheral perfusion (152). Care should be exercised in interpreting changes obtained by pulse oximetry alone (121). Significant desaturation, defined as a reduction in SpO_2 ≥5%, should be confirmed with arterial blood gases (148).

CLINICAL SIGNS AND SYMPTOMS

In a symptom-limited test, it is important to describe and characterize signs and symptoms limiting the test (47): e.g., chest pain, breathlessness, leg fatigue, wheezing, diaphoresis, arrhythmia. Ratings of perceived exertion symptoms (breathlessness, fatigue, chest pain) using the Borg scale (0 to 10) (153) or other rating scores, including visual analog scales (154, 155), should be noted with the physiologic measurements.

Normal Integrative Exercise Response

The graphic representation of the normal cardiopulmonary response of a healthy physically active young person to a symptom-limited maximal incremental exercise test appears in Figure 3.5. The healthy adult responds to the demands for increased O_2 delivery and CO_2 removal by fairly precise regulation of cardiac output, blood flow distribution, and ventilation. Thus for a given work rate on the cycle ergometer, many physiological responses are quite predictable.

$\dot{V}O_2$, $\dot{V}CO_2$, and $\dot{V}E$ increase as work rate increases (Fig. 3.5, upper panel). The increase in $\dot{V}O_2$ is linear with increases in work rate. During the early stages of exercise, $\dot{V}CO_2$ and $\dot{V}E$ also increase linearly with $\dot{V}O_2$ until approximately 50% to 60% of $\dot{V}O_2max$ when $\dot{V}CO_2$ and $\dot{V}E$, which remain closely linked, rise disproportionally to $\dot{V}O_2$ as a consequence of increases in lactic acid (classical ventilatory determined AT). Approaching approximately 70% of $\dot{V}O_2max$, the increase in $\dot{V}E$ is disproportionate to $\dot{V}CO_2$, probably owing to the greater stimulation of hydrogen ions elicited by the increase in lactic acid relative to the ventilatory compensation. The respiratory exchange ratio, the ratio of $\dot{V}CO_2/\dot{V}O_2$, is less than one below the AT and greater than one above the AT.

HR increases linearly and proportionally with increases in work rate. O_2 pulse ($\dot{V}O_2/HR$) likewise increases nearly

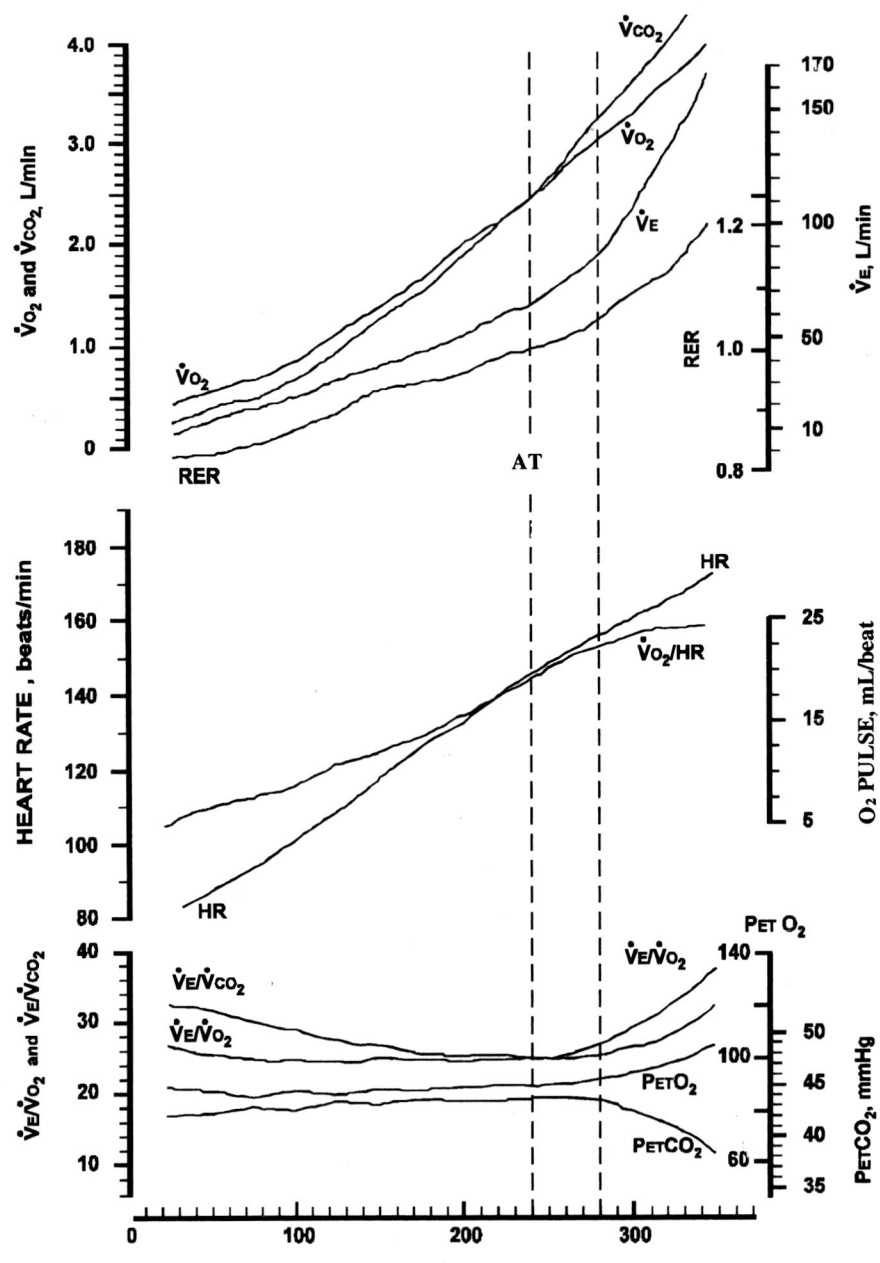

FIGURE 3.5. Normal cardiopulmonary responses to exercise. Shown are the changes in oxygen consumption ($\dot{V}O_2$), carbon dioxide production ($\dot{V}CO_2$), minute ventilation ($\dot{V}E$), respiratory exchange ratio (RER), heart rate (HR), O_2 pulse, ($\dot{V}O_2/HR$), partial pressure of end-tidal CO_2 ($P_{ET}CO_2$), partial pressure of end-tidal oxygen ($P_{ET}O_2$), $\dot{V}E/\dot{V}O_2$, and $\dot{V}E/\dot{V}CO_2$ with incremental work. (From Weisman IM, Zeballos RJ. Clinical exercise testing. *Clin Chest Med* 2001;22:679–701, with permission.)

linearly until a plateau is achieved near maximal exercise, representing the achievement of maximum O_2 extraction and maximum stroke volume (Fig. 3.5, middle panel).

Figure 3.5, bottom panel, illustrates the normal responses of the ventilatory equivalents for $\dot{V}O_2$ ($\dot{V}E/\dot{V}O_2$) and $\dot{V}CO_2$ ($\dot{V}E/\dot{V}CO_2$), as well as the normal response of $P_{ET}O_2$ and $P_{ET}CO_2$. The trend of these variables is a logical consequence of the relation of $\dot{V}E$ to $\dot{V}O_2$ and $\dot{V}CO_2$. The initial response is owing to the hyperventilation caused by the anxiety of exercise and use of the mouthpiece. During moderate exercise, the ventilation is proportional to the metabolic de-

mand of exercise. During heavy exercise, there is a relative hyperventilation for $\dot{V}O_2$; near the end of exercise, a relative hyperventilation for both $\dot{V}O_2$ and $\dot{V}CO_2$.

BREATHING PATTERN AND STRATEGY

This includes the combination of V_T and breathing frequency, breath timing, and variations in end inspiratory and EELV. The normal flow–volume response to exercise in healthy young (average fitness) and older adults (high fitness) are shown in Figure 3.4. In general, V_T increases in a progressive manner along with breathing frequency, until V_T reaches approximately 50% of the vital capacity (usually a twofold to threefold increase in the rest V_T). Subsequently, $\dot{V}_E$ increases primarily by a rise in respiratory rate. Near maximal exercise, some studies have noted an actual fall in V_T as respiratory rate accelerates more quickly. Inspiratory time relative to total time tends to remain at about 0.4 to 0.5 of the breathing cycle throughout exercise, and V_T is increased by encroachment on both of the inspiratory and expiratory reserve volumes. By peak exercise, however, rarely does end inspiratory lung volume (V_T plus functional residual capacity) reach more than 90% of total lung capacity (in average, fit, healthy adults). EELV (volume of air in the lungs at the end of an expiration) falls approximately 0.5 to 1.0 L with moderate-to-heavy exercise. The fall in EELV tends to keep the tidal breath on the linear portion of the pressure–volume relationship of the lung and chest wall and may provide a beneficial lengthening of the inspiratory muscles.

Differences between the healthy young adult and the active older adult are outlined in the legend of Figure 3.4. Both have a similar flow–volume response with mild-to-moderate exercise; however, because of the increased fitness of the older subjects (relative to age), breathing strategy and pattern alter as they approach expiratory flow limitation.

EXERCISE LIMITATION

The major determinants of maximal aerobic capacity appear in Figure 3.6. Clinically, it is increasingly appreciated that exercise limitation or low $\dot{V}o_2$max achieved is multifactorial and, as such, is not typically limited by any single component of the O_2 transport/utilization process but rather by their collective quantitative interaction (55, 99, 102). Although several factors may be involved, one factor often predominates, with variable contributions to exercise intolerance from the other factors. Exercise in normal subjects is mainly limited by the cardiovascular system. Many factors limit exercise in patients (Table 3.5). There are three major categories of exercise limitation with reduced $\dot{V}o_2$max: *cardiovascular limitation,* which includes the heart, pulmonary and systemic circulations, and blood (anemia, HbCO); *respiratory limitation,* which includes ventilatory (mechanical) and gas exchange factors; and *peripheral limitation,* which includes a broad spectrum of neuromuscular- and microvascular-related abnormalities that could impact tissue O_2 conductance, O_2 utilization, and mechanisms of contraction (66, 100). Abnormal symptom perception (e.g., breathlessness, fatigue) is also a factor that must be considered (156). As noted, in many disease states (e.g., heart failure, COPD), the underlying disease etiology may result in severe deconditioning, muscle loss, or wasting, which in turn may become the predominant limiting influence. In addition, patients with heart failure may develop marked pulmonary changes, including abnormalities in pulmonary function and significant pulmonary hypertension, both of which may contribute to reduced exercise tolerance. Similarly, the high right heart pressures may result in a cardiac-related limitation in patients with chronic obstructive lung disease.

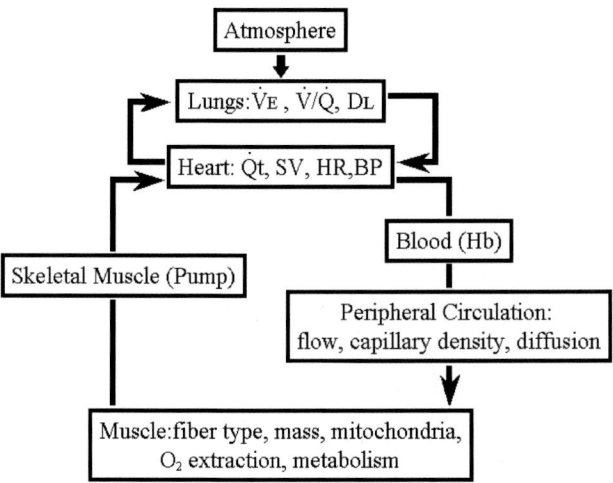

FIGURE 3.6. The schematic demonstrates the major determinants of maximal aerobic capacity ($\dot{V}o_2$max). The oxygen (O_2) transport/utilization processes that contribute to $\dot{V}o_2$max extend from the environment all the way to the muscle capillaries and mitochondria. Clinically, it is increasingly appreciated that exercise limitation or $\dot{V}o_2$max achieved is multifactorial and, as such, is not limited by any single component of the O_2 transport/utilization process but rather by their collective quantitative interaction.

TABLE 3.5. EXERCISE LIMITATION

Exercise Limitation

- Cardiovascular
    - Reduced stroke volume
    - Abnormal heart rate response
    - Abnormal systemic and pulmonary circulation
    - Hemodynamic consequences of dynamic hyperinflation
    - Abnormal blood (anemia, HbCO)
- Pulmonary
    - Ventilatory (mechanical)
        - Respiratory muscle dysfunction (dynamic hyperinflation)
    - Gas exchange
- Peripheral
    - Inactivity (disuse), loss of muscle mass (atrophy), neuromuscular dysfunction
    - Peripheral circulatory abnormalities
    - Reduced skeletal muscle oxidative capacity (metabolic myopathy)
    - Malnutrition
- Deconditioning
- Perceptual
- Motivation
- Environmental

Exercise limitation is often multifactorial
Adapted from Weisman IM, Zeballos RJ. Integrative approach to the interpretation of cardiopulmonary exercise testing. In: Weisman IM, Zeballos RJ, eds. *Clinical exercise testing: progress in respiratory research.* Basel: Karger, 2002:300–322, with permission.)

INTERPRETATION

Interpretative Strategies

Several approaches to interpretation of CPET results should be considered, as there is no consensus on any one interpretative strategy. Approaches that emphasize the mechanism for exercise limitation (i.e., ventilatory limitation to exercise) are limited by their lack of gold standard definition and the realization that exercise limitation is often multifactorial. Algorithms based on key measurements and conceptual framework (52, 157, 158) are limited by excessive reliance on single measurements. Interpretative error may result if that one measurement at a key branch point is wrong for whatever reason (i.e., anaerobic threshold). Standard algorithms are inadequate for the evaluation of patients with early/mild disease, in patients with combined disease (heart-lung), and in patients with variable responses that are borderline. Furthermore, although many interpretative algorithms have been developed, none have been clinically validated (52, 157, 158). Consequently, an integrative approach to CPET interpretation, which emphasizes the interrelationships, trending phenomena, and patterns of key variable responses in a clinical setting, is recommended (22, 39, 142).

Integrative Approach

An integrative approach to the interpretation of CPET is summarized in Figure 3.7 and includes the following: (a) reasons for testing, assessment of overall test quality and subject effort, and reason(s) for exercise cessation; (b) the identification of key measurements: initially $\dot{V}O_2$, then HR, $\dot{V}_E$, and SaO_2 with other measurements evaluated subsequently based on the reasons for which CPET was obtained; (c) determination of whether the measurements are normal or abnormal compared with appropriate (normal) reference values (Table 3.4); (d) attention to trending phenomena (i.e., submaximal through maximal exercise results) as reflected in graphic analysis for important relationships; (e) evaluation of patterns of responses and limitations(s) to exercise, including a determination of physiologic versus nonphysiologic basis; (f) consideration of conditions/clinical entities that may be

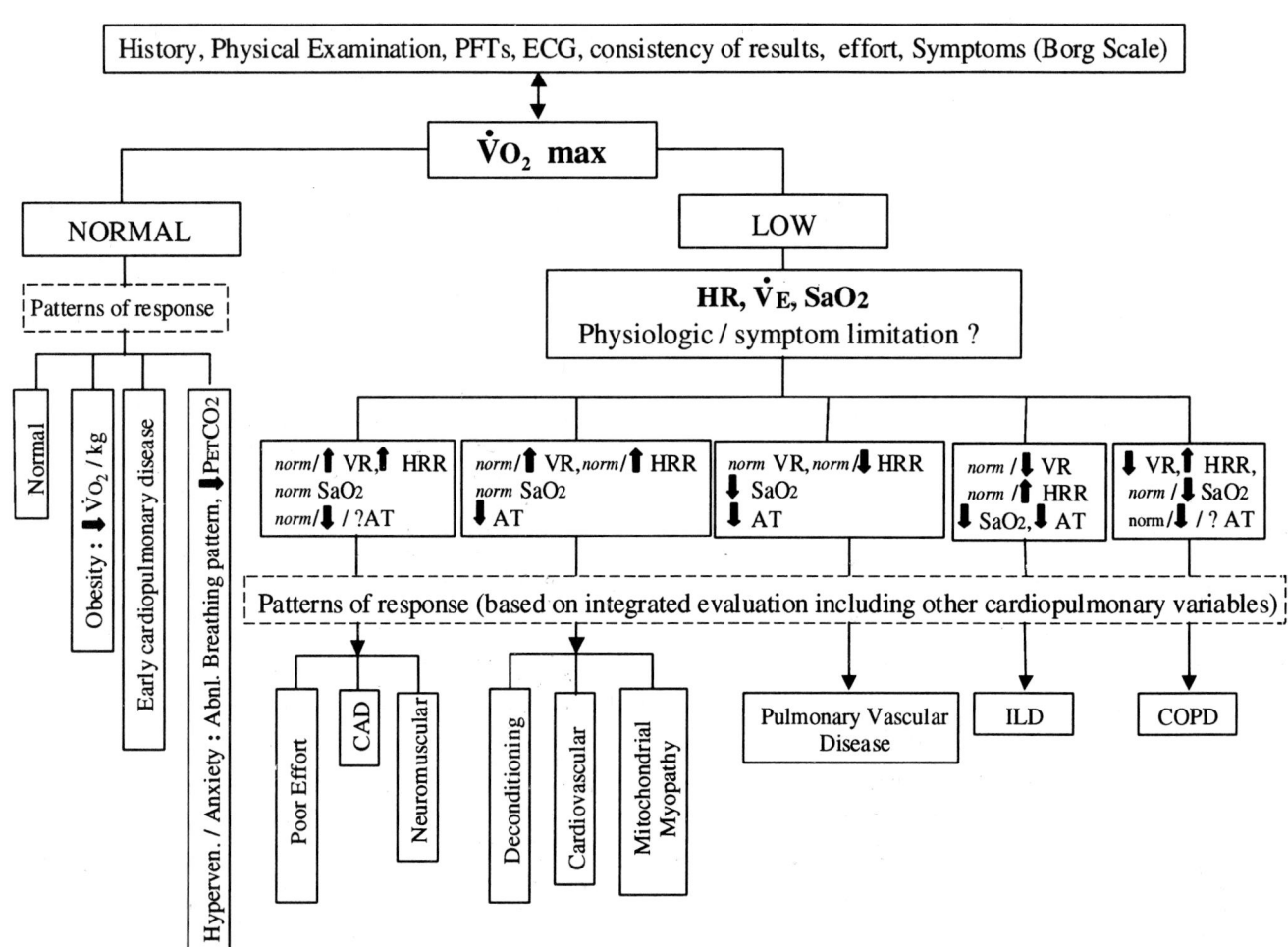

FIGURE 3.7. Integrative approach to interpretation of a cardiopulmonary exercise test. (Adapted from Weisman IM, Zeballos RJ. Clinical exercise testing. *Clin Chest Med* 2001;22:679–701, with permission.)

associated with these patterns; and (g) correlation of exercise results with the patient's clinical information, including level of physical activity and results of other tests (i.e., PFT).

The selection of an appropriate set of reference values should be a function of the patient population, age, height, weight, sex, and physical activity and may vary from laboratory to laboratory (52, 123, 124). Different sets of peak reference values may have a significant impact on the interpretation of CPET results (39).

Evaluation of Cardiopulmonary Exercise Testing Results

A normal $\dot{V}o_2$ peak reflects a normal exercise capacity and provides reassurance that no significant functional abnormality exists. A reduced $\dot{V}o_2$ peak is the starting point in the evaluation of reduced exercise capacity. Typical CPET response patterns for several clinical conditions, including chronic heart failure, COPD, ILD, pulmonary vascular disease, obesity, and deconditioning are presented in Table 3.6. This table is admittedly oversimplified and does not permit the wide range of responses that may be seen for instance within a full spectrum (mild to severe) of patients with COPD or heart disease. It must be clearly appreciated that significant overlap exists in the response patterns of patients with different cardiopulmonary diseases to exercise. Furthermore, wide confidence intervals for exercise responses in normal patients are also noted. In addition, patients often have coexisting conditions (e.g., obesity, deconditioning) that may contribute to exercise intolerance.

Cardiovascular Disease

Many factors contribute to exercise intolerance in patients with cardiovascular disease, including inadequate O_2 delivery, abnormalities in the distribution of the peripheral circulation, skeletal muscle abnormalities (e.g., O_2 utilization, atrophy), deconditioning, and pulmonary abnormalities (63, 159–161). In patients with cardiovascular disease, exercise stops prematurely with attainment of a lower $\dot{V}o_2$ owing to these factors. Early onset metabolic acidosis is manifested by a reduced AT. O_2 pulse, as an indirect measure of reduced stroke volume (assuming normal $Cao_2 - Cvo_2$ content), is reduced and cardiac output is maintained almost exclusively by increases in HR (49). Peak HR may not be attained; however, this may be highly variable and a function of the type and severity of the heart disease (49). The reduced $\dot{V}o_2$ peak and the early exercise cessation are usually associated with a reduced $\dot{V}emax$ but with considerable ventilatory reserve and no arterial desaturation. Increases in Vd/Vt and $\dot{V}e/\dot{V}co_2$ owing to reduced pulmonary perfusion consequent to reduced cardiac output are also observed (162). The presence of a reduced ventilatory reserve (high $\dot{V}e/MVV$) in these patients may signal the presence of combined cardiovascular and respiratory limitation (39, 59).

In some patients with left ventricular dysfunction, mechanical constraints to breathing may be evident without a high $\dot{V}e/MVV$ relationship. Figure 3.8 shows an example of the flow–volume response to exercise in a patient with a history of congestive heart failure. Despite apparent room to increase EELV, in the setting of severe expiratory flow limitation, the patient continues to breathe near residual volume,

TABLE 3.6. USUAL CARDIOPULMONARY EXERCISE RESPONSE PATTERNS

Measurements	Heart Failure	Chronic Obstructive Pulmonary Disease	Interstitial Lung Disease	Pulmonary Vascular Disease	Obesity	Deconditioned
$\dot{V}o_2$max or $\dot{V}o_2$peak	Decreased	Decreased	Decreased	Decreased	Decreased for actual, normal for ideal weight	Decreased
Anaerobic threshold	Decreased	Normal/decreased/ indeterminate	Normal or decreased	Decreased	Normal	Normal or decreased
Peak heart rate	Variable, usually normal	Decreased, normal in mild	Decreased	Normal/slightly decreased	Normal/slightly decreased	Normal/slightly decreased
Oxygen pulse	Decreased	Normal or decreased	Normal or decreased	Decreased	Normal	Decreased
[(Peak $\dot{V}e$/MVV) × 100]	Normal or decreased	Increased	Normal or increased	Normal	Normal or increased	Normal
$\dot{V}e/\dot{V}co_2$ (at AT)	Normal or increased	Increased	Increased	Increased	Normal	Normal
Vd/Vt	Increased	Increased	Increased	Increased	Normal	Normal
Pao_2	Normal	Variable	Decreased	Decreased	Normal/may increase	Normal
$Pao_2 - Pao_2$	Normal	Variable, usually increased	Increased	Increased	May decrease	Normal

Decreased, normal, and increased with respect to normal response.
Modified from multiple sources (39,52,166).
$\dot{V}o_2$, oxygen consumption; $\dot{V}e$, minute ventilation; MVV, maximum voluntary ventilation; $\dot{V}co_2$, carbon dioxide production; AT, anaerobic threshold; Vd/Vt, dead space/tidal volume; Pao_2, arterial blood partial pressure of oxygen; $Pao_2 - Pao_2$, alveolar-arterial partial pressure of oxygen difference.

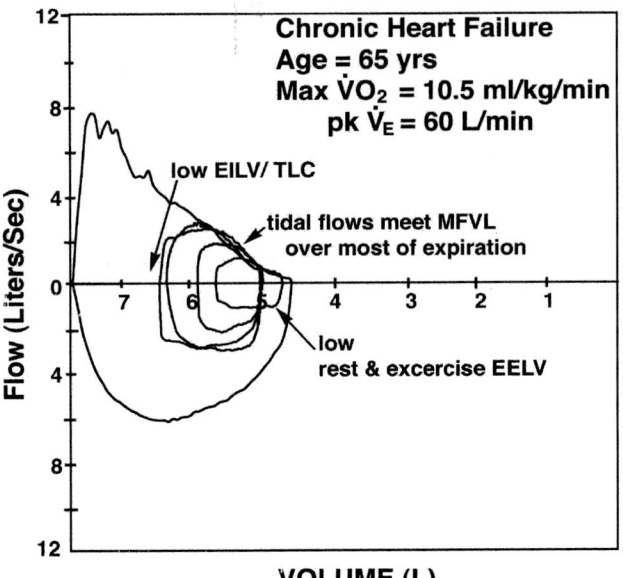

FIGURE 3.8. Flow–volume responses to exercise in a patient with stable congestive heart failure. Shown are rest, mild, moderate, and peak exercise tidal flow–volume loops plotted within the maximal flow–volume envelope obtained after exercise. Despite room to increase the end expiratory lung volume to avoid significant expiratory flow limitation, this subject continued to breathe near residual volume throughout exercise.

even at maximal exercise. This altered breathing strategy may be owing to the less compliant lungs of the patient with congestive heart failure combined with weak inspiratory muscles but may contribute to exercise intolerance (159).

Pulmonary Vascular Disease

Patients with pulmonary vascular disease are likewise usually cardiovascular limited, with a normal ventilatory reserve but with an abnormal breathing strategy consisting of rapid respiratory frequency and low V_T. A spectrum of pulmonary gas exchange abnormalities, including evidence of inefficient ventilation (increased $\dot{V}E/\dot{V}CO_2$), increased dead-space ventilation (abnormal V_D/V_T responses), and arterial desaturation with abnormal widening of the $P_{AO_2} - Pa_{O_2}$, are seen (49, 52, 78–80, 123).

Deconditioning

Physical inactivity for a variety of reasons is the main cause of deconditioning or unfitness (106, 163, 164). In deconditioning, early cessation of exercise is associated with low/low normal $\dot{V}O_2$ peak, normal or early onset of metabolic acidosis (normal/low AT), a reduced O_2 pulse, and little/no HRR but with increased HR at submaximal levels of $\dot{V}O_2$. There is significant ventilatory reserve and no abnormal pulmonary gas exchange. Deconditioning is often difficult to distinguish from early or mild heart disease (49, 52, 58). Although mitochondrial myopathy occurs much less frequently, recent

work has suggested that it also be included within the differential diagnosis (60). Deconditioning commonly coexists in patients with chronic illness, including those with heart and lung disease and in patients with mitochondrial myopathy. Response to an aerobic training regimen with monitoring of responses ($\dot{V}O_2$, O_2 pulse, AT, HR) may help to distinguish between heart disease and deconditioning, but not necessarily between deconditioning and mitochondrial myopathy (60).

Chronic Obstructive Pulmonary Disease

The exercise response pattern in a patient with COPD usually depends on the stage of disease. Consequently, a spectrum of exercise response patterns can be seen. Although patients with mild COPD have an essentially normal exercise response pattern with normal/near normal exercise capacity, patients with moderate/severe COPD will usually have reduced $\dot{V}O_2$ peak and work rate (65, 165, 166). One of the distinguishing features of many patients with COPD is a reduced ventilatory reserve ($\dot{V}Emax/MVV$ approaching or exceeding 100%) with attainment of low $\dot{V}O_2$ peak, suggesting ventilatory limitation to exercise (52). There is usually significant HRR, a reflection that the cardiovascular system has been relatively unstressed. In a retrospective study of patients with COPD categorized as mild, moderate, or severe, as disease severity progressed, $\dot{V}O_2$max and ventilatory reserve decreased and HRR increased (167). Blunted V_T and IC responses owing to dynamic hyperinflation are associated with increased work of breathing and dyspnea (67, 70, 72). Exercise limitation in COPD, however, is multifactorial.

In patients with COPD, the AT response may be normal, low, or indeterminate. Early onset metabolic acidosis (low AT) usually reflects deconditioning owing to physical inactivity and/or skeletal muscle dysfunction, including alterations in exercise-related substrate levels, especially glutamate (163, 168). The O_2 pulse is usually (but not invariably) proportionately reduced to $\dot{V}O_2$max owing to ventilatory limitation, deconditioning, and possibly hypoxemia. Reduction in O_2 pulse, as has been suggested, may also reflect the hemodynamic consequences of dynamic hyperinflation (169). Other respiratory abnormalities include increasing dynamic hyperinflation (IC decreases with exercise), inefficiency of ventilation ($\dot{V}E/\dot{V}CO_2$) owing to increased deadspace ventilation with abnormal V_D/V_T responses, alveolar hypoventilation with Pa_{CO_2} not changing or increasing compared with normal levels, and hypoxemia (52, 58, 65, 123). It has recently been suggested that in advanced COPD, the likelihood of developing CO_2 retention during exercise with marked $\dot{V}/\dot{Q}$ inequalities primarily reflects the severe mechanical constraints on ventilation owing to lung hyperinflation (170). Pa_{O_2} may be variable but is more often reduced in patients with moderate/severe COPD; $P_{AO_2} - Pa_{O_2}$ usually increases abnormally, especially when Pa_{O_2} decreases.

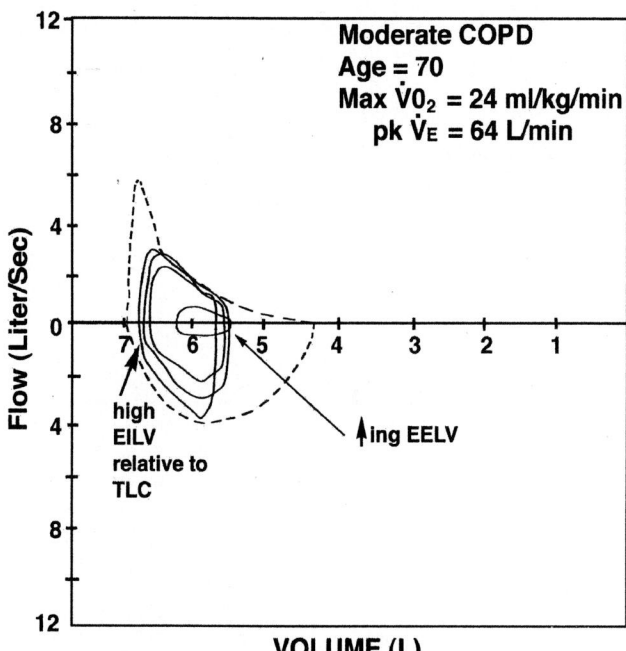

FIGURE 3.9. Flow–volume response to exercise in a patient with moderate COPD. Note unlike the healthy young adult (Fig 3.4) or the older highly fit adult, end expiratory lung volume begins to rise with the onset of exercise, reflecting early expiratory flow limitation. By moderate levels of exercise, the entire tidal breath reaches the maximal expiratory flows available. Thus, little ventilatory reserve is available for increasing ventilation by peak exercise. (From Johnson BD, Beck KC, Zeballos RJ, et al. Advances in pulmonary laboratory testing. *Chest* 1999;116:1377–1387, with permission.)

Figure 3.9 shows an example of the flow–volume responses to exercise in a patient with moderate COPD and average age-related fitness. Unlike the healthy subjects (Fig. 3.4), this patient demonstrates an increase in EELV with the onset of exercise and is constrained by significant expiratory flow limitation and an end inspiratory lung volume that approaches total lung capacity by peak exercise.

Interstitial Lung Disease

$\dot{V}O_2$peak and peak work rate are usually reduced. A spectrum of ventilatory and pulmonary gas exchange abnormalities are seen. A reduced ventilatory reserve (high $\dot{V}E$/MVV) and ventilatory limitation to exercise are often seen in patients with ILD. However, a recent retrospective analysis of patients with interstitial pulmonary fibrosis, has suggested that the ventilatory reserve is normal and that exercise is cardiovascular/pulmonary circulatory limited (171). The AT may be normal or reduced reflecting pulmonary circulatory involvement, skeletal muscle dysfunction, or deconditioning. A combined cardiovascular and respiratory limitation may exist. Rapid shallow breathing (high respiratory rate, low V_T, low IC and, consequently, high V_T-to-IC ratio) occurs commonly as does evidence of inefficient ventilation ($\uparrow \dot{V}E/\dot{V}CO_2$) in response to increases in V_D/V_T. Impressive arterial desat-

uration with abnormal widening of $P_{AO_2} - P_{aO_2}$ is usually seen (44, 61, 75, 76).

Obesity

$\dot{V}O_2$ as percentage of predicted can be normal or low in obese patients; however, when expressed as $\dot{V}O_2$ per kilogram body weight, it is low and with increasing obesity (disproportionately lower). There is an excessive metabolic requirement manifested by an upwardly displaced $\dot{V}O_2$/work rate relationship with a normal slope (172). The $\dot{V}E$ at a given external work rate is higher as a reflection of increased mechanical work, but the ventilatory reserve ($\dot{V}E$/MVV) can be normal or increased. A trend toward abnormally increased respiratory rate and reduced V_T is often seen (173). Recent exercise tidal flow–volume loop analysis suggests that there is ventilatory constraint (flow limitation) during exercise, as obese subjects breathe at low lung volumes (138). HR is increased at submaximal work with attainment of normal or near normal peak HR with little or no HR reserve (174). Resting P_{aO_2} and $P_{AO_2} - P_{aO_2}$ may improve with exercise, reflecting improved V/Q relationships. Obesity is often associated with other conditions in negatively impacting exercise capacity.

SUMMARY/INTERPRETATION

The integrative approach to the interpretation of CPET results is evolving and requires attention to fundamental principles, including a systematic analysis of factors discussed previously (see section "Integrative Approach," Fig. 3.7, and Tables 3.3 through 3.6). Although reasonable, several assumptions used in this approach require additional study. Although widely used, relatively few studies have evaluated the sensitivity, specificity, and positive predictive value of a "patterns-based" approach of evaluating exercise responses for diagnosing and distinguishing different clinical entities. Furthermore, the impact of this approach on clinical decision making in well-established clinical entities remains incompletely characterized.

Well-designed and executed clinical studies that fulfill evidence-based criteria for systematic review of CPET results are becoming available and, hopefully, will provide answers to clinically relevant questions not immediately available.

ACKNOWLEDGMENTS

We would like to thank Renee Blumers for preparation of the manuscript. This work was supported by National Heart Lung and Blood Institute grant HL71478 and Department of Health and Human Services grant M01-RR00585, General Clinical Research Center Division of Research Resources, National Institutes of Health.

REFERENCES

1. Bassett DR, Vachon JA, Kirkland AO, et al. Energy cost of stair climbing and descending on the college alumnus questionnaire. *Med Sci Sports Exerc* 1997;29:1250–1254.

2. Pollock M, Roa J, Benditt J, et al. Estimation of ventilatory reserve by stair climbing: a study in patients with chronic airflow obstruction. *Chest* 1993;104:1378–1383.

3. Girish M, Trayner E Jr, Dammann O, et al. Symptom-limited stair climbing as a predictor of postoperative cardiopulmonary complications after high-risk surgery. *Chest* 2001;120:1147–1151.

4. Olsen GN, Bolton JW, Weinman DS, et al. Stair-climbing as an exercise test to predict the postoperative complications of lung resection. *Chest* 1991;99:587–590.

5. Holden DA, Rice TW, Stelmach K, et al. Exercise testing, 6-min walk and stair climb in the evaluation of patients at high risk of pulmonary resection. *Chest* 1992;102:1774–1779.

6. Brunelli A, Al Refai M, Monteverde M, et al. Stair climbing test predicts cardiopulmonary complications after lung resection. *Chest* 2002;121:1106–1110.

7. American Thoracic Society. ATS statement: guidelines for the six-minute walk test. *Am J Respir Crit Care Med* 2002;166:111–117.

8. Zeballos RJ, Weisman IM. Modalities of clinical exercise testing. In: Weisman IM, Zeballos RJ, eds. *Clinical exercise testing: progress in respiratory research.* Basel: Karger; 2002:30–42.

9. Guyatt GH, Pugsley SO, Sullivan MJ, et al. Effect of encouragement on walking test performance. *Thorax* 1984;39:818–822.

10. Solway S, Brooks D, Lacasse Y, et al. A qualitative systematic overview of the measurement properties of functional walk tests used in the cardiorespiratory domain. *Chest* 2001;119:256–270.

11. Cahalin L, Pappagianopoulos P, Prevost S, et al. The relationship of the 6-minute walk test to maximal oxygen consumption in transplant candidates with end-stage lung disease. *Chest* 1995;108:452–459.

12. Kadikar A, Maurer J, Kesten S. The six-minute walk test: a guide to assessment for lung transplantation. *J Heart Lung Transplantation* 1997;16:313–319.

13. Sciurba FC, Rogers RM, Keenan RJ, et al. Improvement in pulmonary function and elastic recoil after lung-reduction surgery for diffuse emphysema. *New Engl J Med* 1996;334:1095–1099.

14. Criner GJ, Cordova FC, Furukawa S, et al. Prospective randomized trial comparing bilateral lung volume reduction surgery to pulmonary rehabilitation in severe chronic obstructive pulmonary disease. *Am J Respir Crit Care Med* 1999;160:2018–2027.

15. Oga T, Nishimura K, Tsukino M, et al. The effects of oxitropium bromide on exercise performance in patients with stable chronic obstructive pulmonary disease. *Am J Respir Crit Care Med* 2000;161:1897–1901.

16. Roomi J, Johnson MM, Waters K, et al. Respiratory rehabilitation, exercise capacity, and quality of life in chronic airways disease in old age. *Age Ageing* 1996;25:12–16.

17. Redelmeier DA, Bayoumi AM, Goldstein RS, et al. Interpreting small differences in functional status: the six-minute walk test in chronic lung disease patients. *Am J Respir Crit Care Med* 1997;155:1278–1282.

18. Kessler R, Faller M, Fourgaut G, et al. Predictive factors of hospitalization for acute exacerbation in a series of 64 patients with chronic obstructive pulmonary disease. *Am J Respir Crit Care Med* 1999;159:158–164.

19. Miyamoto S, Nagaya N, Satoh T, et al. Clinical correlates and prognostic significance of six-minute walk test in patients with primary pulmonary hypertension: comparison with cardiopulmonary exercise testing. *Am J Respir Crit Care Med* 2000;161:487–492.

20. Bittner V, Weiner DH, Yusuf S, et al. Prediction of mortality and morbidity with a 6-minute walk test in patients with left ventricular dysfunction. *JAMA* 1993;270:1702–1707.

21. Enright PL, Sherrill DL. Reference equations for the six-minute walk in healthy adults. *Am J Respir Crit Care Med* 1998;158:1384–1387.

22. American Thoracic Society/American College of Chest Physicians. Statement on cardiopulmonary exercise testing. *Am J Respir Crit Care Med* 2003;167:211–277.

23. Nohria A, Eldrin L, Warner Stevenson L. Medical management of advanced heart failure. *JAMA* 2002;287:628–639.

24. Stevens D, Elpern E, Sharma K, et al. Comparison of hallway and treadmill six-minute walk tests. *Am J Respir Crit Care Med* 1999;160:1540–1543.

25. Singh SJ, Morgan MD, Scott S, et al. Development of a shuttle walking test of disability in patients with chronic airways obstruction. *Thorax* 1992;47:1019–1024.

26. Singh SJ, Morgan MD, Hardman AE, et al. Comparison of oxygen uptake during a conventional treadmill test and the shuttle walking test in chronic airflow limitation. *Eur Respir J* 1994;7:2016–2020.

27. Morales FJ, Martinez A, Mendez M, et al. A shuttle walk test for assessment of functional capacity in chronic heart failure. *Am Heart J* 1999;138:291–298.

28. American Thoracic Society. Guidelines for methacholine and exercise challenge testing-1999. *Am J Respir Crit Care Med* 2000;161:309–329.

29. Godfrey S. Clinical and physiological features. In: McFadden ER Jr, ed. *Exercise-induced asthma.* New York: Marcel Dekker Inc, 1999:11–45.

30. Cypcar D, Lemanske RF Jr. Asthma and exercise. *Clin Chest Med* 1994;15:351–368.

31. Beck KC, Offord KP, Scanlon PD. Bronchoconstriction occurring during exercise in asthmatic patients. *Am J Respir Crit Care Med* 1994;149:352–357.

32. National Institutes of Health. Expert panel report 2: guidelines for the diagnosis and management of asthma. Bethesda, MD: National Institutes of Health, National Heart, Lung, and Blood Institute; 1997; 97-4051.

33. Sterk PJ, Fabbri LM, Quanjer PH, et al. Airway responsiveness: standardized challenge testing with pharmacological, physical, and sensitizing stimuli in adults: report Working Party Standardization of Lung Function Tests, European Community for Steel and Coal: official statement of the European Respiratory Society. *Eur Respir J* 1993[Suppl];16:53–83.

34. Elliasson AH, Phillips YY, Rajagopal, KR, et al. Sensitivity and specificity of bronchial provocation testing: an evaluation of four techniques in exercise-induced bronchospasm. *Chest* 1992;102:347–355.

35. Zeballos RJ, Weisman IM, Connery SM, et al. Standard treadmill (STE) vs incremental cycle ergometry (IET) in the evaluation of airway hyperreactivity in unexplained dyspnea. *Am J Respir Crit Care Med* 1999;159:A419(abst).

36. ACC/AHA/ACP-ASIM guidelines for the management of patients with chronic stable angina: executive summary and recommendations. *Circulation* 1999;99:2829–2848.

37. ACC/AHA guidelines for exercise testing: a report of the American College of Cardiology/American Heart Association Task Force on practice guidelines (Committee on Exercise Testing). *J Am College Cardiol* 1997;30:260–315.

38. Weisman IM, Zeballos RJ. Clinical exercise testing. *Clin Chest Med* 2001;22:679–701.

39. Weisman IM, Zeballos RJ. Integrative approach to the interpretation of cardiopulmonary exercise testing. In: Weisman IM, Zeballos RJ, eds. *Clinical exercise testing: progress on respiratory research.* Basel: Karger, 2002:300–322.

40. Bye PT, Anderson SD, Woolcock AJ, et al. Bicycle endurance performances of patients with interstitial lung disease breathing air and oxygen. *Am Rev Respir Dis* 1982;126:1005–1012.

41. Carlson DJ, Ries AL, Kaplan RM. Prediction of maximum exercise tolerance in patients with COPD. *Chest* 1991;100:307–311.

42. Dillard TA, Piantadosi S, Rajagopal KR. Prediction of ventilation at maximal exercise in chronic airflow obstruction. *Am Rev Respir Dis* 1985;132:230–235.

43. Dillard TA, Hnatiuk OW, McCumber TR. Spirometric determinants in chronic obstructive pulmonary disease patients and normal subjects. *Am Rev Respir Dis* 1993;147:870–875.

44. Keogh BA, Lakatos E, Price D, et al. Importance of the lower respiratory tract in oxygen transfer: exercise testing in patients with interstitial and destructive lung disease. *Am Rev Respir Dis* 1984;129:S76–S80.

45. Sue DY, Oren A, Hansen JE, et al. Diffusing capacity for carbon monoxide as a predictor of gas exchange during exercise. *New Engl J Med* 1987;316:1301–1306.

46. Ries AL, Farrow JT, Clausen JL. Pulmonary function tests cannot predict exercise-induced hypoxemia in chronic obstructive pulmonary disease. *Chest* 1988;93:454–459.

47. Hamilton AL, Killian KJ, Summers E, et al. Muscle strength, symptom intensity, and exercise capacity in patients with cardiorespiratory disorders. *Am J Respir Crit Care Med* 1995;152:2021–2031.

48. Franciosa JA, Park M, Levine TB. Lack of correlation between exercise capacity and indexes of resting left ventricular performance in heart failure. *Am J Cardiol* 1981;47:33–39.

49. Weber KT, Janicki JS. *Cardiopulmonary exercise testing: physiologic principles and clinical application.* Philadelphia: WB Saunders, 1986.

50. Szlachcic J, Massie BM, Kramer FL, et al. Correlates and prognostic implication of exercise capacity in chronic congestive heart failure. *Am J Cardiol* 1985;55:1037–1042.

51. Punzel, PA, Ries AL, Kaplan RM, et al. Maximum intensity exercise training in patients with chronic obstructive pulmonary disease. *Chest* 1991;100:618–623.

52. Wasserman K, Hansen JE, Sue DY, et al. *Principles of exercise testing and interpretation,* 3rd ed. Philadelphia: Lippincott Williams & Wilkins, 1999.

53. Killian KJ, LeBlanc P, Martin DH, et al. Exercise capacity and ventilatory, circulatory, and symptom limitation in patients with chronic airflow limitation. *Am Rev Respir Dis* 1992;146:935–940.

54. Curtis JR, Deyo RA, Hudson LD. Health-related quality of life among patients with chronic obstructive pulmonary disease. *Thorax* 1994;49:162–170.

55. Jones NL, Killian KJ. Exercise limitation in health and disease. *New Engl J Med* 2000;343:632–641.

56. O'Donnell DE. Breathlessness in patients with chronic airflow limitation. *Chest* 1994;106:904–912.

57. Stelken AM, Younis LT, Jennison SH, et al. Prognostic value of cardiopulmonary exercise testing using percent achieved of predicted peak oxygen uptake for patients with ischemic and dilated cardiomyopathy. *J Am Coll Cardiol* 1996;27:345–352.

58. Weisman IM, Zeballos RJ. An integrated approach to the interpretation of cardiopulmonary exercise testing. *Clin Chest Med* 1994;15:421–445.

59. Weisman IM, Zeballos RJ. Clinical evaluation of unexplained dyspnea. *Cardiologia* 1996;41:621–634.

60. Flaherty KR, Wald J, Weisman IM, et al. Unexplained exertional limitation: characterization in a large cohort discovered to have mitochondrial myopathy. *Am J Respir Crit Care Med* 2001;164:425–432.

61. Martinez FJ, Stanopoulos I, Acero R, et al. Graded comprehensive cardiopulmonary exercise testing in the evaluation of dyspnea unexplained by routine evaluation. *Chest* 1994;105:168–174.

62. Weisman IM, Zeballos RJ. Cardiopulmonary exercise testing. *Pulmonary Crit Care Update Ser* 1995;11:1–8.

63. Mancini DM, Eisen H, Kussmaul W, et al. Value of peak oxygen consumption for optimal timing of cardiac transplantation in ambulatory patients with heart failure. *Circulation* 1991;83:778–786.

64. Stevenson LW, Steimle AE, Fonarow G, et al. Improvement in exercise capacity of candidates awaiting heart transplantation. *J Am Coll Cardiol* 1995;25:163–170.

65. Gallagher CG. Exercise limitation and clinical exercise testing in chronic obstructive pulmonary disease. *Clin Chest Med* 1994;15:305–326.

66. Richardson RS, Sheldon P, Poole DC, et al. Evidence of skeletal muscle metabolic reserve during whole body exercise in patients with chronic obstructive pulmonary disease. *Am J Respir Crit Care Med* 1999;159:881–885.

67. O'Donnell DE, Bertley JC, Chau LKL, et al. Qualitative aspects of exertional breathlessness in chronic airflow limitation. *Am J Respir Crit Care Med* 1997;155:109–115.

68. Belman MJ, Botnick WC, Shin JW. Inhaled bronchodilators reduce dynamic hyperinflation during exercise in patients with chronic obstructive pulmonary disease. *Am J Respir Crit Care Med* 1996;153:967–975.

69. Martinez FJ, Montes de Oca M, Whyte RI, et al. Lung-volume reduction improves dyspnea, dynamic hyperinflation, and respiratory muscle function. *Am J Respir Crit Care Med* 1997;155:1984–1990.

70. O'Donnell DE, Lam M, Webb KA. Measurement of symptoms, lung hyperinflation, and endurance during exercise in chronic obstructive pulmonary disease. *Am J Respir Crit Care Med* 1998;158:1557–1565.

71. O'Donnell DE, Lam M, Webb KA. Spirometric correlates of improvement in exercise performance after anticholinergic therapy in chronic obstructive pulmonary disease. *Am J Respir Crit Care Med* 1999;160:542–549.

72. O'Donnell DE. Exercise limitation and clinical exercise testing in chronic obstructive pulmonary disease. In: Weisman IM, Zeballos RJ, eds. *Clinical exercise testing: progress in respiratory research.* Basel: Karger, 2002:138–158.

73. Harris-Eze AO, Sridhar G, Clemens RE, et al. Oxygen improves maximal exercise performance in interstitial lung disease. *Am J Respir Crit Care Med* 1994;150:1616–1622.

74. Marciniuk DD, Gallagher CG. Clinical exercise testing in interstitial lung disease. *Clin Chest Med* 1994;15:287–303.

75. Risk C, Epler GR, Gaensler EA. Exercise alveolar-arterial oxygen pressure difference in interstitial lung disease. *Chest* 1984;85:69–74.

76. Watters LC, King TE, Schwarz MI, et al. A clinical, radiographic, and physiologic scoring system for the longitudinal assessment of patients with idiopathic pulmonary fibrosis. *Am Rev Respir Dis* 1986;133:97–103.

77. Krishnan BS, Marciniuk DD. Cardiorespiratory responses during exercise in interstitial lung disease. In: Weisman IM, Zeballos RJ, eds. *Clinical exercise testing: progress in respiratory research.* Basel: Karger, 2002:186–199.

78. D'Alonzo GE, Gianotti LA, Pohil RL, et al. Comparison of progressive exercise performance of normal subjects and patients with primary pulmonary hypertension. *Chest* 1987:57–62.

79. Janicki JS, Weber KT, Likoff MJ, et al. Exercise testing to evaluate patients with pulmonary vascular disease. *Am Rev Respir Dis* 1984;129:S93–S95.

80. Sun XG, Hansen JR, Oudiz RJ, et al. Exercise pathophysiology in patients with primary pulmonary hypertension. *Circulation* 2001;104:429–435.

81. Rubin LJ. Primary pulmonary hypertension. *Chest* 1993;104:236–250.

82. Nixon PA, Orenstein DM, Kelasy SF, et al. The prognostic value of exercise testing in patients with cystic fibrosis. *New Engl J Med* 1992;327:1785–1788.

83. Moser C, Tirakitsoontorn P, Nussbaum E, et al. Muscle size and cardiorespiratory response to exercise in cystic fibrosis. *Am J Respir Crit Care Med* 2000;162:1823–1827.

84. Bolliger CT, Perruchoud AP. Functional evaluation of the lung resection candidate. *Eur Respir J* 1998;11:198–212.

85. Gilbreth EM, Weisman IM. Role of exercise stress testing in preoperative evaluation of patients for lung resection. *Clin Chest Med* 1994;15:389–403.

86. Morice RC, Peters EJ, Ryan MB, et al. Exercise testing in the evaluation of patients at high risk for complications from lung resection. *Chest* 1992;101:356–361.

87. Olsen GN. The evolving role of exercise testing prior to lung resection. *Chest* 1989;95:218–225.

88. Bolliger CT, Jordan P, Soler M, et al. Exercise capacity as a predictor of postoperative complications in lung resection candidates. *Am J Respir Crit Care Med* 1995;151:1472–1480.

89. Morice RC, Walsh GL, Ali MK, et al. Redefining the lowest exercise peak oxygen consumption acceptable for lung resection of high risk patients. *Chest* 1996;110:161S.

90. Wyser C, Stulz P, Soler M, et al. Prospective evaluation of an algorithm for the functional assessment of lung resection candidates. *Am J Respir Crit Care Med* 1999;159:1450–1456.

91. Older P, Smith R, Courtney P, et al. Preoperative evaluation of cardiac failure and ischemia in elderly patients by cardiopulmonary exercise testing. *Chest* 1993;104:701–704.

92. Benditt JO, Lewis S, Wood DE, et al. Lung volume reduction surgery improves maximal O$_2$ consumption, maximal minute ventilation, O$_2$ pulse, and dead space–to–tidal volume ratio during leg ergometry. *Am J Respir Crit Care Med* 1997;156:561–566.

93. Cordova F, O'Brien G, Furukawa S, et al. Stability of improvements in exercise performance and quality of life following bilateral lung volume reduction surgery in severe COPD. *Chest* 1997;112:907–915.

94. Ferguson GT, Fernandez E, Zamora MR, et al. Improved exercise performance following lung volume reduction surgery for emphysema. *Am J Respir Crit Care Med* 1998;157:1195–1203.

95. Oswald-Mammosser M, Kessler R, Massard G, et al. Effect of lung volume reduction surgery on gas exchange and pulmonary hemodynamics at rest and during exercise. *Am J Respir Crit Care Med* 1998;158:1020–1025.

96. Sciurba FC. Early and long-term functional outcomes following lung volume reduction surgery. *Clin Chest Med* 1997;18:259–276.

97. Howard DK, Iademarco EJ, Trulock EP. The role of cardiopulmonary exercise testing in lung and heart-lung transplantation. *Clin Chest Med* 1994;15:405–420.

98. Williams TJ, Patterson GA, McClean PA, et al. Maximal exercise testing in single and double lung transplant recipients. *Am Rev Respir Dis* 1992;145:101–105.

99. Dempsey JA, Babcock MA. An integrative view of limitations to muscular performance. *Adv Exp Med Biol* 1995;384:393–399.

100. Evans AB, Al-Himyary AJ, Hrovat MI, et al. Abnormal skeletal muscle oxidative capacity after lung transplantation by 31P-MRS. *Am J Respir Crit Care Med* 1997;155:615–621.

101. Hall MJ, Snell GI, Side EA, et al. Exercise, potassium, and muscle deconditioning post-thoracic organ transplantation. *J Appl Physiol* 1994;77:2784–2790.

102. Wagner PD. Determination of maximal oxygen transport and utilization. *Annu Rev Physiol* 1996;58:21–50.

103. ACCP/AACVPR. PD. Evidence-based guidelines for pulmonary rehabilitation. *Chest* 1997;112:1363–1396.

104. American Thoracic Society. Official statement: pulmonary rehabilitation, 1999. *Am J Respir Crit Care Med* 1999;159:1666–1682.

105. Casaburi R, Patessio A, Loli F, et al. Reductions in exercise lactic acidosis and ventilation as a result of exercise training in patients with obstructive lung disease. *Am Rev Respir Dis* 1991;143:9–18.

106. Gosselink R, Troosters T, Decramer M. Peripheral muscle weakness contributes to exercise limitation in COPD. *Am J Respir Crit Care Med* 1996;153:976–980.

107. Casaburi R. Physiologic responses to training. *Clin Chest Med* 1994;15:215–227.

108. Maltais F, LeBlanc P, Simard C, et al. Skeletal muscle adaptation to endurance training in patients with chronic obstructive pulmonary disease. *Am J Respir Crit Care Med* 1996;154:442–447.

109. Casaburi R, Porszaz J, Burns MR, et al. Physiologic benefits of exercise training in rehabilitation of patients with severe chronic obstructive pulmonary disease. *Am J Respir Crit Care Med* 1997;155:1541–1551.

110. Maltais F, LeBlanc P, Jobin J, et al. Intensity of training and physiologic adaptation in patients with chronic obstructive pulmonary disease. *Am J Respir Crit Care Med* 1997;1997:555–561.

111. Ortega F, Toral J, Dejudo P, et al. Comparison of effects of strength and endurance training in patients with chronic obstructive pulmonary disease. *Am J Respir Crit Care Med* 2002;166:669–674.

112. Weisman IM, Lynch JL, Martinez FJ. Role of physiological assessment in advanced interstitial lung disease. In: Maurer J, ed. *Non-neoplastic advanced lung disease. lung, health, biology series.* New York: Marcel Dekker, 2003;179–247.

113. Cotes JE. Rating respiratory disability: a report on behalf of a working group of the European Society for Clinical Physiology. *Eur Respir J* 1990;3:1074–1077.

114. Smith DD. Pulmonary impairment/disability evaluation: controversies and criticisms. *Clin Pulmon Med* 1995;2:334–343.

115. Sue DY. Exercise testing in the evaluation of impairment and disability. *Clin Chest Med* 1994;15:369–387.

116. Gordon EE. Energy costs of activities in health and disease. *Arch Intern Med* 1958;101:702.

117. American Thoracic Society. Evaluation of impairment/disability secondary to respiratory disorders. *Am Rev Respir Dis* 1986;133:1205–1209.

118. Agostoni P, Smith DD, Schoen RB, et al. Evaluation of breathlessness in asbestos workers. *Am Rev Respir Dis* 1987;135:812–816.

119. Sue DY, Oren A, Hansen JE, et al. Lung function and exercise performance in smoking and nonsmoking asbestos-exposed workers. *Am Rev Respir Dis* 1986;132:612–618.

120. Ortega F, Montemayor T, Sanchez A, et al. Role of cardiopulmonary exercise testing and the criteria used to determine

disability in patients with severe chronic obstructive pulmonary disease. *Am J Respir Crit Care Med* 1994;150:747–751.

121. Beck KC, Weisman IM. Methods for cardiopulmonary exercise testing. In: Weisman IM, Zeballos RJ, eds. *Clinical exercise testing: progress on respiratory research.* Basel: Karger; 2002:43–59.

122. Beaver WL, Wasserman K, Whipp BJ. On-line computer analysis and breath-by-breath graphical display of exercise function tests. *J Appl Physiol* 1973;34:128–132.

123. Jones NL. Clinical exercise testing, 4th ed. Philadelphia: WB Saunders, 1997.

124. Zeballos RJ, Weisman IM. Behind the scenes of cardiopulmonary exercise testing. *Clin Chest Med* 1994;15:193–213.

125. Marciniuk DD, Watts R, Gallagher CG. Reproducibility of incremental maximal cycle ergometer testing in patients with restrictive lung disease. *Thorax* 1993;48:894–898.

126. Zeballos RJ, Weisman IM, Connery SM. Comparison of pulmonary gas exchange measurements between incremental and constant work exercise above the anaerobic threshold. *Chest* 1998;113:602–611.

127. Fletcher GF, Balady G, Froelicher VF, et al. Exercise standards: a statement for healthcare professionals from the American Heart Association. *Circulation* 1995;91:580–615.

128. Myers J, Voodi L, Umann T, et al. A survey of exercise testing: methods, utilizations, interpretation, and safety in the VAHCS. *J Cardiopulm Rehabil* 2000;20:251–258.

129. *ACSM's guidelines for exercise testing and prescription,* 4th ed. Philadelphia: Lea & Febiger, 1991.

130. *ACSM's guidelines for exercise testing and prescription,* 6th ed. Philadelphia: Lippincott Williams & Wilkins, 2000.

131. Cotes JE. *Lung function: assessment and application in medicine,* 5th ed. Oxford: Blackwell Science, 1993:54–58.

132. Astrand PO, Rodahl K. *Textbook of work physiology: physiological bases of exercise,* 3rd ed. New York: McGraw-Hill, 1986.

133. Shephard RJ. Tests of maximum oxygen intake: a critical review. *Sports Med* 1984;1:99–124.

134. Cumming GR, Borysyk LM. Criteria for maximum oxygen uptake in men over 40 in a population survey. *Med Sci Sports Exerc* 1972;14:18–22.

135. Myers J, Walsh D, Buchanan N, et al. Can maximal cardiopulmonary capacity be recognized by a plateau in oxygen uptake? *Chest* 1989;96:1312–1316.

136. Stringer WW, Hansen JE, Wasserman K. Cardiac output estimated noninvasively from oxygen uptake during exercise. *J Appl Physiol* 1997;82:908–912.

137. Babb TG. Mechanical ventilatory constraints in aging, lung disease, and obesity: perspective and brief review. *Med Sci Sports Exerc* 1999;31[Suppl]:S12–S22.

138. Johnson BD, Weisman IM, Zeballos RJ, et al. Emerging concepts in the evaluation of ventilatory limitation during exercise. *Chest* 1999;116:488–503.

139. Johnson BD, Beck KC, Zeballos RJ, et al. Advances in pulmonary laboratory testing. *Chest* 1999;116:1377–1387.

140. Marciniuk DD, Sridhar G, Clemens RE, et al. Lung volumes and expiratory flow limitation during exercise in interstitial lung disease. *J Appl Physiol* 1994;77:963–973.

141. Myers J, Ashley E. Dangerous curves: a perspective on exercise, lactate, and the anaerobic threshold. *Chest* 1997;111:787–795.

142. ERS task force on standardization of clinical exercise testing. Clinical exercise testing with reference to lung diseases: indications, standardization, and interpretation strategies. *Eur Respir J* 1997;10:2662–2689.

143. Sue DY, Wasserman K, Moricca RB, et al. Metabolic acidosis during exercise in patients with chronic obstructive pulmonary disease: use of V-slope method for anaerobic threshold determination. *Chest* 1988;94:931–938.

144. Chua TP, Ponikowski P, Harrington D, et al. Clinical correlates and prognostic significance of the ventilatory response to exercise in chronic heart failure. *J Am Coll Cardiol* 1997;29:1585–1590.

145. Anthonisen NR, Fleetham JA. Ventilation: total, alveolar, and dead space. In: Fishman AP, ed. *Handbook of physiology, the respiratory system: gas exchange.* Bethesda, MD: American Physiological Society, 1987:113–117.

146. Lewis DA, Sietsema KE, Casaburi R, et al. Inaccuracy of noninvasive estimates of V_D/V_T in clinical exercise testing. *Chest* 1994;106:1476–1480.

147. Wagner PD. Ventilation-perfusion matching during exercise. *Chest* 1992;101:S192–S198.

148. AARC clinical practice guideline: exercise testing for evaluation of hypoxemia and/or desaturation. *Respir Care* 1992;37:907–912.

149. Ries AL, Farrow JT, Clausen JL. Accuracy of two ear oximeters at rest and during exercise in pulmonary patients. *Am Rev Respir Dis* 1985;132:685–689.

150. Severinghaus JW, Naifeh KH, Koh SO. Errors in 14 pulse oximeters during profound hypoxia. *J Clin Monitoring* 1989;5:72–81.

151. Zeballos RJ, Weisman IM. Reliability of noninvasive oximetry in black subjects during exercise and hypoxia. *Am Rev Respir Dis* 1991;144:1240–1244.

152. Hansen JE, Casaburi R. Validity of ear oximetry in clinical testing. *Chest* 1987;91:333–337.

153. Borg GAV. Psychophysical bases of perceived exertion. *Med Sci Sports Exerc* 1982;14:377–381.

154. Aitken RC. Measurement of feelings using visual analogue scales. *Proc Roy Soc Med* 1969;62:989–993.

155. Mahler DA, Guyatt GH, Jones PW. Clinical measurement of dyspnea. In: Mahler DA, ed. *Dyspnea: lung biology in health and disease series.* New York: Marcel Dekker, 1998:149–198.

156. Killian KJ, Jones NL. Mechanisms of exertional dyspnea. *Clin Chest Med* 1994;15:247–257.

157. Neuberg GW, Friedman SH, Weiss MB, et al. Cardiopulmonary exercise testing: the clinical value of gas exchange data. *Arch Intern Med* 1988;148:2221–2226.

158. Eschenbacher WL, Mannina A. An algorithm for the interpretation of cardiopulmonary exercise tests. *Chest* 1990;97:263–267.

159. Johnson BD, Beck KC, Olson LJ, et al. Ventilatory constraints during exercise in patients with chronic heart failure. *Chest* 2000;117:321–332.

160. Mancini DM. Pulmonary factors limiting exercise capacity in patients with heart failure. *Prog Cardiovasc Dis* 1995;37:347–370.

161. Mancini D, Reichek N, Chance B, et al. Contribution of skeletal muscle atrophy to exercise intolerance and altered muscle metabolism in heart failure. *Circulation* 1992;85:1364–1373.

162. Myers J, Froelicher VF. Hemodynamic determinants of exercise capacity in chronic heart failure. *Ann Intern Med* 1991;115:377–386.

163. Engelen MPKJ, Schols AMWJ, Does JD, et al. Exercise-induced lactate increase in relation to muscle substrates in patients with chronic obstructive pulmonary disease. *Am J Respir Crit Care Med* 2000;162:1697–1704.

164. Saltin B, Blomquist G, Mitchell JH, et al. Response to exercise after bed rest and after training. *Circulation* 968;38[Suppl 7]:1–78.

165. Babb TG, Viggiano R, Hurley B, et al. Effect of mild-to-moderate airflow limitation on exercise capacity. *J Appl Physiol* 1991;70:223–230.

166. Marciniuk DD, Gallagher CG. Clinical exercise testing in chronic airflow limitation. *Med Clin North Am* 1996;80:565–587.

167. LoRusso TJ, Belman MJ, Elashoff JD, et al. Prediction of maximal exercise capacity in obstructive and restrictive pulmonary disease. *Chest* 1993;104:1748–1754.

168. Maltais F, Simard AA, Simard C, et al. Oxidative capacity of the skeletal muscle and lactic acid kinetics during exercise in normal subjects and in patients with COPD. *Am J Respir Crit Care Med* 1996;153:288–293.

169. Montes de Oca M, Rassulo J, Celli BR. Respiratory muscle and cardiopulmonary function during exercise in very severe COPD. *Am J Respir Crit Care Med* 1996;154:1284–1289.

170. O'Donnell DE, D'Arsigney C, Fitzpatrick M, et al. Exercise hypercapnia in advanced chronic obstructive pulmonary disease. *Am J Respir Crit Care Med* 2002;166:663–668.

171. Hansen JE, Wasserman K. Pathophysiology of activity limitation in patients with interstitial lung disease. *Chest* 1996;109:1566–1576.

172. Whipp BJ, Davis JA. The ventilatory stress of exercise in obesity. *Am Rev Respir Dis* 1992;145:101–105.

173. Sakamoto S, Ishikawa K, Senda S, et al. The effect of obesity on ventilatory response and anaerobic threshold during exercise. *J Med Syst* 1993;17:227–231.

174. Salvadori A, Fanari P, Fontana M, et al. Oxygen uptake and cardiac performance in obese and normal subjects during exercise. *Respiration* 1999;66:25–33.

175. Johnson BD, Badr MS, Dempsey JA. Impact of the aging pulmonary system on the response to exercise. *Clin Chest Med* 1994;15:229–246.

4 Bronchoscopy

Tanya Wiese · Paul A. Kvale

BRONCHOSCOPIC TECHNIQUES

History

The rigid bronchoscope was invented in 1897 by Gustav Killian (1). Early on, bronchoscopes were mainly used by surgeons to treat airway obstruction caused by foreign bodies and tracheal stenosis caused by diphtheria infections. However, by the 1950s bronchoscopes were predominately being used to establish the diagnosis of lung cancer. Then, with the development of the optical properties of glass fibers, the first flexible fiberoptic bronchoscope was used in 1967 by Shigeto Ikeda (2). Today, flexible bronchoscopy has evolved into the most commonly used diagnostic modality for pulmonary disorders (3). Although bronchoscopy has not traditionally been a common therapeutic modality for pulmonary disorders, bronchoscopy has been expanded for use in this area.

Equipment

The basic equipment consists of a flexible bronchoscope attached to a light source, various brushes, biopsy forceps, and extraction tools. The diameter of the flexible bronchoscope varies from a pediatric size of 3.5 mm up to an adult largest size of 6 mm. Ultrathin flexible bronchoscopes are also available, but most practitioners do not commonly use them. The diameter of the working channel (channel used for suctioning, instillation of solutions, and passage of equipment) in standard-size flexible bronchoscopes ranges from 1.2 to 2.8 mm. Brushes vary by length of the bristles. A length that is adequate to obtain a decent sample size, while trying to minimize traumatic bleeding, is the goal when choosing a brush. Biopsy forceps are selected based on operator preference and location of target tissue. Likewise, extraction tools are selected based on type and location of the aspirated foreign body. Fluoroscopic screening is not required during endobronchial biopsies or during transbronchial biopsies in diffuse lung disease, but a C-arm or biplane fluoroscope is essential for accurate and safe biopsies of localized peripheral lung lesions. A fluoroscope is also useful to rule out a pneumothorax after transbronchial biopsies, alleviating the need to obtain a chest radiograph.

The rigid bronchoscope consists of a hollow straight stainless steel tube. A removable telescope with a light source can be placed through the proximal end. Several telescopes (0-, 30-, and 90-degree angled lenses) are needed to visualize the upper lobe bronchi with a rigid bronchoscope. There are also proximal ports for ventilation, a suction catheter, and the passage of various instruments (Fig. 4.1). The barrel comes in various lengths and diameters. The distal end of the barrel is beveled and has side ports for ventilation. The beveled end helps to facilitate atraumatic entry through the vocal cords, cork-screwing through narrowed airways, and coring-out of obstructive lesions.

Indications

There are many indications for flexible bronchoscopy, both diagnostic and therapeutic (Table 4.1). The most common indication is for the diagnosis of suspected lung cancer. Other common indications include evaluation of diffuse lung disease, infiltrates in an immunocompromised patient, cough, and hemoptysis. Indications in the intensive care unit may include evaluation of ventilator-associated pneumonia, removal of mucous plugs, and inspection of endotracheal tube placement. Rigid bronchoscopy has the same indications as those of flexible bronchoscopy, with the exception of assessment of endotracheal tube placement. Rigid bronchoscopy

T. Wiese and **P. A. Kvale:** Division of Pulmonary, Critical Care, Allergy, Immunology, and Sleep Disorders Medicine, Henry Ford Hospital, Detroit, Michigan.

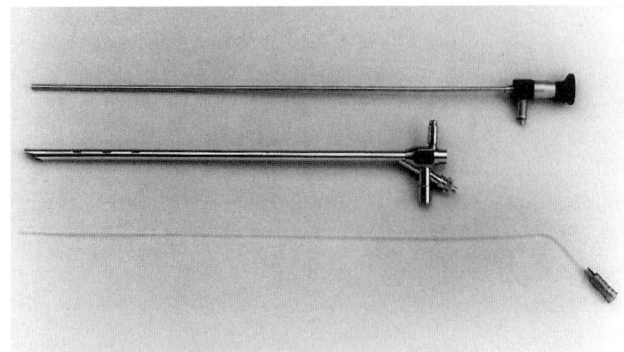

A

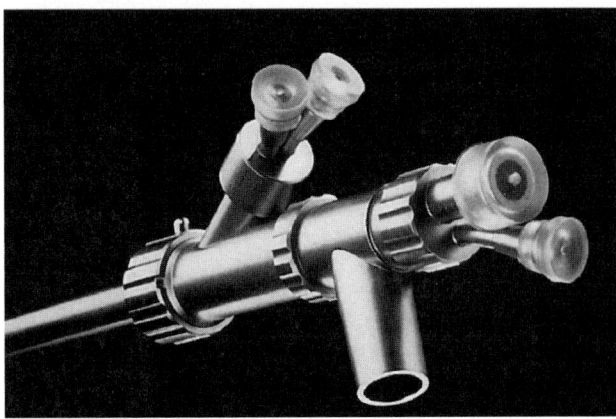

B

FIGURE 4.1. A: Rigid bronchoscope **(middle)** with telescope **(top)** and suction catheter **(bottom). B:** Proximal end of universal head of Dumon bronchoscope, showing ports for suction catheters, laser fiber, telescope, and ventilation. (From Beamis JF Jr. Modern use of rigid bronchoscopy. In: Bolliger CT, Mahtur PN, eds. *Interventional bronchoscopy.* New York: Karger, 1999:23–24, with permission.)

offers advantages over flexible bronchoscopy in certain cases of foreign body extraction, massive hemoptysis, debulking of central airway tumors, and placement of silicone airway stents. This is because the rigid bronchoscope allows for complete airway control and has a much larger lumen for

TABLE 4.1. INDICATIONS FOR BRONCHOSCOPY

Evaluation of abnormal chest radiograph
Cough
Hemoptysis
Localized wheeze
Suspected tracheoesophageal fistula
Chest trauma or inhalation injury
Persistent atelectasis
Localization of bronchopleural fistula
Foreign body aspiration
Delivery of brachytherapy
Evaluation for rejection in a lung transplant recipient
Evaluation of unilateral hyperlucency
Placement or confirmation of endobronchial tube
Unexplained hoarseness or vocal cord paralysis
Research
Delivery of therapeutic modalities (e.g., brachytherapy, bronchoplasty, laser)

removing tissue or foreign bodies and placing large biopsy forceps.

Contraindications

There are very few absolute contraindications for bronchoscopy. Hypoxia that cannot be corrected, in the range of an arterial blood partial pressure of oxygen (Pao$_2$) less than 60 mm Hg, is a contraindication owing to the expected decrease in oxygenation with bronchoscopy. Bronchoscopy can also precipitate ischemia in those with severe cardiac disease, especially a patient with a recent myocardial infarction. Thus, bronchoscopy should generally be avoided in any patient with unstable or severe cardiac disease. On the other hand, it has been demonstrated that flexible bronchoscopy can be performed with relative impunity for emergent reasons (usually hemoptysis) in patients with recent myocardial infarction (4). Bleeding can occur from bronchoscopic trauma to the nasal mucosa, from friable airways, and after biopsies. To avoid significant bleeding, it is generally recommended that oral instead of nasal intubation with the bronchoscope be performed and transbronchial biopsies should be avoided, if the platelet count is less than 50,000/mm^3. Finally, elevated intracranial pressures can occur during bronchoscopy. The bronchoscope can act as a strong stimulus for the cough reflex, which can cause elevation in intracranial pressures. Thus, any conditions in which elevated intracranial pressure puts the patient at risk for intracranial bleed are contraindications for bronchoscopy.

Complications

Flexible bronchoscopy is generally a safe procedure. A review of four major studies shows a morbidity range of 0.08% to 0.8%, with a mortality range of 0% to 0.04% (5–9). The major complications include hypoxia, aspiration, fever, bacteremia, and hemorrhage.

Hypoxia is a common complication, even in patients with normal oxygenation before the procedure. This occurs from ventilation–perfusion mismatching secondary to airway obstruction from the bronchoscope, instillation of solutions or lavage fluid, and suctioning. The other major cause of hypoxia is from hypoventilation secondary to sedatives. Thus, it is recommended that patients be monitored with a pulse oximeter during and after the procedure (10). Sedatives should be used in incremental doses to achieve adequate sedation and amnesia without oversedation. Midazolam, because of its rapid onset, short duration, and anterograde amnestic effects, has become one of the preferred agents for sedation in the outpatient setting (11). It is recommended to give a 1 to 2 mg intravenous bolus of midazolam and then 1 mg intravenous every 2 minutes until adequate sedation is achieved. Flumazenil, a specific benzodiazepine antagonist, should be kept on hand for reversal of oversedation.

Patients are instructed not to eat or drink 4 to 12 hours before the procedure to reduce the risk of aspiration. Another complication of bronchoscopy is fever. A review of four studies showed the rate of fever to be 10% to 30% after bronchoscopy with bronchoalveolar lavage (BAL), 15% with transbronchial biopsies, and 10% with transbronchial needle aspiration (TBNA) (12–14). Another study found transient bacteremia in 6.5% of patients after bronchoscopy, raising the question of whether to give prophylactic antibiotics to patients with asplenia, valvular heart disease, or history of endocarditis (15). The American Heart Association currently recommends prophylactic antibiotics for those with risk factors who are undergoing a rigid bronchoscopy because of the higher likelihood of mucosal damage (16). However, these recommendations are not intended as the standard of care or to take the place of clinical judgment. Another, potentially dangerous complication of bronchoscopy is hemorrhage. Studies have shown that prebronchoscopic coagulation tests can not predict which patients will have a clinically significant bleed and thus are unjustified in patients with no risk factors (17, 18). Patients with increased risk include those with platelet counts less than 50,000/mm^3, pulmonary hypertension, uremia, immunosuppression, liver disease, superior venal caval syndrome, use of antiplatelet medication, and coagulation disorders. A rare complication, which is sometimes seen with bronchoscopy, is a vasovagal reaction.

Standard practice once included the administration of atropine before bronchoscopy, both to prevent vasovagal reactions and to decrease secretions and cough. However, recent studies have shown that there is no reduction in vasovagal response or noticeable advantage of diminished secretions and cough (19, 20). Thus, atropine is no longer recommended to prevent these complications. Topical lidocaine is used to anesthetize the nares, vocal cords, and airways. Toxic dosages can occur with resultant seizures or cardiac arrhythmias. Limiting the total dosage to 8 mg/kg is recommended to avoid these complications. Also, prebronchoscopic aerosolized lidocaine can help reduce the dose of topical lidocaine needed during bronchoscopy (21). Finally, transbronchial biopsies can cause a pneumothorax; thus, either a chest radiograph or fluoroscopic examination of the chest should be performed after these biopsies.

CANCER DIAGNOSIS

Lung cancer has reached epidemic proportions and has become the most common and lethal form of cancer in Western society. Bronchogenic carcinoma can be divided into central (endobronchial) or peripheral lesions. Central lesions may be predicted based on the presence of cough, hemoptysis, pneumonia, or atelectasis. It may also be detected on radiographic images. Although the endobronchial lesion may be readily identified with bronchoscopic inspec-

tion, a complete airway examination should be performed before any diagnostic samples are taken. This will prevent missing other important abnormalities in the remaining airways, if a bleed were to occur from the diagnostic procedures. Forceps biopsy, brushings, washings, and needle aspirations are all techniques that can be performed to help establish a diagnosis.

Forceps biopsies should be performed with a gentle avulsion technique to minimize bleeding. Pulling forcefully on the end of the forceps can cause damage to the delicate linkage mechanisms in the bronchoscope when the forceps is suddenly released from the tissue. Instead the bronchoscopist should gently pull the bronchoscope and forceps back as a unit. This same technique should be used for transbronchial biopsies of peripheral lesions. To obtain the highest diagnostic yields for central lesions (endoscopically visible) at least three biopsy samples should be obtained with either brushings or washings (22).

After brushing a lesion, the brush can be pulled through the working channel of the bronchoscope (withdrawn technique), or the bronchoscope with the brush protruding from the distal end (nonwithdrawn technique) can be removed as a unit to avoid losing tissue sample in the working channel. Although no study has shown statistical superiority of one technique over the other, evidence points in the direction of better samples using the nonwithdrawn method to obtain brush samples (23). Brush samples should then be applied to a slide in a circular motion and immediately put in preservative solution to prevent air-drying. Other methods of processing the brush samples include agitating the brush in saline or a preservative solution, after which cytospin or cell-block preparations can be used for cytologic analysis. Bronchial washings (instillation of small volumes of saline, followed by aspiration of the fluid into a suction trap) is a third type of specimen that can be processed cytologically. Washings are appropriate for central (endoscopically visible) tumors, but they do not add to the overall yield when a combination of biopsies and brushings are performed (24). Bronchoalveolar lavage can be performed for peripheral (endoscopically invisible) lesions, once the bronchoscope is wedged within the target bronchial segment. Aliquots of 20 mL of 0.9% normal saline are instilled into the segment, and then with a negative pressure of about 50 to 80 mm Hg, the lavage fluid is suctioned back into a collection chamber. If suction pressure is too high, the airways will collapse and inhibit adequate return of the lavage. Usually the return is about 40% to 60% of lavage instilled; thus, it may take up to 50 to 75 mL of saline to get an adequate return of 20 to 30 mL.

The diagnostic yield for forceps biopsy, brushing, and washing in central lesions is 76%, 52%, and 49.6%, respectively (25). The combination of forceps biopsy with brushing or washing increases the diagnostic yield to 95%. There is little advantage of performing all three techniques, and thus for cost effectiveness, this should not be done for central lesions (26). In a study that reviewed results of forceps biopsy compared with needle aspiration of a central lesion, the diagnostic yield was 67% to 100% and 65% to 92%, respectively (27). Although this study did not show any advantage of needle aspiration over forceps biopsy for central lesions, there are three conditions in which needle aspiration may be more advantageous: when deeper tissue penetration is needed to avoid surface necrosis, when small cell carcinoma is suspected because crush artifact by forceps can make the diagnosis difficult, and when lesions may have a greater chance of bleeding. Thus, to obtain the highest diagnostic yields for central lesions at least three biopsy samples should be obtained with either brushing or washing.

Transbronchial forceps biopsy, brushing, washing, and TBNA are used for the diagnosis of peripheral lesions. Fluoroscopic imaging and computed tomography (CT) imaging techniques are used to help confirm proper location for biopsies. At least five to six biopsies are recommended (22). The diagnostic yield for transbronchial forceps biopsy, brushing, and washing is 36.5%, 38.1%, and 28.6%, respectively (25). The combination of all three techniques increases the diagnostic yield to 48%, and one study showed that if TBNA was added, the diagnostic yield increases to 69% (28). Other studies have shown even higher diagnostic yields with the use of TBNA, with variability in yields thought to be dependent on the expertise of bronchoscopist and the type of tumor–bronchi relationship (Fig. 4.2). As demonstrated in the Figure 4.2, forceps biopsy, washing, or brushing cannot easily sample type III and IV lesions. Recently, evidence has shown that TBNA has a higher diagnostic yield than transbronchial biopsies alone or in combination with brushing or washing, and that TBNA for peripheral lesions is underused (29–32). Underuse may be in part because of the lack of adequate training and fear of complications.

In addition to the above techniques for the diagnosis of peripheral lesions, there has been new interest in routinely performing blind forceps biopsies of the main carina and upper lobe carina ipsilateral to the lesion at the initial bronchoscopic examination to improve staging. A recent study showed that performing this procedure changed the status of 25% of patients to inoperable (33). As of yet, this procedure has not been recommended as the standard of care.

Optimizing Cancer Diagnoses

It has been generally accepted that the poor prognosis of lung cancer is owing to its advanced stage at presentation. At the time of diagnosis, 80% of all lung cancers are inoperable. And over the past several years, the overall 5-year survival rates have remained around 13% to 15% (34). This has prompted a search for new modalities to help with earlier detection of lung cancer. Autofluorescence bronchoscopy is one new technique that allows detection of carcinoma in situ or high-grade dysplasia in the central airways. The LIFE system (laser-induced fluorescence endoscopy) has recently been approved by the Food and Drug Administration for the early detection of lung cancer. Fluorescence bronchoscopy uses the different absorptive properties of light by normal tissue compared with malignant tissue. On illumination by violet or blue light, normal airway tissues fluoresce strongly green. As tissues become dysplastic, this absorption decreases and the tissues fluoresce brown, purple, or red. This is owing to the decrease in chromophores and increase in angiogenesis in dysplastic tissues. One large worldwide study showed a twofold improvement in the detection rates of cancer with the use of autofluorescence bronchoscopy compared with the standard white-light bronchoscopy (35). Five additional studies comparing white-light bronchoscopy to autofluorescence bronchoscopy, showed a 1.5- to 6.3-fold increase in the detection of high-grade dysplasia or carcinoma in situ (36–40). It has yet to be determined if autofluorescence will have a significant impact on the 5-year survival rates of lung cancer. Currently, there are no established techniques for screening or early detection of lung cancer.

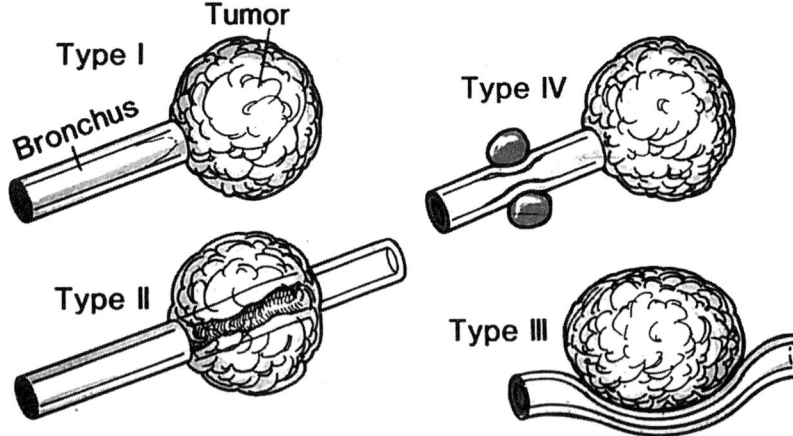

FIGURE 4.2. Tumor-bronchial relationship. (From Schenk DA, Chasen MH, McCarthy MJ, et al. Potential false positive transbronchial needle aspiration in bronchogenic carcinoma. *Chest* 1984;86:649–650, with permission.)

OPTIMIZING CANCER DIAGNOSIS

Summary Statement	Level of Evidence
Combinations of specimens lead to improved diagnostic yields	Multiple case series
Central visible carcinomas: three biopsies, plus one additional specimen (brushings, washings, *or* needle aspiration in the case of submucosal or necrotic tumors)	Multiple case series
Peripheral tumors (not endoscopically visible): six biopsies, plus brushings *and* washings or bronchoalveolar lavage. Fluoroscopic guidance needed for proper instrument placement	Several case series

Staging the Mediastinum Using Transbronchial Needle Biopsy

CT imaging and surgery are used to identify the etiology of mediastinal lesions and for the staging of mediastinal lymph nodes. The American Joint Committee on Cancer and the American Thoracic Society together have developed a classi-fication system of mediastinal lymph nodes to help describe location and to stage lung cancer (Fig. 4.3; see also Color Figure 4.3). Although CT imaging can identify lymph nodes that are less than a centimeter in size, the specificity of this finding is very low. Enlarged lymph nodes (>1 cm) may be owing to infiltration of metastatic bronchogenic carcinoma, but they can also occur as an inflammatory response to cancer, with infection, or with other systemic disorders. Surgery, on the other hand, is 100% specific and 87% sensitive, but it carries a high cost and a 1% morbidity and 0.2% mortality rate (41). Also, mediastinoscopy cannot assess the lymph nodes in the posterior subcarinal or aortopulmonary window. On the other hand, TBNA can be used to stage the mediastinum and has the advantage of a high sensitivity and specificity while being less invasive and costly (42). The first endoscopic puncture of mediastinal lymph nodes across the trachea was performed in the mid-1900s with a rigid bronchoscope. Improved techniques for obtaining cytological and histological samples from mediastinal, hilar, subcarinal, and paratracheal lesions became possible in 1983 with the development of the double-lumen flexible needle. This commonly

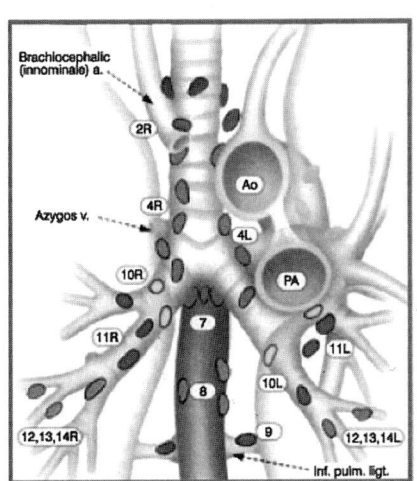

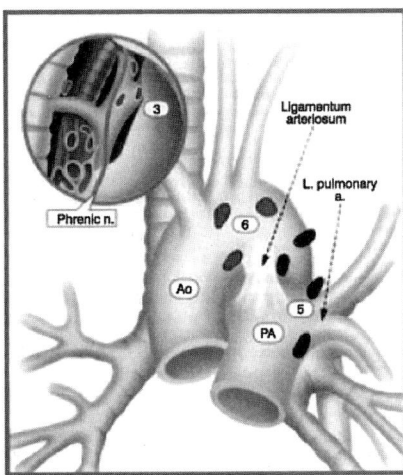

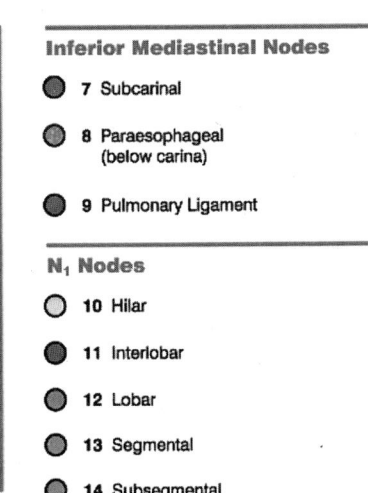

Superior Mediastinal Nodes

1 Highest Mediastinal

2 Upper Paratracheal

3 Pre-vascular and Retrotracheal

4 Lower Paratracheal (including Azygos Nodes)

N_2 = single digit, ipsilateral
N_3 = single digit, contralateral or supraclavicular

Aortic Nodes

5 Subaortic (A-P window)

6 Para-aortic (ascending aorta or phrenic)

Inferior Mediastinal Nodes

7 Subcarinal

8 Paraesophageal (below carina)

9 Pulmonary Ligament

N_1 Nodes

10 Hilar

11 Interlobar

12 Lobar

13 Segmental

14 Subsegmental

FIGURE 4.3. (See also Color Figure 4.3) Regional lymph node classification system. (Mountain/Dresler modifications from Naruke/American Thoracic Society Lung Cancer Staging Map; with permission.)

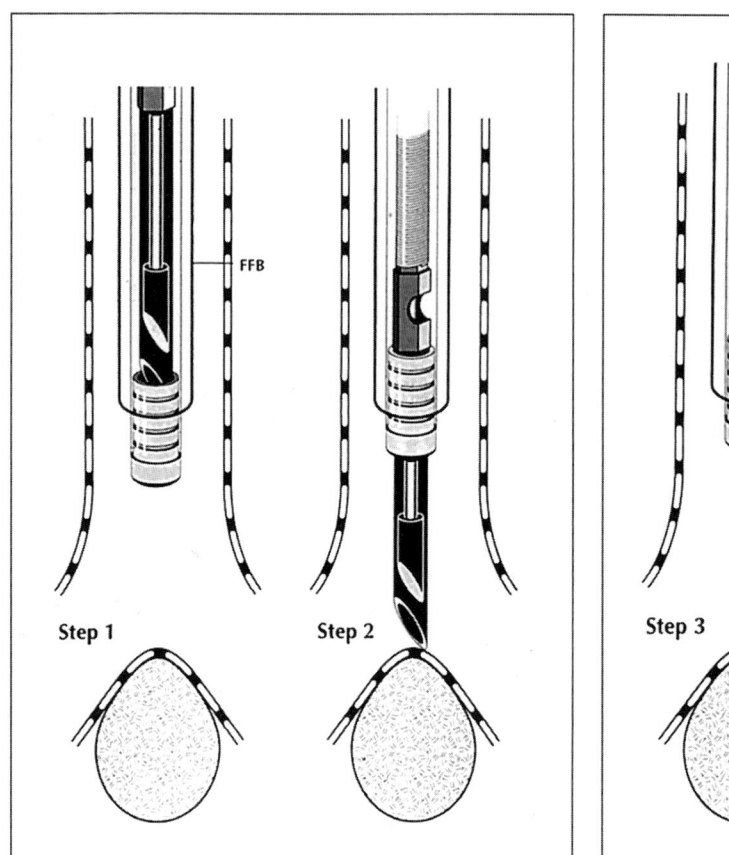
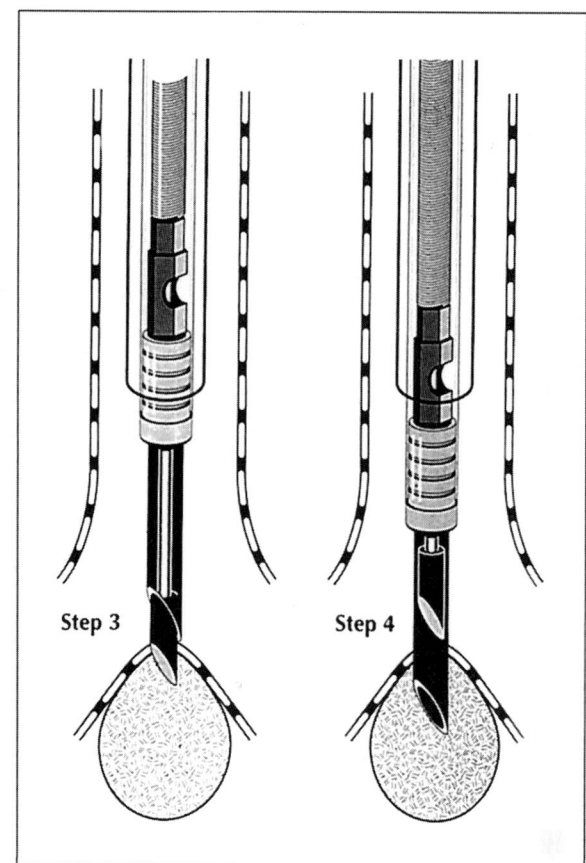

FIGURE 4.4. Transbronchial needle aspiration for histology specimen. (From Mehta AC, Meeker DP. Transbronchial needle aspiration for histology specimen. In: Wang KP, Mehta AC. eds. *Flexible bronchoscopy.* Cambridge: Blackwell Science, 1995:201, with permission.)

consists of a 19-gauge outer needle with a retractable 21-gauge needle housed within its lumen. The inner 21-gauge needle is used to penetrate the tissue and prevent plugging of the 19-gauge needle with the tracheal or bronchial wall material. An intercartilaginous space in the location of the target lymph node is penetrated at a perpendicular angle. Once the inner needle is buried, it is then pulled back into the lumen, leaving the hollow 19-gauge needle in place (Fig. 4.4). Suction is then applied to the needle to help pull and hold any cellular material and tissue specimens within the core of the needle. Also, the absence of blood being suctioned back helps to confirm that the needle has not inadvertently entered a blood vessel. Four to five core biopsies are then obtained. Several different methods have been developed for obtaining these core biopsies (Fig. 4.5). They involve various methods of moving the outer 19-gauge needle in and out of the target tissue. After these core samples have been obtained, it is important to make sure that the needle is back to a neutral position before withdrawing it through the working channel. Failing to obtain neutrality before withdrawing the needle through the working channel has made this procedure the most common cause of damage to the bronchoscope (43).

A review of several studies report sensitivity rates of 61% to 96% for TBNA in staging the mediastinum in bronchogenic carcinoma (44–50). Higher rates correlate with radiological evidence of lymph node enlargement (lymph node >1 cm). To reduce the risk of false positive results, the hilar or mediastinal lymph nodes should be sampled by TBNA before performing biopsies of central or peripheral lesions. This helps to avoid contamination of the proximal airways with distal cellular material. As in the diagnosis of peripheral pulmonary lesions, there is general agreement that TBNA is also underused for staging of the mediastinum. One study found that this is owing to the lack of sufficient training in pulmonary and critical care training programs (51). This lack of training causes lower diagnostic yields and thus less frequent performance of TBNA by the bronchoscopist. Others argue that the complex anatomy within the mediastinum along with motion artifact caused by respirations and pulsations of vessels lead to the low diagnostic yields. However, with an average training of only 24 months, one study showed an increase in diagnostic yields from 21.4% to 47.6% (52).

Experienced bronchoscopists use endobronchial landmarks and mental reconstructions of a preprocedural chest

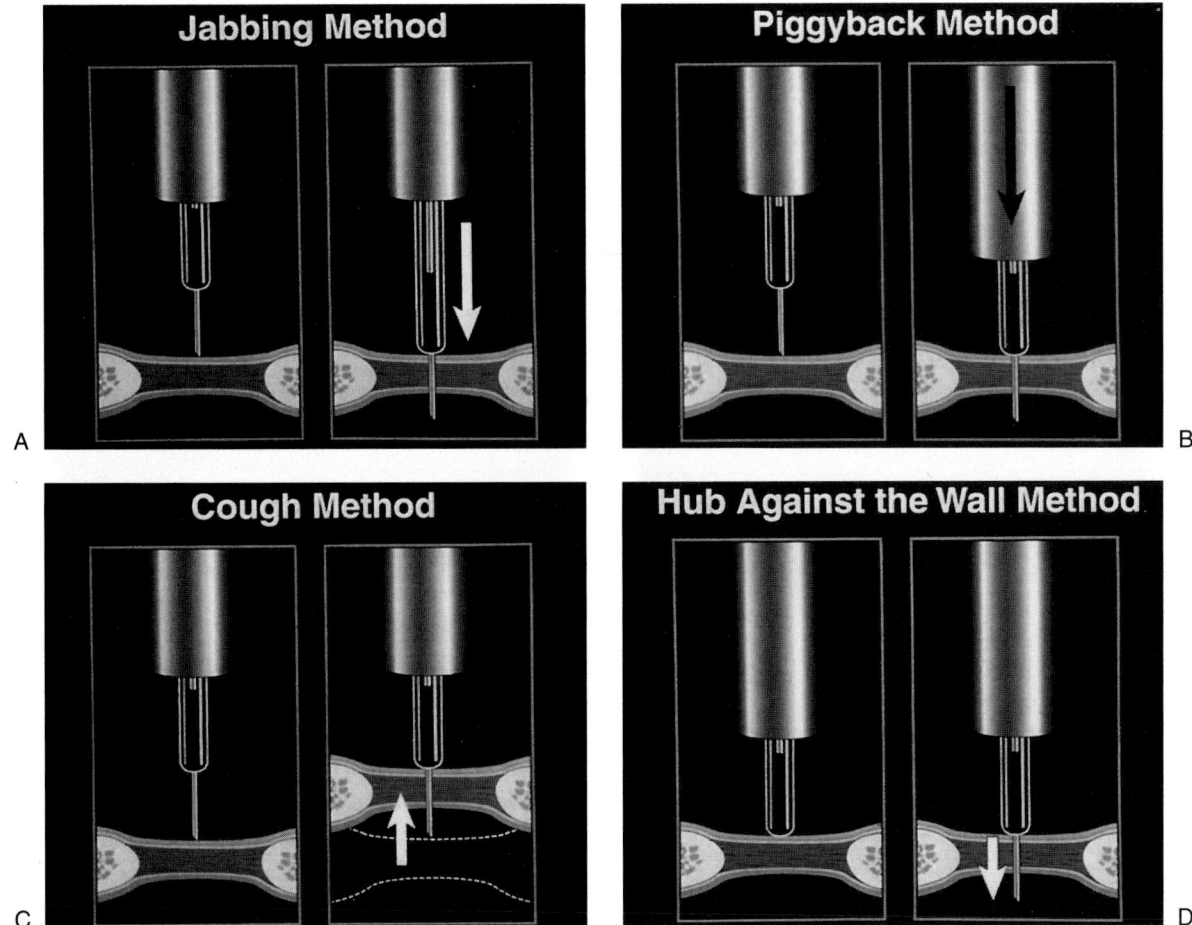

FIGURE 4.5. Different techniques used for tracheobronchial wall penetration by transbronchial needle aspiration: jabbing method **(A)**, piggy-back method **(B)**, cough method **(C)**, and hub-against-the-wall method **(D)**. (From Dasgupta A, Mehta AC, Wang KP. Transbronchial needle aspiration. In: Mathur P, Mehta AC. eds. *Seminars in respiratory and critical care medicine.* New York: Thieme Medical Publishers, 1997:573, with permission.)

CT scan for guidance in locating the target lymph node. However, even the most skilled bronchoscopist will encounter situations in which additional help is needed for localizing the target lesion or lymph node. Endobronchial ultrasound (EBUS) and CT imaging of the chest are two modalities currently being used to help improve the accuracy of TBNA.

EBUS allows for the visualization of vessels and lymph nodes (Fig. 4.6). A miniaturized probe is inserted through the working channel of the flexible bronchoscope. The tip of the probe is a small piezoelectric crystal that is rotated by a mechanical driving unit. Alternating electric current causes vibrations that initiate emission of sound waves. The probe is also constructed with a balloon at the tip, which is filled with water to allow full contact with bronchial wall. This provides a complete 360-degree view of the mediastinal structures. The higher the frequency of ultrasonic waves, the farther the depth of penetration, typically up to 4 to 5 cm beyond the wall of the bronchus or trachea. The lower the frequency of ultrasonic waves, the better the resolution.

EBUS can detect target lymph nodes as small as 3 mm. In addition to aiding in the location of lymph nodes, EBUS can also be used to assess depth of tumor invasion in the central airway (see section "Therapeutic Applications"). This is important because invasion of cancer beyond the cartilaginous layer is usually not amenable to endobronchial therapeutic modalities. To date, there has been no study performed to show that EBUS-guided technology increases the diagnostic yield of TBNA.

CT fluoroscopic–guided TBNA can be done in real or still time. CT fluoroscopy adds the benefit of confirming needle location. Only small studies evaluating CT fluoroscopy with TBNA have been performed thus far, but they have shown up to an 83% diagnostic yield (53). It is very difficult to compare these results with those of TBNA alone because of the variability in skills of those performing the TBNA. However, because it is less costly to perform TBNA alone, it is recommended that TBNA without CT guidance should be performed, except in the more difficult situations such as small lymph node size or a difficult location.

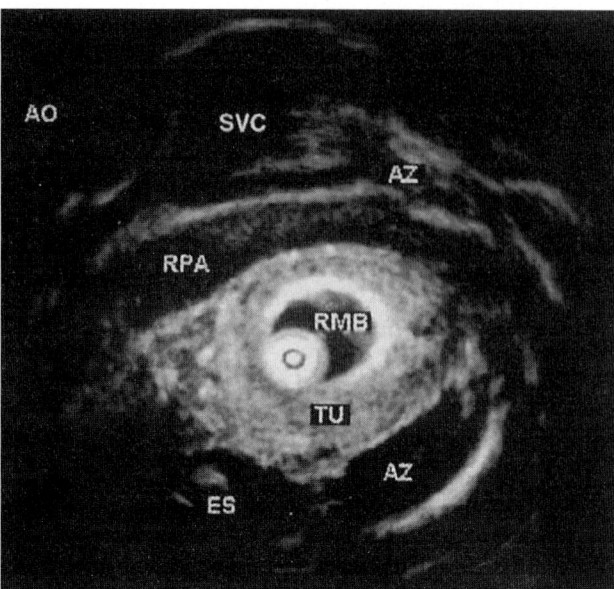

FIGURE 4.6. Endobronchial ultrasound of the right mainstem bronchus. The following structures are identified: aorta *(AO)*, superior vena cava *(SVC)*, azygos vein *(AZ)*, right pulmonary artery *(RPA)*, esophagus *(ES)*, and tumor infiltration *(TU)*. (From Heinrich D. Becker, M.D., Associate Director, Thoraxklinik, Heidelberg, Germany, with permission.)

TRANSBRONCHIAL NEEDLE ASPIRATION

Summary Statement	Level of Evidence
TBNA should be done routinely when lung cancer is suspected and chest CT scans reveal enlarged mediastinal lymph nodes in accessible locations; chest CT scans should be obtained before the initial bronchoscopy	Multiple case series
Histology needles (19 gauge) are associated with improved yields, compared with those for smaller needles	Multiple case series
TBNA samples should be obtained before other samples are collected	Multiple case series
Endobronchial ultrasound or CT guidance improves yield	A few small case series

TBNA, transbronchial needle aspiration; CT, computed tomography.

DIFFUSE PARENCHYMAL LUNG DISEASE IN IMMUNOCOMPETENT PATIENTS

Diffuse parenchymal lung disease (DPLD) is a heterogeneous group of inflammatory and fibrotic disorders of the lower respiratory tract. They may involve interstitial, alveolar, bronchial, or vascular structures and are classified together based on their common clinical, radiographic, physiologic, and pathologic features. There are well over 150 different agents or disorders that can cause DPLD. Although bronchoscopy mainly plays a supportive role in their diagnosis, there are some disorders in which transbronchial biopsy

or BAL can be diagnostic. DPLD can be divided into acute and chronic processes, with the majority of causes being from various infections, drugs, connective tissue disorders, and granulomatous diseases (Table 4.2).

Transbronchial biopsy in DPLD is generally a safe procedure; however, the risk of a clinically significant bleed (>50 mL) is 1.6% to 4.4% of patients, which is slightly higher than for all patients undergoing transbronchial biopsies (54). Overall, the diagnostic yield for transbronchial biopsies in DPLD has been reported between 25% to 50% (28, 55–57). Bronchoscopic procedures in DPLD that have the best diagnostic yield is for sarcoidosis, which is the most common idiopathic cause of DPLD. Studies have shown a 60% to 90% diagnostic yield with transbronchial biopsies. The higher yields are in those with chest radiographic stage II or III (58, 59). Endobronchial forceps biopsy of mucosa that has an abnormal appearance (especially nodularity, yellowish in color) in sarcoidosis has a 45% to 71% diagnostic yield, compared with a 35% diagnostic yield with mucosa that is normal in appearance (58). Also, TBNA of enlarged lymph nodes in sarcoidosis has shown sensitivies up to 90% (59, 60). The combination of endobronchial biopsy,

TABLE 4.2. BRONCHOSCOPY FOR DIFFUSE PARENCHYMAL LUNG DISEASE

Diffuse Parenchymal Lung Disease	Types
Granulomatous disease	Hypersensitivity pneumonitis, some inhalation causes, some drugs, sarcoidosis, Langerhans cell granulomatous, Hand-Schuller disease, Letter syndrome, Wegener granulomatosis, lymphomatoid granulomatosis, Churg-Strauss syndrome, bronchocentric granulomatosis, berylliosis, some infections
Connective tissue disease	Rheumatoid arthritis, systemic lupus erythematosis, scleroderma, Behcet syndrome, mixed connective tissue disease
Inhalation causes	Occupational dusts, gases, fumes, vapors, birds, pets
Inherited causes	Tuberous sclerosis, Hermansky-Pudlak syndrome, neurofibromatosis, metabolic storage disease, hypocalciuric hypercalcemia, Neimann-Pick disease, Gaucher disease, cystic fibrosis
Miscellaneous	Bronchiolitis obliterans, bronchiolitis obliterans organizing pneumonia, eosinophilic pneumonia, some drugs, irradiation, pulmonary alveolar proteinosis, lymphangioleiomyomatosis, amyloidosis, inflammatory bowel disease, graph versus host disease, infections
Malignancy	Bronchoalveolar carcinoma, lymphangitic carcinoma
Idiopathic interstitial pneumonitis	Idiopathic pulmonary fibrosis, nonspecific interstitial pneumonitis, desquamative interstitial pneumonitis, respiratory bronchiolitis, acute interstitial pneumonitis, lymphocytic interstitial pneumonitis

TABLE 4.3. CELLULAR ANALYSIS AND THE RELATIONSHIP TO VARIOUS TYPES OF DIFFUSE PARENCHYMAL LUNG DISEASES

Cellular Analysis	Cause of Diffuse Parenchymal Lung Disease
Lymphocytes >20%	sarcoidosis, drugs, BOOP, LIP, NSIP, HP, berylliosis, lymphoproliferative disorders
Neutrophils >5%	AIP, diffuse panbronchitis, connective tissue disorders, drugs, IPF
Eosinophils >5%	eosinophilic pneumonia, drugs, hypereosinophilic syndrome, IPF, Churg-Strauss syndrome, pulmonary Langerhans granulomatosis

Normal bronchoalveolar lavage cellular analysis shows a differential of 90%–98% macrophages, 5%–15% lymphocytes, 1%–3% polymorphic neutrophils, and <1% eosinophils, mast cells, and squamous epithelial cells. BOOP, bronchiolitis obliterans organizing pneumonia; LIP, lymphoid interstitial pneumonitis; NSIP, nonspecific interstitial pneumonitis; HP, hypersensitivity pneumonitis; AIP, acute interstitial pneumonitis; IPF, idiopathic pulmonary fibrosis.

transbronchial biopsy, and TBNA for chest radiograph stages I and II shows a sensitivity of 90% and a specificity of 100%. The same results can be obtained in chest radiograph stage III disease with just the combination endobronchial and transbronchial biopsies (60).

BAL plays more of a supportive role in the diagnosis of DPLD. Table 4.3 shows a list of disorders causing DPLD in which BAL cellular analysis may be helpful in narrowing the differential diagnosis. In addition to the cellular analysis, there are several other characteristics of the BAL that can be

TABLE 4.4. OTHER FINDINGS FROM BRONCHO-ALVEOLAR LAVAGE THAT MAY ALLOW A DIAGNOSIS IN SPECIFIC DISEASES

Disease	Finding in Bronchoalveolar Lavage Fluid
Pulmonary alveolar proteinosis	Lipoproteinaceous material that looks milky and sandy; stains positive with periodic acid–Schiff
Pulmonary alveolar microlithiasis	Looks milky and sandy; centrifuging will demonstrate sedimentation
Pulmonary Langerhans cell granulomatosis	>5% Langerhans cells (antigen presenting cell distinct from macrophages), Birbeck granules/X bodies (pentalaminar cytoplasmic inclusions seen on electron microscopy)
Asbestosis	Ferruginous bodies (coated fibers)
Silicosis	Dust particles seen by polarized microscopy
Berylliosis	Positive lymphocyte transformation test
Some drugs	Foamy macrophages (not specific)
Diffuse alveolar hemorrhage	Hemosiderin-laden macrophages, progressively bloodier bronchoalveolar lavage aliquots
Lipoid pneumonia	Fat globules in macrophages
Malignancy: bronchoalveolar, lymphoma, lymphangitic carcinomatosis	Malignant cells

helpful in the evaluation of DPLD (Table 4.4). Good examples are pulmonary alveolar proteinosis and pulmonary alveolar microlithiasis. They have a distinct milky white lavage owing to elevated levels of surfactant. Centrifuging the lavage will distinguish the two disorders by demonstrating sedimentation with microlithiasis.

Transbronchial biopsy and BAL are recommended as the initial procedures to evaluate patients with DPLD, especially if there is other evidence to suggest a disorder in which these procedures are known to be helpful (Table 4.4). However, the pathology in DPLD is frequently inhomogeneous and difficult to characterize definitively on the basis of a small transbronchial biopsy. Thus, when a disorder is suspected in which bronchoscopic techniques are known to be of little help, a surgical biopsy should be performed.

OPTIMIZING DIAGNOSIS IN THE IMMUNOCOMPETENT HOST

Summary Statement	Level of Evidence
Best yield for transbronchial lung biopsy in diseases that have specific histologic features, such as sarcoidosis	Multiple case series
For sarcoidosis, combinations of biopsies (transbronchial, mucosal, needle core of mediastinal lymph nodes) improve overall yield	Multiple case series
Selected diseases (e.g., pulmonary alveolar proteinosis, histiocytosis X) can be diagnosed with confidence with bronchoalveolar lavage specimens	A few small case series

INFECTIOUS DISEASES

Currently, community-acquired and nosocomial pneumonia are treated empirically according to well-established guidelines. The role of bronchoscopy in pneumonia remains controversial. Conditions in which bronchoscopy may be beneficial included unresolving pneumonia, ventilator-associated pneumonia, or pneumonia in an immunocompromised patient. Bronchoscopic techniques used for obtaining samples are predominately BAL, and a protected specimen brush that uses a double-sheathed catheter to minimize bacterial contamination from the upper airways. Less commonly used are transbronchial biopsy and TBNA. Quantitative culture techniques are used to increase diagnostic specificity. The threshold for a BAL culture of 10^4 colony-forming units (cfu)/mL and for a protected specimen brush of 10^3 cfu/mL is recommended for improved specificity. These threshold levels are controversial, but most studies have supported these levels as having the most accurate diagnostic yield (61–63). These values, however, do not apply to organisms considered to be strict pathogens such as *Nocardia* or to organisms shown to be significant pathogens in lower numbers such as *Pseudomonas aeruginosa*.

The definition of unresolving or slowly resolving pneumonia is controversial. Some investigators define it as persistent fever, leukocytosis/leukopenia, purulent sputum production, and persistent chest radiographic opacities after 72 hours of antibiotic therapy. The time of 72 hours is arbitrary and lacks precision. Other investigators suggest that unresolving pneumonia should be defined as any pneumonia that persists beyond the expected time course for resolution. Studies examining the role of bronchoscopic techniques in unresolving pneumonia have shown no significant difference in diagnostic yield for BAL, protected brush specimen, or tracheal aspirates (64, 65). Although some reports suggest that bronchoscopy may lead to a more specific microbiologic diagnosis, no study has shown improvement in outcome (65, 66). However, many other noninfectious disorders, as well as uncommon infectious etiologies, need to be considered in the management of unresolving pneumonia (Table 4.5). In these situations, bronchoscopy may still serve a role.

Ventilator-associated pneumonia is defined as pneumonia occurring more than 48 hours after intubation. Clinical and radiographic signs of ventilator-associated pneumonia are nonspecific, and the presence of upper respiratory tract colonization does not necessarily mean infection of lung tissue. Relying on cultures from the upper respiratory tract can lead to the unnecessary use or inappropriate selection of antibiotics, thereby increasing the risk of resistant organisms and, ultimately, mortality. Thus, bronchoscopy has been proposed as a means of increasing diagnostic accuracy and more specific choices among available antibiotics.

Before performing a bronchoscopy on a ventilated patient, certain adjustments to the mechanical ventilator may be required. The inspired oxygen should be 100%, and the mode of ventilation should be in assist control. Maintaining a peak inspiratory flow rate at 60 L/min will help decrease the elevation in peak airway pressures caused by the bronchoscope. In addition, increasing the pressure limit on the ventilator will ensure adequate tidal volumes. Finally, a special swivel connector with a perforated diaphragm, through which the bronchoscope can be inserted, is used to allow continued ventilation and maintenance of positive end expiratory pressure in hypoxic patients.

Studies regarding the beneficial effect of bronchoscopy on the mortality in ventilator-associated pneumonia are con-

TABLE 4.5. DIFFERENTIAL DIAGNOSIS OF UNRESOLVING PNEUMONIA

Inappropriate antibiotics
Sequestered site of infection
Impaired immune defenses
Nonbacterial or uncommon bacteria
Endobronchial obstruction
Noninfectious

flicting. Some studies have shown that bronchoscopic information is commonly obtained too late to make an impact, that the same information can be provided by simpler methods (e.g., tracheal aspirates, blood cultures), that the sensitivity of the diagnostic yield is decreased in the presence of antibiotics, and that highly resistant organisms are often found so that any change in antibiotics will not make a difference on outcome (67). Despite these claims, many studies have shown less organ dysfunction and less inappropriate antibiotic usage when bronchoscopy is used (67–70). One large prospective, randomized study showed that antibiotics were used in only 52% of patients who had a bronchoscopy performed compared with 91% who only had tracheal aspirates collected (71). This same study showed a decrease in 14-day mortality from 26% to 16%. Another study examined the use of Gram stains obtained from bronchoscopy to guide empiric therapy while cultures where pending. Gram-positive stains predicted growth of more than 10^3 cfu/mL on culture from BAL with a 78% sensitivity, which led to improved accuracy of antibiotic coverage (72). In summary, studies have shown that bronchoscopy may be beneficial in ventilator-associated pneumonia because mortality may be reduced by eliminating the use of unnecessary antibiotics and by limiting the inappropriate initial selection of empiric antibiotics (73–75). In summary, further studies are needed to better evaluate the utility of bronchoscopy in ventilator-associated pneumonia.

Although the lung is the most commonly infected tissue in all immunocompromised patients, there are many noninfectious conditions in this patient population that can present like pneumonia. Thus, early diagnosis and specific therapy is the cornerstone to successful treatment. Bronchoscopy is an important tool for obtaining good-quality lower respiratory tract samples in the immunocompromised patient who typically does not produce sputum, even with pneumonia. Also because of the lack of an inflammatory response, a negative chest radiograph is common, especially in those who are neutropenic. This should not have an impact on the decision to perform a bronchoscopy. In this situation, a chest CT scan is often helpful to direct appropriate bronchoscopic sampling, because the chest CT scan will often show lesions that are not appreciated on a chest radiograph. The majority of studies regarding bronchoscopy in immunocompromised patients show convincing evidence of the superiority of invasive (BAL, protected specimen brush, transbronchial biopsy, TBNA) versus noninvasive (blood cultures, sputum cultures, nasal pharyngeal washing, tracheal aspirates) diagnostic techniques on outcome (76–78). Thus, there should be no delay in obtaining bronchoscopic samples in the immunocompromised patient.

There are several additional points that are peculiar to bronchoscopy in immunocompromised patients with *Pneumocystis carinii* pneumonia (PCP), cytomegalovirus (CMV) pneumonia, tuberculosis, or fungal pneumonia. Although the diagnosis of PCP can usually be made with induced sputum samples, the sensitivity of this technique has shown considerable variability (55%–90%) between institutions (79–81). Bronchoscopy with BAL in PCP is known to have a very high diagnostic yield, 90% or higher in almost all reports (82). There is controversy on whether empiric treatment should be started before bronchoscopy for patients with negative sputum examinations for PCP. Also controversial is whether transbronchial biopsies should routinely be performed in suspected cases of PCP. In institutions with good yields from sputum analysis but with negative results on analysis of sputum specimens, bronchoscopy with BAL will provide a definitive diagnosis in 50% of the remaining patients truly infected with *Pneumocystis carinii* (82). A combination of BAL and transbronchial biopsy is reported in some centers to increase the diagnostic yield for all pathogens up to 98% and to help diagnose noninfectious disease processes (83). Because the patient may not have PCP or may become too ill after ineffective therapy, most investigators agree that BAL and transbronchial biopsy should be performed when sputum samples are negative. One additional point needs to be made regarding the effect of pentamidine on diagnostic yields for PCP. Studies have shown that the diagnostic yield is decreased when the patient is on pentamidine unless the upper lobes are sampled (84). Thus, for all patients on pentamidine, BAL should be performed in the upper lobes.

CMV pneumonia is also a consideration in any immunocompromised patient with pulmonary infiltrates. This disease process, however, is complicated by the fact that shedding of CMV is frequently isolated from respiratory secretions without causing disease. A study performed by the National Institutes of Health on 66 individuals showed a positive BAL culture in 47% of asymptomatic volunteers, 72% of patients who had respiratory complaints, and 100% of patients who had CMV retinitis. Only one of the 66 individuals developed clinical signs of CMV pneumonia within the following 3 months (85). Another study showed a positive BAL culture for CMV in 51% of HIV-infected patients who had no hypoxemia, chest radiograph abnormalities, or increase in short-term mortality (86, 87). When BAL cultures for CMV were compared to postmortem lung histopathological samples, results showed only a 61% positive predictive value (88). Thus, because CMV cultures from BAL are not specific, it has been proposed that the diagnosis of CMV pneumonia be limited to patients who have respiratory symptoms with pathological evidence of CMV lung infection (positive BAL or biopsy cultures demonstrating CMV inclusion bodies).

Sputum cultures for tuberculosis have very high diagnostic yields. When compared with results obtained by bronchoscopy, there is little difference (89, 90). Thus, obtaining sputum for smears, cultures, and polymerase chain reaction probes is the preferred route for diagnosis, not only for ease of performance and low cost but also for avoidance of the risk of aerosol transmission of tuberculosis to health care personnel during a bronchoscopy. However, when sputum samples fail to reveal the diagnosis, bronchoscopy with both BAL and transbronchial biopsies should be performed. Studies show that transbronchial biopsies often will lead to a diagnosis when sputum and BAL are negative(91, 92). Also, although mediastinal lymphadenopathy is often absent in the immunocompromised patient, when present it is usually owing to mycobacterial or fungal infections. TBNA may be helpful in these patients.

Fungal pneumonia is a common cause of morbidity and mortality in the immunocompromised host (93). The most commonly recovered species are *Aspergillus, Cryptococcus, Candida,* and *Mucor* species. Bronchoscopy is an important diagnostic tool in fungal pneumonia, because many of these organisms colonize the upper airways in immunocompromised patients, rendering sputum cultures diagnostically unreliable. Overall, studies have shown better sensitivity with improved survival when bronchoscopic techniques are performed in suspected fungal pneumonia (94–96).

DIAGNOSING INFECTIOUS DISEASES

Summary Statement	Level of Evidence
Unresolving pneumonia: value of bronchoscopy is controversial; most helpful to diagnose noninfectious causes	Conflicting reports from multiple case series
Ventilator-associated pneumonia: quantitative cultures needed, may improve specificity of antibiotic choice	Conflicting data from multiple case series; one prospective controlled study
Immunocompromised patients: very high sensitivity and specificity for identification of pathogens; noninfectious diseases can be diagnosed with transbronchial lung biopsy as well	Numerous case series
Tuberculosis: bronchoscopy is a good means to establish a diagnosis, but there is a hazard to the personnel performing the procedure. Sputums should be obtained first	Multiple case series

HEMOPTYSIS

The causes of hemoptysis are diverse and can be subdivided into massive hemoptysis, usually defined as more than 600 mL per 24 hours (Table 4.6). The most common causes of massive hemoptysis in the United States are chronic inflammatory lung diseases and bronchogenic carcinoma, with tuberculosis as the most common cause worldwide (97). Bronchoscopy is used to help establish the site and cause of hemoptysis. It also has several therapeutic applications; however, these will be discussed later (see section "Therapeutic Applications"). A chest CT scan is generally recommended

TABLE 4.6. MAJOR CAUSES OF HEMOPTYSIS

Infectious: especially tuberculosis, fungus ball, lung abscess
Inflammatory: bronchitis, bronchiectasis
Neoplastic: bronchogenic carcinoma, bronchial adenoma, hemangioma
Immune disorders: especially Wegener granulomatosis and
    Goodpasture syndrome
Pulmonary vascular disorders: PE, AVM, mitral valve disease, PA
    catheter, LVD, fistula
Miscellaneous: catamenial, pneumoconiosis, coagulopathy, anticoagulant
    therapy, cocaine, foreign body, endobronchial tumors, broncholith,
    myxoma, DIC, trauma, idiopathic

PE, pulmonary emboli; AVM, arteriovenous malformation; PA, pulmonary
artery; LVD, left ventricular dysfunction; DIC, disseminated intravascular
coagulation.

before bronchoscopy in a stable patient with scant or small amounts of hemoptysis, as it can lead to the diagnosis and/or help to identify the site of bleeding to direct appropriate treatment. Flexible bronchoscopy is preferred in all other situations. It has been found to be 86% accurate for the localization of the bleed, which is more accurate than history, physical examination, or chest radiograph (98). Appropriate timing of bronchoscopy for hemoptysis can be very difficult to determine. Factors that need to be considered in the decision-making process include hemodynamics, volume of bleeding, rapidity of bleeding, and comorbidities of the patient. Early flexible bronchoscopy is usually the rule, as waiting may make localization difficult if bleeding slows; moreover, clinical deterioration can occur very quickly (99, 100). If the site of bleeding is not readily apparent, serial washings of the suspected bronchial segments with aliquots of 15 to 20 mL of 0.9% normal saline may help to identify the location of the bleed. Despite use of all of the available diagnostic techniques for the evaluation of hemoptysis, 5% to 15% of cases will remain unexplained (101).

THERAPEUTIC APPLICATIONS

Although the bronchoscope traditionally has been used for diagnosis, its use as a therapeutic instrument is increasing with the development of newer technologies. Interventional pulmonology is the term used to describe this new field within pulmonary medicine that focuses on the use of advanced bronchoscopic and pleuroscopic techniques for the treatment of a large spectrum of thoracic disorders. The rigid bronchoscope has traditionally been the instrument of choice for these procedures because of its superior suctioning capabilities, airway control, and ability to accommodate the passage of large accessory instruments and the removal of large pieces of tumor or foreign bodies. However, because more physicians are comfortable with the flexible bronchoscope and because it has the ability to better visualize the distal airways, it is also used by many for these new therapeutic applications.

Interventional bronchoscopy is most commonly used to treat airway obstruction owing to endobronchial malignancies. At the time of diagnosis, 80% to 85% of patients with bronchogenic cancer only qualify for palliative care; and of these patients, 30% to 50% have involvement of the central airways (100, 102, 103). Interventional bronchoscopy may function as a palliative treatment strategy in these patients, because surgical resection may not be possible owing to the advanced stage of the cancer or because of the patient's underlying lung disease. Indications for bronchoscopic treatment of malignant disease include life-threatening obstruction of the central airways, symptomatic obstruction, asymptomatic obstruction with an endobronchial diameter narrowed to 50% of its normal diameter, and inoperable early lung cancer. A treatment algorithm for the management of malignancy involving the central airways is seen in Figure 4.7. The different therapeutic modalities as they relate to malignancy, as well as some other pulmonary disorders, are discussed below.

Lasers

Laser (light amplification by the stimulated emission of radiation) therapy is used for ablation of endoluminal benign or malignant tumors, strictures, and granulation tissue. Two types are predominately used, the Nd:YAG (neodymium:yttrium-aluminum-garnet) for bulky endobronchial tumors and carbon dioxide (CO_2) lasers, which are more appropriate for tracheal weblike stenosis. The CO_2 laser has precise cutting abilities, with minimal tissue penetration of 0.1 to 0.5 mm; it can be used only with a rigid bronchoscope. The Nd:YAG laser has less precise cutting abilities but can penetrate tissue to a depth of 3 to 5 mm; it also has far better potential to control bleeding than does a CO_2 laser. Nd:YAG lasers can be used with flexible or rigid bronchoscopes. Lasers are safe; infrequent complications include endobronchial fire, hemorrhage, and the development of a tracheoesophageal or bronchoesophageal fistula or of a tracheal-pulmonary arterial fistula. Recanalization rates for laser therapy in malignant disease have been reported to be greater than 90%; for benign disorders, between 50% to 80% (101, 104–106). In addition, studies have also shown that laser therapy for central airway obstruction can improve dyspnea, ventilation, and survival (107–109). A commonly encountered benign condition for which laser therapy is also being used is a tracheal web. Successful treatments can be performed with radial laser incisions, followed by gentle balloon dilation (110).

Stents

Endoprostheses or airway stents are devices designed to maintain the integrity of the trachea or bronchi. They are used for maintaining patency in airways that are extrinsically compressed by tumor or enlarged lymph nodes. They are also

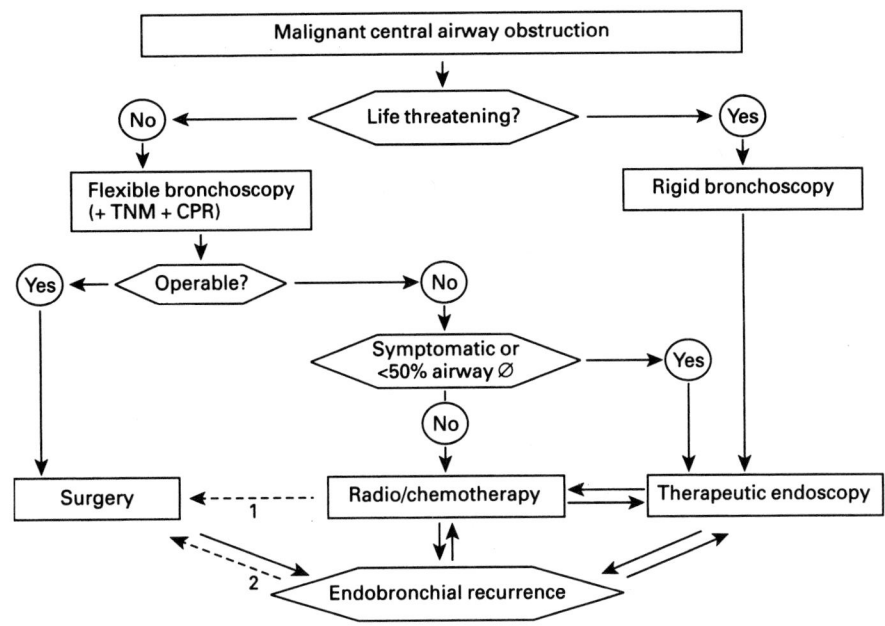

FIGURE 4.7. Algorithm for the management of malignant central airway obstruction. (From Bolliger CT. Statement on interventional pulmonology. *Eur Respir J* 2002;19:356–373, with permission.)

used for residual mucosal tumor after a debulking procedure, for covering tracheoesophageal or bronchoesophageal fistulas, and for tracheobronchomalacia. Stents are made of metal or silicone. Silicone stents must be placed in the airways with a rigid bronchoscope. They are easy to remove but frequently migrate and cause inspissation of secretions. Expandable metallic stents can be placed with a flexible or rigid bronchoscope. They are less likely to migrate, and they have fewer problems with inspissated secretions. However, they are expensive, are difficult to remove, and have higher rates of causing granulation tissue to form. Many studies evaluating the use of stents in the above-mentioned conditions have shown good outcomes (111–114).

Bronchoplasty

Bronchoplasty, or dilation of an airway with a balloon, is used to treat malignant and benign airway stenosis. Bronchoplasty is usually performed before or after placing a stent in the airway, or before placing a brachytherapy catheter. Bronchoplasty can be done with a flexible or rigid bronchoscope. Complications include bronchospasm, chest pain, and perforation of the airway. Most reported series of bronchoplasty are small, have inconsistent lengths of follow-up, and involve various medical conditions. However, most of these studies have shown bronchoplasty to be a safe and beneficial procedure (115–118).

Electrocautery, Cryotherapy, and Argon Plasma Coagulation

Electrotherapy and cryotherapy are used for the treatment of disorders similar to those treated with a laser. However,

these modalities may be better for more distal lesions because they have a lower risk for airway perforation. Both can be used with a flexible or rigid bronchoscope. Electrotherapy can be used with a blunt-tip probe or a snare. The addition of argon plasma coagulation eliminates the need for tissue contact and decreases the risk of perforation, because the tissue penetration depth attained is only 2 to 3 mm. In addition, electrotherapy is an excellent tool for hemostasis. Most studies of electrotherapy have examined its use in the removal of tumors and have shown success rates of between 75% and 95% (119, 120).

Cryotherapy causes tissue necrosis through hypothermic cellular destruction. However, the major disadvantage of this modality is its delayed effects. A repeat bronchoscopy is usually needed a day or two later to remove the sloughed tissue. Also, it does not work on fat, cartilage, bone, connective tissue, or fibrotic tissue. Cryotherapy has its advantage in removing foreign bodies or clots from the airways.

Photodynamic Therapy and Brachytherapy

Photodynamic therapy (PDT) and brachytherapy are used in the treatment of malignancies. PDT is primarily used as a curative treatment for carcinoma in situ or high-grade dysplastic lesions of the central airways and, to a lesser extent, palliative treatment of airway obstruction (121). PDT can treat cancer to a depth of 5 mm. EBUS can sometimes be used to help assess the depth of tumor invasion. PDT involves injecting hematoporphyrin derivatives systemically into the patient. Hematoporphyrins clear from most cells in the body within 72 hours; however, delayed clearance is seen in skin, liver, spleen, and cancer cells. Because hematoporphyrins are photosensitive, a specific laser can be used at the site of cancer to induce a cytotoxic reaction, leading to cell death. Like cryotherapy, the reaction is delayed, and a repeat bronchoscopy needs to be performed a day or two later to clean up the sloughed tissue.

Brachytherapy is the treatment of tumors with radiation delivered directly into the bronchi through radioactive seeds that are temporarily placed in the airways. This is accomplished with bronchoscopic insertion of a thin hollow catheter through a malignant obstruction under fluoroscopic guidance. Radioactive seeds are then inserted into the catheter and left in position for several minutes (high-dose techniques) or for 2 to 40 hours (low-dose techniques). The major complication of endobronchial brachytherapy is hemorrhage. The effects of treatment begin to appear in 2 to 3 weeks. Thus, this modality cannot be used as treatment for emergent obstructions. Studies involving brachytherapy as the treatment for airway obstruction owing to bronchogenic cancer demonstrate a 60% to 90% recanalization rate (122).

Bronchoscopic Control of Hemoptysis

The timing of bronchoscopy and its role in the localization of hemoptysis was discussed earlier (see "Hemoptysis"). The treatment of hemoptysis includes airway protection, volume resuscitation, and correction of any coagulopathy. Bronchoscopic modalities include airway tamponade, electrotherapy, cryotherapy, and instillation of vasoconstrictive medications at the site of bleed. To protect the airway, the bleeding lung should be placed down. If ventilation is at all compromised, the patient should be intubated with a single-lumen 8-mm endotracheal tube or larger so as to accommodate a flexible bronchoscope. Double-lumen endotracheal tubes can also be used, but they are not as useful to manage a major airway bleed as is a single-lumen tube. If the blood is coming from the right lung, the left lung can be electively intubated and ventilated and vice versa. A 14F Fogarty balloon-tipped catheter or a double-lumen bronchus blocker can be used to tamponade the bronchus from which the blood is coming for up to 24 hours while a more definitive treatment is planned. The double-lumen bronchus blocker has the advantage of being able to fit through the working channel of a bronchoscope, and it has an inner channel through which medications can be instilled. The instillation of 1 to 2 mL of 1:20,000 epinephrine may help stop or slow the bleeding (123). Also shown to be beneficial is the instillation of 50 mL aliquots of 4°C iced saline (124). If an endobronchial lesion is identified as the source of bleeding, electrotherapy, laser therapy, or an argon plasma coagulator can be used. Also, cryotherapy can be used to help remove large clots that can impair visualization.

Foreign Bodies

Deaths caused by ingestion of a foreign body have remained greater than 3,000 per year for the past 5 years (125). Factors

that contribute to the ingestion of foreign bodies include alcohol, sedatives, poor dentition, senility, neuromuscular disorders, seizure, and trauma. The most common location for a foreign body is in one of the right lower lobe bronchi. This is because of their larger diameter and more vertical position. Both the flexible and rigid bronchoscope can be used to remove a foreign body. Oral intubation should be performed for easier removal of the foreign body; the nasal airway may be too small. Also, the foreign body cannot be removed through the working channel of a flexible bronchoscope; thus, the foreign body, bronchoscope, and grasping instrument will all need to be removed together. There are a diverse array of instruments that can be used with the flexible or rigid bronchoscope to assist in removal of a foreign body. These include various forceps, baskets, and snares (Fig. 4.8). A 4F to 7F Fogarty balloon can also be used. It is advanced beyond the foreign body and then inflated. Once inflated, it is pulled back toward the bronchoscope in an attempt to dislodge and move the object into a more proximal airway. A laser may be used to cut the object or to ablate granulation

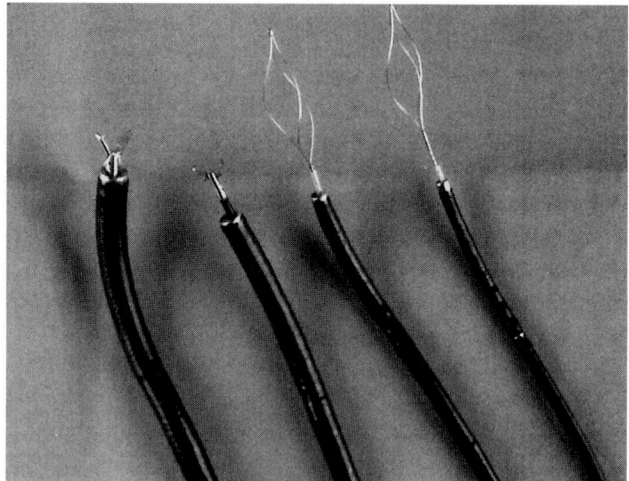

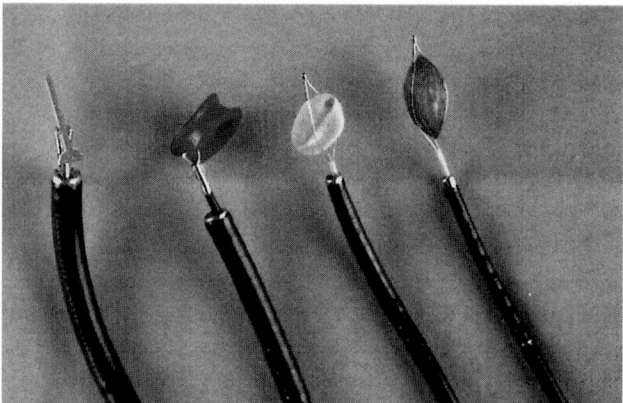

FIGURE 4.8. Tools for foreign body removal (forceps, grasping claws, and baskets) can be passed through flexible bronchoscope, as shown, or through a rigid bronchoscope. (From Marquette CH, Martinot A. Foreign body removal in adults and children. In: Bolliger CT, Mahtur PN, eds. *Interventional bronchoscopy.* New York: Karger, 1999:101, with permission.)

THERAPEUTIC APPLICATIONS

Summary Statement	Level of Evidence
Malignancies causing endobronchial obstruction: quick relief of associated symptoms by using a variety of ablative instruments (laser, electrocautery, argon plasma coagulator). Much slower response from cryotherapy or endobronchial brachytherapy. Either flexible or rigid bronchoscopes, but rigid is better (quicker)	Many case series
Extrinsic compression: balloon dilation and stent insertion often palliate symptoms	Multiple case series
Photodynamic therapy: best application is for carcinoma in situ or high-grade dysplasia. Bulky tumors can be treated this way, but it is not as effective as other ablative devices.	Multiple case series
Foreign bodies: invaluable tool for removal. Rigid generally better than flexible bronchoscope	Has stood the test of more than a century of practice

tissue that may form. Cryotherapy also can be used to freeze the tip of the probe to the object and then remove it.

REFERENCES

1. Killian G. Removal of a bone splinter from the right bronchus with help of direct laryngoscopy. *Proc Southwest German Otorhino* 1897;44: 86.
2. Ikeda S, Yanai N, Ishikawa S. Flexible bronchofiberscope. *Keio J Med* 1968;17:1–16.
3. Prakash UBS, Offord KF, Stubbs SE. Bronchoscopy in North America: the ACCP survey. *Chest* 1991;100:1668–1675.
4. Dweik RA, Mehta AC, Meeker DP, et al. Analysis of the safety of bronchoscopy after recent acute myocardial infarction. *Chest* 1996;110:825–828.
5. Credle WF Jr, Smiddy J, Elliott R. Complications of fiberoptic bronchoscopy. *Am Rev Respir Dis* 1974;109:67–72.
6. Suratt P, Smiddy J, Gruber B. Deaths and complications associated with fiberoptic bronchoscopy. *Chest* 1976;69:747–751.
7. Simpson FG, Arnold AG, Purvis A, et al. Postal survey of bronchoscopic practice by physicians in the United Kingdom. *Thorax* 1986;41:311–317.
8. Pue C, Pacht E. Complications of fiberoptic bronchoscopy at a university hospital. *Chest* 1995;107:430–432.
9. Milman N, Faurschou P, Gorde G, et al. Pulse oximetry during fibreoptic bronchoscopy in local anaesthesia: frequency of hypoxaemia and effect of oxygen supplementation. *Respiration* 1994;61:342–347.
10. Crawford M, Pollock J, Anderson K, et al. Comparison of midazolam with propofol for sedation in outpatient bronchoscopy. *Br J Anaesth* 1993;70:419–422.
11. de Fijter J, Van Der Hoeven J, Eggelmeijer F, et al. Sepsis syndrome and death after bronchoalveolar lavage. *Chest* 1993;104:1296–1297.
12. Rennard SI, Aalbers R, Bleeker E, et al. Bronchoalveolar lavage: performance, sampling procedure, processing, and assessment. *Eur Respir J* 1998;26[Suppl]:135–155.
13. Krause A, Hohberg B, Heine F, et al. Cytokines derived from alveolar macrophage induced fever after bronchoscopy and bronchoalveolar lavage. *Am J Resp Crit Care Med* 1997;155:1793–1797.
14. Witte M, Opal S, Gilbert J, et al. Incidence of fever and bacteremia following transbronchial needle aspiration. *Chest* 1986;89:85–87.
15. Yigla M, Orev I, Beutur Z, et al. Incidence of bacteraemia following fibreoptic bronchoscopy. *Eur Respir J* 1999;14:789–791.
16. Dajani AS, Taubert KA, Wilson W, et al. Prevention of bacterial endocarditis: recommendations by the American Heart Association. *Clin Infect Dis* 1997;25:1448–1458.
17. Bjortuft O, Brosstao F, Boe J. Bronchoscopy with transbronchial biopsies: measurement of bleeding volume and evaluation of the predictive value of coagulation tests. *Eur Respir J* 1998;12:1025–1027.
18. Kozak E, Brath L. Do "screening" coagulation tests predict bleeding in patients undergoing fiberoptic bronchoscopy with biopsy? *Chest* 1994;106:703–705.
19. Hewer RD, Jones PM, Thomas PS, et al. A prospective study of atropine premedication in flexible bronchoscopy. *Aust NZ J Med* 2000;30:466–469.
20. Cowl CT, Prakash UBS, Kruger BR. The role of anticholinergics in bronchoscopy: a randomized clinical trial. *Chest* 2000;118:188–192.
21. Foster WM, Hurewitz AN. Aerosolized lidocaine reduces dose of topical anesthetic for bronchoscopy. *Am Rev Respir Dis* 1992;146:520–522.
22. Popovich J Jr, Kvale PA, Eichenhorn MS, et al. Diagnostic accuracy of multiple biopsies from flexible fiberoptic bronchoscopy. *Am Rev Respir Dis* 1982;125:521–523.
23. Elkus R, Miller M, Kini S, et al. A comparison of withdrawn and nonwithdrawn brushes in the diagnosis of lung cancer. *J Bronchol* 1994;1:269–275.
24. Kvale PA, Bode FR, Kini S. Diagnostic accuracy in lung cancer: comparison of techniques used in association with flexible fiberoptic bronchoscopy. *Chest* 1976;69:752–757.
25. Govert JA, Kopita JM, Matchar D, et al. Cost-effectiveness of collecting routine cytologic specimen during fiberoptic bronchoscopy for endoscopically visible lung tumor. *Chest* 1996;109:451–456.
26. Dasgupta A, Mehta AC. Transbronchial needle aspiration: an underused diagnostic technique. *Clin Chest Med* 1999;20:39–51.
27. Shure D, Fedullo PF. Transbronchial needle aspiration. *Am Rev Respir Dis* 1983;128:1090–1092.
28. Katis K, Inglesos E, Zachariadis E, et al. The role of transbronchial needle aspiration in the diagnosis of peripheral lung masses or nodules. *Eur Respir J* 1995;8:963–966.
29. Baaklini WA, Reinosis MA, Gorin AS, et al. Diagnostic yield of fiberoptic bronchoscopy in evaluating solitary pulmonary nodules. *Chest* 2000;117:1049–1054.
30. Kvale PA. Bronchoscopic biopsies and bronchoalveolar lavage. *Chest Surg Clin N Amer* 1996;6:205–222.
31. Reichenberger F, Weber J, Tamm M, et al. The value of transbronchial needle aspiration in the diagnosis of peripheral pulmonary lesions. *Chest* 1999;116:704–708.
32. Gunen H, Kizkin O, Tahaoglu C, et al. Utility of blind forceps biopsy of the main carina and upper-lobe carina in patients with non-small cell lung cancer. *Chest* 2001;119:632–637.

33. Williams MD, Sandler AB. The epidemiology of lung cancer. *Cancer Treat Res* 2001;105:31–52.

34. Lam S, MacAulay C, leRiche JC, et al. Detection and localization of early lung cancer by fluorescence bronchoscopy. *Cancer* 2000;89[Suppl 11]:2468–2473.

35. Lam S, MacAulay C, Hung J, et al. Detection of dysplasia and carcinoma in situ by a lung imaging fluorescence endoscope device. *J Thorac Cardiovasc Surg* 1993;105:1035–1040.

36. Lam S, MacAulay C, Palcic B. Detection and localization of early lung cancer by imaging techniques. *Chest* 1993;103[Suppl 1]:12S–14S.

37. Lam S, Kennedy T, Unger M, et al. Localization of bronchial intraepithelial neoplastic lesions by fluorescence bronchoscopy. *Chest* 1998;113:696–702.

38. Sato M, Sakurada A, Sagawa M, et al. Diagnostic results before and after introduction of autofluorescence bronchoscopy in patients suspected of having lung cancer detected by sputum cytology in lung cancer mass screening. *Lung Cancer* 2001;32:247–253.

39. Khanavkar B, Gnudi F, Muti A, et al. Basic principles of LIFE-autofluorescence bronchoscopy: results of 194 examinations in comparison with standard procedures for early detection of bronchial carcinoma-overview. *Pneumologie* 1998;52:71–76.

40. Luke WP, Pearson FG, Todd TR. Prospective evaluation of mediastinoscopy for assessment of carcinoma of the lung. *J Thorac Cardiovasc Surg* 1986;91:53–56.

41. Jain P, Arroliga A, Mehta AC. Cost effectiveness of transbronchial needle aspiration in staging of cancer. *Chest* 1996;110[Suppl]:24S.

42. Wang KP, Brower R, Haponik EF, et al. Flexible transbronchial needle aspiration for staging of bronchogenic carcinoma. *Chest* 1983;84:571–576.

43. Harris RJ, Kavuru MS, Mehta AC, et al. The impact of thoracoscopy on the management of pleural disease. *Chest* 1995;107:845–852.

44. Schenk DA, Bower JH, Bryan CL, et al. Transbronchial needle aspiration staging of bronchogenic carcinoma. *Am Rev Respir Dis* 1986;134:146–148.

45. Shure D, Fedullo PF. The role of transcarinal needle aspiration in the staging of bronchogenic cancer. *Chest* 1984;86:693–696.

46. Mehta AC, Kavuru MS, Meeker DP, et al. Transbronchial needle aspiration for histology specimens. *Chest* 1989;96:1268–1232.

47. Bilaceroglu S, Cagiotariotaciota U, Gunel O, et al. Comparison of rigid and flexible transbronchial needle aspiration in the staging of bronchogenic cancer. *Respiration* 1998;65:441–449.

48. Rodriguez de Castro F, Diaz Lopez F, Serda GJ, et al. Relevance of training in transbronchial fine needle aspiration technique. *Chest* 1997;111:103–105.

49. Wang KP. Staging of bronchogenic carcinoma by bronchoscopy. *Chest* 1994;106:588–593.

50. Haponik EF, Shure D. Underutilization of transbronchial needle aspiration: experiences of current pulmonary fellows. *Chest* 1997;112:25–253.

51. Haponik EF, Cappellari JO, Chin R, et al. Education and experience improve transbronchial needle aspiration performance. *Am J Respir Crit Care Med* 1995;151:1998–2002.

52. White CS, Weiner EA, Patel P, et al. Transbronchial needle aspiration: guidance with CT fluoroscopy. *Chest* 2000;118:1630–1638.

53. Mitchell D, Emerson C, Collins J, et al. Transbronchial lung biopsy with the fibreoptic bronchoscope: analysis of results in 433 patients. *Br J Dis Chest* 1981;75:258–262.

54. Zsiray M, Appel J, Lantos A. Transbronchial biopsy in diffuse infiltrative lung diseases. *Orv Hetil* 1999;140:1239–1243.

55. Ahluwalia G, Sharma SK, Datagupta S, et al. Role of transbronchial lung biopsy in diffuse pulmonary disease. *Indian J Chest Dis Allied Sci* 1999;41:213–217.

56. Descombes E, Gardiol D, Levenberger P. Transbronchial lung biopsy: an analysis of 530 cases with reference to the number of samples. *Monaldi Arch Chest Dis* 1997;52:324–329.

57. Shorr AF, Torrington KG, Hnatiuk OW. Endobronchial biopsy for sarcoidosis: a prospective study. *Chest* 2001;120:109–114.

58. Wang KP, Fuenning C, Johns CJ, et al. Flexible transbronchial needle aspiration for the diagnosis of sarcoidosis. *Ann Otol Rhinol Laryngol* 1989;98:298–300.

59. Bilaceroglu S, Perim K, Gunel O, et al. Combining transbronchial aspiration with endobronchial and transbronchial biopsy in sarcoidosis. *Monaldi Arch Chest Dis* 1999;54:217–223.

60. King TE Jr. Interstitial lung disease. In: Feinsilver SH, Fein AM, *Textbook of bronchoscopy.* Baltimore: Williams and Wilkins, 1995;185.

61. Baselski VS, el-Torky M, Coalson JJ, et al. The standardization of criteria for processing and interpreting laboratory specimens in patients with suspected ventilator associated pneumonia. *Chest* 1992;102[Suppl 1]:571S–579S.

62. Chastre J, Fagon JY, Bornet-Lesco M, et al. Evaluation of bronchoscopic techniques for the diagnosis of nosocomial pneumonia. *Am J Respir Crit Care Med* 1995;152:231–240.

63. Ewig S, Torres A. Flexible bronchoscopy in nosocomial pneumonia. *Clin Chest Med* 2001;22:263–279.

64. Niederman MS. Bronchoscopy in nonresolving nosocomial pneumonia. *Chest* 2000;117[Suppl 2]:212S–218S.

65. Pereira Gomes JC, Pedreira WL Jr, Araujo EM, et al. Impact of bronchoalveolar lavage on management of pneumonia with treatment failure. *Chest* 2000;118:1739–1746.

66. Luna CM, Vujacich P, Niederman MS, et al. Impact of BAL data on the therapy and outcome of ventilator-associated pneumonia. *Chest* 1997;111:676–685.

67. Baughman RP. Protected-specimen brush technique in the diagnosis of ventilator- associated pneumonia. *Chest* 2000;117[Suppl 2]:203S–206S.

68. Sanchez-Nieto JM, Torres A, Garcia-Cordoba F, et al. Impact of invasive and noninvasive quantitative culture sampling on outcome in ventilator-associated pneumonia: a pilot study. *Am J Respir Crit Care Med* 1998;157:371–376.

69. Heyland DK, Cook DJ, Marshall J, et al. The clinical utility of invasive diagnostic techniques in the setting of ventilator associated pneumonia: Canadian Critical Care Trials Group. *Chest* 1999;115:1076–1084.

70. Sole-Violan J, Fernandez JA, Benitez AB, et al. Impact of quantitative invasive diagnostic techniques in the management and outcome of mechanical ventilated patients with suspected pneumonia. *Crit Care Med* 2000;28:2737–2741.

71. Guerra LF, Baughman RP. Use of bronchoalveolar lavage to diagnosis bacterial pneumonia in mechanical ventilated patients. *Crit Care Med* 1990;18:169–173.

72. Chastre J, Viau F, Brun P, et al. Prospective evaluation of the protected specimen brush for the diagnosis of pulmonary infections in ventilated patients. *Am Rev Respir Dis* 1984;130:924–929.

73. Chastre J, Fagon JY, Bornet-Lesco M, et al. Evaluation of bronchoscopic techniques for the diagnosis of nosocomial pneumonia. *Am J Respir Crit Care Med* 1995;152:231–240.

74. Broughton WA, Middleton RM 3rd, Kirkpatrick MB, et al. Bronchoscopic protected specimen brush and bronchoalveolar lavage in the diagnosis of bacterial pneumonia. *Infect Dis Clin North Am* 1991;5:437–452.

75. Shelhamer JH, Toews GB, Masur H, et al. NIH conference: respiratory disease in the immunosuppressed patient. *Ann Intern Med* 1992;117:415–431.

76. Rano A, Agusti C, Jimenez P, et al. Pulmonary infiltrates in non-HIV immunocompromised patients: a diagnostic approach using noninvasive and bronchoscopic procedures. *Thorax* 2001;56:379–387.

77. Xaubet A, Torres A, Marco F, et al. Pulmonary infiltrates in immunocompromised patient: diagnostic value of telescoping plugged catheter and bronchoalveolar lavage. *Chest* 1989; 95:130–135.

78. Rafanan AL, Klevjer-Anderson P, Metersky ML. *Pneumocystis carinii* pneumonia diagnosed by non-induced sputum stained with a direct fluorescence antibody. *Ann Clin Lab Sci* 1998;28:99–103.

79. Chouaid C, Housset B, Lebeau B. Cost-analysis of four different strategies for *Pneumocystis carinii* pneumonia in HIV-infected subjects. *Eur Respir J* 1995;8:1554–1548.

80. Kovacs JA, Ng VL, Masur H, et al. Diagnosis of *Pneumocystis carinii* pneumonia: improved detection in sputum with use of monoclonal antibody. *N Engl J Med* 1988;318:589–593.

81. Broaddus C, Dake MD, Stulbarg MS, et al. Bronchoalveolar lavage and transbronchial biopsy for diagnosis of pulmonary infection in the acquired immunodeficiency syndrome. *Ann Intern Med* 1985;102:747–752.

82. Huang L, Hecht FM, Stansell JD, et al. Suspected *Pneumocystis carinii* pneumonia with a negative induced sputum examination: is early bronchoscopy useful? *Am J Respir Crit Care Med* 1995;151:1866–1871.

83. Yung RC, Weinacker AB, Steiger DJ, et al. Upper and middle lobe bronchoalveolar lavage to diagnose *Pneumocystis carinii* pneumonia. *Am Rev Respir Dis* 1993;148:1563–1566.

84. Jules-Elysee KM, Stover DE, Zaman MB, et al. Aerosolized pentamidine: effect of diagnosis and presentation of *Pneumocystis carinii* pneumonia. *Ann Intern Med* 1990;112:750–757.

85. Mann M, Shelhamer JH, Masur H, et al. Lack of clinical utility of bronchoalveolar lavage cultures for cytomegalovirus in HIV infection. *Am J Respir Crit Care Med* 1997;155:1723–1728.

86. Miles PR, Baughman RP, Linnemann CC Jr. Cytomegalovirus in the bronchoalveolar lavage fluid of patients with AIDS. *Chest* 1990;97:1072–1076.

87. Uberti-Foppa C, Lillo F, Terreni MR, et al. Cytomegalovirus pneumonia in AIDS patients: value of cytological culture from BAL fluid and correlation with lung disease. *Chest* 1998:113:919–923.

88. Anderson C, Inhaber N, Menzies D. Comparison of sputum induction with fiber-optic bronchoscopy in the diagnosis of tuberculosis. *Am J Respir Crit Care Med* 1995;152:1570–1574.

89. Conde MB, Soares SL, Mello FC, et al. Comparison of sputum induction with fiberoptic bronchoscopy in the diagnosis of tuberculosis: experience at an acquired immune deficiency syndrome reference center in Rio de Janeiro, Brazil. *Am J Respir Crit Care Med* 2000;162:2238–2240.

90. Charoenratanakul S, Dejsomritrutai W, Chaiprasert A. Diagnostic role of fiberoptic bronchoscopy in suspected smear negative pulmonary tuberculosis. *Respir Med* 1995;89:621–623.

91. Kennedy DJ, Lewis WP, Barnes PF. Yield of bronchoscopy for the diagnosis of tuberculosis in patients with human immunodeficiency virus infection. *Chest* 1992;102:1040–1043.

92. Chen KY, Ko SC, Hsueh PR, et al. Pulmonary fungal infection: emphasis on microbiological spectra, patient outcome, and prognostic factors. *Chest* 2001;120:177–184.

93. von Eiff M, Roos N, Fegeler W, et al. Hospital-acquired candida and aspergillus pneumonia-diagnostic approaches and clinical findings. *J Hosp Infect* 1996;32:17–28.

94. von Eiff M, Roos N, Schulten R, et al. Pulmonary aspergillosis: early diagnosis improves survival. *Respiration* 1995;62:341–347.

95. Reichenberger F, Habicht J, Matt P, et al. Diagnostic yield of bronchoscopy in histologically proven invasive pulmonary aspergillosis. *Bone Marrow Transplant* 1999;24:1195–1199.

96. Cahill BC, Ingbar DH. Massive hemoptysis: assessment and management. *Clin Chest Med* 1994;15:147–167.

97. Simoff MJ. Endobronchial management of advanced lung cancer. *Cancer Control* 2001;4:337–343.

98. Purer ST, Lindskog GE. Hemoptysis. *Am Rev Respir Dis* 1961; 84:329–336.

99. Susanto I. Managing a patient with hemoptysis. *J Bronchol* 2002;9:40–45.

100. Dweik RA, Stoller JK. Role of bronchoscopy in massive hemoptysis. *Clin Chest Med* 1999;20:89–105.

101. Szidon JP, Fishman AP. Approach to the pulmonary patient with respiratory signs and symptoms. In: *Pulmonary disease and disorders.* New York: McGraw-Hill, 1988:346–351.

102. Cavaliere S, Venuta F, Foccoli P, et al. Endoscopic treatment of malignant airway obstruction in 2,008 patients. *Chest* 1996;110:1536–1542.

103. Luomanen RKJ, Watson WL. Autopsy findings. In: Watson WL, ed. *Lung cancer.* St Louis: Mosby, 1968;504–510.

104. Shah H, Garbe L, Nussbaum E, et al. Benign tumors of the tracheobronchial tree: endoscopic characteristics and use of laser resection. *Chest* 1995;107:1744–1751.

105. Otto W, Szlenk Z, Paczkowski P, et al. Endoscopic laser treatment of benign tracheal stenosis. *Otolaryngol Head Neck Surg* 1995;113:211–214.

106. Personne C, Colchen A, Leroy M. Indications and techniques for endoscopic laser resection in bronchology: a critical analysis based on 2,284 resections. *J Thorac Cardiovasc Surg* 1986;91:710–715.

107. Eichenhorn MS, Kvale PA, Miks VM, et al. Initial combination therapy with YAG laser photoresection and irradiation for inoperable non–small cell cancer of the lung: a preliminary report. *Chest* 1986;89:782–785.

108. Kvale PA, Eichenhorn MS, Radke JR, et al. YAG laser photoresection of lesions obstructing the central airways. *Chest* 1985;87:283–288.

109. Desai SJ, Mehta AC, VanderBrug Medendorp S, et al. Survival experience following Nd:YAG laser photoresection for primary bronchogenic cancer. *Chest* 1988;94:939–944.

110. Mehta AC, Lee FY, Cordasco EM, et al. Concentric tracheal and subglottic stenosis: management using the Nd:YAG laser for mucosal sparing followed by gentle dilation. *Chest* 1993;104:673–677.

111. Mehta AC, Dasgupta A. Airway stents. *Clin Chest Med* 1999;20:139–151.

112. Dumon JF, Cavaliere S, Diaz-Jiminez JP, et al. Seven year experience with the Dumon prosthesis. *J Bronchol* 1996;3:6–10.

113. Carrasco CH, Nesbitt JC, Charnsangavej C, et al. Management of tracheal and bronchial stenosis with the Gianturco stent. *Ann Thorac Surg* 1994;58:1012–1018.

114. Hauck RW, Lembeck RM, Emslander HP, et al. Implantation of Accuflex and Strecker stents in malignant bronchial stenosis by flexible bronchoscopy. *Chest* 1997;112:134–144.

115. Keller C, Frost A. Fiberoptic bronchoplasty: description of a simple adjunct technique for the management of bronchial stenosis following lung transplantation. *Chest* 1992;102:995–998.

116. Carre P, Rousseau H, Lombart L, et al. Balloon dilation and self-expanding metal Wallstent insertion: for management of bronchostenosis following lung transplantation: the Toulouse Lung Transplantation Group. *Chest* 1994;105:343–348.

117. Fouty BW, Pomeranz M, Thigpen TP, et al. Dilation of bronchial stenosis due to sarcoidosis using a flexible fiberoptic bronchoscope. *Chest* 1994;106:677–680.

118. Ferretti G, Jouvan FB, Thony F, et al. Benign noninflammatory bronchial stenosis: treatment with balloon dilation. *Radiology* 1995;196:831–834.

119. Carpenter RJ 3rd, Neel HB 3rd, Sanderson DR. Comparison of endobronchial cryotherapy and electrocoagulation of bronchi. *Trans Am Acad Opthalmol Otolaryngol* 1977;84:313–323.

120. Sutedja G, van Kralingen K, Schramel FM, et al. Fibreoptic bronchoscopic electrosurgery under local anaesthesia for rapid palliation in patients with central airway malignancies: a preliminary report. *Thorax* 1994;49:1243–1246.

121. Edell ES, Cortese DA. Bronchoscopic phototherapy with hematoporphyrin derivative for treatment of localized bronchogenic cancer: a 5-year experience. *Mayo Clin Proc* 1987;67:8–14.

122. Seijo LM, Sterman DH. Interventional pulmonology. *N Engl J Med* 2001;344:740–749.

123. Zavala DC. Pulmonary hemorrhage in fiberoptic bronchoscopic transbronchial biopsy. *Chest* 1976;70:584–588.

124. Conlan AA, Hurwitz SS. Management of massive hemoptysis with the rigid bronchoscope and cold saline lavage. *Thorax* 1980;30:901–904.

125. Rafanan A, Mehta AC. Adult airway foreign body removal: what's new? *Clin Chest Med* 2001;22:319–330.

Invasive Pulmonary Diagnostic Procedures: Pleural Diagnostic Procedures

5

Robert Loddenkemper · Wolfgang Frank

THORACENTESIS

Clinical Role

Invasive procedures in the evaluation of pleural disease usually follow a hierarchy of graded invasiveness as required by the clinical course under careful weighing of diagnostic demands versus risks. Because effusion is the prevailing manifestation of pleural disease, sampling of pleural fluid *(thoracentesis)* usually represents a basic step and a clinical platform to decide on the need for further microbiological, histological, or immunological studies. Thoracentesis may suffice to verify a clinical diagnosis with reasonable certainty in about 50% of patients and may allow presumptive diagnosis in another 25%. It will provide information relevant to the clinical decision-making process in more than 90% of patients. Thoracentesis is indicated when there is sufficient effusion for the procedure to be safely performed (i.e., with a fluid film >10 mm in the lateral decubitus position) and when the clinical setting suggests that pleural fluid sampling will likely yield etiologic information into the disease process owing to expected direct pleural involvement. This will usually be reflected by exudative effusion characteristics. In indirect ("innocent-bystander"-type) pleural involvement—as occurs in distant extrapleural disorders like congestive heart failure, hepatic dysfunction, renal disease and hypoproteinemia—thoracentesis is only indicated when the presumptive transudative effusion fails to respond to medical treatment or when discrepant clinical observations such as chest pain or fever suggest local causes. When using this algorithm in a random patient sample, based on current epidemiologic data, less than 60% of all effusions will need to be evaluated by thoracentesis (1). In an intensive care setting, on a cardiac unit, or a postsurgical ward, the odds ratio to face true exudative features in pleural effusion is even lower and may approach 0.25 (2).

Technique

Diagnostic thoracentesis may be performed in a bedside setting or in an endoscopic/radiologic unit. If anxiety of the patient is properly controlled by the operator guidance and explanations, it will usually not require sedative premedication or local anesthesia. A recent chest radiograph is a standard prerequisite to safely perform thoracentesis. Modern ultrasound exploration using linear, convex, or sector scanners has now evolved as a superior imaging technique and has largely replaced fluoroscopy-monitored postural maneuvers for the selection of interest- and safety-defined entry points (3). Ultrasound contributes valuable descriptive clues as to the presence of a trapped or chambered ("multilocular") effusion or of a free flowing ("monolocular") fluid collection. Another asset is the recognition of impeding factors such as pleural thickening owing to membranes and peels. In experienced hands, classical percussion-guided bedside thoracentesis remains an expedient and safe option for thoracentesis, and this is particularly true in profuse and monolocular effusion. The point of entry should then be determined two interspaces below the level of flattening of percussion sound to avoid puncture of the ascending flat part of the fluid collection and, thus, the possibility of accidental lung injury. In trapped or multilocular collections, direct ultrasound-guidance may be extremely helpful to precisely target even minor accessible fluid compartments and to avoid a "dry" puncture.

The patient is usually optimally placed in a sitting or supported position or—in the case of severe debilitation, as in intensive care—in a lateral decubitus position with the side of the effusion dependent. Once the relevant costal

R. Loddenkemper: Professor, Humboldt University; Department of Pneumology II, Zentralklinik Emil von Behring, Lungenklinik Heckeshorn, Berlin, Germany.

W. Frank: Johanniter-Krankenhaus Treuenbrietzen, Pneumologische Klinik III, Treuenbrietzen, Germany.

interspace has been determined with the method of choice, the site should be generously cleaned with a sterile scrubbing technique using a 10% polyvidone-iodine solution. The needle entry point should carefully avoid the vasculature- and nerve bundle-conducting lower rib sulcus, and the penetration should not be too deep. An appropriate needle and a quick but unforceful insertion technique should be used. The discomfort of the patient will hardly exceed that of venipuncture. The needle used should be small and short enough to minimize pain and complications in general, but large and long enough to obtain viscous fluid samples like pus and to overcome eventual pleural thickening. A 19-gauge (1.1-mm) needle of at least 1.5-in. (4 cm) but no longer than 2.4-in. (6 cm) length would appear to usually be an appropriate compromise. For diagnostic thoracentesis, the needle is assembled with a 20-mL syringe, which should be anticoagulant-conditioned (e.g., contain minimal amount of 1:1000 heparin or sodium citrate solution) to avoid clotting artifacts. The initial aspirate portion after needle insertion must be critically scrutinized. In most instances, the recovery of straw- to amber-colored, clear or variably turbid fluid (including frank pus or milky [chyliform] fluid) confirms the correct position of the needle. Problems with the sample not being representative may arise with sanguinous aspirates or frank blood. Artificial hemorrhage and blood contamination by malpuncture may be easily recognized by a changing degree of blood staining occurring during aspiration at different levels of penetration. Sometimes it may suffice to discard the initial contaminated specimen portion and then obtain a representative sample with a second syringe. Another pitfall may be "dry" puncture, suggesting either tough viscous or clotted aspirate, peels, chambers, or a completely dystopic position of the needle. Should malpuncture occur, *multiple* or *parallel thoracenteses* should be considered at different imaging-confirmed safe entry sites. This may even be diagnostically crucial and useful with correct puncture when the representation of a single sample is at doubt, as in multilocular effusion in which the fluid composition may vary from one to another pleural compartment. In other instances— e.g., parapneumonic and paramalignant effusion—the fluid features may change rapidly with the evolution of the disease, giving rise to more or less close follow-up investigations *(serial thoracentesis).*

The optimum amount of fluid aspirate at thoracentesis has been a subject of controversy. No more than 20 to 40 mL fluid is required to meet all analytic demands. In clinical practice, occasionally amounts up to 1 L or more are being recovered with a claim to superior diagnostic power. However, there is no evidence for a proportional gain in sensitivity of diagnostic tests with large fluid amounts, except when these are being centrifuged for microbiologic evaluation (e.g., *Mycobacterium tuberculosis*). Otherwise, large volume diagnostic thoracentesis is not necessary or desirable because it may (a) induce complications (in particular pneumothorax) and (b) create adhesions, thus impeding eventual more powerful endoscopic investigation. Exceptionally, it may still be indicated when simultaneous palliation in compressive effusion is an intention. Even then, fluid removal should be limited, avoiding a one-step removal of fluid amounts larger than 1.5 L to prevent hypotensive circulatory effects and reexpansion pulmonary edema. When palliation is the primary intention, the use of commercially available *thoracentesis kits* is advised. These devices typically include a modified, somewhat larger and longer needle (up to 16 gauge, 3 in.), often housing a spring-loaded blunt internal cannula, a three-way stopcock, a 50- to 100-mL syringe, and a 2-L collection bag, thus preventing trauma to the lung, infectious contamination, and air access to the pleura. The recovered pleural fluid sample is usually divided to different flasks for chemical, immunological, cytological, and microbiological analytic processing. An exception would apply to microbiological studies (in particular when expecting anaerobes). In these instances, the specimen should be kept and delivered cooled in the original syringe for laboratory processing.

Diagnostic Yield

Clinical Clues

These may be directly derived from gross appearance and certain physical properties. The major categories of pleural fluid are (clear or turbid) serous, sanguinous, putrid, chyliform, and hemorrhagic. Although the presence of frank blood, pus, or chyle would appear obvious from appearance, the consequent diagnosis of hemothorax, empyema, or chylothorax may be ambiguous, as these qualities may merge and there is a broad overlap with sanguinous, turbid serous, and chyliform effusions, respectively. Thus, these diagnoses also require biochemical criteria, as set out in the following sections. Abnormal viscosity, as sometimes seen in empyema or hemothorax, should be noted. An offensive foul smell is an unerring sign of (anaerobic) bacterial infection; a (very rare) ammoniacal odor indicates the presence of urinothorax. Transudates occasionally reveal a colorless, almost water-clear, appearance but are otherwise unrecognizable. The differential diagnosis between "true" (biochemical) turbidity, as that occurring in chylothorax and pseudochylothorax, and cell debris–related turbidity, as that occurring in bacterial infection and malignancy, can be readily made by centrifugation. A clearing turbidity and formation of a cell debris supernatant will exclude chylothorax and pseudochylothorax.

Biochemical Categories and Parameters

The most important categorization to be established by thoracentesis is the distinction between a *transudate* and an *exudate.* Although by gross appearance conspicuously cell-rich effusions such as an empyema or hemothorax are by definition exudates, the vast majority of effusions will reveal indiscriminate serous properties and need to be categorized biochemically.

The classical tools—also referred to as *Light's criteria*— consist in the determination of the *protein* and *lactate contents* of the effusion and their ratio compared with serum values (PF/S ratio). The discriminatory sensitivity of this approach has been reported in major series and metaanalyses to be 94% to 98%, the specificity is 77% to 83%, and the overall accuracy is 95% (4–7). Earlier specific gravity determination (</> 1,016) was commonly used, but it was much less reliable than was Light's criteria and has therefore been largely abandoned. More recently, the inclusion of *cholesterol* has shown additional value by increasing specificity (91%) but reducing sensitivity (81%), thus resulting in an overall accuracy of 83% (8). The superior specificity of cholesterol is believed to be related to its low molecular weight, colloid-osmotically neutral properties, and corresponding insensitivity to secondary volume shifts. Numerous additional biochemical and inflammatory markers (acute phase proteins and chemokines) with sometimes promising features like α_2-macroglobulin, α_1-acid glycoprotein, adenosine deaminase (ADA), C-reactive protein, interleukin-8, granulocyte-colony stimulating factor (G-CSF), interleukin-1β (IL-1β), and soluble leukocyte-selectin have been suggested over time but have not achieved clinical significance owing to limiting factors such as general availability, cost, laboratory feasibility, reproducibility, or applicability being restricted to inflammatory exudates. An optimum and pragmatic policy would currently suggest the triad of combined Light's criteria and cholesterol for clinical use, according to the validated reference values given in Table 5.1 and Figure 5.1 (see also color Fig. 5.1), in which the PF/S ratio cut-off values for each parameter will perform slightly superior to the absolute effusion concentrations (4–6). As an adjunct to transudate/exudate distinction in borderline cases, as may occur in so-called *pseudo-exudates* (i.e., transformed long-standing transudates), the determination of the PF/S albumin gradient has been recommended, in which values greater than 1.2 g/dL would favor a transudative mechanism (4).

In addition to protein, lactic dehydrogenase, and cholesterol, determination of pleural *glucose* concentration and *pH* have considerable value in clinical practice. These to-some-extent interrelated parameters may reflect aspects of severity and extension of pleural involvement. Values significantly lower than serum reference values probably result from enhanced local substrate utilization and/or decreased influx to the pleura. Thus, they nonspecifically feature encased and membranous fluid collections, as typically occur in tubercu-

losis, empyema, and rheumatic disease but also in malignant effusions. pH values less than 7.30 and glucose levels less than 60 mg/dL may narrow differential diagnosis to these entities, with the lowest (sometimes undetectable) glucose concentrations being found in empyema and rheumatoid effusions, and the lowest pH-values in esophageal rupture, empyema, and collagen vascular disease. There is some evidence that pH values below 7.30 predict a shorter survival and poor response to pleurodesis in malignant pleurisy (9). In parapneumonic effusion, metaanalysis has identified low pH values with a cut-off of 7.2 as a predictor of progression to empyema, thus necessitating chest drainage intervention (10, 11). Lactic dehydrogenase may also be used as a semiquantitative but nonspecific marker of the intensity of pleural inflammation, in which grossly elevated levels (>1,000 IU/mL) are part of the above-addressed prointerventional algorithm in the management of bacterial pleurisy (10, 11). Chemical determination of single lipid components such as *triglycerides, LDL cholesterol,* and *chylomicrons* by lipid electrophoresis can differentiate between chylothorax (triglycerides >110 mg/dL, presence of chylomicrons) and pseudochylothorax, also termed "cholesterol-pleurisy" (LDL cholesterol >200 mg/dL). Measurement of *amylase* may identify effusions complicating pancreatic disease, but elevated amylase levels are also compatible with adenocarcinoma of the parotid gland or esophagus rupture. *Isoenzyme* determination will then settle the question of a salivary gland or pancreas disease association. Sanguinous pleural effusion as a common finding, typically occurring in malignant effusion (about 50%), may easily be taken as frank blood unless hematocrit and hemoglobin levels are being determined. Although hematocrit levels as low as 5% and hemoglobin values lower than 1 mmol/L may give the impression of blood, the diagnosis of hemorrhagic effusion (true hemothorax) requires both hematocrit and hemoglobin values greater than 50% of the streaming blood.

TABLE 5.1. COMMONLY USED PARAMETERS AND RECOMMENDED CUT-OFF VALUES FOR DISTINGUISHING TRANSUDATES FROM EXUDATES

Parameter	Cut-Off Absolute Values (Transudate < Exudate>)	Cut-Off PF/S-Ratio (Transudate < Exudate>)
Protein	3 g/dL	0.5
Lactic dehydrogenase	200 IU/dL	0.6
Cholesterol	60 mg/dL	0.3

PF/S, pleural fluid/serum.

BIOCHEMICAL DISCRIMINATION BETWEEN EXUDATES AND TRANSUDATES

Summary Statement	Level of Evidence
Value of LIGHT's criteria	Randomized controlled studies
Cholesterol determination improves specificity	Randomized controlled studies
Pleural fluid/serum ratios of biochemical parameters improve both sensitivity and specificity	Randomized controlled studies
Low pH values predict poor pleurodesis response and outcome in malignant effusion	Conflicting results (randomized and nonrandomized studies)
Low pH values in bacterial pleurisy feature empyema or predict progression to empyema in parapneumonic effusion; in addition; they indicate need of drainage therapy	Randomized controlled studies

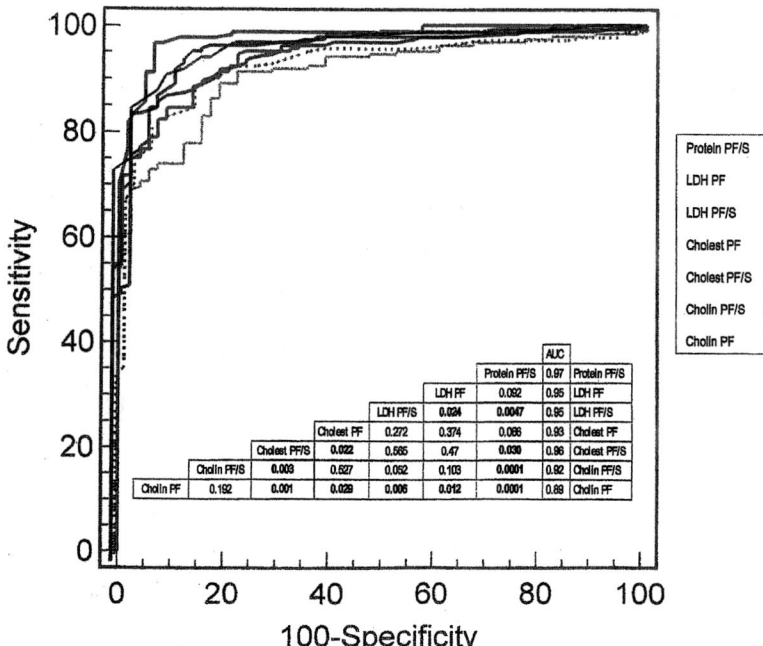

							AUC	
						Protein PF/S	0.97	Protein PF/S
					LDH PF	0.092	0.95	LDH PF
				LDH PF/S	0.024	0.0047	0.95	LDH PF/S
			Cholest PF	0.272	0.374	0.086	0.93	Cholest PF
		Cholest PF/S	0.022	0.565	0.47	0.030	0.96	Cholest PF/S
	Cholin PF/S	0.003	0.527	0.052	0.103	0.0001	0.92	Cholin PF/S
Cholin PF	0.192	0.001	0.029	0.006	0.012	0.0001	0.89	Cholin PF

Legend:
Protein PF/S
LDH PF
LDH PF/S
Cholest PF
Cholest PF/S
Cholin PF/S
Cholin PF

FIGURE 5.1. (See also color Fig. 5.1.) Receiver operating characteristics (ROC) curves of commonly used parameters for distinguishing transudates from exudates adopted from various sources (4–8). Note that the pleural fluid/serum (PF/S) ratio values generally perform superior, and that the highest area under the curve (AUC) values are achieved by protein PF/S values (0.97) and cholesterol PF/S values (0.96), respectively.

Immunological and Molecular Investigations

There is a panel of conventional immunological investigations in pleural fluid, most of which deal with collagen vascular disease and include the *rheumatoid factor, antinuclear antibodies, antineutrophil cytoplasmatic antibodies,* and *components of the complement cascade (C3, C4).* Although these parameters may specifically suggest a systemic immunological disease as causative, their sensitivity is limited. Rheumatoid factor and antinuclear antibodies titers greater than 1:320 with a PF/S ratio greater than 1 are considered highly suggestive of rheumatic effusion; the reported sensitivity of antineutrophil cytoplasmatic antibody determination varies in the literature between 50% and 98% (12). With recent progress in immunologic research of inflammatory mediator and interleukin networking, a variety of highly sensitive and specific inflammatory markers continue to enter the clinical stage. Interleukin-8 and interleukin-1β appear to be powerful inflammatory markers for bacterial pleurisy, in particular empyema, with a reported 100% sensitivity and a specificity as high as 96% in one source (13). ADA, an inflammatory enzyme expressed by sensitized and activated T lymphocytes and macrophages, has evolved as a promising semispecific biochemical marker for inflammatory processes involving T-lymphocyte/macrophage interactive granuloma formation. Thus, ADA has been shown to be particularly sensitive to tuberculous pleurisy, whereas isoenzymes (ADA$_1$) appear to nonspecifically reflect empyema and collagen vascular diseases (14). Excellent results in tuberculous pleurisy are reported in one recent study, with a 100% sensitivity and 95% specificity, using a cut-off of 47 IU/mL (15). Obviously, these data were subject to age-selective and epidemiologic pretest probability bias. In other more representative series, both the sensitivity (91%–100%) and specificity (81%–94%) were distinctly inferior, the positive and negative predictive values ranging from 84% to 93% and 89% to 100%, respectively (16–18). Another single parameter adding substantially to the diagnostic yield in tuberculous pleurisy is interferon-γ. The two largest published series revealed sensitivities and specificities of 99% and 98% and of 95% and 96%, respectively, at cut-off values of 3.7 U/mL and 240 pg/mL (19, 20). These results would place interferon-γ determination similar to ADA as a first-rank minimally invasive diagnostic test for tuberculous pleural effusion. A summary and comprehensive overview of immunologic tests in pleural effusion is provided in Table 5.2.

Microbiological Assessment

The microbiological yield in nonspecific bacterial pleurisy (parapneumonic effusion and empyema) varies largely in the literature, with a mean of 54% and a range of 24% to 94% (21). The responsible factors may include a host of factors such as (a) different patient and etiologic microorganism mix, (b) different rates and intensity of antibiotic pretreatment, and (c) different—and often inappropriate—methods of sample collection and isolate-cultivation, which is especially true for anaerobes.

In tuberculous pleurisy, the diagnostic yield from thoracentesis is virtually zero as far as the smear is concerned, unless large amounts of pleural fluid are being centrifuged or the patient has tuberculous empyema. The cultural yield has been given in collective reviews, with a wide scatter of 8% to 40% around a mean of 25% (22). The use of radiometric or nonradiometric liquid culture systems (BACTEC, MB/BacT, MGIT) will markedly accelerate results and possibly enhance the yield up to 50% when bedside—instead of laboratory—inoculation is chosen (23).

TABLE 5.2. IMMUNOLOGICAL PARAMETERS IN THE DIAGNOSIS OF INFLAMMATORY ETIOLOGIES IN PLEURAL EFFUSION

Etiology/Entity	Parameter	Sensitivity (%)	Specificity (%)
Tuberculosis	ADA (ADA$_2$)	97 (91–100)	9 (81–94)
	Interferon-γ	97 (94–100)	98 (91–100)
Empyema	IL-8/IL-1β	100	96
Rheumatoid arthritis	RF >1:320	80	<90
	(PS/S >1)		
	ANA >1:320	80	100
	(PF/S >1)		
	C3/4	70	<90
Systemic lupus	LE cells	28	100
Paucicellular Immunovasculitis	C/p-ANCA	50–98	95

Means and range from representative sources in the literature (12–20, 32, 42).
ADA, adenosine deaminase; IL, interleukin; RF, rheumatoid factor; ANA, antinuclear antibodies; PF/S, pleural fluid/serum; C3/4, complement cascade; LE, lupus erythematosus.

Molecular methods using a variety of *nucleic acid amplification techniques* have been intensively investigated since their introduction into clinical medicine (1989), with a focus on *M. tuberculosis*. So far, published papers have shown considerable variance of diagnostic yield, which ranged from 20% to 81% in terms of sensitivity, with the specificity being only exceptionally less than 100% (98%) (24–26). An overview of representative data from the past 10 years is given in Table 5.3.

When analyzing the sources of the variation in sensitivity—apart from technical developments and problems—the most important determinant appears to be the number of bacilli in the pleural fluid sample. Thus, regardless of the theoretical advantage of requiring only a single microorganism, nucleic acid amplification techniques may fail to detect *M. tuberculosis* DNA when the pleurisy is paucibacillary correlating with culture negativity (22,

24–26). Extension of sampling material to formalin-fixed and paraffin-embedded tissue specimens apparently does not substantially abolish sensitivity shortcomings (27–30) (Table 5.3). With the use of commercial DNA amplicons (ligand chain *M. tuberculosis* assay or AMPLICOR *M. tuberculosis*), as well as RNA amplicons (amplified *M. tuberculosis* direct test), according to a recent source, the sensitivity of each single technique was 52.8% and 63.2%, respectively, with a 100% specificity each (31) (Table 5.3). The combined sensitivity amounted to 80.7%, which is superior to the 73.7% yield obtained from conventional pleural fluid and biopsy cultures. Again, when conventional and nucleic acid amplification techniques were combined, the yield was 96.5%, the overall diagnostic gain compared with conventional microbiology alone being 22.8%. This emphasizes and illustrates the current role of nucleic acid amplification techniques, which may be defined as

TABLE 5.3. VALUE OF NUCLEIC ACID AMPLIFICATION TECHNIQUES IN THE DIAGNOSIS OF TUBERCULOUS PLEURISY

First Author (Reference)	Case No. TB/Non-TB	Amplicor/Kit	Sensitivity (%)			Specificity (%)
			Overall	Culture-Positive	Culture Negative	
Fluid-based						
DeWit (25)	53/31	336 r.squ.	81	—	—	78
Lassence (24)	14/10	IS 6110	60	100	50	100
		65 XD	20	66	8	100
Querol (26)	21/86	IS 6110	81	100	60	98
Tissue-based						
Salian (27)	25/35	IS 6110	73	—	—	100
Marchetti (28)	26/11	IS 6110	80–87	100	73–82	100
Gamboa (29)	67/97	AMTDT	83	—	—	100
Palacios (30)	18/168	LCxMTB	90.4	—	—	98.5
Ruiz-Manzano (31)	57/17	AMTDT	53	—	—	100
		LCxMTB	63	—	—	100
		combined	80.7	—	—	100

r. squ., repetitive sequence; IS, insertion sequence, AMTDT, amplified *M. tuberculosis* assay; LC × MTB, ligand chain *M. tuberculosis* assay.

(a) improving sensitivity, (b) accelerating conventional microbiologic techniques, and (c) providing excellent specificity. Although further standardizations and optimization of nucleic acid amplification techniques may be expected in the future, some setbacks such as intrinsic sample amplification inhibitors are likely to persist.

Cytology and Neoplastic Markers

Pleural fluid may reveal an enormous spectrum of cytologic findings as regards absolute counts and cell composition. Analysis of cellular pleural fluid constituents is therefore of crucial clinical importance, with a focus on inflammatory and neoplastic disease. Transudates are by definition oligocellular, and the absolute nucleated cell count ($</>10,000 \times \mu L^{-1}$) has been used to discriminate transudates from exudates, but is clearly inferior to biochemical parameters. In the absence of significant inflammation and malignancy, mesothelial cells contribute the overwhelming majority of free pleural cells (>90%). Inflammatory disease is characterized by a highly variable expansion of the inflammatory effector cell pool, the composition of which may reveal more or less typical profiles for a number of etiologies. *Neutrophilia* with the endpoint of gross purulent effusion, *lymphocytosis,* and *eosinophilia* are the basic patterns that need to be analyzed in terms of relevant etiologies, as listed in Table 5.4

TABLE 5.4. DIFFERENTIAL DIAGNOSIS OF PLEURAL FLUID INFLAMMATORY CELL PROFILES (LYMPHOCYTOSIS AND EOSINOPHILIA)

Disease/Condition	Comment
Pleural lymphocytosis	
(>80%)	
Tuberculosis	Most frequent cause
Lymphoma	~100%, in particular, M. Hodgkin
Chylothorax	
Rheumatic effusion	Often associated with trapped lung
Sarcoidosis	Very rare (>90% lymphocytes)
Malignancy	In about 50%, but <70% lymphocytes
Yellow nail syndrome	Very rare
Pleural eosinophilia	
(>10%)	
Pneumothorax	Most common cause, up to 50% Eos.,
Hemothorax	Delayed after precipitating cause
Previous thoracentesis	Pneumothorax; and bleeding related
Pulmonary embolism	May be hemorrhagic
Benign asbestosis (BAPE)	Up to 50% eosinophils
Parasitic disease	Various parasites
Fungal disease	Histoplasmosis, coccidioidomycosis
Allergic and immunologic conditions	Drugs, Wegener granulomatosis
Lymphoma	M. Hodgkin
Carcinoma	Uncommon, even with sanguinolent effusion

Eos., eosinophils; M. Hodgkin, morbus Hodgkin.
Modified from Sahn SA. The diagnostic value of pleural fluid analysis. *Semin Resp Crit Care Med* 1995;16:269–278, with permission.

(32). The timing of the investigation plays a crucial role in inflammatory cell analysis because absolute counts and composition may change rapidly, e.g., between polymorphonuclear and mononuclear predominance. As a general rule, acute injury will enhance neutrophil patterns, whereas prolonged or chronic lesions correlate with lymphocytosis. Clinical examples are tuberculosis, pneumonia, pulmonary infarction and pancreatitis. Pleural eosinophilia, as indicated in Table 5.4, may provide recalcitrant interpretation problems in which (a) common artificial causes are often overlooked; (b) anecdotic occurrence in common conditions, as in tuberculosis, must be considered; and (c) rare etiologies such as fungal infection, parasitosis, and drug hypersensitivity need to be excluded. Unexplained pleural eosinophilia is believed to be an expression of unrecognized benign asbestos-associated pleurisy in many cases (33). Rare cytologic findings include the presence of significant numbers of *plasma cells,* which may be observed nonspecifically in a number of conditions ranging from collagenous vascular disease to congestive heart failure. One should, however, examine the possibility of malignant disease (multiple myeloma) individually.

Cytologic analysis of *neoplastic cells* is a challenging clinical task that requires extraordinary experience to avoid confusion of malignant cells with inflammatorily activated and transformed residential mesothelial cells. The diagnostic yield of conventional morphologic cytology is generally reported with a wide range on the order of 40% to 70%, but sensitivities as high as 87% have been claimed, being probably related to some preselection (32, 34). The yield with advanced immunocytochemistry-supported ancillary techniques is on the order of 70% to 80%, although sensitivities up to 91% at a 100% specificity have been reported (34–36). Here again, advanced case preselection bias might be involved. Empirical panels of commercially available markers—mostly monoclonal antibodies—are now commonly used for specific immune staining of malignant cells and assignment to cell lineage. The main issue in neoplastic pleural cytology consists in the reliable discrimination among (a) reactive (benign) mesothelial cells, (b) autochthonous malignant cells (i.e., mesothelioma), and (c) metastatic adenocarcinoma. A battery of new markers such as thrombomodulin, *N*-cadherin, HBME1, AgNOR (silver staining of nucleolus organizing regions), and nucleic acid amplification techniques for the demonstration of aberrant expression of mucin genes have been developed and evaluated in recent time, but the quest for definitive markers continues (37, 38). A commonly used and suggested panel of sequentially performed immunological markers is shown in Table 5.5 (37, 39). Opinions among pathologists on single markers are often divided, and even with the combined power of marker panels, the overall accuracy for distinguishing mesothelioma from adenocarcinoma does not exceed 90%. Also, importantly, there has not yet been identified a marker or monoclonal antibodies that reliably distinguishes transformed benign mesothelial from malignant cells (39).

TABLE 5.5. IMMUNOCYTOCHEMICAL STAINING IN THE DIFFERENTIAL DIAGNOSIS OF ADENOCARCINOMA VERSUS MESOTHELIOMA

Marker/Monoclonal Antibody	Adenocarcinoma	Malignant Mesothelioma
Cytokeratin	+	+
Epithelial membrane antigen	+	+
Carcinoembryonic antigen	+/−	−
MOC 31	+/−	−
LeuM1	+/−	−
B72.3	+	−
BerEP4	+	−
CA 19-9	+	−
Calretinin	−	+
E-cadherin	−	+/−
HBME1	+	+
AgNOR	−	+

Modified from Fetsch PA, Abati A. Immunocytochemistry in effusion cytology: a contemporary review. *Cancer Cytopathol* 2001;93:293–308; Lozano MD, Panizo A, Toleso GR et al. Immunocytochemistry in the differential diagnosis of serous effusions: a comparative evaluation of eight monoclonal antibodies in Papanicolaou stained smears. *Cancer Cytopathol* 2001;93:68–72.

The value of *soluble*, mainly bronchial, carcinoma-associated *tumor marker* determination in the pleural fluid has been intensively studied. The sensitivity of virtually all currently available markers—such as tissue polypeptide antigen (TPA), carcinoembryonic antigen (CEA), cancer antigen (CA) 15-3, squamous cell carcinoma antigen, cytokeratin fragment (CYFRA)21, and neniune specific enolase (NSE)—never exceed 74%, with specificities varying from 68% to 90% (40, 41). These data do not justify the continued routine use of soluble markers in the pleural fluid for establishing the diagnosis of malignant pleurisy. They may be exceptionally recruited for surveillance of individual clinical courses in malignancy. CEA has maintained some value in the clinically important distinction between diffuse malignant pleural mesothelioma and metastatic adenocarcinomatosis. According to our own data, a CEA value exceeding a 50 ng/mL cut-off will exclude the presence of mesothelioma in malignant effusion with 99% certainty (41).

Complications

There are no absolute and only a few relative contraindications to thoracentesis. Thoracentesis should be avoided or postponed when there is evidence of a hemorrhagic diathesis (e.g., anticoagulation) or when the size of the effusion is small. In patients on mechanical ventilation and in those with critically impaired respiratory performance, thoracentesis is not generally advisable, but a high clinical need for the diagnosis may offset the relative contraindication.

The main complication of thoracentesis is *pneumothorax*, the incidence of which varies widely in the literature, between 3% and 42% depending on the investigator's experi-

OPTIMIZING DIAGNOSTIC YIELD FOR TUBERCULOSIS AND MALIGNANCY

Summary Statement	Level of Evidence
Adenosine deaminase is a useful inflammatory marker in the diagnosis of tuberculous pleurisy	Randomized controlled studies
Interferon-γ is a useful cytokine for the diagnosis of tuberculous pleurisy	Nonrandomized studies
Nuclear acid amplification techniques improve the diagnosis of tuberculous pleural effusion, but sensitivity depends on the pleural bacillary load. Tissue specimen–derived techniques perform similar to fluid specimen–derived techniques	Nonrandomized studies
Conventional microbiologic studies (smear, solid and liquid cultures) are highly specific but moderately sensitive for the diagnosis of tuberculous pleurisy	Uncontrolled and observational studies
Limited conventional cytological yield for the diagnosis of malignancy	Uncontrolled and observational studies
High sensitivity of immunocytochemistry for the diagnosis of malignancy but limited specificity in cell lineage determination	Expert opinion and consensus panel
Pleural fluid soluble tumor marker determination for the screening and diagnosis of malignancy is not routinely justified	Limited number of controlled prospective studies

ence and skill, effusion volume, the use of imaging guidance, the type and size of needle used, the quantity of recovered fluid and predisposing morbidity, and, most importantly, chronic obstructive pulmonary disease (42). Should pneumothorax occur, it will in the majority of cases be limited enough to allow an expectant management. Chest pain and cough may cause considerable discomfort but rarely amount to serious problems. Bleeding and malpuncture involving the liver and spleen, as well as infection, should virtually not occur when highly experienced individuals do the thoracentesis and when imaging control is used in doubtful situations.

PLEURAL BIOPSY AND ENDOSCOPY TECHNIQUES

Clinical Role

Pleural biopsies via closed needle biopsy or thoracoscopy (pleuroscopy) are indicated when there is suspicion of pleural lesions, revealing specific histological patterns and/or microbiologic findings, but imaging techniques and thoracentesis provide inconclusive or conflicting evidence. The main focus of biopsy studies will be suspected malignancy and tuberculosis unless additional rare infectious diseases like fungal and parasitic pleurisy must be taken into consideration. A third entity comprises noninfectious inflammatory lesions expressing more or less specific patterns such as granuloma formation in collagen vascular disease or sarcoidosis. In the presence of effusion, pleural biopsies are usually reserved to exudates and follow the decision sequence shown in Figure 5.2. Before proceeding to unnecessary invasive investigations in the case of borderline low protein exudates one should always consider the possibility of a transformed transudate (so-called pseudo-exudate).

Closed Needle Biopsy

Technique

Closed needle biopsy should be invariably performed as *image-guided* with fluoroscopy or ultrasound regardless whether a solid or circumscribed chest wall lesion is explored or *blind biopsy* is intended in the presence of effusion. Various types of needles have been developed over time. The oldest Abrams and Ramel needles may still be popular but new developments and improvements of these basic types (Radja and Cope needles, respectively) are increasingly used. More recently hollow-cylinder cutting needles (Tru-cut) would appear preferable because of their simpler design, superior handling, and better (i.e., larger) biopsy quality, although they do not allow prior fluid aspiration. Older needles that allow thoracentesis are certainly more versatile, and this feature will also confirm a safe position within the pleura. Image-guided closed needle biopsy may be safely used to explore

pleural changes when the pleural space is intact and a pleural effusion is present. When the pleural space is obliterated, the indication for closed needle biopsy may be expanded to the exploration of deeper structures, including pulmonary lesions adjacent or fused to the pleura.

Safe performance of closed needle biopsy requires the patient to be placed in a stable lateral decubitus position with the side not being investigated dependent in an endoscopic or radiologic unit. Similar to thoracentesis, prior sedative and analgetic medication are not routinely necessary. The site selection for intervention within the ultrasound-verified region of interest must be even stricter than in thoracentesis to avoid the intercostal vascular and nerve bundle. Needle biopsy is distinctly more aggressive than thoracentesis and will be easier and safer when performed in the thin anterolateral to posterolateral region of the chest wall than in the strictly posterior regions, especially the paravertebral area. The immediate parasternal region is a critical location because the internal mammary artery may be dangerously exposed to injury. After skin disinfection with 10% polyvidone iodide, local anesthesia using 1% to 2% lidocaine must be generously applied to the relevant intercostal space, with particular attention to the sensitive upper and lower rib edge. Skin and chest wall penetration with any type of needle will be grossly facilitated if a narrow and sufficiently deep stab incision with a scalpel is being made. Because of the pressure that must be exerted with the active hand to penetrate the chest wall, it is a prudent precaution to use the non-dominant hand protectively to avoid dangerous "overshoot" penetration and this applies especially to thick portions of the thoracic wall. The principle and tissue recovery technique of

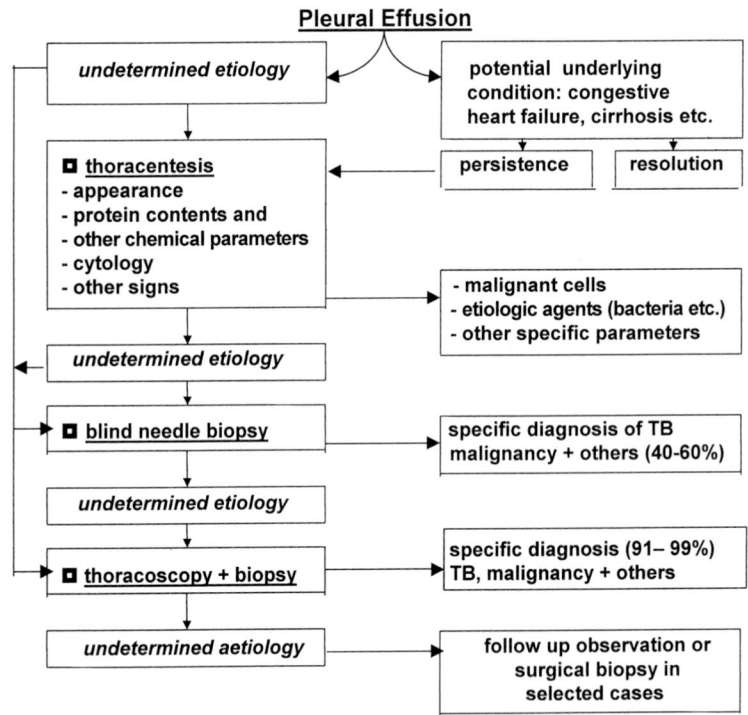

FIGURE 5.2. Flowchart for the clinical use of diagnostic pleural procedures.

different needles is demonstrated in Figure 5.3 (42, 43). At least three separate biopsies should be obtained, because even with optimum technique, they will not regularly contain a representative parietal pleural sample. There is recent evidence that both in malignancy and in inflammatory disease, a total number of six biopsy samples is a desirable optimum to achieve at least two valid pleural samples (44, 45).

Diagnostic Yield

With the premise of at least two valid specimens, needle biopsy is diagnostic in tuberculous pleurisy (combined histology and microbiology) in about 60% of cases (46–49). In one major series (n = 100), the yield was 63%, being composed of 51% positive biopsy specimen and 28% positive fluid culture (50). Reviews of the literature show pleural needle biopsies to have a diagnostic sensitivity of 69%, with a range of 28% to 88%, which includes data for tuberculous pleurisy averaging in high prevalence areas (42). In neoplastic effusion, the maximum possible diagnostic yield of blind closed needle biopsy is on the order of 70%, being usually lower than that of cytology (51), although with image guidance, 86% sensitivity has been reported in mesothelioma (52). The value of needle biopsy may thus be defined as augmenting the yield of pleural fluid cytology, an effect that amounted in our series of 86 cases of malignant pleurisy to a diagnostic gain of 16% (from 58% to 74%) (53). In the large series of the Mayo Clinic (281 patients), in which pleural biopsy identified only 7% additional malignant effusions with negative fluid cytology, this augmenting effect was much less consistent (54).

Contraindications and Complications

As with any biopsy investigation, a bleeding diathesis is an absolute contraindication. Relative contraindications are comparable to thoracentesis and include severe respiratory impairment or a poor imaging representation of the region of interest. Although the overall rate of complications is low, they may be more severe than those in thoracentesis. The main determinants are the site of intervention, the depth of penetration, the type of needle used, and—most of all—the investigator's expertise and skills. Hemorrhage (hemoptysis, hemothorax), pneumothorax, syncope, air embolism, pain, and injury to neighboring organs (liver, spleen) are the most important complications. Their combined incidence has been reported to be 15%, and lethal complications occur in 0.09% (46, 54). Because of a rather unfavorable complication profile and the limited gain in diagnostic yield, the trained physician will tend to bypass blind closed needle biopsy and prefer the higher efficacy of thoracoscopy. The domain of blind needle biopsy is now best restricted to situations with logistic, technical, and clinical obstacles to thoracoscopy (availability, adhesions, contraindications, noncompliance), in addition to solid lesions involving deeper chest wall structures that may be invisible from the internal pleural surface at thoracoscopy.

PROCEDURAL RECOMMENDATIONS	
Summary Statement	**Level of Evidence**
Technical approach and procedural recommendations for closed needle biopsy	Expert opinion and consensus panel
Optimum number of specimen	Nonrandomized studies
Limited diagnostic yield both in inflammatory and neoplastic disease	Uncontrolled clinical series
Safety and complication profile, contraindications for closed needle biopsy	Observational studies and expert opinion

THORACOSCOPY (PLEUROSCOPY)

History and Clinical Glossary

Thoracoscopy would appear in many areas of the world as a rather innovative diagnostic procedure, but was in fact introduced into diagnosis of diseases as early as 1910 by Jacobaeus in Sweden (55). He also "invented" what would become much later a rapidly developing innovative branch of modern thoracic surgery, i.e., *minimal invasive surgical thoracoscopy*, by using the technique of pneumothorax treatment of tuberculosis. Later, with the rediscovery of the diagnostic potential of thoracoscopy, the addition of the term "medical" became necessary to distinguish the procedure from *"video-assisted thoracic surgery" (VATS)*, although the video technique is equally integrated into modern medical thoracoscopy. VATS requires the full facilities of an operating theater, with double-lumen intubation, multiple entry points, and general anesthesia and is clearly less versatile and more expensive than is medical thoracoscopy. Consequently, over time, the ability to use medical thoracoscopy to biopsy any suspicious area of the pleura at a remarkable safety level and with vision

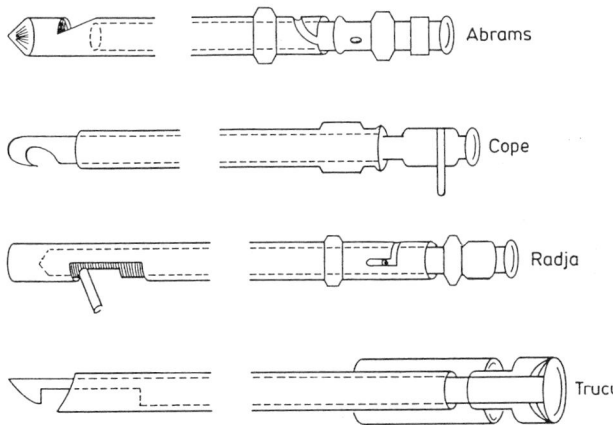

FIGURE 5.3. Examples of commonly used closed biopsy needles.

control in the conscious patient, using only local anesthesia, has established the procedure worldwide as the gold standard technique for the diagnosis of pleural disease (56–58). Based on the consensus experience that pleural effusions predominate the indication spectrum, it has been appropriately suggested to adopt the term *"pleuroscopy"* in the future (59).

Indications

Thoracoscopy (pleuroscopy) allows visualization of most intrathoracic structures and may therefore be used—apart from pleural effusion—to explore a spectrum of diseases, including interstitial lung disease, pneumothorax and localized lesions of the lung, the chest wall, and the diaphragm, as well as the mediastinum. The principle of the investigation is illustrated by the CT simulation in Figure 5.4.

Pleural effusion, as the major classical indication, currently accounts for up to 90% of all investigations. Several studies have tried to determine the diagnostic accuracy of medical thoracoscopy in the setting of undiagnosed pleural effusion, with results varying over a range of 69% to 90%. One well-designed study including follow-up periods of 1 to

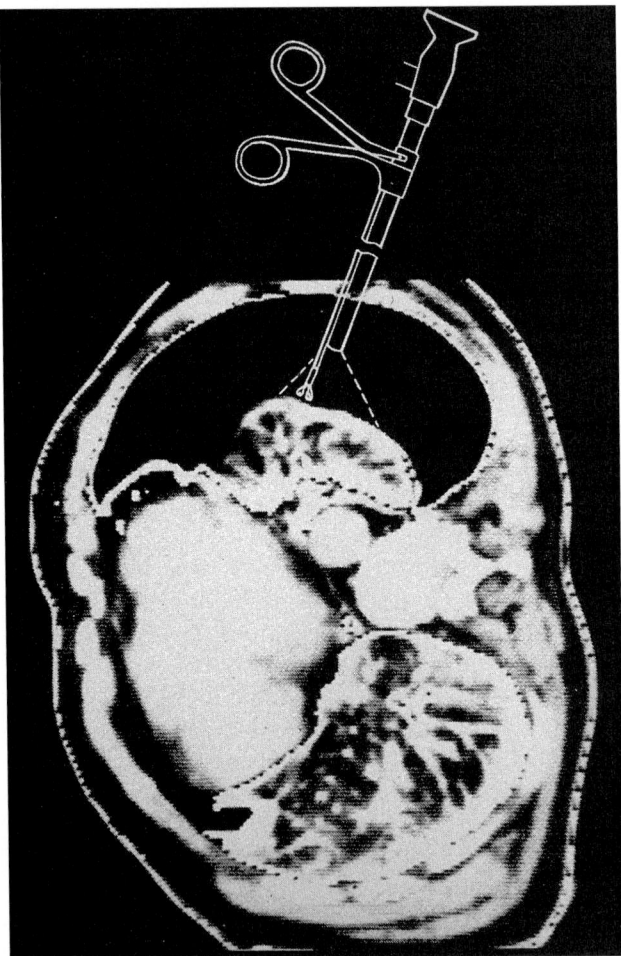

FIGURE 5.4. Computed tomography simulation of medical thoracoscopy (right thoracic cavity in left lateral position).

2 years found a sensitivity of 91%, specificity of 100%, an overall accuracy of 96%, and a negative predictive value of 93% (60). Boutin and colleagues report a false-negative rate of 15% within a 5-year follow-up period (61). Because of its high diagnostic accuracy, thoracoscopy should be performed in almost all cases of exudative effusion in which the etiology remains undetermined after pleural fluid analysis, following the diagnostic flowchart of Figure 5.2. Thoracoscopy is also preferred to closed needle biopsy, unless it is unfeasible owing to technical or clinical obstacles as previously described. The reported diagnostic yield in malignant effusion is 95% and may approach 98% when taken together with fluid cytology and needle biopsy results (53). These figures basically apply to any type of malignancy, including diffuse malignant mesothelioma, lymphoma, and metastatic carcinoma (57). Thoracoscopy will provide a number of additional advantages, such as accurate intrathoracic staging of mesothelioma as a main determinant of therapeutic decisions (surgical versus nonsurgical approaches) and demonstration of etiologic macroscopic findings (62). Examples are certain proliferation features ("grapelike appearance") and the presence of hyaline plaques that may suggest mesothelioma or asbestos exposure, respectively. In the staging of bronchial carcinoma with concomitant effusion, thoracoscopy allows discrimination between paramalignant (i.e., benign) effusion and carcinosis, thus avoiding exploration thoracotomy. Finally, extensive tissue samples can be recovered for additional investigations such as immunohistochemistry and hormone receptor staining (63). Thoracoscopy may have a clinically highly relevant interventional focus with the induction of *talc pleurodesis*, using the dry powder insufflation technique ("poudrage") as the currently best validated conservative treatment option. With the strict observation of thoracoscopy-controlled predictors and prerequisites such as complete fluid removal, agent distribution, and unimpeded lung expansion, success rates of more than 90% are realistic (64, 65).

Thoracoscopy is also very sensitive for the diagnosis of tuberculous pleurisy, identifying immediately 94% of cases by histology. The culture yield from thoracoscopic biopsies in our series (n = 100) was twice as high (78%) as the combined yield of pleural fluid and closed-needle biopsy (39%) and approached 99% with the addition of histology (50). The macroscopic appearance of tuberculous pleurisy can be recognized as fairly specific by the experienced investigator; in addition, the often abundantly present fibrinous membranes and peels may reveal culture positive findings in 87% (50). Thoracoscopy is likely to improve gross therapeutic results by breaking up pockets, improve removal of peels, and improve complete drainage of effusion. Antituberculous drug therapy can be started instantly on the basis of the reasonable histology-based diagnostic certainty. A similar therapeutic benefit can be achieved in nonspecific empyema, with the option of mechanical debridement of fibrinopurulent inflammatory membranes and removal of loculations, including subsequent induction of highly effective fibrinolysis via optimal chest tube placement (66).

The management of pneumothorax benefits considerably from the application of thoracoscopy to visualize cysts, bullae, blebs, or pleural leaks and to permit rational treatment designs (67). Again, thoracoscopy offers the interventional possibility to combine chest drainage with coagulation of blebs and bullae, as well as pleurodesis by talc poudrage (68). Long-term recurrence rates of less than 10% justify a medical thoracoscopic approach, at least in the elderly and in secondary spontaneous pneumothorax. In case of large cysts or adhesions, a decision algorithm may alternatively assign patients to surgery.

Localized lesions of the pleura—basically, those well accessible to thoracoscopy—have now become a rare or third-line indication because these mostly benign lesions can be more appropriately clarified and/or resected by a combined imaging and surgical approach.

Technique

Medical thoracoscopy is usually performed under local anesthesia and conscious sedation in a properly equipped endoscopy suite under sterile conditions (surgical hand-washing, gown, and gloves) with the patient lying—unless otherwise required for exploration of localized lesions—in the lateral decubitus position on the noninvolved side. Most investigators prefer a single entry approach, using a 9- or 11-mm (especially with an interventional option) thoracoscope that accommodates both the scope and accessory instruments (56, 57, 69, 70). Others prefer a 7-mm port for visualization and a separate 5-mm instrumentation port with extended anesthesia demands (neurolept or general anesthesia) (71). The optimum operating team would include the main investigator, an assistant physician, and two specially trained nurses. State-of-the-art thoracoscopy, apart from standard endoscopic equipment, requires the following special components:

- A mobile fluoroscopy and/or ultrasound facility
- Needles for induction of pneumothorax (Denneke, Veress)
- Pneumothorax apparatus or alternative gas insufflator
- Thoracoscopy instruments as shown and specified in Figure 5.5, which are basically rigid and may include angled telescopes (flexible bronchoscopy instruments do not confer advantages and are difficult to sterilize)
- A high-power (>200 W) cold light source
- Electrocautery or laser-coagulation facility
- Video equipment, including a color printer (not mandatory)
- An optional photographic camera system.

The image processing components of the system are optimally integrated into a mobile rack.

The practice of thoracoscopy requires adequate investigational experience of at least 20 previous supervised examinations and continuous performance of 20 investigations or more per year (72). Preinvestigation clinical studies should include a chest radiograph (with or without ultrasonography), arterial or capillary blood gases, an optional spirometry, and electrolyte and blood coagulation tests. The patient needs to be provided with extensive written and verbal information and supportive counseling to minimize apprehension and to give final written consent.

With the use of the more-common single-port technique, thoracoscopy is performed according to the following procedural line:

(1) *Induction of premedication 30 to 45 minutes beforehand.* Most investigators use a combined sedative (midazolam 2–3 mg intramuscularly) and antitussive medication (hydrocodone 7.5–15 mg intramuscularly), but various other protocols including analgesic opiates (morphine 0.2-0.5 mg/kg) and/or neuroleptics (propofol 0.5–1.0 mg/kg) are in use. Dose adjustments may be required in elderly and in cardiorespiratory premorbidity. Anticholinergic premedication is not required in sedative protocols; the patient may even be allowed a bland meal up to 4 hours before the investigation.

(2) *Positioning of the patient,* including cardiorespiratory monitoring systems (ECG, respiratory rate, pulse oximetry) and cautery electrodes; insertion of a venous cannula.

(3) *Induction of artificial pneumothorax* by insufflation of carbon dioxide (CO_2) as the preferred filling gas and special needles (Denneke, Veress) housing a blunt internal cannula and/or side openings to prevent lung injury in the absence of effusion. Induction of a pneumothorax with a regular needle is advisable, even in effusion, to avoid accidental entry of the trocar within unrecognized adhesions. The created pleural gas space, as fluoroscopically verified, should be large enough to allow complete inspection of the pleural cavity. With adhesions, the minimal required cavity for a safe access is an air space of 2-cm depth. It may eventually be enlarged during thoracoscopy.

(4) *Selection of optimum and safe entry site* using fluoroscopy: The fifth-sixth (seventh) intercostal space in the mid to anterior axillary line has evolved as an almost standard entry point, providing an optimum overview of the pleural cavity and free access to all objects of interest. Local adhesions and unusual object localizations may modify the entry point.

(5) *Implementation of local anesthesia* using 1% novocaine or 1% to 2% lidocaine. Previous aspiration of filling gas from the pleural cavity is an ultimate safeguard against inadequate entry points. The needle is then stepwise withdrawn under generous infiltration of the intercostal pleura, the rib edges, and the skin. Inappropriate local anesthesia may be responsible for severe pain and syncope.

(6) *A preparatory deep skin incision* about 1.5 cm long is required to allow subsequent smooth penetration of the trocar. It is prudent to integrate closed needle biopsy at

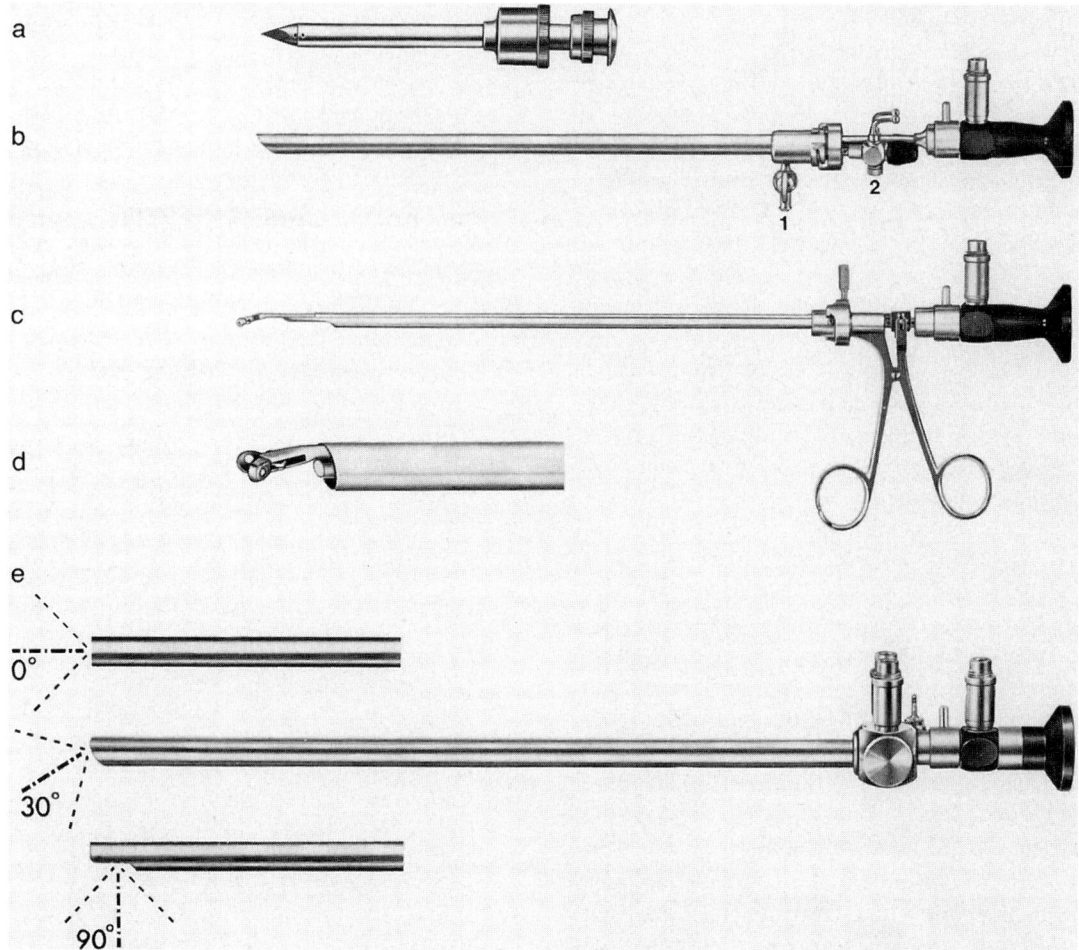

FIGURE 5.5. Basic instrumental set for medical thoracoscopy. **A:** Trocar obturator with integrated valve and sharp internal cannula of 7-, 9-, or 11-mm diameter for single- or two-port technique. **B:** Single incision thoracoscope (9- or 11-mm diameter). **C:** Biopsy forceps with integrated 0°-optical system. **D:** Magnification of optics and forceps in the thoracoscope shaft ready for biopsy. **E:** Various straight and angled vision telescopes for the single-entry technique, with adapted photograph light shaft.

this step because (a) thoracoscopy is blinded at the immediate entry point, and (b) needle biopsy may give cross-sectional information of the chest wall, examining deeper structures than those thoracoscopically visualized.

(7) *Cautious trocar insertion,* avoiding too deep overshoot penetration by controlling the operative with the nondominant hand. Forceful trocar handling is a frequent and potentially dangerous mistake.

(8) *Evacuation of the entire fluid collection* to ensure unimpeded inspection of the pleural space. This can be done without risk with a suction tube, because the open trocar valve will create constant pressure equilibration with the ambient air. Complete evacuation is also essential for optimum pleurodesis by avoiding dilution and postthoracoscopic losses of talcum.

(9) *Introduction of the telescope and visual examination.* The normal pleura presents as a delicate, transparent, light-reflecting surface. A profound knowledge of thoracic anatomy and of vital landmark structures (e.g., peri-

cardium, large vessels, vagus, phrenic nerve, and sympathetic trunk) is indispensable. Angled or terminally flexible telescopes may allow access to remote or concealed locations such as the paravertebral area, the chest apex, the interlobar spaces, and the mediastinal pleura. Descriptive terms of pleural changes include hypervascularity, diffuse ("pachypleuritis") or circumscribed thickening (plaques), granulations, lymphangitis, nodules and nodes, large-scale tumors, blood-derived products (fibrin, septae, membranes, pus, blood), and, finally, adhesions and strands. Those for the pulmonary changes include inflation status and color (hyperinflation, emphysema, atelectasis, anthracosis, congestion, induration) and circumscribed findings (consolidation, tumors. hemorrhage, blebs, bullae, cysts and visible air leaks).

(10) *Optional blunt dissection of impeding adhesions and breaking of septae and membranes* is essential in multiloculated effusions to create a representative overview and to allow biopsy access and full postthoracoscopic

lung expansion. An initially small cavity may be expanded to the full-size pleural space, but organized fibrotic and vascularized adhesions and strands must be spared.

(11) *Video and optional photographic documentation* are important for case documentation and teaching, as well as training purposes.

(12) *Biopsies* are taken from several suspect areas, including the anterior and posterior chest wall and the diaphragm. The intercostal spaces must be clearly identified to prevent accidental too deep biopsy at the inferior rib sulcus. Although biopsies cause a short and sharp pain, no additive anesthesia is needed. Macroscopic visual examination is remarkably sensitive and specific to a number of etiologies such as tuberculosis, carcinosis, and mesothelioma, but may be misleading and should never be relied on solely. Therefore, generous and numerous (at least six) biopsies, even in normal appearing sites, are recommended. To avoid unnecessary air leaks, lung biopsies are not taken routinely, except suspect lesions are confined to the visceral pleura or superficial lung areas. Electrocautery or laser cautery may help to control this problem. In suspected infectious disease, biopsy samples must be divided or additional specimens obtained for culturing. Bleeding is a regular side-effect of biopsy but rarely requires cautery for control. Arterial bleeding (e.g., an intercostal artery) could be particularly serious but is extremely rare with adequate precaution. In the authors' decades of experience with this procedure, a surgical intervention has never been required.

(13) *Assessment of lung expandability* is particularly important when induction of pleurodesis is an intention. The main causes of impeded lung expansion are (inflammatory or malignant) parenchymal entrappings (trapped lung), gross pulmonary consolidation, major air leaks, and lung collapse owing to main bronchus obstruction.

(14) *Optional induction of talc powder pleurodesis* (58, 65).

(15) *Insertion of chest drainage in an optimum apicodorsal direction* or in any desired vision-guided position covering the pulmonary surface. An interlobar mediastinal position is both less effective and less tolerable.

(16) *Suture fixation of the drain at the penetration site,* where, however, pursed string sutures are not needed.

(17) *Cautious lung expansion* is accomplished with low initial suction levels (<10 cm water pressure). The level of further suction and the time setting of lung expansion must take into account risks such as reexpansion pulmonary edema secondary to long-standing compressive effusion and well-recognized impediments (trapped lung, consolidation, air leak). Not all investigators use continuous chest drainage after reexpansion when the lung is intact and has not been biopsied. However, an indwelling drain increases safety and facilitates postthoracoscopic management in effusion. For correct management of pleurodesis, it is indispensable.

(18) *Radiographic confirmation of drain position and correct drain function*

(19) *Removal of drain and clamping/suture of the insertion site* as soon as stable lung expansion and discontinuation of excretions (< 100 mL/day) have been confirmed.

Contraindications and Complications

There are a few absolute and some relative contraindications to thoracoscopy as listed below:

Absolute Contraindications

- Bleeding disorders (partial thromboplastin time >40 seconds, thromboplastin time test [QUICK-test] less than 60% corresponding to international normalized ratio [INR] >2, platelets <40,000/nL)
- Critical cardiac performance (left ventricular ejection fraction <0.35, recent infarction, cardiac arrhythmias less than Lown IVb despite therapy)
- Obliterated pleural space or non-detachment of the lung on pneumothorax induction.

Relative Contraindications

- Critical respiratory performance (partial pressure of oxygen <50 mm Hg, partial pressure of CO_2 >50 mm Hg) unless caused by pneumothorax or effusion
- Critical small pleural cavity to explore and/or impeded difficult access
- Pulmonary hypertension (pulmonary artery pressure >35 mm Hg) and/or critically decreased lung compliance when lung biopsy is being considered

Complications

Taking into account the required level of invasiveness, medical thoracoscopy is a safe procedure. With strict observation of contraindications and precautions, important complications (especially *major bleeding* and *severe dyspnea*) occur in less than 3% of cases, and *lethal complications* have been reported in less than 0.01% (69, 73, 74). Thus, the overall safety level is comparable to that of flexible bronchoscopy. *Infection* (empyema) complicates thoracoscopy in less than 1% of cases. *Mediastinal* and, in particular, *soft tissue emphysema* are more frequent (<7%) but rarely represent a major problem. *Air embolism* is a serious complication but is fortunately extremely rare. The preference of CO_2 as the filling gas, favoring rapid intravascular gas reabsorption, is already part of a prevention strategy. *Persistent air leaks* may require longer-than-usual suction periods of 3 to 5 days, particularly in patients with stiff lungs, but will eventually subside with conservative management. *Malignant seeding* of the chest wall entry site is virtually unique to mesothelioma; preventive local irradiation has been shown to be an effective means of prevention (75). Reexpansion lung edema is a realistic complication that is clearly associated with profuse and longstanding collapse. If risk situations are recognized and preventive strategies observed, such as prolonged lung expansion using low suction, the incidence is less than 0.5% (70). Side effects and complications of pleurodesis are not directly thoracoscopy-related and are discussed elsewhere.

THORASCOPY	
Summary Statement	**Level of Evidence**
Technical approach and procedural recommendations; anesthesiologic setting for medical thoracoscopy	Expert opinion and consensus panel
Superior diagnostic yield in both inflammatory and neoplastic pleural disease	Prospective clinical trials
Superior diagnostic yield of medical thoracoscopy in pneumothorax	Prospective clinical trials
Validity of interventional approaches (talcum pleurodesis) in malignancy and pneumothorax	Prospective clinical trials
Validity of interventional approaches in inflammatory disease (empyema, tuberculosis)	Uncontrolled, observational studies; expert opinion; and consensus panel
Safety and complication profile; contraindications for medical thoracoscopy	Observational studies, one prospective study, and expert opinion

OPEN (SURGICAL) PLEURAL BIOPSY

Surgical biopsy would be an ultimate possibility to explore the pleural space, providing both excellent visualization of target areas and the largest possible biopsy size. In addition, it may be combined with a potentially curative therapeutic approach by partial pleurectomy and/or partial chest wall resection. The fact, however, is that the combined power of modern imaging techniques—such as ultrasound, computed tomography, magnetic resonance, and, very recently, positron emission tomography—in conjunction with thoracoscopic visualization has virtually abolished the need for surgical exploration. There are, however, a few exceptions conceivably related to the issue of diagnosing a paramalignant effusion or an occult malignant mesothelioma in individuals previously exposed to asbestos (56). Others include strictly localized chest wall lesions that may diagnostically and curatively resected within one intervention.

REFERENCES

1. Light RW. Approach to the patient. In: *Pleural diseases,* 3rd ed. Baltimore: Williams & Wilkins, 1995:75–83.
2. Mattison LE, Coppage L, Alderman DF, et al. Pleural effusions in the medical ICU: prevalence, causes and clinical implications. *Chest* 1997;111:1018–1023.
3. Yu CJ, Yang PC, Chang DB, et al. Diagnostic and therapeutic use of chest sonography: value in critically ill patients. *AJR Am J Roentgenol* 1992;159:695–701.
4. Light RW. Diagnostic principles in pleural disease. *Eur Respir J* 1997;10:476–481.
5. Burgess LJ, Maritz FJ, Taljaard FFJ. Comparative analysis of the biochemical parameters used to distinguish between pleural transudates and exudates. *Chest* 1995;107:1604–1609.
6. Romero S, Candela A, Martin C, et al. Evaluation of different criteria for the separation of pleural transudates from exudates. *Chest* 1993;104:399–404.
7. Heffner JE, Brown LK, Barbieri CA. Diagnostic value of tests that discriminate between exudative and transudative pleural effusions. *Chest* 1997;111:970–980.
8. Valdes L, Pose A, Suarez J, et al. Cholesterol: a useful parameter for distinguishing between pleural exudates and transudates. *Chest* 1991;99:1097–1102.
9. Rodriguez-Panadero F, Lopez-Mejas J. Low glucose and pH levels in malignant pleural effusions, diagnostic significance and prognostic value in respect to pleurodesis. *Am Rev Respir Dis* 1989; 139:663–667.
10. Heffner JE, Brown LK, Barbieri CA, et al. Pleural fluid chemical analysis in parapneumonic effusions: a metaanalysis. *Am J Respir Crit Care Med* 1995;151:1700–1708.
11. Light RW. A new classification of parapneumonic effusions and empyema. *Chest* 1995;108:299–301.
12. Light RW. Pleural disease due to collagen vascular disease. In: *Pleural diseases,* 3rd ed. Baltimore: Williiams & Wilkins 1995:208–218.
13. Silva-Mejas C, Gambao-Antinolo F, Lopez-Cortes LF, et al. Interleukin-1β in pleural fluids of different etiologies. *Chest* 1995; 108:942–945.
14. Riantawan P, Chuwalit P, Wongsangiem M, et al. Diagnostic value of pleural fluid adenosine deaminase in tuberculous pleuritis with reference to HIV coinfection and a Bayesian analysis. *Chest* 1999;116:97–103.
15. Valdes L, Alvarez D, SanJose E, et al. Value of adenosine deaminase in the diagnosis of tuberculous pleural effusions in young patients in a region of high prevalence of tuberculosis. *Thorax* 1995; 50:600–603.
16. Burgess LJ, Maritz FJ, Le Roux I, et al. Combined use of adenosine deaminase with lymphocyte/neutrophil ratio. *Chest* 1996; 109:411–419.
17. Valdes L, Alvarez D, San Jose E, et al. Diagnosis of tuberculous pleurisy, a study of 254 patients. *Arch Intern Med* 1998;158:2017–2021.
18. Gilhotra R, Sehgal S, Jindal SK. Pleural biopsy and adenosine deaminase enzyme activity in effusions of different aetiologies. *Lung India* 1989;3:122–124.
19. Villena V, Lopez-Encuentra A, Echave-Sustaeta J, et al. Interferon-γ in 388 immunocompromised and immunocompetent patients for diagnosing pleural tuberculosis. *Eur Respir J* 1996;9:2635–2639.
20. Wongtim S, Silachamroon U, Ruxrungtham K, et al. Interferon-γ for diagnosing tuberculous pleural effusions. *Thorax* 1999;54:921–924.
21. Alfagame I, Munoz F, Pena N, et al. Empyema of the thorax in adults: etiology, microbiologic findings and management. *Chest* 1993;103:839–843.
22. Ferrer J. Tuberculous pleural effusion and tuberculous empyema. *Sem Respir Crit Care Med* 2001;6/22:637–646.
23. Maartens G, Bateman ED. Tuberculous pleural effusions: increased culture yield with bedside inoculation of pleural fluid and poor diagnostic value of adenosine deaminase. *Thorax* 1991; 46:96–99.

24. Lassence A, Lecossier D, Pierre C, et al. Detection of mycobacterial DNA in pleural fluid from patients with tuberculous pleurisy by means of the polymerase chain reaction: comparison of protocols. *Thorax* 1992;47:265–269.

25. DeWit D, Maaertens G, Steyn L. A comparative study of the polymerase chain reaction and conventional procedures for the diagnosis of tuberculous pleural effusion. *Tuber Lung Dis* 1992;73:262–267.

26. Querol JM, Minguez J, Garcia-Sanchez E, et al. Rapid diagnosis of pleural tuberculosis by polymerase chain reaction. *Am J Respir Crit Care Med* 1995;152:1977–1981.

27. Salian NV, Rish JA, Eisenach KD, et al. Polymerase chain reaction to detect mycobacterium tuberculosis in histologic specimens. *Am J Respir Crit Care Med* 1998;158:1150–1155.

28. Marchetti G, Gori A, Catozzi L. Evaluation of PCR in the detection of mycobacterium tuberculosis from formalin-fixed paraffin-embedded tissues: comparison of four amplification assays. *J Clin Microbiol* 1998;36:684–689.

29. Gamboa F, Fernandez G, Pallida E, et al. Comparative evaluation of initial and new versions of the gene-probe amplified mycobacterium tuberculosis in respiratory and non-respiratory specimens. *J Clin Microbiol* 1998;36:684–689.

30. Palacios JJ, Ferro J, Ruiz-Palma N, et al. Comparison of the ligase chain reaction with solid and liquid culture media for routine detection of mycobacterium tuberculosis in respiratory specimens. *Eur J Clin Microbiol Infect Dis* 1998;17:767–772.

31. Ruiz-Manzano J, Manterola JM, Gamboa F, et al. Detection of mycobacterium tuberculosis in paraffin-embedded pleural biopsy specimen by commercial ribosomal RNA and DNA amplification kits. *Chest* 2000;118:648–655.

32. Sahn SA. The diagnostic value of pleural fluid analysis. *Semin Resp Crit Care Med* 1995;16:269–278.

33. Schwartz DA. New developments in asbestos-induced pleural disease. *Chest* 1991;99:191–198.

34. Light RW. Malignant pleural effusions. In: Light RW: *Pleural diseases,* 3rd ed. Baltimore: Williams & Wilkins, 1995:94–116.

35. Sahn SA. Pleural effusion in lung cancer. *Clin Chest Med* 1993;14:189–200.

36. Guzman J, Bross KJ, Costabel U. Malignant pleural effusions due to small cell carcinoma of the lung: an immunocytochemical cell surface analysis of lymphocytes and tumour cells. *Acta Cytol* 1990;497–501.

37. Fetsch PA, Abati A. Immunocytochemistry in effusion cytology: a contemporary review. *Cancer Cytopathol* 2001;93:293–308.

38. Yu CJ, Shew JY, Liaw, YS, et al. Application of mucin quantitative competitive reverse transcription polymerase chain reaction in assisting the diagnosis of malignant pleural effusion. *Am J Respir Crit Care Med* 2001;164:1312–1318.

39. Lozano MD, Panizo A, Toleso GR, et al. Immunocytochemistry in the differential diagnosis of serous effusions: a comparative evaluation of eight monoclonal antibodies in Papanicolaou stained smears. *Cancer Cytopathol* 2001;93:68–72.

40. Romero S, C Fernandez, JM Arriero, et al. CEA, CA 15-3 and CYFRA-21 in serum and pleural fluid of patients with pleural effusions. *Eur Respir J* 1996;9:17–23.

41. Riedel U, Schoenfeld N, Savaser M, et al. Diagnostischer Wert der Tumormarker TPA-M, Cyfra21-1 und CEA bei Pleuraergüssen -Prospektiver Vergleich bei thorakoskopisch untersuchten Peuraergüssen. *Pneumologie* 1999;53:471–476.

42. Light RW. Thoracentesis (diagnostic and therapeutic) and pleural biopsy. In: *Pleural disease,* 3rd ed. Baltimore: Williams & Wilkins, 1995:311–326.

43. Colt HG, Mathur NM. Pleural procedures. In: *Manual of pleural procedures.* Philadelphia: Lippincott Williams & Wilkins, 1999:93–163.

44. Kirsch CM, Kroe DM, Azzi RL, et al. The optimal number of pleural biopsy specimens for a diagnosis of tuberculous pleurisy. *Chest* 1997;112:702–706.

45. Jimenez D, Perez-Rodriguez E, Diaz G, et al. Determining the optimal number of specimens to obtain with needle biopsy of the pleura. *Respir Med* 2002;96:14–17.

46. Chretien J, Daniel CJ. Needle pleural biopsy. In: Chretien J, Bignon J, Hirsch A, et al., eds. *The pleura in health and disease.* New York: Marcel Dekker, 1985:1107–1108.

47. Cope C. A new pleural biopsy needle: preliminary study. *JAMA* 1958;167:1107–1108.

48. Radja GO, Argaval V, Vizoli LD, et al. Comparison of the Radja and the Abrams pleural biopsy needles in patients with pleural effusions. *Am Rev Respir Dis* 1993;147:1291–94.

49. O'Connor S, Yung TA. A comparison of Abrams and Radja pleural biopsy needles. *Aust NZ J Med* 1992;22:237.

50. Loddenkemper R, Grosser H, Mai J, et al. Diagnostik des tuberkulösen Pleuraergusses, prospektiver Vergleich laborchemischer, bakteriologischer, zytologischer und histologischer Untersuchungsergebnisse. *Prax Klin Pneumol* 1983;37:1153–56.

51. Canto-Armengod A, Rivas J, Saumench J, et al. Points to consider when choosing a biopsy method in cases of pleurisy of unknown origin. *Chest* 1983;84:176.

52. Adams R, Gray W, Davies RJO, et al. Percutaneous image-guided cutting needle biopsy of the pleura in the diagnosis of malignant mesothelioma. *Chest* 2001;120:1798–1802.

53. Loddenkemper R, Grosser H, Gabler A, et al. Prospective evaluation of biopsy methods in the diagnosis of malignant pleural effusions: intrapatient comparison between pleural fluid cytology, blind needle biopsy and thoracoscopy. *Am Rev Respir Dis* 1983;127[Suppl 4]:114.

54. Prakash UBS, Reiman HM. Comparison of needle biopsy with cytologic analysis for the evaluation of pleural effusion: analysis of 414 cases. *Chest* 1983;84:176.

55. Jacobaeus HC. Über die Möglichkeit, die Zystoskopie bei Untersuchung seröser Höhlen anzuwenden. *Münch Med Wschr* 1910; 57:2090–92.

56. Mathur PN, Boutin C, Loddenkemper R. Medical thoracoscopy: technique and indications in pulmonary medicine. *J Bronchol* 1994;1:228–239.

57. Loddenkemper R. Thoracoscopy: state of the art. *Eur Respir J* 1998;11:213–221

58. American Thoracic Society. Management of malignant pleural effusions (official statement). *Am J Respir Crit Care Med* 2000; 162:1987–2001.

59. Seijo LM, Sherman DH. Interventional pulmonology. *N Engl J Med* 2001;344:740–749.

60. Menzies R, Charbonneau M. Thoracoscopy for the diagnosis of pleural disease. *Ann Intern Med* 1991;114:271–276.

61. Boutin C, Viallat JR, Cargino C, et al. Thoracoscopy in malignant pleural effusions. *Am Rev Respir Dis* 1981;124:588–592.

62. Boutin C, Frey F, Gouvernet J, et al. Thoracoscopy in pleural malignant mesothelioma: a prospective study of 188 consecutive patients: 1, diagnosis; 2, prognosis and staging. *Cancer* 1993;72:389–404.

63. Levine MN, Young JE, Ryan ED, et al. Pleural effusion in breast cancer: thoracoscopy for hormone receptor determination. *Cancer* 1986;57:324–327.

64. Hartman DL, Gaither JM, Kesler KA, et al. Comparison of insufflated talc under thoracoscopic guidance with standard tetracycline and bleomycin pleurodesis for control of malignant pleural effusion. *J Thorac Cardiovasc Surg* 1993;105:743–748.

65. Rodriguez-Panadero F, Antony VB. Pleurodesis: state of the art. *Eur Respir J* 1997;10:1648–1654.

66. Karmy-Jones R, Sorensen V, Horst M, et al. Rigid thoracoscopic debridement and continuous pleural irrigation in the management of empyema. *Chest* 1997;111:272–274.

67. Vanderschueren RG. The role of thoracoscopy in the evaluation and management of pneumothorax. *Lung* 1990;[Suppl]:1122–1125.

68. Milanez JRC, Vargas FS, Filomeno LTB, et al. Intrapleural talc for the prevention of recurrent pneumothorax. *Chest* 1994;106:1162–1165.

69. Brandt HJ, Loddenkemper R, Mai J. *Atlas of diagnostic thoracoscopy.* New York: Thieme Inc, 1985.

70. Colt HG. Thoracoscopy: window to the pleural space. *Chest* 1999;116:1409–15.

71. Boutin C, Viallat JR, Aelony Y. *Practical thoracoscopy.* New York: Springer-Verlag, 1991.

72. Mares DC, Mathur PN. Medical thoracoscopy: the pulmonologists perspective. *Sem Respir Crit Care* 1997;18:803–816.

73. Viskum K, Enk B. Complications of thoracoscopy. *Poumon-Coeur* 1981;37:25–28.

74. Colt HG. Thoracoscopy: a prospective study of safety and outcome. *Chest* 1995;108:324–329.

75. Boutin C, Rey F, Viallat JR. Prevention of malignant seeding after invasive diagnostic procedures in patients with pleural mesothelioma: a randomised trial of local radiotherapy. *Chest* 1995;108:754–758.

Baum's Textbook of Pulmonary Diseases, 7th ed. Edited by James D. Crapo, Jeffrey Glassroth, Joel Karlinsky, and Talmadge E. King, Jr.
Lippincott Williams & Wilkins, Philadelphia © 2004.

Preoperative Evaluation and Relation to Postoperative Complications

Janine R. E. Vintch · James E. Hansen

6

This chapter is designed to review—for general internists, pulmonologists, and surgeons—the physiologic alterations that result from general anesthesia and surgical procedures and how they relate to postoperative pulmonary complications. It has become increasingly recognized that pulmonary complications contribute to prolonged hospital stays, increased health care expenditures, and postoperative morbidity and mortality (1). Recently, there has been a more concentrated effort to better define the patient population at risk for developing such complications so that clinicians caring for these patients can try to intervene and attempt to minimize these risks if possible. Pulmonary complications are more likely to occur in patients who are older, obese, or current smokers, or in those undergoing thoracic or upper abdominal surgery (2). This chapter will review those complications that have been clearly demonstrated to impact on the patient's clinical postoperative course.

MAJOR POSTOPERATIVE PULMONARY COMPLICATIONS

Atelectasis and Shunting with Hypoxemia

Lung volumes change quickly with the induction of anesthesia, remain reduced throughout the surgical procedure, and may persist into the postoperative period. Figure 6.1 shows the decline in both vital capacity (VC) and forced expiratory volume in 1 second (FEV_1) and the concurrent increases in alveolar-arterial differences in the partial pressure of oxygen (PAO_2-PaO_2) in the week after upper abdominal or thoracic surgery even though no lung was resected (3). During surgery with general anesthesia, the

J. R. E. Vintch and J. E. Hansen: UCLA School of Medicine, Los Angeles, and Harbor-U.C.L.A. Medical Center, Torrance, California.

increases in PAO_2-PaO_2 and alveolar-arterial differences in the partial pressure of carbon dioxide ($PACO_2$-$PaCO_2$) could be attributed to decreases in lung compliance, increased shunting, increased pulmonary dead space, or decreased efficiency of ventilation secondary to ventilation and perfusion mismatching—i.e., mechanisms causing increases in venous admixture (4).

Altered mechanics of the chest wall and diaphragm with a decrease in functional residual capacity (FRC) are the primary cause of the development of areas of atelectasis and secondary hypoxemia. If patchy atelectasis is sought, it can nearly always be demonstrated roentgenographically during general anesthesia for upper abdominal surgery (5). The appearance of these areas of atelectasis during anesthesia in normal individuals correlates positively with the magnitude of shunting and can usually be cleared by the application of positive end-expiratory pressure (PEEP) at 10 cm water (6). Under general anesthesia in the supine position, the diaphragm moves in a cephalad direction, contributing to decreased lung volumes. It has been noted that patients undergoing upper abdominal surgery who have the greatest reduction in FRC postoperatively also have the highest incidence of pulmonary complications (7). It appears that the observed postoperative atelectasis not only is owing to decreased diaphragmatic contractility and splinting owing to postoperative pain but also may be owing to a reflex neural inhibition of the diaphragm itself (8). In addition, ventilation during anesthesia with gas mixtures low in nitrogen may accelerate air space collapse (4). It has also been observed that patients after an abdominal procedure assume a rapid shallow breathing pattern, with a tendency toward paradoxical movements of the abdominal wall, further promoting atelectatic lung segments (5). Finally, some studies have shown that inhalational anesthetics inhibit hypoxic pulmonary vasoconstriction more than intravenous anesthetics do, thus tending to cause more overperfusion of poorly ventilated air spaces

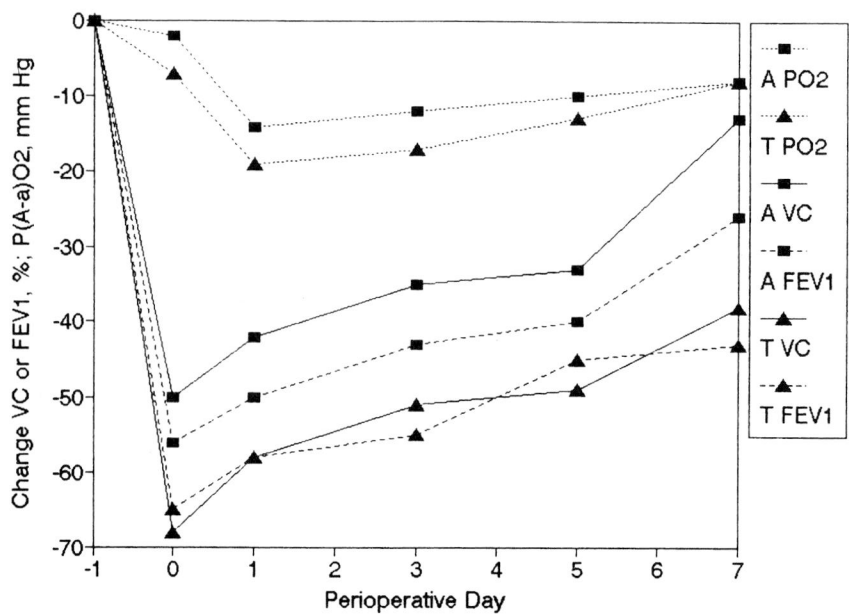

FIGURE 6.1. Average change in spirometric values (%) and alveolar-arterial differences in the partial pressure of oxygen (mm Hg) after thoracic *(T)* or abdominal *(A)* surgical procedures in 34 patients. (Modified from Bryant LR, Preston D, Houck G, et al. Lung perfusion scanning for estimation of postoperative pulmonary function. *Arch Surg* 1972;104:52–55, with permission.)

and subsequent greater hypoxemia (9). This area remains controversial as other studies have not demonstrated these same findings.

Pulmonary hypertension may develop owing to reduction of the pulmonary capillary volume after lung resection in patients with severe underlying lung disease. If right atrial pressures exceed left atrial pressures during the procedure or in the postoperative period, the opening of a foramen ovale may occur causing the shunting of blood from the right to left atria with a widening Pao_2-Pao_2 and a compensatory hyperventilation (10). The diagnosis of a patent foramen ovale can be made by having the patient breath 100% oxygen (O_2) and demonstration of an increased shunt fraction. The venous admixture resulting from the development of a right-to-left shunt reduces the measured Pao_2 in an almost linear fashion proportional to the size of the shunt itself.

Postoperative Pneumonia

Impaired Mucociliary Clearance

Transport of mucus from the lower lobes and trachea is impaired for several days after upper abdominal surgery under general anesthesia, but only minimally after surgery of a lower extremity. Insufflation of the airways with tantalum can demonstrate such slowed transport. This impaired clearance of secretions has been implicated in contributing to pulmonary complications (11). The actual mechanism behind this reduced transport is unclear but may include the effects of inhalational anesthetics and trauma from endotracheal intubation (12). In addition, this transport inefficiency is probably compounded by postoperative immobilization, diaphragmatic dysfunction from the surgical procedure and anesthetic effects, and ineffective coughing. Overall, the in-

ability to properly clear secretions from the airways potentially contributes to the development of pneumonia in these postoperative patients.

Impaired Cough

Coughing to clear secretions is especially difficult in the presence of postoperative chest and abdominal pain because patients tend to suppress their cough in order to avoid or diminish this incisional discomfort pain. In addition, the ability to generate a forceful cough and expel secretions from the airways depends on the generation of an adequate expiratory flow rate. Patients with obstructive lung disease have low expiratory flow rates at baseline and the predisposition for an ineffective cough. As stated previously, the postoperative reduction in FEV_1 contributes to less effective cough generation. Finally, patients undergoing thoracic surgery that disrupts the chest wall musculature may experience decreased chest wall compliance (13). When the muscles responsible for generating expiratory flow rates are damaged, the patient's cough will be temporarily impaired.

Aspiration

Aspiration of oropharyngeal and gastric contents occurs occasionally in normal individuals during sleep. In the perioperative period, such aspiration of gastric or oropharyngeal contents into the tracheobronchial tree may cause pulmonary dysfunction, resulting from acid burns, mechanical obstruction, or bacterial pathogens (14,15). Aspiration can easily occur during induction of anesthesia if the stomach is not emptied properly, or after surgery if extubation occurs prematurely before the gag reflex returns. Aspiration can also occur around the endotracheal tube cuff, whether or not it is inflated properly. Finally, the use of a nasogastric tube, which leads to a continuously patent gastroesophageal junction, may promote an increased risk of pulmonary aspiration (16).

Preexisting Lung Infection

Both clinically evident and subclinical respiratory tract infections are associated with an increased risk for pneumonia. Carrel and colleagues found that pneumonia frequently developed in cardiac patients in whom immediate postsurgical tracheal aspirates were positive for microorganisms, despite perioperative antibiotic therapy (eight of 26), but rarely in those with negative aspirates (one of 72) (17). Thus, it is important to thoroughly preoperatively evaluate patients for possible lower airway infections and to administer antibiotics if clinically indicated to decrease this risk. It may be difficult to discern infection in patients who chronically produce sputum. A low index of suspicion and inquiring about changes in sputum production or color as well as shortness of breath may help identify patients with underlying lung disease and chronic sputum production who would benefit from preoperative antibiotics (18).

Respiratory Failure

Respiratory failure is not a common pulmonary complication in the postoperative period. The actual occurrence of this finding depends on the duration of the surgery, the type of surgical procedure performed, and the characteristics of the underlying patient population (19). When respiratory failure does occur, which is defined in most studies as patients requiring "prolonged mechanical ventilation" for more than 48 hours or reintubation, it is most commonly seen in patients with underlying severe obstructive lung disease undergoing thoracic or upper abdominal surgery. Kroenke and colleagues evaluated 89 patients with severe chronic obstructive pulmonary disease (COPD) undergoing a wide variety of surgical procedures, including both thoracic and upper abdominal surgeries. They found the incidence of ventilatory failure in their patient population was 5.6% (19). Subsequently, Samuels and colleagues in 1998 evaluated patients undergoing coronary artery bypass grafting. Prolonged mechanical ventilation was required in 5.2% of their COPD patients but in only 2.8% in their non-COPD patients (20).

Preoperative carbon dioxide (CO_2) retention, obesity, sepsis, and shock all increase the probability of postoperative respiratory failure. Maeda and colleagues (21) showed that the ratio of abdominal to transdiaphragmatic pressure decreased postoperatively, indicating diaphragmatic weakness. They found that the greatest reduction occurred in four of their 20 patients, who required mechanical ventilation for 2 to 6 days. The decrease in lung volumes and flow rates during the several days after chest or upper abdominal surgery—especially when combined with pain, weakness, and sedation—necessarily reduces the drive and ability

of postoperative patients to ventilate and remove metabolically produced CO_2. The elimination of CO_2 is rarely a problem except in patients with significant lung disease. In these patients, the ability to ventilate may not only be seriously reduced but also inefficient—the latter attributable to an increase in the ratio of physiologic dead space to tidal volume (V_D/V_T). Postoperative infection with fever and increased metabolism causing high CO_2 production and the intraoperative insufflation of CO_2 during abdominal endoscopic procedures are additional causes of acute respiratory acidosis and subsequent respiratory failure (22). In addition, nutritional supplementation, especially with high carbohydrate diets, by increasing the respiratory quotient may contribute to an increase in CO_2 production and ventilatory requirement.

The degree of V_D/V_T abnormality can be calculated from the patient's estimated or measured CO_2 output and measurement of the arterial CO_2 and minute ventilation (23). In patients whose ability to ventilate is compromised, repeated assessments with changes in ventilator settings and body position may be necessary to reduce the V_D/V_T and optimize CO_2 removal.

Pulmonary Embolism

Pulmonary embolism is a common sequela of venous thrombosis in the deep veins of the legs, pelvis, or arms. The risk of upper extremity deep vein thrombosis (DVT) appears to be increasing with the more frequent use of central venous catheters (24). In the perioperative period, the factors that increase patient risk of venous thrombosis and subsequent pulmonary embolism include immobility, venous stasis, vascular trauma, and impaired fibrinolysis (25). These risk factors should be recognized and countered whenever possible.

In one study, the incidence of deep venous thromboses in three groups of hospitalized patients was as follows: (1) 11% in those with none of the risk factors of advanced age, obesity, malignancy, recent surgery, or history of deep venous thrombosis; (2) 50% in those with three risk factors; and (3) 100% in those with four or more risk factors (26). A more recent expert group addressed the risk of thromboembolic disease in surgical patients based on risk factors and found the following estimates: (1) The *highest risk group,* with an approximately 10% to 20% incidence of proximal DVT and 4% to 10% incidence of clinical pulmonary embolism, consisted of patients older than 40 years with a recent history of venous thrombosis, cancer, or hypercoagulable state; patients undergoing major orthopedic surgery of a lower extremity, including hip or knee arthroplasty and hip fracture surgeries; and patients with major trauma or spinal cord injury. (2) The *high risk group,* with an approximately 4% to 8% incidence of proximal DVT and 2% to 4% incidence of clinical pulmonary embolism, consisted of patients older than 60 years or with other additional risk factors undergoing intermediate surgery, or surgery in patients older than

40 years of age without other risk factors. (3) The *moderate risk group,* with a 2% to 4% incidence of proximal DVT and 1% to 2% risk of clinical pulmonary embolism, consisted of patients undergoing minor surgery with additional risk factors; patients 40 to 60 years of age undergoing intermediate surgery without other risk factors; or patients younger than 40 years undergoing a major surgical procedure without additional risk factors. (4) The *low risk group,* with 1% to 2% incidence of proximal DVT and a less than 1% risk of clinical pulmonary embolism, consisted of patients younger than 40 years of age undergoing minor surgical procedures (25).

Despite this known high incidence of disease, even in a well-known academic medical center with a major interest in thromboembolic disease, a correct diagnosis was established before autopsy in only 30% of patients who had a fatal pulmonary embolism (26). The investigators further noted a low incidence of thromboembolic prophylaxis even in high-risk patients, ranging from 9% to 56% in different New England hospitals. The recent American College of Chest Physicians (ACCP) guidelines attribute the lack of prophylaxis among hospitalized and postoperative patients to the belief of many physicians that the overall incidence of venous thromboembolic disease has decreased over the past several decades to the point that it no longer requires prophylaxis, to the fear of bleeding complications from anticoagulant use, to the subjective misperceptions of the magnitude of the problem and effectiveness of prophylaxis based on individual experience, and to the frequent silent nature of the disease process (25).

MAJOR POSTOPERATIVE PULMONARY COMPLICATIONS

Summary Statement	Level of Evidence
Pulmonary atelectasis is a common occurrence during general anesthesia in the supine position.	Prospective nonrandomized trials, prospective model-building studies, and retrospective case reviews
The incidence of postoperative pneumonia is increased in patients with obstructive lung disease, impaired cough, and acute or chronic bronchitis or (lower airway infections).	Prospective nonrandomized trials and prospective model-building studies
After thoracic or upper abdominal surgery, prolonged mechanical ventilation is often required in patients with severe obstructive lung disease, obesity, or sepsis.	Well-designed clinical studies, including retrospective case reviews
The incidence of both detectable and unsuspected postoperative pulmonary embolism is strongly related to the following risk factors: major surgery, advanced age, obesity, malignancy, history of venous thrombosis, and lack of thromboembolic prophylaxis.	Evidence is of high quality for each factor based on well-designed clinical studies, including nonrandomized prospective and retrospective trials and retrospective case reviews.

OTHER RISK FACTORS

Age

The maximal flow rates, FEV_1, VC, FEV_1/VC, and maximum voluntary ventilation (MVV) all decline with age so that normal individuals have less ventilatory reserve and less ability to clear secretions by coughing as they age. Additionally, the PaO_2-PaO_2 increases by approximately 0.4 mm Hg annually (27). Thus, even without pulmonary, neuromuscular, or other organ disease processes, there is a gradual reduction in PaO_2 with aging and less reserve for the increased ventilatory requirements that may be needed postoperatively (28). Hence, aging affects lung mechanics and oxygenation, which puts this patient population at risk of pulmonary complications.

The more frequent occurrence of comorbid diseases with advancing age adds to the likelihood of postoperative problems. Many studies cite advancing age, usually greater than 60 years, as a risk factor for postoperative pulmonary complications. Hall and colleagues (29) evaluated more than 1,000 patients undergoing abdominal surgery and found that the combination of the American Society of Anesthesiologists classification score and age greater than 59 years identified 88% (205 out of 232) of the patients who developed postoperative pulmonary complications. Kroenke and colleagues (30) evaluated 26 COPD patients undergoing a variety of surgical procedures and also found that American Society of Anesthesiologists score and age were the only independent predictors of serious pulmonary and cardiac complications.

Obesity

There is some disagreement as to whether or not obesity causes postoperative *pulmonary* complications. At least two older studies found that after upper abdominal surgery, obesity was the most important risk factor associated with clinically significant atelectasis (7,31). Newer studies also found more pulmonary complications after abdominal procedures in patients with a body mass index (BMI) greater than 25 and 27, respectively (2,29). In contrast, Moulton and colleagues did not find obesity to be a predisposing factor for pulmonary complications in their review of 2,299 patients undergoing cardiopulmonary bypass surgery (32). Similarly, Dales and colleagues did not find a difference in pulmonary complications in their patient population undergoing thoracic surgery when they were stratified based on body mass index (33). The site of surgery may account for these reported differences.

Physiologic alterations associated with obesity clearly have an impact on oxygenation in the postoperative period. The incidence of both preoperative and postoperative hypoxemia increases strikingly with obesity and age and is worse in the supine position (34) (Fig. 6.2). Hypoxemia is primarily a consequence of the high proportion of regions with decreased ventilation without compensatory reduction in perfusion

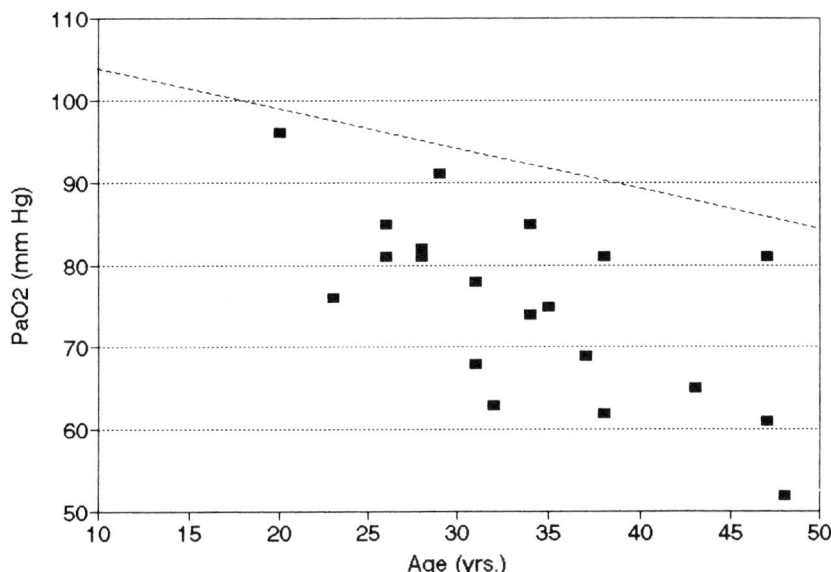

FIGURE 6.2. Effect of age on arterial blood partial pressure of oxygen in morbidly obese, awake, supine patients. The **dotted line** is regressed from data of Sorbini and colleagues for normal adults, with a standard deviation of 4 mm Hg. (Modified from Vaughan RW, Engelhardt RC, Wise L. Postoperative hypoxemia in obese patients. *Ann Surg* 1974;180:877–882, with permission.)

(low VA/Q) at the lung bases. It may also be aggravated by reduced ventilatory drive associated with CO_2 retention or metabolic alkalosis and the increased ventilatory work associated with truncal obesity. Although the VC may remain within normal limits with moderate thoracic or abdominal obesity, the expiratory reserve volume inevitably declines, indicating that the resting position of the diaphragm is elevated. With extreme obesity, the VC and MVV decrease well below predicted values in the absence of intrinsic lung disease and despite normal general muscle strength (35). Thus, the incidence of hypoxemia, hypercapnia, and pulmonary hypertension increases even in patients with moderate obesity.

Additional disadvantages for obese patients are the requirements for larger doses of many anesthetic agents because of their high solubility in fatty tissue, the longer time needed to eliminate anesthetics from the body, the longer period necessary to complete the surgical procedure, the increased acidity of gastric juice, and the increased frequency of aspiration of gastric contents (36). To this list can be added the higher incidence of diabetes mellitus, cardiovascular and thromboembolic diseases, obstructive sleep apnea-hypopnea syndrome, obese hypoventilation syndrome, and the difficulties involved in postoperative ambulation and nursing care.

Smoking

Many studies confirm that smokers, even those without demonstrable pulmonary or cardiovascular disease, are at increased risk for postoperative complications. For example, Wightman found a 15% incidence of postoperative complications, defined in this study as fever, productive cough, and abnormal chest findings, after abdominal surgery in smokers compared with a 6% incidence in nonsmokers (37). Laszlo

and colleagues found a 53% incidence of postoperative complications in smokers versus 22% incidence in nonsmokers (38). Carrel and colleagues prospectively evaluated 100 patients undergoing cardiac surgery and found that the development of postoperative pneumonia was highly correlated with smoking, abnormal spirometry, and positive tracheal aspirates at the time of intubation (17).

It may be difficult to ascertain whether it is smoking itself or the disease processes associated with tobacco use that lead to increased postoperative pulmonary complications. Poor oral hygiene, chronic cough, reduced airway ciliary function, the likelihood of larger numbers of pulmonary bacterial pathogens, elevated carboxyhemoglobin levels, and the effects of nicotine on the cardiovascular system all contribute to the increased morbidity in smokers. More recent data suggest that smoking modulates the antimicrobial and proinflammatory functions of the alveolar macrophages, leading to a limited ability to mount an effective pulmonary immune defense after anesthesia and surgery (39). These findings indicate that smoking imposes a multifactorial impairment to patients undergoing surgery.

Lung Disease

Although postoperative morbidity and mortality cannot be accurately predicted for every patient, patients with significant lung disease undergoing thoracic or abdominal surgery are at higher risk. Obstructive lung disease imposes a greater postoperative risk than does restrictive lung disease, probably because peak flow rates and the ability to clear secretions are reduced more in the former. In 1956, Miller and colleagues (40) introduced a four-quadrant diagram based on the $FEV_{0.5}$ and VC, later modified by others, to categorize disturbed respiratory mechanics (41,42). This diagram

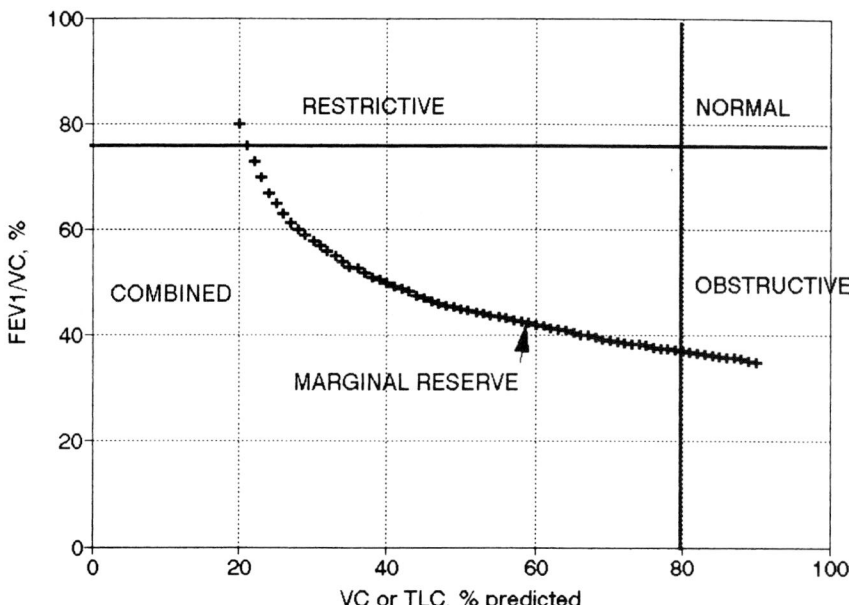

FIGURE 6.3. Four-quadrant diagram for estimation of the relative risk of surgery in patients with lung disease. The upper fourth of the graph includes patients who are normal or have only restrictive lung disease; the lower three fourths includes patients with obstructive disease with or without restrictive lung disease. As a broad generalization, all patients below the marginal reserve line can be expected to require ventilatory support postoperatively. (Modified from Hodgkin JE. Evaluation before thoracotomy. *West J Med* 1975;122:104–109, with permission.)

graphically identifies relative postoperative risk in patients with obstructive, restrictive, and combined lung disorders (Fig. 6.3). All other things being equal, it can be noted in this diagram that the risk for postoperative ventilatory failure might be (1) slightly better than marginal in a patient with an FEV_1/VC of 50% and a VC or total lung capacity (TLC) that is 50% of predicted (i.e., moderate obstruction and moderate restriction); (2) prohibitive in a patient with an FEV_1/VC of 35% and VC or TLC that is 80% of predicted (i.e., severe obstruction and mild restriction); and (3) satisfactory in a patient with an FEV_1/VC of 70% and a VC or TLC that is 45% of predicted (mild obstruction and severe restriction). These differences in risk are logically related to the difficulty encountered by patients with obstructive disease in clearing airway secretions in the postoperative period.

Stein and colleagues noted that a reduced forced expiratory flow ($FEF_{200-1200}$) was a potent predictor of postoperative pulmonary complications (43). Even patients with severe restrictive lung disease, who often have increased lung elastic recoil, can maintain satisfactory peak flow measurements and can clear secretions adequately. On the other hand, patients with severe obstructive lung disease often have a very low $FEF_{200-1200}$ or peak flow readings and an ineffective cough. When either restrictive or obstructive lung disease has progressed to the stage at which CO_2 retention has occurred, the risk of surgery increases markedly. To oversimplify this statement, the "blue bloater" chronic bronchitic patient is likely to be at greater risk than the "pink puffer" for the same severity of airway obstruction. However, newer data, including a study by Kearney and colleagues, did not find alterations on preoperative blood gas analysis, including hypercarbia with a $Paco_2$ greater than 45 mm Hg to be predictive of complications (44).

Kroenke and colleagues published several papers evaluating the risk of postoperative pulmonary complications in patients with underlying chronic obstructive lung disease. In their evaluation of 89 patients with chronic obstructive lung disease undergoing 107 surgical procedures, they found an overall complication rate of 29% (19). They confirmed that the type of procedure was strongly linked to the incidence of pulmonary complications, with the highest rates seen in patients undergoing coronary artery bypass grafting and upper abdominal procedures. Serious complications and death appeared to occur primarily in patients undergoing cardiac surgery. They concluded that surgical procedures, with the exception of cardiac and pulmonary resection procedures, could be safely performed in the majority of patients with COPD. Another study by this same group evaluated 26 "severe COPD" patients, defined as patients with an FEV_1 less than 50% of predicted and found, that for serious pulmonary complications and death, an abnormal chest radiograph and the need for perioperative bronchodilators were predictive of postoperative pulmonary complications, more so then the findings on preoperative spirometry (30). Lawrence and colleagues also found that abnormal findings on lung examination or on the chest radiograph were most predictive of postoperative pulmonary complications (45). In summary, patients with significant lung disease who have abnormal findings at the time of the surgical procedure have the highest risk of postoperative complications.

The risk for complications in the asthmatic patient appears to be inversely related to the adequacy of control of their disease before surgery, with bronchospasm and barotrauma being frequently cited events. Reflex stimulation during intubation and the release of inflammatory mediators induced by some anesthetic agents can lead to bronchospasm (46).

Warner and colleagues (47) found a very low rate of bronchospasm (1.7%, or 12 out of their 706 asthmatic patients undergoing a variety of surgical procedures) compared with other previously quoted retrospective reviews that cited an incidence of bronchospasm ranging from 6% to 24% in patients with asthma. They concluded that the frequency of bronchospasm in patients with well controlled or asymptomatic asthma approaches that of the nonasthmatics. Conversely, poorly controlled asthmatics had a higher frequency of postoperative complications.

Other Organ System Dysfunction

Patients with heart failure, recent myocardial infarction, or arrhythmia are at increased risk for postoperative cardiopulmonary complications, but moderate systemic hypertension does not appear to be a significant risk factor (48). Understandably, damage to the upper airways or rib cage, difficulty with mastication or swallowing, chronic drug or alcohol abuse, psychosis or severe neurosis, recent stroke, degenerative neurologic processes, acute or chronic infections, compromised immunologic status, and chronic toxic or metabolic disorders all increase the likelihood of pulmonary morbidity.

Several groups have proposed indices to predict postoperative pulmonary complications. These indices demonstrate the importance of nonpulmonary organ dysfunction contributing to pulmonary complications. The Cardiopulmonary Risk Index proposed by Epstein and colleagues indicates that cardiac abnormalities are important in contributing to pulmonary outcomes (49). The more recent Postoperative Pneumonia Risk Index includes risk factors related to the patient's general health, immune status, neurologic function, and fluid balance (50). Abnormalities in any of these areas contribute "points" to the patient's overall risk score for postoperative pneumonia.

Surgical and Incisional Site

Evidence is overwhelming that the incidence of postoperative morbidity and mortality is closely linked to the site of the surgical intervention. It should be recalled that with upper abdominal surgery or thoracic surgery without lung resection, the FEV_1 and VC are strikingly reduced as soon as they can be measured postoperatively and do not usually return to preoperative levels within the first week (3). When possible, it is desirable to choose an incisional site in thoracic surgery that is associated with lesser postoperative discomfort (51). Vaughan and Wise found a higher rate of atelectasis and hypoxemia with vertical than with horizontal laparotomies (52). The overall incidence of postoperative cardiopulmonary complications becomes progressively lower in patients undergoing lower abdominal, pelvic, and extremity surgery (53). However, the incidence of venous thrombosis and pulmonary emboli is very high in patients undergoing extremity surgery such as hip and knee arthroplasty or replacement (26).

Resection of Lung Tissue

It is logical to expect that morbidity and mortality would be directly related to the amount of lung tissue resected. In many series, this expectation is obscured by patient selection because those who are not expected to tolerate or survive often do not have lung resected. More important than the amount of lung tissue removed is the ability of the remaining lung tissue to transfer O_2 and CO_2 between blood and environment through the processes of ventilation, diffusion, and perfusion.

Type and Duration of Anesthesia

In choosing a form of anesthesia the following goals are desirable: a smooth induction, adequate control of the airway and ventilation, adequate oxygenation without sudden shifts in acid-base status, reduction in atelectasis during and after surgery, adequate blood and fluid replacement, avoidance of other organ toxicity, and quick recovery from the anesthetic and muscle relaxant agents. There is strong evidence that the duration of the surgical procedure is much more significant than the type or route of administration of anesthesia (7,19).

Because of the many variables that influence selection of anesthetics and postoperative morbidity, it is difficult to compare different types and routes of anesthesia for the same operation. In general, regional anesthesia has little impact on diaphragmatic function because its innervation is derived

OTHER RISK FACTORS	
Summary Statement	**Level of Evidence**
Increasing age, cigarette smoking, severe obstructive lung disease, long duration of surgery, and incisional locations associated with more pain or immobilization all increase the risk of postoperative complications.	Prospective longitudinal studies, retrospective cohort studies, and retrospective case reviews
Abnormal auscultation of the chest, heart failure, arrhythmias, diabetes mellitus, and patients with swallowing disorders are associated with increased risk of postoperative complications.	Small number of clinical studies, including a nested case control study
Obesity, abnormal chest roentgenograms, poorly controlled asthma, severe psychiatric or neurological disorders, and reduced immune status are associated with increased risk of postoperative complications.	A few clinical studies, including retrospective case reviews, and/or a consensus of expert opinion

from the cervical plexus but reduces expiratory ability by affecting abdominal musculature (54). This may lead to an impaired cough reflex and ability to clear secretions postoperatively. In two series of patients with severe obstructive lung disease, there was no difference in arterial oxygenation when general anesthesia was compared with regional anesthesia for lower abdominal surgical procedures (55,56). However, other studies have demonstrated an overall higher frequency of postoperative pulmonary complications after general anesthesia (57). Currently, there is no consensus recommendation on what form of anesthesia to offer patients at risk of postoperative pulmonary morbidity. Each decision must be individualized to the patient, their risk factors, and the proposed surgical procedure.

PREOPERATIVE EVALUATION OF PATIENTS NOT UNDERGOING LUNG RESECTION

History and Physical Examination

It is trite but true that a thorough history and physical examination are extremely cost-effective and essential if unexpected morbidity and mortality are to be avoided. In fact, several studies have pointed out the importance of clinical variables that are readily assessed by history taking and physical examination that can help with determining a patient's postoperative risk without ordering an excessive number of studies.

The preoperative history should include specific questions regarding unexplained dyspnea; current activity level and estimation of exercise tolerance; cough frequency and characteristics; quantity and type of sputum production; intermittent wheezes or noisy breathing; the duration and frequency of smoking; other drug use history; chest pain, tightness, or distress; recent infections involving any organ system; toxin or occupational exposure; recent weight changes; immobility; and venous insufficiency or high susceptibility to pulmonary embolism. Gracey and colleagues found that daily production of 2 oz or more of sputum was a valuable predictor of postoperative complications (58).

The physical examination should focus on abnormalities that could contribute to postoperative pulmonary complication risk. Areas to specifically comment on include body habitus and chest wall abnormalities; oropharyngeal crowding or narrowing; dentition with evidence of poor oral hygiene; signs of airway disease or abnormal lung findings; the duration (in seconds) of a complete forced expiration; and evidence of clubbing, edema, or venous disease. Lawrence and colleagues reported that abnormal findings on physical examination—including decreased breath sounds, prolonged expiration, or adventitial sounds such as rales, rhonchi, or wheezes—were important predictors of complications (45). If the patient's subjective complaints or assessment seems discordant with objective physical findings, further evaluation is necessary.

Wise physicians weigh their assessment of the patient's daily activity, exercise, and symptom status (or lack thereof) along with their physical examination findings against the expected stress of the planned surgical procedure. Some patients are so limited from their advanced heart or lung disease that they do not complain of dyspnea because their level of exertion is so low. We highly regard those clinicians who walk or climb stairs with their patients before major surgery!

Chest Roentgenogram and other Laboratory Tests

The "routine" ordering of a battery of laboratory tests during the preoperative assessment is unwise because it may yield false-positive results that could lead to further testing and even the delay of the surgical procedure. The necessity for laboratory measures, including a hemogram, coagulation studies, urinalysis, blood chemistries, chest roentgenogram, and electrocardiogram (ECG), depends on the surgery contemplated and the findings elicited or suspicions aroused during the history and physical examination.

There is little data to support the utility of obtaining routine preoperative chest radiography in all patients undergoing surgery. Common reasons cited for obtaining these routine x-rays include screening for silent disease, evaluating suspected underlying lung disease, and establishing a baseline for future comparison during the postoperative period (59). A metaanalysis of 21 studies (60) found that 10% of routine preoperative chest films had abnormalities, but only 1.3% of these findings were unanticipated. In addition, these radiographic abnormalities were of sufficient importance to cause a change in patient management only 0.1% of the time. Another review found that chest x-ray findings led to a change in clinical management in 0% to 2.1% of all patients reviewed (61). Thus, both reviews concluded that the cost of routine preoperative chest radiography without relying on the guidance of history and physical examination findings far outweighed its clinical benefit.

Preoperative chest radiography should be considered in patients with signs or symptoms of active pulmonary disease, as well as in patients undergoing intrathoracic surgical procedures. A chest x-ray is not indicated solely on the basis of an individual's age. However, given the higher prevalence of symptoms and signs of chest disease in the aging population, radiography may be ordered more frequently in this age group (59).

Arterial Blood Gas Analysis

An arterial blood gas analysis is indicated for patients suspected of significant lung disease and for patients with neuromuscular disorders. Assessment of gas exchange should also be considered in the obese patient population. These patients may be noted to have varying degrees of hypoxemia and hypercapnia, related to restrictive lung defects;

hypoventilation; and anatomical shunts, related directly to their underlying obesity (62). If these abnormalities are noted preoperatively, then more aggressive perioperative management may be given to avoid serious complications. Earlier studies found that an elevated $Paco_2$, regardless of the cause, was associated with high postoperative risk (41,43,63), but a more recent study did not find that a $Paco_2$ higher than 45 mm Hg was a significant predictor of morbidity in patients undergoing lung resection (44). A Pao_2 significantly below that predicted for the patient's age and body habitus indicates the need for further evaluation. Lastly, unexpected acid-base disturbances may also be detected from analysis of arterial blood gases and pH, which require further work-up or management in the perioperative period.

Spirometry

Spirometry is probably not cost-effective in asymptomatic patients or in mildly symptomatic patients undergoing surgery involving the lower abdomen or an extremity. However, we recommend spirometry for patients undergoing upper abdominal or thoracic surgery who have a history of heavy smoking, those who have symptoms or signs suggesting significant lung disease or heart failure, and those who are moderately to severely obese. The FEV_1, VC, FEV_1/VC, $FEF_{200-1200}$, or peak flow rate and the directly measured MVV for 10 to 12 seconds should be measured. If airway obstruction is present, spirometry should be repeated after inhalation of a bronchodilator. It is important to measure the MVV directly in a patient who appears to be infirm or who is undergoing thoracic or upper abdominal surgery. Inability to perform the MVV maneuver adequately gives warning that the patient may not be able to cooperate, coordinate, learn, or perform the necessary postoperative ventilatory maneuvers.

A review by Zibrak and colleagues criticized the methodology of earlier studies and concluded, in part, that "in upper abdominal surgery, spirometry and arterial blood gas analysis did not consistently have measurable benefit in identifying patients at increased risk for postoperative pneumonia, prolonged hospitalization, and death" (64). They suggested that further critical investigation was required. Similarly, in their review of the literature in 1989, Lawrence and colleagues argue that no study of spirometry before abdominal surgery clearly demonstrated its superior predictive value over less expensive clinical assessment (65). Subsequently, the American College of Physicians (ACP) issued a position paper in 1990 (66) that recognized that although spirometry assists physicians in making decisions regarding lung resection, there is no clear role for routine spirometry for other surgical procedures. They concluded that a thorough history and physical examination may be enough to risk stratify patients with regards to pulmonary complications. Subsequently, Lawrence and colleagues in a study of more than 2,000 patients concluded that spirometry was not helpful in predicting post-

operative pulmonary complications compared with clinical examination and chest radiographic findings (45).

On the other hand, there is significant evidence that preoperative spirometry is valuable in identifying patients at increased risk. Three decades ago, Stein and colleagues prospectively selected, at random, 100 ward patients admitted for surgical procedures (43). Of these patients, 32 did not have surgery because of lack of surgical indication, and five were not operated on because of the severity of their cardiac or pulmonary disease. The 63 remaining patients were divided into two groups on the basis of their respiratory function. Group 1 included patients with essentially normal lung function: $FEF_{200-1200}$ was greater than 200 L/min (3.3 L/s) in 30 and unmeasured in three patients, the single-breath O_2 test was less than 2.5% in 30 and unmeasured in three, and the estimated $Paco_2$ was greater than 41 mm Hg in 28 and unmeasured in five. Group 2 included patients with abnormal lung function: $FEF_{200-1200}$ was less than 200 L/min in 30 patients; the single-breath O_2 test was greater than 2.0% in 18, less than 2.5% in eight, and unmeasured in four; and the estimated $Paco_2$ was greater than 42 mm Hg in nine, less than 41 mm Hg in 18, and unmeasured in three. Respiratory complications occurred in only one patient in group 1 and in 21 patients in group 2. In group 2, seven of nine patients undergoing thoracotomy and 11 of 12 patients undergoing abdominal surgery experienced complications.

In addition, the positive evidence from four other studies should be considered. First, Gracey and colleagues in a prospective study found that six of 35 patients with a mid-expiratory flow rate (FEF_{25-75}) below 50% of predicted and forced VC (FVC) below 75% of predicted (group A) required prolonged mechanical ventilation, whereas only one of 122 patients with values exceeding these (group B) required such ventilation after several types of surgery (58). Four of the six patients in group A died. The total number of complications also differed significantly. Complications occurred in 12 of 35 patients (34%) in group A versus 15 of 122 patients (12%) in group B. Poe and colleagues prospectively examined 209 patients undergoing elective cholecystectomy and postoperatively identified 21 with atelectasis, eight with purulent bronchitis, and two with pneumonia (67). These 31 patients were hospitalized an average of 1.5 days longer than were the others. Abnormal peak flow and the single-breath O_2 test were significant predictors of postoperative pulmonary complications, whereas reduced FVC was a significant predictor of prolonged hospitalization. Vodinh and colleagues prospectively studied 153 patients undergoing nonurgent vascular surgery (51). In comparing 24 clinical and laboratory factors, they found postoperative respiratory complications were significantly higher only in those with a clinical chest abnormality, recent bronchitis, aortic surgery, longer duration of surgery, low FEV_1/VC, and low Pao_2. They concluded that spirometry and blood gas analysis were helpful in assessing risk. Finally, Carrel and colleagues, in a prospective study of patients undergoing cardiac surgery, also demonstrated that the incidence of postoperative pneumonia was correlated with abnormal results of preoperative lung function studies (17).

It is unlikely that any test can ever clearly distinguish between those who will or will not survive or between those who will or will not have a specific complication. We suggest that spirometry and blood gas analyses should not be performed indiscriminately in everyone undergoing abdominal or thoracic surgery without lung resection. These tests are usually indicated for patients with asthma, chronic obstructive lung disease, chronic cough, sputum production, dyspnea, wheezing, poor exercise tolerance, congestive failure, weakness, or morbid obesity. Zibrak and colleagues suggest that "when a general preoperative evaluation uncovers a history of cigarette smoking or other evidence of uncharacterized lung disease, pulmonary function testing may assist in making a specific pulmonary diagnosis, assessing the degree of impairment, and identifying appropriate preoperative therapy." (68) We agree.

Exercise Testing

A patient's capacity to increase oxygen delivery during exercise, which can be evaluated with a cardiopulmonary exercise test using metabolic, ventilatory, gas exchange, blood pressure, and ECG measures, may correlate with their ability to maintain end-organ perfusion and system function after surgery. The determination of the peak Vo_2 and the Vo_2 at the anaerobic threshold (AT) might prove useful in identifying patients at high risk for cardiopulmonary complications. We recommend considering such testing in the elderly, in patients with significant heart or lung disease, and in patients with marginal function who might be deemed inoperable without such physiologic data supporting their ability to possibly tolerate a surgical stress (69).

Because of the high perioperative mortality in elderly patients undergoing elective colorectal surgery or abdominal surgery for aortic aneurysm repair, Older and colleagues began to use noninvasive cardiopulmonary exercise testing with gas exchange measurements to screen patients over the age of 60 years (70). Forty-four of 187 such patients had ECG tracings during exercise that showed changes attributable to myocardial ischemia. The postoperative in-hospital mortality was 7.5%, with 5.9% owing to cardiovascular causes. Mortality from cardiovascular causes was 18% in the 55 patients with an Vo_2 AT of less than 11 mL/(kg · min) but was only 0.8% in the 132 patients with an AT that was less than 11 mL/(kg · min). The association of an AT of less than 11 mL/(kg · min) and preoperative ischemia resulted in a mortality rate of 42%, whereas those with preoperative ischemia and a higher AT had a mortality rate of only 4%. Their further experience, recently reported (71), found that postoperative cardiac failure, rather than myocardial infarction, was the major cause of death. They now routinely use cardiopulmonary exercise testing to preoperatively screen

patients over age 65 years before elective major abdominal surgery. Patients with an AT less than 11 mL/(kg · min) are referred to cardiologists with a view to angiography and possible myocardial revascularization. Remaining patients with a low AT are admitted for preoperative stabilization and are operated on only if there is no alternative. The use of these policies has measurably reduced mortality for patients over 65 years undergoing major abdominal surgery, as nonsurgical postoperative mortality has fallen to 0.5% (71).

Gerson and colleagues also prospectively evaluated a geriatric population of 177 patients undergoing abdominal and noncardiac thoracic surgery and included supine exercise testing in their multivariate analysis (72). They found that a patient's inability to perform 2 minutes of such exercise and raise the heart rate above 99 beats per minute (bpm) was the best single predictor of cardiac (14%), pulmonary (14%), or combined (22%) complications. There were 10 complications (9%) and one death (1%) in the group of 108 patients who could increase their heart rate to greater than 99 bpm, and 29 complications (42%) and five deaths (7%) in the group of 69 patients who were unable to do so.

At institutions in which formal cardiopulmonary exercise testing is unavailable, some investigators have suggested that an estimate of the patients Vo_2 and cardiopulmonary reserve may be obtained with stair climbing. Pollock had demonstrated a linear relationship between peak Vo_2 and the number of stairs climbed when he collected expired gases from 31 patients with chronic obstructive lung disease climbing stairs (73). Girish and colleagues recently prospectively evaluated stair climbing in 83 patients undergoing thoracic and upper abdominal surgery (74). Eight out of nine patients (89%) who were unable to climb any flights of stairs developed postoperative cardiopulmonary complications, whereas no patient able to climb seven flights of stairs had any postoperative problems. Girish and colleagues also noted that the inability to climb two flights of stairs had a positive predictive value of 82% for the development of postoperative complications. The morbidity associated with the inability to climb stairs could be owing to obesity, underlying pulmonary or cardiovascular disease, or other causes. Thus, simply walking patients preoperatively may be able to give the clinician an insight into the patient's preoperative risk status.

Conclusions

Williams-Russo has commented that "preventing cardiac morbidity may be the best approach to reducing pulmonary morbidity." From the viewpoint of the patient, surgeon, and internist, we may unwisely evaluate the risks for morbidity and death by segregating the causes as "cardiovascular" or "pulmonary," as these systems are so clearly interrelated in real life.

In the individual patient, the risk of operative intervention needs to be weighed against the risk of no other therapies for the patient's disorder. It may be wise to delay a nonemergent

TABLE 6.1. SOME FACTORS ASSOCIATED WITH HIGH SURGICAL MORTALITY[a]

Factor or test	Upper abdominal surgery	Lung resection[b]
Age >70 y	+	+
Abnormal electrocardiogram	+	+
FEV_1 <40% predicted	+	++
FEV_1/VC <40%	++	++
$FEF_{200-1200}$ <2 L/s	++	++
MVV <50% predicted	+	+++
D_LCO <50% predicted	+	++
$Paco_2$	++	+++
Pao_2 <60 mm Hg	+	±
$\dot{V}o_2$max <15 mL/(min · kg)	++	+++

±, possible increase in mortality; +, some increase in mortality; ++, considerable increase in mortality; +++, very high increase in mortality; FEV_1, forced expiratory volume in 1 s; VC, vital capacity; MVV, maximum voluntary ventilation; D_LCO, diffusing capacity of carbon monoxide; Pao_2, arterial blood partial pressure of oxygen; $Paco_2$, arterial blood partial pressure of carbon dioxide; $\dot{V}o_2$, maximum oxygen consumption.
[a]None of these factors or values should be used as absolute contraindications to surgery.
[b]Preoperative quantitative perfusion scans with preoperative FEV_1, MVV, D_LCO, and $\dot{V}o_2$max tests values are helpful in predicting same test values postoperatively after lung resection.

surgical procedure when the likely morbidity and mortality of thoracic or upper abdominal surgery can be reduced by active intervention (e.g., through weight loss, anticoagulation, antibiotic or corticosteroid therapy, or intensive bronchodilator therapy). If such delay significantly decreases the patient's chances for recovery or cure of the primary disorder, then only very brief interventions before a decision regarding surgery are warranted. Table 6.1 gives some broad guidelines suggestive of high morbidity and mortality in thoracic and upper abdominal surgery.

PREOPERATIVE EVALUATION WITHOUT LUNG RESECTION

Summary Statement	Level of Evidence
The preoperative history, including estimates of the patient's daily activity, physical examination, electrocardiograms, cardiopulmonary exercise testing with measurements of anaerobic threshold and peak oxygen uptake, and stair climbing ability are useful in identifying patients at increased operative risk.	Prospective consecutive and cohort series, prospective nonrandomized trials, and a nested case control study
In patients with suspicion of abnormality raised by the history or physical examination, the following other tests are helpful in identifying patients at increase operative risk: chest roentgenograms, spirometry, and arterial blood gas and pH analyses.	Prospective nonrandomized trials and a nested case control study

PREOPERATIVE EVALUATION OF PATIENTS UNDERGOING LUNG RESECTION

Initial Preoperative Assessment

All the evaluations considered for patients in whom lung resection is not planned, including diffusing capacity of carbon monoxide (D_LCO) and lung volume measurements, are useful in the patient being evaluated for lung resection. Lobectomy and pneumonectomy are most commonly performed for malignant conditions. However, a similar assessment is indicated for patients with decreased lung function resulting from inflammatory, traumatic, hereditary, or other disorders that require removal of any lung segments. Preoperative roentgenographic examinations will always be more complete in these patients, and bronchoscopy results may be available. Bronchodilator responsiveness becomes important if ventilatory function is significantly reduced, and D_LCO should always be measured. If maximal inspiratory and expiratory pressures are low, preoperative pulmonary rehabilitation may reduce the incidence of postoperative complications (75).

In the earliest of several retrospective studies, Gaensler and colleagues (76) found that the MVV was an important predictor of survival in patients undergoing lung resection for tuberculosis. If the preoperative MVV was less than 50% of predicted, 50% of the patients died, whereas if the MVV was greater than 50% of predicted, only 1% of the patients died. Boushy and colleagues found that advanced age, severity of dyspnea, high residual volume (RV), low gas transfer per lung volume (D_LCO/Va), reduced FEV_1, and reduced MVV were all significant predictors of high morbidity and mortality (77,78). Confirming the value of the MVV maneuver, Didolkar and colleagues, in a retrospective study of resection for lung cancer, found that mortality from cardiopulmonary complications was much higher in those with an MVV that was less than 60% of predicted (79). There were no postoperative deaths in the nine patients older than 70 years who had a normal ECG and an MVV that was greater than 60% of predicted.

Ferguson and colleagues retrospectively reviewed their results for lung resection in 237 patients (203 with malignancies) (80). They considered 38 different preoperative and operative risk factors and found, by logistic regression analysis, that the D_LCO was the most important predictor of postoperative survival and the sole predictor of pulmonary complications. For D_LCO values that were less than 60%, 61% to 80%, 81% to 100%, and greater than 100% of predicted, postoperative mortality was 25%, 8%, 5%, and 0%, respectively. In addition, pulmonary complications were 45%, 33%, 13%, and 11%, respectively, for these patient groups. A subsequent study in 1999 by this same group reviewed pulmonary complications in 40 patients undergoing lung resection by open thoracotomy (81). Again, they confirmed that patients with a lower percentage of predicted D_LCO, in this study less than 65%, had a higher rate of pulmonary complications compared with those with a normal LCO.

Several investigators have used measures of pulmonary arterial pressure, pulmonary vascular resistance, and right ventricular ejection fraction preoperatively and intraoperatively after pulmonary arterial clamping. Evidence from these studies may indicate the presence or the development of severe pulmonary hypertension from the planned resection that would make it unlikely that the patient would survive the contemplated procedure (82,83). Today, these invasive measures are generally less useful than noninvasive exercise testing and quantitative scans in estimating postoperative morbidity and mortality (69).

Predicting Postoperative Function

When preoperative lung function, as measured by spirometry and D_{LCO}, is significantly impaired or when large portions of lung may be removed surgically, it is useful to attempt to predict postoperative lung function. Bronchospirometry and the lateral position tests, introduced in the 1950s and 1960s, were of some assistance in predicting postoperative function but have now been supplanted by newer techniques (84,85).

Quantitative radioisotopic ventilation and perfusion scans are now commonly and effectively used to predict postoperative FEV_1, D_{LCO}, and peak V_{O_2} (86–91) (Figs. 6.4

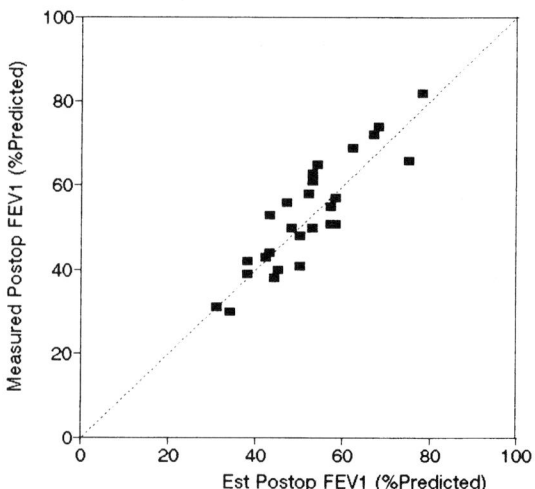

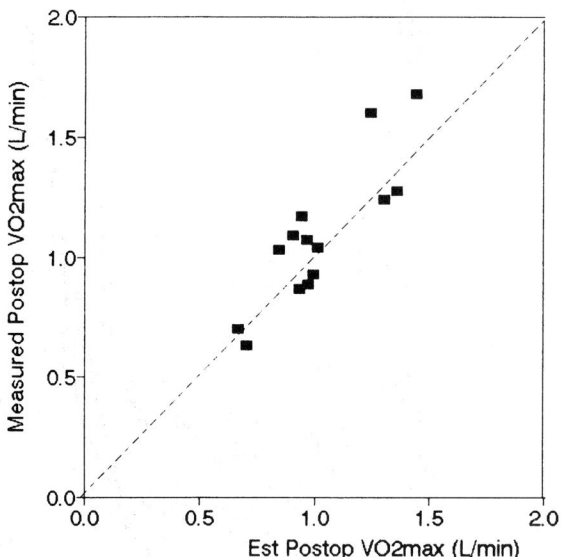

FIGURE 6.4. Comparison of measured postoperative forced expiratory volume in 1 second (FEV_1) and estimated postoperative FEV_1 in 28 patients undergoing pneumonectomy. Estimated postoperative FEV_1 was calculated from preoperative FEV_1 and quantitative technetium ^{99m}Tc perfusion scans. (Modified from Corris PA, Ellis DA, Hawkins T, et al. Use of radionuclide scanning in the preoperative estimation of pulmonary function after pneumonectomy. *Thorax* 1987;42:285–291, with permission.)

FIGURE 6.5. Comparison of measured postoperative maximum oxygen consumption ($V_{O_2}max$) and estimated postoperative $V_{O_2}max$ in 14 patients undergoing pneumonectomy. Estimated postoperative $V_{O_2}max$. was calculated from preoperative $V_{O_2}max$ and quantitative ^{99m}Tc perfusion scans. (Modified with permission from Corris PA, Ellis DA, Hawkins T, et al. Use of radionuclide scanning in the preoperative estimation of pulmonary function after pneumonectomy. *Thorax* 1987;42:285–291, with permission.)

and 6.5). In each case, the predicted postoperative FEV_1, D_{LCO}, or peak V_{O_2} is calculated by multiplying each preoperative value by the measured ratio of expected postoperative lung activity to preoperative total lung activity. For example, if 40% of the quantitatively measured perfusion scan activity occurs in the lung that is to be resected, the calculated postoperative D_{LCO} or peak V_{O_2} will be 60% of the preoperative D_{LCO} or peak V_{O_2}, respectively. Ventilation scans or quantitative computed tomography (CT) can be also used to predict postoperative FEV_1 values (92,93). Similarly, another calculation is based on the preoperative FEV_1 and the amount of lung parenchyma that is expected to be resected. One can then use the assumption that each lung segment constitutes approximately 5.2% of the total lung parenchyma and multiply this by the preoperative FEV_1 to estimate the amount of potential lung function to be lost from the proposed procedure. These types of calculations tends to underestimate the amount of total postoperative lung function, owing to the actual size and function of the segments removed (94).

Markos and colleagues prospectively studied lung function tests and scintigraphy in 55 consecutive candidates for lung cancer resection (95). Fifty-three underwent thoracotomy, with pneumonectomy in 18, lobectomy in 29, and no resection in six. Postoperative FEV_1 and D_{LCO} were well predicted from preoperative measures. There were only three deaths, with all deaths occurring in candidates who had a predicted postoperative FEV_1 of 40% or less. This same year Wahi and colleagues reviewed 197 consecutive cancer patients undergoing pneumonectomy (96). Of the 14 perioperative deaths, 13 occurred in patients undergoing right pneumonectomy, suggesting that loss of the larger lung may be detrimental to patients with borderline lung function. Those patients with a predicted postoperative FEV_1 exceeding 1.65 L had a lower overall mortality rate in this study.

Pierce and colleagues found that the predicted postoperative product, which is the predicted postoperative FEV_1 multiplied by the predicted postoperative D_{LCO}, was the best predictor of surgical mortality in 54 consecutive patients with bronchogenic carcinoma (97). The mean values of their population were as follows: age, 67; FEV_1, 76% of predicted; D_{LCO}, 85% of predicted; and peak V_{O_2}, 18.4 mL/(min · kg). Pneumonectomy was performed in 11, lobectomy in 29, and lesser resection in 14. There were 48 total survivors. Although peak V_{O_2} values did not predict outcome, two of the three patients with peak V_{O_2} values that were less than 14 mL/(min · kg) died in the perioperative period.

Exercise Testing

Recent evidence-based articles suggest that exercise testing with the assessment of the patient's peak V_{O_2} be obtained in all patients believed to be at high risk for lung resection on the basis of the predicted postoperative lung function studies (94). This recommendation is based on a number of studies supporting the importance of this data in determining a patient's postoperative risk. Two earlier studies demonstrated the value of preoperative exercise testing in patients undergoing lung resection. Eugene and colleagues found that among 19 patients, death occurred in three of four patients with a peak V_{O_2} of less than 1 L/min (98). In 22 patients, Smith and colleagues found no deaths and 10% morbidity if peak V_{O_2} exceeded 20 mL/(min · kg), 17% deaths and 67% morbidity with peak V_{O_2} of 15 to 20 mL/(min · kg), and 17% deaths and 100% morbidity if peak V_{O_2} was less than 15 mL/(min · kg) (99).

Bechard and Wetstein prospectively evaluated 50 consecutive patients undergoing lung resection with the surgeon blinded to the preoperative peak V_{O_2} values (100). Candidates for resection were required to have an FEV_1 of >1.7 L for pneumonectomy (10 patients), 1.2 L for lobectomy (28 patients), or 0.9 L for wedge resection (12 patients). Overall mortality was 4%, whereas morbidity was 12%. Both peak V_{O_2} and AT measures predicted mortality and morbidity, whereas age, FVC, FEV_1, and MVV did not. Morice and colleagues found eight of 37 high-risk patients who were considered inoperable based on preoperative or predicted postoperative FEV_1 less than 40% or greater than 33%, respectively, or a $Paco_2$ exceeding 45 mm Hg, had a peak V_{O_2} of greater than 15 mL/(min · kg) (101). These patients were subsequently offered surgical resection, and all eight survived.

Walsh and colleagues prospectively evaluated 66 patients with potentially resectable non–small cell lung cancer. These patients were considered to be high-risk candidates based on a preoperative FEV_1 that was less than 40% of predicted, postoperative FEV_1 that was less than 33% of predicted, resting $Paco_2$ exceeding 45 mm Hg, or at least two criteria indicating cardiac disease (102). In 20 patients with a peak V_{O_2} of greater than 15 mL/(min · kg), there were no perioperative deaths and 40% complications. Among five patients with a peak V_{O_2} of less than 15 mL/(min · kg), there was one death. In this population, only surgical versus medical treatment and peak V_{O_2} greater than 15 mL/(min · kg) significantly predicted survival, whereas age, FEV_1, $Paco_2$, clinical stage, and TNM status did not. In another series of 25 high-risk patients undergoing lung resection (103), lower preoperative or predicted postoperative peak V_{O_2} values correlated with higher morbidity and mortality. Girish and colleagues recently evaluated the ability of stair climbing to predict postoperative cardiopulmonary complications (74) in 40 patients undergoing lung resection, including three total pneumonectomies. In the end, this group found that the patients who were unable to climb any stairs had the greatest complication rate of 89%. They concluded that simple stair climbing could be used to assess a patient's risk of postoperative complications. The climbing of two flights of stairs was established as an important level of exertion to achieve in this study. Patients who could climb more than two flights of stairs are considered at an acceptable risk level for postoperative complications according to these investigators.

Conclusions

Physicians and surgeons are obligated to share information and expectations with patients before making final decisions regarding therapy. Assigning an exact risk to a major surgical procedure in the individual cancer patient can be difficult. Multiple high-risk factors and common sense, however, can dictate against surgical intervention in some cases. Debility and cardiovascular disease always add to this risk assessment. Smoking cessation, vigorous bronchodilator therapy, and rehabilitating exercise therapy instituted preoperatively may help reduce this risk and may make borderline candidates more acceptable for surgical resection of lung parenchyma. In high-risk patients, measures of D_{LCO}, quantitative perfusion-scan, and gas exchange exercise testing are all clearly useful in assessing risk. Because of differences in patient sex, size, and age, both absolute and percentage of predicted values should be considered in making final recommendations. As Bollinger demonstrated in his small study, even patients who are deemed inoperable based on initial lung function assessments can undergo and survive lung resection surgery when their peak V_{O_2} and predicted postoperative V_{O_2} are above an acceptable range (usually >15 mL/[kg · min]) (103).

PREOPERATIVE EVALUATION WITH LUNG RESECTION

Summary Statements	Level of Evidence
In addition to the evaluations identified in the prior table, the following additional tests are useful in identifying perioperative risk and later meaningful physical activity in patients undergoing lung resection: volume of lung to be resected, gas transfer index or diffusing capacity, residual lung volume, maximum voluntary ventilation, and isotopic ventilation and perfusion scans.	Prospective nonrandomized trials, a prospective blinded trial, and retrospective case reviews
Peak oxygen uptake values of <1 L/min or 15 mL/kg are associated with high postresectional morbidity and mortality.	Prospective nonrandomized trials and retrospective case reviews

REDUCTION IN COMPLICATIONS

Preoperative Considerations

The more severe the risk of complications, the more important it is to take effective action during the preoperative period. A number of issues may be identified during the preoperative assessment that will lead to management strategies aimed at decreasing the individual's postoperative complication risk. To demonstrate this, Stein and Cassara compared three groups of patients undergoing abdominal and thoracic surgery: those considered to be of normal risk (group 1); those considered, on the basis of pulmonary function tests, to be high-risk and who were not treated (group 2); and those considered to be high risk and who were treated intensively preoperatively with smoking cessation, bronchodilator drugs, inhalation of humidified gases, chest physiotherapy, and antibiotics when indicated (group 3) (104). Postoperative pulmonary complications occurred in one of 17 patients in group 1, 14 of 20 patients in group 2, and five of 22 patients in group 3. Thus, patients at higher risk had a significantly better outcome when treated aggressively preoperatively.

Smoking Cessation

Patients should stop smoking as soon as it is realized that surgery is likely, even if the patient has normal findings on pulmonary function tests. Cessation for even a few days may be advantageous, as benefits include an expected reduction in cough, improvement in ciliary function and mouth hygiene, reduction in lower airway pathogens, and reduction in carboxyhemoglobin levels. Warner and colleagues, in a blinded prospective study of patients undergoing coronary bypass surgery, found that postoperative pulmonary complications developed in approximately one third of current smokers. Patients who had quit for less than 2 months had complication rates four times that of those who had stopped for more than 2 months. Additionally, patients who had stopped smoking for more than 6 months had complication rates approaching rates of the nonsmoking population (105). This study raised concerns that smoking cessation for less than 8 weeks was associated with a higher risk of complications compared with the risk of the currently smoking population. It has been postulated that the increased complication rate in those patients who had recently quit smoking may be related to nicotine withdrawal and increased mucous secretion in the immediate postcessation period (106). Several investigators have followed up on this study to try to better evaluate this issue. Bluman and colleagues performed a prospective cohort study and found that current smokers, as well as smokers that had decreased their tobacco consumption within 1 month of surgery, had an increased risk of postoperative pulmonary complications compared with that of nonsmokers (107). Nakagawa and colleagues then reviewed 288 consecutive patients undergoing lung resection surgeries and found that at least 4 weeks of abstinence from tobacco use was necessary to reduce the incidence of postoperative pulmonary complications (108).

Weight Reduction

In the obese patient, weight reduction is advisable if surgery can be delayed, especially if the procedure involves the thorax or upper abdomen. In those with hypoventilation and CO_2 retention, a weight loss of 10 to 20 kg may lead to improvement in gas exchange (109). Although weight loss is advocated, it is important to maintain adequate caloric and fluid intake perioperatively.

Treatment of Underlying Lung Disease

Intensive bronchodilator therapy and steroids should be used in symptomatic COPD and asthmatic patients to prevent bronchospasm and to treat any reversible component of airway disease (110). There is little evidence to support the routine use of antibiotics prophylaxis, but suspected pulmonary infections should be investigated, diagnosed, and treated for several days preoperatively if feasible.

Lung Expansion Techniques

Several studies demonstrate that preoperative training in deep breathing respiratory maneuvers reduces postoperative complications and is cost-effective in patients who undergo thoracic or upper abdominal surgery. The modalities most extensively studied have included deep breathing exercises, intermittent positive pressure breathing treatments, and incentive spirometry. Bartlett and colleagues emphasized that frequent inspiratory rather than expiratory maneuvers were essential (111). In a prospective study of 343 cholecystectomy patients, Thoren found roentgenographic atelectasis in 12% of those who performed preoperative and postoperative breathing exercise, 27% of those who performed postoperative breathing exercise only, and 42% of the control group without any exercise (112). In patients undergoing abdominal surgery, Celli and colleagues found that clinical complications and duration of hospital stay were much diminished in patients who had respiratory treatment started 1 day before surgery and continued postoperatively (113). Roukema and colleagues prospectively randomized patients with noncompromised pulmonary status undergoing abdominal surgery into two groups (114). Group 1 consisted of 84 patients with no breathing exercises, whereas group 2 consisted of 69 patients treated with preoperative and postoperative exercises. Pulmonary complications occurred in 60% of group 1 versus 19% of group 2.

Deep Venous Thrombosis Prophylaxis

The prevention of DVTs by pharmacologic or physical methods is cost-effective and life-saving and should be used whenever possible in patients with high-to-moderate risk for thromboembolism. There are a number of options for prophylaxis, depending on the surgical procedure performed and the patient's risk classification for a thromboembolic event. Currently used methods include low-dose unfractionated heparin at 5,000 U subcutaneously every 8 to 12 hours, starting 1 to 2 hours before the operation and continued postoperatively; adjusted dose heparin dosed every 8 hours, with a goal of midinterval activated partial thromboplastin time in the high-normal range; low-molecular-weight heparin (dose and interval depends on the surgical intervention and the agents used); and oral anticoagulants such as warfarin started at a dose of 5 to 10 mg given the day of or the day after surgery and continued postoperatively, with a target prothrombin international normalized ratio in the 2.5 range. Alternatively, prophylaxis can consist of mechanical means to reduce venous stasis using either intermittent pneumatic leg compression or graduated compression stockings. The 2001 ACCP Consensus Conference guidelines can help guide the selection of prophylaxis based on the patient's profile and planned surgical intervention (25).

Management of other Disease States

In patients at risk of aspiration, including obese patients, a course of antacid therapy preoperatively may be beneficial. A study by Taylor and colleagues demonstrated that this intervention tended to minimize the expected pulmonary complications (115).

Cardiovascular disease should be treated aggressively to minimize pulmonary edema, congestive failure, myocardial ischemia, arrhythmias, and significant systemic or pulmonary hypertension.

Intraoperative Considerations

To the best of our knowledge, there is no evidence that the route or type of anesthetic used affects the likelihood of postoperative pulmonary complications. Usually the anesthesiologist, on the basis of skill, training, and experience, selects the most appropriate agents and route for the specific problem at hand. There is no clear evidence that spinal anesthesia is superior to general anesthesia in maintaining intraoperative and postoperative oxygenation, even in patients with severe obstructive lung disease (55,56). It has been proposed that control of the airways may be better with general anesthesia. Among other things, the anesthesiologist attempts to maintain adequate cardiac output, oxygenation, CO_2 removal, and stable fluid and acid-base status, while attempting to minimize arrhythmias, pooling of blood in extremities, microatelectasis, macroatelectasis, and aspiration of oral and gastric contents into the lung.

During laparoscopic cholecystectomy in which CO_2 is used for insufflation, a significant respiratory acidosis may develop in patients with cardiac or pulmonary disease who are not capable of exhaling this added gaseous burden (22). In this clinical situation, $Paco_2$ and pH should be monitored because end-tidal CO_2 pressures may be misleading during such insufflation,

Postoperative Considerations

Gas Exchange

Ventilatory support after recovery from anesthesia may be brief or prolonged. Continuous positive airway pressure (CPAP) or PEEP is usually helpful in improving oxygenation and CO_2 removal by decreasing atelectasis, improving ventilation/perfusion matching, and reducing barotrauma to the lung. Hypoxemia can be reduced and ventilation of the lung bases improved by keeping the patient, especially if obese, in a sitting or semirecumbent position rather than in a supine position (116) (Fig. 6.6).

Lung Expansion Techniques

Aggressive respiratory therapy to minimize atelectasis, increase FRC, improve oxygenation, and clear secretions is valuable and cost-effective. Previously, expiratory resistance and intermittent positive-pressure breathing were used frequently, but these techniques have generally been discarded because of ineffectiveness, high cost, or barotrauma (113,117,118). Bronchodilator aerosol therapy alone is

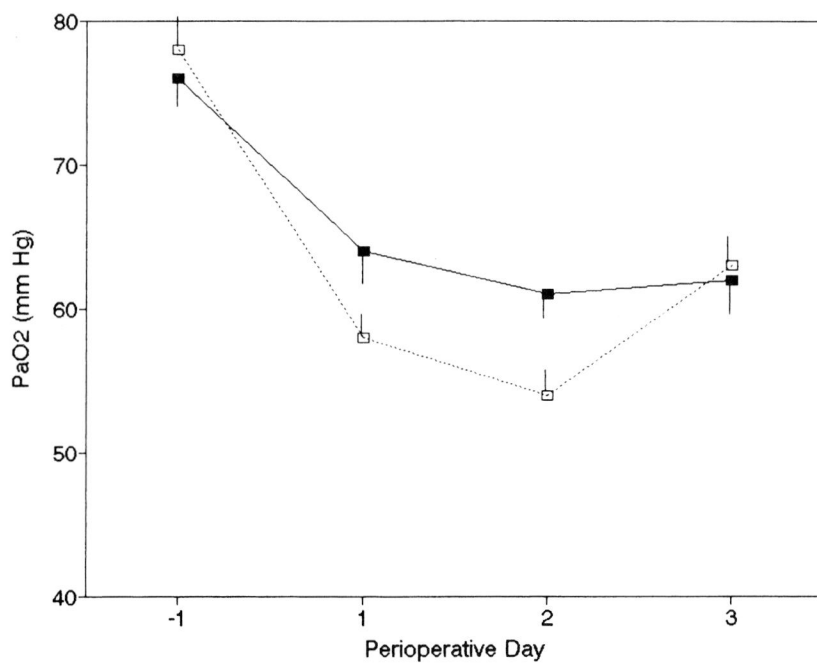

FIGURE 6.6. Effect of body position on arterial blood partial pressure of oxygen after abdominal surgery in 22 markedly obese patients. *Solid symbols* and *solid line* indicate semirecumbent position; *hollow symbols* and *dotted line* indicate supine position. (Modified from Vaughan RW, Wise L. Postoperative arterial blood gas measurements in obese patients: effects of position on gas exchange. *Ann Surg* 1975; 182:705–709, with permission.)

insufficient to improve lung volumes and oxygenation maximally after thoracic or upper abdominal surgery. There are many reports that compare the effectiveness of the following currently recommended modalities: coughing and deep breathing exercises, sustained maximal inspiration or incentive spirometry using one of several available devices, breathing with inspiratory resistance, and CPAP or PEEP by face mask (113,118–120,122). The major disadvantages of coughing and deep breathing, incentive spirometry, and inspiratory resistance are the necessity for patient cooperation and the likely attendant increase in incisional pain. PEEP or CPAP may be more costly and slightly increase the possibility of barotrauma or aspiration, but they hasten improvement in FRC and Pao₂ postoperatively in patients in whom atelectasis tends to develop. These modalities may be detrimental to patients with severe emphysema who are already hyperinflated because of highly compliant lung units.

Pain Control

Nearly all investigators stress the necessity for frequent and vigilant respiratory care in the high-risk population. Because of postoperative pain, analgesics may be necessary to improve coughing and deep breathing. With severe thoracic or abdominal pain, selective and repeated nerve blocks may help the patient's performance of ventilatory maneuvers. In addition to controlling pain, regional analgesic techniques may also help optimize postoperative pulmonary function by decreasing the reflex inhibition of respiratory muscles if the afferent reflex limb is targeted (46).

Aspiration Precautions

It is important to reduce the likelihood of aspiration with optimal endotracheal tube and cuff care, as well as with good technique when giving nutritional support. If a nasogastric tube is necessary, it should be of the smallest caliber possible. Finally, overdistention of the stomach should be avoided.

Deep Venous Thrombosis Prophylaxis

Secondary prophylaxis for thromboembolism is more costly than primary prophylaxis but is still cost-effective and life-preserving. It consists of screening high-risk patients postoperatively with tests specific for venous thromboses (e.g., fibrinogen uptake, Doppler ultrasonography, impedance plethysmography, and venography), followed by full-dose anticoagulant therapy when test results are positive. Secondary prophylaxis should be used when prophylactic anticoagulation is desired but contraindicated (e.g., urgency of surgery, neurosurgery, spinal anesthesia) or when supplementation of primary prophylaxis is required in very high-risk patients.

Conclusions

The perioperative period offers a number of opportunities to reduce the risk of postoperative pulmonary complications. In the preoperative period, smoking cessation, weight loss, and training in lung expansion techniques can be important. Postoperatively, adequate pain control, aspiration precautions, and DVT prophylaxis may decrease morbidity and mortality. These practices are especially important in patients with limited pulmonary and cardiovascular functional reserves.

REDUCTION OF COMPLICATIONS

Summary Statement	Level of Evidence
Postoperative complications are less likely to occur in those patients who have stopped smoking for at least 4 to 8 wk before surgery.	Prospective nonrandomized trials, prospective and retrospective cohort studies, and retrospective case reviews
In patients undergoing thoracic and upper abdominal surgery, pain control and the preoperative and postoperative use of breathing exercises that emphasize inspiratory maneuvers reduce the incidence of postoperative pulmonary complications.	Prospective randomized controlled trials and prospective nonrandomized trials.
In surgical patients at moderate-to-high risk for thromboembolism, the use of pharmacologic and physical methods to reduce deep venous thrombosis is cost-effective and life-saving.	Prospective and retrospective trials and expert consensus panel opinion.

REFERENCES

1. Lawrence VA, Hilsenbeck SG, Mulrow CD, et al. Incidence and hospital stay for cardiac and pulmonary complications after abdominal surgery. *J Gen Int Med* 1995;10:671–678.
2. Brooks-Brunn JA. Predictors of postoperative pulmonary complications following abdominal surgery. *Chest* 1997;111:564–571.
3. Bryant LR, Preston D, Houck G, et al. Lung perfusion scanning for estimation of postoperative pulmonary function. *Arch Surg* 1972;104:52–55.
4. Rehder K, Sessler AD, Marsh HM. General anesthesia and the lung. *Am Rev Respir Dis* 1975;112:541–563.
5. Ford GT, Whitelaw WA, Rosenal TW, et al. Diaphragm function after upper abdominal surgery in humans. *Am Rev Respir Dis* 1983;127:431–436.
6. Tokics L, Hedenstierna G, Strandberg A, et al. Lung collapse and gas exchange during anesthesia: effects of spontaneous breathing, muscle paralysis, and positive end-expiratory pressure. *Anesthesiology* 1987;66:157–167.
7. Meyers JR, Leembeck L, O'Kane H, et al. Changes in functional residual capacity of the lung after operation. *Arch Surg* 1975;110:576–583.
8. Reeve EB, Nanson EM, Rundle FF. Observations on inhibitory reflexes during abdominal surgery. *Clin Sci* 1951;10:65–87.
9. Anjou-Lindskog E, Broman L, Broman M, et al. Effects of intravenous anesthesia on V_A/Q distribution. *Anesthesiology* 1985;62:485–492.
10. Sun XG, Hansen JE, Oudiz RJ, et al. Gas exchange detection of exercise-induced right-to-left shunt in patients with primary pulmonary hypertension. *Circulation* 2002;54–60.
11. Gamsu G, Singer MM, Vincent HH, et al. Postoperative impairment of mucous transport in the lung. *Am Rev Respir Dis* 1976;114:673–679.
12. Warner DO. Preventing postoperative pulmonary complications: the role of the anesthesiologist. *Anesthesiology* 2000;92:1467–1472.
13. Bolton JWR, Weiman DS. Physiology of lung resection. *Clin Chest Med* 1993;14:293–303.
14. Bartlett JG, Gorbach SL. The triple threat of aspiration pneumonia. *Chest* 1975;68:560–566.
15. Little JW. Pulmonary aspiration: medical staff conference, University of California, San Francisco. *West J Med* 1979;131:122–129.
16. Ruggera G, Taylor G. Pulmonary aspiration in anesthesia. *West J Med* 1976;125:411–414.
17. Carrel T, Schmid ER, von Segesser L, et al. Preoperative assessment of the likelihood of infection of the lower respiratory tract after cardiac surgery. *Thorac Cardiovasc Surg* 1991;39:85–88.
18. Hotchkiss RS. Perioperative management of patient with chronic obstructive pulmonary disease. *Int Anesthesiol Clin* 1988;26:134–142.
19. Kroenke K, Lawrence VA, Theroux JF, et al. Operative risk in patients with severe obstructive pulmonary disease. *Arch Intern Med* 1992;152:967–971.
20. Samuels LE, Kaufman MS, Morris RJ, et al. Coronary artery bypass grafting in patients with COPD. *Chest* 1998;113:878–882.
21. Maeda H, Nakahara K, Ohno K, et al. Diaphragm function after pulmonary resection: relationship to postoperative respiratory failure. *Am Rev Respir Dis* 1988;137:678–681.
22. Wittgen CM, Andrus CH, Fitzgerald SP, et al. Analysis of the hemodynamic and ventilatory effects of laparoscopic cholecystectomy. *Arch Surg* 1991;126:997–1001.
23. Selecky PA, Wasserman K, Klein M, et al. A graphic approach to assessing interrelationships among minute ventilation, arterial carbon dioxide tension, and ratio of physiologic dead space to tidal volume in patients on respirators. *Am Rev Respir Dis* 1978;117:181–184.
24. Black MD, French GJ, Rasuli P, et al. Upper extremity deep venous thrombosis. Underdiagnosed and potentially lethal. *Chest* 1993;103;1887–1890.
25. Geerts WH, Heit JA, Clagett, et al. Prevention of venous thromboembolism. *Chest* 2001;119:132S–175S.
26. Wheeler HB, Anderson FA. Prophylaxis against venous thromboembolism in surgical patients. *Am J Surg* 1991;161:507–540.
27. Sorbini CA, Grassi V, Solenas E, et al. Arterial oxygen tension in relation to age in healthy subjects. *Respiration* 1968;25:3–13.
28. Kitamura H, Sawa T, Ikezono E. Postoperative hypoxemia: the contribution of age to the maldistribution of ventilation. *Anesthesiology* 1972;36:244–252.
29. Hall JC, Tarala RA, Hall JL, et al. A multivariate analysis of the risk of pulmonary complications after laparotomy. *Chest* 1991;99:923–927.
30. Kroenke K, Lawrence VA, Theroux JF, et al. Postoperative complications after thoracic and major abdominal surgery in patients with and without obstructive lung disease. *Chest* 1993;104:1445–1451.
31. Latimer RG, Dickman M, Day WC, et al. Ventilatory patterns and pulmonary complications after upper abdominal surgery determined by preoperative and postoperative computerized spirometry and blood gas analysis. *Am J Surg* 1971;122:622–632.
32. Moulton MJ, Creswell LL, Mackey ME, et al. Obesity is not a risk factor for significant adverse outcomes after cardiac surgery. *Circulation* 1996;94[Suppl II]:II-87–II-92.
33. Dales RE, Dionne G, Leech JA, et al. Preoperative prediction

of pulmonary complications following thoracic surgery. *Chest* 1993;104:155–159.

34. Vaughan RW, Engelhardt RC, Wise L. Postoperative hypoxemia in obese patients. *Ann Surg* 1974;180:877–882.

35. Ray CS, Sue DY, Bray G, et al. Effects of obesity on respiratory function. *Am Rev Respir Dis* 1983;128:501–506.

36. Vaughan RW, Bauer S, Wise L. Volume and pH of gastric juice in obese patients. *Anesthesiology* 1975;43:686–689.

37. Wightman JAK. A prospective survey of the incidence of postoperative pulmonary complications. *Br J Surg* 1968;55–85.

38. Laszlo G, Archer GG, Darrell JH, et al. The diagnosis and prophylaxis of pulmonary complications of surgical operation. *Br J Surg* 1973;60:129–134.

39. Kotani N, Hashimoto H, Sessler DI, et al. Smoking decreases alveolar macrophage function during anesthesia and surgery. *Anesthesiology* 2000;92:1268–1277.

40. Miller WR, Wu N, Johnson RL Jr. Convenient method of evaluating pulmonary function with a single breath test. *Anesthesiology* 1956;17:480–493.

41. Hodgkin JE. Evaluation before thoracotomy. *West J Med* 1975;122:104–109.

42. Meneely GR, Ferguson JL. Pulmonary evaluation and risk in patient preparation for anesthesia and surgery. *JAMA* 1960;175:1074–1080.

43. Stein M, Koota GM, Simon M, et al. Pulmonary evaluation of surgical patients. *JAMA* 1962;181:765–770.

44. Kearney DJ, Lee TH, Reilly JJ, et al. Assessment of operative risk in patients undergoing lung resection: importance of predicted pulmonary function. *Chest* 1994;105:753–759.

45. Lawrence VA, Dhanda R, Hilsenbeck SG, et al. Risk of pulmonary complications after elective abdominal surgery. *Chest* 1996;220:744–750.

46. Warner DO. Preventing postoperative pulmonary complications: the role of the anesthesiologist. *Anesthesiology* 2000;92:1467–1472.

47. Warner DO, Warner MA, Barnes RD, et al. Perioperative respiratory complications in patients with asthma. *Anesthesiology* 1996;85:460–467.

48. Goldman, L. Cardiac risks and complications of noncardiac surgery. *Ann Intern Med* 1983;98:504–513.

49. Epstein SK, Faling LJ, Daly BDT, et al. Predicting complications after pulmonary resection: preoperative exercise testing vs a multifactorial cardiopulmonary risk index. *Chest* 1993;104:694–700.

50. Arozullah AM, Khuri SF, Henderson WG, et al. Development and validation of a multifactorial risk index for predicting postoperative pneumonia after major noncardiac surgery. *Ann Intern Med* 2001;135:847–857.

51. Vodinh J, Bonnet F, Touboul C, et al. Risk factors of postoperative pulmonary complications after vascular surgery. *Surgery* 1988;105:360–365.

52. Vaughan RW, Wise L. Choice of abdominal operative incision in the obese patient: a study using blood gas measurements. *Ann Surg* 1975;181:829–835.

53. Jackson CV. Preoperative pulmonary evaluation. *Arch Int Med* 1988;148:2120–2127.

54. Sykes LA, Bowe EA. Cardiorespiratory effects of anesthesia. *Clin Chest Med* 1993;14:211–226.

55. Boutros AR, Weisel M. Comparison of effects of three anesthetic techniques on patients with severe pulmonary obstructive disease. *Can Anaesth Soc J* 1971;18:286–292.

56. Ravin MB. Comparison of spinal and general anesthesia for lower abdominal surgery in patients with chronic obstructive pulmonary disease. *Anesthesiology* 1975;35:319–322.

57. Pedersen T, Viby-Morgensen J, Ringsted C. Anesthetic prac-

tice and postoperative pulmonary complications. *Acta Anesthesiol Scand* 1992;36:812–818.

58. Gracey DR, Diverite MB, Didier EP. Preoperative pulmonary preparation of patients with chronic obstructive pulmonary disease. *Chest* 1979;76:123–129.

59. Tape TG, Mushlin AI. The utility of routine chest radiographs. *Ann Intern Med* 1986;104:663–670.

60. Archer C, Levy AR, McGregor M. Value of routine preoperative chest x-rays: a meta-analysis. *Can J Anaesth* 1993;40:1022–1027.

61. Munro J, Booth A, Nicholl J. Routine preoperative testing: a systematic review of the evidence. *Health Technol Assess* 1997;1:1–62.

62. Flancbaum L, Choban PS. Surgical implications of obesity. *Annu Rev Med* 1998;49:215–234.

63. Tisi GM. Preoperative evaluation of pulmonary function. *Am Rev Respir Dis* 1979;119:293–310.

64. Zibrak JD, O'Donnell CR, Marton K. Indications for pulmonary function testing. *Ann Intern Med* 1990;112:763–771.

65. Lawrence VA, Page CP, Harris GD. Preoperative spirometry before abdominal operations: a critical appraisal of its predictive value. *Arch Intern Med* 1989;149:280–285.

66. American College of Physicians. Preoperative pulmonary function testing. *Ann Intern Med* 1990;112:793–794.

67. Poe RH, Kallay MC, Dass T, et al. Can postoperative complications after elective cholecystectomy be predicted? *Am J Med Sci* 1988;5:29–34.

68. Zibrak JD, O'Donnell CR. Indications for preoperative pulmonary function testing. *Clin Chest Med* 1993;14:227–236.

69. Wasserman K, Hansen JE, Sue DY, et al. Clinical applications of cardiopulmonary exercise testing. *Principles of exercise testing and interpretation.* Maryland: Lippincott Williams & Wilkins, 1999:196–198.

70. Older PO, Smith RER, Courtney PG, et al. Preoperative evaluation of cardiac failure and ischemia in elderly patients by cardiopulmonary exercise testing. *Chest* 1993;104:701–704.

71. Older P, Hall A. Preoperative assessment of elderly surgical patients. In: Wasserman K, ed. *Cardiopulmonary exercise testing and cardiovascular health.* Armonk, NY, 2002,119–133.

72. Gerson MC, Hurst JM, Hertzberg VS, et al. Prediction of cardiac and pulmonary complications related to elective abdominal and noncardiac thoracic surgery in geriatric patients. *Am J Med* 1990;88:101–107.

73. Pollock M, Roa J, Benditt J, et al. Estimation of ventilatory reserve by stair climbing: a study in patients with chronic airflow obstruction. *Chest* 1993;104:1378–1383.

74. Girish M, Trayner E, Dammann O, et al. Symptom-limited stair climbing as a predictor of postoperative cardiopulmonary complications after high-risk surgery. *Chest* 2001;120:1147–1151.

75. Chumillas S, Ponce JL, Delgado F, et al. Prevention of postoperative pulmonary complications through respiratory rehabilitation: a controlled clinical study. *Arch Phys Med Rehabil* 1998;79:5–9.

76. Gaensler EA, Cugell DW, Lindgren I, et al. The role of pulmonary insufficiency in mortality and invalidism following surgery for pulmonary tuberculosis. *J Thorac Surg* 1955;29:163–187.

77. Boushy SF, Helgason AH, Billig DM, et al. Clinical, physiologic, and morphologic examination of the lung in patients with bronchogenic carcinoma and the relation to postoperative deaths. *Am Rev Respir Dis* 1970;101:685–695.

78. Boushy SF, Billig DM, North LB, et al. Clinical course related to preoperative and postoperative pulmonary function in patients with bronchogenic carcinoma. *Chest* 1971;59:383–391.

79. Didolkar MS, Moore RH, Takita H. Evaluation of the risk in pulmonary resection for bronchogenic carcinoma. *Am J Surg* 1974;127:700–703.

80. Ferguson MK, Little L, Rizzo L, et al. Diffusing capacity predicts morbidity and mortality after pulmonary resection. *J Thorac Cardiovasc Surg* 1988;96:894–900.

81. Wang J, Olak J, Ultmann RE, et al. Assessment of pulmonary complications after lung resection. *Ann Thorac Surg* 1999;67:1444–1447.

82. Olsen GN, Block AJ, Swenson EW, et al. Pulmonary function evaluation of the lung resection candidate: A prospective study. *Am Rev Respir Dis* 1975;111:379–386.

83. Olsen GN. Lung cancer resection: who's inoperable? *Chest* 1995;108:298–299.

84. Snider GL, Shaw AR. A critical evaluation of bronchospirometric measurement in predicting loss of ventilatory function due to thoracic surgery. *J Lab Clin Med* 1964;64:321–329.

85. Bergen F. A simple method for determination of the relative function of the right and left lung. *Acta Chir Scand Suppl* 1960;253:58–63.

86. Corris PA, Ellis DA, Hawkins T, et al. Use of radionuclide scanning in the preoperative estimation of pulmonary function after pneumonectomy. *Thorax* 1987;42:285–291.

87. Ali MK, Mountain CF, Ewer MS, et al. Predicting loss of pulmonary function after pulmonary resection for bronchogenic carcinoma. *Chest* 1980;77:337–342.

88. Boysen PG, Harris JO, Block AJ, et al. Prospective evaluation for pneumonectomy using perfusion scanning: follow-up beyond one year. *Chest* 1981;80:163–166.

89. Juhl B, Frost N. A comparison between measured and calculated changes in the lung function after operation for pulmonary cancer. *Acta Anesthesiol Scand Suppl* 1975;57:39–45.

90. Kristersson S, Lindell SE, Svanberg L. Prediction of pulmonary function loss due to pneumonectomy using ^{133}Xe-radiospirometry. *Chest* 1972;62:694–698.

91. Kristersson S, Arborelius M, Jungquist G, et al. Prediction of ventilatory capacity after lobectomy. *Scan J Respir Dis* 1973;54:315–325.

92. Wu MT, Chang JM, Chiang AA, et al. Use of quantitative CT to predict postoperative lung function in patients with lung cancer. *Radiology* 1994;191:257–262.

93. Zeiher BG, Gross TJ, Kern JA, et al. Predicting postoperative pulmonary function in patients undergoing lung resection. *Chest* 1995;108:68–72.

94. Reilly JJ. Evidence-based preoperative evaluation of candidates for thoracotomy. *Chest* 1999;116:474S–476S.

95. Markos J, Mullan B, Hillman D, et al. Preoperative assessment as a predictor of mortality and morbidity after lung resection. *Am Rev Respir Dis* 1989;139:902–910.

96. Wahi R, McMurtrey MJ, DeCaro LF, et al. Determinants of perioperative morbidity and mortality after pneumonectomy. *Ann Thorac Surg* 1989;48:33–37.

97. Pierce RJ, Copland JM, Sharpe K, et al. Preoperative risk evaluation for lung cancer resection: predicted postoperative product as a predictor of surgical mortality. *Am J Respir Crit Care Med* 1994;150:947–955.

98. Eugene J, Brown S, Light R, et al. Maximum oxygen consumption: a physiology guide to pulmonary resection. *Surg Forum* 1982;33:260–262.

99. Smith TP, Kinasewitz GT, Tucker WY, et al. Exercise capacity as a predictor of post-thoracotomy morbidity. *Am Rev Respir Dis* 1984;129:730–734.

100. Bechard D, Wetstein L. Assessment of exercise oxygen consumption as preoperative criterion for lung resection. *Ann Thorac Surg* 1987;44:344–349.

101. Morice RC, Peters EJ, Ryan MB, et al. Exercise testing in the evaluation of patients at high risk for complications from lung resection. *Chest* 1992;101:356–361.

102. Walsh GL, Morice RC, Putnam JB, et al. Resection of lung cancer is justified in high-risk patients selected by exercise oxygen consumption . *Ann Thorac Surg* 1994;58:704–711.

103. Bollinger CT, Wyser C, Roser H, et al. Lung scanning and exercise testing for the prediction of postoperative performance in lung resection candidates at increased risk for complications. *Chest* 1995;108:341–348.

104. Stein M, Cassara EL. Preoperative pulmonary evaluation and therapy for surgery patients . *JAMA* 1970;211:787–790.

105. Warner MA, Offord KP, Warner ME, et al. Role of preoperative cessation of smoking and other factors in postoperative pulmonary complications: a blinded study of coronary artery bypass patients. *Mayo Clin Proc* 1989;64:609–616.

106. Moores LK. Smoking and postoperative pulmonary complications: an evidence-based review of the recent literature. *Clin Chest Med* 2000;21:139–146.

107. Bluman LG, Mosca L, Newman N, et al. Preoperative smoking habits and postoperative pulmonary complications. *Chest* 1998;113:883–889.

108. Nakagawa M, Tanaka H, Tsukuma H, et al. Relationship between the duration of the preoperative smoke-free period and the incidence of postoperative pulmonary complications after pulmonary surgery. *Chest* 2001;120:705–710.

109. Rochester DF, Enson Y. Current concepts in the pathogenesis of the obesity-hypoventilation syndrome. *Am J Med* 1974;57:402–420.

110. Celli BR. Perioperative respiratory care of the patient undergoing upper abdominal surgery. *Clin Chest Med* 1993;14:253–261.

111. Bartlett RH, Gazzaniga AB, Geraghty TR. Respiratory maneuvers to prevent postoperative pulmonary complications. *JAMA* 1973;224:1017–1021.

112. Thoren L. Postoperative pulmonary complications: observations on their prevention by chest physiotherapy . *Acta Chir Scand* 1954;107:193–205.

113. Celli BR, Rodriguez KS, Snider GL. A controlled trial of intermittent positive pressure breathing, incentive spirometry, and deep breathing exercises in preventing pulmonary complications after abdominal surgery. *Am Rev Respir Dis* 1984;130:12–15.

114. Roukema JA, Carol EJ, Prins JG. The prevention of pulmonary complications after upper abdominal surgery in patients with noncompromised pulmonary status. *Arch Surg* 1988;123:30.

115. Taylor G, Pryse-Davis J. The prophylactic use of antacids in the prevention of the acid-pulmonary-aspiration syndrome. *Lancet* 1966;1:288–291.

116. Vaughan RW, Wise L. Postoperative arterial blood gas measurements in obese patients: effect of position on gas exchange . *Ann Surg* 1975;182:705–709.

117. Gold MI. Is intermittent positive pressure breathing necessary in the surgical patient? *Ann Surg* 1976;184:122–124.

118. Scuderi J, Olsen GN. Respiratory therapy in the management of postoperative complications. *Respir Care* 1989;34:281–291.

119. Christensen EF, Schultz P, Jensen OV, et al. Postoperative pulmonary complications and lung function in high-risk patients:

a comparison of three physiotherapy regimens after upper abdominal surgery in general anesthesia. *Acta Anesthesiol Scand* 1991;35:97–104.

120. O'Donahue WJ. National survey of the usage of lung expansion modalities for the prevention and treatment of postoperative atelectasis following abdominal and thoracic surgery. *Chest* 1985;87:76–80.

121. Ricksten SE, Bengtsson A, Soderberg C, et al. Effects of periodic positive airway pressure by mask on postoperative pulmonary function. *Chest* 1986;89:774–781.

122. Stock MC, Downs JB, Gauer DK, et al. Prevention of postoperative pulmonary complications with CPAP, incentive spirometry, and conservative therapy. *Chest* 1985;87:151–157.

7 Pulmonary Aerosols

Lewis J. Smith · Semil Mehta

INTRODUCTION

Pulmonologists must have an understanding of the pharmacokinetics and pharmacodynamics of those medications used to treat pulmonary diseases. *Pharmacokinetics* refers to the relationship between the dose of a drug and its level in the plasma or in the tissue at its site of action (1, 2). It is the quantitative analysis of the processes of drug absorption, distribution, and elimination or clearance. *Pharmacodynamics* refers to the relationship between the concentration of a drug and its pharmacologic effect. Pharmacodynamic properties are determined by the amount of drug reaching the site of action (an important issue for medications delivered by the aerosol route), how avidly the drug binds to its receptor, how rapidly its effect(s) is transduced, and how effectively the drug inhibits other bioactive compounds. *Pharmacogenetics* refers to the relationship between individual genetic variability and the efficacy or toxicity of a drug. Genetic variability can influence drug absorption, metabolism, distribution, and drug-receptor interactions.

In this chapter, we begin by reviewing general pharmacokinetic and pharmacodynamic principles. We will apply these principles to oral and inhaled medications commonly used to treat obstructive lung diseases. Our major focus is on aerosolized medications delivered directly to the airways, which may act locally, as is the case for the treatment of airway disease (β_2-agonists), or at distant sites (insulin). Regardless of the intended site of action, the principles governing drug delivery, absorption, distribution, and clearance apply to both situations. We will also discuss basic information necessary to the understanding of pulmonary drug delivery systems.

L. J. Smith and **S. Mehta:** Division of Pulmonary and Critical Care Medicine, Northwestern University Feinberg School of Medicine, Chicago, Illinois.

General Pharmacokinetic and Pharmacodynamic Concepts

The factors that determine the relationship between drug dose and concentration in plasma and tissue include the mode of drug delivery, the rate of absorption and tissue volume of distribution, the degree of binding to circulating plasma proteins, hepatic and renal function, and the rate of transfer between plasma and tissue. By definition, 100% of a medication administered intravenously is absorbed. In contrast, absorption may vary widely for drugs administered orally or via the airways. This variability may be attributed to a number of factors, including host variability and the specific formulation and properties of the drug.

Distribution via the circulation results in delivery of a portion of the medication to one or more tissues, including the target tissue. The portion delivered to tissues is referred to as the *peripheral volume* of distribution. The remainder stays in the plasma, and this amount is called the *central volume.* The size of the peripheral volume(s) is directly proportional to the tissue solubility of the drug. At steady state, the total volume of distribution equals the central plus the peripheral volumes.

Clearance is defined as the volume that is cleared of drug per unit of time. Clearance of drugs occurs by two major mechanisms: systemic clearance and intercompartmental or distribution clearance. Systemic clearance involves metabolism and excretion of a drug. This form of clearance occurs largely by hepatic and renal mechanisms. Intercompartmental clearance involves movement of a drug from its site of action to another compartment, e.g., movement from the target organ to the plasma. Plasma protein binding will influence drug clearance from the central volume and its subsequent metabolism. Although the lung may clear only a small portion of medications administered orally or intravenously, it clears a major portion of drugs administered via aerosol.

Most drugs are cleared via zero-order kinetics, first-order kinetics, or a combination of the two. A drug with a concentration that decreases at a constant rate (e.g., linearly) exhibits zero-order kinetics. If the concentration of drug (x_0) at one time (t_0) and its rate of change over time (k) are known, the concentration remaining at a subsequent time (x_1, t_1) can be calculated using the following equations and solving for x_1 in the first equation or $x(t)$ in the second equation:

$$(x_1 - x_0)/(t_1 - t_0) = k$$
$$x(t) = x_0 + k(t)$$

When a drug exhibits first-order kinetics, the concentration of the drug decreases in proportion to the amount of drug present at any time. The drug concentration decreases more quickly when the concentration of drug is higher and more slowly when the drug concentration is lower. This relationship is represented by the following equation:

$$x(t) = x_0 \, e^{-kt}$$

The pharmacodynamic properties of a drug are defined by its dose-response relationships, efficacy, and potency. The dose- or concentration-response relationship is a standard tool for illustrating the effect different doses or concentrations of drug have on a measurable outcome. An example of the relationship between dose and physiologic measurement is shown in Figure 7.1 (3). Different doses of zafirlukast were administered to patients with mild-to-moderate asthma, and their effect on the forced expiratory volume in 1 second (FEV_1) was measured. This figure also illustrates

the pharmacokinetics of zafirlukast in that the drug dose is related to the plasma concentration obtained at the end of the 12-hour dosing interval.

Another example is provided by the methacholine dose-response curve (Fig. 7.2). The nebulizer concentration of methacholine is plotted on the x-axis, and the FEV_1, expressed as a percentage of the initial value, is plotted on the y-axis. This figure, which includes idealized results for normal individuals, patients with mild asthma, and patients with more severe asthma, illustrates the variability in response between human subjects.

Drug-receptor interactions contribute to the efficacy and potency of a drug. Efficacy is a measure of the intrinsic ability of a drug to produce a desired physiologic or clinical effect. It is influenced by receptor coupling to G proteins, activation of second messengers, and the ability to finally produce the effect. Drugs that are full agonists (e.g., formoterol) are said to have an efficacy of one; drugs that are partial agonists (e.g., salmeterol) have an efficacy greater than zero but less than one. As observed with these two long-acting β_2-agonists, partial agonists can be as effective as full agonists in producing the desired physiologic effect (e.g., bronchodilation) (4,5).

Potency refers to the quantity of drug that must be given to produce a specific effect. For example, if 10 mg of the leukotriene receptor antagonist montelukast produces the same maximum effect as 40 mg of zafirlukast, then montelukast is 4 times more potent than zafirlukast in producing that effect (e.g., increasing the FEV_1). Thus, a drug with lower potency can be as effective as one of higher potency at a higher dose. However, the toxicity may increase as the dose rises.

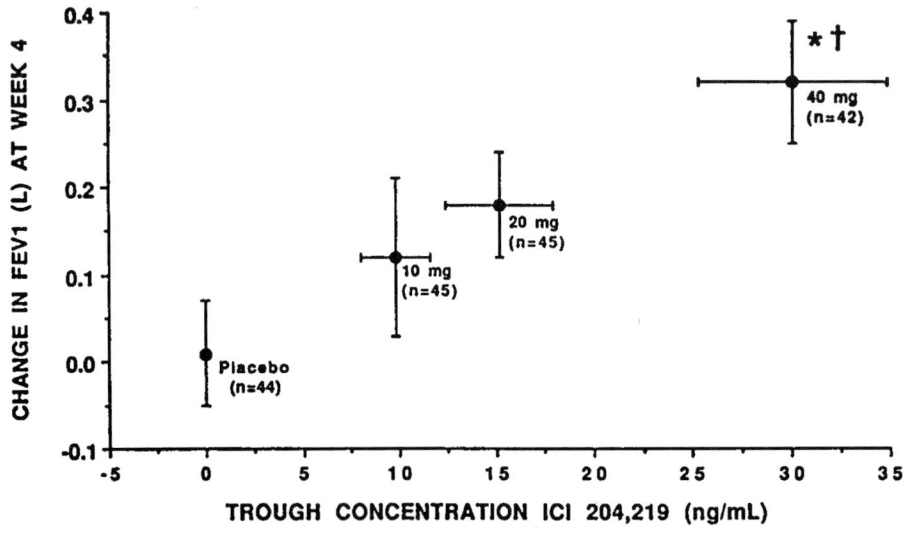

FIGURE 7.1. Association between the change in forced expiratory volume in 1 second (FEV_1; L) and plasma concentrations (ng/mL) of ICI 204,219 (zafirlukast) and placebo at week 4. *$p < .01$ for the change in FEV_1 between 40 mg ICI 204,219 and placebo. †$p < .05$ for the linear trend with dose of ICI 204,219. (From Spector SL, Smith LJ, Glass M, et al. Effect of 6 weeks of therapy with oral doses of ICI 204,219, a leukotriene D$_4$ receptor antagonist, in subjects with bronchial asthma. *Am J Respir Crit Care Med* 1994;150:618–623, with permission.)

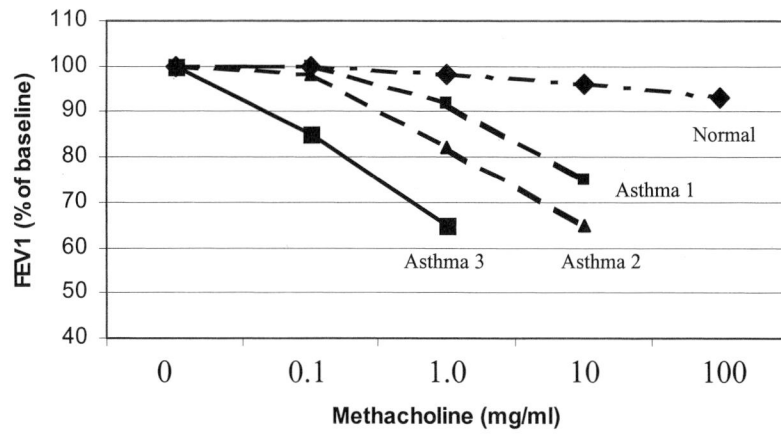

FIGURE 7.2. Relationship between the concentration of methacholine administered by nebulizer and the forced expiratory volume in 1 second (FEV_1), expressed as a percentage of the value after inhaling the diluent.

The therapeutic index describes the relationship between the effectiveness of a drug and its toxicity. In simplest terms, the therapeutic index is the ratio of the dose of drug that produces the desired effect in 50% of the population (ED_{50}) to the dose that kills 50% of the population (LD_{50}). This type of analysis is traditionally performed as part of the preclinical pharmacology and toxicology testing of new therapies. Variations of the therapeutic ratio are used in early phase clinical studies to optimize the dose chosen for testing in later-phase, large-scale clinical trials. Theophylline, dosed to produce clinical bronchodilation, is an example of a drug that has a relatively low therapeutic index. In studies of human subjects, other measures of toxicity are commonly used, such as the number of all adverse effects divided by the number of study subjects or the percentage of patients who develop abnormal liver function or other organ function test results

Systemically Administered Pulmonary Drugs

Because of the difficulty in targeting a medication to a specific organ, many drugs are given orally or intravenously and delivered by the circulation. Several systemically administered drugs are effective in the treatment of airway diseases, including corticosteroids, β-agonists, phosphodiesterase inhibitors such as theophylline, and leukotriene modifiers. With the exception of the leukotriene modifiers, particularly montelukast and zafirlukast, which have little if any currently recognized toxicity when administered via the oral route, the other systemically administered therapies have the potential for substantial toxicity. Fortunately, both β-agonists and corticosteroids are highly effective and less toxic when delivered by the airways. For some therapies used to treat lung diseases, oral or intravenous administration may not be as effective as is aerosol therapy, because the medication is inactivated in the gastrointestinal tract by acid and peptidases or in the liver (first-pass metabolism). This is the case with anticholinergic bronchodilators such as ipratropium bromide and antiallergic drugs such as cromolyn sodium.

Aerosolized Medications

There are advantages to treating airway diseases by the inhaled route. They include direct delivery of drug to the airway and lung, allowing a lower total dose, reduced systemic absorption and distribution, fewer issues with absorption and metabolism, and limited side effects (Table 7.1). All of these features can increase the therapeutic index. An example is provided by a study in which albuterol was given either orally, sublingually, or by aerosol (pressurized metered-dose inhaler [pMDI]) to a group of patients with asthma (6). Albuterol given by the inhaled route produced the most rapid increase in FEV_1 and was not associated with tremor, as was the case with the other two routes of administration.

The amount of drug delivered to the lung is the result of a complex interplay of breathing pattern and inspiratory flow rate, the type and severity of underlying airway or lung disease, the physiochemical properties of the medication, and the exact method of delivery (7–9) (Table 7.2). Problems in any of these areas can render a therapy ineffective. For example, an aerosol may be preferentially delivered to lung units with little disease relative to other highly diseased units in patients with airflow obstruction, compared with normal subjects in whom distribution is uniform (10). Secretions, the area available for drug absorption, and the efficiency of mucociliary clearance vary from patient to patient, particularly in those with diseased lungs. Patients may also differ in their ability to trigger a MDI or to generate an adequate inspiratory flow rate for optimal function of a dry powder inhaler (DPI).

TABLE 7.1. ADVANTAGES OF TREATING AIRWAY DISEASES BY THE INHALED ROUTE

Increased delivery to the site of interest
Use of a lower total dose
Fewer issues with absorption and metabolism
Reduced systemic absorption and distribution
Reduced side effects

TABLE 7.2. FACTORS INFLUENCING DELIVERY OF MEDICATIONS TO THE LUNG

Patient-specific factors (e.g., breathing pattern, normal variations in airway geometry)
Underlying airway or lung disease
Physiochemical properties of the medication
Delivery device

Before discussing these issues and describing specific delivery devices, we will review basic concepts about aerosols and the mechanics of airflow and particle distribution.

AEROSOLS AND THE MECHANICS OF AIRFLOW AND PARTICLE DISTRIBUTION IN THE AIRWAYS

Aerosols are stable suspensions of solid or liquid particles in air (11, 12). Aerosols play several important roles in respiratory medicine (13) (Table 7.3). They can produce lung disease in susceptible individuals (toluene diisocyanate, thermophilic actinomycetes) or worsen preexisting disease (sulfur dioxide or ozone exposures in asthmatics and in those with chronic bronchitis). Aerosols are used to diagnose and assess the severity of certain lung diseases (pulmonary embolism); to measure drug deposition and clearance from the lung in research protocols (14); to induce sputum (hypertonic saline); and, finally, to determine airway reactivity (methacholine or histamine aerosol challenges). Currently, aerosols are widely used in clinical practice as primary therapies for a variety of lung diseases (e.g., asthma, chronic obstructive pulmonary disease, cystic fibrosis, bronchiectasis) and, in the near future, they may be used to treat non-lung diseases such as diabetes mellitus and acute or chronic pain.

The Importance of Particle Size

Aerosols are either of uniform (monodisperse) or varied (heterodisperse) size. Monodisperse aerosols have a geometric standard deviation (σ_g) less than 1.2 (see below). Environmental and therapeutic aerosols used in clinical practice are heterodisperse, with a wide range of particle size. Aerosols found as condensation nuclei are usually between 0.001 and 0.1 μm in diameter, those created by cigarette smoke and

TABLE 7.3. ROLE OF AEROSOLS IN RESPIRATORY MEDICINE

Produce disease in susceptible individuals
Worsen preexisting disease
Diagnose and assess severity of disease
Treat lung diseases
Treat non-lung diseases
Provide anesthesia before bronchoscopy and related procedures
Research tool to define mechanisms of disease

automobile exhaust are between 0.1 and 1 μm, and aerosols formed by pollens and grinding or mining activities are typically between 3 and 20 μm in diameter. Therapeutic aerosols tend to be in the 1- to 5-μm range, as particles of this size have a high likelihood of reaching the airways and distal lung and remaining there (15). In general, very small particles are respirable without being deposited. However, condensation nuclei can grow and coalesce to form particles in the 0.1 to 10 μm size range, which then favors lung deposition. Large particles ($\geq$10 μm) characteristically settle out of aerosols, especially if a holding chamber is used, and hence penetrate poorly into the alveoli.

Heterodisperse therapeutic aerosols may be characterized by a log-normal distribution in which a plot of particle density (number of particles per given size) versus the logarithm of size yields a bell-shaped normal distribution curve (Fig. 7.3) (16). The mass median aerodynamic diameter (MMAD) of an aerosol is the aerodynamic diameter around which the mass is centered. It takes into account aspects of particles that are difficult to measure, such as shape and density, and it is the key determinant of particle deposition in the lung. The aerodynamic diameter (d_a) of an aerosolized particle is related to its actual diameter and its density. The width of the aerosol size distribution is represented by the geometric standard deviation (σ_g), which is the ratio of the size below which 84.13% of the mass resides to that below which 50% of the mass resides. Values of σ_g of 1.2 or less indicate a narrow size distribution and define monodisperse aerosols.

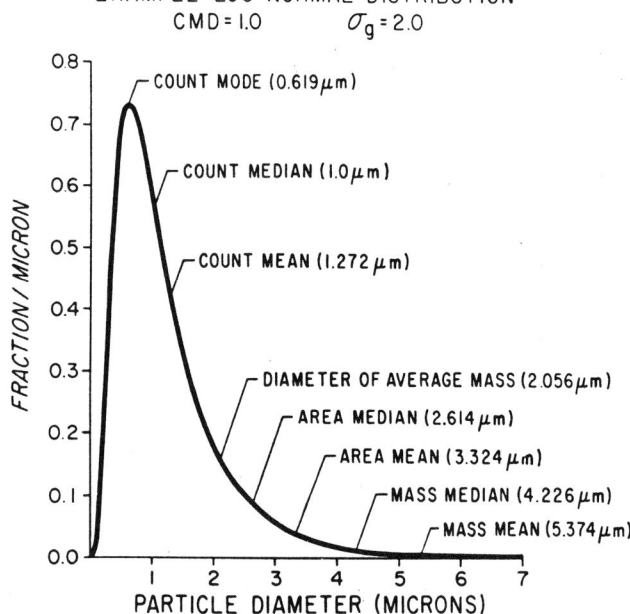

FIGURE 7.3. An example of the log-normal distribution in normalized linear form of aerosol particle sizes for a count median diameter (CMD) equal to 1 mm ($\pm$2 SD). Particle density is on the y-axis, and particle size is on the x-axis. (From Raabe OG. Particle size analysis utilizing grouped data and the log-normal distribution. *Aerosol Sci* 1971;2:289–303, with permission.)

Deposition of Aerosols in the Lung

Aerosols deposit in the lung predominantly by inertial impaction, sedimentation, and diffusion. Electrostatic precipitation and interception also play a role, but mostly under select circumstances. A particle deposits by *impaction* when its inertia is such that it is unable to continue to flow with the air stream as the air stream changes direction. Particle impaction generally occurs in the upper airways at locations at which the air stream curves sharply (nose, pharynx to larynx), and in the lower airways at airway bifurcations. The degree of impaction is proportional to d^2Q, where d is the diameter of the particle and Q is the velocity of the air stream. The number of particles impacting increases with increasing flow rates, with larger particle size, with the acuteness of the angle through which the air stream turns, and with decreasing airway diameter. Turbulent flow, which occurs at airway branch points, is associated with increased particle impaction.

Sedimentation is primarily responsible for the deposition of particles that do not impact a surface when entering the lung. Such particles, usually less than 5 μm in size, are subject to gravitational forces based on the square of their diameter. Sedimentation is enhanced by breath-holding and slow steady breathing. Sedimentation tends to occur where flow is laminar. *Brownian diffusion* is the major mechanism by which particles less than or equal to 0.5 μm in diameter deposit in the lung. These particles deposit in distal, non-airway lung units. They comprise only a small fraction of the total pulmonary deposition of therapeutic aerosols. Deposition of condensation nuclei in the lung occurs mostly by diffusion.

Electrostatic precipitation can contribute to the deposition of very small particles in the lung because most aerosols are charged. Electrostatic precipitation may be most important outside the lung; it is the mechanism by which therapeutic aerosols deposit in narrow plastic tubes and thereby decreases delivery of drug to the lung, especially in the case of DPIs. *Interception* occurs when the distance to a surface is less than the diameter of a particle. It is the major mechanism by which fibers (fiberglass, asbestos) deposit on airway walls but is of little importance in the delivery of therapeutic aerosols.

The therapeutic relevance of particle size and its effects on deposition are apparent from reports indicating that for both ipratropium bromide and albuterol, particle sizes around 2.8 μm provide optimal bronchodilation (17, 18). Larger particles, which would be expected to exhibit greater upper airway impaction, are less effective.

Factors Influencing Aerosol Deposition in the Lung

For the purpose of understanding particle deposition in the lung and the effects of various factors on deposition, the lung can be divided into three compartments: nasopharyngeal, tracheobronchial, and pulmonary. The major determinants of particle deposition are different for each. Inertial impaction is most important in the nasopharyngeal compartment; inertial impaction and sedimentation are both important in the tracheobronchial compartment; and sedimentation and diffusion are important in the pulmonary compartment (Fig. 7.4).

In addition to particle size, other factors that can influence aerosol deposition in the lung include airway geometry, the breathing pattern, particle tonicity, and the presence and severity of airway disease (10, 19–27). Normal subjects have variable airway anatomy. In those with smaller conducting airways, central (tracheobronchial) deposition of aerosols is greater than in those with larger airways. Breathing pattern also influences deposition (24, 25). Rapid inhalation of an aerosol that is injected into the air stream at the middle or end of a rapid inspiration increases central deposition. In contrast, aerosol inhalation at the beginning of a slow inspiration, as well as a breath-hold at the end of inspiration, increases peripheral (e.g., pulmonary) deposition. Increased minute ventilation, as occurs during exercise, increases particle deposition in the lung. However, the deposition pattern may be altered by changes associated with the increased minute ventilation, such as greater inspiratory flow rates and decreased ability to humidify the inspired particles fully, resulting in reduced hygroscopic growth (26). The influence of tonicity on aerosol deposition is a consequence of growth or shrinkage of nonisotonic particles as they pass through humidified airways (27). The resultant change in particle size also alters deposition.

Airway narrowing from any cause—including bronchospasm, airway remodeling, or the presence of secretions—influences particle distribution in the lung. Most obstructive lung diseases are associated with increased central deposition (20). For example, the reduced airway caliber of patients with cystic fibrosis enhances delivery to the tracheobronchial compartment by 200% to 300% (10). A similar phenomenon is seen in patients with asthma and chronic obstructive lung disease from other causes (19–22).

A change in deposition pattern, whether produced by disease or other factors, has potential therapeutic and diagnostic implications that may differ depending on the drug or chemical administered. For example, the β-adrenergic agonist terbutaline has been reported to produce an equivalent degree of bronchodilation and improvement in gas exchange, regardless of whether it is deposited predominantly in the central airways or in the peripheral airways (28). In contrast, in patients with asthma, central deposition of methacholine produces a greater degree of bronchoconstriction than does peripheral deposition (29). Body position may also influence aerosol deposition. The importance of this phenomenon is illustrated by the use of aerosolized pentamidine to prevent *Pneumocystis carinii* pneumonia in immune-compromised patients. If a patient inhales the medication while in an upright position with a normal breathing pattern, less

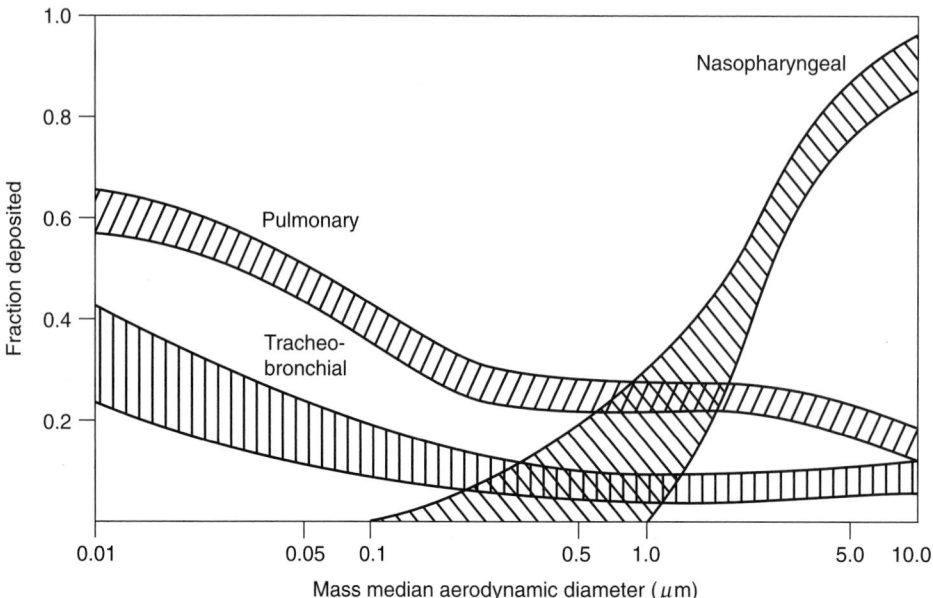

FIGURE 7.4. Particle deposition in the respiratory tract, based on the three-compartment model of the International Committee on Radiation Protection. Each of the shaded areas indicates the variability of deposition for a given mass median (aerodynamic) diameter in each compartment when the geometric standard deviation varies from 1.2 to 4.5 and the tidal volume is 1450 mL. (From Morrow PE. Deposition and retention models for internal dosimetry of the human respiratory tract. *Health Phys* 1966;12:173–207, with permission.)

medication reaches the upper lung zones, and disease preferentially develops there (30).

Nasal or mouth breathing also influences aerosol deposition. Because of the narrow nasal cross-sectional area (which produces a high linear velocity), sharp bends, and hairs, most large particles ($\geq$10 μm) and a high proportion of soluble gases are removed in the nose. Nasal humidification causes growth of hygroscopic particles, further favoring impaction there. Despite the vascular nature of the nasal bed and the high degree of particle deposition in the nasal turbinates, the surface area available for systemic absorption of medications (150–200 cm^2) is limited compared with the area of the lung (75 m^2). Because of these factors, the oral inhaled route is preferred.

It is also important to consider the difference between deposition and retention. Retention equals deposition minus clearance. Clearance mechanisms in the airways, including translocation of deposited particles and removal by the mucociliary system, may have a major effect on the ability of aerosols to cause or treat disease (12, 31).

AEROSOL DELIVERY DEVICES

A number of inhalational devices are available that produce aerosols of respirable particles. They include pMDIs, DPIs, and nebulizers (jet and ultrasonic). Each of these categories comprises several devices with differing characteristics. Production lots of the same device may vary such that particle distribution in the lung and the effects of the material being delivered are altered. When characterizing an aerosol delivery device, one must understand the distinctions between the "metered" dose, the "delivered" dose, and the "respirable" dose. The metered dose is the dose filling and subsequently emptied from the metering device. The delivered dose is the dose exiting the device. The respirable dose is the dose exiting the device with an aerodynamic diameter of 6 μm or less.

Metered-Dose Inhalers

MDIs are the most common delivery system used to administer drugs to patients with airway disease, especially asthma (32). They are convenient to use, small, portable, and safe. In addition, they accurately deliver multiple doses of a drug. The essential components of a MDI are (1) a canister containing the drug mixed with propellant and surfactant, (2) a metering chamber that releases the proper amount of medication, and (3) a mouthpiece that directs the spray of medication (Fig. 7.5). The mouthpiece also serves as the actuator seat for the release of the drug from the device. The drugs in MDIs are either dissolved or suspended as fine crystals in the liquid propellant. The canister in the MDI is pressurized, thus the designation pMDI. When a patient actuates (compresses) the pMDI, a dose of the drug, plus surfactant and propellant, is released as a plume of gas traveling at a speed of about 30 m/s. The propellant immediately begins to evaporate, which generates an aerosol of micrometer-sized particles of the drug suspended in surfactant and the

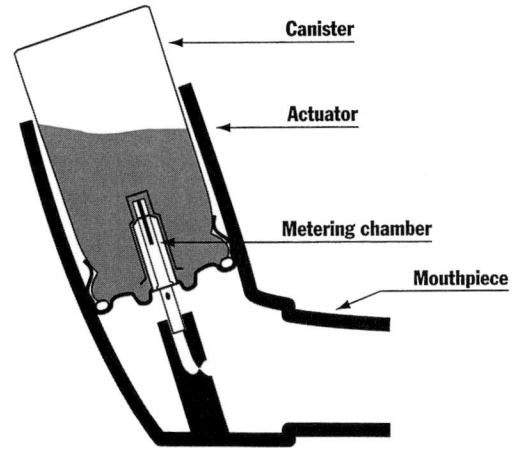

Canister

Actuator

Metering chamber

Mouthpiece

FIGURE 7.5. Typical pressurized metered-dose inhaler. The diagram illustrates the basic components of the device. The canister contains the medication, propellant, and surfactant. The metering chamber ensures delivery of a uniform dose of medication. The mouthpiece directs the aerosol toward the patient's airway.

remaining propellant. When proper technique is used and the patient inhales slowly, the particles are drawn into the airways.

Historically, the propellant used in pMDIs has been a chlorofluorocarbon (CFC), but the concern about ozone depletion and global warming has resulted in a worldwide ban on CFCs. Newer propellants, such as hydrofluoroalkanes (HFAs), are replacing CFCs in pMDIs. Studies using these new propellants illustrate how a change in the propellant can influence the pharmacokinetic and pharmacodynamic properties of an established drug. This was shown by Leach and colleagues when they reported that beclomethasone dissolved in an HFA propellant had a MMAD of approximately 1.1 μm compared with a MMAD of about 3.5 μm when the same corticosteroid was suspended in a CFC propellant (33). A subsequent study of these two preparations demonstrated the significance of this change in particle size. Busse and colleagues reported that a 2.6-fold higher dose of the CFC/beclomethasone preparation was needed to produce the same increase in FEV_1 as the HFA/beclomethasone preparation (34).

Several problems have been recognized with pMDIs. One is that pMDIs are sensitive to technique (e.g., inspiratory flow rate); some individuals have difficulty in coordinating triggering of the device with their breathing pattern. If the pMDI is triggered well after inspiration has begun, less drug reaches the lung and its distribution differs from the distribution that is found when triggering occurs during early inspiration (35). A second problem is the initial rapid velocity imparted to the aerosol as it leaves the device. This can cause discomfort and coughing in some individuals, which may lead to discontinuation of the medication. In addition, a large number of particles deposit in the oropharynx, decreasing the dose available to the lung and increasing the likelihood of developing oral thrush and dysphonia when

using inhaled corticosteroids. It has been estimated that when spacer devices are not used, less than 20% of a drug dose is delivered to the lung from pMDIs, whereas 80% or so is deposited in the oropharynx (36, 37). A less commonly appreciated problem is the effect of environmental temperature on particle size and therefore on lung deposition. Lower temperatures result in larger particles and decreased lung deposition. Keeping the device in an inside pocket rather than a purse and warming it in the hand before using it out of doors in cold weather can minimize this problem.

Several innovations have been devised to deal with some of the problems associated with pMDIs. One is a breath-actuated device (Autohaler and others), which triggers the pMDI valve at the start of inspiration. The initial velocity is lower with some of these devices, reducing oropharyngeal deposition. However, individuals with arthritis or weakness involving the hand muscles may be unable to set the trigger. Further, the device requires sealing the lips around the mouthpiece. This practice is at variance with recommendations by manufacturers of other devices that the pMDI be placed a few inches outside the open mouth.

A second innovation has been spacer or reservoir devices. These come in a variety of sizes and shapes; cost and convenience also vary. All reduce the need to synchronize triggering of the inhaler with the onset of inspiration, while decreasing oropharyngeal and increasing lung deposition (38, 39). Hence, drug bioavailability in the lung is increased and systemic bioavailability is reduced; the extent of each depends on the particular drug (40). Spacers are of greatest benefit in young children, the elderly, and those inhaling corticosteroid or other medications that have the potential to produce adverse effects if deposited in the oropharynx.

Dry-Powder Inhalers

Dry-powder inhalers(DPIs) include the Spinhaler, Rotahaler, and Aerolizer, which deliver a single dose of drug (cromolyn, albuterol, or formoterol); the Diskhaler and Diskus (Fig. 7.6), which deliver multiple doses of drug (salmeterol, fluticasone, salmeterol-fluticasone combination) from a packet containing individual compartments; and the Turbuhaler (Fig. 7.7), which delivers as many doses of drug (budesonide, terbutaline) from a single container as does a typical pMDI.

These devices are highly effective for delivering bronchodilators and corticosteroids to the lungs of patients with airway disease (41–43). The major advantages of DPIs are breath rather than hand actuation, which reduces difficulties with triggering the device at the start of inspiration, and the absence of CFCs or other propellants. Disadvantages are those associated with any breath-actuated device: variable delivery at very low flow rates (typically <30 L/min) and the need to insert the device in the mouth and seal the lips. Spacer devices are not routinely used with DPIs, and most DPIs are unable to accept the commonly available spacers.

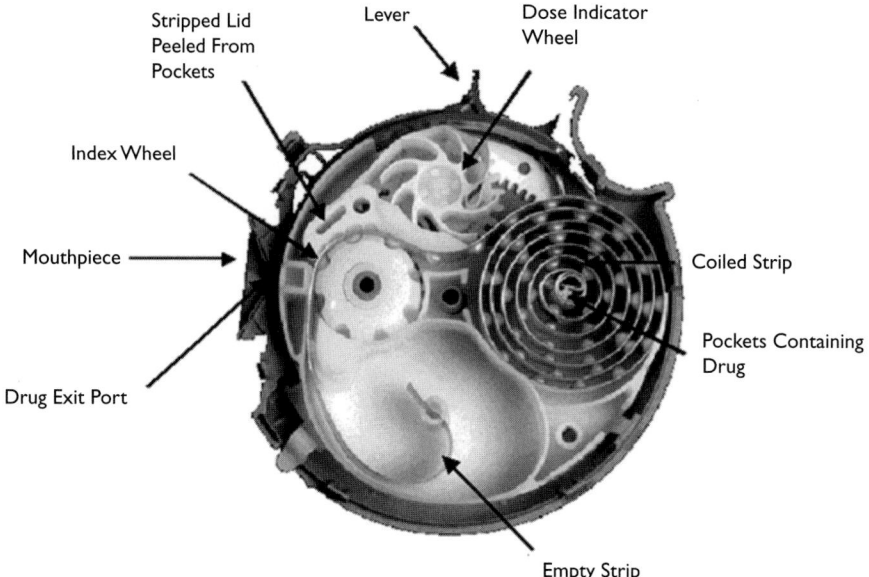

Stripped Lid
Peeled From
Pockets

Lever

Dose Indicator
Wheel

Index Wheel

Mouthpiece

Drug Exit Port

Coiled Strip

Pockets Containing
Drug

Empty Strip

FIGURE 7.6. The Diskus dry powder inhaler device. The diagram illustrates the components of the device, including the coiled strip with multiple pockets that contain individual doses of medication.

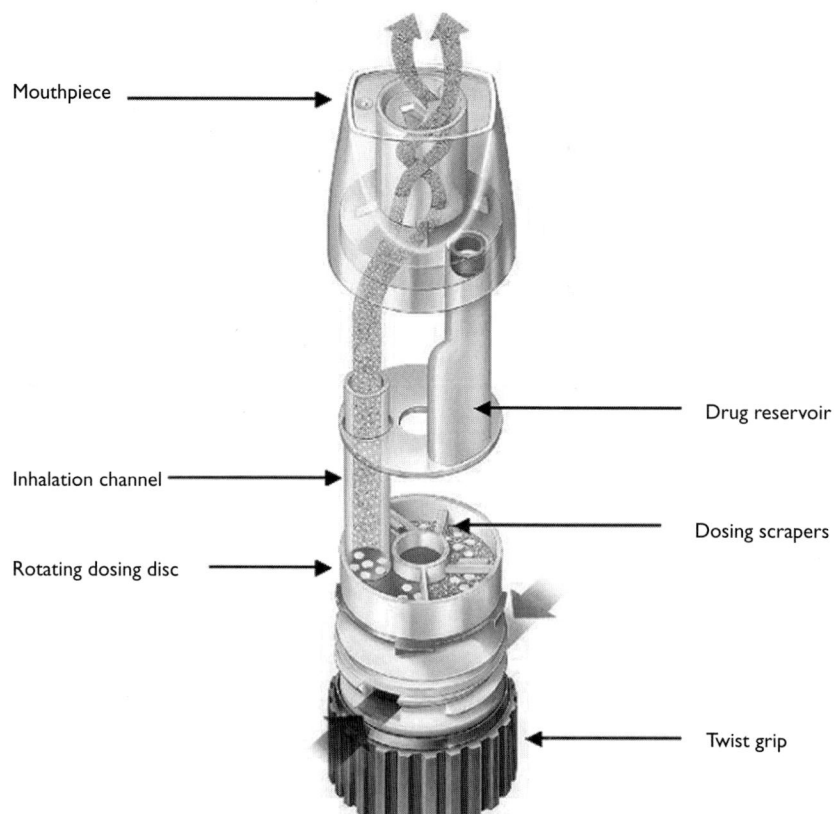

Mouthpiece

Inhalation channel

Rotating dosing disc

Drug reservoir

Dosing scrapers

Twist grip

FIGURE 7.7. The Turbuhaler dry powder inhaler device. The diagram illustrates the components of the device. In contrast to the Diskus device, individual doses of medication are prepared immediately before inhalation by "shaving off" a precise amount of medication from the bulk medication.

The same medication may be available in both a pMDI and a DPI formulation. Several studies have shown that the dose delivered to the lung and its pharmacological effect differ depending on the device. Thorsson and colleagues reported that the lung deposition of budesonide delivered by the Turbuhaler DPI was twice that achieved with a pMDI (41). Borgstrom and colleagues demonstrated a similar result with terbutaline (42). This same group subsequently reported that the difference in pharmacokinetics (lung deposition) corresponded to differences in bronchoprotection against both methacholine and histamine challenges (43). Conversely, increases in lung deposition may be associated with increased systemic bioavailability (41) and the potential for increased toxicity.

Nebulizers

Nebulizers (jet, ultrasonic) are effective when high doses of drugs need to be administered. Drugs typically administered by nebulizer include albuterol, ipratropium, and budesonide. Topical anesthetics such as lidocaine are also given by nebulizer to produce airway anesthesia before performing bronchoscopy. Nebulizers are especially valuable for infants and young children, who cannot use handheld devices. Their major advantages are that coordination with the respiratory cycle is not required, and they are effective even when patients have very low inspiratory flow rates. The major disadvantages are their relatively large size and the need for an external power source. Both of these factors limit a patient's mobility.

Jet nebulizers produce an aerosol by moving a blast of air across a narrow nozzle into which liquid has been drawn (Bernoulli principle). When the air hits the liquid, small droplets are formed. Because the air stream is curved in the nebulizer before the aerosol exits, larger particles (≥ 10 μm) are removed. The distribution of particles generated by a nebulizer and subsequent deposition in the lung depend on the nebulizer (model, lot, and individual unit), the number and size of baffles, the diameter of the exhalation port tubing, the use of vents, gas flow rates, fill volume in the nebulizer reservoir, viscosity and surface tension of the solution, and ambient temperature and humidity. When choosing a nebulizer it is important to know the specific characteristics of the unit being used and to carefully follow the manufacturer's recommendations regarding proper operation.

Ultrasonic nebulizers use a piezoelectric crystal, operating in the range of 1 to 3 MHz, which transforms high-frequency electric oscillations into mechanical oscillations, thereby providing energy for producing an aerosol. Output tends to be greater than that from a jet nebulizer, and the particle size is usually larger. With both types of nebulizers, much of the drug remains in the nebulizer well after the treatment is completed. Further, the concentration of the drug being administered may increase during the time the solution is being nebulized. The advantages and disadvantages of the different delivery devices are summarized in Table 7.4.

TABLE 7.4. DELIVERY DEVICES: ADVANTAGES AND DISADVANTAGES

	pMDI	DPI	Nebulizer
Convenient to use	Yes	Yes	Yes
Small/portable	Yes	Yes	Yes/No (needs power source)
Safe	Yes	Yes	Yes
Accurate	Yes	Yes	Variable
Sensitive to technique	Yes	Yes (at low inspiratory flows)	No
Sensitive to temperature	Yes	No	No
Oropharyngeal deposition (without spacer)	Yes	Limited	Limited

pMDI, pressurized metered-dose inhaler; DPI, dry powder inhaler.

Pharmacokinetics and Pharmacodynamics of Aerosols

Aerosol therapy is generally inefficient. New devices, holding chambers (spacers), and an improved understanding of how other factors, such as breathing pattern, contribute to aerosol delivery to the lung have improved efficiency. Yet, only a small and variable fraction of the drug that leaves the delivery device deposits in the lung (36, 37). The pharmacokinetics of a drug delivered by aerosol to the lung can be more difficult to study than are the pharmacokinetics of a drug delivered by the systemic route. Blood levels, the principle method to determine the pharmacokinetics of a drug, may not be reflective of levels in the lung, especially if care is not taken to minimize absorption from the gastrointestinal tract. Also, assays may not be sufficiently sensitive to measure the low blood levels. Sputum and urine are alternative biologic fluids that may be analyzed. However, some individuals may not be able to produce sputum, and urine levels will not provide the same detailed pharmacokinetic information as does blood. The use of radiolabeled aerosols is another way to measure specific pharmacokinetics. Assuming the radiolabel does not alter the characteristics of the particles, this method provides valuable information about the delivery, distribution, and retention of aerosols in the lung (44–46). Filter paper sampling of airway surface liquid via a transbronchoscopic protected catheter, which has been used to define the pharmacokinetics of amiloride given by ultrasonic nebulizer (47), is an alternative approach. However, the invasive nature of this procedure reduces its general value. Lastly, physiologic measurements (pharmacodynamics) are sometimes used as an alternative to or to complement the direct measurement of a drug in a biologic fluid. By using a combination of these tools, a comprehensive picture can be obtained of the pharmacokinetics of aerosols.

An example of pharmacokinetic profiling of a typical aerosol is provided by Anderson and colleagues, who studied the usual dose of albuterol (180 μg delivered by pMDI) in healthy normal subjects (48). They used charcoal slurries to block gastrointestinal absorption of the drug and measured plasma levels of albuterol using a highly sensitive assay. They found that peak plasma levels of albuterol were reached in 12.6 $\pm$ 2.2 (SD) minutes, which illustrates the rapid delivery of this aerosolized drug to the lung and its rapid entry into the systemic circulation. The mean half-life of distribution was 17.9 $\pm$ 8.2 minutes, and the mean half-life of elimination was 4.4 $\pm$ 1.5 hours. This study and others (49) demonstrate that the peak plasma levels of albuterol, which were reported in earlier studies to occur 2 to 4 hours after inhalation, were owing to the large amount of drug swallowed and its slow gastrointestinal absorption.

Systemic absorption of inhaled particles contributes to the toxicity of medications meant to work in the lung (β-agonists, corticosteroids) (50) and to the therapeutic effectiveness of medications meant to reach a target tissue outside the lung (insulin, morphine) (51,52). The effectiveness of the aerosol also depends on where the particle deposits in the lung (53). Absorption from the periphery of the lung is twice as fast as from the central portions. This is likely owing to the greater thickness of the bronchial epithelium and possibly to the greater surface area of the alveolar epithelium. As a result, drugs given by aerosol for systemic distribution, such as insulin and morphine, should be of smaller size so that they are preferentially delivered to distal regions of the lung. On the other hand, drugs meant to act in the lung will have a greater potential for toxicity when they are delivered to distal lung regions. This paradigm is especially important for inhaled corticosteroids because they may be most effective when they reach the terminal and respiratory bronchioles, in addition to the more proximal airway. They will then have greater systemic availability and the potential for greater toxicity at the same time.

Drug-Drug Interactions

Combining two medications in a single aerosol delivery device is becoming increasingly common. Drug interactions may occur because of changes in pharmacokinetics (absorption, distribution, metabolism), altered pharmacodynamics (drug-receptor binding), and/or direct physical or chemical interactions. In designing combination therapies for the treatment of airway disease, it is important to test for possible interactions before the combination is approved for general use.

Two types of combination aerosol therapies are currently available. One is the combination of a short-acting β-agonist and an anticholinergic (albuterol plus ipratropium either in a pMDI or nebulizer form). The other is the combination of a long-acting β-agonist and an inhaled corticosteroid (salmeterol plus fluticasone either in a pMDI or DPI, or budesonide plus formoterol). The available data and clinical experience indicate that these combinations work at least as well as when

the component medications are taken individually. Some data suggest the beneficial effects may be even greater when the medications are combined than when they are taken separately (54, 55). This may be owing to corticosteroid-induced increased transcription of the β_2-receptor gene (54) and β_2-agonist–induced activation of glucocorticoid receptors (55). In clinical practice the benefit of using a combination product may also relate to improved patient compliance.

Aerosol Delivery during Mechanical Ventilation

Inhaled medications, including bronchodilators, antibiotics, and surfactants, are commonly administered to patients receiving mechanical ventilation. The delivery of aerosolized medications through a ventilator presents several problems that include the addition of the ventilator circuit, a severely diseased lung, different delivery devices, and multiple modes of ventilation. Inadequate attention to these and to other issues unique to this setting can result in poor delivery of a drug to its site of action (56, 57) or in excessive delivery resulting in mucosal ulceration (58).

Studies have been performed to identify the most effective method to deliver inhaled medications, particularly bronchodilators, during mechanical ventilation (56–64). However, the results reported for both nebulizers and pMDIs vary widely. Several studies have compared drug delivery between ambulatory patients and those receiving mechanical ventilation. In one study, a pMDI with spacer resulted in 24% of the drug (fenoterol) being delivered to the airways in ambulatory patients, but only 6% being delivered to mechanically ventilated patients (59). Despite this difference, serum drug levels were similar.

Most currently available pMDIs and nebulizers used with ventilators achieve MMADs of 1 to 5 μm, values similar to those obtained in ambulatory patients. Yet, there is a wide range of efficiency for airway delivery of bronchodilators. For nebulizers, the reported range is 0 to 42%; for pMDIs, the range is 0.3% to 97% (60). Studies using *in vitro* models of mechanical ventilation have provided insight into this variability. Adapters play an important role in the ability of pMDIs to deliver aerosols by mechanical ventilation. For example, elbow devices result in minimal delivery if the timing of drug administration does not coincide with the inspiratory phase (61). Second, important technical differences exist between delivery devices, which when used improperly can influence drug delivery. One study reported that delivery of β_2-adrenergic agonists by pMDI through a spacer is superior to nebulizer delivery under *in vivo* and *in vitro* conditions (62). Another study demonstrated that even large doses of β_2-adrenergic aerosols administered by pMDI to ventilated patients fail to have any appreciable physiologic effects, whereas nebulizers produce significant bronchodilation (63). Third, spacer design is of prime importance for pMDI effectiveness. In addition, the further away the spacer or holding chamber is placed from the endotracheal tube, the greater the drug delivery (64). Fourth, pMDI delivery systems are sensitive to humidity and to synchronization with inspiration. Delivery decreases with increased humidification and increases when the medication is aerosolized during inspiration (61). Fifth, jet nebulizers and pMDI/actuator devices deliver comparable amounts of medication, but the latter require more direct therapist time. Sixth, ventilator settings and endotracheal tube size influence aerosol delivery. Low flow rates, larger tidal volumes, and larger endotracheal tubes increase delivery. On the other hand, kinks and turns in the ventilator circuit favor impaction of respirable particles, which decreases drug delivery to the lung.

A frequent observation is that patients on mechanical ventilation often require higher and more frequent dosing of bronchodilators (63). The reasons for this include severity of disease and reduced drug delivery, for the reasons already outlined. This has led to recommendations that the dose and frequency of inhaled bronchodilators should be titrated to effect. Factors that do not appear to influence aerosol delivery during mechanical ventilation include breath-holding after inspiration and ventilator inspiratory wave form (e.g., sinusoidal, square wave, decelerating) as long as tidal volume, peak inspiratory flow, frequency, and inspiratory-to-expiratory ratio are controlled (60).

Aerosols for Treating Systemic Disease

There is increasing interest in delivering medications to the systemic circulation by the aerosol route. One example of this is insulin, which is currently administered by subcutaneous injection. Because this form of delivery is both inconvenient and painful, alternative means of delivery have been evaluated. The pharmacokinetics of insulin given by the inhaled route has been compared with subcutaneous administration in a small number of healthy subjects and patients with diabetes but without known airway disease (65–68). Using a nebulizer delivery system with a mean particle size of about 5 μm, inhaled insulin achieved peak plasma levels (Tmax) within 15 to 40 minutes in one study and 7 to 20 minutes in another, compared with 60 minutes after subcutaneous injection (65, 66). Interestingly, peak levels are achieved earlier in smokers (65). This may be owing to increased epithelial permeability associated with cigarette smoking.

Bioavailability of inhaled insulin is reported to be between 10% and 20% (65). However, pharmacokinetic and pharmacodynamic parameters are altered by respiratory maneuvers. For example, inhalation during a shallow inspiration results in slower absorption and time to peak effect. Further, a series of forced expiratory maneuvers performed 30 minutes after inhalation results in an immediate increase in serum insulin concentrations (54). Adequate glycemic control has been achieved without significant systemic or pulmonary toxicity (68), although additional experience is needed to confirm the long-term safety of insulin administered by aerosol to the lung.

Other biopeptides designed to reach the systemic circulation, such as leuprolide and calcitonin, also may be effective when administered as an aerosol. Bioavailability will depend on the molecular weight of the particular biopeptide, because that contributes to the ability of a molecule to move across the alveolar epithelium, and on the multiple factors already discussed. There are other medications—including aerosolized iloprost, for the treatment of pulmonary hypertension (69), and morphine (60), for the treatment of pain—that may be effective when given by aerosol. Although technical and clinical issues remain, the aerosol route offers substantial advantages.

Finally, other medications such as recombinant human DNAase and antibiotics are currently being given by aerosol to treat diseases such as cystic fibrosis and pneumonia (71–73). Here, too, the same principles apply. The pharmacokinetic and pharmacodynamic properties of each drug administered by the aerosol route must be carefully studied by using the delivery system and patient population in which it will be given.

REFERENCES

1. Schwinn DA, Shafer SL. Basic principles of pharmacology related to anesthesia. In: Miller RD, ed. *Anesthesia,* 5th ed. Philadelphia: Churchill Livingston, 2000:15–47.
2. Atkinson AJ Jr. Introduction to clinical pharmacology. In: Atkinson AJ Jr, Daniels CE, Dedrick RL, et al., eds. *Principles of clinical pharmacology.* San Diego: Academic Press, 2001:1–6.
3. Spector SL, Smith LJ, Glass M, et al. Effect of 6 weeks of therapy with oral doses of ICI 204,219, a leukotriene D_4 receptor antagonist, in subjects with bronchial asthma. *Am J Respir Crit Care Med* 1994;150:618–623.
4. Palmqvist M, Persson G, Lazer L, et al. Inhaled dry powder formoterol and salmeterol in asthmatic patients: onset of action, duration of effect and potency. *Eur Respir J* 1997;10:2484–2489.
5. Palmqvist M, Ibsen T, Mellen A, et al. Comparison of the relative efficacy of formoterol and salmeterol in asthmatic patients. *Am J Respir Crit Care Med* 1999;160:244–249.
6. Lipworth BJ, Clark RA, Dhillon DP, et al. Pharmacokinetics, efficacy and adverse effects of sublingual salbutamol in patients with asthma. *Eur J Clin Pharmacol* 1989;37:567–571.
7. Witek TJ Jr. The fate of inhaled drugs: the pharmacokinetics and pharmacodynamics of drugs administered by aerosol. *Respir Care* 2000;45:826–830.
8. Suarez S, Hickey AJ. Drug properties affecting aerosol behavior. *Respir Care* 2000;45:652–666.
9. Skoner DP. Pharmacokinetics, pharmacodynamics, and the delivery of pediatric bronchodilator therapy. *J Allergy Clin Immunol* 2000;106:S158–S164.
10. Martonen T, Katz I, Cress W. Aerosol deposition as a function of airway disease: cystic fibrosis. *Pharm Res* 1995;12:96–102.
11. Brain JD, Valberg PA. Deposition of aerosol in the respiratory tract. *Am Rev Respir Dis* 1979;120:1325–1373.
12. Raabe OG. Deposition and clearance of inhaled aerosols. In: Witschi H, Nettesheim P, eds. *Mechanisms in respiratory toxicology,* Vol. 1. Boca Raton, FL: CRC Press, 1982:27–76.
13. Moren F, Newhouse MT, Dolovich MB. *Aerosols in medicine: principles, diagnosis and therapy.* New York: Elsevier, 1985.

14. Beinert T, Brand P, Behr J, et al. Peripheral airspace disease dimensions in patients with COPD. *Chest* 1995;108:998–1003.

15. Morrow PE. Deposition and retention models for internal dosimetry of the human respiratory tract. *Health Phys* 1966;12:173–207.

16. Raabe OG. Particle size analysis utilizing grouped data and the log-normal distribution. *Aerosol Sci* 1971;2:289–303.

17. Zanen P, Go TL, Lammers J-WJ. The optimal particle size for β-adrenergic aerosols in mild asthmatics. *Int J Pharm* 1994;107:211–217.

18. Zanen P, Go TL, Lammers J-WJ. The optimal particle size for parasympathetic aerosols in mild asthmatics. *Int J Pharm* 1995;114:111–115.

19. Lippmann M, Schlesinger RB. Effect of airway size and geometry on particle deposition in the lung: interspecies comparisons of particle deposition and mucociliary clearance in tracheobronchial airways. *J Toxicol Environ Health* 1984;13:441–469.

20. Anderson PJ, Wilson JD, Hiller FC. Respiratory tract deposition of ultrafine particles in subjects with obstructive or restrictive lung disease. *Chest* 1990;97:1115–1120.

21. Melchor R, Biddiscombe MF, Mak VH, et al. Lung deposition patterns of directly labeled salbutamol in normal subjects and in patients with reversible airflow obstruction. *Thorax* 1993;48:506–511.

22. Svartengren K, Philpson K, Svartengren M, et al. Tracheobronchial deposition and clearance in small airways in asthmatic subjects. *Eur Respir J* 1996;9:1123–1129.

23. Touw DJ, Jacobs FAH, Brimicombe RW, et al. Pharmacokinetics of aerosolized tobramycin in adult patients with cystic fibrosis. *Antimicrob Agents Chemo* 1997;41:184–187.

24. Miller FJ, Martonen TB, Menosche MG, et al. Influence of breathing mode and activity level on the regional deposition of inhaled particles and implications for regulatory standards. In: Dodgson J, McCallum RI, Bailey MR, et al., eds. *Inhaled particles.* Oxford: Pergamon Press, 1988:3–7.

25. Kim CS, Hu S-C, DeWitt P, et al. Assessment of regional deposition of inhaled particles in human lungs by serial bolus delivery method . *J Appl Physiol* 1996;81:2203–2213.

26. Hickey AJ, Martonen TB. Behaviour of hygroscopic pharmaceutical aerosols and the influence of hydrophobic additives. *Pharm Res* 1993;10:1–7.

27. Phipps PR, Gonda I, Anderson SD, et al. Regional deposition of saline aerosols of different tonicity. *Eur Respir J* 1994;7:1392–1394.

28. Hultquist C, Wollmer PO, Eklundh G, et al. Effect of inhaled terbutaline sulphate in relation to its deposition in the lungs. *Pulm Pharmacol* 1992;5:127–132.

29. Laube BL, Norman PS, Adams GK. The effect of aerosol distribution on airway responsiveness to inhaled methacholine in patients with asthma. *J Allergy Clin Immunol* 1992;89:510–518.

30. Jules-Elysee KM, Stover DE, Zaman MB, et al. Aerosolized pentamidine: effect on diagnosis and presentation in *Pneumocystis carinii* pneumonia. *Ann Intern Med* 1990;112:750–757.

31. Oberdorster G. Lung clearance of inhaled insoluble and soluble particles. *J Aerosol Med* 1988;1:289–330.

32. Ariyananda PL, Agnew JE, Clarke SW. Aerosol delivery systems for bronchial asthma. *Postgrad Med J* 1996;72:151–156.

33. Leach CF, Davidson PJ, Boudreau RJ. Improved airway targeting with the CFC-free HFA-beclomethasone metered-dose inhaler compared with CFC beclomethasone. *Eur Respir J* 1998;12:1346–1353.

34. Busse WW, Brazinsky S, Jacobson K, et al. Efficacy response of inhaled beclomethasone dipropionate in asthma is proportional to dose and is improved by formulation with a new propellant. *J Allergy Clin Immunol* 1999;104:1215–1222.

35. Dolovich M, Leach C. Drug delivery devices and propellants. In: Busse WE, ed. *Asthma and rhinitis,* 2nd ed. London: Blackwell Science, 2000:1719–1731.

36. Newman SP, Pavia D, Moren F, Sheahan NF, Clarke SW. Deposition of pressurized aerosols in the human respiratory tract. *Thorax* 1981;36:52–55.

37. Dolovich M. Lung dose, distribution, and clinical response to therapeutic aerosols. *Aerosol Sci Tech* 1993;18:230–240.

38. Selroos O, Hulme M. Effect of a volumetric spacer and mouth rinsing on systemic absorption of inhaled corticosteroids from a metered-dose inhaler and dry-powder inhaler. *Thorax* 1991;46:891–894.

39. Vidgren P, Vidgren M, Paronen P, et al. Effects of Inspirease holding chamber on the deposition of metered-dose inhalation aerosols. *Eur J Drug Metab Pharmacokinet* 1991;3:419–425.

40. Hindle M, Chrystryn H. Relative bioavailability of salbutamol to the lung following inhalation using metered-dose inhalation methods and spacer devices. *Thorax* 1994;49:549–553.

41. Thorsson L, Edsbacker S, Conradson TB. Lung deposition of budesonide from Turbuhaler is twice that from a pressurized metered-dose inhaler. *Eur Respir J* 1994;7:1839–1844.

42. Borgstrom L, Derom E, Stahl E, et al. The inhalation device influences lung deposition and bronchodilating effect of terbutaline. *Am J Respir Crit Care Med* 1996;153:1636–1640.

43. Derom E, Borgstrom L, van Schoor J, et al. Lung deposition and protective effect of terbutaline delivered from pressurized metered-dose inhalers and the Turbuhaler in asthmatic individuals. *Am J Respir Crit Care Med* 2001;164:1398–1402.

44. O'Riordan TG, Iacono A, Keenan RJ, et al. Delivery and distribution of aerosolized cyclosporin in lung allograft recipients. *Am J Respir Crit Care Med* 1995;151:516–521.

45. Iacono AT, Keenan RJ, Duncan SR, et al. Aerosolized cyclosporine in lung recipients with refractory chronic rejection. *Am J Respir Crit Care Med* 1996;153:1451–1455.

46. Smaldone JC. Radionuclide scanning, respiratory physiology, and pharmacokinetics. *J Aerosol Med* 2001;14:135–137.

47. Noone PG, Regnis JA, Liu X, et al. Airway deposition and clearance and systemic pharmacokinetics of amiloride following aerosolization with an ultrasonic nebulizer to normal airways. *Chest* 1997;112:1283–1290.

48. Anderson PJ, Zhou X, Breen P, et al. Pharmacokinetics of (R,S)-albuterol after aerosol inhalation in healthy adult volunteers. *J Pharmaceut Sci* 1998;87:841–844.

49. Duarte AG, Dhand R, Reid R, et al. Serum albuterol levels in mechanically ventilated patients and healthy subjects after metered dose inhaler administration. *Am J Respir Crit Care Med* 1996;154:1658–1663.

50. Lipworth BJ. New perspectives on inhaled drug delivery and systemic bioactivity. *Thorax* 1995;50:105–110.

51. Dershwitz M, Walsh JL, Morishige RJ, et al. Pharmacokinetics and pharmacodynamics of inhaled versus intravenous morphine in healthy volunteers. *Anesthesiology* 2000;93:619–628.

52. Farr SJ, McElduff A, Mather LE, et al. Pulmonary insulin administration using the AERx system: physiological and physiochemical factors influencing insulin effectiveness in healthy fasting subjects. *Diabetes Tech Ther* 2000;2:185–197.

53. Brown RA Jr, Schanker LS. Absorption of aerosolized drugs from the rat lung. *Drug Metab Dispos* 1983;11:355–360.

54. Mak JCW, Nishikawa M, Barnes PJ. Glucocorticoids increase β₂-adrenergic receptor transcription in human lung. *Am J Physiol* 1995;12:L41–L46.

55. Eickelberg O, Roth M, Lorx R, et al. Ligand-independent activation of the glucocorticoid receptor by β₂-adrenergic receptor

agonists in primary lung fibroblasts and vascular smooth muscle cells. *J Biol Chem* 1999;274:1005–1010.

56. O'Riordan TG, Greco MJ, Perry RJ, et al. Nebulizer function during mechanical ventilation. *Am Rev Respir Dis* 1992;145:1117–1122.

57. Thomas SH, O'Doherty MJ, Page CJ, et al. Delivery of ultrasonic nebulized aerosols to a lung model during mechanical ventilation. *Am Rev Respir Dis* 1993;148:872–877.

58. Spahr-Schopfer I, Lerman J, Cutz E, et al. Proximate delivery of a large experimental dose from salbutamol MDI induces epithelial airway lesions in intubated rabbits. *Am J Respir Crit Care Med* 1994;150:790–794.

59. Fuller HD, Dolovich MB, Chambers C, et al. Aerosol delivery during mechanical ventilation: a predictive in vitro lung model. *J Aerosol Med* 1992;5:251–259.

60. Dhand R, Tobin M. Inhaled bronchodilator therapy in mechanically ventilated patients. *Am J Respir Crit Care Med* 1997;156:3–10.

61. Diot P, Morra L, Smaldone G. Albuterol delivery in a model of mechanical ventilation: comparison of metered-dose inhaler and nebulizer efficiency. *Am J Respir Crit Care Med* 1995;152:1391–1394.

62. Rau J, Harwood R, Groff J. Evaluation of a reservoir device for metered-dose bronchodilator delivery to intubated adults: an *in-vitro* study. *Chest* 1992;102:924–930.

63. Manthous CA, Hall JB, Schmidt GA, et al. Metered-dose inhaler versus nebulized albuterol in mechanically ventilated patients. *Am Rev Respir Dis* 1993;148:1567–1570.

64. O'Doherty M, Thomas S, Page C, et al. Delivery of a nebulized aerosol to a lung model during mechanical ventilation: effect of ventilator settings and nebulizer type, position, and volume of fill. *Am Rev Respir Dis* 1992;146:383–388.

65. Laube BL, Benedict GW, Dobs AS. Time to peak insulin level, relative bioavailability, and effect of site of deposition of nebulized insulin in patients with non–insulin-dependent diabetes mellitus. *J Aerosol Med* 1998;11:153–173.

66. Farr SJ, McElduff A, Mather LE, et al. Pulmonary insulin administration using the AERx system: physiological and physiochemical factors influencing insulin effectiveness in healthy fasting subjects. *Diabetes Tech Ther* 2000;2:185–197.

67. Heinemann L, Pfutzner A, Heise T. Alternative routes of administration as an approach to improve insulin therapy: update on dermal, oral, nasal, and pulmonary insulin delivery. *Curr Pharm Des* 2001;7:1327–1351.

68. Cefalu W, Skyler J, Kourdes I, et al. Inhaled human insulin treatment in patients with type 2 diabetes mellitus. *Ann Intern Med* 2001;134:203–207.

69. Hoeper, MM. Long-term treatment of primary pulmonary hypertension with aerosolized iloprost, a prostacyclin analogue. *N Engl J Med* 2000;342:1866–1870.

70. Dershwitz M, Walsh JL, Morishige RJ, et al. Pharmacokinetics and pharmacodynamics of inhaled versus intravenous morphine in healthy volunteers. *Anesthesiology* 2000;93:619–628.

71. Fuchs HS, Borowitz DS, Christiansen DH, et al. Effects of aerosolized recombinant human DNase on exacerbations of respiratory symptoms and on pulmonary function in patients with cystic fibrosis. *N Engl J Med* 1994;331:637–642.

72. Ramsey BW, Dorkin HL, Eisenberg JD, et al. Efficacy of aerosolized tobramycin in patients with cystic fibrosis. *N Engl J Med* 1993;328:1740–1746.

73. Smaldone GC, Palmer LB. Aerosolized antibiotics: current and future. *Respir Care* 2000;45:667–675.

The Epidemiology of Asthma

8

Scott T. Weiss · Rosalind J. Wright

INTRODUCTION

Epidemiology involves the study of the distribution and determinants of disease frequency through systematic investigation of different populations in distinct environments, and assessment of exposures and genes causing disease. The application of epidemiologic methodology has provided insight into disease expression that other disciplines cannot offer. The epidemiologist is interested in identifying specific environmental and genetic factors that determine disease in human populations.

Over the past three decades, major contributions to our understanding of the epidemiology of asthma have come from three broad areas of study. The first area arises from longitudinal investigations of the natural history of both asthma and allergy, which have revealed that the majority of asthma cases begin in early childhood. The second is the determination of the frequency and distribution of asthma in population studies. The focal point of epidemiological studies of asthma and allergy has derived from the observation that the prevalence and severity of asthma has increased worldwide since the 1970s, and the question of whether these trends are real or a consequence of biased information. Third, efforts to define the etiologic risk factors for asthma and allergy have intensified in the face of these trends. The new focus on longitudinal studies have prompted investigations into early-life risk factors, with particular attention to the perinatal and early-childhood phenomena underlying development of allergic sensitization and inception of asthma.

In this chapter we will discuss each of these in turn, beginning with a discussion of definitions and methodologic concerns; next addressing the issue of natural history; then considering prevalence, morbidity, and mortality; and finishing with a discussion of emerging risk factors influencing the population trends.

Definitions and Methodologic Concerns

Asthma is defined as "a chronic inflammatory disorder of the airways in which many cells and cellular elements play a role, in particular, mast cells, eosinophils, T lymphocytes, macrophages, neutrophils, and epithelial cells. In susceptible individuals, this inflammation causes recurrent episodes of wheezing, breathlessness, chest tightness, and coughing, particularly at night or in the early morning. These episodes are usually associated with widespread but variable airflow obstruction, which is often reversible either spontaneously or as the result of treatment. The inflammation also causes an increase in the existing bronchial hyperresponsiveness to a variety of stimuli" (1).

It is clear, based on this definition, that asthma is a syndrome without a single defining laboratory test; thus, questionnaire data, or even a physician's diagnosis, has the potential to introduce observation bias and subsequent misclassification into epidemiologic surveys. This bias is greatest at the extremes of life, i.e., before the age of 6 years and after the age of 40 years, when other conditions can mimic asthma with significant frequency and when parental history, smoking, and patient gender tend to greatly influence clinician diagnostic labeling.

One approach to diagnosis has been to include objective measures of disease, such as airway hyperresponsiveness, pulmonary function tests, and atopic markers (i.e., skin-prick tests and serum immunoglobulin E [IgE] antibodies) in population studies. However, because no consensus on a gold standard objective approach to defining asthma has been reached, definition of disease by questionnaire

S. T. Weiss and **R. J. Wright:** Brigham and Women's Hospital, Boston, Massachusetts.

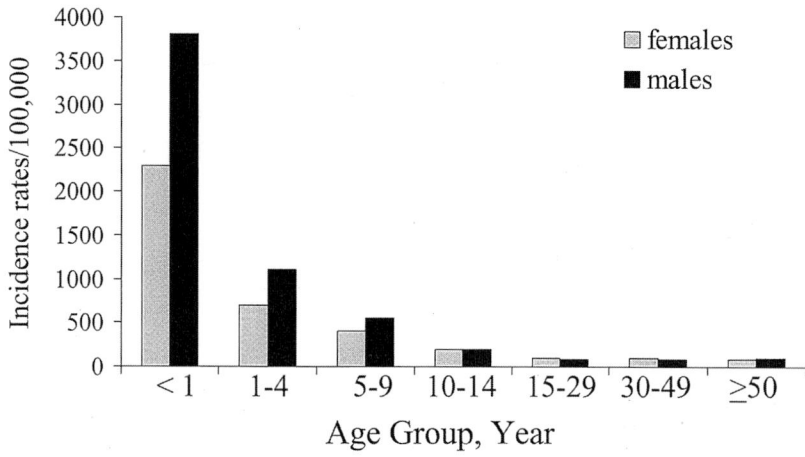

FIGURE 8.1. Annual incidence rates of asthma per 100,000 person-years, stratified by sex and age, among Rochester, Minnesota, residents from 1964–1983. The vast majority of asthmatic subjects are diagnosed before the age of 4 years.

remains the principal method that has been used in large-scale population-based studies around the world.

Allergy is defined as an altered immune state and is often used to denote one particular type of altered immunity, elevations in IgE antibody. Atopy refers to the inherited tendency to develop IgE antibody and refers to three inherited atopic diseases: asthma, atopic dermatitis, and allergic rhinitis. The association between asthma and clinical allergy has long been recognized (2, 3). Several population studies have documented the relationship between asthma and other atopic disorders, including allergic rhinitis and atopic dermatitis. Since the beginning of the 20th century, standard teaching has held that there were two distinguishable forms of asthma: "extrinsic" asthma owing to IgE, and allergen exposure and "intrinsic" asthma felt to be nonallergic and of unknown etiology (4). This notion seemed to be supported by studies demonstrating that many subjects with asthma were not atopic (with atopy identified by a wheal-and-flare reaction to allergy skin testing) (5, 6).

At the present time, epidemiologists believe that although IgE antibody to aeroallergens plays an important role in asthma persistence and in the rise in asthma prevalence; asthma previously considered intrinsic also has an allergic component. Allergy and airway responsiveness are, however, separate phenotypes inherited independently, and the presence of allergy is not necessary to define the asthma phenotype. These intermediate traits can be considered to be overlapping on Venn diagrams. Multiple genes may influence each condition, and they are likely mutually reinforcing. It is clear that asthma may exist without allergy, and the converse is also true.

NATURAL HISTORY

Early Childhood (Birth to Age Six)

It is now an accepted truism that asthma is first apparent and usually diagnosed in early childhood. It is estimated that 90% of all childhood asthma is diagnosed by the age

of six. This estimate has been based on numerous population studies that have observed children prospectively (7). Perhaps the most convincing data comes from Yuninger and colleagues (Fig. 8.1) who surveyed the population of Olmstead County, Minnesota, and asked individuals when they were diagnosed with asthma. These individual self-reports were then checked by review of the patient's medical record. Because all individuals resided in Olmstead County and received their care at the Mayo Clinic and in-migration into the county was negligible, there was an opportunity to compare prospectively collected data (the hospital record with physician diagnosis) with patient memory (patient self-report). It is clear that the distribution as presented in Figure 8.1 from the hospital record is skewed in the direction of younger ages, and the difference between Figure 8.1 and the distribution for self-report (data not shown) can be attributed to recall bias on the part of study participants as to their age at disease onset. This suggests that in older individuals, recall bias may play a prominent role in determining disease onset. The lack of long-term prospective studies, coupled with recall bias, creates a severely distorted picture of the natural history of asthma as a disease.

To summarize this problem, 40% to 50% of children wheeze in the first year of life, and 80% to 90% of all asthma is diagnosed by age six (8). However, respiratory symptoms are intermittent, particularly because as lung function increases, symptoms will tend to decrease. Recall of early life events before the age of six is relatively poor, and hence, older children and adults may not remember even significant wheezing episodes that resulted in hospitalization at an early age. Because clinicians tend to rely on symptoms, rather than on objective measures such as lung function, both in childhood and in adulthood, the discrepancy between symptoms and lung function can be large. Disease may appear incident in adolescence or early adulthood, when it is not truly so. The above clinical construct helps explain the relatively high prevalence of asthma intermediate phenotypes in asymptomatic adults between the ages of 16 and 35 years. In this age range, approximately half of all adults have skin test reactivity, and about 25% will have significant methacholine airways responsiveness (9). An interaction of these intermediate phenotypes with the relevant environmental exposures will produce recrudescent (falsely incident) disease in the absence of knowledge of early life asthmatic events.

The magnitude of recall bias can only be assessed through longitudinal prospective studies. One such study, reported by Sears and colleagues, followed up a cohort of 713 children in Dunedin, New Zealand, who were initially seen at age six, nine, and 12 years. The study evaluated the presence or absence of airways responsiveness and its relationship to asthma symptoms (10). What is remarkable is that although a statistically significant relationship between current asthma and having methacholine responsiveness was demonstrated, almost half of the children in the survey with reported or unreported prior asthma had no current symptoms. Thus, roughly one fourth of all children with asthma in the past failed to recall their diagnosis of asthma 3 years later, suggesting the importance of recall bias. This group of prior asthmatics made up approximately half of all the asthma in this preadolescent group, and 47% had increased airways responsiveness. These prospective data demonstrate the importance of early childhood events and recall bias as important factors in the natural history of asthma.

Figure 8.2 summarizes the natural history of wheezing during the first 6 years of life and identifies a number of distinct groups based on symptoms. There is a group of persistent wheezers who begin wheezing during the first year of life, and continue to wheeze through age six. These persistent wheezers are characterized by early development of allergy, cord blood eosinophilia, wheezing with lower respiratory tract infections, and a family history of asthma and/or atopy (11). They are also characterized by lower lung function at birth. Although this group of persistent wheezers

represents a minority of the children who wheeze in the first year of life, they represent the vast majority of the children diagnosed with asthma at age six, virtually all of whom are atopic and have a parental history of asthma. Thus, certain features of asthma and its persistence emerge in this early childhood group. The greater the duration of symptoms, the stronger the parental history of asthma; the more atopy (presence of other allergic diseases such as atopic dermatitis or allergic rhinitis), the lower the lung function; and the more severe the disease, then the more likely it is to persist. Thus, emergence of allergy at an early age is important in the perpetuation of asthma in early childhood. Although the diagnostic label of asthma may depend on the provider or on access to a health care system, it seems clear from the epidemiologic data that the atopic asthmatic can be identified at a relatively early age.

There is a second group of transient wheezers in whom the major environmental exposure seems to be in utero tobacco smoke exposure. These individuals also have reduced levels of lung function (12). It is important to recognize that although this group may represent a distinct subphenotype, persistent wheezers may also be exposed to tobacco smoke so that there is overlap among transient early and the persistent wheezer.

Later Childhood and Adolescence (Age Seven through 16)

A significant number of early childhood wheezers will have decreases or disappearance of their symptoms in later childhood and adolescence. This is especially true among males. The reasons for this gender effect are unknown, but may possibly relate to the effects of female sex hormones on immune function (13). The degree of skin test reactivity and

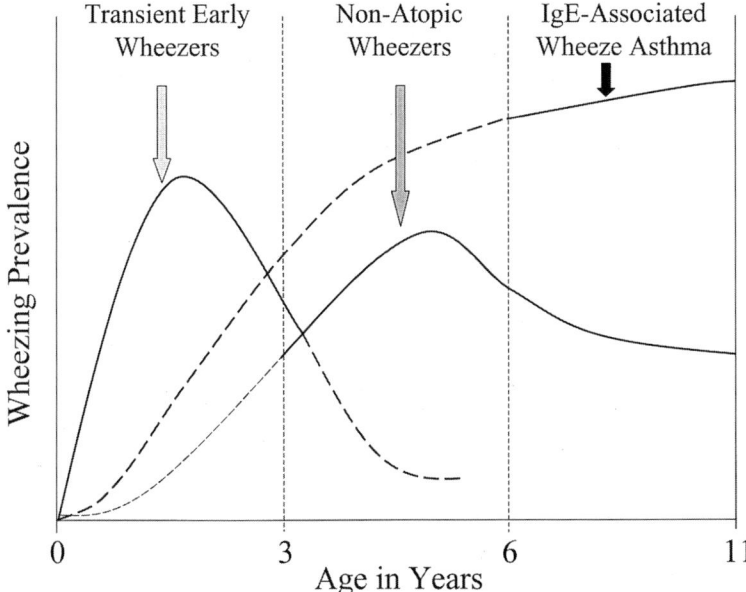

FIGURE 8.2. Histogram of wheeze prevalence vs. age. Three groups are depicted: transient early wheezers, nonatopic wheezers, and atopic wheezers. Note that these three phenotypes are not mutually exclusive.

continued allergen exposure are clearly risk factors for symptom persistence in this age group (14). The presence of allergy is one of the predictive factors for persistent disease. Just as in the early childhood group, those with symptoms will tend to develop more symptoms. It is also a clinical axiom that females with asthma after puberty are unlikely to experience reductions in their symptoms. Recently, it has been shown that obesity is one of the factors associated with asthma persistence in these young women. The mechanism of this association may relate to increased estrogen level with concomitant adverse effects on airway responsiveness and immune function (15).

Another important feature of this age group is the prevalence of cigarette smoking. Active smoking at this age, even smoking as little as one cigarette per day for as short a period as 3 years, can be associated with as much as a 10% reduction in maximal forced expiratory volume in 1 second (EV$_1$) from predicted values (16). The large effect of cigarette smoking during the adolescent growth spurt on pulmonary function contrasts to much smaller effects in later adult life. Finally, the presence of other atopic diseases, such as atopic dermatitis or allergic rhinitis, are also factors that are associated with the persistence of asthma in early adult life.

Early Adulthood (Age 16 to 35)

Maximum increases in FEV$_1$ occurs at about age 14 in females and age 21 in males (X. Wang, personal communication, 1997). Because lung function is maximal at this time, pulmonary symptoms are likely to be minimal. Thus, the model of a large group of subjects with asymptomatic airway hyperresponsiveness and/or allergy who are at risk for airway inflammation given the appropriate environmental exposure seems apt. Figure 8.3 depicts a log-normal population distribution of airway hyperresponsiveness. Susceptible individuals could move in or out of the symptomatic range, depending on particular environmental exposures. Again, in this age group, the presence of persistent symptoms is associated with lower levels of lung function and more severe disease, as emphasized by data from the Melbourne Study on the natural history of asthma (17). Symptom status at age 14 is correlated with lung function status both at age 14 and at age 21, and it is clear that those people with persistent symptoms are more likely to have lower levels of lung function.

The number of individuals in this group progressively decreases with increasing age, as there is a secular trend for symptoms to decrease from early childhood through early adulthood, as a result of lung growth. Prospective studies of individuals in this age range have demonstrated the importance of allergy, cigarette smoking, and airways responsiveness as predictors of the development of "incident" asthma in young adults. As noted earlier, it is likely that these are not truly "incident" cases, and that most of these adults had symptoms and/or the development of the intermediate phenotypes at an earlier age, but now appear incident because of a long lag time since the reporting of prior symptoms. Dodge and colleagues studied more than 1,000 subjects monitored for 12 years who were initially 15 to 19 of age (18). Positive skin prick tests and higher total IgE levels predicted the development of a diagnosis of asthma in this cohort. Carey and colleagues studied a prospective cohort of 281 children, 12 to 18 years of age, followed for 6 years (19). Those who had a positive airway challenge test to either cold air or methacholine were almost four times more likely to wheeze at the next visit compared with unresponsive individuals. Abramson and colleagues performed a cross-sectional study of 553 randomly selected young adults between the ages of 20 and 44 years (20). A family history of asthma (odds

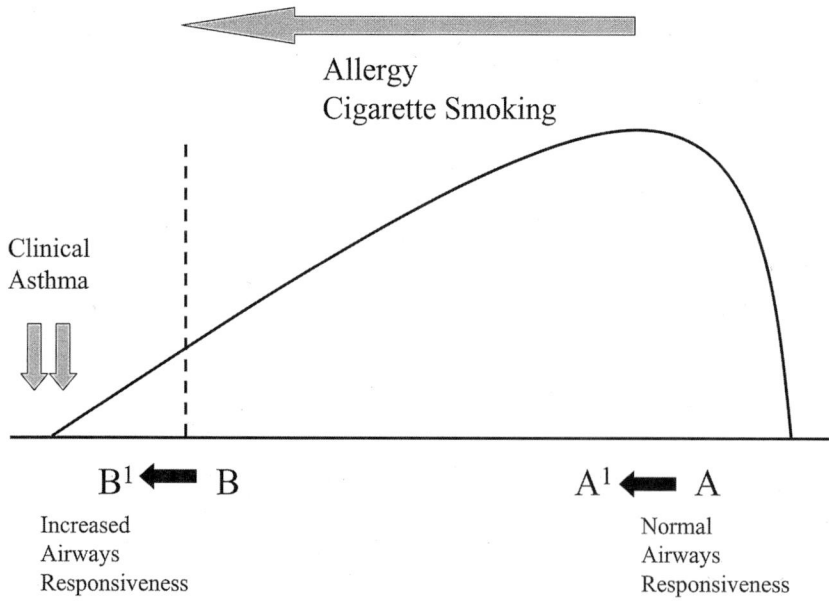

FIGURE 8.3. Schematic representation of risk for developing asthma as a function of genetic susceptibility and environmental exposures. Individuals without genetic susceptibility *(A)* may have some increased airways responsiveness with exposure to environmental factors such as allergic triggers and cigarette smoke *(A to A^1)*, but they do not cross the threshold for clinical asthma. Genetically predisposed individuals *(B)* can cross the threshold to develop clinical asthma *(B^1)* with such environmental exposures.

ratio, 2.4), current smoking (odds ratio, 1.7), and positive skin prick test (odds ratio, 5.9) were all independent predictors of adult asthma. Similar results have been found by Bodner (21). These data strongly support the suggestion that in young adults, smoking is strongly associated with a diagnosis of asthma (22).

Later Life

In the late 1980s, Burrows reported that women with relatively little smoking history were likely to develop severe chronic obstructive pulmonary disease (21). He noted that this fixed airflow obstruction was often associated with airways responsiveness and elevated IgE and positive skin prick tests, suggesting that the fixed airflow obstruction seen in these women was a function of an asthma diathesis interacting with cigarette smoking exposure. Because there is relatively little prospective data on young adults, the relationship of smoking, airways responsiveness, and allergy in this age group is less well described that in any other period of life.

PREVALENCE, INCIDENCE, MORBIDITY, AND MORTALITY: THE ASTHMA EPIDEMIC

Cross-sectional surveys, because they assess exposure and disease at the same point in time, cannot determine whether the exposure precedes disease onset or whether the disease somehow affects the subject's level of exposure. Prevalence (the proportion of the population that has a disease at a measured point in time), determined from these cross-sectional data, depends on both the incidence (the rate of occurrence of new disease during a measured time period) and the duration of the disease from its onset. In this instance, duration reflects both the degree to which atopy and asthma (wheeze syndromes) tend to persist or remit and the mortality associated with the disease. The number of people who die of asthma is relatively small and therefore is not likely to affect the incidence-duration relationship significantly (23).

The National Health Interview Survey reports the 12-month prevalence of asthma on a regular basis in the United States. In the 16-year period 1980 to 1996, the prevalence increased 73.9%, with the latest figure totalling 14.6 million people (Fig. 8.4). Since 1997, the Centers for Disease Control has been using a different reporting set of questions to determine prevalence, and hence, a sufficient time has not elapsed to allow us to know if the trends toward increasing prevalence are continuing. Over the relatively short time period of 1992 to 1999, Emergency Department (ED) visits for asthma increased by 36%, with the highest rates being noted for the youngest children (Fig. 8.5). In contrast to the ED data, the data on hospitalizations from the mid-1980s to the present suggests a decline (Fig. 8.6). Although the rate in the youngest age group had continually increased, it appears to have stabilized after 1998. Substantial regional variation

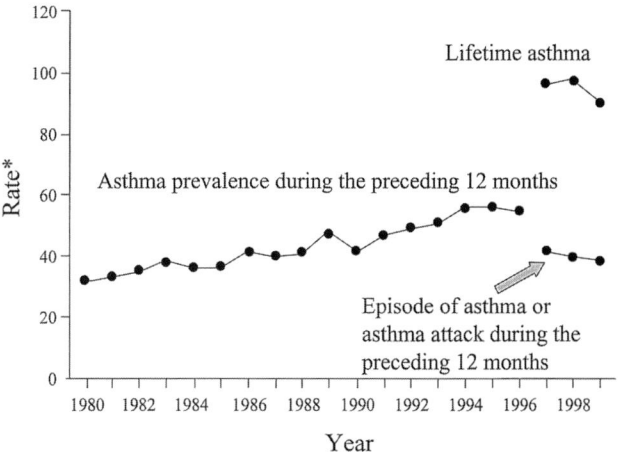

FIGURE 8.4. Estimated annual prevalence of asthma in the United States according to the National Health Interview Survey, 1980–1999. *Per 1,000 population; age adjusted to the 2000 U.S. population. (From Centers for Disease Control *MMWR* 2002;51[Suppl 1]:1–13, with permission.)

remains. Asthma deaths are relatively rare and occur for the most part in older subjects. Deaths increased steadily from 1980 to 1995, at which point they leveled off (Fig. 8.7). It is difficult to infer much meaning with regard to public health trends given that the overall rate is low and deaths have occurred disproportionately in the older population, whereas the prevalence increase has occurred in the young.

Counter-arguments regarding the veracity of these perceived trends introduce issues of potential bias. Diagnostic transfer and diagnostic bias have been central to the controversy. At the same time, increased public awareness of the signs and symptoms of asthma and its association with allergy may have resulted in its more frequent diagnosis by individuals and their health care providers since the 1970s.

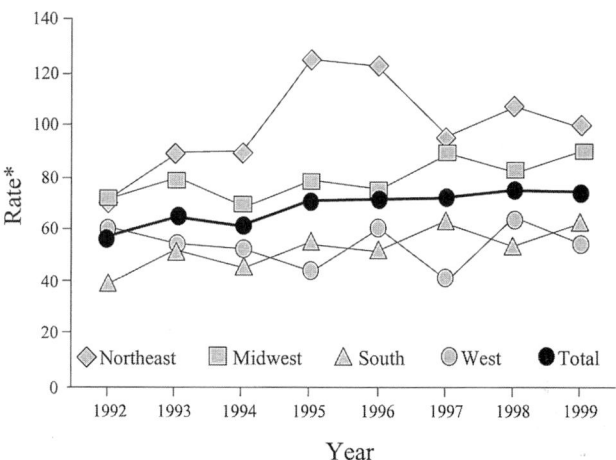

FIGURE 8.5. Estimated annual rate of emergency department visits for asthma as the first-listed diagnosis by region and year according to the National Hospital Ambulatory Medical Care Survey of the United States, 1992–1999. *Per 1,000 population; age adjusted to the 2000 U.S. population. (From Centers for Disease Control *MMWR* 2002;51[Suppl 1]:1–13, with permission.)

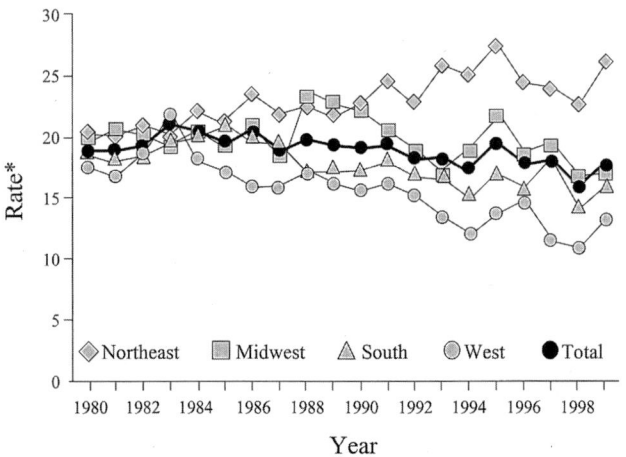

FIGURE 8.6. Estimated annual rate of hospitalization for asthma as the first-listed diagnosis by region and year according to the National Hospital Discharge Survey of the United States, 1980–1999. *Per 1,000 population; age adjusted to the 2000 U.S. population. (From Centers for Disease Control *MMWR* 2002;51[Suppl 1]:1–13, with permission.)

Several lines of evidence address these issues and, in the aggregate, lead to the conclusion that these alternative explanations are highly implausible. Weiss and colleagues considered the impact of diagnostic accuracy and diagnostic transfer on the U.S. data and concluded that although these factors contributed to the observed trends, they did not fully account for the observed prevalence increases (24). As Weiss and colleagues indicate, the International Classification of Diseases (ICD) codes were revised in 1979 such that, under the eighth revision (ICD-8), "bronchitis with mention of asthma" was coded as "bronchitis," whereas this same

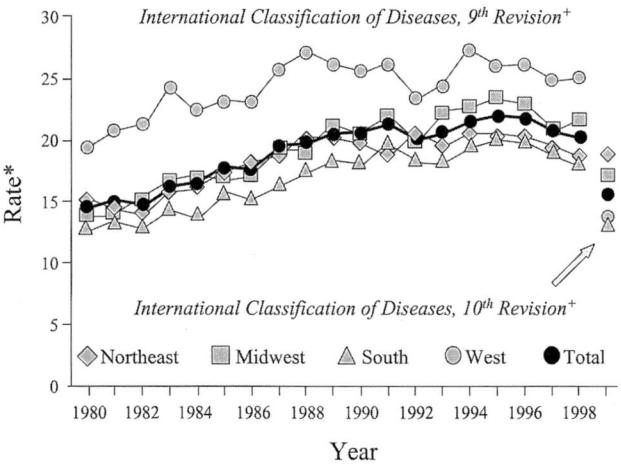

FIGURE 8.7. Annual rate of death for asthma as the underlying cause of death by region and year according to the Mortality Component of the National Vital Statistics System of the United States, 1980–1999. *Per 1,000 population; age adjusted to the 2000 U.S. population. +World Health Organization. *Manual of the international statistical classification of diseases, injuries, and causes of death, 10th revision.* Geneva, Switzerland: World Health Organization, 1999. (From Centers for Disease Control *MMWR* 2002;51[Suppl 1]:1–13, with permission.)

symptom complex was coded as "asthma" under the ninth revision (ICD-9). When hospitalization rates for asthma and bronchitis in children over the decade were examined, changes related to the ICD coding revisions were evident; however, rates for bronchitis remained essentially constant, whereas rates for asthma continued to rise. These data argue against a significant impact of diagnostic transfer from bronchitis to asthma hospitalization rates.

In the United States, it can be argued that diagnostic bias has influenced results in another way. Because it is widely accepted that many young children will "outgrow" their asthma, pediatricians are reluctant to make this diagnosis in early childhood. In addition, families with young children not infrequently transfer from one managed care health plan to another, in which case, asthma as a preexisting condition may make it difficult to obtain continuing health insurance. These American health care phenomena tend to cause under-diagnosis of asthma by pediatricians, especially in the preschool age group (i.e., children <5 years of age), yet this is exactly the population in which we have seen the greatest increase. Thus, the consensus is that diagnostic inaccuracy and increased public awareness have influenced the precision of the increase in the observed rates of asthma but do not fully explain it.

EMERGING RISK FACTORS TO EXPLAIN THE INCREASE IN ASTHMA

The prevalence data show that there has been a clear increase in asthma prevalence in the United States over the past 20 years. The observed increase in atopic diseases, which has occurred over one to three decades, is too rapid to be plausibly attributed to genetic mutation and change in the prevalence of genetic susceptibility alone.

This increase is most noticeable in the youngest age group and has prompted a focus on early-life environmental events that can influence immune system ontogeny in early and intermediate postnatal life, which might impact on genetic susceptibility. In particular, interest has focused on the role of three groups of factors—obesity, diet, and infection broadly (i.e., endotoxin exposure, day care attendance, viral and bacterial infections, vaccinations, antibiotic use)—and their role on immune system development.

The newborn period is dominated by T helper cell type 2 (Th2) reactivity, with both atopic and nonatopic individuals typically developing IgE and immunoglobin G antibodies in response to allergens. It is also evident that the T helper cell type 1 (Th1) memory cells selectively develop shortly after birth (i.e., at 3–6 months of age) and persist into adulthood in non-atopic subjects (25). Strong evidence indicates that the cellular immune response is not truly "naive" at birth (26–28). In a recent study, Holt and colleagues found that more than 80% of full-term babies demonstrate immunological priming (lymphoproliferation) to common allergens (29). Furthermore, accumulating evidence indicates that for most children who become allergic or asthmatic, the polarization of the immune system into an atopic phenotype likely occurs in the first few years of life (30).

DIET

Diet is a major source of allergen exposure in early childhood. Consumption of oily fish is negatively correlated with bronchial hyperreactivity (31) and is associated with a significantly reduced risk of current asthma in children (odds ratio, 0.26; 95% confidence interval, 0.09–0.72; $p <.01$) (32). Low salt intake has been associated with decreased bronchial hyperreactivity, improvement of asthma symptoms (33), and improved peak flows in asthmatic subjects (34) in short-term randomized controlled trials. Two large population-based studies have failed to convincingly show an association between airway responsiveness and 24-hour sodium intake (35). A series of small short-term clinical studies have found a positive association between vitamin C intake and decreased reactivity to methacholine challenge in asthmatics (36) and normal subjects (37, 38). One case control study of 12 asthmatics found an attenuation of exercise-induced bronchospasm as well as an improvement in the measured forced vital capacity with vitamin C intake (39). Other investigators have been unable to demonstrate a relationship between vitamin C intake and similar outcomes (40–42). Of note, studies with negative results tended to use lower doses of vitamin C. The epidemiologic data are also reasonably consistent. The Zutphen Study found that fruit and vegetable intake, a surrogate marker of vitamin C intake, was inversely related to the collective incidence of asthma, bronchitis, and emphysema. Miedema and colleagues found that higher fruit and vegetable intake was associated with approximately a 25% reduction in obstructive airway disease risk (odds ratio, 0.73; 95% confidence interval, 0.53–0.99) (43). Strachan and colleagues found that low levels of fresh fruit consumption was associated with an FEV_1 that was 809 mL lower, on average, than the value associated with regular fruit consumptions (44). Schwartz and Weiss found a relationship between low levels of vitamin C (assessed by 24-hour recall and a food frequency questionnaire) and lower levels of FEV_1 in subjects in the first National Health and Nutrition Examination Survey (45). Congruent with this finding, Britton and colleagues estimated that a 1-SD decrease in vitamin C intake had approximately the same effect as five pack years of cigarette smoking on the measured FEV_1 (46).

However, because these are cross-sectional studies, it is difficult to assess whether the onset of symptoms caused the change in vitamin C intake. Recent interest has focused on polyunsaturated fatty acids, particularly N-3 and N-6 fatty acids, as they may have effects on the developing immune system.

In summary, the study of diet as a risk factor and/or a potential modifier of the effect of other environmental exposures on the inception of asthma is in its early stages. Furthermore, of the few large-scale epidemiologic investigations that have been conducted, most are cross-sectional and focus on adults. The existing data are sufficiently persuasive regarding potentially important associations to warrant further investigation in this area. Given the now-accepted fact that the events of the first decade of life are most important in the inception of asthma and allergy, prospective studies of diet in young children are particularly needed.

OBESITY

From 1960–1994, the prevalence of overweight individuals in the United States has increased from 30.5% to 32% of the population, and the prevalence of overt obesity has increased from 12.8% to 22.5% of the population. Of note is that most of the increase in the prevalence of obesity occurred from 1976–1994, coincident with the asthma epidemic. The impact of increased weight on birth weight trends is less well identified. A variety of studies suggest that obesity influences asthma incidence. Epidemiologic data from the CARDIA Study (47) and the Nurses' Health Study (48) documented that increases in body mass index are associated with the development of "incident" asthma symptoms, particularly among adult women. This hardly explains the asthma epidemic, given the age of onset of the disease in early childhood. Data from the Tucson Epidemiologic Study supports a persistence of asthma symptoms in obese adolescent girls (49). The mechanisms by which obesity could potentially influence asthma are through mechanical factors leading to a decreased functional residual capacity and decreased tidal volume with less smooth muscle stretch, or through inflammatory or immune modification, increases in estrogen, or precipitating gastroesophageal reflux. The interactions of obesity in asthma have been detailed in numerous review articles (50), and these effects may be totally independent from effects of diet and physical activity.

HYGIENE HYPOTHESIS (INFECTION)

These increases in prevalence appear to track with the "westernization" of society. Asthma and atopy are most prevalent in economically developed and affluent parts of the world. Asthma and allergy occur more commonly in Western societies (e.g., the United States, Europe, and Australia) and are notably rare or uncommon in non-Western societies, particularly among children. Studies from the developing world have shown a disparity between rural and urban areas in terms of asthma prevalence in genetically similar populations (51–53). Both the significant increase in prevalence and the geographical variation of prevalence (most notably between developed and undeveloped countries and regions) argue strongly for environmental causes underlying these trends in any given population.

An inverse relation between the number of older siblings in families and the incidence of allergy, first demonstrated by Strachan (44) in British households and supported by data from German reunification (55), led to the theory that increased exposure to certain infections in early childhood may be protective against asthma. This has been termed the hygiene hypothesis.

Shaheen et al. reported a reduction in atopy in relation to a specific childhood viral infection (measles), providing further support for the notion that some early childhood infections may prevent allergic sensitization (56). A documented history of measles infection was associated with a decrease in skin-prick test positivity to dust-mite allergen (odds ratio, 0.20; 95% confidence interval, 0.05–0.81; $p < .02$) (57). Experimental evidence suggests that a high rate of infections early in life can result in up-regulation of the T-cell immune response nonatopic phenotype, selecting for interferon-γ–secreting Th1 cells while inhibiting the development of interleukin-4–secreting Th2 cells (58, 59). No specific infectious agent has been identified that could account for the increase, but day care attendance as a protective factor and reductions in endotoxin exposure as a causative factor are worth mentioning.

Further support for this hypothesis comes from two prospective studies of day care attendance in the first years of life. Ball and colleagues have shown that day care attendance is protective for the development of asthma and allergies at age six in a general population sample (61). Celedon and colleagues confirmed this finding in a prospective birth cohort study of infants of allergic parents and demonstrated that the protective effect was confined to the group of children with a low genetic risk of allergic disease (62). The nature of the protective agent in day care centers is unclear but could be endotoxin or the increased occurrence of colds and infections. Bacterial infections also influence immune system development. Thus, the overall decline in bacterial infections in Western industrialized countries over the past 30 years and/or an increase in antibiotic use could be contributing to a rise in asthma prevalence. No data have yet been collected related to these hypotheses.

Vaccination could be affecting the expression of the Th1/Th2 immune phenotype in childhood and, hence, influencing asthma and allergy risk. In contrast to measles infection, measles vaccination appears not to be protective against asthma (63). In at least one report from Japan, bacille Calmette-Guérin vaccination appeared to be protective against atopy (64). Several studies of vaccination have failed to find either a protective benefit or an increased risk for developing asthma associated with the usual childhood vaccinations. There has also been no association found between vaccination trends in children and the increase in asthma and allergic disease. Thus, vaccination would not appear to be a substantial risk.

Overall, infectious disease influences on immune system development will reflect the sum of an individual's exposures, including viral, bacterial, and parasitic infections, as well as vaccinations. Timing and concomitant exposure to other factors potentially important to the development of asthma or allergy (e.g., dietary components, allergens, cigarette smoke) may also be critical.

A series of epidemiologic reports suggest that there is a decreased frequency of allergy and asthma among children of farmers in Western industrialized countries. This has led investigators to measure endotoxin, a lipopolysaccharide that is a constitutive component of the outer layer of the cell membrane of Gram-negative bacteria. Endotoxin is present in the fecal flora of larger mammals such as cows, horses, pigs, and dogs. The decline in farming and the presence of domestic animals has occurred coincident with the rise in allergies and asthma and, thus, is consistent with the trends seen both internationally and within Western developed countries. Recently, investigators have measured endotoxin levels in mattress dust and found a relationship between higher levels of endotoxin and dust and a decreased frequency of hay fever, allergic asthma, and allergic sensitization in children in both farming and nonfarming households in rural areas of central Europe (60). The exact mechanisms by which endotoxin might decrease allergies and allergic asthma are unknown; however, signaling through the innate immune pathway resulting in a more normal immune system ontogeny in early life is a leading hypothesis that needs to be tested. At low doses, endotoxin is an inducer of interleukin-12 and interferon-γ cytokines that stimulate Th1-mediated immunity. Further studies are needed to assess whether endotoxin or other environmental exposures, such as heat-shock protein or β1-3 glucan, mediate these effects.

STRESS

It has long been speculated that psychologic stress can influence wheeze and asthma in early life (65). Although a causative link has not yet been clearly established, several lines of research suggest that psychologic stress may be a factor contributing to childhood respiratory illness and wheeze (66). Wright and colleagues have recently shown that the perceived stress of the caregiver remained a significant predictor of asthma in the recipient, even after controlling for factors potentially associated with both stress and wheeze (parental asthma, socioeconomic status, race/ethnicity), and for potential mediators through which stress might have influenced wheeze (smoking, breast-feeding, birth weight, lower respiratory infections) (67). They felt that stress in early life was associated with an increased risk of repeated wheeze in a genetically predisposed birth cohort, even after controlling for factors associated with stress and wheeze, as well as for potential mediators through which stress influenced wheeze.

Psychologic stress might impact asthma risk by affecting neuroendocrine and immune processes that promote airway inflammation and obstruction (68). Psychologic stress has been associated with the activation of the hypothalamic-pituitary-adrenal (HPA) axis and disturbed regulation of the HPA system. Some optimal level of mediators is needed to maintain a functional balance, and the absence of appropriate levels of glucocorticoids and catecholamines may allow immune mediators to overreact and increase the risk of inflammatory disorders such as asthma (69). Gestational exposures to maternal stress have been shown to alter the development of humoral immunocompetence in offspring, as well as their hormonal and immunologic responses to postnatal stress (70–72). Evidence in rhesus monkeys indicates that stress experienced during pregnancy impacts the infants' response to antigens at birth (73). Some speculate that stress triggers hormonal production in early life that favors Th2 cell predominance, perhaps through direct influence of stress hormones on cytokines that subsequently modulate the direction of differentiation. A substantial literature exists demonstrating how psychologic stress can influence cell trafficking, T-cell function, and lymphocyte production of cytokines (74). Stress can modulate immune response through pathways connecting the autonomic nervous system, endocrine regulation, and the immune system by triggering the release of hormones and neuropeptides that interact with immune cells (75, 76). This phenomenon includes stress-elicited changes of cytokine production (77, 78).

SUMMARY

In summary, asthma is a disease that begins in early childhood with 90% of all cases diagnosed by the age of 6 years. As a result of this, recall bias is a major problem with regard to incident events later in life. In addition, there is a disconnection between the presence of the intermediate phenotypes of allergy and airways responsiveness and the presence of respiratory symptoms used by physicians to make an asthma diagnosis. Despite these difficulties, asthma prevalence has increased substantially in the United States. There has been an increase in prevalence of almost 75% in the 16-year period 1980–1996. Unfortunately, current reporting does not allow direct comparison between current prevalence and the prevalence in 1996. The current paradigm suggest that factors influencing the immune system ontogeny in early life—i.e., diet, obesity, and infections or infectious agents or their cell wall constituents (endotoxin)—are the primary factors that have changed gradually over a 25- to 30-year period, leading to the increase in allergic diseases.

Work focused on understanding the underlying genetic and pathophysiologic mechanisms by which these environmental exposures influence prevalence is ongoing.

REFERENCES

1. NHLBI/WHO Workshop Report. Global initiative for asthma. Bethesda, MD: National Institutes of Health; 1995;95–3659.
2. Holgate ST. Asthma: a dynamic disease of inflammation and repair. *The rising trends in Asthma.* West Sussex, England: John Wiley & Sons, 1997:5–28.
3. Hennekens CH, Buring JE. *Epidemiology in medicine.* Boston: Little, Brown and Company, 1987:3.
4. Ebell B *The papyrus ebers.* Copenhagen: Levin Munksgaard, 1937.
5. Epstein I. *The babylonian talmud.* London: Soncino, 1935.
6. Rosen Z. Nasal allergy in biblical and talmudic times. *Ann Allergy* 1971;29:260–262.
7. Yunginger JW, Reed CE, O'Connell EJ, et al. A community-based study of the epidemiology of asthma. *Am Rev Respir Dis* 1992;146:888–894.
8. Gold DR, Burge HA, Carey V, et al. Predictors of repeated wheeze in the first year of life: the relative roles of cockroach, birth weigh, acute lower respiratory illness, and maternal smoking. *Am J Respir Crit Care Med* 1999;160:227–236.
9. Weiss ST, Sparrow D, eds. *Airways responsiveness and atopy in the development of the obstructive airways disease.* New York: Raven Press, 1989.
10. Sears MR, Burrows B, Flannery EM, et al. Relation between airway responsiveness and serum IgE in children with asthma and apparently normal children. *N Engl J Med* 1991;325:1067–1071.
11. Wright AL, Sherrill D, Holberg CJ, et al. Breast-feeding, maternal IgE, and total serum IgE in childhood. *J Allergy Clin Immunol* 1999;104:589–594.
12. Martinez FD. Role of respiratory infection in onset of asthma and chronic obstructive pulmonary disease. *Clin Exp Allergy* 1999;54[Suppl 49]:24–28.
13. Weiss ST, Segal MR, Tager IB, et al. Effects of asthma on pulmonary function in children: a longitudinal population-based study. *Am Rev Respir Dis* 1992;145:58–64.
14. Zeiger RS, Dawson C, Weiss ST. Childhood Asthma Management Program (CAMP) Research Group. Relationship between duration of asthma and asthma severity among children in the Childhood Asthma Management Program (CAMP). *J Allergy Clin Immunol* 1999;103:376–387.
15. Castro-Rodriguez JA, Holberg CJ, Morgan WJ, et al. Weight and early puberty are risk factors for increased wheezing in females. *Am J Respir Crit Care Med* 2000;161:A498.
16. Tager IB, Munoz A, Rosner B, et al. Effect of cigarette smoking on the pulmonary function of children and adolescents. *Am Rev Respir Dis* 1985;131:752–759.
17. Kelly WJW, Hudson I, et al. Childhood asthma and adult lung function. *Am Rev Respir Dis* 1988;138:26–30.
18. Dodge R, Cline MG, Lebowitz MD, et al. Findings before the diagnosis of asthma in young adults. *J Allergy Clin Immunol* 1994;94:831–835.
19. Carey VJ, Weiss ST, Tager IB, et al. Airway responsiveness, wheeze onset, and recurrent asthma episodes in young adolescents: the East Boston Childhood Respiratory Disease Cohort. *Am J Respir Crit Care Med* 1996;153:356–361.
20. Abramson M, Kutin JJ, Raven J, et al. Risk factors for asthma among young adults in Melbourne, Australia. *Respirology* 1996;1:291–297.

21. Bodner CH, Ross S, Little J, et al. Risk factors for adult on-set wheeze: a case control study. *Am J Respir Crit Care Med* 1998;157:35–42.

22. Burrows B, Bloom JW, Traver GA, et al. The course and prognosis of different forms of chronic airway obstruction in a sample from the general population. *N Engl J Med* 1987;317:1309–1314.

23. Woolcock AJ. Asthma-disease of a modern lifestyle. *Med J Aust* 1996;165:358–359.

24. Weiss KB, Gergen PJ, Wagener DK. Breathing better or wheezing worse? the changing epidemiology of asthma morbidity and mortality. *Annu Rev Publ Health.* 1993;14:491–513.

25. Holt PG. Immunoprophylaxis of atopy: light at the end of the tunnel. *Immunol Today* 1994;15:484–489.

26. Rinas U, Horneff G, Wahn V. Interferon-γ production by cord-blood mononuclear cells is reduced in newborns with a family history of atopic disease and is independent from cord blood IgE-levels. *Pediatr Allergy Immunol* 1993;4:60–4.

27. Tang MLK, Kemp AS, Thorburn J, et al. Reduced interferon-γ secretion in neonates and subsequent atopy. *Lancet* 1994;344:983–986.

28. Liao SY, Liao TN, Chiang BL, et al. Decreased production of IFN and decreased production of IL-6 by cord blood mononuclear cells of newborns with a high risk of allergy. *Clin Exp Allergy* 1996;26:397–405.

29. Prescott SL, Sly PD, Holt PG. Maturation of immune responses to aeroallergens in the early postnatal period: pediatric asthma: A to Z. San Francisco, CA: American Thoracic Society postgraduate course, May 1997.

30. Yabuhara A, Macaubas C, Prescott Sl, et al. Th-2-polarised immunological memory to inhalant allergens in atopics is established during infancy and early childhood. *Clin Exp Allergy* 1997:1261–1269.

31. Peat JK, Haby M, Spijker J, et al. Prevalence of asthma in adults in Busselton, Western Australia. *BMJ* 1992;305:1326–1329.

32. Hodge L, Salome CM, Peat JK, et al. Consumption of oily fish and childhood asthma risk. *MJA* 1996;164:137–140.

33. Javid A, Cushley MJ, Bone MF. Effect of dietary salt on bronchial reactivity to histamine in asthma. *BMJ* 1988;297;454.

34. Medici TS, Schmidt AZ, Hacki M, et al. Are asthmatics salt sensitive? *Chest* 1993;104:1138–1143.

35. Britton J, Pavord I, Richards K, et al. Dietary sodium intake and the risk of airway hyperreactivity in a random adult population. *Thorax* 1994;49:875–880.

36. Mohsenin V, DuBois AB, Douglas JS. Effect of ascorbic acid on response to methacholine challenge in asthmatic subjects. *Am Rev Respir Dis* 1983;127:143–147.

37. Ogilvy CS, DuBois AB, Douglas JS. Effect of ascorbic acid and indomethacin on the airways of healthy male subjects with and without induced bronchoconstriction. *J Allergy Clin Immunol* 1981;67:363–369.

38. Zuskin E, Lewis AJ, Boubays A. Inhibition of histamine induced airway constriction by ascorbic acid. *Allergy Clin Immunol* 1973;51:218–226.

39. Schacter EN, Schlesinger A. The attenuation of exercise induced bronchospasm by ascorbic acid. *Ann Allergy* 1982;49:146–151.

40. Ting S, Mansfield LE, Yarborough J. Effects of ascorbic acid on pulmonary functions in mild asthma. *J Asthma* 1983;20:39–42.

41. Malo JL, Cartier A, Pineau L, et al. Lack of effects of ascorbic acid on spirometry and airway responsiveness to histamine in subjects with asthma. *J Allergy Clin Immunol* 1986;78:453–458.

42. Hunt HB. Ascorbic acid in bronchial asthma. *BMJ* 1938;1:726.

43. Miedema I, Feskens EJM, Heederik D, et al. Dietary determinants of long term incidence of chronic nonspecific lung disease. *Am J Epidemiol* 1993;138:37–45.

44. Strachan DP, Cox BD, Erzinclioglu SW, et al. Ventilatory function and winter fresh fruit consumption in a random sample of British adults. *Thorax* 1991;46:624–629.

45. Schwartz J, Weiss ST. The relationship of dietary vitamin C intake to level of pulmonary function in the First National Health and Nutrition Survey (NHANES I). *Am J Clin Nutr* 1994;59:110–114.

46. Britton JR, Pavord ID, Richards KA, et al. Dietary antioxidant vitamin intake and lung function in the general population. *Am J Respir Crit Care Med* 1995;151:1383–1387.

47. Beckett WE, Jacobs DR Jr, Xu X, et al. Asthma is associated with weight gain in females but not males, independent of physical activity. *Am J Respir Crit Care Med* 2001;164:2045–2050.

48. Camargo CA Jr, Weiss ST, Zhang S, et al. Prospective study of body mass index, weight change, and risk of adult-onset asthma in women. *Arch Intern Med* 1999;159:2582–2588.

49. Castro-Rodriguez JA, Holber CJ, Morgan WJ, et al. Increased incidence of asthmalike symptoms in girls who become overweight or obese during the school years. *Am J Respir Crit Care Med* 2001;163:1344–1349.

50. Tantisira KG, Weiss ST. Complex interactions in complex traits: obesity and asthma. *BMJ* 2000;320:827–832.

51. Wuthrich B, Schindler C, Leuenberger P, et al. Prevalence of atopy and pollinosis in the adult population of Switzerland (SAPALDIA Study). *Int Arch Allergy Immunol* 1995;106:149–156.

52. Mitchel C, Miles J. Lower respiratory tract symptoms in Queensland schoolchildren. *Aust NZ J Med* 1983;13:264–269.

53. Weiss ST, Tager IB, Weiss JW, et al. Airways responsiveness in a population sample of adults and children. *Am Rev Respir Dis* 1984;129:898–902.

54. Welty C, Weiss ST, Tager IB, et al. The relationship of airways responsiveness to cold air, cigarette smoking and atopy to respiratory symptoms and pulmonary function in adults. *Am Rev Respir Dis* 1984;130:198–203.

55. Burr ML, St. Leger AS, Bevan C, et al. A community survey of asthmatic characteristics. *Thorax* 1975;30:663–668.

56. Burney PGJ, Laitinen LA, Perdrizet S, et al. Validity and repeatability of the IUATLD bronchial symptoms questionnaire: an international comparison. *Eur Respir J* 1984;2:940–945.

57. Shaheen SO, Aaby P, Hall AJ, et al. Measles and atopy in Guinea-Bissau. *Lancet* 1996;347:1792–1796.

58. Centers for Disease Control. Asthma: United States, 1980–1990. *MMWR* 1992;41:733–735.

59. Barbee RA, Dodge PR, Lebowitz ML, et al. The epidemiology of asthma. *Chest* 1985;87:21S–25S.

60. Braun-Fahrlander C, Riedler J, Hertz U, et al. Environmental exposure to endotoxin and its relationship to asthma in school age children. *N Engl J Med* 2002;347:869–877.

61. Ball TM, Castro-Rodriguez JA, Griffith KA, et al. Siblings, day-care attendance, and the risk of asthma and wheezing during childhood. *N Engl J Med* 2000;343:538–543.

62. Celedon JC, Litonjua AA, Ryan L, et al. Day care attendance, respiratory tract illnesses, wheezing, asthma, and total serum IgE level in early childhood. *Arch Pediatr Adolesc Med* 2002;156:241–245.

63. Dodge RR, Burrows B. The prevalence and incidence of asthma and asthma-like symptoms in a general population sample. *Am Rev Respir Dis* 1980;122:567–575.

64. Croner S, Kjellman M-I M. Natural history of bronchial asthma in childhood: a prospective study from birth up to 12-14 years of age. *Allergy* 1992;47:150–157.

65. Minuchin S, Gaker L, Rosman BL, et al. A conceptual model of psychosomatic illness in children. Family organization and family therapy. *Arch Gen Psychiatry* 1975;32:1031–1038.

66. Wright RJ, Rodriguez M, Cohen S. Review of psychosocial stress and asthma: an integrated biopsychosocial approach. *Thorax* 1998;53:1066–1074.

67. Wright RJ, Cohen S, Carey V, et al. Parental stress as a predictor of wheezing in infancy: a prospective birth-cohort study. *Am J Respir Crit Care Med* 2002;165:358–365.

68. Wright RJ, Rodriguez M, Cohen S. Review of psychosocial stress and asthma: an integrated biopsychosocial approach. *Thorax* 1998;53:1066–1074.

69. Sternberg EM. Neural-immune interactions in health and disease. *J Clin Invest* 1997;100:2641–2647.

70. Sobrian SK, Vaughn VT, Ashe WK, et al. Gestational exposure to loud noise alters the development and postnatal responsiveness of humoral and cellular components of the immune system in offspring. *Environ Res* 1997;73:227–241.

71. Coe CL, Lubach GR, Karaszewski JW. Prenatal stress and immune recognition of self and nonself in the primate neonate. *Biol Neonate* 1999;76:301–310.

72. Reyes TM, Coe CE. Prenatal manipulations reduce the proinflammatory response to a cytokine challenge in juvenile monkeys. *Brain Res* 1997;769:29–35.

73. Coe CL, Lubach GR, Karaszewski JW, et al. Prenatal endocrine activation alters postnatal cellular immunity in infant monkeys. *Brain Behav Immun* 1996;10:221–234.

74. Herbert T, Cohen S. Stress and immunity in humans: a meta-analytic review. *Psychosom Med* 1993;55:364–379.

75. Cohen S, Herbert T. Health psychology: psychological factors and physical disease from the perspective of human psychoneuroimmunology. *Annu Rev Psychol* 1996;47:113–142.

76. Kiecolt-Glaser JK, Cacioppo JT, Malarkey WB, et al. Acute psychological stressors and short-term immune changes: what, why, for whom, and to what extent? *Psychosom Med* 1992;54:680–685.

77. Dobbin JP, Harht M, McCain GA, et al. Cytokine production and lymphocyte transformation during stress. *Brain Behav Immun* 1991;5:339–348.

78. Glaser R, Kennedy S, Lafuse WP, et al. Psychological stress-induced modulation of interleukin 2 receptor gene expression and interleukin 2 production in peripheral blood leukocytes. *Arch Gen Psychiatr* 1990;47:707–712.

9 Pathophysiology of Asthma

Peter J. Barnes

Asthma is characterized by a specific pattern of inflammation that is largely driven by immunoglobulin E (IgE)–dependent mechanisms. Genetic factors are an important influence on whether atopy develops, and several genes have now been identified (1). Most of the genetic linkages reported for asthma are common to all allergic diseases (2). However, environmental factors appear to be more important in determining whether asthma develops in an atopic individual, although genetic factors may affect how severely the disease is expressed and the degree of amplification of the inflammatory response.

INFLAMMATION

It has been recognized for many years that patients who die of acute attacks of asthma have grossly inflamed airways. The airway lumen is occluded by a tenacious mucus plug composed of plasma proteins exuded from airway vessels and mucus glycoproteins secreted from surface epithelial cells. The airway wall is edematous and infiltrated by inflammatory cells, which are predominantly eosinophils and lymphocytes. The airway epithelium is invariably shed in a patchy manner, and clumps of epithelial cells are found in the airway lumen. Occasionally, when opportunities have arisen to examine the airways of asthmatic patients who died accidentally, similar although less marked inflammatory changes have been observed (3). More recently, it has been possible to examine the airways of asthmatic patients by fiberoptic and rigid bronchoscopy, bronchial biopsy, and bronchoalveolar lavage (BAL). Direct bronchoscopy reveals that the airways of asthmatic patients are often reddened and swollen, indi-

cating acute inflammation. Lavage has revealed an increase in the numbers of lymphocytes, mast cells, and eosinophils, and examination of the macrophages has revealed that they are activated in comparison with macrophages obtained from controls without asthma. Examination of biopsy material has revealed increased numbers and activation of mast cells, macrophages, eosinophils, and T lymphocytes (4,5). These changes are found even in patients with mild asthma who have few symptoms. All evidence to date suggests that asthma is an inflammatory condition of the airways.

Inflammation is classically characterized by four cardinal signs: *calor* and *rubor* (caused by vasodilation), *tumor* (caused by plasma exudation and edema), and *dolor* (caused by sensitization and activation of sensory nerves). It is now recognized that inflammation is also characterized by an infiltration with inflammatory cells and that the types and numbers of cells differ depending on the type of inflammatory process. Inflammation is an important defense response that defends the body against invasion by microorganisms and against the effects of external toxins. The inflammation in allergic asthma is driven on exposure to allergens through IgE-dependent mechanisms, resulting in a characteristic pattern of inflammation. This allergic inflammatory response consists of an infiltration with eosinophils and resembles the inflammatory process mounted in response to parasitic and worm infections. The inflammatory response not only provides an acute defense against injury but also is involved in the healing and restoration of normal function after tissue damage resulting from infection or exposure to toxins. In asthma, the inflammatory response is activated inappropriately and is harmful rather than beneficial. It is unknown why some allergens, such as house dust mite and pollen proteins, induce a eosinophilic inflammation. Normally, such an inflammatory response would kill the invading parasite (or vice versa) and would therefore be self-limiting, but in allergic disease, the inciting stimulus persists and the acute

P. J. Barnes: Department of Thoracic Medicine, National Heart and Lung Institute, Imperial College, London, United Kingdom.

inflammatory response is converted into a chronic inflammation that may have structural consequences in the airways and skin.

Intrinsic Asthma

Although most patients with asthma have atopy, some exhibit no evidence of atopy, with normal levels of total and specific IgE and negative skin test results. These individuals are said to have "intrinsic" asthma. This entity arises later in life and tends to be more severe than allergic asthma (6). The pathophysiology is very similar to that of allergic asthma, and evidence is increasing for *local* IgE production, possibly directed at bacterial or viral antigens (7).

Inflammation and Airway Hyperresponsiveness

The relationship between inflammation and the clinical symptoms of allergy is not yet clear. Evidence suggests that the degree of inflammation is related to airway hyperresponsiveness, measured by histamine or methacholine challenge. Increased airway responsiveness is an exaggerated airway narrowing in response to many stimuli and is the defining characteristic of asthma. The degree of airway hyperresponsiveness is related to asthma symptoms and the need for treatment. Inflammation of the airways may increase airway responsiveness and thereby allow triggers that would not normally narrow the airways to do so. Inflammation may also directly lead to an increase in asthma symptoms, such as cough and chest tightness, through the activation of airway sensory nerve endings (Fig. 9.1).

Persistence of Inflammation

Although most attention has focused on the inflammatory changes seen during acute episodes of asthma, inflammation persists in most patients for years, making asthma a chronic condition. The mechanisms involved in the persistence of inflammation are poorly understood. Usually, the chronic inflammatory state is punctuated by acute inflammatory episodes that correspond to exacerbations of clinical asthma.

INFLAMMATORY CELLS

Many different inflammatory cells are involved in asthma, but the precise role of each cell type is not yet certain (4). It has become evident that although no single inflammatory cell can account for the complex pathophysiology of allergic disease, certain cells do predominate in asthmatic inflammation.

Mast Cells

Mast cells initiate the acute bronchoconstrictor responses to allergens and probably also to other indirect stimuli, such as exercise and hyperventilation (via osmolality or thermal changes). They also play an important role in inducing symptoms of rhinitis after exposure to allergens, such as grass pollen. Treating asthmatic patients with prednisone results in a decrease in the number of tryptase-positive mast cells (8). Furthermore, mast cell tryptase appears to play a role in airway remodeling because this mast cell product stimulates human lung fibroblast proliferation (9). Mast cells also secrete certain cytokines, such as interleukin-4 (IL-4) and tumor necrosis factor-α (TNF-α), that may be involved in maintaining the allergic inflammatory response (10).

However, questions have been raised about the role of mast cells in chronic allergic inflammation, and it seems probable that other cells, such as macrophages, eosinophils, and T lymphocytes, are more important in chronic inflammatory processes, including airway hyperresponsiveness. Classically, mast cells are activated by allergens through an IgE-dependent mechanism. The importance of IgE in the pathophysiology of asthma has been highlighted by

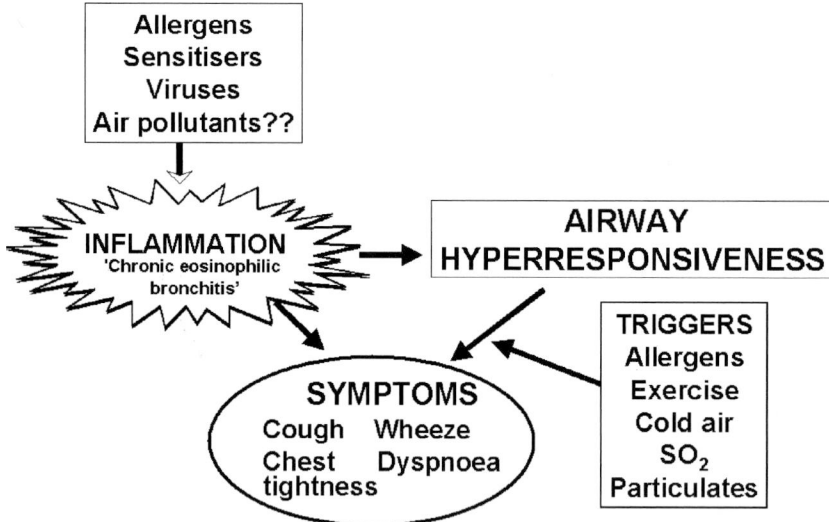

FIGURE 9.1. Inflammation in the airways of asthmatic patients leads to airway hyperresponsiveness and symptoms.

clinical studies with humanized anti-IgE antibodies, which inhibit IgE-mediated effects (11,12). Although anti-IgE antibody reduces circulating IgE to undetectable levels, this treatment produces only minimal clinical improvement in patients with severe, steroid-dependent asthma (13). Interestingly, the anti-IgE monoclonal antibody treatment did allow a reduction of the dose of steroids necessary to control asthma. This observation suggests that the mechanisms whereby IgE leads to airway obstruction are steroid-sensitive, although corticosteroids do not reduce, and may even increase, circulating levels of IgE (14,15).

It is now increasingly recognized that mast cells may also release several other mediators that play a role in the pathophysiology of asthma, including neurotrophins, proinflammatory cytokines, chemokines, and growth factors. This understanding has led to a reevaluation of the role of mast cells, particularly during exacerbations (16).

Macrophages

Macrophages, which are derived from blood monocytes, traffic into the airways and may be activated by allergen via low-affinity IgE receptors ($Fc_\epsilon RII$) (17,18). The enormous immunologic repertoire of macrophages allows these cells to form many different products, including a large variety of cytokines, that help orchestrate the inflammatory response. Macrophages have the capacity to initiate a particular type of inflammatory response through the release of a certain pattern of cytokines. Macrophages may both increase and decrease inflammation, depending on the stimulus. Alveolar macrophages normally have a *suppressive* effect on lymphocyte function, but this may be impaired in asthma after allergen exposure (19). One antiinflammatory protein secreted by macrophages is IL-10, and its secretion is reduced in patients with asthma (20). Macrophages from normal subjects also inhibit the secretion of IL-5 from T lymphocytes, probably through the release of IL-12, but this process is defective in patients with allergic asthma (21). Macrophages may therefore play an important antiinflammatory role by preventing the development of allergic inflammation. Macrophages also act as antigen-presenting cells, which process allergen for presentation to T lymphocytes, although alveolar macrophages are far less effective in this respect than macrophages from other sites, such as the peritoneum (22).

Certain subtypes of macrophages may perform different inflammatory, antiinflammatory, or phagocytic roles in allergic disease. Immunologic markers that distinguish these subpopulations are beginning to emerge (23). However, no differences have been detected between the macrophage population in the induced sputum of allergic asthmatic persons and that in normal subjects (24).

Dendritic Cells

Dendritic cells are specialized macrophage-like cells that have a unique ability to induce a T lymphocyte–mediated immune response and therefore play a critical role in the development of asthma (25). Dendritic cells in the respiratory tract form a network that is localized to the epithelium and act as very effective antigen-presenting cells (26). It is likely that dendritic cells play an important role in the initiation of allergen-induced responses in asthma (27). Dendritic cells take up allergens, process them to peptides, and then migrate to local lymph nodes, where they present the allergenic peptides to uncommitted T lymphocytes. With the aid of costimulatory molecules, such as B7.1, B7.2, and CD40, they program the production of allergen-specific T cells. Animal studies have demonstrated that myeloid dendritic cells are critical to the development of T helper subset 2 (Th2) cells and eosinophilia (28). Immature dendritic cells in the respiratory tract promote Th2-cell differentiation and require cytokines such as IL-12 and TNF-α to promote the normally preponderant Th1 response (29). Dendritic cell–based immunotherapy may be developed in the future to prevent and control allergic diseases.

Eosinophils

Eosinophil infiltration is a characteristic feature of allergic inflammation. Asthma might more accurately be termed *chronic eosinophilic bronchitis* (a term noted as early as 1916). Allergen inhalation results in a marked increase in eosinophils in BAL fluid at the time of the late reaction, and a correlation has been found between eosinophil counts in peripheral blood or BAL fluid and airway hyperresponsiveness. Eosinophils are linked to the development of airway hyperresponsiveness through the release of basic proteins and oxygen-derived free radicals (30,31). Experimentally activated eosinophils have been shown to induce airway epithelial damage, a characteristic of patients with asthma (32).

Several mechanisms are involved in the *recruitment* of eosinophils into the airways (33). Eosinophils are derived from bone marrow precursors. After allergen challenge, eosinophils appear in BAL fluid during the late response, and this is associated with a decrease in peripheral eosinophil counts and with the appearance of eosinophil progenitors in the circulation (34). The signal for increased eosinophil production is presumably derived from the inflamed airway. Eosinophil recruitment initially involves adhesion of eosinophils to vascular endothelial cells in the airway circulation, followed by migration into the submucosa and subsequent activation. The role of individual adhesion molecules, cytokines, and mediators in orchestrating these responses has been extensively investigated. Adhesion of eosinophils involves the expression of specific glycoprotein molecules on the eosinophil cell surface (integrins) and a similar expression on vascular endothelial cells (intercellular adhesion molecule-1 [ICAM-1]) (35,36). An antibody directed at ICAM-1 markedly inhibits eosinophil accumulation in the airways after allergen exposure and also blocks the accompanying airway hyperresponsiveness (37), although results in other species are less impressive (38). However,

ICAM-1 is not selective for eosinophils and cannot account for the selective recruitment of eosinophils in allergic inflammation. Very late antigen-4 (VLA-4), an adhesion molecule expressed on eosinophils that interacts with vascular cell adhesion molecule-1 (VCAM-1), appears to be more selective for eosinophils (39); of note is the fact that IL-4 increases the expression of VCAM-1 on endothelial cells (40). Granulocyte-macrophage colony-stimulating factor (GM-CSF) and IL-5 may be important for the survival of eosinophils in the airways and for "priming" eosinophils to exhibit enhanced responsiveness.

Eosinophils from asthmatic patients show exaggerated responses to platelet-activating factor (PAF) and phorbol esters in comparison with eosinophils from atopic nonasthmatic individuals (41). These responses are increased further by allergen challenge (42), suggesting that eosinophils may have been primed by exposure to cytokines in the circulation.

Several mediators are involved in the migration of eosinophils from the circulation to the surface of the airway. The most potent and selective agents appear to be chemokines such as RANTES (regulated upon activation, normal T-cell expressed and secreted), eotaxins-1, -2, and -3, and macrophage chemoattractant protein-4 (MCP-4), which are expressed in epithelial cells (43). There appears to be a cooperative interaction between IL-5 and chemokines, so that both cytokines are necessary for eosinophilic migration to airways (44). Once recruited to the airways, eosinophils require various growth factors, of which GM-CSF and IL-5 appear to be the most important, to survive (45). In the absence of these growth factors, eosinophils may undergo programmed cell death (apoptosis) (46,47).

A humanized monoclonal antibody to IL-5 has been administered to asthmatic patients (48); as in animal studies, a profound and prolonged reduction in circulating eosinophils was noted. Although the infiltration of eosinophils into the airway after inhaled allergen challenge was completely blocked, no effect on the bronchoconstrictor response to inhaled allergen and no reduction in airway hyperresponsiveness occurred. A clinical study with anti–IL-5 blocking antibody showed a similar profound reduction in circulating eosinophils, but no improvement in clinical asthma (49). These data question the pivotal role of eosinophils in airway hyperresponsiveness and asthma; it is possible that eosinophils may influence the structural changes that occur in chronic asthma through the secretion of growth factors, such as transforming growth factor-β (TGF-β) (50).

Neutrophils

Whereas considerable attention has focused on the role of eosinophils in allergic disease, much less attention has been paid to neutrophils. Although neutrophils are not a predominant cell type in the airways of patients with mild to moderate chronic asthma, they appear to be more prominent in the airways and induced sputum of those with severe asthma (51–53). Large numbers of neutrophils are found in the airways of patients who die suddenly of asthma (54), although this may reflect the more rapid kinetics of neutrophil than of eosinophil recruitment to the airways in airway hyperresponsiveness. The presence of neutrophils in severe asthma may reflect treatment with high doses of corticosteroids; steroids prolong neutrophil survival by inhibiting apoptosis (46,55,56). However, it is possible that neutrophils are actively recruited to the airways in severe asthma because increased concentrations of IL-8 are found in the induced sputum of these patients (52). This in turn may be a consequence of the increased levels of oxidative stress in severe asthma (57). The fact that patients with even greater degrees of neutrophilic inflammation, such as some individuals with chronic obstructive pulmonary disease or cystic fibrosis, do not have airway hyperresponsiveness makes it unlikely that neutrophils alone can increase airway responsiveness. However, it is possible that they are associated with the reduced responsiveness to corticosteroids of patients with severe asthma. Neutrophils may also play a role in acute exacerbations of asthma.

T Lymphocytes

T lymphocytes play a very important role in coordinating the inflammatory response in asthma by releasing specific patterns of cytokines that result in the recruitment and survival of eosinophils and in the maintenance of mast cells in the airways (58). T lymphocytes are coded to express a distinctive pattern of cytokines similar to that described in murine Th2 lymphocytes, which characteristically express IL-4, IL-5, IL-9, and IL-13 (59). The programming of T lymphocytes is presumably stimulated by antigen-presenting cells, such as dendritic cells, which may migrate from the epithelium to regional lymph nodes or interact with lymphocytes resident in the airway mucosa. The naive immune system is skewed to express the Th2 phenotype; data now indicate that children with atopy are more likely than normal children to retain this skewed phenotype (60). Some evidence suggests that infection or exposure to endotoxins early in life may promote predominantly Th1-mediated responses, and that a clean environment or a lack of infection in childhood may favor Th2-cell expression and atopic disease (61–63). Indeed, the balance between Th1 and Th2 cells is thought to be determined by locally released cytokines, such as IL-12, which tip the balance in favor of Th1 cells, or IL-4 or IL-13, which favor the emergence of Th2 cells (Fig. 9.2). Some evidence indicates that steroid treatment may differentially affect the balance between IL-12 and IL-13 expression (64). Data from murine models of asthma strongly suggest that IL-13 is both necessary and sufficient for induction of the asthmatic phenotype (65).

Regulatory T (Tr) cells suppress the immune response through the secretion of inhibitory cytokines, such as IL-10 and TGF-β, and play an important role in immune

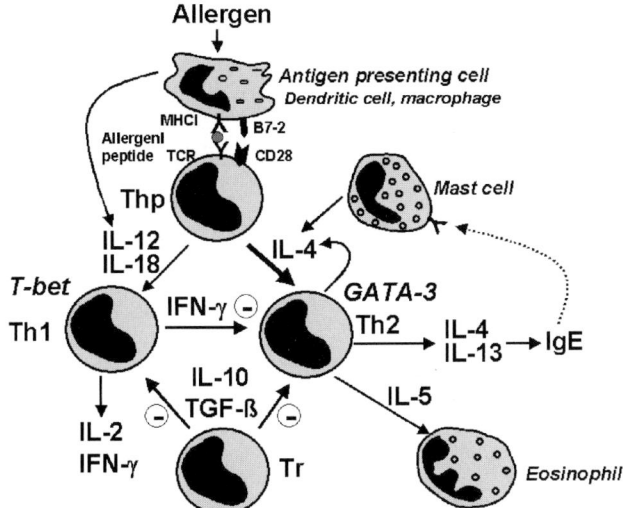

FIGURE 9.2. Asthmatic inflammation is characterized by a preponderance of T helper 2 (Th2) lymphocytes over Th1 cells. The transcription factors T-bet and GATA-3 may regulate the balance between Th1 and Th2 cells. Regulatory T (Tr) cells have an inhibitory effect.

regulation with the suppression of Th1 responses (66,67). However, their role in allergic diseases has not yet been well defined.

B Lymphocytes

B lymphocytes secrete IgE in allergic diseases; the factors regulating IgE secretion are now much better understood (68). IL-4 is crucial in switching B cells to IgE production, and CD40 on T cells is an important accessory molecule that signals through interaction with CD40 ligand on B cells. Evidence is increasing for the local production of IgE, even in patients with intrinsic asthma (see section "Intrinsic Asthma") (6).

Basophils

Basophils have previously been difficult to detect by immunocytochemistry (69). However, with the use of a basophil-specific marker, a small increase in basophils has been documented in the airways of asthmatic patients. The number of basophils further increases after allergen challenge, but basophils are far outnumbered by eosinophils (in a ratio of approximately 10:1) (70,71). The numbers of basophils, and of mast cells, are also increased in induced sputum after allergen challenge (72). The role of basophils, as opposed to that of mast cells, is somewhat uncertain in asthma (73).

Platelets

Some evidence has been found for the involvement of platelets in the pathophysiology of allergic diseases; activated

platelets have been found in the bronchial biopsy specimens of asthmatic patients (74). After allergen challenge, the number of circulating platelets decreases (75). Circulating platelets from patients with asthma may also be activated and release the chemokine RANTES (76). Chemokines associated with Th2 cell–mediated inflammation have recently been shown to activate and aggregate platelets (77).

Structural Cells

Structural cells of the airways, including epithelial cells, endothelial cells, fibroblasts, and even smooth muscle cells, may also be an important source of inflammatory mediators, such as cytokines and lipid mediators, in asthmatic individuals (78–81). Indeed, because structural cells far outnumber inflammatory cells in the airway, they may be the major source of mediators driving chronic inflammation in asthma. Epithelial cells may play a key role in translating inhaled environmental signals into an airway inflammatory response and are probably the major target cell for inhaled glucocorticoids (Fig. 9.3).

INFLAMMATORY MEDIATORS

Many different mediators have been implicated in asthma. They may produce a variety of effects on airways that potentially can account for all the pathologic features of allergic diseases (82) (Fig. 9.4). Mediators such as histamine, prostaglandins, leukotrienes, and kinins contract airway smooth muscle, increase microvascular leakage, increase airway secretion of mucus, and attract other inflammatory cells. Because each mediator has many effects, the role of individual mediators in the pathophysiology of asthma is not yet clear. The multiplicity and redundancy of the effects of mediators make it unlikely that preventing the synthesis or action of a *single* mediator will have a major impact in asthma. However, some mediators may play a more important role if they are upstream in the inflammatory process. The effects of single mediators can be evaluated only through the use of specific receptor antagonists or specific inhibitors of mediator synthesis.

Lipid Mediators

The cysteinyl leukotrienes (leukotriene C_4 [LTC_4], LTD_4, and LTE_4) are potent constrictors of human airways and have been reported to increase airway hyperresponsiveness (83). The introduction of potent specific leukotriene antagonists has made it possible to evaluate the role of these mediators in asthma. Potent LTD_4 antagonists protect (~50%) against exercise- and allergen-induced bronchoconstriction, suggesting that leukotrienes contribute to bronchoconstrictor responses. Long-term treatment with antileukotrienes improves lung function and symptoms in asthmatic patients,

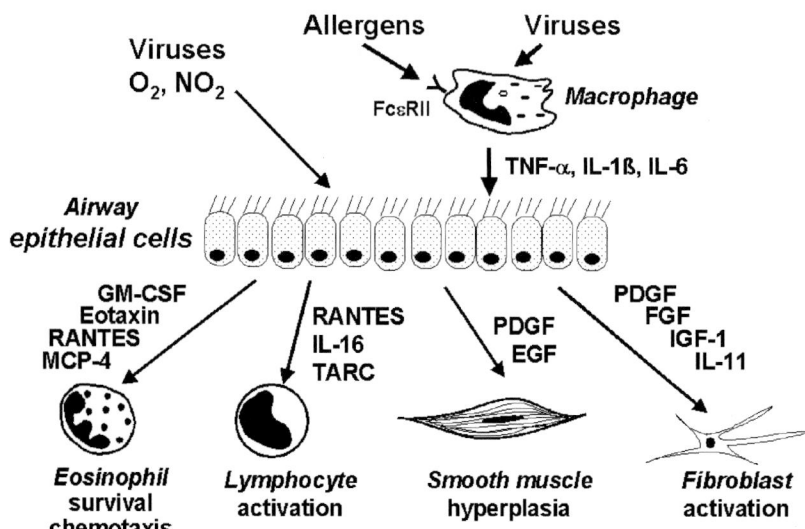

FIGURE 9.3. Airway epithelial cells may play an active role in asthmatic inflammation through the release of many inflammatory mediators, cytokines, chemokines, and growth factors.

although the degree of improvement in lung function is not as great as with inhaled corticosteroids, which have a much broader spectrum of effects (84,85). In addition to their effects on airway smooth muscle and vessels, the cysteinyl leukotrienes have weak inflammatory effects, increasing the number of eosinophils in induced sputum (86). The antiinflammatory effects of antileukotrienes are small (87).

PAF is a potent inflammatory mediator that induces many of the features of asthma, including eosinophil recruitment and activation and induction of airway hyperresponsiveness (88), yet even potent PAF antagonists, such as modipafant, do not control asthmatic symptoms, at least in chronic disease (89–91). A genetic mutation that results in impaired function of PAF acetylhydrolase, the PAF-metabolizing enzyme, is associated with severe asthma in Japan (92), suggesting that PAF may play a role in some forms of asthma.

Prostaglandins have potent effects on airway function, and the expression of the inducible form of cyclooxygenase (COX-2) is increased in asthmatic airways (93). Inhibition of prostaglandin synthesis with cyclooxygenase inhibitors, such as aspirin or ibuprofen, does not have any effect in most patients with asthma. Some patients have aspirin-sensitive asthma, which is more common in certain ethnic groups, such as eastern Europeans and Japanese (94). It is associated with an increased expression of LTC_4 synthase, which results in an increased formation of cysteinyl leukotrienes, possibly because of genetic polymorphisms (95). Prostaglandin D_2 (PGD_2) is a bronchoconstrictor prostaglandin produced predominantly by mast cells. Deletion of the PGD_2 receptors in mice significantly inhibits inflammatory responses to allergen and inhibits airway hyperresponsiveness, suggesting that this mediator may be important in asthma (96). It has also been discovered that PGD_2 activates a novel chemoattractant receptor, chemoattractant receptor of Th2 cells (CRTH2). This receptor, which is expressed on Th2 cells, eosinophils, and basophils, mediates chemotaxis of these cell types and may provide a link between mast cell activation and allergic inflammation (94).

Cytokines

Cytokines are important mediators of chronic inflammation and play a critical role in orchestrating the type of inflammatory response (97) (Fig. 9.5). Many inflammatory cells (macrophages, mast cells, eosinophils, and lymphocytes) are capable of synthesizing and releasing these proteins, and structural cells (epithelial cells, airway smooth muscle cells, and endothelial cells) may also release a variety of cytokines and therefore participate in the chronic inflammatory response (98). Although inflammatory mediators like histamine and leukotrienes may be important in the acute and subacute inflammatory responses and in exacerbations of asthma, it is likely that cytokines play a dominant role in maintaining the chronic inflammatory state in allergic diseases. Depending on conditions, almost every cell is capable of producing cytokines. Research in this area is hampered by a lack of specific antagonists, although important observations

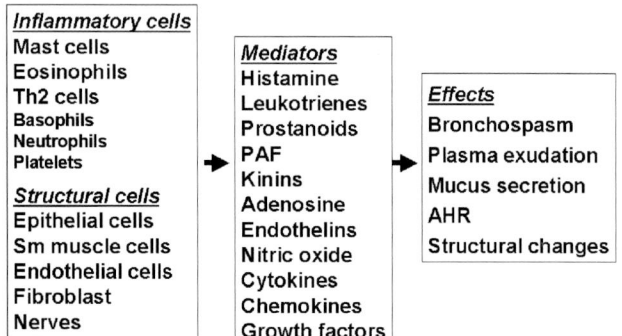

FIGURE 9.4. Many cells and mediators are involved in asthma and have several effects in the airways.

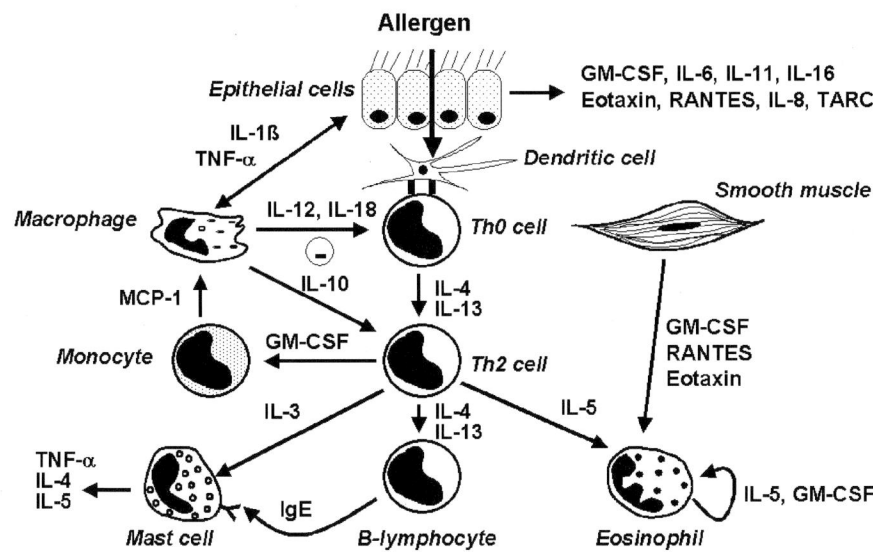

FIGURE 9.5. The cytokine network in asthma. Many inflammatory cytokines are released from inflammatory and structural cells in the airway and orchestrate and perpetuate the inflammatory response.

have been made with the use of specific neutralizing antibodies developed as novel therapies (99).

The cytokines that appear to be of particular importance in asthma include the lymphokines secreted by T lymphocytes: IL-3, which is important for mast cell survival in tissues; IL-4, which is critical in causing B lymphocytes to produce IgE and for the expression of VCAM-1 on endothelial cells; IL-13, which acts similarly to IL-4; and IL-5, which is of critical importance in the differentiation, survival, and priming of eosinophils. The gene expression of IL-5 is increased in the lymphocytes in bronchial biopsy specimens of patients with symptomatic asthma and allergic rhinitis (100). The importance of IL-5 in eosinophil recruitment in humans has been confirmed in a study in which administration of an anti–IL-5 antibody (mepolizumab) to asthmatic patients was associated with a profound decrease in eosinophil counts in their blood and induced sputum (48). Interestingly, in this study, no effect on the physiology of the allergen-induced asthmatic response was noted, and this observation was confirmed in a study of symptomatic asthmatic patients who showed no clinical improvement despite a marked fall in circulating eosinophils (49). These results call into question the critical role of eosinophils in asthma. IL-4 and IL-13 both play key roles in the allergic inflammatory response in that they determine the isotype switching in B cells that results in IgE formation. IL-4, but not IL-13, is also involved in the differentiation of Th2 cells and therefore may be critical in the initial development of atopy, whereas IL-13 is much more abundant in established disease and may therefore be more important in maintaining the inflammatory process (65,101). Another Th2 cytokine, IL-9, may play a critical role in sensitizing responses to the cytokines IL-4 and IL-5 (102,103).

Other cytokines, such as IL-1β, IL-6, TNF-α, and GM-CSF, are released from a variety of cells, including macrophages and epithelial cells, and may be important in amplifying the inflammatory response. TNF-α may be an amplifying mediator in asthma and is produced in increased amounts in asthmatic airways (104). Inhalation of TNF-α increased airway responsiveness in normal individuals (105). TNF-α and IL-1β both activate the proinflammatory transcription factors nuclear factor-κB (NF-κB) and activator protein-1 (AP-1), which then switch on many inflammatory genes in the asthmatic airway.

Other cytokines, such as interferon-γ (IFN-γ), IL-10, IL-12, and IL-18, play a regulatory role and inhibit the allergic inflammatory process (see section "Antiinflammatory Mechanisms," below).

Chemokines

Chemokines are directly involved in the recruitment of inflammatory cells to the lung in asthma (43). More than 50 different chemokines are now recognized, and they activate more than 20 different surface receptors (106). Chemokine receptors are members of the seven transmembrane receptor superfamily of G protein–coupled receptors, so that it is possible to identify small molecule inhibitors; this has not been possible for the classic cytokine receptors (107). Some chemokines appear to be selective for single chemokine receptors, whereas others are promiscuous and mediate the effects of several related chemokines. Chemokines appear to act sequentially and thereby determine the final inflammatory response; inhibitors may be more or less effective, depending on the relative kinetics of each individual reaction (108).

Several chemokines, including eotaxin, eotaxin-2, eotaxin-3, RANTES, and MCP-4, activate a common receptor on eosinophils, CC chemokine receptor-3 (CCR3) (109). A neutralizing antibody against eotaxin reduces eosinophil recruitment and the associated airway hyperresponsiveness in mouse lung after allergen exposure (110). Increased expression of eotaxin, eotaxin-2, MCP-3, MCP-4, and CCR3 has been found in the airways of asthmatic patients and correlates with increased airway hyperresponsiveness (111,112). Several small molecule inhibitors of CCR3, including UCB35625, SB-297006, and SB-328437, are effective in inhibiting eosinophil recruitment in allergen models of asthma (113,114); drugs in this class are currently undergoing clinical trials. Although it was thought that CCR3 is restricted to eosinophils, some evidence has been found for its expression on Th2 cells and mast cells, so that inhibitors may have more widespread effects than on eosinophils alone, making them potentially more valuable in asthma treatment. RANTES, the expression of which is increased in asthmatic airways (115), activates CCR3, and it also has effects on CCR1 and CCR5, possibly affecting T-cell recruitment.

MCP-1 activates CCR2 on monocytes and T lymphocytes. Blocking MCP-1 with neutralizing antibodies reduces the recruitment of both T cells and eosinophils in a murine model of ovalbumin-induced airway inflammation, with a marked reduction in airway hyperresponsiveness (110). MCP-1 also recruits and activates mast cells, an effect that is mediated via CCR2 (116). MCP-1 instilled into the airways induces marked and prolonged airway hyperresponsiveness in mice that is associated with mast cell degranulation. A neutralizing antibody to MCP-1 blocks the development of airway hyperresponsiveness in response to allergen (116). MCP-1 levels are increased in the BAL fluid of patients with asthma (117). These data have led to a search for small molecule inhibitors of CCR2.

CCR4 is selectively expressed on Th2 cells and is activated by the chemokines monocyte-derived chemokine (MDC) and thymus- and activation-regulated chemokine (TARC) (118). Epithelial cells of patients with asthma express TARC, which recruits Th2 cells (119). Increased concentrations of TARC are also found in the BAL fluid of asthmatic patients, whereas MDC is only weakly expressed in the airways (120). TARC may thus induce a sequence of responses resulting in coordinated eosinophilic inflammation (Fig. 9.6). Inhibitors of CCR4 may therefore inhibit the recruitment of Th2 cells to the lung and so reduce persistent eosinophilic inflammation in the airways.

Oxidative Stress

As in all inflammatory diseases, oxidative stress is increased in allergic inflammation because activated inflammatory cells, such as macrophages and eosinophils, produce reactive oxygen species. Evidence for increased oxidative stress in asthma is provided by increased concentrations of 8-isoprostane (a product of oxidized arachidonic acid) in exhaled condensates (57) and increased concentrations of ethane (a product of oxidative lipid peroxidation) in the exhaled breath of asthmatic patients (121). Persuasive epidemiologic evidence indicates that a low dietary intake of antioxidants is linked to an increased prevalence of asthma (122). Increased oxidative stress is related to disease severity and may amplify

the inflammatory response and reduce responsiveness to corticosteroids, particularly in severe disease and during exacerbations. One of the mechanisms whereby oxidative stress may be detrimental in asthma is through the reaction of superoxide anions with nitric oxide to form the reactive radical peroxynitrite, which may then modify several target proteins.

Endothelins

Endothelins are potent peptide mediators that are vasoconstrictors and bronchoconstrictors (123,124). Levels of endothelin-1 are increased in the sputum of patients with asthma; these levels are modulated by allergen exposure and steroid treatment (125,126). Endothelins are also expressed in the nasal mucosa in rhinitis (127). Endothelins induce airway smooth muscle cell proliferation and promote a profibrotic phenotype and may therefore play a role in the chronic inflammation of asthma.

Nitric Oxide

Nitric oxide (NO) is produced by several cells in the airway by NO synthases (128,129). Although the cellular source of NO within the lung is not known with certainty, inferences based on mathematical models suggest that the large airways produce NO (130). Current data indicate that the level of NO in the exhaled air of patients with asthma is higher than the level of NO in the exhaled air of normal subjects (131). The elevated levels of NO are more likely reflective of a poorly defined inflammatory mechanism than of a direct pathogenetic role of this gas in asthmatic individuals (132,133). Recent data suggest that the level of NO in exhaled air may increase in acute exacerbations of asthma as a consequence of a fall in pH (increased acidity) associated

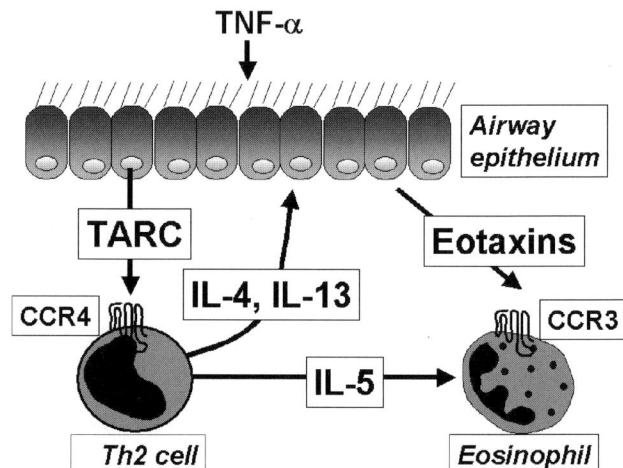

FIGURE 9.6. Chemokines in asthma. Tumor necrosis factor-α (TNF-α) releases thymus- and activation-regulated chemokine (TARC) from epithelial cells, which attracts Th2 cells via the activation of CCR4 receptors. These promote eosinophilic inflammation directly through the release of interleukin-5 (IL-5) and indirectly through the release of IL-4 and IL-13, which induce eotaxin formation in airway epithelial cells.

with inflammation (134). The combination of increased oxidative stress and NO may lead to the formation of the potent radical peroxynitrite and subsequent nitrosylation of airway proteins (135). The measurement of exhaled NO in patients with asthma is increasingly being used as a noninvasive way of monitoring the inflammatory process (136).

EFFECTS OF INFLAMMATION

The acute and chronic allergic inflammatory responses previously outlined directly affect the target cells of the respiratory tract, resulting in the characteristic pathophysiologic changes associated with asthma (Fig. 9.7). Important advances have been made in understanding these changes, although their relation to clinical symptoms is often not clear. Of considerable current interest are the structural changes that occur in the airways of patients with asthma that are loosely termed *remodeling*. It is believed that alterations in airway structure underlie the irreversible changes in airway function that occur in some patients with asthma (137,138). However, many patients with asthma continue to have normal lung function throughout life, so it is likely that genetic factors influence which patients acquire structural changes.

Epithelium

Airway epithelial shedding is a characteristic feature of asthma and may be important in contributing to airway hyperresponsiveness. Ozone exposure, viral infections, chemical sensitizers, and allergen exposures can all lead to epithelial

disruption. Epithelium may be shed as a consequence of exposure to inflammatory mediators, such as eosinophil basic proteins and oxygen-derived free radicals, along with exposure to proteases released from inflammatory cells. Epithelial cells are commonly found in clumps in the BAL fluid or sputum (Creola bodies) of asthmatic patients, suggesting a loss of attachment to the basal layer or basement membrane. Epithelial damage may contribute to airway hyperresponsiveness in a number of ways, including the following: reducing airway barrier function, allowing the penetration of allergens to smooth muscle; decreasing the levels of protective enzymes produced by airway epithelium (neutral endopeptidase) that normally degrade inflammatory mediators; reducing the level of smooth muscle relaxant factor (so-called epithelium-derived relaxant factor); and exposing sensory nerves, thereby causing reflex neural effects on the airway.

As previously discussed (see section "Structural Cells"), epithelial cells appear to be an important source of mediators in allergic inflammation (Fig. 9.3). The release of mediators from epithelial cells may be stimulated by various inhaled substances, resulting in an increased inflammatory response. Epithelial cells may also release growth factors that stimulate structural changes in the airways, including fibrosis, angiogenesis, and the proliferation of airway smooth muscle. These responses may be seen as an attempt to repair the damage caused by chronic inflammation (139).

Fibrosis

By conventional light microscopy, the basement membrane in the airways of asthmatic individuals appears to be

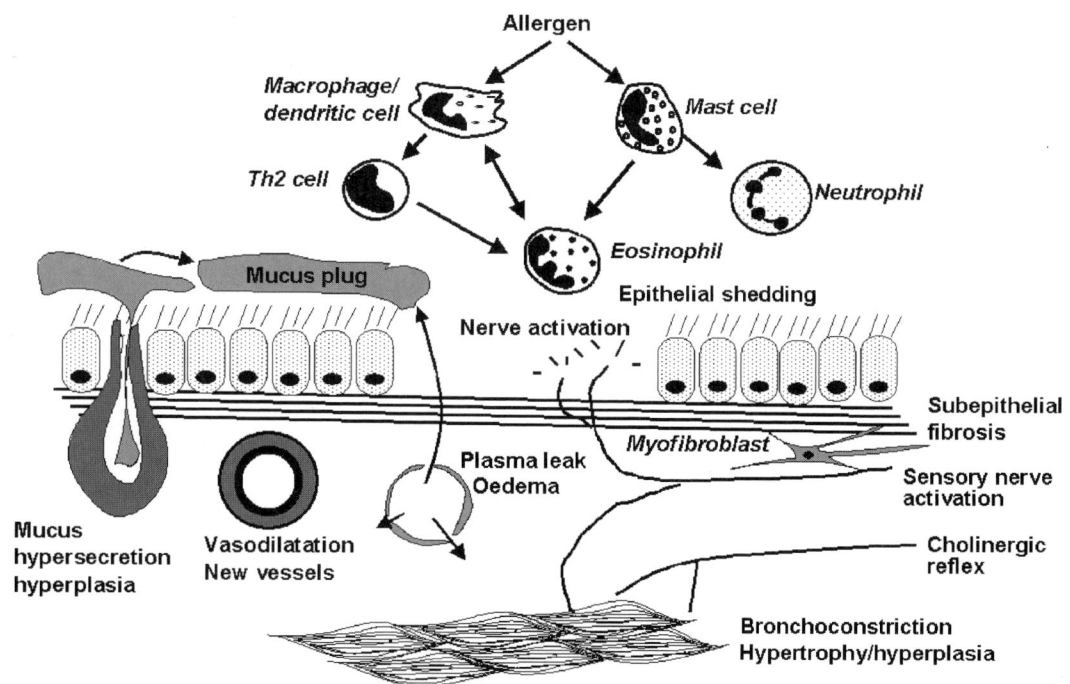

FIGURE 9.7. The pathophysiology of asthma is complex. The participation of several interacting inflammatory cells results in acute and chronic inflammatory effects in the airway.

thickened. By electron microscopy, it has been demonstrated that this apparent thickening is caused by subepithelial fibrosis, with the deposition of types III and V collagen beneath the true basement membrane (140,141). Several profibrotic cytokines, including TGF-β and platelet-derived growth factor (PDGF), and mediators such as endothelin-1 can be produced by epithelial cells or macrophages in the inflamed airway and increase collagen synthesis (140). Even mechanical manipulation can alter the phenotype of airway epithelial cells to release profibrotic growth factors (142). The role of fibrosis in asthma is unclear; subepithelial fibrosis has been observed even in patients with mild asthma at the onset of disease, so it is not certain whether the collagen deposition has any functional consequences or is correlated with disease severity (143,144). Evidence has also been found for fibrosis in airway smooth muscle; deposition in this location is more likely to have functional consequences (145). However, the fact that many asthmatic patients are subject to chronic inflammation through many decades without the development of gross fibrosis of the airways argues that powerful inhibitory mechanisms must prevent a fibrotic reaction to the multiple profibrotic mediators that are produced.

Airway Smooth Muscle

Debate is ongoing about the role of abnormalities of smooth muscle in asthmatic airways. Airway smooth muscle contraction plays a key role in the symptomatology of asthma because many inflammatory mediators released in asthma have bronchoconstrictor effects. It has now been recognized that airway smooth muscle cells have other functions in asthmatic airways (146). *In vitro*, airway smooth muscle from asthmatic patients usually shows no increased responsiveness to spasmogens. Reduced responsiveness to β-adrenergic agonists has been reported in the bronchi of asthmatic patients removed surgically or postmortem; however, the number of β-receptors is not reduced, suggesting that the β-receptors have been uncoupled from G proteins affecting intercellular signaling (147). These abnormalities of airway smooth muscle may be a reflection of the chronic inflammatory process. For example, chronic exposure to inflammatory cytokines, such as IL-1β, down-regulates the response of airway smooth muscle to β_2-adrenergic agonists *in vitro* and *in vivo* (148–150). The reduced β-adrenergic responses in airway smooth muscle could be a consequence of the phosphorylation of the stimulatory G protein coupling β-receptors to adenylyl cyclase. This would result from the activation of protein kinase C in airway smooth muscle cells through stimulation by inflammatory mediators, and from increased activity of the inhibitory G protein (G_i) induced by proinflammatory cytokines (149,151,152).

Inflammatory mediators may also modulate the ion channels that serve to regulate the resting membrane potential of airway smooth muscle cells, thus altering the level of excitability of these cells. Furthermore, modulation of the activation kinetics of other ion channels by key inflammatory mediators can lead to altered contractile characteristics of smooth muscle.

Asthmatic airways are also characterized by *hypertrophy* and *hyperplasia* of airway smooth muscle (153), which is presumably the result of stimulation of airway smooth muscle cells by various growth factors, such as PDGF, or endothelin-1 released from inflammatory cells (140,154). Airway smooth muscle also plays a secretory role in asthma and has the capacity to release multiple cytokines, chemokines, and lipid mediators (81).

Vascular Responses

Allergic inflammation has several effects on blood vessels in the respiratory tract. Vasodilation occurs in inflammation, yet little is known about the role of the airway circulation in asthma, partly because of the difficulties involved in measuring airway blood flow. Studies in which an inhaled absorbable gas was used have demonstrated increased airway mucosal blood flow in asthma (155). An increase in the temperature of exhaled breath has been reported in patients with asthma, which presumably reflects the increased vascularity associated with inflammation (156). The bronchial circulation may also play an important role in regulating airway caliber because an increase in the vascular volume may contribute to airway narrowing. Increased airway blood flow may be important in removing inflammatory mediators from the airway and may be an important mechanism in the development of exercise-induced asthma (157). The number of blood vessels in asthmatic airways may also be increased as a result of angiogenesis secondary to the release of growth factors such as vascular endothelial growth factor (VEGF) and TNF-α (158,159). The increased expression of VEGF in asthmatic airways, particularly in macrophages and eosinophils, is related to the increased vascularity (160).

Microvascular leakage is an essential component of the inflammatory response, and many of the inflammatory mediators implicated in asthma produce this leakage (161,162). The evidence for microvascular leakage in asthma is good, and it may have several consequences on airway function, including an increase in airway secretions, impairment of mucociliary clearance, the formation of new mediators from plasma precursors (such as kinins), and mucosal edema, which may contribute to airway narrowing and increased airway hyperresponsiveness (163,164).

Hypersecretion of Mucus

The hypersecretion of mucus is a common inflammatory response in secretory tissues. Increased mucus secretion contributes to the viscid mucus plugs that occlude asthmatic airways, particularly in fatal cases. Evidence has been found of hyperplasia of the submucosal glands confined to large airways and of increased numbers of epithelial goblet cells in asthmatic airways (165,166). This increased secretory response may be a consequence both of inflammatory mediators acting on submucosal glands and of stimulation of neural elements (167). The Th2 cytokines IL-4, IL-13, and IL-9 have all been shown to induce mucus hypersecretion in experimental models of asthma (165,168–170). The relationship among mediators that results in mucus hyperplasia is not yet fully understood, but evidence suggests that epithelial growth factor (EGF) is a key molecule in initiating mucus secretion of the upper and lower airways (170). Indeed, the production of EGF may be the final common step for many of the factors that stimulate mucus secretion, including IL-13 and oxidative stress (171,172). EGF may stimulate the expression of the mucin gene MUC5AC, which is up-regulated in asthma (165,166).

The functional role of hypertrophy and hyperplasia of the mucosecretory apparatus in asthma is not yet known because it is difficult to quantify mucus secretion in airways. Experimental data indicate that airway hyperresponsiveness and mucus hypersecretion, together with increased MUC5AC expression, are associated with the expression of a specific calcium-activated chloride channel in murine goblet cells, designated gob-5, which has a human counterpart, hCLCA1 (173). Overexpression of gob-5 was associated with marked airway hyperresponsiveness and mucus hypersecretion in mice, indicating that mucus hypersecretion may play a role in airway hyperresponsiveness.

Neural Effects

Interest has been revived in neural mechanisms in asthma and rhinitis, particularly in the context of the relation between symptoms and airway hyperresponsiveness (174). The autonomic nervous control of the respiratory tract is complex; in addition to classic cholinergic and adrenergic mechanisms, nonadrenergic noncholinergic (NANC) neurons and several neuropeptides have been identified in the respiratory tract (175,176). Several studies have investigated the possibility that defects in autonomic control may contribute to airway hyperresponsiveness in asthma, and abnormalities of autonomic function, such as enhanced cholinergic and α-adrenergic responses or reduced β-adrenergic responses, have been proposed. Current thinking suggests that these abnormalities are likely to be secondary to the disease, rather than primary defects (174). It is possible that airway inflammation may interact with the autonomic nervous system by several mechanisms.

There is a close interaction between nerves and inflammatory cells in allergic inflammation. Inflammatory mediators activate and modulate neurotransmission; conversely, neurotransmitters may modulate the inflammatory response. Inflammatory mediators may act on various prejunctional receptors on airway nerves to modulate the release of neurotransmitters (177). Inflammatory mediators may also activate sensory nerves, resulting in reflex cholinergic bron-

choconstriction or the release of inflammatory neuropeptides. Bradykinin is a potent activator of unmyelinated sensory nerves (C fibers) (178), and it also sensitizes these nerves to other stimuli (179).

Inflammatory products may also sensitize sensory nerve endings in the airway epithelium, so that the nerves become hyperalgesic. Hyperalgesia and pain (dolor) are cardinal signs of inflammation, and in the asthmatic airway they may mediate cough and chest tightness, which are classic, characteristic symptoms of asthma. The precise mechanisms of hyperalgesia are not yet certain, but mediators such as prostaglandins, certain cytokines, and neurotrophins may be important. Neurotrophins, released from various cell types in peripheral tissues, may cause proliferation and sensitization of airway sensory nerves (180,181). Neurotrophins, such as nerve growth factor (NGF), may be released from inflammatory and structural cells in asthmatic airways and then stimulate the increased synthesis of neuropeptides, such as substance P, in airway sensory nerves, in addition to sensitizing nerve endings in the airways (182). NGF is released from human airway epithelial cells after exposure to inflammatory stimuli (183). Neurotrophins may play an important role in mediating airway hyperresponsiveness in asthma (184).

Nonadrenergic bronchodilator nerves are prominent in human airways, and it has been suggested that these nerves may be defective in asthma (185). In animal airways, vasoactive intestinal peptide (VIP) has been shown to be a neurotransmitter of these nerves, and a striking absence of VIP-immunoreactive nerves has been reported in the lungs of patients with severe fatal asthma (186). However, no difference in the expression of VIP has been reported in bronchial biopsy specimens from asthmatic patients (187). It is likely that this loss of VIP immunoreactivity in severe asthma can be explained by the degradation by tryptase released from degranulating mast cells in the airways of asthmatics. In human airways, the unique bronchodilator neurotransmitter appears to be NO (188).

Airway nerves may also release neurotransmitters that have inflammatory effects. Thus, neuropeptides such as substance P, neurokinin A, and calcitonin gene–related peptide may be released from sensitized inflammatory nerves in the airways that increase and extend the ongoing inflammatory response (189,190) (Fig. 9.8). Evidence has been found for an increase in substance P–immunoreactive nerves in the airways of patients with severe asthma (191), which may be a consequence of the proliferation of sensory nerves and increased synthesis of sensory neuropeptides as a result of the release of NGFs during chronic inflammation, although this has not been confirmed in patients with milder asthma (187). The activity of enzymes such as neutral endopeptidase, which degrade neuropeptides such as substance P, may also be reduced (192). Evidence has been found for increased gene expression of the receptors that mediate the inflammatory effects (NK1) and bronchoconstrictor effects (NK2) of substance P (193,194). Thus, chronic asthma may be

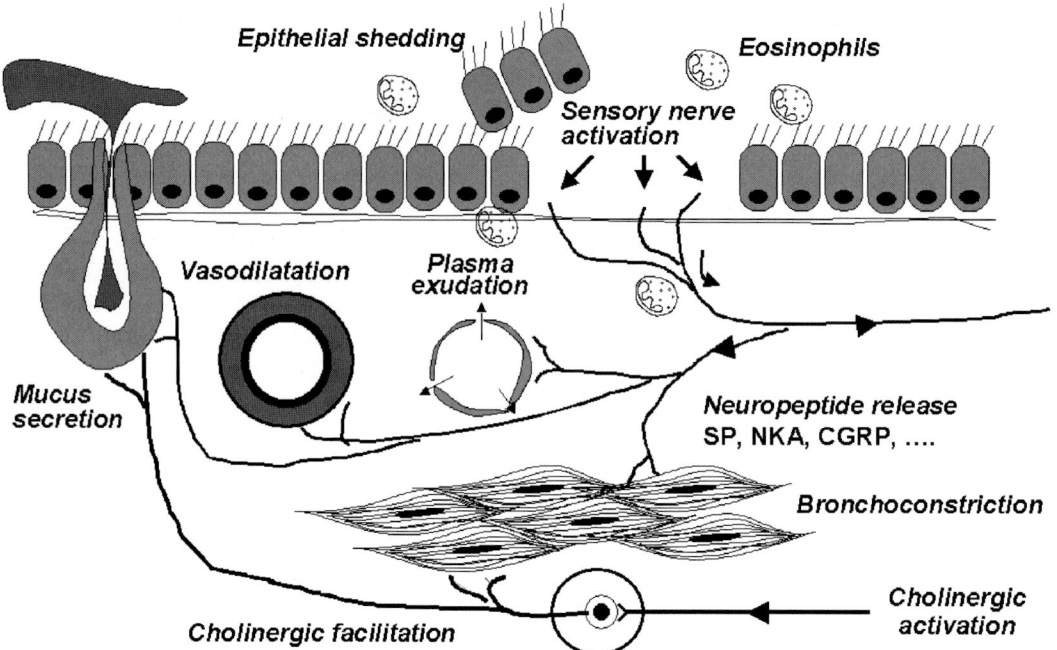

FIGURE 9.8. Possible neurogenic inflammation in asthmatic airways by the retrograde release of peptides from sensory nerves via an axon reflex. Substance P (*SP*) causes vasodilation, plasma exudation, and mucus secretion, whereas neurokinin A (*NKA*) causes bronchoconstriction and enhanced cholinergic reflexes and calcitonin gene–related peptide (*CGRP*) causes vasodilation.

associated with an increase in neurogenically generated inflammation, which may provide a mechanism for perpetuating the inflammatory response even in the absence of initiating inflammatory stimuli. At present, little direct evidence has been found for neurogenic inflammation in asthma, but this is partly because it is difficult to make the appropriate measurements in the lower airways (190).

TRANSCRIPTION FACTORS

The chronic inflammation of asthma is caused by the increased expression of multiple inflammatory proteins (cytokines, enzymes, receptors, adhesion molecules). In many cases, these inflammatory proteins are induced by transcription factors, which are DNA binding factors that increase the transcription of selected target genes (195) (Fig. 9.9). One transcription factor that may play a critical role in asthma is NF-κB, which can be activated by multiple stimuli, including protein kinase C activators, oxidants, and proinflammatory cytokines (e.g., IL-1β and TNF-α) (196). Evidence suggests an increased activation of NF-κB in asthmatic airways, particularly in epithelial cells and macrophages (197,198). NF-κB regulates the expression of several key genes that are overexpressed in asthmatic airways, including proinflammatory cytokines (IL-1β, TNF-α, GM-CSF), chemokines (RANTES, macrophage inflammatory protein-1α [MIP-1α], eotaxin), adhesion molecules (ICAM-1, VCAM-1), and

inflammatory enzymes (COX-2 and inducible NO synthase [iNOS]). The c-Fos component of AP-1 is also activated in asthmatic airways and often cooperates with NF-κB in switching on inflammatory genes (199). Many other transcription factors are involved in the abnormal expression of inflammatory genes in asthma. There may be a common mechanism whereby the activation of inflammatory genes by transcription factors induces the acetylation of core histones around DNA. This unwinds DNA, opening up the chromatin structure, and allows gene transcription to proceed (200,201).

Transcription factors play a critical role in determining the balance between Th1 and Th2 cells. The evidence is persuasive that GATA-3 determines Th2 cell differentiation (202) and is highly expressed in asthmatic patients (203,204). The differentiation of Th1 cells is regulated by the transcription factor T-bet (205). Deletion of the T-bet gene is associated with an asthma-like phenotype in mice, suggesting that it may play an important role in impeding the development of Th2 cells (206).

ANTIINFLAMMATORY MECHANISMS

Although most emphasis has been placed on inflammatory mechanisms, important antiinflammatory mechanisms may be defective in asthma, resulting in increased inflammatory responses in the airways (207). Endogenous cortisol

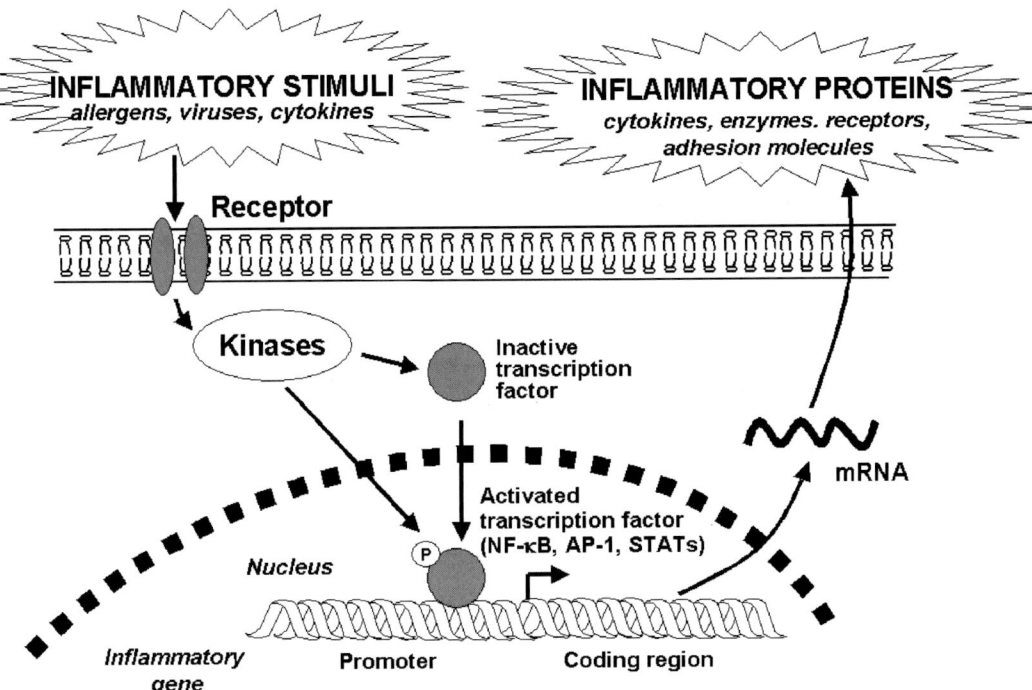

FIGURE 9.9. Transcription factors play a key role in amplifying and perpetuating the inflammatory response in asthma. Transcription factors, including nuclear factor kappa-B (NF-κB), activator protein-1 (AP-1), and signal transduction–activated transcription factors (STATs), are activated by inflammatory stimuli and increase the expression of multiple inflammatory genes.

may be important as a regulator of the allergic inflammatory response, and nocturnal exacerbations of asthma may be related to the circadian fall in plasma cortisol. The blockade of endogenous cortisol secretion by metyrapone results in an increase in the late response to allergen in the skin (208). Cortisol is converted to inactive cortisone by the enzyme 11β-hydroxysteroid dehydrogenase, which is expressed in airway tissues (209). It is possible that this enzyme functions abnormally in asthma or may determine the severity of asthma.

Various cytokines have antiinflammatory actions (210). IL-1 receptor antagonist (IL-1ra) inhibits the binding of IL-1 to its receptors and therefore has potential antiinflammatory effects in asthma. IL-1ra has been reported to be an effective therapy in an animal model of asthma (211). IL-12 and IFN-γ increase the number of Th1 cells and inhibit the production of Th2 cells and also may be useful as asthma therapy. IL-12 promotes the differentiation and thus the suppression of Th2 cells, resulting in a reduction in eosinophilic inflammation (65). IL-12 infusions in patients with asthma do indeed inhibit peripheral blood eosinophilia (212). Some evidence suggests that IL-12 expression may be impaired in asthma (64).

IL-10, which was originally described as cytokine synthesis inhibitory factor, inhibits the expression of multiple inflammatory cytokines (TNF-α, IL-1β, GM-CSF) and chemokines, in addition to inflammatory enzymes (iNOS,

COX-2). Evidence indicates that IL-10 secretion and gene transcription are defective in the macrophages and monocytes of asthmatic patients (20,213); this defect may enhance inflammatory effects in asthma and be a determinant of asthma severity (214) (Fig. 9.10). IL-10 secretion is reduced in the monocytes of patients with severe as opposed to mild asthma (215), and haplotypes associated with decreased production correlate with severe asthma (216).

Other mediators may also have antiinflammatory and immunosuppressive effects. PGE$_2$ has inhibitory effects on macrophages, epithelial cells, and eosinophils. Exogenous PGE$_2$ inhibits allergen-induced airway responses, and its endogenous generation may account for the refractory period after exercise challenge (217). However, it is unlikely that endogenous PGE$_2$ is important in most asthmatic patients because nonselective cyclooxygenase inhibitors worsen asthma in a minority of patients (aspirin-induced asthma). Other lipid mediators may also be antiinflammatory, including 15-hydroxyeicosatetraenoic (HETE) acid, which is produced in high concentrations by airway epithelial cells. 15-HETE acid and lipoxins may inhibit the effects of cysteinyl leukotrienes in the airways (218). Lipoxins are known to have strong antiinflammatory effects by way of modulating the trafficking of key intracellular proinflammatory intermediates (219). The peptide adrenomedullin, which is expressed in high concentrations in lung, has bronchodilator activity (220) and also appears to inhibit the secretion of cytokines from

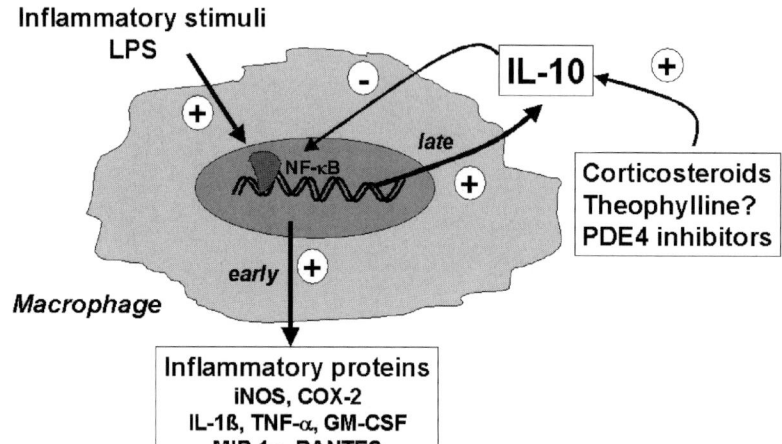

FIGURE 9.10. Interleukin-10 (IL-10) is an antiinflammatory cytokine that may inhibit the expression of inflammatory mediators from macrophages. A deficiency of IL-10 secretion in the macrophages of patients with asthma results in an increased release of inflammatory mediators.

macrophages (221). Its role in asthma is currently unknown, but plasma concentrations are no different in patients with asthma (222).

REFERENCES

1. Cookson WO, Moffatt MF. Genetics of asthma and allergic disease. *Hum Mol Genet* 2000;9:2359–2364.
2. Barnes KC. Evidence for common genetic elements in allergic disease. *J Allergy Clin Immunol* 2000;106:S192–S200.
3. Dunnill MS. The pathology of asthma, with special reference to the changes in the bronchial mucosa. *J Clin Pathol* 1960;13:27–33.
4. Busse WW, Lemanske RF. Asthma. *N Engl J Med* 2001;344:350–362.
5. Bousquet J, Jeffery PK, Busse WW, et al. Asthma. From bronchoconstriction to airways inflammation and remodeling. *Am J Respir Crit Care Med* 2000;161:1720–1745.
6. Humbert M, Menz G, Ying S, et al. The immunopathology of extrinsic (atopic) and intrinsic (non-atopic) asthma: more similarities than differences. *Immunol Today* 1999;20:528–533.
7. Ying S, Humbert M, Meng Q, et al. Local expression of epsilon germline gene transcripts and RNA for the epsilon heavy chain of IgE in the bronchial mucosa in atopic and nonatopic asthma. *J Allergy Clin Immunol* 2001;107:686–692.
8. Bentley AM, Hamid Q, Robinson DS, et al. Prednisolone treatment in asthma. Reduction in the numbers of eosinophils, T cells, tryptase-only positive mast cells, and modulation of IL-4, IL-5, and interferon-gamma cytokine gene expression within the bronchial mucosa. *Am J Respir Crit Care Med* 1996;153:551–556.
9. Akers IA, Parsons M, Hill MR, et al. Mast cell tryptase stimulates human lung fibroblast proliferation via protease-activated receptor-2. *Am J Physiol Lung Cell Mol Physiol* 2000;278:L193–L201.
10. Williams CM, Galli SJ. The diverse potential effector and immunoregulatory roles of mast cells in allergic disease. *J Allergy Clin Immunol* 2000;105:847–859.
11. Fahy JV. Reducing IgE levels as a strategy for the treatment of asthma. *Clin Exp Allergy* 2000;30[Suppl 1]:16–21.
12. Barnes PJ. Anti-IgE therapy in asthma: rationale and therapeutic potential. *Int Arch Allergy Immunol* 2000;123:196–204.
13. Milgrom H, Fick RB Jr, Su JQ, et al. Treatment of allergic asthma with monoclonal anti-IgE antibody. *N Engl J Med* 1999;341:1966–1973.
14. Zieg G, Lack G, Harbeck RJ, et al. *In vivo* effects of glucocorticoids on IgE production. *J Allergy Clin Immunol* 1994;94:222–230.
15. Barnes PJ. Corticosteroids, IgE, and atopy. *J Clin Invest* 2001;107:265–266.
16. Barnes PJ. Are mast cells still important in asthma? *Rev Fr Allergol Immunol Clin* 2002;42:20–27.
17. Lee TH, Lane SJ. The role of macrophages in the mechanisms of airway inflammation in asthma. *Am Rev Respir Dis* 1992;145:S27–S30.
18. Poulter LW, Burke CM. Macrophages and allergic lung disease. *Immunobiology* 1996;195:574–587.
19. Spiteri MA, Knight RA, Jeremy JY, et al. Alveolar macrophage-induced suppression of peripheral blood mononuclear cell responsiveness is reversed by *in vitro* allergen exposure in bronchial asthma. *Eur Respir J* 1994;7:1431–1438.
20. John M, Lim S, Seybold J, et al. Inhaled corticosteroids increase IL-10 but reduce MIP-1α, GM-CSF and IFN-γ release from alveolar macrophages in asthma. *Am J Respir Crit Care Med* 1998;157:256–262.
21. Tang C, Ward C, Reid D, et al. Normally suppressing CD40 coregulatory signals delivered by airway macrophages to TH2 lymphocytes are defective in patients with atopic asthma. *J Allergy Clin Immunol* 2001;107:863–870.
22. Holt PG, McMenamin C. Defence against allergic sensitization in the healthy lung: the role of inhalation tolerance. *Clin Exp Allergy* 1989;19:255–262.
23. Taams LS, Poulter LW, Rustin MH, et al. Phenotypic analysis of IL-10–treated macrophages using the monoclonal antibodies RFD1 and RFD7. *Pathobiology* 1999;67:249–252.
24. Zeibecoglou K, Ying S, Meng Q, et al. Macrophage subpopulations and macrophage-derived cytokines in sputum of atopic and nonatopic asthmatic subjects and atopic and normal control subjects. *J Allergy Clin Immunol.* 2000;106:697–704.
25. Banchereau J, Briere F, Caux C, et al. Immunobiology of dendritic cells. *Annu Rev Immunol* 2000;18:767–811.
26. Holt PG, Stumbles PA. Regulation of immunologic homeostasis in peripheral tissues by dendritic cells: the respiratory tract as a paradigm. *J Allergy Clin Immunol* 2000;105:421–429.
27. Lambrecht BN. The dendritic cell in allergic airway diseases: a new player to the game. *Clin Exp Allergy* 2001;31:206–218.
28. Lambrecht BN, De Veerman M, Coyle AJ, et al. Myeloid dendritic cells induce Th2 responses to inhaled antigen, leading to

eosinophilic airway inflammation. *J Clin Invest* 2000;106:551–559.

29. Stumbles PA, Thomas JA, Pimm CL, et al. Resting respiratory tract dendritic cells preferentially stimulate T helper cell type 2 (Th2) responses and require obligatory cytokine signals for induction of Th1 immunity. *J Exp Med* 1998;188:2019–2031.

30. Gleich GJ. Mechanisms of eosinophil-associated inflammation. *J Allergy Clin Immunol* 2000;105:651–663.

31. Robinson DS, Kay AB, Wardlaw AJ. Eosinophils. *Clin Allergy Immunol* 2002;16:43–75.

32. Yukawa T, Read RC, Kroegel C, et al. The effects of activated eosinophils and neutrophils on guinea pig airway epithelium *in vitro. Am J Respir Cell Mol Biol* 1990;2:341–354.

33. Adamko D, Lacy P, Moqbel R. Mechanisms of eosinophil recruitment and activation. *Curr Allergy Asthma Rep* 2002;2:107–116.

34. Woolley MJ, Denburg JA, Ellis R, et al. Allergen-induced changes in bone marrow progenitors and airway responsiveness in dogs and the effect of inhaled budesonide on these parameters. *Am J Respir Cell Mol Biol* 1994;11:600–606.

35. Tachimoto H, Bochner BS. The surface phenotype of human eosinophils. *Chem Immunol* 2000;76:45–62.

36. Wardlaw AJ. Molecular basis for selective eosinophil trafficking in asthma: a multistep paradigm. *J Allergy Clin Immunol* 1999;104:917–926.

37. Wegner CD, Gundel L, Reilly P, et al. Intracellular adhesion molecule-1 (ICAM-1) in the pathogenesis of asthma. *Science* 1990;247:456–459.

38. Sun J, Elwood W, Haczku A, et al. Contribution of intracellular adhesion molecule-1 in allergen-induced airway hyperresponsiveness and inflammation in sensitised Brown-Norway rats. *Int Arch Allergy Immunol* 1994;104:291–295.

39. Pilewski JM, Albelda SM. Cell adhesion molecules in asthma: homing activation and airway remodeling. *Am J Respir Cell Mol Biol* 1995;12:1–3.

40. Lamas AM, Mulroney CM, Schleimer RP. Studies of the adhesive interaction between purified human eosinophils and cultured vascular endothelial cells. *J Immunol* 1988;140:1500–1510.

41. Chanez P, Dent G, Yukawa T, et al. Generation of oxygen free radicals from blood eosinophils from asthma patients after stimulation with PAF or phorbol ester. *Eur Respir J* 1990;3:1002–1007.

42. Evans DJ, Lindsay MA, O'Connor BJ, et al. Priming of circulating human eosinophils following exposure to allergen challenge. *Eur Respir J* 1996;9:703–708.

43. Blease K, Lukacs NW, Hogaboam CM, et al. Chemokines and their role in airway hyper-reactivity. *Respir Res* 2000;1:54–61.

44. Collins PD, Marleau S, Griffiths-Johnson DA, et al. Cooperation between interleukin-5 and the chemokine eotaxin to induce eosinophil accumulation *in vivo. J Exp Med* 1995;182:1169–1174.

45. Park CS, Choi YS, Ki SY, et al. Granulocyte macrophage colony-stimulating factor is the main cytokine enhancing the survival of eosinophils in asthmatic airways. *Eur Respir J* 1998;12:872–878.

46. Simon HU. Regulation of eosinophil and neutrophil apoptosis-similarities and differences. *Immunol Rev* 2001;179:156–162.

47. De Souza PM, Kankaanranta H, Michael A, et al. Caspase-catalyzed cleavage and activation of Mst1 correlates with eosinophil but not neutrophil apoptosis. *Blood* 2002;99:3432–3438.

48. Leckie MJ, Ten Brincke A, Khan J, et al. Effects of an interleukin-5 blocking monoclonal antibody on eosinophils, airway hyperresponsiveness and the late asthmatic response. *Lancet* 2000;356:2144–2148.

49. Kips JC, O'Connor BJ, Langley SJ, et al. Results of a phase I trial with SCH55700, a humanized anti–IL-5 antibody in severe persistent asthma. *Am J Respir Crit Care Med* 2000;161:A505.

50. Minshall EM, Leung DY, Martin RJ, et al. Eosinophil-associated TGF-beta1 mRNA expression and airways fibrosis in bronchial asthma. *Am J Respir Cell Mol Biol* 1997;17:326–333.

51. Wenzel SE, Szefler SJ, Leung DY, et al. Bronchoscopic evaluation of severe asthma. Persistent inflammation associated with high-dose glucocorticoids. *Am J Respir Crit Care Med* 1997;156:737–743.

52. Jatakanon A, Uasaf C, Maziak W, et al. Neutrophilic inflammation in severe persistent asthma. *Am J Respir Crit Care Med* 1999;160:1532–1539.

53. Gibson PG, Simpson JL, Saltos N. Heterogeneity of airway inflammation in persistent asthma: evidence of neutrophilic inflammation and increased sputum interleukin-8. *Chest* 2001;119:1329–1336.

54. Sur S, Crotty TB, Kephart GM, et al. Sudden-onset fatal asthma: a distinct entity with few eosinophils and relatively more neutrophils in the airway submucosa. *Am Rev Respir Dis* 1993;148:713–719.

55. Cox G. Glucocorticoid treatment inhibits apoptosis in human neutrophils. *J Immunol* 1995;193:4719–4725.

56. Meagher LC, Cousin JM, Seckl JR, et al. Opposing effects of glucocorticoids on the rate of apoptosis in neutrophilic and eosinophilic granulocytes. *J Immunol* 1996;156:4422–4428.

57. Montuschi P, Ciabattoni G, Corradi M, et al. Increased 8-isoprostane, a marker of oxidative stress, in exhaled condensates of asthmatic patients. *Am J Respir Crit Care Med* 1999;160:216–220.

58. Kay AB. Allergy and allergic diseases. *N Engl J Med* 2001;344:109–113.

59. Mosmann TR, Sad S. The expanding universe of T-cell subsets: Th1, Th2 and more. *Immunol Today* 1996;17:138–146.

60. Prescott SL, Macaubas C, Smallacombe T, et al. Development of allergen-specific T-cell memory in atopic and normal children. *Lancet* 1999;353:196–200.

61. Holt PG, Sly PD. Prevention of adult asthma by early intervention during childhood: potential value of new-generation immunomodulatory drugs. *Thorax* 2000;55:700–703.

62. Ball TM, Castro-Rodriguez JA, Griffith KA, et al. Siblings, day-care attendance, and the risk of asthma and wheezing during childhood. *N Engl J Med* 2000;343:538–543.

63. Christiansen SC. Day care, siblings, and asthma—please, sneeze on my child. *N Engl J Med* 2000;343:574–575.

64. Naseer T, Minshall EM, Leung DY, et al. Expression of IL-12 and IL-13 mRNA in asthma and their modulation in response to steroids. *Am J Respir Crit Care Med* 1997;155:845–851.

65. Wills-Karp M. IL-12/IL-13 axis in allergic asthma. *J Allergy Clin Immunol* 2001;107:9–18.

66. Levings MK, Sangregorio R, Roncarolo MG. Human CD25+CD4+ T regulatory cells suppress naive and memory T cell proliferation and can be expanded *in vitro* without loss of function. *J Exp Med* 2001;193:1295–1302.

67. Roncarolo MG, Bacchetta R, Bordignon C, et al. Type 1 T regulatory cells. *Immunol Rev* 2001;182:68–79.

68. Gould HJ, Beavil RL, Vercelli D. IgE isotype determination: epsilon-germline gene transcription, DNA recombination and B-cell differentiation. *Br Med Bull* 2000;56:908–924.

69. Costa JJ, Weller PF, Galli SJ. The cells of the allergic response: mast cells, basophils, and eosinophils. *JAMA* 1997;278:1815–1822.

70. Macfarlane AJ, Kon OM, Smith SJ, et al. Basophils, eosinophils, and mast cells in atopic and nonatopic asthma and in late-phase

allergic reactions in the lung and s_..n. *J Allergy Clin Immunol* 2000;105:99–107.

71. Braunstahl GJ, Overbeek SE, Fokkens WJ, et al. Segmental bronchoprovocation in allergic rhinitis patients affects mast cell and basophil numbers in nasal and bronchial mucosa. *Am J Respir Crit Care Med* 2001;164:858–865.

72. Gauvreau GM, Lee JM, Watson RM, et al. Increased numbers of both airway basophils and mast cells in sputum after allergen inhalation challenge of atopic asthmatics. *Am J Respir Crit Care Med* 2000;161:1473–1478.

73. Holgate ST. The role of mast cells and basophils in inflammation. *Clin Exp Allergy* 2000;30[Suppl 1]:28–32.

74. Herd CM, Page CP. Pulmonary immune cells in health and disease: platelets. *Eur Respir J* 1994;7:1145–1160.

75. Sullivan PJ, Jafar ZH, Harbinson PL, et al. Platelet dynamics following allergen challenge in allergic asthmatics. *Respiration* 2000;67:514–517.

76. Moritani C, Ishioka S, Haruta Y, et al. Activation of platelets in bronchial asthma. *Chest* 1998;113:452–458.

77. Abi-Younes S, Si-Tahar M, Luster AD. The CC chemokines MDC and TARC induce platelet activation via CCR4. *Thromb Res* 2001;101:279–289.

78. Levine SJ. Bronchial epithelial cell–cytokine interactions in airway epithelium. *J Invest Med* 1995;43:241–249.

79. Saunders MA, Mitchell JA, Seldon PM, et al. Release of granulocyte-macrophage colony-stimulating factor by human cultured airway smooth muscle cells: suppression by dexamethasone. *Br J Pharmacol* 1997;120:545–546.

80. Johnson SR, Knox AJ. Synthetic functions of airway smooth muscle in asthma. *Trends Pharmacol Sci* 1997;18:288–292.

81. Chung KF. Airway smooth muscle cells: contributing to and regulating airway mucosal inflammation? *Eur Respir J* 2000;15:961–968.

82. Barnes PJ, Chung KF, Page CP. Inflammatory mediators of asthma: an update. *Pharmacol Rev* 1998;50:515–596.

83. Drazen JM, Israel E, O'Byrne PM. Treatment of asthma with drugs modifying the leukotriene pathway. *N Engl J Med* 1999;340:197–206.

84. Bleecker ER, Welch MJ, Weinstein SF, et al. Low-dose inhaled fluticasone propionate versus oral zafirlukast in the treatment of persistent asthma. *J Allergy Clin Immunol* 2000;105:1123–1129.

85. Kim KT, Ginchansky EJ, Friedman BF, et al. Fluticasone propionate versus zafirlukast: effect in patients previously receiving inhaled corticosteroid therapy. *Ann Allergy Asthma Immunol* 2000;85:398–406.

86. Diamant Z, Hiltermann JT, Van Rensen EL, et al. The effect of inhaled leukotriene D_4 and methacholine on sputum cell differentials in asthma. *Am J Respir Crit Care Med* 1997;155:1247–1253.

87. Pizzichini E, Leff JA, Reiss TF, et al. Montelukast reduces airway eosinophilic inflammation in asthma: a randomized, controlled trial. *Eur Respir J* 1999;14:12–18.

88. Chung KF. Platelet-activating factor in inflammation and pulmonary disorders. *Clin Sci (Colch)* 1992;83:127–138.

89. Freitag A, Watson RM, Mabos G, et al. Effect of a platelet-activating factor antagonist, WEB 2086, on allergen-induced asthmatic responses. *Thorax* 1993;48:594–598.

90. Kuitert LM, Angus RM, Barnes NC, et al. The effect of a novel potent PAF antagonist, modipafant, in chronic asthma. *Am J Respir Crit Care Med* 1995;151:1331–1335.

91. Spence DPS, Johnston SL, Calverley PMA, et al. The effect of the orally active platelet-activating factor antagonist WEB 2086 in the treatment of asthma. *Am J Respir Crit Care Med* 1994;149:1142–1148.

92. Stafforini DM, Numao T, Tsodikov A, et al. Deficiency of platelet-activating factor acetylhydrolase is a severity factor for asthma. *J Clin Invest* 1999;103:989–997.

93. Taha R, Olivenstein R, Utsumi T, et al. Prostaglandin H synthase 2 expression in airway cells from patients with asthma and chronic obstructive pulmonary disease. *Am J Respir Crit Care Med* 2000;161:636–640.

94. Hirai H, Tanaka K, Yoshie O, et al. Prostaglandin D_2 selectively induces chemotaxis in T helper type 2 cells, eosinophils, and basophils via seven-transmembrane receptor CRTH2. *J Exp Med* 2001;193:255–261.

95. Cowburn AS, Sladek K, Soja J, et al. Overexpression of leukotriene C_4 synthase in bronchial biopsies from patients with aspirin-intolerant asthma. *J Clin Invest* 1998;101:834–846.

96. Matsuoka T, Hirata M, Tanaka H, et al. Prostaglandin D_2 as a mediator of allergic asthma. *Science* 2000;287:2013–2017.

97. Chung KF, Barnes PJ. Cytokines in asthma. *Thorax* 1999;54:825–857.

98. Barnes PJ. Cytokines as mediators of chronic asthma. *Am J Respir Crit Care Med* 1994;150:S42–S49.

99. Barnes PJ. Cytokine modulators as novel therapies for asthma. *Ann Rev Pharmacol Toxicol* 2002;42:81–98.

100. Greenfeder S, Umland SP, Cuss FM, et al. The role of interleukin-5 in allergic eosinophilic disease. *Respir Res* 2001;2:71–79.

101. Borish LC, Nelson HS, Corren J, et al. Efficacy of soluble IL-4 receptor for the treatment of adults with asthma. *J Allergy Clin Immunol* 2001;107:963–970.

102. Levitt RC, McLane MP, MacDonald D, et al. IL-9 pathway in asthma: new therapeutic targets for allergic inflammatory disorders. *J Allergy Clin Immunol* 1999;103:S485–S491.

103. Zhou Y, McLane M, Levitt RC. Interleukin-9 as a therapeutic target for asthma. *Respir Res* 2001;2:80–84.

104. Kips JC, Tavernier JH, Joos GF, et al. The potential role of tumor necrosis factor-α in asthma. *Clin Exp Allergy* 1993;23:247–250.

105. Thomas PS, Yates DH, Barnes PJ. Tumor necrosis factor-α increases airway responsiveness and sputum neutrophils in normal human subjects. *Am J Respir Crit Care Med* 1995;152:76–80.

106. Rossi D, Zlotnik A. The biology of chemokines and their receptors. *Annu Rev Immunol* 2000;18:217–242.

107. Proudfoot AE, Power CA, Wells TN. The strategy of blocking the chemokine system to combat disease. *Immunol Rev* 2000;177:246–256.

108. Gutierrez-Ramos JC, Lloyd C, Kapsenberg ML, et al. Non-redundant functional groups of chemokines operate in a coordinate manner during the inflammatory response in the lung. *Immunol Rev* 2000;177:31–42.

109. Gutierrez-Ramos JC, Lloyd C, Gonzalo JA. Eotaxin: from an eosinophilic chemokine to a major regulator of allergic reactions. *Immunol Today* 1999;20:500–504.

110. Gonzalo JA, Lloyd CM, Kremer L, et al. Eosinophil recruitment to the lung in a murine model of allergic inflammation. The role of T cells, chemokines, and adhesion receptors. *J Clin Invest* 1996;98:2332–2345.

111. Ying S, Robinson DS, Meng Q, et al. Enhanced expression of eotaxin and CCR3 mRNA and protein in atopic asthma. Association with airway hyperresponsiveness and predominant co-localization of eotaxin mRNA to bronchial epithelial and endothelial cells. *Eur J Immunol* 1997;27:3507–3516.

112. Ying S, Meng Q, Zeibecoglou K, et al. Eosinophil chemotactic chemokines (eotaxin, eotaxin-2, RANTES, monocyte chemoattractant protein-3 [MCP-3], and MCP-4), and C-C chemokine receptor 3 expression in bronchial biopsies from atopic and nonatopic (intrinsic) asthmatics. *J Immunol* 1999;163:6321–6329.

113. Sabroe I, Peck MJ, Van Keulen BJ, et al. A small molecule antagonist of chemokine receptors CCR1 and CCR3. Potent inhibition of eosinophil function and CCR3-mediated HIV-1 entry. *J Biol Chem* 2000;275:25985–25992.

114. White JR, Lee JM, Dede K, et al. Identification of potent, selective non-peptide CC chemokine receptor-3 antagonist that inhibits eotaxin-, eotaxin-2–, and monocyte chemotactic protein-4–induced eosinophil migration. *J Biol Chem* 2000;275:36626–36631.

115. Berkman N, Krishnan VL, Gilbey T, et al. Expression of RANTES mRNA and protein in airways of patients with mild asthma. *Am J Respir Crit Care Med* 1996;154:1804–1811.

116. Campbell EM, Charo IF, Kunkel SL, et al. Monocyte chemoattractant protein-1 mediates cockroach allergen-induced bronchial hyperreactivity in normal but not CCR2−/− mice: the role of mast cells. *J Immunol* 1999;163:2160–2167.

117. Holgate ST. Cellular and mediator basis of asthma in relationship to natural history. *Lancet* 1997;350[Suppl 2]:S115–S119.

118. Lloyd CM, Delaney T, Nguyen T, et al. CC chemokine receptor (CCR)3/eotaxin is followed by CCR4/monocyte-derived chemokine in mediating pulmonary T helper lymphocyte type 2 recruitment after serial antigen challenge *in vivo*. *J Exp Med* 2000;191:265–274.

119. Berin MC, Eckmann L, Broide DH, et al. Regulated production of the T helper 2-type T-cell chemoattractant TARC by human bronchial epithelial cells *in vitro* and in human lung xenografts. *Am J Respir Cell Mol Biol* 2001;24:382–389.

120. Sekiya T, Miyamasu M, Imanishi M, et al. Inducible expression of a Th2-type CC chemokine thymus- and activation-regulated chemokine by human bronchial epithelial cells. *J Immunol* 2000;165:2205–2213.

121. Paredi P, Kharitonov SA, Barnes PJ. Elevation of exhaled ethane concentration in asthma. *Am J Respir Crit Care Med* 2000;162:1450–1454.

122. Barnes PJ. Reactive oxygen species in asthma. *Eur Respir Rev* 2000;10:240–243.

123. Hay DW, Henry PJ, Goldie RG. Is endothelin-1 a mediator in asthma? *Am J Respir Crit Care Med* 1996;154:1594–1597.

124. Goldie RG, Henry PJ. Endothelins and asthma. *Life Sci* 1999;65:1–15.

125. Chalmers GW, Little SA, Patel KR, et al. Endothelin-1-induced bronchoconstriction in asthma. *Am J Respir Crit Care Med* 1997;156:382–388.

126. Redington AE, Springall DR, Ghatei MA, et al. Airway endothelin levels in asthma: influence of endobronchial allergen challenge and maintenance corticosteroid therapy. *Eur Respir J* 1997;10:1026–1032.

127. Mullol J, Picado C. Endothelin in nasal mucosa: role in nasal function and inflammation. *Clin Exp Allergy* 2000;30:172–177.

128. Barnes PJ, Liew FY. Nitric oxide and asthmatic inflammation. *Immunol Today* 1995;16:128–130.

129. Gaston B, Drazen JM, Loscalzo J, et al. The biology of nitrogen oxides in the airways. *Am J Respir Crit Care Med* 1994;149:538–551.

130. Silkoff PE, Sylvester JT, Zamel N, et al. Airway nitric oxide diffusion in asthma: role in pulmonary function and bronchial responsiveness. *Am J Respir Crit Care Med* 2000;161:1218–1228.

131. Kharitonov SA, Barnes PJ. Exhaled markers of pulmonary disease. *Am J Respir Crit Care Med* 2001;163:1693–1772.

132. Jatakanon A, Lim S, Kharitonov SA, et al. Correlation between exhaled nitric oxide, sputum eosinophils and methacholine responsiveness. *Thorax* 1998;53:91–95.

133. Lim S, Jatakanon A, Meah S, et al. Relationship between exhaled nitric oxide and mucosal eosinophilic inflammation in mild to moderately severe asthma. *Thorax* 2000;55:184–188.

134. Hunt JF, Fang K, Malik R, et al. Endogenous airway acidification. Implications for asthma pathophysiology. *Am J Respir Crit Care Med* 2000;161:694–699.

135. Saleh D, Ernst P, Lim S, et al. Increased formation of the potent oxidant peroxynitrite in the airways of asthmatic patients is associated with induction of nitric oxide synthase: effect of inhaled glucocorticoid. *FASEB J* 1998;12:929–937.

136. Kharitonov SA, Barnes PJ. Clinical aspects of exhaled nitric oxide. *Eur Respir J* 2000;16:781–792.

137. Lange P, Parner J, Vestbo J, et al. A 15-year follow-up study of ventilatory function in adults with asthma. *N Engl J Med* 1998;339:1194–1200.

138. Ulrik CS, Lange P. Decline of lung function in adults with bronchial asthma. *Am J Respir Crit Care Med* 1994;150:629–634.

139. Holgate ST, Davies DE, Lackie PM, et al. Epithelial-mesenchymal interactions in the pathogenesis of asthma. *J Allergy Clin Immunol* 2000;105:193–204.

140. Redington AE. Fibrosis and airway remodelling. *Clin Exp Allergy* 2000;30[Suppl 1]:42–45.

141. Chetta A, Foresi A, Del Donno M, et al. Airways remodeling is a distinctive feature of asthma and is related to severity of disease. *Chest* 1997;111:852–857.

142. Ressler B, Lee RT, Randell SH, et al. Molecular responses of rat tracheal epithelial cells to transmembrane pressure. *Am J Physiol Lung Cell Mol Physiol* 2000;278:L1264–L1272.

143. Kips JC, Pauwels RA. Airway wall remodelling: does it occur and what does it mean? *Clin Exp Allergy* 1999;29:1457–1466.

144. Fish JE, Peters SP. Airway remodeling and persistent airway obstruction in asthma. *J Allergy Clin Immunol* 1999;104:509–516.

145. Wilson JW, Li X. The measurement of reticular basement membrane and submucosal collagen in the asthmatic airway [see Comments]. *Clin Exp Allergy* 1997;27:363–371.

146. Barnes PJ. Pharmacology of airway smooth muscle. *Am J Respir Crit Care Med* 1998;158:S123–S132.

147. Bai TR, Mak JCW, Barnes PJ. A comparison of beta-adrenergic receptors and *in vitro* relaxant responses to isoproterenol in asthmatic airway smooth muscle. *Am J Respir Cell Mol Biol* 1992;6:647–651.

148. Hakonarson H, Herrick DJ, Serrano PG, et al. Mechanism of cytokine-induced modulation of β-adrenoceptor responsiveness in airway smooth muscle. *J Clin Invest* 1996;97:2593–2600.

149. Koto H, Mak JCW, Haddad E-B, et al. Mechanisms of impaired β-adrenergic receptor relaxation by interleukin-1β *in vivo* in rat. *J Clin Invest* 1996;98:1780–1787.

150. Laporte JD, Moore PE, Panettieri RA, et al. Prostanoids mediate IL-1beta–induced beta-adrenergic hyporesponsiveness in human airway smooth muscle cells. *Am J Physiol* 1998;275:L491–L501.

151. Grandordy BM, Mak JCW, Barnes PJ. Modulation of airway smooth muscle β-receptor function by a muscarinic agonist. *Life Sci* 1994;54:185–191.

152. Mak JC, Hisada T, Salmon M, et al. Glucocorticoids reverse IL-1β–induced impairment of β-adrenoceptor–mediated relaxation and up-regulation of G-protein–coupled receptor kinases. *Br J Pharmacol* 2002;135:987–996.

153. Ebina M, Yaegashi H, Chiba R, et al. Hyperreactive site in the airway tree of asthmatic patients recoded by thickening of bronchial muscles: a morphometric study. *Am Rev Respir Dis* 1990;141:1327–1332.

154. Hirst SJ, Walker TR, Chilvers ER. Phenotypic diversity and

molecular mechanisms of airway smooth muscle proliferation in asthma. *Eur Respir J* 2000;16:159–177.

155. Kumar SD, Emery MJ, Atkins ND, et al. Airway mucosal blood flow in bronchial asthma. *Am J Respir Crit Care Med* 1998;158:153–156.

156. Paredi P, Kharitonov SA, Barnes PJ. Faster rise of exhaled breath temperature in asthma. A novel marker of airway inflammation? *Am J Respir Crit Care Med* 2002;165:181–184.

157. McFadden ER. Hypothesis: exercise-induced asthma as a vascular phenomenon. *Lancet* 1990;335:880–883.

158. Kuwano K, Boskev CH, Paré PD, et al. Small airways dimensions in asthma and chronic obstructive pulmonary disease. *Am Rev Respir Dis* 1993;148:1220–1225.

159. Wilson J. The bronchial microcirculation in asthma. *Clin Exp Allergy* 2000;30[Suppl 1]:51–53.

160. Hoshino M, Takahashi M, Aoike N. Expression of vascular endothelial growth factor, basic fibroblast growth factor, and angiogenin immunoreactivity in asthmatic airways and its relationship to angiogenesis. *J Allergy Clin Immunol* 2001;107:295–301.

161. Persson CGA. Plasma exudation and asthma. *Lung* 1988;166:1–23.

162. Chung KF, Rogers DF, Barnes PJ, et al. The role of increased airway microvascular permeability and plasma exudation in asthma. *Eur Respir J* 1990;3:329–337.

163. Persson CG, Andersson M, Greiff L, et al. Airway permeability. *Clin Exp Allergy* 1995;25:807–814.

164. Yager D, Martins MA, Feldman H, et al. Acute histamine-induced flux of airway liquid: role of neuropeptides. *J Appl Physiol* 1996;80:1285–1295.

165. Longphre M, Li D, Gallup M, et al. Allergen-induced IL-9 directly stimulates mucin transcription in respiratory epithelial cells. *J Clin Invest* 1999;104:1375–1382.

166. Ordonez CL, Khashayar R, Wong HH, et al. Mild and moderate asthma is associated with airway goblet cell hyperplasia and abnormalities in mucin gene expression. *Am J Respir Crit Care Med* 2001;163:517–523.

167. Rogers DF. Motor control of airway goblet cells and glands. *Respir Physiol* 2001;125:129–144.

168. Zhu Z, Homer RJ, Wang Z, et al. Pulmonary expression of interleukin-13 causes inflammation, mucus hypersecretion, subepithelial fibrosis, physiologic abnormalities, and eotaxin production. *J Clin Invest* 1999;103:779–788.

169. Temann UA, Prasad B, Gallup MW, et al. A novel role for murine IL-4 *in vivo*: induction of MUC5AC gene expression and mucin hypersecretion. *Am J Respir Cell Mol Biol* 1997;16:471–478.

170. Takeyama K, Dabbagh K, Lee HM, et al. Epidermal growth factor system regulates mucin production in airways. *Proc Natl Acad Sci U S A* 1999;96:3081–3086.

171. Takeyama K, Dabbagh K, Jeong SJ, et al. Oxidative stress causes mucin synthesis via transactivation of epidermal growth factor receptor: role of neutrophils. *J Immunol* 2000;164:1546–1552.

172. Shim JJ, Dabbagh K, Ueki IF, et al. IL-13 induces mucin production by stimulating epidermal growth factor receptors and by activating neutrophils. *Am J Physiol Lung Cell Mol Physiol* 2001;280:L134–L140.

173. Nakanishi A, Morita S, Iwashita H, et al. Role of gob-5 in mucus overproduction and airway hyperresponsiveness in asthma. *Proc Natl Acad Sci U S A* 2001;98:5175–5180.

174. Barnes PJ. Is asthma a nervous disease? *Chest* 1995;107:119S–124S.

175. Barnes PJ, Baraniuk J, Belvisi MG. Neuropeptides in the respiratory tract. *Am Rev Respir Dis* 1991;144:1187–1198, 1391–1399.

176. Joos GF, Germonpre PR, Pauwels RA. Role of tachykinins in asthma. *Allergy* 2000;55:321–337.

177. Barnes PJ. Modulation of neurotransmission in airways. *Physiol Rev* 1992;72:699–729.

178. Fox AJ, Barnes PJ, Urban L, et al. An *in vitro* study of the properties of single vagal afferents innervating guinea-pig airways. *J Physiol* 1993;469:21–35.

179. Fox AJ, Lalloo UG, Belvisi MG, et al. Bradykinin-evoked sensitization of airway sensory nerves: a mechanism for ACE-inhibitor cough. *Nat Med* 1996;2:814–817.

180. Colucci WS, Wright RF, Braunwald E. New positive inotropic agents in the treatment of congestive heart failure. Mechanisms of action and recent clinical developments. *N Engl J Med* 1986;314:349–358.

181. Braun A, Lommatzsch M, Renz H. The role of neurotrophins in allergic bronchial asthma. *Clin Exp Allergy* 2000;30:178–186.

182. Carr MJ, Hunter DD, Undem BJ. Neurotrophins and asthma. *Curr Opin Pulm Med* 2001;7:1–7.

183. Fox AJ, Patel HJ, Barnes PJ, et al. Release of nerve growth factor by human pulmonary epithelial cells: role in airway inflammatory diseases. *Eur J Pharmacol* 2001;424:159–162.

184. Renz H. Neurotrophins in bronchial asthma. *Respir Res* 2001;2:265–268.

185. Lammers JWJ, Barnes PJ, Chung KF. Non-adrenergic, non-cholinergic airway inhibitory nerves. *Eur Respir J* 1992;5:239–246.

186. Ollerenshaw S, Jarvis D, Woolcock A, et al. Absence of immunoreactive vasoactive intestinal polypeptide in tissue from the lungs of patients with asthma. *N Engl J Med* 1989;320:1244–1248.

187. Howarth PH, Springall DR, Redington AE, et al. Neuropeptide-containing nerves in bronchial biopsies from asthmatic and non-asthmatic subjects. *Am J Respir Cell Mol Biol* 1995;13:288–296.

188. Belvisi MG, Stretton CD, Barnes PJ. Nitric oxide is the endogenous neurotransmitter of bronchodilator nerves in human airways. *Eur J Pharmacol* 1992;210:221–222.

189. Barnes PJ. Sensory nerves, neuropeptides and asthma. *Ann N Y Acad Sci* 1991;629:359–370.

190. Barnes PJ. Neurogenic inflammation in the airways. *Respir Physiol* 2001;125:145–154.

191. Ollerenshaw SL, Jarvis D, Sullivan CE, et al. Substance P immunoreactive nerves in airways from asthmatics and non-asthmatics. *Eur Respir J* 1991;4:673–682.

192. Nadel JA. Neutral endopeptidase modulates neurogenic inflammation. *Eur Respir J* 1991;4:745–754.

193. Adcock IM, Peters M, Gelder C, et al. Increased tachykinin receptor gene expression in asthmatic lung and its modulation by steroids. *J Mol Endocrinol* 1993;11:1–7.

194. Bai TR, Zhou D, Weir T, et al. Substance P (NK$_1$)- and neurokinin A (NK$_2$)-receptor gene expression in inflammatory airway diseases. *Am J Physiol* 1995;269:L309–L317.

195. Barnes PJ, Adcock IM. Transcription factors and asthma. *Eur Respir J* 1998;12:221–234.

196. Barnes PJ, Karin M. Nuclear factor-κB: a pivotal transcription factor in chronic inflammatory diseases. *N Engl J Med* 1997;336:1066–1071.

197. Hart LA, Krishnan VL, Adcock IM, et al. Activation and localization of transcription factor, nuclear factor-κB, in asthma. *Am J Respir Crit Care Med* 1998;158:1585–1592.

198. Hart L, Lim S, Adcock I, et al. Effects of inhaled corticosteroid therapy on expression and DNA-binding activity of nuclear factor-κB in asthma. *Am J Respir Crit Care Med* 2000;161:224–231.

199. Demoly P, Basset-Seguin N, Chanez P, et al. c-Fos proto-oncogene expression in bronchial biopsies of asthmatics. *Am J Respir Cell Mol Biol* 1992;7:128–133.

200. Urnov FD, Wolffe AP. Chromatin remodeling and transcriptional activation: the cast (in order of appearance). *Oncogene* 2001;20:2991–3006.
201. Ito K, Barnes PJ, Adcock IM. Glucocorticoid receptor recruitment of histone deacetylase 2 inhibits IL-1β–induced histone H$_4$ acetylation on lysines 8 and 12. *Mol Cell Biol* 2000;20:6891–6903.
202. Zheng W, Flavell RA. The transcription factor GATA-3 is necessary and sufficient for Th2 cytokine gene expression in CD4 T cells. *Cell* 1997;89:587–596.
203. Nakamura Y, Ghaffar O, Olivenstein R, et al. Gene expression of the GATA-3 transcription factor is increased in atopic asthma. *J Allergy Clin Immunol* 1999;103:215–222.
204. Caramori G, Lim S, Ito K, et al. Expression of GATA family of transcription factors in T-cells, monocytes and bronchial biopsies. *Eur Respir J* 2001;18:466–473.
205. Szabo SJ, Sullivan BM, Stemmann C, et al. Distinct effects of T-bet in Th1 lineage commitment and IFN-gamma production in CD4 and CD8 T cells. *Science* 2002;295:338–342.
206. Finotto S, Neurath MF, Glickman JN, et al. Development of spontaneous airway changes consistent with human asthma in mice lacking T-bet. *Science* 2002;295:336–338.
207. Barnes PJ. Endogenous inhibitory mechanisms in asthma. *Am J Respir Crit Care Med* 2000;161:S176–S181.
208. Herrscher RF, Kasper C, Sullivan TJ. Endogenous cortisol regulates immunoglobulin E-dependent late phase reactions. *J Clin Invest* 1992;90:593–603.
209. Schleimer RP. Potential regulation of inflammation in the lung by local metabolism of hydrocortisone. *Am J Respir Cell Mol Biol* 1991;4:166–173.
210. Barnes PJ, Lim S. Inhibitory cytokines in asthma. *Mol Med Today* 1998;4:452–458.
211. Selig W, Tocker J. Effect of interleukin-1 receptor antagonist on antigen-induced pulmonary responses in guinea-pigs. *Eur J Pharmacol* 1992;213:331–336.
212. Bryan S, O'Connor BJ, Matti S, et al. Effects of recombinant human interleukin-12 on eosinophils, airway hyperreactivity and the late asthmatic response. *Lancet* 2000;356:2149–2153.
213. Borish L, Aarons A, Rumbyrt J, et al. Interleukin-10 regulation in normal subjects and patients with asthma. *J Allergy Clin Immunol* 1996;97:1288–1296.
214. Barnes PJ. IL-10: a key regulator of allergic disease. *Clin Exp Allergy* 2001;31:667–669.
215. Tomita K, Lim S, Hanazawa T, et al. Attenuated production of intracellular IL-10 and IL-12 in monocytes from patients with severe asthma. *Clin Immunol* 2002;102:258–266.
216. Lim S, Crawley E, Woo P, et al. Haplotype associated with low interleukin-10 production in patients with severe asthma. *Lancet* 1998;352:113.
217. Pavord ID, Tattersfield AE. Bronchoprotective role for endogenous prostaglandin E$_2$. *Lancet* 1995;344:436–438.
218. Lee HJ, Masuda ES, Arai N, et al. Definition of *cis*-regulatory elements of the mouse interleukin-5 gene promoter. Involvement of nuclear factor of activated T cell–related factors in interleukin-5 expression. *J Biol Chem* 1995;270:17541–17550.
219. Levy BD, Fokin VV, Clark JM, et al. Polyisoprenyl phosphate (PIPP) signaling regulates phospholipase D activity: a 'stop' signaling switch for aspirin-triggered lipoxin A$_4$. *FASEB J* 1999;13:903–911.
220. Kanazawa H, Kurihara N, Hirata K, et al. Adrenomedullin, a newly discovered hypotensive peptide, is a potent bronchodilator. *Biochem Biophys Res Commun* 1994;205:251–254.
221. Kamoi H, Kanazawa H, Hirata K, et al. Adrenomedullin inhibits the secretion of cytokine-induced neutrophil chemoattractant, a member of the interleukin-8 family, from rat alveolar macrophages. *Biochem Biophy Res Commun* 1995;211:1031–1035.
222. Ceyhan BB, Karakurt S, Hekim N. Plasma adrenomedullin levels in asthmatic patients. *J Asthma* 2001;38:221–227.

Diagnosis and Treatment of Asthma

E. Rand Sutherland · Monica Kraft · James D. Crapo

Asthma is one of the most prevalent chronic diseases in the United States. In 1995, an estimated 14,900,000 Americans had asthma, with a self-reported prevalence of asthma of approximately 57 per 1,000 persons. According to 1995 data, asthma accounts for 1,500,000 emergency department encounters, 500,000 acute care hospitalizations, and more than 5,500 deaths each year. The estimated total financial impact of asthma in 1998 alone was $11,300,000,000. Furthermore, the prevalence of asthma has been steadily increasing in all age groups since 1980, and this rise in prevalence has been associated with an increased number of emergency department visits for asthma and either stable or increasing rates of acute care hospitalizations for asthma (1).

Although little evidence indicates that appropriate pharmacologic therapy reduces the incidence or prevalence of asthma, treatment plays a significant role in improving the quality of life. Treatment also reduces the number of physician encounters for acute worsening of asthma and the overall costs of asthma to both individuals and society. A number of therapeutic options are now available to improve the respiratory health of patients with asthma. This chapter reviews important clinical aspects of asthma as they relate to diagnosis and treatment and discusses the characteristics and utilization of drugs currently available for the treatment of asthma. Discussions of the evidence supporting the use of the various agents are included, and references to consensus guidelines for the treatment of asthma are made throughout.

MAKING THE DIAGNOSIS OF ASTHMA

Asthma often presents a diagnostic challenge. In part, this is because asthma is not a single disease entity, but rather a clinical syndrome that results from a combination of airway inflammation, airway responsiveness, and bronchodilator-reversible limitation of expiratory airflow. Because no set of reference standard criteria is available for the diagnosis of asthma, the most commonly utilized definitions of asthma are based on expert panel consensus (2). The National Institutes of Health (NIH) guidelines define asthma as a chronic inflammatory disorder of the airways that, in susceptible individuals, causes signs and symptoms of airflow limitation, including episodic wheezing, breathlessness, chest tightness, and cough. These symptoms occur more frequently at night and in the early morning and are associated with reversible airflow limitation and bronchial hyperresponsiveness (2).

It is likely that a wide variety of both genetic and environmental factors predisposes to the development of asthma, although the exact factors and their importance in the pathogenesis of asthma remain unknown. Furthermore, the symptoms that are common in patients with asthma are also common in many other lung diseases. A differential diagnosis of asthma in adults is provided in Table 10.1.

Much of the information needed to make the diagnosis of asthma is obtained from the history, physical examination, and spirometry. An appropriate diagnostic evaluation allows the physician not only to make the diagnosis of asthma, but also to stage the severity of asthma and detect confounding factors, all of which directly influence asthma therapy. In making the diagnosis of asthma, three criteria are important: (a) Signs or symptoms of episodic airflow limitation must be present; (b) airflow limitation, once documented, must be at least partially reversible with bronchodilator therapy; and (c) pulmonary diseases other than asthma should be excluded (2).

Historical Clues to Asthma

The clinical history is a critical initial element in the evaluation of asthma. Historical factors that should lead the

E. R. Sutherland, M. Kraft, and J. D. Crapo: Department of Medicine, National Jewish Medical and Research Center, Denver, Colorado.

TABLE 10.1. DIFFERENTIAL DIAGNOSIS OF ASTHMA

Other diffuse airways diseases	Chronic bronchitis
	Emphysema
	Cystic fibrosis
	Sarcoidosis
	Bronchiectasis
	Bronchiolitis obliterans
	Postinfectious airways responsiveness
	Congestive heart failure–associated bronchospasm
Focal airway abnormalities	Paradoxical vocal cord dysfunction
	Airway stenoses or strictures
	Endobronchial tumors
	Sarcoidosis
Parenchymal lung diseases	Hypersensitivity pneumonitis
	Sarcoidosis
	Silicosis
	Churg-Strauss syndrome
	Vasculitis
Other diseases	Rhinosinusitis
	Gastroesophageal reflux disease

physician to consider a diagnosis of asthma include episodic wheezing, cough, dyspnea, and chest tightness. These signs and symptoms may worsen at night, resulting in nocturnal awakening. Other factors that can trigger worsening of symptoms in asthmatic patients include exercise, weather changes or exposure to cold air, upper respiratory tract infections, and exposure to tobacco smoke, animals, pollens, or molds (2).

Although these signs and symptoms are taught as the key classic findings in asthma, they may be present only variably and are not reported by all patients with asthma. In 1986, Baumann and colleagues (3) reported that only 36% of patients with asthma had the classic features of cough, dyspnea, and wheezing during bronchoconstriction induced with histamine or house dust mite antigen. Under these same conditions of induced bronchoconstriction, 27% of asthmatic subjects demonstrated no clinical symptoms at all. Burrows and colleagues (4) reported that in a cohort of elderly sub-

jects with newly diagnosed asthma, wheezing was the most commonly reported symptom but was seen in only 50% of subjects. Based on multiple logistic regression, the combination of attacks of dyspnea and wheezing was the best predictor of a subsequent diagnosis of asthma.

In 2001, Sistek and colleagues (5) reported the results of a questionnaire study of 9,651 Swiss adults, 2.3% of whom carried a doctor's diagnosis of asthma and had experienced an asthma exacerbation within the previous year. Wheezing was the most prevalent symptom, reported by 75% of asthmatic subjects. Exertional dyspnea was reported by 69.3% of asthmatic subjects, rest dyspnea by 47.1%, and nocturnal dyspnea by 46.2%. Nocturnal cough was reported by 49.3% of asthmatic subjects, and 21.5% had chronic cough. The best performing indicators of asthma (as measured by the positive predictive value [PPV], which is the probability that an individual actually has asthma given a positive report of a symptom [6]) were the combination of wheezing and dyspnea, which had a PPV of 23.9%, and nocturnal dyspnea, which had a PPV of 21.5% (5) (Table 10.2). Many of these symptoms demonstrated high negative predictive values (Table 10.2), suggesting that asthma is less likely if the symptom is absent.

In summary, the signs and symptoms of airflow limitation are useful in raising the clinical suspicion of asthma. The presence of these symptoms is consistent with, but not diagnostic of, asthma and should prompt further diagnostic evaluation. Finally, the absence of symptoms such as wheezing, exertional dyspnea, and cough should prompt the clinician to consider other diagnoses.

The Physical Examination in Asthma

The reduced airway caliber that occurs as a result of airway inflammation, airway smooth muscle contraction, and mucus plugging leads directly to expiratory airflow limitation and to many of the manifestations of asthma apparent

TABLE 10.2. TEST CHARACTERISTICS OF SELF-REPORTED RESPIRATORY SYMPTOMS IN THE DIAGNOSIS OF ASTHMA

Symptom	Sensitivity (%)	Specificity (%)	Positive Predictive Value (%)	Negative Predictive Value (%)
Wheezing	74.7	87.3	12.4	99.3
Wheezing + dyspnea	65.2	95.1	23.9	99.1
Nocturnal chest tightness	49.3	86.4	8.0	98.6
Dyspnea with exertion	69.3	75.7	6.4	99.0
Dyspnea at rest	47.1	94.9	8.0	98.7
Nocturnal dyspnea	46.2	96.0	21.5	98.7
Chronic cough	21.5	95.2	9.6	98.1
Nocturnal cough	49.3	72.3	4.1	98.4

Source: From Sistek D, Tschopp JM, Schindler C, et al. Clinical diagnosis of current asthma: predictive value of respiratory symptoms in the SAPALDIA Study. Swiss Study on Air Pollution and Lung Diseases in Adults. *Eur Respir J* 2001;17:214–219, with permission.

on physical examination. However, the physical examination findings of a patient with stable chronic asthma may be normal, so that the physical examination is a somewhat limited tool in the asthma diagnostic algorithm.

Physical findings that may increase the clinician's suspicion of asthma include wheezing on auscultation of the thorax, a prolonged expiratory phase, thoracic hyperexpansion, accessory muscle use, and cutaneous manifestations of atopic dermatitis (2). When subjected to rigorous analysis, however, many of these findings are of limited utility in making an unequivocal diagnosis of asthma. They are useful in raising the clinical suspicion of asthma. As a consequence of their comprehensive 1995 review of the literature on the clinical diagnosis of airflow limitation, Holleman and Simel (7) stated that "no single item or combination of items from the clinical examination rules out airflow limitation." They did report that the combination of decreased breath sounds, wheezing, rales, and a prolonged expiratory time is a useful indicator of airflow limitation, with a likelihood ratio of 3.3.

Pulmonary Function Testing in Asthma

The NIH Expert Panel Report 2 (2) recommends that spirometric indices such as the forced expiratory volume in 1 second (FEV_1), measured FEV_1 expressed as a percentage of the predicted FEV_1 value ($FEV_1\%$), forced vital capacity (FVC), and the FEV_1/FVC ratio be measured both before and after the administration of a short-acting β_2-agonist in all subjects in whom asthma is suspected (2). The FEV_1/FVC ratio is the most reliable spirometric value for diagnosing expiratory airflow limitation because of its sensitivity and reproducibility. However, it is difficult to define a fixed lower boundary value for the FEV_1/FVC ratio because it is inversely related to height and age. Age-, race- and gender-specific population-based reference values are commonly used to determine "normal" values of FEV_1, FVC, and the FEV_1/FVC ratio. The American Thoracic Society has suggested that a value that falls two standard deviations outside the reference population mean value be considered abnormal (8).

Spirometry before and after the administration of albuterol is an important component of pulmonary function testing in asthma. To satisfy the criteria for bronchodilator reversibility, a 12% improvement in either the FEV_1 or the FVC should occur after the administration of a bronchodilator such as albuterol (8). The measurement of lung volumes may be useful in the evaluation of asthma to document gas trapping or hyperinflation, and methacholine or other inhalational challenge techniques may be used to document airway responsiveness. Serial measurements of the peak expiratory flow rate may be used in patients with documented asthma to monitor changes in airflow over time and assist patients in recognizing a change in disease status.

Airway responsiveness, an important physiologic component of asthma, can also be diagnosed in the pulmonary function laboratory. The inhalation of bronchoconstrictors such as methacholine, histamine, and cold air may be used in an attempt to induce airway smooth muscle contraction. This narrows the airway luminal diameter, resulting in acute reductions in spirometric indices of airflow, including FEV_1. Airway responsiveness, although common in asthma, is also seen in patients with lung diseases other than asthma and even in persons who do not have asthma (9). Therefore, although airway responsiveness must be present to make the diagnosis of asthma, it is not a specific finding and must be evaluated in the context of clinical and other physiologic findings. A change in the FEV_1 of 20% (PC_{20}) is typically used as the diagnostic threshold for a significant change in airflow as a result of inhalational challenge, and the American Thoracic Society classifies a 20% fall in the FEV_1 occurring at methacholine concentrations between 1 and 4 mg/mL as mild airway responsiveness (9). In addition to methacholine, other inhaled irritants, such as histamine, cold air, and even agents to which a patient is exposed at work, may be used in an attempt to evaluate airway responsiveness.

Other Diagnostic Testing

Other diagnostic tests are useful primarily in excluding alternative diagnoses in patients for whom a diagnosis of asthma is being considered, and their choice should be dictated by the clinical scenario and differential diagnosis. Chest radiography can be used to exclude parenchymal lung disease or other airway diseases, such as bronchiectasis. All patients with asthma should be questioned about their exposure and response to inhaled allergens; if a patient has persistent asthma requiring daily therapy, a careful history of allergen exposure should be taken, and the patient's sensitivity to these allergens and other common environmental allergens should be assessed via skin or *in vitro* testing (2).

CLINICAL PHENOTYPES OF ASTHMA

In 1997, the NIH issued guidelines for classifying the severity of asthma according to both symptomatic and functional criteria. Based on the NIH guidelines, asthma can be classified into four levels (or "steps") of severity that range from mild intermittent asthma (step 1) to severe persistent asthma (step 4). These steps provide a framework for assessing disease severity at the time of initial presentation, determining appropriate therapy, assessing the response to therapeutic interventions, and guiding subsequent changes in therapy. The diagnostic criteria (2) for each step are listed in Tables 10.3 through 10.6. Asthma severity is assessed based on a combination of clinical and physiologic features present before the initiation of therapy, and the most severe feature should be used to determine the stage of disease. The intensity of therapy should be appropriate for the most severe stage for which the patient meets criteria (2).

TABLE 10.3. DIAGNOSTIC CRITERIA FOR MILD INTERMITTENT ASTHMA

Symptoms	Nocturnal Symptoms	Measures of Lung Function
Symptoms 2 times per week	Symptoms 2 times per month	FEV$_1$ or PEFR 80% of predicted value
Asymptomatic with normal PEFR between exacerbations		PEFR variability <20%
Brief exacerbations (hours to days)		

FEV$_1$, forced expiratory volume in 1 second; PEFR, peak expiratory flow rate.
Source: Adapted from Expert panel report 2. *Guidelines for the diagnosis and management of asthma.* Bethesda, MD: National Institutes of Health, National Heart, Lung, and Blood Institute, 1997: NIH Publication No. 97-4051.

Mild Intermittent Asthma

Patients with mild intermittent asthma have symptoms approximately twice a week, are asymptomatic with a normal peak expiratory flow rate (PEFR) between exacerbations, and have exacerbations that last from only a few hours to days. They have nocturnal symptoms approximately twice per month. Their FEV$_1$ or PEFR values are approximately 80% of those predicted, and the circadian variability in their PEFR (the difference between the PEFR measured on awakening and the PEFR measured between 12 p.m. and 2 p.m.) is less than 20% (2) (Table 10.3).

Mild Persistent Asthma

Patients with mild persistent asthma have symptoms more frequently than twice per week, but not as frequently as once per day. Exacerbations may be severe enough to limit activity. Nocturnal symptoms occur more than twice per month. The FEV$_1$ and PEFR values are still approximately 80% of those predicted, but the circadian PEFR variability is 20% to 30% (2) (Table 10.4).

Moderate Persistent Asthma

Patients with moderate persistent asthma have daily symptoms of airflow limitation. These symptoms necessitate the

TABLE 10.4. DIAGNOSTIC CRITERIA FOR MILD PERSISTENT ASTHMA

Symptoms	Nocturnal Symptoms	Lung Function
Symptoms twice weekly, but < once per day.	Symptoms > twice per month	FEV$_1$ or PEFR 80% of predicted value
Exacerbations may reduce maximal activity.		PEFR variability <20%–30%

FEV$_1$, forced expiratory volume in 1 second; PEFR, peak expiratory flow rate.
Source: Adapted from Expert panel report 2. *Guidelines for the diagnosis and management of asthma.* Bethesda, MD: National Institutes of Health, National Heart, Lung, and Blood Institute, 1997: NIH Publication No. 97-4051.

TABLE 10.5. DIAGNOSTIC CRITERIA FOR MODERATE PERSISTENT ASTHMA

Symptoms	Nocturnal Symptoms	Lung Function
Daily symptoms.	Symptoms > once per week	FEV$_1$ or PEFR > 60% but <80% of predicted value
Daily use of inhaled short-acting β_2-agonist.		PEFR variability >30%
Exacerbations may reduce maximal activity.		
Exacerbations 2 times per week, lasting days.		

FEV$_1$, forced expiratory volume in 1 second; PEFR, peak expiratory flow rate.
Source: Adapted from Expert panel report 2. *Guidelines for the diagnosis and management of asthma.* Bethesda, MD: National Institutes of Health, National Heart, Lung, and Blood Institute, 1997: NIH Publication No. 97-4051.

daily use of short-acting bronchodilators, and exacerbations may limit activity. Nocturnal symptoms occur more than once per week. Exacerbations may occur more than twice per week and may last for several days. In these individuals, the FEV$_1$ and PEFR values are between 60% and 80% of those predicted, and the circadian PEFR variability exceeds 30% (2) (Table 10.5).

Severe Persistent Asthma

Patients with severe persistent asthma have continual symptoms of airflow limitation, limited physical activity, and frequent exacerbations. Nighttime symptoms may occur as frequently as every night and disrupt sleep quality. The FEV$_1$ and PEFR values are less than 60% of those predicted, and the circadian PEFR variability is more than 30% (2) (Table 10.6).

SPECIAL CLINICAL SITUATIONS IN ASTHMA

Not every patient with asthma fits neatly into the NIH classification, and any attempt to reduce patients with asthma

TABLE 10.6. DIAGNOSTIC CRITERIA FOR SEVERE PERSISTENT ASTHMA

Symptoms	Nocturnal Symptoms	Lung Function
Continual symptoms	Frequent	FEV$_1$ or PEFR 60% of predicted value
Limited physical activity		PEFR variability >30%
Frequent exacerbations		

FEV$_1$, forced expiratory volume in 1 second; PEFR, peak expiratory flow rate.
Source: Adapted from Expert panel report 2. *Guidelines for the diagnosis and management of asthma.* Bethesda, MD: National Institutes of Health, National Heart, Lung, and Blood Institute, 1997: NIH Publication No. 97-4051.

to a small number of homogeneous groups will not fully represent the spectrum of clinical phenotypes encountered in the evaluation and treatment of this disease. For example, not all patients demonstrate abnormal physiologic test results during the daytime (as is the case in some patients with nocturnal asthma). Fixed airway obstruction may develop in some elderly asthmatic patients with chronic airway inflammation, and they will not respond to inhaled bronchodilators. Additionally, comorbid conditions such as allergic or gastroesophageal reflux disease (GERD) and advanced age can be important factors in determining appropriate therapy.

Nocturnal Asthma

Nocturnal symptoms are frequent in asthmatic individuals, and they are important in determining asthma severity. Nocturnal asthma is a unique clinical phenotype that is associated with specific inflammatory and physiologic substrates. The circadian variation in peak flow or FEV_1 seen in healthy subjects (5%–8%) is markedly accentuated in persons with nocturnal asthma, whose circadian variability may exceed 50% (10) (Fig. 10.1).

In nocturnal asthma, lower airway resistance progressively increases at night. This phenomenon occurs independently of whether patients are awake or asleep, indicating that the circadian changes in airway resistance are independent of sleep. Sleep augments this increase, however, because airway resistance rises further in asthmatic patients during sleep (11). Significant increases in airway resistance during sleep results in airflow limitation that in turn causes nocturnal symptoms in individuals with nocturnal asthma. In 1990, Martin and colleagues (12) demonstrated a significant positive correlation between nocturnal symptoms/awakenings

and overnight fall in PEFR ($r = 0.85$, $P < .001$) (12). This study also revealed significant differences in airways responsiveness between 4 p.m. and 4 a.m., with a decrease in the methacholine PC_{20} (the concentration of methacholine required to provoke a 20% fall in FEV_1) from 1.80 ± 0.75 mg/mL at 4 p.m. to 0.474 ± 0.16 mg/mL at 4 a.m. (mean $\pm$ standard error of the mean [SEM]) (12). These observations of worsening airflow resistance and increased airway responsiveness at night have a direct bearing on asthma therapy and highlight the importance of drug dosing regimens that promote nighttime bronchodilation.

The response to certain forms of controller therapy, particularly glucocorticoids, may be reduced in patients with nocturnal asthma. In 1999, Kraft and colleagues (13) showed that patients with nocturnal asthma have a significantly reduced affinity of the glucocorticoid receptor for glucocorticoids, indicated by an elevated dissociation constant at 4 a.m. versus 4 p.m. This finding was not present in healthy subjects or in asthmatic subjects without nocturnal symptoms. Furthermore, in the nocturnal asthma group, the elevated dissociation constant was inversely correlated ($r = -0.65$, $P = .04$) with the FEV_1 at 4 a.m. (13). This finding is likely caused by an increased expression of the glucocorticoid receptor isoform-β (GR-β), which has been found not to bind glucocorticoids and to antagonize the activity of the normal GR in lung macrophages of patients with nocturnal asthma (14).

Asthma without Bronchodilator Reversibility

Although the effects of long-term airway inflammation are not fully understood, evidence is mounting that over time, both the airways and lung parenchyma undergo structural changes that alter their functional properties (15).

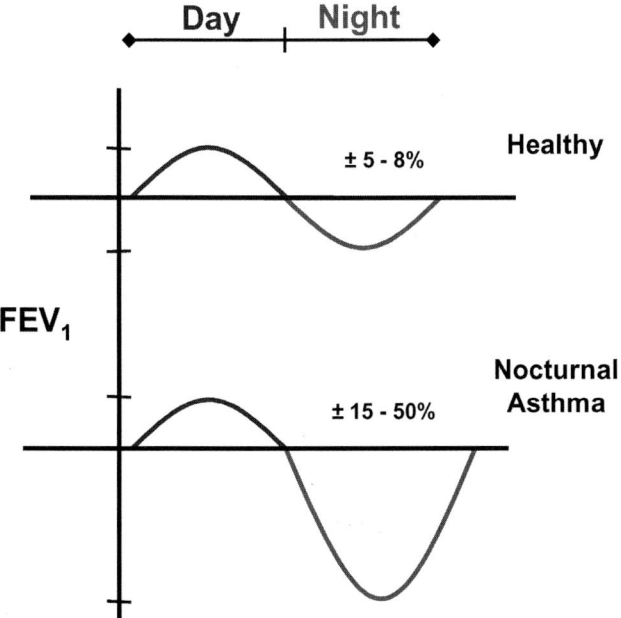

FIGURE 10.1. Circadian variability in forced expiratory volume in 1 second in healthy individuals (**top**) and patients with nocturnal asthma (**bottom**). In healthy individuals, the circadian variability is 5% to 8%, whereas in patients with asthma, variability may exceed 50% (From Martin RJ. Location of airway inflammation in asthma and the relationship to circadian change in lung function. *Chronobiol Int* 1999;16:623–630, with permission).

These changes can lead to irreversible airflow limitation that develops despite appropriate antiinflammatory therapy (16). Some of the pathologic changes resulting from chronic airway inflammation, which as a group may lead to "remodeling" of the airways, include increases in the number of airway mucous glands and goblet cells, airway smooth muscle hypertrophy and hyperplasia, neovascularization of the airways, subbasement membrane thickening, and derangements of submucosal collagen and elastin (17).

In the clinical setting, elderly patients with long-standing asthma comprise a subgroup of patients in whom the effects of airways remodeling may be most important. Cassino and colleagues (18) reported the results of an observational longitudinal cohort study in which elderly subjects (median age, 65 years; range, 60–80 years) were stratified into two groups: one with asthma of long duration, defined as asthma for longer than 26 years (median duration of 40 years), and one with asthma for less than 26 years (median duration of 9 years). Subjects with asthma of long duration had significantly lower $FEV_1\%$ values than did subjects with asthma of short duration (59.5% ± 2.6% vs. 73.8% ± 3.1%; mean ± SEM, $P < .007$), were less likely to attain a normal FEV_1 after bronchodilator administration (18% vs. 50%, $P < .003$), and had a mean $FEV_1\%$ of 65.4% ± 2.9% (mean ± SEM) following bronchodilator administration. Furthermore, an inverse relationship was found between $FEV_1\%$ and duration of asthma, with a longer duration of asthma associated with a lower $FEV_1\%$ ($r = -0.26$, $P < .03$) (Fig. 10.2) and an increased functional residual capacity ($r = 0.38$, $P < .002$) (18).

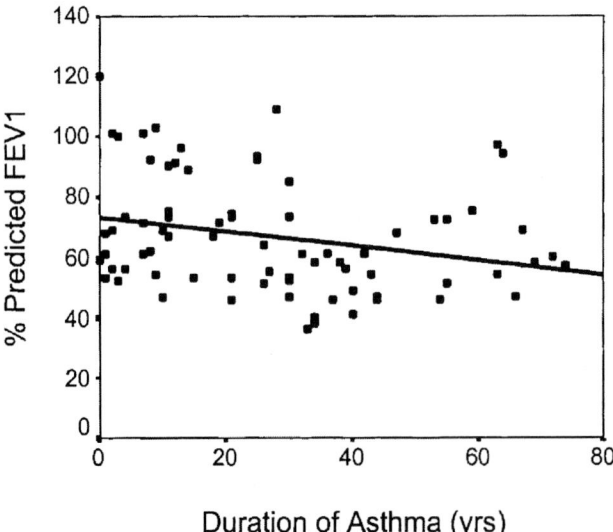

FIGURE 10.2. Regression analysis of the association between asthma duration and percentage of the predicted forced expiratory volume in 1 second ($r = -0.26$, $P < .03$). (From Cassino C, Berger KI, Goldring RM, et al. Duration of asthma and physiologic outcomes in elderly nonsmokers. *Am J Respir Crit Care Med* 2000;162(4 Pt 1):1423–1428, with permission.)

The observations of Cassino and colleagues support the conclusion that long-standing asthma is associated with more severe airflow limitation and a reduction in bronchodilator responsiveness. They also appear to question the utility of bronchodilator responsiveness as a diagnostic criterion in subjects with long-standing asthma. Further research is necessary to determine the clinical importance of these observations.

EVALUATION AND TREATMENT OF COMORBID CONDITIONS

A number of concurrent medical problems can have a significant impact on asthma severity and treatment. Allergic disease, rhinosinusitis, GERD, and advanced age must all be considered as important comorbid conditions in patients with asthma.

Airway inflammation, airway responsiveness, and airflow limitation can worsen in asthmatic patients who are routinely exposed to inhaled allergens to which they are sensitive (19). Furthermore, research suggests that reducing the level of exposure to these allergens can reduce airway inflammation and its sequelae (20,21). For this reason, the current guidelines (2) recommend that all patients with persistent asthma be questioned about their allergenic exposures. Exposure to allergens such as animal dander, molds, cockroaches, trees, and grasses should be investigated by means of interview, and sensitivity to candidate allergens should be evaluated with skin or *in vitro* allergy testing. Once sensitivity has been documented, avoidance measures, such as the removal of animals from the household and dust mite control, should be initiated. Immunotherapy may be considered in cases in which exposure to the allergen is unavoidable or in which avoidance and other forms of medical therapy have failed (2).

Upper respiratory tract inflammation as a result of rhinosinusitis contributes to asthma severity; sinusitis and asthma are common comorbid conditions (22). The treatment of sinusitis with antibiotics (23), nasal corticosteroids, or even surgery (24) may be effective in relieving symptoms and the morbidity related to asthma, although further clinical research is necessary to improve the quality of data regarding this point.

GERD is another important comorbid condition in patients with asthma, and the prevalence of GERD is increased in these individuals. Furthermore, worsening of asthma symptoms is closely associated with episodes of acid reflux. In 1999, Harding and colleagues (25) reported that in asthmatic patients with GERD, approximately 80% of the respiratory symptoms reported during 24-hour esophageal pH monitoring were associated with acid reflux. The close association between low esophageal pH and symptoms was seen even in the subgroup of patients who did not have significant symptoms of reflux, indicating that clinically silent reflux is an important factor and must be considered in the care of these patients. The treatment of GERD with the proton pump inhibitor omeprazole has been shown to relieve asthma-related symptoms and improve measures of airflow (26). All patients with asthma should be carefully queried about GERD symptoms, and medical therapy (either empiric or based on the results of esophageal pH monitoring) should be strongly considered for patients with even mild asthma.

Asthma is a prevalent disease in the elderly. In the Cardiovascular Health Study (27), a prospective cohort study of 4,581 individuals 65 years of age or older, the prevalence of self-reported asthma was 4%; an additional 4% of subjects reported symptoms consistent with undiagnosed asthma. Those subjects who had asthma were more likely to report their general level of health as "fair" or "poor," and they were twice as likely to report symptoms of depression. Only 40% of subjects with a diagnosis of asthma reported that any form of asthma pharmacotherapy had been prescribed, indicating that asthma is undertreated in this age group (27). Furthermore, adverse effects of asthma medications may be more likely to develop in elderly patients, and the increased prevalence of polypharmacy in the elderly increases the risk for drug-drug interactions. Corticosteroids, with their adverse effects of increased fracture risk, cataracts, and myopathy (28), should be used sparingly in elderly patients with asthma. Short- and long-acting β_2-agonists may interact with β-blockers and increase tachycardia and electrolyte abnormalities. Careful attention should be given to treating asthma appropriately in elderly individuals by attempting to avoid drug interactions and other adverse effects of long-term therapies.

INDIVIDUAL PHARMACOLOGIC AGENTS IN THE TREATMENT OF ASTHMA

A number of pharmacologic agents are available for the treatment of asthma. Drugs may be classified as either of two types: "controller" medications, which provide long-term control of airway inflammation, and "reliever" medications, which provide quick relief of symptoms (Table 10.7). Desirable therapeutic outcomes include (a) control or elimination of chronic symptoms such as cough, dyspnea, and nocturnal awakenings; (b) attainment of normal or nearly normal lung function; (c) restoration or maintenance of normal levels of activity; (d) reduction in the number or elimination of recurrent exacerbations; (e) reduction in the number or elimination of emergency department visits and acute care hospitalizations; and (f) elimination or reduction of side effects of medications (2) (Table 10.8).

Inhaled Corticosteroids

Corticosteroids are the mainstay of therapy for patients with all forms of persistent asthma. Corticosteroids inhibit many

TABLE 10.7. CONTROLLER AND RELIEVER MEDICATIONS FOR THE TREATMENT OF ASTHMA

Controller Medications	Reliever Medication
Inhaled corticosteroids (first-line agent)	**Short-acting β-agonists**
Beclomethasone	Albuterol
Budesonide	Bitolterol
Flunisolide	Metaproterenol
Fluticasone	Pirbuterol
Triamcinolone	Terbutaline
Long-acting β-agonists	
Formoterol	
Salmeterol	
Antileukotriene agents	
Montelukast	
Zafirlukast	
Zileuton	
Cromones	
Nedocromil sodium	
Sodium cromoglycate	

of the inflammatory processes at work in the asthmatic airway (29), improve lung function, and reduce the number of asthma exacerbations, the number of acute care hospitalizations for asthma (30), and asthma mortality (31). Corticosteroids administered via inhalation are topically active and have been shown to be as effective in the treatment of asthma as systemically administered glucocorticoids, with less systemic absorption and a more favorable side effect profile. The evidence supporting these multiple beneficial actions of inhaled corticosteroids is summarized in the following paragraphs.

Five different inhaled corticosteroids are currently available in the United States: beclomethasone dipropionate, budesonide, flunisolide, fluticasone propionate, and triamcinolone acetonide. These inhaled corticosteroids have different antiinflammatory potencies. Fluticasone propionate is the most potent. Budesonide and beclomethasone dipropionate are 50% as potent as fluticasone, and flunisolide and triamcinolone acetonide are 25% as potent as fluticasone (32).

TABLE 10.8. THERAPEUTIC GOALS IN THE CARE OF THE PATIENT WITH ASTHMA

Goals of asthma therapy
Reducing symptoms of airflow limitation
Achieving normal or near-normal lung function
Achieving normal activity levels
Reducing recurrent exacerbations
Reducing emergency department visits and acute care hospitalizations
Minimizing or eliminating side effects of pharmacotherapy

Source: Adapted from Expert panel report 2. *Guidelines for the diagnosis and management of asthma.* Bethesda, MD: National Institutes of Health, National Heart, Lung, and Blood Institute, 1997: NIH Publication No. 97-4051.

INHALED CORTICOSTEROIDS IN ASTHMA

Summary Statement	Level of Evidence
Compared with placebo or short-acting β_2- agonist alone, inhaled corticosteroids result in improved peak flows, improved asthma symptom scores, decreased rescue β_2-agonist use, and decreased airway responsiveness.	Randomized, controlled clinical trials
Compared with theophylline, inhaled corticosteroids result in improved peak flows, improved asthma symptom scores, decreased rescue β_2-agonist use, decreased airway responsiveness, and a decreased need for systemic glucocorticoids.	Randomized, controlled clinical trials
Compared with leukotriene modifiers, inhaled corticosteroids result in improved peak flows, improved FEV_1 values, improved asthma symptom scores, decreased rescue β_2-agonist use, and decreased airway responsiveness.	Randomized, controlled clinical trials

FEV_1, forced expiratory volume in 1 second.

Mechanism of Action of Inhaled Corticosteroids

Glucocorticoids exhibit antiinflammatory properties at both the molecular and cellular levels. Inhaled corticosteroids diffuse readily across airway cell membranes to airway smooth muscle cells, where they bind the intracytoplasmic glucocorticoid receptor. This complex is then translocated into the nucleus, where it binds to specific sequences known as *glucocorticoid response elements (GREs)* on DNA upstream from the promoter regions of steroid-responsive genes (33). Up to 100 GRE genes have been identified (34), and either up-regulation or down-regulation of transcription may occur as a result of glucocorticoid binding (35). In some cases, the gene products are proinflammatory cytokines that are down-regulated by glucocorticoid binding to the GRE (36). Glucocorticoids also inhibit the ability of nuclear transcription factors to up-regulate the immune response (37).

At the cellular level, glucocorticoids result in a reduction in the number of eosinophils and activated T lymphocytes in bronchoalveolar lavage fluid and airway epithelium (38,39). This beneficial effect is likely secondary to a reduction in the transcription of proinflammatory cytokine genes.

Evidence for the Clinical Efficacy of Inhaled Corticosteroids

A number of benefits are derived from the antiinflammatory properties of corticosteroids (Table 10.9). Inhaled corticosteroids control the symptoms of asthma, so that the patient's quality of life is improved. Inhaled corticosteroids also improve the spirometric values and other measures of lung function and reduce the rate of acute care hospitalization and asthma mortality. Inhaled corticosteroids may also exert long-term effects on the asthmatic airway by decreasing the

TABLE 10.9. SALUTARY EFFECTS OF INHALED CORTICOSTEROIDS IN ASTHMA

Reduced asthma symptoms
Reduced asthma morbidity
Reduced asthma mortality
Improved quality of life
Improved lung function
Reduced development of fixed airway disease

Source: Adapted from Barnes PJ. Efficacy of inhaled corticosteroids in asthma. *J Allergy Clin Immunol* 1998;102(4 Pt 1):531–538, with permission.

development of irreversible airway changes. They can alter the natural history of asthma by reducing the development of fixed airflow limitation secondary to airway remodeling (although this is a theoretic benefit not yet supported by longitudinal cohort studies).

Inhaled corticosteroids reduce expiratory airflow limitation and airway responsiveness in asthma. In 1991, Haahtela and colleagues (40) published the results of a clinical trial comparing terbutaline (a short-acting β_2-agonist) with inhalation of 600 μg of budesonide twice daily as first-line treatment for newly diagnosed asthma. Subjects treated with inhaled budesonide demonstrated significant improvements in morning peak flow; a mean increase of 32.8 L/min was noted in the budesonide group, compared with 4.8 L/min in the terbutaline-only group ($P < .001$). The evening peak flow also increased significantly in the budesonide group. Furthermore, the budesonide group demonstrated significant decreases in asthma symptoms ($P < .001$) and in the use of rescue β_2-agonists (mean decline in terbutaline use of 70%, $P < .001$). Both groups showed an improvement in airway responsiveness to histamine, but the improvement in the budesonide group was approximately three times that in the terbutaline-only group ($P < .001$) (40).

Lower doses of inhaled corticosteroids confer similar benefits in patients with asthma. Juniper and colleagues (41) reported the results of a trial of inhalation of 400 μg of budesonide daily in subjects with mild asthma. After 1 year of treatment, budesonide resulted in significant decreases in asthma symptoms, number of asthma exacerbations, and the requirement for rescue β_2-agonists in comparison with placebo. These clinical improvements were accompanied by a fourfold improvement in airway responsiveness ($P < .0005$) in the budesonide group (41). The clinical improvement following the initiation of inhaled corticosteroids may be somewhat independent of the effects on airway responsiveness, however, because clinical improvements tend to precede maximal reductions in airway responsiveness (42).

Inhaled corticosteroids not only are superior to placebo or β_2-agonists alone, they also provide advantages when compared with other agents for the treatment of asthma. In 1998, Reed and colleagues (43) compared 84 μg of beclomethasone dipropionate four times daily with sustained-release theophylline (100–300 mg twice daily, titrated to control symptoms) in a 1-year randomized, double-blinded, controlled clinical trial. Beclomethasone treatment resulted in (a) significant improvement in asthma symptom scores ($P = .002$ at 6 months); (b) fewer days in which asthma symptoms were rated as moderately severe or severe; (c) more days in which rescue β-agonist use was not necessary ($P = .038$ at 6 months); (d) less need for systemic glucocorticoid therapy, with 20% of the beclomethasone group requiring one or more courses of systemic glucocorticoids versus 29% of the theophylline group ($P = .009$); (e) improvements in airways responsiveness to methacholine; and (f) a decline in the peripheral blood eosinophil count from 369 ± 291 cells to 286 ± 213 cells per cubic millimeter (mean $\pm$ standard deviation [SD], $P < .001$). A significant decrease in peripheral blood eosinophils was not seen in subjects receiving theophylline alone. In addition, physicians rated the clinical response to beclomethasone better than the response to theophylline (43).

Inhaled corticosteroids are also superior to leukotriene modifiers as a first-line treatment for asthma. In 2001, Busse and colleagues (44) reported the results of a randomized, double-blinded, double-dummy controlled clinical trial in which they compared a low dose of fluticasone propionate (88 μg twice daily) with 10 mg of montelukast once daily in asthmatic subjects with FEV$_1$ values approximately 65.5% of those predicted (65.6% $\pm$ 9.2% vs. 65.4% $\pm$ 8.2% of predicted values, mean $\pm$ SD). When compared with treatment with montelukast, treatment with fluticasone improved both morning PEFR (68.5 vs. 34.1 L/min, $P < .001$) and evening PEFR (53.9 vs. 28.7 L/min, $P < .001$). Greater sustained improvements were observed in the morning pretreatment FEV$_1$ in the fluticasone group than in the montelukast group during the course of treatment (Fig. 10.3). At the end of the study, subjects treated with fluticasone had a greater increase in FEV$_1$ than did subjects treated with montelukast (22.87% $\pm$ 1.41% vs. 14.47% $\pm$ 1.29%, $P < .001$). Furthermore, at the end of the 24-week treatment period, subjects treated with fluticasone had significantly improved asthma symptom scores, significant reductions in the use of rescue albuterol, a significant reduction in the frequency of nocturnal awakenings, and improved asthma-specific quality-of-life scores (44).

Similar physiologic and clinical results were obtained in the study of Bleecker and colleagues (45), which compared the same dose of fluticasone propionate with 20 mg of zafirlukast orally twice daily in subjects with persistent asthma who remained symptomatic despite β_2-agonist monotherapy. Malmstrom and colleagues (46) conducted a randomized, controlled clinical trial comparing 200 μg of beclomethasone inhaled twice daily, 10 mg of montelukast once daily at bedtime, and placebo in subjects with asthma and FEV$_1$ values 50% to 85% of those predicted. They found that although both drugs resulted in clinical improvements, inhaled beclomethasone was superior to both montelukast and placebo; the mean improvement in FEV$_1$ with beclomethasone was 13.1%, versus a 7.4% mean improvement in FEV$_1$ with montelukast ($P < .01$). Asthma symptom scores were also significantly improved with beclomethasone in comparison with both montelukast and placebo (46).

Inhaled Corticosteroids Reduce the Risk for Hospitalization for Asthma

In 1995, asthma accounted for 19.5 hospital discharges per 10,000 people in the United States. These rates of hospitalization reflect a large burden of morbidity in the population

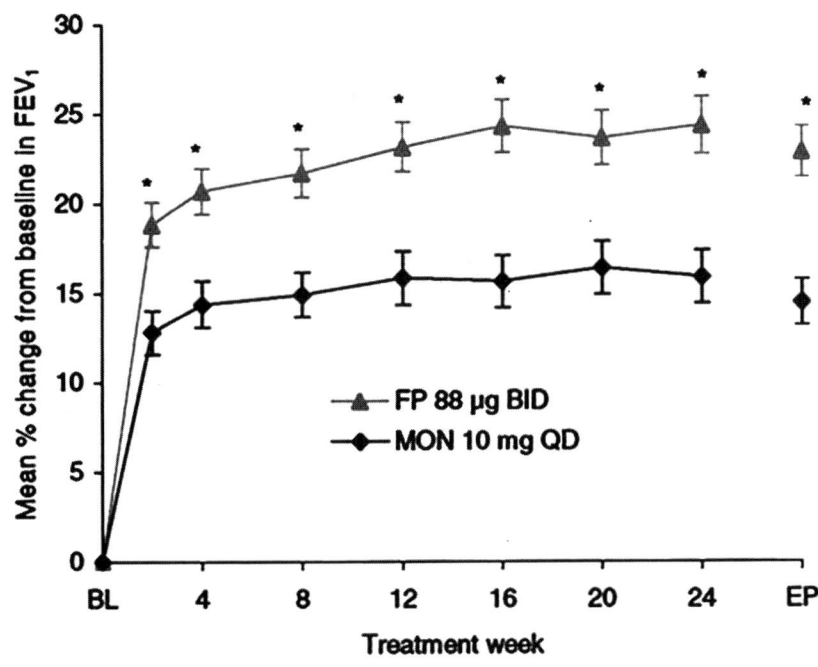

FIGURE 10.3. Mean percentage change in the forced expiratory volume in 1 second in comparison with baseline in subjects treated with 88 μg of fluticasone propionate *(FP)* twice daily and 10 mg of montelukast *(MON)* daily during the 24-week treatment period. *$*P < .001$. *BL,* baseline; *EP,* endpoint. (From Busse W, Raphael GD, Galant S, et al. Low-dose fluticasone propionate compared with montelukast for first-line treatment of persistent asthma: a randomized clinical trial. *J Allergy Clin Immunol* 2001;107:461–468, with permission.)

and account for almost 50% of the direct costs of asthma (1). Hospitalization rates are not commonly reported in studies of inhaled corticosteroids (47), although observational studies (30) have confirmed that inhaled corticosteroids reduce acute care hospitalizations.

In 1997, Donahue and colleagues (30) reported the results of a population-based study of the relationship between inhaled corticosteroid use and the risk for hospitalization in a group of asthmatic subjects cared for in the Harvard Pilgrim Health Care health maintenance organization. The study population consisted of 16,941 subjects with asthma, of whom 40% received a prescription for inhaled corticosteroids. In the study population, 4.4% of subjects were hospitalized for asthma. After adjustment for the dispensing of β_2-agonist medications, the relative risk for hospitalization decreased by 50% among subjects who received inhaled corticosteroids (adjusted relative risk, 0.5; 95% confidence interval [CI], 0.4–0.6). A meaningful dose-response relationship was not observed. The authors also noted that increasing β_2-agonist use was associated with an increased risk for hospitalization, with a fourfold increased risk among subjects who received more than eight β_2-agonist prescriptions per person-year in comparison with subjects receiving no β_2-agonists (30).

Inhaled Corticosteroids Reduce the Risk for Death from Asthma

A number of studies have demonstrated that inhaled corticosteroids are effective in reducing the risk for death from asthma. Although death from asthma is much less common than asthma-related morbidity, it does occur. The asthma-related death rate in the United States has increased more than 50% in recent years, from an age-adjusted rate of 0.93 per 100,000 in 1979–1980 to 1.49 per 100,000 in 1993–1995 (1). In 1992, Ernst and colleagues (48) published the results of a nested case control study conducted in a historical cohort of asthma patients in Saskatchewan, Canada. They demonstrated that after adjustment for other medication- and asthma-related factors, subjects who had been dispensed one or more metered-dose inhalers of beclomethasone per month over a 1-year period had a significantly lower combined risk for fatal and near-fatal asthma, with an odds ratio of 0.1 (95% CI, 0.02–0.6). For design reasons, however, this study was unable to comment on the relationship between beclomethasone dose and morbidity and mortality.

In 2000, Suissa and colleagues (31) reported that the use of inhaled corticosteroids in asthma reduced the risk for death. Their study was a nested case control study of 30,569 subjects conducted in the Saskatchewan Health population-based cohort (age range, 5–44 years) and was designed to evaluate the utility of inhaled corticosteroids in preventing death from asthma. In the cohort, 77 of the 562 deaths were attributed to asthma. Case patients were older, more likely to be men, and as a group had more hospitalizations for

asthma and more asthma-related prescriptions than did the control group. The authors performed a continuous dose-response analysis to evaluate the relationship between the number of canisters of beclomethasone used in the previous year and the risk for asthma. They demonstrated that the rate of death from asthma decreased 21% with each additional canister of inhaled corticosteroids used in the previous year (adjusted rate ratio, 0.79; 95% CI, 0.65–0.97). The benefit increased for each canister used in the 6 months before evaluation (rate ratio, 0.46; 95% CI, 0.26–0.79). Furthermore, asthma mortality rates increased in the first 3 months following discontinuation of therapy in comparison with mortality rates in subjects who continued therapy (rate ratio, 4.6; 95% CI, 1.1–19.1) (31). Although the population-based, nonrandomized nature of this study differentiates it from the controlled circumstances of a clinical trial, the study would be difficult to reproduce in such a form, and the resulting data provide further support for the regular use of inhaled corticosteroids in patients with persistent asthma.

Adverse Effects of Corticosteroids

In many patients with asthma, inhaled corticosteroids are as effective as oral corticosteroids and have a more favorable benefit-risk profile. In general, the use of oral corticosteroids in chronic asthma should be restricted to patients with severe persistent asthma that is not controlled despite aggressive treatment with inhaled corticosteroids, other long-term controller agents, and aggressive treatment of environmental factors and comorbid conditions. In patients with lung disease, the use of oral corticosteroids is associated with a dose-dependent increase in the odds of vertebral, hip, rib, or sternal fracture, cataracts, muscle weakness, easy bruising, and opportunistic infections such as oral candidiasis (28). Although inhaled corticosteroids are much less likely to induce many of these adverse events, they have been associated with the development of dose-dependent accelerated bone loss (49), oral candidiasis (50), and dysphonia (51) and with depression of the hypothalamic-pituitary-adrenal axis (52).

β-Adrenergic Receptor Agonists

Inhaled β_2-adrenergic agonists are the most potent inhaled bronchodilators and the most commonly prescribed medications for the treatment of asthma (53). Formulations with varying durations of action are currently available as options in the treatment of intermittent and persistent asthma.

β-Adrenergic receptors comprise at least three separate groups: β_1-receptors, which are found primarily in cardiac muscle; β_2-receptors, found primarily in airway smooth muscle; and β_3-receptors, found primarily in adipose tissue (54). The β_2-receptor associates with the α subunit of G proteins, facilitating coupling to adenylate cyclase and the mediation of cyclic AMP–induced smooth muscle cell

TABLE 10.10. β-RECEPTOR AGONISTS FOR THE TREATMENT OF ASTHMA

β-Agonist Drug Name	Duration of Bronchodilator Activity (h)
Albuterol	3–6
Bitolterol	3–6
Metaproterenol	3–6
Pirbuterol	3–6
Terbutaline	3–6
Fenoterol[a]	3–6
Formoterol	12
Salmeterol	12

Note: Agents with a duration of 3 to 6 hours are prescribed as "rescue" bronchodilators.
[a] Not currently available in the United States.

relaxation (55). β-Agonist drugs have different affinities for the β₂-receptor, and they also have varying efficacy based on the relative agonist and antagonist properties of the ligand–receptor interaction. Albuterol, for example, has a relatively low affinity for the β-receptor but moderate efficacy (65%–85%), whereas salmeterol has a high affinity for the receptor and a similarly moderate efficacy (65%) (56). As a result of these molecule-specific issues, in addition to issues related to formulation and delivery devices, a variety of β-agonist drugs are available with differing efficacy and duration of action (Table 10.10).

USE OF β₂-AGONISTS IN ASTHMA

Summary Statement	Level of Evidence
Short-acting β₂-agonists are effective bronchodilators and are recommended for the quick relief of asthma symptoms.	Randomized, controlled clinical trials
Long-acting β₂-agonists relieve asthma symptoms and improve physiology when used in concert with antiinflammatory medications.	Randomized, controlled clinical trials
Adding long-acting β₂-agonists to a low or moderate dose of inhaled corticosteroids is as effective as doubling the dose of inhaled corticosteroids.	Randomized, controlled clinical trials
Long-acting β₂-agonists should not be used as single controller medications but should always be used in concert with inhaled corticosteroids.	Randomized, controlled trials and consensus recommendations

Short-Acting β₂-Agonists Are Effective Bronchodilators

Short-acting inhaled β₂-agonist bronchodilators are effective at acutely relaxing airway smooth muscle, thereby reducing airflow limitation in many patients with asthma. As such, they are classified as "reliever" medications. Structural modifications of the epinephrine molecule have led to the development of β-agonist drugs that are β₂-receptor–specific in their action and have a duration of action of approximately

4 to 6 hours; these drugs may be characterized as short-acting β₂-agonists and so can be used as either regularly scheduled or as-needed drugs in the treatment of asthma. Agents in this class include albuterol, bitolterol, metaproterenol, pirbuterol, and terbutaline. Additional modifications have led to the development of agents with an even longer duration (12 hours) of activity.

Short-acting β₂-agonists are used as quick-relief medications in the treatment of asthma and are recommended by the NIH guidelines for use in all stages of asthma severity. However, they are suitable as monotherapy for asthma only in those patients with mild intermittent asthma. Short-acting β₂-agonists do provide significant bronchodilation and can normalize lung function in some patients, but they have no significant antiinflammatory activity (57). Although short-acting β₂-agonists are recommended for all patients with asthma, all adult patients with persistent forms of asthma should be treated with additional daily antiinflammatory medication, along with other long-term controller medications if necessary (2).

Long-Acting β₂-Agonists Are Effective Bronchodilators

Long-acting β₂-agonists (salmeterol, xinafoate, formoterol) are effective and highly selective inhaled β₂-agonists with a longer duration of activity (up to 12 hours) than that of short-acting inhaled bronchodilators. In some cases, however, their onset of action is slower than that of short-acting β₂-agonists, and peak bronchodilation is not achieved until between 2 and 4 hours after administration (58,59). This lengthy time to peak bronchodilation limits their use as short-acting reliever medications for acute symptoms. Long-acting β₂-agonists are therefore classified as long-acting controller medications for the treatment of asthma (2). In addition to being effective bronchodilators, long-acting β₂-agonists confer protection against airway responsiveness to methacholine, and also to nonspecific irritants such as exercise and cold air (60–64). Furthermore, long-acting β₂-agonists appear to protect against allergen-induced airway responsiveness and bronchoconstriction (65).

The use of long-acting β₂-agonists as monotherapy for the long-term control of asthma is not recommended because long-acting β₂-agonists are generally inferior to inhaled corticosteroids as long-term controller medications (66). The current recommendations are that long-acting β₂-agonists be used as second-line controller medications when inhaled corticosteroids alone are inadequate (2). The addition of a long-acting β₂-agonist used twice daily to a regimen of inhaled corticosteroids is at least as effective in the control of asthma as doubling the dose of inhaled corticosteroids (67–70).

Theophylline

Theophylline is a methyl xanthine with multiple potential benefits in the treatment of asthma, including bronchodilation, antiinflammatory activity, bronchial protection, and immunomodulation. The exact mechanism of action of theophylline and other methyl xanthines remains unclear, but it is likely related to phosphodiesterase inhibition, blockade of the adenosine receptor, and effects on calcium flux in airway smooth muscle cells (71). The bronchodilator property of theophylline appears to be mediated through inhibition of phosphodiesterase, but the clinical effect is minimal.

Interest in theophylline has been renewed by increasing evidence of its specific antiinflammatory effects in the airways of asthmatic patients through the modulation of cytokines, including interleukin-4 (IL-4) and IL-5 (72). Finnerty and colleagues (73) demonstrated that theophylline decreases the bronchial mucosal expression of IL-4 and IL-5, and Kosmas and colleagues (74) demonstrated that theophylline decreases the levels of circulating IL-4 and IL-5 in asthmatic subjects classified as having mild atopic asthma. Theophylline also has antiinflammatory effects on lymphocytes and other inflammatory cells. Low-dose theophylline appears to reduce the number of activated lymphocytes in the peripheral blood following allergen challenge (75). In subjects with nocturnal asthma, theophylline significantly reduces the percentage of bronchoalveolar lavage neutrophils and eosinophils at 4 a.m. (76).

USE OF THEOPHYLLINE IN ASTHMA

Summary Statement	Level of Evidence
Theophylline should not be used as a replacement for inhaled corticosteroids in the long-term control of asthma.	Clinical trials
Theophylline has significant *in vitro* antiinflammatory effects.	Experimental studies
The addition of theophylline to inhaled corticosteroids is as effective as doubling the dose of inhaled corticosteroids.	Clinical trials

Theophylline Protects against Airway Responsiveness

A number of randomized controlled trials have evaluated the effects of theophylline in protecting against airway responsiveness in asthma (77–82). In 1984, McWilliams and colleagues (78) reported the results of a randomized clinical trial in which theophylline, dosed to achieve a mean plasma level of 13 mg/L, conferred protection against a 0.9 doubling dose of histamine or a 1.6 doubling dose of methacholine. In 1987, Magnussen and colleagues (77) reported that a similar theophylline dosing scheme protected against a 2.6 doubling dose of histamine and a 1.9 doubling dose of methacholine. This protection against airway responsiveness to histamine and methacholine occurred without significant bronchodilation, however. Conversely, Crescioli and colleagues (80) reported that a 5-day course of sustained-release theophylline resulted in both bronchodilation and decreased airway responsiveness to methacholine.

Theophylline Is Inferior to Inhaled Corticosteroids in the Treatment of Asthma

Despite the antiinflammatory effects of theophylline, the results of multiple clinical trials indicate that methyl xanthines are neither equal nor superior to inhaled corticosteroids in the treatment of chronic asthma. In 1987, Dutoit and colleagues (83) reported the results of a crossover trial in adults who for 3 weeks received either 800 μg of beclomethasone dipropionate per day or theophylline dosed to achieve plasma levels of 10 mg/L. In this study, beclomethasone decreased airway responsiveness and improved control of symptoms, whereas theophylline did not. Other trials in children and adults (43,84) have indicated that inhaled corticosteroids are superior to theophylline as single antiinflammatory agents with regard to outcomes, including airway responsiveness, eosinophilia, the need for rescue β_2-agonists, and the need for systemic corticosteroids to treat exacerbations.

Theophylline Allows a Reduction in the Dose of Inhaled Corticosteroid

Although not suitable as a replacement for inhaled corticosteroids in the monotherapy of chronic asthma, theophylline appears to have additive effects to inhaled corticosteroids. Ukena and colleagues (85) performed a randomized clinical trial comparing 800 μg of beclomethasone daily with 400 μg of beclomethasone daily plus theophylline. Both treatment arms demonstrated significant improvement in clinical indices of asthma control and in physiologic measurements, including peak flow recordings and office spirometry. The concomitant use of theophylline allowed a 50% reduction in the amount of inhaled corticosteroid. The study of Evans and colleagues (86) demonstrated similar findings, although the combination of 800 μg of budesonide per day and low-dose theophylline actually resulted in a greater improvement in FEV_1 than did 1,600 μg of budesonide daily alone. In this study, theophylline was dosed to achieve a mean plasma level of 8.7 μg/mL, and the authors concluded that the strategy of low-dose theophylline in addition to inhaled corticosteroid was equivalent to an increased dose of inhaled corticosteroid (86).

Leukotriene Modifiers

Leukotriene modifiers are currently recommended as second- or third-line long-term controller therapy for patients already receiving inhaled corticosteroids with or without long-acting β_2-agonists. The cysteinyl leukotrienes (leukotriene C$_4$ [LTC$_4$], LTD$_4$, and LTE$_4$) are thought to be important mediators of airway responsiveness, bronchoconstriction, mucus hypersecretion, and airway blood vessel permeability in asthma (87–89). Cysteinyl leukotrienes appear to be ligands for at least two receptors, although most of the biologic effects of cysteinyl leukotrienes are a result of binding to the cysteinyl leukotriene-1 (CysLT$_1$) receptor subtype (90).

In 2001, Figueroa and colleagues (91) used immunohistochemical methods to characterize the lung CysLT$_1$ receptor. They were able to show that the CysLT$_1$ receptor mRNA is distributed throughout normal human lung tissue in airway smooth muscle fibers and that expression of the CysLT$_1$ receptor mRNA coincides with the presence of the receptor protein. The CysLT$_1$ mRNA and receptor protein were also identified in human lung interstitial macrophages, which were closely associated with the smooth muscle cells. Heise and colleagues (92) demonstrated a somewhat different expression of the CysLT$_2$ receptor mRNA in normal human lung, with the strongest expression of the CysLT$_2$ receptor seen in interstitial macrophages, and much weaker expression in airway smooth muscle cells.

Drugs that specifically antagonize the binding of cysteinyl leukotrienes to these receptors (montelukast, pranlukast, zafirlukast) are now available and have been shown to have multiple antiinflammatory effects (93). In addition to cysteinyl leukotriene receptor antagonists, inhibitors of 5-lipoxygenase (zafirlukast) reduce leukotriene production via the arachidonic acid synthetic pathway. They are currently recommended as second-line or alternative controller medications (after inhaled corticosteroids) in the treatment of persistent asthma (2). Given the distribution of CysLT$_1$ and CysLT$_2$ receptors in the airway smooth muscle and interstitium, these agents have significant potential to modify distal lung inflammation.

USE OF LEUKOTRIENE INHIBITORS IN ASTHMA	
Summary Statement	Level of Evidence
Leukotriene modifiers are less effective than inhaled corticosteroids as long-acting controller medications in the treatment of chronic asthma.	Randomized, controlled clinical trials
Leukotriene modifiers are effective in the prevention of exercise-induced bronchospasm.	Randomized, controlled clinical trials
Leukotriene modifiers are effective in protecting against bronchoconstriction in aspirin-induced asthma.	Randomized, controlled clinical trials

Leukotriene Modifiers Are Effective Bronchodilators

In patients with mild to moderate asthma, leukotriene modifiers have been shown to relieve asthma symptoms, reduce the requirements for rescue short-acting β_2-agonists, decrease asthma exacerbations, and improve physiologic measures of airflow, including FEV$_1$ and PEFR.

In 1997, Fish and colleagues (94) reported the results of a 13-week multicenter clinical trial of zafirlukast in symptomatic mild to moderate asthma. Zafirlukast dosed at

20 mg twice daily resulted in significant reductions of daytime asthma symptom scores, nighttime awakenings, and morning asthma symptoms, a reduction in the need for rescue β_2-agonists, and statistically significant, albeit small, improvements in FEV$_1$ and morning peak flow (95).

Montelukast was evaluated in a 12-week controlled clinical trial in which 681 patients were randomized to receive either 10 mg of montelukast orally daily or placebo. In these patients, who had mild to moderate asthma as indicated by an FEV$_1$ value between 50% and 85% of that predicted, treatment with montelukast resulted in significant improvements in FEV$_1$ and morning and evening peak flow, along with a significant reduction in daytime asthma symptom scores (96). Similar results have been shown for the 5-lipoxygenase inhibitor zileuton (97).

COMBINATION THERAPY FOR ASTHMA

Combination therapy can result in better asthma control with lower doses of individual medications and an improved side effect profile. This latter benefit is important for patients who require long-term antiinflammatory therapy, which has side effects that are of real concern (98). Because corticosteroids are first-line therapy for asthma, the following discussion focuses on combinations of medications including inhaled corticosteroids; however, a discussion of other combination therapies is also included.

EQUIVALENT THERAPEUTIC DRUG STRATEGIES IN ASTHMA	
Summary Statement	Level of Evidence
The addition of a long-acting β_2-agonist to a low to moderate dose of inhaled corticosteroids is as effective as doubling the dose of inhaled corticosteroids.	Randomized, controlled clinical trials
The addition of theophylline to inhaled corticosteroids is as effective as doubling the dose of inhaled corticosteroids.	Randomized, controlled clinical trials
The addition of leukotriene modifiers to a high dose of inhaled corticosteroids permits a reduction in the dose of inhaled corticosteroids.	Randomized, controlled clinical trials

Combinations of Inhaled Corticosteroids and β-Agonists

Corticosteroids alone exert very powerful beneficial effects on airway inflammation and responsiveness (39,99–103). Further benefits accrue when inhaled steroids are combined with inhaled β_2-agonists. Steroids have been shown to potentiate the relaxing effect of β_2-agonists in a number of animal studies and also in *in vitro* studies of human bronchial smooth muscle (104). The direct influence on β_2-receptors appears to be mediated by lipocortin through the synthesis of new β_2-receptors, increased coupling between receptors and their functional unit, increased synthesis of catecholamine, and reversal of β_2-receptor dysfunction as a consequence of repeated β_2 stimulation (tachyphylaxis). However, some data suggest that high-dose β_2-agonists may exhibit antiglu-cocorticoid activity (105,106). Further studies are needed to determine the clinical relevance of these data.

Inhaled Corticosteroids and Short-Acting β_2-Agonists

Many studies of combination therapy of inhaled corticosteroids with inhaled β_2-agonists have been conducted since 1989 (107,108). Haahtela and colleagues (108) reported in 1989 that patients inhaling a combination of 100 μg of beclomethasone and 200 μg of salbutamol four times daily exhibited greater improvements in FEV_1, PEFR, and symptom scores than did patients using 400 μg of salbutamol alone four times daily (108). Subsequent studies also demonstrated that the addition of inhaled corticosteroids to inhaled β_2-agonists improved many aspects of asthma control. A 4-year prospective study by Dompeling and colleagues (107) of 56 patients with moderate asthma and 28 patients with chronic obstructive pulmonary disease demonstrated that inhalation of 400 μg of beclomethasone twice daily in addition to inhalation of 400 μg of salbutamol or 40 μg of ipratropium bromide was better than therapy with salbutamol or ipratropium bromide alone. In the asthmatic subjects, the mean before-bronchodilator FEV_1 improved by 562 mL, and the mean after-bronchodilator FEV_1 improved by 201 mL after 6 months of therapy. In addition, the mean residual volume decreased by 0.49 L (95% CI, 0.18–0.80 L). The provocative concentration of histamine producing a fall in FEV_1 of 20% (histamine PC_{20}) increased by three doubling doses per year. Exacerbations fell by 1.3 per year, and the severity of symptoms decreased by 17%. No significant adverse events were noted, although four patients used a spacer because of an increased risk for oral candidiasis.

The question of whether short-acting inhaled β_2-agonists can be used intermittently or regularly in conjunction with inhaled corticosteroid use has been addressed. Tormey and colleagues (109) showed that either regular or intermittent use of β_2-agonists can be combined with the use of an inhaled corticosteroid (500 μg of beclomethasone daily) without significant differences in lung function, histamine PC_{20}, and symptom scores.

Inhaled Corticosteroids and Long-Acting β_2-Agonists

It appears that the addition of a long-acting β_2-agonist to an inhaled corticosteroid confers symptomatic and physiologic benefit greater than that obtained with either drug alone. Van der Molen and colleagues (110) demonstrated that the addition of formoterol to a stable dose of inhaled

corticosteroid (100–3,200 μg/d) improved morning PEFR, relieved symptoms, and decreased short-acting β_2-agonist use. In a double-blinded, randomized, placebo-controlled trial of the addition of salmeterol to an inhaled corticosteroid for 1 year, Wilding and colleagues (111) reported a 17% reduction in the dose of inhaled corticosteroid in subjects receiving salmeterol versus placebo, in addition to improved pulmonary function, reduced symptom scores, and reduced bronchodilator use. Greening and colleagues (68) demonstrated that in patients still symptomatic on 400 μg of beclomethasone or budesonide daily, changing the regimen to 50 μg of salmeterol twice daily together with 200 μg of beclomethasone twice daily was more effective than 500 μg of beclomethasone twice daily. In this study, subjects exhibited improved PEFR, less diurnal variation of PEFR, and fewer symptoms after 21 weeks of treatment (Fig. 10.4).

The addition of a long-acting β_2-agonist may also decrease exacerbations of asthma. Pauwels and colleagues (112) randomized patients with moderate asthma to one of four treatment groups: low-dose budesonide (100 μg twice daily) plus placebo, low-dose budesonide plus formoterol (12 μg twice daily), high-dose budesonide (400 μg twice daily) plus placebo, or high-dose budesonide plus formoterol. Treatment was continued for 1 year. The rates of severe and mild exacerbations in the group as a whole decreased by 26% and 40%, respectively. Patients treated with formoterol and the higher dose of budesonide experienced the greatest reductions (63% and 62%, respectively). There were no signs of worsened asthma control or tolerance to the effects of medication in regard to any clinical or functional variable examined, except for a decrease in the effect of formoterol on the PEFR in the morning after the first 2 days of treatment. The PEFR remained significantly higher than in the budesonide-only groups during the remainder of the 1-year study period. One explanation of these findings is the development of limited tolerance to the bronchodilator effect of formoterol during the early phase of regular treatment, demonstrated in other studies (113–116). The findings of this study suggest, however, that tolerance is of little or no clinical significance.

Dahl and colleagues (117) showed that the combination of inhaled corticosteroids plus the long-acting oral β_2-agonist sustained-release terbutaline reduces nocturnal worsening of asthma better than either used separately. Selby and coworkers (118) compared inhaled corticosteroids plus salmeterol or theophylline in the treatment of nocturnal asthma. Although the overnight falls in PEFR were similar in both groups, subjects experienced fewer nocturnal awakenings while using salmeterol. The authors concluded that in patients with nocturnal asthma, small benefits in sleep quality, quality of life, and daytime cognitive function are appreciated with salmeterol. These data supplement the data of Weersink and colleagues (119), who demonstrated that treatment of nocturnal airway obstruction improves daytime cognitive performance.

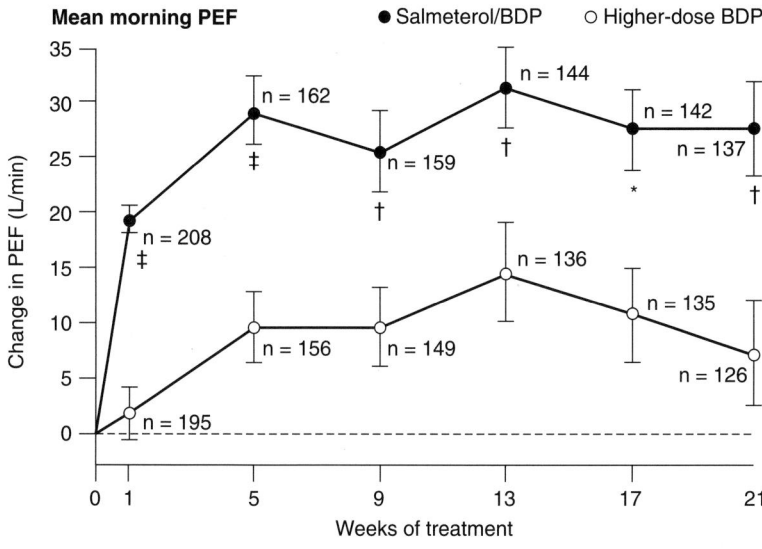

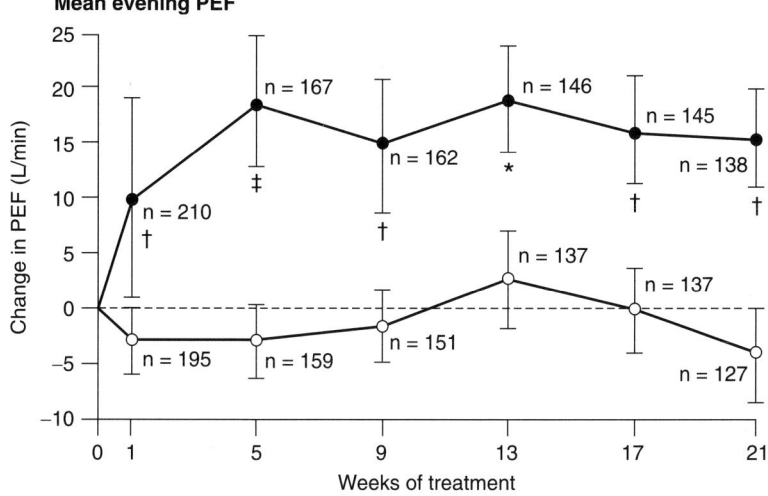

FIGURE 10.4. Mean change in morning and evening peak flow (*PEF*) during 21 weeks with salmeterol plus 200 μg of beclomethasone dipropionate twice daily (*dark circles*) and with 500 μg of beclomethasone dipropionate alone twice daily (*open circles*). (From Greening AP, Ind PW, Northfield M, et al. Added salmeterol versus higher-dose corticosteroid in asthma patients with symptoms on existing inhaled corticosteroid. Allen and Hanbury's Limited U.K. Study Group. *Lancet* 1994;344:219–224, with permission.)

Inhaled Corticosteroids and Theophylline

The use of theophylline preparations as steroid-sparing agents has been examined (85,86). Studies suggest that the combination of inhaled corticosteroids and theophylline is more effective than corticosteroids alone (86). Evans and colleagues (86) treated 62 patients with moderate asthma by adding theophylline (250 or 375 mg twice daily, depending on weight) to inhaled corticosteroids (400 or 800 μg of budesonide twice daily) during a 3-month treatment period. The group receiving the low dose of budesonide plus theophylline exhibited greater improvements in FEV_1 (2.48 $\pm$ 0.18 L to a peak of 2.76 $\pm$ 0.18 L, $P = .002$) than did the group receiving the high dose of budesonide (2.50 $\pm$ 0.14 L to a peak of 2.62 $\pm$ 0.15 L, $P = .37$) (Fig. 10.5). Improvements of similar magnitude were appreciated in the FVC. The authors also evaluated the PEFR and found no differences between the groups, but the theophylline-plus-budesonide group exhibited a reduction in peak flow variability (86).

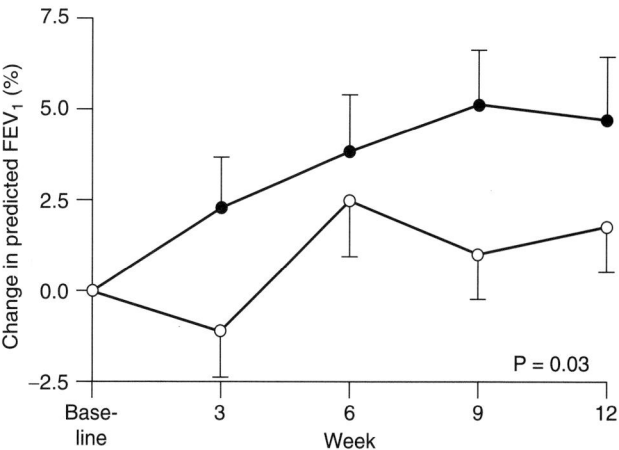

FIGURE 10.5. Mean change in FEV_1% predicted over 12 weeks with 800 μg of budesonide (*open circles*) and with 400 μg of budesonide plus theophylline (*dark circles*). (From Evans DJ, Taylor DA, Zetterstrom O, et al. A comparison of low-dose inhaled budesonide plus theophylline and high-dose inhaled budesonide for moderate asthma. *N Engl J Med* 1997;337:1412–1418, with permission.)

Inhaled Corticosteroids and Cromolyn/Nedocromil

Rebuck and colleagues (120) evaluated the efficacy of nedocromil sodium in patients who had persistent asthma despite inhaled or oral corticosteroids. Two milligrams of nedocromil four times daily or placebo was given to 188 patients for 12 weeks. In addition, 43% of the nedocromil group and 47% of the placebo group used 400 μg of beclomethasone per day. Both groups contained similar proportions of patients taking 800 μg or more of inhaled corticosteroid per day. Thirty-three percent of patients in the nedocromil group took oral corticosteroids, versus 22% in the placebo group. Initial pulmonary function measurements (FEV_1, FVC) showed no significant differences between the two groups. Results demonstrated that morning and evening PEFR values were significantly higher in the nedocromil group during the first 6 to 8 weeks, but these differences diminished by 12 weeks. Symptoms decreased significantly within 4 weeks after the start of nedocromil; no differences in symptom scores were noted within the placebo-treated group. The authors concluded that the addition of nedocromil provides small but important improvements in asthma therapy in this population.

High-dose nedocromil has been studied in combination with inhaled corticosteroids (121). Eight milligrams of nedocromil four times daily or placebo was added to the treatment of 29 asthmatic patients for 6 weeks. All patients were taking inhaled corticosteroids in doses of up to 1,000 μg/d. The morning PEFR increased slightly in the nedocromil group to levels approaching statistical significance ($P = .06$). Daytime asthma symptoms were significantly reduced in the nedocromil group, but nighttime symptoms and bronchodilator use were not different. There was also no difference in the side effect profile. The results suggest that the addition of nedocromil to corticosteroid therapy further relieves symptoms and improves function in individuals with asthma. A study by Svendson and Jorgensen (122) supports these results. The acute administration of cromolyn has also been found to reduce decrements in lung function after challenge with inhalation of 4.5% saline solution in patients treated for 3 months with budesonide (123).

Inhaled Corticosteroids and Leukotriene Modifiers

Cysteinyl leukotrienes (LTC_4, LTD_4, and LTE_4) are released by inflammatory cells in the airways of asthmatic patients. Considerable evidence suggests that these agents are important mediators of asthma (124–128). Two classes of leukotriene modifiers are currently used in the treatment of asthma: zileuton, which is a 5-lipoxygenase enzyme inhibitor, and the LTD_4 receptor antagonists zafirlukast and montelukast. Both classes of leukotriene modifiers have been studied in combination with inhaled corticosteroids in the treatment of asthma (117).

It is now thought that leukotrienes play a central role in aspirin-sensitive asthma (129–133). Consequently, zileuton has been studied in combination with inhaled corticosteroids in patients in whom chronic rhinosinusitis, nasal polyposis, and acute bronchospasm developed when they were given aspirin (134,135). In this study, 600 mg of zileuton four times daily was added to existing therapy, which included medium to high doses of inhaled corticosteroids (average dose, 1,030 μg of beclomethasone or budesonide) or oral corticosteroids (4–25 mg/d). Acute (within 4 hours after ingestion) and chronic improvements in FEV_1 were noted (acute, 12.7% increase with zileuton vs. 6.8% with placebo, $P < .01$; chronic, 7% improvement over placebo at the end of 6 weeks, $P < .01$). These improvements occurred despite reduced rescue bronchodilator use in the zileuton group. Other improvements included higher morning and evening PEFR measurements. Zileuton also diminished nasal dysfunction, one of the cardinal signs of aspirin-sensitive asthma. A return of smell, less rhinorrhea, and a trend toward less congestion were noted. This study suggests that in aspirin-sensitive asthma, the addition of zileuton may effect a greater control of asthma than is achieved by treatment with medium to high doses of corticosteroids alone.

Zafirlukast has been studied in patients whose asthma was not well controlled despite high doses of inhaled corticosteroids (mean dose, 1,600 μg/d) (136). Patients were randomized to receive zafirlukast (80 mg twice daily) or placebo in addition to their usual therapy. After 6 weeks of treatment, the patients who received zafirlukast exhibited significantly higher morning PEFR values than did patients who received placebo (18.7 vs. 1.5 L/min, $P = .001$). Evidence of incremental improvement during each week of the trial was noted in the zafirlukast arm. No evidence was found of any increases in adverse events in the zafirlukast group, and only about half as many patients in the zafirlukast-treated group experienced worsening asthma during the course of the trial that necessitated a change in therapy.

A study evaluated pranlukast and its effect on asthma control during reductions in doses of inhaled corticosteroids (137). Seventy-nine patients requiring high doses of beclomethasone ($>1,500$ μg/d) were treated with either 450 mg of pranlukast twice daily or placebo. At the end of 2 weeks, the doses of inhaled corticosteroids in each group were halved. After 6 weeks, the FEV_1 in the placebo group decreased by 0.33 ± 0.2 L, and the morning and evening PEFR values decreased by 46 ± 7 and 18 ± 6 L/min, respectively. In contrast, these variables were sustained above baseline in the pranlukast group. The use of inhaled β_2-agonists and nocturnal asthma symptoms increased in the placebo group and remained at baseline in the pranlukast group. The authors concluded that pranlukast had prevented the worsening of asthma provoked by the 6-week reduction in the dose of inhaled corticosteroid (137).

CONSENSUS GUIDELINES AND THE MANAGEMENT OF ASTHMA

In 1997, the NIH released *Guidelines for the Diagnosis and Management of Asthma,* a set of clinical practice recommendations for the diagnosis and management of asthma (2). The expert panel assembled to formulate these guidelines was comprised of a multidisciplinary group of clinicians and scientists with extensive knowledge of the pathophysiology and treatment of asthma. The recommendations in the expert panel report were based in large part on results published in the scientific literature, although when studies were not available or the results were conflicting, the recommendations were based on the consensus opinion of the panel. As such, the recommendations contained in this section are based on mixed evidence, some of it high-quality data derived from multiple randomized controlled trials and some of it derived from minimal experimentation.

A major recommendation of the expert panel report is that persistent asthma is most appropriately treated with the daily use of inhaled corticosteroids. Additionally, the expert panel recommends a stepwise approach to pharmacologic therapy, with the clinical severity of asthma dictating the dose of antiinflammatory medications and the frequency of administration. Therapy should be initiated at the highest dose required to establish prompt control; medications are then gradually reduced once control is achieved. Frequent monitoring of airflow and symptoms is the best method for assessing asthma control.

According to the expert panel, mild intermittent asthma does not require the daily use of an inhaled corticosteroid as a long-term controller agent. For rapid relief of symptoms, a short-acting bronchodilator such as an inhaled β_2-agonist is recommended, with the proviso that the use of a short-acting β_2-agonist more than twice weekly may indicate a need for inhaled corticosteroids. In addition to pharmacologic therapy, education about the basic concepts of asthma pathophysiology, the importance and role of different medications, and the appropriate use of metered-dose inhalers is recommended for patients with asthma of all levels of severity, as well as the implementation of self-management and action plans (2).

The treatment of mild persistent asthma in adults is based on the daily use of a low dose of an inhaled corticosteroid as long-term controller therapy (Table 10.11), with use of an inhaled bronchodilator such as albuterol for quick relief of symptoms. The panel notes that an increase in the frequency of inhaled β_2-agonist use or the use of a β_2-agonist more than daily may indicate the need for additional control of inflammation (2). The panel recommends that moderate persistent asthma be treated with medium-dose inhaled corticosteroids or low- to medium-dose inhaled corticosteroids together with a long-acting inhaled β_2-agonist such as salmeterol. Short-acting inhaled β_2-agonists are recommended for quick relief of symptoms, and education remains an important component of comprehensive asthma management (2). The recommended treatment of severe persistent asthma includes a high-dose inhaled corticosteroid in addition to a long-acting inhaled β_2-agonist such as salmeterol, or the use of sustained-release theophylline. Inhaled short-acting β_2-agonists are recommended for the quick relief of symptoms (2). Dose ranges for inhaled corticosteroids in adults are listed in Table 10.11.

Recommendations for adjunctive therapy in asthma include the treatment of concurrent sinus disease (allergic rhinitis and chronic sinusitis) and concomitant GERD, and nonpharmacologic interventions, such as the assessment and control of environmental irritants or allergens and patient

TABLE 10.11. SUGGESTED DAILY DOSES OF INHALED CORTICOSTEROIDS FOR USE IN ADULTS

	Asthma Clinical Phenotype		
Inhaled Corticosteroid	Mild Persistent Asthma (μg)	Moderate Persistent Asthma (μg)	Severe Persistent Asthma (μg)
Triamcinolone acetonide 100 μg/inhalation	400–1,000	1,000–2,000	>2,000
Flunisolide 250 μg/inhalation	500–1,000	1,000–2,000	>2,000
Beclomethasone dipropionate 42 or 84 μg/inhalation	168–504	504–840	>840
Budesonide Turbuhaler 200 μg/inhalation	200–400	400–600	>600
Fluticasone MDI: 44, 110, 220 μg/inhalation or DPI: 50, 100, 250 μg/inhalation	88–264	264–660	>660

Note: These agents are usually administered with one half of the daily dose taken in the morning and one half in the evening. Drugs are in order of increasing potency.
MDI, metered-dose inhaler; DPI, dry powder inhaler.
Source: Adapted from Expert panel report 2. *Guidelines for the diagnosis and management of asthma.* Bethesda, MD: National Institutes of Health, National Heart, Lung, and Blood Institute, 1997: NIH Publication No 97-4051.

education. The expert panel recommends that every available opportunity be taken to teach patients the following: basic facts about asthma, the role of medications in the acute and long-term treatment of asthma, appropriate measures for the control of environmental irritants and allergens, how to use inhaled drugs and devices, and what to do when asthma worsens.

PEAK FLOW MONITORING, SELF-MANAGEMENT, AND THE ASTHMA ACTION PLAN

Each patient should be informed about an appropriate daily self-management plan, with recommendations for daily medication use, the importance of recording daily peak flows and symptoms, and basic steps to be taken when asthma symptoms or peak flow worsens. Daily peak flow monitoring and linking of changes in peak flow to changes in asthma therapy are likely to benefit patients with moderate and severe persistent asthma and those with a history of frequent exacerbations by improving awareness about changes in lung function and allowing changes in therapy to be initiated before a severe exacerbation develops. Peak flows should be measured at the same time each day and with the same peak flow meter over time (2).

All patients should be provided with an asthma action plan that allows them to determine the most appropriate pharmacotherapy for their asthma based on symptoms and PEFR. Recommendations for drug dosing in each situation should be tailored to the individual patient (2). In general, a peak flow between 50% and 80% of the patient's personal best signifies a mild exacerbation that should prompt consideration of an increase in the dose or frequency of administration of both short-acting and long-term controller medications for asthma; a peak flow below 50% of the patient's best indicates a severe exacerbation (2). A peak flow below 50% should prompt the patient not only to increase dosing but also to seek medical attention for further evaluation and instructions (2).

INTEGRATED APPROACH TO ASTHMA MANAGEMENT

These cases are designed to describe for the clinician approaches to asthma of different levels of severity. They represent the "art" of medicine and are not meant to suggest that a described approach is the only correct one. However, they do highlight controversies and possible approaches based on available data.

Mild Persistent Asthma

The approach to mild persistent asthma is relatively straightforward, although the choice of class of medication, inhaled corticosteroid, and initial dose can pose a dilemma for the clinician. These patients exhibit normal lung function ($FEV_1 > 80\%$ of predicted value), use inhaled β_2-agonists more than two times per week, experience fewer than two nocturnal symptoms per month, and demonstrate peak flow variability of less than 20% to 30% (2). The physical examination findings can be normal in these patients, and as previously discussed (see section "Historical Clues to Asthma"), a lack of wheezing does not rule out asthma. One should consider a methacholine challenge if significant bronchodilator responsiveness is not demonstrated.

It is noteworthy that patients may not remain in a specific category; asthma can change from mild to moderate and back depending on exposures and exacerbations. For the purposes of this discussion, the evaluation has determined that the patient has mild but persistent asthma, which underscores the need for daily antiinflammatory therapy. This recommendation is driven by the study by Haahtela and colleagues (40), in which adult patients with mild asthma who were not initially treated with inhaled corticosteroids lost lung function and exhibited increased hyperresponsiveness that did not improve when inhaled corticosteroids were instituted after a 2-year period of observation and treatment with inhaled β_2-agonists alone.

During the evaluation, the presence and role of contributing factors should be considered, such as atopy, sinusitis/rhinitis, GERD, obstructive sleep apnea, and vocal cord dysfunction. The evaluation of these entities includes sinus computed tomography, empiric therapy or pH probe testing to rule out GERD, and an overnight polysomnographic evaluation or pulse oximetry testing. Vocal cord dysfunction can be evaluated by an inspiratory flow-volume loop or laryngoscopy, the latter following a provocative test that may elicit symptoms of variable upper airway obstruction, such as a methacholine or exercise challenge test. Even in mild asthma, these factors may be driving airway inflammation, and proper treatment may significantly reduce the need for medication. The differential diagnosis must always be considered; chronic obstructive pulmonary disease, bronchiectasis, bronchiolitis, heart failure/pulmonary edema, endobronchial lesions, and the use of medications such as β-blockers and angiotensin-converting enzyme inhibitors all must be ruled out.

Peak flow monitoring should be performed during the initial evaluation and also for several weeks after therapy is instituted to determine the patient's best peak flow for use in the asthma action plan. The peak flow can be checked before bedtime and in the morning, because these are relatively convenient times for patients, or in the morning and at midday. It is also helpful, but not always realistic, for patients to record their peak flow during the week before their follow-up appointments.

The NIH guidelines (2) recommend inhaled corticosteroids as first-line therapy for this group of patients. Since the guidelines were published in 1997, results of research have suggested that a leukotriene receptor antagonist can be used as monotherapy in mild persistent asthma (138).

Therefore, the physician must judge whether the patient will comply with inhaled corticosteroid treatment or whether an antiinflammatory medication in the form of a pill will enhance compliance. Some data suggest that compliance may be somewhat improved with the use of a pill, but interestingly, refill rates with either a leukotriene receptor antagonist or inhaled corticosteroids have been suboptimal, so compliance is an important issue regardless of the medication chosen (139). One suggestion would be to define, if possible, whether the patient will use an inhaled corticosteroid daily. If not, a leukotriene receptor antagonist may be a reasonable second choice for this group.

If an inhaled corticosteroid is chosen, then the dose should be in the low to mid range, with plans to taper if possible after a 3-month trial. Spirometry is recommended during the initial evaluation, after the institution of therapy, and at least once every 1 to 2 years or if the patient's symptoms change (2). Because these patients have mild disease, changes in the FEV_1 may not be significant, so the importance of evaluating other parameters, such as exercise tolerance, nocturnal symptoms, and inhaled β_2-agonist use, cannot be overemphasized. Suggested doses for several inhaled corticosteroid preparations for the treatment of mild persistent asthma are listed in Table 10.11.

The actual inhaled corticosteroid chosen is less important than choosing the proper dosage, educating the patient about correct inhaler use, monitoring during therapy, and tapering to the least amount of medication needed to maintain asthma control. The goals of therapy as per the National Asthma Education and Prevention Program expert panel guidelines include no or minimal use of inhaled β_2-agonists (less than once daily), the ability to perform all desired activities, the elimination of nocturnal symptoms, and tight control on the lowest dose of antiinflammatory medication possible. Finally, attention must be paid to the side effects of medication, such as hoarseness and oral candidiasis, and yearly eye examinations are required.

Moderate Persistent Asthma

These patients demonstrate abnormal lung function (FEV_1 > 60% but <80% of the predicted value), experience at least two episodes of nocturnal worsening of asthma per month, exhibit peak flow variability greater than 20% to 30%, and use inhaled β_2-agonists daily. During the initial evaluation, the role of contributing factors should be determined, and these should be managed as discussed previously (see section "Evaluation and Treatment of Comorbid Conditions"). The differential diagnosis should be considered, peak flow monitoring implemented, and an asthma action plan constructed. Inhaled steroids at moderate doses are the mainstay of therapy in this group. Some recommendations for doses are included in Table 10.11.

As in mild asthma, the actual inhaled corticosteroid chosen is less important than ongoing monitoring and tapering to the lowest dose that maintains asthma control.

Because an inhaled corticosteroid alone often will not completely control symptoms (see goals of therapy listed in section "Mild Persistent Asthma"), add-on therapy with a long-acting inhaled β_2-agonist (salmeterol or formoterol), leukotriene receptor antagonist (montelukast or zafirlukast), or theophylline should be considered next. Which is chosen will depend on the willingness of the patient to use another inhaler or a pill because there are no good predictors of response to therapy with any of the add-on agents. Certain data suggest that the addition of a long-acting inhaled β_2-agonist may result in steroid-sparing effects, allowing the physician to reduce the dose of inhaled corticosteroids required to maintain asthma control (68–70). Additional data suggest that inhaled corticosteroids and a long-acting inhaled β_2-agonist may work synergistically to enhance translocation of the steroid receptor complex to the nucleus (140). The fluticasone/salmeterol combination has enhanced convenience and compliance because both medications are now available in the same inhaler. A combination of budesonide and formoterol is currently available outside the United States.

Although the inhaled corticosteroid/long-acting inhaled β_2-agonist combination is popular, data also suggest that the addition of a leukotriene receptor antagonist or theophylline to an inhaled corticosteroid results in steroid-sparing effects (112,136,137). Therefore, the treatment chosen will depend on the physician's notion of the patient's compliance with any of the combinations. Certainly, short-acting inhaled β_2-agonists should continue to be used as rescue therapy for symptoms, and spirometry should be performed initially, after treatment, and then yearly unless the patient's symptoms change. Again, it is helpful if patients can record their peak flow before bed and in the morning for 1 week before their follow-up appointment.

Severe Persistent Asthma

These patients represent a therapeutic challenge because they often require several classes of medications, and their symptoms and lung function may be quite labile. The importance of diagnosing and treating contributing factors in this group cannot be overstated. Attention to the differential diagnosis is also very important; thus, additional evaluation may include high-resolution chest computed tomography to rule out bronchiectasis, emphysema, and signs consistent with allergic bronchopulmonary aspergillosis. The use of pH probe testing should be especially considered because GERD may be silent in these patients yet contribute to ongoing airway inflammation and bronchial constriction. Helpful tests include corticosteroid kinetics to assess absorption of steroids, particularly if the patient is using oral steroids on a long-term basis. If this test is not available, periodic measurements of morning serum cortisol levels and random measurements of blood eosinophil levels should be considered; these should both be suppressed in a compliant patient using oral or high-dose inhaled corticosteroids daily. Additional testing to consider would be close inspection of the flow-volume loop or laryngoscopy to rule out vocal cord dysfunction and a psychiatric evaluation, the latter because the prevalence of stress and psychiatric disease is high in this group (27,141,142).

Once the diagnosis of severe persistent asthma is confirmed (FEV_1 < 60% of predicted value, daily symptoms, peak flow variability >30%, frequent nocturnal symptoms), high-dose antiinflammatory therapy is warranted. Patients may already be taking oral corticosteroids when they present, so the use of high-dose inhaled corticosteroids plus add-on therapy may allow tapering of the oral corticosteroid. Given the number of puffs per day required for some of these inhaled corticosteroid preparations, it is probably more practical to use fluticasone or budesonide initially (Table 10.11).

Add-on therapy will be necessary because it is unlikely that inhaled corticosteroids with or without oral corticosteroids will control asthma symptoms adequately. Additionally, the goal is to taper the oral corticosteroids first, then the inhaled corticosteroids if possible. Therefore, a long-acting β_2-agonist or a leukotriene receptor antagonist should be considered as initial add-on therapy. It is difficult to recommend an oral corticosteroid taper schedule because no data are available; schedules must be individualized, representing the true "art" of medicine. However, one recommendation would be to use a short "burst" of 40 to 60 mg/d in single or divided doses until 80% of the patient's personal best peak flow is achieved. This often takes 3 to 10 days but sometimes longer. If a single dose is to be used, administration at 3 p.m. should be considered because this has been associated with beneficial effects on daytime and nocturnal symptoms and airway inflammation with no increase in adrenal suppression in comparison with morning dosing (143). Further therapy (long-acting β_2-agonist, leukotriene receptor antagonist, theophylline) should be added individually, with at least 1 week allowed to assess the response before the next agent is tried. These should be added while the patient is on oral corticosteroids, and when asthma control is achieved, taper of the steroid should begin. The pace of the taper should reflect the length of time on oral corticosteroids required to achieve asthma control. If 3 to 10 days was required, then a rapid taper should ensue; if a longer period was necessary, then a slower taper should be recommended.

REFERENCES

1. *National Institutes of Health data fact sheet: asthma statistics.* Bethesda, MD: U.S. Department of Health and Human Services, 1999: NIH Publication No. 55-798.
2. Expert panel report 2. *Guidelines for the diagnosis and management of asthma.* Bethesda, MD: National Institutes of Health, National Heart, Lung, and Blood Institute, 1997: NIH Publication No. 97-4051.
3. Baumann UA, Haerdi E, Keller R. Relations between clinical signs and lung function in bronchial asthma: how is acute bronchial obstruction reflected in dyspnoea and wheezing? *Respiration* 1986;50:294–300.
4. Burrows B, Lebowitz MD, Barbee RA, et al. Findings before diagnoses of asthma among the elderly in a longitudinal study of a general population sample. *J Allergy Clin Immunol* 1991;88:870–877.
5. Sistek D, Tschopp JM, Schindler C, et al. Clinical diagnosis of current asthma: predictive value of respiratory symptoms in the SAPALDIA Study. Swiss Study on Air Pollution and Lung Diseases in Adults. *Eur Respir J* 2001;17:214–219.
6. Sackett DL. *Clinical epidemiology : a basic science for clinical medicine,* 2nd ed. Boston: Little, Brown and Company, 1991.
7. Holleman DR Jr, Simel DL. Does the clinical examination predict airflow limitation? *JAMA* 1995;273:313–319.
8. American Thoracic Society. Lung function testing: selection of reference values and interpretative strategies. *Am Rev Respir Dis* 1991;144:1202–1218.
9. Crapo RO, Casaburi R, Coates AL, et al. Guidelines for methacholine and exercise challenge testing—1999 (official statement of the American Thoracic Society adopted by the ATS Board of Directors, July 1999). *Am J Respir Crit Care Med* 2000;161:309–329.
10. Martin RJ. Location of airway inflammation in asthma and the relationship to circadian change in lung function. *Chronobiol Int* 1999;16:623–630.
11. Ballard RD, Tan WC, Kelly PL, et al. Effect of sleep and sleep deprivation on ventilatory response to bronchoconstriction. *J Appl Physiol* 1990;69:490–497.
12. Martin RJ, Cicutto LC, Ballard RD. Factors related to the nocturnal worsening of asthma. *Am Rev Respir Dis* 1990;141:33–38.
13. Kraft M, Vianna E, Martin RJ, et al. Nocturnal asthma is associated with reduced glucocorticoid receptor binding affinity and decreased steroid responsiveness at night. *J Allergy Clin Immunol* 1999;103(1 Pt 1):66–71.
14. Kraft M, Hamid Q, Chrousos GP, et al. Decreased steroid responsiveness at night in nocturnal asthma. Is the macrophage responsible? *Am J Respir Crit Care Med* 2001;163:1219–1225.
15. Tiddens H, Silverman M, Bush A. The role of inflammation in airway disease: remodeling. *Am J Respir Crit Care Med* 2000;162(2 Pt 2):S7–S10.
16. Jeffery PK, Godfrey RW, Adelroth E, et al. Effects of treatment on airway inflammation and thickening of basement membrane reticular collagen in asthma. A quantitative light and electron microscopic study. *Am Rev Respir Dis* 1992;145(4 Pt 1):890–899.
17. Busse W, Elias J, Sheppard D, et al. Airway remodeling and repair. *Am J Respir Crit Care Med* 1999;160:1035–1042.
18. Cassino C, Berger KI, Goldring RM, et al. Duration of asthma and physiologic outcomes in elderly nonsmokers. *Am J Respir Crit Care Med* 2000;162(4 Pt 1):1423–1428.
19. Boulet LP, Cartier A, Thomson NC, et al. Asthma and increases in nonallergic bronchial responsiveness from seasonal pollen exposure. *J Allergy Clin Immunol* 1983;71:399–406.
20. Piacentini GL, Martinati L, Fornari A, et al. Antigen avoidance in a mountain environment: influence on basophil releasability in children with allergic asthma. *J Allergy Clin Immunol* 1993;92:644–650.
21. Peroni DG, Boner AL, Vallone G, et al. Effective allergen avoidance at high altitude reduces allergen-induced bronchial hyperresponsiveness. *Am J Respir Crit Care Med* 1994;149:1442–1446.
22. Slavin RG. Asthma and sinusitis. *J Allergy Clin Immunol* 1992;90(3 Pt 2):534–537.
23. Rachelefsky GS, Katz RM, Siegel SC. Chronic sinus disease with associated reactive airway disease in children. *Pediatrics* 1984;73:526–529.

24. Dunlop G, Scadding GK, Lund VJ. The effect of endoscopic sinus surgery on asthma: management of patients with chronic rhinosinusitis, nasal polyposis, and asthma. *Am J Rhinol* 1999;13:261–265.

25. Harding SM, Guzzo MR, Richter JE. 24-Hour esophageal pH testing in asthmatics: respiratory symptom correlation with esophageal acid events. *Chest* 1999;115:654–659.

26. Harding SM, Richter JE, Guzzo MR, et al. Asthma and gastroesophageal reflux: acid-suppressive therapy improves asthma outcome. *Am J Med* 1996;100:395–405.

27. Enright PL, McClelland RL, Newman AB, et al. Underdiagnosis and undertreatment of asthma in the elderly. Cardiovascular Health Study Research Group. *Chest* 1999;116:603–613.

28. Walsh LJ, Wong CA, Osborne J, et al. Adverse effects of oral corticosteroids in relation to dose in patients with lung disease. *Thorax* 2001;56:279–284.

29. Barnes PJ. Efficacy of inhaled corticosteroids in asthma. *J Allergy Clin Immunol* 1998;102(4 Pt 1):531–538.

30. Donahue JG, Weiss ST, Livingston JM, et al. Inhaled steroids and the risk of hospitalization for asthma. *JAMA* 1997;277:887–891.

31. Suissa S, Ernst P, Benayoun S, et al. Low-dose inhaled corticosteroids and the prevention of death from asthma. *N Engl J Med* 2000;343:332–336.

32. Laurie S, Khan D. Inhaled corticosteroids as first-line therapy for asthma. Why they work and what the guidelines and evidence suggest. *Postgrad Med* 2001;109:44–46, 49–52, 55–56.

33. Luisi BF, Xu WX, Otwinowski Z, et al. Crystallographic analysis of the interaction of the glucocorticoid receptor with DNA. *Nature* 1991;352:497–505.

34. Barnes PJ, Greening AP, Crompton GK. Glucocorticoid resistance in asthma. *Am J Respir Crit Care Med* 1995;152(6 Pt 2):S125–S140.

35. Diamond MI, Miner JN, Yoshinaga SK, et al. Transcription factor interactions: selectors of positive or negative regulation from a single DNA element. *Science* 1990;249:1266–1272.

36. Waage A, Bakke O. Glucocorticoids suppress the production of tumour necrosis factor by lipopolysaccharide-stimulated human monocytes. *Immunology* 1988;63:299–302.

37. Auphan N, DiDonato JA, Rosette C, et al. Immunosuppression by glucocorticoids: inhibition of NF-kappa B activity through induction of I kappa B synthesis. *Science* 1995;270:286–290.

38. Wilson JW, Djukanovic R, Howarth PH, et al. Inhaled beclomethasone dipropionate down-regulates airway lymphocyte activation in atopic asthma. *Am J Respir Crit Care Med* 1994;149:86–90.

39. Laitinen LA, Laitinen A, Haahtela T. A comparative study of the effects of an inhaled corticosteroid, budesonide, and a beta 2-agonist, terbutaline, on airway inflammation in newly diagnosed asthma: a randomized, double-blind, parallel-group controlled trial. *J Allergy Clin Immunol* 1992;90:32–42.

40. Haahtela T, Jarvinen M, Kava T, et al. Comparison of a beta 2-agonist, terbutaline, with an inhaled corticosteroid, budesonide, in newly detected asthma. *N Engl J Med* 1991;325:388–392.

41. Juniper EF, Kline PA, Vanzieleghem MA, et al. Effect of long-term treatment with an inhaled corticosteroid (budesonide) on airway hyperresponsiveness and clinical asthma in non–steroid-dependent asthmatics. *Am Rev Respir Dis* 1990;142:832–836.

42. Vathenen AS, Knox AJ, Wisniewski A, et al. Time course of change in bronchial reactivity with an inhaled corticosteroid in asthma. *Am Rev Respir Dis* 1991;143:1317–1321.

43. Reed CE, Offord KP, Nelson HS, et al. Aerosol beclomethasone dipropionate spray compared with theophylline as primary treatment for chronic mild-to-moderate asthma. The American Academy of Allergy, Asthma, and Immunology Beclomethasone Dipropionate–Theophylline Study Group. *J Allergy Clin Immunol* 1998;101(1 Pt 1):14–23.

44. Busse W, Raphael GD, Galant S, et al. Low-dose fluticasone propionate compared with montelukast for first-line treatment of persistent asthma: a randomized clinical trial. *J Allergy Clin Immunol* 2001;107:461–468.

45. Bleecker ER, Welch MJ, Weinstein SF, et al. Low-dose inhaled fluticasone propionate versus oral zafirlukast in the treatment of persistent asthma. *J Allergy Clin Immunol* 2000;105(6 Pt 1):1123–1129.

46. Malmstrom K, Rodriguez-Gomez G, Guerra J, et al. Oral montelukast, inhaled beclomethasone, and placebo for chronic asthma. A randomized, controlled trial. Montelukast/Beclomethasone Study Group. *Ann Intern Med* 1999;130:487–495.

47. Adams N, Bestall J, Jones P. Inhaled beclomethasone versus placebo for chronic asthma [Cochrane Review]. *The Cochrane Library* 2001.

48. Ernst P, Spitzer WO, Suissa S, et al. Risk of fatal and near-fatal asthma in relation to inhaled corticosteroid use. *JAMA* 1992;268:3462–3464.

49. Israel E, Banerjee TR, Fitzmaurice GM, et al. Effects of inhaled glucocorticoids on bone density in premenopausal women. *N Engl J Med* 2001;345:941–947.

50. Shaw NJ, Edmunds AT. Inhaled beclomethasone and oral candidiasis. *Arch Dis Child* 1986;61:788–790.

51. Toogood JH, Jennings B, Greenway RW, et al. Candidiasis and dysphonia complicating beclomethasone treatment of asthma. *J Allergy Clin Immunol* 1980;65:145–153.

52. Kamada AK, Szefler SJ, Martin RJ, et al. Issues in the use of inhaled glucocorticoids. The Asthma Clinical Research Network. *Am J Respir Crit Care Med* 1996;153(6 Pt 1):1739–1748.

53. O'Byrne PM, Kerstjens HA. Inhaled beta 2-agonists in the treatment of asthma. *N Engl J Med* 1996;335:886–888.

54. Frielle T, Daniel KW, Caron MG, et al. Structural basis of beta-adrenergic receptor subtype specificity studied with chimeric beta 1/beta 2-adrenergic receptors. *Proc Natl Acad Sci U S A* 1988;85:9494–9498.

55. Johnson M. The beta-adrenoceptor. *Am J Respir Crit Care Med* 1998;158(5 Pt 3):S146–S153.

56. Jack D. The 1990 Lilly Prize Lecture. A way of looking at agonism and antagonism: lessons from salbutamol, salmeterol, and other beta-adrenoceptor agonists. *Br J Clin Pharmacol* 1991;31:501–514.

57. Martin RJ, Kraft M, eds. *Combination therapy for asthma and chronic obstructive pulmonary disease.* New York: Marcel Dekker Inc, 2000.

58. Brogden RN, Faulds D. Salmeterol xinafoate. A review of its pharmacological properties and therapeutic potential in reversible obstructive airways disease. *Drugs* 1991;42:895–912.

59. Faulds D, Hollingshead LM, Goa KL. Formoterol. A review of its pharmacological properties and therapeutic potential in reversible obstructive airways disease. *Drugs* 1991;42:115–137.

60. Derom EY, Pauwels RA, Van der Straeten ME. The effect of inhaled salmeterol on methacholine responsiveness in subjects with asthma up to 12 hours. *J Allergy Clin Immunol* 1992;89:811–815.

61. Anderson SD, Rodwell LT, Du Toit J, et al. Duration of protection by inhaled salmeterol in exercise-induced asthma. *Chest* 1991;100:1254–1260.

62. Patessio A, Podda A, Carone M, et al. Protective effect and duration of action of formoterol aerosol on exercise-induced asthma. *Eur Respir J* 1991;4:296–300.

63. Ramsdale EH, Otis J, Kline PA, et al. Prolonged protection against methacholine-induced bronchoconstriction by the

inhaled beta 2-agonist formoterol. *Am Rev Respir Dis* 1991;143(5 Pt 1):998–1001.

64. Simons FE, Soni NR, Watson WT, et al. Bronchodilator and bronchoprotective effects of salmeterol in young patients with asthma. *J Allergy Clin Immunol* 1992;90:840–846.

65. Twentyman OP, Finnerty JP, Harris A, et al. Protection against allergen-induced asthma by salmeterol. *Lancet* 1990;336:1338–1342.

66. Verberne AA, Frost C, Roorda RJ, et al. One-year treatment with salmeterol compared with beclomethasone in children with asthma. The Dutch Paediatric Asthma Study Group. *Am J Respir Crit Care Med* 1997;156(3 Pt 1):688–695.

67. Bouros D, Bachlitzanakis N, Kottakis J, et al. Formoterol and beclomethasone versus higher-dose beclomethasone as maintenance therapy in adult asthma. *Eur Respir J* 1999;14:627–632.

68. Greening AP, Ind PW, Northfield M, et al. Added salmeterol versus higher-dose corticosteroid in asthma patients with symptoms on existing inhaled corticosteroids. *Lancet* 1994;344:219–224.

69. Woolcock A, Lundback B, Ringdal N, et al. Comparison of addition of salmeterol to inhaled steroids with doubling of the dose of inhaled steroids. *Am J Respir Crit Care Med* 1996;153:1481–1488.

70. Lemanske RF Jr, Sorkness CA, Mauger EA, et al. Inhaled corticosteroid reduction and elimination in patients with persistent asthma receiving salmeterol: a randomized controlled trial. *JAMA* 2001;285:2594–2603.

71. Spina D, Landells LJ, Page CP. The role of theophylline and phosphodiesterase 4 isoenzyme inhibitors as anti-inflammatory drugs. *Clin Exp Allergy* 1998;28[Suppl 3]:24–34.

72. Barnes PJ, Pauwels RA. Theophylline in the management of asthma: time for reappraisal? *Eur Respir J* 1994;7:579–591.

73. Finnerty JP, Lee C, Wilson S, et al. Effects of theophylline on inflammatory cells and cytokines in asthmatic subjects: a placebo-controlled parallel group study. *Eur Respir J* 1996;9:1672–1677.

74. Kosmas EN, Michaelides SA, Polychronaki A, et al. Theophylline induces a reduction in circulating interleukin-4 and interleukin-5 in atopic asthmatics. *Eur Respir J* 1999;13:53–58.

75. Sullivan P, Bekir S, Jaffar Z, et al. Anti-inflammatory effects of low-dose oral theophylline in atopic asthma. *Lancet* 1994;343:1006–1008.

76. Kraft M, Torvik JA, Trudeau JB, et al. Theophylline: potential antiinflammatory effects in nocturnal asthma. *J Allergy Clin Immunol* 1996;97:1242–1246.

77. Magnussen H, Reuss G, Jorres R. Theophylline has a dose-related effect on the airway response to inhaled histamine and methacholine in asthmatics. *Am Rev Respir Dis* 1987;136:1163–1167.

78. McWilliams BC, Menendez R, Kelly HW, et al. Effects of theophylline on inhaled methacholine and histamine in asthmatic children. *Am Rev Respir Dis* 1984;130:193–197.

79. Ibanez MD, Laso MT, Alonso E, et al. Effect of theophylline on airway responsiveness to methacholine and on exercise-induced bronchoconstriction. *Ann Allergy* 1994;73:357–363.

80. Crescioli S, Dal Carobbo A, Maestrelli P, et al. Controlled-release theophylline inhibits early morning airway obstruction and hyperresponsiveness in asthmatic subjects. *Ann Allergy Asthma Immunol* 1996;77:106–110.

81. Tinkelman DG, Garcha BS, Lutz CN. Relationship of different serum levels of theophylline on methacholine sensitivity. *J Allergy Clin Immunol* 1990;85:750–755.

82. Page CP, Cotter T, Kilfeather S, et al. Effect of chronic theophylline treatment on the methacholine dose-response curve in allergic asthmatic subjects. *Eur Respir J* 1998;12:24–29.

83. Dutoit JI, Salome CM, Woolcock AJ. Inhaled corticosteroids reduce the severity of bronchial hyperresponsiveness in asthma but oral theophylline does not. *Am Rev Respir Dis* 1987;136:1174–1178.

84. Tinkelman DG, Reed CE, Nelson HS, et al. Aerosol beclomethasone dipropionate compared with theophylline as primary treatment of chronic, mild to moderately severe asthma in children. *Pediatrics* 1993;92:64–77.

85. Ukena D, Harnest U, Sakalauskas R, et al. Comparison of addition of theophylline to inhaled steroid with doubling of the dose of inhaled steroid in asthma. *Eur Respir J* 1997;10:2754–2760.

86. Evans DJ, Taylor DA, Zetterstrom O, et al. A comparison of low-dose inhaled budesonide plus theophylline and high-dose inhaled budesonide for moderate asthma. *N Engl J Med* 1997;337:1412–1418.

87. Adelroth E, Morris MM, Hargreave FE, et al. Airway responsiveness to leukotrienes C$_4$ and D$_4$ and to methacholine in patients with asthma and normal controls. *N Engl J Med* 1986;315:480–484.

88. Dahlen SE, Hedqvist P, Hammarstrom S, et al. Leukotrienes are potent constrictors of human bronchi. *Nature* 1980;288:484–486.

89. Lewis RA, Austen KF, Soberman RJ. Leukotrienes and other products of the 5-lipoxygenase pathway. Biochemistry and relation to pathobiology in human diseases. *N Engl J Med* 1990;323:645–655.

90. Metters KM. Leukotriene receptors. *J Lipid Mediat Cell Signal* 1995;12:413–427.

91. Figueroa DJ, Breyer RM, Defoe SK, et al. Expression of the cysteinyl leukotriene 1 receptor in normal human lung and peripheral blood leukocytes. *Am J Respir Crit Care Med* 2001;163:226–233.

92. Heise CE, O'Dowd BF, Figueroa DJ, et al. Characterization of the human cysteinyl leukotriene 2 receptor. *J Biol Chem* 2000;275:30531–30536.

93. Diamant Z, Sampson AP. Anti-inflammatory mechanisms of leukotriene modulators. *Clin Exp Allergy* 1999;29:1449–1453.

94. Fish JE, Kemp JP, Lockey RF, et al. Zafirlukast for symptomatic mild-to-moderate asthma: a 13-week multicenter study. The Zafirlukast Trialists Group. *Clin Ther* 1997;19:675–690.

95. Suissa S, Dennis R, Ernst P, et al. Effectiveness of the leukotriene receptor antagonist zafirlukast for mild-to-moderate asthma. A randomized, double-blind, placebo-controlled trial. *Ann Intern Med* 1997;126:177–183.

96. Reiss TF, Chervinsky P, Dockhorn RJ, et al. Montelukast, a once-daily leukotriene receptor antagonist, in the treatment of chronic asthma: a multicenter, randomized, double-blind trial. Montelukast Clinical Research Study Group. *Arch Intern Med* 1998;158:1213–1220.

97. Israel E, Cohn J, Dube L, et al. Effect of treatment with zileuton, a 5-lipoxygenase inhibitor, in patients with asthma. A randomized controlled trial. Zileuton Clinical Trial Group. *JAMA* 1996;275:931–936.

98. Barnes PJ, Pedersen S. Efficacy and safety of inhaled corticosteroids in asthma. Report of a workshop held in Eze, France, October 1992. *Am Rev Respir Dis* 1993;148:S1–S26.

99. Laitinen LA, Laitinen A, Heino M, et al. Eosinophilic airway inflammation during exacerbation of asthma and its treatment with inhaled corticosteroid. *Am Rev Respir Dis* 1991;143:423–427.

100. Laursen LC, Taudorf E, Borgeskov S, et al. Fiberoptic bronchoscopy and bronchial mucosal biopsies in asthmatics

undergoing long-term high-dose budesonide aerosol treatment. *Allergy* 1988;43:284–288.

101. Lundgren R, Soderberg M, Horstedt P, et al. Morphological studies of bronchial mucosal biopsies from asthmatics before and after ten years of treatment with inhaled steroids. *Eur Respir J* 1988;1:883–889.

102. Djukanovic R, Wilson JW, Britten KM, et al. Effect of an inhaled corticosteroid on airway inflammation and symptoms in asthma. *Am Rev Respir Dis* 1992;145:669–674.

103. De Baets FM, Goeteyn M, Kerrebijn KF. The effect of two months of treatment with inhaled budesonide on bronchial responsiveness to histamine and house-dust mite antigen in asthmatic children. *Am Rev Respir Dis* 1990;142:581–586.

104. Svedmyr N. Action of corticosteroids on beta-adrenergic receptors. Clinical aspects. *Am Rev Respir Dis* 1990;141:S31–S38.

105. Adcock IM, Stevens DA, Barnes PJ. Interactions of glucocorticoids and β_2-agonists. *Eur Respir J* 1996;9:160–168.

106. Nielson CP, Hadjokas NE. Beta-adrenoceptor agonists block corticosteroid inhibition in eosinophils. *Am J Respir Crit Care Med* 1998;157:184–191.

107. Dompeling E, Van Schayck CP, Van Grunsven PM, et al. Slowing the deterioration of asthma and chronic obstructive pulmonary disease observed during bronchodilator therapy by adding inhaled corticosteroids. A 4-year prospective study. *Ann Intern Med* 1993;118:770–778.

108. Haahtela T, Alanko K, Muittari A, et al. The superiority of combination beclomethasone and salbutamol over standard dosing of salbutamol in the treatment of chronic asthma. *Ann Allergy* 1989;62:63–66.

109. Tormey VJ, Faul J, Leonard C, et al. A comparison of regular with intermittent bronchodilators in asthma patients on inhaled steroids. *Ir J Med Sci* 1997;166:249–252.

110. Van der Molen T, Postma DS, Turner MO, et al. Effects of the long-acting beta agonist formoterol on asthma control in asthmatic patients using inhaled corticosteroids. *Thorax* 1996;52:535–539.

111. Wilding P, Clark M, Coon JT, et al. Effect of long-term treatment with salmeterol on asthma control: a double-blind, randomised crossover study. *BMJ* 1997;314:1441–1446.

112. Pauwels RA, Lofdahl CG, Postma DS, et al. Effect of inhaled formoterol and budesonide on exacerbations of asthma. Formoterol and Corticosteroids Establishing Therapy (FACET) International Study Group. *N Engl J Med* 1997;337:1405–1411.

113. Kalra S, Swystun VA, Bhagat R, et al. Inhaled corticosteroids do not prevent the development of tolerance to the bronchoprotective effect of salmeterol. *Chest* 1996;109:953–956.

114. Bhagat R, Kalra S, Swystun VA, et al. Rapid onset of tolerance to the bronchoprotective effect of salmeterol. *Chest* 1995;108:1235–1239.

115. Cheung D, Timmers C, Zwinderman AH, et al. Long-term effects of a long-acting β_2-adrenoceptor agonist, salmeterol, on airway hyperresponsiveness in patients with mild asthma. *N Engl J Med* 1992;327:1198–1203.

116. Cockcroft DW, Swystun VA, Bhagat R. Interaction of inhaled beta 2 agonist and inhaled corticosteroid on airway responsiveness to allergen and methacholine. *Am J Respir Crit Care Med* 1995;152:1485–1489.

117. Dahl R, Pedersen B, Hagglof B. Nocturnal asthma: effect of treatment with oral sustained-release terbutaline, inhaled budesonide, and the two in combination. *J Allergy Clin Immunol* 1989;83:811–815.

118. Selby C, Engleman HM, Fitzpatrick MF, et al. Inhaled salmeterol or oral theophylline in nocturnal asthma? *Am J Respir Crit Care Med* 1997;155:104–108.

119. Weersink EJ, Van Zomeren EH, Koeter GH, et al. Treatment of nocturnal airway obstruction improves daytime cognitive performance in asthmatics. *Am J Respir Crit Care Med* 1997;156:1144–1150.

120. Rebuck AS, Chapman KR, Abboud R, et al. Nebulized anticholinergic and sympathomimetic treatment of asthma and chronic obstructive airways disease in the emergency room. *Am J Med* 1987;82:59–64.

121. O'Hickey SP, Rees PJ. High-dose nedocromil sodium as an addition to inhaled corticosteroids in the treatment of asthma. *Respir Med* 1994;88:499–502.

122. Svendsen UG, Jorgensen H. Inhaled nedocromil sodium as additional treatment to high-dose inhaled corticosteroids in the management of bronchial asthma. *Eur Respir J* 1991;4:992–999.

123. Anderson SD, Du Toit JI, Rodwell LT, et al. Acute effect of sodium cromoglycate on airway narrowing induced by 4.5 percent saline aerosol. Outcome before and during treatment with aerosol corticosteroids in patients with asthma. *Chest* 1994;105:673–680.

124. Manning PJ, Watson RM, Margolskee DJ, et al. Inhibition of exercise-induced bronchoconstriction by MK-571, a potent leukotriene D_4-receptor antagonist. *N Engl J Med* 1990;323:1736–1739.

125. Cloud ML, Enas GC, Kemp J, et al. A specific LTD_4/LTE_4-receptor antagonist improves pulmonary function in patients with mild, chronic asthma. *Am Rev Respir Dis* 1989;140:1336–1339.

126. Gaddy JN, Margolskee DJ, Bush RK, et al. Bronchodilation with a potent and selective leukotriene D_4 (LTD_4) receptor antagonist (MK-571) in patients with asthma. *Am Rev Respir Dis* 1992;146:358–363.

127. Hui KP, Barnes NC. Lung function improvement in asthma with a cysteinyl-leukotriene receptor antagonist. *Lancet* 1991;337:1062–1063.

128. Impens N, Reiss TF, Teahan JA, et al. Acute bronchodilation with an intravenously administered leukotriene D_4 antagonist, MK-679. *Am Rev Respir Dis* 1993;147:1442–1446.

129. Dahlen B, Nizankowska E, Szczeklik A, et al. Benefits from adding the 5-lipoxygenase inhibitor zileuton to conventional therapy in aspirin-intolerant asthmatics. *Am J Respir Crit Care Med* 1998;157:1187–1194.

130. Yamamoto H, Nagata M, Kuramitsu K, et al. Inhibition of analgesic-induced asthma by leukotriene receptor antagonist ONO-1078. *Am J Respir Crit Care Med* 1994;150:254–257.

131. Christie PE, Tagari P, Ford-Hutchinson AW, et al. Urinary leukotriene E_4 concentrations increase after aspirin challenge in aspirin-sensitive asthmatic subjects. *Am Rev Respir Dis* 1991;143:1025–1029.

132. Israel E, Fischer AR, Rosenberg MA, et al. The pivotal role of 5-lipoxygenase products in the reaction of aspirin-sensitive asthmatics to aspirin. *Am Rev Respir Dis* 1993;148:1447–1451.

133. Nasser SM, Bell GS, Foster S, et al. Effect of the 5-lipoxygenase inhibitor ZD2138 on aspirin-induced asthma. *Thorax* 1994;49:749–756.

134. Dahlen B, Kumlin M, Margolskee DJ, et al. The leukotriene-receptor antagonist MK-0679 blocks airway obstruction induced by inhaled lysine-aspirin in aspirin-sensitive asthmatics. *Eur Respir J* 1993;6:1018–1026.

135. Stevenson DD, Simon RA. Aspirin sensitivity: respiratory and cutaneous manifestations. In: Middleton JE, Reed CE, Silis EF, et al., eds. *Allergy. Principles and practice.* St. Louis: Mosby, 1988:1537–1554.

136. Christian Virchow J, Prasse A, Naya I, et al. Zafirlukast improves asthma control in patients receiving high-dose inhaled corticosteroids. *Am J Respir Crit Care Med* 2000;162:578–585.

137. Tamaoki J, Kondo M, Sakai N, et al. Leukotriene antagonist prevents exacerbation of asthma during reduction of high-dose inhaled corticosteroid. The Tokyo Joshi-Idai Asthma Research Group. *Am J Respir Crit Care Med* 1997;155:1235–1240.

138. Dempsey OJ, Kennedy G, Lipworth BJ. Comparative efficacy and anti-inflammatory profile of once-daily therapy with leukotriene antagonist or low-dose inhaled corticosteroid in patients with mild persistent asthma. *J Allergy Clin Immunol* 2002;109:68–74.

139. Bukstein DA, Henk HJ, Luskin AT. A comparison of asthma-related expenditures for patients started on montelukast versus fluticasone propionate as monotherapy. *Clin Ther* 2001;23:1589–1600.

140. Eickelberg O, Roth M, Lorx R, et al. Ligand-independent activation of the glucocorticoid receptor by beta$_2$-adrenergic receptor agonists in primary human lung fibroblasts and vascular smooth muscle cells. *J Biol Chem* 1999;274:1005–1010.

141. Strunk RC. Death due to asthma. *Am Rev Respir Dis* 1993;148:550–552.

142. Strunk RC, Mrazek DA, Fuhrmann GS, et al. Physiologic and psychological characteristics associated with deaths due to asthma in childhood. A case-controlled study. *JAMA* 1985;254:1193–1198.

143. Beam WR, Weiner DE, Martin RJ. Timing of prednisone and alterations of airways inflammation in nocturnal asthma. *Am Rev Respir Dis* 1992;146:1524–1530.

Epidemiology of Chronic Obstructive Pulmonary Disease

11

Nicholas R. Anthonisen · Jure Manfreda

Although emphysema was first described by Laennec in 1819 (1), it first gained recognition as a major problem in Europe and North America some 50 years ago. For some years, it was called *chronic bronchitis* in the United Kingdom and *emphysema* in North America, although comparative studies show that the terms covered many of the same symptoms and physiologic abnormalities—hence the general descriptive rubric of *chronic obstructive pulmonary disease (COPD)*. Recognition of the magnitude of the problem coincided with prolonged, heavy exposure to tobacco smoke of a large fraction of the male population, and the link between the disease and smoking was soon established (2–5). Ever since, in the developed world, the prevalence of COPD has been largely interpreted as reflecting the smoking habits of the populations concerned. However, clinically apparent COPD develops in only a minority of heavy smokers, so that additional determinants or risk factors must be involved. In this chapter, we review the evidence relating smoking to the development of COPD and the evidence concerning additional risk factors, best described as work still in progress. We limit most of our discussion to the developed world because very little reliable information is available concerning COPD in undeveloped regions and third world countries.

DEFINITIONS

The term *COPD* includes three specific pathologies: chronic bronchitis, peripheral airways disease, and emphysema (6). Chronic bronchitis is usually defined as chronic cough with sputum, "chronic" meaning lasting more than 3 months of the year for 2 years consecutively. Chronic bronchitis is

N. R. **Anthonisen** and J. **Manfreda**: Department of Medicine, University of Manitoba, Winnipeg, Manitoba, Canada.

accompanied by hypertrophy and hyperplasia of the mucus-secreting cells normally present in the large airways, along with some inflammation. Peripheral airways disease involves obstruction of the bronchioles with inflammation, fibrosis, and plugging. Smooth muscle in both the large and small airways may be increased. Emphysema is defined as destruction of the peripheral lung units with loss of gas-exchanging areas. Centrilobular emphysema initially involves the respiratory bronchioles more than the distal alveoli, occurs almost exclusively in smokers, and tends to affect the upper lobes. Panlobular emphysema destroys both the respiratory bronchioles and alveoli and can occur anywhere in the lung. Chronic bronchitis, peripheral airways disease, and emphysema are all strongly related to smoking, and all three are present in many patients with severe COPD, although in varying proportions. Peripheral airways disease and emphysema cause chronic airways obstruction, but it is presently impossible to separate the clinical or physiologic contributions of the two during life. Chronic bronchitis, on the other hand, is not necessarily associated with airways obstruction. Many people have chronic cough with sputum and normal lung function, and in some smokers, severe airways obstruction develops in the absence of cough and sputum. Both emphysema and peripheral airways obstruction may be found in the lungs of individuals who do not have large airways obstruction.

It is because of these complexities that the term *COPD* was coined. COPD is usually defined as chronic airways obstruction that cannot be completely reversed with therapy and is not explained by another, more specific pathology, such as bronchiectasis or cystic fibrosis (7). In the developed world, the term usually implies exposure to tobacco smoke and does not include chronic airways obstruction consequent to asthma (see section "Relationship to Asthma"). Airways obstruction is best defined in terms of decreased maximal expiratory flow rates, and the most efficient test for airways obstruction is measurement of the forced expiratory volume in 1 second (FEV₁), which is relatively simple and reproducible. A reduction in FEV₁ in relation to the forced vital capacity (FVC) defines airways obstruction, and the course of COPD is often described in terms of the rate of decline in FEV₁. The epidemiology of COPD has been largely concerned with factors that influence this index of lung function. Because the FEV₁ is a gross measure of the composite result of a number of pathologic lesions, this approach has obvious drawbacks, but it is better than any alternative that is presently available.

Relationship to Asthma

Asthma also is characterized by airways obstruction. Generally speaking, asthma and COPD present different clinical pictures and have different epidemiologic features and natural histories. Asthma typically begins in childhood and consists of discrete attacks of wheezy dyspnea alternating with periods of normality. Gradually progressive loss of lung function is not the norm. Asthma occurs frequently in nonsmokers. Thus, it is usually not difficult to differentiate asthma from COPD in the clinic. On the other hand, the course of asthma is sometimes unremitting, and irreversible airways obstruction develops in some cases (8). There is good evidence that environmental tobacco smoke is a risk factor for wheezing and perhaps asthma in children. However, it has not been definitively proved that smoking is a causal factor in asthma, and much confusion remains when attempts are made to distinguish between true asthma and symptoms related to smoke exposure. The mechanisms involved in the chronic obstruction of asthma probably differ from those in smoking-related COPD.

Some patients with progressive airways obstruction and significant smoking histories resemble patients with asthma

in that their obstruction can be substantially reversed with inhaled bronchodilators (9). It is unclear whether these patients differ in any important way from COPD patients with less reversibility, especially in that tests of reversibility are not very reproducible. Nevertheless, many clinical trials of COPD therapy have been restricted to patients with little reversibility. We make no attempt to differentiate between COPD patients with and those without reversibility in this chapter.

MORTALITY

Mortality is an important indicator of the incidence of disease because death certificates listing the cause of death are available in most countries for relatively long periods. Methods may vary between jurisdictions and over time, so that comparisons must be made carefully. Mortality reflects not only the incidence but also the severity of a disease. There is no doubt that COPD is an important public health problem in both developed (industrialized) and developing countries. In a World Health Report (10), it was estimated that 2,660,000 deaths were attributed to COPD in 1999 worldwide, which represents 4.8% of all deaths. Slightly more COPD deaths occurred in males (53%) than in females (47%); the proportion of all deaths caused by COPD was also slightly higher for males (4.9%) than for females (4.6%).

Figure 11.1 shows that age-standardized rates of COPD vary substantially between developed countries for both males and females (11). Rates in the United States are higher than in most other countries, and rates for males and females are more similar than elsewhere. Although these rates by country may reflect differences in smoking and environmental exposures, they may also represent differences in the completeness of death certificates and coding practices and conceptual differences about the diagnosis. Viegi and colleagues (12) reported differences between Europe and America in the definition of COPD. Nevertheless, Cooreman and colleagues (13) compared COPD mortality rates between the United States, Canada, and France and concluded that the death rates between 1969 and 1983 were higher in the United States than in either Canada or France, even when an allowance was made for coding practices and revisions in the International Classification of Diseases (ICD).

In 1997 in the United States, 103,595 deaths were attributed to COPD: 80% to chronic airways obstruction, not elsewhere specified (ICD-9 codes 494–496); 13% to emphysema (ICD-9 code 492); and 3% to unspecified causes and chronic bronchitis (ICD-9 codes 490 and 491) (National Institutes of Health, 2000). The age-adjusted mortality rate per 100,000 population was almost one-third higher in males (approximately 52 per 100,000) than in females (approximately 31 per 100,000). Rates for whites were higher than rates for blacks in both males (one third) and females (twice).

DEFINITION AND CHARACTERISTICS OF CHRONIC OBSTRUCTIVE PULMONARY DISEASE

Summary Statement	Level of Evidence
The term COPD includes the clinical entities of emphysema and chronic bronchitis, and some features of asthma as well. The airway obstruction of COPD does not usually respond to bronchodilator therapy.	American Thoracic Society definition
The development of COPD is related to cigarette smoking, although most smokers do not have COPD.	Observational studies
The FEV₁ is a good physiologic proxy for airways obstruction.	Observational studies and clinical practice
Confusion remains regarding the etiologic, pathologic, and clinical overlap between asthma and COPD.	Observational studies

COPD, Chronic obstructive pulmonary disease; FEV₁, forced expiratory volume in 1 second.

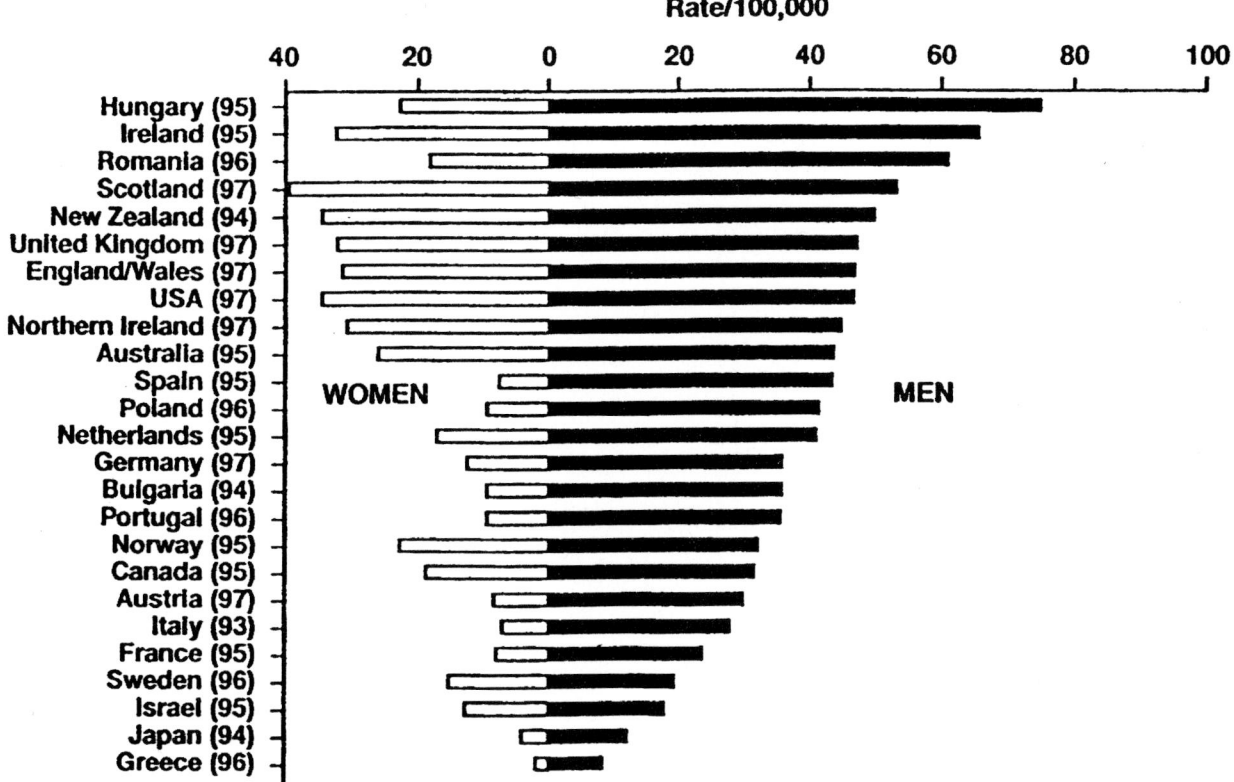

FIGURE 11.1. Age-adjusted mortality rates for chronic obstructive pulmonary disease in women and men ages 35 through 74 in various countries. (From Hurd S. The impact of COPD on lung health worldwide. Epidemiology and incidence. *Chest* 2000;117:1S–4S, with permission.)

COPD mortality increases with age in both genders and races.

COPD is the fourth leading cause of death in the United States. Mannino and colleagues (14) determined that COPD was underreported on death certificates. Between 1979 and 1993, COPD was listed as the underlying cause of death on only 43% of death certificates that listed a COPD diagnosis. Underreporting affected rates for women more than those for men.

In white males, age-adjusted COPD mortality increased in the Unites States between 1960 and 1985 but has been constant since the mid 1980s. In black males, age-adjusted COPD mortality leveled off in the early 1900s. On the other hand, mortality rates of both white and black females have been increasing since 1960. Increases for white females appear to be greater than those for black females (15).

Similar mortality trends were observed in Canada (16,17). In both genders, mortality from COPD varied by birth cohort. Mortality rates increased sooner for male cohorts than for female cohorts, probably because smoking became widely adopted by males earlier than by females. Leveling off of male mortality is primarily a consequence of decreased mortality in cohorts born after 1924. In both the United States and Canada, variation in mortality rates is substantial between states and between provinces, respectively.

It has been predicted that COPD will become the third most common cause of death worldwide by 2020, moving up from sixth place. This prediction is largely based on increased tobacco consumption in the third world (18).

EPIDEMIOLOGY OF CHRONIC OBSTRUCTIVE PULMONARY DISEASE	
Summary Statement	**Level of Evidence**
COPD is the fourth leading cause of death in the United States.	Epidemiologic studies
Worldwide mortality from COPD is predicted to increase because tobacco consumption in third world countries is increasing rapidly.	Observational studies
COPD mortality among women is increasing faster than mortality among men.	Epidemiologic studies

COPD, chronic obstructive pulmonary disease.

PREVALENCE

The third National Health and Nutrition Examination Survey (NHANES III) was conducted between 1988 and 1994

TABLE 11.1. PREVALENCE OF LOW LEVEL OF LUNG FUNCTION AND SYMPTOMS IN THE U.S. POPULATION AGES 17 YEARS AND OLDER BY GENDER, SMOKING STATUS, AND RACE, ESTIMATED BY THE THIRD NATIONAL HEALTH AND NUTRITION SURVEY (1988–1994)

Gender	Smoking Status	Race	Low Lung Function (%)	Cough	Phlegm	Wheezing	Shortness of Breath
Female	Never	Black	2.6	4.5	5.0	10.5	25.8
		White	3.1	5.0	4.3	11.7	20.4
	Former	Black	4.3	2.8	6.6	14.3	28.6
		White	6.8	6.5	4.1	15.3	25.7
	Current	Black	8.6	8.0	9.0	19.9	33.1
		White	13.6	20.6	16.0	31.1	38.7
Male	Never	Black	4.8	4.1	4.3	8.8	14.5
		White	3.3	4.0	5.3	9.4	10.6
	Former	Black	8.4	4.4	5.6	10.8	14.2
		White	6.9	4.7	6.1	15.8	17.3
	Pipe/cigar	Black	7.1	5.4	3.7	15.0	28.8
		White	9.9	13.3	17.3	16.7	9.8
	Current	Black	11.6	10.9	9.7	19.0	21.7
		White	14.2	24.0	20.5	32.2	31.7

Note: FEV_1/FVC ratio <0.70 and FEV_1 < 80% of the predicted value.
Symptoms: Yes to question, Do you usually cough on most days for 3 consecutive months or more per year? for cough; Do you bring up phlegm on most days for 3 consecutive months or more per year? for phlegm; Have you had wheezing or whistling in your chest at any time in the past 12 months? for wheezing; Are you troubled by shortness of breath when hurrying on level ground or walking up a slight hill? for shortness of breath.
FEV_1, forced expiratory volume in 1 second; FVC, forced vital capacity.
Source: Adapted from Mannino DM, Gagnon RC, Petty TL, et al. Obstructive lung disease and low lung function in adults in the United States. Data from the National Health and Nutrition Examination Survey, 1988–1994. *Arch Intern Med* 2000; 160:1683–1689, with permission.

on a multistage probability sample of the population of the United States. Mannino and colleagues (19) used the results of testing of 16,084 individuals from 81 sites to produce the most comprehensive and recent estimate of COPD prevalence for the U.S. population ages 17 years and older. Selected results of their analysis are presented in Table 11.1.

Of the total population of 169.3 million ages 17 years and older, 11.5 million (6.8%) had lung function consistent with COPD: FEV_1/FVC below 0.70 and FEV_1 less than or equal to 80% of the predicted normal value. Approximately one fourth of these (27%) had an FEV_1 value less than 50% of the predicted normal value. Overall, a low level of function was more prevalent in males (8.0%) than in females (6.3%), in whites (7.2%) than in blacks (6.0%), and in current smokers (13.9%) than in former smokers (7.0%) or those who had never smoked (3.5%). To some extent, differences between genders and races were caused by smoking. Of females 17 years of age and older, 54.4% had never smoked, in comparison with 36.7% of males. In the black population, 53.0% had never smoked, in comparison with 44.9% of the white population. Table 11.1 shows the percentages of persons with a low level of lung function according to gender, smoking status, and race. The largest differences are between black and white current smokers of both genders; it is possible that white smokers smoked more each day than black smokers.

Table 11.1 also shows the prevalence of symptoms: cough (coughing for 3 months consecutively or longer during

the year), phlegm (bringing up phlegm on most days for 3 months consecutively or longer during the year), wheezing (at any time in the past 12 months), and shortness of breath (when hurrying on level ground or walking up a slight hill). These symptoms varied by gender and race, with the most powerful determinant being smoking. In former smokers, symptoms were similar to those in never-smokers. This finding was consistent with the Lung Health Study finding that smoking cessation was associated with a substantial reduction in the prevalence of respiratory symptoms (20). Among current smokers in both genders, however, symptoms were more prevalent in whites than in blacks. In never-smokers particularly, the rate of wheezing was high, perhaps a consequence of asthma.

In NHANES III, the overlap between COPD and asthma was substantial. Of an estimated 8.3 million COPD patients, 28% had been told that they had both COPD and asthma (19). Despite a high percentage of people with physician-diagnosed COPD in the population, many also had undiagnosed airflow obstruction. Coultas and colleagues (21) determined that 12% of NHANES III subjects ages 45 years or older had airflow obstruction (FEV_1/FVC below the lower limit of normal according to the equations of Hankinson and colleagues [22]) without physician-diagnosed COPD or asthma. The prevalence of undiagnosed airflow obstruction was higher in males (14.2%) than in females (9.9%). Approximately 10% of the undiagnosed cases of airflow obstruction were of at least moderate severity (i.e., $FEV_1 < 50\%$ of the predicted normal value).

Because of its high prevalence, COPD is a substantial burden for health services and consumes considerable health care resources. In 1997 in the United States, 13.5 million physician office visits were for COPD (ICD-9 codes 490–492 and 494–496). In addition, 634,000 persons were discharged from hospitals with COPD as the first listed diagnosis. The average length of hospital stay was 5.4 days (15). Between 1970 and 1997, hospitalization rates varied substantially in persons ages 45 through 64 years and in those ages 65 and older (15). Sullivan and colleagues (23) estimated that the total cost of COPD in the United States in 1993 was $23.9 billion; of this, the direct cost (hospitalizations, physician fees, medication) was $14.7 billion, or 62% of the total cost.

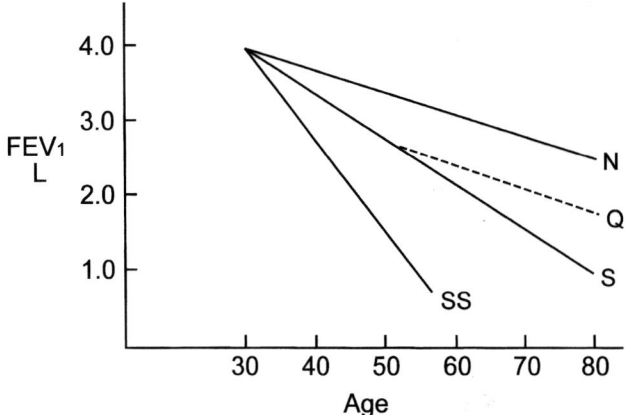

FIGURE 11.2. Schematic model of rate of decline of forced expiratory volume in 1 second in adult men. Trajectories are shown for nonsmokers (*N*), "average" smokers (*S*), "sensitive" smokers (*SS*), and men who quit smoking (*Q*).

RESULTS OF THIRD NATIONAL HEALTH AND NUTRITION EXAMINATION SURVEY	
Summary Statement	**Level of Evidence**
Between 5% and 8% of the U.S. population has COPD as defined by physiologic parameters.	NHANES III
In many individuals, airflow obstruction remains undiagnosed.	NHANES III
COPD is a heavy economic burden to the health care system of the United States.	Single economic study

COPD, chronic obstructive pulmonary disease; NHANES III, third National Health and Nutrition Examination Survey.

SMOKING AND THE NATURAL HISTORY OF CHRONIC OBSTRUCTIVE PULMONARY DISEASE

In the developed world, tobacco smoking accounts for 80% to 90% of the risk for the development of COPD, and this may be an underestimate (24). Smokers have poorer lung function and a more rapid decline in FEV_1 than nonsmokers. Cough, sputum production, and dyspnea are much more common in smokers than in nonsmokers. Deaths ascribed to COPD are much more common in smokers than in nonsmokers. A clear dose-response relationship exists between smoking exposure and the development of COPD. The likelihood of COPD increases with the number of cigarettes smoked per day and the cumulative pack-years of exposure and when smoking is started at an earlier age (25). Pipe and cigar smokers are at less risk for the development of COPD than cigarette smokers but at greater risk than nonsmokers, probably because pipe and cigar smokers inhale less tobacco smoke than cigarette smokers do. Low-tar, filtered cigarettes are apparently associated with less cough and sputum than

unfiltered brands, but the effects of the two types on lung function do not differ (26,27).

Figure 11.2 shows a model of the effects of smoking on lung function that has been adapted from the classic work of Fletcher and colleagues (28) and validated in many subsequent studies (29–37). The decline in FEV_1 starts at about age 30 and is a linear function that may actually accelerate somewhat with age (38). Disability occurs at a value of 1.5 to 2.0 L, and severe disability at a value of 1.0 L. In the average nonsmoker, FEV_1 declines at an annual rate of about 30 mL, slowly enough that disability does not occur during the normal life span. In the average smoker, the FEV_1 declines approximately twice as fast, at an annual rate of about 60 mL. Disability does not occur until quite late in life. A subgroup of smokers are apparently unusually "sensitive" to the effects of tobacco smoke, and their function declines much more rapidly, at annual rates of 100 mL and more. These people become severely disabled in late middle age, in the sixth and seventh decades of life. This "sensitive" subgroup is thought to comprise 15% to 20% of all smokers. Among volunteer smokers ages 35 through 59 who were recruited for the Lung Health Study, some 20% to 30% demonstrated airways obstruction ($FEV_1/FVC < 0.70$) (39).

The effect of smoking cessation in middle age is also shown in Figure 11.2. After smoking is stopped, a minor (50 mL) increase in FEV_1 occurs, but the important effect is that with cessation, the subsequent rate of decline reverts to the normal, nonsmoking rate. This effect was observed repeatedly in people who spontaneously quit smoking, and similar effects were observed in a randomized trial of smoking cessation (29). Clearly, smoking cessation in middle age either prevents or greatly delays the onset of symptomatic disease (Fig. 11.2). Once disability has developed, the benefit of cessation is not as clear. Many COPD patients eventually stop smoking but continue to deteriorate (40), so it is likely that at some point, the basic pathologic processes become independent of continued smoking, as the results of a study imply (41).

PATHOGENESIS OF CHRONIC OBSTRUCTIVE PULMONARY DISEASE

Summary Statement	Level of Evidence
There is a direct relation between the number of cigarettes smoked and the development of COPD in susceptible individuals.	Multiple epidemiologic studies
Pulmonary function is lost at a faster rate in smokers than in nonsmokers. In most people with COPD, symptoms develop in the fifth or sixth decade of life when the FEV_1 falls below 1.0–1.5 L.	Multiple epidemiologic studies
At some point after smoking cessation, pulmonary function begins to fall at a rate approximating that of the nonsmoking population.	Multiple epidemiologic studies
At very low levels of pulmonary function, smoking cessation has very little beneficial effect on preserving remaining function.	Several good clinical studies

COPD, chronic obstructive pulmonary disease; FEV_1, forced expiratory volume in 1 second.

RISK FACTORS

Airways Hyperreactivity

In the 1960s, Dutch investigators proposed that the degree of airways reactivity was an important determinant of the development of COPD (42). According to this argument, chronic airways obstruction would be much more likely to develop in smokers with highly reactive airways than in those with less reactivity. The "Dutch hypothesis" proved difficult to test for several reasons. First, airways hyperreactivity is a hallmark of asthma, and the Dutch investigators tended to include both patients with asthma and those with COPD under the term *chronic nonspecific lung disease*. Thus, many Dutch studies of the influence of airways reactivity on lung function included people who had asthma by North American standards. Second, it was clear that the degree of airways reactivity was inversely proportional to the FEV_1 in people with airways obstruction (43,44), and that the reactivity might be a consequence rather than a cause of the obstruction. In people with reduced airway caliber, a given amount of airway smooth muscle contraction would necessarily be associated with a larger increase in resistance and decrease in expiratory flow than in people with normal airways (45). For this reason, cross-sectional studies of reactivity in people with COPD were of little value in testing the Dutch hypothesis.

Prospective studies of the influence of airways reactivity on the rate of decline in lung function have been carried out in a number of populations. It could be argued that the risk for symptomatic COPD was small in all of them. In a random Dutch sample (46), the degree of reactivity predicted subsequent decline in FEV_1; the effect was evident in the group as a whole, but not in smokers. Asthmatics were apparently not excluded from this study. The Normative Aging Study (47) examined elderly men with excellent lung function who were largely nonsmokers or former smokers and found that responsiveness predicted decline, an effect that was weakened but probably still significant when people with a history of asthma were excluded. Frew and colleagues (48) reported findings in individuals challenged by methacholine and noted that decline in FEV_1 was directly related to responsiveness in smokers, but not in nonsmokers. Tracey and colleagues (49) reported a similar result in a group of elderly British men, again with excellent lung function; reactivity predicted decline in FEV_1 in smokers and former smokers after those with a history of asthma had been excluded. In this study, smoking per se did not affect the rate of decline.

Data from the Lung Health Study (50) provided strong support for the Dutch hypothesis. This study recruited 6,000 nonasthmatic smokers ages 35 through 59 with an FEV_1/FVC ratio below 0.70 and followed them closely for 5 years after a randomly assigned antismoking intervention. At baseline, virtually all participants underwent methacholine challenge. After smoking status, the degree of methacholine responsiveness was the most important predictor of subsequent decline in FEV_1. Methacholine responsiveness was strongly interactive with the variable of smoking; in continuing smokers, reactivity had a powerful effect on loss of lung function, whereas it had much less effect in individuals who had stopped smoking at the beginning of the study. Airways hyperreactivity was an important risk factor in people who continued to smoke but not in those who stopped; smoking cessation was therefore of greatest benefit in individuals with high levels of airways reactivity.

Atopy

Two manifestations of atopy have been thought to be risk factors for loss of lung function and, by implication, for COPD. These are total serum levels of immunoglobulin E (IgE) and skin test reactivity to common allergens. Both are associated with asthma and airways hyperreactivity in healthy people (51). Of the two, IgE levels have received the most attention. For reasons that are unknown, smoking is associated with increased IgE levels (52–54). Given the associations of IgE levels with both smoking and asthma, it is not surprising that the IgE level is inversely related to lung function in cross-sectional studies (55–58). Burrows and colleagues (59) postulated that IgE levels might signify a host factor important in the development of COPD. However, they subsequently found the relationship between IgE and lung function to be largely dependent on the inclusion of asthmatics in the study sample and concluded that IgE was probably not a risk factor for the development of smoking-related COPD (60).

Most longitudinal studies of lung function have not found a relationship between IgE levels and the rate of decline of lung function in smokers (61–64). An exception is the study of Tracey and colleagues (49), who found that besides airways reactivity, IgE levels and skin test allergy predicted the rate of decline of lung function. Analysis of the data from the Lung Health Study also showed no association of IgE levels with the rate of decline of lung function in smokers (unpublished data). Burrows and colleagues were probably correct in concluding that IgE levels are related to asthma and not to COPD.

If asthmatics are excluded, atopy as assessed by skin tests is apparently not related to decline in lung function in either smokers or nonsmokers. This has been demonstrated in one retrospective (62) and two prospective studies (63,64).

Episodes of Acute Bronchitis: Exacerbations

According to the "British hypothesis" of the pathogenesis of COPD, chronic bronchitis predisposed an individual to repeated episodes of chest infection, and these episodes led to irreversible lung damage and airways obstruction (65,66). The hypothesis rested on the observation that many COPD patients had chronic cough and sputum production associated with periodic chest infections that occurred before the onset of dyspnea and disability. Furthermore, even when clinically stable, these patients had bacteria in their sputum (67) that were similar to those recovered during acute episodes (68).

The landmark study of Fletcher and colleagues (28) tested the British hypothesis by following 792 male London transit workers for 8 years with twice-yearly assessments of sputum, chest infections, and FEV_1. They found that neither symptomatic chronic bronchitis nor chest infections correlated with the decline of lung function. They concluded that both chronic bronchitis and airways obstruction were associated with smoking but frequently occurred independently and were not directly related. Acute chest infections were more common in people with chronic bronchitis but were not related to the development of chronic airways obstruction. Their results have been confirmed by other long-term studies (69,70).

For many years, it was thought that acute exacerbations of COPD, with or without acute episodes of bronchitis or pneumonia, had no long-term effect on the course of the disease, although exacerbations undeniably caused short-term decreases in lung function and were important causes of hospitalization and death. Mortality is clearly higher in COPD patients with chronic cough and sputum production than in those without (71,72), probably because exacerbations are more common in patients with these symptoms. Two carefully performed long-term studies have demonstrated that the rate of decline in FEV_1 is higher in smokers with chronic cough and sputum production than in those without symptomatic chronic bronchitis (73,74), so that exacerbations may hasten decline.

New light has been shed on the problem. Many studies had shown that the lung function of patients with exacerbations improved with therapy, but because data from before the exacerbation were not usually available, it was not clear whether recovery was complete. Seemungal and colleagues (75) carefully followed a cohort of COPD patients, characterizing their exacerbations and measuring peak flows before, during, and after the illness. Expected decreases in peak flow were noted with exacerbations of symptoms, but not all patients recovered completely. Indeed, in about 7% of the patients, peak flows were lower 90 days after an exacerbation than they had been before. Thus, exacerbations may have a long-term deleterious effect on lung function in COPD. Retrospective analysis of data from the Lung Health Study (76) supported this argument. A total of 5,887 participants who were followed for 5 years were asked at annual visits if they had seen a doctor for bronchitis, pneumonia, influenza, or chest colds. Positive responses were classified as a lower respiratory infection. Episodes of pneumonia resulting in hospitalization were not included. Participants with chronic cough and sputum production had about twice as many lower respiratory infections as those without. People who quit smoking had fewer lower respiratory infections than those who continued to smoke. In continuing smokers, a single lower respiratory infection was associated with a loss of 7 mL of FEV_1 during the year of the event, and a clear cause-and-effect relationship was noted, in which a greater number of lower respiratory infections was associated with a greater loss. This was true whether or not chronic cough and sputum production were present. In people who stopped smoking, lower respiratory infections had no effect on the rate of decline in FEV_1. Thus, exacerbations of symptoms had a long-term negative effect on lung function, which would be significant if several episodes occurred per year. It is important to note that in individuals with mild or moderate COPD, the effect of a lower respiratory infection depended on continued smoking. Thus, the Lung Health Study data supported both the British and Dutch hypotheses and showed continuing smoking to be crucial in causing exacerbations of COPD and related reductions in lung function.

Gender

COPD has been considered largely a disease of men; patient cohorts recruited in the 1970s in North America were about 80% male (77). This gender distribution reflected differences in smoking habits between men and women, and as the prevalence of female smokers has increased during the last 50 years, so has the prevalence of COPD in women. Women comprised 39% of the participants in the Lung Health Study, which recruited people with relatively mild obstructive disease in 1987 and 1988 (29). There is little question that the

TABLE 11.2. GENDER EFFECTS IN THE LUNG HEALTH STUDY: CHANGE OF FEV$_1$ OVER 11 YEARS

	Women		Men		
	No.	FEV$_1$ (Percentage [%] Predicted)	No.	FEV$_1$ (Percentage [%] Predicted)	P
Sustained quitter	253	−0.05	462	−0.27	<.0001
Intermittent quitter	906	−0.86	1,423	−0.88	.697
Continuous smoker	396	−1.31	644	−1.27	.532

FEV$_1$, forced expiratory volume in 1 second.

prevalence of COPD in women will continue to increase in the foreseeable future.

If gender were an independent risk factor for COPD, COPD would develop at different rates in men and women with the same smoking habits. The effect of smoking on gender-specific lung function has been examined on a number of occasions, with conflicting results. Reviews (78,79) indicate that the results may be related to gender-specific smoking rates and also to gender differences in other types of exposures. In a study from Denmark (80), women were hospitalized more often for COPD than men with similar smoking histories, and this finding was interpreted as indicating greater susceptibility in women.

The Lung Health Study followed a substantial number of women with airways obstruction, and the data from 11 years of follow-up (81) have been examined for gender-specific functional differences. Among the participants who smoked for the full 11 years, men had greater absolute rates of decline in FEV$_1$ (Table 11.2). On the other hand, when function was expressed a percentage of the predicted normal value, rates were quite similar between the genders. Men smokers consumed an average of 25.2 cigarettes per day at the end of the study, and women 22.1, so these results could be interpreted to mean that women are more sensitive than men to cigarette smoke. On the other hand, it could also be argued that women and men smokers have similar susceptibilities to smoke and rates of loss of lung function. It is of interest to note that the rates were similar despite the fact that airways hyperreactivity was considerably more common among the women participants than among the men (82).

Genetic/Hereditary Risk Factors

The observation that COPD develops in only 15% to 20% of smokers strongly indicates that genetic susceptibility to the disease may be involved in its development. Familial aggregation has been documented in COPD, and more cases of the disease than expected have been found in the families of index cases. However, it has been difficult to separate the presumed hereditary effect from the sharing of environmental exposures or lifestyle.

In North America, the effects of familial aggregation and heredity on lung function were examined in at least four cross-sectional community studies. Heritability was estimated as the proportion of the variance in lung function caused by hereditary factors. In Tecumseh, Higgins and Keller (83) examined 9,226 persons, of whom 64% had at least one parent or sibling participating in the study. The FEV$_1$ scores of parents were significantly correlated with those of their children younger than 40 years. The correlation of FEV$_1$ scores was stronger between siblings of the same sex than between siblings of the opposite sex. These correlations were not adjusted for smoking, which also showed a familial aggregation. In Tucson, Lebowitz and colleagues (84) studied 344 nuclear families (mother, father, and at least one natural child) and found a significant correlation between the lung function of parents and their children that disappeared when they controlled for smoking and body build. Chen and colleagues (85) studied 214 nuclear families (799 individuals) in Humboldt, an unpolluted town in rural Canada, and found a significant correlation between parents and children and between siblings for FEV$_1$ after they controlled for smoking and body build. Similarly, Givelber and colleagues (86) studied 1,408 families in Framingham and found that the FEV$_1$ of offspring correlated with that of mothers, fathers, and siblings.

In longitudinal analysis, family history did not independently predict the development of COPD (87). In Framingham, a modest influence of heritability on longitudinal change in lung function (FEV$_1$, FVC, and FEV$_1$/FVC ratio) was found; the significance of this effect increased slightly when only subjects with concordant smoking histories were included in the analysis (88). In Tucson, the decline of FEV$_1$ in siblings was correlated, particularly if they had similar smoking habits (89).

Despite strong inferential evidence for genetic factors in the etiology of COPD, familial aggregation and heritability studies show only a modest effect of such factors. The failure of these studies to show a strong relationship can be explained, at least to some extent, by methodologic problems in conducting such studies that tend to dilute associations.

The only genetic factor that is strongly correlated with the development of COPD is the homozygous ZZ phenotype of α_1-antitrypsin (AAT) deficiency. Even this phenotype leads to substantial obstruction and reduced life expectancy largely in smokers; the effects in never-smokers and those not exposed to environmental hazards are relatively small. Thus, even strong genetic variants must interact with environmental exposure to produce the disease. Because the ZZ phenotype is rare, it accounts for only a small proportion of cases of COPD. Among heterozygous AAT phenotypes, only the more common MZ and SZ phenotypes may interact with smoking and environmental exposure to produce the disease; however, the evidence for their role is not consistent. In the absence of smoking and environmental exposures, these phenotypes do not result in COPD.

It is unlikely that one gene is responsible for COPD susceptibility. COPD is likely a genetically complex disease, being inhomogeneous clinically, pathologically, and physiologically. It is more likely that many genes are involved, mediating different steps in the pathogenesis of the disease and influencing the response to various environmental exposures, including smoking.

The number of new candidate genes is increasing quickly. Blood groups (ABO, ABH secretor status) may play a role in the adhesion of environmental and infectious particles, facilitating the effects of exposure. Deficiencies in AAT, α_1-antichymotrypsin (ACT), and tissue inhibitors of metalloproteinases may facilitate proteolytic damage of the lung parenchyma. Abnormalities of microsomal epoxide hydrolase and heme oxygenase may decrease the capacity to deal with oxidative stress. Certain gene variants may promote inflammatory processes.

α_1-Antitrypsin Deficiency

AAT, a serine glycoprotein, is a strong protease inhibitor of neutrophil elastase. The AAT genotype is determined by a single gene on chromosome 14. There are currently more than 70 genetic variants or AAT phenotypes (Pi types); the most common (90% of the population) is the MM phenotype, which is associated with normal levels of AAT in serum (180–200 mg/dL).

The lowest levels of AAT (15% of the levels in the MM phenotype) are in individuals with the ZZ phenotype. In North America, the frequency of this phenotype has been estimated as 1 in 2,857 blood donors in St. Louis (90), 1 in 3,693 in newborns in New York (91), and 1 in 5,097 newborns in Oregon (92). The ZZ phenotype is more common (1 in 1,666 people) in Sweden (93). Generally, the ZZ phenotype is more common in whites than in blacks or Asians and is more common in northern than in southern Europe.

Since the first report of an association between low levels of AAT and emphysema by Laurell and Erickson (94), it has been shown in numerous studies that the ZZ phenotype is a major risk factor for the development of emphysema. Larsson (95) studied the natural history and life expectancy of 246 individuals with PiZZ. Of these, 109 (44%) had primary emphysema; COPD was also the leading cause of death, responsible for 54 of 91 deaths that occurred during follow-up. The life expectancy of both male and female PiZZ individ-

uals was reduced in comparison with that of the general population, and the reduction was greater for smokers than for nonsmokers. More recently, Seersholm and colleagues (96) studied the life expectancy of 397 ZZ individuals and found that nonindex cases survived longer than index cases. The life expectancy of never-smokers among nonindex cases was similar to that of the general population. This suggests that the worse prognosis experienced by earlier cohorts may have been a consequence of selection bias, with the inclusion of more symptomatic individuals.

The lung function of ZZ subjects varies substantially; many ZZ individuals have relatively normal lung function (97), particularly never-smokers. In addition to smoking, FEV_1 is a strong predictor of life expectancy in both males and females. The life expectancy of those who quit smoking was better than that of continuing smokers (96). Wu and Eriksson (98) studied 158 PiZZ individuals and found FEV_1 to be significantly more reduced in current and former smokers than in never-smokers, suggesting a steeper decline in FEV_1 in smokers. This, however, was not confirmed in the subset of subjects studied longitudinally; the FEV_1 slope was approximately the same in all three smoking groups. Piitulainen and Eriksson (99) studied 608 adult individuals with PiZZ and found that the FEV_1 decline in never-smokers (n = 211) was higher (47 mL annually) than the expected decline in adult never-smokers (20–30 mL annually). The decline in former smokers (n = 351) was similar to that in PiZZ never-smokers (41 mL annually), whereas that of current smokers (n = 46) was substantially greater (70 mL annually).

Nonsmokers in the Swedish AAT deficiency registry were studied to determine the effect of passive smoking, indoor pollution, and occupational exposure on FEV_1 (100). Domiciliary exposure to kerosene heaters and employment in agriculture were found to be independent determinants of FEV_1, whereas environmental tobacco exposure had no effect.

Several heterozygous phenotypes have been examined as possible risk factors for the development of COPD: MS (population frequency, 5%–6%), MZ (2%–3%), and SZ (1%) phenotypes have serum AAT levels approximately 80%, 60%, and 40% of normal, respectively. The evidence of an increased risk for COPD in these phenotypes is not conclusive. Sandford and colleagues (101) reviewed seven case control studies that showed the risk for COPD to be 1.5 to 5.0 times higher in MZ than in normal MM controls. No excess risk was noted for MS and SZ phenotypes. On the other hand, in cross-sectional population studies, little difference was found between MZ or SZ and MM phenotypes with respect to FEV_1, particularly in nonsmoking subjects (102). The most conclusive evidence that the MZ phenotype is associated with an increased risk for COPD in smokers comes from the Lung Health Study. Sandford and colleagues (103) compared smokers with a rapid decline in FEV_1 with nondecliners and found the MZ phenotype to be 2.8 (95% confidence interval [CI], 1.2–7.3) times more frequent than the MM phenotype in the rapid decliners in comparison with the slow decliners. No difference was noted for the MS phenotype.

α_1-Antichymotrypsin

ACT is a serine protease inhibitor (104). Deficiency is inherited in an autosomal-dominant pattern and was detected in 2 (0.7%) of 300 blood donors in Sweden. In one study (105), the deficiency was found in 4 of 100 individuals with COPD and in no controls. Individuals with ACT deficiency had enlarged residual volume, compatible with early emphysema (106).

Matrix Metalloproteinases

Matrix metalloproteinases (MMPs) are a family of proteolytic enzymes whose substrate is connective tissue. Increased levels of MMP-1 and MMP-9 have been described in the lavage fluid of COPD patients (107,108). A number of polymorphisms of human MMP gene promoters occur naturally, and polymorphisms in the MMP-1 and MMP-12 genes, but not MMP-9, have been found to be associated with a rapid decline in FEV_1 (109). A tissue inhibitor of MMP (TIMP) has been described, and two polymorphisms of the TIMP-2 gene were investigated in 88 COPD patients and 40 controls. The GG genotype determined at locus +853 significantly increased the risk for COPD, whereas the GG genotype at locus −418 did so marginally (110).

Vitamin D–Binding Protein

Vitamin D–binding protein (group-specific component) is a serum α_2-globulin encoded by a gene with substantial variability. The three principle alleles are 1F, 1S, and 2. Kueppers and colleagues (111) found phenotype 2-2 to be protective in a comparison of 114 COPD patients with matched controls (1% vs. 5%, $P = .049$). Horne and colleagues (112) compared 104 COPD patients with 413 controls; the relative risk for COPD was decreased in phenotypes carrying allele 2 and increased in those with phenotype 1F-1F. Ishii and colleagues (113) also found an increased risk for COPD associated with homozygote 1F-1F. On the other hand, Kauffmann and colleagues (114) found no difference in the distribution of phenotypes between 45 heavy smokers with high FEV_1 values and 43 never-smokers with low FEV_1 values. These two groups were selected to minimize the confounding effects of smoking and environmental exposures. Similarly, in the Lung Health Study, rapid FEV_1 decliners and nondecliners did not differ with respect to the distribution of vitamin D–binding protein phenotypes (103).

ABO Blood Group Antigens

Cohen and colleagues (115) found significantly more subjects with abnormal FEV_1 values among individuals with

blood group A (22.4%, n = 489) than with B (13.7%, n = 140). This relationship has been confirmed (116). In women, the adjusted loss of FEV_1 was significantly greater in those with allele A (29.22 mL/y) than in those without it (19.77 mL/y). In men, the difference (40.83 mL/y vs. 37.26 mL/y) was not significant. However, the association between ABO group and FEV_1 was not confirmed in the 13-year follow-up of the Cracow study (117), in the Tecumseh study (83), in a study of a rural community in Saskatchewan (118), or in a study of French coal miners (119).

The ability to secrete antigens into body fluids is an autosomal-dominant genetic trait. The approximately 80% of the population who have this ability are termed *ABH secretors*. Cohen and colleagues (120) found that secretors have higher average values of FEV_1 and a lower prevalence of decreased FEV_1 values, suggesting that the ability to secrete antigens has protective effects on lung function. This relationship was observed in all ABO blood groups except AB, although it was significant only in group A. Another study found higher peak expiratory flow rates in secretors than in nonsecretors among current smokers, but not in nonsmokers and former smokers (121). Kauffmann and colleagues (114) found that the nonsecretor status was associated with a low FEV_1 value in never-smokers only in blood group O subjects. In a study of pulp mill workers, no differences in lung function were found between secretors and nonsecretors in any smoking group (122). Moreover, secretor status was not associated with changes in FEV_1 over time in this population (116). Similarly, no association was found in the Tecumseh study (83).

Horne and colleagues (118) found that Lewis-type blood group–negative individuals were at higher risk (relative incidence, 7.18) for airflow obstruction than Lewis-type blood group–positive individuals. Kauffmann and colleagues (119) observed lower FEV_1 scores in Lewis-negative than in Lewis-positive subjects only for those with blood group O.

Microsomal Epoxide Hydrolase

The enzyme microsomal epoxide hydrolase is involved in the metabolism of reactive epoxide intermediates produced in oxidative stress. An exon-3 mutation of the controlling gene reduces the enzyme activity by 50%. Smith and Harrison (123) compared 68 COPD patients with 203 controls and found that the homozygous mutant increased the risk for COPD 3.5-fold (95% CI, 1.5–8.0) and for emphysema 5.6-fold (95% CI, 2.7–11.5). The exon-4 mutant was not significantly associated with an increased risk for COPD. Yim and colleagues (124) compared 83 COPD patients with 76 controls and found no elevated risk for COPD associated with either exon-3 or exon-4 polymorphisms in Koreans.

Heme Oxygenase-I

Heme oxygenase-1 is a lung antioxidant. Yamada and colleagues (125) compared 101 male smokers with emphysema and 100 male smokers without emphysema. Three alleles (L, M, S) of the heme oxygenase-1 gene were assessed; individuals with genotypes containing L were 2.4 times (95% CI, 1.3–5.7) more likely to have emphysema.

Tumor Necrosis Factor-α

Tumor necrosis factor-α (TNF-α) is a multifunctional cytokine, a proinflammatory mediator that is released by epithelial cells and macrophages. Huang and colleagues (126) compared patients who had chronic bronchitis and airflow obstruction with controls who did not have obstruction. The two groups were matched for sex, age, and smoking status. Carriage of the TNF2 allele (polymorphism of the TNF-α gene) was associated with an increased risk for COPD. This finding was not confirmed by Higham and colleagues (127), who compared Caucasian COPD patients with non-COPD smokers as controls. Similarly, in the Lung Health Study, polymorphisms of TNF-α were not associated with the rapid decliner FEV_1 status (103).

Interleukin-1

Interleukin-1 (IL-1), which exists in two forms, is a proinflammatory cytokine associated with airways disease. Both the β form of IL-1 and the IL-1 receptor antagonist (IL-1RN) have naturally occurring genetic polymorphisms that have been studied in COPD (128). Although specific genotypes were not associated with rapid decline of lung function, the distribution of IL-1B/IL-1RN haplotypes differed between smokers with rapid decline and those without.

ETIOLOGIC RISK FACTORS FOR CHRONIC OBSTRUCTIVE PULMONARY DISEASE	
Summary Statement	**Level of Evidence**
Of the multiple risk factors for the development of COPD that have been examined, only cigarette smoking and α_1-antitrypsin deficiency have been proved to be causal.	Multiple observational clinical studies
There are probably host genetic susceptibility risk factors that have yet to be discovered.	Observational clinical studies

COPD, chronic obstructive pulmonary disease.

Occupational Exposures

It has long been known that occupational exposure to dusts can be associated with symptoms and abnormal lung function. However, assessments of the contribution of occupational exposures to the development of COPD have been difficult and results often inconclusive. Epidemiologists must cope with the tendency of people who respond badly to a given exposure to drop out of the workforce, with prob-

lems in quantifying the exposure level, and with the problem that some exposures cause diseases that can be confused with COPD, such as a pneumoconiosis or asthma. Finally, it must be noted that during the past 30 years, the levels of occupational exposure to a variety of dusts have decreased as a result of legislation aimed at workers' protection, so that the current applicability of much of the data in older workers is questionable.

Cross-sectional studies have repeatedly shown occupational exposure to mineral dusts to be associated with chronic cough, sputum production, and reductions in lung function (129); these risks were probably underestimated because of the healthy worker effect. Longitudinal studies of workers exposed to mineral dusts have also shown deleterious effects. The rates of lung function loss are higher in both coal miners and hard rock miners than in controls after correction for the effects of smoking (130–132). Coal mining has been shown to be associated with emphysema in necropsy material (129). The size of the observed effect has varied across studies, with some showing an effect comparable with that of smoking. However, the most recent estimates in coal miners indicate a risk that is at most half that imposed by smoking (132,133).

Other occupational dust exposures have been associated with increased loss of lung function over time. A particularly well-documented instance is exposure to cotton dust in textile workers (134–136). Evidence suggests that relatively low levels of exposure to cotton dust may interact with smoking; exposure-related loss of lung function was evident only in smokers (137). Grain dust exposure has been posited as a risk factor for COPD, but the evidence here is less compelling and complicated by the effects of grain dust in inducing asthma and allergic alveolitis (138).

In cross-sectional studies, exposure to dust had a more pronounced effect on lung function than exposure to gases and fumes, but the latter was associated with some functional deficits (139,140). A special case of fume exposure may be that of smelter workers exposed to cadmium; cadmium is known to cause emphysema in animals. In such workers, the prevalence of airways obstruction and reduced diffusing capacity is high (141). A Norwegian study showed an increased rate of functional decline with exposure to metal fumes and sulfur dioxide, and the rate of decline increased with the number of individual agents to which individuals were exposed, including dusts, vapors, and fumes (142). The excess decline was less than 10 mL yearly, however, even for the most extreme exposures. A Paris study showed a similar effect of a wide variety of occupation-related exposures in smokers and nonsmokers alike (34).

In summary, it is likely that occupation-related exposures to dusts, and to some extent noxious fumes and gases, accelerate loss of lung function. The magnitude of these effects is probably distinctly less than that of smoking, either because tobacco smoke is particularly damaging or because it is administered so efficiently. With the possible exception of people exposed to cadmium and a previous generation of coal miners, it is unlikely that occupational exposure alone causes much COPD, at least in Europe and North America. The situation may differ in other parts of the world, and in these areas, interactive effects between smoking and occupational exposures should be sought.

Air Pollution

Adverse effects of ambient air pollution on respiratory health have been recognized for a long time. Most countries have legislated quality standards for ambient air—that is, levels of air pollution thought not to produce adverse health effects in sensitive population groups. With respect to COPD, the most relevant pollutants are ozone (O_3), nitrogen oxides (NO, NO_2, NOx), sulfur dioxide (SO_2), and particulate matter, a mixture of solid and liquid particles suspended in the air. Nitrogen oxides are produced by reaction between oxygen and nitrogen during combustion in power plants and automobiles. Sulfur dioxide is generated during the combustion of fossil fuels and the smelting of sulfur-containing ore. Nitrogen oxides are precursors of ozone, which is formed by a photochemical reaction between nitrogen oxides and ultraviolet light. In the atmosphere, sulfur dioxide and nitrogen oxides may be transformed into acid aerosols. Particles may be emitted into the air by combustion or abrasion processes; they vary by size (PM10, PM2.5) and by physicochemical composition.

Air pollution is important in regard to public health because of the large number of people exposed. In the 1990s, estimates of the number of people in the United States living in areas that exceeded the National Ambient Air Quality Standard were approximately 70 million for ozone, 9 million for nitrogen dioxide, 5 million for sulfur dioxide, and 22 million for PM10 (143).

In both animal models and laboratory experiments in humans, it has been established that all the pollutants mentioned induce inflammation in the respiratory tract. Furthermore, exposure to these pollutants is associated with acute short-term effects, such as bronchoconstriction and exacerbations of asthma or COPD. It is well established that episodes of severe air pollution are associated with increased rates of hospitalization and mortality, particularly among people with asthma or COPD. Air pollution also affects lung growth and may increase airway hyperresponsiveness.

However, it is less well established whether chronic exposure to air pollution affects the decline in FEV_1. It is difficult to interpret cross-sectional studies, conduct appropriate longitudinal epidemiologic studies, estimate personal exposure levels, test large numbers of individuals, and control for the effects of potential confounders, such as smoking. In addition, people are frequently exposed to several air pollutants concurrently.

In the 1970s, four communities were studied in Los Angeles county in California: Lancaster (low level of air pollutants), Burbank (elevated levels of photochemical oxidants), Long Beach (elevated levels of sulfur dioxide, particulates, and hydrocarbons), and Glendora (elevated levels of pho-

tochemical oxidants, nitric oxide, and sulfates) (144–148). Cross-sectional and longitudinal analyses were performed in both children and adults.

In the cross-sectional analyses of 7- to 17-year-olds, no difference was found between Lancaster and Burbank in the percentage of those with a low FEV_1 (144). In longitudinal analysis, the 5-year change in FEV_1 did not differ between Lancaster, Glendora, and Long Beach for 7- to 18-year-old boys (147,148). However, in girls in this age group, the FEV_1 increased less in Long Beach than in Lancaster (148). The FEV_1 decline for both men and women between the ages of 19 and 24 years was greater in Long Beach than in Lancaster (148).

In cross-sectional analyses of 25- to 59-year-old participants, there was also no difference in the percentage of the population with low FEV_1 values between Lancaster and Burbank (144), and no difference between Lancaster and Glendora for either nonsmokers or current smokers (146). However, the percentage of individuals with low FEV_1 values was significantly higher in Long Beach than in Lancaster (145). In never-smoking females, the FEV_1 decline after 5 years was greater in Glendora (44 ± 2 mL) than in Lancaster (33 ± 3 mL). There was no difference between males (48 ± 6 vs. 46 ± 5, respectively) in the same communities (147). However, the FEV_1 declined significantly more in Long Beach than in Lancaster for both male (66 ± 4 vs. 51 ± 5) and female (50 ± 3 vs. 36 ± 3) never-smokers (148).

Dockery and colleagues (149) and Ware and colleagues (150) found no relationship between FEV_1 and exposure to total particulates, PM15, PM2.5, sulfur dioxide, and nitric oxide in 5,422 children ages 10 to 12 years studied in six U.S. cities.

Peters and colleagues (151) studied 3,293 schoolchildren in grades 4, 7, and 10 in 12 communities in southern California. In 1994, lung function measurements were correlated with air pollution levels estimated for the period between 1986 and 1990 and with the air pollution level measured in 1994. Although no significant relationship between air pollution and FEV_1 was found in boys, FEV_1 values were lower in girls with higher PM10 and nitric oxide exposure between 1986 and 1990 or in 1994. Higher PM2.5 exposure, which was measured only in 1994, was also associated with lower FEV_1 values in girls. Peak or 24-hour average ozone exposures were not associated with lower FEV_1.

In a cross-sectional analysis of data from 3,922 NHANES II participants ages 6 to 24 years, Schwartz (152) found that the FEV_1 adjusted for potential confounders, including smoking, was lower in those with higher levels of exposure to nitric oxide, total particulates, and ozone averaged over the preceding year. The relationship between FEV_1 and either ozone or nitric oxide was stronger than that between FEV_1 and total particulates. No relationship was found between sulfur dioxide exposure and FEV_1.

Abbey and colleagues (153) studied the relationship between lung function measurements obtained in 1993 and exposure to ambient air pollutants during the 20-year period before the survey in 1,391 nonsmokers who were older than 25 years at baseline. In men whose parents had asthma, bronchitis, emphysema, or hay fever, a reduction in FEV_1 could be related to exposure to PM10 and ozone, but no difference was found in other men or in women. On the other hand, an increase of 1.6 $\mu g/m^3$ in sulfur dioxide was associated with a decrease of 1.5% in FEV_1 expressed as a percentage of the predicted normal value in all men.

The relationship between long-term exposure and FEV_1 was studied in 9,651 residents of Switzerland between the ages of 18 and 60 years (154). Increases of 10 $\mu g/m^3$ in the average annual concentrations of PM10, sulfur dioxide, and nitric oxide were associated with significant (1.03%, 0.77%, and 0.68%, respectively) decreases in FEV_1 after adjustments were made for gender, age, smoking, atopy, height, and weight. No consistent relationship with ozone was noted.

Chestnut and colleagues (155) found a significant negative relationship between total particulates and FEV_1 in adult never-smokers in 49 locations in the United States included in NHANES I.

The results of these epidemiologic studies suggest an effect of air pollution on FEV_1. The evidence, however, is not consistent for either younger or older populations. Adverse respiratory effects may not be observed for both males and females in the same location. It is also not clear which pollutants are responsible. Finally, effects on function were seldom as large as those of tobacco smoking.

Environmental Tobacco Smoke

Environmental tobacco smoke (ETS) is emitted as a side stream of smoke into the environment and is added to some of the main stream exhaled by smokers. It is difficult to estimate exposure to ETS; in most studies, it is assessed by questionnaire and expressed as exposure to smokers at home or at work. Usually, never-smokers exposed to smokers (passive smokers) are compared with unexposed persons. Exposure to ETS increases with the number of smokers in the home or workplace, the intensity of their smoking, and the density of people at home or work.

In a 12-year follow-up study of mortality, Sandler and colleagues (156) found an increased risk for dying of emphysema or bronchitis in nonsmoking women exposed to ETS (relative risk, 5.7) but not in men in comparison with unexposed nonsmokers. Most other evidence relating ETS and COPD has been obtained from cross-sectional studies comparing parameters of lung function, particularly FEV_1, between nonsmokers exposed to ETS and nonsmokers not exposed. The results of these studies are inconsistent.

Kauffmann and colleagues (157) found a significant effect of ETS on FEV_1 in French women ages 40 years and older. The average FEV_1 value was approximately 90 mL lower in passive smokers than in unexposed nonsmokers; the difference was not explained by confounding. Similarly, in the

Multiple Risk Factor Intervention Trial in the United States (158), nonsmoking men with smoking wives had FEV_1 values 99 mL lower than those of nonsmokers without smoking wives. In 45- to 64-year-old Scots, Hole and colleagues (159) found the FEV_1 to be 80 mL lower in passive smokers than in unexposed controls. Iranian men and women (160) exposed to ETS at work or at home had significantly reduced FEV_1 values. In Singapore, Ng and colleagues (161) found that passive smoking was significantly associated with a 70-mL reduction in the FEV_1. In China (162), 40- to 69-year-old persons exposed to ETS had FEV_1 values 130 mL lower than those of persons not exposed.

On the other hand, several studies found no relationship between ETS and FEV_1 values. Whereas Kauffmann and colleagues (157) found an effect of ETS exposure on FEV_1 in French women 40 years of age and older, no relationship was found in younger women or in men. No relationship was found between ETS and FEV_1 in women 40 years of age and older in five U.S. cities (163). Schilling and colleagues (164) found no effect of passive smoking on the FEV_1 in adults from 376 American families. White and Froebe (165) compared 400 exposed nonsmokers and 400 unexposed nonsmokers and found no difference in FEV_1 between the groups. Comstock and colleagues (166) compared 78 never-smokers who had at least one smoker in the household with 291 never-smokers who had no smokers in the household and found no difference in FEV_1 between the two groups. Frette and colleagues (167) also did not find any difference in FEV_1 between ETS-exposed and ETS-unexposed nonsmokers in either male or female Californians ages 51 through 95 years. In the Netherlands, Brunekreef and colleagues (168) found no difference in FEV_1 between ETS-exposed and ETS-unexposed nonsmoking women 40 to 60 years of age. In Canada, Masi and colleagues (169) studied younger (ages 15–35 years) men and women and also did not find a difference between those exposed and those not exposed to ETS.

A relationship between ETS and FEV_1 has not been demonstrated in longitudinal studies. In nonsmoking women in the Netherlands, the FEV_1 decline was similar for ETS-exposed and ETS-unexposed groups. Jaakkola and colleagues (170) assessed the effect of ETS on the changes in FEV_1 in 117 Canadian nonsmokers 15 through 40 years old. One cigarette per day was associated with a decline in FEV_1 of 0.53 mL yearly, which was not significant.

These data suggest that although ETS may have an effect on respiratory function and COPD, it is small. In studies that found a difference between ETS-exposed and ETS-unexposed nonsmokers, the difference in FEV_1 was between 70 and 130 mL, too small to produce clinical disease without the presence of other factors. The effect of ETS on FEV_1 was observed more often in Europe and Asia, possibly because of higher levels of ETS exposure as a consequence of more smoking and a greater population density. The effect of ETS was also observed more frequently in people older than 40 years.

Indoor Air Pollution

Indoor air pollution may be an important determinant of health because people spend a substantial proportion of their life indoors, primarily in homes, offices, and other workplaces. Ambient air quality is only one determinant of the indoor air quality; other factors include cigarette smoke, the type and amount of fuel used for cooking and heating, the density of residents, and the type and quality of the ventilation system.

Evidence from developing countries suggests that exposure to wood smoke may be an important determinant of airflow obstruction. In surveys of rural Nepal, Pandey (171) found elevated rates of chronic bronchitis (18.3%), and approximately half of these individuals had airflow obstruction. The prevalence among women was as high as that among men. The high prevalence among women was attributed to their exposure to smoke generated by biomass fuel burned for cooking (172). In Saudi Arabia (173), 50 women and men with spirometrically confirmed COPD were compared with healthy controls. The women, who were almost all never-smokers, were significantly more likely to have been exposed to indoor open fires for more than 20 years than were the controls. No association was found with incense burning. In a hospital-based case control study in Colombia (174), 104 women who had documented COPD were compared with controls who did not have COPD. The COPD patients were 3.9 times more likely to have been exposed to wood smoke. In India, Behera and Jindal (175) surveyed 3,608 nonsmoking women. Those using biomass in chullas for cooking purposes had the lowest mean FEV_1 values. In Mexico (176), women with COPD were compared with four control groups. The odds ratios for exposure to wood smoke were 3.9 (95% CI, 2.0–7.6) for those with chronic bronchitis only, 9.7 (95% CI, 3.7–27) for cases with both chronic bronchitis and chronic airflow obstruction, and 1.8 (95% CI, 0.7–4.7) for those with chronic airflow obstruction only.

Childhood Conditions

Events in childhood could predispose to the development of COPD by a number of mechanisms. Lung growth could be compromised, so that a given amount of subsequent smoking-related loss of lung function would have a greater impact. Childhood events could increase susceptibility to the influences of smoking without altering lung growth, by causing airways hyperreactivity, for example. It is extremely difficult to study longitudinally childhood influences on a disease that develops gradually and becomes apparent only late in adult life, and no such studies are available. Nevertheless, the influences of childhood respiratory infections and exposures to ETS have been investigated.

Burrows and colleagues (177) noted that a history of "childhood respiratory trouble" was an independent predictor of reduced lung function in both smokers and nonsmok-

ers, but they recognized that this might be a consequence of preferential recall on the part of participants with respiratory problems. Samet and colleagues (178) reviewed the topic in 1983 and pointed out that previous respiratory infections were apparently associated with small (2%–7%) decrements in lung function measured at ages 5 through 14 years, but again, recall bias might have played a role in most of the results reported. Some evidence suggested that severe episodes of bronchiolitis, croup, and pneumonia were associated with subsequent airways hyperreactivity in children. Subsequently, in a prospective study, Gold and colleagues (179) showed that pneumonia or hospitalization for a respiratory illness was associated with approximately a 5% decrease in FEV_1 8 years later in nonasthmatic boys, but not girls. Another study (180) prospectively examined the influence of less severe episodes and found that in boys, two or more infections with wheezing in the first 6 years of life were associated with a 10% reduction in FEV_1 at least 2 years later. The effects on girls were less striking and not significant. Respiratory infections not accompanied by wheezing did not influence subsequent lung function. Thus, it appears that early childhood respiratory infections have a demonstrably deleterious effect on subsequent lung function, but the effect is not large, and it is unclear whether it persists into adult life.

ETS generated by parents has been extensively studied and is associated with increased levels of respiratory symptoms and reduced lung function in their offspring. The effect is larger in girls than in boys and is more strongly associated with maternal than with paternal smoking (181). The net effect is small, accounting for a decrease of less than 5% in the FEV_1 at age 20. The effects of ETS and lower respiratory infections in childhood are difficult to separate because the two are clearly associated (182). The reason that girls are apparently more affected by ETS remains unclear, but the work of Tager and colleagues (183) has shown why maternal smoking is more damaging than paternal smoking. Maternal smoking during pregnancy is associated with reductions in lung function in infants, and it is likely that these deficits persist into childhood and adolescence. Again, the effect is small and more prominent in girls than in boys, but it almost certainly contributes to childhood susceptibility to respiratory infections.

In summary, both childhood respiratory infections and ETS exposure cause small reductions in lung function, at least in children. Although these changes per se are not large enough to pose a credible COPD risk factor, it is conceivable that such childhood events increase the susceptibility of smokers to tobacco products.

A specific and promising hypothesis regarding childhood infection and COPD has emerged from the work of Matsuse and colleagues (184), who showed that pieces of the adenoviral genome are commonly present in autopsy lung specimens from smokers with and without COPD. The genetic material is presumably related to previous infection, possibly during childhood, with this agent. They also demonstrated that the

E1A viral segment is present much more often in smokers with airways obstruction than in those without. They subsequently showed that the E1A viral segment may function as a proinflammatory agent (41) and developed an animal model of COPD by combining smoking and adenoviral infection (185). At the moment, this is the most internally coherent and exciting hypothesis regarding the missing "host factor" in COPD.

Dietary Factors

Three groups of dietary factors may play a role in the etiology of chronic obstructive disease: antioxidants, ω-3 fatty acids, and electrolytes. Because studies linking dietary factors with COPD are plagued with methodologic problems, including measuring dietary intake, defining an appropriate COPD outcome variable, and establishing a temporal relationship between exposure and outcome, the evidence from these studies is far from conclusive. On the other hand, because large segments of the population are continually exposed to diets with low levels of antioxidants and ω-3 fatty acids and high levels of some electrolytes, the impact of dietary factors on COPD may be substantial.

Antioxidants

In addition to enzymatic systems that manage the inflammation produced by oxidants, vitamins C and E and β-carotene reduce oxidants and oxidative stress and thus may protect lung tissue from inflammation and injury. Most of the evidence in regard to the protective role of these factors is from cross-sectional studies. For this review, we have considered only studies in which the intake of specific antioxidants was estimated and the FEV_1 was used as an indicator of airways obstruction. In several studies, a greater intake of vitamin C was associated with higher values of FEV_1. Schwartz and Weiss (186) analyzed NHANES I data from 3,478 subjects ages 30 through 74 years and found that those who consumed more than 178 mg of vitamin C per day had FEV_1 values 40 mL higher than those who consumed less than 17 mg. Similar differences in FEV_1 values were found in other studies: a 25-mL increase in FEV_1 was associated with a 40-mg increase in the daily intake of vitamin C (187), a 220-mL increase with an increase of 50 μmol/L in the serum level of vitamin C (188), a 21.6-mL increase with an increase in the daily intake of vitamin C of 100 mg (189), and a 53-mL increase with a 145-mg difference in the intake of vitamin C (190). No satisfactory cohort or follow-up study has been performed in which the association between vitamin C intake and FEV_1 has been confirmed.

Evidence also supports an association of vitamin E, carotenoids, and FEV_1. In the study of Britton and colleagues (187), the association between dietary intake of vitamin E and FEV_1 disappeared after the intake of vitamin C was taken into account. Schünemann and colleagues (191) stud-

ied 1,616 men and women between the ages of 35 and 79 years who were free of respiratory disease. Those in the highest quartile for vitamin E intake had a significantly higher FEV_1 value than those in the lowest quartile (99.4% vs. 95.4% of the predicted normal value). The effect of vitamin E remained significant after vitamin C was included in the model. Higher serum levels of vitamin E were associated with higher values of FEV_1 (192).

In analyzing data from NHANES III, Hu and Cassano (193) concluded that the FEV_1 was higher in those with a higher intake of β-carotene. This observation was supported by findings that higher levels of serum carotenoids are associated with better lung function (192,194,195).

ω-3 Fatty Acids

The balance between ω-3 and ω-6 fatty acids may be important because whereas ω-6 fatty acids are proinflammatory, ω-3 fatty acids are protective. The dietary intake may influence the mix of ω-fatty acids in the body. The primary dietary source of ω-3 fatty acids is fish oil. Schwartz and Weiss (196), in an analysis of NHANES I data, found that the FEV_1 was lowest in individuals who consumed fish less than once per week and highest in those who consumed fish more than once per week. Sharp and colleagues (197) studied 6,346 men 45 to 68 years old and found that smokers who consumed fish more than twice a week had a slightly higher FEV_1 value than those who consumed fish less than twice a week. In a study conducted in England, however, no relationship was found between fish intake and FEV_1 (198).

Electrolytes

No epidemiologic studies have demonstrated a relationship between the dietary intake of sodium or magnesium and FEV_1. However, some studies suggest that bronchial responsiveness is greater in those with a greater intake of sodium, and a greater intake of magnesium may have a protective effect. The level of bronchial responsiveness appears to be a risk factor for COPD in smokers.

OTHER FACTORS INFLUENCING THE DEVELOPMENT OF CHRONIC OBSTRUCTIVE PULMONARY DISEASE	
Summary Statement	**Level of Evidence**
Occupational dust/fume exposures, indoor and outdoor air pollution, environmental factors (side stream tobacco smoke), childhood illness, and dietary factors may play a role in the development of COPD, but their effects, alone or in combination, are much less than that of direct cigarette smoking.	Multiple observational studies

COPD, chronic obstructive pulmonary disease.

REFERENCES

1. Laennec RTH. *A treatise on diseases of the chest.* Translated from French. Published under the auspices of the Library of the New York Academy of Medicine by Harcourt Publishing Co., New York, 1962.

2. Higgins ITT, Oldham PD, Cochrane AL, et al. Respiratory symptoms and pulmonary disability in an industrial town: survey of a random sample of the population. *Br Med J* 1956;2:904–910.

3. Lowell FC, Franklin W, Michelson AL, et al. Chronic obstructive pulmonary emphysema: a disease of smokers. *Ann Intern Med* 1956;45:268–274.

4. Palmer KNV. The role of smoking in bronchitis. *Br Med J* 1954;1:1473–1474.

5. U.S. Department of Health, Education, and Welfare. *Smoking and health: a report to the Advisory Committee to the Surgeon General of the Public Health Service.* Washington, DC: Public Health Service, 1964: Publication No. 1103.

6. Niewoehner DE. Anatomic and pathophysiological correlations in chronic obstructive pulmonary disease. In: Baum GL, Crapo JD, Celli BR, et al., eds. *Textbook of pulmonary diseases,* 6th ed Philadelphia: Lippincott–Raven Publishers, 1998:823–843.

7. Pauwels RA, Buist AS, Calverley PMA, et al. Global strategy for the diagnosis, management, and prevention of chronic obstructive pulmonary disease. *Am J Respir Crit Care Med* 2001;163:1256–1276.

8. Lange P, Parner J, Vestbo J, et al. A 15-year follow-up study of ventilatory function in adults with asthma. *N Engl J Med* 1998;339:1194–2000.

9. Anthonisen NR, Wright EC. Bronchodilator response in chronic obstructive pulmonary disease. *Am Rev Respir Dis* 1986;133:814–819.

10. World health report. Geneva: World Health Organization, 2000. Available from URL *www.who.int/whr/2000/en/statistics.htm*

11. Hurd S. The impact of COPD on lung health worldwide. Epidemiology and incidence. *Chest* 2000;117:1S–4S.

12. Viegi G, Pedreschi M, Pistelli F, et al. Prevalence of airways obstruction in a general population. European Respiratory Society versus American Thoracic Society definition. *Chest* 2000;117:339S–345S.

13. Cooreman J, Thom TJ, Higgins MW. Mortality from chronic obstructive pulmonary diseases and asthma in France, 1969–1983. Comparisons with United States and Canada. *Chest* 1990;97:213–219.

14. Mannino DM, Brown C, Giovino GA. Obstructive lung disease deaths in the United States from 1979 through 1993. An analysis using multiple-cause mortality data. *Am J Respir Crit Care Med* 1997;156:814–818.

15. National Heart, Lung, and Blood Institute. *Morbidity and mortality: chartbook on cardiovascular, lung, and blood diseases.* Bethesda, MD: U.S. Department of Health and Human Services, Public Health Service, National Institutes of Health, 1998. Available from URL *www.nhlbi.nih.gov/nhlbi/seiin//other/cht-book/htm*

16. Manfreda J, Mao Y, Litven W. Morbidity and mortality from chronic obstructive pulmonary disease. *Am Rev Respir Dis* 1989;140:S19–S26.

17. Lacasse Y, Brooks D, Goldstein RS. Trends in the epidemiology of COPD in Canada, 1980 to 1995. *Chest* 1999;116:306–313.

18. Murray CJL, Lopez AD. Alternative projections of mortality and disability by cause 1990–2020: global burden of disease study. *Lancet* 1997;349:1498–1504.

19. Mannino DM, Gagnon RC, Petty TL, et al. Obstructive lung disease and low lung function in adults in the United States. Data from the National Health and Nutrition Examination Survey, 1988–1994. *Arch Intern Med* 2000;160:1683–1689.

20. Kanner RE, Connett JE, Williams DE, et al. Effects of randomized assignment to a smoking cessation intervention and changes in smoking habits on respiratory symptoms in smokers with early chronic obstructive pulmonary disease: the Lung Health Study. *Am J Med* 1999;106:410–416.

21. Coultas DB, Mapel D, Gagnon R, et al. The health impact of undiagnosed airflow obstruction in a national sample of United States adults. *Am J Respir Crit Care Med* 2001;164:372–377.

22. Hankinson JL, Odencrantz JR, Fedan KB. Spirometric reference values from a sample of the general U.S. population. *Am J Respir Crit Care Med* 1999;159:179–187.

23. Sullivan SD, Ramsey SD, Lee TA. The economic burden of COPD. *Chest* 2000;117:5S–9S.

24. U.S. Department of Health, Education, and Welfare. *The health consequences of smoking. Chronic obstructive lung disease.* Rockville, MD: U.S. Department of Health and Human Services, Public Health Service, Office of Smoking, 1984: DHHS (PHS) Publication No. 84-5025.

25. Sherrill DL, Lebowitz MD, Burrows BW. Epidemiology of chronic obstructive pulmonary disease. *Clin Chest Med* 1990;11:375–388.

26. Higenbottam T, Shipley MJ, Clark TJH, et al. Lung function and symptoms of cigarette smokers related to tar yield and number of cigarettes smoked. *Lancet* 1980;1:409–412.

27. Sparrow D, Stefos T, Bosse R, et al. The relationship of tar content to decline in pulmonary function in cigarette smokers. *Am Rev Respir Dis* 1983;127:56–58.

28. Fletcher C, Peto R, Tinker C, et al. *The natural history of chronic bronchitis and emphysema.* Oxford: Oxford University Press, 1976.

29. Anthonisen NR, Connett JE, Kiley JP, et al. Effects of smoking intervention and the use of an inhaled anticholinergic bronchodilator on the rate of decline of FEV_1. The Lung Health Study. *JAMA* 1994;272:1497–1505.

30. Camilli AE, Burrows B, Knudson RJ, et al. Longitudinal changes in forced expiratory volume in one second in adults: effects of smoking and smoking cessation. *Am Rev Respir Dis* 1987;135:794–799.

31. Peat JK, Woolcock AJ, Cullen K. Decline of lung function and development of chronic airflow limitation: a longitudinal study of non-smokers and smokers in Busselton, West Australia. *Thorax* 1990;45:32–37.

32. Wilhelmson L, Orha I, Tibblin G. Decrease in ventilatory capacity between the ages of 5 and 54 in a representative sample of Swedish men. *Br Med J* 1969;3:553–556.

33. Comstock GW, Brownlow WJ, Stone RW, et al. Cigarette smoking and changes in respiratory findings. *Arch Environ Health* 1970;21:50–57.

34. Kauffmann F, Drouet D, Lellouch J, et al. Twelve years' spirometric changes among Paris area workers. *Int J Epidemiol* 1979;8:201–212.

35. Bosse R, Sparrow D, Rose CL, et al. Longitudinal effect of age and smoking cessation on pulmonary function. *Am Rev Respir Dis* 1981;123:378–381.

36. Xu X, Dockery DW, Ware JH, et al. Effects of cigarette smoking on rate of loss of pulmonary function in adults: a longitudinal assessment. *Am Rev Respir Dis* 1992;146:1345–1348.

37. Lange P, Groth J, Nyboe J, et al. Effects of smoking and changes of smoking habits on the decline of FEV_1. *Eur Respir J* 1989;2:811–816.

38. Burrows B, Lebowitz MD, Camilli AE, et al. Longitudinal changes in forced expiratory volume in one second in adults. Methodologic considerations and findings in healthy nonsmokers. *Am Rev Respir Dis* 1986;133:974–980.

39. Connett JE, Bjornson-Benson WM, Daniels KD, for the Lung Health Study Group. Recruitment of participants in the Lung Health Study II: assessment of recruiting strategies. *Control Clin Trials* 1993;14:38S–51S.

40. Intermittent Positive Pressure Trial Group. Intermittent positive pressure breathing therapy of chronic obstructive pulmonary disease. *Ann Intern Med* 1983;99:612–620.

41. Retamales W, Elliott M, Meshi, et al. Amplification of inflammation in emphysema and its association with latent adenoviral infection. *Am J Respir Crit Care Med* 2001;164:469–473.

42. Orie NGM, Sluiter HJ, De Vries K, et al. The host factor in chronic bronchitis. In: Orie NGM, Sluiter HJ, eds. *Bronchitis, an international royal symposium.* Assen, the Netherlands: Royal Van Gorcum, 1961:43–59.

43. Ramsdell JW, Nachtwey FJ, Moser KM. Bronchial hyperreactivity in chronic obstructive bronchitis. *Am Rev Respir Dis* 1982;126:829–832.

44. Bahous J, Cartier A, Pineau L, et al. Nonallergic bronchial hyperexcitability in chronic bronchitis. *Am Rev Respir Dis* 1984;129:216–220.

45. Moreno RH, Hogg JC, Pare PD. Mechanics of airway narrowing. *Am Rev Respir Dis* 1986;133:1171–1180.

46. Rijcken B, Schouten JP, Xu X, et al. Airway hyperresponsiveness to histamine associated with accelerated decline in FEV_1. *Am J Respir Crit Care Med* 1995;151:1377–1382.

47. O'Connor GT, Sparrow D, Weiss ST. A prospective longitudinal study of methacholine responsiveness as a predictor of pulmonary function decline: the Normative Aging Study. *Am J Respir Crit Care Med* 1995;152:87–92.

48. Frew AJ, Kennedy SM, Chan-Yeung M. Methacholine responsiveness, smoking and atopy as risk factors for accelerated FEV_1 decline in male working populations. *Am Rev Respir Dis* 1992;146:878–883.

49. Tracey M, Villar A, Dow L, et al. The influence of increased bronchial responsiveness, atopy, and serum IgE on decline in FEV_1. *Am J Respir Crit Care Med* 1995;151:656–662.

50. Tashkin DP, Altose MD, Connett JE, et al. , for the Lung Health Study Research Group. Methacholine reactivity predicts changes in lung function over time in smokers with early chronic obstructive pulmonary disease. *Am J Respir Crit Care Med* 1996;153:1802–1811.

51. O'Connor GT, Sparrow D, Weiss ST. The role of allergy and nonspecific airway hyperresponsiveness in the pathogenesis of chronic obstructive pulmonary disease. *Am Rev Respir Dis* 1989;140:225–252.

52. Gerrard JW, Heiner DE, Ko CG, et al. Immunoglobulin levels in smokers and non-smokers. *Ann Allergy* 1980;44:261–262.

53. Burrows B, Halonen M, Barbee RA, et al. The relationship of serum immunoglobulin E to cigarette smoking. *Am Rev Respir Dis* 1981;124:523–525.

54. Warren CPW, Holford-Stevens V, Wong C, et al. The relationship between smoking and total immunoglobulin E levels. *J Allergy Clin Immunol* 1982;69:370–375.

55. Jensen EJ, Pedersen B, Schmidt E, et al. Serum IgE in nonatopic smokers, nonsmokers, and recent smokers: relation to lung function, airways symptoms, and atopic predisposition. *J Allergy Clin Immunol* 1992;90:224–229.

56. Burrows B, Lebowitz MD, Barbee RA, et al. Interactions between smoking and immunologic factors in relation to airways obstruction. *Chest* 1983;84:657–661.

57. Annesi I, Orszczyn MP, Frette C, et al. Total circulating IgE and FEV_1 in adult men: an epidemiologic longitudinal study. *Chest* 1992;101:642–648.

58. Omenaas E, Bakke P, Eide GE, et al. Total serum IgE and FEV_1 by respiratory symptoms and obstructive lung disease in adults in a Norwegian community. *Clin Exp Allergy* 1995;25:682–689.

59. Burrows B, Halonen M, Lebowitz MD, et al. The relationship between serum immunoglobulin E, allergy skin tests, and smoking to respiratory disorders. *J Allergy Clin Immunol* 1982;70:199–205.

60. Burrows B, Knudson RJ, Cline MG, et al. A reexamination of risk factors for ventilatory impairment. *Am Rev Respir Dis* 1988;138:829–836.

61. Vollmer WM, Buist SA, Johnson LR, et al. Relationship between serum IgE and cross-sectional and longitudinal FEV_1 in two cohort studies. *Chest* 1986;90:416–423.

62. Taylor RG, Joyce H, Gross E, et al. Bronchial reactivity to inhaled histamine and annual rate of decline in male smokers and ex-smokers. *Thorax* 1985;40:9–16.

63. Parker DR, O'Connor GT, Sparrow D, et al. The relationship of nonspecific airways responsiveness and atopy to the rate of decline of lung function. *Am Rev Respir Dis* 1990;141:589–594.

64. Annesi I, Neukirch F, Orvoen-Frija E, et al. The relevance of hyperresponsiveness but not of atopy to FEV_1 decline. *Bull Eur Pathophysiol Respir* 1987;23:397–400.

65. Stuart-Harris CH. The pathogenesis of chronic bronchitis and emphysema. *Scott Med J* 1965;10:93–107.

66. Fletcher CM. Chronic bronchitis: its prevalence, nature and pathogenesis. *Am Rev Respir Dis* 1959;80:483–494.

67. Laurenzi GA, Potter RT, Kass EH. Bacteriologic flora of the lower respiratory tract. *N Engl J Med* 1961;265:1273–1278.

68. Fisher M, Akhtar AJ, Calder MA, et al. Pilot study of factors associated with exacerbations in chronic bronchitis. *Br J Med* 1969;4:187–192.

69. Howard P. A long-term follow-up of respiratory symptoms and ventilatory function in a group of working men. *Br J Ind Med* 1970;27:326–333.

70. Bates DV. The fate of chronic bronchitis: a report of the 10-year follow-up in the Canadian Department of Veterans Affairs coordinated study of chronic bronchitis. *Am Rev Respir Dis* 1973;108:1043–1065.

71. Annesi I, Kauffmann F. Is respiratory mucus hypersecretion really an innocent disorder? *Am Rev Respir Dis* 1986;134:688–693.

72. Speizer FE, Fay ME, Dockery DW, et al. Chronic obstructive pulmonary disease mortality in six U.S. cities. *Am Rev Respir Dis* 1989;140:S49–S55.

73. Sherman CB, Xu X, Speizer FE, et al. Longitudinal lung function decline in subjects with respiratory symptoms. *Am Rev Respir Dis* 1992;146:855–859.

74. Vestbo J, Prescott E, Lange P, and the Copenhagen City Heart Study Group. Association of chronic mucus hypersecretion with FEV_1 decline and chronic obstructive pulmonary disease morbidity. *Am J Respir Crit Care Med* 1996;153:1530–1535.

75. Seemungal TA, Donaldson GC, Bhowmik A, et al. Time course and recovery of exacerbations in patients with chronic obstructive pulmonary disease. *Am J Respir Crit Care Med* 2000;161:1608–1613.

76. Kanner RE, Anthonisen NR, Connett JE, for the Lung Health Study Research Group. Lower respiratory illnesses promote FEV_1 decline in current smokers but not in ex-smokers with mild chronic obstructive pulmonary disease. *Am J Respir Crit Care Med* 2001;164:358–364.

77. Nocturnal Oxygen Therapy Trial Group. Continuous or nocturnal oxygen therapy in hypoxemic chronic obstructive lung disease. *Ann Intern Med* 1983;99:519–527.

78. Xu X, Weiss ST, Riijcken B, et al. Smoking, changes in smoking habits, and rate of decline in FEV_1: new insights into gender differences. *Eur Respir J* 1994;7:1056–1061.

79. Becklake MR, Kauffmann F. Gender differences in airway behaviour over the human life span. *Thorax* 1999;54:1119–1138.

80. Prescott E, Berg AM, Andersen PK, et al. Gender difference in smoking effect on lung function and risk of hospitalization for COPD: results from a Danish longitudinal population study. *Eur Respir J* 1997;10:822–827.

81. Lung Health Study Research Group. Smoking and lung function of Lung Health Study (LHS) participants after 11 years. *Am J Respir Crit Care Med* 2002;166:675–679.

82. Kanner RE, Connett JE, Altose MD, et al., for the Lung Health Study Research Group. Gender difference in airway hyperresponsiveness in smokers with mild COPD. *Am J Respir Crit Care Med* 1994;150:956–961.

83. Higgins M, Keller J. Familial occurrence of chronic respiratory disease and familial resemblance in ventilatory capacity. *J Chronic Dis* 1975;28:239–251.

84. Lebowitz MD, Knudson RJ, Burrows B. Family aggregation of pulmonary function measurements. *Am Rev Respir Dis* 1984; 129:8–11.

85. Chen Y, Horne SL, Rennie DC, et al. Segregation analysis of two lung function indices in a random sample of young families: the Humboldt family study. *Genet Epidemiol* 1996;13:35–47.

86. Givelber RJ, Couropmitree NN, Gottlieb DJ, et al. Segregation analysis of pulmonary function among families in the Framingham study. *Am J Respir Crit Care Med* 1998;157:1445–1451.

87. Higgins MW, Keller JB, Becker M, et al. An index of risk for obstructive airways disease. *Am Rev Respir Dis* 1982;125:144–151.

88. Gottlieb DJ, Wilk JB, Harmon M, et al. Heritability of longitudinal change in lung function. The Framingham Study. *Am J Respir Crit Care Med* 2001;164:1655–1659.

89. Kurzius-Spencer M, Sherrill DL, Hoberg CJ, et al. Familial correlation in the decline of forced expiratory volume in one second. *Am J Respir Crit Care Med* 2001;164:1261–1265.

90. Silverman EK, Miletich JP, Pierce JA, et al. Alpha-1-antitrypsin deficiency. High prevalence in the St. Louis area determined by direct population screening. *Am Rev Respir Dis* 1989;140:961–966.

91. Spence WC, Morris JE, Pass K, et al. Molecular confirmation of α_1-antitrypsin genotypes in newborn dried blood specimens. *Biochem Med Met Biol* 1993;50:233–240.

92. O'Brien ML, Buist NRM, Murphey WH. Neonatal screening for alpha$_1$-antitrypsin deficiency. *J Pediatr* 1978;92:1006–1010.

93. Sveger T. Liver disease in alpha$_1$-antitrypsin deficiency detected by screening of 200,000 infants. *N Engl J Med* 1976;294:1316–1321.

94. Laurell CB, Erickson S. The electrophoretic α_1-globulin pattern of serum in α_1-antitrypsin deficiency. *Scand J Clin Lab Invest* 1963;15:132–140.

95. Larsson C. Natural history and life expectancy in severe alpha$_1$-antitrypsin deficiency, PiZ. *Acta Med Scand* 1978;204:345–351.

96. Seersholm N, Kok-Jensen A, Dirksen A. Survival of patients with severe α_1-antitrypsin deficiency with special reference to non-index cases. *Thorax* 1994;94:695–698.

97. Silverman EK, Pierce JA, Province MA, et al. Variability of pulmonary function in alpha-1-antitrypsin deficiency: clinical correlates. *Ann Intern Med* 1989;111:982–991.

98. Wu MC, Eriksson S. Lung function, smoking and survival in severe alpha$_1$-antitrypsin deficiency, PiZZ. *J Clin Epidemiol* 1988;41:1157–1165.

99. Piitulainen E, Eriksson S. Decline in FEV$_1$ related to smoking in individuals with severe α_1-antitrypsin deficiency (PiZZ). *Eur Respir J* 1999;13:247–251.

100. Piitulainen E, Tornling G, Eriksson S. Environmental correlates of impaired lung function in non-smokers with severe α_1-antitrypsin deficiency (PiZZ). *Thorax* 1999;53:939–943.

101. Sandford AJ, Weir TD, Pare PD. Genetic risk factors for chronic obstructive pulmonary disease. *Eur Respir J* 1997;10:1380–1391.

102. Turino GM, Barker AF, Brantly ML, et al. Clinical features of individuals with PI*SZ phenotype of α_1-antitrypsin deficiency. *Am J Respir Crit Care Med* 1996;154:1718–1725.

103. Sandford AJ, Chagani T, Weir TD, et al. Susceptibility genes for rapid decline of lung function in the Lung Health Study. *Am J Respir Crit Care Med* 2001;163:469–473.

104. Eriksson S, Lindmark B, Lilja H. Familial α_1-antichymotrypsin deficiency. *Acta Med Scand* 1986;220:447–453.

105. Poller W, Faber J-P, Scholz S, et al. Mis-sense mutation of α_1-antichymotrypsin gene associated with chronic lung disease. *Lancet* 1992;339:1538.

106. Lindmark BE, Arborelius M Jr, Eriksson SG. Pulmonary function in middle-aged women with heterozygous deficiency of the serine protease inhibitor alpha$_1$-antichymotrypsin. *Am Rev Respir Dis* 1990;141:884–888.

107. Finlay GA, Russell KJ, McMahon KJ, et al. Elevated levels of matrix metalloproteinases in bronchoalveolar lavage fluid of emphysematous patients. *Thorax* 1997;52:502–506.

108. Segura-Valdez L, Pardo A, Gaxiola M, et al. Upregulation of gelatinases A and B, collagenases 1 and 2, and increased parenchymal cell death in COPD. *Chest* 2000;117:684–694.

109. Joos L, He J-Q, Shepherdson MB, et al. The role of matrix metalloproteinase polymorphisms in the rate of decline in lung function. *Hum Mol Genet* 2002;11:569–576.

110. Hirano K, Sakamoto T, Uchida Y, et al. Tissue inhibitor of metalloproteinases-2 gene polymorphisms in chronic obstructive pulmonary disease. *Eur Respir J* 2001;18:748–752.

111. Kueppers F, Miller RD, Gordon H, et al. Familial prevalence of chronic obstructive pulmonary disease in a matched pair study. *Am J Med* 1977;63:336–342.

112. Horne SL, Cockcroft DW, Dosman JA. Possible protective effect against chronic obstructive airways disease by the GC 2 allele. *Hum Hered* 1990;40:173–176.

113. Ishii T, Keicho N, Teramoto S, et al. Association of Gc-globulin variation with susceptibility to COPD and diffuse panbronchiolitis. *Eur Respir J* 2001;18:753–757.

114. Kauffmann F, Kleisbauer J-P, Cambon-de-Mouzon A, et al. Genetic markers in chronic air-flow limitation: a genetic epidemiologic study. *Am Rev Respir Dis* 1983;127:263–269.

115. Cohen BH, Ball WC Jr, Brashears S, et al. Risk factors in chronic obstructive pulmonary disease (COPD). *Am J Epidemiol* 1977;105:223–231.

116. Beaty TH, Menkes HA, Cohen BH, et al. Risk factors associated with longitudinal change in pulmonary function. *Am Rev Respir Dis* 1984;129:660–667.

117. Krzyzanowski M, Jedrychowski W, Wysocki M. Factors associated with the change in ventilatory function and the development of chronic obstructive pulmonary disease in a 13-year follow-up of the Cracow study. *Am Rev Respir Dis* 1986;134:1011–1019.

118. Horne SL, Cockcroft DW, Lovegrove A, et al. ABO, Lewis and secretor status and relative incidence of air flow obstruction. *Dis Markers* 1985;3:55–62.

119. Kauffmann F, Frette C, Pham Q-T, et al. Associations of blood group-related antigens to FEV$_1$, wheezing and asthma. *Am J Respir Crit Care Med* 1996;153:76–82.

120. Cohen BH, Bias WB, Chase GA, et al. Is ABH nonsecretor status a risk factor for obstructive lung disease? *Am J Epidemiol* 1980;111:285–291.

121. Haines AP, Imeson JD, Meade TW. ABH secretor status and pulmonary function. *Am J Epidemiol* 1982;115:367–370.

122. Abboud RT, Yu P, Chan-Yeung M, et al. Lack of relationship

between ABH secretor status and lung function in pulp mill workers. *Am Rev Respir Dis* 1982;126:1089–1091.

123. Smith CAD, Harrison DJ. Association between polymorphism in gene for microsomal epoxide hydrolase and susceptibility to emphysema. *Lancet* 1997;350:630–633.

124. Yim J-J, Park GY, Lee C-T, et al. Genetic susceptibility to chronic obstructive pulmonary disease in Koreans: combined analysis of polymorphic genotypes for microsomal epoxide hydrolase and glutathione *S*-transferase M1 and T1. *Thorax* 2000;55:121–125.

125. Yamada N, Yamaya M, Okinaga S, et al. Microsatellite polymorphism in the heme oxygenase-1 gene promoter is associated with susceptibility to emphysema. *Am J Hum Genet* 2000;66:187–195.

126. Huang S-L, Su C-H, Chang S-C. Tumor necrosis factor-α gene polymorphism in chronic bronchitis. *Am J Respir Crit Care Med* 1997;156:1436–1439.

127. Higham MA, Pride NB, Alikhan A, et al. Tumour necrosis factor-α gene promoter polymorphism in chronic obstructive pulmonary disease. *Eur Respir J* 2000;15:281–284.

128. Joos L, McIntyre L, Ruan J, et al. Association of IL-1β and IL-1 receptor antagonist haplotypes with rate of decline in lung function in smokers. *Thorax* 2001;56:863–866.

129. Becklake MR. Chronic airflow limitation: its relation to work in dusty occupations. *Chest* 1985;88:608–617.

130. Love RG, Miller BG. Longitudinal study of lung function in coal miners. *Thorax* 1982;37:193–197.

131. Manfreda J, Johnson B, Cherniack RM. Longitudinal changes of lung function: comparison of employees of hard rock mining industry and general population. *Am Rev Respir Dis* 1984;129:A142.

132. Oxman AD, Muir DC, Shannon HS, et al. Occupational dust exposure and chronic obstructive pulmonary disease. A systematic overview of the evidence. *Am Rev Respir Dis* 1993;148:38–48.

133. Burge PS. Occupation and chronic obstructive pulmonary disease (COPD). *Eur Respir J* 1994;7:1032–1034.

134. Zuskin E, Ivankovic D, Schachter EN, et al. A ten-year follow-up study of cotton textile workers. *Am Rev Respir Dis* 1991;143:301–305.

135. Kamat SR, Kamat GR, Salpekar VY, et al. Distinguishing byssinosis from chronic obstructive pulmonary disease. Results of a prospective five-year study of cotton mill workers in India. *Am Rev Respir Dis* 1981;124:31–40.

136. Berry G, McKerrow CB, Molyneux MKB, et al. A study of the acute and chronic changes in the ventilatory capacity of workers in Lancashire cotton mills. *Br J Ind Med* 1973;30:25–36.

137. Glindmeyer HW, Lefante JJ, Jones RN, et al. Exposure-related declines in the lung function of cotton textile workers. Relationship to current workplace standards. *Am Rev Respir Dis* 1991;144:675–683.

138. Dosman JA, Graham BL, Hall D, et al. Respiratory symptoms and pulmonary function in farmers. *J Occup Med* 1987;29:38–43.

139. Korn RJ, Dockery DW, Speizer FE, et al. Occupational exposures and chronic respiratory symptoms. A population-based study. *Am Rev Respir Dis* 1987;136:298–304.

140. Xu X, Christiani DC, Dockery DW, et al. Exposure-response relationships between occupational exposures and chronic respiratory illness: a community-based study. *Am Rev Respir Dis* 1992;146:413–418.

141. Davison AG, Fayersw PM, Newman-Taylor AJ, et al. Cadmium fume inhalation and emphysema. *Lancet* 1988;1:663–667.

142. Humerfelt S, Gulsvik A, Skjaerven R, et al. Decline in FEV$_1$ and airflow limitation related to occupational exposures in men of an urban community. *Eur Respir J* 1993;6:1095–1103.

143. American Thoracic Society, Committee of the Environmental and Occupational Health Assembly, Bascom R, Bromberg PA, Costa DA, et al. Health effects of outdoor air pollution. Part 1. *Am J Respir Crit Care Med* 1996;153:3–50.

144. Detels R, Rokaw SN, Coulson AH, et al. The UCLA population studies of CORD: I. Methodology and comparison of lung function in areas of high and low pollution. *Am J Epidemiol* 1979;109:33–58.

145. Rokaw SN, Detels R, Coulson AH, et al. The UCLA population studies of CORD: III. Comparison of pulmonary function in three communities exposed to photochemical oxidants, multiple primary pollutants, or minimal pollutants. *Chest* 1980;78:252–262.

146. Detels R, Sayre JW, Coulson AH, et al. The UCLA population studies of CORD: IV. Respiratory effect of long-term exposure to photochemical oxidants, nitrogen dioxide, and sulfates on current and never smokers. *Am Rev Respir Dis* 1981;124:673–680.

147. Detels R, Tashkin DP, Sayre JW, et al. The UCLA population studies of CORD: IX. Lung function changes associated with chronic exposure to photochemical oxidants: a cohort study among never-smokers. *Chest* 1987;92:594–603.

148. Detels R, Taskin DP, Sayre JW, et al. The UCLA population study of CORD: X. A cohort study of changes in respiratory function associated with chronic exposure to SOx, NOx, and hydrocarbons. *Am J Public Health* 1991;81:350–359.

149. Dockery DW, Speizer FE, Stram DO, et al. Effects of inhalable particles on respiratory health of children. *Am Rev Respir Dis* 1989;139:587–594.

150. Ware JH, Ferris BG Jr, Dockery DW, et al. Effects of ambient sulfur oxides and suspended particles on respiratory health of preadolescent children. *Am Rev Respir Dis* 1986;133:834–842.

151. Peters JM, Avol E, Gauderman WJ, et al. A study of twelve southern California communities with differing levels and types of air pollution: II. Effects on pulmonary function. *Am J Respir Crit Care Med* 1999;159:768–775.

152. Schwartz J. Lung function and chronic exposure to air pollution: a cross-sectional analysis of NHANES II. *Environ Res* 1989;50:309–321.

153. Abbey DE, Burchette RJ, Knutsen SF, et al. Long-term particulate and other air pollutants and lung function in nonsmokers. *Am J Respir Crit Care Med* 1998;158:289–298.

154. Ackermann-Liebrich U, Leuenberger P, Schwartz J, et al. Lung function and long-term exposure to air pollutants in Switzerland. *Am J Respir Crit Care Med* 1997;155:122–129.

155. Chestnut LG, Schwartz J, Savitz DA, et al. Pulmonary function and ambient particulate matter: epidemiological evidence from NHANES I. *Arch Environ Health* 1991;46:135–144.

156. Sandler DP, Comstock GW, Helsing KJ, et al. Deaths from all causes in non-smokers who lived with smokers. *Am J Public Health* 1989;79:163–167.

157. Kauffmann F, Tessier JF, Oriol P. Adult passive smoking in the home environment: a risk factor for chronic airflow limitation. *Am J Epidemiol* 1983;117:269–280.

158. Svendsen KH, Kuller LH, Martin MJ, et al. Effects of passive smoking in the Multiple Risk Factor Intervention Trial. *Am J Epidemiol* 1987;126:783–795.

159. Hole DJ, Gillis CR, Chopra C, et al. Passive smoking and cardiorespiratory health in a general population in the west of Scotland. *Br Med J* 1989;299:423–427.

160. Masjedi MR, Kazemi H, Johnson DC. Effects of passive smoking on the pulmonary function of adults. *Thorax* 1990;45:27–31.

161. Ng TP, Hui KP, Tan WC. Respiratory symptoms and lung function effects of domestic exposure to tobacco smoke and cooking

by gas in non-smoking women in Singapore. *J Epidemiol Community Health* 1995;47:454–458.

162. Xu X, Li B. Exposure-response relationship between passive smoking and adult pulmonary function. *Am J Respir Crit Care Med* 1995;151:41–46.

163. Kauffmann F, Dockery DW, Speizer FE, et al. Respiratory symptoms and lung function in relation to passive smoking: a comparative study of American and French women. *Int J Epidemiol* 1989;18:334–344.

164. Schilling RSF, Letai AD, Hui SL, et al. Lung function, respiratory disease, and smoking in families. *Am J Epidemiol* 1977;106:274–283.

165. White JR, Froebe HF. Small-airways dysfunction in nonsmokers chronically exposed to tobacco smoke. *N Engl J Med* 1980;302:720–723.

166. Comstock GW, Meyer MB, Helsing KJ, et al. Respiratory effects of household exposures to tobacco smoke and gas cooking. *Am Rev Respir Dis* 1981;124:143–148.

167. Frette C, Barrett-Connor E, Clausen J. Effect of active and passive smoking on ventilatory function in elderly men and women. *Am J Epidemiol* 1996;143:757–765.

168. Brunekreef B, Fischer P, Remijn B, et al. Indoor air pollution and its effect on pulmonary function of adult non-smoking women: III. Passive smoking and pulmonary function. *Int J Epidemiol* 1985;14:227–230.

169. Masi MA, Hanley JA, Ernst P, et al. Environmental exposure to tobacco smoke and lung function in young adults. *Am Rev Respir Dis* 1988;138:296–299.

170. Jaakkola MS, Jaakkola JJK, Becklake MR, et al. Passive smoking and evolution of lung function in young adults. An 8-year longitudinal study. *J Clin Epidemiol* 1995;48:317–327.

171. Pandey MR. Prevalence of chronic bronchitis in a rural community of the hill region of Nepal. *Thorax* 1984;39:331–336.

172. Pandey MR. Domestic smoke pollution and chronic bronchitis in a rural community of the hill region of Nepal. *Thorax* 1984;39:337–339.

173. Dossing M, Khan J, Al-Rabiah F. Risk factors for chronic obstructive lung disease in Saudi Arabia. *Respir Med* 1994;88:519–522.

174. Dennis RJ, Maldonado D, Norman S, et al. Wood smoke exposure and risk for obstructive airways disease among women. *Chest* 1996;109:115–119.

175. Behera D, Jindal SK. Respiratory symptoms in Indian women using domestic cooking fuels. *Chest* 1991;100:385–388.

176. Pérez-Padilla R, Regalado J, Vedal S, et al. Exposure to biomass smoke and chronic airway disease in Mexican women. A case control study. *Am J Respir Crit Care Med* 1996;154:701–706.

177. Burrows B, Knudson RJ, Lebowitz MD. The relationship between childhood respiratory illness and adult obstructive airway disease. *Am Rev Respir Dis* 1977;115:751–760.

178. Samet JA, Tager IB, Speizer FE. The relationship between respiratory illness in childhood and chronic air-flow obstruction in adulthood. *Am Rev Respir Dis* 1983;127:508–523.

179. Gold DR, Tager IB, Wess ST, et al. Acute lower respiratory illness in childhood as a predictor of lung function and chronic respiratory symptoms. *Am Rev Respir Dis* 1989;140:877–884.

180. Strope GL, Stewart PW, Henderson FW, et al. Lung function in school-age children who had mild lower respiratory illnesses in early childhood. *Am Rev Respir Dis* 1991;144:655–662.

181. Tager IB. "Passive smoking" and respiratory health in children—sophistry or cause for concern? *Am Rev Respir Dis* 1986;133:959–961.

182. Burchfiel CM, Higgins MW, Keller JB, et al. Passive smoking in childhood. *Am Rev Respir Dis* 1986;133:966–973.

183. Tager IB, Ngo L, Hanrahan JP. Maternal smoking during pregnancy. *Am J Respir Crit Care Med* 1995;152:977–983.

184. Matsuse T, Hayashi S, Kuwano K, et al. Latent adenoviral infection in the pathogenesis of chronic airways obstruction. *Am Rev Respir Dis* 1992;146:177–184.

185. Vitalis TZ, Kern I, Croome A, et al. The effect of latent adenovirus 5 infection on cigarette smoke–induced lung inflammation. *Eur Respir J* 1998;11:664–669.

186. Schwartz J, Weiss ST. Relationship between dietary vitamin C intake and pulmonary function in the First National Health and Nutrition Examination Survey (NHANES I). *Am J Clin Nutr* 1994;59:110–114.

187. Britton JR, Pavord ID, Richards KA, et al. Dietary antioxidant vitamin intake and lung function in the general population. *Am J Respir Crit Care Med* 1995;151:1383–1387.

188. Ness AR, Khaw KT, Bingham S, et al. Vitamin C status and respiratory function. *Eur J Clin Nutr* 1996;50:573–579.

189. Hu G, Zhang X, Chen J, et al. Dietary vitamin C intake and lung function in rural China. *Am J Epidemiol* 1998;148:594–599.

190. Grievink L, Smit HA, Ocké MC, et al. Dietary intake of antioxidant (pro)-vitamins, respiratory symptoms and pulmonary function: the MORGEN study. *Thorax* 1998;53:166–171.

191. Schünemann HJ, McCann S, Grant BJB, et al. Lung function in relation to intake of carotenoids and other antioxidant vitamins in a population-based study. *Am J Epidemiol* 2002;155:463–471.

192. Schünemann HJ, Grant GJB, Feudenheim JL, et al. The relation of serum levels of antioxidant vitamins C and E, retinal and carotenoids with pulmonary function in the general population. *Am J Respir Crit Care Med* 2001;163:1246–1255.

193. Hu G, Cassano PA. Antioxidant nutrients and pulmonary function: the third National Health and Nutrition Survey (NHANES III). *Am J Epidemiol* 2000;151:975–981.

194. Chuwers P, Barnhart S, Blanc P, et al. The protective effect of β-carotene and retinal on ventilatory function in an asbestos exposed cohort. *Am J Respir Crit Care Med* 1997;155:1066–1071.

195. Grievink L, DeWaart FG, Schouten EG, et al. Serum carotenoids, α-tocopherol, and lung function among Dutch elderly. *Am J Respir Crit Care Med* 2000;161:790–795.

196. Schwartz J, Weiss ST. The relationship of dietary fish intake to level of pulmonary function in the first National Health and Nutrition Survey (NHANES I). *Eur Respir J* 1994;7:1821–1824.

197. Sharp DS, Rodriguez BL, Shahar E, et al. Fish consumption may limit the damage of smoking on the lung. *Am J Respir Crit Care Med* 1994;150:983–987.

198. Butland BK, Fehili AM, Elwood PC. Diet, lung function, and lung function decline in a cohort of 2,512 middle-aged men. *Thorax* 2000;55:102–108.

COPD: Clinical Manifestations, Diagnosis, and Treatment

Tushar J. Desai · Joel B. Karlinsky

In light of advances in understanding the pathogenesis of chronic obstructive pulmonary disease (COPD), the Global Initiative for Chronic Obstructive Lung Disease (GOLD) committee, a collaborative project of the U.S. National Heart, Lung, and Blood Institute (NHLBI) and the World Health Organization (WHO), has proposed an updated definition of COPD. In the past, COPD had generally been defined as airflow obstruction that is not fully reversible and is caused by either chronic bronchitis or emphysema (1). Chronic bronchitis is defined clinically by the presence of productive cough for 3 months in each of two consecutive years in the absence of other causes for the cough, and emphysema is pathologically defined as the abnormal permanent enlargement of the air spaces distal to the terminal bronchioles, accompanied by destruction of their walls and without obvious fibrosis (2, 3). This previous characterization was conceptually awkward because it combined a physiologic parameter, airflow obstruction, with both a clinical entity, chronic bronchitis, and a pathologic criterion, emphysema. Additionally, in most individuals with COPD, small-airway disease owing to obstructive bronchiolitis as well as reduced lung elasticity and loss of airway tethering due to parenchymal destruction from emphysema both contribute to airflow limitation.

The 2001 GOLD revision emphasizes that COPD represents an underlying active inflammatory disease of the airways that is distinct from asthma and is not merely the manifestation of progressive lung destruction owing to the cumulative toxic effects of cigarette smoke. GOLD defines COPD as "a disease state characterized by airflow limitation that is not fully reversible. The airflow limitation is usually both progressive and associated with an abnormal inflammatory response of the lungs to noxious particles or gases" (4). Airflow obstruction from asthma, believed to be a distinct entity with a different pathogenesis, is specifically excluded from the definition of COPD, except in cases in which the obstruction is not fully reversible, such as in unremitting asthma with airway remodeling, or when these two diseases coexist in an individual.

EPIDEMIOLOGY

Because the epidemiology of COPD is discussed comprehensively in Chapter 11, only the major points will be emphasized here. In the United States, the third National Health and Nutrition Examination Survey (NHANES III), conducted from 1988–1994, found the prevalence of airflow obstruction (defined by forced expiratory volume in 1 second [FEV_1]/forced vital capacity [FVC] < 0.70) in white men to be 14.2% among current smokers, 6.9% among ex-smokers, and 3.3% among never-smokers. Among white women, these prevalence data were 13.6%, 6.8%, and 3.1%, respectively. The prevalence rates of airflow obstruction were similar, but slightly lower, among black men and women (5). An important finding from NHANES III was the significant extent to which chronic airflow obstruction is underdiagnosed in the United States. Over 70% of the surveyed individuals who demonstrated airflow limitation did not have a diagnosis of obstructive lung disease. Even among individuals with an FEV_1 diminished to below 50% of predicted, over 45% did not carry a diagnosis of obstructive lung disease in NHANES III (6). More recent evidence corroborates that primary care physicians continue to underuse spirometry and that a gender bias exists that results in increased underdiagnosis among women (7).

The worldwide prevalence of COPD in 1990 was estimated by the WHO/World Bank Global Burden of Disease

T. J. Desai and **J. B. Karlinsky:** Pulmonary and Critical Care Medicine, VA Boston Healthcare System, West Roxbury, Massachusetts.

Study to be 9.34 per 1,000 in men and 7.33 per 1,000 in women, and many experts believe these data underestimated the true prevalence (8). The death rate attributable to COPD among male Americans in 2000 was 82.6 per 100,000 and among females, 56.7 per 100,000. Although the death rate for men has remained relatively stable, it has been increasing significantly among women, and in 2000, for the first time, the number of women dying from COPD was greater than the number of men (9). Worldwide, the burden of COPD is projected to move up from the 12th leading cause of disability-adjusted life-years in 1990 to fourth in 2020 (10). Data on the health care costs of COPD is unfortunately scant, but according to estimates by the NHLBI, the annual cost to the United States of COPD in 2000 was $30.4 billion (11). Despite its significant and increasing impact in the United States, COPD receives disproportionately less funding from the National Institutes of Health than do other diseases with lower morbidity and mortality (12).

EPIDEMIOLOGY OF CHRONIC OBSTRUCTIVE PULMONARY DISEASE	
Summary Statement	**Level of Evidence**
COPD is underdiagnosed, even in individuals with moderate airflow obstruction.	Observation data
The global economic and health burden of COPD is significant and continues to increase.	Observational data

COPD, chronic obstructive pulmonary disease.

RISK FACTORS FOR CHRONIC OBSTRUCTIVE PULMONARY DISEASE

COPD results from the modulation of external causative factors by host factors inherent in susceptible individuals. Cigarette smoke has been identified as the most important external risk factor for COPD, and the risk is proportional to the cumulative inhaled exposure. Other environmental risk factors include pipe and cigar smoke; occupational dust and chemical exposures, such as those encountered by miners; and indoor air pollution caused by the use of biomass fuel for cooking or heating in the absence of adequate ventilation. Less precisely characterized external risk factors for COPD include a history of severe childhood respiratory infections, HIV infection, outdoor air pollution, and low socioeconomic status. As would be expected, the relevance of particular factors varies significantly between industrialized and developing regions of the world.

Although environmental factors are important, the development of clinically significant COPD requires a susceptible host, as evidenced by the finding that up to 85% to 90% of cigarette smokers may not develop airflow obstruction (13). Identified host risk factors for COPD include airways hyper-responsiveness to methacholine challenge and

TABLE 12.1. RISK FACTORS FOR CHRONIC OBSTRUCTIVE PULMONARY DISEASE

Environmental	Host-Related
Cigarette smoking	Airway hyperresponsiveness
Indoor air pollution from biomass fuel use in setting of inadequate ventilation	Genetic factors (poorly characterized)
Occupational dusts and chemicals	Severe hereditary α_1-antitrypsin deficiency
History of severe childhood respiratory infection	Low birthweight
Pipe/cigar smoking	Maternal cigarette smoking during gestation
HIV infection (118)	
Outdoor air pollution	
Low socioeconomic status	
Intravenous drug use (methylphenidate, methadone, talc granulomatosis (119, 120)	

low birthweight, although the former may be a consequence of smoking rather than an independent risk factor. To date, the best characterized genetic risk factor is severe hereditary α_1-antitrypsin (AAT) deficiency, which accounts for less than 1% of the burden of COPD. The importance of other genetic factors is suggested by familial clustering of early-onset COPD and racial differences in the prevalence of airflow obstruction. The genetic factors associated with the development of COPD with rapid progression of lung function decline are likely to be numerous. This is an intense area of current research that has been enabled by the advent of powerful molecular research tools (14). The hope is that identifying these associations will prove useful in elucidating the specific inflammatory and proteolytic pathways that culminate in emphysema, with the ultimate goal of translating these discoveries into targeted therapy for COPD (15). Table 12.1 lists the external and host-related independent risk factors for COPD.

ETIOLOGY OF CHRONIC OBSTRUCTIVE PULMONARY DISEASE	
Summary Statement	**Level of Evidence**
Chronic obstructive pulmonary disease results from an interaction between a susceptible host and potentially modifiable environmental factors.	Large body of observational data

PATHOPHYSIOLOGY OF CHRONIC OBSTRUCTIVE PULMONARY DISEASE

COPD is a progressive condition characterized by inflammation of airway mucosa associated with mucus gland hypertrophy, hyperplasia of goblet cells, and destruction of alveolar septae with a reduction of diffusing surface area (1). A neutrophilic inflammatory reaction may be found in the mucosa and submucosa of airways as opposed to the lymphocytic reaction found in asthma (4). There may be intraluminal mucus plugging and hypertrophy of airway smooth muscle. The inflammatory reaction that occurs is nonspecific and is similar to that seen in other conditions, such as bronchiectasis and cystic fibrosis. Small respiratory bronchioles (<2 mm diameter) are particularly involved and may eventually become fibrosed. Loss of alveolar septae produces decreases in elastic recoil and reduced tethering of small airways. All the above mechanisms lead to increases in dynamic airway compression and a fixed increase in airflow resistance during the expiratory phase of respiration, which is the characteristic finding of this condition. These physiologic alterations serve to produce the sensation of dyspnea. The relative contributions of loss of elastic recoil and increased airflow resistance to the increase in breathlessness is difficult to assess in any individual. Moreover, there are little data regarding the pathologic correlates of an acute exacerbation of COPD, other than the finding of "bronchiolitis" in 26% of individuals who died during an exacerbation (16).

Pathologically, three subtypes of emphysema have been described: centrilobular, centriacinar, and paraseptal disease. Centrilobular emphysema begins in the center of the anatomical lobule and expands outward to eventually involve the entire structure. It is associated with cigarette smoking and predominantly affects the upper lung zones, reducing recruitable diffusing surface. Centriacinar emphysema begins in the respiratory bronchiole, primarily affects the lower lung zones, and is associated with a higher degree of inflammation than is centrilobular disease. This subtype is the form typically found in individuals with AAT deficiency–associated emphysema. Paraseptal emphysema affects mainly distal, peripheral lung zones, alveolar ducts, and sacs, and is associated with parenchymal fibrous stranding and bullae formation (Fig. 12.1A,B).

In addition to structural alterations in airways and lung parenchyma, skeletal muscle abnormalities contribute to the pathophysiology and symptomatology of COPD (17, 18). Reduction in fat-free muscle mass and atrophy of type I slow and type IIa fast myosin subtypes with concomitant increases in fast type IIb myosin have been identified in the

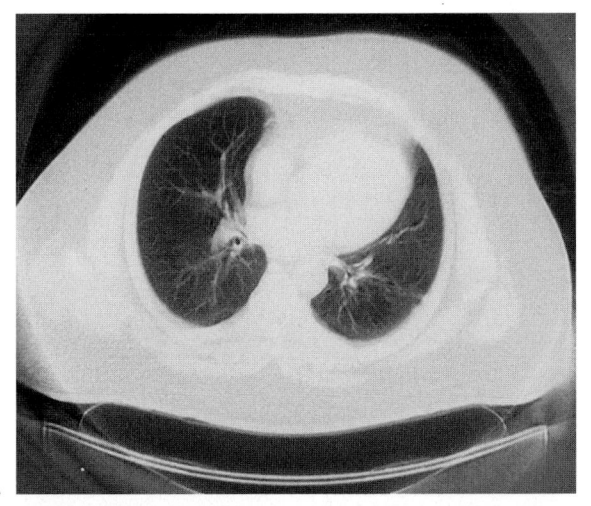

A

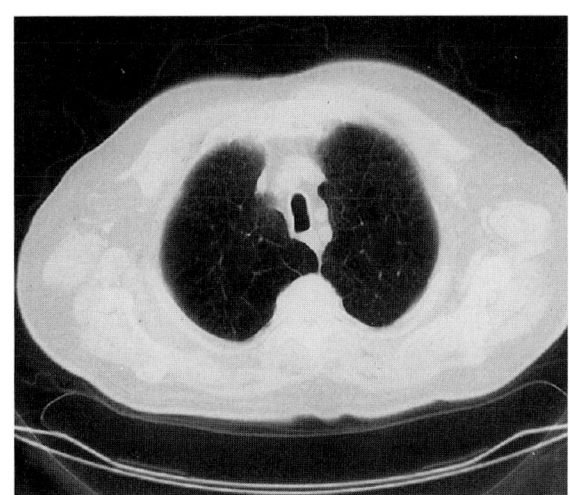

B

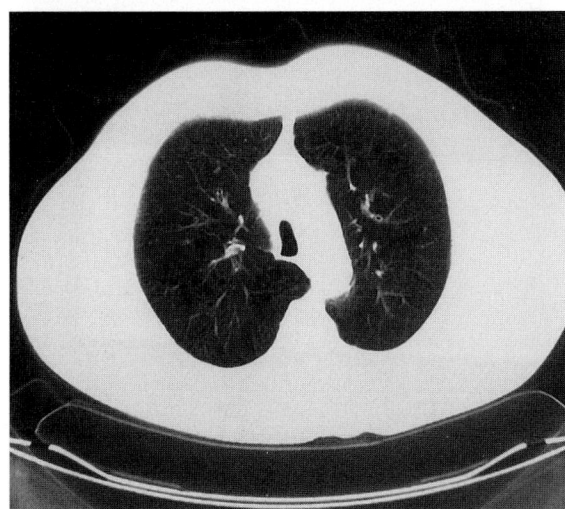

C

FIGURE 12.1. (A) Section of a computed tomography (CT) scan of normal lung with a normal ratio of air to tissue density. There are no enlarged air spaces. **(B)** Section of a CT scan of emphysematous lung revealing enlarged, peripherally located air spaces suggestive of both centrilobular and paraseptal emphysema. **(C)** A more cephalad section of a CT scan of the same emphysematous lung, revealing several small bullae.

peripheral skeletal muscles of individuals with COPD (19). In addition, studies have shown that the density of capillaries in peripheral muscle is also decreased. These changes may occur as muscles adapt to disuse and/or decreases in maximal oxygen delivery during exercise or even perhaps to adapt to nutritional deficiencies (20, 21). As expected, there are associated reductions in muscle strength, with greater decrements found in the lower versus the upper limbs. The data concerning muscle endurance are less clear. A fast-to-slow myosin transformation has been described in the diaphragms of individuals with COPD, which could improve endurance (22).

Diaphragm muscle energetics are also altered with increases in adenosine triphosphate (ATP)-generating capacity relative to ATP utilization having been reported. Muscle breakdown during exercise may be greater in COPD than in normal individuals (23,24). Current research is focused on studying the use of anabolic steroids in conjunction with exercise and nutritional supplementation to increase lower extremity muscle mass, strength, and endurance to reduce exercise-induced dyspnea (25–27).

DIAGNOSIS OF CHRONIC OBSTRUCTIVE PULMONARY DISEASE

Initial Presentation

COPD typically presents in the fifth decade of life with the insidious onset of a chronic cough productive of small amounts of mucoid sputum in the mornings, in association with a history of more than 20 pack-years of cigarette smoking. Such individuals may seek medical attention for an acute chest illness, manifesting with dyspnea, increased sputum production, and possibly wheezing. Others may not present until in their 50s or 60s, with the onset of progressive exertional dyspnea. Patients may report a history of wheezing and prior treatment for asthma.

COPD should be suspected in individuals with appropriate risk factors and respiratory complaints of cough, sputum production, or dyspnea. In such patients, the cumulative pack-years of cigarette smoking, a complete occupational and environmental exposure history, a family history of respiratory disorders, and any personal history of asthma, atopy, sinusitis, nasal polyposis, or respiratory triggers should all be elicited. The patient should also be asked about a history of severe childhood respiratory infections, tuberculosis, and injection drug use or other HIV risk factors.

The review of systems should focus on distinguishing between possible causes of the respiratory symptoms. For example, a report of large volumes of purulent sputum production could indicate bronchiectasis. A history of hemoptysis, although common in COPD from erosion of the airway mucosa, could suggest a space-occupying mass in the proximal airways or a pulmonary embolism. Significant daily variability in symptoms could represent airflow obstruction from

asthma. Episodic dyspnea associated with anxiety in a young adult could indicate a panic attack or vocal cord dysfunction syndrome, also known as laryngeal dyskinesia. A list of common causes of airflow obstruction and clues to their diagnosis is provided in Table 12.2.

Physical examination of the lungs may reveal a prolonged expiratory phase, wheezing, or diminished breath sounds in all lung fields. The anteroposterior diameter of the thorax may be increased from chronic hyperinflation of the lungs ("barrel chest"). In advanced COPD, accessory muscle use, pursed lip breathing, or inward retraction of the lower intercostal muscles on inspiration ("Hoover's sign") may be present. Patients with severe disease often favor sitting in the "tripod position," in which the arms are supported on a fixed surface, thereby enabling the upper thorax to serve as a fulcrum for the strap muscles to assist with inspiration. Peripheral edema could represent right-sided

TABLE 12.2. DIAGNOSIS OF AIRFLOW OBSTRUCTION

Differential Diagnosis of Airflow Obstruction (FEV$_1$/ FVC <70% predicted)	Clues to Diagnosis
Asthma	Reversible to normal with bronchodilators, D$_{LCO}$ normal or high
COPD	>20 pack-years, age >40; D$_{LCO}$ low
Bronchiectasis	Large volumes of purulent sputum
Congestive heart failure	Orthopnea, edema, hepato-jugular reflux
Cystic fibrosis	White, young; extrapulmonary signs
Sarcoidosis	African-American descent; thoracic LAD
BOOP/COP	Nonsegmental, peripheral infiltrates
Obstructive bronchiolar disorders (e.g., OB, respiratory bronchiolitis, panbronchiolitis)	Chest x-ray hyperinflated, mosaic pattern of expiratory air-trapping on chest HRCT
Upper airway obstruction (e.g., subglottic tracheal stenosis, vocal cord paresis)	Localized wheeze on auscultation, flattening of flow-volume loop
Vocal cord dysfunction syndrome	Female >> male; young, episodic symptoms
Postpulmonary tuberculosis (121)	Chest x-ray compatible with prior tuberculosis pneumonia
Post-thoracoplasty	Elderly; history of therapeutic thoracoplasty with or without plombage
Kyphoscoliosis	Observed on physical examination or chest x-ray
Normal/supraphysiologic lung function	Young athlete; FEV$_1$ normal or increased

FEV$_1$, forced expiratory volume in 1s; FVC, forced vital capacity; COPD, chronic obstructive pulmonary disease; D$_{LCO}$, lung diffusing capacity for carbon monoxide; LAD, lymphadenopathy; BOOP/COP, bronchiolitis obliterans organizing pneumonia/cryptogenic organizing pneumonia; OB, obliterative bronchiolitis; HRCT, high-resolution computed tomography.

heart failure, although in patients with COPD, lower extremity edema may be present in the absence of significant pulmonary hypertension (28). The finding of digital clubbing, which is not a feature of COPD, should raise suspicion for an alternative diagnosis such as bronchiectasis or lung carcinoma, and could indicate the presence of a systemic shunt.

The main utility of physical examination lies not in diagnosing COPD but rather in guiding further workup by excluding or suggesting alternate causes for a patient's respiratory symptoms. The clinician should bear in mind that physical findings are both insensitive and nonspecific for diagnosing COPD. In one blinded study involving COPD patients with moderate airflow obstruction, defined by an FEV_1 or FEV_1/FVC less than 60% predicted, the finding of diminished breath sounds was only 65% sensitive, even when combined with a history of self-reported COPD or more than 70 pack-years of smoking (29). In another blinded study, the combined use of an abnormal respiratory history and physical examination in predicting the presence of airflow obstruction yielded a sensitivity and specificity of only 53% and 65%, respectively (30).

DIAGNOSIS OF CHRONIC OBSTRUCTIVE PULMONARY DISEASE	
Summary Statement	**Level of Evidence**
A diagnosis other than COPD should be considered in patients with respiratory symptoms who are <40 y, have less than a 20 pack-year smoking history, or have digital clubbing.	Observational data
Physical examination is of limited utility in diagnosing or excluding COPD, but may help guide further workup by suggesting alternative etiologies for respiratory symptoms.	Several small randomized trials

COPD, chronic obstructive pulmonary disease.

Radiographic Studies

It is generally agreed that a chest x-ray (CXR) should be obtained as part of the initial workup of all patients suspected of having COPD. As is the case with physical examination, the main utility of the CXR lies in excluding or suggesting alternate diagnoses, such as congestive heart failure, that could cause a patient's respiratory symptoms. In individuals with severe emphysema, the CXR may reveal bilateral lung hyperinflation with flattened diaphragms or the presence of bullae, characterized by thin arcuate lines circumscribing areas of radiolucency. It is important to bear in mind, however, that a normal CXR does not exclude the presence of emphysema. In one study, spirometry and chest high-resolution computed tomography (CT) were performed on individuals with more than 30 pack-years of smoking and normal

CXRs. The investigators found that 58% of these individuals had CT evidence of significant emphysema, and there was a positive correlation of pack-years with CT scoring of severity (31).

The CXR may also reveal radiographic changes of pulmonary hypertension in COPD patients with chronic hypoxemia, consisting of enlarged pulmonary arteries, "pruned" or poorly visualized peripheral vasculature, and, on lateral view, right ventricular encroachment into the retrosternal air space. In a relatively young individual of northern European descent with or without a smoking history, CXR findings of basilar-predominant emphysema should raise suspicion for COPD associated with severe hereditary deficiency of AAT. If the CXR suggests significant hyperinflation with upper lobe bullae, consideration should be given to specialty referral for potential lung-volume reduction surgery (LVRS) candidates, discussed in detail later in this chapter. Very rarely, a CXR may reveal giant bullae, for which high-resolution chest CT scanning and physiologic testing could be pursued in selected patients to determine if bullectomy is indicated. In the absence of these or other special indications, there is no role for obtaining a chest CT scan as part of the routine assessment of COPD. Chest high-resolution CT has been demonstrated to be very sensitive in detecting the presence of emphysema, but less reliable in distinguishing between pathologic subtypes (32).

Pulmonary Function Testing

The cornerstone of COPD diagnosis is the demonstration of airflow obstruction by spirometry, usually defined as an FEV_1/FVC ratio of less than 0.7 and an FEV_1 less than 80% predicted. A reduced FEV_1/FVC ratio in conjunction with an FEV_1 within the normal range may indicate early COPD, although this combination can also be observed in athletes with supraphysiologic lung function. It is generally recommended that all patients with COPD perform spirometry with bronchodilator testing to assess for significant reversibility of airflow obstruction. The American Thoracic Society (ATS) defines reversibility as an acute FEV_1 increase after a dose of an inhaled β_2-agonist that is both greater than 12% and more than 200 mL above the pre-dose FEV_1 value. Although bronchodilator therapy should be instituted for symptomatic individuals regardless of the presence or absence of reversibility, testing is useful both in helping to assess for asthma, in which the spirometry may normalize, and because the postbronchodilator FEV_1 is the best predictor of survival in COPD identified to date.

Lung volumes need not be routinely measured in individuals with COPD, but are an important part of the evaluation of patients for LVRS or giant bullae resection. The diffusing capacity of the lung for carbon monoxide (D_{LCO}) likewise does not merit routine measurement, but its severe reduction identifies COPD patients at high mortality risk from surgery involving pulmonary resection, such as LVRS or lobectomy.

The DLCO can also be useful in evaluating COPD patients with oxygen desaturation or dyspnea that is more severe than would be expected based on the degree of airflow limitation. In this clinical setting, a significant reduction in DLCO could represent either primary or secondary pulmonary hypertension, chronic nocturnal hypoxemia from undiagnosed sleep apnea, or possibly chronic pulmonary thromboembolic disease. In cases in which the clinician cannot confidently distinguish between asthma and COPD as the cause of airflow obstruction, an elevated DLCO favors the former diagnosis. This phenomenon of a high diffusing capacity, which can also be observed after recent pulmonary hemorrhage, is not a finding in emphysema.

Additional physiologic testing may be useful for COPD patients in whom concomitant ventilatory impairments are suspected, such as for individuals with dyspnea out of proportion to the degree of airflow limitation. Inspection of repeated flow-volume loops may reveal a sawtooth pattern or reproducible flattening of one or both limbs, suggestive of upper airway obstruction. With clinically significant diaphragm paresis, in addition to the finding of abdominal paradox on physical examination, the vital capacity may be reduced by 20% or more when measured in the supine position compared with the upright position. Diaphragm paresis can be confirmed either with a "sniff test" under fluoroscopy that demonstrates paradoxical diaphragm motion on inspiration, or quantitatively by directly measuring transdiaphragmatic pressure gradients generated during respiratory maneuvers. The latter testing is performed through the use of simultaneous gastric and esophageal balloon manometry.

The maximal inspiratory and expiratory pressures or maximal voluntary ventilation can be obtained as initial evaluation for a systemic myasthenic syndrome or myopathy involving the respiratory muscles, such as that induced by systemic steroids. In clinical practice, however, these measures are effort-dependent and of only limited usefulness. Specialty referral for directed neurologic testing or tissue biopsy may be more appropriate when these diagnoses are a consideration. Finally, cardiopulmonary exercise testing (CPET) can be performed in symptomatic individuals with COPD in whom additional possible etiologies for functional limitation exist, such as cardiac dysfunction, exercise-induced asthma, deconditioning, or a concomitant restrictive ventilatory defect. The CPET results may guide the clinician to direct clinical interventions toward ameliorating the factors responsible for limiting an individual's exercise tolerance, with the goal of improving functional performance.

Ancillary Testing

In the COPD patient with mild airflow limitation (FEV_1 > 60% predicted), no further routine testing is necessary. With moderate or severe obstruction, however, additional tests should be obtained (Table 12.3). Resting pulse oximetry should be checked, and if less than 92%, arterial blood

TABLE 12.3. RECOMMENDED INITIAL WORKUP OF CHRONIC OBSTRUCTIVE PULMONARY DISEASE

Degree of Airflow Limitation	Rationale
All patients	
History and physical examination	Assists with differential diagnosis
Spirometry prebronchodilator and postbronchodilator	If airflow normalizes, indicates asthma
Chest x-ray	Helps to exclude congestive heart failure, bullae, and alternate etiologies for respiratory symptoms
Moderate to severe obstruction:	FEV_1 <50% predicted
Resting and/or exercise pulse oximetry	May suggest need for LTOT
If FEV_1 <1 L, resting oximetry <92%, or hypercapnia suspected (asterixis, h/o morning headaches), obtain arterial blood gas	Assess for degree of hypoxemia and/or baseline hypercapnia
Selected patients	
Hematocrit	LTOT if polycythemic
Electrocardiogram	Cor pulmonale, arrhythmia or prior MI
Cardiac ultrasound	Cardiomyopathy or valvular disease, pulmonary hypertension, cor pulmonale
DLCO	Discriminate from asthma, suggest concomitant pulmonary vascular disease
	Amenability for surgical therapy for emphysema
Lung volume measurements	
Chest HRCT scan	
Serum α_1-antitrypsin level	Characterize distribution of emphysema if potential candidate for LVRS or bullectomy, bronchiectasis
	Early-onset, low environmental risk factors, northern European descent, basilar-predominant emphysema, family history

FEV_1, forced expiratory volume in 1 s LTOT, long-term oxygen therapy; DLCO, diffusing capacity of lungs for carbon monoxide; LVRS, lung-volume reduction surgery.

gas measurement is indicated to assess for hypoxemia. The use of a threshold oximetry value of 92% has demonstrated a sensitivity and specificity of 100% and 86%, respectively, for identifying individuals who should be prescribed long-term oxygen therapy (LTOT) (33). Exercise oximetry can assess if supplemental oxygen is needed with exertion, or to titrate the liter-flow in patients who already require oxygen at rest. An electrocardiogram (ECG) should be obtained if the heart rhythm is irregular or if left-sided heart disease is suspected, because it may reveal atrial fibrillation, left ventricular hypertrophy, or signs of a prior myocardial infarction for which echocardiography or cardiology consultation might be indicated. In COPD patients with pulmonary hypertension, the ECG may suggest right atrial hypertrophy ("P pulmonale," or tall P waves [>2.5 mm] in leads II, III, aVF) or right ventricular hypertrophy (right-axis deviation, dominant R wave in V_1 [≥7 mm], ST depression, and T wave inversions in the right precordial chest leads V_1–V_4). Low-amplitude QRS complexes can be seen in COPD with lung hyperinflation, which can also displace the diaphragm inferiorly and cause clockwise rotation of the heart along its longitudinal axis. This cardiac rotation may manifest on ECG as a "pseudoinfarct" pattern, with poor R-wave progression and deep S waves in the right precordial leads that resemble the QS waves seen after an anterior myocardial infarction. Although up to two thirds of COPD patients have abnormal ECGs, the findings discussed above are not sensitive or specific for right-sided heart disease and therefore should not be relied on to diagnose or exclude cor pulmonale.

If cor pulmonale is suspected based on either ECG, CXR, or clinical findings of right-sided heart failure (such as hepatomegaly, lower extremity edema, or the auscultation of a right-sided S_3 or loud P_2), an echocardiogram can be obtained to confirm the diagnosis. In addition to assessing right heart function and estimating pulmonary artery pressures, a cardiac echo can provide information on left ventricular size and function and rule out significant valvular disease.

If airflow obstruction is severe, with an FEV_1 less than 1 L or if a patient has symptoms or signs potentially owing to hypercapnia (such as morning headache, cognitive impairment, or asterixis), an arterial blood gas (ABG) should be obtained to measure the arterial partial pressure of carbon dioxide ($Paco_2$). In addition to serving as a marker of poor prognosis, the presence of chronic hypercapnia should raise the clinician's vigilance about minimizing the use in that patient of medications that depress respiration, because they could precipitate an acute respiratory acidosis with clinical decompensation. Table 12.3 provides a summary of diagnostic recommendations for initial workup of COPD.

Sleep and Chronic Obstructive Pulmonary Disease

Sleep-disordered breathing in COPD may manifest either as nocturnal hypoventilation with oxygen desaturation in patients with severe airflow obstruction or as coexistent sleep apnea. The physiologic hypoventilation that normally results in mild hypercapnia during sleep is much more significant in COPD patients, particularly during the rapid eye movement (REM) sleep stage, when the ability of intercostal muscles to contribute to ventilation is markedly reduced. Although these mechanisms of hypoventilation have been well-characterized, there are little data on the efficacy of treatment. In one prospective randomized trial involving COPD patients who desaturated to less than 85% during sleep, nocturnal oxygen therapy for 3 years showed no survival benefit over placebo, despite the finding that patients with desaturations during REM sleep had a significantly higher mortality

(34). Studies of respiratory stimulants and theophylline have likewise not demonstrated any convincing evidence of benefit. Based on the limited body of data, the ATS recommends treating COPD patients already receiving daytime LTOT with nocturnal oxygen empirically set at a flow rate of 1 L/min greater than the daytime rate. Alternatively, based on physician preference or for individuals with secondary erythrocytosis or cor pulmonale, overnight oximetry can be performed with oxygen titration to determine the flow rate necessary to maintain saturation greater than 89% during sleep.

The incidence of sleep apnea in COPD patients is estimated to be 10% to 15%, and their coexistence has been termed "the overlap syndrome" (35). Sleep apnea should be considered in COPD patients with a history of snoring, daytime hypersomnolence, obesity or significant weight gain, hypertension, facial features associated with obstructive sleep apnea, or manifestations of hypoxemia, such as cor pulmonale or secondary erythrocytosis that are out of proportion to the awake arterial oxygen tension. If sleep apnea is clinically suspected, full polysomnography should be performed and appropriate therapy instituted if the diagnosis is confirmed.

Staging of Disease

The impact of any disease on an individual's overall state of well-being and prognosis depends on a combination of factors such as the degree of physiologic impairment, symptomatology, rate of disease progression, and interactions of the disease with comorbid conditions. The ideal way to grade disease severity and estimate prognosis would be to integrate these relevant variables into a validated staging system that could be applied to all individuals with the disease. However, because of the lack of a generally accepted staging tool for COPD, the degree of airflow impairment measured by spirometry generally serves as a marker of disease severity. Although suboptimal, because it does not take into account important variables such as smoking status and rate of decline of lung function, the postbronchodilator FEV_1 is the best predictor of mortality in COPD identified to date (36). As examples, in COPD patients age 65 or younger, cumulative survival at 5 years with postbronchodilator FEV_1 50% to 59% predicted is 95%, whereas the 2-year survival with FEV_1 30% to 39% predicted is 83%.

The GOLD committee has proposed classification of COPD severity into four stages based on empiric cutoffs of postbronchodilator FEV_1 expressed as a percentage of the predicted value (Table 12.4). GOLD stage 0, which encompasses individuals with respiratory symptoms but without airflow obstruction, was shown to not be useful in predicting subsequent development of COPD (37). Until a more comprehensive, validated staging system with better predictive ability is developed and gains general acceptance, the postbronchodilator FEV_1 will continue to be used for staging,

TABLE 12.4. GOLD CLASSIFICATION OF SEVERITY

Stage	Severity	Criteria	Associations
0	At risk	Chronic productive cough with normal lung function (FEV_1 >80% predicted)	Smoking
I	Mild	FEV_1/FVC <70% but FEV_1 ≥80% predicted	Chronic cough and sputum production, not dyspneic; do not seek medical attention
IIa	Moderate	FEV_1 = 50%–80% predicted and FEV_1/FVC <70%	Exertional dyspnea; seek medical attention or present with exacerbation
IIb	Moderate	FEV_1 = 30%–50% predicted and FEV_1/FVC <70%	As in stage IIa, but higher frequency of exacerbations
III	Severe	FEV_1 <30% predicted *or* FEV_1 <50% predicted along with either respiratory failure (Pao_2 < 60 mm Hg breathing ambient air at sea level), clinical signs of cor pulmonale and FEV_1/FVC <70%	Functional capacity severely limited owing to dyspnea, usually hypercapnic, on LTOT.

FEV_1, forced expiratory volume in 1 s; FVC, forced vital capacity; Pao_2, arterial blood partial pressure of oxygen; LTOT, long-term oxygen therapy.

despite its limited accuracy in predicting outcomes for individuals with COPD.

MANAGEMENT OF STABLE CHRONIC OBSTRUCTIVE PULMONARY DISEASE

Monitoring of Disease

As is the case for the initial staging of disease, there are no uniformly accepted parameters to use in monitoring COPD progression. Individuals with the same degree of airflow limitation at the time of diagnosis can go on to experience drastically different outcomes. Multiple observational studies have identified predictors of COPD progression, measured in terms of rapidity of subsequent lung function decline and mortality, as outlined in Table 12.5. Relevant monitoring parameters in COPD may be clinical, such as symptoms or respiratory quality of life questionnaires; spirometric, based on progression of airflow limitation; or functional, based on 6-minute walk distance or other indices of exercise capacity.

TABLE 12.5. PREDICTORS OF CHRONIC OBSTRUCTIVE PULMONARY DISEASE PROGRESSION

Variable	Outcome
Peak flow, postbronchodilator FEV_1, low BMI (122), dyspnea level (123), baseline hypercapnia, untreated hypoxemia	Mortality
Cigarette smoking, frequency of lower respiratory infection in current smokers (124), HIV infection (118), methacholine reactivity	Rapid decline in lung function

FEV_1, forced expiratory volume in 1 s; BMI, body mass index.

The postbronchodilator FEV_1, although linked with mortality, does not constitute an assessment of health-related quality of life, which may be more tightly associated with variables such as dyspnea, fatigue, ability to function independently, and frequency of exacerbations. In fact, a low FEV_1 is relatively poorly correlated with lower health status, and gains in health status correlate better with improved exercise performance than with changes in FEV_1 (38).

Sensitive instruments that assess respiratory-related quality of life include the Chronic Respiratory Questionnaire and the St. George Respiratory Questionnaire (SGRQ) (39, 40). The SGRQ has been validated both in discriminating health status levels between individuals with similar degrees of airflow obstruction, and in assessing the effect of therapy on the health status of a given individual. The main role of these tools is for use in population-based trials to assess for the benefit of a therapy on health-related quality of life, which could prove significant even in the absence of a mortality benefit. In assessing for a response to therapy on an individual basis, both the patient's self-assessment of benefit and the clinician's judgment of overall treatment efficacy have been shown to correlate reasonably well with an improvement in SGRQ score. Eliciting specific semiquantitative examples of perceived benefit, such as decreased breathlessness, increased functional capacity, or improved sleep, can also be helpful in assessing for a therapeutic benefit (38).

Health Promotion and Complication Prevention

The primary caregiver should encourage both general and respiratory disease-specific preventive health care measures for all patients with COPD, even for those who continue smoking. Although the adverse health effects of smoking are well characterized and widely known, cigarette smoking remains the leading cause of preventable death in the United States. In addition to COPD, the health risks of smoking include an increased dose-dependent risk of lung cancer and other malignancies, coronary heart disease, and stroke. Observational data from a large British cohort of 35-year-old male physicians who smoked indicated that over the subsequent 35 years, half of the deaths were attributable to smoking (41). From 1995–1999, the U.S. Center for Disease Control estimated the annual health-related economic losses owing to smoking to be approximately $157 billion (42).

Occupational exposures in smokers associated with an augmented risk of lung cancer include arsenic, silica, diesel exhaust, and aromatic amines. Work exposures to asbestos and, in uranium miners, to radon, are particularly significant, because they interact synergistically with smoking to result in a tremendously increased risk of lung cancer. In the case of the former exposure, the risk of lung cancer is markedly increased for smokers who have evidence of interstitial fibrosis from asbestos exposure. Estimates of the risk of cancer owing to cigarette smoking are variable, but a fourfold risk of lung cancer owing to the presence of COPD that is independent of smoking history has also been observed (43).

Fortunately, health benefits from smoking cessation can be achieved from quitting, well into adulthood. One study estimated that smokers who quit at age 35 had a life expectancy that exceeded that of continuing smokers by 6.9 to 8.5 years for men and by 6.1 to 7.7 years for women. Even if quitting smoking occurred at age 65, these gains were 1.4 to 2.0 and 2.7 to 3.7 for men and women, respectively (44). Another epidemiologic survey analyzed data from two large case control studies of smoking prevalence in the United Kingdom, one from 1950 and the other from 1990, in order to elucidate the health impact of continued long-term cigarette smoking and of sustained cessation. The investigators found a cumulative risk of lung cancer by age 75 for men who continued to smoke of 15.9%, compared with 9.9%, 6.0%, 3.0%, and 1.7% in men who stopped around 60, 50, 40, and 30 years of age, respectively. For women, the cumulative risk of lung cancer by age 75 in continued smokers was 9.5%, compared with 5.3% and 2.2% in women who stopped around 60 and 50 years of age, respectively (45).

Although various therapies can improve quality of life for symptomatic individuals at any stage of COPD, smoking cessation is the only intervention that slows the rate of decline of lung function in this disease. The U.S. Public Health Service recommends implementing a five-step program for smoking intervention, the "five A's": *a*sking every patient about tobacco use at every visit, *a*dvising a smoker to quit, *a*ssessing an individual's readiness to initiate quitting, *a*ssisting the patient in quitting, and *a*rranging follow-up on progress, with the understanding that relapse is an inherent part of the quitting process. Although there is a strong association between the intensity of cessation counseling and

its effectiveness, encouragement should be provided even at brief patient encounters, because a 3-minute counseling session has been shown to have a positive impact, resulting in quit rates of 5% to 10% (46, 47) (see Chapter 15).

As regards adjunctive pharmacotherapy, one randomized controlled trial of 9-week treatment with bupropion, nicotine patch, or both in conjunction with group counseling found abstinence rates of 16% for placebo and nicotine monotherapy, versus 30% and 35% with bupropion and with bupropion plus nicotine, respectively, at 12 months (48). Another randomized controlled trial compared bupropion treatment for 7 weeks versus 1 year, finding equivalent abstinence rates of 40% at 2-year follow-up (49). As first-line pharmacotherapy, all individuals wanting to quit smoking who have been unsuccessful on their own should be prescribed a course of bupropion in conjunction with group cessation therapy. If bupropion is contraindicated, as for individuals with a history of seizures, anorexia, or bulimia, patients should be prescribed a form of nicotine replacement therapy, also in conjunction with group counseling. Nicotine appears to be safe in outpatients with known cardiovascular disease, even in patients who smoke concurrent with nicotine replacement (50, 51).

Vaccination recommendations for all patients with COPD include receiving an annual influenza vaccination and a pneumococcal vaccination every 10 years. Observational studies in elderly patients with chronic lung disease have demonstrated significant reductions in rate of respiratory illness, hospitalization, and mortality with the use of influenza vaccination (52). The recommendation for pneumococcal vaccination, in contrast, is based on consensus opinion, because no study has been able to demonstrate a benefit from its use in the COPD population, possibly because of an attenuated immune response to the vaccine. As regards general health care, one report found that elderly patients with COPD were significantly less likely to receive appropriate lipid-lowering medication than were patients with other chronic diseases (53). This finding raises concern that physicians may be neglecting the treatment of unrelated medical disorders in patients with COPD, despite the relatively high prevalence of co-morbidities in this population.

Selected COPD patients with advanced disease and those already on LTOT should be offered preflight counseling to estimate the degree of hypoxemia and the appropriate oxygen flow rate to be used while traveling by airplane. The predicted level of hypoxemia can either be calculated based on standard equations or directly measured with an altitude simulation test. COPD patients with large bullae should also be evaluated by a specialist before flying to assess the potential risk of pneumothorax from bulla expansion owing to reduced ambient pressure in the airplane cabin.

Discussion regarding advance directives for care should be considered for all COPD patients but is particularly relevant for those with advanced disease, who are likely to have a lower quality of life and higher risk for respiratory failure necessitating intubation and mechanical ventilation. One study of physician skills in end-of-life care found that patients with different end-stage diseases valued attributes of emotional support, communication, accessibility, and continuity in their physician. For individuals with COPD, however, concerns regarding the physician's ability to provide patient education in "diagnosis and disease process, treatment, and prognosis, what dying might be like, and advance care planning" stood out as domains of special interest that were unique to this population (54).

HEALTH PROMOTION	
Summary Statement	**Level of Evidence**
Brief counseling regarding smoking cessation at each patient encounter enhances quit rates.	Uncontrolled studies
First-line smoking cessation therapy consists of buproprion in conjunction with a group counseling program.	Randomized controlled trials

MAINTENANCE THERAPIES

β_2-Agonists and Anticholinergics

The pharmacologic treatment of COPD consists of the stepwise addition of medications aimed at alleviating symptoms, because no form of pharmacotherapy has been demonstrated to affect the long-term decline of lung function in this disease. The mainstay of medical therapy consists of β_2-agonists and anticholinergics. The most cost-effective means to administer these medications is by pressurized metered-dose inhaler, because more expensive devices such as dry powder inhalers and nebulizers have not demonstrated better drug delivery (55). These latter devices may be useful for patients unable to carry out the metered-dose inhaler dosing technique effectively. For symptomatic individuals unable to use inhaled therapy, oral β_2-agonists can be prescribed, although they are the least preferred because of increased systemic side effects and a slower onset of action (see Chapter 7).

An inhaled anticholinergic medication should be prescribed on an as-needed basis as first-line therapy for a patient with stable COPD who experiences dyspnea. At this time, the agent of choice in the United States is ipratropium bromide up to four times daily, because tiotropium bromide, which has demonstrated greater bronchodilation with no difference in adverse effects when inhaled once daily, is not yet available here (56). If the dyspnea is not fully controlled, a β_2-agonist that has been shown to have an additive bronchodilatory effect when used with ipratropium in stable COPD should be added. These short-acting agents should be prescribed for use on an as-needed basis, because regularly scheduled use of a β_2-agonist has demonstrated no benefit over as-needed use, yet has resulted in more side effects, twice

the medication use, and increased cost (57). For patients requiring regular bronchodilator use or nocturnal dosing for symptoms during the course of the night, the clinician may add a long-acting β_2-agonist, such as a salmeterol metered-dose inhaler, for scheduled use twice daily.

Although the effect of cardioselective β-blockers in patients with stable COPD has not been well studied, a trial of their use may be considered when indicated for coronary artery disease. A Cochrane systematic review of cardioselective β-blocker use in patients with mild-to-moderate, reversible airway disease found no clinically significant adverse respiratory effects with short-term use over days to weeks. Another Cochrane review pooled data of studies of nonselective β-blockers in patients with reversible airway obstruction and found a statistically significant reduction in FEV_1 without an increase in symptoms or inhaler use, along with a decreased responsiveness to β-agonists. Although some of the analyzed trials included patients with COPD, the application of these results to chronic use in this population is not appropriate, particularly in patients with severe airflow limitation.

Methylxanthines

For stable COPD patients who remain symptomatic despite the use of inhaled bronchodilators, the addition of slow-release theophylline should be considered. Methylxanthines have demonstrated benefit in reduction of dyspnea, increased exercise tolerance, and bronchodilation, particularly when given in combination with inhaled bronchodilators in stable COPD. However, theophylline is not efficacious in all patients, and whether or not an individual will respond cannot be predicted in advance. Its role is further complicated by the fact that therapeutic plasma levels must be individualized for each patient, and dosing requires careful monitoring owing to the narrow therapeutic window of theophylline and its multiple drug interactions. Nonetheless, selected COPD patients can derive significant clinical benefits from regular use of theophylline.

The key to avoiding chronic use of this potentially toxic medication in COPD patients who do not achieve benefit is to assess an individual's clinical response as rigorously as feasible in the ambulatory setting. For patients who are not currently prescribed theophylline, but who are symptomatic on inhaled bronchodilators and without contraindications such as a seizure disorder, the clinician may initiate oral slow-release theophylline at a low dose and may aim to gradually achieve higher plasma levels as tolerated over several weeks. The patient should be assessed for semiquantitative improvement in dyspnea ratings, exercise performance, and airflow obstruction with progressively increasing plasma levels. If the patient has accrued no benefit up to a plasma level that results in adverse effects, theophylline should be discontinued and the individual regarded as a theophylline "nonresponder." On the other hand, if improvement is noted in one or more of the determinants of efficacy at a plasma level that is well tolerated, theophylline therapy should be continued at a dose that maintains this target level.

A different strategy may be used to assess efficacy in COPD patients already prescribed theophylline. In a randomized controlled study involving COPD patients on long-term theophylline who were uncertain if it was beneficial, "n of 1" trials were compared with standard practice in theophylline prescription. The n of 1 trial consisted of a randomized, multiple-crossover comparison of theophylline versus placebo in a single individual over time, and standard practice involved stopping theophylline, resuming it if dyspnea worsened, then continuing it if dyspnea improved with its reintroduction. This trial demonstrated significantly less theophylline use with the n of 1 trial compared with the standard practice group (36% versus 83%) with no decrease in exercise capacity or quality of life (58). The n of 1 trial thus represents a potentially useful tool for the clinician to use in minimizing unnecessary and potentially toxic use of theophylline in COPD patients, by carefully identifying individuals who do and do not derive benefit from its use.

Inhaled Glucocorticosteroids

Despite not being recommended as standard therapy for patients with COPD, inhaled corticosteroids are widely prescribed in this population. Debate about their appropriate indication for this disease continues, in part, because of a lack of data on cost-effectiveness. The effects of inhaled corticosteroids in stable COPD have been well studied in several large, long-term randomized, clinical trials, summarized in Table 12.6. These trials have demonstrated no benefit on the long-term decline in lung function with regular use of inhaled corticosteroids in patients with stable COPD. Some

trials suggest a potential benefit of inhaled steroids in patients with severe COPD in reducing the incidence or severity of exacerbations, but these possible benefits are small, are of questionable clinical significance, and require long-term high-dose therapy.

Unfortunately, there is no reliable way to identify in advance the subset of patients with severe COPD and frequent exacerbations who might benefit from inhaled glucocorticoids. Many individuals may demonstrate an initial gain in FEV_1 over the short term, but the improvement is not durable and is therefore not useful as an indicator of response. Furthermore, even among individuals who are believed by clinicians to have benefitted from the use of oral corticosteroids, the utility of adding inhaled steroids to allow for a reduction in systemic glucocorticoid exposure is uncertain, with no evidence supporting this approach in COPD.

Long-Term Oxygen Therapy

The role of LTOT in COPD has been assessed in several large randomized controlled trials, reviewed in Table 12.7. Significant survival benefits have been demonstrated from administration of oxygen for more than 15 h/d in COPD patients with severe hypoxemia, generally defined as arterial partial pressure of oxygen (Pao_2) of less than 60 mm Hg. An important caveat for the clinician to bear in mind when considering oxygen therapy is that most of these trials excluded patients with significant co-morbidities. Thus, the application of the survival benefit of LTOT to the general COPD population may be limited. No survival benefit of LTOT has been demonstrated in COPD patients with hypoxemia that is mild to moderate in degree. Similarly, COPD patients without daytime hypoxemia but with significant nocturnal

TABLE 12.6. RANDOMIZED CONTROLLED TRIALS OF INHALED CORTICOSTEROIDS IN STABLE CHRONIC OBSTRUCTIVE PULMONARY DISEASE

Trial	Study Population	Treatment	Outcome
Copenhagen City Lung Study (125)	FEV_1/FVC <0.7 Mean FEV_1 = 86% predicted	Budesonide versus placebo over 3 y	No difference in rate of FEV_1 decline, symptoms, or exacerbations
EUROSCOP (126)	Mild COPD, mean FEV_1 = 77% predicted, current smokers	Budesonide versus placebo over 3 y	No difference in rate of FEV_1 decline
ISOLDE (127)	Severe COPD	Fluticasone versus placebo over 3 y	No difference in rate of FEV_1 decline; small reduction in exacerbation frequency and rate of health status decline with fluticasone
Lung Health Study (128)	Moderate COPD Mean FEV_1 = 64% predicted	Triamcinolone versus placebo over 40 mo	No difference in rate of FEV_1 decline; fewer respiratory symptoms and outpatient visits for respiratory symptoms with triamcinolone
Paggiaro et al. (129)	Multicenter trial in 281 patients with COPD, asthmatics excluded	Fluticasone versus placebo over 6 mo	No difference in exacerbation rate; less severe exacerbations and greater improvement in symptoms, FEV_1 and 6-min walk with fluticasone

FEV_1, forced expiratory volume in 1 s; FVC, forced vital capacity; COPD, chronic obstructive pulmonary disease.

TABLE 12.7. RANDOMIZED CONTROLLED TRIALS OF OXYGEN THERAPY IN STABLE CHRONIC OBSTRUCTIVE PULMONARY DISEASE

Trial	Study Population	Treatment	Outcome
Nocturnal Oxygen Therapy Trial, 1980 (87)	Mostly males, average age ~ 65; COPD with Pao_2 <60 mm Hg required	Nocturnal versus continuous oxygen therapy, 1–4 L/min	Significant survival benefit in continuous oxygen group over 24 mo of treatment
Medical Research Council, 1981 (130)	Mostly males, average age ~ 58; COPD with Pao_2 between 40–60 mm Hg and one or more episodes of right-sided heart failure	Oxygen therapy for at least 15 h daily, ≥2 L/min versus no oxygen	Significant survival benefit in oxygen group over 5 y of treatment
Fletcher et al., 1992 (34)	COPD and nocturnal desaturation	Nocturnal oxygen 3 L/min versus nocturnal room air 3 L/min	No difference in survival after 3 y of treatment
Chaouat et al., 1999 (131)	COPD, mild-to-moderate daytime hypoxemia and nocturnal desaturation (excluded if sleep apnea or serious comorbidities)	Nocturnal oxygen, usually 2 L/min versus no nocturnal oxygen	No difference in survival over long-term follow-up
Gorecka et al., 1997 (132)	COPD, moderate hypoxemia; mostly males, mean age ~ 60	Oxygen therapy titrated to maintain Pao_2 >65 mm Hg versus no oxygen	No difference in mortality over 3-y follow-up

COPD, chronic obstructive pulmonary disease; Pao_2, arterial blood partial pressure of oxygen.

desaturations, and who do not have sleep apnea, do not share a survival benefit from long-term nocturnal oxygen therapy. The ATS guidelines for LTOT prescription in COPD reflect this lack of demonstrated efficacy, leaving the detection and correction of nocturnal desaturation with oxygen therapy as optional.

Generally accepted criteria for LTOT prescription in COPD typically mirror criteria for coverage under Medicare and are based primarily on the study findings mentioned above. Table 12.8 outlines the recommended approach for prescribing oxygen.

TABLE 12.8. GUIDELINES FOR LONG-TERM OXYGEN THERAPY IN CHRONIC OBSTRUCTIVE PULMONARY DISEASE

Rationale: LTOT >15 h daily in patients with hypoxemia (Pao_2 <60 mm Hg) has been shown to improve survival in COPD.
Indications: For COPD patients with resting or exertional hypoxemia.
Contraindications: Active smoking or other risk for oxygen ignition
Criteria: Pao_2 ≤55 mm Hg or Sao_2 ≤88% at rest or with exercise
  or Pao_2 56–59 mm Hg or Sao_2 = 88%–89% at rest or with exercise in presence of cor pulmonale, findings of right heart failure, or erythrocytosis (hematocrit >56%)
    or Pao_2 >60 mm Hg or Sao_2 >90% at rest or with exercise with compelling medical justification (e.g., significant CAD, active coronary ischemia)
Therapeutic goals: Titrate to Pao_2 ≥60 mm Hg or Sao_2 ≥90%
Additional information: Specify oxygen source (gas or liquid); method of delivery (e.g., nasal cannula); duration of use (e.g., with exertion, or during daytime); flow rate at rest, during exercise, and during sleep.
Ancillary testing: Obtain PSG to assess for sleep apnea if clinically suspected; if desired, either obtain overnight oximetry with oxygen titration in patients with pulmonary hypertension or instruct patient to increase oxygen rate by 1 L/min during sleep.

LTOT, long-term oxygen therapy; COPD, chronic obstructive pulmonary disease; Pao_2, arterial blood partial pressure of oxygen; Sao_2, arterial oxygen saturation; CAD, coronary artery disease; PSG, polysomnography.

Mucolytics

Evidence for or against the use of mucoactive agents is limited. There is marked global variation in the prescribing pattern for mucolytics. In the United States, where they are little used compared with use in Europe, available agents include oral guaifenesin, saturated solution of potassium iodide, and nebulized acetylcysteine. Guaifenesin is an oral expectorant that acts to increase airway secretions through vagal stimulation and may also reduce mucus viscosity. There is no compelling evidence that its use results in an improvement in lung function or quality of life in patients with COPD. Saturated solution of potassium iodide, which acts to decrease mucus viscosity, is likewise of uncertain benefit and may be associated with side effects such as rash, metallic taste, hypothyroidism, and pancreatitis. A double-blind trial of oral acetylcysteine demonstrated a small, but statistically significant, reduction in the frequency of exacerbations of chronic bronchitis, but it is unclear whether or not its use is cost-effective, and the oral form is not available in the United States (59). Nebulized acetylcysteine, which acts within minutes to liquefy mucus, may also be of benefit, but its use is mainly limited in the United States to direct endobronchial instillation. Because of its ability to induce bronchospasm, nebulized acetylcysteine is typically administered together with a bronchodilator.

Systemic Corticosteroids

There have been no high-quality trials assessing the use of systemic corticosteroids in patients with stable COPD. The limited body of evidence available suggests that most patients will experience no benefit in FEV_1 or exercise capacity from a course of systemic corticosteroids. One metaanalysis found that 10% of COPD patients had a statistically significant improvement in FEV_1 from a course of oral corticosteroids, but the clinical importance of the small gains in lung function is uncertain (60). Furthermore, it is difficult to conduct an adequate evaluation for possible benefit from oral corticosteroids. At the least, the clinician should ensure that the COPD patient is at a stable baseline, obtain spirometry and perform an assessment of functional status, then prescribe a several-week course of oral corticosteroids in the range of 40 mg of prednisone daily. Lung function and exercise performance should be reassessed near the end of this trial, and if there is improvement that the clinician and patient consider clinically significant, the individual may be considered a "corticosteroid responder." Even in this small subpopulation of COPD patients, however, there is no clear evidence of sustained benefit from continuing this therapy, and clinicians may variably choose to discontinue or taper the oral corticosteroids to a low maintenance dose, or to substitute inhaled glucocorticoids. Given the numerous adverse effects associated with corticosteroids, and the absence of any proven benefit from their chronic use in the stable COPD patient, it may be reasonable to restrict such individualized corticosteroid trials to patients in whom asthma is a diagnostic possibility.

As regards the population of COPD patients already maintained chronically on oral corticosteroids, one small, double-blind, controlled trial randomized "steroid-dependent" COPD patients either to continue their usual dose or to have the corticosteroid gradually withdrawn. The discontinuation group demonstrated significantly less corticosteroid use and reduced body weight with no difference in number of COPD exacerbations, spirometry, and health-related quality of life compared with the maintenance group (61). Although this finding should be confirmed in larger trials, clinicians may give consideration to attempting gradual discontinuation of oral corticosteroids in selected COPD patients on chronic therapy.

Adverse Effects of Pharmacotherapy

Both inhaled and systemic corticosteroids are at present widely used in COPD. Assessment of the associated adverse effects has been limited by a lack of prospective well-controlled trials in this specific population, and by uncertainty about the clinical relevance of typically measured outcomes such as changes in bone density (62). The most common adverse effects of inhaled corticosteroids are local, consisting of dysphonia in up to 50% of users, cough or wheezing likely owing to propellant additives and, less commonly, oropharyngeal candidiasis. These effects can be improved by simple measures such as using a spacer and mouth rinsing after inhaler use. Benign cutaneous effects include dermal thinning, and one study found that high-dose inhaled corticosteroids resulted in easy bruising in almost 50% of patients (63). As regards adverse effects from systemic corticosteroid use, most studies have been performed

either in non-COPD patients or in COPD patients with poorly matched controls. These data, although suboptimal, support an association of systemic steroid use with decreases in bone density, particularly affecting skeletal areas with high trabecular bone content, such as the ribs and vertebrae (64). The minimal dose found to be associated with a detectable loss of bone density has been estimated at 6 mg prednisone daily for 9 weeks, and alternate day dosing does not decrease this risk (65).

A metaanalysis of calcitonin found no evidence of fracture reduction in corticosteroid-induced osteoporosis, and there was a high rate of nausea and flushing associated with its use (66). The use of bisphosphonates and the combination of calcium and vitamin D has demonstrated efficacy in reducing bone loss in patients with steroid-induced osteoporosis, but there is no evidence of an accompanying reduction in fracture risk. In addition, the clinical importance of preventing vertebral fractures is uncertain, because many are asymptomatic. A reduction in bone mineral density has been correlated with an increase in fracture risk in postmenopausal osteoporosis, but this association has not been shown in steroid-related osteoporosis, which limits the application of therapeutic trials to the COPD population.

Additional adverse effects of systemic corticosteroid use include cutaneous changes of dermal thinning, purpura, hirsutism, and acne, as well as truncal obesity, moon facies, and buffalo hump. Steroid-unmasked diabetes mellitus may develop during chronic use, and risk of infection may be increased. High doses of systemic corticosteroids may cause skeletal muscle weakness, but the risk of long-term low-dose therapy is less clear.

A dramatic and potentially dangerous adverse effect of systemic corticosteroid therapy is acute psychiatric reactions, manifesting as either psychosis or inappropriate euphoria that resolves with steroid discontinuation or dose reduction. One prospective study found an overall incidence of 3.1% of acute psychiatric disturbances with systemic corticosteroid therapy that was significantly dose dependent, occurring in 1.3% of patients using less than 40 mg prednisone daily, in 4.6% using between 40 and 80 mg daily, and in 18.4% using daily doses greater than 80 mg prednisone (67).

Emerging Therapies

Phosphodiesterase 4 (PDE4) inhibitors have demonstrated both bronchodilatory and anti-inflammatory properties in animal models and in vitro. Several pharmaceutical companies are in the late stages of their development. The most advanced to date, cilomilast, demonstrated improvement of lung function and symptoms over a 6-week phase II study in patients with moderate COPD (68).

Pulmonary Rehabilitation

The most recent ATS guidelines on pulmonary rehabilitation define it as "a multidisciplinary program of care for patients with chronic respiratory impairment that is individually tailored and designed to optimize physical and social performance and autonomy" (69). The expansiveness of this definition reflects the broad scope of pulmonary rehabilitation, of which exercise training, education, behavioral intervention, and psychosocial support are the primary components. It should be underscored that improvement or preservation of lung function is not a goal of such programs, and COPD patients may accrue significant benefits from pulmonary rehabilitation with no change in the degree of airflow obstruction or hyperinflation.

The main goals of pulmonary rehabilitation are to reduce dyspnea, increase endurance, and improve the overall quality of life in any symptomatic COPD patient without regard to the severity of airflow obstruction. Participation in a smoking cessation program is often a requisite for rehabilitation candidates. Although the optimal duration of rehabilitation has not been established, programs typically last 6 to 8 weeks. Benefits have been reported from rehabilitation programs conducted in inpatient, outpatient, and home settings.

During pulmonary rehabilitation, education about the disease process and appropriate use of medications may enhance self-efficacy and should include end-of-life care and nutritional counseling. Behavioral intervention focuses on acquiring practical skills to cope with episodes of dyspnea and associated anxiety, or on learning more general relaxation techniques. Psychosocial support may take the form of group discussions, soliciting and addressing concerns about sexual function, and identifying and treating depression. Physical training involves lower extremity aerobic exercise, and improvement has been demonstrated even in patients with severe COPD and poor exercise performance. Multiple prospective studies have documented benefits of pulmonary rehabilitation on exercise endurance, perception of dyspnea, quality of life, and self-efficacy (70–72). Ongoing trials are investigating the effect of rehabilitation on health care utilization and survival. Pulmonary rehabilitation is discussed in more detail in Chapter 16.

MANAGEMENT OF ACUTE EXACERBATIONS OF CHRONIC OBSTRUCTIVE PULMONARY DISEASE

Overview and Definition of Chronic Obstructive Pulmonary Disease Exacerbation

The natural history of moderate-to-severe COPD is characterized by repeated episodes of acute sustained respiratory deterioration referred to as "exacerbations." The development of appropriate management guidelines has been hampered both by the lack of a consistent definition and by the absence of a consensus regarding an objective scale for classifying exacerbation severity. Most definitions of acute exacerbations of COPD are clinical and include combinations of wors-

ened dyspnea, increased sputum purulence, and increased sputum volume. An operational definition proposed by one workshop required the necessitation of a change in regular medication use (73). In addition, to qualify as a COPD exacerbation, many experts specify that the clinical deterioration cannot be owing to an identifiable diagnosis, such as pulmonary embolism, congestive heart failure, or pneumonia. This exclusion criterion is conceptually appealing, because respiratory decompensation in these already compromised individuals can be the common end result of different pathophysiologic mechanisms for which significantly different treatments are indicated. The inclusion of specific identifiable etiologies under the umbrella term COPD exacerbation because they manifest in part with acute respiratory decline in individuals with pre-existing COPD can be detrimental in practice if it promotes a stereotypical therapeutic approach to these patients.

Evaluation of the Decompensated Chronic Obstructive Pulmonary Disease Patient

The key components of assessing acute respiratory or functional decompensation in individuals with COPD include identifying the cause of the decline, instituting appropriate therapy, and deciding if the patient needs to be hospitalized. Such evaluations typically take place over the telephone, during an office visit, or in the emergency department.

Guidelines regarding the initial assessment of the COPD patient suspected to have an acute exacerbation vary widely between professional societies. One of the two most recent evidence-based reviews, the American College of Chest Physicians and American College of Physicians-American Society of Internal Medicine (ACCP/ACP-ASIM) guidelines, recommends a CXR for patients admitted to the hospital (74). The GOLD guidelines, also published in 2001, recommend obtaining a CXR, ECG, ABG, electrolytes, hematocrit, and, if there is no response to initial empiric antibiotics, sputum culture and susceptibility testing (4). Additional testing should be obtained on an individualized basis as directed by the history and physical examination. Although evaluation for hypoxemia can be performed noninvasively by pulse oximetry, acute respiratory acidosis can only be assessed by ABG measurement. The clinician should maintain a low threshold for obtaining an ABG, because unidentified hypercapnic respiratory failure can prove rapidly fatal. Table 12.9 outlines relevant diagnostic tests the clinician should consider on an individualized basis when evaluating an acutely decompensated COPD patient.

Outpatient Exacerbation Management

Although the majority of exacerbations are mild and managed on an outpatient basis, there have been almost no controlled trials of outpatient management of COPD exacerbations (Table 12.10). Some studies have identified predictors

TABLE 12.9. GUIDELINES FOR EVALUATION OF A CHRONIC OBSTRUCTIVE PULMONARY DISEASE EXACERBATION

Diagnostic Test	Rationale
History and physical examination	May suggest alternate etiology for respiratory deterioration, such as rib fracture or arrhythmia
Pulse oximetry	Assess need for supplemental oxygen
Chest x-ray	Assess for infiltrate, pneumothorax, or congestive heart failure
Electrocardiogram	Assess for arrhythmia, myocardial ischemia, or infarction; may suggest pulmonary embolism if acute right ventricular strain pattern present
Arterial blood gas	Assess for acute respiratory acidosis requiring mechanical ventilation
CT-PA, V/Q scan, pulmonary angiogram	Assess for acute pulmonary embolism requiring heparin therapy
Cardiac telemetry	Monitor heart rate if arrhythmia present requiring medication for ventricular rate control
Serum troponin, serial CK-MB measurement	Assess for myocardial injury or infarction
Serum electrolytes, BUN, creatinine	Assess for renal insufficiency, to adjust medication doses
Sputum culture and sensitivity analysis	To guide antibiotic choice in nonresponders to initial therapy

Definition of COPD exacerbation: an acute, sustained deterioration from baseline respiratory status in an individual with moderate-to-severe COPD, characterized by worsened dyspnea, increase in sputum volume, or increase in sputum purulence, in the absence of a specific identifiable diagnosis that explains the decline in clinical status.
Differential diagnosis: pneumonia, supraventricular arrhythmia with or without rapid ventricular response, myocardial ischemia or infarction, congestive heart failure exacerbation, pneumothorax, pulmonary embolism, or rib fracture.
COPD, chronic obstructive pulmonary disease; CT-PA, computerized tomographic pulmonary angiogram; V/Q, ventilation-perfusion; CK-MB, creatine kinase muscle-brain isotype; BUN, blood urea nitrogen.

of outpatient relapse, usually defined as a return to the emergency department within 14 days of initial assessment. Predictors of relapse include a lower FEV_1 at baseline, increased bronchodilator use in the emergency department, hypoxemia, hypercapnia, and a history of previous relapse. Unfortunately, none of the prediction models of relapse developed to date perform well enough to be useful in clinical decision making. Data-based guidelines for deciding on outpatient versus inpatient management are therefore not available.

For outpatient therapy, most expert panels recommend the scheduled use of inhaled β_2-agonist, inhaled ipratropium, or both, in conjunction with an inexpensive limited-spectrum oral antibiotic, such as amoxicillin or doxycycline, for patients with increased sputum purulence or volume. No firm recommendations are provided on duration of antibiotic therapy, but most courses range from 3 to 14 days. Oral corticosteroids are also generally recommended, starting with the equivalent of prednisone 40 mg daily and tapering off over 8 to 14 days. If the patient clinically worsens or fails to improve during the course of outpatient therapy, the

clinician should consider sending a sputum for culture and sensitivity testing, consider an alternate or supervening diagnosis, and assess the patient for further diagnostic testing and hospital admission. The ACCP/ACP-ASIM position paper on therapy reports an alarming scarcity of high-quality data on the management of COPD exacerbations. They reported that in more than 40 years of research, fewer than 1,100 patients had been enrolled in randomized placebo-controlled trials of antibiotics, fewer than 650 patients had been enrolled in studies comparing corticosteroids with placebo, and virtually no controlled trials had been performed evaluating treatment of outpatient COPD exacerbations (75).

Inpatient Exacerbation Management

The decision to admit a patient to the hospital for management of an acute COPD exacerbation involves attempting to identify individuals at high risk for outpatient failure. Estimation of this risk involves consideration of baseline lung function, relevant co-morbid conditions that could impact on outcome, the individual's fatigue level and remaining physical reserve, and the home resources available to the patient. The ATS recommends considering admission based on multiple factors such as anticipated inability of the patient to perform activities of daily living at home, inadequate response to trial of outpatient management, high-risk co-morbid conditions, and the consideration of physiological markers of altered mentation, worsened hypoxemia, hypercapnia, or cor pulmonale (1). Because a sufficiently accurate tool to assist in individual risk stratification is not available, in the absence of a clear-cut indication for admission such as acute respiratory failure, the caregiver must often rely to some degree on clinical judgment and experience in deciding between inpatient and outpatient settings for exacerbation treatment.

Because the therapeutic principles applying to a COPD exacerbation do not differ based on setting, the main benefit of inpatient care includes provision of nebulized bronchodilators, provision and titration of supplemental oxygen, clinical monitoring for respiratory failure with the capacity to provide mechanical ventilation, assessment for and treating comorbid illnesses, and assistance with activities of daily living. In individuals with cardiovascular disease, continuous telemetry can facilitate management of supraventricular arrhythmias, and serial cardiac enzymes can be measured to assess for myocardial injury or infarct. A large part of the difficulty in arriving at data-based recommendations for management of an exacerbation is the scarcity of high-quality research in this area.

Although data to inform discharge guidelines are lacking, favorable studies have been performed evaluating the use of transitional home nursing care to support early hospital discharge. One randomized, prospective, clinical trial found that home-supported discharge after COPD

TABLE 12.10. THERAPEUTIC OPTIONS FOR CHRONIC OBSTRUCTIVE PULMONARY DISEASE EXACERBATION

Treatment	Regimen	Supporting Evidence
Smoking cessation	Advise quitting during exacerbation; in amenable patient when recovered, prescribe bupropion or nicotine replacement in conjunction with group counseling.	Quitting smoking may reduce exacerbation frequency by approximately one-third (124).
Oxygen	Minimal flow rate necessary to achieve Sao$_2$ $\geq$90%.	Not well studied; may result in mild hypercapnia; benefits of oxygen considered greater than risk (133).
Inhaled bronchodilators	β_2-agonist and/or anticholinergic (ipratropium or glycopyrrolate) via nebulizer or MDI every 4 h.	Equivalent bronchodilation from β_2-agonist or anticholinergic; no evidence of added benefit from combined use (74). Metaanalysis reported no difference in achievable bronchodilation via nebulizer versus MDI (134). Glycopyrrolate may have an additive bronchodilatory effect when used with albuterol (135).
Empiric antibiotic course	Narrow spectrum, inexpensive oral agent (e.g., doxycycline, amoxicillin, trimethoprim/sulfamethoxazole) for 3–10 d.	Reduction in symptom duration, most beneficial among patients with purulent sputum (136). Two metaanalyses of RCTs support antibiotic course if purulent sputum present (74, 137); No evidence on optimal duration of treatment. No evidence to support initial use of newer, more expensive agents, such as fluoroquinolones.
Systemic corticosteroids	Prednisone 40 mg daily (or equivalent) tapered over 8 d–2 wk.	For inpatients, a 15-d course of systemic corticosteroids resulted in more rapid recovery of FEV$_1$, 10% reduction in risk of treatment failure, and reduced hospital stay (138). Another inpatient study found more rapid symptom resolution from a 10-d versus 3-d course (139).
Noninvasive mechanical ventilation	Bilevel positive airway pressure via face or nasal mask, starting with inspiratory and expiratory pressures of 8–12 and 3–5 cm H20, respectively, then adjusted for patient tolerance.	Multiple RCTs have demonstrated greatly reduced intubation rate, shortened hospital stay, and improved survival in selected inpatients with hypercapnic respiratory failure (78, 79, 140). Some trials have reported reduced hospital costs (141).
Invasive mechanical ventilation	Endotracheal intubation and conventional mechanical ventilation.	Considered effective for severe or life-threatening acute respiratory failure.

Sao$_2$, arterial oxygen saturation; MDI, metered-dose inhaler; RCT, randomized clinical trial; FEV$_1$, forced expiratory volume in 1 s.

exacerbation resulted in a significantly shorter duration of hospital stay, decreased total health service cost, and no difference in readmission at 8-week follow-up (76). A similar trial with longer follow-up to 2 months after discharge also found a reduction in hospital days and no difference in readmission or 60-day mortality rates (77).

Acute Respiratory Failure in Chronic Obstructive Pulmonary Disease Exacerbation

An important cause of morbidity and mortality in acute exacerbation is respiratory failure, typically manifesting as an acute respiratory acidosis. Clinical features suggestive of hypercapnic respiratory failure include headache, severe fatigue, and alteration in mental status, ranging from mild confusion to severe lethargy with a decreased level of responsiveness. Associated findings of respiratory compromise may also be present, such as tachycardia, nasal flaring, intercostal muscle retractions, paradoxical abdominal motion, or severe dyspnea. The diagnosis of acute respiratory failure can be confirmed by the finding on ABG of a pH value less than 7.35 associated with a variable degree of hypercapnia, depending on the degree of acute compromise and the patient's baseline Paco$_2$ value.

As regards management of acute respiratory failure in COPD, multiple high-quality trials have shown that the use of noninvasive positive pressure ventilation (NIPPV) in appropriate patients, typically administered as bilevel positive airway pressure via a nasal or face mask, confers large benefits in reducing the need for endotracheal intubation and associated complications, shortening intensive care unit and hospital stay, and improving survival (78–80). Identifying in advance patients who will not benefit from NIPPV and who progress to endotracheal intubation and conventional mechanical ventilation can be difficult, but some clinical trials have found the outcome of these patients to be no worse than those who received endotracheal intubation without a trial of NIPPV (81). The American Association for Respiratory Care recommends that at least two of three selection criteria be present for NIPPV to be considered: respiratory distress with moderate to severe dyspnea as evidenced by the use of accessory muscles or abdominal paradox, pH less than 7.35 with $Paco_2$ greater than 45 mm Hg, and respiratory rate greater than or equal to 25 breaths/min (74). Failure of NIPPV has been associated with a higher severity of acute illness, such as pH less than 7.30 and significantly altered mental status with inability to cooperate with machine-assisted breathing. Cardiovascular instability is also a generally accepted contraindication to the use of NIPPV.

Prognosis following Chronic Obstructive Pulmonary Disease Exacerbation

The frequency of exacerbations is correlated with baseline FEV_1 but may vary significantly between individuals, depending in part on the present smoking status. Almost 50% of patients discharged from hospitals after an acute exacerbation are readmitted more than once in the following 6 months (82). Clinically significant decrements in quality of life can result after recovery from an exacerbation. One study followed a cohort of patients with moderate-to-severe COPD over 2.5 years, finding a median recovery time of approximately 1 week for symptoms and peak expiratory flow rate, although at 35 and 91 days, 25% and 7% of individuals, respectively, had not yet recovered to baseline peak expiratory flow rate.

A prospective study of COPD patients admitted with an exacerbation and hypercapnia, with a $Paco_2$ greater than 50 mm Hg reported an 11% acute hospital mortality, and the 6-month and 1-year mortality were 33% and 43%, respectively (82). The quality of life of survivors was also generally poor, with only 26% reporting a quality of life that was good or better 6 months after the exacerbation. A much larger prospective study reported in-hospital and 1-year mortality rates for COPD patients with acute respiratory failure of 24% and 59%, respectively, with multiorgan failure being an important determinant of outcome (84).

The clinician must bear in mind, however, that no reliable method exists for identifying patients at high risk for either inpatient or 6-month mortality. Thus, the clinical impression regarding the likelihood of in-hospital mortality or probability of achieving extubation should not influence decisions about initiating, continuing, or withdrawing life-sustaining therapies. Rather, clinical factors such as acuity of physiologic dysfunction, baseline lung function, health and nutritional status, and the presence of comorbid illness are more highly predictive of intermediate or long-term prognosis after an episode of respiratory failure (75). The inability of clinicians to predict in-hospital survival in COPD exacerbation holds true regardless of the physician's experience or level of training (85).

In addition, COPD patients surviving mechanical ventilation for an exacerbation have a long-term prognosis that is similar to patients with the same degree of lung dysfunction who have not required ventilation (86). The use of noninvasive mechanical ventilation may represent a treatment option for COPD patients who do not wish to undergo intubation for an exacerbation, although the possibility of a failure of NIPPV treatment must be considered.

As regards oxygen dependency, one observational study found that 20% of COPD patients no longer required oxygen 3 weeks after discharge (87).

α_1-ANTITRYPSIN DEFICIENCY

Severe hereditary AAT deficiency is the best elucidated genetic risk factor for COPD to date. The clinical manifestations, natural history, inheritance, and molecular basis of AAT deficiency have all been well characterized. AAT deficiency is an autosomal-recessive hereditary disorder in which low serum and lung levels of AAT confer a congenital risk of developing panacinar emphysema as an adult and liver disease in childhood. AAT, a serine protease inhibitor synthesized primarily by hepatocytes, acts to inhibit neutrophil elastase. The "elastase/anti-elastase hypothesis" of AAT deficiency proposes that an imbalance between neutrophil elastase and AAT in the lung promotes an unopposed proteolytic state that results in emphysema.

The many identified alleles of the AAT gene are categorized by the protease inhibitor (Pi) system. Each AAT allele is assigned a letter code based on the electrophoretic mobility of the molecule, with the family of normal alleles referred to as M. Because an individual inherits one allele from each parent, the transcription of an AAT phenotype contains two letter codes, such as PiMM for a person with normal serum levels of normally functioning AAT. The serum cutoff level above which there is adequate AAT in the lung and below which an individual has an increased risk for emphysema is 11 μM, which is 35% of the average normal level. The phenotypes associated with serum AAT levels below the protective threshold are PiZZ, PiZ null, Pi null null, and, very rarely, PiSZ heterozygotes. PiZZ is the most common phenotype associated with emphysema, and the Z allele is found in 1% to 2% of the white population in the United States. Estimates of the prevalence of the PiZZ phenotype in North America range from approximately 1:3,500 to 1:1,670, and population data suggest that the overwhelming majority of such individuals with severely reduced AAT levels are unidentified (88). Additionally, one study found a mean delay of more than 7 years between the onset of symptoms and the initial diagnosis, suggesting that AAT deficiency may be under-recognized by physicians as a possible factor in premature emphysema (89).

Because the number of individuals in the general population with a high-risk AAT phenotype is not known, and estimates vary significantly based on the population assessed, it is uncertain what proportion of individuals with the PiZZ phenotype will not develop clinically significant emphysema. One study found that out of almost 1,000 COPD patients, 2% to 3% had severe AAT deficiency (90).

Individuals with severe AAT deficiency and emphysema usually present with typical respiratory symptoms and signs of COPD. Characteristics that may help distinguish this small subgroup from the remainder of the COPD population include a younger mean age of onset and radiographic evidence of basilar hyperlucency owing to bullous emphysema preferentially affecting or limited to the lung bases. Other features that should raise suspicion for severe AAT deficiency in a patient with emphysema include minimal or no tobacco use and a family history of emphysema. The deficiency phenotype is most common in individuals of northern European ancestry, and the Z allele is rare in Asians and blacks.

Nonpulmonary manifestations of AAT deficiency, although uncommon, may also prompt consideration of this diagnosis. Chronic liver disease as a neonate or adult, including persistently elevated liver function tests; cirrhosis; or even hepatocellular carcinoma may occur in up to 12% of patients with the PiZZ phenotype owing to impaired secretion or metabolism of the defective AAT protein (91). More rarely, individuals with AAT deficiency may develop panniculitis.

Workup for AAT deficiency begins with measurement of serum AAT levels, followed by phenotyping of those individuals with low or borderline values. If not already obtained, the clinician should also request CXR, prebronchodilator and postbronchodilator spirometry, and additional studies based on the severity of airflow obstruction, as recommended earlier in this chapter for initial workup of COPD.

Because controlled trials of most therapies have not been performed in the very small subgroup of COPD patients with AAT deficiency, treatment recommendations are primarily based on observational data and expert opinion. By far the most important intervention is smoking cessation, because individuals deficient in AAT are extremely susceptible to rapid declines in FEV_1 induced by cigarette smoke. The ATS guidelines recommend following the same principles of management that apply to the general COPD population, such as smoking cessation, avoidance of respiratory irritants, maximizing bronchodilators, pulmonary rehabilitation, and LTOT as clinically indicated (92). They specifically note the absence of any data on the use of corticosteroids in patients with AAT deficiency. Surgical therapies for severe AAT deficiency include liver or lung transplantation, or possibly even LVRS, although several publications have reported poor outcomes in this population after pneumoplasty.

The ATS also recommends weekly AAT replacement therapy for severely deficient (serum AAT < 11 μM) patients who have airflow obstruction, are not presently smoking, and are deemed willing and able to comply with the regimen of frequent infusions. Specific therapy with human AAT infusion has been shown to raise serum and lung epithelial lining fluid AAT levels above the susceptibility threshold value. Although no upper age or minimal lung function limits are proposed, the guidelines do emphasize that the goal of augmentation therapy is to retard further decline in lung function, and that improvement is not expected. In light of the

sharp rise in the 2-year mortality rate when the FEV_1 falls below 35% of predicted in AAT-associated emphysema, and the lack of suggested benefit from augmentation in observational trials for patients with severely reduced lung function, treatment decisions may be difficult (93). The suggested, but not proven, lack of benefit, the demanding infusion schedule, and the estimated mean annual cost of $40,000 for AAT augmentation therapy must be weighed against withholding a safe well-tolerated treatment with possible benefit for symptomatic patients with limited treatment options (94).

The only randomized trial of replacement therapy to date involved monthly infusions of AAT versus placebo over 3 years in former smokers with moderate airflow obstruction and the PiZZ deficiency phenotype. In this study, there was no benefit of augmentation therapy over placebo on the rate of FEV_1 decline, and only a trend toward reduced loss of lung tissue measured by chest CT that did not reach statistical significance (95). Another prospective trial assessed whether supplementation therapy would result in a reduced rate of urinary excretion of desmosine, a specific marker of elastase degradation. Over the 8-week study period involving 12 AAT-deficient patients with severe COPD, the investigators found no apparent reduction in the baseline elevated rate of elastin degradation (96). To date, the only evidence suggesting clinical benefit from augmentation therapy derives from several large observational studies, of which one noted both a survival benefit and a reduction in the rate of lung function decline in AAT-deficient patients with moderate airflow obstruction, and another reported benefit in lung function decline in patients with mild to moderate airflow obstruction (97–99).

In light of the lack of controlled data on treatment of individuals with severe AAT deficiency and emphysema, the Division of Lung Diseases of the NHLBI formed a patient registry in order to accrue an observational database on which to base therapeutic guidelines. More recently, although acknowledging the difficulties of conducting such a study, the AAT Deficiency Registry Study Group has called for a randomized placebo-controlled trial of augmentation therapy as the best means to resolve the long-standing question of benefit (100).

SURGICAL THERAPY FOR CHRONIC OBSTRUCTIVE PULMONARY DISEASE

Bullectomy

A bulla is generally defined as a localized air space in the lung with a diameter of more than 1 cm. Patients with bullous emphysema have airflow obstruction in conjunction with one or more large bullae, as well as a clinical course characterized by progressive dyspnea and airflow limitation accompanied by enlargement of the bulla. Because no controlled trials of surgical excision for this rare condition have been performed, retrospective analysis of outcomes forms the basis for patient selection guidelines. The clinician must weigh the perioperative morbidity and mortality of undergoing bullectomy against the likelihood of significant benefit in each potential candidate for this palliative procedure.

Generally accepted indications for elective bullectomy include severe dyspnea despite maximal medical therapy in a patient with emphysema and giant bullae occupying at least 30% of the hemithorax, along with CT demonstration of normal lung tissue crowded around the bulla. Individuals with bullae occupying less than 30% of the hemithorax are unlikely to benefit from resection, and several experts recommend at least 50% as optimal. One retrospective study of 25 patients who achieved significant improvement in dyspnea and FEV_1 after bullectomy found preoperative radiographic bulla volume to correlate best with gain in lung function, lending support to this criterion (101). Additional radiographic features suggestive of potential benefit include well-defined large bullae in the absence of diffuse emphysema, expiratory plain films demonstrating good thoracic motion and obscuration of lung tissue around the bulla, and interval bulla enlargement on serial films (102).

Contraindications to bullectomy include vanishing lung syndrome, chronic purulent bronchitis, and frequent respiratory infections. Most surgeons perform resection via thoracotomy, and reported mortality rates vary greatly between series. Common postoperative complications include pneumonia, prolonged air leaks, and acute or chronic respiratory failure. Factors conferring high surgical risk include FEV_1 less than 40% predicted, severe dyspnea, a reduced D_{LCO}, pulmonary hypertension, and hypercapnia.

Lung Volume Reduction Surgery

After their initial report of a small series of patients, in 1996 Cooper and colleagues (103) published the results of 150 consecutive bilateral lung volume reduction procedures performed in a highly selected group of patients with severe emphysema. By using a revision of the pneumoplasty technique developed by Dr. Otto Brantigan in the 1950s, Cooper and colleagues resected 20% to 30% of the volume of each lung using a linear stapler via a median sternotomy approach. The 90-day mortality was 4%, and the major complication was prolonged air leak. The 6-month follow-up included 67% of the initial cohort of patients, reporting mean FEV_1 increased 51% over baseline, residual volume (RV) reduced by 28%, and Pao_2 increased by an average of 8 mm Hg. These physiologic gains were accompanied by a significant reduction in dyspnea and improved quality of life, as measured using validated tools.

In 1995, in anticipation of a massive financial load that would be imposed on Medicare for funding this operation, the Health Care Financing Administration (HCFA) withdrew coverage for LVRS. In conjunction with the NHLBI, the HCFA organized the National Emphysema Treatment Trial (NETT), a multicenter, randomized, clinical trial of medical therapy versus medical therapy plus LVRS for the treatment of severe emphysema (104). The goal of the NETT

was to assess long-term clinical outcomes and to characterize the subgroup of patients with emphysema who might benefit from LVRS. A prospective economic analysis was performed in parallel to determine the cost-effectiveness of LVRS versus medical therapy (105).

The main arguments in favor of the NETT protocol was that the existing database on LVRS was severely limited due to a lack of long-term outcome data demonstrating durability of the short-term gains, heterogeneous short-term results with unreliable characterization of a subset of patients likely to benefit from surgery, and a lack of parallel control groups against whom to compare outcomes (104). Publication bias, whereby unfavorable results are less likely to be reported and published, represented another potentially significant threat to the validity of the LVRS database (106).

While the NETT has been ongoing, additional outcome data on LVRS has accrued. One small, short-term, randomized trial in patients with severe emphysema compared 8 weeks of pulmonary rehabilitation followed by bilateral LVRS versus continued rehabilitation. This study demonstrated significant short-term gains in lung function, quality of life, and gas exchange at 3 months after surgery (107). Another group retrospectively compared outcomes between a group of patients who underwent Medicare-funded LVRS and a well-matched medical cohort group that had been accepted for, but did not undergo, surgery, due to the withdrawal in HCFA funding. The investigators found significant improvement in lung function and decreased supplemental oxygen requirements in the group treated surgically after 2 years, but no difference in survival (108). Other studies reporting follow-up over several years have observed that after peaking within 6 months postoperatively, the subsequent decline in FEV_1 is most rapid in the first year, after which it exponentially decelerates (109). This attenuation of the rate of decline of lung function over time after LVRS may indicate that long-term benefits are more favorable than had been predicted based on the initial extrapolation from short-term data. The longest, prospective follow-up published to date described a cohort of 26 patients who underwent bilateral, upper-lobe LVRS via video-assisted thoracoscopy. Gelb and colleagues (110) found that in this cohort with end-stage emphysema, LVRS provided durable clinical and physiological benefits in nine of 26 patients at 3 years, seven at 4 years, and two at 5 years.

A preliminary report has been issued describing a subgroup of NETT participants who were at high risk for death after LVRS (111). These patients, comprising about 14% of the NETT population, were characterized by an FEV_1 less than 20% predicted in conjunction with either a D_{LCO} less than 20% predicted or a homogeneous distribution of emphysema on chest high-resolution CT. The 30-day mortality in this group was 16%, compared with no mortality in a medically treated cohort, and the 60-day survivors of surgery had only slightly improved functional outcomes and quality-of-life scores. Based on recommendations from the NETT Data and Safety Monitoring Board, the study protocol was revised so that patients meeting these criteria were no longer eligible for enrollment in the trial.

The final results of NETT indicate that overall mortality is not reduced by LVRS, but that improvements in exercise capacity and quality of life were statistically significant (112). However, differential effects of surgery on mortality were noted in different subgroups of patients. Patients with predominantly upper lobe emphysema and low exercise tolerance prior to surgery had a statistically significant lower mortality than did medically treated patients. However, the relative risk of death was statistically greater for individuals with non upper lobe emphysema and good exercise tolerance prior to surgery, and was no different for the other corresponding subgroups than for corresponding medically treated individuals. One problem with the applicability of these results is that the level of "low exercise capacity" was not clearly specified; another problem is with the statistical analysis that was used (multiple-comparisons problem) (112a).

Supporting the NETT findings, the CT emphysema ratio, a quantitative index of the craniocaudal distribution of emphysema, was found to predict post-surgical increased FEV_1 (112b,113). Although the positive predictive value of a high CT emphysema ratio, indicating focal upper-lobe predominant emphysema, was high, this measure was insensitive with a poor negative predictive value, in addition to being poorly predictive of gains in walk distance or reduction in dyspnea. Current recommendations regarding appropriate candidates are summarized in Table 12.11.

Data on the outcome of lung transplantation after LVRS have been published, with one group reporting that LVRS bridged the time to transplant by an average of 28 months, with no increase in post-transplant morbidity or mortality (114). Other published reports describe unexpected benefit of performing chest high-resolution CT during workup for LVRS, from the incidental discovery of early-stage malignant nodules. Additionally, LVRS has been reported in some individuals to improve lung function to the extent that a previously unresectable lung mass could be safely excised. Some surgeons have successfully performed concomitant LVRS and coronary artery bypass grafting in the same operation. Yet another group reported a preliminary trial of nonsurgical lung volume reduction in emphysematous sheep, by using a bronchoscope to administer a fibrin-based glue (115). As exciting as many of these reported outcomes have been, it is important for the clinician to bear in mind that LVRS is a therapeutic modality appropriate for, at best, a small subsegment of the overall COPD population.

Lung Transplantation

Approximately half of all lung transplantations in the United States are performed for treatment of end-stage COPD, including patients with AAT-associated emphysema. Of individuals who received lung transplants in 2000, 47% were between 50 and 64 years of age, 90% were white, and 51% were female (116). Although the absolute number of lung transplants performed in the United States has increased slightly in each recent year, organ availability has been significantly outpaced by the increasing number of patients listed for transplant, with waiting periods now often exceeding 2 years. The United Network Organ Sharing database indicates that 1,053 lung transplants were performed in the United States in 2001, yet approximately 3,800 patients were on the waiting list in 2002. The allocation of donor lungs is based on waiting time without regard for medical urgency, although individuals with idiopathic pulmonary fibrosis are awarded a 90-day credit at the time of listing.

Fifty-six percent of patients undergoing lung transplantation in 1999 required rehospitalization during the first post-transplant year, and the 1-year survival was 77%, with a 5-year survival of 44% for patients that received lung transplants in 1995. Long-term survival at 14 years is 23% (116). No survival benefit from lung transplantation has been demonstrated in the COPD population, in part because

TABLE 12.11. GUIDELINES FOR LUNG-VOLUME REDUCTION THERAPY IN CHRONIC OBSTRUCTIVE PULMONARY DISEASE

Suitability of Disease		Operative Risk Profile	
Favorable	**Unfavorable**	**Favorable**	**Unfavorable**
Heterogeneous distribution of emphysema/upper lobe predominance	Homogeneous, uniform distribution of emphysema	Acceptable cardiac risk stratification	Pulmonary hypertension, hypercapnia
Hyperinflation and air-trapping		Acceptable body mass index	Advanced age, D_{LCO} <20% predicted, FEV_1 <20% predicted

Indications: Palliation of severe emphysema; symptomatic despite maximal medical therapy.
Inclusion criteria: Insurance coverage or willingness to self-pay, able to participate in vigorous pulmonary rehabilitation program, understanding and willingness to accept risks of surgery, abstinence from smoking, suitable disease, and acceptable operative candidate.
Exclusion criteria: Age >75y, baseline copious sputum production or history of recurrent respiratory infections, continued smoking, previous major thoracic surgery, thoracic deformities or pleurodesis, life expectancy ≤2y owing to comorbid condition.
D_{LCO}, diffusing capacity of lungs for carbon monoxide; FEV_1, forced expiratory volume in 1 s.

TABLE 12.12. GUIDELINES FOR LUNG TRANSPLANTATION FOR CHRONIC OBSTRUCTIVE PULMONARY DISEASE

Indication: Palliation of end-stage chronic obstructive pulmonary disease

Inclusion criteria	Exclusion criteria
Predicted life expectancy <2–3 years	Age >65 years
FEV$_1$ <25% of predicted	Ongoing cigarette smoking or substance abuse
Hypercapnia (Paco$_2$ >55 mm Hg)	Unable to comply with medical management
Progressive cor pulmonale	Uncontrolled malignancy
Acceptable cardiac risk stratification	Significant major organ dysfunction

Timing of referral: when predicted life expectancy is ≤3y

FEV$_1$, forced expiratory volume in 1 s; Paco$_2$, arterial partial pressure of carbon dioxide.

of the highly variable and difficult-to-predict survival rates at the end-stage of this disease (117). However, the quality of life in COPD patients was improved at 4 months and maintained at 21 months after lung transplantation for end-stage disease. Table 12.12 outlines the current guidelines for lung transplantation in the treatment of end-stage COPD. This topic is addressed in more detail in Chapter 54.

REFERENCES

1. Standards for the diagnosis and care of patients with chronic obstructive pulmonary disease. American Thoracic Society. *Am J Respir Crit Care Med* 1995;152(5 pt 2):S77–S121.
2. American Thoracic Society. 1962. Chronic bronchitis, asthma, and pulmonary emphysema: a statement by the Committee on Diagnostic Standards for Nontuberculous Respiratory Diseases. *Am Rev Respir Dis* 1962;85:762–768.
3. Snider GL, Kleinerman J, Thurlbeck WM, et al. The definition of emphysema: report of a National Heart, Lung and Blood Institute, Division of Lung Diseases, Workshop. *Am Rev Respir Dis* 1985;132:182–185.
4. Pauwels RA, Buist AS, Ma P, et al. Global strategy for the diagnosis, management, and prevention of chronic obstructive pulmonary disease: executive summary. National Heart, Lung, and Blood Institute and World Health Organization Global Initiative for Chronic Obstructive Lung Disease (GOLD). *Respir Care* 2001;46:798–825.
5. Mannino DM, Gagnon RC, Petty TL, et al. Obstructive lung disease and low lung function in adults in the United States: data from the National Health and Nutrition Examination Survey, 1988–1994. *Arch Intern Med* 2000;160:1683–1689.
6. Petty TL. Scope of the COPD problem in North America: early studies of prevalence and NHANES III data: basis for early identification and intervention. *Chest* 2000;117[5 Suppl 2]:326S–331S.
7. Chapman KR, Tashkin DP, Pye DJ. Gender bias in the diagnosis of COPD. *Chest* 2001;119:1691–1695.
8. *The Global Burden of Disease: a comprehensive assessment of mortality and disability from diseases, injuries and risk factors and 1990 and projected to 2020.* Cambridge: Harvard University Press, 1996.
9. 1998–2001 *MMWR Surveill Summ* 2002;51:1–16.
10. Lopez AD, Murray CC. The global burden of disease, 1990–2001. *Nat Med* 1998;4:1241–1243.
11. National Heart, Lung, and Blood Institute. Morbidity and mortality: chartbook on cardiovascular, lung, and blood diseases. Bethesda, MD: U.S. Department of Health and Human Services, Public Health Service, National Institutes of Health; 2000.
12. Gross CP, Anderson GF, Powe NR. The relation between funding by the National Institutes of Health and the burden of disease. *N Engl J Med* 1999;340:1881–1887.
13. Fletcher CM, Peto R, Tinker C, et al. *The natural history of chronic obstructive lung disease in working men in London.* New York: Oxford University Press, 1976.
14. Sandford AJ, Chagani T, Weir TD, et al. Susceptibility genes for rapid decline of lung function in the lung health study. *Am J Respir Crit Care Med* 2001;163:469–473.
15. Croxton TL, Weinmann GG, Senior RM, et al. Future research directions in chronic obstructive pulmonary disease. *Am J Respir Crit Care Med* 2002;165:838–844.
16. Voelkel NF, Tuder R. COPD: exacerbation. *Chest* 2000; 117[5 Suppl 2]:376S–379S.
17. Skeletal muscle dysfunction in chronic obstructive pulmonary disease: a statement of the American Thoracic Society and European Respiratory Society. *Am J Respir Crit Care Med* 1999;159 (4 pt 2):S1–S40.
18. Casaburi R. Skeletal muscle function in COPD. *Chest* 2000;117[5 Suppl 1]:267S–271S.
19. Maltais F, Leblanc P, Jobin J, et al. Peripheral muscle dysfunction in chronic obstructive pulmonary disease. *Clin Chest Med* 2000;21:665–677.
20. Schols AM, Soeters PB, Mostert R, et al. Physiologic effects of nutritional support and anabolic steroids in patients with chronic obstructive pulmonary disease: a placebo-controlled randomized trial. *Am J Respir Crit Care Med* 1995;152(4 pt 1): 1268–1274.
21. Engelen MP, Wouters EF, Deutz NE, et al. Effects of exercise on amino acid metabolism in patients with chronic obstructive pulmonary disease. *Am J Respir Crit Care Med* 2001;163:859–864.
22. Levine S, Kaiser L, Leferovich J, et al. Cellular adaptations in the diaphragm in chronic obstructive pulmonary disease. *N Engl J Med* 1997;337:1799–1806.
23. Levine S, Gregory C, Nguyen T, et al. Bioenergetic adaptation of individual human diaphragmatic myofibers to severe COPD. *J Appl Physiol* 2002;92:1205–1213.
24. Orozco-Levi M, Lloreta J, Minguella J, et al. Injury of the human diaphragm associated with exertion and chronic obstructive pulmonary disease. *Am J Respir Crit Care Med* 2001;164:1734–1739.
25. Casaburi R. Rationale for anabolic therapy to facilitate rehabilitation in chronic obstructive pulmonary disease. *Baillieres Clin Endocrinol Metab* 1998;12:407–418.
26. Weisberg J, Wanger J, Olson J, et al. Megestrol acetate stimulates weight gain and ventilation in underweight COPD patients. *Chest* 2002;121:1070–1078.
27. Ferreira IM, Brooks D, Lacasse Y, et al. Nutritional support for individuals with COPD: a meta-analysis. *Chest* 2000;117:672–678.
28. Weitzenblum E, Apprill M, Oswald M, et al. Pulmonary hemodynamics in patients with chronic obstructive pulmonary disease before and during an episode of peripheral edema. *Chest* 1994;105:1377–1382.
29. Badgett RG, Tanaka DJ, Hunt DK, et al. Can moderate chronic obstructive pulmonary disease be diagnosed by historical and physical findings alone? *Am J Med* 1993;94:188–196.
30. Mannino DM, Etzel RA, Flanders WD. Do the medical history and physical examination predict low lung function? *Arch Intern Med* 1993;153:1892–1897.
31. Sashidhar K, Gulati M, Gupta D, et al. Emphysema in

heavy smokers with normal chest radiography: detection and quantification by HCRT. *Acta Radiol* 2002;43:60–65.

32. Copley SJ, Wells AU, Muller NL, et al. Thin-section CT in obstructive pulmonary disease: discriminatory value. *Radiology* 2002;223:812–819.

33. Roberts CM, Bugler JR, Melchor R, et al. Value of pulse oximetry in screening for long-term oxygen therapy requirement. *Eur Respir J* 1993;6:559–562.

34. Fletcher EC, Luckett RA, Goodnight-White S, et al. A double-blind trial of nocturnal supplemental oxygen for sleep desaturation in patients with chronic obstructive pulmonary disease and a daytime Pao$_2$ above 60 mm Hg. *Am Rev Respir Dis* 1992;145:1070–1076.

35. Chaouat A, Weitzenblum E, Krieger J, et al. Association of chronic obstructive pulmonary disease and sleep apnea syndrome. *Am J Respir Crit Care Med* 1995;151:82–86.

36. Traver GA, Cline MG, Burrows B. Predictors of mortality in chronic obstructive pulmonary disease: a 15- year follow-up study. *Am Rev Respir Dis* 1979;119:895–902.

37. Vestbo J, Prescott E, Lange P. Association of chronic mucus hypersecretion with FEV$_1$ decline and chronic obstructive pulmonary disease morbidity. Copenhagen City Heart Study Group. *Am J Respir Crit Care Med* 1996;153:1530–1535.

38. Jones PW, Bosh TK. Quality of life changes in COPD patients treated with salmeterol. *Am J Respir Crit Care Med* 1997;155: 1283–1289.

39. Mahler DA, Mejia-Alfaro R, Ward J, et al. Continuous measurement of breathlessness during exercise: validity, reliability, and responsiveness. *J Appl Physiol* 2001;90:2188–2196.

40. Mahler DA. How should health-related quality of life be assessed in patients with COPD? *Chest* 2000;117[2 Suppl]:54S–57S.

41. Doll R, Peto R, Wheatley K, et al. Mortality in relation to smoking: 40 years' observations on male British doctors. *BMJ* 1994;309:901–911.

42. Annual smoking-attributable mortality, years of potential life lost, and economic costs—United States, 1995–1999 *MMWR Morb Mortal Wkly Rep* 2002;51:300–303.

43. Skillrud DM, Offord KP, Miller RD. Higher risk of lung cancer in chronic obstructive pulmonary disease: a prospective, matched, controlled study. *Ann Intern Med* 1986;105:503–507.

44. Taylor DH Jr, Hasselblad V, Henley SJ, et al. Benefits of smoking cessation for longevity. *Am J Public Health* 2002;92:990–996.

45. Peto R, Darby S, Deo H, et al. Smoking, smoking cessation, and lung cancer in the UK since 1950: combination of national statistics with two case-control studies. *BMJ* 2000;321:323–329.

46. Ockene JK, Kristeller J, Goldberg R, et al. Increasing the efficacy of physician-delivered smoking interventions: a randomized clinical trial. *J Gen Intern Med* 1991;6:1–8.

47. Wilson DH, Wakefield MA, Steven ID, et al. "Sick of Smoking": evaluation of a targeted minimal smoking cessation intervention in general practice. *Med J Aust* 1990;152:518–521.

48. Jorenby DE, Leischow SJ, Nides MA, et al. A controlled trial of sustained-release bupropion, a nicotine patch, or both for smoking cessation. *N Engl J Med* 1999;340:685–691.

49. Hays JT, Hurt RD, Rigotti NA, et al. Sustained-release bupropion for pharmacologic relapse prevention after smoking cessation. a randomized, controlled trial. *Ann Intern Med* 2001;135:423–433.

50. Joseph AM, Norman SM, Ferry LH, et al. The safety of transdermal nicotine as an aid to smoking cessation in patients with cardiac disease. *N Engl J Med* 1996;335:1792–1798.

51. Nicotine replacement therapy for patients with coronary artery disease. Working Group for the Study of Transdermal Nicotine in Patients with Coronary artery disease. *Arch Intern Med* 1994;154:989–995.

52. Nichol KL, Goodman M. The health and economic benefits of influenza vaccination for healthy and at-risk persons aged 65 to 74 years. *Pharmacoeconomics* 1999;16[Suppl 1]:63–71.

53. Redelmeier DA, Tan SH, Booth GL. The treatment of unrelated disorders in patients with chronic medical diseases. *N Engl J Med* 1998;338:1516–1520.

54. Curtis JR, Wenrich MD, Carline JD, et al. Patients' perspectives on physician skill in end-of-life care: differences between patients with COPD, cancer, and AIDS. *Chest* 2002;122:356–362.

55. Brocklebank D, Ram F, Wright J, et al. Comparison of the effectiveness of inhaler devices in asthma and chronic obstructive airways disease: a systematic review of the literature. *Health Technol Assess* 2001;5:1–149.

56. van Noord JA, Bantje TA, Eland ME, et al. A randomised controlled comparison of tiotropium and ipratropium in the treatment of chronic obstructive pulmonary disease. The Dutch Tiotropium Study Group. *Thorax* 2000;55:289–294.

57. Cook D, Guyatt G, Wong E, et al. Regular versus as-needed short-acting inhaled β-agonist therapy for chronic obstructive pulmonary disease. *Am J Respir Crit Care Med* 2001;163:85–90.

58. Mahon JL, Laupacis A, Hodder RV, et al. Theophylline for irreversible chronic airflow limitation: a randomized study comparing n of 1 trials to standard practice. *Chest* 1999;115:38–48.

59. Boman G, Backer U, Larsson S, et al. Oral acetylcysteine reduces exacerbation rate in chronic bronchitis: report of a trial organized by the Swedish Society for Pulmonary Diseases. *Eur J Respir Dis* 1983;64:405–415.

60. Callahan CM, Dittus RS, Katz BP. Oral corticosteroid therapy for patients with stable chronic obstructive pulmonary disease: a meta-analysis. *Ann Intern Med* 1991;114:216–223.

61. Rice KL, Rubins JB, Lebahn F, et al. Withdrawal of chronic systemic corticosteroids in patients with COPD: a randomized trial. *Am J Respir Crit Care Med* 2000;162:174–178.

62. McEvoy CE, Ensrud KE, Bender E, et al. Association between corticosteroid use and vertebral fractures in older men with chronic obstructive pulmonary disease. *Am J Respir Crit Care Med* 1998;157(3 pt 1):704–709.

63. Mak VH, Melchor R, Spiro SG. Easy bruising as a side-effect of inhaled corticosteroids. *Eur Respir J* 1992;5:1068–1074.

64. McEvoy CE, Niewoehner DE. Adverse effects of corticosteroid therapy for COPD: a critical review. *Chest* 1997;111:732–743.

65. Goldstein MF, Fallon JJ Jr, Harning R. Chronic glucocorticoid therapy-induced osteoporosis in patients with obstructive lung disease. *Chest* 1999;116:1733–1749.

66. Cranney A, Tugwell P, Zytaruk N, et al. VI. Meta-analysis of calcitonin for the treatment of postmenopausal osteoporosis. *Endocr Rev* 2002;23:540–551.

67. Miyamoto T, Yoshida T, Osawa N, et al. Adrenal response and side reactions after long-term corticosteroid therapy in bronchial asthma. *Ann Allergy* 1972;30:587–594.

68. Compton CH, Gubb J, Nieman R, et al. Cilomilast, a selective phosphodiesterase-4 inhibitor for treatment of patients with chronic obstructive pulmonary disease: a randomised, dose-ranging study. *Lancet* 2001;358:265–270.

69. Pulmonary rehabilitation: 1999. American Thoracic Society. *Am J Respir Crit Care Med* 1999;159(5 pt 1):1666–1682.

70. Goldstein RS, Gort EH, Stubbing D, et al. Randomised controlled trial of respiratory rehabilitation. *Lancet* 1994;344: 1394–1397.

71. Ries AL, Kaplan RM, Limberg TM, et al. Effects of pulmonary rehabilitation on physiologic and psychosocial outcomes in patients with chronic obstructive pulmonary disease. *Ann Intern Med* 1995;122:823–832.

72. Lacasse Y, Wong E, Guyatt GH, et al. Meta-analysis of respiratory rehabilitation in chronic obstructive pulmonary disease. *Lancet* 1996;348:1115–1119.

73. Rodriguez-Roisin R. Toward a consensus definition for COPD exacerbations. *Chest* 2000;117[5 Suppl 2]:398S–401S.

74. Bach PB, Brown C, Gelfand SE, et al. Management of acute exacerbations of chronic obstructive pulmonary disease: a summary and appraisal of published evidence. *Ann Intern Med* 2001;134:600–620.

75. Snow V, Lascher S, Mottur-Pilson C. Evidence base for management of acute exacerbations of chronic obstructive pulmonary disease. *Ann Intern Med* 2001;134:595–599.

76. Skwarska E, Cohen G, Skwarski KM, et al. Randomized controlled trial of supported discharge in patients with exacerbations of chronic obstructive pulmonary disease. *Thorax* 2000;55:907–912.

77. Cotton MM, Bucknall CE, Dagg KD, et al. Early discharge for patients with exacerbations of chronic obstructive pulmonary disease: a randomized controlled trial. *Thorax* 2000;55:902–906.

78. Brochard L, Mancebo J, Wysocki M, et al. Noninvasive ventilation for acute exacerbations of chronic obstructive pulmonary disease. *N Engl J Med* 1995;333:817–822.

79. Kramer N, Meyer TJ, Meharg J, et al. Randomized, prospective trial of noninvasive positive pressure ventilation in acute respiratory failure. *Am J Respir Crit Care Med* 1995;151:1799–1806.

80. Plant PK, Owen JL, Elliott MW. Non-invasive ventilation in acute exacerbations of chronic obstructive pulmonary disease: long term survival and predictors of in-hospital outcome. *Thorax* 2001;56:708–712.

81. Carlucci A, Richard JC, Wysocki M, et al. Noninvasive versus conventional mechanical ventilation: an epidemiologic survey. *Am J Respir Crit Care Med* 2001;163:874–880.

82. Connors AF Jr, Dawson NV, Thomas C, et al. Outcomes following acute exacerbation of severe chronic obstructive lung disease: the SUPPORT investigators (Study to Understand Prognoses and Preferences for Outcomes and Risks of Treatments). *Am J Respir Crit Care Med* 1996;154(4 pt 1):959–967.

83. Seemungal TA, Donaldson GC, Paul EA, et al. Effect of exacerbation on quality of life in patients with chronic obstructive pulmonary disease. *Am J Respir Crit Care Med* 1998;157(5 pt 1): 1418–1422.

84. Seneff MG, Wagner DP, Wagner RP, et al. Hospital and 1-year survival of patients admitted to intensive care units with acute exacerbation of chronic obstructive pulmonary disease. *JAMA* 1995;274:1852–1857.

85. Pearlman RA. Variability in physician estimates of survival for acute respiratory failure in chronic obstructive pulmonary disease. *Chest* 1987;91:515–521.

86. Portier F, Defouilloy C, Muir JF. Determinants of immediate survival among chronic respiratory insufficiency patients admitted to an intensive care unit for acute respiratory failure: a prospective multicenter study. French Task Group for Acute Respiratory Failure in Chronic Respiratory Insufficiency. *Chest* 1992;101:204–210.

87. Continuous or nocturnal oxygen therapy in hypoxemic chronic obstructive lung disease: a clinical trial. Nocturnal Oxygen Therapy Trial Group. *Ann Intern Med* 1980;93:391–398.

88. Silverman EK, Chapman HA, Drazen JM, et al. Genetic epidemiology of severe, early-onset chronic obstructive pulmonary disease: risk to relatives for airflow obstruction and chronic bronchitis. *Am J Respir Crit Care Med* 1998;157(6 pt 1):1770–1778.

89. Stoller JK, Smith P, Yang P, et al. Physical and social impact of α_1-antitrypsin deficiency: results of a survey. *Cleve Clin J Med* 1994;61:461–467.

90. Lieberman J, Winter B, Sastre A. α_1-Antitrypsin Pi-types in 965 COPD patients. *Chest* 1986;89:370-373.

91. Larsson C. Natural history and life expectancy in severe α_1-antitrypsin deficiency, Pi Z. *Acta Med Scand* 1978;204:345–351.

92. Guidelines for the approach to the patient with severe hereditary α_1-antitrypsin deficiency. American Thoracic Society. *Am Rev Respir Dis* 1989;140:1494-1497.

93. Seersholm N, Kok-Jensen A. Survival in relation to lung function and smoking cessation in patients with severe hereditary α_1-antitrypsin deficiency. *Am J Respir Crit Care Med* 1995; 151(2 pt 1):369–373.

94. Mullins CD, Huang X, Merchant S, et al. The direct medical costs of α_1-antitrypsin deficiency. *Chest* 2001;119:745–752.

95. Dirksen A, Dijkman JH, Madsen F, et al. A randomized clinical trial of α_1-antitrypsin augmentation therapy. *Am J Respir Crit Care Med* 1999;160(5 pt 1):1468–1472.

96. Gottlieb DJ, Stone PJ, Sparrow D, et al. Urinary desmosine excretion in smokers with and without rapid decline of lung function: the Normative Aging Study. *Am J Respir Crit Care Med* 1996;154:1290–1295.

97. Survival and FEV$_1$ decline in individuals with severe deficiency of α_1-antitrypsin: the α_1-Antitrypsin Deficiency Registry Study Group. *Am J Respir Crit Care Med* 1998;158:49–59.

98. Seersholm N, Wencker M, Banik N, et al. Does α_1-antitrypsin augmentation therapy slow the annual decline in FEV$_1$ in patients with severe hereditary α_1-antitrypsin deficiency? Wissenschaftliche Arbeitsgemeinschaft zur Therapie von Lungenerkrankungen (WATL) α_1-AT study group. *Eur Respir J* 1997;10:2260–2263.

99. Wencker M, Fuhrmann B, Banik N, et al. Longitudinal follow-up of patients with α_1-protease inhibitor deficiency before and during therapy with IV α_1-protease inhibitor. *Chest* 2001;119:737–744.

100. Schluchter MD, Stoller JK, Barker AF, et al. Feasibility of a clinical trial of augmentation therapy for α_1-antitrypsin deficiency: the α_1-Antitrypsin Deficiency Registry Study Group. *Am J Respir Crit Care Med* 2000;161(3 pt 1):796–801.

101. Baldi S, Palla A, Mussi A, et al. Influence of bulla volume on postbullectomy outcome. *Can Respir J* 2001;8:233–238.

102. Gaensler EA, Jederlinic PJ, FitzGerald MX. Patient work-up for bullectomy. *J Thorac Imaging* 1986;1:75–93.

103. Cooper JD, Patterson GA, Sundaresan RS, et al. Results of 150 consecutive bilateral lung volume reduction procedures in patients with severe emphysema. *J Thorac Cardiovasc Surg* 1996;112:1319–1329.

104. Rationale and design of The National Emphysema Treatment Trial: a prospective randomized trial of lung volume reduction surgery. National Emphysema Treatment Trial Research Group. *Chest* 1999;116:1750–1761.

105. Ramsey SD, Sullivan SD, Kaplan RM, et al. Economic analysis of lung volume reduction surgery as part of the National Emphysema Treatment Trial. NETT Research Group. *Ann Thorac Surg* 2001;71:995–1002.

106. Young J, Fry-Smith A, Hyde C. Lung volume reduction surgery (LVRS) for chronic obstructive pulmonary disease (COPD) with underlying severe emphysema. *Thorax* 1999;54:779–789.

107. Cordova F, O'Brien G, Furukawa S, et al. Stability of improvements in exercise performance and quality of life following bilateral lung volume reduction surgery in severe COPD. *Chest* 1997;112:907–915.

108. Meyers BF, Yusen RD, Lefrak SS, et al. Outcome of Medicare patients with emphysema selected for, but denied, a lung volume reduction operation. *Ann Thorac Surg* 1998;66:331–336.

109. Bloch KE, Georgescu CL, Russi EW, et al. Gain and subsequent loss of lung function after lung volume reduction surgery in

cases of severe emphysema with different morphologic patterns. *J Thorac Cardiovasc Surg* 2002;123:845–854.

110. Gelb AF, McKenna RJ Jr, Brenner M, et al. Lung function 5 years after lung volume reduction surgery for emphysema. *Am J Respir Crit Care Med* 2001;163:1562–1566.

111. Patients at high risk of death after lung-volume-reduction surgery. *N Engl J Med* 2001;345:1075–1083.

112. National Emphysema Treatment Trial Research Group. A randomized trial comparing lung-volume-reduction surgery with medical therapy for severe emphysema. *N Engl J Med* 2003;348(21):2059–2073.

112a. Ware JH. The National Emphysema Treatment Trial—how strong is the evidence? *N Engl J Med* 2003;348(21):2055–2056.

112b. Ingenito EP, Evans RB, Loring SH, et al. Relation between preoperative inspiratory lung resistance and the outcome of lung-volume-reduction surgery for emphysema. *N Engl J Med* 1998;338:1181–1185.

113. Flaherty KR, Kazerooni EA, Curtis JL, et al. Short-term and long-term outcomes after bilateral lung volume reduction surgery: prediction by quantitative CT. *Chest* 2001;119:1337–1346.

114. Burns KE, Keenan RJ, Grgurich WF, et al. Outcomes of lung volume reduction surgery followed by lung transplantation: a matched cohort study. *Ann Thorac Surg* 2002;73:1587–1593.

115. Ingenito EP, Reilly JJ, Mentzer SJ, et al. Bronchoscopic volume reduction: a safe and effective alternative to surgical therapy for emphysema. *Am J Respir Crit Care Med* 2001;164:295–301.

116. Bennett LE, Keck BM, Daily OP, et al. Worldwide thoracic organ transplantation: a report from the UNOS/ISHLT International Registry for Thoracic Organ Transplantation. *Clin Transpl* 2000;31–44.

117. Hosenpud JD, Bennett LE, Keck BM, et al. Effect of diagnosis on survival benefit of lung transplantation for end-stage lung disease. *Lancet* 1998;351:24–27.

118. Diaz PT, King MA, Pacht ER, et al. Increased susceptibility to pulmonary emphysema among HIV-seropositive smokers. *Ann Intern Med* 2000;132:369–372.

119. Goldstein DS, Karpel JP, Appel D, et al. Bullous pulmonary damage in users of intravenous drugs. *Chest* 1986;89:266–269.

120. Sherman CB, Hudson LD, Pierson DJ. Severe precocious emphysema in intravenous methylphenidate (Ritalin) abusers. *Chest* 1987;92:1085–1087.

121. Hnizdo E, Singh T, Churchyard G. Chronic pulmonary function impairment caused by initial and recurrent pulmonary tuberculosis following treatment. *Thorax* 2000;55:32–38.

122. Landbo C, Prescott E, Lange P, et al. Prognostic value of nutritional status in chronic obstructive pulmonary disease. *Am J Respir Crit Care Med* 1999;160:1856–1861.

123. Nishimura K, Izumi T, Tsukino M, et al. Dyspnea is a better predictor of 5-year survival than airway obstruction in patients with COPD. *Chest* 2002;121:1434–1440.

124. Kanner RE, Anthonisen NR, Connett JE. Lower respiratory illnesses promote FEV(1) decline in current smokers but not ex-smokers with mild chronic obstructive pulmonary disease: results from the lung health study. *Am J Respir Crit Care Med* 2001;164:358–364.

125. Vestbo J, Sorensen T, Lange P, et al. Long-term effect of inhaled budesonide in mild and moderate chronic obstruc-

tive pulmonary disease: a randomised controlled trial. *Lancet* 1999;353:1819–1823.

126. Pauwels RA, Lofdahl CG, Laitinen LA, et al. Long-term treatment with inhaled budesonide in persons with mild chronic obstructive pulmonary disease who continue smoking. European Respiratory Society Study on Chronic Obstructive Pulmonary Disease. *N Engl J Med* 1999;340:1948–1953.

127. Burge PS, Calverley PM, Jones PW, et al. Randomised, double blind, placebo controlled study of fluticasone propionate in patients with moderate to severe chronic obstructive pulmonary disease: the ISOLDE trial. *BMJ* 2000;320:1297–1303.

128. Effect of inhaled triamcinolone on the decline in pulmonary function in chronic obstructive pulmonary disease. *N Engl J Med* 2000;343:1902–1909.

129. Paggiaro PL, Dahle R, Bakran I, F et al. Multicentre randomised placebo-controlled trial of inhaled fluticasone propionate in patients with chronic obstructive pulmonary disease. International COPD Study Group. *Lancet* 1998;351:773–780.

130. Long term domiciliary oxygen therapy in chronic hypoxic cor pulmonale complicating chronic bronchitis and emphysema: report of the Medical Research Council Working Party. *Lancet* 1981;1:681–686.

131. Chaouat A, Weitzenblum E, Kessler R, et al. A randomized trial of nocturnal oxygen therapy in chronic obstructive pulmonary disease patients. *Eur Respir J* 1999;14:1002–1008.

132. Gorecka D, Gorzelak K, Sliwinski P, et al. Effect of long-term oxygen therapy on survival in patients with chronic obstructive pulmonary disease with moderate hypoxaemia. *Thorax* 1997;52:674–679.

133. Aubier M, Murciano D, Milic-Emili J, et al. Effects of the administration of O2 on ventilation and blood gases in patients with chronic obstructive pulmonary disease during acute respiratory failure. *Am Rev Respir Dis* 1980;122:747–754.

134. Turner MO, Patel A, Ginsburg S, et al. Bronchodilator delivery in acute airflow obstruction: a meta-analysis. *Arch Intern Med* 1997;157:1736–1744.

135. Cydulka RK, Emerman CL. Effects of combined treatment with glycopyrrolate and albuterol in acute exacerbation of chronic obstructive pulmonary disease. *Ann Emerg Med* 1995;25:470–473.

136. Anthonisen NR, Manfreda J, Warren CP, et al. Antibiotic therapy in exacerbations of chronic obstructive pulmonary disease. *Ann Intern Med* 1987;106:196–204.

137. Saint S, Bent S, Vittinghoff E, et al. Antibiotics in chronic obstructive pulmonary disease exacerbations: a meta-analysis. *JAMA* 1995;273:957–960.

138. Niewoehner DE, Erbland ML, Deupree RH, et al. Effect of systemic glucocorticoids on exacerbations of chronic obstructive pulmonary disease. Department of Veterans Affairs Cooperative Study Group. *N Engl J Med* 1999;340:1941–1947.

139. Sayiner A, Aytemur ZA, Cirit M, et al. Systemic glucocorticoids in severe exacerbations of COPD. *Chest* 2001;119:726–730.

140. Keenan SP, Gregor J, Sibbald WJ, et al. Noninvasive positive pressure ventilation in the setting of severe, acute exacerbations of chronic obstructive pulmonary disease: more effective and less expensive. *Crit Care Med* 2000;28:2094–2102.

141. International Consensus Conferences in Intensive Care Medicine: noninvasive positive pressure ventilation in acute respiratory failure. *Am J Respir Crit Care Med* 2001;163:283–291.

Baum's Textbook of Pulmonary Diseases, 7th ed. Edited by James D. Crapo, Jeffrey Glassroth, Joel Karlinsky, and Talmadge E. King, Jr. Lippincott Williams & Wilkins, Philadelphia © 2004.

13   Cystic Fibrosis

James R. Yankaskas

Cystic fibrosis (CF) is an autosomal-recessive genetic disease that affects the lungs, pancreas, sweat glands, and other epithelium-lined organs. In most patients, symptoms appear in early childhood—mainly malnutrition secondary to exocrine pancreatic insufficiency and progressive respiratory disease related to chronic airway infections. Comprehensive care for the complications of CF has vastly improved the survival and quality of life of these patients. A significant number of patients with CF now reach adulthood, develop productive careers, and have families.

Intensive research in basic science has elucidated many of the pathogenic mechanisms that lead to chronic infection and bronchiectasis in CF. Traditional pharmacologic techniques and high-throughput screenings of compound libraries are identifying drugs that modulate specific pathogenic steps. The efficacy of some new treatments has been tested in controlled clinical trials, and other drugs are now in phase I, II, or III trials. The Cystic Fibrosis Foundation has developed a therapeutic development network to accelerate clinical research and improve care more rapidly. The beneficial effects of the different treatments may be additive, and some may be useful for other airway diseases. These basic and clinical advances are providing hope for patients and their families. Integration of the many therapeutic options requires a good knowledge of the disease and offers fascinating and rewarding challenges to the astute clinician.

EPIDEMIOLOGY

CF is the most common lethal genetic disease in Caucasians (1). This autosomal-recessive disease is caused by mutations

J. R. Yankaskas: Department of Medicine, University of North Carolina, Chapel Hill, North Carolina.

in the CF transmembrane conductance regulator (CFTR) gene located on chromosome 7. A mutated CF gene is carried by 1 in 29 Caucasians, but a mutated gene does not cause symptoms. The carrier rate and incidence vary with ethnic groups. In Caucasians, a case of CF occurs in every 3,300 live births; in Hispanics, in every 9,500; in Native Americans, in every 11,200; in African Americans, in every 15,300; and in Asians, in every 32,100 live births.

When CF was first described in 1938, survival past infancy was rare. Improved treatments for pancreatic insufficiency, lung infections, and other complications increased the median survival from less than 1 year to 18 years by 1972 (2). In 2001, more than 22,700 patients with CF had been identified in the United States, and the median survival was 33.4 years (3). Adults (persons 18 years of age or older) now account for 39.6% of CF patients (3) and include a 78-year-old woman.

PATHOGENESIS

The CFTR gene encodes a 1,480–amino acid protein with 12 membrane-spanning regions, two nucleotide-binding folds, and a regulatory ("R") domain. The mature protein localizes to the apical membranes of the epithelium lining organs affected by the disease, particularly the airways, pancreatic duct, sweat gland ducts, intestines, and reproductive tract. CFTR protein acts as a Cl^- channel (4) and as a regulator of epithelial Na^+ channels (5) and other Cl^- channels (6). More than 1,000 different mutations in the CF gene have been identified along the entire length of the gene. The mutations have been grouped according to their molecular mechanisms. Class I (nonsense) mutations prevent protein production. Class II (trafficking) mutations produce proteins that fail to traffic to the apical cell membrane. The most common CF mutation, $\Delta F508$, is in this class and accounts for 68% of mutations in the United States. Class III (regulatory) mutations traffic properly, but ion channel regulation is defective. Class IV (conductance) mutations traffic properly, but Cl^- conductance is decreased. Some exon splice site mutations have been labeled class V mutations; these permit the transcription of some normal CFTR messenger RNA and confer a less severe clinical phenotype. All classes of mutations alter Cl^- permeability and the regulation of ion transport in the affected epithelial cells.

The pathogenesis of airways disease in CF has been partially elucidated. In bronchial epithelial cells, CFTR mutations decrease Cl^- permeability and increase net Na^+ absorption. As a result, the volume of airway surface liquid is decreased (7,8), mucociliary clearance is impaired, and cough clearance is probably decreased. These alternations in airway defenses facilitate secondary bacterial infection and chronic inflammation. *Pseudomonas* organisms in CF airways tend to form colonies within the mucus and remain intraluminal. As the density of bacteria increases, their quorum-sensing molecules (homoserine lactones) reach an adequate concentration to induce the expression of alginate genes and the formation of biofilms (9). The mucoid bacteria adapt to the nutrient-restricted environment and become resistant to antibiotics and phagocyte destruction (10). These changes may be a consequence of impaired antibiotic penetrance, reduced growth rate, phenotypic changes, or other factors. Nevertheless, chronic inflammation persists and progressively damages the airways. It has also been suggested that CF mutations lead to abnormal sulfation of mucus, abnormal function of peptide antimicrobial molecules (defensins) in the airways, and the accentuation of immune responses. The effects of these mechanisms and CFTR mutations on bronchiolar epithelial cells and submucosal glands are not fully understood. The clinical results are progressive airway destruction, cystic bronchiectasis, and respiratory failure.

CLINICAL FEATURES

CF is classically recognized from the triad of exocrine pancreatic insufficiency, bronchiectatic airways disease, and elevated levels of sweat chloride. In most patients, the onset of cough and chronic respiratory tract infections is during infancy or childhood. Early respiratory tract pathogens include *Staphylococcus aureus, Haemophilus influenzae,* and *Pseudomonas aeruginosa.* It is common to isolate several different bacteria from the sputum of adolescent and adult CF patients. The prevalence of *Pseudomonas* increases to about 80% by the teenage years; the organism usually develops to a mucoid phenotype and becomes the dominant pathogen. Pathologically, inflammation and obstruction of both bronchioles and bronchi develop, with submucosal gland hypertrophy. Bronchiectasis tends to start in the upper lobes and then generalize. Chest x-ray films show hyperinflated lungs, cystic bronchiectasis, and occasionally upper lobe atelectasis.

The clinical course of chronic cough, hypersecretion of mucus, and airway obstruction is progressive and punctuated by pulmonary exacerbations characterized by increased cough, dyspnea, and sputum production. Exacerbations are usually accompanied by a decrease in pulmonary function (i.e., forced expiratory volume in 1 second [FEV_1]). Severe exacerbations may cause anorexia and weight loss, but fevers are uncommon. When exacerbations are effectively treated, pulmonary function may return to the baseline level. With more severe disease, exacerbations tend to become more frequent and less reversible, leading to progressive respiratory failure and culminating in death.

DIAGNOSIS

The diagnostic criteria for CF are evidence of abnormal CFTR function plus characteristic respiratory or gastrointestinal disease (11). CFTR function can be assessed with the sweat chloride test (12), by CFTR mutational analysis, and by *in vivo* measurements of the nasal electric potential difference and its response to selected ion transport modulators (13). The sweat chloride is elevated in more than 98% of patients, but a properly performed sweat test is essential for an accurate diagnosis. Several companies test for many CFTR mutations, including the most common ones. These assays can detect mutations in more than 95% of CF cases. The American College of Obstetrics and Gynecology recommends CF carrier screening for all potential parents. The nasal electric potential difference was developed as a research tool and requires special training. Several research centers sponsored by the Cystic Fibrosis Foundation can provide such testing on a referral basis.

The clinical diagnosis of CF may be suggested by the family history or by the presence of meconium ileus at birth. The latter occurs in approximately 18% of CF cases and has few other causes. Exocrine pancreatic insufficiency occurs in more than 85% of CF patients and usually presents in the first year of life as steatorrhea or failure to gain weight despite a vigorous appetite. Lung disease typically presents with cough or infections with the bacteria previously listed, followed by airway obstruction and bronchiectasis. Of the patients reported to the Cystic Fibrosis Foundation Patient Registry, 51% presented with acute or persistent respiratory symptoms, 43% with failure to thrive or malnutrition, 35% with steatorrhea, and 21% with meconium ileus or intestinal obstruction (3). In about 62% of patients, CF is diagnosed in the first year of life, and in about 4%, it is diagnosed after the age of 18 years. Respiratory and gastrointestinal symptoms are common clues to the diagnosis in adults, whereas chronic pancreatitis, chronic rhinosinusitis, and bilateral absence of the vas deferens are recognized, but less frequent, presentations. Several states have started newborn screening for CF, usually based on the detection of low serum levels of trypsinogen and CFTR mutation analysis (14). Early diagnosis may improve nutrition and delay the onset of *Pseudomonas* infection.

MANAGEMENT

Gastrointestinal System

Pancreatic Insufficiency

Exocrine pancreatic insufficiency can be diagnosed on the basis of steatorrhea and failure to gain weight, and it is confirmed if the fat excreted in a 72-hour stool sample exceeds 7% of the intake. It is treated by administering oral pancreatic enzymes with meals and snacks. Enteric coatings protect the enzymes from gastric acid degradation. The usual adult dose of approximately 500 lipase units per kilogram per meal is titrated to control steatorrhea and maintain weight (15,16). Different brands, especially some generic preparations, have widely different protease and lipase contents and may not be interchangeable (17,18). The suppression of gastric acid production with proton pump inhibitors or histamine H_2 blockers may increase enzyme effectiveness (19). Patients with CFTR mutations that permit exocrine pancreatic function adequate for normal growth may require supplemental enzymes later in life.

Nutrition

The nutritional approach to CF patients changed dramatically in the 1980s. A CF center in Toronto managed patients with a high-protein, high-fat diet and compared their outcomes with those of patients at a similar large CF center in Boston where a low-protein, low-fat diet was used to control symptoms of steatorrhea (20). The two groups were similar in regard to number of patients, sex distribution, and level pulmonary function, but the median survival was 21 years in Boston and 30 years in Toronto. The high-protein, high-fat diet was adopted across the United States, and survival improved accordingly. The key elements are regular nutritional assessment; adequate intake of fat, protein, and calories; and sufficient intake of pancreatic enzymes (15,16). Adequate intake of vitamins, especially vitamins A, D, E, and K (fat-soluble vitamins), is also important. Dietary intake in the form of energy-dense foods, snacks, and commercial oral supplements should be tailored to individual needs. Malnourished patients may also require nocturnal nasogastric or gastrostomy tube feedings, which are preferable to parenteral nutrition (21–23).

Gastrointestinal Complications

Rectal prolapse occurs in about 3.5% of CF patients but is most common in children. Abdominal pain is common (24) and may reflect gastroesophageal reflux disease, gastritis, or other diseases that affect the general population. CF is related to several complications that may occur in adults. Distal intestinal obstruction syndrome develops more frequently in adolescence and adulthood and is manifested by constipation, cramping abdominal pain, and often a "doughy" mass in the right lower quadrant (25). The syndrome is caused by obstruction and irritation of the bowel wall by inspissated stool, commonly near the ileocecal valve. Narcotics, dehydration, inadequate pancreatic enzymes, or dietary changes can precipitate distal intestinal obstruction syndrome. It can often be diagnosed and treated medically with a hypertonic enema, provided that surgical complications such as appendicitis and volvulus have been excluded. Prevention is preferred. Osmotic cathartics counteract the excess salt and water absorption in the colon in CF and can be titrated to prevent recurrences without causing excessive diarrhea (26,27).

Hepatobiliary disease is common in CF patients (28) and often asymptomatic. Liver enzyme levels are elevated in about 25% of cases (29), and progressive inflammation leads to focal biliary cirrhosis. This causes symptomatic portal hypertension in a minority. Ursodeoxycholic acid is effective therapy for primary biliary cirrhosis (30), and clinical trials of its efficacy in CF-related liver disease have been performed (31–33). Complications of portal hypertension, such as bleeding from esophageal varices, are treated with standard measures, including varix banding, transvenous intrahepatic portosystemic shunting, and liver transplantation (34–37). Gallstones requiring surgery occur in about 0.7% of adults per year. Clinical pancreatitis may develop in patients with pancreatic sufficiency (38). This responds to standard medical therapy.

Pulmonary Disease

Airway Clearance

Pulmonary disease is the major form of morbidity in CF and the eventual cause of death in 95% of patients. Daily clearance of airway secretions is essential (39,40). This can be accomplished by chest physiotherapy, which may move secretions from small to larger airways, where cough can be effective. In a study of older children with mild-to-moderate airflow limitation receiving chest physiotherapy on a regular basis, the only documented immediate effect was an increase in the peak expiratory flow rate 30 minutes after therapy. However, after 3 weeks without chest physiotherapy, both the forced vital capacity and flow rates were significantly reduced (41). A metaanalysis of 35 studies concluded that standard chest physical therapy increases sputum production and improves expiratory airflow (FEV_1) (42). Most caregivers prescribe this therapy one to four times a day, depending on the severity of illness. Physical exercise augments airway clearance and improves cardiovascular function (43,44). Several airway clearance techniques have been developed to increase the autonomy of daily care. Special breathing techniques, including forced expiratory technique, autogenic drainage, and active cycle of breathing (45–47), vary the lung volumes and expiratory flows to augment clearance. The specific techniques have been reviewed (48), and a metaanalysis suggests that several can be equivalent to chest physiotherapy (42). Mechanical devices, including the flutter valve (47) and external thoracic compression devices, may improve patient independence, but their efficacy is less well established.

Antibiotics

Antibiotics are used extensively to control the airway infections that contribute to airway damage. Oral antibiotics against *S. aureus* are commonly prescribed, but the benefits of long-term use have not been established (49). Macrolide antibiotics are effective treatment for diffuse panbronchiolitis (50) and have been tested in CF patients. Controlled studies in children in Great Britain (51) and adults in Australia (52) showed better preservation of FEV_1 and fewer pulmonary exacerbations. The mechanisms for these effects have not been established but may be both antimicrobial and antiinflammatory. A larger U.S. study was completed in 2002 and is expected to confirm these findings. The early use of antibiotics for acute bronchitis produces better results than administration delayed until symptoms are advanced. Similarly, *P. aeruginosa* infection has been treated by regularly scheduled courses of intravenous antibiotics (53,54). Data justifying these approaches lack adequate controls.

Pulmonary exacerbations are treated with antibiotics directed at the major pulmonary pathogens, especially *Pseudomonas* species and *S. aureus*. The choice of antibiotics optimally should be based on the results of sputum culture and sensitivity testing during the preceding 1 to 12 months. Because of the high bacterial burden, two antibiotics with different mechanisms of action and with *in vitro* efficacy against each major bacterium are selected. Antibiotic synergy testing is available for Gram-negative bacteria that show resistance to all antibiotics in two of these classes (55). The total body volume of distribution and clearance for β-lactams, aminoglycosides, and sulfa drugs are considerably greater in patients with CF than in others, so that higher doses must be used (56, 57). Aminoglycosides are often dosed at 10 mg/kg per day in two doses. It is essential to titrate the dose to a peak level of 10 to 12 μg/mL with a trough below 2 μg/mL. Some authors advocate a single daily dose despite the risks for ototoxicity and nephrotoxicity (58). Experience also has led many caregivers of CF patients to use longer courses of antibiotics, continued for at least 2 weeks and even 3 to 4 weeks.

Few effective oral antibiotics are available for *Pseudomonas*, so parenteral or preservative-free preparations of aminoglycosides or other antibiotics have been delivered to the lower respiratory tract by aerosol (59). A randomized study demonstrated definite short-term benefits of aerosolized tobramycin (300 mg in a nebulizer) taken twice daily (60). This treatment, administered in alternate months for three cycles, improved lung function, decreased the bacterial burden, and decreased the relative risk for hospitalization. The rate of acquired tobramycin resistance was approximately 7% over 24 weeks in the treated group. Colistin often shows *in vitro* activity against *Pseudomonas,* but with significant toxicity (61). Several case series support its use (62,63), but no controlled studies have been performed. Aerosolized colistin has not been shown to be effective (64).

Bronchodilators

Many CF patients demonstrate bronchial reactivity some of the time. Bronchodilators, particularly β-adrenergic agonists, are safe and may be effective (65). Despite documentation of immediate effectiveness by pulmonary function testing, long-term benefit has not been established (66). Indications for the use of bronchodilators include troublesome wheezing or at least a 15% improvement in the FEV_1. β-Agonists can be nebulized, administered by meter-dose inhalers, or given orally. Theophylline preparations may be effective in selected cases, but CF patients seem to be less tolerant because of frequent gastrointestinal irritation. Ipratropium bromide is at least as effective as β-agonists in CF (67,68). Cromolyn sodium has also been used, but a single study failed to demonstrate efficacy (69).

Mucolytics

Aerosolized Recombinant Human DNase
Recombinant human DNase can lyse viscous DNA in purulent airway secretions and is beneficial in some patients (70). When taken once daily for 6 months, aerosolized DNase reduced the relative risk for respiratory exacerbations by 28% and improved the FEV_1 to approximately 6% above baseline. Not all patients showed an objective improvement in lung function, but symptomatic benefits were noted in many of the treated patients. The long-term effect of DNase on lung function has been evaluated in an open-label multinational study (71).

Other Aerosol Therapy
Other aerosolized solutions may add liquid to inspissated mucous secretions and improve their viscoelastic properties, so that they can be more easily cleared. Normal saline solution (0.9 g/100 mL) is used frequently, but the efficacy of this approach has not been substantiated. Studies from Australia suggest that aerosolized hypertonic saline solution (3–12 g/100 mL) may offer short-term benefit, with acute improvement in lung function and mucociliary clearance (72,73).

N-acetylcysteine reduces disulfide bonds and decreases sputum viscosity *in vitro*. Oral dosing does not produce effective airway concentrations (74), and studies have shown small or no clinical effects (75,76). Aerosolized *N*-acetylcysteine irritates the upper airways and causes bronchospasm. Its efficacy has not been established.

Antiinflammatory Drugs

Corticosteroids

A small double-blinded controlled study of alternate-day oral prednisone administered for 4 years demonstrated better maintenance of pulmonary function and fewer exacerbations of lung disease requiring hospitalization (77). However, a larger multicenter study of prednisone at a dose of 1 or 2 mg/kg every other day failed to confirm efficacy, and this regimen was attended by an unacceptable rate of side effects, including growth suppression and hyperglycemia (78–80). The widespread use of corticosteroids cannot be advocated. Inhaled steroids can reduce systemic toxicity but may not penetrate obstructed airways. Preliminary studies suggest some efficacy (81). Systemic steroids may be used for specific indications, such as allergic bronchopulmonary aspergillosis.

Ibuprofen

A study of high-dose ibuprofen given for 4 years indicated a remarkable slowing of the decline in lung function (eightfold) in young CF patients (younger than 13 years of age) with mild lung disease in comparison with placebo-controlled subjects (82). No effect was documented in patients older than 13 years, even those with the mildest lung

STANDARD THERAPY OF CYSTIC FIBROSIS AIRWAY DISEASE

Summary Statement	Level of Evidence
Regular medical care with frequent spirometry and sputum cultures is recommended.	Consensus of expert opinion
Regular clearance of airway secretions is recommended.	Well-controlled clinical trials
Intermittent use of effective oral antibiotics for subacute exacerbations is recommended.	Consensus of expert opinion
Chronic oral macrolide antibiotics improve pulmonary function and reduce the need for anti-*Pseudomonas* therapy.	Well-controlled clinical trials
Aerosolized tobramycin taken twice daily in alternate months improves lung function and decreases the relative risk for hospitalization.	Well-controlled clinical trials
Aerosolized recombinant human DNase reduces the relative risk for pulmonary exacerbations and improves the FEV_1.	Well-controlled clinical trials
Systemic corticosteroids improve lung function but suppress growth and cause or worsen hyperglycemia.	Well-controlled clinical trials
Lung transplantation is an effective treatment for progressive respiratory failure secondary to cystic fibrosis.	Well-controlled survival studies

FEV_1, forced expiratory volume in 1 second.

disease. Few side effects were noted, but most of the patients were taking antacids or histamine H_2 receptor blockers.

Exacerbations

Pulmonary exacerbations may develop acutely or during several weeks and reflect increased airway inflammation and obstruction. Viral infections, plugging of mucus, or inadequate airway hygiene may precipitate exacerbations. Increased cough or wheezing, dyspnea, a decreased ability to tolerate activity, and anorexia are common symptoms and may be accompanied by decreased pulmonary function, increased hypoxemia, and weight loss. The treatment is intensified airway clearance and the administration of antibiotics directed at the main airway bacteria. Hospitalization is usually required to administer intravenous antibiotics for *Pseudomonas* infection and to intensify physical maneuvers to clear airway secretions.

Antibiotics should be selected on the basis of respiratory tract culture and susceptibility studies during the preceding 1 to 12 months (83). Two anti-*Pseudomonas* drugs from different classes (i.e., aminoglycosides, β-lactams, and fluoroquinolones) are used to reduce the risk for selecting resistant organisms. A third antibiotic may be needed for *S. aureus* or other organisms. Clinical improvements are usually gradual and tend to be slower when airway disease is more severe. A 2-week course generally provides good improvement in pulmonary function (84,85) and more sustained benefit than shorter courses. Treatment for 3 weeks or more may be required for refractory exacerbations. Some advocate intensive therapy until pulmonary function has returned to the recent baseline or until improvement has plateaued. If improvement is not noted, periodic sputum cultures should be obtained to seek new or resistant bacteria. The results of sputum culture may not correlate with the clinical outcome because of heterogeneous lung infections, laboratory sampling, differences between *in vitro* and *in vivo* conditions, and immune responses. The clinical response definitely takes precedence.

Aminoglycosides have been the mainstay of anti-*Pseudomonas* therapy for many years. A major advantage is the ability to titrate the dose to achieve therapeutic blood levels. For gentamicin or tobramycin, the initial dose is 10 mg/kg per day given in two doses and titrated to peaks of 10 to 12 μg/mL and troughs below 2 μg/mL. Patients should be monitored for nephrotoxicity and ototoxicity. The aminoglycoside is usually paired with an effective β-lactam. It is common to isolate several different pseudomonads with different susceptibility patterns. Ideally, two effective antibiotics from different classes should be selected for all the organisms.

Patients with CF, particularly those who are in school or working, may opt to administer intravenous antibiotics at home for all or a portion of the treatment course. Home intravenous antibiotic therapy has cost and convenience advantages, but its clinical efficacy in this setting has not been rigorously established (86). Patients requiring frequent courses or long-term home antibiotic therapy have had central intravenous catheters surgically placed and have used them for prolonged periods.

THERAPY OF PULMONARY EXACERBATIONS IN CYSTIC FIBROSIS	
Summary Statement	**Level of Evidence**
Clearance of airway secretions by multiple daily sessions of chest physical therapy is recommended.	Well-controlled clinical trials and consensus of expert opinion
Two antibiotics from different classes are recommended to maximize efficacy and reduce the incidence of antibiotic resistance.	Consensus of expert opinion
Doses of β-lactam and aminoglycoside antibiotics should be increased because of altered pharmacokinetics and titrated to therapeutic levels.	Pharmacokinetic studies in patients with cystic fibrosis and consensus of expert opinion
Antibiotic treatment should be continued until maximal clinical benefits are achieved.	Consensus of expert opinion

Pneumothorax

Pneumothoraces occur in 0.2% of children and 1.1% of adults with CF per year, and recurrences are common (3). A small and minimally symptomatic pneumothorax can be observed for spontaneous resolution. A large pneumothorax (>20% of the hemithorax volume, compromising ventilation, or causing hypotension) requires tube drainage (87,88). Recurrences may require repeated drainage or multiple chest tubes, or even surgical pleural abrasion (89).

Massive Hemoptysis

The incidence of massive hemoptysis increases from 0.2% annually in children to 1.8% annually in adults with CF (3). Episodes of massive hemoptysis, defined as spitting up more than 240 mL of blood per 24 hours, are managed with antibiotics, transient cough suppression, a reduction in chest physiotherapy, and often bronchial artery embolization (87,90,91). Such therapy is usually effective and does not compromise candidacy for eventual lung transplantation.

Respiratory Failure

Hypercapnic and hypoxemic respiratory failure in CF is caused primarily by progressive obstructive airway disease with alveolar hypoventilation and ventilation-perfusion mismatch. Treatment with antibiotics and the airway clearance

measures previously summarized (see section "Airway Clearance") is essential. Low-flow oxygen is effective at relieving nocturnal, exertional, and resting hypoxemia and does not usually cause significant hypercapnia (92). The use of supplemental oxygen in children has been discouraged (93) because nocturnal oxygen did not improve survival or prevent the development of cor pulmonale in one controlled trial (94). A larger study demonstrated that the development of pulmonary hypertension in adults with CF is strongly correlated with hypoxemia and increased mortality (95). Therefore, supplemental oxygen in accordance with the guidelines established for chronic obstructive pulmonary disease is recommended (96). Diuretics, inotropic agents, and theophylline produce few benefits and are rarely used. Cor pulmonale is a late complication of airway obstruction, and no treatment options beyond those for the primary disease processes are effective.

Ventilatory assistance is effective in CF patients with acute respiratory failure caused by reversible insults (97), but it produces few long-term benefits in patients with respiratory failure secondary to irreversible lung damage caused by CF bronchiectasis (98). Assisted ventilation with the use of nasal or face masks (99,100) or endotracheal tubes can effectively treat patients awaiting lung transplantation (101). The airway disease progresses, however, and long-term ventilatory support is rarely feasible.

Lung Transplantation

The first heart-lung transplant for CF was performed in 1983, and lung transplantation has become an effective form of therapy (102). By 2001, more than 1,270 heart-lung or double-lung transplants (the preferred operation in the United States) for CF had been performed in the United States. Evaluation for transplantation is indicated when natural survival is expected to be slightly longer than the waiting time for donor organ availability, currently about 2 years. The highly variable progression of CF makes prediction difficult, but an FEV_1 value below 30% of the predicted value and increasing functional impairment with frequent hospitalization are accepted referral criteria. The 1- and 5-year survival rates after lung transplantation for CF are 70% and 48%, respectively. These are comparable with the survival rates of patients receiving lung transplants for other diseases. Deaths in the first year are caused primarily by operative complications and infections. After 1 year, most deaths are caused by obliterative bronchiolitis, the pathologic marker of chronic rejection. The scanty number of donor organs limits the availability of lung transplantation, and many patients wait more than 2 years after being accepted as a transplant candidate. Living donor transplantation (sequential transplantation of a lower lung lobe from each of two donors) has become an effective alternative in some centers (103).

Gene Therapy

Transfer of a normal CF gene to CF epithelial cells *in vitro* corrects the ion transport abnormalities and suggests that effective gene therapy can be developed. The potential difficulties include gene packaging and delivery, treating a sufficient number of affected cells, duration of the transferred gene, and local toxicity. A number of clinical trials using adenovirus, adeno-associated virus, and cationic liposomes have been completed. Several demonstrated gene transfer at a low level of efficiency, but none showed clinical efficacy (104).

Reproductive Tract

More than 98% of male patients with CF are infertile because of a bilateral absence of the vas deferens (105). The mechanism has not be established, but some cases suggest obstruction and involution rather than congenital malformation. The fertility of female patients may be decreased because of malnutrition or thickened cervical mucus (106). Concomitant with improved survival, the number of pregnancies reported to the Cystic Fibrosis Foundation Patient Registry has increased to about 180 per year (1.6 live births per year per 100 women ages 13–45 years) (3). Pregnancy increases the respiratory demands in all women, and women with CF-associated severe respiratory impairment (FEV_1 <50% of the predicted value) constitute a high-risk group. The fetal outcomes are comparable with those of the normal population, and pregnancy does not appear to be a significant risk factor for decline in pulmonary function or death (107).

Sweat Glands

The sweat chloride is elevated in most CF patients because of abnormal reabsorption of sodium chloride in the sweat ducts (11). Excessive loss of salt in the sweat predisposes young children to dehydration, especially in the setting of vomiting or diarrhea. These children present with lethargy, anorexia, and hypochloremic alkalosis, particularly in warm, arid zones. Such hypochloremic alkalosis is rare in older children and adults.

Cystic Fibrosis–Related Diabetes

Hyperglycemia secondary to progressive loss of the pancreatic islets in CF can occur at any age but it is generally a problem in the second and third decades of life (108). Ketoacidosis is rarely encountered. When blood glucose levels are only intermittently elevated and glycosuria is not present, no treatment is necessary. If sustained glycosuria develops, insulin treatment should be instituted. Oral hypoglycemic agents, considered ineffective in the past, may be helpful in selected patients. The development of significant hyperglycemia may not affect survival. However, vascular disease of the retinas and kidneys has been documented in CF patients with prolonged hyperglycemia. Therefore, careful control of blood sugar levels is desirable.

Bone Disease

CF predisposes to a low bone mineral density through nutritional limitations and the side effects of some treatments. A low bone mineral density can lead to pathologic fractures, limit the ability to clear airway secretions, and even prevent lung transplant candidacy (109–111). Preventive and symptomatic treatments include excellent nutrition, adequate calcium and vitamin D intake, and exercise. Bisphosphonates to strengthen bone have been tested in adults and shown to be effective (112,113). A committee sponsored by the Cystic Fibrosis Foundation met in 2002 to summarize current knowledge of this topic and is generating consensus recommendations (114–117).

Adult Issues

Psychosocial factors undoubtedly play a prominent role in outcome, but this is difficult to document (118). The role of a supportive family is crucial. Suicide is uncommon. However, it is widely recognized that a substantial number of adolescent and adult patients do not comply fully with their medical regimen because of denial, unresolved dependence-independence issues, and depression. Clearly, attitude and the ability to cope with a fatal illness during maturation and early adulthood can influence quality of life and probably survival.

SUMMARY

As a consequence of improved treatment and increased survival, a large number of adults have CF. Intensive research has identified the main pathogenic factors and permitted the development and testing of treatments that target the pathogenic mechanisms and their secondary effects. The clearance of airway secretions and the administration of antibiotics, supplemented by bronchodilators, mucolytic agents, and other forms of therapy, can modulate chronic disease and treat pulmonary exacerbations.

Clinical research in CF is progressing rapidly. Randomized controlled clinical trials have established the effectiveness of novel treatments, such as aerosolized DNase and tobramycin. The nationwide Cystic Fibrosis Therapeutics Development Network has facilitated and accelerated clinical trials, and subject enrollment is increasing. Novel mechanistic treatments are likely to be developed, tested, and proved effective in the next decade. These may not reverse cystic bronchiectasis, but they are likely to increase survival and improve quality of life further. Their application in children and infants may even prevent the progression of CF airway disease.

REFERENCES

1. Davis PB, Drumm M, Konstan MW. Cystic fibrosis. *Am J Respir Crit Care Med* 1996;154:1229–1256.
2. FitzSimmons SC. The changing epidemiology of cystic fibrosis. *J Pediatr* 1993;122:1–9.
3. Cystic Fibrosis Foundation. *Patient registry 2001 annual report.* Bethesda, MD: Cystic Fibrosis Foundation, 2002.
4. Bear CE, Li C, Kartner N, et al. Purification and functional reconstitution of the cystic fibrosis transmembrane conductance regulator (CFTR). *Cell* 1992;68:809–818.
5. Stutts MJ, Canessa CM, Olsen JC, et al. CFTR as a cAMP-dependent regulator of sodium channels. *Science* 1995;269:847–850.
6. Gabriel SE, Clarke LL, Boucher RC, et al. CFTR and outward rectifying chloride channels are distinct proteins with a regulatory relationship. *Nature* 1993;363:263–266.
7. Matsui H, Grubb BR, Tarran R, et al. Evidence for periciliary liquid layer depletion, not abnormal ion composition, in the pathogenesis of cystic fibrosis airways disease. *Cell* 1998;95:1005–1015.
8. Tarran R, Grubb BR, Parsons D, et al. The CF salt controversy: *in vivo* observations and therapeutic approaches. *Mol Cell* 2001;8:149–158.
9. Costerton JW, Stewart PS, Greenberg EP. Bacterial biofilms: a common cause of persistent infections. *Science* 1999;284:1318–1322.
10. Worlitzsch D, Tarran R, Ulrich M, et al. Effects of reduced mucus oxygen concentration in airway *Pseudomonas* infections of cystic fibrosis patients. *J Clin Invest* 2002;109:317–325.
11. Rosenstein BJ, Cutting GR. *The diagnosis of cystic fibrosis: a consensus statement.* Cystic Fibrosis Foundation Consensus Panel. *J Pediatr* 1998;132:589–595.
12. National Committee for Clinical Laboratory Standards. *Sweat testing: sample collection and quantitative analysis; approved guideline.* Villanova, PA: National Committee for Clinical Laboratory Standards, 1994.
13. Knowles MR, Paradiso AM, Boucher RC. *In vivo* nasal potential difference: techniques and protocols for assessing efficacy of gene transfer in cystic fibrosis. *Hum Gene Ther* 1995;6:445–455.
14. Farrell PM, Kosorok MR, Rock MJ, et al. Early diagnosis of cystic fibrosis through neonatal screening prevents severe malnutrition and improves long-term growth. *Pediatrics* 2001;107:1–13.
15. Ramsey BW, Farrell PM, Pencharz P. Nutritional assessment and management in cystic fibrosis: a consensus report. The Consensus Committee. *Am J Clin Nutr* 1992;55:108–116.
16. Borowitz D, Baker RD, Stallings V. Consensus report on nutrition for pediatric patients with cystic fibrosis. *J Pediatr Gastroenterol Nutr* 2002;35:246–259.
17. Dutta SK, Hubbard VS, Appler M. Critical examination of therapeutic efficacy of a pH-sensitive enteric-coated pancreatic enzyme preparation in the treatment of exocrine pancreatic insufficiency secondary to cystic fibrosis. *Dig Dis Sci* 1988;33:1237–1244.
18. Kraisinger M, Hochhaus G, Stecenko A, et al. Clinical pharmacology of pancreatic enzymes in patients with cystic fibrosis and *in vitro* performance of microencapsulated formulations. *J Clin Pharmacol* 1994;34:158–166.
19. Durie PR, Bell L, Linton W, et al. Effect of cimetidine and sodium

20. Corey M, McLaughlin FJ, Williams M, et al. A comparison of survival, growth, and pulmonary function in patients with cystic fibrosis in Boston and Toronto. *J Clin Epidemiol* 1988;41:583–591.
21. Erskine JM, Lingard CD, Sontag MK, et al. Enteral nutrition for patients with cystic fibrosis: comparison of a semi-elemental and nonelemental formula. *J Pediatr* 1998;132:265–269.
22. Williams SG, Ashworth F, McAlweenie A, et al. Percutaneous endoscopic gastrostomy feeding in patients with cystic fibrosis. *Gut* 1999;44:87–90.
23. Allen ED, Mick AB, Nicol J, et al. Prolonged parenteral nutrition for cystic fibrosis patients. *Nutr Clin Pract* 1995;10:73–79.
24. Littlewood JM. Abdominal pain in cystic fibrosis. *J R Soc Med* 1995;88:9–17.
25. Glick SN, Kressel HY, Laufer I, et al. Meconium ileus equivalent: treatment with Hypaque enema. *Diagn Imaging* 1980;49:149–152.
26. Cleghorn GJ, Stringer DA, Forstner GG, et al. Treatment of distal intestinal obstruction syndrome in cystic fibrosis with a balanced intestinal lavage solution. *Lancet* 1986;1:8–11.
27. Koletzko S, Stringer DA, Cleghorn GJ, et al. Lavage treatment of distal intestinal obstruction syndrome in children with cystic fibrosis. *Pediatrics* 1989;83:727–733.
28. Sokol RJ, Durie PR. Recommendations for management of liver and biliary tract disease in cystic fibrosis. Cystic Fibrosis Foundation Hepatobiliary Disease Consensus Group. *J Pediatr Gastroenterol Nutr* 1999;28[Suppl 1]:S1–13.
29. Modolell I, Alvarez A, Guarner L, et al. Gastrointestinal, liver, and pancreatic involvement in adult patients with cystic fibrosis. *Pancreas* 2001;22:395–399.
30. Poupon RE, Lindor KD, Cauch-Dudek K, et al. Combined analysis of randomized controlled trials of ursodeoxycholic acid in primary biliary cirrhosis. *Gastroenterology* 1997;113:884–890.
31. Colombo C, Crosignani A, Assaisso M, et al. Ursodeoxycholic acid therapy in cystic fibrosis-associated liver disease: a dose-response study. *Hepatology* 1992;16:924–930.
32. Lindblad A, Glaumann H, Strandvik B. A two-year prospective study of the effect of ursodeoxycholic acid on urinary bile acid excretion and liver morphology in cystic fibrosis-associated liver disease. *Hepatology* 1998;27:166–174.
33. Nousia-Arvanitakis S, Fotoulaki M, Economou H, et al. Long-term prospective study of the effect of ursodeoxycholic acid on cystic fibrosis-related liver disease. *J Clin Gastroenterol* 2001;32:324–328.
34. Kerns SR, Hawkins IF, Jr. Transjugular intrahepatic portosystemic shunt in a child with cystic fibrosis. *AJR Am J Roentgenol* 1992;159:1277–1278.
35. Debray D, Lykavieris P, Gauthier F, et al. Outcome of cystic fibrosis-associated liver cirrhosis: management of portal hypertension. *J Hepatol* 1999;31:77–83.
36. Sarin SK, Lamba GS, Kumar M, et al. Comparison of endoscopic ligation and propranolol for the primary prevention of variceal bleeding. *N Engl J Med* 1999;340:988–993.
37. Noble-Jamieson G, Valente J, Barnes ND, et al. Liver transplantation for hepatic cirrhosis in cystic fibrosis. *Arch Dis Child* 1994;71:349–352.
38. Cohn JA, Friedman KJ, Noone PG, et al. Relation between mutations of the cystic fibrosis gene and idiopathic pancreatitis. *N Engl J Med* 1998;339:653–658.
39. Ramsey BW. Management of pulmonary diseases in patients with cystic fibrosis. *N Engl J Med* 1996;335:179–188.
40. Yankaskas JR, Marshall BC, Sufian B, et al. Cystic fibrosis adult

care consensus conference report. *Concepts in care,* vol IX, section 3. Bethesda, MD: Cystic Fibrosis Foundation, 1999:1–50.

41. Desmond KJ, Schwenk WF, Thomas E, et al. Immediate and long-term effects of chest physiotherapy in patients with cystic fibrosis. *J Pediatr* 1983;103:538–542.

42. Thomas J, Cook DJ, Brooks D. Chest physical therapy management of patients with cystic fibrosis. A meta-analysis. *Am J Respir Crit Care Med* 1995;151:846–850.

43. Andreasson B, Jonson B, Kornfalt R, et al. Long-term effects of physical exercise on working capacity and pulmonary function in cystic fibrosis. *Acta Paediatr Scand* 1987;76:70–75.

44. Schneiderman-Walker J, Pollock SL, Corey M, et al. A randomized controlled trial of a 3-year home exercise program in cystic fibrosis. *J Pediatr* 2000;136:304–310.

45. Mahlmeister MJ, Fink JB, Hoffman GL, et al. Positive expiratory pressure mask therapy: theoretical and practical considerations and a review of the literature. *Respir Care* 1991;36:1218–1229.

46. McIlwaine PM, Wong LT, Peacock D, et al. Long-term comparative trial of conventional postural drainage and percussion versus positive expiratory pressure physiotherapy in the treatment of cystic fibrosis. *J Pediatr* 1997;131:570–574.

47. McIlwaine PM, Wong LT, Peacock D, et al. Long-term comparative trial of positive expiratory pressure versus oscillating positive expiratory pressure (flutter) physiotherapy in the treatment of cystic fibrosis. *J Pediatr* 2001;138:845–850.

48. Hardy KA, Anderson BD. Noninvasive clearance of airway secretions. *Respir Care Clin N Am* 1996;2:323–345.

49. McCaffery K, Olver RE, Franklin M, et al. Systematic review of antistaphylococcal antibiotic therapy in cystic fibrosis. *Thorax* 1999;54:380–383.

50. Kudoh S, Azuma A, Yamamoto M, et al. Improvement of survival in patients with diffuse panbronchiolitis treated with low-dose erythromycin. *Am J Respir Crit Care Med* 1998;157:1829–1832.

51. Equi A, Balfour-Lynn IM, Bush A, et al. Long-term azithromycin in children with cystic fibrosis: a randomised, placebo-controlled crossover trial. *Lancet* 2002;360:978–984.

52. Wolter J, Seeney S, Bell S, et al. Effect of long-term treatment with azithromycin on disease parameters in cystic fibrosis: a randomised trial. *Thorax* 2002;57:212–216.

53. Szaff M, Hoiby N, Flensborg EW. Frequent antibiotic therapy improves survival of cystic fibrosis patients with chronic *Pseudomonas aeruginosa* infection. *Acta Paediatr Scand* 1983;72:651–657.

54. Elborn JS, Prescott RJ, Stack BHR, et al. Elective versus symptomatic antibiotic treatment in cystic fibrosis patients with chronic *Pseudomonas* infection of the lungs. *Thorax* 2000;55:355–358.

55. Saiman L, Mehar F, Niu WW, et al. Antibiotic susceptibility of multiply resistant *Pseudomonas aeruginosa* isolated from patients with cystic fibrosis, including candidates for transplantation. *Clin Infect Dis* 1996;23:532–537.

56. de Groot R, Smith AL. Antibiotic pharmacokinetics in cystic fibrosis. Differences and clinical significance. *Clin Pharmacokinet* 1987;13:228–253.

57. Smith A, Cohen M, Ramsey B. Pharmacotherapy. In: Yankaskas JR, Knowles MR, eds. *Cystic fibrosis in adults.* Philadelphia: Lippincott–Raven Publishers, 1999:345–364.

58. Whitehead A, Conway SP, Etherington C, et al. Once-daily tobramycin in the treatment of adult patients with cystic fibrosis. *Eur Respir J* 2002;19:303–309.

59. Ramsey BW, Dorkin HL, Eisenberg JD, et al. Efficacy of aerosolized tobramycin in patients with cystic fibrosis. *N Engl J Med* 1993;328:1740–1746.

60. Ramsey BW, Pepe MS, Quan JM, et al. Intermittent administration of inhaled tobramycin in patients with cystic fibrosis. *N Engl J Med* 1999;340:23–30.

61. Cunningham S, Prasad A, Collyer L, et al. Bronchoconstriction following nebulised colistin in cystic fibrosis. *Arch Dis Child* 2001;84:432–433.

62. Ledson MJ, Gallagher MJ, Cowperthwaite C, et al. Four years' experience of intravenous colomycin in an adult cystic fibrosis unit. *Eur Respir J* 1998;12:592–594.

63. Conway SP, Pond MN, Watson A, et al. Intravenous colistin sulphomethate in acute respiratory exacerbations in adult patients with cystic fibrosis. *Thorax* 1997;52:987–993.

64. Hodson ME, Gallagher CG, Govan JRW. A randomised clinical trial of nebulised tobramycin or colistin in cystic fibrosis. *Eur Respir J* 2002;20:658–664.

65. Eggleston PA, Rosenstein BJ, Stackhouse CM, et al. A controlled trial of long-term bronchodilator therapy in cystic fibrosis. *Chest* 1991;99:1088–1092.

66. Konig P, Poehler J, Barbero G. A placebo-controlled, double-blind trial of the long-term effects of albuterol administration in patients with cystic fibrosis. *Pediatr Pulmonol* 1998;25:32–36.

67. Summers QA, Tarala RA. Nebulized ipratropium in the treatment of acute asthma. *Chest* 1990;97:425–429.

68. Weintraub SJ, Eschenbacher WL. The inhaled bronchodilators ipratropium bromide and metaproterenol in adults with CF. *Chest* 1989;95:861–864.

69. Sivan Y, Arce P, Eigen H, et al. A double-blind, randomized study of sodium cromoglycate versus placebo in patients with cystic fibrosis and bronchial hyperreactivity. *J Allergy Clin Immunol* 1990;85:649–654.

70. Fuchs HJ, Borowitz DS, Christiansen DH, et al. Effect of aerosolized recombinant human DNase on exacerbations of respiratory symptoms and on pulmonary function in patients with cystic fibrosis. The Pulmozyme Study Group. *N Engl J Med* 1994;331:637–642.

71. Rosenstein BJ, Johnson CAC. Long-term follow-up of phase III rhDNase trial. *Pediatr Pulmonol* 1994;10[Suppl]:113–114.

72. Robinson M, Hemming AL, Regnis JA, et al. Effect of increasing doses of hypertonic saline on mucociliary clearance in patients with cystic fibrosis. *Thorax* 1997;52:900–903.

73. King M, Dasgupta B, Tomkiewicz RP, et al. Rheology of cystic fibrosis sputum after *in vitro* treatment with hypertonic saline alone and in combination with recombinant human deoxyribonuclease I. *Am J Respir Crit Care Med* 1997;156:173–177.

74. Cotgreave IA, Eklund A, Larsson K, et al. No penetration of orally administered *N*-acetylcysteine into bronchoalveolar lavage fluid. *Eur J Respir Dis* 1987;70:73–77.

75. Ratjen F, Wonne R, Posselt HG, et al. A double-blind placebo controlled trial with oral ambroxol and *N*-acetylcysteine for mucolytic treatment in cystic fibrosis. *Eur J Pediatr* 1985;144:374–378.

76. Stafanger G, Koch C. *N*-acetylcysteine in cystic fibrosis and *Pseudomonas aeruginosa* infection: clinical score, spirometry and ciliary motility. *Eur Respir J* 1989;2:234–237.

77. Auerbach HS, Williams M, Kirkpatrick JA, et al. Alternate-day prednisone reduces morbidity and improves pulmonary function in cystic fibrosis. *Lancet* 1985;2:686–688.

78. Rosenstein BJ, Eigen H. Risks of alternate-day prednisone in patients with cystic fibrosis. *Pediatrics* 1991;87:245–246.

79. Eigen H, Rosenstein BJ, FitzSimmons S, et al. A multicenter study of alternate-day prednisone therapy in patients with cystic fibrosis. Cystic Fibrosis Foundation Prednisone Trial Group. *J Pediatr* 1995;126:515–523.

80. Lai HC, FitzSimmons SC, Allen DB, et al. Risk of persistent

growth impairment after alternate-day prednisone treatment in children with cystic fibrosis. *N Engl J Med* 2000;342:851–859.

81. Nikolaizik WH, Schoni MH. Pilot study to assess the effect of inhaled corticosteroids on lung function in patients with cystic fibrosis. *J Pediatr* 1996;128:271–274.

82. Konstan MW, Byard PJ, Hoppel CL, et al. Effect of high-dose ibuprofen in patients with cystic fibrosis. *N Engl J Med* 1995;332: 848–854.

83. Cystic Fibrosis Foundation. *Consensus conference. Microbiology and infectious diseases in cystic fibrosis.* Bethesda, MD: Cystic Fibrosis Foundation, 1994:1–26.

84. Redding GJ, Restuccia R, Cotton EK, et al. Serial changes in pulmonary functions in children hospitalized with cystic fibrosis. *Am Rev Respir Dis* 1982;126:31–36.

85. Regelmann WE, Elliott GR, Warwick WJ, et al. Reduction of sputum *Pseudomonas aeruginosa* density by antibiotics improves lung function in cystic fibrosis more than do bronchodilators and chest physiotherapy alone. *Am Rev Respir Dis* 1990;141:914–921.

86. Gilbert DN, Dworkin RJ, Raber SR, et al. Outpatient antimicrobial-drug therapy. *N Engl J Med* 1997;337:829–838.

87. Schidlow DV, Taussig LM, Knowles MR. Cystic Fibrosis Foundation consensus conference report on pulmonary complications of cystic fibrosis. *Pediatr Pulmonol* 1993;15:187–198.

88. Yankaskas JR, Egan TM, Mauro MA. Major complications. In: Yankaskas JR, Knowles MR, eds. *Cystic fibrosis in adults.* Philadelphia: Lippincott–Raven Publishers, 1999:175–193.

89. Egan TM. Thoracic surgery for patients with cystic fibrosis. In: Orenstein DM, Stern RC, eds. *Treatment of the hospitalized cystic fibrosis patient.* New York: Marcel Dekker Inc, 1997:231–281.

90. Fellows KE, Khaw KT, Schuster S, et al. Bronchial artery embolization in cystic fibrosis: technique and long-term results. *J Pediatr* 1979;95:959–963.

91. Brinson GM, Noone PG, Mauro MA, et al. Bronchial artery embolization for the treatment of hemoptysis in patients with cystic fibrosis. *Am J Respir Crit Care Med* 1998;157:1951–1958.

92. Spier S, Rivlin J, Hughes D, et al. The effect of oxygen on sleep, blood gases, and ventilation in cystic fibrosis. *Am Rev Respir Dis* 198;129:712–718.

93. Coates AL. Oxygen therapy, exercise, and cystic fibrosis. *Chest* 1992;101:2–4.

94. Zinman R, Corey M, Coates AL, et al. Nocturnal home oxygen in the treatment of hypoxemic cystic fibrosis patients. *J Pediatr* 1989;114:368–377.

95. Fraser KL, Tullis DE, Sasson Z, et al. Pulmonary hypertension and cardiac function in adult cystic fibrosis: role of hypoxemia. *Chest* 1999;115:1321–1328.

96. Anonymous. Continuous or nocturnal oxygen therapy in hypoxemic chronic obstructive lung disease: a clinical trial. Nocturnal Oxygen Therapy Trial Group. *Ann Intern Med* 1980;93:391–398.

97. Garland JS, Chan YM, Kelly KJ, et al. Outcome of infants with cystic fibrosis requiring mechanical ventilation for respiratory failure. *Chest* 1989;96:136–138.

98. Davis PB, di Sant'Agnese PA. Assisted ventilation for patients with cystic fibrosis. *JAMA* 1978;239:1851–1854.

99. Hodson ME, Madden BP, Steven MH, et al. Noninvasive mechanical ventilation for cystic fibrosis patients: a potential bridge to transplantation. *Eur Respir J* 1991;4:524–527.

100. Piper AJ, Parker S, Torzillo PJ, et al. Nocturnal nasal IPPV stabilizes patients with cystic fibrosis and hypercapnic respiratory failure. *Chest* 1992;102:846–850.

101. Sood N, Paradowski LJ, Yankaskas JR. Outcomes of intensive care unit care in adults with cystic fibrosis. *Am J Respir Crit Care Med* 2001;163:335–338.

102. Yankaskas JR, Mallory GB. Lung transplantation in cystic fibrosis: consensus conference statement. *Chest* 1998;113:217–226.

103. Barr ML, Baker CJ, Schenkel FA, et al. Living donor lung transplantation: selection, technique, and outcome. *Transplant Proc* 2001;33:3527–3532.

104. Griesenbach U, Ferrari S, Geddes DM, et al. Gene therapy progress and prospects: cystic fibrosis. *Gene Ther* 2002;9:1344–1350.

105. McCallum TJ, Milunsky JM, Cunningham DL, et al. Fertility in men with cystic fibrosis: an update on current surgical practices and outcomes. *Chest* 2000;118:1059–1062.

106. Oppenheimer EA, Case AL, Esterly JR, et al. Cervical mucus in cystic fibrosis: a possible cause of infertility. *Am J Obstet Gynecol* 1970;108:673–674.

107. FitzSimmons SC, Fitzpatrick S, Thompson B, et al. A longitudinal study of the effects of pregnancy on 325 women with cystic fibrosis. *Pediatr Pulmonol* 1996;[Suppl 13]:99–101.

108. Moran A, Hardin D, Rodman D, et al. Diagnosis, screening and management of cystic fibrosis-related diabetes mellitus: a consensus conference report. *Diabetes Res Clin Pract* 1999;45:61–73.

109. Grey AB, Ames RW, Matthews RD, et al. Bone mineral density and body composition in adults with cystic fibrosis. *Thorax* 1993;48:589–593.

110. Henderson RC, Spekter BB. Kyphosis and fractures in children and young adults with cystic fibrosis. *J Pediatr* 1994;125:208–212.

111. Aris RM, Renner JB, Winders AD, et al. Increased rate of fracture and severe kyphosis: sequelae of living into adulthood with cystic fibrosis. *Ann Intern Med* 1998;128:186–193.

112. Aris RM, Lester GE, Renner JB, et al. Efficacy of pamidronate for osteoporosis in cystic fibrosis patients following lung transplantation. *Am J Respir Crit Care Med* 2000;162:941–946.

113. Haworth CS, Selby PL, Adams JE, et al. Effect of intravenous pamidronate on bone mineral density in adults with cystic fibrosis. *Thorax* 2001;56:314–316.

114. Hardin DS. The prevalence and clinical manifestations of bone disease in CF. *Pediatr Pulmonol* 2002;[Suppl 24]:175–176.

115. Aris RM. Pathogenesis of CF bone disease. *Pediatr Pulmonol* 2002;[Suppl 24]:177–178.

116. Joseph PM. Screening for CF bone disease. *Pediatr Pulmonol* 2002;[Suppl 24]:178–179.

117. Haworth CS. Treatment of cystic fibrosis bone disease. *Pediatr Pulmonol* 2002;[Suppl 24]:180–181.

118. Abbott J, Dodd M, Bilton D, et al. Treatment compliance in adults with cystic fibrosis. *Thorax* 1994;49:115–120.

14 Bronchiectasis

Anthony W. O'Regan · Jeffrey S. Berman

Bronchiectasis is defined as a permanent dilation of airways that in their normal state are more than 2 mm in diameter (1). The effect of such dilation is to reduce the clearance of mucoid and mucopurulent secretions, and to reduce the expiratory flow of air from the lungs. For this reason, bronchiectasis is categorized as an obstructive lung disease. The true incidence of bronchiectasis is unknown. However, the emergence of high-resolution computed tomography (HRCT) as a noninvasive gold standard in diagnosis has revealed that bronchiectasis has been underdiagnosed. In a British study of patients with chronic obstructive pulmonary disease (COPD) diagnosed by their primary physicians, bronchiectasis was found in 29% (2). It is unclear how much bronchiectasis contributed to the pathophysiology of obstruction or respiratory morbidity in these patients. However, because the treatment of bronchiectasis is different from that of asthma and COPD, it must be differentiated from these more common causes of airways obstruction.

Bronchiectasis is the result of a broad range of pathologic processes, including primary disorders of bronchial structure (cartilage deficiency of Williams-Campbell syndrome); diseases of mucus clearance (cystic fibrosis [CF], disorders of ciliary function); infectious causes (severe childhood pneumonia, immunoglobulin deficiency); and inflammatory diseases (ulcerative colitis) (Table 14.1). In most cases, infection is the primary force behind the ongoing cycle of inflammation, airway damage, and remodeling.

In developed countries, the widespread availability of antibiotics has reduced the impact of childhood infections on the development of bronchiectasis. Patients emigrating from developing countries may still present to the chest physician with classic focal or diffuse bronchiectasis secondary to pulmonary injury sustained during a childhood pneumonia. In a study from the United Kingdom, 150 sequential patients with bronchiectasis were investigated to determine the cause of their disease (3). In 53%, no cause could be found; in an additional 29%, the disease was deemed to be postinfectious. Four patients (3%) were found to have CF, a disease usually thought of as a common cause of diffuse bronchiectasis. These findings highlight the continuing role of infection in the pathogenesis of bronchiectasis in developed countries.

PATHOLOGY AND PATHOPHYSIOLOGY

The major complications of bronchiectasis are related to chronic suppuration in abnormal airways that results in repeated bouts of acute bronchitis and pneumonia. Airway obstruction can lead to dyspnea and respiratory failure. Continuous inflammation secondary to chronic infection worsens bronchial dilation and sets up a "vicious cycle" of repeated infection and airway injury. In addition, chronic inflammation leads to remodeling of the bronchial circulation, causing neovascularization and hypertrophic bronchial vessels, which may result in recurrent and life-threatening hemoptysis, even in patients with focal bronchiectasis.

Pathophysiology of the Airways in Bronchiectasis

Temporary dilation of small bronchi may occur during acute pneumonia, presumably as a consequence of retraction of the surrounding airless lung (4). This generally resolves within a few months after treatment of the pneumonia. Therefore, the diagnosis of bronchiectasis should be made well after the resolution of an acute pneumonia.

Permanent dilation of the airways has been graded according to type and severity (5). The terms *cylindric, varicose,*

A. W. O'Regan and J. S. Berman: Pulmonary Center, Boston University School of Medicine, Boston, Massachusetts.

TABLE 14.1. ETIOLOGY OF BRONCHIECTASIS

Etiology	Percentage (%)
Infection-related bronchial damage	
Postinfectious	30–60
Mycobacteria	
Mycobacterium tuberculosis	
NTMB (MAC)	
Other	
ABPA	10
Swyer-James syndrome	<1
Abnormal host defense	
Local	
Cystic fibrosis	3[a]
Primary ciliary dyskinesia	2
Young syndrome	1–3[a]
Systemic	
B-cell defects	3–9
CGD	<1
HIV infection	
α_1-PI deficiency	
Systemic disease	
IBD	
Collagen-vascular disease	
Relapsing polychrondritis	
Sarcoidosis	
Yellow nail syndrome	
Other causes	
Aspiration	5–10
Bronchial structural defects	
Tracheobronchomegaly	
Williams-Campbell syndrome	
Bronchial obstruction	
Foreign body	5–10
Diffuse panbronchiolitis	<1[a]

[a] Etiology will vary depending on race and population studied.
ABPA, allergic bronchopulmonary aspergillosis; CGD, chronic granulomatous disease; IBD, inflammatory bowel disease; MAC, *Mycobacterium avium* complex; NTMB, nontuberculous mycobacteria; α_1-PI, α_1-protease inhibitor.
Source: Data from Pasteur MC, Helliwell SM, Houghton SJ, et al. An investigation into causative factors in patients with bronchiectasis. *Am J Respir Crit Care Med* 2000;162:1277–1284; Nicotra MB, Rivera M, Dale AM, et al. Clinical, pathophysiologic, and microbiologic characterization of bronchiectasis in an aging cohort. *Chest* 1995;108:955–961.

and *saccular* have been used for 50 years to describe the appearance of airway dilation on bronchographic images or pathologic specimens. However, because these terms do not distinguish between specific causes or pathologic processes and do not change the therapeutic approach, they are probably best avoided. More recently, another grading system has been proposed to stage bronchiectatic areas for surgical excision that is based on the presence or absence of perfusion of the involved area (6). Proponents of this system have suggested that perfused segments participate in gas exchange and thus should be preserved. This staging system has not been extensively validated.

The pathophysiology of bronchial injury in bronchiectasis is poorly understood. It is thought that an initial insult to the bronchial wall, most likely caused by unchecked in-

fection, results in a loss of structural elements, especially cartilage and elastic fibers. Airway wall structural proteins may be disrupted by bacterial exotoxins or proteases, or perhaps by enzymes (elastase, matrix metalloproteases) and free radicals released by neutrophils and macrophages recruited to the lung as part of the inflammatory response. All of these mediators of connective tissue and cellular damage have been detected in the sputum of patients with bronchiectasis during acute exacerbations or at steady state (7–13). Damage to elastic fibers and cartilaginous matrix components is particularly likely to result in permanent structural remodeling of the airway.

The reason that such injury does not occur routinely with infection is not known. It is probable that those who sustain irreversible bronchial injury do so because of increased severity or duration of the infective process. In some cases, unchecked airways infection resulting from local or systemic immunodeficiency is the cause of bronchial injury. In other cases, an enhanced inflammatory response within the airways is the source of bronchial wall damage. Alterations in mucociliary clearance are another important cause of prolonged bronchial infection. These alterations include changes in the volume or viscosity of mucus, as may be seen in CF or even chronic bronchitis or asthma, and abnormal function of the cilia, as may be seen in genetic disorders of ciliary function. Products of bacteria or inflammatory cells may adversely affect the function of cilia and thus mucus clearance.

Some patients with defects in the "antiprotease shield" may also be at risk. One well-known example of this is α_1-protease inhibitor (α_1-PI) deficiency, a heritable condition associated with a risk for emphysema. Although several reports have cited this condition as a risk factor for bronchial wall injury and bronchiectasis, more detailed studies have not suggested a causal role (3). Another protease-antiprotease system is the matrix metalloprotease (MMP)–tissue inhibitor of metalloprotease (TIMP) system. This family of zinc-dependent proteases is of particular interest because of their ability to degrade extracellular matrix, including collagens. MMPs are released by a variety of cells in the airway, including epithelial cells and inflammatory cells. Numerous MMPs have been found in the sputum of patients with bronchiectasis, especially MMP-2, MMP-8, and MMP-9 (7,14,15). MMPs have also been found in the sputum of patients with bronchiectasis, both during acute exacerbations and during steady state, suggesting that these enzymes have a role in causing airway damage. The use of inhibitors of MMPs may be an attractive future therapeutic option in bronchiectasis.

Pathophysiology of Mucociliary Function in Bronchiectasis

The normal mucociliary escalator is the major clearance mechanism of the lung. This system depends on a mucus gel phase that traps particulate matter, a mucus sol phase nearest to the ciliated cells that facilitates movement of the cilia and transmission of work done by the cilia to the gel layer, and proper action of the cilia to propel the mucus cephalad. Finally, effective coughing is necessary to remove cleared materials from the larger airways. The mucociliary escalator is compromised in bronchiectasis. In particular, the retention time of inhaled radioactively labeled materials is significantly increased in patients with bronchiectasis, even during remissions of the disease (16–18). Primary disorders of the clearance system may also predispose patients to the development of bronchiectasis.

The viscosity and production of mucus can be altered in a number of ways. In CF, an abnormal chloride channel reduces the amount of chloride, sodium, and water in the mucous layer; as a result, abnormally dry secretions cannot be transported efficiently by the cilia. In chronic bronchitis and asthma, the production of mucus is increased, and the increased volume of mucus overwhelms ciliary and cough mechanisms. Bacteria and inflammatory cells elaborate products that act as secretagogues, increasing the volume of mucus. The best-known of these secretagogues is elastase, produced by neutrophilic leukocytes and by bacteria (19).

Ciliary function requires the proper assembly and function of the complex motor system of the cilia. Multiple structural abnormalities of ciliary function have been described, all of which lead to inadequate clearance of mucus with resultant sinopulmonary infections and bronchiectasis (see section "Primary Ciliary Dyskinesia"). Acquired abnormalities of ciliary function have also been documented in bronchiectasis. In particular, bronchiectasis sputum and *Pseudomonas* bacterial exotoxins have been found to slow the ciliary beat, which would be expected to decrease the clearance of mucus. Cilia obtained from the respiratory epithelium of patients during acute infections also beat abnormally slowly and in the wrong direction, suggesting that this process is relevant *in vivo* (16).

Finally, cough efficiency may be decreased in bronchiectasis. Effective cough requires an intact rib cage and respiratory muscles that permit the generation of a high forced expiratory flow. In addition, glottic occlusion and release must occur in a coordinated manner. Airflow through the small airways is increased markedly with volume-dependent airways narrowing, sweeping secretions along with the flow of air. In abnormally dilated airways, this narrowing does not occur, and cough efficiency is reduced (20).

Pathophysiology of the Bronchial Circulation in Bronchiectasis

The bronchi are fed by the bronchial arteries, which arise as branches of the thoracic aorta. The arteries follow the branching of the bronchial tree. This systemic high-pressure bronchial circulation is markedly hypertrophic in patients with long-standing bronchiectasis. Feeding arteries are dilated, and neovascularization develops in inflamed areas. Neovascularized areas are prone to bleeding, which may

be severe as a consequence of the high flow rate in the hypertrophic bronchial arteries. The etiology of this vascular remodeling is not known. However, it is reasonable to suggest that ongoing inflammation results in the increased expression of angiogenic factors such as interleukin-8 (IL-8), a chemoattractant cytokine of the CXC chemokine family (21). IL-8 has been found in the sputum of patients with bronchiectasis. The glutamate-leucine-arginine (ELR) motif near the N-terminus of IL-8 has angiogenic activity, and it has been suggested that an imbalance of the chemokines that promote and inhibit angiogenesis during inflammation results in the formation of new vessels and fibrosis. Another angiogenic peptide, endothelin-1, has also been found in bronchiectasis sputum (22,23). Angiogenic factors may represent targets of future therapies aimed at preventing vascular remodeling in patients with bronchiectasis.

CLINICAL FEATURES

The hallmark of bronchiectasis is a chronic cough, lasting months to years, that is productive of large amounts of mucopurulent sputum (24) (Table 14.2). Unlike the cough of chronic bronchitis, that in bronchiectasis is generally constant, with little seasonal variation. Sputum production may exceed 500 mL/d. Some patients with severe bronchiectasis, particularly when it involves the upper lobes, have no sputum production and occasionally no cough. When present, cough and sputum production are worse in the morning, after secretions have pooled during the previous night. Associated symptoms include dyspnea, wheezing, and hemoptysis. Severe disease may be complicated by systemic symptoms of fatigue and weight loss. Patients frequently present with recurrent acute episodes of increased sputum production, pleuritic chest pain, and fevers associated with superinfection and pneumonia involving the diseased lung. Hemoptysis often develops during these infectious exacerbations, and massive hemoptysis is not uncommon, reflecting

TABLE 14.2. CLINICAL FEATURES OF BRONCHIECTASIS IN ADULTS

Clinical Feature	Percentage (%)
Symptoms	
Cough	90
Daily sputum	76
Dyspnea	72
Hemoptysis	56
Pleurisy	46
Physical findings	
Crackles	70
Wheeze	34
Clubbing	3

Source: Data from Pasteur MC, Helliwell SM, Houghton SJ, et al. An investigation into causative factors in patients with bronchiectasis. *Am J Respir Crit Care Med* 2000;162:1277–1284.

TABLE 14.3. ETIOLOGY OF BRONCHIECTASIS AS SUGGESTED BY SPECIFIC CLINICAL AND RADIOGRAPHIC FEATURES

Feature	Etiology
Clinical	
Recurrent otitis media/sinusitis	CF, PCD, Young syndrome, immunoglobulin deficiency
Asthma	ABPA
Nasal polyps	CF, PCD, ABPA
Infertility	CF, PCD, Young syndrome
Family history	CF, PCD, α_1-PI deficiency
Radiographic	
Upper lobes	CF, granulomatous disease, ankylosing spondylitis, ABPA
Central	ABPA, tracheobronchomegaly
Right middle lobe/lingula	MAC
Diffuse/lower lobe	Immunoglobulin deficiency, PCD
Localized	Obstruction, postinfectious

ABPA, allergic bronchopulmonary aspergillosis; CF, cystic fibrosis; MAC, *Mycobacterium avium* complex; PCD, primary ciliary dyskinesia; α_1-PI, α_1-protease inhibitor.

inflamed and hypertrophic bronchial arteries within segments involved by bronchiectasis. Pulmonary crackles are the most common physical examination finding, but wheezing is detected in more than a third of patients and may be the only clinical abnormality. Although finger clubbing is almost universally present in children with CF, it is found in very few adults with bronchiectasis (24). Certain clinical features may be helpful in suggesting the specific cause of bronchiectasis (Table 14.3).

CLINICAL FEATURES OF BRONCHIECTASIS

Summary Statement	Level of Evidence
Characterized by chronic productive cough.	Retrospective case series
Common complications include pneumonia and hemoptysis.	Retrospective case series
Obstructive physiology is seen on pulmonary function testing.	Retrospective studies
Chest x-ray findings are abnormal in 87% of patients but are often nonspecific. High-resolution computed tomography is the diagnostic study of choice, with 97% sensitivity and >93% specificity.	Small prospective studies
H. influenzae and *P. aeruginosa* are the most frequent potential pathogenic microorganisms in sputum, and colonization with *P. aeruginosa* is a poor prognostic marker.	Small prospective studies

Pulmonary Function Tests

Pulmonary function testing in patients with bronchiectasis usually reveals obstructive physiology (24,25). The degree of airway obstruction has varied in several studies, with the ratio of the forced expiratory volume in 1 second to the forced vital capacity (FEV_1/FVC) ranging from 60% to 80% (3,24). The pathophysiology of airflow obstruction in bronchiectasis is unclear. In a study that correlated CT scan findings with pulmonary physiology, airflow obstruction in bronchiectasis was primarily linked to evidence of intrinsic disease in small and medium airways, not to the degree of bronchiectatic dilation in large airways, emphysema, or retained endobronchial secretions (25). Colonization of airways with *Pseudomonas aeruginosa* is associated with more severe impairment of pulmonary physiology (26). In general, pulmonary function testing adds little diagnostic information but is helpful in assessing the severity of illness and response to therapy.

Radiology

The diagnosis of bronchiectasis may be confirmed by radiographic demonstration of bronchial dilation (27–31) (Fig. 14.1). The chest radiographic findings are abnormal in more than 87% of patients with bronchiectasis, but they are usually nonspecific, and the extent and severity of disease are significantly underestimated (24,29). Typical radiographic findings include increases in the number of bronchovascular markings, crowding of bronchi, and in severe cases cystic spaces or linear shadows ("tram tracking"). The latter represent thickened bronchial walls. The plain chest x-ray film is unreliable in determining the exact anatomic distribution of the disease.

Traditionally, bronchography was used to diagnose and anatomically define bronchiectasis (4). The sensitivity and safety of CT have now made bronchography largely obsolete (28,32). High-resolution CT should be performed in patients suspected of having bronchiectasis. A typical protocol visualizes sections 1.5 to 4 mm thick at intervals of 5 to 10 mm. When these parameters are used, CT has a sensitivity of 97% and a specificity of 93% to 100% in diagnosing bronchiectasis (28,32). The increased use of HRCT has led to the realization that bronchiectasis is quite common and often unsuspected (2,28,31,32).

Bronchiectasis is characterized by dilated bronchi with thickened walls extending to the lung periphery on HRCT (Fig. 14.1 B,D). As on chest x-ray films, "tram tracking" may be seen when dilated and thickened bronchioles are oriented horizontally within the CT section. On cross section, the bronchioles in bronchiectasis appear as round, dilated, thick-walled structures accompanied by a pulmonary artery smaller in size than the bronchus (28,33). This creates a "signet ring" appearance, in which the dilated bronchus represents the ring and the pulmonary artery the stone (33) (Fig. 14.2). In bronchiectasis, the bronchus is dilated relative to the hypertrophic pulmonary artery, whereas in normal subjects, the bronchus and the pulmonary artery are of approximately equal size. Mucus within the dilated bronchiole frequently appears as an air-fluid level, and if total mucus plugging is present, as in allergic bronchopulmonary aspergillosis (ABPA), segments involved by bronchiectasis

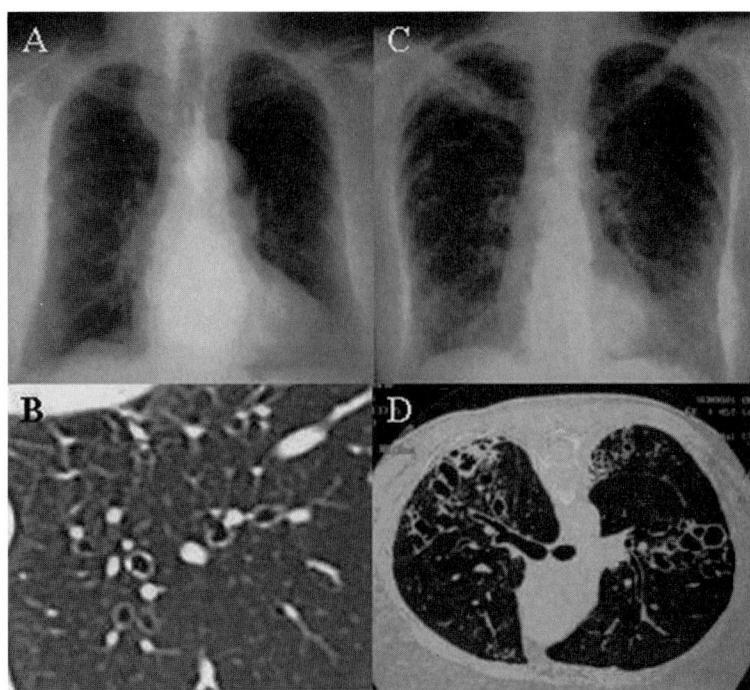

FIGURE 14.1. The spectrum of bronchiectasis. The chest x-ray film (**A**) of a patient with idiopathic bronchiectasis is relatively unremarkable despite the fact that bronchiectasis is seen on an accompanying computed tomographic (CT) scan (**B**). The patient had obstructive lung disease with persistent bilateral basilar crackles. In contrast, the chest x-ray film (**C**) of a patient with postinfectious bronchiectasis shows diffuse dilated air spaces that are also well seen on CT scan (**D**). This patient had cough productive of large volumes of sputum with diffuse crackles and obstructive physiology.

may be mistaken for mass lesions or vascular structures. Cystic lesions unrelated to bronchiectasis often lack thickened walls and are not accompanied by a pulmonary artery (34). The CT findings in bronchiectasis are of limited value in distinguishing between idiopathic and specific types, although certain radiographic patterns of lobar involvement may suggest a specific diagnosis (35) (Table 14.3). As already mentioned (see section "Pathophysiology of the

Airways in Bronchiectasis"), a diagnosis of bronchiectasis should not be made within a few weeks of an acute pneumonia (4).

Microbiology

The lower respiratory tract in normal nonsmokers is sterile. In contrast, in most patients with bronchiectasis,

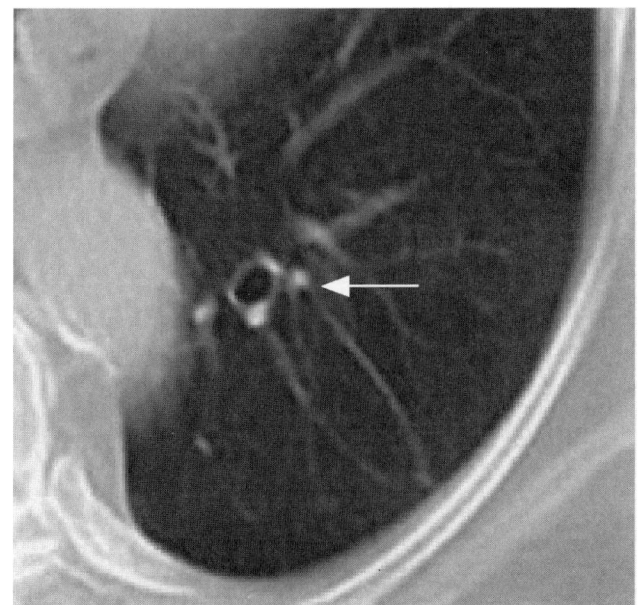
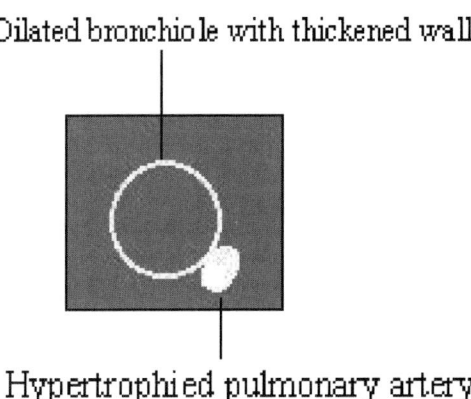

Dilated bronchiole with thickened wall

Hypertrophied pulmonary artery

FIGURE 14.2. The signet ring sign. The diagram shows the relationship of the dilated bronchiole and small accompanying pulmonary artery that form a "signet ring" (indicated by an *arrow* in the computed tomographic scan).

it is colonized with potentially pathogenic microorganisms (3,24,36,37). Colonization of the distal airways with pathogenic organisms can be harmful to the host by causing recurrent pneumonia and persistent inflammation that leads to progressive tissue damage and airway obstruction. The process of chronic colonization, secondary inflammatory reaction, and progressive lung injury represents a vicious cycle and is the reason why an appropriate evaluation of the microorganisms of the distal airways is necessary in patients with bronchiectasis.

The bacteria in bronchiectatic airways have specific survival strategies. For instance, *P. aeruginosa* organisms reside in a biofilm on the bronchiolar surface. In this survival strategy (also exploited by *Burkholderia cepacia*), the organisms use the micromilieu of nutrients but avoid elimination by local phagocytic, antibody, and other immune responses. Frustrated phagocytosis leads to the liberation of proteolytic chemicals, such as elastases and oxygen radicals, that cause further local tissue injury. It has been shown that patients with bronchiectasis who are colonized with *Pseudomonas* species have worse lung function and more progressive disease (26).

The patterns of bacterial colonization in adults with bronchiectasis have been remarkably consistent during the last decade (3,24,36,37) (Table 14.4). Between 66% and 88% of patients have cultures that are persistently positive for at least one organism. Table 14.4 shows the prevalence of various organisms in patients with bronchiectasis. In all studies, *Haemophilus influenzae* (35%–55%) and *P. aeruginosa* (26%–31%) were the most frequently isolated organisms. The presence of *Staphylococcus aureus* should lead the clinician to suspect CF. Risk factors for persistent microbial colonization include an onset of symptoms before the age of 14 years and an FEV_1 value less than 80% of the predicted value (37). From 7% to 14% of patients have mucoid variants of *Pseudomonas,* and these are a poor prognostic marker (24,26,38). Interestingly, *Mycobacterium avium* complex (MAC) infection has been detected in as many as 17% of unselected adults with bronchiectasis, which underscores the potential pathogenic role of MAC in this disease (24).

Approximately 39% of patients are colonized with a single organism, 29% with two, 10% with three, and 8% with four or more (24). Bronchoscopy with protected brush adds little information in comparison with sputum culture alone (36). In contrast, in up to 50% of patients with MAC infection, bronchoscopy is required to document the presence of mycobacteria (3). For these reasons, we recommend routine sputum culture and sensitivity in all patients with bronchiectasis. Bronchoscopy should be reserved for patients in whom MAC infection is likely or in whom the disease is progressive despite optimal therapy.

SPECIFIC CAUSES OF BRONCHIECTASIS

In as many as 50% of adult patients who present with bronchiectasis, a specific cause is not identified (Table 14.1). Still, in the remaining patients, identification of the pathogenesis may aid in the treatment, prognosis, and perhaps genetic counseling. A suggested investigative approach to adults with newly diagnosed bronchiectasis is presented in Figure 14.3.

Infection-Related Bronchial Damage

Postinfectious Bronchiectasis

The occurrence of bronchiectasis following severe or necrotizing pneumonia is well described. Implicated pathogens include *S. aureus, Klebsiella pneumoniae, Mycoplasma pneumoniae, Bordetella pertussis,* influenza virus, adenovirus, and mycobacteria (3,39,40). A history of severe or significant prior pneumonia, measles, or pertussis in found 29% to 65% of adults presenting with bronchiectasis (3,24,37). In one third of these patients, persistent or recurrent upper respiratory tract infection suggests an alternative or additional cause of bronchiectasis. The mechanism of postinfectious bronchiectasis is felt to reflect irreversible scarring of the involved bronchioles. Failure to provide adequate antibiotics together with impairment of host defenses secondary to malnutrition may explain why bronchiectasis is more common in regions with poor access to health care. In addition, potential cofactors may account for differing susceptibilities. Specific cofactors include coinfection with

TABLE 14.4. COMMON MICROORGANISMS ISOLATED FROM PATIENTS WITH BRONCHIECTASIS

Organism	Prevalence (%)		
	U.K.(3)	Spain (37)	Texas (24)
H. influenzae	17	55	30
P. aeruginosa	24	26	31
Mucoid strain	NR	7	14
S. pneumoniae	4	14	10
M. catarrhalis	9	5	5
S. aureus	7	3	8
Coliforms	6	4	13
Aspergillus	2	1[a]	5
Nocardia	NR	1[a]	3
MAC	NR	NR	17
No organism	23	12	36

[a] Only from bronchoscopy specimens.
MAC, *M. avium* complex; NR, not reported.
Source: Data from Pasteur MC, Helliwell SM, Houghton SJ, et al. An investigation into causative factors in patients with bronchiectasis. *Am J Respir Crit Care Med* 2000;162:1277–1284; Angrill J, Agustic, De Celis R, et al. Bronchial inflammation and colonization in patients with clinically stable bronchiectasis. *Am J Respir Crit Care Med* 2002;164:1628–1632; Nicotra MB, Rivera M, Dale AM, et al. Clinical, pathophysiologic, and microbiologic characterization of bronchiectasis in an aging cohort. *Chest* 1995;108:955–961.

Evaluation of Newly-Diagnosed Bronchiectasis

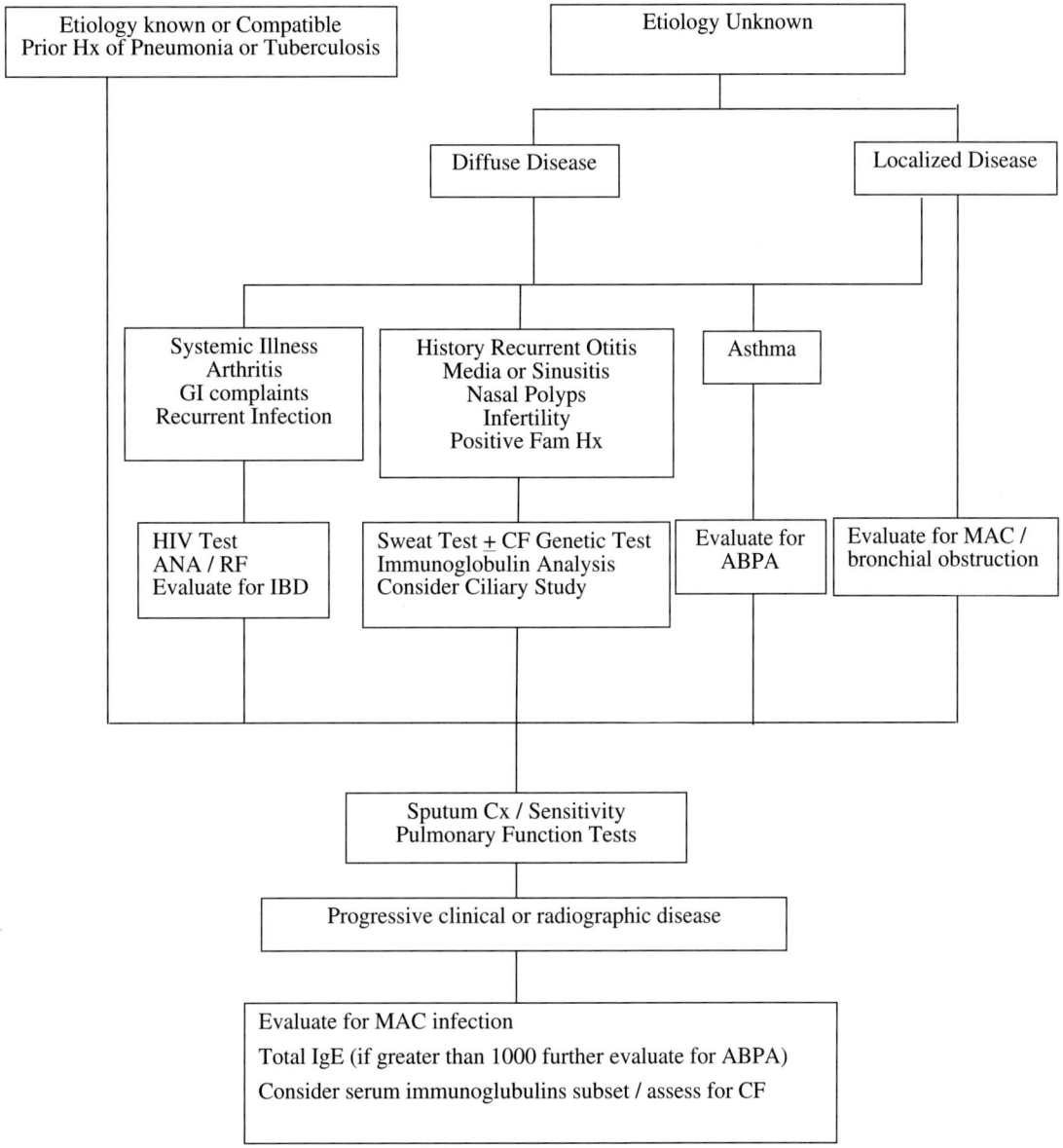

FIGURE 14.3. A flow chart for the suggested evaluation of newly diagnosed bronchiectasis.

other organisms, such as adenovirus or Epstein-Barr virus, or an underlying host susceptibility factor, such as inadequate specific functional antibody responses to certain pathogens (41–44).

Swyer-James-MacLeod syndrome, or unilateral hyperlucent lung syndrome, represents hypoplastic lung development following early childhood bronchiolitis (45). Several viral and bacterial pathogens have been implicated, including adenoviruses 3, 7, and 21, measles virus, and *B. pertussis*. The affected lung is small and hyperlucent as a consequence of hypoplasia of the pulmonary arteries. Bronchiectasis of the central airways that abruptly tapers is seen in more than 25% of cases.

Allergic Bronchopulmonary Aspergillosis (ABPA)

ABPA can cause bronchiectasis, and it is also common for hypersensitivity to *Aspergillus* species to develop in patients with bronchiectasis of another cause. Therefore, the results of studies estimating the prevalence of ABPA in patients with bronchiectasis do not necessarily imply a causative role.

Nevertheless, reports have shown that approximately 7% of unselected patients with bronchiectasis have evidence of primary ABPA (3). The reported prevalence of ABPA in patients with CF ranges from 0.5% to 15%; a study from Spain identified *Aspergillus*-specific immunoglobulin E (IgE) antibodies in 65% of patients with CF (46). Minimal criteria for such a diagnosis are (a) a history of asthma or atopy, (b) immediate skin test reactivity to *Aspergillus fumigatus,* (c) elevated serum total IgE (>1,000 ng/mL), and (d) central bronchiectasis (47). Additional supportive criteria include precipitating serum antibodies to *A. fumigatus,* peripheral blood eosinophilia (>500/mm³) (3), and recurrent pulmonary infiltrates.

Bronchiectasis is detected on HRCT scans in more than 87% of patients with ABPA. Classically, the bronchiectasis is central or proximal with upper lobe predominance in ABPA, but this pattern is not a sensitive diagnostic marker. Indeed, features of bronchiectasis on CT scans fail to differentiate ABPA from other causes of bronchiectasis (35) (Fig. 14.4B). In one study, bronchiectasis affecting three or more lobes, centrilobular nodules, and mucoid impaction in an asthmatic patient were found to be suggestive of underlying ABPA (48). These data would indicate that all patients with a history of asthma and findings of bronchiectasis should be screened for ABPA. It may also be reasonable to screen unselected patients with bronchiectasis for ABPA. A diagnosis of ABPA should prompt aggressive therapy with systemic corticosteroids.

Granulomatous Disease

Tuberculosis and other granulomatous infections and diseases, such as sarcoidosis, frequently cause traction bronchiectasis of the involved lobe, most frequently an upper lobe (49–54). This complication usually reflects distant infection or long-standing disease. Extensive disease can be relatively asymptomatic, presenting either as an incidental finding on chest x-ray films or after an acute event, such as superinfection of the bronchiectatic lung. Hemoptysis is common and may reflect infection, reactivation tuberculosis, scar carcinoma, broncholithiasis, or mycetoma (Fig. 14.5).

In addition to traction bronchiectasis, endobronchial disease or impingement of enlarged lymph nodes on the bronchi can result in obstructive bronchiectasis of the involved segment (54). The right middle lobe is most often compressed by enlarged hilar lymph nodes (55). Endobronchial sarcoidosis is relatively common, affecting up to 37% of patients. A previous report demonstrated bronchial stenosis in 11 patients with sarcoidosis, of whom five had definite bronchiectasis on bronchography (53). Most studies based on HRCT, however, have failed to reproduce these results.

Nontuberculous Mycobacterial Disease

The prevalence of pulmonary nontuberculous mycobacterial disease, most often caused by MAC, is increasing (56). Original reports suggested that nontuberculous mycobacterial infection occurred exclusively in immune-compromised hosts and patients with structural lung diseases, such as COPD, fibrocavitary disease, or bronchiectasis. Nontuberculous mycobacteria in the sputum of patients were often considered "colonizers" and not felt to be pathogenic. In 1989, Prince and colleagues (57) reported a group of elderly female patients without traditional risk factors for nontuberculous mycobacterial disease who had pulmonary MAC infection and nodular bronchiectasis. Since then, this presentation of MAC infection has become well recognized, and true colonization is considered rare. In addition, bronchiectasis of other causes, such as CF, can be complicated by

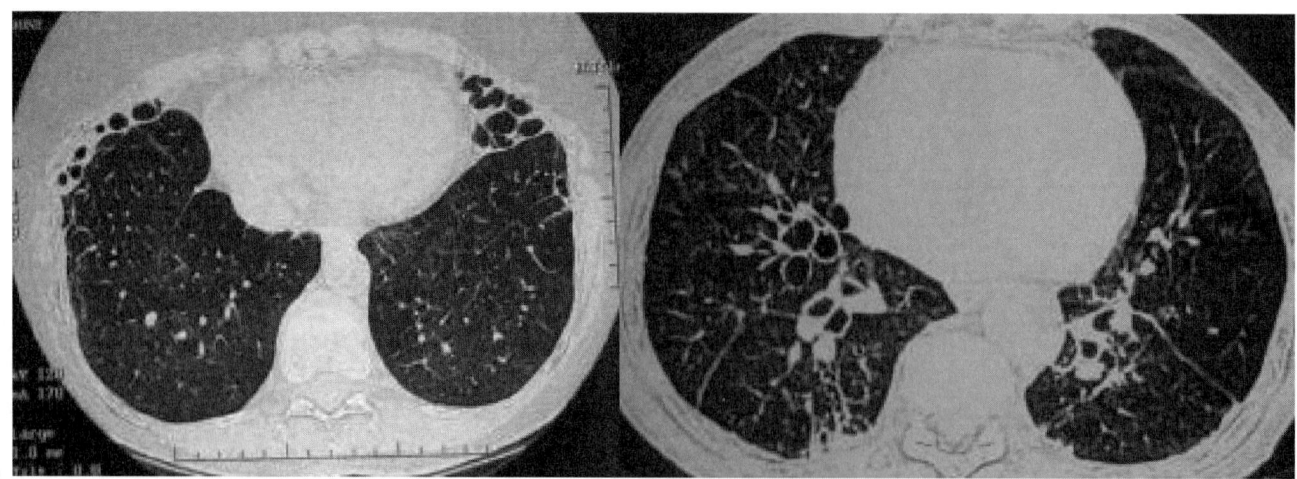

FIGURE 14.4. Specific features on the computed tomographic scan may suggest the cause of bronchiectasis. **A:** Bronchiectasis caused by *Mycobacterium avium-intracellulare* infection. Dilated bronchioles are seen in the right middle lobe and lingula. **B:** Central bronchiectasis as may be seen in allergic bronchopulmonary aspergillosis. This is not a specific sign, however; in this case, the patient had Mounier-Kuhn syndrome.

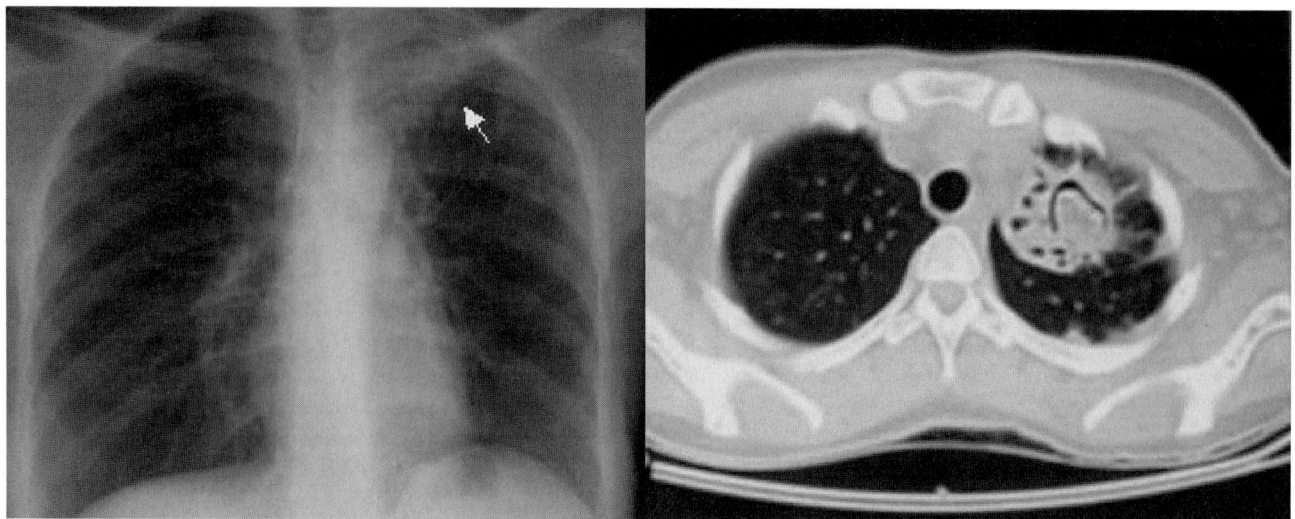

FIGURE 14.5. Posttuberculous bronchiectasis complicated by a mycetoma (*Aspergillus fumigatus*). Note the left upper lobe crescent sign (*arrow*) on the chest x-ray film (**A**), which is confirmed by computed tomography (**B**).

infection with invasive nontuberculous mycobacteria, including rapidly growing mycobacteria such as *Mycobacterium abscessus* (58).

The association of MAC infection with nodular bronchiectasis has typical clinical and radiologic features and has been termed *Lady Windermere syndrome* (59). It typically occurs in elderly white women who are nonsmokers and have no underlying lung disease. Symptoms include chronic cough, sputum production, and fatigue. Studies with HRCT have shown that more than 80% of patients with noncavitary disease caused by MAC have multifocal bronchiectasis, often with associated small pulmonary nodules (<5 mm) (60). Although any lobe can be affected, a predilection for the right middle lobe and lingula has been noted (Fig. 14.4A). The diagnosis requires a combination of typical clinical, radiographic, and bacteriologic criteria from sputum or bronchoscopic samples (Table 14.5). Bronchoscopy or open lung biopsy may be required for diagnosis in up to 45% of the patients because of nondiagnostic sputum cultures (60,61).

The pathogenesis of MAC infection in these patients is uncertain. Although MAC is a common opportunistic pathogen, it is unclear why healthy subjects, mainly elderly women, become infected and why the disease is progressive in some 40% to 50% of patients but not progressive in the remainder. Original reports hypothesized that susceptibility might reflect an underlying anatomic defect characterized by thoracic abnormalities and mitral valve prolapse. Others implicated habitual voluntary cough suppression (hence the name *Lady Windermere syndrome,* after the character in Oscar Wilde's play) causing bronchiectasis in lobes with long narrow bronchi, such as the right middle lobe and lingula. Genetic susceptibility to MAC infection has been suggested by familial disease and associations with certain HLA haplotypes, such as HLA-DR6 (62,63).

The prompt diagnosis of MAC-related nodular bronchiectasis is important because significant morbidity results from progressive bronchiectasis, and new effective antimicrobial therapy is now available (56,64). Treatment is probably indicated in all symptomatic patients or patients with well-defined or progressive lung disease. A macrolide-based regimen is recommended (Table 14.6), and treatment is generally continued for at least 12 months (ideally 10–12 months after sputum conversion) (56). The response to therapy should be monitored based on symptoms, the extent of radiographic disease, and the results of respiratory tract cultures. If medications can be tolerated, response rates exceed

TABLE 14.5. CRITERIA FOR THE DIAGNOSIS OF MAC-RELATED BRONCHIECTASIS

1. Clinical criteria
   Compatible signs and symptoms (cough, sputum, weight loss)
   Reasonable exclusion of other causes of symptoms (tuberculosis, cancer, other causes of bronchiectasis)
2. Radiographic criteria
   Multifocal bronchiectasis with or without small lung nodules on HRCT scan
3. Bacteriologic criteria
   Sputum/bronchial wash
       Three positive cultures/negative AFB smear
   or Two positive cultures with one positive AFB smear
   or One culture with 2+ growth or AFB smear
   Biopsy
       Culture or AFB smear positive
       Granulomatous pathology

Note: It is assumed that the host is HIV-negative. The diagnosis requires that all three criteria be satisfied.
AFB, acid-fast bacillus; HRCT, high-resolution computed tomography.
Source: Adapted from American Thoracic Society guidelines: Anonymous. Diagnosis and treatment of disease caused by nontuberculous mycobacteria. *Am J Respir Crit Care Med* 1997;156:S1–S25.

TABLE 14.6. TREATMENT OF MAC-RELATED BRONCHIECTASIS

Drug	Dose
Macrolide	
Clarithromycin	500 mg twice a day
Azithromycin	250–500 mg three times a week
Rifamycins	
Rifabutin	300 mg/d
Rifamycin	600 mg/d
Ethambutol	15–25 mg/kg

Note: Treat for a minimum of 12 months.
MAC, *Mycobacterium avium* complex.
Source: Adapted from Anonymous. Diagnosis and treatment of disease caused by nontuberculous mycobacteria. *Am J Respir Crit Care Med* 1997;156:S1–S25.

90%, with clinical improvement noted within 3 to 6 months and sputum conversion by 12 months. Unfortunately, more than 50% of patients cannot tolerate these medication regimens (60). Failure to respond should prompt evaluation of noncompliance or macrolide resistance.

Aspiration

Aspiration of food, chemicals, secretions, or gastric contents accounts for between 5% and 15% of cases of bronchiectasis (3). Risks factors include swallowing dysfunction, gastroesophageal reflux disease, seizures, and alcoholism (65,66). Cases have also been described with myopathies predisposing to aspiration and occult tracheoesophageal fistulae (67). One case documented a patient with mitochondrial myopathy that primarily presented with diffuse bronchiectasis (68). Diffuse lower lobe bronchiectasis can also follow the aspiration of chemicals or toxic fumes, such as ammonia.

Abnormal Host Defense

Ineffective or impaired ability to prevent or resolve infections predisposes the host to recurrent pneumonia and bronchiectasis. Specific defects in host defenses may be local, such as ciliary dyskinesia, or systemic, such as hypogammaglobulinemia.

Local Defects

Primary Ciliary Dyskinesia

Primary ciliary dyskinesia (PCD), also called *immotile cilia syndrome,* is characterized by congenital abnormalities of ciliary structure and function (69,70). Normal ciliary function is a critical host defense against respiratory infection. In PCD, complete absence of mucociliary clearance leads to recurrent sinopulmonary infections. Approximately 50% of affected patients have situs inversus or Kartagener syndrome, and infertility is present in all males and 50% of females (70). Overall, PCD accounts for 0.5% to 1% of

cases of bronchiectasis, but most patients with PCD have a normal life span.

The prevalence of PCD is 1 in 20,000 to 1 in 30,000 individuals (70). PCD is an autosomal-recessive disorder affecting all races and both sexes equally. Normal cilia (or sperm flagella) are 6 μm in length and beat 10 to 15 times per second, with a fast forward and a slower recovery stroke. They are composed of central axonemes containing nine pairs of microtubules that form a circle around two central microtubules. Each of the nine doublets has an outer and an inner dynein arm. The dynein proteins are the force-producing element in cilia and require adenosine triphosphate as a source of energy. Although abnormalities of dynein arm structure and function account for most cases of PCD, defects in virtually any polypeptide, matrix, or membrane component of the cilia can result in defective ciliary function. More than 100 different ciliary abnormalities have been described (70).

It is likely that the genes for cilia are widely distributed in the genome and that a large number of chromosomal defects can result in PCD (70). Several specific genetic defects have been localized and characterized, but these account for only a small proportion of the cases of this heterogeneous disorder (70). In the largest study, 25 families were identified with autosomal-recessive PCD that showed allelic segregation compatible with linkage to chromosome 5p containing the dynein gene DNAH5 (71). Ten genetic mutations were identified in these families that resulted in loss of either motor or microtubule binding domains of the outer dynein arms. As is typical of patients with PCD, about 50% of affected individuals had situs inversus (Kartagener syndrome) secondary to a loss of ciliary activity in nodal embryonic cells, which determine normal left-right symmetry (situs solitus) (72). Loss of such function results in randomization of left-right symmetry, with situs inversus in 50% of cases and situs solitus in 50%. Two pairs of monozygotic twins with PCD have been identified; in each pair, one twin had situs inversus and the other situs solitus.

The clinical features of PCD are heterogeneous, with variable organ involvement and severity. Neonatal respiratory distress is common, and the respiratory tract is involved in virtually all patients; recurrent otitis media (100%), nasal polyposis (20%), and bronchiectasis (30%) of the mid and lower lung zones are usually found. Frontal sinus agenesis is common. Spirometry may reveal airway obstruction with variable responsiveness to bronchodilators. Pathogenic organisms include *H. influenzae, Streptococcus pneumoniae, S. aureus,* and less commonly *P. aeruginosa.*

Kartagener syndrome, characterized by situs inversus, is caused by a loss of embryonic nodal cell ciliary function, which is responsible for typical left-right symmetry (situs solitus occurs in 99.9% of the normal population). Hydrocephalus has been described in several patients with PCD; this may reflect defective ciliary function of ependymal cells in the central nervous system. Most affected men have immotile spermatozoa and are infertile. In women, fertility is decreased by impaired movement of ova along the fallopian tubes.

The diagnosis of PCD requires a demonstration of permanent defects in ciliary function (70). Secondary ciliary dyskinesia is seen in a number of inflammatory and infectious respiratory conditions. Assessment of mucociliary transport alone cannot differentiate abnormalities of mucus viscosity, as in CF, from PCD. The demonstration of dynein deficiency by transmission electron microscopy is considered the gold standard for diagnosis, but this deficiency is present only in some patients, and normal ultrastructure does not rule out PCD. Therefore, even when the results of transmission electron microscopy and ciliary function analysis are combined, up to 25% of cases of PCD can be misdiagnosed. Some investigators have reported the usefulness of evaluating ciliogenesis in nasal epithelial cell culture (73). At present, ciliogenesis testing is still experimental and is too expensive and time-consuming to serve as a screening test. If abnormal mucociliary transport is suspected or documented by a radioaerosol study (17), biopsy specimens from the bronchi or nasopharynx can be placed in isotonic saline solution and examined for ciliary motility or placed in glutaraldehyde for ultrastructural investigation to confirm the diagnosis (70).

Persons with PCD generally live an active life and have a normal life span. The rate of decline of lung function is much slower than that in CF. No specific therapy is available.

Young Syndrome

In 1970, Young described 52 men with obstructive azoospermia, of whom half had a history of chronic recurrent lung infections (32). Young syndrome is characterized by obstructive azoospermia (normal spermatozoa in the testis but none in the ejaculate) in association with recurrent sinusitis (50%), otitis media (33%), and bronchiectasis (30%) (74). Unlike sexually transmitted diseases, obstructive azoospermia affects the tail rather than the head of the epididymis. Mucociliary clearance is markedly impaired, but the ciliary ultrastructure and results of tests for CF are normal. In Young syndrome, the mucus appears to be abnormally viscid, leading to inspissated secretions, which might explain the typical constellation of clinical features. The results of studies showing ciliary disorientation but no ultrastructural defects are consistent with this finding, but until the precise defect in the composition of mucus is identified, the cause of the syndrome will remain speculative (75). Some studies have found an association between mercury poisoning and Young syndrome.

Cystic Fibrosis

CF is the most common cause of congenital bronchiectasis in Caucasians and is discussed in detail in Chapter 13 (76). It is inherited as an autosomal-recessive disease, with an allele frequency in certain races as high as 1 in 20 (76,77). Bronchiectasis usually develops in infants, but a late presentation of CF is increasingly described in adults. In several European studies, 3% to 6% of cases of bronchiectasis in adults were caused by CF (3). In non-European populations, the gene frequency is lower, and therefore adult-onset CF is less common (24). Nevertheless, making the diagnosis has important implications in terms of treatment, prognosis, and genetic counseling (76,78). When CF presents late, it is usually associated with mild lung disease and pancreatic sufficiency (79). Bronchiectasis is diffuse and bilateral, often with upper lobe predominance. The presence of *S. aureus* or *P. aeruginosa* in the sputum should alert the clinician to the possibility of CF (39). Diagnostic studies should involve sweat testing and genetic analysis (76).

Immunodeficiency States

Failure of any arm of the immune system can result in recurrent pneumonia and bronchiectasis. Defects may include abnormalities of cell-mediated and humoral immunity in addition to abnormalities of complement, phagocytic, and neutrophil killing systems. In general, many immune deficiency states are associated with the onset of severe recurrent infection in early childhood and a reduced life expectancy. We will limit our discussion to immune defects that present predominantly with recurrent pneumonia and bronchiectasis–namely, humoral or B-cell immune deficiencies.

Humoral or B-Cell Deficiencies

Because of the maternal transmission of antibodies, patients with B-cell deficiency usually present with infection at about 7 to 9 months of life. Recurrent infection is caused by encapsulated bacterial organisms, including *S. pneumoniae* and *H. influenzae*. Major infections include otitis media, sinopulmonary infections, and more rarely gastrointestinal and bone infections. Recurrent fungal, mycobacterial, and viral infections are rare, although chronic enteroviral infections are seen in X-linked (Bruton) agammaglobulinemia. B-cell deficiency is also associated with autoimmune phenomena, such as autoimmune cytopenias, and with chronic diarrhea, particularly involving *Giardia* infection. Unlike T-cell and most other immune defects, humoral deficiencies may present in adulthood, and patients can lead normal lives on replacement immunoglobulin therapy.

Diagnostic studies require a quantitative assessment of serum immunoglobulins and possibly IgG subclasses. In certain cases, it is useful to obtain a qualitative assessment of the immunoglobulin response to isohemagglutinins (IgM antibodies to blood groups A and B) and vaccines such as Pneumovax (IgG2) and *H. influenzae* type b vaccine (IgG1).

The true incidence of immunoglobulin deficiency in patients with bronchiectasis is unknown. Estimates have ranged from 1% to 48% (80). Several studies have suggested that a combined deficiency of subclasses IgG2 and IgG4 is associated with bronchiectasis. Unfortunately, although the normal ranges of the major immunoglobulin groups are known, those for the immunoglobulin subclasses are less clear, with some studies defining normal ranges in cohorts as small as

20 patients. A study from the United Kingdom identified humoral immunodeficiency in 8% of patients with bronchiectasis and IgG subclass deficiency in fewer than 1% (81).

Intravenous immunoglobulin provides safe and effective replacement therapy for B-cell deficiency (82). Dosage regimens range from 200 to 600 mg/kg every 3 to 4 weeks. Higher doses ensure trough levels of IgG in excess of 500 mg/dL and should be considered for patients with established bronchiectasis. Serum IgG trough levels should be monitored after a change in dose, but the clinical response, in terms of number of infections and lung function, is the important index of successful treatment. Allergic reactions and transmission of infection are rare.

Many immune deficiencies are characterized by defects in B-cell development or function. Several, such as X-linked or Bruton agammaglobulinemia and immunodeficiency with hyper-IgM, are associated with profound immunodeficiency and early disease onset. We limit our discussion to defects that are more likely to be encountered in adults.

Common Variable Immunodeficiency. Common variable immunodeficiency comprises a heterogeneous group of disorders involving defects in both B-cell and T-cell function. The predominant manifestation is hypogammaglobulinemia. Patients with common variable immunodeficiency can present in childhood, but most present in the second or third decade of life. In a large study, the average age at first presentation was 25 years, and at definitive diagnosis, it was 28 years (83). The most frequent presentation is recurrent sinopulmonary (100%) and gastrointestinal (50%) infection. Autoimmune cytopenia, rheumatoid disease, or thyroid disease develops in approximately 22% of patients, and malignancy, usually non-Hodgkin lymphoma, in 12%. Immunoglobulin levels are decreased to variable levels, and any or all isotypes can be involved. The number of circulating B cells is normal, and some studies suggest a defect in the terminal differentiation of these cells into plasma cells. The pathogenesis of common variable immunodeficiency is unknown.

Selective Immunoglobulin A Deficiency. IgA deficiency is the most common B-cell immunodeficiency, with an approximate incidence of 1 in 400 to 1 in 700 individuals in the general population. IgA levels are less than 5 mg/dL. Approximately 25% of patients are asymptomatic, 25% have autoimmune phenomena, and 50% have recurrent sinopulmonary and gastrointestinal infections. Coexisting IgG2 and IgG4 subclass deficiency, present in 15% to 20%, may explain the variable presentation and associated sinopulmonary infections. Atopy and allergic reactions to blood products (caused by IgA antibodies) are common.

Immunoglobulin G Subclass Deficiency. The potential role of IgG subclass deficiency in recurrent pyogenic infec-

tions was first reported in 1970. Since then, it has generally been accepted that although the total IgG level may be normal, low levels of certain subclasses of IgG, in particular IgG2, can result in susceptibility to sinopulmonary disease and bronchiectasis. IgG subclass deficiency has been reported in as many as 48% of patients with bronchiectasis (80), but some studies suggest a prevalence of only 1% to 2% (3). Deficiency of an IgG subclass is defined as a serum subclass concentration that is more than two standard deviations below the normal mean for age. The true significance of IgG subclass measurements is controversial, reflecting a lack of well-defined normal values. IgG3 deficiency occurs most commonly; an individual IgG subclass may be decreased, or two or more subclass deficiencies may coexist—for example, IgG2 and IgG4 deficiency. The most frequent clinical problem associated with this disorder is recurrent sinopulmonary infections with encapsulated bacteria and viruses. IgG2 deficiency is associated with recurrent pneumococcal and *H. influenzae* infections and an inability to produce specific antibodies to polysaccharide antigens, such as those in Pneumovax. IgG3 deficiency appears to be associated with a defective response to *Moraxella catarrhalis* and respiratory viruses. In the absence of associated IgG2 deficiency, the significance of decreased IgG4 is controversial.

Occasionally, despite normal serum immunoglobulin and IgG subclass concentrations, selective antibody deficiency to specific polysaccharide antigens may be the basis of increased susceptibility to certain infections. Several cases of recurrent *H. influenzae* infection despite *H. influenzae* type b vaccination have been shown to represent defective antibody responses specifically to *H. influenzae*.

Human Immunodeficiency Virus Infection

The incidence of bronchiectasis in patients with HIV infection is unknown; however, several reports have demonstrated multilobar bronchiectasis in patients with HIV infection and recent pneumonia (84–86). The extent of bronchiectasis exceeded that expected for the localized nature and severity of the pneumonia. Thus, it has been suggested that an accelerated form of bronchiectasis may develop in patients with HIV infection (87). No specific risk factors for bronchiectasis in HIV infection have been identified, but most patients have had advanced disease with low $CD4^+$-cell counts. Predisposing factors include susceptibility to lung infection, severe lung infection, and possible alterations in the baseline inflammatory milieu of the lung. Perhaps reflecting improved therapy for HIV infection, reports of severe bronchiectasis in this population have decreased. This raises questions regarding the significance of the original reports of bronchiectasis in these patients (85).

α_1-Protease Inhibitor Deficiency

α_1-PI deficiency is typically associated with early-onset panacinar emphysema in cigarette smokers. A significant proportion of patients have also been reported to have bronchiectasis, with a prevalence ranging from 2% to 43% (88,89). The association of α_1-PI deficiency with bronchiectasis remains controversial, and in many reported cases, other causes of bronchiectasis have not been ruled out. Prior studies have also suggested that certain α_1-PI allelic variants that are not associated with emphysema may predispose the host to bronchiectasis. However, two studies involving more than 300 patients with well-documented bronchiectasis did not show any clustering of α_1-PI genotypes (3,90). In summary, although α_1-PI deficiency has been associated with bronchiectasis, little evidence supports a causative role for this disorder in bronchiectasis.

SYSTEMIC DISEASE

Certain diseases that have primarily extrapulmonary manifestations are also associated with bronchiectasis (54).

Rheumatologic Diseases

Pleuropulmonary involvement is common in most rheumatologic diseases. Bronchiectasis, one of the many diverse pulmonary pathologic responses encountered in these diseases (Table 14.7), may reflect either the underlying collagen vascular disorder or a side effect, infectious or otherwise, of various treatment strategies. Studies in which HRCT was used have shown that bronchiectasis is more common than previously reported. The clinical significant of these findings is unclear because more than 50% of patients are asymptomatic.

Rheumatoid Arthritis

A clear association has been found between rheumatoid arthritis and bronchiectasis. Bronchiectasis is found in 3.2% to 5.2% of patients with rheumatoid arthritis on plain chest x-ray films, and in 20% to 35% of them on HRCT scans (91,92). Patients with bronchiectasis appear to present at a younger age (19–36 years) and have a higher (fivefold) mortality rate than other patients with rheumatoid arthritis (93). Unlike other pleuropulmonary manifestations of rheuma-

TABLE 14.7. BRONCHIECTASIS IN RHEUMATOLOGIC DISEASE

Disease	Bronchiectasis (%)	
	CXR	HRCT
RA	3–5	20–35
SLE	NR	21
Ankylosing spondylitis	NR	20
Sjögren syndrome	NR	38

Note: Many patients are asymptomatic.
CXR, chest x-ray film; HRCT, high-resolution computed tomography; NR, not reported; RA rheumatoid arthritis; SLE, systemic lupus erythematosis.

toid arthritis, bronchiectasis has not been reported to be associated with rheumatoid factor–positive disease. Bronchiectasis appears to be more common than pulmonary fibrosis in rheumatoid arthritis. The reason for the temporal relationship between bronchiectasis and rheumatoid arthritis is unknown, and in most cases bronchiectasis is not associated with pulmonary fibrosis (traction bronchiectasis) or prior infectious insults. Possible explanations for the association include effects of medication, defective functional antibody responses, associated Sjögren syndrome, or a common genetic predisposition (43,94).

Systemic Lupus Erythematosus

Bronchiectasis was not included among the many thoracic manifestations of systemic lupus erythematosus until HRCT findings in lupus were described by Fenlon and colleagues in 1996 (95). Of 34 patients, one third had bronchial wall thickening and 21% had bronchiectasis. Eighty-two percent of the patients were asymptomatic, and 75% were nonsmokers. No regional predilection was found; bronchiectasis affected all lung zones equally. The chest x-ray findings were considered normal in most cases. The cause of bronchiectasis in systemic lupus erythematosus is unknown.

Other Rheumatologic Conditions

Pleuropulmonary involvement in ankylosing spondylitis is rare (1.2%). The classic finding of apical fibrocavitary disease has been confirmed with the use of HRCT, which also revealed nonapical bronchiectasis in about 20% of cases (96). Similarly, primary Sjögren syndrome has been associated with bronchiectasis, and HRCT has detected bronchiectasis in as many as 38% of patients (97). Bronchiectasis has been described in the setting of other rheumatologic diseases, including Wegener granulomatosis and relapsing polychondritis (54,98).

Inflammatory Bowel Disease

Respiratory involvement is a rare extraintestinal complication of inflammatory bowel disease (IBD). Bronchiectasis, however, is the most common respiratory complication reported in IBD and is found in 23% of cases (54). Before HRCT, bronchiectasis was underdiagnosed in IBD (99). More than 50% of the cases of respiratory illness in these patients involve the airways, and it is likely that previous diagnoses such as chronic suppuration and bronchitis reflected undiagnosed bronchiectasis (100). In the largest study to date, 17 patients (14 with ulcerative colitis, three with Crohn disease) with respiratory symptoms underwent HRCT (101). Bronchiectasis was found in 13 patients (11 with ulcerative colitis, two with Crohn disease). Bronchial disease appears to be more common in patients with ulcerative colitis. In most cases, respiratory symptoms follow the intestinal manifestations of IBD and are more frequent during disease remission. In general, factors other than IBD that might account for bronchiectasis have been absent. The immunopathogenesis of bronchiectasis in IBD is unclear, but morphologic and developmental similarities between airway and colonic epithelium suggest a possible systemic immunologic phenomenon. Several reports have documented dramatic and complete resolution of bronchiectasis after the use of inhaled or systemic steroids. Medium to high doses of inhaled steroid are often required; the dose of prednisone should be 0.5 to 1 mg/kg. The optimal duration of treatment is unknown. Colonic resection does not appear to induce remission and is not recommended for this purpose.

Miscellaneous Causes of Bronchiectasis

Diffuse Panbronchiolitis

Diffuse panbronchiolitis is an idiopathic inflammatory disease characterized by recurrent and persistent sinusitis, suppurative obstructive lung disease, and bronchiectasis (102,103). It is seen predominantly in Japanese, Korean, and Chinese patients and is rare among non-Asian populations. A genetic predisposition is suggested by a strong association with HLA-B54 in Japanese patients. Patients typically present in the second to fifth decades with chronic pansinusitis, cough with purulent sputum, and progressive dyspnea. Radiologic studies reveal evidence of hyperinflation with diffuse nodules and bronchiectasis. On HRCT scans, the disease is seen to progress from stage 1, characterized by tiny nodules (<5 mm), to a "tree in bud" type of bronchiolitis (stage 2) and ultimately to diffuse bronchiectasis (stages 3 and 4). Sputum cultures frequently reveal *H. influenzae* and *P. aeruginosa*. In addition, cold agglutinin titers, rheumatoid factor titers, and serum immunoglobulins may be increased. A lung biopsy will reveal typical features of thickened terminal bronchiole walls with infiltration by lymphocytes, plasma cells, and histiocytes. Erythromycin and other macrolide antibiotics are effective in controlling symptoms and improving lung function and survival. The 5- and 10-year survival rates for untreated persons are 42% and 25%, respectively. With erythromycin therapy, more than 90% of patients are alive after 10 years. The effect of erythromycin in this disease appears to be antiinflammatory rather than antibacterial. A case report of diffuse panbronchiolitis in a Cambodian living in the United States emphasizes that this entity should be considered in Asian-born patients with bronchiectasis (103).

Yellow Nail Syndrome

The association of slowly growing discolored nails and chronic lymphedema was first described as yellow nail syndrome in 1964 (54,104). This is a rare disorder, probably congenital, that is characterized by dilated and hypoplastic lymphatics. Sixty-three percent of patients have pleuropulmonary abnormalities. Pleural effusion is present in 36% of patients, and at least 20% have bronchiectasis (105,106). A long-standing history of chronic sinusitis and bronchitis is typical. No specific treatment is available, and lung disease tends to be irreversible, although the nail discoloration regresses in about 30% of patients.

Abnormalities of the Tracheobronchial Tree

Bronchial Obstruction

Bronchial obstruction can result in bronchiectasis. The pathogenesis involves chronic and probably incomplete obstruction, and therefore bronchogenic carcinoma is rarely if ever associated with bronchiectasis. Typically, the obstructing lesion and associated bronchiectasis are localized. Obstruction can be intrinsic to the bronchus or its wall or represent extrinsic compression. Specific causes include endobronchial tumors, bronchial stenosis and broncholithiasis secondary to tuberculosis and other inflammatory disease, amyloidosis, and foreign body aspiration. Although foreign body aspiration is more common in children, it should also be suspected in adults with unresolving pneumonia or localized bronchiectasis (66). The most common aspirated foreign bodies are dental fragments and bones, which frequently are not detected on plain chest radiographs. Patients often do not recall the aspiration event, and a CT scan showing a dense structure within the bronchial lumen may first suggest foreign body aspiration (107). In addition, right middle lobe syndrome represents a form of localized bronchiectasis (55). It reflects the long narrow nature of the right middle lobe bronchus and probable compression by enlarged lymph nodes. It is seen less often in the era of declining tuberculosis. Right middle lobe syndrome may cause recurrent pneumonic symptoms or be an incidental finding on chest radiographs.

Mounier-Kuhn Syndrome (Tracheobronchomegaly)

Mounier-Kuhn syndrome is a rare disorder characterized by marked dilation of the trachea and main bronchi (108). It typically presents in men in the third or fourth decade of life with chronic sputum production and recurrent infection. Reported tracheal diameters that are diagnostic of the disease have varied from 2.3 to 3 cm and are different in men and women (109). A tracheal diameter exceeding 3 cm on either a plain chest radiograph or CT scan provides a definitive diagnosis. The main bronchi are also dilated, with associated central bronchiectasis. In general, airways distal to the fourth-order bronchi are normal, but retained mucus and recurrent infection may result in diffuse bronchiectasis. Additional findings include tracheal diverticulosis. The pathogenesis is uncertain, but autopsy studies show atrophy of the elastic and smooth muscle tissue of the trachea and main bronchi. In contrast to the Williams-Campbell syndrome, the Mounier-Kuhn syndrome is not characterized by obvious cartilaginous defects. The disease is considered congenital in nature, and a familial form with recessive inheritance has been described. Secondary forms of tracheobronchomegaly have been seen in Ehlers-Danlos syndrome, Marfan syndrome, Kenny-Caffey syndrome, light-chain deposition disease, and various connective tissue diseases and immunodeficiency diseases (108,110). No specific therapy is available.

Other Tracheobronchial Conditions

Williams-Campbell syndrome is a rare condition characterized by congenital absence of annular bronchial cartilage (111,112). Bronchopulmonary sequestration is a congenital anomaly in which a portion of the lung supplied by the systemic circulation develops separately and does not communicate with the normal tracheobronchial tree (113). The terminal bronchioles do not develop, and the proximal airways are dilated in the sequestered segment. Symptoms occur when the sequestered lung communicates with the bronchial tree. Rare cases of bronchiectasis have also been described in association with obliterative bronchiolitis, anorexia nervosa, endometriosis, and celiac disease (114–116).

SPECIFIC CAUSES OF BRONCHIECTASIS

Summary Statement	Level of Evidence
Bronchiectasis is idiopathic in more than 50% of adults despite aggressive investigation.	Prospective and retrospective studies
Chronic infection with MAI causes nodular bronchiectasis and is probably underrecognized.	Retrospective case series
ABPA is a significant primary cause of bronchiectasis and can complicate established bronchiectasis.	Prospective and retrospective studies
Bronchiectasis, often subclinical, is common in inflammatory bowel disease and collagen-vascular disease.	Prospective and retrospective studies
The association of bronchiectasis with HIV infection, α_1-protease inhibitor deficiency, and immunoglobulin subclass deficiency is controversial.	Retrospective case series

ABPA, allergic bronchopulmonary aspergillosis; MAI, *Mycobacterium avium-intracellulare*.

TREATMENT

Antibiotics

Therapy with antibiotics is the cornerstone of medical treatment for bronchiectasis. Antibiotics may be administered orally, intravenously, or by inhalation. Initially, antibiotics are given episodically to treat specific exacerbations of infection, manifested by a change in sputum color or volume, fever, or hemoptysis. The choice of oral or intravenous ther-

apy should be guided by the severity of illness. The choice of antibiotic is usually empiric, and correlation between sputum culture results and antibiotic success are not perfect. For minor exacerbations in outpatients with adequate pulmonary reserve, a 2-week course of an oral broad-spectrum antibiotic covering *S. pneumoniae* and *H. influenzae* is recommended. Frequently used are ampicillin/clavulanic acid, the newer macrolides (azithromycin or clarithromycin), or an oral quinolone (ciprofloxacin, levofloxacin). Trimethoprim/sulfamethoxazole (Bactrim) is another inexpensive antibiotic that may be effective, although its many side effects, including allergy, erythema multiforme, and Stevens-Johnson syndrome, make its use problematic for minor disease flares. In patients colonized or infected with *P. aeruginosa,* therapy aimed at this microbe is required. Orally active drugs against *Pseudomonas* include ciprofloxacin and levofloxacin, although the emergence of resistance is a concern with multiple cycles of antibiotics. For more severely ill patients who require intravenous therapy, dual therapy with an antipseudomonal penicillin plus an aminoglycoside is usually used. One study found a single daily intravenous dose of meropenem (3 g) effective in the treatment of ambulatory patients colonized with *P. aeruginosa* (117). For inpatient or outpatient treatment, inhaled tobramycin is particularly effective in treating infection with *P. aeruginosa* in patients with bronchiectasis. It has been shown to reduce colony counts in sputum and may even result in clearance of organisms from the sputum (see discussion later in this section).

The goal of therapy in acute exacerbations is to reduce sputum purulence and volume and eliminate signs or symptoms of ongoing inflammation, such as fever, weight loss, and night sweats. It is notable that a change in sputum color correlates reasonably well with bacterial colonization and the presence of inflammatory cells. By these measures, antibiotics are clearly effective in relieving an acute infective episode in patients with bronchiectasis. The optimal length of therapy is not known. The length of time between the end of antibiotic therapy and recurrence of symptoms can be quite variable, ranging from a few days to months. Once symptoms return, another course of antibiotics is indicated. The length and frequency of antibiotic therapy must be tailored to the individual patient.

Evidence is increasing that bacterial colonization of the sputum, particularly with *P. aeruginosa,* is associated with an inflammatory response that contributes to ongoing airways damage (37,118,119). Accordingly, some clinicians have promoted the idea of treatment cycles of "rotating" prophylactic antibiotics in patients with stable bronchiectasis to reduce the frequency of exacerbations and the development of drug resistance. Remarkably few trials have compared long-term suppressive antibiotic therapy with episodic antibiotics for exacerbations in patients with PCD or idiopathic bronchiectasis. One study in which low-dose erythromycin (500 mg/d) was given for 8 weeks showed reduction of sputum volume and improvement in pulmonary function (120).

It is not clear whether these improvements were attributable to the antibiotic or anti-inflammatory activity of the drug. It would seem that more long-term trials of this drug are indicated. We reserve long-term oral or inhaled antibiotic therapy for patients in whom symptoms recur within a few days after a course of antibiotics has been stopped.

Inhaled antibiotic therapy is a highly effective way to deliver a high concentration of antibiotic to the airways. Data suggest that the sputum itself is the reservoir of infection in bronchiectasis, and thus delivery of a nonabsorbable antibiotic to the airways is particularly attractive. In patients with CF, an inhaled dose of tobramycin results in serum levels well below acceptable trough levels of the drug, whereas sputum levels are many times the minimal inhibitory concentration for most *Pseudomonas* species. In patients with CF and those with idiopathic bronchiectasis, trials of inhaled tobramycin have shown persistent reduction in bacterial colonization and improvement in general condition, with little emergence of drug resistance (121). Concerns about the safety of long-term use of inhaled tobramycin, in terms of both emergence of resistant species and renal dysfunction or ototoxicity, have not materialized in a large experience in patients with CF.

ANTIBIOTIC TREATMENT OF BRONCHIECTASIS	
Summary Statement	Level of Evidence
Antibiotics are effective for treating acute exacerbations of bronchiectasis.	Extensive clinical experience
Long-term antibiotics can reduce mediators of inflammation in sputum, reduce the number of hospitalizations, and improve quality of life.	Short-term case control trials
Inhaled aminoglycosides (tobramycin, gentamicin) are safe and effective for treating airways disease and colonization, especially in patients colonized with *Pseudomonas aeruginosa*.	Two randomized controlled trials, extensive clinical experience

Bronchodilators

Many patients with bronchiectasis have airways obstruction. In some, the obstruction is not responsive to bronchodilators, whereas others have reactive airways disease. However, in addition to their bronchodilator effects, β-agonists have been reported to stimulate mucociliary clearance (17). This provides a rationale for their empiric use in most patients with bronchiectasis, although they should be used cautiously to avoid the emergence of side effects. Data validating their routine use in patients without airways obstruction are lacking.

Antiinflammatory Therapy

Inflammation, sometimes fueled by bacterial infection, is an important mediator of airway damage. Several studies have indicated that signs of airways inflammation persist after resolution of acute airways infection. These data suggest that the use of antiinflammatory therapy targeted at the airways is warranted. Adequate placebo-controlled trials of systemic steroids in idiopathic bronchiectasis are not available. Steroids are best used as an adjunct to antibiotics and bronchodilators in patients with acute exacerbation who have significant airways obstruction.

Inhaled steroids have shown some benefit in bronchiectasis. A review of randomized trials of inhaled steroids in bronchiectasis found only two acceptable trials, with a total of 54 patients (122). No statistically significant changes in clinical outcome were noted, although there was a trend toward improvement. A 1-month study of high-dose inhaled steroids in 24 patients with severe bronchiectasis found a reduction in "inflammatory mediators" in sputum but no significant change in clinical parameters (123). Further studies are required to examine the effect of high-dose inhaled steroids as an adjunct to antibiotics before they can be recommended as standard therapy.

In contrast to idiopathic bronchiectasis, bronchiectasis secondary to ABPA can be treated with oral corticosteroids. Central bronchiectasis usually represents end-stage and irreversible disease, but asthma and sinus symptoms in addition to the progression of bronchiectasis may be halted by steroids. Oral prednisone is generally given for several weeks at a dosage of 0.5 mg/kg per day and then tapered to every other day. Treatment is usually maintained for 3 months or more, and the response to therapy is monitored by symptoms and the levels of specific antibodies to *Aspergillus*.

A single short-term placebo-controlled trial has suggested that aerosolized indomethacin reduces sputum volume in patients with bronchitis, panbronchiolitis, or bronchiectasis (124). This therapy has not been widely adopted. Similarly, erythromycin and other macrolides have been found in multiple studies to reduce sputum volume and inflammatory mediators in Japanese patients with diffuse panbronchiolitis. This effect was independent of the effect on bacterial load in sputum; some have suggested an antiinflammatory mechanism (120,125,126). Although this remains an active area of clinical investigation, the long-term use of macrolides is not yet standard therapy in bronchiectasis. We reserve macrolides for patients with diffuse panbronchiolitis or those with severe bronchorrhea.

Mobilization of Secretions: Postural Drainage and Chest Physiotherapy

Postural or directed drainage, with or without associated breathing/coughing maneuvers, is helpful in reducing the stasis and pooling of infected secretions in dilated airways not easily drained by gravity in the upright posture. Most of these therapies encourage optimal bronchial hygiene, and although they are not specifically validated in patients with idiopathic bronchiectasis or PCD, they are likely helpful and inexpensive, and they do no harm. The addition of chest physiotherapy (percussion) to postural drainage and coughing maneuvers has not been shown to increase the benefit. Overly vigorous chest physiotherapy can occasionally cause injury in chronically ill, nutritionally depleted patients and requires considerable assistance from another trained person.

External Oscillation

External oscillation of airflow by means of a variable expiratory resistor (flutter device) held to the mouth has been shown to enhance sputum clearance in patients with CF (127–129). The degree of efficacy was similar to that of chest physiotherapy, but a second person was not required to carry out the maneuver. The device is of modest cost (~$50), may be useful, and has not been shown to do any harm. Studies in patients with idiopathic bronchiectasis have not been performed.

Mucolytics

Mucolytic therapy is aimed at reducing the viscosity of mucus in the airways, thereby facilitating their clearance. In addition, some organisms, particularly *Pseudomonas*, live in biofilms associated with mucus and adherent to epithelium and are protected from clearance. Although its goal seems laudable, the efficacy of such treatment has been difficult to document. A notable exception is recombinant human DNAse. This enzyme targets DNA from dead inflammatory cells and bacteria that contributes enormously to sputum viscosity in bronchiectasis. Recombinant human DNAse has been found to be useful as an adjunct treatment for patients with CF. However, one trial found recombinant human DNAse to be "ineffective and potentially harmful" in a group of adults with stable idiopathic bronchiectasis (130). Accordingly, its use is not recommended.

N-acetylcysteine (Mucomyst) has long been used in both aerosolized and oral forms and to liquefy sputum *in vitro* and facilitate laboratory manipulation. Unfortunately, it is rather irritating to the airways, may cause bronchospasm, and requires the concomitant use of bronchodilators. Placebo-controlled trials are difficult to perform because of the characteristic, unpleasant odor of the drug. Several trials in chronic bronchitis have shown a slight benefit from 300 mg of *N*-acetylcysteine orally twice a day in terms of sputum clearance, but convincing data in patients with bronchiectasis are lacking (131,132). Similarly, trials of expectorants such as iodinated glycerol and glyceryl guaiacolate are lacking. Nonetheless, these agents are widely used.

NONANTIBIOTIC THERAPY FOR BRONCHIECTASIS	
Summary Statement	**Level of Evidence**
Human recombinant DNAse is harmful in non-CF bronchiectasis.	One randomized controlled trial of good quality.
N-acetylcysteine is helpful in increasing sputum clearance and improving quality of life in patients with stable bronchiectasis.	Poor quality; few randomized controlled trials.
Inhaled indomethacin reduces sputum volume in bronchiectasis.	One randomized controlled trial.
Inhaled mannitol powder increases sputum clearance in stable bronchiectasis.	One randomized controlled trial.
Mucolytics are helpful in increasing sputum clearance and improving quality of life in patients with acute exacerbations of bronchiectasis.	Several randomized controlled trials.
Chest physiotherapy increases the clearance of sputum more than deep coughing and postural drainage.	One randomized controlled trial did not demonstrate benefit.
Variable expiratory flow device (flutter value) increases sputum clearance in non-CF bronchiectasis.	Evidence is of moderate to poor quality; no potential for harm.

CF, cystic fibrosis.

Surgical Therapy

Resection

As the incidence of bronchiectasis has declined and medical management has improved, resection for bronchiectasis has become increasingly uncommon. However, some patients with bronchiectasis can be significantly helped or even cured by resection of a localized area of damaged lung. Current indications for surgery for bronchiectasis include (a) severe symptoms referable to a localized area of bronchiectasis, especially when caused by an aspirated foreign body; (b) severe or recurrent hemoptysis that can be localized to a resectable segment or lobe in a patient with localized or diffuse bronchiectasis; and (c) resectable disease causing recurrent, severe episodes of infection (133–141). Patients with bronchiectatic involvement of a single segment are particularly good candidates for surgery, provided that the symptoms are severe enough that surgery is warranted. Patients with diffuse bronchiectasis may benefit from surgery if the symptoms are caused primarily by a single segment or lobe. No controlled trials have compared surgical with medical therapy for bronchiectasis.

The selection of patients for resection is extremely important and involves communication between the chest physician and an experienced thoracic surgeon. As in resections for cancer, physiologic measurements should be taken and correlated with HRCT and lung scanning data to ensure adequate postoperative pulmonary function. Considerable effort should be made to ensure optimal nutrition and control of bronchial secretions, hemoptysis, and bronchospasm before surgery. High-resolution CT should be used to determine the extent and location of bronchiectatic segments for resection. Although CT has been shown to correlate well with bronchography and with anatomic pathology in resected specimens (27,28), some surgeons may still require bronchography to map affected areas.

Transplantation

Survival rates following lung transplantation have improved considerably in the past 15 years. Considerable experience has now been acquired at some centers in performing lung transplantation in patients with bronchiectasis, chiefly those with bronchiectasis secondary to CF (142,143). Infectious complication rates among CF patients undergoing transplantation have not been higher than in those undergoing transplantation for other causes, with the exception of those colonized by *B. cepacia*. Such colonization is now viewed as a contraindication to transplantation.

Transplantation therapy for patients with suppurative lung disease is hampered by the shortage of organs available for transplantation and is made more acute by the fact that single lung transplantation is not optimal for patients with bronchiectasis because of the possibility of contamination of the allograft by a residual infected lung. A study of outcomes after heart-lung or double lung transplantation for bronchiectasis with or without CF found no difference in survival rates for these two procedures, suggesting that heart-lung transplantation is not required (144). Survival in this study for either procedure was 84% at 1 year and 76% at 3 years. Currently, double lung transplantation or sequential bilateral lung transplantation is performed in patients with bronchiectasis.

The selection of patients undergoing transplantation for bronchiectasis is similar to that of patients undergoing transplantation for other indications. Generally, they should be at significant risk for dying within 2 years. Established predictors include an FEV_1 less than 30% of the predicted value, a 12-minute walking distance of less than 500 m, hypoxemia

at rest, and signs of cor pulmonale. A report of suture line failures in a patient with Williams-Campbell syndrome suggests that in patients with bronchial cartilage abnormalities, transplantation is not a good choice (145).

COMPLICATIONS AND PROGNOSIS

The morbidity and mortality of patients with bronchiectasis are significantly increased (1,146). One study followed 842 adults with bronchiectasis for 8 to 12.9 years (146). The mortality rate was 24%, and the hospitalization rates were high, although they varied widely among individual patients (between 1 and 51 admissions per patient). Respiratory failure secondary to bronchiectasis was the primary cause of death.

Apart from infectious complications and respiratory failure, patients with bronchiectasis have a high incidence of hemoptysis (146). Studies suggest that 12% to 14% of all patients presenting with hemoptysis have underlying bronchiectasis, and the association is even greater if the hemoptysis is massive (147–149). In one study of patients with hemoptysis but nonlocalizing chest x-ray findings, CT identified underlying bronchiectasis in 24% of them (150). Hemoptysis in bronchiectasis generally occurs when hypertrophic bronchial arteries bleed in the setting of acute infectious exacerbations. Mycetomas are also common, especially in posttuberculous bronchiectasis (Fig. 14.5). In the setting of hemoptysis, emergent bronchoscopy to localize the site of bleeding is useful when radiographic studies are nonlocalizing. In one study of patients with hemoptysis, bronchoscopy successfully localized the bleeding to one lobe in 65% of patients and to one lung in 75% (147). Control of hemoptysis can be achieved at bronchoscopy in some cases, but more invasive approaches are often necessary. Although surgical resection is indicated in localized bronchiectasis with hemoptysis, disease is diffuse in most cases (151). Because underlying lung function may be severely impaired in these patients, we routinely obtain pulmonary function tests at the first clinic visit and annually to gauge the risks of surgical resection if necessary. Lung perfusion studies may also be useful. An alternative management option is bronchial artery embolization (147). No well-controlled trials have assessed the efficacy of this technique specifically in patients with bronchiectasis. However, in studies of patients with hemoptysis, of whom 17% to 47% had bronchiectasis, bronchial artery embolization was technically successful in 65% to 98% of cases and resulted in control of bleeding at 30 days or more in 50% to 85% of the patients who underwent successful embolization (147). Nevertheless, recurrent bleeding is common, and therefore bronchial artery embolization is often a temporizing treatment allowing time for a full assessment of surgical risk.

Other complications of bronchiectasis include ABPA (see section "Allergic Bronchopulmonary Aspergillosis"),

SURGICAL THERAPY FOR BRONCHIECTASIS	
Summary Statement	**Level of Evidence**
Surgical resection of nonfunctional areas of bronchiectasis causing significant symptoms is successful at controlling symptoms and is better than medical therapy for localized bronchiectasis.	Evidence is of moderate or poor quality; numerous surgical series; no randomized controlled trials
Double lung transplantation is successful in bronchiectasis, with a survival similar to that seen in lung transplantation for other causes.	Evidence of moderate quality; mostly extrapolation from the literature on cystic fibrosis

pneumothorax, secondary amyloidosis, and cerebral abscess (3,152–156). The latter two complications are rare, but underlying bronchiectasis should be considered in patients presenting with either clinical syndrome.

REFERENCES

1. Barker AF. Medical progress: bronchiectasis. *N Engl J Med* 2002;346:1383–1393.
2. O'Brien C, Guest PJ, Hill SL, et al. Physiological and radiological characterisation of patients diagnosed with chronic obstructive pulmonary disease in primary care. *Thorax* 2000;55:635–642.
3. Pasteur MC, Helliwell SM, Houghton SJ, et al. An investigation into causative factors in patients with bronchiectasis. *Am J Respir Crit Care Med* 2000;162:1277–1284.
4. Bachman AL, Hewitt WR, Beekly HC. Bronchiectasis: a bronchographic study of 60 cases of pneumonia. *Arch Intern Med* 1953;91:78–98.
5. Reid LM. Reduction in bronchial subdivision in bronchiectasis. *Thorax* 1950;5:233–247.
6. Ashour M. Hemodynamic alterations in bronchiectasis: a base for a new subclassification of the disease. *J Thorac Cardiovasc Surg* 1996;112:328–334.
7. Prikk K, Maisi P, Sepper R, et al. Association of trypsin-2 with activation of gelatinase B and collagenase-2 in human bronchoalveolar lavage fluid *in vivo*. *Ann Med* 2001;33:437–444.
8. Shum DK, Chan SC, Ip MS. Neutrophil-mediated degradation of lung proteoglycans: stimulation by tumor necrosis factor-alpha in sputum of patients with bronchiectasis. *Am J Respir Crit Care Med* 2000;162:1925–1931.
9. Horvath I, Loukides S, Wodehouse T, et al. Increased levels of exhaled carbon monoxide in bronchiectasis: a new marker of oxidative stress. *Thorax* 1998;53:867–870.
10. Wilson CB, Jones PW, O'Leary CJ, et al. Systemic markers of inflammation in stable bronchiectasis. *Eur Respir J* 1998;12:820–824.
11. Loukides S, Horvath I, Wodehouse T, et al. Elevated levels of expired breath hydrogen peroxide in bronchiectasis. *Am J Respir Crit Care Med* 1998;158:991–994.
12. Tsang KW, Chan K, Ho P, et al. Sputum elastase in steady-state bronchiectasis. *Chest* 2000;117:420–426.
13. Amitani R, Wilson R, Rutman A, et al. Effects of human neutrophil elastase and *Pseudomonas aeruginosa* proteinases on human respiratory epithelium. *Am J Respir Cell Mol Biol* 1991;4:26–32.
14. Prikk K, Maisi P, Pirila E, et al. *In vivo* collagenase-2 (MM-8) expression by human bronchial epithelial cells and monocytes/macrophages in bronchiectasis. *J Pathol* 2001;194:232–238.
15. Sepper R, Prikk K, Tervahartiala T, et al. Collagenase-2 and -3 are inhibited by doxycycline in the chronically inflamed lung in bronchiectasis. *Ann N Y Acad Sci* 1999;878:683–685.
16. Rayner CF, Rutman A, Dewar A, et al. Ciliary disorientation in patients with chronic upper respiratory tract inflammation. *Am J Respir Crit Care Med* 1995;151:800–804.
17. Mortensen J, Lange P, Nyboe J, et al. Lung mucociliary clearance. *Eur J Nucl Med* 1994;21:953–961.
18. Houtmeyers E, Gosselink R, Gayan-Ramirez G, et al. Regulation of mucociliary clearance in health and disease. *Eur Respir J* 1999;13:1177–1188.
19. Fahy JV, Schuster A, Ueki I, et al. Mucus hypersecretion in bronchiectasis: role of neutrophil proteases. *Am Rev Respir Dis* 1992;146:1430–1432.
20. McCool FD, Leith DE. Pathophysiology of cough. *Clin Chest Med* 1987;8:189–195.
21. Keane MP, Arenberg DA, Moore BB, et al. CXC chemokines and angiogenesis/angiostasis. *Proc Assoc Am Physicians* 1998;110:288–296.
22. Zheng L, Tipoe G, Lam WK, et al. Endothelin-1 in stable bronchiectasis. *Eur Respir J* 2000;16:146–149.
23. Ahmed SI, Thompson J, Coulson JM, et al. Studies on the expression of endothelin, its receptor subtypes, and converting enzymes in lung cancer and in human bronchial epithelium. *Am J Respir Cell Mol Biol* 2000;22:422–431.
24. Nicotra MB, Rivera M, Dale AM, et al. Clinical, pathophysiologic, and microbiologic characterization of bronchiectasis in an aging cohort. *Chest* 1995;108:955–961.
25. Roberts HR, Wells AU, Milne DG, et al. Airflow obstruction in bronchiectasis: correlation between computed tomography features and pulmonary function tests. *Thorax* 2000;55:198–204.
26. Evans SA, Turner SM, Bosch BJ, et al. Lung function in bronchiectasis: the influence of *Pseudomonas aeruginosa*. *Eur Respir J* 1996;9:1601–1604.
27. Kumar NA, Nguyen B, Maki D. Bronchiectasis: current clinical and imaging concepts. *Semin Roentgenol* 2001;36:41–50.
28. Kang EY, Miller RR, Muller NL. Bronchiectasis: comparison of preoperative thin-section CT and pathologic findings in resected specimens. *Radiology* 1995;195:649–654.
29. Van der Bruggen-Bogaarts BA, Van der Bruggen HM, Van Waes PF, et al. Screening for bronchiectasis. A comparative study between chest radiography and high-resolution CT. *Chest* 1996;109:608–611.
30. Young K, Aspestrand F, Kolbenstvedt A. High-resolution CT and bronchography in the assessment of bronchiectasis. *Acta Radiol* 1991;32:439–441.
31. Grenier P, Maurice F, Musset D, et al. Bronchiectasis: assessment by thin-section CT. *Radiology* 1986;161:95–99.
32. Young D. Surgical treatment of male infertility. *J Reprod Fertil* 1970;23:541–542.
33. Ouellette H. The signet ring sign. *Radiology* 1999;212:67–68.
34. Lee KH, Lee JS, Lynch DA, et al. The radiologic differential diagnosis of diffuse lung diseases characterized by multiple cysts or cavities. *J Comput Assist Tomogr* 2002;26:5–12.
35. Reiff DB, Wells AU, Carr DH, et al. CT findings in bronchiectasis: limited value in distinguishing between idiopathic and specific types. *AJR Am J Roentgenol* 1995;165:261–267.
36. Pang JA, Cheng A, Chan HS, et al. The bacteriology of bronchiectasis in Hong Kong investigated by protected catheter brush and bronchoalveolar lavage. *Am Rev Respir Dis* 1989;139:14–17.
37. Angrill J, Agusti C, De Celis R, et al. Bronchial inflammation and colonization in patients with clinically stable bronchiectasis. *Am J Respir Crit Care Med* 2002;164:1628–1632.
38. Rivera M, Nicotra MB. *Pseudomonas aeruginosa* mucoid strain. Its significance in adult chest diseases. *Am Rev Respir Dis* 1982;126:833–836.
39. Shah PL, Mawdsley S, Nash K, et al. Determinants of chronic infection with *Staphylococcus aureus* in patients with bronchiectasis. *Eur Respir J* 1999;14:1340–1344.
40. Johnston ID, Strachan DP, Anderson HR. Effect of pneumonia and whooping cough in childhood on adult lung function. *N Engl J Med* 1998;338:581–587.
41. Massie R, Armstrong D. Bronchiectasis and bronchiolitis obliterans post respiratory syncytial virus infection: think again. *J Paediatr Child Health* 1999;35:497–498.
42. Bateman ED, Hayashi S, Kuwano K, et al. Latent adenoviral

infection in follicular bronchiectasis. *Am J Respir Crit Care Med* 1995;151:170–176.

43. Snowden N, Moran A, Booth J, et al. Defective antibody production in patients with rheumatoid arthritis and bronchiectasis. *Clin Rheumatol* 1999;18:132–135.

44. Dutz JP, Benoit L, Wang X, et al. Lymphocytic vasculitis in X-linked lymphoproliferative disease. *Blood* 2001;97:95–100.

45. Lucaya J, Gartner S, Garcia-Pena P, et al. Spectrum of manifestations of Swyer-James-MacLeod syndrome. *J Comput Assist Tomogr* 1998;22:592–597.

46. Maiz L, Cuevas M, Quirce S, et al. Serologic IgE immune responses against *Aspergillus fumigatus* and *Candida albicans* in patients with cystic fibrosis. *Chest* 2002;121:782–788.

47. Vlahakis NE, Aksamit TR. Diagnosis and treatment of allergic bronchopulmonary aspergillosis. *Mayo Clin Proc* 2001;76:930–938.

48. Ward S, Heyneman L, Lee MJ, et al. Accuracy of CT in the diagnosis of allergic bronchopulmonary aspergillosis in asthmatic patients. *AJR Am J Roentgenol* 1999;173:937–942.

49. Rilance AB, Gerstl B. Bronchiectasis secondary to pulmonary tuberculosis. *Am Rev Tuberc* 1943;48:8–16.

50. Roberts JC, Blair LG. Bronchiectasis in primary tuberculosis. *Lancet* 1950;1:386–390.

51. Rosenzweig DY, Stead WW. The role of tuberculosis and other forms of bronchopulmonary necrosis in the pathogenesis of bronchiectasis. *Am Rev Respir Dis* 1966;93:769–785.

52. Kim HY, Song KS, Goo JM, et al. Thoracic sequelae and complications of tuberculosis. *Radiographics* 2001;21:839–858.

53. Udwadia ZF, Pilling JR, Jenkins PF, et al. Bronchoscopic and bronchographic findings in 12 patients with sarcoidosis and severe or progressive airways obstruction. *Thorax* 1990;45:272–275.

54. Cohen M, Sahn SA. Bronchiectasis in systemic diseases. *Chest* 1999;116:1063–1074.

55. Kwon KY, Myers JL, Swensen SJ, et al. Middle lobe syndrome: a clinicopathological study of 21 patients. *Hum Pathol* 1995;26:302–307.

56. Anonymous. Diagnosis and treatment of disease caused by nontuberculous mycobacteria. *Am J Respir Crit Care Med* 1997;156:S1–S25.

57. Prince DS, Peterson DD, Steiner RM, et al. Infection with *Mycobacterium avium* complex in patients without predisposing conditions. *N Engl J Med* 1989;321:863–868.

58. Ebert DL, Olivier KN. Nontuberculous mycobacteria in cystic fibrosis. *Infect Dis Clin North Am* 2002;16:221–233.

59. Reich JM, Johnson RE. *Mycobacterium avium* complex pulmonary disease presenting as an isolated lingular or middle lobe pattern. The Lady Windermere syndrome. *Chest* 1992;101:1605–1609.

60. Huang JH, Kao PN, Adi V, et al. *Mycobacterium avium-intracellulare* pulmonary infection in HIV-negative patients without preexisting lung disease: diagnostic and management limitations. *Chest* 1999;115:1033–1040.

61. Tanaka E, Amitani R, Niimi A, et al. Yield of computed tomography and bronchoscopy for the diagnosis of *Mycobacterium avium* complex pulmonary disease. *Am J Respir Crit Care Med* 1997;155:2041–2046.

62. Tanaka E, Kimoto T, Matsumoto H, et al. Familial pulmonary *Mycobacterium avium* complex disease. *Am J Respir Crit Care Med* 2000;161:1643–1647.

63. Kubo K, Yamazaki Y, Hanaoka M, et al. Analysis of HLA antigens in *Mycobacterium avium-intracellulare* pulmonary infection. *Am J Respir Crit Care Med* 2000;161:1368–1371.

64. Wallace RJ Jr, Brown BA, Griffith DE, et al. Clarithromycin regimens for pulmonary *Mycobacterium avium* complex. The first 50 patients. *Am J Respir Crit Care Med* 1996;153:1766–1772.

65. Cook VJ, Coxson HO, Mason AG, et al. Bullae, bronchiectasis and nutritional emphysema in severe anorexia nervosa. *Can Respir J* 2001;8:361–365.

66. Limper AH, Prakash UB. Tracheobronchial foreign bodies in adults. *Ann Intern Med* 1990;112:604–609.

67. Belperio JA, Keane MP, Arenberg DA, et al. CXC chemokines in angiogenesis. *J Leukoc Biol* 2000;68:1–8.

68. Chotmongkol V, Intarapoka B, Mitchai J. Mitochondrial myopathy with respiratory dysfunction: a case report. *J Med Assoc Thai* 2001;84:445–447.

69. Afzelius BA. A human syndrome caused by immotile cilia. *Science* 1976;193:317–319.

70. Afzelius BA. Immotile cilia syndrome: past, present and future prospects. *Thorax* 1998;53:894–897.

71. Olbrich H, Haffner K, Kispert A, et al. Mutations in DNAH5 cause primary ciliary dyskinesia and randomization of left-right asymmetry. *Nat Genet* 2002;30:143–144.

72. Afzelius BA. Asymmetry of mice and men. *Int J Dev Biol* 1999;45:283–286.

73. Jorissen M, Willems T, Van der SB. Ciliary function analysis for the diagnosis of primary ciliary dyskinesia: advantages of ciliogenesis in culture. *Acta Otolaryngol* 2000;120:291–295.

74. Handelsman DJ, Conway AJ, Boylan LM, et al. Young's syndrome. Obstructive azoospermia and chronic sinopulmonary infections. *N Engl J Med* 1984;310:3–9.

75. De Iongh R, Ing A, Rutland J. Mucociliary function, ciliary ultrastructure, and ciliary orientation in Young's syndrome. *Thorax* 1992;47:184–187.

76. Jaffe A, Bush A. Cystic fibrosis: review of the decade. *Monaldi Arch Chest Dis* 2001;56:240–247.

77. Bobadilla JL, Macek M Jr, Fine JP, et al. Cystic fibrosis: a worldwide analysis of CFTR mutations—correlation with incidence data and application to screening. *Hum Mutat* 2002;19:575–606.

78. Shah PL. Update on clinical trials in the treatment of pulmonary disease in patients with cystic fibrosis. *Expert Opin Investig Drugs* 1999;8:1917–1927.

79. Noone PG, Knowles MR. 'CFTR-opathies': disease phenotypes associated with cystic fibrosis transmembrane regulator gene mutations. *Respir Res* 2001;2:328–332.

80. De Gracia J, Rodrigo MJ, Morell F, et al. IgG subclass deficiencies associated with bronchiectasis. *Am J Respir Crit Care Med* 1996;153:650–655.

81. Hill SL, Mitchell JL, Burnett D, et al. IgG subclasses in the serum and sputum from patients with bronchiectasis. *Thorax* 1998;53:463–468.

82. Busse PJ, Razvi S, Cunningham-Rundles C. Efficacy of intravenous immunoglobulin in the prevention of pneumonia in patients with common variable immunodeficiency. *J Allergy Clin Immunol* 2002;109:1001–1004.

83. Cunningham-Rundles C. Clinical and immunologic analyses of 103 patients with common variable immunodeficiency. *J Clin Immunol* 1989;9:22–33.

84. McGuinness G, Naidich DP, Garay S, et al. AIDS-associated bronchiectasis: CT features. *J Comput Assist Tomogr* 1993;17:260–266.

85. King MA, Neal DE, St John R, et al. Bronchial dilatation in patients with HIV infection: CT assessment and correlation with pulmonary function tests and findings at bronchoalveolar lavage. *AJR Am J Roentgenol* 1997;168:1535–1540.

86. Verghese A, Al Samman M, Nabhan D, et al. Bacterial bronchitis and bronchiectasis in human immunodeficiency virus infection. *Arch Intern Med* 1994;154:2086–2091.

87. Bard M, Couderc LJ, Saimot AG, et al. Accelerated obstructive pulmonary disease in HIV-infected patients with bronchiectasis. *Eur Respir J* 1998;11:771–775.

88. King MA, Stone JA, Diaz PT, et al. Alpha 1-antitrypsin deficiency: evaluation of bronchiectasis with CT. *Radiology* 1996;199:137–141.

89. Larsson C. Natural history and life expectancy in severe alpha$_1$-antitrypsin deficiency, Pi Z. *Acta Med Scand* 1978;204:345–351.

90. Cuvelier A, Muir JF, Hellot MF, et al. Distribution of alpha(1)-antitrypsin alleles in patients with bronchiectasis. *Chest* 2000;117:415–419.

91. Walker WC, Wright V. Pulmonary lesions and rheumatoid arthritis. *Medicine (Baltimore)* 1968;47:501–520.

92. Perez T, Remy-Jardin M, Cortet B. Airways involvement in rheumatoid arthritis: clinical, functional, and HRCT findings. *Am J Respir Crit Care Med* 1998;157:1658–1665.

93. Swinson DR, Symmons D, Suresh U, et al. Decreased survival in patients with co-existent rheumatoid arthritis and bronchiectasis. *Br J Rheumatol* 1997;36:689–691.

94. Hillarby MC, McMahon MJ, Grennan DM, et al. HLA associations in subjects with rheumatoid arthritis and bronchiectasis but not with other pulmonary complications of rheumatoid disease. *Br J Rheumatol* 1993;32:794–797.

95. Fenlon HM, Doran M, Sant SM, et al. High-resolution chest CT in systemic lupus erythematosus. *AJR Am J Roentgenol* 1996;166:301–307.

96. Fenlon HM, Casserly I, Sant SM, et al. Plain radiographs and thoracic high-resolution CT in patients with ankylosing spondylitis. *AJR Am J Roentgenol* 1997;168:1067–1072.

97. Koyama M, Johkoh T, Honda O, et al. Pulmonary involvement in primary Sjögren's syndrome: spectrum of pulmonary abnormalities and computed tomography findings in 60 patients. *J Thorac Imaging* 2001;16:290–296.

98. Woywodt A, Goebel U. Bronchial stenosis and extensive bronchiectasis due to Wegener's granulomatosis. *Nephron* 2000;85:366–367.

99. Camus P, Piard F, Ashcroft T, et al. The lung in inflammatory bowel disease. *Medicine (Baltimore)* 1993;72:151–183.

100. Camus P, Colby TV. The lung in inflammatory bowel disease. *Eur Respir J* 2000;15:5–10.

101. Mahadeva R, Walsh G, Flower CD, et al. Clinical and radiological characteristics of lung disease in inflammatory bowel disease. *Eur Respir J* 2000;15:41–48.

102. Fisher MS Jr, Rush WL, Rosado-de-Christenson ML, et al. Diffuse panbronchiolitis: histologic diagnosis in unsuspected cases involving North American residents of Asian descent. *Arch Pathol Lab Med* 1998;122:156–160.

103. Krishnan P, Thachil R, Gillego V. Diffuse panbronchiolitis: a treatable sinobronchial disease in need of recognition in the United States. *Chest* 2002;121:659–661.

104. Samman PD, White WF. The yellow nail syndrome. *Br J Dermatol* 1964;76:153–157.

105. Emerson PA. Yellow nails, lymphedema and pleural effusions. *Thorax* 1966;21:249–253.

106. Wiggins J, Strickland B, Chung KF. Detection of bronchiectasis by high-resolution computed tomography in the yellow nail syndrome. *Clin Radiol* 1991;43:377–379.

107. Zissin R, Shapiro-Feinberg M, Rozenman J, et al. CT findings of the chest in adults with aspirated foreign bodies. *Eur Radiol* 2001;11:606–611.

108. Lazzarini-de-Oliveira LC, Costa de Barros Franco CA, Gomes de Salles CL, et al. A 38-year-old man with tracheomegaly, tracheal diverticulosis, and bronchiectasis. *Chest* 2001;120:1018–1020.

109. Dunne MG, Reiner B. CT features of tracheobronchomegaly. *J Comput Assist Tomogr* 1988;12:388–391.

110. Sane AC, Effmann EL, Brown SD. Tracheobronchomegaly. The Mounier-Kuhn syndrome in a patient with the Kenny-Caffey syndrome. *Chest* 1992;102:618–619.

111. Jones VF, Eid NS, Franco SM, et al. Familial congenital bronchiectasis: Williams-Campbell syndrome. *Pediatr Pulmonol* 1993;16:263–267.

112. Kaneko K, Kudo S, Tashiro M, et al. Case report: computed tomography findings in Williams-Campbell syndrome. *J Thorac Imaging* 1991;6:11–13.

113. Bolman RM, III, Wolfe WG. Bronchiectasis and bronchopulmonary sequestration. *Surg Clin North Am* 1980;60:867–881.

114. Butler H, Lake KB, Van Dyke JJ. Bronchial endometriosis and bronchiectasis. A possible relationship. *Arch Intern Med* 1978;138:991–992.

115. Mahadeva R, Flower C, Shneerson J. Bronchiectasis in association with coeliac disease. *Thorax* 1998;53:527–529.

116. Markopoulou KD, Cool CD, Elliot TL, et al. Obliterative bronchiolitis: varying presentations and clinicopathological correlation. *Eur Respir J* 2002;19:20–30.

117. Darley ES, Bowker KE, Lovering AM, et al. Use of meropenem 3 g once daily for outpatient treatment of infective exacerbations of bronchiectasis. *J Antimicrob Chemother* 2000;45:247–250.

118. Hill AT, Campbell EJ, Hill SL, et al. Association between airway bacterial load and markers of airway inflammation in patients with stable chronic bronchitis. *Am J Med* 2000;109:288–295.

119. Ho PL, Chan KN, Ip MS, et al. The effect of *Pseudomonas aeruginosa* infection on clinical parameters in steady-state bronchiectasis. *Chest* 1998;114:1594–1598.

120. Tsang KW, Ho PI, Chan KN, et al. A pilot study of low-dose erythromycin in bronchiectasis. *Eur Respir J* 1999;13:361–364.

121. Barker AF, Couch L, Fiel SB, et al. Tobramycin solution for inhalation reduces sputum *Pseudomonas aeruginosa* density in bronchiectasis. *Am J Respir Crit Care Med* 2000;162:481–485.

122. Kolbe J, Wells A, Ram FS. Inhaled steroids for bronchiectasis. *Cochrane Database Syst Rev* 2000;CD000996.

123. Tsang KW, Ho PL, Lam WK, et al. Inhaled fluticasone reduces sputum inflammatory indices in severe bronchiectasis. *Am J Respir Crit Care Med* 1998;158:723–727.

124. Tamaoki J, Chiyotani A, Kobyashi K, et al. Effect of indomethacin on bronchorrhea in patients with chronic bronchitis, panbronchiolitis, or bronchiectasis. *Am Rev Respir Dis* 1992;145:548–552.

125. Gorrini M, Lupi A, Viglio S, et al. Inhibition of human neutrophil elastase by erythromycin and flurythromycin, two macrolide antibiotics. *Am J Respir Cell Mol Biol* 2001;25:492–499.

126. Jaffe A, Bush A. Anti-inflammatory effects of macrolides in lung disease. *Pediatr Pulmonol* 2001;31:464–473.

127. Konstan MW, Stern RC, Doerschuk CF. Efficacy of the flutter device for mucus clearance in patients with cystic fibrosis. *J Pediatr* 1994;124:869–893.

128. Gondor M, Nixon PA, Mutich R, et al. Comparison of flutter device and chest physical therapy in the treatment of cystic fibrosis pulmonary exacerbation. *Pediatr Pulmonol* 1999;28:255–260.

129. Dasgupta B, Brown NE, King M. Effects of sputum oscillations and rhDNase *in vitro*: a combined approach to treat cystic fibrosis lung disease. *Pediatr Pulmonol* 1998;26:250–255.

130. O'Donnell A, Barker AF, Ilowite J, et al. Treatment of bronchiectasis with aerosolized recombinant human DNAse I. *Chest* 1998;113:1329–1334.

131. Crockett AJ, Cranston JM, Latimer KM, et al. Mucolytics for bronchiectasis. *Cochrane Database Syst Rev* 2000;CD001289.

132. British Thoracic Society. Statement on *N*-acetylcysteine. *Thorax* 1985;40:832–835.

133. Fujimoto T, Hillejan L, Stamatis G. Current strategy for surgical management of bronchiectasis. *Ann Thorac Surg* 2001;72:1711–1715.

134. Prieto D, Bernardo J, Matos MJ, et al. Surgery for bronchiectasis. *Eur J Cardiothorac Surg* 2001;20:19–23.

135. Corless JA, Warburton CJ. Surgery vs non-surgical treatment for bronchiectasis. *Cochrane Database Syst Rev* 2000;CD002180.

136. Ashour M, Al Kattan K, Rafay MA, et al. Current surgical therapy for bronchiectasis. *World J Surg* 1999;23:1096–1104.

137. Agasthian T, Deschamps C, Trastek VF, et al. Surgical management of bronchiectasis. *Ann Thorac Surg* 1996;62:976–978.

138. Ashour M, Al Kattan KM, Jain SK, et al. Surgery for unilateral bronchiectasis: results and prognostic factors. *Tuberc Lung Dis* 1996;77:168–172.

139. Barker AF. Bronchiectasis. *Semin Thorac Cardiovasc Surg* 1995;7:112–118.

140. Dogan R, Alp M, Kaya S, et al. Surgical treatment of bronchiectasis: a collective review of 487 cases. *Thorac Cardiovasc Surg* 1989;37:183–186.

141. Vejlsted H, Hjelms E, Jacobsen O. Results of pulmonary resection in cases of unilateral bronchiectasis. *Scand J Thorac Cardiovasc Surg* 1982;16:81–85.

142. Charman SC, Sharples LD, McNeil KD, et al. Assessment of survival benefit after lung transplantation by patient diagnosis. *J Heart Lung Transplant* 2002;21:226–232.

143. Rao JN, Forty J, Hasan A, et al. Bilateral lung transplant: the procedure of choice for end-stage septic lung disease. *Transplant Proc* 2001;33:1622–1623.

144. Barlow CW, Robbins RC, Moon MR, et al. Heart-lung versus double-lung transplantation for suppurative lung disease. *J Thorac Cardiovasc Surg* 2000;119:466–476.

145. Palmer SM Jr, Layish DT, Kussin PS, et al. Lung transplantation for Williams-Campbell syndrome. *Chest* 1998;113:534–537.

146. Keistinen T, Saynajakangas O, Tuuponen T, et al. Bronchiectasis: an orphan disease with a poorly understood prognosis. *Eur Respir J* 1997;10:2784–2787.

147. Swanson KL, Johnson CM, Prakash UB, et al. Bronchial artery embolization: experience with 54 patients. *Chest* 2002;121:789–795.

148. Haro EM, Vizcaya SM, Jimenez LJ, et al. Etiology of hemoptysis: prospective analysis of 752 cases. *Rev Clin Esp* 2001;201:696–700.

149. Salajka F. The causes of massive hemoptysis. *Monaldi Arch Chest Dis* 2001;56:390–393.

150. Tak S, Ahluwalia G, Sharma SK, et al. Haemoptysis in patients with a normal chest radiograph: bronchoscopy-CT correlation. *Australas Radiol* 1999;43:451–455.

151. Kutlay H, Cangir AK, Enon S, et al. Surgical treatment in bronchiectasis: analysis of 166 patients. *Eur J Cardiothorac Surg* 2002;21:634–637.

152. Gertz MA, Kyle RA. Secondary systemic amyloidosis: response and survival in 64 patients. *Medicine (Baltimore)* 1991;70:246–256.

153. Grum CM, Lynch JP III. Chest radiographic findings in cystic fibrosis. *Semin Respir Infect* 1992;7:193–209.

154. Wood JR, Bellamy D, Child AH, et al. Pulmonary disease in patients with Marfan syndrome. *Thorax* 1984;39:780–784.

155. Rotheram EB Jr, Kessler LA. Use of computerized tomography in nonsurgical management of brain abscess. *Arch Neurol* 1979;36:25–26.

156. Leibovitch G, Maaravi Y, Shalev O. Multiple brain abscesses caused by *Streptococcus bovis*. *J Infect* 1991;23:195–196.

15 Smoking Cessation

Douglas E. Jorenby · Michael C. Fiore

Tobacco use, and cigarette smoking in particular, claims the lives of more than 400,000 Americans each year through chronic obstructive pulmonary disease; cancer of the lung, throat, bladder, and other sites; stroke; heart disease; sudden infant death syndrome; and complications of pregnancy (1). Therefore, tobacco use is the leading preventable cause of illness and premature death in the United States. Along with the toll in human lives and suffering, tobacco use also results in $50 billion per year in direct medical care costs, and an additional $47 billion in lost productivity and disability (2,3). Despite the volume of information that has accumulated since the 1950s regarding the negative health consequences of smoking, approximately 25% of the adult population in the United States smokes, and some 3,000 children and adolescents become smokers each day (4,5). National rates have not decreased dramatically during the past decade, possibly as a result of two distinct factors: the chronic disease nature of tobacco dependence and limited available clinical interventions to treat tobacco dependence.

MODEL OF CHRONIC DISEASE

Tobacco dependence shares a number of features with other chronic diseases, such as hypertension, dyslipidemia, and diabetes mellitus. Because most smokers begin to use tobacco in childhood or adolescence and continue for decades, tobacco dependence is a long-term condition. It also tends to display periods of remission and relapse or exacerbation. In fact, although the vast majority of U.S. smokers have made at least one attempt to quit, success rates remain

D. E. Jorenby and M. C. Fiore: Department of Medicine, Center for Tobacco Research and Intervention, University of Wisconsin Medical School, Madison, Wisconsin.

quite low for unassisted quitting—on the order of 7% to 12% for sustained cessation (6). A primary cause of this lack of success is the powerfully addictive nature of nicotine, the chief psychoactive agent in tobacco. Nicotine has a variety of effects on mood and attention in human users. It also causes tolerance with repeated use and an aversive withdrawal syndrome on cessation, in the same manner as alcohol, heroin, and cocaine (7). The combination of the psychoactive effects deemed desirable by users, the direct control over nicotine delivery afforded by a cigarette, and aversive symptoms that begin within hours of cessation places smokers at significant risk for relapse, often within days of beginning an attempt to quit. However, clinical intervention can make a positive difference in the probability of relapse. As with other chronic diseases, a combination of clinician counseling and medication can increase rates of long-term cessation.

CLINICAL INTERVENTION

Unfortunately, it appears that opportunities for clinical intervention are often missed. This is not for lack of exposure. Some 70% of smokers visit a physician at least once a year, and also come into contact with other health care professionals, such as nurses, pharmacists, dentists, and physician assistants (8). As noted in the section "Model of Chronic Disease," the vast majority of smokers report that they are interested in cessation; advice from a clinician is a critical factor in deciding to make a quit attempt (9). However, the smoking status of clinic patients is not assessed consistently, and intervention is even less frequent. A survey of a large population reported that fewer than 15% of the people in the sample had received cessation assistance from a clinician, and only 3% had received follow-up support for their cessation efforts (10).

TABLE 15.1. FIVE As FOR BRIEF CLINICAL INTERVENTION

Ask about tobacco use.	Identify and document tobacco use status for every patient at every visit.
Advise to quit.	In a clear, strong, and personalized manner, urge every tobacco user to quit.
Assess willingness to make a quit attempt.	Is the tobacco user willing to make a quit attempt at this time?
Assist in quit attempt.	For the patient willing to make a quit attempt, use counseling and pharmacotherapy.
Arrange follow-up.	Schedule follow-up contact, preferably within the first week after the quit date.

Source: Adapted from Fiore MC, Bailey WC, Cohen SJ, et al. *Treating tobacco use and dependence. Clinical practice guideline.* Rockville, MD: US Department of Health and Human Services, Public Health Service, 2000.

This missed opportunity prompted the Public Health Service expert panel to issue *Treating Tobacco Use and Dependence. Clinical Practice Guideline* (11). The authors of this guideline, an evidence-based product, reviewed the extant tobacco cessation literature from 1975 through 1999, conducted more than 50 metaanalyses, and provided a series of recommendations to guide clinicians in treating tobacco dependence. The recommendations that follow draw heavily on the evidence-based conclusions of this seminal publication.

One of the recommendations of the guideline is a systems-level program to ensure that all tobacco users are identified and receive at least a minimal intervention. The guideline panel promoted a mnemonic, the "five *A*s," to direct systems toward this goal (Table 15.1).

The first step, *a*sking about smoking status, is the most critical one. If a system is not in place that routinely identifies tobacco users at the point of clinical contact, the likelihood of any meaningful intervention drops precipitously. Systems that add questions regarding smoking status to the traditional vital signs, or use some sort of medical record prompt, increased rates of smoker identification more than threefold in comparison with settings in which no screening system was in place, according to a metaanalysis of nine studies (11). A more limited metaanalysis of three studies that related actual patient cessation rates to the presence or absence of formal screening systems suggested that screening doubles cessation rates (odds ratio [OR] of 2.0; OR of 1.0 for the no-screening-system reference group) (11).

Once current tobacco users have been identified, all of them should be *a*dvised to quit in a clear, strong, and personalized manner. This can be done in as brief a statement as telling a patient, "As your clinician, I need to advise you that stopping smoking is the single best thing you can do to protect your current and future health." Of the three elements of brief advice, personalization is the most important. Information that is personally relevant to the patient is more persuasive than abstract information about health risks. For

instance, patients presenting with persistent cough, shortness of breath, poor peripheral circulation, or any of a number of other smoking-related symptoms should be made aware of the connection of these symptoms and signs to tobacco use. Parents with children who have middle ear infections, asthma, and respiratory infections should also be apprised of the connection between these presenting problems and exposure to environmental tobacco smoke. The guideline panel, in a metaanalysis of seven studies, found that brief physician advice (<3 minutes) increased the long-term cessation OR to 1.3 in comparison with no advice (11). More recent research indicates that patients are more satisfied with their care when physicians address smoking, whether the patient is ready to quit or not (12).

The next stage of intervention is *a*ssessing the patient's motivation to quit. Regardless of the level of the clinician's skill, at any given time, a certain number of tobacco users will always be unwilling or unable to make a quit attempt. There is no evidence that trying to force such patients to set a quit date, or providing them with cessation medications, will result in the desired outcome. An alternative is to engage in a brief intervention designed to increase the motivation for tobacco cessation, perhaps at a subsequent clinical contact.

TABLE 15.2. FIVE Rs TO ENHANCE MOTIVATION FOR TOBACCO CESSATION

Relevance	Encourage the patient to indicate why quitting is personally relevant. Motivational information has the greatest impact if it is relevant to a patient's disease status or risk, family or social situation, and other important characteristics.
Risks	Ask the patient to identify potential negative consequences of tobacco use. Examples of risks are the following: ■ *Acute:* Shortness of breath, harm to pregnancy, erectile dysfunction, exacerbation of asthma ■ *Long-term:* Heart attack, stroke, lung and other cancers, chronic obstructive pulmonary disease ■ *Environmental:* Increased risk for sudden infant death syndrome, higher rates of smoking by children as a consequence of modeling, increased risk for lung cancer and heart disease in spouses exposed to environmental tobacco smoke.
Rewards	Ask the patient to identify potential benefits of tobacco use. The most important benefits are the ones most relevant to the patient. Examples might include saving money, setting a good example for children, feeling better physically, improved sense of smell, improved stamina.
Roadblocks	Ask the patient about barriers or impediments to quitting. Examples might include withdrawal symptoms, fear of weight gain after cessation, depression, lack of support, enjoyment of smoking.
Repetition	Patients who have tried to quit before and failed should be informed that most people make several attempts before quitting for good. Repeat motivational interventions as needed at subsequent clinic visits.

Source: Adapted from Fiore MC, Bailey WC, Cohen SJ, et al. *Treating tobacco use and dependence. Clinical practice guideline.* Rockville, MD: US Department of Health and Human Services, Public Health Service, 2000.

In some cases, a specific stressful event, such as starting a new job, may make a patient disinclined to make a quit attempt. In others, it may take several contacts to begin to shift the balance of the perceived benefits and risks of smoking toward quitting. Table 15.2 presents a helpful mnemonic for motivation-enhancing interventions.

For those patients who are willing to make a quit attempt, the clinician can do a number of things to *assist* them in the process of becoming tobacco-free. The guideline panel examined the evidence for and against dozens of elements of tobacco cessation treatment. Strong evidence was found to support the use of five first-line pharmacotherapies and three types of counseling. Each of these is considered in detail.

PHARMACOTHERAPY

The U.S. Food and Drug Administration (FDA) has approved five forms of pharmacotherapy as safe and effective for use in treating tobacco dependence. Four of the therapies are delivery systems for nicotine replacement (nicotine gum, inhaler, nasal spray, and patch); the remaining agent, sustained-release bupropion (bupropion SR), is the only nonnicotine treatment approved to date. The guideline panel found sufficient evidence for the efficacy of these pharmacotherapies to recommend their use in *all* patients willing to make a quit attempt, except in the case of specific contraindications (11). A summary of the clinical guidelines for recommending pharmacotherapy for smoking cessation is provided in Table 15.3.

Sustained-Release Bupropion

Bupropion SR is the only nonnicotine pharmacotherapy to be approved by the FDA to date. The effectiveness of this atypical antidepressant in treating tobacco dependence is thought to be related to blocking the reuptake of dopamine or norepinephrine in the brain. Unlike nicotine replacement

TABLE 15.3. CLINICAL GUIDELINES FOR PRESCRIBING PHARMACOTHERAPY FOR SMOKING CESSATION

Who should receive pharmacotherapy for smoking cessation?	All smokers trying to quit except in special circumstances. Special consideration should be given before using pharmacotherapy in selected populations: those with medical contraindications, those smoking fewer than 10 cigarettes per day, pregnant women, and adolescent smokers.
What are the first-line pharmacotherapies recommended in this guideline?	All five of the FDA-approved pharmacotherapies for smoking cessation are recommended, including bupropion SR, nicotine gum, nicotine inhaler, nicotine nasal spray, and the nicotine patch.
What factors should a clinician consider when choosing among the five first-line pharmacotherapies?	Because of a lack of sufficient data to rank-order these five medications, the choice of a specific first-line pharmacotherapy must be guided by factors such as clinician familiarity with the medications, contraindications for selected patients, patient preference, previous patient experience with a specific pharmacotherapy (positive or negative), and patient characteristics (e.g., history of depression, concerns about weight gain).
Are pharmacotherapeutic treatments appropriate for lighter smokers (e.g., 10–15 cigarettes per day)?	If pharmacotherapy is used for lighter smokers, clinicians should consider reducing the dose of first-line pharmacotherapies.
What second-line pharmacotherapies are recommended in this guideline?	Clonidine and nortriptyline.
When should second-line agents be used for treating tobacco dependence?	Consider prescribing second-line agents for patients unable to use first-line medications because of contraindications or because the first-line medications are not helpful. Monitor patients for the known side effects of second-line agents.
Which pharmacotherapies should be considered for patients particularly concerned about weight gain?	Bupropion SR and nicotine replacement therapies, in particular nicotine gum, have been shown to delay, but not prevent, weight gain.
Which pharmacotherapies should be considered for patients with a history of depression?	Bupropion SR and nortriptyline appear to be effective in this population.
Should nicotine replacement therapies be avoided in patients with a history of cardiovascular disease?	No. Nicotine replacement therapies are safe and have not been shown to cause adverse cardiovascular effects. However, the safety of these products has not been established for use immediately after myocardial infarction or in patients with severe or unstable angina.
Can tobacco dependence pharmacotherapies be used long-term (e.g., 6 months or more)?	Yes. This approach may be helpful in smokers who report persistent withdrawal symptoms during the course of pharmacotherapy or who desire long-term therapy. A minority of individuals who successfully quit smoking use nicotine replacement therapy (gum, nasal spray, inhaler) ad libitum long-term. The use of these medications long-term does not present a known health risk. Additionally, the FDA has approved the use of bupropion SR for a long-term maintenance indication.
Can nicotine replacement pharmacotherapies ever be combined?	Yes. There is evidence that combining the nicotine patch with either nicotine gum or nicotine nasal spray increases long-term abstinence rates over those achieved with a single form of nicotine replacement therapy.

FDA, Food and Drug Administration; SR, sustained release.
Source: Adapted from Fiore MC, Bailey WC, Cohen SJ, et al. *Treating tobacco use and dependence. Clinical practice guideline.* Rockville, MD: US Department of Health and Human Services, Public Health Service, 2000.

therapies, bupropion therapy is initiated 1 to 2 weeks before the quit date; patients most often begin by taking 150 mg in the morning for 3 days, then increasing the dosage to 150 mg twice a day for up to 3 months following the quit date. Two large randomized controlled trials tested the efficacy of bupropion SR in comparison with placebo; the guideline metaanalysis of these trials indicated a cessation OR for bupropion SR of 2.1 (confidence interval [CI], 1.5–3.0) versus placebo (11,13,14). Since the publication of the guideline, an additional randomized controlled trial has demonstrated that extended treatment with bupropion SR (up to 52 weeks) delays the median time to relapse in comparison with extended placebo treatment (15). Bupropion SR is contraindicated in persons with a history of seizure or eating disorder, who have taken a monoamine oxidase inhibitor within the previous 14 days, or are currently using another form of bupropion (Wellbutrin or Zyban). Commonly reported side effects include insomnia and dry mouth. Because bupropion SR is classified as an FDA class B drug, women who are pregnant or nursing should attempt to quit smoking with behavioral methods before considering use of this medication. Bupropion SR may also be combined with nicotine replacement therapy, although more research is needed on optimal combination therapies (14). Bupropion SR may be of particular benefit in patients with a history of depression (11). Detailed prescribing instructions are shown in Table 15.4.

Nicotine Gum

Nicotine gum was the first nicotine replacement therapy to be approved for use in the United States and is one of the most widely studied forms of pharmacotherapy for the treatment of tobacco dependence. In a metaanalysis of 13 studies, the guideline found a long-term cessation OR of 1.5 (CI, 1.3–1.8) for active nicotine gum in comparison with placebo (11). Nicotine gum, available over the counter in both 2- and 4-mg formulations, allows for flexible dosing in response to specific cravings. As with all nicotine replacement therapies, use should begin on the target quit date. Care should be taken to instruct patients in proper use of the gum. Drinking liquids while chewing the gum, or using it within 15 minutes after drinking an acidic beverage (e.g., cola, coffee, citrus juice), diminishes the therapeutic effect. Patients should chew a piece of gum until they feel a tingling sensation or peppery taste; at that point, they should "park" the gum at the side of their mouth until the sensation abates. Using the proper "chew and park" technique not only optimizes the absorption of nicotine through the buccal mucosa but also reduces common side effects, such as hiccups, jaw ache, and mouth soreness. Heavier smokers are likely to be more successful using the 4-mg than the 2-mg strength (16). Detailed instructions for clinical use are presented in Table 15.5.

Nicotine Inhaler

The nicotine inhaler is another nicotine replacement therapy designed to be used as needed. The delivery system consists of a small cartridge containing nicotine that is inserted into a small plastic mouthpiece. As the patient inhales through the mouthpiece, a small amount of nicotine is drawn into the mouth and upper throat. The inhaler mimics the habitual hand-to-mouth action of smoking, but without combustion,

TABLE 15.4. SUGGESTIONS FOR THE CLINICAL USE OF BUPROPION SR

Patient selection	Appropriate as a first-line pharmacotherapy for smoking cessation.
Precautions	*Pregnancy*—Pregnant smokers should be first encouraged to quit without pharmacologic treatment. Bupropion SR should be used during pregnancy only if the increased likelihood of smoking abstinence, with its potential benefits, outweighs the risk of bupropion SR treatment and potential concomitant smoking. Similar factors should be considered in lactating women (class B).
	Cardiovascular diseases—Generally well tolerated; infrequent reports of hypertension.
	Side effects—The most common side effects reported by bupropion SR users were insomnia (35%–40%) and dry mouth (10%).
	Contraindications—Bupropion SR is contraindicated for individuals with a history of seizure disorder, a history of an eating disorder, who are using another form of bupropion (Wellbutrin or Wellbutrin SR), or who have used a monoamine oxidase inhibitor in the past 14 days.
Dosage	Patients should begin with a dose of 150 mg each morning for 3 days, then increase to 150 mg twice daily. Dosing at 150 mg twice daily should continue for 7 to 12 weeks following the quit date. Unlike nicotine replacement therapy, bupropion SR treatment should begin 1 to 2 weeks *before* the patient quits smoking. For maintenance therapy, consider 150 mg of bupropion SR twice daily for up to 6 months.
Availability	**Zyban** (prescription only).
Prescribing instructions	*Cessation before quit date*—Recognize that some patients will lose their desire to smoke before their quit date or will spontaneously smoke less.
	Scheduling of dose—If insomnia is marked, taking the p.m. dose earlier (in the afternoon, at least 8 hours after the first dose) may provide some relief.
	Alcohol—Use alcohol only in moderation.
Cost	$ 3.05/day.

Note: Clinical use approved by the Food and Drug Administration.
SR, sustained release.
Source: Adapted from Fiore MC, Bailey WC, Cohen SJ, et al. *Treating tobacco use and dependence. Clinical practice guideline.* Rockville, MD: US Department of Health and Human Services, Public Health Service, 2000.

TABLE 15.5. SUGGESTIONS FOR THE CLINICAL USE OF NICOTINE GUM

Patient selection	Appropriate as a first-line pharmacotherapy for smoking cessation.
Precautions	*Pregnancy*—Pregnant smokers should be first encouraged to quit without pharmacologic treatment. Nicotine gum should be used during pregnancy only if the increased likelihood of smoking abstinence, with its potential benefits, outweighs the risk of nicotine replacement and potential concomitant smoking. Similar factors should be considered in lactating women (class D).
	Cardiovascular diseases—Nicotine replacement therapy is not an independent risk factor for acute myocardial events. Nicotine replacement therapy should be used with caution in particular cardiovascular patient groups: those who have had a myocardial infarction within the past 2 weeks, those with serious arrhythmias, and those with serious or worsening angina pectoris.
	Side effects—Common side effects of nicotine chewing gum include mouth soreness, hiccups, dyspepsia, and jaw ache. These effects are generally mild and transient and can often be alleviated by correcting the patient's chewing technique (see prescribing instructions).
Dosage	Nicotine gum is available in 2- and 4-mg (per piece) doses. The 2-mg gum is recommended for patients smoking fewer than 25 cigarettes per day, and the 4-mg gum for patients smoking 25 or more cigarettes per day. Generally, the gum should be used for up to 12 weeks with no more than 24 pieces chewed per day. Clinicians should tailor the dosage and duration of therapy to fit the needs of each patient.
Availability	**Nicorette, Nicorette Mint, Nicorette Orange** (over the counter only).
Prescribing instructions	*Chewing technique*—Gum should be chewed slowly until a "peppery" or "minty" taste develops, then "parked" between cheek and gum to facilitate nicotine absorption through the oral mucosa. The gum should be slowly and intermittently "chewed and parked" for about 30 minutes or until the taste dissipates.
	Absorption—Acidic beverages (e.g., coffee, juices, soft drinks) interfere with the buccal absorption of nicotine, so eating and drinking anything except water should be avoided for 15 minutes before and during chewing.
	Scheduling of dose—Patients often do not use enough gum to obtain the maximal benefit; they chew too few pieces per day and do not use the gum for a sufficient number of weeks. Instructions to chew the gum on a fixed schedule (at least one piece every 1–2 hours) for at least 1 to 3 months may be more beneficial than use ad libitum.
Cost	$8.62 for 15 2-mg pieces per day.
	$13.79 for 24 2-mg pieces per day.
	$6.47 for 10 4-mg pieces per day.
	$12.93 for 20 4-mg pieces per day.

Note: Clinical use approved by the Food and Drug Administration.
Source: Adapted from Fiore MC, Bailey WC, Cohen SJ, et al. *Treating tobacco use and dependence. Clinical practice guideline.* Rockville, MD: US Department of Health and Human Services, Public Health Service, 2000.

the user is not exposed to carbon monoxide, tar, or the carcinogens found in tobacco smoke. Absorption is through the buccal mucosa, so the caveats about use of acidic beverages that apply to nicotine gum also apply to the inhaler. The recommended dose is 6 to 16 cartridges per day for the first several months after the quit date, followed by gradually tapered use over 3 months. In a guideline metaanalysis of four studies, the long-term cessation OR was 2.5 (CI, 1.7–3.6) for the nicotine inhaler relative to placebo (11). Commonly reported side effects include coughing, rhinitis, and local irritation of the mouth and throat. Detailed suggestions for clinical use are presented in Table 15.6.

Nicotine Nasal Spray

Nicotine nasal spray is the nicotine replacement therapy that most closely replicates the pharmacodynamics of nicotine delivery via a cigarette, which may explain some of its effectiveness with highly dependent smokers (17). A dose consists of a 0.5-mg squirt in each nostril, used once or twice per hour as needed, up to a total of 40 doses a day. Three studies included in the guideline metaanalysis indicated a cessation OR of 2.7 (CI, 1.8–4.1); however, the side effect profile of the nicotine nasal spray is less favorable than that of other nicotine replacement therapies, with 94% of users reporting nasal irritation of moderate to severe intensity during initial

use (11). The risk for transfer of dependence is also higher than with other nicotine replacement therapies, although the possible health risks of long-term use of nicotine replacement therapy are not comparable with continued tobacco use. Nicotine nasal spray is currently available in the United States by prescription only. Specific prescribing information is summarized in Table 15.7.

Nicotine Patch

The nicotine patch is a nicotine delivery system that was developed in part because of the difficulties patients have in optimizing the use of nicotine gum. Starting on the quit date, the patient applies the patch to an area of the trunk or arms that is not hairy and not irritated. Nicotine is absorbed readily through the skin and distributed throughout the body, reducing withdrawal symptoms and the craving for tobacco. The most common side effect observed with the nicotine patch is skin irritation at the patch site; although this may occur in up to half of users, it is seldom severe enough that treatment must be stopped. Applying the patch on a different site each day may reduce dermal reactions. The guideline conducted a metaanalysis based on 27 studies and concluded that the nicotine patch is significantly superior to placebo (OR, 1.9; CI, 1.7–2.2) (11). Patches may be worn for either 16 (waking) hours or 24 hours with comparable

TABLE 15.6. SUGGESTIONS FOR CLINICAL USE OF THE NICOTINE INHALER

Patient selection	Appropriate as a first-line pharmacotherapy for smoking cessation.
Precautions	*Pregnancy*—Pregnant smokers should be first encouraged to quit without pharmacologic treatment. The nicotine inhaler should be used during pregnancy only if the increased likelihood of smoking abstinence, with its potential benefits, outweighs the risk of nicotine replacement and potential concomitant smoking. Similar factors should be considered in lactating women (class D).
	Cardiovascular diseases—Nicotine replacement therapy is not an independent risk factor for acute myocardial events. Nicotine replacement therapy should be used with caution among particular cardiovascular patient groups: those who have had a myocardial infarction within the past 2 weeks, those with serious arrhythmias, and those with serious or worsening angina pectoris.
	Local irritation reactions—Local irritation in the mouth and throat was observed in 40% of patients using nicotine inhaler. Coughing (32%) and rhinitis (23%) were also common. Irritation was generally rated as mild, and the frequency of such symptoms declined with continued use.
Dosage	A dose from the nicotine inhaler consists of a puff or inhalation. Each cartridge delivers 4 mg of nicotine for 80 inhalations, of which approximately 2 mg is absorbed. The recommended dosage is 6 to 16 cartridges per day. The recommended duration of therapy is up to 6 months. Instruct patient to taper dosage during the final 3 months of treatment.
Availability	**Nicotrol Inhaler** (prescription only).
Prescribing instructions	*Ambient temperature*—Delivery of nicotine from the inhaler declines significantly at temperatures below 40°F. In cold weather, the inhaler and cartridges should be kept in an inside pocket or warm area.
	Duration—Use is recommended for up to 6 months with gradual reduction in frequency of use during the last 6 to 12 weeks of treatment.
	Absorption—Acidic beverages (e.g., coffee, juices, soft drinks) interfere with the buccal absorption of nicotine, so eating and drinking anything except water should be avoided for 15 minutes before and during inhalation.
	Best effects—Best effects are achieved by frequent puffing.
Cost	$9.71 for 10 cartridges per day.
	$15.54 for 16 cartridges per day.

Note: Clinical use approved by the Food and Drug Administration.
Source: Adapted from Fiore MC, Bailey WC, Cohen SJ, et al. *Treating tobacco use and dependence. Clinical practice guideline.* Rockville, MD: US Department of Health and Human Services, Public Health Service, 2000.

TABLE 15.7. SUGGESTIONS FOR CLINICAL USE OF THE NICOTINE NASAL SPRAY

Patient selection	Appropriate as a first-line pharmacotherapy for smoking cessation.
Precautions	*Pregnancy*—Pregnant smokers should be first encouraged to quit without pharmacologic treatment. Nicotine nasal spray should be used during pregnancy only if the increased likelihood of smoking abstinence, with its potential benefits, outweighs the risk of nicotine replacement and potential concomitant smoking. Similar factors should be considered in lactating women (class D).
	Cardiovascular diseases—Nicotine replacement therapy is not an independent risk factor for acute myocardial events. Nicotine replacement therapy should be used with caution among particular cardiovascular patient groups: those who have had a myocardial infarction within the past 2 weeks, those with serious arrhythmias, and those with serious or worsening angina pectoris.
	Nasal/airway reactions—Some 94% of users reported moderate to severe nasal irritation in the first 2 days of use; 81% reported nasal irritation after 3 weeks, although it was rated mild to moderate. Nasal congestion and transient changes in sense of smell and taste were also reported. Nicotine nasal spray should not be used by persons with severe reactive airway disease.
	Dependency—Nicotine nasal spray has a dependence potential intermediate between that of other nicotine-based therapies and that of cigarettes. Fifteen percent to twenty percent of patients reported using the active spray for longer periods than recommended (6–12 months), and 5% used the spray at a higher dose than recommended.
Dosage	A dose of nicotine nasal spray consists of one 0.5-mg delivery to each nostril (total of 1 mg). Initial dosing should be 1 to 2 doses per hour, increased as needed for symptom relief. Minimal recommended treatment is 8 doses per day, with a maximum of 40 doses per day (5 doses per hour). Each bottle contains approximately 100 doses. Recommended duration of therapy is 3 to 6 months.
Availability	**Nicotrol NS** (prescription only).
Prescribing instructions	*Dose delivery*—Patients should not sniff, swallow, or inhale through the nose while dosing because this increases irritating effects. The spray is best delivered with the head tilted slightly back.
Cost	$10.80 for 24 doses per day.
	$18.00 for 40 doses per day at 100 doses per bottle.

Note: Clinical use approved by the Food and Drug Administration.
Source: Adapted from Fiore MC, Bailey WC, Cohen SJ, et al. *Treating tobacco use and dependence. Clinical practice guideline.* Rockville, MD: US Department of Health and Human Services, Public Health Service, 2000.

efficacy (18). They are available as both over-the-counter and prescription products, a distinction that may have important implications for insurance coverage. Generic or house brand patches have recently become available and may be less expensive. Considerations for clinical use are presented in Table 15.8.

Combination Therapy

Combination therapy is a relatively new pharmacotherapeutic innovation for smoking cessation. Although wearing more than one nicotine patch at one time appears to be of little incremental value (19,20), using more than one type of medication may be helpful. The guideline conducted a metaanalysis of three studies examining combination therapy, two in which a nicotine patch was combined with 2-mg nicotine gum and one in which a nicotine patch was combined with nicotine nasal spray. The OR was 1.9 (CI, 1.3–2.6) in comparison with 1.0 for a single nicotine replacement therapy (11); a more recent study in which a nicotine

patch was combined with a nicotine inhaler produced similar results (21). More work is needed in this area to identify optimal combinations. It appears that the combination of a "steady-state" therapy with a therapy to be used as needed may be crucial because combining two different "steady-state" therapies does not appear to confer significant benefit (14).

COUNSELING

Through the years, dozens of behavioral treatments have been proposed as aids to tobacco cessation, including problem solving, affect management, diet programs, hypnosis, acupuncture, social support, contingency contracting, and sensory deprivation. Conceptually, these can be considered in terms of the format of treatment delivery and the content of treatment. The guideline panel evaluated empiric evidence regarding five formats of treatment delivery. The comparison group (no contact) was compared with self-help,

TABLE 15.8. SUGGESTIONS FOR CLINICAL USE OF THE NICOTINE PATCH

Patient selection	Appropriate as a first-line pharmacotherapy for smoking cessation.
Precautions	*Pregnancy*—Pregnant smokers should be first encouraged to quit without pharmacologic treatment. The nicotine patch should be used during pregnancy only if the increased likelihood of smoking abstinence, with its potential benefits, outweighs the risk of nicotine replacement and potential concomitant smoking. Similar factors should be considered in lactating women (class C).
	Cardiovascular diseases—Nicotine replacement therapy is not an independent risk factor for acute myocardial events. Nicotine replacement therapy should be used with caution among particular cardiovascular patient groups: those who have had a myocardial infarction within the past 2 weeks, those with serious arrhythmias, and those with serious or worsening angina pectoris.
	Skin reactions—Up to 50% of patients using the nicotine patch will have a local skin reaction. Skin reactions are usually mild and self-limiting but may worsen during the course of therapy. Local treatment with hydrocortisone cream (1%) or triamcinolone cream (0.5%) and rotating the sites where the patch is applied may lessen such local reactions. In fewer than 5% of patients, such reactions require the discontinuation of nicotine patch treatment.
Dosage	Treatment of 8 weeks or less has been shown to be as efficacious as longer treatment periods.
	Patches worn for 16 or 24 hours are of comparable efficacy. Clinicians should consider individualizing treatment based on specific patient characteristics, such as previous experience with the patch, amount smoked, and degree of addiction. Finally, clinicians should consider starting treatment with a lower-dose patch for patients smoking 10 or fewer cigarettes per day.
Availability	**Nicoderm CQ, Nicotrol** (over the counter)
	Habitrol (prescription)
	Note: Some patches are now available as generic or house brands.

Brand	**Duration**	**Dosage**
Nicoderm CQ and Habitrol	4 weeks followed by	21 mg/24 h
	2 weeks followed by	14 mg/24 h
	2 weeks	7 mg/24 h
Nicotrol	8 weeks	15 mg/16 h
Prescribing instructions	*Location*—At the start of each day, the patient should place a new patch on a relatively hairless location, typically between the neck and waist.	
	Activities—No restrictions while the patch is used.	
	Time—Patches should be applied as soon as the patient wakes on his/her quit day. A patient who experiences sleep disruption should remove the 24-hour patch before bedtime or use the 16-hour patch.	
Cost	Nicoderm CQ—$3.42/day.	
	Nicotrol—$3.68/day.	
	Habitrol—$4.88/day.	

Note: Clinical use approved by the Food and Drug Administration.
Source: Adapted from Fiore MC, Bailey WC, Cohen SJ, et al. *Treating tobacco use and dependence. Clinical practice guideline.* Rockville, MD: US Department of Health and Human Services, Public Health Service, 2000.

proactive telephone counseling, individual counseling, and group counseling in a metaanalysis of data from 58 studies. Self-help materials, such as pamphlets, manuals, and audiotapes and videotapes, were found to be of marginal effectiveness in comparison with no contact (OR, 1.2; CI, 1.02–1.3; it should be noted that a CI that overlaps 1.0 indicates no significant difference from the comparison group) (11). Although these materials can be very efficient ways of conveying information to patients, it appears that by themselves they are not very effective in motivating cessation. Counseling delivered on a one-to-one basis (OR, 1.7; CI, 1.4–2.0) or as part of a traditional smoking cessation group (OR, 1.3; CI, 1.1–1.6) was significantly more likely to promote long-term cessation than no contact (11). Clinicians who have the ability to make referrals to a local specialized cessation program may assist patients in this manner, but the literature indicates that office-based individual counseling is also quite effective. A more recent innovation is proactive telephone counseling. Unlike the older hotline model, in which smokers would call the service *after* experiencing a lapse or relapse to smoking, the proactive model works with smokers before their quit date and also schedules follow-up calls after the quit date. A number of states have established proactive quit lines for their residents with the use of revenues from the Tobacco Master Settlement Agreement. Not only are these programs able to reach smokers in areas that may have limited health care resources, they also appear to be effective (OR, 1.2; CI, 1.1–1.4) (11).

Given that behavioral change can be facilitated effectively through telephone, individual, or group contact, the next logical question to ask is, What counseling content is related to successful cessation? As noted in the section "Clinical Intervention," the guideline panel evaluated dozens of counseling interventions tested in the literature between 1975 and 1999. A metaanalysis of 62 studies identified three types of counseling content associated with higher long-term cessation rates relative to no counseling: problem solving (OR, 1.5; CI, 1.3–1.8), intra-treatment social support (OR, 1.3; CI, 1.1–1.6), and extra-treatment social support (OR, 1.5; CI, 1.1–2.1) (11). Elements of these three counseling contents are shown in Tables 15.9 through 15.11. It is important to note that this pattern of results persisted when trials including FDA-approved pharmacotherapies were removed, suggesting that counseling has an effect on successful cessation that is independent of pharmacotherapy. A strong dose-response relationship is also noted for counseling, such that the more time spent in counseling, the higher the cessation rates. Quit rates are higher than those observed with brief advice, discussed in the section "Clinical Intervention" (11).

The problem-solving approach to counseling is one of the most widely studied and involves two components. The first is providing the patient with basic information, such as the nature of withdrawal symptoms, their likely time course, and the addictive nature of tobacco. The second involves helping

TABLE 15.9. COMMON ELEMENTS OF PRACTICAL COUNSELING (PROBLEM SOLVING/SKILLS TRAINING)

Practical Counseling Problem-Solving/Skills-Training Treatment Component	Examples
Recognize danger situations—Identify events, internal states, or activities that increase the risk for smoking or relapse.	Negative affect. Being around other smokers. Drinking alcohol. Experiencing urges. Being under time pressure.
Develop coping skills—Identify and practice coping or problem-solving skills. Typically, these skills are intended to cope with danger situations.	Learning to anticipate and avoid temptation. Learning cognitive strategies that will reduce negative moods. Accomplishing life style changes that reduce stress, improve quality of life, or produce pleasure. Learning cognitive and behavioral activities to cope with smoking urges (e.g., distracting attention).
Provide basic information—Provide basic information about smoking and successful quitting.	Any smoking (even a single puff) increases the likelihood of full relapse. Withdrawal typically peaks within 1 to 3 weeks after quitting. Withdrawal symptoms include negative mood, urges to smoke, and difficulty concentrating. Smoking is addictive.

Source: Adapted from Fiore MC, Bailey WC, Cohen SJ, et al. *Treating tobacco use and dependence. Clinical practice guideline.* Rockville, MD: US Department of Health and Human Services, Public Health Service, 2000.

TABLE 15.10. COMMON ELEMENTS OF INTRA-TREATMENT SUPPORTIVE INTERVENTIONS

Supportive Treatment Component	Examples
Encourage the patient in the quit attempt.	Note that effective tobacco dependence treatments are now available. Note that half of all people who have ever smoked have now quit. Communicate belief in patient's ability to quit. Ask how patient feels about quitting.
Communicate caring and concern.	Directly express concern and willingness to help. Be open to the patient's expression of fears about quitting, difficulties experienced, and ambivalent feelings.
Encourage the patient to talk about the quitting process.	Ask about the following: Reasons the patient wants to quit. Concerns or worries about quitting. Success the patient has achieved. Difficulties encountered while quitting.

Source: Adapted from Fiore MC, Bailey WC, Cohen SJ, et al. *Treating tobacco use and dependence. Clinical practice guideline.* Rockville, MD: US Department of Health and Human Services, Public Health Service, 2000.

TABLE 15.11. COMMON ELEMENTS OF EXTRA-TREATMENT SUPPORTIVE INTERVENTIONS

Supportive Treatment Component	Examples
Train patient in support solicitation skills.	Show videotapes that model support skills. Practice requesting social support from family, friends, and coworkers. Aid patient in establishing a smoke-free home.
Prompt support seeking.	Help patient identify supportive others. Call the patient to remind him/her to seek support. Inform patients of community resources such as hot lines/help lines.
Clinician arranges outside support.	Mail letters to supportive others. Call supportive others. Invite others to cessation sessions. Assign patients to be "buddies" for one another.

Source: Adapted from Fiore MC, Bailey WC, Cohen SJ, et al. *Treating tobacco use and dependence. Clinical practice guideline.* Rockville, MD: US Department of Health and Human Services, Public Health Service, 2000.

the patient learn to identify likely triggers for the urge to use tobacco. This may be assessed by asking, "When you think of a typical day, when are you most likely to smoke?" Common answers include times of the day (on waking, after meals, during breaks at work), particular events (after finishing a task, while driving, while talking on the telephone), and emotional cues (feeling happy, sad, anxious, stressed). When triggers can be identified, simple distractions or a coping response can be devised to be used when the urge to smoke arises. An example would be someone who reports smoking the first cigarette of the day while drinking coffee and reading the newspaper. On the quit date, this person might plan to leave home as quickly as possible in the morning and have the first cup of coffee in a nonsmoking restaurant, or skip the coffee and newspaper entirely and start the morning with orange juice. The basic idea is to plan ahead and have a distraction ready because most urges to smoke last only a few minutes. Engaging in the distraction helps the patient not to feel helpless in the face of an urge and may actually attack the root cause (e.g., practicing deep breathing while feeling anxious).

The other counseling contents found to be helpful were two different types of social support, intra-treatment and extra-treatment. Both involve communicating encouragement and concern to persons quitting while allowing them to speak openly about their experience. In the case of intra-treatment support, it is the clinician who provides encouragement by pointing out the efficacy of treatment and by being willing to work with the patient to quit successfully. One challenging aspect for the clinician may be listening openly and nonjudgmentally to the patient, particularly when the quit attempt is ambivalent or difficult. In the case of extra-treatment social support, the clinician can help identify

friends or family members who may be sources of support. It may also be helpful to clarify what support means to the patient, so that this can be clearly communicated to others. Some people like to know that others are thinking about them and care about how they are doing. Others find it annoying to be asked on a regular basis how their cessation efforts are going. The clinician should let patients know it is all right to tell others what is or is not helpful for them. As discussed earlier in this section, social support can also be provided through telephone counseling or a formal cessation support group.

Two additional forms of behavioral treatment merit specific mention. Acupuncture was evaluated in a metaanalysis of five studies and was not found to improve results in comparison with a control procedure (OR, 1.1; CI, 0.7–1.6), suggesting that observed benefits may be the result of nonspecific factors (11). The guideline panel was unable to find enough scientifically valid studies to evaluate hypnosis as a treatment for smoking cessation; an independent Cochrane Group Review concluded that hypnosis is not an effective smoking cessation treatment (11,22). Both of these treatments may have some appeal for smokers because of the perception that they work in the absence of a personal motivation to quit. The empiric evidence suggests that this is not the case.

The last of the five *A*s is to *a*rrange follow-up. As discussed earlier in this section, there is a strong dose-response relationship between the amount of contact and success. Timing is also an important factor because most relapses occur soon after the quit date (23). Contact on the quit date, or at least within the first week thereafter, is highly desirable. If the patient has experienced a lapse, it is important not to be punitive or judgmental. Keeping in mind the chronic nature of tobacco use, it is best to deal with the lapse as a learning experience and engage the patient in problem solving to find a different way to cope with the situation. This may help prevent the lapse from becoming a complete return to smoking. Patients should also be praised for success and asked which aspects of cessation have been most rewarding for them.

SUMMARY

Tobacco use is a chronic disease afflicting millions of Americans and exacting a huge price in terms of morbidity, mortality, and cost every year. Although treating tobacco dependence is not an easy task, strong empiric evidence indicates that clinicians and health care systems can provide effective treatment. Systems should assess tobacco use on a routine basis, and all current users should be offered at least a minimal brief advice intervention. For those motivated to make a serious quit attempt, a combination of pharmacotherapy (except when specifically contraindicated) and basic counseling can increase long-term cessation rates to three to four times what they would be without treatment. No other chronic disease presents such a dramatic opportunity for full remission relative to the amount of treatment provided.

REFERENCES

1. US Department of Health and Human Services. *The health benefits of smoking cessation: a report of the Surgeon General.* Atlanta, GA: US Department of Health and Human Services, Public Health Service, Centers for Disease Control, Center for Chronic Disease Prevention and Health Promotion, Office of Smoking and Health, 1990: DHHS Publication No. (CDC) 90-8416.
2. Miller LS, Zhang X, Rice DP, et al. State estimates of total medical expenditures attributable to cigarette smoking, 1993. *Public Health Rep* 1998;113:447–458.
3. Centers for Disease Control and Prevention. Medical care expenditures attributable to cigarette smoking—United States, 1993. *MMWR Morb Mortal Wkly Rep* 1994;43:469–472.
4. Centers of Disease Control and Prevention. Cigarette smoking among adults—United States, 1997. *MMWR Morb Mortal Wkly Rep* 1999;48:993–996.
5. Gilpin E, Choi WS, Berry C, et al. How many adolescents start smoking each day in the United States? *J Adolesc Health* 1999;25:248–255.
6. Centers for Disease Control and Prevention. Smoking cessation during previous year among adults—United States, 1990 and 1991. *MMWR Morb Mortal Wkly Rep* 1993;42:504–507.
7. US Department of Health and Human Services. *The health consequences of smoking: nicotine addiction. A report of the surgeon general.* Atlanta, GA: US Department of Health and Human Services, Public Health Service, Centers for Disease Control, Center for Chronic Disease Prevention and Health Promotion, Office of Smoking and Health, 1988: DHHS Publication No. (PHS)(CDC) 88-8406.
8. Tomar SL, Husten CG, Manley MW. Do dentists and physicians advise tobacco users to quit? *J Am Dent Assoc* 1996;127:259–265.
9. National Cancer Institute. *Tobacco and the clinician: interventions for medical and dental practice.* Monogr Natl Cancer Inst 5, 1-22. NIH Publication No. 94-3693, 1994.
10. Goldstein MG, Niaura R, Willey-Lessne C, et al. Physicians counseling smokers: a population-based survey of patients' perceptions of health care provider–delivered smoking cessation interventions. *Arch Intern Med* 1997;157:1313–1319.
11. Fiore MC, Bailey WC, Cohen SJ, et al. *Treating tobacco use and dependence. Clinical practice guideline.* Rockville, MD: US Department of Health and Human Services, Public Health Service, 2000.
12. Solberg LI, Boyle RG, Davidson G, et al. Patient satisfaction and discussion of smoking cessation during clinical visits. *Mayo Clin Proc* 2001;76:138–143.
13. Hurt RD, Sachs DPL, Glover ED, et al. A comparison of sustained-release bupropion and placebo for smoking cessation. *N Engl J Med* 1997;337:1195–1202.
14. Jorenby DE, Leischow SJ, Nides MA, et al. A controlled trial of sustained-release bupropion, a nicotine patch, or both for smoking cessation. *N Engl J Med* 1999;340:685–691.
15. Hays JT, Hurt RD, Rigotti NA, et al. Sustained-release bupropion for pharmacologic relapse prevention after smoking cessation. *Ann Intern Med* 2001;135:423–433.
16. Herrera N, Franco R, Herrera L, et al. Nicotine gum, 2 and 4 mg, for nicotine dependence. A double-blind placebo-controlled trial within a behavior modification support program. *Chest* 1995;108:447–451.
17. Sutherland G, Stapleton JA, Russell MAH, et al. Randomised controlled trial of nasal nicotine spray in smoking cessation. *Lancet* 1992;340:324–329.
18. Fiore MC, Smith SS, Jorenby DE, et al. The effectiveness of the nicotine patch for smoking cessation: a meta-analysis. *JAMA* 1994;271:1940–1947.
19. Jorenby DE, Smith SS, Fiore MC, et al. Varying nicotine patch dose and type of smoking cessation counseling. *JAMA* 1995;274:1347–1352.
20. Hughes JR, Lesmes GR, Hatsukami DK, et al. Are higher doses of nicotine replacement more effective for smoking cessation? *Nicotine Tobacco Res* 1999;1:169–174.
21. Bohadana A, Nilsson F, Rasmussen T, et al. Nicotine inhaler and nicotine patch as a combination therapy for smoking cessation: a randomized, double-blind, placebo-controlled trial. *Arch Intern Med* 2000;160:3128–3134.
22. Abbot N, Stead L, White ABJ, et al. Hypnotherapy for smoking cessation [Cochrane Review]. *The Cochrane Library* 1999.
23. Westman EC, Behm FM, Simel DL, et al. Smoking behavior on the first day of a quit attempt predicts long-term abstinence. *Arch Intern Med* 1997;157:335–340.

16   Pulmonary Rehabilitation

Barry Make

The major goals of the treatment of any chronic and irreversible disorder are to allay symptoms and minimize the impact of illness by enhancing the patient's ability to perform desirable activities. Pulmonary rehabilitation is a proven, effective therapeutic intervention that can be added to a program of appropriate medications to achieve these goals in patients with lung disease (1–6). Of numerous respiratory conditions, chronic obstructive pulmonary disease (COPD) frequently causes the most chronic, debilitating symptoms, which cannot be completely eliminated or controlled by medications, ambulatory oxygen, and other traditional medical treatments. Because of the severity of the dyspnea associated with activity, COPD frequently impairs the patient's ability to engage constructively in daily activities. Comprehensive pulmonary rehabilitation has also been used successfully in patients with cystic fibrosis and respiratory insufficiency associated with severe neuromuscular disorders. For patients with asthma, comprehensive efforts, including disease management programs to decrease utilization of health care resources, ensure adherence to treatment programs, incorporate health-enhancing behaviors, and enhance collaborative self-management, employ many of the principles of pulmonary rehabilitation.

This chapter defines pulmonary rehabilitation, describes the key components of a comprehensive pulmonary rehabilitation program, discusses the techniques and physiologic basis of the therapies used during rehabilitation, and reviews the evidence-based outcomes that can be achieved with these therapies. Because COPD is the most common chronic respiratory disease and because patients with COPD are the most frequent recipients of pulmonary rehabilitation, this chapter focuses on pulmonary rehabilitation as it is applied in COPD. However, the principles of pulmonary rehabilitation and many of the specific therapeutic modalities and approaches can be successfully used for patients with other respiratory disorders.

DEFINITION AND CONCEPT OF PULMONARY REHABILITATION

Historically, the term *rehabilitation* has been applied to the therapeutic techniques used for patients with limitations resulting from physical impairments such as loss of function of an extremity through injury or a birth defect or loss of function secondary to a neurologic or muscular condition—for example, a spinal cord injury. The principles of rehabilitation are based on the broad goal of restoring individuals to the fullest medical, mental, emotional, social, and vocational potential possible. The term *pulmonary rehabilitation* is used when the recipients of rehabilitation efforts are patients with disorders of the respiratory system; it was originally defined by a committee of the American College of Chest Physicians (ACCP) (7) and later revised by a National Institutes of Health (NIH) workshop (8). A careful evaluation of these definitions of pulmonary rehabilitation provides important insights into this therapy.

The American College of Chest Physicians Definition

The original definition of pulmonary rehabilitation was conceived in an era when little information was available about the efficacy of this form of therapy, and only limited information supporting the physiologic basis for the therapeutic modalities employed. Pulmonary rehabilitation was defined

B. Make: Emphysema Center, National Jewish Medical and Research Center; Department of Medicine, University of Colorado School of Medicine, Denver, Colorado.

as follows:

> "...An art of medical practice wherein an individually tailored, multidisciplinary program is formulated which through accurate diagnosis, therapy, emotional support, and education, stabilizes or reverses both the physio- and psychopathology of pulmonary diseases and attempts to return the patient to the highest possible functional capacity allowed by his pulmonary handicap and overall life situation."

Several important concepts are embodied in this definition.

Individually Tailored

The first implication of the ACCP definition of pulmonary rehabilitation is that the details of the intervention are based on the individual needs of each patient. Not only is a complete assessment of the patient by an experienced pulmonary physician necessary to determine the patient's individual medical needs, but each patient must also provide input to determine his or her individual needs and goals. Because rehabilitation requires the active participation of the recipient, patients must be involved in setting the goals of their efforts.

Multidisciplinary

Second, rehabilitation is not considered to be a single therapy but rather a coordinated program of a number of therapies, most often applied by health care professionals with a variety of backgrounds and with different areas of expertise. Indeed, beneficial results and outcomes have most frequently been demonstrated by comprehensive multimodality pulmonary rehabilitation programs. As noted in the rest of this chapter, the various multifaceted components of pulmonary rehabilitation are not usually within the expertise of a single member of the health care team and often require personnel with knowledge and experience in the following:

- *Exercise* training
- *Psychosocial* evaluation and counseling
- *Respiratory medications* and breathing exercises uniquely used in patients with lung disease
- *Education* of adults with chronic lung disease
- *Nutritional* issues
- *Energy conservation* management techniques
- *Ancillary medical* issues of patients with respiratory disorders.

Improvement in Function

Although individual goals may vary from one patient to another, the objective of pulmonary rehabilitation is to improve the ability of the patient to function to the maximal extent possible given the limitations imposed by the underlying respiratory disorder. Although it may not be possible to reverse the pathologic effects of the disease, the physiologic

and psychologic responses to the disease may be amenable to treatment. For example, although pulmonary rehabilitation does not improve airflow or pulmonary function, the limitations in daily activities imposed by dyspnea and decreased exercise capacity can be lessened. Pulmonary rehabilitation, largely through the benefits of exercise training, results in a reduction in dyspnea and an improvement in exercise capacity, with subsequent improvement in the ability of patients to perform their daily activities. The measurement of patient function, level of dyspnea, and exercise capacity as outcomes of pulmonary rehabilitation is important to determine the effectiveness of this therapy.

The National Heart, Lung, and Blood Institute Definition

A National Heart, Lung, and Blood Institute (NHLBI) workshop formulated another definition of pulmonary rehabilitation:

> "...A multidimensional continuum of services directed to persons with pulmonary disease and their families, usually by an interdisciplinary team of specialists, with a goal of achieving and maintaining the individual's maximum level of independence and functioning in the community" (8).

The NHLBI workshop expanded on the earlier definition by incorporating the scientific basis of pulmonary rehabilitation and integrating the concept of pulmonary rehabilitation into the evolving health care environment in several ways. First, the workshop recognized the evolution of health care delivery, which has increasingly focused on providing care at multiple sites, ranging from the acute care hospital to the home, and to patients at all life stages—a concept referred to as the *continuum of health care delivery*. Second, pulmonary rehabilitation is now seen not as a time-limited therapy used within a defined period to achieve a particular end result but rather as an ongoing program of organized and integrated services provided to the patient to maintain function over the long term. Although this is a laudable goal that will likely improve long-term outcomes, the current reimbursement of health care does not usually recognize the need for long-term outcomes. Thus, pulmonary rehabilitation is most often implemented as a defined program for a limited period of time. Third, the NHLBI definition takes a broader view of pulmonary rehabilitation by recognizing the importance of family members and viewing the patient as functioning and participating within the larger community outside the boundaries of the home. Last, this newer concept of rehabilitation recognizes that although it is usually implemented by a multidisciplinary team, individual elements of pulmonary rehabilitation may be applied in a limited fashion to patients not enrolled in a comprehensive program. For example, prescribing medications always requires that the patient be educated in proper use of the medication. Although education is one of the components of pulmonary rehabilitation, patients should be educated about their medications even when they are not enrolled in a comprehensive rehabilitation program. In recognition of the NHLBI definition, this chapter describes pulmonary rehabilitation as a long-term continuum of a set of comprehensive services provided in an organized manner.

KEY COMPONENTS OF COMPREHENSIVE PULMONARY REHABILITATION

It is generally accepted that a state-of-the-art comprehensive pulmonary rehabilitation program comprises specific key components in (Table 16.1). These include the following: (a) medical evaluation and management; (b) assessment and goal setting; (c) therapeutic interventions, including smoking cessation, exercise training, education, psychosocial counseling, nutritional counseling, and training in daily living and energy management; (d) evaluation of outcomes; and (e) a long-term program.

MEDICAL EVALUATION AND MANAGEMENT

The physician (whether a general practitioner, internist, or pulmonary specialist) who provides primary and ongoing care to the patient with respiratory disease plays an integral role in pulmonary rehabilitation. The physician not only orders pulmonary rehabilitation but also helps to ensure the patient's participation by explaining the rationale and benefits of rehabilitation, integrating rehabilitation into the patient's continuing medical care, and monitoring the patient's short- and long-term adherence to the rehabilitation program.

An appropriate diagnosis and optimal medical treatment of the patient with respiratory disease are prerequisites for the initiation of pulmonary rehabilitation. The goal of evaluation and management by the physician is to minimize the medical impact of the disease on the patient and thereby

maximize the patient's ability to benefit from the pulmonary rehabilitation program. The results of the medical evaluation should be available and communicated to the rehabilitation team. Because patients referred for pulmonary rehabilitation usually have at least moderately severe airflow limitation and significant functional limitations as a result of their illness, it is appropriate for a physician with specialized training in pulmonary medicine to play a major role in confirming the diagnosis and reviewing the medical plan.

As outlined in Table 16.2, medical evaluation and management comprise multiple components. One of the most important elements of the evaluation is the diagnosis of conditions that may limit the patient's ability to participate in and obtain maximal benefit from rehabilitation. For example, COPD patients referred for rehabilitation are usually older and may have concomitant osteoarthritis of the knees, which can impair their ability to engage in walking exercise. Establishing and communicating such comorbidities allows the rehabilitation team to choose exercise programs that minimize stress on the knees. Physician prescription of appropriate medications to reduce inflammation and pain not only ensures that the patient is comfortable but also maximizes participation in the exercise program. The physician should also consider other common diagnoses, such as osteoporosis, particularly in older postmenopausal women and persons with a history of corticosteroid administration. Because patients with COPD are usually older and often have a history of cigarette use that may cause cardiovascular disease, and because the cardiovascular system is stressed during exercise training, cardiac disease should be excluded. A maximal exercise test can be used to screen for ischemic cardiac disease and is also useful to evaluate for the presence of oxygen desaturation with exercise and determine the appropriate dose of oxygen to prevent desaturation during exercise.

TABLE 16.1. COMPONENTS OF A COMPREHENSIVE PULMONARY REHABILITATION PROGRAM

Medical evaluation and management
Assessment and goal setting
Therapeutic modalities
    Smoking cessation
    Exercise training
    Education
    Psychosocial counseling
    Breathing retraining
    Daily activity performance and energy management
    Nutritional counseling
Outcome evaluation
Long-term program

TABLE 16.2. MEDICAL EVALUATION AND MANAGEMENT COMPONENT OF PULMONARY REHABILITATION

Evaluation
Respiratory diagnosis
Severity of respiratory disease
Other conditions potentially interfering with pulmonary rehabilitation
    Arthritis
    Osteoporosis
    Cardiac disorders
Oxygenation at rest and during activity
Safety of rehabilitation (exercise testing)
Management
Reduce airflow limitation
Minimize pulmonary secretions
Eliminate/reduce adverse effects of medication
Promote collaborative self-management
Provide plan to address changes in symptoms
Reduce impact of other conditions on participation in rehabilitation
    program
Provide plan for maintaining continuity of medical care

The medical treatment plan should include prescriptions and specific instructions about the dose and the frequency and route of administration of all medications, particularly those required to reduce airflow limitation. Some patients with COPD have difficulty in clearing respiratory secretions, a condition that leads to dyspnea and increased work of breathing. Although the rehabilitation team can provide assistance with therapies for secretion management, the physician should prescribe antibiotics when necessary to treat acute exacerbations.

The physician should provide a referral to a comprehensive pulmonary rehabilitation program that has the necessary expertise and has demonstrated beneficial outcomes. Because the team providing comprehensive pulmonary rehabilitation will be skilled and experienced in assessing patients to individualize the program for each patient, determine the goals and duration of therapy, and apply each component of rehabilitation, in most cases the physician's order for pulmonary rehabilitation will be very general.

Selection of Patients for Rehabilitation

Based on the definitions, goals, and outcomes of pulmonary rehabilitation, a comprehensive rehabilitation program is recommended for patients who, despite optimal medical management, have functional limitations preventing them from participating fully in daily or vocational activities. As noted in Table 16.3, patients with a variety of respiratory conditions may be candidates for pulmonary rehabilitation. Because of the varied nature of the underlying disorders and

TABLE 16.3. RESPIRATORY DISORDERS SUITABLE FOR PULMONARY REHABILITATION

Obstructive lung disease
Chronic obstructive pulmonary disease
Asthma
Cystic fibrosis
Bronchiectasis

Restrictive lung disease
Interstitial lung diseases
Tuberculosis and other mycobacterial diseases
Restrictive respiratory system disorders

Neuromuscular
After polio
Muscular dystrophy
Guillain-Barré syndrome

Chest wall
Kyphoscoliosis
Thoracoplasty

Other
Before and after lung surgery, including lung volume reduction
Before and after lung transplantation
Lung cancer
Ventilatory dependency
Sleep apnea

the imprecise relationship between pulmonary function and functional capacity, no specific physiologic indices can determine the need for pulmonary rehabilitation. Unfortunately, tools assessing functional capacity, dyspnea, and quality of life have not been widely used as indications for pulmonary rehabilitation. Nevertheless, some general guidelines for patient selection based on the severity of the respiratory impairment can be outlined. In general, patients requiring chronic ambulatory oxygen therapy and those with frequent emergency department visits or hospitalizations are candidates for pulmonary rehabilitation. Pulmonary rehabilitation should be considered for patients with advanced disease as measured by a forced expiratory volume in 1 second (FEV_1) value that is 50% or less of the predicted value. Pulmonary rehabilitation should not be delayed until the patient exhibits very severe physiologic and functional impairment. Based on the demonstrated outcomes of pulmonary rehabilitation (Table 16.4), patients who have significant dyspnea despite optimal medical management, limited tolerance for the activities required for daily life, and a poor quality of life are candidates for pulmonary rehabilitation.

The patient and the physician providing ongoing care, in conjunction with the physician specialist in pulmonary medicine, are in the best position to evaluate the need for pulmonary rehabilitation. It is important to note that third-party payers typically require documentation not only of functional limitations but also of a treatment plan incorporating short- and long-term goals before they will provide reimbursement for rehabilitation.

Oxygen Therapy

The patient's oxygenation status should be assessed either before rehabilitation or during the initial evaluation for pulmonary rehabilitation. To determine the need for the administration of supplemental oxygen during activity, it is recommended that the oxygen saturation (SaO_2) be assessed with pulse oximetry at rest and also during activity and exercise in all patients participating in pulmonary rehabilitation. Although any type of activity performed by the patient on a regular basis can be used for this evaluation, many centers assess pulse oximetry while the patient is walking at a normal pace. The medical aspects of oxygen therapy are covered in greater detail in Chapter 12.

One of the goals of pulmonary rehabilitation is to enhance health-promoting behaviors, and this goal should be pursued in oxygen therapy. When oxygen is prescribed, the patient should receive sufficient education to ensure effective use of this important therapeutic modality. Education should include not only information about the benefits and safe use of oxygen therapy but also details of the specific prescription for oxygen for the individual patient, including the flow rate to be used at rest, with activity, and during sleep. Such education is routinely provided during pulmonary rehabilitation and should include efforts to enhance use of oxygen as prescribed

TABLE 16.4. SUMMARY OF DEMONSTRATED OUTCOMES OF PULMONARY REHABILITATION

Symptom/Rehabilitation Component	Outcome	Grade[a]	Recommendation
Dyspnea	Reduced dyspnea	A	Dyspnea outcomes should be routinely measured.
Lower extremity exercise	Improved exercise tolerance	A	Exercise training of muscles of ambulation is recommended.
Quality of life	Improved quality of life	A	
Health care utilization	Reduced hospitalizations in some uncontrolled studies	B	
Upper extremity exercise	Improved arm function with strength and endurance training	B	Arm exercise is recommended.
Ventilatory muscle training	Improved respiratory muscle strength, but less dyspnea and improved exercise tolerance only in some studies and dyspnea in patients who remain symptomatic despite optimal therapy	B	Not an essential component of pulmonary rehabilitation; may be considered in selected patients with decreased respiratory muscle strength.
Psychosocial function and education	Decreased affective distress	C	Recommended based on expert opinion. Cognitive and behavioral intervention enhance exercise adherence.
Survival	Survival may be improved	C	

[a] Grade, grade of evidence supporting recommendation: A, evidence provided by controlled trials with statistically significant consistent results; B, evidence provided by observational studies or controlled trials with less consistent results; C, expert opinion because of results or lack of controlled trials.
Source: American Thoracic Society. Pulmonary rehabilitation, 1999. *Am J Respir Crit Care Med* 1999;159:1666–1682; British Thoracic Society. Pulmonary rehabilitation. *Thorax* 2001;56:827–834; Lacasse Y, Wong E, Guyatt GH, et al. Meta-analysis of respiratory rehabilitation in chronic obstructive pulmonary disease. *Lancet* 1996;348: 1115–1119; Reis AL, Carlin BW, Carrieri-Kohlman V, et al. Pulmonary rehabilitation: evidence-based guidelines. *Chest* 1997;112:1363–1396.

by the physician. Barriers to use, such as patient fears about the safety of oxygen and the visibility and unsightly nature of the nasal cannula, should be addressed. Patients should be instructed about how to use the specific oxygen system supplied for them, including how to turn the oxygen on and off and how to fill the portable system and obtain additional oxygen and supplies. They should be given the name and phone number of the vendor supplying the oxygen.

The administration of long-term outpatient supplemental oxygen therapy to patients with respiratory disorders may impair mobility and thus quality of life. Despite the benefits of improved exercise capacity and lessened dyspnea with the use of ambulatory oxygen, the size, weight, and limited duration of the portable oxygen supply usually appear to the patient as barriers to achieving the benefits of a greater and more comfortable capacity for activity. Pulmonary rehabilitation can assist in reducing these barriers. For example, patients often feel that oxygen use during activity does not lessen dyspnea. During rehabilitation, it may be helpful to help the patient assess the benefits of oxygen objectively; one method is having the patient walk with and then without oxygen while a health care professional measures the distance walked and the patient quantifies the degree of shortness of breath. In this manner, patients can determine for themselves whether oxygen is beneficial.

During pulmonary rehabilitation, patients should be informed about the different types of portable supply systems available to allow the choice of a system that best meets their needs. One method of overcoming the difficulties associated with the size and weight of the portable oxygen system is to use oxygen conservation devices. The lightest portable oxygen systems have demand delivery oxygen conservers and include cylinders of compressed gas with a device that delivers oxygen only during inspiration and small liquid systems that incorporate a similar conserver.

The physician can initiate discussions with the patient about the types of available oxygen systems and refer the patient to the pulmonary rehabilitation team for the incorporation of oxygen therapy into the daily routine. The physician also serves an important role in writing the prescription for the type of oxygen system that best meets the patient's needs and helps ensure not only patient compliance with the oxygen prescription but also enhanced mobility and quality of life.

INITIAL ASSESSMENT

Probably the most important element of pulmonary rehabilitation is an initial assessment that culminates in the development of goals to guide the rehabilitation process and coordinate the actions of all team members. This element deserves special mention because it is not universally considered a separate component of pulmonary rehabilitation.

The goals of the assessment are the following:

1. Determine the individual needs of the patient.
2. Develop short-term goals for the patient to achieve during the initial rehabilitation program.
3. Provide a baseline to determine if the expected benefits of rehabilitation are realized.
4. Develop long-term goals that may be incorporated into the continuing management of the patient.

This assessment is separate and distinct from the physician's medical evaluation and may be performed by a single pulmonary rehabilitation team member, such as the program coordinator; alternatively, portions of the assessment may be performed by multiple team members. The importance of this process lies in the communication and interaction taking place between practitioners and patients, with the development of mutual trust and respect and the subsequent integration of the health professional's assessments with the patient's needs and desires. From this process flows a therapeutic plan and a set of patient-centered goals that must be agreeable both to the patient and to the rehabilitation team. In addition, short-term goals should be readily achievable within a limited period of time to enhance patient motivation and thus help ensure adherence to continued rehabilitation efforts. Longer-term goals should also be developed and revised as the patient progresses through rehabilitation.

One of the major goals of pulmonary rehabilitation is to improve the patient's level of function. The process of achieving this goal should begin with a careful assessment of all the activities the patient performs every day and what perceived and observed difficulties are encountered in accomplishing these tasks. Activities that are important to the patient include not only the basic activities of daily living, such as bathing, toileting, and dressing, but also vocational, social, and recreational pursuits in both the home and the community. Physical and occupational therapy team members may be very useful in assessing these aspects and developing goals based on the patient's functional ability. Functional assessments may include a history and physical examination, along with evaluation by means of appropriate questionnaires and observation of the performance of functional tasks. Functional goals are important guides for the interventions provided by all pulmonary rehabilitation team members, and most third-party payers require that therapy be based on written functional goals with defined short- and long-term outcomes, including the time frame expected for patients to achieve those goals.

THERAPEUTIC INTERVENTIONS

Smoking Cessation

Although many physicians are averse to referring patients who continue to smoke for pulmonary rehabilitation, there is no consensus that pulmonary rehabilitation should be withheld from such patients. Rather, smoking cessation should be considered an essential part of comprehensive pulmonary rehabilitation, and smoking cessation may be the primary goal for some patients enrolled in pulmonary rehabilitation. When smoking cessation is conducted during a comprehensive rehabilitation program, other positive health-enhancing behaviors, such as exercise, may be substituted for smoking. Additional support and encouragement during the smoking cessation effort can be provided by all rehabilitation team members and also by other patients.

The physician plays a key role in promoting, encouraging, and implementing a smoking cessation program. Smoking cessation is discussed in Chapter 15 (9). As an aid to the routine determination of a patient's smoking habits, it has been suggested that the office staff record the patient's smoking status at every office visit as they do other significant vital signs, such as the heart rate, blood pressure, respiratory rate, and temperature. When recorded in this manner, the smoking status becomes the "fifth vital sign," and this record can serve as a reminder to the physician and office staff to discuss smoking cessation during the visit. Further assistance with smoking cessation should include recommendations for nicotine replacement therapy, such as nicotine gums or patches; such recommendations should include information about the appropriate method of administration, including dose and frequency of use. This is particularly important for nicotine gum, which should be chewed whenever the patient craves a cigarette and then for only a very brief period until tingling develops in the mouth; the gum should then be "parked" between the cheek and the teeth. Because the use of nicotine replacement alone cannot ensure smoking cessation, a program of counseling should accompany all efforts. Written self-help materials are available from many sources, including the NIH, American Lung Association, American Cancer Society, and American Heart Association. Patients can be referred to group programs conducted by local hospitals or nonprofit health organizations for social support. Family members should also be encouraged to assist the patient in smoking cessation. A follow-up visit with the physician should be scheduled to assess the patient's progress and provide ongoing encouragement and support for long-term smoking cessation. The physician should recognize that relapse is common and that many patients require multiple efforts at cessation to achieve long-term abstinence from smoking.

Exercise Training

The most important therapeutic modality in pulmonary rehabilitation is exercise training, and the most important method of exercise training is endurance training of the lower extremities. However, to understand the effects of training, a brief overview of the effects of chronic airflow limitation on exercise capacity is necessary.

Exercise Capacity in Chronic Obstructive Pulmonary Disease

In normal individuals, exercise is limited by the cardiovascular system and the amount of oxygen that can be carried to the exercising muscles. However, in patients with moderate to severe COPD, exercise is usually limited by the respiratory system. This limitation may be caused by one or more of several factors, including abnormal lung mechanics, impaired

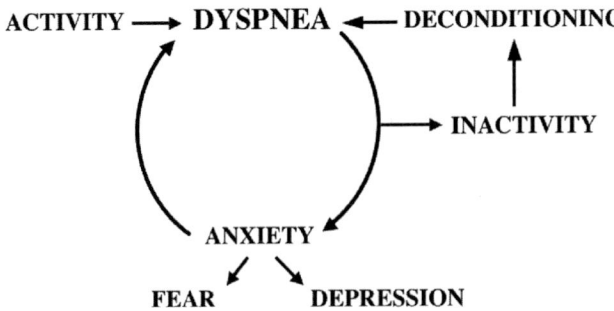

FIGURE 16.1. The vicious cycle of dyspnea. Because increased activity leads to dyspnea in patients with chronic obstructive pulmonary disease, patients learn to prevent dyspnea by reducing their level of activity. Not only is dyspnea provoked by anxiety, it also causes anxiety. (Modified from Make B. COPD: management and rehabilitation. *Am Fam Physician* 1991;43:1315–1324, with permission.)

oxygenation, respiratory muscle dysfunction, and impaired cardiac function.

It is also likely that exercise limitation in COPD is related at least in part to deconditioning, which is in turn related to inactivity resulting from the fear of dyspnea and associated anxiety. It is generally acknowledged that patients with COPD terminate activities performed in the course of daily living because of the uncomfortable and fear-provoking symptom of dyspnea. According to the model of COPD in Figure 16.1, patients with COPD consciously and unconsciously learn to recognize not only that activity leads to dyspnea but also that avoidance of activity prevents shortness of breath. Thus, patients become inactive, and inactivity leads to deconditioning, decreased cardiovascular performance, and reductions in peripheral muscle strength and endurance. This sequence has also been conceptualized as a downward spiral of disease leading to disability, inactivity, and resultant deconditioning. Moreover, anxiety can cause dyspnea even without an increase in physical activity. The anticipatory anxiety associated with the thought of increasing activity, even in the absence of the actual stimulus of the activity, can result in shortness of breath.

Lower Extremity Exercise Training

Pulmonary rehabilitation does not improve lung mechanics, and thus many of the limitations to exercise previously noted (see section "Exercise Capacity in Chronic Obstructive Pulmonary Disease") should not be expected to improve following exercise training. However, multiple other mechanisms may explain the beneficial effects of exercise training in patients with respiratory disease, including increased efficiency in activity performance, enhanced motivation, desensitization to dyspnea, improved cardiovascular function, improved muscle function, and increased aerobic capacity. Because one or more of these mechanisms may occur in a given individual, published evidence indicates that patients with severe COPD can derive a physiologic benefit from ex-

ercise training. It has been demonstrated, for example, that aerobic capacity can be increased in these patients. After training, reduced levels of lactate are seen at a given level of exercise; the reduced lactate production is associated with a reduced minute ventilation, which in turn is associated with a reduced level of dyspnea (Fig. 16.2). In this regard, it has been demonstrated that high-intensity exercise is more effective than low-intensity training (10).

Although the most effective exercise prescription has not been precisely determined, pulmonary rehabilitation programs uniformly incorporate lower extremity aerobic endurance exercise. Following the principles of exercise training for healthy persons, the mode, intensity, duration, and frequency of exercise training should be individually prescribed for each patient based on the baseline exercise capacity.

Mode of Exercise Training

Lower extremity aerobic exercise training is the cornerstone of exercise training during pulmonary rehabilitation. In healthy persons, the effects of exercise training are specific to the muscles that are trained. This concept of the specificity of training implies that leg exercises will improve the performance of the leg muscles and arm exercise will improve the performance of the arms. Because most daily activities require walking and use of the legs, leg exercise improves a patient's functional performance during the activities of daily living. Nevertheless, lower extremity exercise with a stationary bicycle also improves exercise capacity and can be used in training programs. Less information is available concerning the efficacy of other training modalities, such as swimming. Strength training in patients with COPD has also been shown to produce beneficial outcomes.

Exercise Intensity

Although few guidelines are available regarding the optimal intensity of training, it is generally felt that a minimum of intensity is required to achieve benefits. Lactate production, heart rate, and oxygen uptake have been proposed as indicators of the appropriate level of training. Although it has been suggested that healthy persons must exercise at a heart rate that is more than 60% of their predicted maximal heart rate, this rate may not be appropriate for patients whose heart rate is limited by lung disease. Nevertheless, patients who can achieve this heart rate during training are likely to achieve benefits from exercise. Alternatively, it has been suggested that patients should exercise above their anaerobic threshold; however, such an exercise prescription requires a formal exercise test before training to determine the anaerobic threshold. Finally, some investigators recommend training at a predefined level of maximal exercise capacity and have used intensities between 50% and 80% of the patient's maximal exercise capacity. Some training programs simply use continuous walking as long as tolerated and limited by the patient's sensation of dyspnea. Whatever intensity is chosen, the patient's level of dyspnea must be considered. Nevertheless,

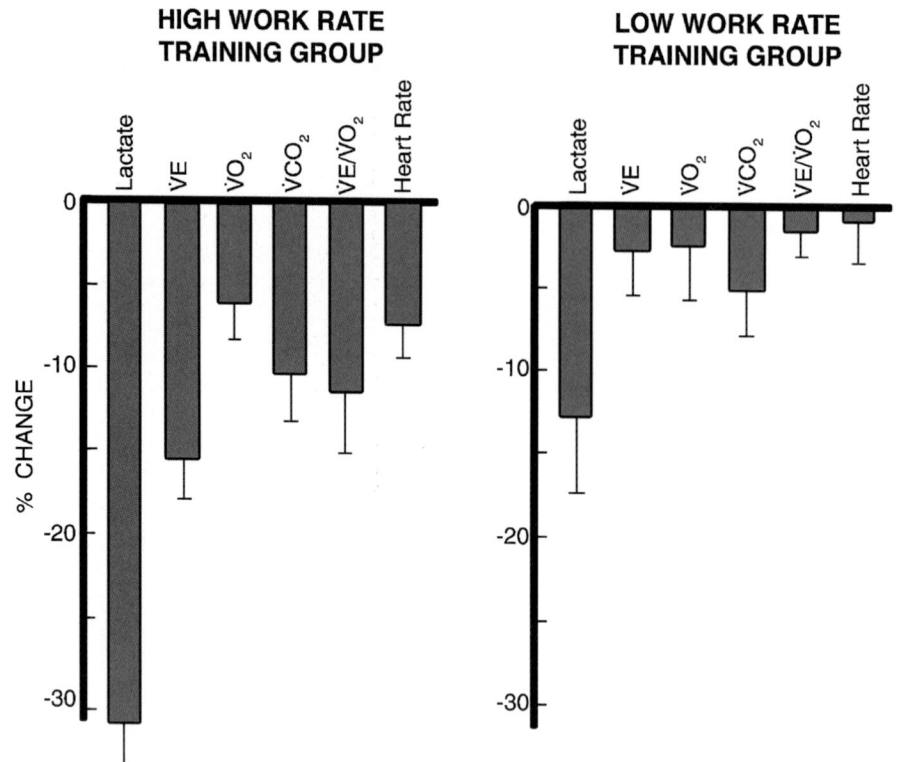

FIGURE 16.2. Changes in physiologic responses to exercise produced by two training strategies in patients with chronic obstructive pulmonary disease (forced expiratory volume in 1 second [FEV₁] 56% of predicted value). **Left panel:** Results in 11 patients trained at a high work rate (60% of the difference between the anaerobic threshold work rate and the maximal work rate) for 45 minutes a day five times a week for 8 weeks. **Right panel:** Results in eight patients who trained at a lower work rate (90% of the anaerobic threshold work rate). Reductions in lactate and minute ventilation (*VE*) were greater with high-work-rate than with low-work-rate training. (From Casaburi R, Patessio A, Ioli F, et al. Reductions in exercise lactic acidosis and ventilation as a result of exercise training in patients with obstructive lung disease. *Am Rev Respir Dis* 1991;143:9–18, with permission.)

with continued encouragement and training, most patients with COPD should be able to reach the higher intensities of exercise required to achieve benefits.

Duration of Training Session

Although the information for recommending a precise duration of training is limited, the exercise sessions should probably last 30 to 45 minutes. Longer sessions may predispose to injury, and based on information from healthy individuals, sessions shorter than 20 minutes are likely to be ineffective. The duration of training should be based on the goals to be achieved. If weight loss is the major goal, longer periods (lasting 45–60 minutes) of activity are likely to be more beneficial than shorter periods. It is generally accepted that aerobic activity should be preceded by a short warm-up period and that stretching exercises should follow the training.

Most programs incorporate a single exercise session each day. Although the efficacy of more frequent daily sessions has not been studied, some patients cannot tolerate continuous exercise. Patients with severe interstitial lung disease may have severe exercise-induced hypoxemia that cannot be corrected with supplemental oxygen therapy. In such cases,

interval training (brief periods of exercise initially for as little as 1 minute followed by rest periods lasting for the same amount of time or longer) may be necessary not only to prevent desaturation but also to limit severe dyspnea.

Frequency of Training

Although benefits may accrue from as little as twice-weekly training sessions, it is generally agreed that training should take place three to five times each week to obtain maximal benefits. This recommended frequency is applicable both to initial training and also to long-term exercise regimens. Daily training is impractical in most cases and probably adds little benefit. Although many rehabilitation programs offer formal supervised training twice a week, patients in such programs should also be expected to exercise on their own.

Duration of Training Program

The optimal duration of the initial training is unknown. In healthy persons in a constant-intensity exercise program, maximal physiologic benefits are achieved in about 3 to 4 weeks. Thus, an initial exercise program might be conducted in as little as 3 weeks. Nevertheless, most rehabilitation programs offer structured training sessions for 6 to 12 weeks in an attempt to achieve maximal benefit from the initial program.

After the initial training component, a long-term exercise program is necessary to retain the benefits of the initial training. Patients may have to restart their exercise program at a lower level following an exacerbation of their underlying lung disease or intercurrent illness that reduces their level of activity. Although lifelong exercise is recommended, few studies have outlined methods to ensure continued patient compliance with an exercise program. Because it is likely that most patients do not continue to exercise following the initial training, education about continued exercise and behavioral approaches to ensure continued patient adherence should be incorporated into the rehabilitation program.

Upper Extremity Exercise Training

Until recently, little emphasis has been placed on training the upper extremities during pulmonary rehabilitation, although many daily functional tasks require use of the arms. In healthy persons, arm work entails a higher metabolic demand than leg work. Thus, for a given workload, upper extremity activity is associated with a higher rate of oxygen uptake and minute ventilation, heart rate, blood pressure, and rate of lactate production than leg exercise. In addition, as individuals age, they tend to lose muscle mass and strength in their arms, which are used to a lesser extent in daily activities than the legs. These factors suggest that upper extremity training may be beneficial in patients with COPD.

In patients with COPD, arm exercise is terminated at a lower level of oxygen consumption than leg exercise. During arm exercise in patients with severe airflow limitation, irregular and dyssynchronous movements of the thorax and abdomen may develop, and even abdominal paradox accompanied by severe dyspnea. It has been suggested that upper extremity exercise places a dual burden on the muscles of the shoulder girdle, requiring them to participate simultaneously in arm activity and ventilatory activity. As a result, an increased demand is placed on the diaphragm to increase its contribution to ventilation, so that shortness of breath is increased.

The simple act of raising the arms without support increases the ventilatory and metabolic demands of patients with COPD. It has been shown that following pulmonary rehabilitation including unsupported arm exercise, the work required for simple arm elevation is reduced.

Based on the available evidence, it appears prudent to include upper extremity exercise during pulmonary rehabilitation, and it has been suggested that both supported and unsupported training may be beneficial. Unsupported exercises may require the patient to lift a dowel to the level of the shoulders, inhaling as the dowel is raised, exhaling as the dowel is lowered, and pacing the activity with a comfortable respiratory rate. Because dyspnea develops rapidly during such exercise, interval training has been recommended, initially with very brief periods of 1 minute of exercise followed by 2 minutes of rest. The exercise intervals may be increased as tolerated, weights may be added to the dowel, and the duration of the session may be increased to a total of 20 to 30 minutes. Supported arm training may also be used.

Strength Training

For patients to participate in an aerobic training program, they must have sufficient strength to perform the exercises. In patients with muscle weakness from age, disuse, deconditioning, or the effects of medications such as oral corticosteroids, strength training may be necessary before an intensive aerobic conditioning program can be initiated. An evaluation with a manual muscle test administered by a trained physical therapist can be helpful in identifying muscle groups that are weak and that consequently may benefit from strength training. Alternatively, equipment for isokinetic muscle testing may provide similar objective information about muscle strength.

Even in patients who demonstrate relatively normal strength, strength training is routinely used in most pulmonary rehabilitation programs to preserve and enhance strength and as an adjunct to aerobic conditioning. Strength training should be carried out 3 to 5 days each week in addition to lower and upper extremity training. Training can be accomplished with either free weights or muscle isolation equipment.

Ventilatory Muscle Training

The inspiratory muscle strength of patients with severe COPD, measured by maximal inspiratory pressure at the mouth, is often reduced. Several mechanisms are likely to account for this finding: reduced diaphragm curvature associated with hyperinflation and consequently reduced force-generating capacity, alterations in the orientation of other respiratory muscles associated with hyperinflation, and possibly diaphragm weakness associated with increased demands imparted by the increased work of breathing. It is also speculated that diaphragm weakness or fatigue may impair ventilation and increase dyspnea in COPD. An attractive hypothesis is therefore that specific training of the inspiratory muscles may improve not only ventilatory muscle strength but also endurance and ventilatory capacity, and reduce dyspnea. However, these additional benefits have not been demonstrated with ventilatory muscle training, so it is not widely used (11).

If ventilatory muscle training is offered, it should follow the principles of intensity, frequency, mode, and duration suggested for the other forms of muscle training. In particular, the training load should be carefully monitored. Training devices with a linear resistance pattern should be used that permit the specified workload to be maintained over a wide range of inspiratory flow rates. With resistors that are not linear, patients may alter their breathing pattern to minimize inspiratory resistance and thus not achieve the desired training load. An initial training resistance that ensures a mouth pressure of about 30% of the maximal inspiratory pressure should be used.

Psychosocial Counseling

Psychologic Issues in Chronic Obstructive Pulmonary Disease

Patients with chronic lung disease frequently exhibit emotional and psychologic concerns related to their illness. Anxiety is a common complaint, particularly in patients with more severe COPD. As noted in Figure 16.1, anxiety may in part be caused by the disabling symptom of dyspnea and be severe enough to be considered panic, which then limits activities. The physical consequence of such an emotional response is often increasing shortness of breath. To avoid this fear-provoking symptom, patients may repress their emotions, a situation described as "emotional straitjacketing."

Depressive symptoms are frequent in patients with COPD and may in part be caused by a reduced functional capacity and resultant impairment in vocational pursuits, recreational interests, and activities of daily living. These changes in life style have been documented to impair the quality of life and consequently diminish the patient's role within the family and community. Patients may express feelings of worthlessness and despair because of their inability to provide financial or emotional support to family members. Depression is the most common emotional consequence of COPD and is more common in this illness than in other chronic medical disorders.

Sexual functioning may also be altered in patients with COPD, with greater impairment in patients with more severe lung disease. Dyspnea may limit intercourse, lead to impotence, alter relationships with spouses or significant others, and lead to a reduced sexual self-image. Physicians should recognize that the impotence and reduced sexual activity of these patients may not be a consequence of advancing age but rather of the effects of lung disease. Educational programs and counseling to address sexual issues are routinely included in most pulmonary rehabilitation programs.

Neuropsychologic deficits may also be seen in patients with COPD. Decreased fine motor speed and coordination, impaired perceptual motor skills, and difficulty with abstracting have been documented. However, memory is usually spared. Neuropsychologic dysfunction is more severe in patients with more severe hypoxemia.

Psychosocial Interventions

Exercise Training

Based on the theory depicted in Figure 16.1, depressive symptoms and anxiety may improve with pulmonary rehabilitation as exercise capacity is improved. The importance of the emotional support and encouragement provided by health professionals during exercise training should not be underestimated. Exercising under the supervision and direct observation of a physical therapist, respiratory therapist, or nurse experienced in the management of patients with respiratory disease and in whom the patient has confidence is an important factor in allaying anxiety and fear and reducing the panic associated with activity.

Antidepressant Medications

If significant clinical depression is confirmed, therapy with antidepressant medications should be considered. The side effects of antidepressants should be kept in mind because patients with COPD tend to be older and may have excessive respiratory secretions and frequently prostatic hypertrophy. Some antidepressants produce sedation and others are associated with activation, and these drugs should be tailored to the needs of individual patients. In patients with hypercapnia, drugs that act centrally and reduce respiratory drive should be avoided. Agents with cholinergic properties are not appropriate for patients with prostatic hypertrophy. Anxiolytic agents may be effective in selected patients with severe agitation and anxiety that is unresponsive to counseling, relaxation, and the other components of pulmonary rehabilitation.

Psychosocial Support

Psychosocial clinicians, including licensed clinical social workers, clinical psychologists, and psychiatrists, may help to structure the psychosocial component of the rehabilitation program and provide psychosocial evaluation and support services. Psychosocial support techniques include group and individual counseling, stress management, relaxation, and enrollment in support groups. Group sessions with the patient and family that incorporate counseling and peer group support are used in many rehabilitation programs. Groups allow patients to see that their feelings are shared by others, and the group may provide insights into methods of coping that have proved effective. Anxiety may be lessened by teaching patients stress management and relaxation techniques to allow them to gain control over their symptoms.

Breathing Retraining

Breathing retraining includes the techniques of pursed-lips breathing, diaphragmatic breathing, and controlled breathing. The goal of these breathing techniques is to reduce dyspnea, and they have the additional benefit of improving respiratory physiologic parameters. Controlled breathing may be practiced during exercise, during daily activities to lessen dyspnea, and whenever the patient experiences increased shortness of breath. These methods may improve oxygenation, slow the respiratory rate, increase tidal volume, decrease air trapping, and reduce the work of breathing.

Pursed-Lips Breathing

Pursed-lips breathing is the most commonly used technique and is often learned and adopted by patients without instruction from health care professionals. Patients breathe in slowly through the nose and then exhale slowly over 4 to 6 seconds or longer through lightly pursed lips. Pursed-lips breathing may be used with diaphragmatic breathing during inspiration. One explanation for the physiologic benefits of pursed-lips breathing is that airway pressure is increased during exhalation, thereby preventing airway collapse in patients with reduced elastic recoil, so that hyperinflation is decreased and oxygenation improved. However, pursed-lips breathing has also been shown to improve oxygenation in patients with interstitial lung disease, whose elastic recoil is increased. In some studies, the work of breathing has been shown to increase with pursed-lips breathing, an effect that may be exaggerated if the lips are pursed too tightly, causing a significantly higher expiratory resistance.

Diaphragmatic Breathing

In this technique, patients are encouraged to use their diaphragm by attempting to push the abdomen outward during inspiration. The technique was originally described for use with the patient supine and the hands placed on the abdomen to facilitate an assessment of outward abdominal motion. The physiologic and clinical benefits of diaphragmatic breathing have been less well studied, and patients often report greater relief of dyspnea with the use of pursed-lips breathing.

Controlled Breathing

During periods of greatly increased effort, most healthy persons tend to hold their breath. During activity, patients with lung disease often exhibit breathing patterns that are irregular and not coordinated with their activity. In controlled or paced breathing, a regular breathing pattern is coordinated with activity. For example, during arm activities, inhalation may be coordinated with raising the arms and exhalation with lowering the arms. During stair climbing, exhalation may be coordinated with raising the body up to the next step. Controlled breathing during exercise training may also increase exercise endurance and delay the onset of shortness of breath.

Daily Activity Performance and Energy Management

Based on the initial patient assessment, appropriate goals of treatment to improve the performance of daily activities include the following: (a) reducing shortness of breath during performance of the basic activities of daily living; (b) applying regular coordinated breathing patterns; (c) increasing functional endurance; (d) using energy and time manage-ment methods; (e) using adaptive equipment; (f) obtaining assistance from others, including family members; and (g) enhancing performance at work. These potential treatment goals are in addition to the goals of reducing stress and providing relaxation, which also decrease energy requirements during the day.

In patients whose functional capacity is limited, energy management techniques can facilitate the performance of desired tasks. Energy management includes using energy conservation techniques, improving work efficiency, using proper body mechanics, and incorporating the principles of time management, pacing, and careful planning. These techniques are not tools that are practiced routinely by healthy persons, so they are not usually self-evident to patients. However, incorporating these principles into daily life can enhance functional performance. For example, it may be impossible for a patient to climb a flight of stairs to a restaurant quickly after walking from a parked car. The stairs may be climbed more easily if the patient leaves home with sufficient time to avoid rushing (planning), is left at the door to the building (planning and energy conservation), rests before climbing the stairs (energy management), walks up the stairs more slowly (pacing), rests on the stairs when needed (energy management), and uses a regular breathing pattern incorporating pursed-lips breathing.

An important part of daily life is recreation and leisure pursuits. The evaluation of leisure function includes an assessment of barriers that limit participation in such activities. Such barriers are potentially related to financial issues (e.g., limited income), physical concerns secondary to dyspnea, and emotional factors (e.g., the fear of dyspnea associated with increased activity). Addressing these barriers and discussing methods of successfully participating in leisure activities may enhance the patient's quality of life.

Education

The traditional goal of education has been to increase cognitive knowledge—that is, to inform patients about their disease. Such education requires that patients acquire an understanding of how the lungs work, the nature of their lung disease and its signs and symptoms, and the actions and side effects of medications, in addition to their names. However, a more appropriate and effective role of education for individuals with chronic illness is to effect a positive behavioral change. For example, the goal of education about inhaled medications is to ensure that the patient uses the prescribed medications to achieve the desired benefits (i.e., reduction of dyspnea and improvement in the ability to perform daily activities). Knowledge about the mechanism of action of inhaled bronchodilators is likely to be less important in achieving this goal than information about the benefits to be derived by the individual patient. In addition, important information about dosing, including the schedule and technique of administration of medications for each individual, may help ensure compliance with the medication regimen.

Based on the health beliefs model, patients and their families should be queried about their perceptions regarding the seriousness of their disease, their susceptibility to further illness and complications, the threat of their disorder, the benefits of treatment, and barriers to therapy. An understanding of the health beliefs of the patient and family will facilitate the educational efforts of the rehabilitation team to modify these beliefs so that the treatment plan will be more readily accepted and compliance with the prescribed therapies improved.

An initial educational evaluation is recommended for all patients enrolled in pulmonary rehabilitation. Because learning styles differ, it is useful to determine whether the patient will learn best by using verbal or visual methods and to provide the educational material in a manner that is most appropriate for the patient's learning style. The patient's educational level, native language, and reading level are also important to assess, along with any difficulty in vision and hearing. Written information should be provided to all patients, particularly when memory problems are evident.

Education may be conducted both formally and informally throughout the comprehensive pulmonary rehabilitation program and should be guided by learning objectives based on the needs of the individual patient. Education begins before the initiation of rehabilitation with explanations of the purpose, goals, expected results, and nature of the rehabilitation program. Formal education may be provided through classes, one-on-one teaching with a health care professional, or written or audiovisual materials. Informal education should take place with every member of the pulmonary rehabilitation team, such as when a physician prescribes a new medication, a respiratory therapist performs a pulmonary function test, a physical therapist performs chest physiotherapy, an occupational therapist evaluates the activities of daily living, or a social worker implements a relaxation program. Patient learning should be assessed both formally and informally to determine whether the learning objectives are being met.

Nutritional Counseling

It is reasonable to assume that for patients to participate in pulmonary rehabilitation that incorporates exercise training, adequate nutritional intake must be ensured, excess weight should be treated, and weight loss should be avoided. Even though the scientific information on the best approaches to nutritional counseling in patients with respiratory disease is limited, recommendations for counseling patients about the common problems of weight loss and dyspnea during meals are outlined in Table 16.5.

A nutritional evaluation should be performed for all patients involved in pulmonary rehabilitation. It is important to elicit a dietary history, including what the patient actually consumes and a history of any weight loss or weight gain. The patient may be asked to recall his or her diet for the last 24 hours or maintain a diary of foods eaten to determine the amount and types of food consumed. Based on the patient's height and age, tables can be used to identify the ideal body weight. However, it is also important to determine lean body mass and fat mass to develop an optimal nutritional program for each patient. A relatively simple way to assess lean body mass involves measuring the skinfold thickness and skeletal circumference at established sites. A goal of nutritional counseling should be to ensure an optimal lean body mass, which includes muscle mass, and minimize excessive fat mass.

In part because of the reduced activity levels associated with severe respiratory disease and the decreased caloric needs associated with advancing age, patients with COPD may be overweight and have excessive fat mass. Individuals who are overweight, particularly those who are obese ($>120\%$ of ideal body weight), may be expected to have a more limited exercise capacity for weight-bearing activity than patients of normal weight. Thus, weight loss in this group of patients is theoretically desirable to reduce the metabolic and thus the ventilatory demands of daily activities. Weight loss should be associated with decreased dyspnea and improved exercise capacity and is an important adjunct to the other elements of pulmonary rehabilitation.

Patients with severe COPD may be underweight ($<90\%$ of ideal body weight). Severe weight loss has several potentially deleterious implications, including decreased diaphragm and respiratory muscle function, decreased hypoxic and hypercapnic ventilatory responses, and decreased

TABLE 16.5. SYMPTOMS AND COUNSELING STRATEGIES FOR NUTRITIONAL THERAPY IN CHRONIC OBSTRUCTIVE PULMONARY DISEASE

Problem	Recommendations
Decreased appetite Weight loss	Eat high-calorie foods first.
	Have favorite foods available.
	Try more frequent small meals and snacks throughout the day.
	Add butter, mayonnaise, sauces, and gravies to add calories.
	Limit liquids in meals; sip liquids an hour after meals.
	Cold foods can give less of a sense of fullness than hot foods.
	Consider anabolic steroids to increase fat-free mass.
Dyspnea	Rest before meals.
	Use bronchodilators before meals.
	Use secretion-clearance strategies if indicated.
	Eat more slowly.
	Use pursed-lips breathing between bites.
	Use tripod position for meals.
	Have readily prepared meals available.
	Evaluate for oxygen desaturation during meals.

Source: Modified from Rogers RM, Donahoe M. Nutrition in pulmonary rehabilitation. In: Fishman AP, ed. *Pulmonary rehabilitation.* New York: Marcel Dekker Inc, 1996:555, with permission.

respiratory clearance and defense mechanisms. It has also been demonstrated that weight loss in patients with COPD is associated with increased mortality. Whether the weight loss in some undefined manner directly causes early mortality or whether it is simply a marker of more severe lung disease has not been determined. Several studies have shown that improved caloric intake and weight gain in persons with COPD does not reduce mortality rates. Anabolic steroids have been shown to increase fat-free mass. Adequate caloric intake can be expected to be helpful in improving muscle strength and endurance in underweight patients, but it may not decrease mortality.

LONG-TERM PROGRAM

It is understandably difficult for older individuals who have been both sedentary and independent their entire lives to incorporate changes learned through rehabilitation into their daily routine. Although the degree of patient adherence to continued exercise and pulmonary rehabilitation is unknown, it is likely that long-term compliance is less than optimal. In studies of patients with chronic illness, rates of lack of adherence vary greatly and are frequently more than 50%.

Little literature is available to guide clinicians and suggest the best methods of ensuring long-term adherence to the key elements of pulmonary rehabilitation. However, it is prudent to incorporate as many techniques as possible to help the patient adhere to a life-long program. It is the responsibility of every pulmonary rehabilitation program not only to provide long-term goals for the patient but also to assist the patient in developing daily routines that incorporate methods of achieving these goals. In addition, barriers to long-term maintenance, such as the site and costs of regular ongoing exercise training, should be addressed and resolved in a cooperative manner by the patient and rehabilitation team. The term *collaborative self-management* has been applied to a long-term cooperative effort by patient and physician to emphasize the importance of the patient's central role in making decisions and choices regarding disease management and the physician's role as educator and facilitator. The role of education in allowing patients to become active participants in their care and to assume responsibility for their own health cannot be overemphasized.

POTENTIAL OUTCOMES OF PULMONARY REHABILITATION

Many of the potential outcomes listed in Table 16.6 can be affected by multidimensional pulmonary rehabilitation programs. Determination of the results, or outcomes, of pulmonary rehabilitation is important for three major reasons. First, a clear and concise description of the expected outcomes of pulmonary rehabilitation can be used to convey the benefits of pulmonary rehabilitation to patients who are considering participation, physicians who refer patients for rehabilitation, and medical benefits providers paying for such services. Information about outcomes that have been documented by other programs can be gleaned from studies published in the medical literature and provide proof of the medical necessity of rehabilitation services. Second, assessment of outcomes of programs within the local community must be used to evaluate results in individual patients to ensure that the desired results are actually achieved. Third, outcomes assessment should be used to guide the development and ongoing evaluation of comprehensive programs. Each pulmonary rehabilitation program should assess outcomes and decide which outcomes are important to measure.

Medical issues are addressed by the first four outcomes listed in Table 16.6. Traditionally, *mortality*, or survival, is the most important outcome of medical care. However, patients with chronic disease frequently indicate that quality of life is much more important to them than quantity of life. *Morbidity* in patients with respiratory disease includes complications of the primary respiratory process. In patients with COPD, pulmonary hypertension with subsequent cor pulmonale, acute exacerbations of COPD, and respiratory tract infections all increase morbidity. Morbidity also includes hospitalizations for acute exacerbations and the need for emergency or urgent medical care related to the respiratory disorder, although these may also be considered as costs.

Respiratory symptoms are prominent complaints in patients with respiratory disorders. The primary symptom of

TABLE 16.6. POTENTIAL OUTCOMES OF MANAGEMENT OF RESPIRATORY DISORDERS

Survival
Morbidity
    Exacerbations
    Hospitalizations
Respiratory symptoms
Physiologic indices
    Pulmonary function
    Exercise tests
Functional capacity
    Walk tests
Neuropsychologic function
Health-promoting behaviors
    Adherence to prescribed treatments
    Smoking cessation
Health-related quality of life (health status)
    Physical functions
    Mental/emotional functions
    Social function
    Role function
    General well-being
Vocational: ability to work
Use of assistive devices
Caregiver burden
Patient satisfaction
Costs of care

respiratory disease is shortness of breath, which may be disabling for patients with severe airflow limitation. Secondary symptoms related to the effects of respiratory disease, such as headaches related to hypoxemia and fatigue, should also be considered.

Physiologic indices in patients with respiratory disorders can be measured by simple spirometry and include the forced vital capacity (FVC) and forced expiratory volume in 1 second (FEV_1). However, in patients with COPD, these physiologic indices, in addition to measures of oxygenation, are not expected to change because the underlying respiratory disorder is not altered by pulmonary rehabilitation. On the other hand, adherence to medications may reduce airflow limitation in patients with reversible disorders, such as asthma. One of the more important physiologic indices is exercise capacity, which can be most objectively evaluated with a cardiopulmonary exercise tolerance test performed in a controlled laboratory setting. Workload, oxygen consumption, heart rate, and minute ventilation are relatively easy to measure with commercially available equipment while the patient exercises on a treadmill or bicycle ergometer according to steady-state or incremental exercise protocols.

The remainder of the potential outcomes of pulmonary rehabilitation listed in Table 16.6 address "nonmedical" issues, which are not considered as important as the "medical" factors. As already mentioned, nonmedical issues are frequently identified as goals by patients and thus are incorporated into rehabilitation programs. Because walking is an important daily activity, functional capacity may be measured as the distance walked in 6 or 12 minutes. This walk test is an outgrowth of the 12-minute run developed to evaluate the fitness of army recruits. Although the run has been shown to correlate with maximal exercise capacity, the walk test is more appropriately considered a functional evaluation tool in patients with respiratory disease. Because encouragement by the tester can increase the distance walked, the walk test should be performed according to a rigid protocol defining the number of walks and methodology to be used by the tester.

Patients with COPD are often hypoxemic and demonstrate associated reductions in neuropsychologic function, which can also be affected by advancing age. Patient adherence to health-related behaviors should be stressed during pulmonary rehabilitation. Cigarette smoking is the major cause of COPD, and efforts at smoking cessation are often incorporated into pulmonary rehabilitation programs. Adherence to medication, oxygen, and exercise prescriptions are other behavioral outcomes that foster continued health and thus should be assessed following pulmonary rehabilitation.

Physical function, mental/emotional function, social function, role function, and perception of well-being are often considered together as "health-related quality of life." Although it is a perception by patients of their own condition, quality of life can nevertheless be measured objectively. *Physical health* is the ability to perform everyday activities, including self-care, and maintain mobility. *Mental/emotional health* incorporates feelings such as anxiety, nervousness, and depression; control over behaviors, feelings, and thoughts; and cognitive functions such as memory, orientation, and alertness. *Social health* incorporates interactions with other individuals in the community. *Role function* refers to the performance of activities such as employment, school, and housework. A global perception of *general well-being* can also be evaluated.

The *ability to work* may be important for younger persons but not as critical for elderly, retired patients. The ability of children to attend school and participate in the full range of school activities should be considered. Time lost from work or school because of illness may also be an important outcome. *Caregiver burden* refers to the effects of the patient's illness on family, friends, and others who may assist with the patient's care. This includes financial issues, such as time lost from work, in addition to psychologic stressors for family members caring for chronically ill patients. Patients with limited function may benefit from the use of assistive technology, such as wheelchairs and vans for people with neuromuscular disorders, which may be lessened by rehabilitation. As health care expenditures are being more tightly controlled, costs are increasingly of concern. Direct costs of medical care include not only the costs of rehabilitation but also those of hospitalizations, emergency medical care, and prescription medications. Indirect costs include lost wages for patients and families and the psychosocial impact of illness on both patients and their families.

TOOLS FOR ASSESSING QUALITY-OF-LIFE OUTCOMES

Because enhancement of the quality of life is one of the major goals of pulmonary rehabilitation, and because assessment of the quality of life is a relatively new field, this section reviews the use of questionnaires to assess health-related quality of life.

Criteria for Quality-of-Life Questionnaires

Before a measurement tool is selected, the intent of the measurement must be defined to ensure that the measurement instrument can adequately assess the desired outcome. Measurement tools can be classified into three types—discriminative, predictive, and evaluative—based on the purpose for which they are used. The measurement of outcomes of pulmonary rehabilitation requires the use of evaluative tools designed to detect a difference over time in a group, such as before and after pulmonary rehabilitation in patients with COPD. An established evaluative measurement tool must meet three fundamental psychometric criteria: reliability, validity, and sensitivity.

The reliability of a measurement tool refers to its accuracy and its lack of change over time. If a scale is used as an example of a reliable measurement tool for weight, repeated measurements of the same object with the same scale should yield the same results. To assess the reliability of a questionnaire, the tool may be administered twice to a group of people who are thought to be stable, and then the results of the two tests are compared, a process known as test–retest reproducibility. Interobserver reliability assesses differences in results obtained by different observers administering the same instrument to the same subject and is important when questionnaires cannot be completed without a trained administrator.

Demonstration of the validity of a quality-of-life instrument is a process of accumulating sufficient evidence to document that the tool actually measures the desired attribute. Because no "gold standard" measure of the quality of life has been agreed on universally, the validity of instruments that measure quality of life is difficult to assess. The development of quality-of-life questionnaires is usually based on expert knowledge and experience of a disease, and the tool is derived from such evidence combined with theories and postulations. However, both the instrument and its underlying theories must be assessed for accuracy.

Pulmonary rehabilitation programs are interested in changes that occur in response to the program intervention and thus must ascertain that they are using tools that can measure change. When evaluative tools are readministered after rehabilitation, they should be able to reflect a clinically relevant difference, a capability referred to as *sensitivity* or *responsiveness*.

General Quality-of-Life Tools

Quality-of-life instruments are structured as either general or disease-specific tools. General health or generic tools are intended to profile comprehensively the areas believed to be affected by any disease or treatment, including physical and emotional function and general well-being. These instruments can be used across cultures, genders, populations, and diseases. General health profiles have the advantage of measuring the global impact of a disease or medical intervention. Three general quality-of-life tools have been used in patients with COPD.

SF-36 Health Survey

The SF-36 Survey contains 36 written questions that can be answered independently by the patient in 5 to 10 minutes. Eight subscale scores are generated: physical functioning, social functioning, role-physical, role-emotional, bodily pain, general health, vitality, and mental health. Each subscale score ranges from 0 to 100, with 100 representing the most desirable score. Two summary scores (physical and mental) have also been described.

Quality of Well-Being Scale

The Quality of Well-Being Scale is a somewhat complex tool requiring administration by a trained interviewer, and a response-coding procedure must be applied before the questionnaire can be scored. The interviewer must keep an elaborate record of the subject's verbal and bodily responses. It contains 50 items and can be administered in about 10 to 15 minutes. Components include mobility, physical activity, social activity, and symptoms, and the results are weighted by general population preferences. The measured general health status is reported on a continuum between optimal functioning (represented by a score of 1) and death (represented by a score of 0). Subjects can be classified into one of 43 states of functioning ranging between 1 and 0; the weight of each state is derived from community surveys to reflect social preference. The Quality of Well-Being Scale can be used to profile a single day or a span of several days, with the interviewer probing health, symptoms, and performance. In addition, the effects of a treatment can be expressed as well-years.

Sickness Impact Profile

The Sickness Impact Profile is designed to assess the impact of illness on behaviors and activities. This questionnaire contains 136 questions, which are grouped into 12 subscales and further summarized into two broad scores and an overall summary score. The general scale of physical activity includes subscales of ambulation, mobility, and body care and movement. The psychosocial score includes subscales of social interaction, communication, alertness, and emotional behavior. Additional subscales include sleep and rest, eating, work, home management, and recreation and pastimes. Although this questionnaire is long, it has been widely used and can be completed independently by the patient.

Quality-of-Life Tools Specific to Respiratory Disease

Although general health surveys can provide useful information, their sensitivity may be limited in patients with severe disease and specific symptom complexes, such as those with COPD. One aspect of health in which this issue is likely to arise is physical activity. For example, a scale of physical functioning that includes questions about running, lawn mowing, or other strenuous activities lacks the sensitivity to differentiate among individuals with extremely limited abilities who are recipients of pulmonary rehabilitation. Moreover, a scale can thwart the detection of differences if it contains a significant proportion of items to which most COPD patients will typically respond in a similar manner, either with or without therapeutic interventions. Some disease-specific tools allow patients to identify individual areas or activities that they feel are most affected, and these patient-selected areas can be reassessed over time. This process allows individuals to determine the impact of disease on their own lives. Although such individualization increases the sensitivity to changes in an individual, comparisons across disease groups or populations are difficult.

St. George's Respiratory Questionnaire

This self-administered questionnaire incorporates 76 items for use in patients with respiratory disease, including COPD and asthma. The questions are weighted according to their importance, and a computerized scoring system is required to obtain a total score and three component scores: respiratory symptoms, performance of activities, and impact of the illness. Normal ranges have been determined, and the instrument appears sensitive to change. This instrument is unique in that clinically significant changes in the scores have been determined.

Chronic Respiratory Disease Questionnaire

One of the more widely used tools to evaluate patients with respiratory disease is the Chronic Respiratory Disease Questionnaire, which was designed to measure the impact of chronic airflow limitation on quality of life. Because different individuals with chronic lung disease often identify different physical tasks that have been adversely affected, this questionnaire allows individual patients to choose the activities in which their performance has been most altered. The interviewer asks each subject to identify five activities most affected by dyspnea, and the patients are queried about these same activities at each subsequent administration of the questionnaire, at which time it is suggested that they be informed about their response to the prior questionnaire. Responses are recorded on a Likert scale ranging from 1, indicating extreme disability, to 7, indicating no disability. This questionnaire includes 15 items measuring dyspnea and fatigue (physical functioning scale), anxiety and depression (emotional functioning scale), and sense of control over respiratory disease (mastery scale). After the initial administration by an interviewer, the patient can complete the questionnaire independently.

OUTCOMES OF PULMONARY REHABILITATION

Improvements in many of the important outcome domains have been demonstrated following pulmonary rehabilitation in patients with COPD (Table 16.6). Although it is not always clear which component of pulmonary rehabilitation is most responsible for a specific outcome, most of the results noted in the next sections have been demonstrated in response to comprehensive multidisciplinary programs. The reader is referred to several evidence-based reviews of pulmonary rehabilitation included in the references that provide documentation of the outcomes of pulmonary rehabilitation.

Survival

Mortality is most closely related to the degree of airflow limitation as measured by the FEV_1, but it is also related to age and possibly to exercise tolerance and perceived physical disability. Because pulmonary rehabilitation does not change the underlying pulmonary disease and FEV_1 in patients with COPD, it might be anticipated that survival would be unchanged following rehabilitation in patients with very severe airflow limitation. On the other hand, in selected groups of patients with COPD who have a decreased exercise capacity and increasingly frequent exacerbations with resultant deconditioning, pulmonary rehabilitation may decrease the frequency of exacerbations, lessen physical disability, and improve exercise tolerance, and thus may improve survival.

Oxygen therapy in patients with COPD and severe hypoxemia has been clearly shown to improve survival. However, conclusive evidence that comprehensive pulmonary rehabilitation decreases mortality is lacking. Based on data from historical control groups and observational studies, several publications have suggested that pulmonary rehabilitation may improve 5-year survival by 13% to 28%, and randomized studies have demonstrated a trend toward improved survival. Nevertheless, further controlled randomized studies are required to address the effects of rehabilitation on survival more completely. The investigations evaluating survival have frequently not incorporated a concurrent control population that did not receive pulmonary rehabilitation. In addition, the available studies include patients with differing degrees of severity of underlying pulmonary disease as measured by the FEV_1 and report divergent survival rates, so that comparisons between studies are difficult.

Morbidity

Several studies have demonstrated a reduction in the number of hospital days in COPD patients following pulmonary rehabilitation programs that used the services of a nurse and other ancillary health care personnel when necessary in the home or other outpatient settings. It is most likely that hospitalizations were decreased in patients with frequent hospital admissions and moderately severe pulmonary disease who were enrolled in a home care program. In the current health care environment, with its focus on cost containment and a reduction in hospitalizations, the role of pulmonary rehabilitation in reducing morbidity and the utilization of expensive health care resources in hospitals and emergency departments is of critical importance.

Because the number of hospital days is reduced, pulmonary rehabilitation can decrease the costs of medical care of patients with COPD. The cost savings associated with reduced hospitalizations following pulmonary rehabilitation are in the range of $2,000 per patient per year. The cost-effectiveness of rehabilitation in patients with COPD has also been evaluated by using the Quality of Well-Being Scale to measure years of quality life (well-years) as an outcome. The cost per additional year of well-being was $24,256, considered cost-effective by current standards in comparison with other therapeutic modalities for other diseases.

Respiratory Symptoms

The respiratory symptom of major concern to patients with COPD is breathlessness. Randomized controlled clinical trials have shown that dyspnea decreases as a result of pulmonary rehabilitation, both when measured by the specific questionnaires assessing breathlessness and when measured by disease-specific quality-of-life questionnaires such as the St. George's Respiratory Questionnaire (Fig. 16.3). A reduction in dyspnea measured during formal exercise tests has also been documented following rehabilitation. A reduction in breathlessness has been noted after rehabilitation applied in different sites, including the home outpatient setting and the inpatient setting. The major component of rehabilitation leading to a reduction in breathlessness is lower extremity exercise training. Breathing retraining, including pursed-lips and diaphragm breathing, is also known to decrease dyspnea. Because of the importance of this cardinal symptom and the frequency with which a reduction in dyspnea is a stated goal of the patient, dyspnea is an important

symptom to monitor and assess in response to pulmonary rehabilitation. The respiratory disease-specific questionnaires (e.g., the Chronic Respiratory Disease Questionnaire and the St. George's Respiratory Questionnaire) incorporate measures of dyspnea. Specific dyspnea questionnaires are also available (e.g., the Baseline and Transitional Dyspnea Indices), and other tools are designed to assess dyspnea during exercise (e.g., the Borg Dyspnea Scale and the Visual Analog Scale).

Functional Capacity

Pulmonary rehabilitation improves both objectively assessed functional capacity and patient-perceived functional status. Some studies have classified patients by their functional ability and demonstrate an improvement in functional classification following rehabilitation. The 6- or 12-minute walk test can also be used to assess functional capacity; walk distance improves about 20% to 25% following rehabilitation in patients with COPD.

Exercise Capacity

It has been repeatedly demonstrated that pulmonary rehabilitation including aerobic exercise training of the lower extremities improves exercise tolerance (Fig. 16.4). Exercise capacity can be measured objectively in the laboratory on a bicycle or treadmill with an incremental maximal test or a steady-state endurance test. During steady-state exercise, declines in oxygen consumption, heart rate, respiratory rate, and minute ventilation and an increase in exercise duration are noted following rehabilitation. Improvement in peak

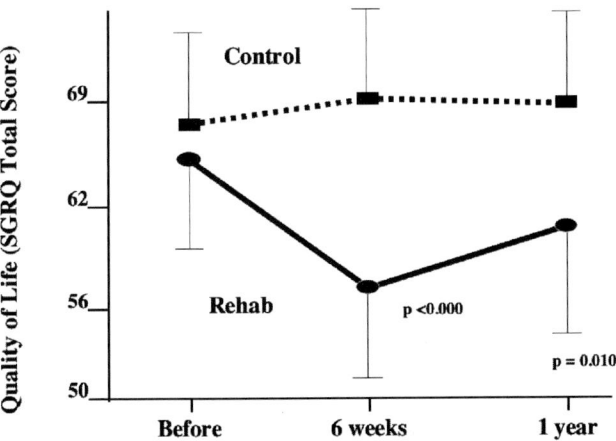

FIGURE 16.3. Disease-specific quality of life (measured by the St. George's Respiratory Questionnaire total score) is improved immediately after rehabilitation (6 weeks) and at 1 year in patients with chronic obstructive pulmonary disease randomized to receive comprehensive pulmonary rehabilitation in comparison with that of patients receiving standard medical management. Note that lower scores indicate improve health status. (Based on data from Griffiths TL, Burr ML, Campbell IA, et al. Results at 1 year of outpatient multidisciplinary pulmonary rehabilitation: a randomized controlled trial. *Lancet* 2000;355:362–368, with permission.)

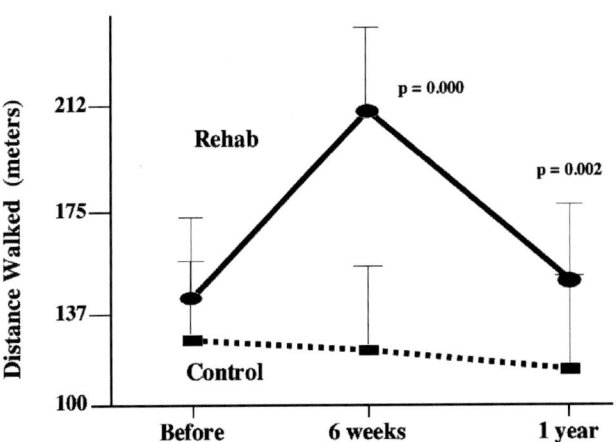

FIGURE 16.4. Shuttle walk distance (meters) is improved immediately after rehabilitation (6 weeks) and at 1 year in patients with chronic obstructive pulmonary disease randomized to receive comprehensive pulmonary rehabilitation in comparison with that of patients receiving standard medical management. (Based on data from Griffiths TL, Burr ML, Campbell IA, et al. Results at 1 year of outpatient multidisciplinary pulmonary rehabilitation: a randomized controlled trial. *Lancet* 2000; 355:362–368, with permission.)

exercise capacity (peak work and oxygen consumption) has also been demonstrated.

Strength Training

Other forms of exercise, including strength training, have also been used, but to a lesser extent. Strength training of the upper and lower extremities has been shown to reduce dyspnea and increase mastery and bicycle exercise endurance time in COPD.

Upper Extremity Training

Training of the upper extremities in COPD is specific for arm function and reduces the increased metabolic demand and ventilation associated with arm elevation and arm work. Upper extremity training does not appear to improve performance in other tests not related to the training, such as lower extremity walking or treadmill exercise. In addition, although upper extremity training increases endurance during arm exercise, improvement in the activities of daily living with arm exercise as the sole intervention has not been documented. A reduction in perceived dyspnea during upper extremity exercise has also been noted. Current recommendations indicate that supported and unsupported upper extremity training should be incorporated into comprehensive pulmonary rehabilitation programs.

Ventilatory Muscle Training

The only modes of respiratory muscle training that increase the strength and endurance of the ventilatory muscles are those that achieve an adequate training load, which underscores the importance of linear resistance characteristics of the training device. With adequate training loads, it appears that the endurance and function of the inspiratory muscles are improved when resistance training is performed with controlled-flow breathing patterns. However, published studies indicate inconsistent results in other outcomes of inspiratory muscle training. For example, exercise capacity and quality of life are not uniformly improved following inspiratory muscle training in patients with COPD, in part because of the lack of an adequate training stimulus. Ventilatory muscle training may be considered as an adjunctive form of therapy to improve exercise capacity and quality of life in selected patients if an adequate training load can be ensured.

Quality of Life

Based on published studies, comprehensive pulmonary rehabilitation should be considered a therapeutic intervention that improves the quality of life of patients with COPD. Although most studies that have evaluated quality of life have demonstrated improvements following comprehensive pulmonary rehabilitation, not all studies have used standard quality-of-life tools or controlled randomized study designs. Nevertheless, several randomized controlled studies in which respiratory disease-specific quality-of-life instruments were used have documented improvements in quality of life. However, some studies in which general health quality-of-life measures were used have not shown improvements in quality of life, which illustrates the importance of choosing quality-of-life instruments that are sensitive to change. Improvements in quality of life have been noted for rehabilitation conducted in an outpatient setting, inpatient setting, or the home.

The precise components of comprehensive rehabilitation that are most responsible for improvements in quality of life are unclear. However, it appears that comprehensive programs that include exercise training may be necessary to improve quality of life. Education alone has not been shown to result in significant quality-of-life benefits.

Ability to Work

It is unclear whether pulmonary rehabilitation can assist patients in returning to gainful employment. It is important to emphasize that this is not generally a goal of pulmonary rehabilitation, particularly for patients with relatively advanced COPD, who are generally older and retired. Pulmonary rehabilitation is generally considered more effective in maintaining employment in younger patients with less advanced disease and thus should be started earlier in the course of COPD. Some investigators have noted poor compliance with vocational rehabilitation, and others have suggested that the success of vocational rehabilitation is related to intelligence test scores. The energy requirements of patients with higher IQs may be smaller because the nature of their employment poses fewer physical demands and so allows better vocational outcomes.

Other Outcomes

Little information is available concerning caregiver burden and outcomes of the use of assistive technology in COPD. An improved ability for self-care and a decreased need for nursing home care have been reported.

Prediction of Beneficial Outcomes

Although it is tempting to predict which patients are most likely to benefit from pulmonary rehabilitation, previous investigations have not consistently been able to identify such individuals. Age and sex do not appear to be predictors of outcome. The ability of baseline functional capacity and airflow limitation to predict outcome is questionable. It has been suggested that patients with less airflow limitation (i.e., a higher FEV_1 value) are more likely to show improvement with rehabilitation, and therefore rehabilitation should be started earlier in the course of COPD to achieve greater cumulative benefits. However, some studies have demonstrated a greater improvement in walk distance (measured as the percentage of increase in walk distance) in patients with the lowest baseline walk distances. Whether these benefits in more functionally limited patients represent the effect of deconditioning or of the degree of airflow limitation before rehabilitation has not been evaluated.

Because it not possible to identify which patients are most likely to benefit from rehabilitation, and because pulmonary rehabilitation reduces dyspnea, increases exercise capacity, improves quality of life, and reduces hospitalizations, it is reasonable to enroll patients with dyspnea, reduced exercise capacity, impaired quality of life, and frequent hospitalizations in comprehensive programs of pulmonary rehabilitation.

SUMMARY

Comprehensive pulmonary rehabilitation programs can improve physiologic measures of exercise capacity, functional capacity, and health-related quality of life. The variety, diversity, and number of potential outcomes of pulmonary rehabilitation suggest that not all outcomes will be of equal importance for all patients with COPD. Based on the nature and needs of the populations and individuals being served, pulmonary rehabilitation programs should determine which outcomes ought to be the focus of their rehabilitative efforts. Periodic assessment of the outcomes achieved by rehabilitation can be used to modify the rehabilitation program, with the goals of improving outcomes and thus enhancing patient care.

ACKNOWLEDGMENT

The author wishes to thank Marie Kindred for her excellent secretarial assistance during the preparation of this manuscript.

REFERENCES

1. American Thoracic Society. Pulmonary rehabilitation, 1999. *Am J Respir Crit Care Med* 1999;159:1666–1682.
2. Bach JR, ed. *Pulmonary rehabilitation: the obstructive and paralytic conditions.* Philadelphia: Hanley & Belfus/Mosby, 1996.
3. British Thoracic Society. Pulmonary rehabilitation. *Thorax* 2001; 56:827–834.
4. Fishman AP, ed. *Pulmonary rehabilitation, lung biology in health and disease.* New York: Marcel Dekker Inc, 1996.
5. Lacasse Y, Wong E, Guyatt GH, et al. Meta-analysis of respiratory rehabilitation in chronic obstructive pulmonary disease. *Lancet* 1996;348:1115–1119.
6. Ries AL, Carlin BW, Carrieri-Kohlman V, et al. Pulmonary rehabilitation: evidence-based guidelines. *Chest* 1997;112:1363–1396.
7. American Thoracic Society. Pulmonary rehabilitation. *Am Rev Respir Dis* 1981;124:663–666.
8. Fishman AP. Pulmonary rehabilitation research: NIH workshop summary. *Am J Respir Crit Care Med* 1994;149:825–833.
9. Fiore MC, Bailey WC, et al. *Clinical practice guideline: treating tobacco use and dependence.* Bethesda, MD: US Department of Health and Human Services, Public Health Service, June 2000.
10. Casaburi R, Patessio A, Ioli F, et al. Reductions in exercise lactic acidosis and ventilation as a result of exercise training in patients with obstructive lung disease. *Am Rev Respir Dis* 1991;143:9–18.
11. Smith K, Cook D, Guyatt GH, et al. Respiratory muscle training in chronic airflow limitation: a meta-analysis. *Am Rev Respir Dis* 1992;145:533–539.

Upper Respiratory Tract Infections

17

Richard J. Blinkhorn, Jr.

INFECTIONS OF THE ORAL CAVITY

Infections of the oral cavity most often are of dental origin, and although they are rare, local spread to the deep fascial spaces may occur, with subsequent life-threatening parapharyngeal, retropharyngeal, or pleuropulmonary extension. It is beyond the scope of this chapter to describe all the potential intraoral infections, so only those infections with complications that commonly involve the upper respiratory tract are reviewed.

The microbiologic aspects of abscesses of dental origin have been extensively studied, and the evidence available suggests that anaerobes play a major role in these infections. The most common microbial isolates include *Fusobacterium* species, *Bacteroides* species, anaerobic streptococci, and the aerobic viridans streptococci (1).

The parapharyngeal space is shaped like an inverted cone, with its base at the skull and its apex at the hyoid bone. Infections of this space may result from peritonsillar abscess, parotitis, mastoiditis, or molar tooth infection. Parapharyngeal abscess may spread to the mediastinum along the carotid sheath or via extension into the retropharyngeal space. Infection may invade the carotid artery or jugular vein, resulting in thrombosis or intravascular sepsis, sometimes with metastatic hematogenous spread and septic pulmonary emboli. The latter is referred to as *Lemierre postanginal sepsis*, and *Fusobacterium necrophorum* has been the leading etiologic agent (2). The characteristic unilateral suppurative thrombophlebitis of the internal jugular vein is often misdiagnosed as cervical lymphadenitis. Thrombosis of the internal jugular vein can be diagnosed noninvasively by ultrasonography, axial computed tomography (CT), or magnetic

resonance angiography of the neck. Pulmonary involvement is reported in up to 85% of cases, in which multiple bilateral necrotic infiltrates are frequently associated with pleural effusion or empyema. The optimal antibiotic regimen is not known. Most authors recommend a combined treatment with high-dose penicillin plus metronidazole or monotherapy with clindamycin for 2 to 6 weeks (2). Ligation of the internal jugular vein was common in the pre-antibiotic area but is no longer considered necessary. The role of anticoagulation has not been adequately studied, and anticoagulation generally has been reserved for cases of thrombosis with retrograde propagation to the cavernous sinus (2).

MANAGEMENT OF INTERNAL JUGULAR SEPTIC THROMBOPHLEBITIS	
Summary Statement	**Level of Evidence**
Antibiotics for 2–6 weeks	Expert opinion
Ligation unnecessary	Expert opinion

The retropharyngeal space is located between the pharynx and prevertebral fascia and extends from the base of the skull into the mediastinum. Infection of this space usually results from lymphatic spread to the retropharyngeal lymph nodes with subsequent suppuration and abscess. Afferent drainage to these nodes arises from the nasopharynx, adenoids, and sinuses. Retropharyngeal abscess is mainly a disease of young children because these lymph nodes atrophy by 3 or 4 years of age. Common causative organisms include *Streptococcus pyogenes* and anaerobic bacteria. Spontaneous rupture into the pharynx may result in aspiration with pneumonia and empyema.

The term *Ludwig angina* has been loosely applied to a heterogeneous array of infections involving the submandibular and sublingual spaces. First described in 1836, this is a diffuse

R. J. Blinkhorn, Jr.: Department of Medicine, MetroHealth Medical Center; Department of Medicine, Case Western Reserve University School of Medicine, Cleveland, Ohio.

bilateral cellulitis of the floor of the mouth and upper cervical areas characterized by toxicity, fever, brawny indurated swelling of the submandibular space, tongue elevation, and dysphagia. A dental source of infection is found in 50% to 90% of reported cases, with the second and third mandibular molars most commonly involved. Rapid progression of infection may result in edema of the neck and glottis, thereby precipitating asphyxiation. Treatment requires parenteral antibiotics (as previously discussed), airway monitoring, early intubation or tracheostomy when necessary, soft tissue decompression, and surgical drainage (3).

RHINITIS

The nonspecific term *acute rhinitis* is used to describe infections of the internal nose. Acute rhinitis may represent the sole or main manifestation of the "common cold," which is a mild, self-limited, catarrhal syndrome that is the leading cause of visits to a physician in the United States. The major respiratory viruses causing colds include rhinovirus, coronavirus, parainfluenza virus, and respiratory syncytial virus. Influenza virus and adenovirus may produce the common cold syndrome but tend to be associated with more severe illness often involving the lower respiratory tract.

The cardinal symptoms are nasal discharge, nasal obstruction, sore throat, and cough. The median duration of illness is 1 week, although almost 25% of cases last up to 2 weeks. The main challenge to the physician is not to establish a specific viral etiology but rather to distinguish the uncomplicated cold from the approximately 0.5% to 2% of cases with secondary bacterial sinusitis or otitis media.

Antibiotics have no place in the management of uncomplicated colds. Controlled clinical trials have demonstrated the effectiveness of antihistamines (reduced sneezing, rhinorrhea, and nasal mucus production) and nonsteroidal antiinflammatory drugs (reduced cough, headache, and malaise) (4,5). More than a dozen well-designed clinical trials have been conducted, and evidence that oral or intranasal zinc is effective in the prevention or treatment of the common cold is lacking (6).

MANAGEMENT OF RHINITIS	
Summary Statement	**Level of Evidence**
Antibiotics are not indicated.	Randomized controlled trials
Give antihistamine and NSAID for symptoms.	Randomized controlled trials
No role for oral/intranasal zinc.	Randomized controlled trials

NSAID, nonsteroidal antiinflammatory drug.

SINUSITIS

The frontal, ethmoid, maxillary, and sphenoid sinuses are paired, mucosa-lined cavities of the anterior portion of the skull. Predisposing factors to sinus disease can be divided into local, regional, and systemic factors. The most common local predisposing cause of suppurative sinusitis is a viral upper respiratory tract infection. Inflammation and edema in the ostiomeatal complex can obstruct the sinus ostium, leading to reduced oxygenation of the sinus, disturbed function of the ciliary and mucus blanket, and diminished local resistance. Other local nasal factors that cause obstruction in the ostiomeatal complex are nasal polyps, allergic rhinitis, foreign bodies, and nasal septal pathology. In hospitalized patients, nasogastric tubes may functionally obstruct sinus ostia, thereby predisposing to nosocomial sinusitis. The immotile cilia syndrome is another local factor predisposing to sinus disease, but it does not involve structural obstruction of sinus ostia. Regional factors include maxillary dental infections, and predisposing systemic factors include malnutrition, diabetes mellitus, long-term corticosteroid therapy, hypogammaglobulinemia, blood dyscrasias, and chemotherapy.

Symptoms associated with bacterial sinusitis include nasal drainage, facial pain or pressure, nasal congestion, hyposomia, fever, cough, fatigue, and ear fullness or pressure. In sphenoid sinusitis, headache is the most common initial symptom.

Symptoms and signs suggesting acute bacterial sinusitis overlap considerably with those of viral upper respiratory tract infection. Contrary to popular belief, a change in the color or characteristics of the nasal discharge is not a specific sign of a bacterial infection (7). A diagnosis of acute bacterial sinusitis may be made in adults with viral upper respiratory tract infection that is no better after 10 days or worsens after 5 to 7 days (8). Sinus aspiration studies in adults demonstrate significant bacterial growth in approximately 60% of patients with symptoms of upper respiratory tract infection lasting at least 10 days (9).

The physical examination is not extremely useful in the diagnosis of bacterial sinusitis. The reproducibility rates of transillumination for assessing disease within the maxillary and frontal sinuses are 60% and 90%, respectively, but transillumination does not differentiate bacterial from viral infection (10). Fiberoptic endoscopy allows visualization of the middle meatus, and direct culture of purulent matter in this region may correlate with culture of aspirates from the maxillary sinus (11). Endoscopy, however, is not necessary in uncomplicated cases. Maxillary sinus puncture should be reserved for the research setting or for patients with unresponsive or complicated infections.

Imaging studies are not recommended for the routine diagnosis of community-acquired sinusitis because of their lack of specificity. Plain radiographs are imprecise in determining the extent of disease. A metaanalysis of six studies demonstrated that positive findings on plain films have moderate sensitivity (76%) and specificity (79%) in comparison with maxillary sinus puncture (12). A negative radiograph has more diagnostic value than either a negative clinical examination or a negative ultrasonogram. CT scans clearly demonstrate abnormalities within the sinuses, but abnormalities are also found in almost 90% of patients with acute viral disease. CT is not indicated, therefore, in uncomplicated acute bacterial sinusitis (13).

Although normal paranasal sinuses have long been believed to be sterile, transient colonization with organisms normally populating the upper airway may occur. Overgrowth of this transient resident flora may produce infection when local clearance mechanisms are impaired. In all studies of acute community-acquired bacterial sinusitis, more than 50% of isolates are either *Streptococcus pneumoniae* or *Haemophilus influenzae*, with *Moraxella catarrhalis*, other streptococci, *Staphylococcus aureus*, and Gram-negative bacteria accounting for the rest. When appropriate anaerobic cultures are performed, anaerobes can be isolated in at least 10% of acute cases, with a higher isolation rate of approximately 50% in chronic sinusitis. A mixed anaerobic infection with *Bacteroides* and anaerobic streptococci would suggest infection of dental origin. Patients with cystic fibrosis or immotile cilia syndrome are predisposed to *Pseudomonas aeruginosa* and *S. aureus* infection. Immunocompromised patients and patients with nosocomial sinusitis have a higher incidence of aerobic Gram-negative bacterial infections. Cultures from patients with chronic sinusitis are often polymicrobial, and at least half harbor anaerobes.

Evidence for clinical improvement after antimicrobial therapy in acute bacterial sinusitis can be found in double-blinded controlled trials of antimicrobial therapy in adults (7,14). By day 10, 86% of patients treated with antimicrobial agents had recovered or felt better, and 86% also showed sinus improvement on CT scan.

The recommendations for antimicrobial treatment have changed as the sensitivity patterns of causative bacteria have evolved, especially as strains of *S. pneumoniae* with intermediate- or high-level penicillin resistance have emerged. Antimicrobial therapy is usually empiric because culture of sinus aspirates is not routinely available or indicated. Treatment should be directed against the expected pathogens. The β-lactam antimicrobial agents that continue to show the best activity against intermediately resistant strains of pneumococci and are also effective against β-lactamase–producing *H. influenzae* and *M. catarrhalis* are amoxicillin/clavulanate, cefpodoxime, cefdinir, and cefuroxime. The new quinolones also show excellent activity against sinusitis pathogens. Although trimethoprim/sulfamethoxazole, doxycycline, and macrolides may be considered, bacteriologic failure rates of 20% are possible.

The symptoms of acute community-acquired sinusitis usually abate after 2 or 3 days of treatment and generally resolve by 10 to 14 days. For patients who do not respond to an initial course of therapy, referral to an otolaryngologist for sinus puncture and lavage is highly recommended to avoid the sequelae of chronic sinusitis.

Ancillary treatment should be directed at drainage of the nasal passages and sinuses and the relief of sneezing, coughing, and systemic complaints. Oral decongestants are pre-ferred to topical preparations because they avoid rebound vasodilation, enhance drainage of the ostiomeatal complex, and avoid pharyngeal irritation. There is no good evidence that topical steroids are effective, and they should be avoided.

MANAGEMENT OF ACUTE BACTERIAL SINUSITIS	
Summary Statement	**Level of Evidence**
Imaging is not useful in uncomplicated cases.	Expert opinion, nonrandomized trials
Antibiotics (high failure rate TMP/SMX, doxycycline, macrolides).	Randomized controlled trials
Use oral decongestants/saline rinses.	Expert opinion
Avoid topical steroids.	Expert opinion

TMP/SMX, trimethoprim/sulfamethoxazole.

Chronic sinusitis can be defined by symptoms persisting for longer than 12 weeks or by abnormal CT changes after 4 weeks of medical therapy. Therapy for chronic sinusitis includes the aforementioned antimicrobial agents, given for 3 to 4 weeks, plus corticosteroids. Patients who fail this approach should be referred for endoscopic sinus surgery, which is reported to result in marked short-term improvement in 85% of patients (15).

MANAGEMENT OF CHRONIC SINUSITIS	
Summary Statement	**Level of Evidence**
Antibiotics for 3–4 weeks.	Expert opinion, nonrandomized trials
Corticosteroids.	Expert opinion, nonrandomized trials
Consider endoscopic sinus surgery, if not resolved after antibiotics and corticosteroids.	Expert opinion

PHARYNGITIS

Acute pharyngitis is an inflammatory condition of the pharynx, and its principal symptom, sore throat, is a frequent accompaniment of many other respiratory illnesses. Many of the known microbial causes of pharyngitis are listed in Table 17.1. For the clinician, it is most important to differentiate viral from streptococcal pharyngitis because of the response of the latter to penicillin therapy, in addition to its potential sequelae of acute rheumatic fever and acute glomerulonephritis.

Viruses account for most cases of pharyngitis in adults, and a mild-to-moderate pharyngeal discomfort frequently accompanies common colds. Sore throat is a major complaint in some patients with influenza, and the

TABLE 17.1. MICROBIAL AGENTS ASSOCIATED WITH PHARYNGITIS

Agents	Clinical Syndrome	Frequency of Occurrence
Viruses		
Respiratory[a]	Common cold	Common (winter)
Adenovirus	Pharyngoconjunctival fever	Common (winter)
Influenza virus	"Flu," pneumonia	Common (winter)
Coxsackievirus A	Herpangina	Occasional (summer, fall)
Epstein-Barr virus	Infectious mononucleosis	Common
Cytomegalovirus	Infectious mononucleosis	Occasional
HIV	Fever, adenopathy, rash	Uncommon
Herpes simplex virus	Gingivostomatitis	Occasional
Bacteria		
Streptococci, group A	Tonsillitis, scarlet fever	Common
Mixed anaerobes	Gingivitis, Vincent angina	Occasional
Corynebacterium diphtheriae	Membranous pharyngitis	Rare
Arcanobacterium haemolyticum	Scarlatiniform rash	Occasional (young adults)
Neisseria gonorrhoeae	Sexually transmitted disease	Occasional
Treponema pallidum	Chancre, syphilis	Rare
Francisella tularensis	Pharyngeal ulcer, tularemia	Rare
Yersinia enterocolitica	Exudative pharyngitis, enterocolitis	Rare
Fungi		
Candida albicans	Thrush, esophagitis	Occasional
Chlamydiae		
C. psittaci	Pneumonia	Rare
C. trachomatis	Sexually transmitted disease	Occasional
C. pneumoniae	Hoarseness, pneumonia	Occasional
Mycoplasmata		
M. pneumoniae	Pneumonia, bronchitis	Occasional

[a]Rhinovirus, coronavirus, parainfluenza virus.

accompanying myalgia, headache, fever, and cough readily suggest the diagnosis. Adenoviral pharyngitis is usually more severe than the illness typical of the common cold, and conjunctivitis is a distinguishing feature present in one third to one half of cases. The presence of vesicles or shallow ulcers of the palate is characteristic of primary infection with herpes simplex virus, although gingivostomatitis is a more common presentation than acute pharyngitis. During the summer and fall months, pharyngitis caused by coxsackievirus, so-called herpangina, can be distinguished by the presence of small vesicles on the soft palate, uvula, and anterior tonsillar pillars. Exudative tonsillitis, fever, cervical adenopathy, and fatigue are characteristic features of Epstein-Barr virus infectious mononucleosis, and approximately half of cases have associated generalized adenopathy or splenomegaly. Febrile pharyngitis with cervical lymphadenopathy and a truncal maculopapular rash has been described as a characteristic feature of primary infection with HIV and may mimic the mononucleosis syndrome (16).

Approximately 15% of all cases of pharyngitis are caused by group A streptococci, which are the most common bacterial pathogen isolated from patients of school age. It is not clear that non–group A β-hemolytic streptococci, such as groups C and G, cause pharyngitis in nonepidemic settings. The severity of infection varies considerably, but gen-

erally marked pharyngeal pain, dysphagia, tender cervical adenopathy, and fever are present. In most cases, an etiologic diagnosis is not possible on clinical grounds alone. Rapid streptococcal antigen testing has replaced throat cultures in general practice, but a negative result should be substantiated by a simultaneous throat culture.

Outbreaks of diphtheria still occur in unvaccinated populations in the United States. Most cases occur in the Southwest among blacks, Mexican Americans, and Native Americans. Pharyngeal diphtheria is characterized by small areas of exudate that coalesce to form a light to dark gray membrane that becomes progressively thicker and more difficult to remove. The condition usually involves little toxicity and only modest temperature elevation. Membranous spread to the larynx and trachea can cause life-threatening respiratory obstruction characterized by inspiratory stridor and cyanosis. Management includes prompt administration of diphtheria antitoxin intravenously, antimicrobial therapy (penicillin or erythromycin), and airway management (intubation or tracheostomy) (17). *Arcanobacterium (Corynebacterium) haemolyticum* has been increasingly identified as a cause of exudative pharyngitis in adolescents and young adults and may be associated with an erythematous maculopapular, sometimes pruritic, skin rash (18). Pharyngitis accompanying sexually transmitted disease caused by

Neisseria gonorrhoeae, Chlamydia trachomatis, or *Treponema pallidum* is not uncommon, but these agents would be rare causes of pharyngitis in an unselected general population. Asymptomatic gonococcal throat colonization is much more common than pharyngitis; in various series, no more than 30% of patients with positive pharyngeal cultures had any clinical manifestations. Ceftriaxone, administered intramuscularly in a single dose of 250 mg, is the drug of choice. Although *C. trachomatis* has been isolated from patients with pharyngitis, asymptomatic throat colonization occurs more often. Rarely, syphilis may present as a primary pharyngeal chancre.

Although exudative pharyngitis with cervical lymphadenopathy may complicate infection with *Yersinia enterocolitica* and *Francisella tularensis,* other manifestations of systemic diseases caused by these agents usually predominate in the clinical picture, and isolated pharyngeal disease is quite rare. Similarly, when *Chlamydia psittaci, Chlamydia pneumoniae,* or *Mycoplasma pneumoniae* infection is associated with pharyngitis, the pharyngeal disease is generally accompanied by tracheobronchitis or pneumonia and seldom occurs as an isolated event.

EPIGLOTTITIS

First described in an adult, epiglottitis is a life-threatening disease observed most frequently in 1- to 6-year-old children, most often during the fall and winter. It is important to emphasize, however, that epiglottitis has been increasingly reported in adults. *Supraglottitis* may be the preferred term because the infection involves the arytenoids, aryepiglottic folds, and epiglottis while sparing the pharynx, true vocal cords, and trachea. The infection can be primary or secondary to adjacent infection or trauma and results in either acute diffuse inflammation, acute ulcerative inflammation, or epiglottitis with abscess formation on the free edge, laryngeal surface, or lingual surface.

Acute epiglottitis develops in either of two distinct forms: a gradual form that develops within days, usually following an upper respiratory tract illness, or an accelerated form that develops within hours. The characteristic early symptoms are sore throat and dysphagia. Odynophagia thereafter becomes the predominant symptom and may be so severe that the patient would rather not eat or drink. The voice tends to be muffled rather than hoarse, and the temperature is usually strikingly elevated. Respiratory distress with tachypnea, dyspnea, and cyanosis occurs late and heralds acute airway obstruction. In this setting, the patient is observed drooling, sitting up, leaning forward, and breathing quite deliberately. The patient should not be examined in the recumbent position. Despite the prominence of pain, the pharynx is usually normal in appearance.

Roentgenograms of the chest often show hyperinflation, and areas of atelectasis or pneumonitis may be present. The epiglottic swelling can be seen on a lateral x-ray film of the neck. Laboratory examination shows an elevated white blood cell count with an increase in mature polymorphonuclear leukocytes and band forms.

Asphyxia and cardiopulmonary arrest are dreaded complications, and several factors contribute to the development of respiratory tract obstruction. Edema of the lingual mucosa of the epiglottis causes the epiglottis to curl posteriorly and inferiorly, narrowing the air space, and edema of the aryepiglottic folds worsens the obstruction. During inspiration, these swollen structures are drawn downward into the airway, further reducing the size of the lumen. In children, airway resistance in the setting of turbulence may vary by as much as the fifth power of the radius. Therefore, reducing the airway diameter by half may increase airflow resistance up to 32 times (19). The potential abrupt airway obstruction in epiglottitis is functional rather than a complete physical obstruction. The airway resistance can simply exceed the patient's ability to overcome it. Inflammation of the supraglottic structures inhibits swallowing, so that an accumulation of secretions and saliva further compromises the airway.

Acute epiglottitis is a bacterial infection; viruses have not been conclusively linked to the disease. In 80% of cases in children, *H. influenzae* type b can be isolated from the epiglottis or bloodstream. In adults, however, the etiologic agent is not always obvious, and blood cultures are negative in 70% to 85% of cases (20). *H. influenzae* type b accounts for 20% to 25% of cases in adults, with *S. pneumoniae,* β-hemolytic streptococci, viridans streptococci, nonencapsulated *H. influenzae, M. catarrhalis,* and *S. aureus* occasionally implicated. In up to 40% of adult cases, no etiologic agent is recovered (20).

The diagnostic and therapeutic approach depends on the clinical presentation. Unstable patients with "classic" epiglottitis (stridor, drooling, dyspnea, and fever) should be taken immediately to the operating room for direct laryngoscopy and nasotracheal or endotracheal intubation. Preparations should be made for emergency cricothyrotomy if intubation is not possible. In most adults and a large number of children, however, the presentation is not classic, and their management is less straightforward. In adults, indirect laryngoscopy or flexible nasoendoscopy is safe in the initial assessment; no complications of this approach have been reported (21). Radiography, however, remains useful in differentiating other upper airway disease (e.g., foreign body or abscess) from epiglottitis. In children, manipulating the upper airway is more hazardous, and radiography should be the initial procedure when epiglottitis is weakly or moderately suspected. In stable children with normal radiographic findings, the epiglottis should be visualized to rule out "normal radiograph" epiglottitis. Whereas intubation or tracheostomy is virtually mandatory in children with epiglottitis, this remains a point of ongoing controversy in the management of adults. It is reasonable in adults to defer airway intervention so long as close follow-up by individuals specifically skilled in emergency airway control can be ensured. Stridor and infection with *H. influenzae* type b appear to increase the likelihood of acute airway obstruction.

Intravenous antimicrobial therapy directed against *H. influenzae* should be administered, and cefotaxime, ceftriaxone, or ampicillin/sulbactam is a reasonable choice. Improvement is generally seen within 12 to 48 hours, and the artificial airway can usually be removed during this period. Before extubation, the patient should exhibit clinical improvement and be afebrile and alert. Evidence of clinical improvement can be corroborated by direct visualization with a fiberoptic laryngoscope (22). Antibiotics should be continued for 7 to 10 days. Although often administered in the hope of diminishing supraglottic edema, corticosteroids have not been conclusively shown to alter the course of the disease. Immunization against *H. influenzae* has reduced the incidence of childhood epiglottitis (23). The risk for the development of invasive *H. influenzae* infection is considerably increased in both the siblings and parents of patients with epiglottitis, and rifampin prophylaxis should be administered to these household contacts. Some experts also recommend prophylaxis for health care workers who have come into especially close contact with a patient's airway or respiratory secretions.

LARYNGOTRACHEOBRONCHITIS

Unlike epiglottitis, which is a bacterial disease, laryngotracheobronchitis (croup) is usually caused by a viral infection. The peak incidence is in late fall, with a smaller peak in late spring; this pattern is related to the prevalence of parainfluenza viruses in the community. The subglottis and trachea are involved, whereas the area above the true vocal cords is spared. In children, croup usually occurs in the first half-decade of life and begins with rhinorrhea. The first sign of spread to the larynx is the gradual development of a harsh, barking cough and hoarse voice. Fever is variable. The major clinical features of croup are related to inflammatory edema and fibrinous exudate in the subglottic area, which narrow the airway and cause inspiratory stridor. Inflammation and edema commonly extend down the trachea and bronchi, producing thick, viscid secretions and ventilation–perfusion mismatch. Involvement of these lower airways, superimposed on the already narrowed subglottic area, results in increased work of breathing and hypoxemia.

Chest roentgenographic findings may be normal or show evidence of hyperaeration and sometimes areas of atelectasis. An anteroposterior radiograph of the neck may show the characteristic subglottic swelling, sometimes referred to as the *"hourglass"* sign. The white blood cell count is usually normal, sometimes with a predominance of lymphocytes. Parainfluenza viruses 1 through 3 have been implicated most frequently, but influenza virus, respiratory syncytial virus, coronavirus, rhinovirus, adenovirus, enterovirus, and cox-

TABLE 17.2. DISTINGUISHING FEATURES: CROUP AND EPIGLOTTITIS

Feature	Croup	Epiglottitis
Patient age	Younger (6 mos–3 ys)	Older (3–6 ys)
Season	Late spring, late fall	All year
Antecedent illness	Rhinorrhea	Uncommon
Clinical appearance	Child lying down	Child sitting
	Nontoxic condition	Toxic condition
	Not drooling	Drooling
Cough	Barking in quality	Absent
Voice	Hoarse	Muffled
Fever	Variable	High-grade
Leukocytosis	Absent	Present
Progression	Usually slow	Rapid
Causative agent	Parainfluenza virus I	*Haemophilus influenzae* type b

sackievirus are all capable of producing the disease. Measles virus is an infrequent cause.

For the clinician, the initial step in management is to distinguish croup from epiglottitis (Table 17.2). Despite a plethora of home therapies for croup, none has proved consistently effective. Although humidification may reduce upper airway secretions, controlled trials have not demonstrated a beneficial effect on subglottic swelling, lower parenchymal abnormalities, or airway resistance (24,25). The arterial oxygen saturation should be continuously monitored with oximetry. Most children with hypoxemia without hypercarbia respond to supplemental oxygen because the hypoxemia results primarily from areas of lung with abnormal ventilation–perfusion mismatch. Nebulized racemic epinephrine has been shown to decrease the need for intubation (26). Corticosteroids have been added to the armamentarium for the treatment of croup because controlled clinical trials have demonstrated a benefit of corticosteroids with various routes of administration (intramuscular, oral, and nebulized) (27). The administration of antibiotics is unwarranted. Intubation should be reserved for patients with worsening hypercarbia despite conservative management (28).

MANAGEMENT OF LARYNGOTRACHEOBRONCHITIS IN CHILDREN

Summary Statement	Level of Evidence
No utility of humidification.	Randomized controlled trials
Nebulized racemic epinephrine.	Randomized controlled trials
Administer corticosteroids; various routes effective.	Randomized controlled trials
Maintain airway.	Expert opinion

Laryngotracheobronchitis is more complex etiologically in adults and in both children and adults compromised by hematologic malignancy or neutropenia. In noncompromised adults, laryngotracheobronchitis is often manifested by hoarseness and substernal pain, frequently of a burning quality. Influenza viruses, parainfluenza viruses, or adenoviruses are the likely offending agents, but in addition, bacteria (particularly *H. influenzae*) and *M. pneumoniae* can produce the syndrome. If the patient is compromised and neutropenic, opportunistic organisms such as *P. aeruginosa, Klebsiella, Serratia,* and *Enterobacter* can be responsible. If the patient has defective cell-mediated immunity and oral thrush, the *Candida* infection may move from the oropharynx to the larynx and trachea. In patients who are receiving immunosuppressive agents, herpesvirus 1 or 2 may cause laryngotracheobronchitis.

Bacterial tracheitis in infants and older children has features of both epiglottitis and croup. Clinically, it is characterized by fever, toxicity, brassy cough, and often inspiratory stridor. In most cases, chest roentgenograms show patchy or focal infiltrates. The epiglottic and arytenoepiglottic folds appear normal on direct examination, but subglottic edema is present. One may see purulent secretions that are often profuse and thick and can obstruct the trachea. The isolated organism is often *S. aureus,* and the response to appropriate antimicrobial agents is satisfactory. Endotracheal intubation is usually required to maintain a patent airway and handle copious secretions.

ACUTE BRONCHITIS (OR TRACHEOBRONCHITIS)

Acute inflammatory disease of the trachea and bronchi can be caused by a variety of stimuli, including the following: constituents of tobacco and cannabis; ammonia; trace metals such as vanadium and cadmium; air pollutants such as sulfur dioxide and nitrogen dioxide; vegetable substances such as bagasse, cotton, flax, hemp, and paprika; and a farrago of infectious agents, including viruses, mycoplasmata, bacteria, and parasites.

Viruses account for the majority of cases, including respiratory syncytial virus, rhinovirus, echovirus, parainfluenza viruses 1 through 3, herpesvirus, coxsackievirus, influenza virus, coronavirus, and adenovirus. It is virtually impossible to separate one virus from another clinically. All those capable of producing pharyngeal and nasal disease also can cause bronchitis.

The bacteria most often recovered in acute purulent bronchitis are *H. influenzae, S. pneumoniae,* and *M. catarrhalis. Bordetella pertussis* is responsible for whooping cough in children. It is less well appreciated that *B. pertussis* and *Legionella* infections may cause acute and subacute bronchitis in adults.

Evidence is increasing that yeasts and fungi may cause bronchitis in the absence of parenchymal disease. This is true of *Candida albicans* and *Candida tropicalis, Cryptococcus neoformans, Histoplasma capsulatum, Coccidioides immitis,* and *Blastomyces dermatitidis.* As serologic analyses have

been performed more regularly, it has become clear that both *M. pneumoniae* and *C. pneumoniae* cause acute bronchitis. Bronchitis also can occur during the migration of *Strongyloides* and *Ascaris* larvae, and a few cases of paroxysmal cough caused by the parasite *Syngamus laryngeus* have been reported in residents of or visitors to Brazil, the Philippines, the West Indies, Puerto Rico, and British Guiana.

Cough is uniformly found in acute bronchitis, and it may be productive of mucoid or purulent sputum. The cough may be accompanied by variable degrees of hemoptysis or substernal pain that is often described as of a burning quality; it is usually accentuated on inspiration. The frequency and duration of cough appear to be prolonged in cigarette smokers. Generally, the temperature is only minimally to moderately elevated. Physical examination often shows harsh breath sounds, rhonchi, and variable degrees of expiratory wheezing.

Wheezy bronchitis is a specific clinical entity occurring for the most part in children who have a tendency to wheeze and a family history of atopy. Viruses appear etiologically related in only a minority of cases; rhinoviruses and respiratory syncytial viruses are the agents that have been most often isolated. The syndrome of intermittent, recurrent wheezy bronchitis in children also may result from reduced esophageal sphincter tone with reflux.

The organisms responsible for bronchitis in a compromised host may be quite different from the agents affecting an uncompromised person. In older persons and immunocompromised hosts, herpes simplex virus 1 may cause tracheobronchitis manifested primarily by bronchospasm. Intravenously administered acyclovir is the treatment of choice. Such patients are also susceptible to Gram-negative infection with species of *Klebsiella, Serratia, Enterobacter,* and *Pseudomonas.* If a Gram-negative superinfection occurs during antibiotic treatment for infection elsewhere, the organisms may be markedly antibiotic-resistant. The pharynx of alcoholics is colonized more frequently than the pharynx of nonalcoholics by enteric Gram-negative organisms, particularly *Enterobacter* species and *Escherichia coli.* Pharyngeal colonization may be followed by aspiration and acute bronchitis.

Treatment in most cases is symptomatic and directed primarily at control of cough. Placebo-controlled clinical trials have demonstrated that nonsteroidal antiinflammatory agents (naproxen, ibuprofen) and first-generation antihistamines are effective in reducing the severity of cough (4,5). For patients with protracted cough following an episode of infectious bronchitis, oral or inhaled corticosteroids are administered in clinical practice, but they have not been adequately studied in clinical trials. Controlled clinical trials comparing antibiotic treatment with placebo have yielded conflicting results, but antibiotics are not generally recommended for the treatment of acute bronchitis in otherwise healthy adults (29). Macrolide or azalide therapy should be considered, however, when *M. pneumoniae, C. pneumoniae,* or *B. pertussis* is suspected on clinical grounds. During annual winter epidemics of influenza, treatment with amantadine, rimantadine, or the newer neuraminidase inhibitors should be administered to patients with suspected influenza-like illness if the duration of the illness is less than 48 hours. Exacerbations of chronic bronchitis in patients with chronic obstructive pulmonary disease are discussed in Chapter 12.

MANAGEMENT OF ACUTE BRONCHITIS	
Summary Statement	**Level of Evidence**
Antibiotics not recommended (excluding certain organisms; see text).	Conflicting results (controlled clinical trials)
Administer first-generation antihistamines.	Randomized controlled trials
Administer NSAID.	Randomized controlled trials

NSAID, nonsteroidal antiinflammatory drug.

BRONCHIOLITIS

In the strictest sense, bronchiolitis, a disease of small airways, should be considered a lower respiratory tract illness. It is so frequently preceded by an upper respiratory tract infection, however, that it is included in the present chapter. Bronchiolitis is a disease of children; the incidence is 6 to 7 cases per 100 children per year, with most cases occurring during the first 2 years of life.

Bronchiolitis was first described as a complication of measles and mumps, but in more recent years, it has been associated with infection by most of the respiratory viruses, especially respiratory syncytial virus. Although most cases of bronchiolitis are caused by viruses, *H. influenzae* type b and *M. pneumoniae* have been implicated in some cases. Outbreaks generally occur in the winter and spring in temperate climates, and epidemics are usually associated with respiratory syncytial virus, influenza virus, adenovirus, or parainfluenza virus.

Airways from 75 to 300 μm in diameter are involved. Following invasion by microorganisms, cellular infiltration and edema develop together with proliferation and necrosis of the bronchiolar epithelium. The secretion of mucus is increased, and the mucus, inflammatory exudate, and cell debris obstruct the bronchioles. Adenoviruses cause a more severe disruption of the mucosa than respiratory syncytial viruses—a necrotizing bronchiolitis with a higher mortality.

The initial symptoms of nasal discharge and cough are indistinguishable from those of the common cold. Within 1 to 2 days, fever and cough become prominent and are soon followed by tachypnea and suprasternal, substernal, and subcostal retraction. To prevent coughing and reduce the work of breathing, infants and children breathe rapidly and shallowly. Deep breaths are accompanied by fine rales

and diffuse expiratory wheezing and usually trigger a paroxysm of coughing. Hypercapnia and cyanosis commonly develop as the work of breathing increases, and infants less than 6 months of age may present with apnea.

The peripheral white blood cell count may be normal or moderately elevated. Blood gas analysis typically shows profound hypoxemia. Chest roentgenograms reveal hyperinflation, increased bronchial markings, and frequently areas of atelectasis or infiltrate. The densities on chest films may be more striking than the degree of clinical or radiographic evidence of small-airway obstruction and so misinterpreted as pneumonia. It should be emphasized, however, that these pulmonary densities represent predominantly areas of atelectasis.

The normal terminal bronchiole of less than 0.1 mm in diameter is beyond the resolving capability of high-resolution computed tomography (HRCT). Together with the dilation and wall thickening that accompany bronchiolar inflammation, a number of abnormalities have been described by HRCT. Most commonly, a nonspecific pattern of linear or nodular peripheral opacities, the "tree in bud" appearance, is present (30). Most experienced clinicians are comfortable establishing the diagnosis of bronchiolitis on clinical grounds, so that HRCT is not generally necessary.

A specific diagnosis often can be made retrospectively by the study of paired sera for antibodies to viruses or mycoplasmata. Nasopharyngeal secretions can be obtained for viral culture, but growth may require up to 14 days. Respiratory syncytial virus infection can be diagnosed rapidly by antigen detection with the use of immunofluorescence techniques or enzyme-linked immunosorbent assays.

The only specific therapy currently available for bronchiolitis caused by respiratory syncytial virus is ribavirin. Ribavirin has been approved only for infants hospitalized with respiratory syncytial virus infection. It is administered as an aerosol for 8 to 12 hours each day, usually for 2 to 5 days. In a number of relatively small placebo-controlled studies, ribavirin has been associated with more rapid improvement in oxygen saturation levels, but a shorter period of hospitalization has not been shown consistently (31,32). Infants who should be considered for therapy with ribavirin include those at risk for complicated respiratory syncytial virus infection, especially if they are premature or have cardiopulmonary disease.

Bronchodilator therapy is perhaps the most frequently used treatment for bronchiolitis despite the lack of evidence supporting the efficacy of these agents. Bronchodilators are generally administered to more than 80% of hospitalized infants with bronchiolitis, and in a 1995 poll of members of the European Society for Paediatric Infectious Diseases, their use was nearly universal (33).

Corticosteroids have been reported to be used in more than 80% of children with bronchiolitis, but their efficacy has not been established (33). Most controlled clinical trials have demonstrated no significant benefit whether they are given parenterally or orally with or without bronchodilators (34,35).

Antibiotics should not be administered routinely to infants with bronchiolitis because bacteria do not play a causative role. Furthermore, secondary bacterial infection is rarely observed as a complication after bronchiolitis (36).

REFERENCES

1. Gill Y, Scully C. Orofacial odontogenic infections: review of microbiology and current treatment. *Oral Surg Oral Med Oral Pathol* 1990;70:155–158.
2. Kristensen LH, Prag J. Human necrobacillosis, with emphasis on Lemierre's syndrome. *Clin Infect Dis* 2000;31:524–532.
3. Chow AW. Infections of the oral cavity, neck, and head. In: Mandell GL, Bennett JE, Dolin R, eds. *Principles and practice of infectious diseases,* 5th ed. Philadelphia: Churchill Livingstone, 2000:689–702.
4. Gwaltney JM Jr, Druce HM. Efficacy of brompheniramine maleate treatment for rhinovirus colds. *Clin Infect Dis* 1997;25:118–119.
5. Gwaltney JM Jr. Combined antiviral and antimediator treatment of rhinovirus colds. *J Infect Dis* 1992;166:776–782.
6. Jackson JL, Lesho E, Peterson C. Zinc and the common cold: a meta-analysis revisited. *J Nutr* 2000;130:1512S–1515S.
7. Wald ER. Purulent nasal discharge. *Pediatr Infect Dis J* 1991;10:329–333.
8. Lanza DC, Kennedy DW. Adult rhinosinusitis defined. *Otolaryngol Head Neck Surg* 1997;117:S1–S7.
9. Gwaltney JM Jr, Scheld WM, Sande MA, et al. The microbial etiology and antimicrobial therapy of adults with community-acquired sinusitis. *J Allergy Clin Immunol* 1992;90:357–461.
10. Williams JW Jr, Simel DL. Does this patient have sinusitis? Diagnosing acute sinusitis by history and physical examination. *JAMA* 1993;270:1242–1246.
11. Gold SM, Tami TA. Role of middle meatus aspiration culture in the diagnosis of chronic sinusitis. *Laryngoscope* 1997;107:1586–1589.
12. AHCPR. *Diagnosis and treatment of acute bacterial rhinosinusitis.* Rockville, MD: Agency for Health Care Policy and Research, 1999.
13. Sinus and Allergy Health Partnership. Antimicrobial treatment guidelines for acute bacterial rhinosinusitis. *Otolaryngol Head Neck Surg* 2000;123:S1–S32.
14. Lindbaek M, Hjortdal P, Johnsen V. Randomized, double-blind, placebo-controlled trial of penicillin V and amoxicillin in treatment of acute sinus infection in adults. *BMJ* 1996;313:325–329.
15. Kennedy D. Prognostic factors, outcomes, and staging in ethmoid sinus surgery. *Laryngoscope* 1992;102:1–18.
16. Kahn JO, Walker BD. Acute human immunodeficiency virus type 1 infection. *N Engl J Med* 1998;339:33–39.
17. MacGregor RR. *Corynebacterium diphtheriae.* In: Mandell GL, Bennett JE, Dolin R, eds. *Principles and practice of infectious diseases,* 5th ed. Philadelphia: Churchill Livingstone, 2000:2190–2198.
18. Karpathios T, Drakonaki S, Zervoudaki, et al. *Arcanobacterium hemolyticum* in children with presumed streptococcal pharyngotonsillitis or scarlet fever. *J Pediatr* 1992;12:735–737.
19. Watts AMI, McCallum MD. Acute airway obstruction following facial scalding: differential diagnosis between a thermal and infective cause. *Burns* 1996;22:570–573.
20. Carenfelt C. Etiology of acute infectious epiglottitis in adults: septic versus local infection. *Scand J Infect Dis* 1989;21:53–57.
21. Mayo-Smith MF, Spinale JW, Donskey CJ, et al. Acute epiglottitis: an 18-year experience in Rhode Island. *Chest* 1995;108:1640–1647.
22. Andreassen UK, Baer S, Nielsen TG, et al. Acute epiglottitis—25 years' experience with nasotracheal intubation, current management policy and future trends. *J Laryngol Otol* 1992;106:1072–1075.
23. Takala AK, Petola H, Eskola J. Disappearance of epiglottitis during large-scale vaccination with *Hemophilus influenzae* type B conjugate vaccine among children in Finland. *Laryngoscope* 1994;104:731–735.
24. Bourchier D, Dawson KP, Fergusson DM. Humidification in viral croup: a controlled trial. *Aust Paediatr J* 1984;20:289–291.
25. Lenny N, Milner AD. Treatment of acute viral croup. *Arch Dis Child* 1978;53:704–706.
26. Waisman Y, Klein BL, Boenning DA, et al. Prospective randomized double-blind study comparing L-epinephrine and racemic epinephrine aerosols in the treatment of laryngotracheitis (croup). *Pediatrics* 1992;89:302–306.
27. Geelhoed GC, Macdonald WBG. Oral and inhaled steroids in croup: A randomized, placebo-controlled clinical trial. *Pediatr Pulmonol* 1995;20:355–361.
28. Schuller DE. Birck HG. The safety of intubation in croup and epiglottitis: an eight-year follow-up. *Laryngoscope* 1975;85:33–46.
29. Mackay DN. Review: antibiotics are ineffective for acute bronchitis. *ACP J Club* 1997;March/April:39.
30. Waitches GM, Stern EJ. High-resolution CT of peripheral airways diseases. *Radiol Clin North Am* 2002;40:21–29.
31. Hall CB, McBride JT, Walsh EE, et al. Aerosolized ribavirin treatment of infants with respiratory syncytial virus infection: a randomized double-blind study. *N Engl J Med* 1983;308:1443–1447.
32. Smith DW, Frankel LR, Mathers LH, et al. A controlled trial of aerosolized ribavirin in infants receiving mechanical ventilation for severe respiratory syncytial virus infection. *N Engl J Med* 1991;325:24–29.
33. Kimpen JL, Schaad UB. Treatment of respiratory syncytial virus bronchiolitis:1995 poll of members of the European Society for Paediatric Infectious Diseases. *Pediatr Infect Dis J* 1997;16:479–481.
34. Springer C, Bar-Yishay E, Vwayyed K, et al. Corticosteroids do not affect the clinical or physiological status of infants with bronchiolitis. *Pediatr Pulmonol* 1990;9:181–185.
35. DeBenedictis FM, Canny GJ, Levison H. The role of corticosteroids in respiratory diseases of children. *Pediatr Pulmonol* 1996;22:44–57.
36. Hall CB, Powell KR, Schnabel KC, et al. The risk of secondary bacterial infection in infants hospitalized with respiratory syncytial virus infection. *J Pediatr* 1988;113:266–271.

Baum's Textbook of Pulmonary Diseases, 7th ed. Edited by James D. Crapo, Jeffrey Glassroth, Joel Karlinsky, and Talmadge E. King, Jr. Lippincott Williams & Wilkins, Philadelphia © 2004.

Pulmonary Infections in the Immunocompromised Host

18

Jean T. Santamauro · Nicholas J. Vander Els

Suzette Garofano · Diane E. Stover

A characteristic of immunocompromised patients is their susceptibility to infection by agents with little virulence. Patients who have cancer, are receiving chemotherapy or immunosuppressive agents, have acquired immune deficiency syndrome (AIDS) or other acquired or congenital immune defects, or have undergone organ transplantation are included in the category of immunocompromised hosts. As a consequence of the use of more intensive therapy for cancer, widespread successful organ transplantation, and the AIDS epidemic, the number of immunosuppressed patients and the spectrum of disorders to which they are susceptible have markedly increased. Survival continues to improve as a result of more effective prophylaxis and treatment options, including the newer antimicrobial agents. Despite these advances, the lungs remain a target for infection in these patients (1–4).

APPROACH TO THE IMMUNOCOMPROMISED HOST WITH SUSPECTED PULMONARY INFECTION

When confronted with an immunocompromised patient who has pulmonary signs or symptoms, the clinician should address three important questions (5–9):

1. What are the important immunologic abnormalities in this patient?
2. What is the radiographic picture?
3. What is the tempo of the disease process?

Other factors that must be considered include environmental exposures, remote and recent travel history, iatro-

genic procedures, recent antimicrobial therapy, both therapeutic and prophylactic, and, when appropriate, specific organ transplantation.

What Are the Important Immunologic Abnormalities?

Simply stated, most immunologic abnormalities can be categorized according to whether they are caused by B-cell, T-cell, or neutrophil dysfunction (10,11). Neutropenia is the most frequent abnormality associated with neutrophil dysfunction and is common in patients with acute leukemia on myelosuppressive treatment and in those who have undergone bone marrow transplantation. The risk for infection is directly related to the duration of the neutropenia and inversely proportional to the degree—that is, when the cell count falls below $1,000/mm^3$, the risk for infection begins to increase significantly (12). Because the neutrophil is the primary defense against bacteria and opportunistic fungi, such as *Aspergillus*, infections caused by these organisms occur most frequently in neutropenic patients (13).

Deficiencies of humoral factors are seen in patients with some lymphoproliferative disorders, especially chronic lymphocytic leukemia and multiple myeloma, and in those receiving drugs, particularly corticosteroids. Deficiencies of humoral factors predispose patients predominantly to infections caused by encapsulated bacteria, such as *Streptococcus pneumoniae, Haemophilus influenzae, Staphylococcus aureus,* and aerobic Gram-negative bacteria. Infections caused by opportunistic organisms, such as *Pneumocystis carinii,* have been reported in this group but remain uncommon.

Cellular immunodeficiencies are encountered in patients who have lymphoproliferative disorders, especially Hodgkin disease and AIDS; those receiving immunosuppressive therapy, including corticosteroids; those who have undergone bone marrow transplantation; and those with renal

J. T. Santamauro, N. J. Vander Els, and D. E. Stover: Department of Medicine, Weill Medical College of Cornell University, New York, New York.

S. Garofano: Department of Medicine, New York University Medical Center, New York, New York.

insufficiency. The broad spectrum of pulmonary pathogens in this category ranges from pathogenic microbes (e.g., tuberculous and nontuberculous mycobacteria, endemic fungi, and *Legionella* species) to opportunistic organisms (e.g., *P. carinii* and *Strongyloides stercoralis*) and viral pathogens, especially cytomegalovirus (CMV).

What Is the Radiographic Picture?

The patterns on chest radiograph or computed tomographic (CT) scan are helpful, not only in focusing the differential diagnosis on a subset of pulmonary infectious agents, but also in guiding the appropriate diagnostic workup and estimating how urgently a specific diagnosis is required. Although many types of radiographic patterns are useful in developing clinicopathologic correlations, initially it is most important to distinguish between a localized process (i.e., one confined to a lobe or segment) and a process that involves multiple lobes bilaterally, commonly described as diffuse. The presence of a segmental or lobar infiltrate, combined with a clinical history that suggests an acute illness, favors the diagnosis of bacterial pneumonia, whereas diffuse infiltrates suggest opportunistic infections, such as *P. carinii* pneumonia (PCP) and viral pneumonia, or noninfectious causes, such as pulmonary edema (both cardiogenic and noncardiogenic), drug-induced lung injury, and lymphangitic spread of tumor (14).

Other Radiographic Patterns Worth Noting

- *Hilar or mediastinal adenopathy* is suggestive of mycobacterial or pathogenic fungal disease.
- *Nodular lesions* are suggestive of *Nocardia* or *Actinomyces*, atypical mycobacteria, and opportunistic fungi.
- *Bilateral pleural effusions* are suggestive of congestive heart failure, whereas unilateral effusions are more often seen with bacterial, mycobacterial, and fungal infections.
- *Cavitation* is nonspecific and may be seen with all types of bacteria, tuberculous and nontuberculous mycobacteria, pathogenic and opportunistic fungi, and septic emboli.

The radiographic pattern can also help guide the management of the patient. For example, patients who present with an acute onset of a febrile illness and a localized infiltrate usually are treated with antibiotics for bacterial pneumonia, whereas patients who present with diffuse infiltrates frequently undergo a diagnostic procedure, such as a bronchoscopy, because diffuse pulmonary infiltrates indicate a much broader range of diagnostic possibilities.

It should be remembered that the chest radiograph in an immunocompromised host with significant pulmonary disease may appear normal because the inflammatory response is depressed. Chest CT is much more sensitive and may reveal abnormalities even when the chest radiographic findings are normal or subtle. CT of the chest can also be helpful in defining the most appropriate invasive procedure and site for optimal sampling. For example, if CT shows a peripheral nodular density, the yield of fine needle aspiration would be greater than that of fiberoptic bronchoscopy (15).

What Is the Tempo of the Disease Process?

The rate of progression of the radiographic pattern and the rate at which the patient's condition deteriorates can influence decisions regarding whether a response to empiric therapy can be awaited or an invasive procedure should be performed immediately. Bacterial infections are usually acute in onset and may be heralded by fever with shaking chills. PCP in a patient who does not have AIDS can also be acute in onset, but in a patient infected with HIV, it may follow a subacute course, with several weeks elapsing before the patient seeks medical attention. CMV pneumonia more commonly evolves during a period of weeks—a tempo similar to that of pulmonary aspergillosis. Some infections can develop during a period of months, mimicking noninfectious processes. Nocardiosis, tuberculosis (TB), nontuberculous mycobacterial disease, and some fungal infections, such as cryptococcosis, can follow this type of insidious course.

Other Considerations

Other important considerations in forming a differential diagnosis include the temporal relationship of the pulmonary disease to the underlying disease or transplant and the history of previous antimicrobial prophylaxis. For example, a patient who has undergone bone marrow transplantation and has a pulmonary infection within the first month after the procedure is more likely to have a bacterial or opportunistic fungal pneumonia. CMV infection usually develops several months after bone marrow transplantation and almost always after engraftment has taken place (16).

In HIV-infected patients, the differential diagnosis of pulmonary disorders depends in part on the CD4$^+$ cell count. When the CD4$^+$ cell count is higher than 500/mm^3, the patient is likely to have bacterial pneumonia or TB, whereas infection with opportunistic agents, such as *P. carinii*, CMV, and *Aspergillus*, develops when the CD4$^+$ cell counts are much lower (17).

Low intermittent doses of trimethoprim/sulfamethoxazole (TMP/SMX), dapsone, or aerosolized pentamidine are commonly administered to patients at risk for PCP. As a result, the incidence of PCP has decreased. In HIV-infected patients, the risk for PCP has further declined with the advent of highly effective antiretroviral therapy.

The physical examination findings at times can be helpful. For example, the presence of bilateral rales in a patient with a unilateral infiltrate would alter the diagnostic spectrum.

More importantly, the physical appearance can convey an immediate sense of how sick the patient is.

GENERAL APPROACH TO PULMONARY INFECTION IN IMMUNOCOMPROMISED HOSTS

Summary Statement	Level of Evidence

Consider the following:
  Immunologic defect
  Radiographic pattern
  Disease tempo
  Environmental exposures
  Travel history
  Iatrogenic procedures
  Antimicrobial therapy
  Organ transplant (when appropriate)
	Observational studies
	and expert opinion

DIAGNOSTIC PROCEDURES

Noninvasive Procedures

Diagnosing a pulmonary infection in an immunocompromised host is often difficult because the spectrum of potential agents is broad. Sputum is often not available, and antibody titers are usually insensitive and nonspecific. Examination of the sputum, either spontaneously produced or induced by inhalation of hypertonic saline solution (3%–5%), may be useful to diagnose mycobacterial disease (spontaneous or induced) or *P. carinii* infection (induced) (18,19). The highest yields from the induction of sputum to diagnose *P. carinii* infection are obtained in HIV-infected patients and range from 55% to 95% (18). If TB is suspected, sputum induction should be reserved for patients who do not expectorate sputum or whose expectorated sputum is negative on smear.

Sputum analysis to diagnose bacterial pneumonia in this patient population is controversial. Finding an acid-fast organism on smear is sufficient evidence to prompt the initiation of anti-TB therapy. Special preparations can be applied to sputum to provide immediate diagnostic information: India ink staining of a wet preparation of sputum can show encapsulated budding yeast forms of *Cryptococcus* species; a wet mount of sputum, the parasitic larvae of *Strongyloides* species; and Giemsa, Gram-Weigert, or toluidine blue O stains of induced sputum, the cyst wall of *P. carinii*. Direct fluorescent antibody staining provides a specific means of identifying *Legionella* species, but its sensitivity is low, whereas immunofluorescent monoclonal antibody staining for *P. carinii* provides some of the highest diagnostic yields (20). Sputum examination is of greatest value when organisms that are not normally present in the oropharynx are seen or isolated in culture. For example, sputum cultures that grow *Cryptococcus* and *Nocardia* organisms are almost always pathogenic in the immunocompromised host, whereas isolation of *Candida* species usually represents contamination or colonization of the upper respiratory tract.

The presence of serum cryptococcal antigen is considered highly useful in the diagnosis of invasive cryptococcosis, and the measurement of *Histoplasma capsulatum* antigen has been helpful in diagnosing histoplasmosis and following the response of HIV patients to treatment. Other skin and serologic testing is of very little value in the diagnosis of acute infections in the immunocompromised host (21).

Polymerase chain reaction (PCR), DNA probes, nucleic acid hybridization, and antigen detection are techniques with the potential for rapidly diagnosing many infections, but the number of available validated assays is limited. Sensitivities and specificities above 90% have been reported for PCR on sputum in the diagnosis of *Mycobacterium tuberculosis* infection (22). Similar results have been reported for PCR on oral washes in the diagnosis of PCP (23).

Noninvasive tests such as gallium scanning, pulmonary function testing, and rest and exercise oximetry are sensitive for the detection of pulmonary disease but are nonspecific for an etiologic diagnosis. These tests are most helpful when the presence of pulmonary disease is in doubt, particularly when the chest radiographic findings are normal or subtle.

Invasive Procedures

The invasive procedures most commonly used to make a specific diagnosis include fiberoptic bronchoscopy (FOB) with transbronchial biopsy (TBB) and bronchoalveolar lavage (BAL), transthoracic (TTNA) or fine needle aspiration (FNA), and video-assisted thoracoscopic surgery (VATS) or open lung biopsy (OLB). The decision to perform an invasive procedure often depends on the therapeutic options (e.g., amphotericin B vs. corticosteroid therapy), the tempo of the disease, the patient's prognosis based on the underlying disease, and lastly, the patient's wishes.

The selection of the optimal invasive procedure is determined by the nature (i.e., focal vs. diffuse) and location of the pulmonary lesions, the patient's underlying medical condition, including clotting parameters, and the facilities and skills available to the treating physician. Diffuse lesions are usually sampled by TBB and BAL, whereas nodules, particularly if they are peripheral in location, are best sampled by CT-guided needle aspiration (TTNA, FNA) or open biopsy procedures (VATS, OLB) (5,24–28).

Flexible Fiberoptic Bronchoscopy

In 1967, Shigeto Ikeda designed and standardized the flexible fiberoptic bronchoscope. Flexible FOB is the single most important technique that has advanced the diagnosis of pulmonary disorders in the immunocompromised host. It is ideal for this patient population because it can be performed safely in the setting of mechanical ventilation and in patients with thrombocytopenia or other platelet dysfunction. Although the sensitivity and specificity of FOB vary with the immunocompromised population, generally bronchoscopy with BAL and TBB has an overall diagnostic yield of 50% to 70% in non–HIV-immunocompromised hosts, and the diagnostic yield may be as high as 90% in HIV-infected patients undergoing the procedure. The yield is higher in infectious than in noninfectious complications, and the infections most commonly diagnosed by bronchoscopy include PCP, CMV infection, and mycobacterial disease. The importance of bronchoscopy in diagnosing CMV pneumonia is declining as a consequence of the use of CMV serum antigen screening in patients at high risk (29). The infectious diseases most commonly missed include fungal disease, especially aspergillosis. When infection other than bacterial pneumonia is considered, investigators have reported sensitivities and specificities ranging from 80% to 90% in non–HIV-infected patients and higher than 90% in HIV-infected patients. Even with TBB, the yields in noninfectious disorders, such as drug-induced lung injury, metastatic disease, and pulmonary hemorrhage, are lower than those in infectious disorders.

Generally to avoid multiple sequential procedures, most experts recommend adding TBB to BAL when possible. However, depending on the patient's underlying immune defect, recent history of therapy and prophylaxis, and likely pulmonary disease, samples obtained from bronchoscopy vary. In HIV-related opportunistic infections, BAL is highly sensitive because large numbers of organisms are present in the lavaged alveoli. In patients with a bone marrow transplant, CMV pneumonia is common, and the finding of CMV antigens in the BAL fluid, even in the absence of histopathologic correlation, is significant. In patients who are likely to have bacterial pneumonia, the specimen should include material from the involved area obtained with a protected catheter. For this technique to have adequate specificity and sensitivity, quantitative bacterial counts must be performed. Concurrent antibiotic therapy markedly blunts the yield. Because of this drawback, the procedure has not gained widespread use in immunocompromised patients.

The obvious limitation of BAL is that it does not provide tissue for histologic examination. Hence, BAL should be supplemented by TBB, especially when a noninfectious etiology is suspected. Biopsy does add to the risk of the bronchoscopic procedure, particularly in patients with an uncorrectable coagulation disorder or pulmonary hypertension. TBB also entails a risk for pneumothorax, which is increased in patients on mechanical ventilation. However, the rates of major complications of bronchoscopy in the immunocompromised population remain low and range from 0.08% to 5%, with mortality rates from 0.01% to 0.5%. Besides bleeding and pneumothorax, other serious complications include respiratory depression and hypotension from sedation, laryngospasm, bronchospasm, and hypoxemia. Fever usually follows bronchoscopy and BAL but is self-limited and not associated with infection. FOB carries a very low risk for infection, and prophylactic antibiotics are not routinely recommended.

Transthoracic (or Fine) Needle Aspiration

The major indication for fluoroscopically or CT-guided TTNA is the presence of pulmonary nodules, especially if they are peripheral and less than 2 cm in size (26). TTNA has the advantage of directly sampling the diseased area, so that a small core of lung tissue or lung fluid can be examined both microbiologically and cytologically. The diagnostic yield for infections ranges from 40% to 90%, with the higher yields reported for nonbacterial infections. The most common complication of TTNA is pneumothorax, which occurs in 10% to 37% of procedures; however, chest tube placement is required in fewer than half of the patients. Other complications include hemoptysis, which is usually self-limited, intraparenchymal hemorrhage, venous air embolism, subcutaneous emphysema, and infrequently hemopericardium when lesions are located near the pulmonary artery. The mortality rate associated with these procedures is about 0.2%. Contraindications to performing TTNA (FNA) include an uncooperative patient, excessive coughing, uncorrectable coagulopathy, and a hydatid cyst. Relative contraindications include severe emphysema, previous pneumonectomy, pulmonary artery hypertension, mechanical ventilation, and a suspected vascular lesion.

Open Lung Biopsy and Video-Assisted Thoracoscopic Surgery

OLB procedures are the most reliable for obtaining lung tissue, and a specific diagnosis is made in 65% to 88% of patients, with a 5% to 8% morbidity rate and 0.5% to 2% mortality rate (27). The major advantage of open procedures is that they can be performed promptly; the diagnosis can be made rapidly and without concern that a process is being overlooked. Additional advantages of open procedures are that the area to be sampled can be selected under direct vision, effective hemostasis can be achieved even in the presence of a coagulopathy, and the procedure can be performed in severely ill patients on mechanical ventilation. Even when a definitive diagnosis is not made, some toxic therapies often can be discontinued by ruling out certain diagnoses. The disadvantages include the requirement for an operating room and general anesthesia, the potential for postoperative infection or chronic air leak, and postoperative pain and chest tube placement.

VATS in this patient population appears to be of equal diagnostic accuracy and may be less invasive than standard thoracotomy, with less postoperative morbidity. In patients

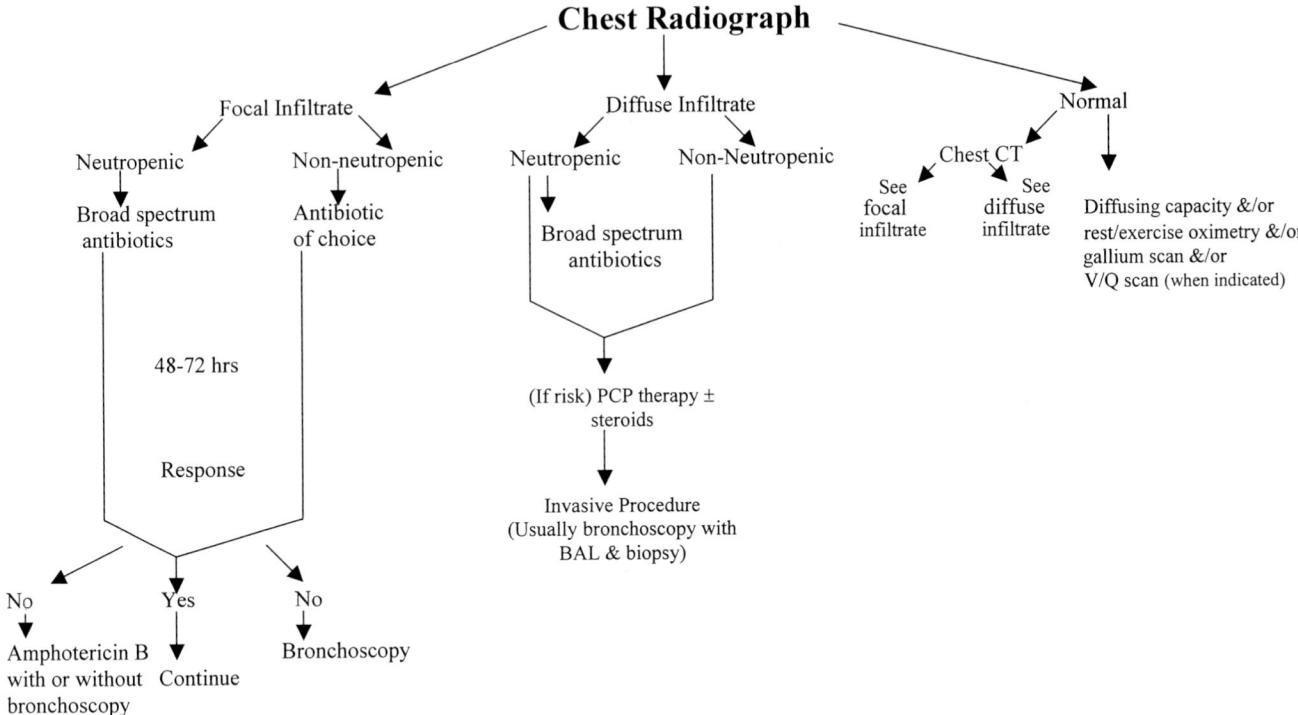

FIGURE 18.1. Algorithm for the approach to immunocompromised patients with suspected pulmonary infections based on presenting chest radiograph/chest computed tomographic scan. In patients with HIV infection, routine stains and culture of sputum for bacteria, fungi, and acid-fast bacilli may be helpful to guide initial therapy, and sputum induction should be considered when *Pneumocystis carinii* pneumonia or tuberculosis is suspected.

who are not immunocompromised, respiratory compromise, pain, chest tube drainage time, and hospital stay are all less after VATS than after conventional thoracotomy. In our experience, the diagnostic yield and complication rate of VATS are similar to those of conventional thoracotomy in immunocompromised patients. VATS also appears to be safe in patients with thrombocytopenia but can be performed only in those who can tolerate single-lung ventilation. Larger studies are necessary to evaluate further the limitations and complication rates of VATS in the immunocompromised patient population.

EMPIRIC THERAPY

Empiric treatment is often initially undertaken based on the nature of the defect in host defenses, the most likely pathogens, and the chest radiographic presentation. If the patient's condition improves, therapy is sometimes continued without a definitive diagnosis. If the patient's condition does not improve or worsens on empiric treatment, a decision then has to be made about performing an invasive procedure or adding other nonspecific therapies. This decision depends on a number of factors, including the diagnostic possibilities, treatment options, toxicity associated with the options, severity and pace of the pulmonary process, and most im-

portantly, the ultimate prognosis and wishes of the patient (Fig. 18.1).

SPECIFIC PATHOGENS

Bacteria

Organisms such as *S. pneumoniae* and *H. influenzae,* which commonly infect immunocompetent patients, are also the most common cause of pneumonia in immunocompromised patients. The humoral immunity of patients with B-cell defects, such as those associated with chronic lymphocytic leukemia, small cell lymphocytic lymphoma, and multiple myeloma, is defective, and they are especially susceptible to infection with these encapsulated organisms. Defects in humoral immunity are also found among patients with common variable immunodeficiency (CVID), a heterogeneous syndrome characterized by hypogammaglobulinemia. The consequence of repeated infection may be the development of bronchiectasis and respiratory insufficiency. Martinez Garcia and colleagues (30) found that bronchiectasis developed in 11 (58%) of 19 patients with CVID. In 8 (41%) of the patients, the involvement was multilobar. Ekdahl and colleagues (31), studying patients admitted for recurrent pneumonias in Sweden, found that 11 (29%) of 38 had some underlying immunoglobulin deficiency.

Susceptibility to infection with encapsulated organisms is not limited to patients with immunoglobulin defects. Patients with defects of complement function, such as sickle cell anemia, are also susceptible, as are patients who have undergone splenectomy.

The spectrum of flora in granulocytopenic patients differs from that in patients with B-cell defects. Carratala and colleagues (32) studied 408 patients with neutropenia and bacteremia and identified 40 with pneumonia. *P. aeruginosa* and *S. pneumoniae* accounted for 73% of the cases (17 and 12 cases, respectively), with significant numbers of *Escherichia coli* and *Streptococcus mitis* (5 and 3 cases, respectively) also seen. Of the streptococcal species, 47% were penicillin-resistant and also showed decreased susceptibility to ceftazidime.

Bacterial pneumonia is more common in HIV-infected patients, and the incidence increases with the progression of immunocompromise. The Pulmonary Complications of HIV Infection Study Group (PCHISG) monitored a cohort of 1,130 HIV-infected patients and 167 HIV-negative adults for 64 months (33,34). In that period, the HIV-infected patients had 237 cases of bacterial pneumonia, a rate of 5.5 episodes per 100 patient-years, compared with 6 episodes for the HIV-negative adults, a rate of 0.9 episodes per 100 patient-years. The rate of pneumonia increased as the $CD4^+$ cell count fell. When patients were stratified into groups with $CD4^+$ cell counts per cubic millimeter above 500, between 200 and 500, and below 200, the rates of pneumonia were 2.3, 6.8, and 10.8 episodes per 100 patient-years, respectively. Cordero and colleagues (35) found a similar trend. In a study limited to 26 HIV-infected patients hospitalized with pneumonia secondary to *H. influenzae* infection, the majority of patients (73%) had a $CD4^+$ cell count below $100/mm^3$. The PCHISG found that regardless of the $CD4^+$ cell count, the incidence of pneumonia was higher in injection drug users than in the other HIV-infected patients.

When hospitalized patients are studied, pseudomonal species become more prominent. Afessa and Green (36) found that bacterial pneumonia accounted for 111 (9%) of 1,225 admissions among HIV-infected patients at the University of Florida. Community-acquired pneumonia accounted for 80 (72%) of 111 cases of pneumonia. The most common pathogen was *P. aeruginosa* (32 admissions), followed by *S. pneumoniae* (22 admissions), *S. aureus* (16 admissions), and *H. influenzae* (11 admissions). Bacteremia occurred in 33 (30%) of the patients and was most commonly a consequence of pneumococcal infection (21 patients).

Antibiotics given as prophylaxis against *P. carinii* and *Mycobacterium avium* complex (MAC) infection are protective against bacterial pneumonias. In the PCHISG study, the use of TMP/SMX was associated with a 67% reduction in bacterial pneumonia, not surprising given that *S. pneumoniae* was their most commonly isolated specimen (36 cultures), followed by *S. aureus* (13 specimens) and *H. influenzae* (12 specimens) (34).

The use of clarithromycin, given as prophylaxis against MAC infection, also provides protection against bacterial pneumonia. Currier and colleagues (37) studied 394 HIV-infected patients for 21 months. The study included bacteremia and the development of deep visceral abscesses as index events, together with bacterial pneumonia, under the heading "serious bacterial infections." Overall, there were 56 such infections, associated with increased mortality. Both clarithromycin and TMP/SMX had significant protective effects.

The effect of highly active antiretroviral therapy (HAART) on bacterial pneumonia in HIV-infected patients is less clear. Some discrepancies in the reports are related to differing methods of patient accrual. Wolff and O'Donnell (38) found PCP to be less prevalent and bacterial infections more common in the post-HAART era. They reviewed pulmonary referrals seen at Georgetown from 1993 to 1995 and compared them with referrals seen from 1997 to 2000. Patients with PCP accounted for 74 (36%) of 204 consultations from the pre-HAART era, compared with 9 (17%) of 51 patients receiving HAART. Conversely, bacterial pneumonia was seen in 59 (29%) of the 204 pre-HAART patients, compared with 24 (47%) of the 51 patients receiving HAART. There is an element of bias in the study in that patients were drawn from the records of consultations with the pulmonary service. The findings seem to contradict those of Sullivan and colleagues (39), who found that years of HAART resulted in a decreased incidence of community-acquired pneumonia. The study of Wolff and O'Donnell included patients with nosocomial pneumonia and was based on patients sick enough to require a pulmonary consult. As such, it reflects the clinical spectrum seen in an inpatient practice.

Immunocompromised hosts are susceptible to infection with a number of less common bacteria, such as *Nocardia* and *Rhodococcus* (40–44). *Nocardia* can infect immunocompetent as well as immunocompromised hosts; it is seen in patients on steroid therapy or with hematologic malignancies in addition to HIV-infected patients. Radiographically, it presents as small nodules and has a predilection for the skin and central nervous system. *Nocardia* is one of the so-called higher bacteria. It is a Gram-positive rod with a complex, branching structure that appears lacy and beaded on Gram stain and acid-fast bacillus (AFB) stain. It is seen better on Fite stain, a modified AFB stain. With the silver stain used for fungi, it appears black and resembles the reticulum strands within the lung. An index of suspicion must exist for the laboratory to find it. *Nocardia* grows on the standard media used for bacterial cultures of respiratory specimens, but it does not always grow before such cultures are discarded. It is our practice to request that specimens from immunocompromised hosts be held for *Nocardia* culture. The treatment of choice is 6 months of TMP/SMX.

Rhodococcus equi is seen mainly in HIV-infected patients, but it may also affect patients with hematologic malignancies and others with severe immunosuppression. It is a

Gram-negative rod generally acquired through proximity to horses. It can cause disseminated disease (42,45). An intracellular organism, it is best treated with erythromycin.

Legionella is a common cause of pneumonia that is difficult to culture. It can colonize the water systems in hospitals, causing nosocomial spread, especially among transplant patients (46,47). It can be removed from the water system by superheating or copper–silver ionization. The clinical presentations are protean, varying from indolent fevers to fulminant respiratory failure. The use of macrolides for treatment is problematic in transplant patients because of the interaction with immunosuppressive agents, especially cyclosporine. Quinolones can be used successfully to treat such patients (48).

Mycobacteria

Tuberculous Mycobacteria

The host response to TB is controlled almost entirely by cell-mediated immunity, primarily involving the macrophage and the $CD4^+$ cell (49). Clinical tuberculosis after infection with *M. tuberculosis* (MTB) develops in fewer than 10% of immunocompetent hosts (50). In the typical sequence of events, an aerosol droplet containing MTB enters a lower lobe alveolus, where it is taken up by an alveolar macrophage. Migration to the hilar and mediastinal lymph nodes follows, after which a bacteremic phase occurs in which MTB encounters host $CD4^+$ cells. Acquired cellular immunity to MTB develops in the form of a clone of $CD4^+$ cells specific for MTB. These cells produce interferon-γ, which activates the macrophages to kill phagocytosed MTB throughout the body, a process less efficient in the apex of the lung (51,52). Immunocompromise may affect any of these steps. Clinical TB may begin if the macrophages fail to inactivate the initial inoculum, in which case primary TB develops in the form of lower lobe infiltrates. Bacteria may multiply in the lymph nodes, causing tuberculous lymphadenitis. The bacteremic phase may lead to disseminated TB. Containment of the initial infection does not preclude reactivation of residual bacteria as postprimary TB at a later date.

One would expect the incidence of clinical disease after infection to be higher in patients with impaired cellular immunity, with increased numbers of cases of primary and disseminated disease. This phenomenon has been best documented in HIV-infected patients (52). The radiographic and clinical presentations change as the $CD4^+$ cell count decreases. In the study of Greenberg and colleagues (53), the radiographs of most HIV-infected patients with TB showed patterns suggestive of primary disease (53). As the $CD4^+$ cell count fell, a normal chest radiograph became as common as a postprimary pattern.

The increased prevalence of primary patterns on chest radiographs reflects the changing epidemiology in the community. Studies from the Bronx and San Francisco charac-

terized MTB isolates by using restriction fragment length polymorphisms to map the spread of disease. In the Bronx, 37% of TB cases represented primary disease, and in San Francisco, 31% of cases were primary disease (54,55). Before the HIV epidemic, only 10% of TB cases were primary disease.

In addition to a higher incidence of primary disease, HIV-infected patients also have a higher incidence of disseminated disease. Jones and colleagues (56) found that 22 (29%) of 75 AIDS patients with TB had positive blood cultures. The proportion increased to 18 (49%) of 37 patients with a $CD4^+$ cell count below $100/mm^3$. In general, extrapulmonary disease becomes more common as the $CD4^+$ cell count falls. It was seen in 5 (28%) of 18 of patients with a $CD4^+$ cell count above $300/mm^3$ and in 30 (70%) of 43 patients with a $CD4^+$ cell count below $100/mm^3$.

Extrapulmonary disease is common in HIV-infected patients. No site that can be sampled should be overlooked. Enlarged extrathoracic lymph nodes are present in 20% of HIV-infected patients with TB, and 77% are positive on smear after aspiration. In combination with culture, the yield of such sampling is 96%. Pleural involvement is common, seen in 10% of HIV-infected patients with TB. The yield on culture of pleural fluid approaches 90% (57).

The collection of sputum for smear and culture remains the cornerstone of diagnosis. In HIV-infected patients, a positive smear is 80% specific for active TB. The high specificity of the AFB smear makes the use of direct amplification tests (DATs) problematic (22,58). These are PCR tests that can be applied to a sputum smear to detect RNA as well as DNA genetic material of MTB. Barnes (58) has postulated a number of scenarios regarding their clinical application. For a patient with a positive AFB smear, DAT has a sensitivity and specificity of 95%. The positive predictive value of these tests is 98%, but the negative predictive value is low, at 37%. Given the urgency of beginning treatment for TB in an AIDS patient with a positive AFB smear, a positive DAT result adds little to the decision to start treatment. On the other hand, a negative DAT result would be insufficient evidence to withhold treatment from such a patient. The use of DAT is also problematic in patients with negative AFB smears. TB can progress rapidly in HIV-infected patients. A negative DAT result would not entirely exclude the diagnosis in a smear-negative patient, and the consequences of discontinuing treatment can be dire.

Bronchoscopy can be effective for the diagnosis of TB, but its use is associated with a risk for infecting the bronchoscopist and support staff (59). Its use is generally limited to patients with negative sputum smears (expectorated or induced) and those unable to produce sputum. Saltzman and colleagues (60) were able to make an early diagnosis in 39% of patients with TB when TBB was included. In 2000, Conde and colleagues (61) compared sputum induction with BAL in 251 patients with suspected TB, 44 of whom were infected with HIV. Patients were included who could not produce expectorated sputum or who had one negative specimen. The sensitivity was the same for both sputum induction and BAL. Of the 25 patients found on long-term follow-up to have had TB, 9 (36%) had a positive smear on sputum induction and 10 (40%) had a positive smear on BAL. The smears agreed in 43 of 44 patients. By culture, both sputum induction and BAL were positive in 15 (60%) of 25 patients. The smear and culture from BAL added little information to a well-performed sputum induction for diagnosing TB. However, not all patients can produce a specimen on sputum induction, and BAL has been found useful for diagnosing nontuberculous infections related to HIV. Saltzman and colleagues (60) found that 16% of their early-diagnosed cases came from the addition of TBB.

The literature regarding TB and other types of immune defects is scant save for descriptions of the groups at risk for reactivation. Kaplan and colleagues (62) at Memorial Sloan-Kettering Cancer Center reviewed 201 patients with TB and cancer. TB was most commonly seen in patients with head and neck cancer (45 patients) and lung cancer (44 patients). Those with lymphoproliferative disorders had the highest mortality (48%). It was noted that TB in patients with head and neck cancer or lung cancer was generally present at the time the cancer was diagnosed, whereas in other patients, especially those with lymphoproliferative disease, TB developed after they had received immunosuppressant therapy. The strongest association was with the use of steroids. These patients were culled from hospital admissions between 1950 and 1971. The results might differ now because significant advances have been made in the chemotherapy of both cancer and TB. Patients treated with bone marrow transplantation may be as profoundly immunocompromised as HIV-infected patients. One would expect a similar pathophysiology, but the records of TB are limited to a few case reports (63,64).

Therapy for TB in HIV-infected patients involves the same drug regimens as those used for patients not infected with HIV. However, the type of antiretroviral therapy prescribed must be considered. Rifampin induces cytochrome P-450 CYP3A, and induction hastens the metabolism of protease inhibitors and nonnucleoside reverse transcriptase inhibitors to subtherapeutic levels (50,52). Therapy is discussed fully in Chapter 20.

The risk for progression to clinical TB after infection with MTB is highest in HIV-infected patients; clinical disease develops in approximately 10% each year, where it develops in 10% of immunocompetent hosts during the course of a lifetime (50). Six months of daily isoniazid given to patients with a purified protein derivative tuberculin skin test result larger than 5 mm reduces progression to clinical disease by 70%. Twelve months of isoniazid reduces the risk by 93%. The current recommendation is for 9 months. An alternative regimen is for 2 months of rifampin and pyrazinamide (50,52,65).

Nontuberculous Mycobacteria

The most common nontuberculous mycobacterial infection in the United States is MAC infection. In HIV-infected patients, the disease is not pulmonary, but disseminated (66). MAC is commonly considered a colonizer of sputum. In the absence of evidence of disseminated disease, the decision to treat is made only after other pulmonary infections have been excluded. Pulmonary disease is more typically seen in older patients or those with underlying chronic lung disease than in HIV-infected immunocompromised patients. Malouf and Glanville (67) found MAC to be a significant pulmonary pathogen among lung transplant patients. Of 261 patients studied, the course of 23 (9%) after transplant was complicated by mycobacterial infection. MAC was the most prevalent cause of pulmonary disease, affecting 13 patients, with MTB a distant second, affecting two patients. These infections responded well to the regimen of clarithromycin, ethambutol, and rifampin. In that same series, five patients had disseminated *Mycobacterium haemophilum* infection, characterized by extensive cutaneous lesions. *M. haemophilum* is an emerging pathogen among severely immunocompromised patients. It is generally seen in patients with HIV infection or those who have received a bone marrow transplant (68). However, rare reports have appeared of disease in immunocompetent hosts (69). Isolation of this organism is simple, but not routine. It will grow on standard media for mycobacteria that have been supplemented with iron. Iron supplementation is not technically difficult, but the pulmonologist must specify that *M. haemophilum* is suspected when sending specimens to the laboratory, so that the appropriate media can be set up. This has become standard procedure in some transplant centers. *M. haemophilum* infection responds to regimens containing isoniazid, rifampin or rifabutin, ciprofloxacin, and amikacin. *Mycobacterium kansasii* has a predilection for patients with hairy cell leukemia, who often present with disseminated disease. Other pathogenic mycobacteria that can be seen in the immunocompromised host but are uncommon include *Mycobacterium xenopi*, *Mycobacterium chelonae*, and *Mycobacterium fortuitum*.

Fungi

Opportunistic Fungi

Aspergillus

Aspergillus is a filamentous fungus widely distributed in nature; it is found in soil, water, and decaying matter. Conidial heads, or spores, exist when the organism is grown in nature and are ubiquitous in the air. *Aspergillus fumigatus* and *Aspergillus flavus* account for the majority of human infections.

Invasive disease occurs in the immunocompromised host after the spores are inhaled from the environment; in a minority of patients, the invasive disease disseminates. Neutrophils and macrophages are the most important components of host defense against invasive *Aspergillus* infection. Persons at risk for invasive *Aspergillus* infection include patients with prolonged neutropenia, on long-term corticosteroid therapy, on prolonged antibiotic therapy or chemotherapy, or with a previous history of *Aspergillus* infection. *Aspergillus* infection has been reported in increasing numbers of patients with HIV infection but without other predisposing conditions. This increase is likely a consequence of defects in B-lymphocyte, neutrophil, and monocyte/macrophage function and the effects of cytokines that develop in HIV-infected patients in the later stages of AIDS in addition to the well-known abnormalities of T helper cells (70).

Classically, invasive aspergillosis is described in patients with hematologic malignancies recently treated with chemotherapy who have prolonged periods of profound neutropenia and have been exposed to broad-spectrum antibiotics. Invasive pulmonary aspergillosis occurs in about 6% of these patients (71). As a consequence of prolonged immunosuppression, invasive aspergillosis is a very frequent complication in patients with bone marrow transplants. Invasive aspergillosis also develops in patients with solid organ transplants, but to a lesser degree than in patients with leukemia or lymphoma. It develops in about 1% of HIV-infected patients, usually those with a CD4$^+$ cell count below 50/mm^3, on corticosteroid therapy, or with neutropenia (72,73)

Pulmonary involvement is the most common presentation of invasive *Aspergillus* infection in the neutropenic or HIV-infected patient. Patients with invasive pulmonary aspergillosis present with fever unresponsive to antibiotics, chest pain, nonproductive cough, and hemoptysis (74). *Aspergillus* tends to invade blood vessels, sometimes causing massive hemoptysis, a rare but well-described and at times fatal complication. The physical examination can be unrevealing, although patients may have a friction rub, localized rales, wheezes, or splinting as a result of significant chest pain. The radiographic findings may be normal, especially in isolated cases of *Aspergillus* bronchitis, but more often they demonstrate single or multiple focal nodular infiltrates that may progress and cavitate. On chest CT, a halo of ground-glass attenuation surrounding a masslike infiltrate is highly suggestive of fungal pneumonia (75). The development of the air crescent sign later in the course of the disease is also highly suggestive of *Aspergillus* pneumonia. The crescent develops as a consequence of necrosis of the lung tissue as the neutrophil count increases in neutropenic patients (76). Invasion of blood vessels by the fungus may produce pulmonary infarcts that present as pleura-based, wedge-shaped infiltrates.

Establishing the diagnosis of *Aspergillus* pneumonia in the immunocompromised host is difficult. Because of profound thrombocytopenia and coagulopathies in large numbers of patients at risk for invasive *Aspergillus* infection, biopsy specimens are often not obtained. Without biopsy material, it is difficult to establish the diagnosis of invasive disease definitively. Patients at high risk for invasive fungal pneumonia with persistent fever unresponsive to antibacterial therapy and suggestive radiographs are often presumed to have invasive fungal disease and are routinely treated empirically. Attempts should be made to establish a diagnosis of *Aspergillus* infection because it may help to tailor therapy. Sputum specimens should be obtained, and if *Aspergillus* is found, the presumptive diagnosis of invasive *Aspergillus* infection can be made in the proper clinical setting (77). Because these patients are at risk for other opportunistic infections and pulmonary complications of their disease and therapy, FOB is often pursued to try to establish a diagnosis. The yield of bronchoscopy with washings and BAL is 50% for *Aspergillus* at our institution, and in the literature it is 30% to 100% (78,79). Serologic studies are unreliable for establishing the diagnosis of aspergillosis in these patients (71,80). Surgical biopsies are rarely undertaken to diagnose aspergillosis.

Only two agents have been approved for the therapy of aspergillosis—amphotericin B and itraconazole. Intravenous therapy is the preferred initial route of administration, especially in acutely ill patients, to ensure absorption. Formerly, amphotericin B was the only intravenous preparation available, but itraconazole now has an intravenous formulation.

Systemic amphotericin B has been the mainstay of therapy for invasive pulmonary aspergillosis, but it has many adverse effects and a suboptimal overall response rate of about 55% (81,82). The response rates vary depending on the underlying disease, extent of infection, and resolution of the underlying immunodeficiency, among other factors. In a review of published case series including a total of 1,223 cases, the response rate to more than 14 days of amphotericin B deoxycholate was 83% in patients with heart and kidney transplants, 54% in leukemic patients, 33% in bone marrow transplant recipients, and 20% in liver transplant recipients (81). HIV-infected patients had a 37% response, and many of them had also received itraconazole (81).

Three new lipid formulations of amphotericin B have been developed and approved; these include amphotericin B lipid complex, amphotericin B cholesteryl sulfate, and liposomal amphotericin B (83). These agents have an improved safety profile in comparison with amphotericin B deoxycholate; a decrease in nephrotoxicity and fewer side effects during infusion allow higher doses of the drug to be delivered (83,84). In addition, higher tissue concentrations of the drug accumulate in the lungs, liver, and spleen (85). In patients with invasive pulmonary aspergillosis or febrile neutropenia, lipid formulations of amphotericin B were found to be as efficacious but not superior to amphotericin B deoxycholate (86–88). A study comparing the toxicities of liposomal amphotericin B and amphotericin B lipid complex favored liposomal amphotericin B (89). These agents are much more expensive than amphotericin B deoxycholate, costing as much as 10 to 20 times more per dose (85). The recommended doses of amphotericin B in invasive disease are 1 to 1.5 mg of amphotericin B deoxycholate per kilogram per day, or the equivalent of 5 mg of the lipid formulations per kilogram per day (90). Indications for the lipid formulations of amphotericin B include renal insufficiency (creatinine >2.5 mg/dL), severe infusion side effects despite adequate premedications, and disease progression after the equivalent of 500 mg of amphotericin B deoxycholate (85).

Itraconazole, the new triazole, has been approved by the Food and Drug Administration for the treatment of aspergillosis. In patients with febrile neutropenia, itraconazole was found to be as effective as conventional amphotericin B, with fewer side effects (91). No controlled trials comparing amphotericin B with itraconazole in invasive pulmonary aspergillosis have been performed, but smaller studies suggest that itraconazole may be a reasonable alternative to amphotericin B deoxycholate, especially in patients with respiratory disease (82). In two studies, oral itraconazole induced a complete or partial response in 39% to 63% of patients (92,93). The recommended dose of oral itraconazole is 200 mg three times daily for 4 days, then 200 mg twice a day. In a study of 31 patients with invasive pulmonary aspergillosis treated initially with intravenous itraconazole for 14 days, then with 12 weeks of oral therapy, 25.8% showed a complete response, 22.6% had a partial response, and 19.4% had stable disease (94). The optimal duration of therapy with itraconazole in invasive pulmonary aspergillosis is unknown, but the suggested duration is 6 to 12 months in non–HIV-immunocompromised patients and for life in AIDS patients (92).

The more expensive lipid formulations of amphotericin B and itraconazole have yet to prove superior to amphotericin B deoxycholate in invasive pulmonary aspergillosis. However, patients who fail or cannot tolerate amphotericin B deoxycholate therapy may respond to these new drugs. Still newer agents, including the triazoles voriconazole, posaconazole, and ravuconazole, the intravenous lipid complex nystatin, and three echinocandin derivatives, have activity against *Aspergillus* and are in various stages of development (90).

Surgical intervention may be indicated for selected patients, including those with progression of invasive pulmonary aspergillosis despite appropriate therapy, with life-threatening hemoptysis and focal disease, or with residual disease, especially mycetomas, requiring prolonged courses of immunosuppression. Despite frequent significant abnormalities in hematologic parameters, surgical intervention can be a high-yield, relatively low-risk procedure (79). A study of 27 neutropenic patients who underwent lung resection for suspected invasive pulmonary aspergillosis confirmed fungal pneumonia in 22 patients, with a 30-day mortality of 11% and a 3-month survival of 77% (79).

Pathogens Causing Mucormycosis

Major pathogens in the order Mucorales include the genera *Mucor, Absidia,* and *Rhizopus.* Pulmonary disease caused by these pathogens, called *mucormycosis,* is very similar to disease caused by *Aspergillus* but much less common (71). These are very difficult infections to diagnose before death. Once the diagnosis has been established, they are also difficult to eradicate. Amphotericin B is the only reliable drug available. Systemic antifungal therapy should be used in conjunction with debridement of necrotic tissue for definitive treatment.

Candida

Candida frequently infects the upper respiratory tract but rarely causes pneumonitis in the immunocompromised host. Candidiasis is the only major deep fungal infection that is not acquired by inhalation. The organism is part of the normal skin and mucous membrane flora. In the setting of neutropenia, *Candida* proliferates and invades the bloodstream through defects in the mucosa or instrumented skin, causing disseminated disease. Pulmonary infection can develop from organisms in the pulmonary arterial blood, but this is exceedingly rare (71). Even in neutropenic patients who aspirate *Candida* organisms into the tracheobronchial system, an acute candidal pneumonitis rarely develops because the alveolar macrophage, not the neutrophil, is the major defense cell against *Candida* pneumonia (71).

In HIV-infected patients, thrush, esophageal candidiasis, and vaginal candidiasis are the common manifestations; disseminated candidiasis is rare except in patients with indwelling catheters (70). In patients with lung transplants, invasive disease with *Candida* is manifested by wound infection and mediastinitis, and mycotic aneurysms of the aortic anastomosis develop in patients receiving combined heart–lung transplants (95).

The definitive diagnosis of invasive *Candida* pneumonia requires lung biopsy because the organism is frequently isolated in respiratory secretions contaminated by oropharyngeal flora. The presumptive diagnosis of *Candida* pneumonia can be made at times in patients with disseminated disease and large numbers of *Candida* organisms isolated from the tracheobronchial tree. Amphotericin B is the drug of choice for the treatment of both disseminated candidiasis and the rare cases of true *Candida* pneumonia.

Pneumocystis carinii

P. carinii causes life-threatening pneumonia in the immunocompromised host. PCP was originally described in malnourished infants in Europe in the 1930s and 1940s. Before the 1980s, PCP was a rare disease, seen in patients who were immunocompromised by chemotherapy or who had intrinsic immunodeficiency syndromes. With the onset of the AIDS epidemic in the early 1980s, the number of cases increased exponentially. With improvements in diagnosis, treatment, and prophylaxis, the number of cases of PCP has now dramatically decreased (96).

P. carinii was originally classified as a protozoan because of its morphologic features, which were similar to those of other protozoans, and because the organism could be treated with antiprotozoal agents. It has recently been reclassified as an atypical fungus because of its yeastlike characteristics, revealed by molecular biologic techniques; its closest relatives appears to be the ascomycetous yeasts, such as *Saccharomyces cerevisiae* and *Candida albicans* (97). Immunologic and molecular studies have demonstrated multiple strains of the organism, each of which can infect only one species (97,98). As an example, human-derived *P. carinii* can infect only humans, and rat-derived *P. carinii* can infect only rats.

Despite its recent reclassification, no reliable long-term *in vitro* culture system is available for *P. carinii*, and as a result, its life cycle and pathogenesis remain obscure. Nonetheless, molecular biologic techniques have identified some of the target enzymes of sulfamethoxazole and trimethoprim, including the genes that encode dihydropteroate synthase and dihydrofolate reductase (96).

The environmental source and modes of transmission of *Pneumocystis* remain uncertain. Because antibodies develop in 80% of the human population during childhood, it is widely believed that after subclinical infection, the organism acts as a lung saprophyte, to be reactivated during immunosuppression (99,100). Some studies suggest that PCP may develop from a new infection from the environment (101,102). Airborne transmission of the organism is the presumed method of naturally acquired infection. Person-to-person transmission has never been documented, although cluster outbreaks have occurred (103).

Abnormal cellular immunity is the major immune defect that predisposes patients to PCP, although patients with isolated B-cell defects rarely have been described (17,100). PCP is most common in patients with AIDS, lymphoma, or acute lymphocytic leukemia; in patients with bone marrow or solid organ transplants; in those on high-dose corticosteroid therapy; and in patients with severe protein malnutrition (104). The attack rates for non–HIV-infected patients without prophylaxis vary from 22% to 43% in patients with acute lymphocytic leukemia to 1.3% in patients with primary brain tumor or metastatic disease to the brain on high-dose corticosteroid therapy (105). In HIV-infected patients, as the CD4$^+$ cell count falls below 200/mm^3, the risk for PCP dramatically increases (17,106). When the AIDS epidemic began, PCP developed in 75% of AIDS patients during the course of their illness. With the use of PCP prophylaxis and HAART, the incidence of PCP has decreased dramatically (107).

Dyspnea, cough, and fever are the most common clinical manifestations of PCP in patients with and without HIV infection (108,109). Some patients are asymptomatic, whereas others present with fulminant respiratory failure. HIV-infected patients tend to present with a more insidious course than non–HIV-infected patients (108). Extrapulmonary *Pneumocystis* infection is rare but can occur in patients with or without HIV infection (110).

The classic chest radiograph in PCP shows bilateral, symmetric interstitial or alveolar infiltrates. Less common radiographic presentations include interstitial and alveolar infiltrates, localized patchy parenchymal consolidation, thin-walled cysts, nodules, pneumothorax, parenchymal cavitation, and honeycomb lesions (108,111,112). Normal chest radiographs have also been reported in HIV-infected patients and non–HIV-infected patients (111,113). High-resolution CT can demonstrate ground-glass attenuation and may better define cystic or cavitary lesions, subpleural disease, and pneumothoraces (112,114).

In HIV-infected patients, the CD4$^+$ cell count is the most important indicator of the risk for PCP, but it is not diagnostic of PCP itself. As the CD4$^+$ cell count falls below 200/mm^3, the risk for PCP increases. In some patients, PCP may develop at higher levels, but the risk is low. Limited data suggest that the CD4$^+$ cell count may also correlate with the risk for PCP in non–HIV-infected patients. The serum lactate dehydrogenase level can be a sensitive but nonspecific test, especially in patients with underlying malignancy or liver dysfunction (115). An abnormal diffusing capacity and oxygen desaturation with exercise are sensitive but nonspecific tests and may aid in the evaluation of a symptomatic patient at risk for PCP who has normal radiographic findings or subtle changes because physiologic abnormalities may predate anatomic changes. Gallium scans have been used in the past to help establish the diagnosis of PCP; these are sensitive but nonspecific tests that are time-consuming and expensive and expose patients to ionizing radiation. Gallium scans, like pulmonary function tests, may be helpful in patients with atypical presentations of PCP, but prophylaxis may also cause atypical scans (116).

The diagnosis of PCP is established by demonstrating the organism in pulmonary secretions or body tissues; *P. carinii* still cannot be reliably cultured. In patients with HIV infection, sputum induction should be the initial diagnostic procedure if available. The sensitivity of sputum induction for diagnosing PCP in HIV-infected patients is 55% to 95% at experienced institutions (18,117–119). The yield of sputum induction in patients without HIV infection has not been well studied, but in our experience it is very low.

FOB is a sensitive, specific, and well-tolerated procedure for diagnosing PCP in patients with and without HIV infection. TBB and BAL are equally sensitive for diagnosing PCP in HIV-infected patients (120). When both BAL and TBB are performed, the overall yield for PCP in HIV-infected patients is 94% to 100%, and 95% in non–HIV-infected patients (5,120). BAL can be used as the sole diagnostic modality because alone it has a yield for PCP of 79% to 98% in HIV-infected patients and 82% to 94% in non–HIV-infected patients (5,120,121). In non–HIV-infected patients, the yield of TBB is 92%, but this modality often cannot be used because of the presence of thrombocytopenia and coagulopathies (5). The use of PCP prophylaxis may decrease the yield of sputum induction, and BAL and TBB may be needed to establish the diagnosis.

In HIV-infected patients, if sputum induction is nondiagnostic, then FOB should be performed. In non–HIV-infected patients, the procedure of choice is FOB with BAL and, if possible, TBB. In the minority of cases in which neither sputum induction nor bronchoscopy is diagnostic, surgical lung biopsy, usually performed via VATS, may be required. The need for surgical biopsy is more common in non–HIV-infected patients, in whom the differential diagnosis is wider and the yield of bronchoscopy is lower.

The organism in fluid and tissues was originally identified with stains specific for the cyst form, including Gomori methenamine-silver, Gram-Weigert, and toluidine blue O, or with Giemsa stain specific for the trophozoite form. In the mid-1980s, monoclonal antibodies with a fluorescent antibody stain that could detect both cysts and trophozoites allowed a rapid diagnosis that was more sensitive (96). Newer molecular techniques such as PCR amplification, which may be even more sensitive and can be used on oral wash specimens, may decrease the need for sputum induction or bronchoscopy in the future (23).

The drugs used to treat PCP are the same for patients with and without HIV infection. The duration of therapy is traditionally 14 days in non–HIV-infected patients and 21 days in HIV-infected patients (104,122). The mainstay of therapy is TMP/SMX (15–20 mg/kg per day based on the trimethoprim component); if this is not tolerated, intravenous pentamidine (3–4 mg/kg per day) is used (122). Limited prospective trials have shown TMP/SMX and pentamidine to be equally effective, and they are the drugs of choice for the treatment of moderate to severe PCP (123–125). Side effects occur frequently with both drugs, especially in patients with HIV infection (122). In non–HIV-infected patients, bone marrow suppression with TMP/SMX can be a concern. Aerosolized pentamidine is not effective therapy (126).

For patients with mild to moderate disease who cannot tolerate TMP/SMX or pentamidine, alternative agents include clindamycin with primaquine, dapsone with trimethoprim, and atovaquone (127–129). Dapsone alone is not recommended for the treatment of PCP (130).

Several studies have shown reduced rates of respiratory failure and mortality in HIV-infected patients with a PaO_2 of 70 mm Hg or less who are given adjunctive corticosteroids within 72 hours after the initiation of PCP therapy (131–134). The recommended steroid regimen is 40 mg of prednisone orally twice daily for 5 days, then 40 mg of prednisone daily for 5 days, then 20 mg until the completion of anti-PCP therapy. The data regarding the use of adjunctive corticosteroid therapy in non–HIV-infected patients, many of whom are already on steroids at the time PCP is diagnosed, are limited. In two small retrospective studies, rates of mortality and intubation were comparable for those patients who received adjunctive corticosteroids (135,136). Pareja and colleagues (135) found an accelerated rate of recovery and a decrease in the duration of intubation, number of intensive care unit admissions, and supplemental oxygen requirement in patients who received adjunctive corticosteroid therapy. Adjunctive corticosteroids for PCP in non–HIV-infected patients may be beneficial and should be considered. At our institution,

adjunctive corticosteroids are added to the therapy of non–HIV-infected patients in whom PCP is diagnosed. For those patients already on steroids, the dose is adjusted to the recommended doses. If the patients are on equivalent or higher doses at the time of diagnosis, the steroid dose is maintained.

Prophylaxis against PCP with TMP/SMX is effective in patients with and without HIV infection (137,138). TMP/SMX is the drug of choice for PCP prophylaxis. HIV-infected patients taking the drug regularly have only a 5% breakthrough rate (139). Because the incidence of adverse effects is high, especially among HIV-infected patients, alternative regimens are available, including dapsone, dapsone with pyrimethamine, atovaquone, clindamycin and primaquine, pyrimethamine and sulfadiazine combinations, and intravenous or aerosolized pentamidine (140–145).

The indications for PCP prophylaxis in the HIV-infected patient are well established and include a $CD4^+$ cell count below 200/mm^3, unexplained fever of 100°F or higher for 2 weeks or more, and a prior episode of PCP (122). Studies have shown that once the $CD4^+$ cell count has been above 200/mm^3 for more than 3 months, PCP prophylaxis can be safely discontinued (146–148). Indications for PCP prophylaxis in the non–HIV-infected patient are less well defined because the exact degree of required immunosuppression is unknown. Traditionally, patients with acute lymphocytic leukemia, Hodgkin disease, or lymphoma and recipients of bone marrow or solid organ transplants are at high risk for PCP and require prophylaxis (105,149). In addition, patients on long-term steroid therapy ($\geq$20 mg of prednisone a day for >4 weeks) with an additional risk factor for immunosuppression, including underlying active solid malignancy or collagen-vascular disease, should be considered for PCP prophylaxis (149). The duration of PCP prophylaxis in the non–HIV-infected patient is the duration of known immunosuppression and varies according to the underlying disease, chemotherapeutic regimen, response to therapy, and duration of corticosteroid therapy (105,149). (See the table at the top of the facing page.)

With the widespread use of prophylactic and therapeutic agents for PCP, the development of resistance to sulfa and atovaquone has become a matter of concern. Because the organism cannot be cultured, traditional sensitivity studies cannot be performed. PCR testing has shown mutations in the dihydropteroate synthase enzyme that is targeted by sulfamethoxazole and dapsone (150–152). Mutations in *P. carinii* cytochrome *b* are much more common in patients exposed to atovaquone, which suggests that resistance may develop (96). The clinical relevance of these mutations is unclear, but some small studies suggest lower response rates of PCP to standard therapy (153,154).

Cryptococcus

Cryptococcus neoformans is a budding yeast and the only pathogenic fungus with a capsule that develops in mammalian tissues (155). The fungus is distributed worldwide

MANAGEMENT AND PREVENTION OF *PNEUMOCYSTIS CARINII* PNEUMONIA

Summary Statement	Level of Evidence
TMP/SMX and pentamidine are equally effective for the therapy of PCP in patients with and without HIV infection.	Randomized controlled trials
Compared with TMP/SMX and pentamidine, alternative therapies for mild to moderate PCP include trimethoprim/dapsone, clindamycin/primaquine, and atovaquone.	Prospective trials, some randomized
Adjunctive corticosteroid therapy reduces the likelihood of respiratory failure from PCP in HIV-infected patients.	Randomized controlled trials and expert opinion
Adjunctive corticosteroid therapy for PCP in non–HIV-infected patients may be beneficial and should be considered.	Very limited data; only small observational studies
PCP prophylaxis is indicated in HIV-infected patients with CD4$^+$ cell counts <200/mm^3, fever ≥100°F for >2 weeks, or prior episode of PCP.	Randomized controlled trials
PCP prophylaxis can be safely discontinued in HIV-infected patients with CD4$^+$ cell counts >200/mm^3 for >3 months.	Randomized controlled trials
PCP prophylaxis is indicated in patients with ALL, Hodgkin disease, lymphoma, BMT, or a solid organ transplant.	Randomized controlled trials
PCP prophylaxis is indicated in non–HIV-infected patients on long-term steroid therapy (≥20 mg of prednisone for >4 weeks) and an additional risk factor for immunosuppression, including active solid malignancy or collagen-vascular disease.	Small observational studies and expert opinion

ALL, acute lymphocytic leukemia; BMT, bone marrow transplant; PCP, *P. carinii* pneumonia; TMP/SMX, trimethoprim/sulfamethoxazole.

and is easily recovered from the environment. The organism grows best in desiccated bird feces, although most patients do not have a known exposure to birds. Without the capsule, the fungus is small enough to be easily inhaled into the alveoli.

In the immunosuppressed host, isolated pulmonary infections are rarely seen. Although the portal of entry is the lung, the pulmonary infection is often silent, and the central nervous system is frequently the site of symptomatic infection, especially in patients with T-cell defects associated with HIV infection, long-term corticosteroid therapy, chronic lymphocytic leukemia, chronic myelogenous leukemia, or Hodgkin disease. In patients with pulmonary disease, with or without disseminated disease, the pulmonary symptoms may be minimal, if present, and include fever, cough, chest pain, and malaise. Radiographic findings may include solitary nodules, multiple nodules, masslike nodular infiltrates, cavities, miliary lesions, diffuse infiltrates, pleural effusions, and mediastinal adenopathy.

The detection of serum cryptococcal polysaccharide capsular antigen is highly sensitive and specific for invasive dis-

ease, but it does not indicate the site of infection. In HIV-infected patients, the sensitivity and specificity of serum cryptococcal antigen are higher than 90% for disseminated disease (156). The presence of disseminated disease may be confirmed by finding the organisms in sterile sites, including cerebrospinal fluid, blood, and urine. The diagnosis of pulmonary cryptococcosis is established by the presence of the organism in smears or tissue specimens from a respiratory source, including sputum, BAL fluid, lung tissue, and pleural fluid.

Disseminated disease requires a course of induction therapy, preferably with 0.5 to 1 mg of amphotericin B per kilogram per day and 100 mg of flucytosine per kilogram per day for 2 weeks. This is followed by maintenance suppressive therapy with 400 mg of fluconazole per day for a minimum of 10 weeks (157). HIV-infected patients may not be able to tolerate flucytosine because of bone marrow suppression. Lifelong suppressive therapy with fluconazole is required for HIV-infected patients. Non–HIV-infected patients with isolated pulmonary cryptococcosis and mild to moderate symptoms can be treated with 200 to 400 mg of fluconazole daily as monotherapy for 6 to 12 months (157). Alternative therapies include lipid formulations of amphotericin B, and for those who cannot tolerate fluconazole, itraconazole can be substituted.

Endemic Fungi

Histoplasma capsulatum
Histoplasmosis is acquired by inhaling the dimorphic fungus *Histoplasma capsulatum,* which is found worldwide and is endemic along the Mississippi, Ohio, and St. Lawrence river valleys in the United States, in the Caribbean, and in Central and South America. In patients with defects of cellular immunity associated with AIDS, corticosteroid therapy, chemotherapy, or solid organ or bone marrow transplantation, histoplasmosis is a disseminated disease (158). In 1995, more than 90% of all cases of disseminated histoplasmosis in the United States occurred in patients with AIDS (159). Histoplasmosis develops in 5% to 27% of HIV-infected patients living in areas of endemicity, most likely as a consequence of the progression of a primary infection (159). However, some cases represent the reactivation of latent infection as immunity decreases.

Isolated pulmonary histoplasmosis is rare in the immunocompromised host, but pulmonary involvement is frequent in patients with disseminated disease, who present with a progressive febrile illness characterized by weight loss, hepatosplenomegaly, and cough. Chest radiographs reveal diffuse reticulonodular infiltrates.

The organism can be seen in the buffy coat layer of peripheral blood after staining with Wright or Giemsa stain and in bone marrow directly examined for rapid diagnosis. Direct smear or culture may also reveal the organism in BAL specimens. In disseminated disease, the yield of fungal cultures of bone marrow is up to 75%, and blood cultures can be positive in 50% of cases (160). In HIV-infected patients, the detection of *Histoplasma* polysaccharide antigen in urine and serum is highly sensitive, and a negative test result virtually excludes the diagnosis of disseminated histoplasmosis (159). The antigen concentration decreases with therapy and increases with relapse and is helpful for monitoring therapy (161).

The treatment of disseminated histoplasmosis in immunocompromised patients requiring hospitalization should begin with amphotericin B. Once the patient is able to take oral medications, itraconazole can be substituted (161). In patients without AIDS, the recommended dosage of itraconazole is 200 mg once or twice per day, and the duration of therapy is 6 to 18 months (161). In patients with AIDS, a 12-week induction period of therapy with 200 mg of either amphotericin B or itraconazole twice a day is followed by lifelong maintenance therapy with 200 mg of itraconazole once or twice per day to prevent relapse (161). Immune reconstitution with HAART may permit discontinuation of maintenance therapy.

Coccidioides immitis

C. immitis is a fungus endemic to the southwestern United States that causes self-limited disease in the immunocompetent host. In patients with T-cell defects associated with AIDS, corticosteroid therapy, chemotherapy, or solid organ or bone marrow transplantation, disseminated disease is the most common presentation, with fever as the predominant symptom. Skin, bone, and central nervous system manifestations predominate, although *C. immitis* can infect any organ (155). Pulmonary symptoms may include cough and dyspnea. The chest radiographic findings may be normal, or diffuse reticulonodular densities may be seen. Coccidioidomycosis is a common opportunistic infection in HIV-infected patients living in areas of endemicity, and risk for the development of active disease is associated with a CD4$^+$ cell count below 250/mm^3 and a diagnosis of AIDS (70). Latent disease can be reactivated in persons previously exposed while in an area of endemicity in whom cellular immunity is subsequently depressed.

Coccidioidomycosis is diagnosed by demonstrating the organism in body fluids or tissues, including sputum or bronchoscopic specimens. Antifungal therapy for disseminated disease begins with amphotericin B and then oral azole therapy for a minimum of a year. For those with profound immunodeficiency, the azole should be continued for lifelong secondary prophylaxis (162).

Blastomyces dermatitidis and *Paracoccidioides brasiliensis*

B. dermatitidis and *P. brasiliensis* are uncommon endemic dimorphic fungi that rarely cause disease in immunocompromised hosts, especially those with T-cell defects. *B. dermatitidis* is found in the same areas as *H. capsulatum* but

causes only 10% as many cases of illness as *H. capsulatum* (159). *P. brasiliensis* is found in Central and South America, especially Brazil, Colombia, and Venezuela. Both of these fungi are inhaled and usually cause pulmonary symptoms, although extrapulmonary spread is common in both diseases. The diagnosis depends on identification of the organisms in fluid or tissue specimens; no reliable serologic methods are available. Treatment for seriously ill patients should begin with amphotericin B followed by maintenance therapy with itraconazole.

Protozoa

P. carinii, previously considered a protozoan, is now classified as a fungus and has been discussed (see section "*Pneumocystis carinii*"). The two most common protozoal infections encountered in immunocompromised patients are those caused by *Strongyloides stercoralis* and *Toxoplasma gondii*. *S. stercoralis* is an intestinal parasite endemic to the southeastern United States, the Caribbean, Central America, the Pacific basin, and Central Africa. Of American veterans returning from Vietnam, 6% were colonized with the parasite (163,164). A hyperinfection syndrome can occur following glucocorticoid therapy, immunosuppressive therapy, or HIV infection (165). The syndrome is often accompanied by polymicrobial sepsis and should be suspected in that setting and in patients who come from areas of endemicity. The diagnosis can be made by examining sputum, stool, small bowel aspirates, and BAL fluid. Treatment may be given with thiobendazole or ivermectin.

T. gondii can cause pneumonia in immunocompetent and immunocompromised patients (166,167). In both patient populations, diffuse bilateral infiltrates are seen. When the diagnosis is made, the mortality is extremely low for immunocompetent patients and 40% for immunocompromised patients. *T. gondii* infection has been well recognized in AIDS patients and has also been described in patients after bone marrow transplantation (168). Treatment is with a combination of pyrimethamine and sulfadiazine.

Viruses

Herpesviruses

CMV is the most important cause of viral pneumonia in the immunocompromised host. The incidence of CMV disease, including pneumonitis, varies with the underlying disease, but CMV disease is most common in patients with impaired cellular immunity, especially recipients of allogeneic bone marrow and solid organ transplants.

In recipients of bone marrow transplants, CMV infection may be caused by reactivation of latent infection, viral transmission from a seropositive marrow donor, or transfusion of CMV-infected blood products. The pathogenesis of CMV pneumonitis has not been well elucidated, but it appears to be more complex than just lung destruction caused by viral replication. A possible immunologically mediated component to the lung injury may progress even without further viral replication. This hypothesis is supported by the finding that CMV pneumonitis typically occurs 8 to 12 weeks after transplantation and does not develop before bone marrow engraftment and leukocyte recovery. The association of CMV pneumonitis with acute graft versus host disease, and the ineffectiveness of single therapy with ganciclovir despite reduction in the lung CMV titers, offer further support for the role of the inflammatory response to the virus in the development of pneumonitis.

The signs and symptoms of CMV pneumonitis are nonspecific and include fever, dyspnea, nonproductive cough, and hypoxemia. Diffuse bilateral interstitial infiltrates are the most common radiographic findings. Solid and multiple nodules and focal consolidation have also been described.

The diagnosis of CMV is usually based on a compatible clinical presentation and the detection of CMV in BAL fluid by cytology or shell-vial culture techniques. In some circumstances, the presence of CMV in BAL fluid does not necessarily indicate active infection, and a definitive diagnosis must be established by the detection of cytomegalic inclusions in TBB or OLB specimens. The utility of CMV immunostaining of BAL fluid with anti-CMV antibodies has been well established (169). In one study, the sensitivity and specificity of immunostaining in the diagnosis of CMV pneumonitis in immunocompromised patients were 89.9% and 98.6%, respectively (170). In many cases, this technique has now supplanted the more invasive biopsy procedures, which are often contraindicated in this population because of abnormal coagulation parameters.

The mortality rate of CMV pneumonitis in bone marrow transplant recipients remains high. Treatment with ganciclovir alone is ineffective. However, the combination of intravenous immunoglobulin and ganciclovir has reduced mortality in some centers from 90% to between 30% and 50% (171). Preemptive therapy of asymptomatic infection with low-dose ganciclovir can prevent progression to symptomatic disease, but the incidence of adverse effects, particularly bone marrow toxicity, is significant. Many centers use semiquantitative PCR or antigenemia assays on peripheral blood leukocytes to identify high-risk patients who require prophylactic ganciclovir therapy (172,173).

Recipients of solid organ transplants begin to manifest symptoms of CMV infection, including pneumonitis, approximately 6 weeks after transplantation. CMV infection after solid organ transplantation can be acquired by the same means as after bone marrow transplantation. Primary CMV infection in this population is associated with a much higher incidence of symptomatic disease than reactivation infection because of the absence of intrinsic immunity against CMV. The patients at greatest risk for primary CMV infection are those who are seronegative before transplantation and receive a graft from a seropositive donor. The incidence and severity

of CMV pneumonia are greater in lung transplant recipients than in recipients of other solid organ transplants, and CMV pneumonia has been associated with chronic graft rejection (174). The clinical presentation, radiographic appearance, and approach to the diagnosis of CMV pneumonia in recipients of solid organ transplants are the same as in recipients of bone marrow transplants.

Various prophylactic strategies have been used in an attempt to reduce the incidence of symptomatic disease in patients at risk for primary infection and in those with infection before the emergence of overt disease. Ganciclovir administered intravenously or orally is the most effective and widely used prophylactic agent. The optimal route, dose, and duration of therapy have not been established. Ganciclovir in combination with intravenous immunoglobulin is the treatment of choice for active CMV disease. CMV pneumonia generally responds to a 2- to 3-week course of therapy followed by 3 to 6 weeks of maintenance treatment (95). The efficacy of this regimen may be augmented by a reduction in immunosuppressive therapy if the clinical circumstances allow.

The clinical importance of CMV pneumonia in HIV-infected patients remains controversial. Multiple studies have demonstrated the frequent recovery of CMV in bronchoscopy specimens in HIV-infected patients without pulmonary disease (175). The presence of CMV has not been associated with hypoxemia, chest radiographic abnormalities, or mortality. When treated for coexisting infection, most patients recover without specific anti-CMV therapy. Additionally, no significant difference in the clinical course has been demonstrated between patients with coexisting CMV and PCP and patients with PCP alone (176,177). Autopsy studies, however, have demonstrated CMV as a cause of pulmonary disease in a small percentage of HIV-infected patients. In one study, 44 of 75 autopsies showed histologic evidence of CMV infection. In 21 of these cases, CMV was considered to be a significant contributor to the pulmonary disease, including five cases in which CMV was the sole isolated pathogen (178).

Although it has not been well established, a few studies suggest some efficacy of ganciclovir therapy for presumed CMV pneumonitis in HIV-infected patients (179–181). The clinical dilemma is how to identify those patients with HIV infection who should be treated for CMV pneumonia. Currently, no markers are available to identify them reliably. Therapy with ganciclovir is generally reserved for patients with evidence of CMV and worsening respiratory failure in the absence of other treatable infections or despite treatment for coexisting infections.

Other herpesviruses are uncommon causes of pneumonia in the immunocompromised host. Herpes simplex virus pneumonia is generally a result of aspiration from the oropharynx or extension from herpetic tracheobronchitis. The chest radiograph most often shows focal infiltrates. Hematogenous dissemination may occur and leads to

MANAGEMENT OF CYTOMEGALOVIRUS PNEUMONIA

Summary Statement	Level of Evidence
Treatment with combined ganciclovir and intravenous immunoglobulin has significantly reduced mortality from CMV pneumonia in non–HIV-immunocompromised hosts.	Several prospective nonrandomized studies
Ganciclovir may be effective therapy for CMV pneumonia in HIV-infected patients.	A few observational studies and prospective nonrandomized studies

CMV, cytomegalovirus.

bilateral interstitial pneumonia (182). Acyclovir is the drug of choice for treatment. Pneumonia caused by human herpesvirus 6 has been reported following bone marrow transplantation (183). Human herpesvirus 6 may account for some cases of pneumonitis previously classified as idiopathic interstitial pneumonia, typically occurring within 3 to 6 months after transplantation.

Other Viruses

Respiratory Syncytial Virus

Respiratory syncytial virus (RSV) has become increasingly recognized as a cause of pneumonia in immunocompromised hosts, particularly bone marrow transplant recipients. RSV infections usually occur during community outbreaks, typically in the fall and winter. Nosocomial transmission has been demonstrated. Infected patients usually present initially with prominent upper respiratory tract symptoms, including cough, rhinorrhea, sinusitis, and otitis (184). The frequency of progression to pneumonia is greatest in recipients of bone marrow transplants before marrow engraftment or less than 1 month after transplantation. Pneumonia has been reported to occur in 70% to 80% of this subset of patients (185). The clinical manifestations of RSV pneumonia include cough, wheezing, and dyspnea. Bilateral interstitial infiltrates are the most common radiographic appearance. RSV pneumonia can be diagnosed by viral culture of respiratory tract specimens. However, isolation of the virus may require several days. Antigen detection techniques provide a rapid means of diagnosis. In the immunocompromised host, the sensitivities of these assays vary with the source of the specimen. BAL has a reported sensitivity of 89%, compared with 15% for nasal washes and throat swabs (186).

The overall mortality from RSV pneumonia is 60% to 80%. Controlled studies are needed to define optimal therapy. Combined treatment with aerosolized ribavirin and intravenous immunoglobulin has been shown to reduce the mortality rate of bone marrow transplant recipients with RSV pneumonia to 31% when administered before the development of respiratory failure requiring mechanical ven-

tilation (185). Data suggest that preemptive therapy at the stage of upper respiratory tract infection can reduce the frequency of progression to pneumonia and mortality rates. One study reported a 29% progression to pneumonia and 14% mortality rate after prompt treatment of RSV upper respiratory tract symptoms with aerosolized ribavirin and intravenous immunoglobulin (187). Immunoglobulin with high RSV titers and RSV monoclonal antibodies have been approved for prophylaxis in high-risk infants and children. Further studies are needed to determine their potential role in prophylaxis or treatment in immunocompromised adults.

Adenovirus

Adenovirus infections have been reported in recipients of bone marrow and solid organ transplants and in HIV-infected patients. In recent years, the role of adenovirus in the morbidity and mortality of bone marrow transplant recipients has become appreciated. Adenovirus can be isolated in 3% to 5% of bone marrow transplant recipients (188,189). The majority of cases of adenovirus infection occur during the first 100 days after transplant. Adenovirus causes a wide spectrum of clinical syndromes, including respiratory disease, hepatitis, enteritis, and hemorrhagic cystitis. Respiratory involvement may present as an upper respiratory tract illness or as an isolated pneumonia. Pneumonia may also occur as part of disseminated disease. Disseminated disease is more common in recipients of allogeneic bone marrow transplants and has been associated with graft versus host disease during concurrent immunosuppressive therapy (188). Chest radiographs typically reveal diffuse interstitial infiltrates.

Mortality rates of 70% to 80% have been reported in bone marrow transplant recipients with adenovirus pneumonia with or without disseminated disease (188). Various therapies, including intravenous ribavirin, have been attempted, but no effective treatment or prophylaxis for adenovirus infection has been established.

Influenza Virus

During community outbreaks, influenza virus must be considered a potential cause of pneumonia in the immunocompromised host. Infection with influenza virus presents as an acute respiratory illness accompanied by systemic signs and symptoms, including fever, headache, myalgias, and malaise. Pneumonia associated with infection may be a primary influenza pneumonia, a secondary bacterial pneumonia, or a pneumonia with features of both. Primary influenza pneumonia manifests radiographically as diffuse interstitial or patchy infiltrates. A secondary bacterial pneumonia often develops after the acute viral syndrome has abated. The most common bacterial pathogens are *S. aureus* and *S. pneumoniae*.

The role of influenza virus as a cause of pneumonia in the immunocompromised host has not been well studied. The severity of disease appears to be related to the degree of underlying immunosuppression. Cell-mediated immunity appears to play an important role in viral clearance. In one prospective study of hospitalized adult bone marrow transplant recipients, influenza A virus was isolated from a respiratory source in 29% of the patients with an acute respiratory illness. The illness was complicated by pneumonia in 75% of these patients, with a mortality of 17% (190). Infection with influenza virus, including pneumonia, has been reported in HIV-infected adults. More severe illness in HIV-infected patients has been suggested in one study that detected an excess mortality from pneumonia or influenza in this population during the influenza season (191). Infection with influenza virus has been reported infrequently in solid organ transplant recipients. A report of three lung transplant recipients with influenza pneumonia noted a possible association between the viral infection and the subsequent development of bronchiolitis obliterans (192).

Influenza pneumonia often cannot be clinically differentiated from pneumonia with other potential causes. Influenza virus can be isolated from respiratory sources in tissue culture within 72 hours (193). Immunofluorescent staining of tissue culture or of cells obtained from nasopharyngeal washings may provide a more rapid means of viral identification. Amantadine and rimantadine are active only against influenza A virus and are effective in decreasing the duration of fever and symptoms when started within 48 hours after the onset of illness. The treatment of influenza pneumonia is primarily supportive. Whether amantadine and rimantadine are effective in treating pneumonia or preventing progression of uncomplicated illness to pneumonia in the immunocompromised host is unknown. Aerosolized and intravenous ribavirin have been used to treat severe influenza virus infection in a small number of immunocompromised patients with variable results. The neuraminidase inhibitors zanamivir and oseltamivir are effective against both influenza A and B virus and have been approved for the treatment of acute uncomplicated infection (194). Annual influenza vaccination with inactive virus is recommended in the immunocompromised patient. Although the vaccine is safe in this population, the ability to mount a protective antibody response is variable. Chemoprophylaxis with amantadine/rimantadine should be considered in addition to vaccination in immunocompromised patients during the influenza season. However, case reports have documented emergence of drug-resistant strains of virus (195).

REFERENCES

1. Masur H, Shelhamer J, Parrillo JE. The management of pneumonias in immunocompromised patients. *JAMA* 1985;253:1769–1773.
2. Rosenow EC III, Wilson WR, Cockerill FR III. Pulmonary disease in the immunocompromised host. *Mayo Clin Proc* 1985;60:473–487.
3. Rosenow EC III, Wilson WR, Cockerill FR III. Pulmonary disease in the immunocompromised host. *Clin Chest Med* 1990;11:55–64.
4. Williams DM, Frick JA, Remington JS. Pulmonary infection in the compromised host: parts I and II. *Am Rev Respir Dis* 1976;114:359–394, 593–627.
5. Stover DE, Zaman MB, Hajdu SL, et al. Bronchoalveolar lavage in the diagnosis of diffuse pulmonary infiltrates in the immunocompromised host. *Ann Intern Med* 1984;101:1–7.
6. Vander Els, Stover DA. Approach to the patient with pulmonary disease. *Clin Chest Med* 1996;17:767–785.
7. Rubin RH, Greene R. Clinical approach to the compromised host with fever and pulmonary infiltrates. In: Rubin RH, Young LS, eds. *Clinical approach to infection in the compromised host,* 3rd ed. New York: Plenum Publishing, 1994:121.
8. Hopewell PC. Evaluation of pulmonary disease in the immunocompromised host. In: Kelley WN, ed. *Textbook of internal medicine,* 3rd ed. Philadelphia: Lippincott–Raven Publishers, 1997:1968–1973.
9. Pizzo PA. Fever in immunocompromised patients. *N Engl J Med* 1999;341:893–900.
10. Matthay RA, Greene WH. Pulmonary infections in the immunocompromised host. *Med Clin North Am* 1980;64:529–551.
11. Singer C, Armstrong D, Rosen PP, et al. Diffuse pulmonary infiltrates in immunocompromised patients: prospective study of 80 cases. *Am J Med* 1979;66:110–120.
12. Bodey G, Buckley M, Sathe Y, et al. Quantitative relationships between circulating leukocytes and infection in patients with acute leukemia. *Ann Intern Med* 1966;64:328–340.
13. Pizzo PA, Robichaud KJ, Gill FA, et al. Empiric antibiotic and antifungal therapy for cancer patients with prolonged fever and granulocytopenia. *Am J Med* 1982;72:101–110.
14. Tenholder MF, Hooper RG. Pulmonary infiltrates in leukemia. *Chest* 1980;78:468–473.
15. Greene R. Transthoracic needle aspiration biopsy. In: Athanazoulis C, Pfister R, Greene R, et al., eds. *International radiology.* Philadelphia: WB Saunders, 1981:587.
16. Fanta CH, Pennington JE. Pulmonary infections in the transplant patient. In: Morris PF, Tilney NL, eds. *Progress in transplantation,* vol 2. New York: Churchill Livingstone, 1985:207.
17. Masur H, Ognibene FP, Yarchoan R, et al. CD4 cells are predictors of opportunistic pneumonias in human immunodeficiency virus (HIV) infection. *Ann Intern Med* 1989;111:223–231.
18. Huang L, Hecht FM, Stansell JD. Suspected *Pneumocystis carinii* pneumonia with a negative induced sputum examination. Is early bronchoscopy useful? *Am J Respir Crit Care Med* 1995;151:1866–1871.
19. Anderson C, Inhaber N, Menies D. Comparison of sputum induction with fiberoptic bronchoscopy in the diagnosis of tuberculosis. *Am J Respir Crit Care Med* 1995;152:1570–1574.
20. Kovacs JA, Ng VL, Masur H, et al. Diagnosis of *Pneumocystis carinii* pneumonia: improved detection in sputum with the use of monoclonal antibodies. *N Engl J Med* 1988;316:589–593.
21. Goodman JS, Kaufman L, Koenig MG. Diagnosis of cryptococcal meningitis: value of immunologic detection of cryptococcal antigen. *N Engl J Med* 1971;285:434–436.
22. Catanzaro A, Davidson BL, Fujiwara PI, et al. Rapid diagnostic tests for tuberculosis. What is the appropriate use? *Am J Respir Crit Care Med* 1997;155:1804–1814.
23. Helweg-Larsen J, Jensen JS, Berfield T, et al. Diagnostic use of PCR for detection of *Pneumocystis carinii* in oral wash samples. *J Clin Microbiol* 1998;36:2068–2072.
24. Williams D, Yungbluth M, Adams G, et al. The role of fiberoptic bronchoscopy in the evaluation of immunocompromised hosts with diffuse pulmonary infiltrates. *Am Rev Respir Dis* 1985;131:880–885.
25. Cazzadori A, Di Perri G, Todeschini G, et al. Transbronchial biopsy in the diagnosis of pulmonary infiltrates in immunocompromised patients. *Chest* 1995;107:101–106.

26. Castellino RA, Blank N. Etiologic diagnosis of focal pulmonary infection in immunocompromised patients by fluoroscopically guided percutaneous needle aspiration. *Radiology* 1979;132: 563–567.

27. Cockerill PR, Wilson WR, Carpenter HA, et al. Open lung biopsy in immunosuppressed patients. *Arch Intern Med* 1985; 145:1398–1404.

28. White DA, Wong PW, Downey R. The utility of open lung biopsy in patients with hematologic malignancies. *Am J Respir Crit Care Med* 2000;161:723–729.

29. Feinstein MB, Mokhtari M, Ferreiro R, et al. Fiberoptic bronchoscopy in allogeneic bone marrow transplantation. *Chest* 2001; 120:1094–1100.

30. Martinez Garcia MA, De Rojas MD, Nauffal Manzur MD, et al. Respiratory disorders in common variable immunodeficiency. *Respir Med* 2001;95:191–195.

31. Ekdahl K, Braconier JH, Rollo FJ. Recurrent pneumonia: a review of 90 adult patients. *Scand J Infect Dis* 1992;24:71–76.

32. Carratala J, Roson B, Fernandez-Sevilla A, et al. Bacteremic pneumonia in neutropenic patients with cancer: causes, empirical antibiotic therapy, and outcome. *Arch Intern Med* 1998;158:868–872.

33. Beck JM, Rosen MJ, Peavy HH. Pulmonary complications of HIV infection. Report of the fourth NHLBI workshop. *Am J Respir Crit Care Med* 2001;164:2120–2126.

34. Hirschtick RE, Glassroth J, Jordan MC, et al. Bacterial pneumonia in patients with HIV infection. Pulmonary Complications of HIV Infection Study Group. *N Engl J Med* 1995;333:845–851.

35. Cordero E, Pachon J, Rivero A. *Haemophilus influenzae* pneumonia in human immunodeficiency virus–infected patients. *Clin Infect Dis* 2000;30:461–465.

36. Afessa B, Green B. Bacterial pneumonia in hospitalized patients with HIV infection: the pulmonary complications, ICU support, and Prognostic Factors of Hospitalized Patients with HIV (PIP) Study. *Chest* 2000;117:1017–1022.

37. Currier JS, Williams P, Feinberg J, et al. Impact of prophylaxis for *Mycobacterium avium* complex on bacterial infections in patients with advanced human immunodeficiency virus disease. *Clin Infect Dis* 2001;32:1615–1622.

38. Wolff AJ, O'Donnell AE. Pulmonary manifestations of HIV infection in the era of highly active antiretroviral therapy (HAART). *Chest* 2001;120:1888–1893.

39. Sullivan JH, Moore RD, Keruly JC, et al. Effect of antiretroviral therapy on the incidence of bacterial pneumonia in patients with advanced HIV infection. *Am J Respir Crit Care Med* 2000;162:64–67.

40. Nenoff P, Kellermann S, Borte G, et al. Pulmonary nocardiosis with cutaneous involvement mimicking a metastasizing lung carcinoma in a patient with chronic myelogenous leukaemia. *Eur J Dermatol* 2000;10:47–51.

41. Jones N, Khoosal M, Louw M, et al. Nocardial infection as a complication of HIV in South Africa. *J Infect* 2000;41:232–239.

42. Akan H, Akova M, Ataoglu H, et al. *Rhodococcus equi* and *Nocardia brasiliensis* infection of the brain and liver in a patient with acute non-lymphoblastic leukemia. *Eur J Clin Microbiol Infect Dis* 1998;17:737–739.

43. Mari B, Monton C, Mariscal D, et al. Pulmonary nocardiosis: clinical experience in ten cases. *Respiration* 2001;68:382–388.

44. Holtz H, Lavery DP, Kapila R. Actinomycetales infection in the acquired immunodeficiency syndrome. *Ann Intern Med* 1985; 102:203–205.

45. Kedlaya I, Ing MB, Wong SS. *Rhodococcus equi* infections in immunocompetent hosts: case report and review. *Clin Infect Dis* 2001;32:E39–E46.

46. Chow JW, Yu VL. *Legionella*: a major opportunistic pathogen in transplant recipients. *Semin Respir Infect* 1998;13:132–139.

47. Kool JL, Fiore AE, Kioski CM, et al. More than 10 years of unrecognized nosocomial transmission of legionnaires' disease among transplant patients. *Infect Control Hosp Epidemiol* 1998;19:898–904.

48. Harris A, Lally M, Albrecht M. *Legionella bozemanii* pneumonia in three patients with AIDS. *Clin Infect Dis* 1998;27:97–99.

49. Danenberg AM. Pathogenesis of pulmonary tuberculosis. *Am Rev Respir Dis* 1982;125(3 Pt 2):42–49.

50. Small PM, Fujiwara PI. Management of tuberculosis in the United States. *N Engl J Med* 2001;345:189–200.

51. Newport MJ, Huxley CM, Huston S, et al. A mutation in the interferon-gamma-receptor gene and susceptibility to mycobacterial infection. *N Engl J Med* 1996;335:1941–1949.

52. Havir DV, Barnes PF. Tuberculosis in patients with human immunodeficiency virus infection. *N Engl J Med* 1999;340:367–373.

53. Greenberg SD, Frager D, Suster B, et al. Active pulmonary tuberculosis in patients with AIDS: spectrum of radiographic findings (including a normal appearance). *Radiology* 1994;193:115–119.

54. Alland D, Kalkut GE, Moss AR, et al. Transmission of tuberculosis in New York City. An analysis by DNR fingerprinting and conventional epidemiologic methods. *N Engl J Med* 1994;330: 1710–1716.

55. Small PM, Hopewell PC, Singh SP, et al. The epidemiology of tuberculosis in San Francisco. A population-based study using conventional and molecular methods. *N Engl J Med* 1994;330:1703–1709.

56. Jones BE, Young SM, Antoniskis D, et al. Relationship of the manifestations of tuberculosis to CD4 cell counts in patients with human immunodeficiency virus infection. *Am Rev Respir Crit Care Med* 1993;148:1292–1297.

57. Shafer RW, Kim DS, Weiss JP, et al. Extrapulmonary tuberculosis in patients with human immunodeficiency virus infection. *Medicine (Baltimore)* 1991;70:384–397.

58. Barnes PF. Rapid diagnostic tests for tuberculosis: progress but no gold standard. *Am J Respir Crit Care Med* 1997;155:1497–1498.

59. Malasky C, Jordan T, Potulski F, Reichman LB. Occupational tuberculosis infections among pulmonary physicians in training. *Am Rev Respir Dis* 1990;142:505–507.

60. Saltzman SH, Schindel ML, Aranda CP. The role of bronchoscopy in the diagnosis of pulmonary tuberculosis in patients at risk for HIV infection. *Chest* 1992;102:143–146.

61. Conde MB, Soares SL, Mello FC, et al. Comparison of sputum induction with fiberoptic bronchoscopy in the diagnosis of tuberculosis: experience at an acquired immune deficiency syndrome reference center in Rio de Janeiro, Brazil. *Am J Respir Crit Care Med* 2000;162:2238–2240.

62. Kaplan MH, Armstrong D, Rosen P. Tuberculosis complicating neoplastic disease: a review of 201 cases. *Cancer* 1974;33:850–858.

63. Martino R, Martinez C, Brunet S, et al. Tuberculosis in bone marrow transplant recipients: report of two cases and review of the literature. *Bone Marrow Transplant* 1996;18:809–812.

64. Aljurf M, Gyger M, Alrajhi A, et al. *Mycobacterium tuberculosis* infection in allogeneic bone marrow transplantation patients. *Bone Marrow Transplant* 1999;24:551–554.

65. Prevention and treatment of tuberculosis among patients infected with human immunodeficiency virus: principles of

therapy and revised recommendations. *MMWR Morb Mortal Wkly Rep* 1998;47(RR-20):1–58.

66. MacDonnell KB, Glassroth J. *Mycobacterium avium* complex and other nontuberculous mycobacteria in patients with HIV infection. *Semin Respir Infect* 1989;4:123–132.

67. Malouf MA, Glanville AR. The spectrum of mycobacterial infection after lung transplantation. *Am J Respir Crit Care Med* 1999;160:1611–1616.

68. Straus WL, Ostroff SM, Jernigan DB, et al. Clinical and epidemiologic characteristics of *Mycobacterium haemophilum,* an emerging pathogen in immunocompromised patients. *Ann Intern Med* 1994;120:118–125.

69. White DA, Kiehn TE, Bondoc AY, et al. Pulmonary nodule due to *Mycobacterium haemophilum* in an immunocompetent host. *Am J Respir Crit Care Med* 1999;160:1366–1368.

70. ATS Statement. Fungal infection in HIV-infected persons. *Am J Respir Crit Care Med* 1995;152:816–822.

71. Jones JM. Pneumonia due to *Candida, Aspergillus,* and Mucorales species. In: Shelhammer J, Pizzo P, Parillo J, et al., eds. *Respiratory disease in the immunosuppressed host.* Philadelphia: JB Lippincott Co, 1991:338–354.

72. Miller WT, Sais GJ, Frank I, et al. Pulmonary aspergillosis in patients with AIDS. Clinical and radiographic correlations. *Chest* 1994;105:37–44.

73. Denning DW, Follansbee SE, Scolaro M, et al. Pulmonary aspergillosis in the acquired immunodeficiency syndrome. *N Engl J Med* 1991;324:654–662.

74. Caillot D, Casasnovas O, Bernard A, et al. Improved management of invasive pulmonary aspergillosis in neutropenic patients using early thoracic computed tomographic scan and surgery. *J Clin Oncol* 1997;15:139–147.

75. Kuhlman JE, Fishman EK, Siegelman SS. Invasive pulmonary aspergillosis in acute leukemia: characteristic findings on CT, the CT halo sign and the role of CT in early diagnosis. *Radiology* 1985;157:611–614.

76. Gefter WB, Albelda SM, Talbot GH, et al. Invasive pulmonary aspergillosis and acute leukemia. Limitations in the diagnostic utility of the air crescent sign. *Radiology* 1985;157:605–610.

77. Horvath JA, Dummer S. The use of respiratory tract cultures in the diagnosis of invasive pulmonary aspergillosis. *Am J Med* 1996; 100:171–178.

78. Freeberg G, Stover DE, Levine S, et al. Spectrum of pulmonary aspergillosis in immunocompromised hosts. *Chest* 1990;98: 31S.

79. Reichenberger F, Habicht J, Kaim A, et al. Lung resection for invasive pulmonary aspergillosis in neutropenic patients with hematologic disease. *Am J Respir Crit Care Med* 1998;158:885–890.

80. Lortholary O, Meyohas MC, Dupont B et al. Invasive aspergillosis in patients with acquired immunodeficiency syndrome: a report of 33 cases. *Am J Med* 1993;95:171–187.

81. Denning DW. Therapeutic outcome in invasive aspergillosis. *Clin Infect Dis* 1996;23:608–615.

82. Terrell C. Antifungal agents. Part II. The azoles. *Mayo Clin Proc* 1999;74:78–100.

83. Wong-Beringer A, Jacobs RA, Guglielmo BJ. Lipid formulations of amphotericin B: clinical efficacy and toxicities. *Clin Infect Dis* 1998;27:603–618.

84. Ng TC, Denning DW. Liposomal amphotericin B (Ambisome) therapy in invasive fungal infections. *Arch Intern Med* 1995;155: 1093–1098.

85. Dismukes WE. Introduction to antifungal drugs. *Clin Infect Dis* 2000;30:653–657.

86. Walsh TJ, Hiemenz JW, Seibel NL, et al. Amphotericin B lipid complex for invasive fungal infections: analysis of safety

and efficacy in 556 cases. *Clin Infect Dis* 1998;26:1383–1396.

87. Walsh TJ, Finberg RW, Arndt C et al. Liposomal amphotericin B for empirical therapy in patients with persistent fever and neutropenia. *N Engl J Med* 1999;340:764–771.

88. White MH, Bowden RA, Sandler ES, et al. Randomized, double-blind clinical trial of amphotericin B colloidal dispersion vs. amphotericin B in the empirical treatment of fever and neutropenia. *Clin Infect Dis* 1998;27:296–302.

89. Wingard JR, White MH, Anaissie E, et al. A randomized double-blind comparative trial evaluating the safety of liposomal amphotericin B versus amphotericin B lipid complex in the empirical treatment of febrile neutropenia. *Clin Infect Dis* 2000;31:1155–1163.

90. Stevens DA, Kan VL, Judson MA, et al. Practice guidelines for diseases caused by *Aspergillus. Clin Infect Dis* 2000;30:696–709.

91. Boogerts M, Winston DJ, Bow EJ et al. Intravenous and oral itraconazole versus intravenous amphotericin B deoxycholate as empirical antifungal therapy for persistent fever in neutropenic patients with cancer who are receiving broad-spectrum antibacterial therapy: a randomized, controlled trial. *Ann Intern Med* 2001;135:412–422.

92. Denning DW, Lee JY, Hostetler JS, et al. NIAID Mycoses Study Group multicenter trial of oral itraconazole therapy for invasive aspergillosis. *Am J Med* 1994;97:135–144.

93. Stevens DA, Lee JY. Analysis of compassionate use itraconazole for invasive aspergillosis by the NIAID Mycoses Study Group criteria. *Arch Intern Med* 1997;157:1857–1862

94. Caillot D, Bassaris H, McGeer A, et al. Intravenous itraconazole followed by oral itraconazole in the treatment of invasive pulmonary aspergillosis in patients with hematologic malignancies, chronic granulomatous disease, or AIDS. *Clin Infect Dis* 2001;33:E83–E90.

95. Trulock EP. Lung transplantation. *Am J Respir Crit Care Med* 1997;155:789–818.

96. Kovacs JA, Gill VJ, Meshnick S, et al. New insights into transmission, diagnosis, and drug treatment of *Pneumocystis carinii* pneumonia. *JAMA* 2001;286:2450–2460.

97. Cushion MT. Taxonomy, genetic organization and life cycle of *Pneumocystis carinii. Semin Respir Infect* 1998;13:304–312.

98. Gutierrez Y. The biology of *Pneumocystis carinii. Semin Diagn Pathol* 1989;6:203–211.

99. Su TH, Martin WJ. Pathogenesis and host response in *Pneumocystis carinii* pneumonia. *Annu Rev Med* 1994;45:261–272.

100. Walzer PD. Pathogenic mechanisms. In: Walzer, ed. *Pneumocystis carinii pneumonia,* 2nd ed. New York: Marcel Dekker Inc, 1994:251–265.

101. LaTouche S, Rabodonirina M, Mazars E. *Pneumocystis:* the 'carrier state': epidemiology and transmission of human pneumocystosis. *FEMS Immunol Med Microbiol* 1998;22:81–86.

102. Chen W, Gigliotti F, Harmsen AG. Latency is not an inevitable outcome of infection with *Pneumocystis carinii. Infect Immun* 1993;61:5406–5409.

103. Sepkowitz KA, Brown AE, Telzak E, et al. *Pneumocystis carinii* pneumonia among patients without AIDS at a cancer hospital. *JAMA* 1992;267:832–837.

104. Sepkowitz KA. Patients with T cell defects: part 2. *Pneumocystis carinii* pneumonia in patients without AIDS. *Clin Infect Dis* 1993;17[Suppl 2]:S416–S422.

105. Sepkowitz KA, Brown AE, Armstrong D. *Pneumocystis carinii* pneumonia without acquired immunodeficiency syndrome: more patients, same risk. *Arch Intern Med* 1995;155:1125–1127.

106. Phair J, Munoz A, Detels R, et al. The risk of *Pneumocystis carinii*

pneumonia among men infected with human immunodeficiency virus type 1. *N Engl J Med* 1990;322:161–165.

107. Hoover DR, Saah AJ, Bacellar H, et al. Clinical manifestations of AIDS in the era of *Pneumocystis* prophylaxis. *N Engl J Med* 1993;329:1922–1926.

108. Kovacs JA, Hiemenz JW, Macher AM, et al. *Pneumocystis carinii* pneumonia: a comparison between patients with the acquired immunodeficiency syndrome and patients with other immunodeficiencies. *Ann Intern Med* 1984;100:663–671.

109. Nuesch R, Bellini C, Zimmerli W. *Pneumocystis carinii* pneumonia in human immunodeficiency virus (HIV)-positive and HIV-negative immunocompromised patients. *Clin Infect Dis* 1999;29: 1519–1523.

110. Telzak E, Cote RJ, Gold JWM, et al. Extrapulmonary *Pneumocystis carinii* pneumonia. *Rev Infect Dis* 1990;12:380–386.

111. Kennedy CA, Goetz MB. Atypical roentgenographic manifestations of *Pneumocystis carinii* pneumonia. *Arch Intern Med* 1992; 152:1390–1398.

112. Boiselle PM, Crans CA, Kaplan MA. The changing face of *Pneumocystis carinii* pneumonia in AIDS patients. *Am J Radiol* 1999;172:1301–1309.

113. Smith DE, Wyatt J, McLuckie A, et al. Severe exercise hypoxemia with normal or near normal x-rays: a feature of *Pneumocystis carinii* infection. *Lancet* 1988;2:1049–1051.

114. Gruden JF, Huang L, Turner J, et al. High-resolution CT in the evaluation of clinically suspected *Pneumocystis carinii* pneumonia: radiographic characteristics, natural history, and complications. *AJR Am J Roentgenol* 1997;169:967–975.

115. Zaman MK, White DA. Serum lactate dehydrogenase levels and *Pneumocystis carinii* pneumonia. *Am Rev Respir Dis* 1988; 137:796–800.

116. Jules-Elysee KM, Stover DE, Zaman MB, et al. Aerosolized pentamidine: effect on the diagnosis and presentation of *Pneumocystis carinii* pneumonia. *Ann Intern Med* 1990;112:750–757.

117. Bigby TD, Margolskee D, Curtis JL, et al. The usefulness of induced sputum in the diagnosis of *Pneumocystis carinii* pneumonia in patients with the acquired immunodeficiency syndrome. *Am Rev Respir Dis* 1986;133:515–518.

118. Pitchenik AE, Ganji P, Torres A, et al. Sputum examination for the diagnosis of *Pneumocystis carinii* pneumonia in the acquired immunodeficiency syndrome. *Am Rev Respir Dis* 1986;133:226– 229.

119. Levine SJ, Masur H, Gill VJ, et al. Effect of aerosolized pentamidine prophylaxis on the diagnosis of *Pneumocystis carinii* pneumonia by induced sputum examination in patients infected with the human immunodeficiency virus. *Am Rev Respir Dis* 1991;144:760–764.

120. Broaddus C, Dake MD, Stulbarg MS, et al. Bronchoalveolar lavage and transbronchial biopsy for the diagnosis of pulmonary infections in the immunodeficiency syndrome. *Ann Intern Med* 1985;102:747–752.

121. Meduri GU, Stover DE, Nash T. Bilateral bronchoalveolar lavage in the diagnosis of opportunistic pulmonary infections. *Chest* 1991;100:1272–1276.

122. Masur H. Prevention and treatment of *Pneumocystis* pneumonia. *N Engl J Med* 1995;327:1853–1860.

123. Hughes WT, Feldman S, Chaudhary SC, et al. Comparison of pentamidine isethionate and trimethoprim-sulfamethoxazole in the treatment of *Pneumocystis carinii* pneumonia. *J Pediatr* 1978;92:285–291.

124. Wharton JM, Coleman DL, Wolfsky CB, et al. Trimethoprim-sulfamethoxazole or pentamidine for *Pneumocystis carinii* in the acquired immunodeficiency syndrome. *Ann Intern Med* 1986;105:37–44.

125. Klein NC, Duncanson FP, Lenoa TH, et al. Trimethoprim-

sulfamethoxazole versus pentamidine for *Pneumocystis carinii* pneumonia in AIDS patients: results of a large, prospective randomized trial. *AIDS* 1992;6:301–305.

126. Soo Hoo GW, Mohsenifar Z, Meyer RD. Inhaled or intravenous pentamidine therapy for *Pneumocystis carinii* pneumonia in AIDS. *Ann Intern Med* 1990;113:195–202.

127. Safrin S, Finkelstein DM, Feinberg J, et al. Comparison of three regimens for treatment of mild to moderate *Pneumocystis carinii* pneumonia in patients with AIDS: a double-blind, randomized trial of oral trimethoprim-sulfamethoxazole, dapsone-trimethoprim, and clindamycin-primaquine. *Ann Intern Med* 1996;124:792–802.

128. Hughes W, Leong G, Kramer F, et al. Comparison of atovaquone (566C80) with trimethoprim-sulfamethoxazole to treat *Pneumocystis carinii* pneumonia in patients with AIDS. *N Engl J Med* 1993;328:1521–1527.

129. Dohn MN, Weinberg WG, Torres RA, et al. Oral atovaquone compared with intravenous pentamidine for *Pneumocystis carinii* pneumonia in patients with AIDS. *Ann Intern Med* 1994;121: 174–180.

130. Safrin S, Sattler FR, Lee BL, et al. Dapsone as single agent is suboptimal therapy for *Pneumocystis carinii* pneumonia. *J AIDS* 1991;4:244–249.

131. Bozzette SA, Sattler FR, Chiu J, et al. A controlled trial of early adjunctive treatment with corticosteroids for *Pneumocystis carinii* pneumonia in the acquired immunodeficiency syndrome. *N Engl J Med* 1990;323:1451–1457.

132. National Institutes of Health-University of California expert panel. Consensus statement on the use of corticosteroids as adjunctive therapy for *Pneumocystis* pneumonia in the acquired immunodeficiency syndrome. *N Engl J Med* 1990;323:1500– 1504.

133. Gagnon S, Boota AM, Fischl MA, et al. Corticosteroids as adjunctive therapy for severe *Pneumocystis carinii* pneumonia in the acquired immunodeficiency syndrome: a double-blinded, placebo-controlled trial. *N Engl J Med* 1990;323:1444–1450.

134. Montaner JS, Lawson LM, Levitt N, et al. Corticosteroids prevent early deterioration in patients with moderately severe *Pneumocystis carinii* pneumonia in the acquired immunodeficiency syndrome (AIDS). *Ann Intern Med* 1990;113:14–20.

135. Pareja JG, Garland R, Koziel H. Use of adjunctive corticosteroids in severe adult non-HIV *Pneumocystis carinii* pneumonia. *Chest* 1998;113:1215–1224.

136. Delclaux C, Zahar R, Amraoui G. Corticosteroids as adjunctive therapy for severe *Pneumocystis carinii* pneumonia in non–HIV-infected patients: retrospective study of 31 patients. *Clin Infect Dis* 1999;29:670–672.

137. Hughes WT, Kuhn S, Chaudhary S, et al. Successful chemoprophylaxis for *Pneumocystis carinii* pneumonitis. *N Engl J Med* 1977;297:419–426.

138. Hoover DR, Saah AJ, Bacellar H, et al. Clinical manifestations of AIDS in the era of *Pneumocystis* prophylaxis. *N Engl J Med* 1993;329:1922–1926.

139. Ionnadis JP, Cappalleri JC, Skolnik PR, et al. A meta-analysis of the relative efficacy and toxicity of *Pneumocystis carinii* prophylactic regimens. *Arch Intern Med* 1996;156:177–188.

140. Masur H, Bozzette SA, Finkelstein DM, et al. A randomized trial of three anti-*Pneumocystis* agents in patients with advanced human immunodeficiency virus infection. *N Engl J Med* 1995;332:693–699.

141. El-Sadr WM, Murphy RL, Yurik TM, et al. Atovaquone compared with dapsone for the prevention of *Pneumocystis carinii* pneumonia in patients with HIV infection who cannot tolerate trimethoprim, sulfonamides, or both. *N Engl J Med* 1998;339:1889–1895.

142. Ena J, Amador C, Pasquau F, et al. Once-a-month administration of intravenous pentamidine to patients infected with human immunodeficiency virus as prophylaxis for *Pneumocystis carinii* pneumonia. *Clin Infect Dis* 1994;18:901–904.

143. Barber BA, Pegram PS, High KP, et al. Clindamycin/primaquine as prophylaxis for *Pneumocystis carinii*. *Clin Infect Dis* 1996;23:718–722.

144. Bessesen MT, Miller LA, Cohn DL, et al. Administration of pyrimethamine/sulfadoxine for prevention of *Pneumocystis carinii* pneumonia in patients with AIDS. *Clin Infect Dis* 1995;20:730–731.

145. Mustafa MM, Pappo A, Cash J, et al. Aerosolized pentamidine for the prevention of *Pneumocystis carinii* pneumonia in children with cancer intolerant or allergic to trimethoprim/sulfamethoxazole. *J Clin Oncol* 1994;12:258–261.

146. Lopez JC, De Quiros B, Miro JM, et al. A randomized trial of the discontinuation of primary and secondary prophylaxis against *Pneumocystis carinii* pneumonia after highly active antiretroviral therapy in patients with HIV infection. *N Engl J Med* 2001;344:159–167.

147. Ledergerber B, Mocroft A, Reiss P, et al. Discontinuation of secondary prophylaxis against *Pneumocystis carinii* pneumonia in patients with HIV infection who have a response to antiretroviral therapy. *N Engl J Med* 2001;344:168–174.

148. Furrer H, Egger M, Opravil M, et al. Discontinuation of primary prophylaxis against *Pneumocystis carinii* pneumonia in HIV-1–infected adults treated with combination anti-retroviral therapy. *Lancet* 1999;353:1293–1298.

149. Sepkowitz KA. *Pneumocystis carinii* pneumonia without acquired immunodeficiency syndrome: who should receive prophylaxis? *Mayo Clin Proc* 1996;71:102–103.

150. Kazanjian P, Lock AB, Hossler PA, et al. *Pneumocystis carinii* mutations associated with sulfa and sulfone prophylaxis failures in AIDS patients. *AIDS* 1998;12:873–878.

151. Ma L, Borio L, Masur H, et al. *Pneumocystis carinii* dihydropteroate synthase but not dihydrofolate reductase gene mutations correlate with prior trimethoprim-sulfamethoxazole or dapsone use. *J Infect Dis* 1999;180:1969–1978.

152. Kazanjian P, Armstrong W, Hossler PA, et al. *Pneumocystis carinii* mutations are associated with duration of sulfa or sulfone prophylaxis exposure in AIDS patients. *J Infect Dis* 2000;182:551–557.

153. Mei Q, Gurunthan S, Masur H, et al. Failure of co-trimoxazole in *Pneumocystis carinii* infection and mutations in dihydropterate synthase gene. *Lancet* 1998;351:1631–1632.

154. Helweg-Larsen J, Benfield TL, Eugen-Olsen J, et al. Effects of mutations in *Pneumocystis carinii* dihydropterate synthase gene on the outcome of AIDS-associated *P. carinii* pneumonia. *Lancet* 1999;354:1347–1351.

155. Drutz DJ. Pneumonia due to endemic fungi. In: Shelhammer J, Pizzo PA, Parillo JE, et al., eds. *Respiratory disease in the immunosuppressed host*. Philadelphia: JB Lippincott Co, 1991:355–385.

156. Eng RH, Bishburg E, Smith SM, et al. Cryptococcal infections in patients with acquired immunodeficiency syndrome. *Am J Med* 1986;81:19–23.

157. Saag MS, Graybill RJ, Larsen RA, et al. Practice guidelines for the management of cryptococcal disease. *Clin Infect Dis* 2000;30:710–718.

158. Wheat LJ, Slama TG, Norton JA, et al. Risk factors for disseminated or fatal histoplasmosis. *Ann Intern Med* 1982;96:159–163.

159. Davies SF, Sarosi GA. Fungal pulmonary complications. *Clin Chest Med* 1996;725–744.

160. Wheat LJ. Histoplasmosis. *Infect Dis Clin North Am* 1989;3:843.

161. Wheat J, Sarosi G, McKinsey D, et al. Practice guidelines for the management of patients with histoplasmosis. *Clin Infect Dis* 2000;30:688–695.

162. Galgiani JN, Ampel NM, Catanzaro A, et al. Practice guidelines for the treatment of coccidioidomycosis. *Clin Infect Dis* 2000;30:658–661.

163. Chu E, Whitlock WL, Dietrich RA. Pulmonary hyperinfection syndrome with *Strongyloides stercoralis*. *Chest* 1990;97:1475–1477.

164. Scowden EB, Schaffner W, Stone WJ. Overwhelming strongyloidiasis: an unappreciated opportunistic infection. *Medicine (Baltimore)* 1978;57:527–544.

165. Kramer MR, Gregg PA, Goldstein M, et al. Disseminated strongyloidiasis in AIDS and non-AIDS immunocompromised hosts: diagnosis by sputum and bronchoalveolar lavage. *South Med J* 1990;83:1226–1229.

166. Pomeroy C, Felice GA. Pulmonary toxoplasmosis: a review. *Clin Infect Dis* 1992;14:863–870.

167. Ortonne N, Ribaud P, Meignin V, et al. Toxoplasmic pneumonitis leading to fatal acute respiratory distress syndrome after engraftment in three bone marrow transplant recipients. *Transplantation* 2001;15:1838–1840.

168. Bonilla CA, Rosa UW. *Toxoplasma gondii* pneumonia in patients with the acquired immunodeficiency syndrome: diagnosis by bronchoalveolar lavage. *South Med J* 1994;87:659–663.

169. Emanuel D, Peppard J, Stover DE, et al. Rapid immunodiagnosis of cytomegalovirus (CMV) pneumonia by bronchoalveolar lavage using human and murine monoclonal antibodies. *Ann Intern Med* 1986;104:476–481.

170. Tamm M, Traenkle P, Grilli B, et al. Pulmonary cytomegalovirus infection immunocompromised patients. *Chest* 2001;119:838–843.

171. Emanuel D, Cunningham I, Jules-Elysee K, et al. Cytomegalovirus pneumonia after bone marrow transplantation successfully treated with the combination of ganciclovir and high-dose intravenous immune globulin. *Ann Intern Med* 1988;109:777–782.

172. Koehler M, St. George K, Ehrlich GD, et al. Prevention of CMV disease in allogeneic BMT recipients by cytomegalovirus antigenemia-guided preemptive ganciclovir therapy. *J Pediatr Hematol Oncol* 1997;19:43–47.

173. Evans MJ, Edwards-Spring Y, Myers J. Polymerase chain reaction assays for the detection of cytomegalovirus in organ and bone marrow transplant recipients. *Immunol Invest* 1997;26:209–229.

174. Duncan RS, Paradis IL, Yousem SA, et al. Sequelae of cytomegalovirus pulmonary infection in lung allograft recipients. *Am Rev Respir Dis* 1992;146:1419–1425.

175. Mann M, Shelhamer JH, Masur H, et al. Lack of clinical utility of bronchoalveolar lavage cultures for cytomegalovirus in HIV infection. *Am J Respir Crit Care Med* 1997;155:1723–1728.

176. Millar AB, Patou G, Miller RF, et al. Cytomegalovirus in the lung of patients with AIDS. Respiratory pathogen or passenger? *Am Rev Respir Dis* 1990;141:1474–1477.

177. Miles PR, Baughman RP, Linnemann CC. Cytomegalovirus in the bronchoalveolar lavage fluid of patients with AIDS. *Chest* 1990;97:1072–1076.

178. McKenzie R, Travis WD, Dolan SA, et al. The causes of death in patients with human immunodeficiency virus infection: a clinical and pathologic study with emphasis on the role of pulmonary diseases. *Medicine* 1991;70:326–343.

179. Salomon N, Gomez T, Perlman DC, et al. Clinical features

and outcome of HIV-related cytomegalovirus pneumonia. *AIDS* 1997;11:319–324.

180. Rodriguez-Barradas MC, Stool E, Musher DM, et al. Diagnosing and treating cytomegalovirus pneumonia in patients with AIDS. *Clin Infect Dis* 1996;23:76–81.

181. Waxman AB, Goldie SJ, Brett-Smith H, et al. Cytomegalovirus as a primary pathogen in AIDS. *Chest* 1997;111:128–134.

182. Ramsey PG, Fife KH, Hackman RL, et al. Herpes simplex virus pneumonia: clinical, virologic and pathologic features in 20 patients. *Ann Intern Med* 1982;97:813–820.

183. Buchbinder S, Elmaagacli AH, Schaefer UW, et al. Human herpesvirus 6 is an important pathogen in infectious lung disease after allogeneic bone marrow transplantation. *Bone Marrow Transplant* 2000;26:639–644.

184. Breese Hall, C. Respiratory syncytial virus and parainfluenza virus. *N Engl J Med* 2001;344:1917–1928.

185. Whimbey E, Champlin RE, Englund JA, et al. Combination therapy with aerosolized ribavirin and intravenous immunoglobulin for respiratory syncytial virus disease in adult bone marrow transplant recipients. *Bone Marrow Transplant* 1995;16:393–399.

186. Englund JA, Piedra PA, Jewell A, et al. Rapid diagnosis of respiratory syncytial virus in immunocompromised adults. *J Clin Microbiol* 1996;34:1649–1653.

187. Ghosh S, Champlin RE, Englund J, et al. Respiratory syncytial virus upper respiratory tract illness blood and marrow transplant recipients: combination therapy with aerosolized rib-

avirin and intravenous immunoglobulin. *Bone Marrow Transplant* 2002;25:751–755.

188. La Rosa AM, Champlin RE, Mirza N, et al. Adenovirus infections in adult recipients of blood and marrow transplants. *Clin Infect Dis* 2001;32:871–876.

189. Shields AF, Hackman RC, Fife KH, et al. Adenovirus infections in patients undergoing bone-marrow transplantation. *N Engl J Med* 1985;312:529–533.

190. Whimbey E, Elting LS, Conch RB, et al. Influenza A virus infections among hospitalized adult bone marrow transplant recipients. *Bone Marrow Transplant* 1994;13:437–440.

191. Lin JC, Nichol KL. Excess mortality due to pneumonia or influenza during influenza seasons among persons with acquired immunodeficiency syndrome. *Arch Intern Med* 2001;161:441–446.

192. Garantziotis S, Howell DN, McAdams HP, et al. Influenza pneumonia in lung transplant recipients—clinical feature and association with bronchiolitis obliterans syndrome. *Chest* 2001;119:1277–1280.

193. Massad MG, Ramirez AM. Influenza pneumonia in thoracic organ transplant recipients. What can we do to avoid it? *Chest* 2001;119:997–999.

194. Gubareva LV, Kaiser L, Hayden FG. Influenza virus neuraminidase inhibitors. *Lancet* 2000;35:827–835.

195. Whimbey E, Englund JA, Couch RB. Community respiratory virus infections in immunocompromised patients with cancer. *Am J Med* 1997;102(3A):10–18.

19 Pulmonary Fungal Infections

Scott F. Davies · George A. Sarosi

This chapter focuses on the clinical manifestations, diagnosis, and treatment of histoplasmosis, blastomycosis, coccidioidomycosis, and cryptococcosis. The first three diseases are the most common of the four major endemic mycoses of the Western Hemisphere. Histoplasmosis and blastomycosis are endemic in much of the north central, central, and south central United States, with the highest rate of disease activity in the Ohio and Mississippi River valleys. Although histoplasmosis and blastomycosis are both endemic in these large areas, the area of endemicity for histoplasmosis extends to the Caribbean islands, Central America, and the St. Lawrence River valley of eastern Canada, whereas the area of endemicity for blastomycosis extends to northern Wisconsin, northern Minnesota, and large areas of central Canada. Coccidioidomycosis occurs in North America (the desert southwest of the United States and adjacent areas of Mexico) and to a lesser extent in South America. Paracoccidioidomycosis occurs exclusively in South and Central America and is not discussed here. Although histoplasmosis and blastomycosis are occasionally diagnosed on other continents, the major areas of endemicity for all these fungal infections are in the Western Hemisphere. The areas where histoplasmosis, blastomycosis, and coccidioidomycosis are endemic have been defined by means of skin tests for *Histoplasma capsulatum* (1) and *Coccidioides immitis* infection (2) and by the tabulation of patients with *Blastomyces dermatitidis* infection (3,4). Cryptococcosis occurs throughout the world and is also discussed in this chapter.

The endemic mycoses share certain characteristics. The causative organisms grow in the soil in a mycelial form (containing hyphae, which are long, ribbonlike strands of fungus that can form a dense, tangled mat). Each fungus has a different ecologic niche, requiring specific nutrients and soil conditions for growth. When temperature, rainfall, and other factors are optimal, fungal growth accelerates, and spores (specialized structures, often very small, initially attached to the hyphae) are formed. If a site harboring active fungal growth is disturbed, the spores are easily aerosolized. If a proximate mammal inhales the aerosolized spores, infection may occur.

After being inhaled into mammalian lungs, these fungi convert to characteristic parasitic forms. This phenomenon is known as *dimorphism* ("two forms"). *H. capsulatum* and *B. dermatitidis* convert to a yeast form at 37°C (thermal dimorphism), and the spores of *C. immitis* convert in tissue to spherules that reach a giant size (to 100 μm) and reproduce by progressive endosporulation with eventual rupture and release of endospores (tissue dimorphism). The parasitic forms of these fungi cannot be killed by pulmonary macrophages or recruited neutrophils (5).

Cryptococcus neoformans is a soil-dwelling, encapsulated yeast that causes disease in both normal and immunosuppressed hosts. Similar to the endemic mycoses, disease is always caused by the inhalation of airborne particles, which in the case of cryptococcosis are likely small, desiccated yeast forms. This organism is not dimorphic; it grows as a yeast in nature and in infected mammalian tissue. *C. neoformans* is widely distributed in nature, and disease caused by the fungus has been recognized throughout the world.

Cryptococcosis also shares certain important characteristics with the endemic mycoses. The disease is acquired by inhalation. The organism does not have a specific parasitic form, but in the infected host, it produces a thick polysaccharide capsule that is antiphagocytic. Control of cryptococcal infection also depends on intact T-cell function. Only with the advent of specific T cell–mediated immunity can

S. F. Davies: Department of Medicine, Hennepin County Medical Center and the University of Minnesota Medical School, Minneapolis, Minnesota.

G. A. Sarosi: Department of Medicine, Indiana University School of Medicine; Medical Service, Indianapolis VAMC, Indianapolis, Indiana.

infection be contained. Immunologically intact persons usually have self-limited primary infections, and diminution of T-cell activity allows progression of primary infection.

Epidemiologic evidence suggests that fungal organisms long dormant within the mammalian host may reactivate when intercurrent illness or immunosuppressive therapeutic agents greatly depress T cell–mediated immunity. Although late reactivation of these infections may occur, it is likely much less common than in tuberculosis (TB). Another important difference between the fungal infections and TB is the lack of person-to-person spread, which is partly a consequence of the dimorphic nature of the endemic fungi. The infecting particles in nature are very small and easily aerosolized. In contrast, the tissue forms of the dimorphic fungi are poorly aerosolized (because of large size or intracellular location) and do not serve as a vector to other humans. *Cryptococcus* has only one form, but it is likely that the yeast particles in established lung infection are larger and have more of a capsule than the infecting particles from the soil. As in the endemic mycoses, person-to-person spread has not been proved.

Another common dimorphic fungus, *Sporothrix schenckii,* is primarily acquired by subcutaneous inoculation of the infecting particles and typically presents with nodules along draining lymph channels. Patients with lung disease, presumably acquired by inhalation, have been reported. Such pulmonary infections are rare and are not discussed in this chapter.

Diseases such as aspergillosis and mucormycosis are caused by opportunistic fungi, and similar but much rarer diseases are caused by a variety of other soil fungi that when inhaled can exploit a severe decrease in phagocyte number or function. Fungi can also colonize lung cavities resulting from TB or other destructive processes and locally invade adjacent, usually abnormal lung tissue. They virtually never infect a structurally normal lung in a normal host. They are discussed briefly here and in greater detail in relation to immunocompromised hosts in Chapter 18. *Candida,* another phagocyte opportunist that is part of the endogenous flora, is also discussed in relation to conditions of immunodeficiency.

HISTOPLASMOSIS

Histoplasmosis is the most common of the endemic mycoses. It is acquired by inhalation and usually presents as a self-limited respiratory infection with mild symptoms of brief duration. For this reason, the vast majority of cases are undiagnosed, hidden within the huge numbers of self-limited respiratory tract infections of all causes. Primary infections come to attention when a point source outbreak involves multiple persons at the same time, when unusual radiographic features such as unilateral hilar adenopathy or diffuse micronodular infiltrates are detected, when sys-

temic manifestations including arthralgias and rashes (e.g., erythema multiforme and erythema nodosum) are prominent, and when complications such as pericarditis develop. Chronic pulmonary histoplasmosis tends to be slowly progressive (like TB) and forces a diagnosis when symptoms or radiographic findings become severe. Progressive disseminated histoplasmosis is often very severe and rapidly progressive, especially in AIDS. Tests are often urgently needed to make a diagnosis and drive specific therapy.

Pathogenesis

The portal of entry for *H. capsulatum* is the lung. After inhalation, the small ($<5\,\mu$m) infectious spores (microconidia) elude nonspecific pulmonary defenses and reach the alveoli. Conversion to the parasitic yeast phase begins immediately. The original cellular response to the infection includes recruitment of neutrophils, followed by a rapid increase in macrophages and monocytes. Neutrophils are unable to kill the yeast. Macrophages ingest the yeast particles, but in their preimmune state, they also cannot kill them. The yeast particles actively multiply within macrophages and disseminate throughout the body. Distant foci of infection are established in tissues rich in reticuloendothelial cells (RE), such as liver, spleen, lymph nodes, and bone marrow (6).

Intracellular proliferation of the fungus continues until specific T-cell immunity develops and checks further proliferation. With the advent of specific immunity, immune lymphocytes move into the lung and other infected organs. These lymphocytes then arm the macrophages, so that their ability to sequester and kill the fungus improves. Granulomas form, and depending on the intensity of the inflammatory process, central necrosis develops that is indistinguishable from that seen in TB. Areas of central necrosis develop in granulomas in the lung and at all distant sites. Fibrous encapsulation contains the central necrotic material, which later may calcify. Calcifications in the lung and draining hilar and mediastinal lymph nodes may be very similar to the classic Ghon complex and are often mistakenly ascribed to remote primary TB (7). Because necrosis also occurs at extrapulmonary sites, calcification can be seen in other organs, especially liver and spleen, of persons who have recovered from self-limited primary histoplasmosis. Small calcifications in spleen and liver are very commonly seen on routine diagnostic computed tomographic (CT) scans performed within areas of endemicity. They reflect the frequency of remote healed histoplasmosis in the population but do not have any clinical significance.

Clinical Manifestations

Primary Pulmonary Histoplasmosis

After inhaling the fungus, most normal persons have a mild primary infection with minimal or no symptoms (6).

Symptoms, when present, are so nonspecific that isolated sporadic cases of primary histoplasmosis are rarely diagnosed. Knowledge about benign, self-limited primary histoplasmosis comes mostly from the careful study of point source outbreaks in which the clustering of cases facilitates diagnosis. Cough and chest pain are the most common symptoms. The intensity of symptoms varies with the size of the infecting dose. Symptoms are often severe if the infection is acquired in a closed space (inoculum likely to be large) but trivial if the infection is acquired in an open area (inoculum likely to be much smaller). The site of exposure in most early outbreaks was often a closed space (cellar, chicken coop, cave), and many patients had severe symptoms (8). Chicken coops no longer exist, and small outbreaks today are often related to excavation, cleaning or demolishing old buildings, and cutting downed trees with a chain saw. Most large outbreaks now occur in urban centers, where heavily treed areas populated by blackbirds provide excellent sites for fungal growth (7). Many outbreaks have occurred in urban areas on the fringe of an area of endemicity where relatively few cases of histoplasmosis were previously recognized, including Mason City, Iowa (10), and Montreal, Canada (10). However, the largest known outbreak was in Indianapolis, Indiana (11), well within the area of endemicity. The usual precipitating event is heavy construction activity, disturbing contaminated soil and creating an infectious aerosol. In community-wide outbreaks, highly symptomatic disease is much less common than in smaller outbreaks associated with heavier exposure in closed spaces. Symptoms, even trivial ones, are reported by fewer than 50% of persons infected in large, open air outbreaks. Asymptomatic patients are identified by the serologic testing of exposed persons and coincidental chest radiography.

The incubation time for acute histoplasmosis is 14 days, with a fairly tight distribution (documented most carefully in open air outbreaks with a well-defined time of exposure). It has been speculated that heavy exposure in a closed space can lead to earlier fever and infiltrates, as can reexposure in previously infected persons.

Symptomatic patients with histoplasmosis have an illness that resembles influenza. The onset is abrupt, with fever, chills, substernal chest pain, and nonproductive cough. Nonspecific headache is common. Myalgias and arthralgias occur in a minority of patients (6). Although respiratory complaints are extremely common, serious impairment of gas exchange is rare. However, with a large infecting dose, rapid progression of illness may lead to diffuse infiltrates and hypoxemia. In extreme cases, hypoxemia is very severe, and the illness manifests as acute respiratory distress syndrome (ARDS).

Even in symptomatic patients, the chest radiographic findings may be negative. More often, the initial chest radiograph shows one or more areas of pneumonitis, usually in the lower lung fields, presumably because of the higher rate of ventilation in that region. Hilar adenopathy is com-

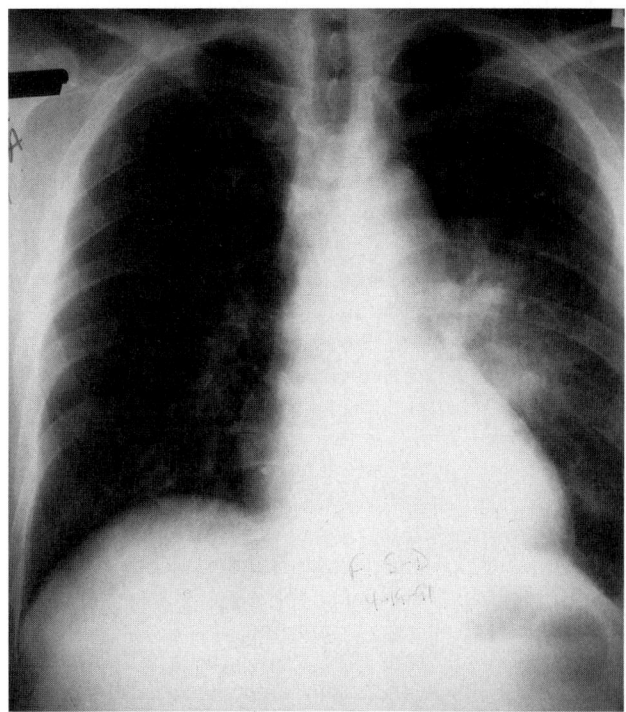

FIGURE 19.1. Primary pulmonary histoplasmosis. Chest radiograph shows massive left hilar adenopathy.

mon and usually ipsilateral (Fig. 19.1). When a patient in an area where the disease is highly endemic has symptoms of a lower respiratory infection and the chest radiograph shows a focal pulmonary infiltrate with enlarged unilateral hilar nodes, the diagnosis of histoplasmosis is relatively easy. However, parenchymal infiltrates are not always accompanied by hilar adenopathy; in that case, the radiograph is very nonspecific. Alternatively, hilar adenopathy may be present without infiltrate, so that the question of lymphoma or sarcoidosis arises. A variety of invasive diagnostic tests are often considered, depending on the radiographic findings. These tests (bronchoscopy, fine needle aspiration, mediastinoscopy, thoracoscopic video-assisted or traditional open lung biopsy) can usually be avoided if histoplasmosis is considered and diagnosed serologically.

The symptoms of primary histoplasmosis last a few days to a few weeks. In some cases, the chest radiographic manifestations clear completely. In others, the primary parenchymal infiltrate fails to resolve. It rounds up, undergoes central necrosis, and is contained by fibrous tissue. These rounded, densely fibrotic lesions later present as coin lesions that are difficult to differentiate from bronchogenic carcinoma. In the absence of specific benign patterns of calcification, the only absolute way to prove that these nodules are benign is surgical resection. Total calcification, dense central (exactly centered) calcification, and multiple concentric rings of calcification are virtually diagnostic of old granulomas, which are almost always histoplasmomas if the patient has a negative tuberculin skin test and lives or has lived in an area of endemicity. In contrast, eccentric clumps of calcification can be seen in benign lesions but also in malignant lesions because necrosis and dystrophic calcification can develop as a malignant tumor grows rapidly. Positron emission tomography (PET) can also be used to distinguish cancers (metabolically active) from old granulomas (metabolically inactive). False-negative results are possible with very small malignant lesions (<1 cm), and false-positive results if the infectious process is acute.

The approach to pulmonary nodules is complex. If old chest radiographs prove size stability for 2 years, the lesion is benign and can be ignored. Small lesions in patients younger than 35 years can be followed with a low but not zero chance of malignancy. If any lesion grows under observation, it should be studied further or removed. A positive PET result in an older patient with a significant smoking history, a large or growing nodule, and a low surgical risk is a strong indication for biopsy and resection if the lesion is malignant or indeterminate. Fine needle aspiration for diagnosis is also reasonable for any large or growing lesion, especially in a patient with a moderate to high surgical risk. The diagnosis of a specific benign condition precludes the need for surgery, a nonspecific result decreases the chance of cancer but does not exclude it, and a positive diagnosis of cancer warrants a more aggressive approach despite increased risk.

Chest CT for lung cancer, used increasingly to screen current and remote smokers for lung cancer, detects large numbers of nodules, especially when performed in patients who live or have lived in areas where histoplasmosis is highly endemic. In a study from Rochester, Minnesota, 66% of the patients had one to six noncalcified, mostly very small nodules (12). The incidence of lung cancer was 1.7%, and the false-positive rate was 98%. These tiny nodules are not fully understood and are not all granulomas. Careful serial follow-up of small and multiple lesions must be undertaken to remove all cancers early and yet avoid thoracotomy for benign disease. The follow-up algorithm recommended by the Mayo Clinic group is very complex (13). Serial studies are required for most patients, usually at 3- to 6-month intervals. Larger lesions discovered on initial screening should be addressed directly, as previously explained.

Hilar and mediastinal lymph nodes may calcify, as in TB. Foci of calcification in histoplasmosis tend to be larger; the whole node may become densely calcified.

A large infecting dose can cause a diffuse micronodular infiltrate. Healing and subsequent calcification of all these tiny nodules can result in "buckshot" calcifications throughout all lung fields. Often discovered on routine chest radiographs, they are highly characteristic of healed primary histoplasmosis (6). Many patients have no history of notable respiratory infection. The calcifications have no effect on pulmonary mechanics or gas exchange.

The physical examination findings during the acute phase of histoplasmosis are usually negative. Hepatosplenomegaly suggests disseminated disease (14). However, several clinical syndromes uncommonly occur with acute histoplasmosis. One is the arthralgia, erythema nodosum, and erythema multiforme complex (13). Arthralgias, when present, develop during the acute phase of the illness and may be severe enough to interfere with walking. They usually resolve quickly. Rarely, the arthralgias are accompanied by erythema multiforme or erythema nodosum, or both. These skin manifestations often occur in just a few patients in a large outbreak, and they frequently provide a clue that histoplasmosis may be the cause of the outbreak. They are most common in Caucasian women and may develop without other manifestations of histoplasmosis. The incidence is estimated at 1 in 200 infections (9).

Pericarditis may develop during the course of acute histoplasmosis. Although rarely mentioned earlier, pericarditis was a relatively common complication of acute histoplasmosis during a large outbreak in Indianapolis (15). Forty-five (6.3%) of 712 patients had pericarditis. Pericardial effusions are usually sterile and result from inflammation in the adjacent lung or mediastinum rather than direct spread of fungal organisms to the pericardium (15). Presumably, sporadic cases in the past were not linked to histoplasmosis and were likely diagnosed as benign pericarditis of presumed viral etiology.

Enlarged intrathoracic lymph nodes (called *mediastinal granulomas* when they are clinically significant) frequently impinge on adjacent mediastinal structures. Enlargement of the peritracheal nodes can cause an irritating cough or dyspnea. Pressure on the esophagus may lead to dysphagia. Enlarged nodes adjacent to the superior vena cava may obstruct the vessel and cause edema of the head and upper extremities. In some patients, the middle lobe syndrome may develop with collapse secondary to compression of the middle lobe bronchus. Large nodes in strategic places can be resected when they are causing severe symptoms, but the back wall of the nodal mass should be left and not dissected off the adjacent structure (overly aggressive attempts to resect the entire nodal mass can injure adherent structures and lead to hemorrhage if the nodal mass is compressing a vascular structure). Although surgery may relieve the symptoms, the natural history tends to be benign, with gradual improvement.

One of the most feared complications of histoplasmosis is exuberant mediastinal fibrosis, which can entrap vital structures and lead to severe functional derangement. The entrapment of bronchi, pulmonary arteries, and pulmonary veins may cause a range of problems, including postobstructive pneumonia, hemoptysis (sometimes from pulmonary venous obstruction), and in the worst cases progressive pulmonary hypertension and death from cor pulmonale. Surgery is dangerous and usually unsuccessful (16). Case reports and small series have documented stenting of individual narrowed arteries, veins, and bronchi. In a few select individuals with highly favorable focal narrowing of these structures, such procedures can result in clinical improvement

(17). Mediastinal fibrosis is a totally different disorder from mediastinal granuloma and does not result from progression of that entity.

Chronic Pulmonary Histoplasmosis

The clinical features of acute pulmonary histoplasmosis are very different in patients with structurally abnormal lungs. Many lifetime smokers have centrilobular emphysema, usually more severe in the upper lung zones. Infiltrates that develop after the organisms are inhaled tend to be located in one or both upper lobes (18). Areas of emphysema within the infiltrate sometimes cause it to appear cavitary. Most of these patients eventually recover, but clearing of the chest radiograph is very slow (19). In approximately 20% of such patients, a progressive destructive upper lobe disease develops that closely mimics TB (19–21) (Fig. 19.2). In fact, such patients were first recognized in TB sanatoriums in Missouri. They were admitted with the presumptive diagnosis of TB but were later shown to have histoplasmosis when multiple sputum cultures were negative for TB but positive for histoplasmosis (22).

The clinical manifestations of chronic pulmonary histoplasmosis resemble those of TB—low-grade fever, anorexia, and weight loss. Usually, the patient has a progressively worsening cough with the production of mucopurulent sputum. Chronic dyspnea is a frequent symptom, mostly caused by the underlying lung disease. Night sweats occur but are usually not as severe as in TB (21). Chronic pulmonary histo-

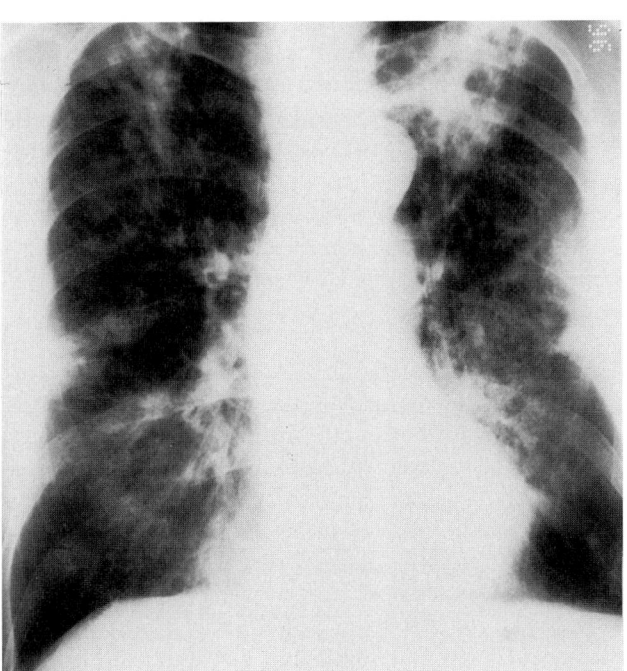

FIGURE 19.2. Chronic pulmonary histoplasmosis in a heavy smoker with moderate chronic obstructive pulmonary disease. Chest radiograph shows bilateral upper lobe fibronodular disease.

plasmosis is also called *chronic cavitary histoplasmosis*. The clinical and radiographic findings are very similar to those of adult reinfection TB, and great care is necessary to differentiate these two illnesses (20,21). Chronic pulmonary histoplasmosis usually smolders in the lung but does not spread to extrapulmonary sites.

Progressive Disseminated Histoplasmosis

During acute pulmonary infection, before the establishment of specific T cell–mediated immunity, the fungus gains access to the circulation through the hilar lymph nodes and spreads hematogenously to RE organs throughout the body. It is likely that benign extrapulmonary spread of the fungus occurs in this manner in most patients. Evidence for such spread comes from careful postmortem studies in Cincinnati, Ohio, in which healed *Histoplasma* granulomas were found in the spleen in more than 70% of patients who died of other causes (7).

Circulating *Histoplasma* yeast is phagocytosed by cells of the fixed RE system. Initially, rapid intracellular multiplication of the fungus takes place. Only with the onset of specific immunity can the armed macrophages check further replication of the ingested fungus. When T cell–mediated immunity fails to develop or is inadequate, the yeast multiplies unchecked. Heavily parasitized RE cells die, and the yeast particles are released but taken up by other macrophages (fixed cells and cells recruited to the area) that in their turn are destroyed by rapid growth of the fungus. In cases of severe T cell–mediated immune deficiency, whether induced by immunosuppressive drugs or by an underlying illness such as AIDS, a severe, progressive systemic illness develops that without treatment eventually kills the patient. This illness is referred to as *progressive disseminated histoplasmosis (PDH)* (14). The term *progressive* is important because it distinguishes unchecked systemic histoplasmosis from the benign extrapulmonary spread that accompanies most primary infections but is quickly limited by the advent of specific immunity (6,23).

PDH is a disease of the RE system in which the organism continues to multiply. Patients with PDH have a high fever and anorexia; this is a rapidly progressive, wasting illness. Respiratory symptoms may or may not be prominent; they are absent in about one third of patients at the onset of the febrile illness. The chest radiographic findings may be entirely normal. The physical examination reveals a febrile, toxic, ill patient. Hepatosplenomegaly is frequently present. Mucocutaneous ulcers may develop (14). The laboratory evaluation may show pancytopenia, abnormal serum liver chemistries, and, in a minority of patients, severe disseminated intravascular coagulation. None of these abnormalities distinguish histoplasmosis from other systemic infections or processes. Although uncommon, a markedly elevated serum ferritin level (≥10,000 ng/mL) has been reported in AIDS patients with PDH, but also in other clinical conditions (24).

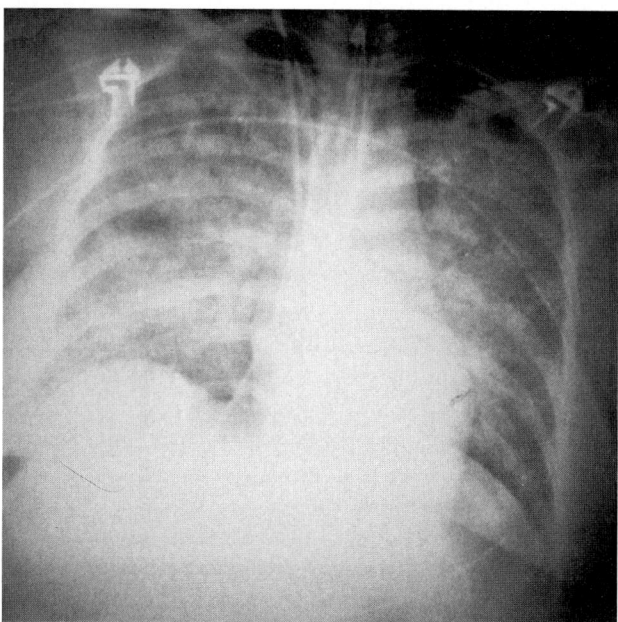

FIGURE 19.3. Progressive disseminated histoplasmosis in a patient with AIDS. Chest radiograph shows diffuse infiltrates.

The initial chest radiograph may show a variety of patterns, ranging from normal to diffusely abnormal with micronodular infiltrates or even diffuse noncardiac pulmonary edema (Fig. 19.3). In all patients with normal chest radiographic findings early in the course of the illness, pulmonary infiltrates develop as the illness progresses. Today, most cases of PDH occur in patients with AIDS (25,26). PDH also complicates organ transplantation and the glucocorticoid and immunosuppressive treatment now used for a wide variety of malignant and nonmalignant conditions.

The clinical onset of PDH may be temporally related to the onset of an immunosuppressive illness or the initiation of immunosuppressive therapy, most commonly high-dose glucocorticoids (27). This temporal relationship suggests that reactivation of previously healed and dormant histoplasmosis may be the mechanism of infection for some patients with PDH, as demonstrated by HIV-infected patients in whom, after many years of residence in areas where histoplasmosis is not endemic, PDH develops under the pressure of severely diminished CD4[+] lymphocyte counts (25). Most AIDS patients in whom PDH is diagnosed who are living in New York City and other cities in the eastern United States where histoplasmosis is not endemic have previously lived in the Caribbean basin, an area where *H. capsulatum* infection is endemic (28). Most AIDS patients in whom PDH is diagnosed who are living in San Francisco and other cities in the far western United States where histoplasmosis is not endemic have previously lived in areas of the central United States where it is highly endemic. *H. capsulatum* isolates from specific patients in New York City and San Francisco have been typed and found to be similar to strains from the

areas of endemicity where they lived before moving to these cities.

Ample evidence also suggests that primary infections in immunosuppressed persons rapidly disseminate. Most of the patients in whom PDH developed during a community-wide outbreak of histoplasmosis in Indianapolis were severely immunocompromised (29). These patients acquired new infections during the outbreak that rapidly progressed in the face of well-established T-cell defects. Study of another, more recent outbreak in the same city revealed that PDH developed in an astonishing one fourth or more of HIV-infected patients during the outbreak (26).

Some patients with PDH have a milder and more chronic illness. Careful evaluation of these patients after recovery reveals no obvious T-cell dysfunction. It is tempting to speculate that these persons may have had a transient T-cell dysfunction, possibly during an acute viral illness, but this hypothesis is unproven (14). In some patients, a chronic wasting disease develops that is similar to chronic TB. The main clinical findings are weight loss and low-grade fever. Ulcers of the mucocutaneous junction and mucosa may be seen in the mouth, pharynx, or rectum and on the glans penis. Extensive granulomatous involvement of the adrenal glands may destroy them and cause adrenal insufficiency. Histopathologic examination of involved tissues shows well-formed epithelioid granulomas with few organisms visible (14,30). An analogy to leprosy suggests that these patients have better T-cell function, well-developed granulomas, and few organisms (the "tuberculoid" form), whereas patients with severe T-cell deficiency, usually as a consequence of HIV infection, have no granulomas and an extremely high density of organisms in infected tissue (the "lepromatous" form).

Involvement of the central nervous system (CNS) by *H. capsulatum* is rare. CNS involvement can present as a space-occupying lesion (e.g., intracranial histoplasmoma) or as chronic meningitis (31). Endovascular infections may involve the valvular endocardium and abdominal aortic aneurysms (32).

Diagnosis

The gold standard for diagnosis is culture of the infecting organism from biologic material, which has perfect specificity. However, this method entails many problems. In primary pulmonary histoplasmosis, the cough is usually nonproductive, so that no specimen is readily available for culture. In mildly ill patients, invasive studies such as bronchoscopy and lung biopsy cannot be justified to obtain material for culture. On the other hand, culture isolation can take several weeks and is too slow for acutely ill patients. Thus, culture is complemented by serodiagnosis and direct histopathology in various forms of histoplasmosis. Histopathology is pathognomonic if the characteristic small intracellular yeast can be visualized in tissue; usually, special stains are required

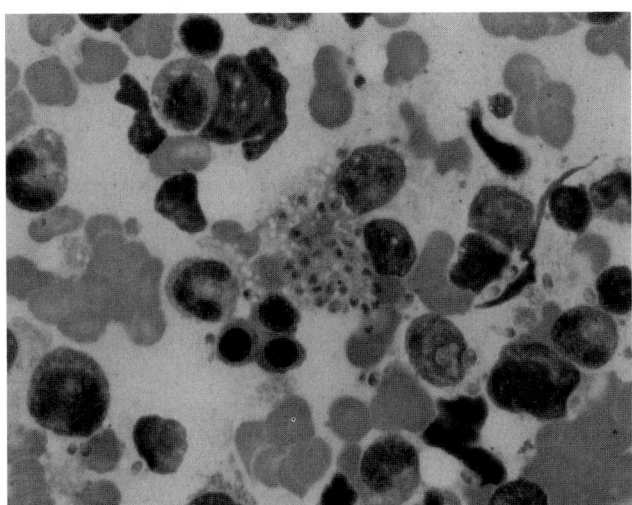

FIGURE 19.4. (See also Color Fig. 19.4.) Bone marrow aspirate from a patient with AIDS and progressive disseminated histoplasmosis. Highly characteristic image shows macrophage filled with 1- to 2-μm yeast cells (Wright stain, original magnification ×400).

(Fig. 19.4). Direct visualization of the organisms in sputum (which is scanty and seldom yields a diagnosis) is not helpful, as it is in blastomycosis and coccidioidomycosis. Characteristic organisms can sometimes be seen directly in blood smears (especially of buffy coat), bone marrow smears, and preparations of bronchoalveolar lavage (BAL) fluid when special stains are used. Visualization of the characteristic organisms, like a positive culture, has perfect specificity.

Most cases of primary histoplasmosis are diagnosed by serology. The disease of only 8% of patients in one large Indiana outbreak was diagnosed by positive sputum culture. In only one study (the outbreak in Orono, Minnesota) were cases identified by a case definition, which allowed a totally independent evaluation of serodiagnostic tests (33). Sensitivity increased with time. At 4 weeks after the onset of clinical illness (6 weeks after exposure), the sensitivity of complement fixation (CF) (to yeast phase antigen at a titer of 1:8 or higher) was 75%, and the sensitivity of immunodiffusion was 50%. The specificity depends on assumptions about the control group. About 5% of patients in areas with a high level of endemicity who have pneumonia of another cause have a histoplasmosis CF titer of 1:8 or higher, likely reflecting recent or remote infections that have resolved; in patients with other fungal infections, TB, or pneumonia of another cause, the incidence of positive CF tests is higher, at least double (34–37). Thus, for a nonspecific respiratory infection in an area where histoplasmosis is highly endemic (if one assumes that 10% of patients with other pneumonias would have a positive test result), the sensitivity of a 1:8 CF titer would be 75%, the specificity 90%, the positive predictive value 88%, and the negative predictive value 78%. If one assumes that 10% of similar infections are caused by histoplasmosis (pretest probability of 10%), then the posttest probability of disease with a positive test result would be 45%, and

the posttest probability of disease with a negative test result would be only 3%. However, in special situations in which the pretest likelihood of histoplasmosis is very high (focal infiltrate with unilateral hilar node, diffuse micronodular infiltrates 14 days after strong exposure history, or a group of multiply exposed persons with compatible history), then the performance of a 1:8 CF titer becomes much better. If the pretest likelihood of primary histoplasmosis is 50% (very likely a conservative estimate in the preceding situations), then the posttest probability is 88% if the test result is positive, and the posttest probability is 22% if the test result is negative. CF titers of 1:32 (or a fourfold titer rise under observation) have a lower sensitivity but a higher specificity. In acute histoplasmosis, about 75% of patients with a positive CF test of any titer reach a titer of 1:32 or higher (35). If one assumes a 1% likelihood of a 1:32 titer in patients with pneumonia of other causes in areas where the disease is heavily endemic, the sensitivity of a 1:32 titer would be 55%, but the specificity would be 99%, with a positive predictive value of 98% and a negative predictive value of 69%. If one uses examples similar to the previous ones, if the pretest probability of histoplasmosis is 10%, then the posttest probability if the test result is positive is 86%, and the posttest probability if the test result is negative is 4%. If the pretest probability of histoplasmosis is 50%, then the posttest probability if the test result is positive is 98%, and the posttest probability if the test result is negative is 31%. A positive immunodiffusion test result, although less sensitive than a 1:8 CF titer, likely has sensitivity and specificity similar to those of a 1:32 CF titer.

Urine *Histoplasma* polysaccharide antigen (HPA) has a low sensitivity in primary pulmonary histoplasmosis (25% in mild disease, increasing to 50% in severe disease) but a good specificity except for cross-reactivity with blastomycosis. Assuming blastomycosis is 10% as common as histoplasmosis and has a 50% cross-reactivity, then the sensitivity of urine HPA in mild acute histoplasmosis is 25%, the specificity is 99%, the positive predictive value is 96%, and the negative predictive value is 57%. Assuming that 10% of all nonspecific pneumonias in an area of heavy endemicity are caused by histoplasmosis, then the posttest probability if the test result is positive is 74%, and the posttest probability if the test result is negative is 8%. The sensitivity of urine HPA in severe acute histoplasmosis is 50%, the specificity is 99%, the positive predictive value is 98%, and the negative predictive value is 66%. Assuming that 10% of all nonspecific pneumonias in an area of heavy endemicity are caused by histoplasmosis, then the posttest probability if the test result is positive is 85% and the posttest probability if the test result is negative is 5%.

For the rare patients with rapidly progressive primary pulmonary infection impairing gas exchange, the diagnostic evaluation should start with urine HPA but often requires escalation to invasive tests ranging from bronchoscopy to video-assisted thoracoscopic open lung biopsy until a specific diagnosis is achieved by histopathology (pathognomonic 1- to 2-μm intracellular yeast particles) or by culture. This escalation of diagnostic tests is necessary to make a specific diagnosis among many possible infectious and immunologic cases of rapidly progressive ARDS.

Chronic cavitary histoplasmosis is easier to diagnosis. Sputum cultures are positive in at least 80% of cases and have perfect specificity. The CF titer is 1:8 or higher in 90% of patients. The sensitivity of a 1:8 CF titer is 90%, the specificity (assuming 10% background positivity in patients from areas of endemicity with similar chronic lung infection of different cause) is 90%, the positive predictive value is 90%, and the negative predictive value is 90%. If the clinical picture is highly suggestive (chronic fibrocavitary infiltrates with negative TB skin test and cultures), the pretest probability may be as high as 50%. With that assumption about pretest probability, the posttest probability if the test result is positive is 90%, and the posttest probability if the test result is negative is 10%. Urine HPA for chronic cavitary histoplasmosis is a very poor test; specificity is very good, but sensitivity is only 15%. For chronic pulmonary histoplasmosis, bronchoscopy and video-assisted thoracoscopic open lung biopsy (in that order, for cultures and histopathology) are seldom needed but can provide a specific diagnosis in difficult cases.

Progressive disseminated histoplasmosis today is most common in patients with AIDS. The burden of organisms is very high, and the diagnosis is usually not difficult. Some very good diagnostic tests have been carefully evaluated. In non-AIDS immunosuppressed patients, the diagnostic tests are generally less sensitive, and more invasive tests are sometimes needed.

Blood cultures (with use of the lysis centrifugation system) are positive in 90% of AIDS patients with PDH. In experienced hands, the intracellular organisms can be seen on the peripheral blood smear in 50% of patients. These tests have perfect specificity. The urine HPA test measures fungal antigen rather than an antibody response. This test is nearly perfect in AIDS patients, in whom the burden of organisms is very high, likely about 1 log higher than in other immunosuppressed patients. In AIDS (assuming the ratio of histoplasmosis to blastomycosis in AIDS is 100:1), HPA has sensitivity of 97%, specificity of 99%, positive predictive value of 99%, and negative predictive value of 99%. Assuming a 10% pretest probability for histoplasmosis in an AIDS patient with high fever and diffuse infiltrates in an area of endemicity, the posttest probability if test positive is 99%, and the posttest probability if test negative is less than half of 1%. The diagnosis in AIDS seldom needs to go beyond these three tests. Other tests that have high sensitivity and specificity include bronchoalveolar lavage and bone marrow biopsy.

In non-AIDS immunosuppressed patients, the sensitivity of blood cultures and peripheral blood smear is much lower. The urine HPA assay still has very good specificity but is less sensitive (50%–75%). More patients ultimately require

bronchoscopy and bone marrow biopsy (for histopathology and culture). The bone marrow biopsy is perhaps the best test in immunosuppressed patients with systemic febrile illness, no localizing symptom, and no response to antibacterial antibiotics. Specificity is perfect for positive cultures and for direct visualization of the characteristic intracellular organisms. Sensitivity is unknown but likely high if the infection is widely systemic and not localized to a specific organ system. Patients with isolated involvement of the skin, gastrointestinal tract, larynx, CNS, or other sites often require target-specific biopsies (38,39). Routine serodiagnostic tests such as CF and immunodiffusion have a lesser role in PDH. The results are often negative. Even when positive, they must be confirmed by more specific tests.

Finally, a word is required about skin testing, which has been a valuable epidemiologic tool but is not a diagnostic test for individual case finding. Intradermal skin testing with histoplasmin has been used extensively in epidemiologic studies and was the tool used to define and map the area of endemicity. Positive reactions are long-lasting. In areas where disease is highly endemic, virtually everyone by the age of 18 has a positive histoplasmin skin test result (40). Thus, a positive skin test result, even in the presence of an active pulmonary infiltrate, is not diagnostic of current histoplasmosis. It is more likely that the pulmonary infiltrate being investigated is the result of another infection and that the positive skin test result is only a relic of remote histoplasmosis. Most patients with PDH have a negative skin test reaction because AIDS or another immunosuppressive condition is causing a generalized T-cell defect (29). In summary, a positive skin test reaction does not prove current histoplasmosis, and a negative skin test reaction does not rule it out. The histoplasmin skin test should be used only as an epidemiologic tool, not for the diagnosis of individual infections (40). The production of histoplasmin has been discontinued, so the skin test may become of historical importance only.

Treatment

The highly effective treatment of fungal diseases began with amphotericin B in 1956. Before that time, patients with serious progressive forms of histoplasmosis generally died. Amphotericin B proved to be very effective therapy for the vast majority of these patients. Placebo-controlled trials were not performed, and dosages and duration of therapy were determined by retrospective analysis of successfully treated patients. A 40- to 50-mg daily dose of amphotericin B to response and then three times weekly to a total dose of 2 g was highly effective and could be given without undue toxicity. Newer agents were compared with amphotericin B, but only in selected groups of patients. (Clinical studies usually were limited to patients with mild to moderate disease not involving the CNS.) Ketoconazole had a higher failure rate and more relapses, even in these selected patients. Itraconazole proved much better, equal to amphotericin B in selected

DIAGNOSIS OF HISTOPLASMOSIS

Summary Statement	Evidence
Primary forms	
Culture has low sensitivity.	Expert opinion
Serology is most useful for diagnosis; CF has greatest early sensitivity; immunodiffusion is less sensitive but more specific.	Observational studies
Urine HPA has good specificity but is relatively insensitive in early-stage disease; it is more sensitive for acute progressive and disseminated disease.	Observational studies
Chronic cavitary	
Sputum culture has high sensitivity.	Expert opinion and
CF is 90% sensitive and highly specific.	observational studies
Urine HPA has low sensitivity.	
Progressive disseminated	
Blood cultures have high sensitivity only in AIDS; bone marrow biopsy/culture is highly sensitive with systemic disease; most tests are more sensitive in AIDS patients.	Expert opinion and observational study
Urine HPA is also highly sensitive, especially in AIDS.	Expert opinion and observational study
Serology has low sensitivity.	

CF, complement fixation; HPA, *Histoplasma* polysaccharide antigen.

patients, and became the standard of oral therapy. Amphotericin B is still used for the most severely ill patients and for all patients with CNS disease (itraconazole has very poor CNS penetration). Fluconazole has better tissue penetration than itraconazole but is likely less effective for histoplasmosis. For example, fluconazole is less likely in AIDS to prevent relapse after initial successful therapy. Voriconazole is the newest agent, showing some promise based on pharmacologic features and the results of *in vitro* testing, but it has not been studied in histoplasmosis and has been introduced at a very high price.

Expert committees of the Mycoses Study Group of the National Institute of Allergy and Infectious Diseases (NIAID) have reviewed in detail the available evidence and made treatment recommendations for the various fungal diseases, including histoplasmosis. Their work was published by the Infectious Diseases Society of America in the April 2000 issue of *Clinical Infectious Diseases* (41,42). The treatment recommendations in this publication represent a then-current consensus of expert opinion. References to published data were very complete. Each treatment recommendation was graded from A through E based on the strength of the recommendation and I, II, or III based on the quality of the evidence. Grades A, B, and C represent strong, moderate, and weak recommendations for treatment, and grades D and E represent moderate or good recommendations against treatment. Grade I evidence required a randomized controlled trial; grade II required well-designed clinical trials without randomization, high-quality analytic studies, or dramatic

results of uncontrolled experiments; and grade III evidence relied on expert opinion, descriptive studies, or committees. The treatment recommendations were mostly strong to moderate. Most of the evidence was of moderate quality. Even when prospective randomized trials compared one treatment with another, the selection criteria for inclusion were often somewhat subjective, and many studies of the oral agents excluded the most severely ill patients. When possible in this chapter, we reference the treatment recommendations of the Mycoses Study Group committees and the grade that they assigned.

Acute pulmonary histoplasmosis generally requires no treatment (E-III). Unusual patients who remain symptomatic for more than 4 weeks can be treated with 200 mg of itraconazole twice daily for 6 to 12 weeks (B-III). Rare patients in whom respiratory failure develops and who require ventilatory support should be treated with amphotericin B (A-III). After clinical improvement, these patients can be switched to 200 mg of itraconazole twice daily for 12 weeks (A-III). Most such patients receive 500 mg to 1,000 mg of amphotericin B before they are switched to oral therapy. Some but not all experts use a short course of corticosteroids as an initial adjunct to amphotericin B for patients who require mechanical ventilation (C-III).

The expert committee recommended a 3-month course of itraconazole for patients with mediastinal fibrosis. Evidence for this recommendation was poor (C-III).

Chronic pulmonary histoplasmosis can usually be treated with 200 mg of itraconazole twice daily for 6 to 18 months (A-II). For the most severely ill patients (in the hospital, in the intensive care unit, actual or impending respiratory failure, requiring mechanical ventilation or close to that point), amphotericin B should be used initially until clinical improvement and stability (usually a course of 500–1,000 mg), followed by 6 to 18 months of itraconazole (A-II).

PDH in AIDS is often a severe illness. Most patients (except those with the mildest cases) should be treated with amphotericin B until clinical improvement is noted—usually to a total dose of 1,000 mg (A-II). At that point, 200 mg of itraconazole twice daily is begun and continued for life (A-II). It is uncertain whether the requirement for lifetime maintenance will change if highly active antiretroviral therapy (HAART) results in a full reconstitution of cellular immunity as judged by a normal $CD4^+$ cell count and undetectable viral load. However, it is clear that patients require lifetime maintenance therapy if their immune system cannot be restored. Since the expert committee report, one study has shown a survival benefit of liposomal amphotericin B in comparison with regular amphotericin B for the initial phase of therapy of PDH in AIDS (43). Based on this single study, liposomal amphotericin B should be considered for induction therapy of PDH in AIDS, but additional confirmatory studies should likely be performed.

PDH in non-AIDS patients should be treated with amphotericin B at the onset if the patient is severely ill and at risk for respiratory failure. After an initial response (usually a total dose of 1,000 mg of amphotericin B), treatment is switched to 200 mg of itraconazole twice daily and continued for 6 to 18 months (A-II). Non-AIDS patients with milder forms of PDH (and even some AIDS patients with mild PDH) can be treated from the onset with 200 mg of itraconazole twice daily for a total course of 12 to 18 months (A-II).

CNS involvement in PDH is most common in AIDS. Amphotericin B should be used for 3 months and followed by 400 to 800 mg of fluconazole per day for at least 12 months (B-III), with lifetime maintenance therapy after that (A-II). Liposomal amphotericin B can be substituted for amphotericin B in patients with renal failure. Liposomal amphotericin B is attractive for CNS disease because of higher brain tissue levels, although additional benefit is theoretic at this time.

TREATMENT OF HISTOPLASMOSIS	
Summary Statement	**Evidence**
Acute pulmonary histoplasmosis	
1. Treatment is generally not required.	1. Expert opinion and observational studies
2. Persistent symptoms (>4 weeks) treat with itraconazole for 4–12 weeks.	2. Expert opinion
3. Progressive to respiratory failure treat with AMB and then itraconazole.	3. Expert opinion
4. Corticosteroids may be used as an adjunct in No. 3.	4. Expert opinion (mixed)
Mediastinal fibrosis	
Itraconazole for 3 months.	Expert opinion (mixed)
Chronic pulmonary histoplasmosis	
1. Itraconazole for 6–18 months.	1. Nonrandomized trials
2. With respiratory failure start with AMB then itraconazole as in No. 1.	2. Nonrandomized clinical trial
Progressive disseminated histoplasmosis	
1. Start with AMB for approximately 1000 mg then itraconazole for 18 months (non-AIDS), for life or until immune reconstitution (AIDS).	1. Expert opinion
2. Corticosteroids may be used adjunctively.	2. Expert opinion (mixed)
3. Liposomal AMB may be superior to AMB; preferred with CNS involvement.	3. Single randomized controlled trial

AMB, amphotericin B; CNS, central nervous system.

BLASTOMYCOSIS

Blastomycosis is concomitantly endemic with histoplasmosis over much of the central and south central regions of the United States. Disease activity extends northward across northern Wisconsin and Minnesota and into central Canada.

As in histoplasmosis, the causative organism is a soil fungus, and the disease is acquired by inhalation. Also as in histoplasmosis, antifungal treatment is highly effective and usually includes amphotericin B, itraconazole, or both. However, many differences exist. Blastomycosis is less common than histoplasmosis, perhaps 10% as common based on frequency of clinically diagnosed cases and frequency of hospitalization. The epidemiology is not as well defined, and the true incidence of subclinical cases is unknown. The area of endemicity has been mapped by tabulation of cases rather than by skin test surveys. The tissue reaction is mixed pyogenic and granulomatous. Patients with pneumonia often cough up pus, and the diagnosis is most often made by direct examination of sputum or other biologic material that shows a pathognomonic large yeast with single broad-based budding and a doubly refractile cell wall (Fig. 19.5). Serodiagnosis is relatively unimportant. Lobar pneumonia and ARDS are more common than in histoplasmosis. Distant spread of infection, when it occurs, is usually to skin and bone rather than to the RE system.

Pathogenesis

At ambient temperatures, the fungus grows in nature as an aerial mycelium. Rising soil temperature favors growth, and rain on the day of exposure enhances the release of fungal spores (44). If the site is disturbed, small (2–5 μm) infecting conidia become airborne, and an infectious aerosol is formed. When the spores are inhaled by humans or other mammals, some may elude nonspecific lung defenses and reach the alveoli. There, they convert to the yeast form. The yeast cells are large (8–20 μm); other features are a doubly refractile cell wall and single budding with a characteristic broad neck of attachment between mother and daughter cells.

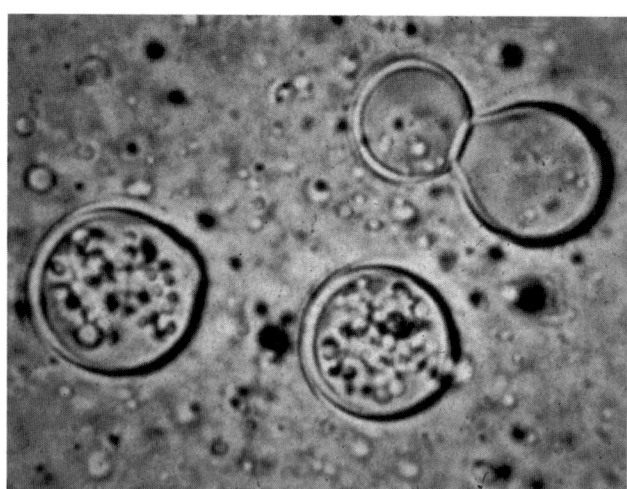

FIGURE 19.5. Pulmonary blastomycosis. Potassium hydroxide preparation of sputum. Highly characteristic organisms show broad-based single budding and a doubly refractile cell wall.

The initial inflammatory response is predominantly neutrophilic. Neutrophils can destroy the conidia, but they are unable to kill the parasitic yeast (5). During the first few days, the nature of the inflammatory exudate changes (45), and macrophages become more prominent. Preimmune macrophages ingest the spores but also cannot kill them. With the development of T cell–mediated immunity, the now-armed macrophages can kill the ingested yeast. Eventually, granuloma formation and healing take place. This process is both similar to and different from that observed in histoplasmosis. Both infections begin as a neutrophil-rich inflammatory exudate, but the neutrophils disappear during the early phases of infection in histoplasmosis. Neutrophils persist as part of the ongoing inflammatory response in blastomycosis. Although the relative proportion of neutrophils to chronic inflammatory cells varies among patients, a mixed pyogenic and granulomatous exudate is always present. In some instances, the neutrophilic component is so predominant that the histopathology mimics that of bacterial infection.

Unlike histoplasmosis, in which benign extrapulmonary spread during the preimmune phase of the infection is universal (1), blastomycosis at an extrapulmonary site is always evidence of true dissemination and always mandates treatment. Involved organs, in decreasing order of frequency, are the skin, bone, male genitourinary system, and meninges. Virtually all other organs may be involved (4).

Clinical Manifestations

In most primary blastomycotic infections, the portal of entry is the lung (26,46). Only rare cases of direct inoculation into subcutaneous tissues have been documented (47,48). After inhalation, the mean incubation time is approximately 45 days, with a wide range of 3 to 15 weeks (31). Outbreaks of infection have occurred in areas of endemicity, related to excavation and outdoor activities near recreational water. Most cases of blastomycosis are sporadic and cannot be linked to any specific exposure. Hunting dogs in areas of endemicity are also prone to blastomycosis. *B. dermatitidis* is very difficult to recover from the soil, even with extensive culturing of soil during investigation of recognized outbreaks.

Pulmonary blastomycosis often mimics bacterial pneumonia. The onset of symptoms is abrupt, with high fever and chills followed by a cough that rapidly becomes productive of purulent sputum (46). Arthralgias and myalgias may occur, but they are not as common as in histoplasmosis. Pleuritic chest pain also occurs in a small minority of patients.

Approximately two thirds of patients with pulmonary blastomycosis have acute pulmonary symptoms resembling bacterial pneumonia. About one third of patients present with a subacute or even chronic illness. Symptoms include low-grade fever, cough productive of mucopurulent sputum,

and weight loss. Clinicians often initially suspect TB or bronchogenic neoplasm (49–51).

The findings on physical examination in acute pulmonary blastomycosis may include crackles and focal signs of consolidation. In many patients, especially those with nodular disease, the results of a chest examination are negative. Erythema nodosum may accompany the onset of pulmonary disease, although it occurs less frequently than in the other endemic mycoses (39,52). Skin involvement may occur early or late. The skin must be examined carefully in every case of pulmonary blastomycosis. Lesions vary from nondescript papules to subcutaneous abscesses to large open ulcerations with indurated borders to crusted lesions of varying size that are somewhat characteristic. The usual areas of skin involvement are the face, hands, and legs. The initial laboratory examination usually shows few abnormalities, but an elevated leukocyte count with a shift to the left may be observed.

The findings on the chest roentgenogram vary widely. Patients with an acute onset of symptoms (including many patients from point source outbreaks) often have bilateral air space disease involving predominantly the lower lung fields, as in the other endemic mycoses. Some patients have a lobar infiltrate closely resembling pneumococcal pneumonia (Fig. 19.6). Patients with severe disease may have diffuse infiltrates that can be interstitial, micronodular, macronodular, or even alveolar (as in ARDS of any cause). In patients with

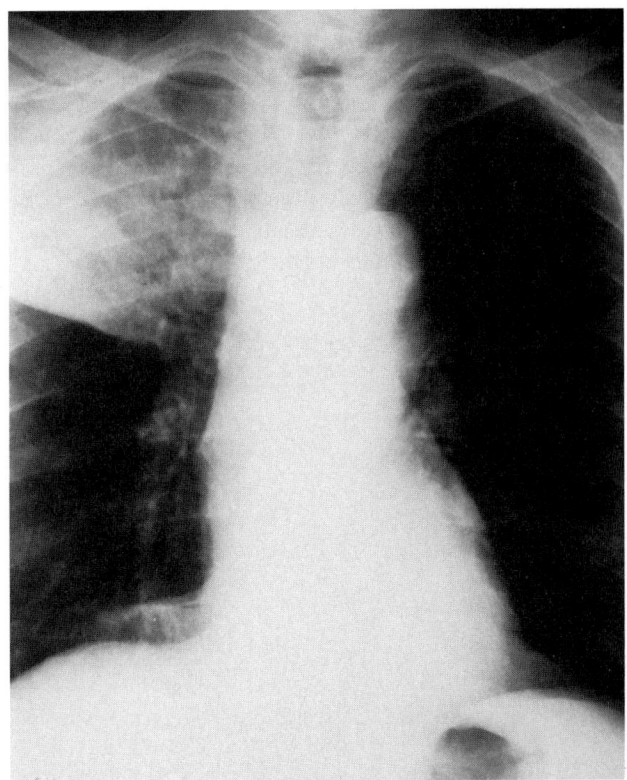

FIGURE 19.6. Pulmonary blastomycosis. Chest radiograph shows right upper lobar pneumonia.

subacute or chronic pulmonary blastomycosis, the lesions vary widely from single or multiple masslike densities to segmental and even lobar consolidation. The combination of alveolar infiltrates with nodules can be a clue to blastomycosis. Juxtahilar infiltrates are common, most often on the right side (53). In these cases, the lateral chest radiograph shows a masslike infiltrate in the apical posterior segment of the right lower lobe. On the posteroanterior film, the infiltrate projects over the right hilum. This presentation mimics bronchogenic carcinoma. Cavitation is uncommon in blastomycosis. Hilar adenopathy is much less frequent than in histoplasmosis or coccidioidomycosis. Calcification in healed pulmonary blastomycosis has been reported but is rare, especially in comparison with histoplasmosis, in which it is very common. Pleural effusions are uncommon but can be a prominent feature in individual cases.

Pulmonary blastomycosis is the most common clinical form of blastomycosis. The exact frequency of the various forms of blastomycosis differs from series to series, heavily influenced by the source of the case material (often hospital-based) and by referral patterns. In a large series of consecutive cases from Mississippi, 107 (87%) of 123 patients had pulmonary involvement (the respiratory distress syndrome developed in nine of them) (54). In contrast, only 47% of a series of 119 patients from the Mayo Clinic with blastomycosis had pulmonary involvement (55). Cutaneous blastomycosis is the second most common form (15%–20% of patients and up to a third of patients in some series), followed by osseous blastomycosis (10%–15% of patients) (Figs. 19.7 and 19.8). Newer series of blastomycosis cases generally have a higher frequency of pulmonary disease and less skin and bone disease than older series, likely because current earlier detection and more effective therapy of pulmonary infections results in cure before distant spread can occur. CNS blastomycosis develops in fewer than 5% of patients.

Extrapulmonary dissemination of the fungus usually occurs early, during the symptomatic phase of the pulmonary

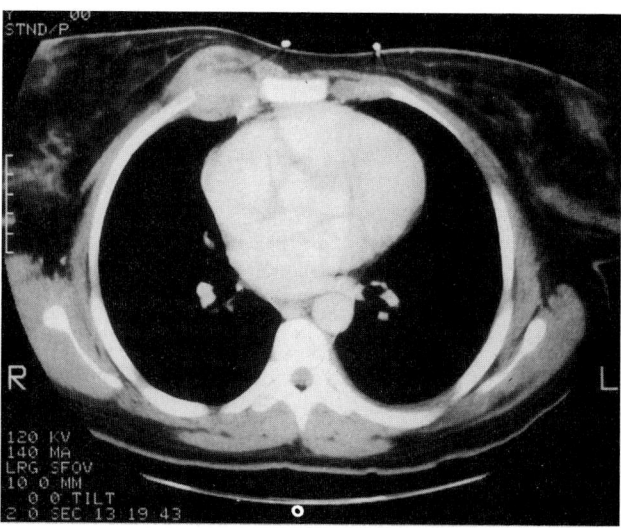

FIGURE 19.7. Bony blastomycosis involving a right anterior rib. Computed tomography shows destruction of the rib and a surrounding mass.

illness. However, distant skin or bone lesions may be the only manifestation of the disease, either because the primary pulmonary process is asymptomatic or because it has already healed. When patients with cutaneous or bony lesions are investigated, a routine chest radiograph may show a totally asymptomatic pulmonary lesion that proves to be blastomycosis. In other cases, the chest radiograph is normal because the pulmonary infiltrate has already cleared (56). Importantly, all blastomycotic skin lesions represent distant spread from the lung, even when the chest radiograph is normal. Cases illustrating this point have been reported (57), in which initial pulmonary blastomycosis (undiagnosed at the time) resolved spontaneously without a diagnosis but blastomycosis recurred as symptomatic extrapulmonary disease months to years later. The patients all underwent diagnostic bronchoscopy to rule out cancer at the time of the initial pulmonary illness, but no cause was established and

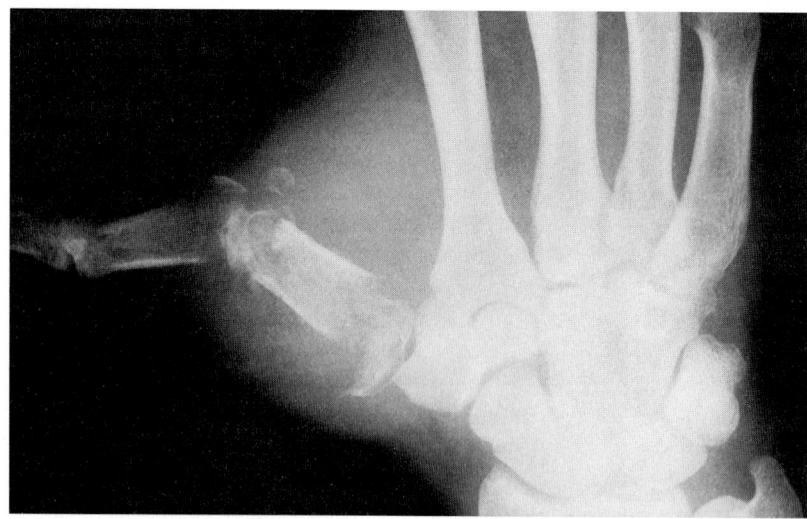

FIGURE 19.8. Bony blastomycosis. Radiograph shows destruction of the proximal first metacarpal bone.

no treatment was given. Careful retrospective evaluation of bronchoscopic material showed characteristic *B. dermatitidis* yeast (not recognized earlier) on the original Papanicolaou-stained cytology slides (57).

Blastomycosis involves the CNS in fewer than 5% of cases. Patterns include basilar meningitis (acute or subacute presentation) or single or multiple parenchymal brain lesions, which can present with seizures or focal deficits.

Most patients with blastomycosis have no obvious immune defects. Nevertheless, in patients with demonstrable T-cell defects, such as organ transplant recipients or those receiving high-dose glucocorticoids, blastomycosis behaves as an opportunist. The pace of the illness is more rapid and the involvement more extensive than in normal hosts (58). In a small number of HIV-infected patients, severe, rapidly progressive blastomycosis develops while they are significantly deficient in T cells as a consequence of HIV infection. In such patients, the disease is usually widespread and aggressive, involving multiple sites (59). Meningitis is common, seen in up to 40% of cases in one series (59). In reported series, mortality has been high, with an average survival of only a few months.

Diagnosis

The gold standard for diagnosis is culture of the infecting organism from biologic material, which has perfect specificity. In a series of cases of pulmonary blastomycosis from the Mayo Clinic, culture of noninvasive specimens (usually sputum) had a sensitivity of 75% per specimen and 86% per patient (55). Culture of bronchoscopy specimens was even better (92%), with culture of bronchial secretions (19 of 19) outperforming culture of BAL fluid (4 of 6). Isolation and identification of the organism by the mycology laboratory is not difficult, but it takes time. Depending on the inoculum size, growth may occur as early as 5 to 7 days after exposure. If the inoculum is small, it may take as long as 30 days to grow the fungus. Formerly, positive identification of the fungus required conversion of the mycelial isolate to the yeast phase and then back again to the mycelial phase. With exoantigen testing, final identification can be made as soon as moderate growth occurs on the culture plate, sometimes within 5 days but more often in a week or two. Because culture results have the disadvantage of slow return, disease in many patients is diagnosed by direct smear while the results of culture are pending. If direct smears are not performed or the results are negative, patients are often sent to undergo more invasive procedures pending the results of culture (ultimately positive) of specimens obtained by less invasive means, especially if the patients are seriously ill and their disease is progressing.

Direct smears are the preferred and most common method of diagnosis in blastomycosis. The advantages are a characteristic yeast form (8- to 20-μm yeast with single broad-based budding), which has the same perfect specificity as a culture identification and a rapid same-day turnaround

(Fig. 19.6). Unfortunately, all the various diagnostic tests have not been performed in one large series, so that the sensitivity, specificity, and the positive and negative predictive value of each technique cannot be determined precisely.

The quickest and simplest way to establish the diagnosis of blastomycosis is to examine sputum or aspirated pus after digestion by 10% potassium hydroxide (KOH). Under reduced light, the characteristic organisms are readily seen. The broad neck of attachment between the mother cell and the single daughter cell is the most important characteristic. The doubly refractile nature of the wall can be revealed by varying the focus, and multiple nuclei are visible. Calcofluor white is a fluorescent stain that may offer some advantages. Another quick and reliable test is routine cytologic examination of the respiratory secretions by means of the Papanicolaou technique. The fungi are large, dark pink- to red-staining organisms, with the characteristic budding and doubly refractile cell wall clearly visible. Cytotechnologists are trained to look for malignancy first; it is relatively easy to overlook *Blastomyces* organisms unless the cytotechnologist is specifically looking for them (60). No study has compared KOH preparation, calcofluor white stain, and the Papanicolaou stain for the diagnosis of blastomycosis. Molecular probes offer promise of greater sensitivity but are much more expensive.

In many centers in areas of high prevalence, direct examination of sputum and other specimens is used extensively and is the method of diagnosis in most cases of blastomycosis. Cultures are usually also positive but are reported later, after the diagnosis has already been made. A study from Mississippi reported the specific tests that first made the diagnosis of blastomycosis in a large series of patients with pulmonary blastomycosis (54). A positive result of KOH digestion of sputum was the diagnostic test 54% of the time. Sputum cytology made the diagnosis 9% of the time, and sputum culture was the first positive test result in another 9% of cases. Bronchoscopy made the diagnosis in 21% of cases (KOH 12%, cytology 7%, and culture 2%). Lung biopsy was the method of diagnosis in 10%, and skin biopsy and bone biopsy in just 1% each. Analysis of another large series showed cytology to be more powerful than KOH digestion for direct morphologic diagnosis (54). In that series, results of cytology were positive in 97% of 69 patients with lung involvement. If direct smears are underutilized, a much higher percentage of cases of disease will be diagnosed by culture (with some delay) or by more invasive means. Referral patterns and patient mix also affect the frequency of the various diagnostic tests. In some series of cases of blastomycosis, skin biopsy is the diagnostic test in a significant minority of patients.

If the results of direct smears are negative or direct smears are not performed, diagnostic testing escalates to tissue biopsy, which shows pyogenic and granulomatous inflammation and also often shows the organism on special stains. Most laboratories use one of several modifications of the silver stain or the periodic acid-Schiff (PAS) stain. The PAS stain better preserves morphologic detail (4).

Three serologic tests are available: CF, immunodiffusion, and enzyme immunoassay. The best data for serodiagnosis come from the Eagle River outbreak (62). Sensitivity was 8% for CF and 27% for immunodiffusion, in comparison with 16% for CF and 40% for immunodiffusion in a Mayo Clinic study (58). Other studies show greater sensitivity but often use serum banks of cases selected in part for positive serodiagnostic test results. At Eagle River, the sensitivity of enzyme immunoassay was 77%. However, because of cross-reactivity with histoplasmosis in areas where both diseases are endemic (and histoplasmosis is much more common), that test has poor specificity. Specificity of the immunodiffusion test is believed to be moderately good, and a positive immunodiffusion test result should always prompt further investigation to prove or disprove blastomycosis (40,62). In clinical practice, serodiagnosis rarely make the diagnosis (none in the large study from Mississippi previously mentioned). The usual diagnostic sequence for pulmonary disease is direct examination and culture of sputum, direct examination and culture of bronchoscopic specimens, then histopathology of bronchoscopic, video-assisted thoracoscopic, or open lung biopsy specimens. For extrapulmonary sites, direct approach to the lesion is best, especially with skin lesions that are readily accessible. Direct examination of any purulent material and then biopsy of the active edge of the lesion will give the best results.

Treatment

The story is very similar to that for histoplasmosis. Highly effective treatment of fungal diseases began with amphotericin B in 1956. Before that time, patients with serious progressive forms of blastomycosis generally died. Amphotericin B proved to be very effective therapy for the vast majority of these patients. Placebo-controlled trials were not performed, and dosages and duration of therapy were determined by retrospective analysis of successfully treated patients. A 40- to 50-mg daily dose of amphotericin B to response and then three times weekly to a total dose of 2 g was highly effective and could be given without undue toxicity. Newer agents were compared with amphotericin B, but only in selected groups of patients. (Clinical studies usually were limited to mild to moderate disease not involving the CNS.) Ketoconazole had a higher failure rate and more relapses than amphotericin B, even in selected patients. Itraconazole proved much better, equal to amphotericin B in selected patients, and became the standard of oral therapy. Amphotericin B is still used for the most severely ill patients and for all patients with CNS disease (itraconazole has very poor CNS penetration). Fluconazole has better tissue penetration than itraconazole but is less effective for blastomycosis. Voriconazole is the newest agent, showing some promise based on pharmacologic features and the results of *in vitro*

testing, but it has not been studied in blastomycosis and has been introduced at a very high price.

An expert committee of the Mycoses Study Group of the NIAID has reviewed in detail the possible treatment options for various forms of blastomycosis (63) (see general discussion in the section on the treatment of histoplasmosis). Amphotericin B and itraconazole are both highly effective treatment. Itraconazole is equal to amphotericin B for the treatment of mild to moderate non-CNS disease (as shown in good randomized studies, with selection criteria excluding life-threatening disease). In clinical practice, more than 80% of all cases of blastomycosis can be successfully treated with this agent. The most severely ill patients were excluded from comparative studies and were treated with amphotericin B. The following recommendations (with some modifications by the authors) represent a current consensus of expert opinion based on variable but generally moderately strong evidence.

Most patients with blastomycosis require treatment. If a pulmonary infection has spontaneously remitted without treatment before the diagnosis is made (usually by late return of cultures of respiratory secretions), the patient can simply be followed closely. All patients with active pulmonary disease at the time of diagnosis and all patients with extrapulmonary disease should be treated.

For all life-threatening disease, including ARDS and edematous lobar pneumonia, and for all cases of meningitis, amphotericin B should be used as initial therapy. A 40- to 50-mg dose is given daily to improvement and then three times weekly. A total dose of 1.5 to 2.5 g is recommended (A-II). Alternatively, once the patient has stabilized (usually after a total dose of amphotericin B of 500–1,000 mg), therapy can be switched to 200 mg of itraconazole twice daily, which is continued for 6 months (B-II). All immunosuppressed patients with blastomycosis should also be treated with amphotericin B followed by itraconazole in similar manner (B-III), but the itraconazole should be continued longer, at least 12 months for transplant recipients and indefinitely for AIDS patients.

Itraconazole is very effective in all immunocompetent patients with mild to moderate pulmonary and extrapulmonary disease excluding CNS disease. The usual dose for pulmonary, cutaneous, osseous, and prostatic blastomycosis is 200 mg twice daily for 6 to 12 months (A-II) (64). Treatment for bony disease should be continued for 12 months. Itraconazole is now used for most cases of blastomycosis. Amphotericin B is still needed only for the most severe cases.

Fluconazole in doses of 200 to 400 mg is not highly effective for blastomycosis. Higher doses of fluconazole (600–800 mg/d) have been used with good success rates. High-dose fluconazole has never been compared directly with standard doses of itraconazole, but it may have similar efficacy and is an option for patients who cannot tolerate or cannot absorb itraconazole (B-III).

Amphotericin B should be used to treat CNS blastomycosis with a total dose of 2 g (A-II). Azoles should not be used for the primary treatment of CNS blastomycosis (E-III). In special circumstances, 800 mg of fluconazole per day can be considered (C-III). (One example is long-term maintenance in AIDS patients who respond to initial amphotericin B therapy.) Liposomal amphotericin B may have a role in patients intolerant of amphotericin B and has the theoretic advantage of better CNS penetration.

BLASTOMYCOSIS

Summary Statement	Evidence
Diagnosis	
Various direct smear techniques (including Papanicolaou) of sputum, BAL fluid, aspirated pus or tissue are rapid, sensitive, and reasonably specific.	Uncontrolled studies, expert opinion
Culture is highly sensitive and specific but can be slow if inoculum is small; exoantigen testing may expedite identification.	Uncontrolled studies, expert opinion
Serologic tests: CF and ID are relatively insensitive; EIA is more sensitive (>75%) but cross-reaction with histoplasmosis lowers specificity.	Uncontrolled studies
Serodiagnosis is generally not helpful in acute disease.	Expert opinion
Treatment	
AMB to total dose of 1.5–2.5 g is the "gold standard."	Observational studies
Itraconazole is deemed equal to AMB for mild or moderate *non-CNS* disease.	Nonrandomized studies
AMB should be used for severe disease; change to itraconazole may be possible after initiation of treatment with AMB.	Nonrandomized studies
Immunosuppressed patients should all receive AMB; if itraconazole is subsequently given, it should used for at least 12 months.	Expert opinion
Liposomal AMB may be useful in AMB-intolerant patients or for CNS disease.	Expert opinion

AMB, amphotericin B; BAL, bronchoalveolar lavage; CF, complement fixation; CNS, central nervous system; EIA, enzyme immunoassay; ID, immunodiffusion.

COCCIDIOIDOMYCOSIS

C. immitis grows in the desert rather than in the great river valleys. In the United States, the areas of greatest endemicity include the San Joaquin Valley, centered in Bakersfield, California, and the central Arizona desert beginning north of Phoenix and extending south to Tucson. Some disease activity extends east to Texas. West of San Antonio, Texas, the areas where coccidioidomycosis and histoplasmosis are endemic are contiguous. Otherwise, the area within the United States where coccidioidomycosis is endemic is totally distinct

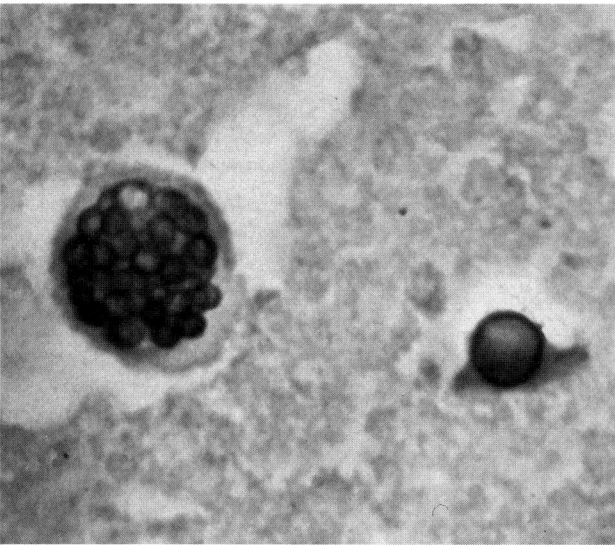

FIGURE 19.9. (See also Color Fig. 19.9.) Giant spherule, highly characteristic of coccidioidomycosis. Structure to the right is a single endospore (Gomori methenamine silver stain, original magnification ×100).

from the areas where histoplasmosis and blastomycosis are endemic. Adjacent desert areas of northern Mexico harbor the fungus, and foci of disease activity exist in Argentina and Paraguay. As in blastomycosis, a characteristic morphology is seen in secretions and tissue—in this case a large spherule (Fig. 19.9). Inflammation is pyogenic and granulomatous, and secretions are often purulent and a good source of specimens for diagnosis by direct examination and culture. Distant spread is to skin and bone, but meningeal involvement is more common. As in histoplasmosis, primary pulmonary infection is common and usually self-limited. Serodiagnosis is the major diagnostic tool for primary infections. One major difference from both blastomycosis and histoplasmosis is that the organism is not as responsive to current antifungal therapeutics, which are less effective in the severe and progressive forms of coccidioidomycosis, which require treatment.

Coccidioidomycosis was first described in Argentina in 1896 (65). Shortly thereafter, it became obvious that the disease was much more common in central California than in Argentina. At first, only the most severe cases were recognized. Anecdotal reports described patients with the severe form of the disease, referring to it as *coccidioidal granuloma*. No one reported milder cases. During the same period (before 1930), practitioners in the San Joaquin Valley in California had recognized several self-limited clinical syndromes of unknown etiology; these included a nonspecific febrile illness ("valley fever"), acute polyarthritis ("desert rheumatism"), and erythema nodosum (the "bumps"). These illnesses were sometimes severe, but usually self-limited. Causation was a mystery.

Dickson and Gifford (66,67) first described primary pulmonary coccidioidomycosis and proved that it could be a benign illness. They carefully studied a laboratory accident and showed that primary coccidioidomycosis was acquired by inhalation. They also demonstrated that "valley fever" and the "bumps" were manifestations of acute pulmonary coccidioidomycosis, which was a very surprising finding at the time.

World War II greatly increased our knowledge of coccidioidomycosis, largely because of the work of C. E. Smith. He carried out extensive epidemiologic studies (including serial skin tests and serial serodiagnostic testing) on the large number of recruits brought to the San Joaquin Valley and central Arizona for flight training. Most recruits whose coccidioidin skin test converted from negative to positive had no symptoms. Most of the minority with symptoms had a nonspecific febrile illness or a self-limited respiratory illness. Only a few had erythema nodosum or the polyarthralgia syndrome. Recruits who entered training with positive skin test results were protected and did not become ill. Only a few (<0.5%) of the documented new infections progressed to dissemination (2). Infections were common in dry weather and dusty areas, and when heavy construction disturbed the soil. The incidence of infection decreased during the cold and wet rainy season. After construction activities on the bases slowed, the grass began to grow, sidewalks were finished, and the frequency of new infections decreased markedly (68).

The U.S. Army required a complete postmortem examination of all soldiers who died (69). This policy provided useful information about the fatal form of coccidioidomycosis. Risk differed among racial groups. The incidence of disseminated disease was higher in blacks than in whites, even though the risk for infection, as measured by skin test conversion, was not significantly different. A racial difference in risk for dissemination was subsequently confirmed in the study of a great California windstorm in 1979 (70).

Pathogenesis

The climatic conditions of the lower Sonoran life zone (typical of the desert southwest of the United States below 3,500 feet of elevation) favor the growth of *C. immitis*. The weather during most of the year is hot, with rainfall occurring in short bursts in the spring. The fungus grows and germinates, especially in areas with a high nitrogen content, including ground squirrel and prairie dog burrows. In desert soil, the fungus grows as an aerial mycelium composed of septate hyphae. In mature hyphae, arthrospores alternate with empty cells. The mycelia break easily, and the arthrospores become airborne. They are small, thick-walled, and barrel-shaped, about 2 to 5 μm long (2). High winds in southern California (the Santa Ana winds) can carry the arthrospores for many miles (under exceptional circumstances as far as 200 miles).

Aerosolized arthrospores are easily inhaled. A few organisms may elude the nonspecific lung defenses and reach the alveoli. Germination begins, and the arthrospores convert to the tissue phase of the fungus, becoming spherules. These large structures are 10 to 80 μm in diameter. Further reproduction occurs by formation of endospores within the spherule. After the spherule matures, it ruptures, and the endospores are released. Each endospore can develop into a new giant spherule.

The initial inflammatory response is neutrophilic. Macrophages also increase in number. Macrophages phagocytose the arthrospores and present antigens to specific T lymphocytes, which then multiply. These T cells recruit and arm more macrophages, completing the cell-mediated specific immune response. Armed macrophages control the infection by killing the organism or walling it off within granulomas. Histopathologically, coccidioidomycosis is a mixed pyogenic and granulomatous infection, more similar to blastomycosis than to histoplasmosis. The development of T cell–mediated immunity and its histopathologic correlate, granuloma formation, are essential for control of the infection.

Most infections are asymptomatic or mildly symptomatic. Although proof is lacking, it appears that in most primary infections the fungus remains localized in the lung and the draining hilar lymph nodes. Involvement of any distant organ is considered proof of disseminated disease (with the possible exception of coccidioidouria during some primary infections). Virtually any organ may be involved, but skin, bone, and meninges are the usual sites.

Clinical Manifestations

Pulmonary Coccidioidomycosis

The usual portal of entry is the lung. Rarely, the organism can be directly inoculated subcutaneously, usually during a surgical or pathologic accident. The cardinal clinical manifestation of acute coccidioidomycosis is a localized area of pneumonia. A pulmonary infiltrate is common, even in asymptomatic patients with disease detected by skin test conversion. Symptomatic disease ranges from a mild respiratory illness to rapidly progressive ARDS. Symptoms are highly variable. Most patients have fever, cough, and pleuritic chest pain. Pleuritic chest pain can be severe and is frequently incapacitating (71). Nonspecific headaches often accompany the acute illness, causing concern because of the potential for meningitis. Spread to the meninges can occur early during the clinical illness. If the headache is severe or unrelenting or if any evidence of meningeal irritation is noted, a lumbar puncture should be performed immediately to exclude coccidioidomycotic meningitis.

A nonspecific "toxic" rash occurs in a small percentage of patients with acute infection. The rash is erythematous and slightly raised but not quite papular. It usually appears early during the illness, about the same time that the skin test becomes positive. Because coccidioidomycosis frequently occurs during the hot summer months, the rash is frequently misdiagnosed as a "heat rash." More characteristic skin manifestations of primary coccidioidomycosis are erythema nodosum and, less commonly, erythema multiforme. These striking findings also develop about the same time as skin test conversion. For many years, the appearance of erythema nodosum was thought to be a highly favorable prognostic sign, portending spontaneous recovery. However, some cases with erythema nodosum progress to life-threatening illness. Erythema nodosum occurs most commonly in adult white women (72).

About three fourths of patients with symptomatic primary pulmonary coccidioidomycosis have abnormal chest radiographic findings. The abnormality usually is a single area of pneumonitis with or without enlargement of the draining hilar lymph nodes. Isolated hilar adenopathy may occur with no obvious infiltrate (73).

The usual clinical course of the primary illness is rapid improvement. After 6 weeks, the chest radiograph has cleared and symptoms have abated. In a few patients, symptoms and roentgenographic abnormalities may persist beyond 6 weeks, a condition referred to as *persistent pulmonary coccidioidomycosis*. The patchy pulmonary infiltrate may gradually harden and round off, producing a coin lesion, which is common in the area of endemicity. The coin lesions of coccidioidomycosis differ from those of histoplasmosis. In histoplasmosis, they are healing granulomas, but in coccidioidomycosis, they are abscesses undergoing resolution (74) (Fig. 19.10). Needle biopsy of *Histoplasma* granulomas rarely shows the organism; needle biopsy of coccidioidal lesions usually does.

Necrotic material is in the center of the rounded lesions, and expectoration of this semisolid material frequently leaves a cavity. The hallmark of persistent pulmonary coc-

cidioidomycosis is a thin-walled cavity that evolves from a solid pulmonary lesion (75). Most cavities are asymptomatic, and the only usual complaint is an occasional bout of scanty hemoptysis. Established cavities remain stable for long periods, and medical intervention is seldom required. Approximately 50% of cavities smaller than 4 cm in diameter close within 2 years (75,76).

Even though the cavitary lesions are usually benign, several complications can occur. The lesions may enlarge subpleurally and eventually rupture into the pleural space, leading to a pneumohemothorax or pyopneumothorax. Rupture into the pleura is a life-threatening complication, and prompt diagnosis and treatment are important (76,77). Hemoptysis is a frequent complication of coccidioidal cavities. Although it is sometimes alarming, it is seldom life-threatening. Fungus balls occasionally develop in the cavities, usually caused by *Aspergillus* species, rarely by *C. immitis*. Bacterial superinfection of the cavities may also occur.

If primary pulmonary coccidioidomycosis fails to resolve and instead progresses within the chest, the condition is called *progressive pulmonary coccidioidomycosis*. Symptoms include fever and cough, and the prognosis is quite poor. Many of these patients have underlying immune defects or belong to racial groups with a higher incidence of severe disease. Serial chest radiographs show progression of the parenchymal infiltrate.

Rarely, pulmonary coccidioidomycosis presents with a TB-like picture, slowly progressive with low-grade fever, night sweats, cough, weight loss, and occasional hemoptysis. The chest radiograph resembles that of the adult form of reinfection TB (Fig. 19.11). The usual patient is older,

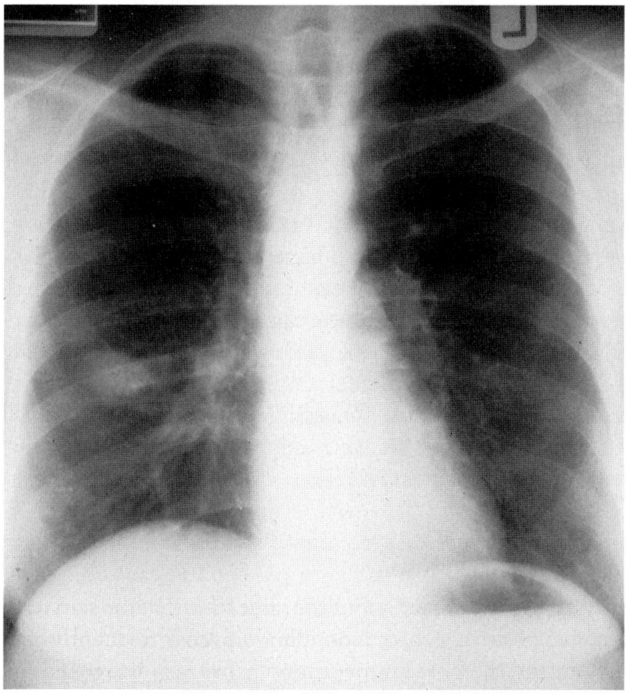

FIGURE 19.10. Residual coccidioidomycotic abscess. Radiograph shows stable round lesion in right lower lobe. Sputum in this case was negative, serology positive, and fine needle aspiration positive.

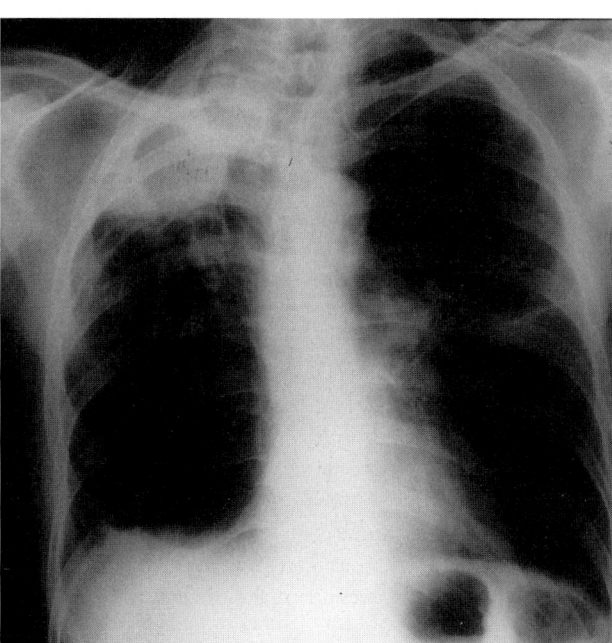

FIGURE 19.11. Chronic pulmonary coccidioidomycosis. Chest radiograph shows chronic right upper lobe infiltrate. Sputum cultures were positive.

and the disease progresses slowly. Treatment is necessary to prevent further pulmonary destruction.

Disseminated Coccidioidomycosis

In most patients, the primary coccidioidomycotic infection is restricted to the lungs and resolves spontaneously. Occasionally, the pulmonary infection persists or slowly progresses. Although a few patients die of coccidioidomycosis limited to the lung, most recover or stabilize. In just a few patients, the fungus disseminates widely throughout the body. A benign fungemia likely develops in the preimmune stage of histoplasmosis. It is unknown whether or how often this occurs in coccidioidomycosis. Documentation of infection at any distant site is considered proof of true dissemination.

Most cases of disseminated disease occur in persons receiving glucocorticoid or cytotoxic therapy (78), in organ transplant recipients (79), and especially in AIDS patients with advanced immunosuppression (80). T-cell immunosuppression is a risk factor; risk is also related to race and sex. Disseminated disease is more likely to occur in blacks and Native Americans than in whites (81,82). Male sex further increases the risk for dissemination. Diabetes mellitus has long been thought to increase the risk for dissemination, but solid data supporting this general impression are lacking. Disseminated coccidioidomycosis is more likely to develop in very young or very old persons. Pregnancy has also long been thought to increase the risk for dissemination, but certain data have cast some doubt on this supposition (83). Nevertheless, many experts feel that coccidioidomycosis in the third trimester of pregnancy is a potentially severe illness with a high risk for dissemination and requires prompt treatment.

The temporal relation of dissemination to the primary infection is seldom established. Most authorities think that dissemination tends to occur early during the course of the disease (84). In many patients, however, the appearance of disseminated disease is the first sign of coccidioidomycosis. It is possible that an asymptomatic primary pulmonary infection resolves without causing any symptoms, preceding eventual dissemination by an unknown interval.

C. immitis can disseminate to any organ of the body, but the skin is the most common site. Single or multiple sites may be involved, and the gross appearance is not diagnostic. Presentations vary from trivial lesions resembling folliculitis to large, draining pustules and ulcers. Skin lesions may heal spontaneously or follow a rapidly progressive course with enlargement and direct spread into underlying tissues. The organism can also spread directly to subcutaneous sites. Subcutaneous abscesses often are associated with sinus tracts to the skin. These drain thick, yellow pus heavily laden with spherules.

Bone is the next most common site of involvement. Many bones can be simultaneously involved in widespread, disseminated illness. At the other extreme, a single bony lesion may represent the entire extent of disease. The vertebrae are most frequently involved, followed by the skull and long bones. Infection of virtually every bone in the body has been documented. The radiographic appearance of coccidioidomycotic osteomyelitis is similar to that of other forms of chronic osteomyelitis, including TB and blastomycosis. Osteomyelitis of the spine usually narrows the disc space and causes sclerosis of the two adjacent vertebrae. The vertebral lesions resemble TB radiographically, but actual formation of a gibbus is unusual (84). With vertebral involvement, large paraspinous abscesses sometimes compromise the spinal cord (85). Paraspinous abscesses should be drained. Because bony lesions are common, every patient with severe or disseminated coccidioidomycosis should undergo a bone scan before treatment is started to search for asymptomatic bony lesions. If asymptomatic skeletal lesions are not recognized before the initiation of therapy, their appearance during therapy may be misconstrued as evidence of treatment failure.

Joint involvement may result from hematogenous dissemination to a joint or from direct extension of a contiguous bony infection. The knees and ankles are most frequently involved. Even though clinical evidence of chronic arthritis is present, the organism is seldom recognized in the fluid by smear or culture. Most patients require synovial biopsy for accurate diagnosis.

The genitourinary system is not a frequent site of dissemination, but coccidioidouria is fairly common and should be sought in all patients suspected of having coccidioidomycosis. Apparently, the presence of *C. immitis* in the urine does not prove disseminated disease. In one report, urine cultures were positive for *C. immitis* in 7 of 29 patients with pulmonary disease. Two of the seven patients with positive urine cultures were not treated, and the disease resolved spontaneously (86).

Involvement of the meninges is the most dreaded complication of coccidioidomycosis. Meningeal involvement occurs in approximately one third of patients with disseminated coccidioidomycosis. These patients often have no other evidence of coccidioidomycosis. Coccidioidomycotic meningitis is a chronic illness, and the dramatic clinical features of acute bacterial meningitis are rarely seen. The usual manifestations are the gradual onset of headache and minimal alteration of higher cortical functions (87,88). In many cases, meningitis is diagnosed only when a lumbar puncture performed for the routine evaluation of a patient with disseminated disease reveals cerebrospinal fluid (CSF) pleocytosis.

Coccidioidomycotic meningitis is a disease of the base of the brain, which explains most of its clinical features. As the disease progresses, a thick, plastic exudate at the base of the brain obstructs the aqueduct of Sylvius and the foramina of the fourth ventricle, causing hydrocephalus. This complication should be suspected if a patient's mental status deteriorates suddenly. In patients whose condition is deteriorating, signs of intracranial hypertension, including papilledema, are frequent.

Examination of the CSF shows the characteristic manifestations of chronic meningitis—a mononuclear cell pleocytosis with only occasional polymorphonuclear leukocytes, an increased protein level, and a decreased glucose level. Many investigators mention CSF eosinophilia as an important finding, but it is not common. Nevertheless, if eosinophils are seen in the CSF of a patient with chronic meningitis, that finding suggests coccidioidomycosis as the likely cause.

Coccidioidomycosis in HIV-infected patients follows a variable course, depending on the timing of the infection relative to the course of the HIV infection. In patients who become infected when their CD4$^+$ cell counts are normal or nearly normal, an illness develops similar to that seen in the general population (80). However, if the CD4$^+$ cell count is 200/mm^3 or lower, a severe, rapidly progressive, disseminated disease develops. The patient has high fever, weight loss, and dyspnea. Physical examination frequently shows evidence of extensive pneumonitis, with crackles and multiple areas of consolidation. Hepatosplenomegaly may occur. The laboratory examination usually reveals hypoxemia, and the chest radiograph shows diffuse micronodular to macronodular infiltrates (Fig. 19.12). Meningeal involvement is common. Approximately 25% of patients with diffuse nodules in the lung have concomitant meningitis. Untreated, the illness progresses rapidly to death (89).

Diagnosis

The gold standard for diagnosis is culture of the infecting organism from biologic material, which has perfect specificity. Recovery of the fungus in culture is not difficult, but

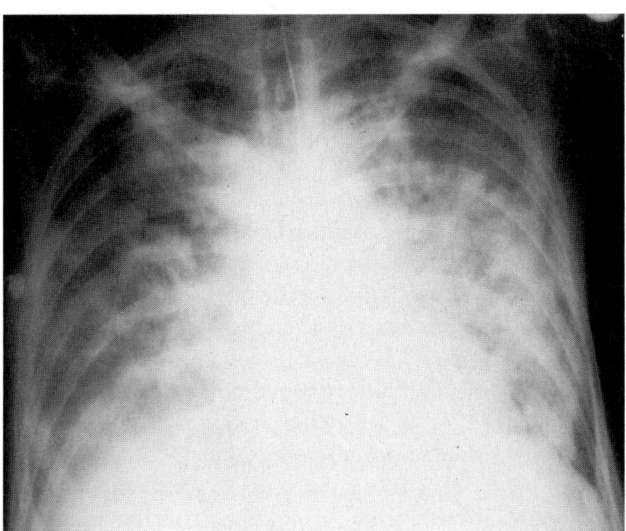

FIGURE 19.12. Disseminated coccidioidomycosis in AIDS. Chest radiograph shows diffuse infiltrates.

extreme caution must be used in handling the specimen because the risk for infecting susceptible laboratory workers is high. When coccidioidomycosis is suspected, the laboratory should be alerted to use slants rather than Petri dishes for culture to reduce the risk for aerosolization. Expert laboratories using exoantigen testing can confirm coccidioidomycosis in 5 to 7 working days (90), but a more usual time frame is one to several weeks. Because culture is hazardous and slow and because in many patients with primary pulmonary coccidioidomycosis sputum production is minimal, serodiagnostic testing is very important in milder cases, and direct examination of biologic material (including direct smears and histopathology) is important in severe and progressive cases.

Most cases of primary coccidioidomycosis are diagnosed by serology. Most laboratories use an immunodiffusion test for immunoglobulin M (IgM) antibodies for screening (the tube precipitin test and the latex particle agglutination test measure similar IgM antibodies). Sensitivity in symptomatic cases is believed to be as high as 90% by 3 weeks after the onset of illness (sensitivity is lower in asymptomatic patients identified in outbreaks). Specificity depends on assumptions about the control group. It is likely that fewer than 5% of patients with pneumonia of other causes in the areas where coccidioidomycosis is most heavily endemic will have a positive screening test result (for this analysis, we will use 2%). Thus, for a nonspecific respiratory infection in an area of endemicity, the sensitivity of a screening test for IgM would be 90%, the specificity 98%, the positive predictive value 98%, and the negative predictive value 91%. Let us assume that 10% of symptomatic respiratory infections in areas where the disease is highly endemic in the proper season are caused by coccidioidomycosis. In that case, the posttest probability of disease with a positive test result would be 83%, and the posttest probability of disease with a negative test result would be only 1%. However, in special situations in which the pretest likelihood of coccidioidomycosis is very high (prominent arthralgias, early toxic rash, erythema nodosum, thin-walled cavity), the positive predictive value of a positive screening test result becomes much better. If the pretest likelihood of primary coccidioidomycosis is 50% (likely a conservative estimate in the preceding situations), then the posttest probability of disease with a positive test is 98%, and the posttest probability of disease with a negative test is 9%.

Perhaps the most important serodiagnostic test is the CF test, which is both diagnostic and prognostic. CF antibodies are IgG antibodies and appear later than IgM antibodies. CF antibodies appear in 3 to 6 weeks and persist for many months. The CF test it is less sensitive than the screening tests for IgM, especially in patients with mild infection. Specificity is good for infection within the previous 1 to 2 years. CF testing remains extremely important in the management of patients with coccidioidomycosis. High or rising titers are associated with a poor prognosis, but no specific titer guarantees a good or bad outcome in a specific patient (90).

Few reports in the medical literature have been as misunderstood as Smith's work on the coccidioidomycosis CF test (91). He performed almost 40,000 CF tests and showed that many patients with high titers (≥1:32) had dissemination or impending dissemination. However, not all patients with disseminated disease had high titers, nor did all patients with high titers have disseminated disease. Any patient whose CF titer is rising under observation or whose previously stable CF titer begins to rise after therapy is completed should be evaluated carefully for evidence of disseminated disease. Another confounding factor is that most laboratories use different techniques and different standardization. Only Pappagianis and colleagues at the University of California at Davis (92) use the exact original method. A high titer was defined as 1:32 in Smith's assay, but titers from other laboratories are usually relatively higher. An immunodiffusion test for IgG antibody is readily available and has the approximate sensitivity and specificity of the more cumbersome CF test. However, it does not provide the same prognostic information.

Direct examination of expectorated sputum, bronchoscopic specimens, or aspirated pus can reveal characteristic spherules, which are diagnostic. This is the fastest way to make the diagnosis and has perfect specificity. If only endospores are seen, it is harder to exclude a number of other fungi (Fig. 19.13). For expectorated sputum and BAL specimens, the best preparation appears to be the Papanicolaou stain. Digestion by 10% KOH can also be used. From a single published comparative study, it appears that the Papanicolaou stain has approximately twice the sensitivity of KOH digestion (93).

Histopathologic examination of tissue biopsy specimens is also helpful. If spherules are seen, the diagnosis of coc-

cidioidomycosis is certain. Unfortunately, intact spherules are uncommon in histopathologic preparations. If only endospores are seen, it is harder to exclude a number of other fungi. Giant spherules are revealed by standard hematoxylin and eosin stain and with special stains. Special stains, including the silver stain and the PAS stain, are especially useful to demonstrate endospores in the tissue. The sensitivity of direct smears and histopathology is different in different forms of coccidioidomycosis and in different patient groups.

Persistent pulmonary coccidioidomycosis can be presumptively diagnosed by serology and confirmed by direct examination and culture of sputum or pus aspirated from an abscess by fine needle.

Chronic fibrocavitary pulmonary coccidioidomycosis can be presumptively diagnosed by serology and confirmed by direct examination and culture of sputum or material obtained at bronchoscopy (washings or BAL fluid).

Disseminated coccidioidomycosis in AIDS can be diagnosed by direct examination (and culture) of sputum or bronchoscopy specimens, or by biopsy of distant sites of infection. In AIDS, the burden of organisms is very high, and the diagnosis is usually not difficult. Endobronchial ulcers are sometimes seen at bronchoscopy and show the organisms on biopsy specimens. Large macronodular diffuse infiltrates on the chest radiograph are sufficiently characteristic to allow a presumptive diagnosis in AIDS patients in areas where the disease is heavily endemic. Serodiagnostic test results are positive in about half of AIDS patients who have disseminated coccidioidomycosis. CNS involvement in AIDS is usually part of widespread disseminated disease. In that setting, any abnormal CSF finding suggests the diagnosis. Results of cultures and CSF serology are often positive.

Disseminated coccidioidomycosis in non-AIDS patients can be more difficult to diagnose. Results of serology (CF or immunodiffusion) are positive in most patients; however, direct biopsy of skin, bone, or other distant sites for culture and histopathology is the preferred approach.

The diagnosis of chronic meningitis secondary to coccidioidomycosis can sometimes be difficult. Cultures of CSF are positive less than 50% of the time. IgG antibodies can be detected in serum in 75% of cases but are not specific for the cause of the abnormal CSF findings. IgG antibodies can be detected in CSF in more than 90% of patients.

Like the histoplasmin skin test, the coccidioidin skin test is valuable mainly for epidemiologic investigation. A positive skin test reaction is long-lasting and may result from a recent or remote infection. In areas of endemicity, where the diagnosis of pulmonary coccidioidomycosis is most likely to be considered, a positive skin test result cannot be assumed to be causally related to the acute clinical illness being evaluated. It may be the marker of remote self-limited coccidioidomycosis in a patient with a current active pneumonia caused by a totally different agent. In addition, many patients with acute pulmonary coccidioidomycosis do not have a positive skin test result because of the considerable time required to

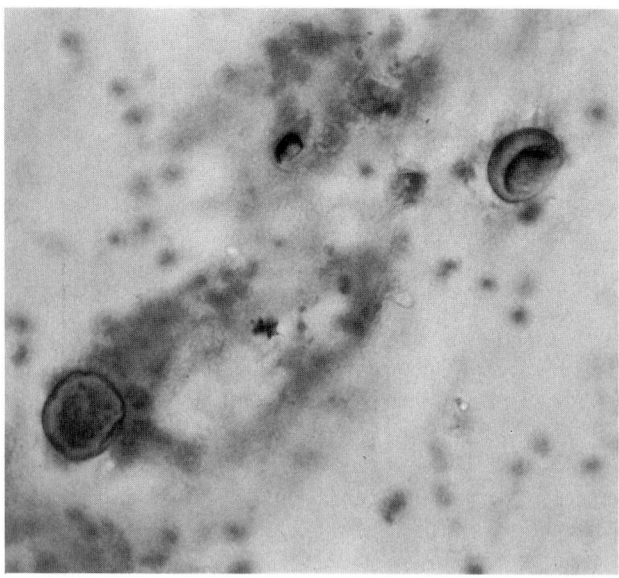

FIGURE 19.13. (See also Color Fig. 19.13.) Disseminated coccidioidomycosis in AIDS. Bronchoalveolar lavage fluid was positive for endospores (Papanicolaou stain, original magnification ×1,000).

develop T cell–mediated immunity. Furthermore, as many as 50% of patients with disseminated coccidioidomycosis have negative skin test results. The skin test is seldom useful for individual case diagnosis.

Treatment

The immune system handles coccidioidomycosis very well, likely as well as histoplasmosis. In both infections, more than 99% of cases are self-limited. However, antifungal treatment for the small number of patients in whom severe progressive forms of the disease develop is not as effective as it is in histoplasmosis, and meningeal spread, which is particularly hard to treat, is relatively more common.

Highly effective treatment of fungal diseases began with amphotericin B in 1956. Before that time, patients with serious, progressive forms of coccidioidomycosis usually died. Whereas amphotericin B was effective in histoplasmosis and blastomycosis, it proved to be only moderately effective therapy for many patients with chronic forms of coccidioidomycosis, including bone, soft tissue, and especially meningeal disease. Placebo-controlled trials were not performed, and dosages and duration of therapy were determined by treatment response. Even higher doses (≥ 1.0 mg/kg per day) and longer courses of treatment (often a total dose of 5 to 7 g given over months to years) were often suppressive rather than curative. Coccidioidal meningitis in particular was almost never cured. Systemic amphotericin B at onset was supplemented by intrathecal amphotericin B for maintenance therapy, administered by either repeated lumbar punctures, repeated cisternal taps, or a reservoir device placed in the lateral ventricle for ease of access. Higher doses of amphotericin B and longer courses of amphotericin B therapy were associated with a higher rate of renal toxicity than the treatment regimens used for histoplasmosis and blastomycosis. Newer agents were compared with amphotericin B but generally were used because they were a less toxic means of long-term therapy, not because they offered better hope of cure. Ketoconazole had a high failure rate and a high relapse rate, even in patients with chronic and subacute disease. Fluconazole is more potent than ketoconazole and much less toxic than amphotericin B. Fluconazole proved a good agent for maintenance therapy after an initial course of amphotericin B and is even used as primary therapy for some patients with mild to moderate disease. Fluconazole is the azole of choice whenever meningitis is proven or suspected. However, itraconazole proved equal to fluconazole in the treatment of chronic, nonmeningeal, progressive forms of disseminated coccidioidomycosis (pulmonary, soft tissue, or skeletal) in a large randomized double-blinded prospective trial (94).

In 2000, an expert committee of the Mycoses Study Group of the NIAID reviewed in detail the possible treatment options for the various forms of coccidioidomycosis (see general discussion in the section on the treatment of histoplasmosis) (95). In many cases, treatment is only moderately successful. Better agents are needed. The following recommendations represent a current consensus of expert opinion based on evidence of variable but generally moderate quality.

Most patients with acute coccidioidomycosis are not treated because in most cases the disease is undiagnosed. The infection is asymptomatic or causes minimal symptoms, so that medical attention is not sought. Most patients in whom mild or moderately symptomatic primary pulmonary coccidioidomycosis ("valley fever") is diagnosed also require no treatment. They do require careful clinical and serologic evaluation to identify those with progressive disease. In areas where the disease is highly endemic, many patients with acute pulmonary coccidioidomycosis are treated with 400 mg of fluconazole per day for weeks to months, based on minimal evidence (C-III).

Patients with unusually severe primary infections and those at high risk for severe infection (HIV-positive, organ transplant recipient, high-dose corticosteroid treatment) should be treated with 400 to 800 mg of fluconazole per day or 200 mg of itraconazole twice daily (A-II). Treatment is usually continued for 3 to 6 months. Primary coccidioidomycosis in the third trimester of pregnancy should be treated with amphotericin B (A-III) (azoles are teratogenic). Patients with diffuse pulmonary infiltrates (usually but not always patients with AIDS) should be treated with amphotericin B to improvement (B-III), then with an azole for at least 1 year (B-III). Secondary prophylaxis with an azole should be continued for life in patients with AIDS (A-II).

In addition to immunosuppressed patients, disseminated disease is believed more likely to develop in blacks and Hispanics (81,82), and possibly in patients with diabetes (78–80). Acute infections in these high-risk patient groups should be treated to prevent dissemination. Oral azoles for 3 to 6 months are frequently used (B-III).

If symptomatic pulmonary disease persists for 6 weeks, spontaneous clearing is less likely. Many such patients have persisting infiltrates. In some cases, a solid round lesion evolves that is a blocked pulmonary abscess. Patients with persistent disease may also be given amphotericin B (total dose of 500–2,000 mg) to reduce the risk for local progression and prevent dissemination. In current practice in areas of endemicity, many high-risk patients with acute infection and many patients with persistent disease are given oral fluconazole therapy for various periods without proof of efficacy. Before the availability of fluconazole, ketoconazole was used in the same way, especially for patients with persistent coccidioidomycosis. Many patients showed clinical improvement, but the relapse rate after cessation of therapy was as high as 50% (96). No controlled studies have evaluated these agents prospectively, nor has any comparison been made of the two oral agents or of the azoles versus amphotericin B in patients with persistent pulmonary symptoms and radiographic abnormalities lasting beyond 6 weeks.

The characteristic thin-walled cavitary lesion of coccidioidomycosis usually does not require treatment. This is a shelled-out abscess but is relatively less active than an infiltrate or solid nodule. About 50% of lesions smaller than 4 cm in diameter resolve under observation within 2 years. If cavities persist beyond 2 years, if they enlarge subpleurally, or if hemoptysis is troublesome, treatment is reasonable. Amphotericin B and the oral azoles have been used, but efficacy has not been carefully evaluated (B-III for both). A pyopneumothorax from a ruptured cavity should be treated with chest tube drainage and antifungal therapy (amphotericin B, fluconazole, and itraconazole have all been used) (C-III). Selected patients (especially young, otherwise healthy patients with persistent air leak or a poor response to antifungal therapy) require lobectomy and decortication (A-III) together with antifungal therapy (C-III). In cases in which the surgical risk is high, the treatment options may be limited to medical therapy as previously outlined (C-III).

Isolated small pulmonary nodules (blocked cavities or coccidioidal abscesses) can be observed initially. If pus (containing spherules) is recovered by fine needle aspiration, most clinicians treat with a course of fluconazole. Many coin lesions are removed surgically to rule out bronchogenic cancer. If the lesions are resected incidentally (under the assumption that they are cancerous), most authorities do not suggest postoperative treatment with amphotericin B (E-III). If the pleural space is contaminated during surgery, most authorities agree that treatment is necessary (77). The optimal total dose and the required duration of therapy are unknown. Early anecdotal experience suggested that a 500-mg course of intravenous amphotericin B given preoperatively and postoperatively helps to provide a therapeutic umbrella for resection of a proven coccidioidal lesion. Although this practice is common and seems reasonable, it also has not been evaluated. Our own practice is not to use antifungal therapy after complete and clean resection of a nodule that proves pathologically to be coccidioidomycosis. If the abscess has been transected and material has spilled into the pleural space, we recommend 500 to 1,000 mg of amphotericin B postoperatively.

Patients with chronic fibrocavitary pneumonia should be treated with azole therapy for at least 1 year (A-II). The relapse rate is high when therapy is stopped (historically, it was highest after ketoconazole therapy, as high as 50%). High-dose fluconazole, amphotericin B, and surgical resection for localized disease can be considered in selected cases (B-III).

Disseminated coccidioidomycosis requires rapid and aggressive treatment. Azoles are recommended for initial therapy (A-II). For nonmeningeal disease, fluconazole and itraconazole are likely equally effective (94). Amphotericin B is an alternative, especially for severely ill patients. Amphotericin B therapy in coccidioidomycosis is not as effective as it is in histoplasmosis and blastomycosis. The standard total dose of amphotericin B in coccidioidomycosis is between 2,500 and 3,000 mg, administered over several months (72).

If the clinical disease is stabilized but not cured, much larger total doses of amphotericin B are given by extending the therapy. One method is to treat patients with up to 50 mg of amphotericin B daily until their condition stabilizes or improves; 50 mg is then given three times weekly on an outpatient basis. Beyond this daily dose, renal failure is almost universal. Because many patients improve with amphotericin B but are not cured, a switch to fluconazole after initial stabilization is often made. Surgical debridement of local areas of infection, including bony lesions (especially spine lesions) and soft tissue lesions, is often required as an adjunct to antifungal therapy. Surgical therapy of coccidioidomycosis must be individualized and requires a great deal of experience.

Disseminated coccidioidomycosis in AIDS is a major therapeutic challenge. As expected, the disease is aggressive and progresses rapidly. In one series, 49% of the patients died within 3 months, with a mean survival of 59 days (90). In such a rapidly progressive disease, amphotericin B should be used for initial therapy. Some patients do respond to amphotericin B. After stabilization of the clinical illness, it is reasonable to switch to oral fluconazole ($\geq$400 mg/d). In the same series (90), all the patients who survived more than 1 year had received a minimum of 1 g of amphotericin B and then continuous suppressive therapy with an oral azole. Maintenance therapy for all the endemic mycoses (and for cryptococcosis) has been required for life in patients with AIDS who respond to initial treatment. With the advent of HAART, the possibility of immune reconstitution in some patients may obviate the need for lifetime maintenance. Until good studies are performed, stopping maintenance therapy for coccidioidomycosis in AIDS patients is not advised.

Coccidioidal meningitis is also a major therapeutic challenge. Historically, standard therapy included systemic amphotericin B (2,500–3,000 mg) plus intensive and long-term intrathecal amphotericin B therapy (72,87). To administer intrathecal treatment, a reservoir was placed in one of the lateral ventricles. Intraventricular amphotericin B in doses between 0.25 and 1.0 mg was injected two or three times weekly until the symptoms abated and the CSF pleocytosis decreased. After clinical improvement and a decrease in the CSF pleocytosis, the frequency of intrathecal injections was gradually reduced from twice weekly, to weekly, to every other week, and finally to monthly. Monthly treatment was continued for years, even for life. Even with this method of treatment, relapses were common, requiring a return to more frequent treatment. With careful management, some patients could be maintained in a good clinical state for a long time, even a decade or more.

Today, therapy with oral fluconazole (400–800 mg/d) is recommended for coccidioidal meningitis (A-II). Itraconazole at a dosage of 400 to 600 mg/d has also been used and has similar efficacy (B-II). Patients who respond to azole therapy should continue this treatment indefinitely (A-III). Cure of the disease should not be expected, but many patients are maintained in a good functional state and can lead essentially normal lives. Intrathecal amphotericin B can be tried in patients who do not respond to azoles. The dose and duration of intrathecal amphotericin B therapy in this circumstance have not been defined, but likely they are similar to the historical regimen previously outlined (C-III). Hydro-

cephalus nearly always requires a shunt for decompression (A-III).

The treatment of coccidioidomycosis remains a difficult clinical problem. None of the standard antifungal agents are highly effective, and the clinical response is not predictable. Many patients die (especially patients with AIDS), and in many others, chronic infections develop that must be managed rather than cured. Each patient's treatment must be individualized. Treatment strategies are evolving with time, and the general approach presented here will not be static.

CRYPTOCOCCOSIS

C. neoformans is a truly cosmopolitan yeast that has been isolated on all continents. Most isolations from nature have come from soils heavily contaminated by bird droppings, especially pigeon droppings. Fresh pigeon dropping do not contain the fungus, but older, dry specimens frequently are teeming with the organism. The pigeons are not infected, but the droppings are an important source of organic nitrogen needed for fungal growth (97). The organism is a 4- to 8-μm yeast with a large carbohydrate capsule. In nature, *C. neoformans* is a desiccated, unencapsulated yeast. It is likely that small, capsule-poor organisms are the infecting particles (98). After the organism enters a human host, the capsule is reconstituted. *C. neoformans* is the only encapsulated yeast that infects humans.

Pathogenesis

As with the dimorphic fungi, the portal of entry is the lung. Once in the alveoli, the large capsule reappears, and the fungus multiplies by binary fission. The capsule is antiphagocytic. Nonencapsulated cryptococcal species are easily ingested and destroyed by neutrophils, but encapsulated *C. neoformans* organisms resist phagocytosis (99). Within the neutrophil, oxidative and nonoxidative pathways accomplish killing of the organism. Patients with chronic granulomatous disease lack effective oxidative metabolism in their neutrophils and kill cryptococci poorly.

After *C. neoformans* gains a foothold in the mammalian lung, T cell–mediated immunity is required for adequate handling of the organism. This requirement was recognized very early because cryptococcal meningitis developed in many patients with Hodgkin disease (100). Since the advent of the HIV pandemic, the importance of intact T cell–mediated immunity has been confirmed (101). *Cryptococcus* infection is the most common fungal disease complicating HIV infection.

In the normal lung, granuloma formation checks further fungal growth (102). Extrapulmonary spread of the organism may occur during the preimmune phase of self-limited pulmonary infection, as in histoplasmosis. The only evidence for this is that all cases of meningitis represent distant spread

COCCIDIOIDOMYCOSIS	
Summary Statement	**Evidence**
Diagnosis	
Stain and culture are sensitive and specific for diagnosis, particularly of established or chronic disease.	Observational studies, expert opinion
Serodiagnosis is important in mild or primary disease (lower sensitivity in immunocompromised/HIV-infected patients). Immunodiffusion for IgM is sensitive and specific in that setting.	Expert opinion
CF has moderate sensitivity and specificity for diagnosis and is most useful for managing patients with disease; high or rising titers suggest progressive or disseminated disease and a poor prognosis.	Observational studies, expert opinion
Treatment	
Most patients with moderately symptomatic primary infection require no treatment; clinical/serologic monitoring for progressive disease is indicated.	Expert opinion
Severe primary disease or disease in setting of immunocompromise should be treated. Fluconazole or itraconazole should be used (except in third trimester of pregnancy or when diffuse infiltrates are present; AMB should then be used).	Observational studies, expert opinion
Acute infections in some groups at high risk for dissemination should be treated with an azole for 3–6 months.	Expert opinion
Patients with presistent primary pulmonary infection should be treated with AMB; some use an azole in this setting.	Expert opinion
Thin-walled/small cavities may be observed; persistent or enlarging cavities should be treated with AMB, and azoles have been used. Surgical resection should be considered if response is poor.	Expert opinion
Fibrocavitary disease should be treated with azoles; localized disease may be considered for resection.	Observational studies, expert opinion
Disseminated disease without CNS involvement should be treated with azoles (fluconazole/itraconazole equivalent).	Observational studies
AMB is used for severe disease or treatment failure. Indefinite maintenance therapy with an azole should be given to AIDS patients treated for cocci pending further studies.	Expert opinion
Oral azoles are first-line treatment for coccidioidal meningitis.	Observational studies
Treatment should be continued indefinitely.	Expert opinion

AMB, amphotericin B; CF, complement fixation; CNS, central nervous system.

from the lung, even though the lung infection has often already cleared by the time meningitis appears.

In patients with suppressed T cell–mediated immunity, granulomas do not form, and growth continues. At surgery or postmortem examination, large masses of cryptococci are seen without any evidence of tissue reaction, producing large gelatinous masses. The most important feature of the pathogenesis of cryptococcal disease is the remarkable tropism of the organism for the CNS. Cryptococcal meningitis is the most commonly recognized form of the illness.

Clinical Manifestations

It is likely that most primary pulmonary infections are subclinical. The diagnosis of isolated pulmonary disease is uncommon; cases of isolated pulmonary disease represent fewer than 10% of all diagnosed cases, even though the portal of entry is always the lung. Campbell (103), in his classic review of cryptococcal pulmonary disease in 1966, identified only 101 cases restricted to the lung. Although no large review has been published since then, isolated pulmonary disease (without extrapulmonary spread) is still uncommon.

Some patients have no pulmonary symptoms and present with an abnormality discovered on a routine chest radiograph. Patients with symptomatic pulmonary cryptococcosis have fever, chest pain, and cough, usually of modest intensity (104). Some patients clear their pulmonary infections uneventfully but later present with meningitis. In fact, 50% to 75% of patients with cryptococcal meningitis (excluding those with AIDS) have normal chest radiographic findings and no history of pneumonia (105).

The findings on the chest radiograph are highly variable, including the size and location of infiltrates. Infiltrates may be single or multiple, and the disease is often confused with other pulmonary infections or neoplasms. Primary TB may be suspected if a peripheral infiltrate with ipsilateral hilar adenopathy is present (106). Occasionally, patients have round masses as large as 10 cm in diameter, which mimic cancer.

Most patients in whom pulmonary or CNS cryptococcosis is diagnosed have abnormal cell-mediated immunity. The natural history of cryptococcal pulmonary infection in immunocompromised patients is dissemination to the meninges (107). However, cryptococcal meningitis can also develop in immunologically intact persons, although the pulmonary disease more often is self-limited.

Meningitis is the most important form of cryptococcal infection. The presentation ranges from asymptomatic meningitis to focal neurologic findings to coma (107,108). The tempo of the CNS involvement is also highly variable. Long life has been reported in patients with proven and untreated cryptococcal meningitis, but the disease can also kill within a few days after onset (83). Some persons may have no meningeal signs despite fulminant meningitis (101,109).

The CSF shows a mononuclear cell pleocytosis. The leukocyte count is highly variable and may be lower than 5/mm^3 or even zero. The protein concentration is usually elevated, and the glucose level is reduced, occasionally to very low levels. A hallmark of cryptococcal meningitis is elevation of the CSF pressure secondary to involvement of the subarachnoid villi, which usually reabsorb CSF. This is seen especially in patients with AIDS. In approximately 60% of AIDS patients with cryptococcal meningitis, the opening pressures are higher than 18 cm H$_2$O. CT of the head often fails to show hydrocephalus because the increased pressure is uniformly distributed throughout the brain. The clinical manifestations of increased pressure are headache and cranial nerve abnormalities—especially the cranial nerves of the eyes (III, IV, and VI), which are anatomically susceptible to increased CSF pressures. Untreated, high pressures lead to coma and death. Treatment involves serial removal of CSF and in some cases shunting.

Other extrapulmonary sites of involvement by cryptococci include the skin, bones, and prostate. Unless evidence is found of direct local inoculation (a chancre and enlarged draining lymph nodes), all forms of cutaneous cryptococcal disease should be assumed to represent dissemination from a central focus, usually the meninges or the lungs (110).

The AIDS epidemic has markedly altered the landscape of cryptococcal infection. Most diagnosed cryptococcal infections (as many as 90%) now occur in AIDS patients. Most AIDS patients have widely disseminated disease in addition to meningitis. Many have diffuse infiltrates. The diagnosis is usually easy, but treatment must include induction therapy to achieve remission and long-term maintenance to prevent relapse. Lasting cure was not possible before the development of HAART. Even with HAART, more study is needed to determine when it is safe to stop maintenance therapy.

Diagnosis

Cryptococcosis was the first disease in which the detection of fungal antigen became the standard diagnostic test. Measuring antigen rather than antibodies to fungus has the advantage of perfect specificity. It does not depend on an intact immune system of the host, as does antibody production. With proper controls, the specificity of the cryptococcal antigen test is 100%. (Problems of cross-reactions with high titers of rheumatoid factor have largely been solved.)

In non-AIDS patients, chronic meningitis is the most common form of the disease. The sensitivity of cryptococcal antigen in CSF is 95% (101). The specificity is 100%. The positive and negative predictive values are both 100%.

In patients with AIDS, the serum is nearly always positive for cryptococcal antigen, usually at a higher titer than the CSF. The serum test is very sensitive (72 of 73 cases in one series) and has perfect positive and negative predictive values. Cryptococcal antigen is present in the CSF of all AIDS patients with meningitis, who comprise the vast majority of cases. However, the serum cryptococcal antigen is present at a higher titer. Serum antigen is also present in the uncommon AIDS patient with pulmonary or nonmeningeal systemic cryptococcosis that has not yet spread to the meninges.

In AIDS, cultures of blood and BAL fluid (and direct smears) are usually positive, as are CSF cultures and CSF India ink preparations (70%), but these tests are seldom necessary for the diagnosis. The serum cryptococcal antigen test outperforms them.

The CSF is positive by culture in 50% to 75% of cases of non-AIDS chronic meningitis. India ink preparations are positive in fewer than half of cases (Fig. 19.14). Both tests are outperformed by the CSF cryptococcal antigen test. The serum is usually negative for cryptococcal antigen.

The diagnosis of isolated cryptococcal pneumonia in non-AIDS patients is more difficult. The serum is usually negative for cryptococcal antigen. Culture (of sputum or broncho-scopic specimens) and histopathology are the mainstays of diagnosis.

C. neoformans grows readily on routine laboratory media. However, positive sputum cultures, even in the presence of radiographic abnormality, must be interpreted carefully. The organism may colonize airways. Most susceptible are patients with chronic bronchitis with a low risk for dissemination (111). In histopathologic sections, the organism appears as a small yeast with single narrow-necked buds. In standard hematoxylin and eosin–stained sections, the unstained capsule appears as a halo surrounding the yeast. A silver stain shows the organism but not the capsule. The mucicarmine stain colors the carbohydrate capsule bright red (Fig. 19.15).

Treatment

In the 1970s, a number of controlled studies documented several effective regimens for the treatment of cryptococcal meningitis. Then the AIDS epidemic began, and within a

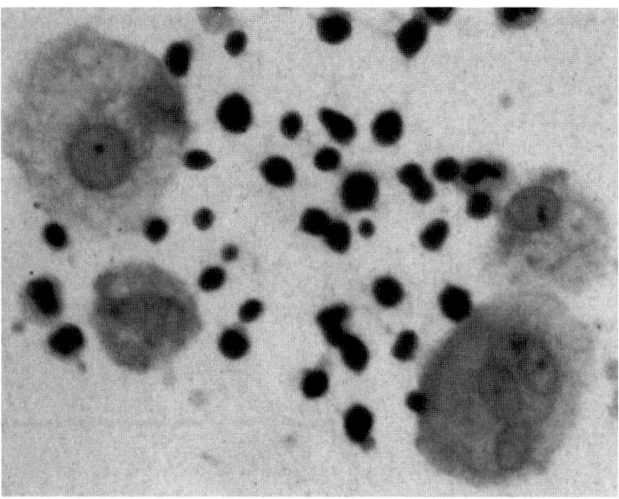

FIGURE 19.15. (See also Color Fig. 19.15.) Disseminated cryptococcosis in AIDS. Bronchoalveolar lavage fluid was positive for encapsulated yeast. Capsular material stains bright red on special stain (mucicarmine stain, original magnification × 400).

short time, 90% of cases of cryptococcal meningitis were in patients with AIDS. Fluconazole also became available, the first azole with excellent CNS penetration. Naturally, most of the investigative energy shifted to determining the best therapy for cryptococcal infection in AIDS. In 2000, the treatment options for all forms of cryptococcal disease were reviewed by an expert committee of the Mycoses Study Group of the NIAID and published as part of a series by the Infectious Diseases Society of America (see general discussion in the section on the treatment of histoplasmosis) (112). The evidence was reviewed and graded. Most of the evidence was of good or moderate quality.

A positive sputum culture should be interpreted with a certain degree of skepticism. Even if the chest radiograph is abnormal, several explanations are possible. The organism may be a contaminant, a colonizer, or the cause of a self-limited pneumonia. Routine bacterial pathogens should be treated first. If the infiltrate persists, isolated cryptococcal pulmonary disease is likely. In the past, asymptomatic immunocompetent patients with this diagnosis were followed without treatment because the natural history is spontaneous improvement. However, a risk for meningeal dissemination, although low, does exist. Because fluconazole is a nontoxic oral agent, treatment with fluconazole (200–400 mg/d for 3–6 months) is reasonable even if the patient is asymptomatic (A-III) (113). Immunocompetent patients with isolated pulmonary cryptococcosis who have symptoms should be treated with 200 to 400 mg of fluconazole per day for 3 to 6 months (A-III) (114). If disease is severe or progressive, amphotericin B (0.4–0.7 mg/kg per day to a total dose of 1–2 g) can be given (B-III).

All patients with positive blood cultures, all patients with a serum cryptococcal antigen titer above 1:8, and all patients with isolated cutaneous and renal disease should be treated with 200 to 400 mg of fluconazole per day for 3 to 6 months.

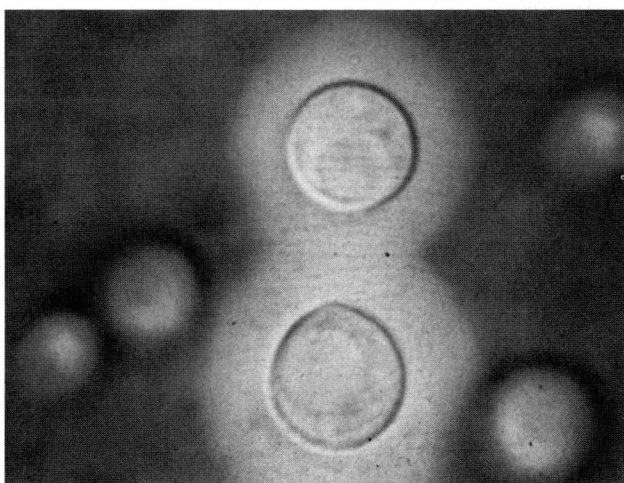

FIGURE 19.14. *Cryptococcus neoformans.* India ink preparation shows halo effect around the yeast, caused by the large capsule.

Bony disease often requires some combination of surgical resection and prolonged antifungal therapy. It should be noted that all patients with cryptococcal infection require a spinal tap to exclude meningitis.

The treatment of non-AIDS immunosuppressed patients (including transplant recipients) with cryptococcal pneumonia is always necessary because the natural history is spread to the meninges. Mild to moderate cases can be treated with 400 mg of fluconazole daily for 6 to 12 months. Severe cases should be treated like CNS disease with 0.7 to 1.0 mg of amphotericin B per kilogram for 2 weeks (with or without 100 mg of 5-flucytosine per kilogram per day in four divided doses) or until clinical improvement, followed by 400 mg of fluconazole per day for 6 to 12 months.

The recommended treatment of cryptococcal meningitis in non-AIDS patients is 0.7 to 1.0 mg of amphotericin B per kilogram with 5-flucytosine (100 mg/kg per day) for 2 weeks, followed by 400 mg of fluconazole per day for at least 10 weeks (A-I). Another regimen is amphotericin B (0.7–1 mg/kg daily) with 5-flucytosine (100 mg/kg daily) for a minimum of 6 to 10 weeks (A-I) (115). Mild to moderate cases of cryptococcal meningitis (normal mental status at diagnosis) in non-AIDS patients can also be treated with amphotericin B alone (total dose of 1–2 g), or shorter courses of amphotericin B followed by fluconazole, or even 400 mg of fluconazole per day started at the onset and continued for 6 to 12 months. No prospective or randomized data are available regarding regimens in non-AIDS patients, including fluconazole, because the vast majority of cases of cryptococcal infections today occur in patients with AIDS. Great care must be taken when 5-flucytosine is used. The drug accumulates rapidly, especially if renal function is reduced. If the serum level is high ($>100 \ \mu g/mL$), 5-flucytosine is toxic to bone marrow. If a rapid turnaround time for 5-flucytosine levels cannot be ascertained, the agent should be avoided.

The treatment of cryptococcal disease in patients with AIDS is a different problem. It is assumed that all AIDS patients with cryptococcal infection at any site either have meningitis or, if untreated, will soon have it. All patients with an isolate from any site and all patients with serum positive for antigen must have a lumbar puncture. All must be treated. No time of cure of the fungal infection has been established. When the standard time-limited regimens previously described were used in patients with AIDS, virtually all of them relapsed. The concept of posttreatment prophylaxis or maintenance therapy was quickly established. The total dose and duration of treatment became less important because everyone had continued to receive either weekly or biweekly suppression with amphotericin B or a daily suppressive azole drug. Fluconazole was the natural choice for oral therapy because of its high penetration into CSF (levels in CSF $\geq 80\%$ of simultaneous serum levels).

Four hundred milligrams of fluconazole per day is a safe and effective treatment for the uncommon cases of non-meningeal disease in AIDS, including isolated cryptococcal lung disease. (A-II). After 3 to 6 months, the dose is reduced to 200 mg/d and continued for life. With HAART for AIDS and the possibility of immune reconstitution in these patients, the duration of therapy is becoming a practical question. Future studies are planned to determine whether it is ever possible to stop therapy for cryptococcal meningitis in selected AIDS patients with high CD4$^+$ cell counts. The results would likely be relevant to pulmonary cryptococcosis in AIDS. Four hundred milligrams of itraconazole per day can be used for AIDS patients with nonmeningeal cryptococcal infection who cannot tolerate fluconazole. Four hundred milligrams of fluconazole per day plus 100 mg of flucytosine per kilogram per day for 10 weeks can be used in severe cases, followed by fluconazole for maintenance.

Most of the focus has been on the treatment of cryptococcal meningitis in AIDS. Because of the lesser toxicity of fluconazole, studies were undertaken to compare amphotericin B with fluconazole for initial therapy. Time to culture negativity in the fluconazole group was longer (116), and at least one study suggested a greater number of early deaths. Nonetheless, both agents were effective and roughly equivalent, especially in patients with normal mental status at onset of therapy. Four hundred milligrams of fluconazole a day for 3 to 6 months followed by 200 mg/d for life is likely a safe and effective treatment for selected mild cases of cryptococcal meningitis in AIDS, although this approach is discouraged by some authorities.

Another study evaluated amphotericin B at a dose of 0.7 to 1.0 mg/kg per day with or without 100 mg of 5-flucytosine per kilogram per day for 2 weeks, followed by fluconazole (117). The short-term results were similar, but those receiving 5-flucytosine showed slightly better results on long-term follow-up.

Current consensus recommendations for cryptococcal meningitis in AIDS include amphotericin B (0.7–1 mg/kg daily) with 5-flucytosine (100 mg/kg per day) for 2 weeks, followed by 400 mg of fluconazole per day for a minimum of 10 weeks, then 200 mg of fluconazole per day for life (A-I). Another effective regimen is 0.7 to 1.0 mg of amphotericin B per kilogram with 5-flucytosine (100 mg/kg per day) for 10 weeks, followed by 200 mg of fluconazole per day for life (A-I). Lipid formulations of amphotericin B can be used when renal function is impaired or deteriorates during amphotericin B therapy. One non–amphotericin B regimen is 400 to 800 mg of fluconazole per day plus 100 to 150 mg of flucytosine per kilogram per day (C-II). This last regimen is toxic, especially in view of the bone marrow depression associated with AIDS and the toxicity of concurrent pharmacotherapy that is required. Careful management of increased intracranial pressure (including serial removal of spinal fluid) is an important adjunct to drug therapy. Initial lumbar drainage is performed to reduce the pressure to 20 cm H_2O or to 50% of the initial opening pressure. This is followed by repeated daily drainage until the opening pressure is stable (A-II).

For maintenance therapy, 400 mg of fluconazole per day was compared with 200 mg of itraconazole orally every 12 hours in a study that lasted for 12 weeks (A-II for both). These treatments were not significantly different. When maintenance therapy was continued beyond 12 weeks with reduced doses of fluconazole and itraconazole, fluconazole was the superior drug, with itraconazole a second choice (118).

In general, the treatment of cryptococcal pulmonary disease is not based on carefully performed prospective studies. Treatment recommendations are based on the large experience with cryptococcal meningitis, on anecdotes, and on opinions.

CRYPTOCOCCOSIS

Summary Statement	Evidence
Diagnosis	
Cryptococcal antigen is highly specific and sensitive for CNS and blood stream dissemination.	Observational studies
Smear, culture, histology usually required for isolated pneumonia in immunocompetent host.	Expert opinion
Treatment	
All pulmonary disease should be treated; CSF should be tested to exclude meningitis.	Expert opinion
Fluconazole is recommended for isolated pulmonary disease.	Expert opinion
AMB is recommended for severe/progressive disease.	Randomized studies
AMB + 5-FC is recommended for initial meningitis treatment; fluconazole may be used to complete therapy and for long-term maintenance therapy in AIDS patients.	Expert opinion
Itraconazole is equivalent to fluconazole for maintenance therapy.	Observational studies
Lipid AMB may be used in the setting of renal dysfunction from AMB.	Expert opinion

AMB, amphotericin B; CSF, cerebrospinal fluid; CNS, central nervous system; 5-FC, 5-flucytosine.

ASPERGILLOSIS

Although the most common form of aspergillosis, disseminated or pyemic aspergillosis, is addressed in Chapter 18, three syndromes caused by *Aspergillus* require brief mention in this chapter.

Aspergilloma

The most common form of aspergillosis worldwide is the aspergilloma, or fungus ball (119). An aspergilloma consists of masses of fungal mycelial mat interspersed with fibrin, mucus, and other tissue debris, along with inflammatory cells.

Aspergillomas develop in preformed lung cavities that most often are the residual of inactive or healed TB. Although TB remains the main cause of residual pulmonary cavities, even in Europe and North America, residual pulmonary cavities caused by fungal infections, sarcoidosis, bronchiectasis, reactive spondyloarthropathy, or cancer represent a sizable number of cavities colonized by *Aspergillus* in North America.

Most aspergillomas are recognized on incidental chest radiographs, and only an occasional fungus ball presents with symptoms, usually hemoptysis. Although the hemoptysis is usually mild, it is sometimes life-threatening. Massive bleeding usually complicates aspergillomas in tuberculous cavities. The frequently mentioned symptom of dyspnea during effort is most likely a consequence of severe underlying lung disease rather than of the aspergilloma.

The diagnosis of aspergilloma is seldom difficult because the fungus ball is readily seen on chest radiographs or CT scans, which show the freely movable intracavitary mass. In most instances, the colonizing fungus is *Aspergillusis fumigatus*.

Treatment remains problematic. Incidentally discovered aspergillomas do not require treatment. Because the response to antifungal agents is not consistent, symptomatic patients require resection of the involved lobe if lung function permits (120). Resection is difficult and may carry significant mortality and morbidity.

When surgery is not possible because of poor underlying lung function and hemoptysis is life-threatening, bronchial artery embolization may allow temporary control of the bleeding.

Allergic Bronchopulmonary Aspergillosis

This syndrome occurs in patients with asthma that is often severe. Allergic bronchopulmonary aspergillosis (ABPA) also develops in about 10% of patients with cystic fibrosis. It is thought that these patients, in addition to cystic fibrosis, have reactive airways disease.

When ABPA is considered on clinical grounds, it is usually because of the occurrence of recurrent, fleeting pulmonary infiltrates, fever, and the reported expectoration of brownish bronchial casts. The chest radiograph is suggestive, especially when distended bronchi are seen radiating from the hilum, giving rise to the "fingers in glove" appearance. At later stages of the disease, central, cylindric bronchiectasis may develop, which can be readily seen on chest CT scans.

Diagnostic criteria have been developed, and the modified criteria of Greenberger and Patterson (121) are used by most authorities. These are listed in Table 19.1.

The standard of care in ABPA is glucocorticoid therapy to reduce airway inflammation (119,122). This usually effects a marked symptomatic improvement. Prednisone is started at 0.5 mg/kg daily for approximately 2 weeks, then can be slowly tapered. Typically, the total serum IgE level is used as

TABLE 19.1. DIAGNOSTIC CRITERIA FOR ALLERGIC BRONCHOPULMONARY ASPERGILLOSIS

Asthma
Immediate skin reactivity to *Aspergillus*
Serum precipitins to *Aspergillus fumigatus*
Increased serum IgE and IgG to *A. fumigatus*
Total serum IgE >1,000 ng/mL
Current or previous pulmonary infiltrates
Central bronchiectasis
Peripheral eosinophilia (1,000 cells per microliter)

Source: From Greenberger PA, Patterson R. Diagnosis and management of allergic bronchopulmonary aspergillosis. *Ann Allergy* 1986;56:444–448, with permission.

the target for tapering, with the dose decreased as the level normalizes. More recently, some have suggested using the cellularity of induced sputum as a marker of bronchiectasis in ABPA, and possibly as a therapeutic target (123). Although in occasional patients ABPA clears completely, many require long-term low-dose suppressive therapy (124). A randomized controlled trial of adjunctive therapy with itraconazole has shown a significant steroid-sparing effect. Itraconazole is given at a dose of 200 mg twice daily for 16 weeks (125). Although it has not been proved, long-term suppressive therapy with 200 mg of itraconazole per day following the initial course of itraconazole may be beneficial.

Chronic Necrotizing Aspergillosis

This relatively rare form of disease has been described in patients without classic forms of immunocompromise, although most have been alcoholic, diabetic, or malnourished. A localized, chronic infiltrative process develops with or without cavitation. Chest pain, weight loss, cough, and fever are common. The condition typically follows a protracted course and is initially mistaken for more common bacterial pneumonias, but it fails to respond to antibiotics. The generally poor underlying condition of the patients makes treatment difficult, even with appropriate antifungal agents, although most survive at least several years and generally succumb to other conditions (126). Newer agents, such as itraconazole, may facilitate their care (127). Other fungi, particularly those of the order Mucorales (*Mucor, Rhizopus, Absidia*), are also rarely associated with a similar presentation.

ACTINOMYCOSIS AND NOCARDIOSIS

Originally considered with the fungi when taxonomy was based entirely on morphology, the organisms that cause both these diseases are now known to be higher-order bacteria. Nevertheless, by custom, they are frequently discussed with the endemic fungi.

Actinomyces israelii is the principal organism causing human disease. The organism is Gram-positive, non–acid-fast, and a facultative or strict anaerobe. In culture, it forms long, delicate, branching, beaded filaments. When pus is expressed from an actinomycotic lesion, it may appear as yellow ("sulfur") granules. The organism usually infects only diseased tissues, such as a periodontal abscess or an area of aspiration pneumonitis. The three main clinical forms of actinomycosis are cervicofacial, thoracic, and abdominal.

Pulmonary actinomycosis usually presents as an indolent, destructive pulmonary process, mostly in patients likely to have aspirated. The organism is moderately aggressive, may cause cavitation, crosses fissures, and on occasion invades the chest wall, frequently mimicking lung cancer (128).

The diagnosis usually involves identification of the organism by culture. When actinomycosis is clinically suspected, the laboratory should be advised to process the specimen anaerobically. Bedside inoculation of the specimen into culture media markedly increases the yield. The distinctive appearance on Gram stain of Gram-positive branching organisms is frequently helpful. In contradistinction to *Nocardia* species, these organisms are not acid-fast.

The drug of choice for the treatment of actinomycosis is penicillin, initially administered intravenously, then orally for 6 to 12 months. Tetracycline, clindamycin, chloramphenicol, and macrolides have also been used, but experience with each of these is limited.

Nocardiosis

Nocardia asteroides is the predominant organism causing human disease. This is a soil-dwelling bacterium. Although direct inoculation may occur, most human disease is the result of inhalation. More than two thirds of all infected persons have some degree of immunosuppression, associated with hematologic neoplasms (especially Hodgkin disease), chronic granulomatous disease, or long-term glucocorticoid therapy. Pulmonary nocardiosis is usually an indolent disease, although in immunosuppressed patients the tempo is generally increased. Neither the symptoms nor the radiologic findings, which may include nodules, infiltrates (sometimes with cavitation), and empyema, are sufficiently specific to suggest the diagnosis (129). Investigation directed at the correct diagnosis is usually triggered by the host's underlying illness or the treatment being administered.

About half of patients have extrapulmonary spread of the disease. The CNS is the most frequently recognized site.

The diagnosis is not difficult once the proper tests have been ordered. Gram stain usually reveals long, slender filaments with a beaded appearance. Most but not all isolates of *Nocardia* are acid-fast when stained with weak acid decolorizing stains, such as the Kinyoun or Ziehl-Neelsen stain. Cultural identification of the organism is not complicated, but not every sputum specimen from an infected patient will yield the organism. Because of the slow growth of the organism, cultures should be kept for at least 30 days.

Treatment usually includes a sulfa-containing agent. Because sulfadiazine is often not available, most modern series have used trimethoprim/sulfamethoxazole in high doses. The key to success is prolonged treatment. Other antimicrobials have also been used, including tetracycline, chloramphenicol, and most recently combinations such as imipenem and amikacin. Experience with these agents is limited.

REFERENCES

1. Goodwin RA Jr, Desires RM. Histoplasmosis: state of the art. *Am Rev Respir Dis* 1978;117:929–956.
2. Drutz DJ, Catanzaro A. Coccidioidomycosis: state of the art. Part I. *Am Rev Respir Dis* 1978;117:559–585.
3. Furcolow ML, Chick ER, Busey JD, et al. Prevalence and incidence studies of human and canine blastomycosis I: cases in the United States 1895–1968. *Am Rev Respir Dis* 1970;102: 60–67.
4. Sarosi GA, Davies SF. Blastomycosis: state of the art. *Am Rev Respir Dis* 1979;120:911–938.
5. Schaffner A, Davis CE, Schaffner T, et al. *In vitro* susceptibility of fungi to killing by neutrophil granulocytes discriminates between primary pathogenicity and opportunism. *J Clin Invest* 1986;78:511–524.
6. Goodwin RA Jr, Loyd JE, DesPrez RM. Histoplasmosis in normal hosts. *Medicine (Baltimore)* 1981;60:231–266.
7. Straub M, Schwarz J. Healed primary complex in histoplasmosis. *Am J Clin Pathol* 1955;25:727–738.
8. Feller AE, Furcolow ML, Larsh HW, et al. Outbreak of an unusual form of pneumonia at Camp Gruber, Oklahoma, in 1944. Follow-up studies implicating *H. capsulatum* as the etiologic agent. *Am J Med* 1956;21:184–192.
9. Sarosi GA, Parker JD, Tosh FE. Histoplasmosis outbreaks: their patterns. In: Balows A, ed. *Histoplasmosis. Proceedings of the second national conference.* Springfield, IL: Charles C Thomas Publisher, 1971;123–128.
10. D'Alessio DJ, Herren RH, Hendricks SL, et al. A starling roost as the source of urban epidemic histoplasmosis in an area of low incidence. *Am Rev Respir Dis* 1965;932:725–731.
11. Wheat LJ, Slama TG, Eitzen HE, et al. A large outbreak of histoplasmosis: clinical features. *Ann Intern Med* 1981;94:331–337.
12. Swensen SJ, Jett JR, Sloan JA, et al. Screening for lung cancer with low-dose spiral computed tomography. *Am J Respir Crit Care Med* 2002;165:508–513.
13. Medeiros AA, Marty SD, Tosh FE, et al. Erythema nodosum and erythema multiforme as clinical manifestations of histoplasmosis in a community outbreak. *N Engl J Med* 1966;274:415–420.
14. Goodman RA Jr, Shapiro JL, Thurman GH, et al. Disseminated histoplasmosis: clinical and pathologic correlations. *Medicine (Baltimore)* 1980;59:1–33.
15. Wheat LJ, Stein L, Corya BC, et al. Pericarditis as a manifestation of histoplasmosis during two large urban outbreaks. *Medicine (Baltimore)* 1983;62:110–118.
16. Goodwin RA Jr, Nickell JD, DesPrez RM. Mediastinal fibrosis complicating healed primary histoplasmosis and tuberculosis. *Medicine (Baltimore)* 1972;51:227–246.
17. Doyle TP, Loyd JE, Robbins IM. Percutaneous pulmonary artery and vein stenting: a novel treatment for mediastinal fibrosis. *Am J Respir Crit Care Med* 2001;164:657–660.
18. Tosh FE, Doto IL, DìAlessio DJ, et al. The second of two epidemics of histoplasmosis resulting from work on the same starling roost. *Am Rev Respir Dis* 1966;94:406–414.
19. Goodwin RA Jr, Snell JD, Hubbard WW, et al. Early chronic pulmonary histoplasmosis. *Am Rev Respir Dis* 1966;93:47–51.
20. Davies SF, Sarosi GA. Acute cavitary histoplasmosis. *Chest* 1978;73:103–105.
21. Goodwin RA Jr, Owens FT, Snell JD, et al. Chronic pulmonary histoplasmosis. *Medicine (Baltimore)* 1976;55:413–452.
22. Bunnell IL, Furcolow ML. A report of ten proven cases of histoplasmosis. *US Public Health Rep* 1948;63:299–316.
23. Paya CU, Roberts GN, Cockerill FR III. Transient fungemia in acute pulmonary histoplasmosis: detection by new blood-culturing techniques. *J Infect Dis* 1987;156:313–315.
24. McKenzie SW, Means RT. Extreme hyperferritinemia in patients infected with human immunodeficiency virus is not a highly specific marker for disseminated histoplasmosis. *Clin Infect Dis* 1997;24:519–520.
25. Johnson PC, Hamill RJ, Sarosi GA. Clinical review: progressive disseminated histoplasmosis in the AIDS patient. *Semin Respir Infect* 1989;4:139–446.
26. Wheat LJ, Connolly-Stringfield PA, Baker RL, et al. Disseminated histoplasmosis in the acquired immunodeficiency syndrome: clinical findings, diagnosis and treatment, and review of the literature. *Medicine (Baltimore)* 1990;69:361–374.
27. Tompsett R, Portera LA. Histoplasmosis: twenty-year experience in a general hospital. *Trans Am Clin Climatol Assoc* 1975;87:214–223.
28. Salzman SH, Smith RL, Aranda CP. Histoplasmosis in patients at risk for the acquired immunodeficiency syndrome in a nonendemic setting. *Chest* 1988;93:916–921.
29. Wheat LJ, Slama TG, Norton JA, et al. Risk factors for disseminated or fatal histoplasmosis. *Ann Intern Med* 1982;96:159–163.
30. Sarosi GA, Voth DW, Dahl BA, et al. Disseminated histoplasmosis: results of long-term follow-up. *Ann Intern Med* 1971;75:511–516.
31. Anaissi E, Fainstein V, Samo T, et al. Central nervous system histoplasmosis. *Am J Med* 1988;84:215–217.
32. Harris RL, Lawne GM, Wheeler TM, et al. Successful management of *Histoplasma capsulatum* infection of an abdominal aortic aneurysm. *Vasc Surg* 1986;1:40–44.
33. Davies SF. Serodiagnosis of histoplasmosis. *Semin Respir Infect* 1986;1:9–15.
34. Wheat LJ. Laboratory diagnosis of histoplasmosis: update 2000. *Semin Respir Infect* 2001;16:131–140.
35. Wheat JL, French MLV, Kohler RB, et al. The diagnostic tests for histoplasmosis: analysis of experience in a large urban outbreak. *Ann Intern Med* 1982;97:680–685.
36. Wheat JL, French MLV, Kamel S, et al. Evaluation of cross-reactions in *Histoplasma capsulatum* serologic tests. *J Clin Microbiol* 1985;23:493–499.
37. Wheat LJ, Kohler RB, French MLV, et al. Immunoglobulin M and G *Histoplasma* antibody response in histoplasmosis. *Am Rev Respir Dis* 1983;128:65–70.
38. Lamps LW, Molina CP, West AB, et al. The pathologic spectrum of gastrointestinal and hepatic histoplasmosis. *Am J Clin Pathol* 2000;113:64–72.
39. Smith JR Jr, Harris JS, Conant NF, et al. An epidemic of North American blastomycosis. *JAMA* 1951;158:641–645.
40. Davies SF, Sarosi GA. Role of serodiagnostic tests and skin tests in the diagnosis of fungal disease. *Clin Chest Med* 1987;8:135–146.
41. Sobel JD, for the Mycoses Study Group. Practice guidelines for the treatment of fungal infections. *Clin Infect Dis* 2000;30:630.
42. Wheat LJ, Sarosi GA, McKinsey D, et al. Practice guidelines for the management of patients with histoplasmosis. *Clin Infect Dis* 2000;30:688–695.
43. Johnson PC, Wheart LJ, Cloud GA, et al. U.S. National Institute of Allergy and Infectious Diseases Mycoses Study Group. Safety

and efficacy of liposomal amphotericin B compared with conventional amphotericin B for induction therapy of histoplasmosis in patients with AIDS. *Ann Intern Med* 2002;137:105–109.

44. Klein BS, Vergeront JM, Weeks RJ, et al. Isolation of *Blastomyces dermatitidis* in soil associated with a large outbreak of blastomycosis in Wisconsin. *N Engl J Med* 1986;314:529–534.

45. Schwarz J, Salfelder K. Blastomycosis. A review of 152 cases. *Curr Top Pathol* 1977;65:165.

46. Sarosi GA, Hammerman KJ, Tish FE, et al. Clinical features of acute pulmonary blastomycosis. *N Engl J Med* 1974;290:540–543.

47. Larsh HW, Schwarz J. Accidental inoculation blastomycosis. *Cutis* 1977;19:334–337.

48. Larson DM, Eckman MR, Alber RL, et al. Primary cutaneous (inoculation) blastomycosis: an occupation hazard to pathologists. *Am J Clin Pathol* 1983;79:253–255.

49. Witorsch P, Utz JP. North American blastomycosis. A study of 40 patients. *Medicine (Baltimore)* 1968;47:169–200.

50. Abernathy RS. Clinical manifestations of pulmonary blastomycosis. *Ann Intern Med* 1959;51:707–727.

51. Kunkel WM Jr, Weed LA, McDonald Jr, et al. North American blastomycosis: Gilchrist's disease. A clinicopathologic study of 90 cases. *Surg Gynecol Obstet* 1954;99:1–26.

52. Miller DD, Davies SF, Sarosi GA. Erythema nodosum and blastomycosis. *Arch Intern Med* 1982;142:1839.

53. Lasky WL, Sarosi GA. The radiologic appearance of pulmonary blastomycosis. *Radiology* 1978;126:351–357.

54. Lemos LB, Guo M, Baliga M. Blastomycosis: organ involvement and etiologic diagnosis. A review of 123 patients from Mississippi. *Ann Diagn Pathol* 2000;4:391–406.

55. Martynowicz MA, Prakash UB. Pulmonary blastomycosis: an appraisal of diagnostic techniques. *Chest* 2002;121:677–679.

56. Sarosi GA, Davies SF, Phillips JR. Self-limited blastomycosis: a report of 39 cases. *Semin Respir Infect* 1986;1:40–44.

57. Laskey WL, Sarosi GA. Endogenous reactivation in blastomycosis. *Ann Intern Med* 1978;88:50–52.

58. Davies SF, Sarosi GA. Clinical manifestations and management of blastomycosis in the compromised patient. In: Warnock DW, Richardson MD, eds. *Fungal infection in the compromised patient*, 2nd ed. New York: John Wiley & Sons, 1991:214–229.

59. Pappas PG, Pottage JC, Powderly WG, et al. Blastomycosis in patients with the acquired immunodeficiency syndrome. *Ann Intern Med* 1992;116:847–853.

60. Sanders JS, Sarosi GA, Nollet DJ, et al. Exfoliative cytology in the rapid diagnosis of pulmonary blastomycosis. *Chest* 1977;72:193–196.

61. Patel RG, Patel B, Petrini MF, et al. Clinical presentation, radiographic findings, and diagnostic methods of pulmonary blastomycosis: a review of 100 consecutive cases. *South Med J* 1999;92:289–295.

62. Klein BS, Vergeront JM, Kaufman L, et al. Serological tests for blastomycosis: assessment during a large point-source outbreak in Wisconsin. *J Infect Dis* 1987;155:262–268.

63. Chapman SW, Bradsher RW Jr, Campbell GD, et al. Practice guidelines for the management of patients with blastomycosis. *Clin Infect Dis* 2000;30:679–683.

64. Dismukes WE, Bradsher RW Jr, Cloud GC, et al. Itraconazole therapy for blastomycosis and histoplasmosis. *Am J Med* 1992;93:489–497.

65. Rixford E, Gilchrist TC. Two cases of protozoan (coccidioidal) infection of the skin and other organs. *Johns Hopkins Hosp Rep* 1896;1:209–265.

66. Dickson EC. Coccidioidomycosis: the preliminary acute infection with fungus *Coccidioides*. *JAMA* 1938;111:1362–1365.

67. Dickson EC, Gifford MA. *Coccidioides* infection (coccidioidomycosis) II. The primary type of infection. *Arch Intern Med* 1938;62:858–871.

68. Smith CE, Beard RR, Rosenberger HG, et al. Effect of season and dust control on coccidioidomycosis. *JAMA* 1946;132:833–839.

69. Forbus WD, Bestebreurtje AM. Coccidioidomycosis. A study of 95 cases of the disseminated type with special reference to the pathogenesis of the disease. *Mil Surg* 1946;99:653–719.

70. Flynn NM, Hoeprich PD, Kawachi MM, et al. An unusual outbreak of windborne coccidioidomycosis. *N Engl J Med* 1979;301:358–361.

71. Goldstein DM, McDonald JB. Primary pulmonary coccidioidomycosis. Follow-up of 75 cases with 10 more cases from a new endemic area. *JAMA* 1944;124:557–561.

72. Drutz DJ, Catanzaro A. Coccidioidomycosis. State of the art. Part II. *Am Rev Respir Dis* 1978;177:727–771.

73. Bayer AS. Fungal pneumonias, pulmonary coccidioidal syndromes (part I). *Chest* 1981;79:575–583.

74. Bayer AS. Fungal pneumonias, pulmonary coccidioidal syndromes (part II). *Chest* 1981;79:686–691.

75. Winn WA. A long-term study of 300 patients with cavitary abscess lesions of the lung of coccidioidal origin. *Dis Chest* 1968;54[Suppl 1]:12–16.

76. Hyde L. Coccidioidal pulmonary cavitation. *Dis Chest* 1968;54[Suppl 1]:17–21.

77. Cunningham RT, Einstein H. Coccidioidal pulmonary cavities with rupture. *J Thorac Cardiovasc Surg* 1982;84:172–177.

78. Deresinski SC, Stevens DA. Coccidioidomycosis in compromised hosts: experience at Stanford University Hospital. *Medicine (Baltimore)* 1975;54:377–395.

79. Cohen IM, Galgiani JN, Potter D, et al. Coccidioidomycosis in renal replacement therapy. *Arch Intern Med* 1982;142:489–494.

80. Fish DG, Ampel NM, Galgiani JN, et al. Coccidioidomycosis during human immunodeficiency virus infection. A review of 77 patients. *Medicine (Baltimore)* 1990;60:384–391.

81. Smith CE, Beard RR, Whiting EG, et al. Varieties of coccidioidal infection in relation to the epidemiology and control of the disease. *Am J Public Health* 1946;36:1394–1402.

82. Pappagianis D, Lindsay S, Beall S, et al. Ethnic background and the clinical course of coccidioidomycosis [Letter]. *Am Rev Respir Dis* 1979;120:959–961.

83. Catanzaro A. Pulmonary mycosis in pregnant women. *Chest* 1984;86:145–185.

84. Dalinka MK, Greendyke WH. The spinal manifestations of coccidioidomycosis. *J Can Assoc Radiol* 1971;22:93–99.

85. Dalinka MK, Dinnenberg S, Greendyke WH, et al. Roentgenographic features of osseous coccidioidomycosis and differential diagnosis. *J Bone Joint Surg Am* 1971;53A:1157–1164.

86. DeFelice R, Wieden MA, Galgiani JN. The incidence and implications of coccidioidouria. *Am Rev Respir Dis* 1982;125:49–52.

87. Winn WA. Coccidioidal meningitis: a follow-up report. In: Ajello L, ed. *Coccidioidomycosis.* Tucson, AZ: University of Arizona Press, 1966:55–61.

88. Bouze E, Dreyer JS, Hewitt WL, et al. Coccidioidal meningitis. An analysis of thirty-one cases and review of the literature. *Medicine (Baltimore)* 1981;60:139–172.

89. Singh VR, Smith DK, Lawrence J, et al. Coccidioidomycosis in patients infected with human immunodeficiency virus: review of 91 cases from a single institution. *Clin Infect Dis* 1996;23:563–568.

90. Standard PG, Kaufman L. Immunological procedure for the rapid and specific identification of *Coccidioides immitis* cultures. *J Clin Microbiol* 1977;5:149–153.

91. Smith CE, Saito MT, Beard RR, et al. Serologic tests in the

diagnosis and prognosis of coccidioidomycosis. *Am J Hyg* 1950;52:1–21.

92. Pappagianis D, Drasnow RI, Beall S. False-positive reactions of cerebrospinal fluid and diluted sera with the coccidioidal latex-agglutination test. *Am J Clin Pathol* 1976;66:916–921.

93. Warlick MA, Quan SF, Sobonya RE. Rapid diagnosis of pulmonary coccidioidomycosis. Cytologic vs. potassium hydroxide preparation. *Arch Intern Med* 1982;143:723–725.

94. Galgiani JN, Catanzaro A, Cloud GA, et al. Comparison of oral fluconazole and itraconazole for progressive, non-meningeal coccidioidomycosis. A randomized double-blind trial. Mycoses Study Group. *Ann Intern Med* 2000;133:676–686.

95. Galgiani JN, Ampel NM, Catanzaro A, et al. Practice guidelines for the treatment of coccidioidomycosis. *Clin Infect Dis* 2000;30:658–661.

96. Galgiani JN, Stevens DA, Graybill JR, et al. Ketoconazole therapy of progressive coccidioidomycosis. Comparison of 400- and 800-mg doses and observations at higher doses. *Am J Med* 1988;84:603–610.

97. Sarosi GA. Cryptococcal pneumonia. *Semin Respir Infect* 1997;12:50–53.

98. Powell KE, Dahl BA, Weeks RJ, et al. Airborne *Cryptococcus neoformans*: particles from pigeon excreta compatible with alveolar deposition. *J Infect Dis* 1972;125:412–415.

99. Bulmer GS, Sans MDF. *Cryptococcus neoformans* II: phagocytosis by human leukocytes. *J Bacteriol* 1967;94:1480–1483.

100. Collins UP, Gellhorn A, Trimble JR. The coincidence of cryptococcosis and disease of the reticuloendothelial and lymphatic systems. *Cancer* 1951;4:883–889.

101. Chuck SL, Sande MA. Infections with *Cryptococcus neoformans* in the acquired immunodeficiency syndrome. *N Engl J Med* 1989;321:794–799.

102. Salyer WR, Salyer DC, Baker RD. Primary complex of *Cryptococcus* and pulmonary lymph nodes. *J Infect Dis* 1974;130:74–77.

103. Campbell GD. Primary pulmonary cryptococcosis. *Am Rev Respir Dis* 1966;94:236–243.

104. Kerkering TM, Duma RD, Shadomy S. The evolution of pulmonary cryptococcosis. *Ann Intern Med* 1981;94:611–616.

105. Lewis JI, Rabinovich SH. The wide spectrum of cryptococcal infections. *Am J Med* 1972;53:315–322.

106. Baker RD. The primary pulmonary lymph node complex of cryptococcosis. *Am J Clin Pathol* 1976;65:83–92.

107. Sarosi GA, Parker JD, Doto IL, et al. Amphotericin B in cryptococcal meningitis. *Ann Intern Med* 1969;71:1079–1087.

108. Mangham D, Gerding DN, Sarosi GA. Fungal meningitis manifesting as hydrocephalus. *Arch Intern Med* 1983;143:728–731.

109. Larsen RA. Cryptococcal meningitis in persons with AIDS. In: Sarosi GA, Davies SF, eds. *Fungal diseases of the lung,* 2nd ed. New York: Raven Press, 1993:237–245.

110. Sarosi GA, Silberfarb PM, Tosh FE. Cutaneous cryptococcosis. A sentinel of disseminated disease. *Arch Dermatol* 1971;104: 1–3.

111. Hammerman KJ, Powell KE, Christianson CS, et al. Pulmonary cryptococcosis: clinical forms and treatment. *Am Rev Respir Dis* 1973;108:1116–1123.

112. Saag MS, Graybill RJ, Larsen RA, et al., for the Mycoses Study Group *Cryptococcus* Subproject. Practice guidelines for the man-

agement of cryptococcal disease. *Clin Infect Dis* 2000;30:710–718.

113. Sarosi GA, Cryptococcal lung disease in patients without HIV [Editorial]. *Chest* 1999;115:610–611.

114. Nunez M, Peacock JE Jr, Chin R Jr. Pulmonary cryptococcosis in the immunocompetent host. Therapy with oral fluconazole: a report of four cases and a review of the literature. *Chest* 2000;118:527–534. *Semin Respir Infect* 2001;16:131–140.

115. Bennett JE, Dismukes WE, Duma RJ, et al. A comparison of amphotericin B alone and combined with flucytosine in the treatment of cryptococcal meningitis. *N Engl J Med* 1979;301:126–131.

116. Powderly WG, Saag MS, Cloud GA, et al., and the NIAID AIDS Clinical Trials Group and the NIAID Mycoses Study Group. A controlled trial of fluconazole or amphotericin B to prevent relapse of cryptococcal meningitis in patients with the acquired immunodeficiency syndrome. *N Engl J Med* 1992;326:793–798.

117. Van der Horst CM, Saag MS, Cloud GA, et al., and the NIAID Mycoses Study Group and the AIDS Clinical Trials Group. Treatment of cryptococcal meningitis associated with the acquired immunodeficiency syndrome. *N Engl J Med* 1997;337:15–21.

118. Saag MS, Cloud GA, Graybille JR, et al., and the NIAID Mycoses Study Group. A comparison of itraconazole versus fluconazole as maintenance therapy for AIDS-associated cryptococcal meningitis. *Clin Infect Dis* 1999;28:291–292.

119. Soubani AO, Chandrasekar PH. The clinical spectrum of pulmonary aspergillosis. *Chest* 2002;121:1988–1999.

120. Park CK, Jheon S. Results of surgical treatment for pulmonary aspergilloma. *Eur J Cardiothorac Surg* 2002;21:918–923.

121. Greenberger PA, Patterson R. Diagnosis and management of allergic bronchopulmonary aspergillosis. *Ann Allergy* 1986;56: 444–448.

122. Vlahakis NE, Aksamit TR. Diagnosis and treatment of allergic bronchopulmonary aspergillosis. *Mayo Clin Proc* 2001;76:930–938.

123. Wark PAB, Saltos N, Simpson J, et al. Induced sputum eosinophils and neutrophils and bronchiectasis severity in allergic bronchopulmonary aspergillosis. *Eur Respir J* 2000;16:1095–1101.

124. Stevens DA, Kan VL, Judson MA, et al. Practice guidelines for diseases caused by *Aspergillus*: Infectious Diseases Society of America. *Clin Infect Dis* 2000;30:696–709.

125. Stevens DA, Schwartz HJ, Lee JY, et al. A randomized trial of itraconazole in allergic bronchopulmonary aspergillosis. *N Engl J Med* 2000;342:756–762.

126. Binder RE, Faling LJ, Pugatch RD, et al. Chronic necrotizing pulmonary aspergillosis: a discrete clinical entity. *Medicine (Baltimore)* 1982;61:109–124.

127. Saraceno JL, Phelps DT, Ferro T, et al. Chronic necrotizing aspergillosis: approach to management. *Chest* 1997;112:541–548.

128. Filice GA. Actinomycosis. In: Sarosi GA, Davies SF, eds. *Fungal diseases of the lung*. Philadelphia: Lippincott Williams & Wilkins, 2000:187–195.

129. Filice GA. Nocardiosis. In: Sarosi GA, Davies SF, eds. *Fungal diseases of the lung*. Philadelphia: Lippincott Williams & Wilkins, 2000:197–212.

Pulmonary Infections Caused by Mycobacterial Species

20

Jeffrey Glassroth · Christopher J. Crnich

DISEASE CAUSED BY *MYCOBACTERIUM TUBERCULOSIS*

Epidemiology

Tuberculosis (TB), which is caused by a complex of organisms, *Mycobacterium tuberculosis, Mycobacterium bovis,* and *Mycobacterium africanum,* is an ancient human disease. Evidence of TB can be found in human remains dating back to Neolithic times. The most recent World Health Organization data estimate that 1.86 billion persons are currently infected with TB. At any time, an estimated 16 million persons worldwide demonstrate active disease, and 8 million new active cases develop each year, of which 3.5 million manifest as the infectious pulmonary form of the disease. This remarkable prevalence of disease is estimated to be responsible for at least 2 million deaths each year, making TB the most frequent infectious cause of death in the world and the seventh most frequent cause of morbidity among all diseases.

The World Health Organization declared TB a world global emergency in 1993; however, economic and political commitment to TB control programs is lacking in many countries, and it is estimated that 95% of new cases of TB occur in countries with limited resources (1). This situation facilitates inappropriate or unsustained TB therapy, which in turn has promoted a rise in the rates of multidrug-resistant TB (MDR-TB) (2). Furthermore, immigration patterns have contributed to increased rates of TB in countries where effective control measures do exist (3–5). Finally, the creation of an enormous pool of immunosuppressed pa-

tients as a consequence of the global HIV/AIDS epidemic has expanded the number of persons with the infectious pulmonary form of the disease, and it is now estimated that nearly 10 million persons worldwide are coinfected (6,7).

Although rates of TB infection in the United States declined an average of 5.3% per year after 1992 to a total 16,377 cases in 2000 (5.8 cases per 100,000) (8), an examination of recent events in the United States is instructive. Reported cases of TB declined from a total of 84,304 cases in 1953 to 22,255 cases in 1984, but in 1985, this trend reversed (3). From 1985 to 1992, the number of reported cases of TB rose 20% (26,673 cases in 1992), and the rate of TB infections per 100,000 persons per year reached 10.5 in 1992 (Fig. 20.1) (9).

During this period, rates of TB varied markedly between segments of the U.S. population. Cases of TB among African Americans increased from 23 to 31.7 per 100,000 persons per year (+37.8%), whereas rates among non-Hispanic whites decreased from 4.5 to 4 cases per 100,000 persons per year (−11.1%). Reported rates of TB in urban and nonurban areas were 22 and 6.5 per 100,000 persons per year, respectively (9), and although average TB rates in the United States were only 4.2 cases per 100,000 persons per year among the highest income groups for the period from 1985 to 1991, rates among the lowest income groups were 33 per 100,000 persons per year (10).

The explosion of TB among homeless persons well demonstrates the interaction between socioeconomic status and TB rates. The average rate of TB among San Francisco's homeless population was 270 cases per 100,000 persons per year between 1991 and 1996, and Moss and colleagues (11) demonstrated clustered patterns of mycobacterial DNA restriction fragment length polymorphism in 60% of active cases, suggesting recent transmission of disease. Similar data

J. Glassroth: Section of Pulmonary Medicine, Department of Medicine, University of Wisconsin Medical School, Madison, Wisconsin.

C. J. Crnich: Section of Infectious Diseases, University of Wisconsin Hospital and Clinics, Madison, Wisconsin.

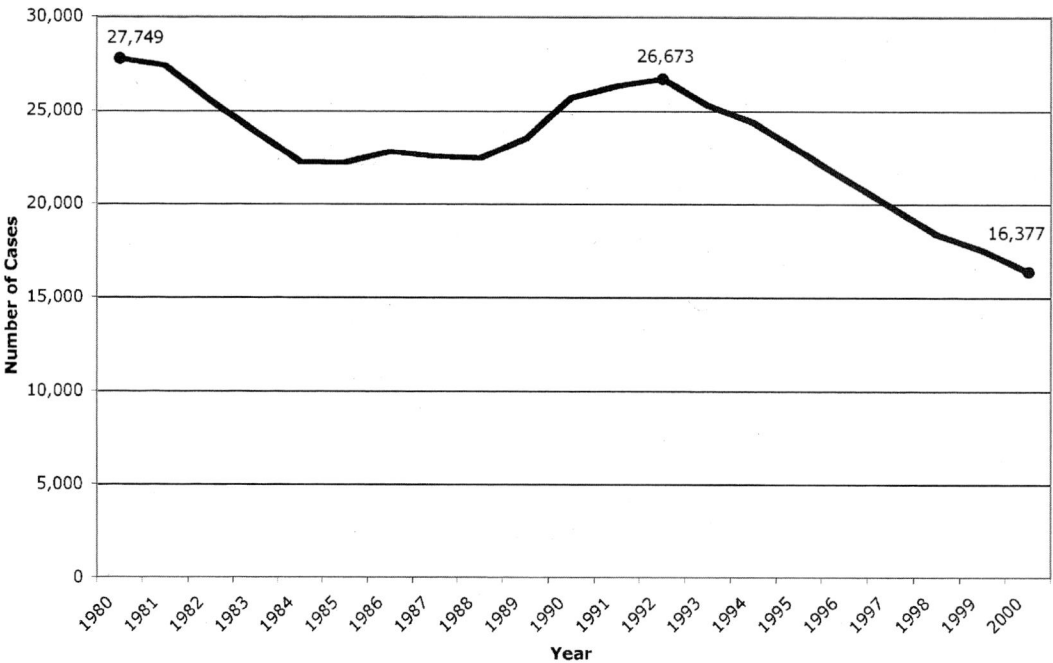

FIGURE 20.1. Reported cases of tuberculosis in the United States from 1980 to 2000. (From Centers for Disease Control and Prevention. *Reported tuberculosis in the United States, 2000.* Available at http://www.cdc.gov/nchstp/tb/surv/surv2000, 2001.)

documenting the failure of treatment programs are available from New York City, where 68% of the TB patients referred to a hospital in Harlem were homeless; 89% of this cohort were lost to follow-up after being discharged on therapy for active TB (12).

Although the rate of TB among native-born persons has dropped markedly since 1990, the rate of TB among foreign-born persons has remained relatively stable, and foreign-born cases now account for about 46% of all cases of TB reported in the United States (8). Most cases of TB in foreign-born persons are reported within 5 years after their arrival in this country (5,13), and studies suggest that reactivation of infection acquired in the native country, rather than recent acquisition, accounts for most of these cases (14,15).

Perhaps no factor has been more important than the HIV epidemic in contributing to the resurgence of TB worldwide and in the United States. The estimated rate of HIV and TB–coinfected injecting drug users (i.e., seropositive and tuberculin-positive) is about 8% (16). A more representative cohort study of 1,130 HIV-positive patients found that the rate of active TB in the years from 1988 to 1990 was 700 cases per 100,000 persons per year (17). Although determining the exact prevalence of HIV infection in patients with TB in the United States is difficult, data from the Centers for Disease Control and Prevention (CDC) based on partial reporting suggest that 10% of persons with TB are coinfected with HIV and that the rate of coinfection is highest (19%) among persons ages 25 to 44 years (8).

The average risk for the development of active TB after exposure is 5% to 10% during the lifetime of an immunocompetent person; however, the risk in HIV-positive persons ranges from 5% to 10% *per year*, and this risk is influenced strongly by the status of the immune system (i.e., $CD4^+$ lymphocyte count) (7). Large cohort studies in the United States and Italy found that the rate of TB was 300 to 500 cases per 100,000 persons per year in patients whose $CD4^+$ cell count was $200/mm^3$ but was 1,200 to 1,300 per 100,000 persons per year when the $CD4^+$ cell count was less than $200/mm^3$ (17,18). In contrast to the commonly held belief that 90% of cases of active TB represent reactivation of latent TB, nearly one half of cases of TB in several HIV-positive patient cohorts demonstrated clustered restriction fragment length polymorphism, suggesting recent acquisition of their infection, including acquisition of second TB infections in persons known to have been previously infected (7,14,15).

The most worrisome aspect of the recent resurgence of TB has been the rising rates of resistance to isoniazid (INH) and rifampin in some areas. MDR-TB reduces the likelihood of treatment success (19), increases costs (20), and more importantly is associated with a mortality of 30% to 40% (19,21). In the United States, rates of INH resistance in 1991 were 9%, rates of MDR-TB were 3.5%, and 14% of all isolates were resistant to at least one anti-TB medication (22). The number of cases of MDR-TB peaked in 1992, and the most recent surveillance data from the CDC show that rates of INH resistance have decreased to 7.7% and that rates of MDR-TB have been reduced to 1.2% of all isolates (8).

Pathogenesis

As few as five *M. tuberculosis* (MTB) bacilli are necessary for human infection (23), but only TB-containing particles small enough to reach the vulnerable environment of the alveolar space (typically <5–10 μm) are considered infectious. After inhalation, these infectious particles deposit preferentially in the dependent lower half of the lung, where they subsequently initiate a primary focus of infection.

Initially, the primary pulmonary infection is a localized process. Unprimed alveolar macrophages rapidly phagocytose inhaled bacilli but are unable to destroy the intracellular organisms, which begin to multiply at an exponential rate. Infected macrophages secrete interleukin-12 (IL-12), which promotes a nonspecific immune response mediated primarily by natural killer cells (24) and γ/δ T cells (25). The nonspecific immune response may retard the local infection but is usually unable to control it (26), and bacilli spread to local lymph nodes, where they may enter the blood (bacillemia). From this point, TB infection is a systemic process characterized by lymphatic and hematogenous spread and the deposition of bacilli in multiple extrapulmonary sites (i.e., bones, meninges, kidney, and the posterior apical segment of the lungs), creating the potential for disease in virtually any anatomic location.

Eventually, MTB antigens in association with the class II major histocompatibility complex are presented to naive CD4$^+$ T cells, heralding the onset of specific anti-TB cell-mediated immunity (T helper subset 1 [Th1] cell immunity). Anti-TB CD4$^+$ T cells coordinate the specific immune response by two routes: (a) secretion of IL-2 supports cytotoxic T-lymphocyte function, allowing these cells to kill other cells already infected with MTB directly (23), and (b) secretion of interferon-γ (IFN-γ) primes uninfected macrophages, allowing them to kill the intracellular pathogen efficiently (27). The onset of the cytotoxic T-lymphocyte response several weeks after infection coincides with the development of caseous necrosis at the site of primary infection and the development of delayed-type hypersensitivity (28). The cytotoxic T-lymphocyte response is bacteriostatic only against MTB bacilli and does not confer immunity to infection. Priming of the macrophage, which occurs somewhat later (4–6 weeks in animal models), is crucial for ultimate control and eradication of the primary infection (29).

The immune response detailed above is able to control the primary infection in most situations; however, in approximately 5% of cases, primary infection is progressive, and in another 5% to 10%, the immune system initially controls the primary infection only to fail at a later time, with resultant endogenous reactivation (30). Progressive pulmonary TB is characterized by liquefaction of the solid caseous core, extracellular proliferation of very high numbers of organisms (10^7–10^9 bacilli), extensive localized tissue necrosis caused by the cytotoxic T-lymphocyte reaction to the high levels of mycobacterial antigens, tubercle wall rupture with subsequent cavity formation, and bronchopneumonia resulting from aspiration of the caseous discharge (23).

The mechanism by which endogenous reactivation takes place remains largely unknown, but most experts feel that it results from a gradual or acute decline in local cell-mediated immunity (31). Such reactivation tends to occur at sites of high oxygen tension that were hematogenously seeded during the primary infection. Thus, endogenous reactivation most commonly develops in the posterior apical segments of the upper lobes of the lung, renal cortex, and endplates of the vertebral bodies. In an immunocompetent individual, local reactivation results in a cell-mediated response that tends to limit systemic involvement, but in persons with altered immunity, such as those with HIV infection, such a response may be inadequate or even absent. In these individuals, endogenous reactivation may be associated with extensive systemic and even miliary disease.

Persons with conditions associated with abnormalities in cell-mediated immunity, such as HIV infection, are clearly at risk for progression of primary infection and endogenous reactivation (Table 20.1). In HIV-positive persons, peripheral blood lymphocytes secrete abnormally low amounts of IFN-γ in response to mycobacterial antigens (32), and the risk for extrapulmonary and miliary TB increases as the level of immunosuppression increases (33).

Progressive primary infection and endogenous reactivation also occur in persons with no apparent immune system abnormality. Differences in the virulence of the infecting organism may explain, in part, why these individuals are unable to control their infection. Animal studies have demonstrated that strains of MTB with a high bacillemic potential are associated with larger primary lung lesions than strains with a low bacillemic potential (29), and rapidly growing TB isolates from humans have been associated with much more extensive communicability than slowly growing TB isolates (34,35).

More important than the virulence of the infecting strain, however, may be genetic differences in the host's immune system. IL-12 is important for the development of cell-mediated immunity (36), and defects in the IL-12 receptor have been associated with disseminated mycobacterial infection following bacille Calmette-Guérin (BCG) vaccination (37,38). Tumor necrosis factor-α (TNF-α) is responsible for granuloma formation and also for the production of reactive nitrogen intermediates needed to kill intracellular bacilli (27), and high rates of active TB have been described following the administration of anti–TNF-α antibodies (39). IFN-α is necessary for the production of TNF-α by macrophages, and genetic absence of the IFN-γ receptor has been associated with disseminated nontuberculous mycobacterial infections in humans (40). Some have hypothesized that subtle alterations in the IFN-γ receptor may be responsible for

TABLE 20.1. CRITERIA FOR TUBERCULIN POSITIVITY BY RISK GROUP

Reaction ≥ 5 mm of Induration	Reaction ≥ 10 mm of Induration	Reaction ≥ 15 mm of Induration
HIV-positive persons	Recent immigrants (i.e., within the last 5 years) from high-prevalence areas	Persons with no risk factors for TB
Recent contacts of TB case patients		
Patients with fibrotic changes on chest radiograph consistent with prior TB	Injection drug users	
	Residents and employees of high-risk congregate settings:	
Patients with organ transplants	Prisons and jails	
Patients receiving ≥ 15 mg of prednisone daily for ≥ 1 month	Nursing homes and other long-term care facilities	
	Hospitals and other health care facilities	
	Residential facilities for patients with AIDS	
	Shelters for the homeless	
	Mycobacteriology laboratory personnel	
	Persons with high-risk clinical conditions:	
	Silicosis	
	Diabetes mellitus	
	Chronic renal failure	
	Hematologic disorders (leukemia and lymphoma)	
	Carcinoma of the head and neck or lung	
	Weight loss ≥ 10% of ideal body weight	
	Gastrectomy	
	Jejunoileal bypass	

Source: Adapted from American Thoracic Society. Diagnostic standards and classification of tuberculosis in adults and children. *Am J Respir Crit Care Med* 2000;161: 1376–1395, with permission.

variations in susceptibility to the development of TB (41). Finally, variability in the HLA-D gene locus, possibly related to a reduced affinity of the class II major histocompatibility complex for mycobacterial antigens (42), in addition to genetic polymorphisms in the natural resistance–associated macrophage protein-1 (NRAMP-1) (43), have been associated with an increased likelihood for the development of clinically apparent disease.

Clinical Presentation

Pulmonary Tuberculosis

Primary TB infection is usually silent and unrecognized by most patients. In those in whom clinically active disease develops, either from progression of primary infection or endogenous reactivation, the disease can manifest in a myriad of ways, depending on the site of involvement and a variety of host factors (Table 20.1).

Generalized symptoms, including fever, night sweats, malaise, weakness, anorexia, and weight loss, accompany TB infection regardless of the site of infection and initially may be the only evidence of active disease. Fever is seen in 40% to 80% of patients with pulmonary TB but is less common in elderly patients (44). Anorexia and weight loss are equally common in all age groups but are often overlooked or attributed to another cause in geriatric patients (45).

Active pulmonary TB may begin with isolated constitutional symptoms; however, cough eventually develops in most patients. Initially mild and nonproductive, cough from active pulmonary TB can become continuous and productive without treatment. In this later stage, cough may be associated with hemoptysis that is usually mild but, rarely, can be massive as a result of ectatic blood vessel rupture in the wall of a TB cavity (Rasmussen aneurysm). Dyspnea is uncommon without extensive parenchymal involvement or preexisting lung disease (44). Pleuritis is also uncommon but suggests extension of the inflammatory process to the pleura and may be associated with pleural effusion and, rarely, empyema.

Other than localized auscultatory changes over the involved areas of the lung, the physical examination findings and routine laboratory test results are nondiagnostic with rare exception. Immunologic phenomena, such as clubbing, erythema nodosum, and erythema induratum, may occur infrequently as a result of active pulmonary infection. Extrapulmonary disease occurs simultaneously with pulmonary disease in nearly 10% of patients (more commonly in HIV-positive patients). In this latter situation, lymphadenopathy or cutaneous manifestations of disseminated disease, such as scrofuloderma or lupus vulgaris, may be present. A normocytic, normochromic anemia in addition to a mild leukocytosis is common, and monocytosis may rarely be present. Hyponatremia related to the syndrome of inappropriate secretion of antidiuretic hormone (SIADH), an elevated sedimentation rate, and hypoalbuminemia are other nonspecific laboratory findings that may be seen.

Tuberculous Pleurisy

In the most recent data from the CDC, 80% of the reported cases of active TB in the United States were of the pulmonary form, whereas 20% of the cases involved extrapulmonary sites (8) (Fig. 20.2). As many as 62% of TB cases in HIV-positive patients may be extrapulmonary (46), and

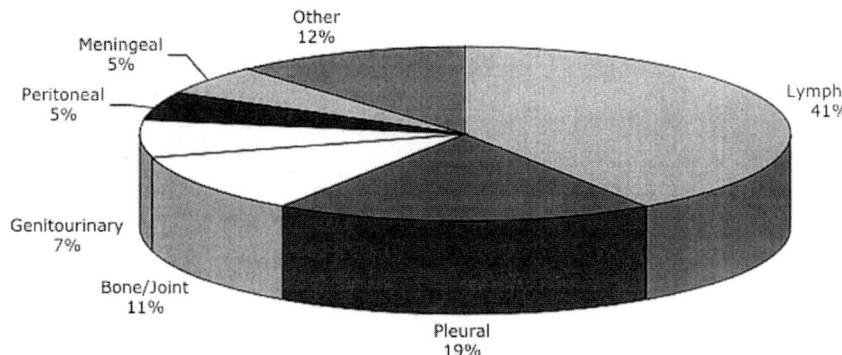

FIGURE 20.2. Reported cases of extrapulmonary tuberculosis by anatomic site, 2000. (Adapted from Centers for Disease Control and Prevention. *Reported tuberculosis in the United States, 2000.* Available at *http://www.cdc.gov/nchstp/tb/surv/surv2000*, 2001.)

studies have shown that the risk for extrapulmonary disease correlates directly with the degree of immunocompromise (47).

The pleura is the second most commonly involved extrapulmonary site (Fig. 20.2), and tuberculous pleurisy can develop with the primary infection or later as an isolated manifestation of endogenous reactivation (48). Patients most commonly present with fever and other constitutional symptoms and are subsequently found to have a pleural effusion, but cough, pleuritic chest pain, and dyspnea may also be presenting symptoms.

The tuberculin skin test (TST) result may be negative in up to a third of HIV-seronegative patients (48) and is negative in 60% of HIV-seropositive patients (49). The pleural fluid is uniformly exudative; the fluid protein concentration is usually more than 4 g/dL and often more than 5 g/dL, and the fluid lactate dehydrogenase concentration is usually more than 500 IU/mL (48,50). Chronic tuberculous pleurisy may rarely present as a pseudochylothorax in which the pleural fluid takes on a milky appearance as a result of the accumulation of cholesterol (51). The cellular composition of the fluid is characterized by a lymphocytic predominance and an "absence" of mesothelial cells (i.e., <5%), although a high neutrophil count may be present early in the disease (48,50). Cultures of the pleural fluid are positive in 30% to 40% of cases (48,50); however, when culture is combined with histologic examination of a pleural biopsy specimen, the diagnostic yield may approach 90% (52).

Miliary Tuberculosis

Miliary TB (Fig. 20.3) is a unique form of extrapulmonary TB that is a result of massive hematogenous dissemination, most often in the setting of primary pulmonary infection but also associated with endogenous reactivation of an extrapulmonary focus. The clinical presentation can vary from isolated fever and malaise (53,54) to fulminant disease characterized by adult respiratory distress syndrome and multiple organ system failure (55). Involvement of multiple organs is common and may influence the presentation. The examination may reveal generalized lymphadenopathy, including hepatosplenomegaly (53,54). Cutaneous manifestations of TB, such as diffuse skin involvement (tuberculosis cutis miliaris disseminata), may also be present (56). Hematologic abnormalities, such as anemia and leukopenia, are common, and patients may have pancytopenia (57). Other laboratory abnormalities, such as hyponatremia and elevated serum liver chemistries, especially alkaline phosphatase, are seen in many patients.

The TST result remains negative in 50% to 75% of cases of miliary TB (53,54). Smears of sputum and bronchoalveolar lavage fluid samples are acid-fast bacillus (AFB)–positive in a third of patients, and culture is positive in up to 75% of cases (53). Smear and culture of gastric aspirates and culture of urine (even in the setting of normal sediment) may be positive, and histologic examination of liver and bone marrow biopsy specimens may demonstrate granulomas in a significant proportion of patients (53). Despite the disseminated

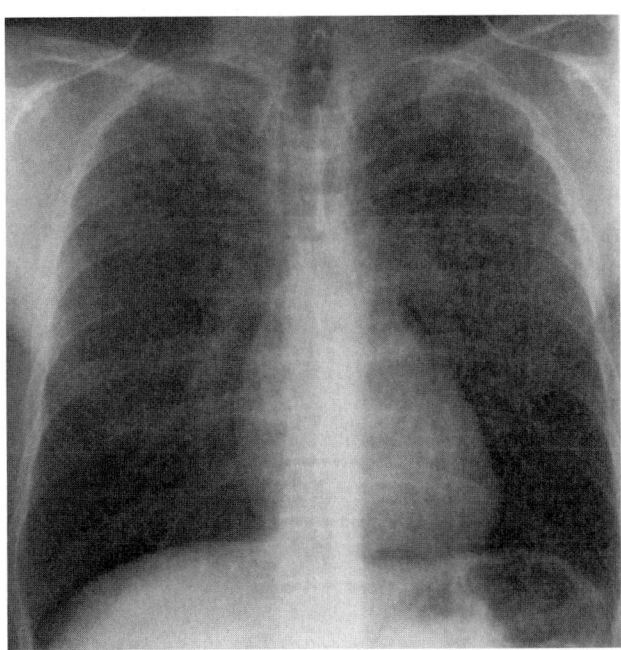

FIGURE 20.3. Chest radiograph (posteroanterior view only) demonstrating the radiographic presentation of miliary tuberculosis.

nature of miliary TB, blood cultures are rarely positive in patients without HIV infection but may be positive in 30% to 40% of patients with HIV coinfection when lysis centrifugation techniques are used (58).

Other Forms of Extrapulmonary Tuberculosis

Tuberculous lymphadenitis, or scrofula, is the most common form of extrapulmonary TB (Fig. 20.2) and typically presents as a cool, enlarging, but painless mass in the head or neck. The anterior cervical nodes are most often involved, and diffuse adenopathy is unusual except in the setting of miliary TB. Intrathoracic lymphadenitis can occur but in the absence of HIV coinfection is more commonly a manifestation of primary infection than of reactivation. Systemic constitutional symptoms are uncommon, seen in about 20% of patients. Fine needle aspiration of the involved node demonstrates granulomatous changes, AFB positivity, and culture positivity in approximately 80%, 40%, and 70%, of patients, respectively (59,60).

Skeletal TB is a disease of older persons and most commonly involves the lumbar or thoracic spine. Patients typically present with pain, and 50% to 80% with neurologic deficits (61); only 40% have constitutional symptoms. The findings on plain films may be normal, but the films typically show anterior vertebral body involvement early in the disease. With progression, the vertebral body takes on a moth-eaten appearance, and kyphosis may develop. Magnetic resonance imaging is a more sensitive imaging test. The epidural space is involved in the majority of patients (61), and extension into adjacent soft tissues causes large abscesses in the psoas muscle or in the retropharyngeal space if cervical disease is present.

Tuberculous arthritis presents as an isolated swollen and painful joint with little in the way of warmth, erythema, or constitutional symptoms. The weight-bearing joints of the hips and knees are most commonly involved. Plain radiographs demonstrate juxtaarticular osteoporosis with peripheral osseous erosions; however, the joint space is relatively preserved early in the disease and becomes narrowed only if the patient goes untreated for a prolonged period of time. Aspiration of the synovial fluid demonstrates an intermediately elevated cell count ($10,000–20,000/mm^3$), but low or high cell counts are occasionally seen ($<100/mm^3$ or $>50,000/mm^3$) (62).

Many patients with genitourinary TB are asymptomatic (63); however, up to half of them have vague urinary symptoms that include frequency, dysuria, back pain, and hematuria. Systemic symptoms of infection are uncommon (63), and radiographs may demonstrate calcification of the kidneys or prostate (64). In more than half of patients, examination of the urine demonstrates a "classic" sterile (for common bacteria) pyuria that is often associated with an acidic pH, proteinuria, and hematuria. Culture of a single urine sample is positive in only 30% to 40% of cases (65); thus, serial culture of three to six first-voided urine samples may be needed to confirm the diagnosis.

Tuberculous peritonitis is a relatively uncommon form of extrapulmonary TB that affects younger rather than older patients and women more than men. It most commonly presents with painful ascites but can present as a fibroadhesive form with minimal peritoneal fluid. Fever and weight loss are more common than in other forms of extrapulmonary TB, and the TST result is positive in up to 70% of patients (66). The protein level in the peritoneal fluid is usually above 2.5 g/dL, and the serum–ascites albumin gradient is usually less than 1.1 unless concomitant portal hypertension is present. Unfortunately, AFB stains of the fluid are rarely positive, and cultures of the fluid with conventional techniques are positive in only 20% to 45% of cases (67) unless a large amount of fluid (>1 L) is cultured (68). The current diagnostic gold standard is laparoscopy/laparotomy with peritoneal biopsy, which confirms the diagnosis in more than 90% of cases (67,69).

Seeding of the meninges and parenchyma of the brain and spinal cord can occur early in primary pulmonary infection. Progressive infection or subsequent reactivation at these sites results in meningitis, tuberculoma formation, or spinal arachnoiditis (70). The clinical presentation depends on the location of disease and may be gradual or acute (71,72). For example, patients with tuberculoma present with headache, seizure, or paralysis as a result of the expanding space-occupying lesion, whereas patients with basilar meningitis present early with apathy, lethargy, personality changes, and fever, which subsequently progress to headache with or without meningismus, cranial nerve palsies, focal neurologic deficits, confusion, and eventually coma. Imaging of the head usually reveals abnormalities such as basal meningeal enhancement, vasculitis with parenchymal infarcts or hydrocephalus in the setting of tuberculous meningitis or tuberculoma, and single or multiple parenchymal ring-enhancing lesions. The cerebrospinal fluid (CSF) may be normal in the case of an isolated tuberculoma; however, in meningitis, a lymphocytic pleocytosis with an elevated protein level and a low glucose level is usually present. The CSF protein concentration typically ranges from 100 to 500 mg/dL but may become markedly elevated in cases of subarachnoid blockage. The CSF glucose level is less than 45 mg/dL in 80% of cases but rarely less than 30 mg/dL (72). Direct examination of the CSF demonstrates AFB-positive organisms in only 12% to 37% of cases (72); however, the percentage of AFB-positive results increases to 45% to 87% if serial examinations (generally four or more) are performed with an adequate amount of CSF (>10 mL). Culture of the CSF is positive in 45% to 86% of cases, and newer diagnostic studies may improve this yield further (72).

Diagnosis

Latent Tuberculosis Infection

Tuberculin Skin Testing

The TST is the standard method for identifying patients with latent TB infection. Currently available test preparations of tuberculin use purified protein derivative (PPD) standardized for potency. Local induration develops within 48 to 72 hours at the site of intradermal PPD injection (Mantoux method) in patients with sensitivity to the antigen. The largest reactions to PPD-tuberculin are expected in persons infected with MTB (73). However, cross-reaction with some nontuberculous mycobacteria takes place, and some persons infected with MTB may be anergic and unable to respond as expected. By lowering or raising the size required to define a "positive" reaction, the sensitivity and specificity of the TST can be modified (Table 20.1).

The TST result typically becomes positive 4 to 7 weeks after primary infection, and testing within this period may result in a false-negative TST result. The TST has an estimated specificity of 99% that is reduced to 95% in populations in which infection with cross-reacting mycobacteria is common—for example, those in the southeastern United States (74). More than 90% of patients undergoing a TST within 8 weeks after receiving the BCG vaccine will have more than 10 mm of skin induration, but the durability of this reaction is poor, and studies of reaction persistence suggest that only 20% of individuals retain their response to the TST more than 10 years after vaccination (75). For these reasons, it is currently recommended that BCG vaccine status not be considered when the results of a TST are interpreted (76).

Both false-negative and false-positive TST results may occur for a variety of reasons (Table 20.2). The delayed-type hypersensitivity response to latent TB infection may wane with time, and it is common for elderly patients with prior reactivity to have a negative TST result. The absence of a delayed-type hypersensitivity response with an initial TST does not necessarily represent the absence of latent TB

infection; subsequent rechallenge with intradermal PPD can sometimes result in a positive TST reaction in certain patients. This so-called booster effect is most common in persons with latent TB infection who are older than 55 years and is the result of an amnestic response to the initial PPD antigen that allows for a full delayed-type hypersensitivity response with a subsequent challenge (77). The booster effect occurs most predictably when rechallenge occurs within 1 to 3 weeks after the initial TST but may last for as long as 1 year. Routinely performing an initial two-step TST in older persons subjected to serial testing (e.g., nursing home residents, hospital employees)—retesting nonreactive patients 2 to 3 weeks after an initial test and recording the reaction to the second TST as the true response—avoids the confusion that may arise with annual skin testing.

Several groups of patients may have a false-negative TST reaction as a result of impaired cell-mediated immunity. For example, data from several HIV cohort studies have shown that HIV-positive persons are half as likely to have a positive TST reaction as age-matched HIV-negative controls, and this disparity increases with the degree of immunosuppression (78). Moreover, active TB infection may be associated with a negative TST reaction in 10% to 25% of individuals (79). This rate may be higher in specific forms of TB, such as pleural and miliary TB; TST reactions were negative in up to 40% of patients with pleural TB and in 60% to 80% of patients with miliary TB (53).

Several groups have clinical disease or an exposure history that puts them at higher risk for active TB (16,17,80,81). Targeted skin testing of these high-risk patients increases the predictive value of the TST and is the basis for the updated American Thoracic Society (ATS) recommendations for testing (76), in which the size of the skin induration that constitutes a positive test result depends on the risk of the individual patient for the development of TB (Table 20.1). Patients who are not at excess risk for active disease or exposure to TB should not be tested because the low prevalence of latent TB infection in this population, estimated to be between 0.01% and 0.1% (74), leads to many more false-positive than true-positive results (Table 20.3).

TABLE 20.2. FACTORS ASSOCIATED WITH A FALSE-NEGATIVE TUBERCULIN SKIN TEST

Host factors
Infections
   Viral (e.g., measles, mumps, HIV)
   Bacterial (e.g., typhoid fever, miliary TB, TB meningitis)
   Fungal (e.g., blastomycosis)
Live viral vaccines
Chronic renal failure
Malnutrition and low protein states
Neoplastic disease (e.g., Hodgkin disease, lymphoma)
Corticosteroids and other immunosuppressants
Booster phenomenon
Severe stress (e.g., trauma, burn victims)
Recent exposure (within 4–7 weeks)

Improper administration
Injection of inadequate volume
Subcutaneous injection
Inexperienced reader

Problems with tuberculin
Improper storage (i.e., exposure to heat and light)
Improper dilution
Contamination

DIAGNOSIS OF LATENT TUBERCULOSIS INFECTION

Summary Statement	Level of Evidence
A positive tuberculin skin test result in high-risk patients is predictive of a high likelihood of developing active disease, and screening of these patients is recommended.	Multiple well-designed clinical trials and cohort studies
Targeted tuberculin skin testing in low-risk patients will yield an excessive number of false-positive results, and screening of these patients is discouraged.	Consensus of expert opinion

TABLE 20.3. POSITIVE PREDICTIVE VALUE OF A TUBERCULIN TEST

Prevalence of TB infection (%)	Positive Predictive Value (%)	
	Specificity of 95%	Specificity of 99%
90	99	99.9
50	95	99
25	86	97
10	67	91
5	50	83
1	16	49
0.1	3	10
0.01	0.2	9

Source: From American Thoracic Society, Diagnostic standards and classification of tuberculosis in adults and children. *Am J Respir Crit Care Med* 2000;161:1376–1395, with permission.

Serum Interferon-γ Levels

Because of the limitations of the TST, efforts to develop tests with better sensitivity and specificity have been pursued. IFN-γ, as noted (see section "Pathogenesis"), plays an integral role in priming alveolar macrophages in the immune response to TB, and an *in vitro* assay has been developed that detects cell-mediated reactivity to MTB and *Mycobacterium avium* by measuring the production of IFN-γ in peripheral blood lymphocytes (obtained by venipuncture) after exposure to TB and avian PPD antigens. Mazurek and colleagues (82) compared the IFN-γ assay with the standard TST in 1,226 patients stratified according to likely latent TB infection, suspected active TB, and treated TB. The overall correlation between the IFN-γ assay and the TST was good (83.1%). The IFN-γ assay result was less likely to be positive in patients with a history of BCG vaccination. Moreover, by assessing the differential IFN-γ responses to TB and avian antigens, the authors found that as many as a fifth of TST responses in patients may be caused by cross-reactivity with nontuberculous mycobacteria. The exact role of IFN-γ testing remains to be defined.

Active Pulmonary Disease

Radiography

Radiographically, primary pulmonary TB classically presents as a segmental or lobar consolidation in any lobe of the lung, although the lower lobes are involved in more than half of cases (83). Involvement of a single lobe is the most common presentation, but multilobular disease is seen in up to a fourth of patients. Ipsilateral hilar and mediastinal adenopathy is more common in children than adults and may be associated with atelectasis of the upper or middle lobes when an adjacent bronchus is compressed (84). Pleural effusion is seen in only 6% to 7% of cases, but pleural effusion in combination with mediastinal adenopathy may be the only evidence of primary infection (85).

In contrast to primary infection, endogenously reactivated pulmonary TB typically results in a chronic consolidation in the apical and posterior segments of the upper lobe or the superior segment of the lower lobe. A cavitary lesion is observed in 40% of adult cases; it may be thick- or thin-walled and typically is without an associated air-fluid level (84) (Fig. 20.4). Endobronchial spread to adjacent segments of the lung can occur, and although an ipsilateral pleural effusion may be seen rarely in reactivation disease, the presence of adenopathy is decidedly rare. Of patients with a fibronodular pattern on chest radiographs, typically interpreted as evidence of "old" TB, 5% to 15% have AFB-positive sputum, and up 5% of patients with a "normal" chest radiograph have microbiologically proven TB; thus, the chest radiograph must never be the sole factor in determining the presence of active or inactive disease.

More recently, investigators using restriction fragment length polymorphism analysis of sputum isolates have suggested that the radiographic difference between primary and reactivated disease may be less than traditionally thought (86).

Miliary TB is most often associated with primary infection (1%–7% of all cases), and nearly two thirds of patients with miliary TB present with the classic "miliary" radiograph, characterized by diffuse, symmetric micronodular infiltrates 1 to 3 mm in size (83,85) (Fig. 20.3). In the absence of a classic miliary pattern, radiographic signs of active or healed pulmonary disease, adenopathy, or pleural effusions are often present, but the chest radiographic findings may be normal in up to 5% of patients.

A number of patterns have been described on chest computed tomography (CT) (87). Of these, the so-called tree in bud is most often associated with early disease and varying degrees of focal bronchiectasis with healed/quiescent foci of remote disease (Fig. 20.5).

The chest radiographic findings are often atypical in HIV-coinfected patients and are correlated with the patient's CD4$^+$ cell count; radiographs in patients with CD4$^+$ cell counts above 200/mm^3 commonly demonstrate patterns consistent with reactive TB, whereas radiographs in patients with CD4$^+$ cell counts below 200/mm^3 more commonly demonstrate patterns consistent with primary TB (88). Other findings that are more common in coinfected patients with advanced AIDS are a miliary pattern, which may seen in 6% to 19% of cases; a normal chest radiograph may be seen in up to 14% of patients with active pulmonary TB (89).

Identification of the Organism

Specimen collection, the number of required samples, and the manner in which they are collected vary according to site of infection, and detailed guidelines for this process have been published (74). For patients with suspected pulmonary TB, at least three freshly expectorated first morning sputum samples should be collected from a deep, productive cough in a sterile container with a wide mouth. Ideally, the volume of each sample should be more than 5 mL (90). Induction of

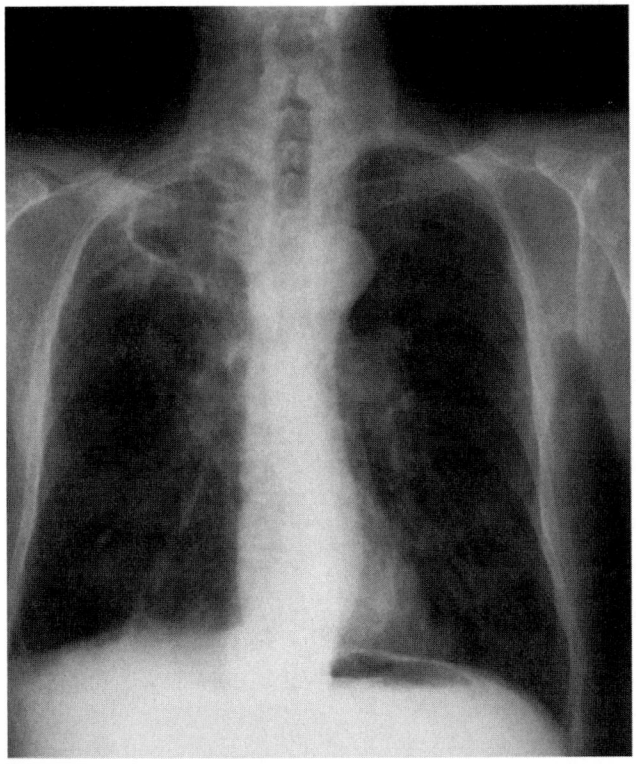
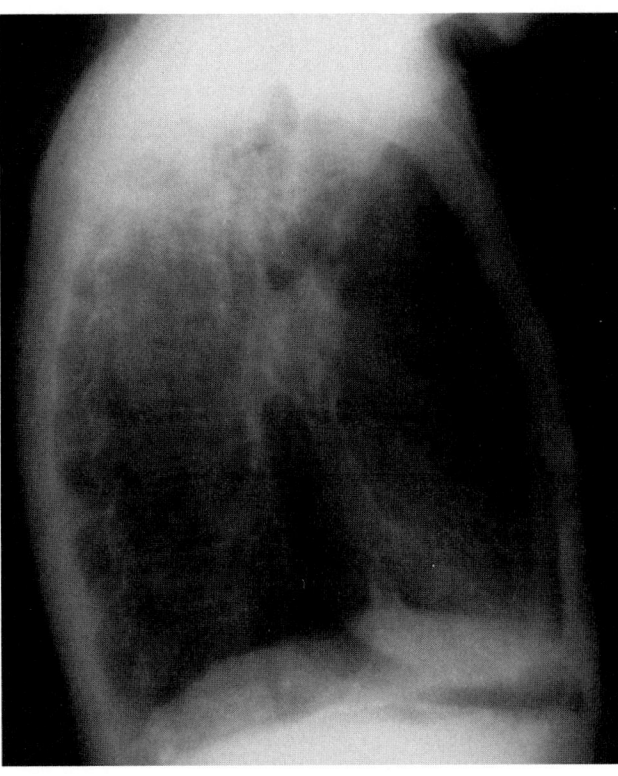

A

B

FIGURE 20.4. Chest radiographs (posteroanterior and lateral views) demonstrating cavitary reactivation of latent tuberculosis infection in the posterior apical segment of the right upper lobe.

sputum with aerosolized hypertonic saline solution may be required if the patient is having difficulty producing sputum; serial morning gastric lavage and bronchoalveolar lavage are alternative methods of obtaining clinical specimens.

Staining for Acid-Fast Bacilli. Examination of stained smears for AFB remains the most rapid and inexpensive method for detecting mycobacteria. Both carbolfuchsin

(Ziehl-Neelson or Kinyoun method) and fluorochrome (auramine–rhodamine) stains are available, but fluorochrome staining is more sensitive and has become the standard staining method used in the United States (91). Staining techniques require the presence of at least 5,000 to 10,000 organisms for a positive result (74). The reported sensitivity of the AFB smear for respiratory samples ranges from 45% to 75%, and specificity is reported to be greater

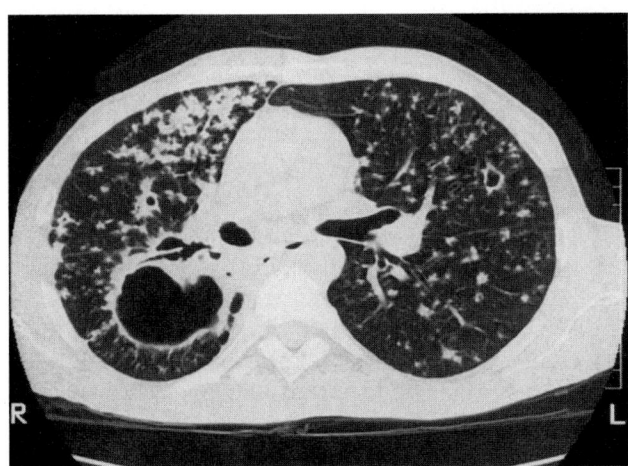
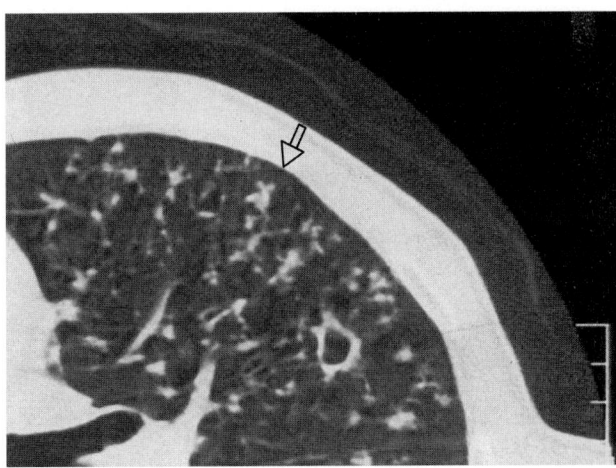

A

B

FIGURE 20.5. A. Computed tomographic scan of a patient with extensive bilateral cavitary tuberculosis. **B:** Enhancement of the left anterior quadrant of the figure demonstrating the "tree in bud" pattern (*arrow*).

TABLE 20.4. REPORTED SENSITIVITIES OF VARIOUS DIAGNOSTIC TESTS FOR PULMONARY AND EXTRAPULMONARY FORMS OF TUBERCULOSIS

Site of Infection	AFB Staining[a] (%)	Culture[a] (%)	Nucleic Acid Amplification[b] (%)
Sputum	45–75	87–95 (broth)	95–96 (AFB$^+$)
		52–80 (agar)	48–53 (AFB$^-$)
		42–77 (egg)	
Lymph node aspirate	25–50	70	80–93
Pleural fluid	9–20	30–40	20–100
Pleural biopsy	17–40	65–75	64
Joint fluid aspirate	20	80	—
Skeletal biopsy specimen	—	83–88	—
Urine	—	80–95	92
Peritoneal fluid	<5	20–45	—
Cerebrospinal fluid	12–37	45–86	33–100

[a] May represent the overall yield of multiple clinical samples.
[b] Based on the use of either the Amplified *Mycobacterium tuberculosis* Direct (MTD) Test or the Amplicor nucleic acid amplification test. Other polymerase chain reaction–based studies excluded.
AFB, acid-fast bacillus.

than 97% in most studies (90). The yield of a single specimen is low and can be improved by submitting multiple samples of adequate volume. For example, Warren and colleagues (90) found that implementing a policy of rejecting sputum samples less than 5 mL in volume increased the sensitivity of AFB smears from 72.5% to 92%. Patients with cavitary TB are more likely to have a positive AFB smear because of the high number of organisms present in this form of TB (92), whereas a positive AFB smear is less likely in most types of extrapulmonary disease given the relatively low numbers of organisms in these forms of TB (Table 20.4).

Culture Methods. The AFB smear is limited by its poor sensitivity and inability to differentiate between MTB, non-tuberculous mycobacterial species, and other acid-fast organisms. Mycobacterial culture is able to detect as few as 10 organisms per milliliter and overcomes many of the limitations of AFB staining. Several types of culture media have been developed for the isolation of mycobacteria, including agar-based media (Middlebrook 7H10-selective 7H11), egg-based media (Lowenstein-Jensen), and liquid media (Middlebrook 7H12). The development of automated broth culture systems, such as BACTEC 460 (Becton Dickinson Microbiology Systems, Sparks, Maryland), BACTEC 960 mycobacterial growth indicator tube (MGIT) systems (Becton Dickinson Microbiology Systems), Septi-Check ESP (Trek Diagnostic Systems, Westlake, Ohio), and MB/BacT (Organon Teknika, Durham, North Carolina), has been a major step in accelerating the diagnosis of MTB; traditional solid media–based systems require 3 to 8 weeks for organism growth, whereas broth culture methods require 1 to 3 weeks (93–95). Published recovery rates are 87% to 95% for broth cultures, 52% to 80% for agar-based techniques, and 42% to 77% for egg-based techniques (96); however, because some species of the MTB complex may grow only on solid media, inoculation of both types of media is recommended (74).

Direct Amplification Techniques. Even with the use of broth-based culture systems, confirming the presence of MTB from the time of specimen collection takes at least a week and more often 2 to 3 weeks. Methods to detect the presence of TB directly from clinical specimens more rapidly have been a significant advance in the treatment of TB (97–103). Current direct methods are based on nucleic acid amplification techniques, and two different tests are commercially available: a transcription-mediated amplification method (Amplified *Mycobacterium tuberculosis* Direct [MTD] Test; Gen-Probe, San Diego, California) and a polymerase chain reaction–based assay (Amplicor; Roche Diagnostic Systems, Branchburg, New Jersey).

The performance of nucleic acid amplification techniques has been most rigorously evaluated in respiratory samples, in which both tests have a sensitivity of about 96% and a specificity of 100% for AFB smear-positive samples when combined with appropriate nucleic acid probes (104). Their performance in AFB smear-negative specimens is significantly less impressive, with sensitivities ranging from 48% to 53%, although their specificity remains high, at 96% to 99% (104–106). The accuracy of nucleic acid amplification testing may be reduced by the concurrent use of antituberculous therapy, and inhibitors in the patient's sputum may also cause a false-negative result.

With these factors taken into account, nucleic acid amplification tests offer the opportunity to diagnose pulmonary TB within several hours, and their application to the first specimen of all clinically suspected cases is recommended (107). Figure 20.6 summarizes the CDC recommendations for the use of nucleic acid amplification tests in the evaluation of patients with suspected pulmonary TB. Some authors have recommended that nucleic acid amplification tests be applied only to AFB smear–negative sputum isolates from patients deemed to be at an especially high risk for TB (108).

NUCLEIC ACID AMPLIFICATION FOR THE DIAGNOSIS OF TUBERCULOSIS

Summary Statement	Level of Evidence
Commercially available nucleic acid amplification/probe techniques are highly sensitive and specific for *M. tuberculosis* in smear-positive specimens.	Multiple well-designed clinical trials
The use of nucleic acid amplification tests on smear-negative specimens and in extrapulmonary tuberculosis may be of adjunctive value.	Subgroup analysis of multiple well-designed clinical trials

Speciation Techniques. Traditionally, the speciation of mycobacterial isolates has been achieved by means of biochemical testing, including niacin production, nitrate reduction, and inactivation of catalase. Unfortunately, such methods are cumbersome and time-consuming. The development of newer diagnostic techniques, including the *p*-nitro-α-acetylamino-β-hydroxypropiophenone (NAP) test (109), high-performance liquid chromatography (HPLC), and nucleic acid hybridization probes, has significantly shortened the time required to speciate an AFB-positive culture.

High-Performance Liquid Chromatography. HPLC is based on the unique production of mycolic acids by different species of mycobacteria. It can differentiate between nearly 50 different mycobacteria species, including the MTB complex, with nearly 99% accuracy, and results are generally available within 6 to 7 hours (110).

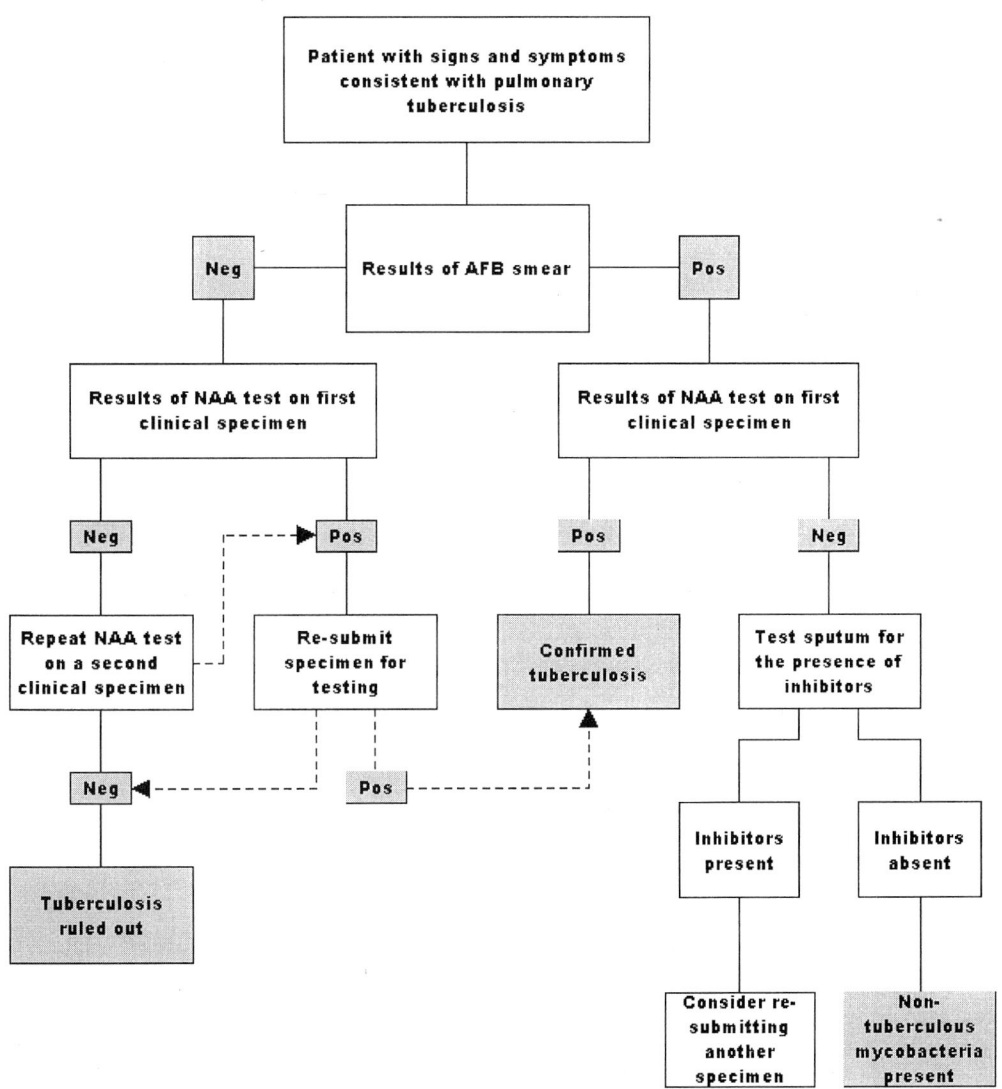

FIGURE 20.6. The use of nucleic acid amplification tests in the diagnostic evaluation of patients with suspected pulmonary tuberculosis.

Nucleic Acid Probes. Nucleic acid probes have been developed that can specifically hybridize with DNA or RNA from MTB, *M. avium, M. intracellulare, M. kansasii,* and *M. gordonae.* The rapidity of this test allows for species identification within 2 hours and has a sensitivity and specificity that approaches 100% for MTB (111). Although the test requires more than 10^5 organisms or the use of an amplification technique to achieve an adequate yield, when it is combined with automated broth culture methods, the time for detecting and identifying MTB can be reduced to as little as 4 to 7 days (112).

Identification of Resistance

The identification of antimicrobial resistance among clinical isolates is necessary to ensure optimal therapy and prevent the spread of these organisms to others. Traditionally, agar- and broth-based methods have been used to detect drug resistance (74). In the agar-based method, organisms are allowed to grow on both a drug-containing medium and a drug-free medium. Growth of the organisms on a medium containing a drug that equals 1% or more of the growth of the organisms on a medium without the drug indicates resistance to that drug (91). Broth-based radiometric methods use a similar process and correlate well with agar-based methods (95%–100%) but allow resistance to be detected much earlier than do solid media (4–7 days vs. 14–21 days) (93). Because of the importance of resistance, it is recommended that both media be used (74).

The continued evolution of molecular technology may soon permit the rapid identification of resistance in clinical isolates in the same way that nucleic acid amplification tests allow the rapid identification of TB. For example, mutations in an 81–base pair segment of the *rpoB* gene are responsible for 97% of cases of clinical resistance to rifamycins, so that molecular identification is technically feasible (111). INH resistance is more complicated because resistance can occur by a variety of mutations on different genes (*katG, inhA,* and *ahpC*). Using a polymerase chain reaction technique, Telenti and colleagues (113) were able to identify all submitted clinical samples with rifampin resistance, although the performance for the detection of INH resistance was only 87%. A commercial rifampin resistance detection kit is currently in use in Europe, but approval in the United States is still pending (114).

Diagnostic Issues in Extrapulmonary Tuberculosis

Adenosine Deaminase

Adenosine deaminase is an enzyme produced by activated T lymphocytes, and measurement of the adenosine deaminase level in certain extrapulmonary body fluids (pleural fluid, ascitic fluid, CSF) has been evaluated as a diagnostic test for TB. In several studies, the sensitivity of the adenosine deaminase level in pleural fluid ranged from 83% to 99%, with a specificity that ranged from 89% to 97% when cutoff levels of 45 to 60 U/L were used (50,115–117); however, many of these studies were based on highly selected populations in areas where TB was endemic. The positive predictive value of the test would be much lower in areas like the United States, where the prevalence of TB and hence the pretest probability are lower (e.g., the positive predictive value is 50% when the pretest probability is 5%) (118).

Nucleic Acid Amplification

The use of nucleic acid amplification tests in the diagnosis of extrapulmonary TB remains controversial (119). The adjunctive value of nucleic acid amplification tests in the diagnosis of tuberculous pleuritis remains largely undefined, although studies of commercially available tests have demonstrated sensitivities ranging from 20% to 100% for pleural fluid and from zero to 100% for pleural biopsy specimens (119,120). The few studies that used commercially available nucleic acid amplification tests (i.e., Amplified MTD Test and Amplicor) in other forms of extrapulmonary TB generally found good correlation with culture of the clinical specimens (Table 20.4). These tests may be of benefit in patients with a high probability of extrapulmonary TB; however, until more data are available, the routine testing of nonrespiratory specimens, particularly AFB smear–negative specimens, cannot be recommended.

Treatment of Active Infection

The effective management of TB encompasses several aspects of patient care, including preventing transmission from potentially infectious patients, prescribing the appropriate combination of anti-TB medications for an appropriate length of time, monitoring patients for potential toxicity, and ensuring that they comply with the prescribed regimen.

Prevention of Transmission

Numerous reports of TB outbreaks in prisons, hospitals, and other health care settings in the early and mid-1990s reminded the health care community of the risk associated with the care of patients with TB (121–123). The likelihood that a susceptible person exposed to a patient with active TB will become infected is a function of the concentration of organisms in the air and the duration of exposure. Factors associated with a higher likelihood of transmission include (a) disease of the lungs, airways, or larynx; (b) cavitary disease on the chest radiograph; (c) cough; (d) failure of patients to cover their mouth during sneezing or coughing; (e) positive AFB smear of sputum; (f) procedures that enhance the aerosolization of organisms (i.e., sputum induction, nebulizer therapy, endotracheal intubation, bronchoscopy); and (g) inappropriate or short duration of chemotherapy for TB (124).

Guidelines for the prevention of nosocomially acquired TB have been published (124) and include (a) prompt isolation and treatment of patients with confirmed or suspected TB; (b) use of rapid diagnostic tests to confirm the diagnosis of TB; (c) use of negative-pressure isolation rooms; and (d) use of personal protection equipment for health care workers in direct contact with patients with confirmed or suspected TB. Implementation of these recommendations in a high-prevalence New York hospital resulted in a decrease in the case rates of MDR-TB from 32% to 14% and a reduction in the TST conversion rate among health care workers from 17% to 5% (125).

Any patient admitted to the hospital with a pulmonary process and one of the epidemiologic risk factors previously discussed (see section "Epidemiology") should be suspected of having TB. Admission to the hospital should be determined by general medical necessity and by the need to isolate patients with suspected active TB who, by the nature of their environment, are likely to expose uninfected persons (i.e., homeless persons and prisoners), but it is not necessary to admit and isolate all outpatients with suspected TB. Patients who are not admitted should be instructed to remain at home and avoid contact with unexposed persons (family members are considered to be exposed) until they have been proved to be noninfectious.

The use of negative-pressure ventilation prevents potentially infectious aerosols from escaping into the rest of the hospital environment, and the installation of ventilation systems that achieve at least six, and preferably 12, complete room air changes per hour is recommended. Air from the isolation rooms should be exhausted to the outside or, if this is impossible, recirculated after passage through a high-efficiency particulate air (HEPA) filter. Ultraviolet germicidal irradiation of upper room air removes aerosolized BCG at a rate equivalent to 10 to 25 complete room air exchanges per hour (126); however, adoption of this technology has been slow because of concerns regarding photodermatitis and keratitis. Despite these concerns, ultraviolet germicidal irradiation may have a role in disinfecting high-risk areas (e.g., bronchoscopy suites) or large rooms, such as hospital waiting or emergency rooms, where enhancing ventilation may be cost-prohibitive or not technologically feasible (127).

Despite a paucity of data demonstrating their benefit in reducing the transmission of TB, the use of personal protection respiratory devices, such as HEPA filter–containing respirators, has been recommended for all health care workers in direct contact with patients with confirmed or diagnosed TB (124). Two cost–benefit analyses found that it would cost between \$1.3 and \$7 million to use HEPA filter–containing respirators to prevent the transmission of a single case of TB (128,129). More recently, the National Institute for Occupational Safety and Health modified its recommendations to include the less efficient (95% vs. >99% for the HEPA filter) but considerably cheaper N95 particulate filter respirator as an acceptable form of personal protection equipment in the care of patients with confirmed or suspected TB. Clearly, adequate ventilation contributes substantially to reducing TB transmission, and the use of personal protection equipment is of greatest benefit in poorly ventilated settings (130).

Principles of Therapy for Active Tuberculosis

Effective therapy for active TB requires (a) drugs that are active against TB in its various phases of growth, (b) the use of drug combinations to prevent the emergence of resistance, and (c) the use of drugs for a prolonged period of time.

The most active anti-TB regimens have bactericidal activity against organisms in all three phases of the growth cycle: (a) actively multiplying in the extracellular environment; (b) growing slowly in the intracellular environment of the macrophage; and (c) residing in a nearly dormant state in the necrotic center of the caseating granuloma. All the primary drugs, with the exception of ethambutol, are bactericidal against MTB in one or more of its phases of growth and are approved for daily and twice- or thrice-weekly dosing regimens (Table 20.5). Salvage or "second-line" drugs are generally only bacteriostatic, must be used daily, and are generally associated with more toxicity than primary agents (Table 20.6).

Resistance develops during therapy for TB as a result of random point mutations in a variety of genes. It is estimated that the rate of mutations conferring resistance to one of the primary anti-TB drugs is 10^{-7} to 10^{-9} per bacterium per cell division, depending on the drug used (131). The use of a single drug in the presence of 10^9 organisms (assuming a mutation rate of 10^{-7}) would result in failure caused by resistance in nearly 100% of cases. In contrast, the use of two drugs, with a rate of spontaneous resistance to *both* drugs of 10^{-14} to 10^{-18} (the product of the individual drug mutation rates), would result in failure caused by the emergence of resistance in about 0.1% of cases. Because the number of organisms in a patient with active TB rarely exceeds 10^9, the routine use of at least two drugs to which the organism is sensitive in any drug regimen should prevent the emergence of drug-resistant TB in the vast majority of patients. In areas of the world where the rate of primary resistance is "high" (usually defined as ≥4%) among TB isolates, the empiric use of additional drugs may be required to ensure that at least two of the drugs in the selected regimen are active.

Anti-TB regimens must incorporate a combination of bactericidal drugs that are given for at least 6 months when INH, rifampin, and pyrazinamide are used and for considerably longer periods, up to 18 months, when these agents cannot be used (132), reflecting the efficiency of different regimens at eradicating MTB in its various phases of growth.

Primary Drugs

Isoniazid

INH inhibits cell wall synthesis by interfering with the synthesis of mycolic acid and is bactericidal against rapidly multiplying extracellular organisms but only bacteriostatic

TABLE 20.5. PRIMARY ANTITUBERCULOSIS DRUGS

Drug	Dosage[a] Daily Regimen		Twice-Weekly Regimen		Thrice-Weekly Regimen		Major Side Effect	Recommended Monitoring
	Children	Adults	Children	Adults	Children	Adults		
Isoniazid	10–20 mg/kg Max 300 mg	5 mg/kg Max 300 mg	20–40 mg/kg Max 900 mg	15 mg/kg Max 900 mg	20–40 mg/kg Max 900 mg	15 mg/kg Max 900 mg	Hepatitis Peripheral neuropathy	Baseline liver enzymes (monitor monthly if values abnormal)
Rifampin	10–20 mg/kg Max 600 mg	10 mg/kg Max 600 mg	10–20 mg/kg Max 600 mg	10 mg/kg Max 600 mg	10–20 mg/kg Max 600 mg	10 mg/kg Max 600 mg	Hepatitis Colors body fluids orange Flulike illness Induction of cytochrome P-450 system	Baseline liver enzymes (monitor monthly if values abnormal)
Pyrazinamide	15–30 mg/kg Max 2 g	15–30 mg/kg Max 2 g	50–70 mg/kg Max 4 g	50–70 mg/kg Max 4 g	50–70 mg/kg Max 4 g	50–70 mg/kg Max 4 g	Hepatitis Polyarthralgias Hyperuricemia	Baseline liver enzymes (monitor monthly if values abnormal) Check baseline uric acid level
Ethambutol	15–25 mg/kg	15–25 mg/kg	50 mg/kg	50 mg/kg	25–30 mg/kg	25–30 mg/kg	Optic neuritis	Measure visual acuity and red–green color perception at baseline and regularly thereafter
Streptomycin	20–40 mg/kg Max 1 g	15 mg/kg Max 1 g	25–30 mg/kg Max 1.5 g	25–30 mg/kg Max 1.5 g	25–30 mg/kg Max 1.5 g	25–30 mg/kg Max 1.5 g	Vestibular toxicity Ototoxicity Nephrotoxicity	Baseline audiometry and renal function tests and regularly thereafter during therapy

[a]Recommendations of the American Thoracic Society and the Centers for Disease Control and Prevention. Max, maximum.

Source: From Bass JB, Farer LS, Hopewell PC, et al. Treatment of tuberculosis and tuberculosis infection in adults and children. American Thoracic Society and the Centers for Disease Control and Prevention. *Am J Respir Crit Care Med* 1994;149:1359–1374, with permission.

TABLE 20.6. SECOND-LINE ANTITUBERCULOSIS DRUGS

Drug	Daily Dose (Adults and Children)[a]	Major Side Effects	Recommended Monitoring
Ethionamide	15–20 mg/kg Max 1 g	Gastrointestinal irritation Hepatotoxicity Metallic taste	Baseline liver enzymes (monitor monthly if abnormal)
Cycloserine	15–20 mg/kg Max 1 g	Psychosis Seizures Headache	Assess mental and psychologic status at baseline and regularly thereafter
Para-aminosalicylic acid	150 mg/kg Max 12 g	Gastrointestinal irritation Hypersensitivity reactions Hepatotoxicity	Baseline liver enxzymes (monitor monthly if abnormal)
Clofaziamine	100–300 mg	Gastrointestinal irritation Orange–brown discoloration of skin	
Capreomycin	15–30 mg/kg Max 1 g	Ototoxicity Vestibular toxicity Nephrotoxicity	Baseline audiometry and renal function and regularly thereafter during therapy
Kanamycin	15–30 mg/kg Max 1 g	Ototoxicity Vestibular toxicity Nephrotoxicity	Baseline audiometry and renal function and regularly thereafter during therapy
Fluoroquinolones (ciprofloxacin, ofloxacin, and levofloxacin)	750 mg bid (ciprofloxacin) 800 mg PO qd (ofloxacin) 500 mg PO qd (levofloxacin)	Gastrointestinal irritation Insomnia Photosensitivity	

[a] Recommendations from the American Thoracic Society and the Centers for Disease Control and Prevention.
Max, maximum.
Source: From Bass JB, Farer LS, Hopewell PC, et al. Treatment of tuberculosis and tuberculosis infection in adults and children. American Thoracic Society and the Centers for Disease Control and Prevention. *Am J Respir Crit Care Med* 1994;149:1359–1374, with permission.

against intracellular organisms. It has excellent oral bioavailability and is metabolized primarily by the liver, with a half-life of 1 to 3 hours. Asymptomatic elevations in hepatic aminotransferases, to three to five times above baseline, occur in 10% to 20% of patients taking INH, but clinically overt hepatotoxicity is seen in only about 1% of patients being treated for active TB (133). Factors associated with an increased risk for hepatotoxicity include advanced age, coexisting alcoholic liver disease, slow acetylator status, pregnancy, and the concurrent use of acetaminophen (134). Peripheral neuropathy is an infrequent complication of INH when it is administered at a standard dose of 300 mg/d, and the risk can be reduced by the simultaneous administration of pyridoxine (10–50 mg/d). Other rare complications of INH therapy include psychosis, seizures, hypersensitivity reactions, and antineutrophil cytoplasmic antibody–associated vasculitis.

Rifamycins

Rifampin is a semisynthetic derivative of rifamycin that inhibits the DNA-dependent RNA polymerase of MTB. It is bactericidal against MTB in all three phases of its growth. Its effectiveness in sterilizing slowly growing organisms has permitted the use of short-course regimens (i.e., 6 and 9 months), and regimens that exclude this agent should be continued for 18 or more months (135). Rifampin is well absorbed orally and is metabolized by the hepatic cytochrome P-450 system. Rifampin colors body fluids orange, including urine, sweat, and tears, which may stain soft contact

lenses. Hepatotoxicity is the major side effect of rifampin, and studies suggest that the risk for hepatotoxicity of regimens that contain both INH and rifampin is approximately double that of regimens that contain only one of the drugs (136). Rifampin administered at high doses can result in a flulike syndrome and can induce hypersensitivity reactions at any dose, which may manifest as fever, rash, hemolysis, or interstitial nephritis (137). A major problem associated with the use of rifampin is its effects on other drug concentrations by virtue of its induction of the P-450 enzymes. Rifampin accelerates the metabolism of the protease inhibitors used in many HIV treatment regimens, so that its use in anti-TB regimens is precluded in these patients.

Other rifamycins that have been studied in the treatment of TB include rifabutin and rifapentine. Rifabutin has become the rifamycin of choice for the treatment of HIV-positive patients with TB because of its reduced effects on the hepatic P-450 system, and its use is discussed later (see section "Treatment of the Patient Coinfected with HIV"). Rifapentine is a newer rifamycin with a long half-life that permits once-weekly dosing. It has been evaluated for the continuation phase of TB therapy in three open-label, randomized clinical trials (138–140). In these trials, the use of once-weekly rifapentine and INH was associated with a relapse rate of 8.2% to 10%, compared with 4% to 5.6% for thrice-weekly INH and rifampin. Further analysis demonstrated that relapse was primarily in patients with cavitary TB and in patients whose sputum failed to sterilize after 2 months of therapy. HIV-infected patients were included only in the study by Bock and colleagues (140), but this arm of the trial was discontinued because of an unacceptably high rate of relapse (10.2%) with rifamycin-resistant organisms (141).

Pyrazinamide

Pyrazinamide is a synthetic derivative of nicotinamide that requires a low pH for activity, which may account for its efficiency in killing organisms within phagocytic cells (131). Six-month anti-TB regimens that include pyrazinamide are more effective than regimens that do not include this drug (142). Its major drawback is hepatotoxicity, yet studies suggest that its inclusion in the first 2 months of an anti-TB regimen does not add to the risk of INH/rifampin regimens (143,144). Other common side effects of pyrazinamide are nongouty polyarthralgias and hyperuricemia, which may rarely result in exacerbations of gout during therapy.

Ethambutol

Ethambutol is a bacteriostatic drug used in anti-TB regimens to prevent the emergence of resistance. Its use should be considered when the local rates of TB resistance are known to be higher than 4% or are not known. Its major side effect is optic neuritis, which may manifest as central scotomata, loss of red and green color vision, or decreased visual acuity. Fortunately, optic neuritis is rare when a daily dose of 15 mg/kg is given, but it may occur in up to 3% of patients who are taking 25 mg of the drug per kilogram (145).

Streptomycin

Streptomycin is an aminoglycoside antibiotic that is bactericidal against organisms in the actively multiplying phase of extracellular growth. It is not absorbed orally and must be given by the parenteral route. Vestibular toxicity, which manifests as dizziness or gait instability, is the most common side effect of streptomycin, although ototoxicity can also occur. Nephrotoxicity is less common than with the other aminoglycosides; however, dosing must be adjusted carefully in patients with renal insufficiency and in the elderly.

Adjunctive Treatment

In patients who are particularly toxic from TB and who are receiving adequate anti-TB therapy, corticosteroids or, more recently, agents that reduce or block TNF-α (e.g., thalidomide, etanercept) may reduce fever, improve appetite, and prevent inflammatory sequelae, such as adhesive arachnoiditis (146,147).

Recommended Regimens

The introduction of rifampin in 1966 opened the doorway to shorter regimens when it was shown that a 9-month regimen of INH and rifampin was as efficacious as 18- and 24-month regimens (148,149). Subsequent studies demonstrated that the use of INH, rifampin, and pyrazinamide in a 2-month bactericidal phase followed by a 4-month continuation phase of INH with rifampin was as effective as longer regimens (144,150). The addition of either ethambutol or streptomycin to the initial regimen did not decrease relapse rates in drug-susceptible cases (151–153) but were beneficial in cases of resistance to one of the primary agents (154). Finally, other studies demonstrated that the drugs could be used twice or thrice weekly during the continuation phase with results similar to those of regimens in which the drugs were given daily (142,155). These intermittent regimens made directly observed therapy (DOT) practical.

Based on the results of these studies, the ATS, CDC, and Infectious Diseases Society of America published guidelines for the treatment of active TB (156) (Table 20.7). These recommendations place more of an emphasis on the total number of doses received than on the duration of therapy, although prolonged interruptions in therapy (14 days) may require reinitiation of the entire treatment regimen. Nine-month regimens are now recommended for all patients with cavitary lung disease on their initial chest radiograph *and* persistently positive sputum cultures after 2 months of therapy. Patients with only one of these risks for relapse should be monitored closely for the first 6 to 12 months after completing treatment. Nine-month regimens that omit pyrazinamide are acceptable for patients without these risk factors if the organism is known to be susceptible to both drugs. If sensitivities are not known, then ethambutol or streptomycin should be added until susceptibility results are available. Short-course regimens may be used in most forms of extrapulmonary TB, except for musculoskeletal, central nervous system, and miliary TB, in which extending the duration of therapy for at least a year has been recommended (132).

DOT programs have been shown to increase the rate of completion of short-course regimens (157), reduce the emergence of resistance during therapy (158), and be cost-effective in comparison with self-administered therapy programs (159). The risk for therapeutic failure or relapse is intrinsically increased in intermittent regimens because the effect of missing doses is higher; therefore, *all* short-course regimens that include intermittent weekly dosing should be administered as DOT (i.e., directly observed therapy—short-course, or DOTs).

Patients undergoing therapy for active TB, regardless of whether they are receiving DOTs, should be monitored regularly for response to therapy and for adverse effects of the treatment regimen. Sputum samples should be sent for smear and culture on a biweekly or monthly schedule, and response to therapy at 2 months should be assessed. Eighty-five percent of patients who comply with therapy will have negative cultures 2 months after initiating treatment (160,161), and patients who have persistently positive sputum cultures beyond this time should receive a prolonged continuation

TABLE 20.7. RECOMMENDED DRUG REGIMENS FOR THE TREATMENT OF ACTIVE TUBERCULOSIS INFECTION IN ADULTS

Regimen	Drugs	Initial Phase Interval and Doses (Minimum Duration)[a]	Regimen	Drugs	Continuation Phase Interval and Doses (Minimum Duration)[a,b]	Total Duration and Doses
1	INH RIF PZA EMB	Seven days per week for 56 doses (8 weeks) or 5 days per week for 40 doses (8 weeks)	1A	INH RIF	Seven days per week for 126 doses (18 weeks) or 5 days per week for 90 doses (18 weeks)	182 or 90 (26 weeks)
			1B	INH RIF	Twice weekly for 36 doses (18 weeks)	92 or 76 (26 weeks)
			1C	INH RPT	Once weekly for 18 doses (18 weeks)	74 or 58 (26 weeks)
2	INH RIF PZA EMB	Seven days per week for 14 doses (2 weeks) or 5 days per week for 15 doses (3 weeks) then twice weekly for 12 doses (6 weeks) or 10 doses (5 weeks)	2A	INH RIF	Twice weekly for 36 doses (18 weeks)	62 or 63 (26 weeks)
			2B	INH RPT	Once weekly for 18 doses (18 weeks)	44 or 43 (26 weeks)
3	INH RIF PZA EMB	Thrice weekly for 24 doses (8 weeks)	3	INH RIF	Thrice weekly for 54 doses (18 weeks)	78 (26 weeks)
4	INH	Seven days per week for 56 doses (8 weeks) or 5 days per week for 40 doses (8 weeks)	4A	INH RIF	Seven days per week for 196 doses (28 weeks) or 5 days per week for 140 doses (28 weeks)	252 or 180 (36 weeks)
	RIF EMB		4B	INH RIF	Twice weekly for 56 doses (28 weeks)	112 or 96 (36 weeks)

[a] When directly observed therapy is used, drugs may be given 5 days per week and the necessary number of doses adjusted accordingly.
[b] Patients with cavitation on initial chest radiograph and positive cultures at completion of 2 months of therapy should receive a 7-month (28-week, either 196 doses [daily] or 56 doses [twice weekly]) continuation phase.
EMB, ethambutol; INH, isoniazid; PZA, pyrazinamide; RIF, rifampin; RPT, rifapentine.
Source: Adapted from American Thoracic Society, Centers for Disease Control and Prevention, and the Infectious Diseases Society of America. Treatment of tuberculosis. *Am J Respir Crit Care Med* 2003;167:603–662, with permission.

phase (7 months vs. the typical 4 months) if their baseline chest radiograph also demonstrates cavitary disease; however, patients without cavitation may also benefit from a longer course of therapy. Additionally, persistently positive sputum cultures should prompt an investigation for problems with adherence or the emergence of resistance. In the latter situation, two anti-TB drugs should be added to the existing regimen because the addition of a single drug risks promoting further resistance. Blood chemistries (particularly creatinine) should be monitored regularly while patients are receiving streptomycin; however, unless the baseline laboratory tests reveal abnormalities, regular testing for other drugs is not recommended. Patients should be educated about the signs and symptoms of the adverse effects associated with each drug they are given and should be able to contact a caregiver if toxicity does develop.

Treatment of the Patient Coinfected with HIV

Studies of patients coinfected with TB and HIV have shown that they are more likely to progress to AIDS (162)

TREATMENT OF ACTIVE TUBERCULOSIS

Summary Statement	Level of Evidence
Six-month short-course regimens that include a rifamycin and pyrazinamide are as efficacious as longer-lasting regimens.	Multiple well-designed clinical trials
A short course of directly observed therapy (DOTs) is effective at reducing noncompliance, treatment failure, and emergence of resistance and should be considered for use in all patients.	Multiple well-designed clinical trials
The patient's sputum should be monitored regularly and documented for conversion to culture-negative at 2 months of therapy.	Consensus of expert opinion
Patients who have baseline cavitary disease and whose sputum cultures fail to sterilize with 2 months of therapy should receive a 7-month continuation course of tuberculosis therapy.	Multiple well-designed clinical trials

and have a higher 1-year mortality rate (20%–35%) than HIV-positive but TB-negative patients (163). The treatment of coinfected patients is complicated by an apparent increased rate of MDR-TB among this population, a potentially higher rate of relapse after treatment is completed, a higher rate of adverse effects of treatment, and a significant risk for interactions between prescribed anti-TB and anti-HIV regimens.

Many of the studies describing outbreaks of MDR-TB in the nosocomial setting involved mostly HIV-positive patients (164–166), and the results of a national resistance surveillance study found a higher rate of drug resistance among HIV-positive patients (167). A higher rate of recent acquisition with progression to active disease in areas with high rates of resistance may partially explain these results (14,15,168).

Studies of coinfected patients have demonstrated that HIV-positive patients respond to short-course anti-TB regimens as well as HIV-negative patients (169–172); however, the risk for relapse after therapy is completed has been an area of controversy. Whereas one study found a higher "relapse" rate in HIV-positive patients than in HIV-negative patients (170), this study failed to differentiate between relapse and reinfection. The CDC has stated that a 6-month regimen (thrice-weekly dosing only; twice-weekly dosing and once-weekly dosing are *not* recommended) is appropriate if carried out as DOT *and* the patient's sputum converts rapidly (<2 months) (163). Patients who do not meet these criteria should receive therapy for a longer period (i.e., 9 months).

The complexity of highly active antiretroviral therapy (HAART) regimens makes the administration of an intensive anti-TB regimen difficult. Moreover, a study by Dean and colleagues (173) found that 54% of HIV-positive patients initiating anti-TB therapy experienced adverse side effects, including peripheral neuropathy (21%), rash (17%), and gastrointestinal upset (10%). Univariate analysis demonstrated that concurrent therapy with HAART was significantly associated with the development of toxicity (odds ratio [OR], 1.88; confidence interval [CI], 1.03–3.42), and based on this finding, the authors suggested that for patients with less advanced HIV (>100 $CD4^+$ cells per cubic millimeter), deferral of HAART during the initial 2 months of anti-TB therapy should be considered.

Rifampin, as noted (see section "Rifamycins"), is a potent inducer of the cytochrome P-450 system and interacts significantly with HAART regimens that include protease inhibitors and nonnucleoside reverse transcriptase inhibitors. Rifabutin has been associated with less induction of the P-450 system and has been studied extensively in coinfected patients (174–176). These studies have established the efficacy of rifabutin-containing regimens for the cure of TB, but their effect on the efficacy of HAART regimens remains unsettled. Because of these residual concerns, rifabutin-containing regimens should be used in patients who cannot safely stop HAART during TB therapy ($CD4^+$ cell count <100/mm^3).

Compared with rifampin, rifabutin carries a lower risk for hepatitis but is associated with a higher risk for arthralgias, neutropenia/leukopenia, and uveitis. Furthermore, although rifabutin interacts less with antiretrovirals than rifampin does, it still cannot be used with delavirdine, and its dose must be adjusted when it is used with the other antiretrovirals (177). Adverse effects and the HIV load should be assessed frequently, and the dose of protease inhibitors may have to be increased 20% to 25% during concurrent therapy.

TREATMENT OF TUBERCULOSIS AND HIV COINFECTION

Summary Statement	Level of Evidence
Patients with HIV and TB coinfection can be safely treated with 6-month short-course regimens *if* they receive DOT *and* their sputum culture converts by 2 months.	Multiple well-designed clinical trials
Patients with HIV and TB coinfection **should not** receive once-weekly (INH with rifapentine) or twice-weekly (INH with rifampin or rifabutin) regimens in the continuation phase of therapy.	Lack of efficacy from multiple well-designed clinical trials
In patients with stable HIV infection ($CD4^+$ cell count > 100/mm^3), antiretroviral therapy should be withheld during the first 2 months of anti-TB therapy.	Single prospective cohort study
Rifabutin should be substituted for rifampin in HIV-positive patients who *require* antiretroviral therapy that includes a protease inhibitor or a nonnucleoside reverse transcriptase inhibitor during anti-TB therapy.	Multiple well-designed clinical trials

DOT, directly observed therapy; INH, isoniazid; TB, tuberculosis.

Treatment of Tuberculosis during Pregnancy

Active TB during pregnancy poses an extreme risk for both mother and fetus and therefore should prompt initiation of therapy regardless of the term (180). INH, rifampin, and ethambutol can all be given safely during pregnancy. Pyrazinamide, however, has not been approved for use during pregnancy and should not be given. Because the rates of relapse in regimens that excluded pyrazinamide have been as high as 7% to 9%, extending the duration of therapy to 9 months (rifampin-based regimens) should be strongly considered.

Treatment of Patients with Negative Smears/Cultures

In some cases, patients present with symptoms and a chest radiograph consistent with "old" TB, typically an upper lobe fibronodular pattern, but have negative sputum smears and cultures. These patients may have "subclinical" active TB or simply latent TB infection with significant scarring.

However, the risk for the development of overtly active TB is higher than in persons without radiographic abnormalities, and treatment is recommended. The initial evaluation should include an aggressive attempt to culture organisms. Although some studies have suggested that smear-negative but culture-positive cases can be treated for a shorter period than smear-positive cases (181), we believe that any patient with a positive sputum culture requires a standard short-course regimen. If initial cultures are negative, several studies have found that combined therapy with INH and rifampin for 4 months reduces the likelihood of the development of overtly active disease as well as 12 months of INH monotherapy (182). The use of four-drug regimens for 4 months has also been studied (181,183), but in the United States, where primary resistance is relatively low, the use of INH and rifampin for 4 months appears to be efficacious and cost-effective (182). The chest radiograph should be followed at least monthly during treatment, and improvement suggests the presence of active disease, whereas failure to improve after 3 months of therapy suggests latent TB infection or an alternative diagnosis.

Treatment of Resistant Mycobacterium tuberculosis Infection

Resistant TB has been defined as an organism that is resistant to a single anti-TB drug, whereas MDR-TB is classically defined as resistance to both INH and rifampin. Although reports of monoresistance to rifampin have been increasing in the literature, primarily in HIV-positive patients (141), most organisms with resistance to rifampin are also resistant to INH, so that the identification of rifampin resistance is a good marker for MDR-TB. While the rates of MDR-TB decreased from nearly 3% in 1993 to 1.2% in 2000, the rates of INH resistance have remained fairly stable (~8.0%) (8).

Intrinsic resistance to anti-TB drugs in wild strains of MTB is rare; resistance is a phenomenon more common in persons who have received prior (usually suboptimal) TB therapy and have acquired resistance, after which the resistant organism can spread to others. Most persons who present for re-treatment of TB have a history of inadequate therapy or noncompliance with therapy, and rates of resistance in this population (secondary resistance) are twice as high as those in patients presenting for initial TB treatment (primary resistance) (22,167). Moreover, in a study from New York, in the 89 cases of MDR-TB (19% of all cases) seen in 1991, prior TB therapy was the strongest predictor of resistance (OR, 5.3; *P* <.001) (184). Other factors associated with MDR-TB include exposure to persons with known MDR-TB and immigrant status (184). Reports differ as to the relationship between HIV infection and MDR-TB (168,185).

Mortality rates in patients with MDR-TB range from 14% to 58% (19,186–188), and response to therapy varies from 50% to 77% (19,186,189). In general, patients should be treated with at least two drugs to which the organism is most susceptible as judged by *in vitro* testing (190,191).

Extensive testing with agents not regularly used for TB may be warranted, and surgery for localized disease should also be considered. Experimental therapies, in particular inhaled IFN-γ and inhaled streptomycin, have shown promise (192,193). Even when these measures are used, successful eradication of infection remains elusive. Goble and colleagues (19) achieved only a 65% cure rate in 171 patients with MDR-TB.

Treatment of Latent Tuberculosis Infection

The treatment of patients with latent TB infection has been shown to reduce the risk for subsequent reactivation. In studies performed in the 1950s and 1960s in HIV-negative patients, the administration of INH to patients with a positive TST result reduced the risk for subsequent TB by 25% to 93% (194). Moreover, a metaanalysis of 11 studies that included nearly 74,000 patients showed that INH therapy in patients with latent TB infection reduces the risk for the development of active TB by 60% (relative risk [RR], 0.40; 95% CI, 0.31–0.52), and this benefit appears to be lifelong (195).

Many of the chemoprophylaxis trials used variable periods of INH therapy, and only one trial was designed to evaluate differences in outcome related to duration of therapy (196). In this trial, a 6-month and a 12-month regimen of INH led to a 65% and a 75% reduction in the development of active disease, respectively. This difference did not reach statistical significance; however, analysis of only those patients who took 80% or more of their medication showed that the 12-month regimen was clearly superior to the 6-month regimen (93% vs. 69%). A subsequent analysis of data from the Alaskan INH chemoprophylaxis trials suggested that 9 months of INH was superior to 6 months of INH, but increasing the duration of therapy to 12 months was of minimal additional benefit (197). Based on the results of these studies, the ATS and CDC now recommend a 9-month INH regimen as the preferred regimen for the treatment of latent TB infection (76).

A surveillance study that included 13,838 patients found that approximately 1% of patients taking INH without monitoring developed hepatotoxicity that was associated with a 5% mortality rate. The risk for hepatotoxicity was higher in patients who drank alcohol on a daily basis (2.6%) and in patients older than 35 years, with a peak incidence (2.3%) around 50 years of age (198). The use of regular clinical monitoring can significantly reduce the risk for INH-associated hepatotoxicity (133,199,200).

Based on these studies, it appears that INH is effective and safe, and the most recent ATS and CDC guidelines recommend initiating therapy for latent TB infection (Table 20.8) in all patients with a positive TST result regardless of age, although the criteria for a positive TST result vary depending on the TB risk (Table 20.1). *In effect, a decision to test is a decision to treat.* All patients receiving therapy for latent TB infection should be clinically assessed on a

TABLE 20.8. RECOMMENDED DRUG REGIMENS FOR THE TREATMENT OF LATENT TUBERCULOSIS INFECTION IN ADULTS

Drug	Interval and Duration	Comments	Rating[a] (Evidence)[b] HIV−	HIV+
Isoniazid	Daily for 9 mo[c,d]	In HIV-infected patients, isoniazid may be administered concurrently with NRTIs, NNRTIs, or protease inhibitors.	A-II	A-II
	Twice weekly for 9 mo[c,d]	DOT must be used with twice-weekly dosing.	B-II	B-II
	Daily for 6 mo[d]	Not indicated for HIV-infected persons, those with fibrotic lesions on chest radiographs, or children.	B-I	C-I
	Twice weekly for 6 mo[d]	DOT must be used with twice-weekly dosing.	B-II	C-I
Rifampin plus pyrazinamide	Daily for 2 mo	May also be offered to persons who are contacts of patients with isoniazid-resistant, rifampin-susceptible TB. In HIV-infected patients, protease inhibitors or NNRTIs should generally not be administered concurrently with rifampin; rifabutin can be used as an alternative for patients treated with indinavir, nelfinavir, amprenavir, ritonavir, or efavirenz, and possibly with nevirapine and soft-gel saquinavir.[e]	B-II	B-I
	Twice weekly for 2–3 mo	DOT must be used with twice-weekly dosing.	C-II	C-I
Rifampin	Daily for 4 mo	For persons who cannot tolerate pyrazinamide. For persons who are contacts of patients with isoniazid-resistant, rifampin-susceptible TB who cannot tolerate pyrazinamide.	B-II	B-III

[a] Strength of recommendation: A, preferred; B, acceptable alternative; C, offer when A and B cannot be given.
[b] Quality of evidence: I, randomized clinical trial data; II, data from clinical trials that were not randomized nor were conducted in other populations; III, expert opinion.
[c] Recommended regimen for children younger than 18 years of age.
[d] Recommended regimens for pregnant women. Some experts would use rifampin and pyrazinamide for 2 months as an alternative regimen in HIV-infected pregnant women, although pyrazinamide should be avoided in the first trimester.
[e] Rifabutin should not be used with ritonavir, hard-gel saquinavir, or delavirdine. When rifabutin is used with a protease inhibitor or NNRTI, dose adjustment of rifabutin may be required.
DOT, directly observed therapy; NNRTI, nonnucleoside reverse transcriptase inhibitor.
Source: Adapted from American Thoracic Society. Targeted tuberculin testing and treatment of latent tuberculosis infection. *MMWR Morb Mortal Wbly Rep* 2000;49:1–51; Centers for Disease Control and Prevention. Update: fatal and severe liver injuries associated with rifampin and pyrazinamide for latent tuberculosis infection, and revisions in American Thoracic Society/CDC recommendations—United States, 2001. *MMWR Morb Mortal Wbly Rep* 2001;50:733–735.

monthly basis, and they should be informed of the signs and symptoms of hepatitis before therapy is initiated. Routine laboratory testing is not necessary for most patients; however, the hepatic transaminases should be measured at baseline and on a regular basis thereafter in patients with chronic liver disease, women who are pregnant, HIV-positive patients, and patients who are likely to continue drinking alcohol while on therapy (76).

Two metaanalyses of the results of treatment of latent TB infection in HIV-positive patients found that INH therapy for the treatment of latent TB infection in HIV-positive patients is associated with a 60% to 76% reduction in the subsequent development of active TB (201,202).

The use of a 2-month regimen of rifampin/pyrazinamide in HIV-positive patients was evaluated in three trials (203–205). Rifampin/pyrazinamide was shown to be equivalent to INH in all three studies, and the 2-month regimen was associated with a higher rate of compliance than INH-containing regimens. Moreover, the rifampin/pyrazinamide regimen was well tolerated in all three trials and was not associated with a higher rate of adverse effects than an INH-

containing regimen. Based largely on the results of these trials, the ATS and CDC approved the use of the 2-month rifampin/pyrazinamide regimen in HIV-positive patients in 2000 (76). However, a subsequent report of 21 cases of severe hepatitis that resulted in five deaths in patients on the 2-month regimen prompted concerns about safety (206), and the ATS and CDC guidelines were revised to indicate that rifampin/pyrazinamide must be used with caution and that the hepatic transaminases of patients should be measured at baseline and every 2 weeks during therapy.

Other preventive regimens, including rifampin only and rifampin/INH, have been less well evaluated in clinical trials. The use of both regimens for 3 months was found to be equivalent to 6 months of INH in a single randomized clinical trial (81), and rifampin/INH for 4 months has been used in England with encouraging results (207). Rifampin-containing regimens are particularly attractive in areas where the rate of INH resistance is high (208); however, a direct comparison with longer INH regimens (>6 months) and between the different types of rifampin regimens has not been published, and their use should be restricted to specific situations (i.e., exposure to a person with known INH-resistant TB, inability to tolerate INH or pyrazinamide).

TREATMENT OF LATENT TUBERCULOSIS INFECTION

Summary Statement	Level of Evidence
All patients with latent TB infection based on interpretation of the skin test reaction (Table 20.1), regardless of age, should receive preventative treatment.	Multiple observational studies
Nine months of INH, given daily or twice daily, is the preferred regimen for the treatment of latent TB infection.	Single randomized clinical trial and post hoc analysis of data from another clinical trial
Rifampin/pyrazinamide for 2 months is an acceptable regimen alternative in patients who cannot take INH but **must be used with caution.**	Multiple randomized clinical studies
A rifampin-only regimen, given for 4 months, may be used in patients who cannot tolerate an INH or rifampin/pyrazinamide regimen.	Single randomized trial and consensus expert opinion
All HIV-positive patients with positive skin test results should be treated for latent TB infection.	Two well-designed metaanalyses

INH, isoniazid; TB, tuberculosis.

Bacille Calmette-Guérin Vaccination

Bacille Calmette-Guérin is an attenuated vaccine that was prepared from a single strain of *M. bovis* in 1921 but today exists as a variety of vaccine strains. Despite sharing a common origin, these vaccines differ phenotypically and genetically as a result of repeated subculture and the use of different culture techniques (209). Studies have demonstrated that BCG vaccination confers a level of resistance to primary TB infection that varies from zero to 80% (210); differences in the protocols and vaccine strains used in individual studies may account for differences in the reported outcomes.

Two metaanalyses regarding the efficacy of the BCG vaccine have been published (211,212). Rodrigues and colleagues (211) found that the heterogeneity of the included studies was too great to allow a determination of the protective efficacy of the vaccine against pulmonary TB, but that the vaccine conferred an 86% level of protection against miliary/meningeal TB. Colditz and colleagues (212) reached a similar conclusion and also determined that the vaccine could prevent up to 51% of cases of pulmonary TB.

The benefit of vaccination in both analyses was primarily assessed in infants, and neither study was able to determine adequately whether BCG vaccination confers a similar level of protection in adults or what the durability of protection might be. Because of variability in the vaccine strains, uncertainty regarding efficacy, the fact that BCG vaccination does nothing in respect to latent TB infection, and the fact

that vaccination often causes skin test conversion, thereby undermining skin testing as a surveillance tool, current expert panels have recommended against the routine use of BCG vaccine in the United States (213). However, BCG vaccination may be warranted in infants and children who cannot be removed from a high-exposure environment (e.g., a caretaker with known active TB) or in health care workers employed in an institution where TB is endemic and the rate of MDR-TB is high.

DISEASE CAUSED BY NONTUBERCULOUS MYCOBACTERIA

More than 50 different species of nontuberculous mycobacteria have been identified; however, only a handful of these have been routinely implicated in human disease. A variety of approaches to classifying nontuberculous mycobacteria have been published, including some based on an organism's responsiveness to antimicrobial therapy (214) or the location of disease (215), but the original system published by Runyon (216) has remained the most commonly cited method for classifying the nontuberculous mycobacteria, although new genetic approaches to classification may alter this. In the Runyon system, nontuberculous mycobacteria are classified according to their physical appearance on agar plates and their rate of growth (Table 20.9). Group I

TABLE 20.9. NONTUBERCULOUS MYCOBACTERIA AS ORIGINALLY CLASSIFIED BY RUNYON

Group	Species
Runyon group I (photochromogens)	*Mycobacterium kansasii*[a] *Mycobacterium marinum*[a] *Mycobacterium simiae*[a] *Mycobacterium asiaticum*[a]
Runyon group II (scotochromogens)	*Mycobacterium scrofulaceum*[a] *Mycobacterium szulgae*[a] *Mycobacterium gordonae* *Mycobacterium flavescens*
Runyon group III (nonchromogens)	*Mycobacterium avium-intracellulare complex*[a] *Mycobacterium xenopi*[a] *Mycobacterium malmoense*[a] *Mycobacterium ulcerans*[a] *Mycobacterium haemophilum*[a] *Mycobacterium gastri* *Mycobacterium terrae* *Mycobacterium triviale*
Runyon group IV (Rapidly growing)	*Mycobacterium fortuitum*[a] *Mycobacterium chelonae*[a] *Mycobacterium abscessus*[a] *Mycobacterium septicum*[a] *Mycobacterium phlei* *Mycobacterium smegmatis* *Mycobacterium vaccae*

[a]Potential human pathogens.
Source: From Runyon EH. Anonymous mycobacteria in pulmonary disease. *Med Clin North Am* 1959;43:273–282, with permission.

(photochromogens) are slow-growing organisms that form pigment when grown in light, group II (scotochromogens) are slow-growing organisms that form pigment when grown in the dark, group III (nonchromogens) are slow-growing organisms that do not form pigment, and group IV are rapidly growing organisms.

Epidemiology

Nontuberculous mycobacteria are free-living saprophytic organisms that have been recovered from such varied environmental sources as surface water, soil, milk and food products, and both domestic and wild animals (217,218). The isolation of various species of nontuberculous mycobacteria from commercial and nosocomial water systems has been well described (218). Although some strains of *M. avium-intracellulare* complex (MAC) possess plasmid-derived virulence factors that enhance their aerosolization (219), patient-to-patient transmission of the nontuberculous mycobacteria has not been well documented, and it is likely that the vast majority of infections caused by these organisms are environmentally acquired, so that the isolation of patients with nontuberculous mycobacterial infection is unnecessary.

Population studies have shown that the geographic distribution of the various species of nontuberculous mycobacteria species varies substantially. For example, *M. malmoense* appears to be restricted to northwestern Europe, whereas MAC is widely distributed throughout the globe (218). However, even MAC varies geographically, as shown in a U.S. study; when population skin testing was performed with PPD-B, derived from an antigen from *M. intracellulare,* it was found that skin reactors tended to be concentrated in the southeastern region of the country (220). In a subsequent study, published by Good and Snider (221), MAC was recovered more commonly in clinical isolates from the southeastern United States, whereas *M. kansasii* was more often recovered in clinical isolates from the central United States.

The exact frequency of disease caused by nontuberculous mycobacteria remains unknown because these infections are not reported, and many isolates are not associated with disease (222–224). O'Brien and colleagues (222) estimated the nationwide rate of nontuberculous mycobacterial infection in the United States to be 1.78 cases per 100,000 persons between 1981 and 1983. Thirty-eight percent of cases reported in this study were felt to represent true infection, and of these, MAC (62.0%), *M. kansasii* (24.0%), *M. fortuitum* (4.6%), *M. chelonae* (3.2%), *M. marinum* (2.5%), and *M. scrofulaceum* (2.2%) accounted for 98.5% of all isolates. Similarly, the study of Tsukamura and colleagues (223) found a rate of nontuberculous mycobacterial infection of 1.73 cases per 100,000 persons, and, as in the United States, MAC (74.5%) and *M. kansasii* (19.6%) accounted for the majority of isolates recovered from clinical specimens. In contrast, Debrunner and colleagues (224) found a lower rate of infection caused by nontuberculous mycobac-

teria in Switzerland (0.9 cases per 100,000) and a wider distribution of disease caused by the specific nontuberculous mycobacterial species: MAC (38.2%), *M. kansasii* (26.5%), *M. xenopi* (11.8%), *M. malmoense* (8.8%), and *M. fortuitum* (5.9%).

The epidemiology of nontuberculous mycobacterial infection in immunosuppressed patients differs from that in immunocompetent patients. First, AIDS patients with nontuberculous mycobacterial infection are much more evenly distributed throughout in the United States than immunocompetent patients with nontuberculous mycobacterial infection (225), and despite the environmental ubiquity of the organisms, infection with nontuberculous mycobacteria in immunosuppressed patients remains an uncommon event in the developing world (218). Second, disseminated nontuberculous mycobacterial infection is much more likely to develop in immunosuppressed than in immunocompetent patients, who typically present with localized infection.

Horsburgh and Selik (225) found that disseminated infection with nontuberculous mycobacteria developed in 5.5% of the AIDS patients diagnosed between 1981 and 1987, the vast majority of which were caused by MAC (96.1%). MAC infection is rare in patients with $CD4^+$ cell counts above $200/mm^3$ and is seen almost exclusively in patients with $CD4^+$ cell counts below $100/mm^3$; it has been estimated that AIDS patients with a $CD4^+$ cell count below this number who do not receive prophylaxis have a 20% chance of acquiring disseminated MAC infection per year (226,227). More than 90% of disseminated MAC infections in HIV-positive patients are caused by *M. avium*, whereas in HIV-negative patients, *M. intracellulare* accounts for 40% of clinical isolates (228).

Pathogenesis

The pathogenesis of nontuberculous mycobacterial infection is similar to that of TB, and inhalation of organisms from the environment is felt to be the primary route of infection in most patients. However, ingestion and direct inoculation are other presumed routes of infection, especially in patients with disseminated infection or with skin and soft tissue infection.

Although most infections caused by nontuberculous mycobacteria occur in patients with impaired immunity, certain populations of patients with pulmonary disease are susceptible (229–231), and rare cases of disseminated nontuberculous mycobacterial infection have been well described in patients without an identifiable immune defect (232). Perhaps an as yet undefined immunodeficiency exists in these patients; abnormal production of IFN-γ, TNF-α, and IL-12 (233,234), in addition to mutations in the IFN-γ receptor (40), have all been reported in "seemingly immunocompetent" patients with disseminated infections caused by nontuberculous mycobacteria.

Clinical Presentation

The spectrum of clinical disease caused by nontuberculous mycobacteria can be separated into four distinct patterns:

- Pulmonary disease
- Lymphadenitis
- Skin and soft tissue infection
- Disseminated disease.

The majority of patients without HIV/AIDS present with pulmonary disease, whereas those with AIDS most commonly present with disseminated disease and only rarely with pulmonary disease.

Pulmonary Disease

The classic form of pulmonary disease caused by nontuberculous mycobacteria occurs most often in middle-aged or older men with a history of alcohol and tobacco abuse associated with underlying obstructive lung disease or another chronic lung disease, such as silicosis or asbestosis (235,236). These patients typically present with chronic cough and dyspnea, weight loss, fatigue, and malaise. Fever and hemoptysis are rare in patients presenting with early disease and are seen only in advanced disease. Radiographically, the patients present with fibronodular or fibroproductive opacities in the apical or posterior segments of the upper lobes that progress to thin-walled cavities in 80% to 95% of cases (237) (Fig. 20.7). Pleural thickening is more common than in TB, but pleural effusions and thoracic adenopathy are uncommon. MAC is the species of nontuberculous mycobacteria

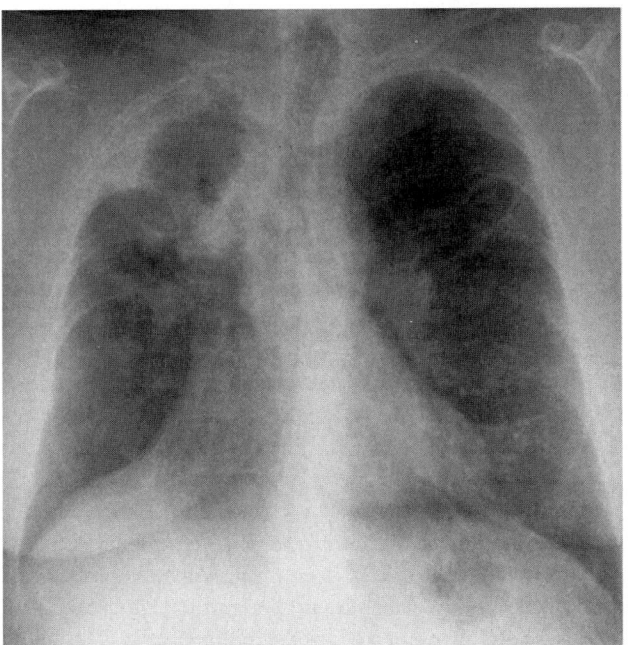

FIGURE 20.7. Pulmonary infection caused by *Mycobacterium avium* complex complicated by cavitation and pleural reaction.

most often isolated from these patients, and *M. kansasii* is the second most common isolate in the United States. In contrast, *M. xenopi* is the second most frequently isolated species in Canada and Europe, and *M. malmoense* is the second most commonly isolated species in Scandinavia (238). Other species of nontuberculous mycobacteria that have less often been implicated in this form of pulmonary disease include *M. abscessus, M. fortuitum, M. szulgae, M. simiae, M. celatum, M. asiaticum,* and *M. shimodii* (238).

In the past decade, it has become increasingly clear that a second form of pulmonary disease is caused by nontuberculous mycobacteria. In contrast to the patients with the classic form of nontuberculous mycobacterial pulmonary disease, most (80%–100%) of the patients presenting with this "nonclassic" pattern of nontuberculous mycobacterial pulmonary infection are thin older women without underlying lung disease (229,239). They most commonly present with a chronic cough in the absence of other pulmonary or constitutional symptoms (229–231), and plain radiographs may demonstrate bilateral nodular or irregular interstitial infiltrates in the lower lung zones, particularly in the right middle lobe or the lingula (237). Studies with high-resolution CT have shown that most of these patients have multiple micronodular infiltrates in addition to cylindric bronchiectasis (240–242). Cavitation is relatively uncommon early in disease but may develop within the pulmonary nodules with advancing disease. MAC has been the only nontuberculous mycobacterial species associated with this form of pulmonary disease; however, this may simply reflect the rarity with which other species of nontuberculous mycobacteria cause pulmonary disease. A subset of patients with this type, the so-called Lady Windermere syndrome (230), may present with consolidation, usually of the right middle lobe or lingula.

Extrapulmonary Disease

Disease of the superficial lymph nodes is the most common form of nontuberculous mycobacterial infection in children; the cervical or facial lymph nodes are involved in the majority of cases (243). In contrast, nontuberculous mycobacterial lymphadenitis is rare in adults, in whom TB causes most cases of lymphadenitis (244). Patients usually present with a painless, enlarging neck or face mass in the absence of constitutional symptoms. Cultures of aspirated or resected material most commonly recover MAC, and *M. scrofulaceum* is the next most commonly isolated organism; however, *M. malmoense* remains a major cause of lymphadenitis in Europe (245).

Localized infection of the skin and soft tissues is most often caused by rapidly growing nontuberculous mycobacteria, including *M. fortuitum, M. chelonae,* and *M. abscessus* (246), or *M. haemophilum* in the immunocompromised host (247). Infection occurs most commonly after traumatic inoculation, and reports of nosocomial outbreaks after surgery (248,249) or the placement of intravascular devices (250) have been published. Superficial and deep soft tissue infection with *M. marinum* following traumatic injury of persons cleaning commercial fish tanks (fish tank granuloma) or handling fish or shellfish has been well described (251). Patients typically present 2 to 3 weeks after inoculation with a papular lesion on the upper or lower extremity that subsequently ulcerates and may rarely progress to involve the local lymphatic system.

Disseminated nontuberculous mycobacterial infection in the absence of AIDS is uncommon, but patients with other inherited or acquired forms of immunosuppression, such as solid organ transplant recipients and patients with leukemia or lymphoma, are most at risk (236,252,253). The most frequently isolated nontuberculous mycobacterial species in disseminated infection is MAC, and in patients with AIDS, a prolonged high-grade fever associated with night sweats and evidence of extensive visceral involvement on examination and laboratory testing is the most common presentation (254). *M. kansasii, M. scrofulaceum, M. genavense,* and *M. haemophilum* cause disseminated infection less often, but the presentation is similar to that of MAC infection. The rapidly growing mycobacteria *M. chelonae* and *M. fortuitum* have also been reported to cause disseminated disease, most commonly in solid organ transplant recipients, in whom infection manifests as fever and diffuse skin involvement (253).

A hypersensitivity pneumonitis-like syndrome has been described caused by exposure to metal-working fluid contaminated with the rapidly growing nontuberculous mycobacterial species *M. immunogenum* (255).

Diagnosis

Given the ubiquity of nontuberculous mycobacteria in the environment, differentiating environmental contamination or colonization from true infection is necessary before a complex and prolonged course of therapy can be initiated. Recommendations for the diagnosis of pulmonary infection caused by nontuberculous mycobacteria have been published and rely on the presence of clinical, radiologic, and bacteriologic criteria (238) (Table 20.10). The microbiologic techniques described for TB should be used (see section "Identification of the Organism"), and liquid broth media are preferred over solid media, although special culture techniques are required in patients suspected of being infected with *M. haemophilum* or *M. genavense* (238).

Drug susceptibility testing is less helpful for nontuberculous mycobacterial infection than for TB, and its routine use in all cases of nontuberculous mycobacterial infection is discouraged (238). Specific situations in which susceptibility testing is of benefit include the following: (a) Isolates from patients with a documented infection caused by MAC who have received prior macrolide prophylaxis or have failed treatment with a regimen that includes a macrolide should be tested for sensitivity to clarithromycin; (b) isolates from pa-

TABLE 20.10. RECOMMENDED CRITERIA FOR DETERMINING THE PRESENCE OF CLINICAL INFECTION CAUSED BY NONTUBERCULOUS MYCOBACTERIA

Criteria[a]	Description
Clinical	1. Compatible signs and symptoms, such as cough and dyspnea
	2. Absence of other diseases, such as tuberculosis or cancer
Radiologic	1. Progressive infiltrates
	2. Cavitation or nodules on plain radiographs
	3. Multiple nodules and bronchiectasis on high-resolution computed tomography
Bacteriologic	1. Repeated strongly positive AFB smears ($\geq 2^+$) or cultures from sputum
	2. Large number of organisms on culture of a bronchial wash
	3. Growth of organisms from culture of a tissue biopsy specimen

[a] One finding from each criterion must be present to arrive at a clinical diagnosis.
AFB, acid-fast bacillus.
Source: From the American Thoracic Society. Diagnosis and treatment of disease caused by nontuberculous mucobacteria. *Am J Respir Crit Care Med* 1997;156: S1–S25, with permission.

tients who have documented infection caused by *M. kansasii* should be tested for susceptibility to rifampin only because sensitivity to other anti-TB medications is predictably high; and (c) isolates from patients with documented infection caused by a rapidly growing mycobacterial species should not be tested against any of the anti-TB medications but instead should be subjected to "routine" antimicrobial susceptibility testing against amikacin, doxycycline, clarithromycin, cefoxitin, sulfonamides, and ciprofloxacin.

The diagnosis of extrapulmonary nontuberculous mycobacterial infection relies on many of the bacteriologic techniques previously described; however, several aspects of the diagnosis deserve mention. Fine needle aspirates of lymph nodes of patients with suspected lymphadenitis are positive on culture in only 50% of cases, and definitive diagnosis often relies on complete excisional biopsy because simple incisional biopsy may result in a chronically draining sinus tract (243). The diagnosis of disseminated MAC infection is often confirmed by isolation from blood cultures (with the use of lysis centrifugation); lymph node or bone marrow biopsy may be required in some cases, particularly those caused by other species of nontuberculous mycobacteria.

Treatment

Recommendations for the treatment of nontuberculous mycobacterial infections have been published by the ATS and are summarized in Table 20.11. In contrast to MTB, only a few NTM species are sensitive to primary anti-TB drugs, and of these, *M. kansasii, M. xenopi, M. malmoense,* and

TABLE 20.11. RECOMMENDED TREATMENT REGIMENS FOR INFECTIONS CAUSED BY NONTUBERCULOUS MYCOBACTERIA

Organism	Recommended Regimen	Alternative Drugs	Duration of Regimen
Mycobacterium avium complex	Clarithromycin 500 mg PO bid + Rifabutin 300 mg PO qd + Ethambutol 25 mg/kg PO qd for 2 months then 15 mg/kg PO qd +/− Streptomycin 25–30 mg/kg PO twice/thrice weekly for first 2–3 months of therapy	Azithromycin 250 mg PO qd Rifampin 600 mg PO qd	Treat for 12 months after sputum cultures have become negative.
Mycobacterium kansasii	Isoniazid 300 mg PO qd + Rifampin 600 mg PO qd + Ethambutol 25 mg/kg PO qd for 2 months then 15 mg/kg PO qd	Clarithromycin 500 mg PO bid Sulfamethoxazole 1 g PO tid[a] + Streptomycin 25–30 mg/kg PO twice/thrice weekly for first 2 months of therapy[a]	Treat for 18 months with at least 12 months of sputum negativity.
Mycobacterium xenopi	Same as for *M. avium* complex		
Mycobacterium malmoense	Same as for *M. avium* complex		
Mycobacterium abscessus[b]	Administer two active drugs concurrently: Amikacin 10–15 mg/kg IV in divided doses Cefoxitin 12 g/d IV in divided doses Imipenem 2–4 g/d IV in divided doses		Treatment for 2–4 week will usually result in improvement, but 4–6 months is probably necessary for cure.
Mycobacterium fortuitum[b]	Administer two active drugs concurrently: Clarithromycin 500 mg PO bid Ciprofloxacin 500 mg PO bid *or* Ofloxacin 400 mg PO qd Doxycycline 100 mg PO bid *or* Minocycline 100 mg PO bid Trimethoprim/sulfamethoxazole 180/800 mg PO bid		Usually, 6–12 months of therapy is necessary for cure.

[a] This combination should be used for rifampin-resistant cases, in which case, high-dose isoniazid (900 mg PO qd) and ethambutol (25 mg/kg) should be administered concurrently.
[b] Initial antimicrobial therapy should always be based on the results of sensitivity testing.
Source: From the American Thoracic Society, Diagnosis and treatment of disease caused by nontuberculous mycobacteria. *Am J Respir Crit Care Med* 1997;156:S1–S25, with permission.

M. szulgai appear to be most susceptible to INH, rifampin, and ethambutol. However, when a patient with *M. malmoense* is treated, streptomycin should be considered as a replacement for INH because INH may be less effective in infections caused by this bacillus. It should be noted that pyrazinamide has no role in the treatment of nontuberculous mycobacterial infections.

The treatment of infections caused by MAC remains difficult despite the introduction of new antimicrobials and varies with the site of infection. Lymphadenitis caused by MAC is best managed by surgical resection because studies of medical therapy have demonstrated failure rates that approach 50% (256). Therapy for disseminated MAC infection is managed by a regimen that includes at least three drugs—clarithromycin, ethambutol, and rifabutin (257). Despite isolated reports of success (258), treatment of pulmonary disease caused by MAC has traditionally been associated with high rates of failure and relapse (259). The introduction of clarithromycin-containing regimens has the potential to revolutionize the management of this difficult infection.

For example, uncontrolled prospective trials have demonstrated that clarithromycin, either alone or in combination with other drugs, sterilizes sputum in 84% to 92% of patients with MAC isolates initially susceptible to clarithromycin and who complete at least 3 to 6 months of therapy (260–262). Although wild strains of MAC are consistently sensitive to clarithromycin, monotherapy is not recommended because high rates of resistance emerge during the course of therapy (256,261).

The management of infections caused by rapidly growing nontuberculous mycobacteria is unique in that these species are nearly uniformly resistant to anti-TB drugs. Instead, the "traditional" antimicrobials, such as sulfonamides, amikacin, cefoxitin, minocycline, imipenem, macrolides, and the fluoroquinolones, appear to be the most active against these organisms. Of the three most commonly isolated species, *M. fortuitum* is most consistently susceptible to available antimicrobials, whereas *M. abscessus* most often displays the highest levels of resistance, with *M. chelonae* somewhere in between. Therefore, it is imperative that isolates from all clinically documented infections caused by these organisms be subjected to susceptibility testing and that empiric regimens include at least two drugs against which the isolate is likely to be susceptible (238).

REFERENCES

1. Raviglione MC, Snider DE, Kochi A. Global epidemiology of tuberculosis. Morbidity and mortality of a worldwide epidemic. *JAMA* 1995;273:220–226.
2. Pablos-Mendez A, Raviglione MC, Laszlo A, et al. Global surveillance for antituberculosis drug resistance, 1994–1997. World Health Organization–International Union against Tuberculosis and Lung Disease Working Group on Antituberculosis Drug Resistance Surveillance. *N Engl J Med* 1998;338:1641–1649.
3. Cantwell MF, Snider DE Jr, Cauthen GM, et al. Epidemiology of tuberculosis in the United States, 1985 through 1992. *JAMA* 1994;272:535–539.
4. Rieder HL, Zellweger JP, Raviglione MC, et al. Tuberculosis control in Europe and international migration. *Eur Respir J* 1994;7:1545–1553.
5. McKenna MT, McCray E, Onorato I. The epidemiology of tuberculosis among foreign-born persons in the United States, 1986 to 1993. *N Engl J Med* 1995;332:1071–1076.
6. Raviglione MC, Harries AD, Msiska R, et al. Tuberculosis and HIV: current status in Africa. *AIDS* 1997;11:S115–S123.
7. Girardi E, Raviglione MC, Antonucci G, et al. Impact of the HIV epidemic on the spread of other diseases: the case of tuberculosis. *AIDS* 2000;14:S47–S56.
8. Centers for Disease Control and Prevention. Reported tuberculosis in the United States, 2000. Available at *http://www.cdc.gov/nchstp/tb/surv/surv2000/*, 2001.
9. Centers for Disease Control and Prevention. Tuberculosis morbidity—United States, 1992. *MMWR Morb Mortal Wkly Rep* 1993;42:696–697, 703–704.
10. Barr RG, Diez-Roux AV, Knirsch CA, et al. Neighborhood poverty and the resurgence of tuberculosis in New York City, 1984–1992. *Am J Public Health* 2001;91:1487–1493.
11. Moss AR, Hahn JA, Tulsky JP, et al. Tuberculosis in the homeless. A prospective study. *Am J Respir Crit Care Med* 2000;162:460–464.
12. Brudney K, Dobkin J. Resurgent tuberculosis in New York City. Human immunodeficiency virus, homelessness, and the decline of tuberculosis control programs. *Am Rev Respir Dis* 1991;144:745–749.
13. Zuber PL, McKenna MT, Binkin NJ, et al. Long-term risk of tuberculosis among foreign-born persons in the United States. *JAMA* 1997;278:304–307.
14. Alland D, Kalkut GE, Moss AR, et al. Transmission of tuberculosis in New York City. An analysis by DNA fingerprinting and conventional epidemiologic methods. *N Engl J Med* 1994;330:1710–1716.
15. Small PM, Hopewell PC, Singh SP, et al. The epidemiology of tuberculosis in San Francisco. A population-based study using conventional and molecular methods. *N Engl J Med* 1994;330:1703–1709.
16. Selwyn PA, Hartel D, Lewis VA, et al. A prospective study of the risk of tuberculosis among intravenous drug users with human immunodeficiency virus infection. *N Engl J Med* 1989;320:545–550.
17. Markowitz N, Hansen NI, Hopewell PC, et al. Incidence of tuberculosis in the United States among HIV-infected persons. The Pulmonary Complications of HIV Infection Study Group. *Ann Intern Med* 1997;126:123–132.
18. Antonucci G, Girardi E, Raviglione MC, et al. Risk factors for tuberculosis in HIV-infected persons. A prospective cohort study. The Gruppo Italiano di Studio Tubercolosi e AIDS (GISTA). *JAMA* 1995;274:143–148.
19. Goble M, Iseman MD, Madsen LA, et al. Treatment of 171 patients with pulmonary tuberculosis resistant to isoniazid and rifampin. *N Engl J Med* 1993;328:527–532.
20. Mahmoudi A, Iseman MD. Pitfalls in the care of patients with tuberculosis. Common errors and their association with the acquisition of drug resistance. *JAMA* 1993;270:65–68.
21. Garcia-Garcia ML, Ponce de Leon A, Jimenez-Corona ME, et al. Clinical consequences and transmissibility of drug-resistant tuberculosis in southern Mexico. *Arch Intern Med* 2000;160:630–636.
22. Bloch AB, Cauthen GM, Onorato IM, et al. Nationwide survey of drug-resistant tuberculosis in the United States. *JAMA* 1994;271:665–671.
23. Dannenberg AM. Pathophysiology: basic aspects. In: Schlossberg D, ed. *Tuberculosis and nontuberculous mycobacterial infections.* Philadelphia: WB Saunders, 1999:17–47.
24. Scott P, Trinchieri G. The role of natural killer cells in host-parasite interactions. *Curr Opin Immunol* 1995;7:34–40.
25. Barnes PF, Grisso CL, Abrams JS, et al. Gamma delta T lymphocytes in human tuberculosis. *J Infect Dis* 1992;165:506–512.
26. D'Souza CD, Cooper AM, Frank AA, et al. An anti-inflammatory role for gamma delta T lymphocytes in acquired immunity to *Mycobacterium tuberculosis. J Immunol* 1997;158:1217–1221.
27. Flynn JL, Chan J. Immunology of tuberculosis. *Annu Rev Immunol* 2001;19:93–129.
28. Smith DW, McMurray DN, Wiegeshaus EH, et al. Host-parasite relationships in experimental airborne tuberculosis. IV. Early events in the course of infection in vaccinated and nonvaccinated guinea pigs. *Am Rev Respir Dis* 1970;102:937–949.
29. Smith DW, Wiegeshaus EH. What animal models can teach us about the pathogenesis of tuberculosis in humans. *Rev Infect Dis* 1989;11:S385–S393.
30. Ellner JJ. Review: the immune response in human tuberculosis—implications for tuberculosis control. *J Infect Dis* 1997;176:1351–1359.
31. Balasubramanian V, Wiegeshaus EH, Taylor BT, et al. Pathogenesis of tuberculosis: pathway to apical localization. *Tuber Lung Dis* 1994;75:168–178.
32. Zhang M, Gong J, Iyer DV, et al. T cell cytokine responses in persons with tuberculosis and human immunodeficiency virus infection. *J Clin Invest* 1994;94:2435–2442.
33. Havlir DV, Barnes PF. Tuberculosis in patients with human immunodeficiency virus infection. *N Engl J Med* 1999;340:367–373.
34. Valway SE, Sanchez MP, Shinnick TF, et al. An outbreak involving extensive transmission of a virulent strain of *Mycobacterium tuberculosis. N Engl J Med* 1998;338:633–639.
35. Zhang M, Gong J, Yang Z, et al. Enhanced capacity of a widespread strain of *Mycobacterium tuberculosis* to grow in human macrophages. *J Infect Dis* 1999;179:1213–1217.
36. Sieling PA, Wang XH, Gately MK, et al. IL-12 regulates T helper type 1 cytokine responses in human infectious disease. *J Immunol* 1994;153:3639–3647.
37. Altare F, Durandy A, Lammas D, et al. Impairment of mycobacterial immunity in human interleukin-12 receptor deficiency. *Science* 1998;280:1432–1435.
38. De Jong R, Altare F, Haagen IA, et al. Severe mycobacterial and *Salmonella* infections in interleukin-12 receptor–deficient patients. *Science* 1998;280:1435–1438.
39. Keane J, Gershon S, Wise RP, et al. Tuberculosis associated

with infliximab, a tumor necrosis factor alpha-neutralizing agent. *N Engl J Med* 2001;345:1098–1104.

40. Newport MJ, Huxley CM, Huston S, et al. A mutation in the interferon-gamma-receptor gene and susceptibility to mycobacterial infection. *N Engl J Med* 1996;335:1941–1949.

41. Dupuis S, Doffinger R, Picard C, et al. Human interferon-gamma–mediated immunity is a genetically controlled continuous trait that determines the outcome of mycobacterial invasion. *Immunol Rev* 2000;178:129–137.

42. Goldfeld AE, Delgado JC, Thim S, et al. Association of an HLA-DQ allele with clinical tuberculosis. *JAMA* 1998;279:226–228.

43. Bellamy R, Ruwende C, Corrah T, et al. Variations in the NRAMP1 gene and susceptibility to tuberculosis in West Africans. *N Engl J Med* 1998;338:640–644.

44. Perez-Guzman C, Vargas MH, Torres-Cruz A, et al. Does aging modify pulmonary tuberculosis?: A meta-analytical review. *Chest* 1999;116:961–967.

45. Couser JI Jr, Glassroth J. Tuberculosis. An epidemic in older adults. *Clin Chest Med* 1993;14:491–499.

46. Small PM, Schecter GF, Goodman PC, et al. Treatment of tuberculosis in patients with advanced human immunodeficiency virus infection. *N Engl J Med* 1991;324:289–294.

47. Jones BE, Young SM, Antoniskis D, et al. Relationship of the manifestations of tuberculosis to CD4 cell counts in patients with human immunodeficiency virus infection. *Am Rev Respir Dis* 1993;148:1292–1297.

48. Epstein DM, Kline LR, Albelda SM, et al. Tuberculous pleural effusions. *Chest* 1987;91:106–109.

49. Relkin F, Aranda CP, Garay SM, et al. Pleural tuberculosis and HIV infection. *Chest* 1994;105:1338–1341.

50. Valdes L, Alvarez D, San Jose E, et al. Tuberculous pleurisy: a study of 254 patients. *Arch Intern Med* 1998;158:2017–2021.

51. Ferrer J. Pleural tuberculosis. *Eur Respir J* 1997;10:942–947.

52. Kirsch CM, Kroe DM, Azzi RL, et al. The optimal number of pleural biopsy specimens for a diagnosis of tuberculous pleurisy. *Chest* 1997;112:702–706.

53. Maartens G, Willcox PA, Benatar SR. Miliary tuberculosis: rapid diagnosis, hematologic abnormalities, and outcome in 109 treated adults. *Am J Med* 1990;89:291–296.

54. Sharma SK, Mohan A, Pande JN, et al. Clinical profile, laboratory characteristics and outcome in miliary tuberculosis. *QJM* 1995;88:29–37.

55. Sydow M, Schauer A, Crozier TA, et al. Multiple organ failure in generalized disseminated tuberculosis. *Respir Med* 1992;86:517–519.

56. Rietbroek RC, Dahlmans RP, Smedts F, et al. Tuberculosis cutis miliaris disseminata as a manifestation of miliary tuberculosis: literature review and report of a case of recurrent skin lesions. *Rev Infect Dis* 1991;13:265–269.

57. Hunt BJ, Andrews V, Pettingale KW. The significance of pancytopenia in miliary tuberculosis. *Postgrad Med J* 1987;63:801–804.

58. Bouza E, Diaz-Lopez MD, Moreno S, et al. *Mycobacterium tuberculosis* bacteremia in patients with and without human immunodeficiency virus infection. *Arch Intern Med* 1993;153:496–500.

59. Lau SK, Wei WI, Kwan S, et al. Combined use of fine-needle aspiration cytologic examination and tuberculin skin test in the diagnosis of cervical tuberculous lymphadenitis. A prospective study. *Arch Otolaryngol Head Neck Surg* 1991;117:87–90.

60. Lau SK, Wei WI, Hsu C, et al. Efficacy of fine needle aspiration cytology in the diagnosis of tuberculous cervical lymphadenopathy. *J Laryngol Otol* 1990;104:24–27.

61. Pertuiset E, Beaudreuil J, Liote F, et al. Spinal tuberculosis in adults. A study of 103 cases in a developed country. *Medicine (Baltimore)* 1999;78:309–320.

62. Wallace R, Cohen AS. Tuberculous arthritis. A report of two cases with review of biopsy and synovial fluid findings. *Am J Med* 1976;61:277–282.

63. Simon HB, Weinstein AJ, Pasternak MS, et al. Genitourinary tuberculosis. Clinical features in a general hospital population. *Am J Med* 1977;63:410–420.

64. Kollins SA, Hartman GW, Carr DT, et al. Roentgenographic findings in urinary tract tuberculosis. A 10-year review. *Am J Roentgenol Radium Therm Nucl Med* 1974;121:487–499.

65. Lattimer JK, Reilly RJ, Segawa A. The significance of the isolated positive urine culture in genitourinary tuberculosis. *J Urol* 1969;102:610–613.

66. Shetty A, Kane GC. Tuberculous peritonitis. In: Schlossberg D, ed. *Tuberculosis and nontuberculous mycobacterial infections.* Philadelphia: WB Saunders, 1999:234–237.

67. Shakil AO, Korula J, Kanel GC, et al. Diagnostic features of tuberculous peritonitis in the absence and presence of chronic liver disease: a case control study. *Am J Med* 1996;100:179–185.

68. Singh MM, Bhargava AN, Jain KP. Tuberculous peritonitis. An evaluation of pathogenetic mechanisms, diagnostic procedures and therapeutic measures. *N Engl J Med* 1969;281:1091–1094.

69. Demir K, Okten A, Kaymakoglu S, et al. Tuberculous peritonitis—reports of 26 cases, detailing diagnostic and therapeutic problems. *Eur J Gastroenterol Hepatol* 2001;13:581–585.

70. Al-Deeb SM, Yaqub BA, Sharif HS, et al. Neurotuberculosis: a review. *Clin Neurol Neurosurg* 1992;94:S30–S33.

71. Kent SJ, Crowe SM, Yung A, et al. Tuberculous meningitis: a 30-year review. *Clin Infect Dis* 1993;17:987–994.

72. Verdon R, Chevret S, Laissy JP, et al. Tuberculous meningitis in adults: review of 48 cases. *Clin Infect Dis* 1996;22:982–988.

73. Al Zahrani K, Al Jahdali H, Menzies D. Does size matter? Utility of size of tuberculin reactions for the diagnosis of mycobacterial disease. *Am J Respir Crit Care Med* 2000;162:1419–1422.

74. American Thoracic Society. Diagnostic standards and classification of tuberculosis in adults and children. *Am J Respir Crit Care Med* 2000;161:1376–1395.

75. Menzies D. What does tuberculin reactivity after bacille Calmette-Guérin vaccination tell us? *Clin Infect Dis* 2000;31:S71–S74.

76. American Thoracic Society. Targeted tuberculin testing and treatment of latent tuberculosis infection. *MMWR Morb Mortal Wkly Rep* 2000;49:1–51.

77. Thompson NJ, Glassroth JL, Snider DE Jr, et al. The booster phenomenon in serial tuberculin testing. *Am Rev Respir Dis* 1979;119:587–597.

78. Markowitz N, Hansen NI, Wilcosky TC, et al. Tuberculin and anergy testing in HIV-seropositive and HIV-seronegative persons. Pulmonary Complications of HIV Infection Study Group. *Ann Intern Med* 1993;119:185–193.

79. Huebner RE, Schein MF, Bass JB Jr. The tuberculin skin test. *Clin Infect Dis* 1993;17:968–975.

80. Steinbruck P, Dankova D, Edwards LB, et al. The risk of tuberculosis in patients with fibrous lesions radiographically diagnosed. *Bull Int Union against Tuberculosis* 1972;47:144–171.

81. Hong Kong Chest Service/British Medical Research Council. A double-blind placebo-controlled clinical trial of three antituberculosis chemoprophylaxis regimens in patients with silicosis in Hong Kong. *Am Rev Respir Dis* 1992;145:36–41.

82. Mazurek GH, LoBue PA, Daley CL, et al. Comparison of a whole-blood interferon-gamma assay with tuberculin skin testing

for detecting latent *Mycobacterium tuberculosis* infection. *JAMA* 2001;286:1740–1747.

83. Choyke PL, Sostman HD, Curtis AM, et al. Adult-onset pulmonary tuberculosis. *Radiology* 1983;148:357–362.

84. McAdams HP, Erasmus J, Winter JA. Radiologic manifestations of pulmonary tuberculosis. *Radiol Clin North Am* 1995;33:655–678.

85. Miller WT. Tuberculosis in the normal host: radiological findings. *Semin Roentgenol* 1993;28:109–118.

86. Jones BE, Ryu R, Yang Z, et al. Chest radiographic findings in patients with tuberculosis with recent or remote infection. *Am J Respir Crit Care Med* 1997;156:1270–1273.

87. Im JG, Itoh H, Shim YS, et al. Pulmonary tuberculosis: CT findings—early active disease and sequential change with antituberculous therapy. *Radiology* 1993;186:653–660.

88. Perlman DC, El-Sadr W, Nelson ET, et al. Variation of chest radiographic patterns in pulmonary tuberculosis by degree of human immunodeficiency virus-related immunosuppression. *Clin Infect Dis* 1997;25:242–246.

89. Greenberg SD, Frager D, Suster B, et al. Active pulmonary tuberculosis in patients with AIDS: spectrum of radiographic findings (including a normal appearance). *Radiology* 1994;193:115–119.

90. Warren JR, Bhattacharya M, De Almeida KN, et al. A minimum of 5.0 mL of sputum improves the sensitivity of acid-fast smear for *Mycobacterium tuberculosis*. *Am J Respir Crit Care Med* 2000;161:1559–1562.

91. Salfinger M, Pfyffer GE. The new diagnostic mycobacteriology laboratory. *Eur J Clin Microbiol Infect Dis* 1994;13:961–979.

92. Greenbaum M, Beyt BE Jr, Murray PR. The accuracy of diagnosing pulmonary tuberculosis at a teaching hospital. *Am Rev Respir Dis* 1980;121:477–481.

93. Roberts GD, Goodman NL, Heifets L, et al. Evaluation of the BACTEC radiometric method for recovery of mycobacteria and drug susceptibility testing of *Mycobacterium tuberculosis* from acid-fast smear-positive specimens. *J Clin Microbiol* 1983;18:689–696.

94. Anargyros P, Astill DS, Lim IS. Comparison of improved BACTEC and Lowenstein-Jensen media for culture of mycobacteria from clinical specimens. *J Clin Microbiol* 1990;28:1288–1291.

95. Kanchana MV, Cheke D, Natyshak I, et al. Evaluation of the BACTEC MGIT 960 system for the recovery of mycobacteria. *Diagn Microbiol Infect Dis* 2000;37:31–36.

96. Wilson ML, Stone BL, Hildred MV, et al. Comparison of recovery rates for mycobacteria from BACTEC 12B vials, Middlebrook 7H11-selective 7H11 biplates, and Lowenstein-Jensen slants in a public health mycobacteriology laboratory. *J Clin Microbiol* 1995;33:2516–2518.

97. Ehlers S, Pirmann M, Zaki W, et al. Evaluation of a commercial ribosomal-RNA target amplification assay for detection of *Mycobacterium tuberculosis* complex in respiratory specimens. *Eur J Clin Microbiol Infect Dis* 1994;13:827–829.

98. Miller N, Hernandez SG, Cleary TJ. Evaluation of Gen-Probe amplified *Mycobacterium tuberculosis* direct test and PCR for direct detection of *Mycobacterium tuberculosis* in clinical specimens. *J Clin Microbiol* 1994;32:393–397.

99. Beavis KG, Lichty MB, Jungkind DL, et al. Evaluation of Amplicor PCR for direct detection of *Mycobacterium tuberculosis* from sputum specimens. *J Clin Microbiol* 1995;33:2582–2586.

100. Zolnir-Dovc M, Poljak M, Seme K, et al. Evaluation of two commercial amplification assays for the detection of *Mycobacterium tuberculosis* complex in respiratory specimens. *Infection* 1995;23:216–221.

101. Bennedsen J, Thomsen VO, Pfyffer GE, et al. Utility of PCR in diagnosing pulmonary tuberculosis. *J Clin Microbiol* 1996;34:1407–1411.

102. Fairfax MR. Evaluation of the Gen-Probe amplified *Mycobacterium tuberculosis* direct detection test. *Am J Clin Pathol* 1996;106:594–599.

103. Portaels F, Serruys E, De Beenhouwer H, et al. Evaluation of the Gen-Probe amplified *Mycobacterium tuberculosis* direct test for the routine diagnosis of pulmonary tuberculosis. *Acta Clin Belg* 1996;51:144–149.

104. American Thoracic Society. Rapid diagnostic tests for tuberculosis: what is the appropriate use? *Am J Respir Crit Care Med* 1997;155:1804–1814.

105. Brown TJ, Power EGM, French GL. Evaluation of three commercial detection systems for *Mycobacterium tuberculosis* where clinical diagnosis is difficult. *J Clin Pathol* 1999;52:193–197.

106. Al Zahrani K, Al Jahdali H, Poirier L, et al. Accuracy and utility of commercially available amplification and serologic tests for the diagnosis of minimal pulmonary tuberculosis. *Am J Respir Crit Care Med* 2000;162:1323–1329.

107. Centers for Disease Control and Prevention. Update: nucleic acid amplification test for tuberculosis. *MMWR Morb Mortal Wkly Rep* 2000;49:593–594.

108. Schluger NW. Changing approaches to the diagnosis of tuberculosis. *Am J Respir Crit Care Med* 2001;164:2020–2024.

109. Warren NG, Body BA. Bacteriology and diagnosis. In: Rossman MD, MacGregor RR, eds. *Tuberculosis.* New York: McGraw-Hill, 1995:35–56.

110. Zheng X, Roberts GD. Diagnosis and susceptibility testing. In: Schlossberg D, ed. *Tuberculosis and nontuberculous mycobacterial infections.* Philadelphia: WB Saunders, 1999:57–64.

111. Hale YM, Pfyffer GE, Salfinger M. Laboratory diagnosis of mycobacterial infections: new tools and lessons learned. *Clin Infect Dis* 2001;33:834–846.

112. Shinnick TM, Good RC. Diagnostic mycobacteriology laboratory practices. *Clin Infect Dis* 1995;21:291–299.

113. Telenti A, Honore N, Bernasconi C, et al. Genotypic assessment of isoniazid and rifampin resistance in *Mycobacterium tuberculosis*: a blind study at reference laboratory level. *J Clin Microbiol* 1997;35:719–723.

114. Cooksey RC, Morlock GP, Glickman S, et al. Evaluation of a line probe assay kit for characterization of *rpoB* mutations in rifampin-resistant *Mycobacterium tuberculosis* isolates from New York City. *J Clin Microbiol* 1997;35:1281–1283.

115. De Oliveira HG, Rossatto ER, Prolla JC. Pleural fluid adenosine deaminase and lymphocyte proportion: clinical usefulness in the diagnosis of tuberculosis. *Cytopathology* 1994;5:27–32.

116. Burgess LJ, Maritz FJ, Le Roux I, et al. Use of adenosine deaminase as a diagnostic tool for tuberculous pleurisy. *Thorax* 1995;50:672–674.

117. Villegas MV, Labrada LA, Saravia NG. Evaluation of polymerase chain reaction, adenosine deaminase, and interferon-gamma in pleural fluid for the differential diagnosis of pleural tuberculosis. *Chest* 2000;118:1355–1364.

118. Riantawan P, Chaowalit P, Wongsangiem M, et al. Diagnostic value of pleural fluid adenosine deaminase in tuberculous pleuritis with reference to HIV coinfection and a bayesian analysis. *Chest* 1999;116:97–103.

119. Ehlers S, Ignatius R, Regnath T, et al. Diagnosis of extrapulmonary tuberculosis by Gen-Probe amplified *Mycobacterium tuberculosis* direct test. *J Clin Microbiol* 1996;34:2275–2279.

120. Pfyffer GE, Kissling P, Jahn EM, et al. Diagnostic performance of amplified *Mycobacterium tuberculosis* direct test with cerebrospinal fluid, other nonrespiratory, and respiratory specimens. *J Clin Microbiol* 1996;34:834–841.

121. Pearson ML, Jereb JA, Frieden TR, et al. Nosocomial transmission of multidrug-resistant *Mycobacterium tuberculosis*. A risk to patients and health care workers. *Ann Intern Med* 1992;117:191–196.

122. Griffith DE, Hardeman JL, Zhang Y, et al. Tuberculosis outbreak among healthcare workers in a community hospital. *Am J Respir Crit Care Med* 1995;152:808–811.

123. Jereb JA, Klevens RM, Privett TD, et al. Tuberculosis in health care workers at a hospital with an outbreak of multidrug-resistant *Mycobacterium tuberculosis*. *Arch Intern Med* 1995;155:854–859.

124. Centers for Disease Control and Prevention. Guidelines for preventing the transmission of *Mycobacterium tuberculosis* in healthcare facilities, 1994. *MMWR Morb Mortal Wkly Rep* 1994;43:1–132.

125. Maloney SA, Pearson ML, Gordon MT, et al. Efficacy of control measures in preventing nosocomial transmission of multidrug-resistant tuberculosis to patients and health care workers. *Ann Intern Med* 1995;122:90–95.

126. Riley RL, Knight M, Middlebrook G. Ultraviolet susceptibility of BCG and virulent tubercle bacilli. *Am Rev Respir Dis* 1976;113:413–418.

127. Nardell EA. Interrupting transmission from patients with unsuspected tuberculosis: a unique role for upper-room ultraviolet air disinfection. *Am J Infect Control* 1995;23:156–164.

128. Adal KA, Anglim AM, Palumbo CL, et al. The use of high-efficiency particulate air-filter respirators to protect hospital workers from tuberculosis. A cost-effectiveness analysis. *N Engl J Med* 1994;331:169–173.

129. Nettleman MD, Fredrickson M, Good NL, et al. Tuberculosis control strategies: the cost of particulate respirators. *Ann Intern Med* 1994;121:37–40.

130. Fennelly KP, Nardell EA. The relative efficacy of respirators and room ventilation in preventing occupational tuberculosis. *Infect Control Hosp Epidemiol* 1998;19:754–759.

131. Gillespie SH. Evolution of drug resistance in *Mycobacterium tuberculosis:* clinical and molecular perspectives. *Antimicrob Agents Chemother* 2002;46:267–274.

132. Bass JB, Farer LS, Hopewell PC, et al. Treatment of tuberculosis and tuberculosis infection in adults and children. American Thoracic Society and the Centers for Disease Control and Prevention. *Am J Respir Crit Care Med* 1994;149:1359–1374.

133. Nolan CM, Goldberg SV, Buskin SE. Hepatotoxicity associated with isoniazid preventive therapy: a 7-year survey from a public health tuberculosis clinic. *JAMA* 1999;281:1014–1018.

134. Wallace RJ. Antimycobacterial agents. In: Mandell GL, Bennett JE, Dolin R, eds. *Principles and practice of infectious diseases.* New York: Churchill Livingstone, 2000:436–448.

135. Espinal MA, Laszlo A, Simonsen L, et al. Global trends in resistance to antituberculosis drugs. World Health Organization–International Union against Tuberculosis and Lung Disease Working Group on Antituberculosis Drug Resistance Surveillance. *N Engl J Med* 2001;344:1294–1303.

136. Steele MA, Burk RF, DesPrez RM. Toxic hepatitis with isoniazid and rifampin. A meta-analysis. *Chest* 1991;99:465–471.

137. Martinez E, Collazos J, Mayo J. Hypersensitivity reactions to rifampin. Pathogenetic mechanisms, clinical manifestations, management strategies, and review of the anaphylactic-like reactions. *Medicine (Baltimore)* 1999;78:361–369.

138. Tam CM, Chan SL, Lam CW, et al. Rifapentine and isoniazid in the continuation phase of treating pulmonary tuberculosis. Initial report. *Am J Respir Crit Care Med* 1998;157:1726–1733.

139. Package insert. Rifapentene (Priftin) data on file. Hoechst Marion Roussel, Kansas City, MO.

140. Bock NN, Sterling TR, Hamilton CD, et al. A prospective, randomized, double-blind study of the tolerability of rifapentine 600, 900, and 1,200 mg plus isoniazid in the continuation phase of tuberculosis treatment. *Am J Respir Crit Care Med* 2002;165:1526–1530.

141. Vernon A, Burman W, Benator D, et al. Acquired rifamycin monoresistance in patients with HIV-related tuberculosis treated with once-weekly rifapentine and isoniazid. Tuberculosis Trials Consortium. *Lancet* 1999;353:1843–1847.

142. Hong Kong Chest Service/British Medical Research Council. Five-year follow-up of a controlled trial of five 6-month regimens of chemotherapy for pulmonary tuberculosis. *Am Rev Respir Dis* 1987;136:1339–1342.

143. Steele MA, Des Prez RM. The role of pyrazinamide in tuberculosis chemotherapy. *Chest* 1988;94:845–850.

144. Combs DL, O'Brien RJ, Geiter LJ. USPHS Tuberculosis Short-Course Chemotherapy Trial 21: effectiveness, toxicity, and acceptability. The report of final results. *Ann Intern Med* 1990;112:397–406.

145. Haas DW, Des Prez RM. Current treatment and management. In: Rossman MD, MacGregor RR, eds. *Tuberculosis.* New York: McGraw-Hill, 1995:187–207.

146. Dooley DP, Carpenter JL, Rademacher S. Adjunctive corticosteroid therapy for tuberculosis: a critical reappraisal of the literature. *Clin Infect Dis* 1997;25:872–887.

147. Holland SM. Cytokine therapy of mycobacterial infections. *Adv Intern Med* 2000;45:431–452.

148. British Thoracic and Tuberculosis Association. Short-course chemotherapy in pulmonary tuberculosis. A controlled trial. *Lancet* 1976;2:1102–1104.

149. Dutt AK, Jones L, Stead WW. Short-course chemotherapy of tuberculosis with largely twice-weekly isoniazid-rifampin. *Chest* 1979;75:441–447.

150. Algerian Working Group/British Medical Research Council. Controlled clinical trial comparing a 6-month and a 12-month regimen in the treatment of pulmonary tuberculosis in the Algerian Sahara. *Am Rev Respir Dis* 1984;129:921–928.

151. East Africa/British Medical Research Council. Controlled clinical trial of four 6-month regimens of chemotherapy for pulmonary tuberculosis. Second report. *Am Rev Respir Dis* 1976;114:471–475.

152. Snider DE, Zierski M, Graczyk J, et al. Short-course tuberculosis chemotherapy studies conducted in Poland during the past decade. *Eur J Respir Dis* 1986;68:12–18.

153. Singapore Tuberculosis Service/British Medical Research Council. Five-year follow-up of a clinical trial of three 6-month regimens of chemotherapy given intermittently in the continuation phase in the treatment of pulmonary tuberculosis. *Am Rev Respir Dis* 1988;137:1147–1150.

154. Hong Kong Chest Service/British Medical Research Council. Controlled trial of 2, 4, and 6 months of pyrazinamide in 6-month, three-times-weekly regimens for smear-positive pulmonary tuberculosis, including an assessment of a combined preparation of isoniazid, rifampin, and pyrazinamide. Results at 30 months. *Am Rev Respir Dis* 1991;143:700–706.

155. Cohn DL, Catlin BJ, Peterson KL, et al. A 62-dose, 6-month therapy for pulmonary and extrapulmonary tuberculosis. A twice-weekly, directly observed, and cost-effective regimen. *Ann Intern Med* 1990;112:407–415.

156. American Thoracic Society, Centers for Disease Control and Prevention, and the Infectious Diseases Society of America. Treatment of tuberculosis. *Am J Respir Crit Care Med* 2003;167:603–662.

157. Chaulk CP, Kazandjian VA. Directly observed therapy for treatment completion of pulmonary tuberculosis. Consensus

statement of the Public Health Tuberculosis Guidelines Panel. *JAMA* 1998;279:943–948.

158. Weis SE, Slocum PC, Blais FX, et al. The effect of directly observed therapy on the rates of drug resistance and relapse in tuberculosis. *N Engl J Med* 1994;330:1179–1184.

159. Burman WJ, Dalton CB, Cohn DL, et al. A cost-effectiveness analysis of directly observed therapy vs self-administered therapy for the treatment of tuberculosis. *Chest* 1997;112:63–70.

160. American Thoracic Society. Treatment of tuberculosis and tuberculosis infection in adults and children. *Monaldi Arch Chest Dis* 1994;49:327–345.

161. Mitchison DA. Assessment of new sterilizing drugs for treating pulmonary tuberculosis by culture at 2 months. *Am Rev Respir Dis* 1993;147:1062–1063.

162. Whalen C, Horsburgh CR, Hom D, et al. Accelerated course of human immunodeficiency virus infection after tuberculosis. *Am J Respir Crit Care Med* 1995;151:129–135.

163. Centers for Disease Control and Prevention. Prevention and treatment of tuberculosis in patients infected with human immunodeficiency virus: principles of therapy and revised recommendations. *MMWR Morb Mortal Wkly Rep* 1998;47:1–58.

164. Edlin BR, Tokars JI, Grieco MH, et al. An outbreak of multidrug-resistant tuberculosis among hospitalized patients with the acquired immunodeficiency syndrome. *N Engl J Med* 1992;326:1514–1521.

165. Fischl MA, Uttamchandani RB, Daikos GL, et al. An outbreak of tuberculosis caused by multiple-drug-resistant tubercle bacilli among patients with HIV infection. *Ann Intern Med* 1992;117:177–183.

166. Coronado VG, Beck-Sague CM, Hutton MD, et al. Transmission of multidrug-resistant *Mycobacterium tuberculosis* among persons with human immunodeficiency virus infection in an urban hospital: epidemiologic and restriction fragment length polymorphism analysis. *J Infect Dis* 1993;168:1052–1055.

167. Moore M, Onorato IM, McCray E, et al. Trends in drug-resistant tuberculosis in the United States, 1993–1996. *JAMA* 1997;278:833–837.

168. Gordin FM, Nelson ET, Matts JP, et al. The impact of human immunodeficiency virus infection on drug-resistant tuberculosis. *Am J Respir Crit Care Med* 1996;154:1478–1483.

169. Kassim S, Sassan-Morokro M, Ackah A, et al. Two-year follow-up of persons with HIV-1- and HIV-2-associated pulmonary tuberculosis treated with short-course chemotherapy in West Africa. *AIDS* 1995;9:1185–1191.

170. Perriens JH, St Louis ME, Mukadi YB, et al. Pulmonary tuberculosis in HIV-infected patients in Zaire. A controlled trial of treatment for either 6 or 12 months. *N Engl J Med* 1995;332:779–784.

171. Sterling TR, Alwood K, Gachuhi R, et al. Relapse rates after short-course (6-month) treatment of tuberculosis in HIV-infected and uninfected persons. *AIDS* 1999;13:1899–1904.

172. Narita M, Hisada M, Thimmappa B, et al. Tuberculosis recurrence: multivariate analysis of serum levels of tuberculosis drugs, human immunodeficiency virus status, and other risk factors. *Clin Infect Dis* 2001;32:515–517.

173. Dean GL, Edwards SG, Ives NJ, et al. Treatment of tuberculosis in HIV-infected persons in the era of highly active antiretroviral therapy. *AIDS* 2002;16:75–83.

174. Gonzalez-Montaner LJ, Natal S, Yongchaiyud P, et al. Rifabutin for the treatment of newly diagnosed pulmonary tuberculosis: a multinational, randomized, comparative study versus rifampicin. Rifabutin Study Group. *Tuber Lung Dis* 1994;75:341–347.

175. McGregor MM, Olliaro P, Wolmarans L, et al. Efficacy and safety of rifabutin in the treatment of patients with newly diagnosed pulmonary tuberculosis. *Am J Respir Crit Care Med* 1996;154:1462–1467.

176. Narita M, Stambaugh JJ, Hollender ES, et al. Use of rifabutin with protease inhibitors for human immunodeficiency virus-infected patients with tuberculosis. *Clin Infect Dis* 2000;30:779–783.

177. Centers for Disease Control and Prevention. Updated guidelines for the use of rifabutin or rifampin for the treatment and prevention of tuberculosis among HIV-positive patients taking protease inhibitors or non-nucleoside reverse transcriptase inhibitors. *MMWR Morb Mortal Wkly Rep* 2000;49:185–189.

178. Chaisson RE, Clermont HC, Holt EA, et al. Six-month supervised intermittent tuberculosis therapy in Haitian patients with and without HIV infection. *Am J Respir Crit Care Med* 1996;154:1034–1038.

179. Schwander S, Rusch-Gerdes S, Mateega A, et al. A pilot study of antituberculosis combinations comparing rifabutin with rifampicin in the treatment of HIV-1–associated tuberculosis. A single-blind randomized evaluation in Ugandan patients with HIV-1 infection and pulmonary tuberculosis. *Tuber Lung Dis* 1995;76:210–218.

180. Snider DE, Layde PM, Johnson MW, et al. Treatment of tuberculosis during pregnancy. *Am Rev Respir Dis* 1980;122:65–79.

181. Hong Kong Chest Service/British Medical Research Council. A controlled trial of 3-month, 4-month, and 6-month regimens of chemotherapy for sputum-smear-negative pulmonary tuberculosis. Results at 5 years. *Am Rev Respir Dis* 1989;139:871–876.

182. Jasmer RM, Snyder DC, Chin DP, et al. Twelve months of isoniazid compared with four months of isoniazid and rifampin for persons with radiographic evidence of previous tuberculosis: an outcome and cost-effectiveness analysis. *Am J Respir Crit Care Med* 2000;162:1648–1652.

183. Goldberg SV, Duchin JS, Shields T, et al. Four-month, four-drug preventive therapy for inactive pulmonary tuberculosis. *Am J Respir Crit Care Med* 1999;160:508–512.

184. Frieden TR, Sterling T, Pablos-Mendez A, et al. The emergence of drug-resistant tuberculosis in New York City. *N Engl J Med* 1993;328:521–536.

185. Chawla PK, Klapper PJ, Kamholz SL, et al. Drug-resistant tuberculosis in an urban population including patients at risk for human immunodeficiency virus infection. *Am Rev Respir Dis* 1992;146:280–284.

186. Turett GS, Telzak EE, Torian LV, et al. Improved outcomes for patients with multidrug-resistant tuberculosis. *Clin Infect Dis* 1995;21:1238–1244.

187. Park MM, Davis AL, Schluger NW, et al. Outcome of MDR-TB patients, 1983–1993. Prolonged survival with appropriate therapy. *Am J Respir Crit Care Med* 1996;153:317–324.

188. Geerligs WA, Van Altena R, De Lange WCM, et al. Multidrug-resistant tuberculosis: long-term treatment outcome in the Netherlands. *Int J Tuber Lung Dis* 2000;4:758–764.

189. Tahaoglu K, Torun T, Sevim T, et al. The treatment of multidrug-resistant tuberculosis in Turkey. *N Engl J Med* 2001;345:170–174.

190. Iseman MD. Treatment of multidrug-resistant tuberculosis. *N Engl J Med* 1993;329:784–791.

191. Gonzalez-Montaner LJ, Palmero D, Montaner JG. Treatment of multiple drug-resistant tuberculosis in patients with the acquired immunodeficiency syndrome. *Clin Pulm Med* 1998;5:343–349.

192. Giosue S, Casarini M, Alemanno L, et al. Effects of aerosolized interferon-alpha in patients with pulmonary tuberculosis. *Am J Respir Crit Care Med* 1998;158:1156–1162.

193. Rikimaru T, Koga T, Sueyasu Y, et al. Treatment of ulcerative endobronchial tuberculosis and bronchial stenosis with aerosolized

streptomycin and steroids. *Int J Tuber Lung Dis* 2001;5:769–774.

194. Ferebee SH. Controlled chemoprophylaxis trials in tuberculosis. A general review. *Adv Tuber Res* 1969;17:28–106.

195. Smieja MJ, Marchetti CA, Cook DJ, et al. Isoniazid for preventing tuberculosis in non-HIV infected persons. *Cochrane Database Syst Rev* 2002:1.

196. International Union against Tuberculosis Committee on Prophylaxis. Efficacy of various durations of isoniazid preventative therapy for tuberculosis: five years of follow-up in the IUAT Trial. *Bull World Health Organ* 1982;60:555–564.

197. Comstock GW. How much isoniazid is needed for prevention of tuberculosis among immunocompetent adults? *Int J Tuber Lung Dis* 1999;3:847–850.

198. Kopanoff DE, Snider DE, Caras GJ. Isoniazid-related hepatitis. A U.S. Public Health Service Cooperative Surveillance study. *Am Rev Respir Dis* 1978;117:991–1001.

199. Salpeter SR. Fatal isoniazid-induced hepatitis. Its risk during chemoprophylaxis. *West J Med* 1993;159:560–564.

200. Millard PS, Wilcosky TC, Reade-Christopher SJ, et al. Isoniazid-related fatal hepatitis. *West J Med* 1996;164:486–491.

201. Bucher HC, Griffith LE, Guyatt GH, et al. Isoniazid prophylaxis for tuberculosis in HIV infection: a meta-analysis of randomized controlled trials. *AIDS* 1999;13:501–507.

202. Wilkinson D. Drugs for preventing tuberculosis in HIV infected persons. *Cochrane Database Syst Rev* 2002:1.

203. Halsey NA, Coberly JS, Desormeaux J, et al. Randomised trial of isoniazid versus rifampicin and pyrazinamide for prevention of tuberculosis in HIV-1 infection. *Lancet* 1998;351:786–792.

204. Mwinga AG, Hosp M, Godfrey-Faussett P, et al. Twice-weekly tuberculosis preventative therapy in HIV infection in Zambia. *AIDS* 1998;12:2447–2457.

205. Gordin F, Chaisson RE, Matts JP, et al. Rifampin and pyrazinamide vs isoniazid for prevention of tuberculosis in HIV-infected persons: an international randomized trial. Terry Beirn Community Programs for Clinical Research on AIDS, the Adult AIDS Clinical Trials Group, the Pan American Health Organization, and the Centers for Disease Control and Prevention Study Group. *JAMA* 2000;283:1445–1450.

206. Centers for Disease Control and Prevention. Update: fatal and severe liver injuries associated with rifampin and pyrazinamide for latent tuberculosis infection, and revisions in American Thoracic Society/CDC recommendations—United States, 2001. *MMWR Morb Mortal Wkly Rep* 2001;50:733–735.

207. Ormerod LP. Rifampicin and isoniazid prophylactic chemotherapy for tuberculosis. *Arch Dis Child* 1998;78:169–171.

208. Polesky A, Farber HW, Gottlieb DJ, et al. Rifampin preventative therapy for tuberculosis in Boston's homeless. *Am J Respir Crit Care Med* 1996;154:1473–1477.

209. Zhang Y, Wallace RJ Jr, Mazurek GH. Genetic differences between BCG substrains. *Tuber Lung Dis* 1995;76:43–50.

210. Brewer TF. Preventing tuberculosis with bacillus Calmette-Guérin vaccine: a meta-analysis of the literature. *Clin Infect Dis* 2000;31:S64–S67.

211. Rodrigues LC, Diwan VK, Wheeler JG. Protective effect of BCG against tuberculous meningitis and miliary tuberculosis: a meta-analysis. *Int J Epidemiol* 1993;22:1154–1158.

212. Colditz GA, Brewer TF, Berkey CS, et al. Efficacy of BCG vaccine in the prevention of tuberculosis. Meta-analysis of the published literature. *JAMA* 1994;271:698–702.

213. Advisory Council for the Elimination of Tuberculosis and the Advisory Committee on Immunization Practices. The role of BCG vaccine in the prevention and control of tuberculosis in the United States. *MMWR Morb Mortal Wkly Rep* 1996;45:1–18.

214. Bailey WC. Treatment of atypical mycobacterial disease. *Chest* 1983;84:625–628.

215. Shinners D, Yeager H. Clinical syndromes and diagnosis: overview. In: Schlossberg D, ed. *Tuberculosis and nontuberculous mycobacterial infections,* 4th ed. Philadelphia: WB Saunders, 1999:341–350.

216. Runyon EH. Anonymous mycobacteria in pulmonary disease. *Med Clin North Am* 1959;43:273–282.

217. Meissner G, Anz W. Sources of *Mycobacterium avium* complex infection resulting in human diseases. *Am Rev Respir Dis* 1977;116:1057–1064.

218. Falkinham JO. Epidemiology of infection by nontuberculous mycobacteria. *Clin Microbiol Rev* 1996;9:177–215.

219. Meissner PS, Falkinham JO. Plasmid DNA profiles as epidemiological markers for clinical and environmental isolates of *Mycobacterium avium, Mycobacterium intracellulare,* and *Mycobacterium scrofulaceum. J Infect Dis* 1986;153:325–331.

220. Edwards LB, Acquaviva FA, Livesay VT, et al. An atlas of sensitivity to tuberculin, PPD-B, and histoplasmin. *Am Rev Respir Dis* 1969;99:1–133.

221. Good RC, Snider DE. Isolation of nontuberculous mycobacteria in the United States, 1980. *J Infect Dis* 1982;146:829–833.

222. O'Brien RJ, Geiter LJ, Snider DE. The epidemiology of nontuberculous mycobacterial diseases in the United States. *Am Rev Respir Dis* 1987;135:1007–1014.

223. Tsukamura M, Kita N, Shimoide H, et al. Studies of the epidemiology of nontuberculous mycobacteriosis in Japan. *Am Rev Respir Dis* 1988;137:1280–1284.

224. Debrunner M, Salfinger M, Brandii O, et al. Epidemiology and clinical significance of nontuberculous mycobacteria in patients negative for human immunodeficiency virus in Switzerland. *Clin Infect Dis* 1992;15:330–345.

225. Horsburgh CR, Selik RM. The epidemiology of disseminated nontuberculous mycobacterial infection in the acquired immunodeficiency syndrome (AIDS). *Am Rev Respir Dis* 1992;139:4–7.

226. Horsburgh CR. *Mycobacterium avium* complex infection in the acquired immunodeficiency syndrome. *N Engl J Med* 1991;324:1332–1338.

227. Nightingale SD, Byrd LT, Southern PM, et al. Incidence of *Mycobacterium avium-intracellulare* complex bacteremia in human immunodeficiency virus-positive patients. *J Infect Dis* 1992;165:1082–1085.

228. Guthertz LS, Damsker B, Bottone EJ, et al. *Mycobacterium avium* and *Mycobacterium intracellulare* infections in patients with and without AIDS. *J Infect Dis* 1989;160:1037–1041.

229. Prince DS, Peterson DD, Steiner RM, et al. Infection with *Mycobacterium avium* complex in patients without predisposing conditions. *N Engl J Med* 1989;321:863–868.

230. Reich JM, Johnson RE. *Mycobacterium avium* complex pulmonary disease presenting as an isolated lingular or middle lobe pattern. The Lady Windermere syndrome. *Chest* 1992;101:1605–1609.

231. Kubo K, Yamazaki Y, Hachiya T, et al. *Mycobacterium avium-intracellulare* pulmonary infection in patients without known predisposing lung disease. *Lung* 1998;176:381–391.

232. Chetchotisakd P, Mootsikapun P, Anunnatsiri S, et al. Disseminated infection due to rapidly growing mycobacteria in immunocompetent hosts presenting with chronic lymphadenopathy: a previously unrecognized clinical entity. *Clin Infect Dis* 2000;30:29–34.

233. Levin M, Newport MJ, D'Souza S, et al. Familial disseminated atypical mycobacterial infection in childhood: a human mycobacterial susceptibility gene. *Lancet* 1995;345:79–83.

234. Frucht DM, Holland SM. Defective monocyte costimulation for

IFN-gamma production in familial disseminated *Mycobacterium avium* complex infection. Abnormal IL-12 regulation. *J Immunol* 1996;157:411–416.

235. Rosenzweig DY. Pulmonary mycobacterial infections due to *Mycobacterium intracellulare-avium* complex: clinical features and course in 100 consecutive cases. *Chest* 1979;75:115–119.

236. Wolinsky E. Nontuberculous mycobacteria and associated diseases. *Rev Infect Dis* 1979;119:107–159.

237. Miller WT. Spectrum of pulmonary nontuberculous mycobacterial infection. *Radiology* 1994;191:343–350.

238. American Thoracic Society. Diagnosis and treatment of disease caused by nontuberculous mycobacteria. *Am J Respir Crit Care Med* 1997;156:S1–S25.

239. Reich JM, Johnson RE. *Mycobacterium avium* complex pulmonary disease. Incidence, presentation, and response to therapy in a community setting. *Am Rev Respir Dis* 1991;143:1381–1385.

240. Hartman TE, Swenson SJ, Williams DE. *Mycobacterium avium-intracellulare* complex: evaluation with CT. *Radiology* 1993;187:23–26.

241. Moore EH. Atypical mycobacterial infection in the lung: CT appearance. *Radiology* 1993;187:777–782.

242. Primack SL, Logan PM, Hartman TE, et al. Pulmonary tuberculosis and *Mycobacterium avium-intracellulare:* a comparison of CT findings. *Radiology* 1995;194:413–417.

243. Wolinsky E. Mycobacterial lymphadenitis in children: a prospective study of 105 nontuberculous cases with long-term follow-up. *Clin Infect Dis* 1995;20:954–963.

244. Lai KK, Stottmeier KD, Sherman IH, et al. Mycobacterial cervical lymphadenopathy. Relation of etiologic agents to age. *JAMA* 1984;251:1286–1288.

245. Grange JM, Yates MD, Pozniak A. Bacteriologically confirmed non-tuberculous mycobacterial lymphadenitis in southeast England: a recent increase in the number of cases. *Arch Dis Child* 1995;72:516–517.

246. Wallace RJ, Swenson JM, Silcox VA, et al. Spectrum of disease due to rapidly growing mycobacteria. *Rev Infect Dis* 1983;5:657–679.

247. Saubolle MA, Kiehn TE, White MH, et al. *Mycobacterium haemophilum:* microbiology and expanding clinical and geographic spectra of disease in humans. *Clin Microbiol Rev* 1996;9:435–447.

248. Hoffman PC, Fraser DW, Robicsek F, et al. Two outbreaks of sternal wound infections due to organisms of the *Mycobacterium fortuitum* complex. *J Infect Dis* 1981;143:533–542.

249. Kuritsky JN, Bullen M, Broome CV, et al. Sternal wound infections and endocarditis due to organisms of the *Mycobacterium fortuitum* complex: a potential environmental source. *Ann Intern Med* 1983;98:938–939.

250. Raad II, Vartivarian S, Khan A, et al. Catheter-related infections caused by the *Mycobacterium fortuitum* complex: 15 cases and review. *Rev Infect Dis* 1991;13:1120–1125.

251. Jernigan JA, Farr BM. Incubation period and sources of exposure for cutaneous *Mycobacterium marinum* infection: case report and review of the literature. *Clin Infect Dis* 2000;31:439–443.

252. Horsburgh CR Jr, Mason UG 3rd, Farhi DC, et al. Disseminated infection with *Mycobacterium avium-intracellulare.* A report of 13 cases and a review of the literature. *Medicine (Baltimore)* 1985;64:36–48.

253. Ingram CW, Tanner DC, Durack DT, et al. Disseminated infection with rapidly growing mycobacteria. *Clin Infect Dis* 1993;16:463–471.

254. Horsburgh CR Jr, Gettings J, Alexander LN, et al. Disseminated *Mycobacterium avium* complex disease among patients infected with human immunodeficiency virus, 1985–2000. *Clin Infect Dis* 2001;33:1938–1943.

255. Respiratory illness in workers exposed to metal-working fluid contaminated with nontuberculous mycobacteria—Ohio, 2001. *MMWR Morb Mortal Wkly Rep* 2002;51:349–352.

256. Chaisson RE, Benson CA, Dube MP, et al. Clarithromycin therapy for bacteremic *Mycobacterium avium* complex disease: a randomized, double-blind, dose-ranging study in patients with AIDS. *Ann Intern Med* 1994;121:905–911.

257. Shafran SD, Singer J, Zarowny DP, et al. A comparison of two regimens for the treatment of *Mycobacterium avium* complex bacteremia in AIDS: rifabutin, ethambutol, and clarithromycin versus rifampin, ethambutol, clofazimine, and ciprofloxacin. *N Engl J Med* 1996;335:377–383.

258. Ahn CH, Ahn SS, Anderson RA, et al. A four-drug regimen for initial treatment of cavitary disease caused by *Mycobacterium avium* complex. *Am Rev Respir Dis* 1986;134:438–441.

259. Griffith DE, Wallace RJ. Treatment of pulmonary *Mycobacterium avium* complex lung disease in non-acquired immunodeficiency syndrome (AIDS) patients in the era of the newer macrolides and rifabutin. *Am J Med* 1997;102:22–27.

260. Dautzenberg B, Piperno D, Diot P, et al. Clarithromycin in the treatment of *Mycobacterium avium* lung infections in patients without AIDS. *Chest* 1995;107:1035–1040.

261. Wallace RJ, Brown BA, Griffith DE, et al. Clarithromycin regimens for pulmonary *Mycobacterium avium* complex. The first 50 patients. *Am J Respir Crit Care Med* 1996;153:1766–1772.

262. Tanaka E, Kimoto T, Tsuyuguchi K, et al. Effect of clarithromycin regimen for *Mycobacterium avium* complex pulmonary disease. *Am J Respir Crit Care Med* 1999;160:866–872.

Anaerobic and Other Infection Syndromes

21

Ronald F. Grossman

ASPIRATION PNEUMONIA

The term *aspiration pneumonia* refers to a condition in which a radiographic infiltrate develops in the setting of either a witnessed episode of gross aspiration or risk factors for aspiration. This is an infectious process that follows the aspiration of infected oropharyngeal secretions. Because aspiration of pathogens from a previously colonized oropharynx is the primary pathway by which organisms gain entrance to the lungs, most pneumonias are to some extent aspiration-related. Aspiration pneumonia is different from aspiration pneumonitis, a condition defined as acute lung injury with diffuse alveolar damage that develops after the inhalation of sterile gastric contents (1). Aspiration pneumonitis is a chemical injury to the lung related to the volume and pH of the aspirated material.

An underlying disease is usually associated with aspiration pneumonia, as with most other respiratory tract infections. Approximately 50% of normal adults aspirate while sleeping without any obvious health effects (2,3). Pneumonia can develop in patients with certain underlying diseases that tend to impair host defenses. Besides host factors, other factors that modify the risk for pneumonia after aspiration include certain characteristics of the aspirated material. The bacterial load, bacterial virulence, pH, tonicity, and volume of the aspirate, in addition to the frequency of aspiration, are all related to the development of pneumonia (4).

Most infiltrates that follow aspiration resolve, but 25% to 50% progress to infectious pneumonia or fulminant acute lung injury. Among patients in a nursing home who were evaluated for aspiration with videofluoroscopy, pneumonia developed in 50% of those with documented aspiration during a 12-month period and in 12.5% of those without aspiration (5). The volume of the aspirate was directly related to the risk for pneumonia; pneumonia developed in 43% of patients with mild aspiration (of thin liquids), and in 67% of patients with severe aspiration (of material of all consistencies at almost every swallow). In a retrospective study, Bynum and Pierce (6) evaluated 50 patients with significant aspiration. Rapid clearing of infiltrates was noted in 62%, usually within 5 days, and adult respiratory distress syndrome (ARDS) with a fatal outcome developed in 12%. Infectious pneumonia developed in the remaining 26% of patients, often after initial improvement.

Risk Factors

Host Factors

Host factors that predispose to aspiration pneumonia either impair host defenses or enhance the risk for aspiration (Table 21.1). A number of conditions, such as diabetes mellitus, congestive heart failure, malnutrition, chronic obstructive lung disease, renal failure, and malignancy, can impair host defenses and have been associated with an increased risk for pneumonia. Many host factors predispose to aspiration as the result of neurologic, mechanical, or contractile dysfunction of the esophagus and upper airway (Table 21.2). They include stroke, dysphagia, gastroesophageal reflux, altered sensorium, placement of a feeding tube, and the postgastrectomy state (7–10). Once material has gained access to the airways, the clinical response depends on the characteristics of the aspirate. If the aspirate is small in volume but highly contaminated with bacteria, then host defenses may be overwhelmed and pneumonia can result. If the aspirate is large in volume but relatively less contaminated, then pneumonia will result only if the aspirated organisms are highly virulent, airway obstruction occurs with subsequent poor

R. F. Grossman: Department of Medicine, University of Toronto, Toronto, Ontario, Canada.

TABLE 21.1. RISK FACTORS FOR ASPIRATION PNEUMONIA

Host Risk Factors	Aspirate Risk Factors
Underlying serious illness	Fluid pH << 2.5
Altered sensorium	Large particles
Stroke	Large volume (1 mL/kg)
Dysphagia	Hypertonic fluid
Gastroesophageal reflux	Bacterial contamination
Postgastrectomy	
Xerostomia	
Feeding tube	
Periodontal disease	

clearance of the aspirated material, or the host defenses are severely abnormal. The oropharyngeal flora can reach extremely high concentrations in the presence of periodontal disease. Whereas normal saliva contains 10^8 organisms per milliliter, saliva from a patient with gingivitis may contain 10^{11} organisms per milliliter. In periodontal disease, anaerobes predominate among the oral flora.

Xerostomia can predispose to aspiration pneumonia (11). Normal saliva flushes the oral cavity and maintains a bacterial level below 7×10^8 organisms per milliliter. In xerostomia, the normal salivary flow rate is diminished and patients are at risk for gingivitis, and these two factors can result in bacterial counts that are higher than normal. When a patient with xerostomia aspirates, the lower respiratory tract is exposed to larger numbers of bacteria than normal, and aspiration pneumonia can result.

When aspiration develops in a hospitalized patient, many of the same host risk factors prevail. However, in the intensive care unit, particular issues to consider in the evaluation of a patient's risk for aspiration include the patient's position,

TABLE 21.2. CONDITIONS THAT INCREASE THE RISK FOR ASPIRATION

Neurologic	Mechanical	Contractile
Unconsciousness	Obesity	Gastroesophageal reflux
Laryngeal nerve damage	Head and neck surgery	Diabetic gastropathy
Advanced age	Bowel obstruction	Critical illness
Acute stroke	Abdominal surgery	Trendelenburg position
Pseudobulbar palsy	Enteral feeding	Protracted vomiting
Seizures	Pregnancy	
Parkinson disease	Endotracheal intubation	
Insulin-induced hypoglycemia	Tracheostomy	
Alcoholism		
Drug abuse		
Cardiac arrest		
Metabolic encephalopathy		

site of enteral feeding (stomach or small bowel), volume of the gastric contents, and size of any feeding tube that is used (12,13). Studies have suggested a reduced risk for aspiration of gastric contents in patients who are maintained in a semierect position.

Characteristics of the Aspirate

The characteristics of the aspirated material play an important role in the pathogenesis of pneumonia. Because only 25% to 50% of all cases of aspiration progress to pneumonia, infection is particularly likely if contaminated material is aspirated. Pneumonia may also develop in persons who aspirate certain types of noninfectious material that injures the lungs.

Aspiration of very toxic, irritant material with high concentrations of hydrogen ion (pH < 2.5) results in a chemical pneumonitis. This initial type of lung injury is typically noninfectious and characterized by a predominance of neutrophils. The magnitude of lung injury is directly related to the volume and hydrogen ion concentration of the aspirated material (14,15). In animal models of aspiration, acid pneumonitis does not develop unless the pH is less than 2.5. The resulting damage renders the mucosal barrier of the lower respiratory tract incompetent and increases the risk for infectious pneumonia as new sites for bacterial binding are created.

The majority of large-volume and large-particle aspirates are composed of vegetable matter, which can mechanically obstruct the lower airways and cause atelectasis, stagnation of secretions, and thus an increased risk for infection. In addition, bacteria can contaminate aspirates containing particulate matter because potentially pathogenic organisms often heavily colonize oral secretions. In hospitalized patients, the stomach can harbor large numbers of enteric Gram-negative bacteria if the gastric pH is more than 3.5 to 4.0 (16). In patients in the intensive care unit, the risk for the development of pneumonia is great when the morning gastric pH is high (>3.5). Enteral feeding, antacids, or histamine H_2 antagonists may elevate the gastric pH. The effect of prophylaxis for intestinal bleeding in the pathogenesis of pneumonia is uncertain, with continuing controversy about the role of the stomach in causing pneumonia (17). In addition, histamine H_2 antagonists have not uniformly led to an increased risk for pneumonia in all studies, and their impact must be considered in relation to gastric volume, patient position, and site of enteral feeding.

Because community-acquired aspiration pneumonia usually involves anaerobic bacteria, it should be viewed as part of a continuum that can progress to cavitation (lung abscess) or even empyema. If aspiration pneumonia is not treated, necrotizing abscesses form within 8 to 14 days, usually in a peripheral location, that are characterized by the expectoration of putrid sputum. When anaerobic lung infection occurs, the pleura is commonly involved, being affected alone or in combination with parenchymal tissue in up to half of all patients.

Bacteriology

The bacteriology of aspiration pneumonia is intimately related to the flora of the oropharyngeal cavity. Under normal circumstances, the saliva of the oral cavity contains 10^8 organisms per milliliter, with a predominance of anaerobic organisms. Persons with poor dental hygiene or gingivitis can have anaerobic bacterial levels of 10^{11}/mL of saliva, and patients with underlying illness who are hospitalized for prolonged periods can become colonized by enteric Gram-negative bacilli (18). Most cases of aspiration pneumonia are caused by anaerobic organisms originating in the oropharynx and are usually polymicrobial, with at least two anaerobic organisms and sometimes a mixture of aerobic and anaerobic pathogens (19–21).

The bacteriology of aspiration pneumonia has not changed much during the last few decades, although the taxonomy of some of the involved pathogens has. For example, some organisms originally classified in the *Peptostreptococcus* genus have now been reclassified in the *Streptococcus* genus (e.g., *Streptococcus intermedius*). With this in mind, many studies in the 1970s and 1980s documented anaerobic streptococci, *Fusobacterium nucleatum*, and *Prevotella melaninogenicus* (formerly classified in the genus *Bacteroides*) as the three major pathogens in aspiration pneumonia. It was once thought that *Bacteroides fragilis* was a significant pathogen in anaerobic lung infections, although recent data make this seem less likely.

Aerobic bacteria are found as either primary pathogens (~10% of cases) or as copathogens (~40% of cases); they include *Streptococcus* species, *Staphylococcus aureus*, *Klebsiella pneumoniae*, *Escherichia coli*, *Enterobacter cloacae*, and *Pseudomonas aeruginosa*. A more recent study examining early aspiration pneumonia in intensive care unit patients documented a more virulent profile of aerobic pathogens (22). In this series, no anaerobes were isolated, but in those patients who had community-acquired early aspiration pneumonia, *Streptococcus pneumoniae*, *S. aureus*, *E. coli*, *E. cloacae*, *Haemophilus influenzae*, *Streptococcus viridans*, and *P. aeruginosa* were isolated alone or in combination. Among those patients who aspirated in the hospital, *S. aureus*, *H. influenzae*, *Serratia marcescens*, *Morganella morganii*, *Candida albicans*, *K. pneumoniae*, *P. aeruginosa*, and *Proteus mirabilis* were isolated alone or in combination by a protected specimen brush. These findings were reproduced in a separate study of 25 patients with gastric aspiration and significant risk factors for gastric colonization (23). These data suggest that the bacteriology in severely ill patients with underlying medical diseases may differ from that of patients with aspiration pneumonia that is not severe. They also raise doubts about the significance of anaerobic organisms, even among patients who aspirate.

Clinical Presentation

Most patients with classic anaerobic lung infections present with an insidious illness characterized by cough, the production of foul-smelling and purulent sputum, low-grade fever, and weight loss, particularly after the onset of tissue necrosis. Most of them have significant risk factors for aspiration, such as alcoholism, seizure, and neurologic and swallowing disorders.

In contrast, patients who have aspirated aerobic organisms present with the abrupt onset of fever, cough productive of purulent but not foul-smelling sputum, hemoptysis, and chest pain. Usually, no evidence of necrosis is found, and the organisms involved depend in part on where the illness was acquired (community or hospital).

The site of the infection is invariably the dependent portions of the lung. Depending on the time course, the patient's underlying state of health, and the organisms involved, lung necrosis, lung abscess, and empyema may develop.

Treatment

The administration of antibiotics and supportive care remain the major modalities of therapy for aspiration pneumonia. In the setting of a witnessed or suspected aspiration, antibiotics are generally started if an infiltrate is present. If the infiltrate clears in 24 to 48 hours, the pneumonitis was likely noninfectious, and therapy can be discontinued. If no infiltrate is present, therapy can be withheld provided that the patient is followed with serial chest radiographs. *In the absence of a witnessed or suspected aspiration, antimicrobial agents should be chosen to cover the usual community-acquired respiratory pathogens, such as* S. pneumoniae, Mycoplasma pneumoniae, Chlamydia pneumoniae, H. influenzae, *and* Legionella pneumophila. Antibiotic therapy for patients with aspiration pneumonia should be based on an assessment of the severity of illness (Table 21.3), where the infection was acquired

TABLE 21.3. FEATURES OF SEVERE ASPIRATION PNEUMONIA

Respiratory rate >30 breaths per minute
Need for mechanical ventilation
Chest radiographic findings
    50% increase in the infiltrate in 48 hours
    Bilateral multilobar involvement
Presence of shock
SIRS (systemic inflammatory response syndrome) or need for
    vasopressors to support blood pressure
Severe lung injury (Pao_2/Fio_2 ratio <<250 mm Hg)
Urine output <<20 mL/h
Acute renal failure requiring dialysis

Fio_2, fraction of inspired oxygen; Pao_2, arterial partial pressure of oxygen.

TABLE 21.4. RISK FACTORS FOR GRAM-NEGATIVE COLONIZATION

Malnutrition
Severe illness
Coma
Intubation
Diabetes
Prior surgery
Lung disease
Renal failure
Prior antibiotic use
Hypotension
Cigarette smoking
Prolonged hospitalization

TABLE 21.5. INITIAL ANTIBIOTIC REGIMEN FOR ASPIRATION PNEUMONIA

Oral Route	Parenteral Route	Hospital-Acquired or Severe Community-Acquired
Penicillin	Penicillin	Clindamycin + fluoroquinolone[a]
Penicillin + metronidazole	Penicillin + metronidazole	Clindamycin + aminoglycoside[a]
Clindamycin	Piperacillin[a]	Clindamycin + third-generation cephalosporin
Amoxicillin/ clavulanate	Imipenem[a]	Imipenem/meropenem
	Clindamycin	Piperacillin/tazobactam
	Ampicillin/sulbactam	Ampicillin/sulbactam
	Ticarcillin/clavulanate	Ticarcillin/clavulanate

[a] If any of the following are present, *Pseudomonas aeruginosa* infection is possible: prior antibiotic use, prolonged hospital course, or severe pneumonia. If *P. aeruginosa* infection is suspected, dual anti-*Pseudomonas* therapy should be initiated with a β-lactam/aminoglycoside or a β-lactam/quinolone combination.

(community or hospital), and the presence or absence of risk factors for Gram-negative colonization (Table 21.4).

If *aspiration* pneumonia has been acquired in the community, then Gram-negative infection is less likely than if the infection has been acquired in the hospital. In community-related aspiration pneumonia, it is reasonable to select an antibiotic regimen directed against the oral anaerobes (e.g., anaerobic streptococci, *F. nucleatum*, and *P. melaninogenicus*). Patients should be treated empirically without collection of sputum for culture by expectoration or invasive aspiration. No evidence indicates that antibiotics directed solely at anaerobes are superior to other regimens. No data from randomized trials with adequate patient numbers are available to guide antimicrobial therapy. *However, clinical experience acquired since the advent of the antibiotic era has led to a consensus that penicillin is the drug of choice for anaerobic lung infections.* For patients strongly suspected of having aspirated mainly anaerobic pathogens (severe periodontal disease, putrid sputum), the initial empiric antibiotic may be penicillin alone, clindamycin, or a combination of penicillin and metronidazole. Some data show a lower failure rate in patients treated with clindamycin than in patients treated with penicillin for anaerobic pleuropulmonary infection, suggesting a primary role for clindamycin in this infection (24). A study of patients with community-acquired lung abscess found resistance rates to penicillin, metronidazole, and clindamycin of 21%, 12%, and 5%, respectively, again supporting a primary role for clindamycin in anaerobic lung infections (25).

The route of antibiotic administration is determined by the severity of the pneumonia and by whether treatment is being administered on an outpatient or inpatient basis. Treatment may be given orally to both outpatients and inpatients, depending on the severity of illness, but initial therapy in severely ill and hospitalized patients is usually by the intravenous route.

The preceding antibiotic regimen must be modified for patients with severe infection, hospital-acquired aspiration, or risk factors for Gram-negative colonization (Table 21.4). In these cases, the likelihood of infection with a virulent Gram-negative bacillus or an aerobic organism is greater, and therefore additional antibiotic coverage is required. Sputum or tracheal aspirate may be helpful in identifying high-risk pathogens, such as *P. aeruginosa*, in intubated patients. After empiric therapy has been started, culture results can be useful to determine the presence or absence of infection with *P. aeruginosa*. Some authors recommend a respiratory fluoroquinolone, such as levofloxacin, gatifloxacin, or moxifloxacin, as single-agent therapy even though anaerobic coverage is relatively poor, especially for levofloxacin (26). Of these agents, moxifloxacin offers the best Gram-positive and anaerobic coverage (27). In more seriously ill patients, especially those with necrotizing pneumonia, piperacillin/tazobactam or imipenem/meropenem or a combination of ciprofloxacin or ceftriaxone plus clindamycin or metronidazole would offer excellent coverage of the most likely pathogens (Table 21.5). If risk factors for infection with *P. aeruginosa* are present, empiric antibiotic therapy with a dual anti-*Pseudomonas* combination until culture results are known is usually recommended (28).

ANAEROBIC PNEUMONIA

Summary Statement	Level of Evidence
Anaerobic bacteria are important pathogens in community-acquired aspiration pneumonia.	Observational studies, expert opinion
Aerobic pathogens are important in hospital-acquired aspiration pneumonia.	Observational studies, nonrandomized studies
Antibiotics with good anaerobic coverage are beneficial in community-acquired aspiration pneumonia.	Randomized and observational clinical studies
Antibiotics with good anaerobic coverage are beneficial in hospital-acquired aspiration pneumonia.	Nonrandomized studies

LUNG ABSCESS

A lung abscess is defined as a localized (usually >2 cm in diameter), suppurative, necrotizing process occurring within the pulmonary parenchyma. Several processes, either respiratory or systemic, can lead to abscess formation. Most abscesses are primary and result from necrosis in an existing parenchymal process, usually untreated aspiration pneumonia. Among the causes of necrotizing pneumonitis, infections and neoplasms are the most frequent. A secondary abscess is one that complicates either a septic vascular embolus (e.g., right-sided endocarditis) or a bronchial obstruction (e.g., aspirated foreign body).

Anaerobes are the most common cause of lung abscess, although aerobic bacilli, fungi, parasites, and mycobacteria may also be responsible (25,29,30). Among neoplastic causes, primary squamous carcinoma of the lung is the malignancy most often associated with abscess formation. Between 8% and 18% of lung abscesses are associated with neoplasms in all age groups, but in patients older than 45 years, the association approaches 30% (31).

The incidence of lung abscess has declined as much as 10-fold during the last few decades, presumably as a result of improved treatment regimens for pneumonia. Accompanying this decrease in incidence has been a decrease in mortality to between 5% and 10%, with one series reporting a mortality rate of 2.4% in community-acquired lung abscess and 66.7% in hospital-acquired abscess (32). Diagnosis and treatment have changed little through the years because lung abscesses are uncommon and it is difficult to obtain enough patients to perform controlled clinical trials. Administration of antibiotics is the most important treatment, as in aspiration pneumonia. The role of the newer antimicrobial agents remains controversial, although they may represent an advance over traditional therapeutic agents (penicillin), especially as drug-resistant bacteria become more prevalent.

Pathogenesis

Infectious agents, such as bacteria, fungi, parasites, and mycobacteria, cause most lung abscesses. In the majority of cases, a mixed bacterial flora can be found, with anaerobes present in approximately 80% of cases. Aerobic bacilli are present in up to 50% of patients, but in most cases they coexist with anaerobes, and in only 10% of cases are they the sole responsible pathogens.

As in aspiration pneumonia, the basis of lung abscess formation is aspiration of infectious oropharyngeal material, usually in a host with inadequate defenses. Persons predisposed to lung abscess formation are those with host defense defects in the setting of risk factors for aspiration (Tables 21.1 and 21.2). Aspiration, as previously described (see preceding section "Risk Factors"), is more likely in patients who have neurologic, mechanical, or muscular dysfunction associated with alcoholism, seizure disorders, drug overdose,

general anesthesia, protracted vomiting, or neurologic disorders such as cerebrovascular accidents, myasthenia gravis, and amyotrophic lateral sclerosis or other bulbar processes.

In addition to having risk factors for aspiration, patients predisposed to the formation of lung abscess are exposed to large concentrations of potentially pathogenic bacteria, usually oral or gingival in origin. Abscess formation is enhanced by poor dentition and gingival disease, two conditions that are associated with bacterial counts in saliva in excess of 10^{11}/mL. Approximately 73% of patients with lung abscess have at least one predisposing factor for aspiration, and many have clinically silent gingival disease (33).

The pathophysiology of lung abscess formation appears to be related to a combination of aspiration, host defense defects, and size of the infectious inoculum. Experimental data suggest that lung abscesses form 8 to 14 days after infectious oral/gingival material has been aspirated. When aspirated in large amounts, a single species of anaerobic bacteria or a combination of organisms can cause a necrotizing pneumonitis that, if progressive or untreated initially, leads to the formation of a lung abscess. The location of the abscess is determined by gravity and body position at the time of aspiration. Lung abscesses are typically located in the basal segments of the lower lobes, the superior segment of the lower lobe, or the posterior segments of the upper lobes, analogous to the location of infiltrates in patients with aspiration pneumonia.

Microbiology

Approximately 90% of lung abscesses are associated with anaerobic bacteria, either as the primary pathogens or in combination with aerobic bacteria. This observation may be explained by the fact that anaerobic bacteria commonly cause necrotizing inflammation. Other bacteria associated with lung abscess include *S. aureus, E. coli, K. pneumoniae, P. aeruginosa,* other Gram-negative bacilli, *Streptococcus pyogenes, Pseudomonas pseudomallei* (melioidosis), *H. influenzae* (especially type b), *L. pneumophila, Nocardia asteroides, Actinomyces* species, and rarely pneumococci. Parasites (*Paragonimus westermani, Entamoeba histolytica*), fungi, and mycobacteria also may cause lung abscess (Table 21.6).

Anaerobes are usually part of a polymicrobial flora, with the average number of organisms isolated being three, either strictly anaerobes or a combination of aerobic and anaerobic bacteria (25).

Classification

Lung abscesses have been categorized by several methods, but the classification into acute versus chronic appears to be the most useful one clinically. This distinction is not absolute, but it can aid the clinician in formulating treatment regimens and identifying patients who may require further diagnostic evaluation, such as bronchoscopy.

TABLE 21.6. CAVITARY LUNG LESIONS

Infectious

Bacterial	*Fungal*	*Parasitic*
Anaerobic abscess	Coccidioidomycosis	Echinococcosis
Aerobic abscess	Histoplasmosis	Amebiasis
Infected bulla	Blastomycosis	
Infected pulmonary infarct	Aspergillosis	
Empyema	Cryptococcosis	
Tuberculosis		
Actinomycosis		

Neoplastic	**Inflammatory**
Bronchogenic carcinoma	Wegener's
Squamous cell carcinoma	granulomatosis
Metastatic carcinoma	Sarcoidosis
Colorectal cancer	
Renal cancer	
Lymphoma	
Hodgkin disease	

A lung abscess is defined as acute if the patient presents with symptoms of less than 2 weeks' duration. Patients with an acute lung abscess are less likely to have an underlying neoplasm but are more likely to have an infection caused by a virulent aerobic bacterial agent, such as *S. aureus*. In a series of patients with acute community-acquired lung abscess, the mean number of bacterial species identified per patient was 2.3, with anaerobes isolated alone in 44% of cases, aerobes alone in 19%, and mixed aerobes and anaerobes in 22%; the remaining cases were caused by an unidentified pathogen or *Mycobacterium tuberculosis* (25). The most common anaerobic pathogens identified were *Prevotella* species, and the most common aerobic pathogens were *S. viridans* and *Staphylococcus* species.

A chronic lung abscess is defined by symptoms lasting for more than 4 to 6 weeks; patients are more likely to have an underlying neoplasm or infection with a less virulent anaerobic agent. Some overlap may occur with this classification scheme because it does not take into account host defense factors or serious comorbidity, but it can be useful during the initial evaluation.

Clinical Features

In most patients with lung abscess, the presentation is insidious, with symptoms lasting at least 2 weeks before evaluation. Signs and symptoms include cough, foul-smelling sputum that forms layers on standing, hemoptysis (25% of patients), fever, chills, night sweats, anorexia, pleuritic chest pain (60% of patients), weight loss, and clubbing. Although most of these signs and symptoms are present, their specificity for lung abscess is low. On the other hand, putrid sputum is a highly specific sign that is pathognomonic for anaerobic infection, although it is present in only 50% to 60% of patients (34). A history of weight loss is common, noted in 60% of patients, with an average loss of between 15 and

20 lb. Historical data usually include risk factors for aspiration, such as alcoholism, drug overdose, seizures, head injury, or stroke, and the absence of such risk factors should prompt a search for a diagnosis other than primary lung abscess.

Nonspecific laboratory data include an elevated erythrocyte sedimentation rate, anemia of chronic inflammation, and leukocytosis. Culture and microbiologic information from sputum are generally not helpful unless agents that are not anaerobic, such as mycobacteria, fungi, or aerobic bacteria, are causing the abscess. If the abscess is associated with an empyema, as is the case 30% of the time, then culture of the empyema fluid may yield reliable bacteriologic data.

More invasive methods of microbiologic diagnosis (transtracheal aspiration and bronchoscopy) are rarely used; the majority of patients are treated empirically. This approach is supported by data showing that most lung abscess pathogens are sensitive to conventional antimicrobial therapy. On the other hand, if the presentation is atypical or the patient is not responding to therapy, then invasive techniques are justified (Table 21.7).

Chest radiography generally shows a solitary cavitary lesion of variable size, more often on the right than on the left side. Some studies report that the size of the cavity is helpful in distinguishing neoplastic from nonneoplastic lung abscesses, but others have not found such a correlation. Minimal inflammation surrounding the abscess on radiographs suggests an underlying neoplasm. Bronchogenic carcinoma and lung abscess may coexist in as many as 12% of cases (34).

Radiographically, empyema and infected bullae are sometimes difficult to distinguish from a lung abscess. Empyema is a purulent infection that in most cases is confined to the pleural space, although it can develop as a complication, or be a cause, of a lung abscess. An infected bulla is pneumonia within a preexisting bullous cavity and does not result from tissue necrosis. Both entities can demonstrate air-fluid levels, but one is parenchymal (infected bulla) and the other is extraparenchymal (empyema). If an empyema contains an

TABLE 21.7. CRITERIA FOR FIBEROPTIC BRONCHOSCOPY IN PATIENTS WITH LUNG ABSCESS

Atypical presentation
    Absence of fever
    White blood cell count $<<$ 11,000/mm^3
    Absence of systemic symptoms
    Fulminant course
    Absence of predisposing factors for aspiration
    Atypical abscess location
    Abscess formation in an edentulous patient
Failure to respond to antibiotics
Mediastinal adenopathy
Suspected underlying malignancy
Suspected foreign body

air-fluid level, then a bronchopleural fistula is present. When the chest radiograph cannot distinguish these two entities from a lung abscess, computed tomography (CT) suggests a lung abscess if a thick, irregular, walled cavity with no associated lung compression is seen. Empyema or an infected bulla usually is characterized by thin, smooth walls with compression of uninvolved lung and, in the case of the infected bulla, minimal surrounding inflammation.

If a lung abscess fails to communicate with a bronchus, the characteristic air-fluid level within a cavity will not be seen radiographically. In this case, the radiographic appearance is one of a focal, ground-glass infiltrate with indistinct borders. *This may be seen early in the disease because it takes 8 to 14 days for tissue necrosis with abscess formation to develop (4). However, tissue breakdown should be evident.* Given the history of this illness and the radiographic picture, the differential diagnosis includes other chronic pulmonary infections, such as postobstructive bacterial pneumonia, nocardiosis, fungal pneumonia, tuberculosis, and actinomycosis. In addition, a variety of noninfectious pulmonary processes can be confused with a noncavitary lung abscess. These include bronchiolitis obliterans organizing pneumonia, radiation pneumonitis, chronic eosinophilic pneumonia, and allergic bronchopulmonary aspergillosis. When a lung abscess presents in this manner, a further diagnostic workup, such as bronchoscopy or lung biopsy, is usually necessary. This is also the case if multiple cavities are seen on the radiograph, a rare finding in an anaerobic process not complicated by immunosuppression, recurrent aspiration, or virulent anaerobe(s) causing a necrotizing pneumonitis.

Treatment

In the pre-antibiotic era, three treatment modalities—namely, supportive care, postural drainage with or without bronchoscopy, and surgery—were available for lung abscess. All three modalities were associated with the same mortality rate of 30% to 35%. Currently, the mainstay of therapy for lung abscess is antimicrobial therapy with intravenous penicillin alone, penicillin plus metronidazole, or clindamycin. Penicillin has historically been the therapy of choice since its first use in the 1950s, with a cure rate of 95%. With the growing concern about penicillin-resistant anaerobes, clindamycin was compared with penicillin in two studies with a prospective design (24,35). Both found clindamycin therapy to be associated with fewer treatment failures and a shorter time to symptom resolution. However, neither study was adequately powered, and the clinical endpoint was assessed very early in the course of treatment. When metronidazole was evaluated as a single treatment modality, it was found to have a 43% failure rate and hence is not recommended as single-agent therapy (36). Metronidazole in combination with penicillin is considered an appropriate treatment regimen for lung abscess because penicillin has activity against the aerobic and microaerophilic

streptococci that are often resistant to metronidazole. Many other antibiotics have *in vitro* activity against oral anaerobes but have never been evaluated in clinical trials to gain Food and Drug Administration approval for use in these infections. These include chloramphenicol, imipenem, erythromycin, azithromycin, clarithromycin, moxifloxacin, and β-lactams with a β-lactamase inhibitor (e.g., ampicillin with sulbactam).

It is usually recommended that patients be treated until the pulmonary infiltrates have resolved or until the residual lesion is small and stable. Initially, antibiotics are given intravenously until the patient is afebrile and shows clinical improvement (4–8 days). Oral medications are then given, usually for a prolonged period, although the length of time needed varies from patient to patient. However, oral therapy can be as effective as parenteral therapy (37). Many patients require a total of 6 to 8 weeks of antimicrobial therapy.

Adequate drainage of the lung abscess is an important part of management. An air-fluid level implies the presence of a communication from the abscess cavity to the tracheobronchial tree. Avoidance of sedating medications, encouragement of cough, and mobilization of secretions are potentially useful interventions. Chest physical therapy and postural drainage may be helpful, although scattered reports of significant pulmonary hemorrhage associated with these modalities have appeared. Bronchoscopy is reserved for patients with an atypical presentation who are suspected of having an underlying malignancy or foreign body (Table 21.7). Bronchoscopy is no longer routinely used for abscess drainage because the majority of abscesses spontaneously communicate with the airways and drain. It is also possible to rupture an abscess during bronchoscopy and contaminate previously uninvolved lung segments.

Criteria for bronchoscopy to exclude an underlying carcinoma in patients with lung cavities are (a) mean oral temperature below 100°F, (b) absence of systemic symptoms, (c) absence of predisposing factors for aspiration, and (d) mean leukocyte count below 11,000/mm³ (31). When more than three of these factors are present in a patient with lung abscess, an underlying carcinoma is likely. Other factors that should prompt bronchoscopic evaluation include an atypical clinical presentation (noncavitary lesion or lesions and fulminant time course), atypical abscess location (especially in the anterior half of the lung), abscess formation in an edentulous patient, failure to respond to antibiotics, and lung abscess associated with mediastinal adenopathy, a finding that is uncommon in anaerobic lung infection.

Before the antibiotic era, distant septic complications such as metastatic brain infection or unrelenting sepsis were infrequent (<10%) but feared problems. Complications of lung abscess include empyema formation resulting from a bronchopleural fistula, massive hemoptysis, spontaneous rupture into uninvolved lung segments, and failure of the abscess cavity to resolve (38,39). Although uncommon, these complications often require prolonged medical therapy in

TABLE 21.8. FACTORS ASSOCIATED WITH FAILURE OF MEDICAL THERAPY IN PATIENTS WITH LUNG ABSCESS

Recurrent aspiration
Large cavity size (>6 cm)
Prolonged symptom complex before presentation
Abscess associated with an obstructing lesion
Presence of thick-walled cavities
Underlying serious comorbidity
Development of empyema

addition to surgical intervention, either with tube thoracostomy in the case of empyema or lung resection in the case of massive hemoptysis.

Surgical treatment of lung abscess is usually reserved for cases with complications such as massive hemoptysis, bronchopleural fistula, and empyema. It is also used in the setting of fulminant infection and in patients who fail medical therapy. Approximately 10% of lung abscesses require surgical intervention. Prognostic factors associated with failure of medical treatment include recurrent aspiration, large cavity size (>6 cm), prolonged symptom complex before presentation, abscess associated with an obstructing lesion, abscess with a thick-walled cavity, advanced age, neoplasm, and other chronic medical conditions (33) (Table 21.8). An alternative to surgical drainage is percutaneous catheter placement. At this time, percutaneous drainage should be reserved for patients who are unresponsive to medical therapy and have lung abscesses located peripherally. Drainage of an abscess is recommended when (a) sepsis persists 5 to 7 days after the initiation of antibiotic therapy, (b) the abscess is larger than 4 cm, or (c) the abscess increases in size while the patient is on medical therapy (40). Placement of a percutaneous catheter can obviate the need for surgery in a significant percentage of patients who have failed medical treatment, with a mean time to abscess resolution of 10 to 15 days and improvement in clinical parameters within 48 hours (41). These patients should also receive intravenous antibiotics during and after percutaneous drainage of a lung abscess.

LUNG ABSCESS

Summary Statement	Level of Evidence
The vast majority of lung abscesses are caused by anaerobic bacteria.	Nonrandomized and observational studies
Treatment should be with penicillin, penicillin plus metronidazole, or clindamycin.	Randomized and observational studies
Clindamycin may be preferable to the other agents.	Randomized clinical studies
Bronchoscopy is not routinely required.	Nonrandomized and observational studies

LIPOID PNEUMONIA

Lipoid pneumonia is a chronic illness of the lower respiratory tract resulting from the accumulation of lipoid material in the alveoli or interstitium; it is not strictly an infectious syndrome. The clinical characteristics of this disease depend on whether the syndrome is exogenous or endogenous. A noninfectious alveolar filling process causes chronic, nonresolving pneumonia, but lipoid pneumonia can be complicated by secondary infection, as in a patient with postobstructive pneumonia secondary to an endobronchial lesion.

Exogenous lipoid pneumonia is the result of aspiration of lipid material such as mineral oil, vegetable oil, and animal fats, with the type of aspirate predicting the underlying pathologic response. As a consequence of fatty acid production, aspiration of animal fat usually causes a severe inflammatory reaction resulting in hemorrhagic pneumonia. On the other hand, aspiration of vegetable oil results in little or no pathologic response, and mineral oils usually cause a foreign body reaction that leads to pulmonary fibrosis. This pathologic response to mineral oil is actually used in animals as a model of pulmonary fibrosis.

In exogenous mineral oil lipoid pneumonia (the most common syndrome), the clinical features include cough, dyspnea, sputum production, occasional hemoptysis, and chest radiographic abnormalities consisting of nonspecific infiltrates in the lower lobes, although any pattern can be seen, including cavitary lung lesions (42). A majority of patients have conditions that predispose them to oil aspiration or inhalation, including gastroesophageal reflux and neurologic or psychiatric illness (43). The most common radiographic abnormalities are alveolar consolidation, ground-glass opacity, and alveolar nodules. Magnetic resonance imaging may allow the detection of pulmonary consolidation of high signal intensity on T1-weighted images, consistent with lipid content (44). Although nonspecific, areas of consolidation with low attenuation and a "crazy paving" pattern are frequently seen on high-resolution CT (44–46). *In the "crazy paving" pattern, the CT scan demonstrates diffuse ground-glass density with thickened intralobular and interlobular septa that produce polygonal shapes.* Ordinarily, patients have minimal or no clinical symptoms and seek medical assistance because of incidental abnormal findings on a chest radiograph. The intratracheal aspiration of mineral oil generally occurs subclinically, and patients are usually without cough, other signs of liquid aspiration, or acute inflammation.

The typical patient who recurrently aspirates mineral oil–based medicinal aids is an elderly person who has used oil-based nose drops or an oil-based laxative for several years. The diagnosis can be made by a history of the use of mineral oil or other oil in a patient with respiratory symptoms and chronic nonresolving pneumonia. Not uncommonly, the diagnosis is made on biopsy because lipoid pneumonia can mimic infectious diseases and lung malignancy. Once exogenous lipoid pneumonia has been diagnosed, treatment consists of removing the cause (e.g., oil-based laxatives) and supportive therapy. Other therapeutic modalities, such as repeated bronchoalveolar lavage and corticosteroids, are available, but their overall clinical usefulness is uncertain.

Endogenous lipoid pneumonia is caused by the accumulation of lipids derived from the breakdown of endogenous products (e.g., cell membranes and surfactant). The material most often associated with this type of lipoid pneumonia is cholesterol, and thus *cholesterol pneumonia* is another name for this entity. The pathologic process is usually localized and limited to an abnormal region of the lung, in contrast to what occurs in exogenous lipoid pneumonia. The most common underlying abnormality resulting in endogenous lipoid pneumonia is an obstructing endobronchial lesion, either lung cancer or a foreign body.

The clinical presentation of patients with endogenous lipoid pneumonia is typically that of the underlying cause. In the case of an obstructing lesion, cough, fever, chills, and a chest radiograph revealing an underlying mass or segmental lesion with a concomitant postobstructive pneumonia are characteristic. In sharp contrast to exogenous lipoid pneumonia, endogenous lipoid pneumonia is not associated with recurrent aspiration or a history of use of an oil-based substance. Like the exogenous type, endogenous lipoid pneumonia is not infectious in origin, but infection secondary to the underlying obstructive process can occur.

LIPOID PNEUMONIA	
Summary Statement	**Level of Evidence**
Removing the cause (e.g., oil-based laxatives) and supportive measures are the recommended treatments.	Observational studies, expert opinion
Bronchoalveolar lavage and corticosteroids have no proven role in management.	Observational studies, expert opinion

ACUTE EXACERBATIONS OF CHRONIC OBSTRUCTIVE PULMONARY DISEASE

Chronic obstructive pulmonary disease (COPD) is defined as irreversible or partially reversible airway obstruction associated with chronic bronchitis or emphysema (47). COPD is the fourth leading cause of death in America, and its prevalence is rising (48–50). In excess of 1 million visits are made to emergency departments annually in the United States by patients with a principal diagnosis of bronchitis, and more than 10 million office visits were made in 1994 for the same diagnosis. Two thirds of patients presenting to ambulatory care physicians with a diagnosis of bronchitis are given an

antibiotic (51), and their more than 6 million prescriptions comprise 11% of all antibiotic prescriptions (52).

Diagnosis

No characteristic laboratory or radiographic features correlate with acute exacerbations of COPD. Clinical criteria (history of increased cough or sputum production, increased purulence of sputum, and dyspnea) in the absence of acute radiographic abnormalities define these episodes (53). The differential diagnosis would include congestive heart failure, pneumonia, pulmonary embolism, and aspiration.

Anthonisen and colleagues (53), in a landmark study, graded patients based on their presenting clinical symptoms. A type I exacerbation was defined as increase in dyspnea, volume of sputum, or purulence of sputum. A type II exacerbation was defined as the presence of two of these symptoms, and a type III exacerbation was the presence of one of the cardinal symptoms plus at least one of the following: upper respiratory tract infection within the past 5 days, fever without any other cause, increase in wheezing, increase in cough, and 20% increase in respiratory or heart rate in comparison with baseline. Patients with a type I or II exacerbation derived a demonstrable benefit from antimicrobial therapy (better outcome, shorter clinical illness, fewer cases of deterioration), which implied a bacterial etiology, whereas the response of patients with a type III exacerbation did not differ from that of patients receiving placebo. Stockley and colleagues (54) pointed out that frank sputum purulence was 94.4% sensitive and 77.0% specific for a high bacterial load in subsequent sputum culture. They suggested that sputum color might be the simplest clinical marker of patients most likely to respond to antibacterial therapy.

Physical Examination

Patients with an acute exacerbation frequently demonstrate rales and expiratory wheezing, both nonspecific findings. Fever is often absent. An elevated temperature and focal chest findings suggest pneumonia as an alternative diagnosis.

Radiography

Most physicians do not obtain a chest radiograph unless they clinically suspect pneumonia or congestive heart failure. In most patients, the chest radiograph is normal or demonstrates increased bronchovascular markings.

Sputum Examination

Sputum examination is not necessary in most patients. Because the upper airway is frequently colonized with commensals, interpreting the results of sputum culture is difficult. In the face of failure of standard empiric therapy, frequent exacerbations, recent previous antibiotic therapy, or severe exacerbation, sputum culture may help identify an unusual or drug-resistant pathogen.

Role of Bacteria

The majority of acute exacerbations of chronic bronchitis are infectious in origin, but exposure to allergens, pollutants, or cigarette smoke may also precipitate a sudden deterioration. Viral and, to a much lesser extent, *Mycoplasma* and *Chlamydia* infections are associated with up to a third of acute exacerbations (55). Approximately half of all exacerbations of COPD can be attributed to bacterial infection. The major pathogens are nontypeable *H. influenzae*, other *Haemophilus* species, *S. pneumoniae,* and *Moraxella catarrhalis* (56). These organisms are often found in the upper respiratory tract of normal persons and can be seen in the expectorated sputum of patients with chronic bronchitis during periods of clinical stability. Exacerbations can be caused by endogenous or exogenous reinfection by *H. influenzae* (57). Among patients with reasonably well-preserved lung function, Gram-positive organisms such as *S. pneumoniae* and common Gram-negative organisms such as *H. influenzae* and *M. catarrhalis* predominate. However, in patients with declining lung function, some evidence has been found of an increasing prevalence of enteric Gram-negative organisms and, in some cases, *P. aeruginosa* (58,59).

Four studies examining lower airway bacteriology in acute exacerbations identified potential pathogens at concentrations consistent with tissue infection (60–63). Monsó and colleagues (60) compared patients with an acute exacerbation and a control group with stable COPD. Bacterial pathogens were isolated twice as frequently at the cutoff concentration of 10^3 organisms per milliliter in the acutely ill group. In these studies, the organisms isolated were similar to those identified in sputum cultures—namely, *H. influenzae*, *S. pneumoniae*, and *M. catarrhalis*.

An increased concentration of inflammatory mediators in pulmonary secretions, including interleukin-8, tumor necrosis factor-α, and neutrophil elastase, is associated with bacterial exacerbations but not exacerbations that are culture-negative. The treatment of purulent exacerbations with antibiotics is also associated with a substantial decline in inflammatory markers (64). Human serum antibodies bactericidal for nontypeable *H. influenzae* have been identified during exacerbations (65,66). These antibodies, directed against the outer membrane protein OMP P2, confer specific immunity against that strain but not against any other strain of *H. influenzae*. Acquisition of a new strain may be associated with clinical deterioration. The development of symptoms depends on the virulence of the newly infecting strain. Similar findings have been demonstrated with *M. catarrhalis*, but studies have not been performed in patients with recently acquired strains of *S. pneumoniae* (67). These data explain, in part, older observations that colonization rates are similar

in the sputum of infected and stable patients. These studies were unable to differentiate among different strains of a potentially pathogenic species. More recent studies examining longitudinal trends in airway colonization suggest that strain changes may explain many but not all exacerbations. *H. influenzae* is capable of invading airway tissue and can be found in subepithelial spaces and within macrophages (68,69). Tissue invasion may explain how these bacteria can persist despite bactericidal antibodies and potent antibiotics.

Role of Antibiotics

The results of randomized placebo-controlled antimicrobial trials conducted in previous decades were inconclusive (70–75) (Table 21.9). Most of the studies were not sufficiently powered to reach a definitive conclusion, but more recent, better-designed studies have concluded that antibiotics are effective. Anthonisen and colleagues (53), in a prospective randomized placebo-controlled trial, demonstrated improved outcomes among patients with the most severe exacerbation, defined previously (see section "Diagnosis"). Allegra and colleagues (76), in another well-designed randomized trial involving a large number of patients, demonstrated the superiority of amoxicillin/clavulanate to placebo. Reanalysis of these data suggests that the greatest benefit of antibiotics is in patients with the worst lung function (77). In a randomized double-blinded placebo-controlled trial of 93 patients with an acute exacerbation associated with respiratory failure, performed by Nouira and colleagues (78), fluoroquinolones, in comparison with placebo, were associated with reductions in mortality, need for additional antibiotics, duration of mechanical ventilation, and hospital stay. A conflicting study by Sachs and colleagues (79) that demonstrated no benefit of antibiotics is flawed by the small number of patients enrolled, the lack of patients with severe disease, and most importantly, the inclusion of patients with asthma. Although the Anthonisen classification is helpful in predicting an antimicrobial response, it has a sensitivity of only 59% and a specificity of 60% in predicting a bacterial exacerbation (80). This would suggest that although it represents an advance, the classification is only moderately successful in predicting a bacterial etiology and confirming the role of antimicrobials. Stockley and colleagues (81) showed that the presence of frankly purulent sputum is adequate in predicting a high bacterial load. Saint and colleagues (82), in a metaanalysis of placebo-controlled trials of patients with acute exacerbations of chronic bronchitis (not including the studies of Allegra and Nouira), demonstrated that antibiotic therapy is associated with a small but statistically significant improvement in clinical outcomes and hastens clinical and physiologic recovery.

Traditionally, an antibiotic such as ampicillin, tetracycline, or trimethoprim/sulfamethoxazole has been the standard treatment choice for acute exacerbations of chronic bronchitis. However, a failure rate of 13% to 25% can be

TABLE 21.9. RANDOMIZED TRIALS OF ANTIBIOTICS IN ACUTE EXACERBATIONS OF CHRONIC BRONCHITIS

Comparators	No. Patients	Outcome of Therapy	Reference
Placebo vs.	37	Treated patients lost half as much time from	Elmes et al., 1957 (70)
oxytetracycline	37	work and exacerbations were shorter.	
Placebo vs.	27	Treated patients recovered sooner and	Berry et al., 1960 (71)
oxytetracycline	26	deteriorated less often.	
Placebo vs.	28	No significant difference in clinical response.	Elmes et al., 1965 (72)
ampicillin	28		
Placebo vs.	10	No significant differences.	Peterson et al., 1967 (73)
physiotherapy vs.	10		
chloramphenicol	9		
Placebo vs.	86	Antibiotic therapy was superior to placebo, but	Pines et al., 1972 (74)
chloramphenicol vs.	84	no differences between antibiotics.	
tetracycline	89		
Placebo vs.	20	100% vs. 100% clinical response.	Nicotra et al., 1982 (75)
tetracycline	20		
Placebo vs. either cotrimoxazole,	180	55% vs.	Anthonisen et al., 1987 (53)
amoxicillin, or doxycycline	182	68% success (P <.01).	
Placebo vs. amoxicillin/	179	50.3% vs.	Allegra et al., 1991 (76)
clavulanate	190	86.4% success (P <.01).	
Placebo vs.	46	45.9% reduction in risk for death and need for	Nouira et al., 2001 (78)
ofloxacin	47	additional antibiotics (P <.0001).	

Source: From Elmes PC, Fletcher CM, Dutton AAC. Prophylactic use of oxytetracycline for exacerbations of chronic bronchitis. *Br Med J* 1957;2:1272–1275; Berry DG, Fry J, Hindley CP, et al. Exacerbations of chronic bronchitis treatment with oxytetracycline. *Lancet* 1960;1:137–139; Elmes PC, King TKC, Langlands JHM, et al. Value of ampicillin in the hospital treatment of exacerbations of chronic bronchitis. *Br Med J* 1965;2:904–908; Peterson ES, Esmann V, Honcke P, et al. A controlled trial of the effect of treatment on chronic bronchitis: an evaluation using pulmonary function tests. *Acta Med Scand* 1967;182:293–305; Pines A, Raafat H, Greenfield JSB, et al. Antibiotic regimens in moderately ill patients with purulent exacerbations of chronic bronchitis. *Br J Dis Chest* 1972;66:107–115; Nicotra MB, Rivera M, Awe RJ. Antibiotic therapy of acute exacerbations of chronic bronchitis. *Ann Intern Med* 1982;97:18–21; Anthonisen NR, Manfreda J, Warren CPW, et al. Antibiotic therapy in exacerbations of chronic obstructive lung disease. *Ann Intern Med* 1987;106:196–204; Allegra L, Grassi C, Grossi E, et al. The role of antibiotics in the treatment of chronic bronchitis exacerbation: follow-up of a multicenter trial. *Ital J Chest Dis* 1991;45:138–148; Nouira S, Marghli S, Belghith M, et al. Once daily oral ofloxacin in chronic obstructive pulmonary disease exacerbation requiring mechanical ventilation: a randomised placebo-controlled trial. *Lancet* 2001;358:2020–2025, with permission.

expected after treatment with first-line antibiotics (amoxicillin, trimethoprim/sulfamethoxazole, tetracycline, erythromycin) (83–85). Patients with significant compromise of lung function tend to require hospitalization and are at risk for the development of respiratory failure. The development of resistance of primary respiratory pathogens to these antibiotics, the recognition of Gram-negative organisms, especially among patients with significant impairment of lung function, and the development of more potent broad-spectrum agents with improved coverage of the major respiratory pathogens has forced a reexamination of the antimicrobial choices.

Resistance to β-lactam antibiotics such as ampicillin can be expected in 20% to 40% of isolated strains of *H. influenzae* and in more than 90% of strains of *M. catarrhalis* (86,87). No clinical features can predict the presence of β-lactamase–producing bacteria except that patients infected with these organisms tend to have had more courses of antibiotics (88). Penicillin resistance is now found in more than 35% of *S. pneumoniae* isolates in some studies and is increasing worldwide (89). Penicillin resistance is also a marker for resistance to other classes of antibiotics, including the cephalosporins, macrolides, β-lactam/β-lactamase inhibitors, trimethoprim/sulfamethoxazole, and tetracyclines

(90,91). Although penicillin or other drug resistance and widespread clinical failure in lower respiratory tract infections have not been linked at this time, this may only be a reflection of the rapidly changing antimicrobial environment. Most organisms demonstrate low levels of penicillin resistance (minimum inhibitory concentrations $\leq 2\ \mu g/mL$). Because the doses of β-lactams usually prescribed achieve high levels in blood, these current levels of resistance can be overcome. If levels of resistance continue to increase, however, the value of many classes of antibiotics, including β-lactams, cephalosporins, macrolides, tetracyclines, and sulfonamides, may diminish. Antibiotic overprescribing for trivial illnesses is a major factor in the emergence of bacterial resistance. Attention must be paid to decreasing antimicrobial prescribing and to identifying those patients who would benefit from aggressive broad-spectrum therapy.

Risk Factors for Treatment Failure

The identification of patients who may fail standard antimicrobial therapy with the usual first-line agents should improve antimicrobial prescribing (Table 21.10). Ball and colleagues (83) enrolled 471 patients with acute exacerbations of chronic bronchitis characterized by increased dyspnea,

TABLE 21.10. RISK FACTORS FOR TREATMENT FAILURE

Reference	Risk Factor
Ball et al. (83)	Cardiopulmonary disease
	More than four chest infections in previous year
Dewan et al. (92)	FEV$_1$ <35% of predicted value
	Use of home oxygen
	Increased frequency of exacerbations
	Use of maintenance steroids
	History of previous pneumonia
Miravitlles et al. (93)	Ischemic heart disease
	Degree of dyspnea
	Number of visits to general practitioner in previous year

FEV$_1$, forced expiratory volume in 1 second.
Source: From Ball P, Harris JM, Lowson D, et al. Acute infective exacerbation of chronic bronchitis. *Q J Med* 1995;88:61–68; Dewan NA, Rafique S, Kanwar B, et al. Acute exacerbations of chronic obstructive lung disease. Factors associated with poor treatment outcomes. *Chest* 2000;117:662–671; Miravitlles M, Murio C, Guerrero T, et al. Factors associated with relapse after ambulatory treatment of acute exacerbations of chronic bronchitis. *Eur Respir J* 2001;17:928–933, with permission.

sputum volume, and purulence. An increased number of chest infections in the previous year and coexistent cardiopulmonary disease were predictors of a return to the physician with a chest problem. Patients with more than four treated exacerbations in the previous year were 2.11 times more likely to fail initial management than patients without this risk factor. Coexistent cardiopulmonary disease increased the odds of failure 2.3 times. Cardiovascular comorbidity and more than four exacerbations in the previous year had a sensitivity of 75% and a specificity of 47% in predicting return to the prescribing physician for further treatment.

In a retrospective study, Dewan and colleagues (92) reviewed the clinical experience with 107 patients in a university Veterans Administration clinic during a 24-month observation period. They noted a 14.7% failure rate within 4 weeks of observation in COPD patients mainly treated with first-line antibiotics. More than half of the patients with exacerbations who failed initial treatment required hospitalization. Independent host factors associated with treatment failure included severe impairment of lung function, the use of home oxygen, frequent exacerbations, a history of pneumonia, and the use of maintenance corticosteroids. When a stepwise logistic regression analysis was performed, the need for home oxygen and frequent exacerbations correctly classified failure in 83% of the patients. In this study, age, the presence of comorbidity, and the choice of antibiotics did not affect treatment outcome.

Miravitlles and colleagues (93) prospectively studied 2,414 patients in Spain and developed a multivariate model to identify risk factors independently associated with treatment failure. In this study, the severity of the underlying disease, number of visits to the primary care physician, and coexistence of ischemic heart disease were predictive of an increased risk for relapse after ambulatory treatment of an

acute exacerbation of chronic bronchitis. The severity of the exacerbation was not predictive of treatment failure.

Risk Factors for Hospitalization

Patients are admitted to the hospital following an inadequate response to outpatient management, an inability to perform the activities of daily living as a consequence of increased dyspnea, or the development of respiratory failure, often in association with comorbidities or inadequate home care resources. Knowledge of the risk factors for hospitalization might allow interventions to prevent this and other unfortunate outcomes (Table 21.11).

In the study of Ball and colleagues (83), significant cardiopulmonary disease was the only predictor of admission to a hospital for further management of an acute exacerbation of chronic bronchitis. Patients with chronic bronchitis for a greater number of years were less likely to be admitted to a hospital. This is in contrast to the findings of Grossman and colleagues (94), who determined that severity of underlying COPD and duration of disease were the best predictors of hospitalization. Patients with severe chronic bronchitis were more than four times more likely to be admitted to a hospital than patients with mild to moderate disease, and the risk was similar for patients who had had disease for more than 10 years. If both risk factors were present, the risk for hospitalization increased almost 20 times. In the study of Kessler and colleagues (95), a small body mass, a limited 6-minute walk test, significant gas exchange impairment, and pulmonary hemodynamic worsening predicted hospitalization. Multivariate analysis indicated that carbon dioxide retention (Paco$_2$ > 44 mm Hg) and pulmonary hypertension (pulmonary artery pressure at rest >18 mm Hg) were the best predictors of hospitalization. Age, comorbidity, and smoking habit were not predictive of hospitalization. Vestbo and colleagues (96) demonstrated in the Copenhagen City Heart Study that chronic mucus hypersecretion was associated with an excess decline in the forced expiratory volume in 1 second (FEV$_1$) and an increased risk for subsequent hospitalization because of COPD. This relationship continued to be significant even after adjustments were made for age, smoking, and the FEV$_1$ value. In a Spanish study with a case control design, three or more COPD admissions in the previous year, a lower FEV$_1$ value, and underprescription of long-term oxygen therapy were predictive of hospitalization for a COPD exacerbation (97).

Risk Stratification

Factors including significant cardiopulmonary and other comorbidity, frequent purulent exacerbations of COPD, advanced age, generalized debility, malnutrition, long-term corticosteroid administration, long duration of COPD, chronic hypersecretion of mucus, undertreatment of cor pulmonale, recurrent hospitalizations for COPD exacerbations,

TABLE 21.11. RISK FACTORS FOR HOSPITALIZATION

Reference	Variable	Odds Ratio	Confidence Interval
Ball et al. (83)	Cardiopulmonary disease	8.89	1.73–45.6
Kessler et al. (95)	$Paco_2$ > 44 mm Hg	2.1	1.4–3.1
	Ppa > 18 mm Hg	2	1.3–3.1
Grossman et al. (94)	Duration of disease	4.6	1.6–13.0
	Severity of disease	4.3	0.8–24.6
	Both	19.8	3.2–120.8
Vestbo et al. (96)	Mucus hypersecretion (men)	2.4	1.3–4.5
	Mucus hypersecretion (women)	2.6	1.2–5.3
Garcia-Aymerich et al. (97)	Three or more COPD admissions in previous year	3.82	1.14–12.75
	Percentage of predicted FEV_1	0.97	0.95–0.99
	Underprescription of long-term oxygen therapy	14.66	1.54–139.75

COPD, chronic obstructive pulmonary disease; FEV_1, forced expiratory volume in 1 second; $Paco_2$, arterial partial pressure of carbon dioxide; Ppa, pulmonary artery pressure at rest.
Source: From Ball P, Harris JM, Lowson D, et al. Acute infective exacerbation of chronic bronchitis. *Q J Med* 1995;88:61–68; Kessler R, Faller M, Fourgaut G, et al. Predictive factors of hospitalization for acute exacerbation in a series of 64 patients with chronic obstructive pulmonary disease. *Am J Crit Care Med* 1999;159:158–164; Grossman RF, Mukerjee J, Vaughan D, et al. A one-year community-based health economic study of ciprofloxacin vs. usual antibiotic treatment in acute exacerbations of chronic bronchitis. *Chest* 1998;113:131–141; Vestbo J, Prescott E, Lange P, et al. Association of chronic mucus hypersecretion with FEV_1 decline and chronic obstructive pulmonary disease morbidity. *Am J Respir Crit Care Med* 1996;153:1530–1535; Garcia-Aymerich J, Monsó E, Marrades RM, et al. Risk factors for hospitalization for a chronic obstructive pulmonary disease exacerbation. Efram Study. *Am J Respir Crit Care Med* 2001;164:1002–1007, with permission.

and severe underlying lung function are associated with failure of therapy with the usual antimicrobial agents, early relapse, and hospitalization (Table 21.11). Patients with these factors may be infected with difficult-to-treat organisms, such as *K. pneumoniae* and *P. aeruginosa*, particularly if their lung function is severely impaired (58,59). Treatment directed toward resistant pathogens with potent bactericidal drugs should improve clinical outcomes and lower overall costs, particularly if hospital admissions and respiratory failure can be prevented. Stratification of patients into risk categories may allow the physician to select targeted antimicrobial therapy to prevent some of these consequences.

This simple classification system divides patients into four groups (Table 21.12). *Group 0* patients present with an acute onset of cough associated with sputum production, often soon after a coryzal illness and fever. Although smokers may be included in this group, the majority of patients have no underlying lung disease. They have acute tracheobronchitis that is usually viral in origin. Because they have no underlying lung disease, the illness of patients in this group is usually self-limited and runs a benign course. In a small number of patients, the course is more protracted. *M. pneumoniae* and *C. pneumoniae* are known etiologic agents of acute tracheobronchitis and may be responsible for illness in those patients not demonstrating a rapid clinical improvement.

Group 1 patients have chronic bronchitis, defined as cough and sputum production for at least 3 months during two consecutive years. With this illness, the cough worsens and the production of purulent sputum increases. However, in general, they are young (age < 65 years), have only mild to moderate impairment of lung function (FEV_1 > 50% of predicted value), experience fewer than four exacerbations per year, and exhibit no significant comorbidity. In this group of patients, the usual pathogens, including *H. influenzae, S. pneumoniae,* and *M. catarrhalis,* are present, although viral infection often precedes bacterial superinfection. Antibiotics have been shown to shorten the clinical illness. Treatment with virtually any antibiotic is usually successful, and the prognosis is excellent. Based on *in vitro* susceptibility data, ampicillin, amoxicillin, cefpodoxime, cefixime, cefdinir, cefuroxime, and trimethoprim/sulfamethoxazole can be recommended. Despite resistance to β-lactams, outcomes in general are acceptable. Until a prospective pharmacoeconomic or clinical study demonstrates some advantage for the use of more potent agents in group 1 patients, this recommendation is based on pharmacokinetic/pharmacodynamic considerations alone.

Group 2 patients tend to be older and have risk factors for treatment failure such as poor underlying lung function (FEV_1 < 50% of predicted value). Their lung function may be only moderately impaired (FEV_1 between 50% and 65% of predicted value), but they have significant comorbidity (diabetes mellitus, congestive heart failure, chronic renal disease, chronic liver disease) or experience four or more exacerbations per year. *H. influenzae, S. pneumoniae,* and *M. catarrhalis* continue to be the predominant organisms. Several studies have indicated that with declining lung function, enteric Gram-negative organisms may be isolated from pulmonary secretions. Treatment with medications directed toward resistant organisms, such as a respiratory

TABLE 21.12. RISK CLASSIFICATION AND SUGGESTED ANTIMICROBIAL THERAPY

Class	Basic Clinical State	Risk Factors	Probable Pathogens	First Choice	Alternatives
0	Acute tracheobronchitis	Cough and sputum without previous pulmonary disease	Usually viral	None unless symptoms persist for > 4–5 days	Macrolide or tetracycline
1	Chronic bronchitis without risk factors	Cough, increased sputum production and purulence	H. influenzae, Haemophilus species, M. catarrhalis, S. pneumoniae	Ampicillin, amoxicillin, cefpodoxime, cefixime, cefdinir, cefuroxime, trimethoprim/sulfamethoxazole	Fluoroquinolone, β-lactam/β-lactamase inhibitor, new macrolide, second- or third-generation cephalosporin
2	Chronic bronchitis with risk factors	As in class 1 plus Severe dyspnea FEV$_1$ < 50% of predicted value Age > 55 years More than four exacerbations per year Significant comorbidity Malnutrition COPD duration > 12 years Long-term oral steroid use	As in class 1 plus Klebsiella species + other Gram-negatives Increased probability of β-lactam resistance	Fluoroquinolone, β-lactam/β-lactamase inhibitor	Second-generation macrolide, some second- and third-generation cephalosporins (cefuroxime or cefprozil, cefixime) May require parenteral therapy Consider referral to a specialist or hospital
3	Chronic suppurative bronchitis	As in class 2 with constant purulent sputum; majority have bronchiectasis	As in class 2 plus P. aeruginosa and multiresistant Enterobacteriaceae and Klebsiella species	Ambulatory patients: ciprofloxacin Hospitalized patients: parenteral therapy usually required; P. aeruginosa common pathogen	

COPD, chronic obstructive pulmonary disease; FEV$_1$, forced expiratory volume in 1 second.

fluoroquinolone or amoxicillin/clavulanic acid, should be more effective than amoxicillin or other first-line agents.

Group 3 patients have chronic bronchial infection with daily production of purulent secretions. They are subject to frequent exacerbations characterized by increased sputum production, sputum purulence, and cough and by worsening dyspnea, often accompanied by hemoptysis. In many cases, evidence of bronchiectasis is found on high-resolution CT. Besides the usual respiratory organisms, other Gram-negative organisms, including Enterobacteriaceae and *Pseudomonas* species, should be considered as potential pathogens. Ciprofloxacin is the oral agent with the most activity against these species and should be considered the agent of choice when they are identified.

DOES EVIDENCE SUPPORT AGGRESSIVE ANTIBIOTIC THERAPY IN HIGH-RISK PATIENTS?

In a decision analysis model, Van Barlingen and colleagues (98) compared macrolides, fluoroquinolones, penicillins, and cephalosporins in the outpatient treatment of acute exacerbations of chronic bronchitis. The key cost drivers were the clinical success/failure rates of first-line treatment and the cost of hospitalization. For patients with less severe disease, they concluded that the differences among the antibiotic classes were not great but slightly favored the macrolides and fluoroquinolones. For patients with more severe acute exacerbations of chronic bronchitis, they concluded that the fluoroquinolones were the most cost-effective. The clinical success rate of the first-line agents was the most important factor in reducing overall costs.

Another economic study pointed out that the clinical success rate of the initial antimicrobial agent is the primary determinant of overall expenditures because of the high cost of treatment failure, particularly if hospitalization becomes necessary (99). The most cost-effective antibiotics are not those with a low acquisition cost but those with a high rate of clinical efficacy.

Following the introduction of ciprofloxacin in the province of Quebec, LeLorier and Derderian (100) examined the role of ciprofloxacin in the treatment of serious lower respiratory tract infections; they noted a decrease in the rate of hospitalizations for asthmatic bronchitis. This decrease was not noted in the province of Saskatchewan, where ciprofloxacin use was severely restricted. A statistically significant correlation was found between increases in ciprofloxacin prescriptions and differences between predicted and observed hospitalization rates.

In the study of Adams and colleagues (101), the rate of recurrence of COPD exacerbations was higher in patients with illness severe enough to present to an emergency department who were treated with ampicillin than in patients who received other antimicrobial therapies. The recurrence rate with ampicillin (54%) was much higher than that with

any other antibiotic examined. This suggests that high-risk patients (presumably anyone requiring treatment in an emergency department for an acute exacerbation of chronic bronchitis) would benefit from aggressive therapy directed toward resistant pathogens.

In a retrospective study by Destache and colleagues (85), the use of antibiotics with broader coverage than that of the usual first-line antibiotics in the treatment of acute exacerbations of chronic bronchitis reduced both the hospitalization rate and the failure rate. Although the acquisition cost of the newer antibiotics (cephalosporins, macrolides, and fluoroquinolones) was higher, the overall costs of the treated patients given these drugs were lower. In particular, the group receiving amoxicillin/clavulanate, azithromycin, or ciprofloxacin had the lowest hospitalization rate, clinical failure rate, and costs in comparison with patients given cephalosporins or first-line therapy.

The hypothesis that aggressive antibiotic therapy should be offered to high-risk patients was tested in a prospective health economic study. Patients with at least three treated exacerbations in the past year were randomized to receive either ciprofloxacin or any non–quinolone-based therapy for their next acute exacerbation of chronic bronchitis (102). Clinical endpoints (days of illness, hospitalizations, time to next exacerbation) were blended with quality-of-life measurements (Nottingham Health Profile, St. George's Hospital Respiratory Questionnaire, Health Utility Index) and total respiratory costs from a societal perspective. Although the overall results indicated no preference for either treatment arm, in patients with risk factors (severe underlying lung disease, more than four exacerbations per year, bronchitis for longer than 10 years, elderly, significant comorbid illness), the use of ciprofloxacin was associated with an improved clinical outcome, better quality of life, and lower costs. The results of this study suggest that aggressive antimicrobial therapy directed especially toward resistant organisms in high-risk patients may be a more effective strategy than no therapy or therapy with older antimicrobials.

Chodosh (103), in a series of double-blinded crossover studies, determined that 0.5 to 1 g of ampicillin four times daily was associated with a low failure rate and an infection-free interval ranging from 117 to 302 days. These studies were conducted in the 1970s, when there were essentially no resistant strains of *H. influenzae* or *M. catarrhalis*. Comparable results were achieved with 750 mg of ciprofloxacin. Tetracyclines, trimethoprim/sulfamethoxazole, and especially cefaclor were associated with higher failure rates and a shorter infection-free interval. Two more recent studies compared 500 mg of ciprofloxacin twice daily with 500 mg of clarithromycin twice daily and 500 mg of cefuroxime axetil twice daily in group 2 patients (104,105). These studies demonstrated similar clinical outcomes, but ciprofloxacin showed a bacterial eradication rate superior to those of the other drugs, and the time to the next exacerbation was shortest for clarithromycin (a poor outcome). In the GLOBE (gemifloxacin long-term outcomes in bronchitis exacerbations) study, 320 mg of gemifloxacin once daily for 5 days was compared with 500 mg of clarithromycin twice daily for 7 days (106). Although the short-term clinical outcomes were similar, gemifloxacin had a significantly better bacteriologic eradication rate and demonstrated faster eradication of *H. influenzae*. Gemifloxacin was superior to clarithromycin in preventing further exacerbations (71.0% vs. 58.5% with no further exacerbations, $P = .016$) and reduced the number of patients hospitalized for respiratory tract infection during 6 months of follow-up (0.023% vs. 0.0625%, $P = .059$). This is the first well-designed clinical trial to demonstrate the clinical superiority of a more potent antimicrobial with the use of clinically relevant outcomes.

Identification of patient risk factors for initial treatment failure and hospitalization is reasonably well developed. This makes it possible to categorize patients into groups that should be predictive of antibiotic efficacy. Given the prevailing resistance patterns of the most prevalent respiratory pathogens, a more rational selection process for antibiotics is possible. The effects of a poor initial treatment choice is

quite clear—significant clinical and economic consequences. Prospective randomized trials properly designed to examine important clinical and economic endpoints are urgently required.

MANAGEMENT OF ACUTE AND CHRONIC BRONCHITIS

Summary Statement	Level of Evidence
Antimicrobial therapy is warranted for patients with an acute exacerbation of chronic bronchitis if they fall into the Anthonisen type I or II category or have frankly purulent sputum.	Randomized and observational studies
A high-risk group of patients can be identified comprising those with significant impairment of lung function (FEV$_1$ ≤ 50% of predicted value), frequent exacerbations (≥ 2–4/y), disease of long duration, significant comorbidity, advanced age, malnutrition, and long-term oral corticosteroid use.	Observational studies, expert opinion
Risk group 0 patients (acute tracheobronchitis) should not be treated with antibiotics unless symptoms persist beyond several days.	Nonrandomized and observational studies, expert opinion
For risk group 1 patients, antimicrobial therapy shortens the clinical illness.	Randomized study
Broad-spectrum potent agents such as respiratory fluoroquinolones and amoxicillin/clavulanate are recommended for group 2 patients.	Randomized study, expert opinion
Group 3 patients at risk for *P. aeruginosa* infection (frequent antimicrobial agents, structural lung damage, long-term corticosteroid treatment) should be treated with an anti-*Pseudomonas* agent (ciprofloxacin).	Expert opinion

FEV$_1$, forced expiratory volume in 1 second.

REFERENCES

1. Mendelson CR. The aspiration of stomach contents into the lungs during obstetric anesthesia. *Am J Obstet Gynecol* 1946;52:191–205.
2. Huxley EJ, Viroslav J, Gray WR, et al. Pharyngeal aspiration in normal adults and patients with depressed consciousness. *Am J Med* 1978;64:544–548.
3. Gleeson K, Eggli DF, Maxwell SL. Quantitative aspiration during sleep in normal subjects. *Chest* 1997;111:1266–1272.
4. Bartlett JG, Gorbach SL. The triple threat of aspiration pneumonia. *Chest* 1975;68:560–566.
5. Croghan JE, Burke EM, Caplan S, et al. Pilot study of 12-month outcomes of nursing home patients with aspiration on videofluoroscopy. *Dysphagia* 1994;9:141–146.
6. Bynum LJ, Pierce AK. Pulmonary aspiration of gastric contents. *Am Rev Respir Dis* 1976;114:1129–1136.
7. Holas MA, DePippo KL, Reding MJ. Aspiration and relative risk of medical complications following stroke. *Arch Neurol* 1994;51:1051–1053.
8. Kidd D, Lawson J, Nesbitt, et al. Aspiration in acute stroke: a clinical study with videofluoroscopy. *Q J Med* 1993;86:825–829.
9. Martin BJ, Corlew MM. The association of swallowing dysfunction and aspiration pneumonia. *Dysphagia* 1994;9:1–6.
10. Marumo K, Homma S, Fukuchi Y. Postgastrectomy aspiration pneumonia. *Chest* 1995;107:453–456.
11. Terpenning M, Bretz W, Lopatin D, et al. Bacterial colonization of saliva and plaque in the elderly. *Clin Infect Dis* 1993;16:S314–S316.
12. Finucane TE, Bynum JPW. Use of tube feeding to prevent aspiration pneumonia. *Lancet* 1996;348:1421–1424.
13. Torres A, Serra-Batles J, Ros E, et al. Pulmonary aspiration of gastric contents in patients receiving mechanical ventilation: the effect of body position. *Ann Intern Med.* 1992;116:540–543.
14. Teabeaut JR. Aspiration of gastric contents: an experimental study. *Am J Pathol* 1952;28:51–67.
15. Exarhos ND, Logan WD Jr, Abbott OA, et al. The importance of pH and volume in tracheobronchial aspiration. *Dis Chest* 1965;47:167–169.
16. Donowitz LG, Page MC, Mileur BL, et al. Alteration of normal gastric flora in critical care patients receiving antacid and cimetidine therapy. *Infect Control* 1986;7:23–26.
17. Cook DJ, Laine LA, Guyatt GH, et al. Nosocomial pneumonia and the role of gastric pH. A meta-analysis. *Chest* 1991;100:7–13.
18. Valenti WM, Trudell RG, Bentley DW. Factors predisposing to oropharyngeal colonization with Gram-negative bacilli in the aged. *N Engl J Med* 1978;298:1108–1111.
19. Bartlett JG, Gorbach SL, Finegold SM. The bacteriology of aspiration pneumonia. *Am J Med* 1974;56:202–207.
20. Lorber B, Swenson RM. Bacteriology of aspiration pneumonia. *Ann Intern Med* 1974;81:329–331.
21. Cesar L, Gonzalez C, Calia FM. Bacteriologic flora of aspiration-induced pulmonary infections. *Arch Intern Med* 1975;135:711–714.
22. Mier L, Dreyfuss D, Darchy B, et al. Is penicillin G an adequate

initial treatment for aspiration pneumonia? A prospective evaluation using a protected specimen brush and quantitative cultures. *Intensive Care Med* 1993;19:279–284.

23. Marik PE, Careau P. The role of anaerobes in patients with ventilator-associated pneumonia and aspiration pneumonia: a prospective study. *Chest* 1999;115:178–183.

24. Bartlett JG, Gorbach SL. Treatment of aspiration pneumonia and primary lung abscess. Penicillin G versus clindamycin. *JAMA* 1975;234:935–937.

25. Hammond JM, Potgieter PD, Hanslo D, et al. The etiology and antimicrobial susceptibility patterns of micro-organisms in acute community-acquired lung abscess. *Chest* 1995;108:937–941.

26. Marik PE. Aspiration pneumonitis and aspiration pneumonia. *N Engl J Med* 2001;344:665–671.

27. Blondeau JM, Felmingham D. *In vitro* and *in vivo* activity of moxifloxacin against community respiratory tract pathogens. *Clin Drug Invest* 1999;18:57–78.

28. Niederman MS, Mandell LA, Anzueto A, et al. Guidelines for the management of adults with community-acquired pneumonia. Diagnosis, assessment of severity, antimicrobial therapy and prevention. *Am J Respir Crit Care Med* 2001;163:1730–1754.

29. Bartlett JG. Anaerobic infections of the lung and pleural space. *Clin Infect Dis* 1993;16[Suppl 4]:S248–S255.

30. Gudiol F, Manresa F, Pallares R, et al. Clindamycin vs. penicillin for anaerobic lung infections: high rate of penicillin failures associated with penicillin-resistant *Bacteriodes melaninogenicus*. *Arch Intern Med* 1990;150:2525–2529.

31. Sosenko A, Glassroth J. Fiberoptic bronchoscopy in the evaluation of lung abscesses. *Chest* 1985;87:489–494.

32. Mori T, Ebe T, Takahashi M, et al. Lung abscess: analysis of 66 cases from 1979–1991. *Intern Med* 1993;32:278–284.

33. Hirshberg B, Sklair-Levi M, Nir-Paz R, et al. Factors predicting mortality of patients with lung abscess. *Chest* 1999;115:746–750.

34. Davis B, Systrom DM. Lung abscess: pathogenesis, diagnosis, and treatment. *Curr Clin Top Infect Dis* 1998;18:252–273.

35. Levison ME, Mangura CT, Lorber B, et al. Clindamycin compared with penicillin for the treatment of anaerobic lung abscess. *Ann Intern Med* 1983;98:466–471.

36. Perlino C. Metronidazole versus clindamycin treatment of anaerobic pulmonary infection. *Arch Intern Med* 1981;141:1424–1427.

37. Weiss W, Cherniack NS. Acute nonspecific lung abscess: a controlled study comparing orally and parenterally administered penicillin G. *Chest* 1974;66:348–351.

38. Barnett TB, Herring CL. Lung abscess. Initial and late results of medical therapy. *Arch Intern Med* 1971;127:217–227.

39. Thoms NW, Wilson RF, Puro HE, et al. Life-threatening hemoptysis in primary lung abscess. *Ann Thorac Surg* 1972;14:347–359.

40. Rice TW, Ginsberg RJ, Todd TR. Tube drainage of lung abscesses. *Ann Thorac Surg* 1987;44:356–359.

41. Ha HK, Kang MW, Park JM, et al. Lung abscesses: percutaneous catheter therapy. *Acta Radiol* 1993;34:362–365.

42. Spickard A, Hirschmann JV. Exogenous lipoid pneumonia. *Arch Intern Med* 1994;154:686–692.

43. Gondouin A, Manzoni Ph, Ranfaing E, et al. Exogenous lipid pneumonia: a retrospective multicenter study of 44 cases in France. *Eur Respir J* 1996;9:1463–1469.

44. Laurent F. Exogenous lipoid pneumonia: HRCT, MR, and pathologic findings. *Eur Radiol* 1999;9:1190–1196.

45. Lee KS, Muller NL, Newell JD, et al. Lipoid pneumonia: CT findings. *J Comput Assist Tomogr* 1995;19:48–51.

46. Lipinski JK, Weisbrod GL, Sanders DE. Exogenous lipoid pneumonitis: pulmonary patterns. *AJR Am J Roentgenol* 1981;136:931–934.

47. American Thoracic Society. Standards for the diagnosis and care of patients with chronic obstructive pulmonary disease. *Am J Respir Crit Care Med* 1995;152:S77–S121.

48. US Bureau of the Census. *Statistical abstract of the United States*, 14th ed. Washington, DC: US Bureau of the Census, 1994:95.

49. Woolcock AJ. Epidemiology of chronic airways disease. *Chest* 1989;96[Suppl 3]:302S–306S.

50. American Lung Association. Trends in chronic bronchitis and emphysema: morbidity and mortality. *www.lungusa.org*.

51. Morrell DC. Expressions of morbidity in general practice. *Br Med J* 1971;2:454–458.

52. Gonzales R, Steiner JF, Sande MA. Antibiotic prescribing for adults with colds, upper respiratory tract infections, and bronchitis by ambulatory care physicians. *JAMA* 1997;278:901–904.

53. Anthonisen NR, Manfreda J, Warren CPW, et al. Antibiotic therapy in exacerbations of chronic obstructive lung disease. *Ann Intern Med* 1987;106:196–204.

54. Stockley RA, O'Brien C, Pye A, et al. Relationship of sputum color to nature and outpatient management of acute exacerbations of COPD. *Chest* 2000;117:1638–1645.

55. Gump DW, Phillips CA, Forsyth BR, et al. Role of infection in chronic bronchitis. *Am Rev Respir Dis* 1976;113:465–473.

56. Chodosh S. Treatment of acute exacerbations of chronic bronchitis: state of the art. *Am J Med* 1991;91[Suppl 6A]:87S–92S.

57. Groeneveld K, Van Alphen L, Eijk PP, et al. Endogenous and exogenous reinfections by *Haemophilus influenzae* in patients with chronic obstructive pulmonary disease: the effect of antibiotic treatment on persistence. *J Infect Dis* 1990;161:512–517.

58. Eller J, Ede A, Schaberg T, et al. Acute infective exacerbation of chronic bronchitis. Relation between bacterial etiology and lung function. *Chest* 1998;113:1542–1548.

59. Miravitlles M, Espinosa C, Fernández-Laso E, et al. Relationship between bacterial flora in sputum and functional impairment in patients with acute exacerbations of COPD. *Chest* 1999;116:40–46.

60. Monsó E, Ruiz J, Rosell A, et al. Bacteria infection in chronic obstructive pulmonary disease. A study of stable and exacerbated outpatients using the protected specimen brush. *Am J Respir Crit Care Med* 1995;152:1316–1320.

61. Fagon J-Y, Chastre J, Trouillet J-L, et al. Characterization of distal bronchial microflora during acute exacerbation of chronic bronchitis. *Am Rev Respir Dis* 1990;142:1004–1008.

62. Soler N, Torres A, Ewig S, et al. Bronchial microbial patterns in severe exacerbations of chronic obstructive pulmonary disease (COPD) requiring mechanical ventilation. *Am J Respir Crit Care Med* 1998;157(5 Pt 1):1498–1505.

63. Pela R, Marchesani F, Agostinelli C, et al. Airways microbial flora in COPD patients in stable clinical conditions and during exacerbations: a bronchoscopic investigation. *Monaldi Arch Chest Dis* 1998;53:262–267.

64. Sethi S, Muscarella K, Evans N, et al. Airway inflammation and etiology of acute exacerbations of chronic bronchitis. *Chest* 2000;118:1557–1565.

65. Musher DM, Kubitschek KR, Crennan J, et al. Pneumonia and acute febrile tracheobronchitis due to *Haemophilus influenzae*. *Ann Intern Med* 1983;99:444–450.

66. Yi K, Sethi S, Murphy T. Human immune response to nontypeable *Haemophilus influenzae* in chronic bronchitis. *J Infect Dis* 1997;176:1247–1252.

67. Murphy TF, Kirkham C, Denardin E, et al. Analysis of antigenic structure and human immune response to outer membrane protein CD of *Moraxella catarrhalis*. *Infect Immun* 1999;67:4578–4585.

68. Van Schilfgaarde M, Eijk P, Regelink A, et al. *Haemophilus influenzae* localized in epithelial cell layers is shielded from antibiotics and antibody-mediated bactericidal activity. *Microb Pathog* 1999;26:249–262.

69. Moller LVM, Times W, Van der Bij W, et al. *Haemophilus influenzae* in lung explants of patients with end-stage pulmonary disease. *Am J Respir Crit Care Med* 1998;157:950–956.

70. Elmes PC, Fletcher CM, Dutton AAC. Prophylactic use of oxytetracycline for exacerbations of chronic bronchitis. *Br Med J* 1957;2:1272–1275.

71. Berry DG, Fry J, Hindley CP, et al. Exacerbations of chronic bronchitis treatment with oxytetracycline. *Lancet* 1960;1:137–139.

72. Elmes PC, King TKC, Langlands JHM, et al. Value of ampicillin in the hospital treatment of exacerbations of chronic bronchitis. *Br Med J* 1965;2:904–908.

73. Peterson ES, Esmann V, Honcke P, et al. A controlled trial of the effect of treatment on chronic bronchitis: an evaluation using pulmonary function tests. *Acta Med Scand* 1967;182:293–305.

74. Pines A, Raafat H, Greenfield JSB, et al. Antibiotic regimens in moderately ill patients with purulent exacerbations of chronic bronchitis. *Br J Dis Chest* 1972;66:107–115.

75. Nicotra MB, Rivera M, Awe RJ. Antibiotic therapy of acute exacerbations of chronic bronchitis. *Ann Intern Med* 1982;97:18–21.

76. Allegra L, Grassi C, Grossi E, et al. The role of antibiotics in the treatment of chronic bronchitis exacerbation: follow-up of a multicenter trial. *Ital J Chest Dis* 1991;45:138–148.

77. Allegra L, Blasi F, De Bernardi B, et al. Antibiotic treatment and baseline severity of disease in acute exacerbations of chronic bronchitis: a re-evaluation of previously published data of a placebo-controlled randomized study. *Pulm Pharmacol Ther* 2001;14:149–155.

78. Nouira S, Marghli S, Belghith M, et al. Once daily oral ofloxacin in chronic obstructive pulmonary disease exacerbation requiring mechanical ventilation: a randomised placebo-controlled trial. *Lancet* 2001;358:2020–2025.

79. Sachs APE, Koeter GH, Groenier KH, et al. Changes in symptoms, peak expiratory flow, and sputum flora during treatment with antibiotics of exacerbations in patients with chronic obstructive pulmonary disease in general practice. *Thorax* 1995;50:758–763.

80. Sethi S, Paluri R, Grant BJB, et al. Prediction models for the etiology of acute exacerbations of COPD. *Am J Respir Crit Care Med* 1999;159:A819(abst).

81. Stockley RA, O'Brien C, Pye A, et al. Relationship of sputum color to nature and outpatient management of acute exacerbations of COPD. *Chest* 2000;117:1638–1645.

82. Saint S, Vittinghoff E, Grady D. Antibiotics in chronic obstructive pulmonary disease exacerbations. A meta-analysis. *JAMA* 1995;273:957–960.

83. Ball P, Harris JM, Lowson D, et al. Acute infective exacerbation of chronic bronchitis. *Q J Med* 1995;88:61–68.

84. MacFarlane JT, Colville A, Guion A, et al. Prospective study of aetiology and outcome of adult lower respiratory tract infections in the community. *Lancet* 1993;341:511–514.

85. Destache CJ, Dewan NA, O'Donohue WJ, et al. Clinical and economic considerations in acute exacerbations of chronic bronchitis. *J Antimicrob Chemother* 1999;43[Suppl A]:107–113.

86. Doern GV, Brueggemann A, Pierce G, et al. Antibiotic resistance among clinical isolates of *Haemophilus influenzae* in the United States in 1994 and 1995 and detection of β-lactamase-positive strains resistant to amoxicillin-clavulanate: results of a national multicenter surveillance study. *Antimicrob Agents Chemother* 1997;41:292–297.

87. Doern GV, Brueggemann A, Pierce G, et al. Prevalence of antimicrobial resistance among 723 outpatients' clinical isolates of *Moraxella catarrhalis* in the United States in 1994 and 1995: results of a 30-center national surveillance study. *Antimicrob Agents Chemother* 1997;40:2884–2886.

88. Sportel JH, Koëter GH, Van Altena R, et al. Relation between β-lactamase–producing bacteria and patient characteristics in chronic obstructive pulmonary disease. *Thorax* 1995;50:249–253.

89. Doern GV, Brueggemann A, Holley HP Jr, et al. Antimicrobial resistance of *Streptococcus pneumoniae* recovered from outpatients in the United States during the winter months of 1994 to 1995: results of a 30-center national surveillance study. *Antimicrob Agents Chemother* 1997;40:1208–1213.

90. Doern GV, Pfaller MA, Kugler K, et al. Prevalence of antimicrobial resistance among respiratory tract isolates of *Streptococcus pneumoniae* in North America: 1997 results from the SENTRY Antimicrobial Surveillance Program. *Clin Infect Dis* 1998;27:764–770.

91. Thornsberry C, Ogilvie P, Kahn J, et al. Surveillance of antimicrobial resistance in *Streptococcus pneumoniae*, *Haemophilus influenzae*, and *Moraxella catarrhalis* in the United States in 1996–1997 respiratory season. *Diagn Microbiol Infect Dis* 1997;29:249–257.

92. Dewan NA, Rafique S, Kanwar B, et al. Acute exacerbations of chronic obstructive lung disease. Factors associated with poor treatment outcomes. *Chest* 2000;117:662–671.

93. Miravitlles M, Murio C, Guerrero T, et al. Factors associated with relapse after ambulatory treatment of acute exacerbations of chronic bronchitis. *Eur Respir J* 2001;17:928–933.

94. Grossman RF, Mukerjee J, Vaughan D, et al. A one-year community-based health economic study of ciprofloxacin vs. usual antibiotic treatment in acute exacerbations of chronic bronchitis. *Chest* 1998;113:131–141.

95. Kessler R, Faller M, Fourgaut G, et al. Predictive factors of hospitalization for acute exacerbation in a series of 64 patients with chronic obstructive pulmonary disease. *Am J Crit Care Med* 1999;159:158–164.

96. Vestbo J, Prescott E, Lange P, et al. Association of chronic mucus hypersecretion with FEV_1 decline and chronic obstructive pulmonary disease morbidity. *Am J Respir Crit Care Med* 1996;153:1530–1535.

97. Garcia-Aymerich J, Monsó E, Marrades RM, et al. Risk factors for hospitalization for a chronic obstructive pulmonary disease exacerbation. Efram Study. *Am J Respir Crit Care Med* 2001;164:1002–1007.

98. Van Barlingen HJJ, Nuijten MJC, Volmer T, et al. Model to evaluate the cost-effectiveness of different antibiotics in the management of acute bacterial exacerbations of chronic bronchitis in Germany. *J Med Econ* 1998;1:210–218.

99. Pechère J-C, Lacey L. Optimizing economic outcomes in antibiotic therapy of patients with acute exacerbations of chronic bronchitis. *J Antimicrob Chemother* 2000;45:19–24.

100. LeLorier J, Derderian F. Effect of listing ciprofloxacin in provincial formularies in hospitalizations for bronchitis and pyelonephritis. *Can J Clin Pharmacol* 1998;5:133–137.

101. Adams S, Melo J, Luther M, et al. Antibiotics are associated with lower relapse rates in outpatients with acute exacerbations of COPD. *Chest* 2000;117:1345–1352.

102. Torrance G, Walker V, Grossman R, et al. Economic evaluation of ciprofloxacin compared with usual antibacterial care for the treatment of acute exacerbations of chronic bronchitis in patients followed for 1 year. *Pharmacoeconomics* 1999;16:499–520.

103. Chodosh S. Treatment of acute exacerbations of chronic bronchitis: state of the art. *Am J Med* 1991;91[Suppl 6A]:87S–92S.

104. Chodosh S, McCarty J, Farkas S, et al. Randomized, double-blind study of ciprofloxacin and cefuroxime axetil for treatment of acute bacterial exacerbations of chronic bronchitis. *Clin Infect Dis* 1998;27:722–729.

105. Chodosh S, Schreurs A, Siami G, et al. Efficacy of oral ciprofloxacin vs. clarithromycin for treatment of acute bacterial exacerbations of chronic bronchitis. *Clin Infect Dis* 1998;27:730–738.

106. Wilson R, Schentag JJ, Ball P, Mandell L. A comparison of gemifloxacin and clarithromycin in acute exacerbations of chronic bronchitis and long-term clinical outcomes. *Clin Ther* 2002;24:639–652.

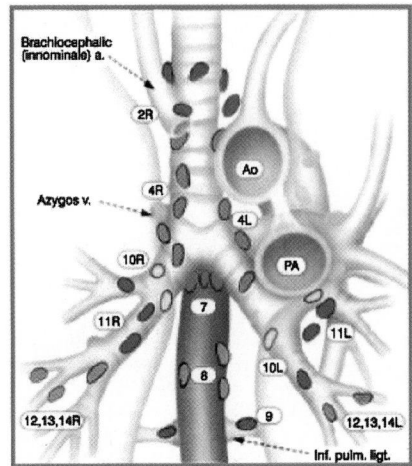

Superior Mediastinal Nodes

- **1** Highest Mediastinal
- **2** Upper Paratracheal
- **3** Pre-vascular and Retrotracheal
- **4** Lower Paratracheal
  (including Azygos Nodes)

N_2 = single digit, ipsilateral
N_3 = single digit, contralateral or supraclavicular

Aortic Nodes

- **5** Subaortic (A-P window)
- **6** Para-aortic (ascending aorta or phrenic)

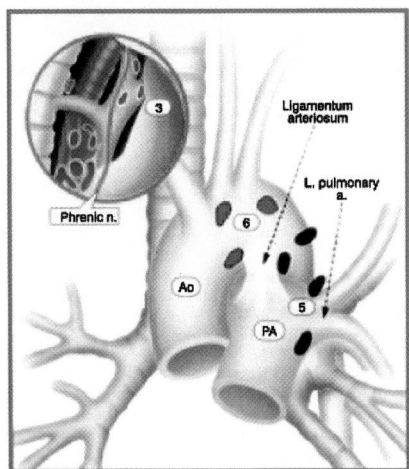

Inferior Mediastinal Nodes

- **7** Subcarinal
- **8** Paraesophageal
  (below carina)
- **9** Pulmonary Ligament

N₁ Nodes

- **10** Hilar
- **11** Interlobar
- **12** Lobar
- **13** Segmental
- **14** Subsegmental

FIGURE 4.3. Regional lymph node classification system. (Mountain/Dresler modifications from Naruke/American Thoracic Society Lung Cancer Staging Map; with permission.)

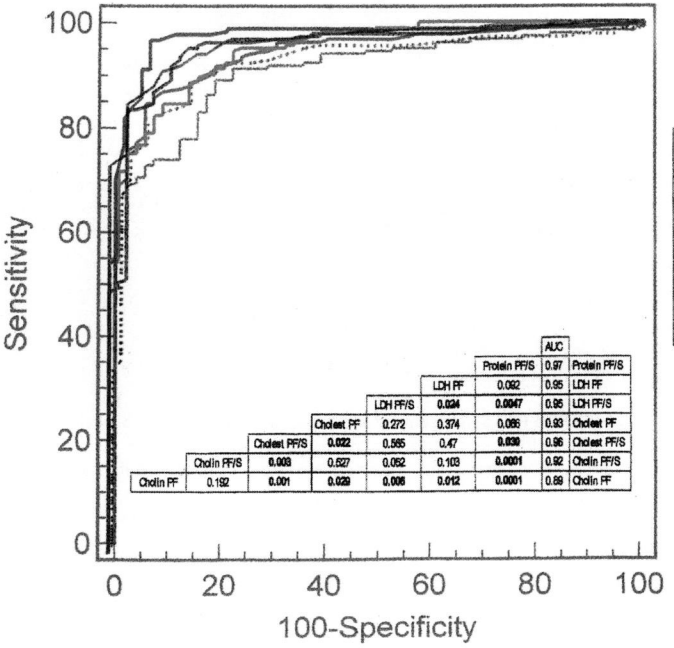

						AUC	
					Protein PF/S	0.97	Protein PF/S
				LDH PF	0.092	0.95	LDH PF
			LDH PF/S	0.034	0.0047	0.95	LDH PF/S
		Cholest PF	0.272	0.374	0.086	0.93	Cholest PF
	Cholest PF/S	0.022	0.565	0.47	0.030	0.96	Cholest PF/S
Cholin PF/S	0.003	0.527	0.062	0.103	0.0001	0.92	Cholin PF/S
Cholin PF	0.192	0.001	0.029	0.006	0.012	0.0001	0.89	Cholin PF

Legend:
- Protein PF/S
- LDH PF
- LDH PF/S
- Cholest PF
- Cholest PF/S
- Cholin PF/S
- Cholin PF

FIGURE 5.1. Receiver operating characteristics (ROC) curves of commonly used parameters for distinguishing transudates from exudates adopted from various sources (4–8). Note that the pleural fluid/serum (PF/S) ratio values generally perform superior, and that the highest area under the curve (AUC) values are achieved by protein PF/S values (0.97) and cholesterol PF/S values (0.96), respectively.

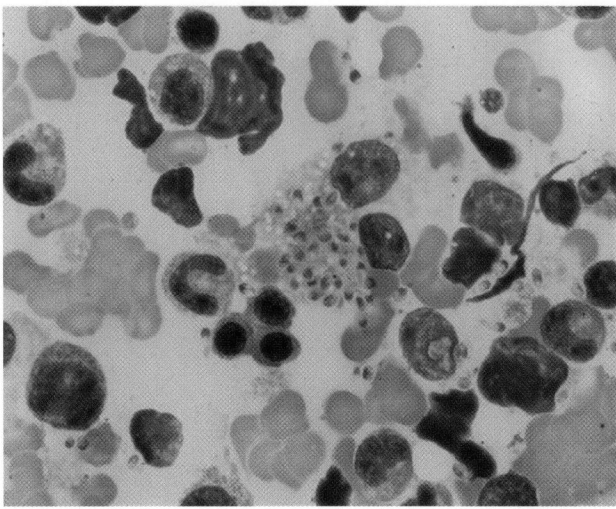

FIGURE 19.4. Bone marrow aspirate from a patient with AIDS and progressive disseminated histoplasmosis. Highly characteristic image shows macrophage filled with 1- to 2-μm yeast cells (Wright stain, original magnification ×400).

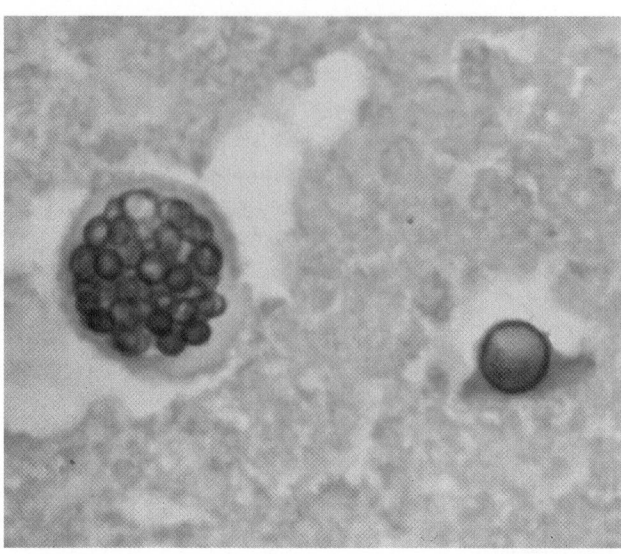

FIGURE 19.9. Giant spherule, highly characteristic of coccidioidomycosis. Structure to the right is a single endospore (Gomori methenamine silver stain, original magnification ×100).

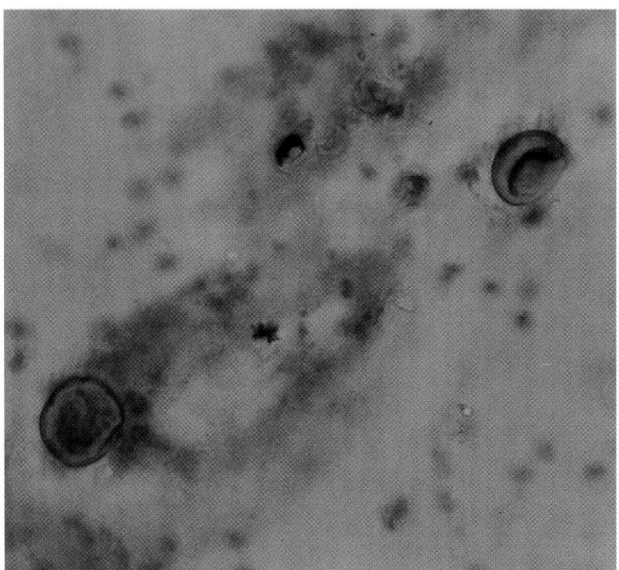

FIGURE 19.13. Disseminated coccidioidomycosis in AIDS. Bronchoalveolar lavage fluid was positive for endospores (Papanicolaou stain, original magnification ×1,000).

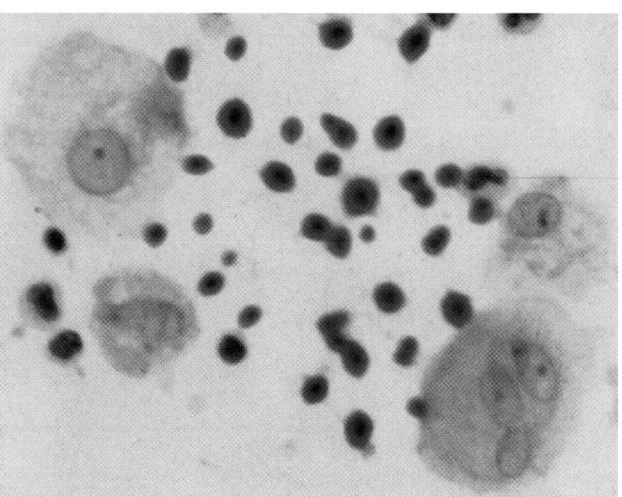

FIGURE 19.15. Disseminated cryptococcosis in AIDS. Bronchoalveolar lavage fluid was positive for encapsulated yeast. Capsular material stains bright red on special stain (mucicarmine stain, original magnification × 400).

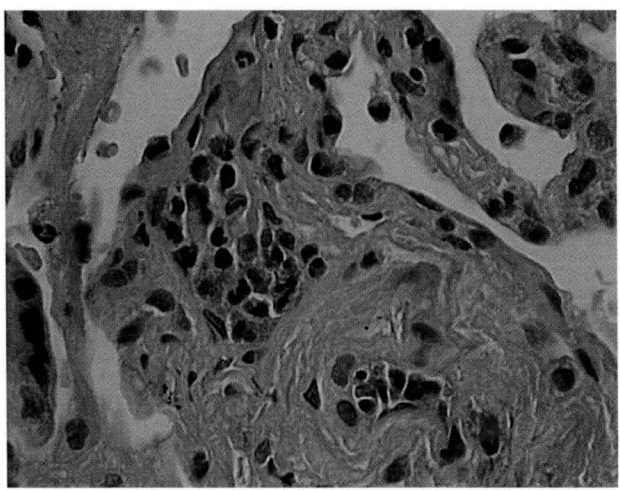

FIGURE 27.4. Lung biopsy specimen from a patient with Churg-Strauss syndrome contains perivascular granulomatous infiltrates with eosinophils.

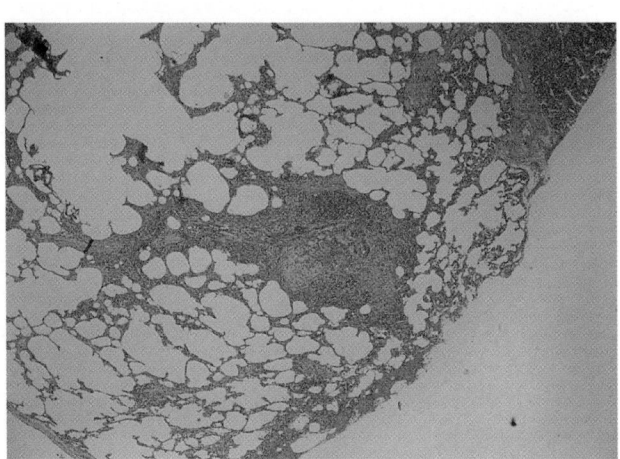

A

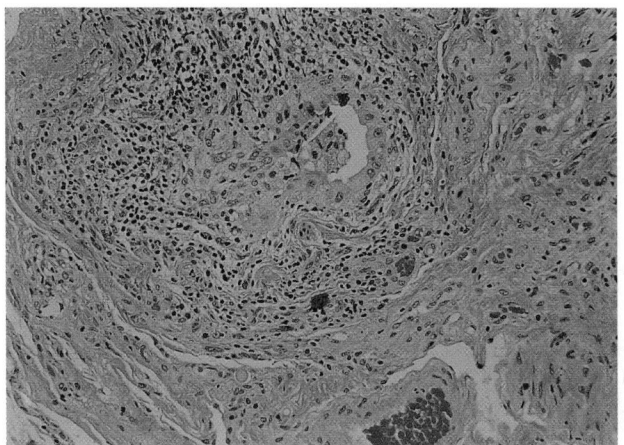

B

FIGURE 29.1. Cellular bronchiolitis. **A:** The lumen of a membranous bronchiole is completely obliterated by intraluminal and parietal inflammation (syncytial respiratory virus bronchiolitis; hematoxylin and eosin, low-power magnification). **B:** The bronchiolar wall is widened by the chronic inflammatory infiltrate. Cuboidal metaplasia of the bronchiolar epithelium (bronchiolitis in a case of hypersensitivity pneumonitis; hematoxylin and eosin, mid-power magnification).

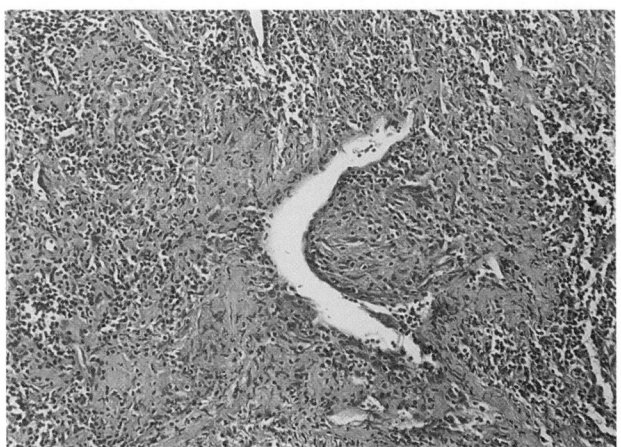

FIGURE 29.2. The lumen of a bronchiole is almost completely occupied by a polyp of granulation tissue (hematoxylin and eosin, mid-power magnification).

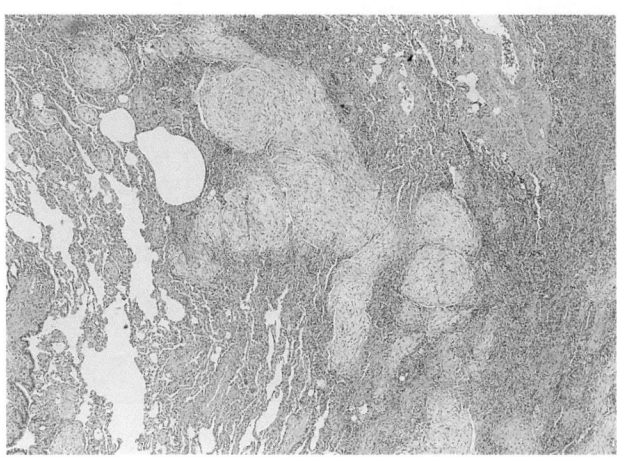

FIGURE 29.3. Bronchiolitis obliterans–organizing pneumonia pattern: serpiginous bundles of pale myxoid material fill the centrilobular air spaces (hematoxylin and eosin, low-power magnification).

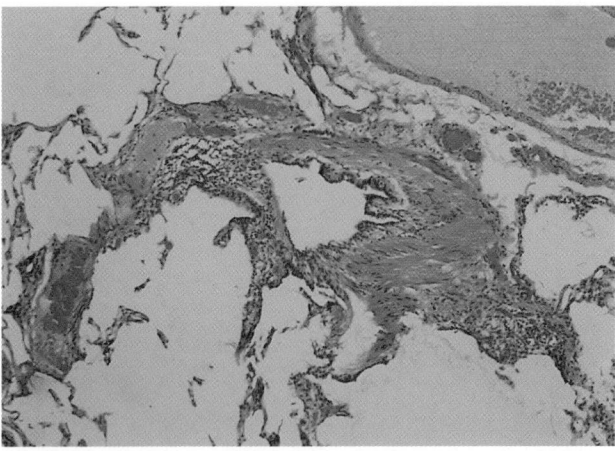

FIGURE 29.4. The lumen of a membranous bronchiole is reduced by concentric acellular fibrosis and scattered intramural inflammatory cells (bronchiolitis obliterans in a patient with graft versus host disease; hematoxylin and eosin, mid-power magnification).

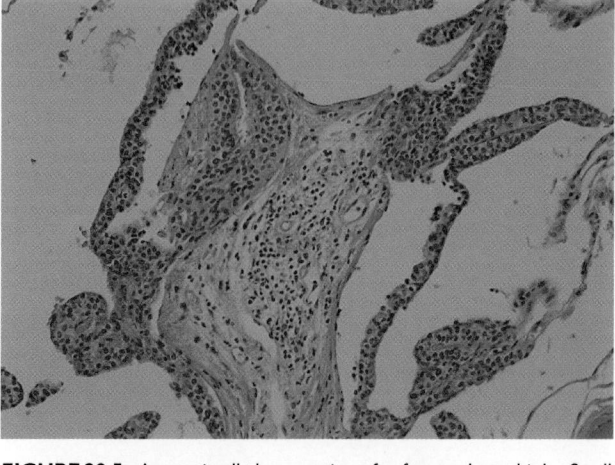

FIGURE 29.5. A scar is all that remains of a former bronchiole. Small neuroendocrine cells proliferate at the periphery (hematoxylin and eosin, mid-power magnification).

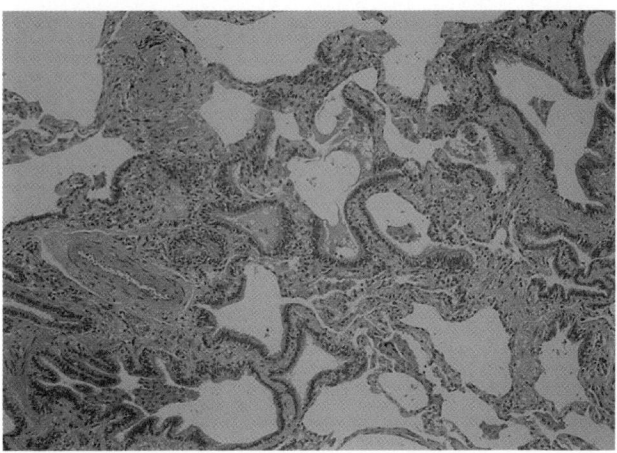

FIGURE 29.6. A bronchiole is evident in the lower left corner. The lumen is slightly reduced, and bronchiolar epithelium extends into the surroundings air spaces ("lambertosis"; hematoxylin and eosin, mid-power magnification).

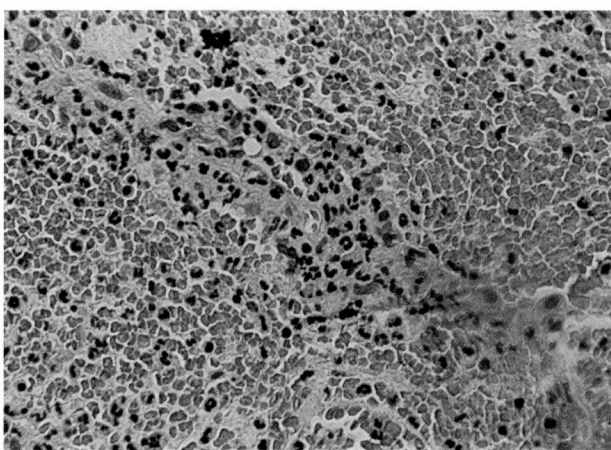

FIGURE 31.1. Diffuse alveolar hemorrhage due to pulmonary capillaritis. The interstitial space is thickened and contains fragmented neutrophils, and the alveolar space is filled with free red blood cells and neutrophils. (From Schwarz MI. Diffuse alveolar hemorrhage. In: Schwarz MI, King TE Jr, eds. *Interstitial lung disease.* Hamilton, Ontario: B.C. Decker, 1998:537, with permission.)

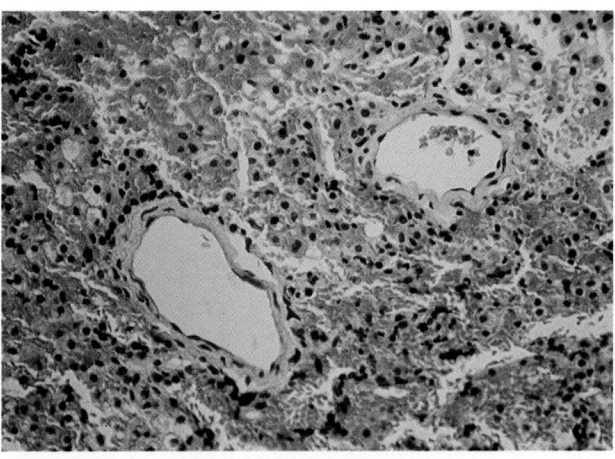

FIGURE 31.2. Diffuse alveolar hemorrhage owing to bland pulmonary hemorrhage in Goodpasture syndrome. Free red blood cells fill the alveolar space, and the interstitium demonstrates the absence of inflammation. Hyperplasia of the type II epithelial cells are noted.

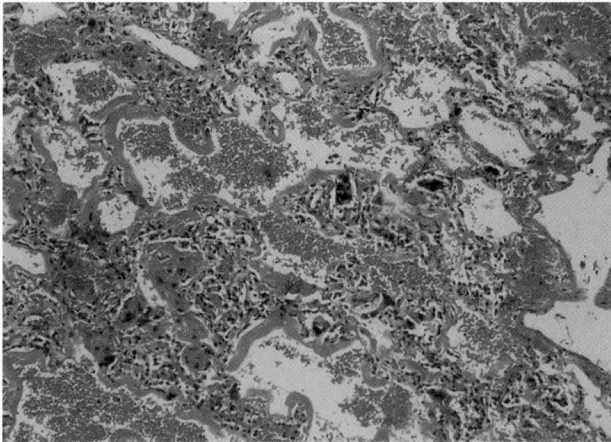

FIGURE 31.3. Diffuse alveolar hemorrhage owing to diffuse alveolar damage. Free red blood cells fill the alveolar space, and prominent hyaline membrane formation is present. (From Schwarz MI: Diffuse alveolar hemorrhage. In: Schwarz MI, King TE Jr, eds. *Interstitial lung disease.* Hamilton, Ontario: B.C. Decker, 1998:538, with permission.)

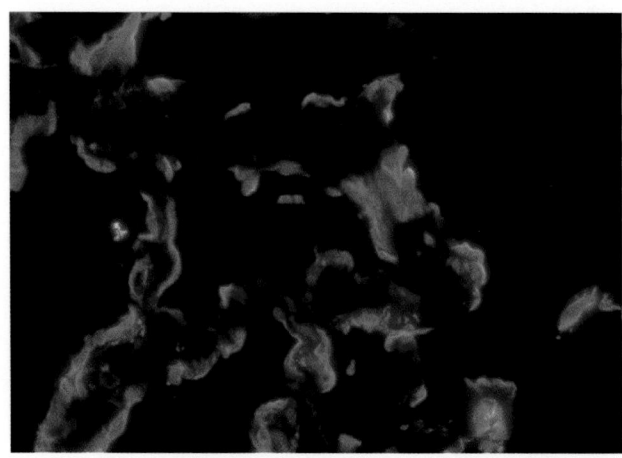 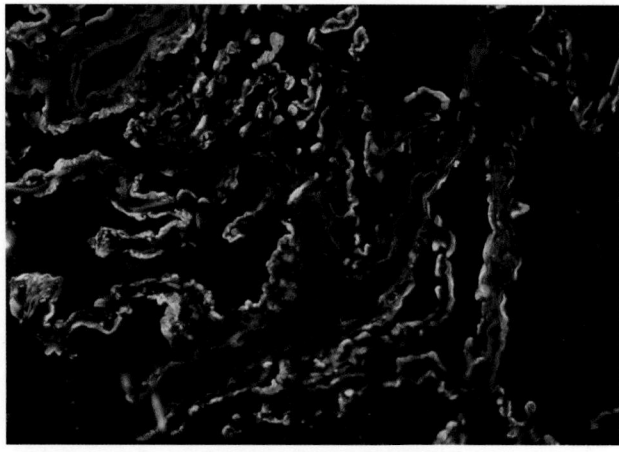

A

B

FIGURE 31.4. Immunofluorescent staining of basement membrane antigens in the alveolus of the lung **(A)** and the glomerulus of the kidney **(B)** in Goodpasture's syndrome. Note the linear deposition of serum antibasement membrane antibody, which characterizes this disease. (From Schwarz MI: Diffuse alveolar hemorrhage. In: Schwarz MI, King TE Jr, eds. *Interstitial lung disease.* Hamilton, Ontario: B.C. Decker, 1998:540, with permission.)

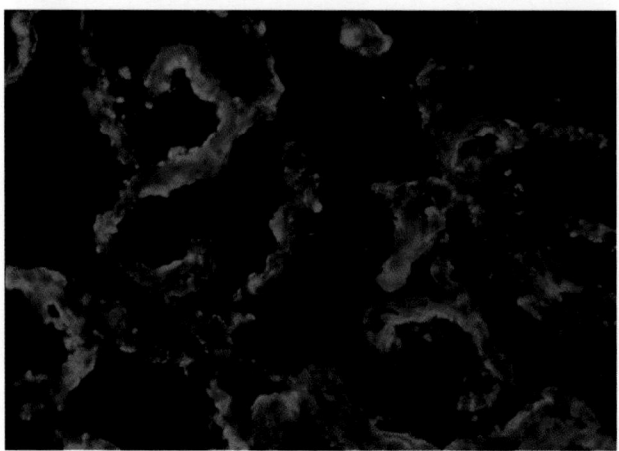

FIGURE 31.5. Immunofluorescent staining of the alveolar basement membrane in a patient with systemic lupus erythematosus. The granular or interrupted deposition of immune complexes easily separates this staining pattern from the continuous staining seen in Goodpasture syndrome. (From Schwarz MI: Diffuse alveolar hemorrhage. In: Schwarz MI, King TE Jr, eds. *Interstitial lung disease.* Hamilton, Ontario: B.C. Decker, 1998:540, with permission.)

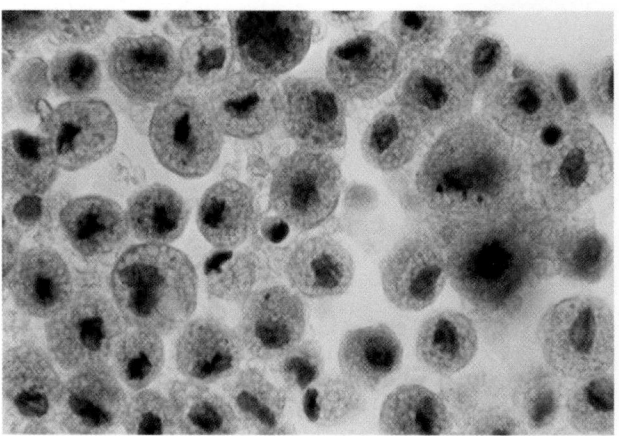

FIGURE 33.2. Amiodarone toxicity. Bronchoalveolar lavage cytologic preparation demonstrating foamy appearance of alveolar macrophages.

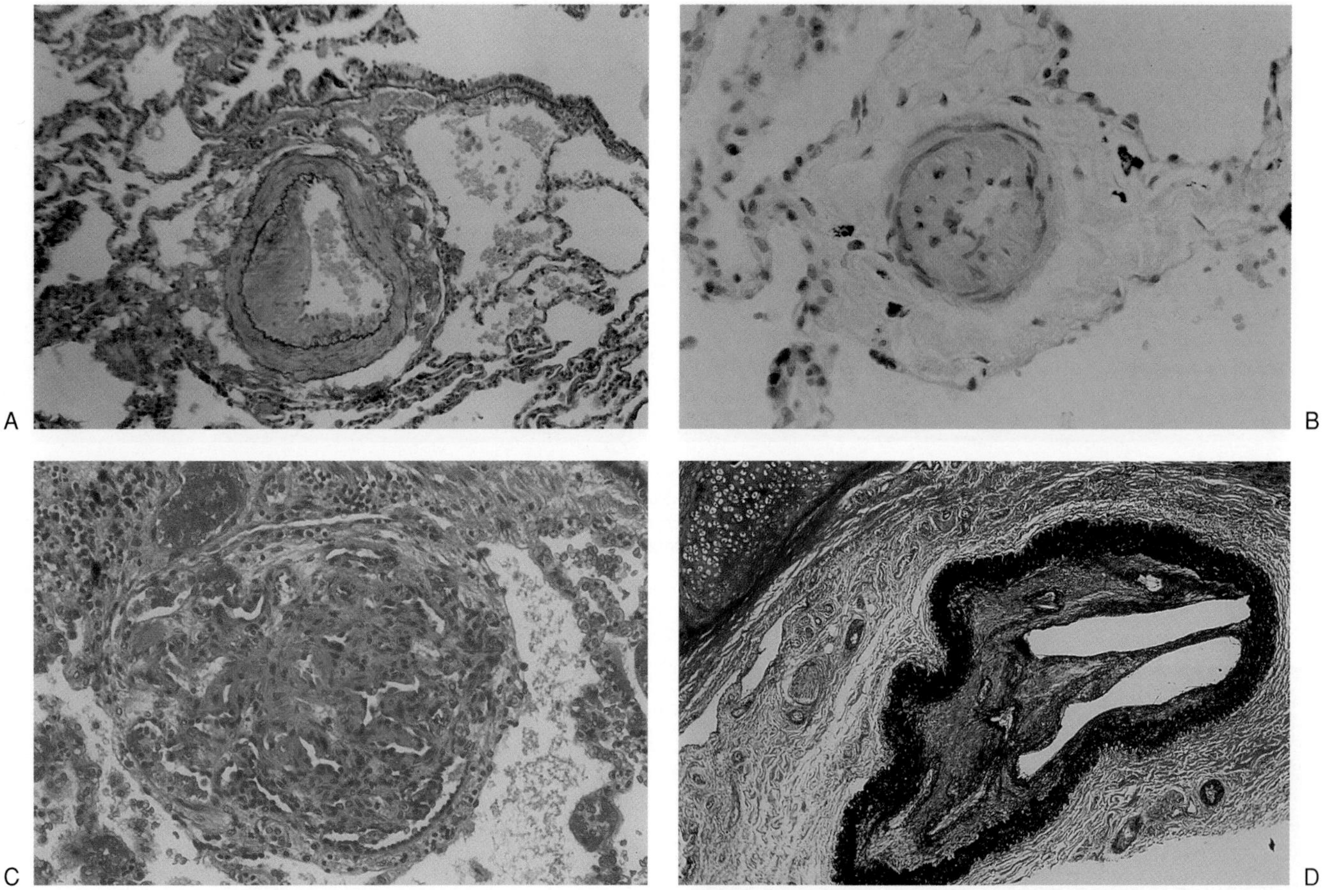

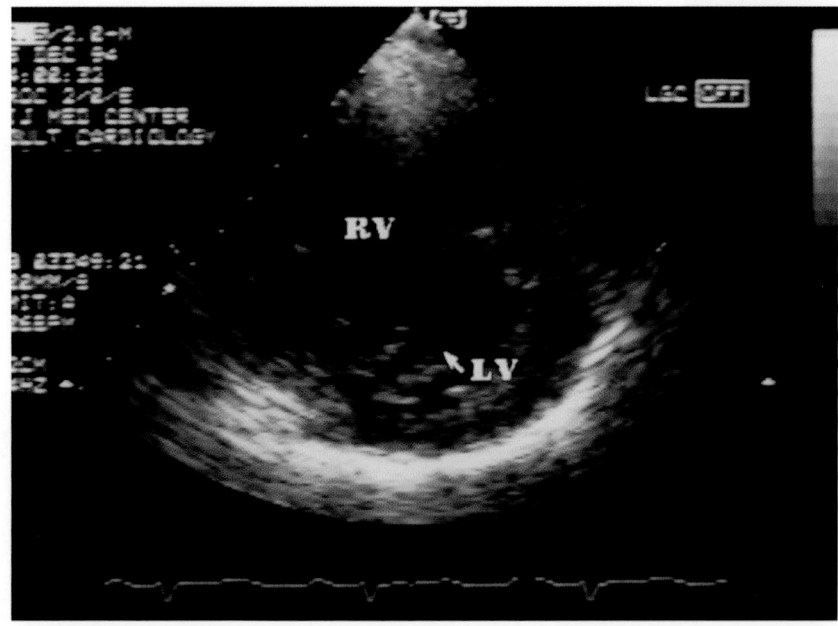

FIGURE 35.3. (A) Eccentric intimal thickening in primary pulmonary hypertension. **(B)** Medial thickening in long-standing mitral stenosis. **(C)** A plexiform lesion in primary pulmonary hypertension (magnification ×600). **(D)** A recanalized, fibrotic thrombus in chronic thromboembolism syndrome. (From Charles Kuhn, with permission.)

FIGURE 38.5. Example of echocardiogram from the patient illustrated in Fig. 38.4 at the time of the most recent chest x-ray. This short-axis view shows severe dilation of the right ventricle (RV), bulging of the septum to the left in diastole, and a small left ventricle (LV) chamber. The RV was noted to be severely hypokinetic. The *arrow* points to the interventricular septum. (From Scott Roth, Division of Cardiology, Long Island Jewish Medical Center, New Hyde Park, New York, with permission.)

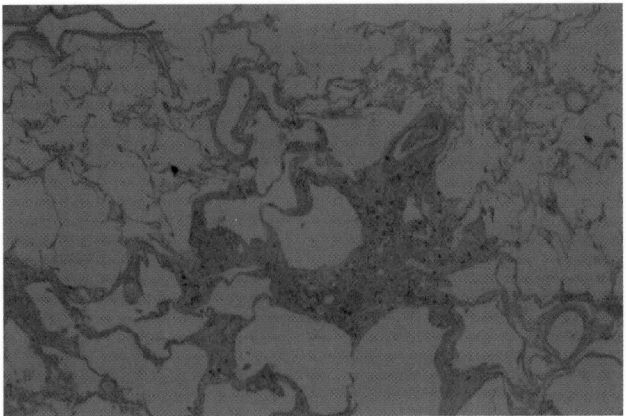

FIGURE 44.1. Asbestos-induced airways disease with alveolar duct fibrosis.

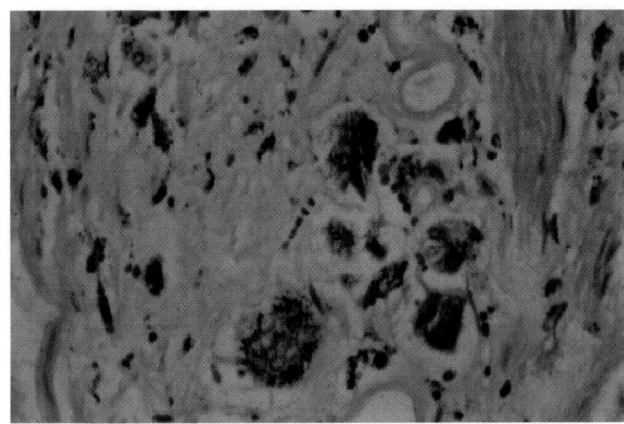

FIGURE 44.2. Asbestos bodies in the wall of an alveolar duct.

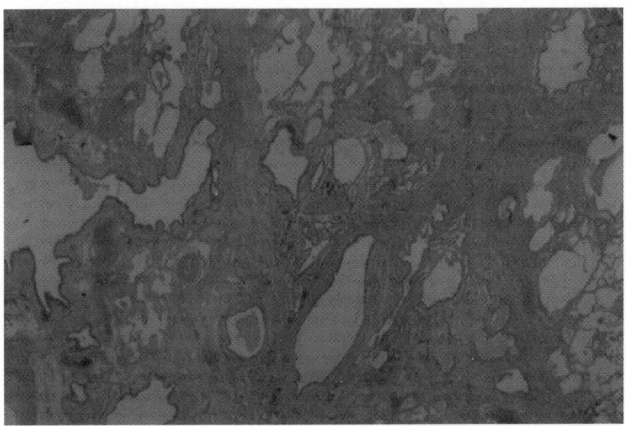

FIGURE 44.3. Severe pulmonary remodeling and honeycombing associated with asbestosis.

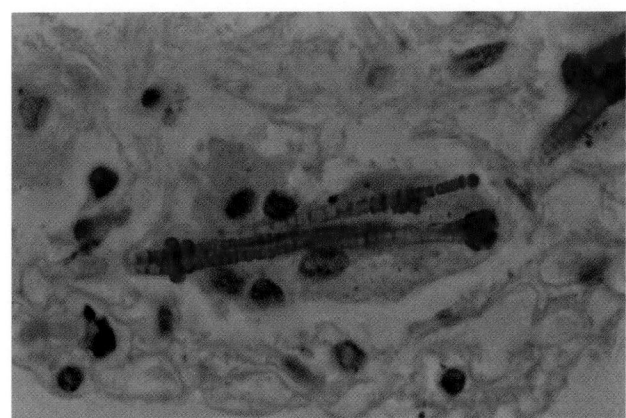

FIGURE 44.4. Photomicrograph of asbestos bodies.

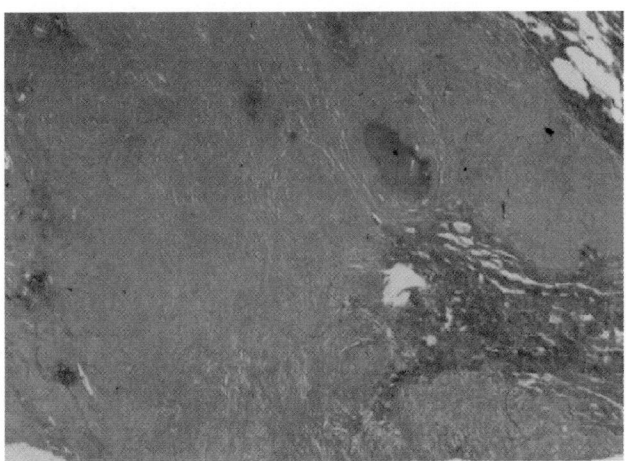

FIGURE 44.5. Progressive massive fibrosis with conglomeration of silicotic nodules.

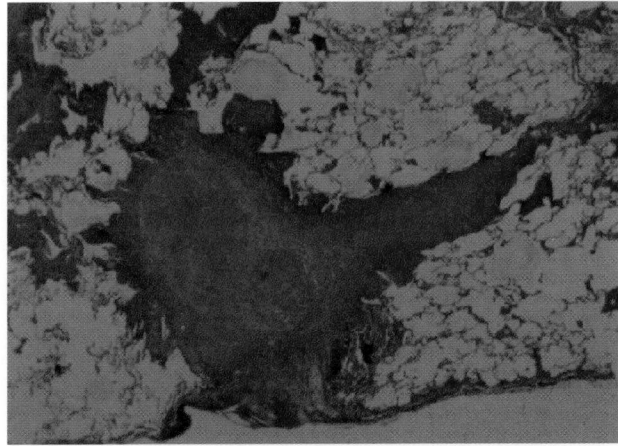

FIGURE 44.6. Early silicotic nodule formation. Nodules are surrounded by dust-filled macrophages.

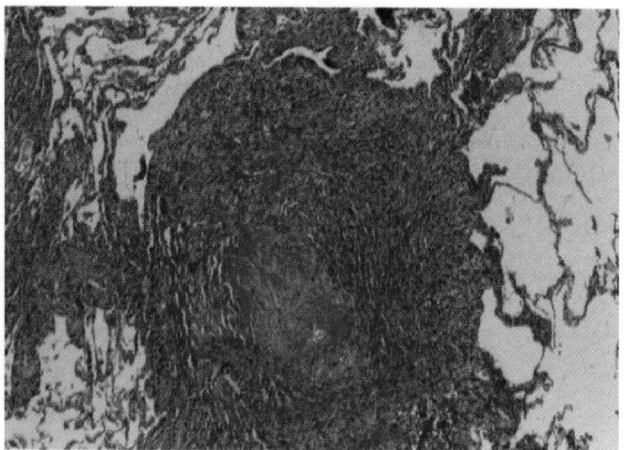

FIGURE 44.7. Early silicotic nodule formation. Nodules are surrounded by dust-filled macrophages (high-power view).

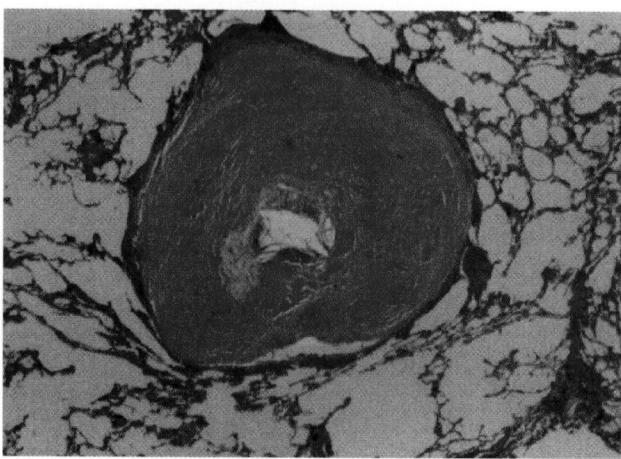

FIGURE 44.8. Classic silicotic nodule.

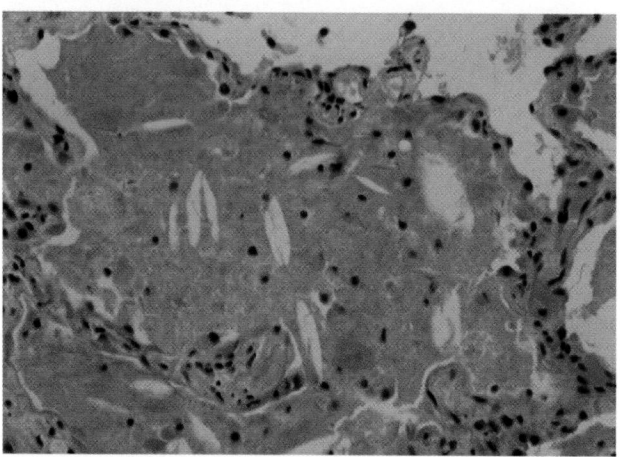

FIGURE 44.9. Acute silicosis ("silicoproteinosis").

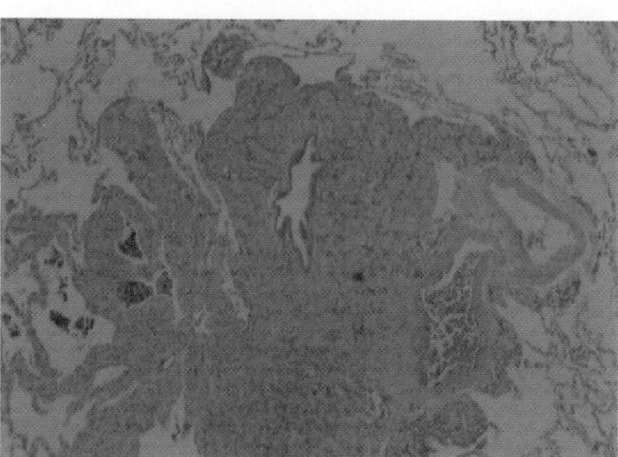

FIGURE 44.10. Peribronchiolar accumulation of macrophages in response to exposure to talc and mixed dust.

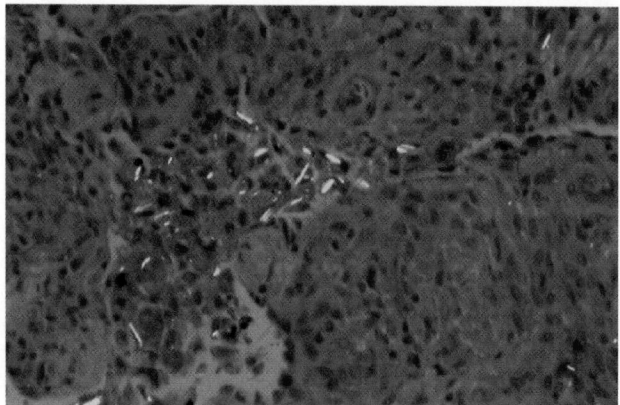

FIGURE 44.11. Partially polarized specimen after exposure to mixed dust showing abundant birefringent silicate material surrounded by macrophages.

Pneumonia, Including Community-Acquired and Nosocomial Pneumonia

22

Michael S. Niederman

Pneumonia is an infection of the gas-exchanging units of the lung, caused most commonly by bacteria but occasionally by viruses, fungi, parasites, and other infectious agents. In the immunocompetent individual, pneumonia is characterized by a brisk filling of the alveolar space with inflammatory cells and fluid. If the alveolar infection involves an entire anatomic lobe of the lung, the condition is termed *lobar pneumonia,* and multilobar illness can be present in some instances. When the alveolar process occurs in a patchy distribution that is adjacent to bronchi, without filling an entire lobe, it is termed a *bronchopneumonia.*

Pneumonia is the sixth leading cause of death in the United States, and the leading cause of death from infectious diseases (1). In hospitalized patients, particularly those who are mechanically ventilated, pneumonia is the leading cause of death from nosocomial infection (2). The infection can develop in persons living in the community (community-acquired pneumonia [CAP]) or in those who are already hospitalized (nosocomial pneumonia [NP]). The most serious form of NP, ventilator-associated pneumonia (VAP), arises in patients who are being mechanically ventilated for other reasons. Presently, the distinction between community and nosocomial infection is less clear because "community" infection includes complicated cases, such as those in patients who have recently been hospitalized, reside in nursing homes, or have chronic diseases that are commonly managed in such facilities as dialysis centers or nursing homes. Although the prognosis and bacteriology in pneumonia vary with the site of origin (CAP, NP, VAP), this variation is probably more a reflection of the types of patients in the community or hospital than of the specific site of onset of illness. This chapter addresses pneumonia arising in and out of the hospital in immunocompetent persons; pneumonia in patients with HIV infection or other forms of immunosuppression (cancer chemotherapy, immunosuppressive medications) is not discussed.

PATHOGENESIS

Pneumonia develops when host defenses are overwhelmed by an infectious pathogen. This may occur because of an inadequate immune response (often the result of underlying comorbid illness such as congestive heart failure, diabetes, renal failure, chronic obstructive lung disease, or malnutrition); anatomic abnormalities (endobronchial obstruction, bronchiectasis); immune dysfunction associated with acute illness (sepsis, extrapulmonary infection); or therapy-induced dysfunction of the immune system (corticosteroids, endotracheal intubation). Pneumonia can also develop in persons with an adequate immune system if the host defense system is overwhelmed by a large inoculum of microorganisms, as often happens in hospitalized individuals (3,4). Outside the hospital, a normal immune system can be overcome by a particularly virulent organism against which a person has no preexisting immunity or cannot mount an adequate acute immune response (3,4).

Bacteria can enter the lung through several routes, but the aspiration of matter from a previously colonized oropharynx is the most common way in which pneumonia develops (5). Although most pneumonias result from microaspiration, patients can also aspirate large volumes of bacteria if the neurologic protection of the upper airway is impaired (stroke, seizure) or if an intestinal illness causes vomiting. Other routes of entry include inhalation (primarily viruses, *Legionella pneumophila,* and *Mycobacterium tuberculosis*); hematogenous dissemination from extrapulmonary sites of infection (e.g., right-sided endocarditis); and direct

M. S. Niederman: Department of Medicine, State University of New York at Stony Brook, Stony Brook, New York; Department of Medicine, Winthrop University Hospital, Mineola, New York.

extension from contiguous sites of infection (e.g., liver abscess). In critically ill hospitalized patients, bacteria can also enter the lung from a colonized stomach (retrograde spread to the oropharynx, followed by aspiration) or a colonized or infected maxillary sinus; they can also enter the lung directly via an endotracheal tube (from the hands of staff members) (6). In critically ill mechanically ventilated patients, large concentrations of bacteria can be harbored in a colonized endotracheal tube and in the tubing of ventilator circuits. Most endotracheal tubes contain a biofilm of bacteria and mucus that forms shortly after intubation, as organisms colonizing the tracheobronchial tree are aerosolized and grow on the inside of the endotracheal tube, free from host defenses or antibacterial therapy. Bacteria in the biofilm can be dislodged when patients are suctioned and enter the lung, causing pneumonia. The presence of a biofilm means that the tracheobronchial tree cannot be sterile once organisms have invaded this site (7).

With this paradigm in mind, it is easy to understand why infection develops in previously healthy persons with virulent pathogens such as viruses, *L. pneumophila, Mycoplasma pneumoniae, Chlamydia pneumoniae,* and *Streptococcus pneumoniae.* On the other hand, chronically ill patients can be infected by these organisms, in addition to organisms that often colonize patients but cause infection only when immune responses are inadequate. These organisms include enteric Gram-negative bacteria (*Escherichia coli, Klebsiella pneumoniae, Pseudomonas aeruginosa, Acinetobacter* species) and fungi.

Studies evaluating the normal lung immune response to infection have shown that in most patients with unilateral pneumonia, the inflammatory response is limited to the site of infection and does not spill over to the uninvolved lung or systemic circulation (3). In patients with localized pneumonia, levels of tumor necrosis factor and interleukins-6 and -8 are increased in the pneumonic lung and generally not increased in the uninvolved lung or serum (8,9). In patients with severe pneumonia, the immune response is characterized by a "spillover" of the immune response into the systemic circulation, reflected by increased serum levels of tumor necrosis factor and interleukin-6 (10). It remains uncertain why localization does not occur in all individuals, and why diffuse lung injury (acute respiratory distress syndrome [ARDS]) or systemic sepsis develops in some patients as a consequence of pneumonia.

COMMUNITY-ACQUIRED PNEUMONIA

Most cases of CAP are managed in the outpatient setting, and the morbidity and mortality of CAP and the greatest part of the cost of its treatment are associated with hospitalization. Thus, the decision about who is hospitalized greatly affects management and costs. The population of elderly patients is increasing in this country, and persons older than 65 years make up about a third of all CAP patients but account for more than half of the cost of this illness. Elderly patients must be hospitalized more often than younger patients, and when hospitalized, they remain in the hospital longer (11) because comorbidity is more common in elderly patients with CAP than in younger ones. In addition, mortality from CAP is higher in the elderly, also because they more often have other illnesses.

Clinical Features

Symptoms and Physical Findings

Patients with CAP and an intact immune system generally have respiratory symptoms, such as cough, sputum production, and dyspnea, along with fever and other symptoms (Table 22.1). Cough is the most common finding and is present in up to 80% of all patients, but it is less frequent in those who are elderly, have serious comorbidity, or reside in a

TABLE 22.1. CLINICAL FEATURES OF COMMUNITY-ACQUIRED PNEUMONIA

Finding	Comment
Fever, chills	May be absent in the elderly or immunosuppressed (including those on corticosteroid therapy)
Dyspnea	Present in only 70%
Worsening of chronic underlying illness	May be only feature in the elderly
Cough and purulent sputum	Appearance of sputum cannot always separate bacterial from nonbacterial infection; cough in up to 80%, 50% with purulence
Duration of symptoms	Tends to be longer in the elderly
Absence of respiratory symptoms	Associated with increased mortality, especially in the absence of pleuritic chest pain
Cardiopulmonary disease, recent antibiotic therapy, age >65 years	Infection with drug-resistant pneumococci and enteric Gram-negatives more likely
Impaired consciousness, poor swallowing	Aspiration risk factors; consider in patients with recurrent infection
Respiratory rate	Rarely <20 if pneumonia; mortality risk increased if >30/min
Bronchial breath sounds or egophony	Suggests air space consolidation
Dullness and reduced breath sounds	May indicate the presence of pleural effusion
Skin rash	*S. aureus, P. aeruginosa, M. tuberculosis,* endemic fungi, *Aspergillus,* varicella-zoster virus, herpes simplex virus, *M. pneumoniae*
Elevated serum liver chemistries	*S. pneumoniae, S. aureus, P. aeruginosa, M. tuberculosis,* Legionella, *H. influenzae, C. immitis, Aspergillus,* herpes simplex virus, varicella-zoster virus, *C. burnetii, M. pneumoniae, C. psittaci*

nursing home (12,13). The elderly generally have fewer respiratory symptoms than younger persons, and the absence of clearly defined respiratory symptoms and an afebrile status have been predictors of an increased risk for death (14). This may be because a lack of respiratory symptoms indicates an impaired immune response; in addition, patients without respiratory symptoms tend to take longer to seek medical attention. Pleuritic chest pain is also common in patients with CAP, and in one study, its absence was identified as a poor prognostic finding (15).

In elderly patients, the presentation of pneumonia can be other than respiratory, with symptoms of confusion, falling, failure to thrive, altered functional capacity, and worsening of a preexisting medical illness, such as congestive heart failure (12–14,16). In one study, delirium or acute confusion was significantly more frequent in elderly patients with pneumonia than in age-matched controls who did not have pneumonia (16). In that study, no association was found between the type of microorganisms isolated and the clinical presentation of CAP, except that pleuritic chest pain was more common in cases of pneumonia caused by bacterial pathogens such as *S. pneumoniae.* Approximately 16% of elderly patients with pneumonia were considered well nourished, in comparison with 47% of controls, with kwashiorkor-like malnutrition the predominant type of nutritional defect and associated with delirium on initial presentation. Several other studies examined the clinical presentation of pneumonia in the elderly and found a substantially higher mortality rate in nursing home residents than in other persons with CAP (32% vs. 14%) (13). These findings may have reflected a higher frequency of comorbid illness and dementia in the nursing home patients. In another study, Metlay and colleagues (12) studied 1,812 patients of all ages and found that with advancing age, the duration of symptoms such as cough, sputum production, dyspnea, fatigue, anorexia, myalgia, and abdominal pain tended to be longer. In general, overall symptoms were less prominent in persons older than 65 years than in those who were younger.

The physical findings of pneumonia include tachypnea, crackles, rhonchi, and signs of consolidation (egophony, bronchial breath sounds, dullness to percussion). Patients should also be examined for signs of pleural effusion. In addition, extrapulmonary findings should be sought to rule out metastatic infection (arthritis, endocarditis, meningitis) or to raise the suspicion of an "atypical" pathogen, such as *M. pneumoniae* or *C. pneumoniae,* which can cause such findings as bullous myringitis, skin rash, pericarditis, hepatitis, hemolytic anemia, and meningoencephalitis.

One of the most important components in the examination of any patient suspected of having pneumonia is measurement of the respiratory rate. In the elderly, an elevated respiratory rate can be the initial presenting sign of pneumonia, preceding other clinical findings by as much as 1 to 2 days. In a prospective study in a long-term care setting,

19 of 21 patients in whom lower respiratory tract infection was diagnosed had a respiratory rate above the normal range of 16 to 25/min, and in general, the elevated rate preceded other clinical findings (17). Although this finding is certainly not specific, it was not present in patients with nonrespiratory infection, and it appears to be a very sensitive indicator of respiratory infection. In another study, tachypnea was the most common finding in elderly patients with pneumonia, present in more than 60% of all patients, and more often in the elderly than in younger patients with pneumonia (12). Measurement of the respiratory rate is not only of diagnostic value but also of prognostic significance. In the evaluation of patients with CAP, a respiratory rate higher than 30/min is one of several factors associated with increased mortality (1).

Radiographic Features

The entry point into most algorithms for CAP is the appearance of a new radiographic infiltrate, but this is not seen in all patients with CAP when they are first evaluated. Even when the radiographic findings are negative, if the patient has appropriate symptoms and focal physical findings, pneumonia may still be present. In one study, 47 patients with clinical signs and symptoms of CAP were evaluated with both chest radiography and a high-resolution computed tomography (CT) of the chest, and CT identified pneumonia in eight patients who had negative findings by chest radiography. In addition, more extensive abnormalities were found by CT; 16 patients had bilateral infiltrates by this technique, but only six by chest radiography (18). Bronchopneumonia was the most common abnormality defined by either technique. The findings of this study underscore the need to repeat chest radiography after 24 to 48 hours in certain symptomatic patients with an initially negative result. The reason for an initially negative chest x-ray film is not clear; some studies have suggested that febrile and dehydrated patients can have a film with normal findings when first admitted with pneumonia, but the idea of hydrating a pneumonia is within the realm of "conventional wisdom" and anecdotal reports (19).

Although a variety of radiographic patterns can be seen in pneumonia, and although the radiographic findings cannot generally be used to predict the microbial etiology in CAP, certain patterns have been associated with specific pathogens (19). Focal consolidation can be seen with infections caused by aspiration (especially in the lower lobes or other dependent segments), pneumococci, *Klebsiella, Staphylococcus aureus, Haemophilus influenzae, M. pneumoniae,* or *C. pneumoniae.* Interstitial infiltrates should suggest viral pneumonia in addition to infection with *M. pneumoniae, C. pneumoniae, Chlamydia psittaci,* and *Pneumocystis carinii.* Lymphadenopathy with an interstitial pattern should raise concerns about *Bacillus anthracis, Francisella tularensis,* and *C. psittaci,* whereas adenopathy can be seen with focal infiltrates in tuberculosis, fungal pneumonia, and bacterial pneumonia. Cavitation can be the result of an aspiration lung abscess or infection with *S. aureus,* aerobic Gram-negatives (including *P. aeruginosa*), *M. tuberculosis,* fungi, *Nocardia,* and *Actinomyces.*

Pleural effusion may appear on the initial chest radiograph, and if present, it is necessary to distinguish empyema from a simple parapneumonic effusion by sampling the pleural fluid. In one study, bilateral pleural effusion was an independent predictor of short-term mortality in CAP (20). Pneumococcal pneumonia is the infection most commonly complicated by effusion (36% to 57% of patients), but other pathogens causing effusion include *H. influenzae, M. pneumoniae, Legionella,* and *M. tuberculosis* (21).

Typical versus Atypical Pneumonia Syndromes

In the past, the clinical and radiographic features of CAP were organized into patterns of either "typical" or "atypical" pneumonia, with the idea that specific patterns could suggest certain etiologic agents. The typical pneumonia syndrome is characterized by the sudden onset of high fever, shaking chills, pleuritic chest pain, lobar consolidation, the appearance of toxicity, and the production of purulent sputum. Although this pattern has been attributed to pneumococci and other bacterial pathogens, these organisms do not always lead to such classic symptoms. The atypical pneumonia syndrome, characterized by a subacute illness, nonproductive cough, headache, diarrhea, and other systemic complaints, is usually the result of infection with *M. pneumoniae, C. pneumoniae, Legionella* species, or viruses. However, patients with impaired immune responses (especially the elderly with chronic illness) may present in this fashion, even if they have bacterial pneumonia. Thus, the ability to use the features at clinical presentation to predict the likely etiologic agents is limited, and attempts are often misleading (1,22–25).

In one study examining the microbial etiology and clinical presentation of CAP, the clinical features were no more than 42% accurate in differentiating among pneumococci, *M. pneumoniae,* and other pathogens (23). In a study of 359 patients with CAP, a comparison of patients with *S. pneumoniae, H. influenzae, L. pneumophila,* or *C. pneumoniae* infection revealed no significant differences in the clinical presentation (24). The limitations of the clinical features in defining the microbial etiology also apply to the radiographic pattern (25). Currently, the syndromic approach to CAP is of limited practical application, particularly among elderly patients with underlying comorbidity (1).

Etiologic Pathogens

Even with extensive diagnostic testing, an etiologic agent is defined in only about half of all patients with CAP, underscoring the limited value of diagnostic testing and the possibility that we do not know all the organisms that can cause CAP (1,24). In the past three decades, a variety of new pathogens for this illness have been identified, including *L. pneumophila, C. pneumoniae,* and hantavirus. In addition, antibiotic-resistant variants of common pathogens such as *S. pneumoniae* have become increasingly common.

Streptococcus pneumoniae

The most common pathogen of CAP in any patient population is *S. pneumoniae,* and this organism may even be responsible for many episodes of infection that go undiagnosed by standard testing. In one study, transthoracic needle aspirates were used to define the cause of CAP in patients with no identified organisms by conventional diagnostic testing (26). Although for many patients a diagnosis was established with the use of polymerase chain reaction probe analysis of transthoracic needle aspirates, in half of the patients in whom the needle provided a diagnosis when other methods had failed, pneumococci were identified.

The organism is a Gram-positive, lancet-shaped diplococcus with 84 different serotypes, each with a distinct antigenic polysaccharide capsule; however, 85% of all infections are caused by one of 23 serotypes that are now included in a vaccine. Infection is most common in the winter and early spring, which may be related to the finding that up to 70% of patients have had a preceding viral illness (27). The organism spreads from person to person and commonly colonizes the oropharynx before it causes pneumonia. Pneumonia develops when colonizing organisms are aspirated into a lung that is unable to contain the aspirated inoculum. Infection is more common in the elderly; those with asplenia, multiple myeloma, congestive heart failure, or alcoholism; after influenza; and in patients with chronic lung disease. Pneumococcal pneumonia with bacteremia is more common in patients with HIV infection than in healthy persons of the same age. The classic radiographic pattern is a lobar consolidation, but bronchopneumonia can also occur and in some series is the most common pattern (28). Bacteremia is present in up to 20% of hospitalized patients with pneumococcal pneumonia, but the impact of this finding on mortality is uncertain (29). Extrapulmonary complications include meningitis, empyema, arthritis, endocarditis, and brain abscess.

In the past decade, antibiotic resistance among pneumococci has become increasingly common, and penicillin resistance, along with resistance to other common antibiotics (macrolides, trimethoprim/sulfamethoxazole, selected cephalosporins), is noted in more than 40% of these organisms (1,30). Fortunately, most penicillin resistance is of the "intermediate" type (penicillin minimum inhibitory concentration [MIC] of 0.1–1.0 mg/L) and not of the high-level type (penicillin MIC $\geq$ 2.0 mg/L). Patients with certain clinical conditions are at increased risk for infection with drug-resistant pneumococci (see section "Predicting Pathogens for Specific Patients"). It is difficult to show a clinical effect of *in vitro* resistance on outcomes such as mortality, but most experts believe that organisms with a penicillin MIC of 4 mg/L can increase the risk for death (1,29,31).

In an early study, Pallares and colleagues (32) were unable to show an effect of resistance on mortality after adjusting for severity of illness in a population of 504 infected patients, 145 of whom were infected with resistant organisms (penicillin MIC > 0.12 mg/L). Turett and colleagues (33) studied a population of 462 patients with pneumococcal bacteremia, of whom more than half were HIV-positive, and found high-level resistance to be a predictor of mortality. Other investigators did not find the risk for death to be increased by infection with resistant organisms, but they did find a greater likelihood of suppurative complications (empyema) and a more prolonged hospital stay (34). The conflicting data in earlier reports may have been the result of studying relatively few patients. Feikin and colleagues (31) studied the effect of pneumococcal resistance in 5,837 patients with bacteremic CAP. They found an increase in mortality with a penicillin MIC of 4 mg/L or higher or with a cefotaxime MIC of 2.0 mg/L or higher. However, this increase in mortality was present only if patients who died within the first 4 days after therapy were excluded from analysis. Fortunately, very few organisms are currently at this level of resistance, but to prevent more organisms of this type from emerging, it may be necessary to identify patients with risk factors for resistance and treat them with highly active antipneumococcal regimens. One limitation of the study of Feikin and colleagues was the failure to account for the severity of illness or therapy choices. More recently, Moroney and colleagues (35), using both cohort study and matched control methods, found that severity of illness, not resistance or accuracy of therapy, was the most important predictor of mortality. Interestingly, in the case control part of the study, illness was more severe in patients without resistant organisms, implying a loss of virulence in organisms that become resistant, a finding noted in another study in which absence of invasive illness was a risk factor for pneumococcal resistance (36).

Atypical Pathogens

Although the term *atypical* does not accurately describe a specific clinical pneumonia syndrome, it can be used to refer to a group of pathogens that includes *M. pneumoniae,* *C. pneumoniae,* and *Legionella.* This group of organisms cannot be reliably eradicated by β-lactam therapy (penicillins and cephalosporins) but must be treated with a macrolide, tetracycline, or quinolone. Some studies have shown that infections with these pathogens are common in patients of all ages, not just young and healthy ones, and the organisms have been reported even among the elderly in nursing homes (1,37,38). In addition, they can be either primary pathogens or part of a mixed infection, along with traditional bacterial pathogens. A mixed infection may lead to a more complex course and a longer hospital stay than an infection with a single pathogen. There may be a particular synergy between

C. pneumoniae and pneumococci, with either sequential or mixed infection with *C. pneumoniae* causing a more severe course of pneumococcal infection (39). The frequency of atypical pathogens has been as high as 60% in some series, with as many as 40% of all CAP patients having a mixed infection (40). Although these high numbers were derived with serologic testing, which is of uncertain accuracy, the importance of the atypical organisms is suggested by studies of inpatients showing a reduced mortality and length of stay when they received empiric therapy that accounted for atypical organisms, rather than regimens that did not account for them (41,42).

Pneumonia caused by atypical organisms may not be a constant phenomenon, and the frequency of infection may vary with time and location. One study showed a variable benefit of empiric therapy directed at atypical pathogens, which was more important in some calendar years than in others (42). The incidence of *Legionella* infection among admitted patients has ranged from 1% to 15% or more, reflecting geographic and seasonal variability in infection rates in addition to the extent of diagnostic testing. To identify *Legionella,* it is necessary to collect both acute and convalescent serologic specimens (43). Atypical pathogens are present in almost 25% of all patients with severe CAP, but the responsible organism may vary over time. In one series, *Legionella* was the most common atypical pathogen leading to severe CAP, but in the same hospital a decade later, it had been replaced by *Mycoplasma* and *Chlamydia* (44).

L. pneumophila is a small, weakly staining, Gram-negative bacillus first characterized after an epidemic in 1976, and infection can occur either sporadically or in epidemic form. At present, 12 different serogroups of the species *L. pneumophila* have been described, and these account for 90% of all cases of Legionnaires disease, with serogroup 1 causing the most cases. The other species that commonly causes human illness is *Legionella micdadei.* The organism is waterborne and can emanate from air conditioning equipment, drinking water, lakes and river banks, water faucets, and shower heads. Infection is generally caused by inhalation of an infected aerosol generated by a contaminated water source. When a water system becomes infected in an institution, endemic outbreaks may occur, as has been the case in some hospitals, particularly in patients receiving corticosteroid therapy (45). In its sporadic form, *Legionella* may account for 7% to 15% of all cases of CAP, being a particular concern in patients with severe forms of illness (1,44).

As mentioned (see section "Typical versus Atypical Pneumonia Syndromes"), it is very difficult to use clinical features to predict the microbial etiology of CAP; however, the classic *Legionella* syndrome is characterized by high fever, chills, headache, myalgias, and leukocytosis. The diagnosis is also suggested by a pneumonia with preceding diarrhea, along with the early onset of mental confusion, hyponatremia, relative bradycardia, and liver function abnormalities, but this syndrome is usually not present. The symptoms are rapidly progressive, and the patient may appear quite toxic, so this diagnosis should always be considered in patients admitted to the intensive care unit (ICU) with CAP.

Gram-Negative Bacteria

The Gram-negative organism most often causing CAP is *H. influenzae*, a frequent pathogen in the elderly and in persons who smoke cigarettes or have chronic bronchitis (1). *H. influenzae* can be either a typeable (encapsulated) or a nontypeable organism and can cause bronchopneumonia and rarely empyema. Enteric Gram-negative organisms are generally uncommon in CAP unless the patients are elderly and have chronic cardiac or pulmonary disease or are alcoholic. These patients can be infected with organisms such as *Escherichia coli* and *K. pneumoniae*. *P. aeruginosa* is an uncommon cause of CAP, but it can be isolated from patients with CAP and bronchiectasis and in those with severe forms of CAP, particularly if they are older than 75 years (1,46).

Other Organisms

CAP is also caused by *S. aureus*, which can be associated with severe illness and cavitary lung infection. This organism can also seed the lung hematogenously from a vegetation in patients with right-sided endocarditis or from a septic thrombophlebitis (secondary to central venous catheter or jugular vein infection). The role of anaerobes in CAP is uncertain, but they may be important in patients with risk factors for aspiration (neurologic illness, impaired swallowing, esophageal disease) and may cause abscess in dependent lung segments. The need to eradicate these organisms when they are part of a mixed infection with aerobic organisms is uncertain (1,47).

An array of other organisms should also be considered in the setting of CAP, depending on the setting, epidemiology, and community patterns of pneumonia. Thus, tuberculosis and, in areas of endemicity, appropriate fungal infections should be considered. In HIV-infected persons, a broad differential diagnosis may be indicated, depending on the degree of immunocompromise thought to be present. A number of viruses and less common pathogens, including some that can be used as agents of bioterrorism, may be considered depending on the circumstances of a patient's presentation. These are discussed in this (see section "Uncommon Causes of Community-Acquired Pneumonia") and other chapters (see Chapters 18–21).

Predicting Pathogens for Specific Patients

Table 22.2 summarizes the pathogens commonly causing CAP in both outpatients and inpatients. The classification is based on the severity of illness and the presence of clini-

TABLE 22.2. COMMON PATHOGENS CAUSING COMMUNITY-ACQUIRED PNEUMONIA

Outpatient, no cardiopulmonary disease or modifying factors
S. pneumoniae, M. pneumoniae, C. pneumoniae (alone or as mixed infection), *H. influenzae*, respiratory viruses, others (*Legionella* species, *M. tuberculosis*, endemic fungi)

Outpatient, with cardiopulmonary disease or modifying factors
All the above plus DRSP, enteric Gram-negatives, and aspirated anaerobes

Inpatient, with cardiopulmonary disease or modifying factors
S. pneumoniae (including DRSP), *H. influenzae, M. pneumoniae, C. pneumoniae*, mixed infection (bacteria plus atypical pathogen), enteric Gram-negatives, aspirated anaerobes, viruses, *Legionella* species, others (*M. tuberculosis*, endemic fungi, *P. carinii*)

Inpatient, with no cardiopulmonary disease or modifying factors
All the above, but DRSP and enteric Gram-negatives not likely

Severe CAP, with no risks for *P. aeruginosa* infection
S. pneumoniae (including DRSP), *Legionella* species, *H. influenzae*, enteric Gram-negative bacilli, *S. aureus, M. pneumoniae*, respiratory viruses, others (*C. pneumoniae, M. tuberculosis*, endemic fungi)

Severe CAP, with risks for *P. aeruginosa* infection
All the pathogens listed, plus *P. aeruginosa*

CAP, community-acquired pneumonia; DRSP, drug-resistant *S. pneumoniae*.
Note: Based on multiple prospective studies of etiology using extensive diagnostic testing and correlation with underlying risk factors.

cal risk factors for infection with specific pathogens, referred to as *modifying factors*. The spectrum of organisms in patients with severe CAP may be slightly different from that in other patients with this illness: patients with severe CAP are frequently infected with pneumococci, atypical pathogens, enteric Gram-negative organisms (including *P. aeruginosa*), *S. aureus*, and *H. influenzae*. The modifying factors for drug-resistant pneumococci are age older than 65 years, β-lactam therapy within the past 3 months, alcoholism, immunosuppressive illness (including therapy with corticosteroids), multiple medical comorbidities, and exposure to a child in day care (1,36,48). The modifying factors for enteric Gram-negatives include residence in a nursing home, underlying cardiopulmonary disease, multiple medical comorbidities, and recent antibiotic therapy. The risk factors for *P. aeruginosa* infection are structural lung disease (bronchiectasis), corticosteroid therapy (>10 mg of prednisone per day), broad-spectrum antibiotic therapy for more than 7 days in the past month, and malnutrition (1). Table 22.3 shows the clinical conditions associated with specific pathogens, and these associations should be considered in all patients when a history is obtained.

Assessment of the Severity of Illness

Decision for Hospitalization

Given the economic and social impact of pneumonia, the decision about the site of initial care is one of the most

TABLE 22.3. CLINICAL ASSOCIATIONS WITH SPECIFIC PATHOGENS

Condition	Commonly Encountered Pathogens
Alcoholism	S. pneumoniae (including PRSP), anaerobes, Gram-negative bacilli (possibly K. pneumoniae)
COPD/current or former smoker	S. pneumoniae, H. influenzae, M. catarrhalis, Legionella
Residence in nursing home	S. pneumoniae, Gram-negative bacilli, H. influenzae, S. aureus, anaerobes, C. pneumoniae; consider M. tuberculosis
Poor dental hygiene	Anaerobes
Bat exposure	H. capsulatum
Bird exposure	C. psittaci, C. neoformans, H. capsulatum
Rabbit exposure	F. tularensis
Travel to southwestern United States	C. immitis, hantavirus in selected areas
Exposure to farm animals or parturient cats	C. burnetii (Q fever)
After influenza pneumonia	S. pneumoniae, S. aureus, H. influenzae
Structural disease of lung (bronchiectasis, cystic fibrosis)	P. aeruginosa, P. cepacia, or S. aureus

COPD, chronic obstructive pulmonary disease; PRSP, penicillin-resistant S. pneumoniae.

important in disease management. Generally, the severity of illness should be determined to define whether the patient should be hospitalized, and a number of prediction models have been developed to guide the admission decision. However, no rule is absolute; the decision to admit a patient should be based on both social and medical considerations and remains an "art of medicine" determination. In general, patients with multiple risk factors for a poor outcome or decompensation of a chronic illness should be observed in the hospital; those who require therapies not easily administered at home (oxygen, intravenous fluids, cardiac monitoring) should also be admitted (1). Risk factors for a poor outcome include a respiratory rate above 30/min, systolic blood pressure below 90 mm Hg, diastolic blood pressure below 60 mm Hg, multilobar pneumonia, confusion, blood urea nitrogen above 19.6 mg/dL, Pao_2 below 60 mm Hg, $Paco_2$ above 50 mm Hg, respiratory or metabolic acidosis, and signs of systemic sepsis (1,49,50). The British Thoracic Society (BTS) rule states that the risk for death is increased 9- to 21-fold if at least two of the following four criteria are present: respiratory rate above 30/min, diastolic BP below 60 mm Hg, blood urea nitrogen above 19.6 mg/dL, and confusion (50).

To make the process more objective, the investigators in the Pneumonia Outcomes Research Team (PORT) study developed a mortality prediction rule that classifies all patients into one of five groups (classes I–V), each with a different risk for death (49). In some CAP management guidelines, this mortality risk score is used to guide the admission de-

cision (47). In the Infectious Diseases Society of America (IDSA) guidelines, admission is recommended for patients in classes IV and V, with predicted mortality risk values of 8.2% to 9.3% and 27% to 31.1%, respectively; outpatient care is recommended for patients in classes I and II, with mortality risk values of 0.1% to 0.4% and 0.6% to 0.7%, respectively (47). Patients in class III are at intermediate risk for death, 0.9% to 2.8%, and the recommendation is that the admission decision be individualized for these patients. In this system, points are calculated based on such factors as age, sex, comorbid medical disease, certain physical findings, and certain laboratory data (49).

When the PORT model was developed, it was validated in large numbers of patients evaluated retrospectively (49). Several prospective studies of the accuracy of the model for the admission decision are now available. In one study, 166 of 826 patients presenting to the emergency department fell into classes I through III, and with application of the admission decision rule, 57% of the low-risk patients were discharged, in comparison with only 42% in a preceding period when clinical judgment was used to define the need for admission (51). However, during the period when the prediction rule was used, 9% of the discharged patients failed outpatient therapy, whereas none did when clinical judgment was used to make this decision. In another study, 70% of low-risk patients were sent home when the admission decision rule was applied, in comparison with approximately 50% when clinical judgment was used (52). However, it is important to remember that the admission decision rule is simply a guide, and that it must be overlooked in certain circumstances. Furthermore, even when it was applied, as many as 30% to 40% of patients in low-risk categories still had to be hospitalized.

One factor that can enhance the admission decision process is an assessment for hypoxemia, with all patients admitted who have an oxygen saturation below 90% on room air, provided they are not on long-term oxygen therapy.

The use of prediction rules is a particular problem in the elderly. Lim and colleagues (53,54) have shown that the BTS rule does not work as well in elderly as in younger patients, reflecting the altered clinical presentations of pneumonia in this population. In one study, the rule had a 66% sensitivity and a 73% specificity for predicting mortality in a population in which 48% of those included were at least 75 years of age. Interestingly, although the BTS rule was not optimal in an elderly population and did not work as well as in other populations, it had a higher sensitivity for predicting mortality than the prognostic scoring index derived from the PORT study (49,53). In the American Thoracic Society (ATS) guidelines for CAP, some of the limitations of using the prognostic scoring index to guide the admission decision were identified, including the fact that age is a heavily weighted variable for defining mortality risk (1). A high risk for mortality is defined as a score above 90 points, and male patients are given one point for each year of age. Thus, an elderly man with any chronic illness will have enough points to fall into a high-risk category and possibly be admitted to the hospital, regardless of the severity of his pneumonic process. On the other hand, a young patient with multilobar pneumonia may never be considered for admission based on the prognostic scoring index unless certain vital sign thresholds are reached (heart rate >125/min, respiratory rate >30/min, systolic blood pressure <90 mm Hg). Thus, the admission decision remains a true clinical judgment, and one that must be made with many clinical and social features taken into consideration.

Need for Intensive Care

No specific rule is available for deciding who should be admitted to the ICU, but in general, the ICU is used for approximately 10% of all CAP patients, and this population has a mortality rate of at least 30%, in comparison with a mortality rate of 12% for all admitted patients and a 1% to 5% mortality rate for outpatients (55). There is some debate about the benefit of intensive care for patients with CAP, but the benefit seems most certain if patients are admitted early in the course of a severe illness (56).

In the 1993 ATS guidelines, 10 criteria from the literature were used to identify patients who might require ICU admission (57). However, when these 10 criteria were used and the presence of any one of them defined severe CAP, the definition was too inclusive, and 65% of all admitted CAP patients (not requiring intensive care) met one of the criteria (58). To define the need for intensive care in CAP better, Ewig (58) and colleagues applied the 10 criteria to 64 patients who were admitted to the ICU and compared their findings with those of 331 patients admitted to the hospital but not the ICU. With this approach, a better definition of severe CAP was derived, with a sensitivity of 78%, specificity of 94%, positive predictive value of 75%, and negative predictive value of 95%. This definition required the presence of either two of three "minor criteria" on admission, or one of two "major criteria" on admission or later in the hospital course. The minor criteria were systolic blood pressure below 90 mm Hg, Pao_2/Fio_2 ratio below 250, or the presence of multilobar infiltrates. The major criteria were a need for mechanical ventilation or the presence of septic shock. As previously discussed (see section "Decision for Hospitalization"), another way to identify patients with more severe illness is to apply the BTS rule, but this approach has not been directly validated to define need for admission to the ICU. In the future, we will have to better define prospectively the criteria for ICU admission.

Diagnostic Testing

Once the history and physical examination have suggested a diagnosis of pneumonia, the diagnosis should be confirmed by chest radiograph (Table 22.4). Although some patients may have clinical findings of pneumonia (focal crackles, bronchial breath sounds) but negative results on the chest radiograph, the need for antibiotic therapy of CAP has been established in patients with a radiographic infiltrate. In some patients with findings of pneumonia but a negative chest radiograph, the correct diagnosis is bronchitis; patients with

TABLE 22.4. DIAGNOSTIC TESTING FOR COMMUNITY-ACQUIRED PNEUMONIA

Test	Sensitivity	Specificity	Comment
Chest radiograph	65%–85%	85%–95%	Computed tomography is more sensitive to infiltrates than routine radiography.
Computed tomography	Gold standard	Not infection-specific	Should not be done routinely, but helpful to identify cavitation and loculated pleural fluid; should also be done for nonresponding patients.
Blood cultures	10%–20%	High when positive	Usually shows pneumococci (in 50%–80% of positive samples) and defines antibiotic susceptibility.
Sputum Gram stain	From 40%–10% depending on criteria	0–100% depending on criteria	Can be correlated with sputum culture to define predominant organism and can be used to identify unsuspected pathogens.
Sputum culture			Use if suspect drug-resistant or unusual pathogen, but positive result cannot separate colonization from infection.
Oximetry or arterial blood gas determination			Both define severity of infection, need for oxygen; if hypercarbia is suspected, a blood gas measurement is needed.
Serologic testing for *Legionella, C. pneumoniae, M. pneumoniae,* viruses			Accurate, but usually requires acute and convalescent titers collected 4–6 weeks apart.
Legionella urinary antigen	50%–80%		Specific to serogroup 1, but the best acute diagnostic test for *Legionella.*

this illness may not require antibiotic therapy if they have no chronic underlying lung disease. However, in other populations, such as the elderly and chronically ill, the clinical diagnosis is difficult; these patients can have pneumonia with only nonrespiratory findings, and for them, a chest radiograph is essential to determine the presence of parenchymal lung infection. Although a radiograph is recommended for all outpatients and inpatients, radiography may be impractical in some settings outside the hospital. A chest radiograph not only confirms the presence of pneumonia but also can be used to identify complicated illness and grade the severity of disease by noting such features as pleural effusion and multilobar illness (1). As previously mentioned (see section "Radiographic Features"), no specific radiographic pattern can be used to define the etiologic pathogen of CAP, but certain findings are associated with specific organisms, such as a cavitary infiltrate with anaerobes and a posterior upper lobe infiltrate with *M. tuberculosis*.

Although defining a specific etiologic agent in CAP allows for focused antibiotic therapy, in most patients, a specific pathogen is not identified, and even if it is, it is identified days or weeks later, when the results of cultures or serologic testing become available. In addition, studies have emphasized the mortality benefit of the prompt initiation of effective antibiotic therapy, with the goal of administering intravenous antibiotics within 8 hours after admission to the hospital to patients with moderate to severe illness (59). Thus, therapy should never be delayed for the purpose of diagnostic testing, and the diagnostic workup should be streamlined, with all patients receiving empiric therapy based on algorithms, as soon as possible. With such empiric regimens, as many as 90% of admitted patients promptly respond to therapy (60).

The recommended testing for outpatients is limited to chest radiography and pulse oximetry, if available, with sputum culture reserved for patients suspected of harboring an unusual or drug-resistant pathogen. For admitted patients, the diagnostic testing should include chest radiography, an assessment of oxygenation (pulse oximetry or blood gas measurement, the latter if retention of carbon dioxide is suspected), routine admission blood work, and two sets of blood cultures (1). If the patient has a pleural effusion, this should be tapped and the fluid sent for culture and biochemical analysis. Although blood cultures are positive in only 10% to 20% of patients with CAP, they can be used to define a specific diagnosis and the presence of drug-resistant pneumococci (29). Sputum culture should be limited to patients suspected of being infected with a drug-resistant or unusual pathogen.

The role of Gram stain of sputum to guide initial antibiotic therapy is controversial. This test is of greatest value in guiding the interpretation of sputum culture and can be used to define the predominant organism in the sample. The role of Gram stain in focusing initial antibiotic therapy is uncertain because the accuracy of the test to predict the culture recovery of an organism such as the pneumococcus depends on the criteria used. If the finding of any Gram-positive diplococcus is used to define a positive test result, then the test will be sensitive but not very specific. On the other hand, the finding of a predominance of Gram-positive diplococci will be specific but not sensitive for predicting the culture recovery of pneumococci (1,61). In one study, the practical limitations of the test were clear: of 116 patients with CAP, only 42 could produce a sputum sample, of which 23 were valid and only 10 were diagnostic; antibiotics were directed to the diagnostic result in only one patient (62). Even if Gram stain findings are used to focus antibiotic therapy, this does not allow for empiric coverage of atypical pathogens that may be present together with pneumococci as part of a mixed infection. Despite these limitations, Gram stain can be used to broaden initial empiric therapy by suggesting the presence of organisms not covered by routine empiric therapy (e.g., *S. aureus*, suggested by clusters of Gram-positive cocci, especially during an influenza epidemic) (1).

Routine serologic testing is not recommended. However, in patients with severe illness, *Legionella* infection can be diagnosed by urinary antigen testing, which is the test most likely to yield a positive result at the time of admission but is specific only for serogroup 1 infection (43). Commercially available tests for pneumococcal urinary antigen have been developed, but their role in the clinical management of CAP has not been defined. Bronchoscopy is not indicated as a routine diagnostic test and should be restricted to immunocompromised patients and selected patients with severe forms of CAP.

Therapy

The goal of empiric therapy in patients with CAP is to target the likely etiologic pathogens according to place where therapy is administered (home, hospital, ICU), the severity of illness, and the presence or absence of cardiopulmonary disease or specific "modifying" factors. With the use of these factors, a set of likely pathogens can be predicted for each patient (Table 22.2), and this information can be used to guide initial empiric therapy. If a specific pathogen is subsequently identified by diagnostic testing, then therapy can be focused.

When empiric therapy of CAP is chosen, certain principles should be followed (1,63). Empiric therapy for outpatients with no cardiopulmonary disease or modifying factors should be with a new oral macrolide (azithromycin or clarithromycin) or a tetracycline. Although erythromycin has been used for these outpatients, its value is limited by a lack of coverage of *H. influenzae* and a higher frequency of intestinal complications (nausea, vomiting) than with the newer macrolides. Therapy with an antipneumococcal quinolone (gatifloxacin, levofloxacin, moxifloxacin) is not necessary in these outpatients because they are not at risk for infection with complicated organisms, such as drug-resistant pneumococci and enteric Gram-negatives. However, outpatients with cardiopulmonary disease or modifying factors should not receive macrolide monotherapy, which has occasionally been associated with therapeutic failure in such populations, primarily because of drug-resistant pneumococci (64). These patients should receive either a selected oral β-lactam with a macrolide or an oral antipneumococcal quinolone (gatifloxacin, levofloxacin, moxifloxacin) alone. Quinolone monotherapy may be easier and less costly than a β-lactam/macrolide combination for these complex outpatients.

For an inpatient who is not in the ICU, therapy can be with an intravenous macrolide (azithromycin) alone, provided that the patient has no underlying cardiopulmonary disease and no risk factors for infection with drug-resistant pneumococci, enteric Gram-negatives, or anaerobes. Although very few patients of this type are admitted to the hospital, macrolide monotherapy has been documented to be effective in this population (65). Most admitted patients have cardiopulmonary disease or modifying factors, and either they can be treated with a selected intravenous β-lactam combined with a macrolide, or they can receive an intravenous antipneumococcal quinolone (gatifloxacin, levofloxacin, moxifloxacin) alone. From the available data, it appears that the two regimens are therapeutically equivalent, and although it has not been proved, it may be useful to use these two types of regimens interchangeably, striving for "antibiotic heterogeneity" in the hospital, so that one regimen is not used exclusively in all patients (1). This type of approach has the theoretic advantage of minimizing the selection pressure for antibiotic resistance. Although oral quinolones may be as effective as intravenous quinolones for admitted patients with moderately severe illness, it is recommended that all admitted patients receive initial therapy intravenously to be sure that the medication has been absorbed (1). Once the patient shows a good clinical response (see section "Evaluation of the Response to Therapy"), oral therapy can be started. Selected inpatients with mild to moderate disease can initially be treated with the combination of an intravenous β-lactam and an oral macrolide, with a switch to exclusively oral therapy once the patient shows a good clinical response.

All patients in the ICU should be treated for drug-resistant pneumococci and atypical pathogens, but only those with appropriate risk factors (see section "Predicting Pathogens for Specific Patients") should be given coverage for *P. aeruginosa* (1). Because the efficacy, dosing, and safety of quinolone monotherapy have not been established for patients with CAP admitted to the ICU, the therapy for such patients, in the absence of risk factors for *Pseudomonas* infection, should be with a selected intravenous β-lactam, combined with either an intravenous macrolide or an intravenous quinolone. For patients with risk factors for *Pseudomonas* infection, therapy can be with a two-drug regimen, an anti-*Pseudomonas* β-lactam (cefepime, imipenem, meropenem, piperacillin/tazobactam) plus ciprofloxacin (the only anti-

Pseudomonas quinolone), or alternatively a three-drug regimen, an anti-*Pseudomonas* β-lactam plus an aminoglycoside plus either an intravenous non–anti-*Pseudomonas* quinolone or macrolide.

The antipneumococcal quinolones have assumed great importance in the therapy of CAP because it is possible with a single drug given once daily to cover pneumococci (including drug-resistant pneumococci), Gram-negatives, and atypical pathogens. Quinolones penetrate well into respiratory secretions and are highly bioavailable; the same serum levels are achieved with oral or intravenous therapy, so that moderately ill outpatients can be managed effectively with oral antibiotics. Although all the antipneumococcal quinolones are available for both oral and intravenous administration and all have been effective therapy for CAP, the available agents differ in their intrinsic activity against pneumococci (1,66,67). On the basis of the MIC, these agents can be ranked as follows from most to least active: moxifloxacin, gatifloxacin, levofloxacin. Some data suggest a lower likelihood of both clinical failures and the induction of pneumococcal resistance to quinolones if the more active agents are used in place of the less active agents (67,68). In addition, treatment failures in pneumococcal pneumonia have now been reported for levofloxacin, and these have occurred in patients who were infected with levofloxacin-resistant organisms after a recent course of quinolone therapy or who acquired resistance during therapy (after infection with an initially sensitive organism) (68,69). Based on these data and on the finding that recent therapy with a macrolide, β-lactam, or quinolone can predispose to resistance to other agents in the same class, a recent history of antibiotic therapy should guide the initial selection of therapy. If the patient has been on any antibiotic in the past 3 months, it may be preferable to choose CAP therapy with an agent in a totally different therapeutic class.

In addition to the general approach to therapy previously outlined, several other therapeutic issues arise in the management of CAP, which are addressed in the next sections.

Timeliness of Initial Therapy of Hospitalized Patients

For inpatients with CAP, timely and accurate therapy is essential to reduce mortality. In patients with severe CAP, survival is improved when the initial empiric therapy is accurate and leads to a rapid clinical response (41,59,70). In one study, when initial therapy led to a clinical response within 72 hours, the mortality of severe CAP was approximately 10%, whereas the mortality rate was 60% when therapy was initially ineffective (70). Another finding is the need to provide intravenous antibiotic therapy within 8 hours after the patient's arrival at the hospital (59). In a large Medicare study of 14,069 patients, mortality at 30 days was significantly reduced for the 75% of patients who received their first dose of therapy within 8 hours after arriving at the hospital (59). Although this has become the target time frame for initial therapy, additional benefit was noted when therapy was given even sooner.

Need to Treat All Populations for Atypical Pathogen Infection

In most available North American guidelines, the initial empiric therapy of CAP provides coverage for atypical pathogens, either as the primary infection or as part of a mixed infection (1,29,47). A high frequency of infection with these organisms has been noted not only in inpatients but also in outpatients (71).

A number of studies of large populations of outpatients and inpatients have shown that when therapy includes a macrolide or a quinolone, outcomes, including mortality, are better than when a β-lactam is used alone (41,42). Although these findings are not definitive, they do support a potentially important role for atypical pathogens. One study reported a greater mortality from bacteremic pneumococcal pneumonia when a single effective agent was used than when dual effective therapy was given (72). Interestingly, in that study, monotherapy with a third-generation cephalosporin was associated with a higher mortality rate than use of the same agent together with an agent that covered atypical pathogens (i.e., a macrolide or quinolone), which implies that coinfection with atypical pathogens may be important even in patients with bacteremic pneumococcal pneumonia.

What Is the Role of Drug-Resistant Pneumococci in Therapy for Community-Acquired Pneumonia?

As previously discussed (see section "Predicting Pathogens for Specific Patients"), both the ATS and IDSA guidelines have identified risk factors for infection with drug-resistant pneumococci, but the IDSA approach is to use these factors to influence therapy only in outpatients, whereas the ATS approach is to consider these factors in deciding on therapy for both outpatients and inpatients (1,47). In the ATS guidelines, if outpatients are at risk for infection with drug-resistant pneumococci, therapy should be with any of the following: oral cefpodoxime, cefuroxime, high-dose amoxicillin, amoxicillin/clavulanate, or an antipneumococcal quinolone, or with parenteral ceftriaxone followed by oral cefpodoxime. Again, if one of the β-lactams is used, a macrolide should be added to cover for atypical pathogens. If an inpatient is at risk for infection with drug-resistant pneumococci, therapy should be with any of the following intravenous agents: cefotaxime, ceftriaxone, ampicillin/sulbactam, high-dose ampicillin, or an antipneumococcal quinolone. When a β-lactam is used, a macrolide is added for the reasons discussed in the previous section. The rationale for using specific agents in patients with risk factors for drug-resistant pneumococcal infection is not only to minimize the risk for treatment failure but also to eradicate pneumococcal organisms with low levels of resistance rapidly

and reliably, so that selection pressure for the emergence of organisms with high-level resistance is reduced.

PRINCIPLES OF ANTIBIOTIC THERAPY OF COMMUNITY-ACQUIRED PNEUMONIA

Recommendation	Evidence
Administer first dose of antibiotics within 8 hours after arrival in hospital.	Observational studies
Treat all patients for the possibility of infection with "atypical pathogens" and pneumococci.	Observational studies of patients > age 65
Monotherapy with a macrolide can be given to outpatients or inpatients with no risk factors for DRSP, Gram-negatives, or aspiration.	Randomized controlled trials
For outpatients and inpatients with risk factors for DRSP or Gram-negatives, use either a β-lactam/macrolide combination or monotherapy with an antipneumococcal quinolone. Quinolone therapy should be used in penicillin-allergic patients.	Randomized controlled trials and observational studies; no strong evidence of one approach being superior to the other
For outpatients at risk for DRSP, the oral β-lactam should be one of the following: cefpodoxime, cefuroxime, high-dose ampicillin, amoxicillin/clavulanate.	*In vitro* susceptibility and expert opinion
For inpatients with clinical risk factors for DRSP, intravenous β-lactam therapy should be with cefotaxime, ceftriaxone, ampicillin/sulbactam, or high-dose ampicillin.	*In vitro* susceptibility and expert recommendation
Limit anti-*Pseudomonas* antibiotics to patients with *Pseudomonas* risk factors; the primary consideration is prevention of resistance, not efficacy.	Expert opinion
Limit the use of vancomycin to empiric therapy of patients with severe illness, especially suspected meningitis (to avoid overuse of this valuable agent).	Expert opinion
Consider the relative activity of the new quinolones for pneumococci (most to least active): moxifloxacin, gatifloxacin, levofloxacin.	
1. Choosing the most active agents can minimize future resistance. 2. Choosing the most active agents provides clinical benefit.	1. Observational studies, expert opinion 2. Expert opinion

DRSP, drug-resistant *S. pneumoniae.*

Evaluation of the Response to Therapy

Most outpatients and inpatients respond rapidly to the empiric therapy regimens previously outlined, with a clinical response usually occurring within 24 to 72 hours. A clinical response for inpatients is defined as relief of the symptoms of cough, sputum production, and dyspnea, along with an improved ability to take medications by mouth, a declining white blood cell count, and an afebrile status on at least two occasions 8 hours apart. When patients have met these criteria for a clinical response, it is appropriate to switch them to an oral therapy regimen and discharge them if they are otherwise medically and socially stable (1,73,74). Observation in the hospital during oral therapy is generally not necessary because patients usually do not deteriorate clinically after reaching signs of stability and after being able to switch to oral therapy (74). Radiographic improvement lags behind clinical improvement, and in a responding patient, a chest radiograph is not necessary until 2 to 4 weeks after the initiation of therapy. In general, 50% of patients with pneumococcal pneumonia show radiographic clearing at 5 weeks, and most show clearing in 2 to 3 months. Of patients with bacteremic disease, 50% have clear chest radiographs at 9 weeks and most by 18 weeks (75,76). Radiographic resolution in CAP is most influenced by the number of lobes involved and the age of the patient. Radiographic clearance of CAP decreases by 20% per decade after the age of 20 years, and multilobar infiltrates take longer to clear than unilobar disease (75).

If a patient fails to respond to therapy within the expected time interval, then it is necessary to consider infection with a drug-resistant or unusual pathogen (*M. tuberculosis, B. anthracis, Coxiella burnetii, Burkholderia pseudomallei, Chlamydia psittaci, Pasteurella multocida,* endemic fungi, or viruses); a pneumonic complication (lung abscess, endocarditis, empyema); or a noninfectious process that mimics pneumonia (bronchiolitis obliterans with organizing pneumonia, hypersensitivity pneumonitis, pulmonary vasculitis, bronchoalveolar cell carcinoma, lymphoma, pulmonary embolus) (1). The evaluation of a nonresponding patient should be individualized but may include CT of the chest, pulmonary angiography, bronchoscopy, and occasionally open lung biopsy.

Prevention

The prevention of CAP is important in all groups but especially the elderly, who are at risk for a higher frequency of infection and a more severe course of illness. Appropriate patients should be vaccinated with both pneumococcal and influenza vaccines, and all at-risk persons should discontinue cigarette smoking.

Pneumococcal Vaccine

Pneumococcal capsular polysaccharide vaccine can prevent pneumonia in otherwise healthy populations, as was initially demonstrated in South African gold miners and American military recruits (77). The benefits in persons of advanced age or with underlying conditions in nonepidemic environments are less clearly defined. The vaccine efficacy has ranged from 65% to 84% in patients with diabetes mellitus, coronary artery disease, congestive heart failure, chronic pulmonary disease, and anatomic asplenia (1,77,78,79). In immunocompetent patients older than 65 years, effectiveness has been documented to be 75%. In immunocompromised pa-

tients, including those with sickle cell disease, chronic renal failure, immunoglobulin deficiency, Hodgkin disease, lymphoma, leukemia, or multiple myeloma, effectiveness has not been proved. A single repeated vaccination is indicated in a person who is 65 years old, initially received the vaccine more than 5 years earlier, and was younger than 65 years at first vaccination. If the initial vaccination was given at the age of 65 years or older, repeated vaccination is not indicated unless the patient has anatomic or functional asplenia or one of the immunocompromising conditions previously listed. For these patients, repeated vaccination is indicated, and the second dose is given at least 5 years after the original dose.

The available pneumococcal vaccine is widely underutilized and could be a vital tool in reducing the mortality

RECOMMENDED USE OF PNEUMOCOCCAL VACCINE	
Populations for Whom Vaccination Recommended (Benefit)	**Evidence**
Patients age 65 years (**>75% protective, especially for bacteremic illness**)	Randomized studies

Persons age <64 years if
• they are living in a special environment, such as a long-term care facility
• they have a chronic illness, such as
   Cardiovascular disease (congestive heart failure)
   Chronic pulmonary disease (COPD, but not asthma)
   Diabetes mellitus
   Alcoholism
   Chronic liver disease (cirrhosis)
   Cerebrospinal fluid leaks
• functional or anatomic asplenia
• they are Alaskan natives or native Americans.
(**Protective in 65%–84% of those with chronic illness**)
	Nonrandomized studies

Immunocompromised patients age <65 years (**try to vaccinate early in the course of chronic illness**): HIV infection, leukemia, lymphoma, Hodgkin disease, multiple myeloma, generalized malignancy, chronic renal disease, nephrotic syndrome, immunosuppressive therapy (including long-term corticosteroids) (**Benefit undetermined**)	Observational studies; expert opinion
Give a single revaccination to anyone 65 years of age who initially received the vaccine >5 years earlier and was age <65 years on first vaccination and to immunocompromised patients after 5 years. (**Uncertain**)	Observational study, expert opinion
Consider vaccination in any hospitalized medical patient before discharge because 60% of patients with CAP have been hospitalized within the preceding 4 years. (**Uncertain**)	Expert opinion

CAP, community-acquired pneumonia; COPD, chronic obstructive pulmonary disease.

and morbidity of CAP. The 23-valent pneumococcal vaccine carries 23 of the 90 known pneumococcal serotypes causing most of the clinical infections in the United States, including 85% of all infections caused by pneumococci. A protein-conjugated pneumococcal vaccine has been licensed and appears more immunogenic than the older vaccine, but it contains only seven serotypes; it is recommended for healthy children but has not yet been adequately tested in adults (80). Hospital-based immunization for most admitted patients could be highly effective because more than 60% of all patients with CAP have been admitted to the hospital for some indication in the preceding 4 years, and hospitalization could be defined as an appropriate time for vaccination (81). Pneumococcal vaccine can be given simultaneously with other vaccines, such as influenza vaccine, but each should be given at a separate site. The vaccine can be given before discharge in patients admitted for CAP.

Influenza Vaccination

Influenza epidemics contribute to morbidity and mortality through both the direct effects and complications of infection. The influenza vaccine preparations are revised annually to account for the changes in the antigenic nature of the virus (antigenic drift) that occur each season. Three strains are represented in each vaccine preparation: two influenza A strains (H3N2 and H1N1) and one influenza B strain. Vaccine should be given to all persons older than 65 years, patients with chronic medical illness (including nursing home residents), and those who provide health care to patients at risk for complicated influenza (1,82). The vaccine is given yearly, usually between September and mid November.

When the vaccine matches the circulating strain, it can prevent illness in 70% to 90% of healthy persons younger than 65 years (1,83). For older persons with chronic illness, the efficacy is less, but the vaccine can still attenuate the influenza infection and decrease the number of lower respiratory tract infections and the morbidity and mortality associated with influenza. In many studies, the vaccine has been shown to be cost-effective and able to prevent severe illness, and it can reduce the occurrence of pneumonia, hospitalization, and death (83).

Uncommon Causes of Community-Acquired Pneumonia

Considerations in the Setting of Possible Bioterrorism

Certain airborne pathogens can cause pneumonia when deliberately disseminated by the aerosol route as a biologic weapon. Victims present with a clinical syndrome of CAP. The pathogens that are most likely to be used in this fashion and can cause severe pulmonary infection are *B. anthracis* (anthrax), *Yersinia pestis* (plague), and *F. tularensis* (tularemia) (47). The Centers for Disease Control and Prevention has classified these agents as category A pathogens because of the high mortality associated with

infection and the potential impact on public health (85). Other pneumonic pathogens that can serve as agents of biologic warfare but with potentially less serious effects are in category B, including *C. burnetii* and *Brucella* species. Certain emerging pathogens are category C agents. These are not widely available as weapons but have the potential to cause high rates of morbidity and mortality; they include hantavirus and multidrug-resistant *M. tuberculosis* (86). Some agents of bioterrorism can be spread via the aerosol route, but infection does not generally present as pneumonia; these include the smallpox virus and the agents of viral hemorrhagic fevers (Ebola virus, Marburg virus).

Anthrax

In the fall of 2001, the United States experienced a series of intentional attacks with the anthrax bacillus that led to 11 confirmed cases of inhalational illness (87,88). *B. anthracis* is an aerobic, Gram-positive, spore-forming bacillus that rarely led to disease in this country before 2001. Particle size determines the infectiousness of the spores, and a size of 1 to 5 μm is necessary for particles to be inhaled into the alveolar space; however, infection generally requires an inoculum of 8,000 to 40,000 spores. The organisms initially enter alveolar macrophages and are transported to mediastinal lymph nodes, where they persist, germinate, and produce two toxins (lethal toxin and edema toxin); illness follows rapidly after germination (87,88). Although respiratory symptoms are often present, anthrax is not a typical pneumonic illness, but rather a disease characterized by hemorrhagic thoracic lymphadenitis, hemorrhagic mediastinitis, and pleural effusion. Whereas the incubation period of anthrax varied from 2 to 43 days in prior outbreaks, in the October 2001 series, the incubation period was from 4 to 6 days (87). In the U.S. experience, all patients had chills, fever, and sweats, and most had nonproductive cough, dyspnea, nausea, vomiting, and chest pain. The chest radiographic findings were abnormal in all of the first 10 patients, and seven had mediastinal widening, eight had pleural effusions (generally bloody), and seven had pulmonary infiltrates (87,88). Blood cultures were positive in all eight patients from whom they were obtained before therapy, but sputum culture and Gram stain are unlikely to be positive. In the U.S. attacks, 5 of 11 patients died.

Therapy includes supportive management and antibiotics, with possibly some role for corticosteroids if meningeal involvement or mediastinal edema is present. The recommended therapy is 400 mg of ciprofloxacin intravenously twice a day or 100 mg of doxycycline intravenously twice a day. Until the patient is clinically stable, one or two additional agents should be added, including clindamycin, vancomycin, imipenem, meropenem, chloramphenicol, penicillin, ampicillin, rifampin, and clarithromycin (87). Therapy should be continued after an initial response with either ciprofloxacin or doxycycline for at least 60 days (87). Postexposure prophylaxis can be carried out with ciprofloxacin or alternatively with doxycycline or amoxicillin for a total of 60 days.

Tularemia

The etiologic agent of this illness, *F. tularensis*, is a small, aerobic, nonmotile, Gram-negative coccobacillus that can infect humans after a bite from an infected arthropod, ingestion of infected food or water, or contact with contaminated soil or animal material. The organism can enter through the skin or mucous membranes, or it can be inhaled. Following inhalational exposure, pneumonic illness can develop after an incubation period of 3 to 5 days (range, 1–14 days) (89). In addition to pneumonia, pharyngitis, bronchiolitis, pleuropneumonitis, and hilar lymphadenitis may develop. Symptoms are not specific and include fever, malaise, and nonproductive cough. Many patients may have a nonspecific systemic illness without pneumonic findings. The chest radiograph can show bronchopneumonia (sometimes ovoid) with or without mediastinal adenopathy or pleural effusion, but the earliest radiographic finding is peribronchial infiltrates. The illness progresses more slowly and is less lethal than anthrax, but it can lead to sepsis and death. The organism can be grown from sputum or blood samples, but special culture and safety methods are required, so if the organism is suspected, the laboratory should be notified. Therapy is with either streptomycin or gentamicin for 10 days, but acceptable alternatives are doxycycline, chloramphenicol, or ciprofloxacin for 14 to 21 days (89).

Plague

This fulminant illness, caused by the Gram-negative bacillus *Y. pestis*, is usually a zoonosis with a rodent host and a flea vector, but it can spread from person to person and be transmitted as an aerosol, causing primary pulmonary infection, or pneumonic plague (85). The bacillus can be destroyed by drying, heat, and ultraviolet light, so it is hard to weaponize, and its potential for bioterrorism is uncertain. Although illness can be contracted through a flea bite, it can also develop following inhalation. The incubation period for pneumonic illness is 2 to 5 days. Symptoms include high fever, chills, headache, severe dyspnea, and a dry cough with blood-tinged sputum, with radiographic evidence of lobar pneumonia (47). The illness is typically fulminant, leading to septic shock and death. The diagnosis is made by culture of the sputum or blood, but because the organism can spread from person to person, health care workers should be warned if the disease is suspected, and the patient and culture samples should be isolated to prevent spread. The patient can spread illness to others during the first 48 hours of therapy. Treatment should be with streptomycin or gentamicin for 10 days; alternative therapies include tetracyclines or quinolones.

Rickettsial Pneumonia

Several rickettsial infections may uncommonly cause CAP. These include Q fever (*C. burnetii*), which occurs worldwide, Rocky Mountain spotted fever, and scrub typhus (*Rickettsia tsutsugamushi*) in Asia and Australia. Transmission typically involves an intermediate vector, often ticks (Q fever, Rocky Mountain spotted fever) or mites (scrub typhus) but also

sheep, cows, and contaminated milk (Q fever). These infections result, after a variable incubation period ranging from days to a few weeks, in febrile syndromes that may have a pneumonic component. Cough is common and usually nonproductive or minimally productive, although blood-tinged sputum may occur in each illness and in Rocky Mountain spotted fever may progress to frank edema and pulmonary hemorrhage associated with pulmonary vasculitis. Constitutional symptoms and dyspnea of varying degrees are often present, and heart failure can develop. The physical examination findings are remarkable for high fever, but with relative bradycardia. The chest findings are variable and can range from rare crackles to signs of frank consolidation. Friction rubs, although rare, may occur. Liver or spleen enlargement is most likely to occur in Q fever but is uncommon even in that setting. A maculopapular rash is relatively common in Q fever and Rocky Mountain spotted fever and may help to suggest the diagnosis of either of these entities. Involvement of the palms and soles with the rash is particularly useful in suggesting Rocky Mountain spotted fever. Chest radiographic abnormalities may be localized, patchy, or diffuse and take the form of alveolar consolidation or interstitial infiltrates. The treatment of choice is doxycycline, and chloramphenicol is an acceptable alternative. Residual weakness with aches and pains for weeks and months after treatment is common, especially after Q fever. Thrombophlebitis, sometimes leading to pulmonary emboli, has been described as a complication of Q fever.

Parasites

Infection with protozoans and helminths can produce lung disease by either an allergic reaction or direct spread to the lung. Loeffler syndrome, which manifests as cough, occasionally fever, patchy pulmonary infiltrates, and a high peripheral blood eosinophil count, has been described in association with intestinal infestation by protozoa and a variety of helminths, particularly nematodes and trematodes. These include *Ancylostoma braziliense*, *Ancylostoma duodenale*, *Entameoba histolytica*, *Enterobius vermicularis*, *Fasciola hepatica*, *Necator americanus*, *Taenia saginata*, *Trichinella spiralis*, and *Trichuris trichiura*. This is usually a benign condition requiring no treatment. Other helminths may cause infiltrates and eosinophilia by direct extension or invasion of the lungs.

Direct invasion of the lungs, including extension from below the diaphragm, may occur with a number of parasites. These include *Schistosoma*, *Echinoccus*, *Strongyloides*, *Ascaris*, *Paragonimus*, and the roundworms *Toxocara canis* and *Toxocara cati*. The clinical picture varies not only with the particular agent involved but also with the stage of infection and the underlying condition of the patient. Thus, in acute schistosomal migration through the lungs, wheezing, dyspnea, and cough are common. In some patients, an acute pneumonic infiltrate may develop weeks to months later and result in severe respiratory distress, hemoptysis, and diffuse infiltrates as an intense inflammatory response to the larvae develops. Later still, pulmonary hypertension and dyspnea may develop as schistosomal ova, produced by adult worms, gain entry to the pulmonary circulation and obstruct arterioles, producing an obliterative vasculitis. Praziquantel is the treatment of choice.

In *Strongyloides* infection, the condition of the host is critical. Normal persons may pass larvae in the stool and sustain reinfection through the perianal skin. Associated migration of larvae through the lungs causes fever, dyspnea, cough, patchy infiltrates, and eosinophilia. This process is usually self-limited, although repeated cycles of so-called exo-autoinfection may occur. The situation may be quite different in immunocompromised hosts. Typically, these persons have received steroids, have advanced HIV coinfection, or are otherwise severely compromised. In this setting, invasion of larvae into the intestinal wall facilitates the translocation of a large inoculum of enteric organisms that cause Gram-negative bacteremia, in addition to larval migration. Diffuse pulmonary infiltrates and respiratory failure/ARDS may occur. Eosinophil counts may be profoundly elevated but may also be normal. Ivermectin or albendazole is recommended for these patients, along with coverage for enteric bacteria. Thiabendazole can also be used.

In a small percentage of patients infected with *Echinococcus granulosus*(rarely with *Echinococcus multilocularis*), spread to the lungs from an abdominal cyst can occur. Disease is most common in the Middle East, Australia/New Zealand, and central Europe. Pockets of disease exist in Latin America, but infection is uncommon in North America. Patients often have a history of exposure to sheep. Typically, the right lower lobes or right pleural space is involved. Patients have cough, hemoptysis, and pleuritic pain. Chest radiographs show single or multiple well-circumscribed nodular infiltrates suggestive of neoplasm. Mediastinal densities can also develop. Surgical resection or percutaneous drainage (sometimes including irrigation with hypertonic saline solution), along with albendazole, is the current treatment for this condition.

Paragonimiasis causes variable symptoms. The flatworm is most prevalent in Southeast Asia and the Philippines and to a lesser extent in Latin America, India, Africa, and the islands of the South Pacific. Lung involvement manifests as cough, occasionally with blood streaking. Pleuritic pain may be present. Crackles are commonly heard on auscultation. Radiographic findings include linear or patchy infiltrates, most often in the lower lung zones. Cystic lesions, sometimes several centimeters in diameter, or inhomogeneous nodular densities may be seen. In a small proportion of patients, pleural effusions or pneumothorax is found. Praziquantel is the treatment of choice. Table 22.5 provides a conceptual classification of these conditions.

Viruses

The incidence of viral pneumonia is difficult to define, but it has been suggested that viruses cause as many as 5% to 15%

TABLE 22.5. CONCEPTUAL CLASSIFICATION OF PARASITIC CONDITIONS

Severity (Eosinophilia)	Class/Example
Acute/life-threatening (−)	Protozoans, nematodes (roundworms), sporozoans/amebiasis, strongyloidiasis, malaria
Acute infiltrate/asthma (+)	Nematodes/ascariasis, ancylostomiasis (hookworm) strongyloidiasis, toxocariasis
Chronic pulmonary disease (+/−)	Nematodes, trematodes (flukes), cestodes (tapeworms)/wuchereriasis, filariasis; paragonimiasis; schistosomiasis; echinococcosis

of cases of CAP. These higher numbers may reflect initial viral syndromes complicated by superinfection with bacteria. During influenza epidemics in particular, viral pneumonia should be considered, but secondary bacterial infection with pneumococci, *S. aureus*, or *H. influenzae* can also occur. Invasive and severe viral disease is most likely in patients who have underlying cardiopulmonary disease or are pregnant.

Adenovirus may cause pneumonia in children and adults that can range from patchy infiltrates to dense lobar consolidation.

Respiratory syncytial virus most commonly infects infants and young children, usually during the winter months. Immunocompromised adults, particularly those receiving bone marrow transplants or treatment for leukemia, or even the institutionalized elderly are vulnerable. Respiratory syncytial virus may cause disease from the upper (croup, sinusitis) to lower (bronchiolitis, pneumonia) respiratory tract. Ribavirin may be useful in severe cases of respiratory syncytial virus infection. The benefit of adding intravenous immunoglobulin to ribavirin is uncertain.

Vaccination has reduced the prevalence of varicella and rubella in normal hosts. Varicella can cause a severe diffuse pneumonia, particularly in immunocompromised persons and pregnant women naive to the virus. The progression of lung infiltrates often parallels the progression of the rash of chickenpox. Acyclovir and corticosteroids can reduce the morbidity and mortality of this condition. A rare syndrome of pneumonitis (especially nodular interstitial disease) has been described in persons who previously received killed measles vaccine and were then exposed to wild-type measles virus or vaccinated with live measles vaccine.

Newly appreciated viral agents may be encountered. Hantavirus, transmitted by aerosols of rodent excrement, has received increasing attention after outbreaks in the southwestern United States and other areas of the country. Hantavirus causes an acute febrile illness that may progress during several days to ARDS. Marked concentration of the blood, an elevated hematocrit, elevated levels of lactate dehydrogenase, and thrombocytopenia may suggest the diagnosis. Ribavirin has been used to treat hantavirus syndrome, although experience is anecdotal to date.

NOSOCOMIAL PNEUMONIA

Epidemiology and Incidence

Hospital-acquired pneumonia, defined as pneumonia beginning within 48 to 72 hours after admission to the hospital, is the leading cause of death from nosocomial infection (2). NP can arise in patients who are on mechanical ventilation, and this form of illness, ventilator-associated pneumonia (VAP), is a common cause of mortality. The frequency of NP increases as mechanical ventilation is prolonged, although the risk is greatest early in the course of ventilation. In a prospective study of 1,014 mechanically ventilated patients performed by Cook and colleagues (90), VAP defined by strict clinical or microbiologic criteria developed in 177 patients. The mean time to onset was 9 days, with a median time to onset of 7 days after ICU admission. However, when the daily hazard rate of infection was calculated, it was estimated to be 3.3% at day 5, 2.3% at day 10, and 1.3% at day 15, figures documenting a dramatic decline in pneumonia risk with time. Because the risk for pneumonia is so high early after intubation, pneumonias beginning within the first 5 days (early-onset infection) account for 50% of all episodes of VAP, and the natural history and pathogens of this infection differ from those associated with VAP of late onset (91). At least 85% of patients in whom pneumonia develops in the ICU are undergoing endotracheal intubation, and the intubation process itself contributes to the risk for infection. When patients with acute respiratory failure are managed with noninvasive ventilation, NP pneumonia is less common (92).

Although NP develops in 50% to 66% of all patients with a tracheostomy, their daily risk (after tracheostomy) is lower than that of patients undergoing short-term endotracheal intubation. The explanation may be the self-selection process of generally healthier patients, who are able to survive long enough to undergo tracheostomy. Kollef and colleagues (93) examined 521 patients requiring mechanical ventilation and compared the 51 who underwent tracheostomy with the 470 who did not. Those requiring a tracheostomy had a higher incidence of NP before tracheostomy, but those who underwent a tracheostomy had a significantly lower hospital mortality rate (13.7%) than those who did not require a tracheostomy (26.4%). This finding suggests that patients who are able to survive their illness and undergo tracheostomy may be better able to recover and resist the development and effects of pneumonia than patients who are too ill to live long enough to undergo tracheostomy.

Attributable Mortality

VAP develops when patients are already acutely and chronically ill, and not all of the 50% of patients who die with this illness die as a direct result of pneumonia; rather, they die of their underlying illness. However, at least a third to a half of all deaths in patients with VAP are caused by the pneumonia, and this "attributable mortality" is greater in medical patients than in surgical patients, in those infected with certain high-risk pathogens (*P. aeruginosa*, *Acinetobacter* species, and *S. aureus*), and in those who receive initially inadequate antibiotic therapy (94–100). The risk factors for mortality from VAP can be categorized as patient factors, bacteriologic factors, and therapy-related risks and are summarized in Table 22.6. In addition to its effect on mortality, hospital-acquired pneumonia increases the length of hospitalization on average by 7 to 9 days per patient (2). The effect of VAP on hospital stay has also been documented in patients with a tracheostomy; in the study of Georges and colleagues (101), the duration of ventilation was increased in patients in whom VAP developed either early or late after tracheostomy (101).

Studies examining the attributable mortality of VAP are difficult to perform and involve a variety of methods, including direct case review, matched cohort studies, and comparisons of observed mortality with the mortality predicted by scoring systems (Acute Physiology and Chronic Health Evaluation [APACHE] or Mortality Prediction Model [MPM]) at the time of admission (100). One study used a matched cohort design to address this question in 85 cases (99), and mortality was similar in both groups: 40% for those with VAP and 38% for the matched controls. The lack of difference may reflect the fact that many of the

TABLE 22.6. RISK FACTORS FOR AN ADVERSE OUTCOME (MORTALITY) FROM VENTILATOR-ASSOCIATED PNEUMONIA

Patient risk factors
  Historical data
    Prolonged mechanical ventilation before pneumonia
    Medical (vs. surgical) diagnosis
    Age >60 years
  Physiologic factors
    Underlying fatal or serious illness
      (APACHE score 11–30)
    Severe pneumonia (with sepsis or ARDS)
    Coma on admission
    Multiple system organ failure
  Laboratory Data
    Bilateral lung infiltrates

Bacteriologic risk factors
  High-risk pathogen
    P. aeruginosa
    Acinetobacter species
    Stenotrophomonas maltophilia
    Methicillin-resistant *S. aureus*
  Antibiotic resistant pathogen, especially if acquired during therapy
  Superinfection after a first course of therapy

Therapy-related risk factors
  Prior antibiotic therapy
  Inadequate initial therapy (organism not sensitive to therapeutic agent)
  Inadequate dose or dosing regimen

APACHE, acute physiology and chronic health evaluation; ARDS, acute respiratory distress syndrome.

patients were surgical patients or trauma victims, not medical patients. In another study with a similar design, in which 177 patients with VAP were compared with a matched cohort of critically ill patients without pneumonia, those with pneumonia had a longer stay (4.3 days longer), a longer duration of mechanical ventilation, and a trend toward increased mortality (~33%) (97). In the same study, attributable mortality was greater for medical patients than for surgical or trauma patients, mortality was increased by certain high-risk organisms (*P. aeruginosa, Acinetobacter, Stenotrophomonas,* and *S. aureus*), and a trend to increased mortality was noted with the use of inappropriate empiric antibiotic therapy. When patients were given adequate therapy for VAP, their attributable mortality rate was only about 20%, versus an attributable mortality of 60% in those who received initially inadequate therapy.

Many retrospective studies have shown that inadequate initial therapy is a major determinant of mortality in patients with VAP (102,103). Thus, the major emphasis in managing these patients is on providing prompt and effective therapy, but this goal is made more difficult by the high frequency of antibiotic-resistant Gram-positive and Gram-negative bacteria that often cause this illness and increase the likelihood that initial therapy will be inadequate. In addition, prospective intervention studies are still needed documenting an effective approach to increasing the number of patients receiving adequate therapy and showing a reduction in mortality with accurate therapy. One such interventional study did show that a protocol for antibiotic use, based on local susceptibility patterns, increased the number of patients given adequate therapy, but no associated reduction in mortality was noted (104).

Relationship of Airway Colonization to Nosocomial Pneumonia

Serious illness of any type can serve as a pathogenic mechanism for pneumonia by leading to Gram-negative bacillary colonization of the respiratory tract (5). As the severity of systemic illness increases, colonization of both the oropharynx and tracheobronchial tree by enteric Gram-negative bacteria becomes more likely, and colonization can serve as the first means of entry of bacteria into the lung and a harbinger of subsequent pneumonia (2,5,105,106).

The oropharynx ordinarily has a microflora, but enteric Gram-negative bacteria are rarely part of this flora in healthy persons. Enteric Gram-negative bacteria are present in the oropharynx of about 6% of healthy persons, but they can be found in the oropharynx of 35% of patients who are moderately ill and in the oropharynx of 73% of critically ill persons (105). The tracheobronchial tree is ordinarily sterile in nonsmokers and rarely harbors enteric Gram-negative bacteria unless they are severely ill. However, tracheobronchial colonization by enteric Gram-negative bacteria occurs in from 45% to 100% of intubated patients, and in those who are

most severely ill and intubated for more than 1 week, *Pseudomonas* species are the predominant pathogens (5). In general, early in the hospital stay, community pathogens colonize the tracheobronchial tree in ventilated patients, but with time, these are replaced by enteric Gram-negatives, including *Pseudomonas* species (2,5,107,108). Although colonization of the oropharynx and tracheobronchial tree by enteric Gram-negative bacteria is commonly associated with VAP, in patients with head trauma, tracheal colonization within 24 hours after admission by *S. aureus, H. influenzae,* or *S. pneumoniae* has been reported to be associated with early-onset VAP (108). In patients with ARDS, preceding tracheobronchial colonization by potentially pathogenic organisms is common, particularly in those with subsequent VAP (109).

The risk factors for oropharyngeal and tracheobronchial colonization with enteric Gram-negative bacteria are similar and include many common comorbidities. In addition to serious illness in general, risk factors for oropharyngeal colonization include renal failure, antibiotic use, the postoperative state, coma, diabetes, advanced age, smoking, malnutrition, acidosis, preexisting lung disease, hypotension, and therapy to neutralize gastric acid (5). Risk factors for tracheobronchial colonization by enteric Gram-negative bacteria include many of the same conditions, in addition to underlying malignancy, cardiac disease, neurologic illness, prolonged hospitalization, corticosteroid therapy, viral infection, and tracheostomy (5).

One of the pathogenic mechanisms that explains how various types of serious illness lead to colonization of a mucosal surface with enteric Gram-negative bacteria is bacterial adherence. Bacteria possess surface appendages, called *adhesins,* that can bind to mucosal receptors via a lock-and-key interaction that is both specific and irreversible (5). Adherence serves as a mechanism of colonization provided that the mucosal site has a receptor for the putative colonizing organism, the organism has the appropriate adhesin for the mucosal site, and the intervening host defenses are sufficiently impaired to allow prolonged contact between bacteria and cells. If all three of these conditions are met, adherence can facilitate bacterial binding to the epithelial surface, and this binding can serve as the first nidus of bacterial colonization. Interestingly, it is known that many of the risk factors for airway colonization enhance the adherence of respiratory tract cells to certain enteric Gram-negative bacteria, particularly *P. aeruginosa* (5,110). *In vitro* studies have correlated changes in oropharyngeal cell adherence with enteric Gram-negative bacterial colonization of this site after exposure of animals or patients to azotemia, endotracheal intubation, general surgery, malnutrition, tracheostomy, or viral infection (5,110). Similarly, airway injury and malnutrition are known to increase tracheal cell bacterial adherence, and changes in this parameter have been correlated with colonization (5,110). One important bacterial binding site in the tracheobronchial tree, in addition to the cell surface itself, is respiratory mucus. Thus, when mucociliary clearance is impaired, colonization can occur because bacteria bound to mucus are not removed, and stagnant mucus acts as a mechanism for propagating organism persistence in the lower respiratory tract (5,111).

Other binding sites for bacteria include injured epithelial surfaces, such as occur at disrupted tight junctions at the basolateral surface of epithelial cells (112). When *P. aeruginosa* binds to these sites, it may become more virulent and secrete the cytotoxic substance exo-U (113). Another important binding site for bacteria in the mechanically ventilated patient is the endotracheal tube itself (7). The endotracheal tube can be colonized by aerosolized bacteria from the tracheobronchial tree, and bacteria at this site are often the same organisms that cause pneumonia; a colonized endotracheal tube can serve as a sequestered nidus of bacteria, unaffected by host defenses or antibiotic therapy. In addition, the tube can traumatize the tracheobronchial surface and cause epithelial cell injury, which favors bacterial adherence because organisms preferentially bind to injured cells and to basement membrane material exposed during tracheobronchial trauma (5). An endotracheal tube also increases the production and stagnation of mucus, thereby providing bacteria with additional binding sites in the lower airway (5).

The sequence of airway colonization is a topic of controversy. In the traditional model of colonization, the oropharynx becomes overgrown with enteric Gram-negative bacteria, which in turn are aspirated into the lung, leading to tracheobronchial colonization. However, two other sites of colonization must be considered: the stomach, which can be an initial site of colonization of bacteria that reach the oropharynx and lung (114), and the tracheobronchial tree, which can be a site of primary colonization (115). The role of the stomach as a site of colonization remains uncertain; many studies show no specific role, but the stomach can serve to "amplify" bacterial growth that begins elsewhere (114). Primary tracheal colonization has been proposed for *P. aeruginosa*, and this organism has a particular ability to adhere to tracheal epithelial cells (115). In some intubated patients, *P. aeruginosa* colonizes the trachea without first colonizing the oropharynx, and this observation may explain why subglottic secretion drainage, which interrupts the oropharyngeal-to-tracheal transfer of bacteria, does not generally prevent late-onset VAP or VAP caused by *P. aeruginosa* (115,116). Not all investigators have found primary tracheal colonization with *P. aeruginosa*, but this organism can arise from exogenous (environmental) sources and enter the lung directly (117,118). In one study, half of all acquisitions of *P. aeruginosa* were from cross-colonization of organisms from other patients in the ICU, whereas the others were from endogenous sources (119). In addition, this organism can persist and recur in tracheal secretions, usually as the consequence of persistence of an infecting strain rather than of acquisition of a new strain (120).

Once systemic illness has led to colonization, pneumonia often follows (105,106). Both oropharyngeal and tracheal colonization have been associated with VAP. Tracheal colonization by community pathogens is a risk factor for early-onset VAP, and colonization by resistant Gram-negatives is a risk factor for late-onset pneumonia (107). The association between colonization and pneumonia is probably the result of two factors: First, colonization exposes patients to large numbers of potential pathogens, and second, colonization can be viewed as a marker of multiple other defects in host respiratory tract defenses that, together with colonization, cause pneumonia. Thus, it is not surprising that the risk factors for colonization and those for NP are similar.

Risk Factors for Illness

As discussed (see section "Epidemiology and Incidence"), prolonged ventilation is a risk factor for VAP, and in one study, the duration of ventilation in patients with pneumonia was 19 days, but only 10 days in those without pneumonia (90). In that study, other risk factors for the development of pneumonia during mechanical ventilation included underlying cardiac disease, respiratory disease, trauma, burns, neurologic disease, emergency admission or admission from the operating room, witnessed aspiration, use of paralytic agents, and nasoenteral feeding. Interestingly, the administration of antibiotics reduced the risk for pneumonia, although this protective effect lasted only 2 to 3 weeks. In another study, in which quantitative bronchoscopic methods were used to define the incidence of VAP, George and colleagues (121) identified risk factors to be low serum albumin (suggesting that impaired host status is important for the development of infection), colonization of the upper respiratory tract by Gram-negative bacteria, absence of antibiotic therapy, and duration of mechanical ventilation. Again, in this study, the risk for pneumonia increased with the duration of ventilation, but that risk was not expressed on a daily basis in a comparison of patients on long-term and short-term ventilation. Clearly, from a number of studies, we can conclude that the risk factors for infection do vary with time. One described entity is pneumonia beginning very early after intubation (within 48 hours), and the pathogenesis may be aspiration during the intubation process, as suggested by the identified risk factors: sedation, absence of antibiotic therapy, and recent cardiopulmonary resuscitation (122). ARDS is another risk factor for pneumonia, but generally that pneumonia is of late onset, and 90% of episodes occur after 7 days of ventilation (123).

Other risk factors for NP in a hospitalized patient include any serious illness that can interfere with host immune defenses and any situation that increases the patient's exposure to large numbers of potentially pathogenic bacteria. Thus, other risk factors for pneumonia include exposure to contaminated respiratory therapy equipment, the use of systemic antibiotics, repeated or difficult endotracheal intubation, the use of total parenteral rather than enteral nutrition, nosocomial sinusitis, supine (rather than semi-erect) positioning, and inadequate endotracheal tube cuff pressure (124–126). The role of the stomach in the pathogenesis of pneumonia is controversial, but manipulations that increase the risk for Gram-negative colonization of the stomach (enteral feeding, histamine H_2 blockers, antacids) or aspiration (large-bore feeding tube, stomach vs. jejunal feeding, large gastric volumes of feedings) are well-identified risk factors for pneumonia (114). Antibiotic use is a particularly important risk factor; it increases the incidence not only of pneumonia, but also of bacteriologically virulent infections, including those caused by resistant Gram-negatives such as *P. aeruginosa* and *Acinetobacter* (127).

When VAP develops after tracheostomy, it may be important to distinguish infection beginning early after the procedure (within 5 days) from that developing later, because each is associated with a unique clinical course and risk factors (101). In one study, early-onset pneumonia after tracheostomy occurred at a mean of 2.7 days after the procedure, and risk factors included heavy colonization of endotracheal aspirates, continued sedation for longer than 24 hours after tracheostomy, and hyperthermia on the day of the procedure. Late-onset pneumonia occurred at a mean of 14.4 days after the procedure, and risk factors included prolonged sedation before tracheostomy and fever on the day of the procedure. The patients in whom VAP developed after tracheostomy had a higher mortality rate (54%) than those in whom it did not (33%), but the direct effect of infection on death was not defined (101).

Diagnostic Issues

Nosocomial pneumonia is diagnosed when a patient has been in the hospital for at least 48 to 72 hours and a new or progressive infiltrate then develops on the chest radiograph, accompanied by at least two of the following: fever, leukocytosis, and purulent sputum (2). Other clinical findings in patients with NP include decreasing oxygenation, pathogens in the sputum, and systemic signs of sepsis. Unfortunately, these clinical findings are sensitive but not specific for pneumonia, and many patients with them can have other conditions, including atelectasis, congestive heart failure, infectious tracheobronchitis, and extrapulmonary infection (sinusitis, central line infection, intra-abdominal infection). The diagnosis is especially difficult in mechanically ventilated patients, who commonly exhibit many clinical features of infection without actually having pneumonia. In addition, the presence of pathogenic organisms in sputum culture is not diagnostic because both oropharyngeal and tracheobronchial colonization with these bacteria occurs in many hospitalized and ventilated patients, so that the mere presence of such organisms does not necessarily indicate infection.

In an effort to enhance the accuracy of clinical tools to diagnose VAP, which is one form of NP, Pugin and colleagues (128) developed a "clinical pulmonary infection score" (CPIS) that weights six variables on a scale from 0 to 2, giving a total score ranging from 0 to 12. The factors included in the CPIS are fever, leukocytosis, purulence of secretions, type of infiltrate, oxygenation, and pathogens in

the sputum. In its original application, a CPIS above 6 correlated well with pneumonia, defined both clinically and by quantitative microbiology. In another study, the CPIS was correlated with autopsy findings of pneumonia, and the score had a sensitivity of 77% and a specificity of 42% (129).

In an effort to make the diagnosis more secure and avoid the excessive administration of antibiotics, some investigators have used quantitative cultures, generally collected by invasive (bronchoscopic) sampling of respiratory secretions, to define pneumonia. Because routine bronchoscopic (or endotracheal) suction samples are often contaminated by oropharyngeal secretions, Wimberley and colleagues (130) developed the double-lumen "protected" specimen brush (PSB). With this method, bronchoscopic samples are cultured quantitatively, and the diagnosis of pneumonia is established if more than 10^3 organisms are isolated per milliliter. Quantitative cultures can also be applied to bronchoalveolar lavage (BAL) or endotracheal aspiration samples, and the threshold is higher, at 10^4/mL or 10^5/mL for BAL, and at 10^6/mL for endotracheal aspiration (102,131,132). Some studies have examined the use of blindly passed nonbronchoscopic catheters for BAL and quantitative culture and have shown this method to be useful, which may be related to the fact that nosocomial bronchopneumonia preferentially develops in dependent lung segments, a site where such sampling is usually performed (133). When BAL has been used, some investigators have also looked at the percentage of cells with intracellular organisms on cytocentrifuge and defined pneumonia by the presence of organisms in 5% to 7% of cells, thereby permitting earlier diagnosis than culture would allow (134,135).

In studies of both animal and human respiratory infection, the sensitivity and specificity of these methods for the diagnosis of VAP have varied widely, with good results in some investigators' hands and less accurate results in others, and with the various methods comparing favorably with one another (136,137). The sensitivity for PSB has varied from as low as 38% to as high as 95% to 100%, with similar results for BAL. The variable sensitivity of these methods may be a consequence of the fact that pneumonia is a patchy process, with some areas involved and others not. Thus, it is possible to collect secretions from an uninvolved area that is adjacent to an infected area and obtain a false-negative result (138). One difficulty in defining the sensitivity and specificity of these methods is the absence of an unequivocal "gold standard," with even autopsy findings interpreted differently by different pathologists (139). Using an autopsy gold standard, Marquette and colleagues (132) found the sensitivity of BAL, PSB, and endotracheal aspiration all to be no higher than 60%. In a similar study, the conclusion was that tracheal aspiration (with a qualitative evaluation) was the most sensitive method for identifying organisms in lung tissue, whereas a sterile BAL sample had the greatest positive predictive value for a sterile culture of lung tissue (139).

When quantitative cultures are used to diagnose VAP, they serve not only to define pneumonia (and whether to start therapy) but also to determine which of the organisms recovered is responsible for infection (and thus which therapy to use). These determinations are made if the quantitative results exceed the previously mentioned threshold concentrations for a potentially pathogenic microorganism. When quantitative cultures are used as a "gold standard," as many as half of all patients with the clinical diagnosis of NP do not have infection. However, the sensitivity of these methods is not 100%, and thus if these tools are used to justify withholding antibiotics until the diagnosis of VAP is absolutely certain, some patients who require therapy will not receive it in a timely fashion. On the other hand, if antibiotics are used too freely, with overly sensitive criteria for the diagnosis of pneumonia, some patients will receive therapy unnecessarily, thereby contributing to the problem of antibiotic resistance.

One practical limitation of quantitative cultures is that patients are often receiving antibiotics at the time of study, and this can lead to both false-positive and false-negative results. Torres (140) compared quantitative cultures with endotracheal aspiration, PSB, and BAL and demonstrated a significant false-positive rate with all three techniques (59% for PSB, 35% for BAL, and 22% for endotracheal aspiration) in patients without respiratory tract infection who had received prior antibiotics. A high false-positive rate was also noted when these techniques were applied to patients with underlying chronic obstructive pulmonary disease (141). Antibiotic therapy can also lead to false-negative results; however, investigators have shown the importance of determining whether a patient had started antibiotics recently (within 24 hours) or had been taking them for more than 72 hours. In the former situation, false-negative results were common, whereas in the latter situation, bronchoscopy often demonstrated a drug-resistant organism (135).

Despite the controversies surrounding bronchoscopic techniques, they are of greatest value in immunocompromised patients, in whom nonbacterial diagnoses are a major concern. However, for patients with VAP, a number of questions about these methods remain, and these must be answered before the techniques are put into widespread clinical use in mechanically ventilated patients. Unanswered questions include the following: Which method (BAL, protected brush) is best? Should testing be performed blindly or bronchoscopically? and most importantly, If clinical decisions are made based on the data these tests provide, will patient outcomes be improved? It is this last question, regarding the effect of invasive methods on the outcomes of patients with VAP, that is most relevant (131,136). Many studies have shown that the most important determinant of outcome is the adequacy of initial antibiotic therapy, and currently no data have shown that invasive methods lead to more accurate empiric therapy than clinical management. If the data from quantitative cultures became available only several days after therapy is started, this might explain why the results of quantitative cultures did not favorably influence the outcome of patients who received initially inaccurate therapy (102,142).

Despite these concerns, one multicenter French study did show a benefit of managing patients with suspected VAP with quantitative cultures. In that study, 413 patients with suspected VAP were randomized to management by either an invasive or a noninvasive approach. In the population managed by the invasive approach, antibiotic therapy was given only if bronchoscopic sampling suggested infection or if a patient had signs of severe sepsis (143). When this strategy was used, antibiotics were never given to 90 of 204 patients. In contrast, therapy was withheld from only 15 of 209 patients managed by clinical judgment. Patients managed with the invasive strategy (which included the group from whom therapy was withheld) had the same 28-day mortality as patients managed by clinical judgment, but a lower 14-day mortality. The differences in mortality may not have been directly related to the diagnostic approach used because the frequency of inadequate empiric therapy was higher in the patients managed by the clinical strategy, for reasons unexplained, than in the patients managed by the invasive strategy. However, this study did show that if appropriate patients are identified, in this case by means of bronchoscopic data, therapy can be safely withheld, potentially reducing the selection pressure for antibiotic resistance.

However, it may be possible to limit the use of antibiotics, and thereby control resistance, but still treat patients with suspected VAP in an aggressive fashion, by applying a clinical rather than a bronchoscopic approach, as suggested by the study of Singh and colleagues (144). In that study, patients with suspected VAP were clinically evaluated with a CPIS based on five components—fever, leukocytosis, appearance of tracheal secretions, radiographic patterns, and oxygenation—to determine the likelihood of pneumonia (144). If the score was higher than 6 (each of the five components was scored 0–2), patients were considered to have pneumonia and were treated for 10 to 21 days. However, those with a score of 6 or less were randomized to "standard care" or 400 mg of ciprofloxacin every 8 hours for 3 days. After 3 days, in the patients treated with ciprofloxacin, the CPIS was measured again, with addition of the criteria of radiographic progression and the results of respiratory cultures, and if the score remained 6 or lower, antibiotics were stopped. When this approach was used, 42 patients with a score of 6 or less received standard therapy, and 39 were randomized to 3 days of ciprofloxacin therapy. Only 11 of the 39 patients required antibiotics for more than 3 days (because the CPIS had risen above 6); in the rest of the group, therapy was stopped after 3 days. The entire group that received a short course of therapy had the same clinical course (CPIS at day 3) and the same mortality as the 42 patients randomized to standard therapy. However, antibiotic resistance was less frequent and therapy was withheld more frequently in the group given a short course of therapy. Thus, the authors demonstrated the safety and feasibility of clinical assessment as a method to limit the use of prolonged antibiotic therapy in patients with suspected

TABLE 22.7. SENSITIVITY AND SPECIFICITY OF PROCEDURES FOR DIAGNOSING VENTILATOR-ASSOCIATED PNEUMONIA

Method	Sensitivity/Specificity[a]	Comment
Bronchoscopic protected specimen brush	33%–100% sensitivity 50%–100% specificity Applies to presence of pneumonia	Assessment limited by absence of gold standard
Bronchoscopic BAL	50%–90% sensitivity 45%–100% specificity Applies to presence of pneumonia	No gold standard
Nonbronchoscopic BAL	Similar to bronchoscopic methods, with close to 90% agreement when both done in the same patient	No gold standard
Quantitative endotracheal aspiration	38%–82% sensitivity 72%–85% specificity	No gold standard
Qualitative endotracheal aspiration	Up to 100% sensitive with specificity as low as <20% for the diagnosis of pneumonia; sensitivity still high (>90%) for presence of etiologic pathogen	
CPIS of at least 6	Sensitivity of up to 90% for presence of pneumonia	May help to guide discontinuation of antibiotics after 3 days if score starts and remains low

[a]All cultures are less accurate if patient is on antibiotics during testing.
BAL, bronchoalveolar lavage; CPIS, clinical pulmonary infection score.

VAP. The diagnostic methods for VAP are discussed in Table 22.7.

To merge these two seemingly conflicting approaches, a management strategy is required that allows patients suspected of having pneumonia to receive prompt and effective therapy yet avoids excessive treatment with antibiotics. This can be accomplished by using an aggressive approach to the empiric use of broad-spectrum antibiotics when pneumonia is clinically suspected, coupled with an equally aggressive approach to narrowing the spectrum, or even discontinuing antibiotic therapy several days later, once culture data and the clinical response to therapy are known. From the data previously discussed, it is clear that the goal of focusing therapy can be achieved if pneumonia is diagnosed either clinically or bronchoscopically, and thus appropriate management should focus on a reevaluation of therapy once the clinical response is observed and bacteriologic data are available. To implement this approach, antibiotic therapy should be started according to the recommendations listed later (see section "Therapeutic Considerations"), modified by a knowledge of local patterns of antibiotic resistance, and a sputum sample or tracheal aspirate (in intubated patients) should be collected before therapy is started. Once the respiratory culture data become available, therapy can be focused on the organisms identified.

Approach to the Diagnosis and Management of Ventilator-Associated Pneumonia

Bacteriology of Nosocomial Pneumonia

Nosocomial pneumonia has traditionally been viewed as a disease caused by enteric Gram-negative bacteria. However, in recent years, the bacteriology has changed, with a Gram-positive organism, *S. aureus*, the second most common cause of NP in the National Nosocomial Infections Surveillance (NNIS) database (145). In addition, antibiotic resistance is an increasing problem for all patients with pneumonia in the ICU, particularly those who are most severely ill. The time of onset of pneumonia is a particularly important factor related to the bacteriology of infection. Fifty-four percent of patients in whom pneumonia develops within the first 5 days of mechanical ventilation (early-onset VAP) are infected by pneumococci, *H. influenzae*, or methicillin-sensitive *S. aureus*, and only 17% of them have a Gram-negative infection, whereas 66% of those with late-onset infection harbor Gram-negative bacteria (91).

All patients are at risk for infection with a group of bacteria referred to as *core organisms*, which include pneumococci, *H. influenzae*, methicillin-sensitive *S. aureus*, and nonresistant Gram-negatives (*E. coli*, *Klebsiella* species, *Enterobacter* species, *Proteus* species, and *Serratia marcescens*) (2). Although these organisms are a concern for all patients, some populations are also at risk for infection with other organisms (particularly drug-resistant pathogens), depending on the presence of risk factors such as prolonged hospitalization, prior antibiotic therapy, witnessed aspiration, corticosteroid therapy, diabetes, and renal failure. Patients who are at risk only for infection with the core organisms are those who have mild to moderate NP (not ventilated) without risk factors, and those who have severe NP (usually VAP) but no risk factors and pneumonia of early onset (beginning within the first 4 days after hospitalization).

In patients who are not intubated, other organisms should be considered if specific risk factors are present.

Although anaerobes are uncommon in patients with VAP, they should be considered in cases of witnessed aspiration or recent abdominal surgery (146). *S. aureus* is a concern in a patient with coma, head trauma, diabetes, or renal failure; resistant Gram-negatives are more likely in a patient with a prolonged hospital stay, corticosteroid therapy, bronchiectasis, tracheostomy, or prior antibiotics. Resistant Gram-negatives include *P. aeruginosa* and *Acinetobacter* species (2). Methicillin-resistant *S. aureus* is a concern in a patient with late-onset pneumonia, especially after prior antibiotic therapy, who is on corticosteroid therapy, or who has underlying chronic obstructive pulmonary disease (147).

Patients who have late-onset VAP (at day 5 of hospitalization or later) and those in whom pneumonia develops after they receive antibiotic therapy for another reason are particularly at risk for infection with resistant Gram-positive (methicillin-resistant *S. aureus*) and resistant Gram-negative bacteria. In one study, 135 patients were stratified on the basis of whether they had received prior antibiotic therapy and whether they had been mechanically ventilated for more than 7 days (148). A total of 22 patients had not received prior antibiotics and were on the ventilator for less than 7 days before the onset of pneumonia, and none had multiresistant pathogens. On the other hand, 84 patients had the two risk factors of prolonged ventilation and prior antibiotic therapy, and 59% were infected with multiresistant Gram-positive or Gram-negative pathogens. Patients with a single risk factor were at intermediate risk for infection with these organisms.

Another described entity is "very-early-onset" VAP, beginning within 48 hours after intubation. Some patients appear to acquire infection by aspirating during an emergent intubation, and they become infected by whatever organisms are colonizing the oropharynx at the time of intubation (122). In one study, antibiotic use at the time of intubation was protective against this form of infection, suggesting that such therapy can eradicate organisms from the lung if it is being given at the time of aspiration.

Although these general patterns apply to a broad group of patients, it is important to recognize that each hospital has its own unique flora and antibiotic susceptibility patterns. Rello and colleagues (149) reported that the specific resistant Gram-negative pathogens in patients with late-onset VAP can vary from one ICU to another. This information is important to consider because antibiotic resistance is frequently a factor contributing to inadequate empiric antibiotic therapy, particularly with organisms such as *P. aeruginosa*, *Acinetobacter* species, and methicillin-resistant *S. aureus* (150). Multiple factors have contributed to the rising frequency of antibiotic resistance in the ICU, but the most important determinants appear to be prior use of antibiotics, prolonged intubation and mechanical ventilation, and underlying severe illness, all common in patients with VAP (2,148).

Therapeutic Considerations

Antibiotic therapy should be given promptly as soon as pneumonia is suspected clinically, and empiric therapy should be dictated by the severity of illness (mild-moderate vs. severe), the risk factors for specific pathogens, and the timing of the onset of infection (early vs. late). In general, patients who are at risk for infection with only the core organisms should receive monotherapy, whereas those with risk factors for infection with other organisms or with relatively severe illness require combination therapy. The recommendations should be adapted to each hospital's unique bacteriology and susceptibility patterns.

One subject of controversy is whether NP can ever be treated with a monotherapy regimen or always requires combination therapy. The advantages of combination therapy include the following: It provides a broader spectrum of coverage than is possible with a single agent; it helps to prevent the emergence of resistance during therapy, which is common in patients who have received monotherapy; and it provides a synergistic effect against *P. aeruginosa* (which is needed if bacteremia is present) (2,151). In the absence of a highly resistant pathogen, monotherapy with certain selected agents has been effective, even for mechanically ventilated patients with VAP. Effective monotherapy in this population has been achieved with imipenem, meropenem, ciprofloxacin, cefepime, and piperacillin/tazobactam (2,152–154). Therapy against *P. aeruginosa* can be with either a quinolone/β-lactam combination or an aminoglycoside/β-lactam combination. Although the combination of an aminoglycoside and a β-lactam is the traditional method of treating *P. aeruginosa* infection, its efficacy has been limited, and nephrotoxicity is possible when an aminoglycoside is used (155). Even when aminoglycosides are dosed once daily, no evidence has been found of a clearly better outcome or a reduced risk for toxicity (156). Another limitation of aminoglycosides is their poor penetration into respiratory sites of infection, which may explain why the addition of one of these agents to a carbapenem was of no benefit in comparison with a carbapenem alone in one clinical trial (155). In addition, many pneumonic areas of lung have an acid pH, and aminoglycosides are not optimally active under these conditions.

When antimicrobial therapy is administered, the dosage must take into account several factors, including mechanism of action, the MIC for the target organism, and penetration into the site of infection. Some antibiotics are bactericidal in a concentration-dependent fashion (aminoglycosides, linezolid, quinolones), whereas others kill in relation to how long the serum concentration exceeds the MIC for the target organism (β-lactam antibiotics, vancomycin) (157). In theory, antibiotics that kill in a concentration-dependent fashion are best administered once daily. This approach achieves a high peak concentration in the serum, which maximizes efficacy, with a low trough concentration, which may minimize the toxicity of agents such as the aminoglycosides.

However, studies of aminoglycosides have not always shown an improved outcome when this approach was used in place of conventional dosing schemes (156). For antibiotics that kill in a concentration-dependent fashion, the area under the drug concentration–time curve can be calculated for 24 hours and then divided by the MIC for the target organism to provide a parameter referred to as the *area under the inhibitory curve (AUIC)*. In the therapy of pseudomonal pneumonia, the optimal AUIC has been observed to be at least 125 (158). When an antibiotic kills in a time-dependent fashion, it has been estimated that the serum concentration should exceed the MIC for the target organism for at least 40% of the dosing interval (159). With this type of agent, the optimal antibacterial effect, with the minimal total dose of antibiotic, can be achieved by continuous infusion, but this approach did not increase the rate of clinical success in the therapy of NP in trauma patients when ceftazidime was administered in this fashion (160).

The antipseudomonal β-lactams include the penicillins piperacillin, azlocillin, mezlocillin, and ticarcillin; the cephalosporins cefepime and ceftazidime; the carbapenems imipenem and meropenem; the monobactam aztreonam; and the β-lactam/β-lactamase inhibitor combinations of piperacillin/tazobactam and ticarcillin/clavulanate. The antipseudomonal aminoglycosides include gentamicin, tobramycin, and amikacin. The other class of antipseudomonal agents is the quinolones, and ciprofloxacin at high doses (typically 400 mg intravenously every 8 hours) is the only active agent in this class. A combination of ciprofloxacin and an antipseudomonal penicillin has been effective in a patient population at risk for infection with *P. aeruginosa* (161).

Patients with severe VAP can also be at risk for infection with methicillin-resistant *S. aureus*, so that some require empiric therapy directed at this organism. Patients most at risk are those with a history of prolonged mechanical ventilation, prior antibiotic therapy, or Gram-positive organisms on tracheal aspiration with Gram stain. Empiric therapy for methicillin-resistant *S. aureus* can be with vancomycin or one of its alternatives, linezolid or quinupristin/dalfopristin. Both alternative agents are equivalent to vancomycin in efficacy, but linezolid is available in an oral form that can achieve the same serum levels as intravenous therapy, and vancomycin is occasionally associated with renal insufficiency (162,163).

Current recommendations suggest that specific at-risk patients should be started on combination therapy with multiple agents for VAP. However, not all such patients will need to complete a full course of therapy with these drugs, and monotherapy can be used in some cases once bacteriologic data become available and it is clear that a patient has had a good clinical response to therapy. A single agent can be effective for patients with NP that is not caused by resistant Gram-positive or Gram-negative organisms. As previously mentioned, only a few agents have been shown to be effective monotherapy for severe VAP, but if one of these agents is included in the initial combination therapy regimen, step-down to monotherapy can be done once appropriate culture data are available. Very few studies have defined the natural history of the resolution of NP or the appropriate duration of therapy (164). In most patients, the clinical findings of pneumonia resolve by day 6, and in one study, a selected group of patients was successfully treated with short-term therapy (as little as 3 days) (144). Although the optimal duration of therapy is unknown, this parameter should probably be individualized, with efforts made to use less than the traditional 10, 14, or 21 days of medication, especially in patients who have had a good clinical and microbiologic response to antibiotics. The safety of combining taper of antibiotics with a shorter course of therapy has been shown in an observational study (104). In that study, patients with VAP were initially treated with a combination of imipenem, ciprofloxacin, and vancomycin, but therapy was readjusted based on culture data after 24 to 48 hours and was stopped after 7 days unless a longer course of therapy was clinically indicated. When this approach was used, in comparison with a period of standard therapy, mortality was similar, but the duration of therapy was shorter, initial therapy was more likely to be adequate, and second episodes of pneumonia were fewer.

The role of aerosolized antibiotics in the therapy of VAP is uncertain, but this form of therapy should be considered for patients who have severe pneumonia, especially with potentially resistant enteric Gram-negatives, and are not responding to systemic antibiotics. Although aerosolized aminoglycosides have been used as sole therapy for infectious tracheobronchitis in intubated patients, they may also have a role as an adjunct to systemic antibiotics in certain patients with VAP (165). The administration of aerosolized antibiotics offers the advantage of achieving high concentrations of antibiotics at the site of infection, thereby overcoming the problem of poor lung penetration of certain agents (aminoglycosides and β-lactams) and providing the high levels of antibiotics needed to kill certain resistant organisms. Locally administered antibiotics are rarely absorbed, and systemic toxicity is minimized. One prospective randomized controlled trial showed no advantage of adding aerosolized tobramycin to systemic antibiotics (166). In that study, 40 mg of tobramycin was injected into the endotracheal tube every 8 hours; the frequency of elimination of bacterial pathogens was higher, but no difference in overall clinical response and no appreciable change in the incidence of antibiotic resistance were noted. However, when this type of therapy was used to prevent VAP, antibiotic resistance was a common complication (167). Smaller series include anecdotal reports of the benefit of adding inhaled aminoglycosides or colistin to systemic antibiotics in patients who are infected with resistant organisms, such as *P. aeruginosa*, and are not responding to conventional therapy (165). Finally, it remains unclear how best to deliver topical antibiotics; some investigators directly inject the medication down the endotracheal tube, whereas others use aerosol delivery devices (168).

Other adjunctive measures that can be used for pneumonia therapy include chest physiotherapy, aerosolized bronchodilators, and mucolytic agents, but the benefits of these therapies are limited, and they must be individualized for each patient.

THERAPEUTIC CONSIDERATIONS IN VENTILATOR-ASSOCIATED PNEUMONIA

Patient Type: Therapy Recommended	Evidence
Mild to moderate pneumonia, no risk factors, onset any time or severe pneumonia, no risk factors, early onset: Monotherapy with any of a group of "core antibiotics": 1. Second-, third-, or fourth-generation cephalosporin (cefuroxime, cefotaxime, ceftriaxone, cefepime) 2. β-Lactam/β-lactamase inhibitor combination (ampicillin/sulbactam, piperacillin/tazobactam) 3. Fluoroquinolone (ciprofloxacin, levofloxacin, gatifloxacin, moxifloxacin) 4. If penicillin-allergic, clindamycin and aztreonam	Observational studies (most studies in this area limited by problems with definition of pneumonia and identification of certain causative organisms)
Mild to moderate pneumonia, with risk factors, onset any time: Use a "core antibiotic" modified for risk factors: *Witnessed aspiration:* Add clindamycin or use β-lactam/β-lactamase inhibitor combination alone. *Coma, head trauma, diabetes, or renal failure:* Use core antibiotic that is active against *S. aureus.* *Corticosteroid therapy:* Add a macrolide if nosocomial *Legionella* infection has occurred. *Prolonged ICU stay, prior antibiotics, corticosteroids, bronchiectasis:* Treat as severe VAP.	Observational studies
Severe VAP with risk factors, any time of onset or severe VAP, late onset, regardless of risk factors: Start with dual anti-*Pseudomonas* therapy and add coverage for MRSA if prior antibiotics or if tracheal aspirate with Gram-positive organisms Ciprofloxacin or aminoglycoside (gentamicin, tobramycin, amikacin) *Plus one of the following:* cefepime, imipenem, meropenem, piperacillin, ticarcillin, ticarcillin/clavulanate, piperacillin/tazobactam, aztreonam *plus* (if suspect MRSA) vancomycin or linezolid or quinupristin/dalfopristin	Observational studies

ICU, intensive care unit; MRSA, methicillin-resistant *S. aureus*; VAP, ventilator-associated pneumonia.

Prevention of Ventilator-Associated Pneumonia

Although no single method reliably prevents pneumonia, multiple small interventions may have benefit. These include avoidance of large inocula of bacteria into the lung (careful handling of ventilator tubing, hand washing), mobilization of respiratory secretions (frequent suctioning, use of rotational bed therapy in selected cases), nutritional support (with enteral feeding preferred to total parenteral nutrition), placement of feeding tubes into the small bowel (to avoid aspiration, which is more likely with stomach tubes), keeping bedridden patients in a semi-erect position (to avoid the risk for aspiration associated with the supine position), and avoidance of large gastric residuals when enteral feeding is given (2,169). In addition, any tube inserted into the stomach or trachea should be placed through the mouth, not the nose, whenever possible to avoid obstructing the nasal sinuses and prevent nosocomial sinusitis, which can cause NP (170). Prophylactic systemic or topical antibiotics have no specific role, but some data suggest that patients with coma secondary to stroke or head trauma and those who may have aspirated during an emergent intubation may benefit from a 24-hour course of systemic antibiotics (171). A regimen of "selective digestive decontamination," which includes systemic and topical intestinal antibiotics, has not proved to reduce the incidence of pneumonia except in highly selected populations, and this approach carries the risk for promoting antibiotic resistance (2,172). In the past, there was controversy about the effects on the incidence of VAP of specific types of agents used as prophylaxis against intestinal bleeding. This issue may be less important than previously thought, especially if efforts are made to minimize the risk for aspiration by paying close attention to patient positioning and the site of placement of enteral feeding (114).

Another issue in prevention is the minimization of antibiotic resistance, which can be achieved by controlling the patterns of antibiotic use. Although resistance to virtually all antimicrobial agents has been identified, data show that patterns of antibiotic use may be related to patterns of resistance, particularly with agents such as vancomycin, the cephalosporins, and the fluoroquinolones. For example, the emergence of Gram-negative bacterial resistance to cephalosporins has been correlated with cephalosporin use, and some studies have shown that resistance can be controlled by restricting the use of these agents. In one survey of antibiotic use and resistance patterns in 10 hospitals, investigators observed a correlation between the use of ceftazidime and the presence of ceftazidime-resistant *P. aeruginosa* and *Enterobacter* species (173). Of the 10 hospitals, the one where the use of ceftazidime was greatest also had the highest rates of resistance, but an inverse correlation was found between the presence of ceftazidime-resistant *Enterobacter* species and the implementation of a policy to control antibiotic use. In another study, a hospital experiencing an outbreak of ceftazidime-resistant *K. pneumoniae* infection was able to reduce the frequency of resistance by restricting the use of ceftazidime, replacing it with imipenem. Although this strategy led to a 44% reduction in the frequency of resistant *Klebsiella* organisms, the frequency of imipenem-resistant *P. aeruginosa* increased (174). These data suggest that controlling the resistance of one pathogen to one antibiotic can result in a new pattern of resistance, which has been referred to as "squeezing the balloon." Although it is uncertain whether antibiotic restriction can be of long-term

benefit in controlling resistance, it is still important to minimize the inappropriate use of antibiotics.

Another factor that promotes resistance is the monotonous use of the same agents for the same indication in all patients. To combat this problem, some investigators have implemented a strategy of "antibiotic rotation" to limit resistance. In this approach, a switch from one antibiotic to another is planned and scheduled for a specific clinical circumstance for a predetermined period, then another regimen is instituted for the same indication for yet another predefined period. The frequency of cycling has varied from monthly to as long as 1 to 2 years (175–177). The design of such regimens is still experimental, with uncertainty not only about how long each cycle should last but also about whether cycling regimens should account separately for Gram-positives and Gram-negatives, which patients should be targeted, which agents should be used, and whether previous regimens should be used again after a specific period. When cycling regimens are used, concurrent bacterial surveillance is required to assess variations in the nosocomial flora and resistance patterns that result from the intervention.

Early studies of this approach were carried out with aminoglycosides, with changes in resistance resulting from the control of specific agents (177). More recently, studies have involved surgical and medical ICU patients, with some benefit. Kollef and colleagues (175) studied a switch from ceftazidime to ciprofloxacin in a cardiac surgical ICU, with each regimen used as empiric therapy for infection, including VAP, for a 6-month period. The rotation from a cephalosporin to a quinolone led to a reduction in the incidence of pneumonia caused by resistant Gram-negative bacteria. The efficacy of a rotation and antibiotic control policy in medical patients has also been documented, but this approach involved changing the empiric antibiotic regimen on a monthly basis (176). More recently, a 2-year study (1 year as baseline, 1 year of intervention) was conducted in surgical patients in which a change of antibiotic therapies for pneumonia and peritonitis was scheduled every 3 months (178). Antibiotic rotation resulted in a significant decrease in crude mortality following infection in comparison with the baseline period (15.5% vs. 38.1%, $P < .0001$), along with a lower frequency of infection with resistant Gram-positive and Gram-negative organisms. All these data suggest a possible role for antibiotic rotation to limit resistance in the ICU, but the procedure remains investigational and requires careful microbiologic surveillance if used.

PREVENTION OF VENTILATOR-ASSOCIATED PNEUMONIA

Strategy/Recommendation	Evidence
Careful handling of ventilator circuits. Wash condensate from patient.	Observational studies
Do not regularly change ventilator circuit.	Randomized studies
Hand washing to control infection and spread of resistant pathogens.	Observational studies
Mobilize secretions to prevent VAP with devices other than suctioning (e.g., lateral rotational bed therapy).	Nonrandomized studies
Use enteral feeding when possible for nutritional support, with attention to patient positioning and tube placement into small bowel, not stomach.	Nonrandomized trials and observational studies
Keep patient in semi-erect position in bed when possible.	Randomized controlled trials and observational studies
Provide continuous aspiration of subglottic secretions.	Randomized controlled trials
Place all tubes through mouth rather than nose to prevent nosocomial sinusitis, which can lead to VAP.	Randomized controlled trials and expert opinion
Do not give prophylactic antibiotics to prevent very early onset of VAP (may be a benefit of 24 hours of therapy after emergent intubation).	Observational studies and single randomized study
Closed suction catheter system may be useful to prevent VAP.	Single randomized study
Do not use selective digestive decontamination (may be useful in some selected populations, which are still poorly defined).	Randomized studies and expert opinion
Maintain adequate endotracheal tube cuff pressure.	Observational studies
Avoid intubation.	Randomized studies (vs. noninvasive ventilation)
Choice of gastrointestinal bleeding prophylaxis probably not a factor in VAP.	Randomized studies (some conflicting data)
Maintain infection control and surveillance program.	Observational studies
Do not use inhaled antibiotics to prevent VAP (use led to antibiotic resistance in organisms).	Randomized studies

VAP, ventilator-associated pneumonia.

EDITOR'S NOTE: SEVERE ACUTE RESPIRATORY SYNDROME

As this book goes to press, an apparently new entity—severe acute respiratory syndrome (SARS)—is being defined. In March 2003, we began to see reports from Asia and elsewhere of a nonspecific initial phase flu-like illness that seemed to progress rapidly to ventilatory failure in a high proportion of patients. Leukopenia/thrombocytopenia and liver enzyme and CPK elevation have been noted. SARS was also associated with a high rate of secondary spread often to healthcare workers (*MMWR* 2003;52:555–556). Definitions have been developed for suspected cases (*MMWR* 2003;52:241–248). These include: fever >39°C; findings of respiratory illness; travel within 10 days of symptom onset to an area with SARS or contact with a person who has respiratory symptoms and has traveled to a SARS area or is suspected of having SARS. The incubation period for SARS is 2 to 7 days. Transmission is likely via droplet-nuclei, though fomites and other mechanisms have not been excluded. A novel coronavirus has been identified as the likely etiologic agent. Treatment with available antiviral agents is not clearly effective. Management involves supportive care. Standard hygiene precautions and isolation of SARS suspects should be used. Until transmission is clarified, airborne (e.g., 14–95 respirator), gown, gloves, and eye protection should be used also.

Jeffrey Glassroth

REFERENCES

1. Niederman MS, Mandell LA, Anzueto A, et al. Guidelines for the management of adults with community-acquired lower respiratory tract infections: Diagnosis, assessment of severity, antimicrobial therapy and prevention. *Am J Respir Crit Care Med* 2001;163:1730–1754.
2. Campbell GD, Niederman MS, Broughton WA, et al. Hospital-acquired pneumonia in adults: diagnosis, assessment of severity, initial antimicrobial therapy, and preventative strategies: a consensus statement. *Am J Respir Crit Care Med* 1996;153:1711–1725.
3. Niederman MS, Ahmed QA. Inflammation in severe pneumonia: act locally, not globally. *Crit Care Med* 1999;27:2030–2032.
4. Welsh DA, Mason CM. Host defenses in respiratory infections. *Med Clin North Am* 2001;85:1329–1347.
5. Niederman MS. Pathogenesis of airway colonization: lessons learned from studies of bacterial adherence. *Eur Respir J* 1994;7:1737–1740.
6. Fleming CA, Balaguera HU, Craven DE. Risk factors for nosocomial pneumonia: focus on prophylaxis. *Med Clin North Am* 2001;85:1545–1563.
7. Feldman C, Kassel M, Cantrell J, et al. The presence and sequence of endotracheal tube colonization in patients undergoing mechanical ventilation. *Eur Respir J* 1996;3:546–551.
8. Dehoux MS, Boutten A, Ostinelli J, et al. Compartmentalized cytokine production within the human lung in unilateral pneumonia. *Am J Respir Crit Care Med* 1994;150:710–716.
9. Boutten A, Dehoux MS, Seta N, et al. Compartmentalized IL-8 and elastase release within the human lung in unilateral pneumonia. *Am J Respir Crit Care Med* 1996;153:336–342.
10. Monton C, Torres A, El-Ebiary M, et al. Cytokine expression in severe pneumonia: a bronchoalveolar lavage study. *Crit Care Med* 1999;27:1745–1753.
11. Niederman MS, McCombs JI, Unger AN, et al. The cost of treating community-acquired pneumonia. *Clin Ther* 1998;20:820–837.
12. Metlay JP, Schulz R, Li Y-H, et al. Influence of age on symptoms at presentation in patients with community-acquired pneumonia. *Arch Intern Med* 1997;157:1453–1459.
13. Marrie TJ, Blanchard W. A comparison of nursing home–acquired pneumonia patients with patients with community-acquired pneumonia and nursing home patients without pneumonia. *J Am Geriatr Soc* 1997;45:50–55.
14. Starczewski AR, Allen SC, Vargas E, et al. Clinical prognostic indices of fatality in elderly patients admitted to hospital with acute pneumonia. *Age Aging* 1988;17:181–186.
15. Fine MJ, Orloff JJ, Arisumi D, et al. Prognosis of patients hospitalized with community-acquired pneumonia. *Am J Med* 1990;88:1N–8N.
16. Riquelme R, Torres A, El-Ebiary, et al. Community-acquired pneumonia in the elderly: clinical and nutritional aspects. *Am J Crit Care Med* 1997;156:1908–1914.
17. McFadden JR, Price RC, Eastwood HD, et al. Raised respiratory rate in elderly patients: a valuable physical sign. *Br Med J* 1982;284:626–627.
18. Syrjala H, Broas M, Suramo I, et al. High-resolution computed tomography for the diagnosis of community-acquired pneumonia. *Clin Infect Dis* 1998;27:358–363.
19. Katz DS, Leung AN. Radiology of pneumonia. *Clin Chest Med* 1999;20:549–562.
20. Hasley PB, Albaum MN, Li YH, et al. Do pulmonary radiographic findings at presentation predict mortality in patients with community-acquired pneumonia? *Arch Intern Med* 1996;156:2206–2212.
21. Sahn SA. Management of complicated parapneumonic effusions. *Am Rev Respir Dis* 1993;148:813–817.
22. Woodhead MA, MacFarlane JT. Comparative clinical laboratory features of *Legionella* with pneumococcal and *Mycoplasma* pneumonias. *Br J Dis Chest* 1987;81:133–139.
23. Farr BM, Kaiser DL, Harrison BW, et al. Prediction of microbial aetiology at admission to hospital for pneumonia from presenting clinical features. *Thorax* 1989;44:1031–1035.
24. Fang GD, Fine M, Orloff J, et al. New and emerging etiologies for community-acquired pneumonia with implication for therapy: a prospective multicenter study of 359 cases. *Medicine (Baltimore)* 1990;69:307–316.
25. Macfarlane JT, Miller AC, Roderick Smith WH, et al. Comparative radiographic features of community acquired Legionnaires' disease, pneumococcal pneumonia, *Mycoplasma* pneumonia, and psittacosis. *Thorax* 1984;39:28–33.
26. Ruiz-Gonzalez A, Falguera M, Nogues A, et al. Is *Streptococcus pneumoniae* the leading cause of pneumonia of unknown etiology? A microbiologic study of lung aspirates in consecutive patients with community-acquired pneumonia. *Am J Med* 1999;106:385–390.
27. Johnson CC, Finegold SM. Pyogenic bacterial pneumonia, lung abscess, and empyema. In: Murray JF, Nadel JA, eds. *Textbook of respiratory medicine*, 2nd ed. Philadelphia: WB Saunders, 1994:1036–1093.
28. Ort S, Ryan JL, Barden G, et al. Pneumococcal pneumonia in hospitalized patients: clinical and radiological presentations. *JAMA* 1983;249:214–218.
29. Mandell LA, Marrie TJ, Grossman RF, et al. , and the Canadian CAP Working Group. Canadian guidelines for the initial management of community-acquired pneumonia: an evidence-based update by the Canadian Infectious Diseases Society and the Canadian Thoracic Society. *Clin Infect Dis* 2000;31:383–421.
30. Plouffe JF, Breiman RF, Facklam RR. Bacteremia with *Streptococcus pneumoniae*. Implications for herapy and prevention.

Franklin County Pneumonia Study Group. *JAMA* 1996;275: 194–198.

31. Feikin DR, Schuchat A, Kolczak M, et al. Mortality from invasive pneumococcal pneumonia in the era of antibiotic resistance, 1995–1997. *Am J Public Health* 2000;90:223–229.

32. Pallares R, Linares J, Vadillo M, et al. Resistance to penicillin and cephalosporin and mortality from severe pneumococcal pneumonia in Barcelona, Spain. *N Engl J Med* 1995;333:474–480.

33. Turett GS, Blum S, Fazal BA, et al. Penicillin resistance and other predictors of mortality in pneumococcal bacteremia in a population with high human immunodeficiency virus seroprevalence. *Clin Infect Dis* 1999;29:321–327.

34. Metlay JP, Hoffman J, Cetron MS, et al. Impact of penicillin susceptibility on medical outcomes for adult patients with bacteremic pneumococcal pneumonia. *Clin Infect Dis* 2000;30:520–528.

35. Moroney JF, Fiore AE, Harrison LH, et al. Clinical outcomes of bacteremic pneumococcal pneumonia in the era of antibiotic resistance. *Clin Infect Dis* 2001;33:797–805.

36. Clavo-Sánchez AJ, Girón-González JA, López-Prieto D, et al. Multivariate analysis of risk factors for infection due to penicillin-resistant and multidrug-resistant *Streptococcus pneumoniae*: a multicenter study. *Clin Infect Dis* 1997;24:1052–1059.

37. Marston BJ, Plouffe JF, File TM Jr, et al. Incidence of community-acquired pneumonia requiring hospitalization. Results of a population-based active surveillance study in Ohio. The Community-Based Pneumonia Incidence Study Group. *Arch Intern Med* 1997;157:1709–1718.

38. Troy CJ, Peeling RW, Ellis AG, et al. *Chlamydia pneumoniae* as a new source of infectious outbreaks in nursing homes. *JAMA* 1997;277:1214–1218.

39. Kauppinen MT, Saikku P, Kujala P, et al. Clinical picture of *Chlamydia pneumoniae* requiring hospital treatment: a comparison between chlamydial and pneumococcal pneumonia. *Thorax* 1996;51:185–189.

40. Lieberman D, Schlaeffer F, Boldur I, et al. Multiple pathogens in adult patients admitted with community-acquired pneumonia: a one-year prospective study of 346 consecutive patients. *Thorax* 1996;51:179–184.

41. Gleason PP, Meehan TP, Fine JM, et al. Associations between initial antimicrobial therapy and medical outcomes for hospitalized elderly patients with pneumonia. *Arch Intern Med* 1999;159:2562–2572.

42. Houck PM, MacLehose RF, Niederman MS, et al. Empiric antibiotic therapy and mortality among Medicare pneumonia inpatients in 10 Western states: 1993,1995,1997. *Chest* 2001;119:1420–1426.

43. Plouffe JF, File TM Jr, Breiman RF, et al. Reevaluation of the definition of Legionnaires' disease: use of the urinary antigen assay. Community-Based Pneumonia Incidence Study Group. *Clin Infect Dis* 1995;20:1286–1291.

44. Ruiz M, Ewig S, Torres A, et al. Severe community-acquired pneumonia: risk factors and follow-up epidemiology. *Am J Respir Crit Care Med* 1999;160:923–929.

45. Stout JE, Yu VL. Legionellosis. *N Engl J Med* 1997;337:682–687.

46. El Solh AA, Sikka P, Ramadan F, et al. Etiology of severe pneumonia in the very elderly. *Am J Respir Crit Care Med* 2001;163:645–651.

47. Bartlett JG, Dowell SF, Mandell LA, et al. Practice guidelines for the management of community-acquired pneumonia in adults. *Clin Infect Dis* 2000;31:347–382.

48. Nava JM, Bella F, Garau J, et al. Predictive factors for invasive disease due to penicillin-resistant *Streptococcus pneumoniae*: a population-based study. *Clin Infect Dis* 1994;19:884–890.

49. Fine MJ, Auble TE, Yealy DM, et al. A prediction rule to identify low-risk patients with community-acquired pneumonia. *N Engl J Med* 1997;336:243–250.

50. Farr BM, Sloman AJ, Fisch MJ. Predicting death in patients hospitalized for community-acquired pneumonia. *Ann Intern Med* 1991;115:428–436.

51. Atlas SJ, Benzer TI, Borowsky LH, et al. Safely increasing the proportion of patients with community-acquired pneumonia treated as outpatients: an interventional trial. *Arch Intern Med* 1998;158:1350–1356.

52. Marrie TJ, Lau CY, Wheeler SL, et al. A controlled trial of a critical pathway for treatment of community-acquired pneumonia. *JAMA* 2000;283:749–755.

53. Lim WS, Lewis S, Macfarlane JT. Severity prediction rules in community-acquired pneumonia: a validation study. *Thorax* 2000;55:219–223.

54. Lim WS, Macfarlane JT. Defining prognostic factors in the elderly with community-acquired pneumonia: a case controlled study of patients aged ≥75 years. *Eur Respir J* 2001;17:200–205.

55. Fine MJ, Smith MA, Carson CA, et al. Prognosis and outcomes of patients with community- acquired pneumonia: a meta-analysis. *JAMA* 1996;275:134–141.

56. Hook EW, Horton CA, Schaberg DR. Failure of intensive care unit support to influence mortality from pneumococcal bacteremia. *JAMA* 1983;249:1055–1060.

57. Niederman MS, Bass JB, Campbell GD, et al. Guidelines for the initial management of adults with community-acquired pneumonia: diagnosis, assessment of severity, and initial antimicrobial therapy. *Am Rev Respir Dis* 1993;148:1418–1426.

58. Ewig S, Ruiz M, Mensa J, et al. Severe community-acquired pneumonia: assessment of severity criteria. *Am J Respir Crit Care Med* 1998;158:1102–1108.

59. Meehan TP, Fine MJ, Krumholz HM, et al. Quality of care, process, and outcomes in elderly patients with pneumonia. *JAMA* 1997;278:2080–2084.

60. Sanyal S, Smith PR, Saha AC, et al. Initial microbiologic studies did not affect outcome in adults hospitalized with community-acquired pneumonia. *Am J Respir Crit Care Med* 1999;160:346–348.

61. Rein MF, Gwaltney JM Jr, O'Brien WM, et al. Accuracy of Gram's stain in identifying pneumococci in sputum. *JAMA* 1978;239:2671–2673.

62. Ewig S, Schlochtermier M, Goke N, et al. Applying sputum as a diagnostic tool in pneumonia: limited yield, minimal impact on treatment decisions. *Chest* 2002;121:1486–1492.

63. Niederman MS. Guidelines for the management of community-acquired pneumonia. Current recommendations and antibiotic selection issues. *Med Clin North Am* 2001;85:1493–1509.

64. Kelley MA, Weber DJ, Gilligan P, et al. Breakthrough pneumococcal bacteremia in patients being treated with azithromycin and clarithromycin. *Clin Infect Dis* 2000;31:1008–1011.

65. Plouffe J, Schwartz DB, Kolokathis A, et al. Clinical efficacy of intravenous followed by oral azithromycin monotherapy in hospitalized patients with community-acquired pneumonia. *Antimicrob Agents Chemother* 2000;44:1796–1802.

66. Niederman MS. Treatment of respiratory infections with quinolones. In: Andriole V, ed. *The quinolones*, 2nd ed. New York: McGraw-Hill, 1998:229–250.

67. Chen DK, McGeer A, De Azavedo JC, et al. Decreased susceptibility of *Streptococcus pneumoniae* to fluoroquinolones in Canada. *N Engl J Med* 1999;341:233–239.

68. Davidson R, Cavalcanti R, Brunton JL, et al. Resistance to levofloxacin and failure of treatment of pneumococcal pneumonia. *N Engl J Med* 2002;346:747–750.

69. Ho PL, Tse WS, Tsang KW, et al. Risk factors for acquisition of levofloxacin-resistant *Streptococcus pneumoniae*: a case-control study. *Clin Infect Dis* 2001;32:701–707.

70. Leroy O, Santre C, Beuscart C. A 5-year study of severe community-acquired pneumonia with emphasis on prognosis in patients admitted to an ICU. *Intensive Care Med* 1995;21:24–31.

71. Marrie TJ, Peeling RW, Fine MJ, et al. Ambulatory patients with community-acquired pneumonia: the frequency of atypical agents and clinical course. *Am J Med* 1996;101:508–515.

72. Waterer GW, Somes GW, Wunderink RG. Monotherapy may be suboptimal for severe bacteremic pneumococcal pneumonia. *Arch Intern Med* 2001;161:1837–1842.

73. Ramirez JA, Vargas S, Ritter GW, et al. Early switch from intravenous to oral antibiotics and early hospital discharge: a prospective observational study of 200 consecutive patients with community-acquired pneumonia. *Arch Intern Med* 1999;159:2449–2454.

74. Rhew DC, Hackner D, Henderson L, et al. The clinical benefit of in-hospital observation in "low risk" pneumonia patients after conversion from parenteral to oral antimicrobial therapy. *Chest* 1998;113:142–146.

75. Mittl RL, Schwab RJ, Duchin JS, et al. Radiographic resolution of community-acquired pneumonia. *Am J Respir Crit Care Med* 1994;149:630–635.

76. Jay S, Johanson W, Pierce A. The radiologic resolution of streptococcal pneumoniae pneumonia. *N Engl J Med* 1975;293:798–801.

77. Breiman, RF, Butler JC, McInnes PM. Vaccines to prevent respiratory infection: opportunities on the near and far horizon. *Curr Opin Infect Dis* 1999;12:145–152.

78. Shapiro ED, Berg AT, Austrian R, et al. The protective efficacy of polyvalent pneumococcal polysaccharide vaccine. *N Engl J Med* 1991;325:1453–1460.

79. Butler JC, Breiman RF, Campbell JF, et al. Pneumococcal polysaccharide vaccine efficacy: an evaluation of current recommendations. *JAMA* 1993;270:1826–1831.

80. American Academy of Pediatrics. Policy statement and technical report: recommendations for the prevention of pneumococcal infections, including the use of pneumococcal conjugate vaccine (Prenevar), pneumococcal polysaccharide vaccine, and antibiotic prophylaxis. *Pediatrics* 2000;106:362–376.

81. Fedson DS, Harward MP, Reid RA, et al. Hospital-based pneumococcal immunization: epidemiologic rationale from the Shenandoah study. *JAMA* 1990;264:1117–1122.

82. Gross PA, Hermogenes AW, Sacks HS, et al. The efficacy of influenza vaccine in elderly persons: a meta-analysis and review of the literature. *Ann Intern Med* 1995;123:518–527.

83. Nichol KL, Margolis KL, Wuorenma J, et al. The efficacy and cost effectiveness of vaccination against influenza among elderly persons living in the community. *N Engl J Med* 1994;331:778–784.

84. Deleted in proof.

85. Darling RG, Catlett CL, Huebner KD, et al. Threats in bioterrorism I: CDC category A agents. *Emerg Med Clin North Am* 2002;20:273–309.

86. Moran GJ. Threats in bioterrorism II: CDC category B and C agents. *Emerg Med Clin North Am* 2002;20:311–330.

87. Bartlett JG, Inglesby TV, Borio L. Management of anthrax. *Clin Infect Dis* 2002;35:851–858.

88. Inglesby TV, O'Toole T, Henderson DA, et al. Anthrax as a biological weapon, 2002: updated recommendations for management. *JAMA* 2002;287:2236–2252.

89. Dennis DT, Inglesby TV, Henderson DA, et al. Tularemia as a biological weapon: medical and public health management. *JAMA* 2001;285:2763–2773.

90. Cook DJ, Walter SD, Cook RJ, et al. Incidence of and risk fac-

tors for ventilator-associated pneumonia in critically ill patients: results from a multicenter prospective study on 996 patients. *Ann Intern Med* 1998;129:433–440.

91. Prod'hom G, Leuenberger P, Koefer J, et al. Nosocomial pneumonia in mechanically ventilated patients receiving antacid, ranitidine, or sucralfate as prophylaxis for stress ulcer: a randomized controlled trial. *Ann Intern Med* 1994;120:653–662.

92. Nava S, Ambrosino N, Clini E, et al. Noninvasive mechanical ventilation in the weaning of patients with respiratory failure due to chronic obstructive pulmonary disease. A randomized controlled trial. *Ann Intern Med* 1998;128:721–728.

93. Kollef M, Ahrens T, Shannon W. Clinical predictors and outcomes for patients requiring tracheostomy in the intensive care unit. *Crit Care Med* 1999;27:1714–1720.

94. Brewer SC, Wunderink RG, Jones CB, et al. Ventilator-associated pneumonia due to *Pseudomonas aeruginosa*. *Chest* 1995;108:1655–1662.

95. Fagon JY, Chastre J, Hance A, et al. Nosocomial pneumonia in ventilated patients: a cohort study evaluation of attributable mortality and hospital stay. *Am J Med* 1993;94:281–288.

96. Fagon JY, Chastre J, Vuagnat A, et al. Nosocomial pneumonia and mortality among patients in intensive care units. *JAMA* 1996;275:866–869.

97. Heyland DK, Cook DJ, Marshall J, et al. The attributable morbidity and mortality of ventilator-associated pneumonia in the critically ill patient. *Am J Respir Crit Care Med* 1999;159:1249–1256.

98. Kollef MH, Silver P, Murphy DM, et al. The effect of late-onset ventilator-associated pneumonia in determining patient mortality. *Chest* 1995;108:1655–1662.

99. Papazian L, Bregeon F, Thirion X, et al. Effect of ventilator-associated pneumonia on mortality and morbidity. *Am J Respir Crit Care Med* 1996;154:91–97.

100. Rello J, Jubert P, Valles J, et al. Evaluation of outcome in intubated patients with pneumonia due to *Pseudomonas aeruginosa*. *Clin Infect Dis* 1996;23:973–978.

101. Georges H, Leroy O, Guery B, et al. Predisposing factors for nosocomial pneumonia in patients receiving mechanical ventilation and requiring tracheotomy. *Chest* 2000;118:767–774.

102. Luna CM, Vujacich P, Niederman MS, et al. Impact of BAL data on the therapy and outcome of ventilator-associated pneumonia. *Chest* 1997;111:676–685.

103. Kollef MH, Sherman G, Ward S, et al. Inadequate antimicrobial treatment of infections: a risk factor for hospital mortality among critically ill patients. *Chest* 1999;115:462–474.

104. Ibrahim EH, Ward S, Sherman G, et al. Experience with a clinical guideline for the treatment of ventilator-associated pneumonia. *Crit Care Med* 2001;29:1109–1115.

105. Johanson WG, Pierce AK, Sanford JP. Changing pharyngeal bacterial flora of hospitalized patients. *N Engl J Med* 1969;281:1137–1140.

106. Johanson WG, Pierce AK, Sanford JP, et al. Nosocomial respiratory infections with Gram-negative bacilli. *Ann Intern Med* 1972;77:701–706.

107. Ewig S, Torres A, El-Ebiary M, et al. Bacterial colonization patterns in mechanically ventilated patients with traumatic and medical head injury: incidence, risk factors, and association with ventilator-associated pneumonia. *Am J Respir Crit Care Med* 1999;159:188–198.

108. Sirvent JM, Torres A, Vidaur L, et al. Tracheal colonization within 24 hours of intubation in patients with head trauma: risk factor for developing early-onset ventilator-associated pneumonia. *Intensive Care Med* 2000;26:1369–1372.

109. Delclaux C, Roupie E, Blot F, et al. Lower respiratory tract colonization and infection during severe acute respiratory distress syndrome. *Am J Respir Crit Care Med* 1997;156:1092–1098.

110. Niederman MS, Merrill WW, Ferranti RD, et al. Nutritional

status and bacterial binding in the lower respiratory tract in patients with chronic tracheostomy. *Ann Intern Med* 1984;100: 795–800.

111. Grant MM, Niederman MS, Poehlman MA, et al. Characterization of *Pseudomonas* binding to cultured hamster tracheal cells. *Am J Respir Cell Mol Biol* 1991;5:563–570.

112. Plotkowski MC, Costa AO, Morandi V, et al. Role of heparan sulphate proteoglycans as potential receptors for non-piliated *Pseudomonas aeruginosa* adherence to non-polarised airway epithelial cells. *J Med Microbiol* 2001;50:183–190.

113. Lee A, Chow D, Haus B, et al. Airway epithelial tight junctions and binding and cytotoxicity of *Pseudomonas aeruginosa*. *Am J Physiol* 1999;277:L204–L217.

114. Niederman MS, Craven DE. Devising strategies for preventing nosocomial pneumonia: should we ignore the stomach? *Clin Infect Dis* 1997;24:320–323.

115. Niederman MS, Mantovani R, Schoch P, et al. Patterns and routes of tracheobronchial colonization in mechanically ventilated patients: the role of nutritional status in colonization of the lower airway by *Pseudomonas* species. *Chest* 1989;95:155–161.

116. Vallés J, Artigas A, Rello J, et al. Continuous aspiration of subglottic secretions in preventing ventilator-associated pneumonia. *Ann Intern Med* 1995;122:179–186.

117. Cardenosa Cendrero JA, Sole-Violan J, Bordes Benitez A, et al. Role of different routes of tracheal colonization in the development of pneumonia in patients receiving mechanical ventilation. *Chest* 1999;116:462–470.

118. Berthelot P, Grattard F, Mahul P, et al. Prospective study of nosocomial colonization and infection due to *Pseudomonas aeruginosa* in mechanically ventilated patients. *Intensive Care Med* 2001;27:503–512.

119. Bertrand X, Thouverez M, Talon D, et al. Endemicity, molecular diversity and colonisation routes of *Pseudomonas aeruginosa* in intensive care units. *Intensive Care Med* 2001;27:1263–1268.

120. Rello J, Mariscal D, March F, et al. Recurrent *Pseudomonas aeruginosa* pneumonia in ventilated patients: relapse or reinfection? *Am J Respir Crit Care Med* 1998;157:912–916.

121. George D, Falk P, Wunderink R, et al. Epidemiology of ventilator-acquired pneumonia based on protected bronchoscopic sampling. *Am J Respir Crit Care Med* 1998;158:1839–1847.

122. Rello J, Diaz E, Roque M, et al. Risk factors for developing pneumonia within 48 hours of intubation. *Am J Respir Crit Care Med* 1999;159:1742–1746.

123. Chastre J, Trouillet J, Vuagnat A, et al. Nosocomial pneumonia in patients with acute respiratory distress syndrome. *Am J Respir Crit Care Med* 1998;57:1165–1172.

124. Rello J, Sonora R, Jubert P, et al. Pneumonia in intubated patients: role of respiratory airway care. *Am J Respir Crit Care Med* 1996;154:111–115.

125. Drakulovic MB, Torres A, Bauer TT, et al. Supine body position as a risk factor for nosocomial pneumonia in mechanically ventilated patients: a randomized trial. *Lancet* 1999;354:1851–1858.

126. Kollef MH. Ventilator-associated pneumonia: a multivariate analysis. *JAMA* 1993;270:1965–1970.

127. Fagon JY, Chastre J, Domart Y, et al. Nosocomial pneumonia in patients receiving continuous mechanical ventilation: prospective analysis of 52 episodes with use of a protected specimen brush and quantitative culture techniques. *Am Rev Respir Dis* 1989;139:877–884.

128. Pugin J, Auckenthaler R, Mili N, et al. Diagnosis of ventilator-associated pneumonia by bacteriology analysis of bronchoscopic and nonbronchoscopic "blind" bronchoalveolar lavage fluid. *Am Rev Respir Dis* 1991;143:1121–1129.

129. Fabregas N, Ewig S, Torres A, et al. Clinical diagnosis of ventilator-associated pneumonia revisited: comparative vali-

130. dation using immediate post-mortem lung biopsies. *Thorax* 1999;54:867–873.

130. Wimberley N, Faling LJ, Bartlett JG. A fiberoptic bronchoscopy technique to obtain uncontaminated lower airway secretions for bacterial culture. *Am Rev Respir Dis* 1979;119:337–343.

131. Sachez-Nieto JM, Torres A, Garcia-Cordoba F, et al. Impact of invasive and noninvasive quantitative culture sampling on outcome of ventilator-associated pneumonia. *Am J Crit Care Med* 1998;157:371–376.

132. Marquette CH, Copin MH, Wallet F, et al. Diagnostic tests for pneumonia in ventilated patients: prospective evaluation of diagnostic accuracy using histology as a diagnostic gold standard. *Am J Respir Crit Care Med* 1995;151:1878–1888.

133. Rouby JJ, DeLassale EM, Poete P, et al. Nosocomial bronchopneumonia in the critically ill: histologic and bacteriologic aspects. *Am Rev Respir Dis* 1992;146:1059–1066.

134. Chastre J, Fagon JY, Soler P, et al. Quantification of BAL cells containing intracellular bacteria rapidly identifies ventilated patients with nosocomial pneumonia. *Chest* 1989;95:190S–192S.

135. Souweine B, Veber B, Bedos JP, et al. Diagnostic accuracy of protected specimen brush and bronchoalveolar lavage in nosocomial pneumonia: impact of previous antimicrobial treatments. *Crit Care Med* 1998;26:236–244.

136. Niederman MS, Torres A, Summer W. Invasive diagnostic testing is not needed routinely to manage suspected ventilator-associated pneumonia. *Am J Respir Crit Care Med* 1994;150:565–569.

137. Baughman RP. Protected-specimen brush technique in the diagnosis of ventilator-associated pneumonia. *Chest* 2000;117:203S–206S.

138. Wermert D, Marquette CH, Copin MC, et al. Influence of pulmonary bacteriology and histology on the yield of diagnostic procedures in ventilator-acquired pneumonia. *Am J Respir Crit Care Med* 1998;158:139–147.

139. Kirtland SH, Corley DE, Winterbauer RH, et al. The diagnosis of ventilator-associated pneumonia. A comparison of histologic, microbiologic, and clinical criteria. *Chest* 1997;112:445–457.

140. Torres A. Accuracy of diagnostic tools for the management of nosocomial respiratory infections in mechanically ventilated patients. *Eur Respir J* 1991;4:1010–1019.

141. Fagon JY, Chastre J, Trouillet JL, et al. Characterization of distal bronchial microflora during acute exacerbation of chronic bronchitis. Use of the protected specimen brush technique in 54 mechanically ventilated patients. *Am Rev Respir Dis* 1990;142:1004–1008.

142. Rello J, Gallego M, Mariscal D, et al. The value of routine microbial investigation in ventilator-associated pneumonia. *Am J Respir Crit Care Med* 1997;156:196–200.

143. Fagon JY, Chastre J, Wolff M, et al. Invasive and noninvasive strategies for management of suspected ventilator-associated pneumonia: a randomized trial. *Ann Intern Med* 2000;132:621–630.

144. Singh N, Rogers P, Atwood CW, et al. Short-course empiric antibiotic therapy for patients with pulmonary infiltrates in the intensive care unit: a proposed solution for indiscriminate antibiotic prescription. *Am J Respir Crit Care Med* 2000;162:505–511.

145. Richards MJ, Edwards JR, Culver DH, et al. Nosocomial infections in medical intensive care units in the United States. *Crit Care Med* 1999;27:887–892.

146. Marik PE, Careau P. The role of anaerobes in patients with ventilator-associated pneumonia and aspiration pneumonia: a prospective study. *Chest* 1999;115:178–183.

147. Rello J, Torres A, Ricart M, et al. Ventilator-associated pneumonia by *Staphylococcus aureus*: comparison of methicillin-resistant and methicillin-sensitive episodes. *Am J Respir Crit Care Med* 1994;150:1545–1549.

148. Trouillet J-L, Chastre J, Vuagnat A, et al. Ventilator-associated pneumonia caused by potentially drug-resistant bacteria. *Am J Respir Crit Care Med* 1998;157:531–539.

149. Rello J, Sa-Borges M, Correa H, et al. Variations in etiology of ventilator-associated pneumonia across four treatment sites: implications for antimicrobial prescribing practices. *Am J Respir Crit Care Med* 1999;160:608–613.

150. Kollef M. Inadequate antimicrobial treatment: an important determinant of outcome for hospitalized patients. *Clin Infect Dis* 2000;31[Suppl 4]:S131–S138.

151. Hilf M, Yu VL, Sharp J, et al. Antibiotic therapy for *Pseudomonas aeruginosa* bacteremia: outcome correlations in a prospective study of 200 patients. *Am J Med* 1989;87:540–546.

152. Fink MP, Snydman DR, Niederman MS, et al. Treatment of severe pneumonia in hospitalized patients: results of a multicenter, randomized, double-blind trial comparing intravenous ciprofloxacin with imipenem-cilastatin. *Antimicrob Agents Chemother* 1994;38:547–557.

153. Sieger B, Berman SJ, Geckler RW, et al. , for the Meropenem Lower Respiratory Tract Infection Group. Empiric treatment of hospital-acquired lower respiratory tract infections with meropenem or ceftazidime with tobramycin: a randomized study. *Crit Care Med* 1997;25:1663–1670.

154. Jaccard C, Troillet N, Harbarth S, et al. Prospective randomized comparison of imipenem-cilastatin and piperacillin-tazobactam in nosocomial pneumonia or peritonitis. *Antimicrob Agents Chemother* 1998;42:2966–2972.

155. Cometta A, Baumgartner JD, Lew D, et al. Prospective randomized comparison of imipenem monotherapy with imipenem plus netilmicin for treatment of severe infections in nonneutropenic patients. *Antimicrob Agents Chemother* 1994;38:1309–1313.

156. Hatala R, Dinh T, Cook DJ. Once-daily aminoglycoside dosing in immunocompetent adults: a metaanalysis. *Ann Intern Med* 1996;124:717–725.

157. Niederman MS. The principles of antibiotic use and the selection of empiric therapy for pneumonia. In: Fishman A, ed. *Pulmonary diseases and disorders*, 3rd ed. New York: McGraw-Hill, 1997:1939–1949.

158. Forest A, Nix DE, Ballow CH, et al. Pharmacodynamics of intravenous ciprofloxacin in seriously ill patients. *Antimicrob Agents Chemother* 1993;37:1073–1081.

159. Craig WA. Does the dose matter? *Clin Infect Dis* 2001;33[Suppl 3]:S233–S237.

160. Hanes SD, Wood GC, Herring V, et al. Intermittent and continuous ceftazidime infusion for critically ill trauma patients. *Am J Surg* 2000;179:436–440.

161. Peacock JE, Herrington DA, Wade JC, et al. Ciprofloxacin plus piperacillin compared with tobramycin plus piperacillin as empirical therapy in febrile neutropenic patients. A randomized, double-blind trial. *Ann Intern Med* 2002;137:77–87.

162. Plouffe JF. Emerging therapies for serious Gram-positive bacterial infections: a focus on linezolid. *Clin Infect Dis* 2000;31[Suppl 4]:S144–S149.

163. Cohen E, Dadashev A, Drucker M, et al. Once-daily versus twice-daily intravenous administration of vancomycin for infections in hospitalized patients. *J Antimicrob Chemother* 2002;49;155–160.

164. Dennesen PJ, Van der Ven AJ, Kessels AG, et al. Resolution of infectious parameters after antimicrobial therapy in patients with ventilator-associated pneumonia. *Am J Respir Crit Care Med* 2001;163:1371–1375.

165. Hamer D. Treatment of nosocomial pneumonia and tracheobronchitis caused by multidrug-resistant *Pseudomonas aeruginosa* with aerosolized colistin. *Am J Respir Crit Care Med* 2000;162:328–330.

166. Brown R, Kruse J, Counts G, et al. Double-blind study of endotracheal tobramycin in the treatment of Gram-negative bacterial pneumonia. *Antimicrob Agents Chemother* 1990;34:269–272.

167. Feely TW, DuMoulin GC, Hedley-Whyte J, et al. Aerosol polymyxin and pneumonia in seriously ill patients. *N Engl J Med* 1975;293:471–475.

168. Palmer L, Smaldone G, Simon S, et al. Aerosolized antibiotics in mechanically ventilated patients: delivery and response. *Crit Care Med* 1998;26:31–39.

169. Kollef MH. The prevention of ventilator-associated pneumonia. *N Engl J Med* 1999;340:627–634.

170. Holzapfel L, Chastang C, Demingeon G, et al. A randomized study assessing the systematic search for maxillary sinusitis in nasotracheally mechanically ventilated patients: influence of nosocomial maxillary sinusitis on the occurrence of ventilator-associated pneumonia. *Am J Respir Crit Care Med* 1999;159:695–701.

171. Sirvent JM, Torres A, El-Ebiary M, et al. Protective effect of intravenously administered cefuroxime against nosocomial pneumonia in patients with structural coma. *Am J Respir Crit Care Med* 1997;155:1729–1734.

172. Gastinne H, Wolff M, Delatour F, et al., and The French Study Group on Selective Decontamination of the Digestive Tract. A controlled trial in intensive care units of selective decontamination of the digestive tract with nonabsorbable antibiotics. *N Engl J Med* 1992;326:594–599.

173. Lesch CA, Itokazu GS, Danziger LH, et al. Multi-hospital analysis of antimicrobial usage and resistance trends. *Diagn Microbiol Infect Dis* 2001;41:149–154.

174. Rahal JJ, Urban C, Horn D, et al. Class restriction of cephalosporin use to control total cephalosporin resistance in nosocomial *Klebsiella. JAMA* 1998;280:1233–1237.

175. Kollef MH, Vlasnik J, Sharpless L, et al. Scheduled change of antibiotic classes: a strategy to decrease the incidence of ventilator-associated pneumonia. *Am J Respir Crit Care Med* 1997;156:1040–1048.

176. Gruson D, Hilbert G, Vargas F, et al. Rotation and restricted use of antibiotics in a medical intensive care unit. Impact on the incidence of ventilator-associated pneumonia caused by antibiotic-resistant Gram-negative bacteria. *Am J Respir Crit Care Med* 2000;162:837–843.

177. Gerding DN, Larson TA, Hughes RA, et al. Aminoglycoside resistance and aminoglycoside usage: ten years of experience in one hospital. *Antimicrob Agents Chemother* 1991;35:1284–1290.

178. Raymond DP, Pelletier SJ, Crabtree TD, et al. Impact of a rotating empiric antibiotic schedule on infectious mortality in an intensive care unit. *Crit Care Med* 2001;29:1101–1108.

Approach to the Patient with Interstitial Lung Disease

23

Talmadge E. King, Jr.

The diffuse parenchymal lung diseases, often collectively referred to as the *interstitial lung diseases (ILDs)*, are a heterogeneous group of lung disorders that are classified together because of similar clinical, roentgenographic, physiologic, or pathologic manifestations (1,2) (Table 23.1). The term *interstitial* is misleading because most of these disorders are also associated with extensive alterations of alveolar, airway, and vascular architecture.

A common pathogenetic sequence likely underlies many ILDs. An initial injury is followed by an influx of inflammatory and immune effector cells (i.e., "alveolitis"). Resolution of the initial inflammatory response leads in many instances to pulmonary fibrosis or scarring. Much has been learned about the role of chronic inflammation in injury and in the initiation of events that result in fibrosis. However, the cellular and molecular mechanisms that underlie the transition from the inflammatory response to tissue repair or irreversible fibrosis remain largely unknown. Pulmonary fibrosis can be a devastating problem, especially idiopathic pulmonary fibrosis (IPF), which is progressive and irreversible (3). Consequently, the management of patients with pulmonary fibrosis is problematic. Current treatments result in no improvement for most patients and only partial or transient suppression of disease progression for many others (4).

INCIDENCE AND PREVALENCE

The exact prevalence and incidence of the ILDs are unknown (5). Studies suggest a prevalence of 80.9 per 100,000 men and of 67.2 per 100,000 women. Similarly, the overall in-

cidence of ILD is slightly more common in men (31.5 per 100,000 per year) than in women (26.1 per 100,000 per year). Both the prevalence and incidence increase with age; for example, among men and women 75 years of age or older, the prevalence of IPF was 250 per 100,000, and the incidence was 160 per 100,000 per year (5).

The vital statistics for pulmonary fibrosis are scant and of limited value. In 1988, an estimated 30,000 hospitalizations (compared with 665,000 hospitalizations for chronic obstructive pulmonary disease [COPD] and asthma) and 4,851 deaths in the United States were attributed to pulmonary fibrosis (6). However, the frequency with which pulmonary fibrosis was listed as the underlying cause of death increased from 48.6 per million in 1979 to 50.9 per million in 1991 among men, and from 21.4 per million in 1979 to 27.2 per million in 1991 among women (6).

CLINICAL ASSESSMENT OF PATIENTS WITH INTERSTITIAL LUNG DISEASE

Patients with ILD commonly come to clinical attention because of the onset of progressive breathlessness with exertion (dyspnea) or a persistent, nonproductive cough. Often, the identification of interstitial opacities on chest roentgenography or lung function abnormalities on spirometry (particularly a restrictive ventilatory pattern) prompts evaluation. Finally, pulmonary symptoms may be associated with another disease, such as a connective tissue disease.

The initial evaluation should include a complete history and physical examination, laboratory investigations, lung function testing, chest imaging, and a histologic examination. The initial laboratory evaluation should include biochemical tests to evaluate liver and renal function and hematologic tests to check for evidence of anemia, polycythemia,

T. E. King Jr.: Department of Medicine, University of California, San Francisco; and Medical Services, San Francisco General Hospital, San Francisco, California.

TABLE 23.1. CLINICAL CLASSIFICATION OF INTERSTITIAL LUNG DISEASES

Fibrotic disorders of unknown etiology (idiopathic interstitial pneumonias) (see Chapter 24: Idiopathic Interstitial Pneumonias)
 I. Idiopathic pulmonary fibrosis/usual interstitial pneumonia
 II. Nonspecific interstitial pneumonia
 III. Cryptogenic organizing pneumonia
 IV. Respiratory bronchiolitis–associated interstitial lung disease/desquamative interstitial pneumonia
 V. Acute interstitial pneumonia
 VI. Lymphocytic interstitial pneumonia
Connective tissue disease associated with interstitial lung disease (see Chapter 26: Connective Tissue Diseases)
Primary or unclassified
 I. Sarcoidosis (see Chapter 28: Systemic Sarcoidosis)
 II. Pulmonary histiocytosis X (eosinophilic granuloma of the lung) (see Chapter 32: Major Pulmonary Disease Syndromes of Unknown Etiology)
 III. Lymphangioleiomyomatosis (see Chapter 32)
 IV. Vasculitides (Wegener granulomatosis, Churg-Strauss syndrome) (see Chapter 30: Pulmonary Vasculitis)
 V. Alveolar proteinosis (see Chapter 32)
 VI. Eosinophilic pneumonia (acute and chronic) (see Chapter 27: Eosinophilic Pulmonary Syndromes)
 VII. Diffuse alveolar hemorrhage (see Chapter 31: Alveolar Hemorrhage Syndromes)
  A. Vasculitides
  B. Collagen-vascular diseases
  C. Drugs
  D. Goodpasture syndrome
  E. Idiopathic pulmonary hemosiderosis
Occupational exposures (see Chapter 44: Occupational Lung Diseases and Chapter 45: Occupational Airway Diseases)
 I. Inorganic dusts
  A. Fibrogenic
   1. Asbestosis
   2. Silicosis
   3. Hard metal dusts (i.e., cadmium, titanium oxide)
  B. Nonfibrogenic
   1. Siderosis (iron)
   2. Stannosis (tin)
   3. Baritosis (barium)
   4. Antimony
  C. Granulomatous/fibrogenic
   1. Berylliosis
 II. Bacterial products (byssinosis)
 III. Chemical sources, gases, fumes, vapors, aerosols, paraquat, radiation
Environmental exposures (see Chapter 25: Hypersensitivity Pneumonitis)
 I. Organic dusts (hypersensitivity pneumonitis or extrinsic allergic alveolitis)
  A. Thermophilic bacteria (i.e., *Micropolyspora faeni, Thermactinomyces vulgaris, T. sacchari*)
  B. Other bacteria (i.e., *Bacillus subtilis, B. cereus*)
 II. True fungi (i.e., *Aspergillus, Crytostroma corticale, Aureobasidium pullulans, Penicillium* species)
 III. Animal proteins (e.g., bird fancier's disease)
Drug-induced lung disease (partial list) (see Chapter 33: Drug-Induced Pulmonary Disease)
 I. Acute onset
  A. Diffuse alveolar damage: crack cocaine, amiodarone, nitrofurantoin, any cytotoxic agent (e.g., bleomycin, carmustine, busulfan, mitomycin, procarbazine, methotrexate)
  B. Noncardiogenic pulmonary edema (probably diffuse alveolar damage): cytosine arabinoside, aspirin and related compounds, narcotics
  C. Diffuse alveolar hemorrhage: crack cocaine, penicillamine, phenytoin, anticoagulants, thrombolytic agents, cytotoxic drugs that cause diffuse alveolar damage
 II. Acute or subacute onset
  A. Eosinophilic pneumonia: nonsteroidal antiinflammatory agents, antibiotics (ampicillin, minocycline, sulfa, nitrofurantoin, sulfasalazine)
  B. Bronchiolitis obliterans–organizing pneumonia: amiodarone, methotrexate, bleomycin
  C. Desquamative interstitial pneumonia: nitrofurantoin, sulfasalazine

or leukocytosis. Serologic studies should be performed if clinically indicated by features suggestive of a connective tissue disease, vasculitis, or hypersensitivity pneumonitis. Complete lung function testing (spirometry, lung volumes, diffusing capacity) should be performed, and the arterial blood gases should be measured with the patient at rest breathing room air. When the diagnosis remains uncertain after chest roentgenography, lung function testing, and clinical assessment, high-resolution computed tomography (HRCT) is the next test of choice and should precede lung biopsy (7). Common diseases, such as COPD, anemia, heart failure, and mycobacterial or fungal disease, can mimic ILD, so they must be ruled out. This process usually identifies the cause of the ILD (8).

Duration of Illness, Age and Sex of the Patient

In the vast majority of patients with ILD, the symptoms and signs are chronic, lasting months to years (e.g., IPF, sarcoidosis, pulmonary histiocytosis X). In some, the onset may be acute (days to weeks) or subacute (weeks to months) (9). These latter processes are often confused with community-acquired pneumonias because many have features of diffuse radiographic opacities, fever, or relapses of disease activity; examples include acute interstitial pneumonia, diffuse alveolar hemorrhage syndromes, bronchiolitis obliterans–organizing pneumonia, some drug-induced ILDs, acute eosinophilic pneumonia, hypersensitivity pneumonitis, and the acute immunologic pneumonia that complicates either systemic lupus erythematosus or polymyositis (9). It is important to review all old chest roentgenograms to assess the tempo of change in disease activity. Radiographic abnormalities may have been present for much longer than symptoms, so that the condition can be identified as chronic. Unfortunately, the time course of many ILDs can vary considerably; for example, cryptogenic organizing pneumonia and eosinophilic pneumonia may present acutely, subacutely, or chronically (7).

The patient's *age* can be helpful, given that the majority of patients with sarcoidosis and connective tissue disease present between the ages of 20 and 40 years. Conversely, most patients with IPF are older than 60 years (10).

The patient's *sex* is important in lymphangioleiomyomatosis, which occurs exclusively in premenopausal women. Also, ILD in the connective tissue diseases is more common in women; the exception is ILD in rheumatoid arthritis, which is more common in men. Because of occupational exposures, men are also more likely to have a pneumoconiosis.

Occupational and Environmental History

A large number of occupational and environmental exposures have been associated with the development of diffuse parenchymal lung diseases. A strict chronologic listing of the patient's lifelong employment must be sought, including specific duties and known exposures to dusts, gases, and chemicals. The degree, duration, and latency of exposure and the use of protective devices should be elicited.

A review of the environment (home and workplace, including those of the spouse and children) is also valuable. It is important to determine if the patient has been exposed to pets (especially birds), air conditioners, humidifiers, hot tubs, evaporative cooling systems (e.g., swamp coolers), or water damage in the home or work environment (11). In hypersensitivity pneumonitis, respiratory symptoms, fever, chills, and abnormalities on the chest roentgenogram are often temporally related to the workplace (farmer's lung) or a hobby (pigeon breeder's disease). Symptoms may diminish or disappear after the patient leaves the place where exposure occurs for several days; similarly, symptoms reappear on return to that place.

Smoking History, Family and Drug History

A history of tobacco use is important because some diseases occur largely in current or former smokers (pulmonary histiocytosis X, desquamative interstitial pneumonitis, IPF, respiratory bronchiolitis) or in never-smokers or former smokers (sarcoidosis, hypersensitivity pneumonitis) (2). Active smoking can lead to complications in some processes, such as Goodpasture syndrome, in which pulmonary hemorrhage is far more frequent in current smokers.

Familial associations (with an autosomal-dominant pattern) have been identified in cases of IPF, sarcoidosis, tuberous sclerosis, and neurofibromatosis (12,13). An autosomal-recessive pattern of inheritance occurs in Niemann-Pick disease, Gaucher disease, and Hermansky-Pudlak syndrome.

A detailed history of the medications taken by the patient, including over-the-counter medications, oily nose drops, and amino acid supplements, is needed to exclude the possibility of drug-induced disease (14). Importantly, lung disease may occur weeks to years after a drug has been discontinued.

Symptoms and Signs

Dyspnea

A sense of shortness of breath (i.e., dyspnea) is common in patients with ILD. The language of dyspnea is often confusing to both clinician and patient (15). Patients with ILD may describe their breathlessness in several different ways, as shown in Table 23.2 (16,17). In most instances, the patient attributes the insidious onset of breathlessness with exertion to aging, deconditioning, obesity, or a recent upper respiratory tract illness. Some patients deny having dyspnea even when questioned, usually because they have so limited their activity that they do not "experience" any significant discomfort. Frequently, a spouse or friend brings the problem to the patient's attention (18). Some patients, especially those with sarcoidosis, silicosis, or pulmonary histiocytosis X, may have extensive parenchymal lung disease radiographically without significant dyspnea, especially early in the course of the disease. A sudden worsening of dyspnea, especially if associated with pleural pain, may indicate a spontaneous pneumothorax (especially in pulmonary histiocytosis X, tuberous sclerosis, lymphangioleiomyomatosis, and neurofibromatosis).

Dyspnea can be measured by clinical instruments, usually questionnaires, that consider various dimensions or components affecting a person's breathlessness and by direct ratings during a physical task or exercise test (19). Dyspnea can be quantified (grades 1–4) in a simple and reliable manner as outlined in the American Thoracic Society Shortness-of-Breath Scale. Various ordinal dyspnea scales, such as the Baseline Dyspnea Index, Medical Research Council Scale,

TABLE 23.2. QUALITATIVE DESCRIPTORS OF EXERTIONAL DYSPNEA

Increased work/effort
   My breathing requires more work.
   My breathing requires effort.
Unrewarded inspiration
   My breath does not go in all the way.
   I feel a need for more air.
   I cannot get enough air in.
Inspiratory difficulty
   My breath does not go in all the way.
   I cannot take a deep breath in.
Heavy breathing
   My breathing is heavy.
   I feel that I am breathing more air.
Shallow breathing
   My breathing is shallow.
Rapid breathing
   I feel that my breathing is rapid.
Tight chest
   My chest feels tight.
   My chest feels constricted.
Expiratory difficulty
   My breath does not go out all the way.
Suffocating feeling
   I feel that I am smothering.
   I feel that I am suffocating.

Source: Modified from Simon PM, Schwartzstein RM, Weiss JW, et al. Distinguishable types of dyspnea in patients with shortness of breath. *Am Rev Respir Dis* 1990;142:1009–1014; O'Donnell DE, Chau LK, Webb KA, Qualitative aspects of exertional dyspnea in patients with interstitial lung disease. *J Appl Physiol* 1998;84:2000–2009, with permission.

and Oxygen-Cost Diagram, also provide semiquantitative information on disease-specific health-related quality of life (HRQL) with good reliability. These measures of dyspnea are significantly associated with physiologic parameters of lung function (see section "Quality-of-Life Evaluation"). Severe breathlessness is correlated with a lower diffusing capacity of the lung for carbon monoxide (D_{LCO}) at rest and an accelerated ventilatory response to exercise. Dyspnea is related to reduced lung compliance and increased elastic work of breathing.

Cough

A dry cough may be particularly disturbing for patients with processes that involve the airways, such as respiratory bronchiolitis, bronchiolitis obliterans, sarcoidosis, hypersensitivity pneumonitis, cryptogenic organizing pneumonia, and pulmonary histiocytosis X. Although a productive cough is unusual in most ILDs, a mucoid, salty-tasting sputum is sometimes reported by patients with diffuse bronchoalveolar cell carcinoma.

Hemoptysis

Spitting of gross blood or blood-streaked sputum occurs in the diffuse alveolar hemorrhage syndromes, lymphan-

gioleiomyomatosis, tuberous sclerosis, pulmonary veno-occlusive disease, longstanding mitral valve disease, and the granulomatous vasculitides. Occasionally, diffuse alveolar bleeding may be present without hemoptysis; the clinical manifestations of dyspnea and an iron deficiency anemia may be present. The new onset of hemoptysis in a patient with known ILD should raise the possibility of a complicating malignancy.

Wheezing

Wheezing is uncommon and has been described in cases of Churg-Strauss syndrome, chronic eosinophilic pneumonia, respiratory bronchiolitis, and lymphangitic carcinomatosis.

Chest Pain

Clinically significant chest pain is uncommon in most ILDs. However, pleuritic chest pain may occur in ILD associated with rheumatoid arthritis, systemic lupus erythematosus, mixed connective tissue disease, and some drug-induced disorders. Substernal chest pain or discomfort is common in sarcoidosis. Chest pain may be an initial manifestation of pneumothorax.

Other Clinical Findings

Clinical findings suggestive of a connective tissue disease (musculoskeletal pain, weakness, fatigue, fever, joint pain or swelling, photosensitivity, Raynaud phenomenon, pleuritis, dry eyes, dry mouth) should be carefully elicited. The specific connective tissue disease may be difficult to define because the pulmonary manifestations occasionally precede the more typical systemic manifestations by months or years (particularly in rheumatoid arthritis, systemic lupus erythematosus, and polymyositis/dermatomyositis). Hematuria may be a presenting manifestation in patients with vasculitis.

Physical Examination

The physical examination findings are commonly not specific, but the examination can be useful because it frequently reveals tachypnea, reduced chest expansion, and bilateral basilar end-inspiratory dry crackles.

Crackles

Crackles ("Velcro rales") are common in most forms of ILD, although they are less likely to be heard in the granulomatous lung diseases, especially sarcoidosis. Crackles may be present in the absence of radiographic abnormalities on the chest radiograph.

Inspiratory Squeaks

Scattered late-inspiratory high-pitched rhonchi, so-called inspiratory squeaks, are often heard during the chest examination in patients with bronchiolitis.

Digital Clubbing

The distal part of the finger is enlarged in comparison with the proximal part. A shiny and smooth appearance of the cuticle with increased sponginess, flattening of the normally obtuse angle on the dorsal surface of the finger at the base of the nail, an increase in the volume of the distal segment of the finger, and an increase in the curvature of the nail in one or both planes are other features. Clubbing is common in some conditions (IPF, asbestosis) and rare in others (sarcoidosis, hypersensitivity pneumonitis, histiocytosis X) (20–22). In most patients, clubbing is a late manifestation that suggests advanced derangement of the lung (21).

Cyanosis

Cyanosis is uncommon and usually a late manifestation of advanced disease.

Cor Pulmonale

The cardiac examination findings are usually normal except in the mid or late stages of the disease, when findings of pulmonary hypertension (i.e., augmented P_2, right-sided lift, and S_3 gallop) and cor pulmonale may become evident. Signs of pulmonary hypertension and cor pulmonale are generally secondary manifestations of advanced ILD, although they may be primary manifestations of a connective tissue disorder (e.g., progressive systemic sclerosis).

Extrapulmonary Physical Findings

These may be helpful in establishing a diagnosis (Table 23.3).

Laboratory Evaluation

The routine laboratory evaluation is often not helpful (Table 23.4). An elevated erythrocyte sedimentation rate and hypergammaglobulinemia are common but not diagnostic. Antinuclear antibodies, anti-immunoglobulin antibodies (rheumatoid factors), and circulating immune complexes are identified in many of these patients, even in the absence of a defined connective tissue disorder. An elevated lactate dehydrogenase level may be noted but is a nonspecific finding common in pulmonary disorders (e.g., alveolar

TABLE 23.3. EXTRAPULMONARY PHYSICAL FINDINGS IN THE INTERSTITIAL LUNG DISEASES

Physical Findings	Associated Conditions
Fever	Infections, eosinophilic pneumonia, drug reactions, vasculitis, connective tissue disease, cryptogenic organizing pneumonia, hypersensitivity pneumonitis, sarcoidosis, lymphoma, lymphangitic carcinoma
Systemic arterial hypertension	Connective tissue disease, neurofibromatosis, some diffuse alveolar hemorrhage syndromes
Skin changes	
Erythema nodosum	Sarcoidosis, connective tissue disease, Behçet syndrome, histoplasmosis, coccidioidomycosis
Maculopapular rash	Drug-induced disease, amyloidosis, lipoidosis, connective tissue disease, Gaucher disease
Heliotrope rash	Dermatomyositis
Telangiectasia	Scleroderma
Raynaud phenomenon	Connective tissue disease (scleroderma)
Cutaneous vasculitis	Systemic vasculitides, connective tissue disease
Subcutaneous nodules	Von Recklinghausen disease, rheumatoid arthritis
Calcinosis	Dermatomyositis, scleroderma
Eye changes	
Uveitis	Sarcoidosis, Behçet syndrome, ankylosing spondylitis
Scleritis	Systemic vasculitis, systemic lupus erythematosus, scleroderma, sarcoidosis
Keratoconjunctivitis sicca	Lymphocytic interstitial pneumonia, Sjögren syndrome
Salivary gland enlargement	Sarcoidosis, lymphocytic interstitial pneumonia, Sjögren syndrome
Peripheral lymphadenopathy	Sarcoidosis, lymphangitic carcinomatosis, lymphocytic interstitial pneumonia, lymphoma
Hepatosplenomegaly	Sarcoidosis, pulmonary histiocytosis X, connective tissue disease, amyloidosis, lymphocytic interstitial pneumonia
Pericarditis	Radiation pneumonitis, connective tissue disease, vasculitis
Myositis	Connective tissue disease, drugs (L-tryptophan)
Muscle weakness	Connective tissue disease
Arthritis	Connective tissue disease, vasculitis, sarcoidosis, Goodpasture syndrome

Source: Adapted from British Thoracic Society. The diagnosis, assessment, and treatment of diffuse parenchymal lung disease in adults. *Thorax* 1999;54[Suppl 1]: S1–S28; Schwarz MI, King TE Jr, Cherniack RM. General principles and diagnostic approach to the interstitial lung diseases. In: Murray JF, Nadel JA, eds. *Textbook of respiratory medicine*, 2nd ed. Philadelphia: WB Saunders, 1994: 1803–1826, with permission.

TABLE 23.4. LABORATORY FINDINGS IN THE INTERSTITIAL LUNG DISEASES

Abnormality	Associated Condition
Leukopenia	Sarcoidosis, connective tissue disease, lymphoma, drug-induced disease
Eosinophilia	Eosinophilic pneumonia, sarcoidosis, systemic vasculitis, drug-induced disease (sulfa, methotrexate)
Thrombocytopenia	Sarcoidosis, connective tissue disease, drug-induced disease, Gaucher disease
Hemolytic anemia	Connective tissue disease, sarcoidosis, lymphoma, drug-induced disease
Normocytic anemia	Diffuse alveolar hemorrhage syndromes, connective tissue disease, lymphangitic carcinomatosis
Urinary sediment abnormalities	Connective tissue disease, systemic vasculitis, drug-induced disease
Hypogammaglobulinemia	Lymphocytic interstitial pneumonitis
Hypergammaglobulinemia	Connective tissue disease, sarcoidosis, systemic vasculitis, lymphocytic interstitial pneumonia, lymphoma
Serum immune complexes	Idiopathic pulmonary fibrosis, lymphocytic interstitial pneumonitis, systemic vasculitis, connective tissue disease, eosinophilic granuloma
Serum angiotensin-converting enzyme	Sarcoidosis, hypersensitivity pneumonitis, silicosis, Gaucher disease
Antibasement membrane antibody	Goodpasture syndrome
Antineutrophil cytoplasmic antibody	Wegener granulomatosis, Churg-Strauss syndrome, microscopic polyangiitis
Serum precipitating antibodies	Hypersensitivity pneumonitis
Surfactant proteins A and B	Idiopathic pulmonary fibrosis, systemic sclerosis
Monocyte chemoattractant protein-1	Idiopathic pulmonary fibrosis
KL-6 (high-molecular-weight glycoprotein)	Idiopathic pulmonary fibrosis, connective tissue diseases
Lymphocyte transfromation test to specific antigens	Chronic beryllium disease, aluminum pot room worker's disease, gold-induced pneumonitis

Source: Adapted from Schwarz MI, King TE Jr, Cherniack RM. General principles and diagnostic approach to the interstitial lung diseases. In: Murray JF, Nadel JA, eds. *Textbook of respiratory medicine,* 2nd ed. Philadelphia: WB Saunders, 1994:1803–1826, with permission.

proteinosis, IPF). An increased level of angiotensin-converting enzyme may be observed in sarcoidosis but is nonspecific because elevated angiotensin-converting enzyme levels have been noted in several interstitial diseases, including hypersensitivity pneumonitis. Antibodies to organic antigens may be helpful in confirming exposure to an antigen when hypersensitivity pneumonitis is suspected, although their presence does not establish causation. The electrocardiographic findings are usually normal in the absence of pulmonary hypertension or concurrent cardiac disease. A number of serum markers suggestive of ILD have been identified, including surfactant proteins A and B (SP-A, SP-B), monocyte chemoattractant protein-1 (MCP-1), and KL-6 (a circulating, high-molecular-weight glycoprotein expressed by type II pneumocytes) (23–25).

Chest Imaging

Chest Roentgenography

The diagnosis of ILD is often suspected initially on the basis of abnormal chest roentgenographic findings. Unfortunately, the chest roentgenogram may be normal in patients with some forms of ILD, particularly hypersensitivity pneumonitis. When a symptomatic patient with a normal chest roentgenogram or an asymptomatic patient with radiographic evidence of ILD is ignored or incompletely evaluated, progression of disease is frequently the result, and the disease may be irreversible by the time the patient seeks additional medical attention.

The most common radiographic abnormality is a reticular or nodular pattern; however, mixed patterns of alveolar filling and increased interstitial markings are not unusual. Most ILDs tend to involve the lower lung zones (Fig. 23.1). As the disease progresses, widespread infiltration is associated with a reduction in lung volume and the development of pulmonary hypertension. A subgroup of ILDs have a predilection for the upper lung zones and are often associated with nodular infiltrates that cause an upward contraction of the pulmonary hilum. With progression of the disease, small cystic structures, representing fibrous replacement of the normal alveolar architecture, and radiographic honeycombing appear. Although the chest roentgenogram is useful in suggesting the presence of ILD, correlation between the roentgenographic pattern and the stage of disease (clinical or histopathologic) is generally poor. Only the radiographic finding of honeycombing (small cystic spaces) correlates with the pathologic findings, and when present, it portends a poor prognosis. Table 23.5 outlines the likely diagnosis for certain radiographic patterns.

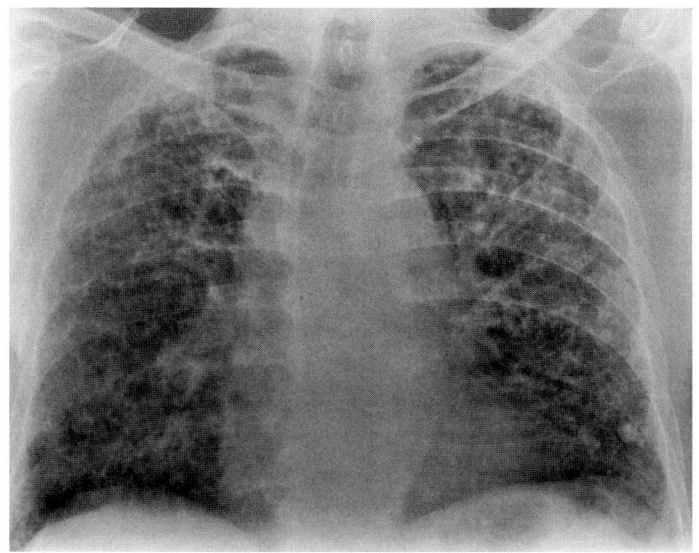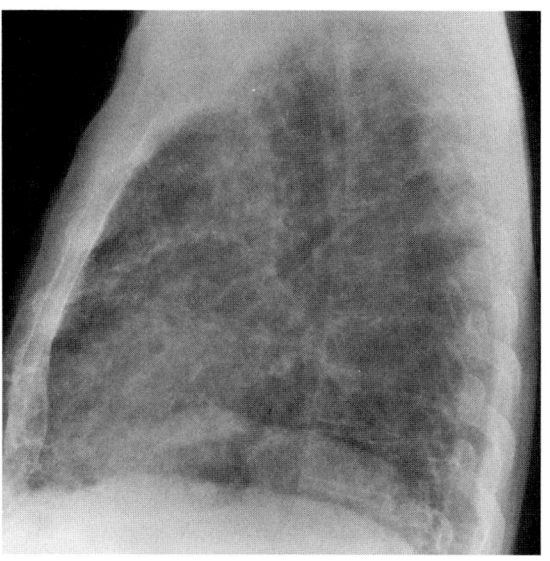

FIGURE 23.1. Posteroanterior (**A**) and lateral (**B**) chest radiographs of a patient with idiopathic pulmonary fibrosis. Diffuse reticular opacities are seen throughout the lung, with somewhat greater involvement peripherally. Cystic honeycombing is apparent in both lower lung fields.

High-Resolution Computed Tomography

HRCT is well suited for the evaluation of diffuse pulmonary parenchymal disease (26) (Fig. 23.2). HRCT enhances pattern recognition in diffuse lung disease because it avoids the problem of superimposition of structures and is exposure-independent. HRCT is more accurate than conventional chest roentgenography in distinguishing air space from ILD. It also offers earlier detection and confirmation of suspected diffuse lung disease, especially in the investigation of a symptomatic patient with normal chest radiographic findings. HRCT better assesses the extent and distribution of disease and often discloses coexisting disease (e.g., occult mediastinal adenopathy, carcinoma, emphysema). HRCT is a specialized technique requiring particular skill in the interpretation of images and a proper understanding of the diffuse parenchymal lung diseases (7,27). In the proper clinical setting, the HRCT findings may be sufficiently characteristic that biopsy is not needed to confirm the diagnosis (7,27–29).

Other Imaging Studies

Lung scanning with ^{67}Ga has been tried as a means of evaluating the inflammatory component of ILD because the isotope is not taken up by normal lung parenchyma. Uptake may be diffuse or patchy and is felt to reflect an increased accumulation of inflammatory cells in the lung. To date, ^{67}Ga scanning has not proved very useful in the diagnosis, staging, or follow-up of ILD (an exception is its occasional value in the assessment of extrapulmonary sarcoidosis) (7,30,31).

The pulmonary clearance of ^{99m}Tc-DTPA (diethylene-triamine pentaacetic acid) aerosol has been evaluated in the diagnosis and assessment of ILD but is not currently recommended as a routine test (32–34).

The usefulness of magnetic resonance imaging (MRI) in the detection and surveillance of interstitial pneumonia has been limited historically by long imaging times and the requirement for careful respiratory gating techniques to minimize artifact from respiratory movements. One of the newer and more sensitive techniques used to image the air spaces of the lung is MRI after the inhalation of hyperpolarized ^{3}He (35). ^{3}He is used because it can be inhaled in relatively large quantities without substantial risk; it is not absorbed by the tissues of the lung. The hyperpolarized ^{3}He is administered as an inhalational "contrast agent" that allows imaging of the airways and air spaces. Normal ventilation is reflected by an almost complete and homogeneous distribution of the hyperpolarized gas, represented by the signal detected. Loss of the signal or an inhomogeneous distribution of the signal represents mass effects and ventilatory abnormalities (35). MRI provides qualitative rather than quantitative information about interstitial pneumonias.

Positron emission tomography (PET) has been used in pilot studies to evaluate the variations in pulmonary vascular permeability seen in IPF. The high cost and restricted availability of PET technology are likely to limit its common use. Neither modality has a role in the routine evaluation or management of IPF at this time.

Pulmonary Function Testing

Lung volume measurement and spirometry are important tests in assessing the severity of lung involvement in patients with ILD. Most of the interstitial disorders have a *restrictive defect*, with a reduced total lung capacity, functional residual capacity, and residual volume. The flow rates are decreased (forced expiratory volume in 1 second [FEV$_1$] and forced vital capacity [FVC]), but the decrease is related to

TABLE 23.5. HELPFUL RADIOGRAPHIC PATTERNS IN THE DIFFERENTIAL DIAGNOSIS OF INTERSTITIAL LUNG DISEASE

Air space opacities
Pulmonary hemorrhage
Chronic or acute eosinophilic pneumonia
Bronchiolitis obliterans–organizing pneumonia
Alveolar proteinosis
Reticular or linear opacities
Peripheral lung zone
  Bronchiolitis obliterans–organizing pneumonia
  Eosinophilic pneumonia
Upper zone predominance
  Granulomatous disease
  Sarcoidosis
  Pulmonary histiocytosis X (eosinophilic granuloma)
  Chronic hypersensitivity pneumonitis
  Chronic infectious diseases (e.g., tuberculosis, histoplasmosis)
  Pneumoconiosis
  Silicosis
  Berylliosis
  Coal miner's pneumoconiosis
  Hard metal disease
  Miscellaneous
  Rheumatoid arthritis (necrobiotic nodular form)
  Ankylosing spondylitis
  Radiation fibrosis
  Drug-induced (amiodarone, gold)
Lower zone predominance
  Idiopathic pulmonary fibrosis
  Rheumatoid arthritis (associated with interstitial pneumonia)
  Asbestosis
End-stage or honeycomb lung
Upper zone predominance
  Sarcoidosis
  Pulmonary histiocytosis X (eosinophilic granuloma)
  Chronic hypersensitivity pneumonitis
  Lymphangiomyomatosis
Lower zone predominance
  Idiopathic pulmonary fibrosis
  Rheumatoid arthritis (associated with usual interstitial pneumonia)
  Asbestosis
Increased lung volumes
Lymphangiomyomatosis
Tuberous sclerosis
Sarcoidosis (stage III)
Pulmonary histiocytosis X (chronic with cyst formation)
Neurofibromatosis
Chronic hypersensitivity pneumonitis
Reticular or nodular opacities, increased lung volumes, and bullous changes
Lymphangiomyomatosis
Tuberous sclerosis
Neurofibromatosis
Chronic sarcoidosis
Pulmonary histiocytosis X
Chronic hypersensitivity pneumonia
End-stage pulmonary involvement in microscopic polyangiitis
Intravenous drug abuse (Ritalin)
Associated with pneumothorax
Pulmonary histiocytosis X (eosinophilic granuloma)
Lymphangiomyomatosis
Tuberous sclerosis
Pleural involvement
Asbestosis

Connective tissue disorders
  Systemic lupus erythematosus
  Rheumatoid arthritis
  Scleroderma
  Mixed connective tissue disease
Lymphangitic carcinomatosis
Lymphangiomyomatosis (chylous effusion)
Drug-induced
  Nitrofurantoin
Sarcoidosis (lymphocytic effusion)
Radiation pneumonitis (chronic with mediastinal lymphatic obstruction)
Hilar or mediastinal lymphadenopathy
Sarcoidosis
Lymphoma
Kaposi sarcoma
Methotrexate-induced lung disease
Lymphangitic carcinomatosis
Berylliosis
Amyloidosis
Gaucher disease
Acute disseminated histoplasmosis or coccidioidomycosis
Eggshell calcification of lymph nodes
Silicosis
Sarcoidosis
Radiation
Associated with Kerley B lines
Lymphangitic carcinomatosis
Chronic left ventricular failure
Mitral valve disease
Lymphoma
Lymphangioleiomyomatosis
Amyloidosis
Subcutaneous calcinosis
Scleroderma (CREST: calcinosis cutis, Raynaud phenomenon, esophageal motility disorder, sclerodactyly, and telangiectasia)
Dermatopolymyositis
Miliary pattern
Sarcoidosis
Silicosis
Hypersensitivity pneumonitis
Bronchiolitis obliterans
Infectious granulomatous disease (tuberculosis, histoplasmosis, coccidioidomycosis)
Metastatic malignant disease
Hypernephroma
Adenocarcinoma of breast
Malignant melanoma
Fleeting or migratory infiltrates
Bronchiolitis obliterans–organizing pneumonia (idiopathic or radiation-induced)
Simple pulmonary eosinophilia (Löffler syndrome)
Hypersensitivity to drugs
Parasitic infections
Fungus-induced, especially allergic bronchopulmonary aspergillosis
Normal[a]
Hypersensitivity pneumonitis (common in population studies, rare in isolated chronic cases)
Sarcoidosis
Connective tissue disease
Bronchiolitis obliterans
Asbestosis
Lymphangioleiomyotosis

[a] High-resolution computed tomography may show abnormal findings in many of these cases.
Source: From Schwarz MI. Radiologic recognition of chronic diffuse lung disease. In: Schwarz MI, King TE Jr, eds. *Interstitial lung disease.* Toronto: BC Decker, 1988:27–36, with permission.

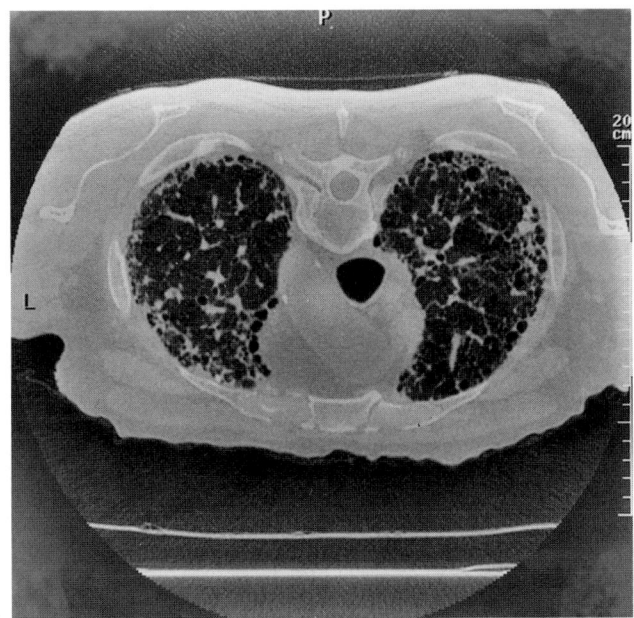

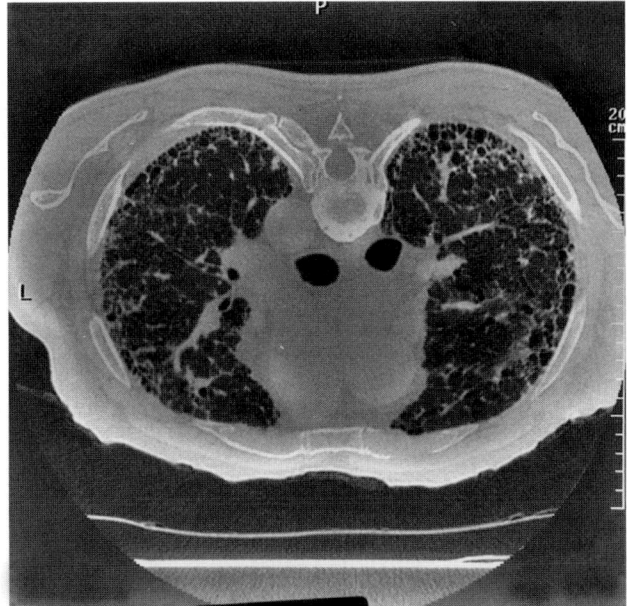

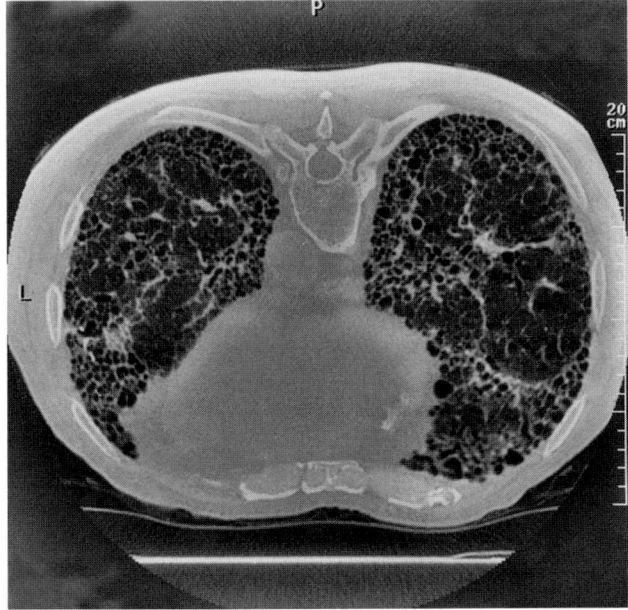

FIGURE 23.2. High-resolution chest computed tomogram (1.5-mm slices) of a patient with idiopathic pulmonary fibrosis. Apical (**A**), mid lung (**B**), and basilar (**C**) cuts are shown. These sections demonstrate marked peripheral fibrotic changes with cystic honeycombing most prominent at the bases of the lungs.

the decreased lung volumes. The FEV_1/FVC ratio is usually normal or increased (Fig. 23.3). The smoking history must be considered in an interpretation of the functional studies (36). A few disorders cause interstitial opacities on chest roentgenograms and obstructive airflow limitation on lung function tests (e.g., sarcoidosis, lymphangioleiomyomatosis, hypersensitivity pneumonitis, tuberous sclerosis, and COPD with superimposed ILD).

A reduction in lung compliance is also common. In symptomatic patients with normal chest radiographic findings and minimal or no restrictive disease, measurement of elastic recoil (pressure-volume curve) may be helpful by identifying lung stiffness (36). Pressure-volume studies often yield a curve that is shifted downward and to the right, consistent with a stiff, noncompliant lung (Fig. 23.3). In general, as the disease progresses, lung compliance decreases and lung volumes fall.

Measurement of Gas Exchange at Rest and During Exercise

Diffusing Capacity

A reduction in the diffusing capacity of the lung for carbon monoxide (D_{LCO}) is common but not specific for a particular type of ILD. The decrease in D_{LCO} is caused, in part, by effacement of the alveolar capillary units but more importantly by the mismatch of ventilation and perfusion in the alveoli.

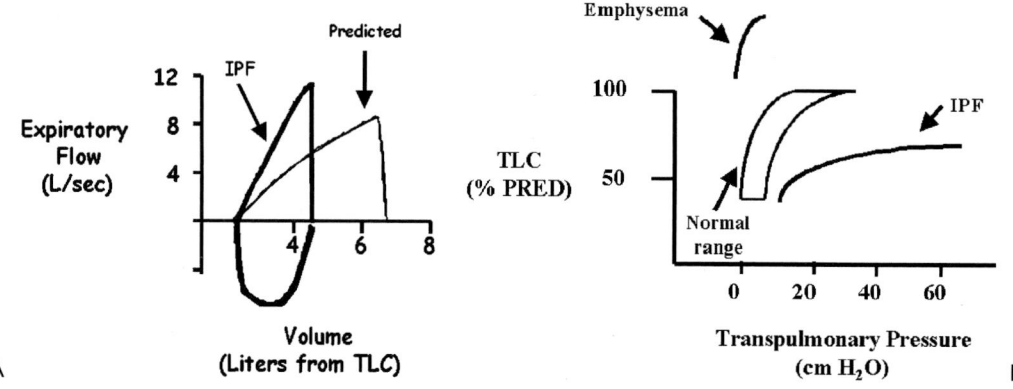

FIGURE 23.3. Maximal expiratory flow volume (MEFV) curve in idiopathic pulmonary fibrosis (IPF). The MEFV curve at presentation of a patient with IPF is shown. The values for the forced expiratory volume in 1 second (FEV_1) and forced vital capacity (FVC) are low relative to the predicted values, but the FEV_1/FVC ratio is increased. However, at any given lung volume, the flow rates are higher than expected because the driving pressure is elevated as a consequence of increased elastic recoil. **Right:** Relationship of the static deflation volume and pressure in a patient with IPF. The percentage of the predicted total lung capacity is plotted against the static transpulmonary pressure (in centimeters of H_2O) for a patient with IPF. The static compliance of the lung (represented by the slope of the pressure-volume curve) is lower than normal.

Lung regions with compliance reduced by either fibrosis or excessive cellularity may be poorly ventilated but still well perfused. The severity of the DLCO reduction does not correlate well with the stage of disease. In some ILDs, especially sarcoidosis, the patient can have considerably reduced lung volumes or severe hypoxemia but a normal or only slightly reduced DLCO. Moderate to severe reductions of the DLCO when lung volumes are normal should suggest ILD with associated emphysema, pulmonary vascular disease, pulmonary histiocytosis X, or lymphangioleiomyomatosis.

Arterial Blood Gases

The resting arterial blood gases may be normal or reveal hypoxemia (secondary to a mismatch of ventilation to perfusion) and respiratory alkalosis. Carbon dioxide retention is rare and usually a manifestation of far-advanced, end-stage disease. Importantly, a normal resting PaO_2 (or O_2 saturation by oximetry) does not rule out significant hypoxemia during exercise or sleep. Furthermore, although hypoxemia with exercise and sleep is very common, secondary erythrocytosis is rarely observed in uncomplicated ILD.

Because resting hypoxemia is not always evident and because severe exercise-induced hypoxemia may go undetected, it is important to perform exercise testing with serial measurement of the arterial blood gases (Fig. 23.4). Arterial oxygen desaturation, a failure to decrease dead space appropriately with exercise (i.e., a high VDS [volume of dead space]/VT [tidal volume] ratio), and an excessive increase in the respiratory rate with a lower than expected recruitment of VT provide useful information regarding physiologic abnormalities and extent of disease. Evidence is increasing that serial assessments of resting and exercise gas exchange are the best way to identify disease activity and responsiveness

to treatment (28,37,38). Oximetry testing is not a reliable method to identify or monitor exercise-induced hypoxemia in patients with ILD.

Bronchoalveolar Lavage

In selected cases, cellular analysis of the bronchoalveolar lavage (BAL) fluid may be useful to narrow the differential diagnostic possibilities between various types of ILD, define the stage of disease, and assess the progression of disease or response to therapy. BAL is useful when malignancy and opportunistic infection are being considered. However, the utility of BAL in the clinical assessment, follow-up, and management of most patients with ILD remains to be established (39–41).

Histopathologic Assessment

In many instances, lung biopsy is indicated because it provides a specific diagnosis that may be difficult to determine from other routine studies (e.g., alveolar proteinosis, sarcoidosis, pulmonary histiocytosis X, respiratory bronchiolitis, lymphangioleiomyomatosis, organizing pneumonia, veno-occlusive disease, vasculitis limited to the lung); occasionally, it identifies a more treatable process than was originally suspected (e.g., hypersensitivity pneumonitis, organizing pneumonia, respiratory bronchiolitis-associated ILD, sarcoidosis) (42). Lung biopsy also excludes neoplastic and infectious processes that occasionally mimic chronic progressive interstitial disease, even when evaluated by physiologic and lung imaging studies. Often, lung biopsy provides the best assessment of disease activity. With a definitive diagnosis, the physician and patient are more comfortable proceeding with therapies that may have serious side effects. Also, a

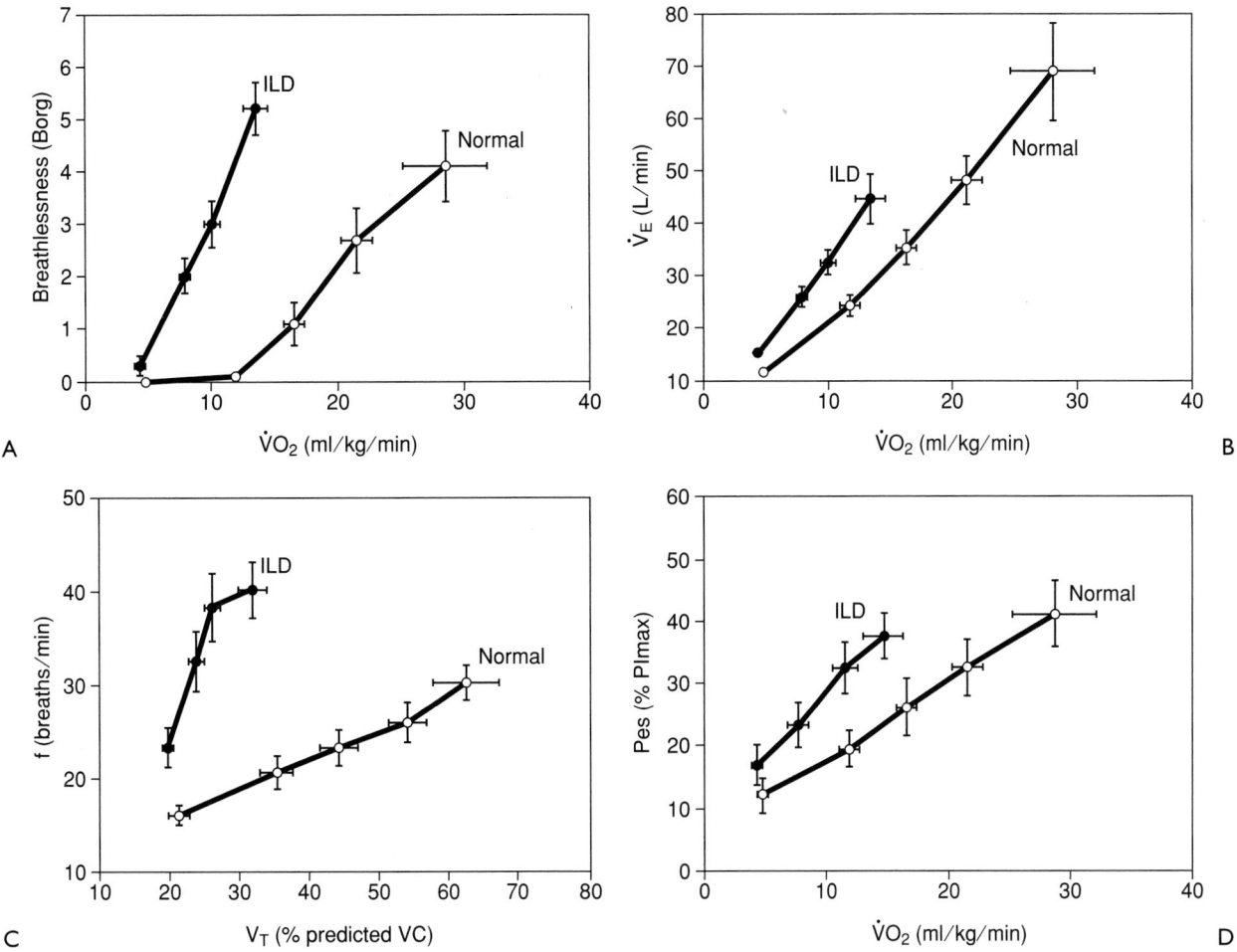

FIGURE 23.4. Responses to exercise in normal subjects and patients with interstitial lung disease (ILD). **A:** Dyspnea. **B:** Minute ventilation ($\dot{V}_E$). **C:** Breathing pattern (breathing frequency [f]). D: Esophageal pressure (*Pes*). Values are means $\pm$ standard error. *Borg*, Borg scale; $\dot{V}_{O_2}$, O_2 uptake; *Vt*, tidal volume; *PI*$_{max}$, maximal inspiratory pressure. All slopes are significantly greater ($P < .05$) in patients with ILD than in normal subjects.

definitive diagnosis prevents confusion (and anxiety) later if the patient is "failing" therapy or experiencing serious side effects of therapy (28). The optimal number, size, and location of lung biopsy specimens depend on the suspected diagnosis and the anatomic distribution of the disease process. The clinician and radiologist should communicate to the thoracic surgeon any specific concerns and suggestions regarding these issues. HRCT may further assist the surgeon in selecting the best location(s) to sample (27,42).

Fiberoptic Bronchoscopy with Transbronchial Lung Biopsy

Fiberoptic bronchoscopy with transbronchial lung biopsy is often the initial procedure of choice, especially when sarcoidosis, lymphangitic carcinomatosis, eosinophilic pneumonia, Goodpasture syndrome, or infection is suspected (41). If a specific diagnosis is not made by transbronchial biopsy, then a surgical lung biopsy is indicated.

Surgical Lung Biopsy

Open lung biopsy is the most definitive method to diagnose and stage the disease so that appropriate prognostic and therapeutic decisions can be made. Open lung biopsy via thoracotomy or video-assisted thoracoscopy is a relatively safe procedure with little morbidity and less than 1% mortality (43). Currently, video-assisted thoracoscopic lung biopsy is the preferred method for obtaining multiple samples of lung tissue for analysis. Relative contraindications to lung biopsy include serious cardiovascular disease, roentgenographic evidence of diffuse end-stage disease (i.e., "honeycombing"), severe pulmonary dysfunction or other major operative risks (especially in elderly patients), and a high likelihood that adequately sized biopsy specimens from multiple sites, usually in two lobes, cannot be obtained (2).

Major Histopathologic Patterns

Several histopathologic patterns found on lung biopsy are useful in confirming the diagnosis; these are described in detail for the individual disorders. Two major histopathologic patterns are seen in ILD. A *granulomatous* process is characterized by an accumulation of T lymphocytes, macrophages, and epithelioid cells organized into discrete structures (granulomas) and results in derangement of the normal tissue architecture (the prototype is sarcoidosis). A chronic *inflammatory and fibrotic process* is characterized by injury to the alveolar walls, changes in the epithelium and thickening of the alveolar walls with fibrosis, and alveolar collapse; it results in marked derangement of the alveolar structures and a loss of functioning alveolar-capillary units (the prototype is usual interstitial pneumonia). Different pathogenetic events take place in other forms of ILD. For example, several diseases are characterized not by inflammation and fibrosis of the alveolar walls but rather by filling of the alveolar space with blood (diffuse alveolar hemorrhage), lipoproteinaceous fluid (alveolar proteinosis), malignant cells (alveolar cell carcinoma), or calcium microliths (alveolar microlithiasis). A hamartomatous proliferation of smooth muscle cells in the alveolar septa, around vessels and lymphatics, and in the pleurae without clearly evident alveolitis is seen in lymphangioleiomyomatosis. Amyloid fibrillary proteins are deposited in the alveolar walls, within the walls of small blood vessels, and in the alveolar capillary basement membrane in pulmonary amyloidosis. In lymphangitic carcinomatosis, tumor cells obstruct both pulmonary lymphatics and muscular pulmonary arteries.

Indications for Referral and Specialized Testing

Patients who have or are suspected of having ILD should be under the direct or joint care of a respiratory physician (7,44) (Table 23.6). The respiratory physician, radiologist, and pathologist (if a lung biopsy has been performed) should meet regularly to evaluate imaging studies and review the histologic findings of patients with diffuse parenchymal lung disease (7,27).

MANAGEMENT OF INTERSTITIAL LUNG DISEASES

The management of most ILDs is difficult, and different approaches may be taken depending on the specific entity (45). Regardless of the cause, end-stage fibrosis is irreversible and untreatable. An extensive and aggressive diagnostic evaluation early on, even in patients with relatively few symptoms, is recommended. Patients with evidence of impaired lung function, progression of disease, or active disease should be treated if no contraindications to therapy exist. Pursuing a diagnosis and instituting appropriate therapy early in the disease course, before extensive fibrosis develops, is likely to improve responsiveness to therapy and, it is hoped, delay or prevent the functional limitation and disability that commonly occur in these patients.

TABLE 23.6. INDICATIONS FOR REFERRAL TO A SUBSPECIALIST

No specific cause of dyspnea or cough can be found.
Symptoms exceed the physiologic or radiographic abnormalities identified.
Empiric management (bronchodilators, diuretics, smoking cessation) has resulted in an atypical or unsatisfactory clinical outcome.
Patient requires impairment or disability evaluation for workers' compensation or another reason.
"Specialized" cardiopulmonary testing is required:
    Fiberoptic bronchoscopy and bronchoalveolar lavage
    Lung tissue to confirm diagnosis (transbronchial, video thoracoscopic, or open lung biopsy)
    Exercise testing with arterial blood gases to determine if physiologic limitation exists and whether its cause is cardiac or pulmonary
    Determination of the pressure-volume relationship in a patient with relatively normal chest x-ray findings or minimal restriction on lung function testing
    Radionuclide scans (e.g., gallium lung scan)
    Catheterization of right side of the heart
    Pulmonary angiography
    Studies of respiratory drive indicated.
Therapeutic immunosuppressive or cytotoxic drug trial is being contemplated.

The major therapies for ILD involve the administration of corticosteroids with or without a cytotoxic agent (cyclophosphamide or azathioprine). More recently, therapies have been aimed at preventing or inhibiting the fibroproliferative response and enhancing normal alveolar reepithelialization. It is hoped that this dual cell targeting will improve outcomes in patients with fibrotic lung disease, especially those with IPF (3).

Many of the patients with ILD are elderly, and the decision to treat elderly patients with immunosuppressive drugs should not be taken lightly because their toxicity and side effects can be substantial. The types and uses of therapy are discussed in the chapters on the specific ILDs.

Quality-of-Life Evaluation

It is important to consider quality of life in an assessment of disease severity and response to therapy in patients with ILD. The sensation of dyspnea and limitations of physical activity are the most important considerations. In addition to dyspnea, other disease-associated factors clearly affect patients' quality of life. The Chronic Respiratory Questionnaire and the St. George's Respiratory Questionnaire evaluate a range of pulmonary symptoms. The SF-36, a short-form health survey with 36 questions, is a generic functional assessment instrument that has been well validated for many chronic illnesses; it has been used to measure HRQL in COPD and correlates well with the Baseline Dyspnea Index. For health outcomes research, a generic instrument such as the SF-36 may be preferred to disease-specific scales for comparing the health states of patients who have pulmonary disease with those of patients who have other chronic conditions. These dyspnea ratings have been shown to correlate with HRQL measurements in patients with IPF (46). It has been assumed that domiciliary oxygen therapy is effective in prolonging survival and improving the quality of life of patients with a diagnosis of ILD and hypoxemia. No data are available to support the assumption that home oxygen therapy has a beneficial effect on survival, but most clinicians believe oxygen therapy has a positive effect on the patient's quality of life (47).

Both dyspnea and quantitative declines in pulmonary function are relevant to the determination of disability. Impairment may be rated by pulmonary function testing, and patients with IPF are much more likely to be impaired, with an FVC of 50% or a D$_{LCO}$ of 40%, than patients with other ILDs.

Indications for Hospitalization and Long-Term Care

Patients with ILD are usually hospitalized because of a sudden worsening of dyspnea or cough. Hospitalization is usually required to rule out or treat acute pneumonia and to manage and monitor the severe hypoxemia that complicates the course of many of these patients. Sudden worsening in association with pleural pain may indicate a spontaneous pneumothorax or pulmonary embolism (45). Few patients with ILD require admission to an intensive care unit during the initial phase of hospitalization (9). Those who do require intensive care for respiratory failure often have associated hemodynamic instability (hypovolemia or sepsis), significant concomitant medical disease (usually cardiovascular disease or renal failure), or severe hypoxemia requiring frequent monitoring of arterial blood gases or mechanical ventilation. Hypercapnia is rare and portends a grave prognosis. Intubation and mechanical ventilation should be introduced only after a careful consideration of the patient's long-term prognosis (48–50). Patients with end-stage lung fibrosis of any cause are difficult to ventilate and are rarely successfully weaned from mechanical ventilation (50). Patients with ILD are rarely candidates for or tolerant of noninvasive ventilation (9).

Many cases of ILD are chronic and irreversible. Consequently, these patients should be encouraged to issue advance directives indicating their wishes with respect to life-sustaining therapies. This issue should be discussed with patients and their families early in the clinical course. Most patients have progressive lung disease and cannot return to full employment after hospital discharge.

Lung transplantation is sometimes offered to patients with end-stage lung fibrosis. It holds promise for young persons without other significant illnesses who have progressive severe disease unresponsive to other forms of treatment. This is a costly procedure, and the guidelines for the selection of patients with ILD for lung transplantation are discussed in Chapter 54.

REFERENCES

1. Schwarz MI, King TE, Jr. *Interstitial lung diseases,* 4th ed. Hamilton, Ontario, Canada: BC Decker, 2003.
2. King TE Jr. Approaches to the patient with interstitial lung diseases. In: Rose BD, ed. *UpToDate.* Wellesley, MA: UpToDate, 2003.
3. Selman M, King TE Jr, Pardo A. Idiopathic pulmonary fibrosis: prevailing and evolving hypotheses about its pathogenesis and implications for therapy. *Ann Intern Med* 2001;134:136–151.
4. Hunninghake GW, Kalica AR. Approaches to the treatment of pulmonary fibrosis. *Am J Respir Crit Care Med* 1995;151:915–918.
5. Coultas DB, Zumwalt RE, Black WC, et al. The epidemiology of interstitial lung disease. *Am J Respir Crit Care Med* 1994;150:967–972.
6. Mannino DM, Etzel RA, Parrish RG. Pulmonary fibrosis deaths in the United States, 1979–1991. An analysis of multiple-cause mortality data. *Am J Respir Crit Care Med* 1996;153:1548–1552.
7. British Thoracic Society. The diagnosis, assessment, and treatment of diffuse parenchymal lung disease in adults. *Thorax* 1999;54[Suppl 1]:S1–S28.
8. Schwarz MI, King TE Jr, Cherniack RM. General principles and diagnostic approach to the interstitial lung diseases. In: Murray JF, Nadel JA, eds. *Textbook of respiratory medicine,* 2nd ed. Philadelphia: WB Saunders, 1994:1803–1826.
9. King TE Jr. Interstitial lung disease. In: Wachter RM, Hollander H, Goldman L, eds. *Hospital medicine.* Philadelphia: Lippincott Williams & Wilkins, 2000:393–404.
10. Wade JF III, King TE Jr. Infiltrative and interstitial lung disease in the elderly. *Clin Chest Med* 1993;14:501–521.
11. Rose C, King TE Jr. Controversies in hypersensitivity pneumonitis. *Am Rev Respir Dis* 1992;145:1–2.
12. Bitterman PB, Rennard SI, Keogh BA, et al. Familial idiopathic pulmonary fibrosis. Evidence of lung inflammation in unaffected family members. *N Engl J Med* 1986;314:1343–1347.
13. Watters LC. Genetic aspects of idiopathic pulmonary fibrosis and hypersensitivity pneumonitis. *Semin Respir Med* 1986;7:317–325.
14. Zitnik RJ, Matthay RA. Drug-induced lung disease. In: Schwarz MI, King TE Jr, eds. *Interstitial lung diseases.* Hamilton, Ontario, Canada: BC Decker, 1998:423–449.
15. Schwartzstein RM. Are you fluent in the 'language' of dyspnea? *J Respir Dis* 1996;17:322–328.
16. Simon PM, Schwartzstein RM, Weiss JW, et al. Distinguishable types of dyspnea in patients with shortness of breath. *Am Rev Respir Dis* 1990;142:1009–1014.
17. O'Donnell DE, Chau LK, Webb KA. Qualitative aspects of exertional dyspnea in patients with interstitial lung disease. *J Appl Physiol* 1998;84:2000–2009.
18. King TE Jr. Interstitial lung diseases: general approaches. In: Parsons PE, Heffner JE, eds. *Pulmonary and respiratory therapy secrets.* Philadelphia: Handley & Belfus, 1997:231–242.
19. Mahler DA, Jones PW. Measurement of dyspnea and quality of life in advanced lung disease. *Clin Chest Med* 1997;18:457–469.
20. Sansores R, Salas J, Chapela R, et al. Clubbing in hypersensitivity pneumonitis. Its prevalence and possible prognostic role. *Arch Intern Med* 1990;150:1849–1851.
21. Scharer L. Clinical description of nail clubbing. *JAMA* 2001;286:1972–1973.
22. Grathwohl KW, Thompson JW, Riordan KK, et al. Digital clubbing associated with polymyositis and interstitial lung disease. *Chest* 1995;108:1751–1752.
23. Kobayashi J, Kitamura S. KL-6: a serum marker for interstitial pneumonia. *Chest* 1995;108:311–315.

24. Hirakata Y, Kobayashi J, Sugama Y, et al. Elevation of tumour markers in serum and bronchoalveolar lavage fluid in pulmonary alveolar proteinosis. *Eur Respir J* 1995;8:689–696.

25. Ohnishi H, Yokoyama A, Kondo K, et al. Comparative study of KL-6, surfactant protein-A, surfactant protein-D, and monocyte chemoattractant protein-1 as serum markers for interstitial lung diseases. *Am J Respir Crit Care Med* 2002;165:378–381.

26. Lynch DA, Newell JD Jr, Lee JS. *Imaging of diffuse lung disease.* Hamilton, Ontario, Canada: BC Decker, 2000:322.

27. American Thoracic Society/European Respiratory Society international multidisciplinary consensus classification of the idiopathic interstitial pneumonias. *Am J Respir Crit Care Med* 2002;165:277–304.

28. American Thoracic Society. Idiopathic pulmonary fibrosis: diagnosis and treatment. International consensus statement. American Thoracic Society (ATS) and the European Respiratory Society (ERS). *Am J Respir Crit Care Med* 2000;161:646–664.

29. Hunninghake G, Zimmerman MB, Schwartz DA, et al. Utility of lung biopsy for the diagnosis of idiopathic pulmonary fibrosis. *Am J Respir Crit Care Med* 2001;164:193–196.

30. Pagniez DC, MacNamara E, Beuscart R, et al. Gallium scan in the follow-up of sarcoid granulomatous nephritis. *Am J Nephrol* 1987;7:326–327.

31. Mochizuki T, Ichijo K, Takehara Y, et al. Gallium-67-citrate scanning in patients with sarcoid uveitis. *J Nucl Med* 1992;33:1851–1853.

32. Mogulkoc N, Brutsche MH, Bishop PW, et al. Pulmonary (99m)Tc-DTPA aerosol clearance and survival in usual interstitial pneumonia (UIP). *Thorax* 2001;56:916–923.

33. Hill C, Romas E, Kirkham B. Use of sequential DTPA clearance and high-resolution computerized tomography in monitoring interstitial lung disease in dermatomyositis. *Br J Rheumatol* 1996;35:164–166.

34. Ishizaka A, Kanazawa M, Suzuki Y, et al. Influence of chest background on pulmonary ^{99m}Tc-DTPA clearance in interstitial lung disease. *J Appl Physiol* 1992;73:1820–1824.

35. Shaw RJ, Djukanovic R, Tashkin DP, et al. The role of small airways in lung disease. *Respir Med* 2002;96:67–80.

36. Hanley ME, King TE Jr, Schwarz MI, et al. The impact of smoking on mechanical properties of the lungs in idiopathic pulmonary fibrosis and sarcoidosis. *Am Rev Respir Dis* 1991;144:1102–1106.

37. King TE Jr, Schwarz MI, Brown K, et al. Idiopathic pulmonary fibrosis. Relationship between histopathologic features and mortality. *Am J Respir Crit Care Med* 2001;164:1025–1032.

38. King TE Jr, Tooze JA, Schwarz MI, et al. Predicting survival in idiopathic pulmonary fibrosis. Scoring system and survival model. *Am J Respir Crit Care Med* 2001;164:1171–1181.

39. Klech H, Pohl W. Technical recommendations and guidelines for bronchoalveolar lavage (BAL). *Eur Respir J* 1989;2:561–585.

40. Klech H, Hutter C. Clinical guidelines and indications for bronchoalveolar lavage (BAL): Report of the European Society of Pneumology Task Force on BAL. *Eur Respir J* 1990;3:937–974.

41. King TE Jr. Interstitial lung disease. In: Feinsilver SH, Fein AM, eds. *Textbook of bronchoscopy.* Baltimore: Williams & Wilkins, 1995:185–220.

42. Collard HR, King TE, Jr. Clinical significance of histopathologic subgroups in the idiopathic interstitial pneumonias: is surgical lung biopsy essential? *Semin Respir Crit Care Med* 2001;22:347–356.

43. Collard HR, King TE Jr. Lung biopsy in patients with usual interstitial pneumonia. *Eur Respir J* 2001;18:895–898.

44. Lok SS. Interstitial lung disease clinics for the management of idiopathic pulmonary fibrosis: a potential advantage to patients. Greater Manchester Lung Fibrosis Consortium. *J Heart Lung Transplant* 1999;18:884–890.

45. Panos RJ, Mortenson R, Niccoli SA, et al. Clinical deterioration in patients with idiopathic pulmonary fibrosis. Causes and assessment. *Am J Med* 1990;88:396–404.

46. Martinez J, Martinez T, Galhardo F, et al. Dyspnea scales as a measure of health-related quality of life in patients with idiopathic pulmonary fibrosis. *Med Sci Monit* 2002;8:CR405–CR410.

47. Crockett AJ, Cranston JM, Antic N. Domiciliary oxygen for interstitial lung disease. *Cochrane Database Syst Rev* 2001;3.

48. Stern JB, Mal H, Groussard O, et al. Prognosis of patients with advanced idiopathic pulmonary fibrosis requiring mechanical ventilation for acute respiratory failure. *Chest* 2001;120:213–219.

49. Fumeaux T, Rothmeier C, Jolliet P. Outcome of mechanical ventilation for acute respiratory failure in patients with pulmonary fibrosis. *Intensive Care Med* 2001;27:1868–1874.

50. Blivet S, Philit F, Sab JM, et al. Outcome of patients with idiopathic pulmonary fibrosis admitted to the ICU for respiratory failure. *Chest* 2001;120:209–212.

Baum's Textbook of Pulmonary Diseases, 7th ed. Edited by James D. Crapo, Jeffrey Glassroth, Joel Karlinsky, and Talmadge E. King, Jr.
Lippincott Williams & Wilkins, Philadelphia © 2004.

Idiopathic Interstitial Pneumonias

24

Sonoko Nagai · Masanori Kitaichi

The idiopathic interstitial pneumonias (IIPs) are a heterogeneous group of entities with overlapping clinical, radiographic, physiologic, and pathologic features. Liebow (1) described the first extensive histopathologic findings in these diseases (Table 24.1). Katzenstein (2) defined the term *interstitial pneumonias* as follows:

"... A diffuse, inflammatory, and often fibrosing process that occurs predominantly within interstices or supporting structures of the lung, as opposed to a lesion in which the predominant reaction takes place within alveolar lumens. The process is usually not exclusively interstitial, however, since some air space abnormalities almost always accompany the interstitial changes; moreover, sophisticated techniques have demonstrated that many processes that appear mainly interstitial by light microscopy actually begin within air spaces."

Usual interstitial pneumonia (UIP) is now recognized to carry a poor prognosis, whereas other histologic patterns of chronic pulmonary fibrosis, such as nonspecific interstitial pneumonia (NSIP), have a more favorable prognosis. The general approach to the diagnosis of interstitial lung disease is described in Chapter 23.

NEW AMERICAN THORACIC SOCIETY/EUROPEAN RESPIRATORY SOCIETY MULTIDISCIPLINARY CLASSIFICATION OF IDIOPATHIC INTERSTITIAL PNEUMONIAS

As a group, the IIPs can be distinguished from other forms of diffuse parenchymal lung disease by a careful consideration of the patient's clinical history, physical examina-

tion findings, chest radiographs, laboratory studies, and lung pathology (3). The new classification comprises the following clinicopathologic entities (in order of relative frequency): idiopathic pulmonary fibrosis (IPF), nonspecific interstitial pneumonia (NSIP), cryptogenic organizing pneumonia (COP), acute interstitial pneumonia (AIP), respiratory bronchiolitis–associated interstitial lung disease (RB-ILD), desquamative interstitial pneumonia (DIP), and lymphocytic interstitial pneumonia (LIP) (Table 24.2).

GENERAL CONSIDERATIONS IN THE DIAGNOSIS OF IDIOPATHIC INTERSITIAL PNEUMONIAS

Epidemiology

Few studies have examined the incidence or prevalence of the IIPs. However, in the case of IPF, the disease incidence has been reported to range from less than 5 to 20.2 per 100,000 males and 13.2 per 100,000 females in the general populations (4,5).

Clinical Presentation

The IIPs can be detected either by diffuse interstitial opacities on chest radiographs or by symptoms such as exertional dyspnea and dry cough. The mode of onset is classified as acute (symptoms or signs lasting from days to weeks), subacute (symptoms or signs for weeks to months), or chronic (symptoms or signs for longer than 1 year). In chronic cases, an acute exacerbation can occur at any time during the clinical course.

Pulmonary Function Testing

Pulmonary function tests commonly show a restrictive dysfunction (reduced vital capacity, reduced total lung capacity,

S. Nagai: Department of Respiratory Medicine, Kyoto University Hospital.
M. Kitaichi: Department of Anatomical Pathology, Kyoto University Hospital, Kyoto, Japan.

TABLE 24.1. PREVIOUS CLASSIFICATIONS OF IDIOPATHIC INTERSTITIAL PNEUMONIAS

Liebow and Carrington (1969)[a]: Chronic Forms	Katzenstein (1997)[b]	Müller and Colby (1997)[c]
Usual interstitial pneumonia	Usual interstitial pneumonia	Usual interstitial pneumonia
Desquamative interstitial pneumonia	Desquamative interstitial pneumonia/ respiratory bronchiolitis interstitial lung disease	Desquamative interstitial pneumonia
Bronchiolitis obliterans interstitial pneumonia and diffuse alveolar damage		Bronchiolitis obliterans–organizing pneumonia
	Acute interstitial pneumonia	Acute interstitial pneumonia
	Nonspecific interstitial pneumonia	Nonspecific interstitial pneumonia
Lymphoid interstitial pneumonia		
Giant cell interstitial pneumonia		

[a]Liebow AA, Carrington CB. The interstitial pneumonias. In: Simon M, Potchen EJ, LeMay M, eds. *Frontiers of pulmonary radiology,* 1st ed. New York: Grune & Stratton, 1969:102–141.
[b]Katzenstein AL. Idiopathic interstitial pneumonia: classification and diagnosis. In: Katzenstein AL, Askin FB, eds. *Surgical pathology of nonneoplastic lung disease.* Philadelphia: WB Saunders, 1997:1–31.
[c]Müller NL, Colby TV. Idiopathic interstitial pneumonias: high-resolution CT and histologic findings. *Radiographics* 1997;17:1016–1022.
Source: From American Thoracic Society/European Respiratory Society international multidisciplinary consensus classification of the idiopathic interstitial pneumonias. *Am J Respir Crit Care Med* 2002;165:277–304, with permission.

increased ratio of the forced expiratory volume in 1 second to the forced vital capacity [FEV_1/FVC]), a reduction in diffusing capacity, and hypoxemia at rest or during exercise.

Chest Imaging Studies

The radiologic features include diffuse interstitial (reticular or nodular) opacities on routine chest radiographs and several nonspecific features on computed tomography (CT), such as reticular or nodular opacities, ground-glass opacities, air space consolidation, traction bronchiectasis, and cystic changes or honeycombing. The distribution of lesions in the lungs may be patchy or diffuse.

High-resolution CT (HRCT) has become an integral part of the evaluation of patients with IIPs (3). When the chest radiograph shows diffuse interstitial opacities and other clinical examination findings support the presence of interstitial pneumonia, HRCT can reveal more critical information: the distribution of the lesions (diffuse, patchy, subpleural, along the bronchovascular bundle), their quality (air space consolidation, ground-glass opacities, traction bronchiectasis, cystic changes with or without honeycombing), and their extent (mild, moderate, severe).

When interpreting the HRCT scan of a patient with diffuse lung disease, the radiologist must first determine the presence or absence of a pattern typical of UIP (Fig. 24.1). In approximately 30% to 50% of cases suspected to be IPF/UIP, the clinical and HRCT features of UIP are sufficiently characteristic that a diagnosis can be made confidently without a lung biopsy. HRCT may also provide clues to non-IIP disorders. Therefore, the primary role of HRCT is to separate patients with UIP from those with non-UIP lesions and those with less specific findings associated with other IIPs (3).

TABLE 24.2. NEW AMERICAN THORACIC SOCIETY/EUROPEAN RESPIRATORY SOCIETY HISTOLOGIC AND CLINICAL CLASSIFICATION OF IDIOPATHIC INTERSTITIAL PNEUMONIAS

Histologic Patterns	Clinical-Radiologic-Pathologic Diagnosis
Usual interstitial pneumonia	Idiopathic pulmonary fibrosis/cryptogenic fibrosing alveolitis
Nonspecific interstitial pneumonia	Nonspecific interstitial pneumonia (provisional)[a]
Organizing pneumonia	Cryptogenic organizing pneumonia[b]
Diffuse alveolar damage	Acute interstitial pneumonia
Respiratory bronchiolitis	Respiratory bronchiolitis–associated interstitial lung disease
Desquamative interstitial pneumonia	Desquamative interstitial pneumonia
Lymphoid interstitial pneumonia	Lymphoid interstitial pneumonia

[a]This is a heterogeneous group with poorly characterized clinical and radiologic features that require further study.
[b]Cryptogenic organizing pneumonia is the preferred term, but it is synchronous with idiopathic bronchiolitis obliterans–organizing pneumonia. Unclassifiable interstitial pneumonia: Some cases are unclassifiable for a variety of reasons (see text).
Source: From American Thoracic Society/European Respiratory Society international multidisciplinary consensus classification of the idiopathic interstitial pneumonias. *Am J Respir Crit Care Med* 2002;165:277–304, with permission.

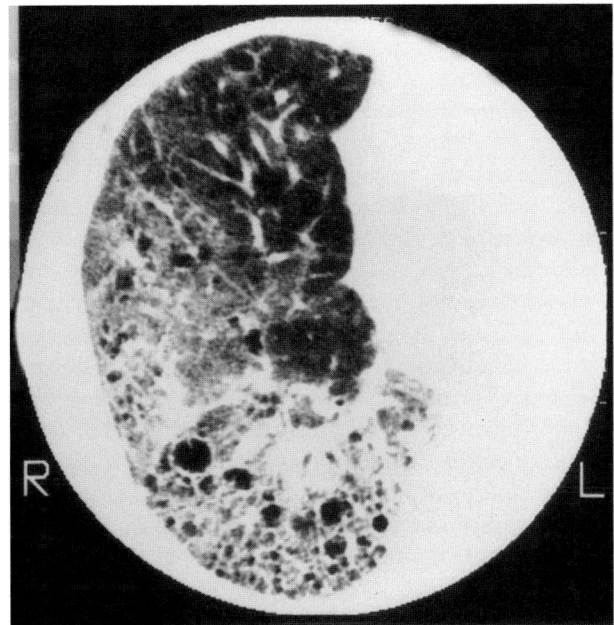 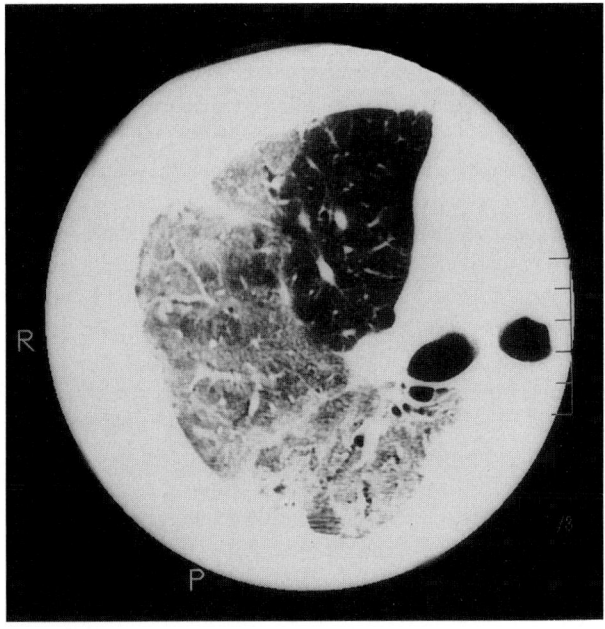

FIGURE 24.1. Appearance of idiopathic interstitial pneumonia on high-resolution computed tomography. **A:** Usual interstitial pneumonia pattern in a patient with idiopathic pulmonary fibrosis. Subpleural cystic changes (honeycombing) and minimal ground-glass opacities. **B:** Nonspecific interstitial pneumonia pattern. Diffuse ground-glass opacities with traction bronchiectasis. Subpleural honeycombing is absent.

Role of Bronchoalveolar Lavage

In the American Thoracic Society (ATS)/European Respiratory Society (ERS) statement, bronchoalveolar lavage (BAL) is not considered imperative for the assessment of all cases of IIP (3) (Table 24.3). The primary use of BAL is to exclude infection, tumor, asbestosis, and other specific diseases, such as alveolar lipoproteinosis (6). The BAL fluid cell profile is strongly influenced by the smoking status; hence, it is difficult to differentiate IIPs in patients with a current smoking habit. Lymphocytosis is characteristically not found in patients with IPF/UIP throughout the clinical course (7,8). In

our experience, BAL fluid cell lymphocytosis, especially an increase in the number of $CD8^+$ T cells, tends to be related to non–UIP-type IIPs and pulmonary fibrosis with temporal homogeneity (9).

Role of Lung Biopsy and Histopathologic Assessment

The role of transbronchial lung biopsy in the diagnosis of IIPs is usually to exclude sarcoidosis, hypersensitivity pneumonitis, neoplasms, alveolar lipoproteinosis, and certain

TABLE 24.3. BRONCHOALVEOLAR LAVAGE FLUID CELLS IN NONSPECIFIC INTERSTITIAL PNEUMONIA AND USUAL INTERSTITIAL PNEUMONIA

Study (Reference)	Lymphocytes (%)		Neutrophils (%)		Eosinophils (%)	
	UIP	NSIP	UIP	NSIP	UIP	NSIP
Nagai et al. (33)	7	37	6	8	3	6
Daniil et al. (35)	8	9	10	8	6	3
Park et al. (51)	3	25	5	12	3	2
Suga et al. (52)	7	21	3	7	2	3

Note: Data are mean values, given as the percentage of total cells.
UIP, usual interstitial pneumonia; NSIP, nonspecific interstitial pneumonia.
Source: Nagai S, Kitaichi M, Itoh H, et al. Idiopathic nonspecific interstitial pneumonia/fibrosis: comparison with idiopathic pulmonary fibrosis and BOOP. *Eur Respir J* 1998;12:1010–1019; Daniil ZD, Gilchrist FC, Nicholson AG, et al. A histologic pattern of nonspecific interstitial pneumonia is associated with a better prognosis than usual interstitial pneumonia in patients with cryptogenic fibrosing alveolitis. *Am J Respir Crit Care Med* 1999;160:899–905; Park CS, Chung SW, Ki SY, et al. Increased levels of interleukin-6 are associated with lymphocytosis in bronchoalveolar lavage fluids of idiopathic nonspecific interstitial pneumonia. *Am J Respir Crit Care Med* 2000;162:1162–1168; Suga M, Iyonaga K, Okamoto T, et al. Characteristic elevation of matrix metalloproteinase activity in idiopathic interstitial pneumonias. *Am J Respir Crit Care Med* 2000;162:1949–1956.

infections. In patients with IIPs, an organizing pneumonia pattern or an organizing diffuse alveolar damage pattern may be detected in the transbronchial biopsy specimens (3). Generally, therefore, transbronchial lung biopsy should be performed before a surgical lung biopsy is undertaken in a patient in whom a clinical-radiologic analysis suggests the possibility of IIPs.

The most important reason for performing a surgical lung biopsy in a patient with ILD is to determine a reasonable treatment option and exclude such conditions as infection, malignancy, and occupational lung disease. A surgical lung biopsy is necessary for a confident clinical-pathologic diagnosis in all cases of IIP not manifesting the typical clinical-radiologic features of IPF/UIP (3). Surgical lung biopsy should be performed before treatment is undertaken to obtain an accurate diagnosis because the histologic findings are nonspecific and can change during treatment and evolution of the inflammatory processes (3).

For patients in whom IPF/UIP is highly likely, it is better to make the diagnosis without a surgical lung biopsy. In a prospective trial of 59 consecutive patients with new-onset untreated disease, Raghu and colleagues (10) concluded that not all patients with new-onset IPF require surgical lung biopsy for a diagnosis, but that a diagnosis of IPF will be missed in nearly one third of cases of new-onset IPF despite evaluation by experts. In this same study, the relatively low sensitivity and specificity for the diagnosis of ILDs other than IPF also strongly suggest that a surgical lung biopsy is indicated in patients with ILD in whom the diagnosis is unclear. In a blinded, prospective study, Hunninghake and colleagues (11) suggested that patients can reasonably be spared lung biopsy if an assessment of the clinical-radiologic

data by experienced pulmonologists and radiologists confidently supports a diagnosis of IPF. However, lung biopsy was very important for patients with an uncertain diagnosis and those in whom IPF was unlikely. In this study, approximately 85% of core pathologic analyses were in agreement regarding the presence or absence of IPF. A specific diagnosis may be difficult in approximately 15% to 20% of patients with ILDs, even when a surgical lung biopsy is performed.

Pathologically, the interstitial pneumonias exhibit either temporal homogeneity or heterogeneity in appearance. In addition, the distribution of the lesions may be patchy or diffuse. The presence or absence of honeycomb cystic changes with destruction of normal parenchymal structures, organization within air spaces, or hyaline membrane formation is important in the differentiation of the individual interstitial pneumonias. These differential points are summarized in Table 24.4 and illustrated in Figure 24.2.

Achieving a correct diagnosis in a patient with findings suggestive of an ILD is a dynamic process. A clinical-radiologic-physiologic approach is always required for differentiation, and histologic differentiation may be essential for a proper diagnosis in many settings. Accordingly, the new ATS/ERS classification defines a set of histologic patterns that provides the basis for a final clinical-radiologic-pathologic diagnosis (Table 24.5). The possibility of sarcoidosis, hypersensitivity pneumonitis, collagen-vascular diseases, drug-induced interstitial pneumonias, occupation-related diseases, infectious processes, and malignancy should be eliminated before it is concluded that a case is idiopathic (3) (Fig. 24.3).

TABLE 24.4. HISTOPATHOLOGIC FEATURES OF IDIOPATHIC INTERSTITIAL PNEUMONIAS

Histopathologic Feature	AIP/DAD	OP/BOOP	NSIP	RB-ILD	DIP	LIP	IPF/UIP
Distribution of lesions	Diffuse	Patchy	Diffuse or patchy	Patchy	Diffuse	Diffuse	Patchy
Hyaline membrane	Present	Absent	Absent	Absent	Absent	Absent	Absent
BOOP	Absent or present	Prominent	Occasional	Absent	Absent	Absent	Absent
Alveolar inflammation	Present	Present	Present	Present	Present	Present	Present
Accumulation of macrophages	Absent or present	Absent	Occasional	Marked	Marked	Occasional	Present (focal areas)
Fibroblastic foci	Diffuse	Intra-alveolar organization	Occasional	Absent	Absent	Absent	Many, usually adjacent to dense fibrosis
Degree of fibrosis	Loose	Loose	Loose or dense	Loose	Loose	Loose	Dense
Interstitial pneumonitis	Mild to prominent	Absent	Mild to prominent	Absent/mild	Mild	Absent/present	Present
Remodeling	Absent/present	Absent	Absent to moderately prominent	Absent/present	Absent/present	Absent/present	Prominent
Honeycomb changes	Absent/present	Absent	Occasional	Absent	Occasional	Occasional	Prominent
Temporal appearance of fibrosis	Homogeneous	Homogeneous	Homogeneous	Homogeneous	Homogeneous	Homogeneous	Heterogeneous

AIP, acute interstitial pneumonia; BOOP, bronchiolitis obliterans–organizing pneumonia; DAD, diffuse alveolar damage; DIP, desquamative interstitial pneumonia; IPF, idiopathic pulmonary fibrosis; LIP, lymocytic interstitial pneumonia; NSIP, nonspecific interstitial pneumonia; RB-ILD, respiratory bronchiolitis–associated interstitial lung disease; UIP, usual interstitial pneumonia.

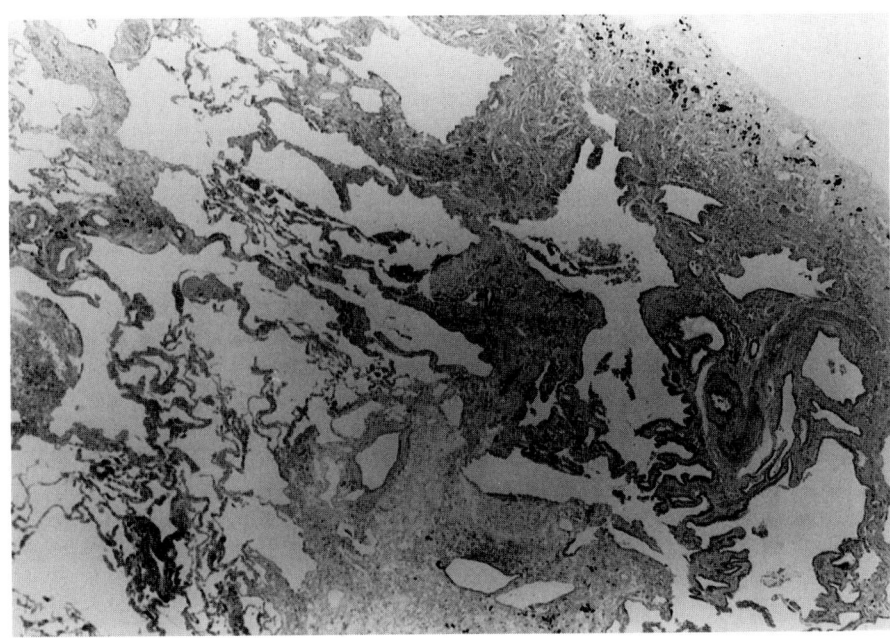

A

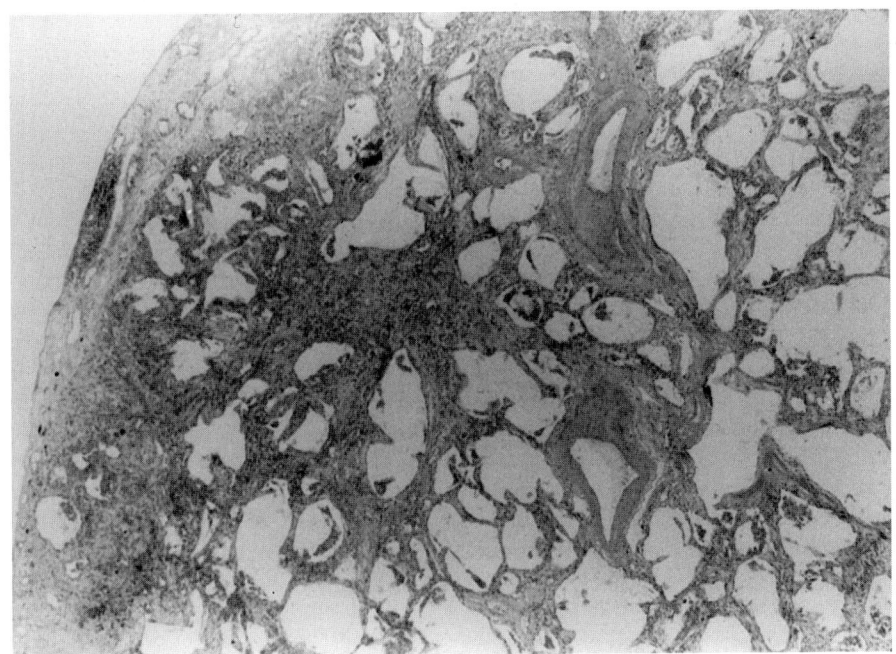

B

FIGURE 24.2. Histologic patterns of idiopathic interstitial pneumonias. **A:** Usual interstitial pneumonia pattern (hematoxylin and eosin). Patchy fibrotic lesions are noted predominantly in the subpleural regions intermingled with normal alveolar walls. The subpleural fibrosis is dense, with smooth muscle proliferation and honeycombing. A few scattered fibroblastic foci are observed. **B:** Nonspecific interstitial pneumonia pattern (hematoxylin and eosin). The interstitial fibrotic changes are diffuse, with multifocal loss of normal alveolar structures caused by fibrotic processes. Granulation tissues in the terminal air spaces are few in number.

Treatment of the Idiopathic Interstitial Pneumonias

Treatments for the IIPs are not well established, partly because of the variety of lesions associated with the IIPs and partly because of the different complications that arise during the progression of disease. The current consensus is that a novel treatment is warranted for patients with IPF/UIP. In the non–UIP-type IIPs, corticosteroids may be expected to have a therapeutic effect, especially when therapy is given relatively early to patients with non-UIP lesions. However, the therapeutic efficacy may depend on differences in the quality and degree of pulmonary fibrosis among the IIPs (Table 24.5).

IDIOPATHIC PULMONARY FIBROSIS

In the 1970s, IPF came to be recognized as a chronic form of IIP, and the Hamman-Rich syndrome came to be seen as an acute form of IIP. In the United Kingdom, IPF was known as *cryptogenic fibrosing alveolitis* (12). The ATS/ERS statement provides criteria for the diagnosis of IPF in the absence of a surgical lung biopsy (Table 24.6).

Clinical Manifestations

The typical patient is 50 to 70 years old and has a history of progressive dyspnea for months to years and a chronic

TABLE 24.5. CLINICAL–RADIOLOGIC–IMMUNOLOGIC–PATHOLOGIC PROFILES OF THE IDIOPATHIC INTERSTITIAL PNEUMONIAS

Disease	Pathologic Pattern	Quality of Fibrosis	BAL Fluid Cell Profiles	HRCT Patterns	Mode of Onset	Prognosis
AIP	DAD	Temporally homogeneous	Neutrophil predominance	Air space consolidation, ground-glass opacities, traction bronchiectasis	Acute	Unfavorable
COP/BOOP	OP	Temporally homogeneous	CD8+ T-cell predominance	Air space consolidation, ground-glass opacities	Subacute	Favorable
NSIP	NSIP	Temporally homogeneous	CD8+ T-cell predominance	Ground-glass opacities, traction bronchiectasis, (air space consolidation, honeycomb changes)	Subacute or chronic	Favorable
DIP	DIP	Temporally homogeneous	Macrophage predominance	Ground-glass opacities, cystic (honeycomb changes)	Chronic	Favorable
RB-ILD	RB	Temporally homogeneous	Macrophage predominance	Centrilobular nodules, ground-glass opacities	Chronic	Favorable
LIP	LIP	Temporally homogeneous	Lymphocyte predominance	Ground-glass opacities, cystic changes	Chronic	Favorable
IPF	UIP	Temporally heterogeneous	No lymphocytosis	Honeycomb changes, traction bronchiectasis, localized ground-glass opacities	Chronic	Unfavorable

AIP, acute interstitial pneumonia; BAL, bronchoalveolar lavage; BOOP, bronchiolitis obliterans–organizing pneumonia; COP, cryptogenic organizing pneumonia; DAD, diffuse alveolar damage; DIP, desquamative interstitial pneumonia; HRCT, high-resolution computed tomography; IPF, idiopathic pulmonary fibrosis; LIP, lymphocytic interstitial pneumonia; NSIP, nonspecific interstitial pneumonia; RB-ILD, respiratory bronchiolitis–associated interstitial lung disease; UIP, usual interstitial pneumonia.

nonproductive cough. The physical examination commonly reveals bilateral basilar fine inspiratory crackles and may show digital clubbing. Pulmonary function testing commonly reveals restrictive lung disease and abnormal gas exchange.

The characteristic HRCT findings include patchy, predominantly basilar, subpleural reticular abnormalities, an absence or limited extent of ground-glass abnormalities, traction bronchiectasis, and honeycombing. A confident HRCT diagnosis of UIP is based on a bilateral, predominantly

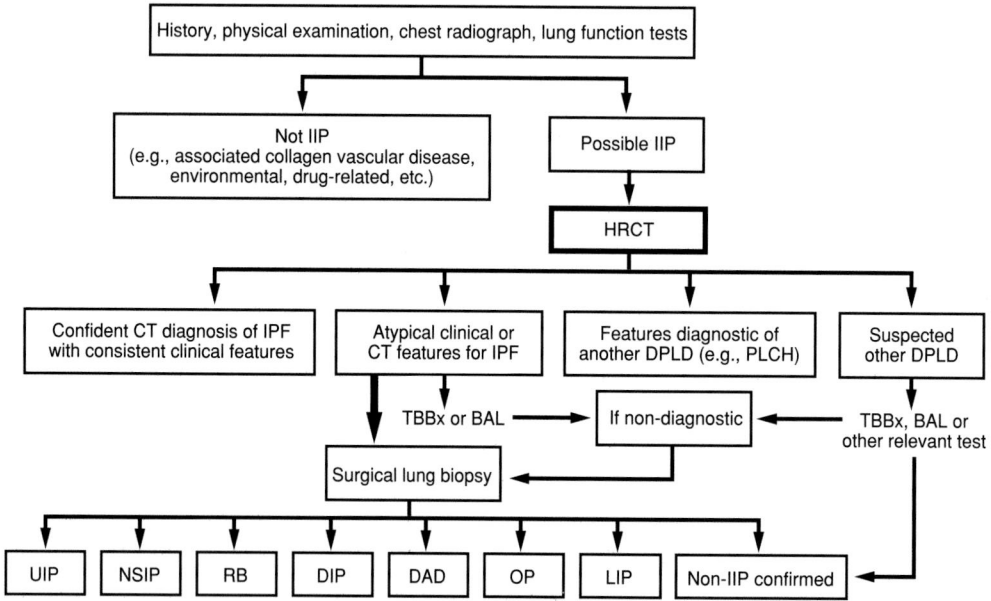

FIGURE 24.3. Diagnostic process in interstitial lung diseases. *IIP,* idiopathic interstitial pneumonia; *CT,* computed tomography; *DPLD,* diffuse parenchymal lung disease; *PLCH,* pulmonary Langerhans' cell histiocytosis; *TBBx,* transbronchial biopsy; see Table 24.5 for definitions of other abbreviations. (*Source:* From American Thoracic Society/European Respiratory Society international multidisciplinary consensus classification of the idiopathic interstitial pneumonias. *Am J Resp Crit Care Med* 2002;165:277–304, with permission.)

TABLE 24.6. CRITERIA SUPPORTING THE CLINICAL DIAGNOSIS OF IDIOPATHIC PULMONARY FIBROSIS

Major criteria (must have all four)
1. Exclusion of other known causes of ILD (e.g., certain drug toxicities, environmental exposures, and connective tissue diseases)
2. Abnormal pulmonary function studies that include evidence of restriction (reduced VC, often with an increased FEV_1/FVC ratio) and impaired gas exchange (increased alveolar-arterial Po_2 gradient with rest or exercise or decreased D_{LCO})
3. Bilateral basilar reticular abnormalities with minimal ground-glass opacities on HRCT scans
4. No transbronchial lung biopsy or bronchoalveolar lavage features to support an alternative diagnosis

Minor criteria (must have at least three of four)
1. Age older than 50 years
2. Insidious onset of otherwise unexplained dyspnea on exertion
3. Duration of illness longer than 3 months
4. Bilateral basilar, inspiratory crackles (dry or "Velcro" type in quality)

D_{LCO}, diffusing capacity of lung for carbon monoxide; FEV_1, forced expiratory volume in 1 second; FVC, forced vital capacity; HRCT, high-resolution computed tomography; ILD, interstitial lung disease.
Source: Adapted from King TE Jr, Costabel U, Cordier J-F, et al. Idiopathic pulmonary fibrosis: diagnosis and treatment. International consensus statement. American Thoracic Society (ATS) and European Respiratory Society (ERS). *Am J Respir Crit Care Med* 2000;161:646–664, with permission.

subpleural reticular pattern that is associated with subpleural cysts (honeycombing) and traction bronchiectasis. The abnormalities gradually become less pronounced on serial scans from the bases to the apices of the lungs. Consolidation and nodules are absent. A radiographic diagnosis of UIP based on these findings is correct in more than 90% of cases (10). A thorough clinical assessment in the diagnosis of new-onset IPF is highly specific (97%) but relatively insensitive (62%); the HRCT features alone have a specificity of 90% but a sensitivity of only 78.5% (10,11).

Histopathologic Findings

The UIP pattern is the histopathologic pattern of IPF. UIP is characterized by a heterogeneous, predominantly subpleural distribution of lesions and temporal heterogeneity, with areas of end-stage fibrosis and honeycombing seen next to areas of active fibroblastic proliferation (fibroblastic foci) and normal lung tissue. Interstitial inflammation is generally minimal, suggesting a primarily fibroproliferative process.

Treatment of Idiopathic Pulmonary Fibrosis/Usual Interstitial Pneumonia

IPF progresses in a relentless and often insidious manner and may be difficult to detect by symptomatology, chest radiographic findings, and spirometry alone (6). Various studies have found a mean survival of 2 to 4 years, far shorter than previously reported (13–16). In IPF/UIP, unfavorable prognostic factors include an absence of BAL fluid lymphocytosis,

a minimum of ground-glass opacities on HRCT with honeycombing at subpleural areas, and variegated fibrosis with temporal heterogeneity and active fibroblastic foci. These findings support the concept that the critical pathway to end-stage fibrosis is not alveolitis but rather the ongoing process of epithelial damage and repair associated with persistent fibroblastic proliferation (17,18). In this regard, we have demonstrated that the histopathologic scores and findings in the early stages of the process are similar to those in the later stages of IPF/UIP (19,20). No pharmacologic therapy has been unequivocally shown to alter or reverse the inflammatory process, and all currently available therapeutic trials are severely limited by uncertainty regarding the natural history of IPF (6,20).

Although no prospective randomized double-blinded placebo-controlled trials have evaluated the efficacy of *corticosteroids* (6), it is widely known that corticosteroid treatment is associated with substantial morbidity in patients with IPF (21). However, patients whose disease remains stable or responds to corticosteroid therapy have a better chance of survival than nonresponders, although whether this difference reflects an effect of treatment or simply less severe disease must be determined in a randomized trial.

Azathioprine or *cyclophosphamide* has been used for steroid nonresponders, patients experiencing serious adverse effects of corticosteroid treatment, and patients at high risk for complications of corticosteroid treatment (22). The combination of azathioprine or cyclophosphamide and corticosteroids has been shown to result in modest improvement and enhanced survival in some patients (22,23). High-dose pulse cyclophosphamide therapy did not have any significant effect on refractory IPF in open trials (24).

Among candidate antifibrotic drugs, *colchicine* has been investigated in a number of studies. Although the efficacy of colchicine has not been established, it appears to be approximately as effective as corticosteroids and without any serious adverse effects (25,26).

In an open, randomized trial performed by Ziesche and colleagues (27), the administration of *interferon-γ-1b* for 1 year in combination with low-dose prednisolone resulted in a greater improvement in pulmonary function than prednisolone alone ($P < .001$).

It has also been reported that *pirfenidone,* a novel antifibrotic drug, may reduce the morbidity and slow progression of advanced IPF (28).

The most frequent cause of death in patients with IPF is respiratory failure (40%); other IPF-associated complications include pulmonary hypertension (30%), heart failure, infection, lung cancer, and pulmonary embolism. In a population-based cohort study of 890 subjects with cryptogenic fibrosing alveolitis and 5,884 control subjects, the incidence of lung cancer was increased in patients with cryptogenic fibrosing alveolitis (relative risk [RR] = 8.25, $P < .001$), and this increase was independent of the effects of cigarette smoking (29).

Indicators of longer survival in patients with IPF include the following: (a) younger age (<50 years) at presentation, (b) female sex, (c) shorter symptomatic period (<1 year) with less dyspnea and relatively preserved lung function, (d) ground-glass and reticular opacities on HRCT, (e) a beneficial response or disease stabilization at 3 to 6 months after initial corticosteroid therapy, and (f) a current smoking habit at the time of diagnosis (30). One study further identified the clinical, radiologic, and physiologic determinants of survival in 238 patients with biopsy-confirmed UIP/IPF; based on the results, the authors introduced a clinical-radiologic-pathologic scoring system for predicting survival in newly diagnosed cases of IPF (31). Using Cox proportional hazard models, they demonstrated that survival was related to age, smoking status (survival was increased in current smokers), clubbing, the extent of interstitial opacities, pulmonary hypertension on chest radiographs, reduced lung volume, and abnormal gas exchange during maximal exercise.

NONSPECIFIC INTERSTITIAL PNEUMONIA

Idiopathic NSIP includes cases of IIP that do not fit into any of the well-defined histologic patterns of IIP. The concept of NSIP has helped to identify a group of IIPs with a better prognosis that must be distinguished from IPF/UIP and also from DIP, AIP, and COP/BOOP (bronchiolitis obliterans–organizing pneumonia) (13,14,32–35). The disease entity of idiopathic NSIP is still being evaluated intensively.

Clinical Findings

Patients typically present between the ages of 40 and 50 years with chronic dyspnea and cough. The duration of symptoms is generally shorter (<6 months) than in IPF. Bilateral basilar fine inspiratory crackles are common, and fever and finger clubbing may occur. Pulmonary function testing shows a restrictive pattern, similar to that seen in IPF. HRCT reveals a predominance of ground-glass abnormalities, most commonly bilateral and subpleural in distribution and associated with volume loss in the lower lobes. Patchy areas of air space consolidation and reticular abnormalities may be present. Honeycombing is unusual.

Histopathologic Findings

NSIP is characterized by varying degrees of inflammation and fibrosis, with some biopsy specimens showing a predominance of inflammatory changes ("cellular" pattern) and others a predominantly fibrotic reaction ("fibrotic" pattern). Although the NSIP pattern may exhibit significant fibrosis, it is usually temporally uniform, and fibroblastic foci and honeycombing, if present, are rare. The temporal uniformity is distinctly different from the temporal heterogeneity of the UIP pattern. However, it can be difficult to distinguish the fibrotic NSIP pattern from the UIP pattern reliably.

Treatment

No prospective data regarding treatment response are available. Retrospective reviews have suggested a generally favorable response to corticosteroids, especially in patients with a primarily cellular NSIP pattern. Several excellent retrospective studies suggest a 5-year survival of 70% to 90% in NSIP (14,15).

CRYPTOGENIC ORGANIZING PNEUMONIA

In the 1980s, Davison and colleagues (36) described the clinicopathologic disease entity known as *COP*. In 1985, Epler and colleagues (37) proposed the same entity under the term *BOOP*. The term *idiopathic BOOP* came into common use to describe cases that presented with a pneumonia-like illness and alveolar opacities on chest radiographs. These patients had a subacute onset of symptoms such as fever, cough, and exertional dyspnea. The process was usually unresponsive to antibiotic therapy. The term *COP* is preferred because it describes the essential pattern of the organizing pneumonia— organization within alveoli, alveolar ducts, and bronchioles with or without organization within bronchioles (polypoid bronchiolitis obliterans). COP/BOOP is discussed in Chapter 29.

ACUTE INTERSTITIAL PNEUMONIA

In 1986, Katzenstein and colleagues (38) proposed the term *AIP* to denote an acute form of IIP, replacing the designation *Hamman-Rich syndrome,* which encompassed both the acute-on-chronic (acute exacerbation of IPF) and acute forms of IIP. Histopathology reveals diffuse alveolar damage, which is a common histopathologic pattern of acute lung injury and the typical finding in patients with acute respiratory distress syndrome (ARDS). The term *AIP* is reserved for cases of unknown cause. Although many have considered AIP fatal, Olson and colleagues (39) showed that nearly 40% of patients with AIP survive.

Clinical Findings

AIP is an acute form of IIP generally characterized by a rapid progression to respiratory failure within days to weeks. The mean age at presentation is 50 years. The patient presents with dyspnea and cough that have developed during a few days to weeks. Fever is occasionally present. Many patients report a viral prodrome consisting of myalgias and upper respiratory symptoms. Diffuse inspiratory crackles are common. Pulmonary function testing shows a restrictive pattern associated with hypoxemia. HRCT reveals ground-glass abnormalities and consolidation, predominantly basilar but often throughout all the lung fields. In early stages of AIP, involvement may be patchy, whereas more advanced cases show diffuse abnormalities. Honeycombing is rarely seen but may be present in advanced cases.

Histopathologic Findings

Diffuse alveolar damage comprises two histopathologic stages: (a) The acute stage is characterized by edema, epithelial necrosis and sloughing, fibrinous exudates in the air spaces, and hyaline membrane formation. The process is usually widespread and temporally uniform. (b) Features of the organizing stage are proliferation of type II pneumocytes, resolution of hyaline membranes and alveolar exudates, and fibroblastic proliferation. Thrombi are commonly present in the small- to medium-sized vessels. This organizing stage is the pattern most often noted at the time of surgical lung biopsy in patients with AIP. With time, end-stage fibrosis develops, and large cystic air spaces are seen to be lined with alveolar epithelium, in contrast to the bronchial epithelium seen in the honeycomb spaces associated with the UIP pattern.

Treatment

No proven treatment for AIP is available. Most reported cases received corticosteroids and antibiotic therapy without any clear benefit. Survival in AIP is worse than in ARDS, with a mortality of more than 50% reported in the literature.

RESPIRATORY BRONCHIOLITIS–ASSOCIATED INTERSTITIAL LUNG DISEASE AND DESQUAMATIVE INTERSTITIAL PNEUMONIA

Myers and colleagues (40) identified the entity of RB-ILD, the clinical manifestation of ILD associated with the pathologic lesions of respiratory bronchiolitis. RB-ILD has been linked to DIP, based on the pathologic similarity of the two diseases and the etiologic link of both to cigarette smoking (3,30,41,42).

Clinical Findings

The mean age at diagnosis is in the third to fourth decade of life. Both RB-ILD and DIP present with chronic, progressive dyspnea and cough. The vast majority of patients are current or former smokers. The physical examination usually reveals bilateral basilar inspiratory crackles. The results of pulmonary function testing are usually normal, or a mildly obstructive pattern may be seen in RB-ILD, likely a consequence of concomitant chronic obstructive pulmonary disease. A restrictive pattern is generally seen in DIP. In patients with RB-ILD, HRCT often reveals central and peripheral bronchial wall thickening (proximal to the subsegmental bronchi), centrilobular nodules, ground-glass opacities, and air trapping. DIP demonstrates more diffuse ground-glass abnormalities, often peripheral in distribution. Honeycombing may be seen but is usually limited.

Histopathologic Findings

The most striking histopathologic feature of both RB-ILD and DIP is the presence of pigment-laden macrophages (macrophages containing dusty brown cytoplasm that often stains with iron stains). An accumulation of pigmented macrophages in the respiratory bronchioles, a common histopathologic pattern in smokers, is called *respiratory bronchiolitis*. In patients with suspected IIP and a predominantly bronchiolar and peribronchiolar distribution on histopathology (i.e., respiratory bronchiolitis), the term *RB-ILD pattern* is used. If the alveolar involvement is more widespread, the term *DIP pattern* is used. The alveolar septa are mildly thickened by inflammatory infiltrate in both conditions.

Treatment

Many cases of RB-ILD and DIP resolve with smoking cessation alone. Corticosteroids are the mainstay of therapy, but no prospective treatment studies have been performed in either condition. The best data on responsiveness to steroids in DIP suggest that about 60% of patients improve. Corticosteroids are generally continued for at least 3 months, as in the other IIPs. The prognosis in both RB-ILD and DIP is good, with survival at 5 years above 70%. Occasionally, some cases progress to chronic pulmonary fibrosis.

LYMPHOCYTIC INTERSTITIAL PNEUMONIA

The term *LIP* was proposed by Liebow and Carrington in 1969 (43) to describe a histologic variant of IIPs characterized by diffuse pulmonary lymphoid hyperplasia with predominantly interstitial changes. With the widespread use of immunohistochemistry and molecular analysis, it is now evident that many of these cases represent lymphoproliferative disorders (44).

Clinical Findings

The clinical presentation of LIP is often indistinguishable from that of the other forms of IIP. Patients with LIP tend to be young (30–50 years old) and are predominantly female. Dyspnea and cough are the most prominent symptoms. Bilateral basilar crackles are common, and lymphadenopathy is occasionally present. Pulmonary function generally reveals restriction. HRCT commonly shows diffuse ground-glass abnormalities, poorly defined centrilobular nodules, thickened bronchovascular bundles, lymph node enlargement, and cysts.

Histopathologic Findings

Tissue examination shows dense interstitial lymphoid infiltrates with variable and usually minor peribronchial involvement. The infiltrates are comprised mostly of T lymphocytes, plasma cells, and macrophages. Type II cell hyperplasia is a frequent association. Lymphoid follicles are often present. Granuloma formation and mild fibrosis may rarely be seen.

Treatment

LIP is generally treated with corticosteroids with or without immunomodulator therapy. The clinical course is quite variable. The condition of most patients with LIP stabilizes or improves, with the 5-year survival estimated at about 60%. A minority of patients progress to diffuse pulmonary fibrosis, lymphoma, and death.

OTHER ISSUES IN GENERAL MANAGEMENT

Lung Transplantation

Patient selection is critical in lung transplantation, and the ATS guidelines stress that intensive medical intervention should be tried first before patients are referred for lung transplantation (6). One study compared the disease management of 54 patients with IPF in an ILD clinic with the disease management of 84 patients with IPF in a general clinic (45). Treatment with drugs such as prednisolone, azathioprine, cyclophosphamide, and cyclosporine was given to 76% of patients in the ILD clinic and 48% of patients in the general clinic. In the ILD clinic, age was an important determinant of outcome. For patients younger than 60 years, the median survival in the ILD clinic was more than 3,700 days, versus 2,535 days in the general clinic ($P = .037$). No difference in survival was found for patients older than 60 years. The authors of this study stress that the current optimal management for IPF involves the identification of potential responders, which promotes intensive immunosuppression and surveillance for opportunistic infection. A strategy of minimalism and early referral for transplant assessment is most appropriate for cases of steroid-unresponsive lung fibrosis (UIP), particularly in patients older than 60 years. In ILD clinics, a good balance between aggressive immunosuppression and minimal intervention may best be achieved by using a variety of surrogate markers of disease progression. Considering the current lack of any evidence-based management protocol advocating the treatment of patients exclusively in tertiary centers, the findings of this study would seem reasonable (i.e., patients with IPF may have a survival advantage if seen in a dedicated multidisciplinary clinic). In addition, we should adopt a minimal therapeutic approach for patients older than 60 years to reduce the incidence of adverse effects during drug therapy.

Long-Term Oxygen Therapy

Long-term oxygen therapy is a good example of a minimal therapeutic approach for patients with IPF/UIP (46). In our clinic, the introduction of long-term oxygen therapy is considered for many IPF patients relatively early because supplemental oxygen during exercise may markedly relieve exercise-induced hypoxemia and improve exercise performance (6). Some patients are treated with a low-dose corticosteroid in conjunction with supplemental oxygen, whereas others are managed with long-term oxygen therapy alone. For patients who have pulmonary hypertension secondary to IPF progression, we feel that long-term oxygen therapy is generally indicated, although no longitudinal data on the effects of long-term oxygen therapy on pulmonary hypertension in patients with IPF are available (47). In one study, 62 patients (49 with IPF and 13 with other forms of fibrosis; mean age, 62 years) were assigned to either of two groups: an oxygen-treated group (n = 37) or a control group (n = 25). The entry criteria were (a) a total lung capacity below 80% of the predicted value and (b) a PaO_2 between 45 and 60 mm Hg. All patients presented with moderate pulmonary hypertension, and the mean pulmonary artery pressure was 33 mm Hg. The patients were followed for 3 years, and only 30% survived until the end of this follow-up period. No difference was found between the survival rate of controls and

IDIOPATHIC INTERSTITIAL PNEUMONIAS: DIAGNOSIS AND TREATMENT	
Summary Statement	**Level of Evidence**
In the absense of contraindications, surgical lung biopsy is advised in patients with suspected IIP who do not show a classic clinical and HRCT picture of IPF/UIP.	Controlled trials, consensus panel
Transbronchial biopsies are not useful in the diagnosis of most of the IIPs.	Observational studies, consensus panel
Bronchoalveolar lavage is not always required in the assessment of the IIPs.	Consensus panel
No data exist that adequately document that any of the current treatment approaches improve survival or quality of life for patients with IPF.	Consensus panel
If therapy is recommended for a patient with IIP, it should be started at the first identification of clinical or physiologic evidence of impairment or documentation of a decline in lung function.	Consensus panel
For smoking-related lesions (e.g., DIP and RB-ILD), cessation of smoking is the best option, and follow-up may show improvement without drug therapy.	Expert opinion
Ambulatory oxygen can help maintain quality of life in the advanced stages of IIP.	Expert opinion

DIP, desquamative interstitial pneumonia; HRCT, high-resolution computed tomography; IIP, idiopathic interstitial pneumonia; IPF, idiopathic pulmonary fibrosis; RB-ILD, respiratory bronchiolitis–associated interstitial lung disease; UIP, usual interstitial pneumonia.

that of the patients treated with oxygen (47). Other studies have reported a similarly poor prognosis for patients with IPF treated with long-term oxygen therapy. In a study by Crockett and colleagues (48), only 10% of patients survived 3 years; Strom (49) reported a 3-year survival rate of 20%, and the ANTADIR (Association Nationale pour le Traitement à Domicile de l'Insuffisance Respiratoire Chronique) group reported a median survival of only 15 months in more than 1,300 patients with IPF (50). However, we agree with the comment of Zielinski (47) that ambulatory oxygen is the best therapeutic option for patients with IPF because it can help maintain their quality of life during the advanced stages of disease.

ACKNOWLEDGMENT

We would like to express our thanks to Professors Takateru Izumi and Talmadge E. King, Jr. for guiding our activities in the field of ILD, and to Mr. Simon Johnson for editorial assistance.

REFERENCES

1. Liebow AA. Definition and classification of interstitial pneumonias in human pathology. *Prog Respir Res* 1975;8:1–33.
2. Katzenstein AL. Idiopathic interstitial pneumonia: classification and diagnosis. In: Katzenstein AL, Askin FB, eds. *Surgical pathology of non-neoplastic lung disease.* Philadelphia: WB Saunders, 1997:1–31.
3. American Thoracic Society/European Respiratory Society international multidisciplinary consensus classification of the idiopathic interstitial pneumonias. *Am J Respir Crit Care Med* 2002;165:277–304.
4. Iwai K, Mori T, Yamada N, et al. Idiopathic pulmonary fibrosis. Epidemiologic approaches to occupational exposure. *Am J Respir Crit Care Med* 1994;150:670–675.
5. Coultas DB, Zumwalt RE, Black WC, et al. The epidemiology of interstitial lung disease. *Am J Respir Crit Care Med* 1994;150:967–972.
6. American Thoracic Society. Idiopathic pulmonary fibrosis: diagnosis and treatment. International consensus statement. American Thoracic Society (ATS) and the European Respiratory Society (ERS). *Am J Respir Crit Care Med* 2000;161:646–664.
7. Klech H, Hutter C. Clinical guidelines and indications for bronchoalveolar lavage (BAL): report of the European Society of Pneumology Task Force on BAL. *Eur Respir J* 1990;3:937–974.
8. Nagai S, Satake N, Shimoji T, et al. Bronchoalveolar lavage (BAL) findings in patients with idiopathic pulmonary fibrosis. In: Takishima T, ed. *Basic and clinical aspects of pulmonary fibrosis.* Boca Raton: CRC Press, 1994:325–336.
9. Nagai S, Kitaichi M, Izumi T. Classification and recent advances in idiopathic interstitial pneumonia. *Curr Opin Pulm Med* 1998;4:256–260.
10. Raghu G, Mageto YN, Lockhart D, et al. The accuracy of the clinical diagnosis of new-onset idiopathic pulmonary fibrosis and other interstitial lung disease: a prospective study. *Chest* 1999;116:1168–1174.
11. Hunninghake G, Zimmerman MB, Schwartz DA, et al. Utility of lung biopsy for the diagnosis of idiopathic pulmonary fibrosis. *Am J Respir Crit Care Med* 2001;164:193–196.
12. Scadding JG, Hinson KFW. Diffuse fibrosing alveolitis (diffuse interstitial fibrosis of the lungs): correlation of histology at biopsy with prognosis. *Thorax* 1967;22:291–304.
13. Bjoraker JA, Ryu JH, Edwin MK, et al. Prognostic significance of histopathologic subsets in idiopathic pulmonary fibrosis. *Am J Respir Crit Care Med* 1998;157:199–203.
14. Travis WD, Matsui K, Moss J, et al. Idiopathic nonspecific interstitial pneumonia: prognostic significance of cellular and fibrosing patterns: survival comparison with usual interstitial pneumonia and desquamative interstitial pneumonia. *Am J Surg Pathol* 2000;24:19–33.
15. Nicholson AG, Colby TV, Dubois RM, et al. The prognostic significance of the histologic pattern of interstitial pneumonia in patients presenting with the clinical entity of cryptogenic fibrosing alveolitis. *Am J Respir Crit Care Med* 2000;162:2213–2217.
16. Hubbard R, Johnston I, Britton J. Survival in patients with cryptogenic fibrosing alveolitis: a population-based cohort study. *Chest* 1998;113:396–400.
17. King TE Jr, Schwarz MI, Brown K, et al. Idiopathic pulmonary fibrosis. Relationship between histopathologic features and mortality. *Am J Respir Crit Care Med* 2001;164:1025–1032.
18. Selman M, King TE Jr, Pardo A. Idiopathic pulmonary fibrosis: prevailing and evolving hypotheses about its pathogenesis and implications for therapy. *Ann Intern Med* 2001;134:136–151.
19. Nagao T, Nagai S, Kitaichi M, et al. Are histological changes found in parallel with the progression of IPF/UIP? *Am J Respir Crit Care Med* 1998;167:A69.
20. Nagai S, Nagao T, Kitaichi M, et al. Clinical courses of asymptomatic cases with idiopathic pulmonary fibrosis and a histology of usual interstitial pneumonia. *Eur Respir J* 1998;11:131s.
21. Flaherty KR, Toews GB, Lynch JP III, et al. Steroids in idiopathic pulmonary fibrosis: a prospective assessment of adverse reactions, response to therapy, and survival. *Am J Med* 2001;110:278–282.
22. Zisman DA, Lynch JP 3rd, Toews GB, et al. Cyclophosphamide in the treatment of idiopathic pulmonary fibrosis: a prospective study in patients who failed to respond to corticosteroids. *Chest* 2000;117:1619–1626.
23. Raghu G, Depaso WJ, Cain K, et al. Azathioprine combined with prednisone in the treatment of idiopathic pulmonary fibrosis: a prospective, double-blinded, randomized, placebo-controlled clinical trial. *Am Rev Respir Dis* 1991;144:291–296.
24. Baughman RP, Lower EE. Use of intermittent intravenous cyclophosphamide for idiopathic pulmonary fibrosis. *Chest* 1992;102:1090–1094.
25. Douglas WW, Ryu JH, Swensen SJ, et al. Colchicine versus prednisone in the treatment of idiopathic pulmonary fibrosis. A randomized prospective study. Members of the Lung Study Group. *Am J Respir Crit Care Med* 1998;158:220–225.
26. Selman M, Carrillo G, Salas J, et al. Colchicine, D-penicillamine, and prednisone in the treatment of idiopathic pulmonary fibrosis: a controlled clinical trial. *Chest* 1998;114:507–512.
27. Ziesche R, Hofbauer E, Wittmann K, et al. A preliminary study of long-term treatment with interferon gamma-1b and low-dose prednisolone in patients with idiopathic pulmonary fibrosis. *N Engl J Med* 1999;341:1264–1269.
28. Raghu G, Johnson WC, Lockhart D, et al. Treatment of idiopathic pulmonary fibrosis with a new antifibrotic agent, pirfenidone: results of a prospective, open-label phase II study. *Am J Respir Crit Care Med* 1999;159:1061–1069.
29. Hubbard R, Venn A, Lewis S, et al. Lung cancer and cryptogenic fibrosing alveolitis. A population-based cohort study. *Am J Respir Crit Care Med* 2000;161:5–8.

30. Yousem SA, Colby TV, Gaensler EA. Respiratory bronchiolitis-associated interstitial lung disease and its relationship to desquamative interstitial pneumonia. *Mayo Clin Proc* 1989;64:1373–1380.

31. King TE Jr, Tooze JA, Schwarz MI, et al. Predicting survival in idiopathic pulmonary fibrosis. scoring system and survival model. *Am J Respir Crit Care Med* 2001;164:1171–1181.

32. Katzenstein AL, Fiorelli RF. Nonspecific interstitial pneumonia/fibrosis. Histologic features and clinical significance. *Am J Surg Pathol* 1994;18:136–147.

33. Nagai S, Kitaichi M, Itoh H, et al. Idiopathic nonspecific interstitial pneumonia/fibrosis: comparison with idiopathic pulmonary fibrosis and BOOP. *Eur Respir J* 1998;12:1010–1019.

34. Cottin V, Donsbeck AV, Revel D, et al. Nonspecific interstitial pneumonia. Individualization of a clinicopathologic entity in a series of 12 patients. *Am J Respir Crit Care Med* 1998;158:1286–1293.

35. Daniil ZD, Gilchrist FC, Nicholson AG, et al. A histologic pattern of nonspecific interstitial pneumonia is associated with a better prognosis than usual interstitial pneumonia in patients with cryptogenic fibrosing alveolitis. *Am J Respir Crit Care Med* 1999;160:899–905.

36. Davison AG, Heard BE, McAllister WAC, et al. Cryptogenic organizing pneumonitis. *Q J Med* 1983;52:382–394.

37. Epler GR, Colby TV, McLoud TC, et al. Bronchiolitis obliterans organizing pneumonia. *N Engl J Med* 1985;312:152–158.

38. Katzenstein ALA, Myers JL, Mazur MT. Acute interstitial pneumonia. A clinicopathologic, ultrastructural, and cell kinetic study. *Am J Surg Pathol* 1986;10:256–267.

39. Olson J, Colby TV, Elliott CG. Hamman-Rich syndrome revisited. *Mayo Clin Proc* 1990;65:1538–1548.

40. Myers JL, Veal CF, Shin MS, et al. Respiratory bronchiolitis causing interstitial lung disease: a clinicopathologic study of six cases. *Am Rev Respir Dis* 1987;135:880–884.

41. Liebow AA, Steer A, Billingsley JG. Desquamative interstitial pneumonia. *Am J Med* 1965;39:369–404.

42. Nagai S, Hoshino Y, Hayashi M, et al. Smoking-related interstitial lung diseases. *Curr Opin Pulm Med* 2000;6:415–419.

43. Liebow AA, Carrington DB. The interstitial pneumonias. In: Simon M, Potchen EJ, LeMay M, eds. *Frontiers of pulmonary radiology.* New York: Grune & Stratton, 1969:102–141.

44. Nicholson AG, Wotherspoon AC, Diss TC, et al. Reactive pulmonary lymphoid disorders. *Histopathology* 1995;26:405–412.

45. Lok SS. Interstitial lung disease clinics for the management of idiopathic pulmonary fibrosis: a potential advantage to patients. Greater Manchester Lung Fibrosis Consortium. *J Heart Lung Transplant* 1999;18:884–890.

46. Crockett AJ, Cranston JM, Antic N. Domiciliary oxygen for interstitial lung disease. *Cochrane Database Syst Rev* 2001;3.

47. Zielinski J. Long-term oxygen therapy in conditions other than chronic obstructive pulmonary disease. *Respir Care* 2000;45:172–176; discussion 176–177.

48. Crockett AJ, Alpers JH, Moss JR. Home oxygen therapy: an audit of survival. *Aust N Z J Med* 1991;21:217–221.

49. Strom K. Experience with an oxygen registry in Sweden. In: O'Donohue W Jr, ed. *Long-term oxygen therapy: scientific basis and clinical applications.* New York: Marcel Dekker Inc, 1995:331–346.

50. Chailleux E, Fauroux B, Binet F, et al. Predictors of survival in patients receiving domiciliary oxygen therapy or mechanical ventilation. A 10-year analysis of ANTADIR Observatory. *Chest* 1996;109:741–749.

51. Park CS, Chung SW, Ki SY, et al. Increased levels of interleukin-6 are associated with lymphocytosis in bronchoalveolar lavage fluids of idiopathic nonspecific interstitial pneumonia. *Am J Respir Crit Care Med* 2000;162:1162–1168.

52. Suga M, Iyonaga K, Okamoto T, et al. Characteristic elevation of matrix metalloproteinase activity in idiopathic interstitial pneumonias. *Am J Respir Crit Care Med* 2000;162:1949–1956.

Hypersensitivity Pneumonitis

25

Mark Schuyler

The term *hypersensitivity pneumonitis (HP),* or *extrinsic allergic alveolitis,* the British term, describes a group of lung diseases caused by inhalation of a wide variety of different molecules that are usually organic and always antigenic. The stereotypic clinical events are transient fever, hypoxemia, myalgias, arthralgias, dyspnea, and cough that occur 2 to 9 hours after exposure and resolve in 12 to 72 hours without specific treatment provided no reexposure takes place.

HP was first clearly described in a doctoral thesis in 1874, as *heykatarr* in Iceland:

"This is a chronic chest disease. I do not know its incidence, as my observations thereupon are incomplete. The disease occurs only in winter, or rather during the time when the animals are kept inside, and is found only in the man whose job it is to loosen the hay in the barn and handle it before it is fed to cattle. The hay is always more or less dusty and has to be shaken to eliminate the dust before it is used as fodder. When this dust is inhaled, especially when the harvesting has been difficult and the hay has moulded in the barn, the man who works with the hay becomes ill with this disease, which lasts as long as he continues the same occupation, but usually disappears in summer. The disease expresses itself by cough, rather scant expectoration, and chest heaviness, especially in the evening (the hay is usually loosened in the afternoon, i.e., when it is intended to be given in the evening and the next morning). When examining the chest of those men, I have on a few occasions found signs of bronchitis, but in most cases I have never found anything abnormal. I have never had the occasion to examine a patient during an acute episode" (1).

Dr. Finsen's description is notable for the association of the illness with a particular environmental exposure, its relationship to the season of the year, its occurrence several

hours after exposure, and the nature of the symptoms and the association with bronchitis. This syndrome was again described in British farmers in the 1930s (2) and designated *farmer's lung disease (FLD).* Many other diseases have since been described that exhibit the same clinical features and are denoted as HP. Despite the terms *hypersensitivity* and *allergic,* HP is not an atopic disease and is not typically associated with an increase in immunoglobulin E (IgE) or eosinophils. Drug reactions are sometimes described as representing HP, usually because certain bronchoalveolar lavage (BAL) fluid findings resemble those in HP. However, these reactions are not HP because the inciting agent is administered systemically and the pathogenetic mechanisms are likely different from those of HP.

Table 25.1 lists currently described examples of HP, the environmental source of antigen associated with the disease, and the likely etiologic agent. Some of these diseases have apparently disappeared from the originally described clinical settings (e.g., bagassosis in Louisiana) but exist in areas with similar agricultural/industrial settings, and other diseases are being newly recognized (e.g., potato riddler's lung and metal-working fluid HP). Both the disappearance of previously described examples of HP and the appearance of new examples are a consequence of changing agricultural and industrial practices that result in exposure of subjects to different antigenic materials that can cause HP. As an example, even small changes in agricultural practices can affect the amount of airborne actinomycetes derived from hay, so that large bales of hay produce more actinomycetes than small bales (3). At the present time, FLD, bird fancier's disease, ventilator lung, and Japanese summer-type HP (in Japan) are the most commonly recognized forms of HP.

The recognition of new examples of HP usually requires a cluster of new cases with a unifying exposure history. Because complete occupational and avocational histories are

M. Schuyler: Department of Medicine, University of New Mexico School of Medicine, Albuquerque, New Mexico.

TABLE 25.1. EXAMPLES OF HYPERSENSITIVITY PNEUMONITIS, THE ENVIRONMENTAL SOURCE OF ANTIGEN ASSOCIATED WITH THE DISEASE, AND THE LIKELY ETIOLOGIC AGENT

Disease	Antigen Source	Probable Antigen
Plant products		
Farmer's lung disease	Moldy hay	Thermophilic actinomycetes
		Saccharopolyspora rectivirgula (*Micropolyspora faeni*)
		Thermoactinomyces vulgaris
		Aspergillus species
		Penicillium species
		Candida species
		Wallemia species
		Fusarium species
		Absidia species
Bagassosis	Moldy pressed sugar cane (bagasse)	Thermophilic actinomycetes
		T. sacchari
		T. vulgaris
Mushroom worker's disease	Moldy compost and mushrooms	Thermophilic actinomycetes
		S. rectivirgula
		T. vulgaris
		Aspergillus species
		Mushroom spores
Suberosis	Moldy cork	*Penicillium* species
Malt worker's lung	Contaminated barley	*Aspergillus clavatus*
Maple bark disease	Contaminated maple logs	*Cryptostroma corticale*
Sequoisis	Contaminated redwood dust	*Graphium* species
		Pullularia species
Soybean lung	Soybeans in animal feed	Soybean hull antigens
Wood pulp worker's disease	Contaminated wood pulp	*Alternaria* species
Wood dust HP	Contaminated wood dust	Pine sawdust
		Bacillus subtilis
		Alternaria species
Compost lung	Compost	*Aspergillus* species
		T. vulgaris
		Lactobacillus species
Cheese worker's disease	Cheese or cheese casings	*Penicillium* species
Wood trimmer's disease	Contaminated wood trimmings, at times in sawmills	*Rhizopus* species
		Mucor species
Thatched roof disease	Dried grasses and leaves	*Saccharomonospora viridis*
Greenhouse lung	Greenhouse soil	*Aspergillus* species
		Penicillium species
		Cryptostroma corticale
Coffee worker's lung	Green coffee dust	Unknown
Potato riddler's lung	Moldy hay around potatoes	Thermophilic actinomycetes
		S. rectivirgula
		T. vulgaris
		Aspergillus species
Tobacco worker's disease	Mold on tobacco	*Aspergillus* species
Wine grower's lung	Mold on grapes	*Botrytis cinerea*
Woodman's disease	Mold on bark and fuel chips	*Penicillium* species
Soy sauce brewer's lung	Fermentation starter for soy sauce	*Aspergillus oryzae*
Domestic allergic alveolitis	Decayed wood	Fungi
		Serpula lacrimans
		Leucogyrophana pinastri
		Paecilomyces variottii
		Aspergillus fumigatus
Riding school lung	Hay in horse stall	Thermophilic actinomycetes
		S. rectivirgula
		T. vulgaris
Stipatosis	Esparto grass (*Stipa tenacissima*) used to make plaster	Esparto grass antigens
		Thermophilic actinomycetes
		S. rectivirgula
		Aspergillus species

(continued)

TABLE 25.1. (Continued)

Disease	Antigen Source	Probable Antigen
Algarroba lung	Livestock feed	Algarroba (legume) antigens
Tiger nut lung	Tiger nuts (Spain)	Tiger nut antigens
El Nino lung	Fungi in basement	*Pezizia domiciliana*
Salami lung	Mold on curing salamis	Fungi
		Penicillium camembertii
Peat moss lung	Mold on peat moss	Fungi
		Penicillium species
		Monocillium species
Animal products		
Pigeon breeder's disease	Pigeon droppings	Altered pigeon serum (probably IgA)
		Pigeon bloom (derived from feathers)
		Pigeon intestinal mucin
Turkey handler's disease	Turkey products	Turkey proteins
Chicken breeder's lung	Chicken feathers	Chicken feather proteins
Bird fancier's lung	Domestic and wild bird products	Bird proteins
Duvet lung	Duvet and pillow	Goose proteins
Laboratory worker's HP	Rat fur	Rat urine protein
Pituitary snuff taker's disease	Pituitary powder	Vasopressin
Shell lung	Oyster or mollusk shell	Shell proteins
Miller's lung	Grain weevils in wheat flour	*Sitophilus granarius* proteins
Sericulturist's lung	Silk worm larvae	Silk worm larvae proteins
Reactive chemicals		
TDI HP	Toluene diisocyanate	Altered proteins (albumin and others)
MDI HP	Diphenylmethane diisocyanate	Altered proteins
HDI HP	Hexamethylene diisocyanate	Altered proteins
TMA HP	Trimetallic anhydride	Altered proteins
Other		
Ventilator lung	Contaminated humidifiers, dehumidifiers, air conditioners, heating systems	Thermophilic actinomycetes
		Thermoactinomyces candidus
		T. vulgaris
		Penicillium species
		Cephalosporium species
		Amebae
		Klebsiella species
		Candida species
		Rhodotorula species
Basement lung	Contaminated basement (sewage or mold)	*Cephalosporium* species
		Penicillium species
Sauna taker's disease	Sauna water	*Aureobasidium* species
Detergent worker's disease	Detergent enzymes	*Bacillus subtilis*
Japanese summer-type HP	House dust	*Trichosporon cutaneum*
	? Bird droppings	*Cryptococcus albidus*
Hot tub lung	Mold on ceiling	*Cladosporium* species
		Mycobacterium avium
Tractor lung	Contaminated tractor cab air conditioner	*Rhizopus* species
Metal-working fluid HP	Contaminated metal-working fluid	*Pseudomonas* species?
		Acinetobacter species?
		Mycobacterium species?
Fertilizer lung	Contaminated fertilizer	*Streptomyces albus*
Sax lung	Saxophone mouthpiece	*Candida albicans*
Smut lung	Japanese handicrafts	*Ustilago esculenta*
Shower curtain lung	Shower curtain	*Epicoccum nigrum*

HP, hypersensitivity pneumonitis.

at times not obtained from patients with "pneumonia," it is likely that substantially more examples of HP exist that have not yet been recognized and described. For example, the introduction of new metal-working fluids led to the recognition of metal-working fluid HP in an auto parts manufacturing facility as the result of a clustering of cases and a common unusual exposure (aerosolized contaminated metal-working fluid) (4). Although it is clear that microbial contamination of the recycled fluid is necessary for the development of metal-working fluid HP, the exact nature of the contamination (mycobacteria, bacteria, fungi) is not clear and may differ between plants (4–9).

EPIDEMIOLOGY

The prevalence of HP is quite variable in different populations, presumably as a consequence of differences in intensity, frequency, and duration of inhalation exposure. Of members of pigeon breeder's clubs who participated in surveys, 8% to 30% exhibited pigeon breeder's disease (PBD) (10–16). Among farmers, 0.5% to 5% have symptoms compatible with FLD (17–24). The prevalence of symptoms is decreased on farms that use hay-drying methods that decrease exposure to the responsible antigens (25), and it is increased following a wet summer season (26).

The population at risk and the season of the year when symptoms occur vary with the type of HP. For example, most cases of FLD occur in cold, damp climates in late winter and early spring (10,24,27) when farmers (usually men) use stored hay to feed their livestock. Pigeon breeder's disease occurs chiefly in men in Europe and the United States and predominantly in women in Mexico because of different patterns of exposure (28), but no seasonal preference is observed in either population. Bird fancier's disease in Europe and the United States occurs in subjects who keep domestic birds and does not show a predilection for either sex. Japanese summer-type HP occurs mostly in women without an occupation outside the home from June to September in warm, moist regions of Japan (29,30).

Unlike other pulmonary diseases, all types of HP show a remarkable predominance (80%–95%) of nonsmokers, whose numbers are substantially higher than the number of nonsmokers in similarly exposed subjects who are nevertheless not ill (12–14,16,19,21,22,30–36). This protection against the development of HP in smokers extends to serum antibody, so that smokers have a lower prevalence of serum antibody than apparently equally exposed nonsmokers (16,18,37,38). The mechanism(s) for these phenomena are unknown but could include the depression of immune responses to antigen delivered to the lung that is well documented in smokers (39,40). These clinical data suggest that active smoking makes the diagnosis of HP less likely; however, it does not exclude it.

An important feature of HP is the great variation in susceptibility among exposed populations and the apparent resistance to illness of most exposed persons. Possible reasons include differences in exposure or in the host, either genetic or acquired. No differences in the prevalence of atopy in exposed subjects with and without HP have been noted. The issue of differences of HLA-A, -B, -C, or -DR haplotypes is not settled. Although most earlier studies indicated no differences of HLA haplotype between patients with HP and exposed subjects without HP (14,21,41–47), evidence suggests that the frequencies of certain HLA-DR

and HLA-DQ haplotypes in patients with PBD differ from those in exposed but not ill subjects and in the general population (48). The same authors demonstrated that a single nucleotide polymorphism (tumor necrosis factor [TNF]-α-308) of the TNF-α promoter is more common in subjects with PBD than in control subjects, although no differences in serum TNF-α were found. Similar findings have been described in FLD (49). Undoubtedly, more polymorphisms will be detected in the future that may relate to the pathogenesis of HP. The involved genes are likely to be cytokines (especially those important in inflammation and its resolution), chemokines, and enzymes that degrade antigens.

CLINICAL PRESENTATION

Several clinical presentations of HP have been described. It is useful to divide the clinical presentation into two major patterns.

Acute Hypersensitivity Pneumonitis

Dyspnea, nonproductive cough, myalgias, chills, diaphoresis, lassitude, headache, and malaise occur 2 to 9 hours after a particular exposure. These symptoms peak typically between 6 and 24 hours and resolve without specific treatment in 1 to 3 days (sometimes longer after a particularly intense exposure). Patients have fever, tachypnea, bilateral basilar crackles, and occasionally cyanosis. Peripheral blood leukocytosis with neutrophilia and lymphopenia, but not eosinophilia, is present, and often hypoxemia. Figure 25.1 illustrates an acute episode of HP.

The acute form of HP can be progressive, resulting in persistent pulmonary symptoms and requiring antigen avoidance and possibly therapy with corticosteroids. This form of HP has been referred to as *subacute HP*. In addition, some forms of acute HP can be nonprogressive and intermittent, with spontaneous improvement after antigen avoidance. To complicate issues further, evidence suggests that some patients have acute nonprogressive HP even with continued exposure to the antigen.

Chronic Hypersensitivity Pneumonitis

Chronic HP presents as progressively more severe dyspnea, nonproductive cough, weight loss, and often anorexia in a patient exposed to a recognized cause of HP. Symptoms are usually present for months to years. Typically, the patient has no fever, but tachypnea and bilateral basilar dry crackles are usually present. Symptoms and signs of cor pulmonale are not uncommon at presentation. In general, clubbing occurs infrequently (50), although Sansores and colleagues (51), using retrospective chart review, reported clubbing in up to 50% of subjects with PBD in Mexico City. Like acute HP,

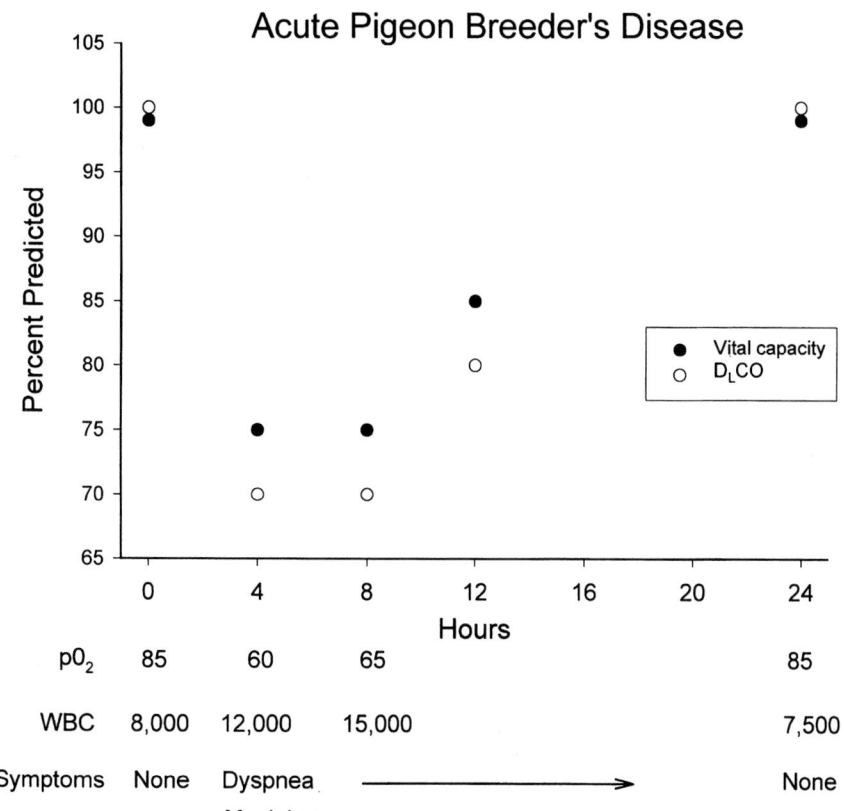

FIGURE 25.1. Diagram of a typical episode of acute pigeon breeder's disease induced by exposure to pigeon serum at 0 hour. $D_{L}CO$, diffusing capacity of lung for carbon monoxide.

chronic HP can present as chronic nonprogressive or chronic progressive HP.

A proportion (20%–40%) of patients with chronic HP present with symptoms of chronic bronchitis (i.e., chronic productive cough) (10–12,17,52,53), some even without radiologic parenchymal densities on standard chest radiographs. Substantial morphologic evidence of bronchitis is found in the large airways of patients with FLD (54,55). Pigeon fanciers also often exhibit clinical evidence of chronic bronchitis and delayed mucociliary clearance (56). Because most patients with HP are nonsmokers without any other reason for the development of chronic bronchitis, these symptoms are likely a result of HP and may correlate with evidence of airway hyperreactivity in patients with chronic HP.

The reasons for the different clinical presentations (i.e., acute and chronic) of HP are not clear but may include differences in intensity and duration of exposure (i.e., low-intensity exposure of long duration tending to cause chronic HP and high-intensity exposure of short duration tending to cause acute HP). This concept is most clearly illustrated in HP caused by exposure to birds. Bird fancier's disease (long-term exposure to small amounts of bird antigens) is associated with chronic HP. PBD presents differently in different geographic areas. Intermittent exposure of pigeon breeders to large amounts of pigeon antigens in the United States and Europe is associated with acute disease and has a good prognosis, whereas long-term exposure to a few household

pigeons in Mexico is associated with chronic disease and has a much poorer prognosis (28). In the United States and Europe, pigeon breeders keep their animals in an enclosure separate from their living areas that they visit only periodically, so that exposure is intermittent. In Mexico, birds are kept in living quarters, so that exposure is continuous. It is of interest that bird antigens can persist in a room for a substantial length of time (>18 months) after the birds have been removed (57); therefore, Mexicans with PBD would be expected to have been exposed to pigeon antigens for prolonged periods of time, even after removal of the pigeons. Thus, PBD in Mexico resembles bird fancier's disease in the United States and Europe in regard to type of exposure, clinical presentation, and prognosis, and differs from PBD in the United States and Europe. Because the relevant antigens are similar in these two examples of bird-associated HP, it is likely that the type of exposure, not antigen characteristics, is important in determining the clinical presentation and prognosis.

Although newly recognized examples of HP are usually acute forms of HP, most patients with well-recognized types of HP present with chronic disease (31). This may be related to the difficulties of establishing a link between chronic disease and long-term exposure, whereas it is relatively easy to associate acute disease with acute exposure.

The preceding discussion indicates that HP, and particularly chronic HP, may be more prevalent than is readily apparent and may be the cause of some cases of chronic pulmonary fibrosis, such as idiopathic pulmonary fibrosis, nonspecific interstitial pneumonia, and bronchiolitis obliterans organizing pneumonia (BOOP). Detailed histories are not always obtained from many patients with idiopathic interstitial pneumonias, serum antibody to the agent responsible for HP tends to wane after cessation of exposure, and high-resolution computed tomographic (HRCT) scans of the chest in patients with chronic HP can resemble those of patients with idiopathic interstitial pneumonia, so it is possible that some patients with idiopathic interstitial pneumonia have chronic HP. The prevalence of HP as a cause of pulmonary fibrosis in a population-based survey was reported to be low (2% of all patients with interstitial fibrosis in Bernalillo County, New Mexico) (58,59). However, most patients did not undergo surgical lung biopsy in this survey of community pulmonologists. Data from referral centers indicate that most patients referred for interstitial lung disease of unknown cause are determined to have chronic HP after a thorough evaluation including lung biopsy, BAL, and an assessment of both the home and work environments (60). Evidence indicates that exposure to wood dust, farming, metal dust, birds, or a moldy environment is associated with idiopathic interstitial pneumonia (61–63). However, because cigarette smoking is a risk factor for many forms of idiopathic interstitial pneumonia, especially idiopathic pulmonary fibrosis (64), and is uncommon in HP, it is unlikely that HP accounts for a large proportion of cases of idiopathic pulmonary fibrosis.

CHEST IMAGING STUDIES

Acute Hypersensitivity Pneumonitis

Chest radiographs demonstrate diffuse, poorly defined nodular opacities, and at times areas of ground-glass opacities or even consolidation. The opacities tend to occur in the lower lobes and spare the apices. Linear opacities (presumably representing areas of fibrosis from previous episodes of acute HP) may also be present (65) (Fig. 25.2). The nodular and ground-glass densities tend to disappear after cessation of exposure, so that the chest radiograph findings may be normal after resolution of an acute episode of HP.

HRCT often demonstrates ground-glass opacities better than chest radiographs and at times reveals a diffuse increase in pulmonary radiodensity (66–68), but the findings may also be normal after resolution of an acute episode (65). In addition to ground-glass opacities, other HRCT features include small, ill-defined nodules (often centrilobular), mosaic attenuation, and relative sparing of disease in the lung bases.

Pleural effusions or thickening, calcification, cavitation, atelectasis, localized opacities (i.e., "coin" lesions or masses), and intrathoracic lymphadenopathy visible on chest x-rays films are rare.

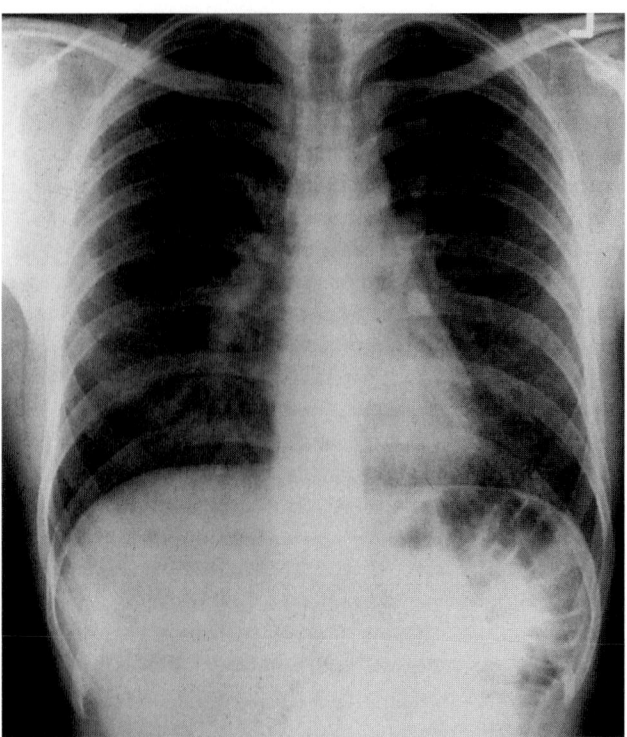

FIGURE 25.2. Chest radiograph of a patient with acute pigeon breeder's disease. Note bilateral lower lobe nodular opacities.

Chronic Hypersensitivity Pneumonitis

Diffuse linear and nodular opacities with upper lobe predominance, sparing of the bases, and volume loss are seen on chest radiographs (69). Pleural effusions and thickening are very unusual, although subcutaneous emphysema (presumably as a consequence of pleural rupture secondary to bronchiolitis and lobular overinflation) has been reported (70).

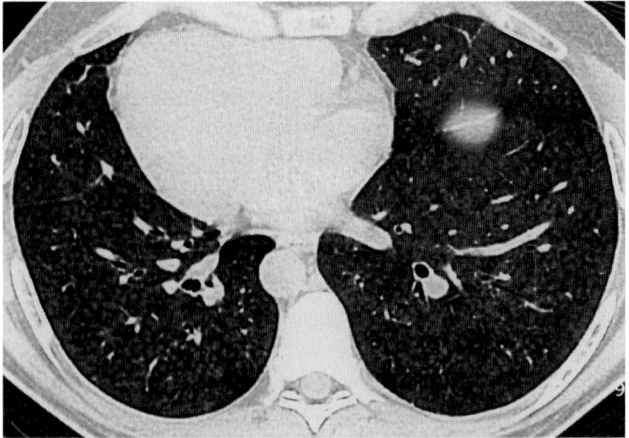

FIGURE 25.3. High-resolution computed tomographic scan of the chest of a patient with hypersensitivity pneumonitis demonstrating bilateral lower lobe centrilobular nodules not associated with bronchovascular bundles.

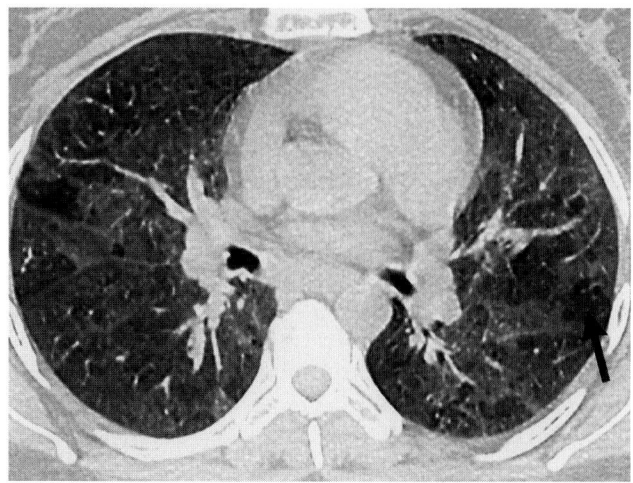

FIGURE 25.4. High-resolution computed tomographic scan of the chest of a patient with hypersensitivity pneumonitis demonstrating bilateral centrilobular nodules (*arrow*), multiple areas of ground-glass densities, and hyperinflation resulting in a mosaic pattern.

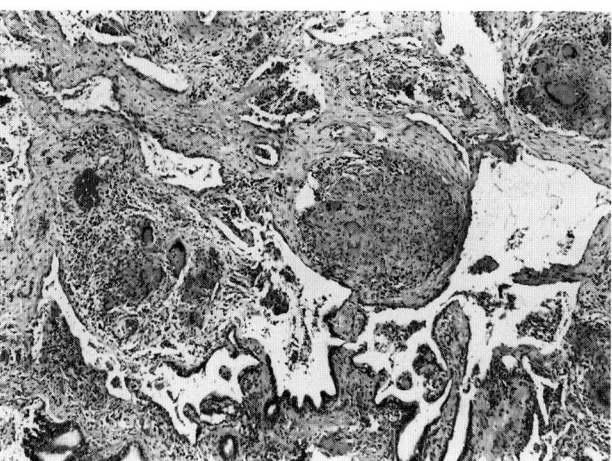

FIGURE 25.5. Histopathology of hypersensitivity pneumonitis. Open biopsy specimen of chronic pigeon breeder's disease. Mostly lymphocytic cellular interstitial infiltrate with epithelioid cells and numerous clearly defined granulomas (original magnification ×450).

HRCT scans of patients with subacute or chronic HP exhibit several patterns. In the most common pattern, ground-glass opacities are present, especially in the lower lobes. In addition, multiple centrilobular nodules, 2 to 4 mm diameter, are frequently distributed throughout the lung fields, often in association with areas of ground-glass opacities (65,67,68,71–74) (Figs. 25.3 and 25.4).s Unlike the nodules in sarcoidosis, these nodules are seldom attached to the pleurae or bronchovascular bundles, and the border between the nodules and the surrounding lung is well demarcated (67,75). Also seen are well-delineated areas of increased radiolucency and evidence of air trapping, which presumably represent hyperinflated pulmonary lobules with partially occluded bronchioles (75–77). The ground-glass opacities and micronodules tend to resolve after cessation of exposure (74,75). Although these findings are suggestive of HP, they are noted in only a subset (50%–75%) of patients with HP, and the HRCT scans of patients with HP can resemble those of patients with idiopathic pulmonary fibrosis (72). The prevalence of mild to moderate emphysema detectable by HRCT is substantial in both nonsmoking and smoking patients with FLD (68,78). HRCT may demonstrate mediastinal adenopathy (68), although this is not evident on chest radiographs. Magnetic resonance imaging is inferior to HRCT in demonstrating anatomic detail but is equal to HRCT in demonstrating ground-glass areas and may be useful in determining the course of ground-glass densities without exposing the patient to radiation (79).

PATHOLOGY

Lung biopsy specimens (almost always from patients with chronic HP) show chronic interstitial inflammation with infiltration of plasma cells, mast cells, histiocytes, and lymphocytes, often with poorly formed, nonnecrotizing granulomas (Fig. 25.5). Bronchiolitis and sometimes (25%–75% of cases) bronchiolitis obliterans are often present (26,80–88) (Fig. 25.6). The airway-centered inflammation merges with the interstitial inflammation in the surrounding alveolar walls. Severe inflammation may result in formation of bronchus-associated lymphoid tissue (89). Organizing pneumonia is also often present, so that 15% to 25% of patients with HP have BOOP. Conversely, in patients with recognized BOOP, HP may be the cause. Interstitial fibrosis is often present to a varying extent. Unlike the interstitial inflammatory cell infiltrate in sarcoidosis, that in HP is both distal and proximal to the granulomas. The granulomas do not occur in groups and are not generally found near the

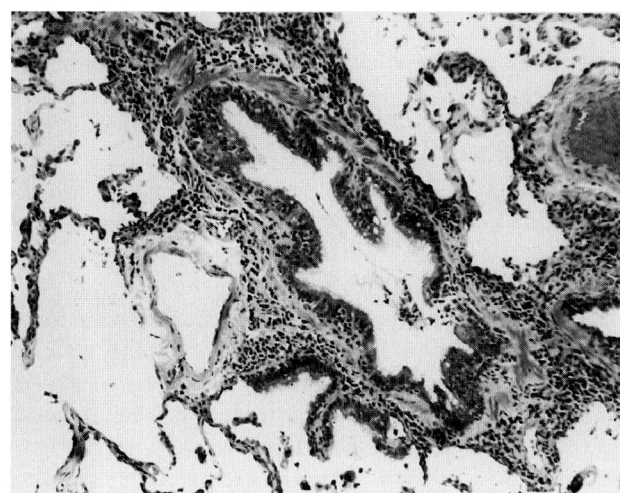

FIGURE 25.6. Histopathology of hypersensitivity pneumonitis. Open biopsy specimen of chronic disease. Bronchiolitis with a mostly chronic inflammation extending into adjacent alveolar walls (original magnification ×200).

bronchi or in subpleural locations, but they are often adjacent to bronchioles and usually single. These characteristics help to differentiate HP from sarcoidosis. Giant cells, at times with Schaumann or asteroid bodies or cholesterol clefts, are present both within and outside the granulomas (90). Foamy alveolar macrophages are often observed in patients with HP caused by bird exposure (86,91). Vasculitis and eosinophils are not evident. Despite the radiologic presence of emphysema in patients with HP (68,78), it is not prominent in lung biopsy specimens.

The specific histologic changes of HP, when present, are quite helpful in indicating the diagnosis. However, the granulomas and respiratory bronchiolitis may not be present years after cessation of exposure, so that only interstitial inflammation and fibrosis remain. Therefore, the classic triad of interstitial inflammation, bronchiolar inflammation, and granulomas is quite specific, but its sensitivity is unknown.

A reclassification of interstitial lung disease has emphasized nonspecific interstitial pneumonitis as a distinct pathologic entity with a relatively good prognosis (92,93). This pathologic pattern may be the only finding in lung biopsy specimens from patients with clinical HP (94), which underscores the value of historical data in addition to pulmonary histology in establishing the diagnosis of HP.

LABORATORY FINDINGS

In addition to peripheral blood leukocytosis with neutrophilia, BAL fluid lymphocytosis (typically 40%–80% of a twofold to fourfold increased number of BAL fluid cells) is usually present when the lungs are lavaged more than 5 days after the last exposure (95,96). Earlier lavage, especially within 48 hours after exposure, is characterized by BAL fluid neutrophilia (95–98). BAL fluid lymphocytosis, at least in dairy farmers, is related to continued antigenic exposure, not to the presence of disease, and does not predict outcome (99–101). In most cases of HP, the BAL fluid lymphocytes are virtually all CD3$^+$ with a relative increase in CD8$^+$ cells, so that the ratio of CD4$^+$ to CD8$^+$ cells is less than 1 (91,102–104). Many of the CD8$^+$ cells express CD57, a marker of cytotoxic cells, and also express CD25 (the interleukin-2 [IL-2] receptor) and other activation markers (103). However, the ratio of CD4$^+$ to CD8$^+$ cells in BAL fluid is greater than 1 in ventilator lung, some cases of bird fancier's disease, and some cases of FLD in Japan (105,106), although the ratio is less than 1 in Japanese summer-type HP (104). These differences between Japanese and non-Japanese patients with some types of HP may be related to differences in type of exposure, time between the last important exposure and BAL, or genetics. In support of the importance of the time between the last exposure and lavage, Soler and colleagues (107) demonstrated that cessation of exposure is associated with an increase of BAL fluid CD8$^+$ cells. Some evidence suggests that an increase in

BAL fluid CD8$^+$ cells is associated with protection against pulmonary fibrosis (106,108). BAL fluid natural killer (NK) cell activity is increased in patients with HP whose exposure to the responsible antigen continues (109,110). The NK cell activity is found in cell populations with characteristics of both NK cells and non-NK cells, including lymphokine-activated killer cells (111). Most of the CD3$^+$ cells are T-cell receptor (TCR)α/β^+, but TCRγ/δ^+ cells are also increased, and some tendency toward T-cell oligoclonality is demonstrated by increased V$_\beta$8, V$_\beta$6, and V$_\beta$5 TCR usage in some patients with HP (112); however, this finding is not universal (113). In comparison with peripheral blood lymphocytes, BAL fluid lymphocytes have characteristics of T helper subset 1 (Th1) cells, including increased high-affinity IL-12 receptor messenger RNA, stimulated increased expression of interferon-γ (IFN-γ), and decreased expression of IL-4 messenger RNA (114). BAL fluid macrophages display many aspects of activation, including spontaneous secretion of TNF-α and IL-1 (110) and expression of CD25 (115). Mast cells, often with ultrastructural markers of degranulation, are increased in both the lung parenchyma and BAL fluid of patients with HP (84,102,107,116,117). Lymphokines, monokines, and chemokines that can activate macrophages, induce lymphocyte proliferation, and cause chemotaxis of CD8$^+$ cells (i.e., macrophage inflammatory protein-1α [MIP-1α], monocyte chemotactic protein-1 [MCP-1], IL-2, and IL-8) are present in the BAL fluid of patients with HP (118–121). Surfactant A is elevated in the BAL fluid of patients with HP (122). The concentrations of IgG, IgM, IgA, and albumin are increased in BAL fluid, presumably as a result of pulmonary inflammation (98). BAL fluid histamine and tryptase are increased in some patients with acute HP (102,107,123).

In some patients with HP, antibody (typically IgG, IgM, and IgA) to the offending material is easily demonstrated in serum and often also in BAL fluid (124,125). A multitude of methods have been used to demonstrate antibody (enzyme-linked immunosorbent assay [ELISA] and variants, indirect immunofluorescence, complement fixation, latex agglutination, counterimmunoelectrophoresis, radioimmunoassay, Western blot). Because most clinical studies have used simple agar diffusion ("Ouchterlony") methods to detect antibody, this is the standard technique, but other methods, such as ELISA, are also acceptable. The key issue is the ability of the antigen to detect antibody in the serum of patients with HP. This varies with the methods of bacterial growth (for bacterial antigens) and of extraction of soluble antigens from either cultured material or material that causes HP (i.e., hay in FLD, bird droppings in bird fancier's disease). Because antigen preparations are not standardized, it is difficult to be confident of the meaning of a negative result unless the antigens have been tested against panels of sera from patients with and without HP, so that specificity and sensitivity can be determined. Therefore, negative results of a commercially available "HP panel" do not exclude the diagnosis of HP (126–128). In addition, the presence of antibody in exposed but not ill subjects means that a positive result of the HP panel does not allow a diagnosis of the patient's illness. At times, it is useful to use antigens prepared from the environment that is suspected to cause HP. This is especially important in patients with ventilator lung (34,129–131).

Serum antibody is also present in many exposed but not ill subjects in virtually the same amounts as in patients with HP (91,132–134), although some data suggest that symptoms are related to the presence of antimucin IgG1 antibody in PBD (135,136). Therefore, the presence of antibody indicates exposure and sensitization, but not necessarily disease (137). Some data indicate that the presence of IgG and IgA antibody to *Trichosporon cutaneum* correlates with symptoms in subjects with Japanese summer-type HP, whereas IgG antibody alone correlates with exposure but no symptoms (138). This correlation of exposure and symptoms with IgA antibody is not found in pigeon breeders (124,139) or farmers (140). In asymptomatic pigeon breeders, the prevalence of antibody to pigeon antigens is 30% to 60% (12,13,15,141). In farmers, the prevalence of anti-*Saccharopolyspora rectivirgula* (anti-*Micropolyspora faeni*) serum antibody is 2% to 27% (18,142,143). The presence of serum antibody is not consistently related to apparent exposure (i.e., hours of exposure or intensity of exposure) in most instances of HP (142,144). This finding may represent a threshold effect, in which most exposures are above the minimum required to induce antibody and increases above that minimum are not associated with increases in the prevalence of antibody. In addition, serum antibody tends to wane after cessation of exposure, so that patients with chronic HP who have not been exposed for some time may not have demonstrable antibody. Approximately 50% of patients with FLD who are initially positive for serum antibody to *S. rectivirgula* lose demonstrable antibody 6 years after cessation of exposure (50,145). Farmers who continue to farm also lose detectable antibody (35%–50% in 5 years) (142,146), and in some asymptomatic farmers who are initially negative for antibody, antibody develops later without FLD (143). In PBD and bird fancier's disease, approximately 50% of patients initially positive for serum antibody to avian antigens lose demonstrable antibody 2 to 3 years after cessation of exposure (147,148). Therefore, it is possible that patients with HP will have no detectable serum antibody, either because an inappropriate antigen is used or because antibody has waned during the time since the last exposure.

Nonspecific markers of inflammation, such as the sedimentation rate and C-reactive protein, are often elevated during an acute episode of HP. Other markers of pulmonary inflammation, such as serum KL-6 (probably associated with regenerating type II cells in the lung), are also elevated in patients with HP (149). A few reports have appeared of an increased prevalence of rheumatoid factor in patients with HP (150,151). Antinuclear antibody and other autoantibodies are not present. The uptake of gallium 67 is increased in the lungs of patients with active HP, which declines as the disease abates (152). Serum angiotensin-converting enzyme levels are not elevated (153), whereas they are in sarcoidosis.

Skin tests (either immediate or delayed type) to detect sensitization to the suspected antigens are not useful because extracts of agents that cause HP induce nonspecific reactions that do not indicate sensitization and do not discriminate between sensitized and nonsensitized subjects (154). In addition, preparations of antigens that cause HP are not readily commercially available. Early reports indicated that some patients with HP demonstrate 4- to 8-hour skin test reactivity ("Arthus" type), which correlates with the presence of serum antibody (155,156). However, the presence of this reaction does not add to information important in the diagnosis of HP because antibody can be readily detected in the serum in patients with Arthus-type skin test reactivity.

Tests designed to detect cell sensitization (most commonly antigen-induced lymphocyte proliferation or lymphokine secretion) are not useful in the clinical diagnosis of HP, although they have been performed in specialized research settings (157–161). Patients with HP have depressed delayed-type skin reactivity to recall antigens (26,162), similar to that observed in patients with sarcoidosis (163).

PULMONARY FUNCTION TESTS

Pulmonary function tests typically demonstrate a restrictive ventilatory defect, with small lung volumes, normal or increased flow rates, increased elastic recoil, and usually decreased diffusing capacity (28,164). A mild obstructive defect and increased airway resistance are frequent findings (165–167), probably related to either bronchiolitis or emphysema. Arterial hypoxemia with hypocapnia reflecting an increased alveolar–arterial oxygen gradient, either at rest or after exercise, is common.

Many (20%–40%) patients with HP exhibit increased nonspecific airway reactivity (31,146,168), which may be related to increases in mast cells and their products in the lungs and BAL fluid or to bronchial epithelial damage (54,55,86), and in some (5%–10%), clinical asthma develops (169). The increased airway reactivity and asthma tend to diminish after cessation of exposure.

DIFFERENTIAL DIAGNOSIS

The symptoms, signs, and laboratory findings of acute HP can resemble those of many other lung diseases, including pulmonary edema, bronchoalveolar cell carcinoma, organic dust toxic syndrome, and some types of pneumoconiosis. Acute HP is most often confused with infectious pneumonia (usually thought to be caused by viruses or mycoplasmata) and at times with psittacosis in subjects exposed to birds.

Organic Dust Toxic Syndrome

Organic dust toxic syndrome has been described in some of the same populations exposed to the materials that cause HP, but organic dust toxic syndrome can occur in a larger proportion of the exposed population than HP. It is characterized by transient fever, dyspnea, nonproductive cough, peripheral blood leukocytosis, and BAL fluid neutrophilia; unlike HP, however, it is not associated with chest radiographic changes, permanent lung damage, or prior sensitization (indicated by the absence of serum antibodies) (170,171). Endotoxin, complement activation, and cytokine release from alveolar macrophages have been implicated as mediators of organic dust toxic syndrome (170). The exposure to antigens of patients presenting with organic dust toxic syndrome tends to be more intense and of shorter duration than that of patients who present with FLD (172).

Inhalation Fever

Another disease resulting from exposure to the same agents that cause ventilator lung is inhalation fever ("Monday morning miseries," "humidifier lung"). This is characterized by the development of fever, chills, myalgias, arthralgias, headache, malaise, cough, dyspnea, peripheral blood leukocytosis, and arterial hypoxemia 4 to 12 hours after exposure. Some investigators report decreased lung volumes with normal flow rates ("restrictive" pattern) and decreased diffusing capacity (173,174), whereas others report normal lung volumes and diffusing capacity (175,176). The clinical syndrome remits after 12 to 24 hours without specific therapy. Symptoms and signs are exaggerated after an exposure that occurs following a period without exposure (e.g., a vacation or a weekend) but then become blunted despite continued exposure ("Monday morning illness"). Monday morning illness with tolerance to apparently the same exposure later in the workweek also occurs in byssinosis and metal fume fever. All signs and symptoms of humidifier fever remit after cessation of exposure, and no permanent physiologic or roentgenologic changes develop. Serum antibodies to thermophilic organisms are rarely present, but antibodies to extracts of humidifier water or slime, Gram-negative and Gram-positive bacteria (*Bacillus, Flavobacterium, Pseudomonas, Streptomyces*), fungi (*Cephalosporium, Penicillium, Sporotrichum, Aspergillus, Fusarium, Mucor, Phoma, Rhizopus*), or amebae are detected (174,175,177–179).

Evidence suggests that some cases of humidifier fever may be caused by endotoxin. Many of the symptoms of humidifier fever can be reproduced by exposure to endotoxin. Rylander and Haglind (180) described a printing factory in which symptoms of humidifier fever developed in 20 of 50 workers. The humidifier water was heavily contaminated with *Pseudomonas* endotoxin, and airborne endotoxin was detected in the factory atmosphere when the humidifier was operating. However, other investigators have not detected endotoxin in humidifier water with use of a pyrogen assay (175), so that the role of endotoxin in humidifier fever is uncertain.

The treatment consists of preventing exposure to contaminated humidifier water by frequently cleaning the humidifier or changing the job location. It is frequently difficult to clean a humidifier permanently because any agent used to clean the water must be removed before the humidifier is put back in use to avoid exposure to the cleaning agent. The prognosis in humidifier fever after exposure is discontinued appears to be excellent because no permanent physiologic or roentgenologic changes develop.

Chronic HP resembles idiopathic pulmonary fibrosis, and in some instances it is impossible to distinguish between the two. The differential diagnoses includes other causes of pulmonary fibrosis (chemotherapy, radiation, inhalation of toxins, sarcoidosis, pneumoconiosis), heart failure, mycobacterial disease (particularly *Mycobacterium avium-intracellulare* infection, especially when associated with hot tubs), desquamative interstitial pneumonitis, and respiratory bronchiolitis–interstitial lung disease.

DIAGNOSIS

A thorough and complete occupational and avocational history is essential to diagnose both forms of HP. The history should seek to establish a link between a particular exposure (at work, home, or some other place) and previous episodes of pneumonia. Knowledge of other exposed persons with similar symptoms should be sought.

If the history suggests a relationship between exposure and pulmonary symptoms, evidence of sensitization should be sought and the nature of the pulmonary inflammatory response determined. Sensitization is indicated by the presence of serum antibody to an agent known to cause HP. A large proportion of lymphocytes in the BAL fluid (usually >40%) is suggestive of HP, although many other pulmonary processes can cause BAL fluid lymphocytosis.

A recurrence of appropriate symptoms and laboratory and radiologic abnormalities associated with exposure to a particular environment is at times sufficient to diagnose HP when the antigen has been well described to cause HP. In questionable instances, a natural exposure (i.e., documentation of appropriate symptoms and laboratory abnormalities after exposure to an environment suspected of causing HP) can be used to diagnose HP. The response to a natural exposure challenge should not be considered positive without objective evidence of a change in temperature, an increase in the alveolar–arterial gradient reflected by the development or worsening of a decrease in the arterial Po_2, a decrease in the total lung capacity or vital capacity (181), an increase in the total peripheral white blood cell count, or appropriate changes on the chest radiograph or HRCT scan.

In some patients, lung biopsy may be required to differentiate HP from other causes of diffuse pulmonary inflammation or fibrosis. Transbronchial lung biopsy specimens often do not provide sufficient material to establish the presence and interrelationship of granulomas, bronchiolitis, and interstitial inflammation (182), so that either open or thoracoscopic lung biopsy is usually required.

The diagnosis of HP can be difficult, especially if the putative antigen has not been well described as a cause of HP. The following is offered as a guide (183). For the diagnosis of HP to be considered, the following should be present (major criteria):

1. Symptoms compatible with HP
2. Evidence of exposure to appropriate antigen by history or detection of serum or BAL fluid antibody
3. Findings compatible with HP on chest radiograph or HRCT scan
4. BAL fluid lymphocytosis (if BAL performed)
5. Pulmonary histologic changes compatible with HP (if lung biopsy performed)
6. Positive response to "natural challenge" (reproduction of symptoms and laboratory abnormalities after exposure to the suspected environment).

The following (minor criteria) make the diagnosis more likely. Although these findings are nonspecific, they are almost always present in HP:

1. Bilateral basilar crackles
2. Decreased diffusing capacity
3. Arterial hypoxemia, either at rest or during exercise.

The diagnosis is confirmed if the patient fulfills four of the major criteria and at least two of the minor criteria, and if other diseases with similar symptoms are ruled out (i.e., sarcoidosis or idiopathic pulmonary fibrosis). Normal chest radiographic findings are acceptable if the pulmonary histology is compatible with HP (183). A normal HRCT scan eliminates the possibility of active acute or chronic HP but is possible between acute episodes (65), so that a normal HRCT scan is acceptable if compatible histologic changes are found in lung tissue obtained between acute episodes.

PATHOGENESIS

Multiple immunologic markers present in subjects with HP suggest that immune mediation is important in the pathogenesis of this syndrome (13,14,16,21,22,133,160). In addition, the necessity for previous sensitization (indicated by the presence of serum antibody in most patients with HP) suggests immune mediation.

The presence of serum antibody in patients with HP and the timing of symptoms after exposure (2–9 hours) led to the hypothesis that HP is an example of immune complex–mediated lung disease (184). However, the presence of antibody in exposed but not ill subjects, the lack of correlation of the presence of serum antibody with pulmonary func-

tion test results (148), the presence of HP in a patient with hypogammaglobulinemia (185), the appearance of HP in a patient with AIDS simultaneously with an increase in CD4$^+$ cells (186), the lack of evidence of complement consumption during acute exposure, pulmonary pathology that includes granulomatous changes, and findings from animal models all strongly suggest that cell-mediated immune processes are very important in HP.

Many of the agents responsible for HP can act as adjuvants and are particulate (promoting retention of antigen within the lung for prolonged periods of time), persistent, and nondegradable. They can interact with humoral mediators (complement and antibody) and cells in the lung to produce inflammation. The agents can induce injury by causing polymorphonuclear leukocytes and macrophages to release phlogistic substances such as reactive oxygen compounds, proteolytic enzymes, and products of arachidonic acid metabolism, including prostaglandins and leukotrienes. The agents can also cause the production and release of IL-1, IL-12, TNF-α, and IL-6 from macrophages and of lymphokines (IL-2 and IFN-γ) from lymphocytes. Injury to the lung caused by these factors could enhance pulmonary exposure to inhaled antigen that might promote immunologic sensitization and subsequent pulmonary damage. Both chemotactic factors (119,187) and adhesion molecules (121,188,189) are increased in the BAL fluid and secreted in increased amounts by the BAL cells of patients with HP (190), providing a mechanism for recruitment and retention of inflammatory cells in the lung. The result of all these processes is pulmonary inflammation.

In animal models, T cells and macrophages are central to the induction and expression of HP. Macrophage-derived cytokines such as IL-1α, IL-6, transforming growth factor-β (TGF-β), TNF-α, and IL-12 appear to play a central role in models that involve the intrapulmonary administration of materials that cause HP (191–194).

Additional factors, such as smoking and viral infections, affect the development of pulmonary inflammation in HP. Convincing evidence indicates that active cigarette smoking protects against the development of HP and suggests that viral infections may increase the likelihood of HP. Both respiratory syncytial virus and Sendai virus increase the expression of HP in mice (195,196). The mechanisms of both these factors may include changes in costimulatory molecules on antigen-presenting cells or T cells (197,198), and a decrease in the ability of alveolar macrophages to suppress inflammation (199).

Adoptive transfer models of HP allow differentiation between direct lung damage (i.e., toxicity), sensitization (the development of antibody and cellular reactivity), and the results of immune reactions (the interaction of antigen with antibody or cells). We have developed such a model in mice that allows the transfer of susceptibility to intratracheally administered *S. rectivirgula* with the use of cultured cells from sensitized animals. Culture of peritoneal exudate, spleen, peripheral, or lung-associated lymph node cells with a soluble extract of *S. rectivirgula,* the agent that causes FLD, confers the ability to induce susceptibility in recipients of transferred cells to increased pulmonary injury 4 days after an intratracheal injection of *S. rectivirgula.* The pulmonary injury is characterized by an increased number of mononuclear cells in the lungs in both perivascular and peribronchiolar locations. This phenomenon is dependent on sensitization of the donor with *S. rectivirgula,* culture with soluble *S. rectivirgula,* and the number of transferred cells, and it persists for at least 8 weeks after cell transfer. Serum from sensitized animals cannot transfer experimental HP. Three different mouse strains (C3H/HeJ, SJL/J, and C57Bl/6) do not differ in response (200). The postculture cells responsible for transfer are CD3$^+$, CD4$^+$, CD8$^-$, and SigM$^-$ T cells (201). The development of cells able to transfer is dependent on the presence of CD3$^+$, CD4$^+$, but not CD8$^+$ cells at the onset of culture. The transferring cells are a mixture of naive and memory (defined by CD44, CD45RB, and LECAM-1 markers) CD4$^+$ cells (202). The presence of recipient CD3$^+$, CD4$^+$, but not CD8$^+$ cells is required for the expression of adoptive experimental HP (203,204). IFN-γ and IL-2 are present in substantial quantities in culture supernatants (205), suggesting a predominance of Th1 CD4$^+$ cells. IL-12 is present in the BAL fluid of animals treated with *S. rectivirgula,* and *S. rectivirgula* causes the secretion of IL-12 from alveolar macrophages (193). Cultured cell lines with the characteristics of Th1 but not Th2 cells can adoptively transfer HP (206). IL-10 suppresses pulmonary inflammation in mice treated with *S. rectivirgula* (207).

Taken together, the human and animal data suggest that HP may be characterized by a predominance of Th1-type immunologic reactivity in the lung that results in pulmonary inflammation. However, the exact details of the mechanisms of HP (i.e., antibody, cell-mediated [Th1 vs. Th2], or innate immunity) are not well delineated. The mechanisms underlying the different degrees of susceptibility of individuals to HP and the resolution of inflammation are also unclear.

PROGNOSIS AND TREATMENT

The prognosis varies considerably with the type of HP and even the geographic location. For example, patients with FLD have a good prognosis in Quebec (208), even farmers who continue to farm. However, FLD in Finland often results in significant physiologic impairment and even death (209). Patients with PBD in the United States and Europe have a good prognosis, whereas patients with the same disease in Mexico have a 5-year mortality of 30% (210). The reasons for these differences are not clear but likely include differences in the antigen and differences in the nature of the exposure.

Eliminating exposure to the offending antigens is usually sufficient to relieve symptoms and physiologic abnormalities

within a few days in acute HP and within a month in chronic HP (169). When symptoms and signs of pulmonary fibrosis persist for more than 6 months, a poor outcome is likely (50). Complete removal from exposure is most effective, but cleaning the environment when removal is impractical (e.g., Japanese summer-type HP) can prevent further episodes of HP (211). In one report, symptoms of HP resolved after the installation of filters in an air conditioning system that greatly lowered the mold colony counts (212). Pigeon lofts in which litter materials designed to absorb pigeon excreta are not used contain a significantly smaller amount of airborne pigeon antigens than lofts in which litter material is used (213). It is not known whether avoidance of litter materials is associated with a decrease in PBD. The application of tannic acid to pigeon lofts does not decrease the amount of bird antigens in dust (214).

Systemic glucocorticoids are sometimes required to treat severe disease, although no formal evidence is available that such treatment is associated with the long-term relief of symptoms or a reduction in radiologic or pulmonary function test abnormalities (146). The usual treatment is 40 to 60 mg of prednisone or prednisolone per day for 2 weeks, followed by a gradual decrease to no treatment during 1 to 2 months, depending on the clinical response. Patients with FLD who are treated with prednisolone, in comparison with those not treated with prednisolone, demonstrated a slightly more rapid resolution of some radiologic abnormalities (ground-glass opacities) and some physiologic abnormalities (slight improvement in diffusing capacity, no difference in lung volumes or arterial Po$_2$). However, no differences were found between the groups 6 months after the diagnosis of HP (146,154,215). This evidence suggests that systemic steroids may slightly increase the rate of resolution of acute pulmonary inflammation but have little or no effects on chronic residua of HP. Nonsteroidal anti-inflammatory agents (e.g., cromolyn, nedocromil) are not indicated in the treatment of HP. Little experience has been reported in the use of systemic immune modulators (e.g., azathioprine, cyclophosphamide) in the treatment of severe, refractory HP. Such patients may require evaluation at referral centers with experience in such treatments. Inhaled glucocorticoids may be effective in the treatment of bird-associated disease (216,217).

If patients are removed from exposure before permanent radiologic or physiologic abnormalities develop, the prognosis is excellent, with little evidence of long-term ill effects (218). If removal from exposure is impossible, the use of efficient masks during exposure can prevent acute HP (219,220) and is associated with an excellent prognosis (221,222). If exposure continues, some patients (the proportion is unclear, but probably 10%–30%) will progress to diffuse pulmonary fibrosis with resultant cor pulmonale and premature death (208,223). Mortality from FLD is associated with an increasing number of episodes and is reported to be between zero and 20%; death usually occurs after more than 5 years of recurrent symptoms (26,224,225), although a few cases of death after acute massive exposure to antigen have been reported (209,226). The prognosis varies considerably with the type of HP. In general, long-term, relatively low-level exposure appears to be associated with a poorer prognosis, whereas short-term, intermittent exposure is associated with a better prognosis. This is well illustrated by PBD. In the United States and Europe, patients with PBD have an excellent prognosis; most of a group of 24 patients with PBD were asymptomatic and all were alive 10 years after diagnosis (227), whereas in patients with PBD from Mexico City, the mortality was 30% after 5 years (210). Unfortunately, many patients with chronic HP present with pulmonary fibrosis and physiologic abnormalities that are only partially reversible after cessation of exposure (228).

Markers of pulmonary inflammation at the time of presentation, such as a high proportion of lymphocytes, neutrophils, or mast cells in the BAL fluid (145,229) or the presence of procollagen III, hyaluronic acid, fibronectin, and fibroblast growth factors in the BAL fluid, do not predict outcome (166).

CONCLUSION

In conclusion, HP is an immunologically mediated lung disease with important roles for T cells and macrophages. It is diagnosed clinically by a careful history and appropriate laboratory tests. Avoidance of exposure is usually associated with a good prognosis. Because of constantly changing environmental exposures, new examples of HP are constantly being described and represent a continuing challenge to astute clinicians.

HYPERSENSITIVITY PNEUMONITIS

Summary Statement	Level of Evidence
Corticosteroids accelerate initial recovery from farmer's lung and bird fancier's lung, particularly in severely ill patients; however, the long-term outcome appears unchanged by corticosteroid treatment.	Randomized controlled trials, observational studies
Efforts must be made to modify or avoid the culprit environment to minimize ongoing exposure.	Observational studies

REFERENCES

1. Schullian D. Notes and events. *J History Med Allied Sci* 1982;37:440–443.
2. Campbell J. Acute symptoms following work with hay. *Br J Ind Med* 1932;2:1143–1144.
3. Ranalli G, Grazia L, Roggeri A. The influence of hay-packing techniques on the presence of *Saccharopolyspora rectivirgula*. *J Appl Microbiol* 1999;87:359–365.
4. Bernstein DI, Lummus ZL, Santilli G, et al. Machine operator's lung. A hypersensitivity pneumonitis disorder associated with exposure to metal-working fluid aerosols. *Chest* 1995;108:636–641.
5. Hodgson MJ, Bracker A, Yang C, et al. Hypersensitivity pneumonitis in a metal-working environment. *Am J Ind Med* 2001;39:616–628.
6. Fox J, Anderson H, Moen T, et al. Metal-working fluid-associated hypersensitivity pneumonitis: an outbreak investigation and case-control study. *Am J Ind Med* 1999;35:58–67.
7. Shelton BG, Flanders WD, Morris GK. *Mycobacterium* sp. as a possible cause of hypersensitivity pneumonitis in machine workers. *Emerg Infect Dis* 1999;5:270–273.
8. Zacharisen MC, Kadambi AR, Schlueter DP, et al. The spectrum of respiratory disease associated with exposure to metal-working fluids. *J Occup Environ Med* 1998;40:640–647.
9. Kreiss K, Cox-Ganser J. Metal-working fluid-associated hypersensitivity pneumonitis: a workshop summary. *Am J Ind Med* 1997;32:423–432.
10. Rodriguez de Castro F, Carrillo T, Castillo R, et al. Relationships between characteristics of exposure to pigeon antigens. Clinical manifestations and humoral immune response. *Chest* 1993;103:1059–1063.
11. Bourke SJ, Carter R, Anderson K, et al. Obstructive airways disease in non-smoking subjects with pigeon fanciers' lung. *Clin Exp Allergy* 1989;19:629–632.
12. Carrillo T, Rodriguez de Castro F, Cuevas M, et al. Effect of cigarette smoking on the humoral immune response in pigeon fanciers. *Allergy* 1991;46:241–244.
13. Banham SW, McSharry C, Lynch PP, et al. Relationships between avian exposure, humoral immune response, and pigeon breeders' disease among Scottish pigeon fanciers. *Thorax* 1986;41:274–278.
14. Christensen LT, Schmidt CD, Robbins L. Pigeon breeders' disease—a prevalence study and review. *Clin Allergy* 1975;5:417–430.
15. Elgerfors B, Belin L, Hanson LA. Pigeon breeder's lung. Clinical and immunological observations. *Scand J Respir Dis* 1971;52:167–176.
16. McSharry C, Banham SW, Boyd G. Effect of cigarette smoking on the antibody response to inhaled antigens and the prevalence of extrinsic allergic alveolitis among pigeon breeders. *Clin Allergy* 1985;15:487–494.
17. Depierre A, Dalphin JC, Pernet D, et al. Epidemiological study of farmer's lung in five districts of the French Doubs province. *Thorax* 1988;43:429–435.
18. Gruchow HW, Hoffmann RG, Marx JJ Jr, et al. Precipitating antibodies to farmer's lung antigens in a Wisconsin farming population. *Am Rev Respir Dis* 1981;124:411–415.
19. Dalphin JC, Debieuvre D, Pernet D, et al. Prevalence and risk factors for chronic bronchitis and farmer's lung in French dairy farmers. *Br J Ind Med* 1993;50:941–944.
20. Madsen D, Klock LE, Wenzel FJ, et al. The prevalence of farmer's lung in an agricultural population. *Am Rev Respir Dis* 1976;113:171–174.
21. Terho EO, Husman K, Vohlonen I. Prevalence and incidence of chronic bronchitis and farmer's lung with respect to age, sex, atopy, and smoking. *Eur J Respir Dis Suppl* 1987;152:19–28.
22. Cormier Y, Belanger J, Durand P. Factors influencing the development of serum precipitins to farmer's lung antigen in Quebec dairy farmers. *Thorax* 1985;40:138–142.

23. Grant IW, Blyth W, Wardrop VE, et al. Prevalence of farmer's lung in Scotland: a pilot survey. *Br Med J* 1972;1:530–534.

24. Smyth JT, Adkins GE, Margaret L, et al. Farmer's lung in Devon. *Thorax* 1975;30:197–203.

25. Vohlonen I, Tupi K, Terho EO, et al. Prevalence and incidence of chronic bronchitis and farmer's lung with respect to the geographical location of the farm and to the work of farmers. *Eur J Respir Dis Suppl* 1987;152:37–46.

26. Emanuel D, Wenzel F, Bowerman C, et al. Farmer's lung. Clinical, pathologic and immunologic study of twenty-four patients. *Am J Med* 1964;37:392–401.

27. Terho EO, Heinonen OP, Lammi S, et al. Incidence of clinically confirmed farmer's lung in Finland and its relation to meteorological factors. *Eur J Respir Dis Suppl* 1987;152:47–56.

28. Sansores R, Perez-Padilla R, Pare PD, et al. Exponential analysis of the lung pressure-volume curve in patients with chronic pigeon-breeder's lung. *Chest* 1992;101:1352–1356.

29. Ando M, Arima K, Yoneda R, et al. Japanese summer-type hypersensitivity pneumonitis. Geographic distribution, home environment, and clinical characteristics of 621 cases. *Am Rev Respir Dis* 1991;144:765–769.

30. Miyagawa T, Hamagami S, Tanigawa N. *Cryptococcus albidus*-induced summer-type hypersensitivity pneumonitis. *Am J Respir Crit Care Med* 2000;161:961–966.

31. Monkare S. Clinical aspects of farmer's lung: airway reactivity, treatment and prognosis. *Eur J Respir Dis Suppl* 1984;137:1–68.

32. Edwards J, Griffiths A, Mullins J. Protozoa as sources of antigen in "humidifier fever." *Nature* 1976;264:438–439.

33. Terho EO, Husman K, Vohlonen I, et al. Serum precipitins against microbes in mouldy hay with respect to age, sex, atopy, and smoking of farmers. *Eur J Respir Dis Suppl* 1987;152:115–121.

34. Baur X, Richter G, Pethran A, et al. Increased prevalence of IgG-induced sensitization and hypersensitivity pneumonitis (humidifier lung) in nonsmokers exposed to aerosols of a contaminated air conditioner. *Respiration* 1992;59:211–214.

35. Warren C. Extrinsic allergic alveolitis: a disease commoner in nonsmokers. *Thorax* 1977;32:567–569.

36. Morgan DC, Smyth JT, Lister RW, et al. Chest symptoms and farmer's lung: a community survey. *Br J Ind Med* 1973;30:259–265.

37. Anderson K, Morrison SM, Bourke S, et al. Effect of cigarette smoking on the specific antibody response in pigeon fanciers. *Thorax* 1988;43:798–800.

38. Baldwin CI, Todd A, Bourke S, et al. Pigeon fanciers' lung: effects of smoking on serum and salivary antibody responses to pigeon antigens. *Clin Exp Immunol* 1998;113:166–172.

39. Finklea J, Hasselblad V, Riggan W, et al. Cigarette smoking and hemagglutination inhibition response to influenza after natural disease and immunization. *Am Rev Respir Dis* 1971;104:368–376.

40. Weissman DN, Bice D, Crowell R, et al. Human lung immunization: impairment of humoral responses in smokers. *Am Rev Respir Dis* 1991;143:A227(abst).

41. Flaherty DK, Braun SR, Marx JJ, et al. Serologically detectable HLA-A, B, and C loci antigens in farmer's lung disease. *Am Rev Respir Dis* 1980;122:437–443.

42. Rodey GE, Fink J, Koethe S, et al. A study of HLA-A, B, C, and DR specificities in pigeon breeder's disease. *Am Rev Respir Dis* 1979;119:755–759.

43. Terho E, Koskimies S, Heinonen O, et al. HLA and farmers' lung. *Eur J Respir Dis* 1981;63:361–362.

44. Selman M, Teran L, Mendoza A, et al. Increase of HLA-DR7 in pigeon breeder's lung in a Mexican population. *Clin Immunol Immunopathol* 1987;44:63–70.

45. Rittner C, Sennekamp J, Mollenhauer E, et al. Pigeon breeder's lung: association with HLA-DR3. *Tissue Antigens* 1983;21:374–379.

46. Muers MF, Faux JA, Ting A, et al. HLA-A, B, C and HLA-DR antigens in extrinsic allergic alveolitis (budgerigar fancier's lung disease). *Clin Allergy* 1982;12:47–53.

47. Richeldi L, Sorrentino R, Saltini C. HLA-DP1 glutamate 69: a genetic marker of beryllium disease. *Science* 1993;262:242–244.

48. Camarena A, Juarez A, Mejia M, et al. Major histocompatibility complex and tumor necrosis factor-alpha polymorphisms in pigeon breeder's disease. *Am J Respir Crit Care Med* 2001;163:1528–1533.

49. Schaaf BM, Seitzer U, Pravica V, et al. Tumor necrosis factor-alpha-308 promoter gene polymorphism and increased tumor necrosis factor serum bioactivity in farmer's lung patients. *Am J Respir Crit Care Med* 2001;163:379–382.

50. Hapke EJ, Seal RM, Thomas GO, et al. Farmer's lung. A clinical, radiographic, functional, and serological correlation of acute and chronic stages. *Thorax* 1968;23:451–468.

51. Sansores R, Salas J, Chapela R, et al. Clubbing in hypersensitivity pneumonitis. Its prevalence and possible prognostic role. *Arch Intern Med* 1990;150:1849–1851.

52. Bourke S, Anderson K, Lynch P, et al. Chronic simple bronchitis in pigeon fanciers. Relationship of cough with expectoration to avian exposure and pigeon breeders' disease. *Chest* 1989;95:598–601.

53. Boyd G, Parratt D. Improved diagnosis of farmer's lung using the fluorescent antibody technique. *Thorax* 1974;29:417–420.

54. Heino M, Monkare S, Haahtela T, et al. An electron-microscopic study of the airways in patients with farmer's lung. *Eur J Respir Dis* 1982;63:52–61.

55. Laitinen LA, Haahtela T, Kava T, et al. Non-specific bronchial reactivity and ultrastructure of the airway epithelium in patients with sarcoidosis and allergic alveolitis. *Eur J Respir Dis Suppl* 1983;131:267–284.

56. Hasani A, Johnson M, Pavia D, et al. Impairment of lung mucociliary clearance in pigeon fanciers. *Chest* 1992;102:887–891.

57. Craig TJ, Hershey J, Engler RJ, et al. Bird antigen persistence in the home environment after removal of the bird. *Ann Allergy* 1992;69:510–512.

58. Coultas DB, Zumwalt RE, Black WC, et al. The epidemiology of interstitial lung diseases. *Am J Respir Crit Care Med* 1994;150:967–972.

59. Mapel DW, Hunt WC, Utton R, et al. Idiopathic pulmonary fibrosis: survival in population-based and hospital-based cohorts. *Thorax* 1998;53:469–476.

60. Jacobs RL, Andrews CP, Coalson J. Organic antigen-induced interstitial lung disease: diagnosis and management. *Ann Allergy Asthma Immunol* 2002;88:30–41.

61. Mullen J, Hodgson MJ, DeGraff CA, et al. Case-control study of idiopathic pulmonary fibrosis and environmental exposures. *J Occup Environ Med* 1998;40:363–367.

62. Hubbard R, Lewis S, Richards K, et al. Occupational exposure to metal or wood dust and aetiology of cryptogenic fibrosing alveolitis. *Lancet* 1996;347:284–289.

63. Baumgartner KB, Samet JM, Coultas DB, et al. Occupational and environmental risk factors for idiopathic pulmonary fibrosis: a multicenter case-control study. Collaborating centers. *Am J Epidemiol* 2000;152:307–315.

64. Baumgartner KB, Samet JM, Stidley CA, et al. Cigarette

smoking: a risk factor for idiopathic pulmonary fibrosis. *Am J Respir Crit Care Med* 1997;155:242–248.

65. Hansell DM, Moskovic E. High-resolution computed tomography in extrinsic allergic alveolitis. *Clin Radiol* 1991;43:8–12.

66. Vincent JM, Flower CD, Shneerson JM, et al. Extrinsic allergic alveolitis: problems in diagnosis and a potential use for computed tomography. *Respir Med* 1992;86:135–141.

67. Akira M, Kita N, Higashihara T, et al. Summer-type hypersensitivity pneumonitis: comparison of high-resolution CT and plain radiographic findings. *AJR Am J Roentgenol* 1992;158:1223–1228.

68. Cormier Y, Brown M, Worthy S, et al. High-resolution computed tomographic characteristics in acute farmer's lung and in its follow-up. *Eur Respir J* 2000;16:56–60.

69. Cook PG, Wells IP, McGavin CR. The distribution of pulmonary shadowing in farmer's lung. *Clin Radiol* 1988;39:21–27.

70. Ichikawa Y, Tokunaga N, Kinoshita M, et al. Subcutaneous and mediastinal emphysema associated with hypersensitivity pneumonitis. *Chest* 1991;99:759–761.

71. Mitani M, Satoh K, Kobayashi T, et al. Hypersensitivity pneumonitis in a pearl nucleus worker. *J Thorac Imaging* 1995;10:134–137.

72. Lynch DA, Newell JD, Logan PM, et al. Can CT distinguish hypersensitivity pneumonitis from idiopathic pulmonary fibrosis? *AJR Am J Roentgenol* 1995;165:807–811.

73. Lynch DA, Rose CS, Way D, et al. Hypersensitivity pneumonitis: sensitivity of high-resolution CT in a population-based study. *AJR Am J Roentgenol* 1992;159:469–472.

74. Patel RA, Sellami D, Gotway MB, et al. Hypersensitivity pneumonitis: patterns on high-resolution CT. *J Comput Assist Tomogr* 2000;24:965–970.

75. Remy-Jardin M, Remy J, Wallaert B, et al. Subacute and chronic bird breeder hypersensitivity pneumonitis: sequential evaluation with CT and correlation with lung function tests and bronchoalveolar lavage. *Radiology* 1993;189:111–118.

76. Buschman DL, Gamsu G, Waldron JA Jr, et al. Chronic hypersensitivity pneumonitis: use of CT in diagnosis. *AJR Am J Roentgenol* 1992;159:957–960.

77. Hansell DM, Wells AU, Padley SP, et al. Hypersensitivity pneumonitis: correlation of individual CT patterns with functional abnormalities. *Radiology* 1996;199:123–128.

78. Erkinjuntti-Pekkanen R, Rytkonen H, Kokkarinen JI, et al. Long-term risk of emphysema in patients with farmer's lung and matched control farmers. *Am J Respir Crit Care Med* 1998;158:662–665.

79. Adler BD, Padley SP, Muller NL, et al. Chronic hypersensitivity pneumonitis: high-resolution CT and radiographic features in 16 patients. *Radiology* 1992;185:91–95.

80. Seal RM, Hapke EJ, Thomas GO, et al. The pathology of the acute and chronic stages of farmer's lung. *Thorax* 1968;23:469–489.

81. Reyes N, Wenzel F, Lawton B, et al. The pulmonary pathology of farmer's lung disease. *Chest* 1982;81:142–146.

82. Sutinen S RK, Huhti E, Darkola P. Extrinsic allergic alveolitis: serology and biopsy findings. *Eur Respir J* 1983;64:271–282.

83. Tukiainen P TE, Korhola O, Valle M. Farmer's lung, needle biopsy findings and pulmonary function. *Eur Respir J* 1980;61:3–11.

84. Kawanami O, Basset F, Barrios R, et al. Hypersensitivity pneumonitis in man. *Am J Pathol* 1983;110:275–289.

85. Reijula K, Sutinen S. Ultrastructure of extrinsic allergic bronchiolo-alveolitis. *Pathol Res Pract* 1986;181:418–429.

86. Barrios R, Fortoul TI, Lupi-Herrera E. Pigeon breeder's disease: immunofluorescence and ultrastructural observations. *Lung* 1986;164:55–64.

87. Perez-Padilla R, Gaxiola M, Salas J, et al. Bronchiolitis in chronic pigeon breeder's disease. Morphologic evidence of a spectrum of small airway lesions in hypersensitivity pneumonitis induced by avian antigens. *Chest* 1996;110:371–377.

88. Coleman A, Colby TV. Histologic diagnosis of extrinsic allergic alveolitis. *Am J Surg Pathol* 1988;12:514–518.

89. Suda T, Chida K, Hayakawa H, et al. Development of bronchus-associated lymphoid tissue in chronic hypersensitivity pneumonitis. *Chest* 1999;115:357–363.

90. Coleman A, Colby TV. Histologic diagnosis of extrinsic allergic alveolitis. *Am J Surg Pathol* 1988;12:514–518.

91. Johnson MA, Nemeth A, Condez A, et al. Cell-mediated immunity in pigeon breeders' lung: the effect of removal from antigen exposure. *Eur Respir J* 1989;2:445–450.

92. Katzenstein A-L, Fiorelli R. Nonspecific interstitial pneumonia/fibrosis. Histologic patterns and clinical significance. *Am J Surg Pathol* 1994;18:136.

93. Katzenstein AL, Myers JL. Idiopathic pulmonary fibrosis: clinical relevance of pathologic classification. *Am J Respir Crit Care Med* 1998;157:1301–1315.

94. Vourlekis JS, Schwarz MI, Cool CD, et al. Nonspecific interstitial pneumonia as the sole histologic expression of hypersensitivity pneumonitis. *Am J Med* 2002;112:490–493.

95. Pesci A, Bertorelli G, Dall'Aglio PP, et al. Evidence in bronchoalveolar lavage for third type immune reactions in hypersensitivity pneumonitis. *Eur Respir J* 1990;3:359–361.

96. Fournier E, Tonnel AB, Gosset P, et al. Early neutrophil alveolitis after antigen inhalation in hypersensitivity pneumonitis. *Chest* 1985;88:563–566.

97. Reynolds SP, Jones KP, Edwards JH, et al. Inhalation challenge in pigeon breeder's disease: BAL fluid changes after 6 hours. *Eur Respir J* 1993;6:467–476.

98. Drent M, Van Velzen-Blad H, Diamant M, et al. Bronchoalveolar lavage in extrinsic allergic alveolitis: effect of time elapsed since antigen exposure. *Eur Respir J* 1993;6:1276–1281.

99. Cormier Y, Belanger J, Laviolette M. Persistent bronchoalveolar lymphocytosis in asymptomatic farmers. *Am Rev Respir Dis* 1986;133:843–847.

100. Leblanc P, Belanger J, Laviolette M, et al. Relationship among antigen contact, alveolitis, and clinical status in farmer's lung disease. *Arch Intern Med* 1986;146:153–157.

101. Cormier Y, Belanger J, Laviolette M. Prognostic significance of bronchoalveolar lymphocytosis in farmer's lung. *Am Rev Respir Dis* 1987;135:692–695.

102. Miadonna A, Pesci A, Tedeschi A, et al. Mast cell and histamine involvement in farmer's lung disease. *Chest* 1994;105:1184–1189.

103. Trentin L, Migone N, Zambello R, et al. Mechanisms accounting for lymphocytic alveolitis in hypersensitivity pneumonitis. *J Immunol* 1990;145:2147–2154.

104. Hamagami S, Miyagawa T, Ochi T, et al. A raised level of soluble CD8 in bronchoalveolar lavage fluid in summer-type hypersensitivity pneumonitis in Japan. *Chest* 1992;101:1044–1049.

105. Suda T, Sato A, Ida M, et al. Hypersensitivity pneumonitis associated with home ultrasonic humidifiers. *Chest* 1995;107:711–717.

106. Murayama J, Yoshizawa Y, Ohtsuka M, et al. Lung fibrosis in hypersensitivity pneumonitis. Association with CD4$^+$ but not CD8$^+$ cell dominant alveolitis and insidious onset. *Chest* 1993;104:38–43.

107. Soler P, Nioche S, Valeyre D, et al. Role of mast cells in the pathogenesis of hypersensitivity pneumonitis. *Thorax* 1987;42:565–572.

108. Mornex JF, Cordier G, Pages J, et al. Activated lung

lymphocytes in hypersensitivity pneumonitis. *J Allergy Clin Immunol* 1984;74:719–727.

109. Trentin L, Marcer G, Chilosi M, et al. Longitudinal study of alveolitis in hypersensitivity pneumonitis patients: an immunologic evaluation. *J Allergy Clin Immunol* 1988;82:577–585.

110. Denis M, Bedard M, Laviolette M, et al. A study of monokine release and natural killer activity in the bronchoalveolar lavage of subjects with farmer's lung. *Am Rev Respir Dis* 1993;147:934–939.

111. Semenzato G, Trentin L, Zambello R, et al. Different types of cytotoxic lymphocytes recovered from the lungs of patients with hypersensitivity pneumonitis. *Am Rev Respir Dis* 1988;137:70–74.

112. Murayama J, Yoshizawa Y, Sato T, et al. A compartmentalized bias for T-cell receptor V beta usage in summer-type hypersensitivity pneumonitis. *Int Arch Allergy Immunol* 1995;107:581–586.

113. Shigematsu M, Nagai S, Nishimura K, et al. Summer-type hypersensitivity pneumonitis. T-cell receptor V gene usage in BALF T-cells from 3 cases in one family. *Sarcoidosis Vasc Diffuse Lung Dis* 1998;15:173–177.

114. Yamasaki H, Ando M, Brazer W, et al. Polarized type 1 cytokine profile in bronchoalveolar lavage T cells of patients with hypersensitivity pneumonitis. *J Immunol* 1999;163:3516–3523.

115. Pforte A, Brunner A, Gais P, et al. Increased levels of soluble serum interleukin-2 receptor in extrinsic allergic alveolitis correlate with interleukin-2 receptor expression on alveolar macrophages. *J Allergy Clin Immunol* 1994;94:1057–1064.

116. Ishida T, Matsui Y, Matsumura Y, et al. Bronchoalveolar mast cells in summer-type hypersensitivity pneumonitis: increase in numbers and ultrastructural evidence of degranulation. *Intern Med* 1995;34:357–363.

117. Haslam PL, Dewar A, Butchers P, et al. Mast cells, atypical lymphocytes, and neutrophils in bronchoalveolar lavage in extrinsic allergic alveolitis. Comparison with other interstitial lung diseases. *Am Rev Respir Dis* 1987;135:35–47.

118. Denis M. Proinflammatory cytokines in hypersensitivity pneumonitis. *Am J Respir Crit Care Med* 1995;151:164–169.

119. Sugiyama Y, Kasahara T, Mukaida N, et al. Chemokines in bronchoalveolar lavage fluid in summer-type hypersensitivity pneumonitis. *Eur Respir J* 1995;8:1084–1090.

120. Dakhama A, Israel-Assayag E, Cormier Y. Role of interleukin-2 in the development and persistence of lymphocytic alveolitis in farmer's lung. *Eur Respir J* 1998;11:1281–1286.

121. Baumer I, Zissel G, Schlaak M, et al. Soluble intercellular adhesion molecule 1 (sICAM-1) in bronchoalveolar lavage (BAL) cell cultures and in the circulation of patients with tuberculosis, hypersensitivity pneumonitis and sarcoidosis. *Eur J Med Res* 1998;3:288–294.

122. Hamm H, Luhrs J, Guzman y Rotaeche J, et al. Elevated surfactant protein A in bronchoalveolar lavage fluids from sarcoidosis and hypersensitivity pneumonitis patients. *Chest* 1994;106:1766–1770.

123. Walls AF, Bennett AR, Godfrey RC, et al. Mast cell tryptase and histamine concentrations in bronchoalveolar lavage fluid from patients with interstitial lung disease. *Clin Sci* 1991;81:183–188.

124. Patterson R, Wang JL, Fink JN, et al. IgA and IgG antibody activities of serum and bronchoalveolar fluid from symptomatic and asymptomatic pigeon breeders. *Am Rev Respir Dis* 1979;120:1113–1118.

125. Sandoval J, Banales JL, Cortes JJ, et al. Detection of antibodies against avian antigens in bronchoalveolar lavage from patients with pigeon breeder's disease: usefulness of enzyme-linked immunosorbent assay and enzyme immunotransfer blotting. *J Clin Lab Analysis* 1990;4:81–85.

126. Patterson R, Greenberger PA, Castile RG, et al. Diagnostic problems in hypersensitivity lung disease. *Allergy Proc* 1989;10:141–147.

127. McClellan JS, Albers GM, Noyes BE, et al. B-lymphocyte aggregates in alveoli from a child with hypersensitivity pneumonitis (bird breeders' lung). *Ann Allergy Asthma Immunol* 1999;83:357–360.

128. Krasnick J, Meuwissen HJ, Nakao MA, et al. Hypersensitivity pneumonitis: problems in diagnosis. *J Allergy Clin Immunol* 1996;97:1027–1030.

129. Robertson AS, Burge PS, Wieland GA, et al. Extrinsic allergic alveolitis caused by a cold water humidifier. *Thorax* 1987;42:32–37.

130. Baur X, Behr J, Dewair M, et al. Humidifier lung and humidifier fever. *Lung* 1988;166:113–124.

131. Patterson R, Mazur N, Roberts M, et al. Hypersensitivity pneumonitis due to humidifier disease: seek and ye shall find. *Chest* 1998;114:931–933.

132. Moore VL and Fink JN. Immunologic studies in hypersensitivity pneumonitis—quantitative precipitins and complement-fixing antibodies in symptomatic and asymptomatic pigeon breeders. *J Lab Clin Med* 1975;85:540–545.

133. Kitt S, Lee CW, Fink JN, et al. Immunoglobulin G4 in pigeon breeder's disease. *J Lab Clin Med* 1986;108:442–447.

134. Fink J, Barboriak J, Sosman A, et al. Antibodies against pigeon serum proteins in pigeon breeders. *J Lab Clin Med* 1968;71:20–24.

135. Baldwin CI, Todd A, Bourke SJ, et al. IgG subclass responses to pigeon intestinal mucin are related to development of pigeon fanciers' lung. *Clin Exp Allergy* 1998;28:349–357.

136. Baldwin CI, Todd A, Bourke SJ, et al. Pigeon fanciers' lung: identification of disease-associated carbohydrate epitopes on pigeon intestinal mucin. *Clin Exp Immunol* 1999;117:230–236.

137. Rodrigo MJ, Benavent MI, Cruz MJ, et al. Detection of specific antibodies to pigeon serum and bloom antigens by enzyme-linked immunosorbent assay in pigeon breeder's disease. *Occup Environ Med* 2000;57:159–164.

138. Ando M, Yoshida K, Soda K, et al. Specific bronchoalveolar lavage IgA antibody in patients with summer-type hypersensitivity pneumonitis induced by *Trichosporon cutaneum*. *Am Rev Respir Dis* 1986;134:177–179.

139. Reynolds SP, Edwards JH, Jones KP, et al. Immunoglobulin and antibody levels in bronchoalveolar lavage fluid from symptomatic and asymptomatic pigeon breeders. *Clin Exp Immunol* 1991;86:278–285.

140. Iranitalab M, Jarolim E, Rumpold H, et al. Characterization of *Micropolyspora faeni* antigens by human antibodies and immunoblot analysis. *Allergy* 1989;44:314–321.

141. Fink JN, Schlueter DP, Sosman AJ, et al. Clinical survey of pigeon breeders. *Chest* 1972;62:277–281.

142. Kusaka H, Homma Y, Ogasawara H, et al. Five-year follow-up of *Micropolyspora faeni* antibody in smoking and nonsmoking farmers. *Am Rev Respir Dis* 1989;140:695–699.

143. Cormier Y, Belanger J. The fluctuant nature of precipitating antibodies in dairy farmers. *Thorax* 1989;44:469–473.

144. McSharry C, Banham SW, Lynch PP, et al. Antibody measurement in extrinsic allergic alveolitis. *Eur J Respir Dis* 1984;65:259–265.

145. Gariepy L, Cormier Y, Laviolette M, et al. Predictive value of BAL cells and serum precipitins in asymptomatic dairy farmers. *Am Rev Respir Dis* 1989;140:1386–1389.

146. Monkare S, Haahtela T. Farmer's lung—a 5-year follow-up of eighty-six patients. *Clin Allergy* 1987;17:143–151.

147. Boyd G. Clinical and immunological studies in pulmonary extrinsic allergic alveolitis. *Scott Med J* 1978;23:267–276.

148. Lee TH, Wraith DG, Bennett CO, et al. Budgerigar fancier's lung. The persistence of budgerigar precipitins and the recovery of lung function after cessation of avian exposure. *Clin Allergy* 1983;13:197–202.

149. Takahashi T, Munakata M, Ohtsuka Y, et al. Serum KL-6 concentrations in dairy farmers. *Chest* 2000;118:445–450.

150. Terho EO, Lindstrom P, Mantyjarvi R, et al. Circulating immune complexes and rheumatoid factors in patients with farmer's lung. *Allergy* 1983;38:347–352.

151. Martinez-Cordero E, Bessudo-Babani A, Trevino-Perez SC, et al. Circulating autoantibodies in patients with pigeon breeder's disease. *Allergol Immunopathol (Madr)* 1989;17:1–6.

152. Vanderstappen M, Mornex JF, Lahneche B, et al. Gallium-67 scanning in the staging of cryptogenetic fibrosing alveolitis and hypersensitivity pneumonitis. *Eur Respir J* 1988;1:517–522.

153. McCormick JR, Thrall RS, Ward PA, et al. Serum angiotensin-converting enzyme levels in patients with pigeon-breeder's disease. *Chest* 1981;80:431–433.

154. Williams J. Inhalation and skin tests with extracts of hay and fungi in patients with farmer's lung. *Thorax* 1963;18:182–196.

155. Fink JN, Sosman AJ, Barboriak JJ, et al. Pigeon breeders' disease. A clinical study of a hypersensitivity pneumonitis. *Ann Intern Med* 1968;68:1205–1219.

156. Freedman PM, Ault B, Zeiss CR, et al. Skin testing in farmers' lung disease. *J Allergy Clin Immunol* 1981;67:51–58.

157. Schatz M, Patterson R, Fink J, et al. Pigeon breeders' disease. II. Pigeon antigen–induced proliferation of lymphocytes from symptomatic and asymptomatic subjects. *Clin Allergy* 1976;6:7–17.

158. Caldwell JR, Pearce DE, Spencer C, et al. Immunologic mechanisms in hypersensitivity pneumonitis. I. Evidence for cell-mediated immunity and complement fixation in pigeon breeders' disease. *J Allergy Clin Immunol* 1973;52:225–230.

159. Hansen PJ, Penny R. Pigeon-breeder's disease: study of the cell-mediated immune response to pigeon antigens by the lymphocyte culture technique. *Int Arch Allergy Appl Immunol* 1974;47:498–507.

160. Schuyler MR, Thigpen TP, Salvaggio JE. Local pulmonary immunity in pigeon breeder's disease. A case study. *Ann Intern Med* 1978;88:355–358.

161. Moore VL, Fink JN, Barboriak JJ, et al. Immunologic events in pigeon breeders' disease. *J Allergy Clin Immunol* 1974;53:319–328.

162. McSharry C, Banham S, Lynch P, et al. Skin testing and extrinsic allergic alveolitis. *Clin Exp Immunol* 1983;54:282–288.

163. Orriols R, Morell F, Curull V, et al. Impaired non-specific delayed cutaneous hypersensitivity in bird fancier's lung. *Thorax* 1989;44:132–135.

164. Dinda P, Chatterjee SS, Riding WD. Pulmonary function studies in bird breeder's lung. *Thorax* 1969;24:374–378.

165. Warren C, Tse K, Cherniack R. Mechanical properties of the lung in extrinsic allergic alveolitis. *Thorax* 1978;33:315–321.

166. Lalancette M, Carrier G, Laviolette M, et al. Farmer's lung. Long-term outcome and lack of predictive value of bronchoalveolar lavage fibrosing factors. *Am Rev Respir Dis* 1993;148:216–221.

167. Allen DH, Williams GV, Woolcock AJ. Bird breeder's hypersensitivity pneumonitis: progress studies of lung function after cessation of exposure to the provoking antigen. *Am Rev Respir Dis* 1976;114:555–566.

168. Freedman PM, Ault B. Bronchial hyperreactivity to methacholine in farmers' lung disease. *J Allergy Clin Immunol* 1981;67:59–63.

169. Kokkarinen JI, Tukiainen HO, Terho EO. Recovery of pulmonary function in farmer's lung. A five-year follow-up study. *Am Rev Respir Dis* 1993;147:793–796.

170. Von Essen S, Robbins RA, Thompson AB, et al. Organic dust toxic syndrome: an acute febrile reaction to organic dust exposure distinct from hypersensitivity pneumonitis. *J Toxicol Clin Toxicol* 1990;28:389–420.

171. DoPico GA. Health effects of organic dusts in the farm environment. Report on diseases. *Am J Ind Med* 1986;10:261–265.

172. Malmberg P, Rask-Andersen A, Rosenhall L. Exposure to microorganisms associated with allergic alveolitis and febrile reactions to mold dust in farmers. *Chest* 1993;103:1202–1209.

173. Friend J, Gaddie J, Palmer K, et al. Extrinsic allergic alveolitis and contaminated cooling water in a factory machine. *Lancet* 1977;1:297–300.

174. Newman Taylor A, Pickering C, Turner-Warwick M, et al. Respiratory allergy to a factory humidifier contaminant presenting as pyrexia of undetermined origin. *Br Med J* 1978;2:94–95.

175. Edwards J, Cockcroft A. Inhalation challenge in humidifier fever. *Clin Allergy* 1981;11:227–235.

176. Solley G, Hyatt R. Hypersensitivity pneumonitis induced by *Penicillium* species. *J Allergy Clin Immunol* 1980;65:65–70.

177. Cockcroft A, Edwards J, Bevan C. An investigation of operating theatre staff exposed to humidifier fever antigens. *Br J Ind Med* 1981;38:144–151.

178. Parrott W, Blyth W. Another causal factor in the production of humidifier fever. *J Soc Occup Med* 1980;30:63–68.

179. Pickering C, Moore K, Lacey J, et al. Investigation of a respiratory disease associated with an air conditioning system. *Clin Allergy* 1976;6:109–118.

180. Rylander R, Haglind P. Airborne endotoxins and humidifier disease. *Clin Allergy* 1984;14:109–112.

181. Ramirez-Venegas A, Sansores RH, et al. Utility of a provocation test for diagnosis of chronic pigeon breeder's disease. *Am J Respir Crit Care Med* 1998;158:862–869.

182. Lacasse Y, Fraser RS, Fournier M, et al. Diagnostic accuracy of transbronchial biopsy in acute farmer's lung disease. *Chest* 1997;112:1459–1465.

183. Schuyler M, Cormier Y. The diagnosis of hypersensitivity pneumonitis. *Chest* 1997;111:534–536.

184. Pepys J. Hypersensitivity diseases of the lungs due to fungi and organic dusts. *Monogr Allergy* 1969;4:1–147.

185. Schkade PA, Routes JM. Hypersensitivity pneumonitis in a patient with hypogammaglobulinemia. *J Allergy Clin Immunol* 1996;98:710–712.

186. Morris AM, Nishimura S, Huang L. Subacute hypersensitivity pneumonitis in an HIV-infected patient receiving antiretroviral therapy. *Thorax* 2000;55:625–627.

187. Oshima M, Maeda A, Ishioka S, et al. Expression of C-C chemokines in bronchoalveolar lavage cells from patients with granulomatous lung diseases. *Lung* 1999;177:229–240.

188. Navarro C, Mendoza F, Barrera L, et al. Up-regulation of L-selectin and E-selectin in hypersensitivity pneumonitis. *Chest* 2002;121:354–360.

189. Shijubo N, Imai K, Shigehara K, et al. Soluble intercellular adhesion molecule-1 (ICAM-1) in sera and bronchoalveolar lavage (BAL) fluids of extrinsic allergic alveolitis. *Clin Exp Immunol* 1995;102:91–97.

190. Lohmeyer J, Friedrich J, Grimminger F, et al. Expression of mucosa-related integrin alphaEbeta7 on alveolar T cells in interstitial lung diseases. *Clin Exp Immunol* 1999;116:340–346.

191. Denis M, Ghadirian E. Transforming growth factor-beta is generated in the course of hypersensitivity pneumonitis: contribution to collagen synthesis. *Am J Respir Cell Mol Biol* 1992;7:156–160.

192. Denis M, Ghadirian E. Murine hypersensitivity pneumonitis:

production and importance of colony-stimulating factors in the course of a lung inflammatory reaction. *Am J Respir Cell Mol Biol* 1992;7:441–446.

193. Schuyler M, Gott K, Cherne A. Mediators of hypersensitivity pneumonitis. *J Lab Clin Med* 2000;136:29–38.

194. Takizawa H, Suko M, Kobayashi N, et al. Experimental hypersensitivity pneumonitis in the mouse: histologic and immunologic features and their modulation with cyclosporin A. *J Allergy Clin Immunol* 1988;81:391–400.

195. Gudmundsson G, Monick MM, Hunninghake GW. Viral infection modulates expression of hypersensitivity pneumonitis. *J Immunol* 1999;162:7397–7401.

196. Cormier Y, Samson N, Israel-Assayag E. Viral infection enhances the response to *Saccharopolyspora rectivirgula* in mice prechallenged with this farmer's lung antigen. *Lung* 1996;174:399–407.

197. Israel-Assayag E, Dakhama A, Lavigne S, et al. Expression of costimulatory molecules on alveolar macrophages in hypersensitivity pneumonitis. *Am J Respir Crit Care Med* 1999;159:1830–1834.

198. Israel-Assayag E, Fournier M, Cormier Y. Blockade of T cell co-stimulation by CTLA4-Ig inhibits lung inflammation in murine hypersensitivity pneumonitis. *J Immunol* 1999;163:6794–6799.

199. Dakhama A, Israel-Assayag E, Cormier Y. Altered immunosuppressive activity of alveolar macrophages in farmer's lung disease. *Eur Respir J* 1996;9:1456–1462.

200. Schuyler M, Gott K, Haley P. Experimental murine hypersensitivity pneumonitis. *Cell Immunol* 1991;136:303–317.

201. Schuyler M, Gott K, Shopp G, et al. CD3+ and CD4+ cells adoptively transfer experimental hypersensitivity pneumonitis. *Am Rev Respir Dis* 1992;146:1582–1588.

202. Schuyler MR, Gott K, Edwards B. Adoptive transfer of experimental hypersensitivity pneumonitis: CD4+ cells are memory and naive cells. *J Lab Clin Med* 1994;123:378–386.

203. Schuyler M, Gott K, Edwards B, et al. Experimental hypersensitivity pneumonitis. Effect of CD4 cell depletion. *Am J Respir Crit Care Med* 1994;149:1286–1294.

204. Schuyler M, Gott K, Edwards B, et al. Experimental hypersensitivity pneumonitis: effect of Thy1.2+ and CD8+ cell depletion. *Am J Respir Crit Care Med* 1995;151:1834–1842.

205. Fei R, Gott K, Edwards B, et al. Experimental hypersensitivity pneumonitis: in vitro effects of interleukin-2 and interferon-gamma. *J Lab Clin Med* 1995;126:485–494.

206. Schuyler M, Gott K, Cherne A, et al. Th1 CD4+ cells adoptively transfer experimental hypersensitivity pneumonitis. *Cell Immunol* 1997;177:169–175.

207. Gudmundsson G, Bosch A, Davidson BL, et al. Interleukin-10 modulates the severity of hypersensitivity pneumonitis in mice. *Am J Respir Cell Mol Biol* 1998;19:812–818.

208. Cormier Y, Belanger J. Long-term physiologic outcome after acute farmer's lung. *Chest* 1985;87:796–800.

209. Kokkarinen J, Tukiainen H, Terho EO. Mortality due to farmer's lung in Finland. *Chest* 1994;106:509–512.

210. Perez-Padilla R, Salas J, Chapela R, et al. Mortality in Mexican patients with chronic pigeon breeder's lung compared with those with usual interstitial pneumonia. *Am Rev Respir Dis* 1993;148:49–53.

211. Yoshida K, Ando M, Sakata T, et al. Prevention of summer-type hypersensitivity pneumonitis: effect of elimination of *Trichosporon cutaneum* from the patients' homes. *Arch Environ Health* 1989;44:317–322.

212. Jacobs RL, Andrews CP, Jacobs FO. Hypersensitivity pneumonitis treated with an electrostatic dust filter. *Ann Intern Med* 1989;110:115–118.

213. Edwards JH, Trotman DM, Mason OF, et al. Pigeon breeders' lung—the effect of loft litter materials on airborne particles and antigens. *Clin Exp Allergy* 1991;21:49–54.

214. Craig TJ, Hershey J, Engler RJ, et al. Tannic acid's effect on bird antigen. *Ann Allergy Asthma Immunol* 1995;75:348–350.

215. Kokkarinen JI, Tukiainen HO, Terho EO. Effect of corticosteroid treatment on the recovery of pulmonary function in farmer's lung. *Am Rev Respir Dis* 1992;145:3–5.

216. Ramírez A, Sansores R, Chapela R, et al. Inhaled beclomethasone versus oral prednisone. A clinical trial in patients with hypersensitivity pneumonitis. *Am J Respir Crit Care Med* 1995;151:A605(abst).

217. Carlsen KH, Leegaard J, Lund OD, et al. Allergic alveolitis in a 12-year-old boy: treatment with budesonide nebulizing solution. *Pediatr Pulmonol* 1992;12:257–259.

218. Zacharisen MC, Schlueter DP, Kurup VP, et al. The long-term outcome in acute, subacute, and chronic forms of pigeon breeder's disease hypersensitivity pneumonitis. *Ann Allergy Asthma Immunol* 2002;88:175–182.

219. Muller-Wening D, Repp H. Investigation on the protective value of breathing masks in farmer's lung using an inhalation provocation test. *Chest* 1989;95:100–105.

220. Hendrick D, Marshall R, Faux J, et al. Protective value of dust respirators in extrinsic allergic alveolitis: clinical assessment using inhalation provocation tests. *Thorax* 1981;36:917–921.

221. Nuutinen J, Terho EO, Husman K, et al. Protective value of powered dust respirator helmet for farmers with farmer's lung. *Eur J Respir Dis Suppl* 1987;152:212–220.

222. Kusaka H, Ogasawara H, Munakata M, et al. Two-year follow-up on the protective value of dust masks against farmer's lung disease. *Intern Med* 1993;32:106–111.

223. Grammer LC, Roberts M, Lerner C, et al. Clinical and serologic follow-up of four children and five adults with bird-fancier's lung. *J Allergy Clin Immunol* 1990;85:655–660.

224. Barbee RA, Callies Q, Dickie HA, et al. The long-term prognosis in farmer's lung. *Am Rev Respir Dis* 1968;97:223–231.

225. Braun SR, DoPico GA, Tsiatis A, et al. Farmer's lung disease: long-term clinical and physiologic outcome. *Am Rev Respir Dis* 1979;119:185–191.

226. Barrowcliff DF, Arblaster PG. Farmer's lung: a study of an early acute fatal case. *Thorax* 1968;23:490–500.

227. Bourke SJ, Banham SW, Carter R, et al. Longitudinal course of extrinsic allergic alveolitis in pigeon breeders. *Thorax* 1989;44:415–418.

228. Ostergaard JR. Reversible pulmonary arterial hypertension in a 6-year-old girl with extrinsic allergic alveolitis. *Acta Paediatr Scand* 1989;78:145–148.

229. Laviolette M, Cormier Y, Loiseau A, et al. Bronchoalveolar mast cells in normal farmers and subjects with farmer's lung. Diagnostic, prognostic, and physiologic significance. *Am Rev Respir Dis* 1991;144:855–860.

26 Connective Tissue Diseases

Thomas J. Gross · Gary W. Hunninghake

The systemic rheumatic disorders are associated with numerous pleuropulmonary manifestations. Table 26.1 outlines the broad spectrum of thoracic diseases associated with rheumatoid arthritis (RA), systemic lupus erythematosus (SLE), Sjögren syndrome, systemic sclerosis (SSc), polymyositis/dermatomyositis (PM/DM), and mixed connective tissue disease (MCTD). Of all the respiratory disorders associated with systemic rheumatic disorders, interstitial lung disease (ILD) is one of the most difficult to diagnose accurately and manage. The true prevalence of the idiopathic interstitial pneumonias in rheumatic disorders is unknown, and estimates vary depending on the diagnostic method used. Plain chest radiographs are the least sensitive, whereas pulmonary function tests detect lung disease at an earlier stage. High-resolution CT (HRCT) and bronchoalveolar lavage (BAL) detect subtler abnormalities not identified by other modalities. Multiple patterns of lung injury may be found in patients with connective tissue disease. Therefore, the gold standard for identifying the type of lesion present remains histologic examination of a surgical lung biopsy specimen.

INTERSTITIAL PNEUMONIA IN RHEUMATIC DISORDERS

Several histologic patterns characteristic of the idiopathic interstitial pneumonias have been described in patients with ILD complicating systemic rheumatic disorders (Table 26.2). Although detailed descriptions can be found in Chapter 24, we present a brief summary here. Usual interstitial pneumonia (UIP) is the pathology that defines idio-

T. J. Gross and **G. W. Hunninghake:** Department of Internal Medicine, Roy J. and Lucille A. Carver College of Medicine, Iowa City, Iowa.

pathic pulmonary fibrosis (IPF) and is an uncommon finding in connective tissue diseases. This pattern is characterized by pleura-based, nonuniform fibrosis with geographic and temporal heterogeneity amid a background of mild inflammation. Foci of active fibroblast proliferation and connective tissue deposition contrast with zones of relatively normal lung. By definition, this pathology implies IPF only in the absence of evidence of a systemic illness (1). A more common finding in biopsy specimens of patients with connective tissue disease–associated ILD is nonspecific interstitial pneumonia (NSIP) (2). NSIP manifests as varying degrees of inflammation and fibrosis uniformly distributed within the interstitium of the lung (3). Areas of acute lung injury are not typical of NSIP. Inflammation tends to be a more prominent feature than in UIP, and dense mononuclear cell infiltrates are present within the alveolar septa. Acute interstitial pneumonia (AIP) features a diffuse fibroproliferative response to a temporally uniform alveolar injury. The histologic features reflect recent diffuse lung injury: proliferating type II pneumocytes; widened interstitial spaces formed by the collapse of denuded alveolar septa; incorporation of alveolar exudates, including remnant hyaline membranes; and diffuse proliferation of fibroblasts and myofibroblasts (4). Cryptogenic organizing pneumonia (COP) (also called *bronchiolitis obliterans–organizing pneumonia,* or *BOOP),* is well described in association with RA and the inflammatory myopathies. In COP, the inflammation is centered on the peribronchial interstitium and alveolar ducts. Characteristic plugs of granulation tissue occlude distal air spaces (5).

The radiographic patterns described for the idiopathic interstitial pneumonias may provide clues to the underlying histopathology in the diffuse parenchymal lung diseases associated with the collagen vascular disorders. The UIP histology correlates with lower lobe, peripheral reticular opacities and honeycomb changes on chest roentgenography. HRCT reveals areas of subpleural cystic change with

TABLE 26.1. RELATIVE FREQUENCY OF PLEUROPULMONARY MANIFESTATIONS OF SYSTEMIC RHEUMATOLOGIC DISORDERS

	RA	SLE	PM/DM	Sjögren Syndrome	SSc	MCTD
Pleural disease	++	+++	−	+	−	+++−++++
Pneumonitis	−	+	−	−	(aspiration)	+
Alveolar hemorrhage	−	+	−	−	−	+
Interstitial pneumonia	+++−++++	++	+++	++−+++	++++	+++
Pulmonary hypertension	+	++	+	−	++++	+++
Airway obstruction	++	−	−	+++	−	+
Bronchiectasis	+++	−	−	++	+	−
Respiratory muscle weakness	−	++	+	−		+

Note: −, not clinically important; +, <5%; ++, 5% to 25%; +++, 25% to 50%; ++++, >50% incidence.
MCTD, mixed connective tissue disease; PM/DM, polymyositis/dermatomyositis; RA, rheumatoid arthritis; SSc, systemic sclerosis; SLE, systemic lupus erythematosus.

traction bronchiectasis and parenchymal distortion, indicating fibrosis. Ground-glass attenuation may be present but is not a prominent feature. Signs of consolidation, pulmonary nodules, or pleural disease suggest another process. The NSIP pattern of ILD often presents as nonspecific bilateral lower lobe opacities with interstitial prominence. HRCT shows large areas of ground-glass opacities with less prominent honeycombing and fibrosis. Subpleural irregular lines may be a prominent finding. AIP presents with dense bilateral consolidation on chest x-ray films, similar to that seen in patients with the acute respiratory distress syndrome. HRCT confirms ground-glass opacities with air bronchograms. As the process progresses, areas of fibrosis may develop, with architectural distortion and traction bronchiectasis. Unilateral or bilateral focal consolidations with air bronchograms characterize COP. HRCT also shows the dense nature of these opacities, along with more subtle ground-glass changes elsewhere. Nodular densities centered on airways are also common. Thus, distinctive radiographic features in the ILDs associated with systemic rheumatic disorders may aid in predicting the underlying pathology.

Although patients with specific pathologic patterns of ILD such as NSIP and COP appear to respond to treatment, no randomized controlled studies have convincingly demonstrated any effective therapy for ILD complicating the rheumatic disorders. Patients with lung pathology characteristic of other forms of ILD (e.g., UIP and AIP) in general do not respond to current therapies.

TABLE 26.2. HISTOLOGIC PATTERNS SEEN IN LUNG BIOPSY SPECIMENS OF PATIENTS WITH INTERSTITIAL PNEUMONIAS ASSOCIATED WITH COLLAGEN-VASCULAR DISEASES

Histologic Pattern	Microscopic Findings	Radiographic Correlates
Usual interstitial pneumonia	Patchy lung involvement	Lower lobe reticular opacities
	Subpleural fibrosis remodeling of lung architecture with frequent "honeycomb" fibrosis	Subpleural honeycombing Traction bronchiectasis
	Proliferating fibroblast foci at edges of dense scars	
	Minimal inflammation	
Nonspecific interstitial pneumonia	Uniform temporal appearance	Lower lobe reticulation
	Intense interstitial inflammation	Ground-glass opacities
	Fibrosis, if present, lacking temporal heterogeneity	
Acute interstitial pneumonia	Diffuse alveolar damage	Dense bilateral opacities
	Uniform temporal appearance	Ground-glass opacities
	Alveolar hyaline membranes	Air bronchograms
	Proliferating pneumocytes	
	Collapse of denuded alveoli	
Organizing pneumonia	Uniform temporal appearance	Focal, patchy consolidation
	Patchy distribution	Ground-glass opacities
	Bronchiolocentric inflammation	Bronchocentric nodules
	Air space granulation tissue plugs	
	Preservation of lung architecture	

RHEUMATOID ARTHRITIS

RA is the most common form of inflammatory arthritis, with a worldwide prevalence of 1%. It affects women more frequently than men, in a ratio of 3:1. RA is a symmetric, inflammatory polyarthritis with a myriad of extraarticular features. The diagnosis of RA is based on the characteristic historical feature of morning stiffness, evidence on physical examination of swollen and tender joints, and supportive laboratory data, including high titers of serum rheumatoid factors and characteristic bone erosion detected by radiography. The American Rheumatism Association has developed classification criteria for RA that are useful in clinical studies (6). RA causes substantial morbidity, predominantly from progressive joint destruction, that results in a work disability rate of 50% after 10 years of active disease. RA also is associated with premature mortality, shortening life expectancy by 8 to 13 years on average. Mortality is most often related to infectious illnesses. RA is strongly associated with an increased frequency of the class II major histocompatibility complex (MHC) serotype HLA-DR4, and specific HLA-DR4 haplotypes (HLA-DRBI*0401 and DRBI*0404) predict more severe RA.

Epidemiology

The pulmonary manifestations in RA range from common (e.g., pleural effusions) to rare (e.g., bronchiolitis obliterans). ILD may be the most common pattern of pulmonary involvement overall, based on series of patients undergoing lung biopsy (7). This entity is commonly referred to as *rheumatoid arthritis–associated interstitial lung disease*

(RA-ILD). The reported prevalence of RA-ILD ranges from 2% to 40% of patients with RA (7–9). The variability in prevalence is related to the different diagnostic modalities used to define this condition. Whereas abnormalities are detected by plain chest radiography in only about 1% to 5% of patients with suspected RA-ILD, the percentage of affected persons increases dramatically if the diagnosis is established by abnormal results of pulmonary function studies (~40% of patients) or abnormal tissue histology (≤80% of patients).

Investigations into risk factors for RA-ILD have yielded disparate results. Although RA is three times more common in women than in men, RA-ILD more frequently affects men (9). Traditional measures of the severity of RA (e.g., serum rheumatoid factor and subcutaneous nodules), Sjögren syndrome, antirheumatic therapies, immunogenetic markers of the severity of disease (HLA-DR4 and HLA-B40), and cigarette smoking all have been identified as potential predictors of RA-ILD, although other studies have failed to confirm these associations (10). The two risk factors that have generated the most interest are cigarette smoking and serum rheumatoid factor. As with IPF, cigarette smoking has a consistently positive association with RA-ILD based on multiple epidemiologic analyses (Fig. 26.1). A positive correlation between the rheumatoid factor titer and abnormal diffusion capacity has been demonstrated, and cigarette smoking is also associated with elevated serum rheumatoid factor. It is uncertain whether rheumatoid factor plays an independent pathogenic role in RA-ILD or is only an epiphenomenon. In conjunction with rheumatoid factor, smoking may synergistically contribute to a diminished diffusing capacity of the lung for carbon monoxide (D_{LCO}). It remains unknown whether cigarette smoking alone is responsible for many

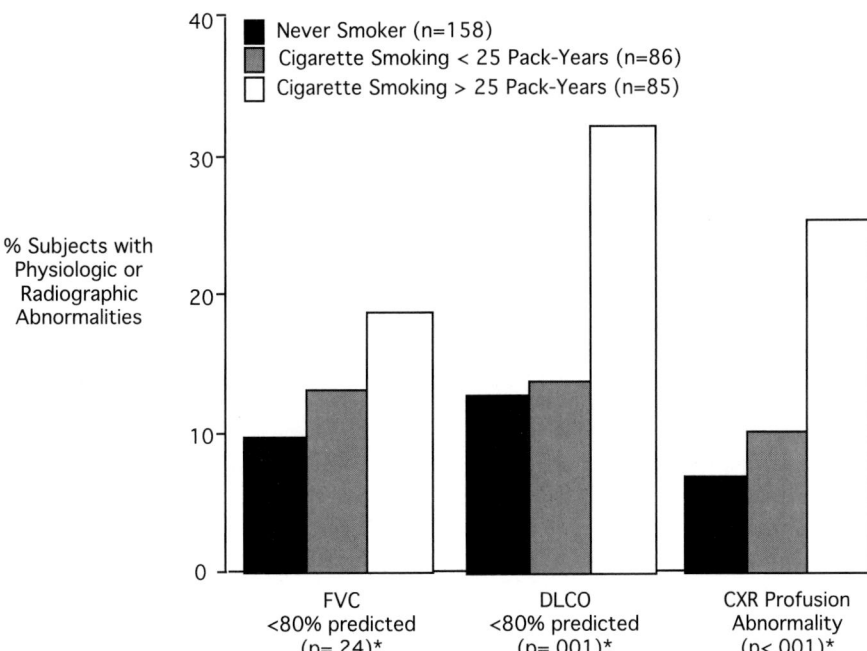

FIGURE 26.1. Cigarette smoking and rheumatoid arthritis–associated interstitial lung disease. Bar histogram demonstrates the association of cigarette smoking (pack-years) with abnormalities in parameters of pulmonary function, including the diffusing capacity of the lung for carbon monoxide (D_{LCO}) and forced vital capacity (*FVC*), and with chest radiograph (*CXR*) profusion abnormalities (interstitial infiltrates). Values for p are the x^2 trend test. (From Saag KG, Kolluri S, Koehnke RK, et al. Rheumatoid arthritis lung disease. Determinants of radiographic and physiologic abnormalities. *Arthritis Rheum* 1996;39:1711–1719, with permission.)

of the pulmonary features of RA (11,12). Very few studies have been large enough to estimate with confidence the confounding risks of occupational exposures or infectious agents. Thus, knowledge about the risk factors for the development of ILD in patients with RA is limited.

Clinical Presentation

RA-ILD commonly follows the development of joint disease, although the time from disease onset to lung involvement is often as short as 5 years. The medical history and physical examination findings are neither sensitive nor specific for the diagnosis of RA-ILD, but certain clinical features are common. In contrast to patients with IPF, many patients report symptoms of pleuritic chest pain. Clubbing has also been detected in some series, but less often than in IPF and usually later in the course of the disease (9,13). Chest crackles are strongly correlated with radiographic changes. Recurrent bronchitis with sputum production may occur in well-established RA-ILD. Of patients with RA-ILD, a surprisingly low percentage report limitations in their level of activity as a consequence of dyspnea. This may be because the physical disability resulting from RA limits patients' functional status and precludes exertional activities strenuous enough to produce pulmonary symptoms.

Physiologic Evaluation

Pulmonary function tests suggest a diagnosis of RA-ILD in a high percentage of cases. An abnormal diffusion capacity is the best predictor of fibrosis on biopsy. A reduction in the diffusion capacity may precede other extraarticular manifestations of RA. Frequently, the coexistence of restrictive and obstructive airway disease in cigarette smokers with RA confounds the interpretation of pulmonary function test abnormalities. Although the patient's lung volumes and flows may normalize because of concurrent airway obstruction and parenchymal restriction, the DLco can be markedly reduced (12,14). Obstructive changes may also result from coexisting rheumatoid airway involvement, such as bronchiectasis or bronchiolitis obliterans (7,15). Because of the high rate of chronic disease–associated anemia in patients with RA, it is often necessary to adjust the DLco reading for the hemoglobin level.

Pulmonary Imaging Findings

Characteristic ILD findings are present on chest radiography in about 12% of patients with RA. The plain radiographic appearance is one of bilateral basilar reticular opacities, often accompanied by nodules and pleural thickening. HRCT can be used to identify very early evidence of RA-ILD, which may not be visible on plain radiographs. HRCT often reveals reticular opacities in the periphery of the lung, in addition

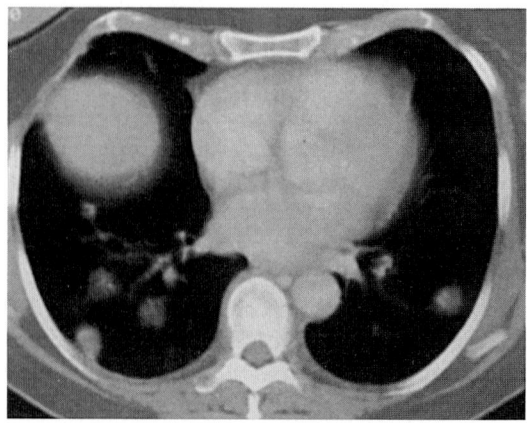

FIGURE 26.2. Multiple bilateral rheumatoid nodules in the lower lung zones. Cavitation is not seen clearly in this computed tomographic image, even though one third of the nodules show cavitation.

to subpleural nodules and cavitations that are unique to RA-ILD (8,13) (Fig. 26.2). Frequently, patients with RA who have abnormalities on pulmonary function testing have abnormalities on HRCT scans but not on plain chest x-ray films. Furthermore, HRCT may aid in the differentiation of RA-ILD from obliterative bronchiolitis in the patient with RA who presents with dyspnea and normal chest radiographic findings (15,16). RA-ILD is characterized by increased septal lines, ground-glass opacities, and honeycomb fibrosis, whereas obliterative bronchiolitis has features of centrilobular nodules and heterogeneous air trapping (8,13,15) (Fig. 26.3). However, the clinician must be aware that the significance of HRCT abnormalities in asymptomatic patients without other diagnostic abnormalities is unclear from both a therapeutic and a prognostic perspective.

Laboratory Studies

No serologic study is sufficiently sensitive or specific to assist in the diagnosis of RA-ILD. As noted, serum rheumatoid

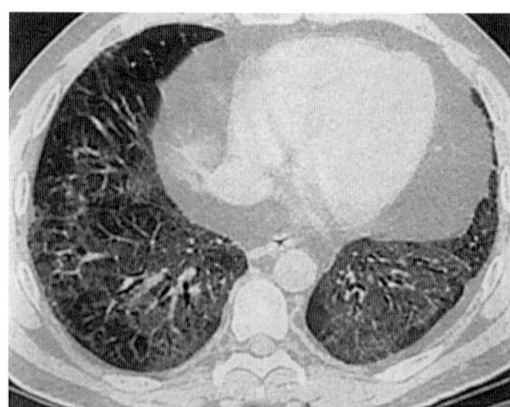

FIGURE 26.3. High-resolution computed tomographic image of basal regions of the lungs in organizing pneumonia associated with rheumatoid arthritis. Diffuse but patchy "ground-glass" opacities are well seen.

factor is a strong predictor of RA-ILD, but it is not a good screening test. Also, serum rheumatoid factor may be detectable in many patients with IPF who, by definition, lack a history of inflammatory arthropathy (1).

Bronchoalveolar Lavage and Lung Biopsy

Although BAL is of greater value in excluding infectious and neoplastic causes of ILD, it may provide usefully prognostic information in RA-ILD. Both neutrophilic and lymphocytic alveolitis has been described in the BAL fluid of patients with RA-ILD (17). As in IPF, elevated lymphocyte counts in BAL occur early in RA-ILD, whereas a neutrophilic predominance is found later in the disease process. Despite the value of BAL, the gold standard in the diagnosis of interstitial fibrosis is the histopathologic examination of open lung biopsy specimens. In the absence of pulmonary nodules that raise the index of suspicion for malignancy, and because the results are unlikely to alter clinical therapy, open lung biopsy is less often performed in RA-ILD than in IPF.

Pathology

The histology of RA-ILD may be nearly indistinguishable from that of UIP, although features of NSIP are more common than the characteristic UIP pattern (Fig. 26.4). Biopsy specimens show thickened alveolar septa and in some cases alveolar cell hyperplasia (18,19). Lymphocytic infiltration of the alveolar wall and cuboidal type I pneumocytes are also present. Features that help differentiate RA-ILD from IPF include a prominent lymphocytic infiltrate, hyperplasia of the lymphoid follicles, and characteristic rheumatoid

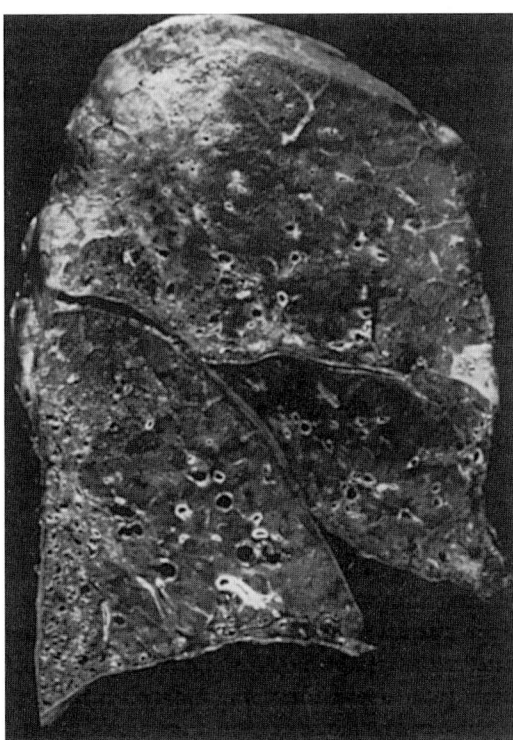

FIGURE 26.4. Gross appearance of chronic interstitial pneumonia in rheumatoid arthritis. Zones of honeycombing can be seen in the posterior subpleural regions. Some contraction and thickening of the lung also are noted, along with pleural thickening.

pulmonary nodules (Fig. 26.5). Rheumatoid nodules in the lung, the only pulmonary lesion specific to RA, impart a better prognosis. Inflammation and fibrosis of the pleura are more common in RA-ILD than in IPF and may help further separate the two entities (Fig. 26.6).

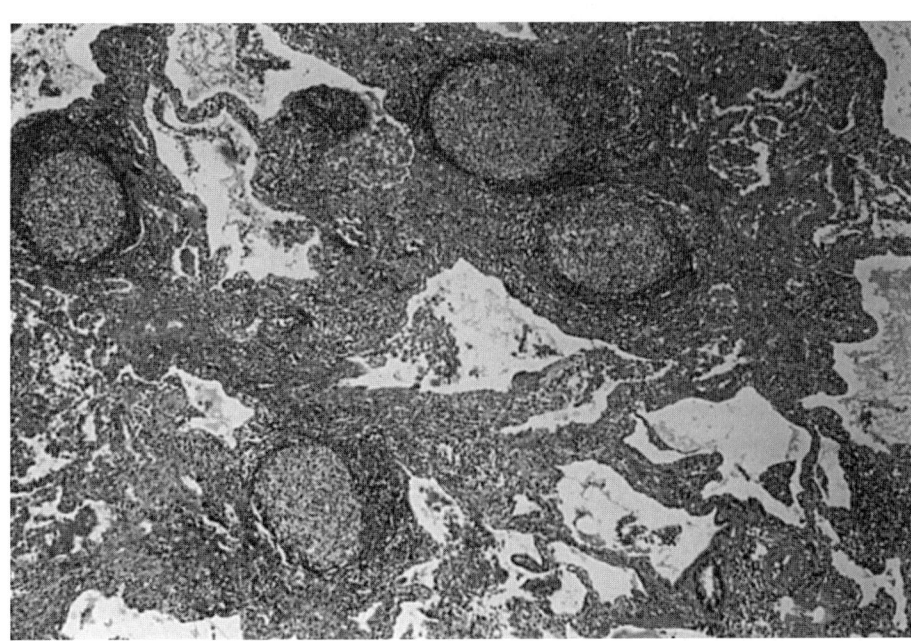

FIGURE 26.5. Chronic fibrosing interstitial pneumonia with associated lymphoid hyperplasia and germinal centers in rheumatoid arthritis. The alveolar architecture is somewhat preserved.

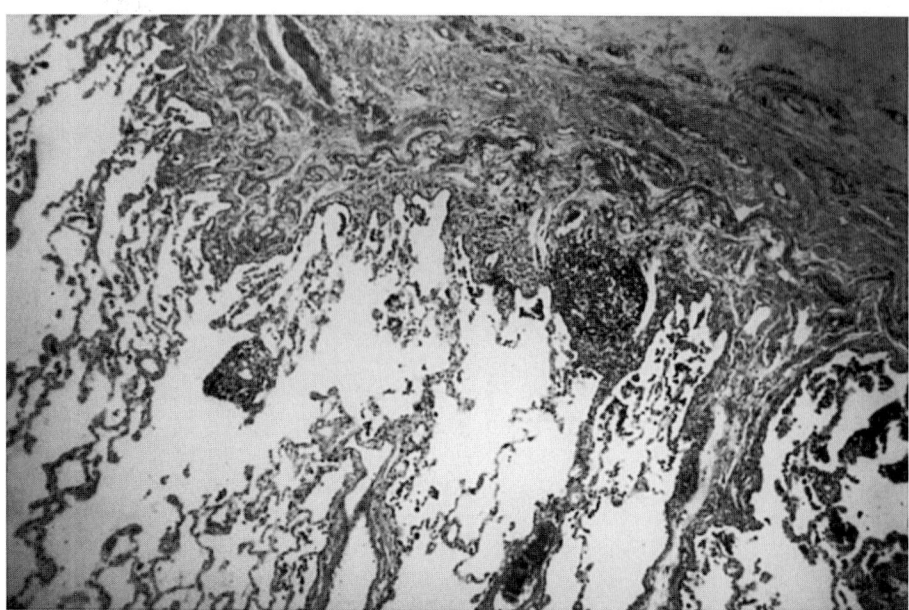

FIGURE 26.6. Pleuropulmonary interphase (**upper right**) in rheumatoid arthritis. Virtually all patients with rheumatoid arthritis show evidence of pleural thickening at autopsy.

Treatment and Prognosis

The treatment of RA-ILD is confounded by the fact that many of the traditional therapies used to manage both the articular and extraarticular manifestations of RA may cause pulmonary toxicity. Intramuscular gold, cyclophosphamide, and methotrexate have all been linked to pneumonitis that may mimic early pulmonary fibrosis. Because methotrexate is currently the most commonly used disease-modifying agent in the treatment of RA, pulmonary toxicity attributable to this therapy is of special concern. Unfortunately, no findings are pathognomonic for methotrexate pneumonitis; like RA-ILD, it may present with nonspecific bilateral reticular or nodular opacities. BAL often reveals a lymphocyte-predominant alveolitis with a variable ratio of T helper to T suppressor cells (20). Although some studies have suggested that methotrexate, gold, and D-penicillamine may be independent risk factors for RA-ILD, most investigations have failed to substantiate these associations (10,21).

Careful monitoring of RA-ILD progression is crucial in guiding therapy because many potential therapeutic agents may cause significant iatrogenic morbidity. Therapy of early, symptomatic RA-ILD consists of high-dose corticosteroids, usually given as 1 mg of prednisone per kilogram of body weight, or the equivalent. Corticosteroids may be more effective if given early in the inflammatory phase; however, more advanced fibrotic disease is often steroid-resistant.

For RA-ILD that is refractory to corticosteroids or necessitates protracted high-dose therapy, cyclophosphamide, methotrexate, and more recently cyclosporine have been used with anecdotal success (22). The newer immunomodulatory therapies aimed at neutralizing tumor necrosis factor have been used successfully in managing the joint manifestations of RA. Whether these agents will alter the course of RA-

ILD remains untested (23). Low-dose macrolide therapy has been reported in case series to improve pulmonary function in RA patients with obliterative bronchiolitis (15,24). No study of this novel treatment in RA-ILD has been reported to date.

THERAPY FOR RHEUMATOID ARTHRITIS–ASSOCIATED INTERSTITIAL LUNG DISEASE	
Summary Statement	**Level of Evidence**
Subjective response to corticosteroids has been anecdotally reported, both with and without objective improvement.	Observational studies (case reports or small case series)
Experience with other immunosuppressive or cytotoxic therapies is limited.	Observational studies (case reports or small case series)

Data about survival for patients with RA-ILD are limited. The prognosis for many patients with mild disease is better than that for patients with IPF (13,25). However, among patients with extensive RA-ILD, the 5-year survival rate is reported to be as low as 39%. The prognosis is significantly improved if a component of the fibrosis appears to be drug-related. Histologic findings of UIP portend a particularly bad prognosis. Likewise, very rare upper lobe fibrosis, akin to ankylosing spondylitis, is a poor prognostic factor. Lastly, bronchogenic carcinoma can complicate RA-ILD. Controversy surrounds the potential independent roles of cigarette smoking, commonly used immunosuppressive agents, and the underlying RA disease process in carcinogenesis.

SYSTEMIC LUPUS ERYTHEMATOSUS

SLE is a heterogeneous multisystem disorder of unknown cause with a predilection for young black and Asian women. SLE is diagnosed on the basis of a constellation of characteristic symptoms, signs, and laboratory abnormalities. Because SLE is a clinical diagnosis and has no pathognomonic features, it is both underdiagnosed and overdiagnosed by many physicians. It is estimated that the average patient with lupus waits for 2 years from the time of symptom onset before a correct diagnosis is achieved. Although some patients, particularly those with discoid skin lesions, have a milder course of disease, involvement of the kidneys, central nervous system, or respiratory tract is associated with significant morbidity and premature mortality.

Epidemiology

The most common form of lupus-associated lung disease is pleurisy with or without pleural effusions (Fig. 26.7); the overall prevalence of pleuropulmonary disease in SLE is about 70% (26–28). In addition, both acute and chronic ILD can develop in SLE. In most cases, ILD occurs in patients who have had other serious SLE-associated organ disease, although it may rarely precede the development of frank SLE. Studies that assess the frequency of lupus-associated lung disease are predominantly small, uncontrolled investigations that suffer from referral and selection bias. Clinically significant ILD occurs in 3% of adult patients with SLE. However, physiologic abnormalities are noted in up to 88% of cases (27,29). Several independent reviews have shown that parenchymal lung disease coincides with other manifestations of SLE in 20% of cases (30). In autopsy series of SLE patients, the majority of pulmonary abnormalities are related to infection, congestive heart failure, coagulopathy, or oxygen toxicity (26). These studies, however, are potentially limited by the selection of specific subsets of SLE patients likely to undergo autopsy and of those seen in referral centers.

Clinical Presentation

Numerous pulmonary syndromes have been described in SLE patients that may be confused with symptomatic ILD. Acute or chronic dyspnea with or without pleurisy is most common. Hemoptysis or respiratory failure is seen with acute lupus pneumonitis or pulmonary vasculitis with alveolar hemorrhage.

Acute Lupus Pneumonitis

This fulminant process develops most often in patients with established SLE. Patients are acutely ill, with the rapid development of tachypnea, dyspnea, fever, cough, and occasionally blood-tinged sputum. The physical examination and laboratory studies demonstrate cyanosis and hypoxemia, and chest radiography reveals prominent alveolar consolidation (Fig. 26.8). The most important differential diagnostic considerations are typical or atypical infectious causes. Of concern, most patients with acute lupus pneumonitis have persistent lung dysfunction after the acute process resolves (28).

Chronic Interstitial Disease

Chronic ILD is uncommon and may develop independently of acute pneumonitis or as its sequela (Fig. 26.9). Dyspnea both at rest and with mild exertion is the predominant symptom (31). Cough and pleuritic chest pain each are

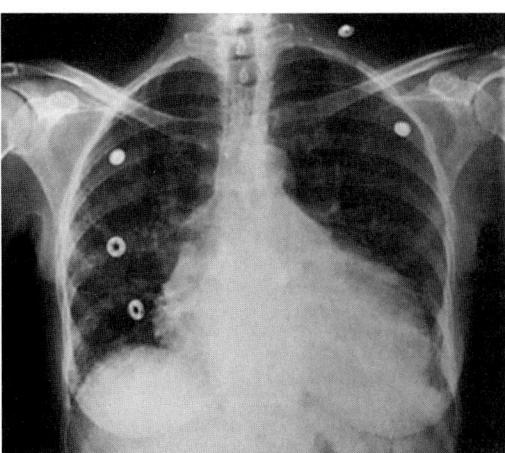

FIGURE 26.7. Chest roentgenogram demonstrates a large pericardial effusion, blunting of the left costophrenic angle, and patchy pulmonary infiltrates in a patient with systemic lupus erythematosus.

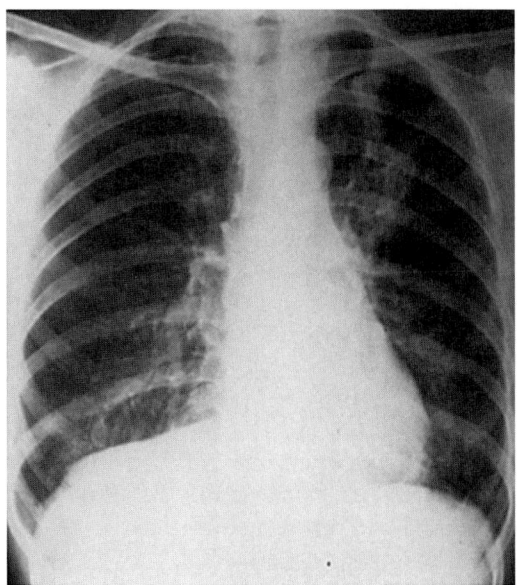

FIGURE 26.8. Acute lupus pneumonitis involving left upper lobe segment. This entity is very rare.

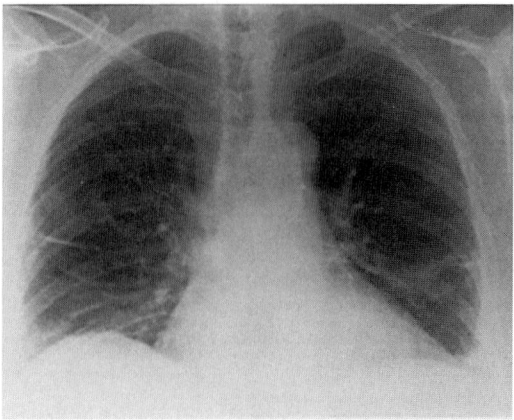

FIGURE 26.9. Discoid or platelike atelectasis, also called *atelectatic pneumonitis*, is perhaps the most common chest roentgenographic finding in patients with chronic systemic lupus erythematosus. A diffuse interstitial process is distinctly uncommon.

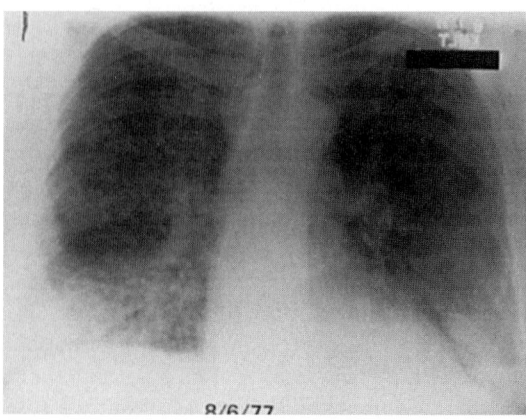

FIGURE 26.10. Pulmonary alveolar hemorrhage in a patient with systemic lupus erythematosus and severe renal involvement. Alveolar opacities are basal and patchy in distribution.

reported in about two thirds of cases. Unlike IPF, chronic ILD is associated with pleuritis in about 40% of cases. Clubbing of the digits is also considerably less common than in IPF and is perhaps secondary to decreased digital perfusion resulting from Raynaud phenomenon. Chronic ILD is more common in the subset of SLE patients who display overlapping features of scleroderma, such as edema of the hands and abnormalities of the nail fold capillaries.

Acute Reversible Hypoxemia

A syndrome of reversible hypoxemia has been observed in hospitalized patients with SLE that is independent of pulmonary parenchymal opacities on chest imaging studies. This presentation has been attributed to pulmonary aggregation of leukocytes in SLE patients who are acutely ill. These white cell clumps lead to substantial ventilation-perfusion mismatching.

Acute Pulmonary Hemorrhage

The sudden development of severe pulmonary insufficiency coupled with hemoptysis and rapidly progressive infiltration should raise strong concerns about pulmonary hemorrhage (Fig. 26.10). Pulmonary hemorrhage may complicate acute lupus pneumonitis or can occur independently. An unexpected elevation in the DLCO, blood visualized by bronchoscopy, or hemosiderin-laden macrophages visible on biopsy all support the diagnosis of this very serious complication.

Shrinking Lung Syndrome

Shrinking lung syndrome is another lupus-associated lung disease that may mimic ILD. Basilar atelectasis is a frequent radiographic finding that can be at least partially attributed to this pathologic process. Shrinking lung syndrome is not an intrinsic pulmonary disorder but rather is caused by diaphragmatic dysfunction and respiratory muscle weakness that result in restrictive physiologic parameters and an elevated diaphragm. Some lupus patients may also demonstrate decreased respiratory muscle strength in the absence of chest radiographic abnormalities.

Physiologic Evaluation

Pulmonary function tests are the most sensitive indicators of chronic ILD in SLE. Diminished lung volumes, a low diffusion capacity, and abnormal compliance occur in both acute and chronic lupus ILD. In one study, the DLCO was reduced in 72% and lung volumes in 49% of all patients with SLE. In a study of younger patients with SLE (mean age, 15.5 years), restrictive pulmonary function test defects were found in 35% and a diminished DLCO in 25% (29,30). A decreased ability to generate inspiratory pressures may be observed in patients with diaphragmatic dysfunction.

Pulmonary Imaging Findings

The plain radiographic findings are often normal early in the course of chronic lupus ILD. In contrast, in both the later stages of chronic lupus ILD and acute lupus pneumonitis, prominent lower lobe opacities are present. Chest radiographs show abnormalities in about 30% of chronic ILD cases. As in other forms of ILD, HRCT may suggest the diagnosis of ILD in a patient with SLE. A ground-glass appearance suggestive of more active inflammation has been correlated with a better response to therapy. In lupus shrinking lung syndrome, CT will show normal parenchyma with dependent atelectasis.

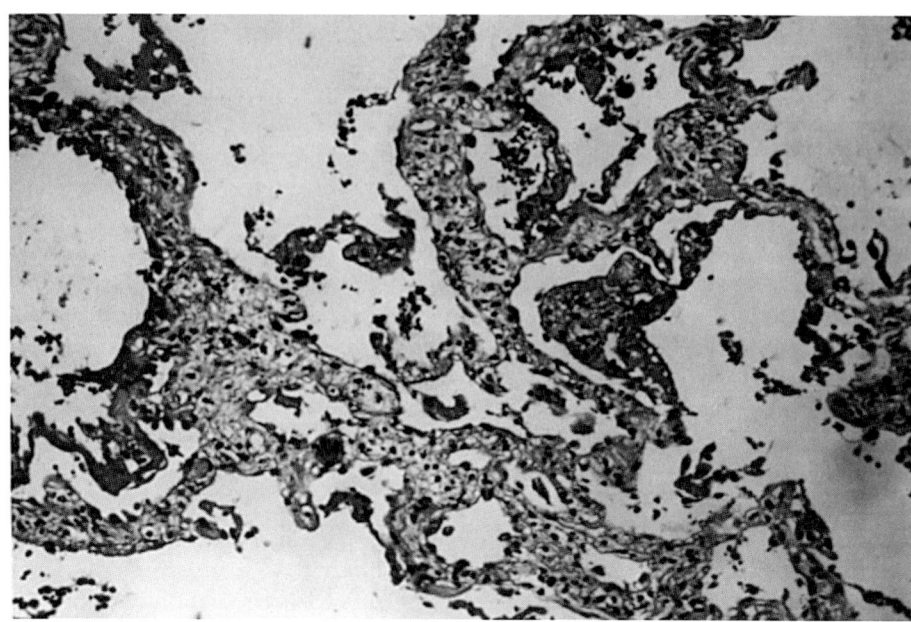

FIGURE 26.11. Lung changes in systemic lupus erythematosus: edema and thickening of the alveolar septa, fibrinous exudate, and hyaline membrane formation in the alveoli.

Laboratory Studies

Antinuclear antibody (ANA) is detectable in the sera of 95% of patients with SLE. The most common ANA pattern is diffuse (also called *homogeneous*), but the peripheral (or rim) pattern is more specific. Although higher levels of antibodies to native (double-stranded) DNA and lower serum complement fractions are associated with more aggressive SLE in some patients, similar associations with lung disease have not been substantiated. Based on small series, the presence of antibodies to U1-RNP (U1 ribonucleoprotein) and to SSA (Sjögren syndrome antigen A) appears to be predictive of chronic restrictive lung disease and a decreased D$_{LCO}$. Because of very poor specificity, assays for immune complexes are not recommended for either the diagnosis or the surveillance of SLE pneumonitis.

Bronchoalveolar Lavage and Lung Biopsy

Particularly with the presentation of acute opacities on chest imaging studies, BAL is necessary to exclude infectious causes. Some authors advocate repeated BAL as a measure of response to therapy, but this approach cannot be strongly advocated in SLE because no evidence has been found of improved management or outcome based on BAL findings.

Pathology

Many of the pathologic lesions of SLE lung disease are at least partially attributable to immune complex deposition. In acute pneumonitis, interstitial edema, hyaline membranes, acute alveolitis, arteriolar thrombosis, intra-alveolar hemorrhage, and alveolar cell hyperplasia are all seen on histology (Fig. 26.11). Immune complexes are identified in alveolar walls and interstitium and near small vessels (Fig. 26.12).

The pathology of chronic ILD is similar to that of other interstitial pneumonias. Chronic inflammatory cell infiltration and the deposition of immunoglobulins and complement are seen in the interstitium. In autopsy series, interstitial inflammatory infiltrates and thickening were ubiquitous, but significant fibrotic changes were not found. The pattern of alveolar septal toss and panacinar emphysema was similar to the fibrosis of SSc. Rarely, lymphocytic interstitial pneumonitis has been seen in SLE (32). Thorough searches for chronic infectious agents as a cause of either acute or chronic lupus lung disease have been consistently unrevealing.

Treatment and Prognosis

After infections have been excluded, the treatment of acute lupus pneumonitis begins with the correction of hypoxemia

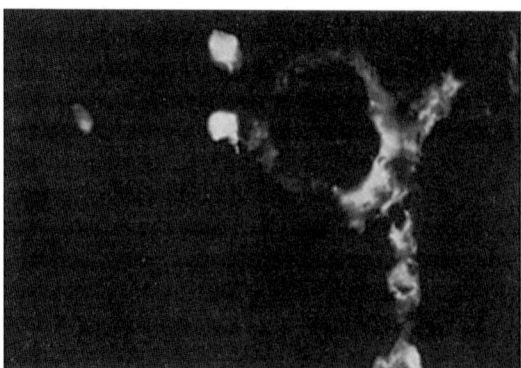

FIGURE 26.12. Immunofluorescence study of lung specimen for immunoglobulin G in systemic lupus erythematosus shows patchy staining of the alveolar wall and a few intra-alveolar cells.

and moderate doses of corticosteroids (typically started at 1 mg of methylprednisolone per kilogram per day in divided doses). If pulmonary disease is refractory to this regimen, pulse methylprednisolone at 1 g/d for 3 days has been advocated, along with the concomitant use of immunosuppressive agents such as intravenous cyclophosphamide. Plasmapheresis also has been used in rapidly deteriorating patients with anecdotal success.

The management of chronic ILD is more controversial. Treatment decisions should be geared toward alleviating symptoms because few data suggest that therapy alters disease progression. Chronic fibrosis indicated by honeycombing on HRCT and the absence of inflammatory alveolitis is poorly responsive to therapy. Pharmacotherapy should be reserved for patients with some evidence of an active inflammatory disease process, which is more likely to respond to the traditional agents. When treatment is indicated, corticosteroids remain the mainstay of the therapeutic armamentarium. They are usually administered as 40 to 60 mg of prednisone equivalent per day. Steroid-sparing therapy with azathioprine, cyclophosphamide, or methotrexate should be considered in refractory cases or when treatment is necessary for a protracted period (33). Careful monitoring of physiologic studies and chest radiographs provides guidance on the response to treatment. No controlled trial has confirmed an effective regimen for the treatment of ILD in SLE.

THERAPY FOR SYSTEMIC LUPUS ERYTHEMATOSUS–ASSOCIATED INTERSTITIAL LUNG DISEASE

Summary Statement	Level of Evidence
Acute lupus pneumonitis: Corticosteroids with or without immunosuppressive agents (cyclophosphamide or azathioprine).	Observational studies and expert opinion
Acute lupus pneumonitis: Plasmapheresis in rapidly deteriorating patients.	Observational studies and expert opinion
Chronic interstitial lung disease: Corticosteroids remain the mainstay of therapy.	Observational studies and expert opinion
Chronic interstitial lung disease: Steroid-sparing therapy with azathioprine, cyclophosphamide, or methotrexate in refractory cases or when treatment is for a prolonged period (>6 months).	Observational studies and expert opinion

Improved chemotherapeutic regimens have increased the survival of patients with nonpulmonary manifestations of SLE. Thus, the long-term outcome of patients who have SLE-associated chronic lung disease often depends on the development of pulmonary hypertension and cor pulmonale. Reports of successful heart-lung transplantation in patients

who have lupus-associated pulmonary hypertension without pulmonary fibrosis raise the hope that this therapy may be successful in patients with end-stage lupus lung disease.

SJÖGREN SYNDROME

Sjögren syndrome is an autoimmune exocrinopathy defined by the constellation of sites of keratoconjunctivitis and xerostomia. Sjögren syndrome occurs both as a primary disorder and as a secondary condition in other rheumatologic disorders—most commonly RA, SSc, and SLE. Although the symptoms of most patients with Sjögren syndrome are limited to the exocrine glands, a myriad of well-described extraglandular features range from renal tubular acidosis to central nervous system lesions. Although Sjögren syndrome is typically a benign lymphoproliferative disorder, progression to pseudolymphoma or frank B-cell lymphoma is an uncommon but well-described disease transformation.

Epidemiology

The most common pulmonary manifestation of Sjögren syndrome is desiccation of the airways (xerobronchia), which leads to chronic cough and recurrent tracheobronchitis (34). Other types of pulmonary abnormalities that have been described include obstructive airway disease, lymphocytic interstitial pneumonitis, chronic interstitial fibrosis, pseudolymphoma, and pulmonary lymphoma (35,36). Pulmonary disease of all types occurs in up to 75% of patients with primary Sjögren syndrome. ILD detected in Sjögren syndrome may begin as a lymphocytic interstitial pneumonia (LIP) but can progress to frank pulmonary fibrosis. More than half of all patients with Sjögren syndrome and LIP also have RA; therefore, it is hard to know which pathologic process is directly responsible for this lung condition. Not surprisingly, pulmonary involvement is both more common and more severe in secondary than in primary Sjögren syndrome. Smoking is not a proven risk factor for the development of pulmonary disease in Sjögren syndrome, as it is in RA-ILD and IPF.

Clinical Presentation

The characteristic clinical features of Sjögren syndrome include sicca symptoms and, less commonly, salivary gland enlargement. Extraglandular tissues that may be involved include those of the central nervous system, gastrointestinal tract (primary biliary cirrhosis), and kidney (type II renal tubular acidosis). In one cross-sectional study, more than 40% of patients with recently diagnosed Sjögren syndrome had respiratory symptoms in the absence of physical signs or radiographic evidence of lung disease (37). Dyspnea on exertion is a common complaint in these patients. Cough and pleuritic chest pain are also reported frequently and correlate with lymphocytosis on BAL. Wheezing is infrequently reported, and clubbing is uncommonly seen except in patients in whom end-stage pulmonary fibrosis develops. The initial presentation of pulmonary Sjögren syndrome may be misdiagnosed as an infectious pneumonia because of fever and the pulmonary symptoms and signs previously noted.

Physiologic Evaluation

The D$_{LCO}$ is diminished in about 19% to 25% of patients with primary Sjögren syndrome, often in the absence of radiographic abnormalities (36). The abnormality of diffusion capacity is more severe if Raynaud phenomenon is present. Positive findings in biopsy specimens of minor salivary glands are correlated with a reduction in lung function (37). Although restrictive pulmonary disease patterns are most commonly reported, tests indicative of abnormalities in small-airway function can be seen in the same patient (38).

Pulmonary Imaging Findings

Bilateral basilar interstitial opacities are the most common plain radiographic finding of LIP. Nodular lesions secondary to atypical lymphoid hyperplasia are seen in the setting of pseudolymphoma. Most nodules represent small areas of peripheral consolidation, frequently containing air bronchograms. Multiple isolated nodules with better-defined margins, a more central location, and mediastinal adenopathy should raise concern about a transformation to a malignant pulmonary lymphoma (39).

Laboratory Studies

Although a variety of autoantibodies are frequently present in the serum of patients with Sjögren syndrome, including rheumatoid factor (found in the majority of both primary and secondary cases), ANA (70% of primary cases), SSA/Ro (70% of primary cases), and SSB/La (50% of primary cases), these serologic markers have very little bearing on the incidence or severity of pulmonary manifestations.

Bronchoalveolar Lavage and Lung Biopsy

The percentage of lymphocytes is higher in the BAL fluid of patients with primary Sjögren syndrome than in that of normal controls, a finding potentially consistent with the underlying disease process.

Pathology

LIP consists mostly of large and small mature B lymphocytes and plasma cells (Fig. 26.13). LIP is analogous to other aspects of Sjögren syndrome; however, instead of the infiltration of exocrine glands, the lungs are invaded by lymphocytes. Chronic LIP may be complicated by amyloidosis. Pulmonary fibrosis can occur late in LIP, although a lymphocytic predominance may persist.

Lymphoproliferation in Sjögren syndrome can progress to pseudolymphoma. Pseudolymphoma is often heralded by a rising level of immunoglobulin M (IgM) and the presence of germinal centers on lung biopsy specimens. If malignant transformation follows, it is associated with a notable decline in the IgM level, generalized hypogammaglobulinemia,

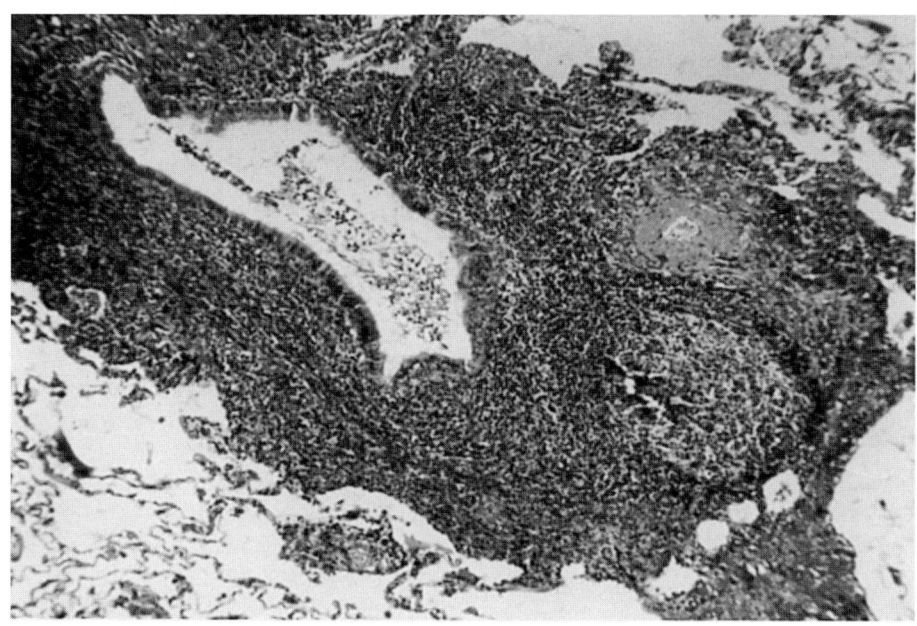

FIGURE 26.13. Chronic bronchiolitis in Sjögren syndrome. Marked chronic inflammation in the wall of the bronchiole is associated with lymphoid hyperplasia with germinal centers (**right**).

and the disappearance of rheumatoid factor. Patients usually have Sjögren syndrome for 15 years or longer before malignant lymphoproliferation develops. If lymphoma occurs, the lungs are involved in at least 20% of cases.

An additional lymphoproliferative disorder that is included in the differential diagnosis of pulmonary Sjögren syndrome is lymphomatoid granulomatosis. Features of this disorder include a proliferation of T lymphocytes (rather than the B lymphocytes seen in Sjögren syndrome) and lesions that infiltrate and destroy blood vessels, frequently involving the upper airways. Rare reports have appeared of concurrent lymphomatoid granulomatosis in patients with preestablished Sjögren syndrome.

Although the cause of Sjögren syndrome and its pulmonary syndromes are unknown, interesting work has focused on the potential role of viruses, such as the Epstein-Barr virus and retroviruses, as possible etiologic agents. The deposition of circulating immune complexes followed by complement activation appears to account partially for the pulmonary manifestations.

Treatment and Prognosis

The standard treatment for ILD associated with Sjögren syndrome is not well established (40,41). In addition to general supportive measures, corticosteroids are often recommended for the treatment of LIP despite an absence of good data to provide clear support for their use. Pseudolymphomatous transformation is believed to merit aggressive chemotherapy with combined corticosteroid and alkylating agent regimens (chlorambucil or cyclophosphamide). When feasible, resection of isolated lymphomatous mass lesions affords another therapeutic option.

THERAPY FOR PULMONARY SJÖGREN SYNDROME	
Summary Statement	**Level of Evidence**
Lymphocytic interstitial pneumonia: Corticosteroids are recommended.	Observational studies
Pseudolymphomatous transformation: Aggressive chemotherapy with combined corticosteroid and alkylating agent regimens (chlorambucil or cyclophosphamide).	Observational studies and expert opinion

SYSTEMIC SCLEROSIS

SSc, also called *scleroderma,* is a rare autoimmune disorder characterized by progressive fibrosis of the skin, vasculature, and internal organs. Estimates of the prevalence of SSc range from as few as 2 to as many as 265 per 100,000 people, and the predominance of women is striking. Hidebound skin

of the digits and distal extremities is the most characteristic finding in this disorder. SSc is subdivided into diffuse (dSSc) and limited (lSSc) variants. Patients with lSSc, or CREST (an acronym for calcinosis, Raynaud phenomenon, esophageal dysmotility, sclerodactyly, and telangiectasia), have a significantly better short-term prognosis, with little proximal skin, renal, and intestinal involvement. However, over the long term, the life span of patients with CREST is also reduced, often because of the development of pulmonary hypertension. In the recent past, the survival of patients with dSSc was decreased most significantly by hypertensive renal crisis and end-stage renal disease. The use of angiotensin-converting enzyme inhibitors has revolutionized the modern approach to dSSc and significantly improved the short-term prognosis. Although skin and gastrointestinal manifestations are more common, pulmonary disease is the most lethal feature of SSc. Interstitial pulmonary fibrosis remains one of the most difficult-to-manage aspects of this disabling and life-shortening disorder.

Epidemiology

Pulmonary disease is estimated to occur in 70% to 85% of patients with SSc (42–44). The exact prevalence of lung disease is difficult to determine because of the rarity of SSc, difficulties with characterization of the SSc subtypes, and the inaccurate diagnosis of the variable pulmonary pathologies. Although the percentage of ILD cases in dSSc is much higher, and although most serious end-stage fibrosis occurs in dSSc, ILD is also described in patients with lSSc. Severe restrictive lung disease appears more likely to develop in African American men with cardiac involvement than in other demographic groups (45).

Intense interest has focused on environmental factors that may predispose to SSc. Of particular interest with respect to lung disease, exposure to silica may increase the risk for SSc 25- to 100-fold (46,47). The putative role of silicone breast implants in the development of SSc has not been supported by large epidemiologic studies.

Clinical Presentation

Sclerodermatous skin changes and Raynaud phenomenon are frequent and striking physical findings that greatly aid in the differential diagnosis. Symptoms of pulmonary disease in SSc include dyspnea on exertion and a dry cough (48). The presence of abnormal nail fold capillary loops with vessel dropout, dilation, and severe ectasia help establish the diagnosis of an underlying connective tissue disorder and predict more severe pulmonary disease, manifested by a diminished D$_{LCO}$ (49). Pulmonary symptoms rarely predate the skin manifestations of SSc, although cases of SSc *sine* scleroderma have been described. Hemoptysis, in some cases secondary to bleeding telangiectases, occurs uncommonly.

SSc is associated with the development of significant impairment; the overall work capacity of patients with SSc is only 50% of the predicted normal. Although pulmonary disease contributes to this functional impairment, myocardial ischemia, ventricular arrhythmia, and limitations in locomotor function are significant cofactors.

Physiologic Evaluation

Abnormalities on pulmonary function testing are detected in up to 70% of patients with CREST, often in the absence of symptoms or chest radiographic evidence of parenchymal disease. A decline in the DLco is more strongly correlated with abnormalities in nail fold capillaries than are decrements in lung volumes (49). Although 20% of patients with SSc who are nonsmokers have an isolated reduction in the DLco, they have a good prognosis overall in regard to pulmonary morbidity and mortality (50). A decline in the DLco in lSSc may be caused by Raynaud phenomenon of the pulmonary vasculature (51). An increase in dead space ventilation is observed in connective tissue diseases associated with Raynaud phenomenon, lending credence to the theory of redistribution of blood flow resulting from pulmonary Raynaud phenomenon. Whether pulmonary Raynaud phenomenon coincides with digital Raynaud phenomenon and how often pulmonary Raynaud phenomenon occurs in SSc are matters of controversy.

Pulmonary Imaging

In dSSc, diffuse or bilateral basilar infiltrates are the typical findings. A bilateral basilar reticulonodular pattern is also seen in cases of lSSc with pathologic evidence of interstitial pneumonia. As in ILD of other causes, the chest radiograph, albeit more specific, is considerably less sensitive for early ILD than are pulmonary function tests.

HRCT has been evaluated as a diagnostic and surveillance tool for ILD in SSc. It is superior to plain radiography in detecting interstitial pulmonary abnormalities that may indicate early disease, such as ground-glass opacities and reticular abnormalities consistent with fibrosis (52,53).

Laboratory Studies

ANA is present in the majority of patients with SSc, most commonly in a speckled pattern on immunofluorescence. Two serologic markers are of particular clinical interest in SSc: antibodies to centromere (ACA), detected in about 50% to 80% of patients with lSSc, and anti–Scl-70 (an antibody to DNA topoisomerase I), seen in one third of patients with dSSc. The finding of anti–Scl-70 predicts restrictive lung involvement and other ominous visceral disease in many studies. Other work has found these markers in the absence of clinical disease (54). In one study, antihistone antibod-

ies, seen commonly in drug-induced lupus, were predictive of more severe pulmonary fibrosis in SSc. Newer work has suggested that serum markers of collagen turnover or airway epithelial injury may correlate with the presence of ILD (55,56). Whether these tests prove to have clinical utility awaits further investigation.

Bronchoalveolar Lavage and Lung Biopsy

BAL is touted by some as a useful tool for accurately identifying patients with SSc and active alveolitis who may respond to aggressive antiinflammatory therapy. Neutrophil influx associated with increased collagen production may be an early pathologic finding in SSc-associated pulmonary fibrosis. Collagenase activity is significantly elevated in patients with BAL neutrophilia, suggesting an increased level of matrix turnover. However, lymphocyte predominance is more frequently seen in many patients, particularly if they have secondary Sjögren syndrome. Increased ratios of lymphocytes to granulocytes may be associated with milder impairment of physiologic parameters. The true utility of BAL information in the management of SSc-associated lung disease is unproven.

Pathology

Interstitial fibrosis, bronchiolectasis with cyst formation, and intimal proliferation with medial hypertrophy of small pulmonary vessels are the classic histologic findings of ILD associated with dSSc (Fig. 26.14). Raynaud phenomenon of the lungs may account for some of the changes noted on pulmonary function studies and may play a role in the development of secondary pulmonary hypertension. Both lung fibrosis and vascular hyperplastic changes are common in

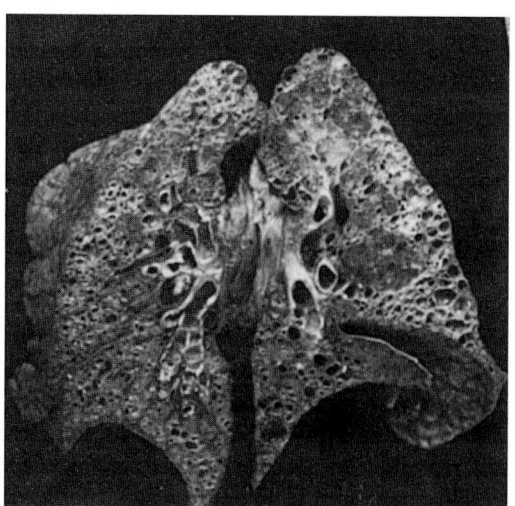

FIGURE 26.14. Gross appearance of the lungs of a patient with severe scleroderma. The lungs show extensive honeycombing.

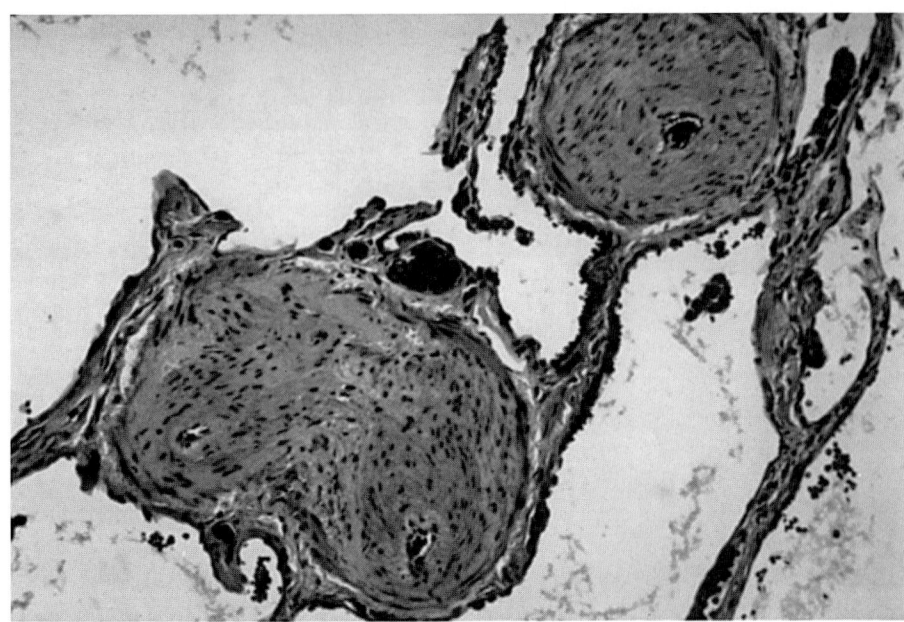

FIGURE 26.15. Pulmonary hypertension in scleroderma, with marked thickening of the muscular walls of the small pulmonary arteries.

SSc and may independently contribute to right-sided heart failure (Fig. 26.15). Patients with lSSc can have pathologic features of NSIP or UIP, particularly those who present with bilateral lower lobe infiltrates (43,57).

Treatment and Prognosis

No pharmacologic agent has been identified that is of unequivocal value in modifying the natural course of lung disease in SSc. Notwithstanding, therapeutic interventions may be indicated for severe pulmonary disease if diagnostic evidence of an active inflammatory process is found. For instance, in patients with rapidly declining lung function and an increased proportion of lymphocytes on BAL, a trial of high-dose corticosteroids and immunosuppressive therapy seems reasonable. This regimen may lead to a decrease in pulmonary inflammation, as assessed by BAL. Based on retrospective data analysis and open-label trials, cyclophosphamide appears to improve the forced vital capacity over time and can be added to corticosteroids in patients with refractory, inflammation-related pulmonary decline (45,58). Large-scale experience with other cytotoxic and antiinflammatory therapies is lacking. Because of its ability to interrupt molecular cross-linking of collagen, D-penicillamine has been of considerable interest to many investigators as a potential disease-modifying agent in SSc. Poor patient tolerance and the hematologic and renal toxicity associated with D-penicillamine have substantially dampened enthusiasm for its use. Furthermore, a long-term study of high- versus low-dose D-penicillamine has been completed and demonstrated no dose-related benefit to patients with dSSc (59).

Based on data from an inception cohort, the estimated 5-year survival rate for all patients with SSc is about 70%

(42). However, the natural history of SSc is highly variable, and a large percentage of patients have a protracted disease course with survival in excess of 20 years. Worsening of ILD in SSc is less rapid than in IPF, and patients with fibrosis secondary to SSc may have a better long-term prognosis than those with other fibrotic lung diseases (60). Isolated impairment of the DLCO (<55% of predicted) does not indicate a poor prognosis. Although abnormalities in static lung compliance and diffusing capacity may worsen over time, the lung volumes did not appreciably deteriorate in one large series of untreated patients followed on average for 3 years (50). Abnormal cardiopulmonary signs in conjunction with severely impaired gas exchange (DLCO < 40% of predicted) are associated with significantly worse survival in several series. Patients with long-term SSc tend to have a rate of decline in pulmonary function tests not substantially different from that of the general population, but this could be partially because of a survival bias.

Death was caused by pulmonary hypertension in 60% of cases in one of the largest prospective series of patients with both dSSc and lSSc (42). Although pulmonary hypertension is a more common outcome in lSSc, secondary pulmonary hypertension may develop in patients with dSSc after years of pulmonary fibrosis. For patients with advanced interstitial disease in whom secondary pulmonary hypertension and cor pulmonale develop, long-term home oxygen therapy may lower the pulmonary vascular resistance and improve quality of life and survival. Once cor pulmonale with peripheral edema has developed, the 5-year mortality rate for patients with SSc is 70% (42). In patients with severe pulmonary vascular changes, rapidly progressive respiratory failure and severe pulmonary hypertension often develop, and these patients die quickly. Although the addition of continuously infused prostacyclin as a regional pulmonary vasodilator has improved physiology and symptom scores (61), the long-term effect on survival remains unclear.

Independently of cigarette smoking, but in relation to pulmonary fibrosis, SSc confers an increased risk for lung cancer estimated at fourfold to 17-fold. Alveolar cell carcinoma in particular, in addition to lymphoma and leukemia, has been reported most commonly. Small cell carcinoma of the lung in the absence of a history of smoking has also been noted.

THERAPY FOR INTERSTITIAL LUNG DISEASE IN SYSTEMIC SCLEROSIS	
Summary Statement	**Level of Evidence**
No pharmacologic agent has been identified to modify the natural course of lung disease in systemic sclerosis. Corticosteroid therapy has been recommended.	Observational studies
Cyclophosphamide may improve lung function in patients with disease refractory to corticosteroids.	Observational studies (retrospective data analysis and open-label trials)
D-Penicillamine does not appear effective and is poorly tolerated because of hematologic and renal toxicity.	Observational studies (open-label trials)

IDIOPATHIC INFLAMMATORY MYOPATHY

The idiopathic inflammatory myopathies (IIMs) comprise a group of illnesses including PM, DM, and inclusion body myositis. The IIMs are rare, with 5 to 10 new cases per million per year occurring in the United States. These related yet distinct disorders all produce nonsuppurative muscle inflammation that leads to weakness and disability. Inclusion body myositis, a disorder of older Caucasian men characterized by both distal and proximal weakness, is the least prevalent of the three conditions; it is seldom associated with respiratory features and is not discussed further here. Despite differing histopathologic findings and putative immunologic mechanisms, PM and DM have many characteristics in common, including a predilection for the proximal musculature and a spectrum of pulmonary disorders.

Epidemiology

Lung disease of all types occurs in up to 50% of cases of DM/PM (62,63). Pulmonary disease in IIM commonly occurs through four processes: (a) aspiration resulting from bulbar weakness, (b) ventilatory insufficiency resulting from myositis of the chest wall and diaphragm, (c) secondary infection, and (d) ILD. Either radiographic or physiologic evidence of ILD is estimated to occur in from 5% to 30% of patients in large series of IIM. Ethnic and racial variation in the prevalence of IIM-associated ILD is uncertain, but in one Japanese series, radiographic evidence of ILD was reported in 81% of cases (64).

Clinical Presentation

Patients with IIM note prominent bilateral proximal weakness that inhibits simple activities of daily living. In patients with DM, a prominent, scaly erythroderma erupts in a V-shaped distribution on the chest and back. Over the knuckles of the proximal interphalangeal and metacarpophalangeal joints of the hands, a scaly rash known as *Gottron papules* is nearly pathognomonic for DM. A heliotrope rash, a purplish edematous discoloration over the eyelids, is also often noted. Constitutional symptoms of fatigue, fevers, and weight loss are additional harbingers of IIM, and it is difficult to determine whether these are caused by myopathy or pulmonary pathology.

In as many as one third of cases, lung disease predates muscle involvement or occurs in patients with only minimal myopathy (65,66). The antisynthetase syndrome, named for the presence of autoantibodies to aminoacyl transfer RNA synthetase (see section "Laboratory Studies" below), is an IIM variant in which seronegative, nonerosive arthritis, fevers, "mechanic's hands," Raynaud phenomenon, and ILD can strongly overshadow a mild or even clinically insignificant myopathy. Clubbing is uncommon in IIM-associated ILD but has been reported.

Physiologic Evaluation

Although ILD associated with IIM frequently causes physiologic abnormalities similar to those of IPF, additional physiologic parameters, such as the maximal ventilatory volume and inspiratory effort, should be measured. Abnormal results of these studies point toward respiratory muscle weakness as an explanation for at least a component of the pulmonary symptoms.

Laboratory Studies

Muscle enzymes such as creatinine kinase and aldolase are usually elevated at some time during the course of an IIM. The diagnosis of PM/DM is ultimately confirmed by characteristic abnormalities on electromyographic recordings and muscle biopsy specimens. Elevations in the erythrocyte sedimentation rate nonspecifically mirror changes in disease activity or herald the development of opportunistic infections. The ANA titer is elevated in a small percentage of cases, often indicative of antisynthetase antibodies. One of the most striking serologic associations is the established relationship between antisynthetase antibodies and IIM-associated ILD.

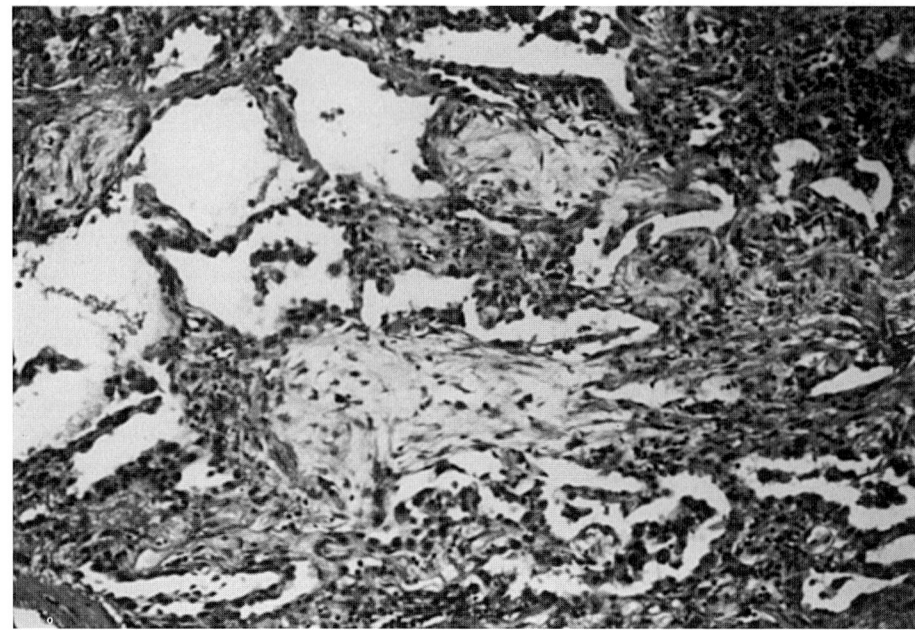

FIGURE 26.16. Patchy organizing pneumonia in polymyositis/dermatomyositis. Two rounded edematous masses of intra-alveolar fibrous connective tissue can be seen in the center of the figure.

Antibodies to histidyl transfer RNA synthetase, known as *anti-Jo-1,* occur in 25% of patients with DM/PM. Of special interest, this antibody is found in 50% of patients with IIM and concomitant ILD. The presence of this antibody in patients with IIM, therefore, should raise concern for concomitant ILD. Additionally, a small percentage of patients have antibodies to signal recognition protein, and they are less likely to have ILD. Autoantibodies to other amino transfer RNA synthetases have also been identified and are variably associated with lung disease (67,68).

Bronchoalveolar Lavage and Lung Biopsy

The need for BAL and lung biopsy is uncertain. Histopathologic and BAL data may predict the therapeutic response, but as in other forms of connective tissue disease–associated ILD, they have not been shown to alter management or outcome significantly.

Pathology

A mononuclear cell infiltration of skeletal muscle and surrounding tissue with fiber degradation, regeneration, and fibrosis is the major systemic feature of PM and DM. Of note, DM is not simply PM with a rash; it is a humorally mediated disease with immune complex deposition in the perimysium and a perivascular vasculitis that is presumed to be responsible for the pathology. PM results from lymphocytic infiltration of the true muscle fibers and is the manifestation of a cell-mediated immune process.

Investigators have identified three major histopathologic forms of IIM-associated ILD that are of prognostic significance: organizing pneumonia, diffuse alveolar damage, and NSIP (Fig. 26.16). Patients with organizing pneumonia appear to have the best prognosis, whereas those with diffuse alveolar damage fare the worst. In a series of patients with IIM and lung disease evaluated by open lung biopsy, more than 80% of the cases had NSIP with a prognosis similar to that of idiopathic NSIP and a survival clearly better than the historical data for IPF (69). Immune complex deposition in the lungs is not usually found in IIM-associated ILD. Cases of pulmonary cryoglobulin deposition have been reported (70).

Treatment and Prognosis

High-dose corticosteroids (1 mg of prednisone per kilogram of body weight) are the starting point for regimens directed at both the muscle disease and newly diagnosed pulmonary involvement. Methotrexate is a commonly used second-line agent for the general manifestations of IIM, and although it is in itself associated with pneumonitis, it is safe to use in IIM-associated ILD. Although some authors question the efficacy of cyclophosphamide in IIM, given its potential value in other types of ILD and reports of its success in IIM, it is prudent to consider this agent if the patient is failing other options (71,72). In uncontrolled case series, cyclosporine led to improvement in patients with steroid-resistant IIM-associated ILD (73–75). Intravenous immunoglobulin has been used effectively for refractory myositis in several case series and controlled trials (76,77). Study endpoints included only measures of motor function, and no mention was made of lung involvement; thus, the role of immunoglobulin therapy in ILD remains unclear.

Adequate control of muscle inflammation is achieved with antiinflammatory agents in many patients. However, a significant percentage continue to require maintenance corticosteroids to avoid relapse. In these patients, sustained morbidity and even mortality may ultimately be caused by the treatment. With respect to IIM-associated ILD, the response to corticosteroids and other immunosuppressive agents is variable. Some studies report very disappointing results, with up to 60% mortality despite aggressive therapy. In another series, the 5-year mortality rate for IIM with ILD was 40%. ILD with minimal myopathy is a poor prognostic sign.

An association between IIM and malignancy has been suspected for many years, and well-conducted population-based studies now fully support both a higher incidence of cancer and a higher rate of mortality from cancer (78,79). Adenocarcinoma (particularly ovarian cancer) is reported most commonly. Some authorities advocate aggressive cancer screening for all patients with newly diagnosed IIM. Based on the need to consider patient comfort and safety, avoid false-positive results that can occur with excessive testing, and constrain health care costs, we recommend a thorough physical examination (including examination of the breasts, genital organs, and rectum) and the prudent use of age-appropriate and clinically directed cancer-screening modalities (i.e., Papanicolaou test, mammography, flexible sigmoidoscopy) for all patients with newly diagnosed IIM.

MIXED CONNECTIVE TISSUE DISEASE

The term *mixed connective tissue disease (MCTD)* was coined in 1972 by Sharp and colleagues (80) to describe a subset of patients with connective tissue disease who have overlapping features of SLE, SSc, and IIM. The initial cases described had a set of common clinical and laboratory features that frequently included, in addition to pulmonary disease, erosive inflammatory arthritis with diffuse hand swelling, esophageal dysmotility, myopathy, Raynaud phenomenon, high titers of speckled ANA, antibodies to U1-RNP, and an absence of antibodies to Smith (Sm) antigen and double-stranded DNA. Not all experts agree that MCTD merits a separate diagnostic label. Physicians experienced in caring for patients with rheumatic diseases recognize that in many cases these disorders have a variable presentation that often does not include the "classic" features of any one particular diagnostic entity (81). As such, it has been suggested that the MCTD paradigm is conceptually flawed because it may not identify a unique patient population, provide direction on specific treatment options, or offer guidance on prognosis.

Epidemiology

Most of the reports on pulmonary involvement in MCTD have focused on pulmonary hypertension. However, ILD may be more frequent and severe in MCTD even than in SSc. In one series, 80% of all patients with MCTD had pulmonary disease, and pulmonary dysfunction was revealed by physiologic testing, chest radiography, or both in 69% of the asymptomatic patients (80).

Clinical Presentation

The most common and worrisome pulmonary feature of MCTD, significant pulmonary hypertension, cannot be accurately predicted based on symptoms, signs, or laboratory data. When ILD occurs in MCTD, it mimics that seen in SSc. As in the other connective tissue disorders, a reduction in the diffusion capacity is the single most sensitive test of physiologic dysfunction in MCTD. Despite abnormal physiology, chest radiographs demonstrate identifiable abnormalities in only 21% of cases (82). A lower lobe predominance of interstitial infiltrates has been described most commonly.

Treatment and Prognosis

Authors report pulmonary improvement in 38% to 86% of patients with MCTD who are treated with corticosteroids, cyclophosphamide, or both (83). Respiratory disease may lead to fatal outcomes, in part because the disease is sometimes not diagnosed until it is far advanced. The pulmonary outcome is worse if the features are more characteristic of SSc.

SERONEGATIVE SPONDYLARTHROPATHIES

This group of heterogeneous disorders includes ankylosing spondylitis, psoriatic arthritis, reactive arthritis (Reiter syndrome), and arthritis associated with bowel inflammation. Although these conditions are in many ways heterogeneous, they share certain features, including inflammatory arthritis of the spine and sacroiliac joints, enthesopathy (inflammation at the insertion of ligaments and tendons into bones), an association with HLA-B27, and a spectrum of mucocutaneous lesions. The occurrence of ILD in ankylosing spondylitis is the best described, although similar changes have been reported in psoriatic arthritis with a lower frequency.

Clinical Presentation

The thoracic involvement in ankylosing spondylitis is often asymptomatic (84). Chest wall and thoracic vertebral involvement may lead to ventilatory restriction, thereby contributing to exercise limitation and dyspnea (85). Patients may present with cough and sputum production if apical fibronodular disease becomes superinfected. Noninfectious fibrobullous disease of the upper lobes of the lungs is nearly pathognomonic for ankylosing spondylitis (86). The abnormality usually appears late in the disease course and does not correlate with the severity of extrapulmonary disease. In a series of 2,080 patients with ankylosing spondylitis seen at the Mayo Clinic, the prevalence was 1.3% (87). The pulmonary process often begins unilaterally, with linear opacities on radiographs (88). As it advances, changes can be seen in both apices, and bullae gradually develop. In advanced cases, pleural thickening and cavitary disease can occur and are commonly confused with tuberculosis.

Pathology

Specimens show intra-alveolar fibrosis, hyalinized connective tissue, and degeneration of elastic fibrils. Despite extensive investigations, no infectious organism has been identified as an etiologic agent for these lesions.

Treatment and Prognosis

Most of the disability associated with ankylosing spondylitis is related to limited mobility rather than respiratory limitation. No studies have demonstrated efficacy for any therapy in the lung disease of ankylosing spondylitis. Secondary infection of bullae with bacteria, mycobacteria, or fungi (particularly *Aspergillus*) may lead to considerable morbidity and mortality.

RELAPSING POLYCHONDRITIS

Relapsing polychondritis is a rare idiopathic disorder. It is an episodic form of inflammatory disease characterized by destructive lesions involving cartilaginous structures of the nose, ears, larynx, tracheobronchial tree, cardiac valves, and joints (89,90). Relapsing polychondritis is a diagnosis of exclusion.

Clinical Presentation

The majority of patients are between the ages of 40 and 60 years, with an equal distribution between the sexes. The disease primarily affects Caucasians. In approximately one third of cases, relapsing polychondritis has been associated with Wegener granulomatosis, RA, SLE, Sjögren syndrome, ankylosing spondylitis, Reiter syndrome, Behçet disease, hypothyroidism, Graves disease, chronic ulcerative colitis, cryptogenic cirrhosis, cryoglobulinemia, or hydralazine therapy. In many patients, these diseases precede the onset of polychondritis by months to years.

Clinical manifestations include iritis, episcleritis, hearing deficit, cataract, aortic valvular insufficiency, anemia, an elevated erythrocyte sedimentation rate, and abnormal liver function.

Biopsy of the affected cartilage is nondiagnostic; only nonspecific cartilaginous destruction is noted. No specific serologic or other tests are available to aid in the diagnosis. If three of the following six criteria are present in the proper clinical setting, then relapsing polychondritis can be suspected: auricular chondritis; nonerosive inflammatory polyarthritis; nasal chondritis; ocular inflammation (conjunctivitis, keratitis, scleritis, episcleritis, uveitis); laryngeal, tracheal, or bronchial chondritis; and cochlear or vestibular damage.

Pulmonary Disease

Recurrent inflammation of the nasal cartilage leads to structural damage and saddle-nose deformity. Respiratory complications develop in more than 50% of patients (89–91). Involvement of the laryngotracheal region portends a poor prognosis (92). Airway pathology includes thickening of the mucosa, loss of elasticity, and the development of stenotic segments. When multiple cartilaginous segments become affected, expiratory collapse of the airway occurs (Fig. 26.17). The resultant weak cough, combined with recurrent infections because of the inability to clear mucus, may cause bronchiectasis.

Flow-volume curves in patients with significant respiratory symptoms demonstrate the plateau patterns of maximal inspiratory or expiratory flows (93).

Tracheal tomography and cine computed tomography may provide further insight into the abnormal anatomy of the major airways. Bronchoscopy is useful in assessing the dynamic function of the airways.

Treatment and Prognosis

Nonsteroidal antiinflammatory agents or corticosteroid (30–60 mg of prednisolone per deciliter) often effectively suppresses acute manifestations. It is not clear whether corticosteroid treatment alters the natural course of this disease. Refractory and recurrent disease has been treated with cyclophosphamide, 6-mercaptopurine, azathioprine, cyclosporin A, and dapsone.

Infection, systemic vasculitis, and malignancy are the most common causes of death (90). Respiratory tract involvement is the cause of approximately 10% of deaths, usually when recurrent attacks lead to the destruction of cartilage in the tracheal and bronchial rings, so that these structures collapse secondary to inflammation, edema, and cicatrization. Major airway stenosis may require the insertion of a tracheobronchial prosthesis or resection if the strictures are localized. Tracheostomy may aggravate the expiratory collapse. Nasal continuous positive airway pressure or similar physiologic stenting may help some patients. Cartilaginous destruction may lead to severe focal or diffuse airway collapse with inadequate ventilation that often is not corrected

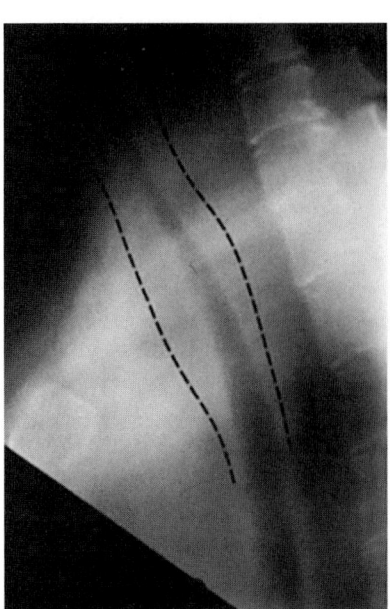
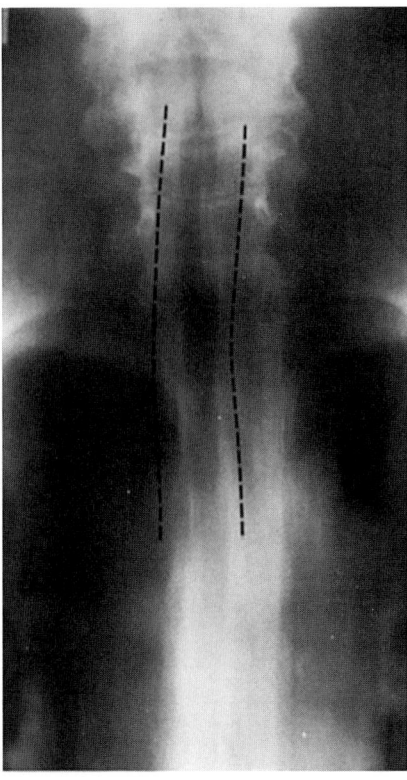

A,B

FIGURE 26.17. Tomogram showing severely narrowed trachea, determined by the size of the air tracheogram in relapsing polychondritis. Anteroposterior (**A**) and lateral (**B**) views delineate the normal dimensions of the trachea.

by tracheostomy and mechanical ventilation. Consequently, death can occur from asphyxiation.

REFERENCES

1. Gross TJ, Hunninghake GW. Idiopathic pulmonary fibrosis: sequential acute lung injury. *N Engl J Med* 2001;345:517–525.
2. Bouros DE, Polychronopoulos V, Conron M, et al. Histopathologic subgroups in patients with fibrosing alveolitis associated with systemic sclerosis. *Eur Respir J* 1999;14[Suppl 30]:272S.
3. Katzenstein A-L, Fiorelli RF. Non-specific interstitial pneumonia/fibrosis: histologic patterns and clinical significance. *Am J Surg Pathol* 1994;18:136–147.
4. Katzenstein A-L, Myers JL, Mazur MT. Acute interstitial pneumonia: a clinicopathologic, ultrastructural, and cell kinetic study. *Am J Surg Pathol* 1986;10:256–267.
5. Epler GR. Heterogeneity of bronchiolitis obliterans organizing pneumonia. *Curr Opin Pulm Med* 1998;4:93–97.
6. Alarcon GS, Blackburn WD, Calvo A, et al. Evaluation of the American Rheumatism Association preliminary criteria for remission in rheumatoid arthritis: a prospective study. *J Rheumatol* 1987;14:93–96.
7. Cervantes-Perez P, Toro-Perez AH, Rodriguez-Jurado P. Pulmonary involvement in rheumatoid arthritis. *JAMA* 1980;243:1715–1719.
8. Dawson JK, Fewins HE, Desmond J, et al. Fibrosing alveolitis in patients with rheumatoid arthritis as assessed by high-resolution computed tomography, chest radiography, and pulmonary function tests. *Thorax* 2001;56:622–627.
9. Roschmann RA, Rothenberg RJ. Pulmonary fibrosis in rheumatoid arthritis: a review of clinical features and therapy. *Semin Arthritis Rheum* 1987;16:174–185.
10. Hyland RM, Gordon DA, Broder I, et al. A systematic controlled study of pulmonary abnormalities in rheumatoid arthritis. *J Rheumatol* 1983;10:395–405.
11. Saag KG, Kolluri S, Koehnke RK, et al. Rheumatoid arthritis lung disease: determinants of physiologic and radiologic abnormalities. *Arthritis Rheum* 1996;39:1711–1719.
12. Westedt ML, Hazes JM, Breedveld FC, et al. Cigarette smoking and pulmonary diffusion defects in rheumatoid arthritis. *Rheumatol Int* 1998;18:1–4.
13. Rajasekaran BA, Shovlin D, Lord P, et al. Interstitial lung disease in patients with rheumatoid arthritis: a comparison with cryptogenic fibrosing alveolitis. *Rheumatology* 2001;40:1022–1025.
14. Schwartz DA, Merchant RK, Helmers RA, et al. The influence of cigarette smoking on lung function in patients with idiopathic pulmonary fibrosis. *Am Rev Respir Dis* 1991;144:504–506.
15. Hayakawa H, Sato A, Imokawa S, et al. Bronchiolar disease in rheumatoid arthritis. *Am J Respir Crit Care Med* 1996;154:1531–1536.
16. Hartley PG, Galvin JR, Hunninghake GW, et al. High-resolution CT-derived measures of lung density are valid indexes of interstitial lung disease. *J Appl Physiol* 1994;76:271–277.
17. Hunninghake GW, Gadek JE, Kawanami O, et al. Inflammatory and immune processes in the human lung in health and disease: evaluation by bronchoalveolar lavage. *Am J Pathol* 1979;97:149–206.
18. Nagai S, Satake N, Kitaichi M, et al. Interstitial pneumonia associated with collagen vascular diseases: histological findings and cells in bronchoalveolar lavage fluid. *Jpn J Thorac Dis* 1995;33:258–263.
19. Yousem SA, Colby TV, Carrington CB. Lung biopsy in rheumatoid arthritis. *Am Rev Respir Dis* 1985;131:770–777.
20. Fuhrman C, Parrot A, Wislez M, et al. Spectrum of CD4 to CD8 T-cell ratios in lymphocytic alveolitis associated with

methotrexate-induced pneumonitis. *Am J Respir Crit Care Med* 2001;164:1186–1191.

21. Gochuico BR. Potential pathogenesis and clinical aspects of pulmonary fibrosis associated with rheumatoid arthritis. *Am J Med Sci* 2001;321:83–88.

22. Ogawa D, Hashimoto H, Wada J, et al. Successful use of cyclosporin A for the treatment of acute interstitial pneumonitis associated with rheumatoid arthritis. *Rheumatology* 2000;39:1422–1424.

23. Agostini C. Cytokine and chemokine blockade as immunointervention strategy for the treatment of diffuse lung diseases. *Sarcoidosis Vasculitis Diffuse Lung Dis* 2001;18:18–22.

24. Kudoh S, Azuma A, Yamamoto M, et al. Improvement of survival in patients with diffuse panbronchiolitis treated with low-dose erythromycin. *Am J Respir Crit Care Med* 1998;157:1829–1832.

25. Hakala M. Poor prognosis in patients with rheumatoid arthritis hospitalized for interstitial lung disease. *Chest* 1988;93:114–118.

26. Haupt HM, Moore GW, Hutchins GM. The lung in systemic lupus erythematosus: analysis of the pathologic changes in 120 patients. *Am J Med* 1981;71:791–798.

27. Keane MP, Lynch JP III. Pleuropulmonary manifestations of systemic lupus erythematosus. *Thorax* 2000;55:159–166.

28. Matthay RA, Schwartz MI, Petty TL, et al. Pulmonary manifestations of systemic erythematosus. *Medicine* 1974;54:397–409.

29. Sant SM, Doran M, Fenelon HM, et al. Pleuropulmonary abnormalities in patients with systemic lupus erythematosus: assessment with high-resolution computed tomography, chest radiography and pulmonary function tests. *Clin Exp Rheumatol* 1997;15:507–513.

30. Silberstein SL, Barland P, Grayzel AI, et al. Pulmonary dysfunction in systemic lupus erythematosus. *J Rheumatol* 1980;7:187–195.

31. Cheema GS, Quismorio FP Jr. Interstitial lung disease in systemic lupus erythematosus. *Curr Opin Pulm Med* 2000;6:424–429.

32. Yood RA, Steigman DM, Gill LR. Lymphocytic interstitial pneumonitis in a patient with systemic lupus erythematosus. *Lupus* 1995;4:161–163.

33. Fink SD, Kremer JM. Successful treatment of interstitial lung disease in systemic lupus erythematosus with methotrexate. *J Rheumatol* 1995;22:967–969.

34. Papiris SA, Maniati M, Constantopoulos SH, et al. Lung involvement in primary Sjögren's syndrome is mainly related to the small airway disease. *Ann Rheum Dis* 1999;58:61–64.

35. Cain HC, Noble PW, Matthay RA. Pulmonary manifestations of Sjögren's syndrome. *Clin Chest Med* 1998;19:687–699.

36. Constantopoulos SH, Papadimitriou CS, Moutsopoulos HM. Respiratory manifestations in primary Sjögren's syndrome: a clinical, functional, and histologic study. *Chest* 1985;88:226–229.

37. Kelly C, Gardiner P, Pal B, et al. Lung function in primary Sjögren's syndrome: a cross-sectional and longitudinal study. *Thorax* 1991;46:180–183.

38. Strimlan CV. Pulmonary function in patients with primary Sjögren's syndrome. *Ann Rheum Dis* 2001;60:429–433.

39. Franquet T, Gimenez A, Monill JM, et al. Primary Sjögren's syndrome and associated lung disease: CT findings in 50 patients. *AJR Am J Roentgenol* 1997;169:655–658.

40. Deheinzelin D, Capelozzi VL, Kairalla R, et al. Interstitial lung disease in primary Sjögren's syndrome. Clinical-pathological evaluation and response to treatment. *Am J Respir Crit Care Med* 1996;154:794–799.

41. Ogasawara H, Sekiya M, Murashima A, et al. Very low-dose cyclosporin treatment of steroid-resistant interstitial pneumonitis associated with Sjögren's syndrome. *Clin Rheumatol* 1998;17:160–162.

42. Lee P, Langevitz P, Alderice CA, et al. Mortality in systemic sclerosis (scleroderma). *Q J Med* 1992;82:139–148.

43. Silver RM. Scleroderma. Clinical problems. The lungs. *Rheum Dis Clin North Am* 1996;22:825–840.

44. Veeraraghaven S, Sharma OP. Progressive systemic sclerosis and the lung. *Curr Opin Pulm Med* 1998;4:305–309.

45. Steen VD, Conte C, Owens GR, et al. Severe restrictive lung disease in systemic sclerosis. *Arthritis Rheum* 1994;37:1283–1289.

46. Nietert PJ, Silver RM. Systemic sclerosis: environmental and occupational risk factors. *Curr Opin Rheumatol* 2000;12:520–526.

47. Pelmear PL, Roos JO, Maehle WM. Occupationally-induced scleroderma. *J Occup Med* 1992;34:20–25.

48. Lalloo UG, Lim S, DuBois R, et al. Increased sensitivity of the cough reflex in progressive systemic sclerosis patients with interstitial lung disease. *Eur Respir J* 1998;11:702–705.

49. Groen H, Wichers G, Ten Borg EJ, et al. Pulmonary diffusing capacity disturbances are related to nailfold capillary changes in patients with Raynaud's phenomena. *Am J Med* 1990;89:34–41.

50. Greenwald GI, Tashkin DP, Gong H, et al. Longitudinal changes in lung function and respiratory symptoms in progressive systemic sclerosis. Prospective study. *Am J Med* 1987;83:83–90.

51. Vergnon J-M, Barthelemy J-C, Riffat J, et al. Raynaud's phenomenon of the lung: a reality both in primary and secondary Raynaud's syndrome. *Chest* 1992;101:1312–1317.

52. Silver RM. Interstitial lung disease of systemic sclerosis. *Int Rev Immunol* 1995;12:281–291.

53. Wechsler RJ, Steiner RM, Spirn PW, et al. The relationship of thoracic lymphadenopathy to pulmonary interstitial disease in diffuse and limited systemic sclerosis: CT findings. *AJR Am J Roentgenol* 1996;167:101–104.

54. Schnitz W, Taylor-Albert E, Targoff IN, et al. Anti-PM/Scl autoantibodies in patients without clinical polymyositis or scleroderma. *J Rheumatol* 1996;23:1729–1733.

55. Diot E, Diot P, Valat C, et al. Predictive value of serum III procollagen for the diagnosis of pulmonary involvement in patients with scleroderma. *Eur Respir J* 1995;8:1559–1565.

56. Nakajima H, Harigai M, Hara M, et al. IL-6 as a novel serum marker for interstitial pneumonia associated with collagen diseases. *J Rheumatol* 2000;27:1164–1170.

57. Yousem SA. The pulmonary pathological manifestations of the CREST syndrome. *Hum Pathol* 1990;21:467–474.

58. Vallance DK, Lynch JP III, McCune WJ. Immunosuppressive treatment of the pulmonary manifestations of progressive systemic sclerosis. *Curr Opin Rheumatol* 1995;7:174–182.

59. Clements PJ, Furst DE, Wong WK, et al. High-dose versus low-dose D-penicillamine in early diffuse systemic sclerosis: analysis of a two-year, double-blinded, randomized, controlled clinical trial. *Arthritis Rheum* 1999;42:1194–1203.

60. Wells AU, Cullinan P, Hansell DM, et al. Fibrosing alveolitis associated with systemic sclerosis has a better prognosis than lone cryptogenic fibrosing alveolitis. *Am J Respir Crit Care Med* 1994;149:1583–1590.

61. Badesch DB, Tapson VF, McGoon MD, et al. Continuous intravenous epoprostenol for pulmonary hypertension due to the scleroderma spectrum of disease. A randomized, controlled trial. *Ann Intern Med* 2000;312:425–434.

62. Schwartz MI, Matthay RA, Sahn SA, et al. Interstitial lung disease in polymyositis and dermatomyositis. *Medicine* 1976;55:89–104.

63. Schwartz MI. The lung in polymyositis. *Clin Chest Med* 1998;19:701–712.

64. Hirakata M, Nagai S. Interstitial lung disease in polymyositis and dermatomyositis. *Curr Opin Rheumatol* 2000;12:501–508.

65. Lampa J, Nennesmo I, Einarsdottir H, et al. MRI-guided muscle

biopsy confirmed polymyositis diagnosis in a patient with interstitial lung disease. *Ann Rheum Dis* 2001;60:423–426.

66. Friedman AW, Targoff IN, Arnett FC. Interstitial lung disease with autoantibodies against aminoacyl-tRNA synthetases in the absence of clinically apparent myositis. *Semin Arthritis Rheum* 1996;26:459–467.

67. Miller FW. Myositis-specific autoantibodies: touchstones for understanding the inflammatory myopathies. *JAMA* 1993;270:1846–1849.

68. Sauty A, Rochat T, Schoch OD, et al. Pulmonary fibrosis with predominant CD8 lymphocytic alveolitis and anti-Jo-1 antibodies. *Eur Respir J* 1997;10:2907–2912.

69. Douglas WW, Tazelaar HD, Hartman TE, et al. Polymyositis-dermatomyositis–associated interstitial lung disease. *Am J Respir Crit Care Med* 2001;164:1182–1185.

70. Lambie PB, Quismorio FP. Interstitial lung disease and cryoglobulinemia in polymyositis. *J Rheumatol* 1991;18:468–469.

71. Takada T, Suzuki E, Nakano M, et al. Clinical features of polymyositis/dermatomyositis with steroid-resistant interstitial lung. *Intern Med* 1998;37:669–673.

72. Tanaka F, Origuchi T, Migita K, et al. Successful combined therapy of cyclophosphamide and cyclosporine for acute exacerbated interstitial pneumonia associated with dermatomyositis. *Intern Med* 2000;39:428–430.

73. Nawata Y, Kurasawa K, Takabayashi K, et al. Corticosteroid-resistant interstitial pneumonitis in dermatomyositis/polymyositis: prediction and treatment with cyclosporine. *J Rheumatol* 1999;26:1527–1533.

74. Oddis CV, Sciurba FC, Elmagd KA, et al. Tacrolimus in refractory polymyositis with interstitial lung disease. *Lancet* 1999;353:1762–1763.

75. Sekigawa I, Ogasawara H, Sugiyama M, et al. Extremely low-dose treatment of cyclosporine for autoimmune diseases. *Clin Exp Rheumatol* 1998;16:352–357.

76. Cherin P, Herson S, Wechsler B, et al. Efficacy of intravenous gamma globulin therapy in chronic refractory polymyositis: an open study with 20 adult patients. *Am J Med* 1991;91:162–168.

77. Dalakas MC. Controlled studies with high-dose intravenous immunoglobulin in the treatment of dermatomyositis, inclusion body myositis, and polymyositis. *Neurology* 1998;51[6 Suppl 5]:S37–45.

78. Buchbinder R, Forbes A, Hall S, et al. Incidence of malignant disease in biopsy-proven inflammatory myopathy: a population-based cohort study. *Ann Intern Med* 2001;134:1087–1095.

79. Hill CL, Zhang Y, Sigurgeirsson B, et al. Frequency of specific cancer types in dermatomyositis and polymyositis: a population-based study. *Lancet* 2001;357:96–100.

80. Sharp GC, Irvin WS, Tan EM, et al. Mixed connective tissue disease—an apparently distinct rheumatic disease syndrome associated with a specific antibody to an extractable nuclear antigen (ENA). *Am J Med* 1972;52:148–159.

81. Ioannou Y, Sultan S, Isenberg DA. Myositis overlap syndromes. *Curr Opin Rheumatol* 1999;11:468–474.

82. Prakash UBS, Luthra HS, Divertie MB. Intrathoracic manifestations in mixed connective tissue disease. *Mayo Clin Proc* 1985;60:813–821.

83. Prakash UBS. Respiratory complication of mixed connective tissue disease. *Clin Chest Med* 1998;19:733–746.

84. Lee-Chong TL Jr. Pulmonary manifestations of ankylosing spondylitis and relapsing polychondritis. *Clin Chest Med* 1998;19:747–757.

85. Seckin U, Bolukbasi N, Gursel G, et al. Relationship between pulmonary function and exercise tolerance in patients with ankylosing spondylitis. *Clin Exp Rheumatol* 2000;18:502–506.

86. Davies D. Ankylosing spondylitis and lung fibrosis. *Q J Med* 1972;164:395–417.

87. Rosenow E, Strimlan CV, Muhm JR, et al. Pleuropulmonary manifestations of ankylosing spondylitis. *Mayo Clin Proc* 1977;52:641–649.

88. Turetschek K, Ebner W, Fleischmann D, et al. Early pulmonary involvement in ankylosing spondylitis: assessment with thin-section CT. *Clin Radiol* 2000;55:632–636.

89. Gibson GJ, Davis P. Respiratory complications of relapsing polychondritis. *Thorax* 1974;29:726–731.

90. Michet CJJ, McKenna CH, Luthra HS, et al. Relapsing polychondritis. *Ann Intern Med* 1986;104:74–78.

91. Burlew BP, Lippton H, Klinestiver D, et al. Relapsing polychondritis: new pulmonary manifestations. *J La State Med Soc* 1992;144:58–62.

92. Faul JL, Kee ST, Rizk NW. Endobronchial stenting for severe airway obstruction in relapsing polychondritis. *Chest* 1999;116:825–827.

93. Krell WS, Staats BA, Hyatt RE. Pulmonary function in relapsing polychondritis. *Am Rev Respir Dis* 1986;133:1120–1123.

The Eosinophilic Lung Diseases

27

James N. Allen

The eosinophilic lung diseases are a diverse group of disorders that are accompanied by eosinophilic infiltration of the airways, alveoli, or interstitium of the lung. Some of these disorders exclusively affect the lung, whereas others are systemic.

Eosinophilic lung diseases were first described as "PIE" (pulmonary infiltrates with [blood] eosinophilia) syndromes. More recently, it has been recognized that in several lung diseases, eosinophilic infiltration in the lungs may be substantial, with little or no increase in the number of eosinophils in the peripheral blood. These diseases may not be correctly diagnosed unless either bronchoalveolar lavage (BAL) or lung biopsy is performed. The most common eosinophilic lung diseases include simple pulmonary eosinophilia, chronic eosinophilic pneumonia, acute eosinophilic pneumonia, Churg-Strauss syndrome, idiopathic hypereosinophilic syndrome, allergic bronchopulmonary aspergillosis (ABPA), bronchocentric granulomatosis, certain parasitic infections, and certain drug reactions (1). Asthma is commonly associated with increased lung eosinophils but is covered in other chapters (see Chapters 8 through 10).

Lung biopsy is the most direct way to verify an increase in the number of lung eosinophils, but biopsy is only occasionally necessary to diagnose the various eosinophilic lung diseases. BAL is frequently used to identify eosinophilic lung disease, and an increased percentage of eosinophils in BAL fluid usually corresponds to an increase in lung tissue eosinophils. A finding of more than 2% eosinophils is abnormal, and a finding of more than 5% eosinophils is most common in drug reactions, parasitic infestation, interstitial lung disease, HIV-associated *Pneumocystis carinii* infection, and the idiopathic eosinophilic pneumonias (2).

Patients presenting with an undifferentiated eosinophilic lung disease can pose a diagnostic challenge, but based on the clinical presentation, radiographic tests, laboratory studies, BAL, and occasionally lung biopsy, one of the specific diseases discussed in this chapter can usually be diagnosed (Table 27.1).

BIOLOGY OF THE EOSINOPHIL

Although often considered white blood cells, many more eosinophils are found in tissues than in the blood. The production of eosinophils is largely regulated by T lymphocytes, particularly those lymphocytes with a T helper subset 2 (Th2) phenotype. The major T-lymphocyte product that controls eosinophils is interleukin-5 (IL-5), although IL-3 and granulocyte-macrophage colony-stimulating factor are also important. The production of each of these cytokines is in turn regulated by other cytokines.

The eosinophil is armed with chemical weaponry within its granules that facilitates host defense against pathogens such as parasites and fungi. Major basic protein, eosinophil cationic protein, eosinophil-derived neurotoxin, and eosinophil peroxidase are all very basic granule contents that can be released by the eosinophil in response to different cytokines and immunoglobulins. Indiscriminate release of these granule contents can result in direct injury to epithelial and endothelial cells and the development of the clinical abnormalities associated with the eosinophilic lung diseases (3).

SIMPLE PULMONARY EOSINOPHILIA

The idiopathic eosinophilic pneumonias can be divided into three distinct clinical entities: simple pulmonary

J. N. Allen: Department of Internal Medicine, Division of Pulmonary and Critical Care Medicine, Ohio State University, Columbus, Ohio.

TABLE 27.1. EOSINOPHILIC LUNG DISEASES

Primary eosinophilic lung diseases
Simple pulmonary eosinophilia
Chronic eosinophilic pneumonia
Acute eosinophilic pneumonia
Churg-Strauss vasculitis
Idiopathic hypereosinophilic syndrome
Allergic bronchopulmonary aspergillosis
Bronchocentric granulomatosis

Secondary eosinophilic lung diseases
Drug-induced pulmonary eosinophilia
Parasite-induced pulmonary eosinophilia
Fungus-induced pulmonary eosinophilia

Diseases occasionally associated with eosinophils
Idiopathic pulmonary fibrosis
Sarcoidosis
Hypersensitivity pneumonitis
Malignancy
Langerhans cell granulomatosis
Bronchiolitis obliterans–organizing pneumonia

eosinophilia, chronic eosinophilic pneumonia, and acute eosinophilic pneumonia (Table 27.2).

Also known as *Löffler syndrome*, simple pulmonary eosinophilia is characterized by patchy, often migratory pulmonary opacities on chest radiographs and an increased blood eosinophil count. Patients with this disorder have few or no respiratory symptoms and are often identified by incidental findings on chest x-ray films or blood counts. Simple pulmonary eosinophilia is frequently caused by parasitic infection or a drug reaction but is sometimes idiopathic. The self-limited opacities and lack of significant symptoms distinguish simple pulmonary eosinophilia from chronic eosinophilic pneumonia and acute eosinophilic pneumonia. Although steroids can hasten the resolution of the pulmonary infiltrates and blood eosinophilia, their use is rarely necessary.

In the original series of Löffler in 1932 (4), most of the patients with simple pulmonary eosinophilia likely had *Ascaris* infection. Currently, in most patients in whom simple pulmonary eosinophilia is initially diagnosed, a parasitic infection or a drug reaction is ultimately identified. However, no cause can be found in up to one third of patients (5). The finding of simple pulmonary eosinophilia should trigger a careful search for occult parasitic infection and for candidate drugs known to cause pulmonary eosinophilia.

The chest x-ray film demonstrates unilateral or bilateral transient, migratory, nonsegmental densities of various sizes that are usually of a combined interstitial and alveolar pattern. They are often peripheral in nature and may appear to be based in the pleura (6).

CHRONIC EOSINOPHILIC PNEUMONIA

Clinical Presentation

Christoforidis and Molnar (7) identified the first patients with chronic eosinophilic pneumonia in 1960, and Carrington and colleagues (8) described the first defining series of patients in 1969. Larger longitudinal series of patients included 19 patients described by Jederlinic and colleagues in 1988 (9) and 62 patients described by Marchand and colleagues in 1998 (10).

Although chronic eosinophilic pneumonia is reported in persons of all ages, the peak incidence is in the fifth decade, and women outnumber men in a ratio of 2:1 (9). Approximately half of the patients have preexisting asthma or atopic disease. Whereas patients with acute eosinophilic pneumonia tend to have a history of smoking, only a very small percentage of patients with chronic eosinophilic pneumonia have a history of cigarette smoking, which raises the question of whether smoking may be protective (9,10).

TABLE 27.2. DISTINGUISHING THE EOSINOPHILIC PNEUMONIAS

	Simple Pulmonary Eosinophilia	Chronic Eosinophilic Pneumonia	Acute Eosinophilic Pneumonia
Etiology	Idiopathic, drugs, parasites	Idiopathic	Idiopathic, tobacco smoke, drugs
Duration of symptoms	1–2 weeks	Several weeks to months	1–5 days
Respiratory failure	Never	Very rare	Frequent
Blood eosinophils	Increased	Increased	Normal
BAL findings	Eosinophils	Eosinophils	Eosinophils, lymphocytes, and neutrophils
Chest radiographic findings	Transient opacities	Peripheral opacities	Diffuse opacities, Kerley B lines
Pleural effusions	Rare	Rare	Frequent
Treatment	Unnecessary	Several years	2–12 weeks
Clinical relapse	Rare	Frequent	Rare

BAL, bronchoalveolar lavage.

The most common symptoms include cough (93%), dyspnea (92%), fever (77%), and weight loss (75%) (10). Rare symptoms include hemoptysis, chest pain, arthralgias, and myalgias. The physical examination findings are most commonly normal, but wheezes, crackles, or both can occasionally be heard during pulmonary auscultation.

Laboratory Tests

The percentage of blood eosinophils and the absolute eosinophil count are elevated in more than 90% of patients. The erythrocyte sedimentation rate is elevated in the majority of patients. The immunoglobulin E (IgE) level is elevated in 50% to 75% of patients, but the value is generally less than 2,000 kIU/L; higher values should raise the possibility of ABPA.

Pulmonary Function Tests

Pulmonary function studies can show a wide variety of findings. The results of spirometry and the lung volumes are normal in one third of patients, show obstruction in one third of patients, and show restriction in one third of patients (9,10). Additionally, the diffusing capacity is low in one half of patients (10). Hypoxemia or an increased alveolar-arterial gradient is present in most patients (9).

Radiographic Features

The conventional chest radiographs of patients with chronic eosinophilic pneumonia typically show peripheral opacities; this appearance has been described as the "photographic negative" of pulmonary edema (7,11). The findings of computed tomography (CT) mirror those of conventional chest radiography: areas of peripheral consolidation, ground-glass opacities, and reticular opacities (12). Honeycombing and traction bronchiectasis are not typical features. The CT appearance of chronic eosinophilic pneumonia may also mimic that of bronchiolitis obliterans–organizing pneumonia (13). On occasion, the opacities may be patchy or even unilateral. Pleural effusions are uncommon but have been reported as a primary radiographic finding (14).

Bronchoalveolar Lavage

The BAL findings in chronic eosinophilic pneumonia are characteristic; an isolated increased percentage of eosinophils is noted in all patients, with an average of 58% (10). In contrast, the percentages of lymphocytes and neutrophils are usually normal or only minimally elevated (10). Macrophages may contain ingested eosinophil granules. Eosinophils in the BAL fluid can be mistaken for neutrophils because alveolar eosinophils frequently have more than the usual two nuclear lobes seen in blood eosinophils, and alveolar eosinophils are frequently degranulated.

Pathology

Although lung biopsy is usually not necessary for the diagnosis of chronic eosinophilic pneumonia, it is sometimes performed when the diagnosis is unclear based on clinical grounds. The main findings are infiltration of the interalveolar septa and alveolar spaces by eosinophils and sometimes intra-alveolar eosinophil microabscess formation (8,15). Alveolar macrophages and neutrophils may contain eosinophil granules and Charcot-Leyden crystals (16). Well-formed granulomas are uncommon, although they have been reported in isolated cases (17); their presence should suggest the possibility of Churg-Strauss syndrome.

Focal areas of bronchiolitis obliterans are seen in some patients, especially those with long-standing eosinophilic pneumonia (18,19). Small- and medium-caliber arteries frequently exhibit infiltration by eosinophils, typically in a segmental fashion. However, true vasculitis is not present. A neutrophilic capillaritis is not a feature of chronic or acute eosinophilic pneumonia; if present, allergic granulomatosis of Churg-Strauss is a more likely diagnosis (20,21).

Fibrosis, although uncommon, is seen on occasion, especially in patients with long-standing disease (22). Because patients sometimes have concurrent asthma, smooth muscle hyperplasia and mucus with Charcot-Leyden crystals and eosinophils may be seen (23).

Following steroid therapy, lung eosinophils rapidly disappear, and the main pathologic findings may be mild septal fibrosis and bronchiolitis obliterans. In this situation, the only clue to the actual diagnosis may be remnant eosinophil granules that have been phagocytosed by macrophages.

Treatment

Although spontaneous resolution has been reported in rare patients (10,24), corticosteroids remain the mainstay of treatment. The clinical response to steroids is usually dramatic, and except for acute eosinophilic pneumonia, no other eosinophilic lung disease responds so completely and so quickly. Most patients have subjective improvement within 48 hours and radiographic resolution within 1 week (8,10). The response to corticosteroids is so characteristic that rapid improvement to a "therapeutic trial" of steroids in the proper clinical and radiographic context can be diagnostic and so obviate the need for biopsy. Effective initial doses of steroids are generally in the range of 40 to 60 mg of prednisone per day, and the steroids can usually be tapered rapidly to a maintenance dose within the first few weeks. Individual variation in the necessary maintenance dose of prednisone is considerable, but in most patients, the disease can be controlled with 5 to 20 mg every day or every other day, with an average dose of 10 mg/d. Recurrent symptoms, abnormalities on chest x-ray films, or peripheral blood eosinophilia can identify relapses.

Although chronic eosinophilic pneumonia responds exceedingly well to corticosteroids, most patients require long-term treatment. Most patients treated for less than 6 months relapse, and the majority of patients require treatment for more than a year, with an average duration of treatment of 82 weeks (10).

Up to half of patients continue to have asthma or show obstructive changes on pulmonary function testing after the chronic eosinophilic pneumonia has resolved (10,24), and residual peribronchial fibrosis has been described (25). In these cases, it is important to distinguish the respiratory symptoms of asthma from those of chronic eosinophilic pneumonia because the latter can be effectively treated with inhaled corticosteroids and bronchodilators, so that systemic corticosteroids are not necessary.

Because chronic eosinophilic pneumonia tends to occur most commonly in middle-aged and older women, osteoporosis is a particular problem with long-term steroid use, and regular bone density evaluation in addition to pharmacologic measures for the primary prevention of osteoporosis is advisable.

CHRONIC EOSINOPHILIC PNEUMONIA	
Summary Statement	**Level of Evidence**
Adequate initial therapy for virtually all patients consists of oral prednisone at a dosage of 40 to 60 mg/d.	Observational studies
Because relapses are common, treatment is maintained for at least 3 months, and usually for 6 to 9 months.	Observational studies
Inhaled corticosteroids (1,000–1,500 μg/24 h) appear to be effective in chronic eosinophilic pneumonia.	Case reports
Relapse is common and does not appear to indicate treatment failure, a worse prognosis, or greater morbidity. Patients with chronic eosinophilic pneumonia continue to be steroid-responsive and respond to prednisone doses at levels similar to those used before the relapse.	Observational studies

ACUTE EOSINOPHILIC PNEUMONIA

Clinical Presentation

Idiopathic acute eosinophilic pneumonia was first recognized as a unique clinical entity in 1989 (26,27). Large case series reported to date include 13 patients reported by Hayakawa and colleagues in 1994 (28) and 15 patients described by Pope-Harman and colleagues in 1996 (29).

All age groups can be affected; the average age of patients is 29 years. Men and women are affected equally, and 40% of patients have a history of smoking cigarettes. Interest-

ingly, there appears to be an association between a recent start of smoking cigarettes and the development of acute eosinophilic pneumonia (30), and it has been speculated that constituents of tobacco smoke may trigger acute eosinophilic pneumonia in susceptible persons. A geographic pattern has not been noted, with cases reported throughout the United States, Europe, and Japan (29). Acute eosinophilic pneumonia has been reported to occur in HIV infection (31), and an acute eosinophilic pneumonia-like syndrome has been reported in association with drug reactions.

The onset is quite rapid; patients usually present within 1 to 5 days after the onset of symptoms (average, 2.3 days) (29). Mild dyspnea can progress to life-threatening respiratory failure in only a few hours (26). Virtually all patients have cough (usually nonproductive), tachypnea, and dyspnea. Fever is invariably present, and the average temperature is 101°F. Chest pain is present in 73% of patients and is usually pleuritic. About half of patients also have myalgias. Crackles are present in 80% of patients, with 13% having both wheezing and crackles. The lungs are clear to auscultation in 20% of patients (29).

An important consideration in the differential diagnosis is *Aspergillus* infection, which can mimic acute eosinophilic pneumonia but requires antifungal antibiotics rather than corticosteroids (32). Patients with exposure to composted organic material and those suspected of having chronic granulomatous disease are at risk.

Laboratory Tests

Hypoxemia is present in all patients, and the average Po_2 value is 57 mm Hg at the time of clinical presentation. Most patients have a respiratory alkalosis secondary to tachypnea. Unlike patients with chronic eosinophilic pneumonia, those with acute eosinophilic pneumonia do not have a striking peripheral blood eosinophilia; the average blood eosinophil count is only 344/mm^3 (29). Hypersegmentation of the blood eosinophil nuclei has been reported and may provide a clue to the diagnosis in the proper clinical context (33). The IgE level can be as high as 2,310 kIU/L (34). When tested, the pleural fluid is exudative, with an increased percentage of eosinophils (29).

Pulmonary Function Studies

Pulmonary function tests are performed before the initiation of treatment in only a few patients, but small-airway obstruction, restriction, and a low diffusing capacity have been reported (34). After treatment, results of pulmonary function studies are normal (35).

Radiographic Features

The radiographic appearance of acute eosinophilic pneumonia differs substantially from that of chronic eosinophilic pneumonia. In patients with acute eosinophilic pneumonia, conventional chest radiographs demonstrate a pattern consistent with pulmonary edema, with extensive air space opacity, interlobular septal thickening (i.e., Kerley B lines), and pleural effusions (35) (Fig. 27.1). The opacities are diffuse and not peripherally based, in contrast to those seen on the radiographs of patients with chronic eosinophilic pneumonia. The pleural effusion tends to accumulate as the parenchymal abnormalities resolve. In one study, the CT findings of patients with acute eosinophilic pneumonia differed substantially from those of patients with chronic eosinophilic pneumonia, such that the two diseases were easily distinguished (12).

Bronchoalveolar Lavage

In the proper clinical setting, the finding of a significantly increased percentage of eosinophils in the BAL fluid can provide a tentative diagnosis of acute eosinophilic pneumonia on which treatment can be based. Because these patients

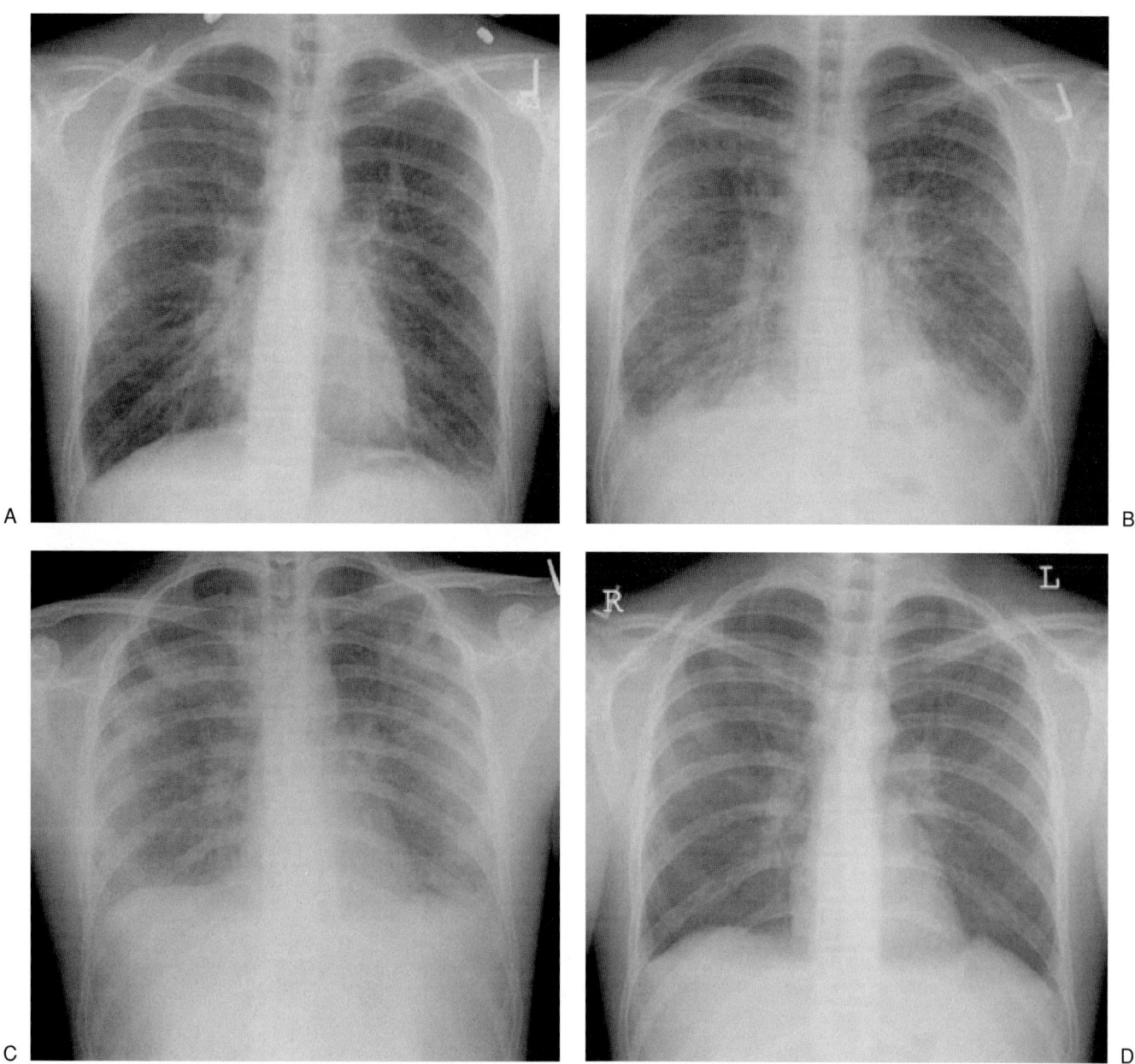

FIGURE 27.1. Chest x-ray films of a patient with acute eosinophilic pneumonia. **A:** Initial presentation showing Kerley B lines and diffuse interstitial opacities. **B:** Film obtained 1 day after admission showing mixed interstitial and alveolar opacities with pleural effusions. **C:** Film obtained 2 days after admission showing diffuse alveolar opacities. **D:** Film obtained during recovery showing resolution of opacities with small residual pleural effusions.

otherwise clinically resemble those with pneumonia or acute respiratory distress syndrome (ARDS), the early performance of BAL in patients with unexplained diffuse pulmonary opacities and respiratory failure is necessary for a prompt diagnosis. In patients with diffuse pneumonia or ARDS, the percentage of neutrophils in the BAL fluid is typically increased, whereas the percentage of eosinophils in these disorders is low.

In acute eosinophilic pneumonia, the increase in eosinophils in the BAL fluid is in striking contrast to the minimal, if any, increase in blood eosinophils. In most patients, eosinophils account for more than 20% of the cells in the BAL fluid, with an average of 37% (29). Like the alveolar eosinophils in chronic eosinophilic pneumonia, the eosinophils in acute eosinophilic pneumonia may be degranulated and have multiple nuclear lobes, so that the distinction between neutrophils and eosinophils can be difficult.

In chronic eosinophilic pneumonia, an isolated increase in BAL fluid eosinophils is noted, with relatively normal percentages of lymphocytes and neutrophils. However, in acute eosinophilic pneumonia, the BAL fluid contains a mixed cellular infiltrate, with a predominance of eosinophils but an average of 20% lymphocytes and 15% neutrophils (29).

Pathology

Lung biopsy is unnecessary for the diagnosis of acute eosinophilic pneumonia in most cases, and consequently relatively few reports have been published. The main purpose of lung biopsy is to exclude other diseases that can mimic acute eosinophilic pneumonia, such as fungal pneumonia (36). Lung biopsy should be performed if the history sug-

gests a risk factor for fungal infection or if the patient fails to improve promptly after the initiation of corticosteroids.

When biopsy is performed, the main findings are a pronounced infiltration of eosinophils in the interstitium and alveolar spaces and features of diffuse alveolar damage (29,37) (Fig. 27.2). Granuloma formation and vasculitis are not characteristic, and if present, they should suggest an alternative diagnosis.

Treatment

The response of patients with acute eosinophilic pneumonia to corticosteroids is rapid and striking. Most patients show significant clinical improvement within 24 to 48 hours, and some within a few hours after the first dose of steroids. Although the optimal dose of corticosteroids is uncertain, commonly used dosages of intravenous methylprednisolone in case series range from 60 to 125 mg every 6 hours until respiratory failure resolves. Thereafter, the patient can be switched to oral prednisone, and the steroids can be tapered over 2 to 12 weeks. The optimal dose and duration of corticosteroids have not been determined (29).

In sharp contrast to patients with chronic eosinophilic pneumonia, those with acute eosinophilic pneumonia do not relapse after completing a short course of corticosteroids. Follow-up chest radiography and BAL performed after the discontinuation of steroid therapy show no abnormalities (29). Recurrence of acute eosinophilic pneumonia later in life is exceedingly rare.

In most patients with acute eosinophilic pneumonia, the cause is unknown, but occasionally an acute eosinophilic pneumonia-like illness can develop as a hypersensitivity

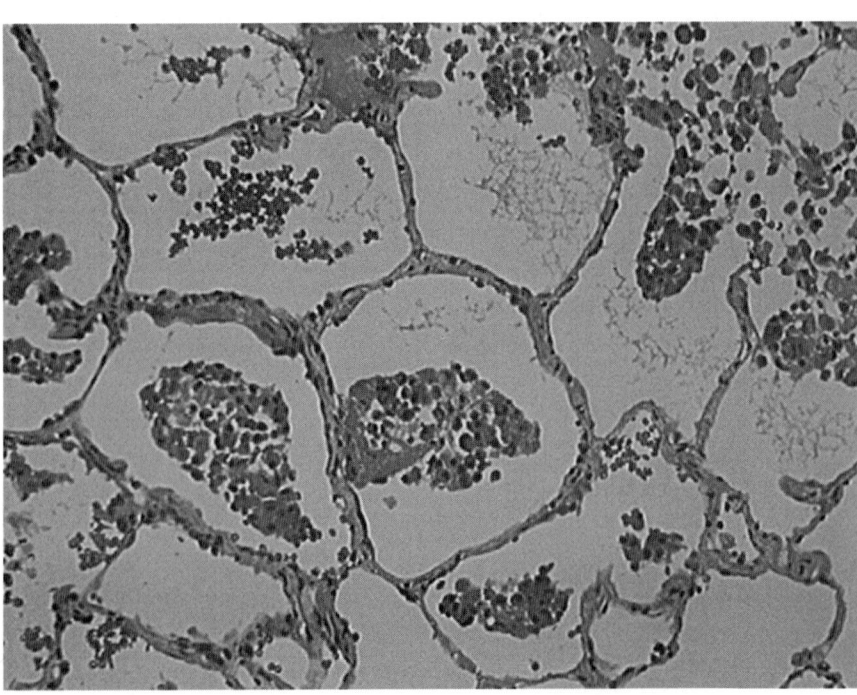

FIGURE 27.2. Lung biopsy specimen from a patient with acute eosinophilic pneumonia. The alveoli are filled with a mixed inflammatory infiltrate composed primarily of eosinophils.

reaction to drugs or tobacco smoke. It is prudent to recommend future avoidance of these substances to such patients because relapse can recur if they resume smoking.

CHURG-STRAUSS VASCULITIS

Clinical Presentation

In the classic scenario, patients usually have a history of allergic disease for 8 to 10 years before presentation; all patients have asthma or a history of asthma, and most have allergic rhinitis (38,39). Dramatic peripheral blood eosinophilia (occasionally as high as 10,000/μL) and infiltration of a variety of tissues with eosinophils follow the appearance of these symptoms. Months to years later, systemic vasculitis develops (40). The mean age at the onset of vasculitis is between 38 and 48 years; men and women are affected equally (41). Interestingly, the symptoms of asthma may diminish as those of vasculitis become more prominent (39). This triad of asthma, eosinophilia, and granulomatous vasculitis is most characteristic of advanced disease, and patients often present before the development of vasculitis with less specific clinical and pathologic findings (42). The lungs and skin are most commonly involved, but any organ system can be affected, including the cardiovascular, gastrointestinal, and central nervous systems (43–45). Churg-Strauss syndrome has been associated with use of leukotriene antagonists in patients with preexisting asthma (46) (see Chapter 30).

Laboratory Tests

The IgE level is elevated, often very much so, and appears to correlate with disease activity (40,45). Low titers of rheumatoid factors can be found in some patients, but complement levels are usually normal (40). The antinuclear antibody (ANA) titer is elevated in 10% of patients (41). Antineutrophil cytoplasmic antibody (ANCA) is present in approximately 50% of patients, usually in the perinuclear (p-ANCA) form (47). Enzyme-linked immunosorbent assay (ELISA) demonstrates that these are antimyeloperoxidase antibodies (41). Most patients have anemia and an increased erythrocyte sedimentation rate (39). The pleural fluid is exudative and may contain high numbers of eosinophils.

The BAL fluid typically shows a very high percentage of eosinophils, with an average of 33% in one study (48).

Pulmonary Function Tests

Pulmonary function tests show obstructive defects (40).

Radiographic Features

Chest x-ray films and CT scans show pulmonary opacities in the majority of patients (Fig. 27.3). These are most often patchy and transient; however, diffuse large and small noncavitary nodules and diffuse interstitial opacities have been reported. Pleural effusions occur in a third of patients, and hilar lymph node enlargement has occasionally been noted. In some patients, angiograms may show hepatic or renal aneurysms resembling those seen in polyarteritis nodosa (40).

Pathology

Because of the systemic nature of Churg-Strauss syndrome, biopsy of a variety of organs may be diagnostic. In all organs, Churg-Strauss syndrome can exist in three pathologic phases. The earliest, prevasculitic phase is characterized by eosinophilic tissue infiltration without vasculitis.

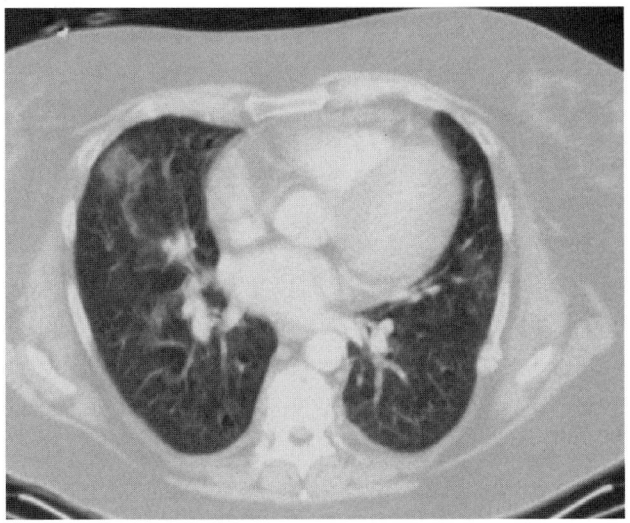
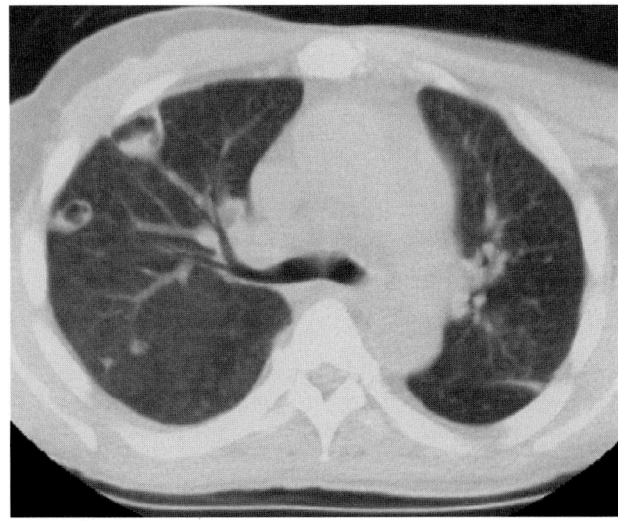

A   B

FIGURE 27.3. Chest computed tomogram of a patient with Churg-Strauss syndrome. **A:** Peripheral pulmonary opacities. **B:** Cavitary nodules.

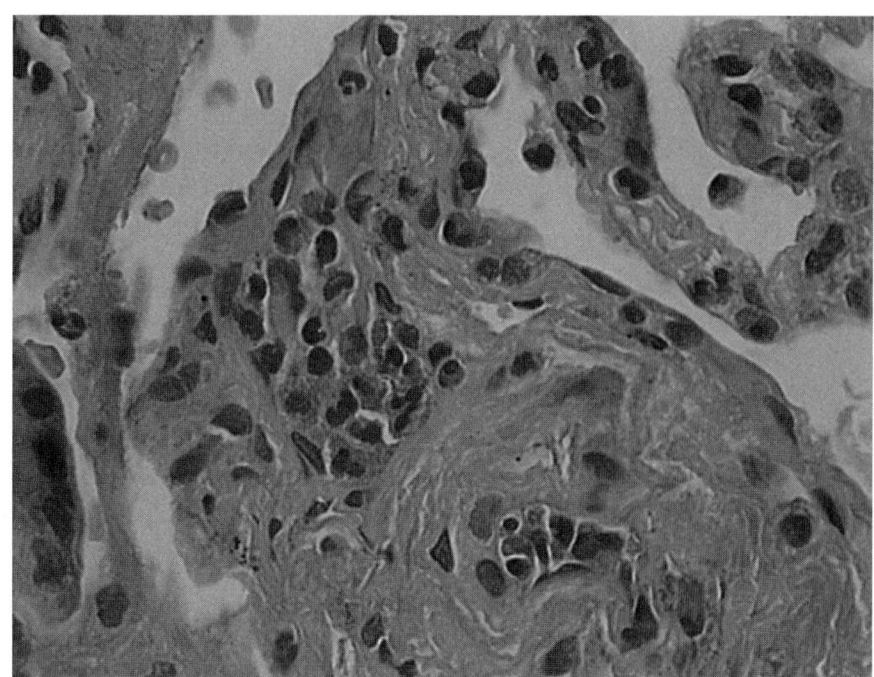

FIGURE 27.4. (See also Color Fig. 27.4.) Lung biopsy specimen from a patient with Churg-Strauss syndrome contains perivascular granulomatous infiltrates with eosinophils.

The vasculitic phase comes later and demonstrates either necrotizing or nonnecrotizing eosinophilic vasculitis, especially of the small arteries and veins (Fig. 27.4; see also Color Fig. 27.4). A late, postvasculitic phase can be seen in patients treated with corticosteroids and is characterized by thrombosed small blood vessels with healed vasculitis (21). Because Churg-Strauss syndrome responds quickly to steroids, histologic specimens may not show eosinophil infiltration if patients have been treated, even for brief periods of time (42). Because lung tissue in the prevasculitic phase can closely resemble that of chronic eosinophilic pneumonia, it can be difficult to distinguish these two diseases on the basis of histology alone, and the diagnosis should always incorporate both clinical and pathologic findings. In this setting, the presence of an antimyeloperoxidase antibody favors Churg-Strauss syndrome. Interstitial and perivascular granulomas are common, and eosinophils accumulate in the blood vessels, interstitial tissue, and alveolar structures (39). Transbronchial biopsy is usually insufficient for the diagnosis because the vascular tissue obtained by this procedure is minimal.

Treatment

Corticosteroids dramatically alter the natural history of Churg-Strauss syndrome (39) (see Chapter 30). In patients who fail to respond to prednisone alone, the addition of cyclophosphamide is often effective (41,49,50). The use of cyclophosphamide as a component of the initial treatment of patients with Churg-Strauss syndrome can reduce the incidence of relapse (51). Patients with myocardial, renal, or gastrointestinal involvement have a worse prognosis (41).

CHURG-STRAUSS SYNDROME

Summary Statement	Level of Evidence
Approximately 50% of untreated patients die within 3 months after the onset of vasculitis. In contrast, a mean survival of 9 years has been reported in patients treated with steroids.	Observational studies
Treatment of concurrent asthma with inhaled steroids may allow a reduction in the dose of oral steroids necessary to control the vasculitis.	Observational studies, expert opinion
Prednisone as a sole agent is usually effective in the prevasculitic phase, whereas prednisone plus cyclophosphamide is frequently necessary in patients with vasculitis.	Observational studies, expert opinion
Plasmapheresis has been shown to be ineffective (52).	Randomized controlled trials
Interferon-α may be effective (53).	Case reports

IDIOPATHIC HYPEREOSINOPHILIC SYNDROME

Clinical Presentation

The idiopathic hypereosinophilic syndrome is characterized by blood eosinophilia ($>1,500/\mu L$) for more than 6 months, an absence of a parasitic or other cause of secondary eosinophilia, and signs or symptoms of end-organ damage related to the increased number of eosinophils (54). The idiopathic hypereosinophilic syndrome may represent several subtypes of disease. The cause is unknown; however, the profound eosinophilia may be lymphocyte-dependent. The finding of an abnormal clonal proliferation of T helper lymphocytes in as many as 25% of patients with the idiopathic hypereosinophilic syndrome indicates that in some patients, the syndrome may be caused by a low-grade T-lymphocyte lymphoma (55–58). Other studies have demonstrated a clonal proliferation of eosinophils in some patients with the idiopathic hypereosinophilic syndrome (59).

The age at onset is usually in the third or fourth decade, although patients as old as 70 years have been reported. A 7:1 male predominance has been noted (60). Common presenting symptoms include night sweats, anorexia, weight loss, pruritus, cough, and fever.

Cardiac involvement, including endocardial fibrosis, restrictive cardiomyopathy, valvular damage, and mural thrombus formation, is perhaps the most important complication of the idiopathic hypereosinophilic syndrome and remains the major cause of morbidity and mortality (61). Pulmonary involvement occurs in up to 40% of patients and typically presents as cough that is often worse at night. Long-standing idiopathic hypereosinophilic syndrome can result in pulmonary fibrosis (54).

Thromboembolic disease, more frequently arterial than venous, occurs in two thirds of patients. Splinter hemorrhages are the most common manifestation; however, renal or splenic infarcts, retinal arteriolar embolism, deep venous thrombosis, femoral artery embolism, cerebrovascular accident, or diffuse small vessel cerebrovascular occlusions can occur and may be refractory to warfarin (60). Peripheral neuropathy occurs frequently in patients with advanced disease (54). Other areas frequently infiltrated with eosinophils and giving rise to symptoms include the gastrointestinal tract, kidneys, joints, skin, and muscles (62).

Laboratory Tests

The most striking finding is profound peripheral eosinophilia, usually 30% to 70% with a total white blood cell count above $10,000/\mu L$ (63). Eosinophils are found in large quantities in the bone marrow, and eosinophilic metamyelocytes and myelocytes may be present in the peripheral blood.

The percentage of eosinophils in the BAL fluid can be very high, up to 73% (64,65).

Radiographic Features

The chest x-ray film typically shows interstitial nonlobar opacities, and approximately 50% of affected patients have pleural effusions (63). Chest CT shows small pulmonary nodules and focal areas of ground-glass opacities, predominantly in the lung periphery (66).

Treatment

In about half of patients, the clinical response to oral corticosteroids alone is good. These patients, in contrast to nonresponders, typically have high levels of IgE, angioedema, and a dramatic reduction in the number of blood eosinophils following the first dose of corticosteroids (67). The treatment regimen suggested by Parrillo and colleagues (67) consists of 60 mg of prednisone per day for 1 week, then 60 mg every other day for 3 months; these authors recommend treatment only for patients with demonstrable end-organ damage from hypereosinophilia. Other drugs have been used successfully, including busulfan, hydroxyurea, cyclophosphamide, azathioprine, interferon-α, cyclosporine, etoposide, vincristine, and 2-chlorodeoxyadenosine (60,63,68–72). Bone marrow transplantation has been used with anecdotal success (73,74).

ALLERGIC BRONCHOPULMONARY ASPERGILLOSIS

Clinical Presentation

ABPA is caused by local airway allergy to *Aspergillus* antigens in patients with either asthma or cystic fibrosis (CF). In ABPA, unlike the other eosinophilic lung diseases, the eosinophilic infiltration is largely confined to the airway. Consequently, the main symptoms are those of asthma, especially difficult-to-treat or steroid-dependent asthma.

ABPA was first recognized in 1952 by Hinson and colleagues (75). Persons of both sexes and all age groups can be affected. The diagnostic criteria for ABPA generally used in the United States are based on those proposed by Rosenberg and colleagues (76) (Table 27.3). Ultimately, this is a clinical diagnosis because no one specific laboratory test finding is unique for ABPA. A determination of the prevalence of ABPA has been hampered by the use of different diagnostic criteria in different studies, so that the reported prevalence rates vary among countries. Although generally associated with *Aspergillus fumigatus*, allergic bronchopulmonary fungal disease has also been reported in association with other fungi (77).

TABLE 27.3. DIAGNOSTIC CRITERIA FOR ALLERGIC BRONCHOPULMONARY ASPERGILLOSIS

Asthma or cystic fibrosis
Peripheral blood eosinophilia
Immediate positive skin prick test result for *Aspergillus* antigens
Serum precipitating antibodies against *Aspergillus* antigens
Increased serum IgE levels
Chest radiographic opacities
Bronchiectasis
Increased *Aspergillus*-specific IgE and IgG

Ig, immunoglobulin.

ABPA progresses through five clinical stages: acute disease, remission, exacerbation, corticosteroid-dependent asthma, and fibrosis (78). The acute stage is characterized by asthma, an IgE level above 2,500 ng/mL, an immediate skin reaction to *Aspergillus* antigen, opacities on chest x-ray films, and proximal bronchiectasis. The administration of corticosteroids at this stage results in resolution of the chest x-ray abnormalities, a decline in the IgE level, and control of the asthma symptoms. The remission stage is characterized by an absence of asthma symptoms with normal chest x-ray findings and IgE levels, and steroids are not required. In the exacerbation stage, disease activity may be marked by symptoms similar to those of the acute stage, an asymptomatic rise in the IgE level, or the appearance of new opacities on chest x-ray films. Patients in the stage of corticosteroid-dependent asthma often have persistently elevated IgE levels and require continuous corticosteroids to control their asthma symptoms. Treatment at this stage should be based on control of symptoms rather than on control of the IgE level (79), and patients should be maintained on the lowest dose of prednisone necessary to control symptoms. In patients with longstanding ABPA, an irreversible fibrotic stage may develop. Because these patients often require long-term moderate-dose corticosteroids, vigilance for opportunistic infection must be maintained. Retrospective studies suggest that the use of long-term corticosteroids in patients with the earlier stages of ABPA may prevent the development of the fibrotic stage (80).

CF is associated with ABPA. In a study of 12,447 European patients with CF, 10% of patients older than 6 years were reported to have ABPA (81). However, of 14,210 patients with CF in the United States, only 2% were reported to have ABPA (82). Reasons for the different incidence rates between Europe and the United States are unclear, but they may be a consequence of underrecognition and the use of different diagnostic criteria in the United States. ABPA was reported to recur in two patients with CF following lung transplantation (83).

CF develops when two genes for the CF transmembrane conductance regulator are abnormal, and persons with two abnormal genes have abnormal levels of sweat chloride. An unusually high incidence of individuals who are heterozygous carriers of this gene and have normal sweat chloride levels has been noted among patients with ABPA (28% vs. 5% in asthmatic controls), which suggests a possible genetic basis for this disease (84). ABPA is additionally associated with HLA-DR2 alleles (85).

Laboratory Tests

The IgE level is probably the most useful laboratory test in ABPA; it correlates well with disease activity, and a normal IgE level in a symptomatic patient virtually excludes the diagnosis (86,87). Total IgE levels above 1,000 ng/mL are usual. In patients with lower total IgE levels who are otherwise suspected of having ABPA, an elevated *A. fumigatus*–specific IgE or IgG antibody is highly suggestive (88).

Other frequent findings include *Aspergillus* organisms in the sputum and a history of expectoration of brown plugs in the sputum.

Pulmonary Function Tests

Most patients have obstruction on spirometry, consistent with the attendant asthma. In contrast to patients with asthma, patients with ABPA frequently also have a low total lung capacity, a low diffusing capacity, or both, similar to other patients with bronchiectasis.

Radiographic Features

Chest radiographs classically demonstrate central bronchiectasis involving the upper lobes; characteristic features are "gloved finger" signs (medium-sized bronchi filled with secretions), ring shadows with or without air-fluid levels within, "tram lines" (parallel linear shadows caused by inflamed and edematous medium-sized bronchi), "toothpaste" shadows (mucoid impaction within bronchi), and consolidation secondary to airway obstruction (89) (Fig. 27.5). Bronchiectasis can occur in patients with asthma; however, bronchiectasis in three or more lobes, centrilobular nodules, and mucoid impaction are much more likely to be seen in ABPA (90,91).

Central bronchiectasis is present in 85% of patients at the time of initial diagnosis (86). Patients lacking central bronchiectasis should not be excluded, however, because it may not yet have developed early in the illness.

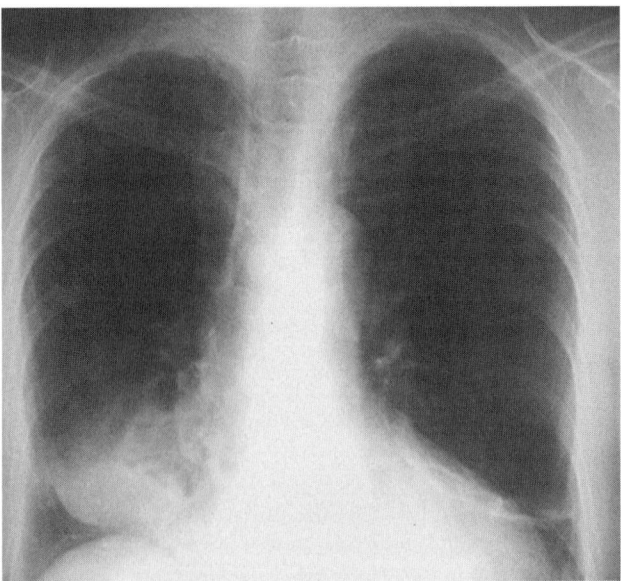

FIGURE 27.5. Chest x-ray film from a patient with allergic bronchopulmonary aspergillosis.

Pathology

Lung biopsy is generally unnecessary to establish a diagnosis, but a biopsy is occasionally performed when lung cancer or interstitial lung disease is being considered in the differential diagnosis. Pathologically, a bronchocentric inflammatory infiltrate composed of eosinophils, lymphocytes, plasma cells, and monocytes is found. *Aspergillus* hyphae can be identified in the lung parenchyma. The blood vessels are largely intact, without destruction of the vessel walls. T lymphocytes may be increased, and a ratio of T helper to T suppressor cells of 2:1 has been reported (92). Other findings that may be seen include bronchocentric granulomatosis, areas of eosinophilic pneumonia, interstitial fibrosis, lymphocytic interstitial pneumonitis, and eosinophilic microabscess formation (93).

Treatment

Corticosteroids are the mainstay of treatment for ABPA, and most patients require prolonged courses of daily steroids. A typical treatment protocol is 0.5 mg of prednisone per kilogram per day for 2 weeks, followed by gradual tapering over a period of several months (86). Additional courses are given as needed to control asthma symptoms; relapses can usually be prevented with doses of prednisone averaging 7.5 mg/day (110). Inhaled steroids were useful to minimize doses of oral steroids in two small, uncontrolled case series (94,95).

Antifungal antibiotics are also useful to minimize the doses of oral corticosteroids. In a nonblinded crossover trial, 200 mg of itraconazole per day for 12 months was found to reduce or eliminate the need for oral steroids and was associated with a reduction in blood eosinophil counts, a reduction in serum IgE levels, and an increase in the forced expiratory volume in 1 second (FEV_1) (96). In a randomized, double-blinded, placebo-controlled trial, 200 mg of itraconazole twice a day for 16 weeks was found to improve overall clinical function (97).

BRONCHOCENTRIC GRANULOMATOSIS

Clinical Presentation

Patients most commonly present with dyspnea or wheezing secondary to airway obstruction (98) (see Chapter 30).

Radiographic Features

The findings are highly variable, with little correlation between the chest x-ray findings and the clinical presentation (99). Nodular or mass lesions, usually solitary, are noted in 60% of patients, and opacities in 20%. Upper lobe and unilateral lung involvement are common. CT scan findings consist of a focal mass or lobar consolidation with atelectasis (100).

Pathology

Lung biopsy specimens demonstrate granulomatous and necrotizing replacement of bronchial epithelium. The surrounding lung parenchyma may exhibit chronic inflammatory changes, tissue eosinophilia with Charcot-Leyden crystals, or aggregated eosinophil granules, but it does not contain granulomas. Granulomatous inflammation of the bronchi can occur in several conditions, including mycobacterial and fungal infection, aspiration, Wegener granulomatosis, and rheumatoid lung disease; therefore, bronchocentric granulomatosis is a diagnosis of exclusion. Tissue samples should be thoroughly examined for infectious pathogens. A helpful point in the differential diagnosis is the fact that the entities mentioned often show extrabronchial granulomatous inflammation, whereas bronchocentric granulomatosis does not.

Patients can be divided into groups. About one third have tissue eosinophilia and tend to have asthma, peripheral eosinophilia, fungal hyphae on biopsy, and sputum cultures positive for *Aspergillus* organisms. This group may have a form of bronchocentric granulomatosis related to ABPA. The remaining two thirds have neutrophils rather than eosinophils in the lung lesions. These patients do not have asthma or microscopic evidence of fungi (101,102).

Treatment

Steroids are effective treatment in many patients; however, they must be used with caution because of the similarity of bronchocentric granulomatosis to invasive mycobacterial and fungal infections. On rare occasions, bronchocentric granulomatosis can present as part of a systemic disease and may require treatment with both corticosteroids and cyclophosphamide (103).

PARASITIC INFECTIONS

Many parasites can cause pulmonary opacities with blood or alveolar eosinophilia (1). A travel history is important because of regional variations in the prevalence rates of infection with various parasites. In the United States, *Strongyloides*, *Ascaris*, *Toxocara*, and *Ancylostoma* are the most common causes of eosinophilic lung disease. Patients infected with one parasite are at risk for infection with multiple parasites. Therefore, the failure of pulmonary symptoms or eosinophilia to resolve despite treatment should prompt a search for additional parasites.

Strongyloides stercoralis infection can be either asymptomatic or accompanied by peripheral blood eosinophilia, rash, and transient pulmonary opacities. The pulmonary opacities may appear before the adult worms develop and consequently before ova can be found in the stool. *Strongyloides* can be missed on direct stool examinations, even when multiple specimens are taken. Serologic studies are more sensitive, but the results do not necessarily imply active infection. *Strongyloides* is capable of reproducing within the body indefinitely, so that patients can present with symptoms decades after the initial infection. Patients who are taking corticosteroids or who are otherwise immunosuppressed are particularly prone to symptoms of massive *Strongyloides* proliferation (the *Strongyloides* hyperinfestation syndrome). The treatment for uncomplicated strongyloidiasis is 25 mg of thiabendazole per kilogram twice a day for 2 days, but for hyperinfestation syndrome, treatment should be continued for at least 2 weeks.

Ascaris lumbricoides is a roundworm that infects 25% of the world's population and is the most frequent cause of peripheral blood eosinophilia with pulmonary opacities in many developing countries. The most frequent symptoms in *Ascaris* pneumonia are self-limited fever and nonproductive cough, often accompanied by chest pain (104). All patients have moderate to extreme blood eosinophilia, and skin rash is common. Chest x-ray films typically reveal bilateral discrete densities up to several centimeters in size, often involving the perihilar regions. Because the pulmonary syndrome occurs before the adult worms mature, the stool examination for ova is usually negative for up to 8 weeks after the onset of respiratory symptoms. The intestinal infection should be treated with 100 mg of oral mebendazole twice daily for 3 days.

Toxocara canis (the dog roundworm) is the cause of visceral larva migrans. Mature worms do not develop in humans; thus, the result of stool examination for ova is negative. Pulmonary involvement is found in 80% of patients with visceral larva migrans and is usually manifested as cough or wheezing. The diagnosis is made serologically. Although toxocariasis is usually self-limited, thiabendazole or mebendazole may relieve symptoms.

"Creeping eruption," caused by infection with the dog hookworm (*Ancylostoma braziliense*), can be associated with pulmonary opacities, peripheral blood eosinophilia, and a serpiginous red rash. In approximately 50% of patients with *Ancylostoma* infection, patchy, migratory opacities appear on chest x-ray films about 1 week after onset of the rash and persist for several weeks. Mature worms do not develop in humans; thus, the result of stool examination for ova is negative. Twenty-five milligrams of thiabendazole per kilogram twice daily for 2 days is effective treatment (105).

Tropical pulmonary eosinophilia is caused by the filarial worms *Wuchereria bancrofti* and *Brugia malayi* (106). Most cases have been reported from India, Africa, South America, and Southeast Asia. The filariae are transmitted to humans by mosquitoes. Patients commonly present with some combination of nocturnal cough, dyspnea, wheezing, fever, weight loss, and malaise. Laboratory findings include very high levels of serum IgE, blood eosinophilia, and BAL fluid eosinophilia. Microfilariae may be demonstrated in the lung, liver, and lymph nodes but not in the blood of affected patients. The diagnosis of tropical pulmonary eosinophilia is established by four main criteria: cough that is worse at night, residence in an area where filarial infection is endemic, an elevated eosinophil count (generally >3,300/mm^3), and improvement after the administration of diethylcarbamazine (6–12 mg/kg per day in three divided doses for 1–3 weeks) (107). The diagnosis is further supported by pulmonary opacities on chest radiographs and an elevated erythrocyte sedimentation rate. Although generally unnecessary for diagnosis, a serum antigen test is available.

Other parasites causing pulmonary eosinophilia include *Schistosoma, Clonorchis sinensis, Opisthorchis, Trichinella spiralis, Paragonimus westermani,* the carnivore tapeworm *Echinococcus granulosus,* and the dog heartworm *Dirofilaria immitis.*

FUNGAL INFECTIONS

Peripheral blood eosinophilia is noted in the majority of cases of primary coccidioidomycosis, and pulmonary eosinophilic infiltrates may be noted on lung biopsy specimens (108) and in BAL fluid (109). A history of travel to areas where coccidioidomycosis is endemic is an important part of the evaluation of any patient presenting with pulmonary opacities associated with either BAL fluid or blood eosinophilia because the eosinophilia can be present early in the infection, when appropriate cultures may be negative. Administration of corticosteroids to patients at this stage can result in acceleration of the infection with fatal dissemination.

An increase in the percentage of BAL fluid eosinophils is noted in 15% of patients with AIDS-associated *P. carinii* pneumonia. BAL fluid eosinophilia is usually not associated with peripheral blood eosinophilia and correlates with the degree of hypoxemia at the time of admission to the hospital (2,110).

Chronic granulomatous disease is an inherited condition caused by defective neutrophils and is associated with recurrent *Aspergillus* infections. During periods of infection, prominent pulmonary eosinophilia may develop, clinically mimicking acute eosinophilic pneumonia. In some adolescents and young adults, the course can be more indolent, and the initial presentation may be that of an eosinophilic lung disease. Chronic granulomatous disease with pulmonary aspergillosis should be suspected in patients in this age group who are presumed to have eosinophilic pneumonia, and lung biopsy should be considered (32,111).

DRUG REACTIONS

Drug reactions are one of the most commonly reported causes of pulmonary opacities in association with blood or alveolar eosinophilia. Unfortunately, most of the literature is in the form of case reports that vary in terms of

TABLE 27.4. DRUGS COMMONLY CAUSING EOSINOPHILIC LUNG DISEASE

Aspirin	Amiodarone
Bleomycin	Captopril
Carbamazepine	Cocaine
G-CSF	GM-CSF
Gold	Hydrochlorothiazide
Iodinated contrast dye	Methotrexate
Minocycline	Nilutamide
Nitrofurantoin	Nonsteroidal antiinflammatory drugs
Penicillamine	Penicillins
Phenytoin	Propylthiouracil
Sulfonamides	Sulfasalazine

G-CSF, granulocyte colony-stimulating factor; GM-CSF, granulocyte-macrophage colony-stimulating factor.

documentation. Many drugs have been associated with pulmonary eosinophilia (1), and a continuously updated list from the University Hospital in Dijon, France, is maintained on the Internet (*www.pneumotox.com*). Table 27.4 lists the drugs most commonly associated with eosinophilic lung disease.

Two causes of drug-induced eosinophilic lung disease warrant special mention because of their historical significance. Eosinophilia-myalgia syndrome (112) resulted from a contaminant found in batches of L-tryptophan made by one manufacturer of the drug in the late 1980s (113). Acute peripheral blood eosinophilia was accompanied by severe myalgias (114), and respiratory symptoms occurred in more than 50% of patients (115). The toxic oil syndrome occurred in Spain in 1981–1982; approximately 20,000 cases of lung disease accompanied by peripheral blood eosinophilia developed when rapeseed oil contaminated with oleoanilide was fraudulently marketed as olive oil (116).

Drug-induced eosinophilic lung disease can vary in presentation from simple pulmonary eosinophilia to an acute eosinophilic pneumonia-like syndrome. Although many cases of drug-induced eosinophilic lung disease remit when the medication is discontinued, in severe or persistent cases, corticosteroids may be necessary.

LUNG DISEASES OCCASIONALLY ASSOCIATED WITH EOSINOPHILS

Idiopathic pulmonary fibrosis is frequently associated with an increase in BAL fluid eosinophils and with peripheral blood eosinophilia (2). Although the eosinophils in BAL fluid usually comprise fewer than 20% of the total number of cells, elevated percentages of BAL fluid eosinophils have been reported in as many as 44% of patients with idiopathic pulmonary fibrosis (117) and are found in both usual interstitial pneumonitis and nonspecific interstitial pneumonitis. Retrospective series have indicated that a percentage of BAL fluid eosinophils above 5% is associated with more severe pulmonary impairment at initial presentation (118) and

predicts a poor response to treatment (119) and more rapid deterioration (120,121). On occasion, the diagnosis of idiopathic pulmonary fibrosis can be difficult because some areas of the lung biopsy specimen of patients with usual interstitial pneumonitis can have features of chronic eosinophilic pneumonia (122). Pulmonary fibrosis associated with collagen-vascular disease can be associated with a mild increase in the number of eosinophils in the BAL fluid in up to 26% of patients (1).

Langerhans cell granulomatosis is associated with an abnormal proliferation of Langerhans cells in the lung and other organs. An increase in tissue eosinophils is noted on open lung biopsy in 81% of patients (123); however, an increase in BAL eosinophils is seen in only 15% of patients (117). Peripheral blood eosinophilia is not present.

The percentage of eosinophils in the BAL fluid is increased in about one fourth of patients with bronchiolitis obliterans–organizing pneumonia; they usually amount to fewer than 20% of the total number of cells in the BAL fluid (124,125). Because many patients with chronic eosinophilic pneumonia have histologic evidence of bronchiolitis obliterans (9), these two clinical entities can on occasion be difficult to distinguish. In fact, it has been suggested that untreated chronic eosinophilic pneumonia may be the cause of some cases of idiopathic bronchiolitis obliterans–organizing pneumonia (126).

Other interstitial lung diseases in which the percentage of eosinophils in the BAL fluid can be mildly elevated include hypersensitivity pneumonitis and sarcoidosis (117).

Several malignancies can be associated with an increase in lung eosinophils. Non–small cell carcinoma can be accompanied by an increase in peripheral blood and tissue eosinophils (127). Tissue eosinophils usually make up a component of the mixed inflammatory infiltrate associated with Hodgkin disease, and an increase in both BAL and blood eosinophils has been reported (2,127). Both non-Hodgkin lymphoma and lymphocytic leukemia can be associated with pulmonary opacities and peripheral blood eosinophilia (128,129). Eosinophilic leukemia can occur in a small subset of patients with myeloblastic leukemia. During periods of extreme eosinophilia, infiltration of the lungs with eosinophils and myeloblasts can cause dyspnea and radiographic opacities (130). Many malignancies that metastasize to the lungs can be associated with peripheral blood eosinophilia, which underscores the importance of a thorough history and physical examination in the initial evaluation of patients.

Other diseases occasionally accompanied by an increase in pulmonary eosinophils include ulcerative colitis, eosinophilic gastroenteritis, respiratory syncytial virus infection, pertussoid eosinophilic pneumonia (a variant of idiopathic simple pulmonary eosinophilia that occurs in infants 3–16 weeks old), tuberculosis, hereditary ataxia-telangiectasia, post-radiation fibrosis, graft versus host disease, scorpion sting, and *Corynebacterium pseudotuberculosis* infection (1).

CLINICAL APPROACH

The history and physical examination remain the most important means of determining the specific cause of eosinophilic lung disease in patients presenting with peripheral blood eosinophilia in conjunction with lung disease, or in patients with an increased number of eosinophils on lung tissue sections or in BAL fluid. A history of asthma may raise the suspicion of Churg-Strauss syndrome, ABPA, or bronchocentric granulomatosis. The travel history may suggest a parasitic infection such as tropical pulmonary eosinophilia, schistosomiasis, or *Paragonimus westermani* infection. Exposure to dogs or cats may suggest *Ancylostoma* or *Toxocara* infection. A careful history should be taken for the use of prescription, nonprescription, and illicit drugs in addition to health food supplements.

In diseases such as Langerhans cell granulomatosis, acute eosinophilic pneumonia, and *P. carinii* pneumonia, and in some cases of drug-induced lung disease, an increase in pulmonary eosinophils may develop without an increase in blood eosinophils. On the other hand, in diseases such as simple pulmonary eosinophilia, chronic eosinophilic pneumonia, parasite infection, some drug-induced lung diseases, ABPA, Churg-Strauss syndrome, fungal infections, and the idiopathic hypereosinophilic syndrome, the number of blood eosinophils is typically high.

Because steroids are used to treat many forms of eosinophilic lung disease and because steroids can worsen fungal and parasitic infection presenting as eosinophilic lung disease, these infections should be considered in all patients presenting with pulmonary eosinophilia. Stool examination for ova and parasites is commonly ordered, but parasites such as *Trichinella*, *Paragonimus*, *Ancylostoma*, *Toxocara*, and *Filaria* cannot be diagnosed by stool examination. Intestinal parasites (e.g., *Ascaris* and *Strongyloides*) may cause pulmonary eosinophilia weeks before ova first appear in the stool, and false-negative stool examination results can be obtained even when adult worms are present in the intestine. In many cases, serologic studies are more sensitive than stool examinations. Fungal infection by *Aspergillus* can be particularly difficult to diagnose, and BAL or lung biopsy is sometimes required.

An elevated IgE level is nonspecific, but very high levels may suggest ABPA. The ANCA and related antimyeloperoxidase antibody are useful in patients with undifferentiated eosinophilic lung disease and support a diagnosis of Churg-Strauss syndrome.

Pulmonary function tests are occasionally useful in evaluating patients with unexplained pulmonary eosinophilia but are generally more helpful in following the course of patients with an established diagnosis.

BAL can be of great value in the assessment of a patient with eosinophilic lung disease. Percentages of BAL fluid eosinophils in excess of 20% are found in acute and chronic eosinophilic pneumonia, hypereosinophilic syndrome, para-

site infections, Churg-Strauss syndrome, and drug reactions. Strongyloidiasis, ascariasis, *Paragonimus* infection, cryptococcosis, coccidioidomycosis, *P. carinii* pneumonia, and *Aspergillus* infection can often be diagnosed by stains of BAL fluid. Fungal cultures are useful in *Aspergillus* infection.

Lung biopsy may be necessary to confirm diseases such as Churg-Strauss syndrome, malignancy, bronchocentric granulomatosis, and some of the interstitial lung diseases. Biopsy is not necessary for the diagnosis of ABPA, hypereosinophilic syndrome, drug reactions, or parasitic infections except in unusual cases. A favorable response to a therapeutic trial of corticosteroids is usually sufficient to confirm acute and chronic eosinophilic pneumonia, but lung biopsy may be necessary if the history suggests fungal infection or if corticosteroids are relatively contraindicated.

The long-term follow-up of patients is desirable because the clinical features of many eosinophilic lung diseases evolve over time. For example, Churg-Strauss syndrome can be indistinguishable from chronic eosinophilic pneumonia early in its course. Similarly, mild forms of chronic granulomatous disease complicated by *Aspergillus* pneumonia may be indistinguishable from uncomplicated acute eosinophilic pneumonia. Gratifyingly, most patients with eosinophilic lung diseases improve substantially, if not completely, with appropriate treatment.

REFERENCES

1. Allen JN, Davis WB. State of the art: the eosinophilic lung diseases. *Am J Respir Crit Care Med* 1994;150:1423–1438.
2. Allen JN, Davis WB, Pacht ER. Diagnostic significance of increased bronchoalveolar lavage fluid eosinophils. *Am Rev Respir Dis* 1990;142:642–647.
3. Allen JN, Davis WB. Eosinophils. In: Crystal RG, West JB, Weibel ER, et al., eds. *The lung: scientific foundations.* Philadelphia: Lippincott–Raven Publishers, 1997:905–915.
4. Löffler W. Zur differential-diagnose der lungeninfiltrierungen. II. Über flüchtige succedan-infiltrate (mit eosinophilie). *Beitr Klin Tuberk* 1932;79:368–392.
5. Ford RM. Transient pulmonary eosinophilia and asthma: a review of 20 cases occurring in 5,702 asthma sufferers. *Am Rev Respir Dis* 1966;93:797–803.
6. Citro LA, Gordon ME, Miller WT. Eosinophilic lung disease (or how to slice P.I.E.). *Am J Roentgenol Radiat Ther Nucl Med* 1973;117:787–797.
7. Christoforidis AJ, Molnar W. Eosinophilic pneumonia: report of two cases with pulmonary biopsy. *JAMA* 1960;173:157–161.
8. Carrington CB, Addington WW, Goff AM, et al. Chronic eosinophilic pneumonia. *N Engl J Med* 1969;280:787–798.
9. Jederlinic PJ, Sicilian L, Gaensler EA. Chronic eosinophilic pneumonia: a report of 19 cases and a review of the literature. *Medicine* 1988;67:154–162.
10. Marchand E, Reynaud-Gaubert M, Lauque D, et al. Idiopathic chronic eosinophilic pneumonia: a clinical and follow-up study of 62 cases. *Medicine* 1998;77:299–312.
11. Gaensler EA, Carrington CB. Peripheral opacities in chronic eosinophilic pneumonia: the photographic negative of pulmonary edema. *AJR Am J Roentgenol* 1977;128:1–13.
12. Johkoh T, Muller NL, Akira M, et al. Eosinophilic lung diseases:

diagnostic accuracy of thin-section CT in 111 patients. *Radiology* 2000;216:773–780.

13. Arakawa H, Kurihara Y, Niimi H, et al. Bronchiolitis obliterans with organizing pneumonia versus chronic eosinophilic pneumonia: high-resolution CT findings in 81 patients. *AJR Am J Roentgenol* 2001;176:1053–1058.

14. Samman YS, Wali SO, Abdelaal MA, et al. Chronic eosinophilic pneumonia presenting with recurrent massive bilateral pleural effusion: case report. *Chest* 2001;119:968–970.

15. Liebow AA, Carrington CB. The eosinophilic pneumonias. *Medicine (Baltimore)* 1969;48:251–285.

16. Kanner RE, Hammar SP Chronic eosinophilic pneumonia. Ultrastructural evidence of marked immunoglobulin production plus macrophagic ingestion of eosinophils and eosinophilic lysosomes leading to intracytoplasmic Charcot-Leyden crystals. *Chest* 1977;71:95–98.

17. Shijubo N, Fujishima T, Morita S, et al. Idiopathic chronic eosinophilic pneumonia associated with noncaseating epithelioid granulomas. *Eur Respir J* 1995;8:327–330.

18. Cooney TP. Interrelationship of chronic eosinophilic pneumonia, bronchiolitis obliterans and rheumatoid disease: a hypothesis. *J Clin Pathol* 1981;149:129–137.

19. Olopade CO, Crotty TB, Douglas WW, et al. Chronic eosinophilic pneumonia and idiopathic bronchiolitis obliterans organizing pneumonia: comparison of eosinophil number and degranulation by immunofluorescence staining for eosinophil-derived major basic protein. *Mayo Clin Proc* 1995;70:137–142.

20. Lai RS, Lin SL, Lai NS, et al. Churg-Strauss syndrome presenting with pulmonary capillaritis and diffuse alveolar hemorrhage. *Scand J Rheumatol* 1998;27:230–232.

21. Katzenstein ALA. Diagnostic features and differential diagnosis of Churg-Strauss syndrome in the lung. *Am J Pathol* 2000;114:767–772.

22. Basset F, Ferrans VJ, Soler P, et al. Intraluminal fibrosis in interstitial lung disorders. *Am J Pathol* 1986;122:443–461.

23. Phunmanee A, Boonsawat W, Charoensiri DJ, et al. Chronic eosinophilic pneumonia: a case report. *J Med Assoc Thai* 2000;83:959–963.

24. Fox B, Seed WA. Chronic eosinophilic pneumonia. *Thorax* 1980;35:570–580.

25. Perrault JL, Janis M, Wolinsky H. Resolution of chronic eosinophilic pneumonia with corticosteroid therapy. Demonstration by needle biopsy. *Ann Intern Med* 1971;74:951–954.

26. Allen JN, Pacht ER, Gadek JE, et al. Acute eosinophilic pneumonia as a reversible cause of noninfectious respiratory failure. *N Engl J Med* 1989;321:569–574.

27. Badesch DB, King TE, Schwarz MI. Acute eosinophilic pneumonia: a hypersensitivity phenomenon? *Am Rev Respir Dis* 1989;139:249–252.

28. Hayakawa H, Sato A, Toyoshima M, et al. A clinical study of idiopathic eosinophilic pneumonia. *Chest* 1994;105:1462–1466.

29. Pope-Harman AL, Davis WB, Christoforidis AJ, et al. Acute eosinophilic pneumonia: a summary of fifteen cases and review of the literature. *Medicine* 1996;75:334–342.

30. Shintani H, Fujimura M, Ishiura Y, et al. A case of cigarette smoking-induced acute eosinophilic pneumonia showing tolerance. *Chest* 2000;117:277–279.

31. Glazer CS, Cohen LB, Schwarz MI. Acute eosinophilic pneumonia in AIDS. *Chest* 2001;120:1732–1735.

32. Trawick D, Kotch A, Matthay R, et al. Eosinophilic pneumonia as a presentation of occult chronic granulomatous disease. *Eur Respir J* 1997;10:2166–2170.

33. Maeno T, Maeno Y, Sando Y, et al. Nuclear hypersegmentation precedes the increase in blood eosinophils in acute eosinophilic pneumonia. *Intern Med* 2000;39:157–159.

34. Ogawa H, Fujimura M, Matsuda T, et al. Transient wheeze: eosinophilic bronchiolitis in acute eosinophilic pneumonia. *Chest* 1993;104:493–496.

35. King MA, Pope-Harman A, Allen JN, et al. Acute eosinophilic pneumonia: radiologic and clinical features. *Radiology* 1997;203:715–719.

36. Ricker DH, Taylor SR, Gartner JC Jr, et al. Fatal pulmonary aspergillosis presenting as acute eosinophilic pneumonia in a previously healthy child. *Chest* 1991;100:875–877.

37. Tazelaar HD, Linz LJ, Colby TV, et al. Acute eosinophilic pneumonia: histopathologic findings in nine patients. *Am J Respir Crit Care Med* 1997;155:296–302.

38. Churg J, Strauss L. Allergic granulomatosis, allergic angiitis, and periarteritis nodosa. *Am J Pathol* 1951;27:277–301.

39. Chumbley LC, Harrison EG, DeRemee RA. Allergic granulomatosis and angiitis (Churg-Strauss syndrome): report and analysis of 30 cases. *Mayo Clin Proc* 1977;52:477–484.

40. Lanham JG, Elkon KB, Pusey CD, et al. Systemic vasculitis with asthma and eosinophilia: a clinical approach to the Churg-Strauss syndrome. *Medicine* 1984;63:65–81.

41. Guillevin L, Cohen P, Gayraud M, et al. Churg-Strauss syndrome: clinical study and long-term follow-up of 96 patients. *Medicine* 1999;78:26–37.

42. Churg A. Recent advances in the diagnosis of Churg-Strauss syndrome. *Mod Pathol* 2001;14:1284–1293.

43. Mouthon L, Le Toumlin P, Andre MH, et al. Polyarteritis nodosa and Churg-Strauss angiitis: characteristics and outcome in 38 patients over 65 years. *Medicine* 2002;81:27–40.

44. Churg J. Allergic granulomatosis and granulomatous-vascular syndromes. *Ann Allergy* 1963;21:619–628.

45. Sale S, Patterson R. Recurrent Churg-Strauss vasculitis with exophthalmos, hearing loss, nasal obstruction, amyloid deposits, hyperimmunoglobulin E, and circulating immune complexes. *Arch Intern Med* 1981;141:1363–1365.

46. Wechsler ME, Garpestad E, Flier SR, et al. Pulmonary infiltrates, eosinophilia, and cardiomyopathy following corticosteroid withdrawal in patients with asthma receiving zafirlukast. *JAMA* 1998;279:455–457.

47. Goeken JA. Antineutrophil cytoplasmic antibody—a useful serological marker for vasculitis. *J Clin Immunol* 1991;11:161–173.

48. Olivieri D, Pesci A, Bertorelli G. Eosinophilic alveolitis in immunologic interstitial lung disorders. *Lung* 1990;168:964–973.

49. Cooper BJ, Bacal E, Patterson R. Allergic angiitis and granulomatosis: prolonged remission induced by combined prednisone-azathioprine therapy. *Arch Intern Med* 1978;138:367–371.

50. MacFadyen R, Tron V, Keshmiri M, et al. Allergic angiitis of Churg and Strauss syndrome. Response to pulse methylprednisolone. *Chest* 1987;91:629–631.

51. Conron M, Huw L, Beynon C. Churg-Strauss syndrome. *Thorax* 2000;55:870–877.

52. Guillevan L, Fain O, Lhote F, et al. Lack of superiority of steroids plus plasma exchange to steroids alone in the treatment of polyarteritis nodosa and Churg-Strauss syndrome: a prospective randomized trial in 78 patients. *Arthritis Rheum* 1992;35:208–215.

53. Tatsis E, Schnabel A, Gross WL. Interferon-alpha treatment of four patients with the Churg-Strauss syndrome. *Ann Intern Med* 1998;129:370–374.

54. Fauci AS, Harley JB, Roberts WC, et al. The idiopathic hypereosinophilic syndrome: clinical, pathophysiologic, and therapeutic considerations. *Ann Intern Med* 1982;97:78–92.

55. Raghavachar A, Fleischer S, Frickhofen N, et al. T-lymphocyte control of human eosinophil granulopoiesis: clonal analysis in an idiopathic hypereosinophilic syndrome. *J Immunol* 1987;139:3753–3758.

56. Cogan E, Schandené L, Crusiaux A, et al. Brief report: clonal proliferation of type 2 helper T cells in a man with the hypereosinophilic syndrome. *N Engl J Med* 1994;330:535–538.

57. Roufosse F, Schandene L, Sibille C, et al. Clonal Th2 lymphocytes in patients with the idiopathic hypereosinophilic syndrome. *Br J Haematol* 2000;109:540–548.

58. Simon HU, Plotz SG, Dummer R, et al. Abnormal clones of T cells producing interleukin-5 in idiopathic eosinophilia. *N Engl J Med* 1999;341:1112–1120.

59. Chang HW, Leong KH, Koh DR, et al. Clonality of isolated eosinophils in the hypereosinophilic syndrome. *Blood* 1999;93:1651–1657.

60. Spry CJF, Davies J, Tai PC, et al. Clinical features of fifteen patients with the hypereosinophilic syndrome. *Q J Med* 1983;205:1–22.

61. Parrillo JE, Borer JS, Henery WL, et al. The cardiovascular manifestations of the hypereosinophilic syndrome. Prospective study of 26 patients, with review of the literature. *Am J Med* 1979;67:572–582.

62. Spry CJF. The hypereosinophilic syndrome: clinical features, laboratory findings, and treatment. *Allergy* 1982;37:539–551.

63. Chusid MJ, Dale DC, West BC, et al. The hypereosinophilic syndrome: analysis of fourteen cases with review of the literature. *Medicine* 1975;54:1–27.

64. Slabbynck H, Impens N, Naegels S, et al. Idiopathic hypereosinophilic syndrome-related pulmonary involvement diagnosed by bronchoalveolar lavage. *Chest* 1992;101:1178–1180.

65. Winn RE, Kollef MH, Meyer JI. Pulmonary involvement in the hypereosinophilic syndrome. *Chest* 1994;105:656–660.

66. Kang EY, Shim JJ, Kim JS, et al. Pulmonary involvement of idiopathic hypereosinophilic syndrome: CT findings in five patients. *J Comput Assist Tomogr* 1997;21:612–615.

67. Parrillo JE, Fauci AS, Wolff SM. Therapy of the hypereosinophilic syndrome. *Ann Intern Med* 1978;89:167–172.

68. Zielinski RM, Lawrence WD. Interferon-α for the hypereosinophilic syndrome. *Ann Intern Med* 1990;113:716–718.

69. Zabel P, Schlaak M. Cyclosporin for hypereosinophilic syndrome. *Ann Hematol* 1991;62:230–231.

70. Smit AJ, Van Essen LH, De Vries EGE. Successful long-term control of idiopathic hypereosinophilic syndrome with etoposide. *Cancer* 1991;67:2826–2827.

71. Ueno NT, Zhao S, Robertson LE, et al. 2-Chlorodeoxyadenosine therapy for idiopathic hypereosinophilic syndrome. *Leukemia* 1997;11:1386–1390.

72. Butterfield JH, Gleich GJ. Interferon-alpha treatment of six patients with the idiopathic hypereosinophilic syndrome. *Ann Intern Med* 1994;121:648–653.

73. Fukushima T, Kuriyama K, Ito H, et al. Successful bone marrow transplantation for idiopathic hypereosinophilic syndrome. *Br J Haematol* 1995;90:213–215.

74. Sigmund DA, Flessa HC. Hypereosinophilic syndrome: successful allogeneic bone marrow transplantation. *Bone Marrow Transplant* 1995;15:647–648.

75. Hinson KFW, Moon AJ, Plummer NS. Broncho-pulmonary aspergillosis. A review and a report of eight new cases. *Thorax* 1952;7:317–333.

76. Rosenberg M, Patterson R, Mintzer R, et al. Clinical and immunologic criteria for the diagnosis of allergic bronchopulmonary aspergillosis. *Ann Intern Med* 1977;86:405–414.

77. Vlahakis NE, Aksamit TR. Diagnosis and treatment of allergic bronchopulmonary aspergillosis. *Mayo Clin Proc* 2001;76:930–938.

78. Patterson R, Greenberger PA, Radin RC, et al. Allergic bronchopulmonary aspergillosis: staging as an aid to management. *Ann Intern Med* 1982;96:286–291.

79. Patterson R, Greenberger PA, Lee TM, et al. Prolonged evaluation of patients with corticosteroid-dependent asthma stage of allergic bronchopulmonary aspergillosis. *J Allergy Clin Immunol* 1987;80:663–668.

80. Capewell S, Chapman BJ, Alexander F, et al. Corticosteroid treatment and prognosis in pulmonary eosinophilia. *Thorax* 1989;44:925–929.

81. Mastella G, Rainisio M, Harms HK, et al. Allergic bronchopulmonary aspergillosis in cystic fibrosis. *Eur Respir J* 2001;17:1052–1053.

82. Geller DE, Kaplowitz H, Light MJ, et al. Allergic bronchopulmonary aspergillosis in cystic fibrosis: reported prevalence, regional distribution, and patient characteristics. Scientific Advisory Group, Investigators, and Coordinators of the Epidemiologic Study of Cystic Fibrosis. *Chest* 1999;116:639–646.

83. Egan JJ, Yonan N, Carroll KB, et al. Allergic bronchopulmonary aspergillosis in lung allograft recipients. *Eur Respir J* 1996;9:169–171.

84. Marchand E, Verellen-Dumoulin C, Mairesse M, et al. Frequency of cystic fibrosis transmembrane conductance regulator gene mutations and 5T allele in patients with allergic bronchopulmonary aspergillosis. *Chest* 2001;119:762–767.

85. Chauhan B, Santiago L, Hutcheson PS, et al. Evidence for the involvement of two different MHC class II regions in susceptibility or protection in allergic bronchopulmonary aspergillosis. *J Allergy Clin Immunol* 2000;106:723–729.

86. Patterson R, Greenberger PA, Halwig JM, et al. Allergic bronchopulmonary aspergillosis: natural history and classification of early disease by serologic and roentgenographic studies. *Arch Intern Med* 1986;146:916–918.

87. Ricketti AJ, Greenberger PA, Patterson R. Serum IgE as an important aid in the management of allergic bronchopulmonary aspergillosis. *J Allergy Clin Immunol* 1984;74:68–71.

88. Krasnick J, Greenberger PA, Roberts M, et al. Allergic bronchopulmonary aspergillosis: serologic update for 1995. *J Clin Lab Immunol* 1995;46:137–142.

89. McCarthy DS, Simon G, Hargreave FE. The radiological appearances in allergic bronchopulmonary aspergillosis. *Clin Radiol* 1970;21:366–375.

90. Mitchell TA, Hamilos DL, Lynch DA, et al. Distribution and severity of bronchiectasis in allergic bronchopulmonary aspergillosis (ABPA). *J Asthma* 2000;37:65–72.

91. Ward S, Heyneman L, Lee MJ, et al. Accuracy of CT in the diagnosis of allergic bronchopulmonary aspergillosis in asthmatic patients. *AJR Am J Roentgenol* 1999;173:937–942.

92. Slavin RG, Bedrossian CW, Hutcheson BA, et al. A pathologic study of allergic bronchopulmonary aspergillosis. *J Allergy Clin Immunol* 1988;81:718–725.

93. Bosken C, Myers J, Greenberger P, et al. Pathologic features of allergic bronchopulmonary aspergillosis. *Am J Surg Pathol* 1988;12:216–222.

94. Seaton A, Seaton RA, Wightman AJ. Management of allergic bronchopulmonary aspergillosis without maintenance oral corticosteroids: a fifteen-year follow-up. *QJM* 1994;87:529–537.

95. Imbeault B, Cormier Y. Usefulness of inhaled high-dose corticosteroids in allergic bronchopulmonary aspergillosis. *Chest* 1993;103:1614–1617.

96. Salez F, Brichet A, Desurmont S, et al. Effects of itraconazole therapy in allergic bronchopulmonary aspergillosis. *Chest* 1999;116:1665–1668.

97. Stevens DA, Schwartz HJ, Lee JY, et al. A randomized trial of itraconazole in allergic bronchopulmonary aspergillosis. *N Engl J Med* 2000;342:756–762.

98. Liebow AA. Pulmonary angiitis and granulomatosis. *Am Rev Respir Dis* 1973;108:1–18.

99. Robinson RG, Wehunt WD, Tsou E, et al. Bronchocentric granulomatosis. Roentgenographic manifestations. *Am Rev Respir Dis* 1982;125:751–756.

100. Ward S, Heyneman LE, Flint JD, et al. Bronchocentric granulomatosis: computed tomographic findings in five patients. *Clin Radiol* 2000;55:296–300.

101. Katzenstein AL, Liebow AA, Friedman PJ. Bronchocentric granulomatosis, mucoid impaction and hypersensitivity reaction to fungus. *Am Rev Respir Dis* 1975;111:497–537.

102. Robinson RG, Wehunt WD, Tsou E, et al. Bronchocentric granulomatosis. Roentgenographic manifestations. *Am Rev Respir Dis* 1982;125:751–756.

103. Wiedemann HP, Bensinger RE, Hudson LD. Bronchocentric granulomatosis with eye involvement. *Am Rev Respir Dis* 1982;126:347–350.

104. Gelpi AP, Mustafa A. *Ascaris* pneumonia. *Am J Med* 1968;44:377–389.

105. Ambrus JL, Klein E. Löffler syndrome and ancylostomiasis brasiliensis. *N Y State J Med* 1988;88:498–499.

106. Ong RK, Doyle RL. Tropical pulmonary eosinophilia. *Chest* 1998;113:1673–1679.

107. Cooray JH, Ismail MM. Reexamination of the diagnostic criteria of tropical pulmonary eosinophilia. *Respir Med* 1999;93:655–659.

108. Lombard CM, Tazelaar MD, Krasne DL. Pulmonary eosinophilia in coccidioidal infections. *Chest* 1987;91:734–736.

109. Whitlock WL, Dietrich RA, Tenholder MF. Acute eosinophilic pneumonia [Letter]. *N Engl J Med* 1990;322:635.

110. Fleury-Feith J, Van Nhieu JT, Picard C, et al. Bronchoalveolar lavage eosinophilia associated with *Pneumocystis carinii* pneumonitis in AIDS patients: comparative study with non-AIDS patients. *Chest* 1989;95:1198–1201.

111. Ricker DH, Taylor SR, Gartner JC Jr, et al. Fatal pulmonary aspergillosis presenting as acute eosinophilic pneumonia in a previously healthy child. *Chest* 1991;100:875–877.

112. Kaufman LD, Seidman RJ, Gruber BL. L-Tryptophan–associated eosinophilic perimyositis, neuritis, and fasciitis. A clinicopathologic and laboratory study of 25 patients. *Medicine* 1990;69:187–199.

113. Philen RM, Hill RH, Flanders WD, et al. Tryptophan contaminants associated with eosinophilia-myalgia syndrome. *Am J Epidemiol* 1993;138:154–159.

114. Kamb ML, Murphy JJ, Jones JL, et al. Eosinophilia-myalgia syndrome in L-tryptophan–exposed patients. *JAMA* 1992;267:77–82.

115. Swygert LA, Maes EF, Sewell LE, et al. Eosinophilia-myalgia syndrome: results of national surveillance. *JAMA* 1990;264:1698–1703.

116. Alonso-Ruiz A, Calabozo M, Perez-Ruiz F, et al. Toxic oil syndrome. A long-term follow-up of a cohort of 332 patients. *Medicine* 1993;72:285–295.

117. Davis WB, Fells GA, Sun XH, et al. Eosinophil-mediated injury to lung parenchymal cells and interstitial matrix: a possible role for eosinophils in chronic inflammatory disorders of the lower respiratory tract. *J Clin Invest* 1984;74:269–278.

118. Watters LC, Schwarz MI, Cherniack RM, et al. Idiopathic pulmonary fibrosis: pretreatment bronchoalveolar lavage cellular constituents and their relationships with lung histopathology and clinical response to therapy. *Am Rev Respir Dis* 1987;135:696–704.

119. Rudd RM, Haslam PL, Turner-Warwick M. Cryptogenic fibrosing alveolitis: relationships of pulmonary physiology and bronchoalveolar lavage to response to treatment and prognosis. *Am Rev Respir Dis* 1981;124:1–8.

120. Hallgren R, Bjermer L, Lundgren R, et al. The eosinophil component of the alveolitis in idiopathic pulmonary fibrosis: signs of eosinophil activation in the lung are related to impaired lung function. *Am Rev Respir Dis* 1989;139:373–377.

121. Peterson MW, Monick M, Hunninghake GW. Prognostic role of eosinophils in pulmonary fibrosis. *Chest* 1987;92:51–56.

122. Yousem SA. Eosinophilic pneumonia-like areas in idiopathic usual interstitial pneumonia. *Mod Pathol* 2000;13:1280–1284.

123. Friedman PJ, Liebow AA, Sokoloff J. Eosinophilic granuloma of the lung. Clinical aspects of primary pulmonary histiocytosis in the adult. *Medicine* 1981;60:385–396.

124. Costabel U, Teschler H, Guzman J. Bronchiolitis obliterans organizing pneumonia (BOOP): the cytological and immunocytological profile of bronchoalveolar lavage. *Eur Respir J* 1992;5:791–797.

125. Izumi T, Kitaichi M, Nishimura K, et al. Bronchiolitis obliterans organizing pneumonia. Clinical features and differential diagnosis. *Chest* 1992;102:715–719.

126. Bartter T, Irwin RS, Nash G, et al. Idiopathic bronchiolitis obliterans organizing pneumonia with peripheral infiltrates on chest roentgenogram. *Arch Intern Med* 1989;149:273–279.

127. Spry CJF. *Eosinophils: a comprehensive review, and guide to the scientific and medical literature.* Oxford: Oxford University Press, 1988.

128. Kawasaki A, Mizushima Y, Matsui S, et al. A case of T-cell lymphoma accompanying marked eosinophilia, chronic eosinophilic pneumonia, and eosinophilic pleural effusion. A case report. *Tumori* 1991;77:527–530.

129. Tan AM, Downie PJ, Ekert H. Hypereosinophilia syndrome with pneumonia in acute lymphoblastic leukaemia. *Aust Paediatr J* 1987;23:359–361.

130. Bentley HP, Reardon AE, Knoedler JP, et al. Eosinophilic leukemia. Report of a case, with review and classification. *Am J Med* 196;30:310–322.

28 Systemic Sarcoidosis

Lynn T. Tanoue · Jack A. Elias

In 1877, Jonathan Hutchinson (1), an English physician/dermatologist, published a description of a coal wharf worker who presented with raised purple skin lesions on the hands and legs that Hutchinson termed "livid papillary psoriasis." This is believed to be the earliest written report of sarcoidosis. In 1889, Besnier (2) described a patient with raised violaceous facial lesions that he called *lupus pernio*. This description was followed by reports by Tenneson (3) and Boeck (4) of the histologic features of these lesions—granulomas consisting of epithelioid cells with a few giant cells. Boeck was struck by the resemblance of the lesions to sarcomas and gave them the name *benign sarcoid*. In the early years of the 20th century, Bittorf and Kuznitsky (5) and Schaumann (6) recognized that sarcoid skin lesions, lupus pernio, and visceral lesions were all part of the same multisystem disorder. This important observation set the stage for the recognition of sarcoidosis as a distinct clinicopathologic entity. In the years since its recognition, sarcoidosis has been the topic of intense investigation. These studies have shed light on some of the clinical manifestations, epidemiologic characteristics, and pathogenic mechanisms of the disease. However, although commonly encountered and frequently diagnosed, sarcoidosis is still poorly understood. Despite decades of study, its etiology remains unknown, and our knowledge of its pathogenesis is incomplete. Furthermore, issues relating to diagnosis and treatment continue to raise controversy. In this chapter, we have attempted to outline the areas of certainty and uncertainty regarding this disorder. We also hope to provide a rational approach that can be used for evaluating and treating affected patients.

DEFINITION

The definition of sarcoidosis remains descriptive (7). Sarcoidosis is a multisystem granulomatous disorder of unknown etiology. Young adults are most frequently affected, but the disease may affect persons of all ages. The organs most commonly involved clinically include the lungs, lymph nodes, skin, and eyes, but the disease may present with manifestations in other organs, including the heart, liver, kidneys, nervous system, spleen, gastrointestinal tract, bones, muscles, and spleen—essentially any and every organ. Consistent immunologic features include depression of delayed-type hypersensitivity, a T helper subset 1 (Th1) cell response at sites of disease activity, and evidence of B-cell hyperactivity and circulation of immune complexes (8–11). The diagnosis is most firmly established when the clinical findings are supported by the histologic demonstration of noncaseating epithelioid granulomas and when other causes of granulomatous inflammation, including local sarcoid reactions, have been excluded (12,13).

EPIDEMIOLOGY

The epidemiology of sarcoidosis has been challenging because of the variable disease presentation, the descriptive definition of the disease, and the lack of specific diagnostic tools. From global epidemiologic studies, it is clear that sarcoidosis can affect persons of every ethnic background and of both sexes (14–16). From data obtained by mass radiographic screening, it is apparent that the prevalence rates vary geographically. For example, rates of 28 cases per 100,000 population and 3 cases per 100,000 population have been reported in Nordic countries and in Japan, respectively (14). Rates as high as 213 cases per 100,000 population are noted among Irish women of childbearing age (17,18).

L. T. Tanoue and **J. A. Elias:** Section of Pulmonary and Critical Care Medicine, Yale University School of Medicine, New Haven, Connecticut.

Disease incidence is also difficult to define in countries and populations in which the rates of other granulomatous diseases with similar presentations, primarily tuberculosis and fungal infection, are high. In the United States, a single population-based study indicated that the incidence rates of sarcoidosis were 5.9 per 100,000 person-years for men and 6.3 per 100,000 person-years for women (19). African Americans and women appear to be at higher risk for disease (14).

Ethnicity appears to play a role in disease presentation. It is widely held that African Americans tend to present with more severe chronic disease than their Caucasian counterparts (13,20,21). Erythema nodosum is more common among Caucasians and relatively uncommon in blacks and is felt to portend a better disease outcome (22). Cardiac sarcoidosis, historically associated with a poor prognosis, is more common in Japan than in the United States (23,24).

Epidemiologic studies of disease clusters have demonstrated that environment, occupation, and genetics are likely contributors to disease incidence. A tendency to occur in the winter and early spring has been noted for sarcoidosis and erythema nodosum (25). Familial clustering has been reported from several regions, suggesting that a genetic predisposition to the development of granulomatous inflammation may exist. Family clusters occur more commonly in blacks, 19% of whom report an affected family member, in comparison with 5% of whites (26). Furthermore, families tend to be exposed to shared environments. Reports of sarcoid clusters in non–blood-related, closely residing persons support the theory that disease occurs in response to environmental antigens (27,28).

ETIOLOGY

The observations of variations in the geographic distribution of disease, clustering of cases that appear to be related to genetics and environment, and the granulomatous nature of the histologic response all support the current hypothesis that sarcoidosis represents an immunologic response to specific environmental antigens in genetically predisposed persons. However, the etiology of sarcoidosis remains obscure despite more than a century of intense observation and investigation.

The granulomatous lesions in sarcoidosis are similar to those caused by infectious agents such as mycobacteria and fungi or inorganic agents such as zirconium and beryllium, and to those seen in hypersensitivity reactions to organic agents such as thermophilic actinomycetes. These similarities have caused many to speculate that infectious agents or organic or inorganic dusts may be etiologic in sarcoidosis. Particular interest has been directed at the possibility that sarcoidosis is the result of an unusual host response to a common agent, or the result of infection by, or inhalation of, a poorly characterized agent. Efforts to test these speculations have been ongoing for many years. Such studies have

failed to observe consistent associations between the occurrence of sarcoidosis and a person's place of birth, place of residence, or personal history of allergies, drug ingestion, exposure to pets, or occupational exposure. In addition, hypotheses that common and exotic infectious agents such as viruses, corynebacteria, fungi, mycobacteria, propionibacteria, and cell wall–deficient organisms and environmental agents such as metals, organic dusts (e.g., pine pollen), and inorganic dusts (e.g., talc) play an etiologic role have not been borne out in repeated studies. Various molecular biologic techniques, including the polymerase chain reaction (PCR), have been used to reinvestigate the role that mycobacteria and other organisms may play in this disorder. Using this technique, some investigators have reported enhanced detection of mycobacterial DNA in patients with sarcoidosis, albeit with an overall high rate of false-positive PCR reactions (29–31). In contrast, others have found mycobacterial DNA in only a small minority of patients with sarcoidosis (32,33). Similarly, quantitative PCR has demonstrated genetic material from propionibacteria in sarcoid granulomas (34). As a result, it cannot be concluded that any infectious agent is etiologic in the majority of cases of sarcoidosis. Indeed, the search for a single etiologic agent in sarcoidosis may be fruitless because its widespread geographic distribution, disparate clinical presentations, and observed clustering suggest that multiple agents may actually be involved.

PATHOLOGY

The histologic features of sarcoidosis consist of varying degrees of granulomatous inflammation and tissue fibrosis.

Granulomatous Inflammation

The epithelioid granuloma is the characteristic lesion of sarcoidosis. These granulomas are usually not necrotic. When necrosis occurs, it is usually minimal and confined to the central portions of the lesion. The granulomas are usually distinct, even when densely clustered. Epithelioid cells and multinucleated giant cells are found in the center of the granulomas. They are intermingled with and surrounded by macrophages, monocytes, and lymphocytes (Fig. 28.1). In some cases, fibroblasts and fibroblast-derived connective tissue products surround the granulomas. The epithelioid cells are derived from tissue macrophages. They have ample, pale-staining cytoplasm, well-defined boundaries, and a central or eccentrically placed oval nucleus. Ultrastructural studies reveal abundant mitochondria, abundant rough and smooth endoplasmic reticulum, large numbers of vesicles, and a well-developed Golgi apparatus, suggesting that these cells have an enhanced secretory capacity. In fact, the epithelioid cells in sarcoid granulomas secrete an abundance of cytokines, enzymes, and other mediators (11,35–39). Multinucleated giant cells form from the fusion of epithelioid

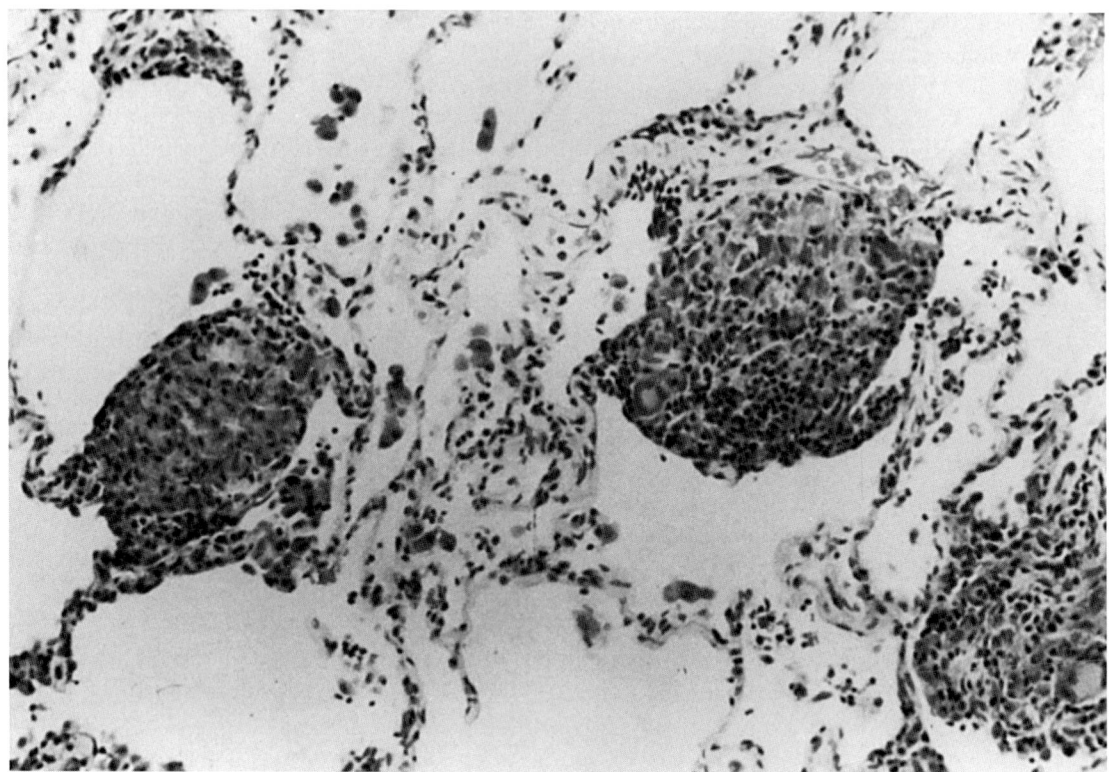

FIGURE 28.1. Lung biopsy specimen demonstrating noncaseating granulomas and interstitial pneumonitis in the lung interstitium.

cells. These giant cells may demonstrate immunoglobulin deposition and inclusion bodies. The latter include Schaumann bodies (which consist of concentric, laminated, calcified structures that result from the lysosomal accumulation of oxidized lipid) and asteroid bodies (which result from the accumulation of cytoskeletal filaments) (40). The lymphocytes in and around the granulomas are often larger and contain more organelles than their circulating counterparts. Characterization with monoclonal antibodies has shown that most of the T cells express the CD4 antigen, which is associated with a helper/inducer phenotype, and a minority express the CD8 antigen, which is associated with a cytotoxic/suppressor phenotype (41–43). As a result, the ratio of helper/inducer lymphocytes to cytotoxic/suppressor lymphocytes (CD4$^+$/CD8$^+$ ratio) in sarcoid granulomas is increased and parallels that noted in cell profiles in bronchoalveolar lavage (BAL) fluid.

Noncaseating granulomas may be found in any organ in the body. In the lung, they tend to be peribronchial, interstitial, and subpleural in location. Perivascular granulomas are also commonly noted. These lesions rarely extend past the vascular adventitia, and luminal distortion and endothelial cell disruption are rare. In the vast majority of cases, true vasculitis is a minor aspect of the lesion. When vasculitis is prominent, alternative diagnostic possibilities should be considered, such as necrotizing sarcoidal vasculitis or Wegener granulomatosis.

Although the epithelioid granuloma is the characteristic lesion of sarcoidosis, it is probably not the first lesion to be present in the lung. The granulomas are preceded by, and then noted in conjunction with, an interstitial pneumonitis characterized by macrophages and lymphocytes, the majority of which are T cells. The macrophages and lymphocytes in these infiltrates appear to be activated because they are larger and contain more organelles than corresponding cells in the circulating pool. The exact relationship between the intensity of the interstitial pneumonitis and the density of granuloma formation is not understood. The possibility that the granulomas are a consequence of the interstitial pneumonitis may explain why most studies find that the granulomas are most prominent when the interstitial pneumonitis is least intense, and vice versa.

Tissue Fibrosis

The interstitial pneumonitis and granulomatous inflammation seen in sarcoidosis are dynamic processes. Some lesions remain cellular for an extended period. In contrast, most resolve, either spontaneously or in response to steroid therapy. Why some lesions vanish entirely while others progress to fibrosis is unknown. The majority of lesions in the lung heal, with preservation of the normal parenchymal architecture. In the rest, the fibroblasts at the periphery of the granulomas proliferate and increase their production of collagen and other matrix molecules. As a result, the granuloma is replaced in a centripetal fashion with scar tissue. In the process, the normal alveolar and bronchial architecture is distorted, and the pulmonary vascular surface area is compromised. Bronchiectasis and cystic parenchymal lesions can result, and in the most severe cases, honeycombing and pulmonary hypertension can occur.

IMMUNOPATHOGENESIS

Sarcoidosis is the prototypic example of a compartmentalized immune response (39,44). Heightened cell-mediated immunity is seen within the lung and at other sites of disease involvement. In contrast, depressed cell-mediated immunity, often with cutaneous anergy, is seen in the peripheral circulation. Studies during the past few decades have added significantly to our understanding of the cellular events involved in the inflammatory and fibrotic phases of this disease. As a result, we have an improved understanding of the state of activation and effector function of the cells in sarcoidal infiltrates, a picture of how these alterations mediate pulmonary inflammation, and a preliminary understanding of the roles that cytokines may play in granuloma formation.

T Cells

In sarcoidosis, T helper lymphocytes accumulate at sites of disease activity. The ratio of helper (CD4$^+$) to suppressor (CD8$^+$) cells is increased in BAL fluid. The T cells that accumulate in the lungs of patients with sarcoidosis and are found in BAL fluid are activated; they express markers of cell surface activation, such as the major histocompatibility complex (MHC) DR antigen, the VLA-1 late activation antigen, and the interleukin-2 (IL-2) receptor (Tac antigen). Unlike unstimulated T lymphocytes, they also spontaneously produce a variety of cytokines, including IL-2, interferon-γ (IFN-γ), monocyte chemotactic factor, and lymphotoxin (9,42,45,46). The IL-2 that is produced by sarcoid T cells appears to bind to the IL-2 receptor and stimulate T-cell proliferation in an autocrine or paracrine fashion, or both. Interestingly, although BAL fluid T cells are spontaneously activated, like peripheral lymphocytes, their response to "recall" antigens such as purified protein derivative and *Candida* is decreased. The reason for this is not clear. This decreased memory function may explain in part the cutaneous anergy observed clinically in some patients with sarcoidosis.

T cells recognize foreign antigens via their T-cell receptors (TCRs). Each T cell expresses a receptor for a unique antigen. The diversity of receptors necessary to encode an appropriately diverse immune repertoire is generated by creating TCRs that differ in the constant (C), joining (J), and variable (V) regions of the two proteins that make up the heterodimeric TCR complex. In an attempt to identify the agents(s) causing the lymphocytosis in sarcoidosis, the

TCRs on the surface of BAL fluid and peripheral blood lymphocytes have been extensively studied. These studies have shown that BAL fluid T lymphocytes are not a clonal population. Some studies have, however, detected a distinct bias for the use of TCRs with the V$_\beta$8 and V$_\alpha$2.3 variable region subtypes and the C$_\beta$1 constant region subtype. Others have reported subgroups of individuals who have sarcoidosis with expression in blood or lung of one or more of a number of V$_\beta$ gene families (V$_\beta$2, 3, 5, 6, 8, 14, 15, 16, 18, 19) (9,47–49). These findings suggest that T-cell activation in sarcoidosis is not a nonspecific process. Instead, the lymphocytosis appears to be a local oligoclonal response associated with a polyclonal expansion of T cells occurring in reaction to exposure to a conventional antigen that is not cleared from the lower respiratory tract.

The majority of T cells in sarcoidosis lesions express α and β TCR proteins (e.g., they are $\alpha\beta$ T lymphocytes). However, a subgroup of individuals with sarcoidosis has been reported in whom the BAL fluid T lymphocytes contain $\gamma\delta$ TCRs. This observation is quite interesting because $\gamma\delta$ T cells may play an important role in the cellular immune response to mycobacterial antigens and mucosal immunity. Immunohistochemical studies, however, have failed to detect $\gamma\delta$ T cells within sarcoid lymph nodes. This discrepancy has not yet been resolved. It may reflect differences in the kinetics of T-cell accumulation because $\gamma\delta$ T cells may be found only at sites of active early alveolitis.

T-Lymphocyte Subsets

Studies of murine, and to a lesser extent human, lymphocytes have demonstrated the existence of subpopulations of cells based on the patterns of cytokines that they produce. Two major subpopulations of CD4 (and other) lymphocytes have been noted—Th1 and Th2 cells. Th1 cells produce IFN-γ and IL-2, cytokines that are important regulators of macrophage function. Th1 cells mediate delayed-type hypersensitivity responses. In contrast, Th2 cells express IL-4, IL-5, and IL-13, cytokines that are important in antibody-mediated responses, IgE class switching, and eosinophilia. Th2 cells are mediators of humorally mediated and eosinophil-mediated disorders, such as atopy and allergy. These lymphocyte subsets also cross-regulate each other, with Th1 cell-derived IFN-γ down-regulating the cytokine production and proliferation of Th2 cells, and Th2-derived IL-4 and IL-10 having similar inhibitory effects on Th1 cells. In addition, the macrophage-derived cytokines IL-10 and IL-12 play an important role in the regulation of these processes, with IL-12 augmenting Th1 responses and IL-10 augmenting Th2 responses.

The Th1-Th2 paradigm provides a theoretic explanation for why cell-mediated immunity predominates in some circumstances, whereas antibody-based responses predominate in others. A variety of lines of evidence suggest that the ratio of Th1 to Th2 cells plays an important role in defining the clinical pattern of sarcoidosis. Many experimental models of granulomatous disease are Th1-mediated and IFN-γ–dependent, emphasizing the importance of Th1 skewing in pathogenesis (50). In addition, studies of BAL fluid from patients with active sarcoidosis have demonstrated increased levels of the Th1 cytokines IFN-γ, IL-2, and IL-12, and often low or undetectable levels of the Th2 cytokines IL-4, IL-5, and IL-10. Similarly, T cells from the lungs of patients with sarcoidosis produce exaggerated amounts of IL-2 and IFN-γ (9,45,46,51,52). As a consequence, active sarcoidosis is now viewed as a Th1-dominated inflammatory disorder. This may, however, not apply to all stages of the disorder because Th2 cytokines have been detected in some patients, and a Th1-to-Th2 shift has been postulated to lead to granuloma resolution with or without fibrosis in this disorder (9,53,54).

Monocytes/Macrophages

Monocytes, macrophages, epithelioid cells, and giant cells are important participants in the inflammatory process in lung tissue from patients with sarcoidosis. The macrophages appear to be activated *in vivo* because, in contrast to the alveolar macrophages of normal persons, they spontaneously release proinflammatory cytokines, such as IL-1, IL-6, tumor necrosis factor (TNF), IL-8, IL-12, IL-15, RANTES (regulated on activation normal T cell expressed and secreted), granulocyte colony-stimulating factor (G-CSF), and granulocyte-macrophage colony-stimulating factor (GM-CSF). They also secrete increased quantities of 1,25-dihydroxyvitamin D, angiotensin-converting enzyme, and reactive oxygen metabolites, such as hydrogen peroxide (51,55–59). Sarcoid macrophages also have an increased capacity to present antigen in comparison with normal macrophages. This may reflect the increased adhesiveness of sarcoid macrophages and lymphocytes. In accord with this concept, sarcoid alveolar macrophages express increased amounts of the cellular surface adhesion molecules leukocyte function–associated antigen-1 (LFA-1) and intercellular adhesion molecule-1 (ICAM-1). In addition to secreting cytokines, these macrophages express cell surface IL-2 receptors and can thus be activated by the IL-2–secreting T cells at sites of inflammation.

Fibroblasts

Investigators are increasingly recognizing the subtleties of fibroblast function in sarcoidosis and other interstitial lung diseases. Traditionally, fibroblasts have been viewed simply as sources of collagen and other extracellular matrix components. The demonstration that IL-1 and TNF regulate fibroblast production of types I and III collagen has added further complexity by showing that dysregulated cytokine production by activated mononuclear cells can lead to fibroblast activation and tissue fibrosis in sarcoidosis. Increasingly, however, a primary immune effector function of fibroblasts is

being appreciated. IL-1 and TNF can induce fibroblast production of a wide variety of cytokines, including IL-6, monocyte chemotactic peptide-1 (MCP-1), IL-8, IL-11, leukemia inhibitory factor, G-CSF, and GM-CSF. IL-6, MCP-1, and the colony-stimulating factors may be particularly important in sarcoidosis. IL-6 activates the acute phase response, B-cell immunoglobulin production, and T-cell proliferation; MCP-1 recruits fresh peripheral blood monocytes to sites of inflammation; and the colony-stimulating factors activate local macrophages. IL-1 and TNF can also increase the adherence of T lymphocytes to lung fibroblasts, a mechanism by which fibroblasts may contribute to the compartmentalized activation of T cells seen in this granulomatous disorder.

Mechanisms of Tissue Inflammation in Sarcoidosis

Inflammatory responses in the sarcoid lung are regulated, at least in part, by a complex network of interacting cytokines. Most of the alveolar macrophages in the lung are derived from circulating blood monocytes. They enter the lung along chemotactic gradients and have a limited but definite capacity to proliferate locally. Sarcoid-inducing infectious agents or antigenic stimuli that reach the lung via the airways are taken up, processed, and presented to T cells in the context of MHC class II. This activates and stimulates the proliferation of CD4+ lymphocytes with appropriate T-cell receptors. These agents also activate resident macrophages to produce TNF, IL-1, IL-6, IL-12, IL-15, transforming growth factor-β (TGF-β), platelet-derived growth factor (PDGF), insulin-like growth factor (IGF), and chemokines such as MCP-1, RANTES, and IFN-γ–inducible protein (IP-10). The chemokines, in conjunction with IL-1, TNF, activated complement fragments, and other chemotactic agents, activate and recruit leukocytes to the lung. This recruitment is at least partially a consequence of cytokine-enhanced expression of endothelial cell adhesion molecules. The cytokines also interact with the antigen-presenting cells (alveolar macrophages and dendritic cells) to activate T lymphocytes. Activated T lymphocytes express high-affinity IL-2 receptors and produce a variety of cytokines, most notably IL-2, IFN-γ, and IL-6. IL-2 and IL-15, as previously noted, act in an autocrine or paracrine fashion to stimulate lymphocyte proliferation. IFN-γ and IL-2 activate local macrophages, and IL-6 contributes to the proliferation and terminal differentiation of B lymphocytes into antibody-producing plasma cells. IL-1, TNF, and presumably other cytokines also stimulate local stromal cells, such as fibroblasts, to produce IL-6, MCP-1, IL-1α, and colony-stimulating factors. These proinflammatory molecules further augment local T-cell and B-cell responses and activate local macrophages. The IL-1, TNF, and IL-6 that are produced also enter the systemic circulation, where they stimulate the production of acute phase proteins and induce fever. In addition, TGF-β, IL-1, PDGF, and IGF may stimulate the fibrotic response; under appropriate circumstances, each can stimulate fibroblast proliferation and collagen production. In addition, in some individuals, a Th1-to-Th2 T-cell shift occurs that augments fibrosis and decreases granulomatous inflammation.

The Kveim-Siltzbach Test

The Kveim-Siltzbach test is a reaction wherein a localized cutaneous nodule develops in a patient with sarcoidosis 2 to 6 weeks after the intradermal injection of an extract of spleen or lymph node from another patient with sarcoidosis (60,61). Biopsy specimens of these Kveim-Siltzbach test lesions exhibit histopathologic similarities to sarcoid granulomas. Moreover, Kveim-Siltzbach lesions and sarcoid granulomas have a similar distribution of CD4$^+$ and CD8$^+$ T cells and a similar distribution of specific V$_\beta$ and T-cell subsets (62). Despite these similarities, the Kveim-Siltzbach reaction cannot be classified as a true immunologic response for several reasons. First, a delayed-type hypersensitivity reaction occurs within 48 to 72 hours and resolves within a week. In contrast, Kveim-Siltzbach nodules develop after 4 to 6 weeks and persist for several months. Second, despite an intensive search, a specific antigen has not been identified in this material. Attempts to induce lymphocytes from patients to proliferate or secrete cytokines after *in vitro* exposure to Kveim material have been largely unrewarding. Unfortunately, Kveim reagent is available at only a few centers, and thus lack of access to the test largely limits its diagnostic utility.

CLINICAL MANIFESTATIONS

The manifestations of sarcoidosis in persons who come to medical attention vary with their ethnic and racial background and the degree to which local medical communities implement chest radiographic screening that detects milder or asymptomatic forms of the disease. Intensive efforts continue at clarifying organ involvement in sarcoidosis, including an organ assessment instrument developed by the steering committee of A Case Control Etiologic Study of Sarcoidosis (ACCESS) in conjunction with the National Heart, Lung, and Blood Institute and the ACCESS clinical centers (63). Sarcoidosis can involve and cause symptoms in virtually any organ in the body. A detailed description of every manifestation is beyond the scope of this chapter. Instead, attention is focused on the major modes of presentation and patterns of organ involvement.

Presentation

As many as 50% of patients with sarcoidosis are asymptomatic at the time of diagnosis. Physicians become aware of these patients as a result of abnormalities noted incidentally on studies, usually chest radiographs, that have been performed for other reasons. Patients who are acutely symptomatic at the time of presentation typically have pulmonary,

TABLE 28.1. FREQUENCY OF SYMPTOMS AT PRESENTATION OF DISEASE

Symptom	Percentage (%)
Asymptomatic	12–50
Systemic	15–40
Fatigue	20–30
Malaise	15
Weight loss	20–30
Fever	15–22
Night sweats	15
Weakness	10
Chills	10–15
Respiratory	15–40
Cough	30–40
Dyspnea	20–30
Sputum production	10–12
Hemoptysis	1–3
Chest pain	15–25
Skin lesions	10–35
Ocular	10–25
Joint	5–17
Neurologic	~5
Cardiac	~5

ocular, dermatologic, or systemic complaints (Table 28.1). Overall, pulmonary symptoms are noted in 15% to 40% of patients presenting with sarcoidosis. Shortness of breath, dyspnea on exertion, cough, and substernal chest pain are common. Between 10% and 32% of patients with sarcoidosis present with skin lesions. Erythema nodosum is seen approximately twice as often as other, more specific skin manifestations and is frequently associated with fever, malaise, and polyarthralgias. The acute presentation of erythema nodosum with fever, polyarthritis, and bilateral hilar adenopathy constitutes Löfgren syndrome. Maculopapular lesions, nodules, and ulcers also can be presenting cutaneous manifestations. Granulomatous infiltration of old scars resulting in swelling, purple discoloration, and occasionally tenderness may cause the patient to seek medical attention. Approximately 10% to 25% of patients present with ocular symptoms, most commonly caused by acute uveitis and consisting of redness of the eye, tearing, cloudy vision, and photophobia. This type of acute ocular involvement is often seen in association with erythema nodosum and bilateral hilar adenopathy. Systemic constitutional symptoms are reported by approximately 40% of patients and are more common in blacks and Asians from the Indian subcontinent. Fever tends to be mild, and weight loss is usually limited to 5 to 15 pounds within the preceding 3 months. However, temperatures as high as 104°F, more severe weight loss, and night sweats, anorexia, fatigue, and myalgias are well described.

Intrathoracic Involvement

Respiratory tract involvement is the most common manifestation of sarcoidosis. Signs and symptoms of respiratory sarcoidosis are present in 90% of patients at some time during the disease (13,64). The true prevalence of respiratory involvement may actually be higher because biopsy specimens from patients with sarcoidosis whose lungs are radiographically and physiologically normal often reveal granulomas. Parenchymal lung involvement and lymph node enlargement are the most common intrathoracic manifestations. Airway disease occurs symptomatically in 20% of patients (65). Clinical pleural disease is uncommon, although well described. Granulomatous vasculitis involving both arteries and veins has been described in patients with sarcoidosis but is generally asymptomatic.

Pulmonary Parenchyma and Intrathoracic Lymph Nodes

By international convention, a staging system for sarcoidosis has been devised based on the appearance of a patient's chest radiograph (Table 28.2). Between 5% and 10% of patients present with stage 0 disease and normal findings on chest radiographs. In these patients, the diagnosis is based on evidence of extrathoracic disease. A high percentage of them have granulomas on lung biopsy, indicating subclinical involvement of the pulmonary parenchyma. Approximately 40% to 60% of patients present with stage I disease (Fig. 28.2A). The chest radiographs of these patients typically demonstrate bilateral hilar lymphadenopathy, with or without paratracheal adenopathy, in the absence of radiographically apparent lung infiltrates. Stage II radiographs are noted in 15% to 30% of patients at the time of diagnosis (Fig. 28.2B). These radiographs demonstrate bilateral hilar adenopathy (with or without paratracheal adenopathy) and associated lung field involvement. The remaining 10% to 15% of patients with sarcoidosis present with stage III radiographs, which show parenchymal lung involvement without evidence of intrathoracic adenopathy (Fig. 28.2C). It should be noted that the severity of lung parenchymal involvement is not indicated by the designation of stages II and III. Physiologic impairment cannot be assumed by classification within these two stages. Patients whose parenchymal involvement is notable for severe pulmonary fibrosis, volume loss, cysts, bullae, and honeycombing are defined as having stage IV disease by most investigators (Fig. 28.2D).

Parenchymal involvement in sarcoidosis can take on a variety of radiographic appearances. It is most commonly symmetric, diffuse and reticular, reticulonodular, or finely nodular in appearance. Symmetric bilateral lesions of the upper lobes or lesions, predominantly in the mid lung fields, are also well documented, as are diffuse alveolar infiltrates. Although unilateral disease, multiple large nodules, and even solitary nodules have been reported, alternative diagnostic possibilities must always be considered when these atypical patterns are noted. When sarcoidosis progresses, the parenchymal infiltrates become coarser and coalesce, with subsequent distortion of the pulmonary architecture. This can cause the development of bronchiectasis, cysts, and bullae. Progressive destruction of the lung parenchyma can result in respiratory failure. In the United States, pulmonary complications are the most common cause of death from sarcoidosis (13,66).

Computed tomography (CT) of the chest is more sensitive than plain chest radiography. Parenchymal abnormalities and occult lymph node enlargement are both more evident by CT. Chest CT is not necessary in the evaluation of patients with abnormalities suggestive of sarcoidosis on simple radiographs. However, in patients with normal chest x-ray findings and atypical presentations in whom the diagnosis of sarcoidosis is entertained, the higher sensitivity of CT in detecting parenchymal and lymph node abnormalities may be useful. It has been suggested that the presence of areas of ground-glass attenuation on high-resolution CT in sarcoidosis and other infiltrative lung diseases may correlate with an inflammatory state likely to be responsive to treatment (67,68). However, like plain chest radiographs, CT cannot definitively confirm the diagnosis.

The architectural distortion that takes place in patients with advanced sarcoidosis predisposes them to a number of complications. Areas of cavitation and bronchiectasis are susceptible to repeated infections. In addition, mycetomas caused by *Aspergillus* (and rarely other fungi) can form in pre-existing cavities and have been reported in as many as 40% of patients with cavitary disease. Progressive pleural thickening in the area around a cavity may be the earliest indication that an aspergilloma is forming. Chest CT is useful in demonstrating these structural abnormalities. The diagnosis requires the presence of immunoglobulin G–precipitating antibodies to the fungus and the demonstration of a mycetoma in the cavity by chest radiography or CT. Although most mycetomas are asymptomatic, they can cause potentially life-threatening hemoptysis. The treatment of patients with mycetoma and massive hemoptysis can be problematic. The presence of the predisposing cavity is usually an indication of underlying advanced lung disease. Surgery has traditionally been the avenue of therapy in such situations. However, underlying respiratory insufficiency precludes surgery for some and increases the risk of surgery for the others. Bronchial arterial embolization or the intracavitary instillation of amphotericin B may be useful, particularly in patients with massive hemoptysis who cannot be treated surgically (69,70). Less commonly, a hypersensitivity reaction may develop to the colonized fungus in patients with mycetoma.

TABLE 28.2. STAGING OF SARCOIDOSIS BY CHEST RADIOGRAPHY

Stage	Radiographic Findings
0	Normal
I	Hilar, mediastinal, or paratracheal adenopathy
II	Hilar, mediastinal, or paratracheal adenopathy with pulmonary parenchymal abnormalities
III	Pulmonary parenchymal abnormalities without adenopathy
IV	Fibrobullous pulmonary parenchymal disease

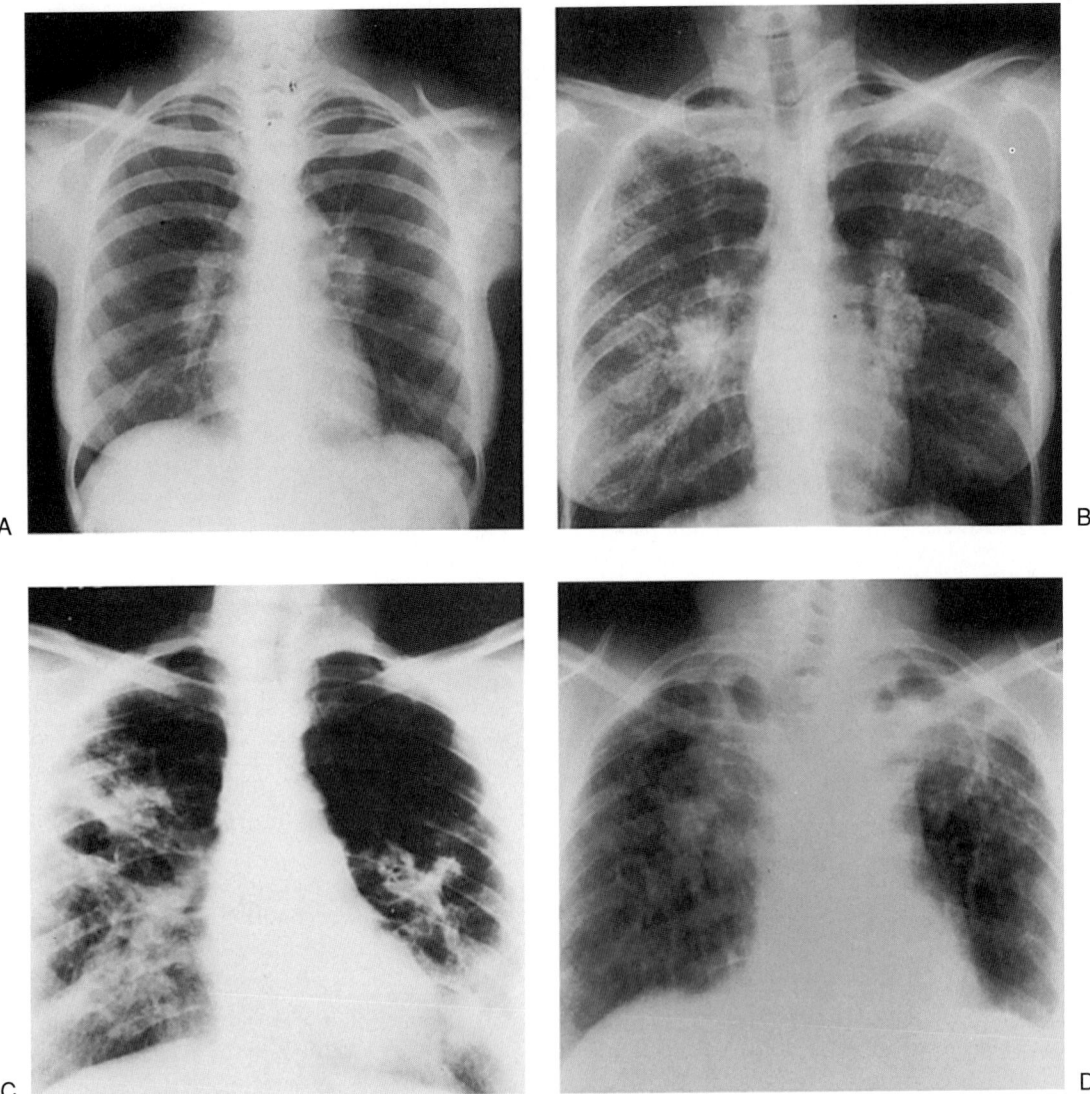

FIGURE 28.2. Radiographs illustrating the different stages of sarcoidosis. **A:** Stage I. Bilateral hilar adenopathy and paratracheal adenopathy with normal lung fields. **B:** Stage II. Bilateral hilar adenopathy with interstitial lung field involvement. **C:** Stage III. Lung field involvement only. **D:** Stage IV. Severely fibrotic lungs with volume loss and cyst formation.

This can be manifested as a bronchospastic disorder with many of the clinical and immunologic characteristics of allergic bronchopulmonary aspergillosis.

Radiographically, bilateral hilar adenopathy is the most common pattern of lymph node involvement in sarcoidosis. This enlargement can be striking, causing some to refer to the lymph nodes as "potato" nodes. Paratracheal adenopathy has been reported in up to 71% of cases. This adenopathy is less common on the left side because the left paratracheal lymph nodes are located more posteriorly, are smaller in size, and are fewer in number than their counterparts on the right. Aortopulmonary window and subcarinal adenopathy can, on rare occasions, cause symptoms by compressing the esophagus and nearby bronchi and vessels. When sarcoidosis causes anterior mediastinal lymph node enlarge-

ment, hilar adenopathy is almost always present. Lymphoma, metastatic malignancy, and other neoplastic conditions must be strongly considered when isolated anterior mediastinal adenopathy is present. Similarly, posterior mediastinal adenopathy and unilateral hilar adenopathy are rare in sarcoidosis and should cause the physician to pursue other etiologic possibilities.

Airways Involvement

Endobronchial biopsy specimens reveal granulomatous infiltration of the airway mucosa and submucosa in 31% to 70% of patients with sarcoidosis. At its mildest, this involvement does not alter the appearance of the bronchial mucosa. When more severe, nodules are seen, described most

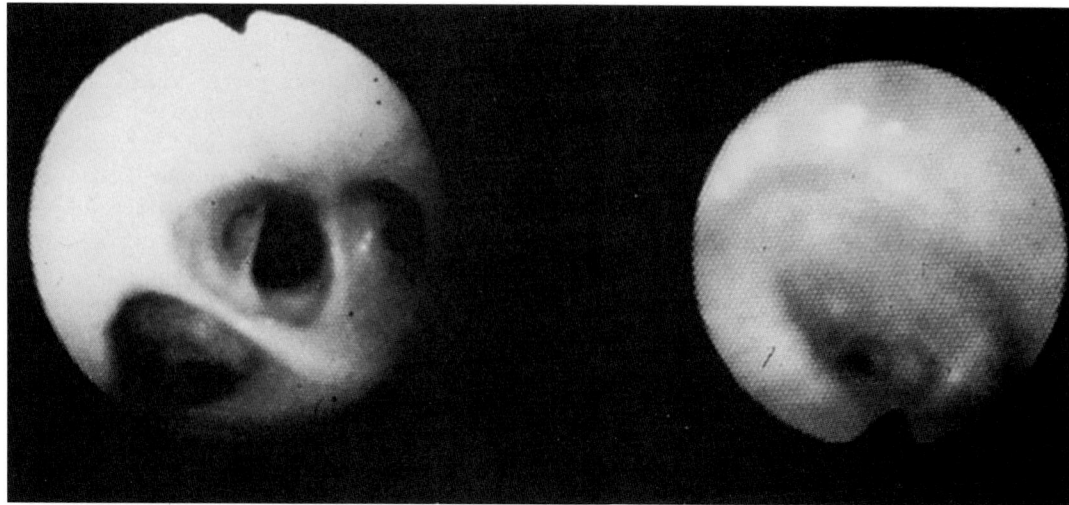

FIGURE 28.3. Comparison of the appearance of a normal endobronchial tree (**left**) and the endobronchial tree of a patient with bronchial stenosis secondary to sarcoidosis (**right**).

frequently as having a "cobblestone" pattern. Up to 20% of patients present with symptoms of airway hyperreactivity, which may mimic asthma (65). As in the interstitium of the lung, granulomatous infiltration in the airways can lead to fibrotic reactions causing fixed lesions. In its most severe form, this may result in bronchial stenosis with bronchial occlusion (71,72) (Fig. 28.3). Endobronchial involvement can be seen in all radiographic stages of the disease. Extrinsic bronchial compression by enlarged lymph nodes and airway architectural distortion resulting from advanced parenchymal fibrosis may also compromise the airway. Such lesions may cause airway narrowing, atelectasis, and ventilation-perfusion mismatching. The clinical manifestations of patients with severe endobronchial involvement often differ from those of the usual patient with parenchymal sarcoidosis. Like patients with asthma, chronic obstructive pulmonary disease, or upper airway obstruction, they may experience dyspnea, stridor, chronic cough, and recurrent episodes of bronchospasm. If bronchial stenosis is present, patients can have repeated episodes of post-stenotic pneumonia and bronchitis, and bronchiectasis may develop (71).

Pleural Involvement

Pleural involvement in sarcoidosis is uncommon, occurring in 2% to 4% of patients (73). This involvement can manifest as pleural thickening, pleural effusion, or spontaneous pneumothorax. Effusions are presumably caused by granulomatous infiltration of the pleura. They are usually small or moderate in size. They occur with equal frequency on the right and left and are bilateral one third of the time. Massive effusions are rare. Vascular compression from mediastinal adenopathy is rarely a cause of pleural effusion in patients with sarcoidosis. The pleural fluid in sarcoidosis can be exudative or transudative and occasionally hemor-

rhagic, and it typically shows a predominance of lymphocytes (74). An increase in eosinophils may also be seen. Effusions have been described in patients with all radiographic stages of sarcoidosis. However, they are more common in patients with widespread parenchymal lung disease and have not been reported as the sole manifestation of disease. A pleural effusion in a patient with sarcoidosis must always be interpreted with caution because this presentation is uncommon. Other causes of pleural disease, including tuberculosis, mycotic or bacterial infections, congestive heart failure, and malignancies, must always be considered. Most sarcoid effusions appear to resolve without residua, either spontaneously or in association with steroid therapy, although progression to chronic pleural thickening has been reported.

Spontaneous pneumothorax in sarcoidosis is usually caused by the rupture of subpleural blebs or by necrosis of subpleural granulomas (75). This occurs most commonly in patients with advanced fibrotic lung disease and upper lobe bullae, but it can also occur in patients with stage 0 or stage I disease.

Upper Respiratory Tract Involvement

Sarcoidosis involves the upper respiratory tract in approximately 2% to 6% of patients. Although occasionally seen in an isolated form, upper respiratory tract involvement is most common in symptomatic patients with manifestations of chronic sarcoidosis, including lupus pernio. The nasal mucosa, pharynx, larynx, nasal bones, and palate can all be involved. Sarcoidosis causes the nasal mucosa to appear erythematous and granular. Epistaxis, stuffiness, crusting, and nasal discharge are common symptoms. In addition, adhesions, polypoid lesions, submucosal nodules, ulcerations, septal perforations, paranasal sinus extension, osteolytic destruction of the nasal bone, and saddle-nose deformities have all been described. In the absence of evidence of sarcoidosis at another site, biopsies of the nasal turbinate can be performed to differentiate sarcoidosis from other nasal disorders.

Pulmonary Physiology

It is well recognized that the presence of chest radiographic abnormalities does not necessarily imply impairment of pulmonary function. Like most other interstitial lung diseases, sarcoidosis, when it involves the pulmonary parenchyma, usually causes a restrictive physiology, manifested by reduced lung volumes and abnormalities in gas exchange (measured by the diffusing capacity of the lung for carbon monoxide [D_{LCO}]) in the absence of abnormalities in large-airway function. Dysfunction of large and small airways resulting from the peribronchial distribution of granulomas may also be clinically evident in patients with sarcoidosis (76). Large-airways obstruction with a decrease in the ratio of the forced expiratory volume in 1 second to the forced vital capacity (FEV_1/FVC ratio) is noted in a minority of patients. It has been described in all radiographic stages of sarcoidosis but is more common in patients with stage III or IV disease. It is usually a consequence of bronchial distortion or bronchiectasis resulting from granulomas, edema, and scarring. Symptoms of wheezing and dyspnea may develop. Some patients may demonstrate bronchial hyperresponsiveness, but large-airway obstruction related to fibrocystic disease, bronchiectasis, or bronchial stenosis is usually irreversible.

Patients with normal or mildly abnormal results on pulmonary function testing usually have normal alveolar-arterial oxygen gradients and arterial blood gas values and normal results on cardiopulmonary exercise testing. Occasionally, exercise testing unmasks modest physiologic abnormalities, even in patients with stage 0 or stage I sarcoidosis. As the disease worsens, the alveolar-arterial oxygen gradient at rest increases. This is followed by exercise-induced oxygen desaturation and then hypoxia at rest. Carbon dioxide retention is uncommon; if noted, it almost always accompanies advanced disease, often with incipient respiratory failure.

The fact that some patients with stage 0 or stage I disease by chest radiography have restrictive physiology demonstrates that pulmonary function tests are more sensitive than chest radiographs in detecting parenchymal lung disease. Increases in the alveolar-arterial oxygen gradient with exercise may be the most sensitive physiologic parameter, followed by the D_{LCO} and vital capacity (56,77). Overall, the degree of physiologic impairment in sarcoidosis correlates somewhat with the radiographic stage of disease. Patients with stage 0 or stage I disease usually have at most mild physiologic derangements, whereas patients with stage IV disease tend to be the most severely restricted (or obstructed). However, the overlap between these categories is large enough to make it difficult and not clinically useful to predict a given patient's pulmonary function from the radiographic stage, with the possible exception of patients with stage IV radiographs.

Studies of structure-function relationships in sarcoidosis have shown that pulmonary function test results generally correlate with the overall severity of the morphologic changes on lung biopsy specimens. Patients with normal or minimally abnormal pulmonary function tend to have mild inflammatory changes with minimal fibrosis on biopsy specimens. Patients with severely abnormal pulmonary function tend to have more extensive inflammatory changes, severe fibrotic changes, or both on biopsy specimens. However, these studies have also shown that the correlation between physiologic abnormalities and pulmonary histology has limitations. Pulmonary function tests may differentiate the extremes of histology but do not accurately differentiate moderate from severe disease. In addition, pulmonary function tests do not indicate the degree to which a defect is caused by interstitial pneumonitis, granulomas, or fibrosis. Thus, for a given patient at a single point in time, pulmonary function tests cannot predict with absolute certainty the severity, character, or reversibility of the histologic lesion that is present. Nevertheless, studies of the natural history of sarcoidosis have demonstrated that pulmonary physiologic alterations over time tend to correlate with changes in the severity and activity of disease. When a patient's parenchymal lesions improve roentgenographically, the vital capacity and diffusing capacity usually also improve. Similarly, when a patient's parenchymal sarcoidosis is radiographically stable or worsening, a decline in the vital capacity, diffusing capacity, or both also usually occurs. The correlations between histologic severity, disease progression, and pulmonary function provide the rationale for the use of pulmonary function tests in the ongoing evaluation of patients with sarcoidosis. It is important to point out, however, that at the present time, no pulmonary function criteria are available that allow the clinician to predict accurately the natural history or response to therapy of a given patient.

Extrathoracic Manifestations

Ophthalmic Features

In 1936, the Heerfordt syndrome of uveitis, salivary gland involvement, seventh cranial nerve palsy, and fever was recognized to be a form of sarcoidosis. Subsequent studies have shown that the eye and its adnexa are involved in 11% to 83% of patients with sarcoidosis (78). Ocular involvement is an important cause of morbidity in this disorder (79). The types of ocular disease noted in patients with sarcoidosis can be classified according to whether they involve the anterior eye, the posterior eye, or the orbit and other structures.

The anterior structures of the eye are involved in 80% to 90% of patients with ophthalmic sarcoidosis. Granulomatous uveitis and granulomatous conjunctivitis are the two most common lesions. Iris nodules, band keratopathy, and interstitial keratitis occur far less frequently. Granulomatous uveitis can be acute or chronic. Patients with acute uveitis can experience the sudden onset of unilateral optic injection, with tearing, blurred vision, and photophobia. Physical examination often reveals circumcorneal ciliary injection, aqueous cells and flares, and "mutton fat" keratitic precipitates. In contrast, chronic uveitis develops more slowly and insidiously. It may be unilateral or bilateral, and when symptomatic, it usually causes pain and blurring of vision. Although keratitic precipitates are often noted, ciliary injection can be absent. Chronic uveitis can lead to adhesions between the iris and lens, glaucoma, cataract formation, and blindness. Chronic uveitis is often seen in association with other manifestations of chronic sarcoidosis, such as lupus pernio, cutaneous plaques, bone lesions, and pulmonary fibrosis. Granulomatous involvement of the conjunctivae occurs in 10% to 60% of patients with ophthalmic sarcoidosis. These conjunctival lesions can appear as tiny, translucent, pale yellow conjunctival follicles. Biopsy specimens of normal-appearing conjunctivae also can show granulomatous inflammation. This involvement can be asymptomatic or cause irritation, resulting in a gritty feeling in the eye.

The posterior structures of the eye are involved in approximately 25% of patients with ocular sarcoidosis. The retina, vitreous, and optic nerve can all be affected. Chorioretinitis, periphlebitis, and chorioretinal nodules are the most frequent lesions. Periphlebitis may be associated with visible evidence of lymphocytic infiltration of the venous walls ("candle wax drippings"). Cellular aggregates (particularly CD4$^+$ T lymphocytes), hemorrhage and opacities in the vitreous, and local neovascularization are less common. Optic nerve involvement in sarcoidosis can take a number of forms and indicates involvement of the nervous system. Papilledema resulting from increased intracranial pressure, optic atrophy, papillitis, optic neuritis, and optic disc granulomas are all well documented. Ninety-five percent of patients with posterior eye involvement also have anterior eye involvement. In addition, the presence of posterior eye involvement should alert the clinician to possible concomitant central nervous system disease because the incidence of central nervous system involvement is increased in these patients.

Granulomatous infiltration of the lacrimal gland is the most common form of orbital involvement, occurring in 5% to 15% of patients with ocular sarcoidosis. It is usually bilateral, often associated with parotid swelling, and can be the sole ocular manifestation. Chronic mass effect from extralacrimal soft tissue involvement may also be seen. Hyposecretion of tears may occur with any of these and can cause a severe sicca syndrome mimicking Sjögren syndrome. Retroorbital granulomas are a less common orbital manifestation of sarcoidosis that have been reported to cause unilateral proptosis and hamper extraocular muscle function.

Lymphadenopathy

Granulomatous infiltration of the lymph nodes is found in up to 95% of patients with sarcoidosis. Although the disease can be solely microscopic, granulomatous involvement may cause palpable adenopathy that is usually symmetric and rarely massive. The nodes tend to be discrete, mobile, and painless and are rarely associated with changes in the overlying skin, ulceration, or sinus formation. All major lymph node groups can be involved. Cervical, axillary, epitrochlear, and inguinal lymphadenopathy may occur in the order noted. The preauricular, postauricular, submaxillary, submental, mesenteric, and retroperitoneal nodes also can be enlarged. Occipital lymphadenopathy is rare. Rarely, massive involvement of retroperitoneal or abdominal lymph nodes can cause abdominal discomfort sufficient to warrant systemic therapy.

Cutaneous Involvement

Skin involvement is seen in 20% to 50% of patients with sarcoidosis and can be divided into two categories: nonspecific, nongranulomatous lesions and specific, granulomatous lesions. Erythema nodosum is the principal nongranulomatous skin lesion, usually occurring in the setting of acute sarcoidosis. Most commonly, it presents as subcutaneous, erythematous, tender, raised nodules that involve the anterior tibial and other extensor surfaces. The onset is usually sudden, and its appearance may herald the beginning of the disease. It may be accompanied by a flulike syndrome with fever, fatigue, polyarthralgia, and bilateral hilar adenopathy (Löfgren syndrome) (80). In addition, it often presents in association with acute uveitis and an elevated sedimentation rate. As the lesions of erythema nodosum resolve, they become ecchymotic (erythema contusiformis) and can leave localized areas of hyperpigmentation. Biopsy specimens of erythema nodosum reveal a septal panniculitis. Erythema nodosum is not specific for sarcoidosis. The clinical picture and histology of erythema nodosum associated with sarcoidosis are indistinguishable from those of erythema nodosum associated with other diseases. However, the presence of erythema nodosum in sarcoidosis appears to have prognostic value. Patients presenting with Löfgren syndrome have a particularly favorable outcome, with at least 90% experiencing a spontaneous resolution of their disease within 6 to 12 months. In addition, in Caucasian patients, the presence of erythema nodosum may correlate with a better prognosis (81).

Granulomatous skin lesions occur in 10% to 35% of patients with sarcoidosis. In general, their presence confers an unfavorable prognosis, suggests a higher likelihood of extensive disease, and may warrant local or systemic treatment. Lupus pernio is a granulomatous lesion that is specific for sarcoidosis and portends a chronic course. It presents as a violaceous, nodular, or plaquelike eruption on the nose, cheeks, and ears (Fig. 28.4) and can be associated with fusiform swelling and mutilation of the fingers. Its onset is usually insidious and the course usually chronic. Lupus pernio can result in significant scarring and deformity. It is more common in African American women between 40 and 60 years of

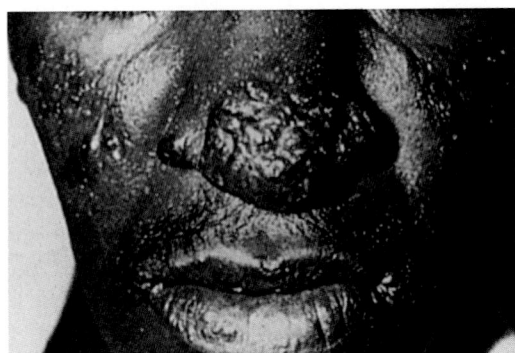

FIGURE 28.4. Raised lesions of lupus pernio.

age and often associated with other manifestations of chronic sarcoidosis, such as pulmonary fibrosis, bone lesions, uveitis, and upper respiratory tract involvement (78,81). Granulomatous infiltration also may cause papules, plaques, nodules, ulcers, ichthyosiform lesions, psoriasis-like lesions, and scarring alopecia.

Neurologic Involvement

Sarcoidosis causes clinically detectable nervous system disease in about 5% of patients (79,82–85). Autopsy studies have shown that subclinical nervous system infiltration occurs in about 14% of patients (86). Of patients with clinical neurosarcoidosis, 50% to 75% have neurologic manifestations as the presenting feature. Multiple neurologic lesions are present in one third of patients. Any structure in the central or peripheral nervous system may be involved, resulting in a wide spectrum of clinical disease. Neurosarcoidosis may cause significant morbidity. It is also associated with a 10% mortality rate, which is approximately twice that of sarcoidosis in general.

Basilar granulomatous meningitis is the most common pathologic lesion in the central nervous system of patients with sarcoidosis. It is clinically apparent in approximately two thirds of patients with neurosarcoidosis and pathologically present in virtually all patients with central nervous system involvement. The predilection for the base of the brain explains the frequent involvement of the cranial nerves, optic chiasm, pituitary, hypothalamus, and periventricular areas. Granulomatous basilar meningitis also can extend along the perivascular space and disrupt the local parenchyma and vascular structures. Meningeal symptoms occur in up to 26% of patients with sarcoidosis (85). In these patients, examination of the cerebrospinal fluid generally shows an elevated protein level and a lymphocytic pleocytosis. In most cases, the glucose levels in the cerebrospinal fluid are normal, but hyperglycorrhachia is described in a minority of patients. Oligoclonal banding can be present (87). Cerebrospinal fluid levels of angiotensin-converting enzyme may be elevated but must be interpreted with caution because similar elevations of angiotensin-converting enzyme may be found in the set-ting of bacterial meningitis and tumors of the central nervous system.

Cranial nerve involvement has been reported in approximately half of patients with neurosarcoidosis. Seventh (facial) nerve involvement is the most common neurologic manifestation of sarcoidosis. It usually presents as a unilateral peripheral lesion but may also occur bilaterally or in association with other cranial nerve abnormalities. The resulting palsy generally resolves spontaneously, but relapses can occur and result in sequelae such as spasms and contractions. The optic nerve is the next most frequently involved cranial nerve; symptoms and signs include decreased or blurred vision, papilledema, optic atrophy, visual field defects, and pupillary abnormalities. Visual evoked potentials may be abnormal in an asymptomatic patient with optic nerve involvement. Cranial nerves IX and X are the next most commonly involved cranial nerve complex in sarcoidosis; their involvement results in dysphagia, hoarseness, an absent gag reflex, an immobile soft palate, and vocal cord dysfunction. The eighth cranial nerve is less commonly affected; involvement can cause deafness, vertigo, and sensory-neural hearing loss.

Peripheral nerve involvement has been noted in approximately 15% of patients with neurosarcoidosis, presenting as a mononeuropathy or polyneuropathy with sensory or motor abnormalities. As a result, pain, paresthesias, muscle weakness, and depression of the tendon reflexes may be found. A Guillain-Barré–like syndrome has also been described.

Hypothalamic-pituitary abnormalities have been noted in approximately 25% of patients with neurosarcoidosis (88). These patients manifest signs and symptoms related to anterior pituitary insufficiency, abnormalities of water metabolism, and compression or infiltration of the nearby optic chiasm. The pituitary and hypothalamus can be separately involved. Most studies show extensive infiltration or mass lesions in the hypothalamus, with a lesser degree of pituitary involvement. Central diabetes insipidus is the most common manifestation of hypothalamic sarcoidosis. Hypothalamic hyperphagia has also been described. Anterior pituitary insufficiency most commonly presents as gonadal dysfunction, with decreased libido, impotence, or amenorrhea, and less commonly as hypothyroidism or adrenal insufficiency. Many of these patients have elevated prolactin levels and normal pituitary responses to hypothalamic releasing hormones, suggesting that the hypothalamus and hypothalamic stalk are the major sites of involvement. The abnormal water metabolism found in most patients with hypothalamic-pituitary sarcoidosis appears to be of multifactorial origin. In some patients, it is the result of partial or complete diabetes insipidus. Other patients appear to have primary abnormalities of thirst. Either or both of these abnormalities may result in chronic hypernatremia.

Granulomatous masses may involve any part of the central nervous system. Whereas most of these are diffuse or infiltrating, some present as space-occupying lesions. The clinical presentation of these lesions is similar to that of mass lesions caused by other processes and can include headaches, seizures, localized neurologic dysfunction, papilledema, and uncal or cerebellar tonsillar herniation. Vascular compromise, manifested as strokes or transient ischemic attacks, rarely occurs in sarcoidosis. This is surprising because perivascular and vascular infiltration of the meningeal and cerebral vessels, often with local infarction, is well described pathologically. Spinal cord involvement is also extremely rare in sarcoidosis; when present, it is caused by local meningeal involvement with extramedullary compression or intramedullary mass formation.

The symptoms that result from central nervous system lesions in sarcoidosis can vary depending on the anatomic site of the infiltrative process and the degree to which intracranial pressure is increased. Increased intracranial pressure can cause headache, nausea, vomiting, lethargy, and cranial nerve palsies. Cortical infiltration can mimic cerebrovascular accidents, and basal ganglion involvement can lead to a wide range of extrapyramidal manifestations, including choreiform movements, hemiballismus, and parkinsonism. Seizures occur in 5% to 22% of patients with neurologic sarcoidosis. Grand mal seizures are most common, but partial, jacksonian, psychomotor, and myoclonic seizures can occur. The presence of seizures is generally associated with a poor prognosis.

The diagnosis of neurosarcoidosis is usually facilitated by evidence of sarcoidosis in other organs. Compatible neurologic findings supported by CT, magnetic resonance imaging (MRI), or cerebrospinal fluid data in the setting of histologic confirmation in other tissues may be adequate for diagnostic purposes (89). Gadolinium-enhanced MRI is currently the preferred diagnostic radiographic procedure for the evaluation of sarcoidosis of the brain and spine (13). The need to obtain nerve tissue may arise in situations in which other etiologies cannot adequately be excluded. In particular, the diagnosis of isolated nervous system sarcoidosis in the absence of other manifestations of sarcoidosis may be extremely difficult.

Hepatic Involvement

Although one can document histologic liver involvement in up to 90% of patients with sarcoidosis, clinically significant hepatic disease is infrequent. Small periportal granulomas are noted most commonly. A nonspecific mononuclear cell infiltrate with varying degrees of fibrosis can also be seen. The majority of patients are asymptomatic and have only low-grade increases in levels of serum alkaline phosphatase, transaminases, or bilirubin. Modest hepatomegaly may be found in a minority of patients. More serious involvement may take the form of chronic hepatocellular injury with secondary cirrhosis, hepatic encephalopathy, portal hypertension, or bleeding esophageal varices. Cases of Budd-Chiari syndrome have been reported. Sarcoidosis may also be associated with chronic intrahepatic cholestasis, which can be difficult to differentiate from primary biliary cirrhosis, and with extrahepatic biliary tract obstruction resulting from granulomatous involvement of the hepatic duct and surrounding lymph nodes.

Hepatic sarcoidosis may also present as fever of unknown origin (90). In patients with hepatic sarcoidosis presenting as fever of unknown origin, the spleen and lymph nodes are also frequently involved.

Splenic Involvement

Like granulomatous infiltration of the liver, granulomatous infiltration of the spleen occurs commonly in patients with sarcoidosis but is usually clinically silent. Splenomegaly develops in 5% to 15% of patients; in a minority of these, complications such as thrombocytopenia, splenic rupture, and abdominal pain develop. Sarcoidosis is only one of many disorders that cause splenic granulomas. Thus, it is important to interpret splenic granulomas in the clinical context in which they are noted.

Cardiac Involvement

Although the most common cardiac presentation of sarcoidosis is secondary cor pulmonale related to severe parenchymal pulmonary disease, primary involvement of the heart does occur. Clinical involvement of the heart is seen in approximately 5% of patients with sarcoidosis (23,24,85,91). At autopsy, granulomas can be found in up to 30% of patients with sarcoidosis. All parts of the heart are susceptible to granulomatous infiltration. The myocardium is most frequently involved, especially the left ventricular free wall (24). In decreasing order of frequency, the ventricular septum, right ventricular free wall, and atria are the areas affected next most often. When the left ventricle is involved, the granulomas are most commonly located in the papillary muscles and the free wall below the papillary muscles. The extent of infiltration and scarring and their proximity to vital structures such as the atrioventricular node and conduction pathways appear to be crucial determinants of the clinical significance of cardiac involvement. The abnormalities that result from these lesions are quite varied and include arrhythmias, conduction system disease, congestive heart failure, mitral regurgitation, ventricular aneurysms, pericardial effusions, and sudden death.

Ventricular tachycardia is the most frequent major arrhythmia in patients with cardiac sarcoidosis. Its appearance usually indicates extensive inflammatory scarring of the heart, although arrhythmias can present in the absence of clinical cardiomyopathy. Ventricular fibrillation and atrial arrhythmias are less commonly noted. When atrial arrhythmias develop, they are usually the result of atrial dilatation arising from left ventricular dysfunction, not the direct result of granulomatous infiltration. Complete heart block and bundle branch blocks also occur and are usually caused by involvement of the cephalic portion of the intraventricular septum near the atrioventricular node and conduction bundles, respectively. Up to 65% of deaths from cardiac sarcoidosis in the past have been attributed to ventricular dysrhythmia or conduction block (24). Such deaths may now be reduced by the availability of implantable defibrillating devices. However, many patients are still likely to succumb to sudden death because ventricular arrhythmia and conduction block may be the presenting symptoms of cardiac sarcoidosis.

Extensive granulomatous infiltration of the myocardium may cause congestive heart failure. In the absence of evidence of systemic sarcoidosis, progressive cardiac sarcoidosis may be indistinguishable from other causes of nonischemic cardiomyopathy. Valvular disease is uncommon but may also cause congestive heart failure. Mitral regurgitation is well described and may be the result of papillary muscle dysfunction caused by infiltration of the papillary muscle or the left ventricular free wall below the papillary muscle. More often, mitral regurgitation is the result of alterations in papillary muscle dynamics caused by left ventricular dilatation or dysfunction. Extensive ventricular involvement can cause cardiomyopathy and congestive heart failure. Ventricular aneurysms can also form and may exacerbate heart failure and arrhythmias.

Establishing a clinical diagnosis of cardiac sarcoidosis may be problematic for two reasons (91). First, the clinical manifestations of the disease—chest pain, palpitations, congestive heart failure, electrocardiographic changes, syncope, and lightheadedness—are also manifestations of other, more common cardiac disorders. Second, when sarcoidosis causes cardiac dysfunction, it often does not cause obvious disease in other organ systems. Thus, many patients with cardiac sarcoidosis do not have overt symptomatic lung, eye, or skin involvement that might lead a physician to suspect this disorder.

As many as half of all patients with cardiac sarcoidosis have electrocardiographic abnormalities. Ventricular arrhythmias are evident in up to 22% of patients (92). For this reason, Holter monitoring has been suggested as part of the routine evaluation of patients with sarcoidosis (23). At a minimum, routine electrocardiography should be performed in all patients. Subclinical cardiac dysfunction can occasionally be detected by cardiopulmonary exercise testing. Endomyocardial biopsies are useful when they yield myocardial granulomas, but a nonspecific lymphocytic myocarditis is commonly encountered. In addition, the diagnostic sensitivity of endomyocardial biopsies is likely quite variable, given the patchy distribution of granulomatous changes in the heart and the inability of the procedure to obtain samples from the ventricular free wall, the area of the heart that is most likely to be involved.

Nuclear imaging may be of limited utility in the diagnosis of cardiac sarcoidosis. A pattern of inhomogeneity of thallium 201 uptake in the myocardium of patients with cardiac sarcoidosis has been described, although its sensitivity and specificity are not clearly defined (93,94). Involved areas are visualized as thallium defects at rest, which then disappear with exercise. This "reverse distribution" pattern is the op-

posite of that seen during thallium imaging in patients with ischemic coronary disease.

Cardiac sarcoidosis should be considered in the differential diagnosis of patients, particularly young patients, who present with arrhythmia or cardiomyopathy in the absence of ischemia, coronary artery disease, or other definable etiology. Untreated conduction system disease or arrhythmia carries a risk for sudden death, which can be potentially minimized with antiarrhythmic medications and implantable defibrillating devices and also with corticosteroids. Similarly, cardiomyopathy from extensive infiltrative disease may respond to medical treatment.

In advanced cases of sarcoid cardiomyopathy, transplantation may be a final option (95).

Renal and Endocrine Abnormalities

Up to 10% of patients with sarcoidosis are hypercalcemic (96,97). The hypercalcemia tends to be episodic in patients with acute sarcoidosis and persistent in patients with chronic disease. It can be mild or severe and life-threatening, and in some patients it is the sole reason for treatment with systemic steroids. Hypercalciuria is more common and often asymptomatic. When clinically evident, it can cause nephrolithiasis, nephrocalcinosis, and renal insufficiency.

The hypercalcemia and hypercalciuria related to sarcoidosis are at least partially a consequence of an increase in the intestinal absorption of calcium. This increase is the result of elevated levels of 1,25-dihydroxy vitamin D caused by the accelerated conversion of 25-hydroxyvitamin D to the active form. The increased 1-hydroxylation occurs independently of parathyroid hormone in the macrophages of sarcoid granulomas. Exposure to sunlight worsens the hypercalcemia of these patients. Increased osteolysis also appears to play a role in the calcium disorder seen in some patients with sarcoidosis. The heightened resorption may be a direct effect of osseous granulomas or of bone-resorbing soluble factor(s) such as osteoclast-activating factor. Other endocrine abnormalities related to pituitary and hypothalamic involvement may occur in the setting of neurosarcoidosis.

Renal insufficiency in sarcoidosis is generally the result of hypercalcemia and hypercalciuria. Granulomatous changes in the kidney are noted in 4% to 40% of sarcoid patients but rarely cause clinically significant renal dysfunction. Granulomatous renal arteritis, glomerulonephritis, and altered renal tubular function can occur but are uncommon.

Musculoskeletal Involvement

Joint signs and symptoms occur in approximately 10% to 35% of patients with sarcoidosis. The major manifestations are an acute and chronic polyarthritis. Acute polyarthritis is typically seen early in the course of the disease. It is usually a symmetric peripheral arthritis that most commonly involves the ankles and knees and less commonly the elbows, wrists, and small joints of the hands and feet. Histologically, a nonspecific inflammatory synovitis is noted. The clinical presentation includes pain, tenderness, restriction of motion, and soft tissue swelling. The joint effusions can be transient and occasionally precede other signs of the disease. This form of joint involvement is frequently seen in association with Löfgren syndrome and generally has a high rate of spontaneous remission. The erythrocyte sedimentation rate may be elevated. In the absence of clinical bone involvement, the radiographic findings are usually normal or reveal soft tissue swelling. Rarely, periarticular osteoporosis is noted.

A relapsing chronic polyarthritis develops in only 3% to 6% of patients with chronic sarcoidosis. Some of these patients have had a previous episode of acute sarcoid polyarthritis, but the majority have not. The shoulders, knees, wrists, ankles, and small articulations of the hands are most commonly involved. Erythema nodosum and fever are uncommon. This involvement can be asymmetric and is rarely monarticular. Radiographic studies reveal soft tissue swelling, periarticular osteoporosis, mild narrowing of the joint space, and well-defined eccentric erosions. In addition, articular destruction and collapse may result from inflammatory extension into subchondral bone. Histologically, the process is characterized by granulomatous inflammation of the synovium, articulations, and tendon sheaths. Synovial fluid analysis reveals increases in protein and leukocytes and occasionally a lymphocytosis.

Radiographic osseous involvement occurs in a small fraction of patients and is generally associated with chronic sarcoidosis. It is more common in African Americans than in Caucasians and is rarely seen without chronic cutaneous lesions (such as lupus pernio), ocular sarcoidosis, and overt lung involvement. Radiographically, sarcoidosis can affect the skeleton in a focal or generalized and usually asymmetric fashion and can cause both osteolytic and, less commonly, osteosclerotic lesions. In all cases, these lesions are not specific for sarcoidosis, radiographically resembling the lesions of other diseases. Osteoporosis, cortical thinning, and well-defined cysts are most common and are usually encountered in the hands; the wrists and feet are less often involved. When diffuse, they can cause a latticework or honeycomb pattern. In general, they are not associated with periosteal reactions or sinus tracts, and the joints are not involved except when bone adjacent to the joint is destroyed. Osseous sarcoidosis is generally asymptomatic except in cases in which soft tissue swelling or bony deformity causes local symptoms. The prognosis for the small number of patients with progressive destructive bony changes is poor because these lesions tend to be unresponsive to treatment.

Hematologic Manifestations

The hematologic manifestations of sarcoidosis include anemia, lymphopenia, eosinophilia, and thrombocytopenia. Of these, peripheral lymphopenia is the most common, occurring in more than half of patients with active disease. However, the T lymphocytes appear to be distributed to active sites. For example, the BAL fluid typically exhibits an increased number of $CD4^+$ T cells while the peripheral blood simultaneously shows a low $CD4^+$ T-cell count (42,98). Examination of the bone marrow may reveal granulomatous infiltration as the cause of cytopenia (99).

ESTABLISHING THE DIAGNOSIS

To establish the diagnosis of sarcoidosis, three criteria must ideally be met: (a) The patient's clinical and radiographic presentation must be compatible with sarcoidosis, (b) a biopsy specimen must demonstrate noncaseating epithelioid cell granulomas, and (c) other causes of granulomatous infiltration must be carefully excluded.

The ease with which the first criterion is met is variable because the clinical presentation of sarcoidosis can be protean, depending on the type and extent of organ involvement. In some cases, the clinical scenario may strongly suggest sarcoidosis. For example, when a patient is found to have bilateral hilar adenopathy in the complete absence of symptoms or physical examination abnormalities, it may be felt that the patient is overwhelmingly likely to have sarcoidosis (100). Similarly, a patient presenting acutely with fever, erythema nodosum, arthralgias, and bilateral hilar adenopathy is highly likely to have sarcoidosis with Löfgren syndrome. In such cases, one could argue that a clinical presentation so strongly suggestive of sarcoidosis might justify observation without histologic confirmation. However, the clinical presentation is more subtle or complicated in most cases, and the diagnosis of sarcoidosis must then be more firmly established. In particular, if treatment with parenteral corticosteroids is anticipated, tissue confirmation of disease should ideally be sought.

Tissue biopsy specimens can be obtained from a number of sites in the body. The optimal site from which to take a specimen depends on the clinical manifestations, the accessibility of an affected site, and the procedures that are performed proficiently at a given institution. The gold standard procedure is surgical lung biopsy (open lung biopsy or video-assisted thoracoscopic biopsy), which yields noncaseating granulomas in more than 90% of patients. Mediastinoscopy in patients with sarcoidosis and mediastinal adenopathy also has a high sensitivity. However, these procedures are invasive and associated with a small but well-recognized incidence of serious complications. Bronchoscopy with transbronchial biopsy is often the procedure of first choice. Because granulomas tend to congregate in the peribronchial area, the diagnostic yield of transbronchial biopsy is high (101). When the procedure is performed with topical anesthesia in an awake patient, it causes minimal discomfort, and the risk for major complications (e.g., pneumothorax, bleeding, respiratory distress) is low. At least four transbronchial biopsy specimens are necessary to obtain an adequate diagnostic yield by bronchoscopy (102). Transbronchial biopsy specimens demonstrate granulomatous inflammation in 70% to

90% of patients with stage I disease, 85% to 95% of patients with stage II disease, and 80% to 90% of patients with stage III disease. The diagnostic yield is more limited in patients with advanced disease because such patients are likely to have fibrotic changes rather than granulomatous inflammation. Bronchoscopy is advantageous in that other specimens can also be collected for cytologic and microbiologic examination, which may help to rule out various conditions. Additionally, many patients demonstrate endobronchial disease with a "cobblestone" appearance to the airway mucosa. Biopsy specimens from these areas may also demonstrate granulomas.

Biopsy of easily accessible sites such as the skin, conjunctivae, salivary glands, and lacrimal glands may also reveal the diagnosis. Skin biopsy is useful only when the skin is clinically involved by lesions other than erythema nodosum. Biopsy specimens of erythema nodosum lesions do not demonstrate granulomatous inflammation and provide no histologic confirmation of the diagnosis. Similarly, specimens of the conjunctivae and salivary and lacrimal glands provide a reasonable yield only if disease is clinically evident in these sites.

The third criterion for diagnosing sarcoidosis is the exclusion of other causes of granulomatous inflammation (Table 28.3). A whole host of infectious, inflammatory, and neoplastic diseases, mostly notably mycobacterial infections, fungal infections, berylliosis, hypersensitivity pneumonitis, granulomatous vasculitis, foreign body granulomas, and granulomatous reactions in lymph nodes draining malignancies, all must be considered in the differential diagnosis. Mycobacterial and fungal infections can usually be excluded by appropriate staining and culture of tissue and secretions.

TABLE 28.3. DIFFERENTIAL DIAGNOSIS OF NONCASEATING GRANULOMAS

Infectious diseases
 Mycobacterial infection
 Fungal disease
 Leprosy
 Syphilis
 Catscratch disease
 Parasitic infection
Inflammatory diseases
 Sarcoidosis
 Berylliosis
 Hypersensitivity pneumonitis
 Granulomatous vasculitides
 Eosinophilic granuloma
 Foreign body reactions
 Biliary cirrhosis
 Crohn disease
Neoplastic diseases
 Lymphoma
 Carcinoma
Other
 Hypogammaglobulinemia

In addition, although up to 50% of patients with sarcoidosis are anergic, patients usually demonstrate cutaneous sensitivity to tuberculin when infected with *Mycobacterium tuberculosis*. A thorough history is essential when berylliosis and hypersensitivity pneumonitis are being considered. The beryllium-induced lymphocyte transformation assay may be used to make a diagnosis of berylliosis. If hypersensitivity pneumonitis is a possibility, the availability of immunoglobulin G–precipitating antibodies to the suspected causal antigen should be investigated. Histologic examination should be adequate to rule out the granulomatous vasculitides, foreign body granulomas, or malignancies. If uncertainty remains, a biopsy specimen from a second site may be required.

The finding of hepatic granulomas is nonspecific and must be considered within the clinical context because it may be impossible to differentiate with confidence chronic intrahepatic cholestasis caused by sarcoidosis from primary biliary cirrhosis. Assays for serum antimitochondrial antibodies can be helpful in these cases because they are positive in 99% of patients with primary biliary cirrhosis and usually negative in sarcoidosis. In addition, the demonstration of extrahepatic granulomas can be used to support a diagnosis of sarcoidosis.

Crohn disease can be difficult to differentiate from sarcoidosis. Both are characterized by the presence of noncaseating granulomas and may be associated with similar dermatologic, hepatic, and ocular lesions. In addition, patients with Crohn disease may have abnormalities on pulmonary function tests and increased numbers of CD4$^+$ T lymphocytes in BAL fluid. At present, these two diseases are probably best distinguished on the basis of clinical differences. Crohn disease is usually localized to the digestive tract. In contrast, sarcoidosis is a systemic disease in which digestive tract manifestations are relatively uncommon.

Gallium 67 scanning, the measurement of serum angiotensin-converting enzyme levels, and BAL with analysis of the recovered cell populations are not sufficiently sensitive or specific to be used alone to establish the diagnosis. Results of gallium scans are positive in two thirds of patients with sarcoidosis, but gallium uptake is increased in many other inflammatory lung disorders. Whereas gallium uptake in the parotid, salivary, and lacrimal glands ("panda" pattern) has been postulated to be helpful in diagnosing sarcoidosis, specificity is lacking (103–107). Serum levels of angiotensin-converting enzyme are elevated in 30% to 80% of patients with sarcoidosis (108). Angiotensin-converting enzyme levels can also be elevated in a wide spectrum of granulomatous and nongranulomatous disorders (Table 28.4), so that the specificity of angiotensin-converting enzyme levels is inadequate for diagnostic purposes. Cell profiles in BAL fluid are also not specific for sarcoidosis and as yet have no role in the clinical arena for either the diagnosis or monitoring of disease (109).

A positive Kveim-Siltzbach test result is felt to be specific for sarcoidosis (110). The test is performed by injecting a

TABLE 28.4. SELECTED DISEASES IN WHICH ELEVATED SERUM LEVELS OF ANGIOTENSIN-CONVERTING ENZYME HAVE BEEN REPORTED

Sarcoidosis
Mycobacterial infection
Histoplasmosis
Lymphoma
Berylliosis
Gaucher disease
Leprosy
Amyloidosis
Multiple myeloma
Farmer's lung
Hyperthyroidism
Alcoholic hepatitis
Silicosis

sterile suspension of sarcoid tissue intradermally. In patients who have sarcoidosis, a nodule forms at the site of the injection in 2 to 6 weeks. The test is then completed by taking a biopsy sample of the nodule and demonstrating that it contains noncaseating granulomas. With properly standardized extract, the test is sensitive and specific for sarcoidosis. However, the result is positive most often in patients with typical sarcoidosis, and the test is far less sensitive in patients with atypical presentations, in whom additional diagnostic studies must be performed. In addition, the test delays a diagnosis by 2 to 6 weeks. Kveim biopsy findings can be difficult to interpret, and patients cannot receive corticosteroid therapy until the test is completed. At present, the lack of readily available standardized antigen extract and the availability of other reliable diagnostic procedures markedly reduce the utility of the Kveim-Siltzbach test.

ASSESSMENT AND DIAGNOSIS

The extent and severity of organ involvement in sarcoidosis must be assessed when the disease is first diagnosed and periodically thereafter. The assessment must be tailored to the individual patient. However, a number of tests should be considered for all patients (Table 28.5). A complete blood cell count and platelet count provide information about the

TABLE 28.5. INITIAL ASSESSMENT IN SARCOIDOSIS

Chest radiography
Complete blood cell count
Serum chemistries: calcium, blood urea nitrogen/creatinine, liver enzymes
Urinalysis
24-Hour urine collection for calcium excretion
Electrocardiography
Tuberculin skin test
Pulmonary function tests
Ophthalmologic examination

patient's hematologic profile. The serum calcium, creatinine, and liver enzyme levels and the blood urea nitrogen should be checked because sarcoidosis can cause hypercalcemia, renal dysfunction, and asymptomatic liver disease. A 24-hour urine calcium collection should be performed to look for hypercalciuria. Periodic chest x-ray studies and pulmonary function testing help to assess a patient's lung involvement. Initial pulmonary function testing should include spirometry, lung volumes, and diffusing capacity. Patients without obstructive physiology can be followed with serial measurements of the vital capacity and diffusing capacity. Tuberculin skin testing should be performed routinely because sarcoidosis and tuberculosis often mimic each other. An electrocardiogram is the minimum initial screening for cardiac involvement in patients without cardiac symptoms. Periodic ophthalmologic slit lamp examinations should be obtained regardless of whether ocular signs or symptoms are present. These tests may be repeated as indicated in monitoring or assessing the therapeutic response.

The majority of patients with sarcoidosis have a good prognosis. In approximately two thirds of patients, the disease resolves spontaneously with minor or no residua. In the other third, the disease smolders or worsens. A number of variables appear to have prognostic value. Those that correlate with a good prognosis include an acute presentation (e.g., Löfgren syndrome), erythema nodosum, acute iritis, a stage I radiograph, and the absence of manifestations of extrathoracic disease. Poor prognostic variables include an insidious disease presentation, African ancestry, a stage III or IV chest radiograph, progressive pulmonary disease, bone involvement, lupus pernio, chronic uveitis, upper respiratory tract or nasal involvement, cor pulmonale, nephrocalcinosis, neurosarcoidosis, and cardiac sarcoidosis. The genetic background also may have prognostic import. For example, African Americans are more likely than whites to present with features of chronic extrapulmonary involvement (81,103,111,112). Overall, 15% to 20% of patients suffer permanent loss of lung function, and approximately 5% die of complications related to sarcoidosis. These deaths are most commonly caused by respiratory failure with cor pulmonale and right-sided heart failure. Hemoptysis secondary to bronchiectasis or aspergillomas, arrhythmias or cardiomyopathy resulting from cardiac involvement, nervous system involvement, and renal failure are less common causes of death from sarcoidosis.

A rough correlation has been found between the radiographic stage and the course of intrathoracic disease (13). Patients with stage I disease have the best prognosis, with approximately 55% to 90% experiencing spontaneous radiographic resolution within 1 to 5 years. Approximately 10% of these patients maintain stage I radiographs for a long time, and 15% to 30% progress to stage II to stage IV disease. Patients presenting with stage II radiographs have a somewhat less favorable prognosis. Approximately 40% to 70% of these patients experience a spontaneous radiographic resolution or remission. The remainder have a chronic stage II radiograph or progress to stage III or stage IV disease. Patients with stage III radiographs have a worse prognosis, with spontaneous radiographic resolution occurring in only 10% to 20% of cases. The remaining patients usually maintain their stage III radiographs, with 5% to 10% progressing to stage IV disease.

The monitoring of disease activity in sarcoidosis has relied on an assessment of the clinical status and physiologic measurements of affected organs. For instance, in lung disease, chest radiographs and pulmonary function tests have been the objective tests usually employed. Disease activity is felt to reflect ongoing granulomatous inflammation. Inflammatory lesions may be reversible, whereas fibrotic lesions are not. Chronic inflammation in sarcoidosis has also been postulated to lead to tissue fibrosis. As a result, it has been assumed that treatment decisions might be made on a more rational basis and patients' responses to antiinflammatory agents might be predicted more accurately if patients with active inflammation could be differentiated from those with largely fibrotic disease. This would allow the physician to identify and treat aggressively the patients at greatest risk for the development of tissue fibrosis and most likely to benefit from the therapeutic intervention. It would also allow the physician to avoid steroid-induced side effects in patients likely to improve spontaneously or not respond to steroid therapy. Unfortunately, objective measurements of inflammation are notably lacking. Several tests have been proposed as potentially reliable but have not proved to be so. The best-known and most readily available of these is the serum angiotensin-converting enzyme level, which tends to correlate with the extent of granulomatous inflammation (108). However, angiotensin-converting enzyme levels can be extremely variable and have not proved to be reliable indicators of disease activity (113). Similarly, other biochemical parameters, including serum lysozyme, soluble IL-2 receptors, and β_2-microglobulin, have not proved to be consistent monitors of disease. BAL fluid cell profiles were felt to be potential indicators of disease activity based on patterns reflecting the degree of alveolitis in sarcoidosis. However, a wide variability of findings related to BAL fluid and a lack of correlation between BAL fluid cell counts or cytokine profiles, clinical abnormalities, and long-term outcomes have been shown in many studies (13,98,109,114–116). Consequently, enthusiasm for the use of BAL measurements as predictors of disease activity has waned.

Thus, an assessment of disease activity in sarcoidosis remains one of clinical evaluation. Effort continues to be directed at identifying objective measurements of inflammation in serum and BAL fluid. It is clear that at some centers and in some patients, these assays, used in serial fashion, have been useful in assessing the prognosis and predicting the therapeutic response. However, the conflicting reports in the literature reflect either a true lack of utility of these tests or differences in the patient populations studied. For the present, disease assessment will continue to rely on the traditional criteria of clinical symptoms and accepted biochemical and physiologic parameters.

TREATMENT

It is not necessary to treat all patients with sarcoidosis. Decisions regarding treatment must be individualized and are best based on specific manifestations of the disease and the clinical course of a given patient.

Extrapulmonary Disease

It is generally agreed that systemic therapy with corticosteroids is indicated for any patient with life- or organ-threatening disease, and for any patient with refractory or progressive organ involvement or symptoms that have not responded to topical or symptomatic therapy. Of the many extrapulmonary forms of disease, cardiac sarcoidosis and neurosarcoidosis in particular are felt to warrant aggressive treatment with corticosteroids. Some of the indications for treatment in extrapulmonary sarcoidosis, in addition to alternatives to corticosteroids, are listed in Table 28.6. Unfortunately, no results of large randomized prospective studies are available on which to base treatment decisions for patients with severe or progressive sarcoidosis. Because the disease can spontaneously remit, some of the "successes" with systemic corticosteroids may be properly attributed not to treatment but to the natural course of the disease. The British Thoracic Society performed a prospective study of 149 patients who had stage II or III sarcoidosis, with the intent of addressing the issue of whether corticosteroids are of benefit in sarcoidosis (117). This study excluded patients who were felt to require corticosteroids for either extrapulmonary sarcoidosis or other pulmonary conditions. One hundred forty-nine patients were enrolled. During a 6-month run-in period before randomization, 33 patients were excluded because of progressive pulmonary disease felt to warrant corticosteroids, and 58 more patients were excluded because of spontaneous remission. The remaining 58 were randomized to treatment or observation and followed for an average of 5 years. Acknowledging that the number of patients left for analysis was small, the study concluded that prolonged treatment with corticosteroids yielded a small but definite advantage in radiographic, functional, and symptomatic measurements. This study and many others highlight several points relevant to the treatment of sarcoidosis. First, a period of observation in patients not felt to require urgent therapy is important for identifying those patients whose disease will spontaneously remit and not require treatment and those whose condition will stabilize or progress and for whom treatment should be considered. Second, corticosteroid treatment is considered standard therapy, even in the absence of randomized controlled trials proving this to be so. The patients in this study

TABLE 28.6. EXTRAPULMONARY SARCOIDOSIS: OPTIONS FOR SYSTEMIC TREATMENT

Affected Organ/Disorder	Clinical Findings	Treatment Options (in Addition to Corticosteroids)
Heart	Arrhythmias, conduction blocks, congestive heart failure	Antiarrhythmics, pacemaker, implantable defibrillating devices should be used when indicated.
Eye	Anterior or posterior chamber involvement	Topical steroids alone may be adequate for anterior disease.
Endocrine	Hypercalcemia, hypercalciuria	Hydration, reduction in calcium and vitamin D intake, and avoidance of sunlight may be sufficient treatment. Ketoconazole may be useful.
Nervous system	Variable	Systemic corticosteroid treatment is usually indicated. Surgical treatment may be necessary in some situations (e.g., for diagnosis of mass lesions, or for hydrocephalus).
Spleen	Cytopenias, massive splenomegaly	Surgery may be indicated for massive splenomegaly.
Pituitary/hypothalamus	Diabetes insipidus, pituitary insufficiency	Hormone replacement, clinical management of water replacement.
Liver	Elevation in transaminases	Patients with asymptomatic elevations in liver transaminases do not require treatment.
Skin	Lupus pernio, skin infiltration with symptomatic or disfiguring lesions	Systemic treatment is indicated if condition is unresponsive to topical or intralesional treatment. Hydroxychloroquine, methotrexate, or thalidomide may be useful.
Musculoskeletal	Acute or chronic polyarthritis	Treatment with antiinflammatory agents is usually adequate and should be tried before parenteral steroids are given.

who were felt to have unstable disease were uniformly offered corticosteroid treatment. Third, a study proposing to enroll, monitor, and follow patients for many years faces formidable challenges. In all likelihood, the answer to the question of whether corticosteroids are truly beneficial in sarcoidosis will not be definitively answered. Because the present "state of the art" is to administer corticosteroids for progressive disease, it seems highly unlikely that a randomized prospective trial of corticosteroid treatment versus observation alone in patients with worsening disease will ever be performed. An extensive literature supports the benefit of corticosteroids, citing such evidence as relief of symptoms, improvements in pulmonary physiologic test results and radiographic findings, and a reduction in measurable disease in extrapulmonary sites (117–122). These benefits presumably reflect the suppression of granulomatous inflammation. However, in some cases, granulomatous disease recurs after treatment is withdrawn, so that treatment must be reinstituted.

The dose of corticosteroids and the duration of treatment should be tailored to the individual patient. When systemic therapy is required for organ-threatening disease, it is usually recommended that treatment be initiated with up to 40 mg of prednisone given orally once each day. Higher initial doses may be required for patients with cardiac sarcoidosis or neurosarcoidosis. Patients should be monitored for a clinical response, which may require 1 to 3 months. At the end of 3 months, the treatment should be reassessed. Patients who have demonstrated no response at this point are unlikely to benefit from continued treatment. Once a clinical response has been achieved, the daily dose can be tapered by 5 to 10 mg monthly. When the daily dose has been reduced to the equivalent of 20 mg of prednisone per day, a schedule of 40 mg on alternate days may be instituted if desired. This dose is slowly tapered, usually over 12 to 18 months, with the rate of taper and ultimate duration of

therapy again tailored to the clinical status of the individual patient. If disease reactivation occurs during dose reduction, the daily or alternate-day dose of prednisone should be increased to the last effective dose, and this dose should be administered for 2 to 3 months before tapering is attempted again. Some patients may require prolonged or even lifelong therapy with low doses of corticosteroids.

It is important to realize that parenteral corticosteroid is not required for all extrapulmonary manifestations of sarcoidosis. Topical steroids are often effective in the treatment of anterior uveitis. Intradermal steroids, hydroxychloroquine, methotrexate, and retinoids may cause sarcoid skin lesions to regress, and nonsteroidal antiinflammatory agents are useful in controlling joint pain and the constitutional symptoms of sarcoidosis. Colchicine may be effective in the treatment of arthralgias related to sarcoidosis. Mild hypercalcemia can often be managed with hydration, a low-calcium diet, and the avoidance of sunlight and vitamin D. Ketoconazole may also be useful in the treatment of hypercalcemia and hypercalciuria because it decreases the synthesis of 1,25-dihydroxyvitamin D.

TREATMENT FOR EXTRAPULMONARY SARCOIDOSIS

Summary Statement	Level of Evidence
Patients with life- or organ-threatening disease should be treated with corticosteroids or appropriate alternate therapy.	Observational studies, consensus recommendations
Alternatives to corticosteroid treatment vary according to the involved site.	Observational studies

Pulmonary Disease

The treatment of patients with pulmonary sarcoidosis remains a subject of considerable controversy. Given the variable clinical course, high rate of spontaneous remission, and lack of reliable prognostic indicators, the criteria for initiating and tapering systemic treatment with corticosteroids remain ill-defined. This controversy is fueled by the realization that although steroids cause radiographic and functional improvement, their ability to alter the natural history of sarcoidosis is difficult to document (73,123,124). Some authors advocate treatment of all patients with pulmonary sarcoidosis, regardless of symptoms or physiologic abnormalities. However, most feel that only patients who are symptomatic or whose condition is deteriorating should be treated (13,125). An approach in accordance with this view is summarized as follows:

1. Patients with stage I disease are often asymptomatic and usually have normal or nearly normal pulmonary function. They should be carefully observed with serial chest radiographs and pulmonary function tests initially every 3 months. If the disease progresses radiographically or if pulmonary function declines significantly (15% decrease in lung volumes or diffusing capacity), treatment with steroids should be considered.
2. Patients with stage II or stage III disease, normal or nearly normal pulmonary function, and minimal symptoms should be followed serially and treated if their disease progresses as described for stage I patients. A period of observation is helpful in identifying patients whose disease may regress spontaneously. Conversely, patients whose disease progresses during the observation period should be treated. Patients presenting at the outset with significantly abnormal pulmonary function (lung volumes or diffusing capacity less than 65% of that predicted) may warrant an empiric trial of steroids. The clinical status and pulmonary function should be monitored and chest radiographs obtained periodically. A response to treatment will usually be evident within 1 to 3 months. If no improvement is seen after 3 months of treatment, it is unlikely that continued medication will be beneficial. Patients with persistent pulmonary function or radiographic abnormalities presumably have irreversible fibrotic changes.
3. Patients presenting with fibrobullous disease (advanced stage III or stage IV) may also warrant an empiric trial of steroids. Although the fibrotic changes are fixed, concomitant pulmonary inflammation may improve significantly with therapy.
4. Patients with severe, end-stage lung disease despite treatment may be candidates for single lung or heart-lung transplantation. Referral to an appropriate transplantation center should be made, preferably before the onset of cor pulmonale.
5. There is little agreement regarding the amount of steroid necessary to treat pulmonary sarcoidosis adequately. Initial doses, the use of daily versus alternate-day regimens,

and schedules for tapering vary among institutions and practitioners. The response (or the lack thereof) of the individual patient largely dictates the regimen. As in extrapulmonary sarcoid, a 40-mg dose of prednisone given every day or every other day can be used from the outset in most cases. The patient is then observed on therapy for up to several months to document improvement or the lack thereof. In patients who appear to respond, the initial dose of prednisone is typically maintained for 3 months and then reduced slowly over months. This usually results in a minimal duration of therapy of about 12 months. In patients who do not respond within the first 3 months, steroids should be tapered and discontinued more rapidly.

Relapses can occur during the treatment period. When this happens, the most recent effective dose should be reinstituted for 2 to 3 months, and then tapering should be reattempted. A minority of patients require lifelong steroid therapy, usually at relatively low doses. In other cases, the disease remits, only to reactivate years later. For these reasons, most patients with sarcoidosis should remain under observation indefinitely, with periodic reassessments of their disease activity.

CORTICOSTEROID TREATMENT FOR PULMONARY SARCOIDOSIS

Summary Statement	Level of Evidence
Patients with stage I disease often do not require treatment and should be observed for changes in clinical or physiologic parameters.	Observational studies, consensus recommendations
Patients with stage II or III disease without significant clinical or physiologic impairment should initially be observed without treatment to assess stability, remission, or progression.	Observational studies, consensus recommendations
Patients whose disease progresses by clinical or physiologic parameters should be treated with corticosteroids.	Observational studies, consensus recommendations
Patients with significantly abnormal pulmonary function or with advanced stage III or IV disease should be considered for an empiric trial of corticosteroids.	Observational studies, consensus recommendations

Alternative Agents

Inhaled corticosteroids are not indicated for patients with advanced pulmonary parenchymal disease. However, they may be effective in patients with lower respiratory tract symptoms related to endobronchial mucosal inflammation (126,127).

The use of cytotoxic agents in the treatment of sarcoidosis is based largely on uncontrolled studies. These agents may be useful in situations in which corticosteroids are associated with intolerable side effects or in which disease is progressing despite treatment with corticosteroids (128). Methotrexate has been used in low doses (e.g., 7.5–25 mg/wk) with some success, particularly in patients with severe skin involvement or refractory pulmonary disease (129). As in other inflammatory diseases, long-term therapy with methotrexate carries a risk for hepatotoxicity. Methotrexate should not be used in patients with renal insufficiency because the drug is cleared by the kidneys. The concomitant use of nonsteroidal antiinflammatory drugs should be avoided because the combination can cause acute renal dysfunction. Cyclophosphamide and azathioprine have also been used in sarcoidosis, as in other inflammatory diseases, and appear to be of limited value. When these drugs are given, their potential toxicities should be kept in mind. The toxicities can be multiple, so physicians and patients must be aware of possible side effects before such treatment is initiated. Hydroxychloroquine has been used primarily to treat cutaneous sarcoidosis but may also be useful in patients with pulmonary disease (130). Thalidomide and pentoxifylline have been reported to be beneficial in cutaneous and pulmonary sarcoidosis (131–133). The choice between these steroid-sparing alternative therapies should be dictated by the clinician's familiarity with each, the patient's clinical presentation, and their individual side effects. In cases in which active sarcoidosis is not adequately treated with high-dose steroids or in which the patient cannot tolerate steroids because of side effects, a trial of one of these agents may be warranted.

Transplantation

End-stage organ failure may develop in patients with severe sarcoidosis. In such situations, the transplantation of solid organs, including lung, heart, liver, and kidney, has been successfully performed (95). The appearance of noncaseating granulomas in lung and heart allografts after transplantation has been well documented (134–136). This recurrence of disease appears to be specific for patients with sarcoidosis and is not observed in the allografts of patients who have undergone transplantation for other diseases. Fortunately, clinically significant disease caused by recurrent sarcoidosis in the transplanted organ is uncommon. This may in part be a consequence of the uniform use of immunosuppressive agents to prevent transplant rejection. Because sarcoid recurrence in allografts appears to be associated with little in the way of clinical symptoms of organ dysfunction, transplantation remains a viable option for patients with sarcoidosis-induced end-stage organ failure.

REFERENCES

1. Hutchinson J. Case of livid papillary psoriasis. In: *Illustrations of clinical surgery.* London: J and A Churchill, 1877:42.

2. Besnier E. Lupus pernio de la face. *Ann Dermatol Syphilol (Paris)* 1889;10:33–36.

3. Tenneson H. Lupus pernio. *Ann Dermatol Syphilol (Paris)* 1889;10:333–336.

4. Boeck C. Multiple benign sarkoid of the skin. *J Cutan Genital Urinary Dis* 1899;17:543–550.

5. Bittorf A, Kuznitsky E. Boeckches Sarkoid mit Beteiligung innerer. *Organe Munch Med Wochenschr* 1915;62:1349.

6. Schaumann J. Lymphogranuloma benigna in the light of prolonged clinical observations and autopsy findings. *Br J Dermatol* 1936;48:399.

7. Yamamoto M, Sharma OP, Hosoda Y. The 1991 descriptive definition of sarcoidosis. In: Izumi T, ed. Proceedings of the XIIth World Congress on Sarcoidosis. *Sarcoidosis* 1992;[Suppl 1]:33–34.

8. Mandel J, Weinberger SE. Clinical insights and basic science correlates in sarcoidosis. *Am J Med Sci* 2001;321:99–107.

9. Conron M, Du Bois RM. Immunological mechanisms in sarcoidosis. *Clin Exp Allergy* 2001;31:543–554.

10. Vourlekis JS, Sawyer RT, Newman LS. Sarcoidosis: developments in etiology, immunology, and therapeutics. *Adv Intern Med* 2000;45:209–257.

11. Kataria YP, Holter JF. Immunology of sarcoidosis. *Clin Chest Med* 1997;18:719–739.

12. James DG. Descriptive definition and historic aspects of sarcoidosis. *Clin Chest Med* 1997;18:663–667.

13. American Thoracic Society. Statement on sarcoidosis. *Am J Respir Crit Care Med* 1999;160:736–755.

14. Hosoda Y, Yamaguchi M, Hiraga Y. Global epidemiology of sarcoidosis. *Clin Chest Med* 1997;18:681–694.

15. Edmondstone WM, Wilson AG. Sarcoidosis in Caucasians, blacks, and Asians in London. *Br J Dis Chest* 1985;79:27–36.

16. Hillerdal G, Nou E, Osterman K. Sarcoidosis: epidemiology and prognosis. A 15-year European study. *Am Rev Respir Dis* 1984;130:29–32.

17. James DG, Hosoda Y. Epidemiology. In: James DG, ed. *Sarcoidosis and other granulomatous disorders.* New York: Marcel Dekker Inc, 1994.

18. Tierstein AS, Lesser M. Worldwide distribution and epidemiology of sarcoidosis. In: Fanburg BL, ed. *Sarcoidosis and other granulomatous diseases of the lung.* New York: Marcel Dekker Inc, 1983.

19. Henke C, Henke EG, Elveback LR, et al. The epidemiology of sarcoidosis in Rochester, Minnesota: a population-based study of incidence and survival. *Am J Epidemiol* 1986;123:840–845.

20. Siltzbach LE, James DG, Neville E, et al. Course and prognosis of sarcoidosis around the world. *Am J Med* 1974;57:847–853.

21. McNichol MW, Luce PJ. Sarcoidosis in a racially mixed community. *J R Coll Physicians Lond* 1985;19:179–183.

22. Rybicki BA, Major M, Popovich J, et al. Racial differences in sarcoidosis incidence: a 5-year study in a health maintenance organization. *Am J Epidemiol* 1997;145:234–241.

23. Iwai K, Sekiguchi M, Hosoda Y, et al. Racial difference in cardiac sarcoidosis incidence observed at autopsy. *Sarcoidosis* 1994;11:26–31.

24. Roberts WC, McAllister HA, Ferrans VJ. Sarcoidosis of the heart: a clinicopathologic study of 35 necropsy patients (group I) and review of 78 previously described necropsy patients (group II). *Am J Med* 1977;63:86–108.

25. Glennas A, Kvien TK, Melby K, et al. Acute sarcoid arthritis occurrence: seasonal onset, clinical features, and outcome. *Br J Rheumatol* 1995;34:45–50.

26. Harrington DW, Major M, Bytbicki B, et al. Familial sarcoidosis: analysis of 91 families. *Sarcoidosis* 1994;11:240–243.

27. Hills SE, Parkes SA, Baker SB. Epidemiology of sarcoidosis in the Isle of Man: 2. Evidence for space-time clustering. *Thorax* 1987;42:427–430.

28. Parkes SA, Baker SB, Boundillon RE, et al. Epidemiology of sarcoidosis in the Isle of Man: 1. A case controlled study. *Thorax* 1987;42:420–426.

29. Saboor SA, Johnson N, McFadden J. Detection of mycobacterial DNA in sarcoidosis and tuberculosis with polymerase chain reaction. *Lancet* 1992;339:1012–1015.

30. Milman N, Andersen AH. Detection of antibodies in serum against *M. tuberculosis* using Western blot technique: comparison between sarcoidosis patients and healthy subjects. *Sarcoidosis* 1995;10:29–31.

31. Mangiapan G, Hance AJ. Mycobacteria and sarcoidosis: an overview and summary of recent molecular biological data. *Sarcoidosis* 1991;12:20–37.

32. Gerdes J, Richter E, Rusch-Gerdes S. Mycobacterial nucleic acids in sarcoid lesions. *Lancet* 1992;339:1536–1537.

33. Ghossein RA, Ross DG, Salomon N. A search for mycobacterial DNA in sarcoidosis using the polymerase chain reaction. *Am J Clin Pathol* 1994;101:733–737.

34. Ishige I, Usui Y, Takemura T. Quantitative PCR of mycobacterial and propionibacterial DNA in lymph nodes of Japanese patients with sarcoidosis. *Lancet* 1999;354:120–123.

35. Bost TW, Riches DWH, Schumacher B, et al. Alveolar macrophages from patients with beryllium disease and sarcoidosis express increased levels of mRNA for tumor necrosis factor-α and interleukin-6 but not interleukin-1β. *Am J Respir Cell Mol Biol* 1994;10:506–513.

36. Daniele RP, Rossman MD, Kern JA, et al. Pathogenesis of sarcoidosis. *Chest* 1986;89:174S–177S.

37. Elias JA, Freundlich B, Kern JA, et al. Cytokine networks in the regulation of inflammation and fibrosis in the lung. *Chest* 1990;97:1439–1445.

38. Girgis RE, Basha MA, Maliarik M, et al. Cytokines in the bronchoalveolar lavage fluid of patients with active pulmonary sarcoidosis. *Am J Respir Crit Care Med* 1995;152:71–75.

39. Muller-Quernheim J, Saltini C, Sondermeyer P, et al. Compartmentalized activation of the interleukin 2 gene by lung T lymphocytes in active pulmonary sarcoidosis. *J Immunol* 1986;137:3475–3483.

40. Sheffield EA. Pathology of sarcoidosis. *Clin Chest Med* 1997;18:741–754.

41. Groen H, Hamstra M, Aalberst R, et al. Clinical evaluation of lymphocyte subpopulations and oxygen radical production in sarcoidosis and idiopathic pulmonary fibrosis. *Respir Med* 1994;88:55–64.

42. Hunninghake GW, Crystal RG. Pulmonary sarcoidosis: a disorder mediated by excess helper T-lymphocyte activity at sites of disease activity. *N Engl J Med* 1981;305:429–434.

43. Vandenplas O, Depelchin S, Delaunois L, et al. Bronchoalveolar lavage immunoglobulin A and G and antiproteases correlate with changes in diffusion indices during the natural course of pulmonary sarcoidosis. *Eur Respir J* 1994;7:1856–1864.

44. Semenzato G, Agostini C, Chilosi M. Immunology and immunohistology of sarcoidosis. In: James DG, ed. *Sarcoidosis and other granulomatous disorders.* New York: Marcel Dekker Inc, 1994:153–180.

45. Pinkston P, Bitterman PB, Crystal RG. Spontaneous release of IL-2 by lung T-cells in active pulmonary sarcoidosis. *N Engl J Med* 1983;308:793–800.

46. Robinson BSW, McLemore T, et al. IFN-γ is spontaneously released by alveolar macrophages and T-lymphocytes in patients with pulmonary sarcoidosis. *J Clin Invest* 1985;75:1488–1495.

47. Bellocq A, Lecossier D, Pierre-Audigier C. T-cell receptor repertoire of T lymphocytes recovered from the lung and blood of patients with sarcoidosis. *Am J Respir Crit Care Med* 1994;149:646–654.

48. Dubois RM. Sarcoidosis. In: Walters EH, Dubois RM, eds. *Immunology and management of interstitial lung disease.* London: Chapman & Hall, 1995.

49. Jones CM, Lake RA, O'Hehir RE. Oligoclonal V gene usage by T lymphocytes in BAL fluid from sarcoidosis patients. *Am J Respir Crit Care Med* 1996;14:470–477.

50. Gudmundsson G, Hunninghake GW. Interferon-γ is necessary for the expression of hypersensitivity pneumonitis. *J Clin Invest* 1997;99:2386–2390.

51. Agostini C, Trentin L, Facco M. Role of IL-2 and IL-15 and their receptors in the development of T cell alveolitis in sarcoidosis. *J Immunol* 1996;157:910–918.

52. Moller DR, Forman JD, et al. Enhanced expression of IL-12 associated with Th1 cytokine profiles in active pulmonary sarcoidosis. *J Immunol* 1996;156:4952–4960.

53. Kunkel SL, Lukacs NW, et al. Th1 and Th2 responses regulate experimental lung granuloma formation. *Sarcoidosis* 1996;13:120–128.

54. Muller-Quernheim J. Sarcoidosis: immunopathogenic concepts and their clinical application. *Eur Respir J* 1998;12:716–738.

55. Blusse van Oud Alblas A, Von Furth R. Kinetics and characteristics of alveolar macrophages in the normal steady state. *J Exp Med* 1979;149:1504–1518.

56. Athos L, Mohler G, Sharma OP. Exercise testing in the physiologic assessment of sarcoidosis. *Ann N Y Acad Sci* 1986;465:491–501.

57. Devergne O, Marfaing-Koka A, Schall TT. Production of the RANTES chemokine in delayed hypersensitivity reactions. Involvement of the macrophages and epithelial cells. *J Exp Med* 1994;179:1689–1694.

58. Hunninghake GW. Release of interleukin-1 by alveolar macrophages of patients with active pulmonary sarcoidosis. *Am Rev Respir Dis* 1984;129:569–572.

59. Muller-Quernheim J, Pfiefer S, Mannel D, et al. Lung-restricted activation of the alveolar macrophage/monocyte system in pulmonary sarcoidosis. *Am Rev Respir Med* 1992;145:187–192.

60. Kveim A. En ny og spesifikk kuran-reaksjon ved Boecks sarcoid. *Nord Med* 1941;9:169–172.

61. Siltzbach L. The Kveim test in sarcoidosis: a study of 750 patients. *JAMA* 1961;178:476–482.

62. Rochester CL, Elias JA. Cytokines and cytokine networking in the pathogenesis of interstitial and fibrotic lung disorder. *Semin Respir Med* 1993;14:389–415.

63. Judson MA, Baughman RP, Teirstein AS. Defining organ involvement in sarcoidosis: the ACCESS proposed instrument; ACCESS Research Group—a case control etiologic study of sarcoidosis. *Sarcoidosis Vasculitis Diffuse Lung Dis* 1999;16:75–86.

64. Romer FK. Presentation of sarcoidosis and outcome of pulmonary changes. A review of 243 patients followed for up to 10 years. *Dan Med Bull* 1982;29:27–32.

65. Bechtel JJ, Starr TD, Dantzker DR, et al. Airway hyperreactivity in patients with sarcoidosis. *Am Rev Respir Dis* 1981;124:759–761.

66. Gideon NM, Mannino DM. Sarcoidosis mortality in the United States 1979–1991: an analysis of multiple-cause mortality data. *Am J Med* 1885;100:423–427.

67. Remy-Jardin M, Giraud F, Remy J, et al. Pulmonary sarcoidosis: role of CT in the evaluation of disease activity and functional impairment and in prognosis assessment. *Radiology* 1994;191:675–680.

68. Murdoch J, Muller NI. Pulmonary sarcoidosis: changes on follow-up CT examination. *Am J Radiol* 1992;159:473–477.

69. Yamada H, Kohne S, Koga H. Typical treatment of aspergilloma

by antifungals: relationship between disease duration and efficacy of therapy. *Chest* 1993;103:1421–1425.

70. Jackson M, Flower CDR, et al. Treatment of symptomatic aspergillomas with intracavitary instillation of amphotericin B through an indwelling catheter. *Thorax* 1993;48:928–930.

71. Udwadia ZF, Pilling JR, Henkins PF. Bronchoscopic and bronchographic findings in 12 patients with sarcoidosis and severe or progressive airways obstruction. *Thorax* 1990;45:272–275.

72. Westcott JL, DeGraff AC. Sarcoidosis, hilar adenopathy, and pulmonary artery narrowing. *Radiology* 1973;108:585–586.

73. Lynch JP, Kazerooni EA, Gay SE. Pulmonary sarcoidosis. *Clin Chest Med* 1997;18:755–785.

74. Nicholls AJ, Friend JA, Legge JS. Sarcoid pleural effusion: three cases and review of the literature. *Thorax* 1980;35:277–281.

75. Soskel NT, Sharma OP. Pleural involvement in sarcoidosis: case presentation and detailed review of the literature. *Semin Respir Med* 1992;13:492–514.

76. Harrison BDW, Shaylor JM, Stokes TC, et al. Air flow limitation in sarcoidosis—a study of pulmonary function in 107 patients with newly diagnosed disease. *Respir Med* 1991;85:59–64.

77. Keogh BA, Hunninghake GW, Line BR, et al. The alveolitis of pulmonary sarcoidosis: evaluation of natural history and alveolitis-dependent changes in lung function. *Am Rev Respir Dis* 1983;128:256–265.

78. Lynch JP, Sharma OP, Baughman RP. Extrapulmonary sarcoidosis. *Semin Respir Infect* 1998;13:229–254.

79. Constantino T, Digre K, Zimmerman P. Neuro-ophthalmic complications of sarcoidosis. *Semin Neurol* 2000;20:123–137.

80. Lofgren S. Erythema nodosum: studies on etiology and pathogenesis in 185 adult cases. *Acta Med Scand* 1946;124:1–197.

81. Israel HL, Karlin P, Menduke H, et al. Factors affecting outcome of sarcoidosis: influence of race, extrathoracic involvement, and initial radiologic lung lesions. *Ann N Y Acad Sci* 1986;465:609–618.

82. Chapelon C, Ziza JM, Piette JC, et al. Neurosarcoidosis: signs, course and treatment in 35 confirmed cases. *Medicine* 1990;69:261–276.

83. Zajicek JP, Scalding NJ, Foster O, et al. Central nervous system sarcoidosis—diagnosis and management. *QJM* 1999;92:103–117.

84. Nowak DA, Widenka DC. Neurosarcoidosis: a review of its intracranial manifestation. *J Neurol* 2001;248:363–372.

85. Sharma OP. Cardiac and neurologic dysfunction in sarcoidosis. *Clin Chest Med* 1997;18:813–825.

86. Ricker W, Clark M. Sarcoidosis: a clinical pathologic review of 300 cases. *Am J Clin Pathol* 1949;19:725–749.

87. McLean BN, Miller D, Thompson EJ. Oligoclonal banding of IgG in CSF, blood-brain barrier function, and MRI findings in patients with sarcoidosis, systemic lupus erythematosus, and Behçet's disease involving the nervous system. *J Neurol Neurosurg Psychiatry* 1995;58:548–554.

88. Sato N, Gordon S, Jung HK. Cystic pituitary mass in neurosarcoidosis. *AJNR Am J Neuroradiol* 1997;18:1182–1185.

89. Christoforidis GA, Spickler EM, Recio MV, et al. MR of CNS sarcoidosis: correlation of imaging features to clinical symptoms and response to treatment. *AJNR Am J Neuroradiol* 1999;20:655–669.

90. Petersdorf RG. Fever of unknown origin. An old friend revisited. *Arch Intern Med* 1992;152:21–22.

91. Sharma OP. Myocardial sarcoidosis: a wolf in sheep's clothing. *Chest* 1994;106:988–990.

92. Sekiguchi M, Numao Y, Imai M. Clinical and histological results of sarcoidosis for the heart and acute idiopathic myocarditis. Concepts through a study employing myocardial biopsy. *Jpn Circ J* 1980;44:249–263.

93. Kinney EL, Caldwell JW. Do thallium myocardial perfusion scan abnormalities predict survival in sarcoid patients without cardiac symptoms? *Angiology* 1990;41:573–576.

94. Haywood L, Sharma OP, Siegel ME. Detection of myocardial sarcoidosis by thallium-201 imaging. *J Natl Med Assoc* 1983;63:478–482.

95. Scott J, Higenbottom T. Transplantation of the lungs and heart for patients with severe complications from sarcoidosis. *Sarcoidosis* 1990;7:9–11.

96. Goldstein RA, Israel HL, Becker KL, et al. The infrequency of hypercalcemia in sarcoidosis. *Am J Med* 1971;51:21–30.

97. Sharma OP. Vitamin D, calcium, and sarcoidosis. *Chest* 1996;109:535–539.

98. Thomas PD, Hunninghake GW. Current concepts of the pathogenesis of sarcoidosis. *Am Rev Respir Dis* 1987;135:747–760.

99. Browne PM, Sharma OP, Salkin D. Bone marrow sarcoidosis. *JAMA* 1978;240:2654–2655.

100. Winterbauer R, Moores KD. A clinical interpretation of bilateral hilar adenopathy. *Ann Intern Med* 1973;78:65.

101. Koerner SK. Transbronchial lung biopsy for the diagnosis of sarcoidosis. *N Engl J Med* 1975;293:268–270.

102. Gilman MJ, Wang KP. Transbronchial lung biopsy in sarcoidosis: an approach to determine the optimal number of biopsies. *Am Rev Respir Dis* 1980;122:721–724.

103. Johns CJ. Tenth International Conference on Sarcoidosis and Other Granulomatous Disorders, September 17–22, 1984, Baltimore, Maryland. *Ann N Y Acad Sci* 1986;465:1–749.

104. Sulavik SB, Spencer RP, Weed DA, et al. Recognition of distinctive patterns of gallium-67 distribution in sarcoidosis. *J Nucl Med* 1990;31:1909–1914.

105. Israel HL, Albertine KH, et al. Whole body gallium 67 scans: role in diagnosis of sarcoidosis. *Am Rev Respir Dis* 1991;144:1182–1186.

106. Baughman RP, Fernandez M, Bosken CH. Comparison of gallium-67 scanning, bronchoalveolar lavage, and serum angiotensin-converting enzyme levels in pulmonary sarcoidosis: predicting response to therapy. *Am Rev Respir Dis* 1984;129:676–681.

107. Mana J. Nuclear imaging. ^{67}Gallium, ^{201}thallium, ^{18}F-labeled fluoro-2-deoxy-D-glucose positron emission tomography. *Clin Chest Med* 1997;18:799–811.

108. Lieberman J. Elevation of serum angiotensin-converting enzyme (ACE) level in sarcoidosis. *Am J Med* 1975;59:365–372.

109. Nagai S, Izumi T. Bronchoalveolar lavage. Still useful in diagnosing sarcoidosis? *Clin Chest Med* 1997;18:787–797.

110. Hirsch JG, Cohen ZA, Morse SI. Evaluation of the Kveim reaction as a diagnostic test for sarcoidosis. *N Engl J Med* 1961;265:827–830.

111. Neville E, Walker AN, James DG. Prognosis factors predicting the outcome of sarcoidosis: an analysis of 818 patients. *Q J Med* 1983;52:525–533.

112. Johns CJ, Schonfeld SA, Scott PP, et al. Longitudinal study of chronic sarcoidosis with low-dose maintenance corticosteroid therapy: outcome and complications. *Ann N Y Acad Sci* 1986;465:702–712.

113. Costabel U, Bois RD, Eklund A. Consensus conference: activity of sarcoidosis. *Sarcoidosis* 1994;11:27–33.

114. Foley NM, Coral AP, Tung K. Bronchoalveolar lavage cell counts as a predictor of short-term outcome in pulmonary sarcoidosis. *Thorax* 1989;44:732–738.

115. BAL Cooperative Group. Bronchoalveolar lavage constituents in healthy individuals, idiopathic pulmonary fibrosis, and selected comparison groups. *Am Rev Respir Dis* 1990;141:S169.

116. Turner-Warwick M, McAllister W, Lawrence R. Corticosteroid treatment in pulmonary sarcoidosis: do serial lavage lymphocyte

counts, serum angiotensin-converting enzyme measurements and gallium-67 scans help management? *Thorax* 1986;41:903–913.

117. Gibson GJ, Prescott RJ, Muers MF, et al. British Thoracic Society Sarcoidosis Study: effects of long-term corticosteroid treatment. *Thorax* 1996;51:238–247.

118. Siltzbach LE. Effects of cortisone in sarcoidosis: a study of 13 patients. *Am J Med* 1952;22:139–160.

119. Israel HL, Fouts DW, Beggs RA. A controlled trial of prednisone treatment of sarcoidosis. *Am Rev Respir Dis* 1973;107:609–614.

120. Young RL, Harkleroad LE, Lordon RE, et al. Pulmonary sarcoidosis: a prospective evaluation of glucocorticoid therapy. *Ann Intern Med* 1971;73:207–212.

121. Harkleroad LE, Young RL, Savage PI, et al. Pulmonary sarcoidosis: long-term follow-up of the effects of steroid therapy. *Chest* 1982;82:84–87.

122. Johns CJ, Zachary JB, Ball WC. A ten-year study of corticosteroid treatment of pulmonary sarcoidosis. *Johns Hopkins Med J* 1974;134:271–283.

123. Winterbauer RH, Kirtland SH, Corley DE. Treatment with corticosteroids. *Clin Chest Med* 1997;18:843–851.

124. Lynch JP III, McCune WJ. Immunosuppressive and cytotoxic pharmacotherapy for pulmonary disorders: state of the art. *Am J Respir Crit Care Med* 1997;155:395–420.

125. Judson MA. An approach to the treatment of pulmonary sarcoidosis with corticosteroids: the six phases of treatment. *Chest* 1999;115:1158–1165.

126. Alberts C, Van der Mark TW, Jansen HM. Inhaled budesonide in pulmonary sarcoidosis: a double-blind, placebo-controlled study.

Dutch Study Group on Pulmonary Sarcoidosis. *Eur Respir J* 1995;8:682–688.

127. Selroos OB. Use of budesonide in the treatment of pulmonary sarcoidosis. *Ann N Y Acad Sci* 1986;465:713–721.

128. Baughman RP, Lower EE. Steroid-sparing alternative treatments for sarcoidosis. *Clin Chest Med* 1997;18:853–864.

129. Baughman RP, Winger DB, Lower EE. Methotrexate is steroid-sparing in acute sarcoidosis: results of a double-blind, randomized trial. *Sarcoidosis Vasculitis Diffuse Lung Dis* 2000;17:60–65.

130. Baltzan M, Mehta S, Kirkham TH. Randomized trial of prolonged chloroquine therapy in advanced pulmonary sarcoidosis. *Am J Respir Crit Care Med* 2000;160:192–197.

131. Carlesimo M, Giustini S, Rossi A, et al. Treatment of cutaneous and pulmonary sarcoidosis with thalidomide. *J Am Acad Dermatol* 1995;32:866–869.

132. Zabel P, Entzian P, Dalhoff K, et al. Pentoxifylline in the treatment of sarcoidosis. *Am J Respir Crit Care Med* 1997;155:1665–1669.

133. Baughman RP, Judson MA, Teirstein AS, et al. Thalidomide for chronic sarcoidosis. *Chest* 2002;122:227–232.

134. Martinez F, Orens JB, Deeb M. Recurrence of sarcoidosis following allogenic lung transplantation. *Chest* 1994;106:1597–1599.

135. Johnson BA, Duncan SR, Ohori NF. Recurrence of sarcoidosis in pulmonary allograft recipients. *Am Rev Respir Dis* 1993;148:1373–1377.

136. Nunley DR, Hattler B, Keenan RJ. Lung transplantation for end-stage pulmonary sarcoidosis. *Sarcoidosis Vasculitis Diffuse Lung Dis* 1999;16:93–100.

Bronchiolar Disease and Bronchiolitis Obliterans– Organizing Pneumonia

29

Venerino Poletti ·Marco Chilosi ·Maurizio Zompatori

The bronchiolar diseases emerged as clinical entities distinct from chronic bronchitis and emphysema in the beginning of the 20th century, when Wilhelm Lange (1) introduced the term *bronchiolitis obliterans*. In 1902, immediately after the histopathology had been recognized, Fraenkel (2) described cases of bronchiolitis obliterans caused by nitrogen oxides. Interest in this topic increased notably about 70 years later, when bronchiolar diseases associated with collagen-vascular diseases and transplantation (3,4) were described and a complete categorization of bronchiolitis obliterans–organizing pneumonia (BOOP) was realized (5). More recently, the development of high-resolution computed tomography (HRCT) has underscored the importance of bronchiolar disorders in pulmonary medicine (6,7). These diseases are rare, and evidence derived from well-conducted cohort studies is still lacking. As a result, many uncertainties remain regarding the epidemiology, pathophysiology, and therapy of these disorders.

ANATOMY AND DEFINITION

The bronchioles are small airways without cartilage in their walls. Their diameter is less than 2 to 3 mm. The last purely conducting bronchiole is the terminal bronchiole. Distal to the terminal bronchiole is the gas-exchanging unit of the lung, the acinus, which comprises respiratory bronchioles (with both alveolar and nonalveolar walls), alveolar ducts, and sacs.

Bronchiolitis is a process occurring in and around the membranous and respiratory bronchioles (with sparing of a

V. Poletti, M. Chilosi, and **M. Zompatori:** Dipartimento di Malattie dell'Apparato Respiratorio e del Torace, Ospedale G. B. Morgagni, Forli; Università di Verona, Verona; Università di Parma, Parma, Italy.

considerable portion of the other parenchymal structures), in which inflammatory cells and mesenchymal tissue are both present (8–10). The differences in the distribution and amount of cellular and mesenchymal components from case to case are responsible for the varied histopathologic, radiographic, and clinical aspects of bronchiolitis.

A clinical definition of bronchiolitis remains elusive. The signs and symptoms are nonspecific and variable. The course is usually chronic but may be acute or subacute. Pulmonary function tests frequently show an obstructive impairment but may also be characterized by a restrictive profile; in the early phases, the results of pulmonary function tests can be normal. Specific laboratory markers for bronchiolitis have not yet been identified. HRCT is clinically useful to confirm a suspected bronchiolar lesion (7). HRCT allows the identification of more specific patterns that correlate with the involvement of small airways.

CLASSIFICATION

Two classification schemes are generally used in defining cases of bronchiolitis. A clinical classification categorizes cases according to their proven or presumed etiology, the pulmonary or systemic diseases with which they are often associated, and the portions of the distal airways primarily involved (conducting airways vs. alveolar airways) (Table 29.1). An etiologic classification may remind the physician when to suspect the presence of bronchiolitis; however, a more useful classification scheme is based on the histologic characteristics. The histologic patterns generally correlate better with the radiologic manifestations and natural history of the disease and the response to therapy. The broad spectrum of inflammatory and fibrotic lesions found in bronchiolitis may be stratified in four main histologic patterns (Table 29.2).

TABLE 29.1. CLINICAL CLASSIFICATION OF BRONCHIOLITIS

Bronchiolitis involving the small conducting airways
Inhalation bronchiolitis
   Toxic fumes
   Irritant gases and mineral dusts
   Organic dusts
Infectious and postinfectious bronchiolitis
Drug-induced bronchiolitis
Collagen-vascular disease–associated bronchiolitis
Inflammatory bowel disease–associated bronchiolitis
Post-transplant bronchiolitis
Paraneoplastic pemphigus–associated bronchiolitis
Neuroendocrine cell hyperplasia with bronchiolar fibrosis
Diffuse panbronchiolitis
Cryptogenic bronchiolitis
Miscellanous
   Lysinuric protein intolerance
   Ataxia-telangiectasia
   Familiar form of immunodeficiency
   Immunoglobulin A nephropathy

Organizing pneumonia (bronchiolitis obliterans–organizing pneumonia)
Idiopathic
Focal
Secondary

TABLE 29.2. HISTOPATHOLOGIC CLASSIFICATION OF BRONCHIOLITIS

Cellular bronchiolitis
   Follicular bronchiolitis
   Diffuse panbronchiolitis
Bronchiolitis with inflammatory polyps or bronchiolitis with intraluminal polyps
   Bronchiolitis obliterans–organizing pneumonia (BOOP) pattern
Constrictive (cicatricial) bronchiolitis
   Neuroendocrine hyperplasia and bronchiolar fibrosis
   Bronchiolar loss
Peribronchiolar fibrosis and bronchiolar metaplasia ("lambertosis")

develops first in the respiratory bronchioles and surrounding alveoli and then in the distal membranous bronchioles, characterized by a mural infiltrate of lymphocytes, plasma cells, and histiocytes and by intraluminal aggregates of neutrophils. Most characteristic is the accumulation of foamy macrophages in the walls and lumina of the respiratory bronchioles and adjacent air spaces. Polyps of granulation tissue may partially occlude adjacent bronchiolar or alveolar lumina. Germinal center hyperplasia can be prominent.

Bronchiolitis with Inflammatory Polyps or Bronchiolitis with Intraluminal Polyps

Inflammatory polyps project into the lumina of the membranous and respiratory bronchioles (Fig. 29.2; see also Color Fig. 29.2). These polyps may have a myxoid or pale-staining matrix (rich in acid mucopolysaccharides) in which elongated fibroblasts are embedded, or they may contain collagen fibers.

When adjacent air spaces are also obliterated by the fibroblastic plugs, a characteristic variation in the shape of the pale-staining intraluminal plugs from round to oval to elongated or serpiginous is noted (Fig. 29.3; see also Color

Cellular Bronchiolitis

The structures of the bronchiole show an increased number of inflammatory cells (Fig. 29.1; see also Color Fig. 29.1). A wide spectrum of pathologic changes are observed in cellular bronchiolitis, including necrosis of epithelial and inflammatory cells (bronchiolar mucosal necrosis), submucosal edema or necrosis, neutrophil microabscesses, and germinal center hyperplasia (follicular bronchiolitis).

Diffuse panbronchiolitis (11) is a peculiar morphologic form of cellular bronchiolitis. Severe chronic inflammation

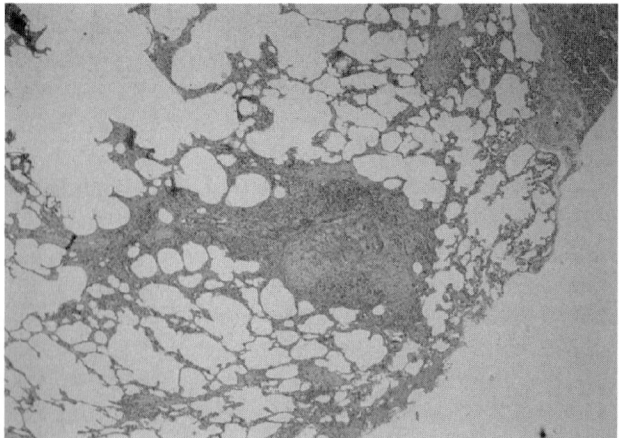

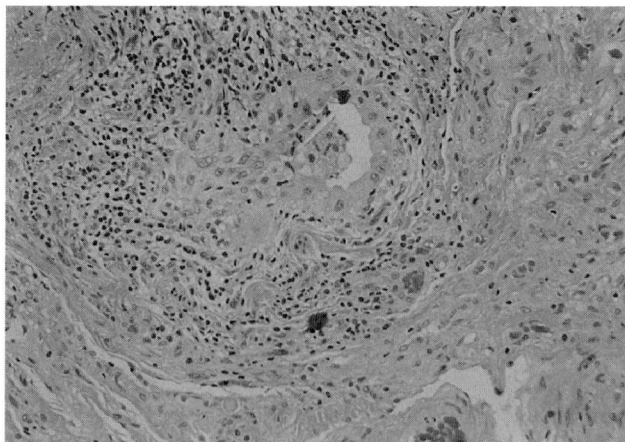

A   B

FIGURE 29.1. (See also Color Fig. 29.1.) Cellular bronchiolitis. **A:** The lumen of a membranous bronchiole is completely obliterated by intraluminal and parietal inflammation (syncytial respiratory virus bronchiolitis; hematoxylin and eosin, low-power magnification). **B:** The bronchiolar wall is widened by the chronic inflammatory infiltrate. Cuboidal metaplasia of the bronchiolar epithelium (bronchiolitis in a case of hypersensitivity pneumonitis; hematoxylin and eosin, mid-power magnification).

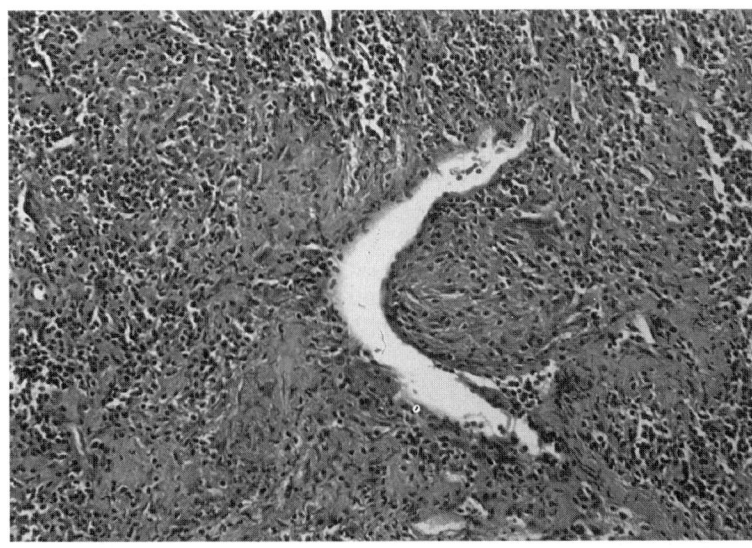

FIGURE 29.2. (See also Color Fig. 29.2.) The lumen of a bronchiole is almost completely occupied by a polyp of granulation tissue (hematoxylin and eosin, mid-power magnification).

Fig. 29.3). This patchy distribution is well-known as *bronchiolitis obliterans–organizing pneumonia.* The surrounding alveolar walls usually show a mild to moderate chronic inflammatory infiltrate with cuboidal alveolar lining cells and foamy intra-alveolar macrophages.

Constrictive or Cicatricial Bronchiolitis

Mural thickening of the membranous bronchioles caused by submucosal collagenization is the morphologic hallmark (Fig. 29.4; see also Color Fig. 29.4). Progressive concentric narrowing is associated with distortion of the lumen, mucus stasis, and patchy chronic inflammation. Bronchiolar ectasis with mucus stasis and bronchiolar smooth muscle hypertrophy may complete the pattern. In some cases, subtle changes or completely distorted and scarred bronchioles can be better appreciated with an elastic tissue stain.

A peculiar form of constrictive bronchiolitis, *neuroendocrine cell hyperplasia with bronchiolar fibrosis,* was reported in 1992 (12). The mildest lesion consists of linear zones of neuroendocrine cell hyperplasia in the bronchiolar mucosa with focal subepithelial fibrosis. In more obvious lesions, a plaque of eccentric fibrous tissue partially occludes the lumen. The most severe stage is characterized by total occlusion of the lumen by fibrous tissue with a few visible neuroendocrine cells (Fig. 29.5; see also Color Fig. 29.5). Small tumors or peripheral carcinoids are frequently observed in the lungs.

Bronchiolar loss (inferred or documented by quantitative methods) results from cicatricial bronchiolitis, which progresses to total fibrous constriction of the bronchioles and their disappearance (9).

Peribronchial Fibrosis and Bronchiolar Metaplasia

Bronchiolar and peribronchiolar scarring is associated with metaplastic bronchiolar epithelium that extends onto the

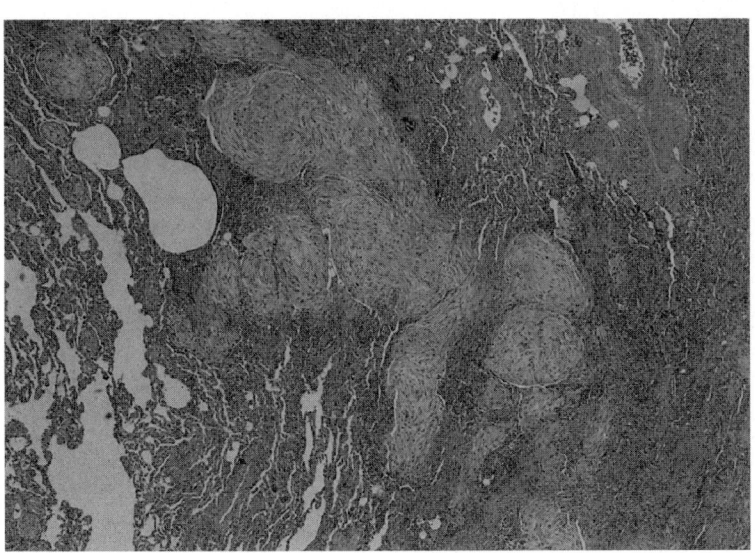

FIGURE 29.3. (See also Color Fig. 29.3.) Bronchiolitis obliterans–organizing pneumonia pattern: serpiginous bundles of pale myxoid material fill the centrilobular air spaces (hematoxylin and eosin, low power magnification).

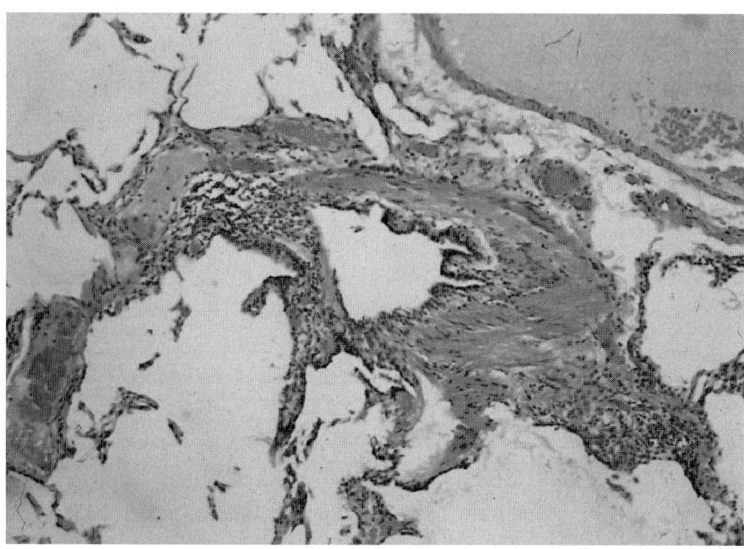

FIGURE 29.4. (See also Color Fig. 29.4.) The lumen of a membranous bronchiole is reduced by concentric acellular fibrosis and scattered intramural inflammatory cells (bronchiolitis obliterans in a patient with graft versus host disease; hematoxylin and eosin, mid-power magnification).

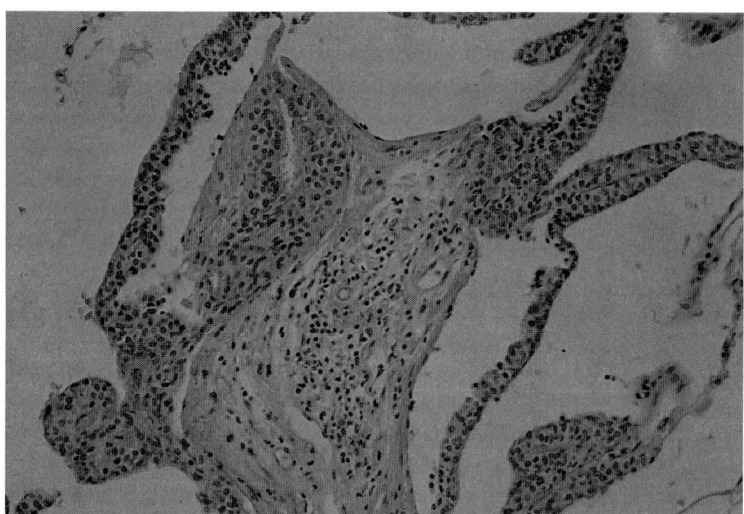

FIGURE 29.5. (See also Color Fig. 29.5.) A scar is all that remains of a former bronchiole. Small neuroendocrine cells proliferate at the periphery (hematoxylin and eosin, mid-power magnification).

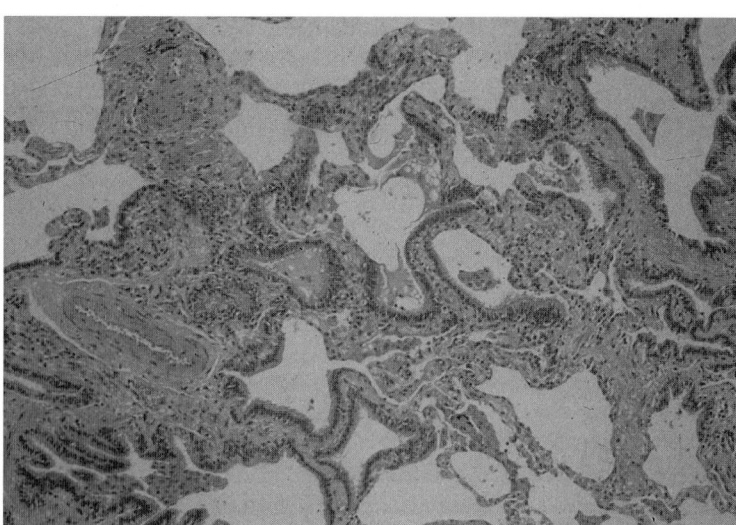

FIGURE 29.6. (See also Color Fig. 29.6.) A bronchiole is evident in the lower left corner. The lumen is slightly reduced, and bronchiolar epithelium extends into the surroundings air spaces ("lambertosis"; hematoxylin and eosin, mid-power magnification).

adjacent fibrotic alveolar walls (so-called lambertosis) (8) (Fig. 29.6; see also Color Fig. 29.6). Inflammatory cells are scanty and usually located in the bronchiolar lumen. In some cases, the pattern consists of respiratory bronchioles that end in multiple fibrous-walled channels covered by cuboidal epithelium, rather than opening into thin-walled alveolar ducts.

RADIOGRAPHIC FINDINGS

The radiographic manifestations of diseases affecting the small airways are manifold (13). The findings range from airways thickened and surrounded by inflammation to manifestations of obstruction at various levels, with or without collateral ventilation. It is evident that the various radiographic patterns can be attributed to bronchiolitis; however, their specificity is low. The chest radiographic findings are often normal in patients with documented bronchiolitis, and the sensitivity of chest radiography in detecting small-airways disease is exceedingly low.

HRCT is currently the best imaging technique for the evaluation of patients suspected of having bronchiolitis. Muller and Miller (7) proposed a classification of the HRCT findings in bronchiolar diseases (Table 29.3). A good correlation between the histopathologic changes and HRCT findings is the basis for this classification.

Centrilobular tubular branching or nodular opacities usually represent abnormal bronchioles filled with fluid, mucus, or pus. This pattern is known as *"tree in bud" opacity* (Fig. 29.7). Poorly defined centrilobular nodular opacities can result from peribronchiolar inflammation or fibrosis. Particularly in cases with an infectious origin, the linear branching and nodules are often accompanied by scattered areas of ground-glass attenuation or consolidation, which reflect the involvement of adjacent alveolar structures and therefore progression to pneumonia.

Ground-glass attenuation (i.e., a hazy increase in opacity that does not obscure normal vessels) or consolidation (i.e., more marked density that obscures vessels) is caused mainly by the alveolar filling that occurs in BOOP (Fig. 29.8).

Mosaic perfusion is caused by decreased vascular perfusion with bronchiolar obstruction and redistribution of flow to normal areas; partial airways obstruction or collateral air drift into the alveoli beyond the obstructed bronchiole typically leads to air trapping, seen best and sometimes only on expiratory scans (dynamic HRCT). Dynamic CT has been

TABLE 29.3. CLASSIFICATION OF HIGH-RESOLUTION COMPUTED TOMOGRAPHIC FINDINGS IN BRONCHIOLAR DISEASES

Centrilobular nodules and branching lines ("tree in bud")
Ground-glass attenuation or alveolar consolidation
Low attenuation (mosaic perfusion) and expiratory air trapping
Mixed patterns

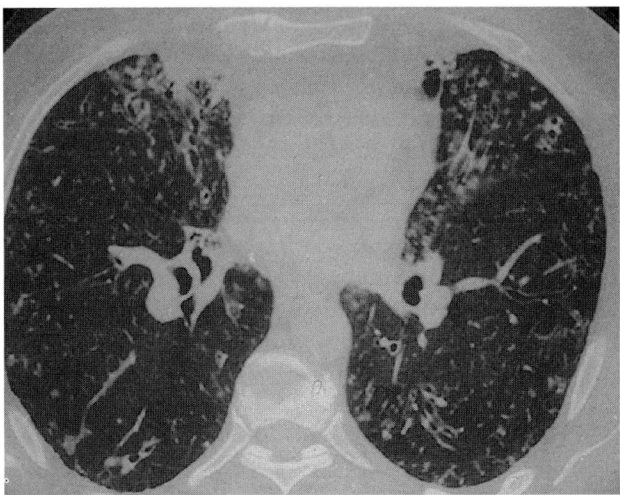

FIGURE 29.7. High-resolution computed tomography. Peripheral centrilobular nodules confluent in the anterior segment of the upper right lobe, dilated bronchioles ("tree in bud" pattern), and peripheral oligemia (diffuse panbronchiolitis).

shown to be more sensitive in detecting regional abnormalities and air trapping (14) (Fig. 29.9). The variations in the attenuation of individual lobules, accentuated when images are obtained after the patient exhales to residual volume, are presumed to be caused by heterogeneous airway involvement that results in patchy airway closure.

A mixed pattern (e.g., a "tree in bud" pattern with mosaic perfusion and expiratory air trapping) can be seen in various entities, such as bronchiectasis and acute bronchopulmonary infections (in particular *Mycoplasma pneumoniae* pneumonia), hypersensitivity pneumonitis, and chronic aspiration (15,16).

Abnormalities of the macroscopic bronchi are a variable feature on HRCT scans but are not unexpected given the anatomic continuity of the macroscopic bronchi

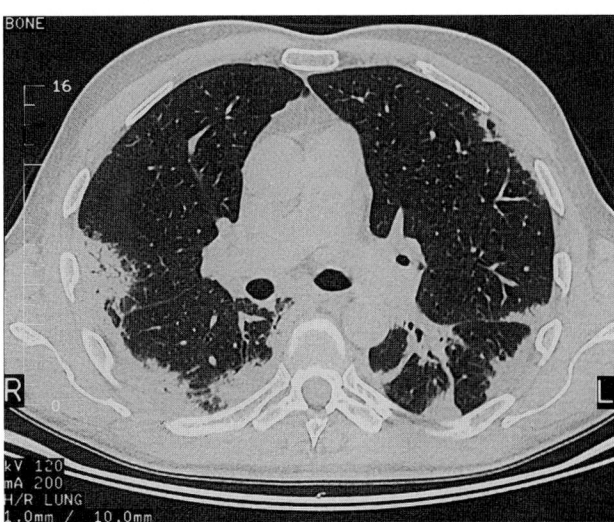

FIGURE 29.8. High-resolution computed tomography. Peripheral subpleural patchy areas of alveolar opacification. Air bronchograms are evident (idiopathic bronchiolitis obliterans–organizing pneumonia).

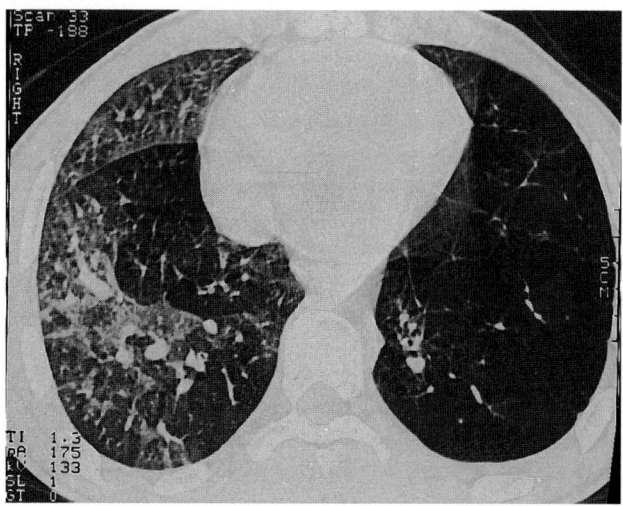

FIGURE 29.9. High-resolution computed tomography. Mosaic oligemia and expiratory air trapping are more evident in the left lung (postinfectious bronchiolitis obliterans).

with the small airways; it appears that bronchial dilatation and bronchial wall thickening are relatively late features of constrictive bronchiolitis and are more frequent in immunologically mediated diseases, such as rheumatoid arthritis, and after transplantation (16).

Ventilation-perfusion scans may be helpful because a markedly abnormal pattern of patchy, matched ventilation-perfusion defects is often seen, even when the plain film is unremarkable (17).

Magnetic resonance imaging with hyperpolarized ^{3}He has made possible the noninvasive reproducible measurement of structure-function relationships in small airways (18).

IMPAIRMENT OF PULMONARY FUNCTION

Pulmonary function tests help to locate the process of inflammation/fibrosis (19). When the membranous bronchioles are involved, an obstructive ventilatory impairment may be evident. Involvement of the "inner area" (between the basement membrane and smooth muscle) of the bronchioles probably correlates best with functional impairment (20). The diffusing capacity is usually normal. The predominant involvement of alveolar structures with relative sparing of the conducting airways is associated with a restrictive ventilatory impairment. In these cases, the diffusing capacity is often reduced.

More sophisticated measurements of small-airways function have been developed (21). Frequency-dependent compliance, density-dependent gas flow studies, measurements of ventilation distribution, and measurements of closing volumes offer more sensitive methods of assessment and may make it possible to identify bronchiolar inflammation or dysfunction earlier. The single-breath washout appears particularly well suited as a screening test because it takes only a few minutes, does not require special operator expertise or patient aptitude, requires only simple equipment, and is noninvasive. However, it is not appropriate for patients with single-lung transplants.

An increased alveolar-arterial oxygen gradient and hypoxemia at rest or during effort are evident in cases in which inflammation/fibrosis is located mainly in the alveolar structures.

SPECIFIC CLINICOPATHOLOGIC FORMS OF DISEASE INVOLVING THE SMALL CONDUCTING AIRWAYS

Bronchiolitis Obliterans Secondary to Inhalation of Irritants

Inhaled gases and fumes can cause severe bronchiolitis with acute ulceration and inflammation. Occlusion of the airways by loose connective tissue follows, and, finally, complete stenosis and occlusion (22,23). Functionally significant bronchiolitis has been reported after exposure to ammonia, oxides of nitrogen, fire smoke, hydrogen selenide, phosgene, hydrogen bromide, sulfur dioxide, chlorine gas, thionyl chloride, grain dust, and "free base" cocaine.

A peculiar form of lymphocytic bronchiolitis and peribronchiolitis with lymphoid hyperplasia has been reported in workers at nylon-flock facilities (24). Workers in the poultry and swine confinement industries experience symptoms of obstructive lung function and bronchiolitis (25). It is likely that many more agents can cause this condition.

The distribution and extent of the lung injury depend on the concentration of the agent, duration of exposure, route and pattern of breathing, solubility and biologic reactivity of the agent, and individual susceptibility. The typical clinical course following exposure to toxic fumes consists of three phases: an acute onset with upper respiratory symptoms and sometimes pulmonary edema; a latent period; and an irreversible obstructive, mixed, or restrictive physiologic picture with dyspnea and cough. The physical examination reveals dry crackles over the lower lobes, particularly during inspiration, and a mid-expiratory squeak. The chest radiographic findings are normal or show hyperinflation and air trapping. Bronchiectasis may coexist. Histologically, a purely constrictive bronchiolitis is seen. The prognosis is poor, and steroids seem to have no beneficial effects.

Infectious and Postinfectious Bronchiolitis in Adults

Bronchiolitis may be a manifestation of acute viral infection in adults, especially in immunocompromised or elderly persons. Cases caused by adenovirus, herpes simplex virus, respiratory syncytial virus, cytomegalovirus, *M. pneumoniae*, acid-fast mycobacteria, *Bordetella pertussis,* and influenza virus have been described (26–29). Uncommon causes of infectious bronchiolitis are the following (28): *Legionella pneumophila, Haemophilus influenzae, Klebsiella pneumoniae, Serratia marcescens, Aspergillus* or *Mucor, Nocardia asteroides,* measles (rubeola) virus, enteroviruses, HIV (30), *Plasmodium* species (malaria), *Cryptosporidium* species (31), and microsporidia (*Encephalitozoon hellem*) (32). The presence of typical inclusions or identification of the offending microorganism with more sophisticated techniques in serum, throat swabs, tracheal aspirates, bronchoalveolar lavage (BAL) fluid, or lung biopsy specimens can help to establish a diagnosis.

Clinically, patients may have fever, cough, sore throat, sinusitis and rhinitis, dyspnea, cough, hypoxemia, and wheezing. Centrilobular and peribronchial nodules, a "tree in bud" pattern, and areas of ground-glass opacity or consolidation are the findings in HRCT scans (33,34). Sometimes, mosaic oligemia and expiratory air trapping are found. Histologically nonspecific, acute or chronic, or granulomatous cellular bronchiolitis is observed in the majority of cases. Follicular bronchiolitis is reported, especially in patients with HIV infection.

Only sporadic cases of fixed airflow obstruction, mosaic oligemia, and expiratory air trapping secondary to infection have been reported in adults (35,36). The agents that have been associated with bronchiolitis include viruses (adenovirus types 3, 7, and 21, respiratory syncytial virus, measles [rubeola] virus, influenza virus, parainfluenza virus, cytomegalovirus) and *M. pneumoniae.* Constrictive bronchiolitis is the most common histopathologic pattern after infection; bronchiolitis with inflammatory polyps has been more rarely reported.

Swyer-James syndrome (28,37) (also termed *MacLeod syndrome, unilateral* or *lobar emphysema,* and *unilateral hyperlucent lung*) is a peculiar variant of postinfectious bronchiolitis. It usually develops as a sequela of viral pulmonary infection in infancy or early childhood and leads to alveolar destruction and obliterative bronchiolitis. Nonviral cases are caused by infections such as *Mycoplasma* pneumonia, tuberculosis, and pertussis and by noninfectious factors such as aspirated foreign bodies, irradiation, and ingested hydrocarbon (10,28). The bronchiolar damage may prevent normal development of the affected lung, resulting in decreased lung volume and decreased blood flow. Radiographically, the condition is characterized by unilateral hyperlucent lung with normal or reduced volume during inspiration and air trapping during expiration; bronchiectasis and bilateral patchy areas of decreased attenuation and air trapping are best seen by HRCT. Typically, patients are asymptomatic. Less commonly, they have exertional dyspnea or repeated respiratory infections. BAL fluid analysis may document an inflammation (with a predominance of neutrophils and CD8$^+$ cells), even in clinically stable patients, which suggests an ongoing active process (38).

Drug-Induced Bronchiolitis Obliterans

Gold compounds, penicillamine, and tiopronin (39–41) have been associated with pure bronchiolitis obliterans. In the cases in which an open lung biopsy was performed, a concentric constrictive bronchiolitis was identified. Most of the patients reported were women. Dyspnea, cough, wheezing, and a high-pitched inspiratory squeak were the symptoms and signs more frequently described. Pulmonary function tests showed a fixed obstruction on expiration. The chest radiographic findings were normal or showed a mild hyperinflation. These patients were also affected by rheumatoid arthritis, so that conclusive proof of an association between these drugs and constrictive bronchiolitis is lacking. This form of bronchiolitis may be characterized by a rapidly deteriorating course and pulmonary insufficiency.

An outbreak of rapidly progressive respiratory distress associated with the consumption of uncooked *Sauropus androgynus,* a vegetable, was reported in Taiwan (42). *S. androgynus* is claimed to be effective in weight control. Most of the patients were young or middle-aged women. Respiratory symptoms (cough and dyspnea) developed about 10 weeks after ingestion of the vegetable juice. Other symptoms included dizziness, insomnia, and palpitations. Laboratory test results were normal except for an increased serum concentration of tumor necrosis factor-α. Although the chest radiographic findings were essentially normal, HRCT of the lung revealed bilateral bronchiolar wall thickening and dilatation and areas of low attenuation with air trapping (43). Pulmonary function tests disclosed severe obstructive ventilation that did not respond to bronchodilators. A moderate to severe reduction in the diffusing capacity was also observed. Histopathologic changes ranged from mild bronchiolar inflammation and fibrosis to severe constrictive bronchiolitis (44). Areas of BOOP, bronchiolitis with inflammatory polyps, and segmental ischemic necrosis of the small bronchi were also reported (45). Neutrophils and to a lesser extent eosinophils were increased in the BAL fluid. Lung transplantation is the only effective treatment reported (46).

Connective Tissue Diseases Associated with Bronchiolitis Obliterans

Diseases involving the conducting small airways have been reported in rheumatoid arthritis and less frequently in lupus erythematosus, polymyositis/dermatomyositis, ankylosing spondylitis, Sjögren syndrome, and scleroderma (3,10). Dyspnea and cough (in some cases with sputum production), often associated with inspiratory rales and mid-inspiratory squeaks, are observed in middle-aged women with seropositive rheumatoid arthritis (less frequently in patients with juvenile rheumatoid arthritis, systemic lupus erythematosus, scleroderma, or Behçet disease) or with evidence of advanced autoimmune exocrinopathy (Sjögren syndrome)

(3,47,48). Pulmonary function tests show fixed airflow obstruction with a normal or nearly normal diffusing capacity. HRCT shows bilateral patchy areas of low attenuation or centrilobular nodules and branching lines. Bronchiectasis may also be documented. The histology is heterogeneous; follicular bronchitis and bronchiolitis, centrilobular clusters of foamy macrophages (diffuse panbronchiolitis-like pattern), constrictive bronchiolitis, and acute epithelial injury often coexist in the same specimen even though a major histologic pattern can be identified (8,49,50). BAL cell analysis reveals a marked increase in the percentage of neutrophils (51). A relationship between bronchiolitis obliterans and penicillamine therapy has been reported in the majority of cases (52,53). Cases with a histology characterized by lymphoid hyperplasia (follicular bronchiolitis) usually respond to corticosteroids or erythromycin (54). Oral prednisone and intravenous cyclophosphamide have been suggested to be effective in some cases (55), but usually the prognosis is poor. Bronchiectasis is detected by HRCT in about 30% of patients with rheumatoid arthritis and less frequently in patients with other collagen-vascular diseases (56). The frequency of heterozygosity for the $\Delta F508$ mutation in the CFTR gene is higher than expected in patients with rheumatoid arthritis and bronchiectasis (57).

Inflammatory Bowel Disease–Associated Bronchiolitis Obliterans

Pulmonary complications occur in an estimated 0.21% of patients with inflammatory bowel disease, ulcerative colitis being the type most often associated with lung problems (58). The most common presentation is large-airway disease, such as tracheobronchitis, chronic bronchitis, or bronchiectasis (59). Bronchiolitis is extremely rare (58,60). Cellular bronchiolitis with an intraluminal accumulation of neutrophils and chronic inflammation of the wall, granulomatous bronchiolitis, cicatricial bronchiolitis, and epithelial ulceration—features similar to those described in diffuse panbronchiolitis—have been reported (58,61). Chronologically, small-airway involvement can develop at any time during the course of inflammatory bowel disease. In about 80% of cases, however, the onset of pulmonary symptoms follows the diagnosis by months to years. The spectrum of HRCT changes is broad; bronchiectasis, mosaic perfusion and air trapping, centrilobular nodules, and branching linear opacities ("tree in bud" appearance) have all been reported (62).

Patients may have cough, dyspnea, or systemic symptoms such as fever and asthenia. Inhaled or oral steroids are the recommended treatment.

Bronchiolitis Obliterans after Organ Transplantation

Obstructive lung disease occurs after allogeneic and rarely autologous bone marrow transplantation and after heart-lung and single- or double-lung transplantation (10,63,64). The clinical, imaging, and functional features are similar in both settings. The prevalence of post-transplant obstructive lung disease has been reported by different centers as between 1.2% and 11% for bone marrow transplantation (10,64,65) and from 20% to 50% for lung transplantation (10,63,66). Risk factors for bone marrow transplant–associated obstructive lung disease include older age, recurrent sinusitis, chronic graft versus host disease, methotrexate prophylaxis for graft versus host disease, and acquired hypogammaglobulinemia. The development of post-transplant obstructive lung disease in patients with a lung transplant is frequently preceded by acute organ rejection. More frequent, more severe, and longer episodes of acute cellular rejection increase the risk for bronchiolitis obliterans syndrome (66). Nonimmunologic inflammatory conditions, such as viral infection and ischemic injury, may also trigger post-transplant obstructive lung disease in patients with lung transplants (66). The peak incidence is between 7 and 12 months after transplantation. Dyspnea with exertion, nonproductive cough, and nasal congestion are the symptoms at presentation. The cough becomes progressively productive in lung transplant patients. The presentation may be acute and mimic a respiratory infection. On physical examination, scattered wheezes and expiratory squeaks are frequently noted. Permanent airway colonization with pathogenic bacteria (*Pseudomonas* and *Staphylococcus* species) and fungi often develops later (67).

Pulmonary function tests show irreversible airflow obstruction. The total lung capacity is lower in patients with lung transplants, and the diffusing capacity of the lung for carbon monoxide (DLCO) may be moderately depressed. The bronchiolitis obliterans syndrome has been divided into four stages based on the decline in the forced expiratory volume in 1 second (FEV_1) from the previously best baseline value. Stage I is associated with at least a 20% decline, stage II with a 35% to 50% decline, and stage III with a decline of more than 50%. Three patterns of progression have been reported in patients with lung transplants (68). The first is characterized by a rapid decline in the FEV_1 that leads to respiratory failure and death within 12 months after diagnosis. The second is characterized by an insidious onset and a slow, progressive decline in the FEV_1 over time. The third pattern consists of an initial rapid decline in the FEV_1 followed by a prolonged period of stability.

Dynamic HRCT can be used to identify the mosaic oligemia pattern and expiratory air trapping when the results of pulmonary function tests are normal (28). Bronchiectasis and bronchial wall thickening may be observed (28). Measurements of the ventilation distribution may detect post-transplant obstructive lung disease at an early stage.

The BAL fluid profile is characterized by an increased total cell count with a substantial neutrophilia, increased levels of granulocyte activation markers (interleukin-8, myeloperoxidase, eosinophil cationic protein) (69,70).

CD8$^+$ lymphocytes may be observed in patients with bone marrow transplants (65).

The pathologic spectrum includes a moderate to severe peribronchial and peribronchiolar mononuclear cell inflammatory infiltrate accompanied by exocytosis into the bronchiolar epithelium (lymphocytic bronchitis/bronchiolitis) (63,71). A lymphocytic infiltrate may be present in the interstitium adjacent to the affected bronchioles. Constrictive bronchiolitis accounts for the luminal narrowing and for bronchiolectasis in the vast majority of cases, but bronchiolitis with intraluminal polyps may also be present in a patchy distribution.

An alveolar component of lung rejection or pulmonary graft versus host disease is more typical of the active phase. The diagnosis can be suspected by HRCT. Histology (surgical lung biopsy is the gold standard) is not required in typical cases. Air trapping as detected in the expiratory phase by HRCT has the best sensitivity (80%–91%) and specificity (80%–94%) (72). In regard to pathogenesis, a leading hypothesis is that this immunologic reaction is a consequence of up-regulation of class II major histocompatibility complex (MHC) antigens on airway epithelium and vascular endothelium (66,67,73). CD4$^+$ and CD8$^+$ lymphocytes are mostly involved, but natural killer cells, Langerhans cells, and cells positive for L26 (a monoclonal antibody of the CD20 cluster; a pre-plasma cell B marker) contribute to the inflammatory infiltrate. Experimental studies suggest that the activation of complement (74) and the production of angiotensin-converting enzyme (75) and RANTES (regulated on activation, normal T cell expressed and secreted) (76) may also contribute to the development of obliterative bronchiolitis. Progression from cellular interstitial pneumonitis to BOOP and cicatricial bronchiolitis has been demonstrated (77). Infections with immunomodulating viruses (cytomegalovirus, Epstein-Barr virus) are also important in up-regulating HLA expression and cytokine production in patients with lung transplants (66,67,73,78). Elevated levels of interleukin-8 (IL-8) and transforming growth factor-β (TGF-β) have been reported in BAL fluid from lung transplant patients; the authors hypothesize that IL-8 and TGF-β may act as key mediators of airway inflammation and fibrous proliferation in the pathogenesis of bronchiolitis obliterans syndrome, with bronchial epithelial cells serving as a source of IL-8 (79). Insulin-like growth factor-1 (IGF-1) and IGF-3 may have a role in the fibrotic process underlying post-transplant obstructive lung disease and are possible early markers of this complication (80). Ischemic injury is also involved because it is associated with bouts of acute inflammation of the airways (67).

Patients are managed primarily by increasing immunosuppression; the administration of azathioprine (1.0–1.5 mg/kg per day) together with steroids and cyclosporine is the most effective approach. Mycophenolate mofetil and thalidomide are other drugs used. Aerosolized bronchodilators and antibiotics are given when deemed appropriate. Evidence suggests that the number of respiratory infections and the aggressiveness with which these infections are treated affect the progression of airflow obstruction (67). Lung transplantation or repeated transplantation is the last resort in well-selected patients.

Paraneoplastic Pemphigus and Constrictive Bronchiolitis

Paraneoplastic pemphigus is an autoimmune disease that occasionally accompanies an overt or occult malignant non-Hodgkin lymphoma and causes blisters (81). It has also been reported in patients with other neoplasms (chronic lymphocytic leukemia, Castleman disease, thymoma, retroperitoneal sarcoma, Waldenström macroglobulinemia). Paraneoplastic pemphigus is characterized by the presence of immunoglobulin G (IgG) autoantibodies that react against desmosomal and hemidesmosomal plakin proteins, desmosomal transmembrane proteins, and an unidentified 170-kd antigen. A complication in about 30% of patients is respiratory failure with clinical features of bronchiolitis obliterans (82–84). The large airways appear to be involved early in the course of the disease. Acantholysis of differentiated ciliary epithelium from the underlying basilar cells is evident in endobronchial biopsy specimens. Later involvement of the small airways leads to respiratory failure and death. Evidence indicates that autoantibodies directed against plakin proteins may be responsible for the acantholytic changes in the bronchial/bronchiolar epithelium observed in these cases (82).

Neuroendocrine Cell Hyperplasia with Bronchiolar Fibrosis

In 1992, Aguayo and colleagues (12) reported six patients, all nonsmokers, with moderate chronic airflow obstruction, three of whom had peripheral carcinoid tumors and three progressive dyspnea. All the patients had foci of neuroendocrine hyperplasia around bronchioles, and this was associated with partial or total occlusion of the lumina by fibrous tissue. Miller and Muller (85) found that 19 (76%) of 25 patients with peripheral carcinoid tumors also had neuroendocrine cell hyperplasia in the airways, mostly bronchioles. Eight of the patients (32%) also had constrictive bronchiolitis. All eight were women, as were all three of the patients of Aguayo and colleagues who had carcinoid tumors. Pulmonary function tests may show a mild to severe airflow obstruction, or the results may be normal. The HRCT findings are quite characteristic (10) (Fig. 29.10): a combination of peripheral nodules, mosaic oligemia, and expiratory air trapping. The hypothesis is that bronchiolar fibrosis is related to one or more peptides secreted by neuroendocrine cells and that these cells are more effective in stimulating fibrosis in women (86). Specific immunostaining for bombesin, a neuropeptide with growth factor–like properties, has been demonstrated within neuroendocrine cells (63).

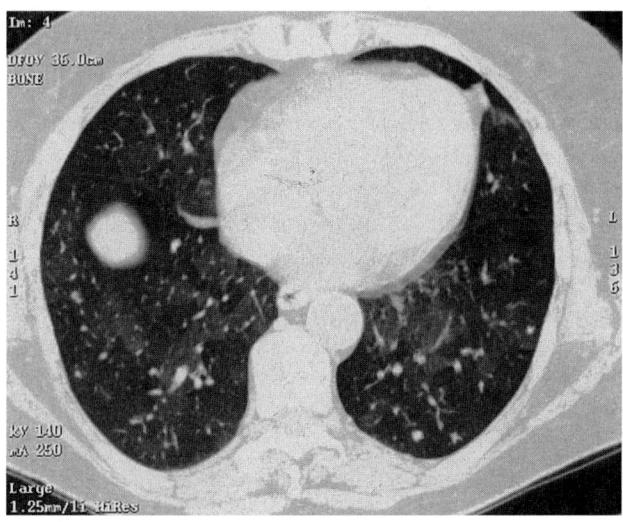

FIGURE 29.10. High-resolution computed tomography. Patchy areas of mosaic oligemia and scattered small nodules in a case of neuroendocrine cell hyperplasia with bronchiolar fibrosis.

Lung transplantation is the only effective treatment reported in cases with severe irreversible airflow obstruction.

Diffuse Panbronchiolitis

Diffuse panbronchiolitis is a distinctive form of small-airway disease with the following diagnostic criteria (87,88): (a) symptoms of chronic cough, sputum, and dyspnea on exertion; (b) physical signs of rales and rhonchi; (c) a chest radiograph showing diffusely disseminated fine nodular shadows, mainly in the lower lung fields, with hyperinflation; (d) lung function studies showing at least three of the following four abnormalities: ratio of the forced expiratory volume in 1 second to the forced vital capacity (FEV_1/FVC) below 70%, vital capacity less than 80% of the predicted value, residual volume more than 150% of the predicted value, and Po_2 below 80 mm Hg. Additional clinical and laboratory findings include chronic paranasal sinusitis (75%–100% of cases), increased cold hemagglutinin titers, increased levels of IgA, and increased serum calcium. Diffuse panbronchiolitis is more prevalent in men (male-to-female ratio, 2:1), and the peak incidence is between the fourth and seventh decades of life. Sinus symptoms often precede chest symptoms by years or decades. Early in the disease course, sputum cultures are unrevealing. Infection or colonization of the airways with *H. influenzae* and occasionally with *Streptococcus pneumoniae, K. pneumoniae,* or *Staphylococcus aureus* follows. Ultimately, these are replaced by chronic infection with *Pseudomonas aeruginosa* or other *Pseudomonas* species. A familial occurrence with a significant increase in HLA-Bw54 has been described (89). Environmental factors also appear important because the disorder is very uncommon in persons of Asian ancestry living abroad. The recurrence of diffuse panbronchiolitis in an African American patient

who underwent bilateral lung transplantation (90) and the association between diffuse panbronchiolitis and rheumatoid arthritis (91,92) suggest the presence of a systemic disorder. Diffuse panbronchiolitis is largely restricted to Japan. It has also been reported from China and Korea. Sporadic case reports and a few short series describing diffuse panbronchiolitis in Western populations have been published (93,94,95).

Pathologically, multiple small gray-white to yellow-tan nodules are confined to the respiratory bronchioles. All layers of the walls of the delicate bronchioles are involved (panbronchiolitis). Histologically, the most distinctive feature of diffuse panbronchiolitis is an accumulation of foam cells in the walls of the respiratory bronchioles, adjacent alveolar ducts, and alveoli (11). An intense T-lymphocytic infiltrate is evident around the bronchiolar lumen; neutrophils are accumulated inside the lumen. Hyperplastic lymphoid follicles are also present around the bronchioles. A marked increase of Langerhans cells in the bronchiolar submucosa associated with a strong expression of granulocyte-macrophage colony-stimulating factor (GM-CSF) protein in the bronchiolar epithelium has been described (96). Advanced disease is manifested by secondary ectasia of the proximal small bronchi.

The HRCT findings are quite characteristic but not pathognomonic (97,98) (Fig. 29.7); nodular shadows are distributed in a centrilobular fashion, often extending to small, branching, linear areas of attenuation ("tree in bud" pattern). Peripheral air trapping is usually confirmed in expiratory films. In addition, dilatation of the airways and bronchial wall thickening are present.

BAL fluid analysis reveals a marked neutrophilia, a decreased ratio of $CD4^+$ to $CD8^+$ cells, and an increase in the absolute number of $CD8^+$ HLA-DR$^+$ cells and $CD3^+$ $\gamma\delta^+$ cells (99,100). Elevated concentrations of IL-8, leukotriene B_4, and defensins have been reported in BAL fluid (101,102). The serum Ca 19-9 level is high and can be a marker of disease activity (103). Diffuse panbronchiolitis is the third disease associated with reduced nasal levels of nitric oxide, the others being cystic fibrosis and primary ciliary dyskinesia syndrome (104).

Low-dose erythromycin (200–600 mg/d) is the therapy of choice (89,105). Macrolides impair neutrophil chemotaxis, neutrophil superoxide production, and neutrophil-derived elastolytic activity; they also significantly reduce the neutrophil count and concentrations of defensins, leukotriene B_4, and IL-8 in BAL fluid and reduce the circulating pool of T lymphocytes bearing HLA-DR (88,105,106). In addition, erythromycin may cause a reduction in mucus production by decreasing glycoconjugate secretion (107). After at least 3 months of therapy, a reduction in the extent of small nodular opacities, the severity of "peri-airways" thickening, and the extent of mucus plugging can be seen on HRCT scans, with a corresponding significant improvement in lung function (108). Nonsteroidal antiinflammatory drugs may have a role in controlling the bronchorrhea associated with this disease by altering airway epithelial ion and water transport. The routine use of β_2-agonists or oxitropium bromide can promote mucociliary clearance and bronchodilation in patients with a component of reversible airway disease. Chronic pulmonary infection secondary to diffuse panbronchiolitis may be associated with p-ANCA (perinuclear form of antineutrophil cytoplasmic antibody) polyangiitis (109,110).

Cryptogenic Bronchiolitis

Cases of cryptogenic bronchiolitis obliterans were first studied by Turton and colleagues (111). Kindt and colleagues (112) in the late 1980s described 16 patients who presented with evidence of airflow limitation and hyperinflation. Most of them were current or former smokers. The pathologic findings were only briefly reported: bronchiolar inflammation, often with an acute component, "bronchiolar obliteration," and excess "mucus" cells in the bronchioles. The BAL fluid profile was characterized by a huge accumulation of neutrophils and neutrophil products. Steroid treatment was beneficial.

Cryptogenic bronchiolitis was reviewed later by Kraft and colleagues (113). They reported four women, 36 to 59 years old, with mild nonspecific symptoms (coryza, cough, dyspnea) and none of the known causes of chronic airflow obstruction. Two patients had crackles on auscultation. The chest roentgenographic findings were normal in one patient, and three had increased bronchial wall thickening. HRCT demonstrated abnormal interstitium in one patient, airway dilatation in another, and minimal upper lobe centrilobular thickening in a third. Pulmonary function testing yielded a variety of results; two patients had increased volumes and airflow limitation, one had a mixed disorder, and the remaining patient had normal pulmonary function. The diffusing capacity was reduced in three patients. These patients showed constrictive bronchiolitis, described as concentric fibrotic narrowing of the lumen of membranous bronchioles accompanied by muscle hyperplasia and "mucus stasis."

A case of bronchiolitis with an intraluminal accumulation of acute inflammatory cells, scattered foamy cells, and HRCT findings suggestive of diffuse panbronchiolitis has been reported (114). This patient's serum level of carbohydrate antigen 19-9 (CA 19-9) was increased. An adult patient with chronic dyspnea, eosinophilic sputum production, centrilobular nodules on HRCT scan, and eosinophilic bronchiolitis has been reported (115). Cases histologically characterized by abundant lymphoid tissue with prominent germinal centers in the wall of bronchioles (follicular bronchiolitis) not associated with autoimmune disorders or infections have been also reported (8). Markopoulou and colleagues (20) described 19 patients with a pathologic diagnosis of obliterative bronchiolitis. The patients had a well-documented exposure to toxic fumes. In a few cases, hypersensitivity pneumonitis in *forme fruste* or a myeloperoxidase-antineutrophil cytoplasmic antibody (MPO-ANCA)–related peribronchiolar

inflammation has been considered. Peribronchiolar fibrosis and bronchiolar metaplasia may be the unique histologic lesion in cases with roentgenologic and clinical features mimicking idiopathic pulmonary fibrosis or chronic hypersensitivity pneumonitis (8).

Cryptogenic bronchiolitis probably represents a heterogeneous group of patients, some with clinical, roentgenologic, and histologic findings suggestive of follicular bronchiolitis or diffuse panbronchiolitis. Exposure to toxic fumes or hypersensitivity pneumonitis must be excluded. Steroids can provide some benefit, and trials of low-dose macrolides should be encouraged.

Miscellaneous Causes of Bronchiolitis Obliterans

Associations between bronchiolitis obliterans and gastroesophageal reflux (116), activated charcoal used to manage a case of medication-related attempted suicide (117), Stevens-Johnson syndrome (118), and primary biliary cirrhosis (119) have been reported. Follicular bronchitis and bronchiolitis have been reported in patients with a familial form of the disease or with immunodeficiency syndromes (120).

Adult patients with lysinuric protein intolerance can present with irreversible respiratory insufficiency and signs of bronchiolitis obliterans (121). Four patients with ataxia-telangiectasia who died of respiratory failure had features of bronchiolitis obliterans in all lobes examined at autopsy (122). Bronchiolitis obliterans in this context may be caused by the underlying immune deficit. A patient with idiopathic bronchiolitis obliterans in whom a rapidly progressive glomerulonephritis secondary to IgA deposits developed has been reported. Extensive deposits of IgA found in the patient's lungs suggested a pathogenetic role for IgA in the tissue injury in both organs (123).

Mimickers of Bronchiolitis Obliterans

The small airways can be more or less involved in the context of specific well-known disorders (124). Furthermore, the clinical and roentgenologic findings of vascular diseases can overlap with those of obstructive bronchiolitis. Asthma and chronic obstructive pulmonary disease are well-recognized diseases of both large and small airways and the most frequent mimickers of specific forms of bronchiolitis.

Centrilobular ground-glass nodules and airflow obstruction may radiographically characterize subacute hypersensitivity pneumonitis. These cases are characterized histologically by cellular bronchiolitis, patchy interstitial alveolar inflammation, foamy intra-alveolar macrophages, intra-alveolar loose fibrotic buds, and poorly formed, scattered, nonnecrotizing granulomas. The definitive diagnosis is usually based on the clinical history, results of laboratory tests for serum precipitins, and BAL fluid findings of marked lymphocytosis. In a few cases, lung biopsy is required.

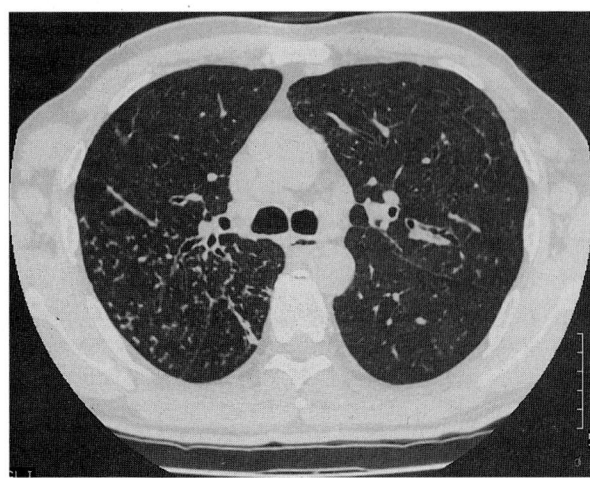

FIGURE 29.11. High-resolution computed tomography. Chronic lymphocytic leukemia in the lung appearing as centrilobular nodules and bronchiectasis and bronchiolectasis in the upper right lobe.

Sarcoidosis can involve primarily the bronchi and bronchioles, causing obstruction, impairment, and wheezing. The incidence of bronchial hyperreactivity is also increased in patients with sarcoidosis.

Carcinomatous lymphangitis has a distinctive HRCT pattern (nodular thickening of the peribronchiolar-vascular spaces of the peripheral lobular septa). However, neoplastic infiltrates associated with a desmoplastic reaction can be prominent in the peribronchiolar-vascular lymphatics; wheezing and dyspnea are the symptoms at onset.

Bronchiolocentric chronic lymphocytic leukemia and small lymphocytic lymphomas, primary in the lungs, have been reported (125) (Fig. 29.11).

Thromboembolism and intravascular neoplastic emboli can all mimic obstructive bronchiolitis.

BRONCHIOLITIS OBLITERANS–ORGANIZING PNEUMONIA

The morphologic pattern of organizing pneumonia (OP) or bronchiolitis obliterans–organizing pneumonia (BOOP) is absolutely nonspecific, being observed more or less predominantly in a variety of pulmonary diseases. A distinct clinical syndrome with features of acute or subacute infectious pneumonia that usually responds noticeably to corticosteroids and in which the unique pathologic hallmark is OP was first reported by Grinblat and colleagues in 1981 (126). In 1983, Davison and colleagues (127) described a similar group of cases as cryptogenic organizing pneumonia. Two years later, Epler and colleagues (5) described similar cases as BOOP. The term *BOOP* is widely used, but the more correct term is *OP* because the process is characterized primarily by intra-alveolar granulation tissue that may extend a short distance into the respiratory or terminal bronchioles. The process

of intra-alveolar organization appears to evolve from acute alveolar epithelial injury with cell necrosis and denudation of the lamina basalis (128,129). Further steps are the accumulation of intra-alveolar fibrinoid inflammatory cell clusters, rich in coagulation factors, and the migration of interstitial fibroblasts through gaps in the injured lamina basalis.

Fibroblasts undergo phenotypic modulation into myofibroblasts and organize into fibrous inflammatory buds with deposition of a loose connective matrix in which tenascin, fibronectin, and type III collagen are abundant. Numerous proteins (tissue factor antigen, adhesive and antiadhesive glycoproteins, IL-8, platelet-derived growth factor, GM-CSF, matrix metalloproteases, gelatinases, stromelysins) have been shown to have a role in these pathogenetic events (130–136). The role of the immune-inflammatory cells (CD8+ cells, neutrophils, eosinophils, mast cells) is evident, although not yet completely understood. Type II pneumocytes, which usually cover the loose fibrotic plugs, can produce a quantity of factors modulating the inflammatory recruitment and intra-alveolar organization (134,137).

The classic clinical profile of OP (or BOOP) is the following (128): acute or subacute onset, dyspnea on effort, cough, rarely hemoptysis, chest pain, bronchorrhea, and systemic symptoms (fever, asthenia, weight loss most common; arthralgia, night sweats uncommon). In about 30% of cases, the symptoms develop over a few weeks after a flulike illness.

Less frequently, patients with rapidly progressive respiratory failure who require mechanical ventilation and asymptomatic subjects with a pseudoneoplastic nodular lesion on chest x-ray films complete the clinical spectrum of this entity (138,139). Laboratory tests show an increase in acute reaction proteins and, in a minority of cases, blood leukocytosis and chemical cholestasis. The serum lactate dehydrogenase level may be increased in a significant percentage of cases. Idiopathic cases are usually negative or only slightly positive for autoantibodies, and the serum level of CA 19-9 is not increased.

The physical examination findings may be normal, but inspiratory crackles are commonly heard over affected areas.

This clinicopathologic syndrome (Table 29.4) can be caused by drugs, radiation, or exposure to paint aerosols, or it may be related to infectious agents or associated with a specific clinical context; more frequently, however, it is idiopathic. In the last setting, men and women are equally affected and are usually between 50 and 60 years of age. A smoking habit is not a predisposing factor. Seasonal cases (late February to early May) with biochemical cholestasis and cases associated with the menstrual cycle have been reported (140).

Pulmonary function is as a rule impaired, with a restrictive pattern the most common finding.

The diffusing capacity is reduced in the majority of patients; hypoxemia and hypocapnia at rest or on exertion and widening of the resting alveolar-arterial oxygen gradient are common abnormalities.

TABLE 29.4. CLINICAL CLASSIFICATION OF ORGANIZING PNEUMONIA/BRONCHIOLITIS OBLITERANS–ORGANIZING PNEUMONIA

Idiopathic
Drugs
    5-Aminosalicylic acid
    Acebutolol
    Amiodarone
    Amphotericin
    Anthracyclins
    Bleomycin
    Busulphan
    Carbamazepine
    Cephalosporin (cefradine)
    Cocaine
    Cytosine arabinoside
    Gold salts
    Hexamethonium
    Interferon-α
    L-Tryptophan
    Mesalazine
    Methotrexate
    Minocycline
    Nilutamide
    Paraquat
    Phenytoin
    Sotalol
    Sulafasalazine
    Tacrolimus
    Trastuzumab
    Vinbarbital-aprobarbital
Acramin FWN (polyamide amine)
Radiation (in patients treated for breast duct carcinoma)
Collagen-vascular diseases
Evans syndrome
Infection
    HIV
    Adenovirus
    Influenza virus
    Respiratory syncytial virus
    Nocardia asteroides
    Mycoplasma pneumoniae
    Legionella pneumophila
    Chlamydia
    Coxiella burnetii
    Aspergillus
    Mucor
    Plasmodium vivax
Sweet syndrome
Chronic thyroiditis
Inflammatory bowel disease
Myelodysplastic syndrome
Lymphoproliferative disorders
Bone marrow transplantation
Lung transplantation/rejection
Common variable immunodeficiency syndrome
Essential mixed cryoglobulinemia

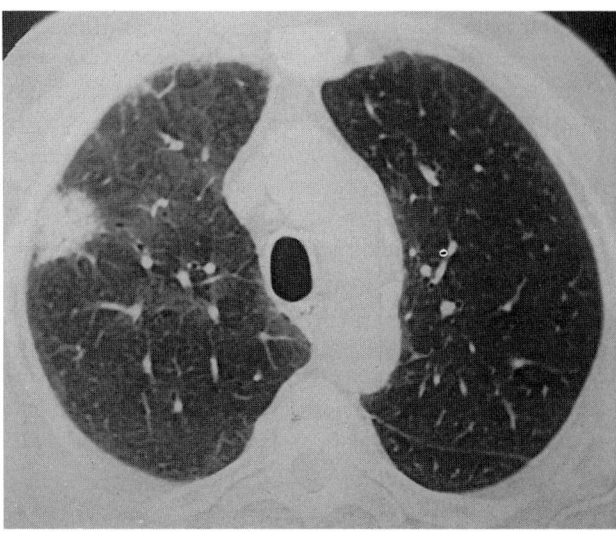

FIGURE 29.12. High-resolution computed tomography. Peripheral subpleural nodular opacity in a histologically proven case of idiopathic bronchiolitis obliterans–organizing pneumonia.

The characteristic imaging profile, best identified by HRCT, includes unilateral or bilateral areas of alveolar opacification or ground-glass attenuation in a patchy subpleural or peribronchial distribution (139,141–147). The lesions predominate in the lower fields. Migration of the lesions is documented in more than 30% of cases. Two other patterns have been reported: diffuse, bilateral, interstitial opacities and a nodular lesion (mimicking bronchogenic carcinoma) (Fig. 29.12). Rarer findings, more frequent in immunocompromised hosts, are multiple nodules or masses without a peripheral distribution mimicking metastases, cavitation of opacities, ring-shaped opacities (the "atoll" sign), and linear shadows. Pleural effusion has been reported in up to 20% of cases. Hilar or mediastinal adenopathy is a rare finding. Honeycombing has been reported in cases not responding to steroids and after multiple relapses (128,138).

The BAL fluid is characterized by an increased total number of cells (but not as many as in hypersensitivity pneumonitis) and a lymphocytosis, usually with a reduced ratio of $CD4^+$ to $CD8^+$ cells and an increase in the number of $CD3^+$ $HLA\text{-}DR^+$ cells (134,139,148). The lymphocytes may have convoluted nuclei with a wider cytoplasm (Lutzner-like cells). The number of neutrophils and eosinophils is also increased. Foamy macrophages, scattered mast cells, and plasma cells complete the BAL fluid profile of OP/BOOP. In a few cases, atypical epithelial cells (probably hyperplastic/dysplastic type II pneumocytes) are also detected (139).

OP/BOOP is by definition a clinicopathologic entity, and therefore the diagnosis is possible when the two patterns are found in the same patient (typical or consistent clinical profile and the histopathologic BOOP pattern). The idiopathic or secondary nature of the process must be identified. The differential diagnosis includes primarily infection, eosinophilic pneumonia, bronchioloalveolar carcinoma, B-cell lymphoma of the MALT (mucosa-associated lymphoid tissue) type primary in the lung, lymphomatoid granulomatosis, Wegener angiitis and granulomatosis, hypersensitivity pneumonitis, nonspecific interstitial pneumonia, acute interstitial pneumonia in an early phase, respiratory bronchiolitis–interstitial lung disease or desquamative interstitial pneumonia, sarcoidosis, lipoid pneumonia, and thromboembolism. The diagnostic workup in suspected cases of OP/BOOP should include testing for autoantibodies and monoclonal serum proteins, an evaluation of the immune status, and a thorough clinical history.

The diagnosis is seldom justified without a biopsy. Transbronchial lung biopsy may be useful, especially when performed with the patient under general anesthesia through a rigid bronchoscope or orotracheal tube. Under fluoroscopic guidance, a large forceps is used to obtain numerous and generous specimens. Step-sectioning of transbronchial biopsy specimens is useful to increase the diagnostic yield. Open lung biopsy should be considered when transbronchial lung biopsy is not diagnostic, in atypical cases at the onset, and in cases with an unusual evolution despite treatment. Because the lung opacities may migrate over time, the biopsy should be performed just a few days after lung CT.

The BAL fluid profile alone may be accepted as a diagnostic proof for a patient who is critically ill if examined by a physician experienced in this procedure in a setting with a laboratory for processing the lavage fluid. BAL (lymphocytosis >25%, CD4$^+$/CD8$^+$ ratio <0.9, foamy macrophages >20%, neutrophils >5%, eosinophils between 2% and 25%) appears to be an effective diagnostic method in typical cases with patchy areas of alveolar opacification (149).

Secondary OP/BOOP is treated by withdrawing the offending agent or administering steroids. Spontaneous improvement is rare. The dose of steroids is not standardized, but a starting dosage of 0.75 mg of prednisone per kilogram per day seems to be effective in most cases. In idiopathic OP/BOOP, spontaneous improvement occurs in a minority of cases. In our experience, remission has occurred in a few cases after a surgical operation (i.e., open lung biopsy) (unpublished data). A therapeutic scheme validated by clinical experience is the following (150): 0.75 mg of prednisone per kilogram of lean body weight daily for 1 month; 0.5 mg of prednisone per kilogram daily for 1 month; 20 mg of prednisone per kilogram daily for 1 month; 10 mg of prednisone daily for 6 weeks; 5 mg of prednisone daily for 6 weeks. Improvement has been reported in some patients after prolonged treatment with erythromycin (128) and methotrexate (151). The response to corticosteroids is impressive, although much less dramatic than in idiopathic eosinophilic pneumonia. Clinical manifestations abate within 48 hours, but complete radiographic resolution usually takes several weeks. BAL lymphocytosis may persist for months after clinical and radiologic resolution.

Some cases with severe disease requiring mechanical ventilation may require higher doses of corticosteroids (up to 250 mg of intravenous methylprednisolone every 6 hours for 3 to 5 days) and the addition of cytotoxic drugs (cyclophosphamide the first choice) as initial treatment. Relapses after steroid withdrawal or when the dose of prednisone is less then 10 mg/d are frequent (>50% of cases). The risk for relapse is increased by delays in starting treatment; mild biochemical cholestasis identifies a subgroup at risk for multiple relapses (150). However, relapses do not appear to affect the outcome in most cases (150).

The prognosis in typical cases of idiopathic OP/BOOP with patchy alveolar opacities is usually excellent after treatment. Factors that appear to be associated with a poor outcome include associated disorders, a predominantly interstitial pattern on imaging, lack of lymphocytosis in the BAL fluid, and a finding on histologic examination of scarring and remodeling of the lung parenchyma in addition to OP (152).

REFERENCES

1. Lange W. Ueber eine eigenthumliche Erkrankung der kleinen und Bronchiolen. *Dtsch Arch Klein Med* 1901;70:342–364.
2. Fraenkel A. Ueber bronchiolitis fibrosa obliterans, nebst bemerkungen ueber lungenhyperaemie und indurirende pneumonie. *Dtsch Arch Klein Med* 1902;73:484–510.
3. Geddes DM, Corrin B, Brewerton DA, et al. Progressive airway obliteration in adults and its association with rheumatoid disease. *Q J Med* 1977;46:427.
4. Ralph DD, Springmeyer SC, Sullivan KM, et al. Rapidly progressive air-flow obstruction in marrow transplant recipients. Possible association between obliterative bronchiolitis and chronic graft-versus-host disease. *Am Rev Respir Dis* 1984;129:641–644.
5. Epler GR, Colby TV, McLoud TC, et al. Bronchiolitis obliterans organizing pneumonia. *N Engl J Med* 1985;312:152–158.
6. Murata K, Itoh H, Todo G, et al. Centrilobular lesions of the lung: demonstration by high-resolution CT and pathologic correlation. *Radiology* 1986;161:641–645.
7. Muller NL, Miller RR. Diseases of the bronchioles. CT and histopathologic findings. *Radiology* 1995;196:3–12.
8. Colby TV. Bronchiolitis. Pathologic considerations. *Am J Clin Pathol* 1998;109:101–110.
9. Miller RR, Muller NL, Thurlbeck WM. Diffuse diseases of the lungs. In: Silverberg SG, ed. *Principles and practice of surgical pathology and cytopathology.* New York: Churchill Livingstone, 1997:1099–1187.
10. Poletti V, Zompatori M, Cancellieri A. Clinical spectrum of adult chronic bronchiolitis. *Sarcoidosis Vasculitis Diffuse Lung Dis* 1999;16:183–196.
11. Iwata M, Colby TV, Kitaichi M. Diffuse panbronchiolitis: diagnosis and distinction from various pulmonary diseases with centrilobular interstitial foam cell accumulations. *Hum Pathol* 1994;25:357–363.
12. Aguayo SM, Miller YE, Waldron JA, et al. Brief report: idiopathic diffuse hyperplasia of pulmonary neuroendocrine cells and airways disease. *N Engl J Med* 1992;327:1285–1288.
13. Friedman PJ. Plain film analysis of diseases of the small airways. In: *Proceedings of the Fleischner Society 26th annual conference on chest disease,* Vancouver, 1996: 169–171.
14. Lucidarne O, Grenier PA, Cadi M, et al. Evaluation of air trapping at CT. Comparison of continuous versus suspended expiration CT techniques. *Radiology* 2000;216:768–772.
15. Webb WR, Muller NL, Naidich DP. *High-resolution CT of the lung.* New York: Lippincott–Raven Publishers, 1996:41.
16. Hansell DM . Small airways diseases: detection and insights with computed tomography. *Eur Respir J* 2001;17:1294–1313.
17. Salmanzadeh A, Pomeranz SJ, Ramsingh PS. Ventilation-perfusion scintigraphic correlation with multimodality imaging

in a proven case of Swyer-James (MacLeod's) syndrome. *Clin Nucl Med* 1997;22:115–118.

18. Altes TA, Powers PL, Knight-Scott J, et al. Hyperpolarized ³He MR lung ventilation imaging in asthmatics: preliminary findings. *J Magn Reson Imaging* 2001;13:378–384.

19. Evans DJ, Grenn M. Small airways: a time to revisit? *Thorax* 1998;53:629–630.

20. Markopoulou KD, Cool CD, Elliot TL, et al. Obliterative bronchiolitis: varying presentations and clinicopathologic correlation. *Eur Respir J* 2002;19:20–30.

21. Estenne M, Van Muylem A, Knoop C, et al. Detection of obliterative bronchiolitis after lung transplantation by indexes of ventilation distribution. *Am J Respir Crit Care Med* 2000;162:1047–1051.

22. Wright JL, Churg A. Diseases caused by gases and fumes. In: Churg A, Green FHY, eds. *Pathology of occupational lung disease.* Baltimore: Williams & Wilkins, 1998:57–75.

23. Douglas WW, Norman G, Hepper G, et al. Silo filler's disease. *Mayo Clin Proc* 1989;64:291–304.

24. Eschenbacker WL, Kreiss K, Lougheed MD, et al. Nylon flock-associated interstitial lung disease. *Am J Respir Crit Care Med* 1999;159:2003–2008.

25. Schwartz DA, Landas SK, Lassie DL, et al. Airway injury in swine confinement workers. *Ann Intern Med* 1992;116:630–635.

26. Wendt CH. Community respiratory viruses: organ transplant recipients. *Am J Med* 1997;102:31–36.

27. Chan ED, Kalayanamit T, Lynch DA, et al. *Mycoplasma pneumoniae*-associated bronchiolitis causing severe restrictive lung disease in adults: report of three cases and literature review. *Chest* 1999;115:1188–1194.

28. Fraser RS, Muller NL, Colman N, et al. Bronchiolitis. In: *Fraser and Parè's diagnosis of diseases of the chest.* Philadelphia: WB Saunders, 1999:2321–2357.

29. Chilosi M, Lestani M, Baruzzi G, et al. Histopathological and immunohistochemical findings in AIDS-associated lung disorders. In: *Eur Respir Monogr* 1995;1:150–185 (Semenzato GP, ed. *AIDS and the lung).*

30. Diaz F, Collazos J, Martinez E, et al. Bronchiolitis obliterans in a patient with HIV infection. *Respir Med* 1997;91:171–173.

31. Travis WD, Schmidt K, MacLowry JD, et al. Respiratory cryptosporidiosis in a patient with malignant lymphoma. Report of a case and review of the literature. *Arch Pathol Lab Med* 1990;114:519–522.

32. Schwartz DA, Visvesvara GS, Leitch GJ, et al. Pathology of symptomatic microsporidial (*Encephalitozoon hellem*) bronchiolitis in the acquired immunodeficiency syndrome: a new respiratory pathogen diagnosed from lung biopsy, bronchoalveolar lavage, sputum, and tissue culture. *Hum Pathol* 1993;24:937–943.

33. Howling SH, Hansell DM, Wells AU, et al. Follicular bronchiolitis: thin-section CT and histologic findings. *Radiology* 1999;212:637–642.

34. Reittner P, Muller NL, Heyneman L, et al. *Mycoplasma pneumoniae* pneumonia. Radiographic and high-resolution CT features in 28 patients. *AJR Am J Roentgenol* 2000;174:37–41.

35. Penn CC, Liu C. Bronchiolitis following infection in adults and children. *Clin Chest Med* 1993,14:645–654.

36. Coultas DB, Funk LM. Postinfectious bronchiolitis obliterans. In: Epler GR, ed. *Diseases of bronchioles.* New York: Raven Press, 1994:215–229.

37. Image interpretation session: 1998. Swyer-James (MacLeod) syndrome. *Radiographics* 1999;19:231–233.

38. Bernardi F, Cazzato S, Poletti V, et al. Swyer-James syndrome: bronchoalveolar lavage in two patients. *Eur Respir J* 1995;8:654–657.

39. Holness I, Tebebaum J, Cooter NB, et al. Fatal bronchiolitis associated with chrysotherapy. *Ann Rheum Dis* 1983;85:593–596.

40. Epler GR, Snider GL, Gaensler EA, et al. Bronchiolitis and bronchitis in connective tissue disease. A possible relationship to the use of penicillamine. *JAMA* 1979;242:528–532.

41. Demaziere A, Maugars Y, Chollet S, et al. Nonfatal bronchiolitis obliterans possibly associated with tiopronin. A case report with long-term follow-up. *Br J Rheumatol* 1993;32:172–174.

42. Lai RS, Chiang AA, Wu MT, et al. Outbreak of bronchiolitis obliterans associated with consumption of *Sauropus androgynus* in Taiwan. *Lancet* 1996,348:83–85.

43. Yang CF, Wu MT, Chiang AA, et al. Correlation of high-resolution CT and pulmonary function in bronchiolitis obliterans: a study based on 24 patients associated with consumption of *Sauropus androgynus. AJR Am J Roentgenol* 1997;168:1045–1050.

44. Chang H, Wang JS, Tseng HH, et al. Histopathological study of *Sauropus androgynus*-associated constrictive bronchiolitis obliterans: a new cause of constrictive bronchiolitis obliterans. *Am J Surg Pathol* 1997;21:35–42.

45. Chang YL, Yao YT, Wang NS, et al. Segmental necrosis of small bronchi after prolonged intakes of *Sauropus androgynus* in Taiwan. *Am J Respir Crit Care Med* 1998;157:594–598.

46. Luh SP, Lee YC, Chang YL, et al. Lung transplantation for patients with end-stage *Sauropus androgynus*-induced bronchiolitis obliterans (SABO) syndrome. *Clin Transplant* 1999;13:496–503.

47. Herzog CA, Miller RR, Hoidal JR, et al. Bronchiolitis in rheumatoid arthritis. *Am Rev Respir Dis* 1981;124:636–639.

48. Wells AU, Du Bois RM. Bronchiolitis in association with connective tissue disorders. *Clin Chest Med* 1993;14:655–666.

49. Kinoshita M, Higashi T, Tanaka C, et al. Follicular bronchiolitis associated with rheumatoid arthritis. *Intern Med* 1992;31:675–677.

50. Yousem SA, Colby TV, Carrington CB. Lung biopsy in rheumatoid arthritis. *Am Rev Respir Dis* 1985;131:770–777.

51. Herer B, De Castelbajac D, Israel-Biet D, et al. Bronchoalveolar lavage in pulmonary involvement in rheumatoid arthritis. *Ann Med Interne (Paris)* 1988;139:310–314.

52. Wolfe F, Schurle DR, Lin JJ, et al. Upper and lower airway disease in penicillamine-treated patients with rheumatoid arthritis. *J Rheumatol* 1983;10:406–410.

53. Tanoue LT. Pulmonary manifestations of rheumatoid arthritis. *Clin Chest Med* 1998;19:667–685.

54. Hayakawa H, Sato A, Imokawa S, et al. Bronchiolar disease in rheumatoid arthritis. *Am J Respir Crit Care Med* 1996;154:1531–1536.

55. Van de Laar MA, Westermann CJ, Wagenaar SS, et al. Beneficial effect of intravenous cyclophosphamide and oral prednisone on D-penicillamine–associated bronchiolitis obliterans. *Arthritis Rheum* 1985;28:93–97.

56. Perez T, Remy-Jardin M, Cortet B. Airways involvement in rheumatoid arthritis: clinical, functional, and HRCT findings. *Am J Respir Crit Care Med* 1998;157:1658–1665.

57. Puechal X, Fajac I, Bienvenu T, et al. Increased frequency of cystic fibrosis deltaF508 mutation in bronchiectasis associated with rheumatoid arthritis. *Eur Respir J* 1999;13:1281–1287.

58. Camus P, Piard F, Ashcroft T, et al. The lung in inflammatory bowel disease. *Medicine (Baltimore)* 1993;72:151–183.

59. Spira A, Grossman R, Balter M. Large airway disease associated with inflammatory bowel disease. *Chest* 1998;113:1723–1726.

60. Ward H, Fisher KL, Waghray R, et al. Constrictive bronchiolitis and ulcerative colitis. *Can Respir J* 1999;6:197–200.

61. Vandenplas O, Casel S, Delos M, et al. Granulomatous bronchiolitis associated with Crohn's disease. *Am J Respir Crit Care Med* 1998;158:1676–1679.

62. Mahadeva R, Walsh G, Flower CD, et al. Clinical and radiological characteristics of lung disease in inflammatory bowel disease. *Eur Respir J* 2000;15:41–48.

63. King TE Jr. Bronchiolitis. In: Schwarz MI, King TE Jr, eds. *Interstitial lung disease.* Hamilton, Ontario: BC Decker, 2003:787–824.

64. Philit F, Wiesendanger T, Archimbaud E, et al. Post-transplant obstructive lung disease ("bronchiolitis obliterans"): a clinical comparative study of bone marrow and lung transplant patients. *Eur Respir J* 1995;8:551–558.

65. Trisolini R, Stanzani M, Lazzari Agli LA, et al. Delayed non-infectious pulmonary complications in allogeneic bone marrow transplant recipients. *Sarcoidosis Vasculitis Diffuse Lung Dis* 2001;18:75–84.

66. Boehler A, Estenne A. Obliterative bronchiolitis after lung transplantation. *Curr Opin Pulm Med* 2000;6:133–139.

67. Paradis I. Bronchiolitis obliterans: pathogenesis, prevention, and management. *Am J Med Sci* 1998;315:161–178.

68. Nathan SD, Ross DJ, Belman ML, et al. Bronchiolitis obliterans in single-lung transplant recipients. *Chest* 1995;107:967–972.

69. Riise GC, Andersson BA, Kjellstrom C, et al. Persistent high fluid granulocyte activation marker level as early indicators of bronchiolitis obliterans after lung transplantation. *Eur Respir J* 1999;14:1123–1130.

70. Reynaud-Gaubert M, Thomas P, Badier M, et al. Early detection of airway involvement in obliterative bronchiolitis after lung transplantation. Functional and bronchoalveolar lavage cell findings. *Am J Respir Crit Care Med* 2000;161:1924–1929.

71. Yousem SA. The histological spectrum of pulmonary graft-versus-host disease in bone marrow transplant recipients. *Hum Pathol* 1995;26:668–675.

72. Leung AN, Fisher KL, Valentine V, et al. Bronchiolitis obliterans after lung transplantation: detection using expiratory HRCT. *Chest* 1998;113:365–370.

73. Poletti V, Salvucci M, Zanchini R, et al. The lung as a target organ in haematologic patients. *Haematologica* 2000;85:855–864.

74. Kallio EA, Lemstrom KB, Hayry PJ, et al. Blockade of complement inhibits obliterative bronchiolitis in rat tracheal allografts. *Am J Respir Crit Care Med* 2000;161:1332–1339.

75. Maclean AA, Liu M, Isher S, et al. Targeting the angiotensin system in posttransplant airway obliteration: the antifibrotic effect of angiotensin-converting enzyme inhibition. *Am J Respir Crit Care Med* 2000;162:310–315.

76. Suga M, Maclean AA, Keshavjee S, et al. RANTES plays an important role in the evolution of allograft transplant-induced fibrous airway obliteration. *Am J Respir Crit Care Med* 2000;162:1940–1948.

77. Trisolini R, Bandini G, Stanzani M, et al. Morphologic changes leading to bronchiolitis obliterans in a patient with delayed non-infectious lung disease after allogeneic bone marrow transplantation. *Bone Marrow Transplant* 2001;28:1167–1170.

78. Hunninghake GW, Monick MM, Geist LJ. Cytomegalovirus infection. *Am J Respir Cell Mol Biol* 1999;21:150–152.

79. Elssner A, Jaumann F, Dobmann S, et al. Elevated levels of interleukin-8 and transforming growth factor-beta in bronchoalveolar lavage fluid from patients with bronchiolitis obliterans syndrome: proinflammatory role of bronchial epithelial cells. Munich Lung Transplant Group. *Transplantation* 2000;70:362–367.

80. Charpin JM, Stern M, Grenet D, et al. Insulin-like growth factor-1 in lung transplants with obliterative bronchiolitis. *Am J Respir Crit Care Med* 2000;161:1991–1998.

81. Allen CM, Camisa C. Paraneoplastic pemphigus: a review of the literature. *Oral Dis* 2000;6:208–214.

82. Nousari HC, Deterding R, Wojtczach H, et al. The mechanism of respiratory failure in paraneoplastic pemphigus. *N Engl J Med* 1999;340:1406–1410.

83. Hasegawa Y, Shimokata K, Ichiyama S, et al. Constrictive bronchiolitis obliterans and paraneoplastic pemphigus. *Eur Respir J* 1999;13:934–937.

84. Takahashi M, Shimatsu Y, Kazama T, et al. Paraneoplastic pemphigus associated with bronchiolitis obliterans. *Chest* 2000;117:603–607.

85. Miller RR, Muller NL. Neuroendocrine cell hyperplasia and obliterative bronchiolitis in patients with peripheral carcinoid tumors. *Am J Surg Pathol* 1995;19:653–658.

86. Cohen AJ, King TE, Gilman LB, et al. High expression of neutral endopeptidase in idiopathic diffuse hyperplasia of pulmonary neuroendocrine cells. *Am J Respir Crit Care Med* 1998;158:1593–1599.

87. Homma H, Yamanaka A, Tanimoto S, et al. Diffuse panbronchiolitis. A disease of the transitional zone of the lung. *Chest* 1983;83:63–69.

88. Tsang KWT. Diffuse panbronchiolitis: diagnosis and treatment. *Clin Pulm Med* 2000;7:245–252.

89. Keicho N, Totunaga K, Nakata K, et al. Contribution of HLA genes to genetic predisposition in diffuse panbronchiolitis. *Am J Respir Crit Care Med* 1998;158:846–850.

90. Baz MA, Kussin PS, Van Trigt P, et al. Recurrence of diffuse panbronchiolitis after lung transplantation. *Am J Respir Crit Care Med* 1995;151:895–898.

91. Homma S, Kawabata M, Kishi K, et al. Diffuse panbronchiolitis in rheumatoid arthritis. *Eur Respir J* 1998;12:444–452.

92. Hayakawa H, Sato A, Imokawa S, et al. Diffuse panbronchiolitis and rheumatoid arthritis-associated bronchiolar disease: similarities and differences. *Intern Med* 1998;37:504–508.

93. Poletti V, Patelli M, Poletti G, et al. Diffuse panbronchiolitis observed in an Italian. *Chest* 1990;98:515–516.

94. Fitzgerald JE, King TE, Lynch DA, et al. Diffuse panbronchiolitis in the United States. *Am J Respir Crit Care Med* 1996;154:497–503.

95. Schulte W, Szrepka A, Bauer PC, et al. Diffuse panbronchiolitis. A rare differential diagnosis of chronic obstructive lung disease. *Dtsch Med Wochenschr* 1999;124:584–588.

96. Todate A, Chida K, Suda T, et al. Increased numbers of dendritic cells in the bronchiolar tissues of diffuse panbronchiolitis. *Am J Respir Crit Care Med* 2000;162:148–153.

97. Akira M, Kitatani F, Yong-Sik N, et al. Diffuse panbronchiolitis. Evaluation with HRCT. *Radiology* 1988;168:433–438.

98. Zompatori M, Poletti V. Diffuse panbronchiolitis. An Italian experience. *Radiol Med (Torino)* 1997;94:680–681.

99. Koga T. Neutrophilia and high level of interleukin-8 in the bronchoalveolar lavage fluid of diffuse panbronchiolitis. *Kurume Med J* 1993;40:139–146.

100. Mukae H, Kadota J, Kohono S, et al. Increase in activated CD8+ cells in bronchoalveolar lavage fluid in patients with diffuse panbronchiolitis. *Am J Respir Crit Care Med* 1995;152:613–618.

101. Oda H, Kadota J, Kohno S, et al. Leukotriene B$_4$ in bronchoalveolar lavage fluid of patients with diffuse panbronchiolitis. *Chest* 1995;108:116–122.

102. Ashitani J, Mukae H, Nakazato M, et al. Elevated concentrations of defensins in bronchoalveolar lavage fluid in diffuse panbronchiolitis. *Eur Respir J* 1998;11:104–111.

103. Mukae H, Hirota M, Kohno S, et al. Elevation of tumor-associated carbohydrate antigens in patients with diffuse panbronchiolitis. *Am Rev Respir Dis* 1993;148:744–751.

104. Nakano H, Ide H, Imada M, et al. Reduced nasal nitric

oxide in diffuse panbronchiolitis. *Am J Respir Crit Care Med* 2000;162:2218–2220.

105. Koyama H, Geddes DM. Erythromycin and diffuse panbronchiolitis. *Thorax* 1997;52:915–918.

106. Lin HC, Wang CH, Liu CY, et al. Erythromycin inhibits beta₂-integrins (CD11b/CD18) expression, interleukin-8 release, and intracellular oxidative metabolism in neutrophils. *Respir Med* 2000;94:654–660.

107. Kondo M, Kanoh S, Tamaoki J, et al. Erythromycin inhibits ATP-induced intracellular calcium responses in bovine tracheal epithelial cells. *Am J Respir Cell Mol Biol* 1998;19:799–804.

108. Akira M, Higashihara T, Sakatani M, et al. Diffuse panbronchiolitis: follow-up CT examination. *Radiology* 1993;189:559–562.

109. Sugiyama Y, Kitamura S. Antineutrophil cytoplasmic antibodies in diffuse panbronchiolitis. *Respiration* 1999;66:233–235.

110. Saku N, Sugiyama Y, Kitamura S, et al. Diffuse panbronchiolitis with p-ANCA–positive arteritis and necrotizing glomerulitis. *Nippon Kyobu Shikkan Gakkai Zasshi* 1996;34:434–438.

111. Turton CW, Williams G, Green M. Cryptogenic obliterative bronchiolitis in adults. *Thorax* 1981;36:805–810.

112. Kindt GC, Weiland JE, Davis WB, et al. Bronchiolitis in adults: reversible cause of airway obstruction associated with airway neutrophils and neutrophil products. *Am Rev Respir Dis* 1988;140:483–492.

113. Kraft M, Mortenson RL, Colby TV, et al. Cryptogenic constrictive bronchiolitis. A clinicopathologic study. *Am Rev Respir Dis* 1992;148:1093–1101.

114. Poletti V, Zompatori M, Boaron M, et al. Cryptogenic constrictive bronchiolitis imitating imaging features of diffuse panbronchiolitis. *Monaldi Arch Chest Dis* 1995;50:116–117.

115. Takayanagi N, Kanazawa M, Kawabata Y, et al. Chronic bronchiolitis with associated eosinophilic lung disease (eosinophilic bronchiolitis). *Respiration* 2001;68:319–322.

116. Rinaldi M, Martinelli L, Volpato G, et al. Gastroesophageal reflux as cause of obliterative bronchiolitis: a case report. *Transplant Proc* 1995;27:2006–2007.

117. Elliott CG, Colby TV, Kelly TM, et al. Charcoal lung: bronchiolitis obliterans after aspiration of activated charcoal. *Chest* 1989;96:672–674.

118. Tsunoda N, Iwanaga T, Saito T, et al. Rapidly progressive bronchiolitis obliterans associated with Stevens-Johnson syndrome. *Chest* 1990;98:243–245.

119. Chatte G, Streichenberger N, Boillot O, et al. Lymphocytic bronchitis/bronchiolitis in a patient with primary biliary cirrhosis. *Eur Respir J* 1995;8:176–179.

120. Yousem SA, Colby TV, Carrington CB. Follicular bronchitis/bronchiolitis. *Hum Pathol* 1985;16:700–706.

121. Parto K, Svedstrom E, Majurin ML, et al. Pulmonary manifestations in lysinuric protein intolerance. *Chest* 1993;104:1176–1182.

122. Ito M, Nakagawa A, Hirabayashi N, et al. Bronchiolitis obliterans in ataxia-telangiectasia. *Virchows Arch* 1997;430:131–137.

123. Hermandez JI, Gomez-Roman J, Rodrigo E, et al. Bronchiolitis obliterans and IgA nephropathy. A new case of pulmonary-renal syndrome. *Am J Respir Crit Care Med* 1997;156:665–668.

124. Shaw RJ, Djukanovic R, Tashkin DP, et al. The role of small airways in lung disease. *Respir Med* 2002;96:67–80.

125. Trisolini R, Lazzari Agli L, Poletti V. Bronchiolocentric pulmonary involvement due to chronic lymphocytic leukemia. *Haematologica* 2000;85:1097.

126. Grinblat J, Mechlis S, Lewitus Z. Organizing pneumonia-like process: an unusual observation in steroid-responsive cases with features of chronic interstitial pneumonia. *Chest* 1981;80:259–263.

127. Davison AG, Heard BE, McAllister WA, et al. Cryptogenic organizing pneumonitis. *Q J Med* 1983;52:382–394.

128. Cordier JF. Organising pneumonia. *Thorax* 2000;55:318–328.

129. Cordier JF, Peyrol S, Loire R. Bronchiolitis obliterans organizing pneumonia as a model of inflammatory lung disease. In: Epler GR, ed. *Diseases of the bronchioles*. New York: Raven Press, 1994:313–345.

130. Svee K, White J, Vailant P, et al. Acute lung injury fibroblast migration and invasion of a fibrin matrix is mediated by CD44. *J Clin Invest* 1996;98:1713–1727.

131. Imokawa S, Sato A, Hayakawa H, et al. Tissue factor expression and fibrin deposition in the lungs of patients with idiopathic pulmonary fibrosis and systemic sclerosis. *Am J Respir Crit Care Med* 1997;156:631–636.

132. Kuhn C, Mason RJ. Immunolocalization of sparc, tenascin, and thrombospondin in pulmonary fibrosis. *Am J Pathol* 1995;147:1759–1769.

133. Carrè PC, King TE Jr, Mortenson R, et al. Cryptogenic organizing pneumonia: increased expression of interleukin-8 and fibronectin genes by alveolar macrophages. *Am J Respir Crit Care Med* 1994;110:100–105.

134. Poletti V, Castrilli G, Romagna M, et al. Bronchoalveolar lavage, histological, and immunohistochemical features in cryptogenic organizing pneumonia. *Monaldi Arch Chest Dis* 1996;51:289–295.

135. Aubert JD, Pare PD, Hogg JC, et al. Platelet-derived growth factor in bronchiolitis obliterans organizing pneumonia. *Am J Respir Crit Care Med* 1997;155:676–681.

136. Edwards DRG, Murphy G, Reynolds JJ, et al. Transforming growth factor-beta modulates the expression of collagenase and metalloproteinase inhibitor. *EMBO J* 1987;6:1899–1904.

137. McCormack FX. Role of pulmonary epithelium and surfactant in the pathogenesis of interstitial lung disease. In: Schwarz MI, King TE Jr, eds. *Interstitial lung disease*. Hamilton, Ontario: BC Decker, 1998:165–180.

138. Cohen AJ, King TE Jr, Downey GP. Rapidly progressive bronchiolitis obliterans organizing pneumonia. *Am J Respir Crit Care Med* 1994;149:1670–1675.

139. Cazzato S, Zompatori M, Baruzzi G, et al. Bronchiolitis obliterans–organizing pneumonia: an Italian experience. *Respir Med* 2000;94:702–708.

140. Mordechai Y, Ofer BI, Solomonov A, et al. Recurrent, self-limited menstrual-associated bronchiolitis obliterans organizing pneumonia. *Chest* 2000;118:253–256.

141. Erasmus JJ, Adams HP, Rossi SE. High-resolution CT of drug-induced lung disease. *Radiol Clin North Am* 2002;40:61–72.

142. Waitches GM, Stern EJ. High-resolution CT of peripheral airways diseases. *Radiol Clin North Am* 2002;40:21–29.

143. Teel GS, Engeler CE, Tashijian JH, et al. Imaging of small airways disease. *Radiographics* 1996;16:27–41.

144. Murphy JM, Schnyder P. Verschakelen J, et al. Linear opacities on HRCT in bronchiolitis obliterans organizing pneumonia. *Eur Radiol* 1999;9:1813–1817.

145. Zompatori M, Poletti V, Battista G, et al. Bronchiolitis obliterans organizing pneumonia (BOOP) presenting as a ring-shaped opacity at HRCT (the atoll sign). A case report. *Radiol Med (Torino)* 1999;97:308–310.

146. Zompatori M, Poletti V, Rimondi MR, et al. Imaging of small airways disease, with emphasis on high-resolution computed tomography. *Monaldi Arch Chest Dis* 1997;52:242–248.

147. Ikezoe J, Johkoh T, Kohno N, et al. High-resolution CT findings of lung disease in patients with polymyositis and dermatomyositis. *J Thorac Imaging* 1996;11:250–259.

148. Costabel U, Teschòer H, Guzman J. Bronchiolitis obliterans organizing pneumonia (BOOP): the cytological and

immunophenotypical profile of bronchoalveolar lavage. *Eur Respir J* 1992;5:791–797.

149. Poletti V, Cazzato S, Minicuci N, et al. The diagnostic value of bronchoalveolar lavage and transbronchial lung biopsy in cryptogenic organizing pneumonia. *Eur Respir J* 1996;9:2513–2516.

150. Lazor R, Vandevenne A, Pelletier A, et al. Cryptogenic organizing pneumonia. Characteristics of relapses in a series of 48 patients. *Am J Respir Crit Care Med* 2000;162:571–577.

151. Egerer G, Witzens M, Spaeth A, et al. Successful treatment of bronchiolitis obliterans organizing pneumonia with low-dose methotrexate in a patient with Hodgkin's disease. *Oncology* 2001;61:23–27.

152. Yousem S, Lohr RH, Colby TV. Idiopathic bronchiolitis obliterans organizing pneumonia/cryptogenic organizing pneumonia with unfavorable outcome: pathologic predictors. *Mod Pathol* 1997;10:864–871.

30 Pulmonary Vasculitis

Joseph P. Lynch, III

Systemic necrotizing vasculitis involves the lung primarily in the context of the granulomatous vasculitis syndromes (e.g., Wegener granulomatosis [1–4], Churg-Strauss syndrome [5–7], lymphomatoid granulomatosis [8,9]) or the pulmonary-renal syndromes (e.g., microscopic polyangiitis, pauci-immune glomerulonephritis [7,10,11]). Pulmonary hemorrhage, usually secondary to capillaritis, is common in microscopic polyangiitis (30%–50%) (7) and rarely complicates Wegener granulomatosis (12,13), Churg-Strauss syndrome (6), Behçet disease (14–17), or Henoch-Schönlein syndrome (18–20). Classic polyarteritis nodosa rarely involves the lung (6, 7). Pulmonary arterial aneurysms are well-recognized complications of Takayasu arteritis (21–23) and Behçet disease (16,24,25). In this chapter, we first review the vasculitides associated with circulating antibodies against the cytoplasmic components of neutrophils and monocytes (i.e., antineutrophil cytoplasmic antibodies), which include primarily Wegener granulomatosis, microscopic polyangiitis, and Churg-Strauss syndrome (7,11,26,27). We next discuss lymphomatoid granulomatosis, a rare entity resembling Wegener granulomatosis that is not a true vasculitis but rather represents a group of lymphoproliferative disorders (including frank malignancies) (28–30). Later, we discuss disorders in which lung involvement is less commonly recognized—Behçet disease (25), Takayasu arteritis (21), and Henoch-Schönlein syndrome (18,19).

ANTINEUTROPHIL CYTOPLASMIC ANTIBODIES

Circulating antineutrophil cytoplasmic antibody (ANCA) is frequently found in necrotizing small vessel vasculitis as-

J. P. Lynch, III: Department of Internal Medicine, University of Michigan, Ann Arbor, Michigan.

sociated with pulmonary capillaritis or glomerulonephritis (7,11,26,27,31). Types of ANCA with differing antigenic specificities have been noted and differ in prognostic and clinical significance (7,27,32). Antibody with antigenic specificity for proteinase-3 (PR3) exhibits a cytoplasmic pattern on immunofluorescence (c-ANCA), whereas antibody with antigenic specificity for myeloperoxidase (MPO) exhibits a perinuclear pattern (p-ANCA) (7,26,27). Antibodies with distinct antigenic determinants are observed in different types of vasculitis. c-ANCA (PR3-ANCA) is detected in 70% to 93% of patients with untreated Wegener granulomatosis (27,32–35) and in 10% to 20% of patients with microscopic polyangiitis or Churg-Strauss syndrome (36–40). More than 50% of patients with microscopic polyangiitis, Churg-Strauss syndrome, or pauci-immune glomerulonephritis demonstrate circulating p-ANCA (MPO-ANCA), whereas p-ANCA is rarely found in Wegener granulomatosis (27,36–40). Detectable ANCA (typically p-ANCA) is present in fewer than 20% of patients with macroscopic polyarteritis nodosa (7,36,41). c-ANCA is relatively specific (>90%) for small vessel vasculitis (7,11), but p-ANCA may be observed in myriad inflammatory disorders in which vasculitis is lacking (e.g., collagen-vascular disease, inflammatory bowel disease) (27).

WEGENER GRANULOMATOSIS

Wegener granulomatosis (WG), the most common of the pulmonary granulomatous vasculitides, typically involves the upper respiratory tract (sinuses, ears, nasopharynx, oropharynx, and trachea), lower respiratory tract (bronchi and lung), and kidneys with varying degrees of disseminated vasculitis (1,2,4,42–44). Major histologic features include a necrotizing vasculitis involving small vessels (arterioles, venules, and capillaries), extensive necrosis, and granulomatous inflammation (1,42,43,45–47). The estimated prevalence of WG is between 13 and 30 cases per million persons per 5-year period (1,48). WG may be more common in northern Europe. Annual incidence rates of WG (per million) are 10.3 in England and 4.1 in Spain (49). A study from Norway cited *annual* incidence rates as high as 12 per million (prevalence of approximately 95 per million) (50). The peak incidence is in the fourth through the sixth decades of life (1,4,48); children or adolescents are rarely affected (51,52). No gender predominance has been noted (2).

Clinical Features

The clinical manifestations are protean, and virtually any organ can be involved. Upper airway symptoms often predominate (1,2,53,54). The lungs are affected in more than two thirds of patients, and glomerulonephritis occurs in 55% to 85% (1,4,42,43,55,56). Although WG usually involves multiple organs, limited variants exist in which only one or two organs are involved (4,57–59). This subset of patients has a more favorable prognosis. DeRemee and colleagues (57) proposed a staging classification based on involvement of ear, nose, throat (E), lung (L), and kidney (K) to stratify patients with single- or multiple-organ involvement. Other major diagnostic criteria (in addition to small vessel vasculitis) proposed by the American College of Rheumatology in 1990 include nasal or oral inflammation, abnormalities on chest radiographs, abnormal urine sediment, and granulomatous inflammation on biopsy specimens (44). Many classic features lacking in the *early* phases of the disease may evolve months or even years after the initial presentation (1,2,4,43). High titers of circulating c-ANCA may support the diagnosis in the appropriate clinical context, even when histologic features are not definitive (27,32–35). However, the specificity of c-ANCA has been challenged (27,60–62).

Upper Airway Involvement

The upper respiratory tract (sinuses, ears, nasopharynx, oropharynx, trachea) is involved in more than 90% of patients (1,2,4,42,43,53,56). Chronic persistent sinusitis, epistaxis, or otitis media is often the presenting and dominant clinical feature of WG but is often mistakenly thought to be of allergic or infectious origin (1,2). Plain sinus radiographs or thin-section computed tomographic (CT) scans reveal abnormalities in more than 85% of patients with WG (1,42,53). Thickening or clouding of the sinuses is a characteristic radiographic feature; erosion or destruction of sinus bones may occur (1,53). Secondary pyogenic sinus infections are common and may be difficult to distinguish from exacerbations of WG (1,2). The ears are involved in 30% to 50% of patients (1,2,53,54). Otalgia and refractory otitis media are common early symptoms of WG (1). Chronic otitis media, chronic mastoiditis, or hearing loss develops in 15% to 25% of patients (1,4,54). The nasopharynx is involved

in 60% to 80% of patients (1,4,53,54). Clinical manifestations include epistaxis, nasal septal perforation, persistent nasal congestion or pain, and mucosal ulcers (1,2). Saddle nose deformity, resulting from destruction of the nasal cartilage, occurs in 10% to 25% of patients (1,4,53,54). Sore throat or hoarseness may reflect ulcerations or granulomatous involvement of the pharynx or vocal cords (1,53,54).

Despite the propensity for WG to affect the upper respiratory tract, histologic confirmation may be difficult. Biopsy specimens of upper airway lesions often demonstrate nonspecific findings of necrosis and chronic inflammation (47,63). The cardinal histologic features of vasculitis and granulomatous inflammation may be lacking. A review of 126 biopsy specimens from upper airway or nasopharyngeal lesions in patients with WG seen at the National Institutes of Health (NIH) revealed the triad of granulomas, vasculitis, and necrosis in only 16% of specimens (47). The combinations of vasculitis plus granulomas and of vasculitis plus necrosis were each noted in 21% of patients (47). Generous biopsy specimens of involved sites or specimens from additional sites are critical to substantiate the diagnosis.

Ocular Involvement

Ocular involvement occurs in 20% to 50% of patients with WG (1,4,42,43,64–67). Manifestations may be superficial (e.g., conjunctivitis, scleritis), but uveitis, vasculitis, or compression of the optic nerve may lead to blindness in 2% to 9% of patients (1,42,43,64–66). Proptosis from a retro-orbital granulomatous inflammatory process has been described in 10% to 22% of patients and may compromise the blood supply to the optic nerve (1,42,66,67). In this context, surgical decompression may be required for patients failing to respond to aggressive medical therapy (66).

Involvement of the Trachea and Bronchi

Stenosis or narrowing of the trachea or major bronchi as a result of granulomatous involvement develops in 10% to 30% of patients with WG (1,2,53,55,68–70). The rate of asymptomatic involvement of major airways is even higher. Tracheal or bronchial involvement is nearly invariably associated with involvement of the nasopharynx or sinuses (53,69). Of 43 patients with subglottic stenosis complicating WG, 47% had saddle nose deformity (69). Tracheal stenosis is usually circumferential and localized, extending for only 3 to 5 cm below the glottis (53,69,70). However, more extensive involvement of the distal trachea or main bronchi may occur (55,70). A study from the Mayo Clinic cited endobronchial abnormalities in 30 (59%) of 51 patients with WG undergoing bronchoscopy (70). Four (13%) had tracheal or bronchial stenosis. Importantly, extensive endobronchial abnormalities were noted in 11 patients with *normal* chest radiographic findings. Ulcerating tracheobronchitis was the most common lesion and led to progressive stenosis in seven patients. Persistent dyspnea or wheezing may reflect scarring at sites of previous endobronchial inflammation. Stridor or wheezing is a clinical clue to the development of large-airway (trachea or main bronchi) stenosis.

Truncation (flow rate limitation) of the inspiratory portion of the flow-volume loop is a sensitive indicator of physiologically significant obstruction of the upper airway (69). When the site of obstruction is fixed, both the inspiratory and expiratory portions are affected (Fig. 30.1). Bronchoscopy or spiral CT more objectively quantifies the degree of airway stenosis (71–73) (Fig. 30.2). A three-dimensional image reconstruction and display technique based on high-resolution CT (virtual bronchoscopy) is a noninvasive means of assessing the presence and extent of airway stenoses with sensitivity at least to segmental bronchi (72).

The histologic confirmation of endobronchial WG is difficult because endobronchial biopsy specimens usually demonstrate nonspecific changes (e.g., necrosis or inflammation). In a study of 26 WG patients with subglottic stenosis, dual features of vasculitis and granulomatous inflammation were present in only 7 (5%) of 140 subglottic biopsy specimens (69). In the Mayo Clinic study, endobronchial specimens fulfilled specific histologic criteria for WG in only 3 of 17 patients (70). Serum titers of c-ANCA did not correlate with endobronchial inflammation (70). Thus, the diagnosis of tracheal or endobronchial involvement in patients with known WG in some cases must be *presumed* in the

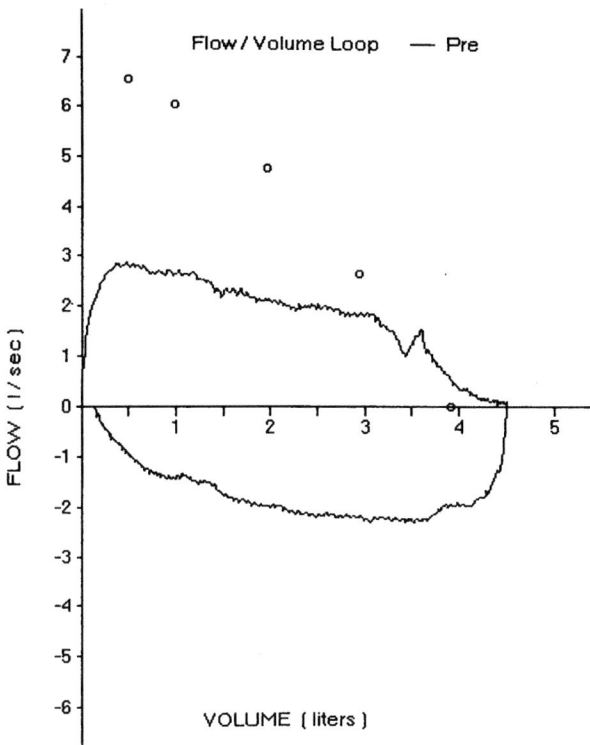

FIGURE 30.1. Wegener granulomatosis. Flow-volume loop from a 34-year-old woman with tracheal (subglottic) stenosis secondary to Wegener granulomatosis. Note the truncation of both the inspiration and expiratory limbs, consistent with fixed obstruction of the upper airway.

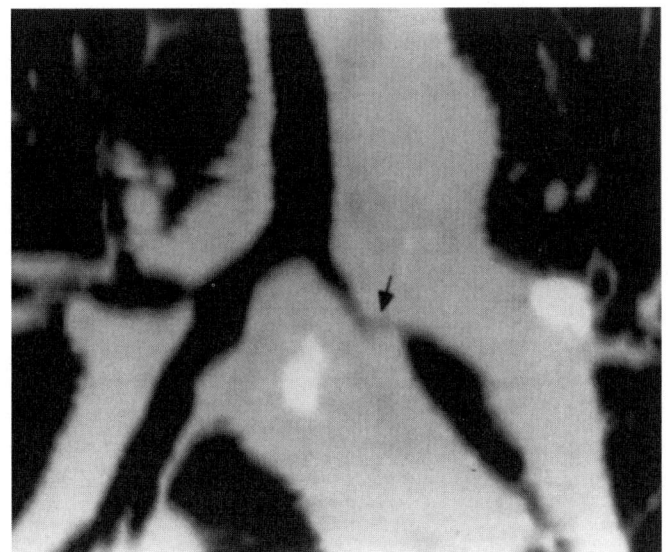

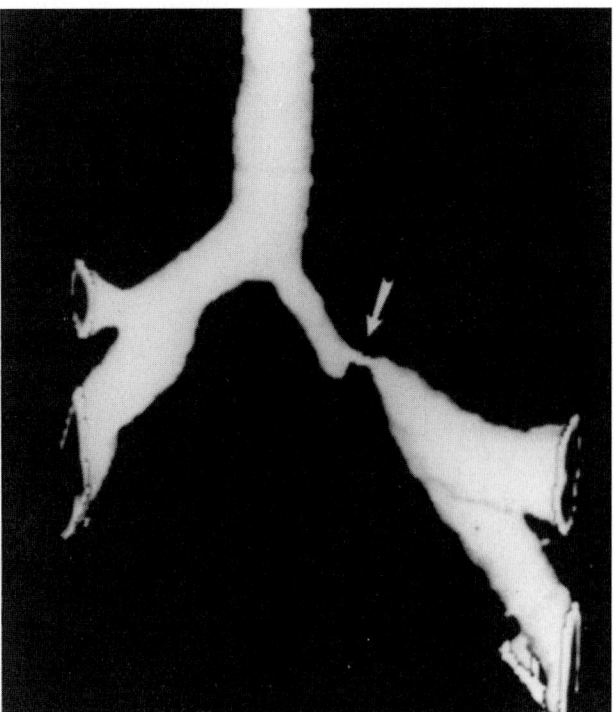

FIGURE 30.2. A: Wegener granulomatosis. Coronal helical computed tomographic reconstruction shows severe stenosis of the left main bronchus (*arrow*) in a patient with Wegener granulomatosis. **B:** Three-dimensional shaded surface display created from helical computed tomographic data shows severe stenosis of the left main bronchus (*arrow*) in a patient with Wegener granulomatosis. (From Lynch JP III, Quint LE. Tracheobronchial and esophageal manifestations of systemic diseases. In: Cummings C, ed. *Otolaryngology head and neck surgery*, 3rd ed. St. Louis: Mosby–Year Book, 1998:2343–2367, with permission.)

appropriate clinical context, even when the histology is less than definitive.

Importantly, progressive subglottic or bronchial stenosis can develop even when the disease is quiescent at other sites (69,70). Severe stenosis of large airways may necessitate treatment with neodymium:yttrium-aluminum garnet (Nd:YAG) laser, dilation, intratracheal corticosteroid injections, or placement of Silastic airway stents (1,53,68–70). Severe obstruction of the upper airway may mandate tracheostomy (69). Tracheal reconstruction has been successfully performed in patients with severe tracheal stenosis refractory to medical therapy, but it is a formidable undertaking (69).

Involvement of the Pulmonary Parenchyma

Pulmonary symptoms (e.g., cough, dyspnea, hemoptysis) are noted in approximately one third to one half of patients with WG and are caused by parenchymal necrosis, endobronchial inflammation and cicatrix formation, and alveolar hemorrhage (1,2,4,42,43,46,55). Pulmonary function tests may demonstrate airflow obstruction (particularly when endobronchial involvement is prominent), restriction, or a mixed pattern (55,74). Despite a relatively low prevalence of clinical symptoms, abnormalities on chest radiographs are noted in more than 70% of patients at some point during the course of the disease (1,2,4,42,55). Single or multiple nodules or nodular opacities are characteristic; cavitation is noted in one fourth (1,42,55) (Fig. 30.3). Other features include focal pneumonic opacities (Fig. 30.4), large mass lesions (Fig. 30.5), pleural effusions, stenosis of the trachea or bronchi, and atelectasis. Hilar or mediastinal lymphadenopathy has only rarely been described (55,75). Extensive alveolar

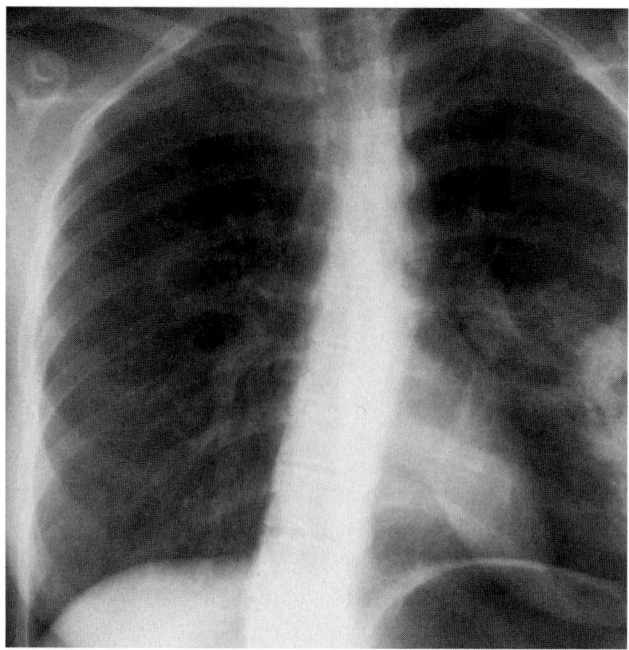

FIGURE 30.4. Wegener granulomatosis. Posteroanterior chest radiograph demonstrates dense focal alveolar opacities in an 18-year-old woman with sinusitis, cough, fever, and cutaneous nodules. The patient's serum was positive for antineutrophil cytoplasmic antibody (c-ANCA titer of 1:1,200). Skin biopsy specimens demonstrated a leukocytoclastic vasculitis. Sinus biopsy specimens revealed a granulomatous necrotizing vasculitis consistent with Wegener granulomatosis. The chest radiographic findings normalized within 2 weeks after the initiation of cyclophosphamide and prednisone therapy.

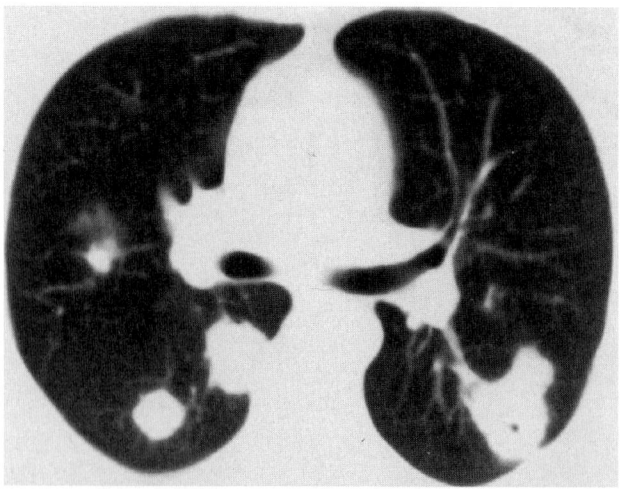

FIGURE 30.3. Wegener granulomatosis. Computed tomographic scan demonstrates multiple focal nodules in a 40-year-old man. Open lung biopsy demonstrated a necrotizing granulomatous vasculitis consistent with Wegener granulomatosis. (From Orens JB, Sitrin RC, Lynch JP III. The approach to nonresolving pneumonia. *Med Clin North Am* 1994;78:1160, with permission.)

or mixed interstitial-alveolar opacities may be seen with pulmonary capillaritis and alveolar hemorrhage (12,76) (Fig. 30.6). Chest CT typically reveals nodules, masses, cavitary lesions, and focal opacities in the context of active disease; additional features on CT that may be missed on conventional chest x-ray films include septal bands, parenchymal scarring, ground-glass opacities, irregular pleural thickening, and stenosis of large airways (73,77,78).

Open (or thoracoscopic) lung biopsy is usually required to substantiate the diagnosis of pulmonary WG. When focal pulmonary opacities or nodules are present, the triad of vasculitis, granulomas, and necrosis is found in more than 90% of patients by surgical biopsy (46). Additional nonspecific features include cryptogenic organizing pneumonia (79), chrondritis involving the bronchial cartilage (80), acute or chronic bronchiolitis (79), interstitial fibrosis (46), and capillaritis (12).

The yield of endobronchial or transbronchial lung biopsy is only 3% to 18% (46,55,70,81). Transthoracic core needle biopsy (guided by CT or fluoroscopy) has been performed in a few patients, but the specificity appears to be low (82).

Massive alveolar hemorrhage is a rare but potentially fatal complication of WG and reflects diffuse injury to the pulmonary microvasculature (12,13). In this setting, rapidly progressive glomerulonephritis is present in more than 90%

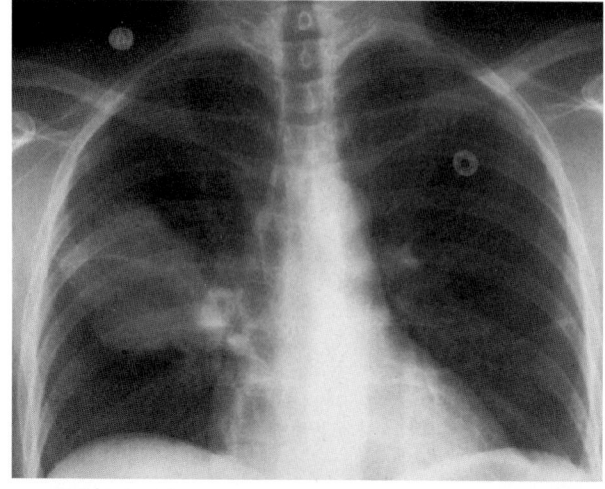

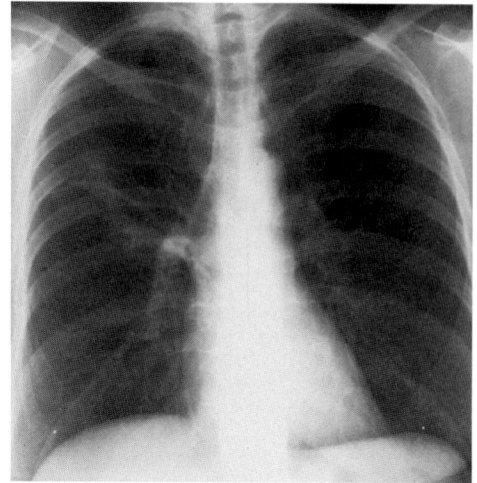

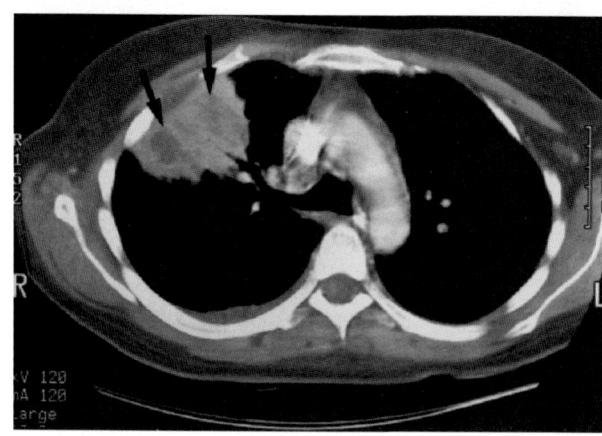

FIGURE 30.5. A: Wegener granulomatosis. Posteroanterior chest radiograph demonstrates a right upper lobe mass in a 36-year-old woman with leukocytoclastic vasculitis, fever, sinusitis, and cough. **B:** Computed tomographic scan from the same patient reveals a mass lesion in the anterior segment of the right upper lobe with focal areas of necrosis (*arrows*). Transbronchial lung biopsy specimens demonstrated a granulomatous vasculitis with extensive necrosis and a polymorphous inflammatory cell infiltrate consistent with Wegener granulomatosis. **C:** Posteroanterior chest radiograph from same patient 5 weeks after the initiation of therapy with cyclophosphamide and prednisone shows nearly complete resolution of the right upper lobe mass.

of patients (12,55,76). By contrast, fewer than 40% manifest upper airway symptoms (76). The role of surgical lung biopsy in the setting of diffuse alveolar hemorrhage is controversial. The histopathologic features are usually nonspecific. Alveolar hemorrhage is the predominant histopathologic finding (12). Inflammation and necrosis of the alveolar capillaries (capillaritis) may be noted, but the granulomatous vasculitis or extensive parenchymal necrosis characteristic of WG at other sites is lacking (12). In cases of severe pulmonary hemorrhage, we believe the risk of surgical lung biopsy outweighs the benefit. A presumptive diagnosis of diffuse alveolar hemorrhage can often be established on the basis of the clinical and radiographic features, the presence of circulating c-ANCA, and the results of bronchoscopy with bronchoalveolar lavage (BAL). Large numbers of hemosiderin-laden macrophages, bloody or serosanguinous BAL fluid, and an absence of infectious causes support the diagnosis of diffuse alveolar hemorrhage (Fig. 30.7). Biopsy of extrapulmonary sites of involvement may substantiate the diagnosis.

Diffuse alveolar hemorrhage is a medical emergency that requires aggressive therapy with intravenous "pulse" methylprednisolone (1 g daily for 3 days) (85) while a diagnostic workup is pursued and the results of biopsies and ancillary laboratory results are awaited. Conventional therapy with

oral cyclophosphamide and a tapered regimen of corticosteroids (42) are appropriate once the diagnosis of WG has been confirmed.

Renal Involvement

Glomerulonephritis (pauci-immune) occurs in 70% to 85% of patients at some point in the course of the disease, but only 11% to 17% of patients exhibit severe renal insufficiency at presentation (1,2,4,42,43,83,84,86). Granulomatous vasculitis is observed in 6% to 15% of renal biopsy specimens from patients with WG (1,42,86,87). The characteristic renal lesion of WG is a segmental focal glomerulonephritis (1,87). In more fulminant forms, a necrotizing, crescentic glomerulonephritis is observed (83,84,87). These histologic findings are nonspecific and can be found in diverse immune-mediated or infectious disorders. Microscopic hematuria or proteinuria precedes detectable abnormalities of renal function (1,83,84).

The clinical course of the renal disease is variable. The patient may progress to renal failure rapidly, within a few days (83,84), or indolently, over months or even years (1,87,88). For patients with crescentic glomerulonephritis, the aggressive and prompt institution of therapy is mandatory to avert

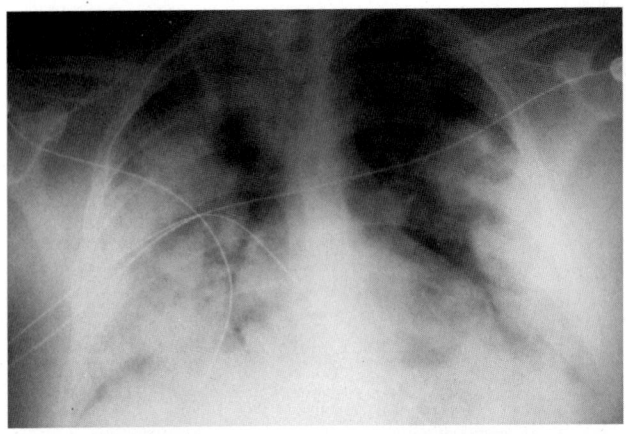

A

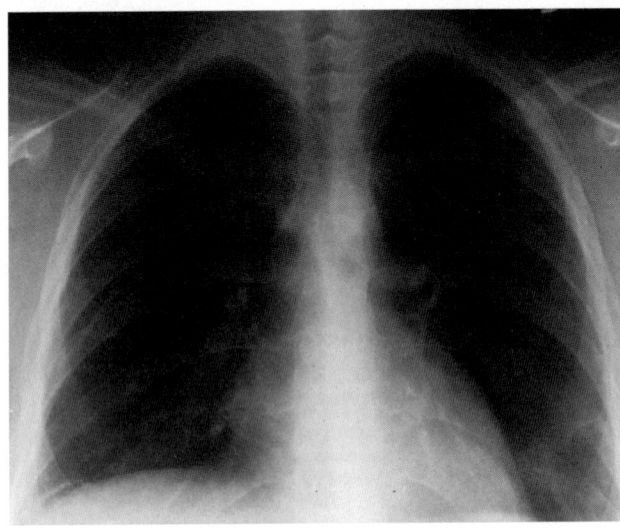

B

FIGURE 30.6. A: Alveolar hemorrhage secondary to Wegener granulomatosis. Posteroanterior chest radiograph from a 13-year-old girl demonstrates extensive, confluent alveolar opacities. She presented with severe dyspnea, fever, and hemoptysis. Urinalysis demonstrated microscopic hematuria and proteinuria. Open lung biopsy demonstrated massive pulmonary hemorrhage and capillaritis, but no granulomas. Review of a prior sinus biopsy specimen demonstrated extensive necrosis and inflammatory exudate with occasional multinucleated giant cells but no definite vasculitis. Pulse methylprednisolone, followed by oral prednisone and cyclophosphamide, was instituted. **B:** Alveolar hemorrhage secondary to Wegener granulomatosis. Posteroanterior chest radiographs from the same patient 3 weeks later demonstrate complete clearing of the alveolar opacities. After institution of therapy, she remained asymptomatic. Cyclophosphamide was discontinued after 15 months, and prednisone was discontinued after 18 months.

irreversible renal damage. Even in oliguric renal failure, substantial recovery of renal function can be achieved in most patients (87). However, end-stage dialysis-dependent renal failure is more common in patients with severe loss of glomeruli on renal biopsy (87,89).

Percutaneous renal biopsy is warranted if the urinary sediment demonstrates microscopic hematuria or if renal insufficiency is present. Rapidly progressive glomerulonephritis that is negative on immunofluorescent staining (i.e., pauci-immune) is characteristic of WG in the context of diffuse alveolar hemorrhage (76,83–85).

Chronic renal failure remains a major cause of death, and 11% to 32% of patients with WG eventually require chronic dialysis (1,84,87,88,90). Renal transplantation has been successfully accomplished in patients with end-stage renal disease and WG in complete remission (88). Recurrence of WG has been rare following transplantation. In anecdotal reports, other rare urologic complications of WG include necrotizing vasculitis of the ureters, penis, or prostate (1).

Central or Peripheral Nervous System Involvement

Central or peripheral nervous system involvement is present in fewer than 4% of patients at initial presentation but even-

tually develops in 10% to 34% (1,42,55,91). In a classic review of 104 patients with WG, Drachman (92) identified three processes of central nervous system involvement: (a) vasculitis; (b) granulomatous lesions resulting from invasion by contiguous nasal, paranasal, or orbital disease; and (c) granulomatous lesions remote from nasal granulomas (involving brain or meninges). Mononeuritis multiplex or polyneuritis accounts for more than 50% of neurologic complications (1,42,91). Other manifestations include the following: cerebral infarction or hemorrhage, cranial nerve palsies, focal deficits or seizures resulting from cerebral mass lesions, diabetes insipidus (secondary to granulomatous involvement of the hypothalamus), quadriparesis or paraparesis (reflecting involvement of the spinal cord microvasculature), generalized seizures (reflecting meningeal involvement) (93), and visual loss (from compression of the optic nerve or vasculitis of the vasculature) (1,42,91,94). Vasculitis of the central nervous system has only rarely been confirmed histologically because of the inaccessible location of lesions and the risks associated with biopsy (95). The diagnosis is usually supported by histologic confirmation at extraneural sites or by noninvasive studies (e.g., electromyography, magnetic resonance imaging [MRI], CT of the brain) in patients with neurologic symptoms and previously documented WG

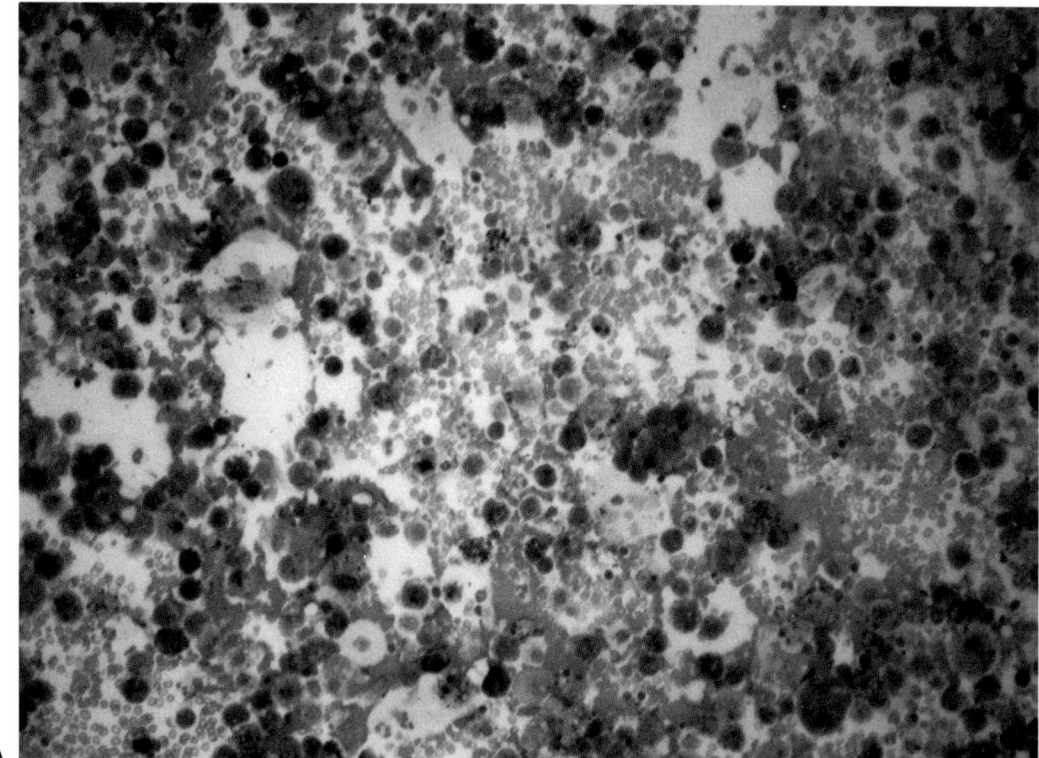

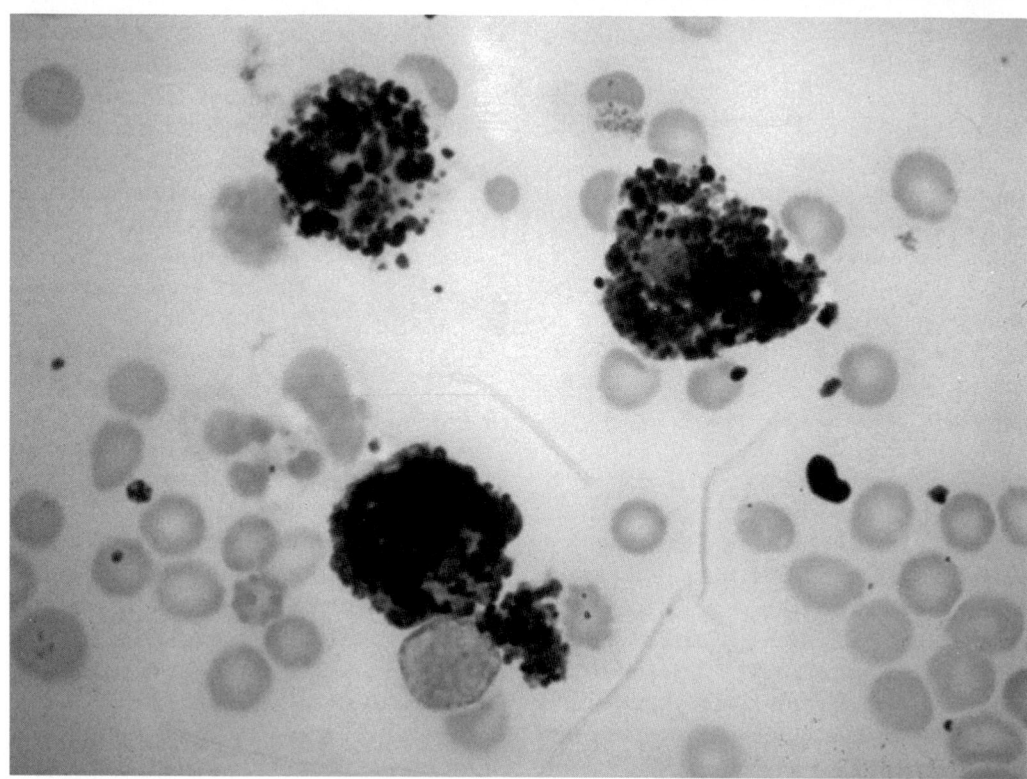

FIGURE 30.7. A: Hemosiderin-laden macrophages. In the photomicrograph, bronchoalveolar lavage fluid contains numerous hemosiderin-laden macrophages with adjacent red blood cells indicating alveolar hemorrhage (Wright stain, low power). **B:** Hemosiderin-laden macrophages. Photomicrograph of bronchoalveolar lavage fluid shows hemosiderin-laden alveolar macrophages stained blue by iron stain (Prussian blue stain, high power).

(96–98). MRI may reveal a wide spectrum of findings, including diffuse or focal dural thickening and enhancement, discrete lesions, infarcts, nonspecific areas of high signal intensity in white matter, enlargement of the pituitary gland with infundibular thickening, and cerebral atrophy (96). Cerebral angiography is ill advised because the small vessels affected in WG are below the sensitivity of angiography. In some patients, the finding on biopsy of the sural nerve or other affected nerves may support the diagnosis (91).

Involvement of Other Organs

Constitutional features (e.g., malaise, fatigue, fever, weight loss) occur in one third or more of patients with WG (1,42). Nondeforming polyarthritis involving medium-size and large joints occurs in two thirds of patients and parallels the activity of the systemic disease (1,42). Articular symptoms usually remit with cytotoxic or corticosteroid therapy.

Cutaneous lesions are present in 20% to 50% of patients during the course of the disease (1,4,42). The manifestations are protean and include palpable purpura, subcutaneous nodules, papules, petechiae, ulcers, and nonspecific erythematous or maculopapular rashes (1,99,100). Skin biopsy specimens may demonstrate granulomatous vasculitis with necrosis but most often show nonspecific changes of leukocytoclastic vasculitis (1,99,100).

Cardiac involvement is rarely documented before death, but prevalence rates of 8% to 15% have been estimated (1,4,101–105). Coronary arteritis and pericarditis are the most common clinical features (101–105). Cardiomy-

opathies, conduction defects, and fatal arrhythmias may reflect necrotizing vasculitis or granulomatous inflammation involving the myocardium or coronary arteries (1,101,102). In one study, valvular abnormalities were detected in eight of nine patients with WG by echocardiography (103), suggesting that asymptomatic cardiac involvement may be common.

Gastrointestinal manifestations (e.g., abdominal pain, diarrhea, hemorrhage, perforation) have been cited in fewer than 5% of patients with WG (1,4). This may in part reflect the inaccessibility of the lesions or the lack of an aggressive diagnostic approach. In two series, gastrointestinal involvement was detected in 4 of 45 (106) and in 4 of 36 patients (107). In a review of the literature, granulomatous or vascular lesions within the gastrointestinal tract were reported in 23 of 59 necropsies in patients with WG (108).

Histopathology

The cardinal histopathologic features of WG include the following: a necrotizing vasculitis affecting arterioles, venules, and capillaries; granulomatous inflammation; geographic parenchymal necrosis; hemorrhagic infarcts; and areas of fibrosis (1,42,45,46). Well-formed sarcoid-like granulomas are uncommon, but multinucleated giant cells, epithelioid cells, and collections of histiocytes are usually evident in involved organs (1,42,45,46). The vascular walls are infiltrated by mononuclear cells and neutrophils, with occasional multinucleated giant cells and eosinophils (Fig. 30.8). Fibrinoid necrosis and thrombosis within vascular lumina are early findings (45). Later, fibrosis of the vascular walls may result in stenosis or obliteration of the lumina. A pronounced

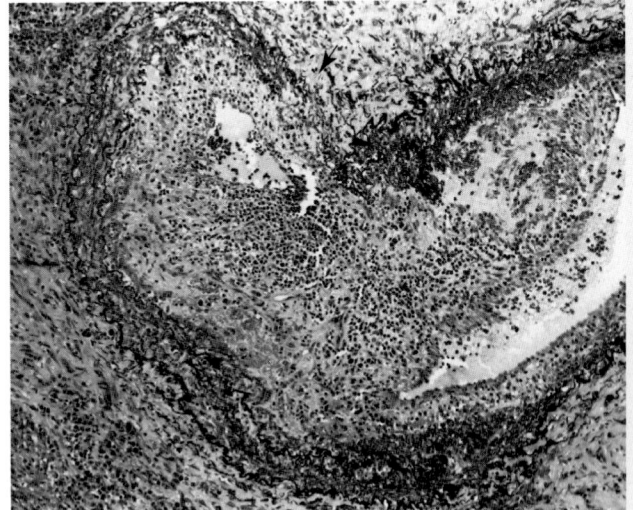
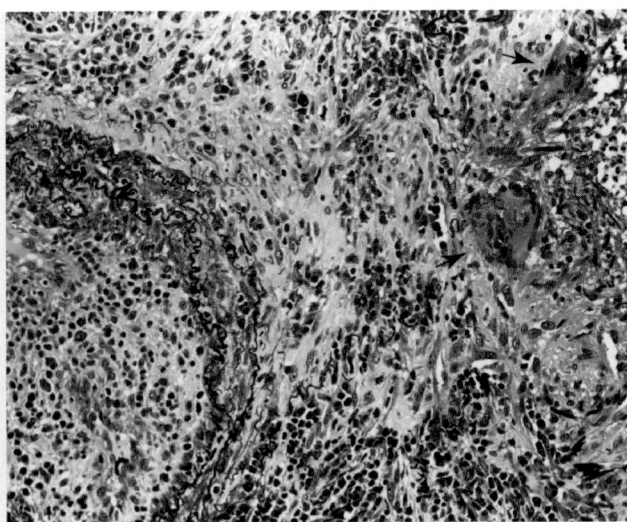

A   B

FIGURE 30.8. A: Wegener granulomatosis. Photomicrograph of lung biopsy specimen demonstrating transmural inflammation of a small vessel with partial destruction of the elastin framework (*arrow*). Note the inflammation of the intima and marked narrowing of the vascular lumen (pentachrome stain). **B:** Wegener granulomatosis. Photomicrograph of lung biopsy specimen demonstrating multinucleated giant cells surrounding necrotic debris (*arrows*). A markedly inflamed blood vessel is visible in the left portion of the field (pentachrome stain). (Courtesy of Andrew Flint, M.D., Department of Pathology, University of Michigan Medical Center.)

fibroblastic component, with concentric rings of collagen and connective tissue matrix, may be present. These histologic features may not be found if small or nonrepresentative biopsy specimens are obtained. Granulomas and inflammation of small vessels may be observed in cases with infection (particularly infection caused by mycobacteria and fungi) (109). Thus, specific staining should be performed in any granulomatous or necrotic lesion to exclude infectious causes.

Laboratory Features

Anemia, thrombocytosis, or leukocytosis has been noted in 30% to 40% of patients with WG (1,2,4,42,55). Leukopenia or thrombocytopenia is rare in the absence of cytotoxic therapy (1,42). Peripheral blood eosinophilia is not a feature of WG. Polyclonal hypergammaglobulinemia occurs in up to 50% of patients (1,42). The serum complement levels are normal or elevated (1,42). Renal function tests (serum creatinine, blood urea nitrogen) and a urinalysis should be performed in all patients initially. Striking increases in the erythrocyte sedimentation rate and C-reactive protein level are characteristic of active, generalized disease (1,83,110,111). However, the erythrocyte sedimentation rate or C-reactive protein level can be normal in active disease, particularly when only a single site is involved (70). Serial determinations of the erythrocyte sedimentation rate or C-reactive protein level are useful in monitoring the disease but are nonspecific because elevations may occur in the presence of coexisting infections (83,110). The c-ANCA titer is helpful in the initial diagnosis of WG and in monitoring the response to therapy (2,27). Increases in c-ANCA have been noted in more than 90% of patients with active generalized WG, and in 40% to 70% of patients with active regional WG (34,112–114). Of WG patients with circulating ANCA, more than 90% have ANCA directed against PR3, a serine protease in azurophilic granules of neutrophils; fewer than 10% have ANCA directed against MPO or other antigenic epitopes (27,60,115,116). Changes in the c-ANCA titer usually correlate with disease activity and are unaffected by intercurrent infection (112,113). However, c-ANCA titers may persist in 30% to 40% of patients even after a complete clinical remission has been achieved (2,112,114,117). Furthermore, increases in the c-ANCA titer do not necessarily presage relapse (26,112,114,117). Serial determinations of the c-ANCA titer provide useful *adjunctive* information in addition to the clinical data, but treatment decisions should not rely *exclusively* on the c-ANCA titer (2,26,31).

Pathogenesis

The cause of WG is unknown. The preponderance of disease in the upper and lower respiratory tract, the intense mononuclear infiltration, and the granulomatous character are consistent with an exaggerated cellular immune response

DIAGNOSIS OF WEGENER GRANULOMATOSIS	
Summary Statement	**Level of Evidence**
The presence of two or more of following clinical criteria have a sensitivity of 88% and a specificity of 92% for the diagnosis: ■ Nasal or oral inflammation (painful or painless oral ulcers or purulent or bloody nasal discharge) ■ Abnormal chest radiograph showing nodules, fixed infiltrates, or cavities ■ Abnormal urinary sediment (microscopic hematuria with or without red cell casts) ■ Granulomatous inflammation on biopsy specimen of an artery or perivascular area	Consensus panel
Nearly all patients with active systemic Wegener granulomatosis test positive for ANCA (range, 65%–>90%). However, the presence c-ANCA is not sufficient to make or exclude the diagnosis accurately.	Nonrandomized trials, observational studies

c-ANCA, cytoplasmic form of antineutrophil cytoplasmic antibody.

to inhaled antigen(s) (2). The granulomatous process in WG is mediated by CD4$^+$ T cells that produce T helper subset 1 (Th1) cell cytokines (e.g., interleukin-2 [IL-2], interferon-γ [IFN-γ], tumor necrosis factor-α [TNF-α]) (118). Increases in serum immunoglobulins, B-cell activity, circulating autoantibody (c-ANCA), and immune complexes suggest that humoral mechanisms are also operative (2). The presence of polymorphonuclear leukocytes in the inflammatory vasculitic process and of circulating autoantibodies directed against neutrophil cytoplasmic components suggest a role for neutrophils and c-ANCA in the pathogenesis and evolution of the disorder (2,119). The binding of PR3-ANCA may activate neutrophils and endothelial cells, eliciting cytokine release and injury (2,120). Exacerbations of WG during intercurrent infections and the frequent relapses observed in patients with WG who are chronic nasal carriers of *Staphylococcus aureus* (121) suggest that infections may amplify the inflammatory process, possibly by eliciting an antibody and acute phase response.

Therapy

Before therapy became available, more than 80% of patients with WG died within 3 years after the onset of symptoms, usually of progressive renal insufficiency (122). Corticosteroids improved survival modestly (123). In the 1970s, the introduction of cyclophosphamide led to a dramatic improvement in prognosis and survival (124). Oral cyclophosphamide (1–2 mg/kg per day) combined with corticosteroids is the treatment of choice for WG. Remissions were achieved in 70% to 93% of patients with this regimen; early mortality was less than 15% (1,4,84,114,122,124). The late sequelae of vasculitis (e.g., cerebrovascular accidents, myocardial infarction, renal failure, hypertension) and complications of cyclophosphamide therapy (e.g., opportunistic infections, neoplasms) contribute to long-term mortality and morbidity (1,3,4,125–128). The dose of cyclophosphamide may have to be adjusted to maintain acceptable blood counts (particularly a leukocyte count > 3,000/mm^3). Corticosteroids relieve many of the inflammatory manifestations of WG and are important as adjunctive therapy. However, corticosteroids are not adequate as *monotherapy*. Of the first 158 patients with WG seen at the NIH, 57 were *initially* treated with corticosteroids (1). Although partial improvement was sometimes cited, none of 45 patients with renal involvement achieved complete remission with corticosteroids *alone*. Furthermore, it should be emphasized that the initial dose of prednisone advocated in the early studies (i.e., 1 mg/kg per day) (1,124) is arbitrary; comparative trials assessing the optimal dose, duration, and rate of taper of corticosteroid therapy are lacking. We individualize the dosing of corticosteroids according to the clinical response and the presence or absence of adverse effects. We attempt to taper to alternate-day prednisone (e.g., 60 mg every other day) within the first 2 to 3 months. Thereafter, we gradually taper the prednisone to a low maintenance dose (e.g., 10–20 mg on alternate days) within 6 to 9 months. Ultimately, corticosteroids are discontinued if remissions are sustained. Excessive cumulative doses of corticosteroids may lead to long-term adverse effects (particularly osteoporosis and opportunistic infections) (3). Similarly, the optimal duration of cyclophosphamide therapy has not been validated in prospective trials. However, because of high relapse rates (30%–70%) following the cessation or tapering of therapy (1,2,4,124), Fauci and Wolff (124) and others (1) advocate continuing cyclophosphamide for a *minimum* of 12 months *after* complete clinical and laboratory remission has been achieved. A shorter duration of therapy has been associated with unacceptably high rates of relapse and late sequelae (84). When relapses occur, reinstitution of therapy is usually efficacious (1,4). Prolonged therapy may be required for patients with a tendency to relapse. Unfortunately, cyclophosphamide is associated with myriad complications. Opportunistic infections (particularly herpes zoster and *Pneumocystis carinii* pneumonia) occur in 20% to 30% of patients receiving cyclophosphamide (2,125–127,129). Other complications include bone marrow toxicity, pulmonary toxicity, alopecia, gastrointestinal symptoms (e.g., nausea, vomiting, diarrhea, hepatotoxicity), stomatitis, infertility, and oligospermia (127). Cyclophosphamide can induce both solid and hematologic neoplasms. Malignant lymphomas or hematologic malignancies have been noted in 1% to 3% of patients with WG receiving cyclophosphamide (1,4). Hemorrhagic cystitis occurs in 12% to 50% of patients but is severe in fewer than 6% of patients (1,4). A long-term study of 146 patients with WG treated with cyclophosphamide cited seven cases of transitional cell carcinoma of the bladder (128). Hematuria preceded the bladder carcinoma in all patients. The risk for blad-

der carcinoma correlated with the duration and total dose of therapy with cyclophosphamide; cigarette smoking may have amplified the risk (128). The incidence of bladder cancer following first exposure to cyclophosphamide was 5% at 10 years and 16% at 15 years (128). However, in a study of 142 WG patients treated with cyclophosphamide, bladder cancer developed in only one (4). Oral mesna (natrium-2-mercaptoethanesulfonate) may protect against bladder toxicity (4), but its role is controversial. The risk for bladder cancer persists for many years after cyclophosphamide has been discontinued (128). Serial urinalyses at 3- to 6-month intervals are advised for patients receiving cyclophosphamide and are sensitive in detecting bladder carcinomas (128). The presence of hematuria (macroscopic or microscopic) warrants cystoscopy.

Intermittent high-dose intravenous (pulse) cyclophosphamide has been used to treat WG, but results have been unimpressive. Early responses were noted in 13 of 14 patients treated with pulse cyclophosphamide in a nonrandomized trial at the NIH (130). However, sustained remissions were achieved in only 3 (21%) of the 14 patients. Pulse cyclophosphamide is less toxic than daily oral cyclophosphamide but is less effective (2,125,126,131–134). The optimal duration of cyclophosphamide therapy (either oral or intravenous pulse) has not been elucidated. Newer treatment strategies advocate initial treatment with cyclophosphamide and corticosteroids for 3 to 6 months (until remissions are achieved), followed by maintenance therapy with less toxic agents (e.g., methotrexate or azathioprine) (4,135,136). These various options are currently being investigated in prospective randomized clinical trials (33).

Methotrexate

Oral or intravenous methotrexate, administered once weekly, can be given to patients in whom serious adverse effects of cyclophosphamide develop or who have *non–life-threatening* WG (135–138). In a prospective (but nonrandomized) study at the NIH, 42 patients with non–life-threatening WG were treated with oral methotrexate *combined with* corticosteroids (137). All patients had active disease at entry into the study, including glomerulonephritis in 21 (50%) and lung involvement in 22 (52%). Patients were excluded if they had acute renal failure, pulmonary hemorrhage, a serum creatinine level above 2.5 mg%, or chronic liver disease. The initial dosage of methotrexate was 0.3 mg/kg once weekly, increased according to tolerance to a maximum of 20 to 25 mg once weekly. Prednisone (1 mg/kg per day) was administered concomitantly and tapered as improvement occurred. Remissions were achieved in 30 (71%) of 42 patients. Relapses occurred in 11 (36%) of the 30 responders at a mean of 29 months. A second remission was induced in six of eight patients following a second course of methotrexate and prednisone. Toxicity was generally mild, but *P. carinii* pneumonia developed in four patients (two of whom died). Long-term follow-up of 21 patients with active glomerulonephritis in that initial study cited durable remissions in 20 patients at a median of 76 months (136). At long-term follow-up, the serum creatinine level was more than 0.2 mg% above baseline in only two patients. Relapses occurred in 11 (55%) of 20 patients. Remissions were achieved in seven patients following re-treatment with methotrexate (136). In a subsequent study by the same group, 31 patients with WG who had experienced remission with conventional therapy (cyclophosphamide plus prednisone) were switched to methotrexate/prednisone for *maintenance of remission* in an open-label trial (139). Methotrexate was added *after remissions had been achieved with cyclophosphamide* at a median of 3 months (range, 1–12 months). Exclusion criteria for methotrexate included a serum creatinine level above 2.5 mg% and chronic liver disease. The dosage of methotrexate was 0.3 mg/kg per week, not to exceed 15 mg weekly. Late relapses occurred in 5 (16%) of 31 patients; all relapses occurred more than 1 year after the initiation of methotrexate. All five patients were taking *only* methotrexate at relapse; all five responded to intensification of therapy. In a similar study, De Groot and colleagues (140) treated patients *initially* with either oral or intravenous pulse cyclophosphamide and then switched them to weekly intravenous methotrexate with or without concomitant corticosteroids *after remissions had been achieved with cyclophosphamide*. The median duration of cyclophosphamide therapy in that study exceeded 24 months. Partial or complete remissions were maintained in 86% of 22 patients who received methotrexate only and in 10 (91%) of 11 of patients who received methotrexate and prednisone. A subsequent report from these investigators documented favorable responses to intravenous pulse methotrexate in 10 (59%) of 17 patients; in that study, low-dose corticosteroids were administered concomitantly (mean prednisone dose < 7 mg/d) (135). All 17 patients had active disease at entry; 11 had received no prior treatment and six had relapsed after initial remission with cyclophosphamide and corticosteroids. By 2000, these same investigators had treated 45 patients with intravenous pulse methotrexate as either initial or maintenance therapy for non–life-threatening WG (4). Patients with impaired renal function were excluded. Among the entire cohort of 155 patients (92% received cyclophosphamide at some point), the overall mortality was only 14% after a median of 5.6 years. These various reports (4,135–138,140) are encouraging and support the use of methotrexate plus prednisone in patients experiencing adverse effects of cyclophosphamide or as *initial* therapy for *mild* WG. Because the kidneys are the major route of methotrexate elimination, toxicity is increased in the presence of renal insufficiency (141). Additionally, the concomitant use of methotrexate and therapeutic doses of 160 mg trimethoprim (TMP)/800 mg sulfamethoxazole (SMX) twice daily has been associated with severe pancytopenia

(138,141). Thrice-weekly TMP/SMX plus methotrexate can be safely administered (139) and should be given as prophylaxis against *P. carinii* pneumonia (137,138,142,143). Additional data are required to determine the role of methotrexate as therapy for more *severe* cases of WG.

Trimethoprim/Sulfamethoxazole

Responses with TMP/SMX have been reported anecdotally (144,145), but data affirming the efficacy of TMP/SMX are lacking. In a nonrandomized clinical trial, DeRemee and colleagues (145) at the Mayo Clinic cited favorable responses with TMP/SMX in a subset of patients who had WG. These investigators added TMP/SMX to a previously failing regimen of cyclophosphamide/prednisone in 31 patients with indolent but progressive WG. Favorable responses were noted in 26 patients; late relapses were observed in four patients in this group. In addition, TMP/SMX was given as *initial* therapy to 15 patients with *limited* WG. In this context, 14 responded; only three experienced late relapses. On the basis of these favorable results, DeRemee and colleagues advocated TMP/SMX (one double-strength tablet twice daily) as initial therapy for patients with limited disease (lacking renal disease or generalized vasculitis) or with progressive disease despite cyclophosphamide and corticosteroids. If no improvement was evident after 8 weeks, prednisone, cyclophosphamide, or both were introduced. Georgi and colleagues (146) cited favorable responses and sustained remissions in all 10 patients treated with TMP/SMX alone for limited, "initial phase" WG. Other investigators cited favorable responses with TMP/SMX, but data are limited. Reinhold-Keller and colleagues (59) prospectively assessed the efficacy of TMP/SMX in *inducing* or *sustaining* remissions in 72 patients with WG. Among 19 patients with initial phase WG confined to the respiratory tract, partial or complete remissions were achieved in 11 (58%) with TMP/SMX alone (one double-strength tablet twice daily). Fifty-three patients with generalized WG were treated with cyclophosphamide plus prednisone; therapy was discontinued 1 year after remissions had been achieved. At that point, patients were subdivided into three groups: TMP/SMX alone (n = 24), no therapy (n = 21), and TMP/SMX plus low-dose prednisone (n = 8). The addition of TMP/SMX did not reduce relapse rates (relapse rates of 42%, 29%, and 100%, respectively). A prospective study at the NIH found that TMP/SMX (alone or combined with corticosteroids) as *initial* therapy for WG *never* induced a complete remission in any of nine treated patients (147). DeGroot and colleagues (140) found that TMP/SMX (alone or combined with prednisone) was less effective than methotrexate (alone or combined with prednisone) in *maintaining* remissions following initial treatment with cyclophosphamide and prednisone (relapse rates of 42%–100% with TMP/SMX and 9%–14% with methotrexate). Nonetheless, a role for TMP/SMX in mitigating the course of the disease is plausible. Stegeman and colleagues (148) evaluated the efficacy of TMP/SMX in preventing relapses in patients with WG who were in remission during or after treatment with cyclophosphamide and prednisone. Patients were randomized to either 160 mg of TMP and 800 mg of SMX twice daily or placebo *in addition to* conventional treatment with cyclophosphamide and prednisone. At 24 months of follow-up, 82% of patients assigned to TMP/SMX were in remission, in comparison with only 60% in the placebo group. The annual rates of respiratory and nonrespiratory tract infections were lower in the TMP/SMX group. Titers of ANCA did not differ between the groups. Although this study did not address TMP/SMX as primary (initial) therapy for WG, TMP/SMX reduced the rate of relapses of WG following conventional treatment with cyclophosphamide/prednisone. Although its mechanism of action is not known, TMP/SMX may suppress autoantibody formation by direct antimicrobial effects or by indirect immunosuppressive or antiinflammatory effects. Relapses of WG are more frequent during respiratory infections or in patients with chronic nasal carriage of *S. aureus* (121). Low-grade bacterial infection may prime neutrophils to express target antigens (e.g., c-ANCA) on the cell surface and may trigger local immune responses (121). As an antimicrobial agent, TMP/SMX may abrogate these effects, limiting neutrophil activation and further tissue damage. Although these data are intriguing, the role of TMP/SMX has not been defined. In view of its low toxicity, TMP/SMX may be considered as adjunctive therapy for persistent, indolent ("grumbling") disease despite cyclophosphamide and corticosteroids. We do not believe that TMP/SMX should supplant conventional therapy with cyclophosphamide and corticosteroids.

Other Therapeutic Options

In view of the rarity of WG, prospective randomized trials assessing therapy have not been performed. Success has been noted anecdotally with other immunosuppressive or cytotoxic agents (e.g., azathioprine, mycophenolate mofetil, chlorambucil), but we consider these to be second-line agents. Chlorambucil was used in early studies of WG with anecdotal reports of success (149,150). However, chlorambucil has many toxic effects (including oncogenicity) (127), and we prefer less toxic agents (e.g., methotrexate, azathioprine, or mycophenolate mofetil) for treating patients with WG who cannot tolerate cyclophosphamide. Azathioprine is clearly less effective than cyclophosphamide in inducing remissions (84,140,149). In an early report from the NIH, cyclophosphamide successfully induced remissions in all 10 patients whose disease had been refractory to therapy with azathioprine (42). However, azathioprine may be effective in *maintaining* remissions following induction with cyclophosphamide and corticosteroids (2,33,124). In two studies, azathioprine successfully main-

tained remissions in 18 of 22 patients initially treated with cyclophosphamide and corticosteroids (124,151). A randomized trial comparing azathioprine with cyclophosphamide as *maintenance* therapy for WG is in progress (33). Mycophenolate mofetil, an inhibitor of purine synthesis, is superior to azathioprine in preventing renal allograft rejection (152) and has been used with anecdotal success in patients with systemic vasculitis and immunoglobulin A (IgA) nephropathy (153), microscopic polyangiitis (154), or WG (154). In one prospective open-label study, 11 patients with pauci-immune glomerulonephritis and generalized WG (n = 9) or microscopic polyangiitis (n = 2) were initially treated with cyclophosphamide and corticosteroids for a minimum of 3 months until remissions had been achieved (154). At that point, cyclophosphamide was discontinued, and mycophenolate mofetil (2 g daily) was added as *maintenance* therapy. After the switch to mycophenolate mofetil, all but one patient remained in remission for a median of 15 months. Relapse occurred in only one of the 11 patients.

Anecdotal responses have been cited with cyclosporin A (155,156), high-dose intravenous immunoglobulin (157–160), monoclonal antibodies targeted against T cells (161–163), Campath-1H (a monoclonal antibody directed against CD52) (164), humanized anti-CD4 antibodies (33), antithymocyte globulin (165), and etoposide (166,167), but data are limited to a few cases in uncontrolled trials. In an open-label trial, 14 patients with active WG were treated with etanercept (a TNF-α receptor antagonist) *combined with* conventional agents (167). The drug was well tolerated, but data are inadequate to assess efficacy. A randomized,

TREATMENT OF WEGENER GRANULOMATOSIS	
Summary Statement	**Level of Evidence**
Daily oral therapy with a cyclophosphamide and corticosteroid combination is favored as the initial treatment.	Nonrandomized prospective studies, expert opinion
Intravenous cyclophosphamide and oral cyclophosphamide appear to be of similar efficacy in terms of inducing remission.	Small prospective randomized trials, metaanalysis
Weekly low-dose methotrexate is an acceptable alternative form of therapy for selected patients who do not have immediately life-threatening disease or who cannot tolerate cyclophosphamide.	Observational studies
Pneumocystis prophylaxis should be provided to all patients who are receiving a cytotoxic agent in combination with corticosteroids.	Observational studies
Plasmapheresis provides no overall benefit for patients with renal disease (patients who are dialysis-dependent at presentation are the exception).	Controlled trials

double-blinded, placebo-controlled trial of etanercept plus standard therapy is ongoing in the United States (167).

POLYARTERITIS NODOSA

Classic (macroscopic) polyarteritis nodosa (PAN) is a necrotizing vasculitis involving small and medium-sized muscular arteries (6,10,36,168). In contrast to WG, PAN spares microscopic vessels (small arterioles, venules, capillaries), and a granulomatous component is lacking (10,168). Macroscopic aneurysms involving the renal, mesenteric, or hepatic arteries can be demonstrated by angiography in more than two thirds of patients (36). Clinical manifestations predominantly affect the kidneys, gastrointestinal tract, central nervous system, skin, heart, and other viscera (36,169). Clinical lung involvement complicates PAN in fewer than 2% of cases (36). Most previously reported cases of PAN with lung involvement were probably either Churg-Strauss syndrome or microscopic polyangiitis (7). These entities are discussed in detail in subsequent sections of this chapter. Circulating ANCA (typically p-ANCA) is present in fewer than 20% of patients with PAN (39). By contrast, circulating ANCA is found in most patients with WG, microscopic polyangiitis, or Churg-Strauss syndrome (27,38,39,170). Most cases of PAN are primary or idiopathic, but secondary forms, caused, for example, by hepatitis B virus (6,41,171) or tumor antigens (36), may occur.

Patients with PAN and hepatitis B antigenemia are usually treated with antiviral therapies in combination with plasmapheresis or immunosuppressive agents (6,41,171). For patients who have PAN without hepatitis B antigenemia, corticosteroids (alone or in combination with cyclophosphamide) are the mainstay of therapy. The 5-year survival exceeds 75% but may be lower in those with adverse prognostic factors (e.g., gastrointestinal tract or central nervous system involvement, renal failure, loss of >10% of body weight, age older than 50 years) (6,172). The optimal dosage of corticosteroids has not been delineated in randomized trials. For mild to moderate cases, initial therapy with prednisone (1 mg/kg per day for 4 weeks), followed by a gradual taper, is reasonable. For more severe or fulminant cases, we initiate therapy with high-dose intravenous methylprednisolone (500–1,000 mg daily for 3 days), followed by oral prednisone (1 mg/kg per day or the equivalent) for 4 to 6 weeks. The dosage of corticosteroids and the rate of tapering must be individualized according to the response and clinical course. Cyclophosphamide is a highly effective drug for PAN, even in corticosteroid-refractory cases. We routinely add oral cyclophosphamide (2 mg/kg per day) to corticosteroid therapy, but some investigators reserve this agent for more severe or steroid-recalcitrant cases. Randomized multicenter trials by the French Vasculitis Group cited higher response rates (and fewer relapses) for regimens of oral cyclophosphamide plus corticosteroids than for regimens of corticosteroids *alone* (173). However, survival did not differ between the groups. Intravenous pulse cyclophosphamide (administered once monthly) may be less toxic than oral cyclophosphamide and appears to be equally efficacious (38). Patients responding to therapy with cyclophosphamide should continue this agent for at least 6 to 12 months after the induction of remission. Substituting a less toxic alternative immunosuppressive agent such as azathioprine or mycophenolate mofetil as *maintenance* therapy after 6 months (as in strategies for WG) (2,33) is reasonable but untested in PAN. Relapses warrant a reinstitution of therapy with corticosteroids plus cyclophosphamide. Plasmapheresis can be considered as adjunctive therapy for *fulminant PAN refractory to conventional therapy* but should not be used routinely. In two randomized trials (including patients with PAN or Churg-Strauss syndrome), the addition of plasma exchange to prednisolone (169) or to prednisolone and pulse cyclophosphamide (174) did not improve the prognosis or reduce mortality.

MICROSCOPIC POLYANGIITIS

Microscopic polyangiitis (MPA, previously termed *overlap polyangiitis syndrome*) has clinical and histopathologic features overlapping with those of classic PAN and Churg-Strauss syndrome (6,7,170,175). The predominant clinical manifestations are glomerulonephritis (90% of patients) and pulmonary capillaritis (manifested as alveolar hemorrhage), but other organs may be involved (6,7,170,175,176). Circulating ANCA, usually MPO-ANCA (p-ANCA) (36,170) but occasionally PR3-ANCA (c-ANCA) (116), is present in 40% to 80% of patients with MPA (22,36,170), suggesting a possible relationship with other ANCA-associated pulmonary vasculitides (WG and Churg-Strauss syndrome) (7,11). MPA is rare, with an estimated prevalence of 2.4 cases per million (range, 0.9–5.3) (177). The mean age at onset is approximately 50 years, but persons of all ages may be affected (6,7,170,175). A slight male predominance has been noted (170,175). As its name implies, MPA involves small vessels (arterioles, venules, capillaries) (7). MPA appears to be identical to what Zeek (178) in 1952 termed *hypersensitivity angiitis*. In the mid-1980s, the term *microscopic polyarteritis* was adopted to distinguish this disorder from macroscopic (classic) PAN. The capillaries are *invariably* involved in MPA, but the arterioles may be spared (7). Thus, the term *microscopic polyangiitis* has replaced *microscopic polyarteritis* (10). The defining criteria for MPA are less crisp than those for either WG or Churg-Strauss syndrome. In 1994, a panel of experts convened at the Chapel Hill Consensus Conference to establish defining criteria for vasculitis (10). MPA and PAN were distinguished primarily by *histologic* features. Small vessels (capillaries, venules, arterioles) are invariably involved in MPA but are always spared in classic PAN (10). Medium-sized or small arteries can be affected in *either* MPA or PAN (7,22,36). Granulomas are absent in both disorders.

Clinical Features

The predominant manifestations of MPA are alveolar hemorrhage and rapidly progressive glomerulonephritis (7,22,36,170,175,179), features rarely seen in classic PAN. The clinical features of MPA were articulated by Savage and colleagues in 1985 (179). A necrotizing, crescentic glomerulonephritis with few or no immune deposits (termed *pauci-immune*) is characteristic of MPA (36,170,175,176,180). Rapidly progressive glomerulonephritis may occur. Consequently, prompt, aggressive treatment is essential to avert end-stage renal failure (176,180). Remissions are achieved with corticosteroids combined with cyclophosphamide in approximately 80% of patients (7,179,180).

Alveolar hemorrhage occurs in 12% to 50% of patients and is often the predominant (and most life-threatening) manifestation (6,36,170,175,179) (Fig. 30.9). Extrapulmonary features (pauci-immune glomerulonephritis, musculoskeletal and constitutional symptoms) are usually evident (175), but *isolated* alveolar hemorrhage without systemic involvement has been described (181,182). Chest radiographs in alveolar hemorrhage reveal bilateral dense alveolar filling (175). Chest CT demonstrates bilateral alveolar opacities, with consolidation in two thirds and ground-glass opacities in 60% (175). In patients who have recurrent episodes of alveolar hemorrhage, CT may reveal a reticular pattern of septal lines without ground-glass opacities (175). The BAL fluid is grossly hemorrhagic in more than 90% of patients; the presence of numerous hemosiderin-laden macrophages supports the diagnosis of alveolar hemorrhage (175). Severe anemia (hemoglobin < 9 g%) is characteristic of massive alveolar hemorrhage (175). Necrotizing glomerulonephritis is found in the kidney biopsy specimens of more than 90% of patients with alveolar hemorrhage (175). Massive alveolar hemorrhage is an important cause of morbidity and mortality in MPA (13,170,175). The diagnosis of alveolar hemorrhage can be made clinically by the constellation of severe anemia, rapidly progressive glomerulonephritis, and bloody BAL fluid with or without circulating ANCA. Surgical lung biopsy is hazardous in cases of severe alveolar hemorrhage and is ill advised. Renal biopsy or the detection of high titers of circulating ANCA may substantiate the diagnosis in the appropriate clinical context. However, video-assisted thoracoscopic biopsy can be considered for patients with isolated alveolar hemorrhage who are not in respiratory failure. Immediate treatment with pulse intravenous methylprednisolone (1 g daily for 3 days, with a corticosteroid taper) is warranted for severe alveolar hemorrhage (175). Cyclophosphamide (intravenous or oral) is administered concomitantly (175). Plasma exchange is reserved for cases of severe alveolar hemorrhage refractory to medical therapy (175). Relapses of alveolar hemorrhage occur in up to 25% to 54% of patients and may be fatal (13,170,175,179). One study of 29 patients with MPA and alveolar hemorrhage cited 1- and 5-year survival rates of 82% and 68%, respectively (175). The requirement for mechanical ventilation at presentation or at any time during the illness was associated with a sixfold higher mortality in comparison with no requirement for ventilation (175). Although pulmonary function usually returns to normal in surviving patients, chronic restrictive or mixed ventilatory defects have been noted in approximately one third (175). Occasionally, pulmonary fibrosis (183) or obliterative bronchiolitis develops in patients with chronic alveolar hemorrhage (184).

A prodromal respiratory illness precedes the onset of vasculitis in one third of patients (6,36,170,175). Arthralgias and myalgias are common (up to 50% of patients) (36,170,175). Involvement of the sinuses or upper airways may occur but is rarely prominent or the presenting feature (6,36,170,175). Oral ulcers have been noted in up to 21% of patients with MPA and may mimic those of WG (6,36,170,175). Ocular involvement, which is frequent in WG, is rare in MPA (<5%) (31,170). Cutaneous involvement (leukocytoclastic vasculitis) is common (170). Renal infarcts, renal vasculitis, and visceral aneurysms, cardinal features of PAN, are rarely observed in MPA (10,36,170,185). In one study of 85 patients with MPA, renal and celiac

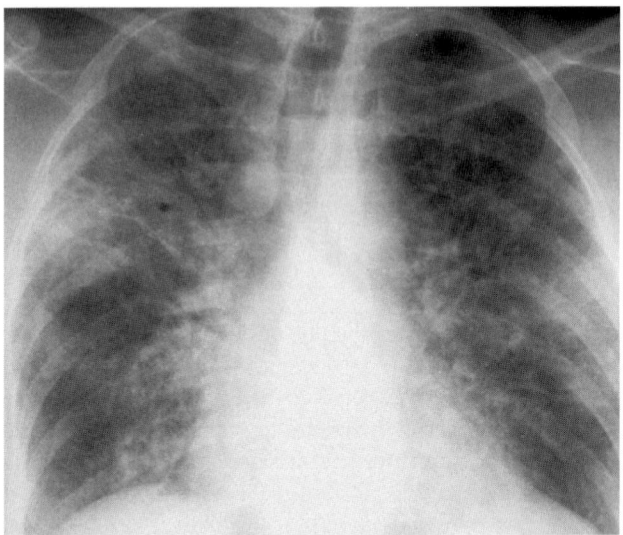

FIGURE 30.9. Alveolar hemorrhage secondary to microscopic polyangiitis. Posteroanterior chest radiograph demonstrates diffuse alveolar infiltrates involving all lobes. Within 24 hours, the opacities worsened, severe respiratory failure developed, and the patient required mechanical ventilatory support and positive end-expiratory pressure of 16 cm H_2O to achieve acceptable oxygenation. Because of the severity of the respiratory failure, no lung biopsy was performed. Urinalysis demonstrated numerous red cells and occasional red cell casts. The serum creatinine level was 1.4 mg%. Pulse prednisolone was initiated at a dosage of 1 g daily for 3 days. Renal biopsy demonstrated glomerulonephritis and a necrotizing vasculitis involving the renal arterioles; no granulomas were present. Cyclophosphamide was instituted at a dosage of 2 mg/kg per day, and corticosteroids were continued. Within 5 days, the opacities had cleared completely, and the serum creatinine level was 0.6 mg%.

angiography was performed in 30 of them, and microaneurysms were detected in four (170). Some authors believe that the presence of "renal infarcts, microaneurysms, and/or stenosis" should be considered "as diagnostic for PAN and exclusionary for MPA, *except when* the patient has clearly established symptoms of MPA, such as glomerulonephritis or alveolar hemorrhage" (170). Peripheral neuropathy, especially mononeuritis multiplex, occurs in 40% to 60% of patients with MAP (7,170). Circulating immune complexes and rheumatoid factor have been noted in 24% of patients with MPA, and antinuclear antibody in 17% (170,175). These nonspecific tests have been supplanted by ANCA (principally p-ANCA), which has been detected in 50% to 90% of patients with MPA (7,170,175). Of 29 patients with MPA and severe alveolar hemorrhage, c-ANCA was detected in 38% and p-ANCA in 48% (175).

Data regarding the role of serial ANCA measurement to assess disease activity in MPA are limited (31), but one study demonstrated higher levels of PR3-ANCA reacting with the pro form of recombinant PR3 in active than in inactive phases of both MPA and WG (116). By contrast, the levels of PR3-ANCA reacting with the mature recombinant PR3 variant did not differ between active and inactive disease. Because most ANCA in MPA is p-ANCA (not c-ANCA), the significance of this finding is not clear. In one study that included both patients with MPA and patients with WG, persistent positivity for ANCA (either c-ANCA or p-ANCA) was associated with active disease, whereas persistently negative test results correlated with sustained remissions (31). We agree with the authors that serial measurement of ANCA (even MPO-ANCA) may be useful in patients with MPA (31). In contrast its high prevalence in patients with MPA, Churg-Strauss syndrome, or WG, ANCA is detected in fewer than 20% of patients with PAN (7). Some authors believe that the presence of ANCA excludes the diagnosis of classic PAN (170).

Several features of MPA (circulating ANCA, small vessel vasculitis, glomerulonephritis, pulmonary capillaritis) may be observed in WG or Churg-Strauss syndrome. These latter vasculitic disorders both exhibit a granulomatous component, which is lacking in MPA (10). Asthma or eosinophilia (in blood or tissue), characteristic of Churg-Strauss syndrome (5,38,40), is not found in MPA. A firm diagnosis of MPA requires the definite exclusion of these alternative diagnoses.

Histopathology

Like the other ANCA-associated vasculitides, MPA principally affects small arterioles, venules, and capillaries (10,170). However, in contrast to Churg-Strauss syndrome and WG, MPA lacks a granulomatous component, and eosinophils are rare or absent (10). Immune complexes are undetectable or present in only small amounts in involved tissue (pauci-immune) (170).

Treatment

Diverse regimens of prednisone, azathioprine, cyclophosphamide, or plasma exchange, alone or in combination, have been used to treat MPA (similar to the treatment regimens for WG and Churg-Strauss syndrome) (36,174,175). Because of the rarity of MPA, few randomized trials have been performed, and optimal treatment has not been elucidated. Most investigators treat MPA with a combination of corticosteroids and cyclophosphamide (36,37,172). The incremental value of cyclophosphamide over corticosteroids was suggested in a retrospective study of 85 patients with MPA; 28 patients (33%) died after a mean follow-up of 70 months (170). However, the mortality rate was lower (24%) in the patients treated with corticosteroids and immunosuppressive therapy than in those treated with corticosteroids *alone* (48%) (170). Several prospective randomized trials of patients with MPA or Churg-Strauss syndrome cited similar survival rates with various regimens, which included corticosteroids alone, corticosteroids plus oral cyclophosphamide, corticosteroids plus intravenous cyclophosphamide, corticosteroids plus plasma exchange, and corticosteroids plus cyclophosphamide plus plasma exchange (36,174,175). Plasmapheresis adds another level of complexity and should be reserved for fulminant or refractory cases. Most investigators use oral cyclophosphamide (2 mg/kg per day) and prednisone (1 mg/kg per day with gradual taper), a regimen similar to that used in WG. Favorable responses are achieved in more than 80% of cases, and 10-year survival exceeds 70% (36,172,179). As in WG, treatment should be continued for a minimum of 1 year after complete clinical and laboratory remission has been achieved. Relapses occur in 20% to 54% of patients, usually as the immunosuppressive therapy is tapered or discontinued (36,172,179,186). The treatment of relapses is similar to the initial induction therapy. Although data on alternative immunosuppressive agents are limited, mycophenolate mofetil has been associated with responses in a few anecdotal cases (153).

CHURG-STRAUSS ANGIITIS (ALLERGIC ANGIITIS AND GRANULOMATOSIS)

Churg-Strauss syndrome, also termed *allergic angiitis and granulomatosis* (38,40), was originally described in 1951 by Churg and Strauss (187), who reported 13 patients with asthma, peripheral eosinophilia, constitutional symptoms, and systemic necrotizing vasculitis. These investigators noted that the syndrome shared histologic features with PAN but was distinct from classic PAN. In 1957, Rose and Spencer (188) identified 32 patients with asthma and features consistent with Churg-Strauss syndrome in a necropsy series of 111 patients with PAN. Only sporadic reports of Churg-Strauss syndrome appeared during the next two decades. In 1977, Chumbley and colleagues (189) reviewed 30 patients with

Churg-Strauss syndrome seen at the Mayo Clinic during a 24-year period. A review of the files of the Armed Forces Institute of Pathology in 1981 revealed only four cases of Churg-Strauss syndrome (190). As of 1982, only 138 cases of Churg-Strauss syndrome had been published (5). In 1984, Lanham and colleagues (5) reported 16 additional patients with Churg-Strauss syndrome (only eight of whom had histologically confirmed vasculitis) seen at a large referral hospital in England during a 6-year period and suggested that the rarity of Churg-Strauss syndrome in part reflected the stringent criteria required for the diagnosis. They suggested that Churg-Strauss syndrome could be diagnosed even when *not all* the classic histologic criteria (necrotizing vasculitis, extravascular granulomas, tissue eosinophilia) were present. They proposed the following criteria for the diagnosis of Churg-Strauss syndrome: evidence of a systemic vasculitis involving two or more extrapulmonary organs, asthma, and peripheral blood eosinophilia ($>1.5 \times 10^9$/L or $>10\%$ of the total leukocyte count) (5). The concept of "limited" forms of Churg-Strauss syndrome, analogous to WG, has also been suggested (191–193). In 1990, the American College of Rheumatology promulgated specific diagnostic criteria for the syndrome (194). A diagnosis of Churg-Strauss syndrome is affirmed by *biopsy evidence of vasculitis and* the presence of at least four of the six following criteria: (a) moderate to severe asthma, (b) peripheral blood eosinophilia ($>10\%$), (c) mononeuropathy or polyneuropathy, (d) non-fixed pulmonary opacities, (e) paranasal sinus abnormality, and (f) a biopsy specimen containing a blood vessel with extravascular eosinophils. Churg-Strauss syndrome can present at any age, but the mean age of patients at onset is 40 to 50 years; no gender predominance has been noted (5,36,38,40,189). The annual incidence of Churg-Strauss syndrome has been estimated at 2.4 to 3.3 cases per million (177,195). The incidence is much higher in persons with asthma (up to 64 cases per million per year) (195).

Pathogenesis

The pathogenesis of Churg-Strauss syndrome has not been elucidated. Several lines of evidence support a role for ANCA (7,40,119). Repeated antigenic stimulation may play a role (38). Repeated vaccination or desensitization has been invoked as a possible etiologic factor (38). Drug-induced vasculitis is a plausible, albeit unproven, mechanism in some cases (38,40). Following the introduction of cysteinyl leukotriene receptor antagonists, such as zafirlukast (196,197), montelukast (198,199), and pranlukast (200), more than 50 cases of Churg-Strauss syndrome were reported worldwide in association with the use of leukotriene receptor antagonists in severe steroid-dependent asthma (201,202). Although a link between the use of leukotriene receptor antagonists and Churg-Strauss syndrome was initially suspected, subsequent reports of cases of Churg-Strauss syndrome in asthmatic patients on inhaled corticosteroids but not leukotriene receptor antagonists (203) suggested that Churg-Strauss syndrome was related to the unmasking of underlying vasculitis concomitant with the withdrawal of systemic corticosteroids rather than to a direct effect of leukotriene receptor antagonists (204,205). The relationship between leukotriene receptor antagonists and Churg-Strauss syndrome (if any) remains controversial (206).

Clinical Features

Asthma *precedes* the diagnosis of Churg-Strauss syndrome in more than 90% of patients and is usually the presenting feature (5,36,38,40). Typically, a history of atopy and asthma precedes the development of vasculitis by months or even years (5,40). A second phase of peripheral blood and tissue eosinophilia ensues (5,36,38). The third phase, vasculitis, develops years after these earlier phases (5,36,38,40). At the time of presentation with vasculitis, a history of hay fever, nasal polyposis, allergic rhinitis, or sinusitis can be elicited in more than two thirds of patients (5,40). Nasopharyngeal manifestations include nasal crusting or nasal polyposis in up to 75% and nasal perforation in 5% (5,38,40). Peripheral blood eosinophilia is prominent during the asthmatic and vasculitic phases. Increasingly severe and more frequent exacerbations of asthma precede the development of necrotizing vasculitis (5).

Pulmonary involvement (characteristically manifested as asthma) is present in virtually all patients (5,36,38,40). Focal alveolar opacities are seen on chest radiographs in 30% to 70% of cases (5,36,38,40); they may be transient. Pleural effusions are noted in up to 30% of patients (5,40,207). Diffuse alveolar hemorrhage is a rare complication (<5%) of Churg-Strauss syndrome and manifests as bilateral dense alveolar consolidation (38). In contrast to WG, Churg-Strauss syndrome is seldom associated with pulmonary nodules or cavitary lesions. Chest CT typically demonstrates focal parenchymal opacities, often with consolidation, in a peripheral distribution (208). Other features include ground-glass opacities, cavitary pulmonary nodules, bronchial wall thickening, centrilobular nodules, thickened interlobular septa, pleural and pericardial effusions, and enlarged hilar or mediastinal lymph nodes (207,208).

Constitutional symptoms are usually prominent in Churg-Strauss syndrome (38). Fever, weight loss, or malaise is noted in more than 90% of patients (5,36,38,40,209). Arthralgias or myalgias occur in 30% to 50% of patients (5,36,38,40). Central or peripheral neurologic involvement occurs in 40% to 78% of patients (5,36,38,40,209,210). Peripheral neuropathy or mononeuritis multiplex predominates; cerebral infarction is uncommon (<10%) (38,40). Cutaneous manifestations (subcutaneous nodules, purpura, petechiae) occur in two thirds of patients (5,36,38). Skin biopsy often demonstrates nonspecific findings of leukocytoclastic vasculitis; when dense eosinophilic infiltrates are noted, the diagnosis of Churg-Strauss syndrome is strongly suggested (38). Cardiac involvement occurs in 15% to 59% of patients with Churg-Strauss syndrome (5,36–38,40). Cardiac involvement accounted for 48% of the deaths in the 50 patients reviewed by Lanham and colleagues (5). Cardiac failure and pericarditis are the most common clinical manifestations. Cardiac involvement may reflect primary coronary vasculitis or eosinophilic endocarditis with associated fibrosis. The abdominal viscera are involved in 30% to 62% of cases (5,36,38). Abdominal pain (caused by eosinophilic gastroenteritis) or perforation of a viscus secondary to ischemia associated with vasculitis may occur (38,40). Renal involvement (typically focal segmental glomerulonephritis) occurs in up to 26% of patients (38), but renal failure is rare (38,40). Hypertension develops in nearly 50% of patients (38,40). Ocular involvement is uncommon (<5%) (5,36,38).

Laboratory studies demonstrate an elevated erythrocyte sedimentation rate and blood eosinophil count in more than 80% of patients during acute exacerbations (5,36–38). The erythrocyte sedimentation rate and blood eosinophil count both usually correlate with disease activity. An elevated level of serum IgE is common (>50%) (5,207). Circulating ANCA (primarily p-ANCA) is present in 40% to 70% patients with Churg-Strauss syndrome (36–40). The antigen causing p-ANCA staining is MPO in 50% of patients (40), but other epitopes (e.g., cathepsin G, lysozyme, glucuronidase, elastase) may be implicated (38,40). The relationship of ANCA titers to disease activity in Churg-Strauss syndrome has not been systemically evaluated (40).

Histopathology

The salient histologic features of Churg-Strauss syndrome include a necrotizing vasculitis of small arteries and veins with eosinophilic and granulomatous components (5,36,38). The

pronounced eosinophilic and granulomatous character distinguishes Churg-Strauss syndrome from the other pulmonary vasculitides (10). The eosinophilic infiltration of vascular walls is usually striking; mononuclear cells, neutrophils, and occasional multinucleated giant cells are also present (191). The presence of granulomas and eosinophils in extravascular tissues is a hallmark of the disorder (10,187). Palisading histiocytes and giant cells surround a central eosinophilic core (187,191) (Fig. 30.10). The diagnosis can be supported even when the histologic features are not definitive provided that the clinical and laboratory features are characteristic (5). The lesions in diffuse alveolar hemorrhage demonstrate nonspecific findings of capillaritis (11,40).

Therapy

Corticosteroids have been the mainstay of therapy for Churg-Strauss syndrome, with remissions achieved in more than 80% of patients (5,36,38). Immunosuppressive and cytotoxic agents have been used for patients with more severe disease (5,36,38). In the 1980s and 1990s, several prospective randomized trials (which enrolled patients with PAN or Churg-Strauss syndrome) were carried out by the French Vasculitis Study Group, a national network comprising 93 centers (38,169,172,173). The medical regimens evaluated included corticosteroids alone, corticosteroids plus oral cyclophosphamide, corticosteroids plus pulse cyclophosphamide, corticosteroids plus plasma exchange, and the combination of corticosteroids, cyclophosphamide, and plasma exchange (38). In the first study, patients were treated with prednisolone (1 mg/kg per day with taper) *plus* 6 months of plasma exchange *or* the same regimen *plus* oral cyclophosphamide (2 mg/kg per day) for 12 months (173). The 10-year survival was similar with both regimens (72% vs. 75%). However, the relapse rate was lower

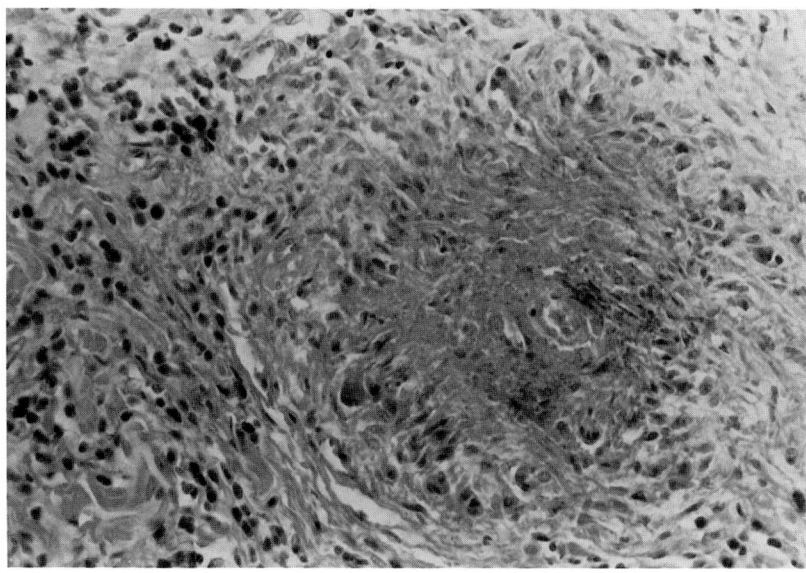

FIGURE 30.10. Churg-Strauss syndrome. Photomicrograph of open lung biopsy specimen demonstrating necrotic lung tissue with palisading histiocytes (hematoxylin and eosin, original magnification ×330). (From Lynch JP III, Fantone J III. Other pulmonary granulomatous vasculitis syndromes. In: Lynch JP III, DeRemee RA, eds. *Immunologically mediated lung diseases.* Philadelphia: JB Lippincott Co, 1991:302–321, with permission.)

in the cohort receiving cyclophosphamide. The second trial randomized patients to prednisolone alone or prednisolone plus plasma exchange (169). The survival and relapse rates were similar in both groups. In the third and fourth trials, the patients were stratified by prognostic factors (38). The third trial randomized patients to prednisolone plus intravenous pulse cyclophosphamide *or* prednisolone plus intravenous pulse cyclophosphamide *plus* plasma exchange (174). This study included *only* patients with one or more criteria *previously* associated with a poor prognosis (renal insufficiency, gastrointestinal tract or central nervous system involvement, cardiomyopathy, age older than 50 years, loss of >10% of body weight) (211). Even in this high-risk group, 5-year survival rates were good and did not differ between the two groups (75% and 88%, respectively) (174). Only four patients died of uncontrolled vasculitis (two in each group). The fourth study compared corticosteroids plus *oral* cyclophosphamide versus corticosteroids plus intravenous *pulse* cyclophosphamide in patients with a good prognosis (38). The response and survival rates were similar with oral or intravenous pulse cyclophosphamide. In summary, in various randomized prospective studies, the survival rates were similar with the various regimens (3-year survival, 80%–90%; 10-year survival, 72%–78%) (36,38,169,172,173).

Relapses occur in 20% to 40% of patients, often as the dose of corticosteroids or cytotoxic drug is reduced (5,36,38,212). During the long-term follow-up of 96 patients with Churg-Strauss syndrome (most of whom were in one of the French vasculitis trials), 23 (24%) of the patients died (38). Poorly controlled vasculitis was responsible for 11 (48%) of the deaths. Factors associated with a worse prognosis by multivariate analysis included myocardial or severe gastrointestinal tract involvement (38). In a previous study of 342 patients with MPA (n = 260) or Churg-Strauss syndrome (n = 82), factors associated with worse survival included proteinuria (>1 g/d), renal insufficiency (serum creatinine > 1.58 mg%), cardiomyopathy, central nervous system involvement, and severe gastrointestinal tract involvement (172). Asthma, polyarthritis, myalgias, ocular signs, weight loss, or cutaneous involvement did not influence the prognosis (172). The authors suggest that more aggressive therapy with corticosteroids plus cyclophosphamide is warranted for patients with adverse prognostic factors (172). A retrospective study of 98 patients with PAN or Churg-Strauss syndrome by the same investigators cited higher mortality rates in patients older than 65 years than in younger patients (6). The 5-year survival rates were 70% and 86% among elderly and younger patients, respectively; the 10-year survival rates were 39% and 76%, respectively (6).

Although the optimal therapy for Churg-Strauss syndrome remains controversial, we believe that treatment can be individualized depending on the acuteness of the presentation and severity of the disease. Mild to moderate cases with no adverse factors can initially be treated with corticosteroids (e.g., 1 mg of prednisone per kilogram per day for 4 weeks, followed by a gradual taper). Oral cyclophosphamide (2 mg/kg per day) is added for more fulminant cases with unfavorable prognostic features or as a steroid-sparing agent (for patients experiencing or at risk for corticosteroid side effects) (172). In fulminant or refractory cases, the disease can be controlled more rapidly with aggressive combination therapies (36). In this context, pulse intravenous methylprednisolone (1 g daily for 3 days) followed by oral prednisone (1 mg/kg per day) combined with cyclophosphamide (2 mg/kg per day) is advised. Plasma exchange is reserved for patients failing or experiencing adverse effects of therapy. Plasmapheresis may be given three times per week for the first 2 to 3 weeks and with decreasing frequency during the next 2 to 4 months (36). It should be emphasized that plasma exchange has not been shown to improve outcome (169), and it increases the risk for infectious complications (36). Because relapses occur in 25% or more of patients with Churg-Strauss syndrome, maintenance therapy may be required for prolonged periods. The optimal regimen for long-term therapy has not been elucidated. Given the potential toxicities associated with long-term cyclophosphamide use (127), azathioprine or mycophenolate may be substituted for cyclophosphamide after 6 months to reduce the cumulative dose of cyclophosphamide (40). Mycophenolate appears to be more effective than azathioprine for other forms of systemic vasculitis (153), but data are limited. Occasionally patients with Churg-Strauss syndrome fail treatment with prednisolone and cyclophosphamide. In this context, responses have been cited anecdotally with IFN-γ (37,213), anti-thymocyte globulin (161,214), and pooled intravenous immunoglobulin (159), but data are sparse.

BRONCHOCENTRIC GRANULOMATOSIS

Bronchocentric granulomatosis was initially described in 1973 by Liebow (215), who reported nine patients exhibiting a striking granulomatous response centered within bronchi and bronchioles that destroyed and obliterated the affected airways. Mild perivascular involvement was evident within the pulmonary vessels contiguous to the granulomatous process, but true vasculitis was absent (215). A sentinel article by Katzenstein and colleagues (216) reviewed the original cases of Liebow and added 14 new cases from several centers. Of the 23 cases of bronchocentric granulomatosis, 10 had asthma, and 9 of these 10 also had peripheral blood eosinophilia and fungal hyphae (primarily *Aspergillus*) within the bronchial lumina or tissue. Dense aggregates of eosinophils predominated in the inflammatory bronchiolar infiltrate. Thus, bronchocentric granulomatosis in these patients represented a hypersensitivity response to fungi, consistent with allergic bronchopulmonary aspergillosis. Of the 13 *nonasthmatic* patients with bronchocentric granulomatosis, two had severe rheumatoid arthritis and four had a history of exposures to potential inhaled toxins. Subsequent reports of cases of bronchocentric granulomatosis in association with tuberculosis, nocardiosis, coccidioidomycosis, echinococcosis, and other infectious disorders suggest that bronchocentric granulomatosis is an unusual host response to inhaled or intrabronchial antigens and should not be considered a primary vasculitis (217,218).

NECROTIZING SARCOID ANGIITIS AND GRANULOMATOSIS

Necrotizing sarcoid angiitis and granulomatosis was initially described in 1973 by Liebow (215) on the basis of 11 patients who exhibited a pulmonary necrotizing granulomatous vasculitis with a sarcoid-like reaction. Confluent, nonnecrotizing granulomas involved the bronchi, bronchioles, and lung parenchyma, consistent with sarcoidosis. A small vessel granulomatous vasculitis, associated with necrosis of the vessel walls, was also present. In 1979, Churg and colleagues (219) reviewed 12 cases of necrotizing sarcoid angiitis and granulomatosis from the pathology files of Stanford University. The histologic features included large masses of confluent granulomas, variable amounts of necrosis and hyalinization, and a prominent granulomatous vasculitis involving arteries and veins, associated with necrosis of the vascular walls (Fig. 30.11). No patient had systemic vasculitis or glomerulonephritis, and extrapulmonary involvement was rare. In two subsequent series comprising 45 patients with necrotizing sarcoid angiitis and granulomatosis, 36 (80%) were asymptomatic, and the prognosis was excellent with or without therapy (220,221). It is likely that most cases of necrotizing sarcoid angiitis and granulomatosis are variants

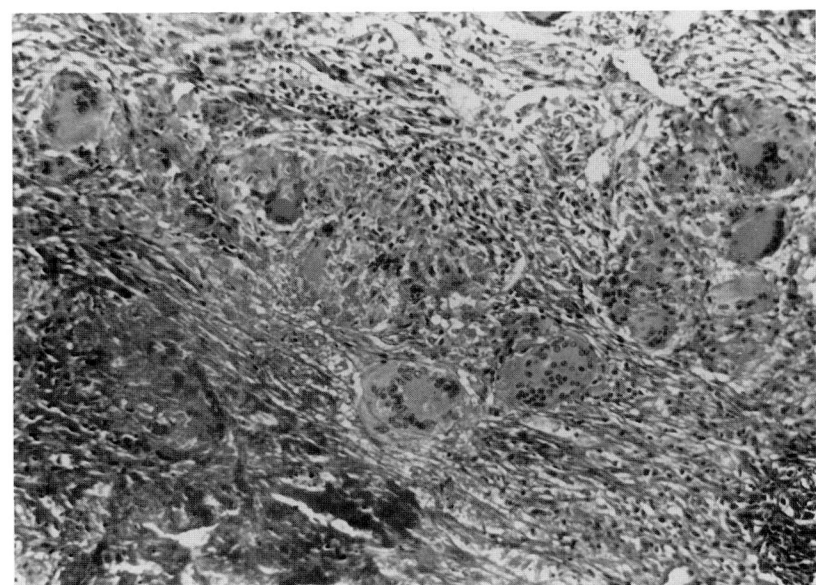

A

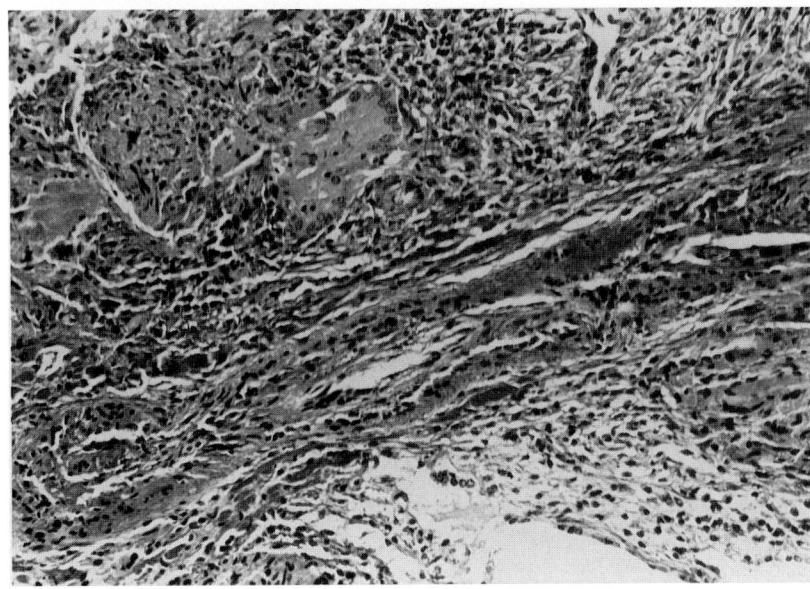

B

FIGURE 30.11. A: Necrotizing sarcoid angiitis and granulomatosis. Photomicrograph of open lung biopsy specimen demonstrating well-formed granulomas, multinucleated giant cells, and chronic inflammatory cells adjacent to a large region of parenchymal necrosis (hematoxylin and eosin, original magnification ×165). **B:** Necrotizing sarcoid angiitis and granulomatosis. Photomicrograph of open lung biopsy specimen from the same patient demonstrates granulomatous vasculitis with destruction of the vessel wall and occlusion of the lumen. Noncaseating granulomas with multinucleated giant cells are in the lung parenchyma (hematoxylin and eosin, original magnification ×165). (From Lynch JP III, Fantone J III. Other pulmonary granulomatous vasculitis syndromes. In: Lynch JP III, DeRemee RA, eds. *Immunologically mediated lung diseases.* Philadelphia: JB Lippincott Co, 1991:302–321, with permission.)

of sarcoidosis, resembling "nodular sarcoid" (222,223). We do not believe that necrotizing sarcoid angiitis and granulomatosis should be considered a true vasculitis.

LYMPHOMATOID GRANULOMATOSIS

Lymphomatoid granulomatosis was initially described in 1972 as a necrotizing vasculitic disorder having several features in common with WG and atypical lymphoma (9). The histologic features included atypical lymphohistiocytic infiltrates surrounding small and medium-sized arteries and veins, associated with pronounced necrosis of the involved organs. The "angiocentric" pattern, multinucleated giant cells, granulomatous component, and mixed inflammatory cellular infiltrates mimicked WG. However, the pronounced cellular atypia resembled a malignant lymphoid disorder

(Fig. 30.12). Subsequent investigations suggested that lymphomatoid granulomatosis represents a spectrum of lymphoid disorders (28,224). A histologic grading system for lymphomatoid granulomatosis distinguishes lesions based on features of cytologic atypia, necrosis, and retention of a polymorphous cellular infiltrate (28). Grade 1 lesions are polymorphous, with little or no atypia or necrosis. Grade 2 lesions are polymorphous with atypical cells and foci of necrosis. Grade 3 lesions exhibit monomorphism, severe atypia, and necrosis and are considered to be malignant "angiocentric" lymphomas. One third of grade 1 lesions and two thirds of grade 2 lesions progress to malignant lymphomas.

The clinical manifestations of lymphomatoid granulomatosis are protean. The lung is nearly always involved; prominent extrapulmonary manifestations affect the central nervous system (30%), skin (30%), and kidneys (30%), but virtually any organ can be involved (8,9,225–227).

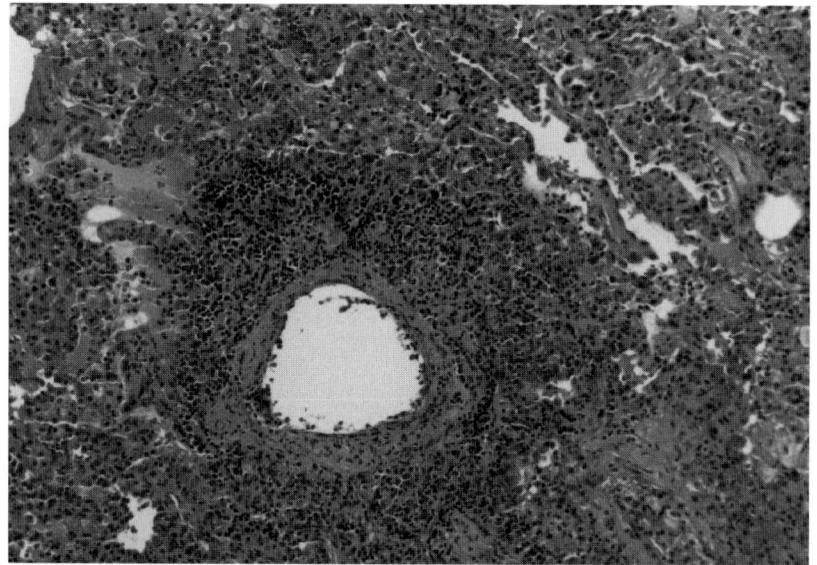

A

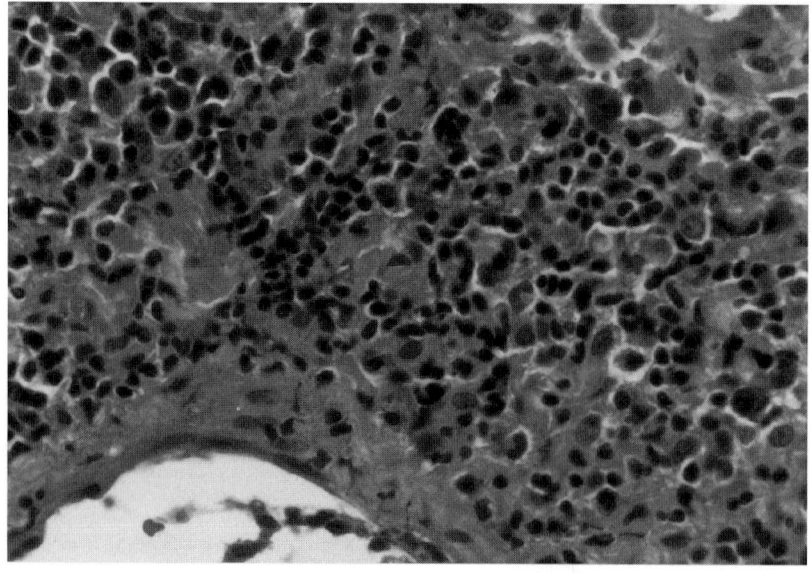

B

FIGURE 30.12. A: Lymphomatoid granulomatosis. Photomicrograph of open lung biopsy specimen demonstrates intense mononuclear infiltrates surrounding a blood vessel (hematoxylin and eosin, high power). **B:** Lymphomatoid granulomatosis. Photomicrograph of specimen from the same patient shows a polymorphous infiltrate composed of atypical lymphoid and histiocytic cells. Granuloma is not a characteristic histologic abnormality, although the name of the entity suggests otherwise (hematoxylin and eosin, oil immersion). (Courtesy of S. Hammar, M.D., University of Washington, Seattle, Washington.)

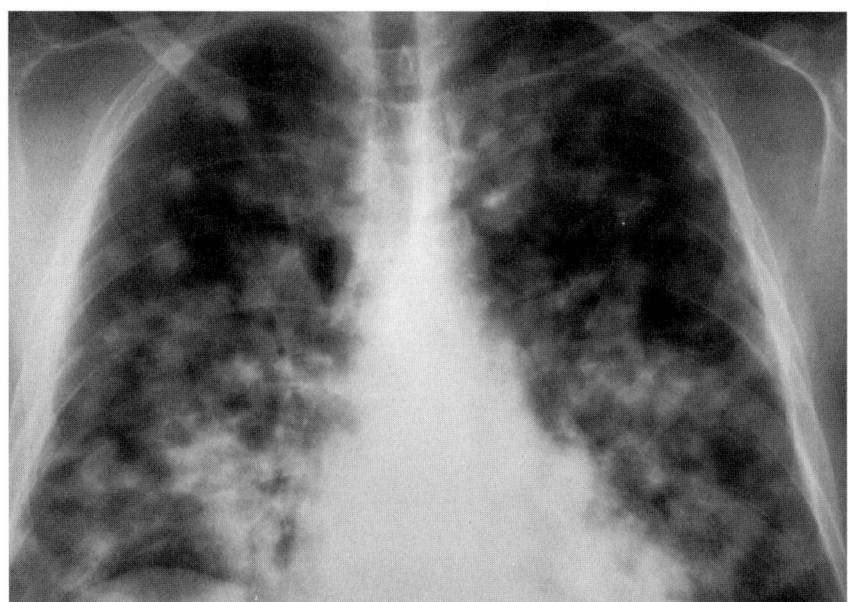

FIGURE 30.13. Lymphomatoid granulomatosis. Posteroanterior chest radiograph demonstrating multiple nodular mass densities throughout both lung fields. Open lung biopsy specimen demonstrating changes consistent with lymphomatoid granulomatosis.

In contrast to other systemic vasculitides, lymphomatoid granulomatosis is rarely associated with glomerulonephritis (8,9,225–227). Involvement of lymph nodes or bone marrow is unusual (8,9,225,227). Aberrations on chest radiographs are nearly invariably present (Fig. 30.13). Multiple nodular lesions are typical, but single mass lesions, alveolar opacities, cavitary lesions, or pleural effusions may be found (225,226,228,229).

Investigations based on molecular biologic and immunohistochemical techniques (e.g., T-cell gene rearrangements, monoclonal stains) suggest that most (if not all) cases of lymphomatoid granulomatosis represent diverse lymphoreticular disorders, including malignant lymphoma, angioimmunoblastic lymphadenopathy, and B- and T-cell lymphomas (29,30,230). Some studies suggest that most cases of lymphomatoid granulomatosis are Epstein-Barr virus–associated B-cell lymphoproliferative disorders (30,230–234). Most *background* lymphocytes are T cells, but the *cytologically atypical* lymphoid cells stain positively for B-cell markers, express Epstein-Barr virus genome, and proliferate at a rapid rate (231,235). Lymphomatoid granulomatosis is more common in immunocompromised patients (236,237), suggesting that deficient regulation of Epstein-Barr virus is critical in the pathogenesis. Furthermore, lymphomatoid granulomatosis may complicate diverse lymphoproliferative disorders, including acute lymphoblastic lymphoma (238) and agnogenic myeloid metaplasia (237). Lymphomatoid granulomatosis should not be classified as a true vasculitis but rather as a stereotypic response to diverse lymphoreticular disorders (29). The term *angioimmunoproliferative lesion/angiocentric lymphoma* has been suggested in lieu of lymphomatoid granulomatosis (28).

The clinical course of lymphomatoid granulomatosis is variable. The disease usually progresses relentlessly, even-

tuating in death (8,9,30,225,227). However, spontaneous remissions have been described. Given the rarity of lymphomatoid granulomatosis, the optimal therapy has not been clarified. In early studies, responses were noted anecdotally to regimens of oral cyclophosphamide and corticosteroids (similar to the treatments for WG) (8). Subsequent studies failed to substantiate benefit from corticosteroids alone or in combination with immunosuppressive or cytotoxic agents (8,28,225,227). Chemotherapeutic regimens of multiple agents for malignant lymphoma or radiation therapy are often used, but results have generally been disappointing (30,225,227,233). Responses to IFN-α2b have been reported anecdotally (239), but the data are limited to a few cases.

BEHÇET DISEASE

Behçet disease is a systemic vasculitis of unknown cause; its major manifestations include oral and genital ulcers, uveitis, phlebitis, and nervous system involvement (25,240,241). The course is characterized by recurrent attacks of acute inflammation (e.g., ulcers, uveitis) rather than chronic, persistent disease (240). Because the symptoms and laboratory features are nonspecific, the diagnosis is based on criteria proposed by the International Study Group for Behçet's Disease in 1990 (242). According to those criteria, recurrent (at least three episodes in a 12-month period) oral ulcers (aphthous or herpetiform) must be present *plus* at least two of the following features: recurrent genital ulceration, eye lesions, skin lesions, or a positive pathergy test result (development of a papule or pustule following a needle prick to the skin) (243).

Although Behçet disease is worldwide in distribution, it is far more common in the eastern Mediterranean Basin, along the ancient Silk Road (240). The highest prevalence is in Turkey, ranging from 80 to 370 per 100,000 (25,240). The prevalence is lower (2–30 cases per 100,000) in other Asian countries, with lower figures (<1 per 100,000) in Europe and the United States (25,240,241). The onset of disease is most commonly in the second, third, or fourth decade of life (25,240). No gender predominance has been noted (25). There is a strong association between HLA-B51 and Behçet disease (25,240). Familial clusters have been described (25). Epidemiologic studies suggest that both genetic and environmental factors (possibly infectious agents) are important in the pathogenesis (25,240).

Oral ulcers are usually the initial manifestation and invariably develop at some time in the course of the disease (25,240). Genital ulcers are present in 65% to 90% of cases, and eye lesions in 35% to 70% (25,241). Arthritis develops in approximately 50% of patients but is not deforming (240,241). Repeated attacks of uveitis can cause blindness (240,241). Small vessel vasculitis is common in Behçet disease (240). Large venous or arterial lesions occur in 7% to 38% of patients (240,241). Occlusion of major arteries or aneurysms may cause bleeding, infarction, or organ failure (240,244). The pathogenesis of aneurysm formation in Behçet disease is active arteritis, followed by thrombosis; rupture may result in massive, even fatal, hemorrhage (244). Recurrent venous thromboses occur in one fourth of patients with Behçet disease (240). Involvement or thrombosis of the superior vena cava, innominate vein, and subclavian veins may occur (240).

Chronic, progressive involvement of the central nervous system occurs in 10% to 20% of patients and may result in permanent neurologic deficits or chronic dementia (25,240,245,246). T_2-weighted MRI may reveal multiple high-intensity focal lesions in the brainstem, basal ganglia, and cerebral white matter (240,241,247). The cerebrospinal fluid demonstrates elevated levels of protein and IgG and a pleocytosis consisting of polymorphonuclear leukocytes and lymphocytes (240,241,247).

A variety of cutaneous lesions may be observed in Behçet disease (25,240). Pustules and acneiform lesions are most common, but erythema nodosum, cutaneous ulcers, and pyoderma gangrenosum may be found (241). Responses to cutaneous trauma manifest as excessive local inflammation, or pathergy (241), which serves as a basis for the diagnosis of Behçet disease. Following venipuncture or abrasion of skin, papules or pustules develop at the site within 24 to 48 hours (241). Pathergy has been demonstrated in up to 80% of Turkish patients with Behçet disease (248) but is less common (<10%) in cohorts of British patients with Behçet disease (241,249).

Other possible sites of involvement in Behçet disease include the gastrointestinal tract, kidneys, heart, and epididymis (25,240,241). Isolated mucosal ulcers may occur at any point in the gastrointestinal tract, but the ileocecal region is most commonly affected (241).

Lung involvement has been cited in only 1% to 7.7% of cases (25,240). Diverse pulmonary manifestations include transient opacities, mass lesions, pleural effusions, hemoptysis, aneurysms of the pulmonary arteries, arterial and venous thromboses, pulmonary infarcts, pulmonary hemorrhage, bronchiolitis obliterans–organizing pneumonia, and recurrent pneumonia (25,240). Massive, fatal hemorrhage may be caused by the rupture or erosion of pulmonary arterial aneurysms (16,244). Pulmonary artery aneurysms augur a poor prognosis, with 30% of patients dying within 2 years (16,25). Sudden hilar enlargement or polylobular, round opacities on chest radiographs may represent pulmonary artery aneurysms (25). Ventilation-perfusion scans are nonspecific; perfusion defects may mimic pulmonary embolism, leading to inappropriate and potentially fatal anticoagulation (241). Helical CT is the preferred method to diagnose pulmonary arterial aneurysms (24,25,250). Noninvasive assessment by spiral CT and MRI can identify pulmonary aneurysms and obviates the need for conventional angiography in the diagnosis and preoperative assessment (250). Aneurysms appear as saccular or fusiform dilatations that fill with contrast simultaneously with the pulmonary artery (25). A mosaic pattern of attenuation (likely reflecting changes in perfusion) has also been noted in some patients with pulmonary aneurysms (24). Pulmonary artery aneurysms are most frequently located in the arteries of the right lower lobe, followed by the right and left main pulmonary arteries (24). MRI is less sensitive than CT (25).

The histologic features of Behçet disease are nonspecific. A necrotizing vasculitis (composed of lymphocytes, plasma cells, and polymorphonuclear leukocytes) involves arteries, veins, and capillaries (25). Intraluminal aggregates of leukocytes are often found within blood vessels, suggesting intravascular leukocyte activation (241). Varying degrees of fibrosis, thrombosis, and necrosis are evident (25). However, frank endothelial cell injury or fibrinoid necrosis is unusual (241). The results of laboratory studies in Behçet disease are nonspecific. Elevations in the erythrocyte sedimentation rate or C-reactive protein are common during flares of the disease but are usually not as high as in other vasculitic disorders (241). The serum complement components are normal, and autoantibodies (e.g., rheumatoid factor, antinuclear antibodies, ANCA) are absent (241). Antiphospholipid antibodies have been cited in 20% of patients (251,252) but are not believed to correlate with the presence of thrombosis (252).

The etiology of Behçet disease is not known (25). Activated neutrophils, deposits of immune complexes and complement in involved tissues, increased expression of several cytokines (e.g., IL-2, IFN-γ, IL-1, IL-6, IL-8, and TNF -α) have been reported (25). Th1 cell proinflammatory cytokines likely play a central role in the pathogenesis (25,253). Oligoclonal T-cell expansion correlates with clinically active disease (254), supporting an antigen-driven immune response. Activated neutrophils with increased chemotaxis and superoxide generation may play a role in the pathogenesis

(25,255). Microbial infection may play a causative role (25). Some investigators believe that ubiquitous antigens, including heat shock protein of microorganisms (256,257), may trigger a cross-reactive autoimmune response in Behçet disease (25). Hormonal factors may play a contributory role in the pathogenesis because the disease is more severe in males (25,258).

The natural history of Behçet disease is characterized by exacerbations and remissions (25,240). The prognosis is worse in males and in patients who are young at the onset of disease (258). Because of the rarity of Behçet disease, few controlled therapeutic trials have been performed. Randomized trials have been carried out only in the context of ocular (259,260) or mucocutaneous (261) disease. Therapy depends on the site(s) and severity of disease. Topical corticosteroids (241), colchicine (262), or thalidomide (261) may be adequate for oral and genital ulcers (240). In a randomized controlled trial, thalidomide (100 or 300 mg/d) was superior to placebo in treating oral or genital ulcerations associated with Behçet disease (261). Although thalidomide appears to more effective than colchicine (261,263), it is teratogenic, may cause peripheral neuropathy (264), and has sedating properties (241), and it should be used with caution (never in women of childbearing age) (241). Colchicine or nonsteroidal antiinflammatory drugs may be adequate to treat arthralgias or erythema nodosum (240,241). Sulfasalazine and corticosteroids may be efficacious for gastrointestinal manifestations (240,247). Acute flares of ocular inflammation can initially be treated with short courses of topical and systemic corticosteroids (240,241). Azathioprine (260,265,266), cyclosporine (259), mycophenolate mofetil (267), or colchicine (260) may be effective to control recurrent flares or corticosteroid-recalcitrant uveitis. In one study, response rates for recurrent uveitis were 50% with corticosteroids, 66% with colchicine, and 71% with azathioprine (260). In another study, cyclosporine was beneficial in more than 70% of patients with recurrent uveitis refractory to corticosteroids, colchicine, or immunosuppressive or cytotoxic agents (259). Data for severe vasculitis are limited to uncontrolled trials. However, involvement of critical organs warrants aggressive treatment with systemic corticosteroids *combined with* immunosuppressive or cytotoxic agents (e.g., cyclophosphamide, chlorambucil, azathioprine, methotrexate, or mycophenolate mofetil) (240,241,247,265–267). Acute, life-threatening conditions (e.g., severe hemoptysis) or severe central nervous system disease mandates treatment with intravenous pulse methylprednisolone and cyclophosphamide (or other cytotoxic agents) (25,240,247,268). Cyclosporine has been used in patients failing corticosteroids and cytotoxic agents with anecdotal responses (240,245,269,270). However, neurologic complications are more common in patients with Behçet disease who are receiving cyclosporine (240,245). Cyclosporine should not be used in patients with neurologic involvement (240). The results of trials of IFN-α for the treatment of Behçet dis-

ease are encouraging (271–274), but data are limited. In one randomized study, the combination of colchicine, IFN-α, and benzathine penicillin was more effective than colchicine and benzathine penicillin in treating ocular manifestations of Behçet disease (273). Anecdotal responses to infliximab (a monoclonal antibody against TNF-α) have been cited for the ocular manifestations (275), orogenital and cutaneous ulcers (276), and gastrointestinal complications (277) of Behçet disease. Anticoagulants and antiplatelet agents have been used to treat deep venous thrombosis (25,241,247), but the risk for bleeding is high when pulmonary vessels are involved (16,240). If thrombi are not extensive, antiplatelet treatment with low-dose aspirin may be sufficient (25), although comparisons with anticoagulants or antiplatelet aggregation therapy have not been made. Aneurysms involving pulmonary arteries or large vessels (e.g., aorta, innominate and subclavian arteries) are potentially lethal and may require resection (16,241,244). However, surgical therapy is often unsuccessful, followed by graft occlusions or new aneurysms (244). Regression or shrinkage of 35 (76%) of 46 pulmonary arterial aneurysms was noted with medical therapy in one study (24). In patients exhibiting improvement, serial helical CT demonstrated thrombosis of the aneurysms, followed by lysis, then total disappearance (24). Others have noted regression of pulmonary arterial aneurysms with corticosteroids or immunosuppressive agents (16,278).

HUGHES-STOVEN SYNDROME

In 1959, Hughes and Stoven (279) described a symptom complex of pulmonary artery aneurysms and recurrent venous thromboses (especially of the vena cava). A review of the literature up to 1981 identified only 12 patients with Hughes-Stoven syndrome; 11 were young males (280). Symptoms included fever, central nervous system symptoms secondary to increased intracranial pressure, hemoptysis, arthralgias, and skin rash. Nine of the 12 patients died of massive hemoptysis resulting from the rupture of pulmonary arterial aneurysms. Surgical resection of the pulmonary aneurysms was accomplished in all three survivors. Cerebral thrombophlebitis was present in 6 of these 12 cases. Histologic examination of the involved tissue demonstrated a necrotizing vasculitis. Most, if not all cases of "Hughes-Stoven syndrome" likely reflect unrecognized pulmonary vasculitis of other causes (particularly Behçet disease).

TAKAYASU ARTERITIS

Takayasu arteritis is a rare vasculitis affecting primarily large vessels (e.g., aorta and its branches); it may cause arterial stenoses, aneurysms, and distal arterial insufficiency (21,23). The most common site of involvement is the subclavian arteries, near their junction with the aorta (21,23). Absent radial pulses gave rise to the term *pulseless disease* (281). Most series have been reported from Japan (282,283), the Orient, and Mexico (284). Takayasu arteritis is rare in the United States and Europe (21,23). Only 32 cases were diagnosed at the Mayo Clinic between 1971 and 1983 (23). The incidence among Caucasians has been estimated at 2.6 cases per million per year (23). Most patients present between the ages of 20 and 30 years; the disease is rare in the elderly. The female predominance is striking (21,23).

Clinical Features

The predominant clinical manifestations are related to cessation of blood flow in the aorta or its branches and include claudication of the arms or legs, dizziness (reflecting occlusion of the carotid or vertebrobasilar arteries), ischemic cardiac disease, visual loss, and back pain (reflecting aortic aneurysms) (21,23). Multiple vascular bruits or absent or reduced pulses are characteristic findings on the physical examination (23). Fever, malaise, weight loss, and anemia are noted in more than one third of patients, and myalgias or arthralgias in nearly 60% (21,23). Elevations in the erythrocyte sedimentation rate may be striking (21,23) and may be a surrogate marker of disease activity (23). Antinuclear antibodies and rheumatoid factor are absent (21,23). Circulating immune complexes have been found in up to 50% of patients with Takayasu arteritis but do not correlate with disease activity (23). Renovascular hypertension occurs in approximately 40% of patients (23). Aortic insufficiency or aneurysms of the root of the aorta, when present, are major causes of death and warrant surgical correction (23).

Pulmonary vasculitis is rarely recognized before death (21,23), but pulmonary arterial aneurysms or stenoses have been documented in up to 50% of patients by pulmonary angiography (284,285) or necropsy (286). In a Japanese study, pulmonary arterial lesions were detected in 12 of 21 cases at necropsy (286). Japanese investigators cited abnormal findings on pulmonary arteriograms in 13 (50%) of 26 of patients with Takayasu arteritis; results of pulmonary perfusion scintigraphy were abnormal in 19 (44%) of 43 cases (285). Abnormalities on pulmonary arteriograms include occlusion, narrowing, irregular lumina, tortuosity, and dilatation (mainly proximal) of the pulmonary arteries (281). The severity of the pulmonary arterial involvement does not necessarily parallel the lesions in the aorta or its main branches (281). Pulmonary hypertension was found in 7 (27%) of 27 patients in whom cardiac catheterization was performed (281). Similarly, a study of 22 patients with Takayasu arteritis in Mexico detected pulmonary angiographic abnormalities in 50%; moderate pulmonary hypertension was present in 73% (284). However, no patient had pulmonary symptoms. Despite the high incidence of pulmonary arterial lesions when angiography or cardiac catheterization techniques are performed, *clinically apparent* pulmonary involvement has rarely been evident in series from the United States. None of 32 patients with Takayasu arteritis seen at the Mayo Clinic

had clinically significant pulmonary arterial involvement at a median follow-up of 5 years (23). A prospective study of 20 patients with Takayasu arteritis at the NIH did not identify clinically significant pulmonary arterial involvement in any patient (21).

The diagnosis of Takayasu disease is usually made on the basis of aortic angiographic findings of occlusions, stenosis, luminal irregularities, tortuosity, or aneurysms in a young woman with arterial occlusive symptoms (281). Dilatation of the aortic root or aortic insufficiency may occur (21,23). Bypass grafting for aortic occlusive lesions has been successfully performed in some patients (21,23). Histopathology is rarely confirmed except at the time of resection or bypass of arterial lesions. Salient features are a granulomatous, sclerosing arteritis that is indistinguishable from giant cell (temporal) arteritis (23).

Therapy

Corticosteroids are the cornerstone of therapy (21,23,281). Most experts initiate therapy with prednisone (1 mg/kg per day) for 4 to 6 weeks, followed by a gradual taper according to the symptoms and sedimentation rate (21). Cyclophosphamide should be considered for severe cases or patients failing corticosteroids (21,23). With aggressive medical therapy, survival exceeds 90%, and severe sequelae can be averted (21,23). Factors associated with increased mortality include severe systemic hypertension, aortic incompetence, and marked aneurysm formation (283). The presence of one of more of these findings was associated with a 5-year survival rate of 74%, whereas 100% of patients *without* such findings survived 5 years (283). Far-advanced stenoses or occlusions associated with inactive, sclerotic lesions are not affected by immunosuppressive therapy. In these circumstances, when symptoms of vascular compromise are evident, angioplasty, surgical reconstruction, or bypass grafting should be performed (21,23).

HENOCH-SCHÖNLEIN SYNDROME

Henoch-Schönlein syndrome (IgA nephropathy) is a necrotizing vasculitis affecting principally children. The major manifestations are palpable purpura, hematuria, arthralgias, and abdominal pain (18–20,287). Persons of all ages may be affected, but the peak incidence is in children 5 years old (287–289). The disease often begins after an upper respiratory tract infection (7). Hematuria and proteinuria are evident in 50% of patients, but only 10% to 20% exhibit renal insufficiency (7,19,20). The hallmark renal lesion is glomerulonephritis; the most common pattern is mesangial proliferative glomerulonephritis without crescents (19). Rapidly progressive renal failure with crescentic glomerulonephritis is rare (18–20). The prognosis of patients with Henoch-Schönlein syndrome is usually good (with or without therapy) (7). However, end-stage renal failure evolves in fewer than 5% of patients (19,20). Factors associated with a worse prognosis in adults at presentation include proteinuria (>1.5 g/d), impaired renal function, and hypertension (19). Lung involvement is exceedingly rare (7,290), but fatal alveolar hemorrhage and capillaritis have been described in a few patients (290,291). Neurologic involvement is rare (292).

Henoch-Schönlein syndrome is caused by circulating immune complexes, with IgA reacting to target antigens in the renal glomeruli, skin, or gastrointestinal tract (7,287). A small vessel vasculitis, associated with pronounced deposition of IgA in glomerular capillaries and affected vessels, is pathognomonic (7). Although ANCA is typically absent in Henoch-Schönlein syndrome, circulating MPO-ANCA was observed in three patients with rapidly progressive IgA nephropathy (18). The role of ANCA in the pathogenesis of a subset of patients with Henoch-Schönlein syndrome is controversial (293).

Henoch-Schönlein syndrome is often self-limited, and patients may not require therapy (19,20). However, progressive renal failure or pulmonary hemorrhage mandates therapy with corticosteroids (alone or combined with immunosuppressive agents) (20,294). Although controlled randomized trials of therapy have not been performed, success has been cited anecdotally with cyclophosphamide (oral or pulse) (294), azathioprine (20), cyclosporine (295), antiplatelet agents (7), and plasma exchange (19,20,294). In one nonrandomized study of children with severe Henoch-Schönlein syndrome nephritis, the combination of azathioprine and corticosteroids (oral or pulse) was associated with a favorable response in 19 of 21 patients (20).

REFERENCES

1. Hoffman GS, Kerr GS, Leavitt RY, et al. Wegener's granulomatosis: an analysis of 158 patients. *Ann Intern Med* 1992;116:488–498.
2. Langford CA, Hoffman GS. Rare diseases. 3: Wegener's granulomatosis. *Thorax* 1999;54:629–637.
3. Lynch JP III, Hoffman GS. Wegener's granulomatosis: controversies and current concepts. *Compr Ther* 1998;24:421–440.
4. Reinhold-Keller E, Beuge N, Latza U, et al. An interdisciplinary approach to the care of patients with Wegener's granulomatosis: long-term outcome in 155 patients. *Arthritis Rheum* 2000;43:1021–1032.
5. Lanham JG, Elkon KB, Pusey CD, et al. Systemic vasculitis with asthma and eosinophilia: a clinical approach to the Churg-Strauss syndrome. *Medicine (Baltimore)* 1984;63:65–81.
6. Mouthon L, Le Toumelin P, Andre M. H, et al. Polyarteritis nodosa and Churg-Strauss angiitis: characteristics and outcome in 38 patients over 65 years. *Medicine (Baltimore)* 2002;81:27–40.
7. Jennette JC, Falk RJ. Small-vessel vasculitis. *N Engl J Med* 1997;337:1512–1523.
8. Fauci AS, Haynes BF, Costa J, et al. Lymphomatoid granulomatosis. Prospective clinical and therapeutic experience over 10 years. *N Engl J Med* 1982;306:68–74.
9. Liebow AA, Carrington CR, Friedman PJ. Lymphomatoid granulomatosis. *Hum Pathol* 1972;3:457–558.
10. Jennette JC, Falk RJ, Andrassy K, et al. Nomenclature of systemic vasculitides. Proposal of an international consensus conference. *Arthritis Rheum* 1994;37:187–192.
11. Schwarz MI, Brown KK. Small vessel vasculitis of the lung. *Thorax* 2000;55:502–510.
12. Travis WD, Colby TV, Lombard C, et al. A clinicopathologic study of 34 cases of diffuse pulmonary hemorrhage with lung biopsy confirmation. *Am J Surg Pathol* 1990;14:1112–1125.
13. Haworth SJ, Savage COS, Carr D, et al. Lung haemorrhage in patients with Wegener's granulomatosis and microscopic polyarteritis. *Br Med J* 1985;290:1775–1778.
14. Stricker H, Malinverni R. Multiple, large aneurysms of pulmonary arteries in Behçet's disease. Clinical remission and radiologic resolution after corticosteroid therapy. *Arch Intern Med* 1989;149:925–927.
15. Raz I, Okon E, Chajek-Shaul T. Pulmonary manifestations in Behçet's syndrome. *Chest* 1989;95:585–589.
16. Hamuryudan V, Yurdakul S, Moral F, et al. Pulmonary arterial aneurysms in Behçet's syndrome: a report of 24 cases. *Br J Rheumatol* 1994;33:48–51.
17. Efthimiou J, Johnston C, Spiro SG, et al. Pulmonary disease in Behçet's syndrome. *Q J Med* 1986;58:259–280.
18. Allmaras E, Nowack R, Andrassy K, et al. Rapidly progressive IgA nephropathy with anti-myeloperoxidase antibodies benefits from immunosuppression. *Clin Nephrol* 1997;48:269–273.
19. Coppo R, Mazzucco G, Cagnoli L, et al. Long-term prognosis of Henoch-Schönlein nephritis in adults and children. Italian Group of Renal Immunopathology Collaborative Study on Henoch-Schönlein purpura. *Nephrol Dial Transplant* 1997;12:2277–2283.
20. Bergstein J, Leiser J, Andreoli SP. Response of crescentic Henoch-Schoenlein purpura nephritis to corticosteroid and azathioprine therapy. *Clin Nephrol* 1998;49:9–14.
21. Shelhamer JH, Volkman DJ, Parrillo JE, et al. Takayasu's arteritis and its therapy. *Ann Intern Med* 1985;103:121–126.
22. Schwarz MI. Nongranulomatous vasculitides of the lung. *Semin Respir Crit Care Med* 1998;19:47–56.
23. Hall S, Barr W, Lie JT, et al. Takayasu arteritis. A study of 32 North American patients. *Medicine (Baltimore)* 1985;64:89–99.
24. Tunaci M, Ozkorkmaz B, Tunaci A, et al. CT findings of pulmonary artery aneurysms during treatment for Behçet's disease. *AJR Am J Roentgenol* 1999;172:729–733.
25. Erkan F, Gul A, Tasali E. Pulmonary manifestations of Behçet's disease. *Thorax* 2001;56:572–578.
26. Girard T, Mahr A, Noel LH, et al. Are antineutrophil cytoplasmic antibodies a marker predictive of relapse in Wegener's granulomatosis? A prospective study. *Rheumatology (Oxford)* 2001;40:147–151.
27. Hoffman GS, Specks U. Antineutrophil cytoplasmic antibodies. *Arthritis Rheum* 1998;41:1521–1537.
28. Lipford EH Jr, Margolick JB, Longo DL, et al. Angiocentric immunoproliferative lesions: a clinicopathologic spectrum of postthymic T-cell proliferations. *Blood* 1988;72:1674–1681.
29. Jaffe ES, Lipford EH Jr, Margolick JB, et al. Lymphomatoid granulomatosis and angiocentric lymphoma: a spectrum of postthymic T-cell proliferations. *Semin Respir Med* 1993;10:167–172.
30. Jaffe ES, Wilson WH. Lymphomatoid granulomatosis: pathogenesis, pathology and clinical implications. *Cancer Surv* 1997;30:233–248.
31. Kyndt X, Reumaux D, Bridoux F, et al. Serial measurements of antineutrophil cytoplasmic autoantibodies in patients with systemic vasculitis. *Am J Med* 1999;106:527–533.
32. Jayne DR, Gaskin G, Pusey CD, et al. ANCA and predicting relapse in systemic vasculitis. *Q J Med* 1995;88:127–133.

33. Jayne DR, Rasmussen N. Treatment of antineutrophil cytoplasm autoantibody-associated systemic vasculitis: initiatives of the European Community Systemic Vasculitis Clinical Trials Study Group. *Mayo Clin Proc* 1997;72:737–747.

34. Rao JK, Weinberger M, Oddone EZ, et al. The role of antineutrophil cytoplasmic antibody (c-ANCA) testing in the diagnosis of Wegener granulomatosis. A literature review and metaanalysis. *Ann Intern Med* 1995;123:925–932.

35. Nolle B, Specks U, Ludemann J, et al. Anticytoplasmic autoantibodies: their immunodiagnostic value in Wegener granulomatosis. *Ann Intern Med* 1989;111:28–40.

36. Lhote F, Guillevin L. Polyarteritis nodosa, microscopic polyangiitis, and Churg-Strauss syndrome. *Semin Respir Crit Care Med* 1998;19:27–45.

37. Gross WL, Schnabel A, Trabandt A. New perspectives in pulmonary angiitis. From pulmonary angiitis and granulomatosis to ANCA-associated vasculitis. *Sarcoidosis Vasculitis Diffuse Lung Dis* 2000;17:33–52.

38. Guillevin L, Cohen P, Gayraud M, et al. Churg-Strauss syndrome. Clinical study and long-term follow-up of 96 patients. *Medicine (Baltimore)* 1999;78:26–37.

39. Guillevin L, Visser H, Noel LH, et al. Antineutrophil cytoplasm antibodies in systemic polyarteritis nodosa with and without hepatitis B virus infection and Churg-Strauss syndrome—62 patients. *J Rheumatol* 1993;20:1345–1349.

40. Conron M, Beynon HL. Churg-Strauss syndrome. *Thorax* 2000;55:870–877.

41. Guillevin L, Lhote F, Cohen P, et al. Polyarteritis nodosa related to hepatitis B virus. A prospective study with long-term observation of 41 patients. *Medicine (Baltimore)* 1995;74:238–253.

42. Fauci AS, Haynes BF, Katz P, et al. Wegener's granulomatosis: prospective clinical and therapeutic experience with 85 patients for 21 years. *Ann Intern Med* 1983;98:76–85.

43. Luqmani RA, Bacon PA, Beaman M, et al. Classical versus nonrenal Wegener's granulomatosis. *Q J Med* 1994;87:161–167.

44. Leavitt RY, Fauci AS, Bloch DA, et al. The American College of Rheumatology 1990 criteria for the classification of Wegener's granulomatosis. *Arthritis Rheum* 1990;33:1101–1107.

45. Mark EJ, Matsubara O, Tan-Liu NS, et al. The pulmonary biopsy in the early diagnosis of Wegener's (pathergic) granulomatosis: a study based on 35 open lung biopsies. *Hum Pathol* 1988;19:1065–1071.

46. Travis WD, Hoffman GS, Leavitt RY, et al. Surgical pathology of the lung in Wegener's granulomatosis. Review of 87 open lung biopsies from 67 patients. *Am J Surg Pathol* 1991;15:315–333.

47. Devaney KO, Travis WD, Hoffman GS, et al. Interpretation of head and neck biopsies in Wegener's granulomatosis: a pathologic study of 126 biopsies in 70 patients. *Am J Surg Pathol* 1990;14:555–564.

48. Cotch MF, Hoffman GS, Yerg DE, et al. The epidemiology of Wegener's granulomatosis. Estimates of the five-year period prevalence, annual mortality, and geographic disease distribution from population-based data sources. *Arthritis Rheum* 1996;39:87–92.

49. Watts RA, Gonzales-Gay M, Garcia-Porrua C, et al. ANCA-associated vasculitis in two European regions. *Clin Exp Immunol* 2000;120[Suppl 1]:60.

50. Koldingsnes W, Nossent H. Epidemiology of Wegener's granulomatosis in northern Norway. *Arthritis Rheum* 2000;43:2481–2487.

51. Rottem M, Fauci AS, Hallahan CW, et al. Wegener granulomatosis in children and adolescents: clinical presentation and outcome. *J Pediatr* 1993;122:26–31.

52. Stegmayr BG, Gothefors L, Malmer B, et al. Wegener granulomatosis in children and young adults. A case study of ten patients. *Pediatr Nephrol* 2000;14:208–213.

53. McDonald TJ, Neel HB 3rd, DeRemee RA. Wegener's granulomatosis of the subglottis and the upper portion of the trachea. *Ann Otol Rhinol Laryngol* 1982;91:588–592.

54. McDonald TJ, DeRemee RA. Wegener's granulomatosis. *Laryngoscope* 1983;93:220–231.

55. Cordier JF, Valeyre D, Guillevin L, et al. Pulmonary Wegener's granulomatosis. A clinical and imaging study of 77 cases. *Chest* 1990;97:906–912.

56. Matteson EL, Gold KN, Bloch DA, et al. Long-term survival of patients with Wegener's granulomatosis from the American College of Rheumatology Wegener's Granulomatosis Classification Criteria Cohort. *Am J Med* 1996;101:129–134.

57. DeRemee RA, McDonald TJ, Harrison EG Jr, et al. Wegener's granulomatosis. Anatomic correlates, a proposed classification. *Mayo Clin Proc* 1976;51:777–781.

58. Carrington CB, Liebow A. Limited forms of angiitis and granulomatosis of Wegener's type. *Am J Med* 1966;41:497–527.

59. Reinhold-Keller E, De Groot K, Rudert H, et al. Response to trimethoprim/sulfamethoxazole in Wegener's granulomatosis depends on the phase of disease. *Q J Med* 1996;89:15–23.

60. Gaudin PB, Askin FB, Falk RJ, et al. The pathologic spectrum of pulmonary lesions in patients with anti-neutrophil cytoplasmic autoantibodies specific for anti-proteinase 3 and anti-myeloperoxidase. *Am J Clin Pathol* 1995;104:7–16.

61. Gaskin G, Savage CO, Ryan JJ, et al. Anti-neutrophil cytoplasmic antibodies and disease activity during long-term follow-up of 70 patients with systemic vasculitis. *Nephrol Dial Transplant* 1991;6:689–694.

62. Hauschild S, Schmitt WH, Csernok E, et al. ANCA in systemic vasculitides, collagen vascular diseases, rheumatic disorders, and inflammatory bowel diseases. *Adv Exp Med Biol* 1993;336:245–251.

63. Del Buono EA, Flint A. Diagnostic usefulness of nasal biopsy in Wegener's granulomatosis. *Hum Pathol* 1991;22:107–110.

64. Newman NJ, Slamovits TL, Friedland S, et al. Neuro-ophthalmic manifestations of meningocerebral inflammation from the limited form of Wegener's granulomatosis. *Am J Ophthalmol* 1995;120:613–621.

65. Bullen CL, Liesegang TJ, McDonald TJ, et al. Ocular complications of Wegener's granulomatosis. *Ophthalmology* 1983;90:279–290.

66. Haynes BF, Fishman ML, Fauci AS, et al. The ocular manifestations of Wegener's granulomatosis. Fifteen years experience and review of the literature. *Am J Med* 1977;63:131–141.

67. Woo TL, Francis IC, Wilcsek GA, et al. Australasian orbital and adnexal Wegener's granulomatosis. *Ophthalmology* 2001;108:1535–1543.

68. Lebovics RS, Hoffman GS, Leavitt RY, et al. The management of subglottic stenosis in patients with Wegener's granulomatosis. *Laryngoscope* 1992;102:1341–1345.

69. Langford CA, Sneller MC, Hallahan CW, et al. Clinical features and therapeutic management of subglottic stenosis in patients with Wegener's granulomatosis. *Arthritis Rheum* 1996;39:1754–1760.

70. Daum TE, Specks U, Colby TV, et al. Tracheobronchial involvement in Wegener's granulomatosis. *Am J Respir Crit Care Med* 1995;151:522–526.

71. Quint LE, Whyte RI, Kazerooni EA, et al. Stenosis of the central airways: evaluation by using helical CT with multiplanar reconstructions. *Radiology* 1995;194:871–877.

72. Summers RM, Aggarwal NR, Sneller MC, et al. CT virtual bronchoscopy of the central airways in patients with Wegener's granulomatosis. *Chest* 2002;121:242–250.

73. Maskell GF, Lockwood CM, Flower CD. Computed tomography of the lung in Wegener's granulomatosis. *Clin Radiol* 1993;48:377–380.

74. Rosenberg DM, Weinberger SE, Fulmer JD, et al. Functional correlates of lung involvement in Wegener's granulomatosis. Use of pulmonary function tests in staging and follow-up. *Am J Med* 1980;69:387–394.

75. George TM, Cash JM, Farver G, et al. Mediastinal mass and hilar adenopathy: rare thoracic manifestations of Wegener's granulomatosis. *Arthritis Rheum* 1997;40:1992–1997.

76. Lynch JP III, Leatherman JW. 1997. Alveolar hemorrhage syndromes. In: Fishman A, ed. *Pulmonary diseases and disorders,* 3rd ed. New York: McGraw-Hill, 1997:1193–1210.

77. Reuter M, Schnabel A, Wesner F, et al. Pulmonary Wegener's granulomatosis: correlation between high-resolution CT findings and clinical scoring of disease activity. *Chest* 1998;114:500–506.

78. Kuhlman JE, Hruban RH, Fishman EK. Wegener granulomatosis: CT features of parenchymal lung disease. *J Comput Assist Tomogr* 1991;15:948–952.

79. Uner AH, Rozum-Slota B, Katzenstein AA. Bronchiolitis obliterans organizing pneumonia (BOOP)-like variant of Wegener's granulomatosis: a clinicopathologic study of 16 cases. *Am J Surg Pathol* 1996;20:794–801.

80. Yousem SA. Bronchocentric injury in Wegener's granulomatosis: a clinicopathologic study of 16 cases. *Am J Surg Pathol* 1991;20:794–801.

81. Lombard CM, Duncan SR, Rizk NW, et al. The diagnosis of Wegener's granulomatosis from transbronchial lung biopsy specimens. *Hum Pathol* 1990;21:838–842.

82. Carruthers DM, Connor S, Howie AJ, et al. Percutaneous image-guided biopsy of lung nodules in the assessment of disease activity in Wegener's granulomatosis. *Rheumatology (Oxford)* 2000;39:776–782.

83. Pinching AJ, Lockwood CM, Pussell BA, et al. Wegener's granulomatosis: observations on 18 patients with severe renal disease. *Q J Med* 1983;52:435–460.

84. Brandwein S, Esdaile J, Danoff D, et al. Wegener's granulomatosis. Clinical features and outcome in 13 patients. *Arch Intern Med* 1983;143:476–479.

85. Leatherman JW. Autoimmune diffuse alveolar hemorrhage. *Clin Pulm Med* 1994;1:356–364.

86. Ten Berge IJ, Wilmink JM, Meyer CJ, et al. Clinical and immunological follow-up of patients with severe renal disease in Wegener's granulomatosis. *Am J Nephrol* 1985;5:21–29.

87. Aasarod K, Bostad L, Hammerstrom J, et al. Renal histopathology and clinical course in 94 patients with Wegener's granulomatosis. *Nephrol Dial Transplant* 2001;16:953–960.

88. Kuross S, Davin T, Kjellstrand CM. Wegener's granulomatosis with severe renal failure: clinical course and results of dialysis and transplantation. *Clin Nephrol* 1981;16:172–180.

89. Bajema IM, Hagen EC, Hermans J, et al. Kidney biopsy as a predictor for renal outcome in ANCA-associated necrotizing glomerulonephritis. *Kidney Int* 1999;56:1751–1758.

90. Andrassy K, Erb A, Koderisch J, et al. Wegener's granulomatosis with renal involvement: patient survival and correlations between initial renal function, renal histology, therapy, and renal outcome. *Clin Nephrol* 1991;35:139–147.

91. Nishino H, Rubino FA, DeRemee RA, et al. Neurological involvement in Wegener's granulomatosis: an analysis of 324 consecutive patients at the Mayo Clinic. *Ann Neurol* 1993;33:4–90.

92. Drachman DA. Neurological complications of Wegener's granulomatosis. *Arch Neurol* 1963;8:145–155.

93. Spranger M, Schwab S, Meinck HM, et al. Meningeal involvement in Wegener's granulomatosis confirmed and monitored by positive circulating antineutrophil cytoplasm in cerebrospinal fluid. *Neurology* 1997;48:263–265.

94. Specks U, Moder KG, McDonald TJ. Meningeal involvement in Wegener granulomatosis. *Mayo Clin Proc* 2000;75:856–859.

95. Cheng TM, O'Neill BP, Scheithauer BW, et al. Chronic meningitis: the role of meningeal or cortical biopsy. *Neurosurgery* 1994;34:590–595; discussion 596.

96. Murphy JM, Gomez-Anson B, Gillard JH, et al. Wegener granulomatosis: MR imaging findings in brain and meninges. *Radiology* 1999;213:794–799.

97. Asmus R, Koltze H, Muhle C, et al. MRI of the head in Wegener's granulomatosis. *Adv Exp Med Biol* 1993;336:319–321.

98. Provenzale JM, Allen NB. Wegener granulomatosis: CT and MR findings. *AJNR Am J Neuroradiol* 1996;17:785–792.

99. Norris MJ, Tomecki KJ, Bergfeld WF, et al. Cutaneous Wegener's granulomatosis: report of a case and review of the literature. *Cleve Clin J Med* 1988;55:181–184.

100. Hu CH, O'Loughlin S, Winkelmann RK. Cutaneous manifestations of Wegener granulomatosis. *Arch Dermatol* 1977;113:175–182.

101. Allen DC, Doherty CC, O'Reilly DP. Pathology of the heart and the cardiac conduction system in Wegener's granulomatosis. *Br Heart J* 1984;52:674–678.

102. Forstot JZ, Overlie PA, Neufeld GK, et al. Cardiac complications of Wegener granulomatosis: a case report of complete heart block and review of the literature. *Semin Arthritis Rheum* 1980;10:148–154.

103. Morelli S, Gurgo Di Castelmenardo AM, Conti F, et al. Cardiac involvement in patients with Wegener's granulomatosis. *Rheumatol Int* 2000;19:209–212.

104. Goodfield NE, Bhandari S, Plant WD, et al. Cardiac involvement in Wegener's granulomatosis. *Br Heart J* 1995;73:110–115.

105. Grant SC, Levy RD, Venning MC, et al. Wegener's granulomatosis and the heart. *Br Heart J* 1994;71:82–86.

106. Haworth SJ, Pusey CD. Severe intestinal involvement in Wegener's granulomatosis. *Gut* 1984;25:1296–1300.

107. Camilleri M, Pusey CD, Chadwick VS, et al. Gastrointestinal manifestations of systemic vasculitis. *Q J Med* 1983;52:141–149.

108. Sokol RJ, Farrell MK, McAdams AJ. An unusual presentation of Wegener's granulomatosis mimicking inflammatory bowel disease. *Gastroenterology* 1984;87:426–432.

109. Ulbright TM, Katzenstein AL. Solitary necrotizing granulomas of the lung: differentiating features and etiology. *Am J Surg Pathol* 1980;4:13–28.

110. Pinching AJ, Rees AJ, Pussell BA, et al. Relapses in Wegener's granulomatosis: the role of infection. *Br Med J* 1980;281:836–838.

111. Hind CRK, Winearis CG, Lockwood CM, et al. Objective monitoring of activity of Wegener's granulomatosis by measurement of serum C-reactive protein concentration. *Clin Nephrol* 1984;21:341–345.

112. Kerr G, Fleisher TA, Hallahan CE, et al. Limited prognostic value of changes in anti-neutrophil cytoplasmic antibody titer in patients with Wegener's granulomatosis. *Arthritis Rheum* 1993;36:365–371.

113. Merkel PA, Polisson RP, Chang Y, et al. Prevalence of antineutrophil cytoplasmic antibodies in a large inception cohort of patients with connective tissue disease. *Ann Intern Med* 1997;126:866–873.

114. Boomsma MM, Stegeman CA, Van der Leij MJ, et al. Prediction of relapses in Wegener's granulomatosis by measurement of antineutrophil cytoplasmic antibody levels: a prospective study. *Arthritis Rheum* 2000;43:2025–2033.

115. Wong RC, Silvestrini RA, Savige JA, et al. Diagnostic value of classical and atypical antineutrophil cytoplasmic antibody (ANCA) immunofluorescence patterns. *J Clin Pathol* 1999;52:124–128.

116. Russell KA, Fass DN, Specks U. Antineutrophil cytoplasmic antibodies reacting with the pro form of proteinase 3 and disease activity in patients with Wegener's granulomatosis and microscopic polyangiitis. *Arthritis Rheum* 2001;44:463–468.

117. Cohen Tervaert JW. The value of serial ANCA testing during follow-up studies in patients with ANCA-associated vasculitides: a review. *J Nephrol* 1996;9:232–240.

118. Ludviksson BR, Sneller MC, Chua KS, et al. Active Wegener's granulomatosis is associated with HLA-DR$^+$ CD4$^+$ T cells exhibiting an unbalanced Th1-type T-cell cytokine pattern: reversal with IL-10. *J Immunol* 1998;160:3602–3609.

119. Jennette JC, Falk RJ. Pathogenesis of the vascular and glomerular damage in ANCA-positive vasculitis. *Nephrol Dial Transplant* 1998;13:16–20.

120. Harper L, Savage CO. Pathogenesis of ANCA-associated systemic vasculitis. *J Pathol* 2000;190:349–359.

121. Stegeman CA, Tervaert JW, Sluiter WJ, et al. Association of chronic nasal carriage of *Staphylococcus aureus* and higher relapse rates in Wegener granulomatosis. *Ann Intern Med* 1994;120:12–17.

122. Hoffman GS. "Wegener's granulomatosis": the path traveled since 1931. *Medicine (Baltimore)* 1994;73:325–329.

123. Walton EW. Giant cell granuloma of the respiratory tract (Wegener's granulomatosis). *Br Med J* 1958;2:265–270.

124. Fauci AS, Wolff SM. Wegener's granulomatosis: studies in 18 patients and a review of the literature. *Medicine* 1973;52:535–561.

125. Guillevin L, Cordier JF, Lhote F, et al. A prospective, multicenter, randomized trial comparing steroids and pulse cyclophosphamide versus steroids and oral cyclophosphamide in the treatment of generalized Wegener's granulomatosis. *Arthritis Rheum* 1997;40:2187–2198.

126. Mahr A, Girard T, Agher R, et al. Analysis of factors predictive of survival based on 49 patients with systemic Wegener's granulomatosis and prospective follow-up. *Rheumatology (Oxford)* 2001;40:492–498.

127. Lynch JP 3rd, McCune WJ. Immunosuppressive and cytotoxic pharmacotherapy for pulmonary disorders. *Am J Respir Crit Care Med* 1997;155:395–420.

128. Talar-Williams C, Hijazi YM, Walther MM, et al. Cyclophosphamide-induced cystitis and bladder cancer in patients with Wegener granulomatosis. *Ann Intern Med* 1996;124:477–484.

129. Cupps TR, Silverman GJ, Fauci AS. Herpes zoster in patients with treated Wegener's granulomatosis. A possible role for cyclophosphamide. *Am J Med* 1980;69:881–885.

130. Hoffman GS, Leavitt RY, Fleisher TA, et al. Treatment of Wegener's granulomatosis with intermittent high-dose intravenous cyclophosphamide. *Am J Med* 1990;89:403–410.

131. Le Thi Huong D, Papo T, Piette JC, et al. Monthly intravenous pulse cyclophosphamide therapy in Wegener's granulomatosis. *Clin Exp Rheumatol* 1996;14:9–16.

132. Reinhold-Keller E, Kekow J, Schnabel A, et al. Influence of disease manifestation and antineutrophil cytoplasmic antibody titer on the response to pulse cyclophosphamide therapy in patients with Wegener's granulomatosis. *Arthritis Rheum* 1994;37:919–924.

133. Haubitz M, Frei U, Rother U, et al. Cyclophosphamide pulse therapy in Wegener's granulomatosis. *Nephrol Dial Transplant* 1991;6:531–535.

134. Drosos AA, Sakkas LI, Goussia A, et al. Pulse cyclophosphamide

135. De Groot K, Muhler M, Reinhold-Keller E, et al. Induction of remission in Wegener's granulomatosis with low-dose methotrexate. *J Rheumatol* 1998;25:492–495.

136. Langford CA, Talar-Williams C, Sneller MC. Use of methotrexate and glucocorticoids in the treatment of Wegener's granulomatosis. Long-term renal outcome in patients with glomerulonephritis. *Arthritis Rheum* 2000;43:1836–1840.

137. Sneller MC, Hoffman GS, Talar-Williams C, et al. An analysis of forty-two Wegener's granulomatosis patients treated with methotrexate and prednisone. *Arthritis Rheum* 1995;38:608–613.

138. Langford CA, Sneller MC, Hoffman GS. Methotrexate use in systemic vasculitis. *Rheum Dis Clin North Am* 1997;23:841–853.

139. Langford CA, Talar-Williams C, Barron KS, et al. A staged approach to the treatment of Wegener's granulomatosis: induction of remission with glucocorticoids and daily cyclophosphamide switching to methotrexate for remission maintenance. *Arthritis Rheum* 1999;42:2666–2673.

140. De Groot K, Reinhold-Keller E, Tatsis E, et al. Therapy for the maintenance of remission in sixty-five patients with generalized Wegener's granulomatosis. Methotrexate versus trimethoprim/sulfamethoxazole. *Arthritis Rheum* 1996;39:2052–2061.

141. Furst DE. Practical clinical pharmacology and drug interactions of low-dose methotrexate therapy in rheumatoid arthritis. *Br J Rheumatol* 1995;34[Suppl 2]:20–25.

142. Stone JH, Tun W, Hellman DB. Treatment of non–life-threatening Wegener's granulomatosis with methotrexate and daily prednisone as the initial therapy of choice. *J Rheumatol* 1999;26:1134–1139.

143. Godeau B, Mainardi JL, Roudot-Thoraval F, et al. Factors associated with *Pneumocystis carinii* pneumonia in Wegener's granulomatosis. *Ann Rheum Dis* 1995;54:991–994.

144. DeRemee RA, McDonald TJ, Weiland LH. Wegener's granulomatosis: observations on treatment with antimicrobial agents. *Mayo Clin Proc* 1985;60:27–32.

145. DeRemee RA. The treatment of Wegener's granulomatosis with trimethoprim/sulfamethoxazole: illusion or vision? *Arthritis Rheum* 1988;31:1068–1074.

146. Georgi J, Ulmer M, Gross WL. Cotrimoxazole in Wegener's granulomatosis—a prospective study [in German]. *Immun Infekt* 1991;19:97–98.

147. Hoffman GS. Immunosuppressive therapy is always required for the treatment of limited Wegener's granulomatosis. *Sarcoidosis Vasculitis Diffuse Lung Dis* 1996;13:249–252.

148. Stegeman CA, Cohen Tervaert JW, De Jong PE, et al. Trimethoprim-sulfamethoxazole (co-trimoxazole) for the prevention of relapses of Wegener's granulomatosis. Dutch Co-Trimoxazole Wegener Study Group. *N Engl J Med* 1996;335:16–20.

149. Israel HL, Patchefsky AS. Treatment of Wegener's granulomatosis of the lung. *Am J Med* 1975;58:671–674.

150. Israel HL, Patchefsky AS, Saldana MJ. Wegener's granulomatosis, lymphomatoid granulomatosis, and benign lymphocytic angiitis and granulomatosis of lung. Recognition and treatment. *Ann Intern Med* 1977;87:691–699.

151. Weiner SR, Paulus HE. Treatment of Wegener's granulomatosis. *Semin Respir Med* 1989;10:156–161.

152. The Mycophenolate Mofetil Renal Refractory Rejection Study Group. Mycophenolate mofetil for the treatment of refractory, acute, cellular renal transplant rejection. *Transplantation* 1996;61:722–729.

153. Nowack R, Birck R, Van der Woude FJ. Mycophenolate

therapy in Wegener's granulomatosis: a pilot study. *J Intern Med* 1992;232:279–282.

mofetil for systemic vasculitis and IgA nephropathy. *Lancet* 1997;349:774.

154. Nowack R, Gobel U, Klooker P, et al. Mycophenolate mofetil for maintenance therapy of Wegener's granulomatosis and microscopic polyangiitis: a pilot study in 11 patients with renal involvement. *J Am Soc Nephrol* 1999;10:1965–1971.

155. Clarke AE, Bitton A, Eappen R, et al. Treatment of Wegener's granulomatosis after renal transplantation: is cyclosporine the preferred treatment? *Transplantation* 1990;50:1047–1051.

156. Allen NB, Caldwell DS, Rice JR, et al. Cyclosporin A therapy for Wegener's granulomatosis. *Adv Exp Med Biol* 1993;336:473–476.

157. Jayne DR, Chapel H, Adu D, et al. Intravenous immunoglobulin for ANCA-associated systemic vasculitis with persistent disease activity. *QJM* 2000;93:433–439.

158. Jayne DR, Esnault VL, Lockwood CM. ANCA anti-idiotype antibodies and the treatment of systemic vasculitis with intravenous immunoglobulin. *J Autoimmun* 1993;6:207–219.

159. Jayne DR, Davies MJ, Fox CJ, et al. Treatment of systemic vasculitis with pooled intravenous immunoglobulin. *Lancet* 1991;337:1137–1139.

160. Richter C, Schnabel A, Csernok E, et al. Treatment of antineutrophil cytoplasmic antibody (ANCA)-associated systemic vasculitis with high-dose intravenous immunoglobulin. *Clin Exp Immunol* 1995;101:2–7.

161. Lockwood CM, Thiru S, Isaacs JD, et al. Long-term remission of intractable systemic vasculitis with monoclonal antibody therapy. *Lancet* 1993;341:1620–1622.

162. Lockwood CM. New treatment strategies for systemic vasculitis: the role of intravenous immune globulin therapy. *Clin Exp Immunol* 1996;104[Suppl 1]:77–82.

163. Lockwood CM, Thiru S, Stewart S, et al. Treatment of refractory Wegener's granulomatosis with humanized monoclonal antibodies. *Q J Med* 1996;89:903–912.

164. Dick AD, Meyer P, James T, et al. Campath-1H therapy in refractory ocular inflammatory disease. *Br J Ophthalmol* 2000;84:107–109.

165. Kool J, De Keizer RJ, Siegert CE. Antithymocyte globulin treatment of orbital Wegener granulomatosis: a follow-up study. *Am J Ophthalmol* 1999;127:738–739.

166. Papo T, Le Thi Huong D, Wiederkehr JL, et al. Etoposide in Wegener's granulomatosis. *Rheumatology (Oxford)* 1999;38:473–475.

167. Stone JH, Uhlfelder ML, Hellmann DB, et al. Etanercept combined with conventional treatment in Wegener's granulomatosis: a six-month open-label trial to evaluate safety. *Arthritis Rheum* 2001;44:1149–1154.

168. Lightfoot RW Jr, Michel BA, Bloch DA, et al. The American College of Rheumatology 1990 criteria for the classification of polyarteritis nodosa. *Arthritis Rheum* 1990;33:1088–1093.

169. Guillevin L, Fain O, Lhote F, et al. Lack of superiority of steroids plus plasma exchange to steroids alone in the treatment of polyarteritis nodosa and Churg-Strauss syndrome. A prospective, randomized trial in 78 patients. *Arthritis Rheum* 1992;35:208–215.

170. Guillevin L, Durand-Gasselin B, Cevallos R, et al. Microscopic polyangiitis: clinical and laboratory findings in eighty-five patients. *Arthritis Rheum* 1999;42:421–430.

171. Mouthon L, Deblois P, Sauvaget F, et al. Hepatitis B virus-related polyarteritis nodosa and membranous nephropathy. *Am J Nephrol* 1995;15:266–269.

172. Guillevin L, Lhote F, Gayraud M, et al. Prognostic factors in polyarteritis nodosa and Churg-Strauss syndrome. A prospective study in 342 patients. *Medicine (Baltimore)* 1996;75:17–28.

173. Guillevin L, Jarrousse B, Lok C, et al. Long-term follow-up after treatment of polyarteritis nodosa and Churg-Strauss angiitis with comparison of steroids, plasma exchange, and cyclophosphamide to steroids and plasma exchange. A prospective randomized trial of 71 patients. The Cooperative Study Group for Polyarteritis Nodosa. *J Rheumatol* 1991;18:567–574.

174. Guillevin L, Lhote F, Cohen P, et al. Corticosteroids plus pulse cyclophosphamide and plasma exchanges versus corticosteroids plus pulse cyclophosphamide alone in the treatment of polyarteritis nodosa and Churg-Strauss syndrome patients with factors predicting poor prognosis. A prospective, randomized trial in sixty-two patients. *Arthritis Rheum* 1995;38:1638–1645.

175. Lauque D, Cadranel J, Lazor R, et al. Microscopic polyangiitis with alveolar hemorrhage. A study of 29 cases and review of the literature. Groupe d'Études et de Recherche sur les Maladies "Orphelines" Pulmonaires (GERM"O"P). *Medicine (Baltimore)* 2000;79:222–233.

176. Hogan SL, Nachman PH, Wilkman AS, et al. Prognostic markers in patients with antineutrophil cytoplasmic autoantibody-associated microscopic polyangiitis and glomerulonephritis. *J Am Soc Nephrol* 1996;7:23–32.

177. Watts RA, Carruthers DM, Scott DG. Epidemiology of systemic vasculitis: changing incidence or definition? *Semin Arthritis Rheum* 1995;25:28–34.

178. Zeek PM. Periarteritis nodosa: a critical review. *Am J Clin Pathol* 1952;22:777–790.

179. Savage CO, Winearls CG, Evans DJ, et al. Microscopic polyarteritis: presentation, pathology, and prognosis. *Q J Med* 1985;56:467–483.

180. Nachman PH, Hogan SL, Jennette JC, et al. Treatment response and relapse in antineutrophil cytoplasmic autoantibody-associated microscopic polyangiitis and glomerulonephritis. *J Am Soc Nephrol* 1996;7:33–39.

181. Akikusa B, Sato T, Ogawa M, et al. Necrotizing alveolar capillaritis in autopsy cases of microscopic polyangiitis. Incidence, histopathogenesis, and relationship with systemic vasculitis. *Arch Pathol Lab Med* 1997;121:144–149.

182. Bosch X, Lopez-Soto A, Mirapeix E, et al. Antineutrophil cytoplasmic autoantibody-associated alveolar capillaritis in patients presenting with pulmonary hemorrhage. *Arch Pathol Lab Med* 1994;118:517–522.

183. Nada AK, Torres VE, Ryu JH, et al. Pulmonary fibrosis as an unusual clinical manifestation of a pulmonary-renal vasculitis in elderly patients. *Mayo Clin Proc* 1990;65:847–856.

184. Brugiere O, Raffy O, Sleiman C, et al. Progressive obstructive lung disease associated with microscopic polyangiitis. *Am J Respir Crit Care Med* 1997;155:739–742.

185. Guillevin L, Lhote F, Amouroux J, et al. Antineutrophil cytoplasmic antibodies, abnormal angiograms and pathological findings in polyarteritis nodosa and Churg-Strauss syndrome: indications for the classification of vasculitides of the Polyarteritis Nodosa Group. *Br J Rheumatol* 1996;35:958–964.

186. Gordon M, Luqmani RA, Adu D, et al. Relapses in patients with a systemic vasculitis. *Q J Med* 1993;86:779–789.

187. Churg J, Strauss L. Allergic granulomatosis, allergic angiitis, and periarteritis nodosa. *Am J Pathol* 1951;27:277–301.

188. Rose GA, Spencer H. Polyarteritis nodosa. *Q J Med* 1957;26:43–81.

189. Chumbley LC, Harrison EG, DeRemee RA. Allergic granulomatosis and angiitis (Churg-Strauss syndrome): report and analysis of 30 cases. *Mayo Clin Proc* 1977;52:477–484.

190. Koss MN, Antonovych T, Hochholzer L. Allergic granulomatosis (Churg-Strauss syndrome): pulmonary and renal morphologic findings. *Am J Surg Pathol* 1981;5:21–28.

191. Lie JT. Diagnostic histopathology of major systemic and

pulmonary vasculitic syndromes. *Rheum Dis Clin North Am* 1990;16:269–292.

192. Nissim F, Von der Valde J, Czernobilsky B. A limited form of Churg-Strauss syndrome: ocular and cutaneous manifestations. *Arch Pathol Lab Med* 1982;106:305–307.

193. Lie JT, Bayardo RJ. Isolated eosinophilic coronary arteritis and eosinophilic myocarditis. A limited form of Churg-Strauss syndrome. *Arch Pathol Lab Med* 1989;113:199–201.

194. Masi AT, Hunder GG, Lie JT, et al. The American College of Rheumatology 1990 criteria for the classification of Churg-Strauss syndrome (allergic granulomatosis and angiitis). *Arthritis Rheum* 1990;33:1094–1100.

195. Reid AJ, Harrison BD, Watts RA, et al. Churg-Strauss syndrome in a district hospital. *Q J Med* 1998;91:219–229.

196. Wechsler ME, Garpestad E, Flier SR, et al. Pulmonary infiltrates, eosinophilia, and cardiomyopathy following corticosteroid withdrawal in patients with asthma receiving zafirlukast. *JAMA* 1998;279:455–457.

197. Katz RS, Papernik M. Zafirlukast and Churg-Strauss syndrome. *JAMA* 1998;279:1949; discussion 1950.

198. Wechsler ME, Finn D, Gunawardena D, et al. Churg-Strauss syndrome in patients receiving montelukast as treatment for asthma. *Chest* 2000;117:708–713.

199. Franco J, Artes MJ. Pulmonary eosinophilia associated with montelukast. *Thorax* 1999;54:558–560.

200. Kinoshita M, Shiraishi T, Koga T, et al. Churg-Strauss syndrome after corticosteroid withdrawal in an asthmatic patient treated with pranlukast. *J Allergy Clin Immunol* 1999;103:534–535.

201. Tuggey JM, Hosker HS. Churg-Strauss syndrome associated with montelukast therapy. *Thorax* 2000;55:805–806.

202. Knoell DL, Lucas J, Allen JN. Churg-Strauss syndrome associated with zafirlukast. *Chest* 1998;114:332–334.

203. Le Gall C, Pham S, Vignes S, et al. Inhaled corticosteroids and Churg-Strauss syndrome: a report of five cases. *Eur Respir J* 2000;15:978–981.

204. D'Cruz DP, Barnes NC, Lockwood CM. Difficult asthma or Churg-Strauss syndrome? *BMJ* 1999;318:475–476.

205. Bili A, Condemi JJ, Bottone SM, et al. Seven cases of complete and incomplete forms of Churg-Strauss syndrome not related to leukotriene receptor antagonists. *J Allergy Clin Immunol* 1999;104:1060–1065.

206. Stirling RG, Chung KF. Leukotriene antagonists and Churg-Strauss syndrome: the smoking gun. *Thorax* 1999;54:865–866.

207. Choi YH, Im JG, Han BK, et al. Thoracic manifestation of Churg-Strauss syndrome: radiologic and clinical findings. *Chest* 2000;117:117–124.

208. Worthy SA, Muller NL, Hansell DM, et al. Churg-Strauss syndrome: the spectrum of pulmonary CT findings in 17 patients. *AJR Am J Roentgenol* 1998;170:297–300.

209. Calabrese LH. Vasculitis of the central nervous system. *Rheum Dis Clin North Am* 1995;21:1059–1076.

210. Sehgal M, Swanson JW, DeRemee RA, et al. Neurologic manifestations of Churg-Strauss syndrome. *Mayo Clin Proc* 1995;70:337–341.

211. Guillevin L, Le Thi Huong D, Godeau P, et al. Clinical findings and prognosis of polyarteritis nodosa and Churg-Strauss angiitis: a study in 165 patients. *Br J Rheumatol* 1988;27:258–264.

212. Calabrese LH, Hoffman GS, Guillevin L. Therapy of resistant systemic necrotizing vasculitis. Polyarteritis, Churg-Strauss syndrome, Wegener's granulomatosis, and hypersensitivity vasculitis group disorders. *Rheum Dis Clin North Am* 1995;21:41–57.

213. Tatsis E, Schnabel A, Gross WL. Interferon-alpha treatment of four patients with the Churg-Strauss syndrome. *Ann Intern Med* 1998;129:370–374.

214. Mathieson PW, Cobbold SP, Hale G, et al. Monoclonal-antibody therapy in systemic vasculitis. *N Engl J Med* 1990;323:250–254.

215. Liebow AA. Pulmonary angiitis and granulomatosis. *Am Rev Respir Dis* 1973;108:1–18.

216. Katzenstein AL, Liebow AA, Friedman PJ. Bronchocentric granulomatosis, mucoid impaction, and hypersensitivity reactions to fungi. *Am Rev Respir Dis* 1975;111:497–537.

217. Koss MN, Robinson RG, Hochholzer L. Bronchocentric granulomatosis. *Hum Pathol* 1981;12:632–638.

218. Lynch JP III, Fantone J III. Other pulmonary granulomatous vasculitis syndromes. In: Lynch JP III, DeRemee RA, eds. *Immunologically mediated lung diseases.* Philadelphia: JB Lippincott Co, 1991:302–321.

219. Churg A, Carrington CB, Gupta R. Necrotizing sarcoid granulomatosis. *Chest* 1979;76:406–413.

220. Koss MN, Hochholzer L, Feigin DS, et al. Necrotizing sarcoid-like granulomatosis: clinical, pathologic, and immunopathologic findings. *Hum Pathol* 1980;11:510–519.

221. Churg A. Pulmonary angiitis and granulomatosis revisited. *Hum Pathol* 1983;14:868–883.

222. Sharma OP, Hewlett R, Gordonson J. Nodular sarcoidosis: an unusual radiographic appearance. *Chest* 1973;64:189–192.

223. Lynch JP 3rd, Kazerooni EA, Gay SE. Pulmonary sarcoidosis. *Clin Chest Med* 1997;18:755–785.

224. Medeiros LJ, Peiper SC, Elwood L, et al. Angiocentric immunoproliferative lesions: a molecular analysis of eight cases. *Hum Pathol* 1991;22:1150–1157.

225. Katzenstein AL, Carrington CB, Liebow AA. Lymphomatoid granulomatosis: a clinicopathologic study of 152 cases. *Cancer* 1979;43:360–373.

226. Patton WF, Lynch JP 3rd. Lymphomatoid granulomatosis. Clinicopathologic study of four cases and literature review. *Medicine (Baltimore)* 1982;61:1–12.

227. Koss MN, Hochholzer L, Langloss JM, et al. Lymphomatoid granulomatosis: a clinicopathologic study of 42 patients. *Pathology* 1986;18:283–288.

228. Lee JS, Tuder R, Lynch DA. Lymphomatoid granulomatosis: radiologic features and pathologic correlations. *AJR Am J Roentgenol* 2000;175:1335–1339.

229. Frazier AA, Rosado-de-Christenson ML, Galvin JR, et al. Pulmonary angiitis and granulomatosis: radiologic-pathologic correlation. *Radiographics* 1998;18:687–710; quiz 727.

230. Nicholson AG, Wotherspoon AC, Diss TC, et al. Lymphomatoid granulomatosis: evidence that some cases represent Epstein-Barr virus–associated B-cell lymphoma. *Histopathology* 1996;29:317–324.

231. Guinee D Jr, Jaffe E, Kingma D, et al. Pulmonary lymphomatoid granulomatosis. Evidence for a proliferation of Epstein-Barr virus–infected B-lymphocytes with a prominent T-cell component and vasculitis. *Am J Surg Pathol* 1994;18:753–764.

232. Katzenstein AL, Peiper SC. Detection of Epstein-Barr virus genomes in lymphomatoid granulomatosis: analysis of 29 cases by the polymerase chain reaction technique. *Mod Pathol* 1990;3:435–441.

233. Myers JL, Kurtin PJ, Katzenstein AL, et al. Lymphomatoid granulomatosis. Evidence of immunophenotypic diversity and relationship to Epstein-Barr virus infection. *Am J Surg Pathol* 1995;19:1300–1312.

234. Taniere P, Thivolet-Bejui F, Vitrey D, et al. Lymphomatoid granulomatosis—a report on four cases: evidence for B phenotype of the tumoral cells. *Eur Respir J* 1998;12:102–106.

235. Guinee DG Jr, Perkins SL, Travis WD, et al. Proliferation and

cellular phenotype in lymphomatoid granulomatosis: implications of a higher proliferation index in B cells. *Am J Surg Pathol* 1998;22:1093–1100.

236. Haque AK, Myers JL, Hudnall SD, et al. Pulmonary lymphomatoid granulomatosis in acquired immunodeficiency syndrome: lesions with Epstein-Barr virus infection. *Mod Pathol* 1998;11:347–356.

237. Mittal K, Neri A, Feiner H, et al. Lymphomatoid granulomatosis in the acquired immunodeficiency syndrome. Evidence of Epstein-Barr virus infection and B-cell clonal selection without myc rearrangement. *Cancer* 1990;65:1345–1349.

238. Bekassy AN, Cameron R, Garwicz S, et al. Lymphomatoid granulomatosis during treatment of acute lymphoblastic leukemia in a 6-year old girl. *Am J Pediatr Hematol Oncol* 1985;7:377–380.

239. Wilson WH, Kingma DW, Raffeld M, et al. Association of lymphomatoid granulomatosis with Epstein-Barr viral infection of B lymphocytes and response to interferon-alpha 2b. *Blood* 1996;87:4531–4537.

240. Sakane T, Takeno M, Suzuki N, et al. Behçet's disease. *N Engl J Med* 1999;341:1284–1291.

241. Pickering MC, Haskard DO. Behçet's syndrome. *J R Coll Physicians Lond* 2000;34:169–177.

242. International Study Group for Behçet's Disease. Criteria for the diagnosis of Behçet's disease. *Lancet* 1990;335:1078–1080.

243. Gul A, Esin S, Dilsen N, et al. Immunohistology of skin pathergy reaction in Behçet's disease. *Br J Dermatol* 1995;132:901–907.

244. Tuzun H, Besirli K, Sayin A, et al. Management of aneurysms in Behçet's syndrome: an analysis of 24 patients. *Surgery* 1997;121:150–156.

245. Kotake S, Higashi K, Yoshikawa K, et al. Central nervous system symptoms in patients with Behçet disease receiving cyclosporine therapy. *Ophthalmology* 1999;106:586–589.

246. Serdaroglu P. Behçet's disease and the nervous system. *J Neurol* 1998;245:197–205.

247. Kaklamani VG, Vaiopoulos G, Kaklamanis PG. Behçet's disease. *Semin Arthritis Rheum* 1998;27:197–217.

248. Yurdakul S, Gunaydin I, Tuzun Y, et al. The prevalence of Behçet's syndrome in a rural area in northern Turkey. *J Rheumatol* 1988;15:820–822.

249. Yazici H, Chamberlain MA, Tuzun Y, et al. A comparative study of the pathergy reaction among Turkish and British patients with Behçet's disease. *Ann Rheum Dis* 1984;43:74–75.

250. Greene RM, Saleh A, Taylor AK, et al. Noninvasive assessment of bleeding pulmonary artery aneurysms due to Behçet disease. *Eur Radiol* 1998;8:359–363.

251. Bergman R, Lorber M, Lerner M, et al. Anticardiolipin antibodies in Behçet's disease. *J Dermatol* 1990;17:164–167.

252. Al-Dalaan AN, Al-Ballaa SR, Al-Janadi MA, et al. Association of anti-cardiolipin antibodies with vascular thrombosis and neurological manifestation of Behçet's disease. *Clin Rheumatol* 1993;12:28–30.

253. Frassanito MA, Dammacco R, Cafforio P, et al. Th1 polarization of the immune response in Behçet's disease: a putative pathogenetic role of interleukin-12. *Arthritis Rheum* 1999;42:1967–1974.

254. Esin S, Gul A, Hodara V, et al. Peripheral blood T-cell expansions in patients with Behçet's disease. *Clin Exp Immunol* 1997;107:520–527.

255. Takeno M, Kariyone A, Yamashita N, et al. Excessive function of peripheral blood neutrophils from patients with Behçet's disease and from HLA-B51 transgenic mice. *Arthritis Rheum* 1995;38:426–433.

256. Direskeneli H, Eksioglu-Demiralp E, Yavuz S, et al. T-cell responses to 60/65-kDa heat shock protein–derived peptides in Turkish patients with Behçet's disease. *J Rheumatol* 2000;27:708–713.

257. Lehner T. The role of heat shock protein, microbial and autoimmune agents in the aetiology of Behçet's disease. *Int Rev Immunol* 1997;14:21–32.

258. Yazici H, Tuzun Y, Pazarli H, et al. Influence of age of onset and patient's sex on the prevalence and severity of manifestations of Behçet's syndrome. *Ann Rheum Dis* 1984;43:783–789.

259. Masuda K, Nakajima A, Urayama A, et al. Double-masked trial of cyclosporin versus colchicine and long-term open study of cyclosporin in Behçet's disease. *Lancet* 1989;1:1093–1096.

260. Kotter I, Durk H, Saal J, et al. Therapy of Behçet's disease. *Ger J Ophthalmol* 1996;5:92–97.

261. Hamuryudan V, Mat C, Saip S, et al. Thalidomide in the treatment of the mucocutaneous lesions of the Behçet syndrome. A randomized, double-blind, placebo-controlled trial. *Ann Intern Med* 1998;128:443–450.

262. Miyachi Y, Taniguchi S, Ozaki M, et al. Colchicine in the treatment of the cutaneous manifestations of Behçet's disease. *Br J Dermatol* 1981;104:67–69.

263. Ehrlich GE. Behçet disease and the emergence of thalidomide. *Ann Intern Med* 1998;128:494–495.

264. Gardner-Medwin JM, Smith NJ, Powell RJ. Clinical experience with thalidomide in the management of severe oral and genital ulceration in conditions such as Behçet's disease: use of neurophysiological studies to detect thalidomide neuropathy. *Ann Rheum Dis* 1994;53:828–832.

265. Hamuryudan V, Ozyazgan Y, Hizli N, et al. Azathioprine in Behçet's syndrome: effects on long-term prognosis. *Arthritis Rheum* 1997;40:769–774.

266. Yazici H, Pazarli H, Barnes CG, et al. A controlled trial of azathioprine in Behçet's syndrome. *N Engl J Med* 1990;322:281–285.

267. Kilmartin DJ, Forrester JV, Dick AD. Rescue therapy with mycophenolate mofetil in refractory uveitis. *Lancet* 1998;352:35–36.

268. Kaklamani VG, Kaklamanis PG. Treatment of Behçet's disease—an update. *Semin Arthritis Rheum* 2001;30:299–312.

269. Vansteenkiste J, Van Haecke P, Demedts M. Long-term treatment with cyclosporin A and coumarin in pulmonary thromboembolic Behçet's disease. *Monaldi Arch Chest Dis* 1998;53:142–143.

270. Sullu Y, Oge I, Erkan D, et al. Cyclosporin-A therapy in severe uveitis of Behçet's disease. *Acta Ophthalmol Scand* 1998;76:96–99.

271. O'Duffy JD, Calamia K, Cohen S, et al. Interferon-alpha treatment of Behçet's disease. *J Rheumatol* 1998;25:1938–1944.

272. Georgiou S, Monastirli A, Pasmatzi E, et al. Efficacy and safety of systemic recombinant interferon-alpha in Behçet's disease. *J Intern Med* 1998;243:367–372.

273. Demiroglu H, Ozcebe OI, Barista I, et al. Interferon alfa-2b, colchicine, and benzathine penicillin versus colchicine and benzathine penicillin in Behçet's disease: a randomised trial. *Lancet* 2000;355:605–609.

274. Zouboulis CC, Orfanos CE. Treatment of Adamantiades-Behçet disease with systemic interferon-alfa. *Arch Dermatol* 1998;134:1010–1016.

275. Sfikakis PP, Theodossiadis PG, Katsiari CG, et al. Effect of infliximab on sight-threatening panuveitis in Behçet's disease. *Lancet* 2001;358:295–296.

276. Goossens PH, Verburg RJ, Breedveld FC. Remission of Behçet's syndrome with tumour necrosis factor-alpha–blocking therapy. *Ann Rheum Dis* 2001;60:637.

277. Hassard PV, Binder SW, Nelson V, et al. Anti-tumor necrosis factor monoclonal antibody therapy for gastrointestinal

Behçet's disease: a case report. *Gastroenterology* 2001;120:995–999.

278. Stricker H, Malinverni R. Multiple, large aneurysms of pulmonary arteries in Behçet's disease. Clinical remission and radiologic resolution after corticosteroid therapy. *Arch Intern Med* 1989;149:925–927.

279. Hughes JP, Stoven PG. Segmental pulmonary artery aneurysms with peripheral venous thrombosis. *Br J Dis Chest* 1959;53:19–27.

280. Durieux P, Bletry O, Huchon G, et al. Multiple pulmonary arterial aneurysms in Behçet's disease and Hughes-Stoven syndrome. *Am J Med* 1981;71:736–741.

281. Kawai C, Ishikawa K, Kato M, et al. "Pulmonary pulseless disease": pulmonary involvement in so-called Takayasu's disease. *Chest* 1978;73:651–657.

282. Ishikawa K. Natural history and classification of occlusive thromboaortopathy (Takayasu's disease). *Circulation* 1978;57:27–35.

283. Ishikawa K. Survival and morbidity after diagnosis of occlusive thromboaortopathy (Takayasu's disease). *Am J Cardiol* 1981;47:1026–1032.

284. Lupi-Herrera E, Sanchez-Torres G, Marcushamer J, et al. Takayasu's arteritis. Clinical study of 107 cases. *Am Heart J* 1977;93:94–103.

285. Ishikawa K, Nakao K, Asai N, et al. Pulmonary circulation in occlusive thromboaortopathy (so-called Takayasu's disease) [in Japanese]. *Blood and Vessel* 1976;7:603.

286. Nasu T. Pathology of pulseless disease: a systemic study and critical review of 21 autopsy cases reported in Japan. *Angiology* 1963;14:225.

287. Mills JA, Michel BA, Bloch DA, et al. The American College of Rheumatology 1990 criteria for the classification of Henoch-Schönlein purpura. *Arthritis Rheum* 1990;33:1114–1121.

288. Michel BA, Hunder GG, Bloch DA, et al. Hypersensitivity vasculitis and Henoch-Schönlein purpura: a comparison between the two disorders. *J Rheumatol* 1992;19:721–728.

289. Dillon MJ, Ansell BM. Vasculitis in children and adolescents. *Rheum Dis Clin North Am* 1995;21:1115–1136.

290. Wright WK, Krous HF, Griswold WR, et al. Pulmonary vasculitis with hemorrhage in anaphylactoid purpura. *Pediatr Pulmonol* 1994;17:269–271.

291. Kathuria S, Cheifec G. Fatal pulmonary Henoch-Schönlein syndrome. *Chest* 1982;82:654–656.

292. Belman AL, Leicher CR, Moshe SL, et al. Neurologic manifestations of Schoenlein-Henoch purpura: report of three cases and review of the literature. *Pediatrics* 1985;75:687–692.

293. Coppo R, Cirina P, Amore A, et al. Properties of circulating IgA molecules in Henoch-Schönlein purpura nephritis with focus on neutrophil cytoplasmic antigen IgA binding (IgA-ANCA): new insight into a debated issue. Italian Group of Renal Immunopathology Collaborative Study on Henoch-Schönlein purpura in adults and in children. *Nephrol Dial Transplant* 1997;12:2269–2276.

294. McGregor D, Lynn KL, Robson R. Rapidly progressive IgA nephropathy with anti-myeloperoxidase antibodies responding to immunosuppression. *Clin Nephrol* 1998;50:64.

295. Schmaldienst S, Winkler S, Breiteneder S, et al. Severe nephrotic syndrome in a patient with Schönlein-Henoch purpura: complete remission after cyclosporin A. *Nephrol Dial Transplant* 1997;12:790–792.

Alveolar Hemorrhage Syndromes

31

Andrew P. Fontenot · Marvin I. Schwarz

The alveolar hemorrhage syndromes represent a group of uncommon disorders characterized by the presence of diffuse intra-alveolar bleeding. This potentially devastating condition occurs primarily because of the disruption of alveolar capillaries and to a lesser extent because of precapillary arterioles or postcapillary venules. The alveolar hemorrhage syndromes must be differentiated from the more common causes of hemoptysis such as bronchiectasis, endobronchial tumors, and bronchitis, which result from disturbances in the bronchial circulation. The clinical features of diffuse alveolar hemorrhage (DAH) include hemoptysis, anemia, diffuse alveolar opacities, and progressive respiratory failure, often necessitating the need for mechanical ventilation. The diagnosis is suggested by the presence of a persistently hemorrhagic bronchoalveolar lavage (BAL). As shown in Table 31.1, a vast number of disorders with differing underlying histopathology can result in DAH. The alveolar hemorrhage syndromes are characterized by the presence of red blood cells and fibrin in the alveolar space followed by the accumulation of hemosiderin-laden macrophages. This chapter will primarily focus on those causes of alveolar hemorrhage syndromes with an underlying immune mechanism. The association of transplant rejection and the development of DAH is discussed in Chapter 54.

CLINICAL MANIFESTATIONS

DAH may occur as the initial manifestation of an underlying systemic disorder. More commonly, patients presenting with DAH have a predisposing condition such as a connective tissue disorder or a systemic vasculitis. Despite the

large number of etiologies that result in DAH, the clinical and radiographic manifestations of this syndrome are similar. Hemoptysis is the cardinal manifestation of DAH and may be present intermittently for weeks before presentation. On the other hand, symptoms and signs of DAH may abruptly develop over several hours, as seen after crack cocaine inhalation (1, 2).

The clinical findings associated with DAH are nonspecific. Cough, fever, chills, and chest pain are common presenting symptoms. Progressive dyspnea and severe respiratory distress necessitating ventilatory support can also be seen. In one third of patients, hemoptysis may be absent at the time of presentation (3). In this setting, the presence of either localized or diffuse alveolar opacities on chest radiographs, a falling hematocrit, and hemorrhagic BAL fluid suggest the diagnosis.

The physical examination is nonspecific and includes the presence of fever, crackles, and signs of alveolar consolidation. Other symptoms and physical findings usually reflect the presence of an underlying systemic disease and include leukocytoclastic vasculitis, arthritis, sinusitis, and/or inflammatory ocular disease.

Despite the nonspecific chest radiographic findings of either patchy or diffuse alveolar filling, certain radiographic abnormalities point to particular diagnoses. For example, the presence of Kerley B lines in the setting of DAH suggests either mitral stenosis or pulmonary veno-occlusive disease. In patients with DAH and an underlying systemic vasculitis or a connective tissue disorder, the presence of Kerley B lines on chest x-ray should suggests the possibility of myocarditis and underlying left ventricular dysfunction. Recurrent episodes of DAH may lead to the development of interstitial fibrosis (4). In addition, recurrent episodes of DAH may lead to hyperinflation and obstructive lung disease (most likely secondary to the development of emphysema) (5, 6).

A. P. Fontenot and **M. I. Schwarz:** Department of Medicine, University of Colorado Health Sciences Center, Denver, Colorado.

TABLE 31.1. CAUSES OF THE ALVEOLAR HEMORRHAGE SYNDROMES BASED ON UNDERLYING HISTOPATHOLOGY

Pulmonary capillaritis
  Connective tissue diseases
    Systemic lupus erythematosus[a]
    Rheumatoid arthritis
    Mixed connective tissue disease
    Scleroderma
    Polymyositis
  Vasculitis
    Wegener granulomatosis
    Microscopic polyangiitis
    Henoch-Schölein purpura
    Behçet syndrome
    Cryoglobulinemia
  Other
    Goodpasture syndrome[a]
    Primary antiphospholipid antibody syndrome
    Isolated pulmonary capillaritis
    Immunoglobulin A nephropathy
    Idiopathic glomerulonephritis
    Acute lung transplant rejection
Bland pulmonary hemorrhage
  Idiopathic pulmonary hemosiderosis
  Goodpasture syndrome[a]
  Systemic lupus erythematosus[a]
  Coagulation disorders
  Trimellitic anhydride
  Isocyanate exposure
  Penicillamine, amiodarone, nitrofurantoin
  Mitral stenosis
  Subacute bacterial endocarditis
  Polyglandular autoimmune syndrome
  Multiple myeloma
Diffuse alveolar damage
  Bone marrow transplantation (idiopathic pneumonia syndrome)
  Crack cocaine inhalation
  Cytotoxic drug therapy
  Systemic lupus erythematosus[a]
  Acute respiratory distress syndrome
Miscellaneous
  Lymphangioleiomyomatosis
  Idiopathic pulmonary fibrosis
  Diphenylhydantoin
  Retinoic acid toxicity
  Autologous bone marrow transplantation
  Myasthenia gravis
  Ulcerative colitis
  Propylthiouracil
  Tuberous sclerosis
  Pulmonary veno-occlusive disease
  Pulmonary capillary hemangiomatosis
  Obstructive sleep apnea

[a]Etiologies with several possible histologic patterns.

A decreasing hemoglobin and nonspecific elevations of the white blood cell and platelet counts are characteristic laboratory findings. Thrombocytopenia in the setting of DAH should suggest the presence of systemic lupus erythematosus (SLE) or the primary antiphospholipid antibody syndrome (7, 8). An elevated erythrocyte sedimentation rate suggests the presence of an underlying systemic vasculitis. Focal segmental necrotizing glomerulonephritis associated with DAH occurs in connective tissue disorders, systemic vasculitis, and Goodpasture syndrome. In this setting, an abnormal urinalysis with proteinuria, microscopic hematuria, and red cell casts associated with an elevated serum creatinine concentration may be seen.

A sequential increase in the diffusing capacity for carbon monoxide (DLco) is a sensitive test for intra-alveolar bleeding, and its measurement can be used to detect more subtle presentations of DAH or early exacerbations in established cases. Unfortunately, repeated testing is often impractical because most patients with alveolar hemorrhage are markedly ill and are not able to perform the testing.

HISTOPATHOLOGY

In the majority of disorders associated with DAH, the underlying histopathology shows capillaritis, bland pulmonary hemorrhage, or diffuse alveolar damage (Table 31.1). Pulmonary capillaritis is the most common histologic pattern associated with the alveolar hemorrhage syndromes and is characterized by the presence of free interstitial red blood cells, fibrinoid necrosis of the alveolar structures, and neutrophil infiltration of the interstitium and adjacent blood vessels (9–11) (Fig. 31.1; see also Color Fig. 31.1). In addition, many of the neutrophils are fragmented (leukocytoclasis) and pyknotic. Other features of pulmonary capillaritis and DAH include capillary and arteriolar thrombosis, organizing pneumonia, and type II epithelial hyperplasia. Pulmonary capillaritis seen in Wegener granulomatosis, microscopic polyangiitis, and isolated pulmonary capillaritis is considered pauci-immune owing to the absence of immune complex deposition. Conversely, immune complex deposition can be detected in the alveolar interstitium of patients with SLE, Henoch-Schönlein purpura, immunoglobulin (Ig) A nephropathy, Goodpasture syndrome, and Behçet disease (15–25).

The most common causes of bland pulmonary hemorrhage include Goodpasture syndrome, SLE, idiopathic pulmonary hemosiderosis (IPH), and coagulation disorders. The histologic appearance of DAH in these disorders includes type II epithelial cell hyperplasia in the absence of inflammation, edema, or necrosis in the alveolar interstitium (Fig. 31.2; see also Color Fig. 31.2). After recurrent episodes of DAH, interstitial fibrosis may occur (26). The pathogenesis of bland pulmonary hemorrhage remains unknown; however, studies in IPH have shown disruption of the integrity of the alveolar-capillary membrane (27–29).

Diffuse alveolar damage is characterized by the presence of alveolar septal edema, capillary microthrombi, and intra-alveolar hyaline membrane formation, as well as the features of DAH (30) (Fig. 31.3; see also Color Fig. 31.3). Diffuse alveolar damage owing to cytotoxic chemotherapy, crack cocaine inhalation, allogeneic bone marrow

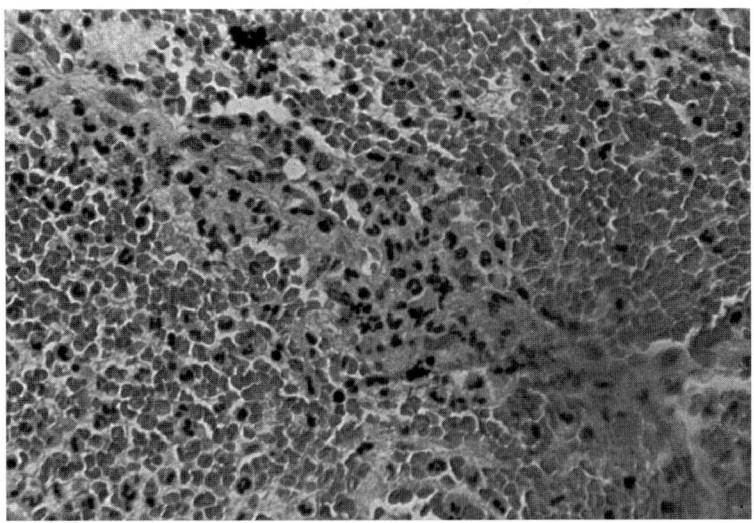

FIGURE 31.1. (See also Color Fig. 31.1.) Diffuse alveolar hemorrhage due to pulmonary capillaritis. The interstitial space is thickened and contains fragmented neutrophils, and the alveolar space is filled with free red blood cells and neutrophils. (From Schwarz MI. Diffuse alveolar hemorrhage. In: Schwarz MI, King TE Jr, eds. *Interstitial lung disease.* Hamilton, Ontario: B.C. Decker, 1998:537, with permission.)

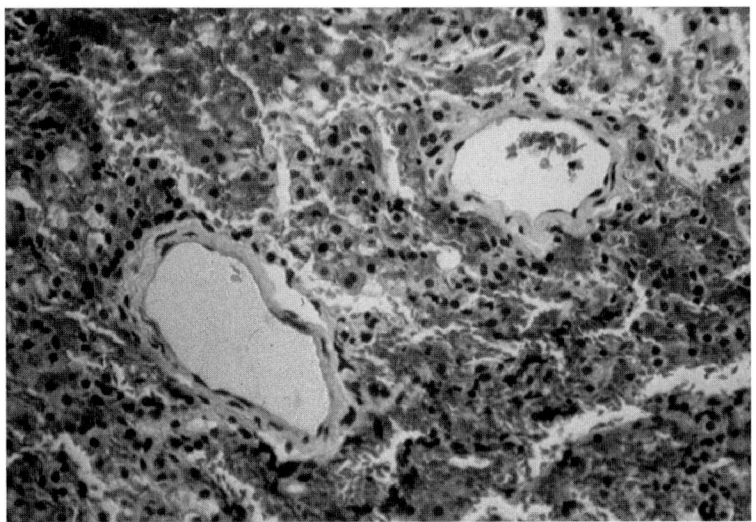

FIGURE 31.2. (See also Color Fig. 31.2.) Diffuse alveolar hemorrhage owing to bland pulmonary hemorrhage in Goodpasture syndrome. Free red blood cells fill the alveolar space, and the interstitium demonstrates the absence of inflammation. Hyperplasia of the type II epithelial cells is noted.

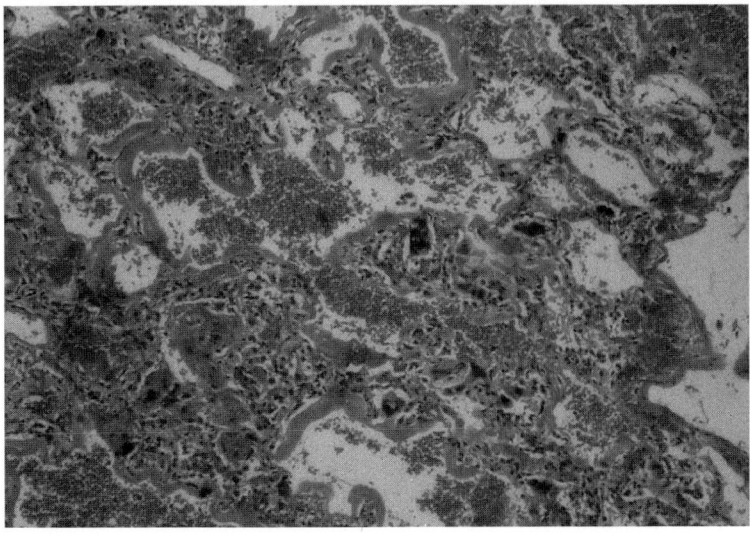

FIGURE 31.3. (See also Color Fig. 31.3.) Diffuse alveolar hemorrhage owing to diffuse alveolar damage. Free red blood cells fill the alveolar space, and prominent hyaline membrane formation is present. (From Schwarz MI: Diffuse alveolar hemorrhage. In: Schwarz MI, King TE Jr, eds. *Interstitial lung disease.* Hamilton, Ontario: B.C. Decker, 1998:538, with permission.)

transplantation, and acute interstitial pneumonia associated with SLE can cause DAH.

DIAGNOSIS

The diagnosis of the alveolar hemorrhage syndromes is supported by the presence of hemoptysis, anemia, and diffuse alveolar opacities on chest imaging studies. In individuals with DAH who present without hemoptysis, a high index of suspicion is required in making the correct diagnosis. A hemorrhagic BAL in a patient without hemoptysis may be the first indication of DAH. Quantitative measurement of macrophage hemosiderin content in the BAL effluent has been suggested as a useful test to determine the degree of alveolar hemorrhage. A better diagnostic test perhaps is the estimation of the percentage of siderophages (hemosiderin-laden macrophages that are at least 20% of the cells) among the total alveolar macrophages recovered by BAL. During BAL, incremental increase in the bloody discoloration of alveolar effluent is one strong indicator of alveolar hemorrhage. However, the possibility of bleeding induced by the procedure itself should be considered.

Thus, in patients who present with nonspecific symptoms and signs, as well as nonspecific radiographic findings, a diagnostic BAL should always be considered early in the evaluation. In Goodpasture syndrome, the diagnosis is confirmed by the presence of serum antibasement membrane antibodies (ABMAs) or by the linear deposition of immunoglobulin and complement in alveolar and glomerular basement membranes (31–33) (Fig. 31.4; see also Color Fig. 31.4). In 5% to 10% of Goodpasture syndrome patients, renal involvement may be absent at the time of DAH (34–37).

DAH in SLE usually occurs in patients with long-standing disease. However, in up to 20% of cases, DAH is the first manifestation of this disease (3, 17, 38). The presence of a decreased serum complement, a positive serum antinuclear antibody, and double-stranded anti-DNA antibodies point to the correct diagnosis. Immune complexes composed of granular deposition of immunoglobulin (Ig) G and complement in pulmonary or renal tissue also support the diagnosis of SLE (15, 17–19) (Fig. 31.5; see also Color Fig. 31.5). Granular deposition of IgA in the lungs and kidneys and serum IgA immune complexes are present in Henoch-Schönlein purpura and IgA nephropathy (20, 21, 39, 40). The presence of recurrent thrombophlebitis and thrombocytopenia suggests the primary antiphospholipid syndrome, and serum anticardiolipin antibodies should be measured (7, 8). Antineutrophil cytoplasmic antibody has emerged as an important diagnostic tool in the evaluation of patients suspected of having vasculitis. The presence of a positive serum antineutrophil cytoplasmic antibody (c-ANCA), which is specific for proteinase 3, strongly supports the diagnosis of Wegener granulomatosis (41–44), whereas a positive antimyeloperoxidase antibody (p-ANCA) suggests either microscopic polyangiitis or pauci-immune idiopathic glomerulonephritis (45, 46). Although the presence of c-ANCA is highly specific for Wegener granulomatosis, the sensitivity of this test is only 63% (47, 48).

GOODPASTURE SYNDROME

Goodpasture syndrome is a rare autoimmune disorder characterized by the presence of alveolar hemorrhage and rapidly progressive glomerulonephritis and is part of a spectrum of diseases known as ABMA diseases. This disorder is owing to the presence of autoantibodies directed against the alveolar and glomerular basement membrane (49, 50). In 60% to 80% of cases, simultaneous involvement of the lungs and

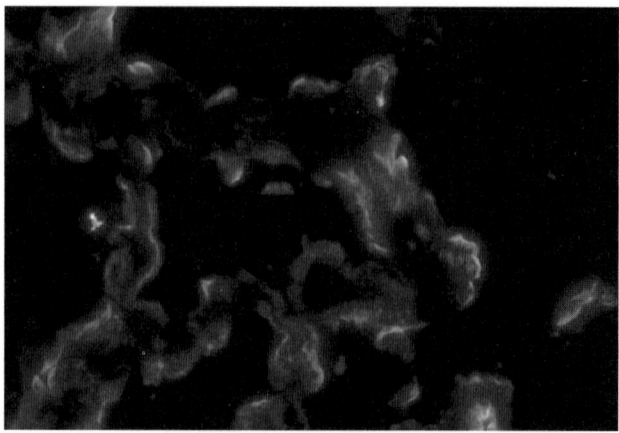
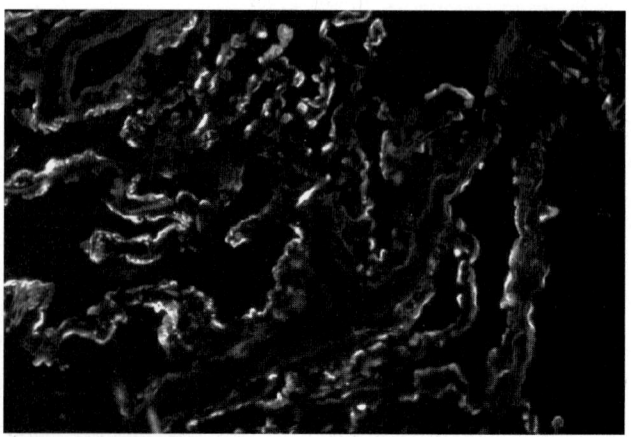

A   B

FIGURE 31.4. (See also Color Fig. 31.4.) Immunofluorescent staining of basement membrane antigens in the alveolus of the lung **(A)** and the glomerulus of the kidney **(B)** in Goodpasture's syndrome. Note the linear deposition of serum antibasement membrane antibody, which characterizes this disease. (From Schwarz MI: Diffuse alveolar hemorrhage. In: Schwarz MI, King TE Jr, eds. *Interstitial lung disease.* Hamilton, Ontario: B.C. Decker, 1998:540, with permission.)

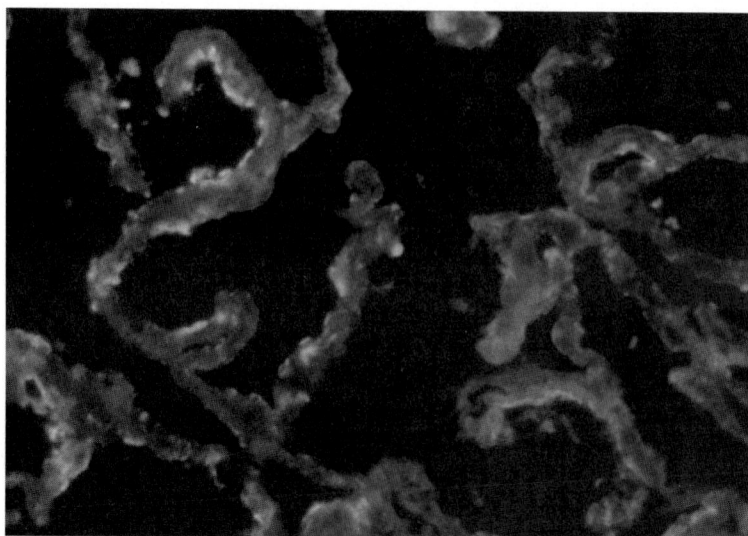

FIGURE 31.5. (See also Color Fig. 31.5.) Immunofluorescent staining of the alveolar basement membrane in a patient with systemic lupus erythematosus. The granular or interrupted deposition of immune complexes easily separates this staining pattern from the continuous staining seen in Goodpasture syndrome. (From Schwarz MI: Diffuse alveolar hemorrhage. In: Schwarz MI, King TE Jr, eds. *Interstitial lung disease.* Hamilton, Ontario: B.C. Decker, 1998:540, with permission.)

kidneys occurs. However, one third of affected patients present with only glomerulonephritis, and in less than 5% of cases, DAH occurs without clinical evidence of renal involvement.

Clinical Manifestations

This disorder predominantly affects the white population, with men being affected slightly more commonly than women. The peak incidence occurs in the second to third decades of life. In older patients, the clinical expression of disease may be limited to the kidney (51). The clinical onset of alveolar hemorrhage has been associated with environmental exposures and viral infections. DAH occurs more commonly in cigarette smokers and after influenza A_2 infection (52, 53). In addition to environmental exposures, genetic susceptibility to disease has been associated with particular alleles of the class II major histocompatibility complex (MHC), including HLA-DR15 and HLA-DR4 (25, 54–56). In particular, almost 80% of affected individuals express HLA-DRB1*1501 (56).

The clinical presentation of Goodpasture syndrome is similar to that of other pulmonary-renal syndromes (see Chapter 58, Table 58.2). Cough, dyspnea, and hemoptysis are the most common symptoms, and fatigue, owing to either iron deficiency anemia or acute renal failure, may be present. Microscopic hematuria, proteinuria, red blood cell casts, and an increased serum creatinine are commonly seen. The chest radiograph is nonspecific, showing patchy or diffuse alveolar opacities (Fig. 31.6). The D_{LCO} is increased during periods of active alveolar bleeding, and an increase in the D_{LCO} of greater than 30% above baseline suggests intra-alveolar hemorrhage (57, 58). The presence of serum or tissue ABMA establishes the diagnosis of ABMA disease in patients with DAH, glomerulonephritis, or both (59). These antibodies are usually IgG, most commonly of the IgG_1 subclass. Both

the radioimmunoassay and enzyme-linked immunosorbent assay for ABMA are sensitive and specific (59, 60). The serum antibody titer does correlate with the severity of the kidney disease, and a decreasing ABMA titer has been associated with improving renal function whereas a rising titer may predict a relapse (59, 61). No correlation exists between the ABMA titer and the severity of lung disease. Serum ANCA is detected in up to 40% of Goodpasture patients (62–64). It is unknown if the presence of serum ANCA in Goodpasture syndrome denotes the presence of underlying capillaritis as the cause of DAH.

Histopathology

As shown in Table 31.1, the DAH in Goodpasture syndrome is secondary to either pulmonary capillaritis or bland alveolar hemorrhage. The renal histopathology demonstrates focal segmental necrotizing glomerulonephritis with crescent formation. This finding is nonspecific and similar to that seen with renal involvement in other rapidly progressive

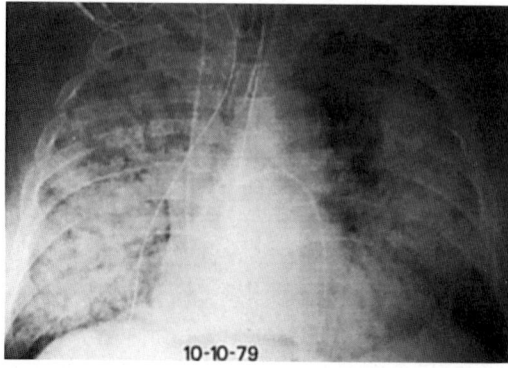

10-10-79

FIGURE 31.6. Extensive dense alveolar opacities secondary to pulmonary alveolar hemorrhage in Goodpasture syndrome. The costophrenic angles are spared. (From Udaya B.S. Prakash, Mayo Medical Center, Rochester, MN, with permission.)

glomerulonephritides. Immunofluorescent staining of both the alveolar and glomerular basement membranes shows an uninterrupted linear deposition of immunoglobulin and complement (see Fig. 31.4A,B).

Pathogenesis

The production of autoantibodies mediates the tissue injury in Goodpasture syndrome as shown by the ability of ABMA from humans to transfer disease to monkeys (65), as well as the therapeutic effect of plasma exchange on disease outcome (66). These autoantibodies are directed against the 230-amino-acid C-terminal noncollagenous domain of the α_3-chain of type IV collagen; a major component of basement membranes (67–69). The tissue-specific involvement in this disease originates from the limited distribution of noncollagenous domain of the α_3-chain of type IV collagen in the body, including the glomerular and alveolar basement membranes. The immunodominant Goodpasture epitope is a conformation-dependent cryptic epitope that has been localized to amino acid residues 17 to 31 in the N-terminal region of noncollagenous domain of the α_3-chain of type IV collagen (67–69). In particular, three hydrophobic residues (alanine at position 18, isoleucine at 19, and valine at 27) are critical for this Goodpasture epitope (70). The gene for human α_3-chain of type IV collagen has mapped to the q35–37 region of chromosome 2 (71).

The important role of cell-mediated immunity in the development of Goodpasture syndrome has only been recently described. In a mouse model of human ABMA disease, Kalluri and colleagues showed that ABMA only facilitate disease in those mouse strains (e.g., those possessing the $H2^s$ MHC haplotype) capable of inducing a Th1-type T cell response (72). In addition, blockade of the costimulatory molecule, CD28, reduces ABMA production and the subsequent development of experimental autoimmune glomerulonephritis in the rat, suggesting the key role of costimulation in the Th1-type T-cell response and the dependence of glomerular injury on cell-mediated mechanisms (73).

How the cryptic Goodpasture antigen is exposed to the circulation, resulting in the development of humoral and cell-mediated immune response, remains unknown. As stated above, certain environmental factors such as influenza A_2 or cigarette smoke may induce injury to the basement membrane, thereby exposing the autoantigen to the bloodstream.

Treatment and Outcome

All of the reported studies of the treatment of Goodpasture syndrome have been uncontrolled trials. Before the introduction of plasmapheresis, the mortality of Goodpasture syndrome ranged from 75% to 90% (49, 66). With the in-

troduction of plasmapheresis combined with corticosteroids and cyclophosphamide, survival has dramatically improved, with an overall 5-year survival of 63% (74–76). In general, plasmapheresis is continued for 2 to 3 weeks. Establishing a prompt diagnosis is essential because the severity of the renal lesion at the time of diagnosis correlates with the recovery of renal function and prognosis (i.e., >85% of glomeruli showing crescents in the initial renal biopsy are associated with a poor prognosis). For example, patients presenting with a creatinine concentration of less than 5.7 mg/dL had a 100% survival and 95% renal survival, whereas dialysis-dependent individuals had a 5-year survival of only 44% (76). On the other hand, patients presenting with severe renal dysfunction (i.e., creatinine concentrations $\geq$ 5.7 mg/dL) do not recover renal function, and renal transplantation should be considered (74, 76–79).

GOODPASTURE SYNDROME	
Summary Statement	**Level of Evidence**
Findings on renal biopsies predict the prognosis.	Observational studies
Earlier therapy is associated with better outcome.	Observational studies
Plasmapheresis is the treatment of choice.	Observational studies

SMALL-VESSEL VASCULITIS

The small-vessel vasculitides represent a diverse group of disorders characterized by the presence of inflammation in the arterioles, capillaries, and venules. Because of the protean clinical manifestations and difficulty in diagnosing a specific form of vasculitis, the Chapel Hill International Consensus Conference developed definitions and classification schemata for the systemic vasculitides based on the size of the involved vessels and the presence or absence of ANCA (80). The small-vessel vasculitides involving the lung are usually systemic in nature and include Wegener granulomatosis, microscopic polyangiitis, and isolated pulmonary capillaritis.

WEGENER GRAUNLOMATOSIS

Wegener granulomatosis was originally described by Klinger in 1931 and represents a necrotizing granulomatous vasculitis involving the upper and lower airways, often associated with glomerulonephritis (41). In 28% of patients, a limited form of the disease occurs with only upper and lower airway involvement (81). Pathologically, a triad of necrosis, granulomatous inflammation, and small-vessel vasculitis is seen (13, 41, 81).

Clinical Manifestations

The incidence of Wegener granulomatosis is unknown, with disease equally distributed between men and women (41, 82). Although the mean age at presentation is 40 years, 15% of patients develop disease before the age of 19 years (41). At initial presentation, 90% of patients have symptoms and signs of upper and lower respiratory tract involvement, including recurrent epistaxis, cough, dyspnea, hemoptysis, mucosal ulcerations, and septal perforation. Other nonspecific findings include fever, fatigue, and weight loss. Tracheobronchial involvement, including subglottic stenosis, occurs in 15% of affected individuals and can result in long-term morbidity. In particular, subglottic stenosis is seen five times more commonly in the pediatric population. DAH owing to small-vessel vasculitis is a rare presenting manifestation of Wegener granulomatosis, occurring in only 5% of patients (83–86). Evidence of renal involvement owing to an underlying focal, segmental, necrotizing glomerulonephritis is usually present in patients presenting with DAH (87). On the other hand, only 20% of patients with Wegener granulomatosis have evidence of renal involvement at presentation (41).

Laboratory findings are nonspecific and include an elevated erythrocyte sedimentation rate, anemia, and leukocytosis. The presence of a serum c-ANCA is highly specific (>95%) for Wegener granulomatosis. However, the sensitivity of the c-ANCA tends to parallel disease activity and may be as low as 70% in patients with inactive disease. This autoantibody is directed against the neutrophil cytoplasmic serine protease, proteinase 3 (47, 48). A positive c-ANCA may also be seen in other disorders such as lymphoma, connective tissue disease, and certain infections. Thus, a positive c-ANCA may narrow the diagnostic possibilities. However, it must always be interpreted in the context of the clinical setting and should supplement, not replace, a tissue diagnosis. The radiographic findings in Wegener granulomatosis include single or multiple pulmonary nodules with or without cavitation, pleural effusions, and diffuse alveolar infiltrates in those presenting with DAH.

Histopathology

The pulmonary histopathology of Wegener granulomatosis is characterized by the triad of vasculitis, parenchymal necrosis, and granulomatous inflammation (81). Other findings include punctate microabscesses and geographic zones of necrosis. In patients presenting with DAH, the underlying pathologic lesion is pulmonary capillaritis (84). Despite the rarity of DAH in patients with Wegener granulomatosis, a small-vessel vasculitis of the lung often coexists with the more typical findings of granulomatous vasculitis. For instance, the frequency of capillaritis ranged from 35% to 47%, always being focal and found adjacent to the granulomatous process (85, 86). The renal histopathology in Wegener granulomatosis is nonspecific, showing focal segmental glomerulonephritis with crescent formation, which is also present in other small-vessel vasculitides and Goodpasture syndrome (88).

Pathogenesis

The etiology of Wegener granulomatosis is unknown. *In vitro* studies suggest a role of ANCA in neutrophil-mediated vascular injury and, thus, in the pathogenesis of Wegener granulomatosis (44, 89). After activation of primed neutrophils and mononuclear phagocytes by ANCA in genetically susceptible individuals, these cells undergo respiratory burst with the release of reactive oxygen species and, therefore, possess the ability to induce endothelial cell cytotoxicity. The proinflammatory chemokines and cytokines induce an influx of monocytes and antigen-specific T cells, which further the inflammatory process. Despite advances in our understanding of the pathogenesis of ANCA-mediated vasculitis, the antigen or autoantigen responsible for the initiation and perpetuation of this disease remains elusive.

Treatment and Outcome

The prognosis of untreated Wegener granulomatosis is poor, with around 90% of patients dying of either respiratory or renal disease within 2 years of diagnosis (41). However, the course of disease has been dramatically improved by the use of cyclophosphamide and prednisone. The recommended regimen consists of cyclophosphamide (2 mg/[kg · d]) and prednisone (1 mg/[kg · d]) with a tapering prednisone dose once a remission is achieved. Cyclophosphamide is continued for 6 to 12 months after the disappearance of symptoms and tapered gradually over the next several months.

With this treatment regimen, a partial remission occurs in 90% of patients, and 75% of patients have a complete remission (41). Approximately 50% of patients who undergo a complete remission suffer one or more relapses. Although this regimen has converted a fatal disease into a treatable disorder with prolonged survival and the potential for a cure, it is associated with significant morbidity. Treatment-related side effects include infections (46% of subjects), hemorrhagic cystitis (50%), bladder cancer (10%), and myelodysplasia (2%) (41, 90). The increased incidence of *Pneumocystis carinii* pneumonia in patients with Wegener granulomatosis has led to the recommendation that all Wegener granulomatosis patients who are receiving daily corticosteroids should be given chemoprophylaxis against *P. carinii* (91). Thus, despite the tremendous advances in the treatment of patients with Wegener granulomatosis, new therapeutic regimens are necessary to alleviate the treatment-related morbidity.

WEGENER GRANULOMATOSIS	
Summary Statement	Level of Evidence
Corticosteroid and cyclophosphamide treatment results in complete remission in >90% of patients.	Observational studies
Pulse cyclophosphamide therapy is effective in patients with moderate disease activity and low titers of c-ANCA.	Observational studies
Pulse cyclophosphamide should not be used as first-line therapy in patients with severe and rapidly progressing disease with high titers of c-ANCA.	Observational studies
Refractory disease has been successfully treated in several cases using high-dose intravenous immunoglobulin.	Observational studies

c-ANCA, antineutrophil cytoplasmic antibody.

MICROSCOPIC POLYANGIITIS

Microscopic polyangiitis is considered a variant of classic polyarteritis nodosa and is a necrotizing small-vessel vasculitis associated with focal segmental glomerulonephritis and often pulmonary capillaritis (92–95). DAH owing to pulmonary capillaritis occurs in one third of patients with microscopic polyangiitis, whereas the classic form of polyarteritis nodosa rarely involves the lung (96–99). This disorder is thought to be one of the most common causes of the pulmonary-renal syndrome (99).

Clinical Manifestations

The average age at the time of disease development is 50 years, and the most common clinical findings include fever, weight loss, and malaise. Other manifestations include arthritis, myositis, mononeuritis multiplex, and gastrointestinal hemorrhage owing to intestinal mucosal vasculitis (93–95). The most common skin lesion is lower extremity purpura, resulting from leukocytoclastic vasculitis (95). Pulmonary involvement is often heralded by the onset of hemoptysis and DAH. Most patients with microscopic polyangiitis have renal involvement owing to focal segmental glomerulonephritis. Greater than 80% of patients with microscopic polyangiitis have a positive serum ANCA, most often it is a p-ANCA (92, 94).

The interval from symptom onset to diagnosis can vary from 2 weeks to 10 years, with 28% of patients having symptoms for longer than 52 weeks (95). In addition, the diagnosis of microscopic polyangiitis is often difficult because this disease shares features of both Wegener granulomatosis and polyarteritis nodosa. The absence of systemic hypertension, the involvement of small vessels, the presence of serum ANCA, and negative serologic tests for hepatitis B assist in the differentiation of microscopic polyangiitis from polyarteritis nodosa (92, 95). Finally, pulmonary involvement, especially

alveolar hemorrhage, is rare in polyarteritis nodosa (100). The differentiation from Wegener granulomatosis can be more difficult because some patients with Wegener granulomatosis can be p-ANCA positive. In this situation, the subsequent development of granulomatous vasculitis helps in the differentiation. However, it is not essential to conclusively distinguish between these related ANCA-associated vasculitides before the initiation of therapy.

Histopathology

The pathologic lesion of microscopic polyangiitis is pauci-immune necrotizing small-vessel vasculitis (pulmonary capillaritis) without the presence of granulomatous inflammation (93, 94). The renal histology is characterized by focal segmental glomerulonephritis with crescent formation, which is present in 80% to 100% of renal biopsies (93).

Treatment and Outcome

Treatment of microscopic polyangiitis is similar to the other systemic vasculitides, consisting of cytotoxic therapy and corticosteroids. With reduction or discontinuation of immunosuppressive therapy, relapses commonly occur. Despite a 5-year mortality rate of 65%, the presence of DAH contributes to the early mortality of about 25% (96). In addition, the main predictors of death are age and the need for mechanical ventilation at the time of diagnosis (95). In ANCA-associated vasculitis, the presence of subclinical alveolar bleeding is a common finding. Schnabel and colleagues (101) found that 95% of patients with ANCA-associated vasculitis had a significantly greater number of hemosiderin-laden macrophages compared with that of patients with connective tissue disease.

ISOLATED PULMONARY CAPILLARITIS

Most cases of pulmonary capillaritis occur in the setting of an underlying systemic vasculitis, a connective tissue disorder, or another autoimmune process (Table 31.1). Isolated pulmonary capillaritis is a pauci-immune small-vessel vasculitis that is confined to the lung without any systemic or serologic findings suggesting another disease process (12, 87, 98, 102, 103). This disorder can occur with or without the presence of a serum p-ANCA. Jennings and colleagues (12) found that isolated pulmonary capillaritis was the most common cause of pulmonary capillaritis in their patient population with DAH, followed by Wegener granulomatosis and microscopic polyangiitis.

Clinical Manifestations

The incidence of isolated pulmonary capillaritis remains unknown. The median age at presentation is 30 years, with men and women being equally affected (12). Cough and dyspnea are the most common presenting symptoms, with pleuritic chest pain and hemoptysis being present in two thirds of patients at presentation. The majority of patients develop acute respiratory failure, requiring mechanical ventilation. Laboratory findings are nonspecific, and the chest radiograph shows diffuse alveolar opacities. In this patient population, no clinical or serologic evidence of a systemic disorder is present.

The diagnosis of isolated pulmonary capillaritis requires tissue confirmation and the absence of granulomatous inflammation and eosinophilia. In the presence of a positive serum p-ANCA, the differentiation of this disorder from lung-limited microscopic polyangiitis can be difficult and only accomplished after the development of extrapulmonary manifestations. In addition, some cases previously diagnosed as IPH may actually represent isolated pulmonary capillaritis.

Histopathology

Capillaritis is characterized by the presence of alveolar hemorrhage in association with interstitial red blood cells, fibrin thrombi occluding capillaries in the alveolar septum, and neutrophils and nuclear dust in the interstitium and adjacent blood vessels (9) (Fig. 31.1). In addition, the absence of immune complex deposition in the lung is a required pathologic finding in this disorder.

Treatment and Outcome

The treatment of isolated pulmonary capillaritis is similar to that of other systemic vasculitides. Clinical remission is achieved in approximately 70% of patients (12). However, recurrent episodes of DAH have occurred in association with the tapering of cytotoxic therapy. With follow-up ranging from 7 to 73 months, Jennings and colleagues (12) noted that none of their surviving patients with isolated pulmonary capillaritis developed a systemic vasculitis or connective tissue disease, suggesting that isolated pulmonary capillaritis indeed represents a true disease entity and not simply an early manifestation of a systemic disorder.

SYSTEMIC LUPUS ERYTHEMATOSUS

SLE is an idiopathic disorder characterized by the presence of autoantibodies directed against a variety of nuclear antigens. These autoantibodies and the resultant immune complexes mediate the manifestations of this disease. Noninfectious pleuropulmonary complications occur during the course of SLE in 50% to 70% of affected patients and include pleuritis and pleural effusion, acute lupus pneumonitis, pulmonary hypertension, and diaphragmatic weakness (3, 104). Alveo-

lar hemorrhage is a life-threatening complication that occurs in approximately 4% of patients, with variable mortality rates (3, 105).

Clinical Manifestations

Alveolar hemorrhage may be the initial manifestation of disease. More commonly, this complication occurs in individuals with well-established SLE and a mean duration of disease at the onset of DAH of 4.5 years (105). The majority of patients who present with DAH also have lupus nephritis (3, 105). Most SLE patients who develop DAH are women, with the age of presentation ranging from 27 to 31 years of age (3, 105). An abrupt onset and short duration of cough, dyspnea, and fever are common. Hemoptysis is only seen in 50% of patients. Thus, the absence of hemoptysis does not exclude the diagnosis, especially in the setting of diffuse alveolar opacities on chest radiograph, a decreasing hematocrit, and a bloody BAL. Laboratory findings are nonspecific with the exception of a low serum complement level and the presence of anti–double-stranded DNA antibodies.

DAH complicating SLE must be differentiated from acute lupus pneumonitis (Fig. 31.7). The clinical and radiographic features of DAH and acute lupus pneumonitis are similar, emphasizing the importance of early BAL in the evaluation of these patients. Unlike DAH, acute lupus pneumonitis is the presenting manifestation of SLE in 50% of the cases, with the underlying histopathology usually showing diffuse alveolar damage.

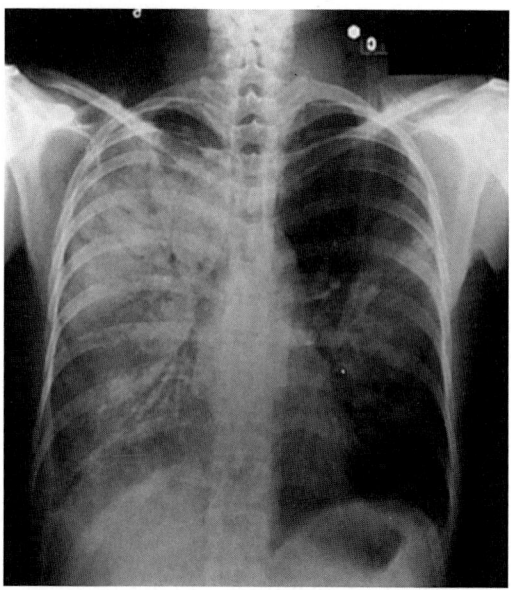

FIGURE 31.7. Marked alveolar opacities in the right lung with only a patchy area of opacity in left midlung. Significant hemoptysis in this patient was caused by systemic lupus erythematosus complicated by renal failure. Not all cases of diffuse alveolar hemorrhage show bilaterally symmetric chest roentgenologic abnormalities. (From Udaya B.S. Prakash, Mayo Medical Center, Rochester, MN, with permission.)

Histopathology

The underlying histopathology of alveolar hemorrhage in SLE may be pulmonary capillaritis, bland pulmonary hemorrhage, or diffuse alveolar damage (3, 15, 17). In a group of 10 SLE patients with DAH, Zamora and colleagues found the predominant histopathologic lesion was pulmonary capillaritis (80% of patients) (3). Immunofluorescence studies have shown that granular deposits of IgG and C3 are present in the alveolar walls, interstitium, and capillary endothelial cells (15, 106) (Fig. 31.5). It has been suggested that the underlying pathogenetic mechanisms of DAH and renal microangiopathy in SLE patients are similar with both owing to microvascular injury related to immune complex deposition and possibly the induction of apoptosis (106).

Treatment and Outcome

Because of the low frequency of alveolar hemorrhage complicating SLE, no controlled trials have been performed. Various combinations of corticosteroids, cytotoxic drugs, and plasmapheresis have been used in the treatment of this condition; however, corticosteroids remain the mainstay of therapy. The role of plasmapheresis in alveolar hemorrhage is unclear despite the presence of immune complexes in the circulation and deposited in tissue (3, 105). Survival rates have markedly varied between the published case reports, ranging from 50% to 100% survival (3, 105, 107, 108). Poor prognostic factors include the need for mechanical ventilation, use of cyclophosphamide, and the presence of infection (3).

OTHER CONNECTIVE TISSUE DISORDERS

Although the development of DAH complicating other connective tissue disorders is an uncommon occurrence, reports of DAH owing to pulmonary capillaritis complicating the course of rheumatoid arthritis, polymyositis, scleroderma, mixed connective tissue disease, and the primary antiphospholipid syndrome have been described (8, 109–113). Similar to the treatment of DAH in SLE, various combinations of corticosteroids, cytotoxic drugs, and plasmapheresis have been used.

DRUG-INDUCED ANTINEUTROPHIL CYTOPLASMIC ANTIBODY–ASSOCIATED VASCULITIS

Recently, a number of case reports of ANCA-associated small-vessel vasculitis induced by the use of certain medications have been published. The drugs most commonly implicated are hydralazine (114) and propylthiouracil (115, 116). Other medications associated with elevated ANCA levels include allopurinol, penicillamine, sulfasalazine, and carbimazole.

Clinical Manifestations

The clinical manifestations in these cases are similar to those of other ANCA-associated small-vessel vasculitides and include sinus involvement, DAH, glomerulonephritis, and leukocytoclastic vasculitis. The majority of these cases are associated with serum p-ANCA positivity. Choi and colleagues (114) found that the prevalence of prior use of hydralazine and propylthiouracil in patients with small-vessel vasculitis and circulating p-ANCA antibodies was 33% and 10%, respectively. Thus, these findings suggest that a substantial proportion of ANCA-associated vasculitis with high titers of p-ANCA are drug-induced.

Histopathology and Pathogenesis

An open lung biopsy in a case of propylthiouracil-induced DAH showed pulmonary capillaritis (115). With the exception of allopurinol, all of the drugs implicated in ANCA-associated vasculitis are also capable of inducing a lupus-like reaction, suggesting a common immunologic mechanism. However, the pathogenesis of drug-induced ANCA-associated vasculitis remains unknown. It is speculated that in the presence of hydrogen peroxide, activated neutrophils release myeloperoxidase, which converts propylthiouracil into cytotoxic products (117). In addition, a direct causal relationship between the use of these drugs and the development of small-vessel vasculitis is suggested by the decline of serum ANCA titers in association with discontinuation of drug therapy and recovery from vasculitis (114).

Treatment and Outcome

The management of drug-induced ANCA–associated vasculitis includes discontinuation of the candidate drug and the institution of corticosteroid therapy. Choi and colleagues (114) reported an overall mortality of 20% in their patient population, with 17% requiring long-term dialysis.

MISCELLANEOUS CAUSES OF ALVEOLAR HEMORRHAGE

Acute Lung Allograft Rejection

After lung transplantation, acute rejection is a common occurrence. Histologically, it is characterized by an infiltration of mononuclear cells in a perivascular distribution. Recently, four cases of DAH with underlying pulmonary capillaritis have been described (118). Hemoptysis was only present in 50% of the cases. This complication developed weeks to months after lung transplantation and was associated with a 40% mortality rate. Treatment consisted of an intensification of the immunosuppressive regimen and plasmapheresis, with recurrence of DAH and capillaritis occurring in 50% of the affected subjects. The investigators hypothesized that this syndrome represents an acute form of vascular rejection at the capillary level (118).

Idiopathic Pulmonary Hemosiderosis

IPH is a rare disorder characterized by recurrent episodes of alveolar hemorrhage associated with the deposition of hemosiderin in the lung and the eventual development of pulmonary fibrosis (119, 120). The incidence of this rare disorder remains unknown. It is predominantly a disease of childhood, occurring before 10 years of age with equal sexual predilection (121). Although the etiology of IPH is unknown, the presence of an elevated serum IgA level in 50% of children with disease, the association with celiac disease, and clinical response in some patients to immunosuppressive therapy suggest an underlying autoimmune mechanism (122, 123).

Clinical Manifestations

The clinical presentation of IPH classically includes the presence of iron deficiency anemia, recurrent episodes of pneumonia, and hemoptysis. As with other causes of DAH, hemoptysis may be absent in up to 40% of subjects (121). In this case, a hemorrhagic BAL and the presence of hemosiderin-laden macrophages suggest the diagnosis of DAH. With recurrent episodes of alveolar hemorrhage, pulmonary fibrosis followed by progressive respiratory insufficiency develops (120)

Histopathology

The diagnosis of IPH requires an open or thoracoscopic lung biopsy in order to exclude all other causes of DAH. Most IPH cases were diagnosed before the availability of a test measuring serum autoantibodies, such as ABMA or ANCA, or antinuclear antibodies. The subsequent development of a systemic disease such as SLE or microscopic polyangiitis has been documented for some cases of adult IPH (124, 125). Thus, it seems likely that most cases of previously diagnosed adult IPH represent isolated pulmonary capillaritis, ANCA-associated vasculitis, or a connective tissue disorder. Histologic examination has shown type II epithelial cell hyperplasia with capillary dilatation and tortuosity and hemosiderin-laden macrophages within both the alveolar space and the interstitium. Electron microscopy has revealed degeneration of type I epithelial cells and a discontinuous capillary basement membrane (119, 126).

Treatment and Outcome

In addition to supportive care, treatment of IPH includes corticosteroids and cytotoxic therapy. Although corticosteroids may improve the clinical course of an acute episode of alveolar hemorrhage, it is unknown whether these drugs alter the natural history of this disease (121, 127, 128). The prognosis of IPH in children is worse than that in adults, with a mean survival of 2.5 years after diagnosis. Despite this poor short-term prognosis, Le Clainche and colleagues (121) reported that 80% of survivors have mild or no respiratory symptoms and lead a normal life.

Diffuse Alveolar Damage

Diffuse alveolar damage occurs as a nonspecific response of the lung to an acute injury and is histologically characterized by the presence of alveolar septal edema and capillary congestion, microvascular thrombi, hyaline membrane formation, and varying degrees of alveolar septal inflammation (1, 30, 129). As a result of the diffuse injury to the epithelium and the alveolar-capillary basement membrane, alveolar hemorrhage often accompanies diffuse alveolar damage, with a hemorrhagic BAL being the only clue to the underlying diagnosis.

The most common cause of alveolar hemorrhage in the setting of diffuse alveolar damage is cytotoxic chemotherapy for the treatment of acute leukemias and solid tumors (130, 131). Although other factors such as infection and previous radiation therapy may play a role, the preconditioning chemotherapeutic regimen in patients undergoing autologous bone marrow transplantation is thought to initiate diffuse alveolar damage (132, 133). The presence of alveolar hemorrhage complicating autologous bone marrow transplantation occurs in 10% to 20% of cases and is associated with a mortality ranging from 50% to 100% (134, 135). The use of high-dose corticosteroids has met with variable rates of success (135).

DAH owing to diffuse alveolar damage after the inhalation of crack cocaine is a completely reversible form of drug-induced DAH (1, 2, 136, 137). Within hours of smoking crack cocaine, hemoptysis and diffuse alveolar opacities on chest x-ray resulting from DAH can occur. Other pulmonary complications include noncardiogenic pulmonary edema, bronchiolitis obliterans organizing pneumonia, eosinophilic pneumonia, and interstitial fibrosis (137, 138). Chronic use can result in a reduction in the diffusion capacity and an increase in alveolar-epithelial permeability (139, 140).

Malignant Diseases

Alveolar hemorrhage is an important complication of pulmonary malignancies (141), especially hematogenous pulmonary metastasis, tumor emboli, or leukemic lung infiltrates. Autopsy studies in patients with leukemia frequently show occult alveolar hemorrhage. Twelve percent of focal and 78% of diffuse pulmonary infiltrates have been attributed to alveolar hemorrhage in leukemic patients. The alveolar hemorrhage is frequently related to other complications such as invasive aspergillosis or zygomycosis, which result from immunosuppression. Occasionally, nonfungal infections can

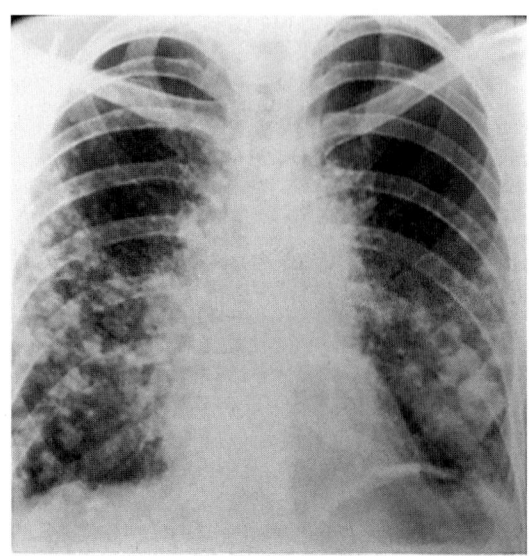

FIGURE 31.8. Diffuse alveolar-nodular opacities caused by hematogenous tumor emboli originating in a hypernephroma resulted in clinically significant alveolar hemorrhage. (From Udaya B.S. Prakash, Mayo Medical Center, Rochester, MN, with permission.)

also produce alveolar hemorrhage. In the majority of the documented cases, thrombocytopenia (platelet count, < 20 × 10^9/L) has been noted. Irrespective of the etiology, alveolar hemorrhage usually is not suspected or diagnosed before death; hemoptysis occurs in less than one fourth of patients. Many patients develop an immunocompromised state because of infections, neoplasms, cytotoxic chemotherapy, or unknown reasons. The incidence of alveolar hemorrhage in this group of patients varies from 3% to 8%.

A high incidence of alveolar hemorrhage with substantial mortality has been noted in patients with Hodgkin and non-Hodgkin lymphoma treated with high-dose radiation and chemotherapy and autologous bone marrow transplantation. Pulmonary alveolar hemorrhage is also common in certain nonhematologic malignancies, e.g., bronchopulmonary Kaposi sarcoma. Hematogenous malignancies with tumor emboli in the pulmonary vessels also cause alveolar hemorrhage (Fig. 31.8). Right atrial myxoma has caused pulmonary hemorrhage.

Other Rare Causes of Alveolar Hemorrhage

Although *mitral valve disease* is now an uncommon cause of alveolar hemorrhage (141) in the developed countries because of prompt surgical therapy, it remains an important etiology of hemoptysis and alveolar hemorrhage in other countries. Earlier publications indicated that hemoptysis in mitral stenosis is caused by the rupture of dilated and varicose bronchial veins. Hemoptysis from this mechanism usually occurs early in the course of mitral stenosis and may be the presenting symptom. Other studies suggest that alveolar hemorrhage is the result of stress failure of pulmonary capillaries; the capillary wall stress greatly increases when

the capillary pressure is raised, and wall damage occurs at pressures of 40 mm Hg and higher. Recurrent episodes of alveolar hemorrhage may result in pulmonary calcification and even true ossification. Pulmonary fibrosis may be seen in some patients.

Ventilator-associated pneumonia is known to produce alveolar hemorrhage. Chest roentgenograms show multiple air bronchograms and bilateral alveolar opacities.

Pulmonary lymphangioleiomyomatosis is an uncommon cause of alveolar hemorrhage syndrome. Hemoptysis occurs as a presenting symptom in 7% of cases and in half the patients during the course of their illness. Alveolar hemorrhage is the result of venous obstruction and capillary hemorrhage caused by proliferation of muscle in the walls of the pulmonary veins.

Pulmonary venoocclusive disease is an uncommon disease and a rare cause of DAH.

REFERENCES

1. Forrester JM, Steele AW, Waldron JA, et al. Crack lung: an acute pulmonary syndrome with a spectrum of clinical and histopathologic findings. *Am Rev Respir Dis* 1990;142:462–467.
2. Haim DY, Lippmann ML, Goldberg SK, et al. The pulmonary complications of crack cocaine: a comprehensive review. *Chest* 1995;107:233–240.
3. Zamora MR, Warner ML, Tuder R, et al. Diffuse alveolar hemorrhage and systemic lupus erythematosus: clinical presentation, histology, survival, and outcome. *Medicine (Baltimore)* 1997;76:192–202.
4. Buschman DL, Ballard R. Progressive massive fibrosis associated with idiopathic pulmonary hemosiderosis. *Chest* 1993;104:293–295.
5. Schwarz MI, Mortenson RL, Colby TV, et al. Pulmonary capillaritis: the association with progressive irreversible airflow limitation and hyperinflation. *Am Rev Respir Dis* 1993;148:507–511.
6. Brugiere O, Raffy O, Sleiman C, et al. Progressive obstructive lung disease associated with microscopic polyangiitis. *Am J Respir Crit Care Med* 1997;155:739–742.
7. Gertner E, Lie JT. Pulmonary capillaritis, alveolar hemorrhage, and recurrent microvascular thrombosis in primary antiphospholipid syndrome. *J Rheumatol* 1993;20:1224–1228.
8. Crausman RS, Achenbach GA, Pluss WT, et al. Pulmonary capillaritis and alveolar hemorrhage associated with the antiphospholipid antibody syndrome. *J Rheumatol* 1995;22:554–556.
9. Mark EJ, Ramirez JF. Pulmonary capillaritis and hemorrhage in patients with systemic vasculitis. *Arch Pathol Lab Med* 1985;109:413–418.
10. Travis WD, Colby TV, Lombard C, et al. A clinicopathologic study of 34 cases of diffuse pulmonary hemorrhage with lung biopsy confirmation. *Am J Surg Pathol* 1990;14:1112–1125.
11. Katzenstein ALA, Askin FA. Miscellaneous pulmonary angiitides. In: Katzenstein ALA, Askin FB, eds. *Surgical pathology of non-neoplastic lung disease.* Philadelphia, WB Saunders, 1990:282–285.
12. Jennings CA, King TE Jr, Tuder R, et al. Diffuse alveolar hemorrhage with underlying isolated, pauciimmune pulmonary capillaritis. *Am J Respir Crit Care Med* 1997;155:1101–1109.
13. Fauci AS, Haynes B, Katz P. The spectrum of vasculitis: clinical, pathologic, immunologic and therapeutic considerations. *Ann Intern Med* 1978;89:660–676.

14. Leavitt RY, Fauci AS. Pulmonary vasculitis. *Am Rev Respir Dis* 1986;134:149–166.

15. Churg A, Franklin W, Chan KL, et al. Pulmonary hemorrhage and immune-complex deposition in the lung: complications in a patient with systemic lupus erythematosus. *Arch Pathol Lab Med* 1980;104:388–391.

16. Eagen JW, Memoli VA, Roberts JL, et al. Pulmonary hemorrhage in systemic lupus erythematosus. *Medicine (Baltimore)* 1978;57:545–560.

17. Myers JL, Katzenstein AA. Microangiitis in lupus-induced pulmonary hemorrhage. *Am J Clin Pathol* 1986;85:552–556.

18. Gould DB, Soriano RZ. Acute alveolar hemorrhage in lupus erythematosus. *Ann Intern Med* 1975;83:836–837.

19. Rodriguez-Iturbe B, Garcia R, Rubio L, et al. Immunohistologic findings in the lung in systemic lupus erythematosus. *Arch Pathol Lab Med* 1977;101:342–344.

20. Kathuria S, Cheifec G. Fatal pulmonary Henoch-Schönlein syndrome. *Chest* 1982;82:654–656.

21. Markus HS, Clark JV. Pulmonary haemorrhage in Henoch-Schönlein purpura. *Thorax* 1989;44:525–526.

22. Lai FM, Li EK, Suen MW, et al. Pulmonary hemorrhage: a fatal manifestation in IgA nephropathy. *Arch Pathol Lab Med* 1994;118:542–546.

23. Beirne GJ, Octaviano GN, Kopp WL, et al. Immunohistology of the lung in Goodpasture's syndrome. *Ann Intern Med* 1968;69:1207–1212.

24. Sisson S, Dysart NK Jr, Fish AJ, et al. Localization of the Goodpasture antigen by immunoelectron microscopy. *Clin Immunol Immunopathol* 1982;23:414–429.

25. Rees AJ, Peters DK, Amos N, et al. The influence of HLA-linked genes on the severity of anti-GBM antibody–mediated nephritis. *Kidney Int* 1984;26:445–450.

26. Lombard CM, Colby TV, Elliott CG. Surgical pathology of the lung in anti-basement membrane antibody–associated Goodpasture's syndrome. *Hum Pathol* 1989;20:445–451.

27. Hyatt RW, Adelstein ER, Halazun JF, et al. Ultrastructure of the lung in idiopathic pulmonary hemosiderosis. *Am J Med* 1972;52:822–829.

28. Gonzalez-Crussi F, Hull MT, Grosfeld JL. Idiopathic pulmonary hemosiderosis: evidence of capillary basement membrane abnormality. *Am Rev Respir Dis* 1976;114:689–698.

29. Yeager H Jr, Powell D, Weinberg RM, et al. Idiopathic pulmonary hemosiderosis: ultrastructural studies and responses to azathioprine. *Arch Intern Med* 1976;136:1145–1149.

30. Haselton PS. Adult respiratory distress syndrome. In: Haselton PS, ed. *Spencers pathology of the lung.* New York: McGraw-Hill, 1996:375–400.

31. Beechler CR, Enquist RW, Hunt KK, et al. Immunofluorescence of transbronchial biopsies in Goodpasture's syndrome. *Am Rev Respir Dis* 1980;121:869–872.

32. Leatherman JW, Davies SF, Hoidal JR. Alveolar hemorrhage syndromes: diffuse microvascular lung hemorrhage in immune and idiopathic disorders. *Medicine (Baltimore)* 1984;63:343–361.

33. Leatherman JW. Immune alveolar hemorrhage. *Chest* 1987;91:891–897.

34. Zimmerman SW, Varanasi UR, Hoff B. Goodpasture's syndrome with normal renal function. *Am J Med* 1979;66:163–171.

35. Carre P, Lloveras JJ, Didier A, et al. Goodpasture's syndrome with normal renal function. *Eur Respir J* 1989;2:911–915.

36. Tobler A, Schurch E, Altermatt HJ, et al. Anti-basement membrane antibody disease with severe pulmonary haemorrhage and normal renal function. *Thorax* 1991;46:68–70.

37. Ekholdt PF, Gulsvik A, Digranes S, et al. Recurrent diffuse pulmonary hemorrhage with minor kidney lesions. *Eur J Respir Dis* 1985;66:353–359.

38. Abud-Mendoza C, Diaz-Jouanen E, Alarcon-Segovia D. Fatal pulmonary hemorrhage in systemic lupus erythematosus:

occurrence without hemoptysis. *J Rheumatol* 1985;12:558–561.

39. Kauffmann RH, Herrmann WA, Meyer CJ, et al. Circulating IgA-immune complexes in Henoch-Schönlein purpura: a longitudinal study of their relationship to disease activity and vascular deposition of IgA. *Am J Med* 1980;69:859–866.

40. Levinsky RJ, Barratt TM. IgA immune complexes in Henoch-Schönlein purpura. *Lancet* 1979;2:1100–1103.

41. Hoffman GS, Kerr GS, Leavitt RY, et al. Wegener granulomatosis: an analysis of 158 patients. *Ann Intern Med* 1992;116:488–498.

42. Gross WL, Ludemann G, Kiefer G, et al. Anticytoplasmic antibodies in Wegener's granulomatosis. *Lancet* 1986;1:806.

43. Andrassy K, Koderisch J, Waldherr R, et al. Diagnostic significance of anticytoplasmatic antibodies (ACPA/ANCA) in detection of Wegener's granulomatosis and other forms of vasculitis. *Nephron* 1988;49:257–258.

44. Harper L, Savage CO. Pathogenesis of ANCA-associated systemic vasculitis. *J Pathol* 2000;190:349–359.

45. Falk RJ, Jennette JC. Anti-neutrophil cytoplasmic autoantibodies with specificity for myeloperoxidase in patients with systemic vasculitis and idiopathic necrotizing and crescentic glomerulonephritis. *N Engl J Med* 1988;318:1651–1657.

46. Walters MD, Savage CO, Dillon MJ, et al. Antineutrophil cytoplasm antibody in crescentic glomerulonephritis. *Arch Dis Child* 1988;63:814–817.

47. Rao JK, Weinberger M, Oddone EZ, et al. The role of antineutrophil cytoplasmic antibody (c-ANCA) testing in the diagnosis of Wegener granulomatosis: a literature review and meta-analysis. *Ann Intern Med* 1995;123:925–932.

48. Rao JK, Allen NB, Feussner JR, et al. A prospective study of antineutrophil cytoplasmic antibody (c-ANCA) and clinical criteria in diagnosing Wegener's granulomatosis. *Lancet* 1995;346:926–931.

49. Duncan DA, Drummond KN, Michael AF, et al. Pulmonary hemorrhage and glomerulonephritis: report of six cases and study of the renal lesion by the fluorescent antibody technique and electron microscopy. *Ann Intern Med* 1965;62:920–938.

50. Sturgill BC, Westervelt FB. Immunofluorescence studies in a case of Goodpasture's syndrome. *JAMA* 1965;194:914–916.

51. Teague CA, Doak PB, Simpson IJ, et al. Goodpasture's syndrome: an analysis of 29 cases. *Kidney Int* 1978;13:492–504.

52. Wilson CB, Smith RC. Goodpasture's syndrome associated with influenza A₂ virus infection. *Ann Intern Med* 1972;76:91–94.

53. Donaghy M, Rees AJ. Cigarette smoking and lung haemorrhage in glomerulonephritis caused by autoantibodies to glomerular basement membrane. *Lancet* 1983;2:1390–1393.

54. Rees AJ, Peters DK, Compston DA, et al. Strong association between HLA-DRW2 and antibody-mediated Goodpasture's syndrome. *Lancet* 1978;1:966–968.

55. Perl SI, Pussell BA, Charlesworth JA, et al. Goodpasture's (anti-GBM) disease and HLA-DRw2. *N Engl J Med* 1981;305:463–464.

56. Fisher M, Pusey CD, Vaughan RW, et al. Susceptibility to anti-glomerular basement membrane disease is strongly associated with HLA-DRB1 genes. *Kidney Int* 1997;51:222–229.

57. Ewan PW, Jones HA, Rhodes CG, et al. Detection of intrapulmonary hemorrhage with carbon monoxide uptake: application in Goodpasture's syndrome. *N Engl J Med* 1976;295:1391–1396.

58. Addleman M, Logan AS, Grossman RF. Monitoring intrapulmonary hemorrhage in Goodpasture's syndrome. *Chest* 1985;87:119–120.

59. Kelly PT, Haponik EF. Goodpasture syndrome: molecular and clinical advances. *Medicine (Baltimore)* 1994;73:171–185.

60. Fish AJ, Kleppel M, Jeraj K, et al. Enzyme immunoassay of

anti-glomerular basement membrane antibodies. *J Lab Clin Med* 1985;105:700–705.

61. Salama AD, Levy JB, Lightstone L, et al. Goodpasture's disease. *Lancet* 2001;358:917–920.

62. Jayne DR, Marshall PD, Jones SJ, et al. Autoantibodies to GBM and neutrophil cytoplasm in rapidly progressive glomerulonephritis. *Kidney Int* 1990;37:965–970.

63. O'Donoghue DJ, Short CD, Brenchley PE, et al. Sequential development of systemic vasculitis with anti-neutrophil cytoplasmic antibodies complicating anti-glomerular basement membrane disease. *Clin Nephrol* 1989;32:251–255.

64. Bosch X, Mirapeix E, Font J, et al. Prognostic implication of anti-neutrophil cytoplasmic autoantibodies with myeloperoxidase specificity in anti-glomerular basement membrane disease. *Clin Nephrol* 1991;36:107–113.

65. Lerner RA, Glassock RJ, Dixon FJ. The role of anti-glomerular basement membrane antibody in the pathogenesis of human glomerulonephritis. *J Exp Med* 1967;126:989–1004.

66. Proskey AJ, Weatherbee L, Easterling RE, et al. Goodpasture's syndrome: a report of five cases and review of the literature. *Am J Med* 1970;48:162–173.

67. Hellmark T, Burkhardt H, Wieslander J. Goodpasture disease: characterization of a single conformational epitope as the target of pathogenic autoantibodies. *J Biol Chem* 1999;274:25862–25868.

68. Gunnarsson A, Hellmark T, Wieslander J. Molecular properties of the Goodpasture epitope. *J Biol Chem* 2000;275:30844–30848.

69. Borza DB, Netzer KO, Leinonen A, et al. The Goodpasture autoantigen: identification of multiple cryptic epitopes on the NC1 domain of the α_3(IV) collagen chain. *J Biol Chem* 2000;275:6030–6037.

70. David M, Borza DB, Leinonen A, et al. Hydrophobic amino acid residues are critical for the immunodominant epitope of the Goodpasture autoantigen: a molecular basis for the cryptic nature of the epitope. *J Biol Chem* 2001;276:6370–6377.

71. Morrison KE, Mariyama M, Yang-Feng TL, et al. Sequence and localization of a partial cDNA encoding the human α_3 chain of type IV collagen. *Am J Hum Genet* 1991;49:545–554.

72. Kalluri R, Danoff TM, Okada H, et al. Susceptibility to anti-glomerular basement membrane disease and Goodpasture syndrome is linked to MHC class II genes and the emergence of T cell–mediated immunity in mice. *J Clin Invest* 1997;100:2263–2275.

73. Reynolds J, Tam FW, Chandraker A, et al. CD28-B7 blockade prevents the development of experimental autoimmune glomerulonephritis. *J Clin Invest* 2000;105:643–651.

74. Lockwood CM, Rees AJ, Pearson TA, et al. Immunosuppression and plasma-exchange in the treatment of Goodpasture's syndrome. *Lancet* 1976;1:711–715.

75. Peters DK, Rees AJ, Lockwood CM, et al. Treatment and prognosis in antibasement membrane antibody-mediated nephritis. *Transplant Proc* 1982;14:513–521.

76. Levy JB, Turner AN, Rees AJ, et al. Long-term outcome of anti-glomerular basement membrane antibody disease treated with plasma exchange and immunosuppression. *Ann Intern Med* 2001;134:1033–1042.

77. Johnson JP, Moore J Jr, Austin HA 3rd, et al. Therapy of anti-glomerular basement membrane antibody disease: analysis of prognostic significance of clinical, pathologic and treatment factors. *Medicine (Baltimore)* 1985;64:219–227.

78. Savage CO, Pusey CD, Bowman C, et al. Antiglomerular basement membrane antibody mediated disease in the British Isles 1980–1984. *Br Med J* 1986;292:301–304.

79. Phelps RG, Rees AJ. The HLA complex in Goodpasture's disease: a model for analyzing susceptibility to autoimmunity. *Kidney Int* 1999;56:1638–1653.

80. Jennette JC, Falk RJ, Andrassy K, et al. Nomenclature of systemic vasculitides: the proposal of an international consensus conference. *Arth Rheum* 1994;37:187–192.

81. Travis WD, Hoffman GS, Leavitt RY, et al. Surgical pathology of the lung in Wegener's granulomatosis: review of 87 open lung biopsies from 67 patients. *Am J Surg Pathol* 1991;15:315–333.

82. Langford CA. Wegener granulomatosis. *Am J Med Sci* 2001;321:76–82.

83. Haworth SJ, Savage CO, Carr D, et al. Pulmonary haemorrhage complicating Wegener's granulomatosis and microscopic polyarteritis. *Br Med J* 1985;290:1775–1778.

84. Travis WD, Carpenter HA, Lie JT. Diffuse pulmonary hemorrhage: an uncommon manifestation of Wegener's granulomatosis. *Am J Surg Pathol* 1987;11:702–708.

85. Myers JL, Katzenstein AL. Wegener's granulomatosis presenting with massive pulmonary hemorrhage and capillaritis. *Am J Surg Pathol* 1987;11:895–898.

86. Colby TV. Diffuse pulmonary hemorrhage in Wegener's granulomatosis. *Semin Respir Med* 1989;10:136–140.

87. Schwarz MI, Brown KK. Small-vessel vasculitis of the lung. *Thorax* 2000;55:502–510.

88. Jennette JC, Falk RJ. The pathology of vasculitis involving the kidney. *Am J Kidney Dis* 1994;24:130–141.

89. Savage CO, Pottinger BE, Gaskin G, et al. Autoantibodies developing to myeloperoxidase and proteinase 3 in systemic vasculitis stimulate neutrophil cytotoxicity toward cultured endothelial cells. *Am J Pathol* 1992;141:335–342.

90. Talar-Williams C, Hijazi YM, Walther MM, et al. Cyclophosphamide-induced cystitis and bladder cancer in patients with Wegener granulomatosis. *Ann Intern Med* 1996;124:477–484.

91. Ognibene FP, Shelhamer JH, Hoffman GS, et al. *Pneumocystis carinii* pneumonia: a major complication of immunosuppressive therapy in patients with Wegener's granulomatosis. *Am J Respir Crit Care Med* 1995;151:795–799.

92. Jennette JC, Falk RJ. Small-vessel vasculitis. *N Engl J Med* 1997;337:1512–1523.

93. Lhote F, Guillevin L. Polyarteritis nodosa, microscopic polyangiitis, and Churg-Strauss syndrome. *Semin Respir Crit Care Med* 1998;19:27–45.

94. Guillevin L, Durand-Gasselin B, Cevallos R, et al. Microscopic polyangiitis: clinical and laboratory findings in 85 patients. *Arthritis Rheum* 1999;42:421–430.

95. Lauque D, Cadranel J, Lazor R, et al. Microscopic polyangiitis with alveolar hemorrhage: a study of 29 cases and review of the literature. Groupe d'Etudes et de Recherche sur les Maladies "Orphelines" Pulmonaires (GERM"O"P). *Medicine (Baltimore)* 2000;79:222–233.

96. Savage CO, Winearls CG, Evans DJ, et al. Microscopic polyarteritis: presentation, pathology and prognosis. *Q J Med* 1985;56:467–483.

97. Zashin S, Fattor R, Fortin D. Microscopic polyarteritis: a forgotten aetiology of haemoptysis and rapidly progressive glomerulonephritis. *Ann Rheum Dis* 1990;49:53–56.

98. Bosch X, Font J, Mirapeix E, et al. Antimyeloperoxidase autoantibody-associated necrotizing alveolar capillaritis. *Am Rev Respir Dis* 1992;146:1326–1329.

99. Niles JL, Bottinger EP, Saurina GR, et al. The syndrome of lung hemorrhage and nephritis is usually an ANCA-associated condition. *Arch Intern Med* 1996;156:440–445.

100. Nick J, Tuder R, May R, et al. Polyarteritis nodosa with pulmonary vasculitis. *Am J Respir Crit Care Med* 1996;153:450–453.

101. Schnabel A, Reuter M, Csernok E, et al. Subclinical alveolar bleeding in pulmonary vasculitides: correlation with indices of disease activity. *Eur Respir J* 1999;14:118–124.

102. Bosch X, Lopez-Soto A, Mirapeix E, et al. Antineutrophil

cytoplasmic autoantibody-associated alveolar capillaritis in patients presenting with pulmonary hemorrhage. *Arch Pathol Lab Med* 1994;118:517–522.

103. Schwarz MI. The nongranulomatous vasculitides of the lung. *Semin Respir Crit Care Med* 1998;19:47–56.

104. Hunninghake GW, Fauci AS. Pulmonary involvement in the collagen vascular diseases. *Am Rev Respir Dis* 1979;119:471–503.

105. Santos-Ocampo AS, Mandell BF, Fessler BJ. Alveolar hemorrhage in systemic lupus erythematosus: presentation and management. *Chest* 2000;118:1083–1090.

106. Hughson MD, He Z, Henegar J, et al. Alveolar hemorrhage and renal microangiopathy in systemic lupus erythematosus. *Arch Pathol Lab Med* 2001;125:475–483.

107. Marino CT, Pertschuk LP. Pulmonary hemorrhage in systemic lupus erythematosus. *Arch Intern Med* 1981;141:201–203.

108. Lee JG, Joo KW, Chung WK, et al. Diffuse alveolar hemorrhage in lupus nephritis. *Clin Nephrol* 2001;55:282–288.

109. Schwarz MI, Zamora MR, Hodges TN, et al. Isolated pulmonary capillaritis and diffuse alveolar hemorrhage in rheumatoid arthritis and mixed connective tissue disease. *Chest* 1998;113:1609–1615.

110. Schwarz MI, Sutarik JM, Nick JA, et al. Pulmonary capillaritis and diffuse alveolar hemorrhage: a primary manifestation of polymyositis. *Am J Respir Crit Care Med* 1995;151:2037–2040.

111. Kallenbach J, Prinsloo I, Zwi S. Progressive systemic sclerosis complicated by diffuse pulmonary haemorrhage. *Thorax* 1977;32:767–770.

112. Griffin MT, Robb JD, Martin JR. Diffuse alveolar haemorrhage associated with progressive systemic sclerosis. *Thorax* 1990;45:903–904.

113. Gertner E. Diffuse alveolar hemorrhage in the antiphospholipid syndrome: spectrum of disease and treatment. *J Rheumatol* 1999;26:805–807.

114. Choi HK, Merkel PA, Walker AM, et al. Drug-associated antineutrophil cytoplasmic antibody-positive vasculitis: prevalence among patients with high titers of antimyeloperoxidase antibodies. *Arthritis Rheum* 2000;43:405–413.

115. Dhillon SS, Singh D, Doe N, et al. Diffuse alveolar hemorrhage and pulmonary capillaritis due to propylthiouracil. *Chest* 1999;116:1485–1488.

116. Harper L, Cockwell P, Savage CO. Case of propylthiouracil-induced ANCA associated small vessel vasculitis. *Nephrol Dial Transplant* 1998;13:455–458.

117. Jiang X, Khursigara G, Rubin RL. Transformation of lupus-inducing drugs to cytotoxic products by activated neutrophils. *Science* 1994;266:810–813.

118. Badesch DB, Zamora M, Fullerton D, et al. Pulmonary capillaritis: a possible histologic form of acute pulmonary allograft rejection. *J Heart Lung Transplant* 1998;17:415–422.

119. Katzenstein ALA. Idiopathic pulmonary hemosiderosis. In: Katzenstein ALA, Askin FB, eds. *Surgical pathology of nonneoplastic lung disorders.* Philadelphia: WB Saunders, 1982:133.

120. Cohen S. Idiopathic pulmonary hemosiderosis. *Am J Med Sci* 1999;317:67–74.

121. Le Clainche L, Le Bourgeois M, Fauroux B, et al. Long-term outcome of idiopathic pulmonary hemosiderosis in children. *Medicine (Baltimore)* 2000;79:318–326.

122. Valassi-Adam H, Rouska A, Karpouzas J, et al. Raised IgA in idiopathic pulmonary haemosiderosis. *Arch Dis Child* 1975;50:320–322.

123. Wright PH, Menzies IS, Pounder RE, et al. Adult idiopathic pulmonary haemosiderosis and coeliac disease. *Q J Med* 1981;50:95–102.

124. Kuhn C. Systemic lupus erythematosus in a patient with ultrastructural lesions of the pulmonary capillaries previously reported in the review as due to idiopathic pulmonary hemosiderosis. *Am Rev Respir Dis* 1972;106:931–932.

125. Leaker B, Cambridge G, du Bois RM, et al. Idiopathic pulmonary haemosiderosis: a form of microscopic polyarteritis? *Thorax* 1992;47:988–990.

126. Irwin RS, Cottrell TS, Hsu KC, et al. Idiopathic pulmonary hemosiderosis: an electron microscopic and immunofluorescent study. *Chest* 1974;65:41–45.

127. Byrd RB, Gracey DR. Immunosuppressive treatment of idiopathic pulmonary hemosiderosis. *JAMA* 1973;226:458–459.

128. Chryssanthopoulos C, Cassimos C, Panagiotidou C. Prognostic criteria in idiopathic pulmonary hemosiderosis in children. *Eur J Pediatr* 1983;140:123–125.

129. Gross NJ. Pulmonary effects of radiation therapy. *Ann Intern Med* 1977;86:81–92.

130. Cooper JA Jr, White DA, Matthay RA. Drug-induced pulmonary disease, part 1: cytotoxic drugs. *Am Rev Respir Dis* 1986;133:321–340.

131. Israel-Biet D, Labrune S, Huchon GJ. Drug-induced lung disease: 1990 review. *Eur Respir J* 1991;4:465–478.

132. Robbins RA, Linder J, Stahl MG, et al. Diffuse alveolar hemorrhage in autologous bone marrow transplant recipients. *Am J Med* 1989;87:511–518.

133. Mulder PO, Meinesz AF, de Vries EG, et al. Diffuse alveolar hemorrhage in autologous bone marrow transplant recipients. *Am J Med* 1991;90:278–281.

134. Jules-Elysee K, Stover DE, Yahalom J, et al. Pulmonary complications in lymphoma patients treated with high-dose therapy autologous bone marrow transplantation. *Am Rev Respir Dis* 1992;146:485–491.

135. Chao NJ, Duncan SR, Long GD, et al. Corticosteroid therapy for diffuse alveolar hemorrhage in autologous bone marrow transplant recipients. *Ann Intern Med* 1991;114:145–146.

136. Murray RJ, Albin RJ, Mergner W, et al. Diffuse alveolar hemorrhage temporally related to cocaine smoking. *Chest* 1988;93:427–429.

137. Thadani PV. NIDA conference report on cardiopulmonary complications of "crack" cocaine use: clinical manifestations and pathophysiology. *Chest* 1996;110:1072–1076.

138. Bailey ME, Fraire AE, Greenberg SD, et al. Pulmonary histopathology in cocaine abusers. *Hum Pathol* 1994;25:203–207.

139. Susskind H, Weber DA, Volkow ND, et al. Increased lung permeability following long-term use of free-base cocaine (crack). *Chest* 1991;100:903–909.

140. Tashkin DP, Khalsa ME, Gorelick D, et al. Pulmonary status of habitual cocaine smokers. *Am Rev Respir Dis* 1992;145:92–100.

141. Parkash UBS. Renal diseases. In: Baum GL, Crapo JD, Celli BR, et al, eds. *Textbook of pulmonary diseases,* Vol. 2. Philadelphia: Lippincott–Raven Publishers, 1998:1111–1132.

Major Pulmonary Disease Syndromes of Unknown Etiology

32

Joseph P. Lynch, III · Ganesh Raghu

The spectrum of clinical, radiographic, physiologic, and histopathologic manifestations of chronic interstitial lung diseases is wide, and significant overlap between these diverse disorders exists. This chapter will discuss four selected major disease syndromes of unknown etiology, which exhibit distinctive clinical, radiographic, or histopathologic features. The clinical features (Tables 32.1 and 32.2), course and treatment of these diverse disorders are variable and will be discussed in detail in the sections that follow.

PULMONARY ALVEOLAR PROTEINOSIS

Pulmonary alveolar proteinosis (PAP), also termed alveolar phospholipidosis, is a rare syndrome of unknown cause originally described by Rosen and colleagues in 1958 (1). The distinctive histological feature is extensive flooding of alveolar spaces with a granular, eosinophilic material composed of surfactant apoproteins; an inflammatory component is lacking (1,2–4). This thick viscid, surfactant-like material fills the alveolar spaces, resulting in cough, dyspnea, and impaired gas exchange.

The estimated incidence of PAP is less than one to four cases per million adults (2,5,6). The disease is two to three times more common in men than in women (2,4). Most cases occur between age 20 and 50 years of age, but all ages may be affected (2,4,7,8). The disease is usually idiopathic (2,3), but secondary forms (termed pseudoproteinosis) complicate

*J. P. Lynch, III: Department of Internal Medicine, University of Michigan, Ann Arbor, Michigan.
Ganesh Raghu: Interstitial Lung Disease, Sarcoid, and Pulmonary Fibrosis Program and Lung Transplant Program, University of Washington Medical Center, Seattle, Washington.
*Supported in part by National Institutes of Health Grant 1P50HL46487.

hematological malignancies (2,9,10), acquired immunodeficiency syndrome (11), or opportunistic infections (2). In these cases, involvement is usually focal and patchy (2,3). The intraalveolar material in pseudoproteinosis may represent necrotic debris and exudate, rather than the surfactant-like material characteristic of PAP (3). Secondary PAP is usually mild and regresses with successful treatment of the underlying disease (2).

In some patients with idiopathic PAP, a history of exposure to chemicals or mineral dusts can be elicited (2,12). Cases of PAP have been described after exposure to titanium (13), aluminum dust (14), silica (15), or chemotherapeutic drugs (e.g., busulfan or chlorambucil) (2). A genetic basis for primary PAP has not been found in adults (2), but rare cases of familial PAP occur in children (7).

Clinical Features

Up to 20% of patients are asymptomatic and never require treatment (2–4). Because of the rarity of PAP and the nonspecificity of symptoms, the mean interval between onset of symptoms and diagnosis often exceeds 1 year (2–4). The clinical features and course of primary PAP are variable (2,4). Symptoms of cough and exertional dyspnea develop insidiously and typically progress over weeks or months (2,4). The cough is usually nonproductive, but some patients expectorate plugs of grayish yellow viscid sputum (3). Hemoptysis is noted in 3% to 24% of patients (2,3). A sensation of chest tightness or heaviness is present in one third of patients. Constitutional symptoms of weight loss, malaise, and fatigue may be present, but extrapulmonary involvement does not occur (2–4). Physical examination reveals rales over involved areas; wheezing is unusual (2,3). Cyanosis is noted in up to 20% of cases; clubbing, in 29% to 40% (2,3).

Serum lactate dehydrogenase (LDH) is increased in 80% of patients (2–4,16). Neutralizing antibodies against

TABLE 32.1. HIGH-RESOLUTION COMPUTED TOMOGRAPHY FEATURES

Pulmonary alveolar proteinosis (PAP)
- Ground-glass opacities
- Consolidation but air-bronchograms uncommon
- Geographical appearance (sharp demarcation of alveolar infiltrates from surrounding normal lung parenchyma)
- Crazy-paving pattern
- No zonal or lobar predominance
- No honeycomb cysts

Pulmonary Langerhans cell histiocytosis (LCH)
- Well-defined cysts (5–>15 mm diameter)
- Peribronchiolar nodules (2–5 mm size)
- Upper and middle lung zone predominance
- No central or peripheral (subpleural) predilection
- Dilated bronchi and bronchioles
- Pneumothoraces ($\pm$)
- Cavitary nodules ($\leq$ 20%)
- Ground-glass opacities ($\leq$ 20%)

Lymphangioleiomyomatosis (LAM)
- Well-defined cysts (5–>15 mm diameter)
- Diffuse; no lung zone predominance
- No nodules
- Pneumothoraces ($\pm$)
- Ground-glass opacities ($\pm$)
- Chylous effusions ($\pm$)
- Abdominopelvic cysts or angiomyolipomas

Pulmonary amyloidosis
- Single or multiple nodular or mass lesions (0.4–15 cm)
- Tracheobronchial amyloidosis: airway wall thickening, irregularly narrowed airway lumens, heterotopic tracheal wall calcifications
- Diffuse interstitial, reticular, or micronodular lesions
- Hilar or mediastinal lymphadenopathy
- Pleural effusions

TABLE 32.2. HISTOPATHOLOGICAL FEATURES

Pulmonary alveolar proteinosis (PAP)
- Filling of alveolar spaces with eosinophilic, granular surfactant-like material
- (+) stains for periodic acid-Schiff (PAS) reagent; (−) alcian blue
- (+) immunohistochemical stains for surfactant apoproteins A and D
- Alveolar architecture preserved
- Minimal or no inflammatory component
- No honeycomb cysts

Pulmonary Langerhans cell histiocytosis (LCH)
- Aggregates of Langerhans cells (cardinal feature)
- Well-defined cysts
- Peribronchiolar nodules; mixed inflammatory cellular infiltrate
- Immunohistochemical stains (+) for CD1a antigen or S100 protein
- Destruction of bronchioles and lung parenchyma
- Stellate pattern of fibrosis
- Respiratory bronchiolitis ($\pm$)

Lymphangioleiomyomatosis (LAM)
- Atypical smooth muscle proliferation (HMB-45 +)
- Well-defined cysts
- Destroyed lung parenchyma
- Hemosiderin-laden macrophages within alveolar spaces or interstitium
- Angiomyolipomas (abdomen or pelvis)

Pulmonary amyloidosis
- Deposits amyloid protein; Congo red (+); green birefringence under polarized light microscopy
- Plaques, nodules of amyloid protein
- Calcified or cartilaginous submucosal nodules (tracheobronchial tree)

granulocyte-macrophage colony-stimulating factor (GM-CSF) are nearly invariably present in sera and bronchoalveolar lavage (BAL) from patients with idiopathic PAP, but not in healthy controls or other lung diseases (17,18). In early reports, opportunistic infections owing to *Nocardia* spp, *Staphylococcus aureus,* mycobacteria, and fungi were cited in up to 20% of patients with PAP (1,2,12). This heightened susceptibility to infections reflects defects in AM chemotaxis (19), phagocytosis, and microbicidal activity (2) and obstruction of the alveolar spaces with the thick debris. Defects in AM function reverse after therapeutic whole-lung lavage. In recent series, infections have been absent or rare (3,4), likely reflecting the impact of therapy.

Chest Imaging Studies

Chest Radiographs

Chest radiographs typically demonstrate symmetrical, fluffy, perihilar alveolar opacities (a bat-wing appearance) (2–4) (Figs. 32.1 and 32.2A). Asymmetrical or even unilateral involvement occurs in 20% of patients (2,3). The opacities

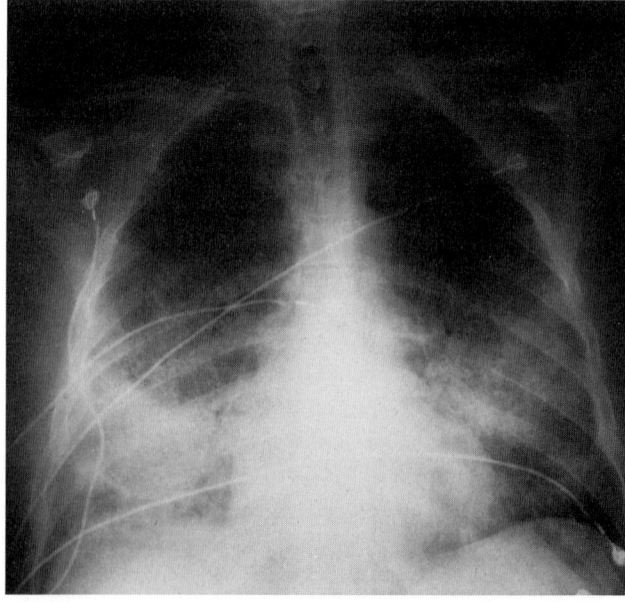

FIGURE 32.1. Pulmonary alveolar proteinosis. Posteroanterior chest radiograph demonstrating bilateral, predominantly bibasilar infiltrates in a 50-year-old man with progressive exertional dyspnea. (From Kuru T, Lynch JP III. Non-resolving or slowly resolving pneumonia. *Clin Chest Med* 1999:20; 623–651,with permission.)

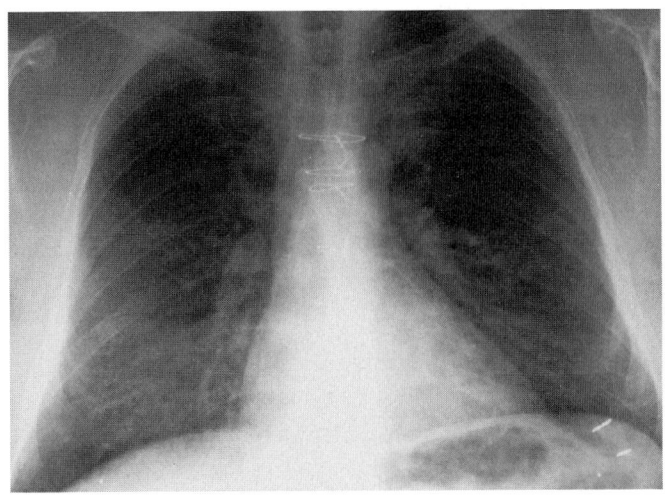
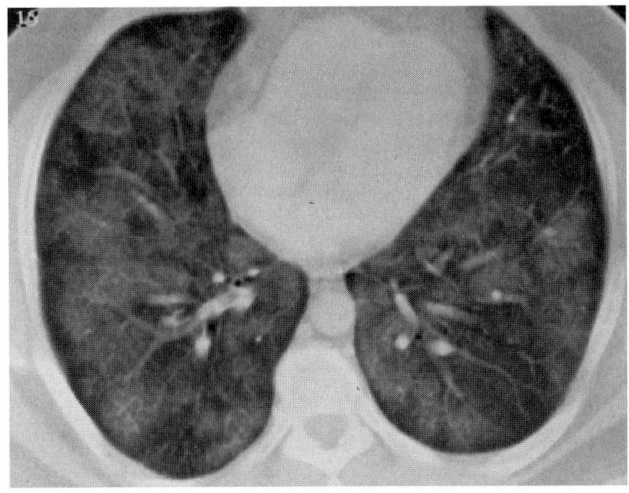

A B

FIGURE 32.2. Pulmonary alveolar proteinosis (PAP). **(A)** Posteroanterior chest radiograph demonstrating bilateral, predominantly bibasilar infiltrates in a 50-year-old man with progressive exertional dyspnea. **(B)** Computed tomographic scan from the same patient demonstrating multiple foci of ground-glass opacification throughout lung parenchyma. Open lung biopsy demonstrating classical features of PAP.

exhibit an alveolar or ground-glass pattern, but mixed reticular and alveolar patterns have been noted. Differential diagnosis includes pulmonary edema (cardiac and noncardiac) and a wide spectrum of interstitial lung diseases, especially, cryptogenic organizing pneumonia, alveolar hemorrhage syndromes, and desquamative interstitial pneumonia (21). Intrathoracic lymphadenopathy, cavitary lesions, or pleural effusions are not features of PAP.

High-Resolution Thin-Section Computed Tomography

High-resolution thin-section computed tomographic (HRCT) scans more clearly reveal the distinctive alveolar involvement, with ground-glass opacities and/or consolidation (2,22) (Fig. 32.2B). The opacities are often clearly delineated with sharp margins surrounded by normal lung (a so-called geographical appearance) (6). Air-bronchograms are uncommon (2,23). Reticular opacities and interlobular septal thickening may be visible in abnormal lung regions (23). There is no specific lobar or zonal predominance (2,23). A distinctive "crazy-paving" appearance (i.e., fine reticular pattern superimposed on areas of ground-glass opacity) is common in PAP (2,22) but is nonspecific (21). These HRCT features may also be observed in bronchioloalveolar cell carcinoma (24) or lipoid pneumonia (25). The extent of alveolar opacities on HRCT or conventional chest radiographs correlate with restrictive physiological impairment (increased forced expiratory volume in one second/forced vital capacity [FEV$_1$/FVC] ratio) and reduced diffusing capacity for carbon monoxide (D$_{LCO}$), and arterial blood partial pressure of oxygen (Pa$_{O_2}$) (23). Although HRCT scans provide superior imaging than do conventional chest radiographs, CT is expensive and is not required to stage or follow PAP (6).

Pulmonary Function Tests

The major physiological aberration is intrapulmonary shunt, resulting in hypoxemia and a widened alveolar-arterial oxygen (A$_{O_2}$-a$_{O_2}$) gradient (2,3). Diffusing capacity is usually reduced, but pulmonary function tests in PAP may be normal (2,3). Vital capacity or lung volumes are only mildly affected (6). Expiratory flow rates and FEV$_1$ are usually normal, but airflow obstruction may be noted in smokers (2). Physiological aberrations improve or normalize after treatment with whole-lung lavage (2,3).

Histological Features

Grossly, the lung is consolidated, and alveolar spaces and respiratory bronchioles are filled with a granular, amorphous acidophilic material (2,3) (Figs. 32.3 A,B). The alveolar septae are usually normal (2). Interstitial inflammation or fibrosis are not found (1). However, hyperplastic type II pneumocytes may be observed. These features bear some resemblance to pneumonia caused by *Pneumocystis carinii*, but lack the interstitial inflammatory component, diffuse alveolar damage, and foamy intra-alveolar exudate seen in that condition (1). The intra-alveolar material in PAP contains phospholipids (surfactant-like material) that stain bright pink with periodic acid-Schiff (PAS) reagent and negative with Alcian blue (2,3). Historically, the diagnosis of PAP was usually established by open lung biopsy, but the diagnosis can often be made by fiberoptic bronchoscopy (2–4). The gross characteristics of BAL fluid are distinctive. The lavage effluent reveals thick, viscid, opaque, yellowish white milky fluid, which sediments into multiple layers on standing (2–4). Positive PAS and negative Alcian blue stains of the foamy BAL fluid may confirm the diagnosis. Large numbers of PAS-positive, eosinophilic acellular bodies,

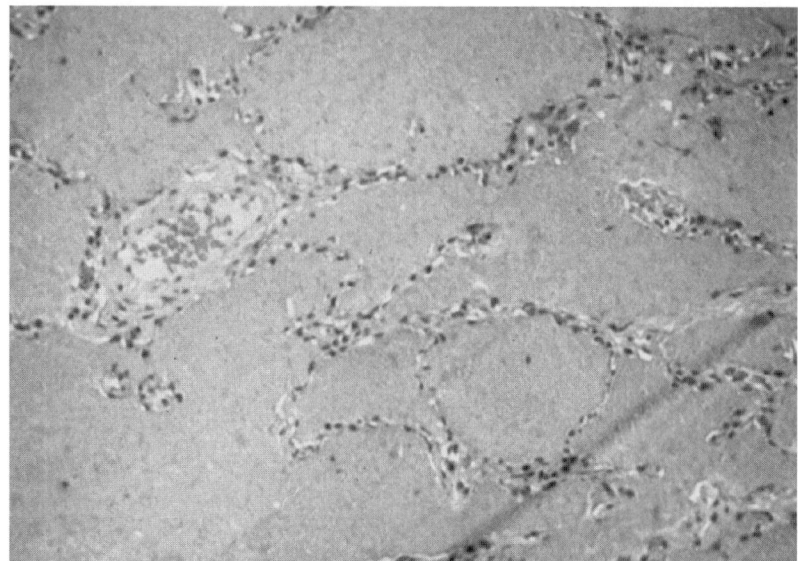

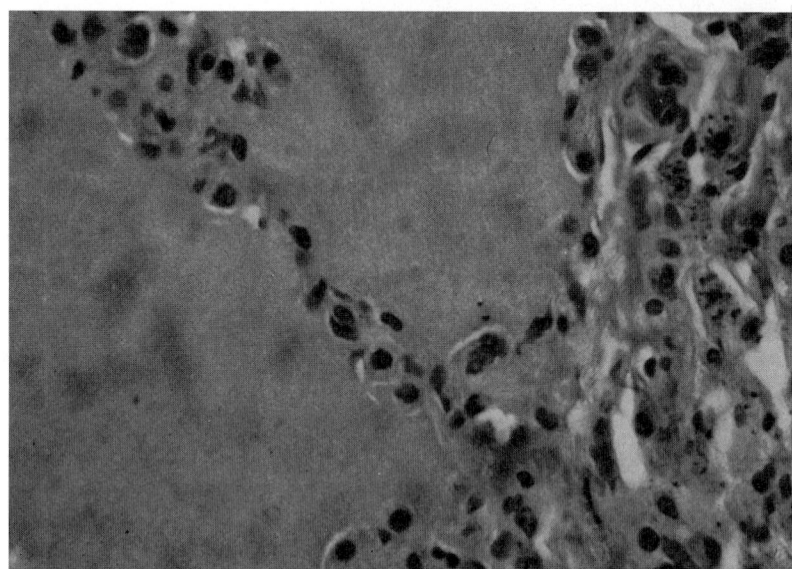

FIGURE 32.3. Pulmonary alveolar proteinosis. Photomicrograph of open lung biopsy demonstrating complete filling of alveolar spaces with a dense proteinaceous exudate. The alveolar architecture is preserved (hematoxylin and eosin; magnification, low power). (From Lynch JP III, Chavis AD. Chronic interstitial pulmonary disorders. In: Victor L, ed. *Clinical pulmonary medicine.* Boston: Little, Brown and Company, 1992, with permission.)

and alveolar macrophages (AMs) containing granular eosinophilic material within phagocytosomes or cytoplasm may be found in BAL fluid (2–4). Surfactant protein (SP)-A is highly glycosylated, which may account for the positive PAS staining. High levels of SP-A (26) and SP-D (27) have been found in BAL fluid from patients with PAP, and stain intensely using immunohistochemical methods. Recent studies noted elevations in tumor markers (28), mucin-like glycoprotein (KL-6) (29), and monocyte chemoattractant protein-1 (30) in serum and BAL fluid in patients with PAP; however, these findings are not specific for PAP. These techniques are limited to a few research laboratories.

Electron microscopy or transmission electron microscopy, performed for research purposes, reveals AMs engorged with phagolysosomes, complex inclusions, lamellar bodies, cholesterol inclusions, and lipid droplets (2,3). Concentric,

laminated lamellar bodies containing phospholipids, tubular myelin, and myelin structures within alveolar spaces or in BAL fluid are pathognomonic for PAP (2,3).

The diagnosis of PAP can be confirmed by bronchoscopy (either BAL or transbronchial biopsy [TBB]), provided that the typical PAS-positive intraalveolar exudate is evident and that clinical and CT features are characteristic (2). For equivocal or nondiagnostic cases, thoracoscopic or open lung biopsies are warranted (3).

Pathogenesis

The pathogenesis of PAP is not known. The massive accumulation of surfactant-like phospholipids within the alveolar spaces could reflect abnormal turnover of phospholipids (e.g., by impaired clearance) or excessive production of surfactant (by type II pneumocytes) (2). Clearance or catabolism of surfactant is in part mediated by AMs; this process is dependent on GM-CSF and other cytokines (2,6). Defects in AM phagocytosis, migration, and phagolysosomal fusion have been noted in patients with PAP (19), and could result in diminished clearance of surfactant (2,6). This could lead to accumulation of surfactant, with subsequent inhibition of AM function (2), resulting in further decrease in surfactant clearance. The pathogenesis of PAP in children (7,8) and adults (2) may differ.

The inciting signals or stimuli for PAP have not been identified, but a history of exposure to hydrocarbons, chemicals, chlorinated resins, fiberglass, aluminum, cadmium, titanium, silica, asbestos, volcanic ash, or a variety of solvents has been elicited in up to 50% of adult patients with idiopathic PAP (2,3). Exogenous dusts or metals may overwhelm the normal clearance mechanisms of the lung. A variety of animal models that resemble PAP were produced by inhalation of fine dust particles (e.g., silica, crushed fiberglass, volcanic ash, bismuth, nickel, aluminum, antimony, titanium) (2,3). In these models, inhaled dust particles elicit an influx of macrophages into the alveolar spaces, followed by proliferation of type II pneumocytes and accumulation of phospholipid. The AMs ingest and become engorged with the phospholipid material. The alveolar spaces become filled with lipoproteinaceous material from the hyperplastic type II pneumocytes and disintegrating phospholipid-laden macrophages. These pathologic features strikingly resemble the lesion of PAP in man.

Chronic ingestion of certain drugs (e.g., amiodarone, chlorphentermine, and iprindole) induce a PAP-like reaction in animals (2,3). Inhibition of phospholipase may be responsible for the excessive accumulation of phospholipids in these affected animals. Cases of drug-induced PAP in humans have not been described, but these animal models provide clues to possible mechanisms for PAP (2,3).

Recent studies suggest that deficiency in GM-CSF may be the pivotal mechanism for the accumulation of surfactant in PAP (6). A possible clue to the pathogenesis of PAP can be gleaned from murine models. Transgenic knock-out mice with a disrupted GM-CSF gene (resulting in a deficiency of GM-CSF) or disrupted β-chain of the GM-CSF/interleukin-3 (IL3)/interleukin-5 (IL5) receptor develop perturbed surfactant homeostasis and lung lesions consistent with PAP (31). These mice exhibit excessive amounts of eosinophilic surfactant-like material in alveolar spaces and BAL fluid, and marked increases in SP-A and SP-B in BAL fluid. PAP in these animals reflects impaired clearance of surfactant rather than exaggerated synthesis (6). GM-CSF has an important role in clearing surfactant. Reconstitution of GM-CSF in the local pulmonary epithelial cells corrected the PAP lesion in GM-CSF–deficient mice (32). Further, bone marrow transplantation and hematopoietic reconstitution of GM-CSF deficiency reverse the lung disease in murine PAP (33). Exogenous administration of aerosolized GM-CSF corrected the lung lesions in the GM-CSF knock-out mice (34). These observations in animals led to recent trials of GM-CSF in patients with PAP, with anecdotal responses (20,35).

Surfactant homeostasis is complex, as diverse cytokines regulate surfactant synthesis and clearance (36,37). Local over-expression of interleukin-4 by lung Clara cells leads to increased surfactant synthesis and a PAP-like syndrome (38). A genetic basis has not been found in adults with PAP (8), but heterogeneous mutations in SP-B gene are responsible for some cases of PAP in infants (7); multiple mutations and phenotypes have been noted (8,39). Interestingly, Dirksen and colleagues described defects in the β_c-receptor for GM-CSF/IL-3/IL-5 (analogous to the murine knock-out model) in three children with idiopathic PAP and normal SP-B levels (39). However, studies in adults with PAP noted normal GM-CSF genes, normal GM-CSF receptors, and normal levels of GM-CSF mRNA (8). Immunoreactive GM-CSF was detected in plasma and bronchoalveolar lavage fluid from 10 patients with PAP; AMs responses to GM-CSF were intact (40). However, adult patients with PAP display a blunted hematologic response to GM-CSF supplementation (20,37, 41). Cultured AMs from a patient with PAP had an intact gene for GM-CSF and expressed mRNA for GM-CSF, but release of the protein from AMs was impaired (42). Neutralization of anti-interleukin-10 antibodies enhanced GM-CSF production (42). The basis for PAP in adults is unknown, but is probably unrelated to a gene deletion or receptor abnormality. Recent reports suggest an autoimmune basis for PAP. Kitamura and colleagues noted neutralizing antibodies of immunoglobulin-G isotype against GM-CSF in BAL fluid and sera from all patients with PAP, but not in healthy controls or other lung disease (17,18). Others confirm the presence of circulating autoantibodies in patients with idiopathic PAP (20). These studies form the basis for repletion of GM-CSF in clinical trials. Although the pathogenesis of secondary PAP is not known, imbalances in cytokines, particularly interleukin-10 and GM-CSF, may lead to abnormal surfactant metabolism (36,37). Defective GM-CSF receptor expression has been observed on leukocytes in acute myeloid leukemia and may explain the high incidence of PAP in this disorder (10). In secondary forms of PAP, remission of the underlying disease is the critical determinant of a successful outcome. Whole-lung lavage, the treatment of choice for primary PAP, is of doubtful value in secondary PAP.

Treatment

Untreated PAP usually progresses indolently over months to years. Some patients manifest a waxing and waning course, over many years (2,4). In early reports, spontaneous remissions were cited in 20% to 30% of cases (1,12). However, a recent review of 303 published cases revealed that spontaneous resolution resulted in normalization of chest radiographs in only 24 patients (8%) and normoxia in only seven (2%) (20). Before availability of therapy, one third of patients died of respiratory failure or infectious complications (1,3,12). Treatment with whole-lung lavage is usually efficacious, and fatalities are rare (2–4). However, relapses occur in 15% to 30% of treated patients (2–4).

Corticosteroids, trypsin, heparin, *N*-acetylcysteine, and pancreatic enzymes have been used to treat PAP, but none are efficacious (2). Whole-lung lavage, introduced by Ramirez and colleagues in 1965 (43), is the treatment of choice for PAP (2–4). Whole-lung lavage physically removes the copious, thick, viscid material, allowing the alveolar spaces to reexpand and participate in gas exchange. When occupational exposure to solvents, chemicals, or dust is suspected as the etiology, withdrawal from that occupation is warranted. Treatment is not required in every patient with PAP, as the disease may be mild and associated with minimal symptoms in some patients (2,4).

Unilateral lung lavage has potential morbidity, and should be performed by individuals with experience with the technique. This is best accomplished under general anesthesia to ensure adequate control of the airway and optimal ventilatory management. A double-lumen endotracheal tube is placed. The most severely involved lung is allowed to deflate, and the opposite lung is ventilated with oxygen and anesthesia. Unilateral lung lavage is then performed with successive aliquots (500 to 1,000 mL) of sterile isotonic saline (warmed to body temperature), and the effluent is immediately suctioned and removed (2). With repetitive instillations, the lavage effluent progressively thins. Chest percussion and rotation of the patient during the procedure may enhance clearance of the thick viscid material (44). The procedure is terminated after the lavage effluent no longer returns significant viscid material or markedly improves. The volume of fluid instilled is considerable, ranging from 20 to 50 L (2–4). The duration of the procedure takes, on average, 3 to 5 hours (2,3). After lavage, the lavage lung is ventilated. Patients can usually be extubated within 1 hour of completion of the procedure. Patients are observed to ensure adequate ventilation. Potential complications of the procedure include pneumothorax, pulmonary edema, spillage of lavage fluid into the contralateral lung, worsening respiratory failure, bronchospasm, and aspiration pneumonia (2). With proper technique and control of the airway, these adverse events occur in fewer than 5% of patients. Most patients can be discharged within 24 hours of completing lavage. Gradual improvement in symptoms, arterial blood gases, and chest radiographs occurs over the next few weeks. We prefer to wait 4 to 6 weeks before performing unilateral lavage of the contralateral lung. However, bilateral sequential lung lavage can be performed in one treatment session (2). For fulminant or severe cases, the contralateral lung can be lavaged immediately after the initial single lung lavage. Whole-lung lavage is highly efficacious. Symptomatic, physiologic, and radiographic improvement is noted in 75% to 95% of patients (2–4). Fatalities are rare (2–4).

Recurrent disease requires re-lavage in 15% to 30% of patients within 1 to 5 years (2,3). Serial chest radiographs, oximetry (or arterial blood gases), and LDH should be monitored at 3-month intervals for the first year to rule out relapse. Thereafter, follow-up at 6- to 12-month intervals is adequate in asymptomatic patients. Recrudescent disease warrants repeat lavage.

Recently, favorable responses were cited in adult PAP patients treated with GM-CSF administered subcutaneously once daily for 12 weeks (6,35,37), but data are sparse. After the seminal report of a favorable response in a single patient treated with subcutaneous GM-CSF (35), a few small series cited benefit in three of four patients (37) and in six of 14 (43%) patients (20). In some patients, improvement was dramatic. Improvement in gas exchange was evident after 4 to 12 weeks of treatment (20,37). The delay in response is consistent with the hypothesis that GM-CSF recruits immature precursor cells to the lung, which later differentiate into functional AMs (6). Aerosolized GM-CSF was beneficial in a single patient (6). These data strongly suggest that a subset of patients with PAP respond to CM-CSF, but optimal dose, route of administration, and duration of therapy have not been elucidated. Further, the durability of remissions is unknown. In one study, five of six responding patients relapsed; three of four responded to retreatment with GM-CSF (20). Finally, patients in whom medical therapy fails may benefit from lung transplantation. Interestingly, recurrence of PAP was cited in one patient after bilateral lung transplantation (45).

PULMONARY ALVEOLAR PROTEINOSIS (PAP)	
Summary Statement	**Level of Evidence**
The most widely accepted and effective form of treatment is therapeutic whole-lung lavage via a double-lumen endotracheal tube	Observational studies
Patients treated with granulocyte-macrophage colony-stimulating factor manifest improvements in pulmonary function, although improvement is of lesser magnitude than with whole-lung lavage	Nonrandomized trials, observational studies

LANGERHANS CELL HISTIOCYTOSIS

Pulmonary Langerhans cell (LC) histiocytosis (LCH, also termed pulmonary eosinophilic granuloma or LC granulomatosis) is a rare disease which may present with cough, dyspnea, and interstitial, reticulonodular, or cystic changes on chest radiographs (46–49). The precise incidence is unknown, but pulmonary LCH accounts for less than 4% of chronic interstitial lung diseases (47), suggesting prevalence rates of one to five cases per million population. Pulmonary LCH is almost exclusively seen in whites, suggesting a genetic predisposition (47,50,51), but a specific genetic defect has not been elucidated. Some studies suggest a male predominance (50,52), but others cite a slight female predominance (46,47,51,53). These variations in sex incidence may reflect differences in smoking habits of the populations studied (49). Pulmonary LCH is rare in children, and typically affects adults between ages 20 and 50 years (46,48,49,51,53). More than 90% of patients with pulmonary LCH are smokers, suggesting an etiological relationship (46–48,50–53).

Clinical Features

Clinical features are variable. Ten percent to 25% of patients with pulmonary LCH are asymptomatic, with incidental findings on chest radiographs (46–50,52,53). Cough or dyspnea are the most common symptoms, noted in 60% to 75% of patients (46–51,53). Symptoms usually develop insidiously, over several weeks or months. Hemoptysis or wheezing occurs in fewer than 10% of patients (47,48). Physical examination is usually unremarkable, but rales, rhonchi, wheezes, or diminished breath sounds may be present (47,49–51). Clubbing is rare (49–51). Pneumothorax, due to rupture of subpleural cysts, occurs in 6% to 20% of patients, and may be the presenting feature (46–51,53,54) (Fig. 32.4). Pneumothoraces frequently recur and may require surgical pleurodesis (50). At thoracotomy, numerous subpleural cysts and blebs are usually evident. Extrapulmonary involvement (particular osteolytic bone lesions or diabetes insipidus from involvement of the pituitary) occurs in 15% to 20% of adults with pulmonary LCH (46,47,49–53). In contrast, LCH in children (typically in children under age 10) is characterized by prominent osseous and extrapulmonary manifestations (55). Constitutional symptoms (e.g., low-grade fever, malaise, weight loss, or anorexia) are present in 15% to 30% of adults with pulmonary LCH (46–51,53). There

are no distinctive blood or serological aberrations in pulmonary LCH (48,49). Blood eosinophil counts are normal (49).

The incidence of bronchogenic carcinoma is increased in pulmonary LCH (47,56–58). In one study of 93 patients with pulmonary LCH, five cases of bronchogenic carcinoma were noted, for an annual risk of 1,040 per 100,000 (58). By contrast, none of 48 patients with LCH in another series developed lung cancer (46). Because virtually all patients with pulmonary LCH are smokers, it is likely that cigarette smoking amplifies the cancer risk. Several studies suggest that the risk of hematological malignancies is also increased in LCH. (47,59–61).

Chest Imaging Studies

Chest Radiographs

Conventional chest radiographs typically reveal diffuse reticular, nodular, or cystic lesions that preferentially involve the mid and upper lung zones, sparing the costophrenic angles (48–51,62) (Fig. 32.5A). Cystic radiolucencies, 5 to 15 mm in diameter, reflect dilated bronchi and bronchioles, with peribronchial thickening, or areas of destroyed lung parenchyma (49). Nodules (typically 2 to 5 mm) are centered around bronchioles and reflect cellular granulomatous lesions. Cavitation of nodules may be evident on HRCT scans but is not evident on conventional chest radiographs (49,54). The combination of pneumothorax, upper lobe cysts, and finely nodular lesions strongly suggests pulmonary LCH. Other chronic interstitial lung disorders with a predilection for upper lobe involvement include sarcoidosis, granulomatous infections, silicosis, ankylosing spondylitis, and chronic eosinophilic pneumonia. Pleural effusions are not features of LCH (48,54,62). Hilar or mediastinal lymphadenopathy is rare (49,51,63).

High-Resolution Thin-Section Computed Tomography Scans

HRCT scans are far more accurate than are conventional chest radiographs in defining the nature and extent of the parenchymal lesions. In several studies of pulmonary LCH, numerous thin-walled cysts were observed in more than 90% of patients; peribronchiolar nodules (typically 1 to 4 mm in diameter) were present concomitantly in 60% to 78% of patients (48,49,54,64,65) (Fig. 32.5B). However, in a recent retrospective study of 29 patients with pulmonary LCH, nodules were the most common feature, noted in 20 patients (69%); lung cysts were detected in only 11 patients (38%) (47). However, consistent with previous reports, the abnormalities predominated in the upper and middle lung fields in 18 patients (60%) (47). The nodules correspond to cellular granulomatous lesions around small bronchioles (66). Coalescence of nodules may result in lesions exceeding 10 mm (54,64,67). This nodular component rarely occurs

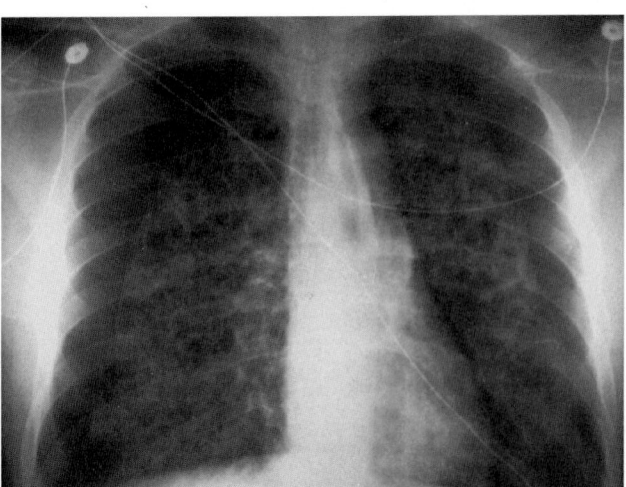

FIGURE 32.4. Langerhans cell histiocytosis (LCH). Posteroanterior chest radiograph demonstrating far advanced cystic changes throughout lung parenchyma and bilateral pneumothoraces in a patient with pulmonary LCH.

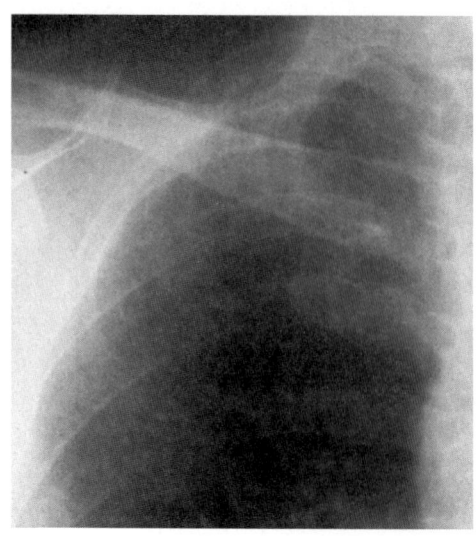
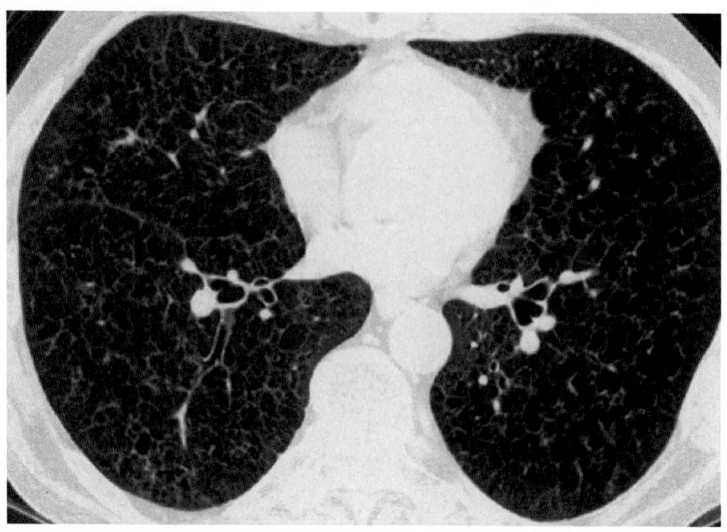

A   B

FIGURE 32.5. Langerhans cell histiocytosis (LCH). **(A)** Coned down view of posteroanterior chest radiograph demonstrating finely nodular and cystic densities throughout lung parenchyma in a 56-year-old man with progressive cough and dyspnea. Transbronchial lung biopsies demonstrated typical histological features of LCH. S100 stains were also positive. **(B)** High-resolution computed tomography scan from the same patient demonstrating multiple well-defined cystic spaces with walls measuring 1 to 2 cm in size. A few ill-defined scattered interstitial nodules are also present but subtle.

in the absence of the cystic lesions. Focal cavitation (owing to necrosis within the peribronchiolar inflammatory nodules) is noted on HRCT in up to 20% of patients but is rarely evident on plain chest radiographs (54,64,66,67). Ground-glass opacities have been described in up to 20% of patients with pulmonary LCH, but are rarely a dominant feature (48,49,54).

As the disease progresses, the nodules cavitate and are replaced by cysts, some of which become confluent (66,67). The cystic lesions correspond to dilated small bronchi and bronchioles or destroyed lung parenchyma. In the early phases, cysts are round and small (<4 mm) but may enlarge and assume distorted shapes. Confluence of cysts may result in bullous lesions exceeding 2 to 3 cm in diameter. The cysts or nodules are associated with areas of intervening normal lung tissue (54,64,66,67). Both the cystic and

nodular lesions have a predilection for the upper and mid lung zones, with relative sparing of the costophrenic angles (54,64) (Figs. 32.6–32.8). There is no central or peripheral predominance. Cystic radiolucencies may be seen in other pulmonary disorders, but the nature and anatomic distribution of the cystic lesions in pulmonary LCH are distinctive. The cysts in pulmonary LCH are thin-walled, often regular in size, and associated with nodules (54,64). Numerous parenchymal cysts are the hallmark of lymphangioleiomyomatosis (LAM) but in LAM, cysts are distributed evenly throughout all lobes and lack the nodular component characteristic of LCH (68). Honeycomb cysts are characteristic features of idiopathic pulmonary fibrosis or of usual interstitial pneumonia (UIP); but in contrast to pulmonary LCH, honeycomb cysts in UIP have a distinctive affinity for subpleural, peripheral, and basilar regions of the lungs (69–71).

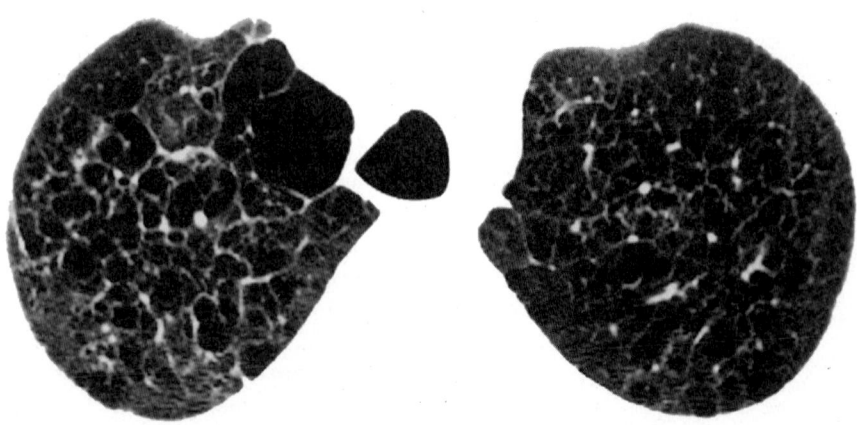

FIGURE 32.6. Langerhans cell histiocytosis. High-resolution computed tomography scan demonstrating multiple well-defined cystic spaces in the upper lobes. A few ill-defined scattered interstitial nodules are also present but subtle.

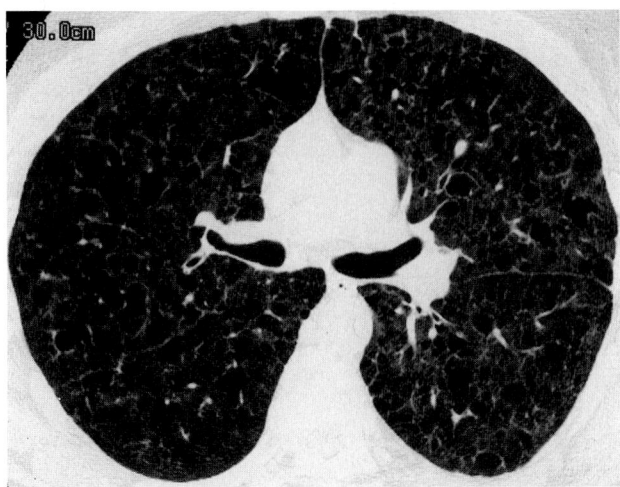

FIGURE 32.7. Langerhans cell histiocytosis. High-resolution computed tomography scan demonstrating extensive cysts involving all areas. Cut is in low lobe. Upper lobes showed even greater degrees of destruction.

Septal bands are evident in idiopathic pulmonary fibrosis or UIP, but are rarely a prominent feature of pulmonary LCH (69–71). In chronic obstructive pulmonary disease, emphysematous "cysts" may be seen, but they are more irregular in size and have a thicker wall compared with that of the cysts of pulmonary LCH (71). The combination of cysts and nodules strongly suggests pulmonary LCH, particularly when the lesions preferentially affect the middle and upper lung zones. Mediastinal or paratracheal adenopathy may be

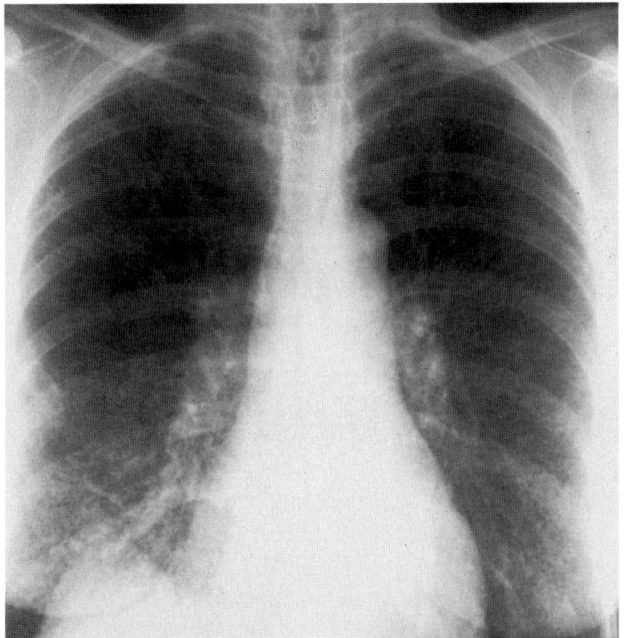

FIGURE 32.8. Langerhans cell histiocytosis (LCH). Posteroanterior chest radiograph demonstrating finely nodular densities throughout lung parenchyma in a 52-year-old woman with progressive cough and dyspnea. Transbronchial lung biopsies demonstrated typical histological features of LCH. S100 stains were also positive.

observed in up to one third of patients with pulmonary LCH by CT (48).

Pulmonary Function

Aberrations in pulmonary function tests are noted in more than 80% of patients with pulmonary LCH (47–51,53,72). The most consistent abnormality is reduced DLCO, noted in 70% to 80% of patients (47–51,53,72). Severe impairment in DLCO is associated with more extensive cystic change and a worse prognosis (47). Vital capacity and/or total lung capacity (TLC) are reduced in 50% to 80% of cases (47–51,53,72). Pure restrictive and mixed obstructive-restrictive patterns may be observed. The mean FEV_1 is often reduced, but the FEV_1/FVC is usually normal or increased (47,48,72). Air trapping (increased residual volume) is noted in nearly 50% of patients with pulmonary LCH, but hyperinflation (TLC > 110% predicted) is uncommon (47,48,72). Pulmonary function tests may not correlate with symptoms or chest radiographs. Serial pulmonary function tests are advised to monitor the course of the disease.

Cardiopulmonary exercise tests in patients with pulmonary LCH usually show reductions in exercise tolerance, maximal workload, oxygen consumption (VO_2 max) and anaerobic threshold, worsening gas exchange and increases in dead space (VD/VT) with exercise (72). Pulmonary hypertension is common in advanced LCH, and reflects a primary proliferative vasculopathy involving muscular arteries and veins (73). Fartoukh evaluated 21 patients with advanced pulmonary LCH referred for lung transplantation (73). Dominant aberrations included reduced DLCO (mean, 27% of predicted), reduced FEV_1 (mean 46% predicted), increased residual volume (mean, 166% predicted), and normal TLC (mean, 95% predicted). Pulmonary hypertension was present in all patients (mean pulmonary artery pressure, 59 mm Hg) and was disproportionate to the degree of pulmonary dysfunction or hypoxemia. Several factors may limit exercise tolerance in pulmonary LCH, including the following: obliteration or loss of the pulmonary microvasculature, impaired pulmonary mechanics, airflow obstruction, and hypoxemia (72,73).

Histopathology

Histologically, pulmonary LCH is characterized by inflammatory, cystic, nodular, and fibrotic lesions distributed in a bronchocentric fashion (47–51,53). The diagnosis often requires surgical lung biopsy, but TBBs can be diagnostic if the salient features are present (46–48,52,74). The disease evolves in distinct phases. Early in the course, proliferation of atypical histiocytes (i.e., LCs) dominates (47,48,51,53). LCs (formerly termed histiocytosis X cells) are moderately large, ovoid histiocytes with pale eosinophilic cytoplasm, indented (grooved) nuclei, inconspicuous nucleoli, and finely dispersed chromatin (48,51,53).

Early lesions form in terminal and respiratory bronchioles, and invade and destroy the bronchial wall (49). As the inflammatory process evolves, bronchioles and alveolar interstitium are destroyed or replaced by fibrotic connective tissue, resulting in dilated distorted bronchioles and alveolar parenchymal cysts (51,53). Cavitation may represent the lumen of the preexisting bronchiole destroyed by the granulomatous process (49).

In the late phases, extensive destruction and fibrosis of lung parenchyma may result. Blebs, subpleural cysts, and interstitial and intraluminal fibrosis may be prominent. The pulmonary microvasculature may be infiltrated or destroyed, even in areas remote from the bronchocentric nodular lesions. In individual patients, all phases of the disorder may be seen concomitantly.

Pulmonary LCH exhibits a distinctive distribution and pattern of lesions on low-power light microscopy. The combination of numerous peribronchiolar nodules and cysts, accompanied by intervening zones of normal lung parenchyma and a stellate pattern of fibrosis, is highly characteristic (48,51,53). Numerous discrete, focal nodules, representing cellular inflammatory lesions, may be seen under low-power magnification (48,51,53). The nodules are centered around bronchioles or may be distributed in subpleural regions. These lesions extend by fingerlike extension into the adjacent alveolar interstitium, resulting in a distinctive star-shaped or stellate pattern (48,51,53) (Fig. 32.9).

Because more than 90% of patients with LCH are smokers, respiratory bronchiolitis is a frequent concomitant finding (48). High-power light microscopy may show intensely cellular granulomatous lesions involving bronchioles and alveolar walls. In some cases, plugs of immature connective tissue within bronchioles, alveolar ducts, and alveolar spaces

resemble cryptogenic organizing pneumonia (53). The granulomatous lesions are comprised of aggregates of LCs (the cornerstone of the diagnosis) admixed with lymphocytes, plasma cells, eosinophils, macrophages, and neutrophils. Aggregates of LCs are found within the peribronchiolar nodules, airspaces, or alveolar interstitium (48,53,75,76) (Fig. 32.10). LCs can usually be recognized under high-power light microscopy, and may comprise more than 50% of cells in the active cellular lesions in some patients (75,76). LCs may be found in normal lung, but rarely constitute more then 4% of cells (53,75,76). Eosinophils may be conspicuous in LCH, but the number of eosinophils is variable and is not a reliable diagnostic criterion. When light microscopic features are nondiagnostic, immunohistochemical stains (e.g., S100 protein and common thymocyte antigen [OKT6 or CD1a]) (53,75–77) or electron microscopy (48,50,51) may substantiate the identification of LCs. These ancillary techniques will be discussed later.

Neither S100 nor CD1a stains are required to diagnose pulmonary LCH, provided the light microscopic features on hematoxylin and eosin stains are distinctive (53). In late phases of pulmonary LCG, the distinctive LC and inflammatory cells may no longer be present, and the lung may be replaced by end-stage honeycomb lung, indistinguishable from other chronic interstitial lung disorders (48,50,51,53). The retention of a nodular or stellate configuration is a clue to the diagnosis (51,53).

Ancillary Diagnostic Techniques

Historically, electron microscopy was used to identify LCs when light microscopy was not definitive. LCs contain distinctive intracytoplasmic rod- or racquet-shape inclusions (termed Birbeck granules or X-bodies), 42 to 45 nm in thickness, which have trilaminar membranes and a central line

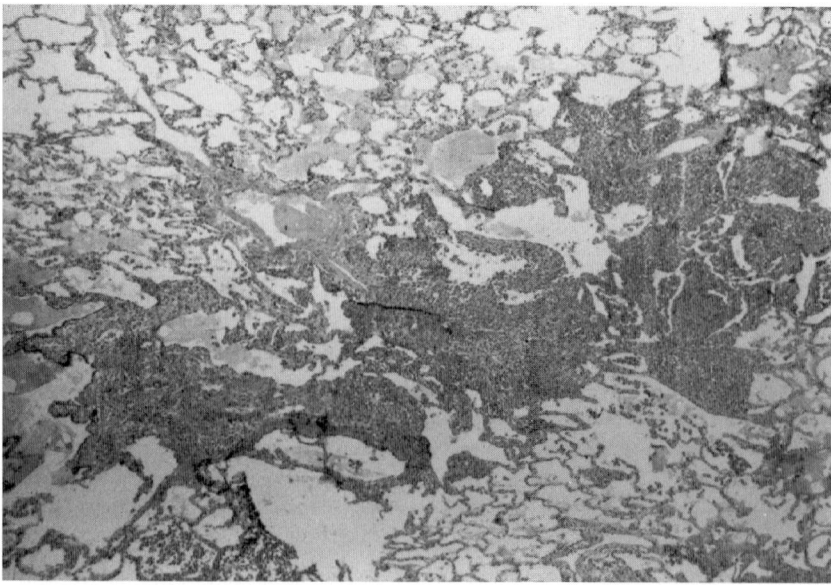

FIGURE 32.9. Langerhans cell histiocytosis. Photomicrograph of open lung biopsy. Low power demonstrating stellate pattern of fibrosis (hematoxylin and eosin). (From Lynch JP III, Chavis AD. Chronic interstitial pulmonary disorders. In: Victor L, ed. *Clinical pulmonary medicine.* Boston: Little, Brown and Company, 1992:243 [Fig. 11–14C], with permission.)

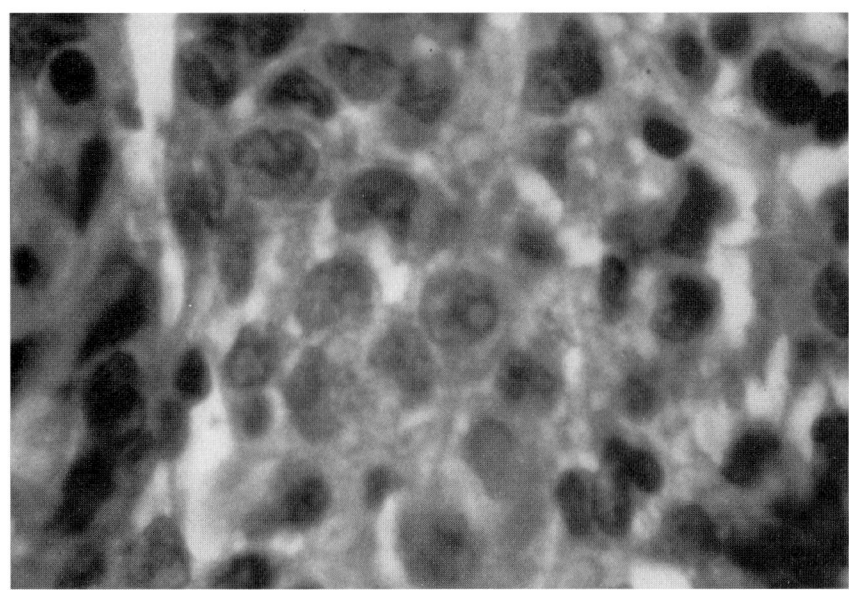

FIGURE 32.10. Langerhans cell histiocytosis. Photomicrograph of open lung biopsy demonstrating an intense cellular infiltrate with multiple Langerhans cells exhibiting the characteristic clefted nuclei (hematoxylin and eosin; magnification, high power).

(48,50,51,53) (Fig. 32.11). Because of the complexity and expense of electron microscopy, immunohistochemical staining for S100 protein or CD1a antigen have supplanted electron microscopy (53,75–78).

Immunostains for S100 protein distinguish LCs from other histiocytes (53,75–78). This technique can be performed in paraffin-embedded biopsies and is less time-consuming and avoids the sampling problems associated with electron microscopy. Large aggregates of S100-positive histiocytes within stellate nodules or granulomatous lesions are virtually pathognomonic of LCH (53,75–78). Staining

for S100 is most intense in the active cellular lesions and diminishes in fibrotic or acellular areas (76,77). LCs may be found in open lung biopsies or BAL fluid in other interstitial lung disorders, but are distributed randomly and in small numbers (rarely exceeding 2% of cells) (77). Lung endocrine cells also stain for S100 protein, but can be distinguished from LCs by histological criteria or by counterstains (e.g., with chromogranin) (76).

LCs also express CD1a, but lymphocytes or monocytes do not (49). Some monoclonal antibodies recognizing the CD1a antigen require fresh or frozen tissue, but anti-CD1a

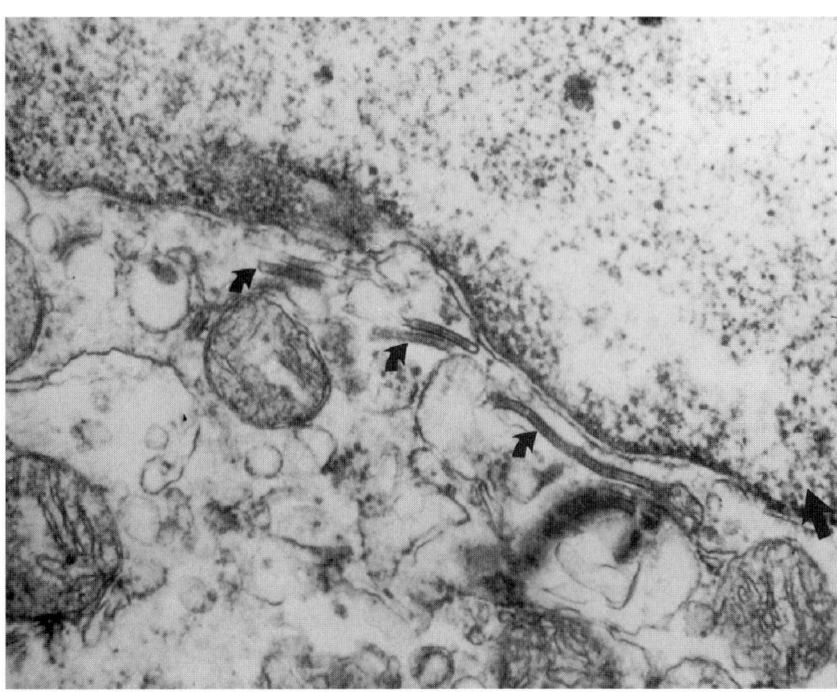

FIGURE 32.11. Langerhans cell histiocytosis. Electron microscopy of Langerhans histiocyte. *Curved arrows* depict Birbeck granules in the cytoplasm. *Straight arrow* points to the nucleus. (From Beals TF, Department of Pathology, Veterans Affairs Medical Center, Ann Arbor, Michigan, with permission.)

O10 recognizes the antigen in fixed and paraffin-embedded tissues (49). Intense staining for CD1a may establish the diagnosis in equivocal cases. In one study, positive immunohistochemical stains to a murine monoclonal antibody (Mab O10) to CD1a were demonstrated in 33 of 34 paraffin-embedded biopsies from patients with LCH (79). Rare CD1a-positive cells may be observed in BAL fluid or lung tissue in patients with diverse pulmonary disorders. However, the mean number of CD1a-positive cells in other conditions is usually less than 0.5% (77). More than 5% of cells staining for CD1a in lung tissue or BAL fluid is relatively specific for LCH (49,77). LCs also express other markers, including HLA-DR, Fc receptor, β_2-integrins (CD11a/CD11c/CD18), adhesins (CD54, CD58), leukocyte common antigen (CD45RO); CD4 antigen, CD1c (marker of a family of antigen-presenting molecules) leucyl-B-naphthylamidase, and B7 molecules (surface markers of activation) (48,49). These latter techniques are limited to research laboratories.

The diagnosis of pulmonary LCH is usually established by conventional histological stains (e.g., hematoxylin and eosin) and light microscopy. Because of the heterogeneous distribution of the lesions, surgical lung biopsy is usually required to confirm the diagnosis. However, TBBs are diagnostic in 10% to 40% of patients (46,48,49,74). Because of the potential for sampling error associated with TBBs (49,74), we perform multiple (four to six) biopsies from both the upper and lower lobes and employ S100 or CD1a stains when LCH is suspected. When TBBs are not definitive, video-assisted thoracoscopic lung biopsy is performed.

Pathogenesis

The pathogenesis of pulmonary LCH is unknown but probably represents an uncontrolled immune response initiated or regulated by LCs (48,49,80). LCs act as accessory cells that drive the immune/inflammatory response. Proliferation of LCs may be a reactive or neoplastic process. Studies using X-linked polymorphic DNA probes in women with disseminated, osseous, or extrapulmonary forms of LCH were consistent with a clonal neoplastic disorder (81). However, the pathogenesis of these nonpulmonary forms of LCH differs from pulmonary LCH, a disease that differs markedly in clinical expression and prognosis.

Pulmonary LCH is polyclonal (82), and likely represents an exuberant immune (reactive) response to inhaled irritants or allergens (49). Tobacco smoke is likely a causative factor, as 90% to 97% of patients with pulmonary LCH are smokers (48,49). The peribronchiolar (bronchocentric) distribution of lesions is consistent with a response to inhaled stimuli (46,53). Cigarette smoke may stimulate and recruit LCs to the lung. Replication of LCs in the alveolar structures perpetuates an alveolitis (46,53,80). Other immune effector cells (e.g., lymphocytes, monocytes, plasma cells, eosinophils) or humoral factors (e.g., immune complexes) play contributory roles in the pathogenesis of pulmonary LCH (48,49). Interactions between these cells, and release of cytokines, may drive the immune and fibrotic response (49,83). The number of pulmonary LCs is increased in asymptomatic smokers (84). Locally secreted cytokines such as tumor necrosis factor-α and GM-CSF may recruit LCs into the lung and facilitate generation of LCs from CD34$^+$ hematopoietic stem cells (48). Increased production of GM-CSF by bronchial epithelial cells may contribute to the recruitment of LCs and may up-regulate lymphostimulatory activity of LCs (85). Immune complexes formed from antibody responses to tobacco antigens may contribute to the inflammatory process (48,49). Tobacco glycoprotein, a potent immunostimulant isolated from cigarette smoke, acts as a T-cell mitogen and stimulates macrophage cytokine production (i.e., interleukin-1 and -6) (48,86). The relevance of tobacco glycoprotein to pulmonary LCH has not been elucidated, but altered peripheral blood lymphocyte responses to tobacco glycoprotein *in vitro* have been noted in pulmonary LCH (86). Cigarette smoking is associated with hyperplasia of pulmonary neuroendocrine cells and increased levels of bombesin-like peptides (BLPs) in the lower respiratory tract (87,88). Bombesin is chemotactic for monocytes and mitogenic for fibroblasts and may play a role in inflammatory or fibrotic responses. Immunohistochemical stains have noted large numbers of bombesin-positive neuroendocrine cells in the lungs of patients with pulmonary LCH (particularly within the airways) (87). Open lung biopsies revealed more than a 10-fold increase in BLPs in pulmonary LCH compared with normal smokers or patients with idiopathic pulmonary fibrosis (87). Cigarette smoke impairs CD10/neutral endopeptidase, an enzyme that plays a role in inactivating BLPs (87). Although neuroendocrine cells or BLPs are not specific for LCH, they provide clues to pathogenetic mechanisms. Hyperplasia of neuroendocrine cells may recruit and activate mononuclear phagocytes and LCs cells to the lung and may stimulate growth of fibroblasts (48). In a murine model, exposure to cigarette smoke evoked interstitial granulomatous inflammation, with features consistent with LCH in humans (89). After cessation of exposure, the density of pulmonary LCs in mice returned to normal levels. These data support the assumption that tobacco products are a major risk factor for pulmonary LCH.

Course and Prognosis

The prognosis of pulmonary LCH is variable. The disease stabilizes or improves in more than two thirds of patients, usually within 6 to 24 months of onset of symptoms (46–51,53). In 15% to 31% of patients, the disease progresses, resulting in destruction of lung parenchyma and irrevocable loss of pulmonary function (46–51,53). Severe late sequelae include pulmonary fibrosis, cor pulmonale, and respiratory failure. Fatality rates range from 6% to 33% (46–51,53). Vassalo and colleagues recently reported their experience with 102 adults with pulmonary LCH seen at the Mayo

Clinic from 1978–1998 (mean follow-up of 4 years; range, 0 to 23) (47). Overall, 33 patients died; 15 deaths were attributable to respiratory failure. Survival rates at 5 and 10 years after diagnosis were 74% and 64%, respectively; median survival was 12.5 years (47). The impact of therapy was not clear. In that study, several variables were predictive of shorter survival by univariate analysis: lower FEV_1, higher residual volume, lower ratio of FEV_1 to FVC, reduced DLCO (47). Earlier retrospective studies cited the following adverse prognostic factors: multisystemic disease, honeycombing on chest radiograph, severe reduction in DLCO, multiple pneumothoraces, a low ratio of FEV_1/FVC, and extremes of age (50,52).

Therapy

Because of the rarity of pulmonary LCH, and the highly variable natural history, the role of therapy is controversial (46–49,51,53). Cessation of cigarette smoking is mandatory (48,90). Corticosteroids and a variety of immunosuppressive and cytotoxic agents (e.g., vinblastine or vincristine, cyclophosphamide, etoposide, methotrexate, or cladribine), have been used in both childhood and adult forms of disseminated LCH, with anecdotal claims for success (49,55,91–96). In a recent study, cyclosporine A was administered alone (10 patients) or in combination with vinblastine, etoposide, prednisolone, and/or antithymocyte globulin in 16 patients with disseminated LCH (97). Complete or partial responses were achieved in only one and three patients, respectively; 22 (85%) failed to respond (97). These agents are of unproven efficacy for pulmonary LCH. Anecdotal responses to corticosteroids have been cited in pulmonary LCH (46,50,52,98), but randomized trials have not been performed. One uncontrolled study cited radiographic improvement in 12 of 14 patients treated with prednisone for progressive pulmonary LCH; the other two patients were stable (98). Another study cited worse survival among LCH patients treated with corticosteroids, but this may reflect a selection bias (52). In the cohort recently reported from the Mayo Clinic, prednisone (alone or combined with immunosuppressive agents) was prescribed in 54 of 102 patients (53%) (47). Although data regarding response to therapy were not provided in that paper, the investigators stated "no specific therapeutic interventions have been shown to prolong survival" (47). Given the paucity of data regarding therapy and the usually good prognosis for adults with localized pulmonary LCH, we reserve therapy for patients with severe, progressive, and debilitating disease. In this context, an empirical trial of corticosteroids for 3 to 6 months is reasonable. Prolonged therapy should be continued only for patients manifesting objective and unequivocal responses. We are reluctant to use cytotoxic or chemotherapeutic agents for pulmonary LCH, because the potential for adverse effects (including oncogenesis) may outweigh the benefit.

Although pulmonary hypertension is a common feature in pulmonary LCH (73), the role of vasodilators has not been studied. However, pulmonary edema developed in two patients with pulmonary LCH treated with intravenous epoprostenol, suggesting that epoprostenol therapy may be contraindicated in patients with pulmonary LCH (73). Single lung transplantation has been successfully accomplished in patients with LCH and end-stage pulmonary fibrosis (99,100). Cessation of cigarette smoking is paramount, as recurrent (ultimately fatal) LCG has been documented in lung allografts among patients who resumed smoking (99,101,102).

LANGERHANS CELL HISTIOCYTOSIS	
Summary Statement	**Level of Evidence**
Cessation of smoking is the treatment of choice.	Observational studies
Prednisone (alone or combined with immunosuppressive agents) does not appear to improve survival.	Observational studies, expert opinion

LYMPHANGIOLEIOMYOMATOSIS

Pulmonary LAM is a rare, idiopathic fibrocystic lung disorder that almost exclusively affects premenopausal women (103–110). LAM rarely occurs in postmenopausal women. Recently, a case of LAM was identified in a male (111). Previous reports of LAM in males likely represented tuberous sclerosis or diffuse pulmonary lymphangiomatosis, disorders that share common clinical and histological features with LAM.

LAM is exceptionally rare (prevalence, 0.4 to three cases per million) (103–105). Published data are derived from a few series (often extracted from consulting pathologists' files) and anecdotal case reports. Silverstein in 1974 (112) and Corrin and colleagues in 1975 (108) described the cardinal features of LAM in two series comprising 32 and 28 patients, respectively. In 1990, Taylor and colleagues reported 32 patients with LAM seen at Stanford and the Mayo Clinic (113). In 1995, Kitaichi and colleagues described 46 patients with LAM from Japan, Korea, and Taiwan (106). In 1999, Urban and colleagues described 69 patients with LAM diagnosed in France from 1973–1996 (105). Johnson and Tatersfield identified 50 patients with LAM in the United Kingdom during a 5-year period (prevalence of one per 1.1 million population) (103). Given the nonspecificity of clinical findings, the prevalence of LAM may be underestimated by historical analyses.

Clinical Features

The classic clinical presentation of LAM is distinctive. Women of childbearing age present with spontaneous pneumothorax, hemoptysis, slowly progressive exertional dyspnea, or chylothorax (103–109,113). The mean age at the onset of symptoms is 30 years of age (103–109). Dyspnea is nearly invariably present, beginning in the third or fourth decade of life, and worsens over years (103–109). Pneumothoraces occur in 50% to 80% of patients with LAM (103–109,113). Chylous effusions, resulting from rupture of involved pleural lymphatics, occur in 7% to 39% of patients; hemoptysis or focal alveolar hemorrhage, owing to obstruction of venules, has been noted in 28% to 40% of patients with LAM (103–109,113).

Pulmonary Function Tests

Pulmonary function tests in LAM typically demonstrate airflow limitation, (often with air-trapping), impaired D_{LCO}, and hypoxemia; lung volumes are normal or increased (103–109,113). In several series, obstructive or mixed obstructive-restrictive defects were noted in 44% to 90% of patients; pure restrictive defects, in only 9% to 36% (103–109,113,114). Airflow obstruction reflects cystic disease with airflow obstruction and air-trapping (114). Airflow obstruction progresses inexorably over the years. Restrictive defects may reflect pleural effusions (typically chylous), smooth muscle proliferation, or pleurodesis. Reductions in D_{LCO} are found in 82% to 97% of patients; hypoxemia, in 50% to 96% (103–109,113,114). Resting arterial blood gases may be normal in the setting of mild disease, but Pa_{O_2} decreases and $A\text{-}a_{O_2}$ gradient widens as the disease progresses (103,107,114). Hypercapnia is uncommon in LAM, but can develop in the terminal phases of the disease.

Exercise performance is impaired. Cardiopulmonary exercise tests demonstrate an excessive ventilatory response and increased V_D (114). Airflow obstruction and impairments in D_{LCO}, exercise capacity, and gas exchange correlate primarily with the extent of airway cystic lesions (114,115). Muscular proliferation in small airways, destruction of pulmonary microvasculature, loss of alveolar support, and loss of parenchymal interdependence may contribute to the physiological aberrations (114). In contrast to pulmonary LCH (73), pulmonary hypertension is uncommon in LAM (100).

In two studies, (106,114), reductions in FEV_1/FVC ratio and increased TLC were associated with worse survival. However, arterial blood gases, $A\text{-}a_{O_2}$ gradient, FVC, and FEV_1 were not predictive of survival (106,114). The rate of progression of airflow obstruction is highly variable (109). In a cohort of 47 patients with LAM, the mean fall in FEV_1 was 118 mL/y, but variability was marked between patients (103).

Chest Imaging Studies

Chest Radiographs

Conventional chest radiographs demonstrate a wide spectrum of abnormalities, including pneumothoraces, bilateral interstitial, reticulonodular, or cystic radiolucencies, pleu-

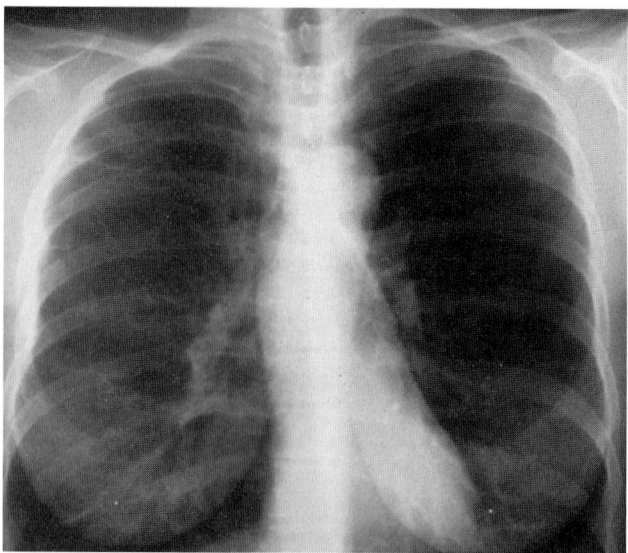

FIGURE 32.12. Lymphangioleiomyomatosis (LAM). Posteroanterior chest radiograph from a 39-year-old woman with LAM demonstrates severe hyperinflation and large cysts and bullous changes. Surgical clips are present on the *right* from a previous thoracotomy and pleurodesis for recurrent pneumothoraces.

ral effusions, or hyperinflation (103–107,109,113). Early in the course of the disease, chest radiographs may be normal (103,105,107,115). As the disease progresses, cystic lesions, reticulonodular infiltrates, or pneumothoraces develop. At the time of presentation, pneumothoraces are noted in 39% to 53% of patients with LAM; reticulonodular infiltrates, in 47% to 85% (103–107,113). As the disease progresses, both of these features are present in more than 80% of patients. Reticular shadows represent the walls of the alveolar cysts (68). Well-defined cystic or bullous lesions are evident in 41% to 58% of patients (103–107,109,113). Hyperinflation develops as the disease worsens and is seen in up to two thirds of patients in the late phases (Fig. 32.12). Pleural effusions (typically chylous) occur in 11% to 29% of patients (103–107,113). Mediastinal or hilar lymphadenopathy are not features of LAM (103,105,106).

High-Resolution Computed Tomography Scans

HRCT scans are highly distinctive in LAM. The cardinal feature is numerous thin-walled cysts (usually <20 mm in diameter) distributed diffusely throughout both lungs; the intervening lung parenchyma is normal (68,105, 107,109,115) (Figs. 32.13–32.15). Cysts are usually round but may assume bizarre shapes as cysts coalesce (68). Semiquantitative and quantitative analyses of extent of disease by HRCT correlate well with physiological parameters (e.g., FEV_1, D_{LCO}, and gas exchange at rest and exercise) (68,115) and exercise performance (116). Cystic lesions may be seen in other pulmonary disorders, (e.g., pulmonary LCH, UIP, emphysema), but the distribution

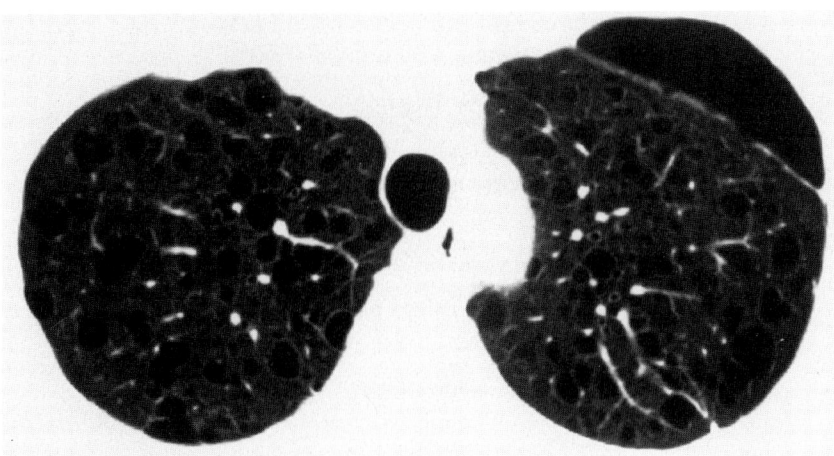

FIGURE 32.13. Lymphangioleiomyomatosis (LAM). Computed tomographic scan from a 41-year-old woman with LAM demonstrating multiple thin-walled cystic radiolucencies in upper lobes bilaterally, with large zones of intervening normal lung parenchyma consistent with LAM.

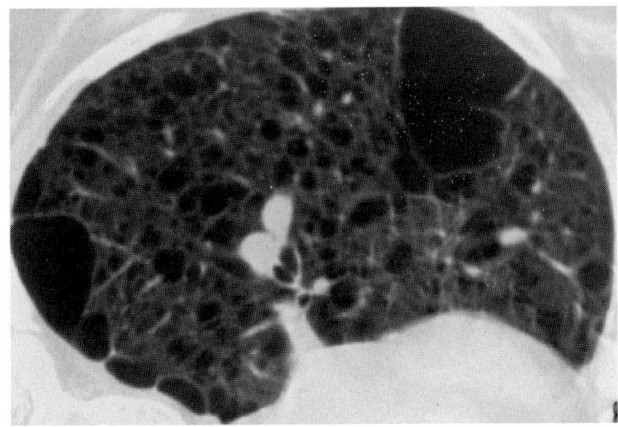

FIGURE 32.14. Lymphangioleiomyomatosis (LAM). Computed tomographic scan from a 44-year-old woman with LAM, demonstrating multiple thin-walled cystic radiolucencies bilaterally. Note the two large lesions, representing confluent cysts.

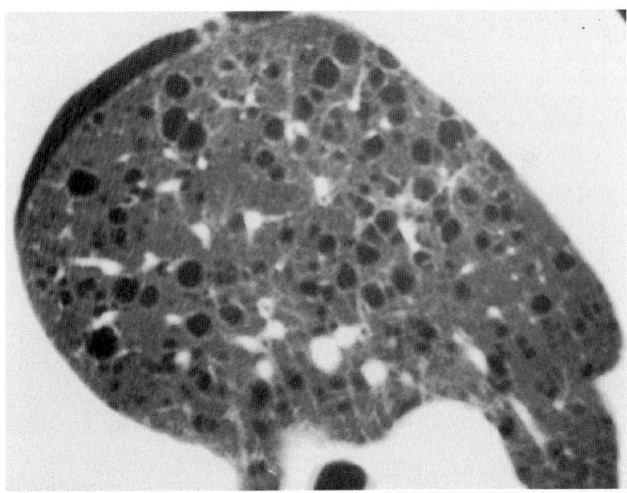

FIGURE 32.15. Lymphangioleiomyomatosis (LAM). Computed tomographic scan demonstrating multiple thin-walled cystic radiolucencies throughout lung parenchyma. Note small associated pneumothorax, a typical finding in LAM. (From Schmidt R, University of Washington, Seattle, Washington, with permission.)

of cysts differs in these disorders. In LAM, the cysts are distributed throughout the lung fields, without predilection for specific regions or lobes (68,115). In pulmonary LCH, the cysts are preferentially distributed in the upper or mid lung zones and are associated with a nodular component (which is lacking in LAM) (54,68,115). Cystic or bullous lesions seen in smokers with emphysema do not have well-formed walls and tend to be more extensive in the upper lobes (68,107,115). Honeycomb cysts are a prominent feature of idiopathic or collagen vascular disease–associated pulmonary fibrosis (69,117). However, in these disorders, the disease is patchy and heterogeneous, and honeycomb cysts are preferentially distributed in the peripheral, subpleural, and basilar regions of the lungs (71). Reticular opacities are prominent associated features in UIP (71), but are absent in LAM (68,115). Focal ground-glass opacities were noted in 12% (eight of 66) (105) and 59% (22 of 37) of patients with LAM in two series (106) and may reflect focal alveolar hemorrhage, pulmonary hemosiderosis, or diffuse proliferation of smooth muscle cells (103,118). Mediastinal or hilar lymphadenopathy is uncommon in LAM (<10% of patients) (106,119), but retrocrural adenopathy was noted in 26% of patients in one series (107). Abdominopelvic CT may reveal cysts or angiomyolipomas in kidney, spleen, or pelvic organs or retrocrural or para-aortic lymphadenopathy (103,107,120, 121).

Ventilation-Perfusion Lung Scans

A recent prospective study cited an unusual "speckling" pattern on ventilation lung scanning in 28 of 39 (72%) of patients with LAM (131). CT scans revealed pulmonary cysts in all 39 patients. Univariate analysis showed that the extent of disease on chest radiographs and CT scans, cyst size, ventilation-perfusion abnormalities, and the degree of speckling correlated inversely with FEV_1, $DLCO$, and ratio of FEV_1/FVC but not with FVC or TLC (131).

Tuberous Sclerosis Complex

Tuberous sclerosis—an autosomal-dominant disorder associated with mental retardation, cranial calcification, and cutaneous manifestations—shares some features with LAM (e.g., extrapulmonary angioleiomyomas; hamartomatous proliferation of smooth muscle, and pulmonary LAM), but the relationship between these disorders is not clear. (122–125).

Retrospective series reported lung cystic lesions indistinguishable from LAM in 1% to 4% of patients with tuberous sclerosis complex (TSC) (124,126). However, a recent prospective study suggest that asymptomatic LAM is far more common in TSC (127). Screening HRCT scans were performed on 48 patients with TSC and no pulmonary symptoms, no prior history of LAM, and normal pulmonary function tests. Pulmonary cysts consistent with LAM were detected in 13 of 38 (34%) women, but in none of 10 men with TSC (127). Similarly, in a retrospective study, 20 of 78 (26%) women with TSC had pulmonary LAM (by CT scan, surgical biopsy, or autopsy) (128). Angiomyolipomas are found in 80% of patients with TSC (68,103,105,125) and in

up to 60% of patients with LAM (119–121,129,130). Angiomyolipomas in both LAM and TSC express the antimelanoma monoclonal antibody HMB-45, suggesting a common origin from a progenitor smooth muscle cell (103,105). Tuberous sclerosis can be distinguished from LAM on clinical grounds, because neurological or cutaneous manifestations are not observed in LAM.

Histopathological Features

LAM is characterized by proliferation of atypical smooth muscle and thin-walled cysts within lung, uterus, kidney, or abdominopelvic lymph nodes (108,109,113,120). Pulmonary LAM is characterized by innumerable small cysts on the lung surface, ranging from a few millimeters to more than 3 cm (108,109,113) (Fig. 32.16A). Light microscopy demonstrates diffuse proliferation of immature/atypical smooth muscle in the walls of the cysts and throughout the peribronchial, perivascular and perilymphatic regions of the lungs (103–107) (Fig. 32.16 B,C). The smooth muscle cells are heterogeneous and, phenotypically,

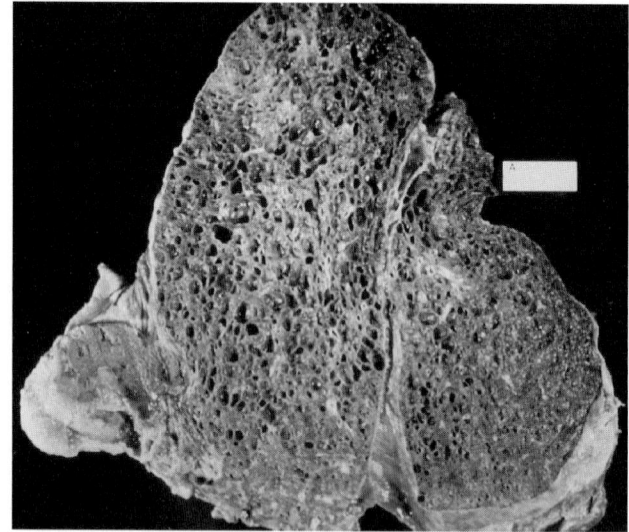

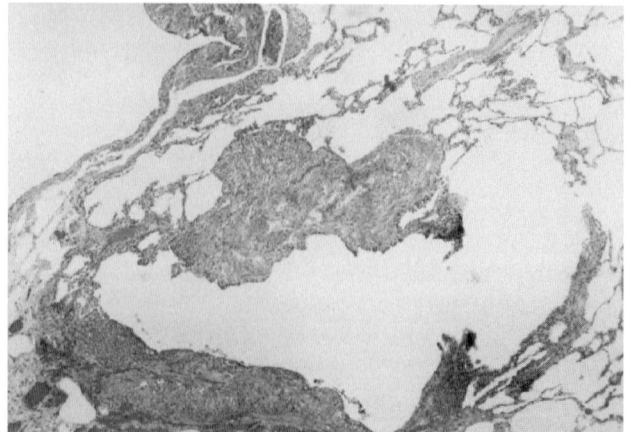

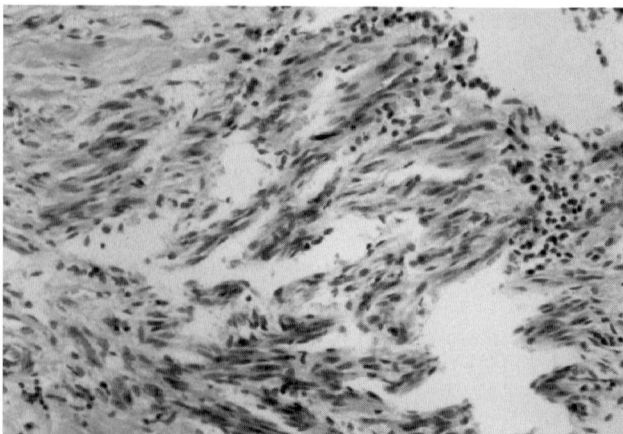

FIGURE 32.16. Lymphangioleiomyomatosis (LAM). **(A)** Photomicrograph of gross appearance of lung removed from a patient with LAM. Note the numerous cysts throughout the lung parenchyma. **(B)** Photomicrograph of lung biopsy, demonstrating aggregates of characteristic smooth muscle bundles in the walls, the cysts, and in the peribronchial areas (hematoxylin and eosin; magnification, low power). **(C)** Photomicrograph of lung biopsy demonstrating aggregates of characteristic smooth muscle bundles with a spindle appearance (hematoxylin and eosin; magnification, high power).

may exhibit features of spindle cells, smaller cells with little cytoplasm, or epithelioid cells (103). The LAM cells grow in a haphazard arrangement, unlike the orderly patterns of organization of normal smooth muscle cells (132). However, these proliferating smooth muscle cells may form nodules or fascicles (103,104,118). These smooth muscle proliferations destroy surrounding lung parenchyma, forming the characteristic LAM cysts (103-106). The diffuse distribution of the muscular and cystic lesions explains the clinical manifestations of LAM. Compression of the conducting small airways results in airflow obstruction and alveolar disruption. Pneumothoraces result from rupture of subpleural cysts (103–106). Obstruction of pulmonary vessels causes venular congestion and disruption, resulting in hemoptysis and hemosiderosis (103,108). Hemosiderin-laden macrophages within alveolar spaces or interstitium may reflect prior episodes of hemorrhage (103,105,106). Hemosiderin-laden macrophages were detected in BAL fluid in 60% to 81% of LAM patients in two studies (105,107). Lymphatic obstruction may cause chylothorax (103). The extent of cystic LAM lesions on open lung biopsy is an important determinant of prognosis. Predominantly cystic lesions suggest a worse survival, whereas the extent of smooth muscle proliferation or hemosiderosis does not correlate with survival (114,106).

Immunohistochemical stains of the proliferating smooth muscle cells in LAM are positive for muscle-specific actin, desmin, and melanoma-related marker (HMB-45) (104,105,133). HMB-45 is never found in normal smooth muscle (104,133). In the absence of melanoma or clear cell tumor of the lung (which also stain for HMB-45), positive staining for HMB-45 in the lung is highly specific (>95%) for LAM (104,133,134). LAM cells also contain increased amounts of matrix metalloproteinases (MMPs), especially MMP-2 but also MMP-1 and MMP-9 (135). These MMPs may play a critical role in the development of the cystic lesions in LAM (135). Progesterone and estrogen receptors are demonstrable in the nuclei of proliferating smooth muscle in some patients (105,113,136), but these findings are not consistent (132).

Electron microscopy (performed for research purposes) of smooth muscle cells in LAM reveal indented round-to-ovoid nuclei with prominent nucleoli, prominent microfilament bundles with dense bodies, a well-developed rough endoplasmic reticulum, and numerous clusters of intracytoplasmic, electron-dense crystalloid granules (137). Similar cells are found in renal or hepatic angiomyolipomas (137).

Historically, the diagnosis of LAM required surgical lung biopsy (108,112,113). The diagnosis was often made inadvertently, at the time of thoracotomy for recurrent pneumothoraces (113). However, TBBs may be adequate in some cases, particularly when HMB-45 stains are positive (105,106,113,134). A diagnosis of LAM can be assumed without lung biopsy, provided HRCT features are characteristic, clinical criteria are consistent, and the following features

are present: typical renal angiomyolipomas, chronic chylous ascites with abdominal lymphadenopathy, and characteristic histopathology on lymph node biopsy (105,107).

Extrapulmonary LAM or cysts may involve the spleen, kidney, liver, abdominal or retroperitoneal lymph nodes, uterus, and ovaries (119–121,130). Expansion of leiomyomas or cysts may cause pain, bleeding, chylous ascites, or compression of contiguous structures (129). Uterine leiomyomas have been cited in up to 41% of patients with LAM (105). Renal angiomyolipomas have been noted in 15% to 60% of patients with pulmonary LAM (105,107,129,130). CT scan is the best screening test for assessing the presence and extent of renal or intra-abdominal cystic or angiomyolipomatous lesions (120,121,129). Ultrasonography and abdominopelvic CT scans have complementary roles in the diagnosis and follow-up of abdominal and pelvic manifestations of LAM (120). Asymptomatic lesions less than 4 cm in size can be followed with annual CT or ultrasonography (129). Larger or symptomatic lesions should be followed more frequently (no less often than 6 months). Expanding or symptomatic lesions more than 4 cm in size should be treated with surgery or embolization (129,138). Partial or total nephrectomy may be required for some complications (e.g., severe pain or hemorrhage) (107,129).

Treatment

The course of LAM is poor, with inexorable progression over 5 to 15 years. Ten-year survival ranges from 21% to 78% (103–109,113). Most deaths are owing to progressive respiratory failure. Earlier publications cited 5- and 10-year survival rates of approximately 60% and 20%, respectively (108,112). Subsequent studies cited improved survival, which could reflect earlier diagnosis or the impact of therapy. In the series from Stanford and the Mayo Clinic, 25 of 32 patients (78%) with LAM were alive a mean of 8.5 years after the onset of disease (113). However, in a study from Asia, only 10 of 26 patients (38%) survived more than 8.5 years (106). A recent study from France of 69 patients with LAM cited 5- and 10-year survival rates of 91% and 79%, respectively (105). Therapy is of unproven value.

Given the rarity of LAM, controlled therapeutic trials have not been performed. Therapy is of unproven benefit (109). Because LAM occurs almost exclusively in women, estrogens are believed to be central to the pathogenesis. Treatment of LAM is directed toward reducing estrogens, either by surgical oophorectomy or antiestrogen regimens (e.g., progesterone, tamoxifen, androgens, luteinizing hormone-releasing agonists) (103–107,109,113). Pregnancy or exogenous estrogens are strongly contraindicated (109). Data regarding therapy are limited by retrospective analyses and small numbers of patients. In the review from Stanford and the Mayo Clinic, oophorectomy was ineffective in all 16 patients (113). All nine treated with tamoxifen deteriorated; two of 19 treated with intramuscular medroxyprogesterone acetate alone stabilized or improved (113). Kitaichi and colleagues retrospectively analyzed diverse therapeutic options in 40 patients with LAM (106). Only two improved; nine stabilized; 29 deteriorated. In that study, oophorectomy alone or progesterone were never effective. The combination of oophorectomy and progesterone was associated with deterioration in nine patients, improvement in one patient, and stabilization in one patient. One patient improved with combined treatment with progesterone, oophorectomy, and tamoxifen. An additional 12 patients treated with tamoxifen (alone or combined with other agents) deteriorated. Gonadotrophin-releasing hormone agonists were ineffective in all six patients. Factors associated with a poor prognosis included worsening airflow obstruction at 2 years after the initial exam; increase in percentage of predicted TLC at 2, 3, and 5 years after the initial examination; predominantly cystic LAM lesions (compared with predominantly smooth muscle proliferation) on open lung biopsy; and higher grades of histologically abnormal areas and cystic lesions on open lung biopsy (106). Urban and colleagues evaluated 57 patients receiving various hormonal therapies; impact of therapy was impossible to ascertain (105). Among 34 patients who had serial pulmonary function tests (PFTs), FEV_1 improved more than 15% in only four patients (12%) (105). Progesterone (oral or intramuscular), alone or combined with oophorectomy, has been used most often to treat LAM (105,107,109,113). In a retrospective study of 50 patients with LAM, Johnson and colleagues cited lower rates of decline in FEV_1 and D_{LCO} among patients treated with progesterone (139). These trends were not statistically significant but suggest that progesterone may slow the course of the disease. Progesterone can be given orally (dose, 10–20 mg/d) or by intramuscular route (medroxyprogesterone acetate 400–800 mg/mo) (105,107,109,113). Parenteral administration achieves higher and more sustained levels (103), but studies comparing these regimens are lacking. Progesterone may be more effective in managing chylous effusions; its efficacy in ameliorating the airway or cystic lesions is unproven (105–107,109,113). Administration of synthetic analogues of luteinizing-releasing hormone was associated with improvement in one patient (140) but was ineffective in two other treated patients (141). Anecdotal case reports cited responses to α_{2b}-interferon (142) and somatostatin (143), but the value of these options is unproven. Unfortunately, current therapeutic regimens for LAM are of limited efficacy. Despite the lack of firm evidence that treatment is effective, the course of LAM is poor, with inexorable progression. However, the rate of progression of LAM varies widely.

Given the poor prognosis of untreated LAM, an empirical trial of therapy with progesterone, gonadotrophin-releasing hormone agonists (e.g., leuprolide acetate), somatostatin, or oophorectomy is reasonable. Because tamoxifen has partial estrogen-agonist activity (103), we believe this agent should not be used in LAM. The decision to treat needs to be individualized, and must take into account the patient's wishes.

The influence of pregnancy on the outcome is not clear, but progression or acceleration of LAM during pregnancy has been noted. We believe pregnancy should be avoided. A trial of β-agonists should be considered in patients with severe airflow obstruction (109).

Chylous effusions refractory to medical therapy may be difficult to manage. Dietary fat restriction, peritoneal-jugular shunts, ligation of the thoracic duct, pleurectomy, and sclerosing agents have been tried, but often are ineffectual (103,105,107,100). Recurrent pneumothoraces may require surgical pleurodesis or pleurectomy (105,107). Unfortunately, pleural sclerosing procedures may preclude subsequent lung transplantation (100). Unilateral or bilateral lung transplantation is an option for incapacitating disease and severe airflow obstruction ($FEV_1 < 30\%$ predicted) or other complications (e.g., refractory, recurrent pneumothoraces) (100,109,144). A retrospective study of 34 patients with LAM cited 1- and 2-year survival rates after lung transplantation of 69% and 58%, respectively (144). Recurrence of LAM in transplanted lung allografts has been noted (145,146), but this appears to be uncommon (one of 29 lung transplant recipients in one review) (144). Hopefully, ongoing research efforts and future studies will shed further light on the pathogenesis of LAM and provide new strategies for curative therapy.

PULMONARY LYMPHANGIOLEIOMYOMATOSIS	
Summary Statement	**Level of Evidence**
Ablate estrogens (oophorectomy, progesterone, gonadotrophin-releasing hormone agonists); therapy is of unproven benefit	Observational studies
Avoid pregnancy	Observational studies
Surgical pleurodesis for recurrent pneumothoraces	Observational studies
Surgical pleurodesis, pleurectomy, ligation of the thoracic duct, peritoneal-jugular shunts (for refractory chylous effusions)	Observational studies

PULMONARY AMYLOIDOSIS

Amyloidosis is a heterogenous group of diseases characterized by deposition of an insoluble β-pleated fibrillar protein in the extracellular matrix of involved tissues (147). Amyloid protein takes up Congo red stain and exhibits apple-green birefringence under polarized microscopy (147) (Fig. 32.17 A,B). Primary amyloidosis, the most common variant, is associated with deposition of the immunoglobulin light chain fragment (amyloid AL), and can be idiopathic or associated with plasma cell dyscrasias (e.g., multiple myeloma) (147). Secondary amyloidosis (amyloid AA) complicates diverse chronic inflammatory conditions (e.g., bronchiectasis, tuberculosis, malaria, chronic infections, and diverse collagen

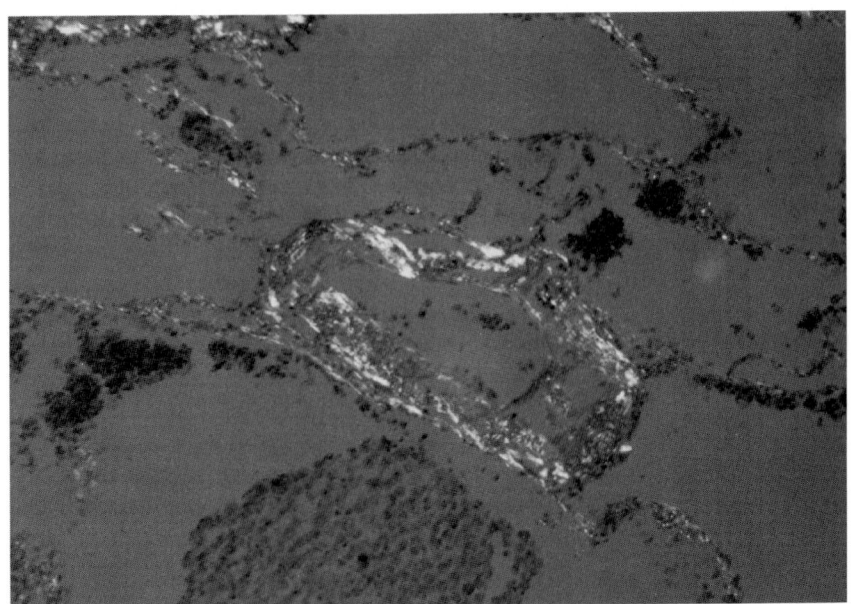

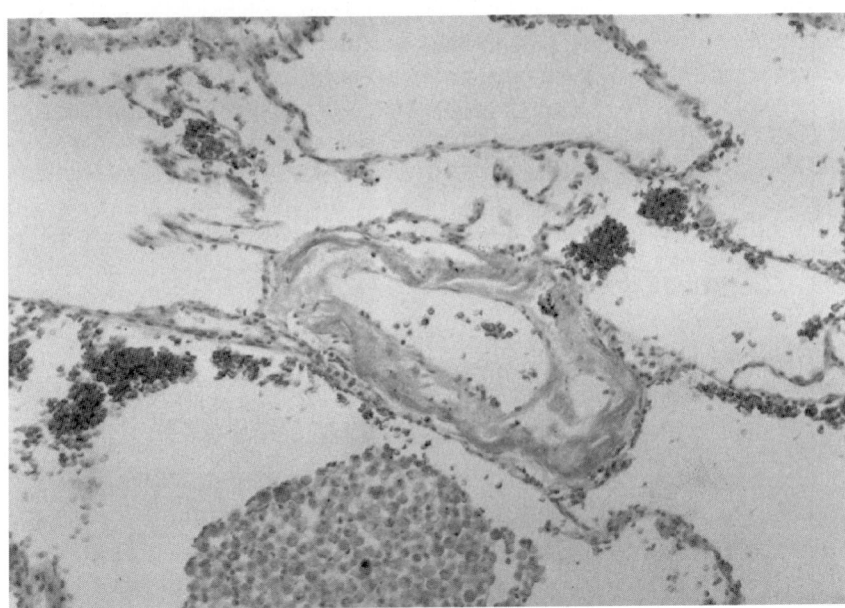

FIGURE 32.17. Amyloidosis. **(A)** Photomicrograph of open lung biopsy demonstrating amyloid deposition within the wall of a pulmonary vessel (hematoxylin and eosin). **(B)** Photomicrograph of open lung biopsy demonstrating amyloid deposition displaying apple-green stain by Congo red stain.

vascular disorders or inflammatory disorders) (147). Amyloid AA protein is an apolipoprotein associated with HDL-3 produced by proteolysis of serum amyloid A proteins (147). With the marked reduction in chronic infectious diseases such as tuberculosis, osteomyelitis, and bronchiectasis in the Western Hemisphere, amyloid AA is rare, but may complicate untreated familial Mediterranean fever, inflammatory bowel disease, or rheumatoid arthritis (147,148). Familial transthyretin-associated (ATTR) amyloidosis also exists; ATTR amyloidosis is 5 to 10 times less common than amyloid AL (147). Additional familial forms owing to diverse mutations have also been described (147). Amyloid protein may be found with advanced age (senile amyloidosis), usually as an incidental finding (147). Prealbumin is associated

with familial and senile forms of amyloidosis. Amyloidosis is exceedingly rare. Only 1,275 to 3,200 new cases of amyloid AL (the most common variant) are diagnosed annually in the United States (147).

Clinical manifestations of amyloid AL are protean. Amyloidosis can affect any organ, but predominant sites of amyloid deposition include heart, kidney, gastrointestinal tract, joints, the tongue, spleen, liver, nervous system, and upper respiratory tract (147). Macroglossia, a classical feature of amyloidosis, occurs in 20% of patients (147). Prognosis of amyloid AL is dictated by extrapulmonary organ involvement. Mean survival in amyloid AL is less than 2 years (149,150). Most deaths are owing to cardiac, renal, neurological, or nonpulmonary causes (149,150). Survival among patients with ATTR amyloidosis varies with the specific mutation and time of diagnosis, but some patients survive more than 15 years from the diagnosis (147). Survival in amyloid AA is influenced by the underlying disease (147).

Clinically significant pulmonary involvement occurs in less than 10% to 20% of patients with amyloid AL (147,148), but amyloid deposits may be observed in up to 90% of patients with amyloid AL at necropsy (149,151–153). Pulmonary involvement is not a significant contributor to death in amyloid AL; median survival of patients with overt lung amyloidosis is similar to systemic amyloid AL (149,154). Lung involvement is rare in amyloid AA amyloidosis (147,148). In one series of 113 cases with amyloid AA, lung involvement was detected in only one patient (152). At the Mayo Clinic, only two cases of pulmonary amyloidosis were identified in patients with amyloid AA over a 14-year period (149). No cases of pulmonary amyloidosis were detected in over 200 patients with systemic AA amyloidosis seen at the Hammersmith Hospital in London (154). "Primary" pulmonary amyloidosis (PPA), a disorder confined to the lungs, tracheobronchial tree, pleura, and/or mediastinal lymph nodes, also exists (149). Utz and colleagues reviewed the Mayo Clinic experience from 1980–1993 and identified 55 patients with pulmonary amyloidosis (149). Thirty-five had amyloid AL, two had amyloid AA, 11 had localized pulmonary amyloid, 6 had senile amyloid, and one had familial amyloid.

Primary Pulmonary Amyloidosis

PPA, or localized pulmonary amyloidosis, is defined as amyloid deposits limited to the lungs and associated structures (i.e., tracheobronchial tree, pleura, and hilar or mediastinal lymph nodes) (151,154–160). In localized forms of amyloidosis, the AL light chains are produced by a clone of lymphoplasmacytics localized in proximity to the amyloid deposits (154). This type of amyloidosis may be nodular in character (154). In contrast, the fibrils in systemic amyloid AL are derived from circulating monoclonal light chains produced by clonal plasma cell dyscrasias (154). Amyloid deposition in the lung owing to secondary or familial amyloidosis is not included in this category. In 1983, Thompson and Citron identified 126 published cases of primary pulmonary amyloidosis in the world's literature (67 tracheobronchial; 59, lung parenchymal) (151). Of the 67 patients with tracheobronchial disease, 57 had multifocal submucosal plaques and 10 had amyloid tumorlike masses.

Tracheobronchial Amyloidosis

Tracheobronchial amyloidosis (TBA) can occur as the only site of involvement, leading to progressive stenosis of trachea or bronchi, leading to progressive respiratory failure (and even death). (154,155). Tracheobronchial amyloidosis is rare; in a recent review of the literature, fewer than 100 cases of TBA had been published (155). Ten cases of TBA were seen at Boston University over a 15-year period (155). Tracheobronchial amyloidosis was never seen in 685 patients with amyloid AL seen at that medical center during that time frame. Investigators at the Mayo Clinic identified 17 cases of TBA between 1973–1999 (159). The diagnosis of TBA may be established by bronchoscopy (155,159). The disease is localized to the airways and spares the lung parenchyma. Relatively flat submucosal plaques of amyloid protein or tracheobronchial nodules may be seen. These may be single, diffuse, or multifocal. Varying degrees of stenosis or encroachment of tracheal or bronchial lumens may be found (155,159). Patients may be asymptomatic or may have hoarseness, wheezing, dyspnea, hemoptysis, cough, atelectasis, recurrent pneumonia, or chronic infections. Respiratory symptoms reflect narrowing or involvement of the nasopharynx, sinuses, larynx, trachea, or bronchi. Some cases of TBA are associated with tracheobronchopathia osteoplastica, a rare disorder of unknown cause that is characterized by calcified or cartilaginous submucosal nodules within the tracheobronchial tree (161,162). Amyloidosis involving the trachea may cause severe (even fatal) airflow obstruction (155). Pulmonary function tests in patients with proximal tracheal stenosis demonstrate severe airflow obstruction. Patients with involvement of distal trachea or bronchi may manifest air trapping; flow rates may be normal or obstructed. The configuration of flow-volume loops can usually distinguish upper airway obstruction from distal stenoses.

Management of TBA may require intermittent bronchoscopic dilatation or debridement, surgical resection, laser therapy, tracheostomy, or tracheal resection (155,159). Resection or biopsy may be complicated by severe bleeding. Data regarding the use of alkylating agents or corticosteroids are sparse. Most centers avoid systemic agents because of the limited disease burden and potential for drug-induced toxicities. Local radiation therapy has been used in a few cases (159). Spiral CT scans are invaluable to quantitatively assess the degree and sites of airway narrowing, and to monitor the course of the disease (163,164). CT scans demonstrate airway wall thickening, irregularly narrowed airway lumens, and heterotopic tracheal wall calcifications in patients with long-standing TBA. The course of TBA is usually slowly progressive; one third of patients with proximal or severe mid airway disease die from progressive respiratory insufficiency within 7 to 12 years after diagnosis (155).

Nodular Amyloid Lesions (Amyloidomas)

Localized pulmonary amyloid nodules (amyloidomas) are uncommon lesions seen in older patients (average age, sixth decade), are usually asymptomatic, and are generally not associated with systemic amyloid AL (154,157,160). Lesions may be single or multiple, ranging in size from 0.4 to

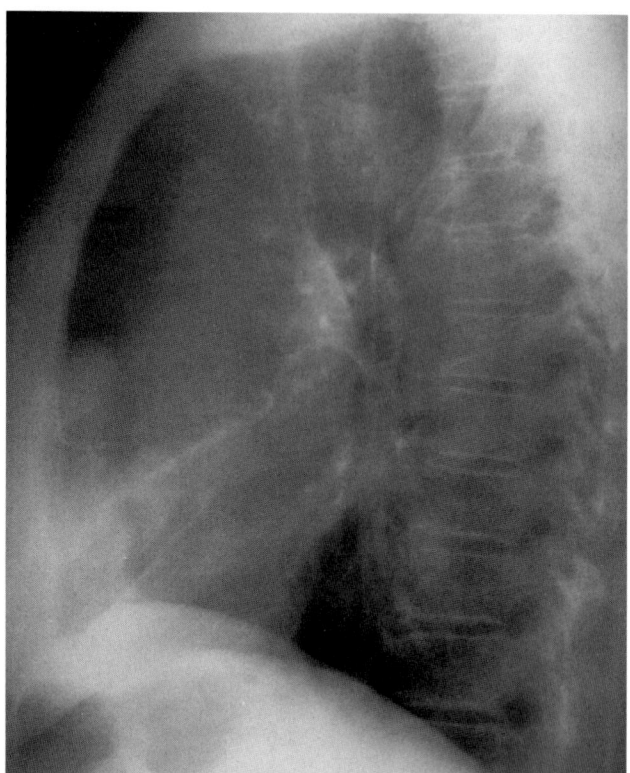

FIGURE 32.18. Amyloidosis. Posteroanterior chest radiograph demonstrates a solitary pulmonary nodule in the retrosternal space. Open lung biopsy demonstrating typical features of amyloidosis. (From Godwin D, University of Washington, Seattle, Washington, with permission.)

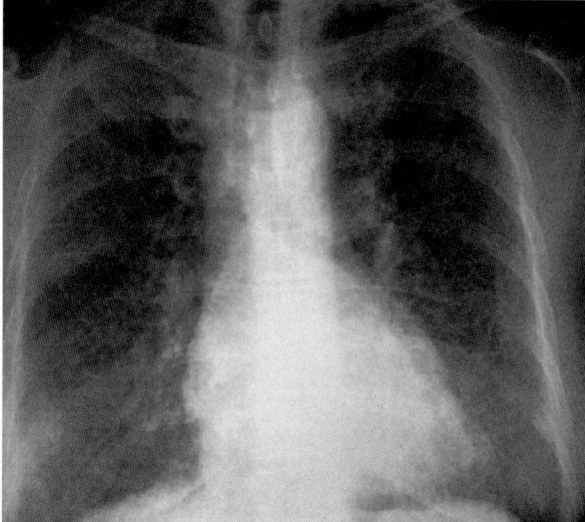

FIGURE 32.19. Amyloidosis. Posteroanterior chest radiograph demonstrates diffuse bilateral reticulonodular infiltrates in a patient with pulmonary amyloidosis. Small bilateral pleural effusions are also present. (From Godwin D, University of Washington, Seattle, Washington, with permission.)

15 cm (154,160). Amyloidomas occur most frequently in the lower lobes and may be asymmetric when multiple nodules are present (154). Amyloidomas may calcify and rarely cavitate (154). Metaplastic bone or cartilage formation may occur. Localized amyloid nodules often present as incidental findings on chest radiographs (154) (Fig. 32.18) or autopsy (160). However, cough or hemoptysis may occur. For solitary nodules causing symptoms, resection may be curative. However, biopsy or resection of nodular mass lesions may cause significant bleeding (165).

Diffuse Interstitial Opacities

Amyloid deposits in the alveolar septae and interstitium may cause reticulonodular or micronodular lesions on chest radiographs or CT scans, as well as physiological aberrations, including restrictive defects, decreased D_{LCO}, widened A_{O_2}-a_{O_2} difference, and pulmonary hypertension (156,157) (Fig. 32.19). Alveolar septal amyloidosis is most commonly seen in amyloid AL and is uncommon in PPA (154). Diffuse interstitial infiltrates were noted in six of 48 patients with PPA reported by Hui and colleagues from the Armed Forces Institute of Pathology (156), but none of 17 patients with PPA recently reviewed by the Mayo Clinic group (149). Because the amyloid deposits and infiltrative process in the alveolar septa often involve the pulmonary vasculature, biopsy or resection of pulmonary lesions may be associated with an increased risk of bleeding.

Senile Pulmonary Amyloidosis

Pulmonary amyloidosis occurring in elderly patients is termed senile pulmonary amyloidosis (149,166). Autopsy studies detected senile pulmonary amyloidosis in approximately 10% of patients older than 80 years of age and in 50% of patients older than 90 years of age (166). These deposits are usually incidental findings and parallel senile cardiac involvement (149,166).

Other Manifestations of Amyloid Deposits

Hilar and mediastinal adenopathy owing to amyloid deposition may occur in conjunction with tracheobronchial amyloidosis and either primary or secondary forms of amyloidosis (167–169). The adenopathy may be unilateral or bilateral (with or without calcification) (149,169). One patient with mediastinal amyloid AL resulting in recurrent laryngeal nerve palsy has been described (167).

Pleural effusions (owing to amyloid deposits along the pleural surface) may occur in amyloid AL or as a complication of PPA (170,171). Amyloid effusions are exudative and may be hemorrhagic PPA (170,171). Transudative pleural effusions may reflect cardiac amyloidosis. Other rare manifestations include obstructive sleep apnea (secondary to involvement of the tongue) and respiratory muscle weakness (owing to amyloid infiltrating the diaphragm) (147). Amyloidosis involving the larynx (with or without systemic involvement) has rarely been described (154,172). Pulmonary marginal zone lymphoma of mucosa-associated lymphoid tissue may be found in association with localized pulmonary amyloidosis (173).

Bleeding Manifestation with Amyloidosis

Hemoptysis may complicate any form of pulmonary amyloidosis (including alveolar septal or tracheobronchial involvement). Focal or diffuse hemorrhage may occur because of amyloid deposits involving vessels. In one retrospective review by Yood and colleagues, 41 of 100 patients with amyloidosis experienced one or more bleeding episodes (three were fatal) (174). Manifestations included petechiae, ecchymoses, gastrointestinal bleeding, hematuria, hemoptysis, and postbiopsy bleeding. Hemoptysis occurred in only two patients. Excessive bleeding associated with amyloidosis may be multifactorial, reflecting amyloid infiltration of blood vessels, hepatic or renal involvement, coagulopathies, or isolated factor-X deficiency (165). In a retrospective review of 337 patients with amyloid AL, 28% manifested abnormal bleeding; abnormal coagulation screens were present in 51% (165). The risk for pulmonary hemorrhage after lung biopsy is concerning, but firm data assessing risks are not available. In one series, TBBs were performed in 11 patients with pulmonary amyloidosis (149). No serious complications ensued, but bleeding more than 100 mL was noted in two patients.

Treatment of Amyloidosis

Optimal therapy for amyloid AL is not clear (147,149). In secondary forms of amyloidosis, aggressive treatment of the underlying disease may delay or reverse the deposition of amyloid protein (147). Alkylating agents (particularly melphalan) may be effective in amyloidosis associated with plasma cell dyscrasias (e.g., multiple myeloma) and improve survival modestly in idiopathic amyloid AL (150,175,176). Colchicine has been used in both amyloid AL and amyloid AA, but its value is doubtful (150). α-Interferon is ineffective (177). High-dose chemotherapy followed by peripheral blood stem-cell transplantation may prolong survival or local symptoms in uncontrolled studies (176,178–180), but randomized trials are lacking. Anecdotal responses were reported with dimethyl sulfoxide (181), vincristine, adriamycin, dexamethasone (176,181), and 4'-iodo-4'-deoxy-doxorubicin, (a new anthracycline), but data are sparse. No proven effective therapy is available for diffuse amyloid infiltrating the tracheobronchial tree or lung parenchyma (154). Resection of localized amyloid deposits surgically (155,159) or by laser (155,159,182,183) may be beneficial in symptomatic foci involving the trachea, larynx, or bronchi. However, recurrence is frequent, and airway compromise may result even with repetitive bronchoscopic techniques (159,183). In rare cases, laryngeal dilatation or tracheostomy is required (155).

External beam radiation therapy was efficacious in one patient with airflow obstruction from tracheobronchial amyloidosis (184).

PULMONARY AMYLOIDOSIS	
Summary Statement	**Level of Evidence**
High-dose chemotherapy followed by peripheral blood stem-cell transplantation may prolong survival or local symptoms.	Observational studies
Secondary AA amyloidosis: treat underlying disease	Observational studies
Tracheobronchial amyloidosis: tracheal dilatation, resection local nodules or plaques, tracheostomy, laser or surgical resection	Observational studies
Localized tracheobronchial amyloidosis may respond to repeated bronchoscopic Nd:YAG or carbon dioxide laser photoresection.	Observational studies

REFERENCES

1. Rosen SH, Castleman B, Liebow AA. Pulmonary alveolar proteinosis. *N Engl J Med* 1958;258:1123–1142.
2. Shah PL, Hansell DM, Lawson PR, et al. Pulmonary alveolar proteinosis: clinical aspects and current concepts on pathogenesis. *Thorax* 2000;55:67–77.
3. Prakash UB, Barham SS, Carpenter HA, et al. Pulmonary alveolar phospholipoproteinosis: experience with 34 cases and a review. *Mayo Clin Proc* 1987;62:499–518.
4. Goldstein LS, Kavuru MS, Curtis-McCarthy P, et al. Pulmonary alveolar proteinosis: clinical features and outcomes. *Chest* 1998;114:1357–1362.
5. Ben-Dov I, Kishinevski Y, Roznman J, et al. Pulmonary alveolar proteinosis in Israel: ethnic clustering. *Israel Med Assoc J* 1999;1:75–78.
6. Mazzone PJ, Thomassen MJ, Kavuru MS. Pulmonary alveolar proteinosis: recent advances. *Semin Respir Crit Care Med* 2002 *(in press)*.
7. Teja K, Cooper PH, Squires JE, et al. Pulmonary alveolar proteinosis in four siblings. *N Engl J Med* 1981;305:1390–1392.
8. Bewig B, Wang XD, Kirsten D, et al. GM-CSF and GM-CSF β_c receptor in adult patients with pulmonary alveolar proteinosis. *Eur Respir J* 2000;15:350–357.
9. Cordonnier C, Fleury-Feith J, Escudiere E, et al. Secondary alveolar proteinosis is a reversible cause of respiratory failure in leukemic patients. *Am J Respir Crit Care Med* 1994;149:788–794.
10. Green D, Dighe P, Ali NO, et al. Pulmonary alveolar proteinosis complicating acute myelogenous leukemia. *Cancer* 1980;46:1763–1746.
11. Ruben FL, Talamo TS. Secondary pulmonary alveolar proteinosis occurring in two patients with acquired immune deficiency syndrome. *Am J Med* 1986;80:1187–1190.
12. Davidson JM, Macleod WM. Pulmonary alveolar proteinosis. *Br J Dis Chest* 1969;63:13–28.
13. Keller CA, Frost A, Cagle PT, et al. Pulmonary alveolar proteinosis in a painter with elevated pulmonary concentrations of titanium. *Chest* 1995;108:277–280.

14. Miller RR, Churg AM, Hutcheon M, et al. Pulmonary alveolar proteinosis and aluminum dust exposure. *Am Rev Respir Dis* 1984;130:312–315.

15. Buechner HA, Ansari A. Acute silico-proteinosis: a new pathologic variant of acute silicosis in sandblasters, characterized by histologic features resembling alveolar proteinosis. *Dis Chest* 1969;55:274–278.

16. Hoffman RM, Rogers RM. Serum and lavage lactate dehydrogenase isoenzymes in pulmonary alveolar proteinosis. *Am Rev Respir Dis* 1991;143:42–46.

17. Kitamura T, Tanaka N, Watanabe J, et al. Idiopathic pulmonary alveolar proteinosis as an autoimmune disease with neutralizing antibody against granulocyte/macrophage colony-stimulating factor. *J Exp Med* 1999;190:875–880.

18. Kitamura T, Uchida K, Tanaka N, et al. Serological diagnosis of idiopathic pulmonary alveolar proteinosis. *Am J Respir Crit Care Med* 2000;162:658–662.

19. Nugent KM, Pesanti EL. Macrophage function in pulmonary alveolar proteinosis. *Am Rev Respir Dis* 1983;127:780–781.

20. Seymour JF, Presneill JJ, Schoch OD, et al. Therapeutic efficacy of granulocyte-macrophage colony-stimulating factor in patients with idiopathic acquired alveolar proteinosis. *Am J Respir Crit Care Med* 2001;163:524–531.

21. Johkoh T, Itoh H, Muller NL, et al. Crazy-paving appearance at thin-section CT: spectrum of disease and pathologic findings. *Radiology* 1999;211:155–160.

22. Godwin JD, Muller NL, Takasugi JE. Pulmonary alveolar proteinosis: CT findings. *Radiology* 1988;169:609–613.

23. Lee KN, Levin DL, Webb WR, et al. Pulmonary alveolar proteinosis: high-resolution CT, chest radiographic, and functional correlations. *Chest* 1997;111:989–995.

24. Tan RT, Kuzo RS. High-resolution CT findings of mucinous bronchioloalveolar carcinoma: a case of pseudopulmonary alveolar proteinosis. *AJR Am J Roentgenol* 1997;168:99–100.

25. Franquet T, Gimenez A, Bordes R, et al. The crazy-paving pattern in exogenous lipoid pneumonia: CT-pathologic correlation. *AJR Am J Roentgenol* 1998;170:315–317.

26. Kuroki Y, Tsutahara S, Shijubo N, et al. Elevated levels of lung surfactant protein A in sera from patients with idiopathic pulmonary fibrosis and pulmonary alveolar proteinosis. *Am Rev Respir Dis* 1993;147:723–729.

27. Honda Y, Kuroki Y, Matsuura E, et al. Pulmonary surfactant protein D in sera and bronchoalveolar lavage fluids. *Am J Respir Crit Care Med* 1995;152:1860–1866.

28. Hirakata Y, Kobayashi J, Sugama Y, et al. Elevation of tumour markers in serum and bronchoalveolar lavage fluid in pulmonary alveolar proteinosis. *Eur Respir J* 1995;8:689–696.

29. Nakajima M, Manabe T, Niki Y, et al. Serum KL-6 level as a monitoring marker in a patient with pulmonary alveolar proteinosis. *Thorax* 1998;53:809–811.

30. Iyonaga K, Suga M, Yamamoto T, et al. Elevated bronchoalveolar concentrations of MCP-1 in patients with pulmonary alveolar proteinosis. *Eur Respir J* 1999;14:383–389.

31. Stanley E, Lieschke GJ, Grail D, et al. Granulocyte/macrophage colony-stimulating factor-deficient mice show no major perturbation of hematopoiesis but develop a characteristic pulmonary pathology. *Proc Natl Acad Sci U S A* 1994;91:5592–5596.

32. Huffman JA, Hull WM, Dranoff G, et al. Pulmonary epithelial cell expression of GM-CSF corrects the alveolar proteinosis in GM-CSF–deficient mice. *J Clin Invest* 1996;97:649–655.

33. Nishinakamura R, Wiler R, Dirksen U, et al. The pulmonary alveolar proteinosis in granulocyte macrophage colony-stimulating factor/interleukins 3/5 β_c receptor-deficient mice is reversed by bone marrow transplantation. *J Exp Med* 1996;183:2657–2662.

34. Reed JA, Ikegami M, Cianciolo ER, et al. Aerosolized GM-CSF ameliorates pulmonary alveolar proteinosis in GM-CSF–deficient mice. *Am J Physiol* 1999;276:L556–L563.

35. Seymour JF, Dunn AR, Vincent JM, et al. Efficacy of granulocyte-macrophage colony-stimulating factor in acquired alveolar proteinosis. *N Engl J Med* 1996;335:1924–1925.

36. Thomassen MJ, Yi T, Raychaudhuri B, et al. Pulmonary alveolar proteinosis is a disease of decreased availability of GM-CSF rather than an intrinsic cellular defect. *Clin Immunol* 2000;95:85–92.

37. Kavuru MS, Sullivan EJ, Piccin R, et al. Exogenous granulocyte-macrophage colony-stimulating factor administration for pulmonary alveolar proteinosis. *Am J Respir Crit Care Med* 2000;161:1143–1148.

38. Ikegami M, Whitsett JA, Chroneos ZC, et al. IL-4 increases surfactant and regulates metabolism *in vivo*. *Am J Physiol* 2000;278:L75–L80.

39. Dirksen U, Nishinakamura R, Groneck P, et al. Human pulmonary alveolar proteinosis associated with a defect in GM-CSF/IL-3/IL-5 receptor common β chain expression. *J Clin Invest* 1997;100:2211–2217.

40. Carraway MS, Ghio AJ, Carter JD, et al. Detection of granulocyte-macrophage colony-stimulating factor in patients with pulmonary alveolar proteinosis. *Am J Respir Crit Care Med* 2000;161:1294–1299.

41. Seymour JF, Begley CG, Dirksen U, et al. Attenuated hematopoietic response to granulocyte-macrophage colony-stimulating factor in patients with acquired pulmonary alveolar proteinosis. *Blood* 1998;92:2657–2667.

42. Tchou-Wong KM, Harkin TJ, Chi C, et al. GM-CSF gene expression is normal but protein release is absent in a patient with pulmonary alveolar proteinosis. *Am J Respir Crit Care Med* 1997;156:1999–2002.

43. Ramirez J, Kieffer RF Jr, Ball WC Jr. Bronchopulmonary lavage in man. *Ann Intern Med* 1965;63:819–828.

44. Hammon WE, McCaffree DR, Cucchiara AJ. A comparison of manual to mechanical chest percussion for clearance of alveolar material in patients with pulmonary alveolar proteinosis (phospholipidosis). *Chest* 1993;103:1409–1412.

45. Parker LA, Novotny DB. Recurrent alveolar proteinosis following double lung transplantation. *Chest* 1997;111:1457–1458.

46. Travis WD, Borok Z, Roum JH, et al. Pulmonary Langerhans cell granulomatosis (histiocytosis X): a clinicopathologic study of 48 cases. *Am J Surg Pathol* 1993;17:971–986.

47. Vassallo R, Ryu JH, Schroeder DR, et al. Clinical outcomes of pulmonary Langerhans' cell histiocytosis in adults. *N Engl J Med* 2002;346:484–490.

48. Vassallo R, Ryu JH, Colby TV, et al. Pulmonary Langerhans'-cell histiocytosis. *N Engl J Med* 2000;342:1969–1978.

49. Tazi A, Soler P, Hance AJ. Adult pulmonary Langerhans' cell histiocytosis. *Thorax* 2000;55:405–416.

50. Basset F, Corrin B, Spencer H, et al. Pulmonary histiocytosis X. *Am Rev Respir Dis* 1978;118:811–820.

51. Friedman PJ, Liebow AA, Sokoloff J. Eosinophilic granuloma of lung: clinical aspects of primary histiocytosis in the adult. *Medicine (Baltimore)* 1981;60:385–396.

52. Delobbe A, Durieu J, Duhamel A, et al. Determinants of survival in pulmonary Langerhans' cell granulomatosis (histiocytosis X): Groupe d'Etude en Pathologie Interstitielle de la Societe de Pathologie Thoracique du Nord. *Eur Respir J* 1996;9:2002–2006.

53. Colby TV, Lombard C. Histiocytosis X in the lung. *Hum Pathol* 1983;14:847–856.

54. Moore AD, Godwin JD, Muller NL, et al. Pulmonary histiocytosis X: comparison of radiographic and CT findings. *Radiology* 1989;172:249–254.

55. Ladisch S, Gadner H. Treatment of Langerhans cell histiocytosis: evolution and current approaches. *Br J Cancer* 1994;23:S41–S46.

56. Tomashefski JF, Khiyami A, Kleinerman J. Neoplasms associated with pulmonary eosinophilic granuloma. *Arch Pathol Lab Med* 1991;115:499–506.

57. Egeler RM, Neglia JP, Puccetti DM, et al. Association of Langerhans cell histiocytosis with malignant neoplasms. *Cancer* 1993;71:865–873.

58. Sadoun D, Vaylet F, Valeyre D, et al. Bronchogenic carcinoma in patients with pulmonary histiocytosis X. *Chest* 1992;101:1610–1613.

59. Neumann MP, Frizzera G. The coexistence of Langerhans' cell granulomatosis and malignant lymphoma may take different forms: report of seven cases with a review of the literature. *Hum Pathol* 1986;17:1060–1065.

60. Burns BF, Colby TV, Dorfman RF. Langerhans' cell granulomatosis (histiocytosis X) associated with malignant lymphomas. *Am J Surg Pathol* 1983;7:529–533.

61. Egeler RM, Neglia JP, Arico M, et al. The relation of Langerhans cell histiocytosis to acute leukemia, lymphomas, and other solid tumors. *Hematol Oncol Clin North Am* 1998;1998:369–378.

62. Lacronique J, Roth C, Battesti JP, et al. Chest radiological features of pulmonary histiocytosis X: a report based on 50 adult cases. *Thorax* 1982;37:104–109.

63. Brambilla E, Fontaine E, Pison CM, et al. Pulmonary histiocytosis X with mediastinal lymph node involvement. *Am Rev Respir Dis* 1990;142:1216–1268.

64. Brauner MW, Grenier P, Mouelhi MM, et al. Pulmonary histiocytosis X: evaluation with high-resolution CT. *Radiology* 1989;172:255–258.

65. Stern EJ, Webb WR, Golden JA, et al. Cystic lung disease associated with eosinophilic granuloma and tuberous sclerosis: air trapping at dynamic ultrafast high-resolution CT. *Radiology* 1992;182:325–329.

66. Soler P, Bergeron A, Kambouchner M, et al. Is high-resolution computed tomography a reliable tool to predict the histopathological activity of pulmonary Langerhans cell histiocytosis? *Am J Respir Crit Care Med* 2000;162:264–270.

67. Brauner MW, Grenier P, Tijani K, et al. Pulmonary Langerhans cell histiocytosis: evolution of lesions on CT scans. *Radiology* 1997;204:497–502.

68. Aberle DR, Hansell DM, Brown K, et al. Lymphangiomyomatosis: CT, chest radiographic, and functional correlations. *Radiology* 1990;176:381–387.

69. Lynch JP III, Wurfel M, Flaherty K, et al. Usual interstitial pneumonia. *Semin Respir Crit Care Med* 2001;22:357–386.

70. Nagai S, Kitaichi M, Itoh H, et al. Idiopathic nonspecific interstitial pneumonia/fibrosis: comparison with idiopathic pulmonary fibrosis and BOOP. *Eur Respir J* 1998;12:1010–1019.

71. Wells A. Clinical usefulness of high resolution computed tomography in cryptogenic fibrosing alveolitis. *Thorax* 1998;53:1080–1087.

72. Crausman RS, Jennings CA, Tuder RM, et al. Pulmonary histiocytosis X: pulmonary function and exercise pathophysiology. *Am J Respir Crit Care Med* 1996;153:426–435.

73. Fartoukh M, Humbert M, Capron F, et al. Severe pulmonary hypertension in histiocytosis X. *Am J Respir Crit Care Med* 2000;161:216–223.

74. Housini I, Tomashefski JF Jr, Cohen A, et al. Transbronchial biopsy in patients with pulmonary eosinophilic granuloma: comparison with findings on open lung biopsy. *Arch Pathol Lab Med* 1994;118:523–530.

75. Webber D, Tron V, Askin F, et al. S-100 staining in the diagnosis of eosinophilic granuloma of lung. *Am J Clin Pathol* 1985;84:447–453.

76. Flint A, Lloyd RV, Colby TV, et al. Pulmonary histiocytosis X. Immunoperoxidase staining for HLA-DR antigen and S100 protein. *Arch Pathol Lab Med* 1986;110:930–933.

77. Chollet S, Soler P, Dournovo P, et al. Diagnosis of pulmonary histiocytosis X by immunodetection of Langerhans cells in bronchoalveolar lavage fluid. *Am J Pathol* 1984;115:225–232.

78. Soler P, Chollet S, Jacque C, et al. Immunocytochemical characterization of pulmonary histiocytosis X cells in lung biopsies. *Am J Pathol* 1985;118:439–451.

79. Emile JF, Wechsler J, Brousse N, et al. Langerhans' cell histiocytosis: definitive diagnosis with the use of monoclonal antibody O10 on routinely paraffin-embedded samples. *Am J Surg Pathol* 1995;19:636–641.

80. Hance AJ. Pulmonary immune cells in health and disease: dendritic cells and Langerhans' cells. *Eur Respir J* 1993;6:1213–1220.

81. Willman CL, Busque L, Griffith BB, et al. Langerhans'-cell histiocytosis (histiocytosis X): a clonal proliferative disorder. *N Engl J Med* 1994;331:154–160.

82. Yousem SA, Colby TV, Chen YY, et al. Pulmonary Langerhans' cell histiocytosis: molecular analysis of clonality. *Am J Surg Pathol* 2001;25:630–636.

83. de Graaf JH, Tamminga RY, Dam-Meiring A, et al. The presence of cytokines in Langerhans' cell histiocytosis. *J Pathol* 1996;180:400–406.

84. Casolaro MA, Bernaudin JF, Saltini C, et al. Accumulation of Langerhans' cells on the epithelial surface of the lower respiratory tract in normal subjects in association with cigarette smoking. *Am Rev Respir Dis* 1988;137:406–411.

85. Tazi A, Bonay M, Bergeron A, et al. Role of granulocyte-macrophage colony stimulating factor (GM-CSF) in the pathogenesis of adult pulmonary histiocytosis X. *Thorax* 1996;51:611–614.

86. Youkeles LH, Grizzanti JN, Liao Z, et al. Decreased tobacco-glycoprotein–induced lymphocyte proliferation *in vitro* in pulmonary eosinophilic granuloma. *Am J Respir Crit Care Med* 1995;151:145–150.

87. Aguayo SM, King TE Jr, Waldron JA Jr, et al. Increased pulmonary neuroendocrine cells with bombesin-like immunoreactivity in adult patients with eosinophilic granuloma. *J Clin Invest* 1990;86:838–844.

88. Aguayo SM. Determinants of susceptibility to cigarette smoke: potential roles for neuroendocrine cells and neuropeptides in airway inflammation, airway wall remodeling, and chronic airflow obstruction. *Am J Respir Crit Care Med* 1994;149:1692–1698.

89. Zeid NA, Muller HK. Tobacco smoke–induced lung granulomas and tumors: association with pulmonary Langerhans cells. *Pathology* 1995;27:247–254.

90. Mogulkoc N, Veral A, Bishop PW, et al. Pulmonary Langerhans' cell histiocytosis: radiologic resolution following smoking cessation. *Chest* 1999;115:1452–1455.

91. Saven A, Burian C. Cladribine activity in adult Langerhans-cell histiocytosis. *Blood* 1999;93:4125–4130.

92. Howarth DM, Gilchrist GS, Mullan BP, et al. Langerhans cell histiocytosis: diagnosis, natural history, management, and outcome. *Cancer* 1999;85:2278–2290.

93. Giona F, Caruso R, Testi AM, et al. Langerhans' cell histiocytosis in adults: a clinical and therapeutic analysis of 11 patients from a single institution. *Cancer* 1997;80:1786–1791.

94. Braier J, Chantada G, Rosso D, et al. Langerhans cell histiocytosis: retrospective evaluation of 123 patients at a single institution. *Pediatr Hematol Oncol* 1999;16:377–385.

95. Zeller B, Storm-Mathisen I, Smevik B, et al. Multisystem Langerhans-cell histiocytosis with life-threatening pulmonary involvement: good response to cyclosporine A. *Med Pediatr Oncol* 2000;35:438–442.

96. Gadner H, Grois N, Arico M, et al. A randomized trial of treatment for multisystem Langerhans' cell histiocytosis. *J Pediatr* 2001;138:728–734.

97. Minkov M, Grois N, Broadbent V, et al. Cyclosporine A therapy for multisystem Langerhans cell histiocytosis. *Med Pediatr Oncol* 1999;33:482–485.

98. Schonfeld N, Frank W, Wenig S, et al. Clinical and radiologic features, lung function and therapeutic results in pulmonary histiocytosis X. *Respiration* 1993;60:38–44.

99. Etienne B, Bertocchi M, Gamondes JP, et al. Relapsing pulmonary Langerhans cell histiocytosis after lung transplantation. *Am J Respir Crit Care Med* 1998;157:288–291.

100. Boehler A. Lung transplantation for cystic lung disease: lymphangioleiomyomatosis, histiocytosis X, and sarcoidosis. *Semin Respir Crit Care Med* 2001;22:509–516.

101. Habbib B, Congelton J, Carr D, et al. Recurrence of Langerhans' cell histiocytosis following bilateral lung transplantation. *Thorax* 1998;53:323–325.

102. Gabbay E, Dark JH, Ashcroft T, et al. Recurrence of Langerhans' cell granulomatosis following lung transplantation. *Thorax* 1998;53:326–327.

103. Johnson S. Rare diseases, 1: lymphangioleiomyomatosis: clinical features, management and basic mechanisms. *Thorax* 1999;54:254–264.

104. NHLBI workshop summary: report of workshop on lymphangioleiomyomatosis. National Heart, Lung, and Blood Institute. *Am J Respir Crit Care Med* 1999;159:679–683.

105. Urban T, Lazor R, Lacronique J, et al. Pulmonary lymphangioleiomyomatosis: a study of 69 patients: Groupe d'Etudes et de Recherche sur les Maladies "Orphelines" Pulmonaires (GERM"O"P). *Medicine (Baltimore)* 1999;78:321–337.

106. Kitaichi M, Nishimura K, Itoh H, et al. Pulmonary lymphangioleiomyomatosis: a report of 46 patients including a clinicopathologic study of prognostic factors. *Am J Respir Crit Care Med* 1995;151:527–533.

107. Chu SC, Horiba K, Usuki J, et al. Comprehensive evaluation of 35 patients with lymphangioleiomyomatosis. *Chest* 1999;115:1041–1052.

108. Corrin B, Liebow AA, Friedman PJ. Pulmonary lymphangiomyomatosis: a review. *Am J Pathol* 1975;79:348–382.

109. Johnson SR, Tattersfield AE. Clinical experience of lymphangioleiomyomatosis in the UK. *Thorax* 2000;55:1052–1057.

110. Oh YM, Mo EK, Jang SH, et al. Pulmonary lymphangioleiomyomatosis in Korea. *Thorax* 1999;54:618–621.

111. Aubry MC, Myers JL, Ryu JH, et al. Pulmonary lymphangioleiomyomatosis in a man. *Am J Respir Crit Care Med* 2000;162:749–752.

112. Silverstein EF, Ellis K, Wolff M, et al. Pulmonary lymphangiomyomatosis. *Am J Roentgenol Radium Ther Nucl Med* 1974;120:832–850.

113. Taylor JR, Ryu J, Colby TV, et al. Lymphangioleiomyomatosis: clinical course in 32 patients. *N Engl J Med* 1990;323:1254–1260.

114. Crausman RS, Jennings CA, Mortenson RL, et al. Lymphangioleiomyomatosis: the pathophysiology of diminished exercise capacity. *Am J Respir Crit Care Med* 1996;153:1368–1376.

115. Muller NL, Chiles C, Kullnig P. Pulmonary lymphangiomy-

116. Crausman RS, Lynch DA, Mortenson RL, et al. Quantitative CT predicts the severity of physiologic dysfunction in patients with lymphangioleiomyomatosis. *Chest* 1996;109:131–137.

117. Lynch JP III, Orens J, Kazerooni EA. Collagen vascular diseases. In: Sperber M, ed. *Diffuse lung diseases: a comprehensive clinical-radiological overview.* New York: Springer-Verlag, 1999:325–355.

118. Hayashi T, Fleming MV, Stetler-Stevenson WG, et al. Immunohistochemical study of matrix metalloproteinases (MMPs) and their tissue inhibitors (TIMPs) in pulmonary lymphangioleiomyomatosis (LAM). *Hum Pathol* 1997;28:1071–1078.

119. Matsui K, Tatsuguchi A, Valencia J, et al. Extrapulmonary lymphangioleiomyomatosis (LAM): clinicopathologic features in 22 cases. *Hum Pathol* 2000;31:1242–1248.

120. Avila NA, Kelly JA, Chu SC, et al. Lymphangioleiomyomatosis: abdominopelvic CT and US findings. *Radiology* 2000;216:147–153.

121. Woodring JH, Howard RS 2nd, Johnson MV. Massive low-attenuation mediastinal, retroperitoneal, and pelvic lymphadenopathy on CT from lymphangioleiomyomatosis: case report. *Clin Imaging* 1994;18:7–11.

122. Peccatori I, Pitingolo F, Battini G, et al. Pulmonary lymphangioleiomyomatosis and tuberous sclerosis complex. *Contrib Nephrol* 1997;122:98–101.

123. Roach ES, Smith M, Huttenlocher P, et al. Diagnostic criteria: tuberous sclerosis complex: report of the diagnostic criteria committee of the National Tuberous Sclerosis Association. *J Child Neurol* 1992;7:221–24.

124. Bonetti F, Chiodera P. Lymphangioleiomyomatosis and tuberous sclerosis: where is the border? *Eur Respir J* 1996;9:399–401.

125. Torres VE, Bjornsson J, King BF, et al. Extrapulmonary lymphangioleiomyomatosis and lymphangiomatous cysts in tuberous sclerosis complex. *Mayo Clin Proc* 1995;70:641–648.

126. Castro M, Shepherd CW, Gomez MR, et al. Pulmonary tuberous sclerosis. *Chest* 1995;107:189–195.

127. Moss J, Avila NA, Barnes PM, et al. Prevalence and clinical characteristics of lymphangioleiomyomatosis (LAM) in patients with tuberous sclerosis complex. *Am J Respir Crit Care Med* 2001;164:669–671.

128. Costello LC, Hartman TE, Ryu JH. High frequency of pulmonary lymphangioleiomyomatosis in women with tuberous sclerosis complex. *Mayo Clin Proc* 2000;75:591–594.

129. Bernstein SM, Newell JD Jr, Adamczyk D, et al. How common are renal angiomyolipomas in patients with pulmonary lymphangiomyomatosis? *Am J Respir Crit Care Med* 1995;152:2138–2143.

130. Maziak DE, Kesten S, Rappaport DC, et al. Extrathoracic angiomyolipomas in lymphangioleiomyomatosis. *Eur Respir J* 1996;9:402–405.

131. Avila N, Chen CC, Chu SC, et al. Pulmonary lymphangioleiomyomatosis: correlation of ventilation-perfusion scintigraphy, chest radiography, and CT with pulmonary function tests. *Radiology* 2000;214:441–446.

132. Matsui K, Takeda K, Yu Z, et al. Downregulation of estrogen and progesterone receptors in the abnormal smooth muscle cells in pulmonary lymphangioleiomyomatosis following therapy: an immunohistochemical study. *Am J Respir Crit Care Med* 2000;161:1002–1009.

133. Chan JK, Tsang WY, Pau MY, et al. Lymphangiomyomatosis and angiomyolipoma: closely related entities characterized by hamartomatous proliferation of HMB-45–positive smooth muscle. *Histopathology* 1993;22:445–455.

134. Guinee DG Jr, Feuerstein I, Koss MN, et al. Pulmonary

lymphangioleiomyomatosis. diagnosis based on results of transbronchial biopsy and immunohistochemical studies and correlation with high-resolution computed tomography findings. *Arch Pathol Lab Med* 1994;118:846–849.

135. Matsui K, Takeda K, Yu ZX, et al. Role for activation of matrix metalloproteinases in the pathogenesis of pulmonary lymphangioleiomyomatosis. *Arch Pathol Lab Med* 2000;124:267–275.

136. Ohori NP, Yousem SA, Sonmez-Alpan E, et al. Estrogen and progesterone receptors in lymphangioleiomyomatosis, epithelioid hemangioendothelioma, and sclerosing hemangioma of the lung. *Am J Clin Pathol* 1991;96:529–535.

137. Kalassian KG, Doyle R, Kao P, et al. Lymphangioleiomyomatosis: new insights. *Am J Respir Crit Care Med* 1997;155:1183–1186.

138. Han YM, Kim JK, Roh BS, et al. Renal angiomyolipoma: selective arterial embolization: effectiveness and changes in angiomyogenic components in long-term follow up. *Radiology* 1997;204:65–70.

139. Johnson SR, Tattersfield AE. Decline in lung function in lymphangioleiomyomatosis: relation to menopause and progesterone treatment. *Am J Respir Crit Care Med* 1999;160:628–633.

140. Rossi GA, Balbi B, Oddera S, et al. Response to treatment with an analog of the luteinizing-hormone–releasing hormone in a patient with pulmonary lymphangioleiomyomatosis. *Am Rev Respir Dis* 1991;143:174–176.

141. Radermecker M, Broux R, Corhay JL, et al. Failure of buserelin-induced medical castration to control pulmonary lymphangiomyomatosis in two patients. *Chest* 1992;101:1724–1726.

142. Klein M, Krieger O, Ruckser R, et al. Treatment of lymphangioleiomyomatosis by ovariectomy, interferon α_{2b} and tamoxifen: a case report. *Arch Gynecol Obstet* 1992;252:99–102.

143. DeBove P, Murris-Espin M, Buscail L, et al. Somatostatin receptors in pulmonary lymphangioleiomyomatosis: therapeutic relevance. *Eur Respir J* 1997;10[Suppl 25]:297S.

144. Boehler A, Speich R, Russi EW, et al. Lung transplantation for lymphangioleiomyomatosis. *N Engl J Med* 1996;335:1275–1280.

145. Bittmann I, Dose TB, Muller C, et al. Lymphangioleiomyomatosis: recurrence after single lung transplantation. *Hum Pathol* 1997;28:1420–1423.

146. Nine JS, Yousem SA, Paradis IL, et al. Lymphangioleiomyomatosis: recurrence after lung transplantation. *J Heart Lung Transplant* 1994;13:714–719.

147. Falk RH, Comenzo RL, Skinner M. The systemic amyloidoses. *N Engl J Med* 1997;337:898–909.

148. Joss N, McLaughlin K, Simpson K, et al. Presentation, survival and prognostic markers in AA amyloidosis. *QJM* 2000;93:535–542.

149. Utz JP, Swensen SJ, Gertz MA. Pulmonary amyloidosis: the Mayo Clinic experience from 1980 to 1993. *Ann Intern Med* 1996;124:407–413.

150. Kyle RA, Gertz MA, Greipp PR, et al. A trial of three regimens for primary amyloidosis: colchicine alone, melphalan and prednisone, and melphalan, prednisone, and colchicine. *N Engl J Med* 1997;336:1202–1207.

151. Thompson PJ, Citron KM. Amyloid and the lower respiratory tract. *Thorax* 1983;38:84–87.

152. Smith RR, Hutchins GM, Moore GW, et al. Type and distribution of pulmonary parenchymal and vascular amyloid: correlation with cardiac amyloid. *Am J Med* 1979;66:96–104.

153. Celli BR, Rubinow A, Cohen AS, et al. Patterns of pulmonary involvement in systemic amyloidosis. *Chest* 1978;74:543–547.

154. Gillmore JD, Hawkins PN. Amyloidosis and the respiratory tract. *Thorax* 1999;54:444–451.

155. O'Regan A, Fenlon HM, Beamis JF Jr, et al. Tracheobronchial amyloidosis: the Boston University Experience from 1984 to 1999. *Medicine* 2000;79:69–79.

156. Hui AN, Koss MN, Hochholzer L, et al. Amyloidosis presenting in the lower respiratory tract: clinicopathologic, radiologic, immunohistochemical, and histochemical studies on 48 cases. *Arch Pathol Lab Med* 1986;110:212–218.

157. Cordier JF, Loire R, Brune J. Amyloidosis of the lower respiratory tract: clinical and pathologic features in a series of 21 patients. *Chest* 1986;90:827–831.

158. Howard ME, Ireton J, Daniels F, et al. Pulmonary presentations of amyloidosis. *Respirology* 2001;6:61–64.

159. Capizzi SA, Betancourt E, Prakash UB. Tracheobronchial amyloidosis. *Mayo Clin Proc* 2000;75:1148–1152.

160. Holmes S, Desai JB, Sapsford RN. Nodular pulmonary amyloidosis: a case report and review of literature. *Br J Dis Chest* 1988;82:414–417.

161. Nienhuis DM, Prakash UB, Edell ES. Tracheobronchopathia osteochondroplastica. *Ann Otol Rhinol Laryngol* 1990;99:689–694.

162. Leske V, Lazor R, Coetmeur D, et al. Tracheobronchopathia osteochondroplastica: a study of 41 patients. *Medicine (Baltimore)* 2001;80:378–390.

163. Quint LE, Whyte RI, Kazerooni EA, et al. Stenosis of the central airways: evaluation by using helical CT with multiplanar reconstructions. *Radiology* 1995;194:871–877.

164. Lynch J P III, Quint L. Tracheobronchial and esophageal manifestations of systemic diseases. In: Cummings CW, ed. *Otolaryngology: head and neck surgery*, 3rd ed. St. Louis: Mosby–Year Book, 1998:2343–2367.

165. Mumford AD, O'Donnell J, Gillmore JD, et al. Bleeding symptoms and coagulation abnormalities in 337 patients with AL-amyloidosis. *Br J Haematol* 2000;110:454–460.

166. Pitkanen P, Westermark P, Cornwell GG III. Senile systemic amyloidosis. *Am J Pathol* 1984;117:391–399.

167. Conaghan P, Chung D, Vaughan R. Recurrent laryngeal nerve palsy associated with mediastinal amyloidosis. *Thorax* 2000;55:436–437.

168. Urschel JD, Urschel DM. Mediastinal amyloidosis. *Ann Thorac Surg* 2000;69:944–946.

169. Khan JA, Shamsi SH, Rana TA, et al. Pulmonary amyloidosis: a case with hilar and mediastinal involvement and a review of the literature. *Clin Pulm Med* 1996;2:66–69.

170. Romero Candeira S, Martin Serrano C, Hernandez Blasco L. Amyloidosis and pleural disease. *Chest* 1991;100:292–293.

171. Kavuru MS, Adamo JP, Ahmad M, et al. Amyloidosis and pleural disease. *Chest* 1990;98:20–23.

172. Thompson LD, Derringer GA, Wenig BM. Amyloidosis of the larynx: a clinicopathologic study of 11 cases. *Mod Pathol* 2000;13:528–535.

173. Lim JK, Lacy MQ, Kurtin PJ, et al. Pulmonary marginal zone lymphoma of MALT type as a cause of localised pulmonary amyloidosis. *J Clin Pathol* 2001;54:642–646.

174. Yood RA, Skinner M, Rubinow A, et al. Bleeding manifestations in 100 patients with amyloidosis. *JAMA* 1983;249:1322–1324.

175. Skinner M, Anderson J, Simms R, et al. Treatment of 100 patients with primary amyloidosis: a randomized trial of melphalan, prednisone, and colchicine versus colchicine only. *Am J Med* 1996;100:290–298.

176. Sezer O, Niemoller K, Jakob C, et al. Novel approaches to the treatment of primary amyloidosis. *Expert Opin Invest Drugs* 2000;9:2343–2350.

177. Gertz MA, Kyle RA. Phase II trial of recombinant interferon

alfa-2 in the treatment of primary systemic amyloidosis. *Am J Hematol* 1993;44:125–128.

178. Dispenzieri A, Lacy MQ, Kyle RA, et al. Eligibility for hematopoietic stem-cell transplantation for primary systemic amyloidosis is a favorable prognostic factor for survival. *J Clin Oncol* 2001;19:3350–3356.

179. Reich G, Held T, Siegert W, et al. Four patients with AL amyloidosis treated with high-dose chemotherapy and autologous stem cell transplantation. *Bone Marrow Transplant* 2001;27:341–343.

180. Dember LM, Sanchorawala V, Seldin DC, et al. Effect of dose-intensive intravenous melphalan and autologous blood stem-cell transplantation on AL amyloidosis–associated renal disease. *Ann Intern Med* 2001;134:746–753.

181. Ichida M, Imagawa S, Ohmine K, et al. Successful treatment of multiple myeloma—associated amyloidosis by interferon-α, dimethyl sulfoxide, and VAD (vincristine, adriamycin, and dexamethasone). *Int J Hematol* 2000;72:491–493.

182. Madden BP, Lee M, Paruchuru P. Successful treatment of endobronchial amyloidosis using Nd:YAG laser therapy as an alternative to lobectomy. *Monaldi Arch Chest Dis* 2001;56:27–29.

183. Mazzantini D, Pazzagli M, Cagno MC, et al. Long-term survival in primary amyloidosis of the laryngotracheobronchial tract by treating complications only. *Monaldi Arch Chest Dis* 2000;55:114–116.

184. Kalra S, Utz JP, Edell ES, et al. External-beam radiation therapy in the treatment of diffuse tracheobronchial amyloidosis. *Mayo Clin Proc* 2001;76:853–856.

Baum's Textbook of Pulmonary Diseases, 7th ed. Edited by James D. Crapo, Jeffrey Glassroth, Joel Karlinsky, and Talmadge E. King, Jr.
Lippincott Williams & Wilkins, Philadelphia © 2004.

Drug-Induced Pulmonary Disease

33

Roberto F. Machado · Raed A. Dweik

Stephen L. Demeter · Muzaffar Ahmad

Since the publication of the first major review of 19 drugs causing pulmonary toxicity in 1972 (1), the lung has been recognized increasingly often as a target organ. Currently, more than 150 pharmacologic agents have been reported to cause adverse pulmonary reactions (2). In drug-induced pulmonary disease, the clinical presentation, radiologic findings, and histologic findings are mostly nonspecific. Therefore, in the appropriate clinical setting, a high index of suspicion should always be maintained.

In this chapter, we provide a brief overview of drug-induced pulmonary disease. We aimed to include the best available evidence regarding diagnostic and treatment recommendations, which are unfortunately, in the majority of cases, not substantiated by prospective controlled trials. A detailed review of the pathophysiology of drug-induced lung disease is beyond the scope of this review. In the first part of the chapter, we discuss various pleuropulmonary patterns of response to drugs (3). The second part addresses the pulmonary effects of different categories of drugs.

Table 33.1 summarizes the more common clinical presentations of pulmonary toxicity induced by noncytotoxic medications, including illicit drugs, and Table 33.2 does the same for pulmonary toxicity induced by cytotoxic agents, including radiation. Some unusual manifestations of drug-induced pulmonary toxicity are listed in Table 33.3. Not all the medications listed in the tables are discussed in the text.

PATTERNS OF RESPONSE

Hypersensitivity-Type Reactions

Pulmonary responses to some drugs may be best thought of in terms of a hypersensitivity reaction (Table 33.1). Typ-

R. F. Machado, R. A. Dweik, and **M. Ahmad:** Department of Pulmonary and Critical Care Medicine, Cleveland Clinic Foundation, Cleveland, Ohio.

S. L. Demeter: Division of Pulmonary Medicine, Northeastern Ohio Universities College of Medicine, Rootstown, Ohio.

ically, the symptoms consist of cough, dyspnea, and fever, with the appearance of an infiltrate on the chest x-ray film. Occasionally, a pleural effusion is seen. In some instances, there may be laboratory manifestations characteristic of hypersensitivity responses, such as peripheral eosinophilia or, more specifically, a positive lymphocyte transformation test response to the offending drug. The adverse response usually remits after cessation of the drug. Corticosteroids may hasten the recovery, although they are generally not needed.

Noncardiogenic Pulmonary Edema

Several factors are responsible for the transvascular flow of fluid. One factor, the filtration coefficient of permeability of the vascular endothelium, is believed to be altered in cases of noncardiogenic pulmonary edema. Overdoses of sedatives and narcotics are most commonly associated with altered permeability of the pulmonary vasculature (4). Most patients with noncardiogenic pulmonary edema also display some degree of central nervous system depression; therefore, it is unclear whether the response represents a drug effect, "neurogenic pulmonary edema," or a combination of the two. Other drugs that cause noncardiogenic pulmonary edema characteristically produce an idiosyncratic response within minutes to hours after absorption.

Interstitial Pneumonitis or Fibrosis

A number of drugs have the potential for causing either an interstitial pneumonitis (acute or chronic inflammatory changes) or an interstitial fibrosis. The interstitial pneumonitis has many of the features of a hypersensitivity state, and the difference may be semantic rather than real. The more common histopathologic finding of interstitial fibrosis is usually manifested by slowly progressive dyspnea and cough in association with progressive reticular opacities in the radiograph.

TABLE 33.1. CLINICAL PRESENTATION OF PULMONARY TOXICITY INDUCED BY NONCYTOTOXIC DRUGS

	PIE	Noncardiogenic Pulmonary Edema	Interstitial Pneumonitis or Fibrosis	Acute Pleural Effusion	Chronic Pleural Effusion	PVD	Parenchymal Hemorrhage	Drug-Induced SLE	BOOP	Asthma
Anorexigens										
Dexfenfluramine						+				
Fenfluramine						+				
Antiinflammatory										
Acetylsalicylic acid		+								+
Colchicine		+								
Gold			+						+	
Interleukin-2		+								
Methotrexate	+		+	+	+				+	
NSAID										+
Penicillamine			+				+		+	
Antimicrobial										
Amphotericin B							+			
Ethambutol	+									
Isoniazid								+		
Nitrofurantoin	+		+	+			+			
Para-aminosalicylic acid	+									
Penicillins	+									
Pentamidine										+
Sulfasalazine	+		+						+	+
Tetracycline	+									
Cardiovascular										
α-Methyldopa								+		
Amiodarone			+	+				+	+	
Anticoagulants				+			+			
β-Blockers										+
Dipyridamole										+
Flecainide			+							
Hydralazine							+	+		
Hydrochlorothiazide	+									
Lidocaine		+								
Procainamide								+		
Propafenone								+		
Tocainide			+							
Illicit drugs										
Cocaine		+					+			+
Heroin		+	+							
Methadone	+									
Methylphenidate						+				
Psychotropic/antiepileptic										
Carbamazepine	+									
Diphenylhydantoin	+									
Phenothiazine		+								
Trazodone	+									
Tricyclics	+									
Miscellaneous										
Bromocriptine				+						
Contrast media										+
Esophageal variceal sclerotherapy agents			+							
Estrogen						+				
Timolol (ophthalmic)										+
Tocolytic agents		+								

PIE, pulmonary infiltrate with eosinophilia; PVD, pulmonary vascular disease; SLE, serum lupus erythematosus; BOOP, bronchiolitis obliterans organizing pneumonia; NSAID, nonsteroidal anti-inflammatory drug.

As expected, this syndrome may be confused with idiopathic pulmonary fibrosis.

Pleural Effusions

An acute pleural effusion in association with drugs has been reported to be part of hypersensitivity reactions or in the setting of drug-induced serum lupus erythematosus. Anticoagulants cause effusion by leading to pleural hemorrhage in the setting of pulmonary infarction or, less commonly, without any predisposing abnormality (5, 6). Chronic pleural effusion develops after long-term use of dantrolene (7), as a manifestation of a retarded hypersensitivity-like response or in association with interstitial fibrosis. Other pleural

TABLE 33.2. CLINICAL PRESENTATION OF PULMONARY TOXICITY INDUCED BY CYTOTOXIC DRUGS AND RADIATION

	Hypersensitivity Infiltrate	PIE	Noncardiogenic Pulmonary Edema	IP-F	Acute Pleural Effusion	Chronic Pleural Effusion	PVD	Parenchymal Hemorrhage	BOOP	Asthma
Azathioprine	+	+						+		
Bleomycin		+		+			+		+	
Busulfan	+			+						
Chlorambucil				+						
Cyclophosphamide				+					+	
Cytosine arabinoside			+							
Fludarabine				+						
Gemcitabine			+							
Melphalan				+						
Methotrexate		+		+					+	
Mitomycin C			+	+	+	+			+	+
Nitrosoureas				+			+			
Paclitaxel				+						+
Procarbazine	+									
Radiation, acute	+	+			+		+	+	+	
Retinoic Acid			+							
Vinca alkaloids (with mitomycin)										+

PIE, pulmonary infiltrate with eosinophilia; IP-F, interstitial pneumonitis or fibrosis; PVD, pulmonary vascular disease; BOOP, bronchiolitis obliterans organizing pneumonia.

manifestations of drug toxicity will be discussed in the next section.

Pulmonary Vascular Responses

Intravenous illicit drugs such as cocaine and amphetamines, as well as their diluents, that are filtered by the pulmonary capillaries are capable of causing angiitis and pulmonary hypertension (8–10). Pulmonary hypertension has also been associated with chronic abuse of inhaled methamphetamine (11).

TABLE 33.3. UNUSUAL MANIFESTATIONS OF DRUG-INDUCED PULMONARY TOXICITY

Presentation	Causative Agent(s)
Alveolar proteinosis	Busulfan
Bronchial necrosis	Radiation therapy, brachytherapy
Bronchospasm (paradoxical)	β_2-adrenergic agonists Intravenous hydrocortisone
Calcification (parenchymal)	Antacids, calcium, phosphorus, vitamin D
Cough	Angiotensin-converting enzyme inhibitors
Goodpasture syndrome	Penicillamine
Lung mass(es) ± cavitation	Amiodarone, bleomycin
Mediastinal lipomatosis	Corticosteroids
Mediastinal widening/ lymphadenopathy	Diphenylhydantoin, methotrexate
Mediastinitis	Esophageal variceal sclerotherapy
Panlobular emphysema	Methylphenidate
Pneumothorax	Nitrosoureas, bleomycin
Pseudosepsis syndrome	Chronic salicylate intoxication

More recently, the anorexic agents fenfluramine and dexfenfluramine have been implicated in the development of pulmonary arterial hypertension. In a case control study (12), the use of anorexic drugs was associated with an odds ratio of 6.3 for the development of pulmonary hypertension. Although the risk was highest with long-term use (>3 months), a case of fatal pulmonary hypertension has been reported in a patient taking a combination of fenfluramine and phentermine for only 23 days (13).

An increase in the risk of venous thromboembolism is seen with oral contraceptive use with both high- or low-dose estrogen preparations (14, 15). The risk may vary, however, depending on the progestin used—being higher with preparations containing desogestrel and gestodene (16, 17). Pulmonary veno-occlusive disease has been reported in association with bis-chloroethylnitrosourea (BCNU), bleomycin, and mitomycin (18–21).

Pulmonary Parenchymal Calcification

Drug-related calcium deposition in the lungs is very rare. It is usually associated with the soft tissue calcification seen in the milk-alkali syndrome or with hypercalcemic states of other causes. Drugs known to have precipitated calcium deposition include antacids (22), calcium (23), phosphorus (24), and high doses of vitamin D (25) (Table 33.3).

Parenchymal Hemorrhage

Hemoptysis as the manifestation of an adverse drug effect is most frequently caused by a drug-related pulmonary embolus, leading to pulmonary infarction. Pulmonary hemorrhage and hemoptysis can be a manifestation of toxicity of a significant number of drugs (Tables 33.1 and 33.2).

Spontaneous pulmonary hemorrhage has been reported in patients who were taking oral anticoagulants, as well as in patients receiving heparin(26, 27) or thrombolytic therapy (28–30). Initial symptoms are dyspnea, hemoptysis, and cough or an infiltrate on the chest roentgenogram.

Mediastinal Manifestations

Although not necessarily representing a pulmonary disease, adverse mediastinal responses appear initially as an abnormality on the chest x-ray film. Diphenylhydantoin occasionally produces a pseudolymphoma syndrome, manifested as peripheral and occasionally mediastinal lymphadenopathy (31, 32) (Table 33.3). Transient hilar adenopathy may accompany a hypersensitivity-like response to methotrexate (33). Mediastinal lipomatosis resulting from chronic corticosteroid use or Cushing syndrome is a well-recognized entity (34, 35).

Drug-Induced Lupus Erythematosus

A number of drugs have been implicated in the syndrome of drug-induced lupus erythematosus, especially those agents that are metabolized by acetylation (Table 33.1). The disease is more likely to develop and to develop sooner in patients who are slow acetylators (36–38).

The lungs and pleurae seem to be involved more frequently in drug-induced than in spontaneous systemic lupus erythematosus (39, 40). Patterns of response include the following: (a) pleural effusion with or without pleuritic pain, (b) pleuritic chest pain with or without effusion, (c) atelectatic pneumonitis, (d) diffuse interstitial pneumonitis, and (e) alveolar opacities. Positive antihistone antibodies are present in greater than 95% of the cases, whereas other autoantibodies are uncommonly present (38). The pleuropulmonary manifestations usually regress with discontinuation of the offending drug.

Drug-Induced Bronchospasm/Asthma

Drug-induced bronchospasm is caused by a variety of agents (Tables 33.1, 33.2). β-Blockers are known to induce bronchospasm in asthmatics (41, 42) and in some patients with chronic obstructive pulmonary disease (43). Bronchospasm can develop even with the administration of timolol ophthalmic solution; it was, however, not demonstrated with betaxolol use (44). Dipyridamole increases the concentration of the bronchoconstrictor adenosine, which can cause significant bronchospasm in some patients with underlying obstructive lung disease. Theophylline is the drug of choice for treatment and/or prophylaxis in these patients.

Vinblastine appears to act synergistically with mitomycin to produce bronchospasm (45). Administration of nebulized or intravenous pentamidine (46, 47) or propellants can further irritate already hyper-reactive airways (48, 49). Paradoxical bronchospasm (Table 33.3) has been reported with the use of nebulized β-agonists (50), as well as intravenous hydrocortisone (not reported with other steroid preparations). There is anecdotal evidence that patients developing paradoxical bronchospasm with β-agonists may benefit from the newly available levo/albuterol preparation. Estrogen therapy may worsen bronchospasm in women with chronic obstructive lung disease or asthma, and estrogen therapy may even be associated with the onset of asthma (51, 52).

Acetylsalicylic acid produces bronchospasm in 0.3% of normal adults (53) and from 4% to 20% of asthmatic patients (54). The acetylsalicylic acid (ASA) triad is a syndrome characterized by asthma, nasal polyposis, and drug sensitivity (55). Furthermore, other nonsteroidal anti-inflammatory agents (NSAIDs) can produce a similar reaction and should be avoided in ASA-sensitive patients(56, 57).

The first manifestation of the syndrome is vasomotor rhinitis with a watery discharge. Typically, this develops in the second or third decade in a person who is not atopic and who has previously taken ASA. The reaction is at first intermittent, later perennial. It is followed by the appearance of nasal polyps, and by midlife, most patients demonstrate an asthmatic response.

The syndrome is not a hypersensitivity response, despite the asthma and angioedema that may be seen after absorption of the drugs. It seems to be mediated by the proinflammatory and bronchoconstrictive properties of active metabolites of arachidonic acid derived through the action of 5-lipoxygenase (58–62). Treatment starts with avoidance of the offending drug. In addition, leukotriene modifiers have been shown to improve pulmonary function and decrease β-agonist use in patients already receiving corticosteroids (63). ASA desensitization can improve refractory upper and lower airway symptoms (64) but is usually reserved to severe cases or when ASA use is absolutely necessary. Nasal polypectomy is reserved for symptoms of nasal obstruction only; it does not alter the response to ASA, and the polyps usually recur.

Bronchiolitis Obliterans Organizing Pneumonia

Bronchiolitis obliterans with organizing pneumonia (BOOP) has been described as a response to a variety of medications (Tables 33.1 and 33.2). Patients frequently have isolated or patchy air space opacities indistinguishable from those of idiopathic BOOP. This reaction is usually reversible with discontinuation of the drug and sometimes requires treatment with corticosteroids.

EFFECTS OF SPECIFIC DRUGS

Anti-Inflammatory Agents and Biologic Response Modifiers

Overdoses of ASA can produce central respiratory stimulation and noncardiogenic pulmonary edema likely owing to increased vascular permeability (65, 66). Risk factors for the development of pulmonary edema include increasing age, history of smoking, chronic salicylate ingestion, and salicylate levels greater than 30 mg/dL. The pulmonary capillary wedge pressure is normal, and although abnormalities on chest x-ray films may take 3 to 8 days to clear, the prognosis is good (66). Chronic salicylate intoxication has been associated with a pseudoseptic syndrome characterized by fever, hyperdynamic shock, and multiorgan failure (67).

Methotrexate is currently used in low doses as an antiinflammatory drug for many conditions, especially rheumatoid arthritis and Wegener granulomatosis. Typically, the patient is given less than 20 mg weekly. The prevalence of pulmonary toxicity in these patients is 3% to 5% (68–70), and most cases occur within 2 years of initiation of therapy. In a case control study (71) increasing age (odds ratio [OR], 5.1), presence of diabetes (OR, 35.6), hypoalbuminemia (OR, 19.5), use of disease modifying antirheumatic drugs (OR, 5.6), and rheumatoid pleuropulmonary involvement (OR, 7.1) were independent predictors for the development of pulmonary toxicity. The onset is insidious and associated with cough, dyspnea, and low-grade fever. Radiographically, the disease most commonly reveals basal or diffuse interstitial opacities that can progress to diffuse air space disease. Pulmonary function studies classically demonstrate a restrictive pattern with a decrease in carbon monoxide diffusing capacity (DLCO). There are, however, some reports suggesting development of airflow obstruction with methotrexate therapy (72, 73). Unfortunately, in a prospective evaluation of 124 patients receiving low-dose methotrexate, surveillance with pulmonary function tests (spirometry, lung volumes, and DLCO) did not allow for detection of toxicity prior to the onset of symptoms (70). Bronchoalveolar lavage fluid demonstrates an increase in CD4$^+$ lymphocytes (74), a nonspecific finding seen in a variety of inflammatory lung diseases. Histologically, changes resembling hypersensitivity pneumonitis (loosely formed granulomas) overlapping with a chronic interstitial pneumonitis are seen in most patients; BOOP and diffuse alveolar damage were also demonstrated in a few cases (68, 75–77). The majority of patients improve with discontinuation of the drug. Corticosteroids have been recommended based on favorable clinical response in case series and expert opinions, but no controlled studies have examined its efficacy.

Penicillamine can cause unique pulmonary complications, including diffuse alveolitis (78, 79), hypersensitivity pneumonitis (80, 81), Goodpasture syndrome (82–84), and obliterative bronchiolitis (85–89). The disease is often fatal in cases of Goodpasture syndrome (three deaths out of five patients reported) or obliterative bronchiolitis (50% mortality in the listed series). The majority of reported patients with alveolitis or hypersensitivity pneumonitis improved with discontinuation of the drug.

A total of 140 cases of *gold-induced* pulmonary toxicity have been reported (90), which manifested as a chronic interstitial pneumonitis, bronchiolitis obliterans, or BOOP. There is no documented relationship between total cumulative dose and the development of lung toxicity (90, 91). Dyspnea and cough are the presenting symptoms. Fever and a concurrent skin rash are seen in 47% and 38% of the cases, respectively. Eosinophilia is seen in about 38% of cases (90). Symptoms usually resolve with discontinuation of the drug. Complete reversal of the pulmonary disease has been demonstrated with corticosteroids in case series (92, 93).

The leukotriene inhibitors *zafirlukast* (94, 95), *montelukast* (96, 97), and *pranlukast* (98) have been associated with the development of Churg-Strauss syndrome in asthmatics. It is not clear whether the syndrome develops because of the use of the leukotriene inhibitors or it is unmasked because of the dose reduction or discontinuation of systemic steroid use achieved by the introduction of the leukotriene antagonists. The latter hypothesis is supported by the occurrence of Churg-Straus syndrome in patients switched from systemic to inhaled corticosteroids (99). However, in one case report the syndrome was reported in one patient given montelukast in the absence of systemic steroid use (100).

Pulmonary edema likely owing to a combination of increased capillary permeability and fluid overload has been reported in association with treatment with *interleukin-2* (101–103). An asymptomatic isolated decrease in diffusing capacity was demonstrated in patients receiving recombinant *tumor necrosis factor* for the treatment of metastatic malignancies (104).

Antimicrobial Agents

Pulmonary toxicity is the most severe adverse effect of *nitrofurantoin* therapy. It seems to be an infrequent complication given the extensive use of the drug. In fact, during a 16-year period, 237 cases of adverse pleuropulmonary reactions were reported in an estimated 44 million courses of the drug (105). Reactions to nitrofurantoin are classified in two types: acute, developing hours to days after the institution of treatment, and chronic, occurring after weeks to years of continuous therapy. The former is more common, being reported in approximately 90% of cases of toxicity in two series (106, 107). In the acute form, fever is seen in approximately 80% of cases in conjunction with cough, dyspnea, rash (20%), and arthralgias (10%–15%) (107). In the patients with the chronic form, fever and rash are not seen, and the respiratory symptoms develop more insidiously. Peripheral blood eosinophilia occurs in 83% of individuals with the acute form (106, 107). Radiographic abnormalities are seen in the vast majority of patients and, most commonly, include diffuse alveolar or interstitial infiltrates. Pleural effusions may be present in conjunction with the parenchymal abnormalities or as an isolated finding.

In the acute form, histologic findings seem to represent a type I hypersensitivity response, including signs of pulmonary vasculitis and interstitial and alveolar monomorphonuclear or polymorphonuclear inflammation with variable presence of eosinophilia (105). Other uncommonly reported findings include diffuse alveolar damage (108), desquamative interstitial pneumonitis–like reaction (107), hypersensitivity pneumonitis–like reaction (109), BOOP (110), and diffuse alveolar hemorrhage (111). A chronic interstitial pneumonia resembling usual interstitial pneumonia is the commonest pathologic finding in patients with chronic nitrofurantoin pulmonary toxicity (107).

Discontinuation of the drug is the mainstay of therapy in both forms of nitrofurantoin pulmonary toxicity. Eighty-eight percent of patients with the acute reactions will have resolution of symptoms within 3 days of discontinuation of the drug. Clinical improvement is slower (weeks to months) in the chronic form (107). Beneficial effects of steroid use have only been demonstrated in case reports (110, 112, 113), and in a series of 447 patients, its use did not accelerate recovery (107). In that same cohort, six cases were fatal, four of which occurred in patients with the chronic form of toxicity.

Sulfasalazine has been reported to cause several pulmonary reactions, including pulmonary infiltrates with eosinophilia (114, 115), hypersensitivity pneumonitis (116), BOOP (117), desquamative interstitial pneumonitis (118), pulmonary fibrosis (115, 119, 120), and bronchospasm (121). Pulmonary function studies can demonstrate both a restrictive or obstructive pattern (114, 120). One patient with bronchospasm (121) and another with bronchiolitis (120) had resolution of their symptoms with steroid use.

A number of *antimicrobials* have been associated with an eosinophilic or hypersensitivity lung reactions, including tetracycline (122), minocycline (123, 124), sulfonamides (125, 126), penicillins (127, 128), para-aminosalicylic acid (129), and ethambutol (130). Fatal pulmonary hemorrhage was demonstrated in 14 of 22 patients receiving amphotericin B in association with granulocyte transfusions (131). Although the effect was not demonstrated in another study (132), a real association cannot be discarded.

Cardiovascular Agents

Amiodarone, an antiarrhythmic drug, can cause pulmonary toxicity in about 6% of patients receiving the drug (133–135). The diagnosis of amiodarone pneumonitis is really one of exclusion. Pulmonary embolism, congestive heart failure, and pneumonia are the main differential diagnoses in pa-

tients suspected of having amiodarone pulmonary toxicity, and they should be excluded first.

Most of the reported patients have received daily doses greater than 400 mg for 2 months or more (133, 136–139). Pulmonary disease can occur with maintenance daily doses less than 400 mg (140–143), but the incidence is lower (1.6%), as reported from combined placebo controlled trials involving 3,439 patients (144). Preexisting lung disease does not seem to increase the risk of development of toxicity, as evidenced by a lack of accelerated decrease in diffusing capacity in patients with COPD receiving amiodarone versus those receiving placebo in a randomized trial (145).

The most common clinical presentation is a chronic interstitial pneumonitis characterized by insidious onset of dyspnea, dry cough, weakness, weight loss, and occasionally fever (133, 135, 136, 140, 146). Organizing pneumonia, presenting more acutely than does chronic interstitial pneumonitis, is seen in 25% of cases (147, 148). A picture suggestive of adult respiratory distress syndrome (ARDS) has been described in patients undergoing general anesthesia for surgical procedures (149–152) or after pulmonary angiography (153). Furthermore, in a retrospective study of 67 patients undergoing map-guided surgical procedures for ventricular tachycardia, the incidence of postoperative acute respiratory failure was 17% in patients previously receiving amiodarone and zero in the patients not exposed to the drug ($P = .03$) (154). Finally, in an unusual presentation, amiodarone pulmonary toxicity may take the form of parenchymal mass lesion(s), which may show cavitation (155, 156) (Table 33.3).

Chest radiographs usually reveal a diffuse reticular pattern or bilateral air space disease and, less commonly, nodular infiltrates or masses, pleural thickening, and pleural effusions (136, 157). Computed tomography (CT) of the lung without the administration of contrast (Fig. 33.1) may be helpful in making the diagnosis. Infiltrates caused by amiodarone toxicity have a high attenuation value (because the drug is an iodinated compound) and appear more dense than do usual infiltrates of other etiologies (158). A positive gallium scan can help differentiate amiodarone pneumonitis from pulmonary embolism or congestive heart failure (in which the gallium scan is negative) as long as infection has been excluded as a cause for the positive scan (159, 160). One important limitation of the gallium scan was evidenced by the lack of resolution of the abnormal uptake in three out of six patients with resolving amiodarone toxicity (161). Pulmonary function studies show restrictive defect and decreased DLco, and abnormal results correlate with exposure to the drug (139, 141). As an example, in a trial of 519 patients, use of amiodarone for 1 year resulted in a significant decrease in DLco in comparison to placebo ($P = .02$) (145). Although an isolated decrease in DLco is a sensitive indicator of toxicity, it lacks specificity. In a prospective study evaluating the diagnostic utility of spirometry and DLco in 91 patients on amiodarone (162), none of the 15 patients who had an asymptomatic decrease in diffusing capacity developed

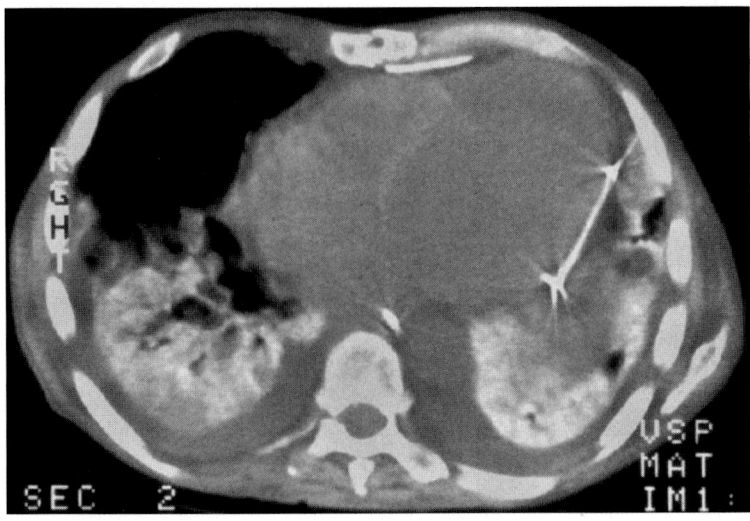

FIGURE 33.1. Non–contrast-enhanced chest computed tomography in amiodarone toxicity. High-attenuation opacities secondary to the presence of iodine in the drug.

pulmonary toxicity despite continuing to take the drug in the 11 months of follow-up. Recently, measurement of serum concentrations of KL-6, a glycoprotein secreted by proliferating type II pneumocytes, has been proposed as a noninvasive marker of amiodarone toxicity. In a small study of 14 men receiving amiodarone (163), KL-6 levels above the upper limit of 520 U/mL were seen in the two patients with pulmonary toxicity as opposed to normal levels in five patients with other pulmonary abnormalities (including pneumonia, congestive heart failure, and bronchogenic carcinoma) and seven asymptomatic individuals.

Histologically, a chronic interstitial pneumonitis associated with accumulation of foamy alveolar macrophages (Fig. 33.2; see also color Fig. 33.2) in the alveolar spaces, hyperplasia of type II pneumocytes, and widening of alveolar septa are the most common findings; diffuse alveolar damage and BOOP are much less common (146, 164). Bronchoalveolar lavage demonstrates the same foamy alveolar macrophages both in patients with or without pulmonary

toxicity, but the absence of this finding makes the diagnosis of toxicity unlikely (164, 165).

Cessation of the drug is the most important aspect of therapy. Corticosteroids have been used in uncontrolled studies and seem to be of greatest value in patients with severe disease and in those in whom the drug cannot be discontinued (166). Furthermore, relapse of toxicity has been demonstrated after withdrawal of steroid therapy (167). Because of its long elimination half-life, amiodarone toxicity can initially progress despite discontinuation of the drug. Overall, the prognosis is favorable, as evidenced in one series by improvement or stabilization in three fourths of patients after discontinuation of the drug with or without steroid treatment (168). However, in patients developing ARDS, mortality can be as high as 50% (164).

Lidocaine used as a local anesthetic caused recurrent noncardiogenic pulmonary edema in one patient (169). *Tocainide* has been associated with the development of interstitial pneumonitis, occurring in average 2 months after initiation of therapy. The majority of patients improve with withdrawal of the drug, although in some cases, steroids were needed to accelerate recovery (170).

Hydrochlorothiazide can cause noncardiogenic pulmonary edema. Patients present with dyspnea, cough, and a low-grade fever within a few hours of taking the medication. The chest roentgenogram shows changes of pulmonary edema; in cases in which the wedge pressure has been measured, it has always been normal. No fatality has been reported. Treatment is supportive, and the patient should avoid the medication thereafter (171).

Angiotensin-converting enzyme (ACE) inhibitors can produce an irritating cough in about 5% to 25% of patients receiving this class of drugs, occurring with all ACE inhibitors and not responding to substitution within the same class (172). The pathogenesis of ACE inhibitor–induced cough likely involves accumulation of kinins and substance P (owing to ACE inhibition), leading to bronchial irritation

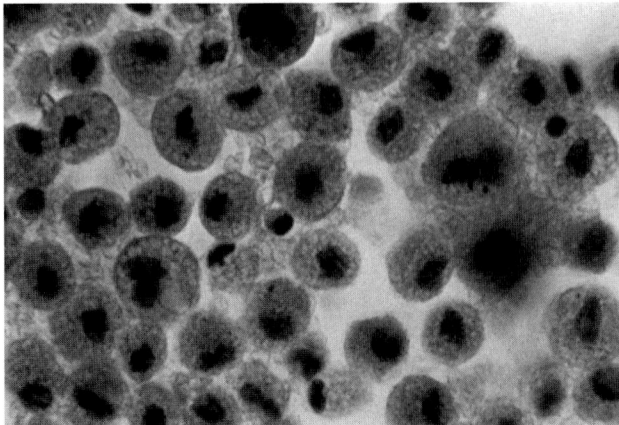

FIGURE 33.2. (See also color Fig. 33.2.) Amiodarone toxicity. Bronchoalveolar lavage cytologic preparation demonstrating foamy appearance of alveolar macrophages.

and cough. Another postulated mechanism is activation of arachidonic acid pathway with consequent elevated levels of thromboxane potentiating the symptoms. In support of this hypothesis in a study using picotamide (an inhibitor of thromboxane synthase and antagonist of the thromboxane receptor) (173), eight of nine patients with cough induced by enalapril had complete resolution of their symptoms. Cough usually completely resolves within 10 days of cessation of therapy (174). *Angiotensin II receptor antagonists,* which do not interfere with the synthesis pathway, are not associated with this side effect and can be used in patients with ACE inhibitor–induced cough (175, 176).

Psychotropic Medications and Anticonvulsants

Overdose of *tricyclic antidepressants* can be associated with pulmonary complications in about one third of cases, usually in the form of noncardiogenic pulmonary edema or aspiration. Treatment is supportive and may include mechanical ventilation. Reported mortality in a series of 82 patients was 6% (177). A series of three cases of *phenothiazine*-induced pulmonary edema has been reported (178). The investigators hypothesized that it is neurogenic in origin, caused by hypothalamic dysfunction. *Trazodone* overdose has been reported to cause eosinophilic pneumonia and respiratory failure (179).

In addition to mediastinal adenopathy, *diphenylhydantoin* has been associated with an acute hypersensitivity reaction characterized by blood and pulmonary eosinophilia and a diffuse reticulonodular pattern on chest radiograph, all of which resolve with discontinuation of the drug (180, 181). A similar presentation is also seen with the use of *carbamazepine* (182, 183).

Illicit Drugs

Opiates and related drugs are well-known causes of pulmonary edema, occurring in 50% to 70% of overdoses (184, 185). It has also been demonstrated with naloxone use, an opiate antagonist (186, 187). Pulmonary edema develops within a few hours of use, and the patient appears with constricted pupils and depressed respiration. The chest radiograph shows alveolar opacities, usually in "bat wing" distribution (188, 189). A high protein concentration in the edema fluid suggests increase in capillary permeability as the etiologic mechanism. The therapy is supportive, with administration of oxygen, narcotic antagonists, and mechanical ventilation if needed.

Cocaine is a highly addictive substance. Pulmonary complications are related to all forms of administration (190, 191). Cough productive of black sputum, dyspnea, chest pain, and hemoptysis occur within minutes of crack cocaine inhalation (192, 193). Pulmonary edema can occur with cocaine regardless of the route of administration, and it has been reported with freebase inhalation (194–196),

intravenous freebase (197), and even "body packing" (smugglers swallowing packets of cocaine, which leak into the gastrointestinal tract). Increased membrane permeability (195) with a possible component of myocardial dysfunction are the mechanisms responsible for the development of pulmonary edema (198). An acute pulmonary syndrome temporally related to inhalation of crack cocaine has also been described and is characterized by fever, hemoptysis, alveolar infiltrates, and respiratory failure (199, 200). Diffuse alveolar damage is the most common pathologic manifestation, and it can be associated with alveolar hemorrhage and eosinophilic infiltration. The patients tend to respond to systemic corticosteroids (200). Other reported complications of smoking freebase cocaine include barotrauma (201), interstitial pneumonitis (199, 200, 202), thermal airway injury (203), bronchospasm (204, 205), and BOOP (206).

Pulmonary edema has been reported with *amphetamine* abuse (207, 208). Early development of panlobular emphysema was described in intravenous abusers of *methylphenidate* (209, 210) and in individuals who inject talc-containing drugs intended for oral use (9).

Miscellaneous Agents

Esophageal variceal sclerotherapy with either *sodium tetradecyl sulfate, ethanolamine, or sodium morrhuate* can cause changes on chest roentgenograms, but these are rarely of clinical significance. Mediastinal widening resulting from noninfectious mediastinitis occurs in 63% of patients (211). Exudative pleural effusion occurs in up to 50% of patients, atelectasis in 16% of patients, and pulmonary infiltrates in 10% of patients (211, 212). Self-limited fever and chest pain are common in the first 24 hours after the procedure. Serious complications, including ARDS and mediastinitis, occur in less than 2% of patients undergoing esophageal sclerotherapy (213), and these should be suspected if the fever and chest pain last for more than 24 hours.

Pleural fibrosis is the most common pleuropulmonary complication of long-term use of *methysergide* (214, 215) or *bromocriptine* (216, 217). In the majority of cases, the abnormalities resolve after discontinuation of the drugs.

Tocolytics (albuterol, terbutaline, ritodrine), used to slow the progression of premature labor, can cause noncardiogenic pulmonary edema in 0.5% to 5% of cases (218, 219). The mechanism of development of pulmonary edema is poorly understood and could involve myocardial depression, postcapillary vasoconstriction, increased capillary permeability, fluid overload, and reduced oncotic pressure (220). Discontinuation of the tocolytics results in rapid resolution of pulmonary edema. Maternal mortality is estimated to be 3% (221).

Antineoplastic Drugs

Delayed adverse effects of cancer treatment is an increasing health problem, as therapeutic regimens for neoplastic diseases evolve and an increased number of long-term survivors is expected. For instance, nearly 30% of long-term survivors of Hodgkin disease complain of dyspnea and have pulmonary function abnormalities (222). Furthermore, in a series of 77 patients who underwent high-dose therapy and autologous bone marrow transplantation, the incidence of drug- or radiotherapy-induced lung toxicity was 16% (223). The adverse pulmonary responses to antineoplastic drugs are usually similar and most often include chronic interstitial pneumonitis/fibrosis, acute hypersensitivity type reactions, and noncardiogenic pulmonary edema (Table 33.2). Typical symptoms of the interstitial pneumonitis/fibrosis develop over weeks to months and include progressive exertional dyspnea, dry cough, and malaise associated with crackles on physical examination. Dyspnea, nonproductive cough, fever, and occasional peripheral blood eosinophilia are the most common features of hypersensitivity type reactions. Symptoms generally occur more rapidly over the course of days. Similarly, patients with noncardiogenic pulmonary edema present with acute respiratory distress. Occasionally, factors such as total cumulative dosage, patient age, or prior use of agents that may act synergistically (e.g., radiation) can be used to anticipate an untoward response.

Interstitial opacities resembling pulmonary fibrosis are the most common roentgenographic findings. Alveolar infiltrates can also be seen in patients presenting with hypersensitivity lung reactions. Pleural effusions are uncommon. Pulmonary function testing is usually consistent with a restrictive ventilatory defect (low vital capacity or total lung capacity) and a reduced DLco; the flow rates are usually preserved.

The list of causes of pulmonary infiltrates in the immunocompromised host always includes infection, which should be excluded as a cause of infiltrates suspected to be owing to drugs. Treatment is discontinuation of the agent. The role of steroids is not well established because no randomized trials have been conducted, but they should probably be tried, especially in severely symptomatic patients.

Azathioprine

Azathioprine has been implicated with acute hypersensitivity-type pneumonitis (224, 225), diffuse alveolar damage (226), and diffuse alveolar hemorrhage (227, 228), with one fatality being reported. All other patients recovered with drug discontinuation and steroids.

Bis-chloroethylnitrosourea (Carmustine)

When used as a single agent, BCNU has been reported to cause pulmonary toxicity in up 20% of patients (229–233). Incidence can be as high as 60% when the drug is used as part of high-dose combination protocols for bone marrow transplantation (234, 235). The incidence of toxicity increases with dose increments. In a series of 93 patients receiving BCNU for the treatment of gliomas, 50% of the individuals receiving 1.5 g/m^2 or more developed pulmonary toxicity (232). In another study, a dose-response relationship was demonstrated with 47% of patients receiving more than 525 mg/m^2 developing toxicity (236). There is also evidence of an increased incidence of toxicity in patients treated before the age of 5 years (237).

Pulmonary fibrosis can develop as an early (within 36 months) or late complication of therapy (up to 17 years) (238). The course of the disease is usually insidious, with progressive cough, dyspnea, and fatigue, although rapidly progressive and fatal presentations have been described (239, 240).

Radiographic findings include bibasilar reticular infiltrates and ground-glass attenuation in the lower lung zones. Less commonly, upper lobe disease, patchy consolidation, and pneumothorax can be seen (241, 242). The radiograph may also be normal even in the presence of histologically proven fibrosis (230). Histologic findings typically include interstitial pneumonitis and fibrosis with atypia of type II cells or diffuse alveolar damage (238).

In patients with early lung toxicity, corticosteroids seem to be helpful. Prednisolone used at doses of 1 mg/kg for 10 days followed by a slow taper resulted in complete recovery in 15 of 17 of patients developing pulmonary toxicity after carmustine-based preparative regimens for bone marrow transplant (243). Some investigators have also recommended discontinuation of therapy and institution of steroids in patients with significant (>10%) decrease in diffusing capacity (235, 243, 244). Steroids are not thought to be beneficial in patients with late-onset fibrosis. The prognosis seems to be more favorable in cases of early-onset fibrosis. A mortality rate of 36% has been reported in 26 patients who developed pulmonary toxicity within 1 year of therapy (236). In a study of 17 survivors of childhood brain tumors who were treated with BCNU, 12% died of lung fibrosis within 3 years of treatment and 47% died after 16 to 20 years of follow-up. Furthermore, all of the long-term survivors had evidence of lung fibrosis (237, 238, 245, 246).

Bleomycin

Bleomycin is deposited in the skin and lungs owing to decreased drug inactivation in these tissues. Thus, the lungs and the skin are the two organs that display the most serious side effects. Approximately 10% of patients receiving bleomycin will develop pulmonary toxicity (247). Interstitial fibrosis is the most commonly mentioned adverse pulmonary response, followed by hypersensitivity pneumonitis (248) and BOOP with parenchymal nodular densities (249, 250). Symptoms usually develop within the first 6 months of therapy and include dry cough and dyspnea. Physical examination reveals tachypnea, basilar crackles, and concomitant hyperpigmentation of the skin. Acute chest pain can also occur in 2.8% of patients during bleomycin infusion, being severe enough to require narcotics and warrant evaluations for myocardial infarction or pulmonary embolism (251).

Factors that appear to increase the toxic potential include age, total cumulative dose, oxygen therapy, renal function, and prior radiation to the thorax (252). In one review (253), the incidence of toxicity was significantly higher in patients older than 70 years (6% in patients 20–70 years versus 15% in those >70 years). Although toxicity can develop with doses as low as 49 U (254, 255), toxicity and fatality sharply increases with doses greater than 450 U (253). Supplemental oxygen administration (fraction of inspired oxygen [F_{IO_2}], 0.35–0.42) was associated with fatal pulmonary toxicity in five patients undergoing surgical procedures, whereas in 12 subsequently operated patients, maintenance of a F_{IO_2} of less than 0.25 resulted in no cases of toxicity (256). In a series of 20 patients with metastatic testicular cancer receiving bleomycin, presence of renal failure was the most significant factor associated with the development of abnormal pulmonary function tests (257). Evidence for the enhancement of toxicity by concomitant use of other antineoplastic agents is inconclusive (247, 258).

In a series of 100 patients, radiographic abnormalities were detected by chest radiograph in 15% of cases and by chest CT in 38% (259). They normally include a nonspecific interstitial pattern, with the most severe changes appearing in the lung bases and subpleural areas. Nodular abnormalities that can be confused with metastatic disease may be encountered. Vital capacity, total lung capacity, and diffusing capacity have been reported to be sensitive markers for detection of early signs of toxicity, but serial measurements were unable to specifically predict development of toxicity (260).

The histologic changes seen in patients with fibrosis are most commonly those of diffuse alveolar damage (261, 262)

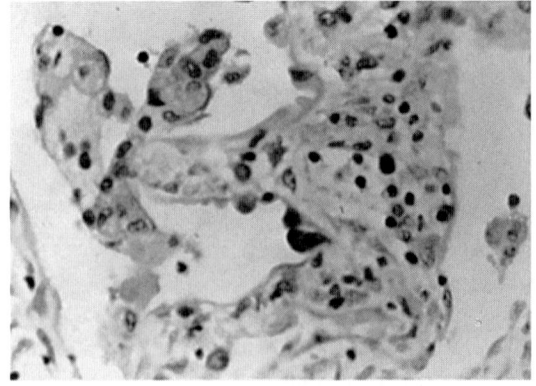

FIGURE 33.3. Bleomycin lung. Hyperplastic alveolar epithelium, septal edema, septal fibrosis, and lymphocytic infiltrates are demonstrated in this open lung biopsy specimen. Hematoxylin and eosin, original magnification ×400. (Photomicrograph from Dr. G. Gephart, Department of Pathology, Cleveland Clinic Foundation, Cleveland, Ohio, with permission.)

(Fig. 33.3). Eosinophilic pneumonia is seen in patients with hypersensitivity pneumonitis(248, 263).

Treatment is discontinuation of the drug. Resolution of interstitial disease has been reported with steroids in case reports (264–266), as well as in cases of hypersensitivity pneumonitis and BOOP (248, 263). If the patient's condition demonstrates reversibility, the roentgenographic findings (Fig. 33.4) and pulmonary function test results usually improve. In a series of 180 patients treated for germ-cell tumors, the mortality related to bleomycin pulmonary toxicity was 2.8% (267).

Busulfan

Busulfan is considered the prototypic drug for cytotoxic drug-induced pulmonary damage. It is estimated to occur in less than 5% of patients taking the drug (268–270). The usual case is one of long-term toxic damage to the lungs, with an insidious onset of symptoms after the patient has taken the drug for 3 to 4 years. Symptoms include cough, dyspnea, fever, and occasionally hyperpigmentation (271).

Diffuse interstitial and alveolar infiltrates are typically seen on the chest x-ray, but nodular densities, pleural effusions, or a normal picture may be seen as well (Fig. 33.5). The pulmonary function tests show restrictive defects and a decrease in diffusing capacity. However, as demonstrated in two studies, pulmonary function studies could not predict development of pulmonary toxicity (272, 273).

Histologic evidence of toxicity may be seen in up to 46% of all patients treated and typically include the presence of large, cytologically atypical type II pneumocytes (268, 272) (Fig. 33.5). Alveolar proteinosis has been reported in a number of patients receiving busulfan (274, 275) (Table 33.3).

Response to steroids has been reported in case series (269). The prognosis is generally poor with a postdiagnosis mean survival of 5% (270, 276).

Chlorambucil

Chronic interstitial pneumonitis secondary to chlorambucil is an uncommon phenomenon despite its wide use as an antineoplastic agent (277–285). Symptoms usually develop 6 months to 3 years after institution of therapy and include the insidious onset of cough and dyspnea. Physical examination reveals fine basilar crackles and fever (279). Recurrent episodes of acute respiratory distress with exposure to the drug have also been described (277, 280, 285).

Chest radiographs demonstrate reticular infiltrates, and diffuse micronodular infiltrates can be seen on CT (284). As expected, pulmonary function studies reveal a restrictive defect and decreased diffusing capacity. Histopathology reveals type II pneumocyte dysplasia, mononuclear cell infiltration, and interstitial fibrosis (279).

The role of steroid treatment in unclear. Approximately 50% of patients succumb to the disease despite treatment.

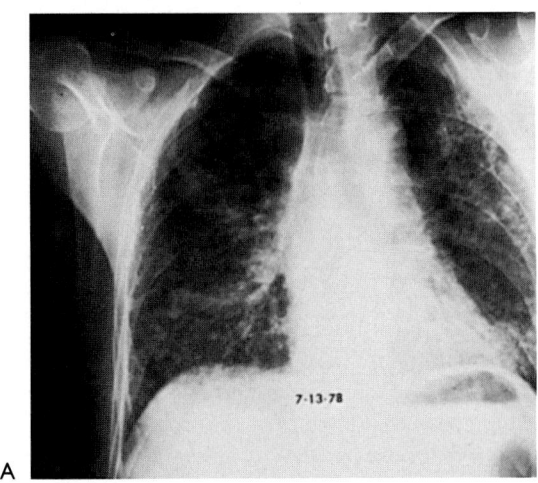
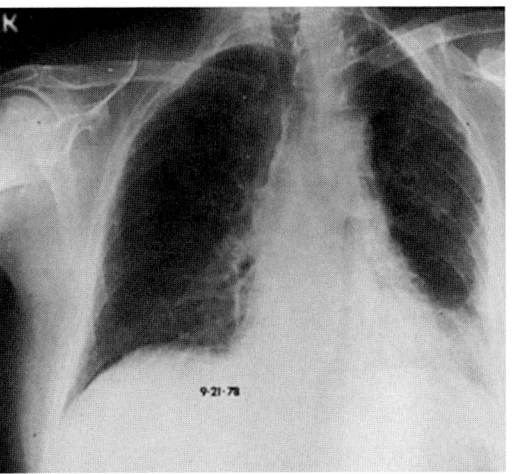

FIGURE 33.4. Bleomycin pneumonitis. **(A)** Posteroanterior chest x-ray film showing bilateral interstitial infiltrates. Total dose of bleomycin was 360 mg during 8 weeks. **(B)** Marked clearing after steroid therapy. (From Brown L, et al. Successful treatment of bleomycin lung. *Cleve Clin Q* 1980;47:99, with permission.)

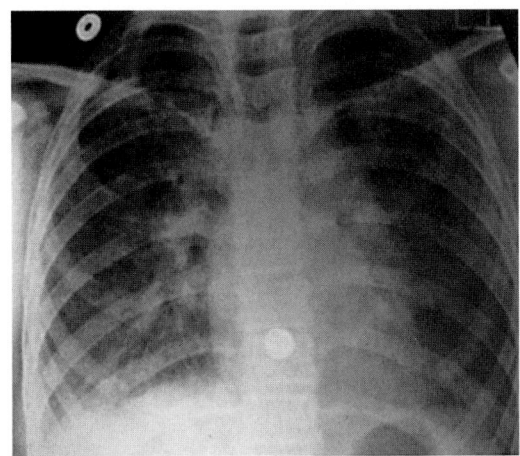

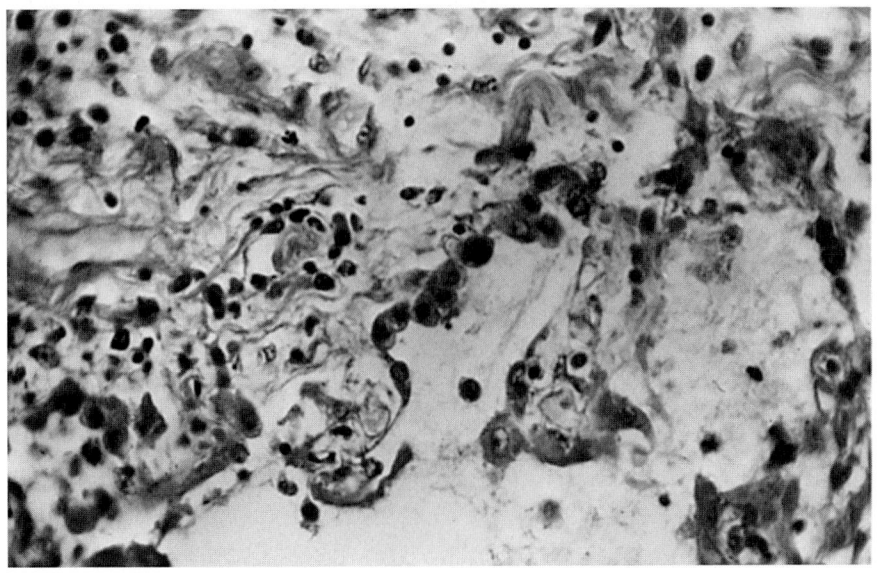

FIGURE 33.5. Cytotoxic pulmonary damage secondary to busulfan in the immunocompromised patient. **(A)** Chest roentgenogram shows diffuse alveolar and interstitial opacities. **(B)** Lung biopsy demonstrates inflammatory changes, fibrosis, and hypertrophy of alveolar lining cells after busulfan therapy.

Cyclophosphamide

Pulmonary toxicity is a rare complication of cyclophosphamide use in either malignant or nonmalignant disorders (286–290). It appears to occur in two distinct forms (291): an early-onset interstitial pneumonitis and a late-onset interstitial pneumonitis with fibrosis, which is seen more frequently. In the early-onset pneumonitis patients present within 1 to 6 months of onset of therapy with dyspnea, cough, fatigue, and frequently fever (287). Insidious and progressive dyspnea and cough occurring months to years after therapy are characteristic findings of the late-onset form. There are no clearly defined risk factors for the development of toxicity.

Interstitial reticular or nodular infiltrates are seen on the chest roentgenogram and, in some cases, in association with bilateral pleural thickening (291). Ground-glass attenuation on high-resolution CT scan has also been reported (292). The pulmonary function tests show restrictive defects and a decreased D$_{LCO}$. Histologic studies typically show organizing diffuse alveolar damage (288, 293, 294) and, less frequently, chronic interstitial pneumonitis (287, 294) and BOOP (295).

Early-onset pneumonitis usually responds to discontinuation of the drug and, in the majority of series, steroids, whereas the course of late-onset pneumonitis is most often progressive and irreversible (287, 291).

Cytosine Arabinoside

Pulmonary toxicity can develop in up to 44% of patients receiving cytosine arabinoside (296). The most common form of presentation is one of noncardiogenic pulmonary edema. Radiographs are abnormal in the majority of patients with interstitial and air space pattern being the most common findings (297). Histologic findings disclose the presence of intra-alveolar proteinaceous edema with minimal inflammatory changes (298). Mortality rates varying from 9% (297) to 69% (298) have been reported.

Gemcitabine

Gemcitabine has been associated with the development of noncardiogenic pulmonary edema (299–303). In a series of 56 patients (304), the incidence of pulmonary toxicity was 7.1%. Chest CT findings include ground-glass attenuation, thickened septal lines, and reticular opacities (303). The majority of patients demonstrated a favorable response to discontinuation of the drug and the use of steroids.

Melphalan

Pulmonary toxicity to melphalan has been reported in eight patients (305–308). Dyspnea and cough insidiously develop over 1 to 4 months after initiation of therapy. Histologic manifestations include interstitial fibrosis, plasma cell interstitial infiltration, and proliferation of bronchiolar and alveolar lining cells (305). Five of the eight reported patients died of respiratory failure.

Methotrexate

The majority of the features of low-dose methotrexate-induced pulmonary toxicity have been discussed earlier in this chapter (see section, "Anti-Inflammatory Agents and Biologic Response Modifiers") and are common to all patients receiving the drug. There is no convincing data to support the hypothesis that higher antineoplastic doses of methotrexate will predispose patients to more pulmonary complications. The pulmonary response to methotrexate may be acute or chronic, and is one of the more reversible of the cytotoxic drug–induced pulmonary reactions. Of note, toxicity has been described after the oral, intravenous, intramuscular, and intrathecal routes of administration (309).

Mitomycin

The incidence of pulmonary toxicity with mitomycin C ranges from 3% to 6% (310–313). Toxicity has been reported with mitomycin alone or in combined treatments, particularly including vinca alkaloids (45, 312, 314, 315). Pulmonary manifestations are somewhat unique and can include bronchospasm, acute and chronic pneumonitis, pleural abnormalities, and hemolytic uremic syndrome (HUS).

Acute bronchospasm occurs in about 5% of patients and is associated with concomitant administration of a vinca alkaloid (45, 314). Acute pneumonitis with concomitant vinca alkaloid administration (312, 315), noncardiogenic pulmonary edema (316), and acute respiratory failure with diffuse alveolar damage (310) comprise the other forms of acute presentation, occurring in average within 3 weeks of the onset of therapy. Chronic interstitial pneumonitis seems to be a less frequent complication, usually occurring in patients receiving more than 30 mg/m^2 of the drug. Pleural disease presenting as exudates or pleural fibrosis seems to occur at a greater frequency with mitomycin than with other antineoplastic agents (313, 317). Finally, a hemolytic/uremic–like syndrome associated with mitomycin has been described. Fifty percent of patients presenting with the syndrome develop ARDS (318).

Radiographic manifestations consist of bilateral reticular infiltrates predominantly in the lower lung zones and are seen in both the acute and chronic forms. Findings consistent with ARDS are also less frequently seen. The D$_{LCO}$ declines by more than 20% in approximately one fourth of patients after they have received three cycles of chemotherapy. Unfortunately, the use of serial D$_{LCO}$ measurements in patients receiving mitomycin cannot predict pulmonary

DRUG-INDUCED LUNG DISEASE

Summary Statement	Level of Evidence
Anorexic agents are associated with the development of pulmonary arterial hypertension.	High-quality case control study
Estrogen increases risk of venous thromboembolism.	Observational studies
Leukotriene modifiers improve lung function in patients with aspirin-induced asthma in patients already receiving corticosteroids.	One randomized, double-blind, placebo-controlled trial
Increasing age, presence of diabetes, hypoalbuminemia, use of disease-modifying antirheumatic drugs, and rheumatoid pleuropulmonary involvement are independent predictors for the development of pulmonary toxicity in patients receiving low-dose methotrexate.	Case-control study
Serial pulmonary functions studies in asymptomatic patients do not help to predict development of pulmonary drug toxicity (drugs studied include amiodarone, bleomycin, busulfan, methotrexate, and mitomycin).	Prospective observational studies
Corticosteroids are beneficial in the treatment of pulmonary drug toxicity, especially of the hypersensitivity type.	Poor-quality case series; expert's opinion
Amiodarone pulmonary toxicity is uncommon with maintenance daily doses of <400 mg.	Randomized placebo-controlled trials
Preexisting chronic obstructive pulmonary disease does not increase risk of development of amiodarone pulmonary toxicity.	Randomized placebo-controlled trials
Increasing age, total cumulative dose, oxygen therapy, decreased renal function, and prior radiation to the thorax are independent predictors for the development of pulmonary toxicity in patients receiving bleomycin.	Observational and retrospective studies

toxicity (313). Histologic findings are typically similar to those found with other cytotoxic agents, (310) and less frequently include BOOP (311). Lung tissue from patients dying from the HUS-like syndrome shows capillary angiomatoid changes (319).

In cases of acute and chronic pneumonitis, prednisone therapy can result in dramatic resolution of both symptoms and roentgenographic abnormalities, as reported in case series (312, 315, 317, 320, 321). Mortality exceeds 70% in cases of HUS (318).

Procarbazine

A hypersensitivity response has been described after the use of procarbazine. It may start within hours of the first dose or may develop after the patient has received the medication for months (322–324). Fever and eosinophilia arise. Diffuse interstitial infiltrates are seen on the chest roentgenogram. The reaction may terminate in respiratory failure. Biopsy shows mononuclear and eosinophilic cell infiltrates and interstitial fibrosis (324). Discontinuation of the drug resolves the symptoms. The clinical picture and histologic findings suggest that the syndrome would respond to steroids.

Paclitaxel

Aside from anaphylactic reactions causing bronchospasm (325), cases of acute pneumonitis have been reported (326, 327). In two cases, toxicity developed in association with doses of 850 mg/m^2 (325). There is also some suggestion of a synergistic toxic effect of paclitaxel and radiotherapy (328, 329).

REFERENCES

1. Rosenow EC 3rd. The spectrum of drug-induced pulmonary disease. *Ann Intern Med* 1972;77:977–991.
2. Rosenow EC 3rd. Drug-induced pulmonary disease. *Dis Mo* 1994;40:253–310.
3. Demeter SL, Ahmad M, Tomashefski JF. Drug-induced pulmonary disease, part I: patterns of response. *Cleveland Clin Q* 1979;46:89–99.
4. Katz S, Aberman A, Frand UI, et al. Heroin pulmonary edema: evidence for increased pulmonary capillary permeability. *Am Rev Respir Dis* 1972;106:472–474.
5. Diamond MT, Fell SC. Anticoagulant-induced massive hemothorax. *N Y State J Med* 1973;73:691–692.
6. Rostand RA, Feldman RL, Block ER. Massive hemothorax complicating heparin anticoagulation for pulmonary embolus. *South Med J* 1977;70:1128–1130.
7. Petusevsky ML, Faling LJ, Rocklin RE, et al. Pleuropericardial reaction to treatment with dantrolene. *JAMA* 1979;242:2772–2774.
8. O'Donnell AE, Pappas LS. Pulmonary complications of intravenous drug abuse: experience at an inner-city hospital. *Chest* 1988;94:251–253.
9. Pare JP, Cote G, Fraser RS. Long-term follow-up of drug abusers with intravenous talcosis. *Am Rev Respir Dis* 1989;139:233–241.
10. Yakel DL Jr, Eisenberg MJ. Pulmonary artery hypertension in chronic intravenous cocaine users. *Am Heart J* 1995;130:398–389.
11. Schaiberger PH, Kennedy TC, Miller FC, et al. Pulmonary hypertension associated with long-term inhalation of "crack" methamphetamine. *Chest* 1993;104:614–616.
12. Abenhaim L, Moride Y, Brenot F, et al. Appetite-suppressant drugs and the risk of primary pulmonary hypertension. International Primary Pulmonary Hypertension Study Group. *N Engl J Med* 1996;335:609–616.
13. Mark EJ, Patalas ED, Chang HT, et al. Fatal pulmonary hypertension associated with short-term use of fenfluramine and phentermine. *N Engl J Med* 1997;337:602–606.

14. Douketis JD, Ginsberg JS, Holbrook A, et al. A reevaluation of the risk for venous thromboembolism with the use of oral contraceptives and hormone replacement therapy. *Arch Intern Med* 1997;157:1522–1530.

15. Bloemenkamp KW, Rosendaal FR, Buller HR, et al. Risk of venous thrombosis with use of current low-dose oral contraceptives is not explained by diagnostic suspicion and referral bias. *Arch Intern Med* 1999;159:65–70.

16. Jick H, Jick S, Gurewich V, et al. Risk of idiopathic cardiovascular death and nonfatal venous thromboembolism in women using oral contraceptives with differing progestogen components. *Lancet* 1995;346:1589–1593.

17. Spitzer WO, Lewis MA, Heinemann LA, et al. Third generation oral contraceptives and risk of venous thromboembolic disorders: an international case-control study. Transnational Research Group on Oral Contraceptives and the Health of Young Women. *BMJ* 1996;312:83–88.

18. Lombard CM, Churg A, Winokur S. Pulmonary veno-occlusive disease following therapy for malignant neoplasms. *Chest* 1987; 92:871–876.

19. Joselson R, Warnock M. Pulmonary veno-occlusive disease after chemotherapy. *Hum Pathol* 1983;14:88–91.

20. Knight BK, Rose AG. Pulmonary veno-occlusive disease after chemotherapy. *Thorax* 1985;40:874–875.

21. Waldhorn RE, Tsou EE, Smith FP, et al. Pulmonary veno-occlusive disease associated with microangiopathic hemolytic anemia and chemotherapy of gastric adenocarcinoma. *Med Pediatr Oncol* 1984;12:394–396.

22. Wermer P, Kushner M, Riley EA. Reversible metastatic calcification associated with excessive milk and alkali intake. *Am J Med* 1953;14:108–115.

23. Cooke C, Hyland JW. Pathological calcifications of the lungs following intravenous administration of calcium. *Am J Med* 1960;29:363–368.

24. Breuer RI, LeBauer J. Caution in the use of phosphates in the treatment of severe hypercalcemia. *J Clin Endocrinol Metab* 1967;27:695–698.

25. Bauer J, Freyberg RH. Vitamin D intoxication with metastatic calcification. *JAMA* 1946;130:1208–1215.

26. Finley TN, Aronow A, Cosentino AM, et al. Occult pulmonary hemorrhage in anticoagulated patients. *Am Rev Respir Dis* 1975;112:23–29.

27. Santalo M, Domingo P, Fontcuberta J, et al. Diffuse pulmonary hemorrhage associated with anticoagulant therapy. *Eur J Respir Dis* 1986;69:114–119.

28. Nathan PE, Torres AV, Smith AJ, et al. Spontaneous pulmonary hemorrhage following coronary thrombolysis. *Chest* 1992;101:1150–1152.

29. Awadh N, Ronco JJ, Bernstein V, et al. Spontaneous pulmonary hemorrhage after thrombolytic therapy for acute myocardial infarction. *Chest* 1994;106:1622–1624.

30. Chang YC, Patz EF Jr, Goodman PC, et al. Significance of hemoptysis following thrombolytic therapy for acute myocardial infarction. *Chest* 1996;109:727–729.

31. Saltzstein SL, et al. Lymphadenopathy induced by anticonvulsant drugs and mimicking clinically and pathologically malignant lymphomas. *Cancer* 1959;12:164–182.

32. Heitzman E. Lymphadenopathy related to anticonvulsant therapy: roentgen findings simulating lymphoma. *Radiology* 1967; 89:311–312.

33. Filip DJ, Logue GL, Harle TS, et al. Pulmonary and hepatic complications of methotrexate therapy of psoriasis. *JAMA* 1971;216:881–882.

34. Bodman SF, Condemi JJ. Mediastinal widening in iatrogenic Cushing's syndrome. *Ann Intern Med* 1967;67:399–403.

35. Santini LC, Williams JL. Mediastinal widening (presumable lipomatosis) in Cushing's syndrome. *N Engl J Med* 1971;284:1357–1359.

36. Fritzler MJ. Drugs recently associated with lupus syndromes. *Lupus* 1994;3:455–459.

37. Grant DM, Morike K, Eichelbaum M, et al. Acetylation pharmacogenetics: the slow acetylator phenotype is caused by decreased or absent arylamine *N*-acetyltransferase in human liver. *J Clin Invest* 1990;85:968–972.

38. Yung RL, Johnson KJ, Richardson BC. New concepts in the pathogenesis of drug-induced lupus. *Lab Invest* 1995;73:746–759.

39. Dubois EL. Procainamide induction of a systemic lupus erythematosus-like syndrome: presentation of six cases, review of the literature, and analysis and followup of reported cases. *Medicine (Baltimore)* 1969;48:217–228.

40. Blomgren SE, Condemi JJ, Vaughan JH. Procainamide-induced lupus erythematosus: clinical and laboratory observations. *Am J Med* 1972;52:338–348.

41. Grieco MH, Pierson RN Jr. Mechanism of bronchoconstriction due to β-adrenergic blockade: studies with practolol, propranolol, and atropine. *J Allergy Clin Immunol* 1971;48:143–152.

42. Williams IP, Millard FJ. Severe asthma after inadvertent ingestion of oxprenolol. *Thorax* 1980;35:160.

43. Popio KA, Jackson DH Jr, Utell MJ, et al. Inhalation challenge with carbachol and isoproterenol to predict bronchospastic response to propranolol in COPD. *Chest* 1983;83:175–179.

44. Dunn TL, Gerber MJ, Shen AS, et al. The effect of topical ophthalmic instillation of timolol and betaxolol on lung function in asthmatic subjects. *Am Rev Respir Dis* 1986;133:264–268.

45. Luedke D, McLaughlin TT, Daughaday C, et al. Mitomycin C and vindesine associated pulmonary toxicity with variable clinical expression. *Cancer* 1985;55:542–545.

46. Gearhart MO, Bhutani MS. Intravenous pentamidine-induced bronchospasm. *Chest* 1992;102:1891–1892.

47. Katzman M, Meade W, Iglar K, et al. High incidence of bronchospasm with regular administration of aerosolized pentamidine. *Chest* 1992;101:79–81.

48. Yarbrough J, Mansfield LE, Ting S. Metered dose inhaler induced bronchospasm in asthmatic patients. *Ann Allergy* 1985;55:25–27.

49. Shim C, Williams MH Jr. Cough and wheezing from beclomethasone aerosol. *Chest* 1987;91:207–209.

50. Nicklas RA. Paradoxical bronchospasm associated with the use of inhaled β-agonists. *J Allergy Clin Immunol* 1990;85:959–964.

51. Collins LC, Peiris A. Bronchospasm secondary to replacement estrogen therapy. *Chest* 1993;104:1300–1302.

52. Troisi RJ, Speizer FE, Willett WC, et al. Menopause, postmenopausal estrogen preparations, and the risk of adult-onset asthma: a prospective cohort study. *Am J Respir Crit Care Med* 1995;152(4 pt 1):1183–1188.

53. Settipane RA, Constantine HP, Settipane GA. Aspirin intolerance and recurrent urticaria in normal adults and children: epidemiology and review. *Allergy* 1980;35:149–154.

54. Zeitz HJ. Bronchial asthma, nasal polyps, and aspirin sensitivity: Samter's syndrome. *Clin Chest Med* 1988;9:567–576.

55. Samter M, Beers RF Jr. Intolerance to aspirin: clinical studies and consideration of its pathogenesis. *Ann Intern Med* 1968;68:975–983.

56. Salberg DJ, Simon MR. Severe asthma induced by naproxen: a case report and review of the literature. *Ann Allergy* 1980;45:372–375.

57. Szczeklik A. Adverse reactions to aspirin and nonsteroidal antiinflammatory drugs. *Ann Allergy* 1987;59(5 pt 2):113–118.

58. Knapp HR, Sladek K, Fitzgerald GA. Increased excretion of leukotriene E$_4$ during aspirin-induced asthma. *J Lab Clin Med* 1992;119:48–51.

59. Ferreri NR, Howland WC, Stevenson DD, et al. Release of leukotrienes, prostaglandins, and histamine into nasal secretions of aspirin-sensitive asthmatics during reaction to aspirin. *Am Rev Respir Dis* 1988 137:847–854.

60. Israel E.A, Fischer R, Rosenberg MA, et al. The pivotal role of 5-lipoxygenase products in the reaction of aspirin-sensitive asthmatics to aspirin. *Am Rev Respir Dis* 1993;148(6 pt 1):1447–1451.

61. Christie PE, Smith CM, Lee TH. The potent and selective sulfidopeptide leukotriene antagonist, SK&F 104353, inhibits aspirin-induced asthma. *Am Rev Respir Dis* 1991;144:957–958.

62. Nasser SM, Bell GS, Foster S, et al. Effect of the 5-lipoxygenase inhibitor ZD2138 on aspirin-induced asthma. *Thorax* 1994;49:749–756.

63. Dahlen B, Nizankowska BE, Szczeklik A, et al. Benefits from adding the 5-lipoxygenase inhibitor zileuton to conventional therapy in aspirin-intolerant asthmatics. *Am J Respir Crit Care Med* 1998;157(4 pt 1):1187–1194.

64. Sweet JM, Stevenson DD, Simon RA, et al. Long-term effects of aspirin desensitization: treatment for aspirin-sensitive rhinosinusitis-asthma. *J Allergy Clin Immunol* 1990;85(1 pt 1):59–65.

65. Hormaechea E, Carlson RW, Rogove H, et al. Hypovolemia, pulmonary edema and protein changes in severe salicylate poisoning. *Am J Med* 1979;66:1046–1050.

66. Heffner JE, Sahn SA. Salicylate-induced pulmonary edema: clinical features and prognosis. *Ann Intern Med* 1981;95:405–409.

67. Leatherman JW, Schmitz PG. Fever, hyperdynamic shock, and multiple system organ failure: a pseudosepsis syndrome associated with chronic salicylate intoxication. *Chest* 1991;100:1391–1396.

68. St Clair EW, Rice JR, Snyderman R. Pneumonitis complicating low-dose methotrexate therapy in rheumatoid arthritis. *Arch Intern Med* 1985;145:2035–2038.

69. Carson CW, Cannon GW, Egger MJ, et al. Pulmonary disease during the treatment of rheumatoid arthritis with low dose pulse methotrexate. *Semin Arthritis Rheum* 1987;16:186–195.

70. Cottin V, Tebib J, Massonnet B, et al. Pulmonary function in patients receiving long-term low-dose methotrexate. *Chest* 1996;109:933–938.

71. Alarcon GS, Kremer JM, Macaluso M, et al. Risk factors for methotrexate-induced lung injury in patients with rheumatoid arthritis: a multicenter, case-control study. Methotrexate-Lung Study Group. *Ann Intern Med* 1997;127:356–364.

72. Dayton CS, Schwartz DA, Sprince NL, et al. Low-dose methotrexate may cause air trapping in patients with rheumatoid arthritis. *Am J Respir Crit Care Med* 1995;151:1189–1193.

73. Beyeler C, Jordi B, Gerber NJ, et al. Pulmonary function in rheumatoid arthritis treated with low-dose methotrexate: a longitudinal study. *Br J Rheumatol* 1996;35:446–452.

74. White DA, Rankin JA, Stover DE, et al. Methotrexate pneumonitis: bronchoalveolar lavage findings suggest an immunologic disorder. *Am Rev Respir Dis* 1989;139:18–21.

75. Elsasser S, Dalquen P, Soler M, et al. Methotrexate-induced pneumonitis: appearance 4 weeks after discontinuation of treatment. *Am Rev Respir Dis* 1989;140:1089–1092.

76. Leduc D, De Vuyst P, Lheureux P, et al. Pneumonitis complicating low-dose methotrexate therapy for rheumatoid arthritis: discrepancies between lung biopsy and bronchoalveolar lavage findings. *Chest* 1993;104:1620–1623.

77. Cannon GW, Ward JR, Clegg DO, et al. Acute lung disease associated with low-dose pulse methotrexate therapy in patients with rheumatoid arthritis. *Arthritis Rheum* 1983;26:1269–1274.

78. Eastmond CJ. Diffuse alveolitis as complication of penicillamine treatment for rheumatoid arthritis. *Br Med J* 1976;1:1506.

79. Scott DL, Bradby GV, Aitman TJ, et al. Relationship of gold and penicillamine therapy to diffuse interstitial lung disease. *Ann Rheum Dis* 1981;40:136–141.

80. Davies D, Jones JK. Pulmonary eosinophilia caused by penicillamine. *Thorax* 1980;35:957–958.

81. Shettar SP, Chattopadhyay C, Wolstenholme RJ, et al. Diffuse alveolitis on a small dose of penicillamine. *Br J Rheumatol* 1984;23:220–224.

82. Sternlieb I, Bennett B, Scheinberg IH. D-Penicillamine-induced Goodpasture's syndrome in Wilson's disease. *Ann Intern Med* 1975;82:673–676.

83. Matloff DS, Kaplan MM. D-Penicillamine-induced Goodpasture's-like syndrome in primary biliary cirrhosis—successful treatment with plasmapheresis and immunosuppressives. *Gastroenterology* 1980;78(5 pt 1):1046–1049.

84. Macarron P, Garcia Diaz JE, Azofra JA, et al. D-Penicillamine therapy associated with rapidly progressive glomerulonephritis. *Nephrol Dial Transplant* 1992;7:161–164.

85. Lyle WH. D-Penicillamine and fatal obliterative bronchiolitis. *Br Med J* 1977;1:105.

86. Epler GR, Snider GL, Gaensler EA, et al. Bronchiolitis and bronchitis in connective tissue disease: a possible relationship to the use of penicillamine. *JAMA* 1979;242:528–532.

87. Stein HB, Patterson AC, Offer RC, et al. Adverse effects of D-penicillamine in rheumatoid arthritis. *Ann Intern Med* 1980;92:24–29.

88. Murphy KC, Atkins CJ, Offer RC, et al. Obliterative bronchiolitis in two rheumatoid arthritis patients treated with penicillamine. *Arthritis Rheum* 1981;24:557–560.

89. Boehler A, Vogt P, Speich R, et al. Bronchiolitis obliterans in a patient with localized scleroderma treated with D-penicillamine. *Eur Respir J* 1996;9:1317–1319.

90. Tomioka R, King TE Jr. Gold-induced pulmonary disease: clinical features, outcome, and differentiation from rheumatoid lung disease. *Am J Respir Crit Care Med* 1997;155:1011–1020.

91. Smith W, Ball GV. Lung injury due to gold treatment. *Arthritis Rheum* 1980;23:351–354.

92. Levinson ML, Lynch JP 3rd, Bower JS. Reversal of progressive, life-threatening gold hypersensitivity pneumonitis by corticosteroids. *Am J Med* 1981;71:908–912.

93. Morley TF, Komansky HJ, Adelizzi RA, et al. Pulmonary gold toxicity. *Eur J Respir Dis* 1984;65:627–632.

94. Wechsler ME, Garpestad E, Flier SR, et al. Pulmonary infiltrates, eosinophilia, and cardiomyopathy following corticosteroid withdrawal in patients with asthma receiving zafirlukast. *JAMA* 1998;279:455–457.

95. Green RL, Vayonis AG. Churg-Strauss syndrome after zafirlukast in two patients not receiving systemic steroid treatment. *Lancet* 1999;353:725–726.

96. Franco J, Artes MJ. Pulmonary eosinophilia associated with montelukast. *Thorax* 1999;54:558–560.

97. Wechsler ME, Finn D, Gunawardena D, et al. Churg-Strauss syndrome in patients receiving montelukast as treatment for asthma. *Chest* 2000;117:708–713.

98. Kinoshita M, Shiraishi T, Koga T, et al. Churg-Strauss syndrome after corticosteroid withdrawal in an asthmatic patient treated with pranlukast. *J Allergy Clin Immunol* 1999;103(3 pt 1):534–535.

99. Le Gall C, Pham S, Vignes S, et al. Inhaled corticosteroids and Churg-Strauss syndrome: a report of five cases. *Eur Respir J* 2000;15:978–981.

100. Tuggey JM, Hosker HS. Churg-Strauss syndrome associated with montelukast therapy. *Thorax* 2000;55:805–806.

101. Conant EF, Fox KR, Miller WT. Pulmonary edema as a complication of interleukin-2 therapy. *AJR Am J Roentgenol* 1989;152:749–752.

102. Vogelzang PJ, Bloom SM, Mier JW, et al. Chest roentgenographic abnormalities in IL-2 recipients: incidence and correlation with clinical parameters. *Chest* 1992;101:746–752.

103. Berthiaume Y, Boiteau P, Fick G, et al. Pulmonary edema during IL-2 therapy: combined effect of increased permeability and hydrostatic pressure. *Am J Respir Crit Care Med* 1995;152:329–335.

104. Kuei JH, Tashkin DP, Figlin RA. Pulmonary toxicity of recombinant human tumor necrosis factor. *Chest* 1989;96:334–338.

105. Hailey FJ, Glascock HW Jr, Hewitt WF. Pleuropneumonic reactions to nitrofurantoin. *N Engl J Med* 1969;281:1087–90.

106. Sovijarvi AR, Lemola M, Stenius B, et al. Nitrofurantoin-induced acute, subacute and chronic pulmonary reactions. *Scand J Respir Dis* 1977;58:41–50.

107. Holmberg L, Boman G. Pulmonary reactions to nitrofurantoin: 447 cases reported to the Swedish Adverse Drug Reaction Committee 1966–1976. *Eur J Respir Dis* 1981;62:180–9.

108. Geller M, Dickie HA, Kass DA, et al. The histopathology of acute nitrofurantoin-associated pneumonitis. *Ann Allergy* 1976;37:275–9.

109. Magee F, Wright JL, Chan N, et al. Two unusual pathological reactions to nitrofurantoin: case reports. *Histopathology* 1986;10:701–706.

110. Cameron RJ, Kolbe J, Wilsher ML, et al. Bronchiolitis obliterans organising pneumonia associated with the use of nitrofurantoin. *Thorax* 2000;55:249–251.

111. Bucknall CE, Adamson MR, Banham SW. Non fatal pulmonary haemorrhage associated with nitrofurantoin. *Thorax* 1987;42:475–476.

112. Hainer BL, White AA. Nitrofurantoin pulmonary toxicity. *J Fam Pract* 1981;13:817–823.

113. Robinson BW. Nitrofurantoin-induced interstitial pulmonary fibrosis: presentation and outcome. *Med J Aust* 1983;1:72–76.

114. Wang KK, Bowyer BA, Fleming CR, et al. Pulmonary infiltrates and eosinophilia associated with sulfasalazine. *Mayo Clin Proc* 1984;59:343–346.

115. Leino R, Liippo K, Ekfors T. Sulphasalazine-induced reversible hypersensitivity pneumonitis and fatal fibrosing alveolitis: report of two cases. *J Intern Med* 1991;229:553–556.

116. Kolbe J, Caughey D, Rainer S. Sulphasalazine-induced sub-acute hyper-sensitivity pneumonitis. *Respir Med* 1994;88:149–152.

117. Gabazza EC, Taguchi O, Yamakami T, et al. Pulmonary infiltrates and skin pigmentation associated with sulfasalazine. *Am J Gastroenterol* 1992;87:1654–1657.

118. Teague WG, Sutphen JL, Fechner RE. Desquamative interstitial pneumonitis complicating inflammatory bowel disease of childhood. *J Pediatr Gastroenterol Nutr* 1985;4:663–667.

119. Davies D, MacFarlane A. Fibrosing alveolitis and treatment with sulphasalazine. *Gut* 1974;15:185–188.

120. Williams T, Eidus L, Thomas P. Fibrosing alveolitis, bronchiolitis obliterans, and sulfasalazine therapy. *Chest* 1982;81:766–768.

121. Collins JR. Adverse reactions to salicylazosulfapyridine (Azulfidine) in the treatment of ulcerative colitis. *South Med J* 1968;61:354–358.

122. Ho D, Tashkin DP, Bein ME, et al. Pulmonary infiltrates with eosinophilia associated with tetracycline. *Chest* 1979;76:33–36.

123. Guillon JM, Joly P, Autran B, et al. Minocycline-induced cell-mediated hypersensitivity pneumonitis. *Ann Intern Med* 1992;117:476–481.

124. Dykhuizen RS, Zaidi AM, Godden DJ, et al. Minocycline and pulmonary eosinophilia. *BMJ* 1995;310:1520–1521.

125. Fiegenberg DS., Weiss H, Kirshman H. Migratory pneumonia with eosinophilia associated with sulfonamide administration. *Arch Intern Med* 1967;120:85–89.

126. Donlan CJ Jr, Scutero JV. Transient eosinophilic pneumonia secondary to use of a vaginal cream. *Chest* 1975;67:232–233.

127. Reichlin S, et al. Loeffler' syndrome following penicillin therapy. *Ann Intern Med* 1953;38:113.

128. Poe RH, Condemi JJ, Weinstein SS, et al. Adult respiratory distress syndrome related to ampicillin sensitivity. *Chest* 1980;77:449–451.

129. Wold DE, et al. Allergic (Loeffler's) pneumonitis occurring during antituberculous therapy: report of three cases. *Am Rev Tuberc* 1956;74:445.

130. Wong PC, Yew WW, Wong CF, et al. Ethambutol-induced pulmonary infiltrates with eosinophilia and skin involvement. *Eur Respir J* 1995;8:866–868.

131. Wright DG, Robichaud KJ, Pizzo PA, et al. Lethal pulmonary reactions associated with the combined use of amphotericin B and leukocyte transfusions. *N Engl J Med* 1981;304:1185–1189.

132. Dana BW, Durie BG, White RF, et al. Concomitant administration of granulocyte transfusions and amphotericin B in neutropenic patients: absence of significant pulmonary toxicity. *Blood* 1981;57:90–94.

133. Rakita L, Sobol SM, Mostow N, et al. Amiodarone pulmonary toxicity. *Am Heart J* 1983;106(4 pt 2):906–916.

134. Martin WJ 2nd, Rosenow EC 3rd. Amiodarone pulmonary toxicity: recognition and pathogenesis (Part 2). *Chest* 1988;93:1242–1248.

135. Martin WJ 2nd, Rosenow EC 3rd. Amiodarone pulmonary toxicity: recognition and pathogenesis (Part I). *Chest* 1988;93:1067–1075.

136. Marchlinski FE, Gansler TS, Waxman HL, et al. Amiodarone pulmonary toxicity. *Ann Intern Med* 1982;97:839–845.

137. Gefter WB, Epstein DM, Pietra GG, et al. Lung disease caused by amiodarone, a new antiarrhythmic agent. *Radiology* 1983;147:339–344.

138. Suarez LD, Poderoso JJ, Elsner B, et al. Subacute pneumopathy during amiodarone therapy. *Chest* 1983;83:566–568.

139. Adams GD, Kehoe R, Lesch M, et al. Amiodarone-induced pneumonitis: assessment of risk factors and possible risk reduction. *Chest* 1988;93:254–263.

140. Cazzadori A, Braggio P, Barbieri E, et al. Amiodarone-induced pulmonary toxicity. *Respiration* 1986;49:157–160.

141. Kudenchuk PJ, Pierson DJ, Greene HL, et al. Prospective evaluation of amiodarone pulmonary toxicity. *Chest* 1984;86:541–548.

142. Ulrik CS, Backer V, Aldershvile J, et al. Serial pulmonary function tests in patients treated with low-dose amiodarone. *Am Heart J* 1992;123:1550–1554.

143. Vorperian VR, Havighurst TC, Miller S, et al. Adverse effects of low dose amiodarone: a meta-analysis. *J Am Coll Cardiol* 1997;30:791–798.

144. Sunderji R, Kanji Z, Gin K. Pulmonary effects of low dose amiodarone: a review of the risks and recommendations for surveillance. *Can J Cardiol* 2000;16:1435–1440.

145. Singh SN, Fisher SG, Deedwania PC, et al. Pulmonary effect of amiodarone in patients with heart failure. The Congestive Heart Failure-Survival Trial of Antiarrhythmic Therapy (CHF-STAT) Investigators (Veterans Affairs Cooperative Study No. 320). *J Am Coll Cardiol* 1997;30:514–517.

146. Kennedy JI, Myers JL, Plumb VJ, et al. Amiodarone pulmonary

toxicity: clinical, radiologic, and pathologic correlations. *Arch Intern Med* 1987;147:50–55.

147. Dean PJ, Groshart KD, Porterfield JG, et al. Amiodarone-associated pulmonary toxicity: a clinical and pathologic study of eleven cases. *Am J Clin Pathol* 1987;87:7–13.

148. Valle JM, Alvarez D, Antunez J, et al. Bronchiolitis obliterans organizing pneumonia secondary to amiodarone: a rare aetiology. *Eur Respir J* 1995;8:470–471.

149. Kay GN, Epstein E, Kirklin JK, et al. Fatal postoperative amiodarone pulmonary toxicity. *Am J Cardiol* 1988;62:490–492.

150. Greenspon AJ, Kidwell GA, Hurley W, et al. Amiodarone-related postoperative adult respiratory distress syndrome. *Circulation* 1991;84[5 Suppl]:III-407–III-415.

151. Saussine M, Colson P, Alauzen M, et al. Postoperative acute respiratory distress syndrome: a complication of amiodarone associated with 100% oxygen ventilation. *Chest* 1992;102:980–981.

152. Van Mieghem W, Coolen L, Malysse I, et al. Amiodarone and the development of ARDS after lung surgery. *Chest* 1994;105:1642–1645.

153. Wood DL, Osborn MJ, Rooke J, et al. Amiodarone pulmonary toxicity: report of two cases associated with rapidly progressive fatal adult respiratory distress syndrome after pulmonary angiography. *Mayo Clin Proc* 1985;60:601–603.

154. Mickleborough LL, Maruyama H, Mohamed S, et al. Are patients receiving amiodarone at increased risk for cardiac operations? *Ann Thorac Surg* 1994;58:622–629.

155. Arnon R, Raz I, Chajek-Shaul T, et al. Amiodarone pulmonary toxicity presenting as a solitary lung mass. *Chest* 1988;93:425–427.

156. Pollak PT, Sami M. Acute necrotizing pneumonitis and hyperglycemia after amiodarone therapy: case report and review of amiodarone-associated pulmonary disease. *Am J Med* 1984;76:935–939.

157. Gonzalez-Rothi RJ, Hannan SE, Hood CI, et al. Amiodarone pulmonary toxicity presenting as bilateral exudative pleural effusions. *Chest* 1987;92:179–182.

158. Nicholson AA, Hayward C. The value of computed tomography in the diagnosis of amiodarone-induced pulmonary toxicity. *Clin Radiol* 1989;40:564–567.

159. van Rooij WJ, van der Meer SC, van Royen EA, et al. Pulmonary gallium-67 uptake in amiodarone pneumonitis. *J Nucl Med* 1984;25:211–213.

160. Zhu YY, Botvinick E, Dae M, et al. Gallium lung scintigraphy in amiodarone pulmonary toxicity. *Chest* 1988;93:1126–1131.

161. Xaubet A, Roca J, Rodriguez-Roisin R, et al. Bronchoalveolar lavage cellular analysis and gallium lung scan in the assessment of patients with amiodarone-induced pneumonitis. *Respiration* 1987;52:272–280.

162. Gleadhill IC, Wise RA, Schonfeld SA, et al. Serial lung function testing in patients treated with amiodarone: a prospective study. *Am J Med* 1989;86:4–10.

163. Endoh Y, Hanai R, Uto K, et al. Diagnostic accuracy of KL-6 as a marker of amiodarone-induced pulmonary toxicity. *Pacing Clin Electrophysiol* 2000;23(11 pt 2):2010–2013.

164. Myers JL, Kennedy JI, and Plumb VJ. Amiodarone lung: pathologic findings in clinically toxic patients. *Hum Pathol* 1987;18:349–354.

165. Liu FL, Cohen RD, Downar E, et al. Amiodarone pulmonary toxicity: functional and ultrastructural evaluation. *Thorax* 1986;41:100–105.

166. Zaher C, Hamer A, Peter T, et al. Low-dose steroid therapy for prophylaxis of amiodarone-induced pulmonary infiltrates. *N Engl J Med* 1983;308:779.

167. Joelson J, Kluger J, Cole S, et al. Possible recurrence of amiodarone pulmonary toxicity following corticosteroid therapy. *Chest* 1984;85:284–286.

168. Coudert B, Bailly F, Lombard JN, et al. Amiodarone pneumonitis: bronchoalveolar lavage findings in 15 patients and review of the literature. *Chest* 1992;102:1005–1012.

169. Howard JJ, Mohsenifar Z, Simons SM. Adult respiratory distress syndrome following administration of lidocaine. *Chest* 1982;81:644–645.

170. Feinberg L, Travis WD, Ferrans V, et al. Pulmonary fibrosis associated with tocainide: report of a case with literature review. *Am Rev Respir Dis* 1990;141:505–508.

171. Kavaru MS, Ahmad M, Amirthalingam KN. Hydrochlorothiazide-induced acute pulmonary edema. *Cleveland Clin J Med* 1990;57:181–184.

172. Israili ZH, Hall WD. Cough and angioneurotic edema associated with angiotensin-converting enzyme inhibitor therapy: a review of the literature and pathophysiology. *Ann Intern Med* 1992;117:234–242.

173. Malini PL, Strocchi E, Zanardi M, et al. Thromboxane antagonism and cough induced by angiotensin-converting-enzyme inhibitor. *Lancet* 1997;350:15–18.

174. Reisin L, Schneeweiss A. Complete spontaneous remission of cough induced by ACE inhibitors during chronic therapy in hypertensive patients. *J Hum Hypertens* 1992;6:333–335.

175. Lacourciere Y, Brunner H, Irwin R, et al. Effects of modulators of the renin-angiotensin-aldosterone system on cough. Losartan Cough Study Group. *J Hypertens* 1994;12:1387–1393.

176. Goldberg AI, Dunlay MC, Sweet CS. Safety and tolerability of losartan potassium, an angiotensin II receptor antagonist, compared with hydrochlorothiazide, atenolol, felodipine ER, and angiotensin-converting enzyme inhibitors for the treatment of systemic hypertension. *Am J Cardiol* 1995;75:793–795.

177. Roy TM, Ossorio MA, Cipolla LM, et al. Pulmonary complications after tricyclic antidepressant overdose. *Chest* 1989;96:852–856.

178. Li C, Gefter WB. Acute pulmonary edema induced by overdosage of phenothiazines. *Chest* 1992;101:102–104.

179. Salerno SM, Strong JS, Roth BJ, et al. Eosinophilic pneumonia and respiratory failure associated with a trazodone overdose. *Am J Respir Crit Care Med* 1995;152(6 pt 1):2170–2172.

180. Fruchter L, Laptook A. Diphenylhydantoin hypersensitivity reaction associated with interstitial pulmonary infiltrates and hypereosinophilia. *Ann Allergy* 1981;47:453–455.

181. Michael JR, Rudin ML. Acute pulmonary disease caused by phenytoin. *Ann Intern Med* 1981;95:452–454.

182. Cullinan SA, Bower GC. Acute pulmonary hypersensitivity to carbamazepine. *Chest* 1975;68:580–581.

183. Barreiro B, Manresa BF, Valldeperas J. Carbamazepine and the lung. *Eur Respir J* 1990;3:930–931.

184. Duberstein JL, Kaufman DM. A clinical study of an epidemic of heroin intoxication and heroin-induced pulmonary edema. *Am J Med* 1971;51:704–714.

185. Wilen SB, Ulreich S, Rabinowitz JG. Roentgenographic manifestations of methadone-induced pulmonary edema. *Radiology* 1975;114:51–55.

186. Flacke JW, Flacke WE, Williams GD. Acute pulmonary edema following naloxone reversal of high-dose morphine anesthesia. *Anesthesiology* 1977;47:376–378.

187. Taff RH. Pulmonary edema following naloxone administration in a patient without heart disease. *Anesthesiology* 1983;59:576–577.

188. Steinberg AD, Karliner JS. The clinical spectrum of heroin pulmonary edema. *Arch Intern Med* 1968;122:122–127.

189. Frand UI, Shim CS, Williams MH Jr. Heroin-induced pulmonary edema. Sequential studies of pulmonary function. *Ann Intern Med* 1972;77:29–35.

190. Heffner JE, Harley RA, Schabel SI. Pulmonary reactions from illicit substance abuse. *Clin Chest Med* 1990;11:151–162.

191. Haim DY, Lippmann ML, Goldberg SK, et al. The pulmonary complications of crack cocaine: a comprehensive review. *Chest* 1995;107:233–240.

192. Itkonen J, Schnoll S, Glassroth J. Pulmonary dysfunction in freebase cocaine users. *Arch Intern Med* 1984;144:2195–2197.

193. Tashkin DP, Khalsa ME, Gorelick D, et al. Pulmonary status of habitual cocaine smokers. *Am Rev Respir Dis* 1992;145:92–100.

194. Kline JN, Hirasuna JD. Pulmonary edema after freebase cocaine smoking: not due to an adulterant. *Chest* 1990;97:1009–1010.

195. Cucco RA, Yoo OH, Cregler L, et al. Nonfatal pulmonary edema after "freebase" cocaine smoking. *Am Rev Respir Dis* 1987;136:179–181.

196. Hoffman CK, Goodman PC. Pulmonary edema in cocaine smokers. *Radiology* 1989;172:463–465.

197. Allred RJ, Ewer S. Fatal pulmonary edema following intravenous "freebase" cocaine use. *Ann Emerg Med* 1981;10:441–442.

198. Moliterno DJ, Willard JE, Lange RA, et al. Coronary-artery vasoconstriction induced by cocaine, cigarette smoking, or both. *N Engl J Med* 1994;330:454–459.

199. Kissner DG, Lawrence WD, Selis JE, et al. Crack lung: pulmonary disease caused by cocaine abuse. *Am Rev Respir Dis* 1987;136:1250–1252.

200. Forrester JM, Steele AW, Waldron JA, et al. Crack lung: an acute pulmonary syndrome with a spectrum of clinical and histopathologic findings. *Am Rev Respir Dis* 1990;142:462–467.

201. Eurman DW, Potash HI, Eyler WR, et al. Chest pain and dyspnea related to "crack" cocaine smoking: value of chest radiography. *Radiology* 1989;172:459–462.

202. Oh PI, Balter MS. Cocaine-induced eosinophilic lung disease. *Thorax* 1992;47:478–479.

203. Taylor RF, Bernard GR. Airway complications from free-basing cocaine. *Chest* 1989;95:476–477.

204. Rebhun J. Association of asthma and freebase smoking. *Ann Allergy* 1988;60:339–342.

205. Rubin RB, Neugarten J. Cocaine-associated asthma. *Am J Med* 1990;88:438–439.

206. Patel RC, Dutta D, Schonfeld SA. Free-base cocaine use associated with bronchiolitis obliterans organizing pneumonia. *Ann Intern Med* 1987;107:186–187.

207. Dowling GP, McDonough ET 3rd, Bost RO. "Eve" and "Ecstasy": a report of five deaths associated with the use of MDEA and MDMA. *JAMA* 1987;257:1615–1617.

208. Nestor TA, Tamamoto WI, Kam TH, et al. Acute pulmonary oedema caused by crystalline methamphetamine. *Lancet* 1989;2:1277–1278.

209. Schmidt RA, Glenny RW, Godwin JD, et al. Panlobular emphysema in young intravenous Ritalin abusers. *Am Rev Respir Dis* 1991;143:649–656.

210. Sherman CB, Hudson LD, Pierson DJ. Severe precocious emphysema in intravenous methylphenidate (Ritalin) abusers. *Chest* 1987;92:1085–1087.

211. Saks BJ, Kilby AE, Dietrich PA, et al. Pleural and mediastinal changes following endoscopic injection sclerotherapy of esophageal varices. *Radiology* 1983;149:639–642.

212. Bacon BR, Bailey-Newton RS, Connors AF Jr. Pleural effusions after endoscopic variceal sclerotherapy. *Gastroenterology* 1985;88:1910–1914.

213. Monroe P, Morrow CF Jr, Millen JE, et al. Acute respiratory failure after sodium morrhuate esophageal sclerotherapy. *Gastroenterology* 1983;85:693–699.

214. Graham JR, Suby HI, LeCompte PR, et al. Fibrotic disorders associated with methysergide therapy for headache. *N Engl J Med* 1966;274:359–368.

215. Hindle W, Posner E, Sweetnam MT, et al. Pleural effusion and fibrosis during treatment with methysergide. *BMJ* 1970;1:605–606.

216. McElvaney NG, Wilcox PG, Churg A, et al. Pleuropulmonary disease during bromocriptine treatment of Parkinson's disease. *Arch Intern Med* 1988;148:2231–2236.

217. Kinnunen E, Viljanen A. Pleuropulmonary involvement during bromocriptine treatment. *Chest* 1988;94:1034–1036.

218. Ingemarsson I, Bengtsson B. A 5-year experience with terbutaline for preterm labor: low rate of severe side effects. *Obstet Gynecol* 1985;66:176–180.

219. Katz M, Robertson PA, Creasy RK. Cardiovascular complications associated with terbutaline treatment for preterm labor. *Am J Obstet Gynecol* 1981;139:605–608.

220. Pisani RJ, Rosenow EC 3rd. Pulmonary edema associated with tocolytic therapy. *Ann Intern Med* 1989;110:714–718.

221. Mabie WC, Pernoll ML, Witty JB, et al. Pulmonary edema induced by β-mimetic drugs. *South Med J* 1983;76:1354–1360.

222. Lund MB, Kongerud J, Nome O, et al. Lung function impairment in long-term survivors of Hodgkin's disease. *Ann Oncol* 1995;6:495–501.

223. Jules-Elysee K, Stover D, Yahalom J, et al. Pulmonary complications in lymphoma patients treated with high-dose therapy and autologous bone marrow transplantation. *Am Rev Respir Dis* 1992;146:485–491.

224. Carmichael DJ, Hamilton DV, Evans DB, et al. Interstitial pneumonitis secondary to azathioprine in a renal transplant patient. *Thorax* 1983;38:951–952.

225. Krowka MJ, Breuer RI, Kehoe TJ. Azathioprine-associated pulmonary dysfunction. *Chest* 1983;83:696–698.

226. Weisenburger DD. Interstitial pneumonitis associated with azathioprine therapy. *Am J Clin Pathol* 1978;69:181–185.

227. Stetter M, Schmidl M, Krapf R. Azathioprine hypersensitivity mimicking Goodpasture's syndrome. *Am J Kidney Dis* 1994;23:874–877.

228. Refaber, L, Sinnassamy P, Leroy B, et al. Azathioprine-induced pulmonary haemorrhage in a child after renal transplantation. *Pediatr Nephrol* 1995;9:470–473.

229. Durant JR, Norgard MJ, Murad TM, et al. Pulmonary toxicity associated with bis-chloroethylnitrosourea (BCNU). *Ann Intern Med* 1979;90:191–194.

230. Selker RG, Jacobs SA, Moore PB, et al. 1,3-Bis(2-chloroethyl)-1-nitrosourea (BCNU)-induced pulmonary fibrosis. *Neurosurgery* 1980;7:560–565.

231. Wolff SN, Phillips GL, Herzig GP. High-dose carmustine with autologous bone marrow transplantation for the adjuvant treatment of high-grade gliomas of the central nervous system. *Cancer Treat Rep* 1987;71:183–185.

232. Aronin PA, Mahaley MS Jr, Rudnick SA, et al. Prediction of BCNU pulmonary toxicity in patients with malignant gliomas: an assessment of risk factors. *N Engl J Med* 1980;303:183–188.

233. Weinstein AS, Diener-West M, Nelson DF, et al. Pulmonary toxicity of carmustine in patients treated for malignant glioma. *Cancer Treat Rep* 1986;70:943–946.

234. Cherniack RM, Abrams J, Kalica AR. Pulmonary disease associated with breast cancer therapy. *Am J Respir Crit Care Med* 1994;150:1169–1173.

235. Chap L, Shpiner R, Levine M, et al. Pulmonary toxicity of high-dose chemotherapy for breast cancer: a non-invasive approach to diagnosis and treatment. *Bone Marrow Transplant* 1997;20:1063–1067.

236. Rubio C, Hill ME, Milan S, et al. Idiopathic pneumonia syndrome after high-dose chemotherapy for relapsed Hodgkin's disease. *Br J Cancer* 1997;75:1044–1048.

237. O'Driscoll BR, Kalra S, Gattamaneni HR, et al. Late carmustine lung fibrosis: age at treatment may influence severity and survival. *Chest* 1995;107:1355–1357.

238. O'Driscoll BR, Hasleton PS, Taylor PM, et al. Active lung fibrosis up to 17 years after chemotherapy with carmustine (BCNU) in childhood. *N Engl J Med* 1990;323:378–382.

239. Patten GA, Billi JE, Rotman HH. Rapidly progressive, fatal pulmonary fibrosis induced by carmustine. *JAMA* 1980;244:687–688.

240. Mitsudo SM, Greenwald ES, Banerji B, et al. BCNU (1,3-bis-(2-chloroethyl)-1-nitrosurea) lung: drug-induced pulmonary changes. *Cancer* 1984;54:751–755.

241. Holoye PY, Jenkins DE, Greenberg SD. Pulmonary toxicity in long-term administration of BCNU. *Cancer Treat Rep* 1976;60:1691–1694.

242. Brown MJ, Miller RR, Muller NL. Acute lung disease in the immunocompromised host: CT and pathologic examination findings. *Radiology* 1994;190:247–254.

243. Alessandrino EP, Bernasconi P, Colombo A, et al. Pulmonary toxicity following carmustine-based preparative regimens and autologous peripheral blood progenitor cell transplantation in hematological malignancies. *Bone Marrow Transplant* 2000;25:309–313.

244. Kalaycioglu M, Kavuru M, Tuason L, et al. Empiric prednisone therapy for pulmonary toxic reaction after high-dose chemotherapy containing carmustine (BCNU). *Chest* 1995;107:482–487.

245. Taylor PM, O'Driscoll BR, Gattamaneni HR, et al. Chronic lung fibrosis following carmustine (BCNU) chemotherapy: radiological features. *Clin Radiol* 1991;44:299–301.

246. Hasleton PS, O'Driscoll BR, Lynch P, et al. Late BCNU lung: a light and ultrastructural study on the delayed effect of BCNU on the lung parenchyma. *J Pathol* 1991;164:31–36.

247. Jules-Elysee K, White DA. Bleomycin-induced pulmonary toxicity. *Clin Chest Med* 1990;11:1–20.

248. Holoye PY, Luna MA, MacKay B, et al. Bleomycin hypersensitivity pneumonitis. *Ann Intern Med* 1978;88:47–49.

249. Glasier CM, Siegel MJ. Multiple pulmonary nodules: unusual manifestation of bleomycin toxicity. *AJR Am J Roentgenol* 1981;137:155–156.

250. Cohen MB, Austin JH, Smith-Vaniz A, et al. Nodular bleomycin toxicity. *Am J Clin Pathol* 1989;92:101–104.

251. White DA, Schwartzberg LS, Kris MG, et al. Acute chest pain syndrome during bleomycin infusions. *Cancer* 1987;59:1582–1585.

252. Catane R, Schwade JG, Turrisi AT 3rd, et al. Pulmonary toxicity after radiation and bleomycin: a review. *Int J Radiat Oncol Biol Phys* 1979;5:1513–1518.

253. Blum RH, Carter SK, Agre K. A clinical review of bleomycin: a new antineoplastic agent. *Cancer* 1973;31:903–914.

254. Jones AW. Bleomycin lung damage: the pathology and nature of the lesion. *Br J Dis Chest* 1978;72:321–326.

255. Bauer KA, Skarin AT, Balikian JP, et al. Pulmonary complications associated with combination chemotherapy programs containing bleomycin. *Am J Med* 1983;74:557–563.

256. Goldiner PL, Carlon GC, Cvitkovic E, et al. Factors influencing postoperative morbidity and mortality in patients treated with bleomycin. *Br Med J* 1978;1:1664–1667.

257. Kawai K, Hinotsu S, Tomobe M, et al. Serum creatinine level during chemotherapy for testicular cancer as a possible predictor of bleomycin-induced pulmonary toxicity. *Jpn J Clin Oncol* 1998;28:546–550.

258. Ngan HY, Liang RH, Lam WK, et al. Pulmonary toxicity in patients with non-Hodgkin's lymphoma treated with bleomycin-containing combination chemotherapy. *Cancer Chemother Pharmacol* 1993;32:407–409.

259. Bellamy EA, Husband JE, Blaquiere RM, et al. Bleomycin-related lung damage: CT evidence. *Radiology* 1985;156:155–158.

260. Wolkowicz J, Sturgeon J, Rawji M, et al. Bleomycin-induced pulmonary function abnormalities. *Chest* 1992;101:97–101.

261. Luna MA, Bedrossian CW, Lichtiger B, et al. Interstitial pneumonitis associated with bleomycin therapy. *Am J Clin Pathol* 1972;58:501–510.

262. Iacovino JR, Leitner J, Abbas AK, et al. Fatal pulmonary reaction from low doses of bleomycin: an idiosyncratic tissue response. *JAMA* 1976;235:1253–1255.

263. Yousem SA, Lifson JD, Colby TV. Chemotherapy-induced eosinophilic pneumonia. Relation to bleomycin. *Chest* 1985;88:103–106.

264. O'Neill TJ, Kardinal CG, Tierney LM. Reversible interstitial pneumonitis associated with low dose bleomycin. *Chest* 1975;68:265–267.

265. McCusker K, Dorman RA, Nicholson DP, et al. Reversible pulmonary injury after a small dose of bleomycin. *South Med J* 1983;76:1447–1449.

266. White DA, Stover DE. Severe bleomycin-induced pneumonitis: clinical features and response to corticosteroids. *Chest* 1984;86:723–728.

267. Simpson AB, Paul J, Graham J, et al. Fatal bleomycin pulmonary toxicity in the west of Scotland 1991–95: a review of patients with germ cell tumours. *Br J Cancer* 1998;78:1061–1066.

268. Heard BE, Cooke RA. Busulphan lung. *Thorax* 1968;23:187–193.

269. Burns WA, McFarland W, Matthews MJ. Busulfan-induced pulmonary disease: report of a case and review of the literature. *Am Rev Respir Dis* 1970;101:408–413.

270. Collis CH. Lung damage from cytotoxic drugs. *Cancer Chemother Pharmacol* 1980;4:17–27.

271. Harrold BP. Syndrome resembling Addison's disease following prolonged treatment with busulphan. *BMJ* 1966;5485:463–464.

272. Littler WA, Kay JM, Hasleton PS, et al. Busulphan lung. *Thorax* 1969;24:639–655.

273. Comhaire F, Van Hove W, Van Ganse W, et al. Busulphan and the lungs: absence of lung function disturbance in patients treated with busulphan. *Scand J Respir Dis* 1972;53:265–273.

274. Miyashita T, Ojima A, Tuji T, et al. Varied pulmonary lesions with intraalveolar large lamellar bodies in an autopsy case with busulfan therapy. *Acta Pathol Jpn* 1977;27:239–249.

275. Aymard JP, Gyger M, Lavallee R, et al. A case of pulmonary alveolar proteinosis complicating chronic myelogenous leukemia: a peculiar pathologic aspect of busulfan lung? *Cancer* 1984;53:954–956.

276. Podoll LN, Winkler SS. Busulfan lung: report of two cases and review of the literature. *Am J Roentgenol Radium Ther Nucl Med* 1974;120:151–156.

277. Rose MS. Busulphan toxicity syndrome caused by chlorambucil. *BMJ* 1975;2:123.

278. Refvem O. Fatal intraalveolar and interstitial lung fibrosis in chlorambucil-treated chronic lymphocytic leukemia. *Mt Sinai J Med* 1977;44:847–851.

279. Cole SR, Myers TJ, Klatsky AU. Pulmonary disease with chlorambucil therapy. *Cancer* 1978;41:455–459.

280. Lane SD, Besa EC, Justh G, et al. Fatal interstitial pneumonitis following high-dose intermittent chlorambucil therapy for chronic lymphocyte leukemia. *Cancer* 1981;47:32–36.

281. Godard P, Marty JP, Michel FB. Interstitial pneumonia and chlorambucil. *Chest* 1979;76:471–473.

282. Giles FJ, Smith MP, Goldstone AH. Chlorambucil lung toxicity. *Acta Haematol* 1990;83:156–158.

283. Carr ME Jr. Chlorambucil induced pulmonary fibrosis: report of a case and review. *Va Med* 1986;113:677–680.

284. Crestani B, Jaccard A, Israel-Biet D, et al. Chlorambucil-associated pneumonitis. *Chest* 1994;105:634–636.

285. Mohr M, Kingreen D, Ruhl H, et al. Interstitial lung disease: an underdiagnosed side effect of chlorambucil? *Ann Hematol* 1993;67:305–307.

286. Alvarado CS, Boat TF, Newman AJ. Late-onset pulmonary fibrosis and chest deformity in two children treated with cyclophosphamide. *J Pediatr* 1978;92:443–446.

287. Mark GJ, Lehimgar-Zadeh A, Ragsdale BD. Cyclophosphamide pneumonitis. *Thorax* 1978;33:89–93.

288. Spector JI, Zimbler H, Ross JS. Early-onset cyclophosphamide-induced interstitial pneumonitis. *JAMA* 1979;242:2852–2854.

289. Spector JI. Zimbler H, Ross JS. Cyclophosphamide and interstitial pneumonitis. *JAMA* 1980;243:1133.

290. Burke DA, Stoddart JC, Ward MK, et al. Fatal pulmonary fibrosis occurring during treatment with cyclophosphamide. *Br Med J (Clin Res Ed)* 1982;285:696.

291. Malik SW, Myers JL, DeRemee RA, et al. Lung toxicity associated with cyclophosphamide use: two distinct patterns. *Am J Respir Crit Care Med* 1996;154(6 pt 1):1851–1856.

292. Padley SP, Adler B, Hansell DM, et al. High-resolution computed tomography of drug-induced lung disease. *Clin Radiol* 1992;46:232–236.

293. Topilow AA, Rothenberg SP, Cottrell TS. Interstitial pneumonia after prolonged treatment with cyclophosphamide. *Am Rev Respir Dis* 1973;108:114–117.

294. Abdel Karim FW, Ayash RE, Allam C, et al. Pulmonary fibrosis after prolonged treatment with low-dose cyclophosphamide: a case report. *Oncology* 1983;40:174–176.

295. Patel AR, Shah PC, Rhee HL, et al. Cyclophosphamide therapy and interstitial pulmonary fibrosis. *Cancer* 1976;38:1542–1549.

296. Rosenow EC 3rd, Myers JL, Swensen SJ, et al. Drug-induced pulmonary disease: an update. *Chest* 1992;102:239–250.

297. Tham RT, Peters G, de Bruine FT, et al. Pulmonary complications of cytosine-arabinoside therapy: radiographic findings. *AJR Am J Roentgenol* 1987;149:23–27.

298. Andersson BS, Luna MA, Yee C, et al. Fatal pulmonary failure complicating high-dose cytosine arabinoside therapy in acute leukemia. *Cancer* 1990;65:1079–1084.

299. Pavlakis N, Bell DR, Millward MJ, et al. Fatal pulmonary toxicity resulting from treatment with gemcitabine. *Cancer* 1997;80:286–291.

300. Marruchella A, Fiorenzano G, Merizzi A, et al. Diffuse alveolar damage in a patient treated with gemcitabine. *Eur Respir J* 1998;11:504–506.

301. Briasoulis E, Froudarakis M, Milionis HJ, et al. Chemotherapy-induced noncardiogenic pulmonary edema related to gemcitabine plus docetaxel combination with granulocyte colony-stimulating factor support. *Respiration* 2000;67:680–683.

302. Linskens RK, Golding RP, van Groeningen CJ, et al. Severe acute lung injury induced by gemcitabine. *Neth J Med* 2000;56:232–235.

303. Boiselle PM, Morrin MM, Huberman MS. Gemcitabine pulmonary toxicity: CT features. *J Comput Assist Tomogr* 2000;24:977–980.

304. Sauer-Heilborn A, Kath R, Schneider CP, et al. Severe non-haematological toxicity after gemcitabine. *J Cancer Res Clin Oncol* 1999;125:637–640.

305. Codling BW, Chakera TM. Pulmonary fibrosis following therapy with Melphalan for multiple myeloma. *J Clin Pathol* 1972;25:668–673.

306. Taetle R, Dickman PS, Feldman PS. Pulmonary histopathologic changes associated with melphalan therapy. *Cancer* 1978;42:1239–1245.

307. Westerfield BT, Michalski JP, McCombs C, et al. Reversible melphalan-induced lung damage. *Am J Med* 1980;68:767–771.

308. Goucher G, Rowland V, Hawkins J. Melphalan-induced pulmonary interstitial fibrosis. *Chest* 1980;77:805–806.

309. Gutin PH, Green MR, Bleyer WA, et al. Methotrexate pneumonitis induced by intrathecal methotrexate therapy: a case report with pharmacokinetic data. *Cancer* 1976;38:1529–1534.

310. Buzdar AU, Legha SS, Luna MA, et al. Pulmonary toxicity of mitomycin. *Cancer* 1980;45:236–244.

311. Gunstream SR, Seidenfeld JJ, Sobonya RE, et al. Mitomycin-associated lung disease. *Cancer Treat Rep* 1983;67:301–304.

312. Rivera MP, Kris MG, Gralla RJ, et al. Syndrome of acute dyspnea related to combined mitomycin plus vinca alkaloid chemotherapy. *Am J Clin Oncol* 1995;18:245–250.

313. Castro M, Veeder MH, Mailliard JA, et al. A prospective study of pulmonary function in patients receiving mitomycin. *Chest* 1996;109:939–944.

314. Kris MG, Pablo D, Gralla RJ, et al. Dyspnea following vinblastine or vindesine administration in patients receiving mitomycin plus vinca alkaloid combination therapy. *Cancer Treat Rep* 1984;68:1029–1031.

315. Thompson CC, Bailey MK, Conroy JM, et al. Postoperative pulmonary toxicity associated with mitomycin-C therapy. *South Med J* 1992;85:1257–1259.

316. Rao SX, Ramaswamy G, Levin M, et al. Fatal acute respiratory failure after vinblastine-mitomycin therapy in lung carcinoma. *Arch Intern Med* 1985;145:1905–1907.

317. Orwoll ES, Kiessling PJ, Patterson JR. Interstitial pneumonia from mitomycin. *Ann Intern Med* 1978;89:352–355.

318. Sheldon R, Slaughter D. A syndrome of microangiopathic hemolytic anemia, renal impairment, and pulmonary edema in chemotherapy-treated patients with adenocarcinoma. *Cancer* 1986;58:1428–1436.

319. Chang-Poon VY, Hwang WS, Wong A, et al. Pulmonary angiomatoid vascular changes in mitomycin C–associated hemolytic-uremic syndrome. *Arch Pathol Lab Med* 1985;109:877–878.

320. Andrews AT, Bowman HS, Patel SB, et al. Mitomycin and interstitial pneumonitis. *Ann Intern Med* 1979;90:127.

321. Chang AY, Kuebler JP, Pandya KJ, et al. Pulmonary toxicity induced by mitomycin C is highly responsive to glucocorticoids. *Cancer* 1986;57:2285–2290.

322. Jones SE, Moore M, Blank N, et al. Hypersensitivity to procarbazine (Matulane) manifested by fever and pleuropulmonary reaction. *Cancer* 1972;29:498–500.

323. Ecker MD, Jay B, Keohane MK. Procarbazine lung. *AJR Am J Roentgenol* 1978;131:527–528.

324. Coyle T, Bushunow P, Winfield J, et al. Hypersensitivity reactions to procarbazine with mechlorethamine, vincristine, and

procarbazine chemotherapy in the treatment of glioma. *Cancer* 1992;69:2532–2540.

325. Weiss RB, Donehower RC, Wiernik PH, et al. Hypersensitivity reactions from Taxol. *J Clin Oncol* 1990;8:1263–1268.

326. Stemmer SM, Cagnoni PJ, Shpall EJ, et al. High-dose paclitaxel, cyclophosphamide, and cisplatin with autologous hematopoietic progenitor-cell support: a phase I trial. *J Clin Oncol* 1996;14:1463–1472.

327. Goldberg HL, Vannice SB. Pneumonitis related to treatment with paclitaxel. *J Clin Oncol* 1995;13:534–535.

328. Reckzeh B, Merte BH, Pfluger KH, et al. Severe lymphocytopenia and interstitial pneumonia in patients treated with paclitaxel and simultaneous radiotherapy for non–small cell lung cancer. *J Clin Oncol* 1996;14:1071–1076.

329. Schweitzer VG, Juillard GJ, Bajada CL, et al. Radiation recall dermatitis and pneumonitis in a patient treated with paclitaxel. *Cancer* 1995 76:1069–1072.

Radiation-Induced Lung Disease

34

John L. Faul · Thomas A. Raffin

Radiation therapy protocols are designed to achieve effective cancer kill while avoiding injury to normal lung. Radiation-induced lung injury encompasses a spectrum that includes acute radiation-induced tracheobronchitis, radiation pneumonitis, radiation-induced bronchiolitis obliterans organizing pneumonia, and radiation-induced lung fibrosis (1–4). Each disorder is iatrogenic and has a characteristic time course, exacerbating feature, and treatment. Much clinical and pathologic data, in addition to controlled experimentation in animal models, have established a good understanding of the temporal progression of tissue injury after irradiation (5, 6). The sequelae of irradiation should be assessed in terms of radiation dose, lung function, and time (7–10). Because the cause of radiation-induced lung disease is known, it is hoped that the clinical sequelae of radiation therapy can be predicted, and severity estimated based solely on a variety of biologic parameters, including prior lung function, radiation dose, concomitant therapy, and treatment intervals (11–15). To date, the interaction between irradiation, chemotherapy, and a variety of biologic response modifiers has made these calculations complex (16, 17). Doses of irradiation that are thought to be safe may prove toxic in combination with other biologic factors (17). In terms of dosage, emphasis is currently placed on the volume of lung irradiated (18). Dose-escalation studies and multicenter studies promise to create accurate models that allow prediction of disease (18, 19).

HISTORICAL PERSPECTIVES

Conrad Roentgen discovered x-rays in 1895. Henri Becquerel discovered x-ray emission from naturally occurring

substances in 1896. The first evidence of pulmonary toxicity was documented in 1898 in a study of guinea pigs by Bergonie and Teissier. With the development of higher-energy x-rays, radiation therapists began to describe lung fibrosis in humans. In 1922, Hines reported two cases of lung fibrosis with autopsy findings. Corticosteroids were first used for the treatment of pulmonary radiation toxicity by Cosgriff and Kligerman and for prophylaxis by Friedenberg and Rubenfeld (20–22).

PRINCIPLES OF RADIATION BIOLOGY

Ionizing radiation does not distinguish between normal cells and cancer cells. Radiation causes ionization of molecules within cells, leading to direct effects in which x-rays actually interact with nuclear DNA (thought to be rare), and to indirect effects in which the ionization of water molecules within a cell creates reactive species $OH, H_2O_2, and O,$ which in turn interact with cell structures, including nuclear DNA (23) (Fig. 34.1). The impact of radiation-induced DNA damage is thought to be greatest at the time of mitotic division (24). Therefore, in general, the impact on tissues with rapidly dividing cells will be greater than the impact on tissues that are quiescent (1).

The conventional term for the energy that leads to damage is termed *ionizing radiation.* In the presence of oxygen, some free radicals oxidize to form organic peroxide, which causes further tissue damage (25). After irradiation of cells *in vitro* or *in vivo* a characteristic dose-response curve is generated (Fig. 34.2). Irradiation may result in sublethal damage (i.e., the amount of radiation absorbed by cells is less than that required to produce a lethal effect). At radiation doses higher than this threshold, the fraction of cells that survive is inversely related to the dose. The amount of sublethal damage that can be repaired has been measured for many cell

J. L. Faul and T. A. Raffin: Division of Pulmonary and Critical Care Medicine, Stanford University Medical Center, Stanford, California.

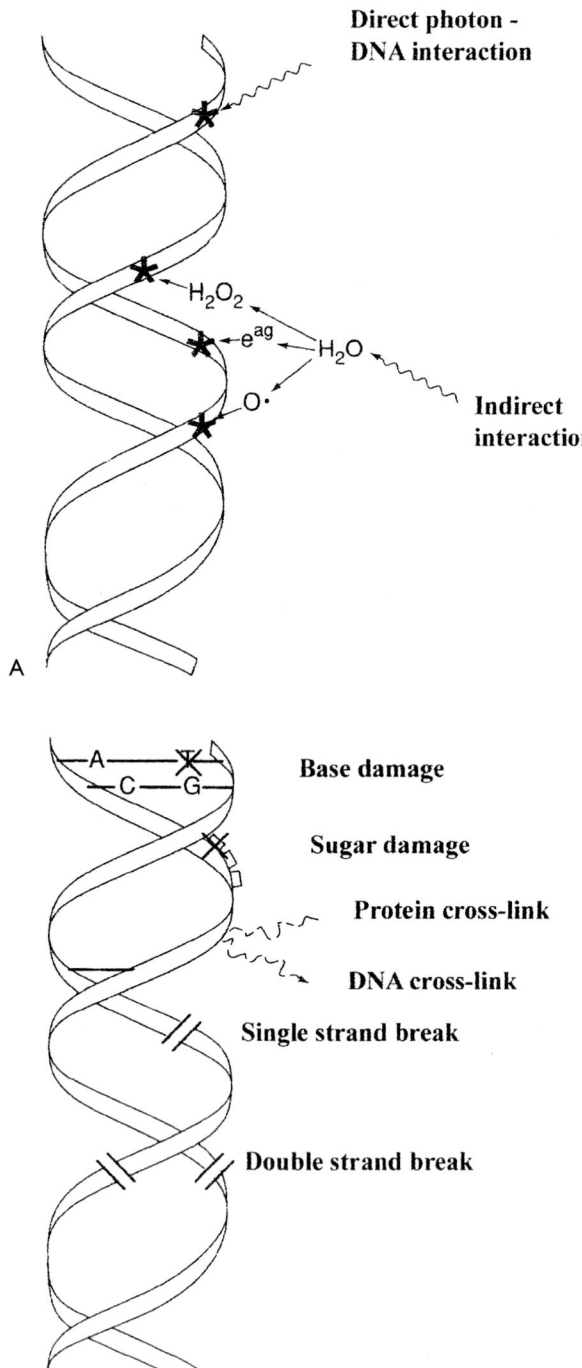

Direct photon - DNA interaction

Indirect interaction

Base damage

Sugar damage

Protein cross-link

DNA cross-link

Single strand break

Double strand break

FIGURE 34.1. Putative mode of damage to DNA during radiation. **(A)** How radiation might interact both directly with the DNA molecule and indirectly by ionizing water to form reactive species that damage DNA. **(B)** Several points at which damage to DNA might lead to DNA mutation. (Adapted from Richter AS. Radiation therapy. In: Abeloff MD, Armitage JO, Lichter AS, et al., eds. *Clinical oncology.* London: Churchill Livingstone, 1995, with permission.)

types, and there are techniques by which it can be measured *in vivo.* Some biologic factors can modify cellular response to injury, including metronidazole, 5-fluorouracil, cisplatin, and hydroxyurea (26–30). The survival curve after a second dose of radiation given after an interval indicates that damage can be accumulated for a lethal effect. In addition, repair can be inhibited, suggesting that repair is an active cellular process (31–34).

The unit of radiation exposure is the roentgen (R). A rad is the unit of absorbed radiation, and it is equal to 100 ergs absorbed energy per gram of tissue. Radiation therapists commonly use the unit gray (Gy), which is equal to 100 rad, or the centigray (cGy), which is equal to 1 rad. The cGy is the amount of energy absorbed per gram of tissue, so that a dose of 50 Gy to a lung is only a fraction of the energy absorbed when 50 Gy is received by the whole body (35).

A variety of mathematical models exist to determine the safe dose an entire organ can receive without producing complications (T5 for whole volume of an organ) or the threshold or tolerance dose for a small boost volume (T5 for partial volume of an organ). These models include Strandqvist lines (36), the nominal standard dose (37), the time-dose factor and cumulative radiation effect (38), and the linear-quadratic survival relationship (α/β ratio) (39) (Fig. 34.3). Currently, emphasis is placed on the volume of lung irradiated, global (whole organ) function, and focal (partial volume) injury as a function of the dose-volume histogram (DVH) (Fig. 34.4). There also appears to be regional variation in the response to radiation. The risk of high-grade pneumonitis is greater in the lower lobes than in the upper lobes (40). There is no single equation that predicts tumor kill or lung damage, because there are a number of assumptions about varying geometry and tissue density that have to be made for each patient by each radiotherapist. In addition, most organ systems are comprised of several key cell types that perform important functions. The most radiosensitive vital cell population will determine organ tolerance and organ failure.

The National Cancer Institute has developed a classification for *s*ubjective, *o*bjective, *m*anagement criteria, and *a*nalytic laboratory and imaging procedures (SOMA). These criteria form a framework for late-effect normal tissue (LENT) expression of radiation-induced lung disease (38, 41). The LENT paradigm suggests an appropriate management plan for patients who undergo radiation therapy. The 10-step process in the clinical management of radiation induced lung disease is as follows.

Clinical Detection

Acute radiation toxicity, including radiation bronchitis, occurs immediately or shortly after radiation treatment (42). Acute radiation toxicity is uncommon and is generally reported only after very high radiation doses (>50–60Gy).

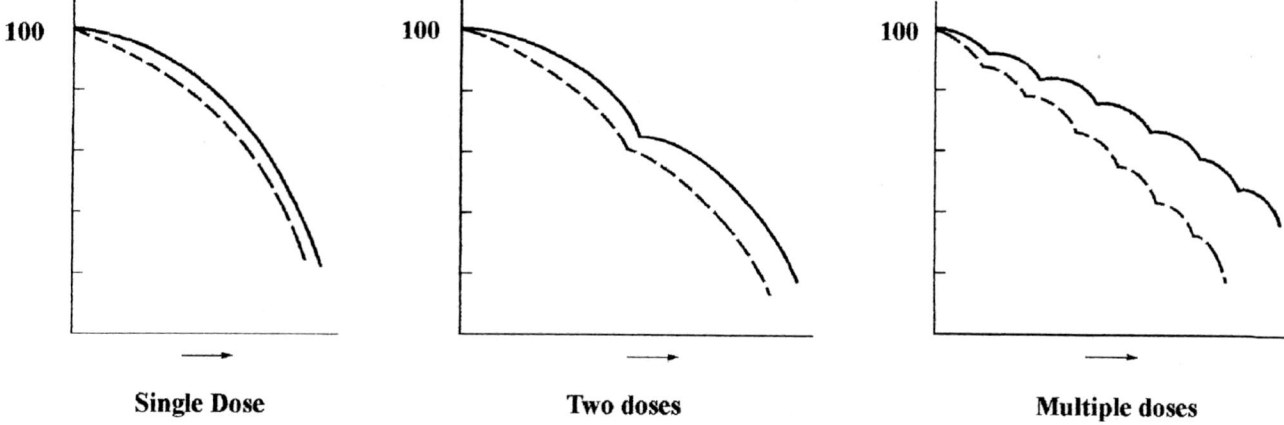

Single Dose **Two doses** **Multiple doses**

FIGURE 34.2. Diagram of the effect of fractionation on cell survival. Cell survival (as a percentage) is represented on the y-axis. The *solid lines* represent cancer cells; *dashed lines,* normal tissue. Small differences in the slopes of the curves are amplified when multiple doses are given. (Adapted from Richter AS. Radiation therapy. In: Abeloff MD, Armitage JO, Lichter AS, et al., eds. *Clinical oncology.* London: Churchill Livingstone, 1995, with permission.)

Damage predominantly involves the tracheobronchial tree. The majority of patients are asymptomatic from a respiratory standpoint immediately after radiation therapy, but some describe an occasional dry cough. If symptoms are severe, the course of treatment should be suspended for a week or two, as much time as for radiation esophagitis. In association with reductions in pulmonary function tests, patients report more coughing, wheezing, and dyspnea (42).

Radiation pneumonitis, rather than lung fibrosis, is acutely life-threatening. Early recognition and diagnosis are important, because early treatment may affect the course of

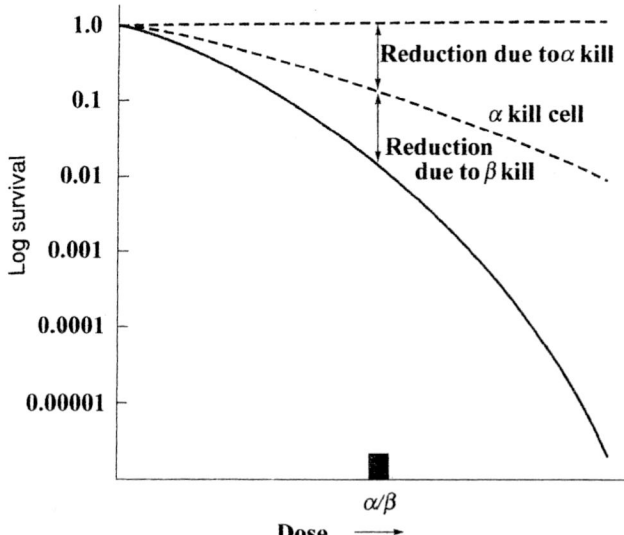

FIGURE 34.3. Illustration of the concept of α/β kill during radiation therapy. Cell killing is comprised of two components. α-Cell kill is irreparable, but β-cell kill can be repaired. The α/β ratio represents the point at which the reduction in cell survival from α and β are equal. (Adapted from Richter AS. Radiation therapy. In: Abeloff MD, Armitage JO, Lichter AS, et al., eds. *Clinical oncology.* London: Churchill Livingstone, 1995, with permission.)

pneumonitis (43). Untoward reactions after radiation can be anticipated by radiologic monitoring and serial lung function testing (44). The appearance of abnormalities does not inevitably lead to pneumonitis. Patients who are at increased risk because of an unavoidable contributory factor should be monitored carefully.

Patients whose symptoms are not severe or those who develop late pneumonitis (i.e., 10–12 weeks after completion of radiotherapy) will probably have a mild clinical course (45). Symptomatic therapy, restriction of activity, cough suppressants, and observation are required. If an early reaction occurs and symptoms progress rapidly, additional therapy, including corticosteroid therapy, may be required.

Radiation pneumonitis develops insidiously (46). Patients commonly present more than 6 to 8 weeks after completion of irradiation, earlier if some contributory factors are present. The most common symptom of radiation pneumonitis is dyspnea. Mild dyspnea occurs on exertion at first, and may progress in the course of a week or two to severe dyspnea on minimal effort. Occasionally, mild dyspnea progresses to severe respiratory failure in only a few days. A dry harsh cough is also common. Small amounts of clear or pink sputum may be seen. Fever and pleuritic chest pain are also common. Physical signs include tachypnea and tachycardia. Examination of the chest may reveal the tattoo marks that outline the treatment field. A comparison between the tattoos and the chest x-ray is highly suggestive of a radiation reaction (47). There is no association between the severity of skin reactions, such as pigmentation and desquamation, and the presence of an underlying lung reaction (48). Pleural friction rubs or rales may be present. Features of respiratory distress syndrome with or without right-sided heart failure are present in severe cases. Radiation pneumonitis typically lasts several weeks or months. Commonly, symptoms persist for a month or more (49).

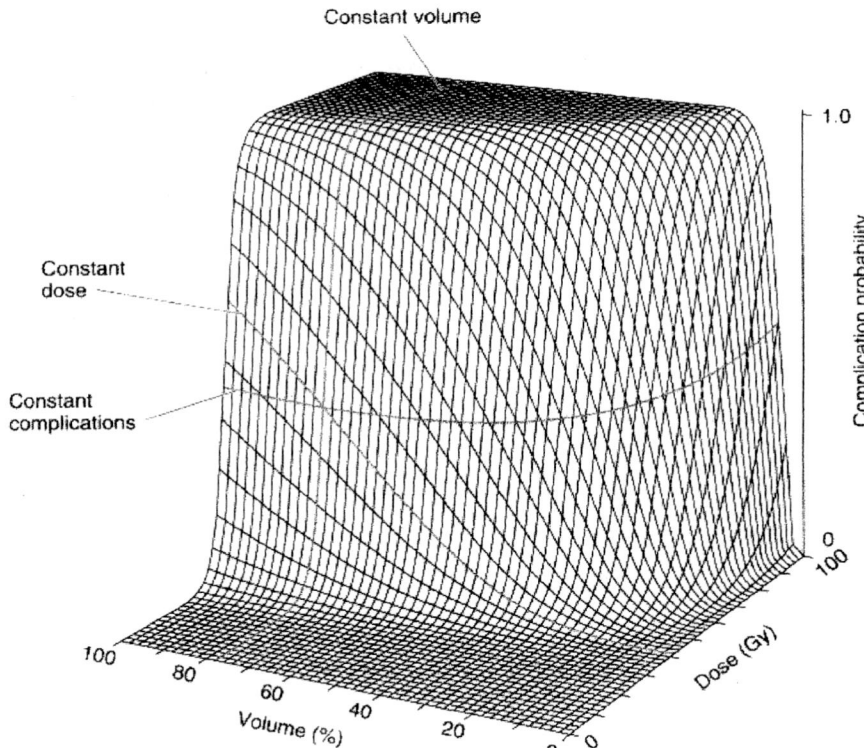

FIGURE 34.4. A three-dimensional representation of the relationship of dose, tissue volume, and complications. (From Burman C, Kutcher GJ, Emami B, et al. Fitting of normal tissue tolerance data to an analytic function. *Int J Radiation Oncol Biol Phys* 1991;21:123–135, with permission.)

The term *radiation fibrosis* is generally used as a clinical, rather than histologic diagnosis. In those who have experienced severe radiation pneumonitis, pulmonary fibrosis results in chronic respiratory failure. Some patients later develop chronic cor pulmonale (Fig. 34.5). Commonly, there is a moderate exacerbation of pre-existing symptoms or reduction in exercise tolerance. Most cases are asymptomatic. Symptoms include low-grade fever, dry cough, and dyspnea. Signs include inspiratory crackles, lung consolidation, and pleural rub. Physical signs are consistent with those of lung restriction, including poor chest expansion, mediastinal shift in the case of unilateral fibrosis, and loss of inspiratory excursion. Finger clubbing may develop. Radiation-induced fibrosis is often a diagnosis of exclusion (50). The workup of patients with radiation-induced fibrosis includes bronchoscopy with bronchoalveolar lavage (BAL). Radiation-induced fibrosis may occur in the presence or absence of prior pneumonitis. Symptoms include exertional dyspnea, orthopnea, chest pain, and cor pulmonale (48). In general, symptomatology is proportional to both the extent and dose

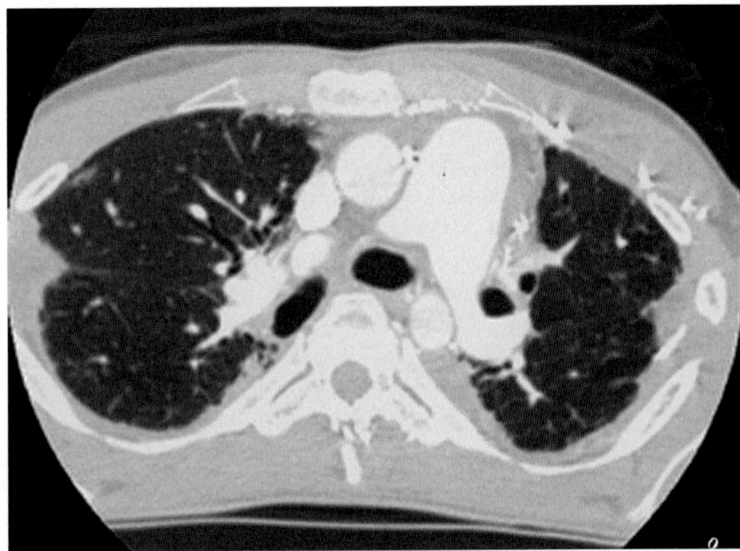

FIGURE 34.5. Thoracic computed axial tomography scan of a 27-year-old man with severe lung restriction, respiratory failure, and pulmonary hypertension, who had received radiation therapy to the chest for Hodgkin disease 10 years earlier. Note the pleural thickening, mediastinal fibrosis, and enlarged pulmonary arterial trunk.

of radiation and pre-existing pulmonary reserve. The volume of irradiated lung is directly associated with the risk of chronic respiratory failure (51).

Time Course

Radiation-induced lung disease generally occurs 1 to 3 months after fractionated and single-dose therapy, although reactions can occur during therapy when combination chemotherapy is used simultaneously (52). Injury to the lung typically occurs during radiation therapy for lung cancer, breast cancer, and thoracic lymphoma. Lung injury is generally divided into three phases: acute, early, and late reactions (53). The two major distinct clinical effects of lung irradiation are conventionally divided into radiation pneumonitis (which occurs after 1–3 months) and radiation fibrosis (which occurs after 2–4 months). Acute pneumonitis generally occurs after radiation exposure of both lungs and occurs with single doses exceeding 7.5 Gy, with a steep dose response up to 10 Gy (which can result in high lethality) (54). Although 5% to 15% of subjects have clinical complaints, more than half have radiographic abnormalities.

Dose/Time/Volume

Are radiation factors consistent with the clinical picture? For single doses to the whole of both lungs, the T5 is about 8 Gy, whereas for fractionated doses of 1.8 to 2.0 Gy with limited volume (>30%), it is 45 to 50 Gy. Strategies to prevent lung injury include three-dimensional (3D) computerized radiation therapy systems to optimize dose and volume. In patients with non–small-cell lung cancer (NSCLC), the risk of lung toxicity is increased when treated with field sizes in excess of the protocol-specified margins (55). It is not the maximum dose that is important but the volume treated to a critical dose. The majority of patients are treated at 1.8 or 2 Gy with each treatment, so fractionation is not as important as it was historically (56).

Many factors—such as fractionation, overall treatment time, and patient specific aspects—are important when estimating the effects of partial lung irradiation. The easy-to-calculate mean lung dose and the volume irradiated to 20 Gy (V_{20}) can both be used to predict the incidence of radiation pneumonitis (57). These parameters represent two extremes in underlying local dose-effect relations for radiation pneumonitis. However, clinically applied treatment plans show a high correlation between the V_{20} and the mean lung dose, so that the decision for the "best" underlying local dose-effect relation should be based on the analysis of additional patient data. Radiation-induced lung injury is also affected by use of various chemotherapeutic agents, in particular, bleomycin, adriamycin, actinomycin D, and carmustine (58). The lung demonstrates a high radiosensitivity. This has been observed in fractionated irradiation exposure as a component of total body irradiation for recipients of bone marrow transplants,

in which many patients suffer fatal pneumonitis. The dose range for a lethal radiation-induced pneumonitis is firmly established at 8.2 Gy for a 5% incidence, 9.3 Gy for a 50% incidence, and 11.0 Gy for an 80% incidence after a single high dose-rate exposure. This dose-response relationship is shifted to the right for protracted low dose-rate radiation as used in total-body irradiation for bone marrow transplants (59, 60).

The relation between lung dose-volume histogram-based factors and symptomatic radiation pneumonitis has been studied in 201 patients with lung cancer who were undergoing 3D radiotherapy planning (61). By using both univariate and multivariate analysis, all dosimetric factors (i.e., mean lung dose, volume of lung receiving greater than 30 Gy, and normal tissue complication probabilities) were associated with the development of radiation pneumonitis. Interestingly, tobacco use at the time of referral for radiation therapy was associated with a reduced risk of developing radiation pneumonitis ($P = .05$) (61). Dosimetric factors appear to be the best predictors of symptomatic radiation pneumonitis after external beam radiation therapy for lung cancer (61). Dubray has demonstrated that after thoracic radiation for Hodgkin lymphoma (35–40 Gy), the risk of radiation fibrosis increases with radiation dose per fraction (62). Roach has demonstrated that the use of a fraction size greater than 2.67 Gy is associated with increased risk of pneumonitis after combined modality therapy for lung cancer (63). In addition, twice-daily dosing is associated with reduced risk of lung injury compared with the same total dose given as a single fraction. (63). Graham and others have demonstrated that a DVH is useful for predicting outcomes as a result of volume loss. V_{20} from DVH may be useful to identify NSCLC patients at risk for pneumonitis when treated with 3D radiation therapy (64).

Chemical/Biologic Modifiers

Several antineoplastic agents potentiate the effects of radiation on the lung (17, 58, 65). Cyclophosphamide, epirubicin, and 5-fluorouracil enhance the toxicity of thoracic radiation (45, 65). In prospective studies, an increased incidence of computed tomography (CT)–observed radiation changes and reductions in lung function have been observed to occur in association with a variety of chemotherapeutic regimes (65, 66). Bleomycin-induced lung injury manifests as an interstitial pneumonitis that can progress to fibrosis. When given in combination with radiation, lung injury is greater than with either agent alone (67). The effect is maximal when bleomycin and radiation therapy are given concurrently. Actinomycin D enhances the adverse effects of radiation therapy on the lung. At equivalent radiation doses, pneumonitis is about 30% more likely to occur in patients who receive concomitant actinomycin D therapy. Patients who receive mechlorethamine, procarbazine, and vincristine have a high incidence of symptomatic radiation pneumonitis compared with that of patients who do not receive chemotherapy. Einhorn reported a high incidence of severe radiation pneumonitis in patients who received concomitant bleomycin, doxorubicin (Adriamycin), cyclophosphamide, and vincristine (68). Patients given chemotherapy alone suffered no pulmonary effects, nor did a further 20 patients who received radiation and the same chemotherapeutic treatment without bleomycin. In another report, fulminant fatal pneumonitis occurred 4 weeks after a course of 4,000 rad to the mantle for Hodgkin disease in a patient who had taken busulfan for polycythemia (69). Doxorubicin has marked effects on the myocardium and may enhance the radiation effects to the lungs. Significant pulmonary toxicity has been associated with actinomycin (0.075 mg/kg of body weight), cyclophosphamide (75 mg/kg), and vincristine (0.5 mg/kg) given 2 hours before irradiation. With actinomycin D, there is a significant increase in toxicity, even when a small dose (0.015 mg/kg) is given 30 days before irradiation. The drugs that potentiate the effects of radiation differ from those that commonly cause pneumonitis in the absence of irradiation (70). There is no obvious relationship between the mode of action of these agents and their toxic effects on the irradiated lung.

When radiation is readministered to the same area, treatment commonly leads to further loss of function. It is unclear whether the phenomenon is a function of the total dose received or whether tissue is more susceptible after the first course (71).

Ataxia telangiectasia, a rare hereditary syndrome characterized by cerebellar ataxia, oculocutaneous telangiectasia, immunologic deficiencies, and an increased incidence of reticuloendothelial malignancy, appears to be associated with abnormal sensitivity to ionizing radiation. Increased radiosensitivity can be demonstrated at the molecular, cellular, and clinical levels (72). Radiotherapy for the malignant complications of the syndrome is likely to be followed by severe radiation toxicity. The radiosensitivity is thought to result from defective DNA repair, because subjects also develop chromosomal instability.

Increased age is associated with a greater loss in lung diffusing capacity (transfer factor) after therapy. There is an age-related increase in the frequency and severity of radio-

logic changes in irradiated breast cancer patients (51). The lungs of children recover better than those of older adults (73).

Radiologic Imaging

Are the findings on the chest x-ray and CT of the thorax consistent with the diagnosis? Radiographic abnormalities are more frequent than are clinical symptoms, and changes are typically confined to the field of irradiation (74, 75) (Table 34.1). Chest radiograph changes include the early onset of diffuse haziness with indistinct vascular markings. These appearances can progress to patchy or homogenous air-space opacification. The radiologic features of fibrosis, including reticular lines, will gradually appear from 6 to 24 months after irradiation and generally persist (76). After several months, reticular shadowing, consistent with fibrosis, typically occurs. This appearance generally remains stable for long periods. Classic findings include linear streaks in the area of previous irradiation, volume loss, pleural thickening, and tenting of the diaphragm consistent with volume loss (77). The progression of radiologic changes occurs in a predictable time course that depends on the dose and interval of radiation therapy. It is estimated that changes appear 8 weeks after treatment with 40 Gy delivered over 4 weeks, but the changes occur 1 week earlier for every 10 Gy over 40 Gy (78). Not only are radiologic changes more commonly seen after lung irradiation, but they generally precede clinical respiratory symptoms. The commonly recognized changes that occur 4 to 8 weeks after radiotherapy are diffuse ground-glass opacification, with indistinct lung markings (79). With evolution, the opacification becomes micronodular with linear branching streaks 1 cm or more in length that resemble Kerley B lines. As nodules and streaks become confluent, the region may become densely opacified, and air bronchograms may appear. Pleural and interlobar effusions may occur. The mediastinum and cardiac silhouettes often become indistinct. The most striking radiologic feature is progressive opacification of the irradiated region (80). This is particularly notable when irradiation was unilateral, because the trachea and mediastinum shift to the irradiated side (accompanied by elevation and tenting of the

TABLE 34.1. THE FREQUENCY OF RADIOGRAPHIC CHANGES AND PNEUMONITIS IN PATIENTS RECEIVING RADIATION THERAPY

Patient Group	Frequency of Radiographic Abnormalities	Frequency of Clinical Pneumonitis	References
Breast cancer	27–40	0–10	Polansky (118)
Lung cancer	~65	5–15	Ikezoe (87)
Mediastinal lymphoma	60–92	0	Shapiro (53)
Miscellaneous	67–87	0–18	Mah (65), Marks (172)

Adapted from McDonald S, Rubin P, Phillips TL, et al. Injury to the lung from cancer therapy: clinical syndromes, measurable endpoints, and potential scoring systems. *Int J Radiat Oncol Biol Phys* 1995;31:1187–1203, with permission.

diaphragm and narrowing of the intercostal spaces) (81). Cavitation does not occur in previously normal lung tissue, although it can occur in irradiated tumors. Hyperlucency of a lung after unilateral x-irradiation owing to hypoplasia of the pulmonary artery has been reported (82). Thoracic irradiation before thoracotomy has been associated with a higher incidence of delayed healing in previously irradiated tissues, leading to bronchopleural fistula and empyema (83).

It is useful to compare chest radiographs before and after therapy, and to observe the skin marks that correspond to the port margins. There is no reported association between the severity of skin pigmentation reactions and the presence of an underlying lung reaction. The diagnosis of radiation pneumonitis can usually be made based on the time course for the development of disease, combined with technical information concerning radiotherapy ports. The early appearance and rapid progression of the radiologic lesion generally signify a more severe clinical episode. The radiologic features of pneumonitis can persist for long periods, even years. Depending on the extent and severity of the lesion, the radiologic changes can resolve or evolve into those of radiation fibrosis. The irradiated region gradually becomes densely opacified within the margins of the treatment port. There may be linear streaks extending outside the port (84, 85). Irradiated regions can adopt a bronchiectatic, cystic, or even honeycomb appearance. Conventional perfusion scans of the lung show reduced perfusion of the irradiated region (86).

Ikezoe has examined the sensitivity of CT scan at evaluating the precise distribution and patterns of infiltrates in 17 patients who received fractionated radiotherapy to the thorax with a large irradiated lung volume. The CT findings were variable; pulmonary infiltrates were homogeneous, patchy, or discrete. CT abnormalities were evident within 16 weeks of radiotherapy in more than 80% of patients; in 13 of 17 patients, abnormalities were detected within 4 weeks (87). CT scan is more sensitive and useful to evaluate precise distribution and patterns of infiltrates (87, 88). Four distinct patterns have been described: ground-glass atten-uation (homogenous opacification involving the irradiated field that preserves the lung architecture), patchy consolidation within irradiated lung that does not conform to the shape of the portals, discrete consolidation that conforms to the shape of the portals but does not outline it uniformly, and consolidation that conforms to and involves the irradiated lung (89, 90). Ventilation-perfusion (V/Q) scans are frequently abnormal, perfusion defects are more common and correspond to the irradiated lung. Perfusion defects are seen in up to 95% of scans in some series, whereas ventilation defects are seen in approximately 35% to 45% of scans (91). Single proton emission CT scan appears to be more sensitive than is planar V/Q, but ^{67}Ga scintigraphy has low sensitivity and specificity (92, 93) (Table 34.2). Magnetic resonance imaging may play a possible role in differentiating radiation-induced changes from tumor recurrence (94).

Laboratory Tests

Are there unique findings or cytokine cascades? Serum assays might be useful indicators to identify patients more likely to develop radiation pneumonitis, but there is no widespread clinical use. Current search is underway for a serum marker that might provide a noninvasive measure of the severity of radiation pneumonitis for use in both clinical trials and oncologic practice. To date, no one marker has proven reliable, but several appear to demonstrate some utility. Serum surfactant apoprotein, soluble intracellular adhesion molecule, and plasma transforming growth factor-β (TGF-β) are being tested (95–98). Abnormalities in the lipid content of BAL are being studied because of the clinical similarity between radiation pneumonitis and acute respiratory distress syndrome (99, 100). At the stage of pneumonitis, (16 weeks after irradiation), most phospholipids in the lung are increased by 50% (101). These increases are probably associated with increased phospholipid turnover. Administration of corticosteroids from 2 to 3 weeks before the onset of pneumonitis increased the phospholipid content in BAL and increased the rate of incorporation of precursors into phospholipids (102).

TABLE 34.2. THE DIAGNOSIS OF RADIATION-INDUCED LUNG INJURY IN PATIENTS RECEIVING RADIATION THERAPY

Diagnostic Tools	Irradiation Dose (Gy)	Time (y) Between Rx and Study	Frequency of Abnormalities[a]	References
Chest x-ray	50–60	< 1–10	40–90 (68)	Bell (74), Polansky (118)
Computed tomography scan	30–54	< 1	39–95 (73)	Mah (65), Frija (76)
Ventilation/perfusion scan				
Ventilation	~30–45	< 1–3	35–45 (40)	Bell (74), Shapiro (53)
Perfusion	~30–45	< 1–3	53–95 (75)	Bell (74), Shapiro (53)
SPECT perfusion	~> 35	< 1–3	84–85 (84)	Bell (74), Marks (172)

[a] Mean is given in parentheses.
SPECT, single photon emission computed tomography.

BAL after lung irradiation sometimes exhibits lymphocytosis (103). In 25% of patients, no lymphocytosis or immune response is detected. Changes in BAL lymphocyte populations, as well as increases in radiolabeled gallium uptake, are seen bilaterally (103). These bilateral findings are thought to result from cytokines released from CD4$^+$ helper T lymphocytes (104), although the incidence of classic hypersensitivity pneumonitis appears to be less than 1%. Corticosteroids also lead to normalization of surface tension properties of alveolar surface lining layer, both *in vitro* and in situ. Total surfactant phospholipids are increased during pneumonitis, whereas their composition remains relatively normal (105). An analysis of surfactant subtype composition shows that the heavy large-aggregate subtype is much more abundant than normal in radiation pneumonitis (106).

Some investigators have observed elevation in serum copper levels in rats after radiation exposure (107). Irradiation of the lung results in an increase in prostaglandin and thromboxane synthesis (108, 109). The effects of γ-interferon have been studied in experimental models. After 35 days, animals that were irradiated and received γ-interferon did not have elevated protein and macrophage counts in lavage fluid (102). Prostacyclin (PGI$_2$) production by the irradiated lung increases progressively from a normal level at 2 months to a level two to three times higher than normal at 6 months after irradiation. This increase coincides with a reciprocal reduction in perfusion of the irradiated lung. Because PGI$_2$ is a potent pulmonary arterial vasodilator, its increased production may reflect a homeostatic response to impaired perfusion in the irradiated lung (110, 111). Variations in levels of markers of free radical activity correlate with pneumonitis (112). Irradiated cells have been shown to have impaired release of plasminogen activator, possibly leading to defective fibrinolysis and in situ thrombosis (113). The current biochemistry of radiation pneumonitis has been extensively studied and is reviewed elsewhere (114).

TGF-β is a multifunctional regulator of cell growth and differentiation (115) that is persistently elevated in plasma at the end of radiation therapy (95) and is associated with increased risk of radiation pneumonitis. Patients with normal or low plasma TGF-β_1 after radiotherapy are at a low risk for pneumonitis (95). Elevated TGF-β during radiotherapy may indicate a higher risk of radiation pneumonitis and of treatment failure in NSCLC patients (95). Soluble intercellular adhesion molecule-1 has also been studied as an early detection marker for radiation pneumonitis (97). Serum surfactant D and interleukin-6 are also reported to be elevated in patients with radiation pneumonitis (116, 117).

Differential Diagnosis

Did you rule out recurrence or metastatic cancer in the first 5 years, other inflammatory diseases in the next 5 to 10 years and second malignant tumors after 10 years? The differential diagnosis of radiation-induced lung disease includes cancer recurrence, infection, drug-induced lung disease, and thromboembolism (118–120). Certain infections and bronchiolitis obliterans organizing pneumonia can also occur in this setting (3, 121, 122). Because of the variety of therapeutic options, an accurate differential diagnosis is important. A diagnosis can usually be made on the basis of clinical features and radiologic appearances. The differentiation of radiation pneumonitis from tumor recurrence is based on the following. Recurrent malignancy is suggested by an interval of more than 4 months after radiation therapy and a gradual progression of radiologic changes. The presence of metastases, anemia, and hemoptysis also suggest recurrent tumor. Lymphangitic spread of tumor is usually associated with very severe dyspnea, and is more marked at the lung bases, where septal lines and long linear streaks are seen. Unlike radiation reactions, tumor recurrence is not usually limited to the field of irradiation. The differentiation of radiation reactions from tuberculosis is difficult, because fever, leukocytosis, and purulent sputum are sometimes absent in cancer patients who have received chemotherapy and/or corticosteroids (123, 124). The diagnosis of infection depends on Gram stains and appropriate cultures of bronchopulmonary secretions and possibly on histologic and microbiologic studies of lung tissue. The diagnosis of radiation reactions is simplified by serial roentgenograms and knowledge of the precise time course of therapy, dose, field margins, and dose schedules.

Pathologic Diagnosis

Was there a biopsy or operative specimen for definitive diagnosis to exclude cancer recurrence? The early (latent) phase occurs between 0 to 2 months after radiation exposure. Early ultrastructural changes include injury to type II pneumocytes (1–7 hours), damage to the capillary endothelium and alveolar epithelium, and hyaline membrane formation composed of a protein-rich exudate with shed cells and macrophages (125, 126). There are declines in levels of angiotensin-converting enzyme (ACE) and PGI$_2$ associated with early surfactant release from type II pneumocytes. Autocrine and paracrine effects of a variety of cytokines and growth factors released influence further changes. The intermediate (exudative) phase occurs 2 to 9 months after radiation exposure and is characterized by progressive organization of intra-alveolar exudates, atypical cells lining alveoli (alteration in type II pneumocytes), and interstitial thickening with edema formation and deposition of collagen (127, 128). The late fibrotic phase occurs more than 9 months after radiation exposure and is characterized by resorption of hyaline membrane and atypical alveolar cells associated with a marked increase in collagen deposition in the interstitium, and the collapse and obliteration of airway and vascular structures (129). Increased numbers of mast cells and mononuclear cells are present in the alveolar septum (interstitial space) early after irradiation (130). Occasionally a brisk inflammatory response has been seen. Fibroblast infiltration can be seen within the first

2 months. Collagen is laid down at about 6 months. At a later stage, dense fibrosis occurs. Conventionally, pneumonitis is thought of as the episode during which the specific effects of lung damage are expressed, and fibrosis is thought of as the subsequent wound-healing phase. High-grade pneumonitis generally develops 80 to 150 days after treatment. After this time, death from radiation is uncommon. In clinical practice, biopsies are only generally performed to diagnose recurrent neoplasms such as Hodgkin disease.

Histologic changes in mice include three consecutive phases (acute, intermediate, and late) (129, 131). The sequence of events starts with morphologic changes in type II pneumocytes that occur at 1 to 7 days, reductions in alveolar macrophages at 1 to 3 weeks, endothelial cell alterations in 1 to 15 days, and fibroblast proliferation at 2 to 6 months. In animal experiments, inhibition of collagen synthesis does not greatly reduce mortality in irradiated rats, suggesting that fibrosis is not a factor in mortality from lung irradiation (132, 133). There is no reason to believe that the pathogenesis of radiation-induced lung disease, including the time course and the contributing factors, is very different in humans and experimental animals.

Fibrosis is very likely to be present in any region of the lung that has received therapeutic doses of radiation, whether or not radiation pneumonitis has occurred. Histologic and physiological alterations combine to indicate that fibrosis begins as early as 2 months after irradiation and may take several months or years to become fully established (134). Some criteria that have been suggested for diagnosis of radiation pneumonitis are (a) the presence within the sample of regions of greatly varying pathologic changes; (b) a combination of atypical alveolar epithelial cells, vascular changes, and widespread hyaline membrane formation; and (c) the absence of much evidence of inflammation and the presence of mast cells adjacent to regions of capillary damage. Reactions are generally not seen outside the irradiated regions, although there may be exceptions. Field placement and biopsy site should overlap. Six months or more after the completion of a course of irradiation, the major abnormality is end-stage lung fibrosis with obliteration of alveolar spaces and vasculature (135).

There is a well described fibroblast response to irradiation that leads to tissue fibrosis. A classic dose-response relationship has been established *in vitro* that allows the prediction of tissue response (136). Even low-dose radiation can lead to pulmonary edema by a loss of endothelial cell–cell integrity and permeability barrier function (136, 137). In humans, several factors commonly predispose to an increased risk of infection, such as underlying lymphoreticular malignancy or the effects of chemotherapy. No particular organisms have been associated with infections after irradiation.

Management

Is restorative, ameliorative, or prophylactic treatment possible? Will it be in the form of medical or surgical intervention? The aim of treatment planning and fractionation schedules is to provide maximal curability with minimal or no toxicity. The development of lung fibrosis after radiation therapy has been altered by a number of agents. Amifostine 340 mg/m² administered daily 15 min before irradiation significantly reduced the incidence of pneumonitis (9% versus 43% in control subjects) and lung fibrosis (28% versus 53% in control subjects) in patients with lung cancer who received radiation therapy (46, 138, 139). Benefits have been demonstrated with agents that affect collagen metabolism: triiodothyronine, colchicine, β-aminopropionitrile (BAPN), and ACE inhibitors (140–142). The best-studied agent is D-penicillamine, a reversible inhibitor of collagen cross-linking and maturation (143–145). Administration of D-penicillamine after irradiation of the rat hemithorax attenuates lung fibrosis in terms of histopathology, hypoperfusion, and collagen accumulation. D-Penicillamine also attenuates the decrease in both ACE and plasminogen activator activity. By using serial lung scans on lung-irradiated rats, Ward and colleagues have shown that progressive hypoperfusion and perfusion defects can be delayed and mitigated by daily penicillamine treatment after irradiation, and recovery from vascular damage can be accelerated, suggesting that this is an active process (145, 146). D-Penicillamine has been used in a number of other disorders in humans, but it has not been given prospective trials in patients undergoing radiation therapy to the lungs.

ACE inhibitors (e.g., captopril) and angiotensin receptor blockers have shown to protect against radiation-induced pneumonitis and fibrosis in murine models (146). A large number of other agents and procedures have been suggested or exposed to trial in the management of radiation pneumonitis. Gross has examined the effect of the administration of nonsteroidal anti-inflammatory drugs 10 to 26 weeks after irradiation on the development of radiation pneumonitis in mice that had received 19 Gy to the thorax (147). A 5-lipoxygenase inhibitor (diethylcarbamazine) and a leukotriene receptor antagonist both reduced mortality in dose-response fashion. Piroxicam and ibuprofen were marginally protective, and indomethacin accelerated mortality. Aspirin reduced mortality in a dose-response fashion (147). L-Triiodothyronine has been given prophylactically to dogs, with small nonsignificant effects on postirradiation thoracic compliance (148). Colchicine (140) and BAPN, an inhibitor of collagen maturation, have been studied as prophylactic agents in experimental models (141). Although an increase in the collagen content of animal lungs was prevented as long as BAPN was administered, mortality was not significantly altered. Surgical pneumonectomy has been performed for severe unilateral radiation pneumonitis (149). Treatment with combined pentoxifylline and tocopherol (vitamin E) can reverse human chronic radiotherapy damage in humans, at least in skin, and should be considered as a therapeutic measure (150,151).

The management of acute tracheobronchitis and radiation-induced pneumonitis includes corticosteroid therapy (152). Ward and colleagues have used a model of bilateral radiation-induced lung disease in the rat to study the effects of corticosteroids. In this model, interstitial edema occurs after 2 weeks, followed by alveolitis and pulmonary edema at 4 weeks. Mast cell density peaks at 7 weeks, and there is a progressive increase in lung collagen (fibrosis) from 5 to 20 weeks. In this model, steroids protected the lung from interstitial edema at 2 weeks, delayed the alveolitis, and significantly reduced alveolar protein leak. However, radiation fibrosis was not attenuated. In rats, corticosteroids reduce the mortality of experimental radiation pneumonitis, when given 10 weeks after irradiation (153). If the corticosteroids are withdrawn during the pneumonitis, the mortality rate returns to that of untreated animals. The effect of treatment coincides with the active phase of radiation pneumonitis (154). The protective effect of corticosteroids on mortality after thoracic irradiation has been demonstrated in mice (155). Methylprednisolone, when given from 11 weeks after gamma irradiation of the thorax, caused an increase in the median lethal dose (11–26 weeks) from 14.3 to 17.6 Gy, a protection factor of 1.2. Withdrawal of steroids at various times during the period of radiation pneumonitis resulted in accelerated mortality in the next 2 to 4 weeks, so that the cumulative mortality "caught up" with that of control animals by 4 weeks after steroid withdrawal. However, after the end of the usual period of pneumonitis, withdrawal of steroids did not result in accelerated mortality, suggesting that the time when steroids are protective corresponds to the duration of pneumonitis. Studies in lethally irradiated mice given steroids after radiation but before pneumonitis show that even moderate doses substantially reduce mortality, provided they are continued through the period when pneumonitis would occur (155).

The use of prophylactic steroid therapy has not been proven and is not used in clinical practice. Nevertheless, steroid withdrawal appears to precipitate radiation pneumonitis. Corticosteroids should be administered either continuously or not at all in the period after radiation. In lethally irradiated mice, deaths were markedly reduced by prophylactic prednisolone, but death occurred rapidly after treatment withdrawal at 160 days (156). The phenomenon may be an unmasking of steroid-responsive pneumonitis or, less likely, as precipitation, by the withdrawal itself, of a reaction that would not have been present at all if steroids had not been given. In one large clinical study, patients received cycles of combination chemotherapy, including corticosteroids (157). Soon after the completion of a cycle, some patients were prone to show signs of radiation pneumonitis, suggesting that latent injury had been suppressed by steroids and unmasked by its withdrawal (157). For more than 30 years, evidence has existed that (158) corticosteroids given just before, during, and after the start of radiation therapy can prevent the obstruction of major airways by swelling of irradiated tumor (156).

Systemic corticosteroids are the mainstay of therapy for radiation pneumonitis. Data from randomized controlled human studies are not available. Clinical experience supports the use of steroids, and most series report response rates of approximately 80% (159,160). The recommended dose is 1 mg/kg followed by a slow taper based on clinical improvement (160). There is no role for prophylactic steroid therapy (161). Corticosteroids are believed to be less beneficial if treatment is delayed. Pneumonitis often appears shortly after withdrawal of steroids, but there is a dramatic response shortly after reinstitution of prednisone, 20 to 80 mg/d. When corticosteroids are given at the onset of pneumonitis, mortality is significantly reduced (162). The early use of steroids prevents further disease progression and may allow repair processes to proceed. This would explain the (a) protective effect of steroids, (b) unmasking of latent injury on steroid withdrawal, (c) abrogation of pneumonitis by early use of corticosteroids, and (d) relative inefficacy of steroids in reversing established pneumonitis. Large doses of corticosteroids for long periods would be required to abolish all pneumonitis; therefore, when symptomatic pneumonitis occurs, and especially if early onset and rapid progression suggest a severe reaction, large doses of corticosteroids (e.g., prednisone, 100 mg/d in an adult) are instituted early, and therapy is continued for several weeks (163). When symptoms are absent, the dose can be carefully reduced but reinstituted if relapse occurs. Tapering generally occurs over several weeks. If respiratory failure occurs, mechanical ventilation and/or supplemental oxygen may be required (164). Corticosteroids are of little benefit to the patient who has severe established respiratory failure. There are many reports in which large doses of corticosteroids fail to prevent the progression of established radiation pneumonitis (159,163). The goal is to recognize pneumonitis early in its course, anticipate its severity, and treat appropriate cases as early as possible with high-dose corticosteroids. The Radiation Therapy Oncology Group acute (within 90 days) radiation morbidity scoring criteria for lung injury is scored as follows: grade 0, no change; grade 1, mild symptoms of dry cough or dyspnea on exertion; grade 2, persistent cough requiring narcotic antitussive agents or dyspnea with minimal effort but not at rest; grade 3, severe cough unresponsive to narcotic antitussive agent, dyspnea at rest, clinical or radiologic evidence of acute pneumonitis, or a requirement for intermittent oxygen or steroids; and grade 4, severe respiratory insufficiency, continuous oxygen, or assisted ventilation (164). The Radiation Therapy Oncology Group/European Organization for Research and Treatment of Cancer late radiation morbidity scoring schema includes the following: grade 0, none; grade 1, asymptomatic or mild symptoms (dry cough) with slight radiographic appearances; grade 2, moderate symptomatic fibrosis or pneumonitis (severe cough), low grade fever, and patchy radiographic changes; grade 3, severe symptomatic fibrosis or pneumonitis and dense radiographic changes; grade 4, severe respiratory insufficiency requiring continuous oxygen or assisted ventilation; and grade 5, death owing to radiation-induced lung injury.

TREATMENT OF RADIATION-INDUCED LUNG INJURY

Summary Statement	Level of Evidence
Corticosteroids prevent mortality in experimental models of radiation pneumonitis.	Multiple controlled scientific studies in animal models
In humans, corticosteroid therapy reduces mortality, improves radiographic appearances, and preserves lung function in patients with radiation pneumonitis.	Observational studies, case series, and cross-sectional analyses

FOLLOW-UP AND PHYSIOLOGIC CHANGES

Patients should be monitored while on corticosteroid therapy (usually several months). The best documentation of physiological deficits in humans has been reported in patients with breast cancer (165) (Table 34.3). Unlike patients with lung cancer, patients with breast cancer, and Hodgkin disease or lymphoma, generally have essentially normal lungs before irradiation. Hassink and colleagues (166) performed pulmonary function tests in 78 patients who had received mantle field irradiation for Hodgkin disease 10 to 18 years previously. The mean values for total lung capacity (95.2%), vital capacity (95.9%), forced expiratory volume in 1 second (FEV_1; 90.6%), and carbon monoxide diffusing capacity per unit alveolar volume (82.7%) were less than predicted (166). By using multiple regression analysis, the normalized total dose of irradiation, the field of irradiation, and the interval since irradiation have been shown to independently lead to negative effects on the test results. Evidence of change in lung perfusion has been obtained by studying ^{131}I-labeled macroaggregates of albumin or [133]Xe. A transient reduction in perfusion has been reported soon after irradiation, particularly after large single doses, but this reduction is of questionable clinical significance (167). In the period from a few days to 14 days after irradiation, some investigators report a decrease in pulmonary perfusion. Pulmonary perfusion is consistently reduced from about 14 days on and is

generally confined to the irradiated region (165). The reduction in perfusion is more severe after 15-MeV neutrons than γ-irradiation and is associated with histological evidence of capillary damage. During pneumonitis, there is a marked reduction in perfusion and a marked increase in permeability of the pulmonary vasculature that results in pulmonary edema (166, 167).

Pulmonary function testing reveals a dose-dependent and time-related reduction in static lung compliance after irradiation. This change occurs at about 40 days, progresses during pneumonitis, and commonly persists indefinitely (168). Restrictive ventilatory deficits depend on three factors: the chest wall, lung parenchyma, and pleura. Studies of excised or exposed lungs of animals show that the fall in chest compliance is entirely owing to a decrease in lung compliance rather than to chest wall compliance (169). In addition, it has been demonstrated that the BAL fluid of irradiated mice behaves abnormally *in vitro,* because it contains a large amount of protein, in particular fibrinogen, which alters surface tension (170). At later stages, reductions in lung compliance appear to result from lung fibrosis and a loss of lung elasticity (171). Regional lung studies have shown that volume loss is confined to the region of irradiation, where decreased perfusion is also present. The changes in lung function are therefore related to the amount of lung irradiated. Airway resistance is generally normal. Consistent with the decrease in lung compliance, the work of breathing is raised, tidal volume is reduced, and breathing frequency increases, resulting in an overall increase in minute ventilation (172, 173).

Within the irradiated region, changes in perfusion outweigh ventilatory changes, resulting in a high V/Q ratio. Generally there is little change in gas transfer, because of redistribution of pulmonary blood flow to other unaffected regions. Therefore, if the volume of irradiated lung is small and the function of unirradiated lung is normal, overall gas transfer (diffusing capacity of carbon monoxide [D_{LCO}]) is not impaired, and blood gases are normal. If the volume of affected lung is large and/or the function of unirradiated lung is impaired, D_{LCO} is reduced (174, 175). Arterial blood gases can show mild to moderate arterial hypoxemia with normal or reduced arterial partial pressure of carbon dioxide and an increased alveolar-arterial oxygen gradient. On average, there is a 20% reduction in vital capacity and FEV_1. The average reduction in D_{LCO} is 10% but is greater in patients

TABLE 34.3. THE FREQUENCY OF DETERIORATING LUNG FUNCTION (EXPRESSED AS PERCENTAGE DECLINE) IN PATIENTS RECEIVING RADIATION THERAPY

Disease Type	FEV_1	FVC	FEV_1/FVC	TLC	VC	D_{LCO}	References
Breast cancer	15	10	5			20	Theuws (178)
Lung cancer	11–18	22		10	20	14–24	Fu (179)
Hodgkin lymphoma	0–10	4–10	0	0–13	5–13	8–34	Theuws (178)

FEV_1, forced expiratory volume in 1s; FVC, forced vital capacity; TLC, total lung capacity; VC, vital capacity, D_{LCO}, diffusing capacity of carbon monoxide.

with radiation pneumonitis. Correlations have been found between reductions in DLco, FEV₁, and the presence of radiation pneumonitis. In more severe degrees of radiation injury, carbon dioxide retention and severe hypoxia occur (174, 177).

In patients with breast cancer and lymphoma, declines in pulmonary function are seen 3 months after radiation therapy, with partial recovery by 18 months (178). In studies of the long-term follow-up of lymphoma patients that received radiation therapy, vital capacity is reported to be approximately 5 to 15% below baseline. In patients with lung cancer, who typically also have a history of heavy tobacco consumption, changes in pulmonary function appear to be dependent on pretherapy lung function (179). When lung compliance is measured, a greater reduction is seen after therapy in children compared with adults (180).

Symptoms of radiation pneumonitis are related to the volume of irradiated lung and are attributable to changes in lung function and associated blood gas abnormalities (180). When only the apex of the lung is irradiated, (postoperative irradiation for breast cancer), the symptomatic and physiological effects are generally less because perfusion is lower at the lung apex (64). Several chemotherapeutic agents cause significant lung toxicity and may amplify radiation toxicity (181–188). Corticosteroids are the therapy of choice for radiation pneumonitis. Amifostine has been shown to ameliorate fibrotic reactions (189). Pentoxifylline and α-tocopherol may prove beneficial in subjects who develop fibrosis (190). Pulmonary function testing that includes lung volumes, diffusion capacity, and arterial blood gas tensions can provide early diagnosis of radiation pneumonitis.

PRINCIPLES OF RADIATION BIOLOGY

Summary Statement	Level of Evidence
Radiation causes tissue injury and cell death that is dependent on total dose, fractions, and oxygen effects	Multiple controlled scientific studies *in vitro* and in animal models
In humans, radiation causes tissue injury that is dependent on the use of chemotherapy and host biologic factors, including underlying disease (ataxia telangiectasia) and patient age	Observational studies, case series, and cross-sectional analyses

REFERENCES

1. Gross NJ. Pulmonary effects of radiation therapy. *Ann Intern Med* 1977;86:81–92.
2. Cherniack RM, Abrams J, Kalica AR. Pulmonary disease associated with breast cancer therapy. *Am J Respir Crit Care Med* 1994;150:1169–1173.
3. Crestani B, Valeyre D, Roden S, et al. Bronchiolitis obliterans organizing pneumonia syndrome primed by radiation therapy to the breast. *Am J Respir Crit Care Med* 1998;158:1929–1935.
4. Siemann DW, Hill RP, Penney DP. Early and late pulmonary toxicity in mice evaluated 180 and 420 days following localized lung irradiation. *Radiat Res* 1982;89:396–407.
5. Down JD, Easton DF, Steel GG. Repair in the mouse lung during low dose-rate irradiation. *Radiother Oncol* 1986;6:29–42.
6. Cuzick J, Stewart H, Rutqvist L, et al. Cause-specific mortality in long-term survivors of breast cancer who participated in trials of radiotherapy. *J Clin Oncol* 1994;12:447–453.
7. Keane TJ, Van Dyk J, Rider WD. Idiopathic interstitial pneumonia following bone marrow transplantation: the relationship with total body irradiation. *Int J Radiat Oncol Biol Phys* 1981;7:1365–1370.
8. McDonald S, Chang AY, Rubin P, et al. Combined Betaseron R (recombinant human interferon β) and radiation for inoperable non–small cell lung cancer. *Int J Radiat Oncol Biol Phys* 1993;27:613–619.
9. McDonald S, Rubin P, Phillips TL, et al. Injury to the lung from cancer therapy: clinical syndromes, measurable endpoints, and potential scoring systems. *Int J Radiat Oncol Biol Phys* 1995;31:1187–1203.
10. Morgan GW, Freeman AP, McLean RG, et al. Late cardiac, thyroid, and pulmonary sequelae of mantle radiotherapy for Hodgkin's disease. *Int J Radiat Oncol Biol Phys* 1985;11:1925–1931.
11. Rubin P, Johnston CJ, Williams JP, et al. A perpetual cascade of cytokines postirradiation leads to pulmonary fibrosis. *Int J Radiat Oncol Biol Phys* 1995;33:99–109.
12. Roach M, Gandara DR, Yuo HS, et al. Radiation pneumonitis following combined modality therapy for lung cancer: analysis of prognostic factors. *J Clin Oncol* 1995;13:2606–2612.
13. Constine LS, Rubin P. Total body irradiation: normal tissue effects. In: Bleehen NM, ed: *Radiobiology in radiotherapy.* New York, Springer-Verlag, 1987:95–121.
14. Rothwell RI, Kelly SA, Joslin CA. Radiation pneumonitis in patients treated for breast cancer. *Radiother Oncol* 1985;4:9–14.
15. Rubin O, Casarett GW. *Clinical radiation pathology,* Vols. 1 and 2. Philadelphia: WB Saunders, 1968:423–470.
16. Ellis F. Dose, time and fractionation: a clinical hypothesis. *Clin Radiol* 1969;20:1–7.
17. Phillips TL, Fu KK. Quantification of combined radiation therapy and chemotherapy effects on critical normal tissues. *Cancer* 1976;37[2 Suppl]:1186–1200.
18. Lyman JT, Wolbarst AB. Optimization of radiation therapy, III: a method of assessing complication probabilities from dose-volume histograms. *Int J Radiat Oncol Biol Phys* 1987;13:103–109.
19. Seppenwoolde Y, Lebesque JV. Partial irradiation of the lung. *Semin Radiat Oncol* 2001;11:247–258.
20. Frame PW. Radioactivity: conception to birth: the Health Physics Society 1995 Radiology Centennial Hartman Oration. *Health Phys* 1996;70:614–620.
21. Rubin P, Casarett GW. *Clinical radiation pathology,* Vols. 1 and 2. Philadelphia: WB Saunders, 1968.
22. Rubin P, Constine LS, Williams JP. Late effects of cancer treatment: radiation and drug toxicity. In: Perez CA, Brady LW, eds. *Principles and practice of radiation oncology,* 3rd ed. Philadelphia: Lippincott–Raven Publishers, 1997.
23. Narayanan PK, Goodwin EH, Lehnert BE. Alpha particles initiate biological production of superoxide anions and hydrogen peroxide in human cells. *Cancer Res* 1997;57:3963–3971.

24. Ross GM. Induction of cell death by radiotherapy. *Endocr Relat Cancer* 1999;6:41–44.

25. Ling CC, Stickler R, Schell MC, et al. The effect of hypoxic cell sensitizers at different irradiation dose rates. *Radiat Res* 1987;109:396–406.

26. Krarup M, Poulsen HS, Spang-Thomsen M. Cellular radiosensitivity of small-cell lung cancer cell lines. *Int J Radiat Oncol Biol Phys* 1997;38:191–196.

27. Ward HE, Kemsley L, Davies L, et al. The pulmonary response to sublethal thoracic irradiation in the rat. *Radiat Res* 1993;136:15–21.

28. Johnston CJ, Piedboeuf B, Baggs R, et al. Differences in correlation of mRNA gene expression in mice sensitive and resistant to radiation-induced pulmonary fibrosis. *Radiat Res* 1995;142:197–203.

29. Webster PJ, Kefford R. Pulmonary toxicity associated with bleomycin. *Med J Aust* 1994;160:584–585.

30. Choi NC, Kanarek DJ, Kazemi H. Prospective study of pulmonary tolerance to radiotherapy or radiotherapy plus multidrug chemotherapy for loco-regional lung carcinoma. *Antibiot Chemother* 1988;41:213–219.

31. Yu YQ, Giocanti N, Averbeck D, et al. Radiation-induced arrest of cells in G_2 phase elicits hypersensitivity to DNA double-strand break inducers and an altered pattern of DNA cleavage upon re-irradiation. *Int J Radiat Biol* 2000;76:901–912.

32. Handschel J, Prott FJ, Sunderkotter C, et al. Irradiation induces increase of adhesion molecules and accumulation of β_2-integrin–expressing cells in humans. *Int J Radiat Oncol Biol Phys* 1999;45:475–481.

33. Seed TM. Hematopoietic tissue repair under chronic low daily dose irradiation. *Adv Space Res* 1996;18:65–70.

34. Sminia P, Schneider CJ, Fowler JF. The optimal fraction size in high-dose-rate brachytherapy: dependency on tissue repair kinetics and low-dose rate. *Int J Radiat Oncol Biol Phys* 2002;52:844–849.

35. Pfalzner PM. Sievert, gray and dose equivalent. *J Can Assoc Radiol* 1983;34:298–300.

36. Ellis F. Relationship between log dose and log time in radiotherapy: the Strandqvist lines. *Br J Radiol* 1976;49:651.

37. Brumm P. On the validity of the NSD concept. *Br J Radiol* 1983;56:957–962.

38. Stone HB, McBride WH, Coleman CN. Modifying normal tissue damage postirradiation. Report of a workshop sponsored by the Radiation Research Program, National Cancer Institute, Bethesda, Maryland, September 6–8, 2000. *Radiat Res* 2002;157:204–223.

39. Denekamp J, Dasu A, Waites A, et al. Hyperfractionation as an effective way of overcoming radioresistance. *Int J Radiat Oncol Biol Phys* 1998;42:705–709.

40. Graham MV, Purdy JA, Emami B, et al. Preliminary results of a prospective trial using three dimensional radiotherapy for lung cancer. *Int J Radiat Oncol Biol Phys* 1995;33:993–1000.

41. Rubin P. Late Effects on Normal Tissues (LENT) consensus conference, including RTOG/EORTC SOMA scales. San Fransisco, California August 26–28, 1992. *Int J Radiat Oncol Biol Phys* 1995;31:1035–1060.

42. Speiser BL, Spratling L. Radiation bronchitis and stenosis secondary to high dose rate endobronchial irradiation. *Int J Radiat Oncol Biol Phys* 1993;25:589–597.

43. Livingston RB, Griffin BR, Higano CS, et al. Combined treatment with chemotherapy and neutron irradiation for limited non–small-cell lung cancer: a Southwest Oncology Group Study. *J Clin Oncol* 1987;5:1716–1724.

44. Chen Y, Williams J, Ding I, et al. Radiation pneumonitis and early circulatory cytokine markers. *Semin Radiat Oncol* 2002;12[1 Suppl 1]:26–33.

45. Wennberg B, Gagliardi G, Sundbom L, et al. Early response of lung in breast cancer irradiation: radiologic density changes measured by CT and symptomatic radiation pneumonitis. *Int J Radiat Oncol Biol Phys* 2002;52:1196–1206.

46. Hernberg M, Virkkunen P, Maasilta P, et al. Pulmonary toxicity after radiotherapy in primary breast cancer patients: results from a randomized chemotherapy study. *Int J Radiat Oncol Biol Phys* 2002;52:128–136.

47. Loyer E, Fuller L, Libshitz HI, et al. Radiographic appearance of the chest following therapy for Hodgkin disease. *Eur J Radiol* 2000;35:136–148.

48. Monson JM, Stark P, Reilly JJ, et al. Clinical radiation pneumonitis and radiographic changes after thoracic radiation therapy for lung carcinoma. *Cancer* 1998;82:842–850.

49. Salinas FV, Winterbauer RH. Radiation pneumonitis: a mimic of infectious pneumonitis. *Semin Respir Infect* 1995;10:143–153.

50. Abratt RP, Morgan GW. Lung toxicity following chest irradiation in patients with lung cancer. *Lung Cancer* 2002;35:103–109.

51. Lind PA, Marks LB, Hardenbergh PH, et al. Technical factors associated with radiation pneumonitis after local ± regional radiation therapy for breast cancer. *Int J Radiat Oncol Biol Phys* 2002;52:137–143.

52. Lamoureux KB. Increased clinically symptomatic pulmonary radiation reactions with adjuvant chemotherapy. *Cancer Chemother Rep* 1974;58:705–708.

53. Shapiro SJ, Shapiro SD, Mill WB, et al. Prospective study of long-term pulmonary manifestations of mantle irradiation. *Int J Radiat Oncol Biol Phys* 1990;19:707–714.

54. Gopal R, Ha CS, Tucker SL, et al. Comparison of two total body irradiation fractionation regimens with respect to acute and late pulmonary toxicity. *Cancer* 2001;92:1949–1958.

55. Byhardt RW, Pajak TF, Emami B, et al. A phase I/II study to evaluate accelerated fractionation via concomitant boost for squamous, adeno, and large cell carcinoma of the lung: report of Radiation Therapy Oncology Group 84-07. *Int J Radiat Oncol Biol Phys* 1993;26:459–468.

56. Lyman JT. Complication probability as assessed from dose-volume histograms. *Radiat Res Suppl* 1985;8:S13–S19.

57. Hurkmans CW, Borger JH, Bos LJ, et al. Cardiac and lung complication probabilities after breast cancer irradiation. *Radiother Oncol* 2000;55:145–151.

58. Phillips TW, Wharam MD, Margolis LW. Modification of radiation injury to normal tissues by chemotherapeutic agents. *Cancer* 1975;35:1678–1684.

59. Salazar OM, Van Houtte P, Rubin P. Once-a-week radiation therapy for locally advanced lung cancer: final report. *Cancer* 1984;54:719–725.

60. Emami B, Lyman J, Brown A, et al. Tolerance of normal tissue to therapeutic irradiation. *Int J Radiat Oncol Biol Phys* 1991;21:109–122.

61. Hernando ML, Marks LB, Bentel GC, et al. Radiation-induced pulmonary toxicity: a dose-volume histogram analysis in 201 patients with lung cancer. *Int J Radiat Oncol Biol Phys* 2001;51:650–659.

62. Dubray B, Henry-Amar M, Meerwaldt JH, et al. Radiation-induced lung damage after thoracic irradiation for Hodgkin's disease: the role of fractionation. *Radiother Oncol* 1995;36:211–217.

63. Roach M 3rd, Gandara DR, Yuo HS, et al. Radiation pneumonitis following combined modality therapy for lung cancer: analysis of prognostic factors. *J Clin Oncol* 1995;13:2606–2612.

64. Graham MV, Purdy JA, Emami B, et al. Clinical dose-volume histogram analysis for pneumonitis after 3D treatment for non–small cell lung cancer (NSCLC). *Int J Radiat Oncol Biol Phys* 1999;45:323–329.

65. Mah K, Keane TJ, Van Dyk J, et al. Quantitative effect of combined chemotherapy and fractionated radiotherapy on the incidence of radiation-induced lung damage: a prospective clinical study. *Int J Radiat Oncol Biol Phys* 1994;28:563–574.

66. Hernberg M, Virkkunen P, Maasilta P, et al. Pulmonary toxicity after radiotherapy in primary breast cancer patients: results from a randomized chemotherapy study. *Int J Radiat Oncol Biol Phys* 2002;52:128–136.

67. Hirsch A, Vander Els N, Straus DJ, et al. Effect of ABVD chemotherapy with and without mantle or mediastinal irradiation on pulmonary function and symptoms in early-stage Hodgkin's disease. *J Clin Oncol* 1996;14:1297–1305.

68. Einhorn L, Krause M, Hornback N, et al. Enhanced pulmonary toxicity with bleomycin and radiotherapy in oat cell lung cancer. *Cancer* 1976;37:2414–2416.

69. Soble AR, Perry H. Fatal radiation pneumonia following subclinical busulfan injury. *AJR Am J Roentgenol* 1977;128:15–18.

70. Phillips TL. Chemical modifiers of cancer treatment. *Int J Radiat Oncol Biol Phys* 1984;10:791–794.

71. Stewart FA. Re-treatment after full-course radiotherapy: is it a viable option? *Acta Oncol* 1999;38:855–862.

72. Woods WG, Byrne TD, Kim TH. Sensitivity of cultured cells to gamma radiation in a patient exhibiting marked in vivo radiation sensitivity. *Cancer* 1988;62:2341–2345.

73. Ried HL, Jaffe N. Radiation-induced changes in long-term survivors of childhood cancer after treatment with radiation therapy. *Semin Roentgenol* 1994;29:6–14.

74. Bell J, McGivern D, Bullimore J, et al. Diagnostic imaging of post-irradiation changes in the chest. *Clin Radiol* 1988;39:109–119.

75. Cazzaniga LF, Bossi A, Cosentino D, et al. Radiological findings when very small lung volumes are irradiated in breast and chest wall treatment. *Radiat Oncol Investig* 1998;6:58–62.

76. Frija J, Ferme C, Baud L, et al. Radiation-induced lung injuries: a survey by computed tomography and pulmonary function tests in 18 cases of Hodgkin's disease. *Eur J Radiol* 1988;8:18–23.

77. Mah K, Poon PY, Van Dyk J, et al. Assessment of acute radiation-induced pulmonary changes using computed tomography. *J Comput Assist Tomogr* 1986;10:736–743.

78. Schratter-Sehn AU, Schurawitzki H, Zach M, et al. High-resolution computed tomography of the lungs in irradiated breast cancer patients. *Radiother Oncol* 1993;27:198–202.

79. Marinus J, Niel CG, de Bie RA, et al. Measuring radiation fibrosis: the interobserver reliability of two methods of determining the degree of radiation fibrosis. *Int J Radiat Oncol Biol Phys* 2000;47:1209–1217.

80. Prato FS, Kurdyak R, Saibil EA, et al. Physiological and radiographic assessment during the development of pulmonary radiation fibrosis. *Radiology* 1977;122:389–397.

81. Teates CD. Effects of unilateral thoracic irradiation on lung function. *J Appl Physiol* 1965;20:628–636.

82. Wencel ML, Sitrin RG. Unilateral lung hyperlucency after mediastinal irradiation. *Am Rev Respir Dis* 1988;137:955–957.

83. Rand RP, Maser B, Dry G, et al. Reconstruction of irradiated postpneumonectomy empyema cavity with chain-link coupled microsurgical omental and TRAM flaps. *Plast Reconstr Surg* 2000;105:183–186.

84. Arbetter KR, Prakash UBS, Tazelaar HD, et al. Radiation-induced pneumonitis in the "nonirradiated" lung. *Mayo Clin Proc* 1999;74:27–36.

85. Satoh H, Yamashita YT, Ohtsuka M, et al. Radiation-induced pneumonitis outside the radiation field. *Mayo Clin Proc* 1999;74:743–744.

86. Freedman GS, Lofgren SB, Kligerman MM. Radiation-induced changes in pulmonary perfusion. *Radiology* 1974;112:435–437.

87. Ikezoe J, Takashima S, Morimoto S, et al. CT appearance of acute radiation-induced injury in the lung. *AJR Am J Roentgenol* 1988;150:765–770.

88. Libshitz HI, Shuman LS. Radiation-induced pulmonary change: CT findings. *J Comput Assist Tomogr* 1984;8:15–19.

89. Phillips TL, Margolis L. Radiation pathology and the clinical response of lung and esophagus. *Front Radiat Ther Oncol* 1972;6:254–260.

90. Park KJ, Chung JY, Chun MS, et al. Radiation-induced lung disease and the impact of radiation methods on imaging features. *Radiographics* 2000;20:83–98.

91. Woel RT, Munley MT, Hollis D, et al. The time course of radiation therapy-induced reductions in regional perfusion: a prospective study with more than 5 years of follow-up. *Int J Radiat Oncol Biol Phys* 2002;52:58–67.

92. Marks LB, Spencer DP, Bentel GC, et al. The utility of SPECT lung perfusion scans in minimizing and assessing the physiologic consequences of thoracic irradiation. *Int J Radiat Oncol Biol Phys* 1993;26:659–668.

93. Kataoka M, Kawamura M, Itoh H, et al. Ga-67 citrate scintigraphy for the early detection of radiation pneumonitis. *Clin Nucl Med* 1992;17:27–31.

94. Sigmund G, Slanina J, Hinkelbein W. Diagnosis of radiation-pneumonitis: recent results. *Cancer Res* 1993;130:123–131.

95. Anscher MS, Murase T, Prescott DM, et al. Changes in plasma TGF β levels during pulmonary radiotherapy as a predictor of the risk of developing radiation pneumonitis. *Int J Radiat Oncol Biol Phys* 1994;30:671–676.

96. Rubin P, McDonald S, Maasilta P, et al. Serum markers for prediction of pulmonary radiation syndromes, part I: surfactant apoprotein. *Int J Radiat Oncol Biol Phys* 1989;17:553–558.

97. Ishii Y, Kitamura S. Soluble intercellular adhesion molecule-1 as an early detection marker for radiation pneumonitis. *Eur Respir J* 1999;13:733–738.

98. Jack CIA, Cottier B, Jackson MJ, et al. Indicators of free radical activity in patients developing radiation pneumonitis. *Int J Radiat Oncol Biol Phys* 1996;34:149–154.

99. Rubin P, Shapiro DL, Finklestein JN, et al. The early release of surfactant following lung irradiation of alveolar type II cells. *Int J Radiat Oncol Biol Phys* 1980;6:75–77.

100. Hallman M, Maasilta P, Kivisaari L, et al. Changes in surfactant in bronchoalveolar lavage fluid after hemithorax irradiation in patients with mesothelioma. *Am Rev Respir Dis* 1990;141(4 Pt 1):998–1005.

101. Rubin P, Siemann DW, Shapiro DL, et al. Surfactant release as an early measure of radiation pneumonitis. *Int J Radiat Oncol Biol Phys* 1983;9:1669–1673.

102. Rosiello RA, Merrill WW, Rockwell S, et al. Radiation pneumonitis: bronchoalveolar lavage assessment and modulation by a recombinant cytokine. *Am Rev Respir Dis* 1993;148:1671–1676.

103. Roberts CM, Foulcher E, Zaunders JJ, et al. Radiation pneumonitis: a possible lymphocyte-mediated hypersensitivity reaction. *Ann Intern Med* 1993;118:696–700.

104. Johnston CJ, Williams JP, Okunieff P, et al. Radiation-induced pulmonary fibrosis: examination of chemokine and chemokine receptor families. *Radiat Res* 2002;157:256–265.

105. Gross NJ. Experimental radiation pneumonitis, III: phospholipid studies on the lungs. *J Lab Clin Med* 1979;93:627–637.

106. Gross NJ. Surfactant subtypes in experimental lung damage: radiation pneumonitis. *Am J Physiol* 1991;260(4 Pt 1):L302–L310.

107. Ward WF, Molteni A, Fitzsimons EJ, et al. Serum copper concentration as an index of lung injury in rats exposed to hemithorax irradiation. *Radiat Res* 1988;114:613–620.

108. Ts'ao CH, Ward WF, Port CD. Radiation injury in rat lung, I: prostacyclin (PGI$_2$) production, arterial perfusion, and ultrastructure. *Radiat Res* 1983;96:284–293.

109. Ts'ao C, Tsao FH, Taylor JM, et al. Annexin I concentration, phospholipase activity and thromboxane synthesis in irradiated rat lung. *Radiat Res* 1995;142:85–90.

110. Ward WF, Molteni A, Ts'ao CH, et al. Radiation pneumotoxicity in rats: modification by inhibitors of angiotensin converting enzyme. *Int J Radiat Oncol Biol Phys* 1992;22:623–625.

111. Ts'ao C, Ward WF, Molteni A, et al. Annexin I concentration and prostacyclin production in rat lung and alveolar macrophages following irradiation. *Prostaglandins Leukot Essent Fatty Acids* 1997;56:99–104.

112. Jack CI, Jackson MJ, Johnston ID, et al. Serum indicators of free radical activity in idiopathic pulmonary fibrosis. *Am J Respir Crit Care Med* 1996;153(6 Pt 1):1918–1923.

113. Ts'ao C, Ward WF. Plasminogen activator activity in lung and alveolar macrophages of rats exposed to graded single doses of gamma rays to the right hemithorax. *Radiat Res* 1985;103:393–402.

114. Morgan GW, Breit SN. Radiation and the lung: a reevaluation of the mechanisms mediating pulmonary injury. *Int J Radiat Oncol Biol Phys* 1995;31:361–369.

115. Vujaskovic Z, Groen HJ. TGF-β, radiation-induced pulmonary injury and lung cancer. *Int J Radiat Biol* 2000;76:511–516.

116. Chen Y, Williams J, Ding I, et al. Radiation pneumonitis and early circulatory cytokine markers. *Semin Radiat Oncol* 2002;12[1 Suppl 1]:26–33.

117. Sasaki R, Soejima T, Matsumoto A, et al. Clinical significance of serum pulmonary surfactant proteins A and D for the early detection of radiation pneumonitis. *Int J Radiat Oncol Biol Phys* 2001;50:301–307.

118. Polansky SM, Ravin CE, Prosnitz LR. Pulmonary changes after primary irradiation for early breast carcinoma. *AJR Am J Roentgenol* 1980;34:101–105.

119. Tefft M. Radiation related toxicities in National Wilms' Tumor Study: number 1. *Int J Radiat Oncol Biol Phys* 1977;2:455–463.

120. Fox AD, Banning AP, Channon K, et al. Saddle embolus of the carotid bifurcation: a late complication of mediastinal radiotherapy. *Eur J Vasc Endovasc Surg* 1999;17:360–362.

121. Van Laar JM, Holscher HC, van Krieken JHJM, et al. Bronchiolitis obliterans organizing pneumonia after adjuvant radiotherapy for breast carcinoma. *Respir Med* 1997;91:241–244.

122. Majori M, Poletti V, Curti A, et al. Bronchoalveolar lavage in bronchiolitis obliterans organizing pneumonia primed by radiation therapy to the breast. *J Allergy Clin Immunol* 2000;105:239–244.

123. Roscoe RJ, Deddens JA, Salvan A, et al. Mortality among Navajo uranium miners. *Am J Public Health* 1995;85:535–540.

124. Zvetina JR, Maliwan N, Frederick WE, et al. *Mycobacterium kansasii* infection following primary pulmonary malignancy. *Chest* 1992;102:1460–1463.

125. Moosavi H, McDonald S, Rubin P, et al. Early radiation dose-response in lung: an ultrastructural study. *Int J Radiat Oncol Biol Phys* 1977;2:921–931.

126. Penney DP, Rubin P. Specific early fine structural changes in the lung irradiation. *Int J Radiat Oncol Biol Phys* 1977;2:1123–1132.

127. Penney DP, Shapiro DL, Rubin P, et al. Effects of radiation on the mouse lung and potential induction of radiation pneumonitis. *Virchows Arch B Cell Pathol Incl Mol Pathol* 1981;37:327–336.

128. Phillips TL. An ultrastructural study of the development of radiation injury in the lung. *Radiology* 1966;87:49–54.

129. Travis EL, Harley RA, Fenn JO, et al. Pathologic changes in the lung following single and multi-fraction irradiation. *Int J Radiat Oncol Biol Phys* 1977;2:475–490.

130. Ward WF, Molteni A, Ts'ao CH, et al. Captopril reduces collagen and mast cell accumulation in irradiated rat lung. *Int J Radiat Oncol Biol Phys* 1990;19:1405–1409.

131. Travis EL. The sequence of histological changes in mouse lungs after single doses of x-rays. *Int J Radiat Oncol Biol Phys* 1980;6:345–347.

132. Song L, Wang D, Cui X, et al. The protective action of taurine and L-arginine in radiation pulmonary fibrosis. *J Environ Pathol Toxicol Oncol* 1998;17:151–157.

133. Karvonen RL, Fernandez-Madrid F, Maughan RL, et al. An animal model of pulmonary radiation fibrosis with biochemical, physiologic, immunologic, and morphologic observations. *Radiat Res* 1987;111:68–80.

134. Rodemann HP, Bamberg M. Cellular basis of radiation-induced fibrosis. *Radiother Oncol* 1995;35:83–90.

135. Basset F, Ferrans VJ, Soler P, et al. Intraluminal fibrosis in interstitial lung disorders. *Am J Pathol* 1986;122:443–461.

136. Onoda JM, Kantak SS, Diglio CA. Radiation-induced endothelial cell retraction in vitro: correlation with acute pulmonary edema. *Pathol Oncol Res* 1999;5:49–55.

137. Hill RP, Rodemann HP, Hendry JH, et al. Normal tissue radiobiology: from the laboratory to the clinic. *Int J Radiat Oncol Biol Phys* 2001;49:353–365.

138. Antonadou D, Coliarakis N, Synodinou M, et al. Randomized phase III trial of radiation treatment ± amifostine in patients with advanced-stage lung cancer. *Int J Radiat Oncol Biol Phys* 2001;51:915–922.

139. Koukourakis MI, Yannakakis D. High dose daily amifostine and hypofractionated intensively accelerated radiotherapy for locally advanced breast cancer: a phase I/II study and report on early and late sequellae. *Anticancer Res* 2001;21(4B):2973–2978.

140. Wang LW, Fu XL, Clough R, et al. Can angiotensin-converting enzyme inhibitors protect against symptomatic radiation pneumonitis? *Radiat Res* 2000;153:405–410.

141. Percarpio B, Fischer JJ. β-Aminopropionitrile as a radiation reaction preventive agent. *Radiology* 1976;121(3 Pt. 1):737–740.

142. Dubrawsky C, Dubravsky NB, Withers HR. The effect of colchicine on the accumulation of hydroxyproline and on lung compliance after irradiation. *Radiat Res* 1978;73:111–120.

143. Ward WF, Molteni A, Ts'ao C, et al. Functional responses of the pulmonary endothelium to thoracic irradiation in rats: differential modification by D-penicillamine. *Int J Radiat Oncol Biol Phys* 1987;13:1505–1513.

144. Percarpio B, Fischer JJ. The effect of penicillamine on radiation-induced pulmonary lethality in mice. *Radiology* 1979;131:791–792.

145. Ward WF, Shih-Hoellwarth A, Tuttle RD. Collagen accumulation in irradiated rat lung: modification by D-penicillamine. *Radiology* 1983;146:533–537.

146. Molteni A, Moulder JE, Cohen EF, et al. Control of radiation-induced pneumopathy and lung fibrosis by angiotensin-converting enzyme inhibitors and an angiotensin II type 1 receptor blocker. *Int J Radiat Biol* 2000;76:523–532.

147. Gross NJ, Holloway NO, Narine KR. Effects of some non-steroidal anti-inflammatory agents on experimental radiation pneumonitis. *Radiat Res* 1991;127:317–324.

148. Tyree EB, Glicksman AS, Nickson JJ. Effect of l-triiodothyronine on radiation-induced pulmonary fibrosis in dogs. *Radiat Res* 1966;28:30–36.

149. Landreneau RJ, Hazelrigg SR, Ferson PF, et al. Thoracoscopic resection of 85 pulmonary lesions. *Ann Thorac Surg* 1992;54:415–419.

150. Delanian S, Balla-Mekias S, Lefaix JL. Striking regression of chronic radiotherapy damage in a clinical trial of combined pentoxifylline and tocopherol. *J Clin Oncol* 1999;17:3283–3290.

151. Kwon HC, Kim SK, Chung WK, et al. Effect of pentoxifylline on radiation response of non–small cell lung cancer: a phase III randomized multicenter trial. *Radiother Oncol* 2000;56:175–179.

152. Khanavkar B, Stern P, Alberti W, et al. Complications associated with brachytherapy alone or with laser in lung cancer. *Chest* 1991;99:1062–1065.

153. Ward HE, Kemsley L, Davies L, et al. The effect of steroids on radiation-induced lung disease in the rat. *Radiat Res* 1993;136:22–28.

154. Gross NJ. Radiation pneumonitis in mice: some effects of corticosteroids on mortality and pulmonary physiology. *J Clin Invest* 1980;66:504–510.

155. Gross NJ, Narine KR. Experimental radiation pneumonitis: corticosteroids increase the replicative activity of alveolar type 2 cells. *Radiat Res* 1988;115:543–549.

156. Castellino RA, Glatstein E, Turbow MM, et al. Latent injury of lungs or heart activated by steroid withdrawal. *Ann Intern Med* 1974;80:593–599.

157. Evans ML, Graham MM, Mahler PA, et al. Use of steroids to suppress cellular response to radiation. *Int J Radiat Oncol Biol Phys* 1987;13:563–567.

158. Cameron SJ, Grant IW, Pearson JG, et al. Prednisone and mustine in prevention of tumour swelling during pulmonary irradiation. *BMJ* 1972;1:535–537.

159. Kwok E, Chan CK. Corticosteroids and azathioprine do not prevent radiation-induced lung injury. *Can Respir J* 1998;5:211–214.

160. Yamada M, Kudoh S, Hirata K, et al. Risk factors of pneumonitis following chemoradiotherapy for lung cancer. *Eur J Cancer* 1998;34:71–75.

161. Gross NJ, Narine KR, Wade R. Protective effect of corticosteroids on radiation pneumonitis in mice. *Radiat Res* 1988;113:112–119.

162. Gibson PG, Bryant DH, Morgan GW, et al. Radiation-induced lung injury: a hypersensitivity pneumonitis? *Ann Intern Med* 1988;109:288–291.

163. Pezner RD, Bertrand M, Cecchi GR, et al. Steroid-withdrawal radiation pneumonitis in cancer patients. *Chest* 1984;85:816–817.

164. Thomas CR Jr, Giroux DJ, Stelzer KJ, et al. Concurrent cisplatin, prolonged oral etoposide, and vincristine plus chest and brain irradiation for limited small cell lung cancer: a phase II study of the Southwest Oncology Group (SWOG-9229). *Int J Radiat Oncol Biol Phys* 1998;40:1039–1047.

165. Dolsma WV, De Vries EG, Van der Mark TW, et al. Pulmonary function after high-dose chemotherapy with autologous bone marrow transplantation and radiotherapy in patients with advanced loco-regional breast cancer. *Anticancer Res* 1997;17:537–540.

166. Hassink EA, Souren TS, Boersma LJ, et al. Pulmonary morbidity 10–18 years after irradiation for Hodgkin's disease. *Eur J Cancer* 1993;29A:343–347.

167. Prato FS, Kurdyak R, Saibil EA, et al. Regional and total lung function in patients following pulmonary irradiation. *Invest Radiol* 1977;12:224–237.

168. Boersma LJ, Damen EM, de Boer RW, et al. Estimation of overall pulmonary function after irradiation using dose-effect relations for local functional injury. *Radiother Oncol* 1995;36:15–23.

169. Penney DP, Van Houtte P, Siemann DW, et al. Long term effects of radiation and combined modalities on mouse lung. *Scan Electron Microsc* 1986;(Pt 1):221–228.

170. Law MP. Vascular permeability and late radiation fibrosis in mouse lung. *Radiat Res* 1985;103:60–76.

171. Emirgil C, Heinemann HO. Effects of irradiation of chest on pulmonary function in man. *J Appl Physiol* 1961;16:331–337.

172. Marks LB, Fan M, Clough R, et al. Radiation-induced pulmonary injury: symptomatic versus subclinical endpoints. *Int J Radiat Biol* 2000;76:469–475.

173. Gogna NK, Morgan G, Downs K, et al. Lung dose rate and interstitial pneumonitis in total body irradiation for bone marrow transplantation. *Australas Radiol* 1992;36:317–320.

174. Villani F, Viviani S, Bonfante V, et al. Late pulmonary effects in favorable stage I and IIA Hodgkin's disease treated with radiotherapy alone. *Am J Clin Oncol* 2000;23:18–21.

175. Ooi GC, Kwong DL, Ho JC, et al. Pulmonary sequelae of treatment for breast cancer: a prospective study. *Int J Radiat Oncol Biol Phys* 2001;50:411–419.

176. Hayakawa K, Mitsuhashi N, Saito Y, et al. Short communication: adverse chronic effects of high-dose irradiation on proximal bronchus in patients treated for bronchogenic carcinoma. *Br J Radiol* 1993;66:477–479.

177. De Vito EL, Quadrelli SA, Montiel GC, et al. Bilateral diaphragmatic paralysis after mediastinal radiotherapy. *Respiration* 1996;63:187–190.

178. Theuws JC, Muller SH, Seppenwoolde Y, et al. Effect of radiotherapy and chemotherapy on pulmonary function after treatment for breast cancer and lymphoma: a follow-up study. *J Clin Oncol* 1999;17:3091–3100.

179. Fu XL, Jiang G, Wang L, Qian H, Fu S, Yie M, Kong F, Zhao S, He S, Liu T. Hyperfractionated accelerated radiation therapy for non–small cell lung cancer: clinical phase I/II trial. *Int J Radiat Oncol Biol Phys* 2001;50:899–908.

180. Boule M, Zucker JM, Gaultier C, et al. Lung function of children treated for malignant extrapulmonary tumors. *Bull Eur Physiopathol Respir* 1984;20:121–126.

181. Block M, Lachowiez RM, Rios C, et al. Pulmonary fibrosis associated with low-dose adjuvant methyl-CCNU. *Med Pediatr Oncol* 1990;18:256–260.

182. Lehne G, Lote K. Pulmonary toxicity of cytotoxic and immunosuppressive agents: a review. *Acta Oncol* 1990;29:113–124.

183. Baker WJ, Fistel SJ, Jones RV, et al. Interstitial pneumonitis associated with ifosfamide therapy. *Cancer* 1990;65:2217–2221.

184. Breen E, Shull S, Burne S, et al. Bleomycin regulation of transforming growth factor-β mRNA in rat lung fibroblasts. *Am J Respir Cell Mol Biol* 1992;6:146–152.

185. Hay J, Shahzeidi S, Laurent G. Mechanisms of bleomycin-induced lung damage. *Arch Toxicol* 1991;65:81–94.

186. Jules-Elysee K, White DA. Bleomycin-induced pulmonary toxicity. *Clin Chest Med* 1990;11:1–20.

187. Kachel DL, Martin WJ 2nd. Cyclophosphamide-induced lung toxicity: mechanism of endothelial cell injury. *J Pharmacol Exp Ther* 1994;268:42–46.

188. Venkatesan N, Chandrakasan G. Cyclophosphamide induced early biochemical changes in lung lavage fluid and alterations in lavage cell function. *Lung* 1994;172:147–158.

189. Komaki R, Lee JS, Kaplan B, et al. Randomized phase III study of chemoradiation with or without amifostine for patients with favorable performance status inoperable stage II-III non–small cell lung cancer: preliminary results. *Semin Radiat Oncol* 2002; 12[1 Suppl 1]:46–49.

190. Lefaix JL, Delanian S, Vozenin MC, et al. Striking regression of subcutaneous fibrosis induced by high doses of gamma rays using a combination of pentoxifylline and α-tocopherol: an experimental study. *Int J Radiat Oncol Biol Phys* 1999;43:839–847.

Pulmonary Hypertension: Pathophysiology and Clinical Disorders

35

Sharon I. S. Rounds · James R. Klinger

The normal pulmonary circulation is a low pressure, high-flow vascular bed, accommodating the entire cardiac output with each heartbeat. Increased cardiac output, a normal response to exercise, does not significantly increase pulmonary arterial pressure. The reasons for the high capacitance of the pulmonary circulation are recruitment of underperfused microvessels and distension of patent vessels in response to increases in blood flow. In addition, tone of the smooth muscle in the media of pulmonary arterioles is lower and the smooth muscle coat of pulmonary resistance vessels is thinner than that of most systemic vascular beds.

Pulmonary hypertension is abnormally elevated pressure in the arterial side of the pulmonary circulation, usually defined as mean pulmonary arterial pressure (PAP) greater than 25 mm Hg at rest or greater than 30 mm Hg with exercise. Most cases of pulmonary hypertension are caused by chronic heart or lung disease. Sustained elevation in PAP secondary to increased pulmonary venous pressure, hypoxic pulmonary vasoconstriction, or increased flow is often referred to as secondary pulmonary hypertension. This type of pulmonary hypertension causes moderate elevation in PAP and is believed to be a physiologic response to sustained elevations in PAP. When pulmonary hypertension is found in the absence of conditions that are known to elevate PAP, it is referred to as idiopathic or primary pulmonary hypertension (PPH). This type of pulmonary hypertension is thought to occur from injury to or abnormal growth response of the pulmonary vasculature itself. PAP becomes elevated secondary to a diseased pulmonary circulation that results in a combination of decreased cross-sectional area and increased arterial tone. PPH typically results in severe elevations in pulmonary pressure and progression to right heart failure and death.

The terminology of PPH and secondary pulmonary hypertension can be confusing, however. Many of the pathological features of PPH and secondary pulmonary hypertension overlap. Also, pulmonary hypertension is seen more frequently in patients with collagen vascular disease, HIV infection, or portal hypertension than in the general population. The pulmonary hypertension that develops in these diseases may be referred to as secondary, but is often clinically and pathologically indistinguishable from PPH.

Because of confusing terminology, the World Health Organization (WHO) offered a modified diagnostic classification of pulmonary hypertensive diseases in 1998 (1) (Table 35.1).

This new classification avoids the major categories of "primary" and "secondary" pulmonary hypertension. Different types of pulmonary hypertension are categorized by the underlying disease or condition with which it is associated. In the WHO classification, the major categories are pulmonary arterial hypertension (PAH), pulmonary venous hypertension, pulmonary hypertension associated with disorders of the respiratory system or hypoxemia, pulmonary hypertension caused by thrombotic or embolic disease, and pulmonary hypertension caused by diseases that directly affect the pulmonary vasculature. The WHO classification of pulmonary hypertension is helpful because it places patients with similar types of pulmonary hypertension in the same groups. It has gained wide acceptance and will be used throughout this chapter. In this chapter, we discuss the pathophysiology of pulmonary hypertension in the context of abnormalities of normal mechanisms of low pulmonary vascular pressure. We survey clinical disorders manifested by pulmonary hypertension, and we review the approach to

S. I. S. Rounds: Pulmonary/Critical Care Section, Providence VA Medical Center; and Department of Medicine, Brown Medical School, Providence, Rhode Island.

J. R. Klinger: Pulmonary and Critical Care Medicine, Rhode Island Hospital; and Department of Medicine, Brown Medical Center, Providence, Rhode Island.

TABLE 35.1. WORLD HEALTH ORGANIZATION DIAGNOSTIC CLASSIFICATION OF PULMONARY HYPERTENSION

1. Pulmonary arterial hypertension
    1.1. Primary pulmonary hypertension
        (a) Sporadic
        (b) Familial
    1.2. Related to
        (a) Collagen vascular disease
        (b) Congenital systemic-to-pulmonary shunts
        (c) Portal hypertension
        (d) HIV infection
        (e) Drugs/toxins
            (1) Anorexigens
            (2) Other
        (f) Persistent pulmonary hypertension of the newborn
        (g) Other
2. Pulmonary venous hypertension
    2.1. Left-sided atrial or ventricular disease
    2.2. Left-sided valvular heart disease
    2.3. Extrinsic compression of central pulmonary veins
        (a) Fibrosing mediastinitis
        (b) Adenopathy/tumors
    2.4. Pulmonary venoocclusive disease
    2.5. Other
3. Pulmonary hypertension associated with disorders of the respiratory system and/or hypoxemia
    3.1. Chronic obstructive pulmonary disease
    3.2. Interstitial lung disease
    3.3. Sleep disordered breathing
    3.4. Alveolar hypoventilation disorders
    3.5. Chronic exposure to high altitude
    3.6. Neonatal lung disease
    3.7. Alveolar-capillary dysplasia
    3.8. Other
4. Pulmonary hypertension owing to chronic thrombotic and/or embolic disease
    4.1. Thromboembolic obstruction of proximal pulmonary arteries
    4.2. Obstruction of distal pulmonary arteries
        (a) Pulmonary embolism (e.g., thrombus, tumor)
        (b) In situ thrombosis
        (c) Sickle cell disease
5. Pulmonary hypertension owing to disorders affecting the pulmonary vasculature directly
    5.1. Inflammatory
        (a) Schistosomiasis
        (b) Sarcoidosis
        (c) Other
    5.2. Pulmonary capillary hemangiomatosis

diagnosis and treatment of pulmonary hypertensive disorders. There has been extraordinary progress in the past 10 to 20 years in understanding of pathogenesis and development (2–4).

PATHOPHYSIOLOGY OF PULMONARY HYPERTENSION

To understand the pathogenesis of pulmonary hypertension, it is necessary to review the determinants of normal pulmonary vascular tone. As illustrated in Figure 35.1, pul-

monary vascular resistance (PVR) is a function of inflow (pulmonary arterial) and outflow (left atrial or pulmonary venous) pressures and is inversely proportional to cardiac output. As noted above, the normal structure and function of pulmonary arterioles are those of a low-resistance circulation. PAP increases with increases in cardiac output and with increases in left atrial pressure. Because of the remarkable capacity of the pulmonary circulation, acute changes in flow and venous pressures do not ordinarily cause significant pulmonary hypertension. However, if these conditions persist in a chronic state (weeks to months), then vasoconstriction, vascular remodeling, and subsequent narrowing of the vessels occurs.

Other factors that modulate PVR are delineated by the Poiseuille law, which describes resistance to flow through rigid tubes (Fig. 35.1). PVR is directly proportional to the viscosity of blood and is inversely proportional to the radius to the fourth power of the aggregate cross-sectional area of the pulmonary vascular bed. Thus, conditions that increase blood viscosity, such as erythrocytosis, may exacerbate pulmonary hypertension. Most importantly, conditions that decrease the luminal area of the pulmonary circulation significantly increase PVR and arterial pressure.

Figure 35.2 illustrates conditions in which the aggregate cross-sectional area of the pulmonary circulation may be diminished. Loss of aggregate cross-sectional area occurs after surgical resection of lung tissue. Ordinarily, even pneumonectomy does not cause resting pulmonary hypertension because of the enormous reserve of the pulmonary circulation. Indeed, more than half of the pulmonary circulation must be removed before pulmonary hypertension is observed at rest. As cardiac output increases with exercise, pulmonary hypertension may be observed with exercise after pneumonectomy. Similarly, if there is some other underlying disorder decreasing pulmonary arterial cross-sectional area, then further loss of area after lung resection may cause resting pulmonary hypertension. Another common cause of loss of pulmonary vascular luminal area is the destructive lung disease emphysema. In emphysema, destruction of alveolar capillary septa results in loss of pulmonary capillaries and microvessels.

The luminal area of the pulmonary circulation may also be decreased by obstruction of vessels, such as occurs after pulmonary thromboembolism. Because of the huge normal cross-sectional area of the pulmonary circulation, acute pulmonary thromboembolism rarely causes sustained pulmonary hypertension, unless there is massive embolization resulting in obstruction of more than half of pulmonary arteries. However, if there is an underlying disorder that has diminished the luminal area, then submassive thromboembolism may cause pulmonary hypertension. Also, recurrent thromboembolism with multiple small clots accumulating over a period of months to years causes sustained pulmonary hypertension.

Widespread narrowing of pulmonary arteries is an important cause of loss of cross-sectional area. Narrowing may be owing to anatomic changes in the vascular wall

PULMONARY VASCULAR RESISTANCE

$$\text{PVR (mmHg/L/min)} = \frac{\overline{\text{PPA}} - \overline{\text{PLA}}}{\text{Q}}$$

POISEUILLE'S LAW

$$R = \Delta P/Q$$

$$R = \frac{8\eta l}{\pi r^4}$$

FIGURE 35.1. The computation of pulmonary vascular resistance (PVR) and Poiseuille's law. PVR in Wood units is calculated from the ratio of differences in pressure across the pulmonary vasculature to blood flow. PPA, mean pulmonary arterial pressure (mm Hg); PLA, mean left atrial (or pulmonary venous) pressure (mm Hg); Q, cardiac output (blood flow, L/min). PVR may also be expressed in units of dyne/(sec • cm^{-5}) by multiplying this ratio by 80. Poiseuille's law describes flow in tubes, such as blood vessels; η, viscosity; l, length of tube; R, aggregate radius of tube(s). (From the American College of Chest Physicians. *Chest* 1984;85:398, with permission.)

structures, such as the vascular remodeling seen after chronic hypoxia or in PPH. Contraction of vascular smooth muscle causes vasoconstriction, another cause of decreased luminal area. Although a variety of mediators cause pulmonary arterial vasoconstriction, the most common cause of pulmonary vasoconstriction is acute alveolar hypoxia. Vasoconstriction and remodeling frequently occur simultaneously, as in conditions characterized by long-standing hypoxia, such as chronic mountain sickness or chronic bronchitis.

Thus, increases in pulmonary blood flow, left atrial or pulmonary venous pressure, and blood viscosity and decreases in pulmonary arterial lumen area all increase PAP. Some of these mechanisms, such as increased blood viscosity, exacerbate pulmonary hypertension, but rarely, if ever, cause clinically significant disease by themselves. In many clinical disorders, more than one mechanism of pulmonary hypertension may be operant. For example, in PPH, vasoconstriction, structural remodeling, and in situ thromboses are all likely contributors to increased PVR. In conditions of sustained increases in pulmonary blood flow, such as congenital left-to-right intracardiac shunts, sustained increases in flow eventually cause increased vasomotor tone and vascular remodeling, which exacerbate and may perpetuate pulmonary hypertension. Thus, regardless of the original insult, the mechanism of sustained pulmonary hypertension is usually multifactorial. In subsequent sections of this chapter, we

REDUCTION

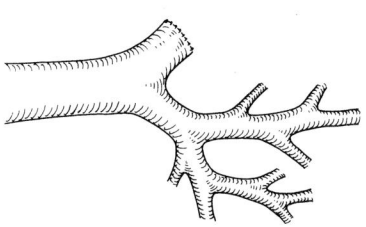

SURGICAL RESECTION

OBSTRUCTION

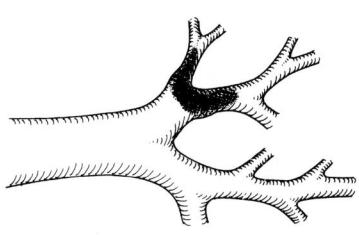

PULMONARY EMBOLISM

RESTRICTION
a. Anatomic

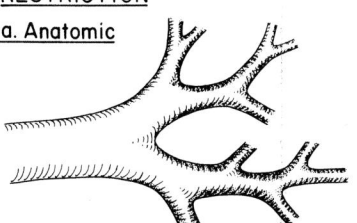

CHRONIC HYPOXIA (REMODELING)

b. Vasoconstriction

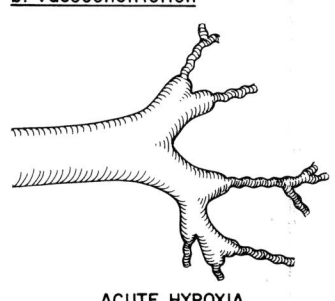

ACUTE HYPOXIA

FIGURE 35.2. Several common causes of decrease in aggregate vascular lumen area. (From the American College of Chest Physicians. *Chest* 1984;85:398, with permission.)

will discuss pulmonary hypertensive disorders in more detail, with correlation of pathologic and physiologic changes and clinical manifestations.

PATHOPHYSIOLOGY OF PULMONARY VASOMOTOR CONTROL

In the healthy pulmonary circulation, pulmonary vascular tone is maintained by numerous factors, including neural stimuli, oxygen tension, potassium channels, and endogenous vasoactive substances. Loss of normal balance among these factors can cause contraction of pulmonary vascular smooth muscle and restriction of the pulmonary vascular bed, resulting in pulmonary hypertension. Whether increased pulmonary vasoconstriction is a primary contributor to the development of pulmonary hypertension or a secondary response of a diseased pulmonary circulation is debatable. However, the demonstration that pulmonary hemodynamics can improve rapidly in response to vasodilators suggests that at least in some patients, abnormally elevated pulmonary vascular tone is an important cause of elevated PAP. Each mechanism is discussed in greater detail below.

Sympathetic Tone

Both the larger proximal pulmonary arteries and more distal resistance vessels contain α- and β-adrenergic receptors that when stimulated result in pulmonary vasoconstriction and vasodilation, respectively (5). Under normal resting tone, β-adrenergic activity predominates over α-adrenergic activity and likely helps to maintain the pulmonary vasculature in a vasodilated state. α-Adrenergic activity increases in response to stress, resulting in pulmonary vasoconstriction. This effect has been best demonstrated for hypoxic pulmonary vasoconstriction. Unfortunately, neither β-adrenergic agonists nor α-adrenergic antagonists have been helpful in the treatment of patients with pulmonary hypertensive diseases. The lack of their success may be owing to pulmonary vascular remodeling that occurs over the course of prolonged α-adrenergic stimulation.

Hypoxia

The pressor response to hypoxia is unique to the pulmonary circulation. Constriction of precapillary arterioles in response to reduced oxygen tension reduces perfusion to poorly ventilated lung units. Local vasoconstrictor responses to hypoxia help to maintain normal ventilation-perfusion ratios (V/Q). However, when a substantial portion of the pulmonary circulation is exposed to hypoxia, as during ascent to high altitude or in chronic lung disease, the result may be sustained pulmonary artery hypertension (6). The mechanism of hypoxic vasoconstriction is not completely understood, but potassium channels appear to play a major role. There is significant variability among individuals in

the magnitude of hypoxic vasoconstriction. This variation, which may be genetic in origin, may explain differences in the degree of pulmonary hypertension–complicating lung diseases. Hypoxic vasoconstriction is enhanced by acidosis and hypercarbia.

Potassium Channels

Like other smooth muscle cells, pulmonary vascular smooth muscle cells require an increase in intracellular calcium levels to contract. There are considerable data to suggest that hypoxic pulmonary vasoconstriction is associated with *trans*-plasmalemmal calcium influx (7) via the opening of voltage-gated L-type calcium channels, and that the opening and closing of these channels is regulated by membrane depolarization via potassium channels (8). The resting membrane potential (Em) of vascular smooth muscle cells is about -55 mV. Inhibition or closing of potassium channels retards the intracellular to extracellular efflux of potassium. As a result, the interior of the cell becomes more positive, or depolarized. Depolarization increases the open probability of the voltage-gated L-type calcium channel, allowing intracellular influx of calcium, activation of actin-myosin, and smooth muscle cell contraction. At least three types of potassium channels have been described in pulmonary vascular smooth muscle, but the major determinant of membrane potential appears to be the voltage-gated potassium (Kv) channel. Several investigators have confirmed that hypoxia reduces potassium currents in pulmonary vascular smooth muscle by inhibiting Kv (9). This effect is unique to pulmonary vascular smooth muscle (10) and likely explains why pulmonary vascular smooth muscle contracts in response to hypoxia, whereas vasodilation is seen in other types of vascular smooth muscle. The Kv channels have also been implicated in sensing oxygen tension in other cell types such as the carotid body. Current research focuses on the identity of the oxygen sensor that allows Kv to sense a decrease in oxygen tension. Whether changes in Kv expression or function are primarily responsible for the development of pulmonary hypertension or whether they are a secondary result of the underlying disease process is uncertain, but it is interesting that pulmonary arteries of patients with PAH have been shown to have decreased potassium currents, increased intracellular calcium levels, and decreased expression of Kv compared with levels in patients with pulmonary venous hypertension or in normal controls (11).

Vasoactive Substances

Numerous vasoactive agents contribute to the modulation of PAP. Some of these help in maintaining basal pulmonary vascular tone. Others are up-regulated in response to stress, such as hypoxia in chronic lung disease or shear stress from increased pulmonary blood flow from congenital left-to-right shunts. The pulmonary vascular endothelium is the primary site of synthesis and/or metabolism of most of these compounds. In addition to their vasoconstrictor effects, some of these agents also act as potent mitogens for pulmonary vascular smooth muscle cells, fibroblasts and endothelial cells. Nitric oxide (NO), endothelin-1 (ET-1), epoprostenol (prostacyclin, or PGI_2), and thromboxane are among the best-described agents currently believed to play major roles in regulating pulmonary vascular tone.

Gene-targeted disruption of endothelial NO synthase (eNOS), the enzyme primarily responsible for constitutive expression of NO in pulmonary endothelial cells, increases PAP only slightly under normoxic conditions but markedly elevates the degree of pulmonary hypertension that develops after exposure to chronic hypoxia (12). Endothelin receptor antagonists blunt the development of hypoxic pulmonary hypertension in animal studies and can partially reverse or retard the development of hypoxia- and monocrotaline-induced pulmonary hypertension when given late in the course of the disease (13). In situ hybridization studies have shown marked decreases in expression of eNOS (14) and increases in expression of ET-1 (15) in the pulmonary vessels of patients with PAH compared with lungs from controls. The decreases in eNOS and increases in ET-1 expression are particularly notable in the endothelial cells and plexiform lesions of the small pulmonary arteries of patients with PPH. Expression of eNOS and ET-1 correlated inversely and directly with pulmonary vascular resistance (PVR), respectively, suggesting that altered expression of these vasoactive agents contribute to the disease process.

PGI_2 and thromboxane A_2 (TxA_2) are products of arachidonic acid metabolism and are secreted by the vascular endothelial cells, including those of the pulmonary circulation. These compounds have opposing effects on pulmonary vascular tone, cellular proliferation, and platelet aggregation. PGI_2 is a vasodilator that inhibits smooth muscle mitogenesis and platelet aggregation, whereas TxA_2 is a potent vasoconstrictor and mitogen. Studies have shown a significantly lower ratio of PGI_2 to TxA_2 in the urine of patients with pulmonary hypertension than in the urine of controls, suggesting that an imbalance in the synthesis and secretion of these agents may contribute to the development of pulmonary hypertension (16). This hypothesis is supported by animal studies showing that mice with gene-targeted disruption of PGI_2 synthase develop more severe pulmonary hypertension than do mice with normal expression of this enzyme (17). Decreased expression of PGI_2 synthase has also been observed in pulmonary vessels of patients with pulmonary hypertension (18).

Serotonin (5-hydroxytryptophan or 5-HT) is a potent pulmonary vasoconstrictor but causes vasodilation in the systemic circulation. Serotonin is secreted primarily by neuroendocrine cells in the gut, and circulating levels are kept extremely low owing to uptake and storage in platelets and hepatic metabolism. Serotonin that reaches the pulmonary circulation causes pulmonary vasoconstriction, proliferation of pulmonary vascular smooth muscles, and platelet

VASOACTIVE AGENTS INVOLVED IN THE PATHOBIOLOGY OF PULMONARY HYPERTENSION

Agent/Effect	Level of Evidence
Nitric oxide (NO): relaxes pulmonary vascular smooth muscle, inhibits pulmonary smooth muscle hypertrophy and hyperplasia, inhibits platelet aggregation	Pulmonary hypertension develops in NO synthase knockout mice. NO synthase expression is decreased in lungs of pulmonary hypertensive patients. Inhaled NO improves pulmonary hypertension in some patients with the disease
Prostacyclin (PGI_2): relaxes pulmonary vascular smooth muscle, inhibits pulmonary smooth muscle hypertrophy and hyperplasia, inhibits platelet aggregation	Pulmonary hypertension develops in mouse PGI_2 synthase knockout models. PGI_2 and PGI_2 synthase expression is decreased in lungs of pulmonary hypertensive patients. Intravenous PGI_2 improves pulmonary hypertension in patients with the disease
Thromboxane (TxA_2): constricts pulmonary vascular smooth muscle, induces pulmonary smooth muscle hypertrophy and hyperplasia, facilitates platelet aggregation and thrombosis	Increases pulmonary vascular smooth muscle hypertrophy/hyperplasia *in vitro*. Evidence of decreased ratio of PGI_2/TxA_2 in patients with pulmonary arterial hypertension
Endothelin-1: potent pulmonary vasoconstrictor, induces pulmonary smooth muscle hypertrophy and hyperplasia, facilitates cardiac hypertrophy	Plasma levels and pulmonary vascular expression are increased in patients with pulmonary hypertension. Endothelin receptor antagonists inhibit development and cause regression of pulmonary hypertension in animals and humans
5-Hydroxytryptophan (serotonin, or 5-HT): potent pulmonary vasoconstrictor, induces hypertrophy/proliferation of pulmonary vascular smooth muscles, facilitates platelet aggregation	Plasma levels increased in some types of pulmonary hypertension. Transporter 5-HT facilitates uptake of anorexigens into pulmonary vascular smooth muscle cells. Evidence of increased 5-HT transporter expression in pulmonary vascular smooth muscle cells in patients with pulmonary arterial hypertension.
Cytokines and chemokines: pulmonary vasoconstrictors, recruit inflammatory cells	Increased plasma levels of cytokines in patients with primary arterial hypertension. Increased expression of chemokines localized to pulmonary vascular endothelial cells in patients with pulmonary hypertension. Chemokine RANTES receptor expression regulated by transforming growth factor-β_1
Angiotensin II: Pulmonary vasoconstrictor, induces hypertrophy of pulmonary vascular smooth muscle and right ventricle	Angiotensin-converting enzyme expression is increased in the heart and lungs of hypoxic rats. Angiotensin II induces pulmonary vascular smooth muscle hypertrophy in vivo
Atrial (ANP) and brain natriuretic peptides: pulmonary vasodilators, inhibit muscularization of pulmonary vessels and right ventricular hypertrophy	Circulating levels correlate with disease severity in patients with pulmonary hypertension. ANP knockout mice have pulmonary hypertension

RANTES, regulated on activation normal T cell expressed and secreted.

aggregation. Serotonin has been implicated in the pathogenesis of pulmonary hypertension for several reasons: (a) serotonin has been reported to be elevated in sporadic cases of PPH (19); (b) amphetamine derivatives such as fenfluramine that have been associated with pulmonary hypertension are substrates for the serotonin transporter (20); and (c) mutations in the 5-HT transporter gene promoter, leading to over-expression of 5-HT transporter and increased uptake of serotonin by pulmonary vascular smooth muscle cells, occur more frequently in pulmonary hypertension patients than in controls (21,22).

Several other vasoconstrictor agents may contribute to the development of pulmonary hypertension by affecting pulmonary tone and vascular smooth muscle growth. Angiotensin II has vasoconstrictor effects on the pulmonary circulation and may contribute to hypertrophy of pulmonary vascular smooth muscle and right ventricular cardiocytes in patients with pulmonary hypertension (23). Plasma levels of atrial and brain natriuretic peptides are elevated in patients with pulmonary hypertension, and gene-targeted disruption of the gene for atrial natriuretic peptide increases PAP in mice (24, 25). Platelet-derived growth factor is released from platelets in the pulmonary circulation and may facilitate pulmonary vasoconstriction. The enzyme 5-lipoxygenase and its activating protein have also been implicated. Finally, inflammation is a well-described cause of pulmonary vasoconstriction in acute lung injury, and increased levels of inflammatory mediators, such as chemokines and interleukin-1 and -6, have been described in patients with pulmonary hypertension (26).

Despite the increased presence of numerous vasoconstrictor agents in the lung of pulmonary hypertensive patients, it is not yet clear if alterations in endothelial cell synthesis of pulmonary vasoactive mediators cause pulmonary hypertension in these patients or if they are merely the result of damage to the pulmonary vascular endothelium.

Another potential cause of abnormal pulmonary vascular tone is enhanced responsiveness of vascular smooth muscle to vasoactive substances. Evidence in support of this idea comes from animal studies that show changes in pulmonary vascular reactivity after lung injuries (27, 28). Depending on the cause of injury, vascular reactivity may be increased or decreased. Thus, not only are vasoactive substances increased in pulmonary hypertension, but also the pulmonary vascular bed may be primed to react more severely to them.

PATHOBIOLOGY OF PULMONARY VASCULAR REMODELING

Pulmonary vascular remodeling is the process resulting in characteristic pathologic changes of pulmonary hypertension. In the past it was thought that pathology was diagnostic of specific causes and clinical progression of pulmonary hypertension (29). However, the most recent world symposium on PPH, sponsored by the WHO (1), recommended that the previous classification system be abandoned in favor of description of the pathologic lesions, and that pathology be used in conjunction with clinical, hemodynamic, and molecular information in arriving at a diagnosis of a specific cause of pulmonary hypertension.

The characteristic pathologic changes of pulmonary hypertension involve thickening of all layers of the vessel wall (30, 31). This thickening is caused by both hypertrophy (cell growth) and hyperplasia (proliferation) of cellular components (endothelial cells, fibroblasts, and smooth muscle cells) and by increased deposition of connective tissue matrix components (collagen, elastin, fibronectin). There are some differences among models and diseases in the degree of endothelial cell injury, inflammatory reactions, and patterns of muscle hypertrophy. However, the process of remodeling is strikingly similar regardless of the inciting stimulus, suggesting a "stereotypical" response to vascular injury.

Unlike large-vessel atheromata in the systemic circulation, remodeling of the pulmonary vasculature occurs primarily in small vessels (diameter, <500 μm). Restriction is caused by both reduction in vessel number and by wall thickening that encroaches on the vascular lumen. Each of the cell types of the vascular wall can participate in the process. Endothelial cell swelling, necrosis, or hypertrophy may narrow the vascular lumen. In addition, endothelial cells may direct the synthesis of noncellular matrix with ensuing increases in intimal thickness (Fig. 35.3A; see also color Fig. 35.3). In situ thromboses also narrow the vascular lumen. Smooth muscle cell hypertrophy and hyperplasia are seen (Fig. 35.3B). This pattern of medial thickening is particularly characteristic of pulmonary hypertension owing to chronic hypoxemia (Table 35.1). A very important role of vascular smooth muscle is the synthesis of matrix material, such as elastin, that contributes to hypertrophy of vascular media. In precapillary segments, differentiation of pericytes and intermediate cells into myofibroblasts causes extension of smooth muscle into partially or nonmuscularized small vessels. These cells undergo phenotype shifts toward smooth muscle cells with characteristic changes in contractile and synthetic properties. Adventitial fibroblasts undergo hyperplasia and markedly increase collagen production, resulting in dramatic increases in adventitial thickness (Fig. 35.3A), which impairs arterial compliance (distensibility).

The plexiform lesion (Fig. 35.3C) may be seen in all types of pulmonary hypertension and, contrary to previous classifications, is not diagnostic of any particular etiologic cause. However, it is most commonly observed in the diseases classified as PAH (32) (Table 35.1). The plexiform lesion is characterized by aneurysmal dilatation of a small muscular pulmonary artery and a network of small blood vessels with downstream angiomatous dilated branches.

In situ thromboses may be seen in small vessels. In pulmonary hypertension owing to chronic thrombotic and/or embolic disease (Table 35.1), clot in proximal vessels may fail to resorb, and residual, fibrotic, organized clot ("webs") may be seen (Fig. 35.3D).

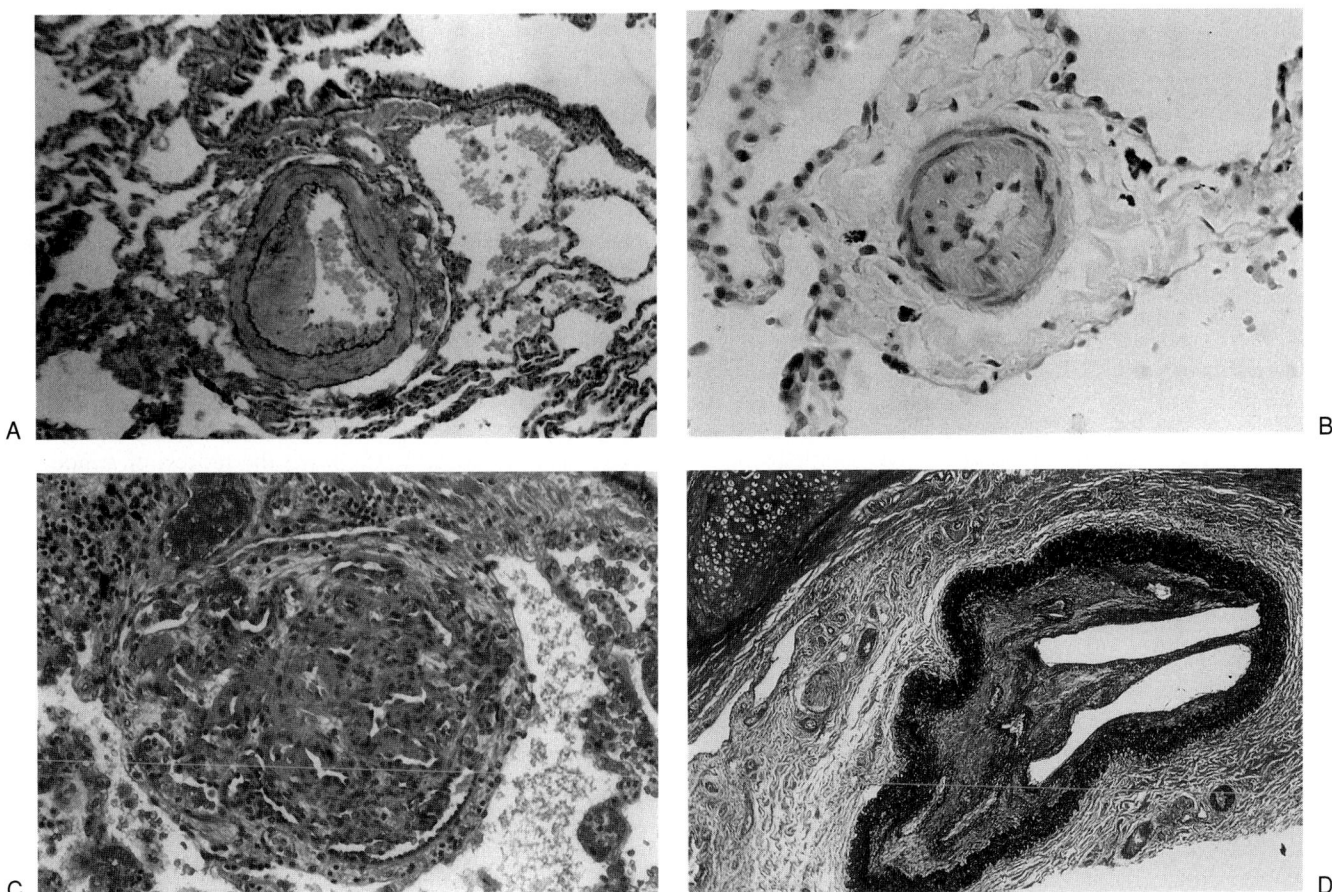

FIGURE 35.3. (See also color Fig. 35.3.) **(A)** Eccentric intimal thickening in primary pulmonary hypertension. **(B)** Medial thickening in long-standing mitral stenosis. **(C)** A plexiform lesion in primary pulmonary hypertension (magnification ×600). **(D)** A recanalized, fibrotic thrombus in chronic thromboembolism syndrome. (From Charles Kuhn, with permission.)

The mechanism of pulmonary vascular remodeling is a subject of intense research interest. It occurs in response to a variety of stimuli, both physical (mechanical stretch, shear stress) and chemical (hypoxia, vasoactive mediators, growth factors). It may also result from lack of apoptosis (programmed cell death) of vascular cells or lack of antiproliferative factors.

Enhanced vasoconstriction predisposes to remodeling, perhaps stimulated by changes in shear forces (33). In addition, several vasoactive mediators, such as angiotensin II (23), ET-1, and 5-hydroxytryptamine (34) also stimulate vascular smooth muscle and fibroblast proliferation. Growth factors, such as transforming growth factor-β (TGF-β), are involved in modulation of extracellular matrix production and of smooth muscle cell proliferation (33). Endothelial cell injury may be an important stimulus to the remodeling response by limiting supply of antiproliferative mediators, such as PGI$_2$ (35). Hypoxia may play a direct role by stimulating production of cytokines, such as vascular endothelial growth factor (VEGF) (36). Inflammatory cells may contribute to remodeling by cytokine (e.g., interleukin-1) production which, in turn, stimulates vascular smooth mus-

cle cell replication (37). Fragmentation of the internal elastic lamina, observed in some patients with pulmonary hypertension, and increased elastase activity may contribute to pulmonary vascular remodeling by enhancing release of matrix-bound growth factors (38). Tenascin-C, an extracellular matrix component, is increased in pulmonary hypertension and amplifies the effects of growth factors, such as fibroblast growth factor and epidermal growth factor (38). Activation of intracellular signaling mechanisms, such as protein kinase C and mitogen-activated protein kinases may also be important in mediating remodeling of vascular smooth muscle and fibroblasts (33).

VEGF is important in the maintenance, differentiation, and function of vascular endothelial cells. The work of Voelkel and Tuder and colleagues suggests that interference with VEGF function may cause pulmonary hypertension (39).

The plexiform lesion is characterized by exuberant endothelial cell growth (40) (Fig. 35.3C), and the work of Voelkel and Tuder and colleagues suggests that in PAH, this lesion may represent abnormal monoclonal endothelial cell proliferation (41). In addition, these investigators have demonstrated up-regulation of genes that may contribute to endothelial cell proliferation (42, 43).

Emerging understanding of the genetic regulation of vascular cell replication and phenotype has stimulated new insights into mechanisms of vascular remodeling. Mutations in the type II receptor for bone morphogenetic protein (BMPR-II) have been shown to underlie many familial and sporadic cases of PPH (see "Genetic Abnormalities Associated with Primary Pulmonary Hypertension" below). BMPR-II is a member of the TGF-β receptor superfamily that mediates the antiproliferative effects of TGF-β on vascular cells (44). BMPR-II is normally localized on pulmonary vascular endothelium with lower expression in vascular smooth muscle (45). BMPR-II expression was decreased in lungs of patients with PPH, regardless of whether the mutation was present, suggesting that abnormal responses to BMP may contribute to pulmonary vascular remodeling (45).

Perpetuation of structural changes, continued cell replication, and matrix accumulation suggest that control of normal reparative processes may be impaired in the process of vascular remodeling. The role of processes causing involution of tissue, such as apoptosis (programmed cell death) or proteolysis of extracellular matrix, is not known at this time.

Approach to Diagnosis

The approach to diagnosis of cause of pulmonary hypertension will be discussed first, following the outline of disease classification in Table 35.1. We subsequently describe features unique to individual disease categories.

The diagnosis of pulmonary vascular disease can be difficult because of its insidious onset, slow progression, and lack of a noninvasive method for accurately assessing PAP. Many of the signs and symptoms of pulmonary vascular disease are not present early in the disease course. Frequently, other diseases are suspected and excluded before the diagnosis of pulmonary hypertension is entertained. For these reasons, it is important to maintain a high level of suspicion and a willingness to entertain the diagnosis of pulmonary hypertension in patients with progressive dyspnea that is not readily explained by other disease processes.

The general approach to diagnosis of the cause of pulmonary hypertension is outlined in Figure 35.4. Pulmonary hypertension is suggested by the physical signs and symptoms described for each type of pulmonary hypertension below. Additional clues may be found on chest x-ray, electrocardiogram, or arterial blood gas levels. Pulmonary function tests should be performed as part of the general

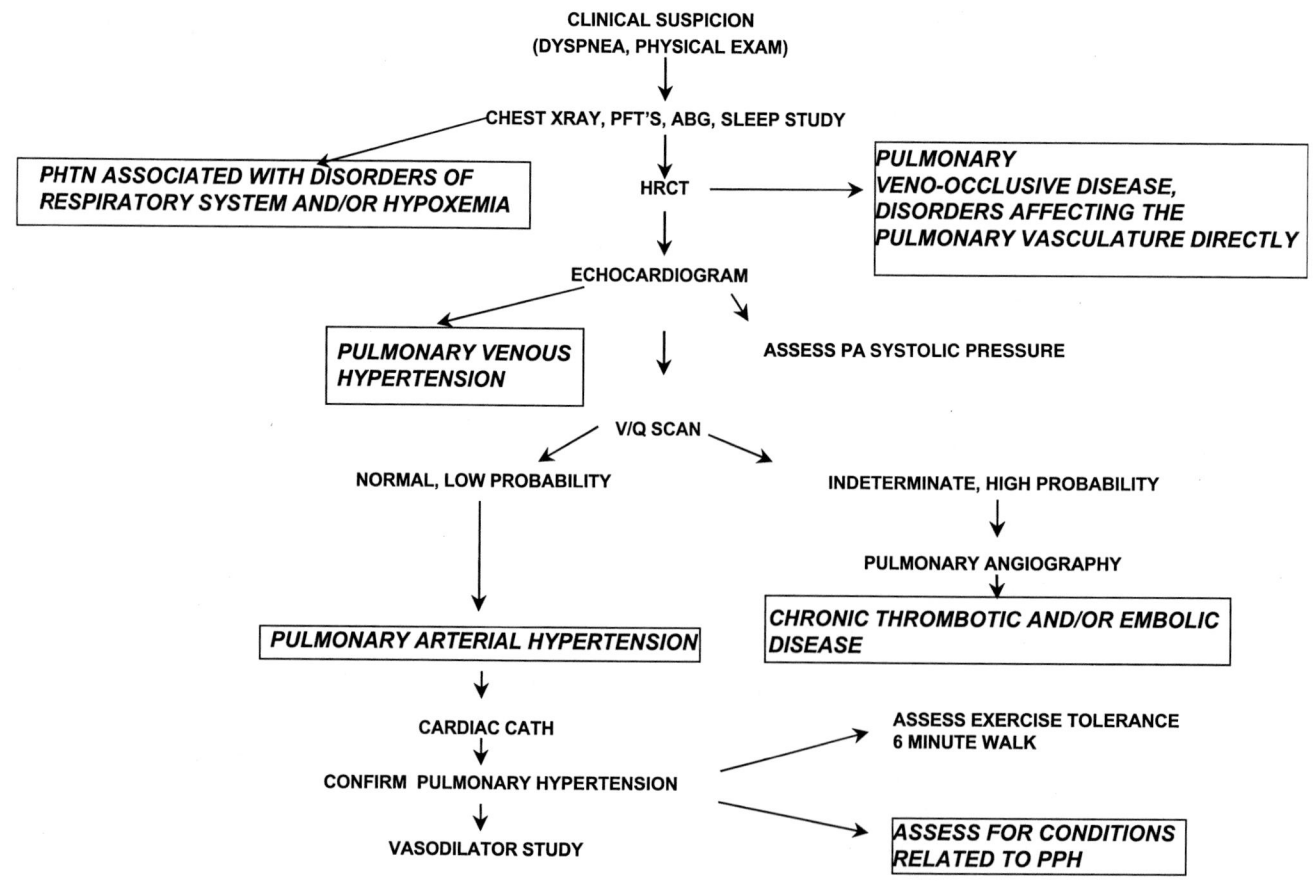

FIGURE 35.4. The approach to diagnosis of the cause of pulmonary hypertension.

work-up of dyspnea and as a component to exclude the presence of significant obstructive or restrictive lung disease. Patients with PPH typically have normal pulmonary function tests or mild restrictive defects. A total lung capacity of less than 60% to 70% of predicted should raise the suspicion of parenchymal lung disease. HRCT scanning may be indicated to exclude the presence of occult interstitial lung disease not seen on chest x-ray, or pulmonary venoocclusive disease (PVOD), pulmonary capillary hemangiomatosis, or other diseases affecting the pulmonary circulation directly. A decrease in the diffusing capacity for carbon monoxide is common in PAH and may reflect obliteration of pulmonary microvessels by the remodeling process. Hemoglobin oxygen saturation should be measured to determine if the pulmonary hypertension is caused by chronic hypoxemia. Patients with pulmonary hypertension may have normal or decreased hemoglobin oxygen saturation at rest. A fall in oxygen saturation with exercise is suggestive of pulmonary vascular disease, including PAH. The role of obstructive sleep apnea in causing pulmonary hypertension continues to be debated but should be screened for and, when present, needs to be adequately treated.

Thromboembolic disease, either chronic or acute, should be excluded by lung scan or other imaging procedures. In patients with PAH, perfusion lung scans may be normal or may reveal diffuse patchy areas of decreased perfusion. The presence of lobar or segmental abnormalities in lung scans should prompt further diagnostic evaluation such as pulmonary angiography. Pulmonary angiography may be necessary to exclude chronic thrombotic and/or embolic pulmonary hypertension (see "Thromboembolic Obstruction of Proximal Pulmonary Arteries" below). Although complications of pulmonary angiography are increased in pulmonary hypertension, the procedure can be performed safely by experienced operators.

Transthoracic echocardiography should be performed to estimate PAP. PAP is estimated by Doppler ultrasound of the regurgitant jet from the tricuspid valve and the assumption that right atrial pressure, which cannot be assessed by echocardiography, is about 10 cm H_2O. Transthoracic echocardiography also provides valuable information on cardiac chamber size and function. Right ventricular enlargement suggests increased end-diastolic pressure and may be the first evidence of right ventricular failure. Paradoxical movement of the interventricular septum toward the left ventricular free wall during diastole suggests severe right ventricular pressure overload. In PAH, left ventricular dimensions are usually normal, although right ventricular pressure overload can impede left ventricular filling and decrease left ventricular end-diastolic volume. In severe cases of PAH, the left ventricle can appear flattened and dysfunctional because of a markedly enlarged right ventricle. Transthoracic echocardiography is important in diagnosing PVH owing to mitral valve disease or impaired left ventricular systolic or diastolic dysfunction. Echocardiography is also useful in identifying an atrial septal defect.

When PAH is diagnosed, a careful search for conditions related to PPH should be undertaken. Screening should be performed for collagen vascular disease, especially the limited form of scleroderma, CREST syndrome, and systemic lupus erythematosus (SLE). Positive tests of "autoimmunity," such as antinuclear antibodies and rheumatoid factor, and the presence of Raynaud phenomenon have been observed in patients with PAH. Whether these findings suggest an "autoimmune" pathogenesis for some cases of PAH or whether they represent PAH associated with subclinical collagen vascular disease continues to be debated. Occasionally, PAH is the initial manifestation of collagen vascular disease.

In some patients, open lung biopsy may be necessary to exclude occult interstitial lung disease or pulmonary vasculitis, or to confirm the presence of veno-occlusive disease.

Once a thorough evaluation has been completed, pulmonary artery catheterization is usually performed to confirm the diagnosis of pulmonary hypertension and to obtain important prognostic data such as right atrial pressure, cardiac index, and response to vasodilators. During catheterization, samples of blood from the superior vena cava, right atrium, right ventricle, and main pulmonary artery should be obtained for measurement of oxygen saturation to exclude left-to-right intracardiac shunt.

Assessment of functional status is crucial in PAH. One common method is to assign the patient to one of four functional classes described by the WHO and modeled after the New York Heart Association (NYHA) classification for heart disease (1). Patients in WHO class I have essentially no limitations to normal activities but are dyspneic with strenuous exercise. Patients in WHO class II have some difficulty with normal activities, but function fairly well. Class III patients have significant functional limitations, including shortness of breath with activities of daily living. Class IV patients are unable to perform nearly any activity without symptoms and may be symptomatic even at rest. A more objective method of functional status is the 6-minute walk test, which requires patients to walk at their own pace on level ground for 6 minutes. Total distance covered is recorded, along with change in heart rate, blood pressure, and oxygen saturation. A dyspnea score, such as the Borg score that rates severity of dyspnea on a scale of one to 10 is recorded at the end of the 6-minute walk. Patients are allowed to stop and rest during the 6 minutes. Several clinical studies have demonstrated that performance on 6-minute walk tests deteriorates over 12 weeks in untreated patients with PAH, but improves in those who are treated (46–48).

CLINICAL SYNDROMES OF PULMONARY HYPERTENSION

Pulmonary Arterial Hypertension

PAH is a group of disorders of differing etiologies, sharing clinical and pathologic characteristics. These disorders present with varying degrees of pulmonary hypertension, but the course of the disease is usually progressive, and outcome is poor without treatment directed at reversal of remodeling changes and/or etiology. The pathology is that of plexogenic arteriopathy with plexiform lesions (Fig. 35.3C), thrombotic lesions, medial hypertrophy with intimal fibrosis (Fig. 35.3A), and medial hypertrophy (Fig. 35.3B).

Clinical Presentation of Pulmonary Arterial Hypertension

Dyspnea on exertion is the most common presenting symptom of patients with PAH, being noted in at least 60% of patients (49). Patients frequently describe relentless progression of their dyspnea over several months to a year, often out of proportion to, or in the absence of, other heart and lung disease. Other symptoms such as chest pain, lightheadedness, and palpitations may also be reported and are usually more common during exertion. Angina-type chest pain and syncope with exertion are particularly worrisome symptoms, as they suggest right ventricular overload and limited cardiac output. Many patients complain of generalized fatigue that often worsens as the day progresses. The degree of impairment as assessed by WHO functional classification and 6-minute walk test in activity is a useful way of monitoring disease progression and response to treatment.

The physical examination of patients with symptomatic PAH usually reveals signs of elevated PAP and right heart overload. The pulmonic component of the S2, heard best in the second intercostal space over the left sternal border, is usually accentuated and may be louder than the aortic component. Right ventricular dilation can cause splitting of the S2 and a holosystolic flow murmur over the right sternal border may occur from tricuspid regurgitation. As the right ventricle enlarges, a right ventricular heave can be felt as a diffuse impulse lifting the sternum with each heart beat, especially at end expiration in the upright position. Chronic right heart failure results in jugular venous distension and peripheral edema. As right ventricular function deteriorates, patients may develop hepatomegaly, hepatojugular reflux, and ascites.

The chest roentgenogram (Fig. 35.5) typically reveals enlargement of the main and hilar pulmonary arteries. A diameter of the right interlobar pulmonary artery greater than 16 mm in adult men or greater than 15 mm in adult women is considered abnormal and suggests pulmonary hypertension (50). "Pruning" of the pulmonary vasculature is often described and refers to a decrease in the number or size of pulmonary vessels as the vascular tree moves toward the lung periphery. Generally, the lung parenchyma is free of infiltrates and congestion in PAH. Right ventricular enlargement may be observed when the right ventricle occupies more than one third of the retrosternal space on the lateral chest x-ray and, when severe, can cause cardiomegaly in the PA projection.

The electrocardiogram may show signs of elevated right heart pressures and right ventricular hypertrophy. Right axis deviation and right atrial enlargement are often present. Increased R-wave amplitude and T-wave inversion or ST segment abnormalities in V_1 through V_3 may indicate right ventricular hypertrophy or ischemia.

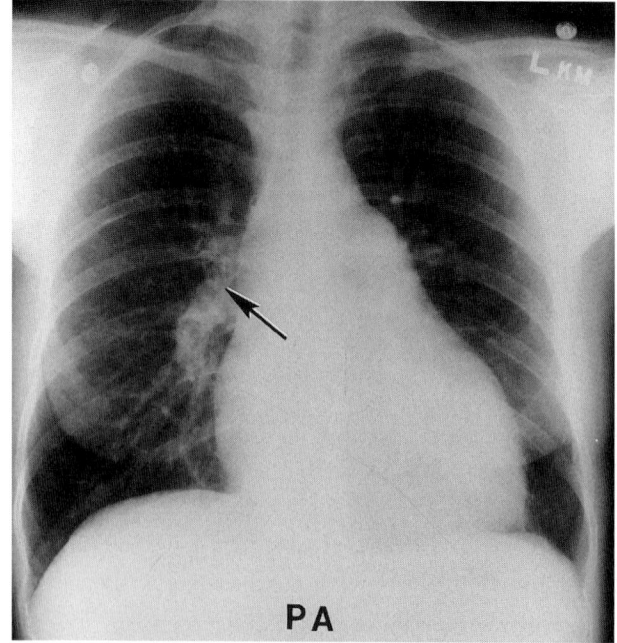
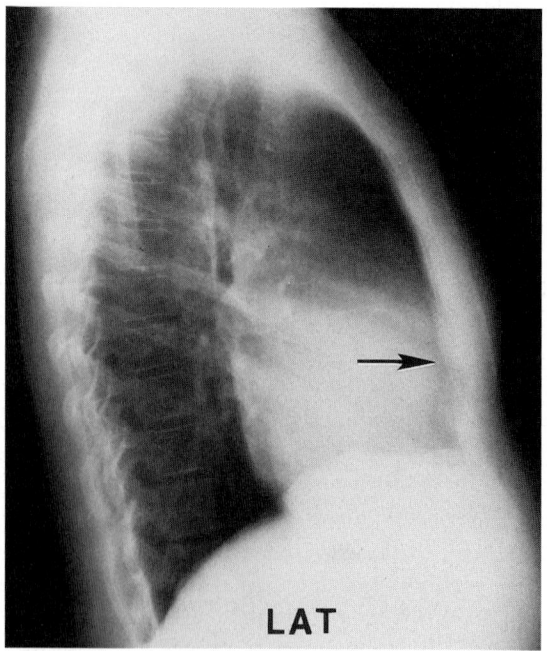

FIGURE 35.5. A chest radiograph from a patient with primary pulmonary hypertension, illustrating enlarged proximal pulmonary arteries and right ventricle *(arrows)*.

Arterial blood gases typically show mild-to-moderate arterial hypoxemia and respiratory alkalosis that is caused by V/Q mismatching (49). Increased right-to-left shunting may occur, particularly in the presence of an atrial septal defect or a patent foramen ovale, as right-sided pressures begin to approximate those of the left.

Hemodynamic Features

Patients with PAH usually have marked elevation of PAP. In severe cases, pulmonary arterial pressures can approximate those of the systemic circulation. Elevation of right atrial pressure and decreased cardiac output are also signs of advanced disease. In the National Institutes of Health patient registry of PPH (49), mean PAP was 60 ± 18 mm Hg (range, 28 to 127 mm Hg), right atrial pressures were 9 ± 6 mm Hg (range, 0 to 29 mm Hg), and mean cardiac index was 2.27 ± 0.9 L/(min $\cdot$ m^2) (range, 0.8 to 7.9 L/[min $\cdot$ m^2]). The pulmonary capillary wedge pressure (PCWP) is usually normal or decreased because of the elevated resistance in the pulmonary arterial and capillary bed. Pulmonary capillary pressure can be estimated by examining the decay curve of the PAP tracing as the balloon is inflated. An increase in the difference between diastolic PAP and PCWP (usually no more than 6 mm Hg) is indicative of PAH and helps differentiate this disease from pulmonary venous hypertension.

Primary Pulmonary Hypertension

PPH is perhaps the best-described and best-studied form of PAH. Although it is a relatively rare disease compared with other types of pulmonary hypertension, it has many of the features common to most types of pulmonary hypertension characterized by intrinsic disease of the small pulmonary arteries. Furthermore, therapies that have been shown to be effective in the management of PPH have also been successful in treating most other types of PAH. In this sense, PPH has served as an excellent model for studying PAH of many causes and pulmonary hypertensive disease, in general.

The first case of PPH was described by Dresdale in 1951 (51); detailed pathologic descriptions were provided by Wagenvoort and Wagenvoort in 1970 (32); and in 1973, WHO described three major pathologic types of disease (29). In 1981, the National Heart, Lung, and Blood Institute (NHLBI) formed the Primary Pulmonary Hypertension Registry and collected important data on the natural history and prognosis of PPH throughout the 1980s (49). Since then, additional information regarding the pathology and pathogenesis has accumulated; however, our understanding of this disease remains incomplete.

Demographics of Primary Pulmonary Hypertension

The incidence of PPH in the general population has been estimated to be about one to two cases per million people per year, and the prevalence of PPH in autopsy studies was 1,300 per million. Thus, PPH is not a common disease (52). However, with improvements in diagnostic techniques and increased awareness of the disease, PPH may be diagnosed more frequently. PPH affects mostly young adults in the third and fourth decade of life, with a female predominance of approximately 1.7:1 (49). PPH has also been reported among the elderly, in whom the diagnosis may be delayed while other more common disorders, such as coronary artery disease or chronic obstructive pulmonary disease (COPD), are entertained and treated (53).

Pathology of Primary Pulmonary Hypertension

The PPH registry sponsored by the NHLBI investigated the pathology of 58 cases meeting clinical criteria for the diagnosis of PPH (54), with 49 patients exhibiting disease in the muscular pulmonary arteries and arterioles, seven exhibiting PVOD, and one with normal pulmonary vessels. Among the histologic patterns observed in the 49 cases of pulmonary arteriopathy were: 25 with plexiform lesions (Fig. 35.3C), 19 with thrombotic lesions, 49 with medial hypertrophy (Fig. 35.3B), and 48 with intimal fibrosis (Fig. 35.3A). Thus, vascular lumina were narrowed by thrombotic, intimal, and medial changes. These results and the work of preceding investigators suggest that in situ or embolic thromboses contribute to remodeling of the pulmonary circulation in PPH. In addition, the association of veno-occlusive changes with pulmonary arteriopathy suggests that venoocclusive disease may be a syndrome resulting from multiple injuries to the entire pulmonary vascular tree rather than a single disease that primarily affects the pulmonary veins (see "Pulmonary Venous Hypertension Owing to Pulmonary Venoocclusive Disease" below).

Subsequent pathologic studies of PPH lungs have revealed increases in adventitial thickness (31) and increased expression of mRNA of the connective tissue protein, collagen (55), and foci of inflammation associated with plexiform lesions (40). Thus, pathologic studies suggest that the pathogenesis of PPH involves sustained cell proliferation, extracellular matrix protein production, inflammation, and thrombosis.

Pathogenesis of Primary Pulmonary Hypertension

PAH indistinguishable clinically from PPH is associated with a variety of disorders or conditions, including familial causes, and exogenous toxins such as the appetite suppressant fenfluramine (see "Pulmonary Arterial Hypertension Related to Drugs/Toxins" below). It may be that PPH is actually a heterogeneous group of disorders of differing pathogenetic sequences, culminating in the recognizable clinical syndrome. There are several factors that play a role in the pathogenesis of PPH. These factors include genetic predisposition,

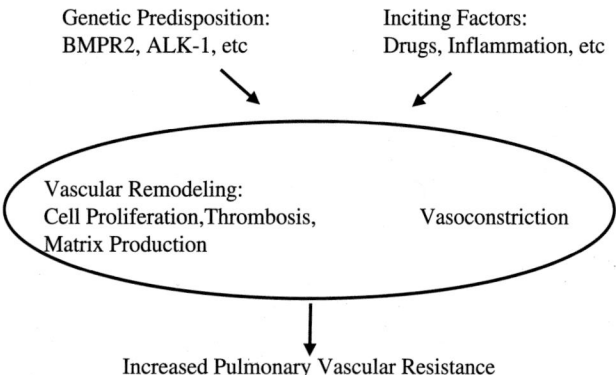

Genetic Predisposition:
BMPR2, ALK-1, etc

Inciting Factors:
Drugs, Inflammation, etc

Vascular Remodeling:
Cell Proliferation, Thrombosis,
Matrix Production

Vasoconstriction

Increased Pulmonary Vascular Resistance

FIGURE 35.6. The pathogenesis of primary pulmonary hypertension.

endothelial cell dysfunction, abnormalities in vasomotor control, thrombotic obliteration of vascular lumen, and vascular remodeling through cell proliferation and matrix production. These complex interactions are illustrated in Figure 35.6. As noted above, several investigators have demonstrated changes in endothelial cell expression of vasoactive mediators such as NO, ET-1, and PGI_2/TxA_2 in patients with PAH, including PPH. This has led to the hypothesis that PPH might originate as an endothelial cell injury or abnormal growth response. In support of this idea, animal models of PPH, such as that caused by monocrotaline, are characterized by endothelial cell dysfunction early in the course of injury. Furthermore, other animal models of repeated endothelial cell injury, such as that related to α-naphthylthiourea, ultimately cause sustained pulmonary hypertension (28). However, altered expression of endothelial cell–derived vasoactive mediators have been reported in pulmonary venous hypertension and in pulmonary hypertension associated with chronic lung disease (15,14). Thus, it is also possible that reported abnormalities of the pulmonary endothelium are not causes of pulmonary hypertension per se, but rather represent injury caused by sustained elevations in PAP or the underlying disease process.

Changes in vasomotor tone and vascular reactivity are thought to contribute to PPH. In support of this is the marked vasodilator response to pharmacologic agents that is observed in some patients with PPH (56). However, most patients with PPH have a minimal response to vasodilators. Although it is possible that "nonresponsive" patients have a more advanced stage of disease, most studies have found that vasodilator response is not well predicted by the degree of elevation of PAP or the histologic grade of findings on lung biopsy (57, 58).

Thrombosis of pulmonary arteries is a frequent finding in patients with PPH, and it is likely that in situ thrombosis plays an important role in the pathogenesis of this disease. Several prothrombotic conditions have been reported in patients with PPH, including an increased prevalence of phospholipid-dependent antibodies, increased endothelial expression of von Willebrand factor, and increased circulating levels of plasminogen activator inhibitor type 1. In ad-

dition, decreased expression of NO and PGI_2 may facilitate platelet aggregation. Interestingly, most of the well-described inheritable coagulopathies—such as deficiencies in protein S, protein C, and antithrombin III or gene mutations in factors V and II—do not appear to be more frequent in patients with PAH (59). Thus, it may be argued that PAH is not caused by hypercoagulable states, but that increased pulmonary vascular thrombosis occurs in response to an injured pulmonary circulation. In either event, active thrombosis appears to contribute to progression of pulmonary hypertensive disease, and anticoagulant therapy has been shown to improve survival in patients with PAH (56).

Finally, vascular remodeling and subsequent restriction of the pulmonary vascular cross-sectional luminal area are believed to contribute heavily to pulmonary hypertension in PPH. The cause of remodeling is not known, but there is evidence to suggest that VEGF may play a role. Other studies suggest that the plexiform lesion in PPH may be a result of abnormal endothelial cell proliferation or disordered angiogenesis. As noted above, PPH is also characterized by monoclonal proliferation of endothelial cells in plexiform lesions in PPH (41), increased expression of angiogenesis-related molecules (42), and microsatellite instability and gene mutations (60). The presence of perivascular inflammatory cell foci in lungs of patients with PPH (40) also suggests that inflammation and inflammatory mediators, such as cytokines and oxidants, are also potential causes or perpetuators of the remodeling response.

Genetic Abnormalities Associated with Primary Pulmonary Hypertension

Several lines of evidence suggest a genetic component to the etiology of PPH. First, the disease is rare, not only in the general population but also in patients with known risk factors such as HIV infection, portopulmonary hypertension, and exposure to fenfluramine. Thus, it appears that a small number of individuals, even in high-risk groups, are more prone to developing the disease than are others. Second, cases of familial pulmonary hypertension are well described and appear indistinguishable from sporadic cases of PPH. Finally, several genetic abnormalities have recently been described in patients with familial and sporadic pulmonary hypertension, providing the first clues as to the underlying abnormalities that predispose these patients to developing this disease.

A hereditary cause of PPH has been suspected almost since the disease was first described. Within a few years of the initial reporting of PPH, Dresdale (61) described a family in which several members were affected with the disease. Since that time, others have described close to 100 American families in which PPH was found in two or more first-degree relatives (62). Originally, familial pulmonary hypertension was thought to constitute only a fraction of patients with PPH. In 1987, Rich and colleagues (49) reported that at least 6% of patients with PPH in a national prospective study had a history of familial pulmonary hypertension. More recent studies (63) suggest that a familial association is often missed, and when carefully screened, as many as 25% of sporadic cases of PPH have family members with PPH and carry genetic mutations similar to those found in familial pulmonary hypertension (64).

Familial PPH is an autosomal-dominant disease with variable penetrance. Only about 10% to 20% of carriers are affected, and the disease has been known to skip entire generations within a family. There is also a gender predilection with a female-to-male ratio of approximately 1.7:1.0. Genetic anticipation (occurrence of the disease at an earlier age in younger generations) has been well described. The genetic defect of familial PPH has been mapped to a 3-cM region on chromosome 2q33 (locus PPH1) (65). In 2000, the affected area was found to involve mutations in the gene that encodes for BMPR-II, a member of the TGF-β family of receptors (64, 66). More than 25 mutations of this gene have been reported, with demonstrated fidelity within affected families. How mutations in BMPR-II facilitate the development of pulmonary hypertension is unknown. The BMPs are a family of growth factors that belong to the TFG-β super-family. Some BMPs appear to be critical for the development of normal lung, but their role in the adult lung is largely unknown (44). Normal BMP signaling (Fig. 35.7) involves binding of BMP either to an accessory protein or TGF-β type III receptor that presents BMP to BMPR-II. Once activated, BMPR-II localizes with and phosphorylates BMPR-I, resulting in activation of the kinase domain of BMPR-I. Activation of BMPR-I leads to phosphorylation of cytoplasmic receptor Smad proteins. Once phosphorylated, these proteins bind to collaborating Smads, and the resulting Smad complex translocates to the nucleus, where it regulates transcription of TGF-β responsive genes. Whether mutations in the BMPR-II gene result in disrupted or dysfunctional BMP signaling is unclear. Many of the defects involve single-amino-acid substitutions and usually result in a protein product that is either severely truncated or that has decreased functionality (haplo-insufficiency) (67). Interestingly, mutations in the gene for activin-receptor–like kinase 1 (ALK-1), a TGF-β type I receptor analogous to BMPR-I, have been linked to pulmonary hypertension in patients with hereditary telangiectasia (68). Thus, defects in either TGF-β type I (ALK-1) or type II (BMPR-II) receptors can predispose to the development of PAH.

Genetic abnormalities affecting 5-HT transport have also been linked to PAH. In a study by Eddahibi and colleagues, 65% of PPH patients, but only 27% of controls, were homozygous for the L-allelic variant of the 5-HT transporter (21). This mutation results in over-expression of 5-HT transporter and accelerated growth of pulmonary artery smooth muscle cells stimulated with 5-HT or serum.

How these various genetic mutations contribute to the development of PPH remains to be elucidated. In the future, they may be used to screen for populations at risk, but more importantly, it is anticipated that further study of these and other genetic abnormalities associated with PPH will enhance our understanding of the pathophysiology of this disease and shed new light on how to treat it.

Survival and Prognosis

Median survival of patients in the PPH registry, before the advent of modern treatment, was 2.8 years, with only 34% of patients alive after 5 years (49). Thus, untreated PPH

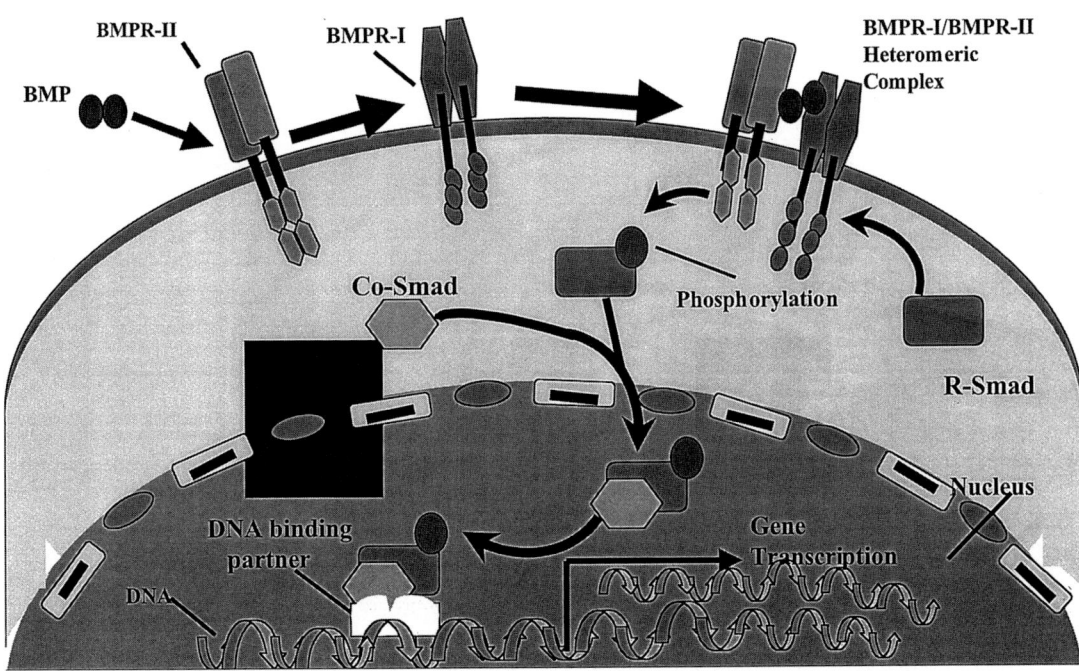

FIGURE 35.7. The cell signaling pathways of the bone morphogenetic protein receptor.

has a poor prognosis. Several factors were associated with poor survival (69). Mortality correlated best with measures of right ventricular hemodynamic function. Mean PAP greater than 85 mm Hg, mean right atrial pressure greater than 20 mm Hg, and cardiac index less than 2 L/(min · m²) were associated with poor survival. Thus, the presence of right ventricular failure indicated a poor prognosis. Accordingly, the risk of death was higher among patients with NYHA functional class III or IV than among those with class I or II function at the time of diagnosis. Indeed, survival was only 6 months for those with class IV function.

Interestingly, the presence of Raynaud's phenomenon was associated with a worse prognosis for unclear reasons. In addition, decreased diffusing capacity also correlated with increased risk of mortality.

The most frequent causes of death in patients with PPH are progressive right ventricular failure and sudden death. Pneumonia is often fatal because alveolar hypoxia may cause pulmonary vasoconstriction and exacerbate pulmonary hypertension, with resulting inadequate cardiac output and cardiogenic shock. Some possible mechanisms for sudden death in PPH include bradyarrhythmias and tachyarrhythmias, acute pulmonary embolus, pulmonary hemorrhage, and sudden right ventricular ischemia.

There have been enormous advances in the past 20 years in the treatment of PPH (see "Vasodilator Therapy" below). Recent studies suggest that the dismal rate of survival in PPH can be improved with modern-day treatment.

Pulmonary Arterial Hypertension Related to Collagen Vascular Disease

Pulmonary hypertension is associated with several connective tissue disorders, including scleroderma, mixed connective tissue disease, SLE, and rheumatoid arthritis. The incidence of pulmonary hypertension varies significantly among connective tissue disorders, but when it occurs it may be devastating. In these disorders, pulmonary hypertension can occur with or without significant parenchymal lung disease.

There is overlap between PPH and PAH associated with connective tissue disease. Female preponderance, similar symptoms on presentation, Raynaud's phenomenon, and elevated rheumatoid factor and antinuclear antibody titers are frequently observed in both types of patients. Despite these similarities, there are notable clinical differences between PPH and PAH associated with connective tissue disease. Patients with connective tissue disease tend to be older women, with a much higher incidence of Raynaud's phenomenon. Pulmonary function tests may demonstrate the presence of restrictive lung disease in patients with connective tissue disease and concomitant parenchymal disease.

Pathology

In addition to the clinical overlap noted above, the connective tissue disease disorders and PPH share similar pathology.

Plexogenic arteriopathy is observed in both groups, suggesting a similar underlying pathogenesis. Intravascular thrombosis, possibly owing to hypercoagulable state(s), may contribute to pulmonary hypertension. An example of such a hypercoagulable state is the presence of circulating antiphospholipid antibodies (70). Vasculitis, with inflammatory cell infiltrate, has been reported in patients with pulmonary hypertension complicating SLE.

Pathogenesis

The pathology of pulmonary hypertension associated with connective tissue diseases suggests that restriction of the pulmonary circulation by remodeling, and obstruction of the microvessels by thromboses, are important in the development of pulmonary hypertension. Acute hypoxic vasoconstriction and compression of pulmonary vessels by associated abnormal lung parenchyma may also contribute to the magnitude of the pulmonary hypertension. Responsiveness to vasodilators and spontaneous fluctuation in levels of pulmonary hypertension in some patients indicate that vasoconstriction may also contribute to increased PVR.

There is little information available concerning the precise mechanisms of pulmonary hypertension at the cellular level. Elevated plasma levels of ET-1 in scleroderma suggest that this potent vasoconstrictor may contribute to pulmonary hypertension in that vasospastic disorder (71). Circulating antiendothelial cell antibodies have been reported in SLE complicated by pulmonary hypertension, suggesting an immunological pathogenesis (72).

Features of Specific Disorders

Systemic sclerosis (scleroderma) is the connective tissue disorder in which pulmonary involvement is most frequent and pulmonary hypertension is most commonly observed, with a prevalence of 9% to 13% (73, 74). The development of severe pulmonary hypertension culminating in cor pulmonale and death is highest in the CREST variant of scleroderma (73). The most common pulmonary parenchymal manifestation in this disease is interstitial fibrosis, but the magnitude of the pulmonary hypertension does not correlate well with the degree of fibrosis. In fact, most notably in the CREST variant, patients may die of malignant pulmonary hypertension without significant pulmonary fibrosis, particularly if it is progressive (74). An isolated decrease in D𝐋co to more than 55% is strongly associated with pulmonary hypertension in scleroderma (75). Endothelial cell injury, intimal and medial cell proliferation, and fibrosis of small arteries and arterioles are the major pathological lesions. Vasculitis is unusual.

Several studies have confirmed that pulmonary vasoconstriction occurs when the hands of scleroderma patients are immersed in cold water (76). This has been described as Raynaud's phenomenon of the pulmonary vasculature and is additional evidence of a generalized disorder of vasospasm in these patients.

Mixed connective tissue disease is a syndrome consisting of features of SLE, scleroderma, Sjögren syndrome, and polymyositis. Pulmonary hypertension and cor pulmonale occur infrequently but may dominate the clinical course, leading to a fatal outcome (77). Although pulmonary function tests commonly suggest the presence of interstitial lung disease, pulmonary vasculopathy is typically more prominent than is interstitial disease on pathological examination of lung tissue. This vasculopathy is characterized by intimal thickening and medial hypertrophy of pulmonary arteries and arterioles and the presence of plexiform lesions.

SLE involves the respiratory system in 50% to 70% of patients, whereas the incidence of pulmonary hypertension is significantly lower, ranging from rare to approximately 14% (78). Noninvasive measurement of PAP by repeated Doppler echocardiography studies in patients with SLE suggests that the prevalence of pulmonary hypertension may increase with time after diagnosis of SLE to as high as 43% (79). When pulmonary hypertension is present, it tends to be mild, with systolic PAP generally less than 40 mm Hg. The pathologic features include intimal and medial hypertrophy and plexiform lesions in more advanced cases. Vasculitis is unusual. The frequent association of antiphospholipid syndrome and SLE suggests that microvascular thrombosis may be an important cause of pulmonary hypertension in SLE.

Rheumatoid arthritis and polymyositis/dermatomyositis may also be complicated by pulmonary hypertension.

Diagnosis

Although decreased diffusing capacity is a sensitive marker for the presence of pulmonary vascular disease, it is also nonspecific, because it may be abnormal in the presence of parenchymal lung disease without a pulmonary vascular component. Because it may be difficult to determine the presence and severity of pulmonary hypertension by clinical assessment and noninvasive laboratory testing alone, right heart catheterization is usually required for definitive diagnosis. Doppler echocardiography is useful as a noninvasive means of estimating PAP in patients with regurgitant tricuspid jets.

Treatment

Small, uncontrolled series of patients have reported benefits of treatment of patients with connective tissue diseases with nifedipine (80), captopril (81), and inhaled NO (82). PGI$_2$ was found to be effective in improving exercise capacity and cardiopulmonary hemodynamics in a randomized, controlled, open-label trial comparing PGI$_2$ infusions to conventional therapy in patients with scleroderma (83). No survival benefit was found in this study. A smaller uncontrolled case series of PGI$_2$ infusion suggests that this drug may also be useful in patients with SLE and severe pulmonary hypertension (84). Inhaled iloprost (85) and subcutaneous treprostinil (86) have also been reported to be useful in pulmonary hypertension owing to connective tissue disease. Because of similar pathological and clinical features of pulmonary hypertension associated with connective tissue disease and PPH, connective tissue disorders have been included with PPH in recent randomized controlled trials, described in the section on PPH (see "Vasoldilator Therapy" below). Although the connective tissue disorders were not analyzed separately, it is generally thought that they respond similarly to PPH.

Pulmonary Arterial Hypertension Related to Systemic-to-Pulmonary Shunts

Pulmonary hypertension is a common manifestation of congenital heart disease. The unifying pathogenetic feature in these congenital abnormalities (ventricular septal defect, atrial septal defect, patent ductus arteriosus, or aortopulmonary window) is that there is a chronic increase in blood flow through the pulmonary vascular bed owing to left-to-right shunting (high-flow states). Over time, if the primary defect is not corrected, PVR progressively increases because of structural changes in the pulmonary arteries. The elevation of PVR ultimately may reverse the direction of shunt blood flow, with subsequent development of cyanosis and severe exercise intolerance, Eisenmenger physiology.

The morphological changes in pulmonary vessels are initiated by the primary pathological increase in pulmonary blood flow through the shunt. There is a progression of pathological changes correlating with the increase in PVR (32). Reversible changes include the development of medial hypertrophy and intimal hyperplasia. As PVR increases, the vascular lumen is occluded by progressive intimal hyperplasia and, ultimately, by formation of plexiform lesions. Plexiform lesions and fibrinoid necrosis represent advanced irreversible changes. The early pathological effects of chronic high-flow states on the pulmonary vasculature are now recognized as changes in the normal pattern of pulmonary vascular growth and development. Medial smooth muscle hypertrophy or extension of vascular smooth muscle into peripheral pulmonary arteries, diminished size and number of peripheral pulmonary arteries, and an increase in intercellular connective tissue proteins in the vessel walls are all different aspects of an altered pattern of pulmonary vascular growth.

A detailed discussion of the treatment of congenital cardiac disease is beyond the scope of this chapter. The basic treatment is surgical repair of the lesion before severe pulmonary hypertension occurs. Surgery halts the progression of the pulmonary vascular disease when performed at an optimum time in most individuals. The rapidity with which pulmonary hypertension develops in these syndromes depends on the anatomic site of the left-to-right shunt. Pulmonary hypertension only develops after many years with atrial septal defects, whereas ventricular septal defects are associated with the development of pulmonary hypertension in early childhood. In addition, variability in the rapidity of the development of pulmonary hypertension with a specific cardiac defect among different patients suggests a genetic predisposition for the risk of development of pulmonary vascular disease. Other factors in addition to blood flow, such as increased pressure and shear stress, probably interact and contribute to the development of pulmonary vascular disease and pulmonary hypertension in this patient population. Detection of congenital cardiac abnormalities before the development of severe pulmonary vascular disease is a key component of care. Patients who have already developed severe pulmonary vascular disease may not be helped by surgery at a late stage of disease. In fact, they may experience further clinical deterioration after surgery related to the presence of advanced pulmonary vascular disease. Rosenzweig and colleagues have reported improvement in hemodynamics and quality of life with long-term PGI$_2$ infusion in an uncontrolled series of 20 patients with severe pulmonary hypertension and associated congenital heart disease (87).

Pulmonary Arterial Hypertension Related to Portal Hypertension

Pulmonary hypertension may be associated with liver disease, frequently in combination with portal hypertension (portopulmonary hypertension). The frequency of this complication of liver disease has been estimated as 2% (88) to 3.1% (89) of patients with cirrhosis: greater than would be expected by chance alone.

The clinical characteristics of portopulmonary hypertension are similar to PPH, but these patients may also present with findings typical of portal hypertension, including significant respiratory alkalosis, elevated cardiac index, and decreased systemic vascular resistance (90). Lung pathologic changes are similar to those seen in PPH (plexogenic arteriopathy). Survival has been reported to vary from 2 to 86 months and appears to be limited by complications of liver disease and portal hypertension (89).

Treatment by liver transplantation has been reported in case reports to result in improvement of pulmonary hypertension (91).

Pulmonary Arterial Hypertension Related to HIV Infection

Pulmonary hypertension was first reported as a complication of HIV infection in 1987 (92). Since then, more than 131 patients have been reported with this complication of HIV infection owing to all causes (93). The estimated incidence of pulmonary hypertension in patients with HIV infection (0.5%) is higher than the estimated incidence of PPH in the general population, suggesting that the viral infection itself is somehow causally linked to the development of pulmonary hypertension (94).

The cause of HIV-related pulmonary hypertension is not known. However, no clear evidence of arterial wall infection with HIV virus has been found in a small number of carefully examined cases (95). It is possible that HIV-induced expression of VEGF or HIV-1/glycoprotein 120–induced stimulation of ET-1 by macrophages may play roles (96). Genetic predisposition may also be important.

In a recent review of published reports, 82% of patients with HIV-associated pulmonary hypertension had pulmonary hypertension that could not be attributed to any other confounding factors (93). Most patients are normoxic and CD4 lymphocyte cell counts may be normal. Thus, pulmonary hypertension is not caused by concomitant respiratory infections and is unrelated to the severity of the HIV infection. Patients with HIV-associated pulmonary hypertension demonstrate pathologic changes similar to PPH, with plexogenic arteriopathy.

Comparison of clinical characteristics of patients with HIV-associated pulmonary hypertension to those of patients with PPH has demonstrated very few distinguishing characteristics (97). Although the magnitude of the pulmonary hypertension may be less severe at the time of presentation in HIV-associated pulmonary hypertension, the presence of Raynaud's phenomenon and the percentage of patients who respond to vasodilator therapy appear to be similar in both groups. Overall survival is poor in both groups of patients. Because of these similarities, HIV testing should be considered in cases of PPH for which no other associated cause is evident.

There has not been sufficient experience in HIV-associated pulmonary hypertension with vasodilator, anticoagulant, or highly active antiretroviral therapy to make any definitive recommendations (93). An uncontrolled case series of six patients with severe HIV-associated pulmonary hypertension showed improvement with long-term PGI$_2$ infusion (98). Obviously, hypoxemia and concomitant lung infections should be treated aggressively.

Pulmonary Arterial Hypertension Related to Drugs/Toxins

In the 1960s, there was a 20-fold increase in the incidence of PAH in western Europe, which occurred after the introduction of the appetite-suppressant aminorex fumarate, with 61% of newly identified patients giving a history of having used this medication (99). The drug was subsequently withdrawn, and the epidemic subsided. However, it was difficult to prove a cause-and-effect relationship because an animal model could not be developed, and there appeared to be little correlation between the severity of the disease and the amount of drug ingested.

Another appetite suppressant, fenfluramine, has also been reported to be associated with PAH (100). In 1985 a fenfluramine derivative, dexfenfluramine, was widely used in western Europe, and in a case control study was found to be associated with PAH with an odds ratio (relative risk estimate) of 6.3, which increased to 23.1 after more than 3 months of use of the drug (101). Increased risk of PPH associated with fenfluramine was confirmed by the Surveillance of North American Pulmonary Hypertension study (102). Fenfluramine was withdrawn from the market in 1997. Although the amphetamine phentermine was commonly used in conjunction with fenfluramine (fen-phen), no clear association between phentermine and PAH has been proven.

Anorexigen-induced PAH has pathologic features consistent with plexogenic arteriopathy and an indistinguishable clinical course. The cause is unclear, but may be related to increased circulating 5-HT, a potent pulmonary vasoconstrictor, stimulant of pulmonary vascular smooth muscle growth, and inducer of platelet aggregation (103).

Treatment of anorexigen-induced pulmonary hypertension is similar to treatment of other plexogenic pulmonary arteriopathies, with emphasis on the use of vasodilators.

In 1981 a disease was reported in Spain that ultimately affected 20,000 individuals and was subsequently termed the toxic oil syndrome by the WHO. The disease was characterized by a pneumonitis, causing acute respiratory distress syndrome, associated with eosinophilia (104). Pulmonary hypertension developed in 20% of patients and spontaneously regressed. Four years after the onset of the syndrome, 1.5% of patients had persistent pulmonary hypertension, indistinguishable from PPH both pathologically and clinically (105). Because this incidence is similar to the reported incidence of PPH at that time, it is thought that perhaps the ingestion of the oil triggered an innate (perhaps genetic) susceptibility to the disease.

Case reports have suggested associations between pulmonary hypertension and other drugs and toxins (amphetamines, L-tryptophan, cocaine), but the associations are less clear.

Pulmonary Arterial Hypertension Related to Persistent Pulmonary Hypertension of the Newborn

Persistent pulmonary hypertension of the newborn (PPHN) is common in neonates with respiratory failure, occurring in 1.9 of 1,000 live births, with a mortality of 11% (106). The syndrome is a failure of adaptation to extrauterine life, characterized by pulmonary hypertension and extrapulmonary right-to-left shunting across a patent ductus arteriosus or foramen ovale, resulting in hypoxemia. The causes of PPHN include underdevelopment of the pulmonary vasculature, as in congenital diaphragmatic hernia or pulmonary hypoplasia; maldevelopment of the pulmonary vasculature with muscularization of peripheral vessels, associated with intrauterine closure of the ductus arteriosus after maternal aspirin or indomethacin ingestion (107); or maladaptation, with persistently increased PVR owing to vasospasm caused by hypoxia,

meconium aspiration, or acidosis (108). Infants with PPHN may have low plasma concentrations of arginine, the NO precursor, and NO metabolites (109). Genetic abnormalities in arginine production may predispose to this syndrome (109).

PPHN is managed by correction of metabolic abnormalities or treatment of infection (108). Inhaled NO (110) or ethyl nitrate (111) inhalation reduce the need for extracorporeal membrane oxygenation.

General Management of Pulmonary Arterial Hypertension

The modern era of treatment of PAH began with studies of vasodilator therapy of PPH. Subsequently, it became apparent that other related diseases classified as PAH were responsive to these treatments. Later, clinical studies have included PPH and other causes of PAH.

Before the onset of modern treatments, median survival after diagnosis of PPH was just under 3 years. This dismal prognosis has been greatly improved with the development of effective pharmacologic therapies. The approach to therapy for PAH consists of symptomatic treatment of right heart failure, anticoagulation, and chronic administration of a selective pulmonary vasodilator. In the past, vasodilators used to treat pulmonary hypertension were nonselective agents such as hydralazine, diazoxide, and calcium channel blockers. These agents usually have a greater vasodilatory effect on the systemic circulation than on diseased pulmonary arteries. As a result, patients occasionally experienced problems with systemic hypotension, syncope, or even death (112, 113). In addition, many systemic vasodilators, such as calcium channel blockers, have negative inotropic effects that can reduce right ventricular contractility and decrease cardiac output. The recent development of several agents with relative selectivity for the pulmonary circulation has led to substantial reduction in the morbidity and mortality of PAH.

Vasodilator Therapy

The rationale for vasodilator therapy in PAH is that pulmonary arterial vasoconstriction is an important component of pulmonary hypertension, and even small reductions in right ventricular afterload may substantially improve cardiac output. As the efficacy of vasodilators in the treatment for systemic hypertension and congestive heart failure became recognized, physicians became interested in using vasodilators for the treatment of PAH. At that time, there was also considerable interest in defining acute vasodilator responsiveness as a measure of severity and as an indication of disease reversibility and overall prognosis. Several lessons were learned from the initial trials of vasodilators for PAH in the 1980s: (a) the severity of the pulmonary hypertension does not predict response to vasodilator therapy (57); (b) vasodilator response does not correlate well with the histologic abnormalities seen on histologic examination of lung biopsy specimens (58); (c) response to one vasodilator does not predict response to another; and (d) the definition of vasodilator response is problematic, because nonselective vasodilators usually increase cardiac output and decrease PVR without decreasing PAP. In fact, the PPH patient registry found that more than half of patients undergoing vasodilator trials had a decrease in total pulmonary resistance alone, but only one third had both an increase in cardiac output and a decrease in mean PAP (57). Although there is no firm definition of a positive vasodilator response, most investigators suggest that both the calculated PVR and the mean PAP should decrease by more than 20%.

There is evidence to suggest that PPH patients with a positive response to acute vasodilator therapy have improved survival compared with that of those who do not respond to vasodilators. Reeves and colleagues reviewed data on 117 patients with PAH receiving acute vasodilator trials and at least 3-month treatment with oral vasodilators (114). They found that 33 of 53 patients (62%) who had an acute vasodilator response (defined as a >30% decrease in PVR) had a favorable clinical response to chronic vasodilator therapy, whereas only four of 64 patients (6%) without an acute vasodilator response improved with long-term vasodilator therapy. Likewise, Rich and colleagues found that 17 of 64 (26%) patients with an positive vasodilator response to calcium channel blockers (defined as a ≥20% decrease in both PVR and mean PAP) had sustained clinical improvement with high-dose calcium channel blockers (56). In addition, they found evidence of partial reversal of right ventricular hypertrophy, and improved 5-year survival (94% versus 55%), compared with that for patients who did not respond initially to calcium channel blockers. Although this was not a randomized controlled trial, the survival rate of the responders was considerably better than the rate of historical controls, suggesting that a positive response to vasodilator therapy identifies a select group of patients with a better prognosis. Unfortunately, only about a one fourth of patients with PPH have a favorable acute response to vasodilators, and thus, another approach is needed for the majority of patients who do not respond.

PGI_2 is a potent vasodilator and inhibitor of platelet aggregation that is produced by the vascular endothelium. In patients with PPH, the ratio of PGI_2 to the potent vasoconstrictor thromboxane is decreased (16), suggesting that inadequate PGI_2 synthesis may contribute to the etiology of PAH (see "Pathogenesis of Primary Pulmonary Hypertension" earlier). In the late 1980s, several investigators examined the effect of continuous intravenous infusion of PGI_2 using a permanent central catheter and portable infusion pump (115, 116). These studies found that long-term administration of PGI_2 resulted in clinical improvement and decreased PVR compared with conventional treatment alone in patients that were refractory to oral vasodilators. In a larger multicenter, randomized, controlled trial, 81 patients with PPH and NYHA class III or IV symptoms were randomized

to receive intravenous PGI_2 or conventional therapy alone (46). After 12 weeks, patients treated with PGI_2 showed a significant increase in distance walked in 6 minutes (32 m), decreases in mean PAP and PVR (8% and 21%, respectively), and improvement in quality of life. This was in contrast to decrease in distance walked (15 m) and increase in PAP and PVR (3% and 9%, respectively) in patients given conventional therapy alone. Eight patients died in the conventional therapy group versus none in the group receiving PGI_2. The beneficial effects of intravenous PGI_2 appear to be sustained during long-term therapy. In one study (117), 26 of the 27 patients had a greater acute vasodilator response to PGI_2 after 12 to 24 months of treatment than at study entry. Interestingly, seven of eight patients who had less than a 20% decrease in PVR during acute vasodilator testing with adenosine, had a significant response to adenosine (mean decrease in PVR, 39%) after long-term PGI_2 therapy. These findings suggest that extended therapy with PGI_2 may lead to improved endothelial function or a partial reversal of pulmonary vascular remodeling, even in patients that do not have a favorable response initially.

Adverse effects of PGI_2 include headache, bone and jaw pain, and diarrhea, but the greatest drawback is the inconvenience of continuous infusion and central line infections at a rate as high as 9% per patient year (117). In an effort to avoid the complications of intravenous therapy, different strategies of PGI_2 administration have been attempted. Treprostinil sodium is a PGI_2 analogue that can be given by subcutaneous infusion, obviating the need for a central venous catheter. In a single randomized controlled trial involving 470 patients with NYHA class II to IV symptoms, treprostinil failed to reach the primary endpoint of an increase in the 6-minute walk test of 55 m (86). However, there was improvement in perceived quality of life. Inhalation of aerosolized PGI_2 or the PGI_2 analogue iloprost has been shown to be effective in the treatment of PPH (85). In a large randomized controlled trial, 203 patients were randomized to receive 2.5 or 5.0 μg of iloprost six or nine times per day or placebo (85). Distance walked in 6 minutes improved by a mean of 36.4 m in the iloprost group as a whole. There were also significant improvements in hemodynamic values compared with those of controls. Unfortunately, the hemodynamic effects of inhaled iloprost may last only 1 to 2 hours, and patients often need to inhale the drug six to eight times daily. An oral form of PGI_2 (beraprost) has been tested in Europe (118). Compared with controls, patients taking beraprost had a 25-m increase in 6-minute walking distance and a 0.94 decrease in Borg dyspnea score after 12 weeks of therapy. Although not all of these drugs are presently available in the United States, it is hoped that multiple options will be available for administration of PGI_2s in the future.

Endothelin receptor antagonists are among the newest therapies of PAH. These agents block the receptors for ET-1, one of the most potent endogenous vasoconstrictors known and a vascular smooth muscle mitogen. As discussed earlier, ET-1 expression is increased in the lungs of patients with PAH and may play an important role in the pathophysiology of this disease. Two types of endothelin receptors have been described, -A and -B. Activation of endothelin receptor-A causes vasoconstrictor effects, whereas vasodilatory and vasoconstrictor effects have been observed with endothelin receptor-B. In a preliminary trial of 32 patients with PAH, 12 weeks of therapy with the nonselective endothelin antagonist bosentan increased distance walked in 6 minutes by 76 m compared with that for placebo (48). There were also significant reductions in PVR and mean PAP. In a larger randomized controlled trial involving 213 patients with PAH, 16 weeks of bosentan increased distance walked in 6 minutes and decreased time to clinical worsening (119). A small trial involving 21 patients given the selective endothelin receptor-A antagonist sitaxsentan has recently been completed (120). Patients had similar improvements in activity and hemodynamics. A multicenter phase III study of sitaxsentan versus placebo was recently completed at the writing of this chapter.

The endothelin antagonists offer a significant advantage over other agents in that they are effective in the majority of patients with PAH and can be taken orally one to two times daily. Reversible increases in liver transaminases have occurred in approximately 11% of patients, however, precluding their use in patients with liver disease and requiring that a diagnosis of PAH be confirmed before starting therapy.

Several investigational therapies also offer promise in the treatment of PAH. Phosphodiesterase inhibitors retard the metabolism of cGMP and thereby potentiate the effects of endogenous pulmonary vasodilators, such as NO and the natriuretic peptides. Recent reports suggest that the phosphodiesterase-5 inhibitor sildenafil acts as a selective pulmonary vasodilator in PAH (121). Large-scale clinical trials are just beginning to evaluate the long-term efficacy of phosphodiesterase inhibitors in the treatment of PAH.

Another investigational agent that has potential for the treatment of PPH is inhaled NO. Several reports have demonstrated that inhaled NO is among the most potent and selective pulmonary vasodilators in PAH (122). Its rapid inactivation by hemoglobin results in virtually no systemic effects when inhaled. Although not approved for long-term use in adult patients, inhaled NO has been approved for the treatment of PPHN and is used by many investigators for acute vasodilator testing in adult patients with PAH. Long-term administration of inhaled NO by nasal cannula increases functional activity in adult patients with PAH (123) and may be especially effective in patients with PAH associated with sarcoidosis (124). Unlike other pulmonary vasodilators that may decrease oxygenation by inhibiting hypoxic pulmonary vasoconstriction, inhaled NO can improve oxygen saturation by decreasing shunt fraction. Thus, it may prove to be helpful to patients with PAH and refractory hypoxemia.

Combination vasodilator therapy in PAH has not been well studied. Preliminary studies have demonstrated additive effects of phosphodiesterase inhibitors and inhaled PGI_2 or inhaled NO, but these agents are still considered investigational. The effectiveness of combining endothelin receptor blockers and PGI_2 analogues is unknown (121, 125). In the future, it is likely that effective treatment of PAH may require the combination of several medications that act via different mechanisms to reverse pulmonary hypertension, just as multiple medications are frequently used to control blood pressure in difficult patients with systemic hypertension.

VASODILATOR THERAPY FOR PULMONARY ARTERIAL HYPERTENSION

Vasodilator/Summary of Effects	Level of Evidence
Calcium channel blockers: decrease pulmonary arterial pressure, decrease pulmonary vascular resistance, improve functional activity by 2 NYHA classes, improve survival.	Nonrandomized trials (historical controls)
Intravenous prostacyclin: decreases pulmonary arterial pressure, decreases pulmonary vascular resistance, improves mean distance walked in 6 min and/or NYHA/WHO class for pulmonary arterial hypertension of PPH, collagen vascular disease and HIV infection. Improves survival in PPH.	Randomized controlled trials and nonrandomized trials
Subcutaneous prostacyclin: decreases pulmonary arterial pressure, improves cardiac output, significant improvement in 6-min walk test. Improvement in perceived quality of life	One randomized clinical trial and expert opinion
Inhaled prostacyclin: decreases pulmonary arterial pressure, improves cardiac output, improves mean distance walked in 6 min and NYHA/WHO functional class	Multiple nonrandomized trials and one randomized controlled trial; limited clinical experience
Oral prostacyclin: increases distance walked in 6 min, decreases Borg dyspnea score. No significant improvement in hemodynamics, possible increase in survival	Randomized controlled clinical trial and nonrandomized trial; limited clinical experience.
Nonselective endothelin receptor antagonist: decrease pulmonary arterial pressure, decreases pulmonary vascular resistance, improves mean distance walked in 6 min and NYHA/WHO class, improved Borg dyspnea score, delays time to clinical worsening	Randomized controlled trials
Selective endothelin receptor A antagonist: decreases pulmonary arterial pressure, decreases pulmonary vascular resistance, improves mean distance walked in 6 min	Single nonrandomized trial of 20 patients

NYHA, New York Heart Association; WHO, World Health Organization; PPH, primary pulmonary hypertension

Other Therapies for Pulmonary Arterial Hypertension

Treatment of right heart failure is aimed at relieving symptoms. Diuretics may relieve peripheral edema and hepatic congestion. One should be careful to avoid development of metabolic alkalosis, which could depress ventilation and thereby exacerbate hypoxemia. In addition, care must be taken to avoid excessive diuresis and decreased venous return to the right ventricle, Because right ventricular function is highly dependent on preload, over diuresis can impede cardiac output and cause loss of responsiveness to vasodilators. Digitalis has been shown to increase cardiac output in some patients (126).

The finding of plexogenic arteriopathy and in situ thrombosis on histologic examination of lung tissue caused many physicians to recommend chronic anticoagulation therapy with coumadin. Indeed, in the study by Rich and colleagues, anticoagulation with coumadin improved survival in subjects who both responded and did not respond to acute vasodilator therapy (56). Long-term anticoagulation continues to be recommended for all patients with PAH unless contraindicated.

Although moderate degrees of hypoxemia have been reported in patients with PPH, there are no firm data that oxygen therapy improves survival with PPH. However, hypoxia may exacerbate pulmonary hypertension via hypoxic vasoconstriction, and hypoxemia is associated with cardiac arrhythmias. Chronic hypoxemia can further exacerbate pulmonary hypertension via secondary erythrocytosis and vascular remodeling. Thus, hypoxemic patients with PPH should be given low-flow oxygen therapy according to guidelines developed for patients with COPD (see Chapter 12).

Some patients with end-stage pulmonary hypertension may benefit from atrial septostomy. In this procedure, a right-to-left interatrial shunt is created by puncturing the atrial septum with a cardiac catheter blade or needle, followed by dilation of the orifice with a balloon catheter. Two techniques are commonly used. Blade balloon atrial septostomy and balloon dilation atrial septostomy. The rationale for this approach is to decompress the overloaded right ventricle by creation of a right to left shunt.

Although first reported by Rich and Lam nearly 20 years ago (127), experience with atrial septostomy in treating PAH is limited. Roughly 80 patients from over a dozen studies have been reported. Findings from these studies are limited because of differences in types of patients that were studied, indications for performing the procedure, and concomitant medical therapies. The results from all but one of these studies were recently analyzed by Sandoval and colleagues (128). In general, the acute hemodynamic effects of atrial septostomy were decreased right atrial pressure and augmented cardiac output. Oxygen delivery usually increased, despite a significant decrease in arterial oxygen saturation. As a group, changes in hemodynamic variables were mild. The mean decrease in right atrial pressure was only 3 mm

Hg. However, cardiac index increased nearly 25%, and the mean decrease in oxygen saturation was greater than 11%. Nearly all patients reported symptomatic improvement after the procedure, including relief of syncope and improved exercise tolerance. In one of the more successful studies involving 14 patients (129), mean NYHA class decreased from 3.57 ± 0.6 to 2.07 ± 0.3, and the distance walked in 6 minutes increased an average of 110 meters. Three year survival was 92% which was considerably better than historical controls (52%).

Enthusiasm for atrial septostomy is tempered by a fairly high peri-procedure mortality rate and the lack of evidence to suggest that it improves underlying pulmonary hypertensive disease (128). Because of the high risk of death, the WHO symposium on PPH recommended that atrial septostomy should be performed only at institutions that are well experienced with the technique, and it should not be performed in patients that have terminal right heart failure on cardiovascular support (1). At the present time, atrial septostomy should be considered as a palliative treatment and reserved for patients who have symptoms of progressive right heart failure despite optimal medical therapy.

Finally, heart–lung transplantation or single-lung transplantation offers the best hope for patients who progress on or fail to respond to optimal medical therapy (130). Unfortunately, limited donor organs make this therapy unavailable to many patients with PPH. It is reasonable to refer patients for lung transplantation if clinical deterioration occurs or if hemodynamic parameters suggest advanced disease. Some physicians prefer to refer patients at the time of diagnosis because the expected waiting period may be extensive. However, optimism regarding transplantation must be tempered with recognition of complications of rejection and the potential for recurrence of PPH in the transplanted lung. Furthermore, many physicians have found that with effective vasodilator therapy, lung transplantation can be delayed indefinitely.

A general approach to treatment in patients with PAH is outlined in Figure 35.8. All patients capable of tolerating long-term anticoagulation should receive it. Symptoms of right heart failure should be treated with diuretics and possibly digoxin. Vasodilator therapy is determined primarily by the patient's response to acute vasodilator testing and by their WHO functional class. Patients in WHO class I or II who respond to acute vasodilators can be managed with calcium channel blockers and careful follow-up. For responders with more advanced disease, WHO class III, endothelin receptor antagonists or subcutaneous infusion of PGI_2 may be a better choice, unless PAP can be returned to near normal levels with calcium channel blockers. Patients who do not respond to acute vasodilators and are in WHO class II or III should be treated with endothelin receptor antagonists or subcutaneous infusion of PGI_2. Nonresponders in WHO class I may be treated or observed, depending on the severity of their pulmonary hypertension. Because of high short-term mortality, patients with WHO class IV symptoms are probably

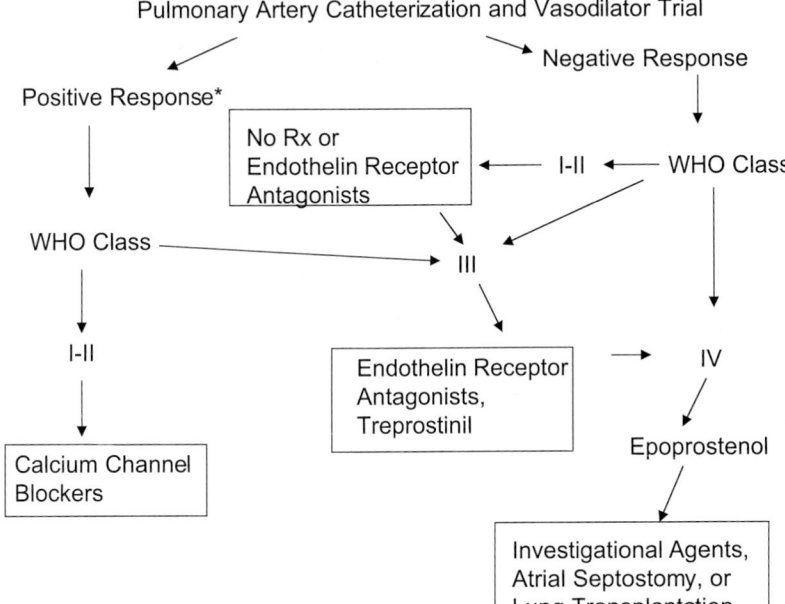

FIGURE 35.8. The approach to treatment of pulmonary arterial hypertension. *A positive response to vasodilator is defined as greater than 20% decrease in calculated pulmonary vascular resistance and in mean pulmonary arterial pressure. WHO, World Health Organization classification of severity of symptoms of pulmonary hypertension (1).

better treated with intravenous PGI_2, as are patients with class III symptoms who progress on endothelin receptor antagonists or subcutaneous PGI_2. Alternative therapies for class III or IV patients who do not respond to conventional therapy include combining endothelin receptor antagonists with subcutaneous or intravenous PGI_2 or investigational agents such as phosphodiesterase inhibitors or inhaled NO. These patients should also be considered for lung transplant. Patients with symptoms of severe heart failure despite optimal medical management may also be considered for atrial septostomy. Female patients with PAH should be counseled to avoid pregnancy.

Pulmonary Venous Hypertension

Pulmonary venous hypertension increases PAP by passive increases in pressure and by narrowing and obstruction of pulmonary arteries owing to remodeling. Pulmonary venous pressure can be elevated by left heart disease, extrinsic compression of pulmonary veins, and venoocclusive disease.

Pulmonary Venous Hypertension Owing to Left-Sided Atrial or Ventricular Heart Disease

Left ventricular failure passively increases PAP because of altered pressure-flow relationships in the pulmonary circulation which occur in stages. The first stage begins with an increase in left ventricular end-diastolic pressure that increases pulmonary blood volume until the pulmonary vascular bed is fully recruited. At this point, any additional increase in left ventricular end-diastolic pressure will increase PAP. If PAP rises to the point at which the critical microvascular pressure (approximately 25 mm Hg) is exceeded, fluid accumulates

in the pulmonary interstitial compartment. As this process continues, the stage of alveolar edema formation begins with loss of lung volume and a further increase in PVR related to compression of small pulmonary vessels by the accumulating alveolar edema fluid. Localized hypoxic vasoconstriction may also contribute to the increase in PAP at this stage. These acute changes are readily reversible with resolution of the primary problem of left ventricular dysfunction, assuming there has been no overt damage to the pulmonary vascular bed.

Pulmonary Venous Hypertension Owing to Left-Sided Valvular Disease

Mitral stenosis causes pulmonary venous hypertension by sustained increases in left atrial pressure. Pulmonary hypertension is owing to passively increased PAP and remodeling of pulmonary arteries and veins. Pathologic changes include medial hypertrophy and fibrosis of pulmonary arteries and veins (Fig. 35.3B). Diagnosis is usually made by echocardiography. Pulmonary hypertension associated with this acquired cardiac condition is usually reversed after relief of valvular obstruction by balloon valvotomy, open commissurotomy, or mitral valve replacement (131). However, if the disease is long-standing, there may not be complete reversal of remodeling changes, and pulmonary hypertension may persist. In one large series, nearly 10% of patients undergoing balloon mitral valvotomy had significant pulmonary hypertension after successfully completing the procedure (132).

Pulmonary Venous Hypertension Owing to Extrinsic Compression of Central Pulmonary Veins

Extrinsic compression of pulmonary veins can be caused by fibrosing mediastinitis, hilar adenopathy or mediastinal tumors. Hilar adenopathy and tumors are usually detected by chest radiography or CT scanning. Fibrosing mediastinitis is an unusual disease that was perhaps best described by Goodwin and colleagues in 1972 as an "exuberant proliferation of fibrous tissue beyond the confines of lymph nodes" (133). Although thought to be the result of an inflammatory response to pulmonary histoplasmosis or tuberculosis, the etiology in most patients is uncertain. Clinical manifestations depend on the size and location of the fibrous tissue within the mediastinum. In descending order of frequency, the structures most often affected are the superior vena cava, esophagus, major bronchi, and pulmonary vessels. Extrinsic compression by the dense fibrous tissue causes pulmonary hypertension by decreasing the cross-sectional area of the proximal pulmonary arterial circulation, the distal pulmonary venous circulation, or both. Pulmonary arteries are affected about as often as pulmonary veins, and the obstruction can be bilateral or unilateral.

The diagnosis of PAH and/or pulmonary venous hypertension can be difficult (134). When the primary involvement is limited to the pulmonary arteries, patients present in a manner similar to chronic thromboembolic disease (see "Thromboembolic Obstruction of Proximal Pulmonary Arteries" below). When the pulmonary veins are the primary source of involvement, patients develop pulmonary venous hypertension and can present with infiltrates and pulmonary edema resembling congestive heart failure or PVOD (see below). Frequently, both pulmonary arterial and pulmonary venous compression are present. Large perfusion defects can be seen on V/Q scanning and pulmonary angiography. The findings of an occluded proximal pulmonary artery in association with signs of pulmonary venous hypertension should suggest the diagnosis. Evidence of hilar or mediastinal enlargement can be seen on chest radiographs in most cases, but the extent of involvement is usually underestimated. CT scan is best able to detect the presence of calcification. The degree of pulmonary vascular involvement is best assessed by contrast-enhanced CT or magnetic resonance imaging (135). Even after extensive evaluation, the diagnosis may be uncertain, necessitating mediastinoscopy and surgical exploration to exclude the presence of other diseases such as sarcoidosis, lymphoma or PVOD.

Treatment of pulmonary hypertension caused by fibrosing mediastinitis is difficult. Steroids and antifungal or antituberculosis medications are generally not effective. The disease is usually progressive and often fatal when vascular structures are involved. Surgical resection may be appropriate in selected patients, but perioperative mortality is high.

Pulmonary Venous Hypertension Owing to Pulmonary Venoocclusive Disease

PVOD is an unusual disorder of unknown etiology that is characterized by clinical and pathologic evidence of occlusion of postcapillary veins and venules (136). PVOD may account for about 10% of pulmonary hypertension cases of unknown etiology. Its rarity has hampered the study of its epidemiology and demographics. Only about 150 cases have been reported in the literature. This idiopathic disorder occurs in children and young adults. Most patients present before age 50, and in adult patients, there has been a male-to-female ratio of approximately 2:1. In addition to the idiopathic form of PVOD, there are sporadic reports of other clinical associations. An acquired variant of this disorder is drug-induced pulmonary vascular disease (e.g., caused by bleomycin, carmustine, or mitomycin) with typical findings of PVOD on pathologic exam. Other reported clinical associations include bone marrow transplantation, malignancy, and an unexplained genetic predisposition for this disorder, suggested by the finding of documented cases of PVOD in siblings.

Pathology

PVOD is characterized by organized and recanalized thrombi in pulmonary veins and venules with eccentric fibrosis of the intima and medial hypertrophy and arterialization of veins. Generally, the small postcapillary pulmonary veins are most affected, but medium and large pulmonary veins can be affected as well. Alveolar capillaries are congested with blood, and hemosiderosis may be noted. There are findings consistent with long-standing hydrostatic pulmonary edema, such as lymphatic dilation and interstitial edema. Because precapillary arterioles may also demonstrate intimal fibrosis and fibrinoid necrosis of media, it is possible that this disease is actually a more generalized obstructive angiopathy. In fact, some investigators have suggested that the disorder be renamed "pulmonary vasoocclusive disease" to reflect its effect on both sides of the pulmonary capillary. However, there is general agreement that the disease primarily effects the pulmonary venous circulation and thus, the term "pulmonary venoocclusive disease" has persisted.

Clinical Presentation and Diagnosis

Patients usually present with dyspnea. The major clinical challenge is establishing the diagnosis of PVOD and distinguishing it from other, more common conditions. PVOD may simulate congestive heart failure with interstitial and alveolar edema and pulmonary vascular congestion. In one series, six out of 11 patients had bibasilar rales, and two had orthopnea and paroxysmal nocturnal dyspnea (137). The chest x-ray frequently provides evidence of pulmonary venous hypertension, including septal thickening, interstitial infiltrates, and pleural effusions (137). The presence of basilar rales and interstitial infiltrates on chest x-ray in some patients with PVOD may lead to an incorrect diagnosis of interstitial fibrosis. The absence of distended upper lobe veins or left ventricular enlargement are important clues to the presence of PVOD as a cause of pulmonary edema. Interlobular septal thickening and patchy ground-glass opacities can be seen on chest HRCT and can be helpful in suggesting the diagnosis (136, 138). Other causes of pulmonary venous obstruction, such as fibrosing mediastinitis and congenital venous atresia or stenosis, should be excluded. V/Q lung scans are generally nonspecific and not thought to be helpful.

Hemodynamic findings may be similar to PAH with elevated PAP and normal PCWP (136). However, in PVOD, PCWP is determined by the degree of clotting involving the venous segments draining the pulmonary artery, which contains the balloon catheter. Because the degree of clotting varies between veins, PCWP readings may differ between different pulmonary arteries. Also, a higher PCWP may be found by wedging the catheter with the balloon down than with the balloon up. This occurs because most of the resistance in PVOD is in the smaller veins that will determine PCWP when the catheter is wedged in a smaller pulmonary artery.

It may be difficult to distinguish PVOD from PPH. Usually, the disease can be suspected by the combination of physical and radiographic findings and the diagnoses pursued with CT scanning, angiography, and careful hemodynamic measurements. In patients in whom the diagnosis is not forthcoming, open lung biopsy is necessary to unequivocally diagnose PVOD.

Treatment

There is no documented effective medical treatment for PVOD. Although case reports have described improvement in some patients treated with calcium channel blockers, inhaled NO, and intravenous or inhaled PGI_2, pulmonary vasodilation in the presence of venous obstruction may cause increased pulmonary microvascular pressures and severe pulmonary edema (136). Most investigators recommend anticoagulants. The definitive treatment remains lung transplantation.

PULMONARY HYPERTENSION ASSOCIATED WITH DISORDERS OF THE RESPIRATORY SYSTEM AND/OR HYPOXEMIA

Disorders of the respiratory system and hypoxemia are very common causes of pulmonary hypertension. Patients with pulmonary hypertension associated with lung disease typically present with symptoms and signs related to the underlying lung disease. This form of secondary pulmonary hypertension is not generally observed until the lung disease is severe, as assessed by pulmonary function testing. The prognosis is generally determined by the underlying respiratory system disorder, although the presence of pulmonary hypertension is an unfavorable prognostic sign (139, 140).

The pathology of pulmonary hypertension associated with disorders of the respiratory system is typical of the primary lung disorder but is particularly characterized by remodeling caused by chronic hypoxia. This includes increases in intimal, medial, and adventitial thickness (Fig. 35.3). In precapillary segments, differentiation of pericytes and intermediate cells into myofibroblasts causes extension of smooth muscle into partially muscularized or nonmuscularized small vessels.

Chronic Obstructive Pulmonary Disease

The degree of pulmonary hypertension in stable COPD is generally mild (mean PAP, 20–42.5 mm Hg) and progresses rather slowly (141). Several mechanisms contribute to the development of pulmonary hypertension in COPD. The most important initiating factor, discussed earlier in this chapter, is alveolar hypoxia, leading to acute hypoxic vasoconstriction and a resultant elevation in PAP and resistance. Global alveolar hypoxia causes generalized vasoconstriction, which may help to recruit additional parts of the underutilized pulmonary vascular space for participation in gas exchange. Sustained alveolar hypoxia causes vascular smooth muscle hypertrophy and remodeling of the pulmonary circulation (Fig. 35.3B). If the elevated PAP is sustained, then sustained increased right ventricular work is required to maintain cardiac output at the same normal level over time.

Several other mechanisms contribute to the development of pulmonary hypertension in COPD (142). Destruction of the pulmonary vascular bed decreases pulmonary cross-sectional area as a direct result of the disease process and thereby contributes to the elevation in PAP. Increased lung volume has complex effects on pulmonary vessels. Pressure in the extra-alveolar vessels (vessels not exposed to alveolar pressure) may actually fall with the increase in lung volume related to the "tethering effect" of being pulled open by the hyperinflated lung. However, the net effect of increased lung volume is increased PAP and PVR owing to compression of alveolar vessels by the raised intra-alveolar pressure. Potentiation of hypoxic vasoconstriction by additional vasoconstrictor stimuli—such as acidosis associated with hypercapnia, increased blood viscosity that may accompany polycythemia, increased platelet aggregation within the pulmonary vasculature, and lung inflammation—may also contribute to pulmonary hypertension.

Pulmonary hypertension in patients with COPD is multifactorial in origin, with sustained alveolar hypoxia being the most important initial stimulus triggering the acute and chronic events culminating in an elevated PAP. In general, pulmonary hypertension in COPD correlates with the severity of the underlying lung disease and resting Pa_{O_2} (142). PAP also increases during exercise, indicating limited ability of the structurally compromised pulmonary vascular bed to accommodate the normal increase in pulmonary blood flow during exercise.

Another factor that may exacerbate the development of pulmonary hypertension in COPD is worsened hypoxemia during sleep (143). Nocturnal oxygen desaturation is very common in this patient population; the most severe episodes occurring during rapid eye movement (REM) sleep. Although the cause of the hypoxemia during sleep is probably multifactorial, the most important contributing factor is centrally mediated hypoventilation during REM sleep. The net result is that diminished alveolar ventilation during sleep may cause profound oxygen desaturation associated with a significantly increased PAP for prolonged times on a recurring basis (episodic hypoxia). In the available studies that have actually measured the changes in pulmonary hemodynamics during sleep, episodes of oxygen desaturation were accompanied by increases in PAP ranging from 10 to 20 mm Hg (143). The increases in PAP were reversed when oxygen saturation returned to baseline, linking oxygen desaturation to the altered pulmonary hemodynamics. Thus, sustained pulmonary hypertension in COPD may be linked to these recurring episodes of oxygen desaturation, which further increase PAP. Studies in animal models lend support to the notion that intermittent cyclical decreases in oxygen saturation may increase PAP more than does continuously decreased saturation. Nevertheless, the overall contribution of alterations in pulmonary hemodynamics during sleep to the magnitude of pulmonary hypertension and the overall clinical course of patients with COPD remain undefined.

Severe pulmonary hypertension in COPD may result in cor pulmonale. The clinical signs of cor pulmonale, including evidence of right ventricular enlargement and pulmonary hypertension, may be obscured by the presence of severe lung disease, specifically hyperinflation. Auscultation of a right-sided S_3 or a loud P_2 may be difficult to appreciate in the patients with overdistended lungs. Similarly, right ventricular enlargement on chest radiograph may be obscured by hyperinflation. Hyperinflation may displace normal liver, which may be mistaken for hepatic enlargement compatible with passive congestion on physical exam.

Interstitial Lung Disease

In this category are diseases of the lung parenchyma—such as idiopathic pulmonary fibrosis, asbestosis, and other pneumoconioses—and other disorders sharing the common feature of loss of lung volume as a direct result of a primary disease process infiltrating the lung parenchyma.

The mechanisms leading to the development of pulmonary hypertension in chronic interstitial lung disease are similar to those discussed above for obstructive disease. Hypoxic vasoconstriction, compression and/or obliteration of lung vessels by fibrosis and loss of lung volume, and destruction of vascular surface area all contribute to pulmonary hypertension. The relationship between lung volume and PVR in parenchymal restrictive lung disease is well defined (144). Typically, vital capacity 50% of predicted is associated with the presence of pulmonary hypertension at rest, whereas vital capacity between 50% to 80% of predicted is associated with the development of pulmonary hypertension only

during exercise. In restrictive parenchymal disease, the major anatomic site of this increase in PAP and PVR is the extraalveolar vessels, which are no longer tethered open as lung volume falls. Acute pulmonary vasodilation in response to inhaled PGI_2 and NO in a small series of patients and long-term clinical improvement in dyspnea with aerosolized PGI_2 (iloprost) suggests that vasoconstriction may play a role in the pathogenesis of pulmonary hypertension in at least some patients with interstitial pulmonary fibrosis (145).

Sleep Disordered Breathing

Many patients with severe obstructive sleep apnea demonstrate periodic elevations in PAP that are preceded by oxygen desaturation (146). These reversible oscillations of PAP are initiated by decreased oxygen tension and, thus, represent examples of acute hypoxic vasoconstriction. Despite these periodic oscillations of PAP, sustained pulmonary hypertension does not develop in the majority of patients with obstructive sleep apnea alone (147). Development of sustained daytime pulmonary hypertension also does not correlate well with the severity of the sleep-related breathing disorder alone (the number or frequency of apneic events). Thus, patients with obstructive sleep apnea who are at greatest risk for the development of resting daytime pulmonary hypertension are patients with underlying obstructive lung disease, hypoxemia and hypercapnia, congestive heart failure, or obesity. However, a subset of obstructive sleep apnea patients with normal pulmonary function have been reported who have mild pulmonary hypertension associated with small-airway closure and heightened pulmonary pressor responses to hypoxia and increased pulmonary blood flow (148).

The most important etiologic factors that contribute to the initiation and maintenance of pulmonary hypertension in obstructive sleep apnea are hypoxic pulmonary vasoconstriction and the added vasoconstrictor stimulus of respiratory acidosis from hypercapnia. Another potential contributor to pulmonary hypertension is increased venous return, caused by generation of significant negative intrathoracic pressure during breathing with a obstructed airway. The development of pulmonary hypertension in obesity hypoventilation syndrome also depends on the development of alveolar hypoxia and acidosis. Correction of the primary process leading to oxygen desaturation and/or hypoventilation improves pulmonary hypertension in these disorders. Nasal continuous positive airway pressure therapy has also been shown to improve pulmonary hypertension in nonhypoxemic patients with obstructive sleep apnea (149).

Alveolar Hypoventilation Disorders

Alveolar hypoventilation is the critical factor in the development of pulmonary hypertension in thoracic cage deformities, diaphragmatic disorders, neuromuscular disease, and spinal cord injury. In all of these disorders, loss of lung volume imposes a mechanical or anatomical limitation on the patient's respiratory system (150). Critical loss of lung volume causes alveolar hypoventilation, with consequent hypoxemia and hypercapnia providing the stimuli for pulmonary vasoconstriction and pulmonary hypertension. Long-standing hypoxia causes remodeling of the pulmonary circulation, as described above, which also contributes to loss of pulmonary vascular cross-sectional area. In addition, superimposed conditions, such as atelectasis or infection, alter V/Q and help to maintain hypoxic vasoconstriction. In many thoracic cage disorders (kyphoscoliosis, thoracoplasty, or restrictive pleural disease), there is compression of lung vessels related to loss of lung volume, which also increases PAP and resistance.

Chronic Exposure to High Altitude

Acute pulmonary hypertension occurs in susceptible individuals within hours of alveolar hypoxia caused by ascension to high altitude (151). Sojourns of weeks at high altitude may result in pulmonary hypertension that is not reversible with oxygen breathing, suggesting remodeling changes (152). High-altitude natives in North and South America have been shown to have moderate pulmonary hypertension at rest, which increases with exercise (153). Interestingly, natives of the Tibetan plateau did not exhibit pulmonary hypertension at rest, with exercise, or during breathing of hypoxic gas (154). These data suggest that prolonged residence at high altitude for many generations may result in acclimatization. There is also considerable interspecies and interindividual variability in pulmonary hypertension associated with high-altitude residence, suggesting that genetic susceptibility may be important (153). Relative hypoventilation and polycythemia may exacerbate pulmonary hypertension, resulting in chronic mountain sickness, characterized by cor pulmonale.

The pulmonary hypertension associated with high-altitude exposure is characterized by remodeling caused by chronic hypoxia. Because it can occur in the absence of underlying heart or lung disease, it is evidence of the important clinical effects of chronic hypoxia. Chronic hypoxia at high altitude may also trigger development of PPH. Treatment of pulmonary hypertension associated with high altitude consists of moving to low altitude.

Neonatal Lung Disease

Neonatal lung diseases associated with pulmonary hypertension and persistence of the fetal pulmonary circulation include meconium aspiration and pneumonia (see Section "Pulmonary Arterial Hypertension Related to Persistent Pulmonary Hypertension of the Newborn").

Alveolar Capillary Dysplasia

Persistent misalignment of pulmonary veins with alveolar capillary dysplasia is an unusual and fatal cause of pulmonary hypertension in the newborn (155). The disorder is char-acterized by paucity of capillaries adjacent to alveolar epithelium, causing impaired gas exchange; anomalous veins within broncho-arterial bundles; and medial thickening of small pulmonary arteries. Patients may be treated with extra-corporeal membrane oxygenation, but it is invariably fatal.

OTHER

Pulmonary Histiocytosis X

Pulmonary histiocytosis X is an interstitial lung disease associated with cigarette smoking and characterized by hyperinflation and/or airway obstruction. Pulmonary histiocytosis X may be complicated by severe pulmonary hypertension, out of proportion to pulmonary function abnormalities, and is generally more severe than the pulmonary hypertension associated with COPD or interstitial pulmonary fibrosis (156). Pathologic changes include intimal fibrosis of both arteries and veins and medial smooth muscle hypertrophy. Venular obliteration and capillary dilatation were also observed. The involvement of pulmonary veins suggests that vasodilator therapy may be contraindicated owing to risk of pulmonary edema.

Treatment of Pulmonary Hypertension Associated with Disorders of the Respiratory System and/or Hypoxemia

Treatment of patients with secondary pulmonary hypertension should be focussed on correction of the underlying respiratory system abnormality and hypoxemia.

Supplemental oxygen can correct arterial hypoxemia and reduce PAP and PVR associated with both obstructive and restrictive lung diseases. The rationale for this therapy emerged from the findings of several studies that demonstrated that the overall prognosis and survival of patients with COPD is correlated with the presence and severity of pulmonary hypertension (139).

The finding that the acute administration of supplemental oxygen to patients with advanced COPD reduces PAP opened a new chapter in the use of oxygen as a therapeutic agent on a chronic basis. The acute administration of oxygen to patients with COPD produces significant moderate reductions in PAP and resistance. PAP does not return to normal immediately in many patients, probably because of morphological changes in the walls of blood vessels and obliteration of the pulmonary vasculature secondary to the disease process. The efficacy of prolonged oxygen therapy for chronic bronchitis and emphysema has been unequivocally established in clinical trials by the Nocturnal Oxygen Therapy Trial Group (157) and the British Medical Research Council Working Party (158). Reductions in PAP, PVR, and long-term mortality were observed in both studies, although the reductions in PVR were modest.

These findings suggest that the survival benefit cannot be attributed solely to changes in pulmonary hemodynamics. The basis for this survival benefit remains undefined, but oxygen therapy is the only approach to date that has been shown to prolong life in COPD. Supplemental oxygen administration does not change lung function. Maximal vasodilatory effects are observed with continuous oxygen administration (>16 h/d), especially during sleep. Prolonged administration of oxygen for weeks further decreases mean PAP, suggesting that supplemental oxygen therapy not only reverses hypoxic vasoconstriction, but may partially reverse some of the morphological changes in the pulmonary vessels.

The long-term efficacy of supplemental oxygen administration in restrictive lung disease has never been validated in prospective clinical trials. There are far fewer patients with advanced restrictive disease who develop pulmonary hypertension and cor pulmonale, perhaps because of advanced underlying lung disease, culminating in death. Many of the mechanisms of pulmonary hypertension are undoubtedly similar. Therefore, in the absence of evidence that this approach is contraindicated or ineffective, it is reasonable to administer supplemental oxygen to appropriately hypoxemic patients with restrictive lung disease.

Obviously, patients with chest wall disorders causing restriction and hypoventilation require treatment of hypoventilation, including (potentially) mechanical ventilation.

There is controversy regarding the benefits of vasodilator treatment of pulmonary hypertension secondary to lung disease. On the one hand, pulmonary hypertension often worsens during an exacerbation of COPD, related to superimposed acute hypoxemia and hypercarbia, and may contribute to the deterioration of right heart function and symptoms of right heart failure. This rationale for pharmacologic treatment of pulmonary hypertension in COPD patients is weakened by lack of selective pulmonary vasodilators and potential for worsening of the matching of ventilation and perfusion, resulting in further decreased arterial oxygen tension. In addition, systemic hypotension and tachycardia may be significant side effects. Thus, vasodilator therapy is not generally recommended for pulmonary hypertension secondary to COPD or restrictive lung disease. However, as selective pulmonary vasodilators, such as aerosolized PGI_2 and inhaled NO, become available, they may be useful in management of pulmonary hypertension due to interstitial pulmonary fibrosis (145).

PULMONARY HYPERTENSION OWING TO CHRONIC THROMBOTIC AND/OR EMBOLIC DISEASE

Thromboembolic Obstruction of Proximal Pulmonary Arteries

Acute pulmonary thromboembolism is normally not associated with significant pulmonary hypertension owing to the abundance of low resistance pulmonary arteries and the ability of the lungs to redirect blood flow to unrecruited vessels.

PAH can be seen with acute pulmonary embolism in patients with underlying pulmonary or cardiac disease or in patients in whom more than half of the pulmonary vascular bed is occluded. Pulmonary hypertension in acute thromboembolic disease is caused not only by vascular obstruction but also by hypoxic vasoconstriction and vasoconstrictive agents released from the pulmonary vascular endothelium and platelets. Typically, PAP is only moderately elevated even with massive pulmonary emboli because the right ventricle is unable to generate systolic pressures much greater than two to three times normal. In the great majority of patients, pulmonary hypertension from acute pulmonary embolism resolves within 3 weeks of the acute event (for a more complete discussion of pulmonary thromboembolism, see Chapters 36 and 37). However, in approximately 0.1% to 0.5% of cases, pulmonary hypertension persists and progresses, owing to impairment of clot resolution or recurrent emboli (159). These patients develop a syndrome referred to as chronic thromboembolic pulmonary hypertension (CTEPH) and often have life-threatening disease. CTEPH occurs in approximately 500 to 2,500 patients each year in the United States (159).

Pathology and Pathogenesis

The etiology of CTEPH in not known. Most patients present late in their disease, often without a history of pulmonary embolism or deep vein thrombosis. Associated abnormalities of the coagulation pathway or the pulmonary endothelium have not been described, although the presence of anticardiolipin antibodies is increased in about 10% of patients (59). The pathology of CTEPH is characterized by incomplete resolution of proximal pulmonary arterial emboli, with residual recanalized clot and/or scarring (Fig. 35.3D). Proximal pulmonary arteries are obstructed by fibrotic (organized) clot, which may extend to more peripheral vessels in a branching pattern. Many patients have significant embolization and thrombosis of small more distal pulmonary vessels, even in areas of lung unobstructed by proximal clot. Although patients generally have greater than 40% of their pulmonary vascular bed occluded, factors other than anatomic obstruction of the vascular bed are likely to play a role. Histologic studies demonstrate many of the features of primary PAH, including plexiform lesions and pulmonary arteriopathy. Some patients progress without evidence of recurrent emboli or in situ thrombosis. Interestingly, changes consistent with pulmonary arteriopathy have been described in lung sections taken from areas that were not affected by pulmonary emboli. Thus, it is likely that CTEPH represents an abnormal response to acute or recurrent emboli, which results not only in persistent thrombosis or recurrent embolism but also in pulmonary vascular remodeling typical of other pulmonary hypertensive diseases.

Obstruction to flow in major arteries from proximal, incompletely resolved clot and also remodeling of small resistance arteries increase PVR, leading to pulmonary hypertension and diminished right ventricular contractility. The specific consequences in an individual patient depend on the presence of preexisting cardiopulmonary disease.

Clinical Presentation

The clinical presentation of patients with CTEPH is relatively nonspecific and resembles that of other types of PAH. A careful history may uncover single or multiple episodes of previous venous thromboembolic disease in either the recent or distant past. Patients may report sudden onset of dyspnea, atrial fibrillation, or syncope, but many patients have no symptoms of previous PE. This may not be surprising, considering that acute pulmonary embolism may be asymptomatic and is frequently misdiagnosed. Physical examination reveals findings associated with PAH and right ventricular overload. Limited cardiac output owing to fixed obstruction of the proximal pulmonary arteries may produce exertional syncope. Bruits over the lung fields have been described in CTEPH and attributed to turbulent blood flow through partially occluded major pulmonary vessels.

Diagnosis

The diagnosis of chronic thromboembolism must be excluded in all patients with PAH. Unlike patients with PPH, in whom V/Q scans are normal or demonstrate only patchy subsegmental defects, the V/Q scan in CTEPH invariably demonstrates at least segmental or larger mismatched defects. However, the degree of pulmonary vascular occlusion can be severely underestimated by V/Q scanning (160). Thus, CTEPH should be considered in patients with PAH who have any segmental defects on V/Q scan. Echocardiography is helpful in evaluating right ventricular function and the degree of pulmonary hypertension. CT pulmonary angiography can be helpful to visualize large clots partially occluding proximal pulmonary arteries, but may miss the diagnosis in patients who have thromboembolic disease primarily in distal vessels. Standard tests for the diagnosis of acute pulmonary emboli, such as V/Q scan, lower extremity Doppler ultrasounds, and CT pulmonary angiography may also have difficulty differentiating between acute and chronic pulmonary emboli. For these reasons, pulmonary angiography is often necessary to make the diagnosis of CTEPH. Findings of pouch defects, webbing, banding, and intimal irregularities of the embolic lesion suggest chronic embolization and recanalization. Pulmonary angiography also provides the best evaluation of the degree of clot burden and whether it is likely to be amenable to surgery.

Pulmonary angiography can be performed safely in experienced hands, even in the setting of increased PAP and right ventricular failure (161). Because the angiographic findings in CTEPH differ from those observed with acute thromboembolic obstruction of the pulmonary circulation, it is helpful to alert the angiographer to the clinical suspicion of CTEPH. Finally, fiberoptic pulmonary angiography can provide direct visualization of the proximal pulmonary arterial tree and is often used in medical centers that specialize in thromboendarterectomy to select patients who are most likely to benefit from surgery.

Treatment

The clinical importance of recognizing CTEPH is that pulmonary thromboendarterectomy can produce dramatic improvement in hemodynamics and functional status in selected patients. Patients in NYHA functional class III or IV status can move to class I or II after operative intervention. However, pulmonary thromboendarterectomy is a technically demanding procedure performed in only a small number of centers. Patients are carefully screened for optimum results. Generally, patients are considered good candidates for thromboendarterectomy if they have a surgically accessible clot and markedly elevated pulmonary hemodynamics at rest or with exercise. In one study, mean PVR before surgery was 800 to 1,000 dyne/(cm $\cdot$ sec^2) (162). Patients with lower PVR may also be considered under special circumstances in which mild impairment of lung function is detrimental, such as residence at high altitude or in a young patient who desires restoration of optimal exercise. To be surgically correctable, the responsible emboli must involve the main, lobar, or proximal segmental arteries (163). The greatest difficulty in determining operability is predicting the degree of hemodynamic impairment caused by surgically removing the clot. Patients with significant thromboembolic disease in distal pulmonary vessels or those with pulmonary hypertension owing to secondary pulmonary arteriopathy may not benefit enough to justify the risk of surgery.

Response to surgical treatment can be dramatic. The average drop in PVR after endarterectomy has been about 65% (163), with some patients experiencing complete normalization of PAP. Most patients improve one or two classes of the NYHA scale, and many return to normal activity. Lifelong anticoagulant therapy is recommended (163) for all patients that can tolerate it, and many receive an inferior vena cava filter. The improvement in exercise tolerance needs to be carefully weighed against the high risk of pulmonary endarterectomy. Overall mortality from this procedure ranges from 4% to 25% (163). Only about 2,000 pulmonary endarterectomies have been performed worldwide, and most have been at a single center. Morbidity and mortality are attributed to cardiac bypass, reperfusion pulmonary edema in areas of clot removal, and right ventricular failure. Pulmonary vascular steal (blood flow diversion to areas of lung opened after thromboendarterectomy) may also contribute to postoperative hypoxemia.

Obstruction of Distal Pulmonary Arteries

Pulmonary Embolism: In Situ Thrombosis or Tumor

Distal pulmonary arteries may be obstructed by thromboembolic clot, tumor emboli, and may be obstructed by in situ thromboses. The latter frequently complicate PAH disorders and are commonly observed on pathologic examination. Distal obstruction of pulmonary arteries may not present with a distinct clinical event, but contributes to slowly developing dyspnea and increased dead space ventilation. These finding may be observed as an incidental finding on pathological examination of the lungs.

Sickle Cell Disease and Other Mixed Hemoglobinopathies

Hemoglobinopathies such as sickle cell disease and mixed hemoglobinopathies (hemoglobin S and C disease, S-β-thalassemia) commonly involve the pulmonary circulation on either an acute or chronic basis. The chronic pulmonary vascular manifestations of this disease are most commonly observed in individuals who are long-term survivors. Retrospective studies have reported up to 40% of patients with sickle cell disease have moderate-to-severe pulmonary hypertension (164). These patients most frequently seek medical attention as a result of the development of the "acute chest syndrome," consisting of fever, pleuritic chest pain, dyspnea, leukocytosis, hypoxemia, and pulmonary infiltrates. Pulmonary vascular occlusions caused by in situ thromboses in the pulmonary microcirculation are a frequent component of this syndrome. Accurate differentiation of infection from pulmonary vascular occlusion and/or infarction may be difficult. Mild pulmonary hypertension in this setting may be related to volume overload as a secondary consequence of chronic anemia and changes in blood viscosity. Survivors of the acute chest syndrome may develop chronic pulmonary disease consisting of pulmonary fibrosis, pulmonary hypertension, and cor pulmonale because of the cumulative effects of pulmonary vascular occlusion. This obstructive vasculopathy is thought to be the end result of several key events, notably chronic hypoxemia, emboli of necrotic bone marrow, in situ thromboses, and endothelial cell damage owing to sequestration of sickle erythrocytes (164). In addition to hydration and prompt treatment of infection, the key principle for management of the pulmonary vascular complications is maintenance of an adequate oxygen tension. Anticoagulants have no documented role in the management of the in situ pulmonary vascular occlusion in these disorders, and may be dangerous because of increased risk of spontaneous bleeding in these patients. Exchange transfusions are often used to treat refractory life-threatening hypoxemia. Individuals with sickle trait rarely develop manifestations of pulmonary vascular complications, although anecdotal reports of an increased risk of sudden death during strenuous exercise highlight the need for further work in this area.

PULMONARY HYPERTENSION DUE TO DISORDERS AFFECTING THE PULMONARY VASCULATURE DIRECTLY

Inflammatory

Schistosomiasis is a common cause of pulmonary hypertension in endemic areas and among immigrant populations. Pulmonary hypertension results from a combination of physical obstruction of the pulmonary vascular bed and vasculitis caused by the immunologic response to the foreign protein of the parasite.

Sarcoidosis is another inflammatory cause of pulmonary hypertension. The prevalence varies, depending on the stage of disease, but may be as high as 50% in stage III sarcoidosis (124). The degree of pulmonary hypertension is also variable; Shorr and colleagues reported mean PAPs of 34 mm Hg among patients with sarcoidosis who were awaiting lung transplant (165). However, Preston and colleagues reported mean PAPs of 55 mm Hg among eight sarcoidosis patients with severe pulmonary hypertension (124). Pulmonary hypertension in sarcoidosis has multiple causes: hypoxia, fibrosis and destruction of vascular bed, extrinsic compression of major pulmonary arteries by enlarged lymph nodes, and granulomatous infiltration of the vascular wall. In addition, acute responsiveness to vasodilators suggests that vasoconstriction plays a role (124).

Pulmonary Capillary Hemangiomatosis

Pulmonary capillary hemangiomatosis is a rare proliferative disorder of the pulmonary capillaries, resulting in compression of pulmonary veins and secondary pulmonary venous hypertension. The disorder presents clinically with pulmonary hypertension, hemoptysis, interstitial lung infiltrates on chest x-ray, pleural effusion, and increased numbers of iron-laden alveolar macrophages in bronchoalveolar lavage or sputum (166). Clear diagnosis requires pathological confirmation, but may be difficult because transbronchial biopsy is contraindicated and open lung biopsy may be hazardous. HRCT is suggestive if poorly defined nodular opacities, septal lines, or pleural effusion are observed (167); indeed, some experts suggest that HRCT scans be obtained in all patients before institution of PGI$_2$ therapy (166). This is because pulmonary edema has been reported to complicate PGI$_2$ treatment of pulmonary capillary hemangiomatosis (166, 167).

SUMMARY AND CONCLUSIONS

The pathophysiology of pulmonary hypertension includes both functional and structural changes in the pulmonary circulation. Functional alterations which increase PVR include increases in blood flow, pulmonary venous pressure, and blood viscosity; increased reactivity of vascular smooth muscle to vasoconstrictor; and decreased reactivity to vasodilator stimuli. Factors that decrease aggregate pulmonary arterial cross-sectional diameter also increase PVR, such as vascular obstruction, vasoconstriction, vessel obliteration, and vascular remodeling. Pulmonary hypertension is the end result of one or more of these pathophysiologic changes that occur in response to primary or secondary pulmonary vascular diseases. Thus, the diagnostic approach to the patient with suspected pulmonary hypertension is to evaluate for underlying heart or lung diseases that might cause pulmonary hypertension. The diagnosis of PPH is made in the absence of secondary causes. Therapy is directed at the underlying heart or lung disease in patients with pulmonary hypertension associated with chronic heart and lung disease. Oxygen is the treatment of choice for hypoxemic patients. Patients with PAH benefit from treatment with anticoagulants, vasodilator therapy, and, in selected cases, lung transplant.

There has been enormous progress in the past 10 to 15 years in understanding of the pathogenesis and treatment of pulmonary hypertensive disorders. The importance of genetic factors in PAH, and probably in other causes of pulmonary hypertension, is just beginning to be understood and represents a new frontier in research in this area.

REFERENCES

1. Rich S. Executive summary: world symposium on primary pulmonary hypertension. Geneva, Switzerland: World Health Organization, 1998: *www.who.int/ncd/cvd/pph.html*.
2. Gaine S, Rubin L. Primary pulmonary hypertension. *The Lancet* 1998;352:719–725.
3. Hoeper M, Galie N, Simonneau G, et al. New treatments for pulmonary arterial hypertension. *Am J Resp Crit Care Med* 2002;165:1209–1216.
4. Rich S, McLaughlin V, eds. *Clinics in chest medicine: pulmonary hypertension,* Vol. 22. Philadelphia: WB Saunders, 2001.
5. Bevan RD. Influence of adrenergic innervation on vascular growth and mature characteristics. *Am Rev Respir Dis* 1989;140:1478–1482.
6. Cutaia M, Rounds S. Hypoxic pulmonary vasoconstriction: physiologic significance, mechanism, and clinical relevance. *Chest* 1990;97:706–718.
7. McMurtry IF, Davidson AB, Reeves JT, et al. Inhibition of hypoxic pulmonary vasoconstriction by calcium antagonists in isolated rat lungs. *Circ Res* 1976;38:99–104.
8. Harder DR, Madden JA, Dawson C. Hypoxic induction of Ca^{2+}-dependent action potentials in small pulmonary arteries of the cat. *J Appl Physiol* 1985;59:1389–1393.
9. Archer SL, London B, Hampl V, et al. Impairment of hypoxic pulmonary vasoconstriction in mice lacking the voltage-gated potassium channel Kv1.5. *FASEB J* 2001;15:1801–1803.
10. Yuan XJ, Goldman WF, Tod ML, et al. Hypoxia reduces potassium currents in cultured rat pulmonary but not mesenteric arterial myocytes. *Am J Physiol* 1993;264:L116–L123.
11. Yuan XJ, Wang J, Juhaszova M, et al. Attenuated K^+ channel gene transcription in primary pulmonary hypertension. *Lancet* 1998;351:726–727.
12. Fagan KA, Fouty BW, Tyler RC, et al. The pulmonary circulation of homozygous or heterozygous eNOS-null mice is hyperresponsive to mild hypoxia. *J Clin Invest* 1999;103:291–299.
13. Cheng HA, Robergs RA, Letellier JP, et al. Changes in muscle proton transverse relaxation times and acidosis during exercise and recovery. *J Appl Physiol* 1995;79:1370–1378.
14. Giaid A, Saleh D. Reduced expression of endothelial nitric oxide synthase in the lungs of patients with pulmonary hypertension. *N Engl J Med* 1995;333:214–221.
15. Giaid A, Yanagisawa M, Langleben D, et al. Expression of endothelin-1 in the lungs of patients with pulmonary hypertension. *N Engl J Med* 1993;328:1732–1739.
16. Christman B, McPherson C, Newman J, et al. An imbalance between the excretion of thromboxane and prostacyclin metabolites in pulmonary hypertension. *New Engl J Med* 1992;327:70–75.
17. Hoshikawa Y, Voelkel NF, Gesell TL, et al. Prostacyclin receptor–dependent modulation of pulmonary vascular remodeling. *Am J Respir Crit Care Med* 2001;164:314–318.
18. Tuder RM, Cool CD, Geraci MW, et al. Prostacyclin synthase expression is decreased in lungs from patients with severe pulmonary hypertension. *Am J Respir Crit Care Med* 1999;159:1925–1932.
19. Herve P, Launay JM, Scrobohaci ML, et al. Increased plasma serotonin in primary pulmonary hypertension. *Am J Med* 1995;99:249–254.
20. Rothman R, Ayestas M, Dersch C, et al. Aminorex, fenfluramine, and chlorphentermine are serotonin transporter substrates: implications for primary pulmonary hypertension. *Circulation* 1999;100:869–875.
21. Eddahibi S, Humbert M, Fadel E, et al. Serotonin transporter overexpression is responsible for pulmonary artery smooth muscle hyperplasia in primary pulmonary hypertension. *J Clin Invest* 2001;108:1141–1150.
22. Fartoukh M, Emilie D, Le Gall C, et al. Chemokine macrophage inflammatory protein-1α mRNA expression in lung biopsy specimens of primary pulmonary hypertension. *Chest* 1998;114[Suppl 1]:50S–51S.
23. Morrell N, Upton P, Kotecha S, et al. Angiotensin II activates MAPK and stimulates growth of human pulmonary artery smooth muscle via AT_1 receptors. *Am J Physiol* 1999;277:L440–L448.
24. Adnot S, Chabrier P, Andrivet P, et al. Atrial natriuretic peptide concentrations and pulmonary hemodynamics in patients with pulmonary artery hypertension. *Am Rev Resp Dis* 1987;136:951–956.
25. Klinger J, Warburton R, Pietras L, et al. Genetic disruption of atrial natriuretic peptide causes pulmonary hypertension in normoxic and hypoxic mice. *Am J Physiol* 1999;276:L868–L874.
26. Humbert M, Monti G, Brenot F, et al. Increased interleukin-1 and interleukin-6 serum concentrations in severe primary pulmonary hypertension. *Am J Respir Crit Care Med* 1995;151:1628–1631.
27. Hill N, Rounds S. Vascular reactivity is increased in rat lungs injured with α-naphthylthiourea. *J. Appl. Physiol* 1983;54:1693–1701.
28. Hill N, O'Brien R, Rounds S. Repeated lung injury due to α-naphthylthiourea causes right ventricular hypertrophy in rats. *J Appl Physiol* 1984;56:388–396.
29. Hatano S, Strasser T, eds. Primary pulmonary hypertension: report on a WHO meeting. Geneva, Switzerland: World Health Organization, 1975.
30. Anderson E, Simon G, Reid L. Primary and thrombo-embolic pulmonary hypertension: a quantitative pathological study. *J Pathol* 1973;110:273–293.

31. Chazova I, Loyd J, Zhdanov V, et al. Pulmonary artery adventitial changes and venous involvement in primary pulmonary hypertension. *Am J Pathol* 1995;146:389–397.

32. Wagenvoort C, Wagenvoort N. Primary pulmonary hypertension: a pathologic study of the lung vessels in 156 clinically diagnosed cases. *Circulation* 1970;42:1163–1184.

33. Jeffrey T, Wanstall J. Pulmonary vascular remodeling: a target for therapeutic intervention in pulmonary hypertension. *Pharmacol Ther* 2001;92:1–20.

34. Fanburg B, Lee S. A new role for an old molecule: serotonin as a mitogen. *Am J Physiol* 1997;272:L795–L806.

35. Wharton J, Davie N, Upton P, et al. Prostacyclin analogues differentially inhibit growth of distal and proximal human pulmonary artery smooth muscle cells. *Circulation* 2000;102:3130–3136.

36. Christou H, Yoshida A, Arthur V, et al. Increased vascular endothelial growth factor production in the lungs of rats with hypoxia-induced pulmonary hypertension. *Am J Respir Crit Care Med* 1998;18:768–776.

37. Cooper A, Beasley D. Hypoxia stimulates proliferation and interleukin-1α production in human vascular smooth muscle cells. *Am J Physiol* 1999;277:H1326–H1337.

38. Rabinovitch M. Pathobiology of pulmonary hypertension. In: Rich S, McLaughlin V, eds. *Clinics in chest medicine pulmonary hypertension,* Vol. 22. Philadelphia: WB Saunders, 2001:433–449.

39. Taraseviciene-Stewart L, Kasahara Y, Alger L, et al. Inhibition of the VEGF receptor 2 combined with chronic hypoxia causes cell death–dependent pulmonary endothelial cell proliferation and severe pulmonary hypertension. *FASEB J* 2001;15:427–438.

40. Tuder R, Groves B, Badesch D, et al. Exuberant endothelial cell growth and elements of inflammation are present in plexiform lesions of pulmonary hypertension. *Am J Pathol* 1994;144:275–285.

41. Lee S-D, Shroyer K, Markham N, et al. Monoclonal endothelial cell proliferation is present in primary but not secondary pulmonary hypertension. *J Clin Invest* 1998;101:927–934.

42. Tuder R, Chacon M, Alger L, et al. Expression of angiogenesis-related molecules in plexiform lesions in severe pulmonary hypertension: evidence for a process of disordered angiogenesis. *J Pathol* 2001;195:367–374.

43. Geraci M, Moore M, Gesell T, et al. Gene expression patterns in the lungs of patients with primary pulmonary hypertension. *Circ Res* 2001;88:555–562.

44. Blobe G, Schiemann W, Lodish H. Role of transforming growth factor β in human disease. *New Engl J Med* 2000;342:1350–1358.

45. Atkinson C, Stewart S, Upton P, et al. Primary pulmonary hypertension is associated with reduced pulmonary vascular expression of type II bone morphogenetic protein receptor. *Circulation* 2002;105:1672–1678.

46. Barst RJ, Rubin LJ, Long WA, et al. A comparison of continuous intravenous epoprostenol (prostacyclin) with conventional therapy for primary pulmonary hypertension: the Primary Pulmonary Hypertension Study Group. *N Engl J Med* 1996;334:296–302.

47. Badesch DB, Tapson VF, McGoon MD, et al. Continuous intravenous epoprostenol for pulmonary hypertension due to the scleroderma spectrum of disease: a randomized, controlled trial. *Ann Int Med* 2000;132:425–434.

48. Channick RN, Simonneau G, Sitbon O, et al. Effects of the dual endothelin-receptor antagonist bosentan in patients with pulmonary hypertension: a randomised placebo-controlled study. *Lancet* 2001;358:1119–1123.

49. Rich S, Dantzker DR, Ayres SM, et al. Primary pulmonary hypertension: a national prospective study. *Ann Int Med* 1987;107:216–223.

50. Chang C. The normal roentgenographic measurement of the right descending pulmonary artery in 1,085 cases. *AJR Am J Roentgenol* 1962;87:929.

51. Dresdale D, Schultz M, Michtom R. Primary pulmonary hypertension: clinical and haemodynamic study. *Am J Med* 1951;11:686–705.

52. McDonnell P, Toye P, Hutchins G. Primary pulmonary hypertension and cirrhosis: are they related? *Am Rev Resp Dis* 1983;127:437–441.

53. Braman SS, Eby E, Kuhn C, Rounds S. Primary pulmonary hypertension in the elderly. *Arch Intern Med* 1991;151:2433–2438.

54. Pietra G, Edwards W, Kay J, et al. Histopathology of primary pulmonary hypertension: a qualitative and quantitative study of pulmonary blood vessels from 58 patients in the National Heart, Lung, and Blood Institute, Primary Pulmonary Hypertension Registry. *Circulation* 1989;80:1198–1206.

55. Botney M, Kaiser L, Cooper J, et al. Extracellular matrix protein gene expression in atherosclerotic hypertensive pulmonary arteries. *Am J Pathol* 1992;140:357–364.

56. Rich S, Kaufmann E, Levy PS. The effect of high doses of calcium-channel blockers on survival in primary pulmonary hypertension. *N Engl J Med* 1992;327:76–81.

57. Rich S, Martinez J, Lam W, et al. Reassessment of the effects of vasodilator drugs in primary pulmonary hypertension: guidelines for determining a pulmonary vasodilator response. *Am Heart J* 1983;105:119–127.

58. Palevsky HI, Schloo BL, Pietra GG, et al. Primary pulmonary hypertension: vascular structure, morphometry, and responsiveness to vasodilator agents. *Circulation* 1989;80:1207–1221.

59. Wolf M, Boyer-Neumann C, Parent F, et al. Thrombotic risk factors in pulmonary hypertension. *Eur Respir J* 2000;15:395–399.

60. Yeager M, Halley G, Golpon H, et al. Microsatellite instability of endothelial cell growth and apoptosis genes within plexiform lesions in primary pulmonary hypertension. *Circ Res* 2001;88:e2–e11.

61. Dresdale D, Michom R, Schultz M. Recent studies in primary pulmonary hypertension including pharmacologic observations on pulmonary vascular resistance. *Bull NY Acad Sci* 1954;30:194–197.

62. Loyd J, Primm R, Newman J. Familial primary pulmonary hypertension: clinical patterns. *Am Rev Resp Dis* 1984;129:194–197.

63. Newman JH, Wheeler L, Lane KB, et al. Mutation in the gene for bone morphogenetic protein receptor II as a cause of primary pulmonary hypertension in a large kindred. *N Engl J Med* 2001;345:319–324.

64. Thomson JR, Machado RD, Pauciulo MW, et al. Sporadic primary pulmonary hypertension is associated with germline mutations of the gene encoding BMPR-II, a receptor member of the TGF-β family. *J Med Genet* 2000;37:741–745.

65. Morse JH, Jones AC, Barst RJ, et al. Mapping of familial primary pulmonary hypertension locus (PPH1) to chromosome 2q31-q32. *Circulation* 1997;95:2603–2606.

66. Deng Z, Morse J, Slager S, et al. Familial primary pulmonary hypertension (gene *PPH1*) is caused by mutations in the bone morphogenetic protein receptor-II gene. *Am J Hum Genet* 2000;67:737–774.

67. Machado RD, Pauciulo MW, Thomson JR, et al. BMPR2 haplo insufficiency as the inherited molecular mechanism for primary pulmonary hypertension. *Am J Hum Genet* 2001;68:92–102.

68. Trembath RC, Thomson JR, Machado RD, et al. Clinical and

molecular genetic features of pulmonary hypertension in patients with hereditary hemorrhagic telangiectasia. *N Engl J Med* 2001;345:325–334.

69. D'Alonzo G, Barst R, Ayres S, et al. Survival in patients with primary pulmonary hypertension. Results from a national prospective study. *Ann Int Med* 1991;115:343–349.

70. Asherson R, Cervera R. Review: antiphospholipid antibodies and the lung. *J Rheumatol* 1995;22:62–66.

71. Morelli S, Ferri C, Polettini E, et al. Plasma endothelin-1 levels, pulmonary hypertension, and lung fibrosis in patients with systemic sclerosis. *Am J Med* 1995;99:255–260.

72. Yoshio T, Masuyama JI, Sumiya M, et al. Antiendothelial cell antibodies and their relation to pulmonary hypertension in systemic lupus erythematosus. *J Rheumatol* 1994;21:2058–2063.

73. Stupi A, Steen V, Owens G, et al. Pulmonary hypertension in the CREST syndrome variant of systemic sclerosis. *Arthritis Rheum* 1986;29:515–524.

74. Macgregor A, Canavan R, Knight C, et al. Pulmonary hypertension in systemic sclerosis: risk factors for progression and consequences for survival. *Rheumatology* 2001;40:453–459.

75. Steen V, Graham G, Conte C, et al. Isolated diffusing capacity reduction in systemic sclerosis. *Arthritis Rheum* 1992;35:765–770.

76. Rozkovec A, Montanes P, Oakley CM. Factors that influence the outcome of primary pulmonary hypertension. *Br Heart J* 1986;55:449–458.

77. Weiner-Kronish J, Solinder A, Warnock M, et al. Severe pulmonary involvement in mixed connective tissue disease. *Am Rev Resp Dis* 1981;124:499–503.

78. Simonson J, Schiller N, Petri M, et al. Pulmonary hypertension in systemic lupus erythematosus. *J Rheumatol* 1989;16:918–925.

79. Winslow T, Ossipov M, Fazio G, et al. Five-year follow-up study of the prevalence and progression of pulmonary hypertension in systemic lupus erythematosus. *Am Heart J* 1995;129:510–515.

80. Alpert M, Pressly T, Mukerji V, et al. Acute and long-term effects of nifedipine on pulmonary and systemic hemodynamics in patients with pulmonary hypertension associated with diffuse systemic sclerosis, the CREST syndrome and mixed connective tissue disease. *Am J Cardiol* 1991;68:1687–1691.

81. Sfikakis P, Kyriakidis M, Vergos C, et al. Cardiopulmonary hemodynamics in systemic sclerosis and response to nifedipine and captopril. *Am J Med* 1991;90:541–546.

82. Williamson D, Hayward C, Rogers P, et al. Acute hemodynamic responses to inhaled nitric oxide in patients with limited scleroderma and isolated pulmonary hypertension. *Circulation* 1996;94:477–482.

83. Badesch D, Tapson V, McGoon M, et al. Continuous intravenous epoprostenol for pulmonary hypertension due to the scleroderma spectrum of disease. *Ann Int Med* 2000;132:425–434.

84. Robbins I, Gaine S, Schilz R, et al. Epoprostenol for treatment of pulmonary hypertension in patients with systemic lupus erythematosus. *Chest* 2000;117:14–18.

85. Olschewski H, Simonneau G, Galie N, et al. Inhaled iloprost for severe pulmonary hypertension. *N Engl J Med* 2002;347:322–329.

86. Simonneau G, Barst RJ, Galie N, et al. Continuous subcutaneous infusion of treprostinil, a prostacyclin analogue, in patients with pulmonary arterial hypertension: a double-blind, randomized, placebo-controlled trial. *Am J Respir Crit Care Med* 2002;165:800–804.

87. Rosenzweig E, Kerstein D, Barst R. Long-term prostacyclin for

pulmonary hypertension with associated congenital heart defects. *Circulation* 1999;99:1858–1865.

88. Hadengue A, Benhayoun M, Lebrec D, et al. Pulmonary hypertension complicating portal hypertension: prevalence and relation to splanchnic hemodynamics. *Gastroenterology* 1991;100:520–528.

89. Yang YY, Lin HC, Lee WC, et al. Portopulmonary hypertension: distinctive hemodynamic and clinical manifestations. *J Gastroenterol* 2001;36:181–186.

90. Kuo P, Plotkin J, Johnson L, et al. Distinctive clinical features f portopulmonary hypertension. *Chest* 1997;112:980–986.

91. Schott R, Chaouat A, Launoy A, et al. Improvement of pulmonary hypertension after liver transplantation. *Chest* 1999;115:1748–1749.

92. Kim K, Factor S. Membranoproliferative glomerulonephritis and plexogenic pulmonary arteriopathy in a homosexual with acquired immunodeficiency syndrome. *Hum Pathol* 1987;18:1293–1296.

93. Mehta N, Khan I, Mehta R, et al. HIV-related pulmonary hypertension. *Chest* 2000;118:1133–1141.

94. Speich R, Jenni R, Opravil M, et al. Primary pulmonary hypertension in HIV infection. *Chest* 1991;100:1268–1271.

95. Mette S, Palevsky H, Pietra G, et al. Primary pulmonary hypertension in association with human immunodeficiency virus infection: a possible viral etiology for some forms of hypertensive pulmonary arteriopathy. *Am Rev Resp Dis* 1992;145:1196–1200.

96. Panther L. How HIV infection and its treatment affects the cardiovascular system: what is known, what is needed. *Am J Physiol* 2002;283:H1–H4.

97. Petipretz P, Brenot F, Azarian R, et al. Pulmonary hypertension in patients with human immunodeficiency virus infection: comparison with primary pulmonary hypertension. *Chest* 1994;89:2722–2727.

98. Aguilar R, Farber H. Epoprostenol (prostacyclin) therapy in HIV-associated pulmonary hypertension. *Am J Resp Crit Care Med* 2000;162:1846–1850.

99. Gurtner H. Aminorex pulmonary hypertension. In: Fishman A, ed. *The pulmonary circulation: normal and abnormal.* Philadelphia: University of Pennsylvania Press, 1990.

100. Douglas J, Munro J, Kitchin A, et al. Pulmonary hypertension and fenfluramine. *Br Medical J* 1981;283:881–883.

101. Abenhaim L, Moride Y, Brenot F, et al. Appetite-suppressant drugs and the risk of primary pulmonary hypertension. *New Engl J Med* 1996;335:609–616.

102. Rich S, Rubin L, Walker A, et al. Anorexigens and pulmonary hypertension in the United States: results from the Surveillance of North American Pulmonary Hypertension. *Chest* 2000;117:870–874.

103. Humbert M, Nunes H, Sitbon O, et al. Risk factors for pulmonary arterial hypertension. In: Rich S, McLaughlin V, eds. *Clinics in chest medicine,* Vol. 22. Philadelphia: WB Saunders, 2001:459–475.

104. Gomez-Sanchez M, Calzada C, Gomez-Pajuelo C, et al. Clinical and pathologic manifestations of pulmonary vascular disease in the toxic oil syndrome. *J Am Coll Cardiol* 1991;18:1539–1545.

105. Gomez-Sanchez M, Juan MM, Gomez-Pajuelo C, et al. Pulmonary hypertension due to toxic oil syndrome: a clinicopathologic study. *Chest* 1989;95:325–331.

106. Walsh-Sukys M, Tyson J, Wright L, et al. Persistent pulmonary hypertension of the newborn in the era before nitric oxide: practice variation and outcomes. *Pediatrics* 2000;105:14–20.

107. Alano M, Ngougmna E, Ostrea E, et al. Analysis of nonsteroidal antiinflammatory drugs in meconium and its relation

of persistent pulmonary hypertension of the newborn. *Pediatrics* 2001;107:519–523.

108. Weinberger B, Weiss K, Heck D, et al. Pharmacologic therapy of persistent pulmonary hypertension of the newborn. *Pharmacol Ther* 2001;89:67–79.

109. Pearson D, Dawling S, Walsh W, et al. Neonatal pulmonary hypertension: urea-cycle intermediates, nitric oxide production, and carbamoyl-phosphate synthetase function. *New Engl J Med* 2001;344:1832–1838.

110. Clark R, Kueser T, Walker M, et al. Low-dose nitric oxide therapy for persistent pulmonary hypertension of the newborn. *New Engl J Med* 2000;342:469–474.

111. Moya M, Gow A, Califf R, et al. Inhaled ethyl nitrite gas for persistent pulmonary hypertension of the newborn. *Lancet* 2002;360:141–142.

112. Buch J, Wennevold A. Hazards of diazoxide in pulmonary hypertension. *Br Heart J* 1981;46:401–403.

113. Packer M, Medina N, Yushak M, et al. Detrimental effects of verapamil in patients with primary pulmonary hypertension. *Br Heart J* 1984;52:106–111.

114. Reeves JT, Groves BM, Turkevich D. The case for treatment of selected patients with primary pulmonary hypertension. *Am Rev Respir Dis* 1986;134:342–346.

115. Rubin LJ, Mendoza J, Hood M, et al. Treatment of primary pulmonary hypertension with continuous intravenous prostacyclin (epoprostenol): results of a randomized trial. *Ann Int Med* 1990;112:485–491.

116. Jones DK, Higenbottam TW, Wallwork J. Treatment of primary pulmonary hypertension intravenous epoprostenol (prostacyclin). *Br Heart J* 1987;57:270–278.

117. McLaughlin VV, Genthner DE, Panella MM, et al. Reduction in pulmonary vascular resistance with long-term epoprostenol (prostacyclin) therapy in primary pulmonary hypertension. *N Engl J Med* 1998;338:273–277.

118. Galie N, Humbert M, Vachiery JL, et al. Effects of beraprost sodium, an oral prostacyclin analogue, in patients with pulmonary arterial hypertension: a randomized, double-blind, placebo-controlled trial. *J Am Coll Cardiol* 2002;39:1496–1502.

119. Rubin LJ, Badesch DB, Barst RJ, et al. Bosentan therapy for pulmonary arterial hypertension. *N Engl J Med* 2002;346:896–903.

120. Barst R, Rich S, Widlitz A, et al. Clinical efficacy of sitaxsentan, an endothelin-A receptor antagonist, in patients with pulmonary arterial hypertension: open-label pilot study. *Chest* 2002;121:1860–1868.

121. Michelakis E, Tymchak W, Lien D, et al. Oral sildenafil is an effective and specific pulmonary vasodilator in patients with pulmonary arterial hypertension: comparison with inhaled nitric oxide. *Circulation* 2002;105:2398–2403.

122. Sitbon O, Brenot F, Denjean A, et al. Inhaled nitric oxide as a screening vasodilator agent in primary pulmonary hypertension: a dose-response study and comparison with prostacyclin. *Am J Respir Crit Care Med* 1995;151:384–389.

123. Channick RN, Newhart JW, Johnson FW, et al. Pulsed delivery of inhaled nitric oxide to patients with primary pulmonary hypertension: an ambulatory delivery system and initial clinical tests. *Chest* 1996;109:1545–1549.

124. Preston IR, Klinger JR, Landzberg MJ, et al. Vasoresponsiveness of sarcoidosis-associated pulmonary hypertension. *Chest* 2001; 120:866–872.

125. Wilkens H, Guth A, Konig J, et al. Effect of inhaled iloprost plus oral sildenafil in patients with primary pulmonary hypertension. *Circulation* 2001;104:1218–1222.

126. Rich S, Seidlitz M, Dodin E, et al. The short-term effects of digoxin in patients with right ventricular dysfunction from pulmonary hypertension. *Chest* 1998;114:787–792.

127. Rich S, Lam W. Atrial septostomy as palliative therapy for refractory primary pulmonary hypertension. *Am J Cardiol* 1983;51: 1560–1561.

128. Sandoval J, Rothman A, Pulido T. Atrial septostomy for pulmonary hypertension. *Clin Chest Med* 2001;22:547–560.

129. Sandoval J, Gaspar J, Pulido T, et al. Graded balloon dilation atrial septostomy in severe primary pulmonary hypertension: a therapeutic alternative for patients nonresponsive to vasodilator treatment. *J Am Coll Cardiol* 1998;32:297–304.

130. Trulock E. Lung transplantation for primary pulmonary hypertension. In: Rich S, McLaughlin V, eds. *Clinics in chest medicine,* Vol. 22. Philadelphia: WB Saunders, 2001:583–593.

131. Carabello B, Crawford F. Valvular heart disease. *New Engl J Med* 1997;337:32–41.

132. Umesan CV, Kapoor A, Sinha N, et al. Effect of Inoue balloon mitral valvotomy on severe pulmonary arterial hypertension in 315 patients with rheumatic mitral stenosis: immediate and long-term results. *J Heart Valve Dis* 2000;9:609–615.

133. Goodwin RA, Nickell JA, Des Prez RM. Mediastinal fibrosis complicating healed primary histoplasmosis and tuberculosis. *Medicine (Baltimore)* 1972;51:227–246.

134. Espinosa RE, Edwards WD, Rosenow EC 3rd, et al. Idiopathic pulmonary hilar fibrosis: an unusual cause of pulmonary hypertension. *Mayo Clin Proc* 1993;68:778–782.

135. Rholl KS, Levitt RG, Glazer HS. Magnetic resonance imaging of fibrosing mediastinitis. *AJR Am J Roentgenol* 1985;145:255–259.

136. Mandel J, Mark E, Hales C. Pulmonary veno-occlusive disease. *Am J Resp Crit Care Med* 2000;162:1964–1973.

137. Holcomb BW Jr, Loyd JE, Ely EW, et al. Pulmonary veno-occlusive disease: a case series and new observations. *Chest* 2000; 118:1671–1679.

138. Swensen SJ, Tashjian JH, Myers JL, et al. Pulmonary venoocclusive disease: CT findings in eight patients. *AJR Am J Roentgenol* 1996;167:937–940.

139. Traver G, Cline M, Burrows B. Predictors of mortality in chronic obstructive pulmonary disease: a 15-year follow-up study. *Am Rev Resp Dis* 1979;119:895–902.

140. Fraser K, Tullis E, Sasson Z, et al. Pulmonary hypertension and cardiac function in adult cystic fibrosis. Role of hypoxemia. *Chest* 1999;115:1321–1328.

141. Kessler R, Faller N, Weitzenblum E, et al. "Natural history" of pulmonary hypertension in a series of 131 patients with chronic obstructive lung disease. *Am J Resp Crit Care Med* 2001;164: 219–224.

142. Scharf A, Iqbal M, Keller C, et al. Hemodynamic characterization of patients with severe emphysema. *Am J Resp Crit Care Med* 2002;166:314–322.

143. Douglas N, Flenley D. Breathing during sleep in patients with obstructive lung disease. *Am Rev Resp Dis* 1990;141:1055–1070.

144. Enson Y, Thomas H, Bosken C, et al. Pulmonary hypertension in interstitial lung disease: relation of vascular resistance to abnormal lung structure. *Trans Assoc Am Physicians* 1975;88:248–255.

145. Olschewski H, Ghofrani H, Walmrath D, et al. Inhaled prostacyclin and iloprost in severe pulmonary hypertension secondary to lung fibrosis. *Am J Resp Crit Care Med* 1999;160:600–607.

146. Niijima M, Kimura H, Hidenori E, et al. Manifestation of pulmonary hypertension during REM sleep in obstructive sleep apnea syndrome. *Am J Resp Crit Care Med* 1999;159:1766–1772.

147. Chaouat A, Weitzenblum E, Krieger J, et al. Pulmonary

hemodynamics in the obstructive sleep apnea syndrome: results in 220 consecutive patients. *Chest* 1996;109:380–386.

148. Sajkov D, Wang T, Saunders N, et al. Daytime pulmonary hemodynamics in patients with obstructive sleep apnea without lung disease. *Am J Respir Crit Care Med* 1999;159:1518–1526.

149. Sajkov D, Wang T, Saunders N, et al. Continuous positive airway pressure treatment improves pulmonary hemodynamics in patients with obstructive sleep apnea. *Am J Resp Crit Care Med* 2002;165:152–158.

150. Bergofsky E. Respiratory failure in disorders of the thoracic cage. *Am Rev Resp Dis* 1979;119:643–669.

151. Kronenberg R, Safer P, Lee J, et al. Pulmonary artery pressure and gas exchange in man during acclimatization to 12,470 ft. *J Appl Physiol* 1971;50:827–837.

152. Groves B, Reeves J, Sutton J, et al. Operation Everest II: elevated high-altitude pulmonary resistance unresponsive to oxygen. *J Appl Physiol* 1987;63:521–530.

153. Naeije R. Pulmonary circulation at high altitude. *Respiration* 1997;64:429–434.

154. Groves B, Droma T, Sutton J, et al. Minimal hypoxic pulmonary hypertension in normal Tibetans at 3.658m. *J Appl Physiol* 1993;74:312–318.

155. Guiterrez C, Rodriguez A, Palenzuela S, et al. Congenital misalignment of pulmonary veins with alveolar capillary dysplasia causing persistent neonatal pulmonary hypertension: report of two affected siblings. *Pediatr Dev Pathol* 2000;3:271–276.

156. Fartoukh M, Humbert M, Capron F, et al. Severe pulmonary hypertension in histiocytosis X. *Am J Resp Crit Care Med* 2000;161:216–223.

157. Nocturnal Oxygen Therapy Trial Group. Continuous or nocturnal oxygen therapy in hypoxemic chronic obstructive lung disease: a clinical trial. *Ann Int Med* 1980;93:391–398.

158. Long-term domiciliary oxygen therapy complicating chronic bronchitis and emphysema: Report of the Medical Research Council Working Party. *The Lancet* 1981;1:681–685.

159. Moser KM, Auger WR, Fedullo PF. Chronic major-vessel thromboembolic pulmonary hypertension. *Circulation* 1990;81:1735–1743.

160. Ryan KL, Fedullo PF, Davis GB, et al. Perfusion scan findings understate the severity of angiographic and hemodynamic compromise in chronic thromboembolic pulmonary hypertension. *Chest* 1988;93:1180–1185.

161. Nicod P, Peterson K, Levine M, et al. Pulmonary angiography in severe chronic pulmonary hypertension. *Ann Int Med* 1987;107:565–568.

162. Hartz RS. Surgery for chronic thromboembolic pulmonary hypertension. *World J Surg* 1999;23:1137–1147.

163. Fedullo PF, Auger WR, Kerr KM, et al. Chronic thromboembolic pulmonary hypertension. *N Engl J Med* 2001;345:1465–1472.

164. Minter K, Gladwin M. Pulmonary complications of sickle cell anemia. *Am J Resp Crit Care Med* 2001;164:2016–2019.

165. Shorr A, Davies D, Nathan S. Outcomes for patients with sarcoidosis awaiting lung transplantation. *Chest* 2002;122:233–238.

166. Humbert M, Maitre S, Capron F, et al. Pulmonary edema complicating continuous intravenous prostacyclin in pulmonary capillary hemangiomatosis. *Am J Resp Crit Care Med* 1998;157:1681–1685.

167. Resten A, Maitre S, Humbert M, et al. Pulmonary arterial hypertension: thin section CT predictors of epoprostenol therapy failure. *Radiology* 2002;222:782–788.

Presentation and Diagnosis of Venous Thromboembolic Disease

36

Victor F. Tapson

The spectrum of venous thromboembolism (VTE) includes deep venous thrombosis (DVT) and pulmonary embolism (PE). This disease is responsible for substantial morbidity and mortality, including the need for recurrent hospitalization, chronic disabling postphlebitic syndrome, chronic thromboembolic pulmonary hypertension, and death from PE. It is often preventable, yet, is likely the most common cause of unexpected death in hospitalized patients. Most commonly, PE results from DVT that develops in the legs, but upper extremity thrombosis is common, particularly in patients with central venous catheters, and these clots may embolize also. PE is identified in at least one third of cases of VTE, and the risk of PE is higher in patients with proximal DVT than in patients with only calf-vein thrombosis (1).

Autopsy studies have repeatedly documented the high frequency with which PE has gone unsuspected and undetected (2). Although diagnostic technology and therapeutic approaches to VTE continue to advance, VTE remains underdiagnosed, and prophylaxis continues to be dramatically underutilized (3). Continued research in this area is essential. An awareness of the potential presenting manifestations of acute VTE and an understanding of appropriate diagnostic strategies are crucial in determining that VTE is present, so it can be managed appropriately. Risk factors are important to review both to optimize appropriate prophylaxis and to add in lowering the threshold for suspecting the diagnosis.

EPIDEMIOLOGY

From various sources using different diagnostic criteria, the annual incidence of VTE in the United States has been reported to be in the range of 125,000 to 400,000 cases an-

nually (4). However, case rates as high as 2 million per year have also been reported (5). Although DVT and, thus, PE are in large part preventable, PE is responsible for as many as 200,000 deaths in the United States every year (6). Patients dying from acute PE may have coexisting terminal illnesses, but it would appear that this disease entity is responsible for the deaths of 50,000 to 100,000 patients with an otherwise good prognosis each year in this country, with many of these deaths probably unnecessary (6). Hospitalized patients are frequently at risk because such individuals have underlying diseases that may increase the risk for VTE, and because they are immobilized to varying degrees, rendering them susceptible. The reason for hospital admission may be the primary focus of the medical or surgical team, and the potential risk and possible presence of VTE may not be appreciated and may not receive adequate attention. Outpatient medical care increasingly involves ill and complex patients, and the risk of VTE would appear to be potentially significant in this group as well.

Although VTE is common in the United States and Europe, it appears that it *may* occur less frequently in other areas in the world, such as parts of Africa and Asia (7).

A study conducted in west Africa (Cote D'Ivoire) suggested a prevalence of VTE of 9.5 per 100,000 in native Africans living there compared with 88 per 100,000 for Europeans living in the same region (8). In a prospective study of 313 patients undergoing major spinal surgery in Seoul, Korea, no prophylaxis was given and a screening ultrasound was performed between days 5 and 7. There was an overall incidence of thrombotic complications of 1.3% with an incidence of symptomatic VTE of 0.3% (9). However, it is known that the sensitivity of ultrasound is low in asymptomatic patients, and some cases may have been missed (10). In California, a very large discharge data set was utilized, and it was determined that the incidence of VTE in Asians and Pacific Islanders discharged from California hospitals

V. F. Tapson: Division of Pulmonary and Critical Care Medicine, Duke University Medical Center, Durham, North Carolina.

was lower than for the age-adjusted white population (11). Although the lower prevalence of factor V Leiden in these patients is one potential explanation for the lower rates, the incidence of idiopathic VTE in African American patients (also with lower incidence of factor V Leiden) was almost 30% higher than in whites, suggesting that another explanation may be needed. Other potential reasons for lower rates might include differences in diet, activity, comorbid disease, and obesity. Genetic differences and poorer access to diagnostic studies might also help to explain the lower incidence of VTE in certain African and Asian countries. Other potential differences in these populations might be higher levels of fibrinolytic activity, lower prothrombin activity, and lower platelet aggregability (12, 13). Interestingly, other recent data suggest that VTE rates could be higher than once suspected and/or increasing in Asia. A randomized trial of 320 Asian patients undergoing colorectal surgery in Singapore revealed a lower rate of postoperative DVT in patients receiving low-molecular-weight heparin prophylaxis compared with those receiving no prophylaxis (14). A postoperative study in Malaysia revealed an incidence of venographically proven DVT of 62.5% in patients after surgery for hip fracture or hip or knee replacement surgery, which is comparable to U.S. rates (15). These findings suggest that additional prophylaxis studies and a careful look at practices in Asian countries are warranted. Asian and African patients with compatible clinical presentations for VTE should undergo appropriate evaluation.

The morbidity and mortality from VTE events is high. In a 25-year, retrospective, one-county cohort study monitoring 2,218 people with DVT and/or PE, approximately 25% of patients died within 7 days of onset of VTE (16). Not surprisingly, early mortality was much higher in patients with PE than in patients with DVT alone. In this study, 36% of the patients with PE who died did so within 1 day of the event. In a hospital-based study in which 59 cases of PE were found in 404 autopsies (14.6%), PE was the direct cause of death in 20 cases; yet, the diagnosis was unsuspected in 14 of those 20 cases (17).

There are substantial long-term sequelae of undiagnosed and untreated (as well as treated) DVT, including postphlebitic syndrome and recurrent thromboembolic events. Postphlebitic syndrome can develop years after the occurrence of symptomatic DVT (18). The morbidity and cost of this entity are difficult to completely grasp but are substantial.

RISK FACTORS FOR VENOUS THROMBOEMBOLISM

Recognizing the risk factors for VTE offers several potential benefits. Their presence, together with compatible symptoms and signs, helps one *suspect* the diagnosis of DVT or PE, as well as helps one be critical in determining appropriate prophylaxis in patients at risk. The role of their presence

in lowering the diagnostic suspicion for VTE is our primary reason for emphasizing them here. Rudolf Virchow described the triad of stasis, venous injury, and hypercoagulability and its association with the development of venous thrombosis when he was 24 years old, nearly 150 years ago (19). This simple concept is perhaps one of the most enduring themes in medicine today, with essentially every risk factor for VTE being derived from this triad. The risk of VTE is significant in both medical and surgical patients, with most surgical scenarios entailing at least some risk of VTE.

One of the most obvious and easily recognized VTE risk factors is major surgery, particularly orthopedic surgery. Based on venographic studies, performed on patients not receiving prophylaxis, the prevalence of DVT at 7 to 14 days after total hip replacement, total knee replacement, and hip fracture surgery is about 50% to 60%, with proximal DVT rates of about 25%, 15% to 20%, and 30%, respectively (20). The leg undergoing the procedure is most commonly affected, but the other leg may be affected in a minority of cases. Patients undergoing other major surgery are also at risk, and associated underlying disease such as cancer may compound this risk. In patients with myocardial infarction, the risk of VTE appears to be approximately 24% in those not receiving antithrombotic treatment and about 55% in patients with lower limb paresis or paralysis (20). Hereditary and acquired thrombophilias increase the risk of VTE but are often not known to the clinician when a patient presents with VTE symptoms.

The presence of other moderate to high-risk conditions should also lower the threshold for considering DVT or PE. Pregnancy and the postpartum period are the most common settings in which women below age 40 develop DVT or PE, and are associated with a fivefold increase in risk (21). Thrombosis appears to be more common in the third trimester and postpartum, but the risk is clearly significant throughout pregnancy (21). Delivery by cesarean section further increases the risk. In patients with respiratory disease, congestive heart failure, or other medical illnesses (such as infection or rheumatic disease) admitted for treatment, the incidence of VTE without prophylaxis may be 15% (22) or higher.

With more serious illness and multiple risk factors, the incidence of VTE increases. In a study based in a medical intensive care unit, 33% of seriously ill patients screened with compression ultrasound had DVT (23). The risk of VTE is high in these patients because of underlying disease, immobility, and veno-invasive catheters and devices. In surgically and medically ill patients, the risk increases with the number of situational, patient-related, and disease-related risk factors present. One population-based epidemiologic study found that 99% of patients with diagnosed VTE had at least one risk factor, and more than 80% had three or more risk factors (24). These data reinforce the importance of identifying VTE risk factors. Results of another population-based case control study identified institutionalization itself as a risk factor; the incidence of VTE was eight times higher in patients confined to a hospital or nursing home than in community controls (25). The frequency with which medical and surgical patients who developed VTE had actually been on prophylaxis was suggested in a recent study involving 384 patients who developed DVT and/or PE while in the hospital or within 30 days after discharge (26). Of interest, more than half of the patients were on medical rather than surgical services: only 201 patients (52%) received prophylaxis and of the 183 patients who did not receive prophylaxis, 110 (60% of this subgroup) were medical patients. Compared with surgical patients, medical patients had a slightly higher risk of VTE but were less likely to receive VTE prophylaxis. The reduced mobility associated with medical illness likely imparts a significant risk for VTE. In addition, the relative immobilization associated with prolonged air travel places individuals at risk for VTE, with the travel distance correlating with the risk of VTE (27). Appropriate preventive approaches in various settings are discussed in Chapter 37.

TABLE 36.1. RISK FACTORS FOR VENOUS THROMBOEMBOLISM*

Clinical factors
Age greater than 40[†]
Prior history of venous thromboembolism
Major surgical procedure/trauma
Hip fracture
Immobilization/paralysis
Varicose veins
Congestive heart failure
Myocardial infarction
Obesity
Pregnancy/postpartum
Oral contraceptive therapy
Cerebrovascular accident
Cancer
Paroxysmal nocturnal hemoglobinemia
Acute medical illness with restricted mobility

Genetic/molecular factors
Antithrombin III deficiency
Factor V Leiden (activated protein C resistance)
Protein C deficiency
Protein S deficiency
Prothrombin gene (G20210A) defect
Heparin cofactor 2 deficiency
Dysfibrinogenemia
Disorders of plasminogen
Elevated factor VIII levels
Elevated factor XI levels
Hyperhomocysteinemia

Acquired factors
Antiphospholipid antibody syndrome
    Lupus anticoagulant
    Anticardiolipin antibodies
Myeloproliferative disease
Hyperhomocysteinemia

*The presence of risk factors may lower the threshold for considering the diagnosis of deep venous thrombosis or pulmonary embolism.
†Although the risk of venous thromboembolism begins to increase at approximately age 40, a more significant increase is noted after approximately age 70.

It is important to consider the diagnosis of DVT or PE in any patient with risk factors when the presenting (but often nonsensitive and nonspecific) symptoms and signs are consistent with these diagnoses. The presence of a lower extremity process, such as cellulitis, or a cardiopulmonary process, such as congestive heart failure or pneumonia, may appear to explain the symptoms and signs, but DVT or PE should still be *considered;* the clinician can determine the extent of evaluation, if any, that is necessary. Risk factors for VTE are listed in Table 36.1.

ACUTE PULMONARY EMBOLISM: THE PHYSIOLOGIC PROFILE

The physiological derangements in acute PE account for the clinical presentation. The severity of symptoms and signs caused by the emboli depend on the extent of obstructed pulmonary vasculature and on the presence or absence of underlying cardiopulmonary disease. Hypoxemia occurs in the majority of patients with PE, and this has been explained by different mechanisms. Ventilation-perfusion (V/Q) mismatch is the most likely general explanation in most cases. In the absence of previous cardiopulmonary disease, regions with low V/Q ratios and shunting secondary to perfusion of atelectatic areas serve as likely mechanisms of hypoxemia. Hypoxemia results in an increase in sympathetic tone with systemic vasoconstriction and an increase in venous return. With submassive emboli, this may actually augment cardiac output.

In patients with massive emboli, there are substantial hemodynamic implications, and these individuals may present with hypotension or sudden death. With such emboli, cardiac output is diminished but may be sustained as the mean right atrial pressure increases. As pulmonary vascular resistance increases, right ventricular outflow is impeded and left ventricular preload decreases. Without previous cardiopulmonary disease, embolic occlusion of 25% to 30% of the pulmonary vascular bed is associated with a rise in pulmonary artery pressure. With increasing obstruction, hypoxemia worsens, stimulating vasoconstriction and a further rise in pulmonary artery pressure. More than 50% obstruction of the pulmonary arterial bed is usually present before *substantial* elevation of the mean pulmonary artery pressure develops. When the extent of obstruction of the pulmonary circulation approaches 75%, the right ventricle must generate a systolic pressure in excess of 50 mm Hg and a mean pulmonary artery pressure of greater than 40 mm Hg to preserve pulmonary perfusion (28). The normal right ventricle cannot achieve this and fails. Patients with underlying cardiopulmonary disease are more inclined to experience more substantial deterioration in cardiac output than are normal individuals in the setting of massive PE. Although supportive measures may sustain a patient with massive PE, any additional increase in embolic load may be fatal.

DIAGNOSING VENOUS THROMBOEMBOLISM: PRELIMINARY TESTING

The key to the diagnosis of DVT and PE is *suspecting* the diagnosis. The diagnostic technology for acute DVT has evolved considerably with the development of convenient and inexpensive techniques such as compression ultrasound, as well as accurate yet more expensive diagnostic modalities such as magnetic resonance imaging (MRI). For PE, VQ scanning followed by pulmonary arteriography has been the gold-standard approach for decades. Spiral (helical) computed tomography (CT) scanning has been used increasingly and, in many hospitals, is the procedure of choice for suspected PE. The presence of risk factors, together with the history and physical examination, generally leads to further diagnostic testing in the setting of suspected VTE. A diagnostic algorithm for acute PE is presented in Figure 36.1.

History and Physical Examination

The clinical diagnosis of both DVT and PE based on the history and physical examination are, unfortunately, insensitive and nonspecific. A number of clinical studies have established that DVT cannot be reliably diagnosed based on the history and physical examination, even in high-risk patients (29, 30). Patients with DVT may or may not experience erythema, warmth, pain, swelling, or tenderness. Homans' sign (pain with dorsiflexion of the foot) is neither sensitive nor specific for DVT. When five clinical studies were compared, the sensitivity of calf pain for acute DVT varied from 66% to 91%; the specificity, from 3% to 87% (29). In six studies that included evaluation for calf tenderness, the range for sensitivity was 56% to 82%, with the range for specificity 26% to 74%. For Homans' sign, the sensitivity varied from 13% to 48%; the specificity, from 39% to 84% (30). The presence of swelling of the calf or leg was also inconsistent, with the sensitivity ranging from 35% to 97%; the specificity, from 8% to 88% (31). When present however, these findings merit further evaluation despite their lack of specificity. It should be stressed that *the clinical evaluation may imply the need for further evaluation but cannot, by itself, be relied on to confirm or exclude the diagnosis of DVT.*

PE should always be considered whenever unexplained dyspnea is present. Dyspnea, pleuritic chest pain, and hemoptysis are common in PE but, again, are nonspecific. Anxiety, lightheadedness, and syncope are all symptoms that

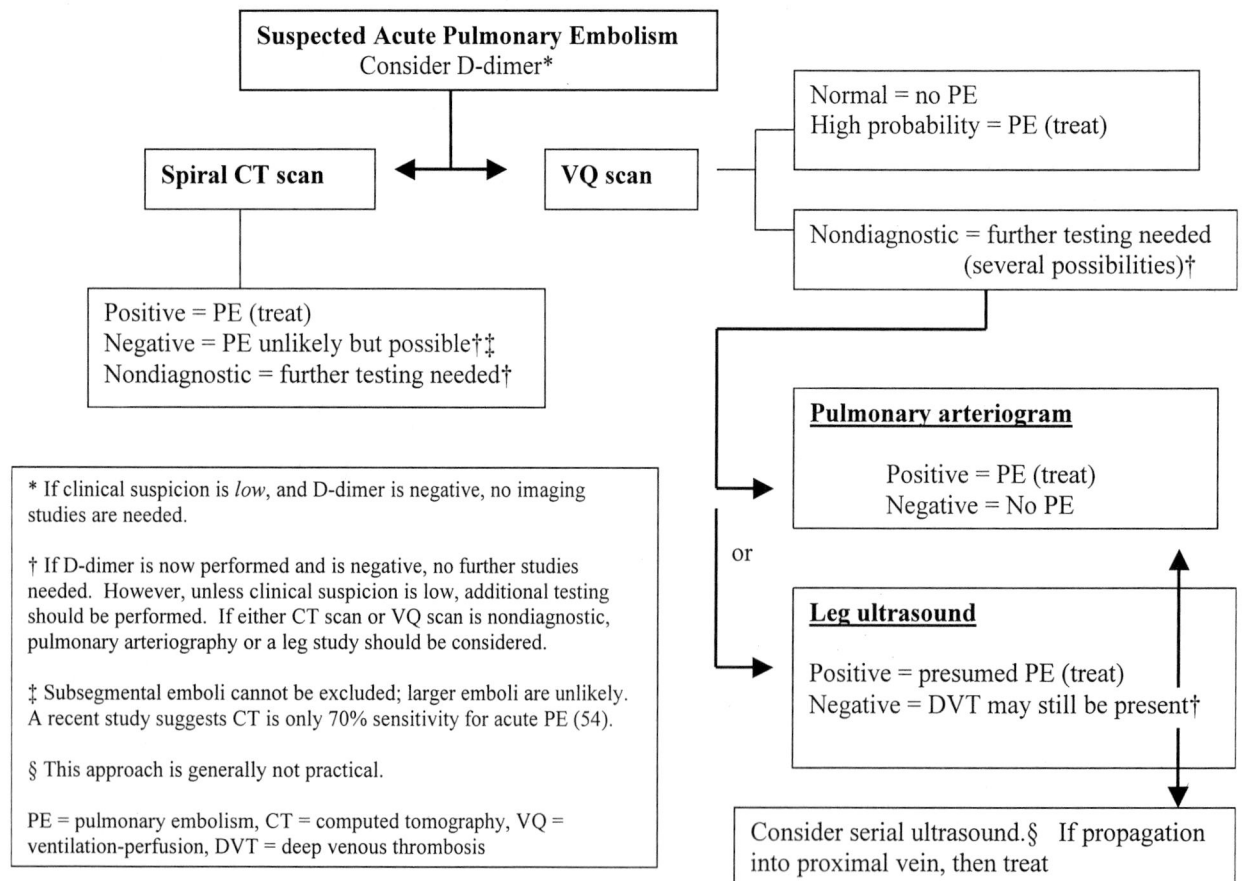

FIGURE 36.1. Algorithm for the diagnostic approach to suspected acute pulmonary embolism.

may be caused by PE but may also result from a number of other disorders that result in hypoxemia or hypotension. Tachypnea and tachycardia are the most common signs of PE but are also nonspecific. PE should always be considered with syncope or sudden hypotension. The cardiac and pulmonary physical examinations are both nonspecific. The index of clinical suspicion does, however, become a more useful parameter when considered in conjunction with V/Q scanning (32). Diagnostic efforts directed at possible PE may be appropriate, despite alternative explanations if risk factors and the clinical setting are suggestive. Dyspnea, tachypnea, clear lung fields, and hypoxemia may be attributed to a flare of chronic obstructive lung disease or asthma when underlying PE is present.

A subset of patients from the Prospective Investigation of Pulmonary Embolism Diagnosis (PIOPED) (32, 33) without preexisting cardiac or pulmonary disease were evaluated in order to determine the frequency of clinical characteristics in patients owing to PE alone. The history, physical examination, chest radiograph, electrocardiogram, and blood gases were evaluated in these individuals. Acute PE was present in 117 patients, and PE was excluded in 248 patients. Among the patients with PE, either dyspnea or tachypnea (respiratory rate, >20 breaths/min) was present in 105 of 117 (90%). Either dyspnea, hemoptysis, or pleuritic pain was present in 107 of 117 (91%). Dyspnea, tachypnea, or pleuritic pain was present in 113 of 117 (97%). Thus, among the patients with PE that were identified, it was a relatively small percentage that did not have at least one of these important manifestations or a combination of them. Clinical evaluation, although nonspecific, is of considerable value in the selection of patients in whom there is a need for further diagnostic studies. Symptoms and signs of acute PE and their frequency based on the Prospective Investigation of Pulmonary Embolism Diagnosis (PIOPED) study are presented in Tables 36.2 and 36.3. The frequency of specific symptoms and signs were similar whether underlying cardiopulmonary disease was present or not, although it is feasible that their severity may vary.

TABLE 36.2. ACUTE PULMONARY EMBOLISM: SYMPTOMS

	All Patients	No Previous Cardiopulmonary Disease
	(n = 383)	(n = 117)
Dyspnea	78%	73%
Pleuritic chest pain	59%	66%
Cough	43%	37%
Leg pain	27%	26%
Hemoptysis	16%	13%
Palpitations	13%	10%
Wheezing	14%	9%
Angina-like pain	6%	4%

From the Prospective Investigation of Pulmonary Embolism Diagnosis [PIOPED] study [32, 33] and modified from Stein PD, ed. *Pulmonary embolism.* Baltimore: Williams & Wilkins, 1996.

TABLE 36.3. ACUTE PULMONARY EMBOLISM: SIGNS

	All Patients	No Previous Cardiopulmonary Disease
	(n = 383)	(n = 117)
Tachypnea (20/min)	73%	70%
Crackles	55%	51%
Tachycardia (>100/min)	30%	30%
Leg swelling	31%	28%
Loud P2	23%	23%
Deep venous thrombosis	15%	11%
Wheezes	11%	5%
Diaphoresis	10%	11%
Temperature (≥38.5)	7%	7%
Pleural rub	4%	3%
Fourth heart sound	—	24%
Third heart sound	5%	3%
Cyanosis	3%	1%
Homans' sign	3%	4%
Right ventricular lift	—	4%

From the PIOPED study [32, 33] and modified from Stein PD, ed. *Pulmonary embolism.* Baltimore: Williams & Wilkins, 1996.

Chest Radiography

Radiographic imaging is essential for the objective diagnosis of DVT and PE. Most patients with PE have an abnormal but nonspecific chest radiograph. Common radiographic findings include atelectasis, pleural effusion, pulmonary infiltrates, and mild elevation of a hemidiaphragm. Classic findings of pulmonary infarction such as Hampton hump or decreased vascularity (Westermark sign) may suggest the diagnosis, but they are infrequent. A normal chest radiograph in the setting of severe dyspnea and hypoxemia without evidence of bronchospasm or anatomic cardiac shunt is strongly suggestive of PE. Under most circumstances, however, the chest radiograph cannot be used to conclusively diagnose or exclude PE. Other processes such as pneumonia, congestive heart failure, pneumothorax, or rib fracture may cause symptoms similar to those of acute PE and should be considered, but the confirmed presence of musculoskeletal or cardiopulmonary disease does not necessarily *exclude* the possibility of acute PE. In the PIOPED study (32), the chest radiograph was abnormal in 98 of 117 (84%) patients, with atelectasis and/or pulmonary parenchymal abnormalities being the most common abnormalities, occurring in 79 of 117 (68%) individuals. Either dyspnea, tachypnea, pleuritic pain, atelectasis, or a parenchymal abnormality on the chest radiograph was present in 115 of 117 (98%).

Electrocardiography

The electrocardiogram cannot be relied on for the diagnosis of acute PE. Findings in acute PE are generally nonspecific and include T-wave changes, ST-segment abnormalities, and left- or right-axis deviation. In the Urokinase Pulmonary Embolism Trial (UPET), electrocardiographic abnormalities were demonstrated in 87% of patients with proven PE without underlying cardiac or pulmonary disease (34). These findings were not specific for PE, however. Even with massive or submassive PE, manifestations of acute cor pulmonale such as the $S_1Q_3T_3$ pattern, right bundle-branch block, P-wave pulmonale, or right-axis deviation only occurred in 26% of patients. The low frequency of specific electrogram changes associated with PE was confirmed in the PIOPED study (32). Nonspecific ST-segment or T-wave change was the most common electrocardiographic abnormality and was noted in 44 of 89 (49%) patients.

Arterial Blood Gas Analysis

Hypoxemia is common in acute PE. Certain individuals, particularly young patients without underlying lung disease, may have a normal arterial blood partial pressure of oxygen (PaO_2). In the PIOPED subset of patients suspected of PE without preexisting cardiopulmonary disease, the PaO_2 and alveolar-arterial difference values were compared (33). Interestingly, patients with and without PE could not be distinguished based upon either of these values. However, the alveolar-arterial difference was increased by more than 20 mm Hg in 76 of 88 (86%) patients with PE. In a retrospective study of hospitalized patients with PE, the PaO_2 was greater than 80 mm Hg in 29% of patients less than 40 years old, compared with 3% in the older group (35). The alveolar-arterial difference was elevated in all patients, that is, the partial pressure of arterial carbon dioxide ($PaCO_2$) was usually low. The diagnosis of acute PE cannot be excluded based on a normal PaO_2, and although the alveolar-arterial difference is usually elevated, it may rarely be normal in patients without preexisting cardiopulmonary disease. It is important to realize that an *elevated* $PaCO_2$ (caused, e.g., by preexisting lung disease or metabolic alkalosis), does *not* rule out the possibility of acute PE!

D-Dimer Testing

D-dimer represents a specific derivative of cross-linked fibrin, and has been extensively evaluated in the setting of suspected acute DVT and PE. A normal enzyme-linked immunosorbent assay appears sensitive in excluding PE. When a positive D-dimer level is considered to be 500 μg/L or greater, the sensitivity and specificity for PE have been shown to be 98% and 39%, respectively (36). Unfortunately, many clinical settings in addition to acute thromboembolism are associated with an elevated D-dimer level. Thus, although the sensitivity of the D-dimer appears high, the specificity is not high enough to be diagnostic.

A negative D-dimer assay together with a respiratory rate of less than 20 breaths/min, and a PaO_2 greater than 80 mm Hg, has proven to be very sensitive in ruling out acute PE (37). Neither symptoms, signs, radiographic findings, electrocardiography, nor the plasma D-dimer measurement can

be considered diagnostic of PE or DVT, and when these entities are suspected, further evaluation with noninvasive or invasive testing is necessary. A recent exhaustive review of the various D-dimer assays and clinical trial results reinforces the above findings (38). Finally, the use of clinical probability scores based on certain simple clinical parameters have been used together with a negative SimpliRED D-dimer test (a rapid red blood cell agglutination D-dimer assay), to help to exclude PE. In a recent prospective clinical trial, the SimpliRED assay was used together with a simple scoring system using scoring parameters that were readily available in the emergency department (39). PE was considered excluded if the patient had been assigned a low clinical pretest probability and had a negative result on D-dimer testing; no imaging procedures were performed in these patients. The physician assigned points for the following: clinical signs and symptoms of DVT, 3.0 points; heart rate greater than 100 beats/min, 1.5 points; immobilization or surgery in the previous 4 weeks, 1.5 points; previous diagnosed DVT or PE, 1.5 points; hemoptysis, 1.0 point; malignancy, 1.0 point; and PE as likely as or more likely than an alternative diagnosis, 3.0 points. For the latter variable, physicians were told to use the clinical information, along with results on chest radiography, electrocardiography, and laboratory tests ordered. The pretest probability of PE was considered low in patients whose score was less than 2.0, moderate if the score was 2.0 to 6.0, and high if greater than 6.0. Of the 437 patients with a negative D-dimer result and low clinical probability, only one developed PE during follow-up; thus, the negative predictive value for the combined strategy of using the clinical model with D-dimer testing in these patients was 99.5%. Another recent study used a different clinical probability prediction score without including the D-dimer (40). This score was based on eight variables, including recent surgery, previous VTE, older age, hypocapnia, hypoxemia, tachycardia, band atelectasis, or elevation of a hemidiaphragm on the chest radiograph. A total of 486 patients (49%) had a low clinical probability of PE, of whom 50 (10.3%) had proven PE. The prevalence of PE was 38% in the 437 patients with an intermediate probability and 81% in the 63 patients with a high probability (40). Although scoring systems appear useful in characterizing patients with suspected PE, they have not yet been used widely in clinical practice.

Different D-dimer assays have been compared in head-to-head studies. In one recent trial, three rapid D-dimer methods were compared in patients with suspected VTE (41). The three D-dimer methods compared were the Accuclot D-dimer, the IL-test D-dimer, and the SimpliRED D-dimer. Of 993 patients, 141 had objectively confirmed DVT or PE. The sensitivity of SimpliRED, Accuclot, and IL-test were 79%, 90%, and 87%, respectively. The three assays gave similar negative predictive values. When combined with pretest probability, all three methods appeared acceptable for use in the diagnosis of VTE.

D-DIMER FOR DIAGNOSIS OF DEEP VENOUS THROMBOSIS/PULMONARY EMBOLISM	
Summary Recommendation	**Level of Evidence**
D-dimer has moderate to good sensitivity but low specificity.	Multiple observational
Test predictive values may be enhanced by combination with common clinical parameters of deep venous thrombosis/pulmonary embolism.	Limited observational study

Cardiac Troponin

Patients with PE sometimes have positive troponin levels. Troponin elevation is specific for cardiac myocyte damage, and the right ventricle appears to be the source of the enzyme elevation in acute PE. Not surprisingly, both cardiac troponin T and troponin I levels have been found to be elevated in acute PE and, in particular, in more massive PE, in which myocyte injury owing to right ventricular strain might be expected. Several studies have suggested that troponin levels may be elevated in acute PE (42–46), and a recent investigation suggested that an elevated level might aid in prognosticating (45). In this study of 38 patients with acute PE, 18 (47%) had elevated cardiac troponin I levels. Of the 18 patients, 12 (67%) had right ventricular dilation/hypokinesis compared with only three of 20 patients (15%) without elevation of cardiac troponin I ($P = .004$). Furthermore, cardiac troponin I–positive patients had significantly higher right ventricular systolic pressures, as well as having a higher chance of developing cardiogenic shock (33% versus 5%, $P = .01$). The odds ratio for the latter was 8.8 (confidence interval, 2.5–21). This information supports earlier data suggesting that cardiac troponin levels are often elevated in acute PE, and although the elevations may occur with smaller PE, they are more common with more massive PE and may be associated with a poorer prognosis. Troponin levels cannot, however, be used like D-dimer testing; i.e., they are not sensitive enough to rule out PE when clinical suspicion is relatively low, without additional diagnostic testing. Despite the above data, however, at present, perhaps the most important aspect of elevated cardiac troponin levels lies in the fact that in a clinically compatible setting, an elevated value might serve as a clue to the diagnosis of PE and result in the diagnosis being pursued.

ACUTE PULMONARY EMBOLISM: SPECIFIC IMAGING STUDIES

Ventilation-Perfusion Scanning and Pulmonary Arteriography

At present, spiral CT scanning and V/Q scanning are the most common specific diagnostic tests used for suspected PE. When the V/Q scan is the initial diagnostic test, and the perfusion scan is normal, the diagnosis of PE is excluded. A high-probability V/Q scan in the setting of clinical suspicion for acute PE is considered diagnostic. Previous PE or chronic PE patients may also have high-probability scans so that the clinical picture is important to consider. Unfortunately, low or intermediate probability (nondiagnostic) scans are commonly found with PE. In the PIOPED study, the utility of V/Q scanning combined with clinical assessment of patients with suspected PE was prospectively evaluated (32). Patients with PE had scans that were high, intermediate, or low probability, but so did most patients without PE. Although the specificity of high-probability scans was 97%, the sensitivity was only 41%. Of interest, 33% of patients with intermediate-probability scans and 12% of patients with low-probability scans were diagnosed definitively with PE by pulmonary arteriography. When the clinical suspicion of PE was considered very high, PE was found to be present in 96% of patients with high-probability scans, 66% of patients with intermediate-probability scans, and 40% of patients with low-probability scans. The diagnosis of PE should be rigorously pursued even when the lung scan is of low or intermediate probability if the clinical scenario suggests PE.

Several potential diagnostic pathways may be appropriate after a nondiagnostic V/Q scan. The gold-standard test (pulmonary arteriography) can be considered, and a nondiagnostic V/Q scan may help guide the arteriogram, limiting the time and amount of contrast required. Arteriography is safe in experienced hands. Another consideration is to do lower extremity studies. If, in the setting of a nondiagnostic V/Q scan, an ultrasound is performed and is positive, no additional studies are needed. When the ultrasound is negative, PE cannot, however, be definitively ruled out because the ultrasound is not sensitive enough when there are no DVT symptoms or signs on exam. Although a negative D-dimer suggests the absence of VTE, additional imaging should be performed when the clinical setting suggests that PE is likely. Another possibility that is sometimes considered, is to perform a contrast-enhanced spiral CT scan. The spiral CT scan is usually ordered as an initial diagnostic test but may sometimes be positive in the face of a nondiagnostic V/Q scan. The specificity and sensitivity of spiral CT are discussed below.

Spiral (Helical) Computed Tomography Scanning

The use of CT scanning for suspected PE has increased significantly over the past decade. A contrast bolus is required for vascular imaging. Spiral CT may reveal emboli in the main, lobar, or segmental pulmonary arteries, with more than 90% sensitivity and specificity. With CT, three-dimensional reconstruction techniques (multiplanar reformation) can be applied to the opacified pulmonary vasculature to better define vessels located within the plane that has been sectioned. Examples of bilateral, central emboli imaged by spiral CT are shown in Figure 36.2. Goodman and colleagues (47) have strongly endorsed the incorporation of CT scanning into diagnostic algorithms for PE. Studies evaluating spiral CT to determine sensitivity and specificity for acute PE have revealed a range of 53% to 100% and 81% to 97%, respectively, for these parameters (48–54). Different study designs, exclusion criteria, levels of experience, and reading protocols have accounted for some of the differences, and most have had readers consider abnormalities proximal to and including the segmental level.

Although some of the studies have been encouraging, others have been less reassuring (53, 54). One recent large, prospective spiral CT study from Switzerland suggested a lower sensitivity for acute PE than given for most previous studies (54). Patients were excluded if they had a negative D-dimer result or contraindications to intravenous contrast. Of the patients enrolled, 118 (39%) had acute PE, and in

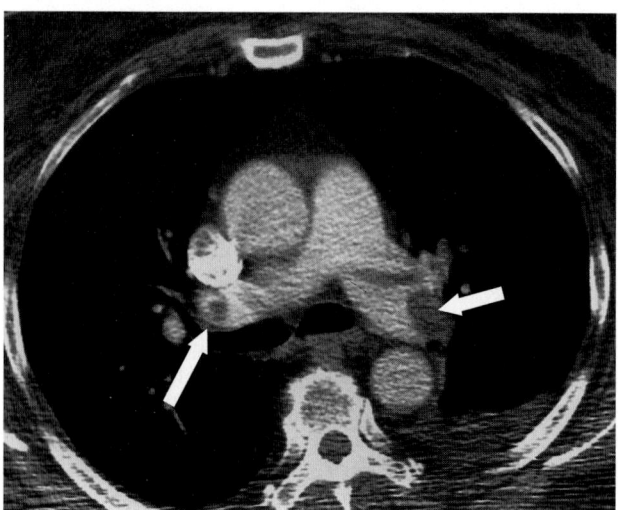

FIGURE 36.2. Bilateral pulmonary embolism *(arrows)* demonstrated by contrast-enhanced spiral computed tomography scan.

12 patients (4%; two with PE), the results of spiral CT were inconclusive. The sensitivity for CT for acute PE was 70%. Results such as this suggest that a negative CT does not exclude all PE, but it would still appear unlikely that large emboli would be missed. The sensitivity for PE in smaller (subsegmental) vessels remains suboptimal, and the importance of such small emboli also creates controversy. A potential concern might be a patient with small, undiscovered subsegmental emboli in whom silent DVT might be present. Not treating such a patient could result in recurrent PE or possibly contribute to the development of postphlebitic syndrome. Thus, considering leg studies in a patient with high clinical suspicion for acute PE and a negative CT would appear prudent. In a prospective study of patients with suspected PE, a negative chest CT, and negative ultrasound of the legs, the outcome was quite good without a significant number of recurrences (55). Thus, perhaps a better measure of the usefulness of a diagnostic technique is whether or not it misses *clinically important* events. A recent study, albeit retrospective, evaluated the clinical outcome of a cohort of 1,512 consecutive patients referred for suspected PE who underwent electron-beam CT (56). Of these patients, 1,010 (67%) had CT scans that were negative for PE. Because 17 patients received anticoagulation, they were excluded. Although 118 of the 993 died, only three died of PE. The 3-month cumulative incidence of overall DVT or PE was 0.5%; of fatal PE, 0.3%. The telephone interviews and mailed questionnaires failed to determine whether or not 19 patients had VTE, but these 19 were known to be alive. This suggests that a negative electron-beam CT scan, *at least in the hands of these investigators/readers,* was very sensitive for acute PE. More long-term problems such as postphlebitic syndrome or chronic thromboembolic pulmonary hypertension might not be detected in such a study.

An important advantage of spiral CT over V/Q scanning in suspected PE is the concomitant ability to define nonvascular pathology such as musculoskeletal abnormalities, airway pathology, lymphadenopathy, lung tumors, and other parenchymal abnormalities, as well as pleural and pericardial disease. In a recent clinical study, the use of CT scanning for suspected PE resulted in 31 new diagnoses other than PE (57). These included diagnoses such as aspiration pneumonia, pulmonary edema, lung cancer, esophageal cancer, and invasive aspergillosis; entities that could not be diagnosed by V/Q scan. Spiral CT scans read as nondiagnostic for PE are much less common than are nondiagnostic V/Q scans; the rate of nondiagnostic CT scans has been reported as 10%, with 4% reported as technically inadequate (58). The most common relative contraindications to performing contrast-enhanced spiral CT scanning are renal insufficiency and allergy to contrast material. The cost-effectiveness of using spiral CT scanning for suspected PE has been studied. The optimal approach remains to be determined, but it would appear that because of the frequency of nondiagnostic V/Q scans, the inclusion of spiral CT scanning may prove to reduce cost.

TABLE 36.4. ADVANTAGES AND LIMITATIONS OF SPIRAL COMPUTED TOMOGRAPHY (CT) SCANNING FOR THE DIAGNOSIS OF ACUTE PULMONARY EMBOLISM

Advantages
   Availability
   Sensitivity for central emboli*
   Specificity*
   Relative rapidity of procedure
   Diagnosis of other disease entities
   Multiplanar reformation (three dimensions)
   Safety
   Advancing technology
   Nondiagnostic readings unusual[†]
   Potential for CT venography
Limitations
   Intravenous contrast required
   Reader expertise required
   Not portable
   Morbid obesity may prevent scanning
Relative contraindications
   Renal insufficiency[‡]
   Contrast allergy

*In clinical trials to date, high sensitivity and specificity have been limited to emboli in the main, lobar, and segmental vessels. Sensitivity is inadequate for subsegmental vessels.
[†]CT scans are read as nondiagnostic in approximately 10% of cases (much lower than for ventilation-perfusion scans).
[‡]Mild renal insufficiency is not a contraindication.

Additional prospective, randomized, clinical trials comparing CT scanning with the standard diagnostic approach to PE are currently underway. In the PIOPED II, sponsored by the National Institutes of Health, more than 1,000 patients with suspected PE are undergoing V/Q scanning, spiral CT, lower extremity ultrasound, and pulmonary arteriography to better assess the appropriate role of the latter modality. A key component of this study is to evaluate the sensitivity and specificity of CT venography. Previous studies suggest the potential for diagnosing either DVT, PE, or both with one contrast injection (60). Advantages and limitations of spiral CT scanning for suspected acute PE are listed in Table 36.4.

SPIRAL COMPUTED TOMOGRAPHY OF CHEST FOR DIAGNOSIS OF PULMONARY EMBOLISM

Summary Recommendation	Level of Evidence
High sensitivity/specificity for main, lobar, and segmental vessels; inadequate sensitivity for subsegmental vessels	Nonrandomized and observational studies
If spiral computed tomography used and negative, addition of negative leg or D-dimer studies adds to negative predictive value for clinically significant pulmonary embolism.	Nonrandomized and observational studies

Magnetic Resonance Imaging

MRI has been used to evaluate clinically suspected PE (51, 61, 62). Although this technique has several potential advantages, including excellent sensitivity and specificity for the diagnosis of DVT (63), potentially allowing simultaneous accurate detection of both PE and DVT, it is often a difficult technique for critically ill patients with respiratory distress to tolerate.

Echocardiography

Other diagnostic techniques sometimes prove useful particularly in the setting of massive PE. Echocardiography, which can often be obtained more rapidly than either lung scanning or pulmonary arteriography, may reveal findings that strongly support hemodynamically significant PE (64). Unfortunately, because patients with PE often have underlying cardiopulmonary disease such as COPD, neither right ventricular dilation nor hypokinesis can be reliably used as indirect evidence of PE in such settings. Direct visualization of massive PE may occasionally be possible, particularly if transesophageal echocardiography is performed. Echocardiography is sometimes used to gauge the extent of right ventricular dysfunction in the setting of proven acute PE (see treatment chapter) (65). Intravascular ultrasound has been used to directly visualize acute PE at the bedside (66). Although this technique appears sensitive for more proximal emboli, it has not achieved widespread use.

MASSIVE PULMONARY EMBOLISM: DIAGNOSTIC CONSIDERATIONS

The presence of suspected massive PE presents both difficulties and potential diagnostic advantages (67). When patients present severely ill with extreme hypoxemia and/or hypotension, the diagnostic evaluation must be performed as quickly as possible. Critically ill patients may be difficult to transport to the radiology department. Portable perfusion scanning may be useful in such individuals because the chances for a diagnostic (high probability) scan are likely to be higher with more massive PE. Similarly, it would be exceedingly unlikely for CT scanning to be negative in the setting of massive PE; larger, more proximal emboli are more likely. Echocardiography would be even more likely to reveal dramatic right ventricular dilation and dysfunction, which in the absence of other potential causes would suggest the possibility of acute PE. Potential therapeutic implications of such findings will be discussed in the chapter on management.

ACUTE DEEP VENOUS THROMBOSIS: SPECIFIC IMAGING STUDIES

As with acute PE, the diagnosis of acute DVT relies upon objective testing. Compression ultrasound is by far the most

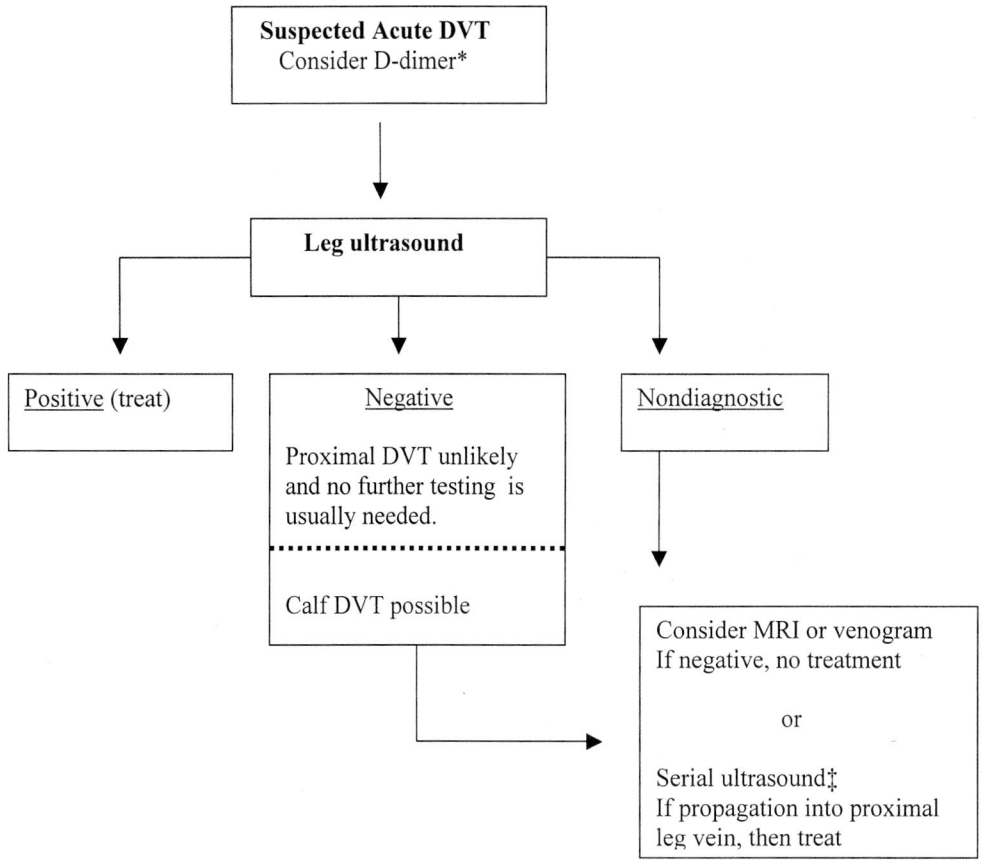

FIGURE 36.3. Algorithm for the diagnostic approach to suspected acute deep venous thrombosis.
*If clinical suspicion is low, and D-dimer is negative, no imaging study needed.
‡Over 7 to 10 days.

common technique used in the setting of suspected DVT. Impedance plethysmography has been studied extensively, and although sensitive for acute proximal DVT, ultrasound has essentially replaced it. It will not be discussed here. An algorithm for the approach to suspected acute DVT is presented in Figure 36.3.

Compression Ultrasound

Although visualization of thrombosis is sometimes possible and although color flow may aid in characterizing abnormal flow, the diagnosis of DVT by the ultrasound technique relies primarily on the lack of compressibility of a thrombosed venous segment. More than a decade ago, the sensitivity and specificity of compression ultrasound for symptomatic proximal DVT proved to be well above 90% (68–70). Innumerable subsequent trials verified this (68). Limitations were also recognized, including the insensitivity for asymptomatic DVT, operator dependence, difficulty in accurately distinguishing acute from chronic DVT in symptomatic patients, and the insensitivity for calf vein thrombosis (71, 72). Certain patient factors such as plaster casts or morbid obesity may affect the sensitivity and ability to visualize the

deep veins. A prospective evaluation of the utility of bilateral color Doppler ultrasound in asymptomatic high-risk (elective unilateral hip or knee replacement) patients revealed that ultrasound was only 38% sensitive for proximal DVT using contrast venography as the diagnostic standard (73). Compared with other technology, it is relatively inexpensive and is the preferred diagnostic modality for straight-forward cases of symptomatic suspected proximal DVT. One approach that has been successfully scientifically tested is that of serial ultrasonography when the initial study is negative in a symptomatic patient (74). Although the rate of VTE with follow-up over 3 months has been exceedingly low, this approach is less than ideal, particularly in outpatients, because of difficulty getting patients to return for serial studies.

Upper extremity thrombosis is common in critically ill or cancer patients and is most frequently related to a central venous catheter. Other settings include compression or invasion by local or metastatic neoplasm, transvenous pacemaker, or effort-induced thrombosis. Each can generally be diagnosed by compression ultrasound and can also result in acute PE (75, 76). Effort-induced (primary subclavian vein) upper extremity thrombosis (Paget-Schroetter syndrome) often affects young, healthy active people and may recur

(77, 78). An exhaustive review of clinical trials examining the sensitivity and specificity of ultrasound techniques for suspected acute DVT is provided in the American Thoracic Society consensus statement on the diagnostic approach to acute venous thromboembolism (68).

Contrast Venography

Contrast venography remains the gold-standard technique for the diagnosis of DVT, but it has been much less commonly performed since the advent of ultrasonography. Although ultrasound has excellent sensitivity for proximal DVT in patients with symptomatic suspected DVT, it is clearly less sensitive than is venography for calf DVT. Venography is an option when noninvasive testing is nondiagnostic or impossible to perform. It is an invasive procedure that may result in superficial phlebitis or hypersensitivity reactions, but it is generally safe and accurate (37).

Magnetic Resonance Imaging and Computed Tomography

MRI is being increasingly used to diagnose DVT and appears to be an accurate noninvasive alternative to venography (63, 79). A major advantage of this technique is the excellent resolution of the inferior vena cava and pelvic veins. Preliminary experience with this technique suggests that it is at least as accurate as contrast venography or ultrasound imaging for proximal DVT and is perhaps more sensitive than either for pelvic vein thrombosis. It offers the opportunity for simultaneous bilateral lower extremity imaging, and it may accurately distinguish acute from chronic DVT (63, 79). However, this technique is not widely used for diagnosing DVT, and as is the case with PE, MRI radiologists with experience are instrumental in maximizing accuracy. Although there are less data evaluating the sensitivity of MRI for calf DVT, a sensitivity of 87% was demonstrated in one prospective study, suggesting that venography may be superior for this location (80). An MRI revealing extensive thrombosis in the iliac vein extending into the inferior vena cava is shown in Figure 36.4.

Finally, spiral CT scanning has been studied for suspected acute DVT. The contrast dye from the bolus injected for lung imaging is followed into the deep veins of the legs for viewing. Initial data are promising (60), and the utility of "CT venography" will be further studied in PIOPED II. These techniques may fit into diagnostic algorithms for DVT and PE, but these algorithms are institution-specific at present, depending on resources and expertise with certain techniques. When a patient with suspected PE has a nondiagnostic lung study and lower extremity imaging is pursued, ultrasound is the most common diagnostic modality used. Although lower extremity MRI might be more sensitive, it has not been prospectively compared in the setting of suspected PE.

DIAGNOSIS OF DEEP VENOUS THROMBOSIS	
Summary Recommendation	**Level of Evidence**
DVT cannot be reliably diagnosed by history and physical examination (they may imply need for further testing).	Multiple observational studies
Compression ultrasound is highly sensitive/specific for symptomatic proximal DVT but has lower sensitivity for asymptomatic DVT.	Multiple observational studies
Contrast venography remains most sensitive test for proximal and distal (calf) DVT but may have limitations in study of pelvic veins.	Multiple observational studies
MRI appears equal to venography for proximal but not distal leg vein studies but may be superior for study of the pelvic vessels.	Limited observational study; expert opinion
Computed tomography venography is promising but of uncertain utility.	Several observational studies; expert opinion

DVT, deep venous thrombosis; MRI, magnetic resonance imaging.

NONTHROMBOTIC PULMONARY EMBOLI

Although the differential diagnosis of acute PE predominantly includes other cardiopulmonary diseases, other nonthrombotic emboli may rarely occur in certain clinical settings. By virtue of venous blood return to the lungs, the pulmonary vascular bed is exposed to a variety of potentially obstructing substances. These substances may be exogenous or endogenous in origin, and may result in various consequences, including dyspnea, chest pain, hypoxemia, and sometimes death. Among these are fat embolism, amniotic fluid embolism, air embolism, schistosomiasis (usually

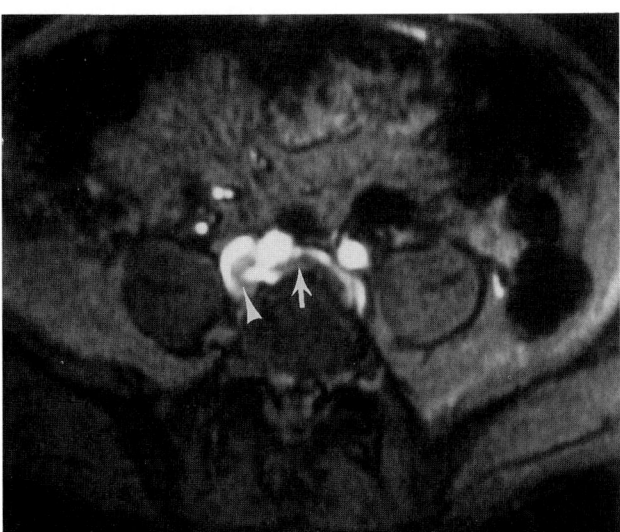

FIGURE 36.4. A magnetic resonance image reveals extensive thrombosis in the left iliac system *(arrow)* extending into the inferior vena cava *(arrowhead)*.

chronic pulmonary hypertension), septic embolism, and tumor embolism (81–85). A detailed discussion of these syndromes are provided elsewhere.

Fat Embolism

Fat embolism most commonly occurs in the setting of the traumatic fracture of long bones (81). This disorder is usually a more impressive clinical syndrome when larger bones and multiple fractures are involved. However, orthopedic procedures and trauma to other fat replete tissues such as the liver or subcutaneous tissue can sometimes result in similar consequences. After the inciting event, there is generally a delay of 24 to 48 hours before symptoms develop. Neutral fat enters the vascular system, and a characteristic syndrome of dyspnea, petechiae, and mental confusion often develops. It is unclear why the syndrome develops in some patients and not in others, even when the extent of injury is comparable. The diagnosis of fat embolism syndrome remains a diagnosis of exclusion and is based on clinical criteria.

The obstruction of numerous vessels by neutral fat particles, as well as the deleterious effects of free fatty acids released from neutral fat by lipases, accounts for the pathophysiologic consequences of fat embolism (81). These free fatty acids cause a diffuse vasculitis with capillary leakage from cerebral, pulmonary, and other vascular beds. The diagnosis is made from the clinical and radiographic findings in the setting of risk factors such as surgery or trauma. Fat droplets (by oil red O stain) in bronchoalveolar lavage fluid may be suggestive of fat embolism, but clinical studies to date suggest that this finding is not sensitive or specific. Treatment is generally supportive, including oxygen and mechanical ventilation, and the prognosis is generally good. Therapy with corticosteroids remains controversial. Steroid prophylaxis in high-risk patients has been suggested by some.

Amniotic Fluid Embolism

Amniotic fluid embolism is uncommon but nonetheless represents one of the leading causes of maternal death in the United States (82). This disorder occurs during or after delivery when amniotic fluid gains access to uterine venous channels and then to the pulmonary and general circulations. The delivery may be either spontaneous or by cesarean section and usually has been without complication. There are no identifiable risk factors in either the patient or the baby. The syndrome is heralded by the sudden onset of severe respiratory distress, and hypotension and death frequently result. The primary mechanism of injury appears to involve the thromboplastic activity of amniotic fluid. Extensive fibrin deposition then develops in the pulmonary vasculature and sometimes in other organs. A consumptive coagulopathy ensues with marked hypofibrinogenemia. An enhanced fibrinolytic state frequently develops after the acute event. Left ventricular dysfunction may result, and a potential role has

been suggested for the myocardial depressant effect of amniotic fluid. The resulting pulmonary edema may be both hydrostatic and noncardiogenic. The differential diagnosis includes pulmonary thromboembolism, septic and hemorrhagic shock, venous air embolism, aspiration pneumonia, congestive heart failure (from acute myocardial infarction or other causes), placentae abruptio, and ruptured uterus. The diagnosis should be suspected based upon the clinical picture. Examination of the pulmonary arterial blood may or may not reveal the amorphous fragments of vernix caseosa, squamous cells, or mucin. Although administration of heparin, antifibrinolytic agents such as aminocaproic acid, and cryoprecipitate have been have been suggested, the primary treatment is supportive, with oxygen and mechanical ventilation. Even with aggressive support, maternal mortality may be as high as 80%.

Air Embolism

The frequency of air embolism reflects the variety of invasive surgical and medical procedures now available, the frequent use of indwelling venous and arterial catheters, and the frequency of thoracic and other forms of trauma (83, 84). The consequences range from minimal to death. With venous embolism in the setting of a patent foramen ovale, embolization to the coronary or cerebral circulation is of the most concern. In the absence of a foramen ovale, the lungs can filter modest amounts of air, but large single or continuous episodes of air embolism can still gain access to the systemic arterial circulation. Symptoms and signs depend on the severity of the episode. Air in the systemic circulation may be difficult to recognize because only small quantities may cause significant symptoms, and intravascular air clears quickly. Dyspnea, wheezing, chest pain, cough, agitation, confusion, tachycardia, and hypotension may be evident. A mill wheel murmur (air in the right ventricle) may sometimes be auscultated. Hypoxemia and hypercapnia are present in more severe cases, and the chest radiograph may reveal pulmonary edema or air-fluid levels. Treatment includes immediate placement of the patient in the Trendelenburg/left lateral decubitus position and administration of 100% oxygen. If a central venous catheter is in place near the right atrium, air aspiration should be attempted. Occasionally, hyperbaric oxygen is indicated. Anticonvulsants are administered in the presence of seizures. Prevention and a high index of suspicion are crucial.

Schistosomiasis

This parasitic disorder causes severe pulmonary vascular obstruction and pulmonary hypertension via both anatomic obstruction by the organism itself and an inflammatory vasculitic response to the organism (85). In endemic areas (e.g., Egypt), schistosomal disease is a common cause of cor pulmonale. The liver is always involved, usually quite extensively, before pulmonary involvement occurs. The disease is refractory to treatment unless it is detected before the development of extensive hepatic and pulmonary inflammation.

Septic Embolism

Intravenous drug abuse is by far the most common cause of septic embolism. Before the drug era, this entity was nearly always a complication of septic pelvic thrombophlebitis owing to both septic abortion and postpartum uterine infection. Infections secondary to indwelling intravenous catheters are increasingly common as well. Subcutaneous injections can cause local infections that subsequently invade veins.

Other Emboli

The lung may be embolized on occasion by a variety of other substances (84). Cancer cells may enter and adhere to pulmonary vessels, occasionally mimicking PE. After head trauma, brain tissue has been discovered in the lungs; as have liver cells after abdominal trauma. Bone marrow has been reported in lung tissue after cardiopulmonary resuscitation.

Noninfectious vasculitic-thrombotic complications also occur in intravenous drug users. Materials, such as talc, used to "cut" the heroin or cocaine, and occasionally the drugs themselves, may provoke vascular inflammation and secondary thrombosis. Perfusion scans occasionally demonstrate segmental or smaller defects. Distinguishing these from emboli caused by DVT can be difficult. Occasionally, repetitive insults lead to chronic pulmonary hypertension.

CONCLUSIONS

VTE is associated with substantial morbidity and mortality. It represents a continuum of DVT and PE, and either or both may be present in a given patient. It is crucial to suspect the diagnosis of either DVT or PE in the setting of consistent, albeit often nonspecific, history and physical examination findings and laboratory tests. The presence of risk factors for VTE should lower the threshold for considering the diagnosis. The diagnosis should be proven objectively with appropriate imaging studies. The diagnostic approach to suspected acute PE is evolving with contrast-enhanced CT scanning being used increasingly. Although nonthrombotic PE can occur, VTE is by far the most common cause of morbidity and mortality. There are several acceptable diagnostic pathways that can be followed for both DVT and PE, but the most important concept should be to *consider the diagnosis,* and if it appears to be a reasonably likely diagnostic possibility, then to pursue it.

REFERENCES

1. Meignan M, Rosso J, Gauthier H, et al. Systematic lung scans reveal a high frequency of silent pulmonary embolism in patients with proximal deep venous thrombosis. *Arch Intern Med* 2000;160:159–164.
2. Lindblad B, Eriksson A, Bergquist D. Autopsy-verified pulmonary embolism in a surgical department: analysis of the period from 1951 to 1988. *Br J Surg* 1991;78:849–852.
3. Bratzler DW, Raskob, GE, Murray CK, et al. Underuse of venous thromboembolism prophylaxis for general surgery patients: physician practices in the community hospital setting. *Arch Intern Med* 1998;158:1909–1912.
4. Silverstein MD, Heit JA, Mohr DN, et al. Trends in the incidence of deep vein thrombosis and pulmonary embolism: a 25-year population-based study. *Arch Intern Med* 1998;158:585–593.
5. Dalen JE, Alpert JS. Natural history of pulmonary embolism. *Prog Cardiovasc Dis* 1975;17:257–270.
6. Anderson FA, Wheeler HB. Venous thromboembolism: risk factors and prophylaxis. *Clin Chest Med* 1995;16:235–251.
7. Cheng XS, Wang Q. Experience of pulmonary embolism in China. In: Morpugo M, ed. *Pulmonary embolism.* New York: Marcel Dekker Inc, 1994.
8. Adoh A, Moncany G, Bogui-Ferron A, et al. Etude de 115 cas de maladies thrombo-emboliques veino-pulmonaires chez le Noir African a Abidjan. *Cardiologie Tropicale* 1989;15:91–96.
9. Mo Lee H, Soo Suk K, Hwan Moon S, et al. Deep vein thrombosis after major spinal surgery: Incidence in an east Asian population. *Spine* 2000;25:1827–1830.
10. Davidson BL, Elliott CG, Lensing AWA. Low accuracy of color Doppler ultrasound in the detection of proximal leg vein thrombosis in asymptomatic high-risk patients. *Ann Intern Med* 1992;117:735–738.
11. White RH, Zhou H, Romano PS. Incidence of idiopathic deep venous thrombosis and secondary thromboembolism among ethnic groups in California. *Ann Intern Med* 1998;128:737–740.
12. Vishudhiphan S, Poolsuppasit S, Piboonnukarintr O. The relationship between high fibrinolytic activity and daily capsicum ingestion in the Thais. *Am J Clin Nutri* 1982;35:1452–1458.
13. Hwang WS. The rarity of pulmonary thromboembolism in Asians. *Singapore Med J* 968;9:269–279.
14. Ho Y-H, Seow-Choen F, Leong AM, et al. Randomized, controlled trial of low molecular weight heparin versus no deep vein thrombosis prophylaxis for major colon and rectal surgery in Asian patients. *Dis Colon Rectum* 1999;42:196–203.
15. Dhillon KS, Askander A, Doraisamy S. Postoperative deep-vein thrombosis in Asian patients is not a rarity: a prospective study of 88 patients with no prophylaxis. *J Bone Joint Surg Br* 1996;78B:427–430.
16. Heit JA, Silverstein MD, Mohr DN, et al. Predictors of survival after deep vein thrombosis and pulmonary embolism: a population-based, cohort study. *Arch Intern Med* 1999;159:445–453.
17. Stein PD, Henry JW. Prevalence of acute pulmonary embolism among patients in a general hospital and at autopsy. *Chest* 1995;108:978–981.
18. Ginsberg JS, Hirsh J, Julian, J, et al. Prevention and treatment of postphlebitic syndrome: results of a three-part study. *Arch Intern Med* 2001;161:2105–2109.
19. Virchow R von. Weitere Untersuchungen ueber die Verstopfung der Lungenarterien und ihre Folge. In: *Traube's Beitraege exp path u Physiol.* Berlin, Germany: 1846:2:21–31.
20. Geerts WH, Heit JA, Clagett GP, et al. Prevention of venous thromboembolism. *Chest* 2001;119:132S–175S.
21. Toglia MR, Weg JG. Current concepts: venous thromboembolism during pregnancy. *N Engl J Med* 1996;335:108–114.
22. Samama MM, Cohen AT, Darmon JY, et al. A comparison of enoxaparin with placebo for the prevention of venous thromboembolism in acutely ill medical patients: Prophylaxis in Medical Patients with Enoxaparin Study Group. *N Engl J Med* 1999;341:793–800.

23. Hirsch DR, Ingenito EP, Goldhaber SZ. Prevalence of deep venous thrombosis among patients in medical intensive care. *JAMA* 1995;274:335–337.

24. Anderson FA Jr, Wheeler HB, Goldberg RJ, et al. A population-based perspective of the hospital incidence and case-fatality rates of deep vein thrombosis and pulmonary embolism: the Worcester DVT Study. *Arch Intern Med* 1991;151:933–938.

25. Heit JA, Silverstein MD, Mohr DN, et al. Risk factors for deep vein thrombosis and pulmonary embolism: a population-based case-control study. *Arch Intern Med* 2000;160:809–815.

26. Goldhaber SZ, Dunn K, MacDougall RC. New onset of venous thromboembolism among hospitalized patients at Brigham and Women's Hospital is caused more often by prophylaxis failure than by withholding treatment. *Chest* 2000;118:1680–1684.

27. Lapostolle F, Surget V, Borron SW, et al. Severe pulmonary embolism associated with air travel. *N Engl J Med* 2001;345:779–783.

28. Benotti JR, Dalen JE. The natural history of pulmonary embolism. *Clin Chest Med* 1984;5:403–410.

29. Wheeler HB. Diagnosis of deep venous thrombosis: review of clinical evaluation and impedance plethysmography. *Am J Surg* 1985;150[Suppl]:7–13.

30. Leclerc JR, Illescas F, Jarzem P. Diagnosis of deep vein thrombosis. In: Leclerc JR, ed. *Venous thromboembolic disorders.* Philadelphia: Lea & Febiger, 1991:176–228.

31. Wheeler HB, Hirsh J, Wells P, et al. Diagnostic tests for deep vein thrombosis: clinical usefulness depends on probability of disease. *Arch Intern Med* 1994;154:1921–1928.

32. Value of the ventilation/perfusion scan in acute pulmonary embolism: results of the prospective investigation of pulmonary embolism diagnosis: The PIOPED investigators. *JAMA* 1990;263:2753–2759.

33. Stein PD, Terrin ML, Hales CA, et al. Clinical, laboratory, roentgenographic and electrocardiographic findings in patients with acute pulmonary embolism and no pre-existing cardiac or pulmonary disease. *Chest* 1991;100:598–603.

34. The Urokinase Pulmonary Embolism Trial: a national cooperative study. *Circulation* 1973;47[Suppl. II]:II-1–II-108.

35. Green RM, Meyer TJ, Dunn M, et al. Pulmonary embolism in younger adults. *Chest* 1992;101:1507–1511.

36. Bounameaux H, Cirafici P, DeMoerloose P, et al. Measurement of D-dimer in plasma as diagnostic aid in suspected pulmonary embolism. *Lancet* 1991;337:196–200.

37. Egermayer P, Town GI, Turner JG, et al. Usefulness of D-dimer, blood gas, and respiratory rate measurements for excluding pulmonary embolism. *Thorax* 1998;53:830–834.

38. Ahearn GS, Bounameaux H. The role of the D-dimer in the diagnosis of venous thromboembolism. *Semin Respir Crit Care Med* 2000;21:521–536.

39. Wells PS, Anderson DR, Rodger M, et al. Excluding pulmonary embolism at the bedside without diagnostic imaging: management of patients with suspected pulmonary embolism presenting to the emergency department by using a simple clinical model and D-dimer. *Ann Intern Med* 2001;135:98–107.

40. Wicki J, Perneger T, Junod A, et al. Assessing clinical probability of pulmonary embolism in the emergency ward: a simple score. *Arch Intern Med* 2001;161:92–97.

41. Kovacs M, MacKinnon KM, Anderson D, et al. A comparison of three rapid D-dimer methods for the diagnosis of venous thromboembolism. *Br J Haematol* 2001;115:140–144.

42. Pacouret G, Schellenberg F, Hamel E, et al. Troponine I dans l'embolie pulmonaire aigue massive: resultants d'une serie prospective. *Presse Med* 1998;27:1627.

43. Giannitsis E, Müller-Bardoff M, Kurowski V, et al. Independent prognostic value of cardiac troponin T in patients with confirmed pulmonary embolism. *Circulation* 2000;102:211–217.

44. Meyer T, Binder L, Hruska N, et al. Cardiac troponin I elevation in acute pulmonary embolism is associated with right ventricular dysfunction. *J Am Coll Cardiol* 2000;36:1632–1636.

45. Mehta NJ, Jani K, Khan IA. Clinical utility and prognostic value of elevated cardiac troponin I in acute pulmonary embolism. *Am Heart J* 2002 *(in press)*.

46. Douketis JD, Crowther MA, Stanton EB, et al. Elevated cardiac troponin levels in patients with submassive pulmonary embolism. *Arch Intern Med* 2002;162:79–81.

47. Goodman LR, Lipchik RJ. Diagnosis of acute pulmonary embolism: time for a new approach. *Radiology* 1996;199:25–27.

48. Remy-Jardin M, Remy J, Wattinne L, et al. Central pulmonary thromboembolism: Diagnosis with spiral volumetric CT with the single-breath-hold technique: comparison with pulmonary angiography. *Radiology* 1992;185:381–387.

49. Remy-Jardin MJ, Remy J, Deschildre F, et al. Diagnosis of acute pulmonary embolism with spiral CT: comparison with pulmonary angiography and scintigraphy. *Radiology* 1996;200:699–706.

50. Goodman LR, Curtin JJ, Mewissen MW, et al. Detection of pulmonary embolism in patients with unresolved clinical and scintigraphic diagnosis: helical CT versus angiography. *AJR Am J Roentgenol* 1995;164:1369–1374.

51. Sostman HD, Layish DT, Tapson VF, et al. Prospective comparison of helical CT and MR imaging in patients with clinically suspected pulmonary embolism. *J Magn Reson Imaging* 1996;6:275–281.

52. Mayo JR, Remy-Jardin M, Muller NL, et al. Pulmonary embolism: prospective comparison of spiral CT with ventilation-perfusion scintigraphy. *Radiology* 1997;205:447–452.

53. Drucker EA, Rivitz SM, Shepard JO, et al. Acute pulmonary embolism: assessment of helical CT for diagnosis. *Radiology* 1998;209:235–241.

54. Perrier A, Howarth N, Didier D, et al. Performance of helical computed tomography in unselected outpatients with suspected pulmonary embolism. *Ann Intern Med* 2001;135:88–97.

55. Ferretti GR, Bosson JL, Buffaz P-D, et al. Acute pulmonary embolism: role of helical CT in 164 patients with intermediate probability at ventilation-perfusion scintigraphy and normal results at duplex US of the legs. *Radiology* 1997;205:453–458.

56. Swensen SJ, Sheedy PF, Ryu JH, et al. Outcomes after withholding anticoagulation from patients with suspected acute pulmonary embolism and negative computed tomographic findings: a cohort study. *Mayo Clin Proc* 2002;77:130–138.

57. Garg K, Sieler H, Welsh CH, et al. Clinical validity of helical CT being interpreted as negative for pulmonary embolism: implications for patient treatment. *AJR Am J Roentgenol* 1999;172:1627–1631.

58. Holbert JM, Costello P, Federle MP. Role of spiral computed tomography in the diagnosis of pulmonary embolism in the emergency department. *Ann Emerg Med* 1999;33:520–528.

59. Gottschalk A, Stein, PD, Goodman LR, et al. Overview of the Prospective Investigation of Pulmonary Embolism Diagnosis (PIOPED II). *Semin Nuc Med* 2002;32:173–182.

60. Loud PA, Katz DS, Klippenstein DL, et al. Combined CT venography and pulmonary angiography in suspected thromboembolic disease: diagnostic accuracy for deep venous evaluation. *AJR Am J Roentgenol* 2000;174:61–65.

61. Meaney JFM, Weg JG, Chenevert TL, et al. Diagnosis of pulmonary embolism with magnetic resonance angiography. *N Engl J Med* 1997;336:1422–1427.

62. Tapson VF. Pulmonary embolism - new diagnostic approaches. *N Engl J Med* 1997;336:1449–1451.

63. Evans AJ, Tapson VF, Sostman HD, et al. The diagnosis of deep venous thrombosis: a prospective comparison of venography and magnetic resonance imaging. *Chest* 1992;102: 120S.

64. Come PC. Echocardiographic evaluation of pulmonary embolism and its response to therapeutic interventions. *Chest* 1992; 101:151S–162S.

65. Goldhaber SZ, Haire WD, Feldstein ML, et al. Alteplase versus heparin in acute pulmonary embolism: randomized trial assessing right ventricular function and pulmonary perfusion. *Lancet* 1993;341:507–510.

66. Tapson VF, Davidson CJ, Kisslo KB, et al. Rapid visualization of massive pulmonary emboli utilizing intravascular ultrasound. *Chest* 1994;105:888–890.

67. Tapson VF, Witty LA. Massive pulmonary embolism: diagnostic and therapeutic strategies. *Clin Chest Med* 1996;16:329.

68. Tapson VF, Carroll BA, Davidson BL, et al. The diagnostic approach to acute venous thromboembolism: clinical practice guideline. American Thoracic Society. *Am J Respir Crit Care Med* 1999;160:1043–1066.

69. Lensing AW, Levi MM, Buller HR, et al. Diagnosis of deep-vein thrombosis using an objective Doppler method. *Ann Intern Med* 1990;113:9–13.

70. Killewich LA, Bedford GR, Beach KW, et al. Diagnosis of deep venous thrombosis: a prospective study comparing duplex scanning to contrast venography. *Circulation* 1989;79:810–814.

71. Burke B, Sostman HD, Carroll BA, et al. The diagnostic approach to deep venous thrombosis: which technique? *Clin Chest Med* 1995;16:253–268.

72. Baxter GM, Duffy P, Partridge E. Colour flow imaging of calf vein thrombosis. *Clin Radiol* 1992;46:198–201.

73. Davidson BL, Elliott CG, Lensing AWA. Low accuracy of color Doppler ultrasound in the detection of proximal leg vein thrombosis in asymptomatic high-risk patients. *Ann Intern Med* 1992;117:735–738.

74. Heijboer H, Buller HR, Lensing AWA, et al. A comparison of real-time compression ultrasonography with impedance plethysmography for the diagnosis of deep-vein thrombosis in symptomatic outpatients. *N Engl J Med* 1993;329:1365–1369.

75. Haire WD, Lynch TG, Lieberman RP, et al. Utility of duplex ultrasound in the diagnosis of asymptomatic catheter-induced subclavian vein thrombosis. *J Ultrasound Med* 1991;10:493–496.

76. Prandoni P, Polistena P, Bernardi E, et al. Upper-extremity deep vein thrombosis: risk factors, diagnosis, and complications. *Arch Intern Med* 1997;157:57–62.

77. Kreienberg PB, Chang BB, Darling RC III, et al. Long-term results in patients treated with thrombolysis, thoracic inlet decompression, and subclavian vein stenting for Paget-Schroetter syndrome. *J Vasc Surg* 2001;S100–S105.

78. Paget J. *Clinical lectures and essays.* London: Longmens Green; 1875.

79. Evans AJ, Sostman HD, Witty LA, et al. Detection of deep venous thrombosis: prospective comparison of MR imaging and sonography. *J Magn Reson Imaging* 1996;6:44–51.

80. Evans AJ, Sostman HD, Knelson MH, et al. *AJR Am J Roentgenol* 1993;161:131–139.

81. Johnson MJ, Lucas GL. Fat embolism syndrome. *Orthopedics* 1996;19:41–48.

82. Martin RW. Amniotic fluid embolism. *Clin Obstet Gynecol* 1996; 39:101–106.

83. Vesely TM. Air embolism during insertion of central venous catheters. *J Vasc Intervent Radiol* 2001;12:1291–1295.

84. King MB, Harmon KR. Unusual forms of pulmonary embolism. *Clin Chest Med* 1994;15:561–580.

85. Morris W, Knauer CM. Cardiopulmonary manifestations of schistosomiasis. *Semin Respir Infect* 1997;12:159–170.

Management of Pulmonary Thromboembolic Diseases

37

Timothy A. Morris

Venous thromboembolism (VTE) is, in theory, an entirely preventable and/or treatable disease. Yet it is a persistent and prevalent cause of morbidity and mortality in modern times. For example, it has been estimated that 50,000 individuals die from pulmonary embolism (PE) each year in the United States, and ten times that number suffer from nonfatal PE. Although important diagnostic and therapeutic developments have occurred in the past decade, it would be ill advised to consider the task completed. Indeed, medical science is at the very beginning of the path to understanding this disease and how to prevent disability and death from it.

PREVENTION OF DEEP VENOUS THROMBOSIS AND PULMONARY EMBOLISM

The best way to reduce the morbidity and mortality of VTE is to prevent it from occurring in the first place. When performed properly, the risks of VTE prophylaxis are small, and the potential benefits are enormous. It is clear that the informed use of VTE prophylaxis can substantially reduce the incidence of death and disability from this disease. The ultimate goal of safely preventing VTE entirely has not yet been achieved and is the focus of a great deal of research.

Theoretically, there are two approaches to the management of VTE: (a) provide prophylaxis or (b) monitor with noninvasive tests and treat if it develops. In virtually all patients, prophylaxis is superior. Deep venous thrombosis (DVT) in asymptomatic patients is not readily detected by current noninvasive tests; yet, clinical complications can develop rapidly (1). More importantly, the first clinically recognized sign of thromboembolic disease can be unexpected and fatal. For example, 70% to 80% of fatal PE is not diagnosed antemortem (2–5). Furthermore, up to 10% of all patients who present "dead on arrival" to hospital emergency departments do so because of previously unsuspected PE (6). Rational prevention of PE should be considered a priority.

Strategies to prevent VTE must address the mechanisms underlying venous thrombi formation and progression to clinically significant disease. The scientific basis of the pathogenesis and natural history of VTE is only partially understood, a fact that is reflected in our inability to thoroughly prevent it. In addition, clinical studies to evaluate prophylactic methods suffer from an incomplete understanding of how best to define and detect clinically significant VTE. These considerations notwithstanding, the prophylactic methods developed and validated thus far have had a tremendous positive impact on reducing the incidence of this disease.

DVT and PE should be viewed as different manifestations of VTE, rather than as separate disorders. The vast majority of clinically significant pulmonary emboli (>95%) arise from deep veins of the lower extremities. Thus, the prevention of PE, for the most part, is really the prevention of lower extremity DVT. Substantial data indicate that clinically apparent emboli are caused only by lower extremity DVT extending into the proximal deep veins (popliteal and above). Thrombi that remain confined to calf veins pose no significant embolic risk: Patients without proximal vein extension in the first week after presentation had excellent outcomes in clinical trials (7,8). It is not known whether these observations reflected the fact that thrombi restricted to the calf veins do not embolize, or that emboli from them are so small that clinical disease does not result. Whatever the case, it is now evident that the key to prevention of PE is the prevention of lower extremity DVT or, failing this, prevention of the extension of calf vein thrombosis into the more proximal venous system.

T. A. Morris: Division of Pulmonary and Critical Care Medicine, University of California, San Diego Medical Center, San Diego, California.

There are two requirements for developing an effective strategy for preventing any disorder: (a) identification of patients at risk, and (b) availability of effective prophylactic modalities. For DVT, both of these requirements have been largely, but incompletely, satisfied. The increased risk for various patient populations have been well defined; yet, we lack an accurate method of assessing risk for individual patients. Likewise, the efficacy and safety of several prophylactic regimens have been established clinically, although these trials are complicated by the difficulties inherent to detecting asymptomatic DVT and controversies over its clinical importance.

The decision to apply prophylaxis involves weighing the risk of venous thrombosis (and therefore PE) versus the risk of the prophylactic regimen. The risk factors are cumulative, and the total clinical picture mandates both the presence and the intensity of prophylaxis. For example, patients undergoing extensive lower extremity orthopedic surgery are at very high risk for DVT, requiring aggressive mechanical and moderate-dose anticoagulant prophylaxis. Younger healthier persons with less severe medical problems and limited immobilization could be adequately prophylaxed with lower doses of anticoagulants or mechanical methods alone.

There are several mechanical and pharmacological approaches to prevent VTE. Many studies have compared different methods or drug regimens for VTE prophylaxis. Although these trials may provide useful clinical guidance, they should be interpreted with some care, considering each trial's sponsorship, scientific rigor, and whether the comparative medication is dosed optimally (or, for mechanical modalities, whether the optimal devices/methods are used).

Mechanical compressive devices prevent venous stasis by inflating a cuff placed around the lower extremities for several seconds of each minute. Some devices compress the calf alone; others compress the calf and thigh sequentially. However, there is little difference in the efficacy between the two (9). Although it is presently unknown whether different pressures and speeds of intermittent cuff inflation will lead to improved prophylactic efficacy, it is clear that the pattern of rhythmic inflation is helpful. Simple elastic stockings have not been shown to be useful unless they are patient-tailored to provide a gradient of pressures. The intermittent compressive devices are safe, effective, and well tolerated (10,11). The only contraindications to their use are the presence of active venous thrombosis (which should be ruled out before their application, if suspected), limb ischemia owing to arterial insufficiency, and the presence of circumstances that prevent their application (e.g., a cast in place). The devices should be applied promptly (e.g., preoperatively) and maintained during the risk period. This approach has particular value in those patient groups for whom antithrombotic drugs are contraindicated (e.g., neurosurgical, head trauma, known hemorrhagic diathesis).

Prophylactic subcutaneous heparin has been studied widely and is a safe and efficacious preventive approach in most patient populations. It is generally administered as a dose of 5,000 to 7,500 U subcutaneously every 8 to 12 hours. This regimen is effective because heparin inhibits the events that occur early in the coagulation cascade, before the elaboration of thrombin. After initial screening studies—platelet count, partial thromboplastin time, prothrombin time, and a careful history—no further coagulation studies are necessary to monitor the patient. Substantial experience has indicated the low bleeding risk associated with this regimen, even in surgical populations.

Low-molecular-weight heparins (LMWHs) represent another option for prophylaxis. These agents include a heterogeneous group of drugs derived by partial depolymerization of heparin and are administered subcutaneously. They possess certain theoretical advantages over (unfractionated) heparin, such as more predictable pharmacokinetics, allowing dose escalation without laboratory monitoring, and a reduced incidence of heparin-induced thrombocytopenia (HIT) during routine use. These medications are 10 times more expensive to use than is heparin and would constitute a great increase in pharmaceutical cost if adopted for all prophylactic needs. The high cost of the various LMWHs would be justified if each drug represented a true clinical advantage over properly dosed heparin.

Warfarin is an alternative effective drug for prophylaxis in high-risk subjects. Several regimens have been studied, particularly in very high risk groups such as those getting hip replacement. One approach is to begin low doses (1–2 mg/d) before surgery and then escalate to a therapeutic range after surgery. Another is to begin warfarin only after surgery with a goal of achieving the desired prothrombin range (international normalized ratio [INR], 2.0–3.0) after several days. It is likely that these regimens do not prevent small calf thrombi but do prevent extension into the popliteal veins and above, thereby sharply reducing embolic risk.

There will remain some patients who are at high risk but in whom neither antithrombotic agents nor venous compression devices can be applied (e.g., patients with extensive trauma). In such patients, prophylactic placement of an inferior vena caval filter should be considered.

The prophylactic approach selected depends on the magnitude of thromboembolic risk and the relative risks inherent to prophylactic methods. In patients at low or moderate risk, either the application of intermittent pneumatic leg compression devices or prophylactic doses of subcutaneous low-dose heparin or warfarin provide adequate protection. Such patients include those who are immobilized for brief periods, are undergoing general surgical procedures (e.g., cholecystectomy), or have suffered an uncomplicated myocardial infarction. However, none of these individual approaches provide optimal protection in patients at high risk, including those with trauma to the pelvis or lower extremities, those undergoing extensive surgical procedures on the lower extremities (e.g., hip or knee replacement) or surgical prostatectomy, and those with multiple risk factors. In these individuals, multiple studies have indicated that the combination of intermittent leg compression with either heparin or warfarin provides optimal protection.

Regardless of the specific regimen selected, it is clear that prophylaxis can, and should, be applied to all patients at risk of VTE. Failure to apply prophylaxis should be specifically justified. Because prevention of DVT is the best means of preventing PE and death owing to embolism, and because the vast majority of venous thrombi arise among hospitalized patients to whom a prophylactic option easily can be applied, widespread use of prophylactic options can, at the current time, considerably reduce the incidence of DVT and PE. Further developments in this field hold the promise of safely preventing it even further, perhaps to the point of eliminating it entirely.

PREVENTION OF DEEP VENOUS THROMBOSIS AND PULMONARY EMBOLISM

Summary Statement	Level of Evidence
Prophylaxis using low doses of heparin, low-molecular-weight heparin or warfarin can help prevent venous thromboembolism in hospitalized patients, with minimally increased risks of bleeding.	Multiple scientific studies
Surveillance for "early" venous thromboembolism, using noninvasive methods, is insensitive and should not be used as a substitute for prophylaxis.	Scientific studies
Prophylaxis against venous thromboembolism can prevent death from pulmonary embolism.	Epidemiological data and scientific studies with low incidences of this outcome

THROMBOEMBOLISM TREATMENT: PHARMACOLOGY

Heparin and Low-Molecular-Weight Heparins

Nearly all (clinically recognized) cases of DVT and PE are treated acutely with either unfractionated heparin (UH) or LMWH. Pharmacological comparisons and contrasts between the two drug types will help to put into perspective the results of disease-specific clinical outcome trials. The two drug types share many structural properties and have multiple mechanisms of action in common. The relative potencies with which the mechanisms are expressed differ between LMWH and UH, and among specific LMWHs. The pharmacokinetics of LMWHs and UH are often compared according to the results of plasma activity against purified factor Xa, although the correlation between anti-Xa assays and the actual mechanisms of action of the drugs is questionable. Animal models of thrombosis give some information regarding the antithrombotic efficacy of different LMWHs compared with UH and to other LMWHs, but the results

are varied and may not be applicable to human thrombosis. Similarly, clinical measurements of clot suppression have yielded conflicting results when the two types of anticoagulants have been directly compared. Numerous clinical outcome studies support the conclusion that subcutaneous regimens of LMWH are at least as effective and safe as intravenous UH for the treatment of clinically stable patients with VTE (12,13). However, subcutaneous UH has also fared better than intravenous UH in clinical trials, suggesting that some of the benefit may be from the subcutaneous administration itself (14). If so, the superiority of one subcutaneous regimen over the others can be established only by the performance of well-planned comparative clinical trials.

All heparins are heterogeneous mixtures of modified polysaccharides (glucose-amino-glycans) derived from animal products that catalyze the blood enzyme antithrombin (also called "antithrombin III") to neutralize activated clotting factors. The various LMWHs are produced by chemically cleaving UH into similarly heterogeneous mixtures of smaller molecules. Each LMWH has its own spectrum of biologic properties, determined by the characteristics of the parent UH and by the effects of the cleavage process on the structures and functions of the low-molecular-weight fragments (15–17). The relative therapeutic "superiority" of the LMWHs, in relationship to each other and to UH itself, is a topic of considerable controversy, which stems in large part from the incomplete knowledge of the mechanisms of each agent's antithrombotic activity (the ability to inhibit the formation and enlargement of blood clots in the body) and of its adverse effects.

UH was discovered by McLean in 1916 and has been used clinically as an antithrombotic agent for several decades. UH is an inexpensive but highly effective drug for the prophylaxis and treatment of various thrombotic disorders, for which it is therapeutic in at least a partially dose-dependent fashion (18). The therapeutic benefits of UH, however, are limited by an increased risk of bleeding, which is also at least partially a dose-dependent phenomenon (19). To optimize the balance between efficacy and bleeding, clinicians have adopted two dosing practices: (a) frequent estimation of UH plasma levels using an *in vivo* marker of anticoagulant activity, the activated partial thromboplastin time (aPTT); and (b) continuous intravenous administration of UH in order to allow multiple rapid dosage adjustments, guided by aPTT values. Although the cost of the aPTT test itself is minimal, the requirement for repeated blood tests and dose adjustments, as well as maintenance of an intravenous catheter, make this method of managing UH so laborious that hospitalization is nearly always required (20), a fact that greatly increases the cost of therapy (21). Although both of these strategies are widely adopted, clinical trials using UH for treatment of VTE have not shown consistent benefits for either aPTT monitoring (22) or intravenous (versus subcutaneous) administration.

LMWHs were developed for clinical use with the intention of overcoming the therapeutic limitations of UH (23). Encouraging preclinical data suggested that LMWH was superior to UH from both biologic and pharmacokinetic standpoints. Biologically, animal experiments suggested that the therapeutic window would be larger for LMWH: it would cause a lower risk of bleeding than an equally effective dose of UH (24). Unfortunately, clinical trials of thromboembolic disease treatment have not demonstrated statistically significant differences in bleeding rates between LMWH and UH (12). From a pharmacokinetic perspective, at least one assay of blood anticoagulant potency, the ability to catalyze the neutralization of activated factor X (see "Activity against Free Factor Xa" below), suggests that LMWH has a more predictable and favorable pharmacokinetic profile than that of UH (25). However, the clinical relevance of this finding depends in large part on the importance of anti-Xa activity to the therapeutic and adverse effects of LMWH and UH.

HEPARIN AND LOW-MOLECULAR-WEIGHT HEPARINS	
Summary Statement	**Level of Evidence**
Heparin and low-molecular-weight heparin have different biological and pharmacokinetic properties.	Multiple scientific studies
Heparin and low-molecular-weight heparin are safe and effective treatments for acute thrombosis.	Multiple scientific studies
Heparin and low-molecular-weight have comparable antithrombotic activities.	Multiple scientific studies

Pharmacokinetics

Comparing the pharmacokinetics of LMWH and UH is conceptually complex. Ordinarily, pharmacokinetic calculations such as clearance and half-life describe the rise and fall of the concentration of a specific drug in the body. However, the "concentration" of UH or LMWH is difficult to define, even before administration. Both of these biologic agents contain mixtures of glycosaminoglycans with various lengths, chemical compositions, and enzymatic activities (15). For example, only about one third of UH molecules contain the specific pentasaccharide sequence necessary for anticoagulant interaction with antithrombin, and an even lower proportion of LMWH molecules contain the sequence (23). Absolute drug levels (i.e., molecular concentrations) are virtually irrelevant to the therapeutic and toxic effects of either drug.

Pharmaceutical preparations of UH and LMWH are measured in terms of their activities in *in vitro* models of anticoagulation. For example, the United States Pharmacopeia unit of heparin is defined as the quantity that prevents 1 mL of sheep plasma from clotting for 1 hour under certain conditions (26). LMWH, on the other hand, is more difficult to measure by clotting tests and is quantified according to the concentration of anti-Xa activity (26). The anti-Xa

activity assay is performed by incubating the drug with an excess of antithrombin, purified (unbound) factor Xa, and a substrate that turns color when cleaved by Xa. The anti-Xa activity is defined as the potency of the drug for causing antithrombin-mediated Xa inactivation (and thereby preventing a color change in the Xa substrate). Although widely used to standardize the manufacture and administration of UH and LMWH, the relationship between either of these two assays and the actual pharmacological activity of the drugs in the body is unclear (18,27). The clinical relevance of this paradox is that the recommended therapeutic doses, measured using these anticoagulation indexes, are different among the individual LMWHs and, of course, between any of them and UH.

The most clinically relevant pharmacokinetic parameters concerning the concentration of active UH and LMWH would be based on measurements of each drug's potential to inhibit *in vivo* thrombosis and to cause bleeding. Unfortunately, no method currently exists to reliably quantitate the *in vivo* antithrombotic activities of anticoagulants in humans. Although clinical indicators of antithrombotic efficacy, such as repeated imaging studies or symptomatic follow-up, provide data useful for patient care, they are inappropriate for use in pharmacokinetic calculations.

Anticoagulation tests, using various *in vitro* models of thrombosis, are often used as surrogate markers of antithrombotic activity, but no single test can be used to compare the concentrations of two distinct medications. Nearly all anticoagulation tests measure the concentration of some aspect of enzymatic activity felt to be relevant to antithrombosis. However, anticoagulation tests have serious limitations in their ability to quantitate the amount of antithrombotic activity in the blood after the administration of LMWH or UH. First, the various preparations of LMWH and UH have markedly distinct potencies of activity with regard to the values measured by different anticoagulation tests (28). Similarly, therapeutic doses of various LMWHs (and of UH), when administered to patients, yield disparate results from one another on various anticoagulation assays (29). Furthermore, depending on what parameter is being measured, the same drug may demonstrate different comparative bioavailabilities, clearances, and half-lives (28). For example, in normal volunteers, the half-life of anti-Xa activity is much longer for subcutaneous enoxaparin (40 mg) than for UH (5,000 U) (30). However, in the same patients, the half-life of anti-IIa activity of both drugs is roughly equivalent (31). In addition, the variably sized molecules that make up UH and LMWH are cleared from the circulation at different rates, and the range of fragment lengths (and the spectrum of activities) of the drugs before administration is different from what is found in the plasma (28). Finally, no single anticoagulation test result is equally applicable to the various LMWHs and to UH for predicting clinical efficacy or bleeding. For these reasons, the validity of using any particular anticoagulation assay to compare the pharmacokinetics of UH to LMWH, or to compare LMWHs to one another, is questionable.

MEASURING THE BIOLOGIC EFFECTS OF LOW-MOLECULAR-WEIGHT HEPARIN

Both the biologic and pharmacokinetic arguments in favor of LMWH over UH (and of one LMWH over another) depend in large part on our understanding of the difference in mechanisms of action between the two drugs. To make matters more complex, UH and the various LMWHs act through multiple mechanisms that are similar among the entire class of anticoagulants. However, each individual drug has its own particular spectrum of potencies for the various biologic mechanisms of action. The relative importance of each proposed mechanism of action to both the antithrombotic efficacy and the risk of bleeding for this class of drugs is fundamental to the question of the clinical superiority of one drug over another.

LMWH and UH have several different mechanisms of action suggested to be responsible for their antithrombotic effect. An exhaustive list of the full spectrum of activities is beyond the scope of this chapter, and excellent descriptions have been published on this topic elsewhere (23,31,32). However, a brief review of several key biologic mechanisms highlights the complexity of measuring and comparing the "activities" of different LMWH preparations and of UH.

Effects Mediated by Antithrombin

A major portion of the clinical effects of UH and of LMWH occur through enhancement of the antithrombotic action of antithrombin. Antithrombin neutralizes activated coagulation factors thrombin, Xa, IXa, XIa, XIIa, and kallikrein, but the major consequences come from the inhibition of thrombin and Xa. In fact, the major biologic difference between LMWH and UH may stem from the relative potency with which each drug stimulates the inactivation of thrombin and of Xa (23). Most of the molecules making up UH enable antithrombin to inactivate both thrombin and Xa, whereas a large proportion of LMWH molecules catalyze Xa inactivation more potently than they do thrombin inactivation. In fact, LMWHs also contain, to varying degrees, proportions of heparin molecules below the critical size necessary to catalyze thrombin inactivation at all, stimulating only inactivation of Xa.

Antithrombin inactivates thrombin and Xa in a similar fashion. Both thrombin and Xa are serine proteases, meaning that they contain serine, histidine, and aspartate residues in reactive sites that form unstable intermediates with target sites on their substrates. The substrates are then cleaved through hydrolysis, whereas the serine proteases return to their original forms, which are able to cleave other substrates. Antithrombin is able to inactivate coagulation enzymes such as thrombin and Xa, but only in the presence of UH or LMWH. Antithrombin inactivates the enzymes by binding irreversibly to the serine protease active sites, a process poetically referred to as *suicide inhibition*.

Both the composition and the size of the individual UH or LMWH molecule bound to antithrombin determine the specificity of the complex for either thrombin or Xa inactivation. A specific pentasaccharide sequence must be present on the UH or LMWH molecule in order to induce antithrombin activity at all. Molecules of UH or LMWH that lack the sequence have no significant effect on antithrombin. In addition, the size of the UH or LMWH molecule affects the specificity of the reaction it catalyzes with antithrombin. Heparin molecules of molecular weight less than 5.4 kd are capable of catalyzing only Xa inactivation. Larger molecules induce antithrombin to inactivate both Xa and thrombin. With increasing size of the heparin molecule, the activity of antithrombin increases against thrombin but remains relatively stable against Xa. The range of sizes of heparin molecules contained within UH or any particular LMWH largely determines the relative activities of the drug against thrombin and Xa (33). For example, UH has a mean MW between 12 and 15 kd (range, 5–30 kd) and has, by definition, equal activities against thrombin and Xa. However, the LMWHs such as enoxaparin (mean molecular weight, 4.5 kd; range, 3–8 kd), dalteparin (5 kd; range, 2–9 kd), and Logiparin (4.5 kd; range, 3–6 kd) have, to varying degrees, relatively more anti-Xa activity than antithrombin activity (23).

Also important, but less well characterized, are the effects on antithrombin specificity of other properties of the heparin molecules, including their degree of sulfation, charge distribution, and characteristics of the terminal saccharide residues. All of these properties differ among different UH and LMWH products (17) and contribute to the particular spectrum of relative activity of each drug against thrombin and against Xa. The optimal spectrum of activity is unclear.

Activity against Free Factor Xa

Factor X activation into factor Xa represents the first step in the final common pathway of the intrinsic and extrinsic coagulation cascades (Fig. 37.1). Factor Xa contributes to the thrombotic process by converting prothrombin into the active enzyme thrombin. Factor Xa, in its free form, slowly converts prothrombin to thrombin. However, when Xa is bound to a phospholipid membrane along with factor Va and calcium (the prothrombinase complex), the reaction proceeds at a much faster rate and accounts for the majority of the thrombin production *in vivo* (34,35). In addition, factor Xa within the prothrombinase complex is much less vulnerable to inactivation by antithrombin than is free factor Xa, regardless of whether antithrombin is stimulated by UH or by LMWH (36). Perhaps for this reason, the plasma assay of anti-Xa activity, which measures only the ability to inactivate free (purified) factor Xa, does not predict the antithrombotic activity of different LMWHs and UH in animal models of thrombosis.

It is clear that inhibition of free Xa is not solely responsible for the anticoagulant action of LMWH. For example, the

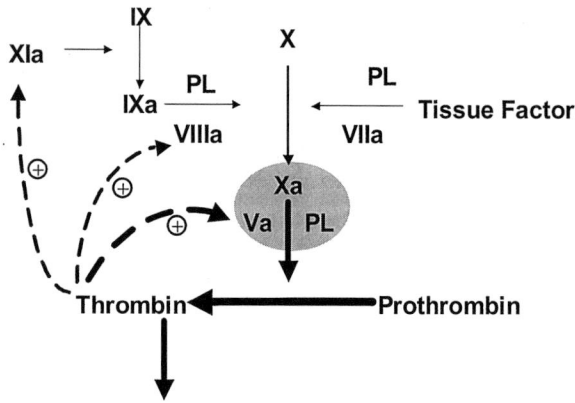

FIGURE 37.1. A simplified outline of the clotting cascade. The final common pathway is the activation of factor X to factor Xa. Factor Xa works primarily on plasma membranes, using factor Va as a coenzyme. While on the membrane, it is relatively resistant to inactivation by heparin or low-molecular-weight heparin. Once thrombosis has begun, the rate-determining reaction is the positive feedback loop, consisting of thrombin-activating pro-coagulant enzymes (primarily factor V), which eventually results in more thrombin generation.

very low-molecular-weight pentasaccharide (which causes antithrombin-mediated inhibition of Xa but not of thrombin) arrested thrombosis in an experimental group of animals only if the plasma anti-Xa activity was several times as high as it was in a similar group given LMWH (37). Likewise, the profile of plasma anti-Xa activities in clinical studies does not correlate well with therapeutic efficacy or complication rates of patients treated with UH or a variety of LMWHs (27,29,38).

Activity against Free Thrombin

Thrombin is responsible for a number of reactions in the coagulation cascade. The most straightforward function is to convert soluble fibrinogen to fibrin, which spontaneously polymerizes to form the structural framework of the blood clot. Thrombin is also involved in numerous positive and negative feedback steps within the coagulation cascade, allowing it to play a major role in controlling the rate of thrombosis. In a striking example of a positive feedback role of thrombin, the thrombin-mediated activation of factor V into Va (a fundamental constituent of the prothrombinase complex) may be the rate-limiting step in the ongoing production of thrombin itself during the initiation and propagation of blood clotting (39). For many reasons, thrombin activity is essential to thrombus enlargement.

The importance of thrombin in the control of coagulation is fundamental to comparisons between LMWH and UH, because it is the higher molecular-weight constituents of both drug types that enable thrombin inactivation (25). In fact, platelet factor 4, a blood protein that binds to and clears higher MW heparin molecules from the circulation, eliminates the antithrombin activity of both LMWH and UH (39). (This interaction forms one of the antigens

responsible for the HIT that complicates treatment with both medications [40].) Perhaps for this reason, the pharmacokinetics of antithrombin activity between subcutaneous injections of UH (5,000 U) and enoxaparin (40 mg) in healthy volunteers are remarkably similar (30).

As was the case with Xa, thrombin has a bound form that retains its thrombotic activity but is resistant to inactivation by antithrombin. As a thrombus is formed, thrombin binds to sites on the fibrin polymer, where it continues to activate the coagulation cascade. Although both UH and LMWH enable antithrombin to inactivate thrombin in its free state, fibrin-bound thrombin is no longer susceptible to the effects of either drug (41). The relative importance of free and fibrin-bound thrombin in the overall kinetics of clot propagation in clinical situations is unknown.

All LMWHs have a high ratio of anti-Xa to antithrombin activity, although the ratio varies widely among different specific drugs. In addition, the anti-Xa activity varies according to different assays (42–44), and the more commonly used assays may overestimate the actual activity of the drugs themselves (42). The ideal ratio is currently unknown, but ongoing clinical trials using newer synthetic drugs with exclusively anti-Xa activity or exclusively antithrombin activity may help determine the relative importance of inhibiting these two coagulation enzymes (45).

Although the currently available assays used for pharmacokinetic comparisons measure only inhibition of free factor Xa (or, less commonly, of free thrombin), the mechanisms of action of UH and LMWH are much more complicated (42). It is unknown whether the actual antithrombin-mediated antithrombotic activity parallels the results of either one of these two assays, or some combination of the two. Because both UH and LMWH consist of variable molecules with different sizes, composition, and clearances, it is plausible that the molecules tracked by any particular assay are not identical to the ones causing the most antithrombin-mediated thrombus inhibition (46). To make matters even more complicated, antithrombotic mechanisms of UH and LMWH that are independent of antithrombin have been recently identified.

Effects Not Mediated by Antithrombin

The release of tissue factor pathway inhibitor (TFPI) is increasingly recognized as an important mechanism of action of LMWH and UH (30,47). When the extrinsic pathway of coagulation is triggered by vascular injury, tissue factor binds to factor VII, and the tissue factor–VII complex activates factor X. TFPI is an important controller of this coagulation step. TFPI binds to and neutralizes the tissue factor–VII complex, suppressing factor X activation and inhibiting clot formation.

TFPI is stored in high quantities on the surface of vascular endothelium. After administration of LMWH or UH, TFPI is released into the circulation (48). Although both drugs cause TFPI release in a dose-dependent fashion, plasma TFPI concentrations do not necessarily parallel the pharmacokinetics of other measurements of heparin activity, such as the aPTT, anti-Xa, antithrombin, or Heptest assays (30). It is even possible that the heparin constituents of LMWH and UH that cause TFPI release have no interaction with antithrombin (46) and would be undetectable by traditional testing. Furthermore, because the antithrombotic mechanism of TFPI release is a postdrug effect, active even after the elimination of the drug from the plasma, the pharmacodynamics of the biologic effects of LMWH and UH may not match their pharmacokinetics (as is the case, e.g., with corticosteroids) (49).

Recent *in vitro* experiments have disclosed a further possible mechanism of LMWH and UH, the enhancement of protein C inactivation of factor Va. Activated protein C inhibits thrombosis by cleaving factor Va, an essential element of the prothrombinase complex, into an inactive form. LMWH and UH augment this antithrombotic property of protein C (50,51). Although firm evidence supports the vital role of protein C in the control of coagulation, the clinical importance of this mechanism to the action of LMWH and UH is currently unknown.

The complexity of the interaction between this class of drugs and numerous coagulation cascade enzymes make it unlikely that any particular anticoagulation assay will enable a valid comparison to be made regarding the efficacy and pharmacokinetics of LMWH and UH.

Antithrombotic Activity

Although LMWHs may have different potencies relative to their multiple mechanisms of action, the ultimate biochemical goal is the same, to prevent thrombin-mediated conversion of fibrinogen to fibrin and, thus, stop thrombus propagation (antithrombosis). Unfortunately, the anticoagulant potencies of these medications, measured by *in vitro* tests of activity such as the aPTT and the plasma anti-Xa activity, do not reliably predict their antithrombotic effects in animal models (52–54).

The antithrombotic activity of different LMWHs and UH regimens has been compared directly in animal experiments. Virtually all of these experiments use some measurement of thrombus propagation on preexisting thrombi, on sites of vascular injury or on a thrombotic substance introduced into the vasculature. Different anticoagulants are then administered, and the ability to suppress thrombus propagation is directly measured. For example, Figure 37.1 describes the results of experiments using a radiolabeled antifibrin antibody, which binds only to newly formed subunits on the fibrin network, to measure the rate of fibrin deposition on preformed thrombi (54). The technique disclosed differences in the antithrombotic activity of the drug regimens used, which were not evident on simultaneous plasma measurements of anti-Xa or antithrombin activity.

Although animal models may disclose substantial differences in antithrombotic activity, the relevance to human therapy is limited by several factors. There may be considerable species-specific differences with humans in physiological aspects such as (a) drug absorption and clearance; (b) thrombus formation, composition, and dissolution; and (c) the sensitivity of thrombus propagation to the action of anticoagulants. In addition, particular characteristics of the model, including the thrombotic stimulus and the method of measuring clot propagation, may affect the relevance to the clinical situation. For example, clot induction by laceration of the jugular vein and insertion of thrombogenic wires may have important pathophysiologic differences with clinical DVT.

Measuring the antithrombotic effects of anticoagulants in humans with VTE is difficult. The most commonly used noninvasive tests for diagnosis of DVT (compression ultrasonography, impedance plethysmography and magnetic resonance imaging) and PE (ventilation-perfusion scanning and helical CT scanning) do not provide sufficiently detailed anatomical information to reliably measure the enlargement of thromboemboli during acute treatment (55). Invasive studies such as contrast venography and angiography, although better at demonstrating gross changes in thrombus size (56), can be painful and are often impractical for monitoring treatment. Furthermore, they may not be able to detect subtle increases in clot dimensions owing to ongoing thrombosis. Finally, all of the anatomical tests described above share the limitation of being unable to differentiate the effects of anticoagulation (preventing clot enlargement) from the effects of the intrinsic fibrinolytic system (reducing clot size).

Attempts to measure antithrombotic activity of LMWHs and UH directly in humans have focused on the ability of these drugs to suppress the formation of serological markers of thrombosis (57). (The popular D-dimer plasma test is actually a marker of plasmin-mediated dissolution of thrombi. Because it remains elevated even during anticoagulation, it is not a valid marker of antithrombotic activity [58].) Potential thrombosis markers primarily consist of biologic by-products of coagulation that have been released into the circulation, such as fragment F1.2 (released as prothrombin is converted to thrombin), thrombin-antithrombin complexes (reflecting thrombin formation, because nearly all free thrombin is eventually inactivated into this complex), and fibrinopeptide A (FPA; released as thrombin cleaves soluble fibrinogen into fibrin) (59). The first two assays, prothrombin F1.2 fragments and thrombin-antithrombin complexes, are serum markers of thrombin activation and are not direct indicators of fibrin(ogen) conversion and polymerization (60). Thus, anticoagulants with different spectra of activity against factor Xa and thrombin (e.g., UH, LMWH, heparin pentasaccharide, and hirudin) would be expected to affect these tests differently, even if their *in vivo* antithrombotic effects were the same.

Fibrinopeptide A, on the other hand, is primarily released during formation of fibrin clots and, theoretically, could be an accurate measure of thrombus propagation (61). FPA is a short-amino-acid sequence situated at the amino termini of the α-chains of soluble fibrinogen. In one of the final steps in the coagulation pathway, thrombin converts soluble fibrinogen to fibrin by cleaving off first FPA, then FPB. Fibrin molecules then polymerize in a semisolid network, whereas the fibrinopeptides remain soluble in plasma. It follows that plasma levels of FPA would reflect the rate and amount of fibrin formation occurring during *in vivo* thrombosis.

Plasma FPA levels are elevated during thrombosis, and this measurement could represent a valid marker for thrombosis and anticoagulation (62). However, FPA is so easily cleaved from fibrinogen that artifactually elevated plasma levels are a common confounding problem. Even when collection tubes are supplemented with proteolytic inhibitors, the sampling procedure itself can cause FPA release. Falsely elevated levels have been associated with factors such as venipuncture techniques (59) and phlebotomy through indwelling catheters (63). One clinical trial suggested that plasma levels of FPA increased during cardiac ischemia and decreased once treatment with UH was initiated (64).

Plasma levels of fibrin monomer are also elevated in patients with thrombosis and can be measured with several available tests (65). In the process of thrombosis, soluble fibrinogen is cleaved by thrombin into fibrin monomers, which spontaneously polymerize with each other into organized (insoluble) networks. When thrombosis occurs on a large scale, fibrin also adheres to soluble fibrinogen itself, and the fibrinogen-fibrin complex remains soluble in the plasma. The presence of large amounts of fibrin monomer (coupled to fibrinogen) in the plasma may indicate the presence of active *in vivo* thrombosis.

Unfortunately, the various assays developed to measure plasma levels of fibrin monomer often yield strikingly different results. The assays differ in the types of fibrin monomers detected ("pure" fibrin versus fibrin partially degraded by plasmin), as well as the methods of detection (antibody tests versus functional assays). As a result, the same plasma sample may measure in the normal range on one assay, but be markedly elevated in another (66). Standardization and calibration between tests is therefore impossible, and the clinical significance of an elevated result can only be determined by comparison to clinical studies using the same assay in an identical manner.

Direct measurement of thrombotic activity in patients would be scientifically valid for comparing the antithrombotic potency of LMWHs to each other and to UH. However, each of the currently available assays of thrombosis markers has serious limitations, preventing its routine use for this purpose. Most importantly, large clinical trials have not confirmed an association between the suppression of these markers and clinical outcome in patients being treated with LMWH for thrombotic disorders (60).

Conclusions

The various LMWHs available for therapeutic use have multiple mechanisms of action, most of which they hold in common with UH. The relative potencies with which the mechanisms are expressed differ between LMWH and UH, and among specific LMWHs. The pharmacokinetics of LMWHs and UH are often measured according to the results of anti-Xa assays, although the correlation between anti-Xa levels and the antithrombotic activities of the drugs is questionable. Animal models of thrombosis give some information regarding the antithrombotic efficacy of different LMWHs compared with UH and with other LMWHs, but the results are not directly applicable to human thrombosis. Unfortunately, no single measure of antithrombosis has been developed in humans whereby the potencies of LMWHs, UH, and other new anticoagulants can be directly compared.

Large clinical outcome studies are expensive and difficult to perform. Perhaps for this reason, different subcutaneous LMWHs have not been compared to each other in this format. Various LMWHs have demonstrated fairly equivalent efficacy and safety to intravenous UH and high-dose subcutaneous UH, and it is reasonable to assume that there would not be large differences in efficacy and safety among different agents. However, the superiority of one subcutaneous regimen over the others can be confirmed (or refuted) only by the performance of well-planned clinical studies.

DEEP VEIN THROMBOSIS AND STABLE PULMONARY EMBOLISM

Summary Statement	Level of Evidence
DVT and stable PE respond well to treatment with either heparin or low-molecular-weight heparin.	Multiple scientific studies
Heparin and low-molecular-weight heparin have similar efficacies and complication rates when used to treat DVT and stable PE.	Multiple scientific studies
Both heparin and low-molecular-weight heparin are safe and efficacious when used in high doses subcutaneously to treat DVT and PE.	Multiple scientific studies
Low-molecular-weight heparin can be given subcutaneously without monitoring in most cases of DVT and PE.	Multiple scientific studies
Heparin doses must be adjusted by repeated activated partial thromboplastin time testing during therapy.	Controversial owing to conflicting epidemiological evidence. No controlled prospective trials to prove benefits of monitoring

DVT, deep venous thrombosis; PE, pulmonary embolism.

DEEP VEIN THROMBOSIS AND STABLE PULMONARY EMBOLISM

In most cases, treatment recommendations for proximal vein DVT and for uncomplicated (hemodynamically normal) PE are similar, reflecting the contention that the two conditions are different manifestations of the same disease process. When patients are systematically examined, many of those with DVT also have (symptomatic or asymptomatic) PE (67,68), and vice versa (69). Furthermore, clinical trials of DVT alone (56,70–76) validated similar treatment regimens to those trials that included patients with DVT and stable PE (77,78), and to those that studied only patients with PE (79,80). None of these treatment trials established the superiority of a regimen for treating stable patients with PE that was substantially different than regimens for patients with DVT.

DVT and PE can be considered different manifestations of the same disease, which require similar, but not necessarily identical, treatment strategies. DVT and PE share the same set of potential clinical sequelae, including death from PE; acute dyspnea, chest pain, and hemodynamic instability from PE; acute leg discomfort from thrombotic occlusion of the deep veins; long-term recurrence of VTE; and other long-term problems such as postphlebitic leg swelling and pulmonary hypertension. A retrospective review of 1,719 patients suggested that the two disorders have the same long-term risk of thromboembolic recurrence (81). On the other hand, patients presenting with PE tend to have a higher short-term mortality (2.3%) than those presenting with DVT (0.5%). Furthermore, the acute mortality for PE patients varies greatly with the stability of the patient during presentation (82). For this reason, unstable PE has a distinct set of treatment strategies and will be discussed separately.

In most cases, the treatment of both DVT and stable PE are identical. From a biologic perspective, the goals of therapy in the acute setting are to reduce the amount of vascular obstruction from PE and DVT, as well as prevent embolization (or further embolization) of DVT. Although the biologic mechanisms relevant to the long-term goals of therapy are incompletely understood, factors such as reducing the damage to the venous wall and valves are likely to be important.

A randomized clinical trial of PE treatment established a dramatic decrease in mortality among patients treated with heparin compared with those not anticoagulated (83). Although (happily) this trial has not been repeated, a wealth of clinical experience has reinforced the benefit of acute treatment with anticoagulants (such as UH and LMWH), which impede ongoing thrombosis directly. By halting thrombus growth, they allow the action of the fibrinolytic system to proceed unopposed. Thus, they indirectly speed the resolution of preexisting DVT and PE and reduce the size of potential emboli.

Acute Anticoagulants

The most commonly used anticoagulants in the acute phase of DVT and stable PE are UH and LMWH. Numerous clinical trials have demonstrated the comparability of UH and LMWHs with respect to safety and efficacy. Metaanalyses of these trials have drawn different conclusions regarding whether LMWH is similar to (12) or superior to (13) UH. However, there is agreement regarding the fact that intravenous administration and dose adjustment using aPTT values make routine UH treatment more complicated and costly than subcutaneous LMWH treatment (21). The merits of these two attributes of UH treatment therefore deserve some discussion.

Subcutaneous Versus Intravenous Heparin

Two heparin regimens are commonly used in the treatment of VTE: continuous intravenous infusion of approximately 18 U/(kg·hr) or twice daily subcutaneous injections of approximately 250 U/kg. Unquestionably, the continuous intravenous regimen has been the most popular. The subcutaneous route allows more mobility and possible outpatient management, and so may gain popularity in the current era of medical cost containment.

Although the most common route of UH administration is intravenous, subcutaneous administration may be just as applicable for UH as it is for LMWH. A metaanalysis of randomized clinical trials comparing therapeutic dose subcutaneous UH (total daily dose of approximately 35,000 U) with intravenous UH also showed the subcutaneous regimens to be more effective and at least as safe as the intravenous ones (14). In fact, only one randomized clinical trial has suggested better outcomes with intravenous UH for DVT treatment; but that trial used low doses of subcutaneous UH (84). Other DVT treatment trials using higher doses in the subcutaneous UH arms reported that this method of administration was more effective (fewer recurrences) and/or safer (less bleeding) than was intravenous UH (85–88). Clinical data actually favor treating stable thromboembolism patients with subcutaneous UH rather than intravenous UH. There is certainly no evidence to suggest that intravenous administration (albeit popular) is necessary for UH treatment.

Is Activated Partial Thromboplastin Time Adjustment Necessary for UH Treatment?

A carefully performed randomized clinical trial has established that a weight-based dosing algorithm achieved a target aPTT value more quickly than did a more subjective method of dose adjustment (89). However, the validity of the aPTT test itself, and the importance of UH dose adjustment by the aPTT test (rather than unadjusted weight-based dosing), is the subject of disagreement among experts.

Fundamental to the question of aPTT validity is the accuracy and repeatability of the test itself. In general, aPTT test results are not repeatable between laboratories. Unlike the prothrombin time, which is standardized across laboratories using the INR, target values for the aPTT are unique to each individual laboratory. Depending on the particular equipment, reagents, and procedures used, the target aPTT ranges for UH treatment may be 47 to 63 seconds in one hospital, but 108 to 158 seconds in another (90). The lack of standardization is not corrected by adjusting heparin to a target aPPT relative to a (pooled normal plasma) baseline: The therapeutic value of this ratio is estimated at 1.5 to 2.5 (84) in some studies and twice that value in others (90). Furthermore, there can be substantial diurnal variation in tests obtained during continuous intravenous infusion of heparin, so that an 8:00 a.m. test does not reliably predict results some hours later.

Clinical data have been used to argue either side of the question over the wisdom of adjusting heparin dose to target aPTT values. In a post hoc analysis of three clinical trials in which DVT was treated with intravenous UH, inadequate initial therapy was associated with both early and long-term recurrence (91). However, a similar post hoc analysis of three clinical DVT treatment trials using intravenous heparin (bolus, 5,000 U; initial rate, 1,250 U/hr) disclosed no significant difference in recurrence rates between patients with subtherapeutic and therapeutic aPTT values (22). Along a similar vein, a prospective multicenter trial of acute VTE treatment disclosed a relationship between the heparin dose and bleeding, independent of the concomitant aPTT results (19). These data suggest that the dose of UH itself, not the aPTT value, determines the outcome of treatment. After an adequate bolus and initial infusion, the clinical benefits of aPTT dose adjustment itself have not been tested in a controlled outcome trial.

The value of aPTT testing is relevant to the issue of the relative cost-effectiveness of LMWH and UH. In current practice, therapy with LMWH is less expensive than that with UH, because the former can more easily be administered subcutaneously to outpatients (21,92). Although therapeutic subcutaneous UH can be administered to outpatients as well (see "Subcutaneous Low-Molecular-Weight Heparin Versus Subcutaneous Unfractionated Heparin" below) (20,93), the dosage adjustment (according to aPTT times) can be time-intensive (20). It is therefore the direct and indirect costs associated with aPTT testing that make LMWH a more financially attractive alternative to UH in current practice.

Is Low-Molecular-Weight Heparin More Effective and Safe than Unfractionated Heparin?

Various formulations of LMWH have been compared to intravenous UH in randomized clinical trials (Table 37.1). The trials used different types and doses of LMWH, differ-

ent endpoints to represent treatment failure (recurrence) and adverse events (significant bleeding), and different statistical tests to define significance. The overwhelming majority of trials disclosed no statistically significant differences in disease recurrence or bleeding between the LMWH regimens and UH.

The numerical results of the comparative trials have been combined in numerous metaanalyses, which suggest that subcutaneous LMWH regimens, as a whole, are clinically superior to intravenous UH (13, 94–96). However, because the individual studies used different outcome definitions, mathematically combining the results may be problematic. Furthermore, the soundness of the metaanalyses depends on the scientific validity of combining all LMWH treatment groups into one large population, with no therapeutically important differences between the groups. In fact, there is growing recognition that each LMWH has a distinct composition and spectrum of biologic activity, and cannot be considered therapeutically identical to other drugs within the same class (15–17,97–101). Even if the superiority of subcutaneous LMWH over intravenous UH was unequivocally established, the subcutaneous route itself may be responsible for the advantages over intravenous UH, as is the case for subcutaneous UH.

Subcutaneous Low-Molecular-Weight Heparin Versus Subcutaneous Unfractionated Heparin

The trends toward improved (or at least not worsened) outcomes with subcutaneous LMWH compared with intravenous UH are similar to the trends observed when subcutaneous UH was compared with intravenous UH. This observation calls into question whether the observed differences were owing to some advantage (pharmacological or practical) to administering the drugs subcutaneously.

Subcutaneous LMWH was directly compared with subcutaneous UH in a randomized clinical trial of DVT treatment. The results disclosed no significant differences in thrombus regression, acute or long-term recurrence, major bleeding, or PE (76). The clinical relevance of this finding depends on such factors as the practicality of outpatient therapy with twice-per-day subcutaneous UH (20) and the related, unsettled issue of the importance of ongoing dose adjustment to achieve aPTT results within target range (18) (see "Is Activated Partial Thromboplastin Time Adjustment Necessary for UH Treatment?" above).

ECONOMICS

Because the two medications are clinically comparable, the relative cost-effectiveness of LMWH and UH may be determined by comparing the total cost of therapy (102). The overall cost of treatment with LMWH or with UH is largely dependent on the setting in which the drugs are used. Although the pharmaceutical costs of LMWH are higher

TABLE 37.1. STUDIES COMPARING UNFRACTIONATED TO LOW-MOLECULAR-WEIGHT HEPARINS

LMWH Regimen (Reference)	Population, n	Double-Blind?	Unstable Patients Excluded?	Measurement of Efficacy	Measurement of Safety (Bleeding)	Statistically Significant Benefit vs. UH? Efficacy	Safety	Thrombocytopenia
Ardeparin, 130 U/kg bid (192)	DVT, 75	No	Yes	Follow-up ultrasound at 6 wk	"Major bleeding" (not otherwise defined)	No	No	—
Certoparin, 8000 U bid (70)	DVT, 257	No	Yes	Improved venogram and V/Q after treatment; symptomatic DVT/PE within 6 months	Fall in hemoglobin > 2.0, 2 U transfusion, intracranial bleed, retroperitoneal bleed	No	No	No
Dalteparin, adjusted dose bid (86)	DVT, 56	Yes	Yes	Improved venograms at 1 wk	"Major bleeding" (not otherwise defined)	No	No	No
Dalteparin IV, adjusted dose (193)	DVT or PE, 194	Yes	Yes	New defects on V/Q or IPG after treatment	Fall in hemoglobin > 2.42, any transfusion, treatment interruption, death	No	No	No
Dalteparin, 120 U/kg bid (194)	DVT, 110	No	Yes	Improved venogram at 1 wk; symptomatic DVT/PE within 12–36 mo	"Bleeding" (not otherwise defined)	No	No	No
Dalteparin, 200 U/kg qd (195)	DVT, 204	No	Yes	Improved venogram after treatment; symptomatic DVT/PE within 6 mo	Fall in hemoglobin > 3.0, intracranial bleed, retroperitoneal bleed or death	No	No	No
Dalteparin, 120 U/kg bid (79)	PE, 60	No	Yes	Symptomatic or asymptomatic PE within 10 d	Fall in hemoglobin > 5.0, 2 U transfusion, intracranial bleed, retroperitoneal bleed, other	No	No	No
Dalteparin, 200 U/kg qd (56)	DVT, 253	No	Yes	Improved venogram after treatment; symptomatic DVT within 6 mo	Fall in hemoglobin > 3.0, any transfusion, death, other	No	No	No
Dalteparin, 200 U/kg qd (73)	DVT, 248	No	Yes	Improved venogram after treatment; symptomatic DVT/PE within 6 mo	Fall in hemoglobin > 3.0, any transfusion, treatment interruption, death	No	No	No
Enoxaparin, 1 mg/kg q12 (196)	DVT, 134	No	Yes	Improved venograms after 10 d; symptomatic DVT/PE within 10 d	Fall in hemoglobin > 2.0, death, intracranial bleed, retroperitoneal bleed	Yes	No	No
Enoxaparin, 1 mg/kg bid (72)	DVT, 500	No	Yes	Symptomatic DVT/PE (or DVT found on IPG screening)	Fall in hemoglobin > 2.0, 2 U transfusion, intracranial bleed, retroperitoneal bleed	No	No	No
Enoxaparin, 1 mg/kg bid or 1.5 mg/kg SC qd (197)	DVT or PE, 900	No	Yes	Symptomatic DVT/PE	Fall in hemoglobin > 2.0, 2 U transfusion; intracranial retroperitoneal or intraocular bleed, death, other	No	No	No
Nadroparin, 200 U/kg bid (74)	DVT, 170	No	Yes	Improved venograms and V/Q after treatment; symptomatic DVT or PE within 6 mo	Fall in hemoglobin > 2.0, 2 U transfusion, intracranial bleed, retroperitoneal bleed, other	No	No	No
Nadroparin, 225 U/kg bid; versus SC UH (76)	DVT, 146	No	Yes	Improved venograms after treatment; symptomatic DVT within 3 mo	Fall in hemoglobin requiring discontinuation of anticoagulation or transfusion, intracranial bleed, retroperitoneal bleed	No	No	No
Nadroparin, 120 U/kg bid (75)	DVT, 400	No	Yes	Symptomatic DVT/PE within 6 mo	Fall in hemoglobin > 2.0, 2 U transfusion, intracranial bleed, retroperitoneal bleed	No	No	No
Reviparin, 6300 U bid (78)	DVT or PE, 1021	No	Yes	Symptomatic DVT or PE within 12 wk	Fall in hemoglobin > 2.0, 2 U transfusion, intracranial bleed, retroperitoneal bleed, intracranial bleed, death, treatment interruption	No	No	No
Sandoparin, 150 U/kg bid (198)	DVT, 50	No	Yes	Improved venograms after treatment, V/Q if PE suspected	"Bleeding" (not otherwise defined)	No	No	No
Tinzaparin, 175 U/kg qd (77)	DVT (PE not excluded), 432	Yes	Yes	Symptomatic DVT/PE within 3 mo	Fall in hemoglobin > 2.0, 2 U transfusion, intracranial bleed, retroperitoneal bleed, other	No	Yes	No
Tinzaparin, 175 U/kg qd (80)	PE, 612	No	Yes	Symptomatic DVT/PE within 90 d	Fall in hemoglobin > 2.0, 2 U transfusion, intracranial bleed, retroperitoneal bleed	No	No	No

LMWH, low-molecular-weight heparin; UH, unfractionated heparin; DVT, deep venous thrombosis; V/Q, ventilation-perfusion; PE, pulmonary embolism; IPG, impedance plethysmography.

than those for UH, a recent analysis calculated that the overall cost of DVT therapy (including, e.g., monitoring, equipment) was lower for subcutaneous LMWH than for intravenous UH, provided that the LMWH is administered to most patients at least partially in an outpatient setting (21). However, if both medications are administered in the hospital, treatment with subcutaneous LMWH has a higher overall cost than that of intravenous UH (and presumably subcutaneous UH) (13). Other cost analyses (103) have yielded different results, and it is recommended that individual institutions perform their own cost comparisons. The cost of outpatient subcutaneous LMWH has not been compared to outpatient subcutaneous UH for DVT treatment. Because LMWH is much more expensive per dose than is UH, the relative cost would depend largely on the frequency of aPTT monitoring and subsequent UH dose adjustments (20).

It is reasonable to conclude that the numerous clinical trials strongly support the conclusion that subcutaneous regimens of LMWH are at least as effective and safe as intravenous UH for the treatment of clinically stable patients with VTE. The immediate economic impact of this finding results from the fact that the LMWHs are effective when given subcutaneously without monitoring. Enormous cost savings are possible if ambulatory patients are treated out of hospital with subcutaneous injections rather than by inpatient intravenous therapy. The true long-term economic impact of this finding depends on the unsettled question of whether subcutaneous, unmonitored outpatient therapy using LMWH is truly superior to the same strategy using UH.

EMBOLIZATION DURING ANTICOAGULATION

When evaluating the benefits of anticoagulants, it must be remembered that they neither prevent thrombi from embolizing nor enhance thrombus resolution directly. Treated patients remain at embolic risk until their DVTs have either dissolved or become organized. Thus, embolization occurring in the first few days of therapy does not reflect drug failure. Only thrombus growth or initiation of a new thrombus during therapy is evidence of heparin (or LMWH) failure. Because nearly half of patients with above-knee acute DVT already have had asymptomatic PE, it is important not to mistake the subsequent discovery of these preexisting emboli for evidence of recurrent thromboembolic disease.

Is it important to prevent such embolizations in stable patients with DVT? Clinical evidence suggests not. In a randomized study of stable patients with DVT and (undefined) risk of PE, inferior vena cava filters resulted in a fivefold reduction in the incidence of PE within the first 12 days of therapy, but had no effect on acute mortality (104). Furthermore, the old practice of strict bed rest to prevent embolization during the initial treatment of stable patients with DVT appears unnecessary in light of the clinical success of

outpatient therapy (105,106). The importance of preventing embolization in unstable patients is addressed in the section "Unstable Pulmonary Embolism."

Bleeding

The major complication of therapy with UH or LMWH is hemorrhage. The initial hope that LMWH would be safer than UH was not borne out in clinical studies; both drugs most likely carry the same risk of bleeding (Table 37.1). In fact, factors other than the type and dose of heparin appear to be far more important in determining bleeding risk, including age (especially beyond the sixth decade), the presence of unsuspected or known bleeding sites (e.g., stomach, bowel, kidney), uremia, and demonstrable hemostatic defects (e.g., thrombocytopenia). Available data indicate that bleeding risk is very low among patients who do not have a significant coexistent disease or coagulopathy. It should also be noted that many hemorrhagic episodes in heparinized patients occur when clotting parameters are in therapeutic range and in the absence of any identifiable risk of hemorrhage.

Heparin-Induced Thrombocytopenia

HIT is among the most serious complications of anticoagulation therapy, often resulting in life-threatening limb ischemia. HIT is often heralded by the unexpected development of thrombocytopenia during therapy. Although more commonly observed after at least 1 week of heparin therapy, the syndrome can occur earlier, especially in patients previously exposed to anticoagulants. The relative risk of developing thrombocytopenia is an important consideration

UNSTABLE PULMONARY EMBOLISM	
Summary Statement	**Level of Evidence**
The risk of death from PE rises dramatically if the patient presents with hemodynamic instability.	Multiple scientific studies
Intravenous heparin reduces mortality from PE.	Based on one scientific study
Inferior vena cava filters reduce mortality in unstable PE.	Controversial, based on assumptions from physiological experiments and uncontrolled clinical data
Thrombolytic medications reduce mortality in unstable PE.	Controversial, based on assumptions from physiological experiments and uncontrolled clinical data
Embolectomy reduces mortality in PE complicated by shock.	Controversial, based on assumptions from physiological experiments and uncontrolled clinical data

PE, pulmonary embolism.

in the choice between LMWHs and standard UH for the acute treatment of VTE. Some current recommendations for VTE treatment are based on the assumption that LMWHs reduce the risk of this complication of VTE treatment, and extend to the recommendation that less frequent platelet monitoring is necessary with LMWH than it is with UH (107). However, high-quality, large, randomized clinical trials (Table 37.1) have not shown significantly lower rates of thrombocytopenia with LMWH than with UH. In fact, considering only medications available in the United States (enoxaparin, dalteparin, and tinzaparin), there is a trend toward a higher incidence of thrombocytopenia with LMWH than with UH. Although the comparative trials did not document the incidence of HIT itself, the results suggest that UH and LMWH require equal consideration of the risk for thrombocytopenia (108).

Unstable Pulmonary Embolism

Although the treatment of PE in very stable patients is generally identical to DVT, several facts specific to PE treatment deserve consideration. The most important issue is that outpatient, subcutaneous treatment regimens have only been tested on the most clinically stable patients with PE. Less healthy patients merit hospital admission. Additional therapeutic issues specific to PE must be considered, including (a) the size of the initial dose of heparin and the dosage regimen during the first 24 hours, (b) the need for cardiopulmonary supportive measures, (c) the role of caval filters and surgery, and (d) the role of thrombolytic agents.

Most patients with PE survive their illness when treated with anticoagulants at doses similar to those used to treat DVT (109). However, a subpopulation of patients with massive PE have a high mortality when treated with standard doses of anticoagulants, even when combined with thrombolytic medications (82). It is generally agreed that those who succumb from PE usually do so because of right ventricular dysfunction and ischemia owing to elevated pulmonary artery resistance (107). However, eventual right ventricular collapse is difficult to predict (110,111), and the pathophysiological mechanisms leading to eventual right ventricular deterioration are not entirely clear. Factors in addition to pure mechanical obstruction are likely to contribute to the increasing load on the right ventricle, because the pulmonary vascular resistance measured in otherwise healthy patients with PE is higher than one would predict from the degree of pulmonary artery occlusion alone (112). For example, ongoing thrombosis on the surface of the emboli may increase pulmonary vascular resistance through mechanisms such as ongoing platelet accumulation and degranulation, as well as microembolization into small pulmonary arteries.

The humoral effects of PE on pulmonary vascular resistance and right heart function have been reviewed comprehensively elsewhere (113,114). PE induces the release of putative mediators of pulmonary artery vasoconstriction from many sources, including platelets, neutrophils, endothelial cells, and autonomic efferent nerve endings (113). Recent attention has been focused on the effects of thromboxane (114), serotonin (114), and endothelin (114–116) on pulmonary artery vasoconstriction. Although the specific role of these mediators is still under investigation, they all may be released in response to stimulation by thrombin or other by-products of active thrombosis (113). It follows that progressive pulmonary artery vasoconstriction would occur in the presence of accelerated thrombosis during pulmonary embolization.

An alternative hypothesis is that clinical deterioration is mediated by factors generated during formation of the thrombus before embolization, and that anticoagulation will have little direct effect once the thrombus has embolized. For example, release from the embolus of vasoactive substances (such as serotonin) discharged by previously trapped platelets could mediate pulmonary vasoconstriction and right ventricular failure. However, platelet degranulation begins immediately on activation by the thrombus, and plasma serotonin levels generally peak by 1 hour (117). By contrast, deterioration after PE is often delayed for hours (118) or even days (119) after the initial event, supporting the argument that active thrombosis induces ongoing mediator production and release.

Clinical Evidence

Unfortunately, a strict evidence-based approach is not often possible when considering therapy for unstable PE. Randomized clinical trials of PE treatment generally exclude unstable patients (78,80,120–122). Unstable PE is generally an unexpected, serious, and rapidly developing event: one that does not lend itself easily to randomized clinical trials. Much of the treatment of PE is, therefore, based on indirect evidence, the interpretation of which varies among experts.

Does Unstable Pulmonary Embolism Necessitate Higher Anticoagulant Doses?

The size of the initial heparin dose required during PE is controversial. Pharmacologically active peptides, released from platelets coating an embolus, may contribute to the initial severity of the cardiopulmonary symptoms by inducing pulmonary vasoconstriction and bronchoconstriction (123). Animal studies have shown that a large initial bolus of heparin is necessary to inhibit platelet aggregation after PE (124), which initiates release of these agents. Based on these data, we recommend a large initial intravenous bolus (15,000–20,000 U) of heparin, followed by a continuous infusion similar to the intravenous regimens discussed above (18 U/[kg·hr]). If dose adjustment is used, it should focus on avoiding low doses/aPTT values during the first 1 to 2 days of therapy. Some clinicians prefer to use larger-dose heparin infusions during the initial 24 hours after massive embolic events, owing to the accelerated generation of thrombin (125) platelet factor IV [which inactivates the antithrombin effect of UH and LMWH (39)] and other substances. No clinical studies are available to compare standard-dose UH to higher-dose UH or LMWH in unstable PE patients.

Cardiopulmonary Support

Cardiopulmonary supportive measures may be indicated for PE treatment, including administration of oxygen if arterial hypoxemia is present. Systemic hypotension, if present, is usually owing to acute right ventricular ischemia and failure (126). Animal experiments suggest that an important mechanism of right ventricular ischemia is low myocardial perfusion pressure (coronary pressure–right ventricular pressure) occurring as the right heart strains to overcome massive pulmonary artery obstruction. Fluid loading may increase right atrial and right ventricular end-diastolic pressure, which, in a small series (13 patients), was associated with an increase in cardiac output from 1.6 ± 0.1 to 2.0 ± 0.1 L/(min·m^2) ($p < .05$) (127). However, the overloaded right ventricle may suffer from decreased coronary perfusion pressure, making right ventricular infarction worse (128). For that reason, fluid loading should be done with caution, and consideration should be given to systemic vasoconstrictive agents, such as phenylephrine, to raise arterial pressure (and coronary pressure) during PE-associated shock (126).

Inferior Vena Cava Filters

Another mode of therapy arose from evidence that many patients who die from PE do so up to 2 weeks after presentation (129). This time frame suggests that a second event, perhaps a subsequent embolization of lower-limb DVT, occurred. During this time frame, it has been established that almost 5% of DVTs will embolize (104). Although stable patients tolerate these incidental emboli quite well, patients who are already hemodynamically compromised may not. In cases of massive embolization, some clinicians (including the author) will place an inferior vena caval filter, which have been shown to decrease the short-term embolization rate by nearly 80% (104). Multiple devices are available to prevent recurrent embolism, but the most sensible ones to use in these situations are those such as the Greenfield (or similar) inferior vena caval filter, which will not decrease venous return and right ventricular filling pressure (130). The devices are rather easy to insert, do not interfere with caval blood flow, and have an excellent (95%) record of long-term patency. Although evidence suggests that filter placement may increase the long-term risk of symptomatic DVT recurrence, it may be a life-saving procedure in the setting of proved massive embolism when a recurrence may be fatal. Because anticoagulation cannot prevent recurrence during the first several days, it is during this period that caval interruption should be considered.

Thrombolytic Therapy

The role of thrombolytic agents in management of PE is unclear. Management decisions must be made on the basis of indirect information rather than by comparative clinical trials in the appropriate patient population.

The Urokinase in Pulmonary Embolism Trial (UPET) (120), the largest trial to randomize patients into thrombolytic or standard heparin therapy, was performed on hemodynamically stable patients. There was a very short-term hemodynamic benefit: Cardiac outputs and pulmonary pressures were improved on the day after thrombolytics. No positive effects on morbidity or mortality were demonstrated, however, nor was the ultimate degree of embolic resolution any greater. By 1 week, the treatment groups were identical (except for an increase in bleeding in the thrombolytic group). Multiple studies have confirmed that these agents promote rapid embolic resolution (131). However, there does not appear to be a long-term benefit to more rapid (but not necessarily more complete) clot resolution (132).

Patients with massive PE have much higher mortality rates than the patients evaluated in UPET. The mortality for patients with high right ventricular pressures and high pulmonary artery pressures is about double the mortality for more stable PE patients. The mortality increases exponentially as patients progress to hypotension, shock, and then the need for cardiopulmonary resuscitation (82). It is likely that the acute hemodynamic benefits of thrombolytics will have a much higher impact on these patients than on the stable patients in UPET. The outcome benefit of thrombolytics in unstable patients has been studied in uncontrolled, retrospective studies. One study reported a lower mortality in patients treated with thrombolytics (82), whereas another reported a higher mortality (owing to bleeding) (111).

A recent study of submassive PE (i.e., with evidence of right ventricular strain) (133) randomized patients either to thrombolytics plus heparin or to heparin plus placebo. The groups were compared on the basis of a combined primary endpoint, including death and escalation of treatment (including subsequent thrombolytic therapy). Although the group receiving thrombolytics had a lower incidence of the combined endpoint, the only actual outcome difference between the groups was that those treated with heparin/placebo received more thrombolytic therapy during the follow-up period. No other outcome, such as death and the need for mechanical ventilation or vasopressors, was different between the groups, begging the question of whether rescue thrombolytic therapy was necessary. Unfortunately, the results did not answer the question of whether thrombolytic therapy is beneficial initially or even during follow-up for patients with evidence of right heart strain.

Thrombolytics are costly and carry significant risks. A review of clinical trials disclosed a 2.1% intracranial hemorrhage rate and 1.6 fatal intracranial hemorrhage rate when thrombolytics were used for thromboembolic disease (134). For this reason, thrombolytics should be reserved for management of the patient with massive embolism and persistent hypotension. Even in this situation, patient selection is difficult, and only physicians quite familiar with the drugs should use them.

Embolectomy

Acute pulmonary embolectomy (by thoracotomy, suction catheter, or balloon catheter) is rarely warranted because medical therapy is so successful, patient selection so difficult, and the results of acute embolectomy so unimpressive. Case series from the 1960s and 1970s documented mortality rates as high as 50% for the procedure (135). However, the mortality reported in subsequent series decreased over time: from 30% (136) to 25% (137) to 11% in a series published in 2002 (138). The improved mortality is most likely owing to a combination of improved surgical and postoperative techniques, as well as selection of less compromised patients for surgery in the more recent series. Unfortunately, there are no large randomized controlled trials to compare the outcome of embolectomy to less invasive strategies for patients with massive PE. Considerable controversy remains about which cases, if any, require embolectomy. However, there are conceivable situations in which massive embolism fails to respond promptly to medical therapy, the diagnosis is certain, and immediate expert surgical intervention is possible.

Echocardiography to Guide Therapy

The appropriate influence of echocardiography on the treatment of PE is controversial. Patients with substantial pulmonary arterial obstruction may have evidence of right ventricular strain on transthoracic echocardiogram (139), such as right ventricular dilatation and septal dyskinesis. (A somewhat more specific finding is evidence of abnormal free wall motion throughout the right ventricle, but with sparing in the area of the apex [140].) In a retrospective series of 121 consecutive PE patients, echocardiographic evidence of right ventricular dysfunction was found in 70% of those with perfusion defects constituting greater than one fifth of the pulmonary vasculature, but in only 31% of those with smaller perfusion defects (141). In the same group of patients, those with echocardiogram findings of right ventricular dysfunction during the acute phase of PE had a greater incidence of in-hospital PE-related mortality (142). Follow-up of these patients after 1 year, however, disclosed no differences in PE-related mortality (143) between those with and without right ventricular failure on echocardiograms. In the former group, 89% had, in fact, normalized the right ventricular function after the first week, and 92% had done so by 1 year. Moreover, in another retrospective series of 170 patients with multilobar PEs, the echocardiographic findings (right ventricular dilatation and septal dyskinesia) in the absence of clinical evidence of shock were not associated with increased mortality, compared with PE patients with more

normal echocardiograms (144). These findings contrast with those of another study, in which three of 65 normotensive patients with echocardiogram evidence of right ventricular strain died from PE, whereas none of the 97 normotensive patients with more normal echocardiograms did (145).

The significance of PE-associated echocardiographic abnormalities themselves on treatment decisions is unclear. The influence of echocardiography and other evidence of right ventricular strain on the decision to use thrombolytics is discussed above. Although evidence of right heart strain may be associated with worse outcomes, there is no clinical data to determine how it would alter the risk/benefit ratios of any of the interventions mentioned in this section. Some experts recommend using echocardiograms in all unstable PE patients, to help identify those in whom additional interventions may become necessary (146). Others recommend that additional interventions be limited to patients with more clinical evidence for cardiopulmonary deterioration (147). Until the issue is clarified by high-quality controlled trials, the decision to perform echocardiography and the influence of the results on management decisions must be individualized according to the judgment of the clinician.

CHRONIC ANTICOAGULATION	
Summary Statement	**Level of Evidence**
Warfarin for at least 3 mo reduces the incidence of recurrence after an episode of DVT or PE.	Multiple scientific studies
Warfarin adjusted to an INR of 2 to 3 optimizes the balance between efficacy and safety during treatment.	Multiple scientific studies
Patients with "unprovoked" DVT or PE have a higher risk of recurrence than those with identifiable (and removable) clinical risk factors.	Multiple scientific studies
In patients at high risk of DVT and PE recurrence, longer durations of warfarin therapy reduce the recurrence rate but increase the risk of bleeding.	Multiple scientific studies
Patients with DVT and/or PE who are heterozygous for factor V Leiden can be treated the same as those with similar presentations without the genetic disorder.	Controversial due to conflicting reports showing equal vs. higher recurrence rates for this population. No controlled trials of short vs long treatment for this population alone
Patients with more severe thrombophilic blood disorders should receive long-term (perhaps indefinite) anticoagulation.	Presumptive, based on data showing high recurrence rates. No controlled trials proving outcome benefits to life-long anticoagulation for this population

DVT, deep venous thrombosis; PE, pulmonary embolism; INR, international normalized ratio.

Chronic Anticoagulation

As soon as the diagnosis of VTE is confirmed, one can assume that follow-up treatment will be required beyond hospitalization. Currently, warfarin is the most practical option; it can be initiated as soon as heparin has been started. Heparin is continued until the prothrombin time has been in range (INR, 2–3) for two consecutive days. At that point, heparin can be discontinued and the patient discharged on warfarin. If, for some reason, warfarin cannot be used, high doses of subcutaneous heparin (adjusted to keep the aPTT greater than 1.5 × control) can be started on day 6 and the patient discharged on this regimen. Both approaches are acceptable; the choice involves the patient's desires (e.g., injections versus the need for regular prothrombin times).

Warfarin

The most commonly used drug for follow-up therapy of VTE disease is warfarin. The antithrombotic activity of warfarin stems from its ability to inhibit the final step in the synthesis of coagulation factors II (thrombin), VII, IX, and X. It is important to realize that warfarin does not inactivate clotting factors that have already been synthesized and activated within the body. In the acute stage, thrombi contain a high concentration of activated clotting factors. For this reason, direct inhibition with heparin or LMWH is necessary to halt the thrombotic process acutely. This principle was confirmed by a clinical trial of DVT treatment in which patients treated exclusively with warfarin had more than three times as many thrombotic complications as did patients in whom warfarin therapy began after an initial course of heparin, with no significant increase in the risk of bleeding (148). A subsequent clinical trial established that in most patients, 5 days of heparin (or, presumably, LMWH) is as effective for initial treatment as is 10 days (149).

Importance of International Normalized Ratio Target Range

Warfarin is adjusted according to the plasma prothrombin time, which is standardized among laboratories as the INR. It is common practice to use a target INR range of two to three for treatment of venous thrombosis. In a 96-patient trial (150), keeping the INR greater than three was no more effective than the two-to-three range, but was associated with a nearly fivefold increase in bleeding rates. In more recent trials (151,152), recurrent thromboembolism was very rare during warfarin treatment when the INR was targeted at two to three: Recurrence occurred only when patients stopped warfarin. Although INR values less than two have been shown to be less effective for a number of cardiovascular diseases, the lower limit for INR has not yet been established in high-quality clinical trials. However, because lower INR ranges have not yet been compared with the (clinically validated) range of two to three, they are not currently recommended for clinical practice (153).

Duration: Clinical Trials

Although follow-up anticoagulation therapy is necessary in almost all cases to prevent recurrence of VTE, the appropriate type and duration of therapy should be tailored to the clinical situation. In patients presenting with DVT or PE, at least 3 months of therapy is necessary: Substantially shorter regimens nearly doubled the recurrence rate in a comparative randomized trial (154). A subgroup analysis suggested that patients who suffered DVT or PE postoperatively may do just as well with 4 weeks of therapy, but the hypothesis has not been proven directly in clinical trials. The duration of follow-up anticoagulation necessary for patients with transient risk factors is controversial. The simple clinical answer is that protection should be continued until the original risk factor(s) has subsided (e.g., the broken leg has healed, and the patient is fully ambulatory).

On the other hand, patients at high risk for recurrence, characterized by having unresolved risk factors for VTE, may require prolonged (possibly lifelong) anticoagulation (152). In some cases, persistent risk factors reflect chronic conditions such as immobility, heart failure, or persistent venous obstruction. In addition, patients with idiopathic VTE have high rates of recurrence and are likely to have persistent hypercoagulable states, based on either known biochemical disorders or on as yet uncharacterized factors.

TREATMENT OF IDIOPATHIC DEEP VEINOUS THROMBOSIS

One double-blinded randomized control trial (152) comparing 3 months (n = 83) to 24 months (n = 79) of therapeutic warfarin for DVT treatment disclosed significantly lower rates of symptomatic recurrence in the group given the longer course of therapy. A subsequent randomized control trial, comparing 3 months to 1 year of anticoagulation, disclosed lower recurrence rates during the first year in the group treated throughout that year. However, during the subsequent year of follow-up (during which anticoagulation was given to neither group), the incidence of recurrent thrombosis was the same in both groups (155). In both studies, the groups given longer durations of anticoagulants also suffered higher bleeding rates. These data suggest that prolonged anticoagulation entails benefits and risks that are manifested only during the treatment period itself. The decision to prolong anticoagulation should be individualized by estimating each patient's particular risks for recurrence and for bleeding.

Treatment of Venous Thromboembolism in the Presence of Thrombophilic Blood Conditions

The recent discovery of specific genetic mutations in large numbers of patients with VTE has greatly increased our understanding of the mechanisms of thrombosis. The most prevalent of those discovered to date is a point mutation in the gene encoding factor V Leiden, which imparts a resistance to the anticoagulant effect of protein C. In certain populations, the heterozygous factor V Leiden genotype is expressed six times more frequently in patients with VTE than in healthy patients (156). The homozygous factor V Leiden genotype, rarely found in healthy individuals, is found in 1% of VTE patients in the same populations. Likewise, a nontranslated mutation in the gene encoding prothrombin (G-20210-A) (157) is found about three times as frequently in VTE patients as in controls (158). The combination of heterozygous factor V Leiden and heterozygous P20210 is more highly associated with recurrent disease than either of the mutations alone (159).

Although the association between factor V Leiden, P20210, and thrombosis is robust, the implications for treating individual VTE patients with these mutations are far from clear. Prospective clinical trails have not consistently demonstrated an increased risk of recurrence in VTE patients heterozygous for factor V Leiden, compared with similar patients without the mutations (152,160–163). Furthermore, there are no randomized clinical trials demonstrating improved outcome when VTE patients with the mutations are anticoagulated for longer periods of time than are clinically similar VTE patients without the mutations.

Although few VTE patients who are homozygous for factor V Leiden have been studied prospectively, they appear to have a much higher risk for recurrent VTE, and prolonged anticoagulation for these patients is reasonable (grade C1 recommendation) (152,162). The combination of heterozygous factor V Leiden and heterozygous P20210 in VTE patients is associated with recurrent disease, but the relative risk (and absolute risk) of recurrent disease is not sufficiently determined to allow risk/benefit analysis of prolonged anticoagulation based on this genetic profile alone (159).

The implications for genetic counseling are even more vague. Relatives of heterozygous factor V Leiden VTE patients who are, themselves, heterozygous for factor V Leiden have a 4.5 times higher annual incidence of VTE than that of relatives without the mutation (164). However, the estimated incidence of VTE in heterozygous relatives is only 0.45% per year (164). The incidence of life-threatening or debilitating disease is even more uncommon.

Other genetic anomalies such as deficiencies of proteins C and S and antithrombin III are less common, and large randomized trials demonstrating the benefits of prolonged anticoagulation for VTE patients with these disorders are lacking. However, clinical experience and case series suggest very high recurrence rates in these patients, and prolonged anticoagulation seems warranted.

The *lupus anticoagulant* is an acquired humoral thrombophilic factor (doubly misnamed because half of occurrences are not associated with connective tissue disorders). The related clinical condition is termed *antiphospholipid antibody syndrome,* characterized by the presence of one or more of a family of acquired autoantibodies (anticardiolipin, antiphospholipid, and others) capable of interfering with factors that maintain the normal balance between thrombosis and antithrombosis (e.g., β_2-glycoprotein, protein C pathway, prothrombin) (165). Risk of VTE is associated with the antiphospholipid antibody syndrome, particularly when the antibodies are present in high titers (166) or when the lupus anticoagulant is present (167). However, the risk of catastrophic recurrent emboli in patients with the syndrome is multifactorial and not entirely dependent on antibody titer. Large retrospective studies of VTE patients with the antiphospholipid antibody syndrome disclosed very high recurrence rates during long-term follow-up, except in those patients treated with indefinite courses of full-dose warfarin (168,169). However, the risk of anticoagulation-associated bleeding in these patients is unclear, and no clinical trial has established improved outcomes using long-term anticoagulation. Furthermore, at least one small prospective trial disclosed no difference in recurrence rates between VTE patients with and without the antiphospholipid antibodies (167). It is reasonable to treat VTE patients with the lupus anticoagulant with long-term anticoagulation. Further study of this topic would enable more definitive recommendations to be made.

The indications for a hypercoagulability workup, and the appropriate influence the results should have on management decisions, are unclear. It seems reasonable that patients with unexplained thrombosis at a young age, those with thromboses in unusual anatomic locations, and those with recurrent thrombosis despite appropriate therapy should be screened. The tests that would have the greatest impact on management decisions would be those associated with very high incidences of recurrence, such as homozygosity for factor V Leiden; antiphospholipid syndrome; and deficiencies of antithrombin, protein C, and protein S. These disorders warrant consideration of long-term (possibly indefinite) durations of anticoagulant therapy.

CHRONIC PULMONARY THROMBOEMBOLIC DISEASE

The vast majority of patients with acute PE resolve their perfusion defects (170) and right ventricular dysfunction (143) within a few weeks of anticoagulant therapy. A small minority of individuals with PE (probably between 1% [171] and 4% [143]) do not resolve the process and subsequently develop pulmonary hypertension. It is worth noting, however, that chronic thromboembolic pulmonary hypertension (like other forms of pulmonary hypertension) is an insidious progressive disease, and the clinical presentation may be subtle in its early stages. In fact, in only about half of cases is a previous history of clinically detected PE elicited. Routine posttreatment ventilation-perfusion scans may be helpful in detecting PE patients prone to develop chronic disease, especially among those who have not fully returned to normal cardiopulmonary function. Among those with abnormal scans, echocardiography can clarify the condition of the right ventricle and, by inference, of the pulmonary vasculature.

Although primary pulmonary hypertension (PPH) and chronic thromboembolic pulmonary hypertension demonstrate similar histologic appearances in the microscopic pulmonary vessels (172) in the latter condition, the primary disorder is most likely obstruction of macroscopic pulmonary arteries by unresolved organized emboli (173). If the obstructing lesions are sufficiently proximal, chronic thromboembolic pulmonary hypertension may be amenable to pulmonary thromboendarterectomy (174). The syndrome should be considered in anyone with unexplained dyspnea on exercise, even if pulmonary function tests reveal mild restriction (175). The most important preliminary diagnostic test is the pulmonary perfusion scan, which nearly invariably discloses perfusion defects, although the size of the perfusion defects frequently underestimates the extent of disease (176). This finding contrasts with scan findings in PPH in which perfusion defects, if present, are minimal. The next step is pulmonary angiography, both to confirm the diagnosis and to determine the accessibility of the large vessel obstruction to surgical endarterectomy. With an experienced surgical and medical team, pulmonary endarterectomy has been shown to result in significant relief of pulmonary hypertension and disability.

Randomized controlled clinical trials of pulmonary thromboendarterectomy for patients with chronic thromboembolic pulmonary hypertension have not been performed because there is no reasonable alternative treatment. However, a cross-sectional survey of 308 patients evaluated at 1 year after pulmonary thromboendarterectomy disclosed dramatic improvements in functional status and quality of life (177).

CHRONIC PULMONARY THROMBOEMBOLIC DISEASE	
Summary Statement	**Level of Evidence**
Chronic pulmonary thromboembolic disease occurs in the minority of patients with pulmonary embolism.	Multiple scientific studies
Pulmonary endarterectomy reduces mortality and improves symptoms in patients with pulmonary hypertension owing to chronic pulmonary thromboembolic disease.	Clinical series with historical controls demonstrating substantial outcome benefits

PRIMARY PULMONARY HYPERTENSION

PPH is treated very differently from chronic thromboembolic disease and from other causes of pulmonary hyperten-

sion. Timely and accurate diagnosis is vital, because mortality is very high without specific treatment. The National Institutes of Health registry of PPH patients, monitored prospectively throughout the 1980s, disclosed a median survival of only 2.8 years after diagnosis (178). However, several therapeutic options are available that may substantially improve the outcome for patients with PPH.

PRIMARY PULMONARY HYPERTENSION	
Summary Statement	**Level of Evidence**
Treatment of primary pulmonary hypertension can dramatically reduce mortality.	Clinical series with historical controls demonstrating substantial outcome benefits
Calcium channel blockade reduces mortality in patients who acutely respond to vasodilatation.	Clinical series with historical controls demonstrating substantial outcome benefits
Prostacyclin and similar medications improve clinical outcome in primary pulmonary hypertension.	Clinical series with historical controls demonstrating substantial outcome benefits
Bosentan and similar medications improves clinical outcome in primary pulmonary hypertension.	Clinical series with historical controls demonstrating substantial outcome benefits

Anticoagulation

Although PPH is not a direct result of VTE, it is likely that in situ thrombosis of the pulmonary vascular bed is at least one of the mechanisms involved in clinical deterioration. It stands to reason that systemic anticoagulants, although incapable of reversing the hypertension per se, would have a beneficial effect on morbidity and mortality. Anticoagulation for PPH has not been tested in large randomized clinical trials. However, retrospective data (179) and a prospective trial referencing historical controls (180) suggest that anticoagulation is associated with improved survival in pulmonary hypertension—especially in those with nonuniform blood flow on perfusion scans.

Calcium Channel Blockers

Up to one fourth of patients with PPH will maintain the ability to dilate the pulmonary arterial bed in response to pharmaceutical stimulation of one type or another. It is important to identify these patients accurately, because patients who acutely respond to vasodilators by substantially decreasing their measured pulmonary pressures are also likely to respond well to long-term vasodilator therapy. In a prospective trial, 64 PPH patients were treated with calcium channel blockade: either nifedipine or diltiazem (180). The 17 (26%) that responded acutely to vasodilator therapy were treated for 5 years and had remarkable outcomes: Their 5-year survival was 94%, compared with 55% for nonresponders and 34% for historical controls (from the National Institutes of Health registry) (178). A dramatic response to vasodilators during a careful hemodynamic study, defined as an acute reduction in pulmonary artery pressures to near normal levels, suggests that calcium channel blockade will result in substantial long-term clinical improvement.

Prostacyclin

Prostacyclin may be beneficial for PPH patients—even those who do not acutely respond to vasodilators. Although prostacyclin is a potent vasodilator, it also has other actions beneficial to PPH patients, such as favorably altering vascular remodeling processes and improving right ventricular contractility. For these reasons, pulmonary hemodynamics improve after chronic prostacyclin administration even in patients who did not acutely respond to vasodilation therapy (181). In a small series, 18 patients with severe PPH who received continuous intravenous prostacyclin and were monitored for a year or more demonstrated improved survival over historical controls (182). In an open clinical trial, 74 patients given continuous intravenous prostacyclin were compared with 24 given standard treatment (anticoagulants with or without calcium channel blockers). Among the more severe patients (with low mixed venous saturations), prostacyclin was associated with a higher event-free survival time (585 days), compared with standard treatment (239 days) (183). In a 12-week prospective trial of 81 patients with severe PPH, the group randomized to receive intravenous prostacyclin had significantly improved exercise capacity, quality of life, and survival (184). Similar improvements were observed when intravenous prostacyclin was given to patients with pulmonary hypertension related to scleroderma (185). These data suggest that continuous intravenous prostacyclin is helpful for patients with PPH and with scleroderma-associated pulmonary hypertension who do not acutely respond to vasodilators.

Bosentan

Endothelin-1 is a potent vasoconstrictor that has been implicated in the development and progression of PPH (186). (In fact, one of the benefits of prostacyclin therapy may be alteration of abnormal pulmonary endothelin-1 homeostasis in PPH [187].) Bosentan, a potent endothelin receptor antagonist, reverses some of the detrimental effects of PPH. The efficacy and safety of bosentan for the treatment of pulmonary hypertension (primary or associated with scleroderma) have been established in clinical trials (188,189). In one double-blind clinical trial (188), 32 patients were randomized to receive either bosentan or placebo for 3 months. Those who received bosentan had significant improvements in cardiac index, pulmonary vascular resistance, relief of dyspnea, and functional class. Perhaps more importantly, the

bosentan group had dramatically improved exercise performance, a parameter that correlates highly with long-term survival (184). These results were confirmed in a multicenter 213-patient, double-blind, placebo-controlled trial, in which patients given bosentan for 3 months had significantly increased exercise performance compared with that of controls (189). The bosentan group also had less dyspnea, better functional class, and fewer episodes of clinical deterioration than did the placebo group.

Surgical Options

Although medical therapy for PPH is improving at a rapid rate, severely advanced cases may still require pulmonary transplantation. In some cases, right ventricular failure may be so severe that atrial septostomy is required to temporarily improve hemodynamics until transplantation is possible. Although randomized controlled trials have not been performed, one small case series showed modest improvement in hemodynamics and clinical performance after percutaneous atrial septostomy in selected patients with severe pulmonary hypertension (190).

Choosing among Agents

At the time of this writing, the numerous therapeutic options have not been compared with each other in high quality controlled trials. However, clinical and pharmacological data may be used to make a reasonable strategy for treatment, as suggested in a recent review (191). Those who have had dramatic responses to vasodilators should be placed on calcium channel blockers. Of the nonresponders, those with mild to moderate symptoms (New York Health Association [NYHA] class I or II) may be treated with anticoagulants and observed. On the basis of their low adverse effect profile, some would recommend endothelin blockers in these patients as well, although this class of drugs has been thoroughly studied only in more symptomatic patients. As they become clinically available, oral prostaglandins may offer another therapeutic choice in this group of patients. Intravenous prostaglandins (prostacyclin or its more stable derivative, iloprost) will have the most immediate and potent effects on hemodynamics and clinical condition. They are also associated with more adverse effects than are the other agents, both on the basis of pharmacology and catheter-related complications. They are best reserved for more severely affected patients, such as those with NYHA class III and especially class IV symptomatology. Intravenous prostaglandins may be life-saving when administered during acute clinical deterioration.

REFERENCES

1. Wicky J, Bongard O, Peter R, et al. Screening for proximal deep venous thrombosis using B-mode venous ultrasonography following major hip surgery: implications for clinical management. *Vasa* 1994;23:330–336.

2. Goldhaber SZ, Hennekens CH, Evans DA, et al. Factors associated with correct antemortem diagnosis of major pulmonary embolism. *Am J Med* 1982;73:822–826.

3. Rubenstein I, Murray D, Hoffstein V. Fatal pulmonary emboli in hospitalized patients. *Arch Intern Med* 1988;148:1425–1426.

4. Karwinski B, Svendsen E. Comparison of clinical and postmortem diagnosis of pulmonary embolism. *J Clin Pathol* 1989; 42:135–139.

5. Stein PD, Henry JW. Prevalence of acute pulmonary embolism among patients in a general hospital and at autopsy. *Chest* 1995; 108:978–981.

6. Silfvast T. Cause of death in unsuccessful prehospital resuscitation. *J Intern Med* 1991;229:331–335.

7. Heijboer H, Buller HR, Lensing AWA, et al. A comparison of real-time compression ultrasonography with impedance plethysmography for the diagnosis of deep-vein thrombosis in symptomatic outpatients. *New Engl J Med* 1993;329:1365–1369.

8. Huisman MV, Buller HR, ten Cate JW, et al. Serial impedance plethysmography for suspected deep venous thrombosis in outpatients: the Amsterdam General Practitioner Study. *New Engl J Med* 1986;314:823–828.

9. Vanek VW. Meta-analysis of effectiveness of intermittent pneumatic compression devices with a comparison of thigh-high to knee-high sleeves. *Am Surg* 1998;64:1050–1058.

10. Chandhoke PS, Gooding GA, Narayan P. Prospective randomized trial of warfarin and intermittent pneumatic leg compression as prophylaxis for postoperative deep venous thrombosis in major urological surgery. *J Urol* 1992;147:1056–1059.

11. Lachiewicz PF, Klein JA, Holleman JBJ, et al. Pneumatic compression or aspirin prophylaxis against thromboembolism in total hip arthroplasty. *J South Orthop Assoc* 1996;5:272–280.

12. Dolovich LR, Ginsberg JS, Dpiletos JD, et al. A meta-analysis comparing low-molecular-weight heparin with unfractionated heparin in the treatment of venous thromboembolism. *Arch Intern Med* 2000;160:181–188.

13. Gould MK, Dembitzer AD, Doyle RL, et al. Low-molecular-weight heparins compared with unfractionated heparin for treatment of acute deep venous thrombosis: a meta-analysis of randomized, controlled trials. *Ann Intern Med* 1999;130:800–809.

14. Hommes DW, Bura A, Mazzolai L, et al. Subcutaneous heparin compared with continuous intravenous heparin administration in the initial treatment of deep vein thrombosis: a meta-analysis. *Ann Intern Med* 1992;116:279–284.

15. Linhardt RJ, Gunay NS. Production and chemical processing of low molecular weight heparins. *Semin Thromb Hemost* 1999;25 [Suppl 3]:5–16.

16. Casu B, Torrington KG. Structural characterization of low molecular weight heparins. *Semin Thromb Hemost* 1999;25 [Suppl 3]:17–25.

17. Jeske W, Fareed J. *In vitro* studies on the biochemistry and pharmacology of low molecular weight heparin. *Semin Thromb Hemost* 1999;25[Suppl 3]:27–33.

18. Anand S, Ginsberg JS, Kearon C, et al. The relation between the activated partial thromboplastin time response and recurrence in patients with venous thrombosis treated with continuous intravenous heparin. *Arch Intern Med* 1996;156:1677–1681.

19. Wester JP, de Valk HW, Nieuwenhuis HK, et al. Risk factors for bleeding during treatment of acute venous thromboembolism. *Thromb Haemost* 1996;76:682–688.

20. Hirsch DR, Lee TH, Morrison RB, et al. Shortened hospitalization by means of adjusted-dose subcutaneous heparin for deep venous thrombosis. *Am Heart J* 1996;131:276–280.

21. Gould MK, Dembitzer AD, Sanders GD, et al. Low-molecular-weight heparins compared with unfractionated heparin for treatment of acute deep venous thrombosis: cost-effectiveness analysis. *Ann Intern Med* 1999;130:789–799.

22. Anand SS, Bates S, Ginsberg JS, et al. Recurrent venous thrombosis and heparin therapy: an evaluation of the importance of early activated partial thromboplastin times. *Arch Intern Med* 1999; 159:2029–2032.

23. Hirsh J, Levine MN. Low molecular weight heparin. *Blood* 1992;79:1–17.

24. Carter CJ, Kelton JG, Hirsh J, et al. The relationship between the hemorrhagic and antithrombotic properties of low molecular weight heparin in rabbits. *Blood* 1982;59:1239–1245.

25. Bendetowicz AV, Beguin S, Caplain H, et al. Pharmacokinetics and pharmacodynamics of a low molecular weight heparin (enoxaparin) after subcutaneous injection, comparison with unfractionated heparin: a three way cross over study in human volunteers. *Thromb Haemost* 1994;71:305–313.

26. Majerus PW, Broze GJ, Miletich JP, et al. Anticoagulant, thrombolytic and antiplatelet drugs. In: Gilman AG, Rall TW, Nies AS, et al., eds. *Godman and Gilman's pharmacological basis of therapeutics.* New York: Pergamon Press, 1990:1311–1331.

27. Leizorovicz A, Bara L, Samama MM, et al. Factor Xa inhibition: correlation between the plasma levels of anti-Xa activity and occurrence of thrombosis and haemorrhage. *Haemostasis* 1993; 23[Suppl 1]:89–98.

28. Brieger D, Dawes J. Production method affects the pharmacokinetic and ex vivo biological properties of low molecular weight heparins. *Thromb Haemost* 1997;77:317–322.

29. Lindhoff-Last E, Mosch G, Breddin HK. Treatment doses of different low molecular weight heparins and unfractionated heparins differ in their anticoagulating effects in respect to aPTT, Heptest, anti-IIa- and anti-Xa-activity. *Lab Med* 1992;16:174–177.

30. Bara L, Bloch MF, Zitoun D, et al. Comparative effects of enoxaparin and unfractionated heparin in healthy volunteers on prothrombin consumption in whole blood during coagulation, and release of tissue factor pathway inhibitor. *Thromb Res* 1993;69:443–452.

31. Hirsh J. Heparin. *N Engl J Med* 1991;324:1565–1574.

32. Hirsh J, Fuster V. Guide to anticoagulant therapy, 1: heparin. American Heart Association. *Circulation* 1994;89:1449–1468.

33. Bendetowicz AV, Pacaud E, Baeguin S, et al. On the relationship between molecular mass and anticoagulant activity in a low molecular weight heparin (enoxaparin). *Thromb Haemost* 1992;67:556–562.

34. Krishnaswamy S, Mann KG, Nesheim ME. The prothrombinase-catalyzed activation of prothrombin proceeds through the intermediate meizothrombin in an ordered, sequential reaction. *J Biol Chem* 1986;261:8977–8984.

35. Bovill EG, Tracy RP, Hayes TE, et al. Evidence that meizothrombin is an intermediate product in the clotting of whole blood. *Arterioscler Thromb Vasc Biol* 1995;15:754–758.

36. Bendetowicz AV, Bara L, Samama MM. The inhibition of intrinsic prothrombinase and its generation by heparin and four derivatives in prothrombin poor plasma. *Thromb Res* 1990;58:445–454.

37. Samama MM, Bara L, Gerotziafas GT. Mechanisms for the antithrombotic activity in man of low molecular weight heparins (LMWHs). *Haemostasis* 1994;24:105–117.

38. Harenberg J, Stehle G, Blauth M, et al. Dosage, anticoagulant, and antithrombotic effects of heparin and low-molecular-weight heparin in the treatment of deep vein thrombosis. *Semin Thromb Hemost* 1997;23:83–90.

39. Padilla A, Gray E, Pepper DS, et al. Inhibition of thrombin generation by heparin and low molecular weight (LMW) heparins in

the absence and presence of platelet factor 4 (PF4). *Br J Haematol* 1992;82:406–413.

40. Suh JS, Aster RH, Visentin GP. Antibodies from patients with heparin-induced thrombocytopenia/thrombosis recognize different epitopes on heparin: platelet factor 4. *Blood* 1998;91:916–922.

41. Weitz JI, Hudoba M, Massel D, et al. Clot-bound thrombin is protected from inhibition by heparin-antithrombin III but is susceptible to inactivation by antithrombin III–independent inhibitors. *J Clin Invest* 1990;86:385–391.

42. Baeguin S, Welzel D, Al Dieri R, et al. Conjectures and refutations on the mode of action of heparins: the limited importance of anti-factor Xa activity as a pharmaceutical mechanism and a yardstick for therapy. *Haemostasis* 1999;29:170–178.

43. Kitchen S, Iampietro R, Woolley AM, et al. Anti Xa monitoring during treatment with low molecular weight heparin or danaparoid: inter-assay variability. *Thromb Haemost* 1999;82:1289–1293.

44. Kovacs MJ, Keeney M, MacKinnon K, et al. Three different chromogenic methods do not give equivalent anti-Xa levels for patients on therapeutic low molecular weight heparin (dalteparin) or unfractionated heparin. *Clin Lab Haematol* 1999;21:55–60.

45. Prager NA, Abendschein DR, McKenzie CR, et al. Role of thrombin compared with factor Xa in the procoagulant activity of whole blood clots. *Circulation* 1995;92:962–967.

46. Barrow RT, Parker ET, Krishnaswamy S, et al. Inhibition by heparin of the human blood coagulation intrinsic pathway factor X activator. *J Biol Chem* 1994;269:26796–26800.

47. Fareed J, Jeske W, Hoppensteadt D, et al. Are the available low-molecular-weight heparin preparations the same? *Semin Thromb Hemost* 1996;22:77–91.

48. Hoppensteadt DA, Walenga JM, Fasanella A, et al. TFPI antigen levels in normal human volunteers after intravenous and subcutaneous administration of unfractionated heparin and a low molecular weight heparin. *Thromb Res* 1995;77:175–185.

49. Kong AN, Ludwig EA, Slaughter RL, et al. Pharmacokinetics and pharmacodynamic modeling of direct suppression effects of methylprednisolone on serum cortisol and blood histamine in human subjects. *Clin Pharmacol Ther* 1989;46:616–628.

50. Peteajea J, Fernaandez JA, Gruber A, et al. Anticoagulant synergism of heparin and activated protein C *in vitro:* role of a novel anticoagulant mechanism of heparin, enhancement of inactivation of factor V by activated protein C. *J Clin Invest* 1997;99:2655–2663.

51. Fernandez JA, Petaja J, Griffin JH. Dermatan sulfate and LMW heparin enhance the anticoagulant action of activated protein C. *Thromb Haemost* 1999;82:1462–1468.

52. Carrie D, Caranobe C, Gabaig AM, et al. Effects of heparin, dermatan sulfate and of their association on the inhibition of venous thrombosis growth in the rabbit. *Thromb Haemost* 1992;68:637–641.

53. Carrie D, Caranobe C, Boneu B. A comparison of the antithrombotic effects of heparin and of low molecular weight heparins with increasing antifactor Xa/ antifactor IIa ratio in the rabbit. *Br J Hematol* 1993;83:622–626.

54. Morris TA, Marsh JJ, Konopka RG, et al. Ability of low molecular weight heparin to inhibit propagation of deep venous thrombosis. *Am J Respir Crit Care Med* 1995;151:A528(abst).

55. Tapson VF, Carroll BA, Davidson BL, et al. The diagnostic approach to acute venous thromboembolism. *Am J Respir Crit Care Med* 1999;160:1043–1066.

56. Fiessinger JN, Lopez-Fernandez M, Gatterer E, et al. Once-daily subcutaneous dalteparin, a low molecular weight heparin, for the initial treatment of acute deep vein thrombosis. *Thromb Haemost* 1996;76:195–199.

57. Ofusu FA, Levine M, Craven S, et al. Prophylactically equivalent doses of enoxaparin and unfractionated heparin inhibit *in vivo* coagulation to the same extent. *Br J Hematol* 1992;82:400–405.

58. Becker DM, Philbrick JT, Bachhuber TL, et al. D-dimer testing and acute venous thromboembolism: a shortcut to accurate diagnosis? *Arch Intern Med* 1996;156:939–946.

59. Miller GJ, Bauer KA, Barzegar S, et al. The effects of quality and timing of venepuncture on markers of blood coagulation in healthy middle-aged men. *Thromb Haemost* 1995;73:82–86.

60. Markers of hemostatic system activation in acute deep venous thrombosis-evolution during the first days of heparin treatment: the DVTENOX Study Group. *Thromb Haemost* 1993;70:909–914.

61. van Hulsteijn H, Brieet E, Koch C, et al. Diagnostic value of fibrinopeptide A and β-thromboglobulin in acute deep venous thrombosis and pulmonary embolism. *Acta Med Scand* 1982;211:323–330.

62. Gando S, Tedo I. Diagnostic and prognostic value of fibrinopeptides in patients with clinically suspected pulmonary embolism. *Thromb Res* 1994;75:195–202.

63. Yung GL, Marsh JJ, Berstein RJ, et al. Fibrinopeptide A levels in primary pulmonary hypertension. *Am J Respir Crit Care Med* 1998;157:A592(abst).

64. Mombelli G, Marchetti O, Haeberli A, et al. Effect of intravenous heparin infusion on thrombin-antithrombin complex and fibrinopeptide A in unstable angina. *Am Heart J* 1998;136:1106–1113.

65. Dempfle CE. The use of soluble fibrin in evaluating the acute and chronic hypercoagulable state. *Thromb Haemost* 1999;82:673–683.

66. Dempfle CE, Pfitzner SA, Dollman M, et al. Comparison of immunological and functional assays for measurement of soluble fibrin. *Thromb Haemost* 1995;74:673–679.

67. Moser KM, Fedullo PF, LitteJohn JK, et al. Frequent asymptomatic pulmonary embolism in patients with deep venous thrombosis. *JAMA* 1994;271:223–225.

68. Nielsen HK, Husted SE, Krusell LR, et al. Silent pulmonary embolism in patients with deep venous thrombosis: incidence and fate in a randomized, controlled trial of anticoagulation versus no anticoagulation. *J Intern Med* 1994;235:457–461.

69. Eze AR, Comerota AJ, Kerr RP, et al. Is venous duplex imaging an appropriate initial screening test for patients with suspected pulmonary embolism? *Ann Vasc Surg* 1996;10:220–223.

70. Kirchmaier CM, Wolf H, Scheafer H, et al. Efficacy of a low molecular weight heparin administered intravenously or subcutaneously in comparison with intravenous unfractionated heparin in the treatment of deep venous thrombosis: Certoparin-Study Group. *Int Angiol* 1998;17:135–145.

71. Lindmarker P, Holmstrom M. Use of low molecular weight heparin (dalteparin), once daily, for the treatment of deep vein thrombosis: a feasibility and health economic study in an outpatient setting. Swedish Venous Thrombosis Dalteparin Trial Group. *J Intern Med* 1996;240:395–401.

72. Levine M, Gent M, Hirsh J, et al. A comparison of low-molecular-weight heparin administered primarily at home with unfractionated heparin administered in the hospital for proximal deep vein thrombosis. *New Engl J Med* 1996;334:677–681.

73. Luomanmaki K, Grankvist S, Hallert C, et al. A multicentre comparison of once-daily subcutaneous dalteparin (low molecular weight heparin) and continuous intravenous heparin in the treatment of deep vein thrombosis. *J Intern Med* 1996;240:85–92.

74. Prandoni P, Lensing AW, Beuller HR, et al. Comparison of subcutaneous low-molecular-weight heparin with intravenous

standard heparin in proximal deep-vein thrombosis. *Lancet* 1992;339:441–445.

75. Koopman M, Prandoni P, Piovella F. Treatment of venous thrombosis with intravenous unfractionated heparin administered in the hospital as compared with subcutaneous low-molecular-weight heparin administered at home. *New Engl J Med* 1996;334:682–687.

76. Lopaciuk S, Meissner AJ, Filipecki S, et al. Subcutaneous low molecular weight heparin versus subcutaneous unfractionated heparin in the treatment of deep vein thrombosis: a Polish multicenter trial. *Thromb Haemost* 1992;68:14–18.

77. Hull RD, Raskob GE, Pineo GF, et al. Subcutaneous low-molecular-weight heparin compared with continuous intravenous heparin in the treatment of proximal-vein thrombosis. *New Engl J Med* 1992;326:975–982.

78. Low-molecular-weight heparin in the treatment of patients with venous thromboembolism: the Columbus Investigators. *New Engl J Med* 1997;337:657–662.

79. Meyer G, Brenot F, Pacouret G, et al. Subcutaneous low-molecular-weight heparin Fragmin versus intravenous unfractionated heparin in the treatment of acute non massive pulmonary embolism: an open randomized pilot study. *Thromb Haemost* 1995;74:1432–1435.

80. Simonneau G, Sors H, Charbonnier B, et al. A comparison of low-molecular-weight heparin with unfractionated heparin for acute pulmonary embolism: the THESEE Study Group. Tinzaparine ou Heparine Standard: Evaluations dans l'Embolie Pulmonaire. *New Engl J Med* 1997;337:663–669.

81. Heit JA, Mohr DN, Silverstein MD, et al. Predictors of recurrence after deep vein thrombosis and pulmonary embolism: a population-based cohort study. *Arch Intern Med* 2000;160:761–768.

82. Kasper W, Konstantinides S, Geibel A, et al. Management strategies and determinants of outcome in acute major pulmonary embolism: results of a multicenter registry. *J Am Coll Cardiol* 1997;30:1165–1171.

83. Barritt DW, Jordan SC. Anticoagulant drugs in the treatment of pulmonary embolism. *Lancet* 1960;1:1309–1312.

84. Hull RD, Raskob GE, Hirsh J, et al. Continuous intravenous heparin compared with intermittent subcutaneous heparin in the initial treatment of proximal-vein thrombosis. *New Engl J Med* 1986;315:1109–1114.

85. Andersson G, Fagrell B, Holmgren K, et al. Subcutaneous administration of heparin: a randomised comparison with intravenous administration of heparin to patients with deep-vein thrombosis. *Thromb Res* 1982;27:631–639.

86. Holm HA, Ly B, Handeland GF, et al. Subcutaneous heparin treatment of deep venous thrombosis: a comparison of unfractionated and low molecular weight heparin. *Haemostasis* 1986;16[Suppl 2]:30–37.

87. Doyle DJ, Turpie AG, Hirsh J, et al. Adjusted subcutaneous heparin or continuous intravenous heparin in patients with acute deep vein thrombosis: a randomized trial. *Ann Intern Med* 1987;107:441–445.

88. Pini M, Pattachini C, Quintavalla R, et al. Subcutaneous vs intravenous heparin in the treatment of deep venous thrombosis: a randomized clinical trial. *Thromb Haemost* 1990;64:222–226.

89. Raschke RA, Reilly BM, Guidry JR, et al. The weight-based heparin dosing nomogram compared with a "standard care" nomogram: a randomized controlled trial. *Ann Intern Med* 1993;119:874–881.

90. Bates SM, Weitz JI, Johnston M, et al. Use of a fixed activated partial thromboplastin time ratio to establish a therapeutic range for unfractionated heparin. *Arch Intern Med* 2001;161:385–391.

91. Hull RD, Raskob GE, Brant RF, et al. The importance of initial heparin treatment on long-term clinical outcomes of antithrombotic therapy: the emerging theme of delayed recurrence. *Arch Intern Med* 1997;157:2317–2321.

92. Hull RD, Raskob GE, Rosenbloom D, et al. Treatment of proximal vein thrombosis with subcutaneous low-molecular-weight heparin vs intravenous heparin: an economic perspective. *Arch Intern Med* 1997;157:289–294.

93. Prandoni P, Bagatella P, Bernardi E, et al. Use of an algorithm for administering subcutaneous heparin in the treatment of deep venous thrombosis. *Ann Intern Med* 1998;129:299–302.

94. Leizorovicz A, Simonneau G, Decousus H, et al. Comparison of efficacy and safety of low molecular weight heparins and unfractionated heparin in initial treatment of deep venous thrombosis: a meta-analysis. *BMJ* 1994;309:299–304.

95. Lensing AWA, Prins MH, Davidson BL, et al. Treatment of deep venous thrombosis with low-molecular-weight heparins: a meta-analysis. *Arch Intern Med* 1995;155:601–607.

96. Siragusa S, Cosmi B, Piovella F, et al. Low-molecular-weight heparins and unfractionated heparin in the treatment of patients with acute venous thromboembolism: results of a meta-analysis. *Am J Med* 1996;100:269–277.

97. Kaiser B, Kirchmaier CM, Breddin HK, et al. Preclinical biochemistry and pharmacology of low molecular weight heparins *in vivo:* studies of venous and arterial thrombosis. *Semin Thromb Hemost* 1999;25[Suppl 3]:35–42.

98. Dietrich CP, Shinjo SK, Moraes FA, et al. Structural features and bleeding activity of commercial low molecular weight heparins: neutralization by ATP and protamine. *Semin Thromb Hemost* 1999;25[Suppl 3]:43–50.

99. Fareed J, Fu K, Yang LH, et al. Pharmacokinetics of low molecular weight heparins in animal models. *Semin Thromb Hemost* 1999;25[Suppl 3]:51–55.

100. Cornelli U, Fareed J. Human pharmacokinetics of low molecular weight heparins. *Semin Thromb Hemost* 1999;25[Suppl 3]:57–61.

101. Nader HB, Walenga JM, Berkowitz SD, et al. Preclinical differentiation of low molecular weight heparins. *Semin Thromb Hemost* 1999;25[Suppl 3]:63–72.

102. Heyland DK, Gafni A, Kernerman P, et al. How to use the results of an economic evaluation. *Crit Care Med* 1999;27:1195–1202.

103. Hull RD, Feldstein W, Pineo GF, et al. Cost effectiveness of diagnosis of deep vein thrombosis in symptomatic patients. *Thromb Haemost* 1995;74:189–196.

104. Decousus H, Leizorovicz A, Parent F, et al. A clinical trial of vena caval filters in the prevention of pulmonary embolism in patients with proximal deep-vein thrombosis. *New Engl J Med* 1998;338:409–415.

105. Koopman MM, Prandoni P, Piovella F, et al. Treatment of venous thrombosis with intravenous unfractionated heparin administered in the hospital as compared with subcutaneous low-molecular-weight heparin administered at home: the Tasman Study Group. *N Engl J Med* 1996;334:682–687.

106. Levine M, Gent M, Hirsh J, et al. A comparison of low-molecular-weight heparin administered primarily at home with unfractionated heparin administered in the hospital for proximal deep-vein thrombosis. *N Engl J Med* 1996;334:677–681.

107. Guidelines on diagnosis and management of acute pulmonary embolism: task force on pulmonary embolism. European Society of Cardiology. *Eur Heart J* 2000;21:1301–1336.

108. Hyers TM, Agnelli G, Hull RD, et al. Antithrombotic therapy for venous thromboembolic disease. *Chest* 1998;114:561S–578S.

109. Douketis JD, Kearon C, Bates S, et al. Risk of fatal pulmonary embolism in patients with treated venous thromboembolism. *JAMA* 1998;279:458–462.

110. Goldhaber SZ, Haire WD, Feldstein ML, et al. Alteplase versus heparin in acute pulmonary embolism: randomised trial assessing right-ventricular function and pulmonary perfusion. *Lancet* 1993;341:507–511.

111. Hamel E, Pacouret G, Vincentelli D, et al. Thrombolysis or heparin in massive pulmonary embolism with right ventricular dilatation: results from a 128-patient, single center registry. *Chest* 2001;120:120–125.

112. McIntyre KM, Sasahara AA. The hemodynamic response to pulmonary embolism in patients without prior cardiopulmonary disease. *Am J Cardiol* 1971;28:288–294.

113. Malik AB, Johnson A. role of humoral mediators in the vascular response to pulmonary embolism. In: Weir EK, Reeves JT, eds. *Pulmonary vascular physiology and pathophysiology.* New York: Marcel-Dekker Inc, 1989:445–468.

114. Smulders YM. Pathophysiology and treatment of haemodynamic instability in acute pulmonary embolism: the pivotal role of pulmonary vasoconstriction. *Cardiovasc Res* 2000;48:23–33.

115. Dschietzig T, Laule M, Alexiou K, et al. Coronary constriction and consequent cardiodepression in pulmonary embolism are mediated by pulmonary big endothelin and enhanced in early endothelial dysfunction. *Crit Care Med* 1998;26:510–517.

116. Sofia M, Faraone S, Alifano M, et al. Endothelin abnormalities in patients with pulmonary embolism. *Chest* 1997;111:544–549.

117. Benedict CR, Mathew B, Rex KA, et al. Correlation of plasma serotonin changes with platelet aggregation in an *in vivo* dog model of spontaneous occlusive coronary thrombus formation. *Circ Res* 1986;58:58–67.

118. Grifoni S, Olivotto I, Cecchini P, et al. Short-term clinical outcome of patients with acute pulmonary embolism, normal blood pressure, and echocardiographic right ventricular dysfunction. *Circulation* 2000;101:2817–2822.

119. Morgenthaler TI, Ryu JH. Clinical characteristics of fatal pulmonary embolism in a referral hospital. *Mayo Clin Proc* 1995;70: 417–424.

120. Urokinase pulmonary embolism trial, phase 1 results: a cooperative study. *JAMA* 1970;214:2163–2172.

121. Blackmon JR, Sautter RD, Wagner HN, et al. Urokinase Pulmonary Embolism Trial. *JAMA* 1970;214:2163–2172.

122. Meyer G, Brenot F, Pacouret G, et al. Subcutaneous low-molecular-weight heparin Fragmin versus intravenous unfractionated heparin in the treatment of acute non massive pulmonary embolism: an open randomized pilot study. *Thromb Haemost* 1995;74:1432–1435.

123. Gurewich V, Cohen ML, Thomas DP. Humoral factors in massive pulmonary embolism: an experimental study. *Am Heart J* 1968;76:784–794.

124. Moser KM, Spragg RG, Bender F, et al. Study of factors that may condition scintigraphic detection of venous thrombi and pulmonary emboli with indium-111–labeled platelets. *J Nucl Med* 1980;21:1051–1058.

125. Morris TA, Marsh JJ, Konopka R, et al. Antibodies against the fibrin β-chain amino-terminus detect active canine venous thrombi. *Circulation* 1997;96:3173–3179.

126. Layish DT, Tapson VF. Pharmacologic hemodynamic support in massive pulmonary embolism. *Chest* 1997;111:218–224.

127. Mercat A, Diehl JL, Meyer G, et al. Hemodynamic effects of fluid loading in acute massive pulmonary embolism. *Crit Care Med* 1999;27:540–544.

128. Vlahakes GJ, Turley K, Hoffman JI. The pathophysiology of failure in acute right ventricular hypertension: hemodynamic and biochemical correlations. *Circulation* 1981;63:87–95.

129. Morgenthaler TI, Ryu JH. Clinical characteristics of fatal pulmonary embolism in a referral hospital. *Mayo Clinic Proc* 1995;70:417–424.

130. Greenfield LJ, Michna BA. Twelve-year clinical experience with the Greenfield vena cava filter. *Surgery* 1988;104:706–712.

131. Meneveau N, Schiele F, Vuillemenot A, et al. Streptokinase vs alteplase in massive pulmonary embolism: a randomized trial assessing right heart haemodynamics and pulmonary vascular obstruction. *Eur Heart J* 1997;18:1141–1148.

132. Meneveau N, Schiele F, Metz D, et al. Comparative efficacy of a two-hour regimen of streptokinase versus alteplase in acute massive pulmonary embolism: immediate clinical and hemodynamic outcome and one-year follow-up. *J Am Coll Cardiol* 1998;31:1057–1063.

133. Konstantinides S, Geibel A, Heusel G, et al. Heparin plus alteplase compared with heparin alone in patients with submassive pulmonary embolism. *N Engl J Med* 2002;347:1143–1150.

134. Dalen JE, Alpert JS, Hirsh J. Thrombolytic therapy for pulmonary embolism: is it effective? Is it safe? When is it indicated? *Arch Intern Med* 1997;157:2550–2556.

135. Mattox KL, Feldtman RW, Beall ACJ, et al. Pulmonary embolectomy for acute massive pulmonary embolism. *Ann Surg* 1982;195:726–731.

136. Gray HH, Morgan JM, Paneth M, et al. Pulmonary embolectomy for acute massive pulmonary embolism: an analysis of 71 cases. *Br Heart J* 1988;60:196–200.

137. Doerge HC, Schoendube FA, Loeser H, et al. Pulmonary embolectomy: review of a 15-year experience and role in the age of thrombolytic therapy. *Eur J Cardiothorac Surg* 1996;10:952–957.

138. Aklog L, Williams CS, Byrne JG, et al. Acute pulmonary embolectomy: a contemporary approach. *Circulation* 2002;105: 1416–1419.

139. Wolfe MW, Lee RT, Feldstein ML, et al. Prognostic significance of right ventricular hypokinesis and perfusion lung scan defects in pulmonary embolism. *Am Heart J* 1994;127:1371–1375.

140. McConnell MV, Solomon SD, Rayan ME, et al. Regional right ventricular dysfunction detected by echocardiography in acute pulmonary embolism. *Am J Cardiol* 1996;78:469–473.

141. Ribeiro A, Juhlin-Dannfelt A, Brodin LA, et al. Pulmonary embolism: relation between the degree of right ventricle overload and the extent of perfusion defects. *Am Heart J* 1998;135:868–874.

142. Ribeiro A, Lindmarker P, Juhlin-Dannfelt A, et al. Echocardiography Doppler in pulmonary embolism: right ventricular dysfunction as a predictor of mortality rate. *Am Heart J* 1997; 134:479–487.

143. Ribeiro A, Lindmarker P, Johnsson H, et al. Pulmonary embolism: one-year follow-up with echocardiography doppler and five-year survival analysis. *Circulation* 1999;99:1325–1330.

144. Vieillard-Baron A, Page B, Augarde R, et al. Acute cor pulmonale in massive pulmonary embolism: incidence, echocardiographic pattern, clinical implications and recovery rate. *Intensive Care Med* 2001;27:1481–1486.

145. Grifoni S, Olivotto I, Cecchini P, et al. Short-term clinical outcome of patients with acute pulmonary embolism, normal blood pressure, and echocardiographic right ventricular dysfunction. *Circulation* 2000;101:2817–2822.

146. Goldhaber SZ. Echocardiography in the management of pulmonary embolism. *Ann Intern Med* 2002;136:691–700.

147. Hyers TM, Agnelli G, Hull RD, et al. Antithrombotic therapy for venous thromboembolic disease. *Chest* 2001;119:176S–193S.

148. Brandjes DP, Heijboer H, Buller HR, et al. Acenocoumarol and heparin compared with acenocoumarol alone in the initial treatment of proximal-vein thrombosis. *N Engl J Med* 1992; 327:1485–1489.

149. Hull RD, Raskob GE, Rosenbloom D, et al. Heparin for 5 days as compared with 10 days in the initial treatment of proximal venous thrombosis. *N Engl J Med* 1990;322:1260–1264.

150. Hull R, Delmore T, Carter C, et al. Adjusted dose subcutaneous heparin versus warfarin sodium in the long-term treatment of venous thrombosis. *N Engl J Med* 1982;306:189–194.

151. Schulman S, Granqvist S, Holmstrom M, et al. The duration of oral anticoagulant therapy after a second episode of venous thromboembolism: the Duration of Anticoagulation Trial Study Group. *N Engl J Med* 1997;336:393–398.

152. Kearon C, Gent M, Hirsh J, et al. A comparison of three months of anticoagulation with extended anticoagulation for a first episode of idiopathic venous thromboembolism. *New Engl J Med* 1999;340:901–907.

153. Hirsh J, Dalen J, Anderson DR, et al. Oral anticoagulants: mechanism of action, clinical effectiveness, and optimal therapeutic range. *Chest* 2001;119:8S–21S.

154. Optimum duration of anticoagulation for deep-vein thrombosis and pulmonary embolism: research committee of the British Thoracic Society. *Lancet* 1992;340:873–876.

155. Agnelli G, Prandoni P, Santamaria MG, et al. Three months versus one year of oral anticoagulant therapy for idiopathic deep venous thrombosis: Warfarin Optimal Duration Italian Trial Investigators. *N Engl J Med* 2001;345:165–169.

156. Rosendaal FR, Koster T, Vandenbroucke JP, et al. High risk of thrombosis in patients homozygous for factor V Leiden (activated protein C resistance). *Blood* 1995;85:1504–1508.

157. Makris M, Preston FE, Beauchamp NJ, et al. Co-inheritance of the 20210A allele of the prothrombin gene increases the risk of thrombosis in subjects with familial thrombophilia. *Thromb Haemost* 1997;78:1426–1429.

158. Souto JC, Coll I, Llobet D, et al. The prothrombin 20210A allele is the most prevalent genetic risk factor for venous thromboembolism in the Spanish population. *Thromb Haemost* 1998;80:366–369.

159. De Stefano V, Martinelli I, Mannucci PM, et al. The risk of recurrent deep venous thrombosis among heterozygous carriers of both factor V Leiden and the G20210A prothrombin mutation. *New Engl J Med* 1999;341:801–806.

160. Eichinger S, Pabinger I, Steumpflen A, et al. The risk of recurrent venous thromboembolism in patients with and without factor V Leiden. *Thromb Haemost* 1997;77:624–628.

161. Simioni P, Prandoni P, Lensing AW, et al. The risk of recurrent venous thromboembolism in patients with an Arg506→Gln mutation in the gene for factor V (factor V Leiden). *New Engl J Med* 1997;336:399–403.

162. Rintelen C, Pabinger I, Knobl P, et al. Probability of recurrence of thrombosis in patients with and without factor V Leiden. *Thromb Haemost* 1996;75:229–232.

163. Ridker PM, Miletich JP, Stampfer MJ, et al. Factor V Leiden and risks of recurrent idiopathic venous thromboembolism. *Circulation* 1995;92:2800–2802.

164. Middeldorp S, Henkens CM, Koopman MM, et al. The incidence of venous thromboembolism in family members of patients with factor V Leiden mutation and venous thrombosis. *Ann Intern Med* 1998;128:15–20.

165. Petri M. Pathogenesis and treatment of the antiphospholipid antibody syndrome. *Med Clin North Am* 1997;81:151–177.

166. Ginsburg KS, Liang MH, Newcomer L, et al. Anticardiolipin antibodies and the risk for ischemic stroke and venous thrombosis. *Ann Intern Med* 1992;117:997–1002.

167. Ginsberg JS, Wells PS, Brill-Edwards P, et al. Antiphospholipid antibodies and venous thromboembolism. *Blood* 1995;86:3685–3691.

168. Schulman S, Svenungsson E, Granqvist S. Anticardiolipin antibodies predict early recurrence of thromboembolism and death among patients with venous thromboembolism following anticoagulant therapy: duration of Anticoagulation Study Group. *Am J Med* 1998;104:332–338.

169. Simioni P, Prandoni P, Zanon E, et al. Deep venous thrombosis and lupus anticoagulant: a case-control study. *Thromb Haemost* 1996;76:187–189.

170. Dalen JE, Banas JS, Brooks HL, et al. Resolution rate of acute pulmonary embolism in man. *N Engl J Med* 1969;280:1194–1199.

171. Fedullo PF, Auger WR, Kerr KM, et al. Chronic thromboembolic pulmonary hypertension. *N Engl J Med* 2001;345:1465–1472.

172. Moser KM, Bloor CM. Pulmonary vascular lesions occurring in patients with chronic major vessel thromboembolic pulmonary hypertension. *Chest* 1993;103:685–692.

173. Moser KM, Auger WR, Fedullo PF. Chronic major-vessel thromboembolic pulmonary hypertension. *Circulation* 1990;81:1735–1743.

174. Jamieson SW, Auger WR, Fedullo PF, et al. Experience and results with 150 pulmonary thromboendarterectomy operations over a 29-month period. *J Thorac Cardiovasc Surg* 1993;106:116–126.

175. Morris TA, Auger WR, Ysrael MZ, et al. Parenchymal scarring is associated with restrictive spirometric defects in patients with chronic thromboembolic pulmonary hypertension. *Chest* 1996;110:399–403.

176. Ryan KL, Fedullo PF, Davis GB, et al. Perfusion scan findings understate the severity of angiographic and hemodynamic compromise in chronic thromboembolic pulmonary hypertension. *Chest* 1988;93:1180–1185.

177. Archibald CJ, Auger WR, Fedullo PF, et al. Long-term outcome after pulmonary thromboendarterectomy. *Am J Respir Crit Care Med* 1999;160:523–528.

178. D'Alonzo GE, Barst RJ, Ayres SM, et al. Survival in patients with primary pulmonary hypertension: results from a national prospective registry. *Ann Intern Med* 1991;115:343–349.

179. Frank H, Mlczoch J, Huber K, et al. The effect of anticoagulant therapy in primary and anorectic drug-induced pulmonary hypertension. *Chest* 1997;112:714–721.

180. Rich S, Kaufmann E, Levy PS. The effect of high doses of calcium-channel blockers on survival in primary pulmonary hypertension. *N Engl J Med* 1992;327:76–81.

181. McLaughlin VV, Genthner DE, Panella MM, et al. Reduction in pulmonary vascular resistance with long-term epoprostenol (prostacyclin) therapy in primary pulmonary hypertension. *N Engl J Med* 1998;338:273–277.

182. Shapiro SM, Oudiz RJ, Cao T, et al. Primary pulmonary hypertension: improved long-term effects and survival with continuous intravenous epoprostenol infusion. *J Am Coll Cardiol* 1997;30:343–349.

183. Higenbottam T, Butt AY, McMahon A, et al. Long-term intravenous prostaglandin (epoprostenol or iloprost) for treatment of severe pulmonary hypertension. *Heart* 1998;80:151–155.

184. Barst RJ, Rubin LJ, Long WA, et al. A comparison of continuous intravenous epoprostenol (prostacyclin) with conventional therapy for primary pulmonary hypertension: the Primary Pulmonary Hypertension Study Group. *N Engl J Med* 1996;334:296–302.

185. Badesch DB, Tapson VF, McGoon MD, et al. Continuous intravenous epoprostenol for pulmonary hypertension due to the scleroderma spectrum of disease: a randomized, controlled trial. *Ann Intern Med* 2000;132:425–434.

186. Giaid A, Yanagisawa M, Langleben D, et al. Expression of endothelin-1 in the lungs of patients with pulmonary hypertension. *N Engl J Med* 1993;328:1732–1739.

187. Langleben D, Barst RJ, Badesch D, et al. Continuous infusion of epoprostenol improves the net balance between pulmonary endothelin-1 clearance and release in primary pulmonary hypertension. *Circulation* 1999;99:3266–3271.

188. Channick RN, Simonneau G, Sitbon O, et al. Effects of the dual endothelin-receptor antagonist bosentan in patients with pulmonary hypertension: a randomised placebo-controlled study. *Lancet* 2001;358:1119–1123.

189. Rubin LJ, Badesch DB, Barst RJ, et al. Bosentan therapy for pulmonary arterial hypertension. *N Engl J Med* 2002;346:896–903.

190. Rothman A, Sklansky MS, Lucas VW, et al. Atrial septostomy as a bridge to lung transplantation in patients with severe pulmonary hypertension. *Am J Cardiol* 1999;84:682–686.

191. Hoeper MM, Galie N, Simonneau G, et al. New treatments for pulmonary arterial hypertension. *Am J Respir Crit Care Med* 2002;165:1209–1216.

192. Goldhaber SZ, Morrison RB, Diran LL, et al. Abbreviated hospitalization for deep venous thrombosis with the use of ardeparin. *Arch Intern Med* 1998;158:2325–2328.

193. Albada J, Nieuwenhuis HK, Sixma JJ. Treatment of acute venous thromboembolism with low molecular weight heparin (Fragmin): results of a double-blind randomized study. *Circulation* 1989;80:935–940.

194. Bratt G, Aberg W, Johansson M, et al. Two daily subcutaneous injections of Fragmin as compared with intravenous standard heparin in the treatment of deep venous thrombosis (DVT). *Thromb Haemost* 1990;64:506–510.

195. Lindmarker P, Holmstreom M, Granqvist S, et al. Comparison of once-daily subcutaneous Fragmin with continuous intravenous unfractionated heparin in the treatment of deep vein thrombosis. *Thromb Haemost* 1994;72:186–190.

196. Simonneau G, Charbonnier B, Decousus H, et al. Subcutaneous low-molecular-weight heparin compared with continuous intravenous unfractionated heparin in the treatment of proximal deep vein thrombosis. *Arch Intern Med* 1993;153:1541–1546.

197. Merli G, Spiro TE, Olsson CG, et al. Subcutaneous enoxaparin once or twice daily compared with intravenous unfractionated heparin for treatment of venous thromboembolic disease. *Ann Intern Med* 2001;134:191–202.

198. Harenberg J, Huck K, Bratsch H, et al. Therapeutic application of subcutaneous low-molecular-weight heparin in acute venous thrombosis. *Haemostasis* 1990;20[Suppl 1]:205–219.

Baum's Textbook of Pulmonary Diseases, 7th ed. Edited by James D. Crapo, Jeffrey Glassroth, Joel Karlinsky, and Talmadge E. King, Jr.
Lippincott Williams & Wilkins, Philadelphia © 2004.

38 Pulmonary Heart Disease

Lewis J. Rubin

The cardiovascular and respiratory systems work together to optimize oxygen (O_2) delivery to peripheral tissues and to excrete gaseous by-products of metabolism. As a result of their interdependence, disorders of one system influence the structure and function of the other. McGinn and White (1) coined the term *acute cor pulmonale* to describe right heart strain resulting from pulmonary hypertension in the setting of acute respiratory insufficiency. *Chronic cor pulmonale* was defined by a committee of the World Health Organization as "an alteration in structure or function of the right ventricle (RV) resulting from disease affecting the structures and function of the lung, except when this alteration results from disease of the left heart or congenital heart disease" (2). Although *cor pulmonale* is often used to describe the presence of right-sided heart failure, this is a late manifestation of pulmonary heart disease (PHD) and need not be present to entertain the diagnosis or institute management.

Although precise estimates of its prevalence are not available, PHD probably constitutes 15% to 20% of all cases of heart failure and 7% to 10% of all heart disease. Approximately 40% of patients with severe chronic obstructive pulmonary disease (COPD) demonstrate clinical or pathologic evidence of PHD, and its presence in the setting of chronic respiratory disease portends an ominous prognosis: The 5-year survival of COPD patients with even modest pulmonary hypertension is similar to that of inoperable lung cancer (3–7).

In this chapter, the factors that characterize acute and chronic PHD are reviewed. Because PHD is primarily a disease of the RV, we briefly describe normal RV function and the response of the RV to imposed mechanical loads. We consider the interactions between the RV and the left ventricle (LV) because these are so important to the normal functioning of the heart. We then consider the pathophysiological and clinical features of acute and chronic PHD.

NORMAL RIGHT VENTRICLE

The RV develops embryologically from two separate components of the primitive cardiac tube. The bulbus cordis is incorporated into the conus (outflow tract), and the sinus venosus is incorporated into the sinus (inflow tract). Normal RV contraction preserves the functional distinction of its dual embryologic origin. RV systole occurs by sequential contraction, beginning at the inflow tract and extending to the outflow tract, and is almost peristaltic in nature, with approximately 25 milliseconds separating contractile activity of the two components. In fact, with increased sympathoadrenal activation, a pressure gradient can develop between the inflow and outflow tracts within the ventricular cavity. This mode of contraction makes the RV ideally suited for its job as a high-volume low-pressure pump.

The RV is normally thin (<0.5 cm thick) and crescent-shaped. Therefore, determination of its volume from the limited numbers of dimensions that can be assessed by using standard imaging techniques is more difficult than for the LV. The difficulty in measuring RV volume using simple imaging techniques is further compounded by the fact that with dilation, its shape becomes more ellipsoidal. Thus, changes in loading conditions can lead to changes in shape. This in turn may be responsible for the fact that in many circumstances there is a poor or nonexistent correlation between end-diastolic and end-systolic pressures and corresponding RV volumes.

L. J. Rubin: University of California, San Diego, La Jolla, California.

RIGHT- AND LEFT-VENTRICLE FUNCTION COMPARED

The fact that the RV free wall may be ablated or surgically replaced with a Dacron patch with no change in resting cardiac output initially led investigators to believe its importance to circulatory homeostasis is minimal. However, when there is an increase in pulmonary arterial pressure or venous return, as with exercise or other stress, normal RV functioning is essential for maintenance of normal circulatory status. Because the RV is capable of generating large increases in cardiac output at extremely low pressures, the RV is considered a volume pump, whereas the LV is a pressure pump. However, compared with its normal physiological pressure range, the RV is capable of increasing maximum pressure generation proportionally to the same degree or even more than that of the LV (8). During acute elevations in pulmonary artery pressure, maximum RV pressure can increase to 55 to 60 torr (almost three times the normal peak systolic pressure) before circulatory failure ensues, and the RV can maintain normal or near-normal cardiac output despite chronic elevations in systolic pressure of four or five times normal (9).

The determinants of both RV and LV function are the same: preload, afterload, and contractility. Figure 38.1 illustrates the pressure-volume history of RV contraction. During diastole, the RV fills along the diastolic or relaxation pressure-volume curve. At end-diastole, isovolumic contraction occurs. The RV pressure increases until the level of pulmonary artery diastolic pressure is reached, at which point shortening occurs. Shortening ceases when the pressure-volume point reaches the curve describing the maximum end-systolic pressure-volume relationship, when isovolumetric relaxation occurs. The point labeled end-diastole in Figure 38.1 represents the stress on the RV at the onset of contraction (preload). The stress on the RV during contraction represents the afterload. The slope of the end-systolic pressure-volume curve represents a load-independent measure of contractility and is sometimes called the *maximum systolic elastance*. These concepts, developed and validated for the LV both in isolated load-clamped heart preparations and in situ preparations, also apply to the RV with some slight modifications. First, pulmonary arterial pressure represents only part of the hydraulic load placed on the RV (afterload) during contraction. A substantial part of the total hydraulic load is represented by the elastance, or input impedance of the pulmonary arterial circulation. Second, end-systole is more difficult to define for the RV than for the LV: End-ejection and end-contraction correspond fairly well for the LV. In contrast, the RV continues to eject for a short time after end-contraction. Further, there are slight differences in end-systolic volume, depending on whether contraction is isovolumetric or isotonic.

Practically speaking, however, these quantitative differences do not negate the concept of the end-systolic pressure-volume curve being an important measure of ventricular contractile function. Often the end-systolic point is defined in terms of a specified time interval, often 100 milliseconds from end-diastole, in analyses of RV mechanics. In general, however, RV and LV contraction behave remarkably similarly. When normalized for peak pressure, the time courses of RV and LV isovolumetric pressure development are practically superimposable. Just as for the LV, RV contraction can be viewed as a series of time-varying elastances, a concept that had been developed for the LV. For the RV, as for the LV, the instantaneous pressure-volume relationship may be expressed as $[P_t = E_t(V_t - V_0)]$, where P_t is the pressure at any given time in the cardiac cycle, E_t is the slope of the pressure-volume curve at time t, V_t is ventricular volume at time t, and V_0 is the volume intercept of the regression line. E_t at end-systole is a measure of ventricular contractility that is relatively independent of preload or afterload.

RIGHT-VENTRICLE RESPONSE TO ACUTELY INCREASED AFTERLOAD: THE PHYSIOLOGY OF ACUTE PULMONARY HEART DISEASE

Investigators have assessed the ability of the RV to tolerate increased afterload by graded occlusions of the pulmonary artery or injection of glass beads or other small particles into the distal pulmonary bed. These two models are not strictly comparable because the hydraulic load produced by main pulmonary arterial constriction is greater than that produced by microvascular embolization. However, the principles governing load tolerance are the same. Relevant clinical conditions include acute massive pulmonary embolism (1) and large increases in lung volume (high levels of positive end-expiratory pressure) in the presence of adult respiratory

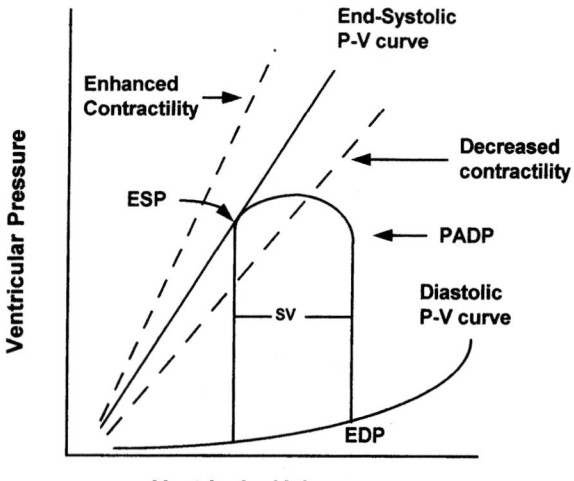

FIGURE 38.1. Ventricular pressure-volume diagram. *EDP,* end-diastolic pressure; *PADP,* pulmonary arterial end-diastolic pressure; *ESP,* end-systolic pressure; *SV,* stroke volume. See text for explanation.

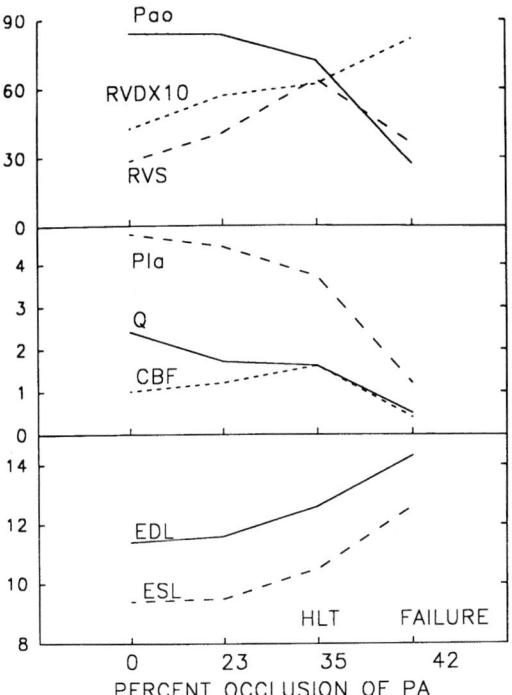

FIGURE 38.2. Summary of hemodynamic changes with acute graded constriction of the pulmonary artery. *Pao*, aortic pressure; *RVD*, right ventricular end-diastolic pressure; *RVS*, right ventricular end-systolic pressure; *Pla*, left atrial pressure; *Q*, cardiac output; *CBF*, coronary blood flow; *EDL*, right ventricular end-diastolic segmental length; *ESL*, right ventricular end-systolic segmental length; *HLT*, highest load tolerable; failure, circulatory collapse. (From Scharf SM. Right ventricular function and cor pulmonale. In: Scharf SM, ed. *Cardiopulmonary physiology in critical care.* New York: Marcel Dekker, 1992:239–247, with permission.)

distress syndrome (10). Figure 38.2 illustrates the results of a typical series of experiments. The RV systolic pressure could be increased to approximately 60 torr with little evidence of circulatory decompensation, although there were decreases in cardiac output and blood pressure. However, a further small increase in the degree of pulmonary arterial constriction brought about sudden and dramatic circulatory collapse accompanied by RV dilation and increased RV end-diastolic pressure. Because RV dilation occurred primarily at the time of circulatory collapse, this might suggest that the Frank-Starling mechanism plays little role in maintaining RV output against an increase in afterload. However, other studies have shown that there is a role for the Frank-Starling mechanism in RV afterload tolerance, although it is not the primary determinant (11). Because the right coronary artery, which supplies the RV free wall, originates in the aorta, coronary blood flow to the RV free wall depends on aortic blood pressure. One hypothesis for the sudden deterioration of the RV with increased afterload is that the balance between RV myocardial O_2 demand and supply suddenly tips in the direction of increased demand, resulting in RV ischemia. Other studies suggest that RV failure does not result from ischemia but, rather, that ischemia is secondary to circulatory collapse. Either way, RV failure with severe pulmonary hypertension

appears to be the result of a vicious cycle in which decreased RV output causes decreased LV output. This in turn leads to decreased aortic pressure, which limits the degree to which coronary flow can increase commensurate with O_2 demand. With inadequate coronary flow relative to O_2 demand, RV contractility decreases, in turn decreasing cardiac output. Limitation of right coronary flow is further enhanced by increased RV intramyocardial pressure during systole, which may produce endocardial ischemia (12,13).

Supportive Therapy of Acute Pulmonary Heart Disease

The issues discussed above have direct clinical relevance to the assessment and treatment of acute PHD. First, sustained RV pressures greater than approximately 60 torr mean that pulmonary hypertension cannot be acute because the normal RV cannot sustain systolic pressures greater than this level. Second, whether or not ischemia is involved, one should view RV failure in the light of the balance between myocardial O_2 supply and demand. Resuscitative maneuvers, such as the administration of isoproterenol or even massive fluid resuscitation, could act to increase RV myocardial O_2 demand and unfavorably influence the supply-demand relationship. Although volume infusion is appropriate when the central venous pressure is low, massive volume infusion when RV afterload is severely elevated may actually worsen failure and produce circulatory decompensation. Support measures should be directed toward maintaining aortic pressure and hence coronary flow. In this setting, vasoconstrictor agents such as phenylephrine or norepinephrine are preferred over agents that increase myocardial contractility and heart rate while producing systemic vasodilation (14). Specific therapies, such as thrombolytic agents in massive pulmonary embolism, should be instituted as rapidly as feasible while supportive measures are being implemented.

Right-Ventricle–Left-Ventricle Interactions

The ventricles exhibit two major types of interactions, series and parallel. A *series interaction* refers to effects of RV output on LV filling and output. *Parallel interaction* refers to those interactions arising from the fact that the two chambers are part of one structure, contain common muscle bands, share a common septum, and are covered by a single pericardial sac. Thus, the function of one ventricle depends on that of the other. When diastolic filling of one ventricle is increased, that of the other is impaired. Although this diastolic interaction is mediated largely through the interventricular septum, it is amplified approximately fourfold by the presence of the pericardium. Conditions that increase the stiffness of the pericardium (pericardial fibrosis, tamponade) increase the degree of diastolic interdependence. These considerations may explain why LV end-diastolic volume decreases and LV end-diastolic pressure either remains the same or increases in response to acute massive overload of the RV. Indeed, bulging of the interventricular septum into the LV is a sign of severe RV overload (see "Echocardiography" below) and is a reflection of diastolic interaction.

The ventricles also interact during systole. This interesting interaction arises because the ventricles share common fiber bundles, contract toward a common center of gravity, are found within a common pericardial sac, and share a common septum. This means that rather than impairing the function of the opposite ventricle, contraction of one ventricle actually enhances the function of the other. Although the low-pressure RV does little to enhance pressure generation in the LV, as much as 40% to 60% of the pressure generated in the RV is attributable to LV contraction. Systolic interaction is mediated largely through the septum but is substantially enhanced by increasing the elasticity of the RV free wall. This is yet another mechanism by which LV systolic pressure increases RV afterload tolerance.

CLINICAL FEATURES OF ACUTE PULMONARY HEART DISEASE

The symptoms of acute PHD are nonspecific and generally reflect those of the underlying disease, such as dyspnea, orthopnea, and cough. Physical examination reveals distended neck veins with prominent *a* and *v* waves, pulsus alternans, and peripheral cyanosis. Cardiac examination may demonstrate a parasternal or subxiphoid heave or a palpable pulmonic valve closure (10). On cardiac auscultation, an S₃ gallop and a loud pulmonic component of the second sound are usually present. A holosystolic murmur along the left parasternal border, accentuated during inspiration, suggests tricuspid regurgitation, often seen with acute or chronic pulmonary hypertension. Auscultation of the lung fields may be normal or may reveal bilateral basilar crackles. Systolic bruits in the lungs are suggestive of chronic thromboembolic pulmonary hypertension, resulting from turbulent flow through partially recanalized vessels (15). Although the patient's history and a carefully performed physical examination may suggest acute PHD, additional diagnostic studies are usually necessary to confirm the diagnosis.

CHRONIC PULMONARY HEART DISEASE

Chronic PHD develops when pulmonary disease is bilateral, diffuse, and chronic. Table 38.1 lists many of the causes of chronic PHD. COPD is by far the most common cause of chronic PHD in the developed world (16,17). PHD is most frequently seen in patients with the features of the "blue and bloated" (type B) syndrome, consisting of hypoxemia, hypercapnia, and peripheral edema (18). Although the exact incidence of chronic PHD is not known, PHD causes 10% to 30% of hospital admissions for congestive heart failure in the

TABLE 38.1. DISEASES ASSOCIATED WITH PULMONARY HEART DISEASE

Diseases affecting airways and lung parenchyma
    Chronic obstructive pulmonary disease
    Cystic fibrosis
    Congenital developmental defects
    Infiltrative or granulomatous defects
    Idiopathic pulmonary fibrosis
    Sarcoidosis
    Tuberculosis
    Pneumoconioses
    Scleroderma
    Mixed connective tissue disease
    Systemic lupus erythematosus
    Rheumatoid arthritis
    Dermatomyositis
    Eosinophilic granuloma
    Radiation
    Diffuse malignant infiltration
    Upper airway obstruction
    Pulmonary resection (provided the lung remnant is abnormal)
Diseases affecting the thoracic cage
    Kyphoscoliosis
    Thoracoplasty
    Neuromuscular disease causing muscle weakness
    Amyotrophic lateral sclerosis
    Muscular dystrophy
    Quadriplegia
Diseases affecting the pulmonary vasculature
    Primary pulmonary hypertension
    Pulmonary venoocclusive disease
    Polyarteritis (pulmonary arteritis)
    Rheumatoid arthritis
    Scleroderma
    Systemic lupus erythematosus
    Acute pulmonary thromboembolism
    Air embolism
    Amniotic fluid embolism
    Fat embolism
    Chronic pulmonary thromboembolic disease
    Portal-pulmonary Hypertension
    Filariasis
    Schistosomiasis
    Sickle cell disease
    Tumor emboli
    Congenital peripheral pulmonary hypertension
    Toxin-induced pulmonary hypertension
        Anorexigens
        Intravenous drug abuse
    Mediastinal tumor external pressure and direct invasion
    HIV Infection
Hypoventilatory disorders
    Sleep apnea syndrome
    Idiopathic alveolar hypoventilation syndrome (Ondine curse)
    Obesity-hypoventilation syndrome
Chronic high-altitude disease

United States. Hypoxemia and subsequent vascular remodeling are the most important correctable features of chronic PHD. Destruction of lung parenchyma with loss of cross-sectional vascular surface area also contributes substantially to increased pulmonary arterial pressure. In patients with COPD, there is a direct correlation between arterial partial pressure of O_2 (Pao_2) and pulmonary arterial pressure, suggesting an additive effect of hypercapnia and acidosis.

Right Ventricle in Chronic PHD

Chronic PHD leads to uniform hypertrophy of the RV. The ventricular wall cross-sectional area increases, as does myocardial fiber thickness. It should be remembered that dilation of the RV may actually be associated with a greater increase in muscle mass than hypertrophy without dilation because of the increase in RV surface area. Baseline coronary flow increases in proportion to muscle mass. Increases in the RV end-diastolic pressure, indicative of the presence of right heart failure, develop only in the later stages of pulmonary hypertension. Because of increased muscle mass, RV myocardial O_2 demand is increased, thus rendering the RV more susceptible to imbalances in demand and supply.

In contrast to acute PHD, RV systolic pressure in chronic PHD can be quite high, occasionally even approaching systemic levels. Cardiac output at rest is usually normal but may be elevated in patients with chronic PHD owing to COPD. This suggests that maintaining peripheral O_2 transport is an important adaptive response to chronic tissue hypoxemia. Polycythemia develops in many patients with chronic PHD and augments peripheral O_2 delivery in the setting of a decreased cardiac output or decreased oxyhemoglobin content. However, severe polycythemia increases blood viscosity and can further increase pulmonary vascular resistance (19).

Patients with chronic PHD frequently experience syncope during or immediately after exercise: Increased venous return during exercise leads to increased RV pressure and volume, thereby increasing O_2 demand. This could produce RV myocardial O_2 supply-demand imbalance and precipitate RV ischemia. In addition, systemic vascular resistance normally decreases during exercise; a decrease in blood pressure will result if cardiac output fails to increase proportionally owing to poor RV function. Decreased systemic arterial pressure could also limit RV coronary blood flow and contribute to circulatory collapse, as well as lead to cerebral hypoperfusion and syncope.

Pathophysiological Features

The pulmonary hemodynamics in COPD have been thoroughly investigated. In the early stages, pulmonary arterial pressure is either normal or only slightly elevated. However, pulmonary arterial pressure almost invariably increases with exercise in patients with PHD owing to the lack of recruitable pulmonary vessels and the inability to further dilate the existing vasculature. As the disease progresses, pulmonary arterial pressure is increased even at rest. Pulmonary arterial pressures increase as hypoxemia worsens with time, even when pulmonary mechanics remain unchanged. The pulmonary arterial pressure increased by a mean of 3 mm Hg/y in patients enrolled in the British Medical Research Council

trial on domiciliary O_2 therapy (20). Although pulmonary hypertension progresses slowly in patients with COPD, its presence is a poor prognostic sign (21). Mortality in patients with COPD and PHD is increased twofold to threefold over that of comparable patients without PHD (6).

The relationship between RV contractile function and clinical features of PHD is not clear. Some investigators have found that RV function deteriorates during exercise in patients with PHD. Others have shown a poor correlation between changes in RV contractile function and clinical features of right heart failure such as peripheral edema, ascites, and increased right atrial pressure. Finally, progressive decreases in systemic arterial pressure have been demonstrated in patients with pulmonary hypertension, which may be the result of worsening hypoxemia and reduced preload to the LV as progressive right heart failure ensues.

Left-Ventricular Function in Chronic PHD

Ventricular interdependence acts to inhibit LV filling with RV dilation, as evidenced by a leftward shift in the interventricular septum on echocardiography, and decreased compliance of the LV has been demonstrated in some patients with chronic PHD. In experimental studies, banding the pulmonary artery in animals leads to combined LV and RV hypertrophy, and LV hypertrophy accompanies RV hypertrophy in approximately 30% of patients with COPD. Depressed LV function has been reported in patients with COPD in the absence of identifiable causes of LV failure such as coronary heart disease, and recent studies have demonstrated LV myocardial fibrosis and cellular hypertrophy in patients with COPD dying of heart failure in whom there was no identifiable cause of LV disease. Hypoxemia, hypercapnia, and increased circulating catecholamine levels could contribute to or produce these changes.

There are a number of causes of impaired LV filling in patients with COPD. Patients with airflow obstruction may generate large negative inspiratory swings in intrathoracic pressure, particularly during exercise. These pressure swings increase venous return during inspiration, further dilating the RV and leading to greater diastolic interdependence, and may explain the early inspiratory decrease in LV preload observed in many studies. This effect is partly or wholly responsible for decreased stroke volume in early inspiration and thus contributes substantially to the pulsus alternans observed in patients with airway obstruction. Patients with COPD usually also manifest pulmonary hyperinflation, and increased lower lobe inflation can compromise LV filling. Finally, hypoxemia itself can impair LV relaxation and produce diastolic dysfunction.

There are several factors that can contribute to LV systolic dysfunction: Large decreases in intrathoracic pressure, especially if sustained, can impair LV ejection by increasing LV afterload. When intrathoracic pressure decreases more than aortic pressure during inspiration, LV systolic transmural pressure—one measure of LV wall stress or afterload—may increase. Although sustained decreases in intrathoracic pressure increase LV afterload, the importance of this mechanism in influencing LV function with intermittent (inspiratory) exaggerated decreases in intrathoracic pressure in obstructive airway disease remains controversial.

Finally, many patients with COPD have concomitant coronary artery, valvular, or hypertensive heart disease. These conditions may affect LV function and secondarily contribute to further deterioration of RV function.

Diagnosis of Chronic PHD

The clinical history and physical examination are critical elements in the diagnosis of PHD. Additionally, there are several noninvasive and invasive modalities that are useful in the assessment of pulmonary hypertension and its cardiac complications.

Clinical Presentation

Patients with chronic PHD exhibit signs and symptoms of the underlying disease. Dyspnea is a frequent symptom and usually is associated with hypoxemia and hypercapnia. However, in many patients, especially those with fibrotic lung disease or vascular obstruction, dyspnea is not necessarily accompanied by resting hypoxemia and is not completely relieved with supplemental O_2 therapy. In these conditions, reflexes originating in the lung parenchyma, vasculature, or chest wall may cause dyspnea.

Patients with severe chronic PHD may present with syncope, especially during exercise, as a result of mechanisms discussed above. Anginal chest pain occurs in some patients with chronic severe PHD. Although it is not usually responsive to nitrates, it is likely that this pain is caused by RV ischemia, resulting from RV O_2 demands outstripping its supply (22).

Hemoptysis occurs in pulmonary hypertension owing to rupture of atherosclerotic or dilated pulmonary vessels. Hemoptysis should not be attributed to PHD until other diagnoses such as tumor, bronchiectasis, or pulmonary infarction are excluded.

Right upper-quadrant fullness, early satiety, nausea, and vomiting are commonly seen in patients with PHD and may indicate the presence of right heart failure with passive congestion of the liver and/or ascites. Neurological symptoms such as headache and mental obtundation are owing to decreased cardiac output and hypoxemia with or without hypercapnia. In severe pulmonary hypertension, hoarseness may result from compression of the left recurrent laryngeal nerve by an enlarged left pulmonary artery.

Tachypnea at rest is a common feature in patients with chronic isolated pulmonary vascular disease or interstitial lung disease, but is usually not seen in patients with stable chronic bronchitis. As in acute PHD, there may be a loud pulmonic component of the S_2, an RV heave, and S_4. An S_3 is indicative of right heart failure. A holosystolic murmur along the left sternal border that is accentuated by inspiration (Carvallo's sign) is characteristic of tricuspid regurgitation. The blowing diastolic murmur of pulmonic insufficiency, heard best at the pulmonic area and left sternal border (Graham-Steele murmur) is indicative of severe pulmonary hypertension. Elevated neck veins with prominent *a* and *v* waves are also indicative of right heart failure.

Peripheral Edema in Pulmonary Heart Disease

Peripheral edema is part of the congestive heart failure syndrome and may extend into the abdominal wall and sacrum. The simplest explanation for edema is that elevated pulmonary artery pressure leads to elevated right atrial, peripheral venous, and capillary pressures, producing an increased hydrostatic gradient for fluid transudation. However, some patients with COPD may experience peripheral edema, despite having a normal right atrial pressure. In this setting, hypoxia can decrease glomerular filtration and filtration of sodium (23). Additionally, retention of bicarbonate by the kidney is a mechanism for maintaining arterial pH in cases of chronic respiratory acidosis, and a parallel increase in sodium reabsorbtion may further contribute to salt and water retention. Hypoxemia may also stimulate the production of arginine vasopressin and lead to decreased free water excretion. Arginine vasopressin production may also be stimulated by the renin-angiotensin system, specifically angiotensin II, which is activated by the reduction in renal blood flow that is seen with hypoxia. Catecholamine levels are often elevated in COPD patients and can also lead to renin release from the kidneys and promote sodium absorption.

Atrial natriuretic peptide (ANP) levels are elevated in patients with COPD and edema. These patients exhibit normal responsiveness to ANP after water loading. However, the response to ANP, which acts to buffer edemagenic mechanisms, is not sufficient to overcome these mechanisms in the most severe patients (24).

Electrocardiogram

The electrocardiographic (ECG) abnormalities in PHD depend on its etiology and severity (25,26). Patients with COPD have a characteristic ECG pattern as a result of major structural changes of the thorax and its contents. The resulting ECG patterns, such as shifts of the P wave and QRS axis, will then be superimposed on the changes caused by right-ventricular hypertrophy. The ECG criteria for PHD listed in Table 38.2 illustrate the common patterns associated with COPD, as well as other parenchymal lung diseases. In general, ECG criteria are fairly specific but not sensitive for the detection of PHD.

Because the electrical activity of the RV is considerably less than that of the LV, small changes in RV forces may be "lost"

TABLE 38.2. ELECTROCARDIOGRAPHIC CHANGES IN COR PULMONALE

ECG criteria for cor pulmonale without obstructive disease of the airways
1. Right-axis deviation with a mean QRS axis > +110°
2. R/S amplitude ratio in V_1 > 1
3. R/S amplitude ratio in V_6 < 1
4. Clockwise rotation of the electric axis
5. P-pulmonale pattern
6. S_1, Q_3 or S_1, S_2, S_3 pattern
7. Normal voltage QRS

ECG changes in chronic cor pulmonale with obstructive disease of the airways
1. Isoelectric P waves in lead I or right-axis deviation of the P vector
2. P-pulmonale pattern (an increase in P-wave amplitude in II, III, AVF)
3. Tendency for right-axis deviation of the QRS
4. R/S amplitude ratio in V_6 < 1
5. Low-voltage QRS
6. S_1, Q_3 or S_1, S_2, S_3 pattern
7. Incomplete (and rarely complete) right bundle-branch block
8. R/S amplitude ratio in V_1 > 1
9. Marked clockwise rotation of the electric axis
10. Occasional large Q wave or QS in the inferior or midprecordial leads, suggesting healed myocardial infarction

in the preponderance of leftward-acting forces. An increase in anteriorly directed forces may occur with RV hypertrophy, but this may also be a sign of posterior LV infarction. Severe RV hypertrophy may lead to Q waves in the precordial leads, falsely suggesting anterior myocardial infarction. However, if the precordial leads are moved down one interspace, Q waves will be abolished in RV hypertrophy but persist with LV anterior wall myocardial infarction.

Cardiac rhythm disturbances may also be present in PHD, ranging from premature atrial contractions to supraventricular tachycardia of all types, including paroxysmal atrial tachycardia, multifocal atrial tachycardia, atrial fibrillation, atrial flutter, and junctional tachycardia. Arrhythmias are particularly observed in chronic PHD patients during an episode of acute respiratory failure. These arrhythmias are usually owing to acute RV pressure overload, electrolyte abnormalities, hypoxemia, and acidosis, but may also be secondary to therapy with β-agonists, methylxanthines, cardiac glycosides, or diuretics. Although the overall incidence of arrhythmias ranges from 20% to 70%, the reported incidence of ventricular arrhythmias is considerably lower (7%–24%). Patients with isolated pulmonary vasculopathy such as primary pulmonary hypertension rarely experience arrhythmias, suggesting that the arrhythmias in COPD are caused by exacerbating factors rather than solely by RV hypertrophy or pulmonary hypertension. Figure 38.3 shows an ECG from a patient with severe PHD.

Chest Roentgenogram

Routine chest radiography demonstrating a right descending pulmonary artery more than 16 mm in diameter or a left artery more than 18 mm in diameter is indicative of pulmonary hypertension. On the posteroanterior view, RV enlargement results in displacement of the cardiac silhouette to the right and in an increased transverse diameter of the heart, often accompanied by attenuation of the peripheral pulmonary vasculature. In the lateral view, RV enlargement leads to filling of the retrosternal air space. However,

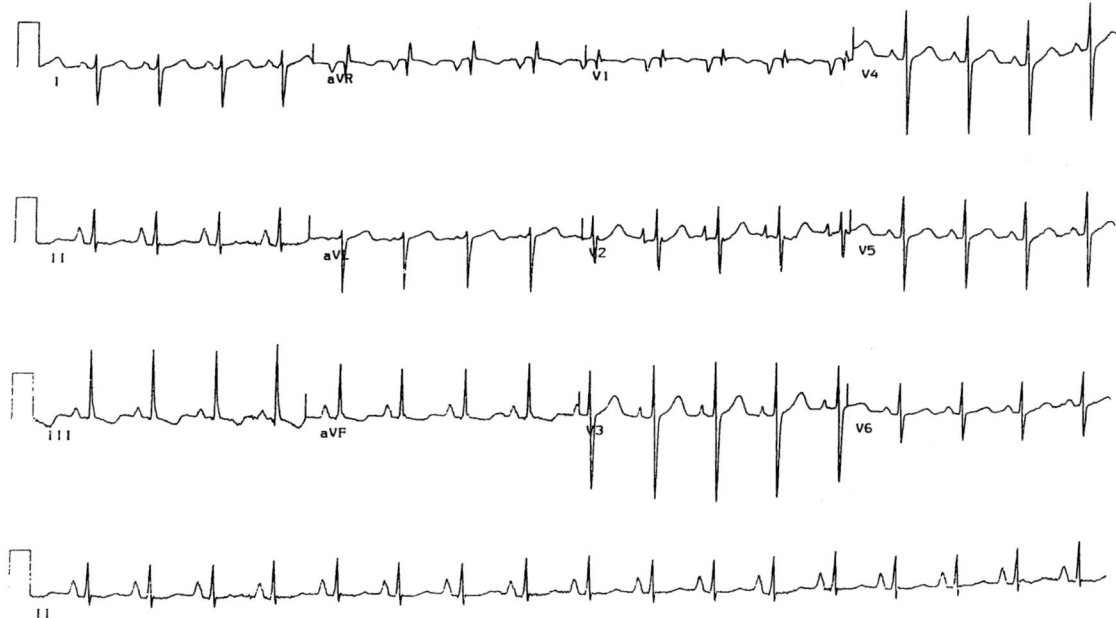

FIGURE 38.3. Example of an electrocardiogram from a 37-year-old woman with chronic pulmonary heart disease related to chronic bronchiectasis. Note right-axis deviation and p-pulmonale in lead 2 along with persistent right axis forces (RS) in the lateral precordium (V_5–V_6).

changes in mediastinal and chest wall configuration in patients with COPD or chest wall deformity may render these radiographic signs unreliable. In the National Institutes of Health Registry on Primary Pulmonary Hypertension, enlarged main pulmonary arteries were observed in 90% of patients, enlarged hilar pulmonary arteries in 80%, and peripheral pulmonary vascular pruning in 51% of patients (27). Heart size was enlarged in 94% of these patients with severe pulmonary hypertension. Figure 38.4 demonstrates typical roentgenographic signs of PHD.

Computed Tomography

Ultrafast, ECG-gated computed tomography scanning has recently been evaluated for studying global and regional systolic and diastolic RV function. Good correlations between

RV and LV stroke volumes have been obtained, and RV ejection fraction (RVEF) can be estimated. Further, the stop-action mode of ultrafast computed tomography yields estimates of RV wall mass that correlate to actual mass in both animal and human studies. As these techniques improve, they may be used increasingly in evaluating the progression of chronic PHD.

Echocardiography

Echocardiography is often the first study that suggests pulmonary hypertension in patients with unexplained dyspnea. However, its utility in COPD is limited owing to pulmonary hyperinflation. Two-dimensional echocardiography provides multiple cross-sectional views of the heart, improves visualization of right-sided cardiac structures, and is

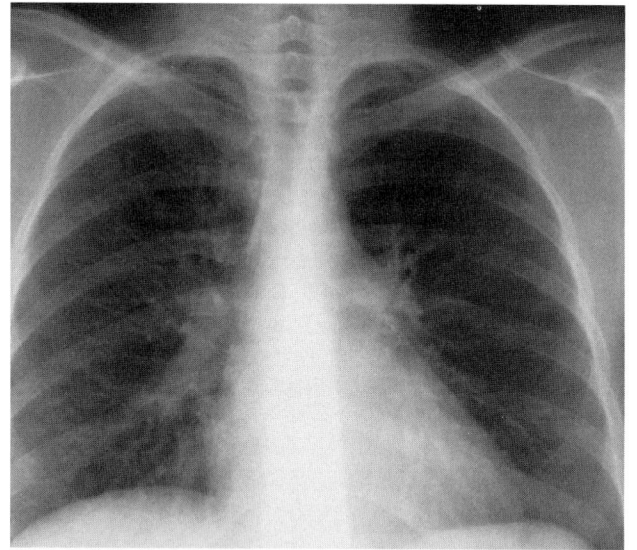

A

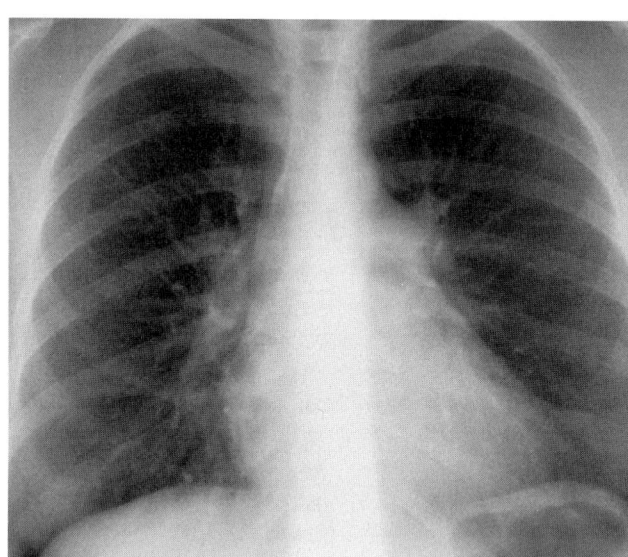

B

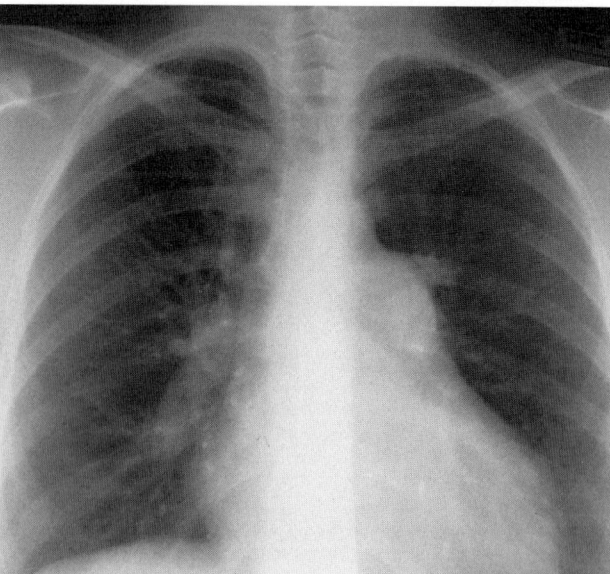

C

FIGURE 38.4. Progression of chest x-ray in a 34-year-old woman with a primary pulmonary hypertension–like syndrome associated with HIV syndrome. Chest x-rays taken in 1991 **(A),** 1992 **(B),** and 1994 **(C).** Note the progressive dilation of the main pulmonary arteries and cardiac dilation over the years.

more useful in assessing RV hypertrophy in patients with PHD than are M-mode techniques. In addition, multiple cross-sectional views can be used to obtain relatively accurate estimations of RV volume using the Simpson's rule approximation technique. Measurements of right atrial and RV size by two-dimensional echocardiography distinguish normal patients from those with RV volume overload and correlate with measurements made at cardiac catheterization.

Correlations between a variety of echocardiographic indices and pulmonary hemodynamics have been attempted. The use of velocity measurements (Doppler echocardiography) has allowed noninvasive estimation of the pulmonary arterial pressure. Because most patients with RV overload develop some degree of tricuspid regurgitation, the pressure gradient across the tricuspid valve during systole can be estimated from the maximum velocity of the regurgitant jet and the modified Bernoulli equation: $PG = 4V^2$, where PG is pressure gradient across the valve, and V is the maximum velocity of the regurgitant jet. Right atrial pressure is estimated by another technique (e.g., by neck vein distention on physical examination or inferior vena cava distention by echocardiography) or a value is assumed, and this value is then added to the value for PG. Thus, RV and pulmonary arterial systolic pressure may be estimated. Other techniques for estimating pulmonary arterial pressure using Doppler measurements of pulmonary arterial velocity also exist and may be used when tricuspid regurgitation is not apparent.

The RV index ($TA \times RVD + AW/BSA$, where TA is the inner tricuspid annulus diastolic dimension, RVD is RV short-axis dimension, AW is RV anterior wall thickness, and BSA is body surface area) also correlates reasonably well with mean pulmonary arterial pressure.

Chronic RV overload leads to RV dilation, especially during inspiration, when venous return is maximized. These changes can result in changes in RV configuration and impairment of LV diastolic filling. Because these effects are mediated through the interventricular septum, they may be detected by echocardiogram. Normally, the septum is concave toward the LV, resulting in a relatively circular LV shape in the axial plane during diastole. During systole, there is symmetric inward motion of the ventricular walls, resulting in constriction of the LV while it maintains its circular shape. Thus, the septum functions as part of the LV during systole. With RV volume overload, the septum may become flattened or even reverse its curvature so as to become concave toward the RV. In extreme cases, the septum may bulge into the LV during diastole. During systole, the septum may demonstrate paradoxic motion, defined as motion away from the LV posterolateral wall and toward the RV free wall. The septum effectively functions as part of the RV in these cases. With a sufficient degree of leftward shift of the septum, LV end-diastolic filling may become compromised and lead to decreased cardiac output. Figure 38.5 shows an example of an echocardiogram in a patient with primary pulmonary hypertension and PHD (see also color Fig. 38.5).

Radionuclide Techniques

The equilibrium-gated blood-imaging technique allows continuous monitoring of RV performance by tagging erythrocytes with ^{99m}Tc. Ejection fraction is calculated by comparing counts at end-systole with those at end-diastole over approximately 10 minutes. Although equilibrium-gated blood pool imaging allows continuous monitoring of RV

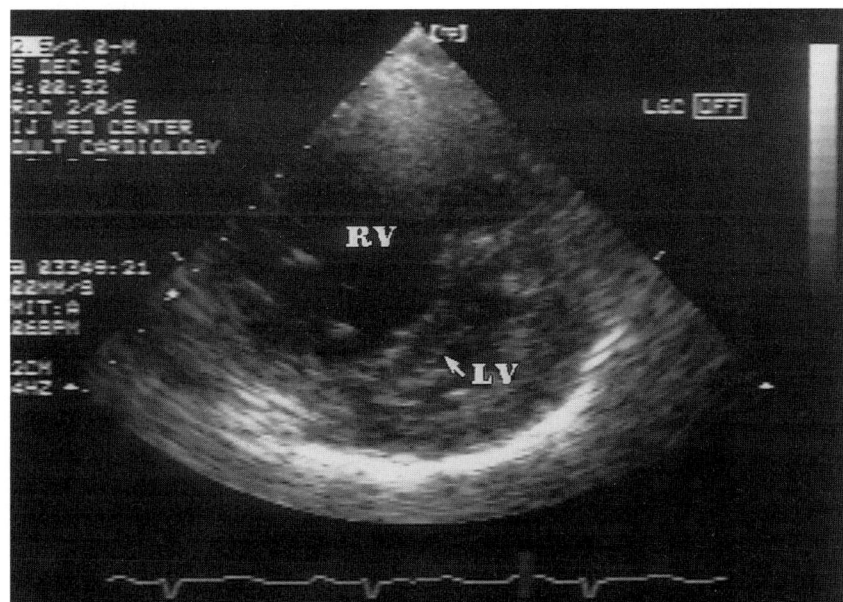

FIGURE 38.5. (See also color Fig. 38.5.) Example of echocardiogram from the patient illustrated in Fig. 38.4 at the time of the most recent chest x-ray. This short-axis view shows severe dilation of the right ventricle (RV), bulging of the septum to the left in diastole, and a small left ventricle (LV) chamber. The RV was noted to be severely hypokinetic. The *arrow* points to the interventricular septum. (From Scott Roth, Division of Cardiology, Long Island Jewish Medical Center, New Hyde Park, New York, with permission.)

performance and provides reliable measurements of RVEF, RV dimensions are difficult to evaluate because the ventricular borders are obscured by the presence of background counts in other cardiac chambers and the lungs. The first-pass technique also involves labeling with ^{99m}Tc but is based on principles of indicator dilution theory, whereby counting is performed sequentially over each cardiac chamber as a function of time. The advantage of the first-pass technique is that data are gathered over only a few heartbeats. Further, the large number of counts relative to background allows definition of the RV borders and estimates of diastolic and systolic size. Both first-pass and equilibrium-gated techniques can be used to evaluate ventricular function at rest and during exercise. The first-pass technique allows patients to be studied in the supine or upright position, which is a major advantage. The 30-degree right anterior oblique position is optimal for assessing the RV. Although radionuclide studies can detect the presence of severely elevated pulmonary arterial pressure, they cannot accurately assess mild pulmonary hypertension.

Right ventricular function in COPD depends on the etiology, duration, and severity of PHD. The correlations between pulmonary arterial pressure and RVEF and, similarly, those between pulmonary vascular resistance and RVEF have generally been weak (28). Exercise studies appear to enhance the detection of decreased RVEF by radionuclide techniques.

^{201}Tl is another radionuclide used for imaging the RV. Thallium is taken up by myocardial tissue, in contrast to technetium, which images the blood pool. Although visualization of the RV at rest is not common in healthy patients, the thickened RV myocardium present in patients with chronic PHD allows RV visualization in these patients. Thallium imaging techniques are most sensitive for detecting RV hypertrophy when mean pulmonary arterial pressure is greater than 30 mm Hg.

Magnetic Resonance Imaging

Magnetic resonance imaging (MRI) allows the noninvasive evaluation of RV free wall mass (29). With this technique, a greater RV free wall mass has been observed in patients with chronic PHD compared with healthy patients. A modified short-axis section of the heart imaged by MRI appears to provide valid clinical configurational information concerning the RV on which the noninvasive diagnosis of PHD may be entertained.

THERAPY OF CHRONIC PULMONARY HEART DISEASE

The mainstay of therapy of chronic PHD is the treatment of the underlying disease process (22). This may include treatment of infection and bronchodilation in COPD, treatment with steroids or other immunosuppressive agents in chronic infiltrative and fibrotic disorders, and anticoagula-

tion in chronic thromboembolic diseases. In this section, we review some of the principles of supportive therapy that apply to cases of chronic PHD.

Oxygen Therapy

O_2 therapy is the only therapeutic modality that has been shown to improve long-term prognosis in patients with hypoxemic COPD (20,30–32). However, the use of O_2 in other causes of PHD has not been firmly established. Although there are no large randomized controlled trials of O_2 therapy in diseases such as pulmonary fibrosis and pneumoconioses as there are for COPD, O_2 therapy provides substantial symptomatic relief in these patients. Additionally, many patients are normoxic at rest (O_2 saturation >92%) but become severely hypoxic either at night or during exercise, and these patients derive functional benefit from the administration of O_2 during periods of hypoxemia. For example, many patients with idiopathic pulmonary fibrosis and exercise-induced hypoxemia will experience increased exercise tolerance and less activity-related dyspnea when portable O_2 is administered during activities of daily living.

Short-Term Effects of Oxygen Therapy

Patients with acute respiratory failure are usually hypoxemic and treatment with O_2 leads to substantial clinical improvement, manifested by diuresis, decreased dyspnea, and improved mentation. The improved arterial O_2 content with short-term O_2 therapy usually translates to improved peripheral O_2 delivery; however, decreased sympathoadrenal stimulation with alleviation of hypoxemia may lead to reductions in cardiac output in some circumstances.

In contrast to its effects on the systemic vasculature, hypoxia causes pulmonary vasoconstriction (33,34), and the presence of pulmonary arterial hypertension is inversely correlated with arterial O_2 saturation in COPD. However, most clinical studies have documented either no change or only slight decreases in pulmonary arterial pressure associated with the acute administration of O_2 to severe COPD patients with acute respiratory failure. This suggests that increased pulmonary vascular resistance is more a result of pulmonary vascular remodeling rather than simply hypoxic vasoconstriction. Similarly, short-term O_2 therapy does not substantially change RV or LV function in most patients with acute respiratory failure. Therefore, the substantial clinical benefits of short-term O_2 therapy appear to derive primarily from effects on peripheral circulatory function rather than improvement in cardiac function.

Long-Term Effects of Oxygen Therapy

The current guidelines for the administration of long-term domiciliary O_2 to patients with COPD derive from two major clinical trials. The British Medical Research Council

Trial randomized 87 patients with severe COPD to O_2 therapy (42 patients) or no therapy (45 patients) (20). The two groups had comparably severe, stable pulmonary function (forced expiratory volume in 1 second, 1.5 L; $Pao_2 = 60$ torr; and peripheral edema with or without hypercapnia). The treatment group was given nasal O_2, 2 L/min, or O_2 sufficient to increase Pao_2 to at least 60 torr, for at least 15 h/d. Survival at 5 years was 50% greater in the O_2-treated group than in the untreated group. Although pulmonary arterial pressure did not decrease in the treated group, it increased by 3 mm Hg/y in the control group. Pulmonary vascular resistance increased by 27% in the untreated patients and decreased by 11% in the treated group, but only after 6 months of treatment. This suggests that chronic supplemental O_2 therapy reversed some of the chronic hypoxemia-induced structural changes in the pulmonary vasculature, and is supported by animal studies demonstrating resolution of structural abnormalities in hypoxia-induced pulmonary hypertension upon removal of the hypoxic stimulus.

The Nocturnal Oxygen Therapy Trial, sponsored by the National Institutes of Health in the United States, compared 24-hour (continuous) with 12-hour (intermittent) O_2 therapy in patients with severe COPD (30). The study was terminated prematurely because a nearly twofold survival benefit was observed in the group receiving continuous O_2 therapy (which actually used O_2 for a mean of 17.7 h/d). Pulmonary vascular resistance increased by 6.5% in the 12-hour group but decreased by 11% in the treated group. Improvement in resting and exercise RV stroke volume and decreased pulmonary vascular resistance predicted long-term survival.

It seems clear from these trials that long-term O_2 therapy in patients with hypoxic COPD improves survival, particularly when it is used nearly continuously. Table 38.3 presents the generally accepted criteria used by physicians and third-party payers for providing long-term domiciliary O_2 in the United States. Because secondary polycythemia, elevations in pulmonary arterial pressure and pulmonary vascular resistance, and peripheral edema are poor prognostic signs, it is reasonable to institute therapy when these are present, even

TABLE 38.3. INDICATIONS FOR LONG-TERM OXYGEN THERAPY IN CHRONIC OBSTRUCTIVE PULMONARY DISEASE

- $Pao_2 \leq 55$ torr or O_2 saturation $\leq 88\%$ on room air at rest in nonrecumbent position
- $Pao_2 > 55$ torr or O_2 saturation $> 88\%$ *with* evidence of secondary polycythemia (hematocrit ≥ 55), p-pulmonale on electrocardiogram, edema, or impaired mental or cognitive function
- $Pao_2 \leq 55$ torr or O_2 saturation $\leq 88\%$ during exercise with demonstrable improvement in exercise performance with O_2 therapy
- $Pao_2 \leq 55$ torr or O_2 saturation $\leq 88\%$ during sleep especially associated with fragmentation of sleep, cardiac arrhythmias or ischemia, or pulmonary hypertension

Pao_2, arterial blood partial pressure of oxygen; O_2, oxygen.

if resting Pao_2 exceeds the strictest criteria. Measurement of O_2 saturation during exercise or sleep provides documentation of arterial desaturation that also warrants the use of supplemental O_2 therapy.

Stability of Respiratory Failure and Long-Term Oxygen Therapy

Long-term O_2 therapy has been shown to be of benefit only in COPD patients with stable chronic respiratory failure. Thus, the decision to institute long-term therapy should not be based on pulmonary function and arterial blood gases taken immediately after a bout of acute respiratory failure. Of course, this does not mean that patients presenting to the hospital who are discharged with resting hypoxemia should not be treated with O_2 for a few weeks while their pulmonary function is allowed to improve. Rather, these patients should be assessed for the need for long-term O_2 use once they have become clinically stable. Studies have demonstrated that after acute respiratory failure, approximately 30% to 40% of patients will improve sufficiently with 3 weeks of standard therapy using bronchodilators and antibiotics to obviate the need for chronic O_2 therapy. Because there are no reliable means of predicting which patients will improve to the point of not needing O_2 therapy, at least 3 weeks of optimum standard care should be instituted in hypoxemic COPD patients before initiation of long-term O_2 therapy.

Patients who smoke should be *required* to stop smoking as a precondition for receiving a prescription for O_2. Aside from the obvious danger and the philosophical concerns of self responsibility, the presence of elevated carboxyhemoglobin in the blood from smoking will largely obviate the effects of O_2 on arterial O_2 content.

Nocturnal Hypoxemia

Many patients with COPD are hypoxic primarily at night and may experience severe desaturation during sleep, especially during rapid eye movement (REM) sleep. Reasons for this include nocturnal hypoventilation, ventilation-perfusion imbalance from loss of tonic skeletal muscle tone, coexisting congestive heart failure with Cheyne-Stokes respiration, and/or concomitant obstructive sleep apnea. Nocturnal alterations in ventilation may contribute to the development of clinical signs of PHD in COPD patients, even when daytime O_2 saturations are in the normal range. Clearly, the combination of COPD and concomitant disease such as obstructive sleep apnea (overlap syndrome) predisposes to severe nocturnal hypoxemia. Both conditions must be dealt with in order to successfully relieve nocturnal hypoxemia.

Clinical PHD is seen in some 5% to 12% of patients with obstructive sleep apnea. Echocardiographic studies have demonstrated an association between RV hypertrophy and the occurrence of obstructive sleep apnea in children and adults. Nocturnal hypoxemia and increases in pulmonary arterial pressure during apneas may contribute to PHD in these patients (5,21,35–37). Another possible mechanism is that during obstructive apneas, there are large increases in venous return during inspiration compared to expiration, which may lead to flow overload of the RV. When upper airway obstruction is relieved in these patients, improvement in RV function is almost always noted.

Exercise Hypoxemia

Some relatively normoxic COPD patients become hypoxemic while exercising. Although this may not lead to increased resting pulmonary arterial pressures or increased mortality, the administration of O_2 during exercise can increase exercise tolerance and thus lead to an improved quality of life. During the Nocturnal Oxygen Therapy Trial, those patients receiving continuous O_2 may have done better not simply because they received O_2 for a greater proportion of the day but because they were better oxygenated during exercise. Similarly, in other hypoxic pulmonary conditions, O_2 administered during exercise may lead to improved quality of life. Exercise testing should be performed to document improved exercise tolerance during administration of O_2 on a case-by-case basis, and O_2 should be prescribed for patients with exercise hypoxemia in whom objective evidence of improved function can be documented.

Pulmonary Vasodilator Therapy in Pulmonary Heart Disease

The demonstrated benefit of pulmonary vasodilator therapy in at least some patients with primary pulmonary hypertension has led to numerous attempts to treat PHD secondary to other conditions, most notably COPD, with vasodilator regimens. This topic has been covered thoroughly elsewhere (38). Various classes of vasodilators, including β-adrenergic blockers, β-agonists, calcium channel blockers, nitrates, and angiotensin-converting enzyme inhibitors, have been tried. In general, vasodilator therapy has failed to demonstrate sustained therapeutic benefit in patients with COPD, and its use is not recommended on a routine basis (22,39–41). Methylxanthines lead to improved RV performance in patients with COPD, perhaps through a vasodilatory mechanism (42). β_2-Specific agonists may also act as pulmonary vasodilators in addition to their well-known effects on bronchomotor tone and mucociliary clearance. At the time of this writing, the Food and Drug Administration has approved three agents for the treatment of pulmonary artery hypertension: two prostanoids—intravenous epoprostenol (Flolan) and subcutaneous trepostinil (Remodulin)—and the oral dual endothelin receptor blocker bosentan (Tracleer). These drugs appear to exert beneficial effects on the pulmonary vascular bed primarily by altering vascular remodeling rather than by vasodilation. None of these agents have been studied ex-

tensively in patients with pulmonary hypertension owing to chronic respiratory disease, and their use cannot be recommended on a routine basis (43). However, a cautious trial may be considered in some patients whose pulmonary hypertension is severe and appears disproportionate to their chronic lung disease. Because the prostanoids also possess potent vasodilator properties, careful monitoring of arterial oxygenation is advised when these agents are administered, because worsening intrapulmonary gas exchange may result from increases in blood flow to poorly ventilated lung units. Newer therapies that are delivered by the inhaled route, such as Iloprost (a stable form of prostacyclin), may ultimately prove to be the preferred approach (44,45).

Cardiac Glycosides

The utility of cardiac glycosides in PHD has been clearly documented only in the presence of concomitant LV dysfunction. There are few data to support therapeutic benefit from cardiac glycosides in isolated PHD. Furthermore, acute hypoxemia increases toxicity of these agents either directly or through secondary mechanisms such as sympathoadrenal stimulation; accordingly, the use of cardiac glycosides for routine treatment of PHD is not recommended (46).

Phlebotomy and Diuretics

Although reduction in intravascular volume could lead to improved RV function, excessive diuresis can reduce mean circulatory pressure and lead to detrimental reductions in cardiac output and renal blood flow. In addition, hypokalemia and metabolic alkalosis can result from overdiuresis and can lead to arrhythmias and decreased respiratory drive, respectively. Accordingly, adequate diuresis for symptomatic edema should be encouraged, but care should be taken to avoid a contracted volume state.

Blood viscosity increases sharply as the hematocrit exceeds approximately 55% and may lead to increased pulmonary vascular and increased RV afterload. Because secondary polycythemia is a compensatory response to hypoxemia, it is usually preventable or treatable with long-term O_2 therapy. However, phlebotomy should be considered when hematocrit is persistently greater than 55%. The improved cardiac output that accompanies a reduction of blood viscosity often increases peripheral O_2 delivery, despite a reduced blood hemoglobin concentration (19).

Lung Transplantation

With the development of effective immune suppression medications and technical advances that have reduced operative and postoperative mortality, the indications and eligibility criteria for lung transplantation have been broadened. Patients with end-stage obstructive, interstitial, and vascular diseases are now considered candidates for single or bilateral lung transplantation. Patients with PHD who undergo lung transplantation may demonstrate normalization of RV function and resolution of pulmonary hypertension (47). Combined heart and lung transplantation is generally reserved for patients with pulmonary vascular disease associated with uncorrectable, complex congenital heart disease. Unfortunately, transplantation remains limited by organ donor availability and by long-term complications, particularly chronic rejection and infections.

Lung Reduction Surgery

Lung reduction surgery for patients with severe pulmonary emphysema is a promising new mode of therapy that may bring improvement in mechanical function of the lungs. Severe PHD is presently considered to be a contraindication for this surgery, primarily because of increased perioperative and postoperative mortality. However, the long-term effects of lung reduction surgery on pulmonary hemodynamics still need to be evaluated. Improved oxygenation and decreased mechanical distortion of pulmonary vessels postoperatively may lead to improved long-term pulmonary hemodynamics.

ACKNOWLEDGMENTS

Thanks go to Steven M. Scharf, MD, who wrote the previous edition of this chapter.

REFERENCES

1. McGinn S, White PD. Acute cor pulmonale resulting from pulmonary embolism. *JAMA* 1935;104:1473–1478.
2. World Health Organization. Definition of chronic cor pulmonale: a report of the expert committee. *Circulation* 1963;27:594–615.
3. Calverley PMA, Howatson R, Flenley DC, et al. Clinicopathological correlations in cor pulmonale. *Thorax* 1992;47:494–498.
4. Fletcher EC, Schaaf JW, Miller J, et al. Long-term cardiopulmonary sequelae in patients with sleep apnea and chronic lung disease. *Am Rev Respir Dis* 1987;135:525–533.
5. Jamal K, Fleetham JA, Thurlbeck WM. Cor pulmonale: correlation with central airway lesions, peripheral airway lesions, emphysema, and control of breathing. *Am Rev Respir Dis* 1990;141:1172–1177.
6. Traver G, Kline M, Burrows B. Predictors of mortality in chronic obstructive pulmonary disease. *Am Rev Respir Dis* 1979;119:895–902.
7. Weitzenblum E, Oswald M, Mirhom R, et al. Evolution of pulmonary hemodynamics in COLD patients under long-term oxygen therapy. *Eur Respir J* 1989;2:669S–673S.
8. Armour JA, Pace JB, Randall WC. Interrelationships of architecture and function of the right ventricle. *Am J Physiol* 1970;218:174–180.
9. Maughan WL, Oikawa RY. Right ventricular function. In: Scharf SM, Cassidy SS, eds. *Heart–lung interactions in health and disease.* New York: Marcel Dekker, 1989:179–220.
10. Dhainaut JF, Aoute P, Brunet FB. Circulatory effects of positive end-expiratory pressure in patients with acute lung injury. In Scharf SM, Cassidy SS, eds. *Heart–Lung Interactions in Health and Disease.* Marcel Dekker: New York, 1989:809–838.
11. Page RD, Harringer W, Hodakowski GT, et al. Determinants of maximal right ventricular function. *J Heart Lung Transplant* 1992;11:90–98.
12. Scharf SM. Right ventricular load tolerance: role of left ventricular function. In: Perret C, Feihl F, eds. *Perspectives en réanimation, les interactions cardio-pulmonaires.* Paris: Société de Réanimation de Langue Français, Arnette, 1994:17–28.
13. Scharf SM, Warner KG, Josa M, et al. Load tolerance of the right ventricle: effect of increased aortic pressure. *J Crit Care* 1986;1:163–173.
14. Ghignone M, Girling L, Prewitt RM. Volume expansion vs. norepinephrine in treatment of a low cardiac output complicating an acute increase in right ventricular afterload in dogs. *Anesthesiology* 1984;60:132–135.
15. Fedullo P, Auger W, Kerr K, et al. Chronic thromboembolic pulmonary hypertension. *N Engl J Med* 2001;345:1465–1472.
16. MacNee W. Pathophysiology of cor pulmonale in chronic obstructive pulmonary disease: part one. *Am J Respir Crit Care Med* 1994;150:833–852.
17. MacNee W. Pathophysiology of cor pulmonale in chronic obstructive pulmonary disease: part two. *Am J Respir Crit Care Med* 1994;150:1158–1168.
18. Schrijen F, Uffholtz H, Polu JM, et al. Pulmonary and systemic hemodynamic evolution in chronic bronchitis. *Am Rev Respir Dis* 1978;117:25–31.
19. Chetty KG, Brown SE, Light RW. Improved exercise tolerance of the polycythemic lung patient following phlebotomy. *Am J Med* 1983;74:415–420.
20. Stuart-Harris C, Flenley DC, Bishop JH. British Medical Research Council Working Party: long-term domiciliary oxygen therapy in chronic hypoxic cor pulmonale complicating bronchitis and emphysema. *Lancet* 1981;1:681–685.
21. Weitzenblum E, Krieger J, Oswald M, et al. Chronic obstructive pulmonary disease and sleep apnea syndrome. *Sleep* 1992;15:S33–S35.
22. Gaine, SP, Rubin, LJ. Medical and surgical treatment options for pulmonary hypertension. *Am J Med Sci* 1998;315:179.
23. Stewart AG, Bardsley PA, Baudouin SV, et al. Changes in atrial natriuretic peptide concentrations during intravenous saline infusion in hypoxic cor pulmonale. *Thorax* 1991;46:829–834.
24. Baudouin SV, Bott J, Ward A, et al. Short term effect of oxygen on renal haemodynamics in patients with hypoxaemic chronic obstructive airways disease. *Thorax* 1992;47:550–554.
25. Nicholas WJ, Liebson PR. ECG changes in COPD: what do they mean? Part I: atrial and ventricular abnormalities. *J Respir Dis* 1987;8:13–18.
26. Nicholas WJ, Liebson PR. ECG changes in COPD: what do they mean? Part II: right ventricular and biventricular hypertrophy and low voltage. *J Respir Dis* 1987;8:103–120.
27. Rich S, Dantzker DR, Ayres SM, et al. Primary pulmonary hypertension: a national prospective study. *Ann Intern Med* 107:216, 1987.
28. Rezai K, Weiss R, Stanford W, et al. Relative accuracy of three scintigraphic methods for determination of right ventricular ejection fraction: a correlative study with ultrafast computed tomography. *J Nucl Med* 1991;32:429–435.
29. Saito H, Dambara T, Aiba M, et al. Evaluation of cor pulmonale on a modified short-axis section of the heart by magnetic resonance imaging. *Am Rev Respir Dis* 1992;146:1576–1581.
30. Nocturnal Oxygen Therapy Trial Group. Continuous or nocturnal oxygen therapy in hypoxemic chronic obstructive airways disease: a clinical trial. *Ann Intern Med* 1980;93:391–398.

31. Stewart AG, Howard P. Indications for long-term oxygen therapy. *Respiration* 1992;59[Suppl 2]:8–13.

32. Timms RM, Khaja FU, Williams GW. The nocturnal oxygen therapy trial group: hemodynamic response to oxygen therapy in chronic obstructive pulmonary disease. *Ann Intern Med* 1985; 102:29–36.

33. Voelkel NF, Tuder RM. Hypoxia-induced pulmonary vascular remodeling: a model for what human disease? *J Clin Invest* 2000; 106:733–738.

34. Wang J, Juhaszova M, Rubin LJ, et al. Hypoxia inhibits gene expression of voltage-gated K channel α subunits in pulmonary artery smooth muscle cells. *J Clin Invest* 1997;100:2347–2353.

35. Davidson WR. Ventricular hypertrophy in sleep apnea. *J Sleep Res* 1995;4[Suppl 1]:176–181.

36. Fletcher EC, Schaaf JW, Miller J, et al. Long-term cardiopulmonary sequelae in patients with sleep apnea and chronic lung disease. *Am Rev Respir Dis* 1987;135:525–533.

37. Tal A, Leiberman A, Margulis G, et al. Ventricular dysfunction in children with obstructive sleep apnea: radionuclide assessment. *Pediatr Pulmonol* 1988;4:139–143.

38. Rubin, LJ. Primary pulmonary hypertension. *N Engl J Med* 1997;336:111–116.

39. Agostoni P, Doria E, Galli C, et al. Nifedipine reduces pulmonary pressure and vascular tone during short-term but not long-term treatment of pulmonary hypertension in patients with chronic obstructive pulmonary disease. *Am Rev Respir Dis* 1989;139:120–125.

40. Evans TW, Tweney J, Waterhouse JC, et al. Almitrine bismesylate and oxygen therapy in hypoxic cor pulmonale. *Thorax* 1990; 45:16–21.

41. Saadjian AY, Phillip-Joet FF, Vestri R, et al. Long-term treatment of chronic obstructive lung disease by nifedipine: an 18-month hemodynamic study. *Eur Respir J* 1988;1:716–720.

42. Matthay RA. Effects of theophylline on cardiovascular performance in chronic obstructive pulmonary disease. *Chest* 1985;88 [Suppl 1]:112S–117S.

43. Badesch DB, Tapson VF, McGoon MD, et al: Continuous intravenous epoprostenol for pulmonary hypertension due to scleroderma spectrum of disease. *Ann Intern Med* 2000;132:425–434.

44. Olschewski, H, Simonneau G, Galie N, et al. Inhaled Iloprost for severe pulmonary hypertension. *N Engl J Med* 2002;347:322–329.

45. Yoshida M, Taguchi O, Gabazza EC, et al. Combined inhalation of nitric oxide and oxygen in chronic obstructive pulmonary disease. *Am J Resp Crit Care Med* 1997;155:526–529.

46. Brown SE, Pakron FJ, Milnen N, et al. Effects of digoxin on exercise capacity and right ventricular function during exercise in chronic airflow obstruction. *Chest* 1984;85:187–191.

47. Pasque MK, Trulock EP, Kaiser LR, et al. Single-lung transplantation for pulmonary hypertension. *Circulation* 1991;84:2275–2279.

39 Lung Cancer

Gary M. Strauss · Ritesh Rathore

Lung cancer is the most deadly of all malignant diseases, both in the United States and worldwide (1,2). According to the American Cancer Society (ACS), bronchogenic carcinoma will be responsible for 157,200 cancer deaths in the United States in 2003 (3). In comparison, it is estimated that 156,200 deaths will be caused by colorectal cancer, breast cancer, pancreatic cancer, and prostate cancer combined, which are the second through fifth leading causes of cancer mortality, respectively (Table 39.1). In 2003, lung cancer was responsible for 28% of all cancer deaths in the United States, and 6.5% of all deaths. An estimated 1.3 million persons succumbed to lung cancer in 2000, comprising approximately 1 million men and more than 300,000 women. Moreover, lung cancer is the most common malignant cause of death in women. Indeed, 73% more women will succumb to lung than to breast cancer in the United States in 2003 (68,800 vs. 39,800). This is true despite the fact that breast cancer was diagnosed in more than two and a half times more women than lung cancer in 2003 (211,300 vs. 80,100).

During the past several decades, rising lung cancer mortality worldwide has made it apparent that we are in the midst of a global lung cancer epidemic. In the United States, an examination of epidemiologic trends demonstrates that sharp rises in lung cancer death rates have been sufficient to account for the increase in overall mortality from cancer in this country (4). It was only during the past decade that lung cancer became the most common cause of cancer death throughout the world.

On the other hand, some encouraging trends have been noted in the United States with regard to age-adjusted incidence and mortality rates, particularly among men. Between 1992 and 1998, lung cancer mortality declined 1.9% per year for men while rates for women increased, but at a much slower pace than was true earlier (5).

Nonetheless, the aging and increasing size of the population have contributed to the grim reality that the absolute number of new cases of lung cancer and the absolute number of lung cancer deaths have steadily increased during at least the past half century. To date, public health measures and therapeutic advances have failed to reverse the inexorable trend of increased lung cancer incidence and mortality throughout the world.

In the United States, effective tobacco control programs have led to some encouraging reductions. However, as Mackay has pointed out (6), as markets for cigarettes have shrunk in developed countries, tobacco companies have greatly expanded sales in the developing world. As antitobacco legislation has reduced cigarette smoking by approximately 20% in the United States during the past decade, the U.S. tobacco industry has increased exports by 260%.

Mackay has estimated that "by 2025, only 15% of the world's smokers will live in developed countries, and it is developing countries that will bear the brunt of the tobacco epidemic in the next century. By 2030, the World Health Organization predicts 10 million people will die annually from tobacco-related diseases, and 70% of these individuals will be from the developing world" (6).

Accordingly, unless death rates decline significantly during the next few years, more people will die of lung cancer during the first 5 years of the 21st century than died in the Holocaust (7). These deaths will be causally related to the most deadly consumer product in the history of humankind, the cigarette.

G. M. Strauss: Department of Medicine, Brown Medical School; Division of Hematology-Oncology, Rhode Island Hospital, Providence, Rhode Island.

R. Rathore: Department of Medicine, Roger Williams Medical Center, Providence, Rhode Island.

TABLE 39.1. AMERICAN CANCER SOCIETY CANCER STATISTICS: 2003

Type	Incidence	Mortality
Lung	171,900	157,200
Colorectal	147,500	57,100
Breast	212,600	40,200
Pancreatic	30,700	30,000
Prostate	220,900	28,900
Cancers of colorectum, breast, pancreas, and prostate combined	611,700	156,200

CIGARETTE SMOKING

Tobacco products were introduced in Europe shortly after the discovery of the New World. In 1604, in "A Counterblast to Tobacco," King James I of England stated that the use of tobacco products represented "a custom loathsome to the eye, hateful to the nose, harmful to the brain, dangerous to the lungs." Nevertheless, lung cancer remained a virtual medical curiosity until the beginning of the 20th century. The development of the ability to mass produce cigarettes and the efficiency with which the American Red Cross and other relief agencies distributed free cigarettes to those serving in World War I greatly contributed to a marked increase in cigarette smoking in men during the early 20th century.

Early Reports of an Association

In 1912, Adler (8) first raised the possibility that lung cancer risk might be associated with cigarette smoking. However, because only 374 cases of lung cancer had been reported in the world literature to date, Adler concluded that "primary malignant neoplasms of the lungs are among the rarest forms of the disease."

In 1928, Lombard and Doering (9) identified a "highly significant" increased rate of tobacco use while comparing 217 cancer patients with 217 controls in Massachusetts. This led them to conclude that "heavy smoking has some relation to cancer in general." However, 73% of "heavy" tobacco users at the time smoked pipes, not cigarettes.

In 1938, Pearl (10) pointed out an association between cigarette smoking and an increased risk for premature death. Through an analysis of mortality patterns among 6,813 men, he found that "the smoking of tobacco was statistically associated with an impairment of life duration, and the amount or degree of this impairment increased as the habitual amount of smoking increased." However, specific causes of smoking-related mortality were not addressed, and no distinction was made between cigarettes and other forms of tobacco exposure.

The first "statistical survey" addressing the relationship between smoking and lung cancer was reported in 1939. Muller (11,12) compared 86 men with lung cancer with

TABLE 39.2. MULLER'S FIRST "STATISTICAL SURVEY" ANALYZING THE RELATIONSHIP BETWEEN SMOKING AND LUNG CANCER

Category	Cases		Controls	
	No.	Percentage	No.	Percentage
Extreme smokers	25	29%	4	5%
Very heavy smokers	18	21%	5	6%
Heavy smokers	13	15%	22	26%
Moderate smokers	27	31%	41	48%
Nonsmokers	3	3%	14	16%
Total	86	100%	86	100%
Proportion of smokers		96.5%		83.7%
P value			<.0001	

Source: From Muller FH. *Z Krebsforschung* 1939;49:57–84; Summary. *JAMA* 1939;1372, with permission.

"the same number of healthy men of the same ages," and the results supported a highly statistically significant relationship between lung cancer and cigarette smoking (Table 39.2). Indeed, if all smoking categories are collapsed together to compare smokers with lifelong nonsmokers, Muller's data demonstrate that lung cancer is five times more likely to develop in smokers than in lifelong nonsmokers (odds ratio [OR], 5.4; 95% confidence interval [CI], 1.4–30.1; $P = .009$).

By the 1940s, it was becoming clear that lung cancer mortality had risen dramatically, particularly among men, during the preceding decades. For example, in 1936, Kenneway and Kenneway (13) reported that lung cancer mortality in England and Wales had increased 5.8-fold in men (from 361 to 2,095) and 3.6-fold in women (from 186 to 680) between 1921 and 1934. This rapid rise contrasted dramatically with the mortality observed between 1911 to 1919, which was stable.

In 1941, Ochsner and DeBakey (14) noted a similarity in the pattern of increasing cigarette sales and increasing incidence of lung cancer in the United States. They expressed a "definite conviction" that cigarette smoking was causally related to lung cancer.

In a follow-up report in 1947, Kenneway and Kenneway (15) pointed out that lung cancer mortality between 1921 and 1945 had increased 16-fold in men and eightfold in women in England and Wales. As in their previous report, their main focus was on risks associated with occupational exposure. Interestingly, the high incidence previously noted in tobacco manufacturers and tobacconists was no longer striking, because "the increasing use of cigarettes has caused the tobacconist to become more and more a vendor of closed packets which can hardly have any occupational effect." Although they made no effort to establish a direct causal relationship, they did point out that "among various possible factors is tobacco smoke; the consumption of tobacco has risen, and so has the percentage of it smoked in the form of cigarettes."

Throughout the 1940s, numerous other reports noted that dramatic increases in lung cancer mortality were appearing, both in Europe and in the United States (16–19). Although such increases were observed in women, lung cancer mortality rates were much higher in men.

However, 1950 was clearly the watershed year, when an unequivocal association between cigarette smoking and lung cancer was established. During that year, two seminal case control studies, one from the United States and the other from the United Kingdom, were published within 4 months of each other.

Case Control Studies: 1950

In May of 1950, Wynder and Graham (20) compared smoking in 684 patients who had lung cancer with smoking in a population comprising 1,332 hospital controls from Saint Louis, Missouri. Modern epidemiologic methods were used to analyze the data (Tables 39.3 and 39.4). With regard to squamous cell, small cell, and undifferentiated carcinomas in men, smokers were at about 13 times greater risk than lifelong nonsmokers (Table 39.3). Indeed, 92% of lung cancers were smoking related. Women smokers had an approximately sixfold greater risk than women nonsmokers, and 83% of the tumors were attributable to smoking. All these differences were highly significant. On the other hand, no evidence was found of an association between smoking and

TABLE 39.3. CASE CONTROL STUDY IN THE UNITED STATES: SQUAMOUS CELL, SMALL CELL, AND UNDIFFERENTIATED CARCINOMAS

	Men		
	Cases	Controls	Total
Smokers	597	666	1,263
Nonsmokers	8	114	122
Total	605	780	1,385
Proportion of smokers	98.7%	85.4%	91.2%
Odds ratio (95% confidence interval)			12.8 (6.2–26.4)
P value			<.0001
Attributable fraction			92%

	Women		
	Cases	Controls	Total
Smokers	15	113	128
Nonsmokers	10	439	449
Total	25	552	577
Proportion of smokers	60.0%	20.5%	22.2%
Odds ratio (95% confidence interval)			5.8 (2.6–13.1)
P value			<.0001
Attributable fraction			83%

Source: From Wynder EL, Graham EA. Tobacco smoking as a possible etiologic factor in bronchogenic carcinoma: a study of 684 proved cases. *JAMA* 1950; 143:329–336, with permission.

TABLE 39.4. CASE CONTROL STUDY IN THE UNITED STATES: ADENOCARCINOMA

	Men		
	Cases	Controls	Total
Smokers	35	666	701
Nonsmokers	4	114	118
Total	39	780	819
Proportion of smokers	89.7%	85.4%	85.6%
Odds ratio (95% confidence interval)			1.5 (0.5–4.1)
P value			.45
Attributable fraction			33%

	Women		
	Cases	Controls	Total
Smokers	2	113	115
Nonsmokers	13	439	452
Total	15	552	567
Proportion of smokers	13.3%	20.5%	20.3%
Odds ratio (95% confidence interval)			0.6 (0–2.4)
P value			0.50
Preventable fraction			40%

Source: From Wynder EL, Graham EA. Tobacco smoking as a possible etiologic factor in bronchogenic carcinoma: a study of 684 proved cases. *JAMA* 1950; 143:329–336, with permission.

adenocarcinoma of the lung in either men or women (Table 39.4). Indeed, a trend toward a reduced risk for adenocarcinoma of the lung was observed in women smokers.

In 1950, Doll and Bradford Hill (21) published a preliminary report comparing 649 men and 60 women who had lung cancer with an age- and gender-matched control group of 709 patients. Although this report did not subdivide lung cancers on the basis of histology, it did demonstrate a highly significant 14-fold increased risk for lung cancer in male smokers in comparison with lifelong nonsmokers. Among women, the lung cancer risk was 2.5-fold higher for smokers, and this difference was also statistically significant. Overall, 94% of smokers with lung cancer smoked cigarettes, and 6% were pipe smokers. Overall, 26% of men and 15% of women with lung cancer were "heavy" or "chain" smokers, in comparison with 13.5% of the male controls and none of the female controls. These findings led to the conclusion that "smoking is an important factor in the cause of carcinoma of the lung."

In 1952, Doll and Bradford Hill (55) reported the results of an expanded study that divided cancers into histologic subtypes. The results for squamous cell carcinoma, small cell carcinoma, and undifferentiated carcinoma demonstrated a highly significant 14-fold increase in risk for smokers in comparison with nonsmokers (Table 39.5). A statistically significant but much weaker relationship between smoking and these histologic subtypes was noted among women. On the other hand, no significant association between smoking and

TABLE 39.5. CASE CONTROL STUDY IN THE UNITED KINGDOM: SQUAMOUS CELL, SMALL CELL, AND UNDIFFERENTIATED CARCINOMAS

	Men		
	Cases	**Controls**	**Total**
Smokers	880	1,296	2,176
Nonsmokers	3	61	64
Total	883	1,357	2,240
Proportion of smokers	99.7%	95.5%	97.1%
Odds ratio (95% confidence interval)			13.8 (4.6–41.7)
P value			<.0001
Attributable fraction			93%

	Women		
	Cases	**Controls**	**Total**
Smokers	45	49	128
Nonsmokers	24	59	449
Total	69	108	577
Proportion of smokers	65.2%	45.3%	53.1%
Odds ratio (95% confidence interval)			2.3 (1.2–4.2)
P value			.0099
Attributable fraction			56%

Source: From Doll R, Bradford Hill A. A study on the aetiology of carcinoma of the lung. *Br Med J* 1952;2:271–1286, with permission.

TABLE 39.6. CASE CONTROL STUDY IN THE UNITED KINGDOM: ADENOCARCINOMA

	Men		
	Cases	**Controls**	**Total**
Smokers	31	1,296	1,327
Nonsmokers	2	61	63
Total	33	1,357	1,390
Proportion of smokers	93.9%	95.5%	95.4%
Odds ratio (95% confidence interval)			0.7 (0.2–3.1)
P value			.67
Preventable fraction			27%

	Women		
	Cases	**Controls**	**Total**
Smokers	5	49	54
Nonsmokers	5	59	64
Total	10	108	118
Proportion of smokers	50%	45%	46%
Odds ratio (95% confidence interval)			1.2 (0.3–4.1)
P value			.78
Attributable fraction			17%

Source: From Doll R, Bradford Hill A. A study on the aetiology of carcinoma of the lung. *Br Med J* 1952;2:1271–1286, with permission.

adenocarcinoma of the lung was found for either men or women (Table 39.6).

Case Control and Cohort Studies: 1950–1955

A remarkable body of information in this area rapidly accumulated during the ensuing years. At least 10 additional retrospective (case control) studies were reported between 1950 and 1954 (22–31). In general, these studies demonstrated a high level of consistency with the results of the first two studies discussed in the preceding section (Tables 39.3 and 39.6).

Moreover, two prospective cohort studies were initiated, and preliminary results for both were published in 1954. One cohort study was based on a questionnaire that was mailed in 1951 to 59,600 physicians in the United Kingdom, of whom 41,024 responded and 40,564 provided useful information. When initial results were reported in 1954 with 29 months of follow-up, a total of 789 deaths had occurred, including 36 lung cancer deaths (32). Because no lung cancer deaths had been reported among nonsmokers, a relative risk could not be calculated. At the time of the second report, in 1956, the relative risk for lung cancer mortality in a comparison of smokers with nonsmokers was 12.8, ranging from 6.7 for moderate smokers to 12.3 for heavy smokers and 23.7 for chain smokers (33).

The second cohort study was an ACS-sponsored study designed to evaluate the relationship between smoking and death rates. Beginning in early 1952, smoking histories were obtained for more than 187,000 men, ages 50 to 70 years;

these men were then followed prospectively. An initial report appeared in 1954, when the average follow-up was 20 months, and a final report in 1958, at which time the average follow-up was 44 months (34,35). In both reports, deaths rates among cigarette smokers were far higher than the rates among lifelong nonsmokers. The overall relative risk for lung cancer mortality was 10.7 times greater in cigarette smokers than in nonsmokers. Indeed, men who smoked more than two packs of cigarettes per day were more likely to die of lung cancer than were lifelong nonsmokers to die of any cancer from all sites (including the lung) combined.

Accordingly, by 1955, a very impressive body of information, based on both retrospective and prospective studies, had become available. These studies clearly demonstrated that the worldwide increase in lung cancer mortality was strongly associated with cigarette smoking. Both retrospective and prospective studies demonstrated a higher rate of lung cancer among cigarette smokers than among nonsmokers, and this increase was proportional to the amount smoked and the duration of smoking (36,37).

Association and Causation

Evidence from these trials clearly demonstrated an extremely powerful statistical association between cigarette smoking and lung cancer. However, as the first Surgeon General's report, in 1964, indicated, "statistical methods cannot establish proof of a causal relationship in an association. The causal significance of an association is a matter of judgment which goes beyond any statement of statistical probability" (38). Thus, despite mounting evidence, questions continued to be raised about whether a true causal relationship existed between cigarette smoking and lung cancer (39–42).

Although even the tobacco industry did not dispute the existence of a statistical association, the industry did its best to dismiss the possibility that the relationship was one of direct cause and effect. For example, in January 1954, the creation of a tobacco industry research committee was announced in response to growing public concern that cigarette smoking might cause lung cancer. To reassure a highly concerned public, the tobacco industry published "A Frank Statement to Cigarette Smokers" in more than 200 newspapers throughout the United States. This statement included the following:

- Recent reports on experiments with mice have given wide publicity to a theory that cigarette smoking is in some way linked with lung cancer in human beings.... We feel it is in the public interest to call attention to the fact that eminent doctors and research scientists have publicly questioned the claimed significance of these experiments. Distinguished authorities point out:
  - that medical research of recent years indicates many possible causes of lung cancer
  - that there is no agreement among the authorities what the cause is
  - that there is no proof that cigarette smoking is one of the causes
- that statistics purporting to link cigarette smoking with the disease could apply with equal force to any one of many other aspects of modern life. Indeed, the validity of the statistics themselves is questioned by numerous scientists.
- We accept an interest in people's health as a basic responsibility, paramount to every other consideration in our business.
- We believe the products we make are not injurious to health.

Of course, it has become very clear during the past decade that the tobacco industry never attempted to inform the public honestly. An enormous body of evidence now exists, primarily from internal tobacco industry documents, that the industry intentionally deceived the public during the 1950s and throughout subsequent decades (43–47).

For example, an internal R. J. Reynolds Tobacco Company report from February 1953 by Claude Teague, entitled "Survey of Cancer Research with Emphasis upon Possible Carcinogens from Tobacco," is probably the most complete and accurate compilation of data that had been collected at the time (48). Unfortunately, the document was never published, nor any action taken.

Nonetheless, it is true that statistical association alone cannot prove causation. However, an enormous body of independent evidence that the relationship between cigarette smoking and lung cancer is indeed one of direct cause and effect has long been available. Such evidence led to the conclusion of a direct causal relationship at the time of the first Surgeon General's Report, in 1964.

Five well-known criteria for the attribution of causality put forth by Bradford Hill were explicitly considered in the 1964 Surgeon General's report (38,49). These five criteria relate to the strength, consistency, specificity, temporality, and coherence of an association. The criteria clearly go well beyond any statistical analysis of the data.

The application of these five criteria to the evidence that existed in 1964 led the Surgeon General to conclude that "cigarette smoking is causally related to lung cancer in men. The magnitude of the effect of cigarette smoking far outweighs all other factors." The 1964 report also added that "the data for women, though less extensive, point in the same direction" (38).

Until relatively recently, the evidence linking cigarette smoking to lung cancer was based primarily on epidemiologic evidence. However, a direct link between tobacco and lung cancer has now been established (50). By means of genetic amplification techniques, it has been demonstrated that a specific metabolite of benzo(a)pyrene, a chemical constituent of tobacco smoke long suspected of being directly involved in carcinogenesis, damages three specific loci on the p53 tumor suppressor gene. These loci are known to be abnormal in about 60% of primary lung cancers.

Although a complete review of this evidence is far beyond the scope of this chapter, it is also clear that early estimates of the harmful effects of cigarette smoking were too conservative. For example, in 1994, Doll and colleagues (51) reported on 40 years of observations from the British doctors cohort and concluded the following: "Results from the first 20 years of this study, and of other studies at that time, substantially underestimated the hazards of long-term use of tobacco. It now seems that about half of all regular cigarette smokers will eventually be killed by their habit."

Recent estimates regarding the relationship between cigarette smoking and lung cancer are that the relative risk for lung cancer mortality is 23.9 for men and 14.0 for women when cigarette smokers are compared with lifelong nonsmokers (52). The magnitude of the absolute lung cancer risk among smokers is somewhat less clear. The lifetime risk for lung cancer among nonsmokers is considerably less than 1%. Peto and colleagues (53) estimate that the risk among continuing smokers up to the age of 75 years is approximately 16% in men and 10% in women.

There is no question that the evidence has long been overwhelming that cigarette smoking causes lung cancer. Indeed, the definitive determination of a causal relationship between cigarette smoking and lung cancer is widely recognized as perhaps the greatest triumph of modern epidemiology (54).

Cigarette Smoking and the Changing Histopathology of Lung Cancer

The relationship between cigarette smoking and squamous cell carcinoma and small cell carcinoma of the lung was established by epidemiologic studies published in the 1950s (20,32,34,55). On the other hand, the relationship between cigarette smoking and both large cell carcinoma and adenocarcinoma of the lung is less clear. A metaanalysis of the

TABLE 39.7. METAANALYSIS: RELATIONSHIP OF CIGARETTE SMOKING AND FOUR MAJOR HISTOLOGIC SUBTYPES OF LUNG CANCER

Histology	Odds Ratio	95% Confidence Interval	Attributable Fraction
Small cell carcinoma	12.9	9.8–17.1	0.92
Squamous cell carcinoma	11.3	9.4–13.5	0.91
Large cell carcinoma	5.6	4.1–7.7	0.82
Adenocarcinoma	3.2	2.6–4.0	0.69

Source: Based on Khuder SA. Effect of smoking on major histological types of lung cancer: a meta-analysis. *Lung Cancer* 2001;31:139–148, with permission.

effect of cigarette smoking on the major histologic types of lung cancer concluded that the association is very strong for squamous cell and small cell carcinoma, but much weaker for large cell carcinoma and adenocarcinoma of the lung (56). The metaanalysis included 27 case control studies and one cohort study published between 1970 and 2000, and it demonstrated highly variable risk ratios associated with smoking and different lung cancer histopathologies (Tables 39.7 and 39.8). This metaanalysis failed to take into account the changing relationship between cigarette smoking and the different histologic subtypes, which is particularly important in the case of adenocarcinoma.

Large Cell Carcinoma

The relationship between cigarette smoking and large cell carcinoma has also been unclear because of changes in the histopathologic classification of lung cancer over time. In reports from the early 1950s, undifferentiated carcinoma was thought to be strongly related to smoking; it is highly likely that most "undifferentiated" carcinomas would be classified as large cell carcinomas today.

However, a multiinstitutional case control study published a decade ago was unable to demonstrate a significant relationship between the number of cigarettes smoked per day and the risk for large cell carcinoma of the lung (57). This may have been related to the small study size; only 156 large cell carcinomas were analyzed (97 men and 59 women).

The authors' skepticism about their own results led them to reexamine this question in the context of a larger study population (58). The expanded series included 382 patients with large cell carcinoma (228 men and 154 women); the smoking patterns of those with large cell carcinoma were compared with the smoking patterns of 4,260 controls (2,545 men and 1,715 women). Only 5% of the patients with large cell carcinomas were lifelong nonsmokers, compared with 37% of the controls (*P* <.0001). The risk for the development of large cell carcinoma increased with

TABLE 39.8. CASE CONTROL STUDY: "CIGARETTE SMOKING AND HISTOLOGIC TYPE OF LUNG CANCER IN MEN, PROVINCE OF TRIESTE (NORTHEASTERN, ITALY)

	Ever Versus Never		Current Versus Never		Former versus Never	
	Ever-Smoker	Never-Smoker	Current Smoker	Never-Smoker	Former Smoker	Never-Smoker
Controls	567	188	362	188	205	188
Squamous cell carcinoma						
Cases	261	6	203	6	58	6
Odds ratio (95% CI)	14.4 (6.5–32.2)		17.6 (7.8–39.4)		8.9 (3.8–20.5)	
Attributable fraction	93%		94%		89%	
Small cell carcinoma						
Cases	212	6	170	6	42	6
Odds ratio (95% CI)	11.7 (5.2–26.2)		14.7 (6.5–33.1)		6.4 (2.7–15.1)	
Attributable fraction	91%		93%		84%	
Adenocarcinoma						
Cases	151	7	109	7	42	7
Odds ratio (95% CI)	7.2 (3.3–15.3)		8.1 (3.8–17.4)		5.5 (2.5–12.3)	
Attributable fraction	86%		88%		82%	
Large cell carcinoma						
Cases	89	1	68	1	21	1
Odds ratio (95% CI)	29.5 (4.1–213.3)		35.5 (4.9–256.3)		19.3 (2.6–144.6)	
Attributable fraction	97%		97%		95%	

Source: From Barbone F, Bovenzi M, Cavallieri F, et al. Cigarette smoking and histologic type of lung cancer in men. *Chest* 1997;112:1474–1479, with permission.

the number of cigarettes smoked in both current and former smokers. Indeed, when only current smokers of more than two packs per day were compared with lifelong nonsmokers, the odds ratio for the development of large cell carcinoma was 37.0 (95% CI, 16.4–83.2) for men and 72.9 (95% CI, 35.4–150.2) for women. The risk for the development of large cell carcinoma was directly related to the number of years of smoking. Among former smokers, the risk decreased with the number of years of abstinence. The authors concluded that "cigarette smoking is the predominant cause of large cell lung cancer" (58). Similarly, a case control study from Italy relating cigarette smoking and lung cancer risk in men demonstrated that the relationship between smoking and large cell carcinoma was stronger than the relationship between smoking and any of the other major histologic types (59). Thus, a strongly positive correlation exists between cigarette smoking and large cell carcinoma of the lung.

Adenocarcinoma

As already stated, the first two case control studies from the early 1950s demonstrated no significant relationship between smoking and adenocarcinoma of the lung (20,55) (Tables 39.4 and 39.6). Moreover, at the time, adenocarcinoma of the lung was uncommon, comprising only about 5% of all primary lung cancers. These and subsequent studies published in the late 1950s and early 1960s concluded that the relationship between cigarette smoking and adenocarcinoma of the lung was "slight, if any" (60,61).

However, during recent decades, adenocarcinoma has become the most common histologic subtype in both men and women (62–66), and a causal relationship between cigarette smoking and adenocarcinoma has been definitively established (67).

The ACS-sponsored Cancer Prevention Study I (CPS-I) recruited more than 1 million participants beginning in 1959, and the Cancer Prevention Study II (CPS-II) recruited more than 1 million participants beginning in 1982. The risk for adenocarcinoma of the lung among persons who smoked cigarettes markedly increased between CPS-I and CPS-II. In CPS-I, in a comparison of cigarette smokers and lifelong nonsmokers, the incidence rate ratio for adenocarcinoma mortality in men was 4.6, and the difference was significant. Among women, the rate ratio was 1.5, although the association was not statistically significant (95% CI, 0.3–7.7) (Table 39.9).

In CPS-II, the risk for mortality from adenocarcinoma of the lung among cigarette smokers was much stronger for both men and women and was highly significant for both sexes. The rate ratio was 19.0 (95% CI, 8.3–47.7) for men and 8.1 (95% CI, 4.5–14.6) for women. These dramatic findings led the authors to conclude that "the ACS studies clearly implicate smoking as the major cause of adenocarcinoma, as well as of other lung cancers" (67). In fact, the mortality from adenocarcinoma of the lung was no different for lifelong nonsmokers when CPS-I was compared with CPS-II, but it increased dramatically for cigarette smokers when the two studies were compared.

The ACS cohort studies demonstrated that the strength of the statistical relationship between smoking and adenocarcinoma of the lung had dramatically increased. Moreover, data from the Connecticut Tumor Registry demonstrated that between 1959 and 1981, the age-adjusted incidence of adenocarcinoma in Connecticut increased approximately 17-fold in women (from 0.9 to 15.2 cases per 100,000 person-years) and 10-fold in men (from 2.4 to 23.2 cases per 100,000 person-years). Although data on individual smoking behavior were not available, these increases followed a clear birth cohort pattern and appeared to reflect gender and generational changes in smoking prevalence, rather than any diagnostic advances: "The increase in adenocarcinoma in the United States since 1950 corresponds temporally with changes in smoking behavior and in

TABLE 39.9. ADENOCARCINOMA OF THE LUNG: AGE-ADJUSTED DEATH RATES AS A FUNCTION OF CIGARETTE SMOKING STATUS IN AMERICAN CANCER SOCIETY COHORT STUDIES

	Men		Women	
	Ever-Smokers	Never-Smokers	Ever-Smokers	Never-Smokers
Cancer Prevention Study I (began 1959)				
Person-time	274,635	180,081	287,220	739,145
Cases	23	5	4	13
Rate ratio (95% CI)[a]	4.6 (1.7–12.6)		1.5 (0.3–7.7)	
Attributable fraction	78%		33%	
Cancer Prevention Study II (began 1982)				
Person-time	201,235	252,731	252,504	708,413
Cases	79	6	42	16
Rate ratio (95% CI)[a]	19.0 (8.3–47.7)		8.1 (4.5–14.6)	
Attributable fraction	95%		88%	

[a] As reported by the authors.
Source: Thun MJ, Lally CA, Glannery JT, et al. Cigarette smoking and changes in the histopathology of lung cancer. *J Natl Cancer Inst* 1997;89:1580–1586, with permission.

cigarette design rather than with diagnostic advances. Adenocarcinoma is now strongly related to cigarette smoking" (67).

Despite the strong relationship between cigarette smoking and adenocarcinoma of the lung, it remains true that of all the major histologic subtypes, adenocarcinoma is most common in nonsmokers (68). Accordingly, the relative risk regarding smoking and adenocarcinoma is weaker than for the other histologies.

Nonetheless, changing distribution of lung cancer histopathology is responsible for the fact that the absolute number of smoking-related deaths is greater for adenocarcinoma than for any other form of cancer in the United States. Based upon the SEER (Surveillance, Epidemiology, and End Results) data on 264,125 lung cancers diagnosed from 1975 to 1999, adenocarcinoma surpassed squamous cell cancer in the 1980s to become the most common form of lung cancer. While relative risk is lower for adenocarcinoma than for squamous cell, large cell, and small cell carcinomas, adenocarcinoma is far more prevalent that the other histologies. Higher prevalence of adenocarcinoma and the dramatic rise in the proportion of adenocarcinomas related to smoking is responsible for the fact that smoking-related adenocarcinoma of the lung is now the most common cause of cancer death in the United States. Based upon the ACS estimate of 157,200 U.S. lung cancer deaths in 2003, mortality from smoking-related adenocarcinoma can be estimated to be approximately 63,000 per year. This compares to 57,100 U.S. deaths that the ACS estimates will be attributed to colorectal cancer in 2003. Moreover, colorectal cancer is second only to lung cancer with regard to total cancer mortality in the United States (Table 39.1). Accordingly, smoking-related adenocarcinoma is now the most common cause of cancer death in the US (69).

The dramatic rise in lung adenocarcinoma and the increased association between cigarette smoking and adenocarcinoma appears to be directly related to the tobacco industry's decision to manufacture, market, and sell what has commonly become known as the "safe cigarette." When the initial studies demonstrating an association between cigarette smoking and lung cancer appeared in the 1950s, unfiltered cigarettes and high tar yields were common. These products were too toxic to allow smokers to inhale deeply into the lungs (70). However, public concern about health hazards led the industry to change cigarette design and increase production of filtered and low-tar cigarettes. Indeed, 97% of cigarettes currently sold in the United States have filters, and the tar yield of cigarettes has declined 60% since the 1950s.

These modifications have not resulted in a safer cigarette. Smokers tend to inhale low-yield filtered cigarettes more deeply than high-yield cigarettes to satisfy their craving for nicotine (66). Accordingly, the periphery of the lung tends to be more heavily exposed to tobacco-related carcinogens, which is the location of most adenocarcinomas. "Widespread use of 'safer and gentler' cigarettes" has ironically led to the dramatic rise in smoking-related adenocarcinoma of the lung during the past few decades (71).

Bronchoalveolar Carcinoma

Bronchoalveolar carcinoma (BAC) is a subtype of adenocarcinoma, and its relationship to cigarette smoking has long been debated (72). One problem with assessing this relationship is that BAC is often not separated from other adenocarcinomas in epidemiologic studies. For example, in the article of Thun and colleagues (67) establishing a relationship between cigarette smoking and adenocarcinoma, data were unavailable regarding the proportion of adenocarcinomas that were BACs. Therefore, few data are available that address this problem directly. Nonetheless, three case control studies do support a powerful association between cigarette smoking and BAC (73,74,74a).

The first case control study was extremely limited by its small sample size (Table 39.10). In this study, 21 patients with BAC diagnosed between 1979 and 1982 were compared with 101 age- and gender-matched controls (74). The results indicated a 2.7-fold increase in the risk for BAC among smokers. However, because the study was underpowered, this difference was not statistically significant. When only heavy smokers were compared with lifelong nonsmokers, a

TABLE 39.10. CASE CONTROL STUDY: CIGARETTE SMOKING AND BRONCHIOLOALVEOLAR CELL CARCINOMA

	Ever-Smokers Versus Lifelong Nonsmokers		
	Cases	Controls	Total
Ever-smokers	18	70	88
Never-smokers	3	31	34
Total	21	101	122
Proportion of ever-smokers	85.7%	69.3%	72.1%
Odds ratio (95% confidence interval)			2.7 (0.8–9.1)
P value			.13
Attributable fraction			62%

	Heavy Smokers Versus Lifelong Nonsmokers		
	Cases	Controls	Total
Heavy smokers[a]	7	10	17
Never-smokers	3	31	34
Total	10	41	51
Proportion of current smokers	70.0%	24.4%	33.3%
Odds ratio (95% confidence interval)			7.2 (1.7–30.8)
P value			.0061
Attributable fraction			86%

[a]One and a half packs per day or more.
Source: From Falk RT, Pickle LW, Fontham ETH, et al. Epidemiology of bronchioloalveolar cell carcinoma. *Cancer Epidemiol Biomarkers Prev* 1992;1:339–344, with permission.

TABLE 39.11. CASE CONTROL STUDY: CIGARETTE SMOKING AND BRONCHIOLOALVEOLAR CELL CARCINOMA

	Ever-Smokers Versus Lifelong Nonsmokers		
	Cases	Controls	Total
Ever-smokers	72	364	436
Never-smokers	15	219	234
Total	87	583	670
Proportion of ever-smokers	82.8%	62.4%	65.1%
Odds ratio (95% confidence interval)			2.9 (1.6–5.1)
P value			.0002
Attributable fraction			65%

	Current Smokers Versus Lifelong Nonsmokers		
	Cases	Controls	Total
Current smokers	36	158	194
Never-smokers	15	219	234
Total	51	377	428
Proportion of current smokers	70.5%	36.9%	45.3%
Odds ratio (95% confidence interval)			3.3 (1.8–6.2)
P value			.0001
Attributable fraction			70%

Source: From Morabia A, Wynder EL. Relation of bronchioloalveolar carcinoma to smoking. *Br Med J* 1992; 304:541–543, with permission.

significant sevenfold increase in BAC was found. A progressive increase was also found in the odds for the development of BAC as the duration of smoking increased (74).

The second case control study compared 87 patients who had BAC with 583 controls (73a). Only 17% of patients with BAC had never smoked, in comparison with 37% of controls. A significant increase in BAC was noted among smokers in comparison with nonsmokers (Table 39.11). The risk increased as the number of cigarettes smoked per day increased. Similarly, a significant reduction in risk followed smoking cessation. Very recently, a third and larger case control study from Rhode Island compared smoking status in 198 patients with BAC to an equal number of controls (74a). It demonstrated an odds ratio of 3.3 for the association of BAC and cigarette smoking (95% CI, 2.0–5.5). An increased risk of BAC was present in both current and former smokers. The study supports the conclusion that while smoking is not the only cause of BAC, approximately 70% of BAC is attributable to cigarette smoking.

Prevalence of Smoking in Adults

Despite increasing lung cancer mortality, the prevalence of smoking among the adult population has been steadily decreasing for decades. A National Cancer Institute (NCI) survey conducted in 1955 demonstrated that nearly 60% of men and 28% of women were current cigarette smokers (75). At

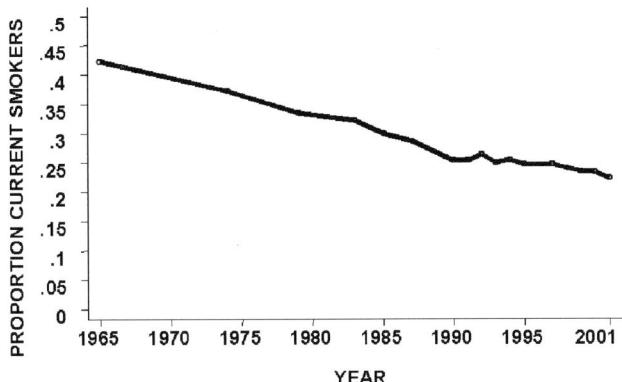

FIGURE 39.1. Prevalence of smoking among adults, United States, 1965–2001.

the time of "Smoking and Health," the first Surgeon General's report, in 1964, 70 million Americans used tobacco products.

In 1965, shortly after the first Surgeon General's report, 42.3% of the U.S. adult population smoked cigarettes (76). This percentage significantly declined during the ensuing decades. The prevalence of smoking steadily decreased in the 1970s and 1980s, although the rate of decline slowed during the 1990s. In 2000, 23.3% of persons older than 18 years were current cigarette smokers (77). Accordingly, the prevalence of smoking among adults had decreased 45% since 1965 (Fig. 39.1). In 1999 in the United States, 46.5 million adults were current smokers (25.7 million men and 22.3 million women), and 45.7 million (25.8 million men and 19.9 million women) were former smokers. Cessation prevented 1.6 million smoking-related deaths between 1964 and 1992, predominantly from cardiovascular disease.

Because 90% of lung cancers are directly attributable to cigarette smoking, the disease is almost completely preventable through tobacco avoidance. However, because many years of smoking abstinence are needed to reduce risk markedly among long-term smokers, lung cancer incidence and mortality rose to epidemic proportions after the first Surgeon General's report (Fig. 39.2). Between 1965 and 2002, the annual lung cancer incidence increased 226% (from 52,000 to 169,400), and mortality rose 230% (from 47,000 to 154,900).

A decrease in the prevalence of smoking, coupled with increases in lung cancer incidence and mortality, suggests that lung cancer is becoming a disease of former smokers. A survey from the Brigham and Women's Hospital demonstrated that of 1,044 patients with newly diagnosed lung cancer seen between 1988 and 1997, 8% were lifelong nonsmokers, 38% were current smokers, and 54% were former smokers (78). Among the former smokers, the median duration of abstinence preceding the diagnosis was 7 years.

These data do not address the magnitude of risk reduction associated with smoking cessation; rather, they describe the smoking behavior of those in whom the disease is diagnosed. The high proportion of former smokers simply reflects the

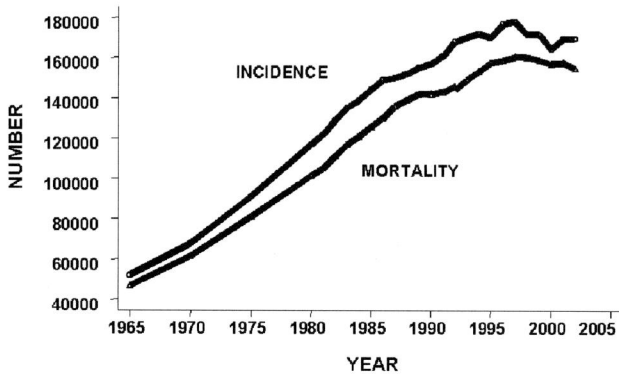

FIGURE 39.2. Annual lung cancer incidence and mortality, United States, 1965–2002.

fact that former smokers greatly outnumber current smokers in age cohorts at greatest risk for lung cancer. However, these data underscore the limitations of smoking cessation as a lung cancer prevention strategy among long-term smokers. Other strategies must receive priority.

Smoking Cessation and Lung Cancer Risk

It is extremely important to understand how smoking cessation influences lung cancer risk among long-term smokers. Five large cohort studies and 10 case control studies have attempted to quantify the magnitude of risk reduction associated with smoking cessation. Many of these data have been summarized in a 1990 Surgeon General's report (79).

Smoking cessation clearly decreases lung cancer risk among former smokers in comparison with those who continue to smoke (79,80). Estimates of the extent of risk reduction over time vary from 20% to 90%, depending on the duration of abstinence. Lung cancer risk in former smokers progressively declines as the duration of abstinence increases. The exception is an apparent increase in lung cancer risk

within the first few years after abstinence, possibly reflecting symptoms of an illness that led to smoking cessation before the diagnosis was made. The reduction in lung cancer risk increases with the duration of abstinence, with risk reduction becoming evident within 5 years after cigarettes have been discontinued. Nonetheless, former smokers continue to have a 10% to 80% greater risk than never-smokers (81).

The five cohort studies include two ACS cancer prevention studies (ACS CP-I and ACS CP-II) (82,83), in addition to studies of British physicians (84), U.S. veterans (85), and Japanese men. In the ACS CP-II study and the studies of British physicians and U.S veterans, former smokers who had been abstinent for more than 15 years sustained an 80% to 90% reduction in risk in comparison with current smokers. In the ACS CP-I study and the Japanese study, the magnitude of risk reduction was slightly lower (79). Data from the ACS CP-II study, a cohort study that included more than 1.2 million subjects, are shown in Table 39.12 (79).

Similarly, case control studies support the conclusion that smoking cessation decreases lung cancer risk. A reduction in lung cancer risk after smoking cessation is observed in both men and women, and for users of filtered or unfiltered cigarettes. The risk for all histologic subtypes of lung cancer is decreased. Nonetheless, lung cancer risk in former smokers remains higher than that in never-smokers, even after prolonged periods of complete abstinence (79). This is in marked contrast to other smoking-related diseases, such as coronary artery disease, in which the beneficial effects of smoking cessation are evident soon after smoking is discontinued.

Although a large number of men quit smoking in the mid-1960s, shortly after the first Surgeon General's report, it took 20 years until the incidence of lung cancer started to decrease in men. As the prevalence of smoking among adults decreases, lung cancer is increasingly becoming a disease of former smokers (86–89).

TABLE 39.12. AMERICAN CANCER SOCIETY CANCER PREVENTION STUDY II

Smoking Status/ Abstinence Duration (y)	Mortality Ratio			
	Men		Women	
	1–20 Cigarettes Per Day	>21 Cigarettes Per Day	1–20 Cigarettes Per Day	>21 Cigarettes Per Day
Never	1.0	1.0	1.0	1.0
Current	18.8	26.9	7.3	16.3
Former				
≤1	26.7	50.7	7.9	34.3
1–2	22.4	33.2	9.1	19.5
3–5	16.5	20.9	2.9	14.6
6–10	8.7	15.0	1.0	9.1
11–15	6.0	12.6	1.5	5.9
≥16	3.1	5.5	1.4	2.6

Note: Lung cancer mortality ratios in men and women for never-, current, and former smokers. Mortality ratio defined as 1.0 for never-smokers.
Source: The health benefits of smoking cessation: a report of the Surgeon General. Washington, DC: U.S. Department of Health and Human Services, Public Health Service, 1990.

Prevalence of Smoking in Children, Adolescents, and Young Adults

The obvious approach to the problem of increasing lung cancer incidence and mortality despite decreasing smoking prevalence in adults is to prevent young people from becoming smokers. Enormous public health and public policy efforts have been directed at preventing smoking among children and adolescents (90,91). Indeed, the prevalence of smoking among young people did undergo a substantial reduction from the mid-1970s to the mid-1980s (92).

Unfortunately, rates of smoking among children, adolescents, and young adults subsequently increased substantially. Between 1991 and 1997, cigarette smoking among high school students increased by 32% (93). Similarly, between 1993 and 1997, smoking among college students increased by 28% (94). In 1997, daily cigarette use among high school seniors was 24.6%, which was the highest it had been since 1979, when the figure was 25.4% (92). It has been estimated that more than 5 million young people now alive will die prematurely of tobacco-related illnesses if current smoking trends are not reversed (95).

In recent years, the smoking prevalence rate among 18- to 24-year-olds, which is 27.9%, has been slightly higher than that among 25- to 44-year-olds, whose rate is 27.5% (96). This represents a significant shift because the prevalence of smoking has historically been significantly lower in this age group than in older adults. It has been suggested that the shift may be attributable to the aging of high school students whose smoking rates were high during the 1990s. However, it has also been suggested that it may indicate increases in the rate of first-time cigarette use in the young adult population. The prevalence of smoking among young adults ages 18 to 24 years increased from 25.8% in 1993 to 27.9% in 1998.

Among adults who smoke, the smoking prevalence rates are highest among young adults. In the most recent data from the Centers for Disease Control and Prevention (77), the prevalence of smoking was 27.9% among persons ages 18 to 24 years (29.5% among men and 26.3% among women). In persons ages 25 to 44 years, the prevalence of smoking was 27.3% (29.6% among men and 25.5% among women). In persons between the ages of 45 and 64 years, the prevalence of smoking was 23.3% (25.8% among men and 21.0% among women). Of persons older than 65 years, only 10.6% were current smokers (10.5% of men and 10.7% of women). The data also indicate that current smoking is related to educational achievement. The prevalence of smoking was highest (40.8%) in those who had earned a general educational development diploma, and lowest (8.5%) in those with a master's, professional, or doctoral degree. The prevalence of smoking was significantly higher in persons living below the poverty level (33.1%) than in those living at or above the poverty level (23.4%).

Efforts at preventing smoking have failed to stem the tide of cigarette smoking among young adults and have failed to stop children and adolescents from starting to smoke. It appears that the prevalence of smoking among young people is not closely linked to the prevalence rates in adults. Higher rates of smoking among young people appear to mirror the intensification of the youth-oriented marketing of cigarettes by cigarette manufacturers (97). As Ling and Glantz (98) have pointed out, "During the critical years of young adulthood, public health efforts dwindle at the same time that tobacco industry efforts intensify.... In spite of the industry's claim that it does not market to nonsmokers, the marketing plan for young adults enables the industry to recruit new smokers between the ages of 18 and 24 years and to encourage light, occasional or experimenting smokers to smoke more regularly. Young adults are also the youngest legal marketing target in an industry that depends on beginning smokers, and they vastly outnumber teen smokers."

The high prevalence of smoking among young adults underscores the need to focus smoking cessation strategies in this population. Unfortunately, smoking cessation among young adults has received little priority and little study (95). As appropriately pointed out by Ling and Glantz, "although important, primary prevention is not the only way to reduce the damage tobacco causes; while never smoking is obviously the most desirable situation, stopping smoking before age 30 eliminates virtually all of the long-term mortality effects" (98).

DETERMINANTS OF LUNG CANCER RISK

Cigarette smoking is such a major determinant of lung cancer risk that the identification of other independent or synergistic factors is complex. Nonetheless, it has been unequivocally demonstrated that certain cigarette smokers are at much greater risk for the development of lung cancer than others. Many studies have demonstrated that susceptibility to lung cancer among cigarette smokers can be substantially modified by a wide variety of environmental agents and host characteristics (99–102). Many of these factors have also been shown to be independent risk factors for the development of lung cancer.

Environmental Tobacco Smoke

Exposure to environmental tobacco smoke is also referred to as *second-hand smoking*, *passive smoking*, or *involuntary smoking*. The concentration of chemical constituents in environmental tobacco smoke is but a small fraction of that in smoke inhaled by a cigarette smoker. Epidemiologic studies estimate that nonsmokers exposed to environmental tobacco smoke have a relative risk for lung cancer of 1.2 in comparison with nonsmokers who have not been exposed (100).

Exposure to environmental tobacco smoke usually begins much earlier in life than direct smoking, and the duration of exposure to carcinogens is longer. A dose-response relationship between intensity of exposure to environmental tobacco smoke and lung cancer risk has been demonstrated.

Occupational and Environmental Carcinogens

Numerous occupational and environmental carcinogens are known to increase the risk for lung cancer in cigarette smokers. Perhaps the best known among these factors are asbestos and radon. However, additional factors include arsenic, bis(chloromethyl) ether, chromium, ionizing radiation, nickel, and polycyclic aromatic hydrocarbons (103).

Asbestos exposure increases lung cancer risk in cigarette smokers (104). Hammond and colleagues (105) demonstrated that the effect of asbestos exposure is greatly magnified by coexisting exposure to tobacco smoke. The risk of asbestos workers for dying of lung cancer was increased 16-fold if they smoked more than 20 cigarettes per day and ninefold if they smoked fewer than 20 cigarettes per day in comparison with the risk of asbestos workers who never smoked regularly. When cigarette smokers were considered as a group, a history of asbestos exposure increased the risk for dying of lung cancer about fivefold.

Moreover, the risk for lung cancer in persons exposed to asbestos and cigarette smoking is multiplicative. If the age-adjusted lung cancer death rate for those without exposure to asbestos or cigarette smoking is arbitrarily defined as 1, then the relative risk for cigarette smokers not exposed to asbestos is 11. For those with asbestos exposure and no smoking history, the relative risk is 6. However, for cigarette smokers with a history of asbestos exposure, the relative risk is 59. For any individual patient, the relative risk fluctuates based on the degree of smoking and the degree of asbestos exposure. The magnitude of the lung cancer risk caused by asbestos depends somewhat on the type of asbestos fiber encountered. Lung cancer risk appears to be considerably higher for workers exposed to amphibole fibers than for those exposed to chrysotile fibers in studies controlling for the amount of exposure (106).

In recent years, considerable public concern has been raised about the possible risks for lung cancer caused by radon exposure in the general population (107). Radon is a decay product of uranium 228 and radium 226 with alpha-emitting progeny that can damage respiratory epithelium. Radon is present in soil, rocks, and groundwater and can accumulate in homes. The risk for lung cancer related to radon exposure has been evaluated in underground uranium miners occupationally exposed to radioactive radon and its decay products. In this setting, an increased risk for lung cancer has been established (108). An interaction between radon exposure and cigarette smoking has also been demonstrated (109).

The risks associated with household exposure remain uncertain. These risks have been assessed in eight case control studies, three of which showed statistically significant associations and five of which did not (110). A metaanalysis of the eight studies reported a greater risk for lung cancer in association with exposure to higher levels of indoor radon. Moreover, the summary exposure-response trend was statistically significant, suggesting that the overall relative risk for lung cancer among persons exposed to household radon is 1.14 (111).

Genetic Determinants and Molecular Epidemiology

Family history has received insufficient attention as a risk factor for lung cancer. One case control study reported that the risk for lung cancer mortality among smoking relatives of lung cancer patients was 2- to 2.5-fold greater than that of smoking relatives of controls (112). Even among nonsmoking relatives, lung cancer risk was higher among relatives of patients than among relatives of controls. Other studies have demonstrated that the first-degree relatives of lung cancer patients have a twofold to threefold higher risk for the development of lung cancer (113,114).

Despite growing evidence for a causal association between cigarette smoking and lung cancer, Fisher in the late 1950s (41) and later others (115,116) suggested a constitutional hypothesis of lung cancer risk. According to this hypothesis, a genetic predisposition to both cigarette smoking and lung cancer is responsible for the association.

However, several studies focusing on smoking discordant twin pairs have effectively refuted the constitutional hypothesis (117–119). The strongest data come from a 24-year study of 1,515 World War II male veteran twin pairs discordant for cigarette smoking. Among monozygotic twins, the relative risk for lung cancer for the smoking in comparison with the nonsmoking twin was 5.0 (95% CI, 2.6–15.0). Among dizygotic twins, the relative risk was 11.0 (95% CI, 4.3–45.0). Although a higher relative risk in smoking-discordant dizygotic than in smoking-discordant monozygotic twins underscores a genetic component to lung cancer risk, these results completely refute the constitutional hypothesis, which maintains that genetic influences rather than smoking are responsible for the relationship between cigarette smoking and lung cancer.

Nonetheless, the genetic component of lung cancer risk is quite important (120). For example, in a study from Louisiana, lung cancer risk was 2.4-fold greater among first-degree relatives of 336 deceased lung cancer probands than in 307 controls (consisting of the probands' spouses) (121). In a case control study from New Mexico, a history of lung cancer in a parent was associated with a 5.3-fold increased risk for the development of lung cancer in the child (122). An excess lung cancer risk in close relatives of lung cancer patients persists even after adjustments have been made for the effects of age, sex, and smoking habits.

Although 90% of lung cancers are smoking related, lung cancer develops in only 10% to 15% of smokers (53). This underscores the enormous variability in individual susceptibility to tobacco-related carcinogens. When the genetic risk for cancer is evaluated, high-penetrance genes such as BRCA1 and BRCA2, which are associated with the development of breast cancer, are usually major genes of interest. However, high-penetrance genes are probably responsible for only a small proportion of adult solid tumors associated with environmental exposures, and no high-penetrance gene has yet been identified for lung cancer (102).

On the other hand, low-penetrance genes are likely to be very important in the molecular pathogenesis of lung cancer. In contrast to high-penetrance genes, low-penetrance genes exert relatively small effects. However, they appear to play a central role in the pathogenesis of most sporadic cancers (102).

Low-penetrance genes modify cancer risk only in conjunction with specific exposures. Accordingly, interactions between low-penetrance genes and environmental exposures, such as cigarette smoking, are likely to be key in the pathogenesis of lung cancer. A growing body of evidence indicates that large numbers of low-penetrance genes are highly associated with lung cancer risk among cigarette smokers (102,123).

The most influential determinants of lung cancer risk may be those that cannot be assessed with current technology. Classic epidemiologic studies attempt to define cancer risk within a population based primarily on such factors as age, sex, ethnicity, family history, and exposure to known carcinogens (124). On the other hand, the burgeoning field of molecular epidemiology uses molecular genetic and biochemical techniques to evaluate cancer risk in individuals (125). Unfortunately, the state of the art in molecular epidemiology is such that existing models have insufficient discretionary power to determine which individuals are destined to acquire the target disease.

Benign Lung Diseases

The coexistence of a number of benign lung diseases (emphysema, bronchitis, pulmonary fibrosis) increases the risk for lung cancer in cigarette smokers. Individuals with diffuse pulmonary interstitial fibrosis have been demonstrated to have a 14-fold increased risk for lung cancer, even when age, sex, and smoking history are taken into consideration (126). In a case control study, chronic obstructive pulmonary disease (COPD) was associated with an overall doubling of the lung cancer risk (122). Similarly, a prospective controlled study demonstrated a statistically significantly higher risk for the development of lung cancer in a group of patients with COPD than in a cohort without COPD (matched for age, sex, occupation, and smoking history) (127). By 10 years, the cumulative lung cancer risk was 8.8% for the cases and 2.0% for the controls ($P = .024$).

An increased risk for lung cancer among persons exposed to asbestos has been discussed (see section "Environmental and Occupational Carcinogens"). However, it appears that lung cancer is much more likely to develop in asbestos workers with asbestosis (interstitial fibrosis) than in those without asbestosis (128–130). In one study of 138 asbestos workers who died of lung cancer, fibrosis was present in all the patients whose lung tissue was examined microscopically (131).

Chemoprevention

Dietary factors have been shown to influence lung cancer risk. An extensive body of literature suggests that certain antioxidant vitamins, particularly derivatives of vitamin A and vitamin E, may help to prevent lung cancer (132). Substantial evidence has been found for a reduction in lung cancer risk associated with the regular ingestion of fruits and vegetables.

More than 100 epidemiologic surveys have demonstrated that persons with high levels of beta-carotene in their diet or blood have a lower risk for cancer in general and lung cancer in particular (133). Case control or cohort studies have consistently demonstrated that certain antioxidant vitamins decrease the risk for lung cancer (134,135). In 30 of 32 studies, the risk for lung cancer was reduced in persons who consumed substantial quantities of fruits, vegetables, or both (136). Existing data suggest that an increased consumption of fruit, green and yellow vegetables, and possibly some micronutrients can meaningfully decrease lung cancer risk among cigarette smokers (137).

Evidence from randomized trials, however, has been much less encouraging. Results of several of these have pointed to effects in the opposite direction. For example, the Alpha-Tocopherol, Beta-Carotene (ATBC) Lung Cancer Prevention Study Group, a population-based randomized trial involving almost 30,000 male cigarette smokers in Finland, demonstrated a statistically significant increase in lung cancer incidence and mortality in those randomized to the beta-carotene arm (138). Similarly, the Beta-Carotene and Retinol Efficacy Trial (CARET), a randomized trial comparing beta-carotene and retinyl palmitate with placebo among more than 18,000 men and women at high risk for lung cancer, also demonstrated a higher incidence and mortality of lung cancer among those in the experimental group (139). In contrast, the Physicians' Health Study, which involved approximately 22,000 male physicians, showed no significant differences in lung cancer or total cancer incidence or mortality between the group randomized to beta-carotene and that randomized to placebo (140). On the other hand, a beneficial effect of beta-carotene on cancer incidence and mortality was demonstrated in the Chinese Cancer Prevention Trial, a randomized trial involving almost 30,000 participants conducted in Linxian County, China (141). Accordingly, these studies provide conflicting information, although the two best-powered studies suggest a detrimental effect.

Results have also been inconsistent with regard to whether chemoprevention strategies can reduce the risk for second lung cancers among persons with a prior history of stage I non–small cell lung cancer (NSCLC). For example, in one trial of patients who had undergone resection for stage I NSCLC, subjects were randomized to either retinyl palmitate or no further treatment. This trial did demonstrate a reduction in the number of second primary lung cancers among those randomized to adjuvant high-dose vitamin A therapy (142). On the other hand, a larger intergoup study demonstrated no significant reduction in second lung cancers among those randomized to isotretinoin (143). In this trial, isotretinoin appeared to have a detrimental effect in current smokers, although a possible beneficial effect was noted among former smokers.

This finding suggests that chemoprevention in former smokers may represent a more fruitful avenue of investigation. Nonetheless, little hard evidence is available at the present time to support this approach (143,144). Although the NCI has given a high priority to investigating this area, there is no reason to use chemoprevention outside the context of a prospective study (145).

SCREENING FOR LUNG CANCER

At the present time, screening for lung cancer is not recommended by any public policy organization in the world. The recommendation against screening for lung cancer is based on the fact that no randomized population trial (RPT) has demonstrated a significant reduction in lung cancer mortality as a result of screening (146).

None of the four RPTs that have evaluated the effectiveness of chest x-ray (CXR) screening, with or without the addition of sputum cytology, have demonstrated a significant reduction in mortality among the screened population. In both the Mayo Lung Project and the Czech Study, the two RPTs that incorporated an assessment of the effectiveness of CXR screening as part of their randomized designs, lung cancer mortality was actually higher in the experimental populations (147–149). Accordingly, if the mortality endpoint provides an accurate measure of the effectiveness of screening, such results support the conclusion that CXR screening is, in reality, detrimental (150). These results have clearly been responsible for the nihilistic view of screening for lung cancer that is so prevalent at this time (151).

In dramatic contrast, the view that computed tomography (CT) represents a major breakthrough in lung cancer screening has been endorsed enthusiastically (152–154). Unquestionably, CT is technologically superior to conventional CXR in detecting small lung nodules. However, the enthusiasm for CT as a screening tool is based primarily on its ability to detect very small tumors in the context of nonrandomized trials. No mortality or survival benefits derived from CT of the chest have been reported.

Chest Roentgenographic Screening

Four RPTs including 37,724 participants have been conducted to evaluate the utility of CXR screening in lung can-

cer. Because they were all initiated in the 1970s, before the epidemic of lung cancer in women, each of these trials was limited to male cigarette smokers. Accordingly, no RPT has evaluated the efficacy of lung cancer screening in women, despite the fact that lung cancer subsequently surpassed breast cancer as the most common cause of cancer death in women.

The NCI sponsored three of these RPTs in the context of the Cooperative Early Lung Cancer Detection Program. In the Memorial-Sloan Kettering Lung Project and the Johns Hopkins Lung Project, participants were randomized at study entry to a "dual-screen" group (in which patients underwent annual chest roentgenography and sputum cytology every 4 months) or to a "single-screen" group (in which CXR screening was performed annually) (155,156). Both trials demonstrated no benefit in adding sputum cytology to annual CXR studies. As randomized comparisons, these trials were designed to assess the benefit of sputum cytology rather than CXR studies.

In this regard, it is informative simply to point out that the long-term survival rates in both the experimental group and the control population in the Memorial Sloan-Kettering and Johns Hopkins studies were approximately threefold superior to that observed in the NCI SEER program for men with disease diagnosed during the same epoch (157). Accordingly, these studies provide some support that annual CXR screening, which all participants underwent, contributed to what may be considered a dramatic improvement in outcome (146).

Mayo Lung Project

The Mayo Lung Project is the most influential RPT focusing on screening for lung cancer (158). The trial results have been interpreted as negative because they failed to demonstrate a significant mortality reduction in the experimental group. On the other hand, significant advantages were noted in stage distribution and long-term survival. An independent analysis of individual patient data from the Mayo Lung Project has been reported (159).

After a usual prevalence screen, which consisted of both a CXR study and sputum cytology, 4,607 male smokers older than 45 years were randomized to an experimental group that underwent a CXR study and sputum cytology every 4 months, and 4,585 were randomized to a control group that underwent no regular screening. The experimental group underwent screening for 6 years on average, followed by 3 years of observation; the controls were followed on average for 9 years (158).

Although the members of the control group were not screened as part of the trial, they did receive a recommendation to undergo an annual CXR study and sputum cytology. This led to significant contamination, reflected by the fact that almost one third of the control cancers were detected by CXR. Nonetheless, despite contamination, significant differences were observed.

TABLE 39.13. MAYO LUNG PROJECT: RESULTS AFTER 9 YEARS

	Experimental Group	Control Group	P Value	Relative Risk (95% Confidence Interval)
Population	4,607	4,585		
Lung cancer incidence and mortality				
Incidence	206	160	.013	1.30 (1.06–1.60)
Mortality	122	115	.62	1.06 (0.83–1.37)
Lung cancer survival and other clinical endpoints				
5-Year survival/9-year survival	34%/29%	13%/13%	0.0021 log rank	
Screen-detected	65%	30%	<.0001	2.15 (1.66–2.78)
Stage I or II	48%	32%	.0019	1.51 (1.15–1.97)
Surgically resected	46%	32%	.0071	1.45 (1.10–1.90)

During the 9-year study period, 366 lung cancers were detected (159) (Table 39.13). The most striking findings were related to the discrepancy between mortality and survival. A modest mortality disadvantage was found for those randomized to screening. On the other hand, a significant survival advantage at both 5 years and 9 years favored the experimental group.

The discrepancy between survival and mortality was possible because the lung cancer incidence was significantly higher in the experimental population. Based on the application of conventional assumptions that underlie the interpretation of early detection in RPTs, survival is assumed to be misleading because of conventional screening biases (160–162).

On the other hand, what the independent analysis demonstrated is that none of the conventional screening biases confounded survival comparisons. Figure 39.3 compares survival for screen-detected and symptom-detected lung cancer in the Mayo Lung Project. It demonstrates a highly significant survival advantage for those with screen-detected disease ($P < .0001$). Although this difference may reflect a screening benefit, it definitely also reflects at least an element of length bias. Because of length-biased sampling, screening tends to detect tumors that grow more slowly. Accordingly, length bias could account for the dramatic survival advantages noted (Fig. 39.3).

Length bias can be excluded by performing an "intent-to-treat" analysis, which respects the integrity of randomization. Figure 39.4 compares the survival of all (screen-detected and symptom-detected) cases in the experimental group with that of all cases in the control group. Because it demonstrates a highly significant survival advantage for those randomized to screening ($P = .0021$), it must be concluded that the observed survival advantage in the experimental group is not attributable to length bias.

However, it has long been understood that improved survival may be "due only to the advancement of the time of diagnosis of cancer and not to the postponement of death" (163). If this occurs, "lead time bias" would lead to a spurious survival advantage. Figure 39.4 represents a traditional survival curve in which survival is measured from the time of diagnosis. It demonstrates that 9-year survival in the experimental group was 29%, compared with 13% in the control group. The question is whether lead time bias could account

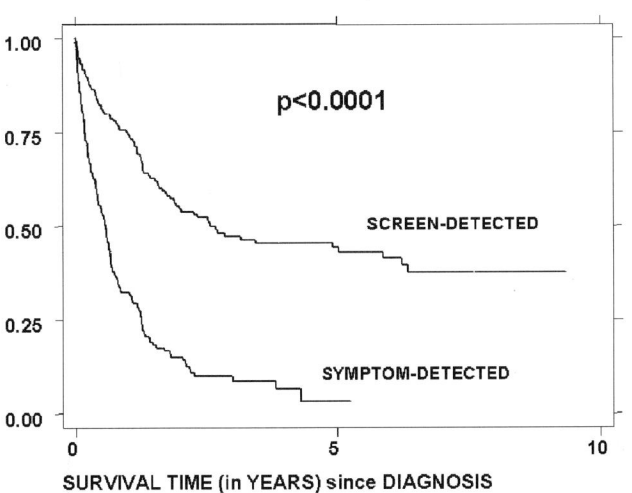

FIGURE 39.3. Survival by method of detection.

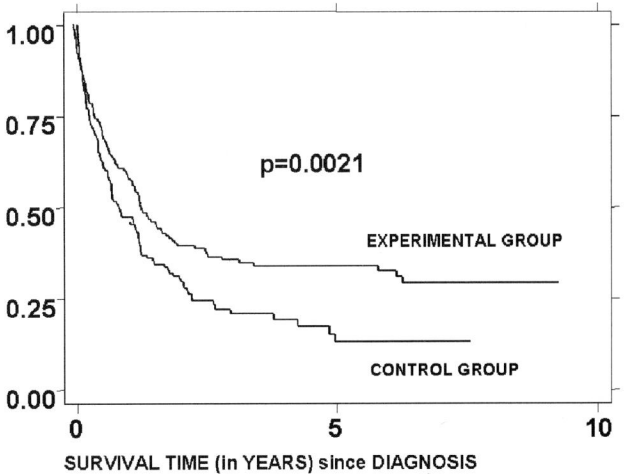

FIGURE 39.4. Kaplan-Meier survival by group (survival time in years since diagnosis).

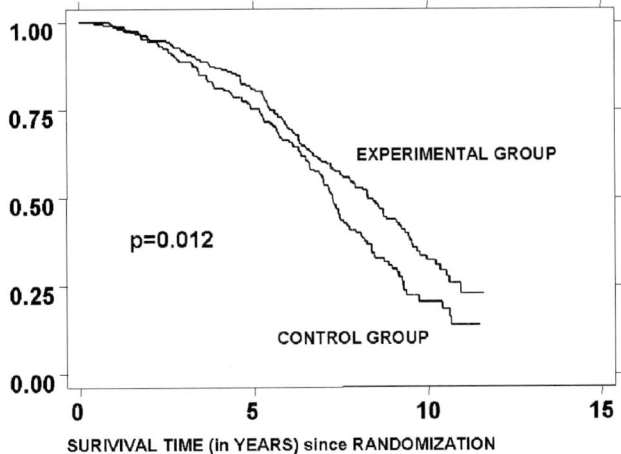

FIGURE 39.5. Kaplan-Meier survival by group (survival time in years since randomization).

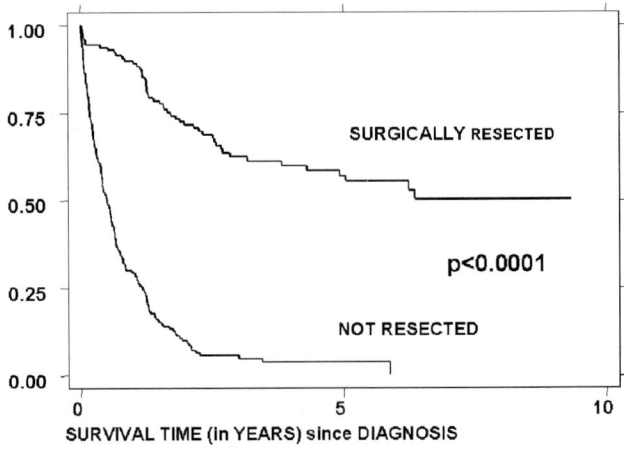

FIGURE 39.6. Kaplan-Meier survival by resectability.

for the survival advantage. This is possible because survival during the asymptomatic, preclinical phase is included in the survival times of the experimental group cases but not in the survival times of the control cases. Although a significant survival advantage that persists 9 years after diagnosis would not be likely to be attributable to lead time bias, it remains possible that the average lead time is so prolonged that longer follow-up is needed for survival curves to converge.

Figure 39.5 shows an analysis in which survival is measured from the time of randomization. It also demonstrates a significant survival advantage favoring the experimental group ($P = .012$). Using randomization as time 0 excludes confounding by lead time bias because the time of diagnosis is no longer a variable when survival between groups is compared. Accordingly, if a significant survival advantage can be shown in an RPT when "intent-to-treat" principles are respected and when survival is measured from randomization, neither length bias nor lead time bias can be responsible for a spurious result.

However, such an analysis does not rigorously exclude confounding by overdiagnosis bias. It is only for this reason that overdiagnosis has been invoked to account for the survival/mortality discrepancy in the Mayo Lung Project (164,165). A "process of elimination" provides the epidemiologic basis for concluding that overdiagnosis accounts for the observed survival/mortality discrepancies (166). In this regard, it is important to be precise about what the term implies. Overdiagnosis exists only if screening detects "pseudodisease, a subclinical condition that would not have produced signs or symptoms before the individual died of other causes" (166).

Univariate testing demonstrated that group assignment, the presence of screen-detected disease, and the presence of surgically resectable disease each significantly reduced the risk for lung cancer mortality (159). When adjustments were made for differences in the resection rates, the presence of screen-detected disease and group assignment were not sig-

nificant. The finding that effective treatment is the only significant multivariate predictor of lung cancer mortality in those with lung cancer indicates that overdiagnosis cannot account for the observed data. Screen detection was important only because it was a predictor of surgical resectability and the ability to carry out "curative" therapy.

Thus, the objective of screening for lung cancer is to identify patients with early-stage lung cancer, who can then undergo curative resection. Figure 39.6 supports the contention that screen detection was important because it predicted for resection, which is the only curative therapy for lung cancer. This conclusion is underscored by the fact that of 185 lung cancer patients who did not undergo curative surgical resection, not one achieved long-term survival. The longest survival in a patient with unresected lung cancer was 70 months. In dramatic contrast, of 181 resected patients, 50% did achieve long-term survival.

Therefore, more than 50% of patients with resected lung cancers were cured of their disease, whereas cure was not achieved in a single patient with unresected cancer. What were the relative contributions of CXR and sputum cytology? As illustrated in Figure 39.7, cytology-detected cases did extremely well and had a survival superior to that of CXR-detected lesions. However, of 181 screen-detected cases, only 18 (10%) were cytology detected, whereas 162 (90%) were CXR detected. Accordingly, CXR was responsible for a favorable outcome in the vast majority of screen-detected cancers in the Mayo Lung Project.

Mortality and Randomization

In addition to eliminating selection bias, randomization must control for confounding (167). Confounding is a distortion that arises when comparisons are made between noncomparable groups. A confounder is an independent risk factor for outcome that is also significantly associated with exposure (168,169).

In the Mayo Lung Project, lung cancer incidence was 30% higher in the experimental group. The finding that excess

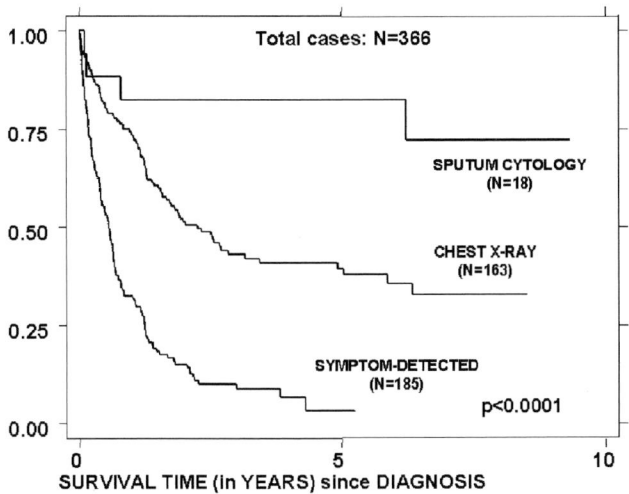

FIGURE 39.7. Kaplan-Meier survival by method of detection.

incidence was not a consequence of overdiagnosis raises the question that incidence discrepancies may reflect an element of randomization failure caused by imbalances in unmeasured or unknown confounders.

Although there were no imbalances in any measured risk factor, randomization in the RPT setting must lead to a balanced allocation for all predictors of cancer development in the general population. We generally assume that if randomization leads to a balanced allocation among measured risk factors, then randomization also leads to a balanced allocation among unmeasured confounders (54,167). However, there is a theoretic basis for questioning this assumption in the RPT setting (146,170).

The suggestion is that randomization failure is more likely in an RPT than in a randomized clinical trial (RCT). In an RCT, randomization need balance only clinical parameters. In cancer, these comprise standard prognostic factors, such as nodal status, tumor size, and histologic grade.

Conversely, in an early-detection RPT in which a cause-specific mortality endpoint is used, randomization must also lead to a balanced allocation for predictors of cancer risk in the general population. Although specific knowledge of these factors is rudimentary, such confounders comprise a broad spectrum of extrinsic exposure and intrinsic genetic susceptibility variables.

The finding that survival was not confounded by conventional screening biases supports the conclusion that the survival advantage noted in the Mayo Lung Project was unbiased (159,171). Accordingly, the presence of a survival/mortality discrepancy confronts us with the need to reconsider our assumptions regarding cause-specific mortality. Obviously, if survival provides an accurate measure of what screening accomplished, there is no alternative to the conclusion that the mortality data were biased.

The controversy surrounding screening for cancer has been based primarily on our uncritical acceptance of cause-specific mortality as the "primary endpoint" (7,146). Mortality can be biased in an RPT, as it was in the Mayo Lung Project. On the other hand, survival can provide definitive evidence for screening efficacy in a mature RPT.

The data support the conclusion that randomization to screening significantly improved lung cancer survival in the Mayo Lung Project. Screen detection led to improved survival because it facilitated surgical resection. It was resection that was directly responsible for the 50% cure rate among those undergoing surgery.

Computed Tomographic Screening

As noted at the beginning of this section, the possibility that screening for lung cancer with low-dose helical CT represents a major breakthrough in lung cancer early detection has been received with enthusiasm (152–154). CT has been heavily promoted and marketed directly to the general public as a screening tool for lung cancer (172). The NCI is currently funding an RPT that will involve 50,000 subjects to compare CT screening with conventional CXR. The trial will use a lung cancer mortality endpoint.

There is little question that CT represents a technologic advance in comparison with conventional CXR. Nonetheless, enthusiasm for CT is largely related to different standards of effectiveness that have driven public perceptions regarding CXR. No randomized trials have been completed, and long-term survival and mortality have not been reported. Enthusiasm for CT is based primarily on its ability to detect early-stage disease in observational trials.

Three nonrandomized trials provide the bulk of the evidence regarding CT screening (173–176). The three studies took place in Matsumoto, Japan, in New York, and at the Mayo Clinic. In both the Japanese trial and the New York Early Lung Cancer Action Project (ELCAP), 84% to 85% of detected cancers were stage IA NSCLC (Table 39.14). The Mayo Clinic study did not confirm such high rates of early disease, although a respectable 51% of cancers had stage IA NSCLC (176–178). Although no comparative data are available, it is highly likely that CT will prove to be more sensitive than conventional CXR in its ability to detect early-stage disease.

A major problem of CT is related to poor specificity and its high false-positive rate. In ELCAP, a noncalcified nodule was identified in 23% of the participants on the initial CT scan (174). However, on repeated screening, false-positive results were obtained in only an additional 23 participants (2.3%) (175). In the Mayo Clinic study, the specificity of CT was remarkably poor; 51% of the subjects had one or more small, noncalcified nodules on the initial CT scan, and 101 (13%) of 1,464 persons who returned for their first repeated CT had nodules that had not been present a year earlier (176).

Although CT screening has generated great excitement, the limitations of the data have been incompletely addressed

TABLE 39.14. NONRANDOMIZED TRIALS OF LUNG CANCER SCREENING WITH COMPUTED TOMOGRAPHY OF THE CHEST

Study (Authors) (Reference)	No. Screened	Lung Cancer No. (%)	Stage IA No. (%)	False Positives No. (%)	Specificity (%)
Japan (Sone et al.) (173)	5,483	19 (0.34)	16 (84)	223 (4.1)	96
ELCAP (Henschke et al.) (174,175)	1,000	27 (2.7)	23 (85)	233 (23.3)	79
Mayo Clinic (Swensen et al.) (176)	1,520	25 (1.6)	13 (52)	782 (51.4)	49

ELCAP, Early Lung Cancer Action Project.

in the literature. The existing observational trials primarily report stage and resectability profiles of prevalence cancers detected by CT (179). Long-term survival results have yet to be reported, and mortality comparisons will not be forthcoming from these nonrandomized trials.

Although survival is likely to be very favorable, survival cannot provide a definite measure of outcome in a nonrandomized trial. Conventional screening biases cannot be eliminated in a nonrandomized trial. Length bias is likely to be a particular problem when the survival of screen-detected tumors discovered on prevalence screening is reported (180,181).

More importantly, selection bias appears to have profoundly influenced the stage distribution findings in these trials, particularly ELCAP. Although such favorable stage distribution profiles demonstrate the ability of CT to detect small tumors, they bear little resemblance to that expected in previously unscreened, high-risk populations.

This problem is illustrated by considering the 31,360 men who underwent CXR screening (with or without sputum cytology) in the context of the initial prevalence screen in the NCI-sponsored randomized trials at the Mayo Clinic, Johns Hopkins Hospital, and Memorial-Sloan Kettering Cancer Center. Of the 223 lung cancers detected, 47% were stage I, 8% stage II, and 45% stage III or IV (182,183). The question is why so few advanced cancers were found in the Japanese study and ELCAP.

In the Japanese series, the absence of advanced cancer might be explained by the fact that participants had previously undergone CXR and sputum cytology screening (173). However, such is not the case with regard to ELCAP. Accordingly, selection bias clearly contributed to this finding and raises major questions about generalizations based on the ELCAP data.

Although CT can detect smaller tumors than conventional CXR, no evidence indicates that the detection of extremely small stage IA lesions provides a survival advantage in comparison with the detection of larger stage IA lesions. Patz and colleagues (184) analyzed 510 patients with stage IA NSCLCs that were subdivided into four size categories. Five-year survival ranged from 80% to 87%; no significant differences in survival based on size were found.

Although CT is probably more sensitive than CXR, CXR is more specific, and it has a lower false-positive rate. Problems with specificity may create insurmountable obstacles with regard to the economic implications of population-based CT screening for lung cancer.

Lung Cancer Screening Reconsidered

For a cancer screening strategy to be recommended as the standard of care, six criteria must be fulfilled (185,186). First, the burden of disease must be sufficient to warrant mass screening. Second, the disease targeted by screening must have a detectable preclinical phase. Third, the screening test should be accurate, with acceptable sensitivity, specificity, and predictive values. Fourth, the test must be acceptable to patients and physicians. Fifth, screening must be effective; the treatment of asymptomatic, early-stage disease should be superior to the treatment of symptomatic disease. Sixth, the cost and cost-effectiveness of screening should be acceptable and should not substantially exceed that of other preventive measures.

The question is whether population-based screening for lung cancer deserves to be recommended on the basis of these factors. From the perspective of burden of disease, there is no question that screening for lung cancer deserves serious consideration. As Parkin and colleagues point out (2), in regard to incidence, mortality, and survival, "Lung cancer is the main cancer in the world today." Moreover, a detectable preclinical phase clearly exists in regard to CXR screening, which provides a window of opportunity for early detection. As for accuracy, two NCI-sponsored randomized trials have demonstrated that the sensitivity of CXR is approximately twofold greater than that of cytology (54% vs. 27%), and the specificity is comparable (186). The positive predictive value of a suspect finding on CXR is superior to that of early detection tools used in other common cancers. The acceptability of CXR to patients and physicians is not in dispute.

The most critical question is whether the evidence supports the conclusion that CXR screening is effective. The answer depends on how "effectiveness" is defined. Results of RPTs consistently demonstrate that CXR screening leads to significant advantages in survival that are also associated with stage and resectability advantages. Moreover, survival advantages cannot be explained on the basis of any conventional screening bias. The evidence is clear that these advantages are not a consequence of overdiagnosis (159,171).

Although cause-specific mortality is assumed to be the most accurate measure of screening effectiveness (160,161, 187), this belief is based on assumptions that have never been validated. Analysis of the data supports the conclusion that survival was unbiased in the Mayo Lung Project and that the mortality endpoint was in fact a biased outcome. Mortality can misrepresent the true effect of screening if randomization fails to create experimental and control populations with an equal probability of cancer. The importance of these issues is in no way limited to the controversy over screening for lung cancer. For example, they are equally relevant to the firestorm of controversy that has recently arisen in regard to population-based screening for breast cancer (188–192).

Finally, what about cost-effectiveness? Cost-effectiveness depends on three variables: the effectiveness of the intervention, the cost of the test, and the size of the target population. Clearly, if mortality is the proper measure of effectiveness, CXR screening for lung cancer is not cost-effective. The cost per life-year saved would be infinite.

On the other hand, if survival reflects an accurate measure of effectiveness, a simple cost-effectiveness analysis suggests a rather different conclusion. A simplified model estimated that annual CXR screening would translate into approximately $7,900 per life-year saved (186). Other analyses support similar conclusions (193,194).

A systematic analysis of the Mayo Lung Project and other RPTs support the conclusion that a survival advantage not related to conventional screening biases represents the best measure of screening effectiveness in the RPT setting. Conversely, the cause-specific mortality endpoint often misrepresents the effects of screening because the mortality endpoint is more sensitive to randomization failure than are survival and other clinical endpoints.

Accordingly, sufficient evidence currently exists to reconsider the standard of care as it relates to screening for lung cancer. It is highly likely that hundreds of thousands of lung cancer deaths could annually be avoided if CXR screening were offered to persons at high risk. Public policy with regard to screening for lung cancer is in urgent need of reconsideration (146,159).

PATHOLOGY AND CLASSIFICATION

The histologic classification of primary lung cancer was initially developed by the World Health Organization (WHO) in 1967. It was subsequently revised in 1981 and most recently 1999. The most recent WHO Histological Classification of Lung and Pleural Tumors, with a focus on epithelial tumors, appears in Table 39.15 (195).

TABLE 39.15. WORLD HEALTH ORGANIZATION 1999 HISTOLOGIC CLASSIFICATION OF LUNG AND PLEURAL TUMORS (ABBREVIATED)

1. Epithelial tumors
  1.1. Benign
    1.1.1. Papillomas
    1.1.2. Adenomas
  1.2. Preinvasive lesions
    1.2.1. Squamous dysplasia/carcinoma in situ
    1.2.2. Atypical adenomatous hyperplasia
    1.2.3. Diffuse idiopathic pulmonary neuroendocrine cell hyperplasia
  1.3. Malignant
    1.3.1. Squamous cell carcinoma
      1.3.1.1. Papillary
      1.3.1.2. Clear cell
      1.3.1.3. Small cell
      1.3.1.4. Basaloid
    1.3.2. Small cell carcinoma
      1.3.2.1. Combined small cell carcinoma
    1.3.3. Adenocarcinoma
      1.3.3.1. Acinar
      1.3.3.2. Papillary
      1.3.3.3. Bronchoalveolar
        1.3.3.3.1. Nonmucinous
        1.3.3.3.2. Mucinous
        1.3.3.3.3. Mixed mucinous and nonmucinous or indeterminate cell type
      1.3.3.4. Solid carcinoma with mucin formation
      1.3.3.5. Adenocarcinoma with mixed subtypes
      1.3.3.6. Variants
    1.3.4. Large cell carcinoma
      1.3.4.1. Large cell neuroendocrine carcinoma
      1.3.4.2. Basaloid carcinoma
      1.3.4.3. Lymphoepithelioma-like carcinoma
      1.3.4.4. Clear cell carcinoma
      1.3.4.5. Large cell carcinoma with rhabdoid phenotype
    1.3.5. Adenosquamous carcinoma
    1.3.6. Carcinoma with pleomorphic sarcomatoid or sarcomatous elements
    1.3.7. Carcinoid tumor
      1.3.7.1. Typical carcinoid
      1.3.7.2. Atypical carcinoid
    1.3.8. Carcinomas of salivary gland type
      1.3.8.1. Mucoepidermoid carcinoma
      1.3.8.2. Adenoid cystic carcinoma
      1.3.8.3. Others
    1.3.9. Others
2. Soft tissue tumors
3. Mesothelial tumors
  3.1. Benign
  3.2. Malignant mesothelioma
4. Miscellaneous tumors
5. Lymphoproliferative diseases
6. Secondary tumors
7. Unclassified tumors
8. Tumorlike lesions

Source: From Travis WD, Colby TV, Corrin B, et al. *World Health Organization international histological classification of tumours: histological typing of lung and pleural tumours,* 3rd ed. Berlin; Springer-Verlag, 1999:1–156, with permission.

The four major histologic subtypes of squamous cell carcinoma, adenocarcinoma, large cell carcinoma, and small cell carcinoma represent approximately 95% of all primary bronchogenic carcinomas. Bronchoalveolar cell carcinoma is classified as a subtype of adenocarcinoma. These four major types of lung cancer are briefly described in the next sections; a full discussion of histologic subtypes is beyond the scope of this chapter. The reader is referred to the most recent WHO publication for further details (195).

Although a specific histopathologic classification is highly desirable, the distinction between small cell lung carcinoma (SCLC) and non–small cell lung carcinoma (NSCLC) is most critical in determining an approach to therapy. Material suitable for definitive histologic diagnosis can come either from biopsy or cytology specimens. Biopsy specimens are most often obtained by bronchoscopy or surgery, including thoracoscopy.

Material suitable for cytologic assessment can come from induced sputum or from bronchial brushings or washings. Moreover, the role of fine needle aspiration (FNA) has increased greatly during the last decade. FNA is an accurate, simple, and relatively inexpensive technique in comparison with invasive surgical techniques. FNA is highly likely to yield a specimen suitable for definitive diagnosis if it is sufficiently cellular. The diagnostic yield of FNA can be enhanced by the ancillary use of immunohistochemistry or electron microscopy.

The relationship between cigarette smoking and the histologic subtypes has been discussed (see section "Cigarette Smoking and the Changing Histopathology of Lung Cancer"). Although the relationship between cigarette smoking and squamous cell carcinoma and small cell carcinoma was completely clarified by the studies reported in the early 1950s, the relationship between smoking and adenocarcinoma and large cell carcinoma was not nearly as well established until the relatively recent past. However, as was explained in detail earlier, the vast majority of adenocarcinomas and large cell carcinomas are clearly causally related to cigarette smoking.

Squamous Cell Carcinoma

In the past, squamous cell carcinoma was the most common histologic subtype of all lung cancers. In the 1970s, squamous cell carcinoma comprised almost 40% of all primary lung cancers, but it now comprises approximately 28% (69). Squamous cell carcinoma occurs almost exclusively in cigarette smokers and is much more common in men than in women.

Approximately two thirds of squamous cell carcinomas occur as central lesions within the lung (Fig. 39.8). They tend to be relatively slowly growing neoplasms. It has been estimated that the average time from the development of carcinoma in situ to a clinically apparent tumor is approximately 3 to 4 years. The tumor spreads along the bronchial

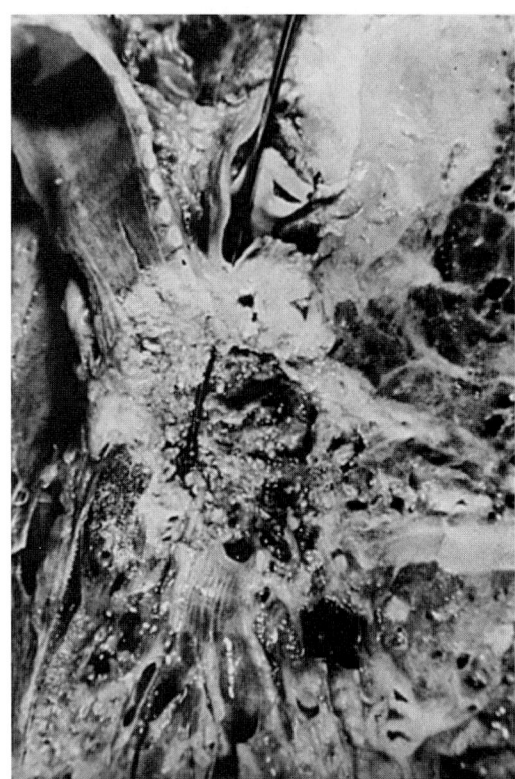

FIGURE 39.8. Central squamous cell carcinoma of left lung with cavitation. This tumor eroded the adjacent pulmonary artery (*probe*), causing fatal hemorrhage. (From Morgan WKC, Hales MR. Bronchogenic carcinoma. In: Baum GL, Wolinsky E, eds. *Textbook of pulmonary diseases*, 3rd ed. Boston: Little, Brown and Company, 1983, with permission.)

wall, directly invading the peribronchial lymph nodes and adjacent pulmonary parenchyma. Peripheral squamous cell carcinomas often directly invade the chest wall. Central tumors tend to arise at the bifurcation of segmental or subsegmental bronchi. Squamous cell cancers tend to become cavitary.

Light microscopically, these tumors are composed of sheets of epithelial cells characterized by keratinization or intercellular bridge formation. Differentiated tumors demonstrate small nest or whorl formation, individual cell keratinization, or keratin pearl formation. They are often preceded sequentially by focal squamous metaplasia, atypical proliferation, desmoplasia, carcinoma in situ, and microinvasion (Figs. 39.9 and 39.10).

Adenocarcinoma

During the past three decades, adenocarcinoma has emerged as the most common histologic subtype of all lung cancers, now accounting for approximately 44% of all lung cancers (69). Adenocarcinomas arise predominantly in the periphery of the lung, often in relation to focal scars or in regions of interstitial fibrosis. They usually do not arise endobronchially and involve the bronchi only through local invasion or submucosal lymphatic spread. Because of their peripheral

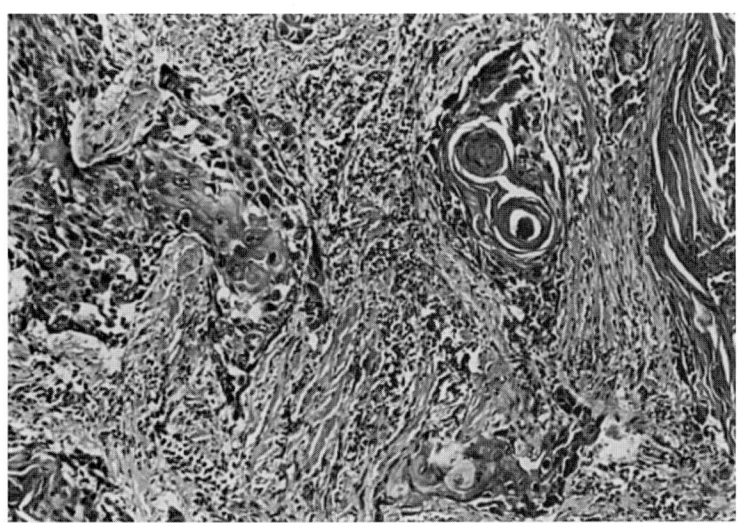

FIGURE 39.9. Well-differentiated squamous cell carcinoma with two keratinized epithelial pearls. Numerous lymphocytes and plasma cells are seen in the desmoplastic stroma. (From Morgan WKC, Hales MR. Bronchogenic carcinoma. In: Baum GL, Wolinsky E, eds. *Textbook of pulmonary diseases*, 3rd ed. Boston: Little, Brown and Company, 1983, with permission.)

location, they are associated with pulmonary symptoms less often than centrally located squamous cell carcinomas. Although adenocarcinomas may present as a solitary pulmonary nodule, they are frequently multicentric.

Adenocarcinomas are the most common histologic subtype in women and in nonsmokers. On the other hand, as previously discussed (see section "Cigarette Smoking and the Changing Histopathology of Lung Cancer: Adenocarcinoma"), the vast majority of adenocarcinomas are now clearly smoking related.

Adenocarcinomas also tend to grow slowly. However, they invade lymphatic and blood vessels relatively early in their

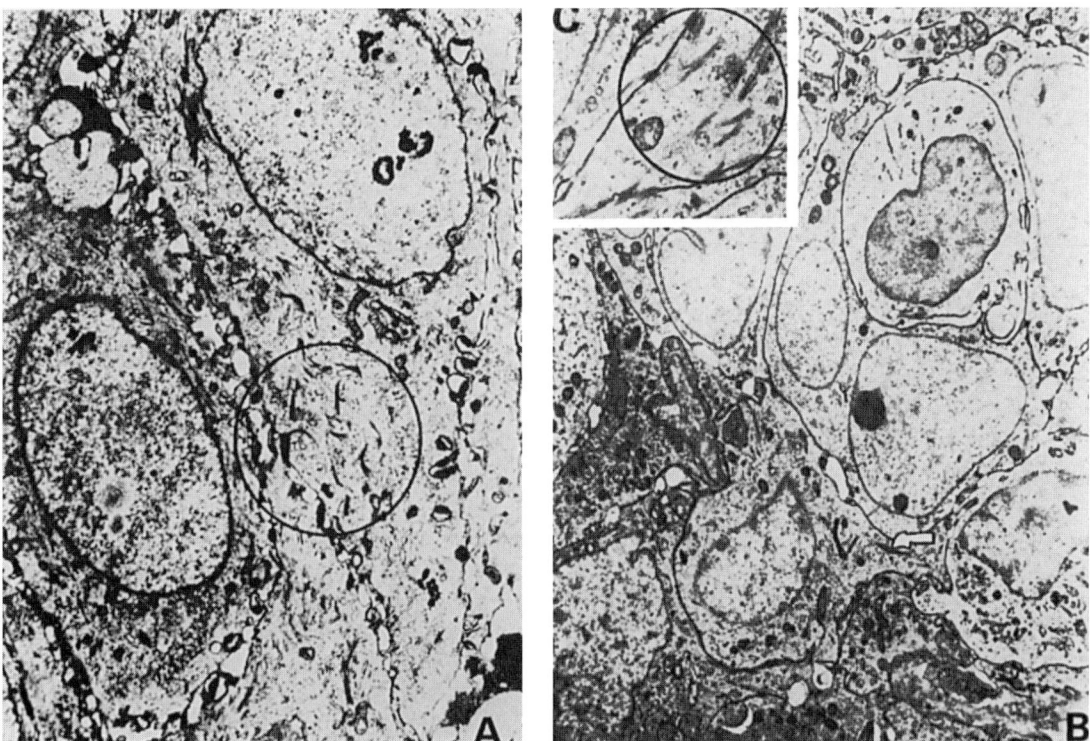

FIGURE 39.10. Overall low-power ultrastructural appearance of a squamous cell carcinoma, with prominent nucleoli and evenly dispersed nuclear chromatin. **A:** Well-formed desmosomes (*within the circle*) join apposing outpouchings of adjacent cells and clusters of tonofilaments in the neighborhood of intercellular junctions, as well as in a paranuclear location (original magnification × 10,000). **B:** Only a few scattered bundles of tonofilaments are identifiable (original magnification ×7,500). **C:** The well-formed desmosomes join apposing cellular membranes and nearby clusters of tonofilaments (original magnification ×22,000). (From Herrera et al. Ultrastructural characterization of pulmonary neoplasms. *Surv Synth Pathol Respir* 1984;3:520, with permission.)

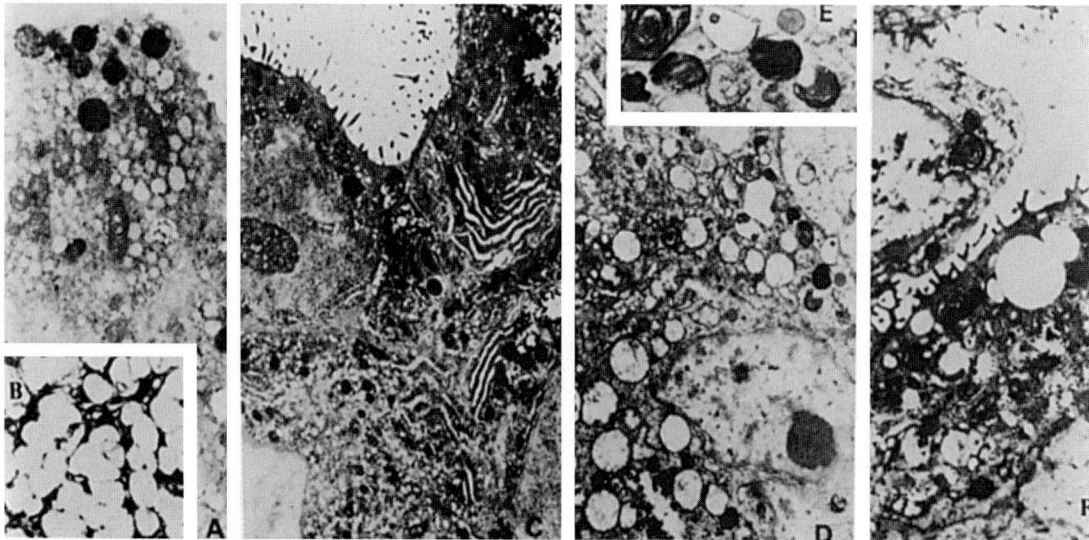

FIGURE 39.11. Adenocarcinomas. **A:** Note the poorly formed surface microvillous border and the collections of coalescent mucin vacuoles (original magnification ×13,000). **B:** Coalescent mucin vacuoles are better illustrated at this magnification (original magnification ×22,000). **C:** Note the dark, electron-dense granules, typical of Clara cell adenocarcinomas. Also note the better-developed microvillous border (original magnification ×10,000). **D:** Note the collections of typical lamellar bodies, indicative of pneumocyte type II differentiation (original magnification ×7,500). **E:** Note the details of the lamellar bodies (original magnification ×28,000). **F:** Note a combination of coalescent mucin vacuoles and Clara cell granules within the same cell, indicative of a mixed adenocarcinoma (original magnification ×13,000). (From Herrera et al. Ultrastructural characterization of pulmonary neoplasms. *Surv Synth Pathol Respir* 1984;3:520, with permission.)

natural history, and for this reason they are more likely than squamous cell carcinomas to metastasize to distant regions. This property helps explain why adenocarcinomas are associated with a poorer survival than squamous cell carcinomas.

By light microscopy, adenocarcinomas exhibit gland formation, a papillary structure, or mucin production (Fig. 39.11). About 10% of the tumors are associated with psammoma body formation. Poorly differentiated adenocarcinomas may produce solid sheets of tumor cells that are weakly associated with small acinar formation. Well-differentiated adenocarcinomas are characterized predominantly by acinar formation, whereas more poorly differentiated adenocarcinomas show less prominent glandular× differentiation. Immunohistochemically, adenocarcinomas express low-molecular-weight cytokeratins, carcinoembryonic antigen (CEA), and epithelial membrane antigen. The major value of CEA is to distinguish adenocarcinomas (which are usually CEA-positive) from mesotheliomas (which are CEA-negative).

The WHO classification divides adenocarcinomas into four major subtypes: acinar, papillary, solid tumor with mucin production, and bronchoalveolar cell carcinoma. Mixed subtypes are also recognized.

When they present as early-stage resectable lesions, solid tumors with mucin production carry the poorest prognosis, whereas bronchoalveolar cell carcinomas carry the most favorable (196).

A number of studies have shown that the frequency of bronchoalveolar cell carcinoma has dramatically increased during the past several decades (63,72,197). Bronchoalveolar cell carcinoma can be defined as an adenocarcinoma with a purely bronchioloalveolar growth pattern, without evidence of stromal, vascular, or pleural invasion. Although a bronchioloalveolar pattern can be recognized on a biopsy specimen, the final diagnosis of bronchoalveolar carcinoma requires a thorough histologic examination of a resected specimen (195). The relationship between cigarette smoking and bronchoalveolar cell carcinoma has already been discussed (see section "Cigarette Smoking and the Changing Histopathology of Lung Cancer: Bronchoalveolar Carcinoma").

Large Cell Carcinoma

Large cell carcinomas constitute approximately 9% of all lung cancers (69). These tumors are so classified because under the light microscope they lack both glandular formation, indicating adenocarcinoma, and keratinization or intracellular bridges, indicating squamous differentiation (Figs. 39.12 and 39.13). In this regard, large cell carcinoma is often a diagnosis of exclusion. However, most large cell carcinomas have ultrastructural features suggestive of either poorly differentiated squamous cell carcinomas or adenocarcinomas (195).

By electron microscopy, some large cell carcinomas show intracytoplasmic tonofilaments, mucin droplets, or electron-dense granules that indicate neuroendocrine differentiation. About 50% of these tumors can be reclassified as poorly differentiated adenocarcinomas or poorly differentiated squamous cell carcinomas.

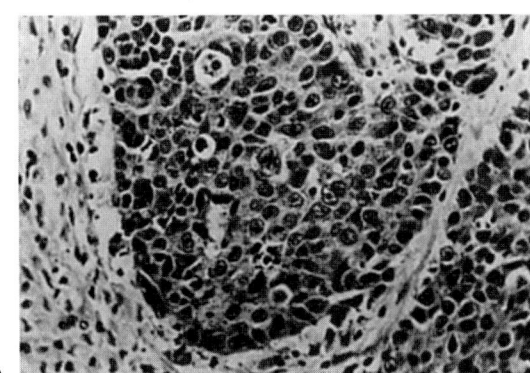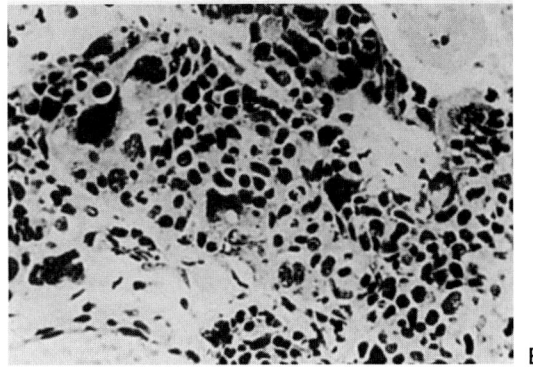

FIGURE 39.12. A: A large cell carcinoma not showing any mucin production or stratification, an example of group 4 in the World Health Organization (1981) classification of undifferentiated large cell carcinomas. **B:** A tumor with large pleomorphic cells. This is another area from the tumor, illustrated as an example of a small cell carcinoma of intermediate type. Such large-celled areas do not preclude the diagnosis of small cell carcinoma, but they may pose problems when a diagnosis is based on small biopsy specimens (hematoxylin and eosin, original magnification ×320). (From Smith JF. *The management of lung cancer*. London: Edward Arnold, 1984, with permission.)

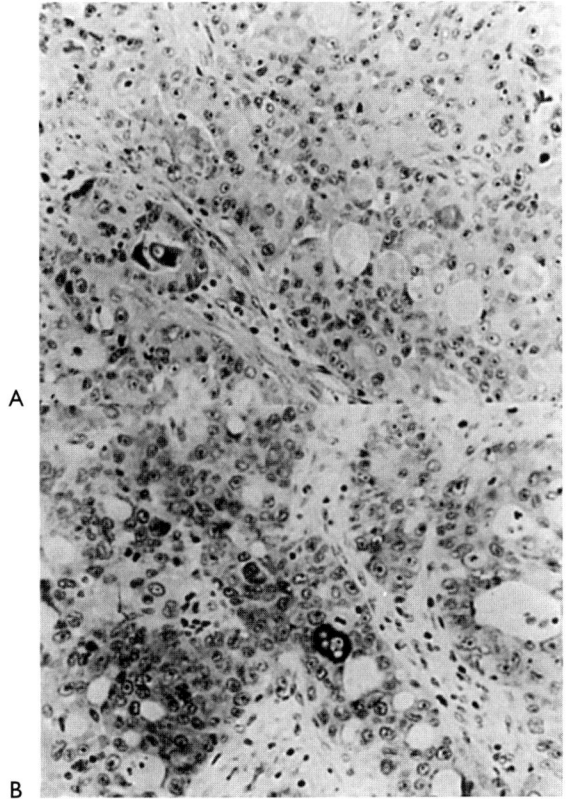

FIGURE 39.13. Photomicrographs of a large-celled anaplastic carcinoma with mucin production. **A:** Most of the mucin was cytoplasmic or in pools, as shown by periodic acid-Schiff staining after diastase digestion. No clear ductal structures or acini were formed. **B:** The same tumor stained immunocytochemically for keratin. Most cells contained keratin-like immunoreactive material, and occasional mononuclear and multinucleated cells were strongly positive (original magnification ×250). (From Carter RL. *Precancerous states*. New York: Oxford University Press, 1984, with permission.)

In recent years, the entity of large cell neuroendocrine carcinoma (LCNEC) has been the focus of considerable interest. It has been recognized that tumors that are otherwise typically squamous cell carcinomas, adenocarcinomas, or large cell carcinomas may show evidence of neuroendocrine differentiation when scrutinized with the electron microscope or through modern immunostaining. LCNECs cannot be distinguished from large cell carcinomas without the use of these special techniques. The prognostic significance of this entity remains controversial. Some evidence indicates that they may respond better to chemotherapy than other large cell carcinomas, although this remains speculative at present.

Large cell carcinomas tend to occur as bulky tumors, most often in the periphery of the lung. They usually present as solitary masses, with associated necrosis but no cavitation. These tumors tend to metastasize widely, in a fashion similar to that of adenocarcinomas.

Small Cell Carcinoma

Small cell carcinomas have consistently comprised 18% to 20% of all lung cancers during the past quarter century (69). The molecular biology of SCLC is quite distinct from that of NSCLC (198).

The very strong association between SCLC and cigarette smoking has been recognized for more than half a century. SCLC tends to occur most frequently in current heavy cigarette smokers; in one case control study, 97 (99%) of 98 patients with SCLC were cigarette smokers and were most likely to be current and heavy smokers. The odds ratios were 109 (95% CI, 15–801) for ever-smokers, 290 (95% CI, 37–2,102) for current smokers, and 31 (95% CI, 4–241) for former smokers. The risk for SCLC rose steeply with the number of pack-years of smoking and decreased greatly as the duration of smoking cessation increased (199). A rise in SCLC among young women who are heavy smokers has also been reported (200,201).

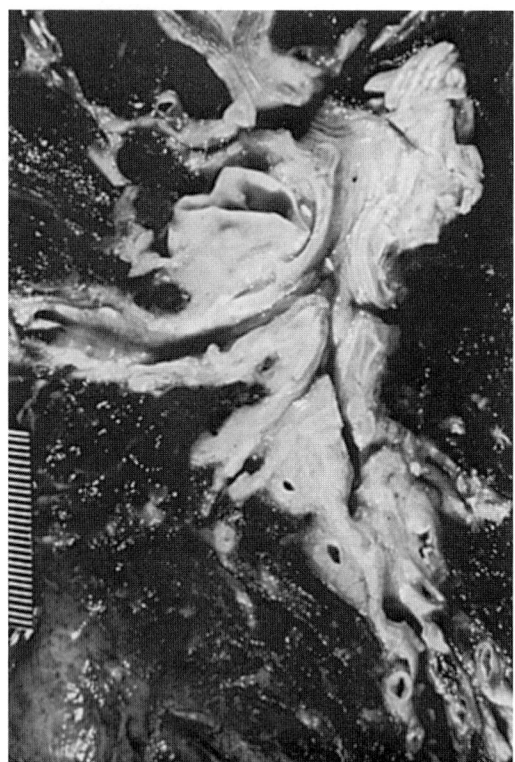

FIGURE 39.14. Small cell anaplastic carcinoma arising in the distal portion of the right intermediate bronchus and extending both proximally and distally along the bronchial vascular rays. Although small in mass, this tumor was responsible for widespread metastases that caused inappropriate secretion of adrenocorticotropic hormone, adrenal cortical hyperplasia, and death from severe, intractable hypokalemia. (From Morgan WKC, Hales MR. Bronchogenic carcinoma. In: Baum GL, Wolinsky E, eds. *Textbook of pulmonary diseases*, 3rd ed. Boston: Little, Brown and Company, 1983, with permission.)

Most SCLCs are located centrally, arising in the peribronchial tissues and infiltrating the bronchial submucosa (Fig. 39.14). They are believed to arise from basal neuroendocrine Kulchitsky cells. However, SCLCs can also arise in the periphery of the lung. SCLC is not known to have a preinvasive phase of carcinoma in situ.

SCLC disseminates early and widely into regional lymph nodes; it is the most common cause of superior vena cava syndrome in adults. It behaves much more aggressively than other lung cancers, with more rapid growth and early dissemination.

SCLC is characterized by a proliferation of highly malignant cells with scant cytoplasm, ill-defined cell borders, finely granular nuclear chromatin, and absent or inconspicuous nucleoli. The nuclei of the cells mold or conform to the cytoplasm of adjacent cells in well-preserved specimens. However, extensive smearing of the fine chromatin of these delicate cells often produces a characteristic "crush" artifact in poorly preserved specimens. Necrosis is common, as are mitotic figures; the average is 60 to 70 mitoses per 10 high-power fields. SCLCs tend to grow in sheets without a specific pattern.

In the past, SCLCs were subdivided into a classic "oat cell" subtype and an intermediate cell type. However, this subclassification has been dropped because of a lack of reproducibility and also a lack of clinical significance of the distinction. The previous category of mixed small cell/large cell has also been deleted.

The only small cell variant that has been retained in the most recent WHO classification is combined small cell carcinoma. This is defined as a mixture of small cell carcinoma and a non–small cell component, including LCNEC.

Spectrum of Neuroendocrine Tumors

An association of SCLC with neuroendocrine differentiation has long been recognized. However, other neuroendocrine cancers arise within the lung. These include LCNEC, typical carcinoids, and atypical carcinoids.

The WHO considered placing neuroendocrine tumors together in the most recent classification. However, because of differences in clinical, epidemiologic, histologic, and molecular characteristics, small cell carcinomas are distinguished from LCNECs and carcinoid tumors within the current WHO classification (Table 39.15). For example, approximately 20% to 40% of typical and atypical carcinoids occur in lifelong nonsmokers, whereas almost all SCLCs and LCNECs occur in cigarette smokers (195).

What most clearly distinguishes SCLCs from carcinoid tumors is their mitotic rate. Typical carcinoids are defined as carcinoid tumors that contain fewer than two mitoses per 10 high-power fields and lack necrosis. Atypical carcinoids are those with between two and 10 mitoses per 10 high-power fields, often in association with punctate necrosis.

A count of 11 or more mitoses per 10 high-power fields is the primary factor that separates SCLCs and LCNECs from atypical carcinoid tumors (195). Clinically, these entities have little in common. Patients with bronchial carcinoids, including atypical carcinoids, have a highly favorable prognosis when treated with complete surgical resection. On the other hand, as is discussed later, SCLC generally has an unfavorable prognosis and is treated primarily with chemotherapy and radiation (see section "Small Cell Lung Cancer").

PROGNOSTIC FACTORS IN NON–SMALL CELL CARCINOMA

The anatomic extent of the cancer, reflected by stage of disease, is the most powerful determinant of the prognosis in lung cancer, particularly in NSCLC. Indeed, the objective of cancer staging is to provide a prognostically useful classification based on the anatomic distribution of disease. Patients with resectable stage I or II NSCLC have a better prognosis than do those with more advanced disease. The significance of most of the nonanatomic determinants of prognosis is dwarfed when considered in the context of distant metastases because stage IV NSCLC is invariably fatal.

Nonetheless, a variety of clinical and pathologic factors can significantly contribute to a prognostic assessment, particularly in patients with resectable disease. Moreover, numerous biologic or molecular markers of prognosis have been identified in recent years. Because a substantial proportion of patients with resectable NSCLC have biologically virulent cancers, prognostic factors can be very useful in assessing the outcome of patients with early-stage disease.

Performance Status and Weight Loss

Although many clinical factors have been reported to be predictive of outcome in lung cancer, the two most important and consistently reported variables are weight loss and performance status (202). It has long been established that a poor performance status predicts a short survival in patients with localized NSCLC (203). Relatively recent reports support the prognostic importance of performance status even in early-stage NSCLC (204,205). In a multivariate analysis of 651 patients, weight loss and poor performance status were significant indicators of an adverse outcome independent of stage, histology, and treatment (206).

Symptomatic Disease

As previously discussed in detail (see section "Screening for Lung Cancer"), screening for lung cancer is not recommended by any public policy organization (207–209). In 1980, the ACS changed a prior recommendation in support of screening when it declared that it "does not recommend any test for the early detection of cancer of the lung, but urges a focus on primary prevention." Because screening for lung cancer is not widely practiced, the vast majority of patients present with symptomatic disease. Unfortunately, when patients present with "signs or symptoms of lung cancer," 85% to 90% already have advanced-stage disease. In one population-based series of 1,539 patients, only 2% were asymptomatic (210). Moreover, 90% to 95% of patients who present with symptomatic lung cancer are destined to die of it, usually within 2 years after the diagnosis (211).

For example, only 6% of 678 lung cancer patients presenting to the Yale–New Haven Hospital or the West Haven Veterans Administration Hospital were asymptomatic at the time of diagnosis. In contrast, 27% of patients had symptoms directly related to the primary tumor, 32% had symptoms of metastatic disease, and 34% had systemic symptoms of cancer (212). The 5-year survival rates of these three groups of symptomatic patients were 12%, 6%, and 0, respectively. In the asymptomatic group, the 5-year survival was 18%. The 5-year survival for the entire group was 7%.

Similarly, only 12% of 702 patients from the Medical University Hospital and the Veterans Administration Hospital in Charleston, South Carolina, were asymptomatic at the time of diagnosis (213). In contrast, 64% of patients presented with cough, 55% with weight loss, 53% with pain, and 44% with sputum production. As in the Yale series, the 5-year survival of the entire group was 7%.

A more recent report from Uppsala, Sweden, indicated the adverse prognostic importance of symptoms at presentation in lung cancer (214). Of 244 lung cancers detected, 28 (11%) were detected by routine CXR, 31 (13%) were found accidentally in asymptomatic persons, and 185 (76%) were detected on the basis of symptoms. The resectability rates of cases detected by routine CXR, by accident, and by symptomatic presentation were 75%, 74%, and 20%, respectively. Most importantly, the 4-year survival for patients whose disease was diagnosed by routine CXR was 39%; for those with an accidental asymptomatic presentation, it was 33%, and for those with a symptomatic presentation, it was 7%. Similarly, in a study of 506 patients with lung cancer diagnosed at Tampere University Hospital in Finland between 1983 and 1987, there were almost no long-term survivors among those with a symptomatic presentation (215).

Lymph Node Involvement

The critical importance of regional node involvement in NSCLC was recognized in the development of the international staging system (ISS), which was introduced for NSCLC in 1986 and modified in 1997. This is discussed in much greater detail later (see section "Staging of Lung Cancer") (216–219). In this system, the classification of disease in stages IIA, IIB, IIIA, and IIIB depends largely on the presence or absence of nodal involvement at specific sites.

The prognostic significance of the level and extent of nodal involvement in NSCLC has led to the development of a thoracic lymph node map (220) (Fig. 39.15). Tumor involvement of specific nodal stations has been shown to have great prognostic significance.

In stage I disease, the regional nodes are not involved. In stage II disease, involvement is limited to the ipsilateral intrapulmonary (hilar, peribronchial, or lobar) nodes. Stage IIIA is defined by the involvement of ipsilateral mediastinal nodes or subcarinal lymph nodes. In stage IIIB disease, contralateral mediastinal or hilar nodes or ipsilateral or contralateral supraclavicular nodes are affected.

Among patients with stage IIIA or IIIB disease, the location of the involved nodal groups may be of prognostic significance. In one Japanese study, patients with resected right-sided lung cancers had a worse prognosis if involved N2 nodes included superior mediastinal nodes as opposed to inferior mediastinal nodes (221). In contrast, for patients with left-sided tumors, the involvement of inferior mediastinal nodes carried a worse prognosis. Patients with single-level mediastinal nodal involvement did better than those with multiple-level metastases.

In addition to the location of involved nodes, the size and number of involved nodes have been shown to be important prognostically. Moreover, extracapsular extension beyond involved nodes is of adverse prognostic significance.

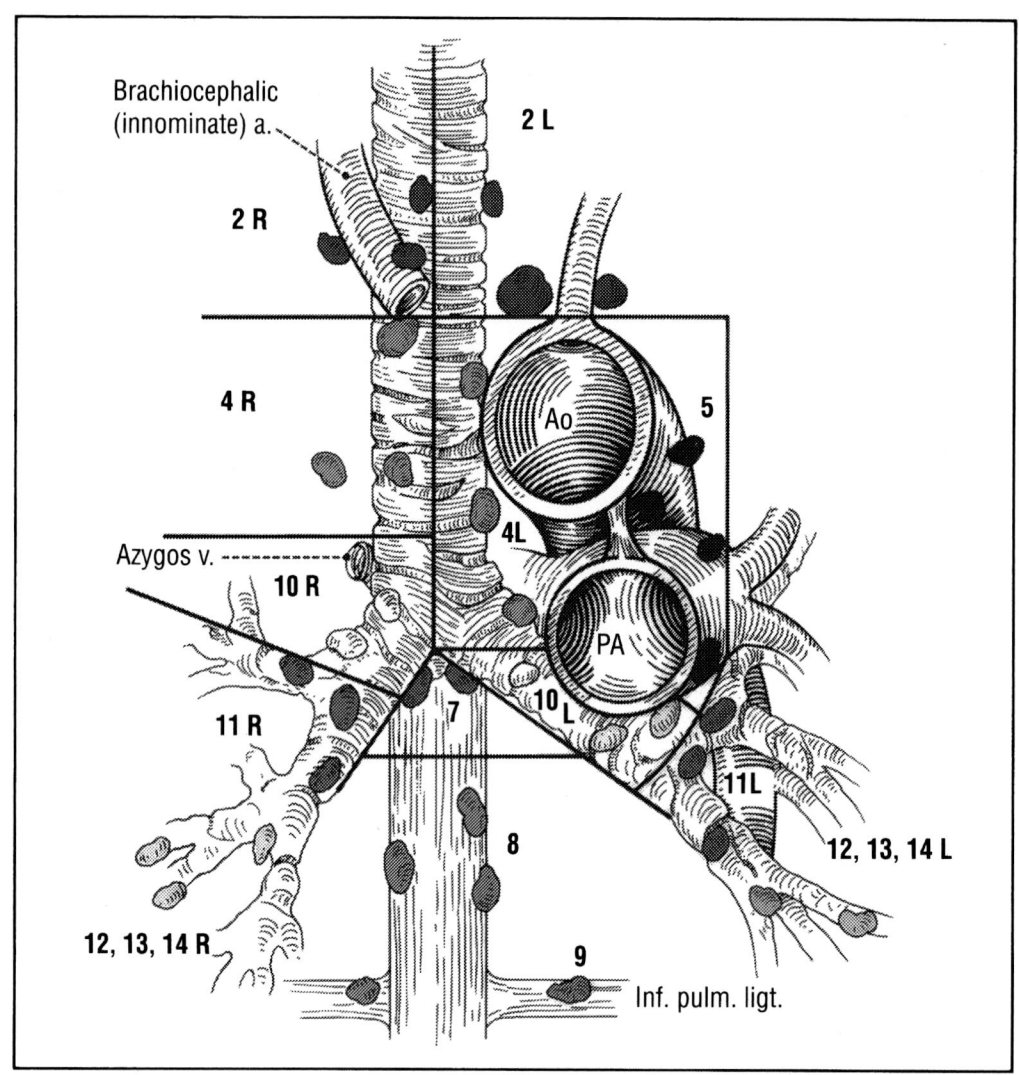

FIGURE 39.15. Classification of mediastinal lymph nodes. (From the Lung Cancer Study Group, courtesy of Bristol-Myers Squibb, with permission.)

For patients with stage II NSCLC, the number or location of involved N1 nodes has also been reported to be a significant determinant of outcome. At the Memorial Sloan-Kettering Cancer Center, the overall 5-year survival was reported to be 39% in stage II NSCLC, although the number of involved N1 lymph nodes was an important predictor of survival (222). In a Japanese series, the overall 5-year survival was 49% in stage II disease (223). However, survival was 65% among patients whose N1 involvement was limited to lobar nodes, but only 40% when hilar nodes were involved ($P = .014$).

Tumor Size

Tumor size has consistently been shown to be an important determinant of outcome in stage I NSCLC. In 10 studies of pathologic stage I NSCLC, a T1 tumor was associated with better survival than a T2 tumor (205,216,224–231) (Table 39.16). Survival among patients with T1 N0 tumors varied from 64% to 85%. Among those with T2 N0 tumors, the variability was greater, with survival ranging from 36% to 68%. Moreover, the magnitude of the differences in survival between T1 or T2 subsets in individual studies varied fairly widely, from 8% to 38%. The survival advantage for patients with T1 tumors was significant in each of the seven studies in which statistical significance was reported.

Despite the consistency of the finding that tumor size is an important prognostic factor, T status may not be a predominant prognostic factor in stage I NSCLC. For example, in one study of 151 patients with stage I disease, a T2 tumor was a highly adverse predictor of survival in univariate analysis ($P = .012$) (228). However, when multivariate analysis was performed to evaluate the relative importance of tumor size and other biomarkers, the predominant factors were found

TABLE 39.16. PROGNOSTIC SIGNIFICANCE OF TUMOR SIZE IN SURGICAL-PATHOLOGICAL STAGE I NON–SMALL CELL LUNG CANCER

Authors	Total No.	Stage IA or T1 Tumor			Stage IB or T2 Tumor			P Value
		No.	Percentage	Years	No.	Percentage	Years	
Mountain	865	429	68%	5 y OS	436	59%	5 y OS	<.01
Naruke	653	281	73%	5 y OS	372	52%	5 y OS	<.01
Gail	392	NR	77%	NR	NR	65%	NR	.004
Pairolero	328	170	70%	5 y DFS	158	58%	5 y DFS	.012
Martini	598	291	82%	5 y OS	307	68%	5 y OS	.009
Ichinose	151	71	85%	5 y OS	80	67%	5 y OS	.012
Harpole	289	173	70%	5 y OS	116	50%	5 y OS	<.001
Lafitte	204	NR	74%	5 y OS	NR	36%	5 y OS	NR
Immerman	77	39	64%	5 y DFS	38	45%	5 y DFS	NR
Van Rens	1,249	416	63%	5 y OS	833	46%	5 y OS	<.0001

DFS, disease-free survival; NR, not reported; OS, overall survival.

to be degree of tumor differentiation (well vs. moderate or poorly differentiated) and DNA ploidy (diploid vs. aneuploid). In multivariate analysis, the T status was no longer a significant determinant of survival ($P = .39$).

Among patients with stage II and III NSCLC, tumor size has not consistently been an important prognostic variable. In a study from Memorial Sloan-Kettering, patients with tumors less than 3 cm in diameter had a significantly better survival than those with tumors more than 5 cm in diameter. In general, once the tumor has progressed beyond the primary site, the presence or absence of nodal or distant metastases is the major determinant of survival, not the size of the primary tumor (232).

Histologic Subtype

Six reports on the prognostic importance of histologic subtype in resectable NSCLC have provided conflicting information with regard to survival implications. In two reports from the Lung Cancer Study Group (LCSG), squamous cell carcinoma appeared to be associated with a better outcome than other histologic subtypes. In one series of 392 patients with stage I disease, the long-term survival was 77% for those with squamous cell carcinoma and 66% for those with adenocarcinoma or large cell carcinoma ($P = .014$) (225). Similarly, among 572 patients with T1 N0 lesions, the recurrence rate was 12% in those with squamous cell carcinoma and 26% in those with adenocarcinoma, large cell carcinoma, or bronchoalveolar cell carcinoma (233). When only squamous cell carcinoma and adenocarcinoma were compared, the probability of recurrence was significantly lower in those with squamous cell carcinoma ($P < .001$).

On the other hand, studies from the Mayo Clinic (226), Memorial Sloan-Kettering (227), Duke University (205), and Japan (228) reported no significant differences in survival based on histologic subtypes of NSCLC. In the Japanese series, 5-year survival trends favored those who had nonsqua-

mous histologies in comparison with those who had squamous cell carcinoma (71% vs. 77%, $P = .076$) (228).

Tumor Differentiation

The data on the prognostic significance of the degree of tumor differentiation are conflicting. In a report from Johns Hopkins, a lack of tumor differentiation was associated with a 5-year survival of 24%, in comparison with 42% for tumors that were better differentiated (234). Similarly, a Japanese study of resected adenocarcinomas of the lung less than 2 cm in diameter reported that the 5-year survival was 78% for those with well-differentiated tumors, 54% for those with moderately differentiated tumors, and 28% for those with poorly differentiated tumors ($P = .001$) (235). In another Japanese study of stage I NSCLC, the 5-year survival among patients with well-differentiated tumors was significantly superior (83%) to the survival of those with moderately differentiated (72%) or poorly differentiated (76%) tumors (228). Survival of those with well differentiated tumors was significantly superior to survival in the other two groups ($P = .035$).

In contrast, a study from Duke University reported no significant differences in survival as a function of the degree of tumor differentiation (205). For tumors that were well, moderately, poorly, and not differentiated, the 5-year survival rates were 60%, 73%, 52%, and 58%, respectively.

Molecular Genetic Markers

During the past decade, advances in molecular biology have provided important information about many molecular genetic markers that are potentially significant determinants of prognosis. These molecular genetic markers can be classified as *oncogenes* and *tumor suppressor genes*.

Oncogenes

Oncogenes are homologues of normal cellular genes in which a mutational change results in constitutive activation and gain of function. Dominant oncogenes such as K-*ras*, the epidermal growth factor receptor (EGFR) oncogene (*erb*-B1), HER-2/*neu*, and *bcl*-2 lead to cellular hyperproliferation by overdriving normal cellular growth.

Expression of K-*ras* Oncogene and p21

The *ras* genes regulate signal transduction pathways that control cell growth and are expressed in virtually all mammalian cells. These genes encode a group of 21-kd proteins, known as *p21*, that are associated with the cell cytoplasmic surface. Mutations at or near the guanosine triphosphate (GTP)–binding domain prevent the inactivation of GTP, thereby resulting in constitutive *ras* activation.

Almost all mutations in NSCLC affect the K-*ras* gene. In one report, K-*ras* mutations occurred exclusively in cancer patients, whereas p53 mutations were present in chronic smokers with no neoplasia (236). In most studies, *ras* mutations are predominantly associated with adenocarcinoma (237–239), although one report found a higher proportion of these mutations in patients with squamous cell carcinoma (240).

Activating mutations of the K-*ras* oncogene may represent an adverse prognostic factor in resectable NSCLC. In one series, a point mutation in the K-*ras* oncogene was noted in 29% of resected specimens (237), and these tumors tended to be smaller, more poorly differentiated, and associated with a significantly worse 3-year mortality rate (63% vs. 32%).

Activating mutations lead to overexpression of p21, the protein product of the *ras* oncogene. In one study, immunohistochemistry in 116 patients with resected NSCLC revealed p21 positivity in 72% of adenocarcinomas and 56% of squamous cell carcinomas (241). The 5-year survival rates among the negatively, moderately, and strongly immunostaining groups were 64%, 38%, and 11%, respectively. Several other series and a metaanalysis have noted a shorter survival in patients with resectable NSCLCs with K-*ras* mutations (240,242–244), but such findings have not been universal (239,245,246).

Expression of *erb*-B1 Oncogene and Epidermal Growth Factor Receptor

EGFR (*erb*-B1 or HER-1) belongs to a family of receptors that includes HER-2/*neu*, HER-3, and HER-4. EGFR is a 170-kd glycoprotein with ligands that include EGF, transforming growth factor-α, β-cellulin, and epiregulin. EGFR is overexpressed in a variety of solid tumors that include lung cancers, predominantly NSCLCs. In a review of multiple studies (247), 84% of squamous cell carcinomas, 65% of adenocarcinomas, and 68% of large cell carcinomas overexpressed EGFR, whereas no SCLC did. Overexpression of EGFR is associated with up-regulation of matrix metalloproteinase-9 (MMP-9), a molecule that regulates tumor invasiveness. It is also associated with other factors involved in cancer cell motility and adhesion. Lung cancers may produce ligands for EGFR that on binding lead to the autocrine and paracrine stimulation of premalignant and malignant cells.

In NSCLC, overexpression of EGFR has been correlated clinically with an advanced stage of disease and a poor prognosis in some but not all studies. In one review, a reduced survival was associated with EGFR expression in only three of nine studies (247). In a study of 121 patients, EGFR expression was associated with reduced survival (248). In a second report, EGFR expression was associated with reduced survival in 290 cases (249). A third study reported that coexpression of MMP-9 and EGFR conferred a poor prognosis in 169 patients with resected stages I through IIIA NSCLC (250). Thus, the adverse effect on prognosis may be small, if any.

Expression of HER-2/*neu* Oncogene and p185

The HER-2/*neu* oncogene encodes a growth factor receptor, p185, that is similar to EGFR (251,252). Overexpression of this protein is thought to confer a growth advantage to tumors and has been associated with an adverse outcome in NSCLC. In a review of multiple studies (253), 41% of adenocarcinomas, 28% of squamous cell carcinomas, and 21% of large cell carcinomas overexpressed p185, whereas none of the cases of SCLC overexpressed p185. In a report of 55 patients, those with adenocarcinoma that overexpressed HER-2/*neu* had a significantly poorer survival, whereas outcome was not affected in patients with squamous cell carcinoma (254). In a second series, 28% of adenocarcinomas overexpressed HER-2/*neu*, but only 2% of squamous cell carcinomas (255). HER-2/*neu* expression was associated with a markedly shorter 5-year survival (30% vs. 52%). Similar data have been reported by other investigators (256–258). In one of these reports, protein overexpression was seen predominantly in patients with node-positive squamous cell carcinomas, whereas it occurred in both node-positive and node-negative adenocarcinomas (256). A third study found that patients whose tumors had HER-2/*neu* tissue values above 350 U/mg had a significantly shorter mean survival (259). The prognostic importance appeared greatest in stage I tumors. However, not all studies associate inferior survival with overexpression of HER-2/*neu* (245).

bcl-2 Oncogene

The *bcl*-2 oncogene encodes a protein, Bcl-2, that suppresses programmed cell death (apoptosis), resulting in prolonged cellular survival in the absence of increased cellular proliferation (260). Positivity for *bcl*-2 has been reported in 22% to 56% of lung cancers (261–266), with a higher expression in squamous cell carcinomas than in adenocarcinomas (263–265).

The association of *bcl*-2 expression and prognosis in NSCLC is unclear. In at least three reports, patients with *bcl*-2–positive lung cancers had a better prognosis than those with *bcl*-2–negative tumors (263,265,266). As an example, in one series of 229 patients with stages I through IIIA NSCLC, the probability of 6-year relapse-free survival was significantly higher for patients whose tumors were *bcl*-2–positive (74% vs. 57%) (266). However, other studies failed to demonstrate a survival advantage with *bcl*-2 positivity (262,263).

Tumor Suppressor Genes

Tumor suppressor genes exert their effect by controlling cell growth. Once these oncogenes are deleted or their function is reduced, normal control mechanisms are inoperative. Examples include p53, the retinoblastoma (Rb) gene, p16INK4A, p15INK4B, and genes on chromosome 3p.

p53 Tumor Suppressor Gene

The p53 gene, located on chromosome 17, encodes a nuclear protein that acts as a transcription factor, blocking the cell cycle late in the G_1 phase. It plays a central role in regulating transcription in the nucleus, particularly in response to DNA-damaging agents such as ionizing radiation and other carcinogens. This has led to its description as the "guardian of the genome" (267).

Deletions and point mutations in the p53 gene lead to a loss of inhibition of proliferation. Thus, p53 appears to function as a tumor suppressor gene. Some p53 mutant proteins also display transforming properties by binding and inactivating available wild-type (normal) p53 protein. The Li-Fraumeni syndrome, in which multiple tumors develop at an early age, is characterized by an inherited germ-line mutation of p53. Soft tissue sarcomas, osteosarcomas, leukemias, brain tumors, adrenocortical malignancies, and early-onset breast cancer develop in affected patients; some form of cancer develops in 50% of carriers by age 30, and in 90% by age 70 (268).

Mutations of p53 are the most common genetic abnormality associated with lung cancer. Mutations occur in approximately 60% of all cases of NSCLC and are more common in squamous cell carcinomas than in adenocarcinomas (269). Loss of heterozygosity (deletion of genetic material from one 17p allele) also occurs in the bronchial tissue of approximately 20% of smokers, possibly identifying a population at high risk for the development of malignancy (270,271). A faulty capacity of DNA to repair tobacco carcinogen–induced damage appears to increase the susceptibility to lung cancer in chronic smokers (272).

The association of p53 mutations with survival in NSCLC is unclear. Abnormalities of p53, in terms of both genetic mutations and protein expression as analyzed by immunohistochemistry, have been reported. Multiple studies in which immunohistochemistry was used as a determinant of p53 status have come to divergent conclusions. One study evaluated p53 abnormalities, both genetic mutations and protein overexpression, in 85 patients with resected NSCLC (273). Overexpression of p53 was detected by immunohistochemistry in 55%, and mutations were noted in 54%, with concordance in only 65% of cases. Overexpression of p53, but not the presence of p53 mutations, was associated with reduced survival. Similar findings have been reported by other investigators (274,275). Contrasting results

were noted in a series of 156 patients with resected NSCLC, 32% of whom had p53 positivity by immunohistochemistry (276). The median survival in the strongly staining group was 65 months, compared with 26 to 33 months in those with weak or no staining. Other reports have found no overall association between p53 expression by immunohistochemistry and survival (245,277–279). However, in one study, p53 expression in 100 patients with adenocarcinoma was associated with worse survival, whereas a survival trend suggesting a better outcome was noted in 88 patients with squamous cell carcinoma (280).

Studies of the prognostic significance of p53 mutations, measured by the polymerase chain reaction, have also resulted in conflicting data. Two studies found no significant association between genetic mutations and survival in NSCLC (245,273). In contrast, a separate report of 120 patients with resected NSCLC identified mutations in 43% of patients, who had a significantly worse 3-year survival than those without mutations (28% vs. 51%) (281).

Retinoblastoma Gene

The retinoblastoma (Rb) gene, located on chromosome 13, is involved in the pathogenesis of retinoblastoma and other solid tumors. The Rb gene encodes a nuclear protein with a tumor suppressor function that was determined by evaluating inheritance patterns in familial retinoblastoma (282). The Rb protein is an important regulator of the cell cycle; its activity depends on its phosphorylation status. Phosphorylation of Rb by cyclin-dependent kinases inactivates it and leads to cell cycle progression. Multiple cyclin-dependent kinase inhibitors have been identified, including p16INK4A, p15INK4B, and p21WAF1/CIP1.

Deletion of the Rb gene has been found in more than 90% of SCLCs and about 15% of NSCLCs. A loss of Rb protein expression is associated with poor prognosis in NSCLC (283,284). In one report, for example, a loss of Rb protein expression was identified in 24% of 101 patients who had undergone successful resection for early-stage NSCLC, and Rb-negative tumors were associated with a significantly shorter median survival (32 vs. 18 months) (283). However, not all studies have shown an association between a loss of Rb protein and a poor outcome (282–285).

Rb mutations may be synergistic with other molecular abnormalities in worsening the prognosis of patients with NSCLC. In one report, the outcome of patients with Rb-negative tumors was worse in the presence of coexisting p53 abnormalities (median survival of 12 months for $Rb^-/p53^+$ tumors vs. 41 months for $Rb^+/p53^-$ tumors) (284). Similar results have been noted in other reports (283,286).

p16INK4A and p15INK4B Genes

Up to 67% of cell lines derived from lung cancers have a characteristic deletion of chromosome 9p21, which implies the presence of one or more tumor suppressor genes in this region (287,288). Through genetic analysis, p16INK4A (p16) and p15INK4B (p15) have been mapped to within 30 kb of each other in this region (289). Both p16 and p15 are candidate tumor suppressor genes in malignancies that contain wild-type Rb protein (288). Both encode proteins that influence cell cycle regulation at the G_1 checkpoint by inhibiting cyclin-dependent kinase-4, thereby preventing progression. Loss of p16 by mutation, deletion, or aberrant promoter methylation (290) frees the cyclin-dependent kinases from inhibition and permits constitutive phosphorylation of Rb and inhibition of growth suppression. Rb-positive NSCLCs have little or no detectable p16 expression, whereas Rb-negative lung cancers have abundant p16 expression (291).

Loss of p16 expression is a common event in early stage NSCLC and correlates with a significantly worse survival (292,293), particularly in squamous cell carcinoma. However, not all reports document a correlation between abnormal p16 and outcome in patients with lung cancer (279,294).

Deletions of 3p

One of the most consistent chromosomal abnormalities in lung cancer is the loss of the short arm of chromosome 3 (3p14-25) (295). The loss of 3p alleles is observed in more than 90% of SCLCs and approximately 50% of NSCLCs (296). Tobacco smoke–induced DNA damage and smoking at an early age appear to induce a loss of chromosome 3p (297). The FHIT gene (for fragile histidine triad), which is involved in the accumulation of diadenosine tetraphosphate, thereby leading to DNA synthesis and proliferation, has been localized to 3p14.2 and is believed to be an important tumor suppressor gene involved in the pathogenesis of lung cancer (298,299). A second postulated tumor suppressor gene, located at 3p21.3, is RASSF1A, which is absent in all SCLCs tested and in 65% of NSCLCs (300,301).

CLINICAL PRESENTATION OF LUNG CANCER

As previously discussed (see section "Screening for Lung Cancer"), screening for lung cancer is neither recommended nor widely practiced. Accordingly, the vast majority of patients are symptomatic at the time of clinical presentation. In one population-based series of 1,539 lung cancer patients from New Hampshire and Vermont, only 28 (2%) were asymptomatic (210). Most asymptomatic patients present incidentally when CXR studies are performed for other reasons. The symptoms and signs of lung cancer are often generally categorized as being caused by local effects of the tumor, metastatic disease, or a paraneoplastic syndrome. Symptoms in the first and second categories are far more common than those in the third.

The most common symptom of lung cancer is cough, occurring in 45% to 75% of all patients (302). Although cough, often with sputum production, is extremely com-

mon, it is a nonspecific symptom because a high proportion of patients with lung cancer have preexisting emphysema or bronchitis, which is often associated with these same symptoms. However, a change in the character of a chronic cough should raise suspicion of a superimposed process.

Large amounts of watery sputum (bronchorrhea) are produced by about 15% of patients with bronchoalveolar cell carcinoma. Bronchoalveolar cell carcinoma is known to present occasionally with a CXR picture more suggestive of pneumonia than a lung tumor (diffuse form) (303). About one third of patients with the diffuse form of bronchoalveolar cell carcinoma present with the production of large quantities of foamy sputum. The infiltrate reflects the interalveolar spread of the tumor (304). Bronchorrhea is extremely rare in any other type of lung cancer.

Dyspnea occurs in about a third to a half of all patients with lung cancer. It is also a nonspecific symptom and may be related to underlying COPD. Shortness of breath in the context of lung cancer can be related to multiple factors, including obstruction of a large airway, obstructive pneumonitis or atelectasis, lymphangitic spread, pleural or pericardial effusion, and thromboembolic disease.

Hemoptysis has been reported in 27% to 57% of patients with lung cancer (302). It should be noted that bronchitis is the most common cause of hemoptysis. Of patients who present with hemoptysis, 19% to 29% have lung cancer. Usually, the volume of blood in the sputum tends to be small. In rare cases, erosion of a bronchial artery by tumor results in massive hemoptysis and death from asphyxiation.

Chest pain occurs in about one fourth to one half of all patients. Some patients have intermittent dull pain on the side of the tumor, which does not necessarily indicate invasion of adjacent structures or preclude resection. On the other hand, persistent severe pain often indicates chest wall or mediastinal invasion and locally advanced disease. Such pain is often associated with rib erosion.

Unilateral localized wheezing is uncommon, but when present, it should raise suspicion of an underlying bronchogenic carcinoma causing fixed obstruction of a major airway. Tracheal obstruction may produce stridor. These symptoms are usually associated with severe dyspnea.

Weight loss has been reported in 8% to 68% of patients with lung cancer. It may be a symptom of local or metastatic disease, or of a paraneoplastic syndrome. Almost all studies demonstrate that weight loss is a negative prognostic factor in lung cancer.

About 70% of patients with lung cancer present with symptoms of intrathoracic or extrathoracic metastases. Dyspnea caused by pleural effusion generally indicates pleural extension. Pericardial effusion can develop by direct extension of the tumor to the pericardium and epicardium.

Hoarseness in patients with lung cancer is most often caused by compression of the recurrent laryngeal nerve and has been reported in 2% to 18% of cases. It is more commonly associated with left-sided tumors because of the circuitous route of the left recurrent laryngeal nerve around the aortic arch.

Superior vena cava syndrome may result from either compression or direct invasion of the great veins of the thoracic inlet by mediastinal nodes or by the tumor itself. It is most often associated with small cell carcinoma. Symptoms of superior vena cava syndrome include headache or a sense of fullness in the head and dyspnea. Physical signs include swelling of the face or upper extremities, plethora, dilated neck veins, and a prominent venous pattern on the chest. In one series of 2,000 patients, 4% had superior vena cava syndrome (305).

Brachial plexopathy is often caused by tumors in the superior sulcus of the lung. Lung cancer presenting as a superior sulcus tumor was first described by Pancoast in 1924 (306). It is characterized by pain in the distribution of the C7, T1, and T2 nerve roots, a Horner syndrome (ptosis, meiosis, anhidrosis), rib destruction, and atrophy of the ipsilateral hand muscles (307).

The organs most commonly involved by distant metastases of lung cancer are the brain, bones, liver, adrenal glands, and skin. Lung cancer can metastasize to virtually any bone, although the vertebrae are most frequently involved. The ribs and pelvic bones are also very often involved. Symptoms include severe pain, which may have a pleuritic component when the ribs are involved. Hepatic metastases most often cause symptoms of weakness and weight loss and carry a very poor prognosis. Headache, nausea and vomiting, focal neurologic symptoms, seizures, confusion, and personality changes may all be manifestations of brain metastases. The lung is the primary site of approximately 70% of cancers that initially present with symptomatic brain metastases (308).

The third group of symptoms are those related to non-metastatic systemic manifestations of the tumor (paraneoplastic syndromes; see Chapter 42). Paraneoplastic syndromes are caused by the production of biologically active substances by the tumor or in response to tumor cells that have distant effects not directly related to tumor dissemination. Often, the mechanism is poorly understood. Overall, clinically significant paraneoplastic syndromes develop in about 10% to 20% of patients with bronchogenic carcinoma.

Some of the paraneoplastic phenomena are associated with specific histologic subtypes of cancer. Hypercalcemia is most strongly associated with squamous cell carcinoma, and digital clubbing and hypertrophic pulmonary osteoarthropathy with adenocarcinoma. Small cell carcinoma is most commonly associated with syndromes related to the ectopic production of hormones, including the syndrome of inappropriate (secretion of) antidiuretic hormone (SIADH) and Cushing syndrome secondary to tumor production of adrenocorticotropic hormone (ACTH). A variety of poorly understood neurologic syndromes also occur, including Eaton-Lambert syndrome (seen almost exclusively in SCLC), peripheral neuropathy, and cortical cerebellar degeneration.

ESTABLISHING THE DIAGNOSIS

Abnormal CXR findings usually prompt a diagnostic investigation for lung cancer (Figs. 39.16 and 39.17). A definitive diagnosis of cancer can be made only by an examination of tissue or exfoliated cells obtained from the tumor. Specific diagnostic techniques include sputum cytology, flexible fiberoptic bronchoscopy, pleural biopsy and fluid analysis, FNA, mediastinoscopy, and open thoracotomy. All patients undergoing a workup for lung cancer should have a CT of the thorax, with contrast when possible, to evaluate the mediastinum for staging purposes. Magnetic resonance imaging (MRI) of the chest (with gadolinium) should be performed if any question arises of invasion of blood vessels by the tumor. Proper staging requires that imaging of the head (CT, MRI) and bones (bone scan) be performed to rule out metastatic disease. An appropriate workup also includes full pulmonary function studies and a cardiac evaluation if symptoms or signs so warrant.

Computed Tomography of the Chest

The use of CT in the evaluation of hilar or mediastinal lymphadenopathy is controversial. CT is quite sensitive for imaging nodes larger than 1.0 cm; its sensitivity ranges from 64% to 79%, with a specificity of 62% to 66%. The false-negative rate is substantial; adenocarcinomas are associated with the highest false-negative rate. Thoracic CT is usually extended to include imaging of the liver, adrenals, kidneys, and upper abdominal lymph nodes because it is the

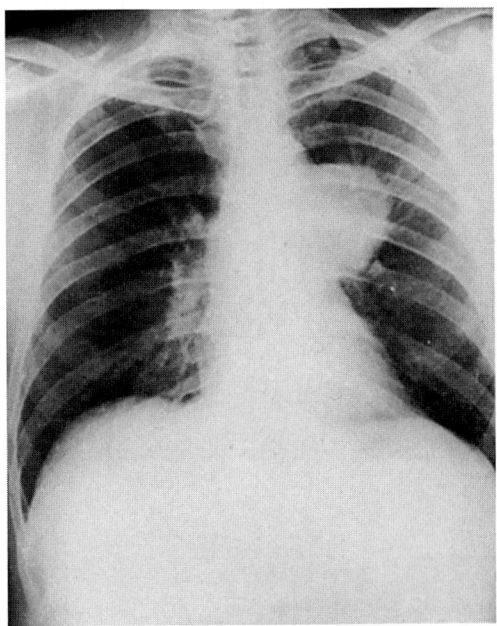

FIGURE 39.16. A large hilar mass caused by carcinoma of the lung. (From Morgan WKC, Hales MR. Bronchogenic carcinoma. In: Baum GL, Wolinsky E, eds. *Textbook of pulmonary diseases*, 3rd ed. Boston: Little, Brown and Company, 1983, with permission.)

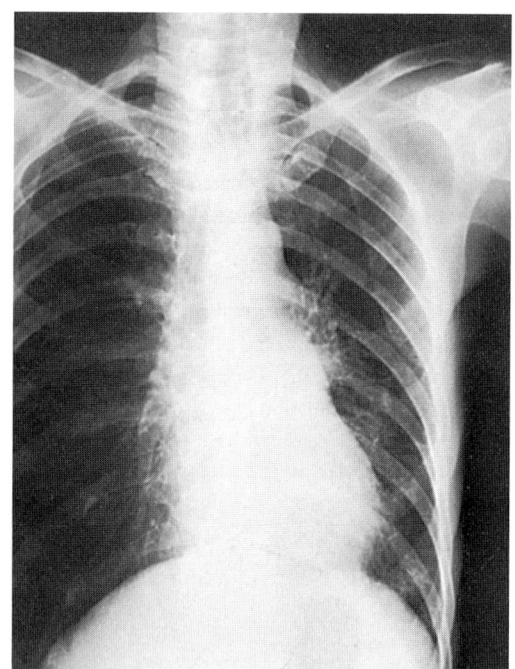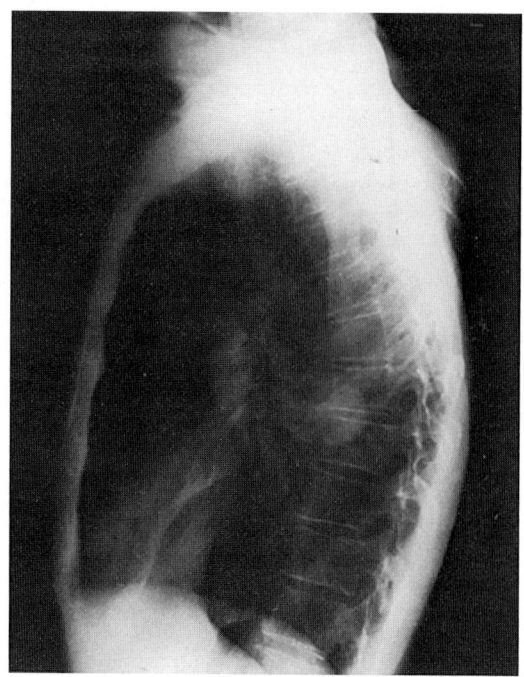

FIGURE 39.17. A: Carcinoma of the lung hidden behind the cardiac silhouette on a posteroanterior roentgenogram. **B:** Lateral view of the chest reveals the carcinoma. (From Morgan WKC, Hales MR. Bronchogenic carcinoma. In: Baum GL, Wolinsky E, eds. *Textbook of pulmonary diseases*, 3rd ed. Boston: Little, Brown and Company, 1983, with permission.)

most effective tool for delineating metastatic disease at these sites.

Sputum Cytology

A specific diagnosis of cancer can be made in approximately 80% of central lesions by cytologic analysis of freshly expectorated and appropriately prepared sputum (Fig. 39.18). A specific cell type can be identified 85% to 95% of the time if malignant cells are seen.

Flexible Fiberoptic Bronchoscopy

Fiberoptic bronchoscopy is a well-tolerated technique that can visualize the central tracheobronchial tree and makes it possible to obtain brushings, washings, and biopsy specimens from any visible lesion. If bronchoscopy is performed under fluoroscopic guidance, more peripheral lesions can be sampled. The diagnostic yield is above 90% when six to 10 biopsy specimens of endoscopically visible carcinomas are obtained. The diagnostic yield of unvisualized peripheral lesions is about 60% if a combination of biopsy and

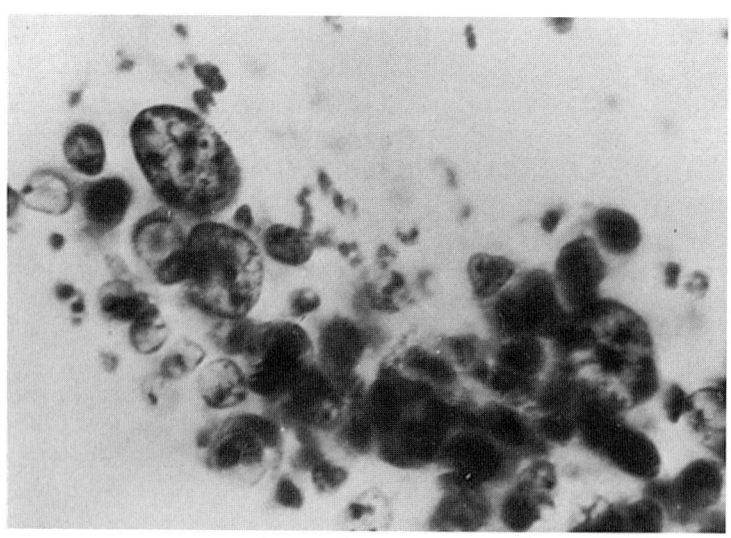

FIGURE 39.18. Photomicrograph of bronchial washings stained by the Papanicolaou technique showing malignant cells. Note the hyperchromatic nuclei with irregularly placed chromatin particles (original magnification ×900). (From Morgan WKC, Hales MR. Bronchogenic carcinoma. In: Baum GL, Wolinsky E, eds. *Textbook of pulmonary diseases*, 3rd ed. Boston: Little, Brown and Company, 1983, with permission.)

brushing is performed. In addition, bronchoscopy is a staging procedure that can exclude contralateral endobronchial (M status) lesions and define the proximal extent of an endobronchial lesion in relation to the main bronchi and trachea (T status). Transtracheal and transbronchial thin needle aspirations (Wang procedure) can be performed to evaluate the paratracheal, precarinal, and subcarinal nodes (N status).

Analysis of Pleural Fluid and Pleural Biopsy Specimens

When a patient has suspected or documented lung cancer and a pleural effusion, analysis of the fluid and a pleural biopsy specimen is also required, either to make the initial diagnosis or to help define the stage. The cytologic accuracy of pleural fluid examinations in the diagnosis of malignant pleural effusion varies from 40% to 87%, depending on the tumor cell type. The accuracy can be increased by examining at least three independently obtained samples. Cytopathologic analysis of both pleural fluid cell blocks and smears should be performed.

Biopsy of the pleura is indicated whenever the cytology of an exudative pleural effusion is nondiagnostic. The specimen will be positive for malignancy 39% to 75% of the time. Analysis of pleural fluid provides a diagnosis of malignancy more often than pleural biopsy.

The presence of a malignant pleural effusion automatically classifies a patient as having an unresectable T4 lesion. Not all malignant effusions reflect pleural involvement by tumor. If the analysis of multiple pleural fluid and tissue samples is nondiagnostic and the fluid is exudative, a thoracoscopic examination of the pleural surface should be performed to help make a diagnosis and stage the patient. A transudative, nonbloody effusion should not be considered in the determination of stage if the result of the cytopathologic examination is negative.

Fine Needle Aspiration

FNA is usually performed transthoracically with CT used to guide placement of the needle within the lesion. The yield from a percutaneous approach is generally higher than the yield from fiberoptic bronchoscopy because placement of the needle within the lesion is much more reliable by a percutaneous approach than placement of a brush or biopsy forceps by an endobronchial approach. The diagnostic yield from percutaneous needle aspiration has been reported to range from 43% to 97% (309).

FNA is more likely to provide a diagnosis than bronchoscopy, particularly when the primary lesion is less than 2 cm in diameter. In this situation, FNA yields a positive diagnosis in more than 60% of malignant lesions. FNA generally involves the aspiration of material for cytology rather than removal of a core of tissue, so that diagnoses other than

malignancy, and especially a specific benign diagnosis, often cannot be made (309).

Transthoracic needle biopsy has become a frequently used method for obtaining tissue for the diagnosis of pulmonary lesions. Berquist and colleagues (310) reported the results from 430 patients who underwent lung FNA from 1968 through 1977 to determine the accuracy and complications of this procedure. A malignant lesion was identified in all but 10 patients. Sufficient tissue for diagnosis was obtained in 82% of cases. The diagnostic yield diminished significantly in the case of central lesions less than 2 cm in size. The most common complications of the procedure were pneumothorax (25%–35%) and minor hemoptysis (1%–10%).

Positron Emission Tomography

Positron emission tomography (PET) is a newer technique that assesses metabolic activity and has been found helpful in predicting the probability of malignancy in a solitary pulmonary nodule (311). Clinical experience with PET remains limited, and its optimal role in the evaluation of pulmonary nodules remains to be defined.

PET for lung cancer commonly uses [^{18}F]fluoro-2-deoxyglucose (^{18}F-FDG). ^{18}F-FDG accumulates rapidly within tumor cells because they take up glucose more rapidly than normal tissue does. Deoxyglucose cannot be metabolized further. It is important to understand that acute hyperglycemia and high levels of glucose can impede ^{18}F-FDG uptake into tumors (312,313).

A number of studies have examined the ability of PET with ^{18}F-FDG to determine whether a solitary pulmonary nodule is a malignant or benign process. Most studies report that the sensitivity of PET is in the range of 95% to 98%, and the specificity is approximately 70% to 78% for detecting malignancy in this setting. The false-negative rate is approximately 8%, and false-negative results are often related to small tumor size, the relatively low level of metabolic activity characteristic of some tumors (e.g., bronchioloalveolar carcinoma, carcinoids), or uncontrolled hyperglycemia. False-positive results can occur in the setting of active infectious or inflammatory processes.

Mediastinoscopy/Anterior Mediastinotomy (Chamberlain Procedure)

These invasive surgical procedures are the most accurate methods for staging the mediastinum and identifying patients with unresectable disease. Contralateral nodal involvement, extranodal extension of cancer, high paratracheal involvement, and a cell type not amenable to surgery (small cell) can all be identified with these techniques. As previously mentioned, many centers use CT as a screening tool to assess the mediastinum before deciding whether to perform a staging surgical procedure.

Lymph nodes larger than 1.0 cm in the short axis are considered abnormal and require sampling by mediastinoscopy.

Patients with an abnormal mediastinum on chest CT should undergo mediastinoscopy or anterior mediastinotomy to obtain tissue to document the presence of malignancy before definitive surgical resection is undertaken. Cervical mediastinoscopy permits direct imaging and sampling of the paratracheal, tracheobronchial, and anterior subcarinal lymph nodes. Anterior mediastinotomy and extended cervical mediastinoscopy allow an assessment of the aortopulmonary window and anterior mediastinal nodes. Mediastinoscopy excludes 30% to 40% of patients initially thought to have surgically resectable tumors by thoracotomy.

Direct Lymph Node Biopsy

Palpable cervical or scalene lymph nodes in the setting of suspected lung cancer should be sampled. Evidence of metastasis usually precludes thoracotomy. In patients with documented lung cancer and palpable scalene nodes, results of biopsy have been positive in 83% of cases; only 20% of nonpalpable nodes were positive for malignancy after biopsy (28).

Thoracotomy

Surgical exploration of the chest is the gold standard for determining the final T and N status of the cancer and permits decision making regarding the surgical procedure required. Thoracotomy should be performed in any patient with a normal mediastinum on CT. All lymph node stations not sampled during mediastinoscopy should be assessed at thoracotomy regardless of the appearance on CT. Samples of nodes from the superior mediastinum and subcarinal, subaortic, peribronchial, and intrapulmonary nodes adjacent to the planned site of bronchial resection should be obtained. The N status often can be determined only at this time.

STAGING OF LUNG CANCER

Once the diagnosis of lung cancer has been established, an assessment of the extent of disease by surgical-pathologic staging provides a basis for determining the appropriate therapy. A TNM (tumor-node-metastasis) staging system for lung cancer has been in use for more than two decades, mainly for NSCLC.

Although the optimal staging of SCLC remains uncertain, a simple two-stage system dividing patients according to whether they have "limited" or "extensive" disease has been widely used. Limited disease either is confined to the hemithorax of origin or may be encompassed within a single radiation portal. Extensive disease has spread beyond the hemithorax of origin.

In regard to NSCLC, the ISS for lung cancer was introduced by Mountain in 1986 and revised in 1997 (216–218). This staging system was subsequently adopted by the American Joint Committee on Cancer. It is based on the principle

TABLE 39.17. INTERNATIONAL STAGING SYSTEM FOR LUNG CANCER

Primary tumor (T)

T1	Tumor < 3 cm in diameter without invasion more proximal than lobar bronchus
T2	Tumor > 3 cm in diameter, or tumor of any size with any of the following:
	Invades visceral pleura
	Atelectasis of less than entire lung
	Proximal extent at least 2 cm from carina
T3	Tumor of any size with any of the following:
	Invasion of chest wall
	Involvement of diaphragm, mediastinal pleura, or pericardium
	Atelectasis involving entire lung
	Proximal extent within 2 cm of carina
T4	Tumor of any size with any of the following:
	Invasion of mediastinum
	Invasion of heart or great vessels
	Invasion of trachea or esophagus
	Invasion of vertebral body or carina
	Presence of malignant pleural effusion

Nodal involvement (N)

N0	No regional node involvement
N1	Metastasis to ipsilateral hilar nodes
N2	Metastasis to ipsilateral mediastinal or subcarinal nodes
N3	Metastasis to contralateral mediastinal or hilar nodes, or ipsilateral or contralateral supraclavicular nodes

Metastases (M)

M0	Distant metastases absent
M1	Distant metastases present

Stage groupings of TNM subsets

Stage IA	T1 N0 M0
Stage IB	T2 N0 M0
Stage IIA	T1 N1 M0
Stage IIB	T2 N1 M0 or T3 N0 M0
Stage IIIA	T3 N1 M0
	T1–3 N2 M0
Stage IIIB	Any T N3 M0
	T4 any N M0
Stage IV	Any T, any N, M1

Source: Based on Mountain CE. Revisions in the international system for staging lung cancer. *Chest* 1997;111:1710–1717, with permission.

of TNM classification and includes seven stage groupings (Table 39.17).

The stage is a highly significant determinant of prognosis in lung cancer (Fig. 39.19). The T stage is a highly significant determinant of survival in patients who undergo resection (314) (Fig. 39.20). However, the most important survival determinant is the presence or absence of distant metastases (Fig. 39.21).

In stages I, II, and IIIA NSCLC, the stages in which resection is a therapeutic option, the prognosis is better when surgical-pathologic staging (pTNM) is performed rather than clinical staging (cTNM) alone (219) (Fig. 39.22). This is because a significant proportion of patients are found to be understaged at surgery despite an extensive preoperative effort.

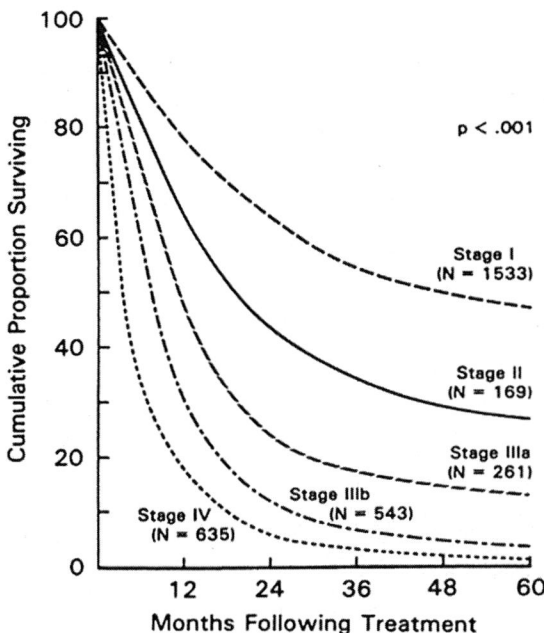

FIGURE 39.19. Cumulative proportion of patients surviving 5 years by clinical stage of disease.

Stage I (T1 N0 or T2 N0) disease is local disease without regional node involvement. In stage II (T1 N1 or T2 N1) disease, regional lymph node involvement is limited to nodes within the substance of the lung itself (peribronchial, lobar, hilar nodes). The current standard of therapy for stages I and II NSCLC is surgical resection. Based on the 1997 modification of the ISS, T3 N0 M0 is characterized as stage IIB disease.

Stage III comprises regionally advanced disease and is subdivided into stage IIIA and stage IIIB. Stage IIIA disease is regionally advanced disease that is nonetheless technically resectable for cure. It comprises T3 N1, T1 N2, and T2 N2 disease. Although stage IIIA NSCLC is technically resectable, the efficacy of surgery is more controversial.

Stage IIIB is regionally advanced and technically unresectable (at least with curative intent) disease (T4 or N3 disease). The treatment for both stage III categories is in

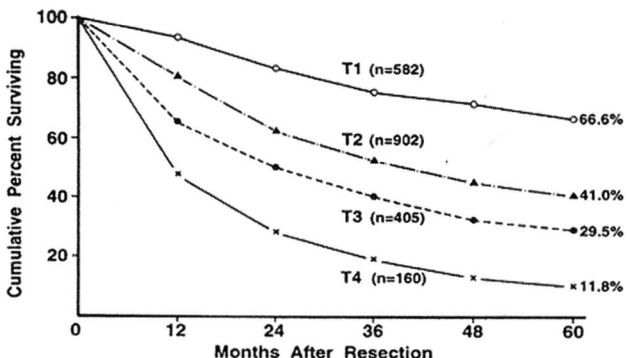

FIGURE 39.20. Survival of 2,055 patients with M0 disease, subdivided by T stage.

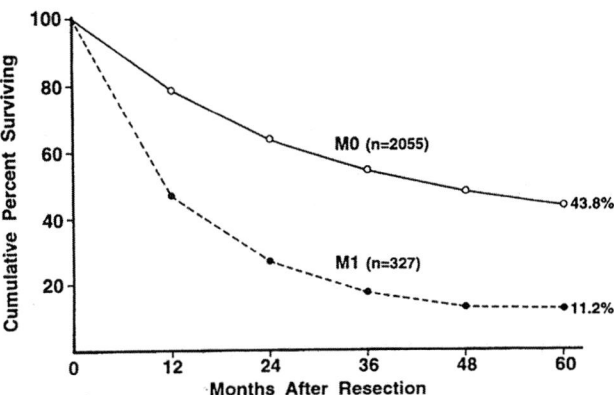

FIGURE 39.21. Survival of 2,383 patients following resection of lung cancer, based on postoperative M classification.

evolution, but most investigative strategies have used multimodality approaches consisting of chemotherapy, radiation, and sometimes surgery.

Stage IV is distant metastatic disease (M1). Treatment generally consists of chemotherapy, palliative radiation, or sometimes no treatment at all.

The proportional stage distribution in NSCLC varies enormously among different series and depends very much on the method of detection. Of the 3,753 patients reported by Mountain whose staging information was used to formulate the ISS, 1,533 (41%) had stage I disease (216). In this series, stage I was by far the most common stage of disease at presentation and was almost two and a half times as frequent as any other stage grouping. However, the proportional stage distribution was clearly skewed toward an overrepresentation of early-stage resectable disease in this referral population.

Perhaps the most accurate data regarding proportional stage distribution at the community level come from the National Cancer Data Base (NCDB) (315). The NCDB contains hospital tumor registry data for 713,043 lung cancer patients collected between 1985 and 1995. The data for the slightly fewer than 500,000 patients for whom stage distribution data are available are depicted in Table 39.18. These patients presented between 1988 and 1995. As shown, 20% had stage I, 7% stage II, 32% stage III, and 41% stage IV disease. Accordingly, 73% of lung cancer patients presented with stage III or IV disease.

TABLE 39.18. STAGE DISTRIBUTION IN LUNG CANCER

Stage	No.	Percentage (%)
I	94,998	20.5
II	30,487	6.6
III	150,293	32.4
IV	187,809	40.5
Total	463,587	

Note: Based on 463,587 lung cancer patients from the National Cancer Data Base, 1988–1995.

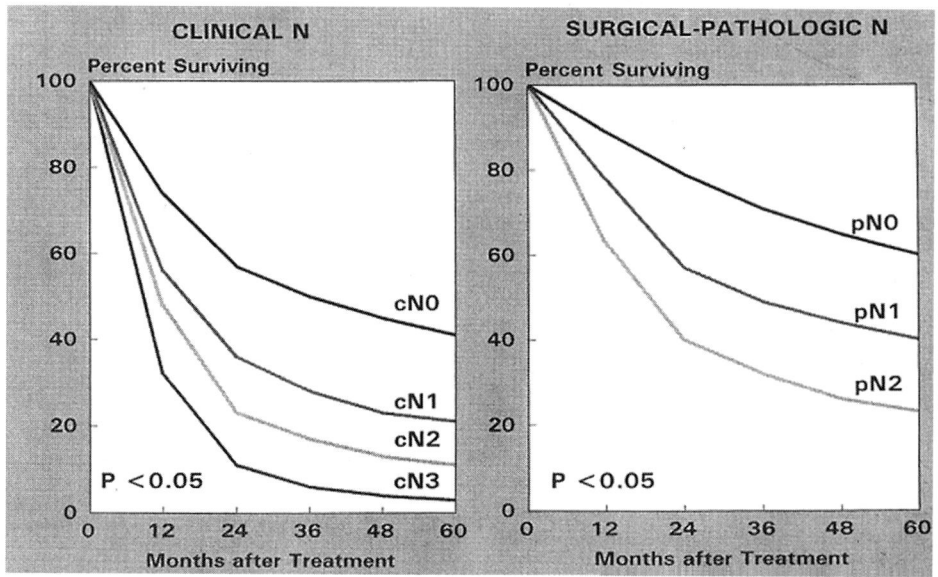

FIGURE 39.22. Survival based on lymph node status, according to both clinical and pathologic staging.

MANAGEMENT OF STAGES I AND II NON–SMALL CELL LUNG CANCER

The therapeutic management of all stages of NSCLC depends on the stage of disease at clinical presentation. Surgical resection is widely recognized as the most effective therapy for patients with stages I and II NSCLC. Only patients who have undergone complete resection are likely to achieve a cure. Adjunctive postoperative radiation therapy and chemotherapy may also be appropriate in some situations.

Surgery

Stage I is the only stage of NSCLC for which a consensus has been reached regarding standard treatment—surgical resection alone. The value of surgical resection has never been established in the context of randomized trials. Nonetheless, the favorable results reported in selected surgical series and the infrequency of long-term survival among patients treated with nonsurgical means clearly establishes surgery as the treatment of choice in resectable early-stage NSCLC.

Lobectomy has generally been accepted as the treatment of choice in both stage I and stage II NSCLC. Lobectomy is usually able to remove all known disease while simultaneously preserving the maximal amount of pulmonary function. With proximal tumors, pneumonectomy may be required, although sleeve resection may be a preferable alternative when experienced operators are available. Sleeve resection preserves pulmonary function while permitting full anatomic removal of tumor.

The role of mediastinal lymph node dissection in patients with early-stage disease remains controversial. There is no question that such a dissection provides the most reliable information regarding the true surgical pathologic stage of disease. A substantial proportion of patients are found to be understaged at surgery despite an extensive preoperative effort (316).

In recent years, advances in video optics have facilitated the development of endoscopic instruments that can be used to perform video-assisted thoracoscopic surgery (VATS), which is characterized as minimally invasive surgery (317). This procedure may be associated with a reduction in surgical morbidity, including postoperative pain. VATS has been used for both diagnosis and staging and also for definitive therapy. In regard to the latter, VATS appears to be very useful in selected patients, particularly elderly patients with significant medical comorbidities.

A Cancer and Leukemia Group B (CALGB) pilot study has demonstrated that VATS lobectomy is feasible and potentially efficacious (318). Currently, no data are available comparing the efficacy of VATS lobectomy with that of standard open lobectomy in stage I NSCLC.

The LCSG conducted an RCT comparing standard lobectomy with limited resection, which consisted of either wedge resection or segmentectomy (319,320). The results demonstrated both an increase in risk for local recurrence and a decrease in survival among patients who underwent limited resection, particularly those with nonsquamous histologies. Based on the results of this trial, it was argued that limited resections should not be routinely used for patients with early-stage tumors, except those unable to tolerate conventional lobectomy. However, in the context of evolving surgical strategies, it may be possible to use minimally invasive techniques as first-line therapy.

The success of surgical therapy for stages I and II NSCLC has varied widely in the literature and clearly depends on the type of staging. In the series of Mountain (216), approximately 50% of patients with clinical stage I NSCLC and 30% of patients with clinical stage II disease survived for 5 years after diagnosis. The 5-year survival rates were 64% and 45%, respectively, for patients with pathologic stages I and II NSCLC. Among patients with pathologic stage I disease, the 5-year survival rates were 69% and 59% for patients with T1 N0 and T2 N0 tumors, respectively. The literature consistently demonstrates a prognostic advantage associated with stage IA in comparison with stage IB NSCLC (Table 39.16). Although the NCDB report did not subdivide stage I disease into stage IA and stage IB, this subdivision may more accurately reflect community practice in the United States. As shown in Figure 39.23, the 5-year survival of stage I patients was 42% (315).

There is no question that the outcomes of patients who undergo surgical therapy of stage I NSCLC are much better than the outcomes reported for the general lung cancer population, which overall achieves a 5-year survival of 10% to 13%. In dramatic contrast, the 5- and 10-year survival rates were 82% and 74% for stage IA NSCLC and 68% and 60% for stage IB disease in 598 patients with stage I disease from the Memorial Sloan-Kettering Cancer Center ($P < .0004$) (232,321). Another large series, from the Netherlands, confirmed these findings, although the results were not quite as favorable. Among 1,249 patients with stage I NSCLC, the 5- and 10-year survival rates for stage IA NSCLC were 63% and 38%, respectively, and for stage IB disease, the figures were 46% and 26% (231).

There has been some debate about how to categorize stage I subsets optimally in terms of tumor size. Patz and colleagues (184) analyzed 510 patients with stage IA NSCLCs that were divided into four size subcategories: 0.27 to 0.96 cm, 0.96 to 1.65 cm, 1.65 to 2.34 cm, and 2.34 to 3.00 cm. The 5-year survival ranged from 80% to 87%, and no significant survival differences based on tumor size were found.

On the other hand, in the Memorial Sloan-Kettering series, tumor size did significantly influence survival. For example, the 10-year survival rates for patients with tumors smaller than 3 cm, between 3 and 5 cm, and larger than 5 cm were 74%, 62%, and 47%, respectively (232,321). Similarly, among 1,020 patients with stage I NSCLC in a multicenter trial, 5-year survival rates of 63%, 56%, 49%, and 38% were found for patients with tumors smaller than 2.0 cm, between 2.1 and 4.0 cm, between 4.1 and 7.0 cm, and larger than 7.0 cm, respectively (322).

The results of surgical resection for stage II NSCLC are considerably less favorable than those of resection for stage I disease. In a review of patients with clinical stage II disease, the 5-year survival was fairly consistent, at about 30% (323). In multiple series reporting outcomes in surgical-pathologic stage II disease, the overall 5-year survival was 41%. However, survival was 52% for patients with stage IIA disease and 39% for those with stage IIB NSCLC. According to the NCDB report, the 5-year survival for patients with stage II disease is only 23% (315) (Fig. 39.23).

The number of involved lymph nodes has been found to be of prognostic importance. Martini and colleagues (222) reported that patients with a single N1 node did better than those with multiple involved nodes. In this series, the distinction between T1 and T2 was not significant, although a significantly superior survival was noted in a comparison of tumors smaller than 3 cm with those larger than 5 cm.

Finally, the histologic subtype may be prognostically important in patients with stage II NSCLC. The LCSG reported that among patients with T1 N1 disease, 5-year survival was 75% for those with squamous cell carcinoma and

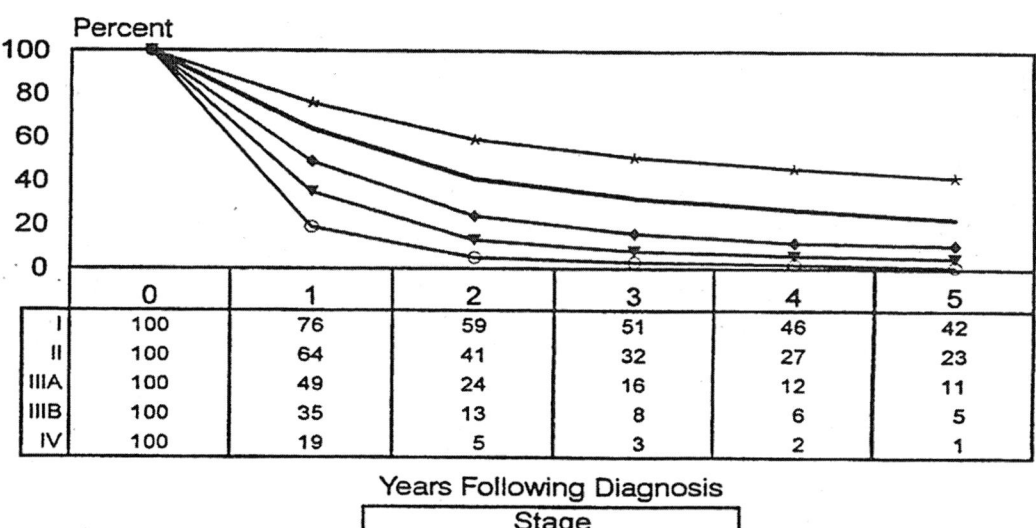

FIGURE 39.23. Cumulative relative survival rates of patients with lung cancer by American Joint Committee on Cancer combined stage at diagnosis.

52% for those with adenocarcinoma (*P* = .04). For patients with T2 N1 tumors, the 5-year survival rates were 53% and 25%, respectively (*P* <.01) (324).

Radiation Therapy

There is little question that surgical resection is the standard of therapy for patients with stages I and II NSCLC. However, radiation therapy has been used in the management of patients with early-stage NSCLC who are not surgical candidates. It has also been used in the postoperative management of patients with resected stage II disease.

A reasonably extensive literature exists for the use of radiation therapy as an alternative to surgery in patients with technically resectable early-stage disease. In general, patients selected for this approach have been those who are elderly, refuse surgical intervention, or have significant medical comorbidities.

Gauden and colleagues (325) retrospectively reviewed the results of 347 patients with clinical stage I NSCLC treated at the Queensland Radium Institute between 1985 and 1992. All patients received at least a 50-Gy tumor dose in 20 fractions over 4 weeks. The overall 5-year survival was 27%, and the median survival was 27.9 months. The 5-year survival among the 167 patients with T1 N0 tumors was 32%, and it was 21% (*P* <.01) for the 180 patients with T2 tumors.

Another series of 84 "medically inoperable" patients with early-stage disease reported a 5-year survival of 31% for clinical stage I NSCLC and of 19% for clinical stage II NSCLC (326). Most patients received 40 Gy of radiation to the primary tumor and mediastinum, with a subsequent boost bringing the dose to 60 to 74 Gy. Tumor size was the most important factor in predicting both local-regional failure and overall survival. Local-regional recurrence developed in 24% of patients with tumors smaller than 5 cm and in 53% of those with larger tumors. Similarly, the 5-year survival was 29% for patients with tumors smaller than 5 cm and 14% for those with tumors larger than 5 cm.

Other series have reported somewhat similar results with radiation therapy alone. A comprehensive review of all reported series concluded that the 5-year survival for patients with stages I and II NSCLC treated with radiation alone is in the range of 15%, and that the median survival is approximately 18 months (327). Accordingly, the available literature strongly suggests that the results of radiation therapy alone are greatly inferior to those achieved with surgical resection.

With regard to postoperative adjuvant therapy following resection, randomized trials have been performed for both stage I and stage II disease. The role of postoperative radiation was studied in a French trial of 132 patients with T2 N0 lesions (229). Patients were randomized to surgery alone or to surgery followed by 45 to 60 Gy of postoperative radiation centered on the hilum and upper mediastinum. The results of the trial demonstrated no advantage for the group undergoing postoperative radiation therapy. In fact,

trends in disease-free survival (*P* = .11) and overall survival (*P* = .049) favored the group without irradiation. The overall 5-year survival was 44% in both groups. The proportion of patients who had local recurrence was 15% in the radiation group and 17% in the control group. The proportion with distant metastases was 37% in the irradiated group and 25% in the group that had surgery alone.

Similarly, a trial from Belgium studied the role of postoperative radiation in 175 evaluable patients with completely resected lung cancer and no nodal involvement. In this trial, 92 patients were randomized to surgery alone and 83 to surgery and 60 Gy of radiation delivered to the mediastinum postoperatively (328). Like the French trial, this study yielded negative results, and survival trends at 5 years also favored the nonirradiated group (24% vs. 43%, *P* = NS). For patients with T2 N0 tumors, a significant survival detriment was actually associated with postoperative radiation (*P* <.05).

Postoperative radiation altered the pattern of tumor recurrence. Among 25 (of 83) patients in the radiation arm who had recurrence, the proportions of recurrences that were exclusively regional, both regional and distant, and exclusively distant were 4%, 12%, and 84%, respectively. In contrast, among 36 (of 92) patients in the surgery arm who had recurrence, 28% of the recurrences were regional only, 25% were regional and distant, and 47% were distant only. Accordingly, radiation decreased the risk for regional recurrence but increased the risk for distant recurrence in this trial.

In stage II NSCLC, the role of postoperative radiation therapy has been best evaluated in LCSG protocol 773. In this trial, 230 patients with completely resected squamous cell carcinoma were randomized to no further therapy or to 50 Gy of postoperative radiation (329). Two thirds of the participants had stage II disease, and the remainder had ipsilateral mediastinal node involvement (stage IIIA). Overall, recurrences were observed in 38 (37%) of 102 in the radiation group and 51 (47%) of 108 in the surgery-only group (*P* = .17). Postoperative radiation also led to a change in the pattern of recurrence. Among irradiated patients who had recurrence, a dramatic reduction in the risk for recurrence to the ipsilateral lung and mediastinum was noted (3% vs. 41%, *P* <.001). However, 37 (97%) of 38 recurrences were distant in the irradiated group, whereas 30 (59%) of 51 recurrences were at distant sites in the surgery-alone group. Survival analysis demonstrated no difference in overall survival between the groups. Accordingly, the results of this trial also demonstrated that postoperative radiation could reduce the risk for local recurrence following resection of squamous cell carcinoma, although the overall recurrence rate and survival were not improved. The results underscore the need for effective systemic therapy to control distant metastatic disease.

A metaanalysis has been published including individual data from 2,128 patients who participated in nine RCTs (330). Overall, the results indicate a statistically significant adverse effect of postoperative radiation on survival (hazard ratio, 1.21; 95% CI, 1.08–1.34). Survival was clearly worse for patients with stages I and II disease. No clear difference was noted for those with stage IIIA N2 disease. It was concluded that postoperative radiation therapy is not warranted for patients with resected stage I or II NSCLC.

Adjuvant Chemotherapy

Because the most common pattern of failure following curative resection of stages I and II NSCLC is distant metastatic disease (230,331), adjuvant chemotherapy is the most rational therapeutic strategy to diminish this risk. However, this area has not been extensively evaluated in the context of randomized trials. Although more than 300 randomized trials of adjuvant chemotherapy of breast cancer have been performed in the past quarter century, fewer than 10% as many trials have focused on adjuvant chemotherapy of lung cancer.

Nonetheless, some important adjuvant trials in resectable NSCLC have appeared, as well as metaanalyses of randomized controlled trials. Based on the bulk of existing data, virtually all authorities have concluded that there is insufficient evidence to recommend adjuvant chemotherapy as the standard of care in any group of resected NSCLC. In dramatic contrast, recent presentation of the results of the International Adjuvant Lung Cancer Trial would appear to support the conclusion that adjuvant chemotherapy deserves consideration in every patient with resectable NSCLC.

Among the most influential adjuvant trials were three studies conducted by the Lung Cancer Study Group (LCSG) in the late 1970s and early 1980s. Each study employed cyclophosphamide, adriamycin, and cisplatin (the CAP regimen) as the adjuvant chemotherapy program. (332,333).

The first study was LCSG 772, which randomized patients with completely resected stage II and III adenocarcinoma and large cell carcinoma to either six cycles of CAP chemotherapy or to immunotherapy with intrapleural bacille Calmette-Guérin and levamisole (334). One hundred forty-one patients were randomized, 45% with stage II and 55% with stage III disease. There was a significant 6-month delay in median time to recurrence favoring the CAP arm, as well as a 15% survival advantage at 1 year (77% vs. 62%). With median follow-up of 8.5 years, survival trends favored the CAP arm, although differences were not significant. Accordingly, this trial does not support routine use of adjuvant chemotherapy.

The second trial (LCSG 791) was for incompletely resected NSCLC of all histologies, and included patients with stages I to IIIA disease (335). Incomplete resection was defined as either the presence of tumor in the highest resected mediastinal node or a margin positive for tumor. One hundred seventy-two patients were randomized to postoperative radiation therapy (40 Gy) or postoperative radiation therapy plus CAP. There were improvements in median survival

(20 vs. 13 months) and median time to recurrence (14 vs. 8 months) favoring the CAP arm. One year after randomization, survival was significantly better in the CAP arm (68% vs. 54%). Unfortunately, after the first year of follow-up, significant differences disappeared. Accordingly, this trial also failed to provide evidence for the effectiveness of adjuvant chemotherapy.

The third study (LCSG 801) was designed for T2 N0 or T1 N1 NSCLC. Of the participants, 85% had T2 N0 and 15% had T1 N1 tumors. A total of 283 patients were randomized to either four cycles of CAP or to no adjuvant therapy (336). Compliance with chemotherapy was problematic, as only 53% of patients received all four cycles of chemotherapy and only 57% of these received the treatment on schedule. The 5-year survival for both groups was 55%, and randomization to adjuvant chemotherapy did not favorably impact on outcome.

Another trial that received considerable attention was reported from Finland (337). In this trial, 110 patients with T1 N0 M0 to T3 N0 M0 NSCLC were randomized to surgery alone or to surgery followed by adjuvant chemotherapy. Of the 110 randomized patients, 99 had stage I disease. Those randomized to chemotherapy received six cycles of CAP chemotherapy (consisting of 400 mg of cyclophosphamide, 40 mg of adriamycin, and 40 mg of cisplatin per square meter). Statistically significant advantages favoring the chemotherapy group were observed with respect to probability of recurrence (31% vs. 48%), 5-year survival (67% vs. 56%), and 10-year survival (61% vs. 48%). However, substantial imbalances appear to have existed in the study because those randomized to surgery alone underwent pneumonectomy more frequently than patients randomized to postoperative chemotherapy. Accordingly, the survival advantage associated with adjuvant chemotherapy in this trial might have been confounded by the fact that the surgery group included more prognostically unfavorable lesions.

Although the results of LCSG 791 suggested that adjuvant chemoradiation is superior to radiation alone, a French Cooperative Group study failed to confirm this finding. In this trial, 267 patients were randomized to either 60 Gy of radiation in 6 weeks or three cycles of adjuvant chemotherapy with cyclophosphamide, doxorubicin, cisplatin, vincristine, and lomustine, followed by a similar radiation protocol (338). Overall, 70% of patients had stage III, 26% had stage II, and 3% had stage I disease. With a 6-year minimum follow-up, no significant differences were noted in disease-free or overall survival.

On the other hand, a Japanese study did show a beneficial effect of chemotherapy in resectable NSCLC. This trial was designed to determine if a "mild" adjuvant chemotherapy program could increase survival in resected NSCLC (339). The regimen consisted of a combination of tegafur plus uracil (UFT) in a molar ratio of 1:4, administered orally. Tegafur (FT) is a derivative of 5-fluorouracil (5-FU) that is well adsorbed following oral administration and converted into 5-FU in vivo.

A total of 323 patients with completely resected stages I to III NSCLC were randomized to the three treatment groups. Overall, 68% had stage I, 12% had stage II, and 20% had stage III disease. One group of 115 patients received adjuvant chemotherapy with one course of cisplatin and vindesine, followed by 1 year of oral UFT. A second group of 108 patients received 1 year of UFT following surgical resection. The control group of 100 patients underwent surgical resection alone. The 5-year survival was 61% in the cisplatin-vindesine-UFT group, 64% in the UFT group, and 49% in the control group. Compliance with the prescribed treatment was good, and toxicity was mild. Statistical evaluation supported a significant difference among the three treatment groups ($P = .044$). When the cisplatin-vindesine-UFT group was compared with controls, the result was not significant ($P = .074$), but a significant difference was observed ($P = .019$) when the UFT group was compared with the control group.

Very recently, the same investigators reported on the results of a randomized, controlled trial comparing UFT to no chemotherapy in resected stage I adenocarcinoma of the lung (339a). A total of 979 eligible patients were randomized. Overall, there was a statistically significant 5-year survival advantage for those randomized to UFT compared to placebo ($P = .036$). Nonetheless, this advantage was associated with an absolute improvement in 5-year survival of only 2.5% (87.9% vs. 85.4%). When considering those with stage IA adenocarcinoma, a significant survival advantage was not observed. However, among those with stage IB adenocarcinoma, there was a greater than 11% absolute improvement in 5-year survival (84.9% vs. 73.5%), and this difference was highly statistically significant ($P = .005$).

In a 1995 metaanalysis of chemotherapy in NSCLC based on data from 14 randomized trials involving 4,357 patients, surgical resection alone was compared with surgery plus adjuvant chemotherapy (340). There were 2,574 deaths. Five of the trials evaluated adjuvant chemotherapy with long-term alkylating agents. In these trials, the hazard ratio favored surgery alone, and the risk for death was 15% higher in those randomized to chemotherapy ($P = .005$).

On the other hand, the hazard ratio estimates favored adjuvant chemotherapy in the eight trials in which a cisplatin-based chemotherapy regimen was used. Overall, a 13% reduction in the risk for death was found in the treated patients ($P = .08$). This translated into an absolute 5% improvement in the probability of long-term survival as a result of adjuvant chemotherapy.

The 5% survival advantage observed in the 1995 metaanalysis provided the rationale for a large randomized trial, known as the International Adjuvant Lung Cancer Trial (IALT). IALT was designed to evaluate the impact on survival of three to four cycles of adjuvant cisplatin-based chemotherapy following complete resection of NSCLC (341). The trial employed a "large simple randomized trial" design proposed by Peto and colleagues (341a).

A total of 1,867 patients were randomized from 148 centers in 33 countries (341). All stages were eligible, and 36% had pathologic stage I, 25% had stage II, and 39% had stage III. Various chemotherapy regimens were permitted, including cisplatin combined with etoposide, vinorelbine, vinblastine, or vindesine. Use of radiation was optional. Overall, survival was significantly superior in those randomized to adjuvant chemotherapy (RR = 0.86; 95% CI, 0.76–0.98; $P < .03$). Two-year survival was 70% in the experimental group compared to 67% among controls, while five-year survival was 45% vs. 40%, respectively. The authors concluded that "the present study supports the use of adjuvant chemotherapy in resected NSCLC."

The question is whether IALT provides definitive evidence for the effectiveness of adjuvant chemotherapy. Indeed, the modest degree of effectiveness demonstrated by this study is plausible and confirms the results of the metaanalysis (340). Accordingly, IALT may be providing an accurate measure of adjuvant chemotherapy in lung cancer.

On the other hand, while the design of the "large simple randomized trial" is appealing, its validity has never been proven. Moreover, if we accept the results of IALT, the state of the art of adjuvant chemotherapy is immediately transformed from unproven in any stage to effective in all resectable stages of NSCLC on the basis of a single study.

A major problem with the "large simple randomized" design in general and IALT in particular is the enormous heterogeneity of both patient population and protocol treatment. Moreover, quality control, which is incorporated into virtually all conventional randomized controlled trials, was not part of IALT. Such quality issues include patient eligibility requirements, uniformity of treatment, adherence to the protocol, central pathology review, and numerous other factors. While proponents of this design maintain that such considerations are unimportant in the context of a large randomized trial, this position is based upon assumption, not evidence.

While the results of randomized trials are almost universally believed to provide the "gold standard" for effectiveness of all medical interventions, the "large simple randomized trial" represents a radical departure from what has become the accepted approach to clinical research. While IALT is likely to change the way lung cancer is treated, it appears that in regard both to the validity of this study design and to adjuvant chemotherapy in NSCLC the jury is still out. Definitive proof must await the results of ongoing well-designed randomized trials which employ specific adjuvant regimens in well defined target populations.

IALT asked the simple question of whether adjuvant cisplatin-based chemotherapy is effective in resectable NSCLC. It is incapable of providing useful information on the value of adjuvant treatment in specific populations with distinct risk profiles.

MANAGEMENT OF STAGES IIIA AND IIIB NON–SMALL CELL LUNG CANCER

The management of regionally advanced NSCLC has evolved rapidly during the past decade. Since the introduction of the ISS in 1986, stage III disease has been subdivided into stages IIIA and IIIB.

Stage IIIA disease is characterized by circumscribed extrapulmonary extension of the primary tumor (implied by the T3 designation) or by N2 nodes. Stage IIIB is characterized by extensive extrapulmonary, although intrathoracic, extension (indicated by the T4 designation) or by nodal disease outside the ipsilateral hemithorax.

Conceptually, stage IIIA was intended to apply to regionally advanced yet potentially resectable disease, whereas stage IIIB was intended to describe regionally advanced and categorically unresectable disease (218,219). Criteria for resectability have been evolving, and the distinction between stage IIIA and stage IIIB disease is often ambiguous. In this era of multimodality therapy, surgery may play a cytoreductive role in the management of stage III disease.

Stage IIIA disease is associated with a better prognosis than stage IIIB disease. According to data presented when the ISS was introduced, stage IIIA has a median survival of 12 months and a 5-year survival of 15%; the corresponding figures for stage IIIB are 8 months and less than 5%. According to the NCDB, the 5-year survival for patients with stage IIIA disease is 11%, compared with 5% for those with stage IIIB disease (315) (Fig. 39.23).

Radiation Therapy in Stage III Non–Small Cell Lung Cancer

Until recently, radiation alone was considered the standard therapy for regionally advanced NSCLC. However, it has long been clear that radiation alone is relatively ineffective as a therapeutic modality in this setting. While effective as a palliative measure, radiation does not provide long-term survival for the vast majority of treated patients (343). The literature on radiation alone in the treatment of regionally advanced stage III NSCLC consistently demonstrates that the median survival achieved is less than 1 year, and 5-year survival rates range between 5% and 8% (344,345).

In the Radiation Therapy Oncology Group (RTOG) protocol 73-01, a four-arm randomized trial, continuous-course radiation was superior to a split-course protocol. Moreover, a radiation dose of 60 Gy was superior to doses of either 50 or 40 Gy (346). The 1- and 3-year survival rates reported with the 60-Gy continuous technique (42% and 15%, respectively) were superior to those of the other arms of the trial. However, by 5 years, survival in all four arms coincided at the 5% level.

Little effort has been made to distinguish stage IIIA from stage IIIB prospectively among patients treated with radiation therapy alone. Curran and Stafford (347) retrospectively assigned a IIIA or IIIB designation to 306 patients treated with standard radiation alone at the Fox Chase Cancer Center between 1978 and 1987. They found no significant differences between the 166 IIIA patients and the 140 IIIB patients in median survival (9.4 vs. 9.8 months) or 2-year survival (17% vs. 18%). Although this analysis is limited because only 28% of patients underwent surgical staging of the mediastinum, the authors concluded that stratification of patients into stage IIIA or IIIB categories has little clinical importance when radiation therapy is used alone.

Local control remains a major problem in most modern radiation series. Schaake-Koning and colleagues (348) reported a 75% local failure rate at 3 years, even among patients with relatively small tumors treated with more than 65 Gy. Local control is not enhanced by increasing the radiation dose when conventional radiation techniques are used. Two series have shown that severe radiation pneumonitis increases as the radiation dose is raised (349,350).

Two randomized trials have suggested that "immediate" radiation therapy delivered at the time of diagnosis prolongs survival little if at all in comparison with "delayed" radiation (given when symptoms supervene) or no radiation. A Veterans Administration trial carried out in the 1960s demonstrated only a very modest 1-year survival advantage (18% vs. 14%) for patients randomized to 40 to 50 Gy of radiation versus placebo in stage III lung cancer (351). Similarly, a Southeast Oncology Group study reported little advantage for immediate radiation therapy (352).

Some evidence indicates that hyperfractionated radiation may be superior to conventional fractionated radiation. The RTOG, in protocol 83-11, performed a five-arm randomized trial in which 848 patients with stage III NSCLC were randomized to one of five different hyperfractionated treatment arms in which 60.0, 64.8, 69.4, 74.4, or 79.2 Gy of radiation was administered (353,354). A survival advantage was reported for a retrospectively identified subgroup of "favorable" patients, defined as those with a Karnofsky performance status of 70% to 100% and a weight loss of less than 6%. Such "favorable" patients who were assigned a dose of 69.4 Gy had a median survival of 13 months and a 2-year survival of 29%, both significantly superior to those achieved with lower radiation doses. No further advantage was noted at higher doses, and no survival advantage was seen in the patients who were not "favorable."

To improve the therapeutic index further, continuous hyperfractionated accelerated radiation therapy, or CHART, has been developed. The objectives are to overcome rapid tumor cell repopulation and decrease late toxicity.

A large RCT in Europe of 563 patients with NSCLC (most of whom had stage III disease) compared conventional radiation therapy (30 once-daily 2-Gy fractions 5 days per week) with CHART (1.5 Gy three times daily on each of

12 consecutive days) (355). CHART was associated with a significantly better 2-year survival (29% vs. 20%) but more frequent dysphagia during the early months of treatment.

CHART has not been widely used in the United States, largely because of logistic constraints. Encouraging preliminary data for an alternative regimen, hyperfractionated accelerated radiation therapy (HART), in which treatment is spaced over 15 days including two weekend breaks, have been reported by the Eastern Cooperative Oncology Group (ECOG) (356). Among 28 patients treated, the median survival was 13 months and the 1-year survival rate was 57%. Based on this encouraging result, an intergroup study is under way in which patients with local-regional NSCLC receive two cycles of chemotherapy followed by either conventional fractionated radiation therapy or HART.

Surgery in Stage III Non–Small Cell Lung Cancer

Because the vast majority of patients with NSCLC who achieve long-term survival have undergone resection, surgery is believed to be the most effective modality in NSCLC. Most cases of stage IIIA NSCLC are technically resectable, and even certain subsets of stage IIIB are amenable to resection. Considerable evidence supports the conclusion that patients with stage IIIA NSCLC should be stratified based on the presence of a T3 primary lesion or N2 regional adenopathy (375).

Patients with T3 tumors comprise a heterogeneous group in which the prognosis varies depending on the basis for the T3 designation. Patients with T3 tumors based on chest wall involvement probably have the most favorable outlook after surgical resection (358). Reports from the Mayo Clinic and the Brigham and Women's Hospital indicate 5-year survivals in excess of 50% for patients with resected T3 N0 lesions of the chest wall (359,360).

Similarly, patients who have superior sulcus (Pancoast) tumors without regional node involvement have respectable long-term survival rates when surgical resection is used (361,362). In the series of Paulson (362), which included such patients treated with radiation followed by resection, the 5-year survival rate was 31%.

Several series demonstrate that 5-year survival rates range from 15% to 29% among highly selected groups of patients undergoing resection of N2 disease (357). A number of factors have been identified that adversely affect survival in patients with resected N2 disease. These include the presence of T3 tumors, nonsquamous histology, high mediastinal nodes, or multiple N2 sites.

The largest experience with surgery in N2 disease comes from Memorial Sloan-Kettering Cancer Center (363). Of 706 patients judged to have N2 disease by either clinical or pathologic criteria (mediastinoscopy was not routinely performed), 404 underwent thoracotomy, and 151 of these

(37% of thoracotomy patients and 21% of all N2 patients) had completely resectable disease. The bulk of mediastinal node involvement significantly affected the likelihood of complete resection. Of 224 patients who were felt by clinical criteria to have N0 or N1 disease but who were found to have otherwise inapparent N2 disease at thoracotomy, 119 (53%) had resectable disease. In contrast, 179 patients had obvious clinical N2 disease, and of these, only 32 (18%) had resectable disease. Approximately 90% of all patients who underwent resection also received postoperative radiation to the ipsilateral hilum and mediastinum (40–45 Gy). The overall 5-year survival for the entire group of patients with resected N2 disease was 30%. For those with clinical N0 and N1 disease, the 3- and 5-year survival rates were 47% and 34%, respectively. Again in contrast, for those with clinically overt N2 disease, the 3- and 5-year survival rates were each 9%; this 9% figure is not very different from that achievable with radiation alone.

A report from the Toronto General Hospital on the surgical treatment of 141 patients with stage IIIA disease demonstrated that cervical mediastinoscopy is extremely useful in selecting patients for surgical resection (364). In contrast to the experience previously cited from Memorial Sloan-Kettering, all the patients in the Toronto study underwent preoperative cervical mediastinoscopy for surgical staging of the mediastinum. In 62 patients, the results of mediastinoscopy were negative, but mediastinal nodal involvement was found at the time of resection. The actuarial 5-year survival in this group was 24%. The results of mediastinoscopy were positive in 79 patients; 67 of these patients underwent resection, but the 5-year survival in this group was only 9%.

Finally, a series from the Netherlands, which included patients with stage IIIA N2 disease, reported 5-year survival rates of 18% among 187 patients with T2 N2 tumors and 7% among 61 patients with T3 N2 lesions (231). In this trial, volume of N2 disease was not reported.

Accordingly, the data support the conclusion that surgical response rates (i.e., resectability) are impressive in certain N2 subsets. Moreover, long-term survival is achieved in some patients. Nonetheless, long-term survival with resection for groups of N2 patients remains modest. Accordingly, there is reason to question whether resection is the most effective modality in stage IIIA NSCLC. This is particularly true for those with clinically overt N2 disease.

Such considerations provide the rationale for an Intergroup Study (INT 0139) designed to evaluate the role of surgery in the context of trimodality therapy in stage IIIA NSCLC (364a). INT 0139 randomized 429 patients with pathologically confirmed N2 disease to either concurrent chemoradiation or to chemoradiation and surgical resection. The chemotherapeutic agents included cisplatin and VP-16.

To date, an advantage in disease-free survival has been reported for those randomized to surgery (median, 14.0 vs.

11.7 months; $P = .02$). However, there was no difference in overall survival (which was approximately 22 months in each group). An obstacle to the ability to demonstrate an overall survival advantage is that there were greater than four times as many early deaths in the group randomized to surgery (14 vs. 3 deaths). In the surgical group, there were more patients alive without progressive disease, but correspondingly more noncancer deaths. Accordingly, the jury is still out as to whether the addition of surgical resection enhances survival in stage IIIA NSCLC.

Combined Surgery and Radiation in Stage III Non–Small Cell Lung Cancer

The rationale for combining radiation and surgery is to improve local-regional control. In theory, better local control improves overall survival, although such has not been observed in most adults with solid tumors. Studies have been carried out in which radiation was used both preoperatively and postoperatively.

Two large randomized trials comparing preoperative radiation therapy followed by surgery with surgery alone were conducted in the 1960s and 1970s. The first was a Veterans Administration study, in which patients were randomized to receive preoperative radiation at 40 to 50 Gy or to immediate surgery (365). In the second study, conducted by NCI, patients were randomized to preoperative radiation with a minimum of 40 Gy or to surgery alone (366). Both trials failed to demonstrate any benefit from preoperative radiation, in terms of either decreased mortality or decreased recurrence. However, modern radiographic and surgical staging was not employed in either study, and patients with SCLC were eligible to participate in these trials.

On the other hand, a report by Sherman and colleagues (367) suggested that preoperative radiation followed by surgical resection may be effective in stage III NSCLC. Fifty-three patients received 30 to 40 Gy of preoperative radiation, after which they underwent resection and postoperative radiation. Forty-six patients underwent thoracotomy, and 38 had resectable disease. The 5-year survival was 18% for the entire cohort but 27% for the 38 resected patients.

The role of postoperative radiation was evaluated in LCSG protocol 773, described previously (see section "Management of Stages I and II Non–Small Cell Lung Cancer: Radiation Therapy") (329). Patients with completely resected stage II or III squamous cell carcinoma were randomized to receive 50 Gy of postoperative radiation or no further therapy. About one third of the patients had stage III NSCLC. Postoperative radiation significantly reduced the incidence of local-regional recurrence in the ipsilateral lung and mediastinum from 41% to 3%. However, this did not translate into a survival advantage. Moreover, as previously noted, the postoperative radiation therapy metaanalysis found postoperative radiation to be deleterious in stage I or II NSCLC, although not in stage IIIA disease (330).

Induction Chemotherapy and Radiation versus Radiation Alone in Stage III Non–Small Cell Lung Cancer

The efficacy of induction chemotherapy and thoracic radiation has been extensively investigated in stage III NSCLC. Although most reports have been of single-arm phase II studies, numerous randomized trials have now also appeared in the literature.

A number of theoretic advantages for the use of induction chemotherapy have been well described (368). These include stage reduction to facilitate local control by radiation, surgery, or both and early treatment of micrometastases. The response rates to identical chemotherapy regimens appear to be higher in stage III than in stage IV disease.

CALGB 84-33 was the first randomized trial to demonstrate a significant benefit of adding chemotherapy to definitive radiation alone (369,370). Eligibility for this trial was limited to patients with prognostically favorable pretreatment characteristics, including a favorable performance status (PS) (ECOG PS of 0 or 1) and minimal weight loss (<5% of body weight in the preceding 3 months). Patients were randomized to receive 60 Gy of radiation over 6 weeks or two cycles of induction chemotherapy with cisplatin and vinblastine followed by an identical radiation program. A total of 78 patients were randomized to chemoradiation, and 77 were randomized to radiation alone. The response rate to the combined treatment was 56%, and to radiation alone it was 43% ($P = .092$). The group randomized to induction chemotherapy showed a significant improvement in median survival (13.7 vs. 9.6 months, $P = .012$) and in the proportions of patients surviving 1, 2, 3, 5, and 7 years (54%, 26%, 24%, 17%, and 13% vs. 40%, 13%, 10%, 6%, and 6%, respectively).

The RTOG and ECOG conducted a confirmatory three-arm trial involving 452 eligible patients randomized to the same two treatment arms used in CALGB 84-33 and to a third arm that included hyperfractionated radiation to a total dose of 69.6 Gy (371). Hyperfractionation had been shown to produce a survival advantage for favorable patients in RTOG protocol 83-11 (353). In preliminary results of the confirmatory trial, the 1-year survival rate and median survival were better in the group randomized to receive induction chemotherapy than in the other two groups ($P = .03$). The 1-year survival rate and median survival for the three groups were as follows: induction chemotherapy and radiation therapy, 60% and 13.8 months; hyperfractionated radiation therapy, 51% and 12.3 months; standard radiation therapy, 46% and 11.4 months.

A metaanalysis evaluated 14 randomized trials comparing chemotherapy and radiation with radiation alone in regionally advanced stage III NSCLC (372). A total of 2,589 patients participated in these trials. Overall, the metaanalysis concluded that combination chemotherapy and radiation reduced the risk for death by 12% at 1 year, 13% at 2 years, and 17% at 3 years. This corresponded to a mean gain in life expectancy of approximately 2 months. The magnitude of the benefit was independent of whether the chemotherapy and radiation were given sequentially or concurrently.

Despite encouraging results of chemoradiation, many important questions remain unanswered. The optimal induction chemotherapy regimen has not been established. The optimal sequence of chemotherapy and radiation remains debatable, as does the role of hyperfractionated radiation. In the past several years, considerable work has been performed with newer chemotherapeutic agents having considerable activity in NSCLC (373). These include the taxanes, such as paclitaxel (Taxol) and docetaxel (Taxotere), in addition to gemcitabine (Gemzar), vinorelbine (Navelbine), and irinotecan (Camptosar). Current investigation has also focused on the dose intensity and timing of radiation, often in combination with the newer chemotherapeutic agents (374).

At present, disease recurs in the vast majority of patients, and they eventually succumb to metastatic NSCLC despite the use of chemoradiation. Local-regional recurrence remains a major impediment to cure. In CALGB 84-33, the group treated with chemoradiation had an 80% incidence of local-regional failure, whereas 90% of those randomized to radiation therapy alone had local-regional failure. Green (375) has emphasized that patterns of failure despite induction chemotherapy and radiation mandate better control of both macroscopic intrathoracic disease and distant micrometastatic disease in the setting of regionally advanced NSCLC.

Concurrent versus Sequential Chemotherapy and Radiation

Another important question relates to the role of concurrent chemoradiation. In two trials by Jeremic and colleagues (376,377), the addition of chemotherapy to hyperfractionated radiation was superior to hyperfractionated radiation alone.

Two randomized trials have suggested that concurrent chemoradiation may be superior to sequential chemoradiation. In 1999, Furuse and colleagues (378) reported the results of a phase III trial in Japan comparing induction chemotherapy followed by thoracic radiation with concurrent chemoradiation. The chemotherapy used was mitomycin, vindesine, and cisplatin. After approximately 3 years of follow-up, the results showed a modest although statistically significant improvement in the overall response rate and in median survival (13.3 months for the sequential arm vs. 16 months for the concurrent arm). Overall survival favored the concurrent arm ($P = .04$). The 2- and 5-year survival rates were 35% and 16% in the concurrent arm versus 27% and 9% in the sequential arm (378).

The RTOG also conducted a randomized comparison of concurrent versus sequential chemoradiation in the context of the three-arm study (RTOG 94-10). Of the 611 patients enrolled, one-third were randomized to receive sequential cisplatin and vinblastine followed by radiation (identical to the regimen of CALGB 84-33). A second group received concurrent cisplatin, vinblastine, and radiation. The third group received concurrent cisplatin, VP-16, and twice-daily hyperfractionated radiation. The median survival for the sequential, concurrent, and hyperfractionation arms were 14.6, 17.0, and 15.6 months, respectively. Four-year survival for the sequential, concurrent, and hyperfractionation arms was 12%, 21%, and 17%, respectively. There was not a significant survival advantage when comparing the hyperfractionation arm to sequential therapy. However, there was a statistically significant survival advantage for concurrent compared to sequential therapy ($P = 0.046$) (379,380).

Phase II Trials: Induction Chemotherapy, Radiation, and Surgery

Numerous phase II trials of trimodality therapy consisting of induction chemotherapy and surgery, and usually also radiation therapy, have been conducted in patients with regionally advanced stage III NSCLC. The design of these trials varies with respect to surgical staging of the mediastinum, delivery of radiation sequentially or concurrently with chemotherapy, specific agents and dosages, radiation dosage, and definitions of resectable disease. Such inconsistencies have led to considerable difficulties in interpreting the trial results.

Table 39.19 lists 10 phase II trials of induction chemotherapy and surgery with or without radiation in stage IIIA NSCLC (381–391). In two of these trials, patients with stage IIIB disease were also eligible to participate (390,391). Each of the trials used a cisplatin-based combination regimen of chemotherapy. The manner in which radiation was used also varied.

Overall, the response rates to induction chemotherapy or chemoradiation were quite high, ranging from 39% to 77%. Resectability rates exceeded 50% in each of these trials and reached 93% in a Massachusetts General Hospital trial that used concurrent chemotherapy and hyperfractionated radiation (387). The median survival was highly variable, ranging from 13 to 32 months. Similarly, the proportion of long-term survivors was highly variable, ranging from 17% to 37%.

As single-arm phase II studies, none of these trials were designed to evaluate the therapeutic role of surgery in the context of regionally advanced disease. However, it does appear that the addition of surgery to chemoradiation improved local control. Local recurrence has generally been observed in fewer than 50% of patients who undergo trimodality therapy. This contrasts with an 80% to 90% rate of persistent or recurrent local-regional disease among those who do not undergo resection.

Group or Institution	Authors (Reference)	No. Patients	Induction Chemotherapy Regimen	Radiation	Response to Induction Therapy	Resectability	Median Survival	Percentage Long-Term Survival
CAP I trial (DFCI)	Skarin et al., 1989 (381)	41	Cisplatin Cyclophosphamide Adriamycin	After induction chemotherapy but before resection (and postoperatively)	53%	88%	32 mo	31% (5y)
CAP II trial (DFCI)	Elias et al., 1994 (382)	54	Cisplatin Cyclophosphamide Adriamycin	Given postoperatively	39%	54%	17.9 mo	22% (5y)
CALGB 8634	Strauss et al., 1992 (343); Strauss et al., 1996 (384)	41	Cisplatin Vinblastine 5-FU	Concurrently with induction chemotherapy (and postoperatively)	51%	61%	15.5 mo	22% (9y)
CALGB 8935	Sugarbaker et al., 1995 (385); Kumar et al., 1996 (386)	74	Cisplatin Vinblastine	Given postoperatively	88% (partial response or stable disease)	62%	15 mo	23% (3y)
MGH	Choi et al., 1997 (387)	42	Cisplatin Vinblastine 5-FU	Twice-daily radiation given concurrently with induction chemotherapy (and postoperatively)	73%	93%	25 mo	37% (5y)
MSKCC	Martini et al., 1993 (388)	136	Mitomycin Vindesine Cisplatin	Not routinely used	77%	65%	19 mo	17% (5y)
Toronto	Burkes et al., 1992 (389)	39	Mitomycin Vindesine Cisplatin	Not routinely used	64%	56%	18.6 mo	26% (3y)
Rush	Reddy et al., 1992 (390)	129 83 stage IIIA 46 stage IIIB	Cisplatin 5-FU ± VP-16	Concurrently with induction chemotherapy	Not reported	72%[a]	17.6 mo	32% (3y)
LCSG	Weiden, 1991	85	Cisplatin 5-FU	Concurrently with induction chemotherapy	56%	52%	13 mo	20% (3y)
SWOG 8805	Albain et al., 1995 (391)	126 75 stage IIIA 51 stage IIIB	Cisplatin VP-16	Concurrently with induction chemotherapy (and postoperatively)	59%	71% 76% stage IIIA 63% stage IIIB	13 mo stage IIIA 17 mo stage IIIB	27% (3y) stage IIIA 24% (3y) stage IIIB

[a]Resectability of 72% achieved among 86 patients deemed "eligible for surgery" at outset. Resectability was 47% among all 129 patients.
CALGB, Cancer and Leukemia Group B; CAP, cisplatin adriamycin, and cyclophosphamide; DFCI, Dana-Farber Cancer Institute; 5-FU, 5-fluorouracil; LCSG, Lung Cancer Study Group; MGH, Massachusetts General Hospital; MSKCC, Memorial Sloan-Kettering Cancer Center; SWOG, Southwest Oncology Group; VP, Vincristine and prednisone.

Accordingly, these phase II trials of induction chemotherapy, surgery, and (usually) radiation lead to a shift in recurrence patterns from both local and distant to predominantly distant. The question is whether overall survival improves.

Phase III Trials: Induction Chemotherapy and Surgery

Reports of several small randomized trials comparing induction chemotherapy followed by surgical resection without systemic therapy have been highly influential in changing our thinking about the role of chemotherapy in the management of regionally advanced NSCLC. The two most influential of these trials were discontinued before their projected accrual goal was reached because of early-stoppage rules in the context of highly encouraging preliminary results (392,393).

In 1994, Rosell and colleagues (392) first reported the results of a randomized study from Barcelona, Spain, in which patients were randomized to induction chemotherapy with cisplatin, mitomycin C, and ifosfamide followed by resection and postoperative radiation therapy (50 Gy) or to resection and the same postoperative radiation therapy. The overall response rate to induction chemotherapy was 60% (including a 7% complete response rate). The resection rates were 85% (23 of 27) in the chemotherapy arm and 90% (27 of 30) in the surgery arm. A dramatic threefold survival advantage was observed in those randomized to receive induction chemotherapy. The median survival of this group was 26 months, whereas it was 8 months ($P < .001$ log rank) in the surgery plus radiation therapy group.

In a similar report by Roth and colleagues (393) from the M. D. Anderson Cancer Center, patients were randomized to induction chemotherapy consisting of three cycles of cyclophosphamide, etoposide, and cisplatin followed by resection or to surgical resection alone. Of note, radiation therapy was given to more than 50% of the patients in both arms. Responses to induction chemotherapy were observed in 35% (including a 4% complete response rate). Resection was achieved in 17 (61%) of 28 patients in the chemotherapy arm and in 21 (66%) of 32 patients in the surgery arm. The group that received chemotherapy achieved an estimated median survival that was almost sixfold greater than that of patients randomized to surgery alone (64 vs. 11 months, $P < .008$). Similarly, the 3-year survival was 56% for the induction chemotherapy group and 15% for the surgery-alone group.

A third randomized trial from the NCI that preceded the other two received much less public attention (394). In this trial of 27 patients, the experimental arm underwent induction chemotherapy with cisplatin and etoposide followed by resection and postoperative chemotherapy. The control group underwent immediate surgical resection and postoperative radiation therapy (54–60 Gy). A response to chemotherapy was observed in 8 (62%) of 13 patients, and resection was achieved in 23 (85%) of 27. The patients treated with induction chemotherapy had a superior survival (28.7 vs. 15.6 months). However, this large difference in survival was not statistically significant because of the small sample size ($P = .095$).

The fourth randomized trial was CALGB 91-34 (395). The experimental arm of this study consisted of two cycles of induction chemotherapy with cisplatin and etoposide followed by resection, two additional cycles of chemotherapy, and subsequent radiation therapy (54 or 60 Gy). The control arm consisted of preoperative radiation therapy (40 Gy), resection, and postoperative radiation therapy (to a total dose of 54 or 60 Gy). The reason preoperative radiation was used in the control arm was concern that the disease of patients with stage IIIA NSCLC randomized to immediate surgery would be unresectable. As previously noted, this concern was not realized in the other three randomized trials.

The original accrual goal for CALGB 91-34 was 250 patients. Unfortunately, the trial had to be closed prematurely after only 57 patients had been entered; a sufficient number of patients could not be accrued because of the inclusion of a no-chemotherapy arm, after enormous enthusiasm for induction chemotherapy had been generated by the encouraging reports from the Barcelona and M. D. Anderson trials.

Nevertheless, with 57 patients, CALGB 91-34 was similar in size to the Barcelona and M. D. Anderson trials. Its results, however, were quite different. The response rate was 46% in the chemotherapy arm (including an 8% complete response rate) and 34% in the radiation arm (including a 13% complete response rate). Overall, the median survival was 18 months for the group undergoing induction chemotherapy and 23 months for the group assigned to preoperative radiation. The trend toward inferior survival in those randomized to induction chemotherapy was not statistically significant ($P = .41$). Thus, the results of CALGB 91-34 directly conflicted with the results of the other three randomized trials.

Although three of the four randomized trials suggested a survival advantage associated with induction chemotherapy, these studies had major shortcomings. One important problem was that the absolute magnitude of the observed survival differences in the M. D. Anderson and Barcelona trials was far greater than could be reasonably expected from the modestly effective chemotherapy regimens used. This discrepancy raises questions about the validity of the findings.

Moreover, each of the four trials was very small. Of the four studies, the largest were the Barcelona and M. D. Anderson trials, each of which enrolled exactly 60 patients. Small randomized trials are likely to have very little statistical power. However, given the large departures from the null observed in the Barcelona and M. D. Anderson trials, there was sufficient statistical power to demonstrate significant differences.

On the other hand, in small randomized trials, randomization may fail to balance all factors that can affect the outcome event of interest. A possible explanation for the magnitude of the differences is that despite randomization, an imbalance of prognostic factors may have existed between the arms.

Some evidence suggests that the results of the Barcelona trial may have been confounded. In this study, the group randomized to surgery alone had a higher proportion of tumors with relatively virulent biologic characteristics (392). For example, a higher proportion of tumors in the surgery arm had K-*ras* mutations (42% vs. 15%, *P* = .096) and were DNA aneuploidy tumors (70% vs. 29%, *P* = .022). Although it is possible that these differences reflected modulation by chemotherapy, it is also possible that an excess of biologically virulent tumors in the group randomized to surgery alone in the Barcelona study was responsible for the observed differences in outcome. No direct evidence has been found of a similar imbalance in the M. D. Anderson trial. However, molecular markers of prognosis were not reported in this trial.

Both studies reported major survival advantages based on short median observation times. The results were not maintained at longer follow-up. Roth and colleagues (396) reported long-term results of the M. D. Anderson study after 82 months of median follow-up. In the combined chemotherapy and surgery arm, 9 (32%) of 28 patients remained alive. After prolonged follow-up, the median survival for those randomized to chemotherapy was only 21 months (compared with 64 months at the time of the initial report). Of those randomized to surgery alone, 5 (16%) of 32 remained alive, and the median follow-up was 14 months. A benefit was seen only among those undergoing complete resection.

Differences after 82 months led the authors to conclude that "the persistent survival difference between the perioperative chemotherapy group and the surgery-alone group supports our original conclusion that patients with resectable stage III NSCLC should no longer be treated with surgery alone." However, it should be pointed out that in the follow-up report, the overall survival difference between the induction chemotherapy and surgery groups was no longer statistically significant (*P* = .056).

Similarly, Rosell and colleagues (397) reported long-term results of the Barcelona trial. The median survival was 22 months (95% CI, 13.4–30.6) in those randomized to induction chemotherapy, and for those randomized to surgery alone, the median survival was 10 months (*P* = .005 log rank). Accordingly, the reported results after 7 years of average follow-up were more similar to those of the earlier report, with an average follow-up of only 2 years. Nonetheless, the results of the Barcelona study are suspect for at least three reasons. First, there is the question of randomization failure, reflected by the higher prevalence of K-*ras* mutations and aneuploidy in the surgery group. Secondly, the surgery arm did extremely poorly. After 7 years, long-term survival in the chemotherapy arm was 20% (6 of 30), whereas it was 0 (0 of 30) in the surgery-alone arm.

Interestingly, the Barcelona group was unable to confirm its own results in a subsequent trial, in which the control arm, consisting of the exact same regimen used in the earlier trial (induction cisplatin, mitomycin C, and ifosfamide), was compared with a regimen containing a higher dose of cisplatin. The median survival for patients on the same regimen was now 11 months, compared with 22 to 26 months in the first trial (398).

Collectively, these four trials provide some information about induction chemotherapy versus surgery alone in stage IIIA N2 NSCLC. However, they perhaps are most informative in regard to the pitfalls of small randomized trials, particularly in the context of early reporting, when the estimated survival time greatly exceeds the actual observation time.

It is also clear that the early reports from the M. D. Anderson and Barcelona trials were grossly misleading in regard to the estimated benefit associated with induction chemotherapy. The actual magnitude of the effect of induction chemotherapy followed by surgery versus that of surgery alone is far less than the early reports suggested.

Conclusions regarding Multimodality Therapy in Stage III Non–Small Cell Lung Cancer

Despite serious limitations in our existing database, particularly with regard to randomized trials of induction chemotherapy and surgery, reasonable evidence indicates that patients with stage IIIA NSCLC derive some survival benefit from induction chemotherapy (with or without radiation therapy) followed by surgical resection. It is also clear that the magnitude of the survival advantages provided by induction chemotherapy was overestimated in the early reports from small, underpowered randomized trials. Numerous phase II trimodality studies support this conclusion. Results for induction chemotherapy with radiation are consistent with those of numerous phase III studies demonstrating that induction chemotherapy with definitive radiation improves outcome in comparison with thoracic radiation therapy alone.

Whether induction chemotherapy deserves to be standard therapy remains highly debatable. Nonetheless, there is a clear suggestion of benefit, and additional randomized clinical trials evaluating this approach will likely be difficult to implement. The evidence appears to be mounting that the concurrent administration of chemotherapy and radiation is better than the sequential use of these modalities (374,399).

The role of resection in stage IIIA disease remains controversial, but local control appears improved in multimodality programs that include resection, and patients in whom N2 nodes are not found at resection do quite well. Results of phase II and phase III trials do provide a basis for optimism that real therapeutic progress is finally being achieved in regionally advanced NSCLC. Further study of therapeutic strategies that incorporate aggressive systemic treatment and maximal local-regional therapy in stage IIIA NSCLC is clearly warranted. The role of newer combination chemotherapy regimens that do not include cisplatin requires further definition. Given the tendency to distant failure of patients with regionally advanced NSCLC, it certainly seems reasonable, particularly in the context of many studies suggesting a role for induction therapy, to incorporate both systemic and local-regional modalities in the management of patients with regionally advanced stage III NSCLC.

MANAGEMENT OF STAGE IV NON–SMALL CELL LUNG CANCER

Stage IV NSCLC is invariably a fatal disease and has proved remarkably resistant to chemotherapy. In 1988, Gralla reviewed 134 phase II trials of single agents in advanced NSCLC and could identify only five (of 48 that were studied) with a response rate exceeding 15% (399a). These were cisplatin, mitomycin C, ifosfamide, vinblastine, and vindesine. Newer agents, such as paclitaxel, docetaxel, gemcitabine, vinorelbine, and irinotecan, all have single-agent response rates above 15%.

The therapeutic options for patients with recurrent or metastatic NSCLC include the following:

1. Best supportive care. All patients presenting with metastatic NSCLC should be given the option of best supportive care with the knowledge that they have an incurable disease and current therapy provides only modest survival benefits.

2. Local-regional therapy. In some instances, patients present with conditions that require local-regional therapy initially (brain metastases, obstructive pneumonia, bone metastases with impending fracture, spinal cord involvement), or they may require it for significant palliation of disabling symptoms and pain control.

3. Systemic chemotherapy. The following principles help guide the use of systemic chemotherapy in patients with advanced NSCLC:

- Patient preference. This is equivalent to treatment planning when the neoplasm is incurable and should be always discussed.
- Performance status (PS). This is the most useful indicator of patient tolerance and likely response to systemic chemotherapy. Patients who are asymptomatic or essentially fully active with symptoms are the best candidates for systemic chemotherapy. Invariably, patients with a PS of 2 (in bed <50% of awake time) have a significantly lower response and higher rates of toxicity and treatment discontinuation.
- Age. Age alone is not a contraindication to therapy, especially if the PS is within acceptable limits. Data support therapy for patients older than 70 years.
- Duration of treatment. Current randomized data suggest a maximum benefit with four cycles of chemotherapy; toxicity is incurred with further therapy.

Active Chemotherapeutic Agents in Non–Small Cell Lung Cancer

Chemotherapeutic agents that have been known for some time to have considerable activity in NSCLC are listed in

TABLE 39.20. ACTIVE CHEMOTHERAPY AGENTS IN NON–SMALL CELL LUNG CANCER

Older Agents	Newer Agents
Cisplatin	Paclitaxel
Carboplatin	Docetaxel
Ifosfamide	Gemcitabine
Mitomycin	Vinorelbine
Etoposide	Irinotecan
Vindesine	Topotecan

Table 39.20. These include the platinum compounds (cisplatin and carboplatin), ifosfamide, mitomycin C, etoposide, and vinblastine. During the 1990s, a number of newer chemotherapeutic agents were identified that are also active in NSCLC. These include vinorelbine (a new vinca alkaloid), the taxanes (paclitaxel and docetaxel), the camptothecins (irinotecan and topotecan), and gemcitabine.

Chemotherapy versus Best Supportive Care

Given the limited activity of combination chemotherapy in stage IV NSCLC, many physicians have come to believe that chemotherapy should not necessarily be used in the setting of advanced disease. NSCLC is unique in that numerous randomized trials have been conducted comparing combination chemotherapy with best supportive care.

Eight randomized trials have compared chemotherapy with best supportive care in patients with advanced NSCLC. Five of them (401,402–405) have been criticized for using substandard chemotherapy. The two best-known individual trials used similar cisplatin-based chemotherapy regimens. The widely cited Canadian study found a statistically significant prolongation of survival from 17 weeks in the control arm to 32.6 weeks in the group receiving cisplatin (100 mg/m^2) and vindesine (406). An Australian study also reported a 17-week median survival in the arm receiving best supportive care, whereas the group receiving cisplatin and vindesine had a median survival of 27 weeks. However, in this study, the survival advantage in the chemotherapy group did not reach statistical significance (407).

Three metaanalyses have been published comparing chemotherapy with best supportive care (408–410). Each one supports the conclusion that combination chemotherapy is associated with a small but significant improvement in survival. In the study of Marino and colleagues (410), the median survival for patients treated with best supportive therapy was 3.9 months, whereas it was 6.7 months for those receiving combination chemotherapy.

Prolongation of life is usually the primary objective of chemotherapy, and survival is very simple to quantify. However, other goals of chemotherapy are important in the setting of advanced disease. Improvement in the quality of life is a potentially valuable surrogate endpoint in addition to overall survival. One study reported that independent of the initial Karnofsky score, 75% of patients treated for advanced

NSCLC reported an improved quality of life (411). Similarly, the metaanalyses demonstrated that chemotherapy improved quality of life.

Despite these advances, chemotherapy has little impact in the setting of advanced disease. Although it may be a reasonable option for many patients, it is certainly not mandatory as the standard of care. Patients with a good PS and minimal weight loss are most likely to respond to chemotherapy in the setting of advanced disease.

Combination Chemotherapy in Advanced Non–Small Cell Lung Cancer

Although combination chemotherapy has been investigated extensively in NSCLC, no single combination has emerged as a standard regimen in advanced NSCLC. Cisplatin was the basis of many of the most effective combination regimens in the past. However, the role of carboplatin has been increasing because of a similar activity level and a toxicity profile more attractive than that of the parent compound. The identification of a wealth of active new agents during the past decade has provided building blocks for many new combinations used in advanced NSCLC, including for the first time active non–platinum-containing regimens.

In a Canadian study performed in the late 1980s, cisplatin and vindesine resulted in higher response rates (25% vs. 15%) and a longer median survival (7.6 months vs. 5.7 months) than an older regimen of cisplatin, doxorubicin, and cyclophosphamide (406). This study helped establish the combination of cisplatin and a vinca alkaloid as standard therapy at the time. Since the early 1990s, the combination regimens of cisplatin plus etoposide and carboplatin plus etoposide have been used widely in advanced NSCLC, with response rates ranging from 25% to 38% and from 29% to 38%, respectively.

A three-arm randomized trial by the ECOG compared cisplatin and etoposide with two other regimens, both containing cisplatin and paclitaxel, in 560 patients (412). Paclitaxel was given by 24-hour continuous infusion, either at a standard dose of 135 mg/m^2 or a higher dose of 250 mg/m^2 (with granulocyte colony-stimulating factor [G-CSF] support). The response rates and median survival times were superior for the two paclitaxel-containing regimens in comparison with the etoposide arm. However, no differences were found between the higher- and lower-dose paclitaxel-containing regimens with respect to response rate (32.1% vs. 26.5%) or median survival time (10.0 vs. 9.6 months). A randomized trial by the Southwest Oncology Group (SWOG) compared cisplatin alone with cisplatin and vinorelbine in 412 patients (413). An advantage was noted for the vinorelbine-containing arm with respect to response rate (25% vs. 10%), median survival time (7 months vs. 6 months), and 1-year survival rate (33% vs. 12%).

In the late 1990s, large trials incorporating some of the newer chemotherapy agents were initiated, and the results of these studies have begun to be reported. A randomized trial

by SWOG compared the older reference regimen of cisplatin and vinorelbine with the newer regimen of carboplatin and paclitaxel in 408 patients (414). The objective response rates with these regimens were 28% and 25%, respectively. The 1-year survival rates were 36% and 38%, respectively, and the median survival time with both regimens was 8 months. The older regimen was significantly more toxic and was associated with a much higher rate of treatment discontinuation. An economic analysis of this trial revealed a much higher cancer-related cost per patient for the regimen of carboplatin and paclitaxel, with a mean difference of $8,648, which could be attributed to higher drug costs (415).

A landmark ECOG study evaluated 1,207 patients who had advanced NSCLC with either the reference regimen of cisplatin plus paclitaxel or one of three experimental regimens: cisplatin and gemcitabine, cisplatin and docetaxel, or carboplatin and paclitaxel (416). The response rate for all evaluable patients was 19%, with a median survival time of 7.9 months, a 1-year survival rate of 33%, and a 2-year survival rate of 11%. The response rate and survival did not differ significantly between patients assigned to receive cisplatin plus paclitaxel and those assigned to receive any of the other regimens. Patients with a moderately impaired PS (2 on the ECOG scale) had a significantly lower survival rate than those with a mildly impaired or normal PS. One of the major conclusions of this study is the obvious lack of superiority of any of the commonly used chemotherapy regimens in terms of survival benefit. Any of these regimens may be considered standard therapy, and individual regimens can be chosen based on the organ function profile of the patient and the toxicity profile of each particular regimen.

One of the current approaches in advanced NSCLC has been to move away from traditional platinum-based chemotherapy so as to avoid the significant toxicity entailed. Toward this end, newer regimens containing combinations of the taxanes and gemcitabine have been evaluated in randomized settings. A study by the European Organization for Research and Treatment of Cancer randomized 480 patients to receive either cisplatin and paclitaxel or an experimental regimen of cisplatin and gemcitabine or gemcitabine and paclitaxel (417). The nonplatinum regimen of gemcitabine and paclitaxel was well tolerated but showed a trend toward lower median, 1-year, and progression-free survival rates. However, the results of two other similar randomized trials from Europe have indicated that the combination of gemcitabine and docetaxel and that of gemcitabine and paclitaxel are as effective in terms of response rates and 1-year survival as the standard platinum- and taxane-containing regimens (418,419). In one of these trials, the regimen of docetaxel and gemcitabine was found to have a more favorable toxicity profile than the standard chemotherapy arm.

In a review of 22 years of randomized trials of combination chemotherapy in this setting, 33 phase III trials performed between 1973 and 1994 were evaluated (420). Only five trials showed a difference in survival outcomes, with a median prolongation of the median survival of 2 months. The increase in median survival in patients treated in the earlier part of the analysis (1973–1983) versus the later part (1984–1994) was 2.6 weeks. Multivariate analysis revealed that cisplatin-based therapy was the major independent variable significantly associated with improved median survival. This review did not include results of trials performed after 1994 and thus excluded data for the newer active agents (taxanes, gemcitabine, camptothecins). It is clear that newer therapeutic approaches are urgently needed.

Investigational Therapy in Advanced Non–Small Cell Lung Cancer

Considerable progress has been made in the development of specific targeted therapies aimed at disrupting the molecular aspects of cancer growth and metastasis in NSCLC. Some of these agents include the following:

1. EGFR inhibitors. This class of agents consists of oral inhibitors of EGFR tyrosine kinase (ZD1839, OSI774) and monoclonal antibodies to EGFR (C225, ABX-EGF). The best studied of these is the oral compound ZD1839, which has been shown to result in significant improvement in quality-of-life endpoints when used as second-line and third-line therapy in patients with metastatic NSCLC.
2. Anti-angiogenesis inhibitors. These include vascular endothelial growth factor receptor (VEGFR) inhibitors and MMP inhibitors. VEGFR targeting by tyrosine kinase inhibitors (SU5416) and monoclonal antibodies (bevacizumab) is being tested in phase III trials in combination with cytotoxic chemotherapy. MMP inhibitors have failed to show a benefit in SCLC and in completed phase III trials of advanced NSCLC. They are currently being evaluated for earlier-stage NSCLC.
3. Farnesyl transferase inhibitors. These target the post-translational modification critical to membrane attachment and *ras* oncogene function. These agents (tipifarnib, lonafarnib, BMS-214662) are in early clinical trials.

Conclusions Regarding the Management of Stage IV Non–Small Cell Lung Cancer

Advanced NSCLC essentially remains incurable. For patients with a good PS of 0 or 1, systemic chemotherapy should be offered. Ideally, patients should be enrolled in an investigational protocol, and if they decline participation or if such therapy is unavailable, then conventional chemotherapy should be assigned according to the organ function. Currently, numerous regimens can be considered standard therapy, including doublet combinations of taxanes, gemcitabine, vinorelbine, and carboplatin, as previously discussed (see section "Combination Chemotherapy in Advanced Non–Small Cell Lung Cancer").

Second-line chemotherapy is not as well established in NSCLC as in SCLC. Typical candidates include patients who responded to first-line chemotherapy and have a good PS and whose disease is progressing after 3 months or more on first-line chemotherapy. The only agent approved for second-line chemotherapy in the United States is docetaxel, which prolonged life and improved quality of life in comparison with best supportive care in the randomized setting. Because palliation with second-line therapy may improve quality of life, second-line chemotherapy can be considered in these selected patients. It is also not unreasonable to consider other unused agents, such as gemcitabine and vinorelbine, in this setting because most patients are exposed to taxanes as first-line therapy today.

Up to a third of patients with NSCLC are older than 70 years, so that the treatment of elderly patients is an important issue. An Italian study showed a benefit of single-agent vinorelbine in comparison with best supportive care, noting improvements in 1-year survival (32% vs. 14%) and median survival (7 vs. 5 months) (421). Quality-of-life measurements indicated a reduction in cancer pain and improved functioning with treatment. A larger Italian study comparing the combination of vinorelbine and gemcitabine with vinorelbine alone found no improvement in response or survival with the addition of gemcitabine (422).

We have reached a therapeutic plateau in the treatment of advanced NSCLC with combination chemotherapy. The current regimens differ in their toxicity profiles, and they all are good choices as first-line therapy in appropriately selected patients. Novel agents able to target and disrupt the specific and key molecular steps in neoplastic transformation, proliferation, and metastasis are currently being evaluated in clinical trials. The results of trials of these target therapies, either as single agents or in combination with traditional chemotherapy, are eagerly awaited and promise to be the next step forward in the therapy of advanced NSCLC.

SMALL CELL LUNG CANCER

SCLC is a clinicopathologic entity that is biologically and clinically distinct from NSCLC. It is distinguished by rapid growth and the early development of widespread metastases. Although it is extremely sensitive to both chemotherapy and radiotherapy, relapse usually occurs despite treatment within 2 years. Overall long-term survival continues to be dismal, with 5-year survival rates of approximately 3% to 8% (423).

Of the lung cancers diagnosed annually, 20% to 25% are SCLCs. Cigarette smoking is the primary risk factor and accounts for more than 90% of cases (424). In one series, only 2% of 500 patients with SCLC had no history of smoking (425). SCLC is also the most common histologic subtype among uranium miners and probably results from exposure to radioactive radon, a by-product of uranium decay (426).

Clinical Presentation, Staging, and Prognostic Factors

Most signs and symptoms in SCLC are comparable with those of NSCLC, except for certain less common paraneoplastic syndromes. Because of the usual central location of the neoplasm, patients with SCLC typically present with cough, shortness of breath, hemoptysis, wheezing, local chest pain, or postobstructive pneumonitis. Large hilar and mediastinal adenopathy, pneumonitis, and atelectasis are more common in SCLC than in NSCLC. A peripheral location, chest wall involvement, and pleural effusions are less common than in NSCLC. Cavitation is very uncommon. A small cohort of patients with SCLC occasionally present with an apparent solitary pulmonary nodule.

Hemoptysis is less common in SCLC because the tumors tend to arise submucosally. Mediastinal extension is almost invariable and causes regional symptoms, including superior vena cava syndrome. This syndrome results from extrinsic compression of the superior vena cava and secondary intraluminal thrombosis and is present at diagnosis in approximately 10% of cases. Survival is not significantly altered by the presence of superior vena cava syndrome (427).

In most cases, systemic dissemination of the tumor has already developed at the time of clinical diagnosis. In a small series, autopsy data from patients with SCLC who had a non–cancer-related death less than 30 days after apparently curative resection revealed metastases in 69% of cases, and 63% of these were distant metastases (428). Sites commonly involved by metastases include the bones, liver, central nervous system (CNS), adrenal glands, and bone marrow. Hepatic metastases cause laboratory abnormalities in 50% to 60% of cases, with severe impairment in only a few. The part of the central nervous system most frequently involved is the brain, and most patients have neurologic symptoms. Bone metastases are usually not painful, and pathologic fractures are uncommon. Extensive bone marrow involvement results in cytopenias, and patients require red blood cell transfusions during chemotherapy.

Paraneoplastic Syndromes

The paraneoplastic syndromes commonly associated with SCLC include SIADH, ectopic Cushing syndrome, Lambert-Eaton myasthenic syndrome, and rare neurologic syndromes, including subacute peripheral neuropathy, cerebellar ataxia, and retinal degeneration. SCLC is frequently associated with elevated levels of polypeptide hormones, although the clinical syndromes associated with these hormones are much less common. In a large series, 11% of the patients had laboratory evidence of SIADH at presentation, but only 27% of them had symptoms of hyponatremia (429). SIADH was not related to disease stage or prognosis. Clinically evident ectopic Cushing syndrome was present at diagnosis in 4.5% of patients in a large series and was asso-

ciated with a short survival, poor response to chemotherapy, and high infection rate (430). SCLC is the malignancy most commonly associated with Lambert-Eaton myasthenic syndrome, which manifests before the cancer itself is diagnosed. Lambert-Eaton myasthenic syndrome is caused by immunologic cross-reactivity between tumor-associated antigens and calcium-gated ion channels. The clinical course of all the neurologic syndromes is generally unrelated to that of the underlying cancer. The endocrinologic syndromes related to peptide production, however, usually abate after effective therapy of the cancer has been initiated.

Extrapulmonary Disease

In about 4% of cases, patients with SCLC do not have any obvious primary pulmonary tumor, nor do they have hilar or mediastinal adenopathy (431). A small fraction of these patients present with either nodal or visceral metastases and no evident primary site, but more often, an obvious primary site is found for extrapulmonary tumors arising in the uterine cervix, esophagus, larynx, pharynx, colon, rectum, prostate, and paranasal sinuses. Histologically, these tumors often resemble SCLC and often contain neurosecretory granules. They behave aggressively and are usually treated with chemotherapy regimens similar to those used for SCLC.

Staging Evaluation

The accurate staging of SCLC is challenging in view of its tendency to disseminate early and its association with paraneoplastic syndromes. Rather than the TNM system used for NSCLC, investigators use a simple two-stage system developed by the Veterans Administration Lung Group.

The Veterans Administration Lung Group grade has been recognized as an independent prognostic indicator in clinical studies (432). Disease is classified as either limited or extensive. Limited disease is confined to the hemithorax of origin and regional lymph nodes (hilar and mediastinal), with or without involvement of the ipsilateral supraclavicular lymph nodes. The disease may be incorporated within a single radiation portal; thus, patients with involved contralateral mediastinal or hilar lymph nodes can be classified as having limited disease. In general, limited disease corresponds to ISS stages I through IIIB. Extensive disease is overt extrathoracic metastatic disease, and approximately 70% of patients with SCLC present with extensive disease. An ipsilateral malignant pleural effusion is generally considered to indicate extensive disease (203,433). The disease stage is clearly of prognostic significance and identifies a subset of patients eligible to receive thoracic irradiation as a component of their treatment plan.

The diagnosis is made after material suitable for histologic or cytologic analysis has been obtained by bronchoscopy, FNA, or mediastinoscopy, as previously discussed (see section "Establishing the Diagnosis"). Chest CT provides a precise determination of the extent of parenchymal, mediastinal, and pleural disease. CT of the upper abdomen with attention to the liver and adrenals is indicated, although a significant number of adrenal glands appearing normal on CT scans may show metastatic disease on a review of biopsy material. Radionuclide bone scans can identify sites of osseous metastases, with skeletal radiographs used to exclude benign bone and joint disease. CT of the brain is indicated in patients with neurologic symptoms. All asymptomatic patients should undergo CT of the brain if prophylactic cranial irradiation is planned. MRI may be used to resolve lesions of questionable significance after CT.

Routine bone marrow aspiration and biopsy is often performed as part of the initial evaluation of SCLC. Outside clinical trials, this is not mandatory in patients without a cytopenia or elevated level of lactate dehydrogenase. The bone marrow is the only site of metastasis in fewer than 5% of patients. The yield of a bilateral bone marrow biopsy can be 10% greater than that of unilateral testing.

Because SCLC progresses rapidly, staging should proceed expeditiously, and long delays in initiating chemotherapy must be avoided. Although extensive staging procedures are often carried out, it is not clear that any advantage is obtained by conducting a more complete staging procedure than is necessary to document extensive disease. A possible exception is CT or MRI of the brain; early treatment of brain metastases is associated with a reduced rate of chronic neurologic disability.

Prognostic Factors

Determinants of an adverse prognosis in SCLC include a poor PS, weight loss, and male sex. Overt distant metastases are by far the worst prognostic feature. Central nervous system or hepatic involvement is particularly unfavorable in comparison with metastatic disease at other sites. Among patients with limited disease, the absence of mediastinal and supraclavicular adenopathy is considered favorable. Paraneoplastic syndromes are generally believed to be associated with an adverse outcome. Elevated lactate dehydrogenase and alkaline phosphatase levels are considered unfavorable. Patients whose tumors progress during chemotherapy have a particularly poor prognosis.

Treatment Aspects of Small Cell Lung Cancer

In the treatment of limited SCLC, the overriding goals are local tumor control and the treatment of micrometastatic disease. With the evolution of combination chemotherapy regimens, complete remission rates continue to increase, but local recurrences are very common. Additional modalities of local therapy, including radiotherapy and surgery, should be considered. The effort to eradicate micrometastatic disease, except in the case of prophylactic cranial irradiation, has concentrated on investigational schedules and intensities of chemotherapy, the investigation of newer immunologic approaches, and more recently maintenance therapy with new agents. Most current approaches are based on integrated multimodality therapy to achieve prolonged complete remissions.

Historical Perspectives

SCLC is a systemic process early in its development. Thus, it is not surprising that historical experience has revealed the futility of managing this disease with local-regional modalities alone. Given the superior responsiveness of all stages of SCLC to chemotherapy, it is natural that the mainstay of therapeutic planning is systemic chemotherapy. In comparison with NSCLC, SCLC is much more responsive to chemotherapy. Moreover, complete responses are quite common in SCLC.

In a 1960s trial conducted before the introduction of systemic chemotherapy, the median survival times for patients with unresectable limited disease and those with extensive disease were approximately 12 weeks and 5 weeks, respectively (434). A British study from the same era, in which 144 patients with apparently resectable SCLC were randomized to either surgery or radiation therapy, demonstrated extremely poor survival in both treatment arms. The median length of survival and the 1-year and 5-year survival rates were 6.5 months, 21%, and 1%, respectively, for those randomized to surgery. Among those treated with definitive radiation, the figures were 10 months, 22%, and 4%, respectively (435). In recent years, thoracic irradiation has seldom been administered alone, and the impact of such therapy on outcomes is difficult to quantify.

In a single-institution report of patients seen between 1931 and 1971, only 7% had resectable tumors, and only two patients survived for 5 years (436). Similarly, among 368 surgically treated patients with SCLC, fewer than 1% survived for 5 years after resection (437). This contrasted with a 5-year survival of 15% to 25% for patients with the other three major histologic subtypes. A review of patients thought to have surgically resectable SCLC could find absolutely no advantage for including surgery in the treatment regimen (438).

In 1969, the first report of an improvement in survival in SCLC with the use of chemotherapy was reported. The Veterans Administration Lung Cancer Study Group trial showed that three cycles of cyclophosphamide could more than double median survival in comparison with supportive care in patients with extensive SCLC (439). Subsequently, data from many small studies showed that chemotherapy could significantly improve survival at 2 years when used in an adjuvant fashion after surgical resection. Similarly, in randomized trials, the addition of chemotherapy to thoracic irradiation improved median survival. The results of these trials rapidly established combination chemotherapy as the mainstay of therapy for both limited and extensive SCLC by the early 1970s.

TABLE 39.21. ACTIVE CHEMOTHERAPY AGENTS IN SMALL CELL LUNG CANCER

Older Agents	Newer Agents
Cyclophosphamide	Irinotecan
Ifosfamide	Topotecan
Doxorubicin	Paclitaxel
Methotrexate	Docetaxel
Etoposide	Gemcitabine
Vincristine	Vinorelbine
Cisplatin	
Carboplatin	

Chemotherapeutic Approaches

Active Single Agents

Numerous agents have shown considerable activity in SCLC (Table 39.21). The active single agents used in the earliest phase of the development of combination chemotherapy included cyclophosphamide, mechlorethamine, doxorubicin, methotrexate, etoposide, and vincristine. Of these, etoposide had an impressive response rate of 40% to 80% in previously untreated patients (440), but in the setting of relapse, a large report showed only a 9% response rate. In the 1980s, cisplatin, ifosfamide, carboplatin, teniposide, epirubicin, and vindesine were documented as having significant activity. Cisplatin was evaluated as a single agent mostly in previously treated patients and showed a response rate similar to that of carboplatin, about 60%, in previously treated patients (441).

The 1990s saw the introduction of a range of new chemotherapeutic agents, including the topoisomerase I inhibitors (topotecan, irinotecan), the taxanes (paclitaxel, docetaxel), vinorelbine, and gemcitabine, as active single agents in the therapy of SCLC. Topotecan had response rates of 39% and 25% among previously untreated and treated patients, respectively (442,443). Irinotecan had response rates of 33% to 47% in previously treated patients and 50% in untreated patients (444). Paclitaxel had a response rate of 34% to 41% in untreated patients in cooperative group phase II trials (445), and docetaxel had a 25% response rate in previously treated patients (446). Vinorelbine had a response rate of 13% to 16% in two small trials (447,448). Gemcitabine had a 29% response rate in previously untreated patients (449).

Impressive response and survival rates were reported with the use of oral etoposide as a single agent in elderly patients with extensive disease (450). Accordingly, single-agent chemotherapy was considered as an option for elderly patients or those with a poor PS. However, two randomized trials comparing oral etoposide with intravenous multiple-agent chemotherapy showed palliation of symptoms to be the same or slightly worse with oral etoposide (451,452). In addition, both trials showed a small but significant survival benefit associated with multiple-agent chemotherapy. Thus, combination chemotherapy remains the standard of care for the vast majority of patients with SCLC.

Combination Chemotherapy

Although few randomized trials have been conducted to address this point, the results achieved with combination chemotherapy appear to have significant advantages in comparison with those achieved with single-agent chemotherapy (453). In the early 1980s, a consensus report concluded that optimal results in the treatment of SCLC could be achieved only with combination chemotherapy (454). Commonly used combination chemotherapy regimens include cisplatin and etoposide (EP), carboplatin and etoposide (EC), and cyclophosphamide, doxorubicin, and vincristine (CAV).

In patients with limited disease, modern chemotherapy regimens are capable of producing overall response rates of 70% to 80%, which include complete response rates of more than 50%. Median survival times of 12 to 16 months have been regularly observed, and 2-year survival rates of 15% to 25% are possible. In extensive disease, the response rate and duration of median survival are clearly inferior to those observed in limited disease. Overall response rates are slightly inferior to those observed in limited disease. Complete response rates are considerably lower, in the range of 15% to 25% in most trials. Median survival times vary from 7 to 11 months, and 2-year survival is seen in fewer than 5% of patients with extensive disease. As is discussed later (see section "Thoracic Irradiation in Small Cell Lung Cancer"), thoracic radiation improves local control rates from 10% to about 40% to 60% in patients with limited disease and increases survival.

The optimal combination chemotherapy regimen in SCLC is not clear. The CAV regimen was widely used in the late 1970s and 1980s. It repeatedly resulted in the optimal response rates and median survival times previously outlined and was considered by many to be the standard regimen. In the 1980s, when etoposide became established as an active agent, trials were conducted to determine if the addition of etoposide to CAV (CAVE regimen) or the substitution of etoposide for vincristine or doxorubicin improved outcome (455). Of three trials that compared CAV with CAVE, two found greater response rates with CAVE (456–458), which did not translate into improved overall survival. Median survival in patients with extensive disease was prolonged modestly with the substitution of etoposide for either vincristine or doxorubicin, but no improvement was seen in patients with limited disease. These studies did not demonstrate a superiority of etoposide over existing regimens.

The EP combination was shown to be highly synergistic in preclinical studies (459). In previously treated patients, the EP regimen produced response rates approaching 50% in early studies (459). Subsequently, the use of EP as first-line therapy led to acceptable results in patients with both limited and extensive disease; response rates as high as 95% were reported. In a pooled analysis of 294 previously treated patients with SCLC who were treated with EP, the overall response rate was 47% (460). Regimens substituting carboplatin for cisplatin in combination with etoposide (EC regimen) in SCLC appeared to have efficacy similar to that of EP, with reduced gastrointestinal toxicity but increased myelosuppression (461).

The EP regimen was directly compared with the CAV regimen in two randomized studies (462,463). In a Japanese study including patients with limited and extensive disease, the overall survival was the same in the CAV and EP arms. The Southeastern Cancer Study Group trial of patients with previously untreated extensive disease showed no difference in response rates or overall survival between CAV and EP. However, EP was twice as effective in relapsing patients previously treated with CAV, whereas CAV was relatively ineffective as a second-line regimen. Less neutropenia and fewer infections were associated with EP than with CAV in these randomized trials. Although CAV appears to be comparable to EP, it has not proved superior, and EP, with its favorable toxicity profile, remains the treatment of choice for patients with limited disease in the United States. In extensive SCLC, carboplatin is routinely substituted for cisplatin in many centers.

Alternating Chemotherapy

One strategy to develop more effective chemotherapy regimens has been to use alternating "non–cross-resistant" chemotherapy, which has theoretic advantages in terms of tumor cell killing according to the mathematical model described by Goldie and Coldman (464). This method potentially overcomes drug resistance by exposing tumors to an increased number of active cytotoxic agents.

Three randomized trials have attempted to prove this theory. A Canadian trial in patients with extensive disease showed better overall response rates and survival with alternating CAV/EP than with CAV alone, but it could not be definitively ascertained whether the improvements were a consequence of alternation or of the superiority of EP over CAV (465). In a Japanese study of 288 patients with both limited and extensive disease, overall response rates in the EP and CAV/EP arms were superior to those in the CAV arm. The larger Southeastern Cancer Study Group trial of 437 patients with extensive disease demonstrated no difference in either observed responses or overall survival between CAV, EP, and alternating CAV/EP. A consensus conference concluded that alternating chemotherapy regimens could not be recommended on the basis of existing randomized trials (466).

Early Dose Intensification

Another approach involves increasing the dose intensity of chemotherapy to enhance response rates and survival. Several randomized trials evaluated dose-response relationships in SCLC. In the late 1970s and 1980s, five studies tested doxorubicin or alkylating agent–based chemotherapy, and only one study demonstrated a modest survival advantage with early dose intensification. Cisplatin-based chemotherapy was evaluated in patients who had limited disease in randomized trials with conflicting results. In a French study,

105 patients received chemotherapy consisting of cisplatin, cyclophosphamide, doxorubicin, and etoposide. The treatment arms differed in cycle 1 only, with the dose-intense regimen containing higher doses of cisplatin and doxorubicin. The 2-year survival rates were 43% and 26% in the dose-intense and standard arms, respectively, whereas no difference in toxicity was found between the two arms (467). A second study at the NCI randomized 90 patients to high-dose or standard-dose EP (468). No difference in overall survival was reported between the two arms, although patients in the dose-intense arm had a higher rate of hematologic toxicity. A comprehensive metaanalysis of 60 trials could show no demonstrable effect on response rate or survival of an increase in dose intensity (469).

Intensive Weekly Dosing

Another approach to dose intensification has been the rapid sequencing of a regimen incorporating several active agents over a short period. One thoroughly studied regimen, CODE, consists of weekly dosing of cisplatin, vincristine, doxorubicin, and etoposide, with alternation of the myelosuppressive and nonmyelosuppressive agents. CODE was designed to increase the dose intensity of these four agents in comparison with CAV/EP. A Canadian pilot study reported a 94% overall response rate and a 40% complete response rate in 48 patients with extensive disease (470). The median survival was 61 weeks, but grade 4 neutropenia developed in 56% patients, and 58% patients required blood transfusions. A phase III Japanese trial randomized patients to CODE plus G-CSF versus CAV/EP and failed to demonstrate any advantage in response rates or survival (471). A confirmatory National Cancer Institute Canada/SWOG trial was prematurely closed because of an excess number of toxic deaths in the CODE arm. Again, no survival benefit was seen with dose intensification.

Dose Intensification with Cytokine Support

Dose intensification with the concomitant use of colony-stimulating factors potentially reduces the development of excessive myelosuppression. Studies in which G-CSF was used demonstrated modest improvements in delivered dose intensity and a reduction in febrile neutropenia without survival benefits. A randomized study of granulocyte-macrophage colony-stimulating factor (GM-CSF) in patients with limited disease showed a significantly increased incidence and duration of life-threatening thrombocytopenia and toxic deaths (472). The preponderance of evidence from randomized trials indicates that comparisons of "high-dose" and "standard-dose" regimens using the same agents do not produce consistent survival advantages, and toxicity, particularly myelosuppression, is greater.

Late Intensification with High-Dose Chemotherapy

SCLC is an appropriate disease to study in the context of late intensification with high-dose chemotherapy and autologous hematopoietic support. Multiple small studies in the

1980s demonstrated an enhanced rate of complete responses without obvious survival benefits. In the only randomized trial reported, 45 patients who had responded to induction chemotherapy were randomized to conventional or high-dose chemotherapy with marrow support (473). Disease-free survival was enhanced, and a trend toward higher median and long-term survival was observed in the high-dose arm. A serious problem with this study was the high toxic death rate of 18%.

In a phase II study of patients with limited SCLC who achieved a complete or nearly complete response with conventional chemotherapy followed by high-dose cyclophosphamide, carmustine, and cisplatin with hematopoietic stem cell support, then by thoracic and prophylactic cranial irradiation, the median progression-free survival was 21 months, and the toxic death rate was 8% in 36 treated patients (474). The overall 2- and 5-year progression-free survival rates were 53% and 41%, respectively. In the patients who were in complete or nearly complete remission before high-dose therapy, these rates were 57% and 53%, respectively. In a feasibility study by the European Group for Blood and Marrow Transplantation, 69 patients received one to three courses of high-dose ifosfamide, carboplatin, and etoposide with stem cell support (475). The rates for toxic death and febrile neutropenia were 9% and 66%, respectively. The response rate was 86% (51% complete response rate). The median survival in patients with limited disease was 18 months, with a 2-year survival of 32%; in patients with extensive disease, the corresponding rates were 11 months and 5%.

During the past decade, the morbidity and mortality associated with high-dose chemotherapy have declined substantially, and the upper age limit for eligible patients in many centers has increased to 65 years. Patients with SCLC are at additional risk for complications secondary to smoking-associated lung damage. Ongoing randomized trials will assist in determining the role of high-dose therapy in patients with limited SCLC and good responses to induction chemotherapy.

Recent Trials of Chemotherapy

The results of the current generation of randomized trials incorporating the newer chemotherapeutic agents into combination regimens have been mixed. A Japanese study in patients with extensive SCLC was prematurely closed because response rates and overall survival were better with cisplatin plus irinotecan than with the standard EP regimen (476). In the final analysis, among the 154 patients randomized, significant differences were found between the experimental and standard arms in terms of response rates (84% vs. 68%), median overall survival (12.8 vs. 9.4 months), and 2-year survival (19.5% vs. 5%). On the other hand, trials in which topotecan or paclitaxel was added to standard regimens failed to show benefit over existing therapy but did show an increase in toxicity with the addition of the third drug (477,478). The current standard chemotherapeutic regimen in SCLC, outside a clinical trial, remains EP or EC. The combination

of cisplatin plus irinotecan can be considered an alternative option.

Summary of Chemotherapy for Small Cell Lung Cancer

The introduction of combination chemotherapy as standard therapy for both limited and extensive SCLC has contributed to significant improvements in survival. Unfortunately, the initial enthusiasm generated by these significant therapeutic advances has waned with the realization that a plateau has been reached and no further major increments in survival have been achieved. Although a number of chemotherapy regimens may be equivalent to EP or EC, alternating and dose-intense regimens have not gained widespread acceptance. Four to six cycles of EP or EC without maintenance therapy appear sufficient by today's standards.

Chemotherapy for Relapsed Disease

The overall survival of patients with relapsed SCLC is 2 to 4 months; second-line chemotherapy may significantly palliate symptoms and prolong survival in some patients. Even though most patients relapse after first-line chemotherapy, the treatment-free interval is variable. It is evident that the likelihood of a response to second-line chemotherapy depends on the length of this interval. Patients who respond to first-line chemotherapy for a period longer than 3 months are thought to be more sensitive to second-line chemotherapy and may have a major response with the same combination of drugs, indicating the presence of sensitive cell clones. Such patients generally have a good PS, which is thought to be an important predictor of response to second-line therapy. On the other hand, disease that has never responded to initial chemotherapy or has progressed within 3 months after the end of initial therapy is thought to be refractory, and the chance of a significant response to second-line chemotherapy is small in such cases. In a review of 1,749 patients, the cumulative response rate to multiple-drug regimens was 21%, and that to single agents was 19% (479).

For patients treated with alkylator- or anthracycline-based regimens, EP is recommended as second-line therapy. However, no standard chemotherapy salvage regimen is available for patients relapsing after EP chemotherapy; the current approach in this setting is to enroll patients in trials incorporating newer active agents. In a randomized trial, sensitive patients with relapsed SCLC were randomized to topotecan or CAV; most of them had received EP as first-line chemotherapy. The response rates and median survival in this study did not differ statistically between the two arms, although patients in the topotecan arm experienced better relief of symptoms (443).

Surgery for Small Cell Lung Caner

As previously discussed (see section "Historical Perspectives"), studies in the 1960s demonstrated that surgical resection alone is not a reasonable option for the management of SCLC. The question arises whether surgery is reasonable in the context of combined modality therapy for this disease.

It has been proposed that surgery be incorporated into the multimodality management of SCLC for the following theoretic reasons: Surgery improves the staging process and thereby provides prognostic information; it may reduce local recurrences; it does not limit the intensity of chemotherapy; and unlike radiotherapy, it does not cause myelosuppressive side effects. A fair collection of data, mostly uncontrolled in nature, is available regarding surgery followed by adjuvant chemotherapy, or induction chemotherapy followed by surgery.

Surgery Followed by Adjuvant Chemotherapy

Of lung cancers presenting as a single lesion smaller than 6 cm in diameter (solitary pulmonary nodule), 4% to 12% were SCLCs in one report (480). In a single-institution report, 15 (4%) of 408 of patients with SCLC presented with a solitary pulmonary nodule (481). About two thirds of SCLC solitary pulmonary nodules are of the "intermediate cell" histologic subtype; in marked contrast, about two thirds of SCLCs presenting in the usual manner are classic "oat cell" subtypes. Although no controlled data are available, the long-term survival rates of patients with SCLC solitary pulmonary nodules who undergo surgical resection are impressive in relation to those of other groups of SCLC patients. Pooled data from available studies show that 40% to 53% of patients with a stage I SCLC solitary pulmonary nodule treated with surgical resection survive for 5 years (480). The role of postoperative therapy in such patients is unclear. Although most patients who undergo resection receive postoperative chemotherapy, some do not and still have a prolonged disease-free survival. Nonetheless, in recognition of the systemic nature of most SCLCs, most authorities recommend that patients with a resected SCLC solitary pulmonary nodule receive adjuvant chemotherapy with an established combination regimen. However, no controlled data are available to establish this point definitively. Similarly, no data are available regarding the efficacy of thoracic radiation or prophylactic cranial irradiation (PCI) in this setting, although it is reasonable to consider such therapy in the context of potentially curative therapy for such patients.

Other studies have also reported impressive long-term survival rates for patients with SCLC undergoing surgical resection. The data suggest that patients with stage I or II SCLC have a 27% to 42% chance of 5-year survival following resection. Long-term survival is less common among patients with more advanced disease. In a prospective evaluation of postoperative adjuvant EP, excellent survival rates were observed for stage I patients, and survival rates in stage II and IIIA disease were not inferior to those achieved with chemoradiation (482). Whether the encouraging trends in resectable SCLC reflect a beneficial effect of the surgery itself or a reduced tumor burden in patients with resectable disease remains unknown. Such data support continued investigation of the role of surgical resection followed by chemotherapy and possibly radiotherapy in early-stage SCLC.

Chemotherapy Followed by Surgery

Surgical resection following induction chemotherapy has been evaluated, with most of the data coming from small phase II trials. In a review of the results of nine trials including 260 patients with limited disease treated with induction chemotherapy followed by consideration of resection in responders to initial therapy, approximately 60% of patients were taken to surgery, and about 80% of these underwent complete resection (approximately 50% of those entering the trials). For patients with completely resected pathologic stage I SCLC, the 5-year survival approached 70%. For patients with stage II or IIIA SCLC, the survival was less favorable, but some cohorts achieved long-term disease-free survival.

These results led to a randomized study by the LCSG evaluating the role of resection in patients with limited SCLC (ISS stages I–IIIB) (483). Patients received five cycles of CAV chemotherapy, and those with disease judged to be suitable for resection were then randomized to surgery followed by thoracic radiation and PCI, or to an identical regimen of radiation treatment without surgery. Of 340 patients, 66% responded to induction chemotherapy (28% complete response rate and 38% partial response rate). A total of 144 (42%) of the patients were randomized, 68 to the surgery arm and 76 to no surgery. No significant differences in median or overall survival were observed between the two groups. The median survival of all patients was 14 months, but it was 18 months for the patients who were randomized. The actuarial 2-year survival was 20% in both arms. Accordingly, the study failed to provide any support for surgical resection in limited SCLC.

Presently, surgery cannot be considered standard for any subgroup of patients with SCLC. However, available evidence from nonrandomized studies does support a role for resection in well-staged patients with ISS stage I and possibly for some patients with stage II disease. Surgery should not currently be included in the management of patients with ISS stages IIIA and IIIB limited disease. Unfortunately, such patients comprise the vast majority of those with limited disease. Accordingly, at the present time, surgery is not indicated for most patients with limited SCLC.

Thoracic Irradiation in Small Cell Lung Cancer

In SCLC, thoracic irradiation alone produces a response in up to 90% of patients. Although disseminated extrathoracic metastases have traditionally been the major site of failure in SCLC, local-regional failure within the chest occurs in up to 80% of patients with limited disease treated with chemotherapy alone (484). This high rate of local failure provides a rationale for the use of thoracic irradiation, with the objectives of improving local control and overall survival. Several randomized trials have been conducted, and a review of these studies has led to certain conclusions regarding chemotherapy and thoracic irradiation. In almost all studies, thoracic irradiation significantly decreased the rate of local failure in SCLC, and therapy with a combination of modalities invariably increased hematologic, pulmonary, and esophageal complications.

The role of thoracic irradiation in SCLC was assessed comprehensively in two metaanalyses published in 1992 (485,486). Thirteen randomized trials comprising more than 2,100 patients with limited disease were included in the larger metaanalysis (486). Chemotherapy regimens differed between studies, as did radiation doses and schedules. In both reports, the addition of thoracic irradiation was associated with a 5% to 7% improvement in 2- and 3-year survival rates. Local control rates were impressively improved by 25%. Overall, local control was observed in 23% of patients receiving chemotherapy alone, and in 48% of patients treated with chemoradiation. The survival benefit was greatest for patients who were less than 55 years of age and was achieved at the cost of increased toxicity.

Optimal Chemotherapy with Thoracic Irradiation

Combined-modality protocols in randomized studies have evaluated alkylator-based, doxorubicin-based, and platinum-based regimens administered concurrently with thoracic irradiation. The EP regimen is more mucosa-sparing and less myelosuppressive, and it is associated with less cardiac and pulmonary toxicity. Several pilot trials with this approach suggested an improvement in long-term outcome in comparison with trials included in the metaanalyses. Results of Japanese and American randomized studies of thoracic irradiation in combination with EP showed a consistent and significant improvement in survival rates in excess of 40% at 2 years. In some centers, carboplatin is used in place of cisplatin because it is more easily administered and appears to cause less toxicity. Equivalent response and survival results have been obtained for EP and EC. Currently, however, the reference arms for most clinical trials continue to use the EP regimen.

Building on the improvements in long-term outcome with EP and concurrent radiotherapy, the current emphasis is on evaluating the possibility of enhancing results by adding newer cytotoxic drugs to the existing regimens. For example, newer drugs such as the taxanes are added to standard chemotherapy regimens. Early reports have noted increased local-regional control at the cost of increased esophageal toxicity. It remains to be seen whether these results translate into long-term survival better than that obtained with EP and radiation.

Timing of Radiation

Methods of combining radiotherapy with chemotherapy include the following:

1. Radiotherapy is given with the initiation of chemotherapy.
2. Induction chemotherapy is followed by radiotherapy during subsequent courses.
3. Chemotherapy is followed sequentially by radiotherapy.
4. Radiotherapy is split between cycles of chemotherapy.

Previous randomized trials specifically addressing this issue have yielded conflicting results. Trials have compared EP or EC with radiation in the second versus the sixth cycle of chemotherapy (487), in the first versus the third cycle (488), and in the first cycle versus sequentially following the fourth cycle (489). The current weight of evidence favors concurrent thoracic irradiation initiated relatively early, with the first or second cycle of platinum-based chemotherapy.

Volume of Radiation

The recommendation for standard radiation portals is based on retrospective studies and includes the original tumor volume with a 1.5- to 2.0-cm free margin. A randomized trial addressing this issue did not reveal any differences in the intrathoracic recurrence rate in a comparison of wide-volume radiotherapy with reduced-volume radiotherapy. Conflicting data from retrospective studies suggest a twofold to threefold increase in thoracic recurrences with reduced-volume radiotherapy. It is not certain whether radiation portals should be designed based on the original tumor volume and uninvolved nodes, or on the reduced volume left after chemotherapy. A review of this issue found no compelling evidence supporting either strategy (490).

Dose of Radiation

For the past three decades, the commonly used dose of thoracic radiotherapy in limited SCLC has been 40 to 50 Gy. Presumably because SCLC is typically much more responsive to radiotherapy than NSCLC, lower doses are used. Most of the data addressing this issue are in the form of retrospective analyses. One retrospective study found that local failure rates for doses below 40 Gy were more than 50%, whereas those for doses between 40 and 50 Gy were 30%. Current U.S. cooperative group trials have started to use higher doses of 60 to 63 Gy.

Radiation Fractionation

In conventional fractionation, radiation is administered as 1.8- to 2.0-Gy fractions daily for a 5-week period. In contrast, in hyperfractionation, twice-daily fractions of lower doses of radiation are administered for a shorter period of 3 weeks. This approach reduces late-effect injury and increases the damage to rapidly proliferating subpopulations of cancer cells that divide within the 24-hour time interval. A number of phase II studies have suggested that hyperfractionation schedules may produce an advantage in terms of local control and possibly survival in comparison with standard once-daily fractionation schedules.

Results of two large, randomized trials provide supporting data for dose-intensive radiation as a means of improving both local-regional control and long-term overall survival. In a large intergroup trial in which twice-daily accelerated radiation (45 Gy over 3 weeks) was given concurrently with cycle 1 of EP to 417 patients with limited disease, the overall survival was 47% at 2 years and 26% at 5 years (491). Survival rates in patients treated with standard once-daily radiation

(45 Gy over 5 weeks) were 41% at 2 years and 19% at 5 years. After a median follow-up of 8 years, median survival times in the twice- and once-daily groups were 23 and 19 months, respectively. The incidence of grade 3 esophagitis was higher with accelerated radiotherapy. Interestingly, survival rates in both arms were better than the 2-year survival of 23% revealed in the metaanalyses.

The other randomized study compared concurrent twice-daily, split-course irradiation with conventional once-daily irradiation in patients with limited disease responding after three cycles of EP (492). A break of 2 1/2 weeks after 24 Gy of hyperfractionated radiotherapy resulted in a similar dose intensity of radiation in both arms, with 48 to 50 Gy delivered over 6 weeks. No differences were found in regard to local-regional control, median survival, and overall survival at 3 years. It is therefore possible that the superior outcomes in the intergroup trial were actually a manifestation of acceleration radiation rather than of hyperfractionation itself.

Accelerated hyperfractionated radiotherapy is an interesting approach to the management of limited SCLC. Improvements in local control and survival are achieved at the cost of increased early but decreased late toxicity, so that it is difficult to incorporate this technique as a standard of care in the community setting. However, further trials with the use of radioprotective agents such as amifostine may be useful in assigning a definite role for this approach in the future.

Current Perspective: Thoracic Irradiation

Thoracic irradiation is firmly established as an integral component of combined-modality therapy for limited SCLC, improving local control and overall survival. Issues of timing, volume, and optimal chemotherapy have been largely addressed by the available data. Ongoing investigation into hyperfractionation, dose increase, additional chemotherapy, and the use of mucoprotective agents will lead to significant refinements in the current standard delivery of thoracic irradiation in the future.

A practical approach is to consider the early integration of thoracic irradiation (from the first or second cycle of chemotherapy onward) with systemic platinum-based chemotherapy. The delivery of a standard dose of 45 to 50 Gy to the original tumor volume is an acceptable start. The use of hyperfractionated radiotherapy or larger doses of radiotherapy, outside the setting of clinical trials, has not yet been adopted, even though it is associated with promising long-term outcomes.

Prophylactic Cranial Irradiation

Shortly after the introduction of successful chemotherapy in SCLC, it was recognized that the CNS is an extremely common site of initial relapse, and frequently the only site of relapse. Most of the commonly used chemotherapeutic agents do not effectively penetrate the blood–brain barrier; accordingly, the brain serves as a sanctuary. In a retrospec-

tive study of 48 patients achieving a complete response to chemotherapy, CNS metastases developed in 38% of them, none of whom had received PCI. In 17% of the patients, the brain was an isolated site of failure (493). Others have reported that the brain may be a first or solitary site of failure in 9% to 14% of patients with SCLC who achieve complete remission. Moreover, the probability of brain metastases increases with the length of survival. The cumulative risk for CNS metastases has been estimated to be 58% to 80% by 2 years after diagnosis (494). Based on these observations, the use of PCI to decrease the rate of CNS failure and improve survival has been studied extensively in SCLC.

Recent Randomized Trials

The results of three large randomized trials including more than 800 patients that were conducted to address the value of PCI have been published. In the PCI85 French trial, 300 patients with SCLC (80% with limited disease) achieving a complete response to chemotherapy were randomized to receive either 24 Gy in eight fractions or no radiation (495). At 2 years, the rate of CNS failure was 67% for those who did not receive PCI and 40% for those who did. Although survival trends favored the group receiving PCI, no significant difference was found at 2 years (29% vs. 21%, $P = .14$). In the PCI88 French trial, 211 patients in complete remission were randomized to PCI of 24 to 30 Gy or to no PCI (496). At 4 years, the survival rates did not differ significantly between the PCI group and the control group (22% vs.16%, $P = .25$). The incidence of brain metastases did not differ between the two groups. Similarly, in a U.K. study involving 314 patients, the CNS failure rate at 3 years was 55% among those who did not receive PCI and 37% among those who did (497). Although survival trend favored the PCI group in this trial, no statistically significant survival differences were found.

The effects of PCI on survival were evaluated in a metaanalysis of 987 patients in seven randomized trials (498), including trials in which patients had a complete response with systemic chemotherapy with or without thoracic irradiation. According to these accumulated data, the relative risk for death was reduced in patients receiving PCI (relative risk, 0.84; 95% CI, 0.73–0.97); this corresponded to an absolute increase of 5.4% in the 3-year survival rate. The rate of disease-free survival increased (relative risk for recurrence or death, 0.75), and the cumulative incidence of brain metastases decreased (relative risk, 0.46). Larger doses of radiation were associated with a greater reduction in the risk for brain metastases.

Neurologic Toxicity

Perhaps the most powerful argument against the routine use of PCI in patients with limited SCLC is related to the toxicity of PCI, particularly potentially disabling late neurologic and intellectual impairment (499). It has been shown that such abnormalities are more frequent in patients who have received PCI. However, it has also been shown that not all approaches to CNS radiation treatment are equally likely to be associated with neurologic sequelae. Two randomized studies of PCI in SCLC prospectively monitored patients for the development of CNS toxicity by neuropsychologic assessment. The PCI85 French trial also performed CT (495). Significant cognitive impairment related to PCI was not documented in either study. On the other hand, it was found that up to 25% to 60% of patients had cognitive impairment before PCI.

Dose and Timing of Radiation

Issues of optimal radiation dosing in PCI have not been resolved. In the British PCI study, the 24 Gy of radiation delivered in 12 fractions was found to be ineffective. Instead, 24 Gy delivered in eight fractions, as in the French trials, may be an acceptable regimen. A regimen commonly used in clinical practice is 30 Gy delivered in 10 fractions. At this time, a dose schedule of 36 Gy in 18 fractions is also an established alternative with clear evidence of a clinical effect. The conventional practice is to introduce PCI as early as possible in the course of treatment after a response to chemotherapy. The metaanalysis demonstrated a significant trend toward a greater reduction in brain metastases in patients who received PCI earlier. It is important, though, to avoid the concurrent administration of chemotherapy and to introduce PCI at the end of induction therapy.

Current Perspective: Prophylactic Cranial Irradiation

A large body of literature based on randomized comparisons indicates that PCI not only decreases the rate of CNS recurrence but also has a small but absolute favorable effect on overall survival. The survival benefit is similar to that seen with thoracic radiotherapy in patients with SCLC, documented by the metaanalyses of thoracic radiotherapy published in the early 1990s. The vast majority of patients, including those with limited disease, eventually succumb to their disease, and systemic failure is the predominant cause of death. PCI can only favorably affect the survival of patients in whom systemic chemotherapy and thoracic radiation control all gross and microscopic sites of disease.

Moreover, if the objective of treatment in limited SCLC is to cure the disease in the highest possible number of patients, the avoidance of CNS metastases becomes a major priority. In recent years, while the survival of patients with SCLC has increased as more effective chemotherapy is combined with thoracic radiotherapy, the cumulative risk for brain metastases has also increased. Because the length of survival is approximately 4 to 5 months after the detection of brain metastases, the overriding objective is prevention. Moreover, an improved quality of life with PCI is always possible.

Based on current evidence, PCI should be incorporated into the primary management of completely responding patients with limited SCLC; it significantly diminishes the risk for CNS recurrence, and evidence suggests that it can be safely administered without a substantial risk for significant neurologic disability. It should be given sequentially following chemotherapy; concurrent chemotherapy and PCI should be avoided. Although the proper dose and schedule of PCI continue to be debated, a total dose of 30 to 36 Gy may be optimal. It is important that the baseline and subsequent neuropsychologic status be assessed. It is also reasonable to consider PCI therapy for patients with SCLC and a good PS who achieve a complete remission with systemic chemotherapy.

Summary of Small Cell Lung Cancer

Combination chemotherapy has contributed to significant improvements in local control and survival in both limited and extensive SCLC. The initial enthusiasm generated by these significant therapeutic advances has waned with the realization that a plateau has been reached, and no additional increments in survival have been gained in the last decade. Although a number of chemotherapy regimens may be equivalent to EP or EC, alternating regimens or dose-intense regimens have not gained widespread acceptance. The roles of thoracic irradiation and PCI in limited SCLC have been firmly established. What remains to be determined is whether chemotherapy combinations incorporating some of the newer active agents will help us move beyond the therapeutic plateau.

REFERENCES

1. Murray CJL, Lopez AD, eds. *The global burden of disease: a comprehensive assessment of mortality and disability from diseases, injuries, and risk factors in 1990 and projected to 2020.* Cambridge, MA: Harvard University Press, 1996.
2. Parkin DM, Pisani P, Ferlay J. Global cancer statistics. *CA Cancer J Clin* 1999;49:33–64.
3. Jemal A, Murray T, Samuels A, et al. Cancer statistics, 2003. *CA Cancer J Clin* 2003;53:5–26.
4. Devesa S, Blot W, Stone B, et al. Recent cancer trends in the United States. *J Natl Cancer Inst* 1995;87:175–182.
5. American Cancer Society. *Cancer facts and figures—2002.* Atlanta, GA: American Cancer Society, 2002:1–48.
6. Mackay J. International aspects of U.S. Government tobacco bills. *JAMA* 1999;281:1849–1850.
7. Strauss GM, Dominioni L. Perception, paradox, paradigm: Alice in the wonderland of lung cancer prevention and early detection. *Cancer* 2000;89:2422–2431.
8. Adler L. *Primary malignant growth of the lungs and bronchi: a pathological and clinical study.* New York: Longmans, Green, & Co, 1912.
9. Lombard HL, Doering CR. Cancer studies in Massachusetts. *N Engl J Med* 1928;198:481–487.
10. Pearl P. Tobacco smoking and longevity. *Science* 1938;87:216–217.
11. Muller FH. Tabakmissbraunch und lungencarcinom. *Z Krebsforschung* 1939;49:57–84.
12. Muller FH. Tabakmissbraunch und lungencarcinom. *JAMA* 1939;1372.

13. Kenneway NM, Kenneway EL. A study of the incidence of cancer of the lung and larynx. *J Hyg* 1936;36:236–267.

14. Ochsner A, DeBakey M. Carcinoma of the lung. *Arch Surg* 1941;42:209–258.

15. Kenneway NM, Kenneway EL. A further study of the incidence of cancer of the lung and larynx. *Br J Cancer* 1947;1:260–298.

16. Schairer E, Schoniger E. Lungendrebs und Tabakverbrauch. *Z Krebsforschung* 1943;54:261–269.

17. Potter EA, Tully MR. The statistical approach to the cancer problem in Massachusetts. *Am J Public Health* 1945;35:485–490.

18. Clemmesen J, Busk T. On the apparent increase in the incidence of lung cancer in Denmark 1931–1945. *Br J Cancer* 1947;1:253–259.

19. American Cancer Society. *Statistics on cancer.* Atlanta, GA: American Cancer Society, Statistical Research Division, 1949.

20. Wynder EL, Graham EA. Tobacco smoking as a possible etiologic factor in bronchogenic carcinoma: a study of 684 proved cases. *JAMA* 1950;143:329–336.

21. Doll R, Bradford Hill A. Smoking and carcinoma of the lung: preliminary report. *Br Med J* 1950;2:739–748.

22. Levin ML, Goldstein H, Gerhardt PR. Cancer and tobacco smoking: a preliminary report. *JAMA* 1950;143:336–338.

23. Schrek R, Mills CA, Porter MM. Tobacco smoking habits and cancer of the mouth and respiratory system. *Cancer Res* 1950;10:539–542.

24. Rienhoff W. A clinical analysis of a follow-up study of 502 cases of carcinoma of the lung. *Dis Chest* 1950;17:33–54.

25. Ariel IM, Avery EE, Kanter L. Primary carcinoma of the lung: a clinical study of 1205 cases. *Cancer* 1950;3:229–239.

26. McConnel RB, Gordon KCT, Jones T. Occupational and personal factors in the aetiology of carcinoma of the lung. *Lancet* 1952;2:651–656.

27. Sadowsky DA, Gilliam AG, Cornfield J. The statistical association between smoking and carcinoma of the lung. *J Natl Cancer Inst* 1953;13:1237–1258.

28. Wynder EL, Cornfield J. Cancer of the lung in physicians. *N Engl J Med* 1953;248:441–444.

29. Koulumies M. Smoking and pulmonary cancer. *Acta Radiol* 1953;30:255–260.

30. Breslow L, Hoaglin L, Rasmussen F, et al. Occupations and cigarette smoking as factors in lung cancer. *Am J Public Health* 1954;44:171–181.

31. Watson WL, Conte AJ. Smoking and lung cancer. *Cancer* 1954;7:245–249.

32. Doll R, Bradford Hill A. The mortality of doctors in relation to their smoking habits. *Br Med J* 1954;1:1451–1455.

33. Doll R, Bradford Hill A. Lung cancer and other causes of death in relationship to smoking: a second report on the mortality of British doctors. *Br Med J* 1956;2:1071–1081.

34. Hammond EC, Horn D. Relationship between human smoking habits and death rates: follow-up study of 187,766 men. *JAMA* 1954;155:1316–1328.

35. Hammond EC, Horn D. Smoking and death rates—report on forty-four months of follow-up of 187,783 men. II. Death rates by cause. *JAMA* 1958;166:1294–1308.

36. Cutler SJ, Loveland DB. The risk of developing lung cancer and its relationship to smoking. *J Natl Cancer Inst* 1954;15:201–211.

37. Cutler SJ. A review of the statistical evidence on the association between smoking and lung cancer. *J Am Stat Assoc* 1955;50:267–282.

38. *Smoking and health: report of the Advisory Committee to the Surgeon General of the Public Health Service.* Washington, DC: U.S. Department of Health, Education, and Welfare, 1964: PHS publication No. 1103.

39. Smithers DW. Facts and fancies about cancer of the lung. *Br Med J* 1953;1:1235–1239.

40. Hueper WC. The cigarette theory of lung cancer. *Curr Med Digest* 1954;21:35–39.

41. Fisher RA. *Smoking—the cancer controversy: some attempts to assess the evidence.* Edinburgh: Oliver and Boyd, 1959:1–47.

42. Brownlee KA. A review of "Smoking and Health." *J Am Stat Assoc* 1965;60:722–729.

43. Glantz SA, Slade J, Bero LA, et al. *The cigarette papers.* Berkeley, CA: University of California Press, 1996:1–539.

44. Cummings K, Pollay R. Exposing Mr. Butts' tricks of the trade. *Tobacco Control* 2002;11[Suppl 1]:i1–i4.

45. Cummings K, Morley C, Hyland A. Failed promises of the cigarette industry and its effect on consumer misperceptions about the health risk of smoking. *Tobacco Control* 2002;11[Suppl 1]:i110–i117.

46. Pauly J, Mepani A, Lesses J, et al. Cigarettes with defective filters marketed for 40 years: what Philip Morris never told smokers. *Tobacco Control* 2002;11[Suppl 1]:i51–i61.

47. Kessler D. *A question of intent: a great battle with a deadly industry.* New York: Public Affairs, 2001:1–492.

48. Teague C. *Survey of cancer research with emphasis upon possible carcinogens from tobacco.* Winston-Salem, NC: R. J. Reynolds Tobacco Company, 1953:1–19.

49. Bradford Hill A. The environment and disease: association or causation? *Proc R Soc Med* 1965;58:295–300.

50. Denissenko MF, Pao A, Tang M, et al. Preferential formation of benzo(a)pyrene adducts at lung cancer mutational hotspots in p53. *Science* 1996;274:430–432.

51. Doll R, Peto R, Wheatley K, et al. Mortality in relation to smoking: 40 years' observations on male British doctors. *Br Med J* 1994;309:901–911.

52. Doll R. Uncovering the effects of smoking: historical perspective. *Stat Methods Med Res* 1998;7:87–117.

53. Peto R, Darby S, Deo H, et al., Smoking, smoking cessation, and lung cancer in the U.K. since 1950: combination of national statistics with two case-control studies. *Br Med J* 2000;321:323–329.

54. Hennekens CH, Buring JE. Epidemiology in medicine. Boston: Little, Brown and Company, 1987:1–383.

55. Doll R, Bradford Hill A. A study on the aetiology of carcinoma of the lung. *Br Med J* 1952;2:1271–1286.

56. Khuder SA. Effect of smoking on major histological types of lung cancer: a meta-analysis. *Lung Cancer* 2001;31:139–148.

57. Morabia A, Wynder EL. Cigarette smoking and lung cancer cell types. *Cancer* 1991;68:2074–2078.

58. Muscat JE, Stellman SD, Zhang Z, et al. Cigarette smoking and large cell carcinoma of the lung. *Cancer Epidemiol Biomarkers Prev* 1997;6:477–480.

59. Barbone F, Bovenzi M, Cavallieri F, et al. Cigarette smoking and histologic type of lung cancer in men. *Chest* 1997;112:1474–1479.

60. Doll R, Bradford Hill A, Kreyberg L. The significance of cell type in relation to the aetiology of lung cancer. *Br J Cancer* 1957;11:43–48.

61. Kreyberg L. Histological lung cancer types: a morphological and biological correlation. *Acta Pathol Microbiol Scand Suppl* 1962;157:1–92.

62. Vincent R, Pickren J, Lane W, et al. The changing histopathology of lung cancer. *Cancer* 1977;39:1647–1655.

63. Auerbach O, Garfinkel L. The changing pattern of lung adenocarcinoma. *Cancer* 1991;68:1973–1977.

64. Perng D, Perng R, Kuo B, et al. The variation of cell type

distribution in lung cancer: a study of 10,910 cases at a medical center in Taiwan between 1970 and 1993. *Jpn J Clin Oncol* 1996;26:229–233.

65. Charloux A, Quiox E, Wolkove N, et al. The increasing incidence of lung adenocarcinoma: reality or artefact? A review of the epidemiology of lung adenocarcinoma. *Int J Epidemiol* 1997;26:14–23.

66. Franceschi S, Bidoli E. The epidemiology of lung cancer. *Ann Oncol* 1999;10[Suppl 5]:S3–S6.

67. Thun MJ, Lally CA, Glannery JT, et al. Cigarette smoking and changes in the histopathology of lung cancer. *J Natl Cancer Inst* 1997;89:1580–1586.

68. Osann K. Epidemiology of lung cancer. *Curr Opin Pulm Med* 1998;4:198–204.

69. Strauss GM, Cummings KM. Smoking-related adenocarcinoma of the lung: Now the most common cause of cancer death in the United States. *Proc Am Soc Clin Oncol* 2003;22:638 (abst 2567).

70. *Risks associated with smoking cigarettes with low machine-measured yields of tar and nicotine.* Bethesda, MD: National Institutes of Health, National Cancer Institute, 2001: monograph 13 (smoking and tobacco control monographs; Burns DM, ed.).

71. Gazdar AF, Minna JD. Cigarettes, sex, and lung adenocarcinoma. *J Natl Cancer Inst* 1997;89:1563–1565.

72. Barkley JE, Green MR. Bronchoalveolar carcinoma. *J Clin Oncol* 1996;14:2377–2386.

73. Morabia A, Wynder EL. Relation of bronchioloalveolar carcinoma to smoking. *Br Med J* 1992;304:541–543.

74. Falk RT, Pickle LW, Fontham ETH, et al. Epidemiology of bronchioloalveolar cell carcinoma. *Cancer Epidemiol Biomarkers Prev* 1992;1:339–344.

74a. Rolen K, Fulton J, Tamura D, Strauss G. Bronchoalveolar carcinoma (BAC) of the lung is related to cigarette smoking: A case-control study from Rhode Island. *Proc Am Soc Clin Oncol* 2003;22:674 (abst 2711).

75. *Strategies to control tobacco use in the United States: a blueprint for public health action in the 1990s.* Washington, DC: U.S. Department of Health and Human Services, Public Health Service, 1991: publication No. 92-3316 (smoking and tobacco control monographs; Shopland DR, et al., eds.).

76. *Health, United States 1996–1997.* Hyattsville, MD: National Center for Health Statistics, Public Health Service, 1997:182.

77. Cigarette smoking among adults—United States 1999. *MMWR Morb Mortal Wkly Rep* 2001;50:869–873.

78. Strauss GM, DeCamp MM, Burns DM, et al. Lung cancer and former smokers: implications for smoking cessation, smoking prevention, and early detection. *Proc Am Soc Clin Oncol* 1997;16:483a(abst 1739).

79. *The health benefits of smoking cessation: a report of the Surgeon General.* Washington, DC: U.S. Department of Health and Human Services, Public Health Service, 1990.

80. Samet JM. Health benefits of smoking cessation. *Clin Chest Med* 1991;12:669–679.

81. Newcomb PA, Carbone PP. The health consequences of smoking: cancer. *Med Clin North Am* 1992;76:305–331.

82. Hammond EC. Smoking in relation to the death rates of one million men and women. In: Haenszel, ed. *Epidemiological approaches to the study of cancer and other chronic diseases.* Washington, DC: U.S. Department of Health, Education, and Welfare, Public Health Service, 1966:127–204.

83. Stellman SD, Garfinkle L. Smoking habits and tar levels in a new American Cancer Society prospective study of 1.2 million men and women. *J Natl Cancer Inst* 1986;76:1057.

84. Doll R, Peto R. Mortality in relation to smoking: 20 years' observations on male British doctors. *Br Med J* 1976;2:1525.

85. Higgins IT, Mahan CM, Wynder EL. Lung cancer among cigar and pipe smokers. *Prev Med* 1988;17:116.

86. Tong L, Spitz MR, Fueger JJ, et al. Lung cancer in former smokers. *Cancer* 1996;78:1004–1010.

87. Strauss G, DeCamp M, DiBiccaro E, et al. Lung cancer diagnosis is being made with increasing frequency in former cigarette smokers! *Proc Am Soc Clin Oncol* 1995;14:362(abst 1106).

88. Halpern MT, Gillespie BW, Warner KE. Patterns of absolute risk of lung cancer mortality in former smokers. *J Natl Cancer Inst* 1993;85:457–464.

89. Sobue T, Suzuki T, Fujimoto I, et al. Lung cancer rise among ex-smokers. *Jpn J Cancer Res* 1991;82:283–289.

90. *Preventing tobacco use among young people: a report of the Surgeon General.* Atlanta, GA: U.S. Department of Health and Human Services, Public Health Service, Centers for Disease Control and Prevention, National Center for Chronic Disease Prevention and Health Promotion, Office on Smoking and Health, 1994.

91. *Reducing tobacco use: a report of the Surgeon General.* Atlanta, GA: U.S. Department of Health and Human Services, 2000.

92. Effective educational strategies to prevent tobacco use among young people. In: *Reducing tobacco use: a report of the Surgeon General.* Atlanta, GA: U.S. Department of Health and Human Services, 2000:59–94.

93. Tobacco use among high school students—United States 1997. *MMWR Morb Mortal Wkly Rep* 1998;47:229–233.

94. Wechsler H, Rigotti N, Gledhill-Hoyt J, et al. Increased levels of cigarette use among college students: a cause for national concern. *JAMA* 1998;284:699–705.

95. Youth Tobacco Cessation Collaborative, National Blueprint for Action. *Youth and young adult tobacco use cessation.* Washington, DC: Center for Advancement for Health, 2000:1–40.

96. Cigarette smoking among adults—United States 1997. *MMWR Morb Mortal Wkly Rep* 1999;48:993–996.

97. Nelson DE, Giovino GA, Shopland DR, et al. Trends in cigarette smoking among U.S. adolescents. *Am J Public Health* 1995;85:34–40.

98. Ling P, Glantz S. Why and how the tobacco industry sells cigarettes to young adults: evidence from industry documents. *Am J Public Health* 2002;92:908–916.

99. Shields P, Harris C. Molecular epidemiology and the genetics of environmental cancer. *JAMA* 1991;266:681–687.

100. Samet JM, ed. *Epidemiology of lung cancer.* New York: Marcel Dekker Inc, 1994:1–543.

101. Shields PG. Molecular epidemiology of lung cancer. *Ann Oncol* 1999;10[Suppl 5]:S7–S11.

102. Shields PG, Harris CC. Cancer risk and low-penetrance susceptibility genes in gene-environment interactions. *J Clin Oncol* 2000;18:2309–2315.

103. LaDou J. *Occupational and environmental medicine,* 2nd ed. Stamford, CT: Appleton & Lange, 1997:1–845.

104. McDonald JC. Asbestos-related disease: an epidemiologic review. In: Wagner MC, ed. *Biological effects of mineral fibers.* Lyon: IARC, 1980:587–602.

105. Hammond EC, Selikoff IJ, Seidman H. Asbestos exposure, cigarette smoking, and death rates. *Ann N Y Acad Sci* 1979;330:473–490.

106. Hughes JM, Weill H. Asbestos and man-made fibers. In: Samet JM, ed. *Epidemiology of lung cancer.* New York: Marcel Dekker Inc, 1994:185–205.

107. Hughson WG, Fedoruk MJ. Occupational and environmental causes of lung cancer and esophageal cancer. In: Aisner J, et al., eds. *Comprehensive textbook of thoracic oncology.* Baltimore: Williams & Wilkins, 1996.

108. Lubin JH, Boice JD, Edling C, et al. *Lung cancer and radon: a joint analysis of 11 underground miner studies.* Bethesda, MD:

National Cancer Institute, 1994: DHS publication No. (NIH) 94-3644.

109. Samet JM. Radon and lung cancer. *J Natl Cancer Inst* 1989;81:745–757.

110. Samet JM. Indoor radon exposure and lung cancer: risky or not?—all over again. *J Natl Cancer Inst* 1997;89:4–6.

111. Lubin JH, Boice JD. Lung cancer risk from residential radon: meta-analysis of eight epidemiologic studies. *J Natl Cancer Inst* 1997;89:49–57.

112. Tokuhata G. Familial factors in human lung cancer and smoking. *Am J Public Health* 1964;54:25–32.

113. Law MR. Genetic predisposition to lung cancer. *Br J Cancer* 1990;61:195–206.

114. Amos CI, Caporaso NE, Weston A. Host factors in lung cancer: a review of interdisciplinary studies. *Cancer Epidemiol Biomarkers Prev* 1992;1:505–513.

115. Burch PR. Smoking and lung cancer. Tests of a causal hypothesis. *J Chronic Dis* 1980;33:221–238.

116. Eysenck HJ. The respective importance of personality, cigarette smoking and interaction effects for the genesis of cancer and coronary heart diseases. *Personality and Individual Differences* 1988;9:453–460.

117. Friberg L, Lundman T, Olsson H. Mortality in smoking-discordant monozygotic and dizygotic twins: a study of the Swedish Twin Registry. *Arch Environ Health* 1970;21:508–513.

118. Kaprio J, Koskenvuo M. Twins, smoking, and mortality: a 12-year prospective study of smoking-discordant twin pairs. *Social Sci Med* 1989;29:1083–1089.

119. Kaprio J, Koskenvuo M. Cigarette smoking as a cause of lung cancer and coronary heart disease: a study of smoking-discordant twin pairs. *Acta Genet Med Gemellol* 1990;39:25–34.

120. Mabry M, Nelkin BD, Baylin SB. Lung cancer. In: Vogelstein B, Kinzler KW, eds. *The genetic basis of human cancer.* New York: McGraw-Hill, 1998:671–680.

121. Ooi WL, Chen VW, Bailey-Wilson JE, et al. Increased familial risk for lung cancer. *J Natl Cancer Inst* 1986;76:217–222.

122. Samet JM, Humble CG, Pathak DR. Personal and family history of respiratory disease and lung cancer risk. *Am Rev Respir Dis* 1986;134:466–470.

123. Bepler G. Lung cancer epidemiology and genetics. *J Thorac Imaging* 1999;14:228–234.

124. Spitz M, Hsu TC. Genetic predisposition and risk models. In: *American Society of Clinical Oncology educational book.* Dallas, TX: American Society of Clinical Oncology, 1994:352–354.

125. Perera FP. Molecular epidemiology: insights into cancer susceptibility, risk assessment, and prevention. *J Natl Cancer Inst* 1996;88:496–509.

126. Turner-Warwick M, Lebowitz M, Burrows B, et al. Cryptogenic fibrosing alveolitis and lung cancer. *Thorax* 1980;35:496–499.

127. Skillud DM, Offord KP, Miller RD. High risk of lung cancer in chronic obstructive pulmonary disease: a prospective, matched, controlled study. *Ann Intern Med* 1986;105:503–507.

128. Churg A. Lung cancer cell type and occupational exposure. In: Samet JM, ed. *Epidemiology of lung cancer.* New York: Marcel Dekker Inc, 1994:413–436.

129. Hughes JR. Asbestosis as a precursor of asbestos-related lung cancer. *Br J Cancer* 1991;48:229–233.

130. Sluis-Cremer GK, Bezuidenhout BN. Relation between asbestosis and bronchial cancer in amphibole asbestos miners. *Br J Ind Med* 1989;46:537–540.

131. Kippen H, Lilis R, Suzuki Y, et al. Pulmonary fibrosis in asbestos insulation workers with lung cancer: a radiological and histopathological evaluation. *Br J Ind Med* 1987;44:96–100.

132. Boone CW, Kellof GJ, Malone WE. Identification of candidate cancer chemopreventative agents and their evaluation in animal models and human clinical trials: a review. *Cancer Res* 1990;50:2–9.

133. Nowak R. Beta-carotene: helpful or harmful? *Science* 1994;264:500–501.

134. Ziegler RG. A review of epidemiologic evidence that carotenoids reduce the risk of cancer. *J Nutr* 1989;119:116–122.

135. Kvale G, Bjelke E, Gatt JJ. Dietary habits and lung cancer risk. *Int J Cancer* 1983;31:397–405.

136. Block G. Fruits, vegetables, and health. In: Bernstein E, ed. *Medical and health annual.* Chicago: Encyclopaedia Britannica, 1994:418–424.

137. Doll R. The lessons of life: keynote address to the nutrition and cancer conference. *Cancer Res* 1992;52[7 Suppl]:2024s–2029s.

138. The Alpha-Tocopherol Beta Carotene Lung Cancer Prevention Study Group. The effect of vitamin E and beta carotene on the incidence of lung cancer and other cancers in male smokers. *N Engl J Med* 1994;330:1029–1035.

139. Omenn GS, Goodman GE, Thornquist MD, et al. Effects of a combination of beta carotene and vitamin A on lung cancer and cardiovascular disease. *N Engl J Med* 1996;334:1150–1155.

140. Hennekens CH. Antioxidant vitamins and cancer. *Am J Med* 1994;97[Suppl 3A]:2S–4S.

141. Blot WJ, Li J-Y, Taylor PR, et al. Nutrition intervention trials in Linxian, China: supplementation with specific vitamin/mineral combinations, cancer incidence, and disease-specific mortality in the general population. *J Natl Cancer Inst* 1993;85:483–492.

142. Pastorino U, Infante M, Maioli M, et al. Adjuvant treatment of stage I lung cancer with high-dose vitamin A. *J Clin Oncol* 1993;11:1216–1222.

143. Lippman SM, Lee JJ, Karp DD, et al. Randomized phase III intergroup trial of isotretinoin to prevent second primary tumors in stage I non–small cell lung cancer. *J Natl Cancer Inst* 2001;93:605–618.

144. Omenn GS. Chemoprevention of lung cancer is proving difficult and frustrating, requiring new approaches. *J Natl Cancer Inst* 2000;92:959–960.

145. *Chemoprevention of tobacco-related cancers in former smokers.* Rockville, MD: National Cancer Institute, 2001.

146. Strauss GM. Randomized population trials and screening for lung cancer: "breaking the cure barrier." *Cancer* 2000;89:2399–2421.

147. Fontana RS. The Mayo Lung Project: a perspective. *Cancer* 2000;89:2352–2355.

148. Marcus PM, Bergstralk EJ, Gagerstrom RM, et al. Lung cancer mortality in the Mayo Lung Project: impact of extended follow-up. *J Natl Cancer Inst* 2000;92:1308–1316.

149. Kubik AK, Parkin DM, Zatloukal P. Czech Study on Lung Cancer Screening. Post-trial follow-up of lung cancer deaths up to year 15 since enrollment. *Cancer* 2000;89:2363–2368.

150. Manser R, Irving L, Stone C, et al. Screening for lung cancer [Cochrane Review]. *The Cochrane Library* 2002 (Oxford, updated software).

151. Porter JC, Spiro SG. Detection of early lung cancer. *Thorax* 2000;55:S56–S62.

152. Jett JR. Spiral computed tomography screening for lung cancer is ready for prime time [Pro/Con Editorials]. *Am J Respir Crit Care Med* 2001;163:812–813.

153. Patz EF, Goodmand PC. Low-dose spiral computed tomography screening for lung cancer: not ready for prime time [Pro/Con Editorials]. *Am J Respir Crit Care Med* 2001;163:813–815.

154. Henschke CI, Yankelevitz DF. CT screening for lung cancer. *Radiol Clin North Am* 2000;38:487–495.

155. Melamed MR. Lung cancer screening results in the National Cancer Institute New York Study. *Cancer* 2000;89:2356–2362.

156. Tockman MS. Survival and mortality from lung cancer in a screened population: the Johns Hopkins Study. *Chest* 1986;89:325S–326S.

157. Myers MH, Gloeckler Ries LA. Cancer patient survival rates: SEER program results for 10 years of follow-up. *CA Cancer J Clin* 1989;39:21–39.

158. Fontana R, Sanderson DR, Woolner LB, et al. Lung cancer screening: the Mayo program. *J Occup Med* 1986;28:746–750.

159. Strauss GM. The Mayo lung cohort: a regression analysis focusing on lung cancer incidence and mortality. *J Clin Oncol* 2002;20:1973–1983.

160. Patz EF, Goodman PC, Bepler G. Screening for lung cancer. *N Engl J Med* 2000;343:1627–1633.

161. Prorok P, Kramer B, Gohagan J. Screening theory and study design: the basics. In: Kramer B, Prorok P, Gohagan J, eds. *Cancer screening: theory and practice.* New York: Marcel Dekker Inc, 1999:29–53.

162. Black WC. Lung cancer. In: Kramer B, Prorok P, Gohagan J, eds. *Cancer screening: theory and practice.* New York: Marcel Dekker Inc, 1999:327–377.

163. Cole P, Morrison AS. Basic issues in population screening for cancer. *J Natl Cancer Inst* 1980;64:1263–1272.

164. Bailar JC. Screening for lung cancer: where are we now? *Am Rev Respir Dis* 1984;130:541–542.

165. Eddy D. Screening for lung cancer. *Ann Intern Med* 1989;111:232–237.

166. Black WC. Overdiagnosis: an unrecognized cause of confusion and harm in cancer screening. *J Natl Cancer Inst* 2000;92:1280–1282.

167. Rothman KJ, Greenland S. *Modern epidemiology,* 2nd ed. Philadelphia: Lippincott-Raven Publishers, 1998:1–738.

168. Weinberg CR. Toward a clearer definition of confounding. *Am J Epidemiol* 1993;137:1–8.

169. Pearl J. *Causality: models, reasoning, and inference.* Cambridge, UK: Cambridge University Press, 2000:1–384.

170. Dempster A. Logicist statistics: models and modeling. *Stat Sci* 1998;13:248–276.

171. Strauss GM. Screening for lung cancer [Letter]. *J Clin Oncol* 2002;20:3931–3934.

172. Lee T, Brennan R. Direct-to-consumer marketing of high-technology screening tests. *N Engl J Med* 2002;346:529–531.

173. Sone S, Takashima S, Li F, et al. Mass screening for lung cancer with mobile spiral computed tomography scanner. *Lancet* 1998;351:1242–1245.

174. Henschke CI, McCauley DI, Yankelevitz DF, et al. Early Lung Cancer Action Project: overall design and findings from baseline screening. *Lancet* 1999;354:99–105.

175. Henschke CI, Naidich D, Yankelevitz DF, et al. Early Lung Cancer Action Project: initial findings on repeat screening. *Cancer* 2001;92:153–159.

176. Swensen S, Jett JR, Sloan J, et al. Screening for lung cancer with low-dose spiral computed tomography. *Am J Respir Crit Care Med* 2002;165:508–513.

177. Jett JR, Swensen SJ, Midthun DE, et al. Screening for lung cancer: Mayo Clinic study with low-dose spiral CT scan (SCT) and sputum cytology (prevalence screen). *Am J Respir Crit Care Med* 2000;161:A13.

178. Jett JR, Swensen SJ, Midthun DE, et al. Screening for lung cancer with low-dose spiral CT scan (SCT): the Mayo Clinic trial. *Am J Respir Crit Care Med* 2001;163:A484.

179. Smith IE. Screening for lung cancer: time to think positive. *Lancet* 1999;354:86–87.

180. Morrison AS. *Screening in chronic disease,* 2nd ed. New York: Oxford University Press, 1992.

181. Smith RA. Screening fundamentals. *Monogr Natl Cancer Inst* 1997;22:15–19.

182. Berlin NI, Buncher CR, Fontana RS, et al. The National Cancer Institute Cooperative Early Lung Cancer Detection Program: results of the initial screen (prevalence). *Am Rev Respir Dis* 1984;130:545–549.

183. Early Lung Cancer Cooperative Study Group. Early lung cancer detection: summary and conclusions. *Am Rev Respir Dis* 1984;130:565–570.

184. Patz EF, Rossi S, Harpole DH, et al. Correlation of tumor size and survival in patients with stage IA non–small cell lung cancer. *Chest* 2000;117:1568–1571.

185. Smith RA. Principles of successful cancer screening. *Surg Oncol Clin North Am* 1999;8:587–609.

186. Strauss GM. Screening for lung cancer: an evidence-based synthesis. *Surg Oncol Clin North Am* 1999;8:747–774.

187. Kramer BS, Gohagan J, Prorok PC. A randomized study of chest x-ray screening for lung cancer as part of the Prostate, Lung, Colorectal, and Ovarian (PLCO) Trial. *Lung Cancer* 1994;11[Suppl]:82–83.

188. Gotzsche PC, Olsen O. Is screening for breast cancer with mammography justifiable? *Lancet* 2000;355:129–134.

189. Olsen O, Gotzsche PC. Cochrane review on screening for breast cancer with mammography. *Lancet* 2001;358:1340–1342.

190. Duffy S, Tabar L, Smith RA. The mammographic screening trials: commentary of the recent work by Olsen and Gotzsche. *CA Cancer J Clin* 2002;52:68–71.

191. Sox H. Screening mammography for younger women: back to basics. *Ann Intern Med* 2002;137:361–362.

192. Goodman S. The mammography dilemma: a crisis for evidence-based medicine? *Ann Intern Med* 2002;137:363–365.

193. Baba Y, Takahashi M, Tominguchi S, et al. Cost-effectiveness decision analysis of mass screening for lung cancer. *Acad Radiol* 1998;5:S344–S346.

194. Caro JJ, Klittich WS, Strauss GM. Could chest x-ray screening for lung cancer be cost-effective? *Cancer* 2000;89:2502–2505.

195. Travis WD, Colby TV, Corrin B, et al. *World Health Organization international histological classification of tumours: histological typing of lung and pleural tumours,* 3rd ed. Berlin: Springer-Verlag, 1999:1–156.

196. Sorensen JB, Olsen JE. Prognostic implications of histopathologic subtyping in patients with surgically treated stage I or II adenocarcinoma of the lung. *J Thorac Cardiovasc Surg* 1989;97:245–251.

197. Barsky SH, Cameron R, Osann KE, et al. Rising incidence of bronchioloalveolar lung cancer and its clinicopathologic features. *Cancer* 1994;73:1163–1179.

198. Wistulba I, Minna J. Molecular genetics of small cell lung carcinoma. *Semin Oncol* 2001;28:3–13.

199. Osann K, Lowery J, Schell M. Small cell lung cancer in women: risk associated with smoking, prior respiratory disease, and occupation. *Lung Cancer* 2000;28:1–10.

200. Thompson S, Pearson M. Changing patterns of lung cancer histology with age and gender. *Thorax* 1998;53[Suppl 4]:A10.

201. Kmietowic Z. Women at double risk of small cell lung cancer. *Br Med J* 1998;317:1614.

202. Feinstein AR. Symptomatic patterns, biologic behavior, and prognosis in cancer of the lung. *Ann Intern Med* 1964;61:27–43.

203. Zelen M. Keynote address on biostatistics and data retrieval. *Cancer Chemother Rep* 1973;4:31–42.

204. Sorensen JB, Badsberg JH. Prognostic factors in resected stage I and II adenocarcinoma of the lung. *J Thorac Cardiovasc Surg* 1990;99:218–226.

205. Harpole DH, Herndon JE, Young WG, et al. Stage I non–small cell lung cancer: a multivariate analysis of treatment methods and patterns of recurrence. *Cancer* 1995;76:787–796.

206. Pater JL, Loeb M. Nonanatomic prognostic factors in

carcinoma of the lung: a multivariate analysis. *Cancer* 1982;50:326–331.

207. American Cancer Society. Report on the cancer-related health checkup: cancer of the lung. *CA Cancer J Clin* 1980;30:199–207.

208. Smith RA, Cokkinides V, Von Eschenbach AC, et al. American Cancer Society guidelines for the early detection of cancer. *CA Cancer J Clin* 2002;52:8–22.

209. U.S. Preventive Services Task Force. Screening for lung cancer. In: *Guide to clinical preventive services.* Baltimore: Williams & Wilkins, 1996:135–139.

210. Chute CG, Greenberg R, Baron J, et al. Presenting conditions of 1539 population-based lung cancer patients by cell type and stage in New Hampshire and Vermont. *Cancer* 1985;56:2107–2111.

211. Strauss GM. Bronchogenic carcinoma. In: Baum JD, et al., eds. *Textbook of pulmonary diseases.* Philadelphia: Lippincott–Raven Publishers, 1998:1329–1381.

212. Carbone PP, Frost JK, Feinstein AR, et al. Lung cancer: perspectives and prospects. *Ann Intern Med* 1970;73:1003–1024.

213. Cromartie RS, Parker EF, May JE, et al. Carcinoma of the lung: a clinical review. *Ann Thorac Surg* 1980;30:30–35.

214. Hillerdal G. Long-term survival of patients with lung cancer from a defined geographical area before and after radiological screening. *Lung Cancer* 1996;15:21–30.

215. Hakama M, Holli K, Visakorpi T, et al. Low biological aggressiveness of screen-detected lung cancers may indicate overdiagnosis. *Int J Cancer* 1996;65:1–5.

216. Mountain CF. A new international staging system for lung cancer. *Chest* 1986;89:225S–233S.

217. Mountain CF. The new international staging system for lung cancer. *Surg Clin North Am* 1987;67:925–935.

218. Mountain CF. Revisions in the international system for staging lung cancer. *Chest* 1997;111:1710–1717.

219. Mountain CF, Dresler CM. Regional lymph node classification for lung cancer staging. *Chest* 1997;111:1718–1723.

220. Naruke T, Suemasu K, Ishikawa S. Lymph node mapping and curability at various levels of metastasis in resected lung cancer. *J Thorac Cardiovasc Surg* 1978;76:832–839.

221. Watanabe Y, Hayashi Y, Shimuzu J, et al. Mediastinal nodal involvement and the prognosis of non–small cell lung cancer. *Chest* 1991;100:422–428.

222. Martini N, Burt M, Bains M, et al. Survival after resection of stage II non–small cell lung cancer. *Ann Thorac Surg* 1992;54:460–466.

223. Yano T, Yokoyama H, Inoue T, et al. Surgical results and prognostic factors of pathologic N1 disease in non–small-cell carcinoma of the lung. Significance of N1 level: lobar or hilar nodes. *J Thorac Cardiovasc Surg* 1994;107:1398–1402.

224. Naruke T, Goya T, Tsuchiya R, et al. Prognosis and survival in resected lung carcinoma based on the new international staging system. *J Thorac Cardiovasc Surg* 1988;96:440–447.

225. Gail M, Eagan RT, Feld R, et al. Prognostic factors in patients with resected stage I NSCLC: a report from the Lung Cancer Study Group. *Cancer* 1984;54:1802–1813.

226. Pairolero PC, Williams DE, Bergstralh EJ, et al. Postsurgical stage I bronchogenic carcinoma: morbid implications of recurrent disease. *Ann Thorac Surg* 1984;38:331–338.

227. Martini N, Bains MS, Burt ME, et al. Incidence of local recurrence and second primary tumors in resected stage I lung cancer. *Proc Am Assoc Thorac Surg* 1994:42.

228. Ichinose Y, Hara N, Ohta M, et al. Is T factor of the TNM staging system a predominant prognostic factor in pathologic stage I non–small-cell lung cancer? *J Thorac Cardiovasc Surg* 1993;106:90–94.

229. Lafitte JJ, Ribet ME, Prevost BM, et al. Postresection irradiation for T2 N0 M0 non–small cell carcinoma: a prospective, randomized study. *Ann Thorac Surg* 1996;62:830–834.

230. Immerman SC, Vanecko RM, Fry WA, et al. Site of recurrence in patients with stages I and II carcinoma of the lung resected for cure. *Ann Thorac Surg* 1981;32:23–27.

231. Van Rens M, De la Riviere A, Elbers H, et al. Prognostic assessment of 2,361 patients who underwent resection for non–small cell lung cancer, stages I, II, and IIIA. *Chest* 2000;117:373–379.

232. Martini N, Ginsberg RJ. Treatment of stage I and II disease. In: Aisner J, et al., eds. *Comprehensive textbook of thoracic oncology.* Baltimore: Williams & Wilkins, 1996:339–350.

233. Thomas PA, Piantadosi S. Postoperative T1 N0 non–small cell lung cancer: squamous versus nonsquamous recurrences. *J Thorac Cardiovasc Surg* 1987;94:349–354.

234. Lipford EH III, Eggleston JC, Lillemoe KD, et al. Prognostic factors in surgically resected limited-stage, non–small cell carcinoma of the lung. *Am J Surg Pathol* 1984;8:357–365.

235. Takise A, Kodama T, Shimosato Y, et al. Histopathologic prognostic factors in adenocarcinomas of the peripheral lung less than 2 cm in diameter. *Cancer* 1988;61:2083–2088.

236. Kersting M, Friedl C, Kraus A, et al. Differential frequencies of p16(INK4a) promoter hypermethylation, p53 mutation, and K-ras mutation in exfoliative material mark the development of lung cancer in symptomatic chronic smokers. *J Clin Oncol* 2000;18:3221–3229.

237. Slebos RJ, Kibbelaar RE, Dalesio O, et al. K-ras oncogene activation as a prognostic marker in adenocarcinoma of the lung. *N Engl J Med* 1990;323:561–565.

238. Rodenhuis S, Slebos RJ. Clinical significance of ras oncogene activation in human lung cancer. *Cancer Res* 1992;52[Suppl]:2665s–2669s.

239. Graziano S, Gamble G, Newman N, et al. Prognostic significance of K-ras codon 12 mutations in patients with resected stage I and II non–small-cell lung cancer. *J Clin Oncol* 1999;17:668–675.

240. Rosell R, Li S, Skacel Z, et al. Prognostic impact of mutated K-ras gene in surgically resected non–small cell lung cancer patients. *Oncogene* 1993;8:2407–2412.

241. Harada M, Dosaka-Akita H, Miyamoto H, et al. Prognostic significance of the expression of ras oncogene product in non–small cell lung cancer. *Cancer* 1992;69:72–77.

242. Huncharek M, Muscat J, Geschwind J. K-ras oncogene mutation as a prognostic marker in non–small cell lung cancer: a combined analysis of 881 cases. *Carcinogenesis* 1999;20:1507–1510.

243. Mitsudomi T, Steinberg SM, Oie H, et al. Ras gene mutations in non–small cell lung cancers are associated with shortened survival irrespective of treatment intent. *Cancer Res* 1991;51:4999–5002.

244. Nelson H, Christiani D, Mark EJ, et al. Implications and prognostic value of K-ras mutation for early-stage lung cancer in women. *J Natl Cancer Inst* 1999;91:2032–2038.

245. Greatens TM, Niehans G, Rubins J, et al. Do molecular markers predict survival in non–small cell lung cancer? *Am J Respir Crit Care Med* 1998;157:1093–1097.

246. Schiller J, Feins R, et al. Lack of prognostic significance of p53 and K-ras mutations in primary resected non–small-cell lung cancer on E4592: a laboratory ancillary study on an Eastern Cooperative Oncology Group prospective randomized trial of postoperative adjuvant therapy. *J Clin Oncol* 2001;19:448–457.

247. Franklin W, Veve R, Hirsch F, et al. Epidermal growth factor receptor family in lung cancer and premalignancy. *Semin Oncol* 2002;29[1 Suppl 4]:3–14.

248. Volm M, Rittgen W, Drings P. Prognostic value of ERBB-1,

VEGF, cyclin A, FOS, JUN and MYC in patients with squamous cell lung carcinomas. *Br J Cancer* 1998;77:663–669.

249. Ohsaki Y, Tanno S, Fujita Y, et al. Epidermal growth factor receptor expression correlates with poor prognosis in non–small cell lung cancer patients with p53 overexpression. *Oncol Rep* 2000;7:603–607.

250. Cox G, Jones J, O'Byrne K. Matrix metalloproteinase 9 and the epidermal growth factor signal pathway in operable non–small cell lung cancer. *Clin Cancer Res* 2000;6:2349–2355.

251. Stern DF, Heffernan PA, Weinberg RA. A product of the neu proto-oncogene is a receptor-like protein associated with tyrosine kinase activity, p185. *Mol Cell Biol* 1986;6:1729–1740.

252. Yamamoto T, Ikawa S, Akiyama T, et al. Similarity of protein encoded by the c-erbB-2 gene to epidermal growth factor receptor. *Nature* 1986;319:230–234.

253. Raben D, Helfrich B, Chan D, et al. ZD1839, a selective epidermal growth factor receptor tyrosine kinase inhibitor, alone and in combination with radiation and chemotherapy is a new therapeutic strategy in non–small cell lung cancer. *Semin Oncol* 2002;29[1 Suppl 4]:37–46.

254. Kern JA, Schwartz DA, Nordberg JE, et al. P185 neu expression in human lung adenocarcinomas predicts shortened survival. *Cancer Res* 1990;50:5184–5191.

255. Tateishi M, Ishida T, Mitsudomi T, et al. Prognostic value of c-erbB-2 protein expression in human lung adenocarcinoma and squamous cell carcinoma. *Eur J Cancer* 1991;27:1372–1375.

256. Shi D, He G, Cao S, et al. Overexpression of the c-erbB-2/neu–encoded p185 protein in primary lung cancer. *Mol Carcinog* 1992;5:213–218.

257. Harpole DH, Herndon JE, Wolfe WG, et al. A prognostic model of recurrence and death in stage I non–small cell lung cancer utilizing presentation, histopathology, and oncoprotein expression. *Cancer Res* 1995;55:51–56.

258. Hsieh C, Chow K, Fahn H, et al. Prognostic significance of HER-2/neu overexpression in stage I adenocarcinoma of the lung. *Ann Thorac Surg* 1998;66:1159–1163.

259. Bennett W, Hussain S, Vahakangas K, et al. Molecular epidemiology of human cancer risk: gene-environment interactions and p53 mutation spectrum in human lung cancer. *J Pathol* 1999;187:8–18.

260. Hockenbery D, Nunez G, Milliman C, et al. Bcl-2 is an inner mitochondrial membrane protein that blocks programmed cell death. *Nature* 1990;348:334.

261. Fleming M, Guinee D, Chu W, et al. Bcl-2 immunohistochemistry in a surgical series of non–small cell lung cancer patients. *Hum Pathol* 1998;29:60.

262. Ohmura Y, Aoe M, Andou A, et al. Telomerase activity and Bcl-2 expression in non–small cell lung cancer. *Clin Cancer Res* 2000;6:2980.

263. Laudanski J, Chyczewski L, Niklinska W, et al. Expression of bcl-2 protein in non–small cell lung cancer: correlation with clinicopathology and patient survival. *Neoplasma* 1999;46:25–30.

264. Groeger AM, Caputi M, Esposito V, et al. Bcl-2 protein expression correlates with nodal status in non–small cell lung cancer. *Anticancer Res* 1999;19:821–824.

265. Pezzella F, Turley H, Kuzu I, et al. Bcl-2 protein in non–small cell lung carcinoma. *N Engl J Med* 1993;329:690–694.

266. Silvestrini R, Costa A, Lequaglie C, et al. Bcl-2 protein and prognosis in patients with potentially curable non–small-cell lung cancer. *Virchows Arch* 1998;432:441–444.

267. Lane DP. p53, guardian of the genome. *Nature* 1992;358:15–16.

268. Malkin D. p53 and the Li-Fraumeni syndrome. *Cancer Genet Cytogenet* 1993;66:83–92.

269. Tammemagi M, McLaughlin J, Bull S. Meta-analyses of p53 tumor suppressor gene alterations and clinicopathological features in resected lung cancers. *Cancer Epidemiol Biomarkers Prev* 1999;8:625.

270. Mao L, Lee JS, Kurie JM, et al. Clonal genetic alterations in the lungs of current and former smokers. *J Natl Cancer Inst* 1997;89:857–862.

271. Wistuba II, Lam S, Behrens C, et al. Molecular damage in the bronchial epithelium of current and former smokers. *J Natl Cancer Inst* 1997;89:1366–1373.

272. Wei Q, Cheng L, Amos C, et al. Repair of tobacco carcinogen–induced DNA adducts and lung cancer risk: a molecular epidemiologic study. *J Natl Cancer Inst* 2000;92:1764–1772.

273. Carbone D, Minna J. Molecular biology of lung cancer. *Mol Found Oncol* 1991;339–366.

274. Quinlan DC, Davidson AG, Summers CL, et al. Accumulation of p53 protein correlates with a poor prognosis in human lung cancer. *Cancer Res* 1992;52:4828–4831.

275. Fujino M, Dosaka-Akita H, Harada M, et al. Prognostic significance of p53 and ras p21 expression in non–small cell lung cancer. *Cancer* 1995;76:2457–2463.

276. Lee JS, Yoon A, Kalapurakal SK, et al. Expression of p53 oncoprotein in non–small-cell lung cancer: a favorable prognostic factor. *J Clin Oncol* 1995;13:1893–1903.

277. McLaren R, Kuzu I, Dunnill M, et al. The relationship of p53 immunostaining to survival in carcinoma of the lung. *Br J Cancer* 1992;66:735–738.

278. Fuchs CS, Colditz GA, Stampfer MJ, et al. A prospective study of cigarette smoking and the risk of pancreatic cancer. *Arch Intern Med* 1996;156:2255–2260.

279. Geradts J, Fong K, Zimmerman P, et al. Correlation of abnormal RB, p16ink4a, and p53 expression with 3p loss of heterozygosity, other genetic abnormalities, and clinical features in 103 primary non–small cell lung cancers. *Clin Cancer Res* 1999;5:791–800.

280. Nishio M, Koshikawa T, Kuroishi T, et al. Prognostic significance of abnormal p53 accumulation in primary, resected non–small-cell lung cancers. *J Clin Oncol* 1996;14:497–502.

281. Mitsudomi T, Oyama T, Kusano T, et al. Mutation of the p53 gene as a predictor of poor prognosis in patients with non–small cell lung cancer. *J Natl Cancer Inst* 1993;85:2018–2023.

282. Knudson AJ. The ninth Gordon Hamilton-Fairley Memorial Lecture. Hereditary cancers: clues to mechanisms of carcinogenesis. *Br J Cancer* 1989;59:661–666.

283. Xu HJ, Quinlan DC, Davidson AG, et al. Altered retinoblastoma protein expression and prognosis in early stage non–small cell lung carcinoma. *J Natl Cancer Inst* 1994;86:695–699.

284. Xu H, Cagle PT, Hu SX, et al. Altered retinoblastoma and p53 protein status in non–small cell carcinoma of the lung: potential synergistic effects on prognosis. *Clin Cancer Res* 1996;2:1169–1176.

285. Volm M, Koomagi R, Rittgen W. Clinical implications of cyclins, cyclin-dependent kinases, RB and E2F1 in squamous-cell lung carcinoma. *Int J Cancer* 1998;79:294–299.

286. Dosaka-Akita H, Fujino M, Harada M, et al. Prognostic significance of p53 and ras p21 expression in non–small cell lung cancer. *Proc Annu Meeting Am Assoc Cancer Res* 1995.

287. Merlo A, Gabrielson E, Askin F, et al. Frequent loss of chromosome 9 in human primary non–small cell lung cancer. *Cancer Res* 1994;54:640–642.

288. Shapiro G, Rollins B. p16INK4A as a human tumor suppressor. *Biochim Biophys Acta* 1996;1242:165.

289. Hannon G, Beach D. P15INK4B is a potential effector of TGF-beta–induced cell cycle arrest. *Nature* 1994;371:257–261.

290. Gazzeri S, Gouyer V, Vourch C, et al. Mechanisms of

p16INK4a inactivation in non–small-cell lung cancers. *Oncogene* 1998;16:497–504.

291. Shapiro G, Edwards C, Kobzik L, et al. Reciprocal Rb inactivation and p16INK4 expression in primary lung cancers and cell lines. *Cancer Res* 1995;55:505–509.

292. Kratzke R, Greatens T, Rubins J, et al. Rb and p16INK4a expression in resected non–small cell lung tumors. *Cancer Res* 1996;56:3415–3420.

293. Taga S, Osaki T, Ohgami A, et al. Prognostic value of the immunohistochemical detection of p16INK4 expression in non–small cell lung carcinoma. *Cancer* 1997;80:389–395.

294. Hommura F, Dosaka-Akita H, Kinoshita I, et al. Predictive value of expression of p16INK4A, retinoblastoma and p53 proteins for the prognosis of non–small-cell lung cancers. *Br J Cancer* 1999;82:374–380.

295. Hibi K, Takahashi T, Yamakawa K, et al. Three distinct regions involved in 3p deletion in human lung cancer. *Oncogene* 1992;7:445–449.

296. Otterson G, Lin A, Kay F. Genetic etiology of lung cancer. *Oncology (Huntingt)* 1992;6:97–104.

297. Hirao T, Nelson H, Ashok T, et al. Tobacco smoke–induced DNA damage and an early age of smoking initiation induce chromosome loss at 3p21 in lung cancer. *Cancer Res* 2001;61:612–615.

298. Sozzi G, Veronese ML, Negrini M, et al. The FHIT gene at 3p14.2 is abnormal in lung cancer. *Cell* 1996;85:17–26.

299. Geradts J, Fong K, Zimmerman P, et al. Loss of FHIT expression in non–small cell lung cancer: correlation with molecular genetic abnormalities and clinicopathologic features. *Br J Cancer* 2000;82:1191–1197.

300. Burbee D, Forgacs E, Zochbauer-Muller S, et al. Epigenetic inactivation of RASSF1A in lung and breast cancers and malignant phenotype suppression. *J Natl Cancer Inst* 2001;93:691–699.

301. Dammann R, Li C, Yoon J, et al. Epigenetic inactivation of a RAS association domain family protein from the lung tumor suppressor locus 3p21.3. *Nat Genet* 2000;25:315–319.

302. Midthun DE, Jett JR. Clinical presentation of lung cancer. In: Pass HI, et al., eds. *Lung cancer: principles and practice*. Philadelphia: Lippincott–Raven Publishers, 1996:421–435.

303. Doyle L, Aisner J. Clinical presentation of lung cancer. In: Roth J, Ruckdeschel J, Weisenburger T, eds. *Thoracic oncology*. Philadelphia: WB Saunders, 1989:52–76.

304. Patel A, Jett J. Clinical presentation and staging of lung cancer. In: Aisner J, et al., eds. *Comprehensive textbook of thoracic oncology*. Baltimore: Williams & Wilkins, 1996:293–318.

305. Hyde L, Hyde CI. Clinical manifestations of lung cancer. *Cancer* 1974;65:299–306.

306. Pancoast HK. Importance of careful roentgen-ray investigations of apical chest tumors. *JAMA* 1924;83:1407.

307. Pancoast HK. Superior pulmonary sulcus tumor: tumor characterized by pain, Horner's syndrome, destruction of bone, and atrophy of hand muscles. *JAMA* 1932;99:1391.

308. Merchut MP. Brain metastases from undiagnosed systemic neoplasms. *Arch Intern Med* 1989;149:1076.

309. Weinberger S. Differential diagnosis and evaluation of the solitary pulmonary nodule. *Up-to-Date in Medicine* 2002.

310. Berquist T, Bailey P, Cortese D, et al. Transthoracic needle biopsy: accuracy and complications in relation to location and type of lesion. *Mayo Clin Proc* 1980;55:475–481.

311. Stark P. Thoracic positron emission tomography. *Up-to-Date in Medicine* 2002.

312. Laking G, Price P. 18-Fluorodeoxyglucose positron emission tomography (FDG-PET) and the staging of early lung cancer. *Thorax* 2001;56[Suppl II]:ii38–ii44.

313. Detterbeck F, Rivera M. Clinical presentation and diagnosis. In: Detterbeck F, et al., eds. *Diagnosis and treatment of lung cancer: an evidence-based guide for the practicing physician*. Philadelphia: WB Saunders, 2001:45–72.

314. Naruke T, Tsuchiva R, Kondo H, et al. Implications of staging in lung cancer. *Chest* 1997;112:242S–248S.

315. Fry WA, Phillips JL, Menck HR. Ten-year survey of lung cancer treatment and survival in hospitals in the United States: a National Cancer Data Base report. *Cancer* 1999;86:1867–1876.

316. Bulzebruck H, Bopp R, Drings P, et al. New aspects of staging of lung cancer. prospective validation of the International Union Against Cancer TNM classification. *Cancer* 1992;70:1102–1110.

317. Mentzer SJ, DeCamp MM, Harpole DH, et al. Thoracoscopy and video-assisted thoracic surgery in the treatment of lung cancer. *Chest* 1995;107:298S–301S.

318. Swanson S, Herndon J, D'Amico A, et al. Results of CALGB 39802: feasibility of video-assisted thoracic surgery (VATS) lobectomy for early stage lung cancer. *Proc Am Soc Clin Oncol* 2002;21:290a(abst 1158).

319. Ginsberg RJ, Rubinstein L, Lung Cancer Study Group. A randomized comparative trial of lobectomy versus limited resection for patients with T1 N0 non–small cell lung cancer. *Lung Cancer* 1991;7[Suppl]:83(abst 304).

320. Ginsberg RJ. The role of limited resection in the treatment of early stage lung cancer. *Lung Cancer* 1994;11[Suppl 2]:35–36.

321. Martini N, Bains MS, Burt ME, et al. Incidence and local recurrence and second primary tumors in resected stage I lung cancer. *J Thorac Cardiovasc Surg* 1995;109:120–129.

322. Lopez-Encuentra A, Duque-Medina J, Rami-Porta R, et al. Staging in lung cancer: is 3 cm a prognostic threshold in pathologic stage I non–small cell lung cancer? A multicenter study of 1,020 patients. *Chest* 2002;121:1515–1520.

323. Detterbeck F, Egan T. Surgery for stage II non–small cell lung cancer. In: Detterbeck F, et al., eds. *Diagnosis and treatment of lung cancer: an evidence-based guide for the practicing physician*. Philadelphia: WB Saunders, 2001:177–190.

324. Holmes EC. Treatment of stage II lung cancer (T1 N1, T2 N1). *Surg Clin North Am* 1987;67:945–949.

325. Gauden S, Ramsay J, Tripcony L. The curative treatment by radiotherapy alone in stage I non–small cell carcinoma of the lung. *Chest* 1995;108:1278–1282.

326. Hayakawa K, Mitsuhanshi N, et al. Definitive radiation therapy for medically inoperable patients with stage I and II non–small cell lung cancer. *Radiat Oncol Invest* 1996;4:165–170.

327. Johnson H, Halle J. Radiotherapy for stage I, II non–small cell lung cancer. In: Detterbeck F, et al., eds. *Diagnosis and treatment of lung cancer: an evidence-based guide for the practicing physician*. Philadelphia: WB Saunders, 2001:198–205.

328. Vanhoutte P, Rocmans P, Smets P, et al. Postoperative radiation therapy in lung cancer: a controlled trial after resection of curative design. *Int J Radiat Oncol Biol Phys* 1980;6:983–986.

329. Lung Cancer Study Group. Effects of postoperative mediastinal radiation on completely resected stage II and stage III epidermoid cancer of the lung. *N Engl J Med* 1986;315:1377–1381.

330. PORT Meta-analysis Trialists Group. Postoperative radiotherapy in non–small cell lung cancer: systemic review and meta-analysis of individual patient data from nine randomized controlled trials. *Lancet* 1999;352:257–263.

331. Feld R, Rubenstein LV, Weisenburger TH. Sites of recurrence in resected stage I non–small-cell lung cancer: a guide for future studies. *J Clin Oncol* 1984;2:1352.

332. Lad TE. Postsurgical adjuvant therapy in stages I, II, and IIIA non–small cell lung cancer. *Hematol Oncol Clin North Am* 1990;4:1111–1119.

333. Holmes EC. Postoperative chemotherapy for non–small cell lung cancer. *Chest* 1993;103:30S–34S.

334. Holmes EC, Gail M, the Lung Cancer Study Group. Surgical adjuvant therapy for stage II and stage III adenocarcinoma and large-cell undifferentiated carcinoma. *J Clin Oncol* 1986;4:710–715.

335. Lad T, Rubinstein L, Sadeghi A, the Lung Cancer Study Group. The benefit of adjuvant treatment for resected locally advanced non–small-cell lung cancer. *J Clin Oncol* 1988;6:9–17.

336. Feld R, Rubinstein L, Thomas PA. Adjuvant chemotherapy with cyclophosphamide, doxorubicin, and cisplatin in patients with completely resected stage I non–small cell lung cancer. *J Natl Cancer Inst* 1993;85:299–306.

337. Niranen A, Niitamo-Korhonen S, Kouri M, et al. Adjuvant chemotherapy after radical surgery for non–small-cell lung cancer: a randomized study. *J Clin Oncol* 1992;10:1927–1932.

338. Dautzenberg B, Chastang C, Arriagada R, et al. Adjuvant radiotherapy versus combined sequential chemotherapy followed by radiotherapy in the treatment of resected non–small cell lung carcinoma. *Cancer* 1995;76:779–786.

339. Wada H, Hitami S, Teramatsu T, West Japan Study Group for Lung Cancer Surgery. Adjuvant chemotherapy after complete resection in non–small cell lung cancer. *J Clin Oncol* 1996;14:1048–1054.

339a. Kato H, Tsuboi M, Ohta E, et al. A randomized phase III trial of adjuvant chemotherapy with UFT for completely resected pathologic stage I (T1N0M0, T2N0M0) adenocarcinoma of the lung. *Proc Am Soc Clin Oncol* 2003;22:621 (abst 2498).

340. Non–Small Cell Lung Cancer Collaborative Group. Chemotherapy in non–small cell lung cancer: a meta-analysis using updated data on individual patients from 52 randomized clinical trials. *Br Med J* 1995;311:899–911.

341. Le Chevalier T, for the IALT Investigators. Results of the randomized International Adjuvant Lung Cancer Trial (IALT): cisplatin-based chemotherapy versus no chemotherapy in 1867 patients with resected non–small cell lung cancer. *Proc Am Soc Clin Oncol* 2003;22:2 (abst 6).

341a. Collins R, Peto R, Gray R, Parish S. Large scale randomized evidence: trials and overviews. In: Warrel D, Cox T, Firth J, Benz E, eds. *Oxford textbook of medicine*. Oxford: Oxford University Press, 2003:24–36.

342. Feld R. Chemotherapy as adjuvant therapy for completely resected non–small cell lung cancer: have we made progress? *J Clin Oncol* 1996;14:1045–1047.

343. Strauss GM, Langer MP, Elias AD, et al. Multi-modality treatment of stage IIIA non–small cell carcinoma of the lung: a critical review of the literature and strategies for future research. *J Clin Oncol* 1992;10:829–838.

344. Hilaris BS, Nori D. The role of external radiation and brachytherapy in unresectable non–small cell lung cancer. *Surg Clin North Am* 1987;67:1061–1071.

345. Perez CA, Stanley K, Grundy G. Impact of irradiation technique and tumor extent in tumor control and survival of patients with unresectable non–oat cell carcinoma of the lung: report by the Radiation Oncology Group. *Cancer* 1982;50:1091–1099.

346. Perez CA, Bauer M, Edelstein S, et al. Impact of tumor control on survival in carcinoma of the lung treated with irradiation. *Int J Radiat Oncol Biol Phys* 1986;12:539–547.

347. Curran W, Stafford P. Lack of apparent difference in outcome between clinically staged IIIA and IIIB non–small cell lung cancer treated with radiation therapy. *J Clin Oncol* 1990;8:409–415.

348. Schaake-Koning C, Schuster-Uitterhoeve L, Hart G, et al. Prognostic factors of inoperable localized lung cancer treated by high-dose radiotherapy. *Int J Radiat Oncol Biol Phys* 1983;9:1023–1028.

349. Perez C, Pajak T, Rubin P, et al. Long-term observations of the patterns of failure in patients with unresectable non–oat

cell carcinoma of the lung treated with definitive radiotherapy: report by the Radiation Therapy Oncology Group. *Cancer* 1987;59:1874–1881.

350. Choi N, Doucette J. Improved survival of patients with unresectable non–small cell bronchogenic carcinoma by an innovated high-dose en bloc radiotherapeutic approach. *Cancer* 1981;48:101–109.

351. Roswit B, Patno ME, Rapp R, et al. The survival of patients with inoperable lung cancer: a large-scale randomized study of radiation therapy versus placebo. *Radiology* 1968;90:688–697.

352. Johnson DH, Einhorn LH, Bartolucci A, et al. Thoracic radiotherapy does not prolong survival in patients with locally advanced, unresectable non–small cell lung cancer. *Ann Intern Med* 1990;113:33–38.

353. Cox JD, Azarnia N, Byhardt RW, et al. A randomized phase I-II trial of hyperfractionated radiation therapy with total doses of 60.0 Gy to 79.2 Gy: possible survival benefit with more than 69.6 Gy in favorable patients with Radiation Therapy Oncology Group stage III non–small cell lung carcinoma: report of Radiation Therapy Oncology Group 83-11. *J Clin Oncol* 1990;8:1543–1555.

354. Cox JD, Azarnia N, Byhardt RW, et al. N2 (clinical) non–small cell carcinoma of the lung: prospective trials of radiation therapy with total doses 60 Gy by the Radiation Therapy Oncology Group. *Int J Radiat Oncol Biol Phys* 1991;20:7–12.

355. Saunders M, Dische S, Barrett A, et al. Continuous hyperfractionated accelerated radiotherapy (CHART) versus conventional radiotherapy in non–small cell lung cancer: a randomised multicenter trial. *Lancet* 1997;350:161–165.

356. Mehta M, Tannehill S, Adak S, et al. Phase II trial of hyperfractionated accelerated radiation therapy for nonresectable non–small cell lung cancer: results of Eastern Cooperative Oncology Group 4593. *J Clin Oncol* 1998;16:3518–3523.

357. Ginsberg RJ, Goldberg M, Waters PF. Surgery for non–small cell lung cancer. In: Roth J, Ruckdeschel J, Weisenburger T, eds. *Thoracic oncology*. Philadelphia: WB Saunders, 1989:177–199.

358. Pairolero P, Trastek V, Payne W. Treatment of bronchogenic carcinoma with chest wall invasion. *Surg Clin North Am* 1987;67:959–964.

359. Piehler J, Pairolero P, Weiland L, et al. Bronchogenic carcinoma with chest wall invasion. Factors affecting survival following en bloc resection. *Ann Thorac Surg* 1982;34:684–691.

360. Sleckman B, Harpole D, Strauss G, et al. Multimodality therapy for chest wall invasive lung cancer. In: *Proceedings of the 47th Annual Cancer Symposium, Society of Surgical Oncology*, 1994.

361. Grover F, Komaki R. Superior sulcus tumors. In: Roth J, Ruckdeschel J, Weisenburger T, eds. *Thoracic oncology*. Philadelphia: WB Saunders, 1989:263–279.

362. Paulson D. Carcinomas of the superior sulcus. *J Thorac Cardiovasc Surg* 1975;70:1095–1104.

363. Martini N, Flehinger BJ. The role of surgery in N2 lung cancer. *Surg Clin North Am* 1987;67:1037–1049.

364. Pearson F, Delarue N, Ives R, et al. Significance of positive superior mediastinal nodes identified at mediastinoscopy in patients with resectable cancer of the lung. *J Thorac Cardiovasc Surg* 1982;83:1–11.

364a. Albain K, Scott C, Rusch V, et al. Phase III comparison of concurrent chemotherapy plus radiotherapy (CT/RT) and CT/RT followed by surgical resection for stage IIIA (pN2) non–small cell lung cancer (NSCLC): Initial results from intergroup trial 0139 (RTOG 93-09). *Proc Am Soc Clin Oncol* 2003;22:621 (abst 2497).

365. Shields TW. Preoperative radiation therapy in the treatment of bronchial carcinoma. *Cancer* 1972;30:1388–1393.

366. Collaborative Study. Preoperative irradiation of cancer of the lung: final report of a therapeutic trial. *Cancer* 1975;3:914–925.

367. Sherman DM, Neptune W, Weishselbaum R, et al. An aggressive approach to marginally resectable lung cancer. *Cancer* 1978;41:2040–2045.

368. Green MR. Multimodality therapy for solid tumors. *N Engl J Med* 1994;330:206–207.

369. Dillman RO, Seagren S, Propert K, et al. A randomized trial of induction chemotherapy plus high-dose radiation versus radiation alone in stage III non–small cell lung cancer. *N Engl J Med* 1990;323:940–945.

370. Dillman RO, Herndon J, Seagren SL, et al. Improved survival in stage III non–small cell lung cancer: seven-year follow-up of Cancer and Leukemia Group B (CALGB) 8433 Trial. *J Natl Cancer Inst* 1996;88:1210–1215.

371. Sause W, Scott C, Taylor S, et al. Radiation Therapy Oncology Group (RTOG) 88-08 and Eastern Cooperative Oncology Group (ECOG) 4588: preliminary results of a phase III trial in regionally advanced, unresectable non–small cell lung cancer. *J Natl Cancer Inst* 1995;87:198–205.

372. Pritchard RS, Anthony SP. Chemotherapy plus radiotherapy compared with radiotherapy alone in the treatment of locally advanced, unresectable, non–small cell lung cancer. *Ann Intern Med* 1996;125:723–729.

373. Belani C, Ramanathan R. Combined-modality treatment of locally advanced non–small cell lung cancer: incorporation of novel chemotherapeutic agents. *Chest* 1998;113:53S.

374. Gordon GS, Vokes EE. Chemoradiation for locally advanced, unresectable NSCLC. New standard of care, emerging strategies. *Oncology* 1999;13:1075–1088.

375. Green MR. Multimodality therapy in unresected stage III non–small cell lung cancer: the American Cooperative Groups' experience. *Lung Cancer* 1995;12[Suppl 1]:S87–S94.

376. Jeremic B, Shibamoto Y, Acimovic L, et al. Randomized trial of hyperfractionated radiation therapy with or without concurrent chemotherapy for stage III non–small cell lung cancer. *J Clin Oncol* 1995;13:452–458.

377. Jeremic B, Shibamoto Y, Acimovic L, et al. Hyperfractionated radiation therapy with or without concurrent low-dose daily carboplatin/etoposide for stage III non–small-cell lung cancer: a randomized study. *J Clin Oncol* 1996;14:1065–1070.

378. Furuse K, Fukuoka M, Kawahara M, et al. Phase III study of concurrent versus sequential thoracic radiotherapy in combination with mitomycin, vindesine, and cisplatin in unresectable stage III non–small cell lung cancer. *J Clin Oncol* 1999;17:2692–2699.

379. Curran W, Scott C, Langer C, et al. Phase III comparison of sequential vs concurrent chemoradiation for patients with unresected stage III non–small cell lung cancer (NSCLC): initial report of the Radiation Therapy Oncology Group (RTOG) 9410. *Proc Am Soc Clin Oncol* 2000;19:484a(abst 1891).

380. Curran W, Scott C, Langer C, et al. Long-term benefit is observed in a phase III comparison of sequential vs concurrent chemo-radiation for patients with unresected stage III NSCLC: Radiation Therapy Oncology Group (RTOG) 9410. *Proc Am Soc Clin Oncol* 2003;22:621 (abst 2499).

381. Skarin A, Jochelson M, Sheldon T, et al. Neoadjuvant chemotherapy in marginally resectable stage III M0 non–small cell lung cancer: long-term follow-up in 41 patients. *J Surg Oncol* 1989;40:266–274.

382. Elias AD, Skarin AT, Gonin P, et al. Neoadjuvant treatment of stage IIIA non–small cell lung cancer: long-term results. *Am J Clin Oncol* 1994;17:26–36.

383. Elias AD, Skarin AT, Leong T, et al. Neoadjuvant therapy for surgically staged IIIA N2 non–small cell lung cancer (NSCLC). *Lung Cancer* 1997;17:147–161.

384. Strauss GM, Herndon JE, Sherman DD, et al. Induction chemoradiation followed by surgery in stage IIIA non–small cell carcinoma of the lung (NSCLC): long-term results of Cancer and Leukemia Group B Protocol 8634. *Proc Am Soc Clin Oncol* 1996;15:376(abst 1121).

385. Sugarbaker DJ, Herndon J, Kohman LJ, et al. Results of Cancer and Leukemia Group B Protocol 8935: a multiinstitutional phase II trimodality trial for stage IIIA (N2) non–small cell lung cancer. *J Thorac Cardiovasc Surg* 1995;109:473–485.

386. Kumar P, Herndon J, Langer M, et al. Patterns of disease failure after trimodality therapy of non–small cell lung carcinoma pathologic stage IIIA (N2). *Cancer* 1996;77:2393–2399.

387. Choi NC, Carey RW, Daly W, et al. Potential impact on survival of improved tumor down-staging and resection rate by preoperative twice-daily radiation and concurrent chemotherapy in stage IIIA non–small cell lung cancer. *J Clin Oncol* 1997;15:712–722.

388. Martini N, Kris M, Flehinger B, et al. Preoperative chemotherapy for stage IIIa (N2) lung cancer: the Sloan-Kettering experience with 136 patients. *Ann Thorac Surg* 1993;55:1365–1374.

389. Burkes RL, Ginsberg RJ, Sheperd FA, et al. Induction chemotherapy with mitomycin, vindesine, and cisplatin for stage III unresectable non–small cell lung cancer: results of a Toronto phase II trial. *J Clin Oncol* 1992;10:580–586.

390. Reddy S, Lee MS, Bonomi P, et al. Combined modality therapy for stage III non–small cell lung cancer: results of treatments and patterns of failure. *Int J Radiat Oncol Biol Phys* 1992;24:17–32.

391. Albain KS, Rusch VW, Crowley JJ, et al. Concurrent cisplatin/etoposide plus chest radiotherapy followed by surgery for stages IIIA (N2) and IIIB non–small cell lung cancer: mature results of Southwest Oncology Group Phase II Study 8805. *J Clin Oncol* 1995;13:1880–1892.

392. Rosell R, Gomez-Codina J, Camps C, et al. A randomized trial comparing preoperative chemotherapy plus surgery with surgery alone in patients with non–small cell lung cancer. *N Engl J Med* 1994;330:153–158.

393. Roth JA, Fossella F, Komaki R, et al. A randomized trial comparing perioperative chemotherapy and surgery with surgery alone in resectable stage IIIA non–small cell lung cancer. *J Natl Cancer Inst* 1994;86:673–680.

394. Pass HI, Pogrebnick HW, Steinberg SM, et al. Randomized trial of neoadjuvant therapy for lung cancer: interim analysis. *Ann Thorac Surg* 1992;53:992–998.

395. Elias A, Kumar P, Herndon J, et al. Radiotherapy versus chemotherapy plus radiotherapy in surgically staged and treated IIIA N2 non–small cell lung cancer (NSCLC). *Clin Lung Cancer* 2002;4:95–103.

396. Roth JA, Atkinson EN, Fossella F, et al. Long-term follow-up of patients enrolled in a randomized trial comparing perioperative chemotherapy and surgery with surgery alone in resectable stage IIIA non–small-cell lung cancer. *Lung Cancer* 1998;21:1–8.

397. Rosell R, Gomez-Codina J, Camps C, et al. Preresectional chemotherapy in stage IIIA non–small-cell lung cancer: a 7-year assessment of a randomized controlled trial. *Lung Cancer* 1999;26:7–14.

398. Felip E, Rosell R, Alberola V, et al. Preoperative high-dose cisplatin versus moderate dose cisplatin combined with ifosfamide and mitomycin in stage IIIA (N2) non–small lung cancer. *Clin Lung Cancer* 2000;1:287.

399. Strauss GM, Baldini EH. Multimodality therapy for stage IIIA and stage IIIB non–small cell carcinoma of the lung. In: Skarin A, ed. *Multimodality treatment of lung cancer*. New York: Marcel Dekker Inc, 2000:207–224.

399a. Gralla R, Kris M. Chemotherapy in non–small cell lung cancer: results of recent trials. *Semin Oncol* 1988;15:2–5.

400. Perez-Soler R, Fosella FV, Glisson BS, et al. Phase II study of topotecan in patients with advanced NSCLC previously untreated with chemotherapy. *J Clin Oncol* 1996;14:503–513.

401. Kaasa A, Lund E, Thorod E, et al. Symptomatic treatment versus combination chemotherapy in patients with non–small cell lung cancer, extensive disease. *Cancer* 1991;67:2443–2447.

402. Cellerinor, Tummarello D, Guidi D, et al. A randomized trial of alternating chemotherapy versus best supportive care in advanced non–small cell lung cancer. *J Clin Oncol* 1991;9:1453–1461.

403. Corimer Y, Bergeron D, LaForge J, et al. Benefit of polychemotherapy in advanced non–small cell lung bronchogenic carcinoma. *Cancer* 1982;50:845–849.

404. Ganz P, Figlin R, Haskell C, et al. Supportive care versus supportive care and continuation chemotherapy in metastatic non–small cell lung cancer: does chemotherapy make a difference? *Cancer* 1989;63:1271–1278.

405. Quoix E, Dieteman A, Charbonneau J, et al. Disseminated non–small cell lung cancer: a randomized trial of chemotherapy versus palliative care. Congress of IASLC, Interlaken. *Lung Cancer* 1988;4:181.

406. Rapp E, Pater J, Willan A, et al. Chemotherapy can prolong survival in patients with advanced non–small cell lung cancer—report of a Canadian multicenter randomized trial. *J Clin Oncol* 1988;6:633–641.

407. Woods R, Williams C, Levi J, et al. Is chemotherapy worthwhile in advanced non–small cell lung cancer? A perspective randomized trial. *Br J Cancer* 1990;61:608–611.

408. Souquet P, Chauvin F, Boissel J, et al. Polychemotherapy in advanced non–small cell lung cancer: meta-analysis. *Lancet* 1993;342:19–21.

409. Grilli R, Oxman A, Julian J. Chemotherapy for advanced non–small cell lung cancer: how much benefit is enough? *J Clin Oncol* 1993;11:1866–1872.

410. Marino P, Pampallona S, Preatoni A, et al. Chemotherapy vs supportive care in advanced non–small-cell lung cancer. *Chest* 1994;106:861–865.

411. Ganz P, Haskell C, Figlin R, et al. Estimating the quality of life in a clinical trial of patients with metastatic lung cancer using the Karnofsky performance status and the functional living index. *Cancer* 1988;61:849–856.

412. Bonomi P, Kim K, Chang A, et al. Phase III trial comparing etoposide-cisplatin versus Taxol with cisplatin-G-CSF versus Taxol-cisplatin in advanced non–small cell lung cancer. An Eastern Cooperative Oncology Group (ECOG) trial. *Proc Am Soc Clin Oncol* 1996;15:382(abst 1145).

413. Wozniak AJ, Crowley JJ, Balcerzak GR, et al. Randomized phase III trial of cisplatin vs cisplatin plus Navelbine in the treatment of advanced non–small cell lung cancer: report of a Southwest Oncology Group Study (SWOG 9308). *Proc Am Soc Clin Oncol* 1996;15:374(abst 1110).

414. Kelly K, Crowley J Jr, et al. Randomized phase III trial of paclitaxel plus carboplatin versus vinorelbine plus cisplatin in the treatment of patients with advanced non–small-cell lung cancer: a Southwest Oncology Group trial. *J Clin Oncol* 2001;19:3210–3218.

415. Ramsey S, Moinpour C, Lovato L, et al. Economic analysis of vinorelbine plus cisplatin versus paclitaxel plus carboplatin for advanced non–small-cell lung cancer. *J Natl Cancer Inst* 2002;94:291–297.

416. Schiller JH, Harrington A, Belani C, et al. Comparison of four chemotherapy regimens for advanced non–small cell lung cancer. *N Engl J Med* 2002;346:92–98.

417. Giaccone G, EORTC. Early results of a randomized phase III trial of platinum-containing doublets versus a nonplatinum doublet in the treatment of advanced non–small cell lung cancer: European Organization for Research and Treatment of Cancer 08975. *Semin Oncol* 2002;29[3 Suppl 9]:47–49.

418. Georgoulias V, Papadakis E, Alexopoulos A, et al. Platinum-based and non–platinum-based chemotherapy in advanced non–small-cell lung cancer: a randomised multicentre trial. *Lancet* 2001;357:1478–1484.

419. Kosmidis P, Mylonakis N, Nicolaides C, et al. Platinum-based and non–platinum-based chemotherapy in advanced non–small-cell lung cancer: a randomised multicentre trial. *J Clin Oncol* 2002;20:3578–3585.

420. Breathnach OS, Freidin B, Conley B, et al. Twenty-two years of phase III trials for patients with advanced non–small cell lung cancer: sobering results. *J Clin Oncol* 2001;19:1734–1742.

421. Gridelli C. The ELVIS Trial: a phase III study of single-agent vinorelbine as first-line treatment in elderly patients with advanced non–small cell lung cancer. Elderly Lung Cancer Vinorelbine Italian Study. *Oncologist* 2001;6[Suppl 1]:4–7.

422. Gridelli C, Perrone F, Cigolari S, et al. The MILES (Multicenter Italian Lung Cancer in the Elderly Study) phase 3 trial: gemcitabine + vinorelbine vs vinorelbine and vs gemcitabine in elderly advanced NSCLC patients. *Proc Am Soc Clin Oncol* 2001;20:308a.

423. Seifter EJ, Ihde DC. Therapy of small cell lung cancer: a perspective on two decades of clinical research. *Semin Oncol* 1988;15:278–299.

424. Mulshine J, Treston A, Brown H, et al. Initiators and promoters of lung cancer. *Chest* 1993;103[Suppl 1]:4S–11S.

425. Ihde DC, Pass HI, Glatstein EJ. Small cell lung cancer. In: DeVita V, Hellman S, Rosenberg S, eds. *Cancer: principles and practice of oncology.* Philadelphia: JB Lippincott Co, 1993:723–758.

426. Archer VE, Saccomanno G, Jones JH. Frequency of different histologic types of bronchogenic carcinoma as related to radiation exposure. *Cancer* 1974;34:2056–2060.

427. Sculier JP, Evans WK, Feld R, et al. Superior vena cava syndrome in small cell lung cancer. *Cancer* 1986;57:847–851.

428. Matthews MJ, Kanhouwa S, Pickren J, et al. Frequency of residual and metastatic tumor in patients undergoing curative surgical resection for lung cancer. *Cancer Chemother Rep* 1973;4:63–67.

429. List AF, Hainsworth JD, Davis BW, et al. The syndrome of antidiuretic hormone in small cell lung cancer. *J Clin Oncol* 1986;4:1191–1198.

430. Shepherd F, Laskey J, Evans W, et al. Cushing's syndrome associated with ectopic corticotropin production and small-cell lung cancer. *J Clin Oncol* 1992;10:21–27.

431. Remick SC, Hafez GR, Carbone PP. Extrapulmonary small cell carcinoma: a review of the literature with emphasis on therapy and outcome. *Medicine* 1987;66:457–471.

432. Sagman U, Evan WK, Warr D, et al. Small cell carcinoma of the lung: derivation of a prognostic staging system. *J Clin Oncol* 1991;9:1639–1649.

433. Albain KS, Crowley JJ, LeBlanc M, et al. Determinants of improved outcome in small-cell lung cancer: an analysis of the 2,580 patient Southwest Oncology Group Data Base. *J Clin Oncol* 1990;8:1563–1574.

434. Medical Research Council of Great Britain. Working party on the evaluation of different methods of therapy in carcinoma of the bronchus: comparative trial of surgery and radiotherapy for primary treatment of small celled or oat celled carcinoma of the bronchus. *Lancet* 1966;2:979–986.

435. Fox W, Scadding JG. Medical Research Council comparative trial of surgery and radiotherapy for primary treatment of small

cell or oat cell carcinoma of the bronchus: ten-year follow-up. *Lancet* 1973;2:63–65.

436. Martini N, Wittes RE, Hilaris BS. Oat cell carcinoma of the lung. *Clin Bull* 1975;5:144–148.

437. Mountain CF, Carr DT, Anderson WA. A system for clinical staging of lung cancer. *Am J Roentgenol* 1974;120:130–138.

438. Mountain CF. Clinical biology of small cell carcinoma: relationship to surgical therapy. *Semin Oncol* 1978;5:272–278.

439. Green RA, Humphrey E, Close H, et al. Alkylating agents in bronchogenic carcinoma. *Am J Med* 1969;46:515–525.

440. Grant S, Gralla R, Kris M, et al. Single-agent chemotherapy trials in small-cell lung cancer 1970 to 1990: the case for studies in previously treated patients. *J Clin Oncol* 1992;10:484–498.

441. Smith I, et al. Carboplatin: a very new active cisplatin analog in the treatment of small cell lung cancer. *Cancer Treat Rep* 1985;69:43.

442. Schiller J, Kim K, Hutson P, et al. Phase II study of topotecan in patients with extensive-stage small-cell carcinoma of the lung: an Eastern Cooperative Oncology Group trial. *J Clin Oncol* 1996;14:2345–2352.

443. Pawel JV, Schiller J, Sheperd F, et al. Topotecan vs cyclophosphamide, doxorubicin, and vincristine for the treatment of recurrent small cell lung cancer. *J Clin Oncol* 1999;17:658–667.

444. Masuda N, Fukuoka M, Kusunoki Y, et al. CPT-11: a new derivative of camptothecin for the treatment of refractory or relapsed small-cell lung cancer. *J Clin Oncol* 1992;10:1225–1229.

445. Kirschling R, Jung S, Jett J. A phase II trial of Taxol and GCSF in previously untreated patients with extensive stage small cell lung cancer (SCC) [Meeting Abstract]. *Proc Annu Meeting Am Soc Clin Oncol* 1994;13:A1076.

446. Smyth J, Smith T, Sessa C, et al. Activity of docetaxel (Taxotere) in small cell lung cancer. *Eur J Cancer* 1994;30A:1058–1060.

447. Jassem J, Karnicka-Mlodkowska H, Pottelsberghe CV. Phase II study of vinorelbine in previously treated small cell lung cancer patients. *Eur J Cancer* 1993;29A:1720–1722.

448. Furuse M, Kubota K, Kawahara M, et al. Phase II study of vinorelbine in heavily previously treated small cell lung cancer. Japan Lung Cancer Vinorelbine Study Group. *Oncology* 1996;53:169–172.

449. Cormier Y, Eisenhauer E, Muldal A, et al. Gemcitabine is an active new agent in previously untreated extensive small cell lung cancer (SCLC). A study of the National Cancer Institute of Canada Clinical Trials Group. *Ann Oncol* 1994;5:283–285.

450. Carney DN, Grogan L, Smit EF, et al. Single agent oral etoposide for elderly small cell lung cancer patients. *Semin Oncol* 1990;17[Suppl 2]:49–53.

451. Girling D. Comparison of oral etoposide and standard intravenous multidrug chemotherapy for small-cell lung cancer: a stopped multicentre randomised trial. Medical Research Council Lung Cancer Working Party. *Lancet* 1996;348:563–566.

452. Souhami R, Spiro S, Rudd R, et al. Five-day oral etoposide treatment for advanced small-cell lung cancer: randomized comparison with intravenous chemotherapy. *J Natl Cancer Inst* 1997;89:577–580.

453. Lowenbraun S, Bartulucci A, Smalley RV, et al. The superiority of combination chemotherapy over single agent chemotherapy in small cell lung carcinoma. *Cancer* 1979;44:406–413.

454. Aisner J, Alberto P, Bitran J, et al. Role of chemotherapy in small cell lung cancer: a consensus report of the International Association for the Study of Lung Cancer Workshop. *Cancer Treat Rep* 1983;67:37–43.

455. Berlin J, Schiller JH. Chemotherapy of small cell carcinoma of the lung. In: Johnson BE, Johnson, DH, eds. *Lung cancer.* New York: Wiley-Liss, 1995:247–261.

456. Jett J, Everson L, Therneau T, et al. Treatment of limited-stage small-cell lung cancer with cyclophosphamide, doxorubicin, and vincristine with or without etoposide: a randomized trial of the North Central Cancer Treatment Group. *J Clin Oncol* 1990;8:33–38.

457. Case L, Zekan P, et al. Improvement of long-term survival in extensive small-cell lung cancer. *J Clin Oncol* 1988;6:1161–1169.

458. Messeih A, Schweitzer J, Lipton A, et al. Addition of etoposide to cyclophosphamide, doxorubicin, and vincristine for remission induction and survival in patients with small cell lung cancer. *Cancer Treat Rep* 1987;71:61–66.

459. Evans WK, Shepherd FA, Feld R, et al. VP-16 and cisplatin as first-line therapy for small-cell lung cancer. *J Clin Oncol* 1985;3:1471–1477.

460. Aisner J, Abrams J. Cisplatin for small cell lung cancer. *Semin Oncol* 1989;16:2–9.

461. Bishop JF, Raghavan D, Stuart-Harris R, et al. Carboplatin (CB-DCA, JM-8) and VP-16-213 in previously untreated patients with small cell lung cancer. *J Clin Oncol* 1987;5:1574–1578.

462. Roth BJ, Johnson DH, Einhorn LH, et al. Randomized study of cyclophosphamide, doxorubicin, and vincristine versus etoposide and cisplatin versus alternation of these two regimens in extensive small-cell lung cancer: a phase III trial of the Southeastern Cancer Study Group. *J Clin Oncol* 1992;10:282–291.

463. Fukuoka M, Furuse K, Saijo N, et al. Randomized trial of cyclophosphamide, doxorubicin, and vincristine versus cisplatin and etoposide versus alternation of these regimens in small cell lung cancer. *J Natl Cancer Inst* 1991;83:855–861.

464. Goldie J, Coldman A. A mathematical model for relating sensitivity of tumors to their spontaneous mutation rate. *Cancer Treat Rep* 1979;63:1727–1733.

465. Evans W, Feld R, Murray N, et al. Superiority of alternating non–cross-resistant chemotherapy in extensive small cell lung cancer. A multicenter, randomized clinical trial by the National Cancer Institute of Canada. *Ann Intern Med* 1987;107:451–458.

466. Bunn PA, Curren M, Fukuoka M, et al. Chemotherapy in small cell lung cancer: a consensus report. *Lung Cancer* 1989;5:127–134.

467. Arriagada R, Chevalier TL, Pignon J, et al. Initial chemotherapeutic doses and survival in patients with limited small-cell lung cancer. *N Engl J Med* 1993;329:1848–1852.

468. Ihde D, Mulshine J, Kramer B, et al. Prospective randomized comparison of high-dose and standard-dose etoposide and cisplatin chemotherapy in patients with extensive-stage small-cell lung canc. *J Clin Oncol* 1994;12:2022–2034.

469. Klasa RJ, Murray N, Coldman AJ. Dose intensity meta-analysis of chemotherapy regimens in small cell carcinoma of the lung. *J Clin Oncol* 1991;9:499–508.

470. Murray N, Osoba D, Shah A, et al. Brief intensive chemotherapy for metastatic non–small cell lung cancer: a phase II study of the weekly CODE regimen. *J Natl Cancer Inst* 1991;83:190–194.

471. Furuse K, Fukuoka M, Nishiwaki Y, et al. Phase III study of intensive weekly chemotherapy with recombinant human granulocyte colony-stimulating factor versus standard chemotherapy in extensive-disease small-cell lung cancer. The Japan Clinical Oncology Group. *J Clin Oncol* 1998;16:2126–2132.

472. Bunn P, Crowley J, Kelly K, et al. Chemoradiotherapy with or without granulocyte-macrophage colony-stimulating factor in the treatment of limited-stage small-cell lung cancer: a prospective phase III randomized study of the Southwest Oncology Group. *J Clin Oncol* 1995;13:1632–1641.

473. Humblet Y, Symann M, Bosly A, et al. Late intensification chemotherapy with autologous bone marrow transplantation in selected small-cell carcinoma of the lung: a randomized study. *J Clin Oncol* 1987;5:1864–1873.

474. Elias A, Ibrahim J, Skarin A, et al. Dose-intensive therapy for limited-stage small-cell lung cancer: long-term outcome. *J Clin Oncol* 1999;17:1175–1184.

475. Leyvraz S, Perey L, Rosti G, et al. Multiple courses of high-dose ifosfamide, carboplatin, and etoposide with peripheral-blood progenitor cells and filgrastim for small-cell lung cancer: a feasibility study by the European Group for Blood and Marrow Transplantation. *J Clin Oncol* 1999;17:3531–3539.

476. Noda K, Nishiwaki Y, Kuwahara M, et al. Irinotecan plus cisplatin compared with etoposide plus cisplatin for extensive small-cell lung cancer. *N Engl J Med* 2002;346:85–91.

477. Mavroudis D, Papadakis E, Veslemes M, et al. A multicenter randomized clinical trial comparing paclitaxel-cisplatin-etoposide versus cisplatin-etoposide as first-line treatment in patients with small-cell lung cancer. *Ann Oncol* 2001;12:463–470.

478. Schiller J, Adak S, Cella D, et al. Topotecan versus observation after cisplatin plus etoposide in extensive-stage small-cell lung cancer: E7593—a phase III trial of the Eastern Cooperative Oncology Group. *J Clin Oncol* 2001;19:2114–2122.

479. Huisman C, Postmus P, Giaccone G, et al. Second-line chemotherapy and its evaluation in small cell lung cancer. *Cancer Treat Rev* 1999;25:199–206.

480. Kreisman H, Wolkove N, Quoix E. Small cell lung cancer presenting as a solitary pulmonary nodule. *Chest* 1992;101:225–231.

481. Quoix E, Fraser R, Wolkove N, et al. Small cell lung cancer presenting as a solitary pulmonary nodule. *Cancer* 1990;66:577–582.

482. Suzuki K, Tsuchiya R, Ichinose Y, et al. Phase II trial of postoperative adjuvant cisplatin/etoposide (PE) in patients with completely resected stage I-IIIA small cell lung cancer (SCLC): the Japan Clinical Oncology Lung Cancer Study Group Trial (JCOG9101). *Proc Am Soc Clin Oncol* 2000;19.

483. Lad T, Thomas P, Piantadosi S, the Lung Cancer Study Group. Surgical resection of small cell lung cancer: a prospective randomized evaluation. *Proc Am Soc Clin Oncol* 1991;10:224(abst 835).

484. Cohen MH, Ihde DC, Bunn PA, et al. Cyclic alternating combination chemotherapy for small cell bronchogenic carcinoma. *Cancer Treat Rep* 1979;62:163–170.

485. Warde P, Payne D. Does thoracic radiation improve survival and local control in limited-stage small-cell carcinoma of the lung? *J Clin Oncol* 1992;10:890–895.

486. Pignon JP, Arriagada R, Ihde DC, et al. A meta-analysis of thoracic radiotherapy for small-cell lung cancer. *N Engl J Med* 1992;327:1618–1624.

487. Murray N, Coy P, Pater JL, et al. Importance of timing for thoracic irradiation in the combined modality treatment of limited stage small cell lung cancer. *J Clin Oncol* 1993;11:336–344.

488. Jeremic B, Shibamoto Y, Acimovic L, et al. Initial versus delayed accelerated hyperfractionated radiotherapy and concurrent chemotherapy in limited small-cell lung cancer: a randomized study. *J Clin Oncol* 1997;15:893–900.

489. Goto K, Nishiwaki Y, et al. Final results of a phase III study of concurrent versus sequential thoracic radiotherapy in combination with cisplatin and etoposide for limited-stage small cell lung cancer: the Japan Clinical Oncology Group Study. *Proc Am Soc Clin Oncol* 1999;18:468a.

490. Lichter A, Turrisi A. Small cell lung cancer: the influence of dose and treatment volume on outcome. *Semin Radiat Oncol* 1995;5:44–49.

491. Turrisi A, Kynugmann K, Blum R, et al. Twice-daily compared with once-daily thoracic radiotherapy in limited small-cell lung cancer treated concurrently with cisplatin and etoposide. *N Engl J Med* 1999;340:264–271.

492. Bonner J, Sloan J, Shanahan T, et al. Phase III comparison of twice-daily split-course irradiation versus once-daily irradiation for patients with limited stage small-cell lung carcinoma. *J Clin Oncol* 1999;17:2681–2691.

493. Rosen ST, Makuch RW, Lichter AS, et al. Role of prophylactic cranial irradiation in the prevention of central nervous system metastases in small cell lung cancer: potential benefit restricted to patients with complete response. *Am J Med* 1983;74:615–624.

494. Nugent JL, Bunn PA, Matthews MJ, et al. CNS metastases in small cell bronchogenic carcinoma: increasing frequency and changing patterns with lengthening survival. *Cancer* 1979;44:1885–1898.

495. Arriagada R, Le Chevalier T, Borie F, et al. Prophylactic cranial irradiation for patients with small cell lung cancer in complete remission. *J Natl Cancer Inst* 1995;87:183–190.

496. Laplanche A, Monnet I, Santos-Miranda J, et al. Controlled clinical trial of prophylactic cranial irradiation for patients with small-cell lung cancer in complete remission. *Lung Cancer* 1998;21:193–201.

497. Gregor A, Cull A, Stephens J, et al. Effects of prophylactic cranial irradiation (PCI) in small cell lung cancer (SCLC): results of UKCCCR/EORTC randomized trial. *Proc Am Soc Clin Oncol* 1996;15:381(abst 1139).

498. Auperin A, Arriagada R, Pignon J, et al. Prophylactic cranial irradiation for patients with small-cell lung cancer in complete remission. Prophylactic Cranial Irradiation Overview Collaborative Group. *N Engl J Med* 1999;341:476–484.

499. Lee JS, Umsawasdi T, Lee Y, et al. Neurotoxicity in long-term survivors of small cell lung cancer. *Int J Radiat Oncol Biol Phys* 1986;12:313–321.

Solitary Pulmonary Nodule and Lung Tumors Other Than Bronchogenic Carcinoma

40

Robert J. Kruklitis · Anil Vachani · Mitchell L. Margolis

In this chapter, we will address issues of importance for the practicing physician that relate to lung neoplasms, excepting the major lung cancer subtypes of squamous cell, large cell, small cell, and adenocarcinoma addressed in the previous chapter. We begin with a discussion of the solitary pulmonary nodule (SPN), a frequent and formidable clinical problem. Our second major focus is metastatic disease to the lung, by far and away the most common cause of pulmonary malignancy. Third, we address bronchoalveolar carcinoma (BAC), an increasingly prevalent and important lung malignancy that can be considered "nonbronchogenic," despite being classified as a subset of adenocarcinoma in the World Health Organization (WHO) lung cancer schema. Fourth, we describe tumors uncommonly seen in clinical practice, i.e., neuroendocrine tumors, hamartomas, and inflammatory pseudotumors. We conclude with brief descriptions and key references pertaining to what can arbitrarily be termed truly rare lung tumors, such as salivary gland type tumors and pulmonary sarcomas. Tumors of the lung that usually arise as part of a systemic disorder (such as lymphoma and rheumatoid arthritis) and pseudotumors (such as those caused by interlobar fluid collections or rounded atelectasis) are discussed elsewhere in this textbook.

SOLITARY PULMONARY NODULE

Diagnosis and Management

The SPN, defined as a nodule less than 3 cm in diameter completely surrounded by pulmonary parenchyma without evidence of adenopathy or atelectasis, is a common occurrence in clinical practice. SPNs are identified in one to two

R. J. Kruklitis, A. Vachani, and M. L. Margolis: Pulmonary, Allergy, and Critical Care Division, University of Pennsylvania, Philadelphia, Pennsylvania.

of every 1,000 chest roentgenograms, resulting in a prevalence of approximately 150,000 SPNs annually in the United States (1). Given their frequent occurrence and malignant potential, proper evaluation and management are crucial. A variety of benign and malignant entities, including many nonbronchogenic tumors, may present as an SPN. These lesions share many radiographic characteristics and a typically asymptomatic presentation. The significance of these nodules, however, varies greatly depending on the precise etiology. A major goal in the management of pulmonary nodules is to minimize morbidity in the evaluation of benign lesions while simultaneously facilitating early diagnosis and definitive treatment of those lesions that are malignant. Towards this end, clinicians must use available historical, clinical, and radiographic clues to help predict the probability that a given nodule is malignant. This prediction significantly influences the diagnostic and management plan for a given nodule.

History

There are several historical clues that can help distinguish between benign and malignant SPNs. Cigarette smoking is the major risk factor for the development of malignant lung tumors; 85% of all bronchogenic carcinomas occur in current or former smokers. Furthermore, the number of cigarettes smoked daily directly correlates with the likelihood that a nodule will be malignant (2). Other environmental agents, such as asbestos or radon, can also greatly increase the risk of malignancy. Age is also a helpful risk factor, as malignancy is rare in patients less than 35 years old (1). In contrast, the rate of malignancy is significantly increased in patients older than 50 (2). A history of chronic obstructive pulmonary disease, even controlling for cigarette usage, is also associated with increased risk of malignancy (3,4). Finally, SPNs presenting as either solitary metastases in patients with a history of malignancy or as new primary lesions are much more likely to be malignant than benign.

Clinical Examination

Usually the clinical examination contributes little to the diagnosis of an isolated pulmonary nodule. However, one can sometimes identify clues that may indirectly suggest the diagnosis. For example, the presence of classic joint deformities of rheumatoid arthritis would suggest a diagnosis of a rheumatoid nodule, whereas the presence of telangiectasias would heighten concern for an arteriovenous malformation. Special attention should also be paid to identifying possible sites of metastatic tumor, especially when the nodule is suspicious for malignancy. Finally, physical examination might also reveal signs of significant comorbid illness, such as severe COPD or heart disease, that influence evaluation and management.

Radiographic Features

There are several radiographic criteria that may be used to help ascertain the likelihood of malignancy for a given SPN. It should be noted, however, that only rarely are the radiographic findings pathognomonic; more often they are only suggestive of an etiology. Nonetheless, the radiographic assessment often greatly impacts the management of SPNs.

The size of a lesion greatly affects the likelihood of malignancy, with larger lesions being more likely malignant. Several studies have documented that lesions larger than 3 cm in diameter are malignant in greater than 80% of cases, whereas nodules less than 2 cm are malignant in only 20% (5–7). However, one recent study of nodules less than 1 cm in diameter disclosed malignancy in 57% of cases (8). Therefore, it would be a serious mistake to assume a nodule benign purely on the basis of its size.

The growth rate of a nodule has also been used to predict malignancy. It is often stated that nodules that double in size either very quickly (<30 days) or very slowly (>500 days) are almost certainly benign. In clinical practice, this rule is often true but by no means absolute. There are many examples of malignancies with doubling times of less than 30 days or greater than 500 days (9); thus, this clinical rule should be used with caution. Nonetheless, growth rate is an important criterion to help determine the probability of malignancy. For instance, nodules that have remained completely stable over a period of years are much more likely to be benign; unfortunately this dictum also is not absolutely reliable (9). However, obtaining old radiographic studies for size comparison can be quite helpful in the evaluation and management of SPNs and should be done whenever possible.

Several other radiologic features of SPNs are noteworthy. In general, benign lesions tend to have smooth and regular borders, whereas malignant nodules are often irregularly shaped, shaggy, or spiculated. The appearance of fine linear streaks emanating outward from a nodule, the "corona radiata" sign, is helpful in predicting malignancy. In two separate studies, the presence of the corona radiata sign alone was able to accurately predict malignancy in 88% and 94% of cases, respectively (7,10). Calcifications may be present within both malignant and benign nodules. The pattern of calcification, however, can be helpful; laminated, central, diffuse, and popcorn patterns are predictive of benignancy, whereas stippled and eccentric patterns suggest malignancy (1). Specifically, the laminated pattern is associated with granulomas, whereas the popcorn pattern is almost exclusively associated with hamartomas. The presence of central fat within a nodule is essentially diagnostic of a benign hamartoma (11,12), whereas the demonstration of bubble-like lucencies within a nodule is highly suggestive of malignancy, seen most often in BAC (12).

Computed Tomography

Although SPNs are often discovered and monitored using routine conventional chest roentgenograms, specific nodular characteristics are better visualized by computed tomography (CT). CT scans are superior to chest roentgenograms because they provide better spatial resolution and more anatomical detail. High-resolution chest CT is particularly useful because the thin cuts optimize resolution and detection of calcium and fat densities within a nodule. Overall, this equates to more accurate size and growth measurements, a better visualization of edge and border characteristics, and improved detection of calcifications. Additionally, CT scanning can be used to assess for contrast enhancement of nodules; enhancing lesions are more likely to be malignant owing to their greater vascularity (13,14). Quantitative enhancement measurements of pulmonary nodules have a sensitivity of 95% to 100% and a specificity of 70% to 93% for predicting malignancy (15).

Positron Emission Tomography

Positron emission tomographic (PET) scanning to help evaluate SPNs is becoming increasingly useful. PET scans take advantage of the enhanced uptake of [^{18}F]fluorodeoxyglucose by tissues with high glucose metabolism (malignant tumors). Several studies have confirmed that lung tumor cells have increased uptake of [^{18}F]fluorodeoxyglucose compared with that of normal lung parenchyma (16,17). Unfortunately, this technique has several important limitations. False-positive PET scans may result from infectious processes or active granulomas (Fig. 40.1), as these too have enhanced glucose metabolism (18). Furthermore, malignant tumors with relatively low metabolic rates, such as BAC (19) and carcinoid tumors (20), may be falsely PET negative. Small malignant nodules are also problematic, as they may be PET negative owing to the modest spatial resolution of current scanners (21). Thus, the

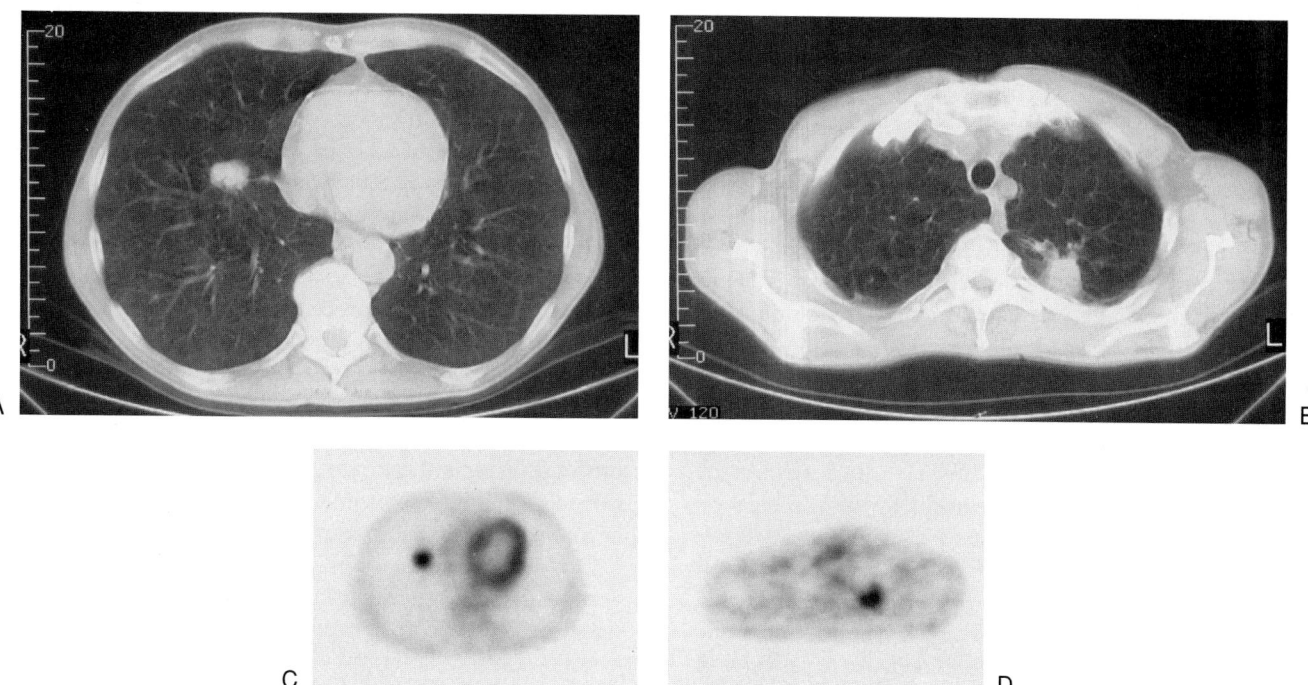

FIGURE 40.1. CT scan showing concomitant right lower lobe mass **(A)** and left upper lobe mass **(B)** in a single patient. Positron emission tomography scan demonstrated true positive uptake for the right lower lobe mass **(C)**, which proved to be a squamous cell carcinoma, and false-positive uptake for a left upper lobe mass **(D)**, which proved to be an active granuloma.

results of PET scans performed on smaller nodules should be interpreted with caution. Other limitations to PET include its expense and relative unavailability at many medical centers. Despite these potential drawbacks, PET scanning can be a useful diagnostic test. A recent metaanalysis evaluated the accuracy of PET scanning for the diagnosis of pulmonary nodules and masses. Together, the results of 40 studies revealed that PET scanning had an overall sensitivity of 97% and specificity of 78% for predicting malignancy (22).

Differential Diagnosis

Approximately 40% to 60% of all biopsied SPNs are malignant in most series, and this number may be increasing (23). The exact percentage of malignant SPNs will vary, depending on the characteristics of the group being examined. Bronchogenic carcinoma accounts for more than 90% of all malignant SPNs, especially the adenocarcinoma and squamous cell carcinoma subtypes. Bronchoalveolar cell carcinoma, carcinoids, lymphomas, sarcomas, and solitary metastasis account for the majority of malignant nonbronchogenic SPNs. Benign tumors can also cause SPNs. Although hamartomas are a relatively common benign cause of SPNs (see "Hamartoma" below), other benign tumors are unusual, accounting together for fewer than 0.5% of all SPNs.

There are many additional causes of SPNs other than benign or malignant lung neoplasms. Overall, infectious or noninfectious granulomas are the most frequent cause of SPNs. The most common infectious etiologies include tuberculosis, histoplasmosis, and coccidioidomycosis, whereas the noninfectious causes include rheumatoid nodules, Wegener granulomatosis, and sarcoidosis.

Remaining causes are rare and are often grouped into a miscellaneous category. Examples of such lesions include arteriovenous malformations (24), pulmonary infarctions (25), mucoid impaction (26), amyloidosis (27), and bronchogenic cysts (28). Infection with *Dirofilaria* often results in a SPN (29), whereas *Pneumocystis carinii* (30) and cytomegalovirus (31) rarely do so.

Management

The management of patients with SPNs is complex, and no one single approach is applicable to all patients. Instead, a multitude of factors must be considered on an individual basis in order to provide specific recommendations. Factors to be weighed include the probability of malignancy and the patient's preference and performance status. If the nodule is almost certainly benign, then observation over time, making certain that the clinical and radiographic characteristics do not change to favor malignancy, should be strongly considered. In contrast, definitive therapy aimed at a cure should be pursued early with nodules that are almost certainly malignant. Surgical resection is the treatment of choice for non–small cell bronchogenic carcinoma and for most of the malignant nonbronchogenic tumors presenting as SPNs.

In addition, resection is the most reliable way to establish a definitive diagnosis. Therefore, surgical resection with both diagnostic and therapeutic intent should be strongly considered for nodules having a high likelihood of malignancy.

Perhaps the most difficult clinical situation is the management of nodules with an intermediate probability of malignancy. In such cases, the burden is on the clinician to prove that the nodule is not malignant. This often leads to a variety of tests and biopsies such as transthoracic needle aspiration (TTNA) and bronchoscopy with transbronchial biopsy (TBB). Biopsies are especially helpful if they can provide definitive evidence of a benign process, such as hamartoma or granuloma, as they would then prevent unnecessary surgery. Biopsies can also provide a malignant diagnosis, which may be vital when patients are not ideal surgical candidates or are extremely reluctant to undergo surgical biopsy or resection.

The diagnostic yield of these techniques depends on the skill of the operator and the size and location of the nodule. The diagnostic yield using fiberoptic bronchoscopy with TBB greatly depends on size, with a 40% to 69% yield in lesions greater than 2 cm in diameter (32,33). This yield drops considerably to only 10% to 33% for nodules less than 2 cm in diameter (34). Location also influences the results, as lesions located in the apical or basilar segments have lower yields (33). Conversely, the bronchus sign, CT evidence of a bronchus leading directly into a nodule, increases the yield of TBB to 60% to 80% (35). On the other hand, TTNA yield is also related to size, but the yield is much higher, particularly for peripheral lesions, with an overall yield of 85% to 95% (36). Unfortunately, negative results most often do not prove that a lesion is benign, given the uncertainties of precise needle placement into small lesions and sparse samples of aspirated cells. In fact, a definitive diagnosis by TTNA is made in only 4% to 14% of benign nodules (37,38). Repeated sampling, the use of larger cutting needles capable of obtaining histological specimens, and the presence of on-site cytopathology all increase the yield (39,40).

Sometimes a definitive diagnosis cannot be made using either TBB or TTNA. Previously, establishing a diagnosis in such cases would require a thoracotomy in order to obtain an adequate tissue specimen. Peripherally located pulmonary nodules can now be resected via video-assisted thoracoscopic surgery (41–44). If a malignancy is found, the operation can be converted to a formal thoracotomy, allowing a definitive cancer operation. However, if the nodule is benign, the procedure is terminated, sparing the patient thoracotomy with its inherent morbidity.

An alternative strategy that can be used with the indeterminate nodule is close observation, or the "watch and wait" strategy. The basis of close observation is to watch a nodule prospectively over time with serial chest x-rays or CT scans, hoping to establish roentgenographic stability or a growth rate that will help with subsequent management. One can easily calculate the time required to double in volume (dou-

bling time) for a given SPN. If spherical, a nodule will double its volume when its diameter increases by only 26%. Thus, small changes in diameter can equate to large volumetric increases. Some of the many pitfalls to this approach were mentioned above. Another major drawback to the observation strategy is the resultant delay in the resection of nodules that ultimately prove to be malignant, thereby allowing tumor growth and the possibility for metastatic spread. In fact, the long-term survival may be enhanced with resection of smaller rather than larger malignant nodules (45), although major controversy exists on this point, especially for very small lesions. Recent advances in imaging technology now permit a detailed three-dimensional characterization of pulmonary nodules. This allows a more precise characterization of subtle changes that could not be detected with standard roentgenograms or conventional two-dimensional CT. This technology, which allows early detection of nodular growth (46), may decrease the time a patient under observation goes without definitive therapy. Hence, monitoring a nodule with three-dimensional imaging might address a major drawback of the observation strategy.

Two additional factors must be considered before implementing a management algorithm: performance status/comorbid illnesses and patient preference. Patients with severe cardiac or pulmonary disease may not be candidates for treatment, especially surgical intervention, regardless of the diagnosis. Finally, the patient's preference can and should influence this process considerably, particularly because decision analysis indicates that the choice of a management strategy is often a "close call" (47). Many patients are completely adverse to any treatment unless it is known with certainty that the nodule is malignant. Conversely, others request surgery irrespective of whether the diagnosis is known with certainty. Some individuals refuse surgery even if it is the optimal choice, based on fears of tumor growth when the chest is opened and the tumor is exposed to air. Many patients can be offered radiotherapy with curative intent for SPNs once a definitive diagnosis of malignancy is achieved by biopsy.

SOLITARY PULMONARY NODULE

Summary Statement	Level of Evidence
A wide variety of imaging tests are useful in diagnosis, particularly when serial tests are performed, but definitive diagnosis usually requires invasive tissue sampling.	Numerous retrospective studies
Any of three initial nonmutually exclusive management strategies (excision, biopsy, or observation) may be acceptable, depending on numerous clinical variables and patient preference.	Minimal experimental evidence; decision analysis, case series, consensus, "standard of care"

TUMORS METASTATIC TO THE LUNG

Metastasis refers to spread of a primary tumor to other organs and distant sites. The lungs are a common site of metastatic disease, with various autopsy series demonstrating an incidence of 20% to 54% in all patients who have cancer (48–50). Pulmonary metastases can manifest as one of several distinct clinical syndromes, including single or multiple nodules, lymphangitic carcinomatosis, endobronchial spread, or metastatic pleural effusions. However, considerable overlap exists, and multiple types of lung metastases may be present in an individual patient. Although chest roentgenogram has been the standard means of detection and monitoring, it has recently been supplanted by CT scanning. The presence of pulmonary metastases is often a grave prognostic sign and has significant therapeutic implications.

Pathogenesis

Metastatic cells most commonly reach the lungs via the pulmonary arteries (48). Metastases can also occur via the bronchial arteries, pulmonary lymphatics, across the pleural space, or through endobronchial spread. Tumors with venous drainage that passes directly through the lungs—including cancers of the head and neck, thyroid, kidneys, testis, melanoma, and osteosarcoma—are particularly susceptible to hematogenous spread (51).

The metastatic cascade involves a sequence of events that includes tumorigenesis, angiogenesis, invasion, embolization via the bloodstream, arrest, extravasation, and proliferation at the metastatic site (52,53). After the initial growth of the primary neoplasm, the tumor recruits its own blood supply via the release of angiogenic factors and suppression of angiogenesis inhibitors (52). A subpopulation of cells within the primary tumor then acquires an invasive phenotype (54). Alterations in cell adhesion and the release of proteolytic enzymes lead to the disruption of the extracellular matrix and access to the stromal compartment (55–58), including both lymphatic and vascular channels, resulting in circulating tumor cells that reach the lung. Fewer than 0.1% of tumor cells in the circulation will produce metastasis (59), as tumor cell viability depends on multiple tumor and tissue microenvironmental factors.

The ultimate appearance of pulmonary metastases depends on the movement pattern of tumor cells. Movement of cells beyond the endothelial cell barrier into the parenchyma will likely produce discrete nodules. However, extension of cells into the perivascular space may lead to spread along lymphatic channels, yielding the classic appearance of lymphangitic carcinomatosis (60). Less frequently, lymphangitic spread can occur by retrograde spread from affected lymph nodes (48).

Patterns of Pulmonary Metastases

Parenchymal Nodules

Pulmonary metastatic disease most commonly presents as a single nodule (Fig. 40.2) or with multiple nodular lesions (Fig. 40.3) within the lung parenchyma. The presence of multiple pulmonary nodules (MPNs) in a patient with known malignancy almost always reflects metastatic disease (61). Even in patients without a known primary malignancy, this finding reflects metastatic disease in the majority of cases (61). Other possible etiologies of MPNs include infection, pulmonary embolic disease, vasculitis, sarcoidosis, lymphoma, rheumatoid arthritis, and arteriovenous malformations. The majority of metastatic nodules are small, usually less than 1 cm (50). However, in the setting of MPNs, the likelihood of malignancy increases with both nodule size and number, particularly with lesions greater than 2.5 cm (cannonball) in diameter or number greater than 10 (61). Most metastatic nodules are located in the periphery of the lung, primarily in a subpleural location (50,62), and are asymptomatic. In addition, most studies show a predominance of nodules in the lower lung zones, reflecting the increased blood flow to the lung bases (50, 63).

Although classically described as smooth and well circumscribed, metastatic nodules demonstrate varied appearance on CT scans, including smooth, poorly defined, or irregular margins (64). The "halo sign," the presence of central soft tissue attenuation surrounded by a region of so-called ground glass, usually indicates hemorrhage (65). Other important CT findings may include calcification (as with osteosarcoma metastases) and cavitation, which may be seen in 4% to 6% of cases, especially metastatic squamous cell carcinoma (66). Metastatic nodules can also form calcifications or cavitation after chemotherapy or radiation therapy (67, 68).

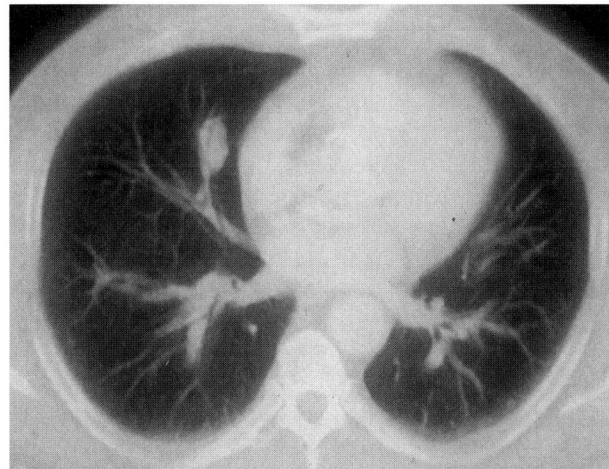

FIGURE 40.2. Solitary pulmonary metastases from malignant melanoma, right middle lobe. Diagnosis made by fiberoptic bronchoscopic biopsy of endobronchial component.

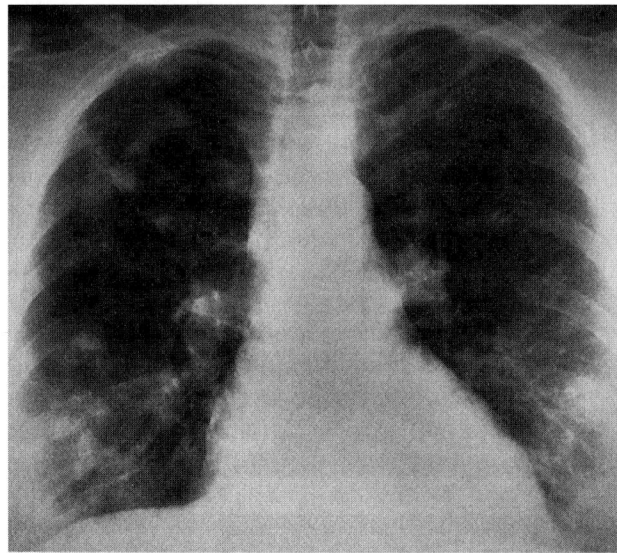
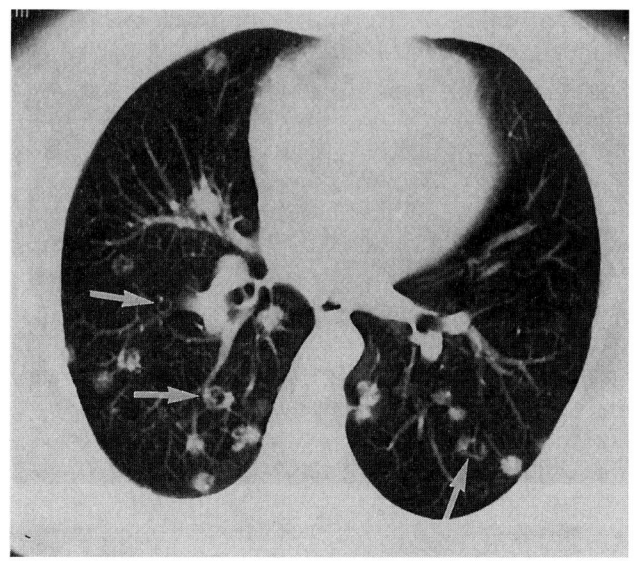

A

B

FIGURE 40.3. Multiple pulmonary metastases from uterine cervical carcinoma. **(A)** Posteroanterior chest radiograph shows multiple bilateral pulmonary nodules, some of which are fairly well circumscribed. **(B)** Computed tomography scan shows well-circumscribed nodules, many of which are cavitary *(arrows)*.

Diagnosis is often based on typical chest films in a patient with known previous cancer, particularly in the case of MPNs. However, sometimes histologic proof is required and may be obtained via bronchoscopy (69,70), TTNA (71), or video-assisted thoracoscopy (72). For solitary nodules that may be metastatic, it is important to consider the potential primary source. In general, a new solitary lesion is likely to represent a primary lung tumor in a patient with previous breast or head and neck cancer, equally likely to represent a primary lung tumor or solitary metastasis in a patient with prior colon cancer, and much more likely to represent a metastasis in a patient with previous sarcoma or melanoma.

Lymphangitic Carcinomatosis and Pulmonary Tumor Microembolism

Lymphangitic spread of tumor is a common manifestation of metastatic disease and carries an extremely poor prognosis. A large autopsy series demonstrated an incidence of 55% in patients who died of cancer (73), but radiographically demonstrable lymphangitic disease is much less common (66), because chest x-rays are normal in 30% to 50% of patients with pathologically proven cases (74). Primary tumors most likely to demonstrate lymphangitic spread include lung, breast, stomach, pancreas, prostate, and thyroid (66,74).

Plain radiographic findings of lymphangitic carcinomatosis include linear markings radiating from the hilum (Kerley A lines) and/or thickening of the interlobular septae (Kerley B lines) superimposed on a background of increased reticular markings (64). Hilar adenopathy and pleural effusions are present in a minority of cases (74,75). High-resolution CT scanning is more sensitive than is plain

radiography in the detection of lymphangitic spread (76). The characteristic high-resolution CT appearance consists of smooth or nodular thickening of interlobular septae (64, 66) (Fig. 40.4).

In patients with a known primary malignancy, the presence of the characteristic radiographic pattern likely reflects the presence of lymphangitic spread, particularly in patients with compatible symptoms such as dyspnea and dry cough. However, other possible etiologies, including pulmonary edema, diffuse infection, or drug-induced (chemotherapy) reactions, must be considered. Further diagnostic testing,

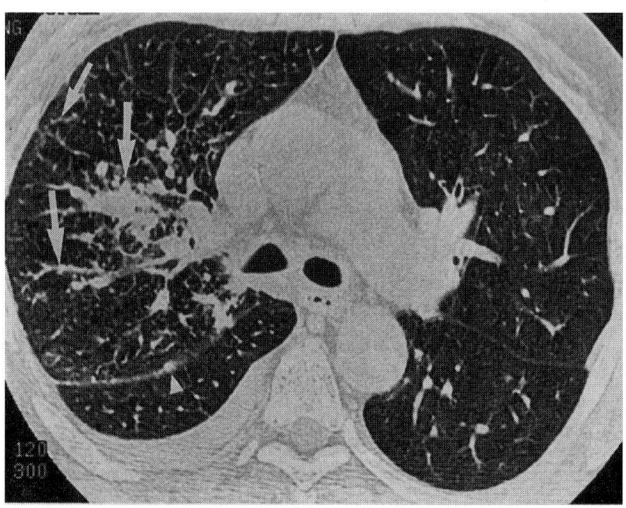

FIGURE 40.4. Lymphangitic carcinomatosis. High-resolution computed tomography shows unilateral nodular thickening of the central and peripheral interstitial compartments *(arrows)*, and a malignant right pleural effusion. Note nodular involvement of the subpleural lymphatics adjacent to the right major fissure *(arrowhead)*.

including bronchoscopy (especially using bronchoalveolar lavage ([77]), pulmonary microvascular cytology (78), or thoracoscopic lung biopsy may be required for definitive diagnosis.

A closely related syndrome, pulmonary tumor microembolism, also presents with dyspnea and cough in patients with metastatic cancer, especially of the breast, lung, and prostate (73,79). In this entity, the pulmonary vascular cross-sectional area is partially occluded by accretions of tumor cells in pulmonary arterioles, often admixed with other thromboembolic constituents, thereby contributing to a clinical picture of subacute progressive pulmonary hypertension. The exact relationship between pulmonary tumor microembolism and lymphangitic carcinomatosis remains problematic, and premortem diagnosis and effective treatment elusive (73,79).

Endobronchial Spread

Endobronchial metastases may be asymptomatic or cause cough, hemoptysis, or shortness of breath. The incidence varies widely in the literature; if one looks only at gross endobronchial spread, the incidence has ranged from 2% to 28% (80–82). However, when microscopically evident endobronchial disease is included, the incidence is as high as 50% (83). The most frequent sources of endobronchial metastases are carcinomas of the breast, kidney, colon, rectum, pancreas, and malignant melanoma of the skin.

On plain radiographs, endobronchial lesions are most often suspected only after evidence of partial or total bronchial obstruction has developed, resulting in postobstructive pneumonia or atelectasis. Growths within the airway are best visualized with CT scanning (84) or bronchoscopy. Furthermore, bronchoscopic biopsy may help differentiate between metastatic disease and a primary bronchogenic carcinoma when endobronchial disease presents in a patient with a known prior malignancy.

Surgical Therapy

Early autopsy studies noted that patients who die of pulmonary metastases often lack metastatic disease at other sites (85,86). This finding suggested that resection of pulmonary metastases may improve survival. In fact, the first patient to undergo resection of a pulmonary metastasis at some distance from the primary tumor, performed in 1883 by Kronlein, went on to live for 7 years before succumbing to her disease (87).

Generally accepted criteria for pulmonary metastasectomy include control of the primary tumor, adequate pulmonary function, absence of extrapulmonary metastases, and complete resectability of the metastases; however, these criteria have been recently questioned (88). Although wedge resection is deemed satisfactory in most cases, substantial controversy persists over appropriate patient selection, the number of lesions that should be removed, the role of ad-

juvant chemotherapy, and prognostic factors relating to the cell type of the primary tumor (89,90). A major limitation has been the lack of prospective randomized trials comparing the efficacy of surgery with other treatment modalities or even with palliative care.

To at least partly address these concerns, the International Registry of Lung Metastases, launched in 1990 at 18 different institutions, collected data on more than 5,000 cases of pulmonary metastasectomy (91). Complete metastasectomy, achieved in 88% of patients, yielded a survival of 36% at 5 years, 26% at 10 years, and 22% at 15 years. Primary germ cell and Wilms tumor demonstrated the best prognosis, whereas melanoma had the worst prognosis. In addition, a disease-free interval of greater than 36 months and single metastasis were also clearly good prognostic markers.

Metastatic Disease from Selected Primary Tumors

Bronchogenic Carcinoma

Primary lung cancers can metastasize to the lung as a secondary neoplasm or even as tertiary metastases from secondary involvement at other sites (86). When a primary lung cancer is found, the presence of a distinct nodule elsewhere in the parenchyma is particularly vexing, in light of recent changes in the lung cancer staging system. The nodule may represent a synchronous primary tumor or a solitary metastasis. For a lesion to be definitively considered synchronous, it must have distinct histological features, but advances in genetic markers promise a more precise method for discrimination of synchronous primary tumors from intrapulmonary metastases (92).

Other rare manifestations include lymphangitic spread, which can result in respiratory failure (93) and diffuse miliary disease, possibly resulting from a shower of tumor emboli originating from bony metastases (94).

Breast Cancer

Routine chest films in early stage (I and II) breast cancer detect asymptomatic pulmonary metastasis in only 0.1% of patients (95). Thus, screening chest x-rays to detect lung metastases after primary therapy for breast cancer are not recommended (96). Nevertheless, pulmonary metastases from breast cancer is a substantial problem, usually presenting as discrete nodules, lymphangitic carcinomatosis, and, less commonly, endobronchial lesions (97).

The presence of a SPN in a patient with breast cancer presents a significant diagnostic challenge. The lesion may be benign, a primary lung malignancy, or metastatic. In studies evaluating synchronous lung lesions in patients with breast cancer, the incidence of primary lung cancer has varied from 20% to 80% (98,99). If a biopsy reveals squamous cell or small cell carcinoma, the lesion represents a primary bronchogenic carcinoma. If, however, the histologic pattern is one of adenocarcinoma, additional testing is required to definitively determine the source of the lesion. The most common confirmatory test used in this circumstance is the use of estrogen and progesterone receptor assays, but additional tumor markers are currently being evaluated (100).

Although no randomized controlled trials have been conducted to evaluate the role of metastasectomy, retrospective studies demonstrate a 5-year survival of 36% to 62% (101–104). Staren and colleagues retrospectively compared surgery with systemic therapy and found a statistically significant improvement in mean survival (55 versus 33 months) (101) in the metastasectomy group. The ultimate role of surgery and chemotherapy in the management of pulmonary metastasis in individuals with breast cancer continues to evolve, but metastasectomy likely has a role in selected patients.

Unusual, recently described manifestations of metastatic breast cancer to lung include diffuse airway narrowing from submucosal metastases (105) and recurrence 40 years after radical mastectomy, with a further 3-year remission after lung metastasectomy combined with chemotherapy (106). Another recent report associated lung metastases in this disease with cigarette smoking, suggesting a preventive role for smoking cessation (107).

Colorectal Carcinoma

The lungs are the most common site of extra-abdominal metastasis in patients with colon cancer, occurring in 10% to 20% of patients after resection (108,109). However, only 2% of all recurrences are limited to the lungs (110).

A major controversy exists over the surgical management of colorectal metastases. As with other solid tumors, pulmonary metastasectomy has been offered to patients who meet appropriate criteria. Although no prospective studies have been performed, several relatively large, contemporary, retrospective studies demonstrate a 5-year survival of 30% to 50% in those undergoing resection (111–115). Unfortunately, substantial uncertainty remains as to the importance of the initial stage of the colon lesion, the number of lesions that should be resected, and many other aspects of surgical case selection. The level of prethoracotomy carcinoembryonic antigen has been found to be a significant prognostic factor, however (88,116).

Less common, recently described presentations include bulky endobronchial metastases that may benefit from laser debulking (117) and bronchorrhea from diffuse lymphangitic metastases (118).

Renal Cell Carcinoma

This tumor is of special interest because removal of the primary renal tumor has been associated with regression of histologically proven pulmonary metastases (119,120).

Benign Metastasizing Leiomyoma

This extraordinarily rare entity, featuring cytologically bland-appearing lesions composed of smooth muscle (121), probably represents late metastases of low-grade, well-differentiated uterine leiomyosarcomas (122). The lesions appear as single or multiple nodules, which seem to be hormonally dependent. Reports have documented growth during pregnancy (123) and regression of lesions after oophorectomy (124).

TUMORS METASTATIC TO LUNG	
Summary Statement	**Level of Evidence**
Diagnosis is often achieved with adequate clinical certainty by radiographic means but may require invasive tissue sampling, depending on myriad clinical circumstances.	Numerous retrospective and autopsy series
Surgical extirpation is the preferred management of certain highly selected subgroups with solitary and multiple lung metastases.	Multiple uncontrolled case series, registry data, consensus and expert opinion

BRONCHOALVEOLAR CELL CARCINOMA

BAC (also referred to as bronchioloalveolar cell or alveolar cell carcinoma) is a primary lung cancer that arises in the distal airways and alveoli and exhibits distinctive clinical, biologic, and perhaps etiologic features. In this sense BAC can be viewed as a "nonbronchogenic carcinoma," despite its classification as a subtype of adenocarcinoma in the WHO lung cancer schema (125). Historically, BAC was felt to represent 5% of all primary lung cancers. More recent data, however, suggest a substantial rise in the incidence of BAC, which may contribute significantly to the overall increase in adenocarcinoma (126,127). In one study, BAC accounted for 24% of all primary lung cancers (126).

Etiology

Although the exact etiology of BAC is unclear and probably multifactorial, several risk factors have been proposed. Cigarette smoking is a predisposing factor for BAC. However, compared with the other primary lung cancers, BAC is the least tightly linked with tobacco use, as up to 30% of patients with BAC are lifelong nonsmokers (126). Additional postulated risk factors include the presence of pulmonary parenchymal damage and poorly characterized occupational exposures, including sugar cane farming and carpentry (128–130). Infectious agents have also been proposed as a possible etiologic factor, especially with the recent discovery of papilloma virus DNA in a few BAC samples (131). Additionally, there is a striking histological and clinical resemblance

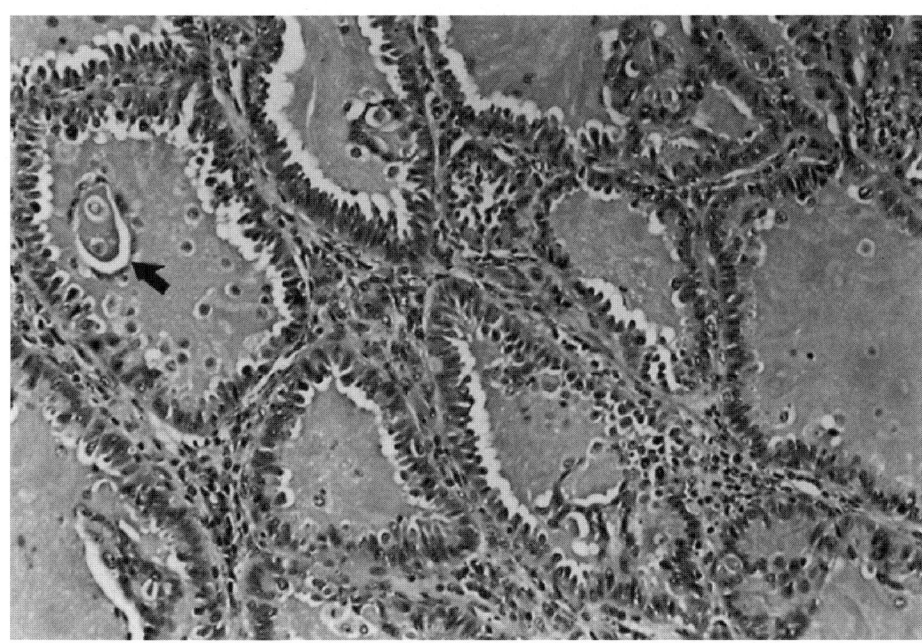

FIGURE 40.5. Bronchoalveolar carcinoma showing tall columnar cells and small nests of tumor floating within mucin (*arrow*). (From Gordon Honda, Department of Pathology, University of California, San Francisco, California, with permission.)

between BAC and Jäagsiekte, a contagious retroviral disease of sheep (132). These similarities suggest the intriguing possibility that BAC may be virally mediated.

Genetic analysis of BAC tissue has revealed frequent mutations in the K-*ras* oncogene, a gene that is intimately involved in cell growth and differentiation. There is a particularly strong association between certain subtypes of BAC and K-*ras,* with mutations occurring in nearly all cases (133). Additionally, mutations of *p53* (131) and other tumor suppressor genes and oncogenes may play a role in the pathogenesis of BAC.

Histology

Histologically, BAC is characterized by the growth of malignant cells along the alveolar and bronchiolar walls (lepidic growth). Malignant cells frequently project into the alveoli but do not distort or invade the pulmonary interstitium. The appearance is sufficiently distinctive as to provide a basis for histopathologic recognition (Fig. 40.5). Nevertheless, small areas of bronchioloalveolar differentiation are frequently noted in adenocarcinomas in general, giving rise to an overlap category of "adenocarcinoma with BAC differentiation." The classic pathologic definition includes the absence of a primary adenocarcinoma elsewhere in the body, the absence of a central bronchogenic source, a peripheral location, and intact pulmonary interstitium.

BAC is divided into two subtypes, mucinous and nonmucinous, with distinct histopathological and clinical profiles. Previously, a sclerotic subtype of BAC was felt to exist. However, as this is nearly identical histologically to the nonmucinous subtype, most investigators now group these subtypes together. The more common nonmucinous sub-

type is felt to originate from type II pneumocytes or nonciliated Clara cells. The malignant cells are cuboidal or columnar with a "hobnail" appearance. They contain prominent nucleoli and eosinophilic inclusions. In contrast, the less frequent mucinous subtype is derived from tall columnar bronchial mucous (goblet) cells. Electron microscopy of these cells reveals numerous cytoplasmic vacuoles rich in mucin. There are no pathognomonic clinical or radiographic findings that reliably distinguish the subtypes of BAC. Although a wide range of findings and patterns can be observed with each subtype, some trends and tendencies can be found (Table 40.1).

Clinical Findings

BAC can present with a wide range of manifestations in a variety of clinical settings. The mean age of diagnosis is

TABLE 40.1. CHARACTERISTICS OF BRONCHOALVEOLAR CARCINOMA SUBTYPES

	Mucinous	Nonmucinous
Cell[s] of origin	Goblet cells	Type II pneumocytes Bronchiolar [Clara] cells
Mucin production	Marked	Scant
Frequency	Less common	More common
Symptoms	Dyspnea Weight loss Bronchorrhea (20%)	Often asymptomatic
Metastases	More common	Less common
Prognosis	Worse 0%–26% 5-year survival Often recurs after resection	Excellent with resection 52%–72% 5-year survival

59 years, with men and women being equally affected. Up to 75% of patients are completely asymptomatic (134), with the diagnostic workup being initiated only after the incidental discovery of a lesion on an abnormal radiograph. Such patients have stage I or II disease. In contrast, patients with advanced disease often complain of dyspnea, cough, chest pain, and constitutional symptoms, including fatigue and weight loss. Hemoptysis was reported in 8.5% of cases in one series (135). Additional rare clinical presentations include pulmonary hypertension, pneumothorax, and pericardial tamponade. Although these are all nonspecific findings, one especially distressing symptom is somewhat more specific for BAC. Bronchorrhea, the production of copious amounts of thin watery sputum, is found in up to 20% of patients, especially in those with advanced mucinous BAC. When bronchorrhea develops, it often dominates the clinical picture with disabling cough and dyspnea; dehydration and severe electrolyte abnormalities may occur (136). Another unusual feature is severe hypoxemia, which is also typically associated with the mucinous subtype. This may relate to flooding of the alveoli with mucus and tumor cells, resulting in shunt physiology. Surgical resection of the diseased lobe has been attempted in exceptional cases and rarely results in improved oxygenation (137). Another unusual characteristic of BAC is its tendency to occur in multiple locations simultaneously. Up to 25% of BAC presents with multifocal disease, compared with less than 5% of other primary lung tumors. It has long been postulated that this multifocality is due to the intrapulmonary aerogenous spread of BAC. However, Barsky and colleagues (138) have shown that

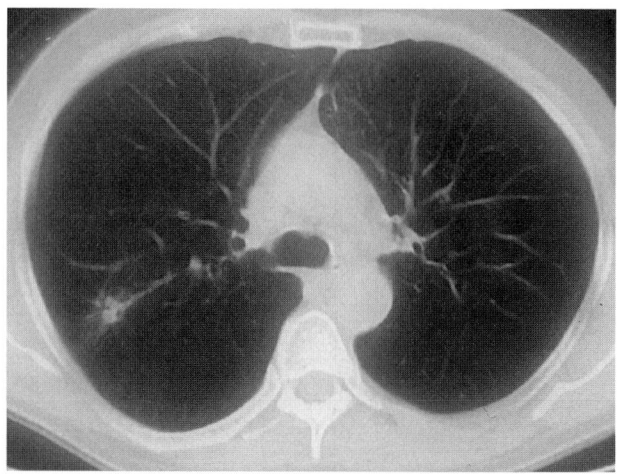

FIGURE 40.6. Solitary nodular bronchoalveolar carcinoma, right upper lobe. Diagnosis made by fiberoptic bronchoscopy with transbronchial biopsy.

multifocal BAC may be multiclonal, which suggests that independent primary tumors have arisen in separate distinct sites.

Radiographic Findings

Traditionally, BAC presents as one of four radiographic patterns on chest roentgenograms and CT: SPN or mass (Fig. 40.6), local consolidation (Fig. 40.7A), diffuse consolidation (Fig. 40.7B), or diffuse nodules (139,140). The

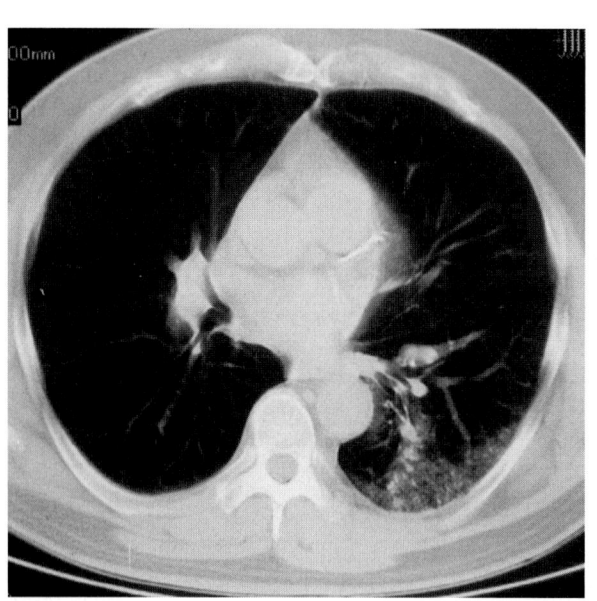

A

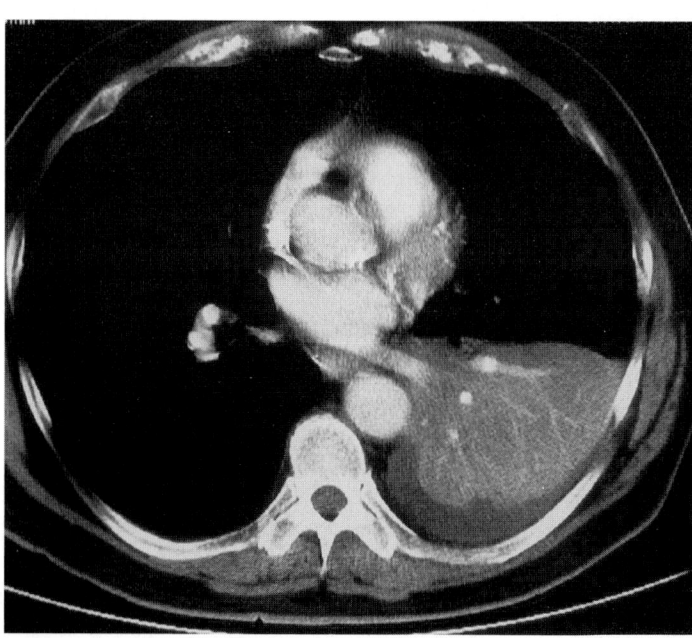

B

FIGURE 40.7. Infiltrative bronchoalveolar carcinoma. **(A)** Infiltrative bronchoalveolar carcinoma involving left lower lobe. Diagnosis made by fiberoptic bronchoscopic brush biopsy. **(B)** Further progression to complete left lower lobe consolidation.

diffuse radiographic presentation typically correlates with the mucinous histologic subtype, whereas localized lesions are more likely to correspond to the nonmucinous subtype. Overall, a solitary nodule or mass is the most frequent radiographic finding, accounting for up to 50% of all cases. These lesions range from subcentimeter nodules to masses greater than 10 cm in diameter. They are typically located in the lung periphery and may have a spiculated appearance. Rarely, a small nodule owing to BAC can appear to grow very slowly or not at all over several years. In less than 10% of cases, internal bubblelike lucencies (once referred to as "Cheerios™ in the chest"), cavitation, and pleural tags are seen, along with calcifications. Localized consolidation often contains cystic air spaces and air-bronchograms (139). The "angiogram sign," which refers to the outlining of a branching vessel by surrounding consolidation caused by low attenuation mucin on CT scanning, is also characteristic (141). Finally, the bulging fissure sign has also occasionally been noted in association with lobar consolidation. Diffuse consolidative disease is the multifocal radiographic analog of localized consolidation. Localized and diffuse consolidation each account for approximately 20% of BAC cases. Diffuse nodules, unlike solitary nodules, are often calcified and may cavitate. The diffuse nodular pattern is the most infrequent of the four major radiologic patterns of BAC, accounting for less than 10% of all cases. With time, BAC may progress radiographically from localized disease to diffuse disease (140), although the frequency of this progression is unknown.

In view of the emerging importance of BAC, its failure to demonstrate enhanced glucose metabolism, often resulting in a false-negative PET scan (19) (see section "Positron Emission Tomography"), represents a potentially significant limitation of this technology for this tumor.

Diagnosis

As BAC most frequently presents as a small peripheral nodule or mass, definitive diagnosis can be problematic. In this situation, cytological analyses of sputum, bronchoalveolar lavage fluid, and bronchial brush specimens are most often nondiagnostic. Transbronchial forceps or needle aspiration biopsies are also typically negative with very small peripheral nodules. In contrast, transthoracic fine needle aspiration has a diagnostic yield of greater than 90% for peripheral mass lesions (142). Furthermore, the cytomorphologic features are sufficiently unique to differentiate BAC from primary or metastatic adenocarcinoma in most cases (142,143). The diagnosis is also made frequently via thoracotomy or video-assisted thoracoscopic resection. For the diffuse infiltrative form of BAC, the diagnostic yield of sputum cytology is much higher and fiberoptic bronchoscopy is extremely useful, especially if transbronchial biopsy and bronchoalveolar lavage are performed as part of the procedure (144).

Treatment

The vast majority of data regarding treatment and prognosis of BAC have grouped the mucinous and nonmucinous subtypes together. Like other forms of non–small cell lung cancer, surgical resection is the treatment of choice for BAC when technically feasible. In general, patients with stage I or II lesions should be considered for surgical excision, whereas those with stage IIIB or IV lesions are not surgical candidates. Stage IIIA remains a controversial area for which multimodality approaches are being actively investigated. The optimal operative procedure has been debated. However, a segmentectomy should be the minimal procedure performed, as it offers an improved prognosis over wedge resection alone (134). In general, lobectomy remains the definitive cancer operation for patients with BAC.

Optimal treatment for patients with more advanced, nonsurgical disease remains to be standardized. Although chemotherapy and radiation therapy have been used, the results have been mixed (145,146). For the latter stages of diffuse infiltrative BAC, palliative measures frequently become the mainstays of therapy. Oxygen, morphine, and antitussives can often provide some measure of relief. In addition, agents such as indomethacin, erythromycin, and external-beam radiation, have been utilized in an attempt to control disabling bronchorrhea (147,148). Unfortunately, a reliable treatment has not been identified to date.

A handful of patients have undergone bilateral lung transplantation for BAC. Although there have been a few long-term survivors, transplant may ultimately be limited because BAC has recurred in the transplanted lung (149).

Prognosis

The overall 5-year survival of surgically resected patients with BAC is 30% to 40%, which is quite similar to that of non–small cell lung cancer in general. Factors that favor improved survival at the time of diagnosis include the absence of symptoms and lower-grade histologic lesions. For example, patients with stage I disease can expect a 5-year survival of up to 75%, whereas those with stage III disease have a 5-year survival of less than 10% (135,150,151). Whether histologic subtype has prognostic significance is still debated; some investigators suggest that the nonmucinous subtype is associated with an improved survival (126,135,151), whereas others have found that there is equivalent survival irrespective of subtype (134). Patients with radiographically diffuse disease do worse compared with those with localized disease (135). This may simply reflect the more advanced stage of the diffuse tumors. Likewise, hilar or mediastinal lymphadenopathy, although occurring in fewer than 20% of cases, adversely affects survival.

Up to 60% of patients who have undergone complete surgical resection will develop recurrent disease. Recurrences occur most frequently in the lungs, but also can occur in the lymph nodes or at distant metastatic sites. The mean time to recurrence was 21 months, with a range from 1 to 71 months in one recent review (135).

Bronchoalveolar Cell Adenoma

Occasionally one or more small adenomatous nodules of uncertain malignant potential are found in resected lobe specimens from patients with lung cancer, especially BAC. Although the significance of these nodules is uncertain, they do not appear to affect prognosis and are not known to transform into conventional BAC.

BRONCHOALVEOLAR CELL CARCINOMA	
Summary Statement	**Level of Evidence**
Diagnosis is usually made by needle biopsy or surgery for the localized form; bronchoscopy, especially with bronchoalveolar lavage and/or transbronchial biopsy, is often recommended for the diffuse form.	Experimental data; multiple case series
A definitive cancer operation is the treatment of choice for bronchoalveolar carcinoma, preferably lobectomy.	Experimental data; multiple case series, "standard of care," expert opinion

NEUROENDOCRINE CARCINOMAS

Lung tumors with neuroendocrine differentiation comprise a diverse group of clinical entities that are linked by their cellular origin. These tumors share the capacity to produce a range of neuropeptides (neuron specific enolase, chromogranin, synaptophysin, serotonin, and bombesin) that are stored within and released from cytoplasmic neuroendocrine granules. Additionally, the cells of these tumors tend to be arranged in ordered structures such as nests, trabeculae, or rosettes. The WHO has classified neuroendocrine tumors into four types, from most to least differentiated: typical carcinoid, atypical carcinoid, large cell neuroendocrine carcinoma, and small cell carcinoma (125). Small cell carcinoma is considered a major subtype of bronchogenic carcinoma and is discussed elsewhere. Despite the above schema, there remains considerable controversy over the exact classification of these tumors, and ambiguity exists as to whether certain histopathologic distinctions correspond to meaningful clinical differences.

Bronchial Carcinoid: Typical

Typical bronchial carcinoid is a well-differentiated low-grade malignant neuroendocrine tumor comprising up to 2% of all lung cancers. The name is an anglicized version of *karzinoide,* a term used by Oberndorfer in 1907 to describe tumors with more indolent behavior than the usual adenocarcinoma. The previously favored term, bronchial adenoma (with its incorrect implication of benignity), has rightly been discarded.

There is a slight female predominance, and although peak incidence is in the fifth decade, carcinoids have been described in the first through ninth decades of life. There are no known predisposing risk factors. Specifically, cigarette smoking has not been associated with the development of carcinoid tumors (152,153). Most are found in the central airways, with approximately 75% in lobar bronchi, 10% in main-stem bronchi, and almost none in the trachea. The remaining tumors, up to 20% in some series (153–155), are peripheral lung lesions that likely originate in distal airways. An unusually wide spectrum of clinical presentations has been described in patients with bronchial carcinoid tumors.

Carcinoids most often give rise to obstructive or postobstructive symptoms, as would be expected given their endobronchial location. Specifically, patients often complain of wheezing, cough, and dyspnea. Hemoptysis is also common, owing to the vascular nature of the lesion, and may be the presenting symptom in 15% to 25% of patients (153). In addition, a variety of paraneoplastic syndromes have been reported. The most frequently observed syndromes include the carcinoid syndrome from 5-hydroxytryptophan or serotonin secretion, Cushing syndrome from adrenocorticotropic hormone secretion, and acromegaly from growth hormone–releasing hormone secretion.

The carcinoid syndrome consists of episodic flushing, wheezing, and diarrhea, sometimes accompanied by fibrous thickening of the right-sided heart valves. The resulting stenotic and regurgitant valvular lesions can produce significant right-sided heart failure, and are believed to result from chemical trauma to the endocardium from circulating serotonin and other biogenic amines normally detoxified by the liver (156). The carcinoid syndrome seldom occurs (<5%) with bronchial tumors (157) and is exceedingly rare in the absence of hepatic metastases (153,158). Finally, many patients with carcinoid tumors are completely asymptomatic. Some series suggest that approximately 50% of patients with carcinoids are asymptomatic at diagnosis, and up to 10% are found incidentally at autopsy (159).

The chest roentgenographic findings, although nonspecific, may be suggestive of carcinoid. Up to 90% of patients will have abnormal findings on plain chest roentgenograms (156,160). Most often, there is evidence of volume loss or complete segmental or lobar atelectasis owing to endobronchial obstruction. Occasionally, when the carcinoid tumor is located in the lung periphery, it presents as a SPN. Although the CT appearance of carcinoid is also nonspecific, several findings when present should enhance clinical suspicion. Both central and peripheral lesions often have diffuse or punctate calcifications and typically uniformly contrast enhance, owing to their vascularity. The CT is also occasionally useful for identifying a small peripheral carcinoid in a perplexing patient with ectopic Cushing syndrome and a normal chest roentgenogram, or when carcinoid-induced Cushing syndrome must be distinguished from pituitary-dependent Cushing syndrome, which can be very difficult to do by tests of endocrine function alone.

Several diagnostic approaches can be considered, but flexible fiberoptic bronchoscopy is the most frequently successful. Bronchoscopic examination often reveals a reddish, fleshy, and smooth endobronchial lesion. Endobronchial biopsy has a diagnostic yield of approximately 85% (159–161). Concerns regarding hemorrhage after biopsy, owing to the vascular nature of these tumors, have probably been overstated, and endobronchial biopsy can be performed safely in most patients if proper technique and precautions are used (160). Alternative diagnostic strategies are typically less fruitful. Sputum cytology is rarely diagnostic, because few cells are shed into the tracheobronchial tree owing to the intact mucosal surface overlying most carcinoids. Fine needle aspiration of either central or peripheral lesions can occasionally provide diagnostic cytologic samples; however, the yield is much lower than that with bronchoscopy (160,162). Furthermore, examination of needle aspirates can lead to confusion between carcinoid and small cell carcinoma owing to their similar cytological appearance. Finally, if the carcinoid syndrome is suspected, elevation of a urinary serotonin metabolite, 5-hydroxyindoleacetic acid, can confirm the presence of a carcinoid tumor and is a useful diagnostic aid.

Histologically, carcinoids appear to arise in the bronchial submucosa from Kulchitsky cells (159,163). In general, the tumor cells are small and polygonal, with eosinophilic cytoplasm, finely stippled chromatin, and round nuclei. They are classically grouped into orderly nests (Fig. 40.8). Characteristically, carcinoids will exhibit positive immunohistochemical staining for neuron-specific enolase, chromogranin, synaptophysin, and serotonin (164). Typical carcinoids, which comprise approximately 90% of all carcinoids, are well-differentiated tumors with few mitotic figures.

The treatment of choice, when feasible, is conservative resection, consisting of wedge or segmental resection. A resection margin of 0.5 cm is usually deemed sufficient, as these tumors invade adjacent tissue less than most other lung cancers. Adequate resection has resulted in low recurrence rates and excellent long-term survival (156). Sometimes scarring and bronchiectasis of distal lung, from postobstructive infection, mandates lobectomy. In general, endobronchial resection is not a curative procedure, owing to the submucosal invasion of the tumor; however, there may be a small subset of patients with typical intraluminal carcinoid who can be cured using only endobronchial techniques (165). At present, most authorities recommend that endobronchial resection be reserved for palliation in patients not suitable for surgery. Overall, surgical resection results in a 5-year survival rate of approximately 90% to 97% for patients with typical carcinoids (155,166,167).

Immunochemical therapy takes advantage of the fact that somatostatin receptors are found in up to 80% of carcinoid tumors (168). Congeners of somatostatin, such as octreotide, have recently proven useful both in imaging and in controlling the clinical manifestations of tumors. This strategy has proven especially useful for patients with metastatic carcinoid and the carcinoid syndrome (156).

Atypical Carcinoids

Atypical carcinoids are much less common, higher-grade tumors that are less well differentiated, with increased mitotic activity, nuclear atypia, and evidence of necrosis (125,154). The histologic criteria with the widest acceptance currently are the presence of necrosis or 2 to 10 mitoses per 10 high-power fields. Clinically, atypical carcinoids occur about a decade later than do typical carcinoids, demonstrate a higher rate of metastasis at presentation (40%–50%), and result in a much lower 5-year survival rate (25%–69%) compared with

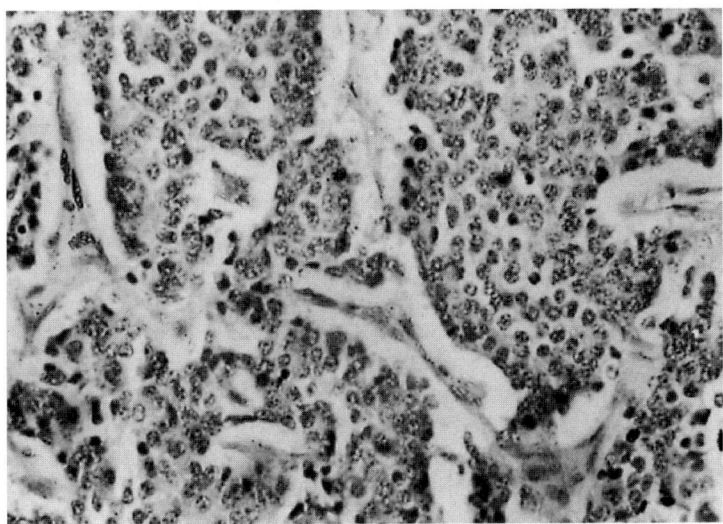

FIGURE 40.8. Bronchial carcinoid tumor. Nests of uniform cells are separated by a delicate connective-tissue stroma. There are round nuclei with evenly dispersed coarse chromatin and pale cytoplasm. (From Miriam Lurie, Department of Pathology, Carmel Hospital, Haifa, Israel, with permission.)

rates for patients with typical carcinoids. There does appear to be a strong correlation with smoking. Whether surgical resection alone is sufficient treatment for the more aggressive atypical carcinoids is a matter of debate. Some investigators advocate adjuvant chemotherapy in addition to lobectomy for these tumors (160,169). Unfortunately, standard chemotherapy and radiation therapy have generally yielded poor results (170,171).

Tumorlets

Occasionally, small foci of well-differentiated neuroendocrine cells are found in the periphery of the lung. These foci, known as carcinoid tumorlets, often occur in association with chronic inflammation, bronchiectasis, or other carcinoid tumors (172). Typically, these tumorlets are subradiographic and discovered only incidentally after resection, but in rare instances have been associated with corticotropin release, resulting in Cushing syndrome (173), or with peribronchial lymph node metastases (174). The natural history of these tumorlets is uncertain, but when they achieve a size greater than 0.5 cm, they are arbitrarily classified as carcinoid tumors (172).

Large Cell Neuroendocrine Carcinoma

Large cell neuroendocrine carcinoma (also referred to as neuroendocrine carcinoma of intermediate cell type) (175) is an uncommon lung tumor that is derived from neuroendocrine cells. This designation is reserved for tumors with neuroendocrine features that do not meet criteria for either carcinoid or small cell carcinoma (125). Their coarsely granular chromatin contrasts with the more finely granular and uniform chromatin of an atypical carcinoid. These tumors are composed of groups of dysplastic cells with neuroendocrine features. Large cell neuroendocrine carcinoma is an aggressive neoplasm found almost exclusively in smokers and has many clinical features in common with atypical carcinoid. Tumors may occur either centrally or peripherally. Overall, patients with large cell neuroendocrine carcinoma have a poor prognosis (176). Although there are no controlled trials available to definitively guide therapy, expert opinion would support surgical resection when possible and combination chemotherapy for advanced disease.

Large Cell Carcinoma of the Lung with Neuroendocrine Differentiation

This term invites confusion with large cell neuroendocrine carcinoma but is actually used to refer to a distinct entity, i.e., large cell bronchogenic carcinoma by light microscopy that demonstrates neuroendocrine differentiation by immunohistochemistry or electron microscopy (125). This tumor seems to be more chemotherapy responsive than are other large cell carcinomas of the lung.

HAMARTOMA

Hamartoma is the most common benign neoplasm of the lung, accounting for up to 8% of all primary tumors (177). Its pathogenesis is currently believed to involve clonal proliferations of mesenchymal elements. Tumors are typically composed of cartilage, fibromyxoid stroma, and adipose tissue, along with incorporated bronchiolar epithelium and less common diverse elements such as bone or hair (178,179). Hamartomas occur more frequently in men, and the mean age at presentation is the sixth decade, with only rare cases described before the third decade of life (180). Overall, the prevalence of hamartomas in the general population is 0.25% (180); however, many cases go unrecognized and are found only at autopsy.

Hamartomas typically present as a SPN, usually discovered incidentally on chest films or during the course of a surgical procedure for another indication (181). Most patients are completely asymptomatic. An exception is the endobronchial hamartoma, which represents fewer than 20% of cases (178,181). Patients with endobronchial hamartomas often complain of cough, dyspnea, wheezing, and occasionally hemoptysis. The rare mesenchymal cystic variant is also typically symptomatic (182).

Radiographically, hamartomas are usually solitary, but multiple nodules have been reported in up to 3% of cases (178,183). The nodules are typically smooth, lobulated, peripheral lesions, approximately 0.5 to 3 cm in diameter. These tumors grow very slowly, with a mean increase in diameter of 3 to 5 mm/yr (184,185), occasionally enlarging to 10 cm in diameter. Classically, hamartomas have an eccentric "popcorn" calcification pattern on plain chest radiographs. Unfortunately, this pattern is seen in only 10% of cases (185). Calcification can been seen more frequently and to better advantage by CT. These scans may also reveal central fat within the lesion, a distinctive and characteristic finding in hamartoma (186) (Fig. 40.9).

Definitive diagnosis is important to exclude malignancy. However, an argument for close observation can be made in nonsmokers with the classical radiographic features of hamartoma described above. If a diagnostic workup is pursued, then transthoracic needle aspiration should be performed, as it has a proven diagnostic yield of greater than 85% (187).

Biopsy-proven hamartomas can be safely observed without specific therapy. Excision is warranted when patients have symptoms or when lesions demonstrate significant growth. Lung-sparing surgical resection is the treatment of choice, because hamartomas rarely recur (185). No additional adjuvant therapy is required for the typical case. Rarely, hamartomas are found in association with a bronchogenic carcinoma (187,188). Although the presence of a hamartoma was associated with an increased relative risk of developing bronchogenic carcinoma in some studies (189,190), this finding was not confirmed in a recent large series (180).

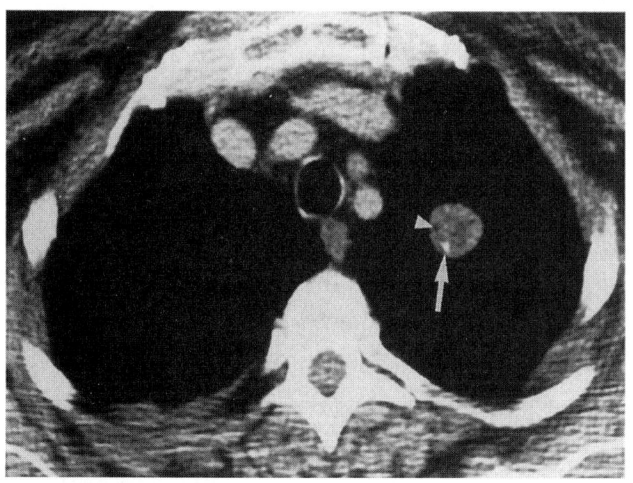

FIGURE 40.9. Computed tomography scan after intravenous contrast demonstrates the presence of calcifications *(arrow)* and fat *(arrowhead)* within the hamartoma.

INFLAMMATORY PSEUDOTUMOR

Inflammatory pseudotumor (IPT) of the lung is an uncommon lesion of unknown cause. Considerable controversy attends even the most basic questions regarding this entity, such as whether it is a localized inflammatory response or a low-grade primary lung neoplasm. As a result of such uncertainty, various names have been applied to this lesion, including plasma cell granuloma, histiocytoma, xanthoma, and fibroxanthoma. Most recently, the term myofibroblastic tumor has been used, emphasizing its general low-grade neoplastic behavior (191).

From a clinical standpoint, IPT is remarkably diverse. There is no sex or racial predisposition; most patients are less than 40 years of age. Although symptoms have been reported in 26% to 78% of patients with IPT, this is likely an overestimate, given that some asymptomatic patients may never come to medical attention. When present, symptoms may include cough, fever, dyspnea, wheezing, chest pain, or hemoptysis. With or without symptoms, IPT is an important mimic of bronchogenic carcinoma, especially given its many radiographic guises, including mass lesions 1 to 10 cm in diameter that may be accompanied by hilar and mediastinal adenopathy, pleural effusion, and/or airway involvement with distal atelectasis (192). The diagnosis is most often made via surgical biopsy for what was thought to be a lung cancer; bronchoscopy and TTNA are rarely helpful. Several series have described invasion of other adjacent structures such as pulmonary vessels, diaphragm, pericardium, esophagus, and thoracic vertebrae (191,193–195); a paraneoplastic dermatomyositis-like presentation has also been recognized on occasion (196).

The etiology of IPT remains controversial. The finding of an antecedent upper respiratory infection in up to one half of all patients has led some to believe IPT represents an aberrant response to tissue injury (192,197). However, the presence of local invasion in up to 50% of cases and evidence of clonal chromosomal abnormalities support a neoplastic origin (197–199).

Treatment is primarily surgical, although some lesions have been known to regress spontaneously. Local recurrence, although uncommon, has been attributed to incomplete excision of the primary lesion (193). The overall prognosis is excellent; in those few cases in which the lesion is not amenable to excision, there may be a role for medical therapy, including radiation, chemotherapy, or steroids (200,201).

VERY RARE TUMORS OF THE LUNG

Many lung tumors are exceedingly rare; therefore, relevant evidence-based clinical guidelines are especially difficult to formulate. In this section, we briefly summarize salient clinical features and cite key recent references that pertain to these tumors. More detailed treatment may be found in several excellent texts (125,192,202).

Several classification schemes have been proposed; none has achieved widespread acceptance. We have chosen a purely clinical approach based on the predominant clinical presentation of each tumor. However, it is recognized that for individual tumors, there may be considerable clinical overlap and variability in biologic behavior, as well as controversy as to histogenesis and nosology.

Some rare lesions may be termed bronchogenic; these typically present with manifestations of endobronchial infiltration and/or obstruction, including hemoptysis, localized wheeze, dyspnea, cough, atelectasis, and obstructive pneumonitis. Such features may allow for earlier diagnosis and somewhat better prognosis. Treatment may entail laser photoresection, stenting, radiation therapy, or bronchoplastic/sleeve resection, depending on the patient's overall condition and on whether the goal of treatment is palliative or curative. Occasionally, the distal lung is bronchiectatic and subject to recurrent infection, necessitating lung resection as well. On the other hand, other very rare tumors originate predominantly in the periphery of the lung, and may attain large size before they produce symptoms. They are usually discovered either incidentally on routine chest x-ray (often as a SPN or mass) or when they involve adjacent thoracic structures, thereby producing symptoms, at which point they may be unresectable. Chemotherapy and/or radiation therapy may be used in such cases (203). It should also be noted that a few tumors, such as pulmonary leiomyoma (204, 205), seem to occur with about equal frequency in the proximal bronchi and parenchyma.

The clinical scenario typically triggers a preoperative workup for suspected "usual" bronchogenic carcinoma, as outlined in the previous chapter. The specific diagnosis of a very rare lung tumor is usually unexpected and often only made postoperatively by the pathologist, because (lipomas and hamartomas excepted) there are no diagnostic roentgenologic signs and because evaluations of bronchoscopic or needle biopsy specimens can be misleading. Frequently, consultation with an expert pulmonary pathologist and specialized techniques such as immunohistochemical staining and electron microscopy are important in establishing a final diagnosis.

With few exceptions, surgery is the treatment of choice to remove potentially lethal lesions and to relieve symptoms. Even benign tumors often require extirpation to treat local manifestations and/or to remove a possible malignant component. In general, conservative resection is the rule for benign lesions, using modern bronchoplastic or thoracoscopic techniques, depending on the site of the lesion. Malignant lesions often require a standard cancer operation, such as thoracotomy with lobectomy and lymph node dissection.

Predominantly Endobronchial Tumors

Papilloma

In adults, a solitary lesion is typical, presenting as a less than 1.5-cm endobronchial tumor in a segmental or lobar bronchus. Alternatively, a polypoid inflammatory mass may be seen, related to exuberant granulation tissue secondary to chronic irritation, as from an embedded foreign body (206). Cellular atypia and the uncertain risk of carcinomatous degeneration have been cited to justify the usual advice for surgical extirpation (207). Recent data suggest some relationship to human papillomavirus, especially for the squamous cell type (207). Glandular and mixed lesions have also been described, sometimes with columnar epithelium (207,208).

Granular Cell Tumor

Granular cell tumor (209) is a sessile or polypoid benign growth usually located within the trachea or a central bronchus. Previously termed myoblastoma, this tumor is now believed to originate from Schwann cells. Multiple tracheobronchial lesions are increasingly recognized (210). Histologically, the outstanding feature is numerous fine, acidophilic, cytoplasmic granules, which appear similar to lysosomes under electron microscopy.

Adenoid Cystic Carcinoma

This malignant tumor usually originates from mucous glands of the trachea (accounting for approximately 20% to 40% of primary tracheal tumors) or main-stem bronchus (often causing atelectasis of an entire lung). Histologically, the tumor is composed of mucous gland cells that form duct-like tubules (hence, the older name cylindroma), along with mucin-containing glands and cysts, indistinguishable from salivary gland tumor. The achievement of surgical cure with clean margins is notoriously difficult owing to occult submucosal infiltration and perineural invasion. This may necessitate tracheal carinal resection or standard lobectomy or pneumonectomy. Local recurrences may occur, usually because of underestimation of intramural spread. Even though adenoid cystic carcinoma is relatively radio-resistant, postoperative radiation should be administered when lymph node metastases have occurred or invasion of perineural lymphatics has been demonstrated in the surgical specimen (211,212).

Mucoepidermoid Carcinoma

This low-grade malignancy also arises from salivary gland-like elements in the central airways. A mixture of epithelial, mucin-secreting, and intermediate cells is seen microscopically. The biologic behavior depends on the histologic appearance; tumors with increased mitoses, necrosis, and nuclear pleomorphism are considered high grade and are usually lethal. The majority are low grade and curable via a lung-sparing operation (213).

Other Salivary Gland-Type Tumors

This group includes acinic cell carcinoma (Fechner tumor), of which only 15 cases had been reported as of 1999 (214); mixed tumor (215); and oncocytoma (215).

Carcinosarcoma

Carcinosarcoma is usually found in older men, commonly in the upper lobes. Histologically, a mixture of carcinoma (usually squamous cell) admixed with heterologous sarcomatous elements such as bone, cartilage, or skeletal muscle is seen. The epidemiology and biologic behavior are typical of non–small call carcinoma of the lung. Extensive endobronchial spread occurs with central tumors, which comprised 62% of cases in one series (216), whereas distant metastatic disease is common at presentation with large peripheral lesions. The prognosis is poor.

Other Predominantly Endobronchial Tumors

Benign tumors in this category include mucous gland adenoma (bronchial cystadenoma) (217), lipoma (218), schwannoma (219), angiomyxoma, and myofibroblast tumor (220). Malignancies include epithelial-myoepithelial carcinoma of the bronchus (221), malignant myxoid tumor (222), and malignant nerve sheath tumor (223).

PREDOMINANTLY PARENCHYMAL TUMORS

Epithelioid Hemangioendothelioma

This low-grade malignant sarcoma of vascular endothelial origin usually presents as small, asymptomatic, bilateral pulmonary nodules (224). Over 80% of patients are female, and about half are less than 40 years of age. Most patients are asymptomatic, although alveolar and intrapleural hemorrhage may occur. These tumors tend to have an indolent but progressive course. Intrapulmonary spread is not uncommon, and extension of tumor to the pleura and pericardium may occur. No effective therapy is available, although radiotherapy may provide some palliation, and excision of the rare solitary lesion is recommended.

Blastoma

This malignant tumor demonstrates a bimodal age distribution, with an initial peak during the first decade and a later peak in the seventh decade. The tumor may be found centrally, but most often presents as a large peripheral mass, with or without symptoms. Histologically, the key feature is undifferentiated embryonic glandular epithelium simulating fetal lung at 10 to 16 weeks of gestation. In biphasic blastoma, a malignant mesenchymal stroma is also present, and the prognosis is considerably worse (225).

Chemodectoma

This benign tumor can rarely occur as a solitary tracheal or pulmonary parenchymal lesion, but occasionally, multiple minute chemodectomas are found as asymptomatic incidental findings, especially in women. Grossly, they appear as 1- to 3-mm nodules on the pleura or within the lung. The histogenesis remains uncertain (226).

Chondroma

Chondromas are benign tumors of cartilage chiefly notable for their association with extra-adrenal paraganglioma and gastric stromal sarcoma in Carney syndrome (227), a peculiar, indolent, and possibly familial condition seen mostly in young women.

Malignant Melanoma

Extrapulmonary malignant melanoma frequently spreads to the lungs and/or bronchi, rendering the diagnosis of primary malignant melanoma of the lung problematic (228). In addition, cutaneous melanomas may regress spontaneously after having metastasized, masking the true primary site. The cell of origin for primary lung lesions is also unclear, because melanin-containing cells are not present in the normal tracheobronchial tree. Suggested diagnostic criteria are controversial and include no previously removed pigmented skin lesions, no melanomas in other organs, and no history of excised ocular tumors (229). A few cases may benefit from surgical resection.

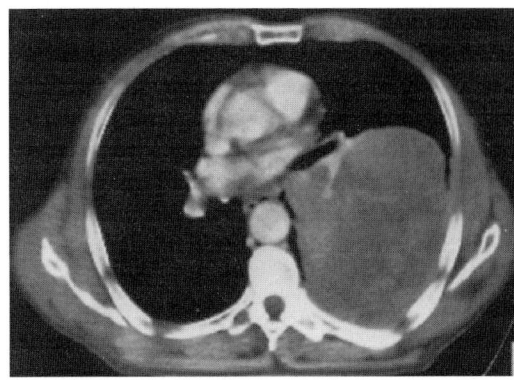

FIGURE 40.10. Primary fibrosarcoma arising from the left main stem bronchus.

Other Sarcomas of the Lung

Pulmonary sarcomas may originate within a main-stem (Fig. 40.10) or lobar bronchus, peripherally within the pulmonary parenchyma, or from major vessels. By far the most common sarcoma of the lung is metastatic; primary sarcomas of the lung comprise a jumble of extraordinarily rare lesions. The most prominent of these is AIDS-related Kaposi sarcoma, a fascinating tumor recently associated with human herpes virus 8 infection. Other prominent primary lung sarcomas include malignant fibrous histiocytoma (230), fibrosarcoma (231), and leiomyosarcoma (232). These tumors are usually large and solitary and may or may not be symptomatic. Chondrosarcoma (233), liposarcoma (234), myxosarcoma (235), rhabdomyosarcoma (236), synovial sarcoma (237), neurogenic sarcoma (238), so-called malignant triton tumor (239), Ewing sarcoma (240), and osteogenic sarcoma (241) also may occur as primary lung neoplasms.

Pulmonary vascular sarcomas are of special interest because of their tendency to mimic chronic thromboembolic disease, sometimes with additional features of weight loss, anemia, and fever (242, 243). Diagnosis may be facilitated by CT and MRI scans, allowing for occasional surgical cures (244).

Malignant fibrous histiocytoma of the lung is an aggressive sarcoma, usually presenting as a solitary mass. The tumor is characterized by a mixture of fibroblasts and histiocytes. Surgery is the treatment of choice, and the role of adjuvant therapy remains undefined (230).

Other Predominantly Parenchymal Tumors

Among other usually benign tumors in this category are sclerosing hemangioma (245), hyalinizing granuloma (246), clear cell (sugar) tumors (247), fibroma (248), myxoma (249), glomus tumor (250), meningioma (251, 252), teratoma (253), neurofibroma (254), a variety of adenomas (255, 256), and miscellaneous lesions arising from ectopic tissues in the lung (257). Malignancies include plasmacytoma (258), clear cell carcinoma (259), hemangiopericytoma

(260,261), choriocarcinoma (262), ependymoma (263), and "lymphoepithelioma-like" carcinoma (264).

REFERENCES

1. Lillington GA. Management of solitary pulmonary nodules. *Dis Month* 1991;37:271–318.
2. Cummings SR, Lillington GA, Richard RJ. Estimating the probability of malignancy in solitary pulmonary nodules: a Bayesian approach. *Am Rev Respir Dis* 1986;134:449–452.
3. Skillrud, DM. Higher risk of lung cancer in chronic obstructive pulmonary disease: a prospective, matched, controlled study. *Ann Intern Med* 1986;105:503–507.
4. Tockman MS, Anthonisen NR, Wright EC, et al. Airways obstruction and the risk for lung cancer. *Ann Intern Med* 1987;106:512–518.
5. Proto AV, Thomas SR. Pulmonary nodules studied by computed tomography. *Radiology* 1985;156:149–153.
6. Rubins JB, Rubins HB. Temporal trends in the prevalence of malignancy in resected solitary pulmonary lesions. *Chest* 1996;109:100–103.
7. Zerhouni EA, Stitik FP, Siegelman SS, et al. CT of the pulmonary nodule: a cooperative study. *Radiology* 1986;160:319–327.
8. Munden RF, Pugatch RD, Liptay MJ, et al. Small pulmonary lesions detected at CT: clinical importance. *Radiology* 1997;202:105–110.
9. Yankelevitz DF, Henschke CI. Does 2-year stability imply that pulmonary nodules are benign? *AJR Am J Roentgenol* 1997;168:325–328.
10. Huston J 3rd, Muhm JR. Solitary pulmonary opacities: plain tomography. *Radiology* 1987;163:481–485.
11. Siegelman SS, Khouri NF, Leo FP, et al. Solitary pulmonary nodules: CT assessment. *Radiology* 1986;160:307–312.
12. Zwirewich CV, Vedal S, Miller RR, et al. Solitary pulmonary nodule: high-resolution CT and radiologic-pathologic correlation. *Radiology* 1991;164:719–722.
13. Littleton JT, Durizch ML, Moeller G, et al. Pulmonary masses: contrast enhancement. *Radiology* 1990;177:861–871.
14. Swensen SJ, Brown LR, Colby TV, et al. Lung nodule enhancement at CT: prospective findings. *Radiology* 1996;201:447–455.
15. Zhang M, Kono M. Solitary pulmonary nodules: evaluation of blood flow patterns with dynamic CT. *Radiology* 1997;205:471–478.
16. Dewan NA, Gupta NC, Redepenning LS, et al. Diagnostic efficacy of PET-FDG imaging in solitary pulmonary nodules: potential role in evaluation and management. *Chest* 1993;104:997–1002.
17. Patz EF Jr, Lowe VJ, Hoffman JM, et al. Focal pulmonary abnormalities: evaluation with F-18 fluorodeoxyglucose PET scanning. *Radiology* 1993;188:487–490.
18. Lewis P, Griffin S, Marsden P, et al. Whole-body ^{18}F-fluorodeoxyglucose positron emission tomography in preoperative evaluation of lung cancer. *Lancet* 1994;344:1265–1266.
19. Higashi K, Ueda Y, Seki H, et al. Fluorine-18-FDG PET imaging is negative in bronchioloalveolar lung carcinoma. *J Nucl Med* 1998;39:1016–1020.
20. Erasmus JJ, McAdams HP, Patz EF Jr, et al. Evaluation of primary pulmonary carcinoid tumors using FDG PET. *AJR Am J Roentgenol* 1998;170:1369–1373.
21. Goldsmith SJ, Kostakoglu L. Nuclear medicine imaging of lung cancer. *Radiol Clin North Am* 2000;38:511–524.
22. Gould MK, Maclean CC, Kuschner WG, et al. Accuracy of positron emission tomography for diagnosis of pulmonary nodules and mass lesions: a meta-analysis. *JAMA* 2001;285:914–924.
23. Rubins JB, Rubins HB. Temporal trends in the prevalence of malignancy in resected solitary pulmonary lesions. *Chest* 1996;109:100–103.
24. Webb WR. CT of solitary pulmonary vascular lesions. *Semin Roentgenol* 1984;19:189–198.
25. Miller JI, Harrison EG Jr, Bernatz PE. Surgically treated unsuspected pulmonary infarction. *Ann Thorac Surg* 1972;14:181–188.
26. Mintzer RA, Neiman HL, Reeder MM. Mucoid impaction of a bronchus. *JAMA* 1978;240:1397–1398.
27. Scott PP, Scott WW Jr. Isolated nodular pulmonary amyloidosis: diagnosis by percutaneous needle aspiration biopsy. *South Med J* 1985;78:467–470.
28. Shin MS, Buchalter SE, Ho KJ. Intrapulmonary bronchogenic cyst: spontaneous dissolution? *Ala Med* 1990;59:20–22.
29. Risher WH, Crocker EF Jr, Beckman EN, et al. Pulmonary dirofilariasis: the largest single-institution experience. *J Thorac Cardiovasc Surg* 1989;97:303–308.
30. Barrio JL, Suarez M, Rodriguez JL, et al. *Pneumocystis carinii* pneumonia presenting as cavitating and noncavitating solitary pulmonary nodules in patients with the acquired immunodeficiency syndrome. *Am Rev Respir Dis* 1986;134:1094–1096.
31. Ravin CE, Smith GW, Ahern MJ, et al. Cytomegaloviral infection presenting as a solitary pulmonary nodule. *Chest* 1977;71:220–222.
32. Shure D, Fedullo PF. Transbronchial needle aspiration of peripheral masses. *Am Rev Respir Dis* 1983;128:1090–1092.
33. Chechani V. Bronchoscopic diagnosis of solitary pulmonary nodules and lung masses in the absence of endobronchial abnormality. *Chest* 1996;109:620–625.
34. Katis K, Inglesos E, Zachariadis E, et al. The role of transbronchial needle aspiration in the diagnosis of peripheral lung masses or nodules. *Eur Respir J* 1995;8:963–966.
35. Gaeta M, Russi EG, La Spada F, et al. Small bronchogenic carcinomas presenting as solitary pulmonary nodules: bioptic approach guided by CT-positive bronchus sign. *Chest* 1992;102:1167–1170.
36. Shaham D. Semi-invasive and invasive procedures for the diagnosis and staging of lung cancer, I: percutaneous transthoracic needle biopsy. *Rad Clin N Am* 2000;38:525–534.
37. Calhoun P, Feldman PS, Armstrong P, et al. The clinical outcome of needle aspirations of the lung when cancer is not diagnosed. *Ann Thorac Surg* 1986;41:592–596.
38. Khouri NF, Stitik FP, Erozan YS, et al. Transthoracic needle aspiration biopsy of benign and malignant lung lesions. *AJR Am J Roentgenol* 1985;144:281–288.
39. Lucidarme O, Howarth N, Finet JF, et al. Intrapulmonary lesions: percutaneous automated biopsy with a detachable, 18-gauge, coaxial cutting needle. *Radiology* 1998;207:759–765.
40. Noppen MM, De Mey J, Meysman M, et al. Percutaneous needle biopsy of localized pulmonary, mediastinal, and pleural diseased tissue with an automatic disposable guillotine soft-tissue needle. Preliminary results. *Chest* 1995;107:1615–1620.
41. Miller DL, Allen MS, Deschamps C, et al. Video-assisted thoracic surgical procedure: management of a solitary pulmonary nodule. *Mayo Clin Proc* 1992;67:462–464.
42. Bernard A. Resection of pulmonary nodules using video-assisted thoracic surgery: the Thorax Group. *Ann Thorac Surg* 1996;61:202–204; discussion 204–205.
43. Allen MS, Deschamps C, Lee RE, et al. Video-assisted thoracoscopic stapled wedge excision for indeterminate pulmonary nodules. *J Thorac Cardiovasc Surg* 1993;106:1048–1052.

44. Landreneau RJ, Hazelrigg SR, Ferson PF, et al. Thoracoscopic resection of 85 pulmonary lesions. *Ann Thorac Surg* 1992;54: 415-419; discussion 419–420.

45. Gail MH, Eagan RT, Feld R, et al. Prognostic factors in patients with resected stage I non–small cell lung cancer: a report from the Lung Cancer Study Group. *Cancer* 1984;54:1802–1813.

46. Yankelevitz DF, Reeves AP, Kostis WJ, et al. Small pulmonary nodules: volumetrically determined growth rates based on CT evaluation. *Radiology* 2000;217:251–256.

47. Cummings SR, Littington GA, Richard RJ. Managing solitary pulmonary nodules: the choice of strategy is a "close call." *Am Rev Resp Dis* 1986;134:453–460.

48. Spencer H. Secondary tumours in the lung. In: Spencer, H. *Pathology of the lung,* 4th ed. New York: Pergamon Press, 1985:1085–1096.

49. Willis RA. *Spread of tumors in the human body,* 3rd ed. Woburn: Butterworth-Heineman, 1973.

50. Crow J, Slavin G, Kreel L. Pulmonary metastasis: a pathologic and radiologic study. *Cancer* 1981;47:2595–2602.

51. Coppage L, Shaw C, Curtis AM. Metastatic disease to the chest in patients with extrathoracic malignancy. *J Thorac Imaging* 1987;2:24–37.

52. Stetler-Stevenson WG, Kleiner DE. Molecular biology of cancer: invasion and metastases. In: DeVita V Jr, Hellman S, Rosenberg SA, eds. *Cancer: principles and practice of oncology.* Philadelphia: Lippincott Williams & Wilkins, 2001:123–136.

53. Pass HI, Temeck BA. Biology of metastatic disease. *Chest Surg Clin N Am* 1998;8:1–11.

54. Fidler IJ. The biology of cancer invasion and metastasis. *Adv Cancer Res* 1978;28:149–250.

55. Liotta LA, Steeg PS, Stetler-Stevenson WG. Cancer metastasis and angiogenesis: an imbalance of positive and negative regulation. *Cell* 1991;64:327–336.

56. Stetler-Stevenson WG, Aznavoorian S, Liotta LA. Tumor cell interactions with the extracellular matrix during invasion and metastasis. *Annu Rev Cell Biol* 1993;9:541–573.

57. Ahmad A, Hart IR. Biology of tumor micrometastasis. *J Hematotherapy* 1996;5:525–535.

58. Dabbous MK, Walker R, Haney L, et al. Host cells and matrix degradation at sites of tumor invasion in rat mammary adenocarcinoma. *Br J Cancer* 1986;54:459–465.

59. Fidler IJ. Metastasis: quantitative analysis of distribution and fate of tumor emboli labeled with ^{125}I-s-iodo-2deoxyurindine. *J Natl Cancer Inst* 1970;45:773–782.

60. Fidler IJ. Invasion and metastases. In: Abeloff MD, Armitage JO, Lichter AS, et al, eds. *Clinical oncology.* New York: Churchill Livingstone, 1995:55.

61. Gross BH, Glazer GM, Brookstein FL. Multiple pulmonary nodules detected by computed tomography, diagnostic implications. *J Comput Assist Tomogr* 1985;9:880–885.

62. Scholten ET, Kreel L. Distribution of lung metastasis in the axial plane. *Radiol Clin North Am* 1977;46:248–265.

63. Hirakata K, Nakata H, Nakagawa T. Appearance of pulmonary metastases on high resolution CT scans: comparison with histopathological findings from autopsy specimens. *AJR Am J Roentgenol* 1993;161:7–43.

64. Snyder BJ, Pugatch RD. Imaging characteristics of metastatic disease to the chest. *Chest Surg Clin N Am* 1998;8:29–48.

65. Primack SL, Hartmann TE, Lee KS, et al. Pulmonary nodules and the CT halo sign. *Radiology* 1994;182:513–515.

66. Herold CJ, Bankier AA, Fleischmann D. Lung metastases. *Eur Radiol* 1996;6:596–606.

67. Chai J, Patz, E. CT of the lung: patterns of calcification and other high attenuation abnormalities. *AJR Am J Roentgenol* 1994;162:1063–1066.

68. Maile C, Rodan B, Godwin JD, et al. Calcification in pulmonary metastases. *Br J Radiol* 1982;55:108–113.

69. Poe RH, Ortiz C, Israel RH, et al. Sensitivity, specificity, and predictive values of bronchoscopy in neoplasm metastatic to lung. *Chest* 1985;88:84–88.

70. Argyros GJ, Torrington KG. Fiberoptic bronchoscopy in the evaluation of carcinoma metastatic to the lung. *Chest* 1994;105:454–457.

71. Patz EF, Fidler J, Knelson M, et al. Significance of percutaneous needle biopsy in patients with multiple pulmonary nodules and a single known primary malignancy. *Chest* 1995;107:601–604.

72. Lewis RJ, Caccavale RJ, Sisler GE. Imaged thoracoscopic lung biopsy. *Chest* 1992;102:60–62.

73. Soares FA, Pinto APFE, Landell AM, et al. Pulmonary tumor embolism to arterial vessels and carcinomatous lymphangitis: a comparative clinicopathological study. *Arch Pathol Lab Med* 1993;117:827–831.

74. Janower ML, Blennerhassett JB. Lymphangitic spread of metastatic to the lung: a radiologic-pathologic classification. *Radiology* 1971;101:267–273.

75. Munk PL, Muller NL, Miller RR, et al. Pulmonary lymphangitic carcinomatosis: CT and pathologic findings. *Radiology* 1988;66:705–709.

76. Davis, SD. CT evaluation for pulmonary metastases in patients with extrathoracic malignancy. *Radiology* 1991;180:1–12.

77. Levy H, Horak DA, Lewis MI. The value of bronchial washings and bronchoalveolar lavage in the diagnosis of lymphangitic carcinomatosis. *Chest* 1988;94:1028–1030.

78. Masson RG, Ruggieri J. Pulmonary microvascular cytology: a new diagnostic application of the pulmonary artery catheter. *Chest* 1985;88:908–914.

79. Bassiri AG, Haghighi B, Doyle RL, et al. Pulmonary tumor embolism. *Am J Respir Crit Care Med* 1997;155:2089–2095.

80. Braman SS, Whitcomb ME. Endobronchial metastasis. *Arch Intern Med* 1975;135:543–547.

81. King DS, Castleman B. Bronchial involvement in metastatic pulmonary malignancy. *J Thorac Surg* 1943;12:305–315.

82. Shephard MP. Endobronchial metastatic disease. *Thorax* 1982;37:362–365.

83. Rosenblatt MB, Lisa JR, Trinidad S. Pitfalls in the clinical and histologic diagnosis of bronchogenic carcinoma. *Dis Chest* 1966;49:396–404.

84. Ikezoe J, Johkoh T, Takeuchi N, et al. CT findings of endobronchial metastasis. *Acta Radiologica* 1991;32:455–460.

85. Viadora E, Brass IDJ, Pickren JW. Cascade spread of bloodborne metastases in solid and nonsolid cancers of the humans. In: Weiss L, Gilbert HA, eds. *Pulmonary metastases.* Boston: GK Hall, 1978:142–167.

86. Dail DH. Metastases to and from the lung. In: Dail DH, Hammer SP, eds. *Pulmonary pathology,* 2nd ed. New York: Springer-Verlag New York, 1994:1581–1615.

87. Martini N, McCormack PM. Evolution of the surgical management of pulmonary metastases. *Chest Surg Clin N Am* 1998;8:13–28.

88. Sakamoto T, Tsubota N, Iwanaga K, et al. Pulmonary resection for metastases from colorectal cancer. *Chest* 2001;119:1069–1072.

89. Matthay RA, Arroliga AC. Resection of pulmonary metastases. *Am Rev Resp Dis* 1993;148:1691–1696.

90. Girard P, Baldeyrou P, Le Chevalier T, et al. Surgical resection of pulmonary metastases: up to what number? *Am J Respir Crit Care Med* 1994;149:469–476.

91. Pastorino U, Buyse M, Friedel G, et al. Long-term results of metastasectomy: prognostic analyses based on 5206 cases: the

International Registry of Lung Metastases. *J Thorac Cardiovasc Surg* 1997;113:37–49.

92. Matsuzoe D, Hideshima T, Ohshima K, et al. Discrimination of double primary lung cancer from intrapulmonary metastasis by *p53* gene mutation. *Br J Cancer* 1999;79:1549–1552.

93. Fujita J, Yamagishi Y, Kubo A, et al. Respiratory failure due to pulmonary lymphangitis carcinomatosis. *Chest* 1993;103:967–996.

94. Umeki S. Association of miliary lung metastases and bone metastases in bronchogenic carcinoma. *Chest* 1993;104:948–950.

95. Chen EA, Carlson EA, Coughlin BF, et al. Routine chest roentgenography is unnecessary in the work-up of stage I and II breast cancer. *J Clin Oncol* 2000;18:3503–3506.

96. American Society of Clinical Oncology 1998 update of recommended breast cancer surveillance guidelines. *J Clin Oncol* 1999;17:1080–1082.

97. Kreisman H, Wolkove N, Finkelstein HS, et al. Breast cancer and thoracic metastases: review of 119 patients. *Thorax* 1983;38:175–179.

98. Harvey JC, Lee K, Beattie EJ. Surgical management of pulmonary metastases. *Chest Surg Clin N Am* 1994;4:55–66.

99. Vogt-Moykopf I, Krysa S, Bylzebruck H, et al. Surgery for pulmonary metastases: the Heidelberg experience. *Chest Surg Clin N Am* 1994;4:85–112.

100. Bodzin, GA, Staren E, Faber LP. Breast carcinoma metastases. *Chest Surg Clin N Am* 1998;8:145–156.

101. Staren ED, Salerno C, Rongione A, et al. Pulmonary resection for metastatic breast cancer. *Arch Surg* 1992;127:1282–1284.

102. Simpson R, Kennedy C, Carmalt H, et al. Pulmonary resection for metastatic breast cancer. *Aust N Z J Surg* 1997;67:717–719.

103. Lanza LA, Natarajan G, Roth JA, et al. Long-term survival after resection of pulmonary metastases from carcinoma of the breast. *Ann Thorac Surg* 1992;54:244–248.

104. Friedel G, Linder A, Toomes H. The significance of prognostic factors for the resection of pulmonary metastases of breast cancer. *J Thorac Cardiovasc Surg* 1994;42:71–75.

105. Taichman DB, Tino G, Aronchick J, et al. Diffuse airway narrowing from carcinoma metastatic to the bronchial submucosa: identification by chest CT. *Chest* 1998;114:1217–1220.

106. Pikoulis E, Varelas PN, Lechago J, et al. Metastatic breast disease 40 years after the initial diagnosis. *Chest* 1998;114:639–641.

107. Murin S, Inciardi J. Cigarette smoking and the risk of pulmonary metastasis from breast cancer. *Chest* 2001;119:1635–1640.

108. Galandiuk S, Wieand HS, Moertel CG. Patterns of recurrence after curative resection of carcinoma of the colon and rectum. *Surg Gyn Obs* 1992;174;27–32.

109. Gilbert JM, Evans JM, Kark AE. Sites of recurrent tumor after "curative" colorectal surgery: implications for adjuvant therapy. *Br J Surg* 1984;71;203–205.

110. McCormack PM, Ginsberg RJ. Current management of colorectal metastases to lung. *Chest Surg Clin N Am* 1998;8:119–126.

111. McCormack PM, Burt ME, Bains MS, et al. Lung resection for colorectal metastases. 10 year results. *Arch Surg* 1992;127:1403–1406.

112. McAfee MK, Allen MS, Trastek VF, et al. Colorectal lung metastases: results of surgical excision. *Ann Thorac Surg* 1992;53:780–785.

113. Okimura S, Kondo H, Tsubai M, et al. Pulmonary resection for metastatic colorectal cancer: experience with 159 patients. *J Thorac Cardiovasc Surg* 1996;112:867–874.

114. van Halteren HK, van Geel AN, Hart AAM, et al. Pulmonary resection for metastases of colorectal origin. *Chest* 1995;107:1526–1531.

115. Sakamoto T, Tsubota N, Iwanaga K, et al. Pulmonary resection for metastases from colorectal cancer. *Chest* 2001;119:1069–1072.

116. Girard P, Ducreux M, Baldeyrou P, et al. Surgery for lung metastases from colorectal cancer: analysis of prognostic factors. *J Clin Oncol* 1996;14:2047–2053.

117. Carlin BW, Harrell JH, Olsen LK, et al. Endobronchial metastases due to colorectal carcinoma. *Chest* 1989;96:1110–1114.

118. Shimura S, Takishima T. Bronchorrhea from diffuse lymphangitic metastasis of colon carcinoma to the lung. *Chest* 1994;105;308–310.

119. Kavoussi LR, Levine SR, Kadmon D, et al. Regression of metastatic renal cell carcinoma: a case report and literature review. *J Urol* 1986;135:1005–1007.

120. Vogelzang NJ, Priest ER, Borden L. Spontaneous regression of histologically proved pulmonary metastases from renal cell carcinoma: a case with 5 year follow-up. *J Urol* 1992;148:1247–1249.

121. Suster S. Pulmonary metastases of extrapulmonary tumors. In: Saldana MJ, ed. *Pathology of pulmonary diseases.* Philadelphia: JB Lippincott Co, 1994:701–710.

122. Wolff M, Kaye G, Silva F. Pulmonary metastases (with admixed epithelial elements) from smooth muscle neoplasms: report of nine cases, including three males. *Am J Surg Pathol* 1979;3:325–342.

123. Horstmann JP, Pietra GG, Harman JA, et al. Spontaneous regression of pulmonary leiomyomas during pregnancy. *Cancer* 1977;39:314–321.

124. Banner AS, Carrington CB, Emory WB, et al. Efficacy of oophorectomy in lymphangioleiomyomatosis and benign metastasizing leiomyoma. *N Engl J Med* 1981;305:204–209.

125. Travis WD, Colby TV, Corrin B, et al. *Histological typing of lung and pleural tumours,* 3rd ed. New York: Springer-Verlag New York, 1999.

126. Barsky SH, Cameron R, Osann KE, et al. Rising incidence of bronchioloalveolar lung carcinoma and its unique clinicopathologic features. *Cancer* 1994;73:1163–1170.

127. Auerbach O, Garfinkel L. The changing pattern of lung carcinoma. *Cancer* 1991;68:1973–1977.

128. Rothschild H, Mulvey JJ. An increased risk for lung cancer mortality associated with sugarcane farming. *J Natl Cancer Inst* 1982;68:755–760.

129. Morton WE, Treyve EL. Histologic differences in occupational risks of lung cancer incidence. *Am J Ind Med* 1982;3:441–457.

130. Falk RT, Pickle LW, Fontham ET, et al. Epidemiology of bronchioloalveolar carcinoma. *Cancer Epidemiol Biomarkers Prev* 1992;1:339–344.

131. Nuorva K, Soini Y, Kamel D, et al. p53 protein accumulation and the presence of human papillomavirus DNA in bronchioloalveolar carcinoma correlate with poor prognosis. *Int J Cancer* 1995;64:424–429.

132. Nobel TA, Perk K. Bronchiolo-alveolar cell carcinoma. Animal model: pulmonary adenomatosis of sheep, pulmonary carcinoma of sheep, pulmonary carcinoma of sheep (jäagsiekte). *Am J Pathol* 1978;90:783–786.

133. Marchetti A, Buttitta F, Pellegrini S, et al. Bronchioloalveolar lung carcinomas: K-*ras* mutations are constant events in the mucinous subtype. *J Pathol* 1996;179:254–259.

134. Okubo K, Mark EJ, Flieder D, et al. Bronchoalveolar carcinoma: clinical, radiologic, and pathologic factors and survival. *J Thorac Cardiovasc Surg* 1999;118:702–709.

135. Regnard JF, Santelmo N, Romdhani N, et al. Bronchioloalveolar lung carcinoma: results of surgical treatment and prognostic factors. *Chest* 1998;114:45–50.

136. Hidaka N, Nagao K. Bronchioloalveolar carcinoma accompanied by severe bronchorrhea. *Chest* 1996;110:281–282.

137. Sarlin RF, Schillaci RF, Georges TN, et al. Focal increased lung perfusion and intrapulmonary veno-arterial shunting in bronchiolo-alveolar cell carcinoma. *Am J Med* 1980;68:618–623.

138. Barsky SH, Grossman DA, Ho J, et al. The multifocality of bronchioloalveolar lung carcinoma: evidence and implications of a multiclonal origin. *Mod Pathol* 1994;7:633–640.

139. Trigaux JP, Gevenois PA, Goncette L, et al. Bronchioloalveolar carcinoma: computed tomography findings. *Eur Respir J* 1996;9:11–16.

140. Hill CA. Bronchioloalveolar carcinoma: a review. *Radiology* 1984;150:15–20.

141. Im JG, Han MC, Yu EJ, et al. Lobar bronchioloalveolar carcinoma: "angiogram sign" on CT scans. *Radiology* 1990;176:749–753.

142. Tao LC, Weisbrod GL, Pearson FG, et al. Cytologic diagnosis of bronchioloalveolar carcinoma by fine-needle aspiration biopsy. *Cancer* 1986;57:1565–1570.

143. Gupta RK. Value of sputum cytology in the differential diagnosis of alveolar cell carcinoma from bronchogenic adenocarcinoma. *Acta Cytol* 1981;25:255–258.

144. Polletti V, Romagna M, Allen KA, et al. Bronchoalveolar lavage in the diagnosis of disseminated lung tumors. *Acta Cytol* 1995;39:472–477.

145. Greco RJ, Steiner RM, Goldman S, et al. Bronchoalveolar cell carcinoma of the lung. *Ann Thorac Surg* 1986;41:652–656.

146. Harpole DH, Bigelow C, Young WG Jr, et al. Alveolar cell carcinoma of the lung: a retrospective analysis of 205 patients. *Ann Thorac Surg* 1988;46:502–507.

147. Krawtz SM, Mehta AC, Vijayakumar S, et al. Palliation of massive bronchorrhea. *Chest* 1988;94:1313–1314.

148. Suga T, Sugiyama Y, Fujii T, et al. Bronchioloalveolar carcinoma with bronchorrhea treated with erythromycin. *Eur Respir J* 1994;7:2249–2251.

149. Paloyan EB, Swinnen LJ, Montoya A, et al. Lung transplantation for advanced bronchioloalveolar carcinoma confined to the lungs. *Transplantation* 2000;69:2446–2448.

150. Manning JT Jr, Spjut HJ, Tschen JA. Bronchioloalveolar carcinoma: the significance of two histopathologic types. *Cancer* 1984;54:525–534.

151. Daly RC, Trastek VF, Pairolero PC, et al. Bronchoalveolar carcinoma: factors affecting survival. *Ann Thorac Surg* 1991;51:368–376; discussion 376–377.

152. Davila DG, Dunn WF, Tazelaar HD, et al. Bronchial carcinoid tumors. *Mayo Clin Proc* 1993;68:795–803.

153. Fink G, Krelbaum T, Yellin A, et al. Pulmonary carcinoid: presentation, diagnosis, and outcome in 142 cases in Israel and review of 640 cases from the literature. *Chest* 2001;119:1647–1651.

154. Arrigoni MG, Woolner LB, Bernatz PE. Atypical carcinoid tumors of the lung. *J Thorac Cardiovasc Surg* 1972;64:413–421.

155. Okike N, Bernatz PE, Woolner LB. Carcinoid tumors of the lung. *Ann Thorac Surg* 1976;22:270–275.

156. Kulke MH, Mayer RJ. Carcinoid tumors. *N Engl J Med* 1999;340:858–868.

157. Ricci C, Patressi N, Massa R, et al. Carcinoid syndrome in bronchial adenoma. *Am J Surg* 1973;126:671–677.

158. Kvols LK, Moertel GC, O'Connell MJ. Treatment of the malignant carcinoid syndrome. *N Engl J Med* 1986;315:663–666.

159. McGaughan BC, Martini N, Bains MS. Bronchial carcinoids: review of 124 cases. *J Thorac Cardiovasc Surg* 1985;89:8–17.

160. Chughtai TS, Morin JE, Sheiner NM, et al. Bronchial carcinoid: 20 years experience defines a selective surgical approach. *Surgery* 1997;122:801–808.

161. Martensson H, Bottcher G, Hambraeus G, et al. Bronchial carcinoids: an analysis of 91 cases. *World J Surg* 1987;11:356–364.

162. Brandt B, Heintz SE, Rose EF, et al. Bronchial carcinoid tumors. *Ann Thorac Surg* 1984;38:63–65.

163. Sheppard MN. Neuroendocrine differentiation in lung tumors. *Thorax* 1991;46:843–850.

164. Vadasz P, Palffy G, Egervary M, et al. Diagnosis and treatment of bronchial carcinoid tumors: clinical and pathological review of 120 operated patients. *Eur J Cardiothorac Surg* 1993;7:8–11.

165. Sutedja TG, Schreurs AJ, Vanderschueren RG, et al. Bronchoscopic therapy in patients with intraluminal typical bronchial carcinoid. *Chest* 1995;107:556–558.

166. Thomas CFJ, Tazelaar HD, Jett JR. Typical and atypical pulmonary carcinoids. Outcome in patients presenting with regional lymph node involvement. *Chest* 2001;119:1143–1150.

167. Froudarakis M, Fournal P, Burgard G, et al. Bronchial carcinoids: a review of 22 cases. *Oncology* 1996;53:153–158.

168. Reubi JC, Kvols LK, Waser B. Detection of somatostatin receptors in surgical and percutaneous needle biopsy samples of carcinoids and islet cell carcinomas. *Cancer Res* 1990;50:5969–5977.

169. Marty-Ane C, Costes V Pujol J, et al. Carcinoid tumors of the lung: do atypical features require aggressive management? *Ann Thorac Surg* 1995;59:78–83.

170. Chakravarthy A, Abrams RA. Radiation therapy in the management of patients with malignant carcinoid tumors. *Cancer* 1995;75:1386–1390.

171. Saltz L, Lauwers G, Wiseberg J. A phase II trial of carboplatin in patients with advanced APUD tumors. *Cancer* 1993;72:619–622.

172. Colby TV, Wistuba II, Gazdar A. Precursors to pulmonary neoplasia. *Adv Anat Pathol* 1998;5:205–215.

173. Arioglu E, Doppman J, Gomes M, et al. Cushing's syndrome caused by corticotropin secretion by pulmonary tumorlets. *N Engl J Med* 1998;339:883–886.

174. D'Agati VD, Perzin KH. Carcinoid tumorlets of the lung with metastasis to a peribronchial lymph node: report of a case and review of the literature. *Cancer* 1985;55:2472–2476.

175. Warren WH, Faber LP, Gould VE. Neuroendocrine neoplasms of the lung: a clinicopathologic update. *J Thorac Cardiovasc Surg* 1989;98:321–332.

176. Hammond ME, Sause WT. Large cell neuroendocrine carcinomas of the lung: clinical significance and histopathologic definition. *Cancer* 1985;56:1624–1629.

177. Jones RC, Cleve EA. Solitary circumscribed lesions of the lung. *Arch Intern Med* 1954;93:842–851.

178. Poirier TJ, Van Ordstand HS. Pulmonary chondromatous hamartomas. *Chest* 1971;59:50–55.

179. Gabrail NY, Zara BY. Pulmonary hamartoma syndrome. *Chest* 1990;97:962–965.

180. Gjevre JA, Myers JL, Prakash UBS. Pulmonary hamartomas. *Mayo Clin Proc* 1996;71:14–20.

181. Fudge TL, Ochsner JL, Mills NL. Clinical spectrum of pulmonary hamartomas. *Ann Thorac Surg* 1980;30:36–39.

182. Mark EJ. Mesenchymal cystic hamartoma. *N Engl J Med* 1986;315:1255–1259.

183. King TEJ, Christopher KL, Schwarz MI. Multiple pulmonary chondromatous hamartomas. *Hum Pathol* 1982;13:496–497.

184. Jensen KG, Schiodt T. Growth conditions of hamartoma of the lung: a study based on 22 cases operated on after radiographic observation for from one to 18 years. *Thorax* 1958;13:233–237.

185. Palnaes-Hansen C, Holtveg H, Francis D, et al. Pulmonary hamartoma. *J Thorac Cardiovasc Surg* 1992;104:674–678.

186. Siegelman SS, Khouri NF, Scott WW. Pulmonary hamartoma: CT findings. *Radiology* 1986;160:313–317.

187. Ribet M, Jaillard-Thery S, Nuttens MC. Pulmonary hamartoma and malignancy. *J Thorac Cardiovasc Surg* 1994;107:611–614.

188. Higashita R, Ichikawa S, Ban T, et al. Coexistence of lung cancer and hamartoma. *Jpn J Thorac Cardiovasc Surg* 2001;49:258–260.

189. Crouch JD, Keagy BA, Starek PJK, et al. A clinical review of patients undergoing resection for pulmonary hamartoma. *Am Surg* 1988;54:297–299.

190. Karasik A, Modan M, Jacob CO et al. Increased risk of lung cancer in patients with chondromatous hamartoma. *J Thorac Cardiovasc Surg* 1980;80:217–220.

191. Pettinato G, Manivel JC, De Rosa N, et al. Inflammatory myofibroblastic tumor (plasma cell granuloma): clinicopathologic study of 20 cases with immunohistochemical and ultrastructural observations. *Am J Clin Pathol* 1990;94:538–546.

192. Hasleton PS. Benign lung tumors and their malignant counterparts. In: Hasleton PS, ed. *Spencer's pathology of the lung,* 5th ed. New York: McGraw-Hill, 1996:875–986.

193. Cerfolio RJ, Allen MS, Nascimento AG, et al. Inflammatory pseudotumors of the lung. *Ann Thorac Surg* 1999;67:933–936.

194. Urschel JD, Unruh HW. Plasma cell granuloma of the lung. *J Thorac Cardiovasc Surg* 1992;104:870–875.

195. Abdul-Karim FW, Slim MS, Melhem RE, et al. Pulmonary inflammatory pseudotumor with esophageal obstruction: report of a case and review of the literature. *Pediatr Surg Int* 1986;1:138–142.

196. Alam M, Morehead S, Weinstein MH. Dermatomyositis as a presentation of pulmonary inflammatory pseudotumor (myofibroblastic tumor). *Chest* 2000;117:1793–1795.

197. Jubrail D, Charalambos Z, Niki A, et al. Inflammatory pseudotumor: a controversial entity. *Eur J Cardiothoracic Surg* 1999;16:670–673.

198. Snyder CS, Dell'Aquila M, Haghighi P, et al. Clonal changes in inflammatory pseudotumor of the lung: a case report. *Cancer* 1995;76:1545–1549.

199. Bisseli R, Ferlini C, Fattorossi A, et al. Inflammatory myofibroblastic tumor (inflammatory pseudotumor): DNA flow cytometric analysis of nine pediatric cases. *Cancer* 1996;77:778–784.

200. Imperato JP, Forkman J, Sagerman RH, et al. Treatment of plasma cell granuloma of the lung with radiation therapy: a report of two cases and a review of the literature. *Cancer* 1986;57:2127–2129.

201. Bando T, Fujimura M, Noda Y, et al. Pulmonary plasma cell granuloma improves with corticosteroid therapy. *Chest* 1994;105:1574–1575.

202. Dail DH. Uncommon tumors. In: Dail DH and Hammer SP. *Pulmonary pathology,* 2nd ed. New York: Springer-Verlag New York, 1994:1279–1462.

203. Miller DL, Allen MS. Rare pulmonary neoplasms. *Mayo Clin Proc* 1993;68:492–498.

204. Vera-Romm JM, Sobonya RE, Gomez-Garcia JL, et al. Leiomyomas of the lung: literature review and case report. *Cancer* 1983;52:936–941.

205. Ayabe H, Tsuji H, Tagawa Y, et al. Endobronchial leiomyoma: report of a case treated by bronchoplasty and a review of the literature. *Surg Today* 1995;25:1057–1060.

206. Greene JG, Tassin L, Saberi A. Endobronchial epithelial papilloma associated with a foreign body. *Chest* 1990;97:229–230.

207. Flieder DB, Koss MN, Nicholson A, et al. Solitary pulmonary papilloma in adults: a clinicopathologic and in-situ hybridization study of 14 cases combined with 27 cases in the literature. *Am J Surg Pathol* 1998;22:1328–1342.

208. Basheda S, Gephardt GN, Stoller JK. Columnar papilloma of the bronchus: case report and literature review. *Am Rev Respir Dis* 1991;144:1400–1402.

209. de Montpreville TV, Dulmet EM. Granular cell tumours of the lower respiratory tract. *Histopathology* 1995;27:257–262.

210. Redjaee B, Rohatgi PK, Herman MA. Multiple endobronchial granular cell myoblastoma. *Chest* 1990;98:945–948.

211. Moran CA, Suster S, Koss MN. Primary adenoid cystic carcinoma of the lung: a clinicopathologic and immunohistochemical study of 16 cases. *Cancer* 1994;73:1390–1397.

212. Kawashima O, Hirai T, Kamiyoshihara M, et al. Primary adenoid cystic carcinoma in the lung: report of two cases and therapeutic considerations. *Lung Cancer* 1998;19:211–217.

213. Vadasz P, Egervary M. Mucoepidermoid bronchial tumors: a review of 34 operated cases. *Eur J Cardiothorac Surg* 2000;17:566–569.

214. Ukoha OO, Quartararo P, Carter D, et al. Acinic cell carcinoma of the lung with metastasis to lymph nodes. *Chest* 1999;115:591–595.

215. Moran CA. Primary salivary gland-type tumors of the lung. *Semin Diag Pathol* 1995;12:106–122.

216. Koss MN, Hochholzer L, Frommelt RA. Carcinosarcomas of the lung: a clinicopathologic study of 66 patients. *Am J Surg Pathol* 1999;23:1514–1526.

217. England DM, Hochholzer L. Truly benign "bronchial adenoma": report of 10 cases of mucous gland adenoma with immunohistochemical and ultrastructural findings. *Am J Surg Pathol* 1995;19:887–899.

218. Moran CA, Suster S, Koss MN. Endobronchial lipomas: a clinicopathologic study of 4 cases. *Mod Pathol* 1994;7:212–214.

219. Tsukada H, Osada H, Kojima K, et al. Bronchial wall schwannoma removed by sleeve resection of the right stem bronchus without lung resection. *J Cardiovasc Surg* 1998;39:511–513.

220. Wang NS, Morin J. Recurrent endobronchial soft tissue tumors. *Chest* 1984;85:787–791.

221. Fulford LG, Kamata Y, Okudera K, et al. Epithelial-myoepithelial carcinomas of the bronchus. *Am J Surg Pathol* 2001;25:1508–1514.

222. Nicholson AG, Baandrup U, Florio R, et al. Malignant myxoid endobronchial tumour: a report of two cases with a unique histologic pattern. *Histopathology* 1999;35:313–318.

223. McCluggage WG, Bharucha H. Primary pulmonary tumours of nerve sheath origin. *Histopathology* 1995;26:247–254.

224. Erasmus JJ, McAdams HP, Carraway MS. A 63-year-old woman with weight loss and multiple pulmonary nodules. *Chest* 1997;111:236–238.

225. Bini A, Ansaloni L, Grani G, et al. Pulmonary blastoma: report of two cases. *Surg Today* 2001;31:438–442.

226. Torikata C, Mukai M. So-called minute chemodectoma of the lung: an electron microscopic and immunohistochemical study. *Virchows Arch A Pathol Anat Histopath* 1990;417:113–118.

227. Carney JA. Gastric stromal sarcoma, pulmonary chondroma, and extra-adrenal paraganglioma (Carney triad): natural history, adrenocortical component, and possible familial occurrence. *Mayo Clin Proc* 1999;74:543–552.

228. Bagwell SP, Flynn SD, Cox PM, et al. Primary malignant melanoma of the lung. *Am Rev Resp Dis* 1989;139:1543–1547.

229. Ost D, Joseph C, Sogoloff H, et al. Primary pulmonary melanoma: case report and literature review. *Mayo Clin Proc* 1999;74:62–66.

230. Halyard MY, Camoriano JK, Culligan JA, et al. Malignant fibrous histiocytoma of the lung: report of four cases and review of the literature. *Cancer* 1996;78:2492–2497.

231. Logrono R, Filipowicz EA, Eyzaguirre EJ, et al. Diagnosis of primary fibrosarcoma of the lung by fine-needle aspiration and core biopsy. *Arch Pathol Lab Med* 1999;123:731–735.

232. Yu H, Ren H, Miao Q, et al. Pulmonary leiomyosarcoma. *Chin Med Sci J* 1997;12:129–131.

233. Hayashi T, Tsuda N, Iseki M, et al. Primary chondrosarcoma of the lung: a clinicopathologic study. *Cancer* 1993;72:69–74.

234. Krygier G, Amado A, Salisbury S, et al. Primary lung liposarcoma. *Lung Cancer* 1997;17:271–275.

235. Inayama Y, Hayashi H, Ogawa N, et al. Low-grade pulmonary myxoid sarcoma of uncertain histogenesis. *Pathol Int* 2001;51:204–210.

236. Comin CE, Santucci M, Novelli L, et al. Primary pulmonary rhabdomyosarcoma: report of a case in an adult and review of the literature. *Ultrastruct Pathol* 2001;25:269–273.

237. Terasaki H, Niki T, Hasegawa T, et al. Primary synovial sarcoma of the lung: a case report confirmed by molecular detection of SYT-SSX fusion gene transcripts. *Jpn J Clin Oncol* 2001;31:212–216.

238. Caves PK, Jacques J. Primary intrapulmonary neurogenic sarcoma with hypertrophic osteoarthropathy with asbestosis. *Thorax* 1971;26:212–218.

239. Moran CA, Suster S, Koss MN. Primary malignant triton tumour of the lung. *Histopathology* 1997;30:140–144.

240. Palmer RN, Saini N, Guccion J. Ewing's-like sarcoma appearing as a primary pulmonary neoplasm. *Arch Pathol Lab Med* 1981;105:277–278.

241. Sievert LJ, Elwing TJ, Evans ML. Primary pulmonary osteogenic sarcoma. *Skeletal Radiol* 2000;29:283–285.

242. Cox JE, Chiles C, Aquino SL, et al. Pulmonary artery sarcomas: a review of clinical and radiologic features. *J Comput Assist Tomogr* 1997;21:750–755.

243. Parish JM, Rosenow III EC, Swensen SJ, et al. Pulmonary artery sarcoma: clinical features. *Chest* 1996;110:1480–1488.

244. Mayer E, Kriegsmann J, Gaumann A, et al. Surgical treatment of pulmonary artery sarcoma. *J Thorac Cardiovasc Surg* 2001;121:77–82.

245. Devouassoux-Shisheboran M, Hayashi T, Linnoila RI, et al. A clinicopathologic study of 100 cases of pulmonary sclerosing hemangioma with immunohistochemical studies: TF-1 is expressed in both round and surface cells, suggesting an origin from primitive respiratory epithelium. *Am J Surg Pathol* 2000;24:906–916.

246. Yousem SA, Hochholzer L. Pulmonary hyalinizing granuloma. *Am J Clin Pathol* 1987;87:1–6.

247. Gal AA, Koss MN, Hochholzer L, et al. An immunohistochemical study of benign clear cell (sugar) tumor of the lung. *Arch Pathol Lab Med* 1991;115:1034–1038.

248. Shah AA, Chitis AS, Khubchandani SR. Pulmonary fibroma: a rare tumour. *J Assoc Physicians India* 1995;43:61–62.

249. Littlefield JB, Drash EC. Myxoma of the lung. *J Thoracic Surg* 1959;37:745–749.

250. Gaertner EM, Steinberg DM, Huber M, et al. Pulmonary and mediastinal glomus tumors: report of five cases including a pulmonary glomangiosarcoma: a clinicopathologic study with literature review. *Am J Surg Pathol* 2000;24:1105–1114.

251. Kaleem Z, Fitzpatrick MM, Ritter JH. Primary pulmonary meningioma: report of a case and review of the literature. *Arch Pathol Lab Med* 1997;121:631–636.

252. Prayson RA, Farver CF. Primary pulmonary malignant meningioma. *Am J Surg Pathol* 1999;23:722–726.

253. Iwasaki T, Iuchi K, Matsumura A, et al. Intrapulmonary mature teratoma. *Jpn J Thorac Cardiovasc Surg* 2000;48:468–472.

254. Batori M, Lazzaro M, Lonardo MT, et al. A rare case of pulmonary neurofibroma: clinical and diagnostic evaluation and surgical treatment. *Eur Rev Med Pharmacol Sci* 1999;3:155–157.

255. Fantone JC, Geisinger KR, Appelman HD. Papillary adenoma of the lung with lamellar and electron dense granules: an ultrastructural study. *Cancer* 1982;50:2839–2844.

256. Burke LM, Rush WI, Khoor A, et al. Alveolar adenoma: a histochemical, immunohistochemical, and ultrastructural analysis of 17 cases. *Hum Pathol* 1999;30:158–167.

257. Marchevsky AM. Lung tumors derived from ectopic tissues. *Semin Diagn Pathol* 1995;12:172–184.

258. Wise JN, Schaefer RF, Read RC. Primary pulmonary plasmacytoma. *Chest* 2001;120:1405–1407.

259. Yamamato T, Yazawa T, Ogata T, et al. Clear cell carcinoma of the lung: a case report and review of the literature. *Lung Cancer* 1993;10:101–106.

260. Katz DS, Lane MJ, Leung AN, et al. Primary malignant pulmonary hemangiopericytoma. *Clin Imaging* 1998;22:192–195.

261. Kiefer T, Wertzel H, Freudenberg N, et al. Long-term survival after repetitive surgery for malignant hemangiopericytoma of the lung with subsequent systemic metastases: case report and review of the literature. *J Thorac Cardiovasc Surg* 1997;45:307–309.

262. Canver CC, Voytovich MC. Resection of an unsuspected primary pulmonary choriocarcinoma. *Ann Thorac Surg* 1996;61:1249–1251.

263. Crotty TB, Hooker RP, Swensen SJ, et al. Primary malignant ependymoma of the lung. *Mayo Clin Proc* 1992;67:373–378.

264. Chen FF, Yan JJ, Lai WW, et al. Epstein-Barr virus-associated non–small cell carcinoma: undifferentiated "lymphoepithelioma-like" carcinoma as a distinct entity with better prognosis. *Cancer* 1998;82:2334–2342.

41

Tumors of the Mediastinum, Pleura, Chest Wall, and Diaphragm

Ali I. Musani · Daniel H. Sterman

TUMORS OF THE MEDIASTINUM

Anatomy of the Mediastinum

The mediastinum is situated in the center of the thoracic cavity, bordered by the two pleural cavities laterally, the diaphragm inferiorly, and the thoracic inlet superiorly (Fig. 41.1). The mediastinum may be further divided into anterior, middle, and posterior compartments, based on lateral chest radiographs rather than on anatomic planes, to assist in the localization of tumors and other conditions (1). The anterior mediastinum is surrounded by the sternum anteriorly and by the heart and brachiocephalic vessels posteriorly. It extends from the thoracic inlet superiorly to the diaphragm inferiorly and contains the thymus gland, fat, and lymph nodes. The middle mediastinum is bounded by the pericardial sac and extends superiorly to the fourth thoracic vertebra. It contains the heart and pericardium, ascending and transverse aorta, brachiocephalic vessels, vena cava, main pulmonary arteries and veins, trachea, bronchi, and lymph nodes. The posterior mediastinum is bordered anteriorly by the heart and trachea and posteriorly by the thoracic vertebrae. It contains the descending thoracic aorta, esophagus, azygos vein, autonomic ganglia and nerves, thoracic lymph nodes, and fat.

Epidemiology of Mediastinal Tumors

Approximately two thirds of all mediastinal tumors are benign in nature. Whereas more than two thirds of asymptomatic patients with mediastinal tumors have benign lesions, almost two thirds of symptomatic patients with mediastinal tumors have malignant lesions.

Approximately half of all mediastinal tumors are found in the anterior mediastinum (2). Masses in the anterior mediastinum are more likely to be malignant than masses in the other compartments. In a report of 400 patients with primary cysts and neoplasms of the mediastinum, the authors noted malignancy in 59%, 29%, and 16% of the anterior, middle, and posterior mediastinal masses, respectively (3) (Table 41.1).

The patient's age provides a clue to the likely causes of a mediastinal mass. Thymomas, thymic cysts, and neurogenic tumors are more common in adults. Hodgkin and non-Hodgkin lymphomas and germ cell tumors are most common between the second and fourth decades of life; thus, the probability of a mediastinal tumor being malignant is greater in this age group.

Signs and Symptoms

In a study of 400 patients with primary mediastinal lesions, 62% were symptomatic at the time of diagnosis (3). As expected, symptoms were more prevalent in those with a malignant neoplasm (85%) than in those with a benign neoplasm (46%). Among the most common symptoms at presentation were chest pain (30%), dyspnea (16%), cough (60%), and fever/chills (20%). Seventy-five percent of the patients with anterosuperior mediastinal masses were symptomatic, in comparison with 45% of those with middle mediastinal masses and 50% of those with posterior mediastinal masses.

Systemic manifestations are common in patients with mediastinal tumors. A classic example is hypercalcemia caused by a parathyroid adenoma (Tables 41.2 and 41.3). Locally, mediastinal tumors may impinge on other structures, causing

A. I. Musani: Department of Pulmonary, Allergy, and Critical Care Medicine, and Interventional Pulmonology Program, Hospital of the University of Pennsylvania, Philadelphia, Pennsylvania.

D. H. Sterman: Interventional Pulmonology Program, Thoracic Oncology Gene Therapy Program, Pulmonary, Allergy and Critical Care Division, University of Pennsylvania Medical Center, Philadelphia, Pennsylvania.

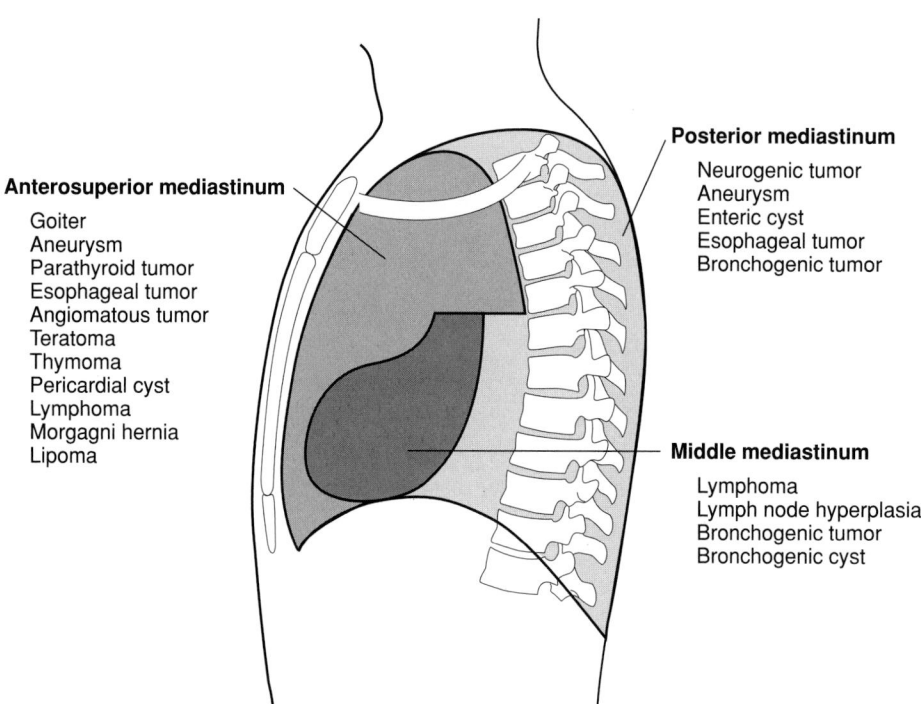

Anterosuperior mediastinum

Goiter
Aneurysm
Parathyroid tumor
Esophageal tumor
Angiomatous tumor
Teratoma
Thymoma
Pericardial cyst
Lymphoma
Morgagni hernia
Lipoma

Posterior mediastinum

Neurogenic tumor
Aneurysm
Enteric cyst
Esophageal tumor
Bronchogenic tumor

Middle mediastinum

Lymphoma
Lymph node hyperplasia
Bronchogenic tumor
Bronchogenic cyst

FIGURE 41.1. Common possible diagnoses of mediastinal masses. The differential diagnosis of a mediastinal mass depends on the anatomic compartment in which it arises. (Modified from Baue AE, et al., eds. *Glenn's thoracic and cardiovascular surgery*, 5th ed. Norwalk, CT: Appleton & Lange, 1991, with permission.)

signs and symptoms. Common signs and symptoms include the following (4):

- Airway compression causing respiratory complications (e.g., airway obstruction/postobstructive pneumonia, atelectasis, hemoptysis)
- Esophageal compression causing dysphagia
- Compression of the spinal cord and vertebral column causing paralysis
- Phrenic nerve injury causing paralysis of the diaphragm
- Recurrent laryngeal nerve injury causing hoarseness and vocal cord paralysis
- Stellate ganglion involvement causing Horner syndrome
- Compression of the superior vena cava causing superior vena cava syndrome.

Diagnostic Evaluation

Appropriately selected imaging techniques can facilitate the differential diagnosis. Routine posteroanterior and lateral chest radiography is a useful diagnostic procedure in the workup of a patient with a suspected mediastinal mass because it can demonstrate size, anatomic location, density, and any calcification. Good localization can help narrow the list of possible diagnoses (4) (Table 41.1).

However, because the mediastinum contains many overlapping structures of similar radiodensities, computed tomography (CT) is required for the exact delineation of a mass and a determination of any involvement of surrounding structures, such as vertebrae and ribs. CT identifies cystic,

TABLE 41.1. USUAL LOCATIONS OF MEDIASTINAL TUMORS

Anterior	Middle	Posterior
Thymoma	Lymphoma	Neurogenic tumor
Teratoma, seminoma	Pericardial cyst	Bronchgenic cyst
Lymphoma	Bronchogenic cyst	Enteric cyst
Carcinoma	Metastatic cyst	Xanthogranuloma
Parathyroid adenoma	Systemic granuloma	Diaphragmatic hernia
Intrathoracic goiter		Meningocele
Lipoma		Paravertebral abscess
Lymphangioma		
Aortic aneurysm		

TABLE 41.2. SYSTEMIC SYNDROMES SECONDARY TO ENDOCRINE FUNCTION OF MEDIASTINAL TUMORS

Syndrome	Tumor
Cushing disease	Carcinoid, thymoma
Gynecomastia	Germ cell tumor
Hypertension	Pheochromocytoma, ganglioneuroma, chemodectoma
Diarrhea	Ganglioneuroma
Hypercalcemia	Parathyroid adenoma, lymphoma
Thyrotoxicosis	Intrathoracic goiter
Hypoglycemia	Mesothelioma, teratoma, fibrosarcoma, neurosarcoma

TABLE 41.3. SYSTEMIC SYNDROMES ASSOCIATED WITH PRIMARY MEDIASTINAL TUMORS AND CYSTS

Syndrome	Tumor
Myasthenia gravis	Thymoma
Pure red cell aplasia	
Hypogammaglobulinemia	
Whipple disease	
Megaesophagus	
Collagen-vascular disease	
Malignancy	
Myocarditis	
Multiple endocrine adenomatosis	Carcinoid, thymoma
Osteoarthropathy	Neurofibroma, neurilemoma, mesothelioma
Vertebral anomalies	Enteric cysts
Fever of unknown origin	Lymphoma
Alcohol-induced pain	Hodgkin disease
Opsomyoclonus	Neuroblastoma

fatty, vascular, and soft tissue structures and the relation of a mass to surrounding tissues (4).

Rarely, studies such as fluoroscopy, barium swallow, angiography, CT angiography, and three-dimensional reconstruction are needed to provide additional information. The role of magnetic resonance imaging (MRI) in the diagnostic workup of a patient with a mediastinal mass is primarily to rule out suspected neurogenic tumors when the contrast media necessary for CT are contraindicated. MRI is very useful for delineating the invasiveness of neurogenic tumors (dumbbell tumors) in the spinal column (5). MRI is also very useful when vascular invasion is suspected or when cardiac imaging is required.

The role of ultrasonography has diminished since the advent of contrast-enhanced CT and MRI. Transthoracic or transesophageal cardiac ultrasonography (echocardiography) can provide important information when mediastinal tumors are close to the heart or involvement of the pericardium or myocardium is suspected. Scanning with a radioactive isotope of iodine is often used to help diagnose a substernal thyroid tumor. Similarly, gallium scanning can be used to stage lymphoma (4). Positron emission tomography (PET) is a new and exciting diagnostic modality with broad applications, particularly in the diagnosis and management of cancer. [18F]Fluorodeoxyglucose (18F-FDG) is the tracer most frequently used for scanning tumors (6). Although most widely applied currently in pulmonary medicine for the diagnosis and staging of lung cancer, PET with 18F-FDG is also beneficial in the evaluation of mediastinal masses. In particular, 18F-FDG PET is quite sensitive and specific in the diagnosis of lymphoma (7). For example, PET can identify more sites of disease than conventional imaging during initial staging and can demonstrate a reduction in uptake after successful therapy. PET is also useful in determining whether residual masses seen on CT are scar tissue or active disease (8).

Biochemical Studies

The detection of certain biochemical markers in the serum can be helpful when a specific diagnosis is in question. Examples include thyroid function studies for retrosternal goiter; measurement of serum levels of calcium, phosphate, and parathyroid hormone for parathyroid tumors; and measurement of α-fetoprotein (AFP) and β-human chorionic gonadotropin (β-hCG) levels for nonseminomatous germ cell tumors (3).

Tissue Diagnosis and Management

All patients with a mediastinal mass require a precise tissue diagnosis before treatment is planned. When a mass is thought to be benign after a clinical and radiographic evaluation, it may be surgically treated without a biopsy diagnosis if it is causing symptoms. Various options include needle aspiration of a benign cystic mass, removal of a bronchogenic cyst or localized neurogenic tumor by video-assisted thoracoscopic surgery (VATS), and transcervical resection of a benign thymoma. Conversely, the mass may be observed over time. If a mass is thought to be malignant, diagnostic biopsy specimens may be obtained by transthoracic or transbronchoscopic needle aspiration, mediastinoscopy, anterior mediastinotomy, or VATS, as indicated by the anatomic location and radiographic appearance of the lesion.

Tumors of the Anterior Mediastinum

Primary neoplasms of the anterior mediastinum comprise a group of tumors arising from different embryonic cell layers (Table 41.1). Fifty-nine percent of these tumors are malignant (3).

Thymoma

Thymomas are the most common primary tumors of the anterior mediastinum (9–11). Twenty percent of all adult mediastinal neoplasms are thymomas, and they are rarely seen in children (12,13). Thymomas occur with equal frequency in men and women in the third and fourth decades of life.

Pathology

Thymomas are classified as lymphocytic, epithelial, or spindle cell variants according to the predominant cell type. However, the cell type does not determine course, invasiveness, response to therapy, or prognosis (14,15). The visualization of characteristic tonofibrils and desmosomes by electron microscopy helps to distinguish thymomas from other tumors with a similar appearance that can arise in the thymus, such as carcinoid tumors, Hodgkin lymphomas, and seminomas. Cytokeratin staining is a diagnostic marker. Immunostaining of the epithelial cells plays a pivotal role in differentiating thymomas from nonepithelial malignancies, such as lymphomas and sarcomas. Immunohistochemical staining of the lymphocytes is not useful in the diagnosis of thymoma.

Most thymomas are solid tumors, but up to one third exhibit necrosis, hemorrhage, and cystic areas (10,16). Most are completely surrounded by a fibrous capsule; however, 34% may invade through the capsule into the pleura, pericardium, great vessels, right atrium, or lung (11,17–20). The term *invasive thymoma* is preferred to *malignant thymoma* because "invasive" thymomas lack the histologic features of malignancy and are microscopically identical to encapsulated thymomas (19).

Transdiaphragmatic extension into the abdomen and metastasis into the ipsilateral pleura and pericardium can occur (9,11,18). Lymphogenous and hematogenous metastasis is rare (16,17).

Classification

The new (as of 1999) World Health Organization classification of thymic tumors recognizes the prognostic significance of the cytologic similarities between the normal thymic epithelium and the neoplastic cells. The five types of thymoma currently identified are the following (21):

1. Type A B: spindle cell, medullary
2. Type AB B: mixed
3. Type B1 B: lymphocyte-rich, lymphocytic, predominantly cortical, organoid
4. Type B2 B: cortical
5. Type B3 B: epithelial, atypical, squamous, well-differentiated thymic carcinoma.

Staging

The most widely used staging system (Masaoka clinical staging) takes into consideration invasion of the tumor through the capsule into the surrounding structures (22).

1. Stage 1: Complete encapsulation macroscopically and no capsular invasion microscopically
2. Stage 2: Invasion into the surrounding fatty tissue or mediastinal pleura macroscopically or invasion into the capsule microscopically
3. Stage 3: Invasion into neighboring organs (i.e., pericardium, great vessels, or lung) macroscopically
4. Stage 4a: Pleural or pericardial dissemination
5. Stage 4b: Lymphogenous or hematogenous metastasis.

Clinical Findings

More often than not, thymoma is an incidental finding on chest radiography performed for unrelated indications in an asymptomatic patient (13,23,24). One third of patients experience chest pain, cough, dyspnea, or other symptoms related to the compression or invasion of adjacent structures (16). Parathymic syndromes such as myasthenia gravis, hypogammaglobulinemia, and pure red cell aplasia are seen in up to half of patients (17).

Approximately 30% to 50% of patients with a thymoma have myasthenia gravis, whereas only 15% of patients with myasthenia gravis have a thymoma (25). Therefore, the serum anti-acetylcholine receptor antibody level should be measured in all patients with a suspected thymoma to rule out myasthenia gravis before surgery, even if they are asymptomatic (26,27). Uncommonly, myasthenia gravis manifests after thymectomy and can be diagnosed by an anti-acetylcholine receptor antibody titer (10,11). Other parathymic syndromes, such as hypogammaglobulinemia and pure red cell aplasia, are present in 10% and 5% of patients with a thymoma, respectively (10).

Thymoma is also associated with various other autoimmune disorders, such as systemic lupus erythematosus, polymyositis, and myocarditis (3,10,18,28).

Pleural or pericardial effusion is the most common form of metastatic involvement. Extrathoracic metastases occur in fewer than 7% of patients, most commonly to the kidney, extrathoracic lymph nodes, liver, brain, adrenal gland, thyroid, and bone. Metastases to the ipsilateral lung are unusual (17).

Diagnosis

As mentioned previously (see section "Clinical Findings"), thymomas are usually found incidentally during chest radiography; the tumor appears as a well-defined lobulated mass in the anterosuperior mediastinum. Although thymomas are usually located in the chest anterior to the aortic root, they can develop anywhere from the neck to the cardiophrenic angle (10,18). Contrast-enhanced thoracic CT typically reveals an encapsulated, well-defined, homogeneous or heterogeneous soft tissue mass, often with hemorrhage, necrosis, or cyst formation (Fig 41.2). Infiltrative lesions, vascular compromise, or an irregular interface with the adjacent lung suggest invasiveness (29). MRI is the best imaging modality when vascular invasion is suspected. Thymoma can mimic malignant mesothelioma by diffusely involving the pleura and encasing the lung (10,19,30). Nevertheless, pleural effusions are uncommon (18).

Surgical excision provides the definitive diagnosis in an appropriate clinical and radiographic setting. However, experience with ultrasonography and CT-guided fine needle aspiration is increasing. Anderson and colleagues (31) reported a success rate of 95% (27 of 28 patients) using ultrasonographically guided fine needle aspiration of anterior mediastinal masses. In one patient, a malignant lymphoma was falsely identified as connective tissue remnant. They concluded that ultrasonographically guided fine needle aspiration is a safe, cost-effective, and reliable alternative to thoracotomy and mediastinoscopy.

In establishing a diagnosis of thymoma, fine needle aspiration and mediastinotomy are preferred to mediastinoscopy because the violation of tissue planes is minimized and the risk for tumor spillage is reduced. Therefore, mediastinoscopy is only rarely used for direct biopsy. Although

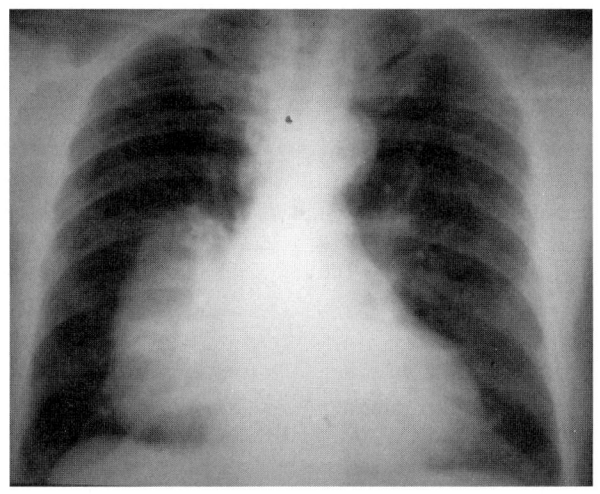
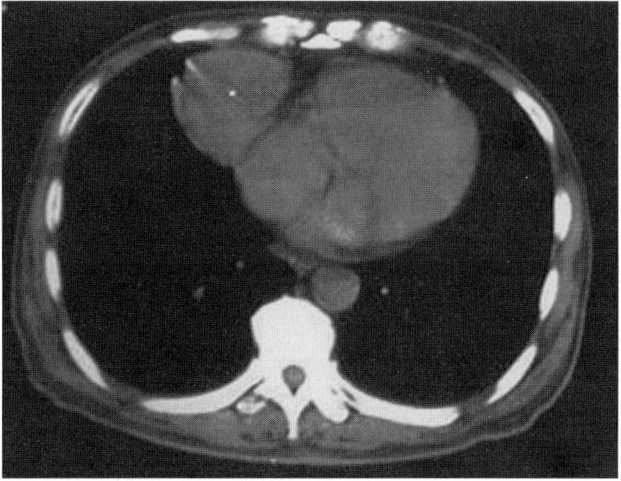

FIGURE 41.2. Chest radiograph and computed tomographic image of a 68-year-old man with a large mediastinal benign thymoma. (From *http://home.kimo.com.tw/2chiu/dd-mediastinaltumor.html*, with permission.)

thoracoscopy has also been used to diagnose thymoma, mediastinotomy is generally preferred if fine needle aspiration is unsuccessful (32). A definitive diagnosis need not be established before surgical resection if thymoma is strongly suspected on the basis of the clinical information and imaging features consistent with the lesion. The surgical diagnosis and therapy of thymoma can be rendered simultaneously through excisional biopsy (32).

Treatment

Complete surgical resection offers the best prognosis in cases of either invasive or noninvasive nonmetastatic thymoma. The extent of local invasion into neighboring structures such as pericardium and pulmonary parenchyma determines the boundaries of surgical resection. Resection of these structures is sometimes required to achieve complete control with histologically negative margins. Resection of the phrenic nerve resection is sometimes necessary because of involvement by tumor.

In a series of 147 female and 136 male patients (ages, 16–90 years; mean age, 52 years) with thymoma treated at the Mayo Clinic, the tumors were locally invasive at operation in 32%, including 6% that were metastatic to lung or pleura. Intrathoracic recurrence was noted postoperatively in 15% of those who had undergone total excision, and distant metastases developed in 3% of the patients. Thymoma was the cause of death in 13%, and myasthenia gravis in 16%. The overall 5-year survival was 67%, and the 10-year survival was 53%. Poor prognostic factors included tumor-related symptoms, large tumor size, local invasion or metastasis at the initial operation, and predominantly epithelial histologic features. Although true thymomas are composed of cytologically benign elements, they show a propensity for local invasion and intrathoracic recurrence. They rarely metastasize beyond the thorax (32).

Adjunctive chemotherapy and radiation therapy play an important role in the treatment of locally advanced or metastatic disease. Radiation therapy is a viable option for patients whose tumors are unresectable because of local invasion/advanced or metastatic disease and for patients with postoperative residual or invasive disease.

In a review of 117 patients, 14 cases were excluded because of a lack of the histologic criteria for a thymic tumor, and the remaining 103 were classified according to a staging system as follows: stage I, completely encapsulated (43 patients); stage II, extension through the capsule or pericapsular fat invasion (21 patients); stage III, invasion of adjacent structures (36 patients); and stage IV, thoracic dissemination or metastases (3 patients). The 5-year actuarial survival and relapse-free survival rates were 67% and 100% for stage I, 86% and 58% for stage II, and 69% and 53% for stage III, respectively. No recurrences developed in patients with stage I disease after total resection without radiotherapy. However, in 8 of 21 patients with invasive (stage II or III) thymomas, the mediastinum was the first site of recurrence after total resection without radiotherapy. The 5-year actuarial mediastinal relapse rate of 53% in this group compared unfavorably with the mediastinal relapse rate of patients with stage II or III disease after total resection with radiotherapy (0) and with that of patients with stage II or III disease after subtotal resection/biopsy with radiotherapy (21%). Despite attempted salvage therapy, five of eight patients with mediastinal relapse following total resection alone died of progressive disease. No significant difference was observed between the local relapse rates, overall relapse rates, and survival rates of the patients who underwent biopsy and radiotherapy and those of the patients who underwent subtotal resection and radiotherapy for invasive thymomas (stages II and III). Total resection alone appears to be inadequate therapy, with an unacceptably high rate of local failure and poor results of salvage therapy (33).

Thymoma is generally a chemotherapy-sensitive tumor. In locally invasive or bulky disease, preoperative cisplatin-based chemotherapy regimens with or without postoperative radiotherapy may offer the best disease-free survival (34). In one study, 23 patients with locally advanced, unresectable disease underwent three courses of induction chemotherapy with cisplatin, doxorubicin, cyclophosphamide, and prednisone (35). The objective response rate was 77%. Of the 21 patients who underwent attempted resection, postoperative radiation (50–60 Gy), and adjuvant chemotherapy (three cycles of the same regimen), 19 completed the entire course of treatment. The 7-year disease-free and overall survival rates of these 19 patients were 77% and 79%, respectively (35).

Patients with recurrent or metastatic thymoma should be referred for enrollment in clinical trials. Several combinations of novel chemotherapeutic agents, such as carboplatin and paclitaxel, are being evaluated at multiple centers around the country under the auspices of the National Cancer Institute (*www.cancer.gov*) in a phase II study of patients with advanced thymoma or thymic carcinoma.

Prognosis

Thymomas are slowly growing tumors, and a patient's prognosis is adversely affected by invasion through the capsule into the surround fat, pleura, or pericardium. Other poor prognostic factors include metastasis, a large tumor size (>10 cm), tracheal or vascular compression, age younger than 30 years, epithelial or mixed histology, and the presence of a hematologic paraneoplastic syndrome. The presence of other, nonhematologic paraneoplastic syndromes is not associated with a poor outcome per se, possibly because of earlier detection (36).

The Masaoka staging system appears to correlate well with the observed 5-year survival rates (22,37).

Stage	*Survival*
Stage I	96%–100%
Stage II	6%–95%
Stage III	56%–69%
Stage IV	11%–50%

Thymic Carcinoma

Thymic carcinomas are a heterogeneous group of aggressive epithelial malignancies. They tend to be locally invasive and metastatic (2). Unlike thymomas, thymic carcinomas typically are not associated with myasthenia gravis or other paraneoplastic syndromes. They may be classified into low- and high-grade histologic types. The squamous cell carcinoma and lymphoepithelioma-like variants are the most common cell types (38).

Incidence

Primary thymic carcinomas are rare. They usually occur in middle-aged men with a mean age of 46 years (38,39).

Clinical and Radiographic Features

Most patients have chest pain and cough. They may have symptoms of superior vena cava syndrome, in addition to constitutional symptoms such as fatigue, weight loss, and anorexia (40). Thymic carcinoma most commonly presents as a large, firm, infiltrating mass with frequent areas of cystic change and necrosis. Tumors are encapsulated in 15% of cases or fewer (40). Radiologically, thymic carcinomas are frequently associated with pleural and pericardial effusions.

Histology

In contrast to thymomas, thymic carcinomas are cytologically malignant, determined by the ubiquitous presence of cellular necrosis, atypia, and mitoses. These histologic findings are rarely found during the microscopic examination of thymomas (40).

Differential Diagnosis

The main differential diagnosis for thymic carcinoma is that of carcinoma metastatic to the mediastinal lymph nodes. The exclusion of a primary tumor is mandatory, especially a lung cancer. Confusion commonly arises in the differentiation of thymic carcinoma from thymoma. Besides having distinctive histologic and cytologic features, thymic carcinoma is rarely associated with paraneoplastic syndromes.

Treatment and Prognosis

The treatment and prognosis depend on the histologic grade and stage of thymic carcinoma. Certain morphologic features that portend a poor prognosis include infiltration of the tumor margin, the absence of a lobular growth pattern, the presence of high-grade atypia and necrosis, and the presence of more than 10 mitoses per high-power field (22). Complete surgical resection is the treatment of choice for thymic carcinoma and can be curative in cases of encapsulated squamous cell carcinoma (41). Combination chemotherapy with etoposide and cisplatin and concurrent radiotherapy are considered a reasonable treatment approach for patients who are not good candidates for surgical resection. When patients are unable to tolerate simultaneous chemotherapy and radiotherapy, sequential therapy can be used (33,35,42).

Of five patients with thymic carcinoma treated with cisplatin-based combination chemotherapy at Indiana University Hospital, three responded, two of them completely. This form of chemotherapy merits additional study. The optimal regimen remains unclear (43).

The overall 3- and 5-year survival rates for patients with thymic carcinoma are 40% and 33%, respectively. The 5-year survival rate for patients with high-grade tumors is 15% to 20%, whereas it is 90% for those with low-grade tumors (38).

Thymic Carcinoid

Thymic carcinoid is a malignant tumor, histologically similar to carcinoid tumors at other sites. It is most common in the fourth and fifth decades of life (40). Certain endocrinologic abnormalities are commonly associated with thymic carcinoid, such as Cushing syndrome, which results from the ectopic production of adrenocorticotropic hormone, and the multiple endocrine neoplasia syndrome (10). Regional lymph node and distant metastases develop in two thirds of patients with thymic carcinoids (44).

Thymic carcinoid presents as a large, lobulated, invasive mass of the anterior mediastinum with or without hemorrhage and necrosis (44). The treatment is complete surgical resection, if possible. For a locally invasive tumor, radiotherapy and chemotherapy are often used, although this tumor is highly resistant to both modalities (44,45).

Thymolipoma

Thymolipoma is a rare, benign, slowly growing tumor of the thymus gland that affects young adults of both sexes with equal frequency (2). It presents as a large tumor of the anterior mediastinum. CT and MRI show a characteristic fat density. The treatment of choice is surgical excision.

Nonneoplastic Thymic Cysts

Thymic cysts are rare tumors of unclear etiology. They can be congenital or acquired, associated either with inflammation or with an inflammatory neoplasm, such as Hodgkin disease (46). Congenital thymic cysts are thought to be remnants of the thymopharyngeal duct (47). Inflammatory cysts probably arise from inflamed thymic parenchyma. Thymic cysts associated with neoplasia are more likely to cause symptoms. Microscopically, inflammatory thymic cysts may be identical to cystic thymic neoplasms, so that thorough sampling and examination are essential (48). Surgical excision is curative (Fig 41.3).

Mediastinal Germ Cell Tumors

Mediastinal germ cell tumors (GCTs) are a heterogeneous group of neoplasms thought to originate from primitive germ cells that fail to migrate completely during early embryonic development (49–51). These tumors account for 15% of anterior mediastinal neoplasms in adults. GCTs are usually diagnosed in young adults with a mean age of 27 years (2). Malignant GCTs are much more common (>90%) in men (48). A mediastinal GCT should prompt a search for a primary gonadal malignancy. Serologic studies for AFP and β-hCG, which are associated with nonseminomatous GCTs, can assist in the diagnostic workup (2).

The classification of GCTs is based on cell type. Although many neoplasms have a mixed cellularity, mediastinal GCTs are classified as benign teratomas, seminomas, or embryonal tumors. The embryonal tumors, also called *malignant teratomas* or *nonseminomatous GCTs*, are diverse and include choriocarcinomas, yolk sac carcinomas, embryonal carcinomas, and teratocarcinomas (52).

Mediastinal Teratomas (Benign)

Benign teratomas are the most common mediastinal GCTs (53). They contain tissues that arise from at least two of the three primitive germ layers (i.e., ectoderm, mesoderm, and endoderm). Ectodermal tissues, which usually predominate, can include skin, hair, sweat glands, and sebaceous material or toothlike structures. Mesodermal tissues, such as fat, cartilage, bone, and smooth muscle, and endodermal tissues, such as respiratory or intestinal epithelium, are less commonly encountered (54).

The vast majority of mediastinal teratomas are mature—that is, they are histologically well differentiated and benign (53). A teratoma rarely contains fetal tissue and is then classified as an immature teratoma, which carries a good prognosis

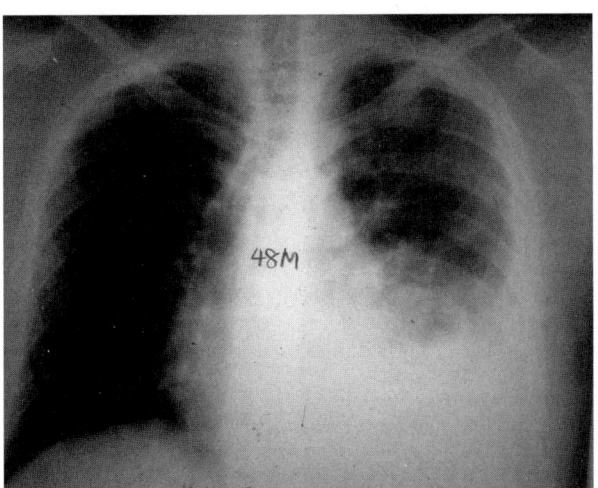
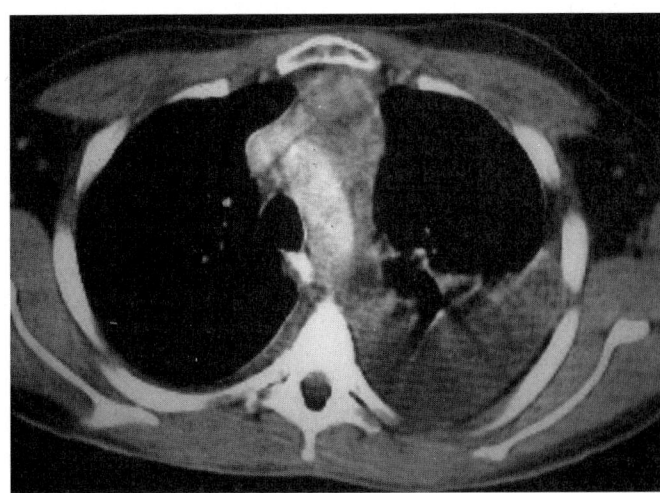

FIGURE 41.3. Chest radiograph and computed tomographic images of a 25-year-old man with a thymic lymphoma of the anterior mediastinum. (From *http://home.kimo.com.tw/2chiu/dd-mediastinaltumor.html*, with permission.)

in children but may recur or metastasize (55). Regardless of the degree of cellular differentiation, mediastinal teratomas have little malignant potential in infants. However, in patients 15 years of age or older, malignant degeneration is associated with immature histology (56). Primary immature mediastinal teratomas presenting in adults carry a poor prognosis.

Clinical Findings. Mature teratoma occurs most frequently in children and young adults, equally in both sexes. Most patients are asymptomatic. Large tumors may cause symptoms, including chest pain, dyspnea, and cough, by compressing and obstructing the surrounding organs. Digestive enzymes secreted by intestinal mucosa or pancreatic tissue in the tumor can lyse tissue and cause rupture of the bronchi, pleura, pericardium, or lung (2). Expectoration of hair (trichoptysis) or sebum is a rare but pathognomonic sign of ruptured mediastinal teratoma (57,58).

Diagnosis. On a chest radiograph, these tumors appear as well-defined round or lobulated masses of the anterior mediastinum. Up to 26% are calcified, and they may display recognizable bone or teeth (59). CT and MRI are helpful in delineating the spatial relationship of the tumor to surrounding structures (Fig. 41.4). They can also characterize densities within the lesion suggestive of fat, sebaceous material, or cystic elements, which support the diagnosis (60,61).

Treatment. Regardless of the histologic maturity, surgical resection is the treatment of choice. Subtotal resection is performed to relieve compression when the tumor cannot be removed completely without jeopardizing surrounding vital structures.

A Japanese group retrospectively studied 11 patients with immature teratomas. The patients were divided into survivors and nonsurvivors. The survivor group had undergone complete resection of the teratoma with preoperative or postoperative chemotherapy, whereas the nonsurvivor group had undergone incomplete resection without chemotherapy. The study concluded that when complete resection is combined with chemotherapy, long-term survival can be expected. Conversely, unless both treatments are offered, the outcome is very poor (62).

Mediastinal Seminoma

Primary mediastinal seminomas are uncommon, representing only 2% to 4% of all mediastinal masses, but they comprise 25% to 50% of malignant mediastinal GCTs. The tumor occurs predominantly in young men between the ages of 20 and 40 years and is usually symptomatic. Mediastinal seminoma can rarely occur in women with normal ovaries (63). It is unusual for this primary genitourinary seminoma to metastasize to the mediastinum in the absence of retroperitoneal lymph node involvement (50). Nonetheless, all pa-

tients with a mediastinal seminoma should undergo a testicular examination, including ultrasonography.

A heterogeneous tumor containing other cellular components, such as embryonal carcinoma, yolk sac carcinoma, and teratocarcinoma, portends poor prognosis. Heterogeneous mediastinal seminomatous tumors behave more like nonseminomatous germ cell malignancies by virtue of their aggressive course and resistance to radiation therapy.

Clinical Findings. Patients with mediastinal seminomas come to medical attention because of their symptoms, which include substernal pain, dyspnea, weakness, cough, fever, gynecomastia, and weight loss. Ten percent of patients with this tumor present with superior vena cava syndrome (63).

Diagnosis. Radiologically, seminomas are bulky, lobulated, homogenous masses of the anterior mediastinum. They uncommonly invade adjacent structures but can metastasize to regional lymph nodes and bone (2). Serum markers such as β-hCG and AFP are helpful in differentiating between seminomas and nonseminomatous GCTs. The level of β-hCG is elevated in more than 80% of patients with a nonseminomatous GCT but in only 34% of those with a mediastinal seminoma (64). The AFP level is elevated in 80% to 85% of patients with a nonseminomatous GCT but almost never in those with a pure seminoma.

Staging. Seminomas are staged according to the American Joint Committee on Cancer tumor-node-metastasis (TNM) staging system as 0, I, II, or III. The details of the staging system are beyond the scope of this chapter.

Routine CT of the chest and abdomen is essential to evaluate the extent of the primary mediastinal tumor and assess the retroperitoneal lymph nodes. Gallium scanning can also be useful. The spread of seminoma beyond the mediastinum indicates a need for systemic chemotherapy.

Treatment. Seminomas are very sensitive to external beam radiation therapy, which is the treatment of choice for localized tumors. Thirteen patients with localized disease were treated with definitive megavoltage radiotherapy at the Stanford University Medical Center. The actuarial survival at 10 years was 69%, with a relapse-free survival of 54%. No patient receiving more than 4,700 rads to the primary lesion had local or systemic relapse (65).

Small, localized tumors may be treated with primary resection followed by radiotherapy. Six hundred thirty-five patients with extragonadal GCTs were studied retrospectively (64). These patients were treated consecutively at 11 centers in the United States and Europe during the era of cisplatin-based chemotherapy between 1975 and 1996. Fifty-two (50%) of them had primary retroperitoneal GCTs and 51 (49%) had primary mediastinal GCTs of purely seminomatous histology. The treatment consisted of platin-based chemotherapy in 77 patients (74%), radiotherapy in

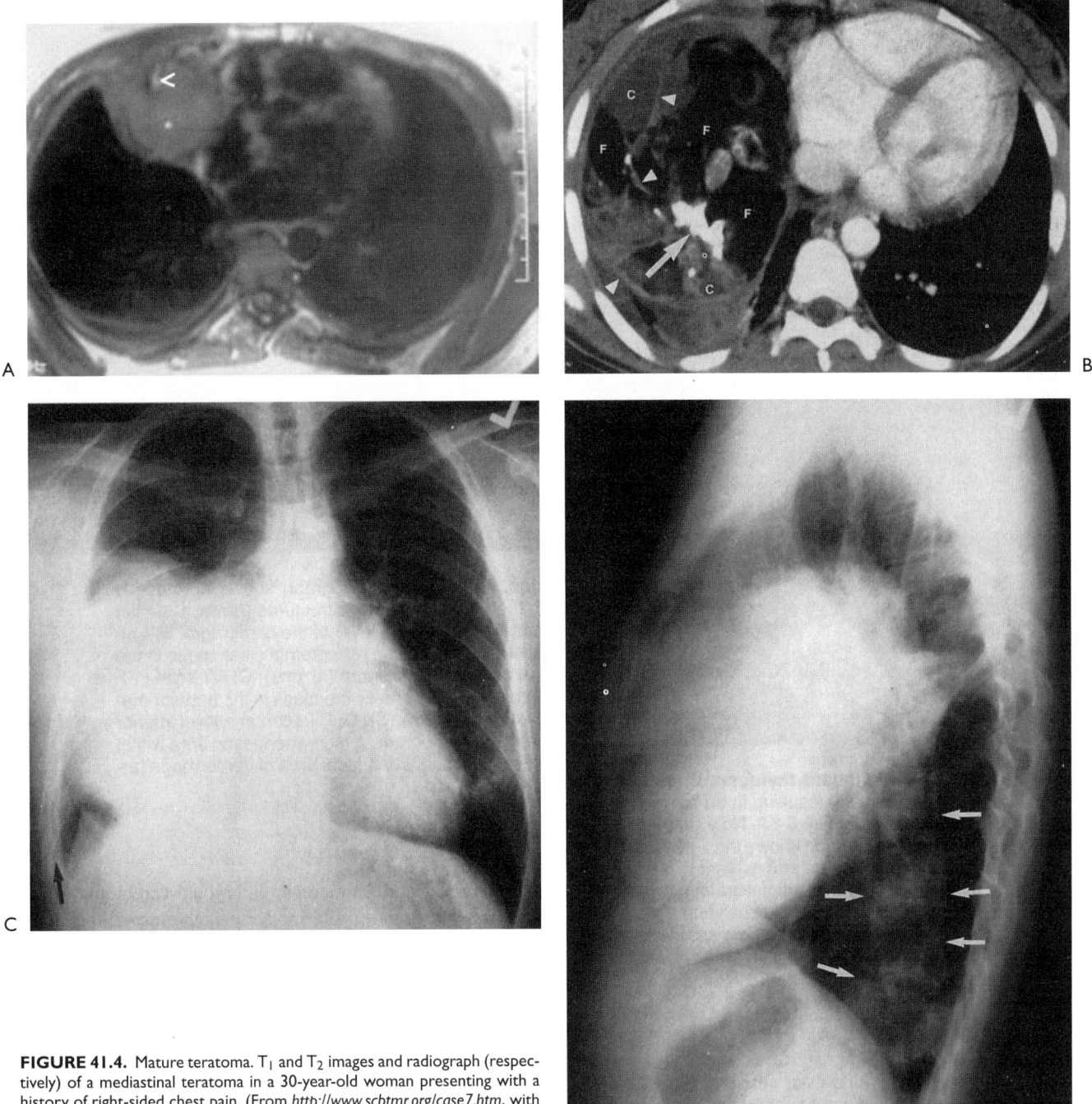

FIGURE 41.4. Mature teratoma. T$_1$ and T$_2$ images and radiograph (respectively) of a mediastinal teratoma in a 30-year-old woman presenting with a history of right-sided chest pain. (From *http://www.scbtmr.org/case7.htm*, with permission.)

9 patients (9%), and combined modality in 18 patients (17%). A favorable response to primary therapy was achieved in 92% of the patients (95% confidence interval, 87%–97%). After a median follow-up of 61 months (range, 1–211 months), 18 patients (17%) had recurrent disease: 14% of those who had received chemotherapy and 67% of those who had received radiation therapy. The 5-year progression-free survival rate favored the chemotherapy group; it was 87% for the chemotherapy group but 33% for the irradiation group (P = .006). The overall survival rates were equal (90% vs. 67%, P = .13). No differences in overall survival or progression-free survival were observed between the patients with primary retroperitoneal seminoma and those with mediastinal seminoma. Prognostic factors that appeared to influence survival negatively were liver metastases (P = .01) and two or more metastatic sites (P = .04). The study concluded that in patients with extragonadal seminoma, a survival rate of more than 90% at 5 years can be achieved

with adequate cisplatin-based chemotherapy. No difference in long-term survival was noted between patients with primary retroperitoneal or mediastinal seminomas and patients with nonseminomatous extragonadal GCTs. The study also concluded that primary radiotherapy appears to be associated with a significantly higher rate of disease recurrence, although most patients can be salvaged with subsequent chemotherapy (64).

For patients with locally advanced disease, the preferred treatment protocol involves systemic chemotherapy followed by surgical resection of residual disease. The Southwest Oncology Group performed a prospective trial of combination chemotherapy followed by surgical removal of residual disease in patients with extragonadal germ cell neoplasms (66). Cycles of vinblastine, bleomycin, and cisplatin were alternated with cycles of etoposide, bleomycin, doxorubicin, and cisplatin. Four cycles of therapy were followed by surgical removal of residual disease when appropriate: Of the 24 patients with mediastinal tumors, complete response rates (chemotherapy and surgery) were noted 18 (75%); at 2 years, the disease-free survival rate for all patients was 87%. The toxicity of the chemotherapy regimen was substantial, with neutropenic fever developing in 41% of the patients during treatment. Additional side effects included nausea and vomiting (76%), mucositis (27%), and pulmonary toxicity (5%). This prospective trial of chemotherapy in patients with extragonadal GCTs demonstrated a significant response in patients with mediastinal tumors and a 4-year survival rate of more than 60% (66).

Mediastinal Nonseminomatous Germ Cell Tumors

The nonseminomatous malignant GCTs include embryonal cell carcinomas, endodermal thymus tumors, choriocarcinomas, and mixed GCTs with heterogeneous cellular components. These malignant and frequently symptomatic tumors usually affect young men (2). They are often associated with hematologic malignancies, and 20% of patients have Klinefelter syndrome (67,68).

Clinical Findings. Eighty-five percent of patients are symptomatic at the time of diagnosis. Symptoms include chest pain, hemoptysis, cough, and fever or weight loss. The superior vena cava syndrome is occasionally seen. Gynecomastia can develop as a consequence of β-hCG secretion by these tumors (52,69).

Diagnosis. The AFP and β-hCG levels are frequently elevated (>80%). However, 10% of patients may have normal concentrations of both markers (52,69).

An elevated AFP level is highly suggestive of endodermal sinus tumor or embryonal carcinoma and is sufficient, in the presence of a mediastinal mass, to establish the diagnosis of a nonseminomatous malignant GCT (52,69).

Radiologically, these are large, irregular masses of the anterior mediastinum, often with central necrosis and hemor-

rhage or cyst formation (70). Invasion of adjacent structures and metastasis to regional lymph nodes and distant sites may occur. Pleural and pericardial effusions are common (53,70).

Treatment. Currently, the standard treatment for a primary mediastinal malignant GCT is chemotherapy. Surgical resection is indicated in the case of a residual mass, especially if the concentrations of tumor markers are normal (66).

In a single institutional experience lasting from 1993 to 1998, 20 male patients with primary nonseminomatous mediastinal GCTs were treated with intensive chemotherapy, followed by radical surgery in those who responded to the neoadjuvant regimen (71). Thirteen patients (65%) had metastatic disease at the time of presentation. Eleven patients had received no prior treatment (initial group), and nine had been referred for salvage therapy after tumor progression despite treatment at other facilities (salvage group). Preoperative chemotherapy consisted of alternating cycles of combinations of three or more drugs, including cisplatin, bleomycin, etoposide, vincristine, methotrexate, actinomycin, cyclophosphamide, and doxorubicin. An average of 10 cycles of chemotherapy was given to the patients in the initial group, and an average of six cycles to those in the salvage group. After chemotherapy, 11 patients underwent surgery, with 10 complete resections of residual mediastinal tumors. No perioperative deaths occurred. The 2-year survival was 72% in the initial group and 42% in the salvage group. The study concluded that an aggressive multidisciplinary approach of alternating cycles of chemotherapy, followed by complete surgical resection of all remaining disease in patients whose marker levels normalize, can be associated with prolonged survival in patients with primary nonseminomatous mediastinal GCTs (71).

In contrast to pure seminoma, nonseminomatous GCT carries a poor prognosis; these patients have a 5-year progression-free survival of 41% and an overall 5-year survival of 48%. Patients with mediastinal seminomas, no distant metastases, and normal serum marker levels have a 5-year progression-free survival of 82% and an overall 5-year survival of 86%. Patients with mediastinal seminomas, nonpulmonary visceral metastases, but normal serum marker levels have a 5-year progression-free survival of 67% and an overall 5-year survival of 72% (72).

Mediastinal Goiter

Mediastinal goiter is reported in 1% to 15% of patients undergoing thyroidectomy (73). Usually, it is found in the anterosuperior mediastinum. However, cervical goiters extending into the middle and posterior mediastinum behind the trachea are also seen, although infrequently. These tumors are almost always benign and are found incidentally in asymptomatic women with a palpable cervical goiter. Virtually all patients with mediastinal goiter are euthyroid. Occasionally, patients present with symptoms such as local fullness, choking, stridor, or dysphagia.

Radiologically, mediastinal goiters are encapsulated, lobulated, heterogeneous tumors (2). The diagnostic radiologic feature on chest CT is continuity between the cervical and mediastinal components of the thyroid. The mass typically shows intense enhancement with intravenous contrast. If the goiter contains functional thyroid tissue, scintigraphy with a radioactive isotope of iodine (^{131}I or ^{123}I) can be diagnostic (2). Surgical resection is now favored for both symptomatic and asymptomatic patients with substernal goiter.

The conclusion of the University of Michigan Medical Center experience of 872 thyroidectomies performed between 1972 and 1982 was that a substernal goiter is in itself an indication for operation (74). In this study, 50 patients (5.7%) were found to have substernal goiters, 42 of which were benign and 8 (16%) malignant. Symptoms included airway compression (22 patients), dysphagia (13 patients), hoarseness (4 patients), weight loss (3 patients), and thyrotoxicosis (10 patients). Five patients with symptoms of compression, four of whom had benign disease, had superior vena cava syndrome. Most of the patients were elderly women (mean age, 66 years; female-to-male ratio, 3.2:1) with long-standing goiters (mean duration, 16 years). All but one operation was performed through a cervical incision. No intraoperative deaths occurred. Complications were pneumonia (1 patient), wound hematoma (1 patient), transient hypocalcemia (2 patients), and atrial fibrillation (2 patients) (74).

Based on this experience, a rationale for operative management was developed: (a) No other treatment is available for large multinodular goiters of long duration; (b) treatment with ^{131}I, the alternative to operation for patients with large thyrotoxic goiters, can precipitate acute reactions in the elderly that can result in respiratory distress; (c) a long history of a large multinodular goiter precludes neither malignancy, hyperfunction, nor complications such as tracheal or esophageal compression; (d) malignancy develops in a significant number of these lesions, which are inaccessible to needle biopsy; (e) nearly all substernal goiters can be removed through a cervical incision (74).

Mediastinal Parathyroid Adenoma

The mediastinum is the most frequent location for ectopic parathyroid tumors. Overall, approximately 20% of parathyroid tumors originate in the mediastinum (75). Most mediastinal parathyroid tumors (80%) are in the anterior mediastinum, although some (20%) are in the superoposterior mediastinum. (Mediastinal parathyroid adenomas are most commonly found in older women who continue to have manifestations of hyperparathyroidism despite cervical parathyroidectomy.)

These tumors are encapsulated, round, small (<3 cm) structures that frequently escape detection on chest radiography and contrast-enhanced CT. Their appearance on CT can resemble that of a normal lymph node (2). MRI can detect abnormal parathyroid tissue in the majority of cases. The characteristic appearance of parathyroid adenomas on MRI involves increased signal intensity on T_2-weighted and gadolinium-enhanced T_1-weighted images (76). Parathyroid adenomas can also be diagnosed by the uptake of radioactive ^{99m}Tc and ^{201}Ti. ^{99m}Tc is more sensitive than ^{201}Ti in detecting parathyroid adenomas (77).

Primary Mediastinal Lymphoma

Lymphoma is one of the most common mediastinal neoplasms and may be found in any mediastinal compartment. Most thoracic lymphomas, however, develop in the anterior mediastinum. Primary mediastinal lymphoma is rather uncommon, accounting for fewer than 10% of mediastinal lymphomas in adults. More frequently, mediastinal lymphoma occurs as a part of Hodgkin disease (50%–70%) or non-Hodgkin lymphoma (15%–25%) (78,79).

The nodular sclerosing subtype of Hodgkin disease is the most common variant to affect the thymus and other structures of the anterior mediastinum. The other subtypes of Hodgkin disease typically do not involve the mediastinum (80). The two variants of non-Hodgkin lymphoma that most often involve the anterior mediastinum are B-cell lymphoma and lymphoblastic lymphoma (80).

Hodgkin Disease (Lymphoma)

Hodgkin disease in the mediastinum is usually of the nodular sclerosing variety, which occurs most commonly in young women (female-to-male ratio, 2:1) predominantly in the third and fourth decades of life (81).

Clinical Findings
The majority of patients with Hodgkin disease present with constitutional (B) symptoms such as fever, night sweats, and weight loss. Local symptoms secondary to compression of the adjacent viscera are infrequent but may include pain, stridor, dyspnea, and superior vena cava syndrome. Pleural effusion frequently accompanies mediastinal Hodgkin disease (81).

Pathology
The pathologic hallmark of mediastinal Hodgkin disease is the classic Reed-Sternberg cell, which has bilobed nuclei containing prominent eosinophilic nuclei. The characteristic immunohistochemical profile is positivity of the cells for CD15 and CD30, and negativity for keratin effectively excludes thymoma (82).

Diagnosis
The chest radiographic findings are abnormal in 67% to 76% of patients with Hodgkin disease, often showing enlargement of the prevascular and paratracheal nodes (83–85). Direct invasion of the lung may occur in 12% of patients

with Hodgkin disease and is almost always associated with hilar adenopathy (85). Evidence of thoracic lymph node involvement is found on the chest CT scan in 71% to 85% of patients with Hodgkin disease. The lymph nodes appear as rounded soft tissue masses, either separate or coalescent (80). Mediastinal visceral and vascular invasion is well delineated by CT. Fibrotic scar after therapy of bulky Hodgkin disease may be difficult to distinguish from residual disease on CT. In these situations, tumor may be differentiated from fibrosis on T_2-weighted MRI by the presence of increased signal intensity in comparison with baseline (83).

Treatment

The modified (Cotswold) Ann Arbor staging system for Hodgkin disease anatomically distinguishes patients who may benefit from radiation alone from those who require both chemotherapy and external beam radiation (86). Patients with surgical stage I or II nonbulky tumors can be treated with radiation alone. Patients with bulky disease or disease requiring extensive radiation of normal tissue are treated with chemotherapy followed by radiation therapy (86). Patients with stages III and IV Hodgkin disease receive chemotherapy, occasionally in combination with radiation. For patients with large mediastinal masses, radiation after chemotherapy is favored by most experts (86).

In a randomized multicenter trial, three regimens of primary systemic therapy for newly diagnosed advanced Hodgkin disease in stages IIIA2, IIIB, and IVA or IVB were compared: (a) MOPP (mechlorethamine, oncovin [vincristine], procarbazine, prednisone) alone for 6 to 8 cycles, (b) MOPP alternating with ABVD (adriamycin [doxorubicin], bleomycin, vinblastine, dacarbazine) for 12 cycles, and (c) ABVD alone for 6 to 8 cycles (87). Patients in a first relapse after radiation therapy were eligible. No additional radiation therapy was given. Patients who did not have a complete response or who had a relapse with either MOPP alone or ABVD alone were switched to the opposite regimen. Of 361 eligible patients, 123 received MOPP, 123 received MOPP alternating with ABVD, and 115 received ABVD alone. The patients were stratified according to age, stage, previous radiation, histologic features, and performance status. The overall response rate was 93%, with complete responses in 77%: 67% in the MOPP group, 82% in the ABVD group, and 83% in the MOPP-ABVD group ($P = .006$ for the comparison of MOPP with the other two regimens, both of which contained doxorubicin). The rates of failure-free survival at 5 years were 50% for MOPP, 61% for ABVD, and 65% for MOPP-ABVD. Age, stage (III vs. IV), and regimen influenced failure-free survival significantly. Overall survival at 5 years was 66% for MOPP, 73% for ABVD, and 75% for MOPP-ABVD ($P = .28$ for the comparison of MOPP with the doxorubicin regimens). MOPP had more severe toxic effects on bone marrow than ABVD and was associated with greater reductions in the prescribed dose. The conclusions of this trial were as follows: ABVD therapy for 6 to 8 months was as effective as

12 months of MOPP alternating with ABVD, and both were superior to MOPP alone in the treatment of advanced Hodgkin disease. ABVD was less myelotoxic than MOPP or ABVD alternating with MOPP (87).

Prognosis

Patients in stage IA and IIA have cure rates of more than 90% with radiation alone. Patients in stage IIIA have a cure rate of 30% to 90% with chemotherapy and radiation therapy. Patients in stage IIIB have a cure rate of 60% to 70%, and those in stage IV have a cure rate of 50% to 60% (80,86). Hodgkin disease ultimately recurs in half of the patients; however, recurrent disease is still potentially curable (86,87).

In a trial sponsored by the National Cancer Institute, 107 patients with Hodgkin disease relapsing after combination chemotherapy were studied (88). The purpose of the study was to evaluate clinical prognostic factors, the probability of response to therapy, the duration of the response, and the overall survival of patients with Hodgkin disease relapsing after a chemotherapy-induced complete remission. Results were as follows: Half of the relapses occurred within the first year after complete remission had been achieved; of patients in remission 5 years or longer, only 4% relapsed. The overall survival of patients with relapse was projected to be 17% at 20 years. The primary treatment regimen, presence of B symptoms, stage, sex, liver involvement, pleural involvement, marrow involvement, and histologic subtype did not affect the survival of patients with relapse. Only the age at diagnosis (older or younger than 30 years) and length of initial remission (shorter or longer than 1 year) had a significant effect on survival. Patients whose initial remission was longer than 1 year had significantly higher complete response rates to salvage therapy, significantly more durable second remissions, and significantly longer survival rates than patients whose initial remission was shorter than 1 year. Patients with a long initial remission had an 85% complete response rate to MOPP, with a disease-free survival rate of 45% at 20 years. Acute leukemia and other treatment-related complications lowered the survival rate in this subset (88).

In an outcome study of 115 patients with refractory or relapsed disease among 415 patients treated with alternating or hybrid MOPP-ABVD followed by radiotherapy (25–30 Gy) to initial bulky sites (median follow-up, 91 months), 39 (34%) of the 115 patients had disease progression while on primary treatment (induction failures), 48 relapsed after complete remissions that lasted 12 months or less, and 28 relapsed after complete remissions that lasted more than 12 months after the end of all treatments (89). At 8 years, the overall survival rate was 27%; it was 54% in patients whose initial complete remission was longer than 12 months, 28% in patients whose initial complete remission was shorter than 12 months, and 8% in patients who failed induction therapy ($P < .001$). The response to first-line chemotherapy and the extent of disease at first progression significantly influenced the long-term results and the incidence and duration of complete remission. The study confirmed the previous observations that the main prognostic factors after salvage treatment are duration of the response to first-line therapy and extent of disease at relapse. The results indicated that the prognosis of patients with relapse after the alternating MOPP-ABVD regimen is similar to that of patients with relapse after a four-drug regimen (MOPP or ABVD alone). Re-treatment with initial chemotherapy appears to be the treatment of choice for patients who relapse after an initial complete remission that lasts longer than 12 months, whereas the real effect of high-dose chemotherapy or new regimens should be assessed in patients with resistant disease (89).

Non-Hodgkin Lymphoma

Mediastinal non-Hodgkin lymphoma is one of the malignant tumors most frequently affecting the mediastinum. Because 98% of mediastinal non-Hodgkin lymphomas are of lymphocyte origin, they often referred to as *mediastinal lymphocytic lymphomas* (90). Overall, non-Hodgkin lymphoma is more common in males and whites than in females and blacks, and it affects all age groups, from childhood through 80 years. The mean age at the time of diagnosis for all patients with non-Hodgkin lymphoma is approximately 55 years (90). In contrast, the median age of patients with primary mediastinal large B-cell lymphoma is 35 years, and that of patients with lymphoblastic lymphoma is 28 years. The majority of these patients present with advanced disease, evidenced by generalized lymphadenopathy, constitutional symptoms, and extensive extranodal involvement. Large B-cell lymphomas tend to affect more females than males. Occasionally, rapidly growing mediastinal masses cause acute obstructive pathology, including superior vena cava syndrome (80) (Fig. 41.5).

Lymphoblastic lymphoma affects adolescents and young adults, and a marked preponderance of male patients has

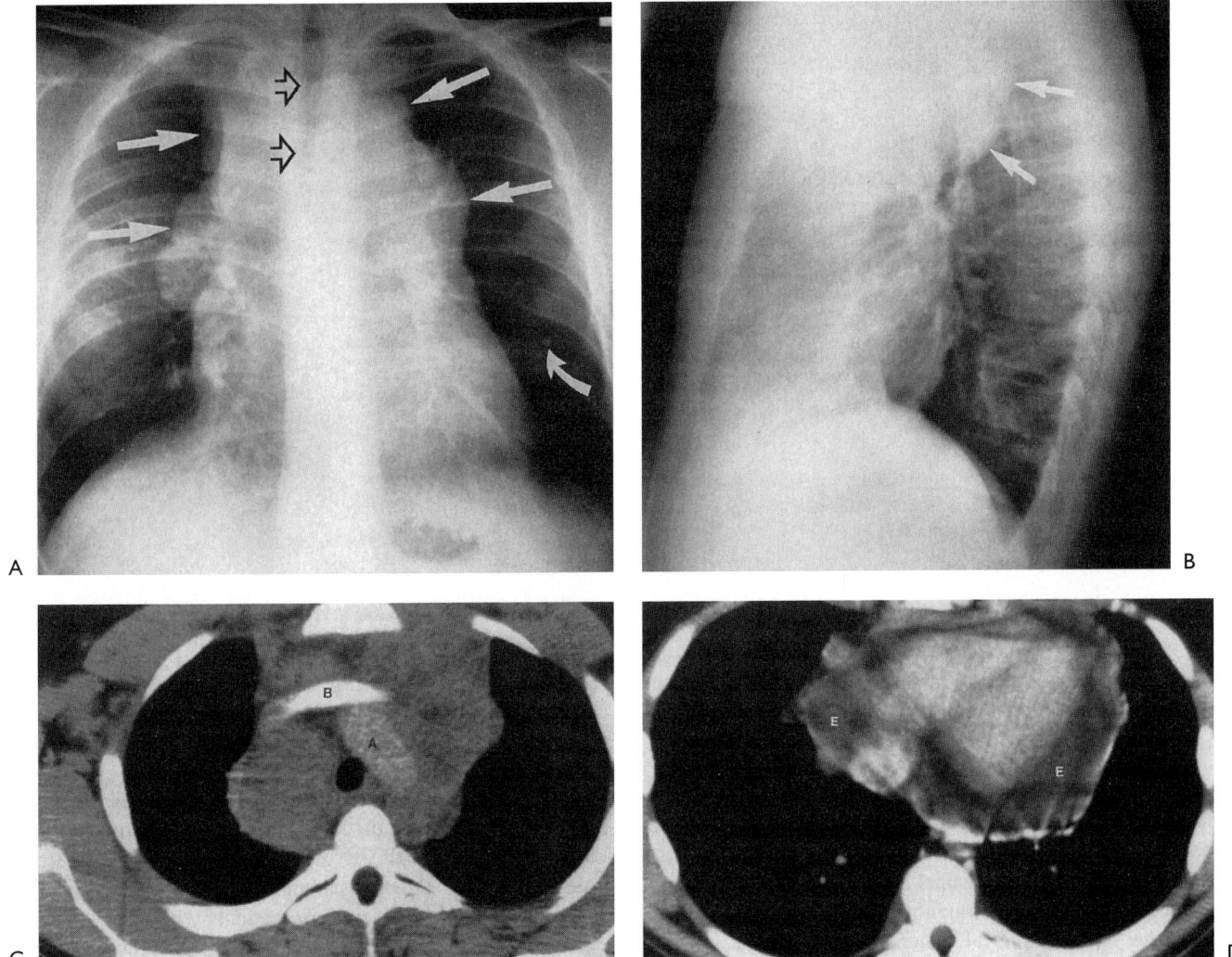

FIGURE 41.5. Chest radiograph and computed tomographic images of an 11-year-old boy with a large lymphoma of the anterior mediastinum causing tracheal and vascular compression. (From *http://home.kimo.com.tw/2chiu/dd-mediastinaltumor.html*, with permission.)

been noted. It is a rather aggressive, high-grade lymphoma. Progression to acute lymphocytic leukemia is a frequent phenomenon (90).

Diagnosis

Chest CT is critical in delineating the extent of disease and compromise of the surrounding structures (Fig. 41.5). The middle and posterior mediastinal lymph nodes tend to be involved more often than the anterior mediastinal nodes (80). The initial diagnosis of non-Hodgkin lymphoma usually requires an excisional lymph node biopsy for precise classification; this is often achieved via transcervical mediastinoscopy or a paramedian sternotomy (Chamberlain procedure) (91). Mediastinal non-Hodgkin lymphoma can also be diagnosed via transthoracic or transbronchoscopic fine needle aspiration or core needle biopsy. A definitive and specific diagnosis of mediastinal non-Hodgkin lymphoma should be made with the assistance of flow cytometry and cytogenetic analysis (91).

Treatment

The current therapy for mediastinal non-Hodgkin lymphoma depends on the stage, histologic subtype, and extent of disease (Fig. 41.6). In a retrospective analysis of 177 patients with stage I (n = 73, 41%) and stage II (n = 104, 59%) follicular small cleaved cell and follicular mixed small cleaved cell and large cell non-Hodgkin lymphoma treated at Stanford University between 1961 and 1994, the data were as follows (92): The histology was follicular small cleaved cell

lymphoma in 101 (57%) of the cases and follicular mixed small cleaved cell and large cell lymphoma in 76 (43%) of the cases. Forty-five (25%) of the patients underwent a staging laparotomy; 34 (19%) had extranodal involvement. All patients had received radiotherapy, either to one side of the diaphragm (involved or extended field) or to both sides (total lymphoid irradiation or subtotal lymphoid irradiation). The doses of radiotherapy ranged from 35 to 50 Gy. The results were as follows: The median follow-up was 7.7 years. The longest follow-up was 31 years. The actuarial survival rates at 5, 10, 15, and 20 years were 82%, 64%, 44%, and 35%, respectively. The median survival time was 13.8 years. At 5, 10, 15, and 20 years, 55%, 44%, 40%, and 37% of the patients, respectively, were free of relapse. Recurrence later developed in only 5 of the 47 patients who had reached 10 years without relapse. Rates of survival and freedom from relapse were significantly worse for older patients. Relapse rates were lower following treatment on both sides of the diaphragm or staging laparotomy. Univariate analysis showed that youth and staging laparotomy were associated with significantly better survival, and that the rate of freedom from relapse was better following treatment on both sides of the diaphragm or laparotomy. From these observations, it was concluded that radiotherapy is the treatment of choice for early-stage low-grade follicular lymphomas and that patients who remain free of disease for 10 years are unlikely to relapse (92).

In a long-term follow-up of 66 patients with stage III follicular lymphoma treated with primary radiotherapy (total

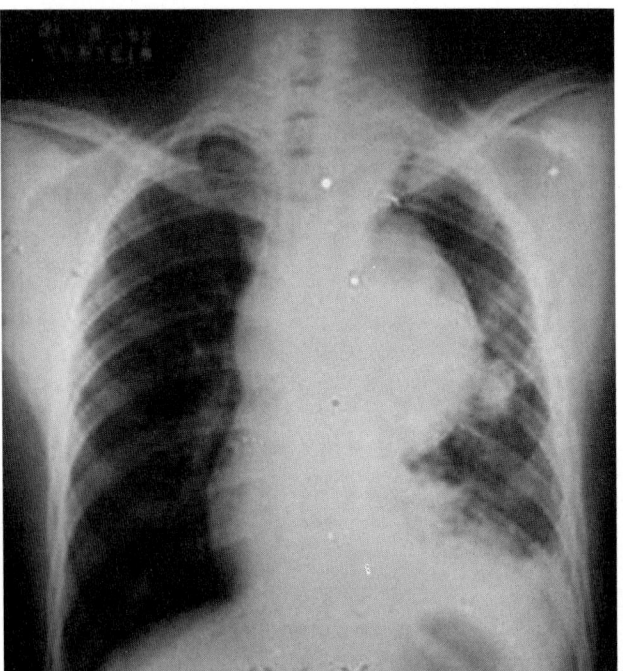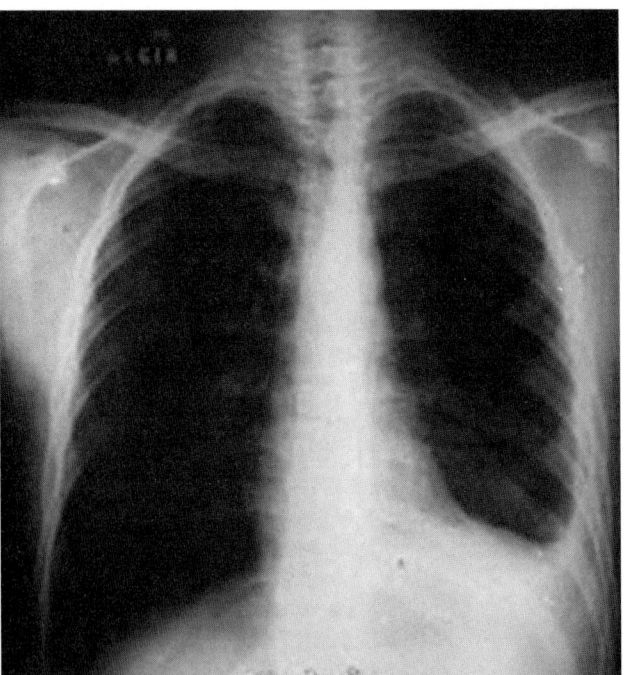

A   B

FIGURE 41.6. Chest radiographs of a malignant mediastinal lymphoma before and after treatment demonstrating dramatic reduction in size of the mediastinal mass and parenchymal nodules in the left lung. (From *http://home.kimo.com.tw/2chiu/dd-mediastinaltumor.html*, with permission.)

lymphoid irradiation in 61 patients and whole-body irradiation in five patients) at Stanford University, of whom 13 received adjuvant chemotherapy, median overall survival, cause-specific survival, freedom from relapse, and event-free survival were 9.5, 18.9, 7.1, and 5.1 years, respectively (93). Age of the patient and the number of diseased sites were the two strongest predictors of overall survival. Patients with limited stage III disease had an 88% rate of freedom from relapse and a 100% rate of cause-specific survival during up to 23.5 years of follow-up. These data are comparable with those for other modalities in the treatment of stage III follicular lymphoma (93).

Persistent or recurrent disease is common. It is usually treated with a combination of chemotherapy and radiation therapy. Bone marrow transplantation may improve survival (83). Large B-cell lymphoma is potentially curable (80,83). Patients with lymphoblastic lymphoma, when treated aggressively, can have long-term disease-free survival (80).

Mediastinal Cysts

Collectively, congenital cysts account for approximately 20% of mediastinal masses (4). The incidence of mediastinal cysts is the same in children and adults. However, mediastinal cysts are more often symptomatic in children because compression of the tracheobronchial tree and esophagus is more likely in a small mediastinum. Conversely, mediastinal cysts in adults are often incidental radiographic findings.

Congenital cysts of the foregut are the most common type of mediastinal cyst. Bronchogenic cysts account for 50% to 70% of all mediastinal cysts, and enterogenous cysts account for 7% to 15%. The remaining 20% of foregut cysts are nonspecific in terms of histologic features. Foregut cysts are classified according to their histologic features rather than their location. Bronchogenic cysts are lined with respiratory epithelium, whereas enterogenous cysts, which arise from the dorsal foregut, histologically resemble the alimentary tract. Foregut cysts affect male and female subjects equally. Although most adults are asymptomatic, symptoms, usually of an obstructive nature, eventually develop in two thirds (80).

Bronchogenic Cysts

Bronchogenic cysts account for 60% of all mediastinal cysts. They are lined with ciliated, pseudostratified, columnar (respiratory) epithelium and contain bronchial glands and cartilaginous plates. Bronchogenic cysts may become filled with serous fluid, mucus, pus, "milk of calcium," and blood (80). Progressively enlarging bronchogenic cysts can compress the airway and cause cough, dyspnea, and wheezing. Complications such as infection and rupture into bronchus, pericardium, or pleura are uncommon.

On radiographic studies, bronchogenic cysts are usually spherical, homogeneous, well-marginated masses measuring from 2 to 10 cm in diameter and typically located in the paratracheal or subcarinal regions. Occasionally, air-fluid levels are seen within the cysts on chest CT and are a consequence of communication with the tracheobronchial tree. Bronchogenic cysts are characteristically nonenhancing on contrast CT. MRI is of some assistance in the diagnosis of bronchogenic cysts and can distinguish them from other mediastinal lesions.

After initial radiographic studies, a presumptive diagnosis of bronchogenic cyst can be established by tracheobronchial, endoscopic, or thoracoscopic needle aspiration of the cyst to obtain mucus and bronchial epithelium. Foregut cysts are generally treated with complete surgical excision, whether or not they are causing symptoms, to prevent future complications (80). Bronchoscopic or thoracoscopic needle drainage offers a palliative alternative for poor surgical candidates. The prognosis of patients with surgically excised cysts is excellent, although bronchogenic cysts can recur locally if incompletely resected. On occasion, asymptomatic patients with bronchogenic cysts may be followed without any intervention.

Enterogenous Cysts

Enterogenous cysts arise from the dorsal foregut and are lined by squamous or enteric (alimentary) epithelium. They may contain gastric mucosa and pancreatic tissue. Esophageal duplication cysts are located in or are attached to the esophageal wall. Twelve percent of patients with esophageal duplication cysts have associated malformations, mostly of the gastrointestinal tract (94).

Esophageal duplication cysts may produce compressive symptoms in children. Secretions of gastric mucosal and pancreatic tissue in the cyst can cause hemorrhage or rupture of the cyst.

Radiologically, enterogenous cysts closely resemble bronchogenic cysts except for the presence of calcifications, which can be seen in esophageal duplication cysts. The management of esophageal cysts is similar to that of bronchogenic cysts, with surgical excision the primary treatment modality. Simple cysts are enucleated, whereas duplication cysts are excised. Previously, a posterolateral thoracotomy was required to remove simple or duplication cysts; however, thoracoscopy is currently used to enucleate cysts and resect duplications and is the procedure of choice (95).

Neuroenteric Cysts

Neuroenteric cysts are characterized by the presence of both enteric and neural tissue in surgical specimens (96). The vast majority of neuroenteric cysts form in the posterior mediastinum above the level of the main carina. The close proximity of foregut and notochord during embryogenesis possibly explains this anatomic location. Neuroenteric cysts are associated with multiple vertebral anomalies, such as scoliosis, spina bifida, hemivertebra, butterfly vertebrae, and vertebral fusion. Neuroenteric cysts are more common in boys than in girls, and almost all are discovered by the age of 1 year as symptoms of tracheobronchial compression develop (80). Neurologic symptoms are also caused by intraspinal extension.

The radiographic appearance of neuroenteric cysts is very similar to that of bronchogenic and esophageal duplication cysts, although the anatomic location is often different. Contrast-enhanced MRI of the thorax is invaluable in the assessment of intraspinal extension. The management of neuroenteric cysts is complete surgical excision (97).

Pericardial Cysts

Pericardial cysts are uncommon. They are generally thin-walled and lined with mesothelial cells arising from the pericardium. For the most part, they are considered to be congenital; however, some may be acquired (80). They are almost always asymptomatic and are identified in the fourth to fifth decade of life. Rarely, symptoms of hemodynamic compromise develop in association with cardiac compression (82). Radiographically, pericardial cysts are well-marginated spherical or teardrop-shaped masses that characteristically abut the heart, anterior chest wall, and diaphragm (80). They usually measure 5 to 8 cm in diameter. The most common site of these cysts is the right cardiophrenic angle (70%), followed by the left cardiophrenic angle (22%) (98). The CT appearance of a pericardial cyst is typically that of a unilocular, nonenhancing mass.

Asymptomatic pericardial cysts are generally followed clinically. Cysts that have an atypical radiographic appearance or are producing symptoms are resected to exclude cystic mediastinal tumors and foregut cysts.

Neurogenic Tumors

Neurogenic tumors arise from tissue of neural crest origin, including cells of the peripheral, autonomic, and paraganglionic nervous systems. They are classified on the basis of cell type (e.g., nerve sheath, ganglionic, neuroblastoma) and comprise approximately 12% to 21% of all mediastinal tumors (99). Ninety-five percent of mediastinal neurogenic tumors occur in the posterior compartment (99). In infants and adults, 50% to 75% of posterior mediastinal neoplasms are neurogenic, whereas in older children, lymphoma is the most common tumor of the posterior mediastinum. From 70% to 80% of neurogenic tumors are benign, and approximately 50% cause no symptoms (100,101).

Nerve Sheath Tumors

These benign, slowly growing tumors comprise 40% to 65% of neurogenic mediastinal masses. They are often asymp-

tomatic and discovered incidentally in men and women in the third or fourth decade of life. Neurilemomas or schwannomas constitute 75% of this group. Grossly, the tumors appear as firm and encapsulated masses, and on histologic sectioning, they consist of Schwann cells. In contrast to neurilemomas, neurofibromas are nonencapsulated, soft, and often friable. They constitute 20% to 25% of nerve sheath tumors and are associated with Von Recklinghausen neurofibromatosis (102,103).

Radiographically, neurilemomas and neurofibromas appear as sharply marginated spherical or lobulated masses in the paraspinal region. They can cause pressure erosion and deformity of the ribs and vertebral bodies. Low attenuation on CT indicates hypocellularity, cystic changes, and hemorrhage and lipid within myelin (80).

Ten percent of neurilemomas and neurofibromas grow through the adjacent intervertebral foramina and extend into the spinal canal in a dumbbell or hourglass configuration (104). Ninety percent of dumbbell tumors originate from nerve sheath cells and are benign (99). MRI is extremely useful to rule out intraspinal extension.

Complete surgical resection via video thoracoscopy or thoracotomy is the treatment of choice. If complete resection cannot be performed, postoperative radiation or chemotherapy may be indicated. Potential postoperative neurologic complications resulting from the resection of nerve sheath tumors include Horner syndrome, partial sympathectomy, recurrent laryngeal nerve injury, and paraplegia (99).

Malignant Tumors of Nerve Sheath Origin

Malignant nerve sheath tumors are a group of rare spindle cell sarcomas of the posterior mediastinum; they include malignant neurofibromas, malignant schwannomas, and neurogenic fibrosarcomas. They affect men and women equally in the third to fifth decade of life and are closely associated with neurofibromatosis. Of note, the incidence of sarcomatous degeneration in patients with neurofibromatosis is approximately 5% (105). Pain and nerve deficits are common heralding symptoms. The optimal treatment approach is surgical; postoperative radiation or chemotherapy is administered to patients with unresectable tumors.

Autonomic Ganglionic Tumors

Tumors of the autonomic nervous system arise from neuronal cells rather than cells of the nerve sheath. They form a continuum ranging from benign encapsulated ganglioneuroma to aggressive malignant nonencapsulated neuroblastoma. Tumors arise in both the sympathetic ganglia and the adrenal glands, but ganglioneuromas and ganglioneuroblastomas arise mostly in the sympathetic ganglia of the posterior mediastinum (106). Fifty percent of neuroblastomas arise in the adrenal glands and up to 30% in the mediastinum (106,107).

Ganglioneuroma

Ganglioneuromas are composed of one or more mature ganglionic cells. They appear as homogeneous, elongated, encapsulated masses (80). Two thirds of the patients are younger than 20 years of age. Half of them are asymptomatic (108). Symptoms are caused mainly by compression or intraspinal tumor extension.

Radiographically, the tumors appear as oblong, well-marginated masses, usually along the anterolateral aspect of the spine. They typically span between three and five vertebrae (108). On chest CT, a ganglioneuroma can manifest as either a homogeneous or heterogeneous mass. MRI is useful in delineating the extent of intraspinal tumors (109). Complete surgical resection is the treatment of choice.

Ganglioneuroblastoma

Ganglioneuroblastomas have histologic features of both ganglioneuromas and neuroblastomas. They are the least common type of neurogenic tumor. The prognosis depends on the exact histologic appearance, and the tumors may produce catecholamines (80). Ganglioneuroblastomas affect both sexes equally in the first decade of life (110). A large tumor size, intraspinal extension, and metastasis can lead to symptoms. Ganglioneuroblastoma and neuroblastoma are staged and managed in similar fashion, as described in the next section.

Neuroblastoma

Neuroblastomas are neoplasms comprised of small round cells arranged in sheets or pseudorosettes (111). They are nonencapsulated lesions, often exhibiting hemorrhage, necrosis, or cystic degeneration. Ninety percent of neuroblastomas occur in children younger than 5 years of age (107,112). The majority of patients in whom a neuroblastoma is diagnosed have symptoms, usually caused by distant metastases. These may include pain, neurologic deficits, Horner syndrome, respiratory distress, and ataxia (111,112). Neuroblastomas, more than ganglioneuroblastomas and ganglioneuromas, can produce catecholamines and vasoactive intestinal peptides that cause hypertension, flushing, and diarrhea (106). The detection of homovanillic acid and vanillylmandelic acid (catecholamine by-products) in the urine can be helpful for diagnosis and follow-up after treatment (106).

Grossly, a neuroblastoma appears as an elongated paraspinous mass, sometimes impinging on adjacent structures and causing skeletal damage (113,114). On CT, 80% of these tumors have various types of calcification (e.g., cloudlike, stippled, ring-shaped, solid) (114). MRI can delineate intraspinal extension and invasion of other adjacent structures (109). Radionuclide imaging with [^{123}I]MIBG (metaiodobenzylguanidine) can also be used to detect primary and metastatic neuroblastoma (115).

Neuroblastomas and ganglioneuroblastomas are staged as follows:

Stage	Characteristic
Stage I	Well-circumscribed, noninvasive ipsilateral tumors
Stage II	Local invasion without extension across the midline, ipsilateral regional lymph node involvement, or both
Stage III	Tumor extension across the midline and involvement of bilateral regional lymph nodes
Stage IV	Metastatic disease
Stage IV S	Clinical stage I or II and metastatic disease limited to the liver, skin, and bone marrow.

The treatment of choice for patients with limited-stage neuroblastoma and ganglioneuroblastoma is complete resection. For patients with stage I disease, resection is usually curative. For patients with stage II and III disease, every effort should be made to resect the tumor completely. In cases of residual disease secondary to incomplete resection, chemotherapy and radiation therapy are used. Poor prognostic factors in neuroblastoma include large tumor size, poorly differentiated cell type, advanced stage, extrathoracic origin, and presentation in an elderly patient (103). Intraspinal tumor extension does not portend a poor prognosis (116).

Paraganglionic Tumors

Paraganglionic tumors can arise from sympathetic or parasympathetic cells. They may be biologically inactive (e.g., chemodectoma arising from nonchromaffin cells) (99).

Peripheral Neurogenic Tumors

These tumors often have features similar to those of Ewing sarcoma and rhabdomyosarcoma. They are thought to have a neuroectodermal or neuroendocrine origin. Tumors occurring in the thoracic-pulmonary region in children are called *Askin tumors* (99).

TUMORS OF THE PLEURA

A vast majority of the tumors found in the pleura are metastatic, usually arising from the lung or breast, or are lymphomatous in origin. Benign primary tumors rarely arise from the pleura; these include lipomas, endotheliomas, and cysts. Tumors of the pleura are usually detected during plain radiography or CT of the chest. The diagnosis is established in the appropriate clinical setting with or without biopsy/resection. Mesothelioma is the most important tumor of the pleura and is discussed here in detail.

Solitary Fibrous Tumor of the Pleura ("Benign Mesothelioma")

Solitary fibrous tumors of the pleura, often called *benign mesotheliomas*, are believed to arise from submesothelial fibroblasts. They can arise from the pleura, peritoneum, and tunica vaginalis testis (117). Solitary fibrous tumors are not associated with asbestos exposure. They can arise in any age group, although the peak incidence is in the fourth to sixth decade. In stark contrast to malignant mesotheliomas, solitary fibrous tumors more often affect women; the female-to-male ratio is 2:1 (118).

Grossly, these tumors are well circumscribed, partially encapsulated, and attached to the mesothelial surface of organs by a thin strip of tissue on a stalk that contains hypertrophic arteries and veins. Occasionally, calcification, hemorrhage, or central necrosis is present (119). Approximately 80% of solitary fibrous tumors of the pleura originate on the visceral pleural surface (117). They vary considerably in size, ranging from 2-cm nodules to large masses 30 cm in diameter. Some reports have described solitary fibrous tumors involving the entire pleural cavity and hemithorax (118).

Histologically, these neoplasms are composed of bland, spindle-shaped cells and show a wide range of cellular density and vascularity (120). They are fibrocellular or sarcomatous in character. Occasionally, a component of epithelium-like cells is observed in a papillary pattern with minimal nuclear pleomorphism and no mitoses. Ultrastructural analysis reveals both fibroblasts and mesothelial cells (117).

Solitary fibrous tumors are usually asymptomatic at presentation and found serendipitously on routine roentgenography. However, some patients present with symptoms caused by enlarging masses, metabolic abnormalities, and paraneoplastic syndromes. Large pleural tumors can give rise to pain and a wide spectrum of symptoms and conditions, such as progressive dyspnea, atelectasis, pneumonia, and superior vena cava syndrome (117).

Several paraneoplastic syndromes have been noted in patients with solitary fibrous tumors, especially larger growths. Manifestations of hypoglycemia may be secondary to tumor production of insulin-like growth factors (IGF-1, IGF-2), or hyponatremia may be caused by the ectopic production of antidiuretic hormone (119). In approximately 25% of patients with solitary fibrous tumors of the pleura, extrathoracic signs are seen, such as pulmonary hypertrophic osteoarthropathy and digital clubbing. The affected long bones show periosteal proliferation and new subperiosteal bone formation. These systemic signs and symptoms typically resolve after resection of the solitary fibrous tumor.

Most solitary fibrous tumors should be removed surgically. Plain radiography, CT, and MRI are all usable options to visualize and delineate the extent of tumor before resection. If solitary fibrous tumors are resected before extensive intrathoracic or intra-abdominal growth occurs, the complete cure rate is high (117). These tumors cause death only in cases of late diagnosis or unresectable recurrence. The best indicator of a good prognosis is a pedicle supporting the tumor. Local recurrence has been reported as long as 17 years after surgery (119).

Malignant Mesothelioma

Mesotheliomas are neoplasms arising from the serosal membranes of the body cavities, including pleura, peritoneum, pericardium, tunica vaginalis testis, and ovarian epithelium. They are often insidious in presentation and refractory to therapy. Eighty percent of mesotheliomas originate in the pleural space, and malignant mesothelioma is the most common primary tumor of the pleural cavity. Mesotheliomas are generally classified as diffuse malignant, localized benign, or localized malignant. Ten percent of localized mesotheliomas are malignant, but these tumors are often low-grade and potentially resectable (118,121). Diffuse mesotheliomas account for the vast majority of primary pleural tumors.

Etiology

Eighty percent of malignant mesotheliomas are caused by the inhalation of asbestos. In rare cases, mesothelioma has been associated with exposure to other inorganic etiologic factors, such as the silicate zeolite in Turkey (122), the inhalation of organic fibers of sugar cane in Louisiana, human infection with simian virus-40, and radiation therapy. Familial clustering of malignant mesothelioma supports the possibility of a genetic predisposition (oncogenes, tumor suppresser genes) (123).

Epidemiology

In the United States, an estimated 2,500 cases are diagnosed annually, which represents a steady rise in the past decade. The incidence is also increasing worldwide. The male-to-female ratio for this disease is 5:1 (122).

Pathology

Early-stage malignant mesothelioma appears as many small gray nodules on the surface of the parietal pleura, often in association with a pleural effusion. Later stages are characterized by diffuse involvement of the visceral and parietal pleura. The tumor eventually encases the entire lung with a layer of malignant tissue that has a thickness of several centimeters. Areas of necrosis and hemorrhage are often seen. The tumor frequently invades the chest wall and mediastinum, eventually involving the contralateral hemithorax. The gross appearance of diffuse malignant mesothelioma is often indistinguishable from that of metastatic adenocarcinoma of the pleura (122,124,125).

Malignant mesothelioma is typically classified into three histologic subtypes—epithelial, sarcomatoid, and biphasic. Patients with epithelial mesothelioma have a significantly better prognosis than those with the sarcomatoid and biphasic forms (122). Ultrastructural analysis with electron microscopy has traditionally been considered the gold standard for the diagnosis of malignant mesothelioma. Well-differentiated epithelial mesotheliomas are characterized by the presence of long, thin, "bushy" microvilli over much of the free cell surface, in addition to prominent desmosomes and numerous tonofilaments.

Clinical Presentation

Malignant pleural mesothelioma most commonly presents in the fifth to seventh decade of life, reflecting the 20- to 40-year period of latency between exposure to asbestos and the development of tumor-related symptoms. A comprehensive occupational history, including questions about the intensity, duration, and type of asbestos exposure, is critical both medically and legally.

The most frequent presenting symptoms of pleural mesothelioma are dyspnea (60%–70%) and nonpleuritic chest pain of insidious onset (50%–70%) (126). In 10% of patients, the disease is discovered when asymptomatic abnormalities, such as small, unilateral pleural effusions, are noted on routine chest roentgenograms. The symptoms of patients presenting in the later stages of disease may include weight loss (25%–30%), cough (27%), fever (33%), weakness (33%), and anorexia (10%) (126).

Significant ventilation-perfusion mismatching develops as deoxygenated blood is shunted into lung and trapped by tumor and effusions; this causes hypoxemia that is often refractory to supplemental oxygen. Five percent of patients present with an acute onset of excruciating chest pain and dyspnea; radiographic evaluation reveals a spontaneous pneumothorax or hemothorax (127). Transdiaphragmatic involvement with intraperitoneal dissemination can lead to bowel obstruction (122,124,125).

Tachycardia and palpitations may reflect pericardial involvement. Involvement of the great vessels of the mediastinum can cause superior vena cava syndrome. Growth into the epicardium may result in right-sided heart failure and arrhythmias that cause death in 10% of patients. Infiltration of the vertebral column causes cord compression and paraplegia. Apical tumor growth may lead to a Pancoast-like syndrome, with recurrent laryngeal nerve paralysis, brachial plexopathy, and a Horner syndrome (124).

The most debilitating symptom is nearly constant pain in the chest wall; this results from tumor invasion of the heavily innervated parietal pleura and eventual invasion of the intercostal nerves and muscles and ribs. The pain is often severe and characteristically resistant to analgesics. If long-acting and rescue narcotics fail to control the pain, intercostal and paravertebral block may be necessary.

Several paraneoplastic syndromes have been described in the setting of mesothelioma, including disseminated intravascular coagulation, migratory thrombophlebitis, thrombocytosis, Coombs-positive hemolytic anemia, hypoglycemia, and hypercalcemia associated with secretion of a parathyroid hormone-like peptide (122).

Physical Examination Findings

The pleural effusion or pleural mass causes local signs and symptoms. The later stages of disease may be associated with signs of mediastinal invasion, such as superior vena cava syndrome, vocal cord paralysis, cyanosis, and involvement of the clavicular and cervical nodes. Tumor encasement of the lung with resultant significant loss of the hemithoracic volume may be manifested by ipsilateral tracheal deviation and thoracic scoliosis. As the disease progresses, patients may demonstrate clubbing, cachexia, and muscle wasting. Signs of extrathoracic involvement are uncommon at presentation, occurring in fewer than 10% of cases (128).

Imaging/Diagnosis

The radiographic diagnosis of pleural mesothelioma requires a high degree of clinical suspicion. The most common radiologic presentation (40%–95% of cases) is a large, unilateral pleural effusion that may completely opacify the hemithorax. Only 10% of patients present with bilateral effusions (129). The other common radiographic finding in malignant pleural mesothelioma (60%–100% of cases) is diffuse, circumferential pleural thickening, usually associated with varying amounts of calcified pleural plaque and effusions. Plaques are the most common manifestation of prior asbestos exposure but do not necessarily denote the presence of mesothelioma (129).

Almost all pleural plaques are detected by CT, whereas most are missed by plain films (130). CT of the chest is the most accurate noninvasive method for assessing the stage and progression of mesothelioma, and for planning treatment (131,132) (Fig. 41.7A). Initially, CT should always be performed with a contrast medium to distinguish tumor from the vascular mediastinal structures.

On CT scans, malignant mesothelioma has a spectrum of appearances: focal nodular masses or lesions; pleural effusions; diffuse pleural thickening; parenchymal tumor spread; invasion of ribs, mediastinum, and hemidiaphragm; and distant hematogenous spread (133).

PET with ^{18}F-FDG is an emerging modality in the evaluation of pleural mesothelioma that may be able to document and quantify the extent of pleural disease, establish mediastinal lymph node involvement, and estimate tumor aggressiveness (134) (Fig. 41.7B).

Tissue sampling must be carried out to diagnose malignant pleural mesothelioma correctly. The most reliable measure of diagnostic accuracy is the method of sample

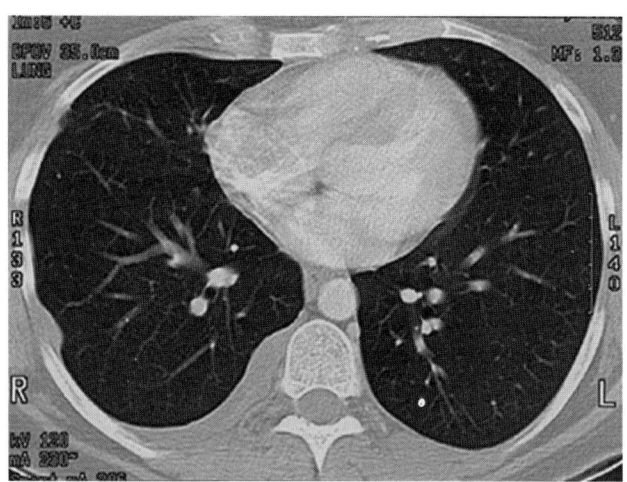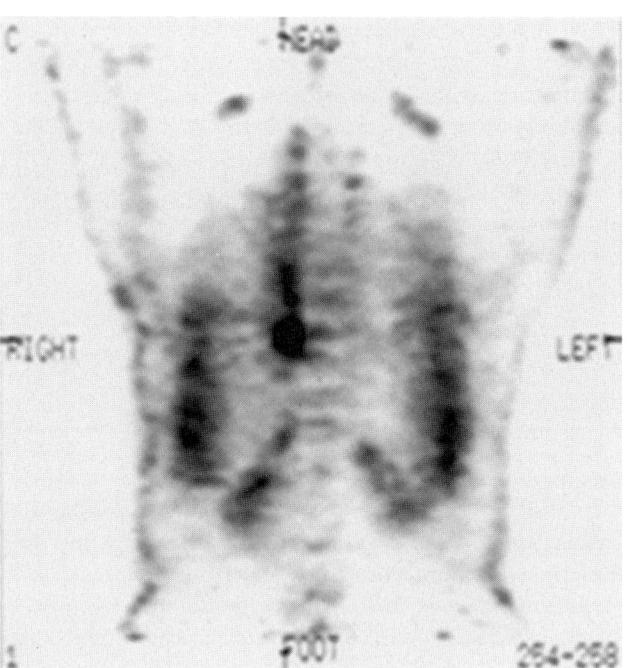

FIGURE 41.7. A: Chest computed tomographic image, axial section, from a young woman with a right-sided stage I malignant pleural mesothelioma. Diagnostic thoracoscopy demonstrated tumor along the parietal, diaphragmatic, and mediastinal pleural surfaces. **B:** [^{18}F]Fluorodeoxyglucose positron emission tomographic image, coronal section, shows intense uptake of the radioactive pharmaceutical at the right cardiophrenic angle, consistent with the findings at thoracoscopy.

collection: thoracentesis (26%), needle biopsy (21%), combined thoracentesis and needle biopsy (39%), and thoracoscopy (98%) (135).

Up to 80% of patients present with an effusion, and an effusion develops in 95% at some time during the course of their disease (126,136).

Staging

The staging of malignant mesothelioma is important prognostically and for guiding treatment. To consolidate the various staging systems then in existence, the International Mesothelioma Interest Group (IMIG) in June of 1994 devised a new TNM staging system based on emerging information about the effects of local tumor extent and nodal status on survival; much of this information was derived from thoracoscopic assessment of the pleural cavity (137) (Table 41.4). The new staging system emphasizes delineation of the early tumor stage, dividing the T1 category of the International Union against Cancer into T1a and T1b (and stage I into Ia and Ib). T1a mesotheliomas are limited to the parietal and diaphragmatic pleura, whereas T1b tumors demonstrate nonconfluent involvement of the visceral pleura. T2 mesotheliomas show diffuse involvement of the visceral pleural, extension into the pulmonary parenchyma, or both. T3 tumors are locally advanced but potentially resectable, with only focal involvement of the chest wall. T4 tumors are locally advanced and

technically unresectable because of diffuse invasion of the chest wall, mediastinum, and diaphragm. Perhaps the most important advance of the IMIG system is the identification of lymph node involvement as an important negative prognostic indicator. In the new system, a patient with a

TABLE 41.4. INTERNATIONAL MESOTHELIOMA INTEREST GROUP STAGING SYSTEM

T1		
	T1a	Ipsilateral parietal pleura only
	T1b	Ipsilateral parietal pleura, with scattered visceral pleural foci
T2	All ipsilateral pleural surfaces, diaphragmatic or parenchymal invasion	
T3	Involvement of the endothoracic fascia, mediastinal fat; solitary, resectable chest wall focus, or nontransmural pericardial invasion	
T4	Diffuse extension into chest wall, peritoneum, spine, mediastinal organs, contralateral pleura, internal surface of pericardium or myocardium	
N0	No regional lymph node metastasis	
N1	Metastases in the ipsilateral bronchopulmonary or hilar nodes	
N2	Metastases in the subcarinal or ipsilateral mediastinal nodes	
N3	Metastases in the contralateral mediastinal or internal mammary lymph nodes, or any supraclavicular node metastasis	

STAGING

Stage I		
	Ia	T1a N0 M0
	Ib	T1b N0 M0
Stage II		T2 N0 M0
Stage III		T3 N0 M0, any N1, N2
Stage IV		Any T4, N3, M1

T1a tumor but positive hilar lymph nodes is classified as stage III.

Prognosis

The overall prognosis of patients with malignant mesothelioma is poor. Most patients die of complications of local extension of this disease. Death is often caused by respiratory failure, pneumonia, pulmonary emboli, or obstruction of the small bowel. The mean survival of all patients with mesothelioma is between 6 and 18 months from the time of diagnosis and is not significantly affected by the standard therapeutic interventions currently available.

Therapeutic Approaches

No particular therapy has emerged as superior to supportive therapy alone in terms of survival. The median survival of patients given no treatment is 6 to 8 months, quite similar to that of patients given therapy (127,128,137–145). The most favorable outcomes reported have been in uncontrolled, nonrandomized studies of multimodality treatment involving surgery, chemotherapy, and radiation therapy in highly selected groups of patients. At the present time, however, no standard of care for patients with pleural mesothelioma is widely accepted.

Chemotherapy

Despite the multiple trials of single-agent and combination chemotherapy in patients with mesothelioma carried out during the past two decades, there is currently little indication for routine, off-protocol use of this treatment modality. Response rates to single-agent chemotherapy have been dismal, ranging from 0 to 20%. Anthracyclines and antimetabolites have shown the greatest promise, with doxorubicin, the most extensively studied agent, achieving an average partial response rate of 20% (146–152). Newer agents currently under investigation include gemcitabine, which has demonstrated some activity against mesothelioma in limited phase I studies, and p30 protein (Onconase), a novel ribonuclease isolated from leopard frog eggs. Several other agents, including detorubicin, high-dose methotrexate, edatrexate, and carboplatin, an analogue of cisplatin, have been studied as single agents and in combination.

In one series, cisplatin and gemcitabine were administered to 21 patients with advanced mesothelioma (153). A partial response was achieved in 10 (48%), and the median duration of the response was 25 weeks. Ninety percent of the responders experienced significant relief of symptoms. A somewhat lower response rate of 16% was reported by others using this combination (154,155), and a response rate of 26% was reported for gemcitabine with carboplatin (156). The combination of cisplatin and irinotecan was studied in 15 patients with previously untreated pleural mesothelioma (157). Four partial responses were noted with a median duration of 26 weeks, and 39% of the patients were alive at

1 year. The combination of cisplatin, fluorouracil, mitomycin, and etoposide was evaluated in 45 patients with stage II mesothelioma (158). A partial response was documented in 17 (38%), and the median duration of the response was 12 months. Preliminary studies suggest that the combination of raltitrexed and oxaliplatin may be efficacious in advanced mesothelioma. In a combined phase I/II trial with raltitrexed, 15 (32%) of 47 patients had a partial response (159).

High-dose methotrexate was combined with interferon-α and interferon-γ in one study of 24 evaluable patients with advanced mesothelioma. Seven (29%) had a partial response, and the 1- and 2-year survival rates were 62% and 31%, respectively (160).

Because the success of systemic chemotherapy has been minimal in mesothelioma, several investigators have evaluated the direct intrapleural delivery of chemotherapy, with the rationale of achieving high local concentrations of drug while reducing systemic toxicity. Agents that have been evaluated in intracavitary treatment to date include cisplatin, cytosine arabinoside, doxorubicin, and mitomycin C (161–164).

Radiation Therapy

External beam radiation therapy, like chemotherapy, has proved ineffective in prolonging the survival of patients with mesothelioma, although several studies have demonstrated some degree of regression of gross disease (165). Palliative radiotherapy with an attempt to treat the entire involved pleural surface is technically difficult and associated with a high risk for radiation pneumonitis, myelitis, hepatitis, and myocarditis. Mesothelioma is more responsive to radiation therapy than non–small cell lung cancer, but it is not as sensitive as small cell carcinoma. Nevertheless, radiation can provide effective local palliation in up to 50% of patients (166). Radiation therapy, given either by external beam or by brachytherapy (direct intrapleural administration of radioactive isotopes), may be effective as an adjunct to surgical resection, with the goal of improving local control of disease. Anecdotal reports have appeared of long-term survival following high-dose external beam irradiation and even the intrapleural administration of radioactive isotopes. Most studies have shown no significant effect on overall survival in patients with mesothelioma (167). However, radiation therapy may play a role by preventing chest wall recurrences after thoracoscopy/thoracotomy and by improving local control after pleurectomy or extrapleural pneumonectomy (124,167).

Surgery

Surgery for pleural mesothelioma is playing an increasingly vital role in the therapeutic armamentarium, particularly in association with the use of video thoracoscopy to diagnose earlier stages of disease. Surgical intervention includes primarily pleurectomy or pleuropneumonectomy for early-stage, potentially resectable disease and palliation via pleurodesis or decortication for later-stage, unresectable disease. Parietal pleurectomy (i.e., open surgical stripping of the pleura and pericardium from the apex of the lung to the diaphragm) is more successful than talc pleurodesis in reducing the recurrence of pleural effusion in mesothelioma. However, pleurectomy alone has not been shown to prolong survival. More recently, thoracoscopic pleurectomy has been used to achieve results similar to those obtained with the open procedure, but with less morbidity (168). Extrapleural pneumonectomy is a radical surgical procedure involving complete removal of the ipsilateral lung along with the parietal and visceral pleura, the pericardium with portions of the phrenic nerve, and most of the hemidiaphragm. This procedure alone is an excellent means of palliating the profound dyspnea and orthopnea associated with the severe ventilation-perfusion mismatch resulting from lung encasement by tumor. However, extrapleural pneumonectomy has not been shown to prolong survival significantly without adjuvant therapy (169).

Combined Modality Approach

Chemotherapy, radiation therapy, or surgical interventions alone have failed to improve survival beyond a few months. The multimodality approach is being investigated vigorously. Several groups are trying sequential postoperative chemotherapy and adjuvant radiotherapy to the postoperative hemithorax, with improvement in median survival depending on the stage and cell type of the tumor.

Some investigators have evaluated the combination of parietal pleurectomy with postoperative intrapleural therapy or external beam irradiation, or both, demonstrating a median survival of 22.5 months and a 2-year survival rate of 41% in a select group of 27 patients, predominantly with the epithelial subtype (167,170,171). Although uncontrolled, these results are better than the usual 6- to 18-month median survival (124,167). However, further evaluation of this single institution's experience with pleurectomy/decortication did not confirm a better survival for patients who underwent pleurectomy than for those treated with extrapleural pneumonectomy (172).

The Thoracic Surgical Oncology Group at the Dana-Farber Cancer Institute in Boston has achieved improved short- and long-term survival in highly selected patients with mesothelioma by using the combined modality approach of extrapleural pneumonectomy followed by radiation therapy and combination chemotherapy (170,173,174). The operative mortality for the extrapleural pneumonectomy group was 4%, with a major morbidity rate of 24%. Overall survival rates were 36% at 2 years and 14% at 5 years. However, the 2- and 5-year survival rates for patients with epithelial cell tumors were 52% and 21%, respectively; for those with sarcomatoid or mixed histology, they were 16% and 0, respectively. Extrapleural nodal involvement was a significant negative prognostic factor: 2- and 5- year survival rates were

42% and 17% for patients without, and 23% and 0 for those with, positive extrapleural nodes. Patients with tumor-free resection margins had 2- and 5-year survival rates of 44% and 25%, respectively; in those with positive resection margins, the rates were 33% and 9%, respectively. The few highly selected patients who had epithelial mesothelioma, no mediastinal lymph node involvement, and negative resection margins at extrapleural pneumonectomy had a remarkable 5-year survival rate of 46%. Despite these promising results, disease recurred in most patients even after an aggressive trimodality approach to therapy (175). One third of the recurrences were in the ipsilateral hemithorax, and one third were abdominal. Distant metastases were rare in the patients with recurrent disease.

Experimental Therapies

Photodynamic Therapy. Photodynamic therapy is the systemic administration of light-sensitive molecules (photosensitizers); these localize in neoplastic cells and produce toxic oxygen free radicals when activated by light of a particular wavelength. Hematoporphyrin derivative (porfimer sodium, Photofrin), the most common photosensitizer in clinical use, selectively lyses neoplastic cells when exposed to 630-nm laser light (175a). Primary side effects of hematoporphyrin derivative include prolonged photosensitivity of the skin secondary to the deposition of photosensitizer in cutaneous tissues.

Moderate success has been achieved with the use of hematoporphyrin derivative photodynamic therapy as an adjuvant to surgery in good-risk patients with a small tumor burden (176–178). Pass and Donington (179) at the National Cancer Institute conducted a phase I trial of maximal surgical debulking and escalating doses of photodynamic therapy with hematoporphyrin derivative in 42 patients with mesothelioma. Patients with isolated pleural malignancies (mesothelioma or lung adenocarcinoma) of the hemithorax were prospectively entered into the trial in groups of three to receive doses of light between 15 to 35 J/cm^2 2 days after the systemic delivery of hematoporphyrin derivative. No significant toxicities were related to the adjuvant photodynamic therapy. A follow-up phase III randomized trial of surgical debulking followed by chemoimmunotherapy with or without hematoporphyrin derivative photodynamic therapy demonstrated no benefit in regard to survival or local control for photodynamic therapy with this first-generation photosensitizer (179). Other attempts to use hematoporphyrin derivative photodynamic therapy as an adjuvant to maximal surgical cytoreduction in mesothelioma have shown limited therapeutic benefit and a high morbidity rate, with several reports of mortality related to bronchopleural fistulae, esophageal perforations, and empyemas (180–182).

Immunotherapy. Immunotherapy has no standard role in the current management of mesothelioma. Historically, mesothelioma has been resistant to immune-mediated destruction. The efficacy of the systemic or intrapleural administration of several cytokines, including transforming growth factor beta-1 (TGFβ-1), interferon-γ (IFN-γ), granulocyte-macrophage colony-stimulating factor, and interleukin-2, is being studied in Europe. The most impressive clinical results of cytokine therapy in mesothelioma have been achieved with the intrapleural delivery of IFN-γ, a lymphokine produced by T lymphocytes in response to specific antigenic or mitogenic stimuli. IFN-γ shares the antiproliferative effects of other interferons and is a potent activator of macrophage antitumor cytotoxicity. In a study of 89 patients treated with the intrapleural delivery of IFN-γ, the overall response rate was 20%, with good tolerance of the cytokine. Eight patients with stage I disease had thoracoscopically and histologically confirmed complete remissions, and nine had partial responses, with more than a 50% reduction in tumor volume. Most of the significant responses were in patients with disease confined to the parietal and diaphragmatic pleura. Overall, patients with stage I disease had a response rate of 45% (183,184). Combination trials with chemotherapeutic agents are also being carried out.

Gene Therapy. In the absence of other reliably effective therapies for malignant mesothelioma, several groups are investigating the evolving technology of gene therapy. Several characteristics of mesothelioma make it an attractive target for gene therapy. The first is the lack of any effective standard therapy. Second is the unique accessibility of the pleural space for vector delivery, biopsy, and subsequent analysis of treatment effects. Third, local extension of disease, rather than distant metastases, is responsible for much of the morbidity and mortality associated with this neoplasm. Thus, small increments in local control might significantly improve palliation or survival in patients with mesothelioma, which is not the case in patients with other, more widespread neoplasms. Accordingly, a number of trials of gene therapy in mesothelioma with a wide variety of approaches have been conducted or are in the planning stages.

A promising approach in current experimental cancer gene therapy is the introduction of a toxic or "suicide" gene into mesothelioma cells to facilitate their destruction (molecular chemotherapy). One such "suicide" gene approach involves the transduction of a neoplasm with a complementary DNA encoding the enzyme herpes simplex thymidine kinase (HSV*tk*) to render its cells sensitive to a "benign" drug, ganciclovir (185). HSV*tk* catalyzes ganciclovir to ganciclovir monophosphate, which is then rapidly converted by mammalian kinases to the triphosphate form. Ganciclovir triphosphate is a toxic analogue that is a potent inhibitor of DNA polymerase and competes with nucleosides for DNA replication (186). A "bystander" effect, in which neighboring, nontransduced tumor cells are also killed, appears to be an important component of this system.

We conducted a series of phase I clinical trials involving the intrapleural delivery of a recombinant, replication-incompetent adenoviral (Ad) vector containing the HSV*tk* gene (Ad.RSV*tk*), followed by systemic treatment with ganciclovir, in 34 patients with malignant pleural mesothelioma. After treatment at dose levels up to 5×10^{13} viral particles, evidence was found of a dose-dependent but superficial intratumoral *tk* gene transfer, in addition to significant immune responses to the Ad vector and the tk protein. Minimal toxicities were seen, and no maximally tolerated dose of Ad.RSV*tk* was established. Preliminary evidence of radiographic and clinical responses was noted in 5 of 34 patients; two patients were alive more than 4.5 years after treatment with evidence of only minimal, stable disease (187).

Immunomodulatory Approach. The use of gene therapy to augment the immune response to tumors is another area under active investigation. This strategy is based on two principles: first, that the immune system can recognize and destroy tumor cells through diverse mechanisms (i.e., cytotoxic T lymphocytes, natural killer cells, macrophages, and eosinophils), and second, that tumor cells have somehow escaped from normal immune surveillance. The systemic or intrapleural administration of cytokines may partially overcome the resistance of mesothelioma to immune destruction, but clinical applications are limited by significant associated toxicity. Another immunomodulatory approach to gene therapy in mesothelioma that is under intense investigation is the intratumoral delivery of a gene encoding the bacterial heat shock protein HSP-65, one of the most immunogenic molecules known.

Localized Malignant Mesothelioma

Localized malignant mesothelioma is the rarest of the three categories of mesothelioma: diffuse malignant, benign fibrous ("localized benign"), and localized malignant. Only one of every six localized mesotheliomas is malignant (121). These tumors have been known to arise in the pleural and peritoneal space (188). Grossly, they resemble solitary benign fibrous tumors (188). Histologically, immunohistochemically, and ultrastructurally, they are identical to diffuse epithelioid and biphasic malignant mesotheliomas. Patients rarely survive more than 2 years (121). When resected, the tumors may appear benign; however, they quickly recur. Recurrences are often characterized by multiple nodules rather than the diffuse pleural rind typical of most malignant mesotheliomas (188). Occasionally, with meticulous resection, cures have been achieved (118,121).

CHEST WALL TUMORS

Primary tumors of the chest wall are a heterogeneous group of tumors that develop in the soft tissue and bones of the thoracic wall. Tumors that invade or metastasize to the chest wall may originate in lung, pleura, mediastinum, muscle, or breast. Primary tumors of the chest wall account for approximately 2% of all tumors of the chest wall. Of these, 50% to 80% are malignant (189). Chest wall tumors grow slowly. Pain is the heralding symptom in most patients with malignant chest wall tumors but is present in only two thirds of those with benign tumors.

Diagnosis

A careful history and physical examination followed by chest radiography or chest CT is almost always diagnostic. MRI is considered superior by most investigators for its ability to delineate the various tissue planes and distinguish nerves and vessels from tumors (189). Radiographic or physical evidence of rapid growth, cortical destruction, and invasion of surrounding tissue suggests a malignant tumor (190). A tissue diagnosis is preferably obtained by open biopsy. With smaller tumors, an excisional biopsy is usually performed (189). Needle aspiration is used in cases of suspected metastatic disease.

Treatment

Both benign and malignant tumors of the chest wall are best treated by surgical resection. The extent of resection may vary depending on the benign, malignant, or metastatic nature of the lesion.

Primary Bone Tumors

Primary bone tumors are rare but are usually malignant in nature.

Benign Tumors of the Rib

Osteochondroma

Osteochondroma is the most common benign tumor of bone, accounting for half of all benign rib tumors (102). It is found mostly in children, with a male-to-female ratio of 3:1 (189). Malignant transformation is unusual. This tumor arises from the metaphyseal region of the ribs as a bony protuberance. The treatment of choice is complete surgical resection.

Chondroma

Chondromas account for fewer than 25% of all the benign neoplasms of the rib cage (189). This tumor affects people of all ages and both sexes. The radiologic appearance of chondroma is indistinguishable from that of chondrosarcoma. Chondroma presents as a lobulated mass that is microscopically composed of lobules of hyaline cartilage. Chondroma should be considered malignant and treated with wide resections (189).

Fibrous Dysplasia

Fibrous dysplasia is a slowly growing painless tumor of the rib cage. It affects children of both sexes, often in infancy. It usually escapes detection until a first chest radiograph is obtained in an otherwise healthy young adult. Fibrous dysplasia is a nonneoplastic cystic lesion that leads to fibrous replacement of the medullary cavity of the rib. Multiple lesions should raise suspicion of Albright syndrome (multiple bone cysts and areas of skin pigmentation and precocious puberty in girls).

Histiocytosis X

Bony lesions are common in histiocytosis X (eosinophilic granuloma, Hand-Schiller-Christian disease, Letterer-Siwe disease); 10% to 20% of them occur in ribs (189). Radiographically, histiocytosis X appears as an expansile lesion causing destruction of the bony cortex. Because of associated findings of fever, malaise, and leukocytosis, osteomyelitis is often considered in the differential diagnosis. The diagnosis is generally established by excisional biopsy. Solitary lesions are treated with excision. Multiple bony lesions are associated with eosinophilic granuloma and are treated with low-dose radiation therapy (189).

Malignant Tumors of the Rib

Multiple Myeloma

Myeloma accounts for one third of all chest wall tumors and is the most common primary malignant tumor of the rib cage (191). Most patients with myeloma of the rib cage have systemic disease. Multiple myeloma usually affects men in the fifth through seventh decades. The clinical picture includes pain, anemia, an elevated sedimentation rate, hypercalcemia, proteinuria, and an abnormal protein electrophoresis.

Radiographically, myeloma appears as punched-out, osteolytic lesions with cortical thinning. Pathologic fractures are not uncommon. Local excision is usually performed to confirm the diagnosis. Radiotherapy is used with chemotherapy for multiple lesions, and alone for solitary lesions. Survival is poor (189).

Chondrosarcoma

Chondrosarcoma, a tumor of the anterior chest wall, accounts for approximately 30% of all primary malignant bone neoplasms. It usually affects men in their 30s and 40s. A chondrosarcoma grows slowly into a large lobulated mass that invades structures anteriorly across the muscle planes and posteriorly across the pleura. Differentiation from chondroma can be difficult unless an experienced pathologist reviews the tissue. There is a questionable association between trauma and the development of chondrosarcoma.

Radiographically, chondrosarcoma appears as a lobulated mass arising from the medullary portion of the bone. The cortex is usually destroyed, and mineralization of the matrix is common. CT can be helpful. Excisional biopsy is a preferred method for establishing the diagnosis and definitively differentiating the lesion from chondroma. Histologic differentiation between the two may be difficult. Wide resection is the treatment of choice. The cure rate is 97%, but recurrence and metastasis are possible (189).

Ewing Sarcoma

Ewing sarcoma accounts for 12% of all primary malignant neoplasms of the rib cage (189). It affects boys in early childhood and adolescence twice as often as girls. The usual clinical picture includes fever, anemia, an elevated sedimentation rate, and leukocytosis. Radiographically, Ewing sarcoma is characterized by both lytic and blastic lesions. An onionskin appearance of the bony surface is caused by elevation of the periosteum and subperiosteal bone formation. This feature is also seen in other bony tumors. The presence of radiating spicules on the surface of the bone makes it difficult to distinguish Ewing sarcoma from osteogenic sarcoma (189).

Grossly, Ewing sarcoma is an unencapsulated whitish gray lesion. Metastatic lesions to the lung and other bones are common. The diagnosis is established by a generous biopsy. Radiation therapy is the mainstay of treatment because of the radiosensitive nature of the tumor. Adjuvant chemotherapy may be necessary (189).

Osteogenic Sarcoma

Osteogenic sarcoma accounts for 6% of all primary malignant bone neoplasms. It occurs in teenage boys more often than in girls. This is a rapidly growing, painful, malignant tumor that carries a poor prognosis. Bony destruction is evident radiographically. Calcifications create a typical sunburst appearance. The mainstay of therapy is wide surgical resection. Chemotherapy and radiation therapy are not useful, and the prognosis is poor.

Radiation-Associated Malignant Tumors

Osteosarcoma and soft tissue sarcoma are the most common tumors of the chest wall following radiation (189). The frequency of these tumors is on the rise. The treatment is wide surgical excision, and the prognosis is similar to that of patients with tumors arising de novo.

Tumors of the Manubrium, Sternum, Scapula, and Clavicle

Tumors of the manubrium and sternum constitute approximately 75% of all primary chest wall tumors and include chondrosarcoma, myeloma, malignant lymphoma, and osteogenic sarcoma (191). Most of these lesions are malignant. The sternum is also a common site of metastases. The scapula is a site of origin of primary bone neoplasms that are similar in nature to the tumors of the rib cage (2.8%) (191). The clavicle is an uncommon site of primary neoplasms, accounting for fewer than 1% of all such lesions. Of these, two thirds are malignant and include myeloma lesions and Ewing sarcoma. Metastatic lesions are found more often than

primary lesions. The treatment of choice for lesions of these bones is wide surgical resection (192).

Primary Soft Tissue Tumors

Benign Soft Tissue Tumors

Several soft tissue tumors of the chest wall have been reported, including fibromas, lipomas, giant cell tumors, neurogenic tumors, vascular tumors, and tumors of the connective tissue. All should be treated with local excision. The prognosis is generally good.

Desmoid Tumors

Desmoids are benign tumors that commonly affect the shoulder and chest wall of men and women from puberty through the fourth decade of life (189). The clinical presentation usually consists of paresthesias, neuromuscular weakness, and vascular compromise secondary to involvement of nerve plexuses and vascular structures in both the neck and mediastinum. These tumors are considered benign fibromatoses. The treatment is wide resection to avoid recurrence.

Malignant Soft Tissue Tumors

Malignant Fibrous Histiocytoma

Most malignant fibrous histiocytomas occur in men in their 50s through 70s. Generally, these tumors are slowly growing, painless, lobulated masses. Some literature supports an association between exposure to radiation and their development (193). The treatment of choice is wide surgical resection. Radiation and chemotherapy have no role in the management of these tumors (189).

Rhabdomyosarcoma is the second most common malignant soft tissue tumor of the chest wall (189). It usually manifests in children and young adults and arises from striated muscle tissue, growing rapidly and painlessly. Current therapies include wide surgical resection followed by irradiation and chemotherapy and result in good 5-year survival rates (189).

Liposarcoma

Liposarcoma affects mostly men in the fourth through sixth decades. This is an encapsulated and lobulated structure that requires wide excision.

Neurofibrosarcoma

Neurofibrosarcoma affects men and women between the ages of 20 and 50 years. These tumors develop along the intercostal nerves and are frequently associated with Von Recklinghausen disease. Although neurofibrosarcoma is an encapsulated tumor, it must be treated with a wide excision (189).

Leiomyosarcoma

Most leiomyosarcomas occur in adult women and present as slowly growing, painful masses. Leiomyosarcomas are lobulated and require wide surgical excision (189).

REFERENCES

1. Fraser RS, Paré JAP, Fraser RG, et al. The normal chest. In: Fraser RS, Paré JAP, Fraser RG, et al, eds. *Synopsis of diseases of the chest,* 2nd ed. Philadelphia: WB Saunders, 1994:1–116.
2. Strollo DC, Rosado-de-Christenson ML, Jett JR, et al. Primary mediastinal tumors, part 1. Tumors of the anterior mediastinum. *Chest* 1997;112:511.
3. Davis RD Jr, Newland Oldham H Jr, Sabiston DC Jr. Primary cysts and neoplasms of the mediastinum: recent changes in clinical presentation, methods of diagnosis, management and results. *Ann Thorac Surg* 1987;44:229–237.
4. Silverman NA, Sabiston DC Jr. Mediastinal masses. *Surg Clin North Am* 1980;60(4):757–777.
5. Grillo HC, Ojemann RG, Scannell JG, et al. Combined approach to "dumbbell" intrathoracic and intraspinal neurogenic tumors. *Ann Thorac Surg* 1983;36:402–407.
6. Barrington SF. Whole body applications of positron emission tomography in oncology. *Imaging* 2001;13:185–196.
7. Moog F, Bangerter M, Diederichs C, et al. Extranodal malignant lymphoma: detection with FDG PET versus CT. *Radiology* 1998;206:475–481.
8. Gupta N, Gill H, Graeber G, et al. Dynamic positron emission tomography with F-18 fluorodeoxyglucose imaging in differentiation of benign from malignant lung/mediastinal lesions. *Chest* 1998;114:1105–1111.
9. Wychulis AR, Payne WS, Clagett OT, et al. Surgical treatment of mediastinal tumors. *J Thorac Cardiovasc Surg* 1972;62:379–391.
10. Rosai J, Levine GD. Tumors of the thymus. In: Firminger HI, ed. *Atlas of tumor pathology,* series II, fascicle 13. Washington, DC: Armed Forces Institute of Pathology, 1976:34–212.
11. Lattes R. Thymoma and other tumors of the thymus: an analysis of 107 cases. *Cancer* 1962;15:1224–1260.
12. Mullen B, Richardson JD. Primary anterior mediastinal tumors in children and adults. *Ann Thorac Surg* 1986;42:338.
13. Gerein AN, Srivastava SP, Burgess J. Thymoma: a ten-year review. *Am J Surg* 1978;136:49–53.
14. Appelquist P, Kostianen L, Franssia K, et al. Treatment and prognosis of thymoma: a review of 25 cases. *J Surg Oncol* 1982;20:265.
15. Gray GF, Cutowski WT. Thymoma, a clinico-pathologic study of 54 cases. *Am J Surg Pathol* 1979;3:235.
16. Wilkins EW Jr, Edmunds L Jr, Castleman B. Cases of thymoma of the Massachusetts General Hospital. *J Thorac Cardiovasc Surg* 1966;52:322–330.
17. Lewis JE, Wick MR, Scheithauer BW, et al. Thymoma: a clinicopathologic review. *Cancer* 1987;60:2727–2743.
18. Verstandig AG, Epstein DM, Miller WT, et al. Thymoma—report of 71 cases and a review. *Crit Rev Diagn Imaging* 1992;33:201–230.
19. Zerhouni EA, Scott WW, Baker RR, et al. Invasive thymomas: diagnosis and evaluation by CT. *J Comput Assist Tomogr* 1982;6:92–100.
20. Yokoi K, Miyazawa N, Mori K, et al. Invasive thymoma with intracaval growth into right atrium. *Ann Thorac Surg* 1992;53:507–509.
21. Muller-Hermelink HK, Marx A. Thymoma. *Curr Opin Oncol* 2000;12:426–433.
22. Masaoka A, Monden Y, Nakahara K, et al. Follow-up study of thymomas with special reference to their clinical stages. *Cancer* 1981;48:2485–2492.
23. Shamji F, Pearson FG, Todd TR, et al. Results of surgical treatment for thymoma. *J Thorac Cardiovasc Surg* 1984;87:43.
24. Cohen DJ, Ronnigan LD, Graeber GM, et al. Management of patients with malignant thymoma. *J Thorac Cardiovasc Surg* 1984;87:301.
25. Osserman KE, Genkins G. Studies in myasthenia gravis: review of a 20-year experience in over 1200 patients. *Mt Sinai J Med* 1971;38:497–537.
26. Lennon VA, Jones G, Howard F, et al. Auto antibodies to acetylcholine receptors in myasthenia gravis. *N Engl J Med* 1983;308:402–403.
27. Howard FM Jr, Lennon VA, Finley J, et al. Clinical correlation of antibodies that bind, block or modulate human acetylcholine receptors in myasthenia gravis. *Ann N Y Acad Sci* 1987;505:526–538.
28. Souadjian JV, Enriquez P, Silverstein MN, et al. The spectrum of diseases associated with thymoma. *Arch Intern Med* 1974;134:374–379.
29. Rosado-de-Christenson ML, Galobardes J, Moran CA. Thymoma: radiologic-pathologic correlation. *Radiographics* 1992;12:151–168.
30. Moran CA, Travis WD, Rosado-de-Christenson ML, et al. Thymomas presenting as pleural tumors. *Am J Surg Pathol* 1992;16:138–144.
31. Anderson T, Lindgren PG, Elvin A. Ultrasound-guided tumor biopsy in the anterior mediastinum. *Acta Radiol* 1992;33:310–311.
32. Morgenthaler TI, Brown LR, Colby TV, et al. Symposium on intrathoracic neoplasms—part IX. *Mayo Clin Proc* 1993;68:1110–1123.
33. Curran WJ Jr, Kornstein MJ, Brooks JJ, et al. Invasive thymoma: the role of mediastinal irradiation following complete or incomplete surgical resection. *J Clin Oncol* 1988;6:1722–1727.
34. Thomas CR, Wright CD, Loehrer PJ. Thymoma. *J Clin Oncol* 1999;17:2280–2289.
35. Kim ES, Putnam JB, Komaki R, et al. A phase II study of a multidisciplinary approach with induction chemotherapy (IC), followed by surgical resection (SR), radiation therapy (RT), and consolidation chemotherapy for unresectable malignant thymoma. *Proc Am Soc Clin Oncol* 2001;20:310(abst).
36. Gamondes JP, Balawi A, Greenland T, et al. Seventeen years of surgical treatment of thymoma: factors influencing survival. *Eur J Cardiothorac Surg* 1991;5:124–131.
37. Schneider PM, Feelbaum C, Fink U, et al. Prognostic importance of histomorphologic subclassification for epithelial thymic tumors. *Ann Surg Oncol* 1997;4:46.
38. Suster S, Rosai J. Thymic carcinoma: a clinicopathologic study of 60 cases. *Cancer* 1991;67:1025–1032.
39. Snover DC, Levine GD, Rosai J. Thymic carcinoma: five distinctive histological variants. *Am J Surg Pathol* 1982;6:451–470.
40. Truong LD, Mody DR, Cagle PT, et al. Thymic carcinoma. A clinicopathologic study of 13 cases. *Am J Surg Pathol* 1990;14:151–166.
41. Ritter JH, Wick MR. Primary carcinoma of the thymus gland. *Semin Diagn Pathol* 1999;16:18.
42. Loehrer PJ, Kim KM, Aisner SC, et al. Cisplatin plus doxorubicin plus cyclophosphamide in metastatic or recurrent thymoma. *J Clin Oncol* 1994;12:1164–1168.

43. Weide LG, Ulbright TM, Loehrer PJ Sr, et al. Thymic carcinoma. A distinct clinical entity responsive to chemotherapy. *Cancer* 1993;71:1219–1223.

44. Wick MR, Bernatz PE, Carney JA, et al. Primary mediastinal carcinoid tumors. *Am J Surg Pathol* 1982;6:195–205.

45. Economopoulos GC, Lewis JW Jr, Lee MW, et al. Carcinoid tumors of the thymus. *Ann Thorac Surg* 1990;50:58–61.

46. Graeber GM, Thompson LD, Cohen DJ, et al. Cystic lesions of the thymus. *J Thorac Cardiovasc Surg* 1984;87:295–300.

47. Indeglia RA, Shea MA, Grage TB. Congenital cysts of the thymus gland. *Arch Surg* 1967;94:149–152.

48. Suster S, Rosai J. Multilocular thymic cyst: an acquired reactive process. *Am J Surg Pathol* 1991;15:388–398.

49. Parker D, Holford CP, Begent RH. Effective treatment for malignant mediastinal teratoma. *Thorax* 1983;38:897.

50. Bohle A, Studor UK, Sonntag RW, et al. Primary or secondary extragonadal germ cell tumor? *J Urol* 1986;135:939.

51. Recondo J, Libshitz HI. Mediastinal extragonadal germ cell tumors. *Urology* 1978;11:369.

52. Javadpour N. Significance of elevated serum alpha fetoprotein (AFP) in seminoma. *Cancer* 1980;45:2166–2168.

53. Nichols CR. Mediastinal germ cell tumors: clinical features and biologic correlates. *Chest* 1991;99:472–479.

54. LeRoux BT. Mediastinal teratoma. *Thorax* 1960;15:333–348.

55. Crussi-Gonzalez F. Extragonadal teratomas. In: Hartmann WH, ed. *Atlas of tumor pathology,* series II, fascicle 18. Washington, DC: Armed Forces Institute of Pathology, 1982:77–94.

56. Carter C, Bibro MC, Touloukian RJ. Benign clinical behavior of immature mediastinal teratoma in infancy and childhood. *Cancer* 1982;49:398.

57. Adebonojo SA, Nicola ML. Teratoid tumors of the mediastinum. *Am Surg* 1976;42:361.

58. Thompson DP, Moore TC. Acute thoracic distress in childhood due to spontaneous rupture of large mediastinal teratoma. *J Pediatr Surg* 1969;4:416.

59. Lewis BD, Hurt RD, Payne WS, et al. Benign teratoma of the mediastinum. *J Thorac Cardiovasc Surg* 1983;86:727–731.

60. Graeber GM, Shriver CD, Albur, RA, et al. The use of computed tomography in the evaluation of mediastinal tumors. *J Thorac Cardiovasc Surg* 1986;91:662.

61. Mueller KH, Rosado-de-Christenson ML, Templeton DA. Mediastinal mature teratoma: imaging features. *AJR Am J Roentgenol* 1997;169:985.

62. Arai K, Ohta S, Suzuki M, et al. Primary immature mediastinal teratoma in adulthood. *Eur J Surg Oncol* 1997;23:64–67.

63. Polansky SM, Barwick KW, Revie CE. Primary mediastinal seminoma. *AJR Am J Roentgenol* 1979;132:17.

64. Bokemeyer C, Droz JP, Horwich A, et al. Extragonadal seminoma: an international multicenter analysis of prognostic factors and long-term treatment outcome. *Cancer* 2001;91:1394–1401.

65. Bush SE, Martinez A, Bagshaw MA. Primary mediastinal seminoma. *Cancer* 1981;48:1877–1882.

66. Bukowski RM, Wolf M, Kulander BG, et al. Alternating combination chemotherapy in patients with extragonadal germ cell tumors. A Southwest Oncology Group study. *Cancer* 1993;71:2631–2638.

67. Dexeus FH, Logothetis CJ, Chong C, et al. Genetic abnormalities in men with germ cell tumors. *J Urol* 1988;140:80–84.

68. Nichols CR, Hoffman R, Einhorn LH, et al. Hematologic malignancies associated with primary mediastinal germ cell tumors. *Ann Intern Med* 1985;102:603–609.

69. Hori K, Uematsu K, Yasoshima H, et al. Testicular seminoma with human chorionic gonadotropin production. *Pathol Int* 1997;47:592–599.

70. Lee KS, Im JG, Han CH, et al. Malignant primary germ cell tumors of the mediastinum: CT features. *AJR Am J Roentgenol* 1989;153:947–951.

71. Walsh GL, Taylor GD, Nesbitt JC, et al. Intensive chemotherapy and radical resections for primary non-seminomatous mediastinal germ cell tumors. *Ann Thorac Surg* 2000;69:337–343; discussion 343–344.

72. International Germ Cell Cancer Collaborative Group. International germ cell consensus classification: a prognostic factor–based staging system for metastatic germ cell cancers. *J Clin Oncol* 1997;15:594–603.

73. Kathic M, Wang C, Grillo H. Substernal goiter. *Ann Thorac Surg* 1985;39:391.

74. Allo MD, Thompson NW. Rationale for the operative management of substernal goiters. *Surgery* 1983;94:969–977.

75. Clark O. Mediastinal parathyroid tumors. *Arch Surg* 1988;123:1096.

76. Hopkins CR, Reading CC. Thyroid and parathyroid imaging. *Semin Ultrasound CT MR* 1995;16:279–295.

77. Oates E. Improved parathyroid scintigraphy with Tc 99m MIBI, a superior radio tracer. *Appl Radiol* 1994;23:37–40.

78. Strickler JG, Kurtin PJ. Mediastinal lymphoma. *Semin Diagn Pathol* 1991;8:2–13.

79. Lichtenstein AK, Levine A, Taylor CR, et al. Primary mediastinal lymphoma in adults. *Am J Med* 1980;68:509–514.

80. Strollo DC, Rosado-de-Christenson ML, Jett JR. Primary mediastinal tumors, part II. *Chest* 1997;112:1344.

81. Vaeth JM, Moskowitz SA, Green JP. Mediastinal Hodgkin's disease. *AJR Am J Roentgenol* 1976;126:123.

82. Kornstein MJ, DeBlois GG. *Pathology of the thymus and mediastinum,* 1st ed. Philadelphia: WB Saunders, 1995.

83. Costello P, Jochelson M. Lymphoma of the mediastinum and lung. In: Taveras JM, Ferrucci JT, eds. *Radiology: diagnosis, imaging, intervention,* vol 1. Philadelphia: Lippincott–Raven Publishers, 1996:1–13.

84. Keller AR, Kaplan HS, Lukes RJ, et al. Correlation of histopathology with other prognostic indicators in Hodgkin's disease. *Cancer* 1968;22:487–499.

85. Castellino RA, Blank N, Hoppe RT, et al. Hodgkin disease: contributions of chest CT in the initial staging evaluation. *Radiology* 1986;160:603–605.

86. DeVita VT, Maack PM, Harris NL. Hodgkin's disease. In: DeVita VT, Hellman S, Rosenberg SA, eds. *Cancer: principles and practice of oncology,* 5th ed. Philadelphia: Lippincott–Raven Publishers, 1997:2242–2283.

87. Canellos GP, Anderson JR, Propert KJ, et al. Chemotherapy of advanced Hodgkin's disease with MOPP, ABVD, or MOPP alternating with ABVD. *N Engl J Med* 1992;327:1478–1484.

88. Longo DL, Duffey PL, Young RC, et al. Conventional-dose salvage combination chemotherapy in patients relapsing with Hodgkin's disease after combination chemotherapy: the low probability for cure. *J Clin Oncol* 1992;10:210–218.

89. Bonfante V, Santoro A, Viviani S, et al. Outcome of patients with Hodgkin's disease failing after primary MOPP-ABVD. *J Clin Oncol* 1997;15:528–534.

90. Sutcliff SB. Primary mediastinal malignant lymphoma. *Semin Thorac Cardiovasc Surg* 1992;4:55.

91. Cheson BD. Hodgkin's disease and the Non-Hodgkin's lymphomas. In: Lenhard RE Jr, Osteen RT, Gansler T, eds. *Clinical oncology.* Atlanta, GA: American Cancer Society, 2001:497–516.

92. MacManus MP, Hoppe RT. Is radiotherapy curative for stage I and II low-grade follicular lymphoma? Results of a long-term follow-up study of patients treated at Stanford University. *J Clin Oncol* 1996;14:1282–1290.

93. Murtha AD, Knox SJ, Hoppe RT, et al. Long-term follow-up of patients with stage III follicular lymphoma treated with primary radiotherapy at Stanford University. *Int J Radiat Oncol Biol Phys* 2001;49:3–15.

94. O'Neill JA. Foregut duplications. In: Fallis JC, Filler RM, Lemoine G, eds. *Current topics in general thoracic surgery: an international series.* New York: Elsevier Science, 1991:121–123.

95. Cioffi U, Bonavina L, De Simone M. Presentation and surgical management of bronchogenic and esophageal duplication cysts in adults. *Chest* 1998;113:1492–1496.

96. Superina RA, Ein SH, Humphreys RP. Cystic duplications of the esophagus and neurenteric cysts. *J Pediatr Surg* 1984;19:527–530.

97. Rescorla FJ, Grosfeld JL. Gastroenteric cysts and neurenteric cysts in infants and children. In: Shields TW, LoCicero J III, Ponn RB, eds. *General thoracic surgery,* 5th ed., vol 2. Philadelphia: Lippincott Williams & Wilkins, 2000:2415–2422.

98. Feigin D, Fenoglio JJ, McAllister HA, et al. Pericardial cysts: a radiologic-pathologic correlation and review. *Radiology* 1977;125:15–20.

99. Reeder LB. Neurogenic tumors of the mediastinum. *Semin Thorac Cardiovasc Surg* 2000;12:261–267.

100. Shapiro B, Orringer MB, Gross MD. Mediastinal paragangliomas and pheochromocytomas. In: Shields TW, LoCicero J III, Ponn RB, eds. *General thoracic surgery,* 5th ed., vol 2. Philadelphia: Lippincott Williams & Wilkins, 2000:2333–2355.

101. Saenz NC. Posterior mediastinal neurogenic tumors in infants and children. *Semin Pediatr Surg* 1999;8:78–84.

102. Wain JC. Neurogenic tumors of the mediastinum. *Chest Surg Clin N Am* 1992;2:121–136.

103. Shields TW, Reynolds M. Neurogenic tumors of the thorax. *Surg Clin North Am* 1988;68:645–668.

104. Aughenbaugh GL. Thoracic manifestations of neurocutaneous diseases. *Radiol Clin North Am* 1984;22:741–756.

105. Ducatman BS, Scheithauer BW, Piepgras DG, et al. Malignant peripheral nerve sheath tumors: a clinicopathologic study of 120 cases. *Cancer* 1986;57:2006–2021.

106. Gale AW, Jelihovsy T, Grant AF, et al. Neurogenic tumors of the mediastinum. *Ann Thorac Surg* 1974;17:434–443.

107. Davis S, Rogers MAM, Pendergrass TW. The incidence and epidemiologic characteristics of neuroblastoma in the United States. *Am J Epidemiol* 1987;126:1063–1074.

108. Benjamin SP, McCormack LJ, Effler DB, et al. Primary tumors of the mediastinum. *Chest* 1972;62:297–303.

109. Wang YM, Li YM, Sheih CP, et al. Magnetic resonance imaging of neuroblastoma, ganglioneuroblastoma, and ganglioneuroma. *Acta Paediatr Surg* 1995;36:420–424.

110. Adams A, Hochholzer L. Ganglioneuroblastoma of the posterior mediastinum: a clinicopathologic review of 80 cases. *Cancer* 1981;47:373–381.

111. Page DL, DeLellis RA, Hough AJ. Tumors of the adrenal. In: *Atlas of tumor pathology,* series II, fascicle 23. Washington, DC: Armed Forces Institute of Pathology, 1986:219–260.

112. Grosfeld JL, Baehner RL. Neuroblastoma: an analysis of 160 cases. *World J Surg* 1980;4:29–38.

113. Bar-Ziv J, Nogrady MB. Mediastinal neuroblastoma and ganglioneuroma: the differentiation between primary and secondary involvement on the chest roentgenogram. *AJR Am J Roentgenol* 1975;125:380–390.

114. Stark DD, Moss AA, Brasch RC, et al. Neuroblastoma: diagnostic imaging and staging. *Radiology* 1983;148:101–105.

115. Hoefnagel CA. Radionuclide therapy in children with neuroblastoma. *Hell J Nucl Med* 2002;2:107–110.

116. Carlsen NLT, Christensen IJ, Schroeder H, et al. Prognostic factors in neuroblastomas treated in Denmark from 1943 to 1980. *Cancer* 1986;58:2726–2735.

117. Briselli M, Mark EJ, Dickersin GR. Solitary fibrous tumors of the pleura: eight new cases and review of 360 cases in the literature. *Cancer* 1981;47:2678–2689.

118. Robinson LA, Reilly RB. Localized pleural mesothelioma. The clinical spectrum. *Chest* 1994;106:1611–1615.

119. Okike N, Bernatz P, Woolner L. Localized mesothelioma of the pleura. Benign and malignant variants. *J Thorac Cardiovasc Surg* 1978;75:363–372.

120. Hammar SP. Pleural diseases. In: Dail DH, Hammar SP, eds. *Pulmonary pathology,* 2nd ed. New York: Springer-Verlag, 1994:1487–1579.

121. Obers VJ, Leiman G, Girdwood RW, et al. Primary malignant pleural tumors (mesotheliomas) presenting as localized masses. Fine needle aspiration cytologic findings, clinical and radiologic features and review of the literature. *Acta Cytol* 1988;32:567–575.

122. Antman KH. Natural history and epidemiology of malignant mesothelioma. *Chest* 1993;103:373S.

123. Roggli VL, McGavran MH, Subach J, et al. Pulmonary asbestos body counts and electron probe analysis of asbestos body cores in patients with mesothelioma: a study of 25 cases. *Cancer* 1982;50:2423–2432.

124. Antman KH, Pass HI, Li FP, et al. Benign and malignant mesothelioma. In: DeVita VT Jr, Hellman S, Rosenberg SA, eds. *Cancer: principles and practice of oncology,* 4th ed. Philadelphia: JB Lippincott Co, 1993:1489–1508.

125. Pisani RJ, Colby TV, Williams DE. Malignant mesothelioma of the pleura. *Mayo Clin Proc* 1988;63:1234.

126. Adams VI, Unni KK, Muhm JR, et al. Diffuse malignant mesothelioma of pleura: diagnosis and survival in 92 cases. *Cancer* 1986;58:1540–1551.

127. Antman KH. Clinical presentation and natural history of benign and malignant mesothelioma. *Semin Oncol* 1981;8:313–320.

128. Chailleux E, Dabouis G, Pioche D, et al. Prognostic factors in diffuse malignant pleural mesothelioma. A study of 167 patients. *Chest* 1988;93:159–162.

129. Miller BH, Rosado-de-Christenson ML, Mason AC. From the archives of the AFIP. Malignant pleural mesothelioma: radiologic-pathologic correlation. *Radiographics* 1996;16:613–644.

130. Rabinowitz JG, Efremidis SC, Cohen B, et al. A comparative study of mesothelioma and asbestosis using computed tomography and conventional chest radiography. *Radiology* 1982;144:453–460.

131. Tammilehto L, Maasilta P, Kostiainen S, et al. Diagnosis and prognostic factors in malignant pleural mesothelioma: a retrospective analysis of sixty-five patients. *Respiration* 1992;59:129–135.

132. Maasilta P. Deterioration in lung function following hemithorax irradiation for pleural mesothelioma. *Int J Radiat Oncol Biol Phys* 1991;20:433–438.

133. Leung AN, Mäller NL, Miller RR. CT in differential diagnosis of diffuse pleural disease. *AJR Am J Roentgenol* 1990;154:487–492.

134. Bénard F, Sterman DH, Smith RJ, et al. Metabolic imaging of malignant pleural mesothelioma with fluorine-18-deoxyglucose positron emission tomography. *Chest* 1998;114:713–722.

135. Boutin C, Rey F. Thoracoscopy in pleural malignant mesothelioma: a prospective study of 188 consecutive patients—part 1: diagnosis. *Cancer* 1993;72:389–393.

136. Renshaw AA, Dean BR, Antman KH, et al. The role of cytologic evaluation of pleural fluid in the diagnosis of malignant mesothelioma. *Chest* 1997;111:106–109.

137. Rusch VW. A proposed new international TNM staging system for malignant pleural mesothelioma from the International Mesothelioma Interest Group. *Lung Cancer* 1996;14:1–12.

138. Huncharek M, Kelsey K, Mark EJ, et al. Treatment and survival in diffuse malignant pleural mesothelioma; a study of 83 cases from the Massachusetts General Hospital. *Anticancer Res* 1996;16:1265–1268.

139. Falkson G, Alberts AS, Falkson HC. Malignant pleural mesothelioma treatment: the current state of the art. *Cancer Treat Rev* 1988;15:231–242.

140. Alberts AS, Falkson G, Goedhals L, et al. Malignant pleural mesothelioma: a disease unaffected by current therapeutic maneuvers. *J Clin Oncol* 1988;l6:527–535.

141. Harvey JC, Erdman C, Pisch J, et al. Diffuse malignant pleural mesothelioma: options in surgical treatment. *Compr Ther* 1995;21:13–19.

142. Chahinian AP, Pajak TF, Holland JF, et al. Diffuse malignant mesothelioma. Prospective evaluation of 69 patients. *Ann Intern Med* 1982;96:746–755.

143. Harvey JC, Fleischman EH, Kagan AR, et al. Malignant pleural mesothelioma: a survival study. *J Surg Oncol* 1990;45:40–42.

144. Law MR, Hodson ME, Turner-Warwick M. Malignant mesothelioma of the pleura: clinical aspects and symptomatic treatment. *Eur J Respir Dis* 1984;65:162–168.

145. Ruffie P, Feld R, Minkin S, et al. Diffuse malignant mesothelioma of the pleura in Ontario and Quebec: a retrospective study of 332 patients. *J Clin Oncol* 1989;7:1157–1168.

146. Ryan CW, Herndon J, Vogelzang NJ. A review of chemotherapy trials for malignant mesothelioma. *Chest* 1998;113:66S–73S.

147. Ong ST, Vogelzang NJ. Chemotherapy in malignant pleural mesothelioma. A review. *J Clin Oncol* 1996;14:1007–1017.

148. Solheim OP, Saeter G, Finnanger AM, et al. High-dose methotrexate in the treatment of malignant mesothelioma of the pleura. A phase II study. *Br J Cancer* 1992;65:956–960.

149. Harvey VJ, Slevin ML, Ponder BA, et al. Chemotherapy of diffuse malignant mesothelioma. Phase II trials of single-agent 5-fluorouracil and adriamycin. *Cancer* 1984;54:961–964.

150. Vogelzang NJ, Schultz SM, Iannucci AM, et al. Malignant mesothelioma. The University of Minnesota experience. *Cancer* 1984;53:377–383.

151. Lerner HJ, Schoenfeld DA, Martin A, et al. Malignant mesothelioma. The Eastern Cooperative Oncology Group (ECOG) experience. *Cancer* 1983;52:1981–1985.

152. Rossof AH. Treatment II: chemotherapy in the management of malignant mesothelioma. In: Kittle CF, ed. *Mesothelioma: diagnosis and management*. Chicago: Year Book Medical Publishers, 1987:73–78.

153. Byrne MJ, Davidson JA, Musk AW, et al. Cisplatin and gemcitabine treatment for malignant mesothelioma: a phase II study. *J Clin Oncol* 1999;17:25.

154. Nowak A, Byrne M, Williamson R, et al. Multicentre phase II study of cisplatin (C) and gemcitabine (G) in malignant mesothelioma. *Ann Oncol* 2000;11:109(abst).

155. Van Haarst JW, Burgers JA, Manegold CH, et al. Multicenter phase II study of gemcitabine and cisplatin in malignant pleural mesothelioma. *Lung Cancer* 2000;29:18(abst).

156. Aversa SM, Favaretto AG. Carboplatin and gemcitabine chemotherapy. *Clin Lung Cancer* 1999;1:73.

157. Nakano T, Chahinian AP, Shinjo M, et al. Cisplatin in combination with irinotecan in the treatment of patients with malignant pleural mesothelioma: a pilot phase II clinical trial and pharmacokinetic profile. *Cancer* 1999;85:2375.

158. Kasseyet S, Astoul P, Boutin C. Results of a phase II trial of combined chemotherapy for patients with diffuse malignant mesothelioma of the pleura. *Cancer* 1999;85:1740.

159. Fizazi K, Caliandro R, Soulie P, et al. Combination raltitrexed (Tomudex[R])-oxaliplatin: a step forward in the struggle against mesothelioma? The Institut Gustave Roussy experience with chemotherapy and chemo-immunotherapy in mesothelioma. *Eur J Cancer* 2000;36:1514.

160. Halme M, Knuuttila A, Vehmas T, et al. High-dose methotrexate in combination with interferons in the treatment of malignant pleural mesothelioma. *Br J Cancer* 1999;80:1781.

161. Colleoni M, Sartori F, Calabro F, et al. Surgery followed by intracavitary plus systemic chemotherapy in malignant pleural mesothelioma. *Tumori* 1996;82:53–56.

162. Sauter ER, Langer C, Coia LR, et al. Optimal management of malignant mesothelioma after subtotal pleurectomy: revisiting the role of intrapleural chemotherapy and postoperative radiation. *J Surg Oncol* 1995;60:100–105.

163. Figlin R, Mendoza E, Piantadosi S, et al. Intrapleural chemotherapy without pleurodesis for malignant pleural effusions. LCSG Trial 861. *Chest* 1994;106:363S–366S.

164. Lerza R, Esposito M, Vannozzi M, et al. High doses of intrapleural cisplatin in a case of malignant pleural mesothelioma. Clinical observations and pharmacokinetic analyses. *Cancer* 1994;73:79–84.

165. Davis SR, Tan L, Ball DL. Radiotherapy in the treatment of malignant mesothelioma of the pleura, with special reference to its use in palliation. *Australas Radiol* 1994;38:212–214.

166. De Graaf-Strukowska L, Van der Zee J, Van Putten W, et al. Factors influencing the outcome of radiotherapy in malignant mesothelioma of the pleura—a single institution experience with 189 patients. *Int J Radiat Oncol Biol Phys* 1999;43:511.

167. Aisner J. Current approach to malignant mesothelioma of the pleura. *Chest* 1995;107:332S.

168. Waller DA, Morritt GN, Forty J. Video-assisted thoracoscopic pleurectomy in the management of malignant pleural effusion. *Chest* 1995;107:1454.

169. Sterman D, Kaiser L, Albelda S. Advances in the treatment of malignant pleural mesothelioma. *Chest* 1999;116:504–520.

170. Sugarbaker DJ, Jaklitsch MT, Liptay MJ. Mesothelioma and radical multimodality therapy: who benefits? *Chest* 1995;107:345S.

171. Rusch VW. Pleurectomy/decortication and adjuvant therapy for malignant mesothelioma. *Chest* 1993;103:382S.

172. Rusch VW, Venkatraman ES. Important prognostic factors in patients with malignant pleural mesothelioma managed surgically. *Ann Thorac Surg* 1999;68:1799.

173. Sugarbaker DJ. Extrapleural pneumonectomy, chemotherapy and radiotherapy in the treatment of diffuse malignant pleural mesothelioma. *J Thorac Cardiovasc Surg* 1991;102:10.

174. Sugarbaker DJ, Flores RM, Jaklitsch MT, et al. Resection margins, extrapleural nodal status, and cell type determine postoperative long-term survival in trimodality therapy of malignant pleural mesothelioma: results in 183 patients. *J Thorac Cardiovasc Surg* 1999;117:54.

175. Baldini EH, DeCamp MM Jr, Katz MS, et al. Patterns of recurrence and outcome for patients with clinical stage II non–small cell lung cancer. *Am J Clin Oncol* 1999;22:8.

175a. Henderson BW, Dougherty TJ. How does photodynamic therapy work? *Photochem Photobiol* 1992;55:145–157.

176. Koren H, Schenk GM, Jindra RH, et al. Hypericin in phototherapy. *J Photochem Photobiol B* 1996;36:113–119.

177. Ris HB, Altermatt HJ, Nachbur B, et al. Intraoperative photodynamic therapy with *m*-tetrahydroxyphenylchlorin for chest malignancies. *Lasers Surg Med* 1996;18:39–45.

178. Pass HI, Temeck BK, Kranda K, et al. Phase III randomized trial of surgery with or without intraoperative photodynamic therapy and postoperative immunochemotherapy for malignant pleural mesothelioma. *Ann Surg Oncol* 1997;4:628–633.

179. Pass HI, Donington JS. Use of photodynamic therapy for the management of pleural malignancies. *Semin Surg Oncol* 1995;11:360–367.

180. Takita H, Mang TS, Loewen GM, et al. Operation and intracavitary photodynamic therapy for malignant pleural mesothelioma: a phase II study. *Ann Thorac Surg* 1994;58:995–998.

181. Temeck BK, Pass HI. Esophagopleural fistula: a complication of photodynamic therapy. *South Med J* 1995;88:271–274.

182. Luketich JD, Westkaemper J, Sommers KE, et al. Bronchoesophagopleural fistula after photodynamic therapy for malignant mesothelioma. *Ann Thorac Surg* 1996;62:283–284.

183. Boutin C, Viallat J, Van Zandwijk N, et al. Activity of intrapleural recombinant gamma-interferon in malignant mesothelioma. *Cancer* 1991;67:2033–2037.

184. Boutin C, Nussbaum E, Monnet I, et al. Intrapleural treatment with recombinant gamma-interferon in early stage malignant pleural mesothelioma. *Cancer* 1994;74:2460–2467.

185. Tiberghien, P. Use of suicide genes in gene therapy. *J Leukoc Biol* 1994;56:203–209.

186. Matthews T, Boehme R. Antiviral activity and mechanism of action of ganciclovir. *Rev Infect Dis* 1988;10:S490–S494.

187. Albelda SM, Wiewrodt R, Sterman DH. Gene therapy for lung neoplasms. *Clin Chest Med* 2002;23:265–277.

188. Crotty TB, Myers JL, Katzenstein A-LA, et al. Localized malignant mesothelioma. *Am J Surg Pathol* 1994;18:357–363.

189. Pairolero PC. Chest wall tumors. In: Shields TW, LoCicero J III, Ponn RB, eds. *General thoracic surgery*, 5th ed., vol 2. Philadelphia: Lippincott Williams & Wilkins, 2000:589–598.

190. Sabanathan S, Shah R, Mearm AJ. Surgical treatment of primary malignant chest wall tumors. *Eur J Cardiothorac Surg* 1999;11:1011–1016.

191. Dahlin DC, Unni KK. *Bone tumors: general aspects and data on 8542 cases.* Springfield, IL: Charles C Thomas Publisher, 1986.

192. Arnold PG, Pairohero PC. Chondrosarcoma of the manubrium. Resection and reconstruction with pectoralis major muscle. *Mayo Clin Proc* 1978;53:54.

193. Weiss SW, Enzinger FM. Malignant fibrous histiocytoma: an analysis of 200 cases. *Cancer* 1978;41:2250.

Extrapulmonary Syndromes Associated with Tumors of the Lung

42

Catherine B. Niewoehner

In 1928, Brown described unexpected adrenal hyperactivity in a bearded woman with diabetes who had oat cell carcinoma of the lung (1). More reports of hormone activity associated with lung cancer followed, but it was not until 1941 that Albright and Reifenstein suggested a possible mechanism for the association (2). They proposed that tumors secrete hormone-like substances that produce clinical syndromes. This was confirmed 20 years later when high adrenocorticotropin (ACTH) concentrations were discovered in the plasma of patients with bronchogenic carcinoma and adrenal hyperactivity (3,4).

Syndromes due to hormone production by tissues not normally associated with hormone secretion were originally termed ectopic ("out of place") hormone syndromes and were thought to be rare events. Since then, better methods of cell culture, immunostaining, and hormone extraction; better assays; and advances in molecular genetics have revealed that peptide hormones are produced by all cancers (5). Tumors that cause hormonal syndromes usually arise from cells that normally produce the hormones. For example, ACTH-producing lung cancers arise from lung cells that normally produce ACTH. Therefore, increased peptide hormone production by lung neoplasms is quantitatively abnormal, but not truly ectopic.

The list of hormones produced by lung tumors includes almost all peptide hormones (Table 42.1) but not steroid hormones or thyroid hormones. Peptide hormones are products of single genes, but synthesis of steroid hormones and thyroid hormones requires expression of a series of genes. Lymphomas produce $1,25(OH)_2D_3$, but activation of the precursor, $25(OH)D_3$, requires only one enzyme.

C. B. Niewoehner: Endocrinology Section, Veterans Administration Medical Center, Minneapolis, Minnesota.

EVIDENCE FOR TUMOR HORMONE PRODUCTION

Criteria for establishing tumor hormone production are listed in Table 42.2. The first four criteria can be established clinically. The rest of the criteria require an invasive procedure or a research laboratory. Rigorous (in vitro) evidence that a circulating hormone is produced by the tumor usually is not available for a given patient. However, in the case of bronchogenic carcinomas, enough evidence has been obtained to establish that they do indeed produce the hormones that cause the syndromes described below.

PROPOSED MECHANISMS FOR TUMOR HORMONE SECRETION

It is unlikely that hormone production by tumors is due to random activation of areas of the genome that normally are repressed. This would not account for the strong association of some hormonal syndromes with specific lung and other carcinomas and the fact that tumors express the same hormones as the tissues from which they arise.

Tumors generally produce proteins that are present in the fetus, such as carcinoembryonic antigen (CEA) or α-fetoprotein (αFP), or hormones that are present in immature cells, such as human chorionic gonadotropin (hCG). There is, however, no evidence supporting a "dedifferentiation hypothesis" of tumor hormone expression. Baylin and colleagues have developed an elegant model that suggests that different types of epithelial bronchogenic carcinomas arise through clonal expansion of a particular cell type during a continuum of differentiation events. Clonal expansion of cells at a less differentiated stage or clonal expansion of rare hormone-secreting cells would result in increased hormone expression (6–8).

TABLE 42.1. HORMONES ASSOCIATED WITH BRONCHOGENIC CARCINOMA PARANEOPLASTIC SYNDROMES

Adrenocorticotropic hormone (ACTH) and proopiomelanocortin (POMC)
Antidiuretic hormone (ADH)/arginine vasopressin
Atrial natriuretic factor
Calcitonin
Corticotropin-releasing hormone
Follicle-stimulating hormone (FSH)
Gastrin-releasing peptide (GRP)
Gonadotropin-releasing hormone (GnRH)
Growth hormone (GH)
Growth hormone-releasing hormone (GHRH)
Human chorionic gonadotropin (hCG)
Human placental lactogen
Luteinizing hormone (LH)
Parathyroid hormone (PTH)
Parathyroid hormone–related protein (PTHrP)
Prolactin
Renin
Somatostatin
Vasoactive intestinal peptide (VIP)

Many neuroendocrine cells have the capacity to make bioamines and store them in neurosecretory granules. These cells sometimes are referred to as amine precursor uptake and decarboxylation (APUD) cells (9). They do not always arise from the primitive neural crest as originally proposed; instead, some are derived from endoderm. APUD cells are found in normal bronchial mucosa, and bronchial carcinoid tumors and small cell lung carcinomas (SCLCs) often are composed of these neuroendocrine cells. Tumors arising from APUD cells are the most likely to secrete biologically active hormones associated with clinical syndromes.

Proto-oncogenes are normal genes that control expression of growth factors or growth factor receptors, or cell systems coupled to growth factor receptors. Transformation to malignancy involves aberrant forms of these genes, called oncogenes. It is likely that some bronchogenic tumor hormone production is linked to activation of oncogenes. SCLC produces and secretes gastrin-releasing peptide (GRP) that stimulates growth via specific receptors (10). Lung cancers also produce insulin-like growth factors (IGFs), neurotensin, and β-endorphin that act locally (autocrine action) to stimulate mitosis and tumor growth.

TABLE 42.2. CRITERIA FOR TUMOR HORMONE PRODUCTION

1. Association of the tumor with a hormonal syndrome or elevated hormone concentration
2. Failure of normal feedback mechanisms to suppress hormone levels
3. Reduced hormone or syndrome if cancer therapy is successful
4. Recurrence of the syndrome with recurrence of the tumor
5. Demonstration of the hormone in tumor tissue
6. Increased hormone concentration across the tumor capillary bed
7. Expression of hormone messenger RNA by tumor
8. Synthesis and release of hormone by tumor tissue *in vitro*

TUMOR VERSUS ENDOCRINE HORMONE PRODUCTION

Many tumor hormones are secreted as inactive, high-molecular weight polypeptide precursors, owing to abnormal post-translational modifications or to abnormal secretory processes. Recognizable clinical syndromes result only if neoplastic tissue is able to metabolize the precursor to a bioactive hormone (5).

Tumors may produce analogs of endocrine hormones. For example, squamous cell lung carcinoma causes hypercalcemia by producing parathyroid hormone (PTH)-related protein rather than PTH.

Tumor hormone secretion often does not respond to normal feedback mechanisms. Pituitary ACTH remains somewhat responsive, even in patients with Cushing disease, but bronchogenic tumor ACTH usually cannot be stimulated by corticotropin-releasing hormone or suppressed by high-dose dexamethasone. Lack of response to dexamethasone may be owing to tumor-associated mutations in the glucocorticoid receptor (11). Bronchial carcinoid tumors are an exception. They retain some typical hormone feedback response.

INCIDENCE OF TUMOR HORMONE PRODUCTION AND HORMONE SYNDROMES

The true incidence of hormone production associated with lung carcinomas is difficult to determine. Surveys probably reflect the minimum incidence. Tumors secrete peptides sporadically, and changes in tumor peptide production occur with time, but tumor markers frequently are measured only once. Metastases may produce peptides that are different from those in the primary neoplasm. Excess hormone secretion sometimes occurs only in response to a stimulus, and provocative tests for hormone responsiveness usually are not performed. Finally, hormone assays vary from laboratory to laboratory.

Tumor hormone secretion is not always accompanied by the expected symptoms and signs, but lung cancers, especially SCLC and bronchial carcinoid tumors, have the highest reported incidence of clinical syndromes owing to tumor hormone expression (5). Hormone-induced syndromes are listed in Table 42.3.

SPECIFICITY OF TUMOR HORMONE PRODUCTION

No single peptide hormone is specific for a given bronchogenic carcinoma. Many tumors produce an array of peptide hormones. Changes in tumor peptide concentration can signal changes in tumor metabolism or malignant potential. Fluctuations in the concentration of peptides

TABLE 42.3. BRONCHOGENIC CARCINOMA HORMONES CAUSING CLINICAL SYNDROMES

Hormone	Tumor Type	Symptoms/Syndrome
ACTH	SCLC	weakness, hypertension, hypokalemia
ACTH	carcinoid	Cushing syndrome
ACTH	several	hyperpigmentation (Nelson syndrome)
PTHrP	squamous cell	humoral hypercalcemia of malignancy
PTH[a]	SCLC, carcinoid	hyperparathyroidism
ADH	SCLC, others	hyponatremia
Unknown[a]	SCLC	osteomalacia, hypophosphatemia
GH, GHRH[a]	carcinoid	acromegaly
VIP[a]	SCLC	watery-diarrhea-hypokalemia-achlorhydria syndrome
Renin[a]	carcinoid	hyperaldoseronism
Insulin[a]	carcinoid	hypoglycemia
5-HTP	carcinoid	carcinoid syndrome
hCG[a]	squamous cell	uterine bleeding

[a]Rare. Case reports only.
ACTH, adrenocorticotropic hormone; SCLC, small cell lung carcinoma; PTHrP, parathyroid hormone–related protein; PTH, parathyroid hormone; ADH, antidiuretic hormone; GH, growth hormone; GHRH, growth hormone–releasing hormone; VIP, vasoactive intestinal peptide; 5-HTP, 5-hydroxytryptamine (seratonin); hCG, human chorionic gonadotropin.

elaborated by bronchogenic carcinomas sometimes reflect the clinical course of these tumors (12,13), but not always (14–16). Peptide production may be better correlated with tumor differentiation than with tumor mass (6,7).

TREATMENT OF PARANEOPLASTIC SYNDROMES

Most treatment for hormonal and metabolic paraneoplastic syndromes is the same as the treatment for the syndromes in an endocrine setting. Randomized controlled trials of treatment of paraneoplastic syndromes are rare. This is due, in part, to the fact that paraneoplastic syndromes are detected less frequently than are endocrine syndromes. Also, many paraneoplastic syndromes occur when the tumor is far advanced, and short life expectancy precludes randomized trials.

HORMONAL AND METABOLIC SYNDROMES

Adrenocorticotropin and Corticotropin-Releasing Hormone

The ACTH concentration in normal lung is only 0.000003% to 0.00005% of that in the pituitary gland. Tissue extracts from lung carcinomas of all types contain a large-molecular-weight, biologically inactive form of ACTH

(proACTH), which can be converted to bioactive ACTH (17,18). Normal lung and all lung carcinomas also contain the precursor peptide pro-opiomelanocortin (POMC) and its component peptides: pro-ACTH and β-lipotropin, a hormone with weak lipotrophic and melanocyte-stimulating activity. POMC also is cleaved to melanocyte-stimulating peptide fragments, β-endorphin, and corticotropin-like intermediate lobe peptide (CLIP), a peptide that has no known function. In normal lung, the concentration of POMC mRNA is only 0.008% to 0.08% of that in the pituitary gland, and smaller forms of POMC mRNA predominate. These do not code for a signal sequence, so the POMC peptides cannot be secreted (19). However, lung carcinomas contain large amounts of full-length POMC mRNA, and can secrete enough POMC-derived peptides to produce clinical syndromes (20). Why so many lung carcinomas produce excess POMC-derived peptides remains an enigma. If the POMC gene product β-endorphin functions as a significant autocrine growth factor, lung cancers overexpressing POMC might have a selective advantage (21). Excess CLIP is produced by lung carcinomas but not by pituitary tumors. If the CLIP assay were readily available, the CLIP/CLIP + ACTH ratio could be used to confirm a nonpituitary source of ACTH.

Ectopic ACTH secretion occurs in 50% of patients with SCLC (22), but only 5% (range, 1.8%–11% in retrospective studies of 840, 545, 345, and 90 patients) (23–26) have clinical and/or biochemical manifestations of Cushing syndrome. Some patients are asymptomatic, even though morning cortisol concentrations are high and the normal diurnal variation of cortisol is absent. Plasma 11-deoxycorticosterone and dehydroepiandrosterone sulfate concentrations and urine free cortisol, 17-hydroxysteroid, and 17-ketosteroid levels also are high.

Patients with SCLC rarely develop the full clinical spectrum of Cushing syndrome, because progression of the disease is so rapid. Effects of high ACTH on electrolyte flux develop more rapidly than do effects on lipid and carbohydrate metabolism. In a study of 23 patients with SCLC and Cushing syndrome (24), the most common clinical features were pretibial and ankle pitting edema (83%), severe proximal muscle weakness (61%), buffalo hump and truncal obesity (35%), and hypertension, hyperpigmentation, and psychoses (22%). All patients had high plasma cortisol, loss of cortisol diurnal variation, and high 24-hour urine free cortisol. Hypokalemia with metabolic alkalosis (serum bicarbonate usually >30 mmol/L and pH >7.45) was found in 96%, and 59% of patients had hyperglycemia. Hyperpigmentation (Fig. 42.1) is the result of the excess lipotropin or melanocyte-stimulating fragments of POMC.

The prognosis for patients with SCLC and Cushing syndrome is terrible. Cortisol excess fosters opportunistic infections that frequently are fatal. These are thought to be responsible for the poor response to chemotherapy, even in patients who are not neutropenic. In one study (26), nine

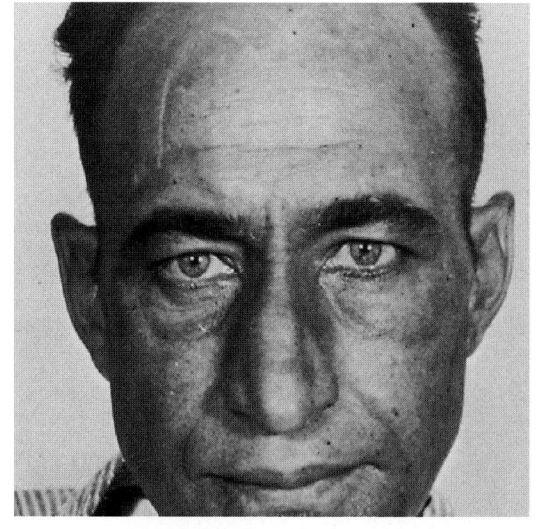

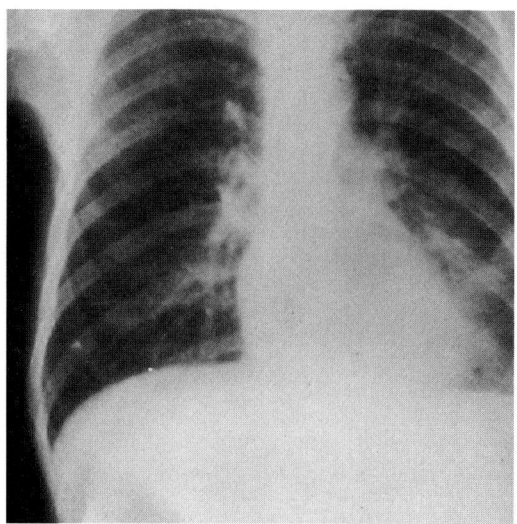

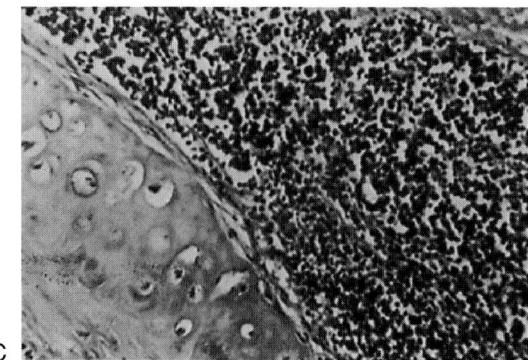

FIGURE 42.1. (A) This patient with carcinoma of the lung complained of darkening of the skin. Note the hyperpigmentation under his eyes and around his mouth. **(B)** His chest film revealed an area of infiltration along the left cardiac border. Scalene node biopsy was positive for anaplastic carcinoma. The patient had increased 17-ketosteroids, total 17-ketogenic steroids, and 17-hydroxycorticosteroids, but had no clinical Cushing syndrome. **(C)** Small cell anaplastic carcinoma arising in the left lower lobe bronchus was found at postmortem examination. Note the marked variation in the size and shape of the deeply staining nuclei (magnification ×450).

of 11 patients with Cushing syndrome died within 14 days of initiation of chemotherapy compared with 19 of 77 control patients who had SCLC without Cushing syndrome. The two patients with Cushing syndrome who survived the initial chemotherapy were treated with metyrapone to control hypercortisolism before chemotherapy was begun. In another study of 10 patients with Cushing syndrome and SCLC (25), hypercortisolism was controlled by chemotherapy in the three patients who survived more than 6 months.

Treatment options include inhibitors of steroid biosynthesis such as metyrapone, ketoconazole, and aminoglutethimide, but all have serious side effects, and overall response is poor. Patients with SCLC usually require high doses of these agents, sometimes in combination. Mifepristone, a drug that blocks steroid action at the receptor level, has been used successfully, but the drug is not available in the United States except for research protocols. The adrenocorticolytic drug mitotane is not useful, because the onset of action is slow and several weeks are required to control cortisol secretion. Potassium and spironolactone can be given to control hypokalemia.

Patients with other types of lung cancers, particularly bronchial carcinoid tumors, also develop Cushing syndrome. These tumors grow more slowly than does SCLC, and

patients develop classic features of Cushing syndrome, including moon facies, truncal obesity, purple abdominal striae, hirsutism, psychosis, hypertension, edema, osteoporosis, and hyperglycemia (Fig. 42.2). Differentiating bronchial carcinoid ACTH production from pituitary tumor ACTH production can be difficult. In patients with SCLC, plasma ACTH and cortisol concentrations usually are not suppressed by high-dose dexamethasone, but partial suppression can occur with carcinoid tumors. In some patients, ACTH and 11β-deoxycortisol increase appropriately after metyrapone administration (27,28).

Occasionally, patients with bronchial carcinoid tumors develop Cushing syndrome owing to tumor corticotropin-releasing hormone that induces pituitary hyperstimulation and bilateral adrenal hyperplasia. These tumors are even more difficult to differentiate from pituitary adenomas by biochemical testing than are bronchial carcinoid tumors that produce ACTH.

If surgical resection of the bronchial carcinoid tumor is not possible, the same drugs used to treat hypercortisolism in patients with SCLC are used for patients with the more indolent bronchial carcinoid tumors (29,30). Smaller doses or a combination of drugs can reduce the side effects of each. The somatostatin analog octreotide has been used for

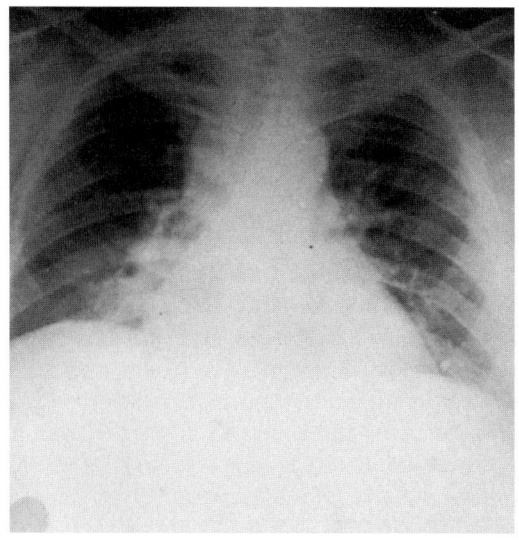

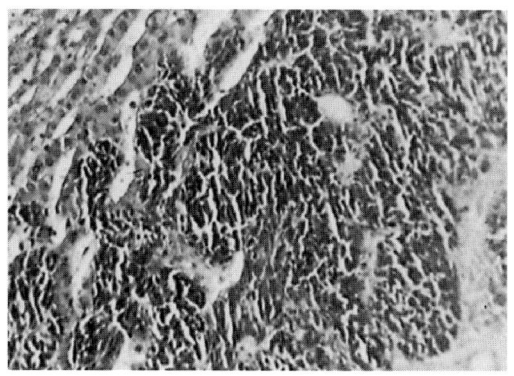

FIGURE 42.2. (A) Chest roentgenogram showing an area of increased density along the right cardiac border. The patient was a 34-year-old man with truncal obesity, edema, hypertension, hypokalemic alkalosis, polycythemia, and the typical urinary steroid values of Cushing syndrome. **(B)** A liver biopsy was obtained at abdominal exploration. A large nest of anaplastic carcinoma cells metastatic from the lung is seen adjacent to cords of liver cells (magnification × 450).

these patients, although paradoxical increases in ACTH after octreotide and lanreotide, a slow release somatostatin analog, have been reported (31). There is one report of suppression of carcinoid tumor ACTH by bromocriptine (32). Bilateral adrenalectomy is effective if medical therapy fails.

BRONCHOGENIC CARCINOMA AND ADRENOCORTICOTROPIN PRODUCTION	
Summary Statement	**Level of Evidence**
Bronchogenic carcinoma produces adrenocorticotropin.	Observational studies
Patients with small cell lung carcinoma–associated hypercortisolism develop weakness and signs of mineralocorticoid excess but do not develop Cushing syndrome.	Case reports and small observational studies
Patients with bronchial carcinoid tumor–associated hypercortisolism develop all clinical features of Cushing syndrome.	Case reports and observational studies

Antidiuretic Hormone (Arginine Vasopressin) and Atrial Natriuretic Factor

In 1938, Winkler and Cranshaw described a patient with the combination of lung cancer, hyponatremia, and excessive urinary sodium loss (33). Almost 20 years later, Schwartz and colleagues observed that despite an increased extracellular fluid volume and hypotonic plasma, the urine of similar patients was hypertonic (34). They proposed that the fluid and electrolyte imbalance seen in these patients was a consequence of inappropriate secretion of antidiuretic hormone (ADH, or arginine vasopressin). ADH subsequently was found in tumor extracts, and synthesis of ADH was demonstrated by tumor tissue *in vitro*. Elevated or inappropriate plasma ADH concentrations have been found in 40% to 50% of patients with SCLC and somewhat less often with other types of lung cancer (35–37).

Tumor-associated ADH is indistinguishable chemically and immunologically from ADH released from the posterior pituitary gland. Pituitary ADH is stored in association with another polypeptide, a neurophysin, and both are secreted together. Tumor neurophysin is detectable in only 70% of patients with SCLC. Inappropriate ADH secretion may precede evidence of the tumor mass by several months. The highest and most persistent ADH concentrations occur in patients with extensive or rapidly progressing tumors (38), but neither plasma nor cerebrospinal ADH concentrations can be used to assess disease progression or response to therapy (39). Radioactive neurophysin antibodies are being tested to see if they can be used for localizing tumors or to monitor the response to therapy.

The clinical response to tumor ADH (syndrome of inappropriate ADH, or SIADH) depends on the degree of water loading (40). Given normal thirst mechanisms, patients will have normal serum sodium levels if water intake is not excessive. If water intake is too high, the ensuing hyponatremia can be severe. Hyponatremia can be exacerbated by chemotherapy, particularly cyclophosphamide, radiation therapy, or prostaglandin inhibitors (prostaglandins of the E_2 series are inhibitors of ADH action) (38). Most patients are asymptomatic if the serum sodium is more than 120 mmol/L, and usually no treatment is necessary. If the serum sodium falls below 120 mmol/L, patients are likely to develop headache, lethargy, generalized weakness, confusion, and somnolence. If severe hyponatremia develops rapidly, patients may present with nausea and vomiting. When serum sodium falls below 110 mmol/L, the risk of seizures, hypothermia, coma, and death increases markedly.

Treatment of tumor-induced SIADH is similar to the treatment of SIADH in other settings (41). Fluid restriction to an intake less than insensible water loss often restores the sodium concentration. If the hyponatremia is severe, hypertonic saline infusion can be coupled with furosemide administration and replacement of urinary electrolyte losses until the serum sodium concentration increases. Demeclocycline, which produces reversible ADH resistance at the kidney (reversible nephrogenic diabetes insipidus), 600 to 1200 mg/d, can be added if fluid restriction alone is not sufficient. Lithium also produces nephrogenic ADH resistance, but the side effects of lithium are greater, unpredictable, and sometimes permanent.

Lung cancer patients with hyponatremia also produce abundant atrial natriuretic factor (42,43). It usually is impossible to determine whether tumor production of atrial natriuretic factor is the primary cause of the hyponatremia or whether atrial natriuretic factor is increased in response to expanded plasma volume caused by inappropriate ADH.

BRONCHOGENIC CARCINOMA AND ANTIDIURETIC HORMONE PRODUCTION	
Summary Statement	**Level of Evidence**
Bronchogenic carcinomas produce ADH. Tumor ADH is indistinguishable from pituitary ADH and causes equivalent hyponatremia.	Observational studies and *in vitro* confirmation of tumor ADH production.
Treatment is usually unnecessary unless serum sodium is <120 mEq/L. If hyponatremia is severe, hypertonic saline may be necessary acutely. Fluid restriction and demeclocycline are the mainstays of treatment.	Clinical studies in patients with excess pituitary ADH; observational studies and case reports in patients with bronchogenic cancer ADH

ADH, antidiuretic hormone.

Calcium-Regulating Hormones: Humoral Hypercalcemia of Malignancy

The association of hypercalcemia and hypophosphatemia with solid tumors without evidence of bony metastases has been known since 1923. The syndrome is referred to as humoral hypercalcemia of malignancy (HHM) (44). HHM is associated most often with tumors of the lung, particularly

squamous cell carcinoma. In the 1980s, PTH-related protein (PTHrP), the agent responsible for most lung cancer–associated hypercalcemia, was isolated from a lung tumor (45), and the cDNA has been cloned (46,47). PTHrP has 70% homology with the 13 N-terminal amino acids of PTH and exerts its calcemic effects by binding to the PTH receptor, resulting in stimulation of adenyl cyclase and phospholipase C.

PTHrP also is expressed widely in normal fetal and adult tissues (48). It plays a paracrine role in regulating cartilage differentiation and bone formation, tooth development, growth and differentiation of skin, breast and pancreatic islets, transepithelial calcium transport in placenta, breast and distal nephron, smooth muscle relaxation in many tissues, and immune function (44). However, circulating concentrations of PTHrP normally are very low.

In HHM, circulating concentrations of PTHrP are high. Hypercalcemia, hypophosphatemia, hypercalciuria, and hyperphosphaturia are the results of markedly increased osteoclastic bone resorption uncoupled from bone formation, associated with increased renal tubular resorption of calcium. Even though PTHrP combines with the PTH receptor, circulating 1,25-dihydroxyvitamin D and intestinal calcium absorption usually are low in patients with HHM (49). Now that an accurate immunoradiometric assay for PTH is available, it is clear that in the absence of renal failure, PTH levels in patients with HHM are low or low-normal, suppressed by the hypercalcemia. Other differences between HHM and primary hyperparathyroidism are shown in Table 42.4. It is possible that tumor cytokines such as interleukin (IL)-1 and IL-6, tumor growth factor-α, and tumor necrosis factor-α (TNF-α) modify the usual effects of PTHrP.

In most patients with HHM, it is unnecessary to order a PTHrP level. The tumor is obvious, and the life expectancy is only 1 to 3 months, with very few living longer than 6 months (50). The low PTH level eliminates most other causes of hypercalcemia.

Patients with mild hypercalcemia often are asymptomatic. Serum calcium concentrations of 2.75 to 3.0 mmol/L

TABLE 42.4. DIFFERENCES BETWEEN HUMORAL HYPERCALCEMIA OF MALIGNANCY AND PRIMARY HYPERPARATHYROIDISM

	HHM	HPT
PTH (plasma)	↓	↑↑
PTHrP (plasma)	↑↑	↓
Bone resorption	↑↑	↑
Bone formation	↓	↑
Intestinal calcium absorption	↓	↑
1,25-dihydroxyvitamin D (serum)	↓	↑
Tubular absorption of HCO_3	↑	↓
Chloride (serum)	↓	↑

HHM, humoral hypercalcemia of malignancy; HPT, primary hyperparathyroidism; PTH, parathyroid hormone; PTHrP, parathyroid hormone–related protein; HCO_3, bicarbonate.

(11 to 12 mg/dL) may be associated only with mild anorexia, constipation, myalgia, or lethargy. Patients who become dehydrated owing to fever, anorexia, or vomiting, as well as patients who have increased bone resorption owing to immobilization or chemotherapy, are at increased risk for developing severe hypercalcemia. If hypercalcemia is severe, patients may develop nausea and vomiting, abdominal pain, polyuria, dehydration, and weakness and become confused or obtunded. Patients do not live long enough to develop band keratitis, uremia, and renal calculi.

Hypercalcemia symptoms improve with treatment. If rapid calcium lowering is needed, intravenous normal saline restores volume, increases glomerular filtration, and decreases sodium and calcium reabsorption in the proximal tubule. If necessary, furosemide can be added to correct the hypernatremia caused by hypercalcemia-induced resistance to ADH. Calcitonin in doses of 200 to 400 IU subcutaneously every 12 hours also helps to lower calcium acutely. The effect usually is transient (48 hours), possibly owing to down-regulation of receptors. Nausea, vomiting, and rash are the main side effects.

The bisphosphonates, pamidronate or zoledronate, given intravenously, increase osteoclast apoptosis and reduce osteoclast-mediated bone resorption. They are the treatments of choice for HMM. The plasma calcium concentration begins to fall within 48 hours; the nadir is reached at 5 to 7 days. In a dose-response study, infusions of 30, 60, or 90 mg of pamidronate in a 24-hour period normalized serum calcium in 30%, 61%, and 100% of patients, respectively (51). In two multicenter, double-blind trials, a total of 287 patients with moderate to severe HHM were given zoledronate (4 mg infused over 15 min) or pamidronate (90 mg infused over 4 hours). Normocalcemia was achieved in 82.6% versus 65.6% of patients at 7 days, respectively. The duration of the response was 32 versus 18 days (52). Most common side effects included transient, low-grade fever (1°C), and hypocalcemia (usually asymptomatic). Small increases in creatinine occurred in some patients. Fever after intravenous pamidronate is associated with a transient decrease in lymphocyte and leukocyte count and with increases in circulating IL-6, TNFα, and C-reactive protein (53). Renal insufficiency (creatinine clearance <35 mg/mL) is the major contraindication to bisphosphonate treatment.

Once achieved, the major problem is maintaining the lower calcium level. Effects of PTHrP on renal tubular resorption of calcium continue even after osteoclast activity is suppressed. Dietary calcium restriction, oral phosphate, and glucocorticoid administration are effective only transiently, if at all. This is not surprising because calcium absorption from the gastrointestinal tract is not increased in HHM. Oral bisphosphonates such as alendronate and risedronate are poorly absorbed from the gastrointestinal tract and cannot be given in sufficiently high doses to overcome the effects of PTHrP without causing esophageal ulceration or gastroin-

testinal distress. However, patients can be retreated with the intravenous bisphosphonates when symptomatic hypercalcemia recurs.

PTHrP is not responsible for all hypercalcemia associated with lung cancers. Hypercalcemia owing to documented secretion of PTH by SCLC has been reported (54). Most hypercalcemia associated with SCLC probably reflects unidentified bone metastases or concomitant hyperparathyroidism, because both bronchogenic cancer and primary hyperparathyroidism are common diseases.

BRONCHOGENIC CARCINOMA AND HYPERCALCEMIA	
Summary Statement	**Level of Evidence**
The association between squamous cell cancer production of PTHrP and HHM is firmly established.	Multiple laboratory studies
Intravenous bisphosphonates (pamidronate and zoledronate) control hypercalcemia by suppressing osteoclast-mediated bone resorption, but the prognosis for these patients is poor.	Randomized, placebo-controlled trials

PTHrP, parathyroid hormone–related protein; HHM, humoral hypercalcemia of malignancy.

Oncogenic Osteomalacia: Renal Phosphate Wasting

Oncogenic osteomalacia has been described in several patients with SCLC although it usually occurs with small mesenchymal tumors that are notoriously difficult to locate (55–57). All patients had marked hypophosphatemia with renal phosphate wasting (low tubular resorption of phosphorus), inappropriately low or low-normal 1,25-dihydroxyvitamin D concentrations, elevated alkaline phosphatase, and osteomalacia or increased osteoid on bone biopsy.

The biochemical picture is very similar to that of X-linked hypophosphatemic rickets. Tumor production of a substance that causes proximal renal tubule phosphate wasting and inhibition of renal 25-hydroxyvitamin D-1-α hydroxylase is thought to be responsible. A substance with these properties that is heat labile and lipid insoluble and presumed to be a peptide has been found in tumor extracts. The substance is *not* PTH or PTHrP, even though tumor extracts stimulate PTH-responsive renal adenylate cyclase. Serum calcium is normal or only slightly decreased; this substance may not react with bone receptors. Serum 25-hydroxyvitamin D and calcitonin levels are normal as well. Renal phosphate handling improves only if chemotherapy induces a remission. Patients may have a partial response to calcium, phosphate salts, and 1,25-dihydroxyvitamin D.

Calcitonin and Calcitonin Gene-Related Peptide

Calcitonin inhibits bone resorption and decreases renal tubular resorption of calcium and phosphorus, but the precise role of calcitonin in normal human physiology is uncertain. The highest concentration of calcitonin is found in the parafollicular cells of the thyroid gland, but calcitonin is produced by neuroendocrine cells in many tissues. The lungs contain more calcitonin, albeit at a lower concentration, than does the thyroid gland. Precursor peptides (procalcitonin) are secreted in response to inflammatory cytokines. Serum and urine calcitonin levels are increased in smokers and in chronic COPD, and may be a sign of lung injury (58). Calcitonin has been found in extracts of neoplasms of all types, particularly SCLC (59,60). Increased serum calcitonin response to pentagastrin stimulation has been described in lung cancer patients whose basal calcitonin concentrations were normal (61). Both serum and urine calcitonin concentrations have been correlated positively with lack of tumor differentiation and increased disease activity in some (62–64) studies, but not all (58). One group reported that calcitonin concentrations decreased in patients who responded to therapy, and increased with relapse or tumor progression (64).

Lung tumors secrete high-molecular-weight forms of calcitonin, indicating lack of prohormone processing capacity in tumor cells (65,66). There are no clinical consequences of calcitonin production by bronchogenic carcinoma. Serum calcium, inorganic phosphate, and vitamin D concentrations remain normal. Patients do not develop diarrhea.

Alternative intranuclear splicing of mRNA yields either the mRNA for calcitonin or for calcitonin gene-related peptide (CGRP) (67). CGRP is a potent vasodilator and is found in pulmonary neuroendocrine cells. CGRP messenger RNA has been detected in lung tumor cell lines by several groups (68), but CGRP may not be produced by lung tumor cells *in vivo* (58,69).

Gonadotropins

Human chorionic gonadotropin (hCG) has been found in extracts of a wide range of normal tissues, including the lung, and in extracts of all types of carcinomas (70). At least three different molecules can be measured in lung cancer patients: intact hCG, free hCG β-subunit or hCG β-core fragment (β-CF) (71). High serum hCG is found in 12% to 30% of lung cancer patients (5,12). Because tumor hCG is poorly glycosylated, tumor hCG may not be bioactive and may be degraded too rapidly to be measured in most patients (72). Approximately 50% of patients with lung cancers of all types have elevated levels of β-CF in their urine, whether or not serum values are high. The more advanced cases are more likely to have high urine β-CF, but even with stage IV cancers, urine β-CF is elevated only 72% of the time (73). The α-subunit, which is common to thyroid-stimulating hormone (TSH), follicle-stimulating hormone (FSH), luteinizing hormone (LH) and hCG, has been found in 33% of men with lung cancer (5,74). Attempts to create a vaccine exploiting the C-terminal peptide of hCG are in progress (75).

The hCG concentration does not reflect the extent of the underlying tumor (12). Tumor hCG is not suppressed by administration of androgens, estrogens, or progestins, and whether tumor hCG is biologically active is uncertain. One group reported that serum estradiol in a group of men with lung cancer was correlated with tumor mass and hCG concentration (76). In another series of patients with lung cancer and high serum hCG, testosterone levels were lower in the cancer patients than in the control group (12). None of the male patients had gynecomastia. Gynecomastia is very common in men over 50 years of age and is correlated with body weight. Because gynecomastia usually is not reported as part of the physical examination, it is difficult to determine whether gynecomastia reported in lung cancer patients is of recent onset, and whether its absence reflects weight loss owing to disease.

There is one case report of a young woman with a large squamous-cell lung carcinoma associated with very high serum levels of hCG and β-hCG and dysfunctional uterine bleeding. Tumor immunostaining was strongly positive for hCG. Dysfunctional uterine bleeding stopped, and hCG and β-hCG levels returned to normal after tumor resection (77).

Although the association of lung cancer and increased hCG seems well established, there is only one case report of a step-up in the arteriovenous gradient of FSH across a bronchogenic carcinoma capillary bed (78). Serum concentrations of both FSH and LH were elevated before tumor resection and decreased postoperatively. In all other cases in which lung tumors have been associated with gonadotropin production, either the gonadotropin proved to be hCG or the immunoassay was not sufficiently specific to exclude hCG.

Human Placental Lactogen and Prolactin

Increased serum levels of human placental lactogen (12,79) and prolactin (80) have been reported in a few patients with bronchogenic carcinoma, but no clinical consequences of either human placental lactogen or prolactin have been found.

Growth Hormone, Growth Hormone–Releasing Hormone, and Somatostatin

Small amounts of human growth hormone (GH) are found in all normal human tissues and in extracts of lung carcinomas of all histologic types (81,82). Immunoreactive GH-releasing hormone (GHRH) is present in SCLC and in bronchial carcinoid tumors (83). Rare bronchial carcinoid tumors secrete enough GHRH to cause acromegaly (83,84). Pituitary enlargement on MRI, the pattern of GH secretion, and acromegalic features are the same whether a GHRH-producing tumor arises in the hypothalamus or the lung. Plasma GHRH concentrations are high only when GHRH is produced by lung tumors, because hypothalamic tumors secrete GHRH directly into the hypothalamic-hypophyseal portal system (83).

Clinical improvement in soft tissue features of acromegaly occurs after carcinoid tumor resection (85) or successful treatment with chemotherapy (86). If these measures are unsuccessful, synthetic analogs of the hypothalamic hormone somatostatin reduce circulating GH and IGF-1 concentrations and symptoms and signs of acromegaly just as they do in patients with pituitary tumors (87). Tumors lacking somatostatin receptors 2 or 5 do not respond. Treatment with the somatostatin analog octreotide may be started at a subcutaneous dose of 50 μg three times a day; the dose is increased if necessary. Patients who respond can be transferred to a longer-acting octreotide preparation, Sandostatin-LAR, at a intramuscular dose of 20 mg every 4 weeks. Sixty-seven percent of pituitary tumors respond to this regimen with normalization of GH and IGF-1. Responses to lanreotide, another somatostatin analog unavailable in the United States, are similar (88). Somatostatin analogs decrease tumor secretion but have little effect on tumor size.

Dopamine agonists such as bromocriptine, cabergoline, and pergolide are less effective, normalizing GH and IGF-1 in 10% to 20% of patients with acromegaly due to pituitary tumors (89). An altered form of GH that binds to the GH receptor and acts as a GH antagonist in patients with pituitary tumors (90) is now available.

Somatostatin, a tetradecapeptide that inhibits release of many hormones, including GH, is found in all bronchial carcinoid tumors and in 25% to 40% of small cell carcinomas (88,91,92). Paracrine and autocrine effects such as inhibition of local growth factors or bombesin-like peptides have been proposed. No clinical sequelae of tumor somatostatin production are known.

Somatostatin receptors were once thought to be expressed only by bronchial carcinoid tumors and SCLC, but non-SCLCs also express somatostatin receptors, albeit fewer of them. Scintigraphic labeling of the somatostatin receptor by ^{111}In-pentetreotide does not identify tumor type, but has been used to locate small tumor masses (88).

Gastrointestinal Hormones

Bombesin-like Peptides

GRP has considerable homology with bombesin, a tetradecapeptide first found in amphibians, and the slightly smaller peptide neuromedin C. All of the bombesin-like peptides have similar actions. They modulate central nervous system activity, especially in the hypothalamus. They lower body temperature, increase the pain threshold, cause satiety, increase gastrointestinal motility, and affect respiration, in addition to stimulating release of gastrin and glucagon and increasing plasma glucose. Peak levels in pulmonary neuroendocrine cells occur shortly after birth, indicating a role for bombesin-like peptides in fetal lung development (93).

Most small cell carcinomas produce GRP, but only 5% of patients with small cell carcinoma have elevated serum levels (94). GRP also is found in carcinoid tumors and adenocarcinomas (93). A role for GRP as an autocrine stimulator of small cell carcinoma growth has been proposed, because GRP stimulates clonal growth and DNA synthesis in small cell carcinoma cell lines. An antibody directed against the GRP binding site prevents growth of tumor cells. No clinical manifestations of GRP produced by a bronchogenic carcinoma are known.

Gastrin is also found in small cell carcinomas and in bronchial carcinoid tumors, but no clinical consequences are known (5).

Vasoactive Intestinal Peptide

Vasoactive intestinal peptide (VIP) was first discovered as a smooth muscle relaxant and vasodilator in lung tissue and was then isolated from the intestine and many other tissues. VIP is a neuropeptide with a wide central and peripheral distribution. It has structural similarity to a many-peptide family and multiple actions, including regulation of blood flow, relaxation of smooth muscle, and stimulation of electrolyte and water secretion (95). Patients with small cell carcinomas with VIP hypersecretion develop the watery diarrhea-hypokalemia-achlorhydria syndrome usually associated with vipomas. Stools do not contain blood, mucus, or excess fat. The hypokalemia can produce profound weakness. Loss of bicarbonate in the stool results in acidosis. Hyperglycemia is caused by VIP-induced glycogenolysis and decreased insulin secretion caused by hypokalemia. Treatment includes fluid and electrolyte replacement. Prednisone may reduce the volume of diarrhea. Case reports indicate that the somatostatin analog octreotide and its long-acting form, Sandostatin-LAR, inhibit VIP secretion and improve symptoms (96). Treatment is initiated with subcutaneous octreotide 100 μg three times a day. The dose can be increased; total daily doses seldom exceed 450 μg/d. Responders can be transferred to the longer-acting analog as for treatment of acromegaly (see "Growth Hormone, Growth Hormone–Releasing Hormone, and Somatostatin" above) or carcinoid syndrome (see "Hormonal Syndromes Associated with Bronchial Carcinoid Tumors" below).

Renin

Most tumors secreting renin are of renal origin. Renin usually is secreted in the form of a large inactive precursor, suggesting that the tumor is unable to carry out normal post-translational processing. However, occasional bronchial carcinoid tumors and SCLCs secrete enough active renin to produce hyperaldosteronism, hypertension, and hypokalemia (93). The hypertension may be severe, resulting in retinal hemorrhage, and is poorly responsive to treatment, including treatment with β-blockers and angiotensin-converting enzyme inhibitors.

Hypoglycemic Factors

Most tumor-associated hypoglycemia occurs in patients with large retroperitoneal tumors, but hypoglycemia has been reported with intrathoracic tumors, including bronchogenic carcinoma (97,98). Increased glucose utilization by the tumor mass cannot account for the hypoglycemia. In most cases, circulating insulin concentrations are low. IGF-I, IGF-II, and other peptides with insulin-like bioactivity not suppressible by antibodies directed against insulin are almost never associated with bronchogenic carcinoma. The mechanism responsible for most hypoglycemia associated with bronchogenic carcinoma is unknown. Hypoglycemia usually develops when patients are fasting. Food ingestion may not be sufficient to relieve symptoms in patients with very severe hypoglycemia. Rare bronchial carcinoid tumors produce insulin.

HORMONAL SYNDROMES ASSOCIATED WITH BRONCHIAL CARCINOID TUMORS

Carcinoid Syndrome and 5-Hydroxytryptamine (Serotonin)

Carcinoid tumors arise from a population of neuroendocrine cells found mostly in the submucosa of the intestine and the bronchi. Carcinoid tumors traditionally have been classified according to the part of the primitive gut from which they are derived, by whether or not they take up and reduce silver salts and whether they produce 5-hydroxytryptophan (5-HTP) or 5-hydroxytryptamine (5-HT) (serotonin) from tryptophan (99). Carcinoid tumors arising in tissues derived from the primitive foregut usually produce 5-HTP. Carcinoid tumors arising from the primitive midgut usually produce 5-HT. Tumors arising from the hindgut do not secrete 5-HTP or 5-HT. 5-HT is metabolized by monoamine oxidase to 5-hydroxyindole acetic acid, which is excreted in the urine.

Carcinoid tumors, like SCLC, are characterized by secretory granules containing an array of hormones, biogenic amines, and markers of neuroendocrine tissue such as neuron-specific enolase (NSE). They also express many peptide receptors on the cell membrane, enabling them to respond to several growth factors. Bronchial carcinoid tumors are classified as well-differentiated tumors with small cells, minor atypia, and rare mitoses (typical carcinoid) or poorly differentiated neuroendocrine carcinomas with more atypia, increased mitoses, and areas of necrosis (atypical carcinoid). The well-differentiated tumors usually are perihilar and rarely produce 5-HT (100). The poorly-differentiated tumors usually are larger, more peripheral, and more aggressive.

Release of enough 5-HT and other vasoactive products such as kallikrein, prostaglandins, histamine, and substance P into the circulation can result in carcinoid syndrome, characterized by episodic flushing, diarrhea, paroxysmal bronchospasm, and valvular disease of the right heart. Most bronchial carcinoid tumors contain 5-HTP, but the carcinoid syndrome occurs in less than 5% of patients (101). Diversion of tryptophan to 5-HTP production can lead to nicotinic acid deficiency and a pellagra-like syndrome.

If the carcinoid tumor cannot be removed, treatment is directed toward the symptoms of carcinoid syndrome. The hypothalamic hormone somatostatin inhibits secretion of many substances, and a somatostatin analog is the treatment of choice. Somatostatin receptors (type 2) are expressed on more than 80% of carcinoid tumors. Flushing and diarrhea were promptly relieved in 22 of 25 patients with carcinoid syndrome treated with subcutaneous octreotide 150 μg three times a day; 5-hydroxyindole acetic acid excretion was reduced by 50% in 18 of 25 patients (102). Octreotide has been shown to retard colon transit and reduce circulating concentrations of peptide YY, neurotensin, VIP, and substance P (103). A randomized trial in 79 patients with carcinoid syndrome compared, double-blinded doses of 10, 20, or 30 mg of long-acting octreotide LAR given intramuscularly every 4 weeks with open-label subcutaneous octreotide100 to 300 μg given three times day (104). Treatment results were similar in all groups and were comparable with those in the previous study.

The longer-acting analog lanreotide is equally effective. An open multicenter crossover study of subcutaneous octreotide 200 μg given two or three times a day and intramuscular lanreotide 30 mg given every 10 days in 33 patients with carcinoid syndrome found no difference in the responses to the two drugs. Flushing and diarrhea disappeared or improved in 14 of 26 and 10 of 22 on lanreotide and in 17 of 27 and 11 of 22 on octreotide. The drugs were equally effective in reducing plasma 5-HT levels and urinary excretion of 5-hydroxyindole acetic acid (105). In a multicenter study of 39 patients with carcinoid syndrome, intramuscular lanreotide 30 mg was given every 14 days for 6 months. Lanreotide resulted in at least a 50% decrease in flushing in 56% and a 50% decrease in bowel movements in 54%. A 50% reduction in 5-hydroxyindole acetic acid secretion was present in 42% of patients at 6 months. No tumor regression was seen (106).

Patients with carcinoid syndrome should be started on subcutaneous octreotide 100 μg three times a day. The dose can be titrated up to 500 μg three times a day as needed. If symptoms are controlled, after 2 weeks, patients can be transferred to the longer-acting form, Sandostatin-LAR, at a intramuscular dose of 20 μg given every 4 weeks. Patients continue to take octreotide for two more weeks until Sandostatin-LAR has had time to take effect. The dose of Sandostatin-LAR can be increased to 30 μg if necessary. Patients may have episodic recurrences of diarrhea. If so, treatment with octreotide is reinstated until the exacerbation subsides. Nicotinamide supplementation may be necessary to prevent a pellagra-like syndrome if tryptophan is severely depleted.

Anesthetics, surgery, and chemotherapy can precipitate a carcinoid crisis with severe flushing, hypotension, tachycardia, arrhythmias, and wheezing if large amounts of amines enter the circulation. This can be treated with an intravenous bolus of 50 to 100 μg of octreotide, which is continued as an infusion (50 μg/h) for 24 to 48 hours (107). Glucocorticoids and antihistamines also may help.

Additional Bronchial Carcinoid–Associated Syndromes

Bronchial carcinoid tumors are remarkable because they can secrete many other hormones (108). Carcinoid corticotropin-releasing hormone or ACTH causes 1% of all cases of Cushing syndrome. ACTH and/or melanocyte-stimulating hormone can produce hyperpigmentation (Nelson syndrome). GHRH causes acromegaly. Bronchial carcinoid tumors can produce enough PTH to cause hypercalcemia, enough ADH to cause hyponatremia, enough insulin to cause hypoglycemia, and enough VIP to cause the watery diarrhea-hypokalemia-achlorhydria syndrome. Carcinoid tumors also are associated with multiple endocrine neoplasia type 1 (109). Immunoperoxidase staining reveals additional hormones that do not cause clinical syndromes: calcitonin, hCG and its α-subunit, GnRH, somatostatin, gastrin, and GRH. As many as eight to 10 hormones may be found in a single tumor. Treatment depends on the hormone secreted (see above).

CARCINOID SYNDROME	
Summary Statement	**Level of Evidence**
Bronchial carcinoid tumor secretion of 5-hydroxytryptamine and other vasoactive peptides is associated with episodic flushing, diarrhea, paroxysmal bronchospasm, and valvular disease of the right heart in ≤5% of cases.	Multiple clinical studies
Treatment with somatostatin analogs reduces or relieves symptoms in >50% of cases.	Several small randomized clinical trials with consistent results

ADDITIONAL PEPTIDE/PROTEIN PRODUCTS OF BRONCHOGENIC CARCINOMAS

Oncofetal Antigens

Glycoproteins such as CEA and αFP normally are found in high concentrations in the developing fetus but in low concentrations in adult tissues. Increased CEA has been found in smokers, in patients with nonneoplastic pulmonary disease, and in all types of lung tumors (110–112). Attempts to locate tumors with scintigraphic CEA (113) and to use serum CEA concentrations to monitor tumor progression (111,114,115) or to differentiate benign from malignant pleural effusions (112,116) have been unsuccessful.

αFP is seldom produced by lung tumors. Immunoreactivity against this antigen is found in less than 3% of cases (112).

Neuron-Specific Enolase

NSE is found in normal neurons and in neuroendocrine cells that contain secretory granules and store and secrete peptides and biogenic amines. Carcinoid tumors and SCLCs, which are derived from these cells, express NSE. NSE is elevated in less than 15% of patients with other types of lung carcinoma. Trump and colleagues have proposed that NSE might be a useful marker for detecting and monitoring SCLC and for separating atypical carcinoid tumors from epidermoid tumors, large cell tumors, and adenocarcinomas (112). NSE levels have been reported to correlate with the tumor burden in patients with small cell carcinoma (117,118). The transient increase in serum NSE after initial chemotherapy is thought to reflect tumor cell destruction (119,120).

Additional Proteins

High levels of creatine kinase BB are found in the serum of 25% to 62% of patients with small cell cancer and have been reported to provide prognostic information about patient survival. Alkaline phosphatase, amylase, thymidine kinase, ferritin, pancreatic oncofetal antigen, calmodulin, β-microglobulin, keratin and other cytoskeletal markers have been reported to be elevated in association with bronchogenic carcinoma. Their concentrations are too erratic and too nonspecific to use as tumor markers.

NEUROLOGIC SYNDROMES

Denny-Brown described a sensory neuropathy associated with bronchogenic carcinoma in 1948 (121). Since then, neurologic syndromes accompanying lung cancer, primarily SCLC, have been shown to be quite common. In a prospective survey of 150 patients with SCLC, definite paraneoplastic syndromes occurred in 3% (122). These syndromes can involve any part of the central or peripheral nervous system (Table 42.5) and often are evident before the underlying malignancy is discovered. There is little correlation between the size of the tumor burden or the rate of progression of the tumor and the severity of the neurologic disease. Unfortunately, most neurologic syndromes do not remit if the malignancy is removed.

A role for the immune system seems well established, based on a strong association between a neurologic syndrome and a specific antibody in cancer patients but not

TABLE 42.5. NEUROLOGIC PARANEOPLASTIC SYNDROMES ASSOCIATED WITH BRONCHOGENIC CARCINOMA

Central nervous system
  Paraneoplastic encephalomyelitis
  Paraneoplastic cerebellar degeneration
  Cancer-associated retinopathy
  Necrotizing myelopathy

Peripheral nervous system
  Subacute sensory neuropathy
  Peripheral sensorimotor neuropathy

Autonomic neuropathy
  Chronic intestinal pseudoobstruction

Paraneoplastic vasculitic neuropathy

Neuromuscular junction syndromes
  Lambert-Eaton syndrome

in controls. It is not clear how the antibodies gain access to neuronal cells. Paraneoplastic syndromes occur when antibodies to tumor tissue cross-react with neuronal antigens. Kornguth has proposed that the immunologic response to the tumor initially protects the patient by slowing tumor growth (123). Data compatible with this hypothesis were obtained by Galanis and colleagues who looked for a correlation between the type or titer of circulating neuronal antibodies and the extent of SCLC dissemination at presentation, the development of neuropathy during cisplatin therapy, and survival time in 58 patients with newly diagnosed SCLC (124). Neuronal autoantibodies were significantly more frequent in patients with limited disease (41%) than in those with extensive disease (17%) at presentation. Neuronal antibodies of nuclear or cytoplasmic specificity were found in 50% of seropositive patients with limited disease but were not found in seropositive patients with extensive disease. Titers fell progressively during cisplatin therapy and did not increase afterward. Seropositivity for autoantibodies did not affect development of cisplatin neuropathy or survival time. The data are compatible with destruction of a protective preexisting antitumor immune response by immunosuppressive chemotherapy.

Most paraneoplastic neurologic syndromes do not respond to immunosuppression, plasmapheresis, chemotherapy, or radiotherapy. Even if serum antibody titers are reduced, cerebrospinal fluid titers remain elevated, and there is no clinical improvement. Occasional cases with milder syndromes remain stable for months (22,125,126).

Central Nervous System Syndromes

Paraneoplastic Encephalomyelitis

Paraneoplastic encephalomyelitis (PEM) is an umbrella term covering limbic encephalitis, brainstem encephalitis, myoclonus-opsoclonus (chaotic, involuntary eye movements), and cerebellar degeneration. These disorders are characterized by perivascular inflammation and neuronal degeneration. Patients present with a variety of psychiatric disorders, memory loss, dementia, and seizures. Brainstem encephalitis may result in ophthalmoplegia, bulbar palsy, involuntary movements, and evidence of bilateral pyramidal tract lesions, depending on the location involved. Patients with cerebellar disease present with ataxia of varying severity. PEM frequently is associated with the paraneoplastic subacute sensory neuropathy described below.

PEM is one of the paraneoplastic syndromes associated with antineuronal nuclear autoantibodies, known as ANNA-1 or anti-HU antibodies, which bind selectively to neuronal tissue. These antibodies can be found in serum and cerebrospinal fluid in patients with SCLC, and in tumor extracts and tumor cell lines. Whether the antibodies are responsible for the development of the neuronal syndromes is not certain.

The effect of immune suppression on patients with PEM and anti-HU antibodies was examined retrospectively in 51 patients (42 with SCLC). Twenty five patients were given immunotherapy. PEM patients with SCLC also were compared with patients with SCLC who did not have PEM. Immunotherapy did not modify PEM or tumor outcome. Complete tumor response to chemotherapy was the only predictor of PEM stabilization (odds ratio, 7.07; 95% confidence interval, 1.68–29.76; $P = .006$). Median survival was similar in patients with or without PEM, although patients with PEM were more likely to survive for 30 months (odds ratio, 5.26; 95% confidence interval, 1.0004–27.6902; $P = .03$) (127).

In a clinical study of 71 patients with PEM associated with the presence of anti-HU (ANNA-1), the presence of the antibody prompted the search for cancer in 60% of patients. In these patients, most of whom had SCLC, there was no response to plasmapheresis, glucocorticoids, or other immunosuppressants (128).

Paraneoplastic Cerebellar Degeneration

Paraneoplastic cerebellar degeneration occurs in patients with SCLC, but it occurs far more often in patients with breast cancer. The clinical presentation usually begins with ataxia, with nystagmus, dysmetria, or tremor and dysarthria developing later. Purkinje cell degeneration is diffuse and is coupled with thinning of other molecular layers, but there are few inflammatory lesions (129). This is in contrast to the inflammatory cerebellar degeneration associated with anti-HU antibodies and paraneoplastic encephalitis.

Paraneoplastic cerebellar degeneration is associated with specific serum and cerebrospinal fluid immunoglobulins that bind to Purkinje cell cytoplasm and proximal dendrites in a characteristic pattern (130). A group of cerebellar proteins that react with the anticerebellar antibodies has been identified (131). The proteins and the antibody recognition do not occur in patients with cerebellar degeneration but no malignancy. The gene coding for one of the paraneoplastic cerebellar degeneration target antigens has been cloned and the mRNA identified in cerebellar tissue and in the RNA isolated from tumor tissue (132). These results support the concept that paraneoplastic neurologic syndromes are the result of shared brain-tumor antigens.

The neurologic deficits usually progress to severe disability over a period of several weeks and then stabilize. With a few exceptions, paraneoplastic cerebellar degeneration follows a course independent of the underlying tumor and does not remit with immunotherapy (129).

Cancer-Associated Retinopathy

Cancer-associated retinopathy is characterized by the triad of scotomatous visual field loss, photosensitivity, and retinal arteriolar narrowing, which may precede discovery of the SCLC. Patients present with rapid visual loss, color loss, and night blindness (133). Patients develop circulating antibodies to components of retinal cells and optic nerve. These antibodies primarily are directed at the photoreceptor cell protein recoverin (134). An antibody to heat shock cognate protein 70 was described recently in four patients with cancer-associated retinopathy (135). Histologic examination reveals loss of the photoreceptor cell layer. Cancer-associated retinopathy is unlike the other paraneoplastic neurologic syndromes, because it sometimes responds to immunosuppressive therapy, particularly prednisone.

Necrotizing Myelopathy

Necrotizing myelopathy is a rare paraneoplastic syndrome associated with ANNA-1 or anti-HU antibodies. The syndrome presents with bilateral loss of motor, sensory, and sphincter function but little pain. Most patients deteriorate rapidly, with ascending paraplegia resulting in death (129).

Peripheral Nervous System Syndromes

Subacute Sensory Neuropathy

Subacute sensory neuropathy, like paraneoplastic encephalitis, is associated with the ANNA-1 or anti-HU antibodies (136). The two syndromes often occur together and may mimic Guillain-Barré syndrome. Subacute sensory neuropathy occurs most often in women with SCLC, and neuropathy usually precedes diagnosis of the tumor by several months. Patients initially develop symmetrical numbness and paresthesias, especially in the lower limbs. Painful dysesthesias develop later. Vibration and position sense are impaired most often, but all sensory modalities are involved. Later in the course, patients frequently are unable to walk owing to pain and loss of proprioception. Pathological findings include loss of sensory neurons of the dorsal root ganglia and degenerative changes in the remaining cells. Some investigators suggest serologic testing for ANNA-1 in elderly smokers

with a peripheral sensory neuropathy of unknown cause, and screening for occult cancer if the antibody is present (129). However, there is no treatment advantage accompanying early diagnosis. Subacute sensory neuropathy does not respond to immunosuppressive therapy or to regression of SCLC with treatment.

Peripheral Sensorimotor Neuropathy

A heterogeneous group of sensorimotor peripheral neuropathies can occur alone or in combination with other paraneoplastic neuropathies and may antedate the diagnosis of malignancy. An axonal form is seen most often in patients with SCLC. Lower neuron symptoms and signs predominate and are symmetrical; symptoms progress at a variable rate. The etiology is unknown.

Autonomic Neuropathy: Chronic Intestinal Pseudoobstruction

Pseudoobstruction is characterized by early satiety, nausea and vomiting, abdominal pain, gastroparesis, small and large bowel dilatation, constipation, and weight loss. Some patients have other signs of abnormal autonomic nervous system function. This paraneoplastic syndrome may be present for months to years before the SCLC is diagnosed (137,138). Pseudoobstruction results from degeneration of neurons in the myenteric plexus. Autopsy studies reveal axonal degeneration in the intestine, infiltration of plasma cells and lymphocytes, and proliferation of Schwann cells of the myenteric plexus.

Pseudoobstruction is associated with high serum titers of the same antineuronal nuclear antibodies (ANNA-1 or anti-Hu) associated with paraneoplastic encephalitis and paraneoplastic subacute sensory neuropathy (139). In one series, very high titers of ANNA-1 were found in four of five patients with SCLC with chronic pseudoobstruction, but not in 29 patients with SCLC without pseudoobstruction or in patients with idiopathic intestinal pseudoobstruction (140).

Twelve patients with cancer and gastrointestinal motor dysfunction (including nine with SCLC and one with anaplastic lung cancer) were identified at the Mayo Clinic from 1985–1996. Symptoms were present for months (mean, 8.7 months; range, 1–24 months) before SCLC was diagnosed. ANNA-1 was present in the eight of nine SCLC patients tested, but not in the other cancer patients. Gastric emptying was delayed in the eight of nine patients tested; esophageal motility was abnormal in four of five patients (141).

The ANNA-1 antibody titer seems to be useful for diagnosis in cases of unexplained chronic pseudoobstruction. It is unclear whether treatment of SCLC ameliorates symptoms. Pharmacologic approaches to increase bowel motility usually are unsuccessful. Total parenteral nutrition and supportive therapy are the primary treatments.

Paraneoplastic Vasculitic Neuropathy

Paraneoplastic vasculitic neuropathy occurs with both SCLC and adenocarcinoma. The syndrome is characterized by asymmetric sensorimotor peripheral neuropathy. Nerve conduction studies reveal either no response or slowed conduction, indicating axonal disease. In most cases, the sedimentation rate is high. In contrast to the other paraneoplastic neurologic syndromes, with which it often occurs, spinal fluid protein is high. The diagnosis is confirmed by nerve biopsy showing microvasculitis and axonal degeneration (142). One case showing improvement after cyclophosphamide treatment directed against the vasculitis has been reported (143).

Neuromuscular Junction Syndromes: Lambert-Eaton Syndrome

Lambert-Eaton syndrome (LES) occurs in 2% to 5% of patients with SCLC, in patients with other cancers, and in patients with autoimmune disorders. Patients complain of easy fatigability and weakness that affects pelvic and shoulder girdle muscles, more than distal strength and bulbar function. Examination reveals proximal muscle weakness, reduced or absent deep tendon reflexes, and autonomic system dysfunction (dry mouth, constipation, and impotence). LES differs from myasthenia gravis, in that muscle strength improves with exercise and the response to edrophonium chloride is poor.

LES is the result of a presynaptic defect in the calcium-dependent release of acetylcholine from nerve terminal stor-

age vesicles (144). Acetylcholine release requires influx of calcium through voltage-gated channels, and SCLC cell lines contain these channels (145). Lennon and colleagues have found P/Q-type calcium channel antibodies in 32 of 32 cancer patients with LES and in 91% of patients without cancer with LES (146). The best evidence that these antibodies cause LES comes from passive transfer experiments. The syndrome has been transferred to mice by administration of purified immunoglobulin G (IgG) from the sera of patients with LES (147,148).

Patients improve if the underlying SCLC responds to treatment. Symptoms also respond to immunosuppressive treatment, including prednisone 40 to 60 mg/d and plasmapheresis.

OTHER SYSTEMS AFFECTED BY NONMETASTATIC BRONCHOGENIC CARCINOMA

Other organ systems affected by nonmetastatic bronchogenic carcinoma are listed in Table 42.6.

Rheumatologic, Connective Tissue, and Osseous Systems

Hypertrophic Osteoarthropathy and Clubbing

Hypertrophic osteoarthropathy (HOA) is characterized by symmetrical proliferative subperiostitis, primarily along the shafts of long bones, and increased blood flow in long

PARANEOPLASTIC NEUROLOGIC SYNDROMES	
Summary Statement	**Level of Evidence**
Antineuronal antibodies are more prevalent in patients with lung cancer and a neurologic syndrome than in lung cancer patients without a neurologic syndrome.	Population studies and case reports
LES is the only neuronal syndrome for which the underlying mechanism is known. Antibodies directed at P/Q-type calcium channel cause a defect in calcium-dependent acetylcholine release from nerve terminals.	Scientific studies
In most cases, the neurologic syndromes do not respond to immunosuppressive therapies or to plasmapheresis and do not improve even if the tumor is treated successfully. Cancer-associated retinopathy and LES are the exceptions, both respond to prednisone (40–60 mg/d).	Case reports and observational studies

LES, Lambert-Eaton syndrome.

TABLE 42.6. OTHER ORGAN SYSTEMS AFFECTED BY NONMETASTATIC BRONCHOGENIC CARCINOMA

Rheumatologic and connective tissue and osseous systems
    Hypertrophic osteoarthropathy and clubbing
    Cancer polyarthritis
    Dermatomyositis and polymyositis
    Systemic sclerosis
    Systemic vasculitis

Skin
    Acanthosis nigricans
    Erythema gyratum repens
    Additonal cutaneous syndromes

Vascular system
    Venous thrombosis
    Nonbacterial endocarditis
    Fibrinogen deficiency

Hematologic system
    Anemia
    Leukemoid and leukoerythroblastic reactions

Gastrointestinal system
    Chronic intestinal pseudo-obstruction
    Biliary tract dilatation

Kidney
    Nephrotic syndrome

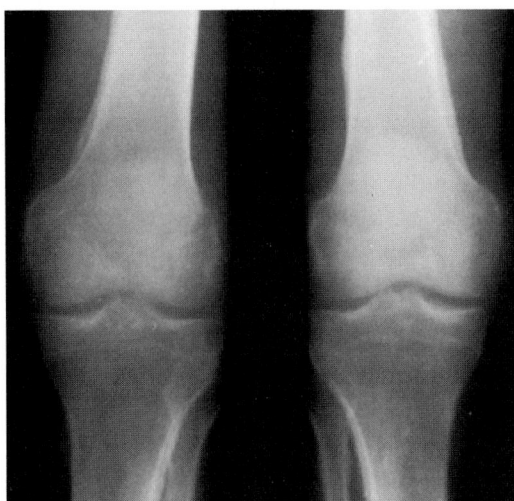

FIGURE 42.3. Roentgenogram of knees shows pulmonary hypertrophic osteoarthropathy. Note the periosteal thickening along the distal shaft of the femur and proximal shaft of the tibia and fibula.

bones, digits, and occasionally periauricular tissue (149). Patients develop bone pain and painful swelling and effusions in the elbows, wrists, knees, and ankles that may be mistaken for rheumatoid arthritis. Radiographic changes occur most often in the tibia and fibula, followed in order of frequency by the femur, ulna, and phalanges (Fig. 42.3). Bone scans show increased uptake in the cortices of affected bones.

HOA is usually accompanied by clubbing, a painless, symmetrical, uniform swelling of soft tissues at the ends of the digits (Fig. 42.4). The earliest changes occur at the base of the nail, where the skin becomes shiny and tense, and the nail rocks more easily on its bed. Later the nail becomes curved, and the angle between the nail and the soft tissues at the base is obliterated. At a more advanced stage, soft tissue hypertrophy develops. The transverse diameter of the distal phalanx increases (acropachy), and the digit resembles a drumstick. Histologic examination of the clubbed digits reveals dilated engorged vessels in the nail bed, edema, and new collagen deposition. Clubbing can occur independently of HOA. When clubbing does occur with HOA, the time of onset may be quite different, and severity may not be proportional to the bone and joint changes.

HOA and clubbing frequently are associated with lung malignancies and may develop long before the underlying tumor becomes apparent. Clubbing was found in 29% of 111 consecutive patients with lung cancer presenting to a tertiary hospital cancer center. Clubbing was more common in women than in men (40% versus 19%). Clubbing occurred more often in patients with non-SCLC than in patients with SCLC (35% versus 4%) (150). HOA also has been associated with mesothelioma.

HOA sometimes is accompanied by thickened, deeply furrowed, oily facial skin; broadening of the nose; and promi-

nent nasolabial folds. When this occurs in the setting of malignancy, the condition is termed pachydermoperiostosis.

The mechanisms underlying HOA and clubbing are uncertain. Studies in humans and dogs have shown that vagotomy decreases peripheral blood flow and abolishes HOA (151). Increased blood flow is thought to be mediated by afferents traveling via the vagus nerve, with release of a growth factor or factors normally inactivated in the lungs. HOA is associated with endothelial cell and platelet activation. Plasma levels of vascular endothelial growth factor were measured in 24 patients with HOA, seven of whom had lung cancer, and 28 individuals without HOA, nine of whom had lung cancer. Vascular endothelial growth factor concentrations were significantly higher in patients with HOA (median, 46.2; range, 19.4–398.8 pg/mL) compared with healthy controls (median, 7.4; range, 0–26.1) and were higher in lung cancer patients with HOA (median, 411.4; range, 164.2–959.5) than in lung cancer patients without HOA (median, 74.5; range, 13.2–205.4) (152).

HOA and clubbing respond to removal of the tumor or to radiation or chemotherapy with reduced joint swelling and partial regression of the bony changes. Prostaglandin synthetase inhibitors such as indomethacin, aspirin, and glucocorticoid therapy may provide symptomatic relief of joint pain and effusion. In one series, eight of 10 patients responded favorably but not completely to aspirin or nonsteroidal antiinflammatory drugs. Thoracotomy produced a complete response (153).

Cancer Polyarthritis

Patients whose polyarthritis precedes or coincides with the diagnosis of nonmetastatic SCLC and other lung cancers have been the subjects of several case reports (154,155). An immune process is assumed to be involved, but the exact mechanism is unknown. Patients with cancer polyarthritis can resemble patients with rheumatoid arthritis, presenting with painful symmetrical polyarthritis of the metacarpophalangeal joints or the proximal interphalangeal joints, hand weakness, and morning stiffness. More typical features include older age, sudden onset, asymmetric joint involvement, predominant lower extremity involvement, no rheumatoid nodules, no increase in rheumatoid factor, and no family history of rheumatoid disease. Serum anti-nuclear antibodies (ANA) may be positive. Cancer-associated arthritis usually is refractory to nonsteroidal antiinflammatory drugs or to corticosteroids, but has responded to successful treatment of the underlying malignancy.

Dermatomyositis and Polymyositis

Approximately 15% of persons with dermatomyositis have an underlying malignancy, including bronchogenic carcinoma (156,157). A population-based cohort study of 788 Swedish patients with a diagnosis of dermatomyositis or polymyositis found a relative risk of bronchogenic carcinoma

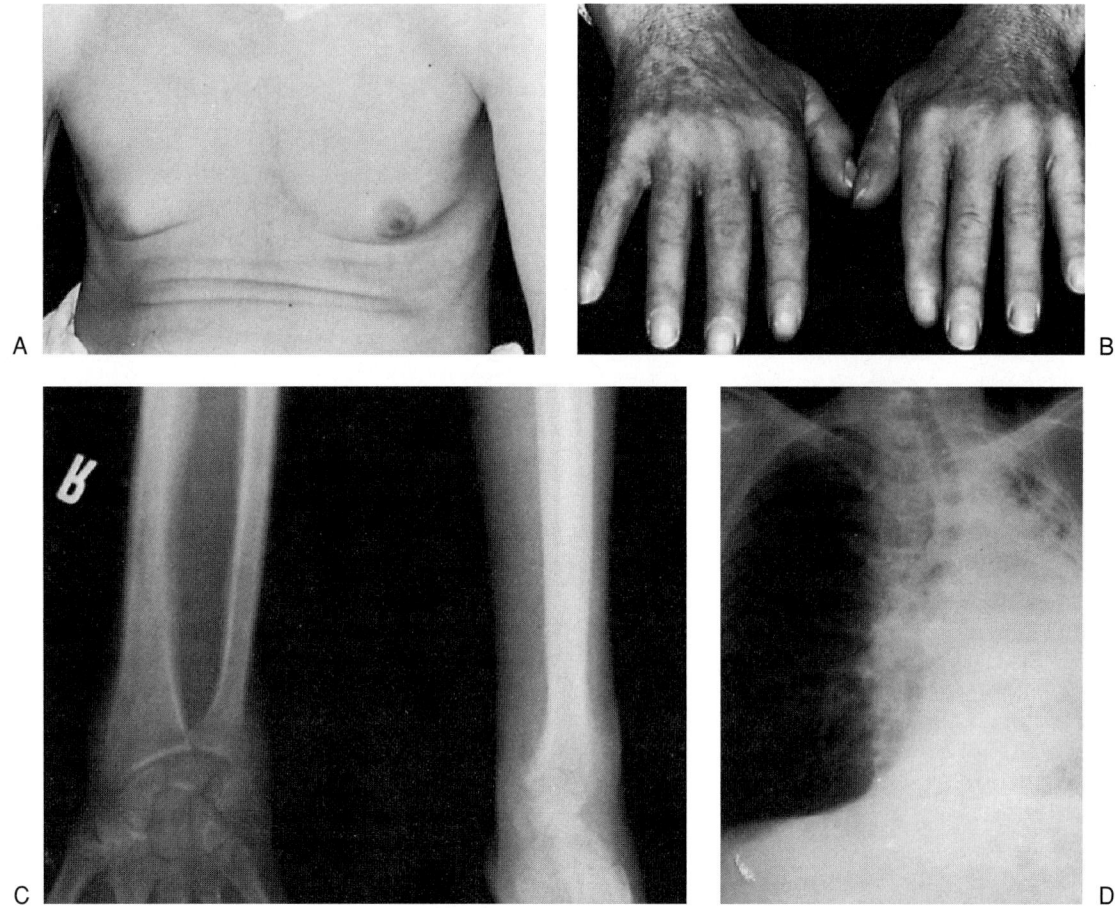

FIGURE 42.4. A 64-year-old man presented with dyspnea, gynecomastia **(A)**, clubbing of the fingers **(B)**, and tender wrists. **(C)** Roentgenogram of the forearm and wrist shows hypertrophic osteoarthropathy. Note the periosteal thickening of the long bones. **(D)** Chest roentgenogram shows complete atelectasis of the left lung. A scalene node biopsy was positive for anaplastic carcinoma.

of 5.6 in men with dermatomyositis (95% confidence interval, 2.2–11.4) and a relative risk of 4.1 (95% confidence interval, 0.5–14.7) in women with dermatomyositis (156). The percentage was higher in persons older than 50 years. Among the 396 patients with polymyositis, risk was increased significantly only for lung cancer and only in men (relative risk, 5.6; 95% confidence interval, 2.2–11.4). Manifestations of dermatomyositis often precede overt appearance of the tumor. The risk of developing polymyositis was increased only in the 1- to 5-year period after diagnosis of the tumor (156,158).

Classic findings of dermatomyositis include proximal muscle weakness and atrophy, usually beginning with the pelvic girdle and progressing to other areas. Skin lesions include erythematous scaly patches over the backs of the hands and other extensor surfaces; pruritic, photosensitive, erythematous lesions on the truck, face, and extremities; periorbital edema; and telangiectasia of the eyelids, producing a violaceous rash on the face and heliotrope eyelids. The mechanism underlying the development of this disorder is unknown.

The skin changes may or may not resolve when the malignancy is treated. Corticosteroids and immunosuppressive drugs may improve the weakness, but not necessarily the skin lesions, when treatment for the underlying tumor is not possible.

Systemic Sclerosis

An association of systemic sclerosis and lung cancer has been described. Lung cancer usually has been diagnosed after the patients have had systemic sclerosis for several years and may be more associated with the pulmonary fibrosis than with the systemic sclerosis. No histologic subtype of cancer predominates. The overall risk for cancer of any kind in patients with systemic sclerosis is 1.5 to 2.4 (159–161).

Systemic Vasculitis

Case reports suggest that occasionally vasculitis can be considered a paraneoplastic syndrome, possibly related to formation of immune complexes of tumor-associated antigens and antibodies. Most cases are associated with hematologic malignancies, but there are a few cases associated with solid tumors, including bronchogenic carcinoma. In most patients the diagnosis of vasculitis preceded the diagnosis of lung cancer. Three case reports describe Henoch-Schönlein purpura that remitted after resection of SCLC; another described relapse of purpura with relapse of oat cell carcinoma (162). Disseminated systemic vasculitis in a patient with SCLC responded to chemotherapy (163). Vasculitis associated with other types of malignancy has improved with prednisone therapy (162).

Skin

Acanthosis Nigricans

Acanthosis nigricans is characterized by bilateral, symmetrical, darkly pigmented, velvety piling up of skin associated with many tiny papillomatous overgrowths. Acanthosis nigricans is found in flexural areas, including the axillae; on the back and sides of the neck; on the antecubital fossae; beneath the breasts or folds of abdominal fat; behind the knees; between the thighs; and in the perianal region. Occasionally, it occurs on the face around the mouth and nose. Mucous membranes also may be involved. Histologic examination reveals thickened layers of the epidermis with an increase in the pigmented basal layers and papillary hypertrophy.

In the absence of malignancy, acanthosis nigricans primarily is associated with obesity, insulin resistance, and autoimmune syndromes. When acanthosis nigricans is associated with malignancy, patients usually are older and may not be obese. Most tumors associated with acanthosis are intraabdominal, but about 5% of patients have adenocarcinoma of the lung (164,165). Detection of acanthosis nigricans may precede detection of the underlying tumor, but the tumor and the skin disorder tend to progress together. Removal of the tumor may lead to regression of the skin changes. The circulating factors(s) responsible for the epidermal overgrowth is (are) unknown.

Erythema Gyratum Repens

Erythema gyratum repens is a slow-moving, erythematous, gyrate macular eruption that gives the skin a knotty-pine appearance. This is a rare condition usually found in association with cancer, especially with bronchogenic cancer (166). This condition is thought to develop in response to altered organ proteins produced by tumor necrosis. Immunoglobulin deposits are found at the basement membrane zone of the skin and in the lung tumor, and antibodies to basement membrane also appear in the circulation (167). The mechanism of the migration is unknown, but has been compared with the movement of amoebae in agar. Resection of the tumor results in disappearance of the cutaneous stigmata (168).

Additional Cutaneous Conditions Associated with Lung Cancers

A number of nonspecific dermatitides have been associated with lung cancers, including hyperpigmentation, erythema, bullous and eczematous rashes, ichthyosis, and hypertrichosis (167–170).

Tripe palms (cutaneous paraneoplastic keratoderma) are thickened palms with hyperkeratosis and acanthosis and exaggerated skin markings that are associated with lung and gastric malignancies. The palm contours supposedly resemble the surface of tripe. The pathogenesis is unknown (171).

Cases of pemphigoid (172) and cutaneous leukocytoclastic vasculitis (173) thought to represent paraneoplastic syndromes associated with lung cancer have been reported.

Vascular System

Venous Thrombosis

The association of venous thrombosis and malignancy, overt or occult, has been reported repeatedly since the first description by Trousseau in 1868 (perhaps the earliest report of a paraneoplastic syndrome). Approximately 20% of patients with untreated cancer have clinical evidence of hemorrhage or thrombosis. Almost all patients with advanced cancer have laboratory evidence of abnormal coagulation. Possible mechanisms—in addition to thrombocytosis, increased platelet adhesiveness, venous stasis, and mechanical obstruction by the tumor—include release of procoagulants from tumor cells, production of clotting factors in response to inflammatory cytokines, dysfibrinogenemia, decreased antithrombin III, and hypercalcemia (175). Twenty percent of cases of venous thrombosis associated with cancer are attributed to lung cancers. Thrombosis is associated particularly with mucin-producing adenocarcinoma (174).

Clinical complications of thrombosis include superficial thrombophlebitis that may be migratory or bilateral, involving the extremities and neck, deep vein thrombosis (DVT), pulmonary embolism, arterial thrombosis, nonbacterial thrombotic endocarditis, gangrene, and priapism.

Several studies indicate that pulmonary embolism, with or without overt DVT, may precede appearance of the neoplasm by months or years. One prospective study monitored 153 patients with acute DVT but no history of previous DVT, obvious risk factors, or cancer. Sixteen percent developed cancer within 2 years (176). Most of the cancers were detected in those who had a second DVT. Another study screened patients with a first DVT aggressively—using tumor markers (CEA, cancer antigen 125, prostate-specific antigen), chest x-ray, pelvic and abdominal computed tomography scans, and gastrointestinal endoscopy—and found a 23% incidence of underlying malignancy (177). The positive predictive value of DVT for cancers of all types was approximately 20%, but only one patient in each series had unsuspected lung cancer. A more recent study in 152 patients with DVT (178) suggests that a comprehensive medical history, physical examination, routine laboratory testing, and chest x-ray are appropriate for detecting cancer in patients with DVT, and that additional testing should be performed only as directed by abnormal results on the initial evaluation.

In contrast to the studies cited, a prospective study at the Mayo Clinic did not find DVT or PE predictive of malignancy (179). Thrombosis was increased in patients with clinically obvious malignancy, but there was no difference in new cancer occurrence over the next 3 years in patients in whom venograms, lung scans, or pulmonary angiography confirmed thrombosis and those in whom the studies were negative. It is therefore not clear whether more aggressive screening and earlier diagnosis would have any impact upon survival in patients with lung cancer.

Treatment is problematic if the tumor cannot be removed. Anticoagulants may be effective in acute situations and can be used to prevent pulmonary emboli, but thromboses often recur despite apparently adequate anticoagulation.

Nonbacterial Thrombotic Endocarditis

Nonbacterial thrombotic endocarditis is often found at autopsy in patients with malignancy but is a rare overt complication in patients with bronchogenic cancer. Accumulation of fibrin and platelets results in sterile vegetations, usually on the mitral and aortic valves. The most severe complications are strokes, myocardial infarctions, and mesenteric ischemia, but emboli can cause pain elsewhere, particularly in the extremities (180).

Fibrinogen Deficiency

Fibrinogen deficiency has been reported in association with bronchogenic carcinoma, but is more common with carcinoma of the prostate (181). Fibrinogen deficiency may be owing to widespread intravascular clotting, but elaboration of a circulating fibrinolysin also is possible.

Hematologic System

Anemia

Anemia in the absence of blood loss is common in malignancy. Most anemias are due to nonparaneoplastic causes such as iron deficiency, impaired iron utilization and erythrocyte formation, chemotherapy, and bone marrow infiltration. However, rare cases of autoimmune hemolytic anemia have been reported in association with lung carcinoma. The underlying tumor antigen is unknown.

Leukemoid and Leukoerythroblastic Reactions

Profound eosinophilia with eosinophilic infiltration in many tissues is associated with production of eosinophilic colony-stimulating factor and eosinophilic chemotactic factor (182). The frequency of eosinophilia reported in patients with bronchogenic carcinoma ranges from 4.7% to 11.4% (183,184), mostly in association with non-SCLC. Circulating eosinophilia is not always associated eosinophilia within the tumor. Successful resection of the tumor results in resolution of the eosinophilia (185).

Lung cancer is associated with neutrophilia and thrombocytosis resulting from production of many colony-stimulating factors (186,187). Humoral hypercalcemia of malignancy is frequently accompanied by leukocytosis, particularly in patients with squamous cell carcinoma (44). The leukocytosis has been linked to colony stimulating factors and cytokines, including IL-6, IL-1, and TNF (188).

Gastrointestinal System

Chronic Intestinal Pseudoobstruction

See sections "Neurologic Syndromes" and "Autonomic Neuropathy."

Biliary Tract Dilatation

Three cases of biliary tract dilatation associated with adenocarcinoma of the lung have been described. None of these patients had biliary symptoms, but they had high levels of alkaline phosphatase, modestly increased total and direct bilirubin, and increased γ-glutamyl transferase. All had dilatation of the entire biliary tree confirmed by computed tomography scan and endoscopic retrograde cholangiopancreatography. None of these patients had any other explanation for biliary tree dilatation. There was no anatomic obstruction; no evidence of metastases to the liver, bile ducts, or bone; and no evidence of any other infiltrative process or gallstones. These patients had no evidence of hepatitis, no use of drugs or medications associated with liver disease, and no history of surgery or other systemic disease to explain the biliary tract dilatation. Biliary manometry and liver biopsies were not performed (189).

Kidney

Nephrotic Syndrome

Nephrotic syndrome presenting in adult patients, especially older adult patients, is reported to be associated with bronchogenic carcinoma in approximately 3% of cases. In most cases involving bronchogenic carcinoma, the nephrotic syndrome is caused by membranous glomerulonephritis, with deposition of immune complexes including tumor antigen and IgG or immunoglobulin A (IgA) on the glomerular basement membrane (190). The nephrotic syndrome regresses in 75% of cases if the tumor responds to surgery or chemotherapy. It also regresses if an unresectable bronchogenic carcinoma responds to radiation therapy (191).

OTHER PARANEOPLASTIC SYNDROMES

Summary Statement	Level of Evidence
Bronchogenic carcinomas produce effects on many organ systems which are either very rare or are largely unrecognized (Table 42.6). Many of these disorders often appear well before the lung tumor becomes apparent.	Case reports
The relationships of hypertrophic osteoarthropathy, dermatomyositis, and polymyositis, and venous thrombosis to malignancy, including lung cancer, are well established.	Observational studies

In summary, it is important to recognize that many endocrine syndromes are associated with lung cancer and, indeed, may be harbingers of the disease. Identification of these syndromes may be helpful in directing the workup and plan for patients, especially if symptoms and signs are not responding readily to usual treatment. However, there is no evidence at this time that increased awareness of the association of these syndromes with lung cancer, and earlier recognition of the malignancy when the tumor burden is smaller, would prolong survival in an individual patient.

REFERENCES

1. Brown WH. A case of pluriglandular syndrome: diabetes of bearded women. *Lancet* 1928;2:1022–1023.
2. Albright F. Case 27461: case records of the Massachusetts General Hospital. *N Engl J Med* 1941;225:789–791.
3. Borstein P, Nolan JP, Bernanke D. Adrenocortical hyperfunction in association with anaplastic carcinoma of the respiratory tract. *N Engl J Med* 1961;264:363–371.
4. Christy NP. Adrenocorticotrophic activity in the plasma of patient with Cushing's syndrome associated with pulmonary neoplasms. *Lancet* 1961;1:85–86.
5. Odell WD, Wolfsen AR, Yoshimoto Y. Ectopic peptide synthesis: a universal concomitant of neoplasia. *Trans Assoc Am Physicians* 1977;40:204–227.
6. Baylin SB, Mendelsohn G. Ectopic (inappropriate) hormone production by tumors: mechanisms involved and the biological and clinical implications. *Endocr Rev* 1980;1:45–77.
7. Baylin SB, Jackson RD, Goodwin G, et al. Neuroendocrine-related biochemistry in the spectrum of human lung cancers. *Exp Lung Res* 1982;3:209–223.
8. Goodwin G, Shaper JH, Abeloff MD, et al. Analysis of cell surface proteins delineates a differentiation pathway linking endocrine and nonendocrine human lung cancers. *Proc Natl Acad Sci U S A* 1983;80:3807–3811.
9. Pearse AGE. The cytochemistry and ultrastructure of polypeptide hormone producing cells of the APUD series and the embryologic, physiologic, and pathologic implications of the concept. *J Histochem Cytochem* 1969;17:303–313.
10. Sporn MB, Todaro CJ. Autocrine secretion and malignant transformation of cells. *N Engl J Med* 1980;303:878–880.
11. White A, Clark AJL. The cellular and molecular basis of the ectopic ACTH syndrome. *Clin Endocrinol* 1993;39:131–141.
12. Gropp C, Havemann K, Scheuer A. Ectopic hormones in lung cancer patients at diagnosis and during therapy. *Cancer* 1980;46:347–354.
13. Kasurinen J, Syrjanen KJ. Peptide hormone reactivity and prognosis in small-cell carcinoma of the lung. *Respiration* 1986;49:61–67.
14. Hansen M, Hammer M, Hummer L. ACTH, ADH, and calcitonin concentrations as markers of response and relapse in small-cell carcinoma of the lung. *Cancer* 1980;46:2062–2067.
15. Hansen M, Bork E. Peptide hormones in patients with lung cancer. *Recent Results Cancer Res* 1985;99:180–186.
16. Hansen M, Pedersen AG. Tumor markers in patients with lung cancer. *Chest* 1986;89[Suppl]:219S–224S.
17. Gewirtz G, Schneider B, Krieger DT, et al. Big-ACTH conversion to biologically active ACTH by trypsin. *J Clin Endocrinol Metab* 1974;38:227–230.
18. Gewirtz G, Yalow RS. Ectopic ACTH production in carcinomas of the lung. *J Clin Invest* 1974;53:1022–1032.
19. DeBold CR, Menefee JK, Nicholson WE, et al. Proopiomelanocortin gene is expressed in many normal human tissues and in tumors not associated with ectopic adrenocorticotropin syndrome. *Mol Endocrinol* 1988;2:862–870.
20. White A, Clark AJL, Stewart MF. The synthesis of ACTH and related peptides by tumours. *Ballieres Clin Endocrinol Metab* 1990;4:1–27.
21. White A, Clark JL. The cellular and molecular basis of the ectopic ACTH syndrome. *Clin Endocrinol* 1993;39:131–141.
22. Schiller JH, Jones JC. Paraneoplastic syndromes associated with lung cancer. *Curr Opin Oncol* 1993;5:335–342.
23. Delisle L, Boyer MJ, Warr D, et al. Ectopic carcinoma syndrome and small-cell carcinoma of the lung. *Arch Intern Med* 1993;153:746–752.
24. Shepherd FA, Laskey JL, Evans WK, et al. Cushing's syndrome associated with ectopic corticotropin production and small-cell lung cancer. *J Clin Oncol* 1992;10:1021–1027.
25. Collichio FA, Woolf PD, Brower M. Management of patients with small cell carcinoma and the syndrome of ectopic corticotropin secretion. *Cancer* 1994;73:1361–1367.
26. Dimopoulos MA, Fernandez JF, Samaan NA, et al. Paraneoplastic Cushing's syndrome as an adverse prognostic factor in patients who die early with small cell lung cancer. *Cancer* 1992;69:66–71.
27. Limper AH, Carpenter PC, Scheithauer B, et al. The Cushing syndrome induced by bronchial carcinoid tumors. *Ann Intern Med* 1992;117:209–214.
28. Malchoff CD, Orth DN, Abboud C, et al. Ectopic ACTH syndrome caused by a bronchial carcinoid tumor responsive to dexamethasone, metyrapone and corticotropin-releasing factor. *Am J Med* 1988;84:760–764.
29. Pass HI, Doppman JL, Nieman L, et al. Management of the ectopic ACTH syndrome due to thoracic carcinoids. *Ann Thorac Surg* 1990;50:52–57.
30. Farwell AP, Devlin JT, Stewart JA. Total suppression of cortisol excretion by ketoconazole in the therapy of the ectopic adrenocorticotropic hormone syndrome. *Am J Med* 1988;84:1063–1066.

31. Rieu M, Rosilio M, Richard A, et al. Paradoxical effect of somatostatin analogues on the ectopic secretion of corticotropin in two cases of small cell lung carcinoma. *Horm Res* 1993;39:207–212.

32. Reith P, Monnot E, Bathija PJ. Prolonged suppression of a corticotropin-producing bronchial carcinoid by oral bromocriptine. *Arch Intern Med* 1987;147:989–991.

33. Winkler AW, Crankshaw OF. Chloride depletion in conditions other than Addison's disease. *J Clin Invest* 1938;17:1–6.

34. Schwartz WB, Hainsworth J, Sismani A, et al. A syndrome of renal sodium loss and hyponatraemia probably resulting from inappropriate secretion of antidiuretic hormone. *Am J Med* 1957;23:529–542.

35. Comis RL, Miller M, Ginsberg SJ. Abnormalities in water homeostasis in small cell anaplastic lung cancer. *Cancer* 1980;45:2414–2421.

36. Mauer LH, O'Donnell JF, Kennedy S, et al. Human neurophysins in carcinoma of the lung: Relation to histology, disease stage, response rate, survival, and syndrome of inappropriate antidiuretic hormone secretion. *Cancer Treat Rep* 1983;76:971–976.

37. Winklemann W, Deuss U, Allolio B, et al. Adrenocorticotropin, calcitonin and antidiuretic hormone as tumor markers in patients with bronchogenic carcinoma of various histologic types. *Klin Wochenschr* 1985;62:1018–1024.

38. List AF, Hainsworth JD, Davis BW, et al. The syndrome of inappropriate secretion of antidiuretic hormone (SIADH) in small-cell cancer. *J Clin Oncol* 1986;4:1191–1198.

39. Pederson AG, Hammer M, Hansen M, et al. Cerebrospinal fluid vasopressin as a marker of central nervous system metastases from small-cell bronchogenic carcinoma. *J Clin Oncol* 1985;3:48–53.

40. Moses AM, Scheinman SJ. Ectopic secretion of neurohypophyseal peptides in patients with malignancy. *Endocrinol Metab Clin North Am* 1991;20:489–506.

41. Androgue HJ, Nadias NE. Hyponatremia. *N Engl J Med* 2000;342:1581–1590.

42. Gross AJ, Steinberg SM, Reilly JG, et al. Atrial natriuretic factor and arginine vasopressin production in tumor cell lines from patients with lung cancer and their relationship to serum sodium. *Cancer Res* 1991;53:67–74.

43. Shimiziu K, Nakano S, Nakano Y, et al. Ectopic natriuretic peptide production in small cell lung cancer with the syndrome of inappropriate antidiuretic hormone secretion. *Cancer* 1991;68:2284–2288.

44. Mundy GR, Guise TA. Hypercalcemia of malignancy. *Am J Med* 1997;103:134–145.

45. Moseley JM, Kubota M, Diefenbach-Jagger H, et al. Parathyroid-related protein purified from a human lung cancer cell line. *Proc Natl Acad Sci U S A* 1987;84:5048–5052.

46. Broadus AE, Mangin M, Ikeda K, et al. Humoral hypercalcemia of cancer. *New Engl J Med* 1988;319:556–563.

47. Martin T, Moseley J, Gillespie M. Parathyroid hormone-related protein: biochemistry and molecular biology. *Crit Rev Biochem Mol Biol* 1991;26:377–395.

48. Strewler G. The physiology of parathyroid-related protein. *N Engl J Med* 2000;342:177–185.

49. Schilling T, Pecherstorfer M, Blind E, et al. Parathyroid hormone-related protein(PTHrP) does not regulate 1,25 dihydroxyvitamin D serum levels in hypercalcemia of malignancy. *J Clin Endocrinol Metab* 1993;76:801–803.

50. Ralston SH, Allacher SJ, Patel U, et al. Cancer-associated hypercalcemia: morbidity and mortality. *Ann Intern Med* 1990;112:499–504.

51. Nussbaum SR, Younger J, Vandepol CJ, et al. Single-dose intravenous therapy with pamidronate for the treatment of hypercalcemia of malignancy: comparison of 30-, 60-, and 90-mg dosages. *Am J Med* 1993;95:297–304.

52. Major P, Lortholary A, Hon J, et al. Zoledronic acid is superior to pamidronate in the treatment of hypercalcemia of malignancy: a pooled analysis of two randomized, controlled clinical trials. *J Clin Oncol* 2001;19:558–567.

53. Sauty A, Pecherstorfer M, Zimmer-Roth I, et al. Interleukin-6 and tumor necrosis factor-α levels after bisphosphonates treatment *in vitro* and in patients with malignancy. *Bone* 1996;18:133–139.

54. Yoshimoto K, Yamasaki R, Sakai H, et al. Ectopic production of parathyroid hormone by small cell lung cancer in a patient with hypercalcemia. *J Clin Endocrinol Metab* 1989;68:976–981.

55. Taylor HC, Falloon MD, Velasco ME. Oncogenic osteomalacia and inappropriate antidiuretic hormone secretion due to oat-cell carcinoma. *Ann Intern Med* 1984;101:786–788.

56. Robin N, Gill G, van Heyningen C, et al. A small cell bronchogenic carcinoma associated with tumoral hypophosphataemia and inappropriate antidiuresis. *Postgrad Med J* 1994;70:746–748.

57. Shaker JL, Brickner RC, Divgi AB, et al. Case report: renal phosphate wasting, syndrome of inappropriate antidiuretic hormone, and ectopic corticotropin production in small cell carcinoma. *Am J Med Sci* 1995;310:38–41.

58. Kelley MJ, Becker KL, Rushin JM, et al. Calcitonin elevation in small cell lung cancer without ectopic production. *Am J Respir Crit Care Med* 1994;149:183–190.

59. Becker KL. The endocrine lung. In: Becker KL, ed. *Principles and practice of endocrinology and metabolism.* Philadelphia: Lippincott–Raven Publishers, 1990:1343–1347.

60. Roos BA, Lindall AW, Baylin SB, et al. Plasma immunoreactive calcitonin in lung cancer. *J Clin Endocrinol Metab* 1980;50:659–666.

61. Samaan NA, Castillo S, Schultz PN, et al. Serum calcitonin after pentagastrin stimulation in patients with bronchogenic and breast cancer compared to that in patients with medullary thyroid carcinoma. *J Clin Endocrinol Metab* 1980;51:237–241.

62. Becker KL, Nash DR, Silva OL, et al. Urine calcitonin levels in patients with bronchogenic carcinoma. *JAMA* 1980;243:670–672.

63. Mulder H, Hackeng WHL, Silberbusch J, et al. Value of serum calcitonin estimation in clinical oncology. *Br J Cancer* 1981;43:786–792.

64. Wallach SR, Royston I, Taetle R, et al. Plasma calcitonin as a marker for disease activity in patients with small cell carcinoma of the lung. *J Clin Endocrinol Metab* 1981;53:602–606.

65. Zajac JD, Martin TJ, Hudson P, et al. Biosynthesis of calcitonin by human lung cancer cells. *Endocrinology* 1985;116:749–755.

66. Cate CC, Pettengill OS, Sorenson GD. Biosynthesis of procalcitonin in small cell carcinoma of the lung. *Cancer Res* 1986;46:812–818.

67. Symes AJ, Craig RK, Brickell PM. Loss of transcriptional repression contributes to the ectopic expression of the calcitonin/aCGRP gene 4 in human lung carcinoma cell line. *FEBS Lett* 1992;306:229–233.

68. Edbrooke MR, Parker D, McVey JH, et al. Expression of the human calcitonin CGRP gene in lung and thyroid carcinoma. *EMBO J* 1985;4:715–724.

69. Hoppener JWM, Steenbergh PH, Moonen PJJ, et al. Detection of mRNA encoding calcitonin, calcitonin gene related peptide and proopiomelanocortin in human tumors. *Mol Cell Endocinol* 1986;47:125–130.

70. Wilson TS, McDowell EM, McIntire KR, et al. Elaboration of

human chorionic gonadotropin by lung tumors. *Arch Pathol Lab Med* 1981;105:169–173.

71. Fukiyama M, Hayashi Y, Koike M, et al. Human chorionic gonadotropin in lung tumors: immunochemical study on unbalanced distribution of subunits. *Lab Invest* 1986;55:433–443.

72. Yoshimoto Y, Wolfsen AR, Odell WD. Glycosylation: a variable in hCG production by cancers. *Am J Med* 1979;76:414–420.

73. Yoshimura M, Nishimura R, Murotani A, et al. Assessment of urinary β-core fragment of human chorionic gonadotropin as a new tumor marker of lung cancer. *Cancer* 1994;73:2745–2752.

74. Nishimura R, Hamamoto T, Morimoto N, et al. The characterization of α-subunit of glycoprotein hormone produced by undifferentiated carcinoma. *Endocrinol Japon* 1982;29:11–19.

75. Triozzi PL, Stevens VC. Human chorionic gonadotropin as a target for cancer vaccines. *Oncol Rep* 1999;6:7–17.

76. Kirschner MA, Cohen FB, Jesperson D. Estrogen production and its origin in men with gonadotropin-producing neoplasms. *J Clin Endocrinol Metab* 1974;39:112–118.

77. Yoshida J, Nagai K, Nishimura M, et al. Secretion of hCG/β-hCG by squamous cell carcinoma of the lung in a 31-year-old female smoker. *Jpn J Clin Oncol* 2000;30:163–166.

78. Faiman C, Colwell JA, Ryan R, et al. Gonadotropin secretion from a bronchogenic carcinoma: demonstration by radioimmunoassay. *N Engl J Med* 1967;277:1395–1399.

79. Harach HR, Skinner M, Gibbs AR. Biological markers in human lung carcinomas: an immunopathological study of six antigens. *Thorax* 1983;35:937–941.

80. Turkington RW. Ectopic production of prolactin. *N Engl J Med* 1971;285:1455–1458.

81. Sonkson PH, Ayres AB, Braimbridge M, et al. Acromegaly caused by bronchial carcinoid tumors. *Clin Endocrinol* 1976;5:503–513.

82. Sparagana M, Phillips G. Hoffman C, et al. Ectopic growth hormone syndrome associated with lung cancer. *Metabolism* 1971;20:730–736.

83. Doga M, Bonadonna S. Burattin A, et al. Ectopic secretion of growth hormone-releasing hormone (GHRH) in neuroendocrine tumors; relevant clinical aspects. *Ann Oncol* 2001;12[Suppl 2]:S89–S94.

84. Frohman LA, Szabo M, Berelowitz M, et al. Partial purification and characterization of a peptide with growth hormone releasing activity from extrapituitary tumors in patients with acromegaly. *J Clin Invest* 1980;65:43–54.

85. Boizel R, Halimi S, Labat F, et al. Acromegaly due to a growth hormone releasing hormone-secreting bronchogenic carcinoid tumor: further information on the abnormal responsiveness of the somatotroph cells and their recovery after successful treatment. *J Clin Endocrinol Metab* 1987;64:304–308.

86. Harris PE, Bouloux PM, Wass JA, et al. Successful treatment by chemotherapy for acromegaly associated with ectopic growth hormone releasing hormone secretion from a carcinoid tumor. *Clin Endocrinol* 1990;32:315–321.

87. Melmed S, Ziel FH, Braunstein GD, et al. Medical management of acromegaly due to ectopic production of growth hormone-releasing hormone by a carcinoid tumor. *J Clin Endocrinol Metab* 1988;67:395–399.

88. Giutsi M, Ciccarelli E, Dallabonzan D, et al. Clinical results of long-term slow-release lanreotide treatment of acromegaly. *Eur J Clin Invest* 1997;27:277–284.

89. Ben-Shlomo A, Melmud S. Acromegaly. *Endocrinol Clin N Am* 2001:30:565–583.

90. Trainer PJ, Drake WM, Katznelson L, et al. Treatment of acromegaly with the growth hormone-receptor antagonist pegvisomant. *N Engl J Med* 2000;342:1171–1177.

91. Penman E, Wass JA, Besser GM, et al. Somatostatin secretion by lung and thymic tumors. *Clin Endocrinol* 1980;13:613–620.

92. Szabo M, Berelowitz M, Pettengill OS, et al. Ectopic production of somatostatin-like immuno- and bioactivity by cultured human pulmonary small cell carcinoma. *J Clin Endocrinol Metab* 1980;51:978–987.

93. Russell PJ, O'Mara SM, Raghavan D. Ectopic hormone production by small cell undifferentiated carcinomas. *Mol Cell Endocrinol* 1990;71:1–12.

94. Roth KA, Evans CJ, Weber E, et al. Gastrin-releasing peptide-related peptides in a human malignant lung carcinoid tumor. *Cancer Res* 1983;43:5411–5415.

95. Said SI, Faloona G. Elevated plasma and tissue levels of vasoactive intestinal polypeptide in the watery-diarrhea syndrome due to pancreatic, bronchogenic and other tumors. *N Engl J Med* 1975; 293:155–160.

96. Farthing MJ. The role of somatostatin analogues in the treatment of refractory diarrhea. *Digestion* 1996;57[Suppl 1]:107–113.

97. Maier HC, Barr D. Intrathoracic tumors associated with hypoglycemia. *J Thorac Cardiovasc Surg* 1962;44:321–329.

98. Touyz R, Plitt M, Rumbak M. Hypoglycemia associated with a lung mass. *Chest* 1986;89:289–290.

99. Williams ED, Sandler M. The classification of carcinoid tumors. *Lancet* 1963;1:238–239.

100. Kulke MH, Mayer RJ. Carcinoid tumors. *New Engl J Med* 1999;30:858–868.

101. Rea F, Binda R, Spreafico G, et al. Bronchial carcinoids: a review of 60 patients. *Ann Thorac Surg* 1989;47:412–414.

102. Kvols LK, Moertel CG, O'Connell MJ, et al. Treatment of the malignant carcinoid syndrome: evaluation of a long-acting somatostatin analogue. *N Engl J Med* 1986;315:663–666.

103. Saslow SB, O'Brien MD, Camilleri M, et al. Octreotide inhibition of flushing and colonic motor dysfunction in carcinoid syndrome. *Am J Gastroenterol* 1997;92:2250–2256.

104. Rubin J, Ajani J, Schirmer W, et al. Octreotide acetate long-acting formulation versus open-label subcutaneous octreotide acetate in malignant carcinoid syndrome. *J Clin Oncol* 1999:17:600–606.

105. O'Toole D, Decreux M, Bommelaer G, et al. Treatment of carcinoid syndrome: a prospective crossover evaluation of lanreotide versus octreotide in terms of efficacy, patient acceptability, and tolerance. *Cancer* 2000;88:770–776.

106. Ruscniewski P, Ducreux M, Chayvialle JA, et al. Treatment of the carcinoid syndrome with the long-acting somatostatin analogue lanreotide: a prospective study in 39 patients. *Gut* 1996;39:279–283.

107. Caplin ME, Buscombe JR, Hilson AJ, et al. Carcinoid tumor. *Lancet* 1998;352:799–805.

108. Davila DG, Dunn WF, Tazelaar HD, et al. Bronchial carcinoid tumors. *Mayo Clin Proc* 1993;68:795–803.

109. Dong Q, Debenelenko LV, Chandrasekharappa SC, et al. Loss of heterozygosity at 11q13: analysis of pituitary tumors, lung carcinoids, lipomas, and other uncommon tumors in subjects with familial multiple endocrine neoplasia type 1. *J Clin Endocrinol Metab* 1997;82:1416–1420.

110. Merrill WW, Bondy PK. Production of biochemical marker substances by bronchogenic carcinomas. *Clin Chest Med* 1982;3:307–320.

111. Harach HR, Skinner M, Gibbs AR. Biological markers in human lung carcinomas: an immunopathological study of six antigens. *Thorax* 1983;35:937–941.

112. Trump BF, McDowell EM, Shamsuddin AKM, et al. Preneoplasia and neoplasia of the bronchus, esophagus, and colon: the use of markers in determining phenotypes and classification. *Monogr Pathol* 1985;26:101–139.

113. Deland FH, Kim EE, Goldenberg DM. Lymphoscintigraphy with radionuclide-labeled antigens to carcinoembryonic antigen. *Cancer Res* 1980;40:2984–3000.

114. Gropp C, Havemann K, Scheuer A. The use of carcinogenic antigen and peptide hormones to stage and monitor patients with lung cancer. *Int J Radiat Oncol Biol Phys* 1980;6:1047–1053.

115. Krauss S, Macy S, Ichiki AT. A study of immunoreactive calcitonin (CT), adrenocorticotropic hormone (ACTH) and carcinoembryonic antigen (CEA) in lung cancer and other malignancies. *Cancer* 1981;47:2485–2492.

116. Vladutiu AO, Brason FW, Adler RH. Differential diagnosis of pleural effusions: clinical usefulness of cell marker quantitation. *Chest* 1981;79:297–301.

117. Sheppard MN, Corrin B, Bennett MH, et al. Immunocytochemical localization of neuron specific enolase in small cell carcinomas and carcinoid tumors of the lung. *Histopathology* 1984;8:171–181.

118. Jorgensen LG, Osterlind K, Hansen HH, et al. The prognostic influence of serum neuron-specific enolase in small cell lung cancer. *Br J Cancer* 1988;58:805–807.

119. Bork E, Hansen M, Urdal P, et al. Early detection of response in small cell bronchogenic carcinoma by changes in serum concentrations of creatine kinase, neuron-specific enolase, calcitonin, ACTH, serotonin and gastrin releasing peptide. *Eur J Cancer Clin Oncol* 1988;24:1033–1038.

120. Fischbach W, Schwarz-Wallrauch C, Jany B. Neuron-specific enolase and thymidine kinase as an aid to diagnosis and treatment monitoring of small-cell lung cancer. *Cancer* 1989;63:1143–1149.

121. Denny-Brown D. Primary sensory neuropathy with muscular changes associated with carcinoma. *J Neurol Neurosurg Psychiatry* 1948;2:73–87.

122. Elrington GM, Murray NM, Spiro SG, et al. Neurological paraneoplastic syndromes in patients with small cell lung cancer. a prospective survey of 150 patients. *J Neurol Neurosurg Psychiatry* 1991;764–767.

123. Kornguth SE. Neuronal proteins and paraneoplastic syndromes. *N Engl J Med* 1989;321:1607–1608.

124. Galanis E, Frytak S, Rowland KM Jr, et al. Neuronal autoantibody titers in the course of small-cell lung carcinoma and platinum-associated neuropathy. *Cancer Immunol Immunother* 1999;48:85–90.

125. Hildebrand J. Signs, symptoms, and significance of paraneoplastic neurological syndromes. *Oncology* 1989;3:57–61.

126. Chad DA, Recht LD. Neuromuscular complications of systemic cancer. *Neurol Clin* 1991;9:901–914.

127. Keime-Guigert F, Graus, F, Broet P, et al. Clinical outcome of patients with anti-Hu–associated encephalomyelitis after treatment of tumor. *Neurology* 1999;53:1719–1723.

128. Dalmau J, Graus F, Rosenblum MK, et al. Anti-Hu–associated paraneoplastic encephalomyelitis/sensory neuropathy. *Medicine* 1992;71:59–72.

129. Dropcho EJ. The remote effects of cancer on the nervous system. *Neurol Clin* 1989;7:579–602.

130. Jaeckle KA, Graus F, Houghton AN, et al. Autoimmune response of patients with paraneoplastic cerebellar degeneration to a Purkinje cell cytoplasmic protein antigen. *Ann Neurol* 1985;18:592–600.

131. Cunningham J, Graus F, Anderson N, et al. Partial characterization of Purkinje cell antigens in paraneoplastic cerebellar degeneration. *Neurology* 1986;36:1163–1168.

132. Dropcho EJ, Chen YT, Posner JB, et al. Cloning of a brain protein identified by autoantibodies from a patient with paraneoplastic cerebellar degeneration. *Proc Natl Acad Sci U S A* 1987;84:4552–4556.

133. Thirkill CE, Keltner JL, Tyler NK, et al. Antibody reactions with retina and cancer-associated antigens in 10 patients with cancer-associated retinopathy. *Arch Ophthalmol* 1993;111:931–937.

134. Adamus G, Guy J, Schmied JL, et al. Role of anti-recoverin autoantibodies in cancer-assisted retinopathy. *Invest Ophthalmol Vis Sci* 1993;34:2626–2633.

135. Ohguro H, Ogawa K, Nakagawa T. Recoverin and Hsc 70 are found as autoantigens in patients with cancer-associated retinopathy. *Invest Ophthalmol Vis Sci* 1999;40:82–89.

136. Graus F, Elkon KB, Cordon-Cardo C, et al. Sensory neuropathy and small cell lung cancer: antineuronal antibody that also reacts with the tumor. *Am J Med* 1986;80:45–52.

137. Sodhi N, Camilleri M, Camoriano JK, et al. Autonomic function and motility in intestinal pseudoobstruction caused by paraneoplastic syndrome. *Dig Dis Sci* 1989;34:1937–1942.

138. Liang BC, Albers JW, Sima AAF, et al. Paraneoplastic pseudo-obstruction mononeuropathy multiplex and sensory neuropathy. *Muscle Nerve* 1994;17:91–96.

139. Kiers L, Altermatt HJ, Lennon VA. Paraneoplastic anti-neuronal nuclear IgG autoantibodies (type 1) localize antigen in small cell lung carcinoma. *Mayo Clin Proc* 1991;66:1209–1216.

140. Lennon VA, Sas DF, Busk MF, et al. Enteric neuronal autoantibodies in pseudoobstruction with small cell lung carcinoma. *Gastroenterology* 1991;100:137–142.

141. Lee, HR, Lennon VA, Camilleri, et al. Paraneoplastic gastrointestinal motor dysfunction: clinical and laboratory characteristics. *Am J Gastroenterol* 2001;96:373–379.

142. Greer JM, Longley S, Edwards N, et al. Vasculitis associated with malignancy: experience with 13 patients and literature review. *Medicine* 1988;67:220–230.

143. Oh SJ, Slaughter R, Harrell L. Paraneoplastic vasculitic neuropathy: a treatable neuropathy. *Muscle Nerve* 1991;14:152–156.

144. Vincent A, Lang B, Newsom-Davis J. Autoimmunity to the voltage-gated calcium channel underlies the Lambert-Eaton myasthenic syndrome, a paraneoplastic disorder. *Trends Neurosci* 1989;12:496–502.

145. Pancrazio JJ, Oie HK, Kim YI. Voltage-sensitive calcium channels in a human small-cell lung cancer line. *Acta Physiol Scand* 1992;144:463–468.

146. Lennon, VA, Kryzer, TJ, Griesmann GE, et al. Calcium-channel antibodies in the Lambert-Eaton syndrome and other paraneoplastic syndromes *N Engl J Med* 1995;332:1467–1474.

147. Fukunaga H, Engel AG, Lang B, et al. Lambert-Eaton myasthenic syndrome with IgG from man to mouse depletes the presynaptic membrane active zones. *Proc Natl Acad Sci U S A* 1983;80:7636–7640.

148. Lambert EH, Lennon VA. Selected IgG rapidly induces Lambert-Eaton myasthenic syndrome in mice: complement independence and EMG abnormalities. *Muscle Nerve* 1988;11:1133–1145.

149. Segal AM, Mackenzie AH. Hypertrophic osteoarthropathy: a 10 year retrospective analysis. *Semin Arthritis Rheumatism* 1982;12:220–232.

150. Sridhar KS, Lobo CF, Altman RD. Digital clubbing and lung cancer. *Chest* 1998;114:1535–1537.

151. Holling HE, Brodey RS, Boland HC. Pulmonary hypertrophic osteoarthropathy. *Lancet* 1961;2:1269–1274.

152. Silveira LH, Martinez-Lavin M, Pineda C, et al. Vascular endothelial growth factor and hypertrophic osteoarthropathy. *Clin Exp Rheumatol* 2000;18:57–62.

153. Davies RA, Darby M, Richards MA. Hypertrophic pulmonary osteopathy in pulmonary metastatic disease: a case report and review of the literature. *Clin Radiol* 1991;43:268–271.

154. Caldwell DS, McCallum RM. Rheumatologic manifestations of cancer. *Med Clin North Am* 1986;70:385–417.

155. Stummvoll GH, Aringer M, Machold KP, et al. Cancer

polyarthritis resembling rheumatoid arthritis as a first sign of hidden neoplasms. *Scand J Rheumatol* 2001;30:40–44.

156. Sigurgeirsson B, Lindelof B, Edhag O, et al. Risk of cancer in patients with dermatomyositis or polymyositis. *N Engl J Med* 1992;326:363–367.

157. Zantos D, Zhang Y, Felson D. The overall and temporal association of cancer with polymyositis and dermatomyositis. *J Rheumatol* 1994;21;1855–1889.

158. Chow SF, Gridley G, Mellemkjar L, et al. Cancer risk following polymyositis and dermatomyositis: a nationwide cohort study in Denmark. *Cancer Causes Control* 1995;6:119–130.

159. Peters-Golden M, Wise RA, Hochberg M, et al. Incidence of lung cancer in systemic sclerosis. *J Rheumatol* 1985;12:1136–1139.

160. Rosenthal AK, McLaughlin JK, Linet MS. Incidence of cancer among patients with systemic sclerosis. *Cancer* 1995;79:910–914.

161. Leandro MJ, Isenberg DA. Rheumatic diseases and malignancy: is there an association?. *Scan J Rheumatol* 2001;30:185–189.

162. Sanchez-Guerrero J, Gutierrez-Urena S, Vidaller A, et al. Vasculitis as a paraneoplastic syndrome: report of 11 cases and review of the literature. *J Rheumatol* 1990;17:1458–1462.

163. Ponge T, Boutoille D, Moreau A, et al. Systemic vasculitis in a patient with small-cell neuroendocrine bronchial cancer. *Eur Respir J* 1998;12:1228–1229.

164. Rigel DS, Jacobs ML. Malignant acanthosis nigricans: a review. *J Dermatol Surg Oncol* 1980;6:923–927.

165. Bottoni U, Dianzani C, Pranteda G, et al. Florid cutaneous and mucosal papillomatosis with acanthosis nigricans revealing a primary lung cancer. *J Eur Acad Derm Venereol* 2000;14:205–208.

166. Boyd AS, Nelder KH, Menter A, et al. Erythema gyratum repens: a paraneoplastic eruption. *J Am Acad Dermatol* 1992;26:757–762.

167. Caux F, Lebbe C, Thomine E, et al. Erythema gyratum repens: a case studied with immunofluorescence, immunoelectron microscopy and immunohistochemistry. *Br J Dermatol* 1994;131:102–107.

168. Lomholt H, Thestrup-Pedersen K. Paraneoplastic skin manifestations of lung cancer. *Acta Derm Venereol* 2000;80:200–202.

169. Hovenden AL. Acquired hypertrichosis lanuginosa associated with malignancy and pruritus. *Arch Intern Med* 1987;147:2013–2019.

170. Winkelmann RK. Dermatologic clinics, 1: comments on pruritus related to systemic disease. *Mayo Clin Proc* 1961;36:187–196.

171. Krahn G, Greulich KM, Bezold G, et al. Receptor tyrosine kinase and p/16/CDKN2 expression in a case of tripe palms associated with non–small-cell lung cancer. *Dermatology* 1999;199:290–295.

172. Setterfield J, Shirlaw PJ, Lasarova Z, et al. Paraneoplastic cicatricial pemphigoid. *Br J Dermatol* 1999;14:127–131.

173. Odeh M, Misselevich, I, Oliven A. Squamous cell carcinoma of the lung presenting with cutaneous leukocytoclastic vasculitis; a case report. *Angiology* 2001;52:641–644.

174. Fisher MM, Hochberg LA, Wilensky ND. Recurrent thrombophlebitis in obscure malignant tumor of the lung: report of four cases. *JAMA* 1951;147:1213–1216.

175. Sons HU. Pulmonary embolism and cancer; predisposition to venous thrombosis and embolism as a paraneoplastic syndrome. *J Surg Oncol* 1989;40:100–106.

176. Prandoni P, Lensing AWA, Buller HR, et al. Deep vein thrombosis and the incidence of subsequent symptomatic cancer. *N Engl J Med* 1992;327:1128–1133.

177. Monreal M, Lafoz E, Casals A, et al. Occult cancer in patients with deep venous thrombosis. *Cancer* 1991;67:541–545.

178. Cornuz J, Pearson SD, Creager MA, et al. Importance of findings on the initial evaluation for cancer in patients with symptomatic idiopathic deep vein thrombosis. *Ann Intern Med* 1996;125:785–793.

179. Griffin MR, Stanson AW, Brown ML, et al. Deep venous thrombosis and pulmonary embolism: risk of subsequent malignant neoplasms. *Arch Intern Med* 1987;147:1907–1911.

180. Sack GH, Levine J, Bell WR. Trousseau's syndrome and other manifestations of chromic disseminated coagulopathy in patients with neoplasms: clinical, pathophysiologic and therapeutic features. *Medicine* 1977;56:1–37.

181. Fountain JR, Holman RL. Acquired fibrinogen deficiency associated with carcinoma of the bronchus. *Ann Intern Med* 1960;52:459–463.

182. Kodama T, Takada, K, Kamaya T, et al. Large cell carcinoma of the lung associated with marked eosinophilia. *Cancer* 1984;4:2313–2317.

183. Dellon AL, Hume RB, Chretien PB. Eosinophilia in bronchogenic carcinoma. *N Engl J Med* 1974;291:207–208.

184. Healy TM. Path MRC. Eosinophilia in bronchogenic carcinoma. *N Engl J Med* 1974;291:794.

185. Diot P, Guimard Y, Besnier JM, et al. Pulmonary solitary mass with a "crescent sign" and blood eosinophilia. *Eur J Med* 1992;1:58–59.

186. Ascensao JL, Oken MM, Ewing SL, et al. Leukocytosis and large cell lung cancer: a frequent association. *Cancer* 1987;60:903–905.

187. Adachi N, Yamaguchi K, Morikana T, et al. Constitutive production of multiple colony-stimulating factors in patients with lung cancer associated with neutrophilia. *Br J Cancer* 1994;69:125–129.

188. Yoneda T, Nakei M, Moriyama K, et al. Neutralizing antibodies to human interleukin-6 reverse hypercalcemia associated with human squamous carcinoma. *Cancer Res* 1993;53:737–740.

189. Yapp RG, Siegel JH. Unexplained biliary tract dilatation in lung cancer patients. *Endoscopy* 1992;24:593–595.

190. Keur I, Krediet RT, Arisz L. Glomerulopathy as a paraneoplastic phenomenon. *Netherlands J Med* 1989;34:270–284.

191. Shikata Y, Hayashi Y, Yamazaki H, et al. Effectiveness of radiation therapy in nephrotic syndrome associated with advanced lung cancer. *Nephron* 1999;8:160–164.

Industrial Hygiene for the Pulmonologist

43

John Martyny · Cecile Rose

For most lung diseases, the scope of work for the pulmonologist primarily involves accurate diagnosis and adequate treatment. In contrast, for occupational lung diseases, the pulmonologist must consider not only diagnosis and treatment but also issues of exposure and prevention. The pulmonologist who recognizes a lung disease that is related to work must consider not only the immediate treatment of the patient but also whether or not the patient will be able to return to work or may require workplace modification to avoid worsening symptoms. The treating pulmonologist must also consider those workers sharing the same exposure environment as the affected patient who may be at risk for lung disease. Thus, the field of occupational and environmental lung diseases requires both a medical approach and a public health approach. Inherent in these approaches is a willingness to tackle complex problems of causation and exposure identification. To do so requires collaboration with professionals in a number of other fields, the most essential being the profession of industrial hygiene. The industrial hygienist is dedicated to the recognition, evaluation, and control of workplace and other environmental hazards. Too often, the languages of industrial hygiene and medicine are opaque to those outside the fields, limiting efforts to accurately identify and, when necessary, mitigate exposures causing lung disease. This chapter focuses on the conceptual framework and language of industrial hygiene, with the intent that practicing pulmonologists who recognize exposure-related lung disease will be better prepared to address the challenges and experience the rewards of collaborating with their industrial hygiene partners.

OVERVIEW OF INDUSTRIAL HYGIENE

Industrial hygiene is the science and art devoted to the anticipation, recognition, evaluation, and control of chemical, biologic, and physical stressors in the workplace environment (1). Since the early 1990s, industrial hygienists have also become more involved with environments outside of the workplace, and a growing number of industrial hygienists are specifically involved with exposures to the general public.

To carry out their mission, most industrial hygienists are educated in a number of fields. They receive training in toxicology, chemistry, biology, engineering, environmental health, occupational health, ergonomics, aerosol physics, and other disciplines that are necessary to perform the specific job duties required. The typical industrial hygienist has a bachelor's degree in an environmental sciences field and a master's degree in industrial hygiene. This training is designed to enable the industrial hygienist to evaluate an environment for health and safety hazards, quantify those hazards, understand the effects of exposure to the hazards, and, if necessary, control exposure to the hazards. Based on this training, the industrial hygienist can provide valuable information and input into an integrated health management team, and in fact, many industrial hygienists are assigned to the medical departments of companies for which they work. Industrial hygienists are also integral members of public health teams in both federal and local governments, and a growing number also teach in schools of public health and medical schools. Industrial hygienists complement the expertise of physicians, occupational health nurses, safety professionals, and other professionals in the safety and health team.

Although industrial hygiene professionals were present before the enactment of the Occupational Safety and Health Act of 1970, their role was enhanced by the promulgation of this act. The act formed the Occupational Safety and Health

J. Martyny and **C. Rose:** Department of Medicine, National Jewish Medical and Research Center, Denver, Colorado.

Administration (OSHA) and required businesses to comply with a number of regulations related to hazardous exposures and to control those exposures to specific levels. In general, employers were charged to provide a work environment that was free from recognized hazards that are or may be able to cause serious injury or death. To comply with these regulations, many large companies found it necessary to hire industrial hygienists. Government agencies also found that they needed to hire a number of industrial hygienists to enforce the newly formed regulations (2).

At the same time, the National Institute for Occupational Safety and Health (NIOSH) was formed as part of the Centers for Disease Control and Prevention and charged to provide OSHA with technical information regarding occupational safety and health through both intramural and extramural research programs (2). NIOSH was also charged to develop a training program for industrial hygienists and to provide grant money to institutions of higher education to increase the numbers of industrial hygienists available in the workforce. A number of education and research centers were established throughout the United States to train not only industrial hygienists but also occupational medicine physicians, occupational health nurses, safety professionals, ergonomists, and other health professionals to function as teams in worker protection. NIOSH also provides technical assistance to industry and government regarding occupational exposures through its health hazard evaluation program (1).

The title of industrial hygienist has not been protected by law in most states, and therefore, anyone may call themselves an industrial hygienist. This raises some concern regarding individuals who use the title without formal experience and training in the field of industrial hygiene. A number of industrial hygienists are registered as certified industrial hygienists (CIHs). This title is copyrighted by the American Board of Industrial Hygiene (ABIH), which certifies industrial hygienists based on education, experience, and performance on a certification test. The requirements to become a CIH include graduation from an approved college or university with specific course work and at least 5 years of experience as an industrial hygienist. An applicant must also have been mentored by a CIH during this time period. After meeting the experience requirement, the individual takes a certification test designed to test knowledge in 16 areas of common industrial hygiene practice (3).

The CIH is expected to have comprehensive knowledge of the practice of industrial hygiene. Because some industrial hygienists work and have experience in very limited areas, ABIH provides special certification for these individuals. The certified associate industrial hygienist (CAIH) is an individual with a bachelor's degree from an acceptable university with specific course work in science and industrial hygiene. The individual has also worked for 4 years in an area of industrial hygiene and has passed a comprehensive examination. Both CIHs and CAIHs must complete a specified number of continuing education requirements within a defined time period in order to maintain their certification (3).

A number of industrial hygiene professional organizations exist. The two largest groups are the American Industrial Hygiene Association (AIHA) and the American Conference of Governmental Industrial Hygienists (ACGIH). Both organizations are open to any industrial hygienist, although regular member status in the ACGIH is open only to governmental industrial hygienists and industrial hygienists employed by educational institutions. The ACGIH also establishes threshold limit values (TLVs), which will be discussed later in this chapter. Both organizations provide a significant body of literature regarding industrial hygiene and allied disciplines.

CHARACTERISTICS OF RESPIRATORY HAZARDS

Respiratory hazards of concern to industrial hygienists and pulmonologists may be chemical, physical, or biologic hazards. They may occur in the form of liquid, vapor, gas, or particulate hazards. Both the type and form of hazard dictate how easily the hazard can be identified and controlled, as well as its health effects. Some compounds and their associated pulmonary health effects are listed in Table 43.1.

Chemicals are widely used in all aspects of our lives and are extremely common in the occupational environment. Synthetic chemicals are present in outside air, air within homes, and air in business settings at easily detectable levels. Chemicals may exist as liquids, vapors, gases, or particles in the form of dusts or fumes. Biologic hazards are primarily particulates, although biotoxins and biologically generated volatile organic compounds can be gases or vapors.

Liquids are one of the most common chemical hazards, including acids, bases, solvents, aldehydes, and other

TABLE 43.1. PULMONARY HEALTH EFFECTS OF SOME COMMON COMPOUNDS

Effect	Gases	Liquid	Particulate
Irritant	Chlorine, ammonia, bromine	Nitric acid, acrolein	Fiberglass
Sensitizer	—	Isocyanates	Beryllium, fungi, cobalt
Fibrogen	—	—	Silica, asbestos, coal
Carcinogen	Ethylene oxide	Formaldehyde	Asbestos, arsenic
Asphyxiants	Carbon monoxide	Methylene chloride	

compounds that are liquids at room temperature. In general, these compounds do not present a respiratory risk as long as they remain in a container in a liquid form. The primary hazards associated with liquids are contact hazards; that is, the chemical may be absorbed through the skin or the chemical may cause damage to the skin itself. The primary method of determining uptake from skin exposure is through measurement of absorbed dose by sampling blood, urine, breath, or some other biologic material (4).

A concern for many liquids is their failure to remain in the container. In many cases the liquid has a vapor pressure that, at room temperature, allows the liquid to evaporate and form a vapor. The liquid may also be mechanically agitated to produce a liquid aerosol. In both cases, the liquid becomes airborne as a vapor or a mist, creating a potential respiratory hazard. Many of the chemicals used in industry and in nonindustrial settings form both aerosols and vapors and become respiratory hazards. One example is styrene used in fiberglass operations. Styrene has a high vapor pressure at room temperature that allows the liquid to vaporize and take on the attributes of a gas. The vapor will quickly occupy any area available and can easily be inhaled by unprotected workers. Styrene is also mixed mechanically with other materials to bind the fiberglass, and an aerosol of very small droplets is formed during the mixing process. In this situation, styrene presents a skin hazard, because it can be absorbed through the skin, and a respiratory hazard, because it is present in the air as a vapor and a mist (5).

The two primary factors that determine the site of deposition of a liquid, vapor, or aerosol are solubility and droplet size. In the case of liquid aerosols, droplet size is a major determinant of where the droplet will be deposited in the lungs. Aerosols with droplets that range from 5 μm to 100 μm in diameter are mostly deposited in the nasopharynx by impaction owing to the abrupt change in direction of a high-velocity airflow. Aerosols that range in size from 1.0 to 10 μm in diameter are primarily deposited in the airway by impaction or interception by the mucous-coated respiratory tract. Droplets of less than 1.0 μm in diameter enter the alveolar portion of the lung, where diffusion into the bloodstream may occur. Solubility also influences where a material is deposited and what areas of the body are affected. Compounds that are soluble in both water and lipids are most likely to penetrate the skin barrier and enter the blood (6,7). Water-soluble aerosols are more likely to be absorbed in the upper airway, whereas insoluble materials are more likely to penetrate further into the lungs. In addition, water-soluble materials may be more readily removed from the body than are fat-soluble materials that may be stored in adipose tissue (6,7).

Gases may cause a number of hazards in industrial and in noncommercial environments. Gases rapidly expand to fill whatever space is available and are easily taken up by the respiratory system. They can be immediately transported into the distal lung and, in some cases, can quickly diffuse through the alveoli and into the blood. Highly soluble gases diffuse quickly through the alveoli and into the blood, whereas less soluble gases may take much more time to penetrate the lungs and may not pose as much of a hazard. Highly soluble gases may also affect the upper respiratory track more than will less soluble gases. Compressed gases may cause problems unrelated to their toxicity but related to their compressed state, resulting in cryogenic damage to the body when the gas is released.

Airborne particles are generally deposited in the lung in the same manner as are liquid aerosols, with the smaller particles penetrating deeper into the lung. Particulate exposure has become a major concern in both industrial and nonindustrial environments. Particulate air pollution, especially particles with a diameter of less than 2.5 μm, concerns both outdoor and indoor air quality specialists. For example, particles with a diameter of less than 1 μm result in a higher risk of sensitization among beryllium workers than does exposure to larger-diameter beryllium aerosols (8,9). Particles may dissolve or be carried to other portions of the body, or they may stay in the lungs and cause injury to the lung tissue itself. Particles may have either toxic or allergic effects or both. Particles formed from the boiling and condensation of metals during welding or casting are called fumes and are generally less than 0.1 μm in diameter (10).

DETERMINING THE HAZARD TO WORKERS

A number of approaches are taken by industrial hygienists to determine the potential hazards to which workers may be exposed. The first step is to determine the potential exposures through an initial survey. Once the spectrum of potential exposures is defined, sampling may be undertaken to determine the magnitude of exposure. Sampling results are frequently compared with published standards, and recommendations are made to reduce exposures if they exceed allowable levels.

THE INITIAL SURVEY

The initial step in determining the hazards to which workers, or anyone else, are exposed is to survey the company, building, home, or workplace for chemical, physical, or biologic hazards. This initial survey determines the job or duties of the individuals involved and how that job is accomplished. The survey is best conducted when the industrial hygienist is accompanied by someone familiar with the processes, the chemicals used, and the maintenance and the layout of the facility. In industrial situations, the initial survey is frequently conducted with the plant operations manager or the plant safety and health specialist. The survey usually involves following the process from the introduction of the raw materials to the shipping of the finished product. All of the chemicals involved in the process, as well as how the chemicals are used, must be noted, with an eye to potential specific exposures.

In surveys that involve nonindustrial settings, such as indoor air quality investigations in commercial buildings, the industrial hygienist generally conducts a walk-through of the entire building, looking for processes that may result in exposures or chemicals that are used within the building. The investigator assesses how airflow within the building is controlled and how well the ventilation system has been maintained. Specific observations on the location of outside air intakes, the presence and type of filters, maintenance of air handlers, type of ductwork, air movement, and exhaust air locations are noted. Processes that use chemicals should be noted, as well as locations that may allow microbial growth owing to moisture intrusion into the building. The design of the building and any modifications should be determined. For example, a building once used as a slaughterhouse was converted into an office area and was found to have biologic contamination, resulting in high fungal exposures. Warehouse areas that have been changed to offices are prone to poor air circulation and indoor air quality complaints.

During a survey, it is important to observe and discuss with employees how they normally conduct their operations and how the operations may change over time. It is important to observe what personal protective equipment is normally used and what equipment is being used at the time of the survey. The types and use of existing exposure control measures should be noted, as well as when and why they were installed. This initial walk-through is also a good time to observe employee/employer relationships and to determine how easily communication occurs between the different groups.

The goal of the initial survey is to determine the potential exposures that could occur within the building. During this initial phase, all potential chemical or biologic exposures, the amounts of materials involved, and which individuals may be exposed are documented. It is impossible to analyze for all chemicals in any sampling program, and without identification of the materials involved, an appropriate sampling approach cannot be recommend. Specific exposure pathways are also noted because even the most toxic compound is not of concern if a potential exposure is not observed.

CHEMICAL IDENTIFICATION

The composition and characteristics of chemicals used in the workplace can usually be obtained from information contained on the label, the material safety data sheet (MSDS) for that chemical, or one of a number of health and safety databases. The chemical label on any chemical considered to be hazardous must provide the name of the compound, the type of warning (e.g., carcinogen, poison, acid), the target organ or toxic effect information, the prohibited uses, and the emergency treatment in case of accidental exposure. In most cases, the label provides only basic information owing

to its size and the need to include directions for use and other data. In addition, it is not unusual to find that a label has worn off or is no longer in a readable condition. For chemicals that are used in hobbies and crafts, an adequate label is not necessarily provided. In addition, chemicals that are received in bulk and divided into smaller quantities frequently do not have the label attached to the smaller containers. In general, labels are not the best method for determining the toxicity of chemicals.

Material Safety Data Sheets

Chemicals that are used in commercial facilities are required by OSHA to come with a MSDS. The MSDS for a chemical must include the following information (11):

- Name and contact information for the supplier
- Identification of the product
- Hazardous materials contained within the product
- Physical data for the product (e.g., molecular weight, density, boiling point)
- Fire and explosion hazard data (e.g., flash point, firefighting procedures)
- Health hazard data
- Reactivity data (stability, incompatibility)
- Spill or leak procedures
- Special protection information (e.g., respiratory protection, gloves, eye protection)
- Special precautions.

The hazardous materials section typically lists components considered to be hazardous. For each of the hazardous components, the MSDS should provide the chemical abstract number, the percentage of the total mixture for that component, the OSHA permissible exposure level (PEL) and the ACGIH TLV. The chemical abstract number is essential because it can be used to determine the chemical used and to link the MSDS to computer databases. In some cases, the hazardous component section is simply labeled as trade secret. In this case, the manufacturer must be contacted to determine components of the compound. Such information is usually provided when a medical question has arisen regarding the use of the compound.

The health hazard portion of the MSDS includes information on the toxicology of the compound and may actually cite published references. In most cases, this portion provides information on the expected symptoms should an overexposure occur. It also provides information regarding first aid for injured individuals and, in some cases, the risk of chronic disease from exposure to the chemical. The MSDS does not provide detailed medical information, and it typically does not provide any information regarding treatment after exposure, other than first aid treatment.

Although MSDSs help convey information regarding hazardous compounds to workers, there are limitations that must be considered before simply taking the information as fact. The information on the MSDS is typically provided by the company that manufacturers or mixes the material, and the information may not be correct. Some MSDS exaggerate the risks of exposure, whereas others understate the risks of illness after exposure. To be confident of the actual exposure risks, a secondary source of information may need to be consulted. A major challenge for companies using chemicals is the need to maintain MSDS that are up-to-date and that accurately reflect the products in use. A product by another company or an older product may have different ingredients than those of the product actually in use. Another problem is that the MSDS may apply only to the concentrated product and not to the dilution that is actually used. It is important to note whether or not a compound is diluted before use.

Although a section on personal protective equipment is contained in the MSDS, it frequently results in misunderstanding. Words similar to "use an approved respirator" or "use only in adequate ventilation" may not provide enough information to allow safe use of the material. An environment that appears to be well ventilated may not actually be adequate to prevent overexposure.

Online Databases

A number of online databases are available either to obtain MSDS information on specific products or to check the information provided on a specific MSDS. The National Library of Medicine manages several databases in the Medical Literature Analysis and Retrieval System (MEDLARS) system that can be searched by using the chemical abstract number to obtain information regarding the chemical and its toxicological properties. Chemline provides information on the chemical properties of a number of chemicals, whereas Toxline and Medline provide information on exposure and resulting disease risks. The hazardous substances database in the MEDLARS system also provides information such as exposures, routes of entry, and persistence for a number of compounds. NIOSH and OSHA maintain databases concerning chemical use and exposure in industry. There are also many private databases that can be searched for exposure information.

EXPOSURE DETERMINATION

After the initial survey has been conducted and the industrial hygienist has identified the potentially hazardous materials used within the facility, it may be important to determine actual exposures to employees or personnel occupying the area. The most common approach is to conduct sampling, although in some cases simple observation may be adequate. For example, if visible mold is present within a building, remediation is required regardless of sampling results. In fact, sampling is not recommended by the ACGIH if visible mold is present because current fungal sampling techniques are not well developed and the visible mold itself indicates a need for remediation (12). In most cases, environmental sampling is the best method with which to determine potential employee exposures to a specific chemical.

Sampling for exposure assessment involves dividing the workforce into groups called similar exposure groups (SEGs). A SEG is a group of employees with similar exposure to a specific chemical or group of chemicals. Employees with similar job duties are then sampled to quantify exposures of interest, and the results of the sampling examined using statistical methods. In many instances, all employee exposures are evaluated, even if the exposure is expected to be trivial, until a statistical model of the exposures within the group is determined. Sampling may then be reduced to a simple surveillance mode until new processes are implemented or job duties change. In this manner, exposures to specific chemicals can be predicted for all individuals within the facility and not just for those individuals who are exposed at levels approaching the current standard (13).

Environmental sampling may also be conducted under a number of specialized circumstances. It is common to conduct sampling to determine the efficacy of a newly installed engineering control method or the level after a change in industrial process. New processes that may be hazardous are frequently sampled first in a controlled area to determine if the exposures are acceptable before the actual implementation of the process. In some circumstances, previously used processes are simulated in order to determine past exposures.

A number of different sampling procedures are available, including breathing zone sampling, area sampling, real-time sampling, grab sampling, and surface sampling. Each of these approaches are described in some detail below.

Breathing Zone Sampling

Breathing zone samples provide the best information regarding individual exposure and are the most commonly collected airborne samples. Breathing zone samples are generally obtained by putting a sampling device within a foot of the nose of the individual to be sampled (Fig. 43.1). In most cases, the sampling device is put on the lapel of an individual, hence the term lapel samples. A list of advantages and disadvantages of breathing zone samples is contained in Table 43.2.

In some cases, breathing zone samples are taken as "grab" samples; i.e., samplers are put into the breathing zone of an individual for a short time during what is expected to be an average exposure period. Although this is a reasonable method to examine exposure during a process that lasts only a short time, it has many shortcomings in exposure assessment efforts. In most cases, it is desirable to have a breathing zone sample that represents the exposure during the entire workday for the employee. Full-shift sampling is therefore desirable because it documents exposure from the

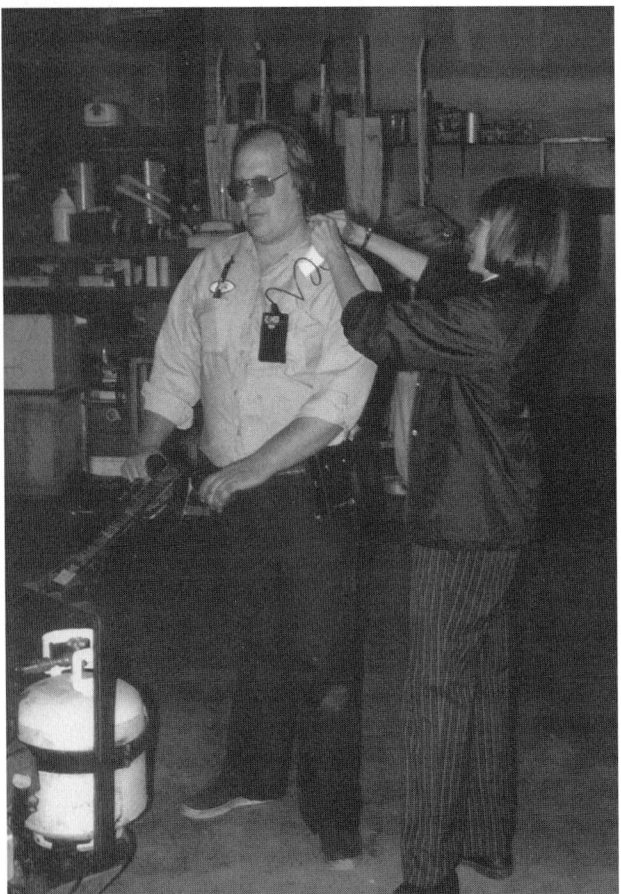

FIGURE 43.1. Industrial hygienist placing a breathing zone sampler on a worker.

time that employee came to work until the employee left to go home. Full-shift sampling thus includes exposures during cleaning, maintenance, and other tasks often not reflected in grab samples.

Grab samples are commonly used to identify where the major exposure occurred during the shift. In this case, samples can be taken when exposures are thought to be the worst. Results can be compared with full-shift samples to determine if they are the worst conditions or if other conditions yield higher exposures. Grab samples may also be used to

TABLE 43.2. ADVANTAGES AND DISADVANTAGES OF BREATHING ZONE SAMPLES

Advantages
    Best representation of actual exposures
    Can be used to assess nonroutine tasks
    Represents entire work shift exposure
    Provides individual exposures

Disadvantages
    Will not show peak exposures
    Limit of detection may be high
    Reason for high results may not be known
    Unsupervised and can be tampered with

determine the worst exposures and to assess efforts to lower those exposures through engineering controls.

Area Samples

Before the use of portable sampling pumps, large-volume samplers were used to determine the exposures within a specific area. The employees were then observed, and a time and motion study was completed for each employee group. The time that an employee spent in each area was multiplied by the measured exposure in that area and divided by the total exposure time. In this manner, a "daily weighted-average exposure" could be obtained for each employee. This approach generally results in exposure estimates that are lower than corresponding measurements taken by using lapel samplers. Area sampling fails to capture circumstances in which the worker closely approaches a process or does something different from standing at a work station. In addition, area sampling cannot be used for less predictable jobs such as maintenance or janitorial work.

Area samples are frequently used to determine exposures from processes that last only a short time. They are also used to take samples for characterizing exposures in a large general area. In some situations, area samplers are the only reliable method by which samples can be collected with a low enough detection level to document low exposures. Area samples are also obtained when sampling devices are not small enough to be worn by an employee. It is important to realize that area samples may not be representative of an employee's actual exposure.

Area samplers are frequently used to determine worst-case exposure conditions (Fig. 43.2). The sampler may be installed near the point of operation, assuming that the sampling results will indicate the highest level of exposure. In most cases, this sample would represent the worst case, but in some cases, it may not. For example, point of operation

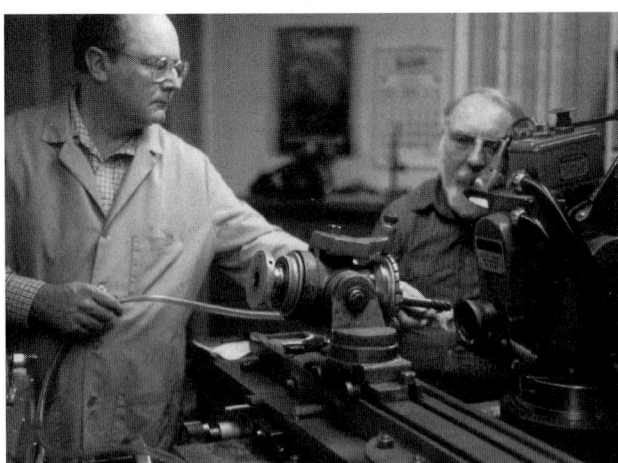

FIGURE 43.2. Industrial hygienist conducting area worst-case sampling at a machining operation.

TABLE 43.3. ADVANTAGES AND DISADVANTAGES OF AREA SAMPLES

Advantages
  May have a low limit of detection
  Difficult to tamper with
  Easy to set up and conduct
  Specialized apparatus may be used

Disadvantages
  May not represent actual employee exposure
  Typically supervised so employee may work differently than usual
  May not be acceptable to Occupational Safety and Health
    Administration
  May not reflect individual exposures

samples may be lower than breathing zone samples owing to a plume coming off a machine that was missed by the area sampler. An individual may move to another machine for a short time and increase exposure. In general, area samples are useful in some circumstances, but care should be taken in interpreting results. A list of advantages and disadvantages of area samples appears in Table 43.3.

Real-Time Samplers

The most desirable type of sampler can provide accurate and precise exposure information instantaneously–a real-time analyzer. Many air samples taken by industrial hygienists must be collected in a special tube filled with a material designed to collect the compound of interest, which is sent to a laboratory for analysis. The time between taking the sample and receiving the results may range from a few days to several months. This delay hinders the use of sampling to determine new exposures at a facility because either employees must be provided personal protective equipment or the process must be shut down until the results arrive. Sampling in cases of public protection after accidental spills are also hampered because the exposures will not be known for some time.

Real-time analyzers have many advantages. Portable gas chromatograph/mass spectrometers, as well as infrared spectrophotometers, are now available for use in measuring a wide variety of compounds. Many other instruments that use chemical cells are available to measure materials such as carbon monoxide, solvents, and hydrogen sulfide. Real-time monitors do have several attributes that may be of concern during use, especially in emergency situations. The monitors must be calibrated before use, and their ability to detect a known quantity of the chemical for which they are to be used must be demonstrated. Failure to do this may result in dangerous exposures to individuals, depending on the instruments. Many real-time instruments also react to a number of compounds other than the compound of interest. Some chemicals will interfere with the detection of another chemical. These properties must be known before the instrument is used for monitoring, especially in emergency situations.

Dust Samples

In settings with metal exposures, dust samples can be taken to determine the amount of toxic metals present in the settled dust of a facility. This information may indicate that the metal dust of concern has been airborne and that an exposure to workers has likely occurred. There is also the possibility that individuals working in the area will resuspend the dust, sustaining the exposure. Many factors influence whether or not the dust can be resuspended in air. Dust in an oily matrix will not be resuspended as readily as will dust in a dry powder with a small particle size. It is important, therefore, to realize that a high metal level in settled dust may not, by itself, indicate high airborne exposures to that metal.

Dust samples are commonly used to determine if clean-up procedures are adequate. Dust samples will also tell the industrial hygienist if the metal of concern has moved from the area where it is machined to other areas of the plant. In fact, sampling for residual dust levels in automobiles has been used to determine if employees are practicing good hygiene after finishing work or if residues of the toxic metal may inadvertently be contaminating their homes. This is accomplished by taking settled dust samples from the workers' automobiles or clothes (14).

Bioaerosol Sampling

Sampling for bioaerosols in both commercial and residential buildings has become a common specialized sampling technique. The capability to detect an airborne biological entity varies significantly, depending on the type of material to be identified. Major gains have been made in determining the levels of airborne mold spores, whereas detection of viruses and some allergens is extremely limited. Currently, most bioaerosol sampling is conducted while looking for fungal spores or bacteria in air. Samples may also be taken to determine the number of spores or bacteria in settled dust or to determine the species of a specific mold.

Two types of bioaerosol sampling are typically conducted, viable sampling and nonviable sampling. Viable sampling requires that the organism be grown in culture and identified. Viable sampling may be as simple as pressing agar plates to a surface and incubating the plate to determine what organisms are present, or may be as complex as air sampling using a microbial impactor. The use of settling plates (agar plates that are placed uncovered around a building) is discouraged because airborne concentrations cannot be accurately determined. The most common viable air sampling method uses a microbial impactor designed to capture fungal spores or bacteria on an agar plate (Fig. 43.3). The pump used to sample is calibrated for a specific flow rate and is run for a specified period of time so that a known volume of air has been sampled. The plate is sent to a laboratory for incubation, and the number and types of organisms are determined. With the amount of air sampled known, a concentration of organisms

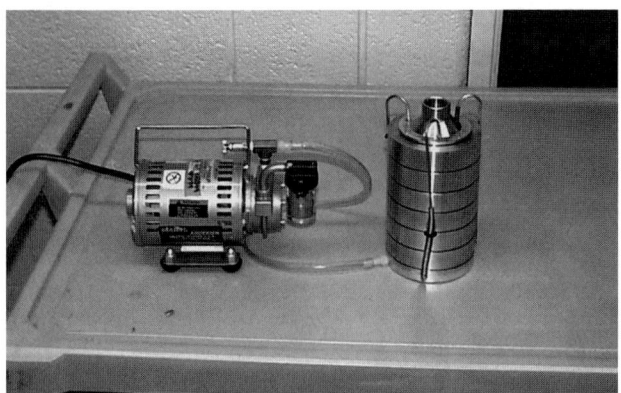

FIGURE 43.3. Anderson cascade impactor used for viable bioaerosol sampling.

per unit of air can be calculated. Results are usually reported as colony-forming units per cubic meter of air (CFU/m³) (12).

Although viable bioaerosol air samples can tell a great deal about the biological constituents of a building, it is easy to misinterpret the results. For example, if the media used was not the best growth media for the organisms present, detection may be limited even though an organism was present in great abundance. The media may not have been incubated at the ideal temperature for an organism, or it may not have been incubated long enough for an organism to grow. In either case, the most predominant environmental organism may not be identified, and a false assumption made that no significant bioaerosol is present.

Nonviable bioaerosol samples are obtained by using a greased slide apparatus that forces air at high speed onto a greased slide. The grease collects particles in the air, which then are stained and observed by using a light microscope. This method works well with fungal spores and pollen but does not work well for bacteria, viruses, and other material not easily identified with a light microscope. A commonly used device is called an Aer-o-cel cassette, a cassette that holds a greased slide. Other spore sampling devices are also available. The advantage of nonviable sampling is that the organism does not need to be grown in culture, avoiding the problems of determining the best media, incubation temperature, and growth period. The disadvantage is that many different spore species are difficult to identify, and many spores cannot be identified to genus.

Nonviable surface samples may be obtained by using sticky tape to determine the number of spores present on a surface such as a desktop or window sill. Dust samples may also be taken using a hand vacuum, and the number of spores per gram of dust determined by using either viable or nonviable methods. In all cases, these dust samples must be evaluated carefully because microbial contaminants are ubiquitous in the environment, and differentiating between a problem area and a nonproblem area is difficult.

In general, bioaerosol sampling results are difficult to interpret because bioaerosols are present in the air of all buildings to some degree. The ACGIH has published guidelines on a bioaerosol investigations and interpretation of results (12). Bioaerosol samples must be planned so that enough samples are taken in enough areas to determine if levels are higher inside a building than outside. It is also useful to determine if concentrations of specific species are higher inside a building than outside. Currently, there are no regulatory standards for bioaerosol concentrations within a building (12).

EXPOSURE EVALUATION

Once samples have been obtained and workplace exposures documented, the results can be compared to a number of standards or values to determine the degree of hazard to the worker. Exceeding an OSHA standard may result in sanctions such as fines and/or legal actions. In other cases, such as the ACGIH TLVs, there is no legally enforceable standard, but exposure may result in risk of illness in the workforce.

Occupational Safety and Health Administration Permissible Exposure Levels

The OSHA PELs are promulgated by OSHA in the U.S. Department of Labor. They are published in the U.S. Code of Federal Regulations, 29, part 1910 and have the force of law in that violation of the PEL may result in fines and/or other legal actions. Most of the PELs concern air exposures to chemicals and are expressed as an 8-hour time-weighted average. That is, the PEL is the 8-hour average airborne exposure beyond which an employee may not be exposed. For example, the PEL for 1,1,1-trichloroethane is 350 ppm, which means that a worker cannot be exposed to more than an average of 350 ppm of trichloroethane over an 8-hour shift. The worker could be exposed to an average of slightly less than 700 ppm over a 4-hour period and still be in compliance with the regulations.

The 8-hour average is determined through the use of the following formula: [measured concentration × hours exposed]/8 hours.

For the above example, the equation would be as follows:

$$[699 \text{ ppm} \times 4 \text{ hours}]/8 \text{ hours}$$
$$= [2,796 \text{ ppm-hours}]/8 \text{ hours} = 349.5 \text{ ppm}.$$

In this example, the employee would not exceed the PEL for 1,1,1-trichloroethane, even though the individual was exposed to levels exceeding the PEL for 4 hours. The PEL does not, therefore, protect the employee against short-term high exposures.

For some compounds, OSHA has established a "ceiling concentration" to regulate the maximum amount of material to which a worker may be exposed during any part of the 8-hour shift. If the concentration of a chemical with a ceiling level can be monitored on a real-time basis, then the levels can never exceed the ceiling level. If the concentration can only be determined by concentrating the sample on a collection media, then the shortest period of time that it would take to detect the ceiling level of a compound would be sampled.

When a worker is exposed to a mixture of similar acting compounds, the formula for the mixture PEL would be as follows: [(concentration A/PEL for A) + (concentration B/PEL for B) + (concentration C/PEL for C)].

If the result of the equation meets or exceeds unity, then the PEL is exceeded. For example, if chemical A has a concentration of 50 and a PEL of 100, chemical B has a concentration of 25 with a PEL of 50, and chemical C has a concentration of 40 with a PEL of 50, the results of the equation would be [(50/100) + (25/50) + (40/50)] = [0.5 + 0.5 + 0.8] = 1.8.

In this case, the PEL for the mixture has been exceeded, and the employees should be provided with some means of protection.

Most of the OSHA PELs were determined by using the ACGIH TLVs existing at the time that the standard was set. In many cases, the standards are based on TLVs from 1969. Although many other standards have been enacted since then, OSHA PELs are generally higher than are the ACGIH TLVs. A court decision regarding a benzene standard promulgated in 1978 required that OSHA show not only a reduction in adverse health effects associated with a lower standard but also the reduction in adverse health effects be commensurate with the cost of achieving the lower levels by industry. Thus, OSHA PELs should not be considered "safe levels" but rather legal levels not to be exceeded. Some individuals may not be protected at chemical concentrations that are less than the OSHA PEL.

American Conference of Governmental Industrial Hygienists Threshold Limit Levels

ACGIH TLVs are determined by the TLV committee of the ACGIH. They are published annually in *Threshold Limit Values for Chemical Substances and Physical Agents and Biological Exposure Indices* by the ACGIH. In the statement of use contained at the beginning of the TLV document, the ACGIH indicates that the TLVs are only guidelines published to assist in the control of health hazards. They are to be applied by trained industrial hygienists and are not to be used as legal standards (4).

TLVs are airborne concentrations of chemicals to which it is believed that nearly all workers may be exposed on a routine work day without developing significant adverse health effects. It is recognized that some individuals are hypersusceptible owing to variables such as sex, age, genetics, and personal habits and may not be protected at the TLV level. TLVs should not be used to evaluate community exposures,

exposures that exceed a normal workday, and continuous exposures or to define exposures that will or will not cause disease. They should also not be considered as a fine line between safe and unsafe, nor do they suggest the relative toxicity of a substance. Overall, TLVs are guidelines to be used by industrial hygienists, recognizing it is always best to control exposures to levels that are as low as readily achievable (4).

Similar to the OSHA PELs, TLVs are calculated on an 8-hour average basis, with the TLV being the average exposure over an 8-hour period. In addition to the TLV, many substances also have an established short-term exposure limit (STEL). The STEL is that concentration of a chemical to which a worker may be continuously exposed for a 15-minute period without suffering any irritation, chronic or irreversible tissue damage, or significant narcosis. This level does not take the place of the TLV, and in fact, the TLV still must be met. Exposures to the STEL should not occur for more that 15 minutes; they should not occur more than four times per day; and there should be at least 60 minutes between successive exposures (4).

ACGIH also publishes a ceiling level that is similar to the OSHA ceiling level, the concentration of a chemical that should not be exceeded during the workday. Ceiling limits provide a definite exposure boundary for those chemicals that have fast-acting effects at lower concentrations at which a long time-weighted average may not be protective (4).

Two other factors for chemicals are published in the TLV booklet. Some chemicals have a "skin notation." This designation indicates that the chemical is able to penetrate skin and that a potential contribution to the worker's dose may come from skin contact. The skin designation does not indicate that the chemical will damage the skin, but rather, it will penetrate the skin. Exposures to chemicals with a skin notation may not be determined by air sampling alone if skin contact is possible. In fact, exposures to chemicals that can penetrate the skin may be very difficult to document as long as there is a potential for skin contact. The OSHA PELs may also carry a "skin designation," indicating that a compound may penetrate the skin (4).

A second notation in the TLV publication is the "sensitizer notation," which indicates that the chemical has been found to produce immunologic sensitization in either animals or humans. Chemicals with a sensitizer notation may cause problems at very low levels for some individuals, and these chemicals may need more effective exposure control than do the majority of chemicals.

Other Standards

Although the OSHA PELs and the ACGIH TLVs are the most widely used and most familiar occupational standards, a number of other organizations also provide standards for chemical exposures. The American Society of Heating, Refrigeration, and Air-Conditioning Engineers (ASHRAE) publishes consensus standards addressing indoor air quality and ventilation in public buildings. The AIHA publishes the workplace environmental exposure levels (WEELs) that are similar to the ACGIH TLVs but less widely used.

NIOSH provides OSHA with recommendations regarding exposure levels to environmental agents. In fulfilling that requirement, NIOSH publishes recommended exposure limits (RELs) for a number of agents. The RELs, unlike the OSHA PELs, are not legal limits. In addition, RELs reflect health effect information without consideration of cost-benefit issues. NIOSH RELs are generally lower than OSHA PELs and frequently are lower than the ACGIH TLVs (15).

NIOSH also publishes immediately dangerous to life or health (IDLH) concentrations for a number of compounds. The IDLH concentration is that likely to cause death, serious permanent health effects, or incapacitation in less than 30 minutes. An exposure at this level may make escape impossible, and entry into environments with exposure concentrations at or above the IDLH should be conducted with only the highest degree of respiratory protection (15).

EXPOSURE CONTROL

Once a potential hazardous exposure has been identified, quantified, and compared with the legal and/or consensus standards, protection of employees can be undertaken. Exposure control is generally effected by using five methods: elimination, substitution, engineering controls, administrative controls, or personal protective equipment. The methods used will depend on a number of factors, including cost, type of exposure, and source of the exposure. The goal of exposure control is to reduce airborne exposures to workers to levels as low as reasonably achievable.

Elimination

Exposure elimination is the best control method available. If the exposure is no longer present, then the workers will no longer have exposure risks. This control method does not rely on worker compliance because the process resulting in the hazardous exposure has been eliminated. Elimination of an exposure may be difficult in that the process may be necessary for product manufacture.

Substitution

Substitution is the replacement of a toxic material with a less toxic material. An excellent example of substitution was described by Valway and colleagues in a study of highway patrol trainees, in which it was found that the use of lead bullets resulted in elevated blood lead levels from airborne lead exposures at a firing range. With a change to copper-jacketed bullets, airborne lead exposures dropped to less than 50 μg/m^3, and blood lead levels did not rise during the subsequent training period (16).

As with elimination, substitution does not rely on employee compliance to reduce exposure, and therefore, exposures will generally remain low. Exposures to the substitute chemical may also produce hazards that are less well recognized. The more that is known about the chemical to be substituted, the better a substitute chemical is likely to be.

Engineering Controls

The use of engineering controls to limit workplace exposures is the best control measure short of elimination or substitution. Engineering controls can be designed to reduce the need for worker compliance, thus limiting the circumstances in which the effectiveness of control measures is reduced by improper training or use. Engineering controls are generally divided into three categories: general dilution ventilation, local exhaust ventilation, and enclosure.

The use of enclosures to contain a process or to isolate a worker from a surrounding process can be extremely effective. In fact, many machines are now being manufactured with an enclosure. Newer enclosed machines contain the mists generated from machining fluids and implicated in risk of hypersensitivity pneumonitis among machinists (Fig. 43.4). The exposure of greatest concern when machines are enclosed occurs during the period in which a worker must enter the machine to clean-up or conduct preventive maintenance. In these circumstances, the worker enters a confined space, and exposures may be high. When appropriate, workers must be provided with respiratory protection during clean-up periods. Another example of an enclosure is the use of glove boxes for the isolation of especially dangerous hazards such as radioactive materials or toxic dusts (Fig. 43.5).

In some cases, enclosures can be used to enclose the employee and prevent exposure to a large process. This type of enclosure is used when the process can be automated and operated remotely by workers. The workers are contained

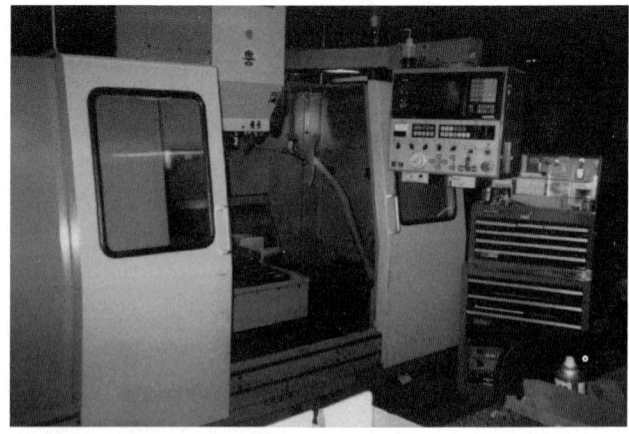

FIGURE 43.4. Enclosed milling machine designed to reduce worker exposure to machining fluids and metal aerosols.

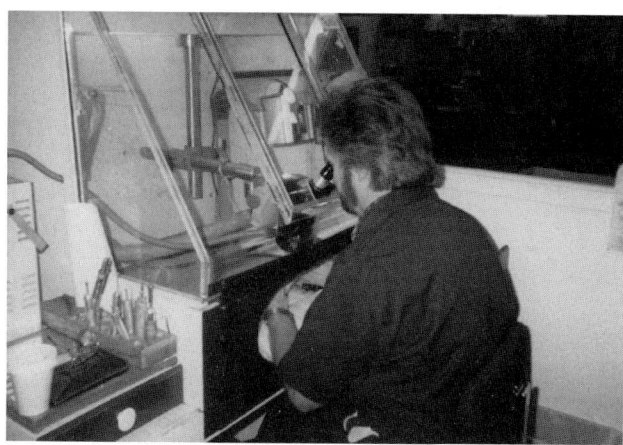

FIGURE 43.5. Glove box used to prevent worker exposure to beryllium dust during deburring operations.

in a booth or room that is isolated from the process and is separately ventilated. This type of enclosure may be used to isolate workers from very noisy areas as well. Enclosures can be of great value when workers do not need to be at the point of operation of a process for extended periods of time.

Local exhaust ventilation is the next best engineering method to reduce worker exposures. Local exhaust ventilation is designed to remove effluents from a process before they enter the air in a room. An effective local exhaust ventilation system can capture all of the emitted materials and eliminate worker exposures to the material of concern (Fig. 43.6). It is important, however, that the correct local ventilation system be used for a specific application. Particles generated by a grinding process are moving at a very high speed, and it may take a very high air movement rate to capture and evacuate the particle. Hot processes must be captured by a hood located over the process to take advantage of the upward movement of hot materials. Many hood

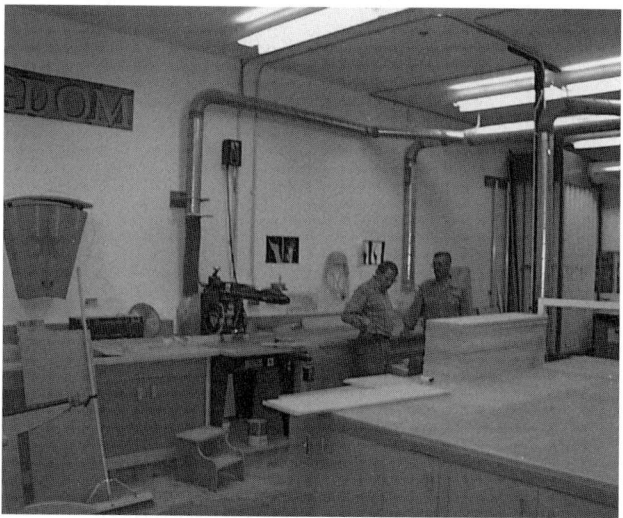

FIGURE 43.6. Dust collection system in a wood shop.

designs that can be applied to specific processes are described in the ACHIH publication *Industrial Ventilation*. Fitting the correct design to the application is essential (17).

Room dilution ventilation is the least desirable type of engineering control in most settings. This approach involves increasing the ventilation rate in a room to a level that reduces exposure to workers. However, because the worker is usually near the process, it is common for the worker to have higher exposures than the general room concentration of the material. Because this method usually requires the movement of large amounts of air, the cost of system operation can be high in temperate climates where outside air must usually be cooled or heated. Room dilution ventilation is usually an option only for materials that have a relatively low toxicity used in relatively small rooms (17).

Personal Protective Equipment

Personal protective equipment is one of the less desirable methods of worker protection owing to the need for individual compliance. It is also the most highly used method of worker protection owing to the initially low cost of implementation. In some cases, other types of controls cannot be used because of the need for worker mobility. Emergency service workers such as firemen are a good example of workers who must use personal protective equipment. Personal protective equipment may consist of gloves, eye protection, protective clothing, foot protection, head protection, and respiratory protection.

Respirators are used to protect individuals from a wide variety of exposures, including chemicals, bioaerosols, radiation, toxic dusts, metal fumes, and low oxygen situations (18,19). There are many different types of respirators available, each with specific uses and limitations (Table 43.4).

Respirators can be divided into four specific types: air supplying, air purifying, tight fitting, and loose fitting (18). The choice of respirator is determined by the exposure from which the individual is to be protected, the facial characteristics of the individual, and the characteristics of the job (19–21). In situations involving low oxygen environments or environments in which the concentrations or types of chemicals are unknown, only the highest degree of protection is allowed (15,18,19). In these situations, the only acceptable type of respiratory protection is a positively pressured self-contained breathing apparatus (SCBA) (15,18). Exposure to a nuisance dust, on the other hand, may require only the use of a half-face disposable respirator. There is usually some type of respirator available for most potential exposures.

Air-supplying respirators provide the greatest degree of protection (18,19). These respirators supply a breathing atmosphere to the wearer and can therefore protect the individual from most exposures. These respirators are normally worn by hazardous materials teams and emergency response crews when dangerous or unknown exposures are likely (19).

TABLE 43.4. CHARACTERISTICS OF SPECIFIC RESPIRATOR TYPES

Category	Respirator Type	NIOSH Protection Factor[a]	Use for Unknown Exposures and Concentrations	Uses Specific Cartridges	Required Maintenance	Eyeglass Interference	Can Be Worn with Facial Hair
Air supplying	Pressure demand, self-contained breathing apparatus	10,000	Yes	No	High	Yes	No
	Supplied air (air line)	10–2,000[b]	No[c]	No	High	Yes	Yes (with loose fitting device only)
Air Purifying	Tightfitting PAPR	50	No	Yes	High	Yes	No
	Loose-fitting PAPR	25	No	Yes	High	No	Yes
	Full-face cartridge	50	No	Yes	Moderate	Yes	No
	Half-face cartridge	10	No	Yes	Moderate	Maybe	No
	Half-face disposable	10	No	No	Low	Maybe	No

[a]National Institute for Occupational Safety and Health (NIOSH) assigns a numeric, theoretical protection factor that can be attained by types of respirators.
[b]Depends on the type of mask used (e.g., half-face, full-face).
[c]Not approved unless an escape-bottle self-contained breathing apparatus is attached.
PAPR, powered air purifying respirator.

This high degree of exposure protection comes at a cost. An SCBA can weigh over 30 lbs and contain only enough air for 30 minutes of time in the exposure area (19). In some cases, just suiting up can take 30 minutes, and the weight, combined with a sealed suit and high temperatures, may exact a heavy toll on the wearer's endurance.

Air-purifying respirators are lighter and easier to use (22). This respirator is the type most commonly used and, consequently, is also the most misused respirator. To reliably use an air-purifying respirator, it is important to know the type and concentration of the exposure to ensure that the respirator will provide adequate protection (22). A respirator designed to protect an individual against a very small particulate, such as asbestos, may provide no protection against a gas, such as arsine gas. The use of an improper respirator may result in injury or death to the wearer. It is also important when using air purifying respirators to be able to determine when the respirator is no longer working. For this reason, air-purifying respirators should only be used when the chemical has properties (irritation or smell) that will let the wearer know that the respirator is failing and leaving the area of exposure is necessary (22).

Disposable respirators are widely used owing to the high comfort level and relatively higher degree of verbal communication they allow (Fig. 43.7). Disposable respirators are most commonly used for particulate exposures, such as exposure to bioaerosols in medical situations (23). The primary limitation of the half-face disposable respirator is the facial fit of the respirator (23). In general, the most comfort and least breathing resistance is obtained using a loose-fitting respirator. Because of leakage, these respirators may not provide the necessary protection. It is important that the primary criterion for the choice of respirator be protection against the potential exposure and not comfort. Typically, this protection level is determined by the assignment of a "protection factor" by NIOSH, the theoretical reduction that should be attained by that respirator. For example, a protection factor of 10 should reduce the concentration inside the respirator to at least one-tenth of the outside concentration (18).

To ensure that the best respirator is chosen, that it is maintained properly, and that the individual is trained to use the respirator properly, a respiratory protection policy should be implemented (20). This type of program is mandated by OSHA and should be in use even if an individual is not covered by OSHA. A respiratory protection program should first ensure that the individual can medically wear a respirator, and then fit the person to the respirator that will best protect yet still let the individual perform the necessary tasks. Respirator choice can be made by using any number of algorithms available in the literature. These algorithms consider, among other criteria, the exposure, job tasks, and oxygen level. Once the respirator type is determined, the individual

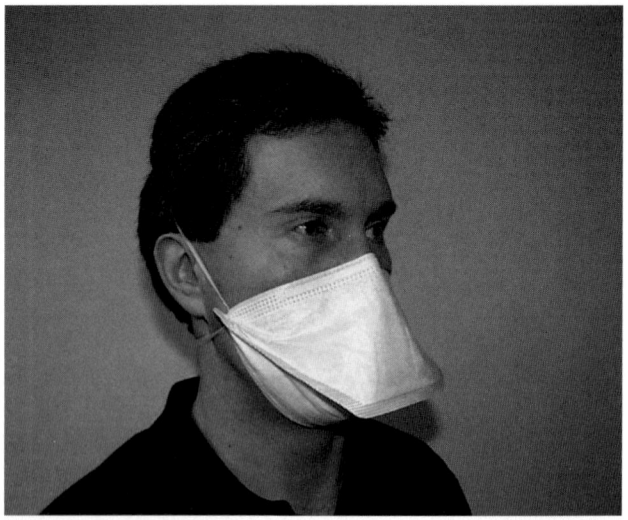

FIGURE 43.7. Employee wearing an N-95 disposable respirator approved for particulate exposures.

should be fit-tested using either qualitative or quantitative testing to determine which size and/or brand of respirator will ensure the best fit. Because most respirators were initially designed for average male workers, women and persons with unusual facial features may require different respirators (21). In addition, individuals with facial hair will not obtain an adequate fit with respirators designed to seal to the face (20).

Training in the use of respirators is extremely important. Events in which individuals use an air-purifying respirator to enter a confined space and then die in the space are reported every year. Individuals must be informed about the limitations of their respirator, as well as the importance of cleaning, inspecting, and changing filters when necessary (18,24). Simply storing a respirator in the wrong place can negate its efficacy. For example, storing a respirator with charcoal filters in an area with solvents will consume the adsorption capability of the respirator. The types of cartridges used with respirators can vary, with many cartridges having multiple media and therefore multiple uses. There is, however, no cartridge that will work for all exposures or under all conditions.

THE PHYSICIAN/INDUSTRIAL HYGIENIST TEAM

Physicians and industrial hygienists working together can contribute more to worker safety and health than can either working alone. Without a diagnosis of a disease or a list of possible causes of illness, an industrial hygienist may have difficulty knowing what exposures to measure. Knowledge of the workplace exposures present and their magnitude may help the physician arrive at a diagnosis and adequate treatment plan for a patient. Input from a physician may help an industrial hygienist determine the best type of control measures for a given process, as well as help to determine the efficacy of the controls. In the case of unknown illnesses occurring in an industry or community, the industrial hygienist and physician, along with epidemiologists, may have a better chance of determining the cause than would any alone.

HOW AND WHERE TO FIND AN INDUSTRIAL HYGIENIST

Finding an industrial hygienist can be accomplished in a number of ways. The AIHA has an extensive list of industrial hygiene consulting firms by state and by areas of expertise. The list can be searched on the AIHA Web site at *www.aiha.org*. A listing of CIHs can be obtained by contacting the American Board of Industrial Hygiene at *www.abih.org*. In some cases, contacting the nearest state university will enable referral to the industrial hygiene department located in the environmental health or public health department.

Industrial hygiene assistance can be obtained from a number of governmental agencies, including NIOSH and OSHA. NIOSH contacts can be made through the Centers for Disease Control and Prevention Web site, with most of the NIOSH industrial hygienists based in Cincinnati, Ohio. OSHA offices are located throughout the country and can be a helpful source of information. Some states also have their own OSHA programs, and industrial hygienists are almost always associated with these programs. Many state and some local health departments provide some industrial hygiene services to state businesses.

REFERENCES

1. Plog BA. Overview of industrial hygiene. In: *Fundamentals of industrial hygiene,* 5 ed. Itasca, IL: National Safety Council, 2002:1–32.
2. US House of Representatives, 91st Congress. Public law 91-596, section 2193, Occupational safety and health act. Washington, US Government Printing Office; 1970.
3. American Board of Industrial Hygiene Web site. Available at: *http://www.acgih.org.* Accessed July 2002.
4. American Conference of Governmental Industrial Hygienists. *2002 threshold limit values for chemical substances and physical agents and biological exposure indices.* Cincinnati: American Conference of Governmental Industrial Hygienists, 2002.
5. Proctor NH, Hughes JP. *Chemical hazards of the workplace.* Philadelphia: JB Lippincott Co, 1978:449–450.
6. Doull J, Klaassen CD, Amdur MO, eds. *Casarett and Doull's toxicology: the basic science of poisons.* New York: Macmillan, 1980.
7. Kelly RJ. Particles. In: Plog BA, ed. *Fundamentals of industrial hygiene,* 5th ed. Itasca, IL: National Safety Council, 2002:1–32.
8. Martyny J, Hoover M, Mroz M, et al. Aerosols generated during beryllium machining. *J Occup Environ Med* 1999;42:8–18.
9. McCawley MA, Kent MS, Berakis MT. Ultrafine beryllium number concentration as a possible metric for chronic beryllium disease risk. *Appl Occup Environ Hyg* 2001;16:631–638.
10. Johnson D, Swift D. Sampling and sizing particles. In: DiNardi SR, ed. *The occupational environment: its evaluation and control.* Fairfax, VA: American Industrial Hygiene Association, 1997:244–261.
11. US Department of Labor, Occupational Safety and Health Administration. Hazard communication. *Federal Register* 29, part 1910.1200.
12. Macher J, ed. *Bioaerosols: assessment and control.* Cincinnati: American Conference of Governmental Industrial Hygienists, 1999.
13. Mulhausen JR, Damiano JD, eds. *A strategy for assessing and managing occupational exposures.* Fairfax, VA: American Industrial Hygiene Association, 1998.
14. Sanderson W, Henneberger P, Martyny J, et al. Beryllium contamination inside vehicles of machine shop workers. *Appl Occup Environ Hyg* 1999;14:223–230.
15. National Institute of Occupational Safety and Health. *Pocket guide to chemical hazards.* Washington, DC: US Department of Health and Human Services, 1994.
16. Valway SE, Martyny JW, Miller JR, et al. Lead absorption in indoor firing range users. *Am J Public Health* 1989;79:1029–1032.
17. American Conference of Governmental Industrial Hygienists. *Industrial ventilation: a manual of recommended practice.* Cincinnati: American Conference of Governmental Industrial Hygienists, 1984.

18. NIOSH National Institute for Occupational Safety and Health. *NIOSH guide to industrial respiratory protection.* Washington: US Dept. of Health and Human Services, 1987: 289.

19. NIOSH National Institute for Occupational Safety and Health. *Occupational safety and health guidance manual for hazardous waste site activities.* Washington: US Dept. of Health and Human Services, 1985.

20. Occupational Safety and Health Administration. *Respiratory protection* (29 CFR part 1910.134). Washington: Occupational Safety and Health Administration, 1998.

21. Gross S, Horstman S. Half-mask respirator selection for a mixed worker group. *Appl Occup Envin Hyg* 1990;5:229–235.

22. Colton C, Nelson T. Respiratory protection. In: DiNardi SR, ed. *The occupational environment: its evaluation and control.* Fairfax, VA: American Industrial Hygiene Association, 1997:1365.

23. Centers for Disease Control and Prevention. Guidelines for preventing the transmission of *Mycobacterium tuberculosis* in health-care facilities, 1994. *MMWR* 1994;43(RR-13):132.

24. American National Standards Institute. *American national standard for respirator protection.* New York: American National Standards Institute, 1992.

Occupational Lung Diseases Caused by Asbestos, Silica, and Other Silicates

44

Jason Kelley

The lung diseases caused by the inhalation of asbestos, silica, and the other silicates are the most prevalent pneumoconioses. The industrial revolution in the Western nations was responsible for widespread exposure during the 19th century. These diseases have caused significant morbidity and mortality, especially during the early part of the 20th century. The resulting cohort of patients with particularly severe manifestations of disease drove epidemiologic and clinical research to define patterns of dust exposure, safe thresholds of exposure, mechanisms of toxicity, and approaches to avoidance and abatement.

However, by the end of the 20th century, the epidemiology of the life-threatening pneumoconioses had undergone global shifts. Dust-induced diseases have become more problematic in emerging nations as a consequence of their rapidly expanding and underregulated industrial base. This shift has occurred just as strict control of dusts in the workplace has gradually reduced disease in advanced nations. Despite the shift, the residual burden of disease in the postindustrial world, including the United States, continues to result in significant morbidity and mortality. Data from death certificates indicate that more than 4,000 to 8,000 deaths occur annually in which pneumoconioses are a contributing or primary cause (1). Most of these deaths are attributable to coal worker's pneumoconiosis, silicosis (2), and asbestosis.

In advanced nations with regulations in place, cases of pneumoconiosis that continue to develop under conditions of rigorous control often present with incidental radiographic findings not associated with disability or premature mortality. Under these conditions, clinicians face a daunting challenge in that they must recognize the subtle or atypical radiographic features of exposure. Such cases are com-plicated by the minimal extent of disease (often apparent only radiographically) and a history of exposure to multiple mineral dusts that leads to cryptic radiographic patterns. To these factors must be added the confounding variable of cigarette smoke–induced lung disease in the exposed population. Moreover, former miners and industrial workers often migrate from regions of high incidence to retirement areas where the low incidence of dust-induced disease makes it unlikely that their radiographic abnormalities will be recognized. Finally, those cases of severe pneumoconiosis that continue to occur despite appropriate industrial hygiene measures tend to be limited to ever smaller groups of workers subjected to intense but brief exposures to dusts, often at sites not appropriately monitored by regulatory agencies (3).

OCCUPATIONAL HISTORY

The most important step in the diagnosis of unsuspected pneumoconiosis is to elicit a detailed work history (4). Specifics of the job and the minerals or materials in the environment must be sought. Often, the subject's past or present occupation may not immediately suggest mineral dust exposure. In this era of a mobile work force, it is always important to seek a detailed account of the subject's remote employment. Increasingly, pneumoconioses can be traced to exposures outside the workplace; hence, it is important to ask the subject about unusual activities and hobbies. Because some pneumoconioses develop after only brief but intense dust exposures, it is important to inquire about part-time or transient employment.

The specific type of work done may provide clues to the severity of exposure. When the interviewer is unfamiliar with the terms used—such as bagger, miller, weaver, pipe fitter, fettler, and tunneler—it may be wise to seek a layperson's description of the actual working habits. The worker

J. Kelley: Department of Medicine, University of Louisville, Louisville, Kentucky.

may provide samples of suspected dusts or materials brought from the workplace; alternately, an inspection of the workplace (if permitted) may be called for. Additional questioning should be directed at whether the worker exposed to mineral dusts had access to a respirator or other protective equipment. The patient should be asked about having been alerted to potential hazards through notices or similar illnesses in coworkers.

Although employment patterns are changing, men have far outnumbered women in the blue collar work force and therefore have borne the burden of exposure to mineral dusts. The rates of cigarette smoking in the blue collar workforce have consistently been very high. Rates as high as 80% have been recorded among miners and hard rock workers. Cigarette smoking can have a particularly devastating impact on workers exposed to mineral dusts. For the clinician/epidemiologist studying the pneumoconioses, the coexistence of smoking effects invariably confounds population studies. In patients with mineral dust diseases causing minimal impairment, the deleterious effects of smoking usually far overshadow those attributable to the dust.

The diagnostic approach to suspected mineral dust diseases differs from the evaluation of other interstitial lung disorders in that issues of potential liability for injury are at stake. The extent of disease and its causality are also relevant to determinations of disability and workers' compensation.

In the proper setting, a history of duration and intensity of exposure coupled with characteristic radiographic findings is adequate for a diagnosis. Lung biopsy via bronchoscopy, video-assisted thoracoscopy, or open thoracotomy is reserved for complex cases. Given the lack of efficacious therapies for the pneumoconioses, typical reasons for performing a biopsy include an atypical presentation, an unusually rapid course of disease, and suspicion of coexisting carcinoma or treatable diseases such as occult infections. Sometimes, biopsy is advocated for liability evaluations. Perhaps most biopsies are performed when pneumoconiosis is unsuspected or when it is included in a longer differential diagnosis of possible infiltrative lung disorders.

ASBESTOSIS

Possibly no mineral has been associated with more social and political controversy during the past century than asbestos. Asbestos (from the Greek $\alpha\varsigma\beta\epsilon\varsigma\tau o\varsigma$, "unquenchable") comprises a group of ductile, fire-resistant mineral silicates with wide commercial applications. During crushing and milling, members of the major asbestos groups, the serpentines and the amphiboles, break into fibers rather than dust. They share the properties of being nearly indestructible, heat- and acid-resistant minerals. In the middle of the 20th century, an epidemic of asbestos-related disease afflicted many heavily exposed workers. Following the recognition of the various lethal clinical disorders resulting from asbestos ex-

TABLE 44.1. MINERAL FORMS OF ASBESTOS

Amphiboles	Serpentines
Crocidolite ("blue asbestos")	Chrysotile
Amosite ("brown asbestos")	
Tremolite	
Actinolite	
Anthophyllite	

posure came legislation, litigation, and often the bankruptcy of large producers.

Asbestos exists in multiple forms, all of them fibrous silicate minerals (Table 44.1). They are variably resistant to heat and to destruction by acids and other chemicals. All forms of asbestos share a fibrous structure, which makes them suitable for use in woven fabrics. The chemical elements present in addition to silicon include magnesium, calcium, iron, and sodium. All forms of asbestos can be classified as either of two mineralogic types, the serpentines (of which chrysotile is the sole example) and the multiple amphiboles. Chrysotile is the most commercially important of the asbestos minerals. Long chrysotile fibers have a curled appearance; the amphiboles have more needle-shaped fibers. Common amphiboles include crocidolite, amosite, anthophyllite, tremolite, and actinolite.

Commercial Uses of Asbestos

Chrysotile accounts for the preponderance (>95%) of asbestos mined and used in the world. Asbestos has been widely mined since the end of the 19th century, primarily in eastern Canada, the New England states of the United States, Finland, and Russia. Crocidolite ("blue asbestos") comes chiefly from South Africa and was also previously mined in western Australia. However, with recognition of its enhanced toxicity, the demand for crocidolite has greatly decreased in recent decades. The European Union has made plans to ban the use of asbestos entirely by the year 2005.

Monitoring and regulatory efforts by government agencies such as the Environmental Protection Agency in the United States have greatly cut down on the use of asbestos. Between 1920 and 1970, world asbestos production rose more than 25-fold. For many years, the sheathing and insulation used in the construction of office buildings and houses consisted largely of products reinforced and rendered heat-resistant with asbestos fibers. Asbestos was used to line furnaces and lag pipes, as friction material in brakes, in spray paints to prevent fire, and as a binder and strengthener for cement pipes. During times of war, it was extensively used in warships for insulation and as a fire retardant. During the 1950s, asbestos was even briefly marketed as a component of cigarette filters. The exposure of workers in the United States continued to be high until legislation and litigation against asbestos producers in the 1970s forced the development of alternate products.

Historical Aspects and Effects of Exposure to Asbestos

Asbestos exposure can lead to several distinct serious pleural and pulmonary conditions: asbestosis, nonmalignant pleural disease (pleural effusion, pleural thickening, pleural plaques), rounded atelectasis, lung cancer, and mesothelioma. Each of these distinct clinical entities may occur alone or in combination.

Asbestosis is a progressive and diffuse remodeling disease of the lung parenchyma characterized by dyspnea, inspiratory crackles, and diffuse bilateral, irregular linear opacities on chest radiographs. It was first recognized as a distinct disease entity at the beginning of the 20th century (5). The magnitude of the hazard and the exposure-effect relationship were worked out in studies published during the subsequent several decades. The development of asbestosis results from cumulative, continuous high-level exposure to airborne asbestos. A definite dose-effect relationship has been established (6).

Recommendations for improved industrial hygiene practices were developed as a result of these seminal studies. The risk to users of finished asbestos products became more generally apparent after the Second World War, when exposure to finished products in shipbuilding and other trades peaked. Before that, sporadic case reports of asbestosis occurring in pipe fitters, welders, and others had been reported. Most such instances suggested that the condition had developed in exposed workers as the result of an exceptional and unusual exposure. Population-based studies made it clear that a significant risk existed in users of the finished product. Furthermore, it became clear from these studies that the prevailing regulatory statutes were not protecting the workforce from asbestos-induced disease.

Standards of Asbestos Exposure

Ever stricter limits of exposure to asbestos were promulgated throughout the 20th century in response to epidemic disease and disability. Precise standards vary somewhat between industrialized nations. In the United States, the regulated standard has been progressively reduced to 0.1 fibers per cubic centimeter. To allow for frequent changes in ambient dust levels in the workplace, this standard refers to an 8-hour time-weighted average (TWA). Asbestos fibers 5 μm and larger harbor most of the toxicity and are therefore the focus of regulatory standards. To account for the different toxicities of different fiber types, some jurisdictions apply more rigorous standards for the amphiboles. Exposure-effect relationships are useful for developing safe "threshold limit values" (TLVs), below which dust levels are unlikely to result in disease during a worker's life span. The accepted TLV below which asbestosis is thought not to develop is 25 fibers-years per cubic centimeter (7–9).

For many years, asbestos was measured as the number of particles per cubic centimeter of ambient air. Asbestos content is usually determined by trapping airborne particles on filters. Fiber size and number are then determined by phase-contrast microscopy. Only fibers longer than 5 μm are measured because smaller fibers are cleared from the lungs and are not likely to lead to pulmonary disease or malignancy. Neither particle nor fiber counting distinguishes other particles or fibers from those of asbestos. Although this does not matter much in asbestos textile factories, where most of the airborne fibers are asbestos, in other occupational settings the percentage of asbestos may be low. Under such circumstances, optical counts obtained with a microscope can be misleading, and when it is imperative to separate asbestos fibers from nonasbestiform fibers, more definitive techniques, such as transmission or scanning electron microscopy, must be used to identify the nature of the fiber correctly.

As a result of regulatory efforts in the industrialized nations of the world, the incidence of asbestosis has decreased during the past several decades. Subjects with established asbestosis are thus becoming an increasingly elderly population. Moreover, as the ambient levels have fallen in the workplace, the period of latency between exposure and the appearance of asbestosis has lengthened. For example, a report from 1938 showed that asbestosis was present after exposures as short as 5 years. At that time, dust levels could be as high as 400 particles per cubic centimeter. During and after the Second World War, the average duration of exposure before the development of asbestosis rose from between 10 and 12 years to in excess of 20 years. Since then, regulatory efforts have become considerably more stringent; it is reasonably certain that few new cases of asbestos-related lung diseases will develop under current standards. Based on long-term follow-up studies, asbestosis was reported to develop in as many as half of all workers exposed during the middle of the 20th century.

Specific Occupational Risks

It has been estimated that as many as 27 million workers in the United States were subjected to a significant exposure to asbestos during the middle four decades of the 20th century. Of these, it is estimated that as many as 6 million Americans are still alive with a significant past exposure to asbestos. Environmental exposure to asbestos and other minerals can occur at each stage of extraction and use: extraction (miners), purification and production (weavers), and use of the finished product (plumbers, laggers, insulation layers). Workers involved in removal of the used product from buildings, ships, and other sites may be exposed to heat-exposed insulation products. Certain industries present greater or lesser risks of disease that can be traced to the mineral type, particle size, and manner of exposure. Somewhat surprisingly, for instance, miners of asbestos have generally been found to be at lower risk for disease than millers and weavers. Regardless of the context of exposure, exposure to the serpentine chrysotile carries significantly less risk than exposure to the amphiboles.

Examples abound of workforces in which certain jobs carry a much higher risk than others performed in equal proximity. Close contact appears to be a critical determinant of risk. Thus, disabling disease develops in pipe fitters that is not often shared by welders working in the same area.

Asbestos-related disease as a result of exposure outside the workplace does occur but is very infrequent and again requires substantial exposure. Stories of wives washing their worker husbands' asbestos-laden clothing are more than apocryphal but are less frequently documented as regulations have been enforced. Low levels of asbestos fibers are found in ambient air in the urban environment. Sources include demolished equipment and buildings. These levels continue to drop as regulatory measures are implemented.

Acute asbestos exposure in lower Manhattan was an immediate concern following the destruction of the World Trade Center towers in September 2001 (10). Close monitoring of environmental asbestos fibers began immediately in conjunction with search efforts and demolition activities. The findings of a survey conducted by the Centers for Disease Control and Prevention documented that the ambient air did not appear to be contaminated with asbestos or crystalline silica to an extent that posed an occupational health hazard.

Undoubtedly, asbestos continues to be an important health concern. As the occupationally induced diseases have abated somewhat in prevalence and severity, concern for nonoccupational indoor exposures has grown. In postindustrial areas of the world, more than 70% of people's time is spent indoors. People who work or live in older buildings containing low levels of asbestos are not at significant risk because the asbestos is largely immobilized in the building materials (11). Worries about vulnerable groups such as schoolchildren and office workers have consequently grown, often not based on sound scientific principles. Indoor levels of exposure in such populations have been estimated to be 1/100,000 the levels of asbestos exposure in industry workers for whom historical risk estimates are available. One study indicated that public buildings contain as few as 0.002 fibers per cubic centimeter, far below the regulated standard (12). Finally, asbestos occurs as a natural pollutant of air and water in certain regions of the world where surface deposits are a prominent feature of the landscape.

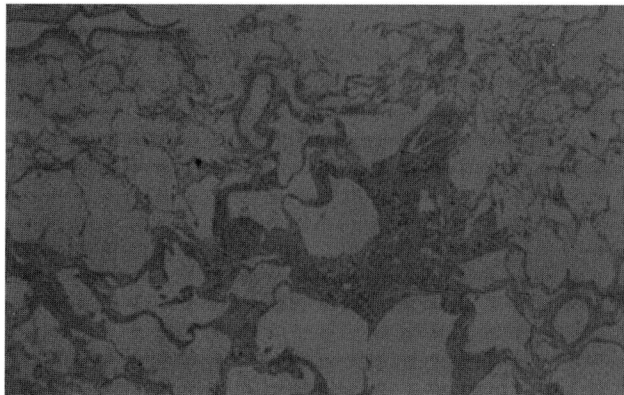

FIGURE 44.1. (See also Color Fig. 44.1.) Asbestos-induced airways disease with alveolar duct fibrosis.

Pathology of Asbestosis: Inhalation and Deposition

The inhalation of airborne asbestos particles is the route of primary exposure. Inhaled asbestos fibers that elude the defense mechanisms of the upper airway are deposited on bifurcations of the respiratory and terminal bronchioles. Lesser degrees of deposition occur in the alveoli. Somewhat paradoxically, it is the longer fibers that have the potential to reach the distal lung and exert toxic effects. Straight fibers as long as 60 μm, a size not normally considered to be in the respirable range, can evade impaction in the large airways. Their exaggerated length-to-width ratio allows penetration into the small airways, from which they can migrate into the pulmonary interstitium. Fibers that elude the mucociliary escalator can elicit a peribronchial inflammatory reaction in small airways and proximal alveolar duct regions with resultant wall thickening and fibrosis (Figs. 44.1 and 44.2). Retained particles migrate into the interstitial spaces of the distal lung, where they encounter and activate phagocytic cells such as interstitial and alveolar macrophages. Fiber processing and migration differ for the different asbestos types, with resultant fundamental differences in the histologic and

ASBESTOS EXPOSURE	
Summary Statement	**Level of Evidence**
Asbestos exposure standards	Nonrandomized, historical and expert opinion
Specific occupational risks	Nonrandomized, historical and expert opinion
Asbestos interaction with smoking	Historical and expert opinion, case series

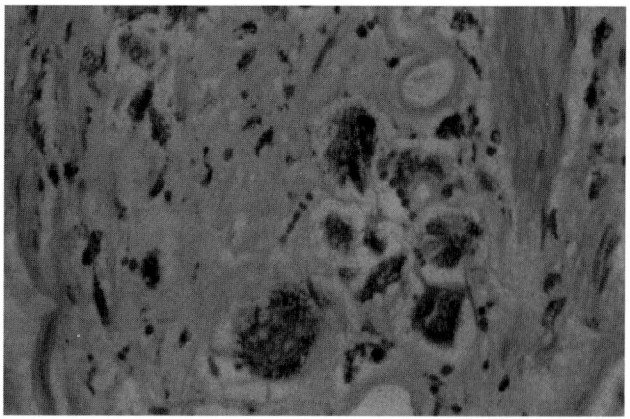

FIGURE 44.2. (See also Color Fig. 44.2.) Asbestos bodies in the wall of an alveolar duct.

ultrastructural effects caused by chronic inhalation of the amphibole crocidolite and the serpentine chrysotile (13).

After ingestion by macrophages, asbestos fibers undergo a process of chemical leaching and partial dissolution. This phenomenon occurs more readily with chrysotile asbestos; the amphiboles are more resistant to macrophage ingestion and leaching. Once deposited, amphibole fibers have a much longer half-life. As a result, amphibole enrichment tends to develop over time in the lungs of subjects with mixed dust exposures. Fibers that cannot be cleared via the mucociliary escalator up the airway lumen move into the alveolar interstitium and can migrate to the regional lymph nodes. The lung can clear chrysotile asbestos more rapidly than the amphibole asbestos forms. All types of asbestos are considered fibrogenic, although crocidolite appears to be more carcinogenic.

The issue of variation in susceptibility to asbestosis and other pneumoconioses in workers with comparable exposures has long interested investigators. The best available evidence suggests that the retention and accumulation of dust in the lungs is more important than the absolute level of exposure. Lung and airway size correlates with the presence or absence of disease in workers exposed to asbestos, silica, and other dusts. Airway caliber in particular seems to be a major determinant of individual susceptibility.

Smokers may be at greater risk for the development of asbestosis as a consequence of delayed and inefficient clearing of asbestos particles from the lung via the mucociliary escalator pathway. As a result, cigarette smoking enhances fiber retention in the lung. The longer residence time and greater burden of fibers in the lungs of smokers allow uptake of fibers by epithelial and other structural cells.

The high incidence of smoking in dust-exposed workers has additional consequences for the management of these subjects. Radiologic patterns are confusing because of the presence of variant features of both disorders; similarly, pathologic findings on biopsy specimens are difficult to ascribe to each disorder specifically. Smoking and its resulting pathologic effects may affect the biology of dust deposition, inflammatory reaction, chemical processing, and particle transport (14,15).

Symptoms and Signs of Asbestosis

Asbestosis is a diffuse fibrotic remodeling of the lungs caused by the inhalation of respirable forms of asbestos. The common presenting symptoms of asbestosis are dyspnea and dry cough. Like persons with other pulmonary disorders, exposed workers often do not seek medical advice until the condition is fairly disabling. If the original exposure was intense, disabling symptoms may continue to progress despite removal from further exposure.

Early in the disease process, bilateral basilar rales are heard in middle to late inspiration. As the disease progresses, they become more widespread. Tachypnea is almost always present by the time the disease has reached the symptomatic

stage. Cyanosis may be visible. Clubbing of the fingers, when present, usually signals advanced disease and a poor prognosis. Signs consistent with right-sided heart failure also become apparent later in the course. Depending on the specific presentation, the differential diagnosis may include usual interstitial pneumonitis, sarcoidosis, chronic pulmonary infections, and other pneumoconioses or toxic inhalation disorders.

Radiographic Features of Asbestosis

The development of irregular linear shadows in the mid zones and bases of the lung on the chest radiograph characterizes the parenchymal remodeling process referred to as *asbestosis*. To assist in standardizing the interpretation of radiographs, the International Labor Office (ILO) developed a classification based on plain radiographs. The ILO classification has some value in predicting life expectancy in exposed populations. Training in ILO classification is rigorous, and periodic updating through review of a set of standard chest films is required.

In the ILO system, small, irregular shadows of increasing size are described as s, t, and u opacities. Round shadows (typical in silicosis) are p, q, and r shadows. As the number or profusion of small, round or irregular shadows increases, they are graded as 0, 1, 2, or 3. When the reader is uncertain about the grade, intermediate grades can be indicated with a slash mark. For example, a reading graded between 1 and 2 would be 1/2, the first number being the one the reader believes to be correct and the second the one the reader is leaning toward. In asbestosis, the smaller s and t shadows predominate over the larger u shadows. A significant percentage of smokers who have had no asbestos exposure have scanty irregular shadows on their chest radiograph, so that their presence is less specific. As in other interstitial lung disorders, these small irregular shadows tend to blur the margins of normal anatomic structures such as the diaphragm and the cardiac, mediastinal, and bronchovascular markings. Initially, the small irregular shadows appear in the lower zones, the site of the most intense asbestos inhalation. With the progression of disease, the upper lung zones become more obviously involved. The use of computed tomography (CT) to detect disease in exposed workers with normal chest radiographs is possible (16) but remains controversial as a mass screening tool. In asbestos-exposed subjects with normal chest radiographic findings but significantly reduced lung function indicative of restrictive lung disease, abnormalities can commonly be identified by high-resolution CT (HRCT).

Pleural thickening may confound the evaluation of the character and profusion of irregular parenchymal shadows. Specifically, thickening of the anterior and posterior pleura, when viewed en face on a posteroanterior chest view, can be mistaken for parenchymal disease. CT is particularly helpful in clarifying this issue.

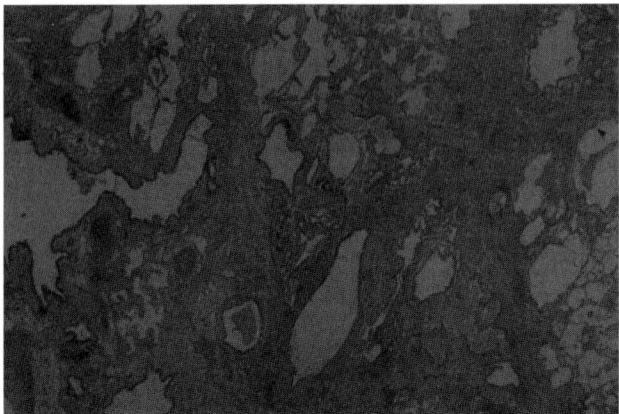

FIGURE 44.3. (See also Color Fig. 44.3.) Severe pulmonary remodeling and honeycombing associated with asbestosis.

With advanced disease, irregular linear shadows give way to more complex radiographic features. As in other forms of fibrotic remodeling, a pattern of "honeycombing," radiographically apparent cystic spaces in the lung, may develop (Fig. 44.3). Honeycombing is incontrovertible evidence of advanced and irreversible lung remodeling. Its appearance is therefore usually associated with severely disabling disease. In late disease, the CT scan shows features similar to those of other forms of usual interstitial pneumonitis. An enlarged right ventricle and prominent pulmonary arteries appear late in the disease process, when pulmonary hypertension and cor pulmonale develop. Rarely, large conglomerate masses in the upper lung zones, such as are seen in coal worker's pneumoconiosis and silicosis, are seen in asbestosis. However, these generally occur in subjects with concomitant silica exposure or in conjunction with rheumatoid arthritis (Caplan syndrome; see section "Inflammatory and Immune Disorders Associated with Pneumoconioses").

The presence of irregular shadows that are not profuse in the lower zones is not specific for asbestosis. Exposure to fibrous dusts other than asbestos may cause small irregular shadows in the lung bases, particularly in smokers and the elderly. When they occur, the irregular shadows are not profuse.

CT of the chest has added a new dimension to our ability to image the pneumoconioses. However, the improved sensitivity provided by CT has not yet been translated into clinically useful standards. This needed transition will require the correlation of imaging studies with careful exposure histories.

Rounded atelectasis ("folded lung") is a distinctive radiographic pattern nearly unique to asbestosis. It probably develops as an exuberant focal pleural reaction that entraps subjacent lung tissue, including distal airways and extrapleural fat, in a swirl of pleural inflammatory reaction. It is important to recognize rounded atelectasis because it may be mistaken on the plain chest radiograph for a peripheral lung mass and lead to an unnecessary search for a cancer. The pathophysiology of rounded atelectasis remains uncertain.

The accepted hypothesis is that an initial focus of injury at the visceral pleural surface leads to local inflammation and collagen deposition, resulting in focal volume loss with torsion of the more compliant underlying parenchyma and bronchovascular structures.

When rounded atelectasis is suspected, CT or magnetic resonance imaging showing the characteristic swirl ("comma") of atelectatic lung tissue and distorted bronchovascular markings can easily confirm it. Although the resolution of rounded atelectasis after decortication has been reported, periodic imaging of the lesion is the only management required. Rounded atelectasis is most often noted in the lingua and the middle and lower lobes; although usually a single lesion, multiple and bilateral shadows may be seen.

Pulmonary Function Studies

Symptomatic asbestosis is associated with changes in the mechanical properties of the lungs that resemble those seen in other forms of fibrotic lung remodeling. As the process progresses and fibrotic remodeling becomes more severe, the lungs become regionally less compliant, and all lung volumes are reduced. The diffusing capacity may be reduced before the lung volumes are overtly lowered. A notable increase in the respiratory rate, a decrease in the tidal volume, and an absolute increase in the minute volume occur as the ventilation-perfusion relationship becomes less efficient. Tests of regional lung function have shown impaired ventilation of the lower zones. As a result of the altered ventilation-perfusion relationship, hypoxemia and hypercapnia may be severe in advanced disease, particularly during exercise. In short, the respiratory impairment has the same characteristics as that of pulmonary remodeling. A number of attempts have been made to detect the disease at a presymptomatic stage and in the absence of overt radiographic abnormalities. Most such efforts have focused on measurements of lung mechanics. It has been possible to show a lower maximal expiratory flow for a given transpulmonary pressure in subjects with normal chest radiographs but significant dust exposure. However, because these approaches require invasive studies and attention to calibration and are relatively cumbersome, measurements of lung mechanics are not feasible in field studies of exposed populations.

The potential importance of small-airways disease in asbestos exposure remains unclear. Certainly, the early lesions in asbestos exposure are localized to the respiratory and terminal bronchioles, and tests of small-airways disease detect flow limitation in small airways before the results of other pulmonary function tests become abnormal. However, asbestos-induced small-airways disease may be independent of the other abnormalities of asbestosis.

Diffuse pleural thickening can cause impairment of pulmonary function independently of the other manifestations of asbestos-related disease, as determined in a cohort of 54 men with occupational exposure to asbestos (17). Individuals with diffuse pleural thickening demonstrated a reduced forced vital capacity (FVC) ($P = .002$) and diffusing capacity for carbon monoxide ($P = .002$) in comparison with matched controls. No such difference was found for the forced expiratory volume in 1 second (FEV$_1$) or the FEV$_1$/FVC ratio. Diffuse pleural thickening in conjunction with either interstitial fibrosis or pleural plaques resulted in a significantly lower vital capacity than was found with fibrosis or pleural plaques alone. The presence of rounded atelectasis and pleural thickening did not worsen the restriction induced by pleural thickening alone. Thus, diffuse pleural thickening is associated with restrictive pulmonary function and a reduced diffusing capacity independently of the other manifestations of asbestos-related disease.

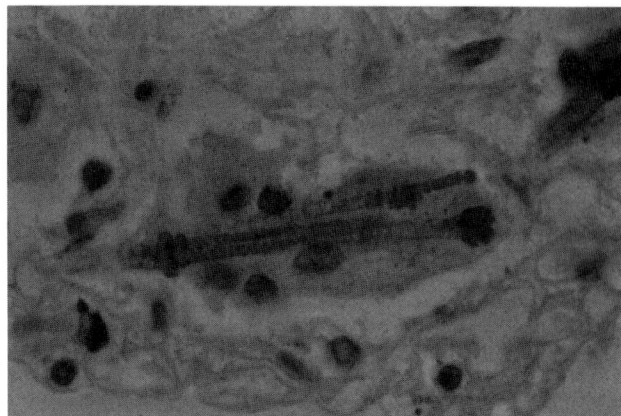

FIGURE 44.4. (See also Color Fig. 44.4.) Photomicrograph of asbestos bodies.

IMAGING PATTERNS AND PULMONARY FUNCTION IN ASBESTOSIS	
Summary Statement	**Level of Evidence**
Chest radiographic patterns	Case series, expert opinion, nonrandomized
Chest computed tomographic patterns	Case series, expert opinion
Pulmonary function tests	Case series, nonrandomized

Diagnosis of Asbestosis

The diagnosis of asbestosis is based on a history of exposure in conjunction with compatible radiographic changes (ILO category > 1/1) and a reduced diffusing capacity and restriction on pulmonary function testing. The American Thoracic Society has published these criteria and the supporting evidence for their acceptance (18). They include a reliable history of significant exposure, an appropriate interval of at least a decade since the initiation of exposure, bilateral persistent rales, compatible radiographic findings, and volume restriction and a reduced diffusing capacity on pulmonary function testing. These criteria have not been updated to include radiographic features detected by CT.

It is difficult to diagnose suspected asbestosis when the usual radiographic changes are not present or are confounded by coexisting lung diseases. Lung biopsy via bronchoscopy, thoracotomy, or video-assisted thoracoscopy is only rarely required or justified in making the diagnosis because no specific therapy is available. Biopsy is usually justified to exclude other, more treatable forms of lung remodeling. No blood tests assist with the diagnosis of asbestosis.

Pathology of Asbestosis

Visual inspection of the lungs of persons with chronic asbestos exposure reveals thickened visceral pleural membranes (19). The cut surfaces of the shrunken lungs exhibit the honeycombing and remodeling of usual interstitial pneumonitis (20).

At the microscopic level, a hallmark of asbestosis is the asbestos body (Fig. 44.4). Asbestos bodies are elongated, golden-brown structures beaded with proteinaceous mate-

rial; their length corresponds to the individual asbestos fibers that form their cores (21). Because of their high iron content, they stain particularly well with iron stains. Early in the disease process, asbestos fibers are found within the cytoplasm of macrophages recruited to the area of deposition. The intracellular portions of the fibers may become leached and fragment to a smaller size. The characteristic beading of the fiber results from biologic modification, with beaded deposition of proteinaceous material rich in ferritin (22). After the macrophage dies, the coated fiber can be recognized under the microscope as an extracellular asbestos body.

The minimum number of asbestos bodies in lung samples required for a certain diagnosis of asbestosis remains unclear despite considerable research. One study has shown that the lungs of urban dwellers with no occupational exposure to asbestos should contain only one asbestos body for every hundred sections of lung tissue examined. Evidence of parenchymal inflammation (early) and fibrotic remodeling (later) should also be present for the diagnosis to hold.

With a few notable exceptions, asbestos bodies are found regularly in patients with asbestosis; conversely, the absence of asbestos bodies is a reliable sign that the disease is not present. In any case, large tissue samples are required for a certain diagnosis; for example, biopsy material obtained by bronchoscopic biopsy is inadequate to identify the infrequent asbestos bodies.

Pleural plaques are almost unique to persons with asbestos exposure and certain other silicate pneumoconioses. They are shiny, white, slightly raised patches on the parietal pleural surfaces that consist of coarse collagen fibers. Calcification is frequently present and often most evident at the periphery of the lesions, at least on the chest radiograph. Histologic examination, however, usually shows that the center of the plaque is also calcified.

Pathogenesis of Asbestosis

A characteristic inflammatory lesion appears to be the earliest tissue response to inhaled asbestos. Experimental studies in animals exposed to asbestos show that the first inflammatory lesions develop at the bifurcations of small airways and alveolar ducts, the sites of the most intense impaction and retention of fibers. A macrophage-dominant inflammatory process eventually involves the lumina of the small airways and extends into the alveoli. Because the macrophage is central to dust phagocytosis, it can be assumed to modulate many of the subsequent pathologic events. In this regard, it is important to note that activated macrophages release a range of inflammatory mediators and proinflammatory cytokines. These include chemotactic cytokines and peptides and growth modulators such as insulinlike growth factor-1, epidermal growth factor, transforming growth factor-β, interleukin-1α, and tumor necrosis factor-α. Also in the armamentarium of macrophages are enzymes catalyzing the rapid generation and release of active oxygen species such as peroxides, hydroxyl radicals, and superoxide anions. These in turn directly oxidize the lipids of cellular membranes and damage DNA and proteins. In conjunction with the effects of proteolytic enzymes such as elastases and cathepsins, these reactions result in the injury and death of adjacent structural lung cells, including epithelial cells, endothelial cells, and interstitial fibroblasts (23,24).

A second step in the pathogenesis of asbestos lesions involves the direct interaction of fibers with various structural lung cells, including epithelial cells and fibroblasts. Undegraded asbestos fibers cross the epithelial cells by endocytosis and are transported along the intracellular microtubular network. From the basolateral surfaces of the cells, the fibers migrate into the interstitium and can directly interact with interstitial fibroblasts.

With time, the inflammatory process results in the laying down of pathologic amounts of extracellular matrix proteins such as collagen, elastin, and proteoglycans. As a consequence of this changing biochemical composition, the lungs lose air space volume and the normal pressure-volume relationship. The anatomic distribution of the pathologic changes favors the lower lung zones, reflecting the proportionally greater particle burden in the bases.

Most of the beaded elongated bodies found in lung specimens are indeed asbestos bodies. However, the inhalation of certain other fibrous minerals, such as glass wool, fibrous alumina, and silicon carbide, may induce the formation of similar elongated structures. Because their core is composed of fibers other than asbestos, these beaded elongated bodies are more accurately referred to as *ferruginous bodies*. Specific mineralogic identification of the fibers by means of electron microscopy and x-ray energy spectroscopy may be required to distinguish between asbestos and the other fibrous minerals.

Workers who have been exposed to asbestos often have asbestos and asbestos bodies in their expectorated sputum, even years after exposure has ceased. Asbestos bodies can also be found in samples of alveolar lavage fluid recovered by bronchoscopy. The finding of asbestos bodies in sputum or lavage fluid confirms exposure but does not confirm the diagnosis of asbestosis. Moreover, the specificity of the finding of "asbestos bodies" is limited by the observation that other mineral fibers may present as "pseudoasbestos bodies" (25). Most residents of industrialized areas have some asbestos bodies in their lungs. However, their presence cannot be construed to represent clinical asbestosis because they are not associated with clinical manifestations of disease. Critical evaluation of the lavage-based quantification of the lung asbestos burden indicates that it is of limited utility (26–28).

When ferruginous bodies are detected in the lungs or respiratory secretions of subjects who report no occupational exposure, the types of asbestos most often found are chrysotile and tremolite. Tremolite may be inhaled during the cosmetic application of facial powder composed of talc contaminated with small amounts of this asbestiform mineral.

Chrysotile is particularly susceptible to biologic leaching and partial degradation; with time, the number and size of chrysotile fibers decline notably. In contrast, amphiboles are more resistant to chemical leaching and tend to persist in the lungs. The intracellular modification and coating of fibers to form asbestos bodies may inactivate the fibers and prevent further toxicity. In chrysotile-induced asbestosis, numerous asbestos bodies and uncoated fibers may be found for prolonged periods despite the leaching process.

From the preceding discussion, it is apparent that the number of fibers and ferruginous bodies found in respiratory secretions and lung tissue examined postmortem can vary considerably, depending on the exposure history and other factors. Urban dwellers without any specific occupational exposure have relatively few fibers; subjects with clear occupational exposures and clinical manifestations of intense asbestosis have a much larger number of fibers.

The hazards of asbestos exposure, namely asbestosis, pleural thickening and plaques, bronchogenic carcinoma, and mesothelioma, can be related to the extent of exposure. The density of fibers found in the dried lung samples of various population groups depends on the intensity of exposure and varies enormously. Although subjects with no occupational exposure have detectable fiber counts, it is important to keep in mind that the numbers of coated and uncoated fibers are hundreds of times lower than in exposed healthy workers and thousands of times lower than in workers with apparent lung disease. Urban dwellers without occupational exposures have fewer than 1,000 fibers per gram of dry lung tissue. Fiber counts in lung samples of patients with established asbestosis and mesothelioma usually exceed 80 million per gram of dried tissue. In subjects with lung cancer, the fiber counts are more difficult to relate to disease risk because of the dominant carcinogenic effect of the components of cigarette smoke.

Measuring Asbestos Fibers in Tissues

Semiquantitative analysis of the dust content of the lungs of exposed workers requires tissue biopsy. Most of the asbestos in the lungs of exposed workers is in the form of short (<5 μm) translucent fibers that do not take up histologic stains. Hence, most of the asbestos burden in lung tissue is invisible by standard light microscopy but can be seen by phase-contrast or electron microscopy techniques. Only small portions of the longer fibers evolve into more conspicuous asbestos bodies. To overcome this problem, various groups have provided standardized scientific approaches for evaluating the asbestos burden (29).

Current pathologic technology allows a determination of the precise mineral composition of asbestos fibers detected in tissue. Transmission electron microscopes equipped with energy-dispersive spectrometers and phase-contrast microscopes can detect and differentiate between chrysotile, tremolite, amosite, and crocidolite (30–32).

The minimum criteria for the histologic diagnosis of asbestosis include the identification of peribronchiolar scarring and at least two asbestos bodies in tissue sections. The number of fibers can be determined by counting the fibers in a digest of tissue. However, enumerating asbestos bodies in tissue sections is a more familiar and convenient approach for general pathologists. It turns out that the agreement between the number of asbestos bodies in tissue sections and the number in digests of tissue is excellent. An average of two asbestos bodies on 2 × 2-cm sections of lung tissue is the equivalent of approximately 200 asbestos bodies per gram of wet fixed tissue.

Pleural Effusion, Diffuse Pleural Thickening, and Plaques

The pleural surfaces are particularly susceptible to the remodeling effects of asbestos, even at low levels of exposure. Visceral pleural thickening develops in response to levels of exposure that typically do not induce parenchymal asbestosis. Benign exudative pleural effusions are usually the earliest evidence of asbestos exposure and can occur within the first decade after exposure.

Evolving pleural disease may be entirely asymptomatic or manifest as acute pleurisy, sometimes accompanied by severe constitutional symptoms (33). The radiographic appearance of asbestos-induced pleural effusions is nonspecific. Because most such effusions are not associated with signs of established asbestosis, diagnostic thoracentesis is often required. The pleural exudate usually contains both polymorphonuclear leukocytes and mononuclear cells; infrequently, the fluid is overtly bloody. Asbestos fibers are hard to find in the fluid; biopsy specimens of the pleura show only a chronic, nonspecific pleural reaction. Because of the cryptic nature of asbestos-induced effusions, they can be a diagnostic dilemma when the exposure history is not clear.

Most asbestos-induced effusions resolve spontaneously. Sometimes, the effusion may linger for several months and lead to diffuse pleural thickening or a fibrothorax. In some instances, the fibrothorax leads to appreciable restric-

tive impairment. When a substantial fibrothorax develops, clinicians tend to consider surgical decortication; however, asbestos-induced pleural thickening and fibrothorax generally resolve gradually during the course of several years and can safely be observed without intervention if the cause is recognized. Despite the heightened concern that they trigger, pleural effusions and thickening usually do not portend the rare development of mesothelioma. Pleural effusions associated with mesothelioma are generally unilateral and notably do not produce mediastinal shift, even when they reach a large size.

Radiographic evidence of pleural thickening is found in many workers with mild to moderate exposure to asbestos. It is characteristically most prominent in the mid zones of one or both hemithoraces. In most cases, thickening is the only manifestation of asbestos exposure, and like plaques, thickening does not necessarily auger parenchymal disease.

Calcified pleural plaques are a characteristic radiographic feature of more prolonged asbestos exposure. These benign plaques are usually bilateral and located on the parietal pleura of the basilar posterolateral chest wall. Their pathogenesis is distinct from the development of effusion and fibrothorax. They are a characteristic marker of asbestos exposure but do not in themselves constitute a disease process, nor do they portend later pulmonary impairment. They develop in more than half of highly exposed workers after a latency of one to two decades. Sometimes, they are seen only on the anterior or posterior chest wall. Pleural plaques, usually on the diaphragm, can be found at autopsy in most subjects who have worked for more than 5 years with asbestos. Other causes of pleural thickening or calcification include prior thoracotomy, tuberculosis (TB), chest trauma, and prior hemothorax. Asbestos pericardial calcification may also occur and can occasionally lead to constrictive pericarditis. Diffuse pleural thickening is often associated with fibrothorax and restrictive ventilatory impairment.

A study based on HRCT analysis showed no correlation between the total surface area of pleural plaques and lung function (34). The study focused on 73 workers who had worked for 23 to 27 years in an asbestos cement factory. Their estimated mean cumulative exposure to asbestos was 26.3 fiber-years per milliliter. Plaques were imaged in 70% of the subjects but in none of a group of unexposed control subjects. No correlation was found between plaque surface area and cumulative asbestos exposure. In those with pleural plaques, the surface of the pleural lesions was not related to cumulative asbestos exposure, smoking history, or time elapsed since the first exposure. Neither the presence nor the extent of the plaques correlated with lung function.

Pleural plaques are seen more frequently after exposure to the amphiboles than after exposure to the serpentine chrysotile. Calcification usually appears in plaques that have been present for three or more decades and is more readily detected on CT scans of the chest than on plain films. It is a common mistake to assume that the mere presence of plaques portends the certain development of mesothelioma or lung cancer.

When viewed *en face* on the posteroanterior chest film, plaques can be mistaken for parenchymal shadows and disease. In such cases, several clues should alert the astute reader to the presence of pleural thickening. These include the absence of obvious parenchymal disease on the lateral chest film and difficulty in ascribing an anatomic lobar localization of the presumed shadows. Finally, CT of the chest makes it clear that the shadows are generated by pleural rather than parenchymal changes.

Clinical Course of Asbestosis

Asbestosis usually has an indolent course and may be present radiographically years before dyspnea or crackles are detected. More severe asbestosis may advance to physiologic deterioration, disability, and death. By the end of the 20th century, the number of deaths attributable to asbestos appeared to have reached a plateau in the United States. Death is the result of respiratory failure with or without associated right-sided heart failure, or of respiratory malignancies. The major reduction in deaths caused by asbestos during recent years in the wake of labor union campaigns and government regulations can be traced to the relatively milder extent of disease in the aging worker population. No effective therapy for established asbestosis has been developed; hence, avoidance remains the only reasonable public health measure to protect workers (35). Treatment of the symptoms—bronchodilators if obstruction is present, long-term low-flow oxygen therapy for hypoxemia, and cardiac medications if right-sided heart failure develops—may provide symptomatic relief.

Asbestos as a Carcinogen

No aspect of asbestos is more controversial than its association with malignancy (36). The recognition of asbestos as a carcinogen dates from debates beginning in the 1930s and 1940s. However, the issue remained controversial until 1955, when Doll (37) published a classic article presenting the statistical evidence required to confirm the association. Doll described the increased risk for lung cancer only in subjects with coexisting asbestosis and did not consider asbestos exposure in the absence of remodeling as a potential cause of lung cancer.

Although the association between exposure to asbestos and the risk for malignancy has been apparent for the past half century, the relationship has been difficult to analyze. Asbestosis, like the other interstitial lung disorders, is associated with a high incidence of pulmonary malignancies (38). At intense levels of exposure, the dose-response relationship is approximately linear. What remains difficult to pin down is the precise risk of asbestos exposure relative to that of other carcinogens and the exact mechanisms of tumor induction. Simultaneous exposures to other dusts and chemicals, in addition to tobacco and other carcinogens, have confounded

the analyses of even relatively large groups of exposed workers. One analysis suggested that lung cancer may account for as many as 26% of deaths in some groups of asbestos workers, a risk three to five times higher than that expected in other workers. In some case surveys, bronchogenic cancer has developed in as many as a fourth of all exposed asbestos workers (39).

The components of asbestos and tobacco smoke are both carcinogens in their own right. In addition, the effect is synergistic in that cigarette smoking alters the processing and clearance of inhaled asbestos fibers (40). In one small study, cigarette smoking was shown to enhance the accumulation of both amosite and chrysotile in the airway mucosa (41,42).

In epidemiologic studies, the excess mortality of lung cancer becomes apparent after at least a decade of exposure, and the risk climbs progressively thereafter. The risk is somewhat dependent on industrial exposure because the incidence of lung cancer is higher in asbestos textile workers than in cement workers, who in turn have more malignancies than asbestos miners. In most such comparative studies, the populations were exposed to chrysotile fibers only; the amphiboles are considered more carcinogenic than chrysotile. Bronchoalveolar cell carcinoma and adenocarcinoma are the types most frequently detected. Asbestosis is usually but not invariably present in cases of bronchogenic carcinoma (43). Human epidemiologic studies, experimental studies of animal implantation and inoculation, and lung burden studies show that fibers wider than 1 μm are not implicated in lung cancer or mesothelioma. Fibers thinner than a few tenths of a micrometer and longer than 5 to 10 μm must be abundant in a fiber population if they are to cause mesothelioma (44).

The presence of pleural plaques on the chest roentgenogram indicates significant exposure to asbestos and thus an increased risk for mesothelioma and possibly also for bronchial carcinoma. A Swedish study that addressed this issue was based on radiographic studies of 1,596 men with pleural plaques. Patients with radiologic asbestosis were overrepresented among those with bronchial carcinoma. The risk for patients with pleural plaques but without asbestosis was also significantly increased, to 40% above the expected rate. Mesotheliomas were 10 times more prevalent than expected. The mean period of latency from the first exposure to the diagnosis of bronchogenic cancer was 44 years, and for mesothelioma, it was 48 years. Any person found to have plaques on a chest roentgenogram should be informed of them and should be persuaded to stop smoking (45).

With progress toward the control of asbestos exposure in the workplace, cigarette smoking may now have become the dominant determinant of lung cancer risk in exposed workers. In this regard, lung cancer has developed in relatively few nonsmoking workers with significant asbestos exposures. A number of questions remain unanswered. The extent to which nonsmoking asbestos workers are at risk for lung cancer through exposure to secondhand smoke is not clear. It is imperative to counsel asbestos-exposed workers strongly to undertake smoking cessation and to emphasize that this is the only clear preventive option they have to lower their risk for the development of lung cancer.

There has long been a question of whether any nonpulmonary malignancies are more likely to develop in response to asbestos exposure. The prolonged inhalation of asbestos fibers has been said to be associated with an increased risk for laryngeal, ovarian, gastrointestinal, and renal carcinomas. However, these malignancies remain rare, and the evidence for such associations remains correspondingly weak.

The minimum level of asbestos exposure or disease that puts an individual at risk for pulmonary malignancy remains uncertain. Backward extrapolation of the concentration that applies to workers with heavy exposures may not be scientifically justified; there are too few reliable data among subjects with lower levels of exposure. Chrysotile ("blue asbestos") has a reputation for being more carcinogenic than crocidolite.

Uncontrolled studies have suggested that lung cancers induced by asbestos tend to develop in the lower lobes, whereas those that arise in association with cigarette smoking tend to develop in the upper lobes. An excess of adenocarcinomas has also been reported among cases not exposed to cigarette smoke and among those exposed to asbestos. In multivariable logistic regression analysis (46), a longer time since smoking exposure remained a statistically significant predictor of adenocarcinoma, but a history of asbestos exposure did not predict tumor histology.

Malignant Mesothelioma

In the late 1950s, an association was made between malignant pleural mesothelioma and asbestos exposure. The risk for the development of mesothelioma, like that for asbestosis and lung cancer, is concentration-related and particularly associated with crocidolite exposure. Severe, unremitting local chest pain and weight loss are invariable features of the disease. In most cases, the disease is present for 6 months or longer before a diagnosis is made.

Pleural mesotheliomas can occur as either benign or malignant tumors. The benign form, which is not associated with asbestos exposure, is frequently accompanied by hypertrophic pulmonary osteoarthropathy. In contrast, malignant mesothelioma is an aggressive, uniformly fatal diffuse cancer arising from the pleura and sometimes the peritoneum. Contrary to popular notion, asbestos pleural effusion is not a harbinger of malignant mesothelioma.

Most malignant mesotheliomas develop after a long latency and can be traced to previous exposure to asbestos or the nonasbestiform fibrous mineral erionite. As mentioned previously, most asbestos-induced mesotheliomas develop only after intense exposure; they almost never develop after the minimal exposure experienced by urban dwellers. The diagnosis may be delayed because the histopathology of mesotheliomas is often cryptic, even when relatively large resected samples are available for pathologic examination. It is not uncommon for controversy regarding the diagnosis to continue even after the postmortem examination.

Malignant mesothelioma remains an extremely rare cancer, and evidence indicates that the rate will decrease about 20 to 30 years after occupational hygiene control reduces high levels of occupational exposure. In the United States, no more than several thousand cases are reported annually, and this number is now declining. Because of a latency of three to four decades after the first exposure to asbestos, most cases develop in the seventh or eighth decade of life. Rare cases develop earlier in response to particularly intense exposure. The median survival time is only 10 months.

EFFECTS OF ASBESTOS	
Summary Statement	**Level of Evidence**
Asbestos as a lung carcinogen	Nonrandomized, historical and expert opinion
Asbestos causing mesothelioma	Historical and expert opinion, case series
Asbestos causing nonrespiratory neoplasms	Historical opinion, case series

SILICOSIS

Pulmonary silicosis develops when free crystalline silica or silicon dioxide is inhaled. Silicon forms the greater part of the earth's crust and is the second most abundant element on the planet. It is therefore ubiquitous in the human environment, and some exposure to silicon dioxide and the silicates is a fact of life. Silicosis results from the inhalation and deposition in the lung of crystalline or free silica, usually as quartz. The disease may have occurred in paleolithic times, as soon as humans began to make stone tools. The term *silicosis* is derived from the Latin word *silex*, meaning flint. Intense exposure leading to disease occurs in miners and in workers in industries in which the mineral is used, such as the manufacture of ceramics, pottery, and bricks. However, as with asbestosis, public health regulations have significantly reduced the number of cases of silicosis in the industrialized world.

Silicon can exist free—that is, not chemically combined with other elements—or form silicates by combining with various cations. Silicon dioxide exists in crystalline and amorphous forms, and also in mixed forms. The crystalline forms include cristobalite, tridymite, and quartz. All can cause fibrotic pulmonary disease, with quartz somewhat less potent in this respect than the others. The amorphous silicas include diatomite, formed from the skeletons of oceanic diatoms, and vitreous silica, a man-made product of heated silica. The amorphous forms are generally nonfibrogenic. Mixed forms, deposits containing crystalline and amorphous features, include chert and flint.

Many of the silicates, salts of silicic acid, are also variably fibrogenic. With the obvious exception of asbestos, the silicates tend to be less toxic than the free crystalline forms of silica. Sandstone and flint are composed of almost pure quartz; granite contains between 15% and 70% free silica by weight, slate 30% to 45%, and shale about 10%. Silica flour, finely ground silica used as a filler for cosmetics, abrasives, and paint extenders, is a particularly hazardous form of silica.

Sources of Exposure

The harmful effects of hard rock mining have been known for millennia. In Roman times, Pliny the Elder wrote about them. In the 16th century, Agricola correctly associated most of the lung disease of metal miners with the continued inhalation of mine dust in his *De Re Metallica*. Later, Ramazzini pointed out that many diseases originated from the workers' occupation and that mining was particularly dangerous. He noted that stonecutters were particularly at risk for the development of lung disease. In the 19th century, grinding, the manufacture of pottery, and trades in which flint and slate were used emerged as particularly hazardous.

Occupations that bring workers in contact with respirable silica include underground and surface mining, foundry work, railroad work, boiler scaling, metal grinding and polishing, shipbuilding, and the manufacture of abrasives, soaps, and detergents. Sandblasting, which generates large amounts of airborne silica, is a particularly high-risk occupation. Sandblasting has been used in the production of tombstones, the cleaning of stone facing on urban buildings, and the removal of rust in maritime sites (ship repair, offshore oil field equipment). The use of silica for this purpose has ceased under regulatory pressure in many advanced nations. In nations such as the United States, where its use persists despite National Institute for Occupational Safety and Health (NIOSH) recommendations, sandblasting remains the most frequent cause of a characteristic form of acute pulmonary silicosis. In nations where sandblasting with silica is still permitted, sandblasters should work only when wearing a carefully tested positive pressure respirator with its own air supply.

Definitive regulatory efforts in the industrialized nations have resulted in a major decrease in silicosis during the past half century. New cases of silicosis tend to be sporadic rather than epidemic. In contrast to the situation in advanced countries, the pneumoconioses present a growing problem in recently industrialized nations, where they persist as a public health menace in workers in coal and metal mines, sandblasting, ceramics refractories, and foundries.

Exposure-Response Relationships

Precise figures on the prevalence and incidence of silicosis are not available. As many as a million Americans may have been subjected to significant exposure to silica in the workplace. It is certain, however, that the prevalence of silicosis has fallen very significantly in recent decades. This drop has been best

documented in the small but well-studied Vermont granite industry, where careful records kept before and after landmark state legislation in the late 1930s have documented the subsequent decline in respiratory disease (47) and associated silicotuberculosis.

Although large groups of workers exposed to free silica have undergone surveillance for many years, few attempts have been made to derive an exposure-response relationship. Currently, studies are under way in the United States, South Africa, and Canada to establish the relationship between the development of silicosis and cumulative dust levels. The current evidence suggests that an air quality standard for free silica of 0.1 mg/m^3 should protect the vast majority of the workforce. Chronic forms of clinically important silicosis are seldom seen before a decade of moderately intense exposure.

The exposure-response relationship for crystalline forms of silica in the development of silicosis remains unclear. An extensive epidemiologic investigation of workers exposed to diatomaceous earth, composed primarily of respirable crystalline silica (cristobalite form), examined this relationship with radiographic scoring (48). Fewer than 5% of 1,809 workers, most of whom were exposed to the lower dust levels prevailing after 1950, were judged to have dust-related opacities on chest radiographs. The age-adjusted relative risk for opacities increased significantly with cumulative exposure to crystalline silica. These findings indicate an exposure-response relationship between cumulative exposure to crystalline silica and radiographic opacities. The relationship was substantially steeper among workers exposed at the highest mean concentrations of crystalline silica.

SILICA EXPOSURE	
Summary Statement	**Level of Evidence**
Exposure standards	Nonrandomized, historical and expert opinion
Exposure-response relationship	Historical and expert opinion, case series

Clinical Features of Silicosis

For clinical purposes, silicosis has traditionally been divided into chronic, subacute, and acute forms. Chronic silicosis can be further divided into simple and complicated forms based on the radiographic appearance (Table 44.2). Simple silicosis is characterized by small, round shadows that usually appear first in the upper lobes and later throughout all the lung zones. Complicated silicosis is said to be present when shadows on the chest radiograph expand to more than 1 cm in diameter (conglomerate masses).

Simple silicosis by itself does not cause respiratory symptoms. Typically, the patient with simple silicosis is discovered only through radiographic screening. The chest radiograph shows a striking profusion of small, round nodules that are

TABLE 44.2. CLINICAL CLASSIFICATION OF SILICA-INDUCED SYNDROMES

Chronic silicosis
    Simple silicosis
    Complicated silicosis
        Conglomerate shadows ("progressive massive fibrosis")
        Silicotuberculosis
        Caplan syndrome (rheumatoid pneumoconiosis)

Acute silicosis (silicoproteinosis)

Other silica-related syndromes
    Irritant bronchitis
    Small-airways disease
    Emphysema

not associated with symptoms. If dyspnea is present at this stage, it is more likely the result of a coexisting disorder, such as chronic obstructive pulmonary disease. In general, simple silicosis does not progress after exposure ceases, and the exposed worker can be assured that functional disability will not occur.

In complicated silicosis, the large radiographic shadows slowly become bigger during a period of years, even without further exposure to dust. Risk factors for complicated silicosis include high levels of dust exposure and coexisting lung disease, such as TB. The earlier the onset of complicated silicosis, the greater the likelihood that it will progress and become disabling. As the size of the conglomerate masses increases, the symptoms of breathlessness, cough, and sputum production progress. Pulmonary function tests demonstrate a worsening restrictive pattern. When cor pulmonale develops, it is not related so much to hypoxia as to a generalized decrease in the pulmonary vascular bed. Thus, pulmonary hypertension and overt cor pulmonale develop late in the disease process.

Pulmonary Function in Silicosis

Perhaps because of their location, the silicotic nodules that are distributed throughout the lung parenchyma have surprisingly little effect on lung function. The pathways of removal of silica particles into the pulmonary interstitium and regional nodes bypass the distal airways and alveoli, minimizing any deleterious effects on gas flow or mechanics. In studies of simple silicosis, a small but statistically significant decrement in the FVC can be detected when exposed population groups are studied and contrasted with unexposed control subjects. These changes have no clinical significance and are not associated with symptoms. Because they are numerically small, the changes cannot routinely be detected in individual subjects. The lung volumes in simple silicosis are nearly always normal. Indices of gas exchange, such as the diffusing capacity and arterial oxygen concentration, are generally normal. Pulmonary compliance may be reduced even though the spirometric values are normal. The extent of the mechanical changes, although somewhat more accu-

rate than the spirometric values, can be related only roughly to the radiographic score.

Studies defining the rate of decrement in pulmonary function among exposed workers have been used to justify the current standards for ambient dust levels. Cross-sectional studies of workers in the Vermont granite industry provided the most comprehensive picture of the impact of any respirable dust on pulmonary function. Results suggested that exposure to granite dust leads to a small loss of vital capacity of only 2 mL per year, which can be compared with a decline of 30 mL per year as a consequence of aging. The studies served as the basis for the NIOSH recommendation that the permissible exposure limit be halved from 0.10 to 0.05 mg/m^3. A later study significantly suggested much more rapid rates of decline in the same population but proved to be technically flawed. An additional longitudinal study in the same workers found no difference in the rates of decline in function and no difference in the changes between granite workers and unexposed blue collar workers from the same region. At this time, no compelling evidence exists that exposure to quartz at levels at or below the current standard of 0.1 mg/m^3 results in a loss of pulmonary function.

Without a doubt, pulmonary mechanics and volumes decline more rapidly in workers with complicated silicosis. Altered pulmonary function accounts for much of the disability and death in severe cases. With changes in regional compliance, ventilation-perfusion mismatching leads to progressive hypoxemia. Airflow obstruction, when present, appears to be caused by torsion and distortion of the large airways and is usually associated with some bullous emphysema and marked overdistention. Pulmonary hypertension develops as a consequence of both hypoxemia and obliteration of the pulmonary vascular bed.

The presentation of acute silicosis is one of rapidly progressing respiratory insufficiency. Both the lung volumes and the diffusing capacity are markedly reduced. The reductions are generally proportional to the extent of the conglomerate shadows. Lung compliance is markedly reduced, and marked hypoxemia is caused by ventilation-perfusion mismatch.

Radiographic Changes in Silicosis

In simple silicosis, the chest radiograph shows a profusion of small (1–3 mm), round shadows in the upper lobes. These round densities actually represent multiple small silicotic nodules superimposed on one another. Indeed, with the higher resolution of chest CT, this summation is lost, and simple silicosis may appear less impressive than on plain frontal chest films.

In complicated silicosis, larger round nodular shadows (type r shadows) become more profuse than the p and q shadows. However, these radiographic changes resemble those of many other advanced nodular pneumoconioses, including coal worker's pneumoconiosis. Symmetric enlargement of the hilar lymph nodes may be noted. Eggshell calcification,

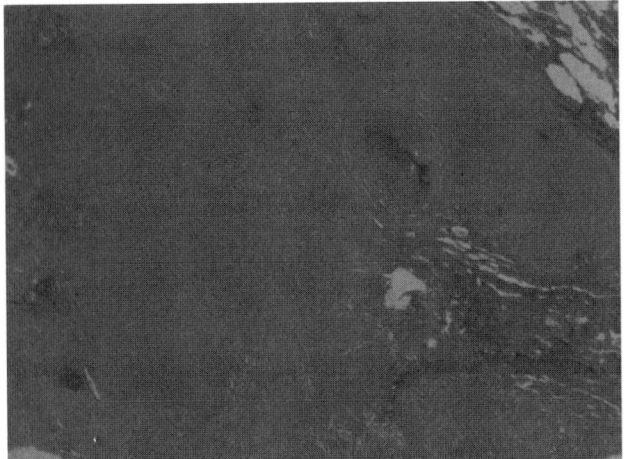

FIGURE 44.5. (See also Color Fig. 44.5.) Progressive massive fibrosis with conglomeration of silicotic nodules.

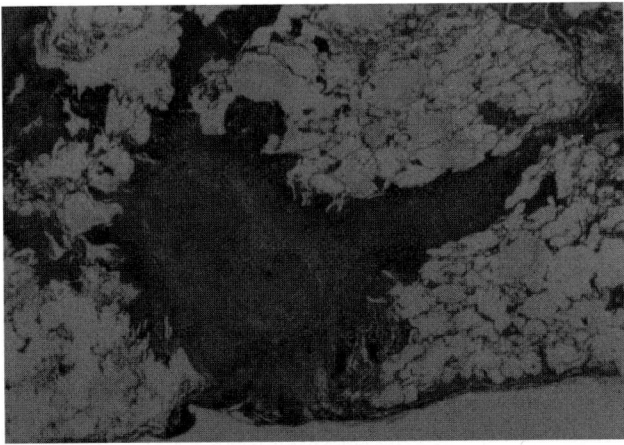

FIGURE 44.6. (See also Color Fig. 44.6.) Early silicotic nodule formation. Nodules are surrounded by dust-filled macrophages.

a characteristic thin rim of calcium around the nodes that is a nearly pathognomonic radiographic feature of silicosis, occurs in 5% to 10% of cases. In severe cases, progressive volume loss in the upper lobes results in upward traction of the hilar shadows and emphysematous overdistention of the lower lobes.

The conglomerate shadows that form in complicated silicosis (Fig. 44.5) are not specific to silicosis and resemble those seen in coal worker's pneumoconiosis. They typically appear in the periphery of the upper lobes first, later migrating toward the hilum. HRCT detects them before they are seen on the chest radiograph.

An important aspect of the management of patients with profuse shadows of silicosis is the difficulty of screening for other lung disorders and the variant features of silicosis. Cavitation of conglomerate shadows may occur and in some cases represents superinfection with TB. Pleural plaques can develop in silicosis but are infrequent. Conglomerate shadows themselves often pose a diagnostic dilemma because malignancy and TB must be ruled out.

Efforts have been made to standardize the use of chest CT in early silicosis (49). In 13 silica-exposed workers (41%) with normal high-quality, high-kilovoltage chest films, CT detected features consistent with early silicosis. CT of a smaller number of subjects with positive findings on chest films raised questions about the specificity of the diagnosis. This small study clearly calls for larger, population-based studies.

IMAGING PATTERNS AND PULMONARY FUNCTION IN SILICOSIS

Summary Statement	Level of Evidence
Chest radiographic patterns in silicosis	Case series, expert opinion, nonrandomized
Pulmonary function tests in silicosis	Case series, nonrandomized

Pathology of Silicosis

The lungs of silicotic subjects adhere to the chest wall, and the pleural surfaces are thickened (50). Calcified pleural plaques may be present on the visceral pleural surfaces. The cut surface of the lungs is studded with round, grayish nodules (Figs. 44.6 and 44.7), usually more numerous in the upper lobes, and calcification may be present. In some instances, individual nodules may have aggregated into conglomerate masses. These masses may cavitate as a result of ischemic necrosis or superinfection with TB.

Under the microscope, the hallmark of simple pulmonary silicosis is the silicotic nodule, a pathognomonic feature. The nodule begins as an aggregation of dust-laden macrophages within the interstitium, particularly near respiratory bronchioles, pulmonary vessels, and pleura. The mature nodule has a central area that gradually becomes acellular and is composed of connective tissue in a concentric onionskin pattern. The central area may eventually become necrotic (Fig. 44.8). The periphery is populated with inflammatory

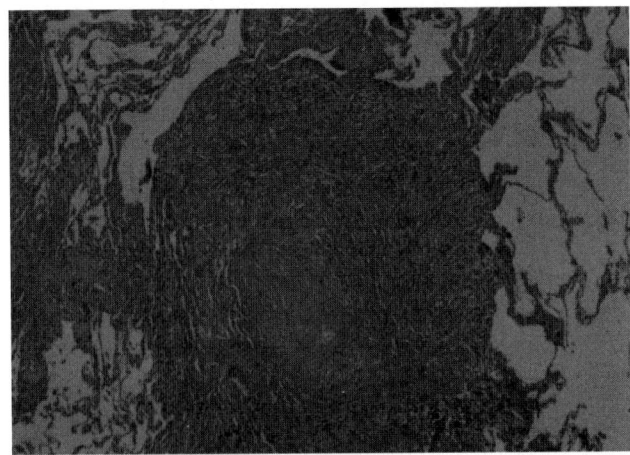

FIGURE 44.7. (See also Color Fig. 44.7.) Early silicotic nodule formation. Nodules are surrounded by dust-filled macrophages (high-power view).

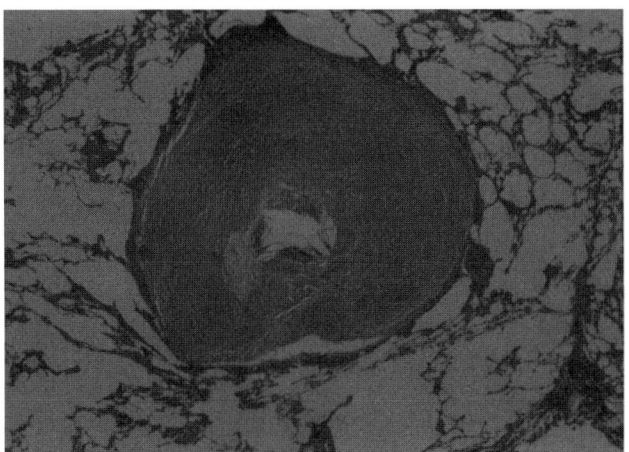

FIGURE 44.8. (See also Color Fig. 44.8.) Classic silicotic nodule.

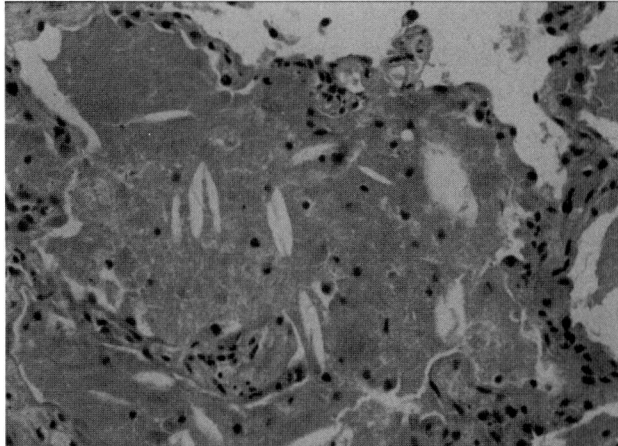

FIGURE 44.9. (See also Color Fig. 44.9.) Acute silicosis ("silicoproteinosis").

cells, particularly lymphocytes and dust-laden macrophages. The nodules may actually assume a granulomatous appearance. Accompanying these changes may be some interstitial thickening in the alveolar wall and a proliferative response of type II pneumocytes in areas of epithelial denudation.

As simple disease progresses to complicated silicosis, the small nodules enlarge and coalesce into large masses of hyalinized tissue. One sees a whorled nodule consisting of a complicated center, through which course fibers of hyalinized collagen. More peripherally, granulation tissue and some palisading of epithelioid cells are seen. The primary nodules are most prominent around pulmonary arterioles and respiratory bronchioles. The pulmonary vascular bed becomes obliterated as the nodule increases in size. Smaller vessels become incorporated into the evolving nodule. Expanding conglomerate masses eventually engulf the larger segmental and lobar arteries, which then undergo thrombosis as they are engulfed by the fibrotic tissue mass. The center of the silicotic nodules, when viewed microscopically under polarized light, contains birefringent silica particles. These tend to be located at the periphery of the nodule, away from the acellular center. Complicated silicosis usually develops in the upper lobes, which become fibrotic and atelectatic. The lower lobes in turn become overdistended, and the hila shift cephalad.

In acute silicosis, the alveoli are diffusely filled with a homogenous pinkish exudate (Fig. 44.9); the interstitium is infiltrated with mononuclear cells. The alveoli are lined with degenerating pneumocytes and abundant quantities of birefringent material. The interstitium is thickened, and fibrosis is apparent. Mixed pathologic patterns containing features of both acute and chronic silicosis are occasionally seen.

Cellular Pathogenesis of Silicosis

Free silica is not biodegradable and presents a toxic burden to a wide variety of lung cells; it is therefore not surprising that many cellular constituents of the lung are involved in silicosis. Because the ingestion of silica particles by macrophages is

such a prominent feature of the disease, their potential role in pathogenesis has been carefully studied. Ingested silica particles appear in the phagosomes of macrophages, which then fuse with and damage lysosomal membranes. When these rupture, the macrophages die and disgorge the silica particles. Along with the silica particles (which are available to be ingested by other phagocytic cells), the macrophages releases cytokines, oxidant species, proteolytic enzymes, and other mediators of cellular toxicity.

Alveolar lining cells (type I pneumocytes) have also been implicated as early targets of silica toxicity. The death of type I cells denudes the alveolar wall, exposing interstitial cells such as fibroblasts to come in contact with fibrogenic mediators and growth-promoting cytokines. Proliferation of these cells and their migration into the damaged alveolar space may result in effacement of the distal air spaces by extracellular matrix components.

Biophysical and biochemical interactions between the negatively charged surfaces of silica particles may be central effectors. It has been proposed that deposited silicates result in the local generation of oxidants in the lung. The surface of all silicates contains silanol (SiOH) groups. These dissociate, resulting in a net negative charge on the particle surface that allows the adsorption of organic and inorganic cations. In particular, ferric ions react and complex with the silanol group. Silanol groups on silicates have the ability to attract ferric ions, forming silicate-iron complexes.

The reduction of iron in the complex results in the generation of hydroxyl radicals (51). These in turn oxidize cellular proteins and lipids, presumably causing the observed cytotoxicity. Thus, the surface of the ingested silicate particle brings together chelated iron, hydrogen peroxide, and a reductant such as superoxide to allow cytotoxicity to proceed. Experimentally, coating the particles before exposing susceptible cells has mitigated the toxicity of silica. In support of this theory, agents such as aluminum or polyvinyl pyridine-*N*-oxide, by changing the charge properties of the silica surface, block or markedly reduce cellular toxicity. This theory also appears to account for the observation that different forms of silica exhibit different toxicities.

Various inflammatory mediators have been implicated in the development of silicosis. Tumor necrosis factor-α is produced by macrophages in response to silica exposure in animal models, and antibodies to this particularly toxic cytokine block the progression of disease in animals. Some of the effects of silica may represent reparative responses to the ongoing cellular injury. For example, hyperplasia of type II pneumocytes helps to repopulate the alveolar surfaces. The mitogenic cytokine transforming growth factor-α released by macrophages has been implicated as a driver of this process.

The effects of inhaled silica are not limited to the lungs. They notably involve the immune system, with both cellular and humoral immune responses markedly altered. In patients who have been exposed to silica and have silicosis, the levels of circulating autoantibodies, such as antinuclear antibodies, are frequently elevated. Rheumatoid factor is usually not elevated. The autoantibodies are thought to represent a systemic response to continued tissue damage and the release of nuclear components from dying lung cells. Further studies have shown no reduction in the number or function of circulating T or B lymphocytes. Delayed hypersensitivity to antigens remains intact. A postulated decrement in the function of T suppressor cells has been invoked to explain the prevalence of autoantibodies in silicosis. To understand the genetic factors involved in the development of silicosis, HLA phenotyping has been carried out in silica-exposed workers, mostly with inconclusive results.

Diagnosis of Silicosis

The occupational history and characteristic findings on a chest radiograph almost always suffice to make the correct diagnosis of simple or complex silicosis without resort to tissue biopsy. The differential diagnosis of the diffuse parenchymal nodular shadows may include sarcoidosis, eosinophilic granuloma, and miliary TB. Prominent hilar adenopathy may raise concern for chronic infection, metastatic malignancy, or lymphoma. The intensity and duration of the occupational exposure should correlate with the changes noted on chest radiograph or CT scan.

Biopsy may be justified in cases of mixed dust exposure when concomitant disease complicates the classic radiographic features. Biopsy may also be helpful in cases of suspected acute silicosis because this disease progresses so rapidly to respiratory failure and shares radiographic features with alveolar proteinosis, diffuse infections, and other treatable entities. If coexisting infection with *Mycobacterium tuberculosis* is suspected, bronchoscopy may be performed to collect cultures of organisms not found in sputum samples. No blood tests specifically aid in the diagnosis of silicosis. An increased frequency of elevated levels of immunoglobu-

lins, rheumatoid factor, and antinuclear antibody has been documented in patients with silicosis.

Treatment and Prevention of Silicosis

In the early part of the 20th century, the mortality of men with occupational exposure to silica was documented to be two to 12 times higher than that of men in the general population. Much of the mortality then was the result of silicotuberculosis. Seminal epidemiologic surveys identified specific risks in granite quarrying and the scouring powder industry, in which employees were exposed to finely pulverized respirable quartz.

No effective treatments for silicosis are available, nor have any randomized clinical trials of pharmacologic agents ever been undertaken in this disorder. The palliative measures are those offered to any patient with a severe restrictive pulmonary disorder and cor pulmonale. Low-flow oxygen is provided in cases of rest or exercise hypoxemia; however, no studies have been carried out to determine the efficacy of oxygen supplementation in prolonging life or improving its quality in patients with silicosis.

No promising drug therapies for silicosis have been developed. Steroid therapy has been of no benefit. Aluminum lactate has been tried in animal models (52). Isolated reports suggesting dramatic responses to long-term steroid therapy may represent patients with silicosis and a second pulmonary disorder that is indeed steroid-responsive. Lung transplantation is a costly and rarely available approach to disabling silicosis. Only 1% of lung transplants recorded in the United States have been carried out in patients with respiratory failure secondary to various pneumoconioses.

Preventive measures are based on dust control through avoidance of the generation of respirable dust and adequate ventilation at the work site. Respirator masks may be used, but it is far preferable to provide adequate ventilation to remove airborne dust.

Irritant Bronchitis and Emphysema in Silicosis

Cough is uncommon in simple silicosis because silica inhalation does not directly affect the larger airways. Cough, when prominent, is usually the result of concomitant smoker's bronchitis or industrial bronchitis. Rarely, cough in complicated silicosis can result from traction bronchiectasis or broncholithiasis.

Questions have been raised as to whether silicosis may be associated with an increased incidence of emphysema. This issue has been difficult to study, given the very high incidence of smoking among workers exposed to silica. One Canadian study based on CT analysis suggested a significant excess of emphysema in both smokers and nonsmokers working with silica. Radiographically evident emphysema was associated with lung dysfunction, both in those with pneumoconioses and in smokers with silica exposure. In nonsmoking miners,

CT detected radiographic evidence of emphysema only in cases with evidence of established pneumoconiosis.

Acute Silicosis

Intense exposure to very high ambient concentrations of silica for a short time leads to the characteristic syndrome of acute silicosis. Because acute silicosis shares pathologic features with alveolar proteinosis, it has also been referred to as *silicolipoproteinosis*. Certain exposed workers, including sandblasters, ceramic workers, and surface coal miners who drill holes to place explosives, are at particular risk for the development of acute silicosis. The production of silica flour may be associated with intense exposure leading to the development of acute silicosis. The duration of exposure to silica in such cases is usually only a matter of months. In the United States, the most notorious epidemic of acute silicosis involved miners, mostly migrant African American workers, who were constructing a hydroelectric tunnel through a sandstone mountain, the Hawk's Nest Tunnel at Gauley Bridge, West Virginia, during the Great Depression. In what was one of the worst industrial disasters in the United States, nearly 500 miners died of acute silicosis, and most of the rest were permanently disabled.

The clinical features of acute silicosis are not specific to the disease and include severe dry cough, fever, intense dyspnea, and weight loss. Hypoxemia may be profound. Pulmonary hypertension and cor pulmonale develop rapidly. The radiograph often shows coalescent shadows in the lower lung zones. Once acute silicosis becomes established, hypoxic respiratory failure develops inexorably. Patients who survive for more than a few months with acute silicosis may be particularly susceptible to infection with various intracellular respiratory pathogens, such as mycobacteria and fungi. Antiinflammatory agents and drugs to prevent remodeling, such as corticosteroids, have proved completely ineffective. Lung transplantation may be the only effective therapy.

Silicotuberculosis

Of the pneumoconioses, silicosis is unique in predisposing to TB and infection with atypical mycobacteria. Miners and other workers with significant exposures to silica have long been known to have a high incidence of TB. Those parts of the world in which TB infection and disease rates have declined to low levels have seen a commensurate decline in silicotuberculosis. In contrast, in the emerging industrialized nations, silicotuberculosis remains a significant problem among exposed workers.

The presenting manifestations of silicotuberculosis are identical to those of TB and include anorexia, weight loss, fever, and cough. The radiographic features of the infection may be difficult to detect at an early stage, superimposed as they are on features of silicosis. Later, the appearance is quite similar to that of classic TB. Silicotuberculosis may progress to cavitation quite rapidly.

The inhalation of silica has long been recognized specifically to impair the phagocytic functions of macrophages. Because monocytes and macrophages are key effector cells in host defenses against *M. tuberculosis* and other intracellular organisms, TB tends to progress rapidly in the silicotic lung. Enhanced susceptibility to TB can be demonstrated in several ways in experimental animals: Initial infection can be established with relatively smaller numbers of organisms than are required to produce disease in unexposed animals, the counts of recovered organisms are higher, and the propensity for spread from subcutaneous inoculation sites to the lungs is greater.

Under conditions of laboratory culture, no evidence has been found that silica alters the growth properties or infectivity of the tubercle bacillus itself, nor do the inhalation and deposition of silica appear to interfere with other components of the immune response. Indeed, greater humoral and cell-mediated immune responses develop in animals exposed to silica than in control animals. It has been suggested that the increased incidence of TB in silicate workers results from the accumulation of iron complexed to silicate dust particles in the lung. According to this hypothesis, silicate particles may act as a local reserve of iron that can be used by dormant mycobacteria as a virulence factor.

Mycobacteria other than *M. tuberculosis* have also been associated with silicosis. *M. avium-intracellulare* and *M. kansasii* have frequently been isolated in subjects with silica exposure, even before overt disease is apparent on the chest radiograph. When these atypical mycobacteria are detected in sputum samples, efforts must be made to determine whether they represent true pathogens or are simply colonizing organisms.

The basic precepts for treating silicotuberculosis are the same as those for treating TB in the absence of pneumoconiosis. However, several important distinctions should be made. First, in severe cases of pneumoconiosis, the radiographic appearance may be dominated by the silicosis rather than by the TB infection itself. As a result, radiographic improvement during the course of successful chemotherapy can be expected to be minimal. Second, because macrophage phagocytic and killing functions are permanently impaired in silicosis, mycobacterial relapse is common despite the use of appropriate drugs and an adequate duration of therapy. Hence, greater vigilance for relapse is in order after a full course of chemotherapy. The eradication of organisms from the sputum may be somewhat slower than in conventional TB.

All subjects with silicosis should be monitored with tuberculin skin tests. Those with positive tuberculin skin test results but no mycobacteria in their sputum should receive routine isoniazid chemoprophylaxis. Unfortunately, single-drug chemoprophylaxis may not be as effective a preventative measure as it is in the general population. Some public health experts have therefore recommended that isoniazid be continued indefinitely if possible in cases of silicosis.

A double-blinded placebo-controlled trial of anti-TB chemoprophylaxis was undertaken in 679 silicotic subjects in Hong Kong, where the prevalence of both silicosis and TB is high. During the 5-year study, active TB developed in 27% of the placebo-treated workers and in 13% of those who received any of three equally effective chemoprophylaxis regimens. Thus, although chemoprophylaxis halved the proportion of patients in whom TB developed, this proportion was still substantial. No evidence was found that chemoprophylaxis leads to the selection of drug-resistant strains of bacilli. These data reaffirm the decreased resistance of silicotic workers to TB and reaffirm the need for more effective anti-TB chemoprophylaxis regimens in this population. A reduction in the prevalence of TB in the general population has greatly reduced this problem in advanced industrial nations.

TREATMENT OF SILICOSIS	
Summary Statement	**Level of Evidence**
Pharmacologic therapy of silicosis	Expert opinion, nonrandomized
Medical support of advanced silicosis	Expert opinion, case series

DISEASES CAUSED BY NONASBESTOS SILICATES: THE SILICATOSES

Silicates

The silicates (e.g., talc, mica, kaolin, and vermiculite) are ubiquitous on the surface of the earth and occur in fibrous and nonfibrous forms. The nonfibrous silicates are referred to as *phyllosilicates* because of their leaflike structure. Fibrous and nonfibrous silicates induce pneumoconioses but are generally far less fibrogenic than quartz. Perhaps because the silicates are less toxic, descriptions of the clinical syndromes they induce are less clear-cut than those of asbestosis or silicosis. No substantial evidence has been found that the nonfibrous silicates are in any way carcinogenic except when contaminated by asbestos.

Talc is a hydrated magnesium silicate that occurs in both fibrous and nonfibrous forms. It is mined in several parts of the United States, including Vermont, New York, Texas, and Montana. Talc has also been produced in Canada, Norway, Italy, France, the United Kingdom, and China. Talc deposits in the United States are often contaminated with nonasbestiform fibrous silicates, including tremolite, actinolite, and anthophyllite.

Talc and mica have a platelike morphology that permits them to slide easily over each other. This property makes them of value as dry powder lubricants and as a base for cosmetic powders. Talc is generally mined as soapstone, then milled and calcined. The latter process involves reduction of the milled material to a powder through heating at high temperatures (1,200–1,400°C).

Industrially, talc is used to produce paints and ceramics and in roof felting. Industrial exposure has been prominent in the rubber industry, where talc is frequently dusted into tire molds, a process that allows the finished tire to be removed more easily. It is also important in the production of pharmaceuticals and in the cosmetic industry, in which it is used as a face powder and in talcum powder. High-grade talc from Italy, Vermont, and China is preferred for cosmetic purposes. Finely ground talc is also used in the production of glossy paper. Low-grade talc is used in the fertilizer industry for its anticaking properties and as a refractory filler.

Talc Pneumoconiosis

Clinical Features of Talcosis

Talcosis, like silicosis, appears to occur in both simple and complicated forms. It was first recognized as a distinct clinical entity at the end of the 19th century. Like simple silicosis, simple talcosis causes few or no symptoms. Dyspnea and productive cough, when present, are usually the result of cigarette smoking, industrial bronchitis, or lung disorders other than the talcosis. However, conglomerate shadows can develop, at which time the subject becomes increasingly and disablingly dyspneic. Talc alone, not its contaminants, is responsible for the pneumoconiosis seen in exposed miners. Nevertheless, talc is far less fibrogenic than silica. Disabling complicated talcosis with conglomerate shadows is now a rare entity in North America.

The radiographic appearance of chronic talc pneumoconiosis depends on the nature of the talc deposits to which the worker has been exposed. When pure talc is involved, the pattern is generally a mixture of round (q and r) and irregular (t and u) shadows located in the middle zones, usually in a perihilar distribution. As the disease progresses, the shadows extend peripherally from the hila to involve the upper and lower zones. Small irregular shadows in the lower lobes are often seen, particularly in cigarette smokers.

Like asbestos, talc can induce pleural plaques, even when it is not contaminated by asbestos. Pleural thickening is also seen in workers exposed to other silicates, such as sepiolite, wollastonite, kaolin, and zeolite. Such plaques often undergo calcification and are otherwise indistinguishable from those induced by asbestos.

In the absence of cigarette smoking, talc pneumoconiosis results in little or no functional impairment as determined on pulmonary function tests. In advanced cases of simple talcosis, mild restrictive ventilatory impairment may be found. Only with the rare development of large conglomerate shadows is the affected worker likely to experience dyspnea. The well-delineated plaques that develop in chronic cases are not associated with significant respiratory impairment.

Pathology of Talcosis

The chronic inhalation of talc initially produces a mild alveolar inflammatory process that infrequently progresses

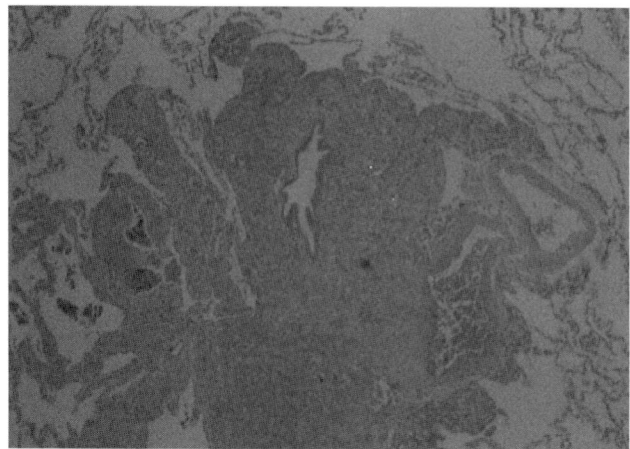

FIGURE 44.10. (See also Color Fig. 44.10.) Peribronchiolar accumulation of macrophages in response to exposure to talc and mixed dust.

to parenchymal remodeling. Inhaled talc particles are constantly removed by alveolar macrophages and cleared from the parenchyma by the defense mechanisms of the lung. Over time, dust macules form (Fig. 44.10). These are aggregations of dust-laden macrophages, foreign body giant cells, and epithelioid cells within the walls of the respiratory bronchioles. They resemble foreign body granulomas rather than the typical whorled nodules of silicosis. When they enlarge, small nodules may appear in the interstitial tissue in the same anatomic pattern of distribution as silicotic nodules. Polarizing microscopy easily identifies an abundance of birefringent particles in the nodules (Fig. 44.11). The importance of contaminating silicates or asbestos in more severe cases of talcosis has been modeled and confirmed in animal exposure studies showing that the response to pure talc is minimal. The potential of industrial talc to induce cancer remains difficult to document; large epidemiologic studies have both supported and refuted the carcinogenicity of talc.

An unusual form of talc granulomatous lung disease has been recorded in intravenous drug users; direct intravenous

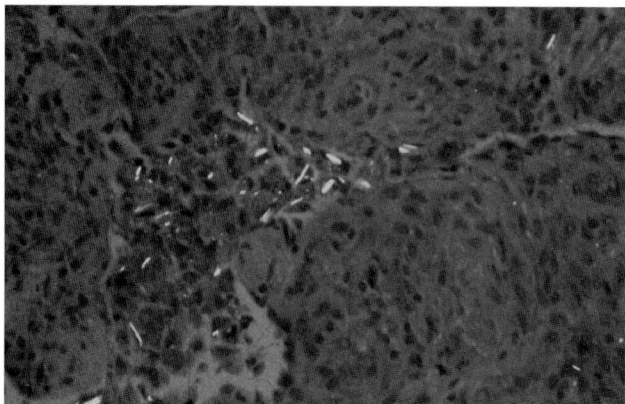

FIGURE 44.11. (See also Color Fig. 44.11.) Partially polarized specimen after exposure to mixed dust showing abundant birefringent silicate material surrounded by macrophages.

introduction of medicinal talc used as a vehicle in illicit drug preparation results in talc embolism in the pulmonary vascular bed.

Nontalc Silicatoses

Kaolinosis

Kaolin pneumoconiosis was first reported in 1936 in the United Kingdom (53). Kaolinite, a complex hydrated aluminum silicate, is used for the manufacture of ceramics (china clay), glossy paper, soap, and toothpaste, and in the pharmaceutical industry during the manufacture of pills. Like silicosis, kaolin pneumoconiosis exists in both simple and complicated forms. The simple form is characterized by the development of nodular shadows in the lung (54). Complicated kaolinosis evolves slowly and mimics silicosis radiographically. Although kaolin is usually contaminated with silica, it is clear that it is the kaolin that is responsible for the pneumoconiosis. In the United States, kaolin is mined in the southeastern regions of the country. Intense exposure to kaolin is most likely to occur during the processing stages (drying and bagging). The simple and complicated pneumoconioses noted in shale miners may in part be a consequence of the kaolin content of shale.

The pathologic picture in the lungs varies somewhat from that of silicosis and includes both interstitial and nodular changes, in addition to mild thickening of the alveolar wall. In simple kaolin pneumoconiosis, the lungs show grayish nodular lesions that are less prominent than those seen in silicosis. Simple kaolinosis is usually not associated with symptoms or alterations in pulmonary function tests. However, as simple kaolinosis progresses to the complicated form, the exposed worker notes the development of dyspnea. In complicated kaolinosis, a restrictive ventilatory pattern is present. Even more so than in silicosis, the profusion of radiographic shadowing is more prominent than the degree of impairment.

Fuller's Earth Pneumoconiosis

Fuller's earth is a fine-grained absorbent clay that was originally used to remove unwanted grease and oil from wool, a process referred to as *fulling*. It has found use in oil refining and as a binder in foundry molding sands, and it has been proposed for use in decontaminating the skin of chemical attack victims. It is also occasionally used in filtration processes and in cosmetic preparations. The various fuller's earths are finely grained calcium montmorillonite clays, attapulgite (palygorskite), and bentonite. Contaminating silica may be responsible for the development of pneumoconiosis because fuller's earth itself is innocuous. Fuller's earth is obtained by opencast and underground mining. It is then dried, crushed, and milled. It is produced in the United Kingdom, Germany, and in the midwestern United States and Georgia (attapulgite).

Fuller's earth pneumoconiosis is a rare and little studied clinical entity. It appears to occur in both simple and complicated forms. As with talcosis, only complicated cases appear to lead to impairment and disability. In the few autopsy-based studies available, the lungs contain large black nodules, usually in the upper zones. These are in a peribronchial distribution. Microscopically, there is a relative paucity of cellular reaction around the birefringent particles. The very few reports of fuller's earth pneumoconioses that have been published suggest a benign course with little risk for symptomatic disease. Secondary users of materials containing fuller's earths are not at risk for disease.

Bentonite Pneumoconiosis

Bentonite is a fine clay consisting mostly of calcium montmorillonite. It swells inordinately when hydrated, having a high capacity for water absorption. It is this property that makes it so useful as a muddy slurry in oil well drilling and also in the refining of petroleum products. Its most prominent domestic application is as cat litter. Much of the world mining of bentonite takes place in Wyoming by means of opencast methods; it is also found in the nations of the northern rim of the Mediterranean. Bentonite is variably contaminated with quartz, shale, and sandstone.

Crushing and drying in ovens creates dust and presents a hazard to workers. Bentonite pneumoconiosis can develop rapidly, be disabling, and result in fatal respiratory failure. Although bentonite is not fibrogenic, it can induce abnormal pathologic changes consisting of foamy macrophages that contain a periodic acid–positive material. This pneumoconiosis is in large part a response to the cristobalite content of the product.

Anhydrous Aluminum Silicates

The anhydrous aluminum silicates include sillimanite, kyanite, and andalusite. They find important uses in the manufacture of refractory materials and porcelain-containing materials such as spark plugs. Dust can be released during the preparation of these natural minerals, and the processes can add contaminating amounts of cristobalite. In general, radiographic changes have been minimal, but some parenchymal fibrosis appears to have developed in a few subjects. It is generally agreed that contaminating quartz is the underlying cause of the very few cases of mild pneumoconioses reported in sillimanite workers.

Miscellaneous Silicates

Mullite is a rare aluminum silicate that can cause pneumoconiosis. It occurs naturally but is also artificially produced for refractory construction. Additionally, it finds use in mortars, kilns, and furnaces. Prolonged exposure to mullite may cause mild pulmonary remodeling, but probably only when the exposed worker has been subjected to a mixed dust exposure.

Zeolites

The zeolites, which include fibrous erionite, are a group of hydrated aluminum silicates quarried from deposits of volcanic lava (tuffs). Because of their marked adsorptive properties, they are well suited for use as molecular sieves, in gas chromatography, in the separation of radioactive gases, and as fillers in paper products.

Zeolites do not cause pneumoconiosis. However, during recent decades, they have been implicated in the high rates of pleural scarring, plaques and calcification, and premature malignant mesothelioma in Turkey. The main fiber type in these deposits is tremolite mixed with lesser amounts of chrysotile. As many as half of the deaths in this region have been caused by mesothelioma and lung cancer. In addition, pleural plaques, calcification, and fibrosis have been noted but have not resulted in deaths. Although initially the epidemic was thought to be the consequence of exposure to asbestos, more recent investigations have shown that ambient levels of fibrous zeolite are responsible.

Erionite, a nonasbestos mineral fiber that belongs to the zeolite group that occurs in volcanic tuffs, has been reported to cause lung and pleural diseases in several villages of Cappadocia, Turkey. Erionite is composed of long, thin mineral fibers and is extensively used in local building materials and stucco. Fibers of erionite have been found in the lungs of patients from the two villages affected. Asbestos soil (white soil) finds many domestic uses in whitewash, plaster, and roofing insulation. Sweeping, stuccoing, and whitewashing in homes leads to elevated levels of airborne fibers. Farming activities such as plowing provide ample exposure to asbestos contained in the soil. Moreover, erionite has proved to be a particularly potent inducer of pleural disease in animal exposure studies. Of hypothetical interest is the observation that many houses in the western United States and southern Mexico contain measurable amounts of locally mined erionite. Environmental tremolite-related diseases are also prevalent in Greece, Cyprus, Corsica, Afghanistan, and New Caledonia.

Other Natural Fibrous Minerals

Attapulgite

Naturally occurring clays such as attapulgite are composed of small, elongated, fiberlike particles that have not been shown to be harmful. Attapulgite is used as cat litter and in paints and fertilizers, and it is also pumped into oil wells to remove moisture during the drilling process. Palygorskite is a chemically related mineral consisting of longer, thinner fibers. It is quarried mainly in eastern Europe. Animal experiments have shown that palygorskite is capable of inducing mesothelioma in animals, in addition to having other effects induced by the amphiboles or asbestos.

Wollastonite

Wollastonite is a fibrous calcium silicate ($CaSiO_3$) that is sometimes contaminated with quartz. It is used in ceramics and paints. In recent decades, it has found an expanding market as a substitute for asbestos in insulation, wallboard, and brake linings. It is mined in the United States, Mexico, and Finland. An extensive survey of the wollastonite mines of the Adirondack Mountain region of New York State, one of the major production areas of the world, found no exposure-effect relationship. No evidence of fibrotic pulmonary disease or pleural disease was detected over time.

Vermiculite

The vermiculites are a group of hydrated laminar magnesium aluminum silicates containing iron. More than 20 varieties occur in deposits that are quarried from opencast mines. Vermiculite deposits are often contaminated by silica, talc, tremolite, or actinolite. These, rather than vermiculite itself, account for the pleural effusions and plaques found in vermiculite workers. Several studies have assessed the deleterious respiratory effects of exposure to vermiculite in mining. Both positive and negative results have been reported. Studies suggesting increased morbidity and mortality may reflect the contamination of vermiculite deposits by asbestiform minerals.

Artificial Fibers

During the past several decades, efforts have been made to replace asbestos with a number of fiberglass and other artificial mineral fibers. Fiberglass is composed of continuous filaments and is therefore not respirable unless modified. Insulation wool is made from metal slag, igneous rocks, and glass, which are mixed and then melted down and spun into a fibrous mat. Many of the fibers produced in this process are in the respirable range. Ceramic fibers are manufactured from molten kaolin or from a combination of alumina and silica.

Most of the artificial mineral fibers cause little or no toxicity, and they do not appear to be carcinogenic. Although they may induce mesothelioma when implanted directly in the pleural or peritoneal cavity of experimental animals, they do not induce pulmonary scarring or tumors when inhaled. Moreover, fiberglass has been shown to undergo leaching and fragmentation and can therefore be removed from the lungs. Although a preponderance of evidence speaks against any increased risk from the use of artificial fibers, caution remains in order. The mineralogic structure of these agents is quite similar to that of fibers known to be carcinogens.

Several factors limit the potential of artificial fibers to induce pneumoconioses. First, the manufacturing process generates relatively few respirable fibers in the workplace environment; second, inhaled and deposited fibers are susceptible to fragmentation and leaching by lung cells.

Silicates as Potential Carcinogens

In recent years, concern has reemerged that silica may be a carcinogen, although the possibility has long been recognized. Theoretic considerations consistent with this notion are derived from our nascent understanding of the molecular biology of the interaction between silica and cell surfaces. Reactions between silanol groups on the surface of silica particles, ferric iron, and cell surface components may be expected to activate intracellular signaling pathways leading to oncogene expression. However, little compelling evidence has been found that even advanced silicosis is associated with lung cancer. Indeed, during the early part of the 20th century, when complex silicosis was much more prevalent, no association with carcinoma was apparent. Many studies have been unable to separate the effects attributed to silica alone from those of other carcinogenic agents to which people are exposed in the workplace, such as organic compounds, radon, and cigarette smoke, including second-hand exposure to smoke. Animal studies are of limited value in answering these questions, given the relatively short term and high intensity of exposure necessary to elicit malignant responses in target species.

In sum, the evidence for an association between lung cancer and either silicosis or mere silica exposure remains controversial. If such an association exists, it is likely that the carcinogenic potential of silica is weak in comparison with that of recognized carcinogens, such as cigarette smoke.

INFLAMMATORY AND IMMUNE DISORDERS ASSOCIATED WITH PNEUMOCONIOSES

In 1953, Caplan (55) described a syndrome of progressive massive fibrosis and rheumatoid arthritis in Welsh coal miners with pneumoconiosis. Caplan syndrome has occasionally been reported in association with silicosis and less commonly with asbestosis. However, in the latter case, the association may simply be the result of mixed exposure to silica or coal dust. Most reports of Caplan syndrome come from the United Kingdom; for unclear reasons, the disorder seems to be rare in North America. Caplan syndrome may occur in workers with elevated serum levels of rheumatoid factor who do not have manifestations of arthritis.

Rheumatoid arthritis and other connective disorders have long been thought to be associated with silicosis. This association would not be surprising given the regional and systemic alterations of the immune system that develop in silicosis. Patients with silicosis often have elevated levels of serum antinuclear activity. However, this activity may simply be a marker of ongoing tissue damage rather than a sign of rheumatologic disease. Systemic sclerosis has long been posited to develop more frequently following silica exposure, although this remains to be established at a statistical level. Despite the possible associations between silica exposure and rheumatologic disorders, the majority of disabled workers have osteoarthritis as a consequence of the heavy mechanical work performed during their careers. Glomerulonephritis has also been reported in conjunction with silica exposure.

ACKNOWLEDGMENT

Photomicrographs have been provided courtesy of Dr. Thomas V. Colby, Mayo Clinic, Scottsdale, Arizona.

REFERENCES

1. National Institute for Occupational Safety and Health. *Work-related lung disease surveillance report, 1996.* Washington, DC: US Government Printing Office, 1996 (Department of Health and Human Services, National Institute for Occupational Safety and Health publication No. 96-134).
2. Bang KM, Althouse RB, Kim JH, et al. Silicosis mortality surveillance in the United States, 1968–1990. *Appl Occup Environ Hyg* 1995;10:1070–1074.
3. Wright RS, Abraham JL, Harber P, et al. Fatal asbestosis 50 years after brief high-intensity exposure in a vermiculite expansion plant. *Am J Respir Crit Care Med* 2002;165:1145–1149.
4. Bégin R, Christman JW. Detailed occupational history. The cornerstone in diagnosis of asbestos-related lung disease. *Am J Respir Crit Care Med* 2001;163:598–599.
5. Murray R. Asbestos: a chronology of its origins and health effects. *Br J Ind Med* 1990;47:361–365.
6. Gaensler EA, Jederlinic PJ, Churg A. Idiopathic pulmonary fibrosis in asbestos-exposed workers. *Am Rev Respir Dis* 1991;144:689–696.
7. Occupational Safety and Health Administration (OSHA). Occupational safety and health standards, toxic and hazardous substances. *Federal Register* (1998) (codified at 29 CFR 1910.1001).
8. American Conference of Governmental Industrial Hygienists (ACGIH). *1999 TLV's and BEIs. Threshold limit values for chemical substances and physical agents, biological exposure indices* . Cincinnati, OH: American Conference of Governmental Industrial Hygienists, 1999.
9. National Institute for Occupational Safety and Health (NIOSH). *Pocket guide to chemical hazards.* Cincinnati, OH: Department of Health and Human Services, Public Health Service, Centers for Disease Control and Prevention, 1997.
10. Occupational exposures to air contaminants at the World Trade Center disaster site—New York, September–October, 2001. *MMWR Morb Mortal Wkly Rep* 2002;51:453–456.
11. Gaensler EA. Asbestos exposure in buildings. *Clin Chest Med* 1992;13:231–242.
12. Upton AC, Barrett JC, Becklake MR, et al. *Asbestos in public and commercial buildings: a literature review and synthesis of current knowledge.* Cambridge, MA: Health Effects Institute—Asbestos Research, 1991.
13. Oghiso Y, Kagan E, Brody AR. Intrapulmonary distribution of inhaled chrysotile and crocidolite asbestos: ultrastructural features. *Br J Exp Pathol* 1984;65:467–484.
14. Bégin R, Filion R, Ostiguy G. Emphysema in silica- and asbestos-exposed workers seeking compensation. A CT scan study. *Chest* 1995;108:647–655.
15. Becklake MR, Toyota B, Stewart M, et al. Lung structure as a risk factor in adverse pulmonary responses to asbestos exposure. *Am Rev Respir Dis* 1983;128:385–389.
16. Staples CA, Gamsu G, Ray CS, et al. High-resolution computed tomography and lung function in asbestos-exposed workers with normal chest radiographs. *Am Rev Respir Dis* 1989;139:1502–1508.
17. Kee ST, Gamsu G, Blanc P. Causes of pulmonary impairment in asbestos-exposed individuals with diffuse pleural thickening. *Am J Respir Crit Care Med* 1996;154:789–793.
18. American Thoracic Society. The diagnosis of nonmalignant disease related to asbestos. *Am Rev Respir Dis* 1986;134:363–368.
19. Craighead JE, Abraham IL, Churg A, et al. The pathology of asbestos-associated diseases of the lungs and pleural cavities: diagnostic criteria and proposed grading scheme. *Arch Pathol Lab Med* 1982;106:542–596.
20. Gibbs AR, Attanoos RL. ACP Best Practice No.161. Examination of lung specimens. *J Clin Pathol* 2000;53:507–512.
21. Roggli VL, Pratt PC. Numbers of asbestos bodies on iron-stained tissue sections in relation to asbestos body counts in lung tissue digests. *Hum Pathol* 1983;14:355–361.
22. Churg AM, Warnock ML. Asbestos and other ferruginous bodies: their formation and clinical significance. *Am J Pathol* 1981;102:447–456.
23. Mossman BT, Churg A. Mechanisms in the pathogenesis of asbestosis and silicosis. *Am J Respir Crit Care Med* 1998;157:1666–1680.
24. Kamp DW, Weitzman SA. The molecular basis of asbestos-induced lung injury. *Thorax* 1999;54:638–652.
25. Dumortier P, Broucke I, De Vuyst P. Pseudoasbestos bodies and fibers in bronchoalveolar lavage of refractory ceramic fiber users. *Am J Respir Crit Care Med* 2001:164:499–503.
26. Sebastien P, Armstrong B, Monchaux G, et al. Asbestos bodies in bronchoalveolar lavage fluid and in lung parenchyma. *Am Rev Respir Dis* 1988;137:75–78.
27. Teschler H, Friedrichs KH, Hoheisel GB, et al. Asbestos fibers in bronchoalveolar lavage and lung tissue of former asbestos workers. *Am J Respir Crit Care Med* 1994;149:641–645.
28. Schwartz DA, Galvin JR, Burmeister LF, et al. The clinical utility and reliability of asbestos bodies in bronchoalveolar fluid. *Am Rev Respir Dis* 1991;144:684–688.
29. Gibbs AR, Pooley FD. Analysis and interpretation of inorganic mineral particles in "lung" tissues. *Thorax* 1996;51:327–334.
30. Dufresne A, Bégin R, Churg A. Mineral fiber content of lungs in patients with mesothelioma seeking compensation in Québec. *Am J Respir Crit Care Med* 1996;153:711–718.
31. Churg A, Wright JL, Vedal S. Fiber burden and patterns of asbestos-related disease in chrysotile miners and millers. *Am Rev Respir Dis* 1984;148:25–31.
32. Dufresne A, Bégin R, Massé S, et al. Retention of asbestos fibres in lungs of workers with asbestosis, asbestosis and lung cancer, and mesothelioma in Asbestos township. *Occup Environ Med* 1995;53:801–807.
33. Mukherjee S, De Klerk N, Palmer LJ, et al. Chest pain in asbestos-exposed individuals with benign pleural and parenchymal disease. *Am J Respir Crit Care Med* 2000;162:1807–1811.
34. Van Cleemput J, De Raeve H, Verschakelen JA, et al. Surface of localized pleural plaques quantitated by CT scanning: no relation with cumulative asbestos exposure and no effect on lung function. *Am J Respir Crit Care Med* 2001;163:705–710.
35. American Thoracic Society. Environmental controls in lung disease. *Am Rev Respir Dis* 1990;142:915–939.

36. Bégin R. Asbestos exposure and pleuropulmonary cancer. *Rev Mal Respir* 1998;15:723–730.
37. Doll R. Mortality from lung cancer in asbestos workers. *Br J Ind Med* 1955;12:81–86.
38. Bouros D, Hatzakis K, Labrakis H, et al. Association of malignancy with diseases causing interstitial pulmonary changes. *Chest* 2002;121:1278–1289.
39. Hammond EC, Selikoff IJ, Seidman H. Asbestos exposure, cigarette smoking, and death rates. *Ann N Y Acad Sci* 1979;330:473–491.
40. Sluis-Cremer GK, Bezuidenhout BN. Relation between asbestosis and bronchial cancer in amphibole asbestos miners. *Br J Ind Med* 1989;46:537–540.
41. Churg A, Stevens B. Enhanced retention of asbestos fibers in the airways of human smokers. *Am J Respir Crit Care Med* 1995;151:1409–1413.
42. Becklake MR, Toyota B, Stewart M, et al. Lung structure as a risk factor in adverse pulmonary responses to asbestos exposure. *Am Rev Respir Dis* 1983;128:385–389.
43. Egilman D, Reinert A. Lung cancer and asbestos exposure: asbestosis is not necessary. *Am J Ind Med* 1996;30:398–406.
44. Wylie AG, Bailey KF, Kelse JW, et al. The importance of width in asbestos fiber carcinogenicity and its implications for public policy. *Am Ind Hyg Assoc J* 1993;54:239–252.
45. Hillerdal G. Pleural plaques and risk for bronchial carcinoma and mesothelioma. A prospective study. *Chest* 1994;105:144–150.
46. Lee BW, Wain JC, Kelsey KT, et al. Association of cigarette smoking and asbestos exposure with location and histology of lung cancer. *Am J Respir Crit Care Med* 1998;57:748–755.
47. Graham WG, Weaver S, Ashikaga T, et al. Longitudinal pulmonary function losses in Vermont granite workers. A reevaluation. *Chest* 1994;106:125–130.
48. Hughes JM, Weill H, Checkoway H, et al. Radiographic evidence of silicosis risk in the diatomaceous earth industry. *Am J Respir Crit Care Med* 1998:158:807–814.
49. Bégin R, Ostiguy G, Filion R, et al. Computed tomography scan in the early detection of silicosis. *Am Rev Respir Dis* 1991;144:697–705.
50. Silicosis and Silicate Disease Committee. Diseases associated with exposure to silica and nonfibrous silicate minerals. *Arch Pathol Lab Med* 1988;112:673–720.
51. Ghio AJ, Kennedy TP, Schapira RM, et al. Hypothesis: is lung disease after silicate inhalation caused by oxidant generation? *Lancet* 1990;336:967–969.
52. Dubois F, Bégin R, Cantin A, et al. Aluminum inhalation reduces silicosis in a sheep model. *Am Rev Respir Dis* 1988;137:1172–1179.
53. Morgan WKC, Donner A, Higgins ITT, et al. The effects of kaolin on the lung. *Am Rev Respir Dis* 1988;138:813–820.
54. Lapenas D, Gale P, Kennedy T, et al. Kaolin pneumoconiosis. Radiologic, pathologic, and mineralogic findings. *Am Rev Respir Dis* 1984;130:282–288.
55. Caplan A. Certain unusual radiological appearances in the chest of coal-miners suffering from rheumatoid arthritis. *Thorax* 1953;8:29–37.

45 Occupational Airway Diseases

R. John Looney · William S. Beckett · Mark J. Utell

OCCUPATIONAL ASTHMA

Occupational asthma may be defined as reversible airway obstruction caused by specific agents in the workplace. It should be distinguished from pre-existing asthma that may be worsened by workplace exposures. The focus of this chapter is primarily on new-onset asthma induced by workplace exposures.

Occupational asthma may be immunologic or nonimmunologic in origin and may be caused by a wide spectrum of low- and high-molecular-weight substances delivered as vapors, gases, or particles. Different classifications are useful when various aspects of occupational asthma are considered (Table 45.1). One classification divides immunologically mediated occupational asthma into subsets based on type of antigen (high- versus low-molecular-weight agents; Table 45.2). A second classification divides occupational asthma into subsets based on pathophysiologic mechanisms. Typically, immunologically mediated asthma is associated with a latency period; in contrast, irritant-induced asthma (e.g., reactive airway dysfunction syndrome [RADS]) occurs without any latency (1–3).

Epidemiology and Prevalence

Occupational asthma is now the most common form of occupational lung disease in many industrialized countries. In the United Kingdom and France, the number of claims for occupational asthma exceeds that of pneumoconioses. In the United States, asthma prevalence is increasing, involving approximately 5% of the population; recent studies indicate that 5% to 10% of adult asthma is attributable to workplace exposures.

It is difficult to estimate the true incidence or prevalence of occupational asthma. Many surveys have used questionnaire responses only, which may not accurately reflect airway hyperreactivity or its etiology. Cross-sectional studies of workers may underestimate asthma prevalence because of the dropout of workers who become sensitized at work. Individuals who remain may reflect a healthy worker effect. Other workers may refuse to participate in epidemiologic studies for fear of losing their jobs.

The prevalence of asthma can be as high as 50% for workers exposed to platinum salts and only 5% among workers exposed to either isocyanates or wood dust from western red cedar. Among 2,500 asthmatic subjects, age 20 to 44 years, studied in a large young-adult Spanish population, the highest risk for occupational asthma was observed among laboratory technicians, spray painters, bakers, plastics and rubber workers, and welders; the risk for asthma attributed to occupational exposures after adjusting for age, sex, residence, and smoking status ranged from 5% to 7%, depending on the definition of asthma (4).

Several risk factors that influence the development of disease have been identified (5). Genetic factors such as atopy predispose to the development of occupational asthma in industries that use high-molecular-weight antigens; the significance of atopy with low-molecular-weight compounds is less clear. In some studies, cigarette smoking has been linked to an increased risk for occupational asthma with some high-molecular-weight substances (e.g., laboratory animals). The relationship between pre-existing airway hyperreactivity and development of occupational asthma is unclear but is under investigation.

MECHANISMS

Asthma is a common disease affecting as many as 20 million individuals in the United States. Workplace exposures may

R. J. Looney, W. S. Beckett, and M. J. Utell: Departments of Medicine and Environmental Medicine, University of Rochester School of Medicine, Rochester, New York.

TABLE 45.1. CLASSIFICATION OF OCCUPATIONAL ASTHMA

Antigens
   High-molecular-weight antigens
      Protein derived from domestic animals, insects, fungi, or vegetable
         matter
      Dextrans
   Low-molecular-weight antigens
      Haptens such as platinum and other metal salts
      Penicillin and other drugs
      Toluene diisocyanate and other reactive chemicals
Pathophysiology
   Immunologic: characterized by a latency
      IgE-mediated (seen with both high- and low-molecular-weight
         antigens)
      Non–IgE-mediated (seen only with low-molecular-weight antigens)
   Nonimmunologic: no latency
      Pharmacologic: mast cells, sensory neurons, or smooth muscle as
         targets
      Irritants and toxins (reactive airway dysfunction syndrome)

exacerbate symptoms in persons with pre-existing asthma (work-aggravated asthma) or trigger new disease. The mechanisms by which occupational agents induce asthma are similar to those that are operative in nonoccupational asthma. Important mechanisms include reflex bronchoconstriction, acute inflammation, and immunologic sensitization. For some agents, responses may be triggered through several pathways, whereas for others the mechanism by which the material causes asthma is undefined.

Work-Aggravated Asthma: Nonimmunologic Mechanisms

Work-aggravated asthma is defined as concurrent asthma worsened by gaseous or particulate irritants or physical stimuli in the workplace. Exposure to numerous industrial agents can cause reflex bronchoconstriction in asthmatic workers with hyperreactive airways. Sulfur dioxide (SO_2), acidic aerosols, environmental tobacco smoke, chemicals, and automobile exhaust can precipitate cough or wheezing by stimulating irritant receptors. A striking example of an acute exposure occurs with the gas SO_2, which induces bronchoconstriction in exercising asthmatic individuals at a concentration less than 1.0 ppm after exposures lasting only 5 minutes. In contrast, inhalation of SO_2 at concentrations of 5 ppm causes only small decrements in airway function in normal subjects. Lung function responses to SO_2 in asthmatic persons are greater when SO_2 exposure is accompanied by increased ventilation, usually stimulated by physical labor or exercise. SO_2-induced bronchoconstriction can be further intensified by breathing cold air and/or dry air (6). Thus, the irritant response can be enhanced by conditions in the workplace.

At times, it may be difficult to draw a clear distinction between work-aggravated and de novo occupational asthma.

This is particularly true in the case of atopic individuals who may become sensitized to allergens at work. The pathogenic mechanisms, and perhaps even the genetic predisposition, are similar for the work-related and non–work-related allergen exposure. For example, the physician may encounter an atopic asthmatic individual with baker's asthma who is sensitized to aeroallergens outside the workplace, such as house dust mites, and also to aeroallergens encountered at work, such as protein antigens in flour. The severity of disease is determined by a combination of immunologic sensitivity and level of exposure to both work-related and non–work-related aeroallergens. The management of such cases needs to address both exposures or risk the possibility of inappropriate attribution; that is, residual symptoms of house dust mite exposure or other nonoccupational allergens may be blamed on responses induced by exposure to flour antigens at work. On the other hand, a specific material may act as both an irritant and immunologically specific antigen. For example, isocyanates can cause cough or irritation to the eyes at high concentrations, but immunologic sensitization can also result, causing asthma at extremely low levels.

A second type of nonimmunologic or irritant-induced asthma is RADS (7). In 1981, 13 workers in whom symptomatic and physiologic evidence of bronchoconstriction developed within hours after a single toxic inhalation exposure were reported. The symptoms were persistent, lasting at least 3 months and averaging 3 years after the time of initial exposure. A case of RADS was defined in the American College of Chest Physicians consensus statement *Assessment of Asthma in the Workplace,* as meeting the following criteria: (a) a documented absence of preceding respiratory complaints; (b) onset of symptoms after a single exposure incident or accident; (c) exposure to gas, smoke, fume, or vapor with irritant properties present in very high concentrations; (d) onset of symptoms within 24 hours after the exposure, with persistence of symptoms of at least 3 months; (e) symptoms consistent with asthma, such as cough, wheeze, and dyspnea; (f) presence of airflow obstruction on pulmonary function tests; (g) presence of nonspecific bronchial hyperresponsiveness; and (h) other pulmonary diseases ruled out (8).

Histopathologic studies in RADS are limited but have shed light on the pathogenic mechanisms. In general, bronchial biopsy specimens have demonstrated only a mild inflammatory response, with sparse lymphocytes and polymorphonuclear cells and no eosinophils. However, biopsy results are variable, depending presumably on type and severity of exposure, type of treatment, and time from injury to biopsy.

Although the acute symptoms after toxic inhalation are related to the resulting airway inflammation, the basis for the persistent bronchial hyperresponsiveness is not well explained. Hypotheses under investigation include altered receptor thresholds in the airways, increased airway

TABLE 45.2. CAUSES OF OCCUPATIONAL ASTHMA

High-Molecular-Weight Material		Low-Molecular-Weight Compounds	
Plants		**Isocyanates**	
Grain dust	grain workers, millers, dock workers	Toluene diisocyanate	polyurethane, plastics
Flour	bakers, millers	Methylene diphenyldiisocyanate	foundries
Soybean	farmers, dock workers	Hexamethylene diisocyanate	spray paint, plastics
Castor bean	dock workers, fertilizer workers	**Acid anhydrides**	
Coffee bean	dock workers, food processors	Phthalic anhydride	plastics, epoxy resins
Tea	food processors	Trimellitic anhydride	plastics, epoxy resins
Hops	brewers	Tetrachlorophthalic anhydride	epoxy resins
Tobacco leaf	farmers, manufacturers	Himic anhydride	fire retardants
Latex	health care and laboratory workers	Hexahydrophthalic anhydride	plastics, epoxy resins
Cottonseed	bakers, fertilizer workers, manufacturers	**Metals**	
Flaxseed	manufacturers	Platinum	refining
Linseed	manufacturers	Nickel	metal plating
Animals		Chromium	tanning, cement
Laboratory animals	laboratory workers	Cobalt	hard metal workers
Birds	pigeon breeders, poultry workers	**Wood dust**	
Eggs	food processors	Western red cedar	carpenters, sawmill workers
Milk	farmers, daily workers	California redwood	carpenters, sawmill workers
Crabs	food processors	Cedar of Lebanon	carpenters, sawmill workers
Prawns	food processors	African maple	carpenters, sawmill workers
Insects		Oak	carpenters, sawmill workers
House dust mites	office workers	Mahogany	carpenters, sawmill workers
Grain mites	farmers, grain workers, dock workers, bakers	African zebra wood	carpenters, sawmill workers
Fowl mites	poultry workers	Central American walnut	carpenters, sawmill workers
Silkworms	sericulture	**Soldering fluxes**	
Mealworms	bait workers	Colophony	electronics
Cockroaches	laboratory workers	Aminoethylethanolamine	aluminum solderers
Honeybees	beekeepers	**Drugs**	
Enzymes		Penicillin	pharmaceuticals
Papain		Cephalosporins	pharmaceuticals
Subtilisin		Spiramycin	pharmaceuticals
Bromelin		Tetracycline	pharmaceuticals
Pancreatin		Piperazine HCl	pharmaceuticals
Pepsin		Phenylglycine acid chloride	pharmaceuticals
Trypsin		Psyllium	pharmaceuticals
Fungal amylase		**Miscellaneous**	
Vegetable gums		Formalin	hospital staff, fur tanning, insulation
Acacia	printers	Ethylenediamine	beauty, plastic, rubber
Tragacanth	printers	Ammonium thioglycolate	beauty parlor
Karaya	hairdressers		
Guar	carpet manufacturers		

permeability, smooth-muscle dysfunction as a result of massive mediator release, and persistent airway inflammation. The treatment of the patient with established RADS is no different from that of any other asthmatic patient.

Immunologically Mediated Occupational Asthma

Two observations suggest that immunologic mechanisms are involved in most cases of occupational asthma. First, there is clinical evidence of sensitization; that is, individuals do not experience respiratory symptoms when first exposed to an antigen, but repeated exposures begin to precipitate symptoms. Moreover, with repeated exposures, symptoms occur at extremely low concentrations. Second, there is immunologic evidence of sensitization. This is most easily seen with agents that induce an immunoglobulin E (IgE) response in which specific antibodies can be detected by immediate skin tests or radioallergosorbent test (RAST) and correlated with the development of allergic symptoms such as conjunctivitis and rhinitis in addition to asthma.

Antigens involved in occupational asthma fall into two categories. The first category consists of macromolecular antigens derived from animals, plants, microbes, and even recombinant DNA technology. These antigens resemble those responsible for atopic asthma and are mainly proteins.

They are complete antigens containing both T- and B-cell epitopes, and they induce and elicit an immune response by themselves. Asthma secondary to these macromolecular agents is closely related to atopic/extrinsic asthma, as it is IgE-mediated. Indeed, atopy is a risk factor for the development of occupational asthma with at least some of these agents. Allergen-specific IgE is invariably found with occupational asthma caused by exposure to high-molecular-weight allergens. The second category consists of molecules of low molecular weight. These low-molecular-weight antigens are incomplete antigens; that is, they first haptenate macromolecules before they induce an immune response and therefore must themselves be chemically reactive molecules or metabolized to reactive intermediates. Asthma induced by some low-molecular-weight molecules is IgE-mediated. However, atopy is generally not a risk factor. Other risk factors have been sought and include, e.g., cigarettes, which increase the risk for both immunologic sensitization to and occupational asthma with platinum salts. It is interesting that some low-molecular-weight molecules induce immunologically mediated asthma in which IgE antibodies appear to play no role. The mechanisms of non–IgE-mediated asthma are poorly understood (9).

Patterns of Cytokine Production

The importance of bronchial inflammation in asthma has become clear (10,11). Eosinophilic and lymphocytic infiltration is present in bronchial biopsy specimens of even mildly asthmatic subjects. A variety of proinflammatory substances are released into the airway tissues of asthmatic subjects, including lipids, proteases, bioamines, neurotransmitters, and cytokines. Of these mediators, cytokines are unique because they are primary effector mechanisms for T cells. The pattern of cytokine secretion appears to differ in the major categories of nonoccupational asthma. Studies of cytokine production at the mRNA and protein levels indicate that in extrinsic asthma (allergic asthma) interleukin (IL)-4 is produced by mast cells and CD4 lymphocytes; IL-5 is produced by these cells and eosinophils. Intrinsic asthma (nonallergic asthma) has not been as extensively studied. Nonetheless, IL-5 and interferon-γ are found, but not IL-4. These patterns of cytokines fit with the immunopathology (12–14). IL-5 is essential for eosinophil production in the marrow and is able to attract, activate, and enhance the survival of mature eosinophils. In both intrinsic and extrinsic asthma, IL-5 is produced in the airway mucosa, and both conditions are associated with prominent bronchial tissue eosinophilia. In extrinsic asthma, IL-4 is produced in the airways; in intrinsic asthma, interferon-γ is produced instead of IL-4. IL-4 is essential for IgE synthesis, whereas interferon-γ inhibits IgE production. Thus, extrinsic or atopic asthma is associated with a pattern of cytokines promoting IgE production, whereas the pattern of cytokines in intrinsic nonallergic asthma inhibits the production of IgE.

TABLE 45.3. IMMUNOGLOBULIN E- VERSUS NON–IMMUNOGLOBULIN E-MEDIATED OCCUPATIONAL ASTHMA

	IgE-mediated	Non–IgE-mediated
Eosinophilic bronchitis	++	++
T-cell infiltration of airways	++	++
Predominant T-cell subset	CD4	CD8
MHC presentation	Class II	Class I
Interleukin-5	++	++
Interleukin-6	++	–
Interferon-γ	–	++

MHC, major histocompatibility complex.

The results of studies of IgE-mediated and non–IgE-mediated occupational asthma are remarkably congruous with those of studies of extrinsic and intrinsic nonoccupational asthma (Table 45.3). In both IgE-mediated and non–IgE-mediated occupational asthma, airway inflammation is a predominant feature, and as in nonoccupational asthma, eosinophils and lymphocytes infiltrate the tissue. Analysis of cytokine production in occupational asthma has been limited. In one interesting study, lymphocytes were harvested from bronchoalveolar lavage (BAL) fluid and grown *in vitro* after exposure to toluene diisocyanate (TDI), an agent that induces non–IgE-mediated occupational asthma. These TDI-elicited T cells were 80% CD8-positive and produced large quantities of IL-5 and interferon-γ but no IL-4 (15). Challenge studies with nonoccupational agents that induce IgE-mediated asthma elicit predominantly CD4 cells producing IL-5 and IL-4 but no interferon-γ. BAL studies have not been performed for IgE-mediated occupational asthma but presumably would be similar to those for IgE-mediated nonoccupational asthma. Thus, the two major differences between IgE-mediated and non–IgE-mediated asthma are the T-cell subset involved and the pattern of cytokine induced.

The preponderance of CD8 cells in BAL fluid after challenge with TDI was surprising, because previous studies of BAL fluid in asthmatic patients reported a predominance of CD4 cells. However, these previous studies used protein antigens, such as house dust mite or pollens. Exogenous protein antigens do not enter the cytoplasm of antigen-presenting cells and are therefore not presented via class I molecules to CD8 T cells. Instead, exogenous protein antigens are taken up into cytoplasmic vesicles, where they become bound to class II molecules and are then returned to the cell surface for presentation to CD4 T cells (16). Because TDI is not a protein but a reactive chemical, it can form covalent bonds with a variety of macromolecules. These macromolecules include self-proteins in the cytoplasm of the cell and even the class I molecules themselves. TDI-modified self-peptides from cytoplasmic proteins or TDI-modified class I molecules would be presented to CD8 T cells. It is interesting to note that although many low-molecular-weight antigens, such as TDI, western cedar, or colophony, induce asthma by non–IgE-mediated mechanisms, another group of low-molecular-weight antigens, such as platinum salts and acid anhydrides, induce antigen-specific IgE. It is tempting to hypothesize that a crucial difference between the chemicals that induce non–IgE-mediated versus IgE-mediated asthma may be presentation of antigen via class I or class II antigens, respectively.

Pathophysiology of Airway Responses

Classically, inhaled protein allergens such as those from cats or mites induce an immediate hypersensitivity response with an early- and/or late-phase pulmonary response in patients who have asthma caused by these agents (Fig. 45.1). Both the early and late phase depend on allergen-specific IgE on the surface of mast cells. The early phase begins within minutes of exposure and typically wanes in an hour. Bronchospasm in the early phase is mediated by soluble factors produced by mast cells. The late-phase response occurs after several hours and then wanes by 12 to 24 hours. It is accompanied by a cellular infiltrate: granulocytes, especially eosinophils, initially and mononuclear cells later. Bronchospasm in the late phase is mediated by soluble factors produced by the infiltrating cells. The vast majority of patients with atopic asthma have an early-phase response, and asthmatic patients with a se-

vere early-phase reaction are more likely to have a late phase. An isolated late-phase response occurs in 10% of atopic persons with asthma. Protein allergens that induce occupational asthma are associated with the same airway changes as protein allergens that cause atopic asthma in the general population; typical IgE-mediated early- and late-phase responses are seen in challenge studies. The pattern of airway response is much more complicated in non–IgE-mediated occupational asthma. Although early- and late-phase responses occur, atypical patterns are also common. These can include isolated late responses, responses that peak early and then persist, responses that begin early and become progressively more severe, and responses that persist for several days (Fig. 45.1) (17).

The pathophysiology of acute bronchospasm induced by TDI and similar agents in the absence of antigen-specific IgE is not well understood. TDI has direct biochemical effects, including the induction of substance P secretion. Moreover, TDI can induce the release of histamine-releasing factor by peripheral blood mononuclear cells from sensitized patients (18). However, neither of these effects provides an adequate explanation for TDI-sensitized patients with immediate bronchospastic responses. The direct effects on substance P or other mediators should not differentiate TDI asthma from asthma of other causes. In addition, histamine-releasing factor is produced slowly and is associated with the

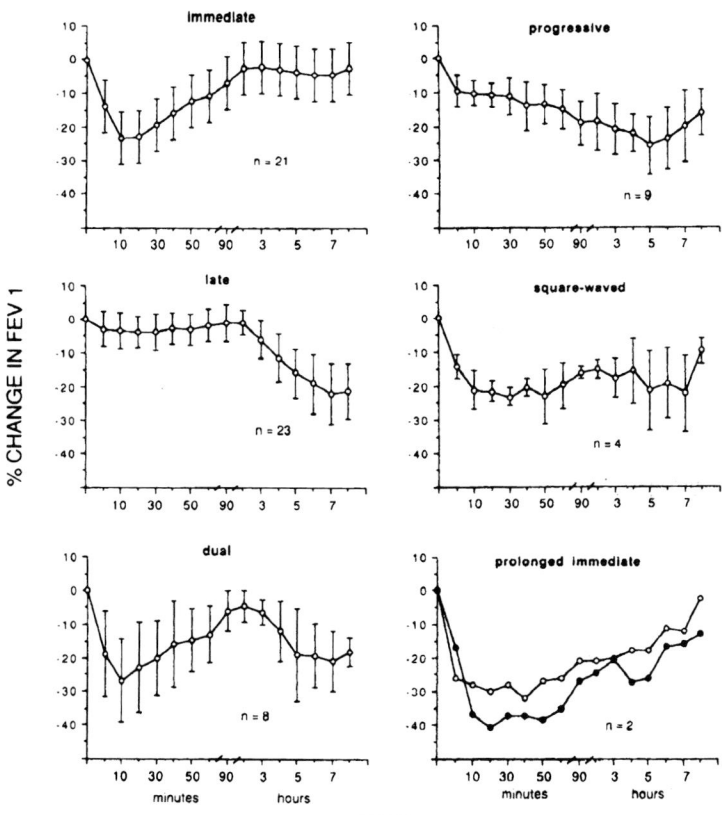

FIGURE 45.1. Patterns of airway response to antigen challenge. (Adapted from Perrin B, Cartier A, Ghezzo H, et al. Reassessment of the temporal patterns of bronchial obstruction after exposure to occupational sensitizing agents. *J Allergy Clin Immunol* 1991;87:630–639, with permission.)

late-phase rather than with the early-phase response. Clearly, additional work is needed to clarify the pathophysiology of non–IgE-mediated occupational asthma.

DIAGNOSIS OF OCCUPATIONAL ASTHMA

The two general requirements for a diagnosis of occupational asthma are (a) a diagnosis of asthma and (b) documentation that the asthma is work-related. Although fulfillment of these criteria is conceptually simple, in practice it is often not straightforward. Several important diagnostic considerations may confound the evaluation of occupational asthma. First, other diagnoses, some of which may also be occupationally related, need to be considered. Second, pulmonary function test results vary considerably, depending on whether the patient is currently exposed. Third, many factors in the workplace may act as nonspecific triggers in patients who have hyperreactive airways. Such individuals have work-aggravated asthma, and their management and prognosis differ from those of individuals with de novo occupational asthma. Finally, the diagnosis has important consequences for both worker and employer. Indeed, patients may either underreport or overreport symptoms for other than medical reasons. Our approach to the workup of occupational asthma is detailed below and illustrated in Figure 45.2.

Defining the Problem

A complete medical history and physical examination are essential in the workup of occupational asthma. The four primary goals are to (a) establish that occupational asthma is sufficiently likely to require further workup, (b) identify

alternative diagnoses, (c) assess the severity of illness and the need to eliminate further workplace exposure, and (d) identify likely etiologic agents. In other clinical situations, interventions might be started with just the data provided by the history and physical examination, but in the setting of occupational asthma, additional objective documentation is usually required.

History of the Present Illness

The interview should be open-ended, allowing the patient to raise concerns, and then focused on identified problems. A chronologic history of symptoms should be elicited, including both work-related and unrelated episodes. Particular attention is given to whether symptoms existed before the current job was started. Preceding asthma is rarely work-related except in the case of a common agent in the environment outside work or a previous work environment. Where and when in the workplace symptoms occur are important in tracking down an etiologic agent; e.g., does the patient have problems only in certain areas, or are symptoms associated with a specific process or incidents, such as spills or other accidents? The temporal relationship between work and the occurrence or exacerbation of symptoms should be understood. Do symptoms begin immediately when the patient arrives at work, or do they appear only toward the end of the shift? Do they resolve after the patient has left work? Do they persist during the whole workweek but disappear during weekends or holidays? Are there eye or nasal symptoms, and how do these symptoms change in relationship to work? Are there known precipitants outside the work environment, such as a cat or another animal, damp basements, or seasonal exacerbations? The severity and progression of

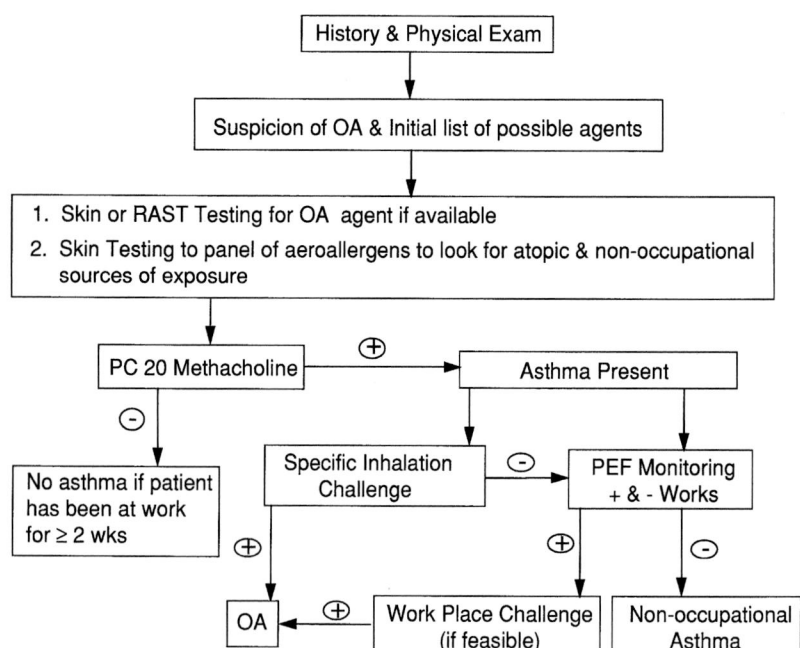

FIGURE 45.2. Algorithm for the workup of occupational asthma. OA, occupational asthma; PEF, peak expiratory flow.

symptoms determine the scope of the workup and whether continued exposure can be tolerated. Evidence of airway hyperreactivity, such as sensitivity to cold air or exercise, and the presence of symptoms that do not support a diagnosis of asthma, such as fever, weight loss, or peripheral edema and orthopnea, are important.

Past Medical History

The past history includes both the personal and occupational medical history. Previous medical records can be especially helpful in ascertaining whether symptoms developed before current workplace exposure. A history of smoking and atopy should be specifically elicited. Childhood respiratory problems such as bronchitis, asthma, frequent colds, hay fever, sinus problems, and allergies point to an atopic predisposition but do not rule out a diagnosis of occupational asthma. A listing of hospitalizations, medical emergencies, and medications should be obtained. Time lost from work and the course of recovery from prior illness may provide insight into how the patient copes with illness. A family history for atopy and other inherited respiratory diseases (e.g., cystic fibrosis) should be obtained.

Occupational History

Identification of potential etiologic agents for occupational asthma begins with characterization of present and past work-related exposures. This includes a general characterization of the types of potential allergens (chemicals, drugs, metals, animal- or plant-derived proteins, recombinant proteins, or organic dust) and respiratory irritants, as well as a general description of the job and the type of job site exposure. Some jobs, such as spray painting or handling animals, necessarily involve exposure to potential allergens. Precautions taken at the workplace, including use of protective gear and ventilation, may mitigate such exposure but can be offset by inadequacy, noncompliance, and accidents. The intensity and duration of exposure should be noted. The clinician should also determine if other workers at the same work site have had work-related respiratory illnesses. Problems with ventilation and humidification systems, including contamination with microbes, are common sources of respiratory complaints in the workplace and should be carefully queried. Dampness, particularly when cloth such as carpeting or decaying organic material is involved, may lead to overgrowth of molds or even allergenic mites. Infesting rodents or cockroaches are also potential sources of allergen.

Nonoccupational Environmental History

Environmental factors outside the workplace need to be investigated. The nature and type of housing, type of heating and floor covering, and the presence of any new construction or excessive dampness should be determined. In addition, household pets and rodents or roaches are potential sources of sensitization. Hobbies may involve exposure to chemicals that are sensitizers.

Physical Examination

Normal findings on physical examination are compatible with a diagnosis of occupational asthma. Wheezing and irritation of the conjunctiva or nasal mucosa are the more common positive findings. Nevertheless, determination of vital signs, including the rate and pattern of respiration; examination of the skin, head and neck heart, extremities, and abdomen; and a screening neurologic examination should be performed in all cases. The primary purpose of this examination is not to make the diagnosis of asthma but instead to exclude other diagnoses.

Confirmation of Asthma

Pulmonary function tests are essential for documenting airway obstruction and reactivity (Table 45.4). In some cases, the patient will have substantial abnormalities in baseline spirometry, and the diagnosis of asthma can be confirmed by demonstrating a 15% improvement in forced expiratory volume in 1 second (FEV_1) with inhaled bronchodilators. More commonly, the results of baseline flow studies are normal. In these cases, assessment of bronchial airway hyperreactivity to methacholine, carbachol, or histamine should be undertaken. Guidelines for methacholine and exercise challenge testing have been published by the American Thoracic Society and are available online (19). Doubling concentrations

TABLE 45.4. CONFIRMATION OF OCCUPATIONAL ASTHMA

	Ease	Availability	Sensitivity	Specificity	Comments
Skin prick tests and RAST	++	++	+++	+	Poor correlation with bronchial reactivity. Usefulness and availability depend on antigen.
Spirometry	++++	++++	+	++	Often normal unless illness is severe.
PEFR, serially	++	+++	+++	+++	Very useful with cooperative patient, but compliance is a problem.
Bronchial reactivity (nonspecific)	++	++	++++	+	Very sensitive, standardized. Not specific for etiology.
Bronchial challenge (specific)	+	+	+++	++++	Potentially hazardous. Dose poorly controlled, but reproduces actual exposures.

PEFR, peak expiratory flow rate; RAST, radioallergosorbent test.

of methacholine (0.031, 0.0625, 0.125, 0.25, 0.5, 1, 2, 4, 8, and 16 mg/mL) are administered as an aerosol via nebulizer for 2 minutes at each dose. A practical problem with this protocol is that the large number of doses requires substantial time in the asthmatic patient with mild or moderate reactivity; often, shorter protocols are used. A major variable in these studies is the nebulizer itself. Use of the same nebulizer in an individual for repeated measurements helps reduce variability. The endpoint for testing is generally a 20% decrease in FEV_1, and the results are expressed as the provocative dose, or PD_{20}. Use of bronchodilators and ingestion of compounds containing bronchodilator agents (e.g., beverages containing caffeine) are stopped before testing. Short-acting bronchodilators can simply be withheld for 8 hours, but other agents require longer periods of abstinence; e.g., ipratropium and leukotriene modifiers should be held for 24 hours, whereas salmeterol, long-acting oral theophyllines, or nedocromil should be stopped 48 hours in advance. If the patient is still working (i.e., has been going to work regularly for at least 2 weeks) and is still having work-related symptoms, then an absence of airway hyperreactivity essentially excludes the diagnosis of occupational asthma, and other diagnoses should be entertained. If the worker has been away from the work site for some time or if symptoms have been intermittent (perhaps because of the intermittent presence of the etiologic agent in the workplace), then the absence of bronchial hyperresponsiveness does not exclude asthma, and additional studies are required. One caveat is that the presence of bronchial hyperresponsiveness does not unequivocally mean asthma, because there are asymptomatic individuals with hyperactive airways. In addition, normal individuals may have bronchial hyperreactivity lasting for several months after a respiratory viral infection, such as influenza.

Identification of Potential Agents

Exposure assessment and immunologic testing are the primary tools in identifying potential agents. Exposure assessment begins with a careful history (see section "Diagnosis of Occupational Asthma" above). Additional sources of information include data from an industrial hygiene program, health and safety personnel, material safety data sheets, other workers, labels from containers at the workplace, and, in some cases, a visit to the work site. When contamination with microbes or mites is suspected, air and/or dust may be sampled for culture, microscopic identification, assays for endotoxin, mycotoxins, and chemicals, or immunoassays for aeroallergens.

Identification of the causative agent occasionally involves an immunologic assessment, because immunologic tests are available for only a few common allergens (Table 45.4). Asthma with a latency period is immunologically mediated. In immunologically mediated asthma, the immune response induces inflammation in the airways, and this inflammation results in nonspecific airway hyperresponsiveness. In some instances, it has been impossible to demonstrate immune

sensitization by skin testing or *in vitro* assays. This has been particularly difficult with low-molecular-weight antigens, especially those that induce asthma via non–IgE-mediated mechanisms. With both high-molecular-weight antigens and low-molecular-weight antigens that sensitize via IgE, skin testing is still the most sensitive assay for demonstration of immediate hypersensitivity. The problem in many cases is that the skin testing materials for these antigens are not standardized and frequently unavailable commercially. The investigators may then be faced with the task of manufacturing skin test reagents and/or verifying that they are active.

With some low-molecular-weight sensitizers, manufacture of material for skin testing may involve conjugating haptens to human serum albumin and measuring the extent of derivation. Allergen-specific IgE can be measured *in vitro* by using RAST with some allergens. The ability of RAST to quantify results and determine the degree of sensitization may be helpful. False negatives are more common with RAST, and false positives may occur in patients with very high total IgE levels. As with airway challenge testing, a database for the individual testing facility can be instrumental in validating skin test or RAST results. Although these tests document immunologic sensitization, sensitization does not prove a diagnosis of occupational asthma or confirm the test antigen as the cause of symptoms. Generally, more individuals have positive skin test results and no symptoms than have positive skin test results with symptoms. Nevertheless, demonstration of positive immediate skin test results and increased nonspecific bronchial hyperresponsiveness in a patient with both appropriate symptoms and exposure is highly predictive of a positive result on airway challenge with a specific antigen. Moreover, negative skin test results with a valid skin test reagent is strong evidence against involvement of that agent in asthma. For many low-molecular-weight antigens, no skin test reagent has been developed, either because the asthma is not IgE-mediated or because the appropriate carrier or metabolite has not been identified. Skin testing to a limited panel of common nonoccupational aeroallergens (in the Northeastern United States a routine panel includes cat, dog, *Dermatophagoides farinae*, *D. pteronyssinus*, cockroach, mouse, mixed grasses, mixed trees, ragweed, *Alternaria, Helminthosporium, Aspergillus, Penicillium*, and any other pet) can be quite useful in the evaluation of patients suspected to have occupational asthma. Results of this panel are used to define atopic status and determine if nonoccupational aeroallergens may play a role. *In vitro* testing for IgG antibodies may also be performed in selected cases, but the presence of IgG antibodies is more helpful in the diagnosis of hypersensitivity pneumonitis than of asthma.

Establishing a Relationship to Work

Monitoring pulmonary function over time and challenges in the laboratory or at the work site are important in relating the workplace exposure to symptoms and physiologic changes and may help to identify the specific agent. Although pulmonary function monitoring to document changes related to work site exposure seems straightforward, there are many potential pitfalls. Perhaps the most significant problem is patient cooperation and compliance. With a highly motivated and reliable individual, useful data can be obtained by measuring peak flows periodically (every 2 hours in most studies, four times a day in some) for 2 weeks. Two studies have evaluated monitoring of peak flows using airway challenge as the gold standard. Peak flow monitoring in these studies was 86% and 87% sensitive and 89% and 84% specific. These results are excellent, but other studies provide evidence that patients are often unreliable and results are fabricated up to 25% of the time. The use of computerized meters that record time and results automatically may improve the reliability of peak flow monitoring (20). Other problems with peak flow monitoring include instances in which exposure may be highly erratic and unpredictable, such as with accidents or equipment failure. In addition, when exposure results in prolonged or delayed respiratory problems, it may be necessary for the worker to be away from the job or on the job for several weeks before a change in function can be seen. Criteria for defining a positive response have often been subjectively based on visual assessment of the record. Objective criteria that have been proposed include (a) diurnal variation in peak flow of 20% or more, (b) occurrence of changes more frequently on days at work than on days not at work, and (c) designation of indeterminate recording when a 20% diurnal change occurs only once or when changes occur over several days rather than daily. By these criteria, 26% of recordings were indeterminate, and the specificity and sensitivity of the remaining recordings were 90% and 93%, respectively. However, "subjective" assessment of the record was essentially equivalent to the more "objective" reading.

Airway challenges with specific antigens remain the gold standard for the diagnosis of occupational asthma. Under most circumstances, challenges are not necessary because of good correlation between positive skin test results plus nonspecific airway responsiveness or peak flow monitoring and airway challenges. In selected situations, however, challenge can be a valuable tool. For example, in the patient with a history highly suggestive of sensitivity to a specific agent but in whom monitoring has been indeterminate or unreliable, airway challenge may clarify the issue. Malo and colleagues (21) reported that in the initial clinical assessment, the predictive value of a history that suggested that occupational asthma was highly probable was only 63% (65 of 104), whereas the predictive value of a history indicating that occupational asthma was unlikely or absent was 83% (19 of 23). The investigators concluded that objective means, including specific inhalation challenge, was at times required to distinguish between individuals with and without occupational asthma. Similarly, if the suspected agent has not previously been reported to cause asthma or if the worker has been away from work for a long time, then airway challenge will document sensitization in a physiologically meaningful sense. Because of practical difficulties, airway challenges with specific anti-

TABLE 45.5. LABORATORY CHALLENGE

Day 1: No exposure
    Baseline PFTs
    FEV_1 fluctuation <10%

Day 2: Exposure to control material

Day 3: Exposure to specific antigen
    For high-molecular-weight material:
        Increase doses of antigen every 20 min.
        Check FEV_1 every 10 min.
    For low-molecular-weight material:
        Increase doses of antigen on successive days.
        Check FEV_1 every 10 min for 1 h, then every 30 min for another
          2 h, then every 1 h for the rest of the 8-h session.

PFT, pulmonary function test; FEV_1, forced expiratory volume in 1 sec.

gens are rarely performed in clinical practice and therefore remain mainly as a research tool.

The overwhelming consideration in these specific challenges is safety. Laboratory challenges should be performed in specialized centers with trained personnel, often in an investigative setting. An intravenous line should be in place to provide access for medications. Oxygen, inhaled bronchodilators, steroids, and equipment for intubation and resuscitation should be at hand. Laboratory challenge involves several days of observation (Table 45.5). On the first day, bronchodilator medications are stopped, and clinical status, baseline pulmonary function, and fluctuation of FEV_1 during several hours are determined. If the variation in FEV_1 is more than 10%, then the patient should return when more stable. On the second day, the subject is exposed to aerosolized diluent. Finally, on the third day, exposure to test material is begun. With high-molecular-weight materials, the patient can be exposed to progressively greater amounts of material throughout the course of the day (every 15 to 30 minutes), as isolated late-phase responses are unusual with this type of allergen. During these repeated exposures, FEV_1 should be measured every 10 minutes. With low-molecular-weight materials, isolated late-phase responses and atypical patterns of response are common. Therefore, the patient should be exposed to progressively greater amounts of test material only on successive days. On each of these test days, FEV_1 should be measured every 10 minutes for the first hour after exposure, then every 30 minutes for 2 hours, and finally every hour for the rest of the 8-hour session. The starting dose of test material has to be individualized based on the material to be tested, the severity of the reaction by history, and the patient's nonspecific airway hyperresponsiveness. A 20% fall in FEV_1 is considered a positive response.

If laboratory challenges are not feasible and peak flow monitoring is unreliable, it may be possible to have the patient return to the work site for progressively longer periods of time, with spirometry, and potential determination of airway responsiveness, performed before and after the exposures. If travel distance permits, these measurements should be made in the pulmonary laboratory. Rarely, it may be necessary for a technician to visit the job site.

Although specific challenge tests may be considered the gold standard, false-negative and false-positive interpretations may result. Sources of false-negative results include testing with the wrong material or using an inadequate dose. In addition, nonspecific airway responsiveness decreases with time away from exposure, and a point may be reached at which several exposures are necessary before airway pathology is re-induced and a drop in FEV_1 occurs. Therefore, if there is no change in FEV_1 with exposure, nonspecific airway responsiveness can be measured at the end of the day and the next day to identify subtle changes. Such changes may be an indication for additional exposures. False-positive test results also occur; these may be caused by nonspecific irritation by the test substance or active asthma with a drop in FEV_1 that is independent of exposure. Suggestion may also play a role in airway responses. Indeed, there is some evidence that mast cell degranulation can be conditioned both in animals and humans. Thus, in some circumstances, blinding of both technicians and patient to the test substance may be an important consideration.

MANAGEMENT AND FOLLOW-UP

The goals of medical treatment of occupational asthma are rapid control of symptoms, reversal of airway hyperresponsiveness, and prevention of irreversible changes to the airways that lead to long-term persistence of symptoms.

In the management of occupational asthma, avoidance is the most important intervention. Once a person becomes immunologically sensitized, even infrequent low-level exposure may cause symptoms to persist. Therefore, patient and employer have to be advised that removal from the work site is essential. Interventions short of complete removal should be contemplated only if there is to be close follow-up and documentation of resolution of airway hyperresponsiveness. Such stringent environmental management may not be required in cases of work-aggravated asthma, i.e., persons who do not have immunologic sensitization to workplace allergens. For these people, moderate improvements in workplace air quality may be sufficient to control work-related symptoms, especially if their nonoccupational asthma is well managed.

Inhaled glucocorticoids are the cornerstone of the pharmacologic treatment of airway inflammation associated with chronic asthma. In a placebo-controlled trial, inhaled steroids have been shown to reverse the airway hyperresponsiveness that otherwise persists for many months after removal from exposure to TDI (22). It is too early to know whether the benefits of such treatment continue once the drug is stopped. However, if inflammation is the essential process in the development of irreversible changes in the airways, the sooner inflammation is eliminated, the lower the likelihood that permanent damage will result. At this point, it would seem prudent to treat occupational asthma aggressively with inhaled steroid for 6 months and then reassess;

it may be reasonable to stop medication at that time and monitor symptoms and airway reactivity.

Finally, it needs to be reemphasized that a large number of diseases may mimic occupational asthma, and these need to be considered whenever the question of occupational asthma is raised. Such illnesses include asthma unrelated to occupational exposures, occupational or nonoccupational rhinitis, occupational or nonoccupational bronchitis, RADS, bronchiolitis obliterans, hypersensitivity pneumonitis, sinus disease, adductor spasm of the glottis, and other causes of extrathoracic obstruction. These alternative diagnoses need to be carefully excluded.

SPECIFIC AGENTS OF OCCUPATIONAL ASTHMA

Low-Molecular-Weight Materials

With asthma induced by low-molecular-weight compounds (Table 45.2), atopy is not a risk factor. In these cases, IgE-mediated sensitization is unpredictable and may or may not be found. Because the antigens are incomplete antigens and need to haptenate a protein carrier, reagents for immunologic testing are often difficult to find. Several examples of asthma resulting from exposure to low-molecular-weight materials are considered below.

Isocyanates

Diisocyanates (TDI, diphenylmethane diisocyanate, hexamethylene diisocyanate, naphthalene diisocyanate) are used in spray painting, plastic molding, foundry work, and the manufacture of polyurethane foams. Asthma occurs in 5% to 10% of exposed workers. Diisocyanate-induced asthma does not appear to be mediated by IgE. Although RAST or skin testing will detect specific IgE in some workers, these tests do not predict clinical sensitization. Airway hyperresponsiveness to histamine or methacholine and eosinophilic inflammation of the airways are consistently found in sensitized workers. Once airway hyperresponsiveness has been established, it may persist for many years (23,24). Early detection of sensitization and removal from exposure are essential to prevent this long-term sequela (25). In addition to removal from exposure, treatment of sensitized workers with inhaled glucocorticoids accelerates resolution of airway hyperresponsiveness and inflammation. Airway challenge with diisocyanates frequently results in an isolated late-phase response. Atypical delayed and persistent responses are also common. Thus, in contrast to challenges with allergens that induce IgE-mediated sensitization, airway challenges with diisocyanates cannot be immediately repeated with an increased dose when an early-phase response is not observed. Hypersensitivity pneumonitis with pulmonary infiltrates has also been reported with diisocyanates (TDI, hexamethylene diisocyanate, and diphenylmethane diisocyanate). In these individuals, specific IgG precipitins can be demonstrated.

Acid Anhydrides

Acid anhydrides (phthalic anhydride, trimellitic anhydride, hexahydrophthalic anhydride, himic anhydride, tetrachlorophthalic anhydride) function as hardening agents in the manufacture of epoxy resins used in adhesives, encapsulating agents, surface coatings, and plastics. Workers are exposed to these reactive compounds as fumes from heated resins, dust generated during the grinding of resins, and powdered chemicals added to reaction chambers.

Acid anhydrides are potent irritants that may cause eye, respiratory tract, and skin symptoms; permissible exposure limits for phthalic anhydride have been developed on this basis (6 mg/m^3). IgE-mediated allergic sensitization also occurs, and the permissible exposure level does not account for this. Conjugates of acid anhydride and human serum albumin are sensitive reagents for skin testing, and RAST can also be performed. Results of airway challenge with acid anhydrides are typical of IgE-mediated sensitization; both an early-phase and a late-phase reaction are frequently seen. Specific IgE can persist for years after exposure. Acid anhydrides (trimellitic anhydride) are also associated with a late-onset respiratory systemic syndrome or with a syndrome of pulmonary hemorrhage and hemolytic anemia. These nonasthmatic pulmonary syndromes are associated with elevated levels of specific IgG.

Metals

Platinum salts can induce the production of specific IgE in a high proportion of heavily exposed workers, and this sensitization may lead to the development of skin rashes, eye and nasal symptoms, or asthma. Skin testing with platinum salts can be used to document sensitization, but high concentrations of platinum salts can cause nonspecific mast cell degranulation in unexposed controls. A RAST using malic dehydrogenase as a protein carrier has been developed. Asthma caused by exposure to a number of other metals has also been reported, including nickel, chromium, vanadium, cobalt, and fumes from steel welding and smelting of aluminum. There is evidence for an IgE mechanism with cobalt, chromium, and nickel in some cases, but the mechanisms involving vanadium or fumes from steel or aluminum are unknown.

Wood Dust

A wide variety of woods have been associated with occupational asthma, but the best studied example is western red cedar. In red cedar asthma, sensitization is to plicatic acid, a reactive compound found in red and white cedar. Although specific IgE can be found in many workers, asthma appears to be non–IgE-mediated, and bronchial challenge is the only reliable test for immunologic sensitization. Delay in removal from exposure after the development of symptoms, particularly in older workers, has been linked with persistent airway hyperresponsiveness and dyspnea (26).

Solder

Colophony is used as flux in soldering, and electrical workers can become sensitized to colophony, with development of asthma (27). Colophony is a derivative of pine tree resin in which several reactive chemicals are found, namely abietic, pimaric, and dihydroabietic acids. As with wood dust, sensitization is not IgE-mediated, and airway challenge is the only reliable test for sensitization. Prolonged symptoms after removal from exposure have also been reported for colophony. Another component of solder flux, aminoethanolamine, can cause isolated late or dual responses.

Drugs

Occupational asthma can develop in workers exposed in the manufacture or use of a number of drugs (e.g., penicillin). Typically, these reactions are IgE-mediated and can be demonstrated with skin testing or RAST.

High-Molecular-Weight Materials

Atopy *is* a risk factor for sensitization to high-molecular-weight materials (Table 45.2). Typically, the sensitization is IgE-mediated. Because these materials are complete antigens, reagents for skin testing or RAST are usually available.

Foods

Asthma is a frequent occupational disease among bakers. Grain allergens are the usual cause, but sensitization to contaminants such as mold spores or grain mites has also been reported. Other foods causing occupational asthma include coffee beans, tea, soybeans, eggs, snow crabs, and cocoa (28). Castor beans containing the toxin ricin appear to be a special problem, and epidemics of asthma in nearby residents, as well as workers, have occurred.

Latex

Latex allergy among health care workers has become a significant occupational problem. Although contact sensitivity is frequently caused by chemicals used in manufacturing, occupational asthma and other IgE-mediated reactions result from sensitization to protein antigens in native latex. Occupational sensitization to latex may have severe consequences for the health care worker who becomes a patient. Sensitized individuals should wear a medical alert bracelet. Use of powder-free, low-latex gloves should be advocated for all individuals. Sensitized individuals and other employees who might expose them to latex may need to use nonlatex gloves.

Animals

Asthma caused by animal proteins in dander, saliva, or urine frequently develops in laboratory workers, farmers, and other people who handle animals. Such sensitization can occur to any warm-blooded animal.

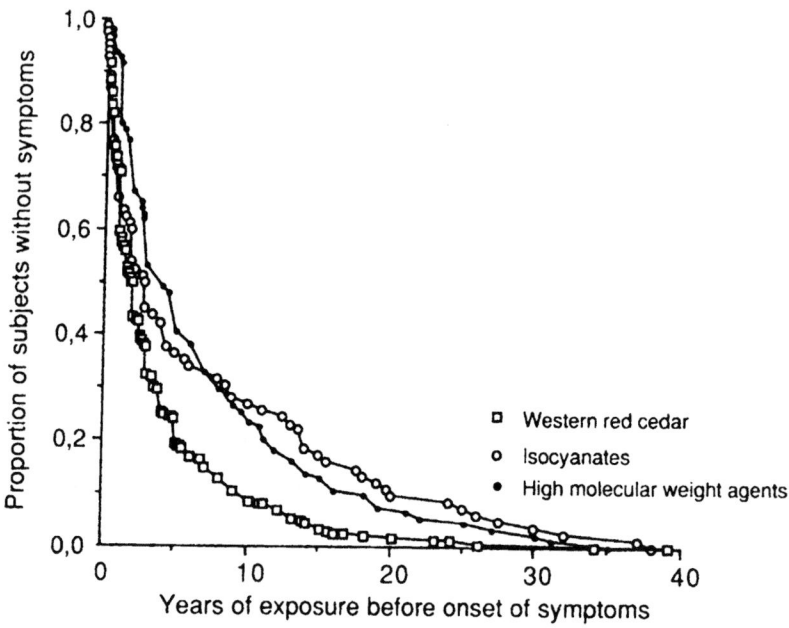

FIGURE 45.3. Proportion of patients without symptoms as a function of exposure interval. (Modified from Malo JL, Ghezzo H, D'Aquino C, et al. Natural history of occupation asthma: relevance of type of agent and other factors in the rate of development of symptoms in affected subjects. *J Allergy Clin Immunol* 1992;90:937–944, with permission.)

Insects

Sensitization to the insects used in their work can develop in bee workers and bait workers. Less obvious exposures include sensitization of farmers, grain handlers, or bakers to storage mites, and sensitization of poultry workers to fowl mites.

Vegetable Gums

Vegetable gums represent another, less obvious source of allergens that may cause occupational asthma in workers in a variety of occupations, including printing, carpet manufacturing, and hairdressing.

Enzymes

Proteolytic enzymes used in detergents, meat tenderizer, and various manufacturing processes are potent sensitizers.

COURSE OF OCCUPATIONAL ASTHMA

Occupational asthma allows investigators to view the entire natural history of asthma in response to a single, clearly defined etiologic agent. This perspective provides insight into the pace and variability of asthma development, and also an opportunity to look at the resolution of asthma as workers are removed from exposures. Thus, occupational asthma provides a unique opportunity to study the pathophysiology of asthma. There have been several surprising findings in terms of the natural history of occupational asthma.

The variability in latency—i.e., the time from initial exposure to development of symptoms—is well demonstrated in studies of occupational asthma (Fig. 45.3). The onset of symptoms follows an exponential curve. For example, the latency period for 50% of cases of sensitization to high-molecular-weight antigens is 3 years, but it takes 9 years to get to 75% of cases. There are even cases of occupational asthma developing in some workers after 30 years of exposure (29).

Another unexpected finding in occupational asthma is that symptoms are often not reversible when the worker is removed from exposure (Table 45.6). Even years after removal, airway hyperresponsiveness and inflammation persist in the majority of patients with occupational asthma studied in large series (23,26–28). The prognosis is worse for workers who stay on the job after onset of asthma and better for those workers who leave as soon as symptoms develop. These findings suggest a window of opportunity to remove the worker before irreversible changes take place. Although these results have been criticized because pre-exposure airway responses were often not available, in several workers with normal baseline function before exposure, airway hyperresponsiveness persisted long after removal from exposure. The relationship of inflammation to the irreversible stage of asthma is still controversial (30). However, an essential component of these irreversible changes may be the development of inflammation in the absence of exogenous antigen. Treatment with inhaled steroids induces resolution

TABLE 45.6. IRREVERSIBLE ASTHMA AFTER SPECIFIC OCCUPATIONAL EXPOSURE

Agent	No. of Patients	Percentage with Residual Asthma	Follow-up
Toluene diisocyanate	50	82%	>4 y
Red cedar	136	60%	4.3 y
Colophony	20	90%	29 mo
Snow crab	31	61%	1 y

of inflammation and the hyperresponsiveness that persists after removal from exposure to TDI. At this point, there is no compelling reason to believe that occupational and nonoccupational asthma differ in regard to pathogenesis of chronic effects. The only real difference may be that it is easier to define the long-term effects in occupational asthma because symptoms persist despite removal from ongoing exposure.

IRREVERSIBLE ASTHMA AFTER OCCUPATIONAL EXPOSURE

Summary Statement	Level of Evidence
Persistent asthma often occurs despite removal from exposure.	Epidemiologic and clinical studies. Better established for toluene diisocyanate and western red cedar than other agents.
Treatment with inhaled glucocorticoids enhances resolution.	Single controlled clinical trial.
Early detection and removal from exposure prevents chronic asthma.	Observational studies and consensus expert opinion.

OCCUPATIONAL CHRONIC OBSTRUCTIVE PULMONARY DISEASE

Inhaled occupational substances may cause chronic airflow obstruction (here defined as a fixed reduction in FEV_1 with a reduction FEV_1/forced vital capacity ratio on spirometry). This may occur de novo in the absence of cigarette smoking, or there may be an interaction between cigarette smoking and inhaled occupational substances causing a greater degree of airflow obstruction. Such disease may occur together with chronic bronchitis (chronic cough with mucous expectoration, four or more days out of the week, three or more months per year, for two or more consecutive years) or in the absence of chronic bronchitis. Mild chronic airflow obstruction may by asymptomatic, but the more severe it becomes, the more likely the patient will require medication, need medical attention, require hospitalization, or experience premature mortality as a result of the lung disease. Selected specific occupational substances now known to cause chronic airflow obstruction are listed in the table below (34–39). This table includes substances for which there are one or more large, well-conducted, and conclusive epidemiological studies in which a significant exposure effect on a large working population is seen, and in which bias or confounding seem highly unlikely to explain the effect. In addition, biological plausibility exists for causation.

The causation of chronic obstructive pulmonary disease (COPD) is multifactorial. The observation that most lifetime cigarette smokers do not develop clinically significant COPD suggests that other predisposing factors must be present in those individuals who smoke and do develop significant disease. Multiple genetic and environmental factors

may contribute. Homozygosity for the Z allele of the α_1-antitrypsin gene is the only well-established specific genetic risk factor for COPD, although heterozygosity for this allele may also confer increased risk. Although only a small minority of patients with COPD carry this allele, it is clear that interaction of its associated diminished protease inhibition with either cigarette smoking or possibly occupational exposures (31) may lead to a worse degree of airflow obstruction. Other genes now being investigated as candidate "susceptibility genes" for COPD include genes coding for other antiproteases, xenobiotic metabolizing substances, antioxidants, inflammatory mediators, and factors related to mucociliary clearance (32). In societies in which cigarette smoking is highly prevalent, smoking is often the most important preventable cause of COPD morbidity, but occupational factors may also contribute a significant fraction of disease, which may have clinically significant clinical impact with regard to chronic disability and premature death, and which may have important economic consequences in health care costs and lost productivity (33). Factors that may raise the suspicion of occupational COPD include disease in a nonsmoker, unusually severe disease at a relatively young age, or prolonged exposure to visible dust of fume. Further investigation by high resolution computed tomography scan of the chest may sometimes reveal a parenchymal pneumoconiosis or evidence of hypersensitivity pneumonitis that was not appreciated on plain chest radiograph. Treatment for COPD related to occupational exposures is not different from usual treatment, except that it important to notify the employer or health officials of a potential risk to others.

OCCUPATIONAL CAUSES OF CHRONIC AIRFLOW OBSTRUCTION

Summary Statement	Level of Evidence
Coal dust causes emphysema with nodular fibrosis.	Epidemiological and autopsy studies
Crystalline silica causes chronic airflow obstruction and nodular fibrosis.	Epidemiological and autopsy studies
Cotton dust causes chronic airflow limitation in those with prolonged occupational exposures.	Epidemiological studies
Cadmium dust exposure causes airflow obstruction and emphysema in some of those with prolonged occupational exposure.	Epidemiological and autopsy studies; toxicologic study support
Toluene diisocyanate causes or contributes to chronic airflow obstruction in some of those with prolonged occupational exposure.	Prospective cohort epidemiological study
Welding fume may cause chronic airflow limitation, midflow-reduction, or increased residual volume with many years of heavy exposure; the effect is much greater in smokers or seen only in smokers.	Cross-sectional studies and one prospective cohort epidemiological study

REFERENCES

1. Bardana E Jr. Occupational asthma and related respiratory disorders. *Dis Mon* 1995;3:144–199.

2. Chan-Yeung M, Lam S. Occupational asthma. *Am Rev Respir Dis* 1986;133:686–703.

3. Chan-Yeung M, Malo JL. Occupational asthma. *N Engl J Med* 1995;333:107–112.

4. Kogevinas M, Anto JM, Soriano JB, et al. The risk of asthma attributable to occupational exposures: a population-based study in Spain. *Am J Respir Crit Care Med* 1996;154:137–143.

5. Panhuysen CIM, Meyers DA, Postma DS, et al. The genetics of asthma and atopy. *Allergy* 1995;50:863–869.

6. Sheppard D, Saisho A, Nadel JA, et al. Exercise increases sulphur dioxide–induced bronchoconstriction in asthmatic subjects. *Am Rev Respir Dis* 1981;123:486–491.

7. Alberts WM, doPico GA. Reactive airways dysfunction syndrome. *Chest* 1996;109:1618–1626.

8. Chan-Yeung M. American College of Physicians consensus statement: assessment of asthma in the workplace. *Chest* 1995;108:1084–1117.

9. Mapp CE, Saetta M, Maestrelli P, et al. Mechanisms and pathology of occupational asthma. *Eur Respir J* 1994;7:544–554.

10. Frew AJ, Chan H, Lam S, et al. Bronchial inflammation in occupational asthma due to western red cedar. *Am J Respir Crit Care Med* 1995;151:340–344.

11. Saetta M, DiStefano A, Maestrelli P, et al. Airway mucosal inflammation in occupational asthma induced by toluene diisocyanate. *Am Rev Respir Dis* 1992;145:160–168.

12. Virchow JC Jr, Kroegel C, Walker C, et al. Cellular and immunological markers of allergic and intrinsic bronchial asthma. *Lung* 1994;172:313–334.

13. Walker C, Bode E, Boer L, et al. Allergic and non-allergic asthmatics have distinct patterns of T-cell activation and cytokine production in peripheral blood and bronchoalveolar lavage. *Am Rev Respir Dis* 1991;146:109–115.

14. Walker C, Bauer W, Braun RK, et al. Activated T cells and cytokines in bronchoalveolar lavages from patients with various lung diseases associated with eosinophilia. *Am J Respir Crit Care Med* 1994;150:1038–1048.

15. Maestrelli P, Del Prete GF, De Carli M, et al. CD8 T-cell clones producing interleukin-5 and interferon-γ in bronchial mucosa of patients with asthma induced by toluene diisocyanate. *Scand J Work Environ Health* 1994;20:387–381.

16. Janeway CA, Travers P, Walport M, et al., eds. *Immunobiology: the immune system in health and disease.* New York: Garland Publishing, 2001.

17. Perrin B, Cartier A, Ghezzo H, et al. Reassessment of the temporal patterns of bronchial obstruction after exposure to occupational sensitizing agents. *J Allergy Clin Immunol* 1991;87:630–639.

18. Herd AL, Bernstein DI. Antigen-specific stimulation of histamine-releasing factors in diisocyanate-induced occupational asthma. *Am J Respir Crit Care Med* 1994;150:988–994.

19. American Thoracic Society. Guidelines for methacholine and exercise challenge testing. Available at: *http://www.thoracic.org/adobe/statements/methacholine.*

20. Quirce S, Contreras G, Dybuncio A, et al. Peak expiratory flow monitoring is not a reliable method for establishing the diagnosis of occupational asthma. *Am J Respir Crit Care Med* 1995;152:1100–1102.

21. Malo JL, Ghezzo H, L'Archeveque J, et al. Is the clinical history a satisfactory means of diagnosing occupational asthma? *Am Rev Respir Dis* 1991;143:528–532.

22. Maestrelli P, DeMarzo N, Saetta M, et al. Effects of inhaled beclomethasone on airway responsiveness in occupational asthma. *Am Rev Respir Dis* 1993;148:407–412.

23. Mapp CE, Corona PC, DeMarzo N, et al. Persistent asthma due to isocyanates: a follow-up study of subjects with occupational asthma due to toluene diisocyanate (TDI). *Am Rev Respir Dis* 1988;137:1326–1329.

24. Paggiaro PL, Vagaggini B, Dente FL, et al. Bronchial hyperresponsiveness and toluene diisocyanate. *Chest* 1993;103:1123–1128.

25. Lozewicz S, Assoufi BK, Hawkins R, et al. Outcome of asthma induced by isocyanates. *Br J Dis Chest* 1987;81:14–22.

26. Chan-Yeung M, MacLean L, Paggiaro PL. Follow-up study of 232 patients with occupational asthma caused by western red cedar *(Thuja plicata)*. *J Allergy Clin Immunol* 1987;79:792–796.

27. Burge PS. Occupational asthma in electronics workers caused by colophony fumes: follow-up of affected workers. *Thorax* 1982;37:348–353.

28. Hudson P, Cartier A, Pineua L, et al. Follow-up of occupational asthma caused by crab and various agents. *J Allergy Clin Immunol* 1985;76:682–688.

29. Malo JL, Ghezzo H, D'Aquino C, et al. Natural history of occupational asthma: relevance of type of agent and other factors in the rate of development of symptoms in affected subjects. *J Allergy Clin Immunol* 1992;90:937–944.

30. Saetta M, Maestrelli P, DiStefano A, et al. Effect of cessation of exposure to toluene diisocyanate (TDI) on bronchial mucosa of subjects with TDI-induced asthma. *Am Rev Respir Dis* 1992;145:169–174.

31. Mayer AS, Stoller JK, Bartelson B, et al. Occupational exposure risks in individuals with Pi*Z α_1-antitrypsin. *Am J Respir Crit Care Med* 2000;162:553–558.

32. Sandford AJ, Joos L, Pare P. Genetic risk factors for chronic obstructive pulmonary disease. *Curr Opin Pulmon Dis* 2002;8:87–94.

33. Leigh JP, Roman PS, Schenker MB, et al. Costs of occupational COPD and asthma. *Chest* 2002;121:264–272.

34. Hendrick DJ. Occupation and chronic obstructive pulmonary disease (COPD). *Thorax* 1996;51:947–955.

35. Hnizdo E, Sluis-Cremer GK, Abramowitrz JA. Emphysema type in relation to silica dust exposure in South African gold miners. *Am Rev Respir Dis* 1991;143:1241–1247.

36. Christiani DC, Ye TT, Wegman DH, et al. Cotton dust exposure, across-shift drop in FEV, and five-year change in lung function. *Am J Respir Crit Care Med* 1994;150:1250–1255.

37. Davison AG, Fayers PM, Taylor AJ. Cadmium fume inhalation and emphysema. *Lancet* 1988;1:663–667.

38. Weill H, Butcher B, Dharmarajan V, et al. Respiratory and immunologic evaluation of isocyanate exposure in a new manufacturing plant: technical report. Cincinnati, OH: National Institute for Occupational Safety and Health; 1981; Contract No. 210-75-0006.

39. Cotes JE, Feinmann EL, Male VJ, et al. Respiratory symptoms and impairment in shipyard welders and caulker/burners. *Br J Ind Med* 1990;47:83–90.

Occupational Pulmonary Neoplasms

46

David R. Graham · Robert B. Reger

W. Keith C. Morgan

Although the incidence of lung cancer is increased in certain occupations, the most important cause of this disease is still cigarette smoking. Even if one considers those cancers associated with a particular trade, the occupational risk is small compared with that of smoking. The reduction and possible elimination of certain types of occupational risk for cancer have been accepted for years, and in this regard much has been done, but there is still some way to go. Sustained effort is necessary for the prevention of occupational lung cancer, and equally imperative is the need to control the concept that every new "chemical" that is introduced is per se a carcinogen.

The first neoplasm noted to be related to a particular occupation was cancer of the scrotum. In 1775, Percival Pott observed that the disease characteristically occurred in chimney sweeps and concluded that it seemed to derive from lodgment of soot in the rugae of the scrotum (1). Tumors of the skin were later described in cotton workers, shale oil workers, and aniline dye workers.

Harting and Hesse were the first to recognize cancer of the lung as a frequent cause of death in miners of copper, iron, and silver in Schneeberg (2). It was many years later that the cause was found to be radioactive air in the mines. This same problem was identified in uranium mines, where the presence of radon daughters was shown to be associated with bronchogenic carcinoma. In more recent years, the risks associated with several other materials used in industry have been recognized. Lung cancer has been shown to be associated with the inhalation of asbestos, arsenic, chromates, iron

D. R. Graham: University of Liverpool Medical School, Liverpool, United Kingdom.

R. B. Reger: Physician Assistant Program, Alderson-Broaddus College, Philippi, West Virginia.

W. K. C. Morgan: Professor Emeritus, University of Western Ontario Medical School, London, Ontario, Canada.

ore, coal gas, chloromethyl ethers, nickel, and chromium salts (Table 46.1). Many other substances have been suspected, but not proven, to be carcinogens (Table 46.2).

CARCINOGENESIS: DEFINITION AND INCEPTION

The Occupational Safety and Health Administration (OSHA) defines a carcinogen as "any substance that has validly been shown to produce tumors, either benign or malignant, in animals, or which decreases the latent period between exposure and the development of such tumors." This definition places much reliance on animal experiments, and moreover, the production of tumors in any species suffices for the substance to be labeled as a carcinogen. The induction of cancer in experimental animals, with certain recognized exceptions, is uncertain and unpredictable. The likelihood of a tumor developing is predicated on the route of administration of the agent being tested, its dose, the duration of exposure, the species of the animal, and the age, diet, and sex of the animals used. At the present time, around 175 to 210 substances are recognized as carcinogens by OSHA, but the acceptance of the development of tumors in any one of the vast variety of species in a myriad of differing circumstances, including tumors that may develop spontaneously, increases the number of substances accepted as carcinogens 30 to 40 times.

There is much support for the hypothesis that most cancer originates as a result of alteration in somatic DNA (3,4). Furthermore, most carcinogens are also mutagens. Hence, it is often assumed that the carcinogenic potential of a particular substance or chemical is related to its ability to damage DNA. There are those, however, who find the fervor of the proponents of the mutagenic supposition unconvincing, and who suggest that genetic transposition is of more importance.

TABLE 46.1. OCCUPATIONAL HAZARDS KNOWN TO CAUSE RESPIRATORY TRACT CANCER

Agent	Occupation	Tumor
Asbestos	Mining, weaving, utilization	Lung cancer, mesothelioma
Radioactivity	Uranium metal mining	Lung cancer
Nickel	Refining	Lung, nasal cancer
Chromates	Electroplating, tanning pigments, chemical industry	Lung cancer
Chloromethyl ethers	Fungicides, chemical industry	Lung cancer
Arsenic	Metal refining, sheep dip	Lung, skin cancer
Fossil fuels	Coal, coke, gas furnaces	Lung cancer
Mustard gas	Manufacture	Lung cancer

The layman and the neophyte scientist often pose the question, "What is the cause of cancer?" In doing so, they imply that (a) cancer is a uniform entity of only one type, and (b) it has a single cause. There are those who attribute all cancers to environmental pollution, whereas others favor viruses or life style. Clearly, all points of view are an oversimplification, and a number of considerations need to be borne in mind.

The origin of cancer cannot be explained entirely by the hypothesis that damage to a DNA strand in the chromosome of a somatic cell can, given that the damage occurs at a susceptible region, cause the development of a clone of cancer cells. This hypothesis has a meretricious veneer of plausibility in that it accommodates a wide range of carcinogens, including radiation and various chemicals. These carcinogens can induce physical damage or react with DNA molecules with a similar result. Such a hypothesis cannot account for the variation in the length of the incubation period of most cancers. When damage occurs at a single position on a DNA strand, why does the affected cell not become an instant nidus for a cancerous clone of cells? Why is it that, as Cairns has observed, chromosomes of cancer cells are most often grossly abnormal in various ways suggesting a gross rearrangement rather than an effect at a single point (5)? Although there are plausible explanations to accommodate these observations, the overall likelihood that there is a single cause of cancer is remote.

TABLE 46.2. OTHER SUBSTANCES THOUGHT BY INTERNATIONAL AGENCY FOR RESEARCH INTO CANCER TO BE RESPIRATORY CARCINOGENS

Agents
Beryllium and compounds
Cadmium and compounds
Formaldehyde
Silica

The observation that persons affected with xeroderma pigmentosum are prone to skin cancer and melanoma is consistent with a simple model, because ultraviolet light is known to damage DNA molecules. The inherent defect in this condition involves the biochemical response that is called into play to repair damaged DNA molecules. The question, however, arises as to why persons with this disease are not susceptible to other kinds of cancer caused by carcinogenic agents. It is evident from Cairns' work that human cancer and its cause are not yet understood (6). The present approach to the problem is best categorized as *hysteron proteron;* i.e., it is difficult to talk about causes when basic mechanisms have still to be elucidated. Until such time as they are understood, it is out of place to presume a single cause, viz., clinical carcinogens, and to postulate that all cancers will respond to a single mode of treatment.

International Agency for Research on Cancer

The International Agency for Research into Cancer (IARC) has devised a rather elaborate rating system for considering the carcinogenicity of various agents and materials. The agency considers the evidence, both in man and in animals, in terms of

- Sufficient evidence of carcinogenicity
- Limited evidence of carcinogenicity
- Inadequate evidence of carcinogenicity
- Evidence suggesting lack of carcinogenicity.

After review of all animal and human data relating to the carcinogenicity of an agent, IARC uses an evaluation technique that places the agent into one of five categories:

1. The agent is carcinogenic to humans.
2. (a) The agent is probably carcinogenic in humans, or (b) the agent is possibly carcinogenic in humans.
3. The agent is not classifiable as to its carcinogenicity to humans.
4. The agent is probably not carcinogenic to humans.

Clearly, groups 2a and 2b are a source of concern and pose difficult problems for exposed workers, industry, and regulatory agencies. Thus, an agent may be placed in group 2a (probably carcinogenic to humans) when there exists only finite evidence of carcinogenicity in humans, but which is accompanied by sufficient evidence of carcinogenicity in experimental animals. In this instance, limited evidence (in humans) is present when a positive association has been observed between exposure to the agent and cancer for which a casual interpretation is considered to be credible, but chance, bias or confounding, cannot be excluded with confidence. Sufficient evidence in animals relates to an increased incidence of the development of malignant tumors in (a) multiple species, (b) multiple experiments, or (c) an atypical manner.

Polychlorinated biphenyls (PCBs), dioxin, and a host of other agents are placed in this category, even though the evidence that, e.g., PCBs are carcinogenic in humans is far from compelling and indeed is tenuous. Unfortunately, the prevailing philosophy of many governmental agencies is to accept positive animal experimentation over negative human studies.

CAUSATION

The assumption of a cause and effect relationship between exposure to a certain agent and the development of disease needs to be considered meticulously and should not be accepted without methodical validation. Observation may suggest or propound that certain happenings regularly follow other events or circumstances; from then on, there is often intuitive inference that remains essential to confirm. Moreover, causation is seldom related to a single factor or exposure, but depends on a series of influences, a concatenation of events or circumstances. Thus, in lung cancer there may be multiple exposures to, e.g., asbestos, cigarette smoke, and radon daughters, whereas other factors such as heredity and diet may also be important. Tolstoy realized the distinction between association and cause and effect when he wrote in *War and Peace,* "Whenever I look at my watch and see the hands pointing to 10, I hear the bells begin to ring in the church close by; but I have no right to assume that the movement of the bell is caused by the position of the hands of my watch."

In considering statistical evidence relating to a set of data and any inferences drawn from them, Bradford Hill recommended that the evidence be assessed in such a way as to answer the crucial question, "is there any other explanation for the happenings or facts before us?" To assess whether there is indeed a cause and effect relationship, Bradford Hill recommended nine criteria that should be used to assess the evidence (7). These can be shortened to six, and include consistency, strength, specificity, chronological relationships, dose response, and biologic plausibility.

Consistency

The presence of one study purporting to show that a particular agent is harmful is insufficient, and there must be multiple studies with comparable results. Thus, almost every investigation that has been performed on lung cancer has shown a preeminent effect of cigarette smoking in the development of the tumor.

Strength

Slight increases in relative risk or the standard mortality rate (SMR) in lung cancer or other respiratory diseases for a par-

ticular type of occupation need to be evaluated with caution. For example, a SMR that is greater than 100 but less than 200 cannot necessarily be regarded as significant without the most careful exclusion of other factors, some of which may not have been considered. This is usually difficult and often impossible.

Specificity

Lung cancer is most commonly related to cigarette smoking; however, it is known that the presence of asbestosis in conjunction with cigarette smoking greatly increases the risk. Similarly, exposure to radon daughters in the absence of cigarette smoking can cause lung cancer, but the risk increases greatly in smokers. It is therefore necessary to ascertain whether there has been a specific exposure or multiple exposures that may explain the development of the particular type of cancer.

Chronological Relationships

There must be an incubation period from the time of first exposure to the time of development of a particular disease. It is illogical to assume that 1 year of exposure to asbestos, even in a cigarette smoker, will lead to the development of lung cancer within 2 to 3 or even 5 years. In general, lung cancer presents only after at least 15 years of smoking, whereas the incubation period for mesothelioma is, for the most part, 25 to 40 years after first exposure.

Dose Response

There is little doubt that many conditions require a cumulative exposure before the disease develops. Thus, there is reliable evidence to indicate that asbestos and excess lung cancer will not develop in workers exposed to less than 1 fiber/cm^3 of asbestos over a working life of 35 to 40 years. Although some casual associations may not show an apparent trend with exposure, most of the etiological agents that cause lung cancer (e.g., asbestos, nickel, and uranium) show an effect that increases with cumulative exposure.

Biologic Plausibility

If the disease can be also produced in animals and has similar features to those that occur in humans, this can be regarded as credible evidence to support a cause and effect relationship. Thus, the development of disease must be in accord with existing biologic facts. Clearly, it is inappropriate to perform experiments in humans that might lead to serious disease such as cancer. Jenner's initial experiment on Billy Phelps, on whom he tested the efficacy of cowpox vaccination for the control of smallpox, may pass muster as a human experiment, and similarly, John Snow's removal of the Broad Street pump handle to control a cholera epidemic also might be classified as a human experiment.

EPIDEMIOLOGICAL STUDIES

Epidemiological studies in humans might be classified as (a) historical cohort studies, (b) case control studies, (c) studies of subjects with a particular condition, and (d) record linkage of etiological studies. For the most part, cohort studies have greater power and are most likely to produce valid results. Simple case series, studies of proportional mortality, and studies of cancer morbidity are less reliable and may be misleading.

Despite the clear-cut criteria established by Bradford Hill, there is little doubt that many human studies purporting to show an increased risk of cancer in various occupations, as well as in particular lung cancer, are of dubious validity. This is particularly true of many of the investigations that have attempted to relate exposure to silica, or other fibroses produced by the dust, to the development of lung cancer. Thus, studies performed on those who have been compensated for a particular disease, e.g., silicosis, are much more likely to have symptoms, and it is the symptoms that make them seek medical attention and undergo the necessary examinations. In the case of chest disease, the particular symptoms that are a cause of concern are cough, sputum, and shortness of breath, and the commonest cause of all three is cigarette smoking. The study of Ng and colleagues from Singapore in which a cohort of subjects was selected from the Singapore Silicosis Register is a classic example (8). The prevalence of smoking in their cohort of silicotics was 91% compared with 60% in the general male population of Singapore. Thus, the excessive lung cancer SMR in their cohort was derived by comparing smoking silicotics with the general male population of Singapore without taking into account the different smoking habits of the two groups.

The epidemiological investigation of occupational lung cancer requires large numbers of subjects, relevant information re smoking, and exposure to the suspected agents. It is these data that are most likely to incriminate the suspected agent.

EXTENT OF RISK: OCCUPATION VERSUS SMOKING

When a substance causing cancer in the human has been identified and proven to be causally related, then it either must be avoided or used as little as possible. This assumes that no suitable substitute is available. The portion of the blame that can be attached to various environmental agents thought to be carcinogens has been a topic of debate for the past three decades. Most of the epidemiological investigations have relied on the incidence and prevalence of occupational

and other cancers that have occurred in various countries and populations.

It has been suggested by those who dwell in never-never land that environmental factors account for 80% of human cancers. The leading advocate of the environment as the main cause of cancer is Epstein, but his views are too radical and unrealistic to be accepted, except by himself (9). Bridbord and colleagues at the National Cancer Institute and the National Institute of Occupational Safety and Health (NIOSH) claimed that occupational cancers comprised between 23% and 38% of all cancers (10). This figure is excessive and is mainly related to the fact that Bridbord and colleagues were mostly interested in asbestos-related cancers, neglecting other causes of cancer. These investigators were particularly concerned with the exposure to, and duration of, asbestos exposure; factors that cannot be assessed reliably. Bridbord and colleagues assumed a constant exposure of the same level of airborne asbestos, when in reality the threshold limit value (TLV) significantly decreased over the years. During the past several decades industrial hygiene in North America and Europe as a whole has greatly improved. Coke ovens, power stations, nickel smelters, etc., have restricted the level of their effluents. By far the best monograph relating to occupational cancer, despite its dotage, is that of Doll and Peto. This was published in 1981 in its entirety in the *Journal of the National Cancer Institute* (11).

Large differences in lung cancer rates between occupations exist and are best explained by the prevalence and intensity of smoking habits. The frequency of smoking varies greatly according to job, religion, and other factors. In an ancient but still pertinent *Lancet* editorial entitled "What Proportions of Cancers are Related to Occupation?," the author pointed out the problems associated with comparing the mortality from malignant disease in Britain according to social class (12). The Registrar General's decennial supplement on occupational mortality records the mortality from malignant diseases by five social classes. These range from unskilled workers to the professions. The 1978 supplement showed an increasing gradient of mortality from malignant neoplasms for skilled, semiskilled, and nonskilled workers. Skilled manual workers had a SMR of 113, whereas skilled nonmanual workers had a SMR of 91. The gradient risk is not as steep as one might anticipate, particularly in view of the fact that occupation is only one of the factors that determines social class mortality. Smoking, in particular, and other habits play a far more important role. By determining the risk of lung cancer for various levels of smoking and relating these to social class, it was possible to show that manual laborers had a lung cancer risk that was 22% higher than that of administrative and clerical workers. Because at that time lung cancer in Britain in men was responsible for just under two fifths of the deaths from all cancers (the incidence of lung cancer in these groups increased over the next 10 years), the effects of smoking and the increased rate of lung cancer would increase the risk for manual workers of all cancers by 9%. Since 1978, there has been a decline in smoking among all classes, but the decline has been least in blue collar workers. Although certain occupations are undoubtedly associated with an increased risk for lung cancer, it is fallacious to assume that occupational exposures to carcinogens are necessarily responsible for most lung cancers, and there is no doubt that the most common carcinogen to which blue collar workers are exposed is cigarette smoke.

A further consideration is the effect of the combination of smoking and exposure to a known occupational carcinogen. A good example of this is the much more frequent occurrence of lung cancer in those with asbestosis and who are cigarette smokers. There are those who maintain that asbestos alone is a carcinogen, but the evidence for this is tenuous and will be discussed in more detail later. Similar effects have been observed in uranium miners, those working in coke ovens, and those exposed to effluents from nickel smelters. The smoking habit vastly increases the number of occupational cancers and, in addition, reduces the age at which cancer develops.

A prospective study of cancer mortality by Shopland and colleagues of over 1.2 million men and women was published in the *Journal of the National Cancer Institute* in 1991 (13). The American Cancer Society projected that cigarette smoking alone would contribute slightly more than 154,000 of the total 514,000 cancer deaths occurring in the United States in 1991. At that time, smoking directly contributed to 25% of all cancer deaths in women and 45% of all cancer deaths in men. Since then, the rate of lung cancer has increased to around 35% to 40% in women, whereas the rate in men has fallen to around 40%. Lung cancer had displaced coronary heart disease as the leading cause of excess mortality among smokers in the United States. Considering that very few women work with asbestos or in coke ovens, uranium mines, etc., it becomes abundantly clear that the vast majority of men and women who develop lung cancer do so from smoking without any interaction from other carcinogens.

INVESTIGATION OF OCCUPATIONAL LUNG CANCER

The investigation of a potential occupational carcinogen can be effected in two ways: laboratory testing and epidemiological surveys. There is a place for both methods, although some agencies tend to give more weight to laboratory testing of animals than to epidemiology. This is a little surprising because the majority of discoveries relating to occupational lung cancer have been made by astute observation, backed by epidemiological confirmation. This approach, not only led to the description of the first occupational neoplasm but also was used by others to identify the association between asbestos and lung cancer and mesothelioma, nickel with lung and nasal cancer, and the making of furniture with nasal cancer.

Laboratory studies also have an important place, particularly when a carcinogen is suspected, not because of an increased incidence in a certain trade, but because a particular chemical has a structure similar to that of a known carcinogen. Thus, the experimental approach was used to confirm the carcinogenicity of the chloromethyl ethers.

Laboratory Testing

If suspicion arises concerning a particular substance that physically or chemically resembles a known carcinogen, the approach should be to use *in vitro* testing, and if the suspicion is warranted, progression to animal exposure studies is appropriate. *In vitro* tests are the quickest and cheapest method of examining potential carcinogens; however, their use is limited because their only function is to show whether or not a particular substance has any effect on DNA. They can be used as a screening test for new materials and are used to show that one carcinogen is more dangerous than another. During *in vitro* testing, the ability of a substance to transform mammalian fibroblasts into particular colonies with malignant characteristics is sought, or as in the Ames test, a change in the rate of mutation of a nutritionally deficient strain on *Salmonella typhimurium* may be demonstrated. When such tests are used, known carcinogens will produce positive results nine times out of 10; however, false-positive and false-negative results occur. No test is yet available that shows whether there is a threshold below which a suspected carcinogen is innocuous in humans.

Animal studies provide data that are more readily applied to humans. Besides ethical considerations, there are important limitations; the production of tumors in animals is uncertain and unpredictable and depends not only on variations between species but also on factors such as sex, diet, and age. Most animal experiments consist of a relatively short exposure of small rodents to substances at inordinately higher concentrations than those that are encountered in the work place. Although valuable information can be obtained from animal experiments, as was the case with chloromethyl ethers, the results of carcinogenesis in animals should not be applied without thought to humans.

The problem with laboratory studies as a determinant of carcinogenic properties lies in the process of carcinogenesis itself. Some time ago, it was felt that certain compounds act as initiators and induce mutation in the DNA or target cells (irradiation, halo ethers, mustard gas). Others such as asbestos were responsible for the second phase of carcinogenesis and were said to act as promoters that induced increased cell multiplication. The initiator/promoter concept is by no means proven but has appeal. Most compounds act directly on DNA; however, nickel interferes with replication, whereas benzpyrene requires activation by the host before carcinogenic properties develop. As mentioned earlier, it is all too evident that the basic mechanisms of carcinogenesis are incompletely understood, and for this reason, laboratory testing is, at best, a rough estimate of the risks that can be involved. Laboratory tests should not be used to declare a compound safe or unsafe, but rather should be used as an indicator of whether protection, surveillance, and further research is required. Animal and other laboratory tests should not be rated more highly than well-designed human epidemiological studies.

PREVENTION OF OCCUPATIONAL LUNG CANCER

Prevention is the most effective method of treating lung cancer, but the prevention of occupational pulmonary neoplasia cannot be realistically separated from the prevention of lung cancer as a whole. Most lung cancers are avoidable by avoiding exposure to the known carcinogens. The American Cancer Society records a prevalence of lung cancer of around 150,000 to 160,000 deaths per year, and although approximately 5% to 10% are associated for the most part with smoking and exposure to occupational and other carcinogens, the majority are a result of smoking alone (13). Fewer than 5% of lung cancers are unrelated to smoking. In any discussion of prevention, these facts must be considered.

The responsibility for reducing the incidence of carcinoma rests with the medical profession, industry, government, and workers. The medical profession must make the facts available to all of the above. Those involved in medicine and science must continue epidemiologic surveillance and research to identify new hazards, and study must be accomplished with the available financial resources. Industry must accept advice from informed sources and do its utmost to protect workers. Government must act responsibly, with its first priority being the health of the work force. Workers must be informed of the risks and must use all protective methods necessary. The pre-eminent reality is that workers must be aware of the risk of smoking, especially in the setting of an occupation with a known hazard.

Surveillance

Although prevention is the best approach to occupational cancer, another, albeit a less effective, alternative exists, namely, the detection of early cases of disease in the hope that prognosis can be improved. There has been much debate concerning the value of screening for occupational cancer, and although the concept of medical monitoring has been received enthusiastically, it must be remembered that the value of screening programs is based on the assumption that early diagnosis is beneficial. Although this is true for most infections, it is not necessarily the case for lung cancer. Is the early detection of mesothelioma beneficial when neither palliation nor cure is available? Similarly, many such early detection studies do not take into account "lead time." Suppose a patient presents in 2002 with lung cancer. The cancer is found to be operable with no overt evidence of metastases.

The patient has a lobectomy, but in 2006 has a recurrence and dies. Thus, the survival time was 4 years. Had the patient had a computed axial tomography scan and cytological examination in 1998, the tumor would probably have been detected and removed. Nonetheless, the patient would still have died in 2006. Thus, survival time increased to 8 years, but the patient died at exactly the same time.

In 1968, the World Health Organization (WHO) published guidelines for screening programs (14). These still apply today. Although most of the criteria are relevant to occupational neoplasia, three of them require special mention. First, there should be an acceptable form of treatment for patients with recognizable disease; second, the cost of case finding needs to be balanced economically in relation to possible expenditure for medical care as a whole; and third, the benefits accruing to persons with true-positive findings should outweigh the harm done as a result of false-positive diagnoses. Added to the required standards of the screening program, the tests chosen must be accurate, sensitive, and specific and have predictive value.

The two tests most easily available for screening occupational lung cancer are the chest radiograph and sputum cytology. Although both these techniques are useful in detecting cancer, in practice many problems still arise. Studies using serial radiography have not improved survival or, at best, have had only a minimal effect. A particular problem is the case of patients with positive sputum cytology but no detectable tumor at fiberoptic bronchoscopy. Segmental bronchial lavage can be performed in an attempt to localize the tumor to a particular segment, but malignant cells can often be retrieved from several sites and from both lungs, presumably as a result of spillover.

The results of an extensive three-center study on screening for lung cancer were published in 1984. The studies left little doubt that cancers could be detected earlier. The radiograph was the most sensitive method, with 40% of cancers identified as stage I (American Joint Committee on Cancer), whereas sputum cytology was effective only in the detection of early squamous cell carcinomata. Despite early detection, it was not clear that there was any subsequent decrease in mortality (15).

Finally, the cost of screening needs to be considered. In one reported experience, the cost per person per year was $135, and as the prevalence of detectable lung cancer is very low (one in 2,000 to 3,000), the cost-to-benefit ratio becomes prohibitive. In an earlier series using the chest radiograph, the cost of detection of each cancer by bronchoscopy and sputum examination was $25,000, with no increase in life expectancy. High-resolution computed axial tomography scanning is being used frequently for early detection of lung cancer, but it is yet unknown whether cure is more frequent. A detailed and rewarding review of the findings of the three-center study is to be found in *Pulmonary Diseases* (sixth edition), which is published by Lippincott–Raven Publishers (15).

Management

The treatment of occupational lung cancer is no different from that in the nonoccupational setting. In general, the disease is incurable, but surgical resection is the treatment of choice and, if successful, affords the patient a 20% to 30% chance of surviving 5 years. The prognosis in occupational lung cancer is slightly worse for two reasons. First, there is a preponderance of small cell carcinoma and adenocarcinomata, both of which have a worse prognosis than that of the squamous cell type. Second, many workers have concurrent lung disease, such as fibrosis, which may make surgery less feasible.

A relatively new concept is chemoprevention, although at this time no proven chemopreventative method exists. Recently, antioxidants and retinols (vitamin A–like compounds) have been used for the prevention and treatment of lung cancer, with little or no success. Numerous drugs and other agents have been used in the hope of either avoiding the development of lung cancer or extending life. Most have been ineffective.

DEFINITE CAUSES OF OCCUPATIONAL LUNG CANCER

Arsenic

Arsenic has been recognized as a carcinogen for many years. As early as 1820, it was thought to cause scrotal cancer, and somewhat later, its therapeutic administration was recognized as a cause of skin cancer. In 1934, lung and skin cancer were found in workers who were involved in making sheep dip containing arsenic. Subsequently, it became evident that most of those involved with the manufacture of sheep dip developed the manifestations of arsenic poisoning, namely hyperpigmentation, warts, and hyperkeratosis (16).

Exposure to arsenic is relatively rare in Europe and North America, but a risk still exists in the preparation of pesticides and metal refining and in the chemical industry (17).

Asbestos

The inhalation and deposition of asbestos in sufficient quantities leads to the development of lung cancer and mesothelioma of the pleura, peritoneum, and tunica vaginalis. The latter is rare and may not be related to asbestos exposure.

Occupational Risks of Exposure to Asbestos

In former times, those who worked in asbestos mills were at a high risk of developing asbestosis (18,19). This was particularly true of carders and weavers. There are few asbestos mills now in North America or in Europe, with the exception of Russia and its immediate neighbors. By way of contrast, the risks associated with asbestos mining have been, and still

are, appreciably fewer. This is true of the chrysotile miners in Quebec and applies not only to mesothelioma but also to the development of asbestosis and lung cancer. An exception is the relatively high risk of miners of crocidolite, with particular emphasis on the now closed down Wittenoom mine in West Australia.

Welders, pipe fitters, and laggers, especially those who used band saws at one time were initially thought not to be at increased risk, but Selikoff proved that asbestos lagging was a major hazard in ship building (20). However, asbestos is now rarely used for the insulation of pipes. Much the same can be said for railway repair shed workers whose job it was to line the furnaces of steam locomotives. Garage mechanics working with brake linings do not appear to be at risk, as the chrysotile is changed to fosterite and rendered innocuous as a result of the immense heat that is generated when brakes are applied. Although new cases of asbestosis are rare, it must be borne in mind that there are still many workers who were exposed to asbestos 20 to 40, or more, years ago and are still at risk of developing mesothelioma. New cases of asbestosis are now rare in North America.

Asbestos as a Carcinogen

Asbestos used to be termed a co-carcinogen, but it was the fact that those who were smokers, and who also had asbestosis, were most prone to the greatly increased incidence of lung cancer. Lung cancer rarely, if ever, occurred in nonsmokers, whether or not they had asbestosis.

It has been estimated in the United States that 430,000 construction workers and 650,000 workers involved in manufacturing asbestos had in the past been "significantly" exposed to asbestos. These estimates were based on a National Institute for Occupational Safety and Health study that calculated that asbestos plays a role in approximately 3% of all lung cancers that occur in the United States, (i.e., 2,501 deaths/y), with the major contribution to the induction of lung cancer being cigarette smoking (21). Over the past three decades, a number of studies have shown that provided the level of asbestos in the air is kept below 1 fiber/cm^3, the risk of the developing asbestosis is negligible (22–26). Similarly, at exposure levels below 1 fiber/cm^3, there is no increased risk of lung cancer developing over a 35- to 40-year working life. In most of these studies, the workers were only exposed to chrysotile. It needs to be borne in mind that lung cancer has been diagnosed in only about 30 or so lifelong nonsmoking workers with asbestosis. Were the smoking histories in these few subjects inaccurate, as is often the case when compensation is being claimed, the incidence in nonsmokers would completely disappear.

Great differences exist between the calculated relative risks of lung cancer obtained by different investigators. Such differences are to be expected in the absence of uniform and consistent protocols. It is generally accepted that the risk for development of lung cancer is related to the cumulative dose;

however, the selection of subjects for epidemiological studies has differed greatly, with some including only workers with prolonged exposure to asbestos ($\geq$20 years), whereas other investigators accepted any exposure of 6 months or longer. Clearly, these variables greatly influence the incidence of asbestosis. The excess risk of lung cancer developing over the period 1960–1990 did not occur until the subject had been exposed to asbestos for at least 15 years and had evidence of asbestosis, this being accepted as the latent period. The development of lung cancer in a subject who has worked with asbestos for only 5 years before the development of his cancer indicates that the tumor is not a consequence of asbestos exposure.

Fiber Type

Fiber type is of great importance in that the risks of the use of certain fibers are greater than risks for others. The likelihood of developing asbestosis, mesothelioma, or lung cancer is much less with chrysotile than it is with amosite or crocidolite. The fibers of chrysotile gradually leach out of the lungs, unlike those of the amphiboles. There is some doubt about whether chrysotile itself ever causes lung cancer. It is certainly true that lung cancer occurs in those exposed to chrysotile, but the subjects who have developed lung cancer have also been exposed to tremolite, the latter being an amphibole known to cause mesothelioma and lung cancer. Amosite is also associated with the risk of lung cancer and, in particular, mesothelioma, but amosite is less hazardous than is crocidolite. Anthophyllite rarely, if ever, causes mesothelioma.

Although asbestosis is declining rapidly in North America, mesothelioma is still present and, if not increasing, is holding steady as far as new cases are concerned. It is likely, however, that with the decline in the use of crocidolite and amosite in North America, there will be a decline in the incidence of mesothelioma, but it may take another 5 to 10 years before this becomes evident.

In their review of the death rates in asbestos insulation workers, Seidman and Selikoff stated that "crocidolite was not used by the insulation workers studied by us" (27). The statement was made so as to indicate that the mesotheliomata that were occurring in the New Jersey shipyards were caused by chrysotile and not by crocidolite, as indicated by Mossman and others (28). The Seidman and Selikoff pronouncement contradicts a number of statements that have appeared in the *Annals of the New York Academy of Sciences* (volume 132), which happened to be edited by the late Dr. Selikoff himself. Thus Hendry, a Johns Mansville geologist, noted that in 1963, 17,000 tons of crocidolite were used in the United States for the manufacture of filters, packing, insulation, and certain types of lagging (29). Selikoff and colleagues later stated in the monograph that crocidolite was found in a number of magnesia insulating blocks (30). It is quite evident that the main cause of mesothelioma in the

United States was, and still is, crocidolite, with amosite being second. There is little evidence to indicate that chrysotile is responsible for the induction of mesothelioma.

Dose-Response Relationships: Type of Work Exposure

A number of studies have been performed to estimate the effects of cumulative asbestos exposure on the induction of lung cancer, along with the level of risk. For the most part, an approximately linear trend has been shown with increasing cumulative exposure, providing allowance is made for a latency period of 15 to 20 years. Lung cancer risk is expressed either as a ratio of observed lung cancers to those expected or as an SMR. The estimated risk varies considerably from study to study. A number of reviews in which the estimated slopes and the various factors that might influence the steepness of the slopes have been analyzed (31, 32). McDonald and colleagues performed a follow-up study in Quebec chrysotile miners, millers, and in some asbestos factories (33). They took into account dust exposures and cigarette smoking in the presence of asbestos. The SMR for lung cancer rose nonsignificantly from 1.25 to 1.39, although deaths from mesothelioma increased from eight to 25. The mortality rates from asbestos and mesothelioma were strongly associated with exposure. There was no evidence to suggest that transient exposures of a month or so could lead to the development of mesothelioma as has been suggested.

In regard to the development of lung cancer in exposed workers, the assumption that there is a linear relationship has received wide but uncritical acceptance. Such a hypothesis is convenient and simple, but is not necessarily valid. It is equally inappropriate to infer that the line of identity must pass through the zero point. Deductions based on the observations of the risk of lung cancer in subjects with high exposure cannot be relied on to predict the response to low or trivial exposures. Back extrapolation of the regression line to a zero intercept in many instances is contrived, and although it demonstrates a neat and pleasing appearance to the eye, it has little statistical justification. It needs to be borne in mind that there are few or no excess deaths that occur with the lower exposures, and Liddell and Hanley and others have shown that the intercept varies significantly according to certain mathematical assumptions, and to variations of estimates of cumulative exposure (31,32). There is much mathematical justification, in most instances, for projecting the progression line so that it has either a negative or positive intercept (Fig. 46.1).

The evidence that chrysotile is less of a risk in regard to lung cancer than are the amphiboles is suggestive but not completely conclusive. The added risk of chrysotile causing lung cancer is around 20%. For mixed exposures of chrysotile and the amphiboles, the figure is 50%; for amphiboles only, from 100% to 380% (34,35). There are many statements to

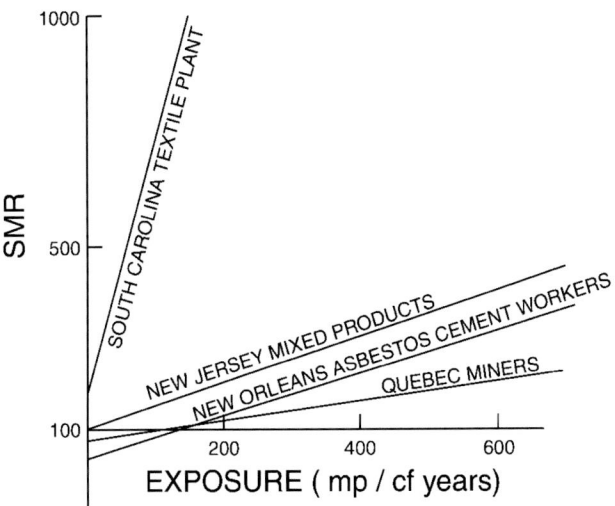

FIGURE 46.1. The standard mortality rate for lung cancer in various exposed populations, showing a lesser risk in asbestos miners. *mp/cf* years, million particles/cubic foot/years.

the contrary, but there is no evidence that asbestos exposure leads to cancer of the larynx or colon (36,37).

Erionite

Erionite is a zeolite and has a fibrous configuration. It is a hydrated alumina silicate and, similar to perlite, originates from volcanic activity. Its crystalline lattice structure makes it useful for molecular sieves, and catalysts. It is found in Oregon, Cappadocia, and New Zealand.

A high incidence of mesothelioma has been found in Cappadocia. This has been traced to exposure to fibers of erionite that have been inhaled. The symptoms of mesothelioma are similar to those induced by asbestos, and similar to the latter, erionite-induced mesothelioma is often preceded by a pleural effusion (38). Many families have built their own house by using local rock contaminated by erionite. The fibers of the latter are also present in much of the soil in Cappadocia. The evidence suggests the almost indefinite persistence of erionite fibers in lung tissue.

Chloroethers

Chloroethers are alkylating agents that have been used in industrial processes as intermediates in organic synthesis, organic solvents, bactericides, fungicides, and cross-linking agents. An alkylating agent with a definite carcinogenic potency is *bis*-(bischloromethyl ether) (BCME), also known as bischlorodimethylether. BCME is unique among causes of human bronchial carcinoma, and activity was first demonstrated in animal experiments (39). This led to epidemiological studies that showed a considerable risk of oat cell cancer in humans (40,41). The carcinogenicity of BCME was first demonstrated in 1968 by painting the skin of mice and by subcutaneous injection in rats. It was also noted that of the

30 mice treated with BCME, papillomata developed in 13, 12 of which progressed to squamous cell carcinomata. The results were confirmed by additional experiments in newborn mice.

Because industrial exposure to BCME usually occurs as a result of inhalation rather than subcutaneous injection, several animal inhalation experiments were undertaken. This led to the development of lung cancer in a significant proportion of rats, around 30% to 40%. Human studies by Figueroa and colleagues (40) and Lemen (41) showed that the incidence of lung cancer was similar, around 3% to 5% among manufacturing workers. This was less than the 12% found by Sakabe in a study in which five subjects developed lung cancer among the 32 who were exposed to BCME (42). The predominance of small cell carcinomata noted in these studies was significant.

Coke Production

In 1775, Pott provided the initial evidence that indicated that carcinogenic agents are produced during the carbonization or combustion of bituminous coal. Since that time, a great amount of information linking excess cancers to several sites among workers in coal combustion or carbonization occupations has been noted. These included excess cancer rates in chimney sweeps and in several categories of gas work employees. The lung cancer rates for gas stokers and coke oven workers were about three times the expected rate (43).

Workers involved in the destructive distillation of coal, i.e., coke production, have been shown by Lloyd to have an increased risk of bronchial cancer (44). The lung cancer mortality rates were twice that expected among all coke oven workers, and the rate increased 10-fold among those employed full time for five or more years on oven tops. Similar studies showed the same increased death rate in British coke workers (45); however, the risk of death was somewhat lower than that found by Lloyd (44). The studies in the United States were extended to evaluate exposure relationships for coal tar pitch volatiles and lung cancer (46). Steps were taken to cut back on the exposure from coke oven fumes and coal tar pitch volatiles. Over the past 20 or so years, the death rates have fallen appreciably.

Chromates

Exposure to certain hexavalent chromium compounds, mainly those that are water insoluble, is related to an increased risk of lung cancer in certain selected workers. By way of contrast, the trivalent chromium compounds are not carcinogenic in either humans or animals. These water-soluble hexavalent chromium compounds, such as chromic acid mist and chromate dusts, can be severe irritants to the nasopharynx, lungs, and skin.

The earliest association for lung cancer owing to exposure to chromium was made by Alwens and Jonas, who noted an excessive frequency of lung cancer among workers involved in the heavy metal industry in Germany (47). Similar findings originated from studies in six major U.S. factories that produced chromates. High rates of lung cancer were found, and the evidence suggested that 16 monochromates, (as opposed to dichromates and trivalent chromates) were likely responsible. These results were confirmed by Baetjer, Mancuso, and Hueper, who studied the mortality rates of workers of a chromate plant and found that the proportional of mortality rate for lung cancer was 15 times the expected rate in the general population (48).

Those chromate workers who died from lung cancer had a high chromium content in their lungs. The average chromium content in six patients with lung cancer who were chromate workers was found to be 36.7 μg of chromium per gram of lung tissue, whereas an nonexposed lung cancer case would have only around 0.21 μg of chromium per gram of lung tissue (49). Without doubt, excessive exposure to insoluble hexavalent chromium compounds is related to increased lung cancer rates. Workers involved in chromate production and the chromate pigment industry are at the highest risk. In addition, it has been suggested that exposure to certain soluble hexavalent chromium compounds, including chromium trioxide in electroplating operations, also increases the risk of bronchogenic cancer as the chromium content increases. Workers involved in a chromate pigment industry are at the greatest risk.

Nickel

The earliest nickel refinery was established in Birmingham in 1900 by Langer and Mond. The first observation of a relationship between nasal cancer and nickel exposure was contained in a report from the chief inspector of factories in the United Kingdom (50). Although 10 cases of nasal cancer were initially identified among the refinery workers, further follow-up resulted in a total of 52 cases of nasal cancer and 93 cases of lung cancer (51). Doll and colleagues studied workers in the same refinery and reported that the deaths from lung cancer were five to 10 times higher among men hired before 1925 (52). Deaths from nasal cancer were more than 100 times greater than expected.

The study of lung cancer deaths and nickel exposure in the United Kingdom was undertaken by Kreyberg (53), who included the findings of others in his evaluation (54). Most lung cancers were of the small cell, anaplastic, and epidermoid types. As expected, the excess lung cancers were particularly prevalent among cigarette smokers, but the role of tobacco smoke in nickel-induced lung cancer remains unclear.

Part of the problem relates to the fact that it has not been possible to identify which nickel compounds are human carcinogens. It appears that the cancer risk is associated mostly with early stages of nickel refining, with lung and nasal sinuses being the target organs most affected (54). It has been suggested that nickel subsulfides and oxides are the most likely carcinogenic agents (55).

A report of an international committee on nickel carcinogenesis proved to be enlightening (56). Ten cohort studies were reviewed and indicated that the excess risk only occurred in nasal sinuses and the lungs. Excess cancer occurred in workers exposed predominantly to soluble nickel. It was also shown that pure nickel powder seemed to be devoid of the risk. The current TLVs are set at 1 mg/m^3 for soluble nickel and 10 mg/m^3 for insoluble nickel. The current TLV appears to offer an increase in the safety factor relative to current exposures. The number of lung cancer deaths occurring in Ontario nickel miners have decreased and seem to be around the general rate to be expected in the population. The decline could be owing to, in part, a decrease in cigarette smoking.

Fluorspar

This mineral, calcium fluoride, is used as a flux in steel making and in the production of aluminum and ceramics. It is a source of fluorine for the chemical industry. The use of fluorspar is worldwide. Certain fluorspar deposits in Newfoundland, which had been worked since the 1930s, were found to be associated with a vastly increased risk of lung cancer (57). Studies showed that the fluorspar miners in this region had a death rate 29 to 30 times greater than that of the unexposed population. The difference could not be attributed to cigarette smoking or pneumoconiosis, and environmental investigation found that the mine air was as radioactive as most uranium mines; however, no radioactive ore was present in the mines. The radioactivity was later shown to emanate from radon daughters dissolved in water that had seeped into the mines. Steps were taken to eliminate the seepage of the affected water.

Uranium and Radioactive Elements

Uranium occurs as an oxide, as pitchblende or as a compound oxide with vanadium and potassium, known as carnotite. The ore contains amounts of silica varying from 5% to 50%, and as a result, uranium mining entails a risk of silicosis. Uranium mining is prevalent in Slovakia, the United States, the Congo, Canada, and Australia. Both surface and deep mining are used, along with drilling and blasting techniques similar to those used in hard rock mining.

The ore that is removed is crushed at the mill, often on the site of the mine. The uranium is then extracted in the form of an uranite, which is also known as yellowcake. This is packed into drums for transportation to the user. The dust is liable to be liberated during these two processes. Uranium is now used principally for production of atomic energy for both peaceful and military purposes and, to some extent, in the ceramics and chemical industries. Laboratory workers who handle uranium are at particular risk from toxic effects that may cause lung cancer.

Fatal lung cancer was first described in miners working in the Erz Mountains in central Europe (58). The excess mortality in the Schneeberg metal mines caused by lung cancer was likely related to the same radioactivity (2). Further similar risks were discovered in association with radioactivity in uranium mines in Colorado and Utah, in hard rock miners in the United States (59), in hematite miners in Cambria, Great Britain (60), and in fluorspar miners in Newfoundland, as described earlier (57).

The most detailed study of the effects of uranium mining on the lungs was performed in the United States from 1950–1967. The mortality rate was related to the calculated cumulative exposure expressed in working months. A working level month is defined as an exposure of 170 working hours to a level of radon daughters of 1 L of air resulting in the emission of 1.3×10^5 MeV of potential alpha energy.

Uranium itself is not dangerous from a biologic point of view, in that it emits mainly gamma rays that are of such high energy that they pass through the human body. The problem occurs as the uranium decays (Fig. 46.2). The first step in the decay series is from ^{238}U to ^{226}Ra, which in turn decays to ^{222}Rn. This element, which is one of the noble gases, decays into its daughters ^{218}Po and ^{214}Po, ^{214}Pb, and ^{214}Bi. Because these radon daughters are ionized metal atoms, they become attached to dust and water vapor. Thus, the radon daughters can be inhaled into the respiratory tract, where they emit alpha radiation. Of particular importance are those daughters that have a short half-life and, as a result, cannot be cleared from the respiratory tract before their energy is emitted. The alpha particles have a range of 40 to 70 λ sufficient at the site of impact to damage the mucosal cells and initiate carcinogenesis.

The interaction between cigarette smoking and radiation is important. Initially, the incidence of smoking was extremely high in the Colorado miners, so high that it was initially believed that smoking was a prerequisite for cancer in uranium miners. Further studies have shown that although uranium miners who smoke have a high risk, nonsmoking miners are by no means immune from having a fourfold increase. Exposure to workers can be prevented by reducing atmospheric levels of radon daughters to a minimum, and providing ventilation and sealing off high risk areas, and controlling water seepage. The work force should be monitored on an individual basis, and exposures should be controlled according to defined standards. In the United States, this is 4 working-level months (WLM) per year with actual exposure levels being 1 to 2 WLM per year.

Coal Tar Derivatives

In addition to coke ovens, there is an excess risk of lung cancer in those who are exposed to fuels such as coal, coal gas, and coal tar, all of which have been shown to have an increased incidence of coal tar. It can be assumed that the same agents that cause cancer in coke oven workers and coal tar pitch volatiles are involved in causing lung cancer in gas works employees, stokers, and possibly selected foundry workers (43,61).

Other recognized agents include mustard gas. Those who manufacture the gas are prone to develop lung cancer. Mustard gas is an alkylating agent and has an effect on cells similar to radiation exposure. Wada and colleagues studied mustard gas production workers in Japan and determined that 33 deaths from respiratory tract carcinomata had occurred since 1952 (62). The findings on the rest of the population used for comparison cancer rates showed a threefold to 40-fold excess. The neoplasms that developed were either squamous or undifferentiated and appeared to be located centrally (63).

A number of other agents have been suggested as carcinogens. These include vinyl chloride, which is certainly

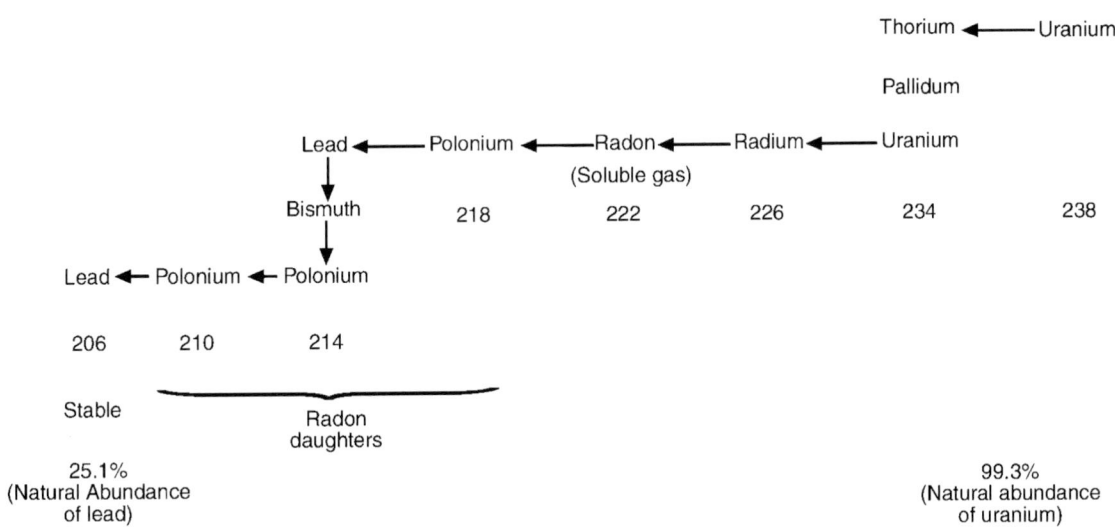

FIGURE 46.2. Simplified natural decay series of uranium.

involved in the development of angiosarcoma of the liver and has also been suggested as being a cause of lung cancer. The association is weak, and other studies have attributed the problem to smoking.

Silica, Alleged Carcinogen

"Inhaled crystalline silica in the form or quartz or cristobalite is carcinogenic to humans. Amorphous silica is not classifiable as to its carcinogenicity in humans," so reads IARC monograph volume 68 (64). This was the conclusion of the IARC working committee on the evaluation of carcinogenic risks in humans, which took place in Lyon on October 15–22, 1996. It must be pointed out that those who voted for the motion that silica is a carcinogen only just prevailed, because nearly as many able physicians and scientists voted against the motion.

The evidence that silica is a carcinogen is tenuous. Numerous different groups of workers are exposed to crystalline silica, including metal miners, roof bolters and drillers in coal mines to some extent, granite shed workers, and those working in quarries. Other exposures occur in those working with tiles and clays, pottery workers, glass manufacturers, stonecutters, nonmetallic minerals, foundry workers, refractory workers, and those who dig tunnels and sandblast. Many workers will state that they have a particular occupation, but it is often difficult to know exactly what they do; it is therefore important to have a detailed description of their activities. Aside from those who work with crystalline silica, some persons are exposed, sometimes unknowingly. Persons who live in the desert and along the sea coast are exposed to some silica. Most of the particles to which they are exposed probably can not be inhaled. However, those who work on seashore golf links are also exposed to considerable amounts of respirable silica. In addition, there is evidence that Bedouins may occasionally develop silicosis, presumably after the repeated sandstorms encountered in the Sahara and deserts of the Middle East (65). Surface coal miners used to be, and still are to a limited extent, exposed to respirable quartz, particularly those who work as drillers and blasters (66). Nevertheless, coal miners, despite their exposure to silica, have a lower SMR for lung cancer than that of the general population (67,68). Moreover, the SMR deficit for lung cancer dates back to the 1940s, 1950s, and 1960s, no matter that analyses of coal miners' lungs show a significantly increased quartz content compared with that for many other occupations (69). Over the past 25 to 30 years, there has been a decrease in the exposure of coal miners not only to coal dust but to silica; nevertheless, the incidence of lung cancer increased from the 1940s to the 1980s, presumably because of the increase in smoking.

Many of the publications that have endeavored to demonstrate that silica is a carcinogen were able to demonstrate slight increases in the SMR for lung cancer. Other papers have had completely negative results. One needs to compare and review the studies that show an association between cigarette smoking and lung cancer with those papers relating exposure to quartz to the development of lung cancer in nonsmokers. It is difficult to find any publication in workers exposed to crystalline silica that shows a greatly increased SMR. Most of the SMRs are below 200, and slight increases could well be owing to inaccurate smoking histories (70, 71).

The possible association between silica exposure (silicosis) and bronchogenic cancer should not necessarily be regarded as a contemporary issue. The debate dates back to the work of Merewether in 1949, who reported large excesses of lung cancer among patients with asbestosis (72). The controls that Merewether used in his necropsy series were patients with silicatosis, who had not developed lung cancers at an excessive rate. Moreover, it is important to bear in mind that Sir Richard Doll's somewhat dated, but relevant, review of occupational lung cancer suggested that some groups of industrial workers appear to be immune from the risk of bronchogenic cancer (73). One such group consisted of workers exposed to silica and who were at risk of developing silicosis. He concluded that "where there is an industrial hazard of lung cancer it is due to some specific characteristics of the industry, and not to a nonspecific effect of pneumoconiosis."

Much of the problem originates from the fact that many cohort and case control studies rely on data from silicosis registers or from claimants who are applying for, or who have already have been granted, workers compensation. As such, many have worked in other occupations in which they have been only slightly exposed to silica. Furthermore, many of the investigators assume that disability claimants are representative of the entire work force. Nothing is further from the truth. Similarly, to obtain reliable smoking data, it is essential to rely on a prospective smoking history. This is best effected at the initial physical examination that the worker undergoes before starting work. The likelihood of obtaining reliable histories from disabled workers, or by questioning surviving relatives of deceased workers, is remote. Of interest is the observation in "occupational mortality" in England and Wales (1970–1972), that the SMR for stomach cancer in quarrymen and non-coal miners was 150, being significantly increased, whereas the SMR for lung cancer was 100 (74).

One of the proponents of silica as a carcinogen has been Checkoway (75). In his first study, he performed a survey of two diatomite mines in California. The workers were exposed to both amorphous and crystalline silica, with the latter being in the form of cristobalite. This form of crystalline silica is produced during calcining of diatomaceous earth. Checkoway's cohort included 2,570 workers, of whom 533 were Hispanic and 2,037 were of non-Hispanic origin. All had to have been employed for at least 1 year (75). The vital status of 91% of the cohort was determined. The SMR for all causes were slightly increased at 112, whereas the SMR for lung cancer was 143. In Checkoway and his colleague's opinion, the SMR was felt to be excessive. Unfortunately, smoking histories were not available except in a minority, many of which were taken from surviving relatives. The investigators demonstrated a relationship between lung cancer and a derived index of exposure to silica; however, the silica index and cigarette smoking were co-linearly related. An attempt to control the confounding effects of smoking was made by calculating the death rates from other cigarette smoking–induced cancers, i.e., laryngeal, bladder, esophageal, renal, and pancreatic. All of these cancers occur more frequently in cigarette smokers than in nonsmokers, but they do not occur as frequently as does lung cancer. Moreover, other habits such as alcohol consumption are of particular importance in laryngeal and esophageal cancer and suggest that smokers were more numerous than the figures given by Checkoway and colleagues. The relationship between laryngeal, bladder, renal, and pancreatic cancer is far weaker than is the association between smoking and lung cancer or between smoking and chronic obstructive pulmonary disease. The SMR for emphysema in Checkoway's cohort of workers was 180, significantly higher than the SMR for lung cancer. The small number of subjects with other smoking related cancers limited the power of his statistical analysis and made it impossible to draw any conclusions in regard to the number of deaths caused by the other malignancies. In contrast, emphysema and chronic obstructive pulmonary disease are almost always caused by cigarette smoking and never by the inhalation of quartz. Over the past 10 years or so, Checkoway and colleagues have published further papers relating to the cohort. All have involved "fine adjustments" to his data (76,77).

The flood of publications attempting to prove that silica is a carcinogen has been overwhelming. Moreover, the authors of the various papers have reworked their statistics frequently in an attempt to obtain further grants and funds so that they can rehash their data in the hope of proving that they are correct. In some instances, uranium miners were working with silica and were also exposed to radon daughters and cigarettes (59). As such, many of the relationships could be explained by other carcinogens.

Two recent reviews have been published that are objective and have critically reviewed the methods used in the many publications that have appeared (70,78). Many of the papers that were reviewed have been found wanting. A thorough review of the various publications, conferences, and regulatory considerations of the relationship of crystalline silica and lung cancer came to the conclusion that the evidence for incriminating silica as a carcinogen is lacking. Most published studies incriminating silica have, in reality, been weakly positive. Silica is not genotoxic and is a pulmonary carcinogen only in the rat, an animal that develops lung cancer on its own without any exposure to carcinogen.

Additional studies assessed the prevalence of radiographic silicosis in a group of 600 retired granite workers who were on a pension (78). Files of regional clinics and hospitals were searched for chest radiographs of the 600 retired workers. A total of 470 films were located and were found suitable for interpretation. Three experienced readers interpreted the film according to the International Labour Organisation classification. Dust exposures were estimated for the workers hired after 1940, with the dust standard of 10^6 particles per cubic foot, equivalent to 0.1 mg/m³. The dust control standard was put into effect by the Vermont Division of Industrial Hygiene. Dust levels were initially high, but gradually declined from 1940–1954, after which a mean dust exposure of around 0.05 to 0.06 mg/m³ came into effect. Nevertheless, about 10% to 15% of samples after 1954 exceeded 0.1 mg/m³. Of the 408 radiographs available, 58 were taken on workers hired before dust controls were instituted in 1940, and 25.9% of them were positive with a profusion of 1/0 or greater. A total of 350 radiographs were taken after 1940, and these showed a prevalence of 5.7%. The radiographic changes in workers hired after 1940 were likely owing to excessive exposures that occurred during the first 15 years of dust control. The death rates from silicosis before measures taken to control dust were significantly greater than those that occurred after 1954. By way of contrast, the less the exposure to silicosis, the greater the number of deaths owing to lung cancer. This presumably occurred as the dust levels started to decrease. The proportion of smokers started to increase in the 1940s and continued to do so until about 5 years ago, leading to an increased SMR from smoking.

Other Suspected Carcinogens

Diesel Exhaust

There have been numerous studies performed on diesel exhaust fumes. A number of studies have shown an increased incidence of lung cancer in those who has been exposed to diesel exhaust; however, when one takes into account smoking, it is evident that most persons who are exposed to diesel exhaust, in particular truck drivers and those who formerly drove diesel locomotives for the railroad, were invariably found to be the heaviest smokers. As far as truck drivers were concerned, many imbibed alcohol freely.

Diesel exhaust is not composed of one or two constituents, but of many components, including gaseous elements, the products of carbon combustion, water, and carbon dioxide, as well as the products of incomplete combustion (carbon monoxide, the oxides of nitrogen, various hydrocarbons, and partially oxidized hydrocarbons such as aldehydes, ketones, phenols, and various sulfur compounds). When compared with a gasoline engine, diesel engines produce far less carbon monoxide but a greater volume of oxides of nitrogen and aldehydes. There is no evidence that these gases, fumes, and other components are carcinogens. Because diesel fumes are a "witch's brew," one cannot infer that the cocktail of components is necessarily carcinogenic (79).

A series of the agents and chemicals have been suggested as carcinogens, but no proof of carcinogenicity has been demonstrated. These include beryllium, formaldehyde, cadmium, dry cleaners, and isopropanol (is associated with nasal cancer), but there is no confirmatory evidence of lung cancer. Although dated, the surgeon general's report of 1985 remains one of the most useful references in regard to cancer in the workplace (80).

CODA

The ready and uncritical acceptance of certain forms of treatment, the assumption that all environmental pollutants are harmful and the instant credence that is given to pronouncements that label relatively innocuous agents as carcinogens (such as PCBs, agent orange, and coffee) have come about as a result of what has been termed the Gold effect (81). This phenomenon was named after Professor T. Gold who first described it as "an effect that usually comes into play following a contrived concatenation of circumstances."

When one or two persons suddenly develop a notion that a particular new treatment is beneficial or that a common well-known agent is harmful, e.g., the Vineberg operation for myocardial ischemia or the concept that diesel fumes are carcinogenic, the interested parties, be they physicians or scientists, devise some method to further the concept. In doing so, they enlist the help of the Green party or other environmentalists in order to provide "moral" and financial support for their preconceived ideas and plans. Their first ploy is to try to interest the more gullible members of the media in publicizing the tenuous hypothesis that is being publicized. The unjustified attention given to such publicity seekers often succeeds in engendering the performance of a number of hastily devised and poorly carried out studies. Such investigations frequently yield equivocal or contradictory results but suffice to suggest a possible relationship between exposure to the particular agent and the development of impairment or of disease, be it cancer, hypertension, atherosclerosis, or fetal abnormalities.

Encouraged by the indefinite and the dubious, a few gullible and usually tendentious medical or scientific adherents of the proposition that virtually everything with which we come in contact is harmful, decide to organize a symposium. Many of the proponents subscribe to the view that all, or nearly all, cancer results from occupational or environmental exposures. Unfortunately, the disinterested and the objective shun the meeting, and most of those who attend are the radical rump of the environmentalists and sundry other visionaries. Subsequently, the proceedings of the symposium are disseminated with great fanfare, with prominence being given to those pessimists of the doomsday genus.

A clique or sect is then established to disseminate the concept that the particular agent under study is harmful. As a consequence, numerous gullible, and usually youthful, investigators who are characterized by extreme naiveté and intellectual egotism are encouraged to perform their own investigations. Most mimic and adopt the same flawed methods used by the original investigators and, in doing, so predictably come to the same erroneous conclusions. As more papers and investigations are published, the consensus undergoes transmogrification into an overwhelming majority. Metaanalyses are carried out and often conclude or state that there seems to be evidence of a definite association, but the authors of such analyses forget that negative findings seldom appear in journals and when they do, they are ignored by the reader. Many of those who know better dismiss the published investigations as inconsequential and fail to take them seriously and, in doing so, do not bother to voice their concerns. Once the hypothesis or concept has been accepted in a "reputable" journal, it becomes almost impossible to eradicate. Orthodoxy and conformity are the criteria by which most articles are accepted for publication, and in no time, the tyranny of the majority reigns supreme. What journals are interested in publishing negative results? As soon as the hypothesis receives the acceptance and blessing of "informed opinion," the clique resorts to ex cathedra pronouncements. What started as a vagary rapidly becomes generally accepted and, in short order, progresses to established fact before finally becoming an incontrovertible self-evident verity. Those courageous enough to differ from the accepted opinion are regarded as industry's eccentric reactionaries or as antisocial misfits with a vested interest in the perpetuation of hazards. Many would say this is crass exaggeration, but in practice, it is little removed from reality.

Finally it must be borne in mind that although great harm can result by failing to diagnose a disease, making a diagnosis of a disease where none exists can have exceedingly dire consequences. The same principle functions in the designation of carcinogens. Workers told that they have been exposed to a carcinogen and are likely to develop cancer, when this is not the case, have been done an appalling disservice. In this context, Thomas Huxley's apothegm reigns supreme: "Blind faith is the one unpardonable sin, skepticism is the supreme virtue."

REFERENCES

1. Pott P. *Chirurgical works,* Vol. 3. London: 1808.
2. Harting FH, Hesse ER. Lungenkrebs die Bergkrankheit in der Schneeburger Gruben. *Vjschr Gericht Med* 1879;31:102.
3. Meselson M, Russell K. Screening for carcinogens: In: Hiatt HH, Watson JD, Winston JA, eds. *Origins of human cancer.* Cold Spring Harbor, NY: Cold Spring Harbor Laboratory Press, 1977:1473–1481.
4. Paterson MC. Environment carcinogenesis and imperfect repair of DNA in *Homo sapiens.* In: Griffin AC, Shaw CR, eds. *Carcinogenesis: identification and mechanisms of action.* New York: Raven Press, 1979:251–286.
5. Cairns J. The origin of human cancers. *Nature* 1981;289:353–357.

6. Saracci R. The IARC monograph program on the evaluation of carcinogenic risk of chemical to humans as a contributor to the identification of occupational carcinogens. In: Peto R, Schneiderman M, eds. *Quantification of occupational cancer.* Cold Spring Harbor, NY: Cold Spring Harbor Laboratory Press, 1981.

7. Bradford Hill A. *A short textbook of medical statistics.* Seven Oaks, UK: Hodder and Stoughton, 1977:285–296.

8. Ng TB, Chan SI, Lee J. Mortality of a cohort of men in a silicosis register: further evidence of an association with lung cancer. *Am J Ind Med* 1990;17:163–171.

9. Epstein S, Schwartz JB. Fallacies of lifestyle cancer theories. *Nature* 1981:289;127–130.

10. Bridbord K, Decoufle P, Fraumeni J, et al. Estimates of the fraction of cancer in the United States related to occupational factors. Washington, DC: National Cancer Institute and National Institute of Occupational Safety and Health, 1978.

11. Doll R, Peto R. The causes of cancer. *J Natl Cancer Inst* 1981;66:1196–1308.

12. What proportion of lung cancers are due to occupation? *Lancet* 1978;2:1238–1240.

13. Shopland DR, Eyre HJ, Pechacek TF. Smoking attributable cancer mortality in 1991. *J Natl Cancer Inst* 1991;83:1142–1148.

14. Wilson MM, Jungner G. *Principles of screening for disease.* Geneva: World Health Organization, 1968.

15. Strauss GM. Chapter 68. In: Baum GL, Crapo JD, Celli BR, et al., eds. *Textbook of occupational diseases,* 6th ed. Philadelphia: Lippincott–Raven Publishers, 1997:1334–1353.

16. Hill AB, Fanning EI. Studies of the inevidence of cancer in a factory handling inorganic compounds: mortality experience in the factory. *Br J Ind Med* 1948;5:1–6.

17. Lee AM, Fraumeni JH Jr. Arsenic and respiratory cancer in men. *J Natl Inst* 1969;42:1045–1052.

18. Merewether ERA, Price CW. *Report of the effects of asbestos dust on the lungs and dust suppression in the asbestos industry.* London: His Majesty's Stationery Office, 1930.

19. Dreesen WC, Dallavalle, JM, Edwards T, et al. A study of asbestosis in asbestos textile industry. Washington, DC: US Government Printing Office; 1938; Public Health Bulletin 241.

20. Selikoff IJ, Churg J, Hammond EC. The occurrence of asbestosis among insulation workers in the United States. *Ann N Y Acad Sci* 1965;132:139–155.

21. National Institute of Occupational Safety and Health Hazard Surveys. Rockville, Maryland, 1973.

22. Thomas HF, Benjamin IT, Elwood PC, et al. Further follow up of workers from an asbestos cement factor. *Br J Ind Med* 1982;39:273–276.

23. Ohlson CG, Hogstedt C. Lung cancer among asbestos cement workers: a Swedish cohort study and a review. *Br J Ind Med* 1985;42:397–402.

24. Hodgson JT, Jones RD. Mortality of asbestos workers in England and Wales: 1971–1981. *Br J Ind Med* 1986;43:158–164.

25. Gardner MJ, Winter PD, Pannett B, et al. Follow up study of workers manufacturing chrysotile asbestos cement products. *Br J Ind Med* 1986;43:726–732.

26. Neuberger M, Kundi MI. Individual asbestos exposure: smoking and mortality: a cohort study in the asbestos cement industry. *Br J Ind Med* 1990;47:615.

27. Seidman H, Selikoff IJ. Decline in death rates among asbestos insulation workers 1967–1986 associated with diminution of work exposure to asbestos. *Ann N Y Acad Sci* 1990;609:300–317.

28. Mossman BT, Bignon J, Corn M, et al. Asbestos, scientific developments and implications for public policy. *Science* 1990;247:294–301.

29. Hendry NW. The geology occurrences and major uses of asbestos. *Ann N Y Acad Sci* 1965;132:12–21.

30. Selikoff IJ, Churg J, Hammond, E. The occurrence of asbestosis among insulation workers in the United States. *Ann N Y Acad Sci* 1965;132:139–155.

31. Liddell FDK, Hanley JA. Relations between asbestos exposure and lung cancer SMRs in occupational cohort studies. *Br J Ind Med* 1985;42:389–396.

32. Acheson AD, Gardner MJ. Health and Safety Executive (UK) Asbestos: the control limit for asbestos. In: *Health and Safety Commission: an update of the ill effects of asbestos upon health.* London: Her Majesty's Stationery Office, 1983.

33. McDonald JC, Liddell FDK, Dufresne A, et al. The 1891–1920 birth cohort of Quebec chrysotile mines and millers: mortality 1970–1988. *Br J Ind Med* 1993;50:1073–1081.

34. Churg A. An analysis of lung asbestos content. *Am Rev Resp Dis* 1991;48:649–652.

35. Hughes JM. Epidemiology of lung cancer in relation to asbestos exposure. In: Liddell FDK, Miller K, eds. *Mineral fibres and health.* Boca Raton, FL: CRC Press, 1991:136–141.

36. Liddell FDK. Laryngeal cancer and asbestos. *Br J Ind Med* 1990;47:289–291.

37. Edelman DA. Exposure to asbestos and the risk of gastrointestinal cancer: a reassessment. *Br J Ind Med* 1988;45:75–82.

38. Boris YI, Sahim AA, Ozesmi M, et al. An outbreak of pleural mesothelioma and chronic pleurisy in the village of Karain Urgup in Anatolia. *Thorax* 1978;33:181–192.

39. Nelson N. Carcinogenicity of halo ethers. *N Engl J Med* 1973;288:1123–1124.

40. Figueroa WG, Raszowski R, Weiss W. Lung cancer in chloromethyl ether workers. *N Engl J Med* 1973;288:1096–1097.

41. Lemen RA, Johnson WM, Wagoner JK, et al. Lung cancer in chloromethyl ether workers. *Ann N Y Acad Sci* 1976;271:71–80.

42. Sakabe H. Lung cancer due to exposure to *bis* (chloromethyl) ether. *Ind Health* 1973;11:145–148.

43. Doll R, Vessey MP, Beasley RWR, et al. Mortality of gas workers: a final report of a prospective study. *Br J Ind Med* 1972;29:394–406.

44. Lloyd JW. Long term mortality in steel workers: respiratory cancer in coke plant workers in Britain. *J Occup Med* 1983;13:53–68.

45. Hurley JF, Archibald RM, Collings PL, et al. The mortality of coke workers in Britain. *Am J Ind Med* 1983;4:691–704.

46. Redmond CK. Cancer mortality among coke oven workers. *Env Health Perspectives* 1983;52:67–73.

47. Alwens W, Jonas W. Der Chromat-Lungen Krebs. *ACTA unio Internationalis Contra-Cancrum* 1938;3:103–118.

48. Baetjer AM. Pulmonary carcinoma in chromate workers, I: a review of the literature and report of cases. *Arch Ind Hyg Occup Med* 1950;2:487–504.

49. Tsuneta Y, Onsaki Y, Kim, WAK, et al. Chromium content of lungs with chromate workers with lung cancer. *Thorax* 1980;35:294–297.

50. Chief Inspector of Factories. Annual report for the year 1932. London: His Majesty's Stationery Office, 1933:33.

51. Chief Inspector of Factories. Annual report for the year 1950. London: Her Majesty's Stationery Office, 1952:145.

52. Doll R, Morgan LG, Speizer FE. Cancers of the lung and nasal sinuses in nickel workers. *Br J Ind Med* 1970;24:623–632.

53. Kreyberg L. Lung cancer in workers in a nickel refinery. *Br J Ind Med* 1978;35:109–116.

54. Loken AC. Lung cancer in nickel workers. *Tidsskr Nor Laegeforen* 1950;70:376–378.

55. Committee of Medical Biologic Effects of Environmental Pollutants (CMBEFEP). Nickel. Washington, DC: Natural Academy of Sciences, 1975.

56. A report of the international committee on nickel carcinogenesis in man. *Scand J Work Environ Health* 1990;6:1–82.

57. De Villiers AJ, Windish JP. Lung cancer in a fluorspar mining community. *Br J Ind Med* 1964;21:94–99.

58. Agricola AC. *De Re Metallica: 1557 AD*. London: Dover Publications, 1950. Hoover HC, translator.

59. Archer VE, Wagoner JK, Lundin, FE. Uranium mining and cigarette smoking effects on man. *J Occup Med* 1973;15:204–211.

60. Boyd JT, Doll R, Faulds JS, et al. Cancer of the lung in ore (haematite) mines. *Br J Ind Med* 1970;27:97–105.

61. Kennaway EL, Kennaway NM. A further study of the incidence of cancer of the lung. *Br J Cancer* 1947;1:260–298.

62. Wada S, Miyanishi M, Nishimoto Y, et al. Mustard gas as a cause of respiratory neoplasia in man. *Lancet* 1968;1:1161–1163.

63. Manning KP, Skegg DCG, Stell PM, et al. Cancer of the larynx and other occupational hazards of mustard gas workers. *Clin Otolaryngol* 1981;6:165–170.

64. *IARC monographs for the evaluation of carcinogenic risks to humans*, Vol. 68. Lyon, France: International Agency for Research into Cancer, 1997:211.

65. Bar-Ziv J, Goldberg CM. Simple siliceous pneumoconiosis in Negev Bedouins. *Arch Environ Health* 1974;29:121–126.

66. Banks DE, Bamed MA, Castellan RM, et al. Silicosis in surface coal mine drillers. *Thorax* 1983;38:275–278.

67. Liddell FDK. Mortality of British coal miners in 1961. *Br J Ind Med* 1973;30:15–24.

68. Costello J, Ortmeyer J, Morgan WKC. Mortality from lung cancer in U.S. coal miners. *Am J Public Health* 1974;64:222–224.

69. Sweet DV, Crouse WE, Crable JV. Chemical and statistical studies of contaminants in urban lungs. *Am Ind Hyg Assoc J* 1978;39:515–526.

70. Hessel PA, Gamble JF, Gee JBL, et al. Silica, silicosis, and lung cancer. *J Occup Envir Med* 2000;42:704–720.

71. Morgan WKC, Reger RB. Silica exposure and risk of lung cancer. *Thorax* 1996;51:772.

72. Merewether ERA. Annual report of the chief inspector of factories for the year 1947. London: His Majesty's Stationery Office, 1949.

73. Doll R. Occupational lung cancer: a review. *Br J Ind Med* 1959;16:103–108.

74. Occupational Mortality. *1970–1972 Decennial Supplement*. London: Her Majesty's Stationery Office, 1978:70–71.

75. Checkoway H, Heyer NJ, Demers PA, et al. Mortality among workers in the diatomaceous earth industry. *Br J Ind Med* 1993;50:586–597.

76. Checkoway H, Heyer NJ, Demers PA, et al. Reanalysis of mortality from lung cancer among diatomaceous earth industry workers, with consideration of potential confounding by asbestos exposure. *Occup Environ Med* 1996:53;645–647.

77. Checkoway H, Heyer NJ, Seixas NS, et al. Dose-response associations of silica with non-malignant respiratory disease and lung cancer in the diatomaceous earth industry. *Am J Epidemiol* 1997;145:680–688.

78. Graham WGB, Vacek PM, Morgan WKC, et al. Radiographic abnormalities in long tenure Vermont granite workers and the permissible exposure limit for crystalline silica. *J Occup Environ Med* 2001;43:412–417.

79. Morgan WKC, Reger RB, Tucker DM. Health effects of diesel emissions. *Ann Occup Hyg* 1997;41:643–658.

80. The health consequences of smoking, cancer, and chronic lung disease in the workplace: a report of the surgeon general. Rockville, MD: U.S. Department of Health and Human Services, Office of Smoking and Health, 1985.

81. Lyttleton RA. The Gold effect. In: Duncan R, Weston-Smith M, eds. *Lying truths: a critical scrutiny of current beliefs and conventions*. Oxford, UK: Pergamon Press, 1979:182–198.

Adaptation and Maladaptation to High Altitude

47

Colin K. Grissom · Robert B. Schoene

Oxygen delivery to the tissues depends on an adequate supply of oxygen at each step of the oxygen transport chain, from the inspired air to the mitochondria. The atmospheric pressure and inspired partial pressure of oxygen decrease predictably with increasing altitude above sea level (Table 47.1). Humans at high altitude, therefore, must overcome the disadvantage of ambient hypoxia by making a number of adaptations to optimize the availability of oxygen to the tissues. A large majority of travelers and high-altitude dwellers are successful in adapting to high altitude, but some do not adapt well and suffer from acute and chronic altitude illness. This chapter first reviews what is known about both acute and chronic adaptation to high altitude and then reviews the illnesses that occur when the body maladapts.

ADAPTATION

Abrupt exposure to high altitude ($>3,000$ m) can result in illness and even death. On the other hand, gradual ascent to these same heights permits a number of physiological adaptations to take place that allow some humans to function quite well. Populations have lived for centuries as high as 5,000 m, and brief forays above 8,000 m, at which the atmospheric pressure is a third of that at sea level, are well documented and are a tribute to the resilience of human physiology.

To optimize oxygen delivery, important compensations take place at each step of the oxygen cascade, which has a number of components: ventilation, matching of ventilation with blood flow, diffusion of oxygen from the air to the blood,

circulation of the blood, diffusion of oxygen from the red blood cell to the tissue, and oxidative metabolism in the mitochondria. The first portion of this chapter reviews each of these steps, beginning with the lung.

Pulmonary Adaptation

Ventilation

An increase in alveolar ventilation occurs immediately on ascent to a high altitude. The partial pressures of oxygen (P_{AO_2}) and carbon dioxide in the alveolus reflect the degree of hyperventilation that attempts to preserve oxygen partial pressure. For instance, at an extreme altitude (summit of Mount Everest, 8,848 m, 253 mm Hg), alveolar ventilation in a climber increases to maintain a P_{AO_2} of about 32 mm Hg and of carbon dioxide of about 8 to 10 mm Hg [1,2]. Lower altitudes have a proportionately lower degree of ventilation.

The increase in ventilation is a result of a complex interaction of physiological events, mediated largely by the hypoxic stimulus to the carotid body. The course of the ventilatory response is what constitutes ventilatory acclimatization. There is individual variation in this response, but essentially, the pattern of any given level of high altitude is one of an abrupt increase in ventilation followed by a more gradual increase for at least a fortnight or longer depending the altitude [3,4] (Fig. 47.1). An arterial alkalemia is present owing to the respiratory alkalosis, but early investigations suggested that a cerebrospinal fluid (CSF) acidosis persisted and resulted in the gradual increase in ventilation over days at high altitude [5]. More recent investigations, however, have shown that in humans and animals, both blood and CSF alkalosis develop in parallel during the respiratory alkalosis of acclimatization [6].

Ventilation increases with acute ascent to high altitude, but after 15 to 25 minutes of acute hypoxic exposure, ventilation decreases 25% to 30% owing to central suppression

C. K. Grissom: Pulmonary and Critical Care Division, Department of Medicine, LDS Hospital and the University of Utah School of Medicine, Salt Lake City, Utah.

R. B. Schoene: Pulmonary and Critical Care Division, Department of Medicine, University of Washington, Seattle, Washington.

TABLE 47.1. U.S. STANDARD ATMOSPHERE: ALTITUDE, BAROMETRIC PRESSURE, AND INSPIRED PARTIAL PRESSURE OF OXYGEN

| Altitude | | Barometric Pressure (mm Hg) | Inspired P_{O_2} (mm Hg) |
Meters	Feet		
0	0	760.0	159.1
1000	3,280	674.4	141.2
2000	6,560	596.3	124.9
3000	9,840	525.8	110.1
4000	13,120	462.8	96.9
5000	16,400	405.0	84.8
6000	19,680	354.0	74.0
8000	26,240	267.8	56.1
8848	29,028	253.0	53.0

Values except 8848 are taken for midlatitude (45°N). There is greater variation at higher latitudes. Modified from Altman PL, Dittmer DS, eds., *Respiration and Circulation.* Bethesda, MD, 1971: Federation of American Societies for Experimental Biology, with permission.

from the action of neurotransmitters and a decrease in the metabolic rate in the brain. Further stay at a high altitude for the sojourner results in an improvement in arterial oxygen saturation secondary to a gradual increase in ventilation over a fortnight or so. At extreme altitude, ventilatory adaptation may take weeks or months or may never be complete (7). The sensitivity of the carotid body increases and plays an important role in the progressive hyperventilation. Carbon dioxide sensitivity, which is mediated primarily in the central chemosensors, also increases and may, therefore, interact with the carotid body to effect an increase in ventilation (8).

Alveolar ventilation and hypoxic chemosensitivity decrease in most lifelong residents of high-altitude regions (9–11) (Fig. 47.1). This decrease in hypoxic drive occurs despite a hypertrophy of the carotid bodies and is proportional to both the altitude and the duration of habitation (12). Because the mechanics of breathing entail a metabolic cost, it is conceivable that well-adapted high-altitude natives have invoked other mechanisms to improve oxygen transport to the mitochondria while minimizing the metabolic cost with lower alveolar ventilation. On the other hand, in

some high-altitude populations, especially in South America, the relative hypoventilation compared with that of sojourners may predispose some populations to chronic mountain sickness (CMS), which involves more profound hypoxemia, pulmonary hypertension, polycythemia, and decreased cerebral function (see section "Chronic Mountain Sickness"). Natives of the Tibetan and Nepalese Himalayas, in whom CMS is very rare, are reported to have less blunted alveolar ventilation and hypoxic chemosensitivity than that of the high-altitude dwellers in the Andes. This intriguing difference suggests an evolutionary influence; wherein, the Tibetans who have lived at a high altitude much longer than have the South Americans have physiological characteristics that have led to more successful tolerance of high altitude (13).

Lung Mechanics

Lung mechanics are affected at least transiently on ascent to a high altitude. Increased blood flow and central blood volume and a possible increase in interstitial fluid may lead to a decreased vital capacity, an increased residual volume, and decreased lung compliance. This explanation remains speculative. High-altitude dwellers in South America, on the other hand, have large chests on physical examination, accompanied by larger vital capacities, in comparison to low-altitude dwellers. The younger the age that the subjects begin living at a high altitude, the more pronounced is this characteristic (13,14).

The increased ventilation at high altitude results in a greater work of breathing for any given workload compared with that at sea level despite the lower gas density encountered at high altitude (15). At high levels of exercise, this cost of an increased work of breathing may be paid for by a diversion of blood flow to the muscles of respiration, resulting in a "steal" of blood flow from the other working muscles and a limit on work output (16,17).

Gas Exchange

The increased ventilation on ascent to high altitude results in an increased P_{AO_2}, but the arterial oxygen content depends on the transfer of oxygen from the alveolus to the capillary and red blood cells. This step requires matching of ventilation ($\dot{V}_A$) to perfusion ($\dot{Q}$) and the diffusion of oxygen to hemoglobin in the red blood cell.

The increase in ventilation is matched in part by an increase in cardiac output and pulmonary blood flow. Alveolar hypoxia leads to pulmonary vasoconstriction, which at rest improves the $\dot{V}_A/\dot{Q}$ match primarily by increasing blood flow to the underperfused portions of the lung, which are usually areas of high $\dot{V}_A/\dot{Q}$ (18). This redistribution of blood flow results in greater homogeneity of $\dot{V}_A/\dot{Q}$.

The next step in gas exchange relies on diffusion of oxygen to the blood. This transfer depends on a pressure gradient

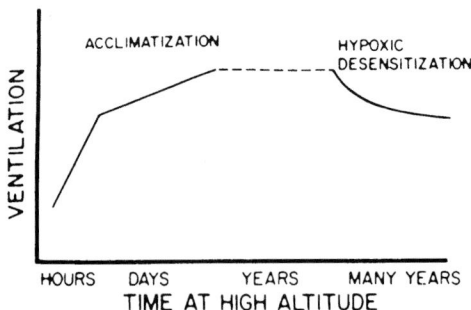

FIGURE 47.1. The time course of ventilatory adaptation to high-altitude exposure. (From Weil JV. Ventilatory control at high altitude. In *Handbook of physiology: the respiratory system,* Vol. 2. Bethesda, MD: American Physiological Society, 1986, with permission.)

for oxygen from the alveolus to the capillary, diffusion capacity of the alveolar–capillary interface (DM), capillary blood volume (VC), and the surface area for gas exchange. A true diffusion limitation for oxygen transfer exists at high altitudes. This phenomenon occurs for several reasons. With increasing altitude, the lower P_{AO_2} results in a lower alveolar–capillary oxygen pressure gradient. Full equilibration of oxygen to the blood also depends on the transit time of the red blood cell across the pulmonary capillary, which at high altitude may not permit full equilibration, especially during exercise, when an increased cardiac output shortens transit time. For example, the circumstances at the summit of Mount Everest, where the barometric pressure is about 250 mm Hg, are expressed by a model for this diffusion limitation with given values for hemoglobin concentration, oxygen consumption ($\dot{V}O_2$), diffusion capacity (DM), acid-base status, and capillary transit time as shown in Figure 47.2 (19–21).

An important factor in this process at extreme altitude may be relatively high oxygen-hemoglobin affinity secondary to respiratory alkalosis found in some high-altitude animals and in climbers at extreme altitudes. In high-altitude natives, the diffusion capacity of the lung (DL) may be more optimal secondary to either an increased capillary surface area (DM) or pulmonary blood volume (VC) (22).

Cardiovascular Adaptation

Cardiac Response

At high altitude, heart rate increases, which results in a greater cardiac output. An accompanying elevation of catecholamines suggests that they mediate the increase in chronotropic effect on the heart (23). Subsequently, over the next few days, resting heart rate decreases as other compensatory mechanisms are invoked. Stroke volume decreases secondary to either a lower plasma volume or an increased pulmonary vascular resistance (24).

During exercise at high altitudes, the relationship between cardiac output and work is maintained, but both maximal work rates and cardiac output achieved at sea level are not reached at high altitudes. Both stroke volume and maximal heart rate are lower at high altitudes (25). There may be an impairment of stroke volume secondary to increased pulmonary vascular resistance, a decrease in left ventricular volumes secondary to right-to-left septal deviation from pulmonary hypertension, a decrease in myocardial contractility, or general constriction from the pericardium (26). The lower maximal heart rate is more marked in sojourners; may be secondary to hypervagal tone, hypoxic myocardial depression, or dysfunction of electrical conduction; and may be a major factor in the decrease in maximal exercise at high altitude. There are, however, few data in sojourners to support these possibilities, and it is now generally thought that the cardiac response is appropriate for the amount of work that is being done (27).

Acute exposure to high altitudes results in an increase in systemic blood pressure and systemic vascular resistance both at rest and during exercise, whereas the dweller at a high altitude may actually develop a lower systemic blood pressure, perhaps secondary to microcirculatory vasodilation.

Pulmonary Vascular Response

Pulmonary artery pressure and pulmonary vascular resistance increase acutely at high altitudes, and this is secondary to

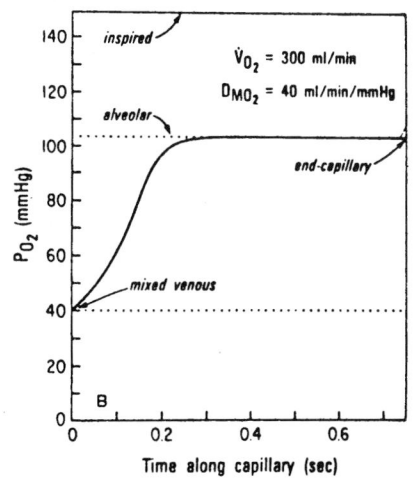
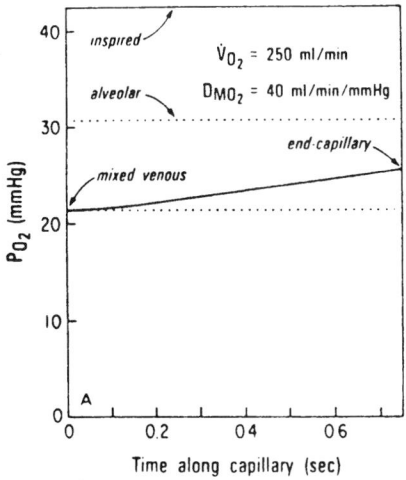

FIGURE 47.2. Comparison of the calculated time course of partial pressure of oxygen in the pulmonary capillary of a climber at rest at sea level **(left)** (barometric pressure [PB] = 760 mm Hg) and at the summit of Mount Everest **(right)** (PB = 250 mm Hg). Adequate time for equilibration is available at sea level, whereas at 8,848 m, full equilibration is not possible. $\dot{V}O_2$, oxygen consumption; DM_{O_2}, diffusion capacity of oxygen at the alveolar–capillary interface. (From West JB, Wagner PD. Predicted gas exchange on the summit of Mount Everest. *Respir Physiol* 1980;42:1, with permission.)

the hypoxic pulmonary vasoconstrictive response (HPVR). The HPVR increases at a Pao_2 of 60 mm Hg or less, and as with the ventilatory response to hypoxia, there is individual and interspecies variation of HPVR. Adaptation of the pulmonary vasculature may be accompanied by an increased secretion of nitric oxide (NO), which is produced in the endothelium and vasodilates the pulmonary vascular bed. Prolonged exposure to hypoxia may lead to fixed pulmonary hypertension. Smooth muscle hypertrophy, fibroblast proliferation, and fibrosis of the intima, which may not be reversible, have been found in high-altitude dwellers. There is evidence that some high-altitude natives who have adapted well to high altitude may have normal pulmonary artery pressures and no hypertrophy of the smooth muscle of the pulmonary arterioles (28).

Hematologic Adaptations

Hemoglobin carries oxygen in the vascular compartment to tissues where oxygen is consumed. At high altitudes, two major adaptations of the carrier mechanism take place to facilitate delivery: (a) the number of red blood cells is increased by the process of erythropoiesis, and (b) the configuration of the hemoglobin molecule changes to alter the affinity of hemoglobin for oxygen in order to optimize the loading and unloading of oxygen.

Erythropoiesis

The decrease in Pao_2, and subsequently in oxygen content, that occurs with progressive hypobaria at high altitude is counterbalanced in part by an increase in hemoglobin concentration and subsequent oxygen-carrying capacity. The increase over the first day or so is secondary to hemoconcentration from a diuresis, whereas the continued increase over the ensuing 2 to 3 weeks is a result of increased red blood cell production stimulated by erythropoietin. Erythropoietin levels increase rapidly with a hypoxic stimulus and then decline in the face of a continued rise in hemoglobin. Erythropoiesis stops abruptly on descent, and hemoglobin concentrations return to sea-level values in approximately 3 weeks (29–31).

A striking feature of the erythropoietic response is the variability between individuals and between different highland populations, which may reflect less-than-optimal adaptations to comparable hypoxic stress. For instance, in the Himalayas at 3,600 m, hemoglobin levels of 16.1 ± 1.2 g/dL have been documented, whereas in the Andes at the same altitude, the values are 18.2 to 19.0 g/dL (32,33). Although the increase in hemoglobin concentration augments arterial oxygen content, an actual decrease in oxygen delivery may ensue if hyperviscosity of the blood limits perfusion to the microvasculature of the exercising muscle. Climbers on Mount Everest undergoing isovolemic phlebotomy to decrease their hematocrits from 60% to 50% had an increase in psychometric function but did not experience a decrease in

aerobic capacity (34). Hemodilution in high-altitude natives of the Andes, achieved by decreasing the hematocrit 20%, resulted in an improved exercise performance (35). Excessive polycythemia in the highland dweller is discussed later.

Oxygen-Hemoglobin Affinity

The role of oxygen-hemoglobin affinity in oxygen delivery at high altitude is not fully understood. Conditions of stress, such as fever and acidemia, are associated with a rightward shift of the oxygen-hemoglobin dissociation curve, or low oxygen and hemoglobin affinity, presumably to facilitate the unloading of oxygen to the tissues, whereas conditions such as hypothermia and alkalosis have opposite effects. At sea level, at which there is an excess of oxygen in healthy individuals, shifts in the oxygen-hemoglobin curve make little difference in oxygen delivery, but at a high altitude, shifts in the curve may have a significant effect.

On acute ascent to a high altitude, hypoxia and the resultant hypocapnic alkalosis stimulate production of 2,3-diphosphoglycerate (2,3-DPG) within the red blood cell, which shifts the curve to the right (36). At the tissue level, production of carbon dioxide and hydrogen ions also improves the unloading of oxygen from hemoglobin (the Bohr effect).

At moderate altitude, the rightward shifts may be an advantage, but the ease of unloading oxygen must be weighed against the potential disadvantage at higher altitudes of loading oxygen onto hemoglobin at the pulmonary capillary level (37). A leftward shift would theoretically convey an advantage to loading oxygen at altitudes at which the partial pressure of the inspired oxygen is so low that the diffusion gradient from air to blood is small. High-altitude animals and birds, such as the bar-headed goose, that migrate over the Himalayas have left-shifted curves, presumably from the marked hypocapnic alkalosis, as well as an inherently left-shifted hemoglobin. Other experimental animal models bear out the advantage of a leftward shift during acute exposure at very high altitudes. An optimal model may exist in the llamas and alpacas of the Andes, who have a left-shifted curve at the lung level and a right-shifted curve at the peripheral tissues.

Humans, on the other hand, have not lived long enough at high altitudes to evolve a characteristic hemoglobin that would be most suitable for high-altitude survival. A number of workers have found a modest leftward shift of the curve in humans living at high altitudes (38). Increased levels of 2,3-DPG have been found in these humans, but a leftward shift of the oxygen-hemoglobin curve was found probably because of the counter-effect of the respiratory alkalosis. A group of climbers after 2 months at 6,300 m or higher on Mount Everest were found to have a respiratory alkalosis, a modest polycythemic response (mean hematocrit of 54.4% ± 4.01%), and a persistently left-shifted curve despite an increased level of 2,3-DPG (39) (Fig. 47.3). The

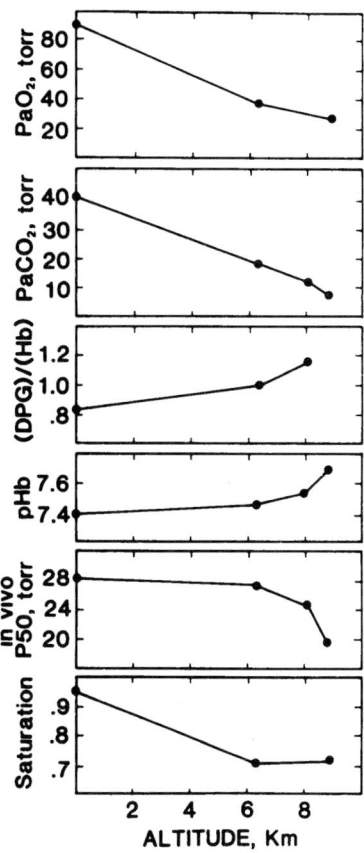

FIGURE 47.3. Effect of altitude on oxygen-hemoglobin affinity. P_{50}, oxygen half-saturation pressure of hemoglobin; DPG, diphosphoglycerate. (From Winslow RM. Red cell function at extreme altitude. In West JB, Lahiri S, eds. *High altitude and man.* Bethesda, MD: American Physiological Society, 1984:59–72, with permission.)

advantages of a left-shifted curve at extreme altitudes, therefore, are at least suggested by the preceding data.

Tissue Alterations

The final stages of oxygen delivery involve the diffusion of oxygen from the blood across the muscle capillary and muscle cell membrane to the cytoplasm and ultimately to the mitochondrion, where oxidative phosphorylation takes place. This process depends on a critical pressure gradient and radial distance for diffusion of oxygen from the blood to the cell. The critical pressure gradient is probably about 5 to 6 mm Hg from the blood into the cytosol and a mere 2 to 3 mm Hg from the cytosol to the mitochondria, but ultimate delivery depends on a number of factors, not the least of which is blood flow, to ensure oxygen flux (40).

Structural morphologic changes at the tissue or cellular level may decrease the distance for diffusion of oxygen from the blood to the mitochondrion. Formation of new capillaries and a recruitment of pre-existing capillaries in response to a hypoxic stimulus are strategies that can achieve that goal. There is ongoing controversy about the effect of hypoxia

on an increase of capillary density because quantification of this response is difficult because muscle cell atrophy also occurs during prolonged (weeks, months) stays at high altitudes (41). The adaptation of the mitochondria to hypoxia is not well defined either; previous studies report that mitochondria may be increased, unchanged, or decreased at high altitudes. Human studies at very high altitudes, on the other hand, have shown a decrease in mitochondria concentration (42).

Several biochemical mechanisms occur and improve oxygen metabolism. Myoglobin, an intracellular protein that binds oxygen at a very low tissue partial pressure of oxygen, facilitates diffusion of oxygen to muscle mitochondria and is increased in animals exposed to and native to high altitude. The enzymes of oxidative metabolism also upgrade their function in response to exposure to and living at high altitudes. Succinic and lactate dehydrogenase, part of the glycolytic pathway, increase at high altitudes, but the changes in these studies were not consistent and depended on the degree of exposure, the tissue involved, and the stress itself. In human studies, results suggest that fatty acid metabolism, which contributes to exercise endurance, is enhanced, whereas glycolytic metabolism, which is responsible for high levels of aerobic work, is decreased (43).

Central Nervous System

The brain is the organ most sensitive to hypoxic stress. The historic flight of the *Zenith* in 1875, a hot-air balloon that carried three Italian scientists to over 8,000 m, during which two of the scientists died, is a testament to the catastrophic effects of acute severe hypoxia on the brain.

The defenses of the brain to the stress of hypoxia are both acute and chronic. The initial decrease in cerebral blood flow that occurs with hypocapnia secondary to hypoxia secondary to the respiratory alkalosis is outweighed by the increase in cerebral blood flow from the hypoxic stimulus. Blood flow increased 33% after 12 hours at 3,800 m and decreased as respiratory adaptation continued, but still was 13% greater than control values after 5 days (44). The net result is that oxygen supply to the brain is probably well preserved despite profound hypoxemia. Despite augmented blood flow, varying degrees of cerebral dysfunction occur, depending on the acuity, duration, and degree of hypoxic stress. The higher one goes, the more that motor, sensory, and complex cognitive abilities are affected. Learning is impaired at 3,000 m, and at 6000 m sensation, perception, and motor skills are diminished.

Several studies have addressed the question of prolonged or permanent effects of hypoxic exposure on central nervous system function. Some investigators found no residual psychometric deficits in climbers who had been above 5,100 m in the Himalayas (45), but two other studies of individuals who had been at a high altitude for 10 months found residual motor incoordination and impaired speech, which resolved within a year (46,47). There was individual variation in these findings, which was also documented in a study of Polish alpinists who had climbed to 5,500 m. All had some impairment noted by psychological testing, and 11 of 30 had electroencephalogram abnormalities (48). A later study showed transient deficits in learning, memory, and verbal expression in two groups of individuals, one that had been on an expedition to Mount Everest, and one that had been exposed to a simulated similar altitude for 40 days in a hypobaric chamber. Fine-motor skills remained abnormal for up to 1 year in many. Unexpectedly, individuals with a high ventilatory response to hypoxia who have higher arterial oxygen saturations and who usually perform better physically had the greatest deficits. The investigators speculated that those who hyperventilated more had greater hypocapnic cerebral vasoconstriction and thus lower oxygen delivery to the brain (49).

Sleep

Periodic breathing, which was described as far back as 1886, occurs during early exposure to high altitudes but decreases as acclimatization ensues. The degree of periodic breathing varies among individuals and may be a function of individual hypoxic chemosensitivity. Findings in both sojourners and high-altitude natives during sleep, when cortical input is minimized, suggest that individuals with high hypoxic chemosensitivity have ventilatory overshoot, resulting in hypocapnic alkalosis, suppression of ventilation, and periodicity of respiration. These oscillations persist throughout sleep and can result in profound arterial oxygen desaturation during the hypopneic and apneic phases. The resulting hypoxemia may contribute to some of the aspects of altitude illness.

Carbonic anhydrase inhibitors eradicate periodic breathing, which may be a result of drug-induced tissue acidosis and subsequent ventilatory stimulation. Discussion of their therapeutic efficacy follows in the section "Acute Mountain Sickness, Prevention."

Exercise

Although a number of observations of the effect of hypoxia on oxygen transport during exercise have been made, an understanding of exercise limitation at high altitudes remains elusive. One thing is certain: Oxygen consumption and, subsequently, exercise performance predictably decrease with ascent to high altitudes (50) (Fig. 47.4).

The increased metabolic rate of exercise and hypoxia of high altitude interact synergistically to augment exercise hyperpnea. The increase in exercise ventilation is proportional to the degree of hypoxia (Fig. 47.5). The degree of exercise hyperpnea is also influenced by the individual's hypoxic ventilatory response, measured at sea level or at high altitude, and extraordinary levels of exercise ventilation may be augmented by the lower gas density. The study on Mount Everest

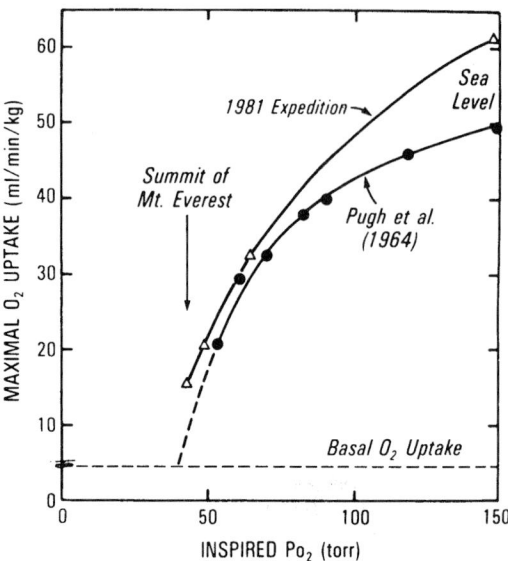

FIGURE 47.4. Maximal oxygen consumption ($\dot{V}O_2$max) against inspired partial pressure of oxygen. There is a predictable decrease in $\dot{V}O_2$max at higher altitudes. The more recent data demonstrate that a low amount of work is possible on the summit of Mount Everest. (From West JB, et al. Maximal exercise at extreme altitudes on Mount Everest. *J Appl Physiol* 1983;55:688, with permission.)

demonstrated that climbers with higher hypoxic chemosensitivity had greater exercise ventilation, less arterial oxygen desaturation, and better climbing performance (51). These data supported studies suggesting that climbers at extreme altitudes (>7,500 m) benefited from a brisk high ventilatory response (52–54). It is, therefore, the ventilatory response at high altitudes that is primarily responsible for the preservation of P_{AO_2} and arterial oxygen partial pressure. On the other hand, in the high-altitude dweller, a lower exercise ventilation is accompanied by a lower alveolar-arterial gradient, suggesting a genetic or adaptive increase in D_L for oxygen that results in improved oxygen transport from the air to the blood (22,55,56).

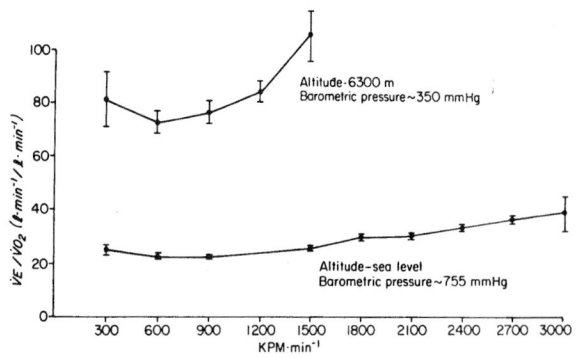

FIGURE 47.5. The ventilatory equivalent ($\dot{V}E/\dot{V}O_2$) for given workloads in a group of climbers at sea level *(lower line)* and at 6,300 m *(upper line)*. The data demonstrate the stimulation of ventilation by hypoxia. (From Schoene RB. Hypoxic ventilatory response and exercise ventilation at sea level and high altitude. In: West JB, Lahiri S, eds. *Man at high altitude*. Bethesda, MD: American Physiological Society, 1984:19–30, with permission.)

Arterial oxygen saturation in sojourners decreases with exercise at high altitude. This desaturation is largely secondary to a diffusion limitation for oxygen from the air to the blood, but some $\dot{V}/\dot{Q}$ heterogeneity contributes to this phenomenon. This $\dot{V}/\dot{Q}$ heterogeneity may be secondary to interstitial lung water, whereas the diffusion limitation is a result of a decreased driving pressure of oxygen from air to blood compounded by a decrease in transit time of blood across the alveolar-capillary membrane (18, 57).

At submaximal work loads during acute exposure, cardiac output is moderately higher than output at sea level, but after a week or so of exposure, heart rate and cardiac output are matched for comparable sea-level work loads (25). On acute high-altitude exposure, maximum cardiac output is the same as at sea level, but it decreases 20% to 30% after 2 months above 4,300 m (58,59). This decrease is a result of a decrease in both maximum heart rate and stroke volume. The decrease in maximum heart rate is more pronounced in sojourners than in high-altitude natives. On the other hand, cardiac output remains appropriate for oxygen consumption, and myocardial contractility, as measured by echocardiography, is preserved even at extreme altitudes (60). Although pulmonary artery pressures are very high during exercise at extreme altitudes, the increase in pulmonary vascular resistance in healthy sojourners does not seem to limit exercise.

MALADAPTATION

Overview

Modern transportation allows millions of people each year to ascend rapidly to high altitudes for travel or recreation. All persons ascending to high altitude undergo the physiologic adaptation response of acclimatization, some more successfully than others. Millions of people also reside at altitudes above 2,500 m, and a certain percentage of those individuals develop chronic altitude disorders. With the previous notes on formal adaptation as a guide, it is the purpose of this section to deal with both acute mountain sickness (AMS) and CMS.

Illnesses of Sojourners to High Altitudes

Acute ascent above 8,000 m can lead to death, whereas, as has been repeatedly achieved in the 20th century, climbers can gradually ascend to these altitudes and live and work for short periods of time quite effectively. In unacclimatized persons ascending to high altitude, failure of the body to adapt to the stress of hypobaric hypoxia may lead to the cerebral and pulmonary syndromes of high-altitude illness. AMS and high-altitude cerebral edema (HACE) refer to the cerebral disorders; high-altitude pulmonary edema (HAPE), to the pulmonary abnormalities. Although there is a great deal of individual variability and overlap in these disorders, this section deals with them separately.

Acute Mountain Sickness

Clinical Picture

AMS is a neurologic syndrome, with headache as the prominent feature associated with one or more nonspecific symptoms. The Lake Louise Consensus Group defined AMS as the presence of headache in an unacclimatized person who has recently ascended to high altitude and who also has one or more of the following: gastrointestinal symptoms (anorexia, nausea, or vomiting), fatigue or weakness, dizziness or lightheadedness, or difficulty sleeping (61). The headache usually begins shortly after ascent (6–24 hours), is more severe in the morning, and is usually treatable with mild analgesics. Some persons show signs of fluid retention with facial or peripheral edema (62,63), or focal crackles on lung auscultation (63), although these signs may also be present in the absence of AMS after ascent to high altitude. Resting heart rate is elevated in AMS (62), and body temperature is mildly elevated (64). Tachypnea is not a distinguishing feature of AMS because it occurs in all persons after ascent to high altitude. All these signs and symptoms usually abate over several days as acclimatization ensues and rarely require more than rest and mild analgesics. Although symptoms of AMS usually resolve without sequelae, AMS can progress to HACE and/or HAPE, which can be life-threatening.

AMS may occur after acute ascent to altitudes greater than 2,000 m. Susceptibility to AMS increases with higher altitude and faster rates of ascent (Table 47.2). On Mount

TABLE 47.2. INCIDENCE OF HIGH-ALTITUDE ILLNESS

Study Group	Sleeping Altitude (meters)	Maximum Altitude Reached (meters)	Average Rate of Ascent to Sleeping Altitude (days)	AMS (%)	HAPE or HACE (%)	Reference
Colorado skiers	2000–3000	3500	1–2	25	0.01	66,117
Mt. Everest trekkers	3000–5200	5500	1–2 (fly)	47	0.05	13,63,89
			10–13 (walk)	23		
Mt. Rainier climbers	3000	4392	1–2	67	0.1	65
Mt. McKinley climbers	3000–5000	6195	4–7	30	1–3	13,116

Modified from Schoene RB, Hackett PH, Hornbein TF. High altitude. In: Murray JF, Nadel JA, eds. *Textbook of Respiratory Medicine*. 3rd ed. New York: W.B. Saunders, 2000, with permission.

Rainier, nearly two thirds of climbers who rapidly ascend from sea level to the summit at 4,400 m over 1 to 3 days develop AMS (65). In Summit County, Colorado, 25% of travelers who ascend from low altitude to ski resorts at 2,000 to 3,000 m develop AMS (66). A prior history of AMS, residence at altitudes below 900 m, and obesity all increase susceptibility to AMS (66). Physical fitness is not protective of AMS (67). Men and women are equally susceptible to AMS (68), and incidence in children is similar to that in adults (69). The elderly, however, are less susceptible to AMS (66,70).

Pathophysiology

In high-altitude illness, neurohumoral and hemodynamic responses occur in the brain, lungs, and peripheral tissues, which result in fluid retention, overperfusion of microvascular beds, and extravasation of fluid into the extravascular space. Symptoms of AMS suggest a primary neurologic syndrome, and current concepts of pathophysiology emphasize a cerebral etiology. By using various neuro-imaging techniques, brain edema has been observed in severe AMS (71,72), suggesting that AMS is the precursor to HACE. In milder cases of AMS, however, edema has not been observed on brain computed tomography (72). A recent study using magnetic resonance imaging suggests that brain swelling occurs in all persons on ascent to high altitude irrespective of development of AMS (73). One hypothesis to explain these discrepancies suggests that persons who develop AMS have less ability to compensate for swelling of the brain that occurs on ascent to high altitude. Those with a lower ratio of cranial CSF–to-brain volume are less able to compensate for swelling through the displacement of CSF and are more likely to have AMS (71). Cerebral blood flow increases on ascent to high altitude, probably because the stimulating effect of hypoxemia dominates the flow-depressant effect of hypocapnia, which results from hyperventilation. Increased cerebral blood flow may increase brain volume and contribute to AMS. Symptoms of AMS, however, have not been shown to correlate with increased cerebral blood flow (74,75).

Systemic fluid retention and weight gain also occur in AMS (76). Individuals who are susceptible to AMS have an exaggerated aldosterone and antidiuretic hormone (ADH) response on ascent that is different from well-acclimatizing individuals who have low ADH and a diuresis (77). A shift of fluid from the extracellular space to the interstitial and intracellular compartments occurs normally during the initial few days at high altitude, but it may be accentuated and prolonged in persons with hypoventilation and AMS (78). Fluid shifts also may explain the pulmonary dysfunctions of relative hypoxemia and mechanical dysfunction in AMS, which may be precursors of overt HAPE.

Pulmonary pathophysiology in AMS includes hypoventilation (78,79), gas-exchange abnormalities (80,81), de-

creased diffusing capacity (82), and pulmonary mechanical dysfunction (65). Individuals with a blunted hypoxic ventilatory response may be more predisposed to fluid retention and AMS (78,79). Climbers at 4,200 m on Mount McKinley, Alaska, who were more hypoxemic than other normally acclimatizing climbers were more likely to get AMS higher on the mountain (83). This suggests that individuals who do not mount a sufficient ventilatory response are more hypoxemic and are more likely to develop AMS.

Prevention

The best strategy for the prevention of AMS is a gradual ascent to allow time for acclimatization. Suggested guidelines are to limit the increase in sleeping altitude to a 600-m elevation gain over a 24-hour period once above 2,500 m and to add an extra day for acclimatization, without an increase in sleeping altitude, after every 600 to 1,200 m gained (84). In one study a gradual ascent over 4 days to 3,500 m, compared with a 1-hour ascent, decreased the incidence and severity of AMS by 41% (85). Pharmacological prophylaxis using acetazolamide or dexamethasone is well proven to prevent AMS, but is recommended only for persons who experience recurrent AMS on ascent to high altitude or for persons who must ascend rapidly—such as in a rescue operation (Table 47.3).

Acetazolamide, a carbonic anhydrase inhibitor, is the primary drug recommended for aiding acclimatization and preventing AMS. Acetazolamide eradicates periodic breathing and arterial oxygen desaturation during sleep at high altitudes (86,87) at a low dose of 125 mg before bedtime, which is sufficient to stimulate ventilation (88). The drug also stimulates ventilation at rest and during exercise by inducing a renal excretion of bicarbonate, causing a metabolic acidosis with compensatory hyperventilation, which may facilitate acclimatization. Acetazolamide also lowers CSF pressure by decreasing CSF formation. Which of these effects is responsible for the drug's efficacy is not known, but it is effective and safe. Side effects of acetazolamide are minimal and include peripheral, self-limited paresthesias, polyuria, and altered taste. A rare side effect is visual disturbance with myopia, which is reversible on discontinuation. Multiple studies have demonstrated the efficacy of acetazolamide in the prevention of AMS (65,89–91). The appropriate dose of acetazolamide for the prevention of AMS is controversial. Two hundred fifty milligrams three times a day is clearly efficacious (92); however, many experts suggest that a lower dose of 125 to 250 mg twice a day is efficacious and results in fewer side effects (84,93). Individuals who are allergic to sulfa drugs should not take acetazolamide.

Multiple studies have demonstrated the efficacy of dexamethasone in prevention of AMS (94–97). Four milligrams of dexamethasone taken two or three times a day is recommended; lower doses have not been shown to be effective (97,98). Dexamethasone taken in combination with acetazolamide may be more effective at preventing AMS than

TABLE 47.3. ACUTE MOUNTAIN SICKNESS (AMS) PREVENTION

Agent	Dose	Comments
Gradual ascent	Average gain of 600 m altitude per day above 2500 m	Sleeping altitude is more important than daytime altitude for risk of AMS
Acetazolamide	250 mg orally two to three times a day starting the day before ascent	Recommended only for those persons with a history of recurrent AMS on ascent to altitude, contraindicated with sulfa allergy
Dexamethasone	4 mg orally two to three times a day starting the day before ascent	Alternative to acetazolamide, recommended if rapid ascent to altitude is required, such as in rescue operations
Ginkgo biloba	80–120 mg orally twice daily starting 3–5 days before ascent	Advantage of essentially no side effects as compared to acetazolamide and dexamethasone

either drug alone (99,100), and this combination might be considered in situations in which rapid ascent to high altitude is required in unacclimatized persons, such as in rescue operations. Because there are no data to suggest that dexamethasone facilitates acclimatization, discontinuation of the drug while the patient is still at a high altitude may result in a rebound of altitude illness (98). The mechanism of dexamethasone in preventing AMS is not known, but it may stabilize the endothelium of the microvascular circulation and prevent capillary leak.

A newer, and less studied, alternative for pharmacological prophylaxis of AMS is *Ginkgo biloba,* which in two randomized controlled studies was effective in preventing AMS (101,102), and in another randomized controlled study was effective in reducing severity of AMS (103). The mechanism for efficacy of *Ginkgo biloba* is unknown but may involve modulation of neurotransmitters and mitochondrial ATP production, promotion of neuronal glucose uptake, reduction of edema, or increase in erythrocyte deformability. In one randomized controlled trial, aspirin was effective at preventing high altitude headache (104).

Treatment

Successful management of AMS involves recognition and appropriate treatment (Table 47.4). If the awareness of and suspicion for AMS are keen enough, then AMS usually will not progress and can be treated with conservative measures, such as rest and mild analgesics (aspirin, acetaminophen, codeine, prochlorperazine). Sedatives, narcotics, and alcohol should be avoided because they may suppress ventilation and mask worsening symptoms. If the subject seems more ill with worsening headache or any other clear neurologic signs, especially ataxia, then this situation should be considered serious, and the patient should descend from high altitude as quickly as possible. Even a few hundred meters may be helpful. If conditions do not permit descent, then oxygen, if available, is a good temporizing measure. Lightweight (15 lb) portable hyperbaric bags operated with a foot pump and capable of pressurizing to about 2 psi are also available for treatment of AMS. These provide a physiologic descent of about 2,000 m. In multiple studies, portable hyperbaric bags have been shown to improve symptoms of AMS (105–108). Short-term pressurization, however, provides no long-term

TABLE 47.4. ACUTE MOUNTAIN SICKNESS (AMS) TREATMENT

Agent	Dose	Comments
Descent	Decrease altitude until symptoms resolve	Recommended if AMS symptoms progress to ataxia or an altered level of consciousness
Oxygen	Low flow nasal cannula to keep $SaO_2 > 90\%$	Simulates descent, may be used for sleep as an adjunct to treatment of mild to moderate AMS
Acetazolamide	250 mg orally two to three times a day	Contraindicated with sulfa allergy
Dexamethasone	4 mg orally three times a day	Alternative to acetazolamide, recommended for more severe symptoms of AMS
Portable hyperbaric bag	30 to 60 minutes of pressurization, or until symptoms resolve	Effective at relieving symptoms of AMS by simulating descent of about 5,000 ft., but rebound AMS usually occurs within hours after treatment

benefit, because once pressurization ceases rebound AMS usually occurs. Still, in remote areas the portable hyperbaric bag provides an excellent reusable alternative to oxygen.

Both acetazolamide and dexamethasone are effective for treating AMS. A small, randomized, placebo-controlled study showed that 250 mg acetazolamide in two doses 8 hours apart reduced severity of AMS within 24 hours (81). Another study that used a higher dose of 1,000 to 1,500 mg of acetazolamide for treatment of AMS also showed improvement in symptoms but with significant side effects, including a worsening of headache in 28% of the subjects (109). Acetazolamide at a dose of 250 mg every 8 to 12 hours is therefore recommended for treatment of AMS. Several randomized controlled studies have shown dexamethasone to be effective for treating AMS (72,108,110), and a dose of 4 mg every 6 hours is recommended. Ibuprofen is effective for treating headache at high altitude (111,112).

The best treatment is prevention, and slow gradual ascent still works. Adequate calories in carbohydrates and maintenance of fluids to ensure a normal urine output are time-honored tactics. The notion that overhydration is beneficial in AMS has no scientific basis and may lead to hyponatremia and worsening AMS or even HACE.

PREVENTION AND TREATMENT OF ACUTE MOUNTAIN SICKNESS

Summary Statement	Level of Evidence
Prevention of acute mountain sickness with acetazolamide, dexamethasone or Ginkgo biloba	Randomized controlled trials
Treatment of acute mountain sickness with descent, oxygen, acetazolamide, dexamethasone and/or portable hyperbaric bag	Randomized controlled trials

---

High-Altitude Cerebral Edema

HACE usually occurs at altitudes greater than 4,000 m and is less common than is HAPE; however, severe HAPE and HACE commonly occur simultaneously. HACE is characterized by progression of global cerebral signs and symptoms in a person with AMS or HAPE. Focal neurologic signs may occur but should also prompt consideration of another diagnosis. Because the symptoms of AMS are similar yet milder than those of HACE, it is reasonable to assume that HACE is the severe progression of AMS pathophysiology. The progression of severe AMS to HACE is distinguished by severe headache and an altered level of consciousness associated with ataxia. HACE may rapidly progress from confusion to obtundation and coma, followed by death, and therefore, lifesaving immediate treatment with descent is mandatory. In addition to descent, treatment with supplemental oxygen and dexamethasone is recommended.

Autopsies have shown cerebral edema with herniation and small petechial hemorrhages in HACE victims (76,113).

Computerized tomographs in HACE show small ventricles, disappearance of sulci, and a diffuse low density appearance of the entire cerebrum, indicating cerebral edema (114). More recently, magnetic resonance imaging studies in seven of nine patients with HACE after evacuation from high altitude showed intense T2 signal in white matter areas, especially the splenium of the corpus callosum, and no gray matter abnormalities (115). These findings suggest that the predominant pathophysiologic mechanism in HACE is vasogenic cerebral edema with movement of fluid and protein out of the vascular compartment likely owing to increased permeability of the blood–brain barrier. In this study, all patients completely recovered, and repeat magnetic resonance imaging in the four patients available for follow-up showed complete resolution of changes.

Early recognition is absolutely essential because HACE, more than any other altitude illness, can progress rapidly to death. Evacuation of a person with HACE is easier and safer for the whole party if HACE is recognized early while the victim is still ambulatory and can aid in his or her own descent. Symptoms improve with descent, although neurologic abnormalities, particularly ataxia, may be slow to recover after descent. Anecdotal experience suggests that oxygen and dexamethasone (8 mg by any route available immediately, then 4 mg every 6 hours until symptoms resolve) may give symptomatic relief until descent can be achieved or may be used as adjunctive therapy with descent. Oxygen and dexamethasone have been lifesaving measures for treatment of HACE at 4,200 m on Mount McKinley in situations in which descent by helicopter evacuation was delayed because of weather. A portable hyperbaric bag may also be helpful but should never delay descent if the patient is ambulatory or transportable. A problematic feature of the portable hyperbaric bag for treatment of HACE in the field is loss of access to a patient with an abnormal mental status. Mannitol and furosemide may be useful for treatment of severe cerebral edema with impending herniation, although no clinical studies have evaluated these drugs for treatment of HACE. Any pharmacologic treatment should be considered as an adjunct to descent for treatment of HACE (Table 47.5).

HIGH-ALTITUDE CEREBRAL EDEMA

Summary Statement	Level of Evidence
Treatment of high-altitude cerebral edema with descent, oxygen, dexamethasone and/or portable hyperbaric bag	Case reports

---

High-Altitude Pulmonary Edema

Clinical Picture

HAPE is a noncardiogenic pulmonary edema that afflicts susceptible persons who ascend to altitudes above 2,500 m and remain there for 24 to 48 hours or longer. Onset of

TABLE 47.5. HIGH-ALTITUDE CEREBRAL EDEMA (HACE)

Agent	Dose	Comments
Descent	Descend in altitude until symptoms resolve	Descent is mandatory and may be lifesaving, early recognition of HACE is essential so that descent may be undertaken while the patient is still ambulatory
Oxygen	Titrate flow to keep SaO$_2$ > 90%	Useful treatment adjunct to descent and simulates descent in situations where descent is delayed
Dexamethasone	8 mg by any route available, then 4 mg every 6 hours	Useful treatment adjunct to descent
Portable hyperbaric bag	Pressurization until descent is possible	May be an effective temporizing treatment if descent is delayed because of weather or terrain conditions

symptoms is within a few days after ascent to high altitude and may be preceded by AMS. As HAPE progresses, incidence of concurrent HACE increases. The incidence of HAPE increases with faster ascent rates and higher altitude and has been reported as high as 15% in Indian troops airlifted from sea level to altitudes between 3,500 m and 5,500 m (76). A lower 2% incidence is reported in climbers making a more gradual ascent to 6,150 m on Mount McKinley in Alaska (116), and a 0.01% rate is reported in visitors to ski resorts in the Rocky Mountains at altitudes of 2,500 to 3,000 m (117). Factors contributing to the development of HAPE include exertion, cold ambient tem-

perature, pre-existing upper respiratory infection, or a prior history of HAPE. HAPE is more common in men than in women (118). Typical symptoms of HAPE are dyspnea, decreased exercise tolerance, and a dry cough that progresses to a cough productive of pink frothy sputum in severe cases. Frank hemoptysis is uncommon. Headache and nausea, typical symptoms of AMS, are common. Signs include cyanosis, tachycardia, tachypnea, low-grade fever, and crackles on lung auscultation (119). The chest radiograph shows patchy bilateral, or unilateral in early HAPE, linear and confluent opacities with a normal cardiac silhouette (119,120) (Fig. 47.6). The degree of hypoxemia depends on the altitude

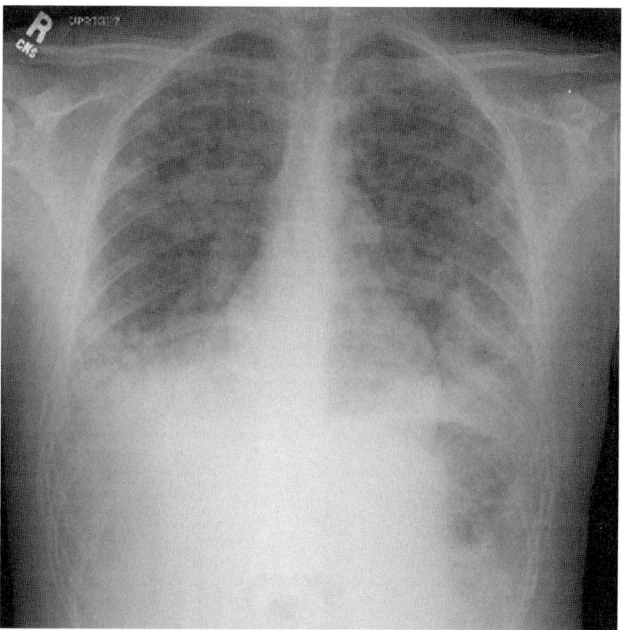 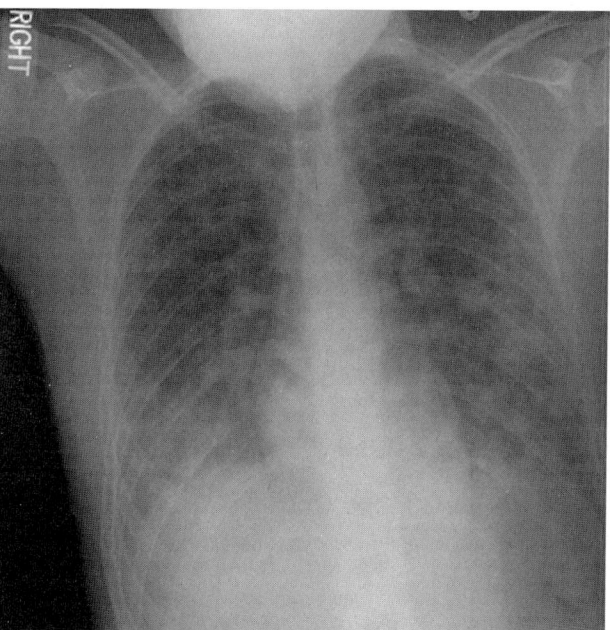

A B

FIGURE 47.6. (A) Chest x-ray film of a 15-year-old boy after helicopter evacuation from an altitude of 11,000 ft for high-altitude pulmonary edema. The chest x-ray shows dense bilateral patchy alveolar infiltrative change and normal cardiac and mediastinal width. **(B)** Chest x-ray from the same patient after one day of treatment with supplemental oxygen delivered by nasal cannula at a flow rate of 4 L/min. The chest x-ray shows improvement in bilateral infiltrates.

at which HAPE occurs. In patients with HAPE at 2,928 m, mean arterial oxygen saturation was 74% (range, 38%–93%) (119), whereas climbers with HAPE at 4,200 m had a mean arterial oxygen saturation of 64% (range, 50%–75%) compared with healthy climbers at that altitude with a mean and standard deviation arterial oxygen saturation of 86% ± 3% (121,122). If symptoms are recognized early enough, while the patient is still ambulatory, descent is a very effective treatment. Most patients recover fully, and many are able to re ascend to high altitude within a fortnight. This observation is important, as it implies that the lung architecture is preserved even after severe edema.

HAPE may be an extension of the normal process of accumulation of lung interstitial edema that occurs on acute ascent to altitude (123). In addition, many asymptomatic individuals have crackles on chest auscultation that resolve with further acclimatization. These findings suggest any person may develop HAPE if exertion, ascent rate, and altitude are great enough. Immunogenetic factors (124), exaggerated hypoxic pulmonary vasoconstriction (125,126), or a blunted hypoxic ventilatory response (127), however, make some persons more susceptible to HAPE.

Pathophysiology

HAPE was described as a unique clinical syndrome in 1960 (128,129), and subsequent studies showed that HAPE is a form of noncardiogenic pulmonary edema associated with pulmonary hypertension (130). Persons susceptible to HAPE have a blunted hypoxic ventilatory response (118) and an exaggerated hypoxic pulmonary vasoconstrictor response that leads to elevated pulmonary artery pressures at high altitude (125,126). HAPE-susceptible persons have augmented sympathetic activation (131), increased release of the pulmonary vasoconstrictor endothelin-1 (132), and decreased synthesis of the pulmonary vasodilator NO (133,134). Exaggerated pulmonary vasoconstriction in HAPE-susceptible persons also leads to redistribution of blood flow in the lungs from the bases to the apices (135). The concept that overperfusion of a vasoconstricted pulmonary vascular bed contributes to the pathophysiology of HAPE is supported by the high susceptibility for HAPE in persons with congenital absence of the right pulmonary artery (136). The role of pulmonary hypertension in HAPE is supported by the efficacy of nifedipine in prevention (137) and inhaled NO in treatment (138). The importance of sympathetic tone in the pulmonary vascular bed in HAPE is supported by the finding that intravenous phentolamine, a short-acting α-adrenergic blocker, decreases pulmonary vascular resistance and improves gas exchange in persons ill with HAPE (139).

Hypoxic pulmonary vasoconstriction, overperfusion, and increased pulmonary artery pressure are clearly associated with the pathophysiology of HAPE. A recent study also suggests that in HAPE-susceptible persons, pulmonary capillary pressure is elevated and pulmonary capillary wedge pressure is normal (140). Increased pulmonary capillary pres-

sure may occur because of pulmonary venular vasoconstriction. Alternatively, an early theory proposed that uneven hypoxic pulmonary vasoconstriction leads to recruitment and overdistension of some parts of the pulmonary vascular bed (141), which would also result in increased pulmonary capillary pressure.

It has been debated whether hypoxic pulmonary vasoconstriction, pulmonary hypertension, overperfusion, and increased pulmonary capillary pressure result in a high pressure (transudative) edema or permeability edema owing to injury of the endothelium. Proponents of HAPE as a hydrostatic edema report objective measures that do not show increased capillary permeability early in HAPE (141,142). In established cases of HAPE, however, high concentrations of proteins in bronchoalveolar lavage (BAL) fluid clearly indicate an exudative edema owing to increased pulmonary capillary permeability (121,143–145) (Fig. 47.7). Initial increases in pulmonary capillary pressure may result in early hydrostatic lung edema, but stress failure secondary to increased capillary transmural pressure may occur, resulting in mechanical injury to pulmonary capillary endothelial cells and increased capillary permeability (146). Increased pulmonary capillary pressure and stress failure of pulmonary endothelial cells in a patchy, rather than diffuse, pattern likely

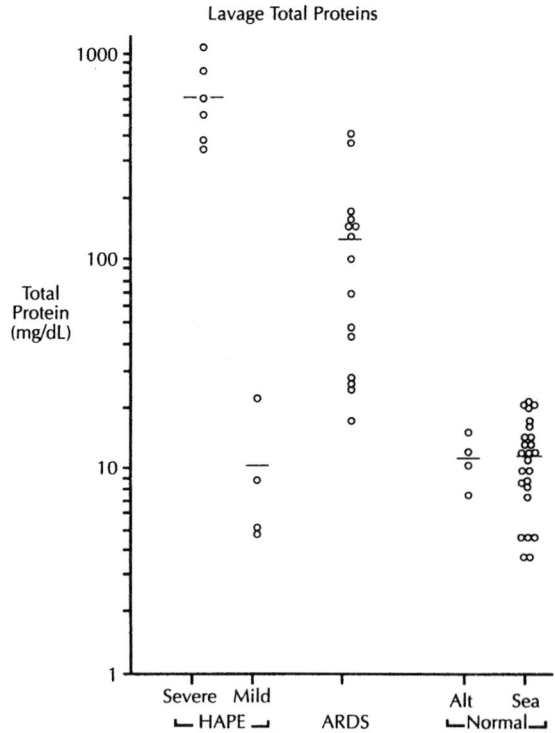

FIGURE 47.7. Protein concentration in bronchoalveolar lavage fluid in patients with **(left to right)** high-altitude pulmonary edema (HAPE), acute mountain sickness with mild arterial oxygen saturation, adult respiratory distress syndrome (ARDS), and two control populations. (From Schoene RB, et al. The lung at high altitude: bronchoalveolar lavage in acute mountain sickness and pulmonary edema. *J Appl Physiol* 1988;64:2605, with permission.)

occurs very early in the course of HAPE and is sufficient to cause alveolar hemorrhage (147,148).

An inflammatory response likely follows mechanical injury to pulmonary capillary endothelial cells in HAPE. Inflammatory markers in BAL fluid from climbers with HAPE include increased leukocytes, primarily macrophages; and increased markers of inflammation including thromboxane B$_2$, a mediator of pulmonary hypertension, and leukotriene B$_4$, a potent chemotactic factor for leukocytes (121,143), and increased concentrations of IL (interleukin)-1β, IL-6, and IL-8 and of tumor necrosis factor-α in BAL fluid (144,145). Increased urinary leukotrienes have also been reported in persons with HAPE (149). The inflammatory response likely follows mechanical pulmonary endothelial cell injury in HAPE because urinary leukotrienes and other inflammatory markers in BAL fluid are not increased early in the course of HAPE (148,150).

Preliminary evidence shows that HAPE-susceptible individuals may have impairment of sodium and fluid clearance from alveoli (151), which would lead to a predisposition for development and retention of alveolar edema. Alternatively, a theory describing the very high protein content in BAL fluid in HAPE, higher than that observed in ARDS (Fig. 47.7), proposes a healthy and intact alveolar epithelium that actively pumps water out of flooded alveoli faster than protein via the Na$^+$-K$^+$ ATPase (152). In both cardiogenic and noncardiogenic pulmonary edema, increased alveolar protein concentration is associated with better outcome, presumably because injury to the alveolar epithelium is limited (153). In HAPE, endothelial cell injury may be limited to isolated areas of overperfused pulmonary capillaries. Therefore, areas of capillary permeability are patchy rather than extensive, and the alveolar epithelium is relatively spared. This is consistent with the easy reversibility of HAPE with appropriate therapy compared with reversibility of ARDS, in which inflammation and endothelial permeability undergo a prolonged course of recovery.

Studies of the leukocyte adhesion molecules, E-selectin and P-selectin, in plasma and BAL fluid in HAPE suggest that endothelial cell activation, platelet activation, and neutrophil recruitment in the lung in HAPE is not as extensive as in ARDS. Plasma concentrations of soluble E-selectin are mildly elevated after ascent to high altitude and in HAPE (122). P-selectin is not elevated in plasma (122) or BAL fluid (144) in HAPE but is markedly elevated in ARDS (154), suggesting that endothelial cell injury and platelet activation in HAPE are not as extensive as in ARDS. In early HAPE, compared with ARDS, the initial process appears to be patchy rather than diffuse and the initial inflammatory response consists of predominately macrophages rather than neutrophils.

An inflammatory response in the lung may cause increased capillary permeability and allow leakage of fluid into alveoli at lower hydrostatic pressures. Animal studies suggest that inflammation may predispose the lung to increased capillary permeability at high altitude. Rats injected with endotoxin have increased lung edema after exposure to high altitude (155), and rats pretreated with dexamethasone are protected from lung leak on exposure to high altitude (156). A pre-existing respiratory infection during ascent to high altitude is known to increase susceptibility to HAPE in humans (157). Inflammation, therefore, may "prime" the pulmonary endothelium to mechanical injury and increase susceptibility to HAPE on ascent to high altitude.

Autopsy studies clearly show inflammation in terminal HAPE. Autopsy specimens from persons who died of HAPE show diffuse lung edema, neutrophilic alveolitis, focal alveolar hemorrhages, thrombi in small pulmonary arteries, and alveolar hyaline membranes (158). Right ventricular and atrial dilation with a normal left ventricle and atrium were also observed. Histologically, these findings are consistent with diffuse alveolar damage, the hallmark of ARDS. Terminal HAPE, therefore, has much in common with ARDS, and two cases of HAPE progressing to ARDS are reported in the literature (159).

Prevention and Treatment

The best way to prevent HAPE is to allow sufficient time for acclimatization. Even HAPE-susceptible individuals can dramatically reduce the incidence of HAPE by ascending gradually over days (160). It is not always possible, however, for climbers, trekkers, or tourists to ascend at a pace that is slow enough to prevent HAPE. Therefore, HAPE will remain an important clinical problem for physicians to recognize and treat.

Because of the low incidence and unpredictability of HAPE, controlled clinical studies and pharmacological trials have been difficult to conduct (Table 47.6). No studies exist that used acetazolamide or dexamethasone in the prevention or treatment of HAPE. One randomized controlled study has shown nifedipine to be effective in preventing HAPE (137). Nifedipine has also been studied for treatment of HAPE, in which it improved gas exchange in some, but not all, subjects (161). Another randomized controlled study showed that an inhaled long-acting β-agonist (salmeterol) was effective in preventing HAPE in susceptible persons (151). The investigators suggested that β-adrenergic stimulation of alveolar transepithelial sodium transport improved fluid clearance from alveoli. In light of these studies, HAPE-susceptible individuals who have to ascend quickly to high altitude should take an extended release preparation of nifedipine and use an inhaled β-agonist.

The most important step in the treatment of HAPE is its early recognition. In remote settings, individuals should descend while they are still able to walk. A descent of 500 to 1,000 m may be all that is necessary to prevent progression of this potentially fatal disease and may actually result in resolution. Oxygen administration, if available, and rest are also helpful but should not delay descent. Careful administration of nifedipine may be a useful adjunctive therapy in

TABLE 47.6. HIGH-ALTITUDE PULMONARY EDEMA (HAPE)

Agent	Dose	Comments
Descent	Descend in altitude until symptoms resolve	Treatment of choice in mountaineering or trekking situations
Oxygen	Titrate flow to keep $SaO_2 > 90\%$	Simulates descent, may be used as the primary treatment at moderate altitude where medical care is available (ski resorts)
Nifedipine	30 to 60 mg sustained release preparation once a day starting the day before ascent for prevention, same dose once a day as an adjunct for treatment	Effective in preventing HAPE in persons with a prior history of HAPE. For treatment of HAPE, useful only as an adjunct to definitive treatment with descent or oxygen
Salmeterol	125 micrograms inhaled twice a day starting one day prior to ascent	May be useful for prevention of HAPE in susceptible persons
Portable hyperbaric bag	Pressurization until descent is possible	May be an effective temporizing treatment if descent is impossible because of weather or terrain conditions

addition to descent or oxygen. In remote areas where supplemental oxygen is unavailable or in limited supply, and when rapid descent may be impossible because of terrain or weather conditions, treatment with pressurization in a portable hyperbaric bag may be lifesaving (162).

In areas where medical help is available, such as recreational ski locations, some patients with HAPE may be treated with supplemental oxygen rather than evacuation to a lower altitude. Patients whose clinical presentation is of the mild or moderate degree, whose oxygen saturation can be improved to greater than 90% by the administration of oxygen, and who have family or friends to watch them can stay at high altitude by using low-flow oxygen therapy and rest (119). Daily follow-up is recommended for patients treated with supplemental oxygen at the same altitude at which HAPE occurred.

Persons with a prior history of a single episode of HAPE should ascend more gradually to high altitude and be aware of symptoms so that HAPE may be treated with early descent. Nifedipine is advised for prophylaxis of HAPE in persons with a prior history of HAPE. Persons with a history of more than one episode of HAPE, or HAPE occurring at under 2,500 m, should have an evaluation for causes of pulmonary hypertension, increased pulmonary vascular resistance, or intrapulmonary or intracardiac right-to-left shunt.

Reentry Pulmonary Edema

Long-time residents at high altitudes may be more susceptible to high-altitude pulmonary edema if they descend to a low altitude and ascend again. Young people (children and teenagers) may be more susceptible, especially if descent and ascent are rapid. Cases have been reported from South America (6.4% incidence) (163) and Leadville, Colorado

(164), but none from Asia. The reasons for this difference are not clear, but it may be secondary to the logistic imposition of a slower ascent in the Himalayas or to the overall better adaptive capabilities of the Tibetan descendants. The cause of reentry HAPE is not known, but it may be secondary to a hypermuscularization and subsequent hyperreactivity of the pulmonary vasculature to hypoxia on reascent (13).

HIGH-ALTITUDE PULMONARY EDEMA

Summary Statement	Level of Evidence
Treatment of high-altitude pulmonary edema with descent and/or oxygen	Case reports and non-randomized clinical studies
Prevention and/or treatment of high-altitude pulmonary edema with nifedipine, salmeterol and/or portable hyperbaric bag	Case reports and small number of randomized clinical studies

Illnesses of High-Altitude Residents

Subacute Mountain Sickness

Two syndromes of pulmonary hypertension and right-sided heart failure have been described in lowlanders who move to high altitude. Subacute infantile mountain sickness was described in Han Chinese infants who were born at low altitude and then moved to Lhasa, Tibet (3,600 m) (165). The adult syndrome was reported in Indian soldiers posted for over 3 months at altitudes over 5,800 m (166). In both syndromes, congestive heart failure and severe pulmonary hypertension inevitably led to death unless the victim was removed to a lower altitude. Polycythemia is not a feature of the disease in children but was present in the adults. In addition to the pulmonary hypertension, pathogenic features in adults include myocardial dysfunction, fluid and salt retention, and impaired renal function.

Chronic Mountain Sickness

Prolonged hypoxic stress at altitudes above 5,000 m limits human habitation. Even though some environments could permit human habitation above 5,000 m, no human civilization has settled above this altitude, probably because acclimatization is never adequate to prevent chronic deterioration owing to hypoxia. Millions of people, however, live between 3,000 and 5,000 m and are exposed to prolonged hypoxic stress. Some individuals residing at high altitudes develop deleterious manifestations of chronic hypoxic stress—polycythemia, pulmonary hypertension, mental slowing, and cor pulmonale. This constellation of findings is termed *chronic mountain sickness* and was first described by Monge in 1928, who noted the sickness in high-altitude natives of the South American Andes (167). Interestingly, although CMS has been observed in all mountain ranges, some populations, especially inhabitants of the Tibetan plateau and women, do not seem very susceptible to CMS (168–170). Populations of lowland natives who move to high altitudes develop CMS over the ensuing years. An interesting study on the Tibetan plateau showed a 13% incidence of CMS in relocated Chinese men, a 1.6% incidence in Chinese women, and a 1% incidence in Tibetan men (171). One could speculate that the Tibetans, who have lived at high altitudes for over 250,000 years, have evolved more successful mechanisms to improve oxygen transport and cope with the hypoxic stress than have Andean natives, who have lived at high altitudes for less than 15,000 years (13).

Clinical Picture

Andean villages have many individuals suffering from CMS. The plethoric male with both mental and physical torpor is classic. Neurologic findings include mental dullness, lethargy, and poor memory. The subjects have polycythemia and cyanosis and resemble, in many respects, the sea-level dweller with cor pulmonale, polycythemia, and sleep disorders with marked nocturnal oxygen desaturation. There may be underlying lung disease as well.

Most of the clinical manifestations can be attributed to hypoventilation, which is associated with a blunted hypoxic chemosensitivity and subsequent relatively greater hypoxemia and greater pulmonary hypertension, which may lead to right-sided heart failure and cor pulmonale. A high-frequency, low-tidal-volume pattern of ventilation may contribute to a low $\dot{V}/\dot{Q}$ ratio, contributing further to the hypoxemia. An increase in red cell mass relative to plasma volume results in a true hyperviscous polycythemia. Hematocrit levels as high as 80% have been described. Hypoventilation, therefore, may be one of the key factors that allows CMS to develop. Other underlying problems, such as lung disease

and an inordinate erythropoietic response, may contribute to the development of CMS (172).

Treatment

The mainstay of treatment is improvement of arterial oxygenation, which should decrease the polycythemia and pulmonary hypertension, and improve cerebral function. If possible, the individual should move to a lower altitude and stop cigarette smoking. Often a relocation is not logistically or culturally possible, and most victims of CMS languish away in remote high-altitude villages. On the other hand, some therapeutic interventions are beneficial. Phlebotomy improves cor pulmonale and increases cardiac output and oxygen transport, but the erythropoiesis eventually returns. Low-flow oxygen, especially at night, is also helpful but not always logistically feasible. Medications that stimulate ventilation and result in a marked improvement in nocturnal oxygen saturation are also beneficial. Acetazolamide is particularly effective, as is medroxyprogesterone acetate, although to a lesser degree (173). Other respiratory stimulants have not been tried.

REFERENCES

1. West JB, Hackett PH, Maret KH, et al. Pulmonary gas exchange on the summit of Mt. Everest. *J Appl Physiol* 1983;55:678–687.
2. Sutton JR, Reeves JT, Wagner PD, et al. Operation Everest II: oxygen transport during exercise at extreme simulated altitude. *J Appl Physiol* 1988;64:1309–1321.
3. Sato M, Severinghaus JW, Powell FL, et al. Augmented hypoxic ventilatory response in men at altitude. *J Appl Physiol* 1992;73:101–107.
4. Goldberg SV, Schoene RB, Haynor D, et al. Brain tissue pH and ventilatory acclimatization to high altitude. *J Appl Physiol* 1992;72:58–63.
5. Severinghaus JW, Mitchell RA, Richardson BW, et al. Respiratory control at high altitude suggesting active transport regulation of CSF pH. *J Appl Physiol* 1963;18:1155–1166.
6. Dempsey JA, Forster HV, Chosy LW, et al. Regulation of CSF (HCO^{3-}) during long-term hypoxic hypocapnia in man. *J Appl Physiol* 1978;44:175–182.
7. Schoene RB, Roach RC, Hackett PH, et al. Operation Everest II: ventilatory adaptation during gradual decompression to extreme altitude. *Med Sci Sports Exerc* 1990;22:804–810.
8. Smith CA, Dempsey JA, Hornbein TF. Control of breathing at high altitude. In: Hornbein TF, Schoene RB, eds. *High altitude: an exploration of human adaptation.* New York: Marcel Dekker Inc, 2001:139–173.
9. Weil JV, Byrne-Quinn E, Sodal I, et al. Acquired attenuation of chemoreceptor function in chemically hypoxic man at high altitude. *J Clin Invest* 1971;50:186–195.
10. Sorensen SC, Severinghaus JW. Irreversible respiratory sensitivity to acute hypoxia in men born at high altitude *J Appl Physiol* 1968;25:217–220.
11. Lahiri S, DeLaney RB, Brody JS, et al. Relative role of environmental and genetic factors in respiratory adaptation to high altitude. *Nature* 1976;261:133–135.
12. Heath D, Edwards C, Harris P. Postmortem size and structure of the human carotid body: its relation to pulmonary disease and cardiac hypertrophy. *Thorax* 1970;25:129–140.

13. Schoene RB, Hackett PH, Hornbein TF. High altitude. In: Murray JF, Nadel JA, eds. *Textbook of respiratory medicine*, 3rd ed. New York: WB Saunders, 2000:1915–1950.

14. Milic-Emili J, Gautier H, Kayser B. Mechanics of breathing. In: Hornbein TF, Schoene RB, eds. *High altitude: an exploration of human adaptation.* New York: Marcel Dekker Inc, 2001:175–198.

15. Cibella F, Cuttitta G, Romano S, et al. Respiratory energetics during exercise at high altitude. *J Appl Physiol* 1999;86:1785–1792.

16. Harms CA, Babcock MA, McClaran SR, et al. Respiratory muscle work compromises leg blood flow during maximal exercise. *J Appl Physiol* 1997;82:1573–1583.

17. Schoene RB. Limits of human lung function at high altitude. *J Exp Biol* 2001;204:3121–3127.

18. Gale GE, Torre-Bueno JR, Moon RE, et al. Ventilation-perfusion inequality in normal humans during exercise at sea level and simulated altitude. *J Appl Physiol* 1985;58:978–988.

19. Wagner PD, Sutton JR, Reeves JT, et al. Operation Everest II: pulmonary gas exchange during simulated ascent of Mt. Everest. *J Appl Physiol* 1987;63:2348–2359.

20. West JB, Wagner PD. Predicted gas exchange on the summit of Mt. Everest. *Respir Physiol* 1980;42:1–16.

21. Wagner PD. Gas exchange. In: Hornbein TF, Schoene RB, eds. *High altitude: an exploration of human adaptation.* New York: Marcel Dekker Inc, 2001:199–234.

22. Schoene RB, Roach RC, Lahiri S, et al. Increased diffusion capacity maintains arterial saturations during exercise in the Quechua Indians of the Chilean Altiplano. *Am J Hum Biol* 1990;2:663–668.

23. Cunningham WL, Becker EF, Krueger F. Catecholamines in plasma and urine at high altitude. *J Appl Physiol* 1965;20:607–610.

24. Vogel JA, Harris CW. Cardiopulmonary responses of resting man during early exposure to high altitude. *J Appl Physiol* 1967;22:1124–1128.

25. Vogel JA, Hartley H, Cruz JC, et al. Cardiac output during exercise in sea level residents at sea level and high altitude. *J Appl Physiol* 1974;36:169–172.

26. Alexander JK, Grover RF. Mechanism of reduced stroke volume at high altitude. *Clin Cardiol* 1983;6:301–303.

27. Wolfel EE, Levine BD. The cardiovascular system at high altitude. In: Hornbein TF, Schoene RB, eds. *High altitude: an exploration of human adaptation.* New York: Marcel Dekker Inc, 2001:235–292.

28. Reeves JT, Stenmark KR. The pulmonary circulation at high altitude. In: Hornbein TF, Schoene RB, eds. *High altitude: an exploration of human adaptation.* New York: Marcel Dekker Inc, 2001:293–342.

29. Knaupp W, Khilnani S, Sherwood J, et al. Erythropoietin response to acute normobaric hypoxia in humans. *J Appl Physiol* 1992;73:837–840.

30. Milledge JS, Coates PM. Serum erythropoietin in humans at high altitude and its relation to plasma renin. *J Appl Physiol* 1985;59:360–364.

31. Sanchez C, Merino C, Figallo M. Simultaneous measurements of plasma volume and cell mass in polycythemia of high altitude. *J Appl Physiol* 1970;28:775–778.

32. Arnaud J, Quilici JC, Gutierrez N, et al. Methemoglobin and erythrocyte reducing systems in high altitude natives. *Ann Hum Biol* 1979;6:585–592.

33. Beall CM, Reischman AB. Hemoglobin levels in a Himalayan high altitude population. *Am J Phys Anthropol* 1984;63:301–306.

34. Sarnquist FH, Schoene RB, Hackett PH. Exercise tolerance and cerebral function after acute hemodilution of polycythemic

mountain climbers. *Aviat Space Environ Med* 1986;57:313–317.

35. Winslow RM, Monge CC. Bloodletting. In: *Hypoxia, polycythemia, and chronic mountain sickness.* Baltimore: Johns Hopkins University Press, 1987:172–202.

36. Lenfant C, Torrance JD, Reynafarje C. Shift of the O_2-Hb dissociation curve at altitude: mechanism and effect. *J Appl Physiol* 1971;305:625–631.

37. Grover RF, Bartsch P. Blood. In: Hornbein TF, Schoene RB, eds. *High altitude: an exploration of human adaptation.* New York: Marcel Dekker Inc, 2001:493–523.

38. Winslow RM, Monge CC, Statham NJ, et al. Variability of oxygen affinity of blood: Human subjects native to high altitude. *J Appl Physiol* 1981;51:1411–1416.

39. Winslow RM, Smaja M, West JB. Red cell function at extreme altitude on Mount Everest. *J Appl Physiol* 1984;56:109–116.

40. Schoene RB. Gas exchange in lung and muscle at high altitude. In: Roca J, Rodrigues-Roisin R, Wagner PD, eds. *Pulmonary and peripheral gas exchange in health and disease.* New York: Marcel Dekker Inc, 2000.

41. Green HJ, Sutton JR. The effects of altitude on skeletal muscle. In: Hornbein TF, Schoene RB, eds. *High altitude: an exploration of human adaptation.* New York: Marcel Dekker Inc, 2001;443–492.

42. MacDougall JD, Green HJ, Sutton JR, et al. Operation Everest II: structural adaptations in skeletal muscle in response to extreme simulated altitude. *Acta Physiol Scand* 1991;142:421–427.

43. Green HJ, Sutton JR, Wolfel EE, et al. Altitude acclimatization and energy metabolic adaptations in skeletal muscle during exercise. *J Appl Physiol* 1992;73:2701–2708.

44. Severinghaus JW, Chiodi H, Eger EL II, et al. Cerebral blood flow in man at high altitude: role of cerebrospinal fluid pH in normalization of flow in chronic hypocapnia. *Circ Res* 1966;19:274–282.

45. Clark CF, Heaton RK, Wiens AN. Neuropsychological functioning after prolonged high altitude exposure in mountaineering. *Aviat Space Environ Med* 1983;54:202–207.

46. Sharma VM, Malhotra MS. Ethnic variations in psychological performance under altitude stress. *Aviat Space Environ Med* 1976;47:248–252.

47. Sharma VM, Malhotra MS, Baskoran AS. Variations in psychomotor efficiency during prolonged stay at high altitude. *Ergonomics* 1975;18:511–516.

48. Ryn Z. Psychopathology in alpinism. *Acta Med Pol* 1976;12:453–467.

49. Hornbein TF, Townes B, Schoene RB, et al. The cost to the central nervous system of climbing to extremely high altitude. *N Engl J Med* 1989:321;1714–1719.

50. West JB, Boyer SJ, Graber DJ, et al. Maximal exercise at extreme altitudes on Mount Everest. *J Appl Physiol* 1983;55:688–702.

51. Schoene RB, Lahiri S, Hackett PH, et al. Relationship of hypoxic ventilatory response to exercise performance on Mount Everest. *J Appl Physiol* 1984;56:1478–1483.

52. Schoene RB. The control of ventilation in climbers to extreme altitude. *J Appl Physiol* 1982;53:886–890.

53. Oelz O, Howald H, diPrampero PE, et al. Physiological profile of world-class high-altitude climbers. *J Appl Physiol* 1986;60:1734–1742.

54. Masuyama S, Kimura H, Sugita T, et al. Control of ventilation in extreme-altitude climbers. *J Appl Physiol* 1986;61:500–506.

55. Dempsey JA, Reddun WG, Birnbaum ML, et al. Effects of acute through life-long hypoxic exposure in exercise pulmonary gas exchange. *Respir Physiol* 1971;13:62–89.

56. Lahiri S, Kao FF, Velasquez T, et al. Respiration of man during

exercise at high altitude: highlanders vs. lowlanders. *Respir Physiol* 1970;8:361–375.

57. Torre-Bueno JR, Wagner PD, Saltzman HA, et al. Diffusion limitation in normal humans during exercise at sea level and simulated altitude. *J Appl Physiol* 1985;58:989–995.

58. Saltin B, Grover RF, Blomqvist CG, et al. Maximal oxygen uptake and cardiac output after two weeks at 4,300 meters. *J Appl Physiol* 1968;25:400–409.

59. Pugh LGCE. Cardiac output in muscular exercise at 5,800 meters. *J Appl Physiol* 1964;19:441–447.

60. Reeves JT, Groves BM, Sutton JR, et al. Operation Everest II: preservation of cardiac function at extreme altitude. *J Appl Physiol* 1987;63:531–539.

61. Roach RC, Bartsch P, Hackett PH, Oelz O, et al. The Lake Louise acute mountain sickness scoring system. In: Sutton JR, Houston CS, Coates G, eds. *Hypoxia and molecular medicine.* Burlington, VT: Charles S. Houston, 1993:272–274.

62. Bartsch P, Shaw S, Franciolli M, et al. Atrial natriuretic peptide in acute mountain sickness. *J Appl Physiol* 1988;65:1929–1937.

63. Hackett PH, Rennie ID. Rales, peripheral edema, retinal hemorrhage and acute mountain sickness. *Am J Med* 1979;67:214–218.

64. Maggiorini M, Bartsch P, Oelz O. Association between raised body temperature and acute mountain sickness: cross sectional study. *BMJ* 1997;315:403–404.

65. Larson EB, Roach RC, Schoene RB, et al. Acute mountain sickness and acetazolamide: clinical efficacy and effect on ventilation. *JAMA* 1982;248:328–332.

66. Honigman B, Theis MK, Kosiol-McLain J, et al. Acute mountain sickness in a general tourist population at moderate altitudes. *Ann Intern Med* 1993;118:587–592.

67. Honigman B, Read M, Lezotte D, et al. Sea-level physical activity and acute mountain sickness at moderate altitude. *West J Med* 1995;163:117–121.

68. Bartsch P, Roach R. Acute mountain sickness and high-altitude cerebral edema. In: Hornbein TF, Schoene RB, eds. *High altitude: an exploration of human adaptation.* New York: Marcel Dekker Inc, 2001:731–776.

69. Pollard AJ, Niermeyer S, Barry P, et al. Children at high altitude: an international consensus statement by an ad hoc committee of the International Society for Mountain Medicine, March 12, 2001. *High Altitude Med Biol* 2001;2:389–403.

70. Roach RC, Houston CS, Honigman B, et al. How well do older persons tolerate moderate altitude? *West J Med* 1995;162:32–36.

71. Hackett PH. High altitude cerebral edema and acute mountain sickness: a pathophysiological update. In: Roach RC, Wagner PD, Hackett PH, eds. *Hypoxia: into the next millennium,* Vol. 474. New York: Kluwer Academic Publishers, 1999:23–45.

72. Levine BD, Yoshimura K, Kobayashi T, et al. Dexamethasone in the treatment of acute mountain sickness. *N Engl J Med* 1989;321:1707–1713.

73. Morocz IA, Zientara GP, Gudbjartsson H, et al. Volumetric quantification of brain swelling after hypobaric hypoxia exposure. *Exp Neurol* 2001;168:96–104.

74. Baumgartner RW, Spyridopoulos I, Bartsch P, et al. Acute mountain sickness is not related to cerebral blood flow: a decompression chamber study. *J Appl Physiol* 1999;86:1578–1582.

75. Jensen JB, Wright AD, Lassen NA, et al. Cerebral blood flow in acute mountain sickness. *J Appl Physiol* 1990;69:430–433.

76. Singh I, Khanna PK, Srivastava MC, et al. Acute mountain sickness. *New Engl J Med* 1969;280:175–184.

77. Bartsch P, Maggiorini M, Schobersberger W, et al. Enhanced exercise-induced rise of aldosterone and vasopressin preceding mountain sickness. *J Appl Physiol* 1991;711:136–143.

78. Hackett PH, Rennie,ID, Hofmeiser SE, et al. Fluid retention and relative hypoventilation in acute mountain sickness. *Respiration* 1982;43:321–329.

79. Moore LG, Harrison GL, McCullough RE, et al. Low acute hypoxic ventilatory response and hypoxic depression in acute altitude sickness. *J Appl Physiol* 1986;60:1407–1412.

80. Sutton JR, Bryan AC, Gray GW, et al. Pulmonary gas exchange in acute mountain sickness. *Aviat Space Environ Med* 1976;47:1032–1037.

81. Grissom CK, Roach RC, Sarnquist FH, et al. Acetazolamide in the treatment of acute mountain sickness: clinical efficacy and effect on gas exchange. *Ann Intern Med* 1992;116:461.

82. Ge Ri-Li, Matsuzawa Y, Takeoka M, et al. Low pulmonary diffusing capacity in subjects with acute mountain sickness. *Chest* 1997;111:58–64.

83. Roach RC, Greene ER, Schoene RB, et al. Arterial oxygen saturation for prediction of acute mountain sickness. *Aviat Space Environ Med* 1998;69:1182–1185.

84. Hackett PH, Roach RC. High altitude Illness. *N Engl J Med* 2001;345:107–114.

85. Purkayastha SS, Ray US, Arora BS, et al. Acclimatization at high altitude in gradual and acute induction. *J Appl Physiol* 1995;79:487–492.

86. Sutton JR, Houston CS, Mansell AL, et al. Effect of acetazolamide on hypoxia during sleep at high altitude. *N Engl J Med* 1979;301:1329–1331.

87. Hackett PH, Roach RC, Harrison GL, et al. Respiratory stimulants and sleep periodic breathing at high altitude: almitrine versus acetazolamide. *Am Rev Respir Dis* 1987;135:896–898.

88. Swenson ER, Leatham KL, Roach RC, et al. Renal carbonic anhydrase inhibition reduces high altitude periodic breathing. *Respir Physiol* 1991;86:333–343.

89. Hackett PH, Rennie D, Levine HD. The incidence, importance, and prophylaxis of acute mountain sickness. *Lancet* 1976;2:1149–1155.

90. Gray GW, Bryan AC, Frayser R, et al. Control of acute mountain sickness. *Aerospace Med* 1971;42:81–84.

91. Greene MK, Keer AM, McIntosh IB, et al. Acetazolamide in prevention of acute mountain sickness: a double blind controlled cross-over study. *BMJ* 1981;283:811–813.

92. Dumont L, Mardirosoff C, Tramer MR. Efficacy and harm of pharmacological prevention of acute mountain sickness: quantitative systematic review. *BMJ* 2000;321:267–272.

93. Ried DL, Carter KA, Ellsworth A. Acetazolamide or dexamethasone for prevention of acute mountain sickness: a meta-analysis. *J Wilderness Med* 1994;5:34–48.

94. Johnson TS, Rock PB, Fulco CS, et al. Prevention of acute mountain sickness by dexamethasone. *N Engl J Med* 1984;310:683–686.

95. Ellsworth AJ, Meyer EF, Larson EB. Acetazolamide or dexamethasone use versus placebo to prevent acute mountain sickness on Mt. Ranier. *West J Med* 1991;154:289–293.

96. Ellsworth AJ, Larson EB, Strickland D. A randomized trial of dexamethasone and acetazolamide for acute mountain sickness prophylaxis. *Am J Med* 1987;83:1024.

97. Rock PB, Johnson TS, Larsen RF, et al. Dexamethasone as prophylaxis for acute mountain sickness, effect of dose level. *Chest* 1989;95:568–573.

98. Hackett PH, Roach RC, Wood RA, et al. Dexamethasone for prevention and treatment of acute mountain sickness. *Aviat Space Environ Med* 1988;59:950–954.

99. Bernhard WN, Schalick LM, Delaney PA, et al. Acetazolamide plus low-dose dexamethasone is better than acetazolamide alone to ameliorate symptoms of acute mountain sickness. *Aviat Space Environ Med* 1998;69:883–886.

100. Zell SC, Goodman PH. Acetazolamide and dexamethasone

in the prevention of acute mountain sickness. *West J Med* 1988;148:541–545.

101. Roncin JP, Schwartz F, D'Arbigny P. EGb 761 in control of acute mountain sickness and vascular reactivity to cold exposure. *Aviat Space Environ Med* 1996;67:445–452.

102. Maakestad K, Leadbetter G, Olson S, et al. *Ginkgo biloba* reduces incidence and severity of acute mountain sickness. *Wilderness Environ Med* 2001;12:51(abst).

103. Gertsch JH, Seto TB, Mor J, et al. Ginkgo biloba for the prevention of severe acute mountain sickness (AMS) starting one day before rapid ascent. *High Altitude Med Biol* 2002;3:29–36.

104. Burtscher M, Likar R, Nachbauer W, et al. Aspirin for prophylaxis against headache at high altitudes: randomised, double blind, placebo controlled trial. *BMJ* 1998;316:1057–1058.

105. Bartsch P, Merki B, Hofstetter D, et al. Treatment of acute mountain sickness by simulated descent: a randomised controlled trial. *BMJ* 1993;306:1098–1101.

106. Kasic JF, Yaron M, Nicholas R, et al. Treatment of acute mountain sickness: hyperbaric versus oxygen therapy. *Ann Emerg Med* 1991;20:1109–1112.

107. Kayser B, Herry JP, Bartsch P. Pressurization and acute mountain sickness. *Aviat Space Environ Med* 1993;64:928–931.

108. Keller HR, Maggiorini M, Bartsch P, et al. Simulated descent v dexamethasone in treatment of acute mountain sickness: a randomised trial. *BMJ* 1995;310:1232–1235.

109. Wright AD, Winterborn MH, Forster PJ, et al. Carbonic anhydrase inhibition in the immediate therapy of acute mountain sickness. *J Wilderness Med* 1994;5:49–55.

110. Ferrazzini G, Maggiorini M, Kriemler S, et al. Successful treatment of acute mountain sickness with dexamethasone. *BMJ* 1987;294:1380–1382.

111. Broome JR, Stoneham MD, Beeley JM, et al. High altitude headache: treatment with ibuprofen. *Aviat Space Environ Med* 1994;65:19–20.

112. Burtscher M, Likar R, Nachbauer W, et al. Ibuprofen versus sumatriptan for high altitude headache. *Lancet* 1995;346:254–255.

113. Dickinson J, Heath D, Gosney J, et al. Altitude-related deaths in seven trekkers in the Himalayas. *Thorax* 1983;38:646–656.

114. Kobayashi T, Koyama S, Kubo K, et al. Clinical features of patients with high altitude pulmonary edema in Japan. *Chest* 1987;92:814–821.

115. Hackett PH, Yarnell PR, Hill R, et al. High altitude cerebral edema evaluated with magnetic resonance imaging, clinical correlation and pathophysiology. *JAMA* 1998;280:1920–1925.

116. Hackett PH, Roach RC, Schoene RB, et al. The Denali medical research project, 1982–1985. *Am Alpine J* 1986;28:129–137.

117. Sophocles AM. High-altitude pulmonary edema in Vail, Colorado, 1975–1982. *West J Med* 1986;144:569–573.

118. Schoene RB, Swenson ER, Hultgren HN. High altitude pulmonary edema. In: Hornbein TF, Schoene RB, eds. *High altitude: an exploration of human adaptation.* New York: Marcel Dekker Inc, 2001:777–814.

119. Hultgren HN, Honigman B, Theis K, et al. High altitude pulmonary edema at a ski resort. *West J Med* 1996;164:222–227.

120. Vock P, Gretz C, Franciolli M, et al. High altitude pulmonary edema: findings at high altitude chest radiography and physical examination. *Radiology* 1989;170:661–666.

121. Schoene RB, Swenson ER, Pizzo CJ, et al. The lung at high altitude, bronchoalveolar lavage in acute mountain sickness and pulmonary edema. *J Appl Physiol* 1988;64:2605–2613.

122. Grissom CK, Zimmerman GA, and Whatley RE. Endothelial selectins in acute mountain sickness and high-altitude pulmonary edema. *Chest* 1997;112:1572–1578.

123. Cremona G, Asnaghi R, Baderna P, et al. Pulmonary extravascular

fluid accumulation in recreational climbers: a prospective study. *Lancet* 2002;359:303–309.

124. Hanaoka M, Kubo K, Yoshitaka Y, et al. Association of high altitude pulmonary edema with the major histocompatibility complex. *Circulation* 1998;97:1124–1128.

125. Hultgren HN, Grover RF, and Hartley LH. Abnormal circulatory responses to high altitude in subjects with a previous history of high altitude pulmonary edema. *Circulation* 1971;44:759–770.

126. Kawashima A, Kubo K, Kobayashi T, et al. Hemodynamic responses to acute hypoxia, hypobaria, and exercise in subjects susceptible to high altitude pulmonary edema. *J Appl Physiol* 1989;67:1982–1989.

127. Hackett PH, Roach RC, Schoene RB, et al. Abnormal control of ventilation in high altitude pulmonary edema. *J Appl Physiol* 1988;64:1268–1272.

128. Houston CS. Acute pulmonary edema of high altitude. *N Engl J Med* 1960;263:478–480.

129. Hultgren H, Spickard W. Medical experiences in Peru. *Stanford Med Bull* 1960;18:76–95.

130. Hultgren HN, Lopez CE, Lundberg E, et al. Physiologic studies of pulmonary edema at high altitude. *Circulation* 1964;29:393–408.

131. Duplain H, Vollenweider L, Delabays A, et al. Augmented sympathetic activation during short term hypoxia and high altitude exposure in subjects susceptible to high altitude pulmonary edema. *Circulation* 1999;99:1713–1718.

132. Sartori C, Vollenweider L, Loffler BM, et al. Exaggerated endothelin release in high altitude pulmonary edema. *Circulation* 1999;99:2665–2668.

133. Duplain H, Sartori C, Lepori M, et al. Exhaled nitric oxide in high altitude pulmonary edema: role in the regulation of pulmonary vascular tone and evidence for a role against inflammation. *Am J Respir Crit Care Med* 2000;162:221–224.

134. Busch T, Bartsch P, Pappert D, et al. Hypoxia decreases exhaled nitric oxide in mountaineers susceptible to high-altitude pulmonary edema. *Am J Respir Crit Care Med* 2001;163:368–373.

135. Hanaoka M, Tanaka M, Ge RL, et al. Hypoxia induced pulmonary blood redistribution in subjects with a history of high altitude pulmonary edema. *Circulation* 2000;101:1418–1422.

136. Hackett PH, Creagh CE, Grover RF, et al. High altitude pulmonary edema in persons without the right pulmonary artery. *N Engl J Med* 1980;302:1070–1073.

137. Bartsch P, Maggiorini M, Ritter M, et al. Prevention of high-altitude pulmonary edema by nifedipine. *N Engl J Med* 1991;325:1284–1289.

138. Scherrer U, Vollenwelder L, Delabays A, et al. Inhaled nitric oxide for high-altitude pulmonary edema. *N Engl J. Med* 1996;334:624–629.

139. Hackett PH, Roach RC, Hartig GS, et al. The effect of vasodilators on pulmonary hemodynamics in high altitude pulmonary edema: a comparison. *Int J Sports Med* 1992;13:S68–S71.

140. Maggiorini M, Melot C, Pierre S, et al. High altitude pulmonary edema is initially caused by an increase in capillary pressure. *Circulation* 2001;103:2078–2083.

141. Hultgren HN. High altitude pulmonary edema. In: Staub N, ed. *Lung water and solute exchange.* New York: Marcel Dekker Inc, 1978:437–469.

142. Kleger GR, Bartsch P, Vock P, et al. Evidence against an increase in capillary permeability in subjects exposed to high altitude. *J Appl Physiol* 1996;81:1917–1923.

143. Schoene RB, Hackett PH, Henderson WR, et al. High altitude pulmonary edema, characteristics of lung lavage fluid. *JAMA* 1986;256:63–69.

144. Kubo K, Hanaoka M, Yamaguchi S, et al. Cytokines in

bronchoalveolar lavage fluid in patients with high altitude pulmonary oedema at moderate altitude in Japan. *Thorax* 1996;51: 739–742.

145. Kubo K, Hanaoka M, Hayano T, et al. Inflammatory cytokines in BAL fluid and pulmonary hemodynamics in high altitude pulmonary edema. *Respir Physiol* 1998;111:301–310.

146. West JB, Colice GL, Lee Y-J, et al. Pathogenesis of high-altitude pulmonary oedema: direct evidence of stress failure of pulmonary capillaries. *Eur Respir J* 1995;8:523–529.

147. Grissom CK, Albertine KH, Elstad MR. Alveolar haemorrhage in a case of high altitude pulmonary oedema. *Thorax* 2000;55:167–169.

148. Swenson ER, Maggiorini M, Mongovin S, et al. Pathogenesis of high-altitude pulmonary edema, inflammation is not an etiologic factor. *JAMA* 2002;287;2228–2235.

149. Kaminsky DA, Jones K, Schoene RB, et al. Urinary leukotriene E$_4$ levels in high-altitude pulmonary edema. *Chest* 1996;110:939–945.

150. Bartsch P, Eichenberger U, Ballmer PE, et al. Urinary leukotriene E$_4$ levels are not increased prior to high altitude pulmonary edema. *Chest* 2000;117:1393–1398.

151. Sartori C, Allemann Y, Duplain H, et al. Salmeterol for the prevention of high-altitude pulmonary edema. *N Engl J Med* 2002;346:1631–1636.

152. Grissom CK, Elstad MR. The pathophysiology of high altitude pulmonary edema. *Wilderness Environ Med* 1999;10:88–92.

153. Matthay MA, Wiener-Kronish JP. Intact epithelial barrier function is critical for the resolution of alveolar edema in humans. *Am Rev Resp Dis* 1990;142:1250–1257.

154. Sakamaki F, Ishizaka A, Handa M, et al. Soluble form of P-selectin in plasma is elevated in acute lung injury. *Am J Respir Crit Care Med* 1995;151:1821–1826.

155. Ono S, Wesctcott JY, Chang SW, et al. Endotoxin priming followed by high altitude causes pulmonary edema in rats. *J Appl Physiol* 1993;74:1534–1542.

156. Stelzner TJ, O'Brien RF, Sato K, et al. Hypoxia-induced increases in pulmonary transvascular protein escape in rats. *J Clin Invest* 1988;82:1840–1847.

157. Durmowicz AZ, Noordeweir E, Nicholas R, et al. Inflammatory processes may predispose children to high-altitude pulmonary edema. *J Pediatr* 1997;130:838–840.

158. Hultgren HN, Wilson R, Kosek JC. Lung pathology in high-altitude pulmonary edema. *Wilderness Environ Med* 1997;8:218–220.

159. Zimmerman GA and Crapo RO. Adult respiratory distress syndrome secondary to high altitude pulmonary edema. *West J Med* 1980;133:335–337.

160. Bartsch P. High altitude pulmonary edema. *Med Sci Sports Exerc* 1999;31:S23–S27.

161. Oelz O, Maggiorini M, Ritter M, et al. Nifedipine for high altitude pulmonary edema. *Lancet* 1989;2:1241–1244.

162. Hackett PH, Roach RC, Goldberg S, et al. A portable, fabric hyperbaric chamber for treatment of high altitude pulmonary edema. In: Sutton JR, Coates G, Remmers JE, eds. *Hypoxia: the adaptations.* Philadelphia: BC Decker, 1990:291(abst).

163. Hultgren HN, Marticorena EA. High altitude pulmonary edema: epidemiologic observations in Peru. *Chest* 1978;74:372–376.

164. Scoggin CH, Hyers TM, Reeves JT, et al. High altitude pulmonary edema in the children and young adults of Leadville, Colorado. *N Engl J Med* 1977;297:1269–1273.

165. Sui GJ, Liu YH, Cheng XS, et al. Subacute infantile mountain sickness. *J Pathol* 1988;155:161–170.

166. Anand IS, Malhotra RM, Chandrashekhar Y, et al. Adult sub-acute mountain sickness: a syndrome of congestive heart failure in man at very high altitude. *Lancet* 1990;335:561–565.

167. Monge CM. La enfermedad de las Andes: sindromes eritremicos. *Ann Fac Med Univ San Marcos (Lima)* 1928;11:1–316.

168. Huang SY, Ning XH, Zhou ZN, et al. Ventilatory function in adaptation to high altitude. In: West JB, Lahiri S, eds. *Studies in Tibet: high altitude and man.* Bethesda, MD: American Physiological Society, 1984:173–177.

169. Monge CC, Leon-Velarde F, Arregui A. Chronic mountain sickness in Andeans. In: Hornbein TF, Schoene RB, eds. *High altitude: an exploration of human adaptation.* New York: Marcel Dekker Inc, 2001:815–838.

170. Kryger M, McCullough R, Doekel R, et al. Excessive polycythemia of high altitude: role of ventilatory drive and lung disease. *Am Rev Respir Dis* 1978;118:659–666.

171. Xie CF, Pei SX. Some physiological data on sojourners and native highlanders at three different altitudes in Xizang. In: Shang LD, ed. *Proceedings of Symposium on Tibet Plateau.* New York: Gordon and Breach Science Publishers, 1981:1449–1452.

172. Kryger MH, Grover RF. Chronic mountain sickness. *Semin Respir Med* 1983;5:164–168.

173. Kryger M, McCullogh RE, Collins D, et al. Treatment of excessive polycythemia of high altitude with respiratory stimulant drugs. *Am Rev Respir Dis* 1978;117:455–464.

Diving Medicine and Near Drowning

48

Claude A. Piantadosi

For physicians in pulmonary and critical care medicine, medical illnesses associated with underwater immersion and diving are a special interest. These illnesses are associated with important mechanisms of pathophysiology and may lead to serious respiratory problems such as hypoxemia, pneumonia, and acute respiratory distress syndrome (ARDS). Caring for patients who suffer accidents underwater, including problems of breath-hold diving and diving with compressed air or other breathing mixtures, requires specialized knowledge and resources. Because of the enormous recent growth in the popularity of aquatic sports, including recreational scuba (self-contained underwater breathing apparatus) diving, familiarity with these activities and the medical problems they encompass is highly desirable for the specialist in respiratory diseases and critical care medicine.

Aquatic and underwater environments are deceptively dangerous, and physical skill, experience, and common sense are needed to enjoy them safely. Too often, swimmers, boaters, or divers ignore signs of danger and find themselves in hazardous situations. Some individuals impair their faculties with alcohol or other drugs, or inadvertently encounter an aquatic environment for which they are not prepared or, as for small children, without proper supervision. These mistakes translate to a large number of incidents, sometimes with disastrous consequences.

DROWNING AND NEAR DROWNING

Three fourths of the earth's surface is covered by water, yet humans lack the innate ability to swim. Without swimming skills, even brief submersion, sometimes in very shallow

C. A. Piantadosi: Department of Medicine, Duke University Medical Center, Durham, North Carolina.

water, can result in drowning [1]. As a result, drowning is second only to motor vehicle accidents as a cause of accidental death in the United States. In addition, most near-drowning victims are young, and death by drowning occurs most frequently in children [2,3]. These accidents occur with greatest frequency in coastal areas and inland regions with abundant natural recreational waters; however, swimming pools, bathtubs, home wells, and even cleaning buckets are sites of drowning.

Incidence and Risk Factors

Of approximately 80,000 submersion incidents each year in the United States, 7,000 to 9,000 deaths are reported. Half of the victims are under age 18 (one fourth less than 5 years), and among the younger group of children, toddlers have the highest rate of drowning [2,3]. Young boys drown five to 10 times more often than young girls and show a biphasic age-related incidence in drowning deaths with peaks at ages 2 and 18 years, whereas the female incidence peaks at 1 year. This gender difference appears to be related to several factors, including boldness and lack of adult supervision in the younger children, whereas more frequent aquatic exposures, greater alcohol consumption, and greater risk-taking behavior are factors in teenage boys.

Apart from young age and male sex, other populations are at risk for drowning, including black children and people who do not swim. Other risk factors include consumption of drugs or alcohol at water recreation sites and water-related injuries such as head trauma and cervical spine dislocation from diving headfirst into shallow water. Pre-existing medical illnesses such as seizure disorders, vagal syncope, and cardiac arrhythmias also predispose to drowning accidents. Drowning is an occupational hazard for maritime workers, including commercial watermen and fishermen, particularly those working in or around cold waters.

The importance of alcohol consumption as a risk factor in drowning cannot be over-emphasized. Alcohol intoxication contributes to one third of drowning incidents in adolescents and young adults. Alcohol impairs alertness, judgment, and coordination and predisposes to hypothermia by interfering with vasoconstriction and body heat conservation. In addition to alcohol, illegal and prescription drugs may play important roles in drowning in adolescents and adults, and toxicological testing is appropriate in unexplained cases.

Terminology

Drowning is defined as death by asphyxia after submersion underwater. The term *near drowning* is used to describe an adverse submersion incident from which the victim survives long enough to receive medical attention (1,4). Thus, near-drowning syndromes in the acute setting represent a continuum from aspiration of a small amount of water to cardiopulmonary arrest. In most near-drowning incidents, the victim aspirates water, particularly when the glottis relaxes after loss of consciousness from cerebral hypoxia. This is sometimes referred to as *wet drowning*. In approximately 15% of victims, however, the lungs contain no water and the drowning is dry. *Dry drowning* appears to be related to persistent laryngospasm, which excludes water from the lower respiratory tract. *Delayed or secondary* drowning syndromes occur when the victim appears to have survived the initial insult but then develops ARDS or severe pneumonia. This is also called *postimmersion syndrome*.

Immersion, the Diving Response, and the Sudden Immersion Syndrome

Immersion of the body in water produces prompt adjustments in respiratory, cardiovascular, renal, and endocrine physiology (5). The important immediate physiological responses are an increase in thoracic blood volume, a sustained increase in cardiac output, a decrease in thoracic gas volume, and an increase in urine output, resulting in dehydration. These responses occur owing to hydrostatic pressure and the high density of water relative to air. During immersion, water supports the extrathoracic blood vessels, and the body is exposed to a hydrostatic pressure gradient proportional to its vertical height. The hydrostatic pressure surrounding the body compresses the abdomen relative to the thorax, causing negative pressure breathing of approximately -20 cm of water. These hydrostatic effects displace the diaphragm upward and decrease the thoracic gas volume and expiratory reserve volume. The pressure gradient across the diaphragm created by immersion, together with the hydrostatic decrease in venous capacitance in the legs, increases the volume of blood in the thoracic vessels, including the heart. The high density of water also facilitates the increase in thoracic blood volume with immersion. Central blood volume may be aug-

mented by peripheral arterial vasoconstriction if the water temperature is below thermoneutrality (34°C, 93.2°F). The increase in central blood volume during immersion distends the cardiac chambers and enhances ventricular diastolic filling, which increases the cardiac output. The increase in cardiac output is attributable almost entirely to stroke volume, which may increase twofold. The elevated cardiac output is persistent and occurs with no measurable increase in systemic oxygen (O_2) uptake. The mechanism of the increase in stroke volume is primarily an increase in cardiac preload.

Cardiovascular distention during immersion activates cardiac mechanoreceptors, which respond to hypervolemia. Although there is no immediate change in total blood volume, the apparent hypervolemia is detected at the hypothalamus via vagal afferents. The ensuing immersion response has two components: diuresis and natriuresis. Peak diuresis occurs in the first 1 to 2 hours of immersion, whereas peak natriuresis occurs after 4 to 5 hours. Fluid restriction and antidiuretic hormone (ADH) administration before immersion prevent diuresis but do not affect natriuresis. The amount of distention of the central circulatory organs correlates with excretion of urinary sodium. The mechanism of the response to increased water loss during immersion is suppression of ADH release. This is also known as the Gauer-Henry response. The natriuresis is related to decreased tubular reabsorption of sodium and not to an increase in filtered sodium. The important factors in the natriuresis appear to be aldosterone suppression (related to decreased renin-angiotensin activity), increased release of atrial natriuretic factor and renal prostaglandins, and decreased sympathetic activity.

The mammalian diving response so integral to the physiology of seals and other diving mammals is also present in humans, but it is not very pronounced except in young children (6). The breath-hold dive invokes a complex response related to apnea and facial immersion that is augmented by cold water. Stimulation of facial receptors by cold water reflexively redistributes blood away from the peripheral tissues and gut toward the heart and brain. Strong vagal stimulation by the diving response produces its primary manifestation, bradycardia. In diving mammals, this response conserves O_2, protects the brain from hypoxia, and lengthens the underwater dive. This interpretation of the response is also reasonable for humans, who show more gradual arterial desaturation during a breath-hold in water than with dry apnea. The magnitude of the diving response varies among individuals, and it becomes more pronounced with training.

The contribution of the human diving response to survival in near-drowning incidents in cold water is not clear. This uncertainty has both a physiological and practical basis. The amount of O_2 stored in the body, primarily in the lungs, is very limited, and panic or struggling underwater rapidly depletes the supply. In children, the diving response is more pronounced, and it may be contribute to survival in cold water drowning because the brain cools rapidly. Young children have recovered with normal neurological function after more than 1 hour submerged in cold water.

In some instances of immersion in very cold water, the victim disappears very suddenly. This is known as the *sudden disappearance syndrome* or the *sudden immersion syndrome*. This syndrome has been attributed to cardiac arrest after sudden facial contact with very cold water. The mechanism of cardiac arrest is often related to strong vagal stimulation resulting in profound bradycardia, and to adrenergic stimulation. This can precipitate ventricular arrhythmias, including ventricular fibrillation, and both have been implicated in the syndrome. Individuals with the long QT syndrome are at increased risk for sudden immersion syndrome.

Shallow water blackout refers to loss of consciousness on ascent to the surface from a breath-hold dive (5). This is a common cause of unconsciousness and near drowning in skin (snorkel) divers and swimmers who hyperventilate and then conduct a breath-hold with exercise. The pathophysiology of shallow water blackout is relatively simple. The main stimulus to breathe at the end of a breath-hold is the partial pressure of carbon dioxide (CO_2) in the blood. This is known as the *breakpoint*. During a breath-hold dive in the water, pre-dive hyperventilation may prolong the time to the breakpoint; however, the consumption of O_2 during the breath-hold continues at the normal rate. When the diver feels the need for air and ascends towards the surface, the thorax re-expands and the partial pressure of O_2 (Po_2) in the alveolus falls owing to the increase in alveolar volume. Thus, the diver may suffer sudden arterial desaturation and extreme cerebral hypoxia near the surface and lose consciousness. It is emphasized that hyperventilation followed by breath-hold is dangerous and is the main factor responsible for shallow water blackout. Hyperventilation therefore should not be used before breath-hold diving or as training technique in water sports.

Pathophysiology of Near Drowning

The immediate medical consequences of near drowning are caused by asphyxia (1,2,4,7–10). Effective pulmonary gas exchange ceases, and the victims suffer the effects of hypoxia and acidosis. The systems most frequently injured by near drowning are the lungs, heart, brain, and kidneys. Complications such as rhabdomyolysis, hemolysis, and coagulopathy may also occur, but they are rare. Initially, the outcome is determined by the presence or absence of cardiopulmonary arrest; if the patient survives the initial insult, the neurological status correlates with prognosis. The other major complications, including ARDS and pneumonia, tend to resolve with appropriate treatment.

Pulmonary Complications

The pathophysiology of lung injury in near drowning is complex (1,4). When either fresh water (FW) or seawa-

ter (SW) contacts the lower respiratory tract, it produces laryngospasm and airway obstruction. If the duration of immersion is brief, laryngospasm may prevent flooding of the lungs. Although 10% to 15% of drowning victims aspirate a trivial amount of water, some of them develop sufficient hypoxia from laryngospasm to produce ventricular arrhythmias or hypoxic encephalopathy. Aspiration of either SW or FW also induces small-airway obstruction, which is aggravated by bronchoconstriction, mucosal edema, water, and debris (e.g., plant matter, sand, mud, teeth, and gastric contents).

Aspiration of small quantities of either SW or FW is sufficient to cause an immediate dramatic decrease in lung compliance and areas of shunt and low ventilation-perfusion ratio ($\dot{V}/\dot{Q}$). Therefore, aspiration may produce more durable hypoxemia than does simple laryngospasm. In animals, some of the early changes in pulmonary gas exchange have been attributable to loss of surfactant activity, injury to alveolar epithelium and capillary endothelium, and alveolar flooding. In many human drowning victims, vomiting and aspiration of stomach contents aggravate airway and alveolar epithelial injury. The alveolar flooding, loss of surfactant function, atelectasis, and alveolar damage may give rise to severe intrapulmonary shunting, which may reach 70% of cardiac output. Severe injury may culminate in ARDS hours to days after the event, and has been reported in up to 40% of the victims. Fortunately, ARDS after near drowning is more readily reversible than other causes of ARDS.

Cardiac Complications

The heart of the near-drowning victim is irritable, and arrhythmias, particularly ventricular fibrillation, occur in severe episodes. These arrhythmias are caused by cardiac ischemia and hypoxia, and excessive stimulation by catecholamines. Hypothermia may also play a role in some cases. Experiments in animals found hemolysis and large shifts in blood electrolyte concentrations after instillation of FW and SW into the lungs, which correlated with the development of ventricular arrhythmias. Human studies have failed to confirm significant electrolyte changes even in patients with ventricular fibrillation, except in drowning in the Dead Sea, which has a much higher mineral content than that of normal SW. Dead Sea drowning causes hypernatremia, hyperchloremia, hypermagnesemia, and hypercalcemia because of absorption of electrolytes from the gastrointestinal tract after swallowing water during the episode. These electrolyte changes can be associated with fatal ventricular fibrillation. Human drowning victims rarely aspirate enough water to produce significant electrolyte changes.

Pathological examinations in humans dying from SW and FW drowning demonstrate cardiac myocyte contraction and hypereosinophilic sarcomeres characteristic of catecholamine excess. Myocardial infarction is also common in drowning victims. These pathological findings suggest that intense adrenergic stimulation is partly responsible for the arrhythmias of drowning. Thus, ventricular fibrillation most likely develops from hypoxia, ischemia, and acidosis in the presence of excessive catecholamine release.

Neurological Complications

The brain injury after drowning differs little from other etiologies of global anoxia or severe hypoxia (1,4,8,9). Prolonged anoxia or hypoxia produces diffuse neuronal damage, which if severe, compromises the function of the blood–brain barrier and leads to cerebral edema. As edema develops, the intracranial pressure (ICP) may rise, further decreasing cerebral perfusion and exacerbating neuronal hypoxia. In severe cases, this may result in uncal herniation. Profound increases in ICP are uncommon but tend to appear more than 24 to 48 hours after successful resuscitation in patients who show evidence of persistent neurological dysfunction. ICP greater than 20 mm Hg is associated with a poor prognosis. A progressive increase in ICP is primarily an indicator of the severity of brain injury that was sustained rather than a source of further damage.

The major differences between drowning and cerebral anoxia of other etiologies are the presence of the diving response and body cooling. Near drowning in cold water slows cerebral metabolism, thereby delaying the deleterious effects of anoxia (4,6,9,11). These factors are associated with a better prognosis after a severe drowning episode in some patients. However, hypothermia can be quite profound and complicate the management of the other aspects of the drowning, particularly if the patient has suffered a circulatory arrest in very cold water.

Renal Complications

Renal insufficiency after drowning is less frequently encountered than is lung, brain, or myocardial damage. The most common renal complication is oliguria from acute tubular necrosis. Acute tubular necrosis in this setting is usually related to hypoxemia and hypotension; however, drowning may be complicated by rhabdomyolysis and hemolysis with disseminated intravascular coagulation, which may contribute to acute tubular necrosis. Patients with acute tubular necrosis may require dialysis; however, long-term recovery of renal function is good in most of these patients.

Management of Near Drowning

The initial care of the patient after near drowning requires a search for the common predisposing factors and complicating injuries. These factors are easily overlooked in the unconscious, critically ill patient, but must be sought because they may affect treatment and prognosis. Alcohol and other central nervous system (CNS)–altering drugs are commonly

implicated in adult drowning incidents, and toxic drug and alcohol blood levels should be measured in patients admitted to the intensive care unit. In particular, sedatives and alcohol may complicate the patient's stay in the intensive care unit by worsening mental status, depressing respiratory drive, and contributing to hypothermia and hypotension.

Another important consideration in evaluating these patients is the discovery of events that compromise the otherwise unimpaired adult swimmer (1). Myocardial infarction, cardiac arrhythmias, seizures, and cerebrovascular accidents have been implicated in many near-drowning episodes. Electrocardiography is recommended because the heart is a major target of hypoxemia. Serial measurements of cardiac enzymes are useful in confirming the diagnosis of myocardial infarction. Stroke and/or status epileptics may need to be excluded in patients whose course is complicated by neurological dysfunction. Recompression and hyperbaric O_2 (HBO) therapy should be considered in scuba divers with coma or other neurological deficits in the setting of near drowning (see section "Diving Medicine").

Injuries to the spine and skull commonly occur in near-drowning victims who have dived into shallow water, striking the head on the bottom or on a submerged object. Another common situation occurs in motor vehicle accidents that have left a passenger submerged in a body of water. Cervical fractures and quadriplegia are encountered in these instances. Additionally, skin, ear, or sinus trauma sustained during the episode may serve as portals of entry for infection.

The primary indications for admitting near-drowning patients to the intensive care unit are respiratory failure, cardiac arrest or arrhythmia, and altered mental status. These patients are often intubated in the emergency department. On examination, the patient may show tachycardia, cyanosis, hypotension or hypertension, hypothermia, respiratory distress with pulmonary edema, crackles, and/or wheezing. Laboratory tests often reveal a lactic acidosis and arterial hypoxemia. Serum electrolytes, with the exception of a decreased bicarbonate concentration, are rarely disturbed. Hypoglycemia is common. Hemolysis and rhabdomyolysis tend to occur early, unless they are the result of sepsis. Electrocardiogram abnormalities include evidence of ischemia or injury and ventricular and atrial arrhythmias. Initial chest radiographic findings are nonspecific, ranging from minor atelectasis or patchy infiltrates to diffuse air space disease, which may progress over hours to days. Radiographic evidence of local volume loss suggests aspiration of a foreign body.

Mechanical ventilation can be a major challenge in the near-drowning victim. Profound atelectasis and pulmonary edema from the loss of surfactant and epithelial damage with intrapulmonary shunting are encountered in drowning of all kinds. ARDS and bronchoconstriction predispose to pulmonary barotrauma and air embolism. High airway pressures can be complicated by the presence of aspiration foreign bodies or debris. Use of sedation and paralysis are best minimized in these patients because they impair the ability to assess the neurological status. They may be necessary to provide adequate mechanical ventilation in agitated or asynchronous patients and may decrease airway pressures and the risk of barotrauma in difficult patients. The use of positive end-expiratory pressure to decrease intrapulmonary shunt in the presence of severe hypoxemia is indicated even in the presence of brain injury. Treatment of children with ARDS after near drowning with artificial surfactant has been studied and has not been found to improve outcome. Bronchodilator therapy with inhaled β-agonist agents may benefit patients with significant shunt or diffuse wheezing. Patients with localized wheezing or atelectasis that fails to improve with effective ventilation should undergo fiberoptic bronchoscopy to check for a foreign body.

Many drowning accidents occur in water contaminated with human or animal waste or naturally pathogenic microbes. The lungs are the common portals of entry for a variety of such organisms. Bronchitis or pneumonia are heralded by typical signs that include fever, leukocytosis, and worsening air space disease on chest radiograph 2 to 7 days after the event. These clinical findings should prompt sputum and blood cultures and initiation of antibiotic therapy. Prophylactic antibiotics do not improve outcome, and their routine use is not indicated. Unusual infections and infection by more than one organism is common, and some aquatic organisms may have growth requirements not provided for in standard in hospital microbial cultures.

Brain resuscitation therapy for the drowning victim is controversial and limited by the lack of predictive information about the factors that govern brain injury and recovery (1,4,9,12). Important variables include the age of the victim, water temperature, and submersion time. In general, the younger the patient, the colder the water, and the shorter the immersion time, the better the prognosis (2,7,10). On presentation to the hospital, poor prognostic signs include the presence of hypotension, cardiac arrest, or severe metabolic acidosis (pH <7.10). Outcome prediction is also complicated by pre-existing illness and concurrent injuries. Uncertainty about brain recovery after a drowning incident requires a full attempt at cardiopulmonary resuscitation, including adequately rewarming the hypothermic patient.

The patient's neurological examinations 2 to 6 hours after resuscitation also provide a general assessment of prognosis. A reasonable neurological outcome prediction can be made by classifying patients after resuscitation into categories; however, in general, the more severe the functional deficit at 6 hours, the less likely the patient is to recover.

Claims of complete or near complete neurological recovery in association with specific therapeutic interventions after prolonged immersion are difficult to confirm. Specific brain resuscitation regimens, e.g., HYPER therapy, have not been found to improve outcome in drowning victims. HYPER was designed to treat the hyperhydration, hyperpyrexia, hyperexcitability, and hyper-rigidity noted in some patients and thought to have adverse consequences. HYPER therapy consists of corticosteroids, osmotic diuretics, hyperventilation, mild hypothermia, barbiturate coma, and muscle relaxants administered to minimize cerebral edema and reduce ICP. The increase in ICP that develops after 24 to 48 hours in some of these patients is usually the result of the neuronal injury rather than its cause. Critical assessment and experience with HYPER therapy failed to confirm its efficacy and indicated potentially harmful effects. In retrospect, patients treated with HYPER appear to have an increased incidence of sepsis and multiple organ failure in association with hypothermia. This may result from cold-induced immune suppression, cold-induced bronchorrhea, and impaired mucociliary clearance. However, milder levels of hypothermia or regional brain hypothermia have not been tested adequately. Corticosteroids are of no proven benefit in reducing brain edema associated with drowning. In the absence of evidence that corticosteroids reduce edema or ICP, or that reduction of ICP improves neurological outcome after near drowning, corticosteroids should be avoided because they are immunosuppressive and predispose to gastrointestinal bleeding. Attempts to decrease ICP by osmotic diuresis also have not been shown to improve outcome after drowning and may cause hyperosmolarity and renal insufficiency. Routine use of osmotic agents is not advocated in these patients. Mild hyperventilation is a comparably benign intervention to reduce ICP temporarily, and ICP monitoring may help direct therapy in the subset of near-drowning patients with elevated ICP and poor prognosis. Aggressive cerebral monitoring and interventions based on ICP, such as the measures above and barbiturate coma, have shown no clinical benefit to date.

Most drowning patients who live until they arrive at a hospital emergency department will recover and return home. Approximately 10% of these patients will succumb to the incident. Cardiac arrest, hypotension, and prolonged need for hemodynamic support carry the poorest prognosis. In the absence of these factors, the probability of full recovery is close to 90%. The remaining patients suffer permanent neurological sequelae.

DIVING MEDICINE

The incredible beauty of the underwater world and the elegant simplicity of modern scuba have attracted thousands of participants to recreational diving in recent years. The opportunity for safe enjoyment of diving as a sport is a direct result of research in diving physiology, life-support equipment, and safe diving procedures by the world's navies and commercial diving interests (13). As a result, the number of underwater dives by civilian sports and technical divers in the United States greatly exceeds the number of military and commercial exposures each year. Most of the diving accidents and fatalities also come from the civilian diving population. According to the statistics published by the Divers

Alert Network, recreational diving accidents account for approximately 100 deaths and 1,000 cases of decompression illness each year in the United States (14). This rest of this chapter will summarize the basic principles of underwater diving and the medical problems most likely to be encountered by specialists in respiratory diseases.

Physics of Diving Environments

The biologic responses to underwater environments are consequences of the physical behavior of gases and the mechanical effects of hydrostatic pressure (15). Pressure measurements, force per unit area, can be expressed in a variety of ways (Table 48.1). Normal atmospheric pressure is approximately 760 mm Hg or 14.7 lb/in^2 (psi). The pressure of a column of water varies linearly with its height and must be added to the normal atmospheric pressure to obtain absolute pressure (ATA pressure). Any ambient pressure greater than 1 ATA pressure is called *hyperbaric* pressure. As shown in Table 48.1, a column of SW 33 ft deep exerts the same pressure as the normal atmosphere at sea level. A diver immersed in SW at 33 feet deep is exposed to a total external pressure of two atmospheres (ATA). When diving with compressed gas, the pressure of the diver's breathing gas must be increased in proportion to the absolute pressure in order to inhale against the pressure of the water column. As a result, more gas molecules must occupy the lungs and other gas-containing cavities of the body to maintain constant volume at a given temperature. The relationships of pressure (P), volume (V), and temperature (T) to the number of moles of gas *(n)* is described by the *ideal gas law:* $PV = nRT$, where R is the universal gas constant. The special gas laws relevant to diving can be derived easily from the ideal gas law. Three special cases of the ideal gas law, where one of three variables is held constant, are known as the Boyle law ($P_1V_1 = P_2V_2$), the Charles law ($P_1/T_1 = P_2/T_2$) and the Guy-Lussac law ($V_1/T_1 = V_2/T_2$). Air and other breathing gases are mixtures of O_2 and other molecules. In a mixture of gases, the total pressure is equal to the sum of the partial pressures of each of the gases (the Dalton law). This means that each component of the mixture behaves as though it alone occu-

pies the available space. The uptake of gas by body tissues is determined primarily by the diffusion of gas into or out of blood from the alveolar spaces. The amount of a gas dissolved in liquid at any temperature, e.g., blood or tissues or the body at 37°C (98.6°F), is also proportional to its partial pressure (the Henry law). This gas is carried into the tissues by the circulation. The tissue gas concentration is related to the partial pressure times its solubility coefficient.

In general, the physiological effects of diving gases, such as inert gas narcosis, correlate directly with the partial pressure of inert gas in the tissues (13,16). The amount of gas taken up by the tissues also relates to the risk of decompression sickness (DCS) when the diver ascends to the surface. Slow ascent or decompression is required to provide time for the circulation to eliminate inert gas from the tissues and avoid the problem of supersaturation, which predisposes to bubble formation in tissues and DCS.

Diving Modes, Equipment, and Conditions

There are several diving modes with vastly different operational requirements, capabilities, and associated medical problems (17). The oldest and most common diving mode is the breath-hold or free dive, which can be done using a mask, fins, and snorkel or without equipment. This is also called skin diving. Breath-hold diving is practiced primarily in shallow water, usually less than 60 ft deep of SW; however, much deeper descents are possible by experienced individuals. The most important medical problems of skin diving are shallow water blackout and untoward effects of hydrostatic pressure, including sinus and ear barotraumas (squeeze) and thoracic squeeze.

Scuba diving utilizes a tank of compressed air or other breathing gas and a two-stage regulator to match the inspired gas pressure with the hydrostatic pressure around the diver's body. The first, or high-pressure, stage of the regulator is fitted to the tank, which is pressurized with clean air to 2,000 psi or more. The regulator reduces the pressure to approximately 60 psi over the ambient water pressure; then the second stage, located in the diver's mouthpiece, equalizes the inspired pressure with the water pressure. The gas is exhaled into the water; hence, the apparatus is said to be open circuit. Scuba diving is limited to a safe depth of approximately 135 ft SW.

Advanced forms of scuba diving using semiclosed or closed circuit apparatus that rely on CO_2 removal canisters and special gas mixtures available to navies and commercial diving companies for many years are becoming available in civilian technical diving. In particular, the use of O_2-enriched air or Nitrox containing 32% or 36% O_2 has become popular recently because it reduces inert gas uptake, thereby extending the dive time and reducing decompression obligation. No matter what the breathing gas, the most important medical problems of scuba are untoward effects of hydrostatic pressure, including ear, sinus, and pulmonary barotrauma

TABLE 48.1. COMMON UNITS OF PRESSURE IN UNDERWATER ENVIRONMENTS

Depth	ATA	PSIA	Absolute (mm Hg)	Po$_2$ (mm Hg)
0	1	14.7	760	159
33	2	29.4	1,520	318
66	3	44.1	2,280	477
99	4	58.8	3,040	635
132	5	73.5	3,800	794
165	6	88.2	4,560	953

ATA, atmospheres absolute; PSIA, pounds per square inch, absolute; Po$_2$, partial pressure of oxygen.

(pneumothorax and pneumomediastinum); DCS; and arterial gas embolism (AGE).

In surface-supplied diving, the diver is tethered to a ship or other surface platform by an umbilical that contains a gas supply hose from a pressurized volume reservoir on the vessel. The reservoir may be pressurized with air or a suitable mixed breathing gas that contains O_2 in combination with various amounts of nitrogen, helium, or hydrogen. The surface gas supply delivers breathing gas at the appropriate pressure for the depth of the dive. Surface-supplied diving is very old and dates to the invention of the air compressor in the early 19th century. The dry or hardhat helmet and umbilical allow communication with the surface and provide a safety margin by protecting against running out of air. The famous brass or bronze helmets of the past have been replaced by modern lightweight plastic or fiberglass helmets with panoramic faceplates. Surface-supplied diving makes it easier to support the diver with special breathing gases or mixed gas, which is generally made in large quantities and stored aboard the ship. The medical problems associated with surface-supplied diving are the same as for the scuba diver.

The most technologically advanced form of diving is known as saturation diving (15). The principles of saturation diving are relatively straightforward. As indicated above, during an underwater excursion, the body tissues gradually take up inert gas, e.g., nitrogen. During ascent or decompression, this gas must be eliminated slowly to avoid formation of bubbles and decompression illness. After 12 to 24 hours underwater, the tissues of the body stop taking up inert gas because they have become saturated at that pressure. Thus, the time needed for decompression becomes constant, i.e., independent of the length of time the diver has been underwater. For instance, a diver "saturated" at 100 ft SW for 1 day has the same decompression obligation as the diver who has been at that depth for a month or more. This means the divers can live and work safely underwater for very long periods of time and then slowly ascend to the surface after completing their task. They remain at risk for barotrauma and DCS and have heightened problems with thermal stress and effects of atmosphere contamination relative to other divers.

The only solution to the physiological problems of breathing compressed air or other gases underwater is to avoid them by using submersibles or one-atmosphere diving suits. These systems have a solid hull or hard shell to prevent exposing the occupants to changes in hydrostatic pressure. The internal environment is maintained at 1 ATA, no matter how deep the system descends underwater. Furthermore, there is no danger from barotrauma or DCS because the internal pressure is constant.

Decompression Principles and Procedures

The most important aspect of diving safety is the use of proper diving techniques, particularly safe decompression practice (18). In diving with compressed air or mixed gases, appropriate decompression is essential for preventing the most serious medical complications of diving: DCS and AGE. Safe decompression practice requires the use of decompression schedules that have been tested for efficacy in many divers. These schedules or tables allow the elimination of inert gas from the tissues by the circulation so that gas tensions do not rise to the point of critical supersaturation, which can result in bubble formation. Decompression tables usually provide specific ascent rate schedules, including safety stops, for different depth-time profiles. Many cases of DCS occur in divers who ascend too rapidly or have omitted a portion of their decompression obligation. However, the occurrence of DCS is a probabilistic event; inherently, there is a finite risk of DCS whenever descending deeper than about 25 ft deep in SW for more than a few minutes.

Historically, the U.S. Navy decompression tables have been used widely for recreational diving because they have a good safety record (15). More recently, automatic, wrist-worn decompression computers have been developed that record time and pressure and calculate a "safe" decompression schedule based on an algorithm (19). These algorithms estimate the tissue nitrogen uptake for the actual dive profile and compute an appropriate decompression profile. Dive computers have become popular because they optimize use of the dive time by frequently updating the decompression schedule, but this also means that they usually do not have the built-in conservative safety margin inherent in the use of standard decompression tables. Whether or not decompression computers are as safe as dive tables is currently unknown; however, many more cases of decompression illness occur in divers who use computers than in divers who use tables. This may be related to more extensive use of computers than of tables today, or to other characteristics of divers who use computers that are independent of the device.

Dysbaric Illnesses

The most important medical problems of diving are related to the adverse effects of a change in pressure on the body. The pathophysiological effects of pressure fall under the terms *dysbarism* or *dysbaric illness*. The most important dysbaric illnesses include various types of barotrauma, AGE, and DCS, which are discussed below. In some texts, the term *decompression illness* is used to describe AGE and DCS because of the diagnostic uncertainty and overlap in presentation in some cases. Most other dysbaric illnesses, such as dysbaric bone necrosis, are less common, nonacute, and beyond the scope of this chapter.

Barotrauma

The pressure in the gas-filled spaces of the body is normally in equilibrium with atmospheric pressure. During a change in barometric pressure, e.g., with descent underwater or ascent to high altitude, the pressure in the gas space equilibrates with the outside environment. If the route of gas movement is obstructed during the pressure change, a pressure difference builds up between the gas-filled cavity and the environment. This differential pressure may damage the tissues surrounding the air space and produce signs and symptoms. This tissue damage, known as barotrauma, is the most common form of injury in diving and it may occur during either descent or ascent (13,20,21). Barotrauma may occur in any tissue location where gas is trapped in a closed space, including inside a face mask, the skin under a gas-filled suit, the middle or external ear spaces, the paranasal sinuses, the lungs, and the gastrointestinal tract. When the barotrauma is associated with an increase in external pressure relative to the body compartment, it is often referred to as squeeze. Thus, the common types of barotrauma of descent are suit, mask, ear, and sinus squeeze. Only ear and sinus squeeze, however, are clinically significant. In very deep breath-hold diving or surface-supplied diving with a rapid descent, lung squeeze can occur, but it is rare. Barotrauma of ascent is most often associated with the ears, sinuses, and lungs.

The most common problem for which divers seek medical attention is *barotitis media* or middle ear squeeze (20,22,23). Barotitis media occurs as a direct result of the Boyle law, wherein during a descent, the volume of air in the middle ear space is compressed by the increase in external pressure. Unless the eustachian tubes function properly and allow more gas into the space, the pressure in the ear space becomes lower than ambient (relative vacuum), which causes the tympanic membrane (TM) to retract inward causing pain. If this problem persists and descent continues, the relative vacuum will pull serum and blood into the middle ear space, the TM will rupture, or both. If rupture occurs, the pressure equalizes and the symptoms are relieved. The incidence of middle ear squeeze is most pronounced near the surface, and usually occurs in the first ten feet of the water column, where according to the Boyle law, the volume change for a given pressure change is the greatest.

The diagnosis of barotitis media can usually be made by clinical history. The appearance of the TM by otoscopic examination, usually confirms the diagnosis. The severity of the squeeze is often graded, e.g., by Teed grade, where grade 0 is symptoms only, grade I is erythema of the TM over the malleus, grade II is erythema over the malleus with focal hemorrhage, grade III is extensive TM hemorrhage, grade IV is free blood in the middle ear space, and grade V is blood in the middle ear space with rupture of the TM. Patients with grades III, IV, and V squeeze may have mild conductive hearing loss and show bloody drainage of the nose or hypopharynx. In severe cases, middle ear barotrauma is associated with inner ear barotrauma, particularly when excessively strong Valsalva maneuvers are used to try to equalize the pressure in the middle ear space during descent. Inner

ear barotrauma can cause labyrinthine rupture of either the round or oval windows with attendant tinnitus, vertigo, and loss of hearing.

The best approach to middle ear squeeze is prevention, and learning proper ear-clearing techniques, appropriately using nasal decongestants, and avoiding diving with upper respiratory infection and allergies are important measures (20,22,23). Barotitis media is treated with nasal decongestants, oral decongestants, and analgesia. Antihistamines should not be used unless an allergic component is present. Antibiotics are not indicated unless more conservative measures fail and there is evidence of middle ear infection. Large defects in the TM should be referred to an otolaryngologist. Diving and flying should be avoided until healing is complete and the patient is able to autoinflate the ear using a gentle Valsalva maneuver.

The incidence of sinus barotrauma in diving is significant but less common than is middle ear barotrauma. The mechanism is essentially identical with middle ear barotrauma. The symptoms of sinus barotrauma are primarily pain or a feeling of pressure over the affected sinus, and relief of pain is associated with filling of the sinus with blood or mucous or, on ascent, with dispelling the sinus contents into the nose or hypopharynx. As with middle ear barotrauma, avoidance is the best approach to sinus barotrauma. The management is also similar.

The most dangerous form of barotrauma is the *pulmonary overpressurization syndrome,* which occurs on ascent when the expanding gas in the lung is unable to escape and ruptures the pulmonary parenchyma, usually at the level of the acini (21,24,25). This produces a range of pulmonary findings, including the typical signs, symptoms, and radiological findings of pulmonary interstitial emphysema, mediastinal emphysema, or pneumothorax. In severe cases, pulmonary overpressurization may allow gas entry into the pulmonary capillaries and lead to *arterial gas embolism* (15,21,26,27). Pulmonary overpressurization is encountered commonly in very shallow water because the greatest change in gas volume for a given change in pressure occurs near the surface (Fig. 48.1). Because pulmonary elastic tissue can undergo rupture at a transpulmonary pressure of less than 100 cm H_2O, pulmonary overpressurization can occur in less than 4 ft of water.

Most victims of pulmonary overpressurization give a history of an uncontrolled ascent owing to an underwater emergency. In some cases, the individual has made a breath-hold ascent while breathing compressed air. In other cases, the ascent is rapid, but no other predisposing factors are apparent. In the latter circumstance, pulmonary overpressurization may occur because of overinflation of a small region of the lung where secretions, bronchospasm, aspirated water, or a pre-existing defect has blocked airflow.

The treatment of the complications of pulmonary overpressurization syndrome is primarily symptomatic unless pneumothorax or AGE is present. A diver with a

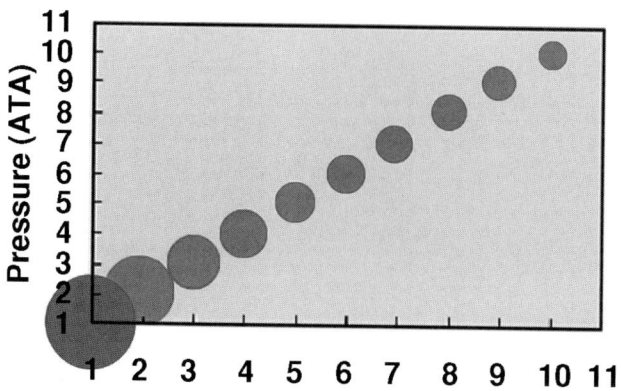

FIGURE 48.1. Relationship of gas bubble volume to pressure during ascent. The graph shows plot of 1/bubble volume against pressure at atmospheric absolute. Bubble size determined by the Boyle law indicates that the greatest increase in volume occurs as the diver approaches the surface. This principle has important implications for both arterial gas embolism and decompression sickness.

pneumothorax should not be placed in a hyperbaric chamber for treatment of DCS or gas embolism until arrangements have been made to place a thoracostomy tube. If serious AGE with neurological deficit is present, the patient may be recompressed provided a plan is in place to vent the pleural space before the chamber is decompressed.

Arterial Gas Embolism

AGE is the most deadly complication of diving with compressed gases (18,21,25,27–29). Although it is rare, AGE has a high morbidity and mortality in diving. Statistics from the Divers' Alert Network indicate that AGE accounts for approximately 5% of dysbaric incidents but 25% of the deaths in recreational divers (14). AGE is caused by the entry of air into the pulmonary venous circulation during pulmonary overpressurization. The mechanism involves rupture of pulmonary capillaries and venules, which fail under the stress of high transpulmonary pressures. Bubbles of gas enter the pulmonary venous blood and are carried to the left heart, where they are disseminated throughout the systemic circulation and obstruct distal blood flow. The amount of gas disseminated into the circulation can be quite large because its volume continues to expand as the diver approaches the surface. These vascular bubbles not only obstruct blood flow but also damage vascular endothelium and activate local coagulation and cellular inflammatory processes. Pathological examination of tissues of patients dying after AGE usually shows evidence of ischemic damage in the distribution of the affected vessels. When the brain has been showered with multiple small bubbles, a diffuse geographic pattern is sometimes seen.

The most important *clinical manifestations* of AGE occur in the heart and the brain. Bubbles can enter the coronary arteries and cause myocardial ischemia, infarction, or arrhythmias. It is also common for bubbles to enter the carotid

arteries and produce symptoms and signs of cerebral gas embolism. The neurological manifestations are sudden and usually occur during ascent or within 15 minutes of surfacing from a dive. A delay in symptom onset of more than 15 minutes indicates another diagnosis, such as DCS. The clinical presentation is also not distinguishable from other types of acute cerebrovascular accidents, which are sometimes precipitated by exertion or straining. The main presenting features of cerebral gas embolism include headache, sudden loss of consciousness, seizures, confusion, ataxia, blindness, and focal motor or sensory deficits. On neurological examination, however, the physical findings of AGE often do not fall into the territory a single vessel because the bubbles have been distributed heterogeneously.

The *laboratory evaluation* for suspected AGE should include a chest radiograph, electrocardiogram, cardiac isoenzymes, complete blood count, electrolytes, blood urea nitrogen, creatinine and glucose. A brain computed tomography scan or magnetic resonance imaging study should be postponed until after recompression therapy unless the history of AGE is not convincing (3,26,28). Although intracerebral gas can sometimes be detected on imaging studies, it adds nothing to the history and physical examination in the appropriate clinical setting. Brain imaging should be postponed if possible until after initial recompression therapy. The imaging studies, as in other forms of acute cerebral ischemia, generally show the most pronounced abnormalities at 4 to 7 days after the injury (30).

The *emergency treatment* of suspected AGE is to remove the patient from the water as quickly as possible and administer high-flow O_2 continuously by face mask. AGE incidents that occur while in the water are often complicated by near drowning, and the patient may require more aggressive resuscitation measures, including cardiopulmonary resuscitation. The victim should be kept supine, but not in a head-down position, which does not prevent dispersal of arterial gas and may worsen cerebral edema. Sedatives and benzodiazepine drugs should be avoided unless the patient is having seizures, because these drugs interfere with the neurological assessment. Isotonic intravenous fluids should be administered and a good urine output maintained because these patients are often dehydrated and suffer from hemoconcentration owing to vascular endothelial injury.

The *definitive treatment* for AGE is prompt recompression with HBO. The standard treatment protocol is the U.S. Navy Treatment Table 6 or 6A (15). For diving-related AGE, most centers use U.S. Navy Table 6A and initially recompress to 165 ft SW by using 50% Nitrox instead of air. This provides extra O_2 and limits further uptake of nitrogen during the recompression. When the quantity of air in the vessels is modest, use of the 60 ft SW recompression table with 100% O_2 (U.S. Navy Table 6) is usually adequate. The earlier that recompression treatment is instituted, the more likely is the patient to have a clinical response and a good outcome. The best responses occur when a recompression chamber is present at the diving site. A delay in treatment of more than 6 hours is likely to result in little or no clinical response to HBO, but a few cases have been reported in which substantial clinical improvement has occurred after initial treatment delays of 12 to 24 hours. Predictably, the prognosis varies according to the amount of gas that enters the cerebral vessels and the delay to treatment (21,24,26–29,31). In general, patients with evidence of severe global anoxia after AGE, or after cardiopulmonary arrest, have a very poor prognosis, whereas those with mild or moderate diffuse injury have an intermediate prognosis, and those with small focal neurological deficits have the best prognosis.

Decompression Sickness

DCS is caused by the formation of bubbles of inert gas in the tissues after the dissolved gas has been supersaturated by a decrease in the ambient pressure (15,28,32–34). The situation is often likened to opening a bottle of carbonated beverage and releasing CO_2 gas from solution. DCS is encountered in divers; in individuals exposed to high pressure inside chambers, tunnels, or caissons; and in aviators or astronauts who travel to high altitude and are exposed to very low atmospheric pressures. In general, the so-called critical supersaturation for bubble formation occurs at a differential pressure of about 1.75 ATA of hyperbaric pressure and 0.5 ATA of hypobaric pressure. The former corresponds to a depth of approximately 25 ft SW; the latter, to an altitude of approximately 18,000 ft. The presence of bubbles produces local effects in the tissues, which through a poorly understood sequence of biochemical events, lead to the symptoms and signs of DCS. In addition, some of these bubbles escape from the tissues and enter the venous circulation, through which they travel to the lungs. The lung is generally an excellent filter for bubbles, and most of the gas in them is eliminated by normal pulmonary gas exchange. Thus, the essential difference between the etiology of DCS and AGE is that the vascular gas in AGE originates in the lung and is disbursed to the systemic tissues, whereas in DCS, the bubbles originate in the tissues and are disbursed to the lungs.

During decompression, clinically silent venous bubbles often occur that can be detected and graded by precordial Doppler ultrasound. In clinically apparent cases, the venous bubble grade correlates roughly with the appearance of symptoms and signs of DCS. If the release of bubbles from the tissues is extensive, the capacity of the lung to handle the gas is exceeded, and severe pulmonary DCS, called chokes, can be produced. In the presence of a patent foramen ovale, venous bubbles can cross from the right side of the heart into the systemic circulation and produce the same symptoms and signs as AGE (35–37).

The incidence of DCS in recreational scuba diving is unknown; however, it has been estimated to be less than about one in 5,000 dives. This number depends on the depth and time profile, and most cases of DCS occur at depths of

TABLE 48.2. CLASSIFICATION OF MAJOR DYSBARIC ILLNESSES

Problem	Signs and Symptoms
Arterial gas embolism	Headache, visual disturbances, loss of consciousness, seizures, altered mental status, focal neurological findings, pleuritic pain, hemoptysis, anginal chest pain
Mild DCS (type 1)	
Skin	Mottling, urticaria, pruritus, niggles
Musculoskeletal	Limb pain (bends), usually in large joints; patchy numbness or dysesthesia, edema, mild erythema
Serious DCS (type 2)	
Skin	Lymphatic obstruction (cutis marmorata)
Cerebral	Loss of consciousness, ataxia, vertigo, aphasia, hemiparesis
Audiovestibular	Vertigo, nystagmus, auditory symptoms, including deafness
Spinal cord	Back or abdominal pain; paraparesis; sensory level, bladder, bowel or sexual dysfunction
Cardiopulmonary	Cough, retrosternal pain, tachypnea, asphyxia (chokes)
Systemic	Extreme fatigue, hypovolemic shock

DCS; decompression sickness.

60 ft SW or greater. The number of deaths reported to the Divers' Alert Network in divers that receive recompression therapy averages about 100 per year, less than 10% mortality (14). Among all diving fatalities, drowning is implicated as a proximate cause of death in approximately half of the cases.

The most important *clinical manifestations* of DCS are shown in Table 48.2. The symptoms and signs are diverse and range from mild joint pain to circulatory shock (38). Traditionally, DCS has been divided into two types: mild, or type I, DCS and serious, or type II, DCS (15,38). Type I DCS consists of musculoskeletal pain only, often but not necessarily restricted to one joint and is called bends, whereas type II DCS has evidence of neurological involvement, e.g., spinal paralysis, or systemic illness. Type I DCS is often said to be more common than type II, but the reporting of DCS in recreational divers indicates that a greater percentage of type II DCS (60%) are treated in civilian chambers than is type I DCS (25%) in the United States.

The utility of the standard DCS classification is less than it would appear at first glance, for pain and neurological involvement occur commonly together, and in some instances, the pain precedes the appearance of neurological findings. The onset of symptoms of DCS may be abrupt or gradual; however, the symptoms usually begin at the end or shortly after the dive. Symptom onset is within 12 hours of the dive in more than 75% of the cases. Initial symptoms that appear more than 24 hours after the dive are rarely caused by DCS unless the patient is exposed to altitude, e.g., flying after diving.

The diagnosis of DCS is clinical and established by history and physical examination (15,26,28,32,39). Currently, there are no diagnostic laboratory tests for DCS. For uncomplicated limb bends, the most important diagnostic distinction to be made is between DCS and trauma. The joint pain of DCS often feels deep within the joint and is made worse with movement. Unfortunately, the quality and characteristics of the pain are nonspecific. In some instances, the pain is accompanied by patchy dysesthesia or numbness around the joint, which should not be confused with type II disease. Mild erythema, warmth, and swelling may be present. In some patients, the application of gentle pressure around the affected limb alleviates the pain. This test can be performed with inflation of a blood pressure cuff to arterial pressure over the area of pain for 1 to 2 minutes (40). If the pain is relieved but recurs after the pressure is released, the probability of DCS is very high. The lack of a response is not helpful for ruling out the presence of DCS, and when the diagnostic uncertainty is great, the patient should be given a "trial of pressure" for 10 to 15 minutes in the recompression chamber to determine if there is any relief of symptoms.

The diagnosis of neurological DCS is not difficult if the physician keeps in mind the diverse heterogeneous nature of the clinical presentation. This heterogeneity is owing to the unpredictability of sites of bubble formation in the nervous system. Hence, DCS may involve the CNS, including brain and spinal cord, or the peripheral nervous system or both. Involvement of the spinal cord is a relatively uncommon, but particularly troublesome, form of DCS. The reason that the spinal cord is susceptible to DCS is not entirely clear, but appears to relate to autochthonous bubble formation in the parenchyma (34) and gas in the epivertebral venous plexus. Spinal cord DCS classically affects the lower thoracic or lumbar cord, although DCS has been reported at all levels of the cord. In serious cases, the patients often present with low back or bandlike abdominal pain, heaviness, weakness, or paralysis of the lower extremities and various sensory findings. The area of involvement may involve the cord at several vertebral levels. Loss of bladder and/or bowel function is present in severe cases. Other serious forms of neurological DCS involve the brain, retina, and inner ear (staggers) (15).

The *laboratory evaluation* for DCS should include a chest radiograph, complete blood count, electrolytes, blood urea nitrogen, creatinine and glucose. Additional studies such as the electrocardiogram, cardiac isoenzymes, and urinalysis are indicated when warranted by the clinical presentation. An elective echocardiogram with a microcavitation study is recommended to determine the presence of right-to-left shunt in patients with serious DCS, particularly when cerebral signs and symptoms are present. As in AGE, neuroimaging studies should be deferred until after initial recompression therapy unless the diagnosis is in question. Imaging studies are useful primarily to evaluate residual or concurrent neurological deficits.

The *emergency treatment* of DCS consists of administration of fluids and high-flow O_2 by face mask. The patient should be transported to a hyperbaric chamber for recompression therapy as soon as feasible. Air travel should be avoided because altitude will exacerbate DCS by allowing expansion of gas in tissues. If transportation requires air travel, the patient should be flown at low altitude or in a 1-ATA cabin while breathing supplemental O_2. In some cases, sea-level O_2 completely relieves DCS; however, it may recur or progress after the O_2 is discontinued. Thus, all patients with presumed DCS should receive recompression therapy to prevent recurrence of symptoms, unless the symptoms are extremely mild and relieved completely by surface O_2 and a recompression chamber is not readily accessible.

The *definitive treatment* for DCS is prompt recompression with HBO (41). The patient should be transported to the nearest available chamber as quickly as possible because the outcome of treatment is strongly influenced by the time between the onset of symptoms and therapy. The standard of care today is to use HBO recompression tables at 2.5 to 3.0 ATA. This therapy optimizes the elimination of inert gas by expanding the O_2 *window*, or the P_{O_2} difference between arterial and venous blood. This principle is illustrated in Figure 48.2. The most widely used O_2 recompression tables are the U.S. Navy 2.8 ATA (60 ft SW) Table 5 for mild and Table 6 for serious DCS. These treatment tables can be found in the U.S. Navy diving manual (15). For altitude bends, often recompression requires only returning to sea level and breathing O_2 for 2 to 4 hours, but U.S. Navy Table 5 may be necessary in refractory cases. In most cases of only DCS, a single treatment is usually sufficient to relieve the condition. Many specialists prefer U.S. Navy Table 6 for routine treatments because recurrence rate is lower.

If the patient's symptoms do not resolve promptly, U.S. Navy Table 6 may be extended at both 60 and 30 ft SW to provide two additional O_2 breathing periods at each depth. In serious cases of neurological DCS, such as those involving the brain or spinal cord, saturation treatment tables may be used, such as the U.S. Navy Table 7, or other saturation treatment tables, such as the Catalina Table. Alternatively, multiple daily treatments with U.S. Navy Table 6 can be performed until the patient's neurological examination reaches a plateau. This usually occurs after 5 to 10 treatments. Emergency consultation about chamber availability, patient transportation, and treatment of dysbaric illnesses can be obtained 24 hours a day, 7 days a week through the Divers' Alert Network by calling 919-684-8111 and asking for the physician on call.

Adjunctive therapy for DCS is very limited. Adequate hydration is important, but little else is indicated routinely. On the basis of experimental studies of AGE, some specialists have recommended intravenous infusion of lidocaine for 24 to 48 hours for treatment of cerebral or spinal DCS (31). This recommendation is not yet supported by randomized, controlled clinical trials. The use of high-dose corticosteroids

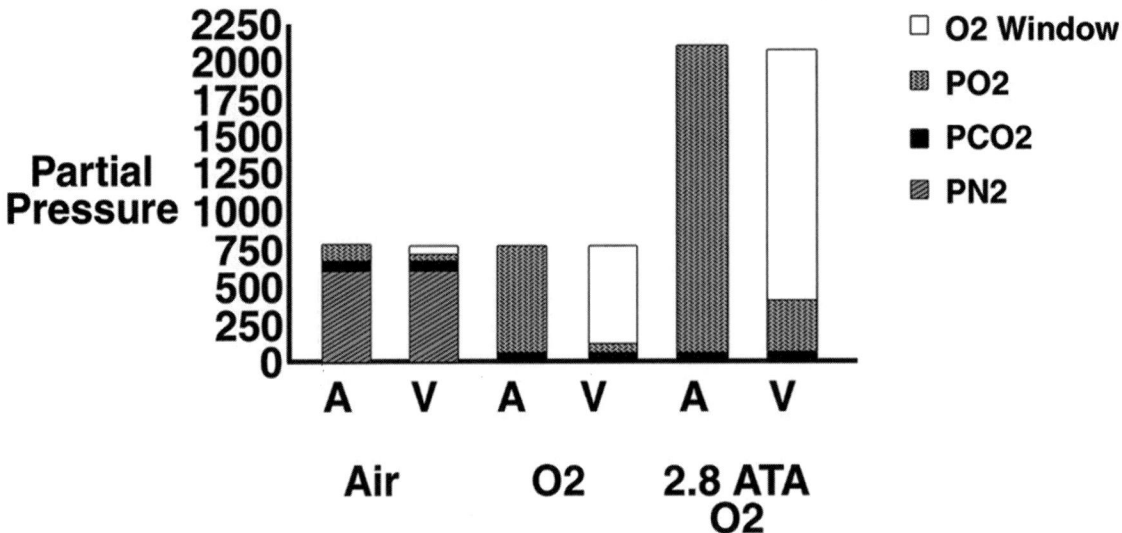

FIGURE 48.2. The oxygen (O_2) window. The sum of the gas partial pressures on the arterial side of the circulation is normally higher than on the venous side because the venous partial pressure of O_2 is lowered by O_2 consumption in tissues. This difference, or O_2 window, allows a gradient for the elimination of other gases, e.g., nitrogen, from tissues. The use of both 100% O_2 and hyperbaric O_2 expand the oxygen window and hasten inert gas elimination.

for the treatment of spinal cord DCS has been advocated in the past on the basis of studies involving spinal cord trauma. However, the use of steroids in neurological DCS remains unproven and is not recommended. Patients who are immobilized by neurological DCS are at risk for deep venous thrombosis and pulmonary thromboembolism and should receive prophylactic anticoagulation routinely.

The prognosis of patients treated for DCS with O_2 recompression therapy is quite good, even with a delay to treatment of several hours (42). The initial resolution rate after O_2 recompression therapy is approximately 75%. The majority of patients (>95%) eventually have complete resolution of their signs and symptoms, although neurological improvement, much like stroke, may be slow. More severe neurological forms of DCS have a higher residual deficit rate, particularly if the delay to recompression has been 12 hours or more (28,33,42). However, even patients with severe spinal cord involvement who show only limited functional recovery after recompression will continue to show gradual improvement for up to 2 years after the injury.

Flying after Diving

The issue of when it is safe to fly after diving arises frequently because many remote dive locations are for all practical purposes, only accessible by air. Commercial aircraft fly at a cabin pressure equivalent to 6,000 to 8,000 ft of altitude, which is sufficiently high to increase the risk of DCS in someone who has been recently diving and still has increased inert gas in body tissues. The reduction in atmospheric pressure in the aircraft cabin is sufficient to cause critical supersaturation of gas, leading to bubble formation and DCS. Flying after

diving is clearly an important cause of DCS in recreational divers, but the frequency at which it occurs is unknown. In approximately 5% of the DCS cases reported to the Divers Alert Network, symptom onset is reported either while flying or while driving over mountains. The risk of DCS after flying is related to the number and type of diving exposure before the flight and the preflight surface interval. Although exact data are scarce, a variety of recommendations have been offered for an adequate preflight surface interval. A minimum wait of 12 hours is usually recommended between the end of the last dive and a flight. If the dives have been of sufficient depth and duration to require decompression stops or if the diving has involved multiple or repetitive dives each day on 2 or more days, then a surface interval before flying of at least 18 hours is advisable. A number of well-documented cases of DCS, however, have been reported during altitude exposure more than 24 hours after diving.

Medical Consequences of Breathing Exotic Gases

Divers who use compressed air or other breathable gas mixtures are sometimes exposed to unusual physiological effects of components of the gases. These physiological effects are related to the partial pressures of the individual gases in the mixture such as O_2, nitrogen, CO_2, or trace contaminants such as carbon monoxide (CO) or hydrocarbons. In open-circuit diving apparatus, such as used for recreational scuba, CO_2 retention is not a problem because the breathing gas is not recycled. In closed-circuit or semiclosed-circuit underwater breathing apparatus, however, all or part of the gas is recycled through a CO_2 scrubbing canister and returned to the diver. Use of these underwater breathing apparatuses may lead to dyspnea, anxiety, narcosis, or unconsciousness owing to CO_2 retention if the CO_2-absorbing material fails.

Oxygen Toxicity

Breathing compressed air and other gas mixtures using open-circuit scuba invariably results in exposure of the diver to elevated Po_2 because gas of a fixed composition is delivered to the lungs at increased pressure. Thus, the inspired Po_2 increases linearly with the total pressure. In closed or semi-closed underwater breathing apparatuses, the Po_2 may be regulated at a constant level by an O_2 sensor system. The Po_2 of these systems can be set anywhere between 0.21 and 1.0, and some allow Po_2 at depth to rise to as high as 1.3 ATA. However, most are usually regulated between 0.3 and 0.5 ATA. In addition, HBO therapy exposes the body to profound hyperoxia. Therefore, it is not unusual for divers to be exposed to inspired Po_2 values of 1.0 to 1.6 ATA; and patients receiving HBO therapy, to 2 to 3 ATA. For example, a scuba diver breathing compressed air at 99 ft SW is exposed to a total atmospheric pressure of 4 ATA. Because air is 20.9% O_2, the diver is breathing the sea level equivalent of 83.6% O_2.

Prolonged exposure to very high Po_2 produces O_2 toxicity mediated by the generation of reactive O_2 species. Although O_2 is toxic to all living systems if Po_2 is high enough, O_2 toxicity in mammalian systems is most pronounced in the lungs, brain, and retina of the newborn (retrolental fibroplasia). In each organ system, the dose-time curve has the shape of a rectangular hyperbola, i.e., the O_2 tolerance time decreases as a function of an increasing O_2 dose (43,44). Because these curves are hyperbolic, there is an asymptote for the curve below which the O_2 is nontoxic. For the human lung, this limit appears to be approximately 0.5 ATA, and the appearance of pulmonary toxicity at 0.6 ATA requires a week or more. At 1.0 ATA, pulmonary symptoms appear within a day and at 3 ATA within a few hours. Thus, in scuba diving, in which exposures tend to be less than 2 hours in duration and less than 132 ft SW (5 ATA) in depth, pulmonary O_2 toxicity is not a significant problem.

The use of inspired Po_2 in the range of 2 to 3 ATA for recompression treatment of DCS and AGE or other indications for HBO can be associated with signs and symptoms of pulmonary O_2 toxicity. The symptoms, usually consisting of retrosternal chest pain, dry cough, and dyspnea on exertion, precede changes in forced vital capacity, airflow, and pulmonary gas exchange. Initially, the physiological changes are rapidly and fully reversible when O_2 is discontinued, but prolonged exposure eventually leads to irreversible impairment of mechanical function and gas exchange. In practice, pulmonary O_2 toxicity can be postponed by interspersing short breaks of air breathing (45). In clinical treatments, 5-minute air breaks are usually given for every 20 to 30 minutes of O_2 breathing.

In divers and patients exposed to O_2 at 1.6 ATA or greater, CNS O_2 toxicity is a potentially serious problem because it can result in sudden grand mal seizures (15,44). CNS O_2 toxicity occurs more readily in underwater divers because immersion, cold, exertion, and CO_2 retention greatly increase the risk of convulsions, which, if they occur underwater, can have dire consequences. Thus, O_2-breathing divers at or below 1.6 ATA (20 ft SW), air-breathing divers at 8 ATA (231 ft SW), or divers breathing O_2-enriched air at 4.4 to 5 ATA (114–132 ft SW) are at risk. The occurrence of CNS O_2 toxicity in HBO therapy is relatively rare because the patients are dry and at rest and do not retain CO_2. The seizures are self-limited and resolve quickly after discontinuing HBO.

Nitrogen Narcosis

Nitrogen narcosis, also called rapture of the deep, is the intoxicating effect of breathing inert gases at elevated partial pressures (16). All inert or noble gases produce a narcotic effect, which is closely related to their solubility in lipids. At high-enough partial pressures, the inert gas acts like a gaseous anesthetic and induces general anesthesia by a similar mechanism. The narcotic effects of nitrogen and other noble gases can be reversed by very high pressure. This effect, called pressure-reversal of anesthesia, has been interpreted as evidence that the effects of inert gases and hydrostatic pressure on the CNS are exactly opposite to each other. In fact, very rapid compression to depths of 600 ft SW or greater, or gradual application of extremely high hydrostatic pressure (usually >1,000 ft SW) produce a syndrome called the high-pressure neurological syndrome, which is characterized by tremor, electroencephalogram abnormalities and micro-sleep. High-pressure neurological syndrome can be ameliorated by addition of a small amount of inert gas to the breathing mixture, but the use of high pressure to alleviate narcosis is not possible.

Nitrogen narcosis is characterized by euphoria, impaired awareness of time and surroundings, and tendency to lose concentration, which lead to overconfidence and errors in judgment. The manifestations of nitrogen narcosis usually begin to appear at 50 to 100 ft SW and progress as the depth increases. At extremely great depth, severe narcosis occurs, sometimes including visual and auditory hallucinations, and culminates in unconsciousness at depths of 360 ft SW or greater. The effects of nitrogen narcosis dissipate rapidly and completely on ascent, but at depth, it has been directly responsible for or contributed to many diving accidents. As a result, the maximum recommended depth for recreational scuba diving is generally 135 ft SW. True physiological adaptation to narcosis has not been demonstrated, but experience with the effect is helpful in dealing with it.

Gas Contamination

The use of compressed gas in diving requires that the tanks be filled from a source of pure air because the biologic effects of toxic contaminants are increased in proportion to the total pressure at which the gas is breathed. For example, air that contains 20 ppm CO in air will still contain 20 ppm at 5 ATA, but the body will be exposed to an amount of CO equivalent to 100 ppm at sea level. CO is particularly dangerous in diving gases because it is tasteless, odorless, and colorless and is a product of incomplete combustion. Thus, air compressors that operate on gasoline or other fossil fuels can contaminate the breathing gas with CO and other combustion products if the seals of the compressor are not maintained properly. Other important breathing gas contaminants include CO_2, irritating hydrocarbons including aldehydes, and oil mist from compressor lubricants, which may cause lipoid pneumonia.

Medical Fitness to Dive

The issue of determining medical fitness to dive has become more difficult in recent years because of advances in equipment safety and portability and interest in recreational diving of the very young, elderly, and those with chronic medical conditions or physical disabilities (35,46–48). Candidates for courses in scuba diving are required to have a current physical examination to be certain they are free of disqualifying medical conditions. Generally, children under age 14 years are not considered for eligibility to dive; otherwise, age is not a consideration. Pregnant women should not dive because the fetus may be at increased risk of decompression stress. The history and physical examination should emphasize otolaryngology, pulmonary, cardiovascular, and neurological systems. In addition, the person's maturity and psychological stability should be considered in the evalua-

tion. Persons under age 40 years should have a physical every 3 years, and those over 40 years should be examined annually and have an electrocardiogram. Because diving is a strenuous physical activity, persons over 35 years with a strong family history or other major risk factors for early coronary disease should have a functional cardiac evaluation, e.g., exercise stress test, before being cleared for diving.

Many medical conditions are absolute contraindications to diving because they prevent appropriate equalization of pressure, increase danger to the individual underwater, or increase the risk of DCS. The most important absolute contraindications are listed in Table 48.3. Many absolute contraindications involve serious cardiopulmonary diseases. It is important to state that a patent foramen ovale (PFO) is not a contraindication to diving, but individuals who have had neurological DCS and are found to have a PFO should reconsider their diving status.

From the perspective of the specialist in respiratory diseases, frequent questions arise about diving in young asthmatics because of the risk of air trapping and pulmonary overpressurization syndrome. Persons with acute asthma or chronic asthma requiring steroid therapy (including inhaled steroids) or with exercise-induced asthma should not participate in scuba diving. Persons with mild seasonal asthma or postviral reactive airway dysfunction requiring periodic use of β-2 agonists can be cleared to dive provided they are free of symptoms and they have a normal chest radiograph and pulmonary function tests. Finally, individuals who have had a spontaneous pneumothorax should not be cleared for diving for 6 months and until a chest computed tomograph indicates there are no structural abnormalities that would predispose to another episode.

In addition to absolute medical contraindications to diving, there are numerous relative contraindications and a number of conditions that are temporary disqualifications. The most important of these are listed in Table 48.3.

TABLE 48.3. MEDICAL CONTRAINDICATIONS TO DIVING

Absolutely Disqualifying Conditions	Possibly Disqualifying Conditions	Disqualifying Until Resolution
Inability to equalize pressure in the middle ear by autoinflation	Middle ear surgery	Perforation of the tympanic membrane
History of epilepsy or other seizure disorder	Migraine and other vascular headaches	Upper respiratory infections
Insulin-dependent diabetes mellitus	Hypertension	Post–upper respiratory infection airway hyper-reactivity
Symptomatic coronary artery disease	Decreased visual acuity	Pregnancy
Sickle-cell diseases or traits		Poor physical fitness
Emphysema		History of previous overpressure diving accident
Chronic bronchitis		Unexplained syncope
Drug or alcohol abuse		Pneumothorax in association with trauma or other physical forces
Recurrent spontaneous pneumothorax		
Placement of prosthesis in the middle ear conduction chain		

TABLE 48.4. SUMMARY OF TREATMENT OPTIONS

Condition	Treatment

Near Drowning
  Brain Injury
 	
  Lung Injury
	1. Hyperventilation
	2. Corticosteroids
	3. Hypothermia
	4. Antibiotic prophylaxis (not recommended)

Cerebral arterial gas embolism	1. Oxygen 2. Oxygen recompression 3. Lidocaine

Decompression sickness
  (types I and II)
	1. Fluids (types I and II)
	2. Oxygen (types I and II)
	3. Oxygen recompression (types I and II)
	4. Prophylactic heparin (type II with
	   immobility only)
	5. Lidocaine (type II only)

Additional information about fitness to dive can be obtained by consultation with a diving medicine physician at the Divers Alert Network by calling 919-684-2948 during normal work hours.

SUMMARY

For a summary of treatment options, see Table 48.4.

REFERENCES

1. Modell JH. Drowning. *N Engl J Med* 1993;328:253–256.
2. Biggart MJ, Bohn DJ. Effect of hypothermia and cardiac arrest on outcome of near-drowning accidents in children. *J Pediatr* 1990;117:179–183.
3. Warren LP, Djang WT, Moon RE, et al: Neuroimaging of scuba diving injuries to the CNS. *AJR Am J Roentgenol* 1988;142:1003–1008.
4. Smyrnios NA, Irwin RS. Current concepts in the pathophysiology and management of near drowning. *J Intensive Care Med* 1991;6:26–35.
5. Stolp BW, CEG Lundgren, Piantadosi CA. Diving and immersion. In: RG Crystal, JB West, Barnes PJ, et al., eds. *The lung: scientific foundations,* 2nd ed. Philadelphia: Lippincott–Raven Publishers, 1997:2699–2712.
6. Schaefer KE, Allison RD, Dougherty JH, et al: Pulmonary and circulatory adjustments determining the limits of depths in breath-hold diving, *Science* 1968;162:1020–1023.
7. Bohn DJ, Biggar WD, Smith R, et al. Influence of hypothermia, barbiturate therapy, and intracranial pressure monitoring on morbidity and mortality after near-drowning. *Crit Care Med* 1986;14:529–534.
8. Modell JH, Graves SA, Ketover A. Clinical course of 91 consecutive near-drowning victims. *Chest* 1976;70:231–238.
9. Ornato JP. The resuscitation of near-drowning victims. *JAMA* 1986;256:75–77.
10. Waugh JH, O'Callaghan MJ, Pitt WR. Prognostic factors and long-term outcomes for children who have nearly drowned. *Med J Aust* 1994;161:594–599.
11. Danzl DF, Pozos RS. Current concepts: accidental hypothermia. *N Engl J Med* 1994;331:1756–1760.
12. Nussbaum E, Maggi JC. Pentobarbital therapy does not improve neurological outcome in nearly drowned, flaccid-comatose children. *Pediatrics* 1988;81:630–634.
13. Edmonds C, Lowry C, Pennefather J, et al. *Diving and subaquatic medicine* 4th ed., Oxford: Edward Arnold Publishers, 2001.
14. Divers Alert Network. *Report on decompression illness and diving and fatalities.* Durham, NC: Divers Alert Network, 2002.
15. *U.S. Navy Diving Manual,* Vols. 1 and 2, Rev. 4. Washington, DC: Naval Sea Systems Command, 1999; 0910-LP-708-8000.
16. Bennett PB. Inert gas narcosis. In Bennett PB, Elliott DH, eds. *The physiology and medicine of diving,* 4th ed. London: WB Saunders, 1997.
17. Phillips JL. *The bends: compressed air in the history of science, diving and engineering.* New Haven, CT: Yale University Press, 1998.
18. Melamed Y, Shupak A, Bitterman H. Medical problems associated with underwater diving. *N Engl J Med* 1992;326:30–35.
19. McGough EK, De Santeles DA, Gallagher TJ. Dive computers and decompression sickness: a review of 83 cases. *J Hyperbaric Med* 1990;5:159.
20. Farmer JC, Thomas WG: Ear and sinus problems in diving. In: Strauss RH, ed. *Diving medicine.* New York: Grune & Stratton, 1976.
21. Leitch DR, Green RD. Pulmonary barotrauma in divers and the treatment of cerebral arterial gas embolism. *Aviat Space Environ Med* 1986;7:931–938.
22. Green SM, et al. Incidence and severity of middle ear barotrauma in recreational scuba diving. *Wilderness Med* 1993;4:270.
23. Parell GJ, Becker GD. Conservative management of inner ear barotrauma resulting from scuba diving. *Otolaryngol Head Neck Surg* 1985;93:393.
24. Dutka AJ. A review of the pathophysiology and potential application of experimental therapies for cerebral ischemia to the treatment of cerebral gas embolism. *Undersea Biomed Res* 1985;12:403.
25. Kizer KW. Dysbaric cerebral air embolism in Hawaii. *Ann Emerg Med* 1987;16:535.
26. Dick APK, Massey EW. Neurological presentation of decompression sickness and air embolism in sport divers. *Neurology* 1985;35:667.
27. Neuman TS, Hallenbeck JM. Barotraumatic cerebral air embolism and the mental status examination: a report of four cases. *Ann Emerg Med* 1987;16:220.
28. Greer HD, Massey EW. Neurologic injury from undersea diving. *Neurol Clin* 1992;10:1031–1044.
29. Raymond LW. Pulmonary barotrauma and related events in divers. *Chest* 1995;107:1648–1652.
30. Hodgson M, Beran RG, Shirtley G. The role of computed tomography in the assessment of neurologic sequelae of decompression sickness. *Arch Neural* 1988;45:1033.
31. Cogas WB. Intravenous lidocaine as adjunctive therapy in the treatment of decompression illness. *Ann Emerg Med* 1997;29:284.
32. Aharon-Peretz J, Adir Y, Gordon CR, et al. Spinal cord decompression sickness in sport diving. *Arch Neurol* 1993;50:753–756.
33. Ball R. Effect of severity time to recompression with oxygen, and re-treatment on outcome in 49 cases of spinal cord decompression sickness. *Undersea Hyperbaric Med* 1993;20:133.
34. Francis TJ, Pezeshkpour GH, Dutka AJ, et al. Is there a role for the autochthonous bubble in the pathogenesis of spinal cord decompression sickness?. *J Neuropathol Exper Neurol* 1988;47:475–487.
35. Cross SJ, Evans SA, Thomson LF et al. Safety of subaqua

diving, with a patent foramen ovale. *BMJ* 1992;1304:481–482.

36. Moon RE, Camporesi EM, Kisslo JA. Patent foramen ovale and decompression sickness in divers. *Lancet* 1989;1:513.

37. Wilmhurst PT, Byme JC, Webb-Peploc MM. Relation between interatrial shunts and decompression sickness in divers. *Lancet* 1989;2:1302.

38. Rivera JC. Decompression sickness among divers: an analysis of 935 cases. *Military Med* 1964;129:314.

39. Wilmhurst PT, Byme JC, Webb-Peploc MM. Neurological decompression sickness. *Lancet* 1989;1:731.

40. Rudge FW, Stone JA. The use of the pressure cuff test in the diagnosis of decompression sickness. *Aviat Space Environ Med* 1991;62:266.

41. Thalmann, ED. Principles of U.S. Navy recompression treatments for decompression sickness. In: RE Moon, PJ Sheffield, eds. *Treatment of decompression illness: 45th workshop of the undersea and hyperbaric medical society.* Kensington, MD: Undersea and Hyperbaric Medical Society, 1996:75–95.

42. Kizer KW. Delayed treatment of dysbarism: a retrospective review of 50 cases. *JAMA* 1983;247:2555.

43. Clark JM, Lambertson CJ. Pulmonary oxygen toxicity: a review. *Pharmacol Rev* 1971;23:37.

44. Donald KW. Oxygen poisoning in man. *BMJ* 1947;1:667.

45. Hendricks PL, Hall DA, Hunter WL, et al. Extension of pulmonary O_2 tolerance in man at 2 ATA by intermittent O_2 exposure. *J Appl Physiol* 1977;42:593–599.

46. Bove AA. *Medical examination of sports scuba divers.* Flagstaff, AZ: Best Publishing Co, 1997.

47. Jenkins C, Anderson SD, Wong R, et al. Compressed air diving and respiratory disease. *Med J Aust* 1993;158:275–279.

48. Neuman TS, Bove AA, O'Connor RD, et al. Asthma and diving. *Ann Allergy* 1994;73:344–349.

49 Medical Legal Aspects of Environmental/Occupational Disability Evaluation

Gary R. Epler

Pulmonary clinicians in an active practice are sometimes asked about the medicolegal aspects of environmental and occupational disorders. They are asked to quantity functional impairment for use in determination of pulmonary disability and to make a determination of a causal relationship between an exposure and a lung disease. Patients needing these evaluations may come from the practice, or claimants may be referred from governmental agencies, insurance companies, or attorneys. This chapter will review the methods used to make the determination of pulmonary impairment and develop a framework to establish a cause and effect association.

An accurate diagnosis is the basis of the evaluation. The pulmonary clinician generally establishes the pulmonary disease diagnosis by using appropriate clinical, radiographic, and physiologic data. A lung biopsy is rarely needed to establish the diagnosis of an environmental or occupationally related disorder, although biopsy material may be available because the tissue was obtained to rule out a chronic infectious or neoplastic process.

The determination of disability begins with the definition of two important terms, impairment and disability. Impairment is a medical term defined as a functional abnormality resulting from a medical condition (1,2). Impairment is defined by the American Medical Association (AMA) guidelines (3) as "a loss, loss of use, or derangement of any body part, organ system, or organ function." An impairment is considered permanent when it has reached maximal medical improvement, which means that it is stabilized and unlikely to change substantially in the next year. The term impair-

ment in the AMA guidelines refers to permanent impairment. The Social Security Administration (SSA) uses the term medically determinable impairment, which is defined as an "impairment that results from anatomical, physiological, or psychological abnormalities which can be shown by medically acceptable clinical and laboratory diagnostic techniques" (4).

Disability is a general term that indicates the "total effect of impairment on a patient's life" (1,2). This is affected by such diverse factors as age, education, social environment, and energy requirements of the occupation. Two individuals with an identical impairment may be differently affected in their life situation. The AMA defines disability as an alteration of an individual's capacity to meet personal, social, or occupational demands because of an impairment (3). For the SSA, the "law defines disability as the inability to engage in any substantial gainful activity by reason of any medically determinable physical or mental impairment, which can be expected to result in death or which has lasted or can be expected to last for a continuous period of not less than 12 months (4)."

The rating of pulmonary impairment falls within the purview of a physician's expertise, whereas the determination of disability is an administrative and judicial decision that requires consideration of both nonmedical and medical variables.

Determination of whether there is an association between an exposure and a specific lung disease can be complex. The answer may be straightforward for the pneumoconiosis because of specific radiographic findings and appropriate exposure information, whereas cause and effect for disorders of the airways can be difficult, especially when in association with cigarette smoking and patients with asthma. The approach to establishing cause-and-effect relationship is discussed at the end of this chapter.

G. R. Epler: Department of Medicine, Harvard Medical School, Cambridge, and Pulmonary and Critical Care Medicine, Brigham and Women's Hospital, Boston, Massachusetts.

ESTABLISHING THE CLINICAL PROFILE AND DATABASE

The evaluation of the patient for pulmonary disability begins in the traditional manner of gathering clinical information. A thoroughly validated respiratory questionnaire is available and suitable for systematically recording the history (5). Categorizing the degree of dyspnea is an important first step because it is often the principal manifestation of impairment. Dyspnea can be coded as 0 (none) to grade 4 (very severe), as shown in Table 49.1.

Although dyspnea can be quantified, the degree of dyspnea cannot be used as a sole criterion for pulmonary disability determination. This conclusion is based on several factors. There are many causes of the feeling of dyspnea, some not related to pulmonary dysfunction. Dyspnea is a subjective finding. The amount of dyspnea experienced by individuals with the same degree of measurement pulmonary impairment varies greatly. These differences may be owing to variable degrees of verbal expression and understanding, unrelated to the extent of the pulmonary disease. A longitudinal study of 1,784 individuals in The Netherlands found that "unfavorable changes in physical functioning were low income and excessive alcohol consumption" (6). There were also effects of "marital status, degree of urbanization, and smoking."

Other pulmonary symptoms such as cough, sputum production, and wheezing should be characterized and quantified as much as possible. For example, frequency and duration of cough and sputum can be categorized by recording the following: (a) whether these symptoms occur in the morning only or throughout the day, (b) the number of days per week these symptoms occur, and (c) whether the cough and sputum have been present for three or more consecutive months. The timing and duration of wheezing should be documented in the same manner. It should be noted whether the cough, sputum production, or wheezing are by themselves disabling by limiting the person's capacity to function in daily work activities.

Information concerning occupations and hazardous exposures is helpful to adjudicators for assessment of the workplace environment and to physicians for determination of causation. The optimal questionnaire continues to be developed (7). Generally, data collection begins with the date and place of birth. This sets the historic tone for beginning the process. After that, the information proceeds through childhood and summer employment, military service, and a chronological list of jobs. Detailed job descriptions should be obtained because titles such as plasterer, fireman, or engineer may be of little value, as the titles may remain the same while job activities and hazardous exposure may change dramatically. In some situations, eliciting the parents' or spouse's jobs and exposures may be helpful. After completing the chronological list of jobs, the employee should be questioned about hazardous exposures to specific types of dusts, chemicals, gases, or fumes. When such an exposure is found, it is important to document the following indices: (a) year first exposed to the agent, (b) total years exposed, (c) estimation of the exposure level, and (d) years since last exposure.

Additional information regarding causation includes amount of cigarette smoking or tobacco use. Individuals can be classified as nonsmokers (never or less than five lifetime packs), ex-smokers (stopped for a least 1 year), or present smokers. The type of smoking such as cigarette, cigar, or pipe should be noted. The age first started and stopped, as well as the average number of packs of cigarettes smoked daily, should be recorded. The number of cigars daily or amount of pipe tobacco used should be noted, as well as the use and amount of chewing tobacco.

Other clinical data that may be useful in situations of multiple impairments or for causation include detailed characterization of other medical problems, previous pulmonary illnesses, family history of pulmonary diseases, and current medications along with the names, dosage, and duration.

The physical examination should include a description of the patient's breathing, the presence of finger clubbing or cyanosis, the presence of lymphadenopathy, the quality of breath sounds, the presence of crackles or wheezes, cardiac findings, and the presence of lower extremity edema. Details concerning the patient's breathing include the use of accessory muscles, paradoxical movement between the rib cage and the abdomen, the use of pursed lips during exhalation, labored breathing at rest, or the inability to speak complete sentences.

Abnormal physical findings may indicate disabling lung disease, but their relationship to severe impairment and disability is variable. For example, crackles are heard in more than three fourths of patients with chronic interstitial pneumonia who are severely impaired, yet crackles are heard almost as often in patients with early disease with minimal impairment. Crackles also occur in a small percentage of individuals with no lung disorder and no pulmonary impairment.

Signs of cor pulmonale should be noted, e.g., neck vein distension, dependent edema, increased liver size, increased intensity of the second heart sound, and the presence of a right-ventricular early diastolic gallop that increases with

TABLE 49.1. DYSPNEA CAN BE CODED AS 0 (NONE) TO GRADE 4 (VERY SEVERE)

Grade	Degree	Description
0	None	Not troubled with breathlessness except with strenuous exercise
1	Slight	Troubled by shortness of breath when hurrying on the level or walking up a slight hill
2	Moderate	Walks more slowly on the level than do people the same age, because of breathlessness
3	Severe	Stops for breath after walking about 100 yd or after a few minutes on the level
4	Very severe	Breathless when dressing or undressing; too breathless to leave the house

inspiration. The presence of documented cor pulmonale usually indicates severe pulmonary impairment (1). For Social Security disability, the presence of chronic and irreversible cor pulmonale requires documentation of signs and laboratory findings of right ventricular overload or failure such as increased pulmonary artery pressure measured by right heart catheterization (4).

CHEST RADIOGRAPH AND CHEST COMPUTED TOMOGRAPHY SCAN

The chest radiograph should be obtained for individuals being evaluated for disability. In diseases of airflow obstruction, such as asthma and emphysema, the appearance of the chest radiograph may indicate no relation to severity of disease. The chest film may be entirely normal in the presence of severe obstruction. For this large group of diseases, no correlation between work status and radiographic findings has been noted. However, as part of an overall evaluation for disability, the chest radiograph should be described in terms of lung size, presence of bullae, flattened diaphragm, increased posterior-anterior diameter, and findings consistent with cor pulmonale, such as an increased size of the pulmonary artery.

For the interstitial lung diseases, the radiographic findings can be quantified on a scale of mild, moderate, and severe (or on a scale of one through three, respectively). Even though quantification of these disorders can be determined, correlation of radiographic severity and impairment is poor. This is especially true for the reticular nodular opacities of the granulomatous diseases such as sarcoidosis. The radiograph may be categorized as severe, yet individuals may have no respiratory symptoms and have normal pulmonary function studies. The explanation for this discrepancy is that granulomas with no associated scarring may appear radiographically, but the lung in between them is normal, resulting in no abnormal physiological consequence.

The same situation occurs with small rounded opacities, such as in coal worker's pneumoconiosis or noncomplicated silicosis, in which there is a poor correlation between radiographic and physiologic abnormalities. However, the development of progressive massive fibrosis generally indicates impairment. In addition, the greater the amount of progressive massive fibrosis, the greater the degree of impairment.

There is also a poor radiographic correlation between the severity of small irregular opacities and pulmonary impairment associated with the chronic interstitial pneumonias including asbestosis. However, the correlation is opposite: the radiographic findings usually underestimate the degree of pulmonary impairment. There are two reasons for this discrepancy. First, linear opacities are present in all chest radiographs, and an abnormal amount of these opacities is not recognized until later in the disease process. Second, the lung between the opacities is not normal. There is diffuse scarring of the lung, potentially causing a severe decrease in pulmonary function, especially the diffusing capacity. Re-

gardless of these limitations, a classification of mild, moderate, and severe remains important.

The findings of the chest computed tomography (CT) or high-resolution CT (HRCT) should also be noted. These findings are helpful for establishing a diagnosis, especially the presence of honeycombing noted by high-resolution chest CT. This finding suggests the diagnosis of pulmonary fibrosis, often usual interstitial pneumonia (8). The presence of enlarged pulmonary arteries should also be noted as a possible diagnosis of pulmonary hypertension or cor pulmonale. The findings of mediastinal or hilar lymphadenopathy or other abnormalities may also be useful for causation.

PULMONARY FUNCTION TESTING

The clinical database and radiographic findings are useful as part of the overall evaluation of impairment and disability; however, symptoms, physical findings, and radiographic abnormalities are often inconsistent or nonspecific. The poor correlation of such information explains the emphasis on physiological studies. Three initial screening tests are used for determination of pulmonary impairment. These are the forced vital capacity (FVC) for volume, the forced expired volume in 1 second (FEV_1) for airflow, and the single-breath diffusing capacity (D_{SB}) for gas exchange.

FVC is the most valuable screening test for volume determination. It is performed routinely with the FEV_1, requires minimal time and effort, and is both valid and reliable; the variance is small; and adequate regression equations for predicted normal values are readily available.

FEV_1 is the single best test for determining severe impairment in patients with airflow obstruction. FEV_1 has found acceptance throughout the world, is simple to perform, is not excessively fatiguing, and does not place excessive demands on instrumentation, and cooperation is generally such that there is little difference between first and subsequent trials.

The D_{SB} is noninvasive and suitable for rapid screening, requires little cooperation or effort, and is a well-standardized test, and adequate regression equations for prediction of normal values are available. It is important that standardized equipment and standardized techniques are used to perform these studies (9,10).

Numerical limits to delineate degrees of impairment are necessary for use as guidelines by administrative personnel. However, such limits pose certain philosophical questions. For example, the Social Security Administration has published tables of lower limits for actual values of FVC and FEV_1 based on height without regard to sex or age (4). It could be concluded that these tables tend to favor elderly individuals, whereas values expressed as percentages of the predicted values do not favor older workers because the respiratory cost of a given task remains unchanged with advancing age. However, the use of percentage of predicted values is generally preferred because physicians charged with rating impairment should compare organ function or function of the whole person to that of a comparable, similarly aged, healthy person. That elderly persons cannot perform strenuous work as well as younger individuals do must be considered by administrative personnel charged with judging disability.

Pulmonary exercise testing can also be used for determination of pulmonary impairment for specific situations. A test designed for direct measurement of work capacity seems desirable for evaluation of pulmonary disability, but it is often not possible to reproduce the specific type of exertion required for various occupations in the laboratory and it is not possible to mimic duration of effort required for regular work. Most occupations in a highly mechanized society are nearly sedentary, and constant maximum oxygen consumption is not required. The main distress associated with work, as experienced by patients with severe pulmonary impairment, is related to long duration of low-level activity and the exertion, frustration, and discomfort experienced in travel to and from the job.

The cycle ergometer and treadmill are both suitable for exercise testing. A higher oxygen consumption and heart rate can be achieved on a treadmill owing to the larger muscle mass employed, whereas arterial sampling and complex ventilatory studies are more easily performed with the patient seated on a cycle ergometer. Cycling is not as universal as walking, and elderly patients find it easy and comfortable to walk on the treadmill.

Steady-state testing for 5 minutes at each level, or incremental studies with minute-by-minute or continuous increases of exercise levels, can be used. Incremental studies are popular because of the ease and short duration of the test, although the steady-state method is useful for disability evaluation because most elderly patients can complete a 5-minute level and because it best reflects work-related activities.

Actual measurement of oxygen consumption (Vo_2) is recommended. The estimated Vo_2, or determination of metabolic equivalents, during a cardiology stress test is not recommended. For disability evaluation, it is important that patients perform the exercise test to an adequate level. Subjective findings noted by the patients, as well as the observers' impressions, should be recorded; however, this is insufficient documentation for defining an adequate or maximal test. Cardiac and pulmonary findings can be used as objective criteria. The heart rate is used as the cardiac criterion because it is part of routine exercise monitoring. The value of 80% of predicted ($210 - \text{age} \times 0.65$) is suggested as a minimal limit. For subjects not attaining this requirement, a ventilation measurement can be used. This is referred to as the maximal expired minute volume (MEV), which is determined by multiplying the actual FEV_1 value by 35. A value of 50% can be used as a minimal limit. Thus a pulmonary exercise study can be deemed adequate if the subject attains a heart rate of at least 80% predicted or an MEV of a least 50% of predicted.

The maximal oxygen uptake gives an excellent estimate of an individual's aerobic fitness; i.e., the ability to perform a task with well-defined aerobic demands (11). A worker involved in manual labor, who is more or less free to set the work pace, normally accepts working with an energy output of approximately 40% of the maximum aerobic power. During shorter periods of time, an individual can work without fatigue at about 50% of the Vo_2max. Therefore, if an individual can exercise for a least 5 minutes with a rate of work resulting in a Vo_2 of 35 mL/(kg · min), work requiring a Vo_2 of 15 mL/(kg · min) could probably be continued for hours. Thus, an individual who can attain an O_2 uptake of 25 to 35 mL/(kg · min) should be able to perform most moderate and heavy work; however, if 15 mL/(kg · min) cannot be achieved, the worker should be considered disabled for most types of labor (1,3).

DETERMINATION OF PULMONARY IMPAIRMENT

A useful method for determining pulmonary impairment consists of recording the respiratory symptoms with quantification, occupational information, physician examination findings, and quantification of the chest radiographic findings, but most importantly, determining the physiological findings. This consists of using the three screening tests: FVC to describe volume, FEV_1 to characterize flow-rate, and diffusing capacity to describe the lung surface area and gas exchange.

If these pulmonary function tests are entirely normal, the patient is not "disabled" because of pulmonary impairment. If the tests show severe impairment, there is pulmonary

PULMONARY IMPAIRMENT	
Summary Statement	**Level of Evidence**
The lower limit of normal is recommended as an abnormal value	Statistically valid value of a 95% confidence interval rather than an arbitrary 80% predicted value. Statistically correct, yet no correlation with symptoms
Reference values for FVC, FEV_1, FEV_1/FVC, and diffusing capacity	Statistically significant number of individuals among a healthy reference population
Mild to moderate degrees of pulmonary impairment	Finding that respiratory symptoms begin to occur at <60% predicted
Severe degree of pulmonary impairment	Some epidemiological studies showing FVC values of ≤50%; FEV_1 and Ds_B values of ≤40% indicate severe impairment and inability to work in patients with airflow obstruction and interstitial disease

FEV_1, forced expiratory volume in 1s; FVC, forced vital capacity; Ds_B, single-breath diffusing capacity.

TABLE 49.2. BASED ON THE 2001 AMERICAN MEDICAL ASSOCIATION GUIDELINES

Pulmonary Function Test	No Pulmonary Impairment*	Mild Pulmonary Impairment	Moderate Pulmonary Impairment	Severe Pulmonary Impairment
FVC	>lower limit of normal	60% predicted to lower limit	51%–60% predicted	≤50% predicted
FEV$_1$	>lower limit of normal	60% predicted to lower limit	41%–60% predicted	≤40% predicted
FEV$_1$/FVC ratio	>lower limit of normal			
Diffusing capacity	>lower limit of normal	60% predicted to lower limit	41%–59% predicted	≤40% predicted
Maximal exercise oxygen consumption	≥25 mL/(kg · min}	20 to 24 mL/(kg · min)	15 to 19 mL/(kg · min)	<15 mL/(kg · min)

FVC, forced vital capacity; FEV$_1$, forced expiratory volume in 1 s.
*The lower limit of normal is based on the 95% confidence interval values from tables in Chapter 5: the respiratory system. In: Cocchiarella L, Andersson G, eds. *Guides to the evaluation of permanent impairment,* 5th ed. Chicago, American Medical Association, 2001;87–116, and from regression formulas in Crapo RO, Morris AH. Standardized single breath normal values for carbon monoxide diffusing capacity. *Am Rev Respir Dis* 1981;123:185–190 and Crapo RO, Morris AH, Gardner RM. Reference spirometric values using techniques and equipment that meet ATS recommendations. *Am Rev Respir Dis* 1981;123:659–664.

dysfunction of such severity that it alone precludes gainful employment, and no further studies are needed. With lesser degrees of impairment, exercise studies may be useful. If a Vo$_2$ of 15 mL/(kg · min) cannot be attained during an appropriate exercise study, the individual will probably not be able to engage in most types of labor (1,3). Above this level, light to moderate labor may be performed, and toward the upper end of the spectrum (e.g., a Vo$_2$ of greater than 25 mL/(kg · min)), virtually all types of labor could probably be performed. Table 49.2 is based on the 2001 AMA guidelines (3).

SPECIAL CONSIDERATIONS

Asthma is considered individually because of its episodic yet disabling nature. Methods developed by the American Thoracic Society and AMA use a scoring system based on the postbronchodilator actual FEV$_1$ value, the change in the post-FEV$_1$ value or change in postmethacholine FEV$_1$ value, and the amount of medication (2,3) (Tables 49.3 and 49.4).

The Social Security Administration defines permanent and total disability from asthma as "attacks in spite of pre-scribed treatment and requiring physician intervention, oc-curring at least once very two months or at least six times a year. Each in-patient hospitalization for longer than 24 hours for control of asthma counts as two attacks, and an evalua-tion period of at least 12 consecutive months must be used to determine the frequency of attacks" (4).

Individuals with *lung cancer* should be considered severely impaired at the time of diagnosis (3). If the person is found to be free of all evidence of tumor recurrence at reevaluation 1 year after the diagnosis, then the individual is evaluated according to the pulmonary impairment criteria. If there is still evidence of tumor, the individual is considered to be severely impaired. A four-grade scale can also be used to quantify the capabilities of individuals with lung cancer (Table 49.5).

PULMONARY IMPAIRMENT FOR ASTHMA

Summary Statement	Level of Evidence
Postbronchodilator FEV$_1$ scores	Committee opinion
Methacholine dose <8 mg/mL indicates airway responsiveness.	Epidemiological studies
Methacholine dose scores	Consensus of committee opinion
Minimum medication scores	Consensus of committee opinion

FEV$_1$, forced expiratory volume in 1 s.

TABLE 49.3. IMPAIRMENT CLASSIFICATION FOR ASTHMA SEVERITY

Score	Post FEV$_1$	% Change Post-FEV$_1$	Methacholine (mg/mL)	Minimum Medication
0	>lower limit of normal	<10%	>8 mg/mL	None
1	≥70% predicted	10% to 19%	8–>0.6 mg/mL	Occasional nondaily use of inhaler
2	60%–69% predicted	20% to 29%	0.6–>0.125 mg/mL	Daily bronchodilator or low-dose inhaled corticosteroid
3	50%–59% predicted	30% or more	≤0.125 mg/mL	Daily high-dose inhaled corticosteroid or one to three courses of systemic steroid
4	<50% predicted			Daily high-dose inhaled corticosteroid and daily or every other day systemic corticosteroid

FEV$_1$, forced expiratory volume in 1 s.

TABLE 49.4. IMPAIRMENT RATING FOR ASTHMA

Total Asthma Score	Impairment Class	Impairment of Whole Person
0	1	None
1–5	2	10%–25%
6–9	3	26%–50%
10–11 or FEV_1 <50% despite >20 mg/d of prednisone	4	51%–100%

FEV_1, forced expiratory volume in 1 s.

TABLE 49.5. GRADE SCALE OF CAPABILITIES FOR SUBJECTS WITH CANCER

Grade	Description of Capabilities
0	Fully active, able to carry on activities without restrictions
1	Restricted in strenuous activity, able to carry out light tasks in the home or office
2	Requires occasional to considerable care for most needs
3	Only capable of limited self-care; confined to bed or chair at least half of waking hours
4	Almost totally impaired; cannot care for self; totally confined to bed or chair.

CAUSATION

A framework for the determination of cause and effect is useful. First, establish the diagnosis. Second, find out everything possible about the exposure. Third, determine whether the exposure can result in this specific disease. Fourth, confirm the cause-and-effect association by evaluating epidemiological studies and meeting the requirements of established criteria.

As a basis, it is important to establish the diagnosis with as much diagnostic information as possible, including respiratory symptoms, other symptoms, other medical conditions, cigarette smoking use, physical findings, pulmonary function test results with prebronchodilator and postbronchodilator studies and diffusing capacity, radiographic findings, and sometimes biopsy material. It is then important to obtain as much exposure information as possible. This information includes the specific name and nature of the suspected agent (material safety data sheets [MSDS] are useful as an initial source of information), amount of exposure, timing of the exposure, duration of the exposure, and the temporal relationship between exposure and the disease.

Searching the literature and evaluating epidemiological studies are then used to determine whether an exposure causes the disease. The strength of the association can be evaluated by thoroughly understanding the techniques, characteristics of the study populations, and results of epidemiological studies. Determine if these epidemiological studies indicate a gradient of risk such that increasing exposure results in increasing risk. Determine if the risk decreases after

TABLE 49.6. IS THE ASSOCIATION CAUSAL OR NOT? BRADFORD HILL'S CRITERIA

1. Strength of the association
2. Does-response effect
3. Lack of temporal ambiguity
4. Consistency of the findings
5. Biological plausibility
6. Coherence of the evidence
7. Specificity of the association

From Hill AB. The environment and disease: association and causation. *Proc R. Soc Med* 1965;58:295–300, with permission.

intervention to reduce exposure. Make a determination as to whether there is a more likely cause or explanation for the diagnosis. Finally, determine whether the association could be due to chance.

There are several criteria that can be used to determine whether an association is unrelated or whether the association is one of cause and effect. Bradford Hill has suggested criteria that can be useful after considering all the epidemiological evidence about a relationship between exposure and disease (14). A surgeon general advisory committee of the United States Public Health Service recommended fewer but similar criteria (15) (Tables 49.6 and 49.7).

CAUSATION

Summary Statement	Level of Evidence
Criteria for determination of causation	Consensus of expert opinion

In conclusion, patients will sometimes need to be evaluated for pulmonary disability, and determination of whether an association between an exposure and a lung disease is a cause-and-effect association. Obtaining pulmonary function studies and classifying degrees of dysfunction can be used to determine pulmonary impairment. Determining the consistency, strength, specificity, temporal, and coherence of the association between an exposure and a lung disorder can be used to determine the cause-and-effect relationship.

TABLE 49.7. IS THE ASSOCIATION CAUSAL OR NOT? SURGEON GENERAL/USPHS CRITERIA

1. Consistency of the association
2. Strength of the association
3. Specificity of the association
4. Temporal relationship
5. Coherence of the association

From Parkes WR. Appendix VI: proof of a causal relationship between a specific exogenous agent and disease. *Occupational lung disorders*; 3rd ed. St. Louis, Butterworth-Heinemann Medical, 1994:874, with permission.

REFERENCES

1. Evaluation of impairment/disability secondary to respiratory disorders: American Thoracic Society. *Am Rev Respir Dis* 1986;133:1205–1209.
2. Guidelines for the evaluation of impairment/disability in patients with asthma: American Thoracic Society. *Am Rev Respir Dis* 1993;147:1056–1061.
3. Chapter 5: the respiratory system. In: Cocchiarella L, Andersson G, eds. *Guides to the evaluation of permanent impairment,* 5th ed. Chicago: American Medical Association, 2001:87–116.
4. Social Security Administration. Disability evaluation under Social Security: 3.00 respiratory system. Baltimore, MD: Social Security Administration; 2001; 64-039, ICN 468600.
5. Ferris BG. Epidemiology standardization project: American Thoracic Society. *Am Rev Respir Dis* 1978;118(pt 2):1–120.
6. Mackenbach JP, Borsboom GJ, Nusselder WJ, et al. Determinants of levels and changes of physical functioning in chronically ill persons: results from the GLOBE study. *J Epidemiol Community Health* 2001;9:631–638.
7. Engel LS, Keifer MC, Zahm SH. Comparison of a traditional questionnaire with an icon/calendar-based questionnaire to assess occupational history. *Am J Ind Med* 2001;40:502–511.
8. Idiopathic pulmonary fibrosis: diagnosis and treatment. International consensus statement. American Thoracic Society (ATS), and the European Respiratory Society (ERS). *Am J Respir Crit Care Med* 2000;161:646–664.
9. Standardization of spirometry, 1994 update: American Thoracic Society. *Am Rev Respir Dis* 1995;152:1107–1136.
10. American Thoracic Society. Single breath carbon monoxide diffusing capacity: recommendations for a standard technique, 1995. *Am J Respir Crit Care Med* 1995;152:2185–2198.
11. Astrand P, Rodahl K. *Textbook of work physiology.* New York: McGraw-Hill, 1977.
12. Crapo RO, Morris AH. Standardized single breath normal values for carbon monoxide diffusing capacity. *Am Rev Respir Dis* 1981;123:185–190.
13. Crapo RO, Morris AH, Gardner RM. Reference spirometric values using techniques and equipment that meet ATS recommendations. *Am Rev Respir Dis* 1981;123:659–664.
14. Hill AB. The environment and disease: association and causation. *Proc R Soc Med* 1965;58:295–300.
15. Parkes WR. Appendix VI: proof of a causal relationship between a specific exogenous agent and disease *Occupational lung disorders,* 3rd ed. St. Louis: Butterworth-Heinemann Medical, 1994: 874.

Baum's Textbook of Pulmonary Diseases, 7th ed. Edited by James D. Crapo, Jeffrey Glassroth, Joel Karlinsky, and Talmadge E. King, Jr.
Lippincott Williams & Wilkins, Philadelphia © 2004.

50 Acute Respiratory Failure

Christine Reardon · John J. Marini · Laurel A. Wright

The primary purpose of the respiratory system is to provide fresh gas from the environment to the alveolus, where the capillary blood can exchange oxygen (O_2) for carbon dioxide (CO_2) across a thin gas-permeable membrane. Provision of O_2 is fundamental to sustaining aerobic metabolism, whereas CO_2 elimination, acting through the bicarbonate buffer system, helps maintain pH homeostasis.

Respiratory failure may be thought of as a problem in one or more of the steps necessary to sustain O_2 availability for mitochondrial energy production. Dysfunction of the respiratory system may occur in ventilation (the movement of gases between the environment and the lungs), in intrapulmonary gas exchange (the process in which mixed venous blood releases CO_2 and becomes oxygenated), in gas transport (the delivery of adequate quantities of oxygenated blood to the metabolizing tissue), or in tissue gas exchange (the extraction or utilization of O_2 and release of CO_2 by the peripheral tissues). The latter two steps in this process may fail independently of the performance of the lung or ventilatory pump.

This discussion examines one primary manifestation of acute respiratory insufficiency-oxygenation failure. The aim is to describe an approach to management that flows from an understanding of the underlying pathophysiology. Ventilatory failure, the second major manifestation of acute respiratory insufficiency, is discussed in Chapters 12 and 53.

C. Reardon: Department of Medicine, Pulmonary Center, Boston, Massachusetts.

J. J. Marini: Department of Medicine, Division of Pulmonary and Critical Care Medicine, University of Minnesota, Minneapolis, Minnesota.

L. A. Wright: Pulmonary and Critical Care Medicine, Park Nicollet Clinic, St. Louis Park, Minnesota.

OXYGENATION FAILURE

Definitions

Tissue O_2 delivery, also known as O_2 transport (Do_2), depends not only on the partial pressure of arterial O_2 (Pao_2) but also on nonpulmonary factors—cardiac output ($\dot{Q}T$), hemoglobin (Hgb) concentration, and the ability of Hgb to take up and release O_2: $Do_2 = \dot{Q}T \times$ concentration of arterial O_2 (Cao_2), and $Cao_2 = 1.36 \times$ Hgb $\times$ saturation of arterial O_2 (Sao_2) $+ 0.003$ (Pao_2). Cardiogenic shock, anemia, and carbon monoxide poisoning provide clinical examples of O_2 transport failure. Laboratory abnormalities characteristic of such conditions are lactic acidosis and reduced O_2 content of mixed venous blood (even in the face of adequate arterial O_2 tension).

Failure of O_2 uptake refers to the inability of tissue to extract and use O_2 for aerobic metabolism. The clearest clinical examples of a derangement in this terminal phase of the O_2 transport chain are cyanide poisoning, in which cellular cytochromes (key enzymes in the electron transport process) are inhibited, and septic shock. During sepsis, there is failure of an often generous cardiac output to distribute appropriately and/or an inability of the tissues themselves to make use of the O_2 available. Unlike transport insufficiency, failure of tissue uptake is distinguished by normal or high values for mixed venous O_2 tension, saturation, and content. Thus, some indices that are helpful in other forms of oxygenation failure—i.e., cardiac output, arterial O_2 tension, and mixed venous O_2 saturation ($S\bar{v}o_2$)—may not reflect impaired tissue O_2 uptake; lactic acidosis may be the sole laboratory indicator. Therapy directed at failure of the O_2 transport and uptake mechanisms is discussed in detail elsewhere. The present discussion focuses on the processes that affect the performance of the lung in oxygenating the arterial blood.

MECHANISMS OF ARTERIAL HYPOXEMIA

Six mechanisms may contribute to arterial O_2 desaturation.

1. Inhalation of a hypoxic gas mixture or severe reduction of barometric pressure
2. Hypoventilation
3. Impaired alveolar diffusion of O_2
4. Ventilation-perfusion ($\dot{V}/\dot{Q}$) mismatching
5. Shunting of systemic venous blood to the systemic arterial circuit
6. Abnormal desaturation of systemic venous blood.

Low Inspired Oxygen Fraction

A decrease in the partial pressure of inhaled O_2 (P_{IO_2}) occurs in toxic fume inhalation, in fires that consume O_2, and at high altitude because of reduced barometric pressure.

Hypoventilation

Hypoventilation causes the partial pressure of alveolar O_2 (P_{AO_2}) to fall when alveolar O_2 is not replenished quickly enough in the face of its ongoing removal by the blood. Although P_{AO_2} may fall much faster than partial pressure of arterial carbon dioxide (P_{aCO_2}) rises during the initial phase of hypoventilation or apnea, the steady-state concentration of P_{AO_2} is predicted by the alveolar gas equation:

$$P_{AO_2} = P_{IO_2} - P_{aCO_2}/R$$

In this equation, P_{IO_2} is at the tracheal level (corrected for water vapor pressure at body temperature), and R is the respiratory exchange ratio, i.e., the ratio of CO_2 production to O_2 consumption at steady state. This value usually approximates 0.8., because normally the rate of O_2 consumed by the tissues exceeds that at which CO_2 is produced. Transiently, however, R can fall to very low values, as O_2 is taken up faster than CO_2 is delivered to the alveolus. Such a mechanism explains posthyperventilation hypoxemia and the hypoxemia that accompanies hemodialysis across membranes that remove CO_2.

Impaired Diffusion

Impaired O_2 diffusion prevents complete equilibration of alveolar gas with pulmonary capillary blood. Although this mechanism has uncertain clinical importance, many factors that adversely influence diffusion are encountered clinically: an increased distance between alveolus and erythrocyte, a decreased O_2 gradient for diffusion, and a shortened transit time of the red cell through the capillary (high cardiac output with limited capillary reserve).

Ventilation-Perfusion Mismatching

Ventilation-perfusion ($\dot{V}/\dot{Q}$) mismatching is the most frequent contributor to clinically important O_2 desaturation.

Lung units that are poorly ventilated in relation to perfusion cause desaturation (low $\dot{V}/\dot{Q}$ units). High $\dot{V}/\dot{Q}$ units contribute to physiological dead space but not to hypoxemia. The relationship of C_{aO_2} to P_{aO_2}, like that of P_{aO_2} to Hgb saturation, is curvilinear. At normal barometric pressure, little additional O_2 can be loaded onto blood with already saturated Hgb, no matter how high the O_2 tension in the overventilated alveolus may rise. Because samples of blood exiting from different lung units mix gas contents (not partial pressures), overventilating some units in an attempt to compensate for others that are underventilated does not maintain P_{aO_2} at a normal level. Hence, when equal volumes of blood from well-ventilated and poorly ventilated units mix, the blended sample will have an O_2 content halfway between them but a P_{aO_2} disproportionately weighted toward that of the lower $\dot{V}/\dot{Q}$ unit. Even though total expired $\dot{V}$ and $\dot{Q}$ may be absolutely normal, regional $\dot{V}/\dot{Q}$ mismatching will cause P_{aO_2} to fall.

Supplemental O_2 will reverse hypoxemia when $\dot{V}/\dot{Q}$ mismatching, hypoventilation, or diffusion impairment is the cause. (The P_{aO_2} of even poorly ventilated units climbs high enough to achieve full saturation.) After a sufficient period of time has been spent breathing 100% O_2, only perfused units that are totally unventilated (shunt units) contribute to hypoxemia. When hypoxemia is caused by alveolar units with very low $\dot{V}/\dot{Q}$ ratios, high concentrations of inspired O_2 must be given before a substantial increase in the P_{aO_2} is observed.

Shunting

The term *shunt* refers to the percentage of the total systemic venous blood flow that bypasses the gas-exchanging membrane and transfers venous blood unaltered to the systemic arterial system. Changes in fractional concentration in inspired O_2 (F_{IO_2})—either upward or downward—have very little influence on P_{aO_2} when the true shunt fraction, as measured on pure O_2, exceeds 30% (Fig. 50.1). In contrast, venous admixture of similar magnitude is variably responsive to the extent that low $\dot{V}/\dot{Q}$ units account for the hypoxemia. Shunting can be intracardiac, as in cyanotic right-to-left congenital heart disease, opening of a patent foramen ovale because of right ventricular overload, or result from passage of blood through abnormal vascular channels within the lung, e.g., pulmonary arteriovenous communications. However, by far the most common cause of shunting is pulmonary disease characterized by totally unventilated lung units that cannot respond to O_2 therapy. After an extended exposure to an F_{IO_2} of 1.0, all alveoli that remain open are filled with pure O_2. Hence, the percentage of shunt can be calculated from the following formula:

$$\dot{Q}s/\text{tidal cardiac output } (\dot{Q}_T) = [C_{cO_2} - C_{aO_2})/ (C_{cO_2} - C_{\bar{v}O_2})] \times 100$$

In this equation, $\dot{Q}s$ denotes physiologic shunt, C_{cO_2}, concentration of end-capillary O_2; $C_{\bar{v}O_2}$, concentration of mixed venous blood O_2. In making such calculations,

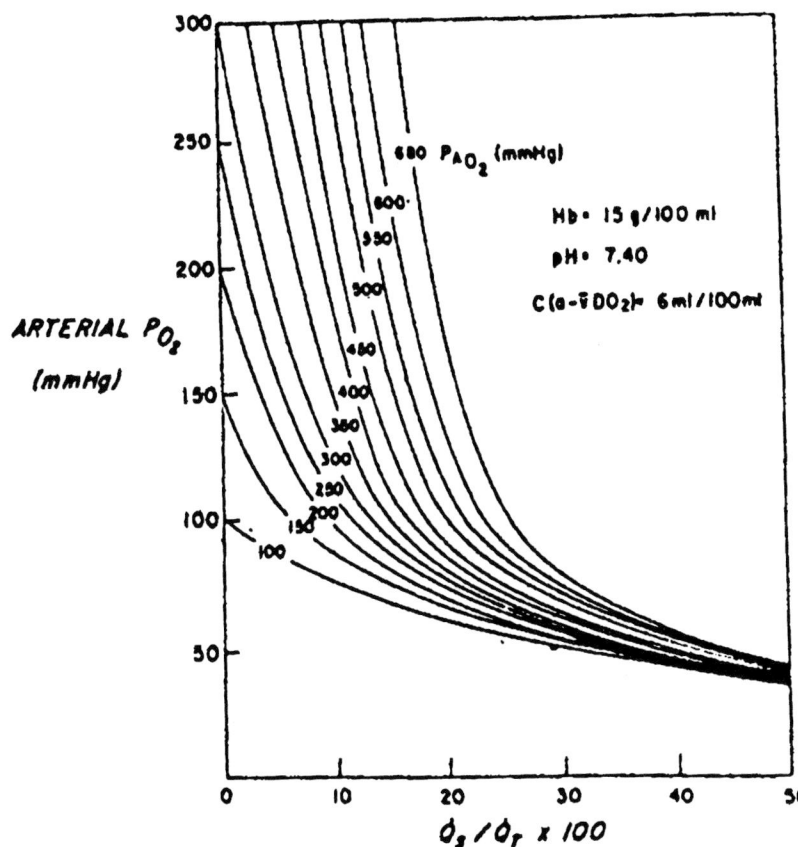

FIGURE 50.1. Relationship of arterial oxygen tension (Pa_{O_2}) to true shunt fraction (Qs/QT) for a range of alveolar oxygen tensions (PA_{O_2}) that are achieved by varying fractions of inspired oxygen (FI_{O_2}) from room air to pure oxygen. Variations of FI_{O_2} exert negligible effects on PA_{O_2} when true shunt exceeds 30%. (From Pontoppidan, Geffin B, Lowenstein E. Acute respiratory failure in the adult. *N Engl J Med* 1972;287:743–752, with permission.)

end-capillary and calculated alveolar O_2 tensions are assumed equivalent. For a patient breathing pure O_2, shunt fractions less than 25% can be estimated rapidly by dividing the alveolar-to-arterial O_2 tension difference ($PA_{O_2} - Pa_{O_2}$) by 20, assuming also that the Pa_{CO_2} and $C\bar{v}_{O_2}$ are normal. Note that some absorption atelectasis may occur in very low $\dot{V}/\dot{Q}$ areas when pure O_2 is breathed, adding to the measured shunt. In the clinical setting, however, the magnitude of this artifact is usually small.

At inspired O_2 fractions less than 1.0, true shunt cannot be estimated reliably by an analysis of O_2 contents, but venous admixture or physiological shunt can. (Note that many authors refer to a venous admixture from any cause as shunt.) Any degree of arterial O_2 desaturation can be considered as if it all originated from true shunt units. To calculate venous admixture, Cc_{O_2} in the shunt formula is estimated from the ideal PA_{O_2} at that particular FI_{O_2}.

Many indices have been devised in an attempt to characterize the efficacy of O_2 exchange across the spectrum of FI_{O_2}. Although no index is completely successful, the Pa_{O_2}/PA_{O_2} ratio and $PA_{O_2} - Pa_{O_2}$ are often used. Both, however, are affected by changes in $S\bar{v}_{O_2}$, even when the lung tissue itself retains normal ability to transfer O_2 to the blood. Another imprecise but commonly used indicator of gas exchange is the Pa_{O_2}/FI_{O_2} ratio (the P/F ratio). In healthy adults, this ratio normally exceeds 400, whatever the FI_{O_2} may be. Hypoventilation and changes in the inspired O_2 concentration minimally alter these ratios in the absence of FI_{O_2}-related absorption atelectasis or cardiovascular adjustments. Whatever index is used, it should be emphasized that the end-expiratory lung volume and mean alveolar pressures can exert a profound influence. For this reason, many centers utilize an oxygenation index that incorporates the mean airway pressure when assessing the efficiency of transpulmonary O_2 transfer under conditions of controlled mechanical ventilation.

Abnormal Desaturation of Systemic Venous Blood

The admixture of abnormally desaturated venous blood is an important mechanism acting to lower Pa_{O_2} in patients with impaired pulmonary gas exchange and reduced cardiac output. Cv_{O_2}, the product of Hgb concentration and Sv_{O_2}, is influenced by $\dot{Q}$, Sa_{O_2}, and O_2 consumption ($\dot{V}_{O_2}$):

$$S\bar{v}_{O_2} \sim Sa_{O_2} - [\dot{V}_{O_2}/(Hgb \times \dot{Q})]$$

It is clear from this equation that $S\bar{v}_{O_2}$ is directly influenced by any imbalance between $\dot{V}_{O_2}$ and O_2 delivery. Thus, anemia uncompensated by an increase in cardiac output or a cardiac output too low for metabolic needs can cause both $S\bar{v}_{O_2}$ and Pa_{O_2} to fall when the venous admixture percentage is abnormal.

Fluctuations in Sv_{O_2} exert a more profound influence on Pa_{O_2} when the shunt is fixed, as in regional lung diseases (e.g.,

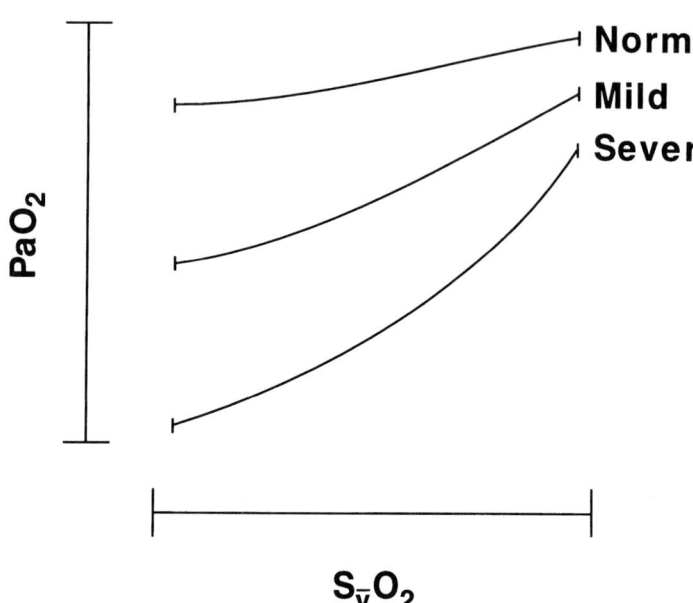

FIGURE 50.2. Influence of mixed venous oxygen saturation (S$\bar{v}$O$_2$) on partial pressure of arterial oxygen (PaO$_2$) in patients with mild and severe lung disease. Variations in S$\bar{v}$O$_2$ related to an oxygen consumption/delivery imbalance have minimal effects on PaO$_2$ in normal subjects but may profoundly affect PaO$_2$ in patients with extensive lung disease. (From Marini JJ, Wheeler AP. *Critical care: the essentials,* 2nd ed. Baltimore: Williams & Wilkins, 1997, with permission.)

atelectasis), than when the shunt varies with changing cardiac output, as it tends to do in diffuse lung injury (acute respiratory distress syndrome [ARDS]) (Fig. 50.2). Even when S$\bar{v}$O$_2$ is abnormally low, PaO$_2$ will remain unaffected if all mixed venous blood gains access to well-oxygenated, well-ventilated alveoli. A marked decline in SvO$_2$ without arterial hypoxemia occurs routinely during heavy exercise in healthy subjects. Thus, abnormal $\dot{V}/\dot{Q}$ matching or shunt is necessary for venous desaturation to be a contributing mechanism in hypoxemia.

COMMON CAUSES OF HYPOXEMIA

Oxygenation crises are conveniently categorized by their radiographic appearances, which give important clues to the appropriate management approach. Lung collapse (atelecta-

sis), diffuse or patchy parenchymal infiltration, hydrostatic edema, localized or unilateral infiltration, and a clear chest x-ray are common patterns (Fig. 50.3).

Atelectasis

Variants of Atelectasis

There are several morphologic types and mechanisms of atelectasis. Regional microatelectasis spontaneously develops in a healthy lung during shallow breathing when it is not periodically stretched beyond its usual tidal range. Plate-like atelectasis may be an exaggeration of this phenomenon caused by regional hypodistention (i.e., pleural effusion or impaired diaphragmatic excursion). Both micro and plate-like atelectasis occur most commonly in dependent lung regions. Lobar collapse usually results from gas absorption in an

A Clear	B Diffuse	C Lobar	D Unilateral
Intracardiac shunt	Bronchopneumonia	Infarction	Aspiration
Pulmonary vascular shunts	BP dysplasia	Occlusion (drowned lung)	Pleural effusion
AV malformation	Hemorrhage	Lobar pneumonia	Mass and drowned lung
Cirrhosis	ARDS		Infarction
Asthma/obstructive lung disease	Hydrostatic edema		Main bronchus intubation
Pulmonary embolism	Aspiration		Mucus plug
Pneumothorax			Contusion
Head injury			Re-expansion edema
Desaturated mixed venous blood			Contralateral pneumothorax
Obesity/airway closure			Pneumonia
			Decubitus position/ hydrostatic edema

FIGURE 50.3. Classification of oxygenation failure by radiographic pattern. (From Marini JJ, Wheeler AP. *Critical care: the essentials,* 2nd ed. Baltimore: Williams & Wilkins, 1997, with permission.)

airway plugged by retained secretions, a misplaced endotracheal tube, or a central mass. External bronchial compression and regional hypoventilation are important in some patients. Micro and platelike atelectasis occur routinely in patients at prolonged uninterrupted bed rest and in postoperative patients who have undergone upper abdominal incisions.

Potential consequences of acute atelectasis are worsened gas exchange, pneumonitis, and increased work of breathing. The PaO_2 drops precipitously to its nadir within minutes to hours of a sudden bronchial occlusion, but it then improves steadily over hours to days as hypoxic vasoconstriction and mechanical factors increase pulmonary vascular resistance through the local area. Whether an individual patient manifests hypoxemia depends heavily on the vigor of the hypoxic vasoconstrictive response, the abruptness of collapse, and the tissue volume involved. If small areas of atelectasis develop slowly, hypoxemia may never surface as a clinical problem.

Diffuse microatelectasis may be radiographically silent but detectable on physical examination by dependent (posterior or basilar) end-inspiratory rales that improve after several sustained deep breaths (sighs) or coughs. Plate atelectasis yields similar physical findings plus tubular breath sounds and egophony over the involved area. Lobar atelectasis gives a dull percussion note and diminished breath sounds if the bronchus is occluded by secretions, but gives tubular breath sounds and egophony if the central airway is patent. (The latter findings correlate well with the presence of air bronchograms on chest x-ray.) Plate atelectasis most frequently develops at the lung base above a pleural effusion or above a raised, splinted, or immobile hemidiaphragm. Lobar atelectasis most commonly occurs in patients with copious airway secretions and limited power to expel them. Acute upper lobe collapse is less common and tends to resolve quickly because of comparatively good gravitational drainage. Collapse of the left lower lobe is more frequent than is collapse of the right lower lobe, perhaps because of its retrocardiac position and its smaller-caliber, sharply angulated bronchus. Lobar atelectasis may be complete or partial, but in either case, it is radiographically recognized by opacification, displaced fissures, compensatory hyperinflation of surrounding tissue, and obliterated air–soft tissue boundaries. Small amounts of pleural fluid are a natural concomitant of lobar collapse and do not necessarily signify an additional pathologic process.

Management of Atelectasis

Prophylaxis

Effective prevention of atelectasis in high-risk patients promotes deep breathing and improves secretion removal. Obesity, chronic bronchitis, increase in secretion volume and viscosity, neuromuscular weakness, pain, and advanced age are predisposing factors. Atelectasis is to be expected whenever the patient is prevented from taking a deep breath by pain, splinting, or weakness. Upper abdominal, thoracic, and lower abdominal incisions are associated with the highest incidence of postoperative atelectasis (in that order). Preoperatively, the airways should be maximally dilated and free of infection. Postoperatively, patients should be encouraged to breathe deeply, to sit upright, and to cough vigorously. Pain should be relieved, but alertness preserved. Frequent turning and early mobilization are among the most important prophylactic maneuvers. Continuous positive airway pressure may be helpful, especially in intubated patients. Respiratory therapy techniques such as airway suctioning, incentive spirometry, and chest physiotherapy are prophylactically (as well as therapeutically) effective in selected patients.

Treatment

Whenever possible, mobilization is the best treatment. Periodic deep breathing effectively reverses plate and microatelectasis. Sustained deep breaths are particularly effective. Whether a higher lung volume is achieved by positive airway pressure or by negative pleural pressure is immaterial, assuming that a similar extent and distribution of distention occurs in both cases. Although rational, the place of positive end-expiratory pressure (PEEP) in treatment of established collapse has not been clarified. Relief of chest wall pain helps to reduce splinting and enables more effective coughing. Intercostal nerve blocks with anesthetic agents such as bupivacaine may be effective for 8 to 12 hours. Intrapleural instillation of lidocaine or bupivacaine (via catheter) can occasionally be effective, but pleural anesthesia may induce temporary ipsilateral diaphragmatic paralysis. Epidural narcotics may also be effective in certain settings. Retained secretions must be dislodged from the central airways. In the non-intubated patient, effective bronchial hygiene is inconsistently accomplished with blind tracheal suctioning alone. Pharyngeal airways certainly help, but they are not well tolerated in conscious patients and are not intended for extended care. Vigorous respiratory therapy initiated soon after the onset of lobar collapse can reverse most cases of atelectasis secondary to airway plugging within 24 to 48 hours. As a general rule, fiberoptic bronchoscopy should be reserved for patients with symptomatic lobar collapse who lack central air bronchograms and who cannot undergo (or fail to respond to or tolerate) 48 hours of vigorous respiratory therapy (e.g., external chest physiotherapy, internal percussive ventilation at pulmonary resonant frequency). Even whole-lung collapse usually merits at least one respiratory therapy treatment before bronchoscopy is performed. After reexpansion, a prophylactic respiratory therapy program should be initiated to prevent recurrence. Adjunctive measures (e.g., bronchodilators, hydration, frequent turning) should be implemented.

Diffuse Pulmonary Infiltration

When fluid or cellular infiltrates cause alveolar flooding or collapse, severe refractory hypoxemia may result. Fluid confined to the interstitial spaces may cause hypoxemia as a result of peribronchial edema, $\dot{V}/\dot{Q}$ mismatching, and microatelectasis; however, interstitial fluid itself does not interfere with O_2 exchange. Very few processes are confined exclusively to the air spaces or to the interstitium. Radiographic signs of alveolar filling include segmental distribution, coalescence, fluffy margins, air bronchograms, rosette patterns, and silhouetting of normal structures. A diffuse infiltrate is said to be largely interstitial if these signs are largely absent and the infiltrate parallels the vascular distribution. Any diffuse interstitial process will appear more radiodense at the bases than at the apices, in part because there is more tissue to penetrate and because vascular engorgement tends to be greater there. Alveoli are also less distended at the bases, so the ratio of aerated volume to total tissue volume declines.

The major categories of acute disease that produce diffuse pulmonary infiltration and hypoxemia are pneumonitis (infection and aspiration), cardiogenic pulmonary edema, intravascular volume overload, and ARDS. From a radiographic viewpoint, these processes may be difficult to distinguish; however, a few characteristic features are helpful.

Hydrostatic Edema

Perihilar infiltrates (sparing the costophrenic angles), a prominent vascular pattern, and a widened vascular pedicle suggest volume overload or incipient cardiogenic edema (Fig. 50.4). A gravitational distribution of edema is highly consistent with well-established left-ventricular failure (or long-standing severe volume overload), especially when accompanied by cardiomegaly and a widened vascular pedicle. Patchy peripheral infiltrates that lack a gravitational predilection and show reluctance to change with position suggest ARDS. Interestingly, septal (Kerley) lines and distinct peribronchial cuffing are very seldom seen in classical ARDS. On the other hand, prominent air bronchograms are quite unusual with hydrostatic etiologies but occur commonly in permeability edema (ARDS) and pneumonia.

Variants of Hydrostatic Edema

Hydrostatic edema (high-pressure edema) may occur in multiple settings that have different implications for prognosis and treatment. The most familiar form of high-pressure edema accompanies left-ventricular failure. In this setting, signs of systemic hypoperfusion and inadequate cardiac output often accompany oxygenation failure. However, high-pressure edema can develop even with a normally well-compensated ventricle during transient heart dysfunction (ischemia, hypertensive crisis, arrhythmias). When the myocardium fails to relax fully during diastole (diastolic dysfunction), superimposed loading or temporary disturbances of left heart contractility (e.g., ischemia), mitral valve functioning, or heart rate or rhythm may cause rapid transient alveolar flooding known as flash pulmonary edema. In this setting, extensive radiographic infiltrates may both develop and resolve with impressive speed.

Acute Lung Injury and Acute Respiratory Distress Syndrome

ARDS was originally called *adult respiratory distress syndrome*. The incidence of ARDS is estimated at 150,000 cases a year in the United States, with a mortality range of 40% to 60% (1). The most recent definition and clinical criteria for ARDS were summarized at the American-European Conference on ARDS in 1994 (1). Acute lung injury (ALI) is a syndrome of inflammation and increased permeability that is associated with a constellation of clinical, radiologic, and physiologic abnormalities that cannot be explained by, but may coexist with, left atrial or pulmonary capillary hypertension. The clinical criteria for ALI include an acute onset of pulmonary failure indicated by a Pao_2/Fio_2 ratio of less than 300 mm Hg, bilateral infiltrates on chest x-ray, and a pulmonary capillary wedge pressure of less than 18 mm Hg or no clinical evidence of increased left atrial pressure. ARDS is a more severe manifestation of ALI in which the same clinical criteria are required, but the Pao_2/Fio_2 ratio is less than 200 mm Hg.

ALI/ARDS can be precipitated by a direct pulmonary injury such as aspiration, pneumonia, near drowning, blunt chest trauma, and toxic inhalation, which all injure the alveolar epithelium. The syndrome can also be caused by an indirect lung injury such as sepsis, transfusions, and pancreatitis in which the systemic inflammatory response creates an injury to the endothelial-alveolar interface. The injured alveolar-capillary interface is more permeable and allows seepage of protein-rich fluid into the interstitial and alveolar

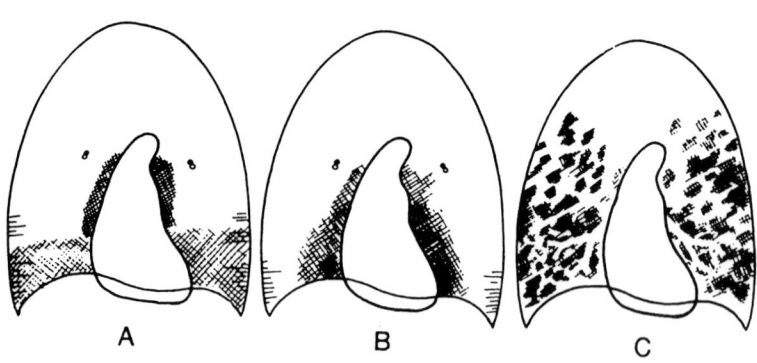

FIGURE 50.4. Radiographic patterns in patients with impaired oxygenation as a result of congestive heart failure **(left),** vascular congestion caused by volume overload **(middle),** and acute respiratory distress syndrome **(right).** Kerley lines, widened vascular pedicle, costophrenic angle sparing, blurred hilar structures, and paucity of air bronchograms help distinguish congestive heart failure from ARDS. (From Milne EN, Pistolesi M, Miniati M, et al. The radiologic distinction of cardiogenic and noncardiogenic edema. *AJR Am J Roentgenol* 1985;144:879–894, with permission.)

A   B   C

spaces. Such fluids inhibit surfactant function, contributing to widespread atelectasis. In addition, the injury to the alveolar epithelium results in less surfactant production, which contributes to the decrease in lung compliance seen in ARDS. Although wedge pressure usually remains normal, increased pulmonary vascular resistance and some degree of pulmonary hypertension are almost invariable in the latter stages of severe disease. Extreme pulmonary hypertension is a very poor prognostic sign.

ALI/ARDS progresses through stages that are defined by the pathologic appearance. The exudative phase demonstrates infiltration of inflammatory cells that cause endothelial and alveolar injury with pulmonary edema. This progresses to the proliferative phase in which fibroblasts infiltrate and begin the process of remodeling. The fibrotic phase results in consolidation and fibrosis of the lung parenchyma. In general, the exudative phase occurs during the first 48 hours after the lung injury, the proliferative phase is usually from day 2 until day 7, and the fibroproliferative phase ensues after day 7 (2).

Rapidly Resolving Noncardiogenic Edema

A few disorders that fall loosely under the heading of ARDS are worth noting because of their fundamentally different pathophysiology and clinical course. In certain settings, transient disruption in the barrier function of the pulmonary capillary can occur without overt endothelial damage. For example, neurogenic and heroin-induced pulmonary edema are two processes in which a transiently elevated pulmonary venous pressure is believed to open epithelial tight junctions, allowing extravasation of proteinaceous fluid. However, resealing and resolution of edema occur promptly without widespread endothelial damage or protracted inflammation. A similar process may be seen in settings such as severe metabolic acidosis and cardiopulmonary resuscitation. From the alveolar side, certain inhalational injuries (e.g., limited chlorine gas or ammonia exposure) can produce a dramatic initial picture, only to clear rapidly over a brief period.

Hypoxemia with a Clear Chest X-Ray

It is not uncommon for patients to present with life-threatening hypoxemia without major radiographic evidence of infiltration. In such cases, occult shunting and severe $\dot{V}/\dot{Q}$ mismatching are the most likely mechanisms (see section "Mechanisms of Arterial Hypoxemia"). Intracardiac or intrapulmonary shunts, asthma and other forms of airway obstruction, low lung volume superimposed on a high closing capacity (i.e., bronchitis in a supine obese patient), pulmonary embolism, and occult microvascular communications (such as occur in patients with cirrhosis) are potential explanations. Hypoxemia is amplified by profound desaturation of mixed venous blood, by reversal of hypoxic vasoconstriction with therapeutic vasoactive agents (i.e., nitroprusside, calcium channel blockers, and dopamine), and by the

severe $\dot{V}/\dot{Q}$ imbalance consequent to acute head injury. (The acute oxygenation crisis after head trauma has been termed *nonedematous respiratory distress syndrome*).

Unilateral Lung Disease

Unilateral infiltration or marked asymmetry of radiographic densities suggests a confined set of etiologic possibilities, most of which occur in highly characteristic clinical settings (Fig. 50.3). Marked asymmetry of radiographic involvement should prompt an especially careful search for an unaddressed and readily reversible cause of hypoxemia. In some cases, especially in the presence of pneumonitis or airway plugging, precautions (i.e., positioning, careful airway suctioning) should be taken against generalization of the process.

Techniques to Improve Tissue Oxygenation

Basic Therapeutic Principles

Although atelectasis, fluid overload, and infection (Table 50.1) often yield to specific measures, the treatment of diffuse lung injury remains largely supportive. The primary therapeutic aims are to maintain O_2 delivery, to relieve an excessive breathing workload, and to establish electrolyte balance while preventing further damage from O_2 toxicity, barotrauma, infection, and other iatrogenic complications. To these ends, the clinician should bear in mind a few fundamental principles.

Minimize the Risk/Benefit Ratio

Positive airway pressure, O_2, and vasoactive drugs are potentially injurious. Therefore, there should be frequent reassessment of the need for current levels of PEEP, F_{IO_2}, and for the use and intensity of ventilator support. An O_2

TABLE 50.1. TECHNIQUES TO IMPROVE TISSUE OXYGENATION

Increase F_{IO_2}
Increase mean lung volume and alveolar pressure
  PEEP/Auto-PEEP
  Extend inspiratory time fraction
Decubitus, upright, or prone positioning
Bronchodilation
Improve O_2 delivery/consumption ratio
  Reduce O_2 requirements
    Work of breathing
    Fever
    Agitation
  Increase cardiac output
  Increase hemoglobin
Remove pulmonary vasodilators (e.g., nitroprusside)
Consider adjunctive support
  Vibration
  Nitric oxide or inhaled prostacyclin

F_{IO_2}, fraction of inspired oxygen; PEEP, positive end-expiratory pressure; O_2, oxygen.

saturation of 85% may be acceptable if the patient has adequate O_2-carrying capacity and circulatory reserve without signs of O_2 privation (e.g., lactic acidosis, cardiac ischemia, arrhythmia, and cerebral dysfunction). In contrast, a reduced O_2 saturation may stimulate ventilatory drive and increase dyspnea in a patient with ventilatory insufficiency. Allowing $Paco_2$ to climb slowly (buffering pH, if necessary, with $NaHCO_3$) may minimize the ventilatory requirement and reduce the risk of barotrauma. Mean intrathoracic pressure can be reduced by allowing the patient to provide as much ventilatory power as possible, compatible with ventilatory capability and comfort.

Prevent Therapeutic Accidents

Patients should be kept under direct observation at all times by well-trained personnel prepared to intervene appropriately, 24 h/d. Paralyzed patients must be watched with special care, as ventilation is totally machine-dependent. Furthermore, the hands must be restrained in semiconscious, agitated, confused, or disoriented patients who receive mechanical ventilation; abrupt ventilator disconnections and extubations can produce lethal bradyarrhythmias, hypoxemia, asphyxia, or aspiration. Special caution is warranted in orally intubated patients, who tend to self-extubate readily. In the setting of pulmonary edema, the interruption of PEEP for even brief periods (suctioning, tubing changes) may cause profound, slowly reversing desaturation as lung volume falls and the airways rapidly flood with edema fluid. The stomach should be decompressed in most recently intubated patients who demonstrate air swallowing or ileus. In mechanically ventilated patients, the clinician must stay alert to the possibility of tension pneumothorax, especially in patients with radiographic evidence of pneumomediastinum or subcutaneous emphysema. Because of the very high incidence of tissue rupture, prophylactic chest tubes may be indicated for patients who form tension cysts that evolve on serial films.

Optimize Extrapulmonary Management

Intravascular volume must be carefully regulated. Although excessive administration of fluids must clearly be avoided to minimize lung water and improve O_2 exchange, severe fluid restriction may compromise perfusion of gut and kidney. The National Institutes of Health ARDS Network is conducting a prospective, randomized, multicenter trial of fluid-conservative versus fluid-liberal management strategies on lung function, nonpulmonary organ function, mortality, and the need for mechanical ventilation. Results from this study may provide new information for fluid management in ARDS. General supportive measures should include appropriate levels of nutritional support, prophylaxis for deep venous thrombosis, prevention of skin breakdown, and prophylaxis for gastric stress ulceration for all mechanically ventilated or immobile patients.

Improving Tissue Oxygen Delivery

In the setting of ALI, the goal is to maintain an adequate O_2 delivery/consumption ratio while allowing time for the underlying lung pathology to reverse. O_2 delivery is the product of cardiac output and the O_2 content of each milliliter of arterial blood. (O_2 content [mL/dL] $= 1.36 \times$ the product of Hgb concentration [g/dL] and percentage saturation/100, plus $0.003 \times Pao_2$.) The O_2-carrying capacity can be improved by increasing Hgb concentration and optimizing its dissociation characteristics. Both factors may be important. Increasing Hgb tends to increase Sao_2, as it reduces the need for any rise in cardiac output compensatory to anemia. Both of these actions (lower cardiac output and higher Sao_2) tend to reduce venous admixture. Hgb performance is improved by reversing alkalemia to facilitate O_2 offloading. As Hgb concentration rises, blood viscosity increases, retarding passage of erythrocytes through capillary networks. Thus, actual O_2 delivery can be impaired as hematocrit rises over 50%. The optimal Hgb concentration for patients with ALI/ARDS is not currently known; there is no large prospective randomized controlled study that has demonstrated that a specific Hgb level improves outcome.

A very high percentage of the O_2 contained in blood is bound to Hgb; the proportion solubilized in plasma is very small (3%) at ambient pressure. However, in severe anemia, the Hgb-bound fraction is disproportionately small, so that total O_2-carrying capacity is significantly boosted when 100% O_2 is used, and breathing pure O_2 helps dissociate carbon monoxide from Hgb. After carbon monoxide exposure, high partial pressures of O_2 (particularly those delivered under hyperbaric conditions) can deliver life-sustaining quantities of dissolved O_2.

Because extravascular water accumulates readily in the setting of permeability edema, fluids should be used judiciously to keep the wedge pressure as low as feasible, consistent with adequate O_2 delivery. Liberal use of inotropes and other vasoactive drugs can occasionally be helpful, especially in certain postoperative or post-trauma settings. Driving the cardiac output to supraphysiological levels, however, appears not to improve the mortality rate of medical patients with ARDS.

Oxygen Therapy

Increasing the Fio_2 improves Pao_2 in all instances in which shunt is not responsible for desaturation. The goal is to increase the saturation of Hgb to 85% to 90% or more without risking O_2 toxicity. O_2 toxicity is both concentration- and time-dependent. As a general rule, very high inspired fractions of O_2 can safely be used for brief periods as efforts are made to reverse the underlying process. Sustained elevations in Fio_2 greater than 0.60 result in inflammatory changes and eventual fibrosis in experimental models; therefore, efforts should be made to keep Fio_2 at less than 0.60 during the support phase of ALI.

Positive End-Expiratory Pressure

PEEP has been used as a technique to improve oxygenation and reduce the fractional O_2 requirement. PEEP prevents end-expiratory bronchiolar collapse, which reduces the amount of derecruitment of the lung. The best level of PEEP in the management of ARDS remains controversial. Heterogeneity in the compliance of the alveolar units in ARDS produces different responses to the same level of PEEP. The ideal PEEP level minimizes the cyclic recruitment/derecruitment of the lung during the respiratory cycle. The best PEEP would also minimize overinflation of alveolar units that can cause volutrauma or ventilator-induced lung injury. The lower inflection point of the elastic pressure-volume curve of the respiratory system has been used as a guide for setting the optimal PEEP level in patients with ARDS. The lower inflection point was thought to represent the pressure required to open collapsed alveoli; thus, PEEP was set 2 cm H_2O above the lower inflection point in an attempt to prevent derecruitment (3). Work has shown that the lower inflection point is a poor predictor of alveolar closure (4). There has not been a randomized controlled study examining optimization of PEEP and mortality outcome in ARDS. There is also no data to show that PEEP prevents the development of ARDS.

The optimal PEEP level is not known at this time. Recommendations at this time would be to increase PEEP incrementally while monitoring mean airway pressure, hemodynamics, and oxygenation. The best PEEP would be the level that allows a reduction in FiO_2, improves oxygenation, has no significant effect on hemodynamics, and does not cause overinflation.

Recruiting Maneuvers

A recruitment maneuver may be performed in an attempt to open a collapsed lung and keep it open. Patients receiving lung protective ventilation with small tidal volumes (VT) may be at risk for alveolar derecruitment. The recruitment maneuver requires the application of continuous positive airway pressure of 35 to 40 cm H_2O for 40 seconds and then reinstitution of PEEP. In the ARDS Network trial, recruitment maneuvers did not show a sustained improvement in gas exchange (5,6). Recruitment maneuvers are not recommended for the routine management of ALI/ARDS.

RECRUITMENT MANEUVERS IN ACUTE RESPIRATORY DISTRESS SYNDROME	
Summary Statement	**Level of Evidence**
Recruitment maneuvers are not recommended for the routine treatment of acute lung injury/acute respiratory distress syndrome.	Randomized controlled clinical trial

Secretion Management and Bronchodilation

Although ARDS is often regarded as a problem of parenchymal injury; airway edema, bronchospasm, and secretion retention often contribute to hypoxemia. Retained secretions pose an overlooked problem that increases endotracheal tube resistance, infection risk, the hazard of barotrauma, and maldistribution of ventilation. In some patients with diffuse lung injury, profound bradycardia develops during ventilator disconnections, discouraging airway suctioning. Although hypoxemia occasionally contributes, this bradycardia is usually reflex in nature and responds to prophylactic (parenteral) atropine or reapplication of positive airway pressure. Circuits that do not interrupt PEEP during suctioning may offer some advantage.

Reducing Oxygen Requirements

Reducing the tissue demand for O_2 can be as effective as improving O_2 delivery. Fever, agitation, overfeeding, vigorous respiratory activity, shivering, sepsis, and a host of other commonly observed clinical conditions can markedly increase VO_2. Fever reduction may have therapeutic value, but shivering must be prevented in the cooling process. Sedation and the use of antipyretics rather than cooling blankets make good therapeutic sense. (Although phenothiazines may prevent shivering, their use may inhibit the cutaneous vasodilation necessary for rapid heat loss.)

Paralysis is a valuable adjunct to reduce O_2 consumption and improve PaO_2 in patients who remain agitated or fight the ventilator despite more conservative measures. Although paralysis is helpful in the first hours of machine support, protracted paralysis must be avoided for several reasons. Paralysis places the entire responsibility for achieving adequate oxygenation and ventilation with the medical team. Furthermore, the patient is defenseless in the event of an unobserved ventilator disconnection. Paralysis also silences the coughing mechanism and creates a monotonous breathing pattern that encourages secretion retention in dependent regions. Finally, protracted and unmonitored paralysis may cause weakness or devastating neuromyopathy.

Mechanical Ventilation in Acute Lung Injury and Acute Respiratory Distress Syndrome

Conventional Approach to Ventilatory Support

The basic principles of managing ALI are well accepted. The primary objective is to accomplish effective gas exchange at the least FiO_2 and pressure cost. On the basis of recent experimental and clinical information, an objective of crucial importance is to establish and maintain patency of all potentially recruitable lung units. The relative hazards of O_2 therapy, high-pressure ventilatory patterns, and abnormal target values for arterial blood gases, pH, and cardiac output continue to be debated (Table 50.2).

TABLE 50.2. APPROACHES TO ACUTE RESPIRATORY DISTRESS SYNDROME VENTILATION

Conventional	Lung Protective
Large tidal volume	Small tidal volume
Minimum PEEP	"Sufficient" PEEP
Normalize $Paco_2$	Permissive hypercapnia
Unrestrained P_{aw}	Pressure limitation

PEEP, positive end-expiratory pressure; $Paco_2$, arterial partial pressure of carbon dioxide; P_{aw}, airway pressure.

TABLE 50.3. CHARACTERISTICS OF EARLY- AND LATE-PHASE ACUTE RESPIRATORY DISTRESS SYNDROME

Early Phase (0–3 Days)	Late Phase (>7 Days)
Structural collagen intact	Collagen degraded and resynthesized
Atelectasis prevalent	Atelectasis less prevalent
Edema prevalent	Edema less prevalent
Mechanics heterogeneous	Mechanics less heterogeneous
Ventilator lung injury (edema, hemorrhage)	Ventilator lung injury (pneumothorax, cystic barotrauma)

Most traditional ventilatory strategies used in intensive care evolved directly from anesthetic and surgical postoperative practice. When the lungs are normal and their capacity to expand is intact (as is common in the perioperative period), large V_T of 10 to 15 mL/kg generates only modest end-inspiratory transalveolar pressure. In fact, large V_T prevents the microatelectasis that accompanies monotonous shallow breathing and is needed by many spontaneously breathing patients to satisfy high ventilatory demands (i.e., metabolic acidosis). Postoperatively, the mandatory respiratory rate is usually adjusted to normalize pH and/or $Paco_2$, and sufficient PEEP is used to achieve acceptable O_2 delivery at what is assumed to be a nontoxic Fio_2. (An $Fio_2 < 0.65$ is commonly targeted.) Typically, airway pressures are monitored but not rigidly constrained.

With few modifications, this high-V_T, normoxic, normocapnic ventilation paradigm developed as the standard approach to supporting most critically ill patients as well. Consequently, V_T that exceeds 800 mL and end-tidal (plateau) alveolar pressures greater than 50 cm H_2O are still common in many intensive care units when dealing with ARDS. How best to select optimal PEEP remains controversial, but many practitioners advocate using the least PEEP consistent with accomplishing acceptable arterial oxygenation. Others rely on computations of systemic O_2 delivery or best tidal compliance to make their selections of PEEP and V_T. Unfortunately, the machine settings that achieve all important clinical objectives do not invariably coincide. A relatively small but growing number of practitioners are now shifting first priority from optimizing gas exchange, O_2 delivery, or respiratory system compliance to a strategy that minimizes the potentially injurious effects of mechanical ventilation.

Ventilator-Induced Lung Damage

Implications of Evolving Histology

Histologic findings evolve continuously (but heterogeneously) over the course of ALI (Table 50.3). It is reasonable to assume that all lung regions sustain the initial insult more or less simultaneously and that, in the most severe cases, proliferation, organization, remodeling, and fibrosis sequentially follow an initial phase of edema and atelectasis. Although parenchymal damage is widespread, the nature, severity, pace of evolution, and perhaps even stage of injury

vary from site to site within the damaged lung. Early in the course of ARDS, gravitation-dependent areas are extensively consolidated and atelectatic, whereas nondependent regions tend to aerate better. Regional blood flows and vascular pressures also vary (Fig. 50.5). Changes of body position alter lung (or chest wall) mechanics, influence the radiographic findings, and affect gas exchange. Although counterexamples occasionally occur, perhaps 60% to 70% of patients respond to prone positioning by improving Pao_2 significantly during this early phase of ARDS. The efficacy of PEEP in improving O_2 exchange relates directly to the reversal of atelectasis and the redistribution of lung water. It is not surprising, therefore, that the effectiveness of PEEP in improving O_2 exchange tends to decline as time passes.

The collagen framework of the normal lung remains relatively intact during the first days of injury but later weakens as inflammation gradually degrades structural protein and nonuniformly remodels the architecture of the lung. Therefore, the same pressures that were tolerated well initially may cause alveolar disruption after the disease is well established. This may explain the tendency for radiographically detectable barotrauma to occur late in the course of the disease—often well after gas-exchange abnormalities have noticeably improved and ventilatory pressures have declined.

Dangers of Excessive and Insufficient Lung Volumes

After acute injury, only a fraction of the injured lung is accessible to gas; in severe cases, no more than one third of all alveoli remain patent. Because well-ventilated lung units may retain nearly normal elastance and fragility, the apparent stiffness of the lung in the early phase of ALI is explained better by fewer functioning alveoli than by a generalized increase in recoil tension. Increased tissue recoil contributes more significantly later on, when cellular infiltration is intense, edema has been reabsorbed or organized, atelectasis is less extensive, and fibrosis is under way. Because the reduced functional compartment of the lung must accommodate the entire V_T, large (conventional) V_T's may cause overdistention, local hyperventilation, and inhibition or depletion of surfactant. Moreover, during rapid inflation to high transalveolar pressures, intense shearing forces may

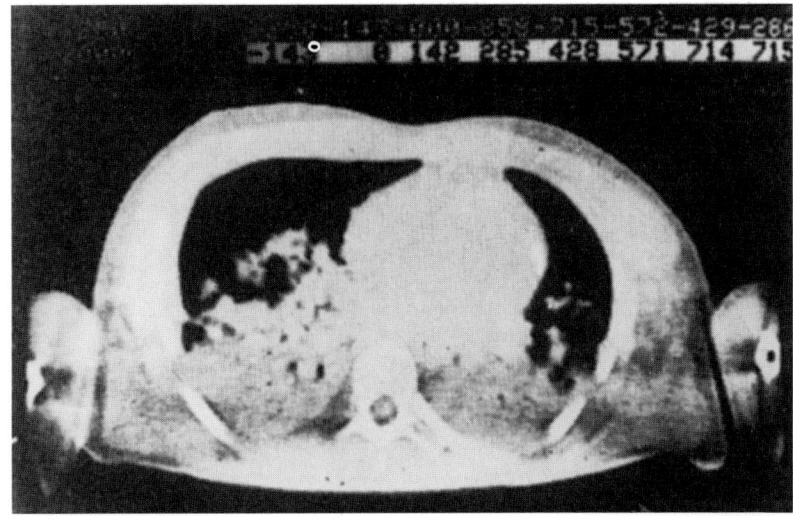

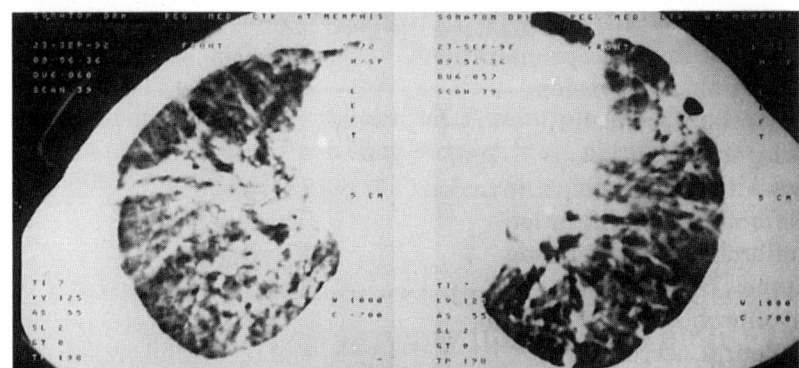

FIGURE 50.5. Computed tomography (CT) appearance of the chest in early **(A)** and late **(B)** phases of ARDS. Although on chest radiographs the lungs appear to be diffusely and uniformly affected in the early stage, the CT image demonstrates a preponderance of atelectasis in the dependent (dorsal) regions. Later, infiltrates are more widely distributed, and cystic spaces often form. In this stage, atelectasis is less prevalent, and infiltrates are more evenly distributed in the transverse plane, as seen in this CT image. (From Gattinoni L, Pelosi P, Vitale G, et al. Body position changes redistribute lung computed tomography density in patients with acute respiratory failure. *Anesthesiology* 1991;74:15–23 **[A]**, and Meduri G. Late adult respiratory distress syndrome. *New Horizons* 1993;1:563–577 **[B]**, with permission.)

develop at the junctions of structures that are mobile (aerated lung units) with those that are immobile (collapsed or consolidated alveoli, distal conducting airways).

Tidal pressures within the alveolus must neither rise too high at any time during the disease course nor fall too low during the first 3 to 5 days of treatment. Experimental damage resulting from overdistension of the alveolar-capillary membrane has been convincingly documented. The absolute value of peak inflation pressure is not the stretching pressure or the true causative variable of barotrauma; rather, peak transalveolar pressure (roughly approximated by the difference between alveolar and pleural pressures) is the relevant variable. The plateau pressure is perhaps the best clinical correlate of peak alveolar (but not necessarily transalveolar) pressure. The severity of stretch injury appears greatest when maximum transalveolar pressures exceed 25 to 30 cm H_2O and insufficient PEEP cannot keep dependent lung units fully recruited. Failure to maintain a certain minimum alveolar volume in the early phase of ALI may induce or accentuate lung damage. Unsupported by PEEP, certain collapsible alveoli may pop open and then close with every tidal cycle, generating shearing stresses within junctional tissues and tending to deplete surfactant. Increases in cycling frequency and duration of exposure to adverse ventilatory patterns ac-

centuate any tendency for damage. The magnitude of blood flow in these stressed areas may also play an important role.

Bronchiolar dilation, cystic changes, and/or microabscesses can be demonstrated in the large majority of patients with ALI who are ventilated for lengthy periods with peak airway pressures considered modest by traditional clinical standards. Such airway damage not only impairs gas exchange but also predisposes to secretion retention and pulmonary infection.

Importance of Cycling Frequency

At levels of minute ventilation and V_T that are traditionally accepted, the ventilator may cycle in excess of 30,000 times per day (20 breaths/min × 60 min/h × 24 h/d). Even if the tidal pressure profile is only slightly damaging, the cumulative effect can be severe. It is very important to reduce V_E requirements and cycling frequency whenever high cycling pressures are in use.

Lower Inflection Region and the Choice of PEEP

A lower inflection (P_{flex}) region on the static pressure-volume curve of the passive respiratory system suggests the existence of a population of alveoli at risk for excessive tidal stresses (Fig. 50.6). Not all patients exhibit a lower P_{flex} region,

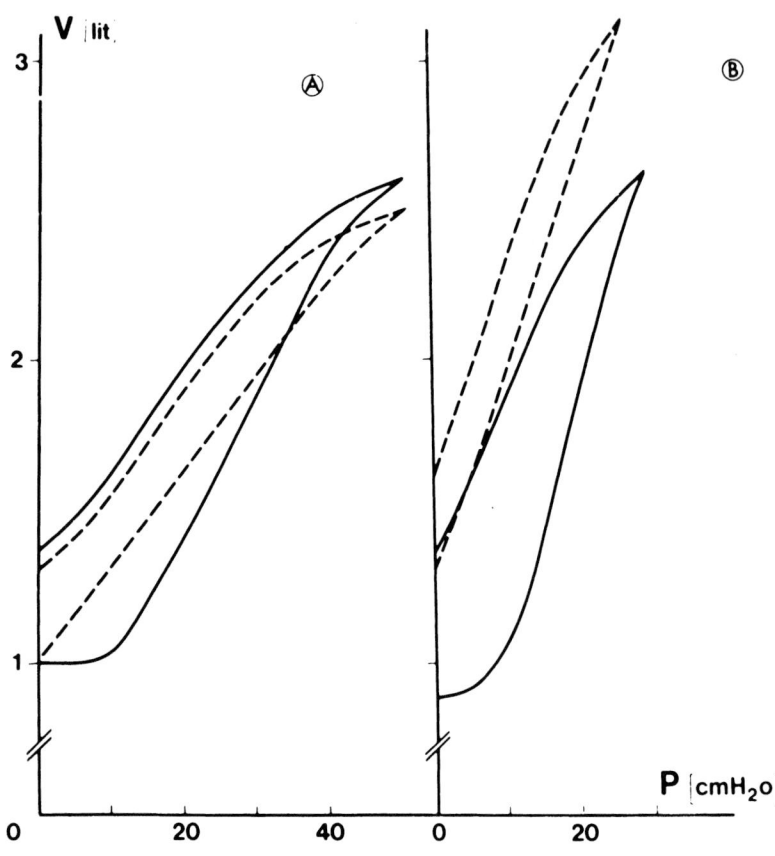

FIGURE 50.6. Pressure-volume curves of the respiratory system from two patients in the earlier and late stages of ARDS. In the earlier stage of ARDS *(solid lines)*, distinct lower inflection and upper deflection limbs are prominent. Later *(dashed lines)*, the inflection and deflection zones are less well demarcated, and hysteresis is reduced. (From Matamis D, Lemaire F, Harf A, et al. Total respiratory pressure-volume curves in the adult respiratory distress syndrome. *Chest* 1984;86:58–66, with permission.)

but those who do are likely to experience extensive end-expiratory atelectasis at lower levels of PEEP. Indeed, arterial oxygenation often improves markedly as the end-expiratory pressure range just below P_{flex} is exceeded. Many investigators currently believe that tidal excursions into the lower inflection range must be avoided. Sufficient PEEP or disease improvement over time obliterates the "P_{flex} point" as well as narrows the hysteresis of the static pressure-volume curve. In contrast, in late-stage ARDS, high PEEP levels may simply add to the risk of lung rupture, or when peak pressure is capped (out of a concern for barotrauma), increasing PEEP may reduce the safe operating V_T.

As a composite of the behaviors of all alveoli within the heterogeneous lung, the contours of the static pressure-volume curve obscure very important regional differences. Alveoli in dependent regions are most susceptible to collapse, and those in nondependent regions are vulnerable to overdistention. This variability of opening pressures helps account for the *zones* (rather than *points*) of lower and upper inflection.

Implications of Pressure Limitation for Tidal Volume

The values for V_T that correspond to the restricted range of safe ventilating pressures are generally approximately 4 to 8 mL/kg of lean weight, or 300 to 600 mL for a 75-kg patient. However, because values for lung and chest wall compliance vary through wide ranges in different patients, unique values for V_T that are consistent with desirable pressure limits cannot be prespecified. Therefore, when a flow-controlled volume-cycled mode of ventilation is used, V_T should be adjusted with guidance by plateau pressure and the response of O_2 exchange to increments of V_T.

A Pressure-Targeted Approach to Ventilating Acute Lung Injury and Acute Respiratory Distress Syndrome

A pressure-targeted approach to ventilation in ALI/ARDS recognizes that several mechanically distinct alveolar populations coexist within the acutely injured lung, that a poorly chosen ventilatory pattern can be damaging, and that the underlying pathophysiology changes over time. This approach gives higher priority to controlling maximal and minimal transalveolar pressures than to achieving normocapnia. Establishing and maintaining full alveolar recruitment while avoiding lung overdistention is the primary guiding principle (Table 50.4).

Once O_2 and ventilatory demands have been minimized and fluid balance and cardiac function have been optimized, the essential strategic elements are as follows.

First, sufficient end-expiratory transalveolar pressure must be used to avert tissue damage resulting from surfactant depletion or stresses associated with persistent collapse or

TABLE 50.4. A LUNG PROTECTIVE STRATEGY FOR VENTILATING ACUTE RESPIRATORY DISTRESS SYNDROME

Tailor ventilatory strategy to the phase of the disease (generous PEEP in early stage; withdraw PEEP later)

Minimize oxygen demands

Minimize pulmonary vascular pressures

Control alveolar pressure, not $Paco_2$

Maintain total alveolar PEEP (PEEP + auto-PEEP) several centimeters of water above P_{flex}. In general, this will be >7 cm H_2O but <20 cm H_2O

Avoid large V_T and use least alveolar pressure required to meet unequivocal therapeutic goals

Hold transalveolar pressure <35 cm H_2O

Consider making necessary increases in mean airway pressure by changing T_I/T_T

Consider specialized adjunctive measures to improve gas exchange and oxygen delivery[a]

[a] In addition to such standard measurements as skillful management of pulmonary vascular pressure, repositioning, and use of cardiotonic agents, specialized adjunctive measures might include (where available) such experimental methods as extracorporeal carbon dioxide removal, inhaled nitric oxide or prostacyclin, partial liquid ventilation, and intravenous or intratracheal catheter-assisted gas exchange.

PEEP, positive end-expiratory pressure; $Paco_2$, arterial partial pressure of carbon dioxide; P_{flex}, lower inflection point of the static pressure-volume relationship of the respiratory system; V_T, tidal volume; T_I/T_T, fractional inspiratory time.

repeated opening and closure of collapsible units during the tidal breathing cycle. The total PEEP applied (the sum of PEEP and auto-PEEP) should be sufficient to obliterate any lower inflection "point" of the pressure-volume curve of the respiratory system, which, at V_T of 7 to 8 mL/kg, generally occurs at a pressure of 10 to 15 cm H_2O in the early phase of ARDS. (For a patient with a stiff chest wall, the PEEP required may be considerably higher.) In truth, there is an inflection *range* rather than a single inflection point, as dependent alveoli in the lower regions of the lung require a greater end-expiratory alveolar pressure to maintain patency than do those regions above them. Improved arterial oxygenation tends to parallel effective recruitment, and CO_2 retention is a consequence of alveolar overdistension. Although actual construction of the pressure-volume curve (by any of a variety of static or dynamic methods) is theoretically appealing, in some patients it is inadvisable to eliminate spontaneous breathing efforts. One simple way to select PEEP (with or without spontaneous efforts) is first to choose the operating V_T (4–7 mL/kg), initially setting PEEP at 8 to 10 cm H_2O. The PEEP is then increased in small (2 cm H_2O) steps, looking for (a) an increase in peak static (plateau) pressure that substantially exceeds the previous PEEP increment (by 2 cm H_2O), signaling overdistension; and (b) markedly improved oxygenation that corresponds to obliteration of the P_{flex} point. (Under certain circumstances, a reasonable alternative to the empirical PEEP step approach is gradually to extend the inspiratory time fraction to create auto-PEEP.) Failure of oxygenation to improve significantly after two successive PEEP steps and a recruitment maneuver strongly suggests that nearly full recruitment had been achieved with the

V_T at a lower PEEP value. The PEEP should be lowered accordingly.

Second, because alveolar subpopulations with nearly normal elastic properties may coexist alongside flooded or infiltrated ones, the clinician must avoid applying transalveolar pressures greater than normal lung tissue is able to sustain at its maximum capacity (30–35 cm H_2O). This pressure generally corresponds to end-inspiratory static airway pressures (plateau pressures) of 35 to 50 cm H_2O, depending on the stiffness of the chest wall. Pressures in this range are generally sufficient to reopen closed airways. Whatever the appropriate maximal pressure setting might be for an individual patient, it seems wise to avoid the upper inflection range of the static pressure-volume curve whenever possible. Incursion into this zone is signaled by deterioration of tidal compliance and, in a passively inflated patient, by convexity of the inspiratory airway pressure curve to the horizontal (time) axis during constant-flow ventilation.

Relatively small V_T often results from imposing these upper and the lower bounds on ventilatory pressure. Therefore, periodic recruiting breaths (e.g., pressures of 35–45 cm H_2O sustained for 5–15 seconds every 10 minutes) may be needed in some patients to maintain adequate lung volume and avoid hypoxemia. One interesting approach to making selections of PEEP and V_T when using pressure-controlled ventilation is to fix maximal airway pressure at approximately 30 to 35 cm H_2O and begin with PEEP of 8 cm H_2O. (Somewhat higher maximum and minimum pressures are more appropriate for a patient with an inflexible chest wall.) PEEP is then increased gradually while maximal airway pressure remains constant (allowing V_T to fall) until the point at which calculated tidal compliance begins to decline—one definition of the optimum PEEP value.

Third, under conditions of passive inflation (no spontaneous efforts), the practitioner should adjust mean airway opening pressure ($\bar{P}_{aw}$) to achieve acceptable pulmonary O_2 exchange by extending the duty cycle (fractional inspiratory time [T_I/T_T]) or by raising PEEP. Cardiac output is supported as necessary to offset any detrimental effects of rising $\bar{P}_{aw}$. Extending the duty cycle improves the distribution of ventilation and may help to recruit or hold open otherwise collapsible lung units. Raising PEEP (and preserving a well-tolerated T_I/T_T) may be the preferred option, however, when the patient retains control of the breathing rhythm.

Fourth, when not contraindicated, hypercapnia should be accepted from the onset of therapy (buffered, when necessary, by judiciously infused sodium bicarbonate or other buffer) in preference to violating the guidelines of controlling alveolar pressure. Pharmacologic buffering may also be needed to allow hypercapnia when deep sedation and/or paralysis is not used. The strategy of permissive hypercapnia may be difficult to implement in the presence of metabolic acidosis. Other measures (i.e., dialysis) may be needed adjunctively.

The largest multicenter, randomized trial evaluating the safety and effectiveness of low V_T ventilation was conducted by the ARDS Network. The trial compared traditional ventilation treatment, defined as an initial V_T of 12 mL/kg of predicted body weight and a plateau pressure of 50 cm H_2O or less, with ventilation at a lower V_T, defined as an initial V_T of 6 mL/kg of predicted body weight and a plateau pressure of 30 cm H_2O or less. The trial was stopped early after the enrollment of 861 patients because the interim analysis demonstrated that the mortality rate was lower in the group of patients treated with low V_T ventilation compared with the conventional treatment group (31.0% versus 39.8%). Additionally, the low V_T ventilation group spent fewer days on mechanical ventilation compared with that of the conventional ventilation group (6).

The data from this large trial support the recommendation that patients with ALI and ARDS should be mechanically ventilated with a lower V_T, leading to decreased mortality and fewer ventilator days.

VENTILATION STRATEGY IN ACUTE RESPIRATORY DISTRESS SYNDROME

Summary Statement	Level of Evidence
Mechanical ventilation with a low tidal volume of 6 mL/kg and plateau pressure <30 cm H_2O reduces mortality and increases the number of ventilatory-free days.	Multicenter, randomized, controlled clinical trial Randomized clinical trial, one center

---

Modes of Mechanical Ventilation in Acute Respiratory Distress Syndrome

Patients with ALI/ARDS can be successfully supported using either pressure-limited or volume-limited modes of ventilation. Pressure-limited modes are used when it is more important to control airway pressures, and volume-limited is used when it is necessary to guarantee a specified V_T. Both modes of ventilation can provide a lung protective ventilatory strategy by delivering a target V_T of 6 mL/kg and maintaining a goal plateau pressure less than 30 cm H_2O. The data showing improved mortality in ARDS with low V_T strategy were collected by using the volume control mode (6). At this time, there is no similar study examining pressure-limited ventilation. A multicenter randomized trial compared pressure-controlled ventilation and volume-controlled ventilation in 79 ARDS patients. The main finding in this study was that in patients with ARDS requiring mechanical ventilation, the method of ventilation that deliberately reduced the inspiratory plateau pressure to less than 35 cm H_2O—by decreasing either V_T in volume control mode or inspiratory pressure in pressure control—did not independently influence mortality (7). It is reasonable to expect pressure-limited ventilation delivered in a manner to provide a target volume of 6 mL/kg, and maintaining a plateau pressure of less than 30 cm H_2O would also provide a mortality benefit similar to that in the ARDS Network trial.

Another mode of ventilation that has been tried in ALI/ARDS is inverse ratio ventilation, implemented as either a pressure control or volume control mode. In this mode, mean airway pressure is increased by increasing the inspiratory time. The inspiratory time can be extended to either equal (1:1 ratio) or exceed the expiratory time (2:1 ratio). The rationale is that ARDS is a heterogeneous disease, and different lung units may require a longer inflation time in order to ventilate. Increasing the inflation time may allow more lung units to open and provide better gas exchange, with a resultant improvement in oxygenation. Complications seen with this type of ventilation include the development of auto-PEEP, pneumothorax, and hypotension. There has not been a randomized controlled study to determine the effect of inverse ratio conventional mechanical ventilation in ARDS. A small series of 20 patients with severe ARDS were switched to inverse ratio ventilation from volume control if they failed to have an O_2 saturation greater than 90% with peak inspiratory pressure greater than 35 cm H_2O, $FIO_2 = 60\%$, and PEEP of 10 cm H_2O. The results demonstrated an improvement in the peak inspiratory pressure, mean airway pressure, and oxygenation (8). This study was not powered to detect mortality benefit because of the small sample size, and there was no control group.

MODES OF VENTILATION IN ACUTE RESPIRATORY DISTRESS SYNDROME

Summary Statement	Level of Evidence
1. Volume-controlled mode of ventilation with low tidal volume of 6 mL/kg and plateau pressure <30 cm H_2O reduces mortality	Multicenter, randomized, controlled clinical trial Randomized clinical trial, one center
2. Pressure-controlled mode of ventilation maintaining a plateau pressure <30 cm H_2O and targeting a tidal volume of 6 mL/kg reduces mortality	Multicenter randomized clinical trial
3. Inverse ratio ventilation may improve oxygenation	Uncontrolled case series

---

Alternative Ventilatory Strategies

Permissive Hypercapnia

CO_2 retention may be an inevitable consequence of a lung-protective strategy that tightly restricts applied pressure and maintains a certain minimum (end-expiratory) lung volume. Maintaining normocapnia may not be appropriate if the cost is impaired lung healing and a heightened risk of extending tissue damage. Permissive hypercapnia is a strategy that allows deliberate hypoventilation in an attempt to reduce peak ventilatory pressures with the secondary effect of $Paco_2$ elevation. Patients ventilated with a low V_T develop hypercapnia because the minute ventilation is decreased and the dead space/V_T ratio is increased. This strategy has been used primarily in ARDS and status asthmaticus.

TABLE 50.5. CONSEQUENCES OF HYPERCAPNIA

System	Effect[a]
Respiratory	Reduced P_{AO_2}
	Rightward shift of oxygen/hemoglobin curve
	Impaired diaphragm function
	Pulmonary vasoconstriction
	Worsened $\dot{V}/\dot{Q}$ mismatching
Renal	Enhanced bicarbonate reabsorption
Central nervous system	Cerebral vasodilation
	Increased intracranial pressure
	Depressed consciousness
	Biochemical changes
Cardiovascular	Reduced cardiac contractility[b]
	Stimulation of sympathoadrenal axis
	Lower systemic vascular resistance

[a] Most effects wane with time as cellular and extracellular pH readjust.
[b] Only if not offset by adrenergic reflex compensation.
P_{AO_2}, alveolar partial pressure of oxygen; $\dot{V}/\dot{Q}$, ventilation-perfusion.

The physiologic effects of CO_2 retention are determined by the severity of hypercapnia and the rate of its buildup (Table 50.5). Except in the most severe cases or those complicated by extraordinary CO_2 production, the CO_2 retention that results from the pressure-targeted ventilation itself is generally modest ($P_{aCO_2} < 70$ mm Hg). Chronic hypercapnia of this magnitude appears to have few notable side effects apart from the reduction in ventilatory drive attendant to compensatory metabolic alkalosis. Although gradual elevations of P_{aCO_2} (<5 mm Hg/h) are often tolerated remarkably well, the rapid development of respiratory acidosis can evoke impressive sympathetic discharge. Allowing hypercapnia may not be advisable for all patients with ALI, i.e., patients with coexisting head injury, recent cerebral vascular accident, seizure disorder, or significant cardiovascular dysfunction (Table 50.6). Acute elevations in P_{aCO_2} increase sympathetic activity, raise cardiac output, heighten pulmonary vascular resistance, alter bronchomotor tone, impair skeletal muscle function, dilate cerebral vessels, and impair central nervous system function. CO_2 retention may be poorly tolerated by patients with autonomic insufficiency, β-blockade, or other conditions interfering with sympathetic

TABLE 50.6. CONTRAINDICATIONS TO PERMISSIVE HYPERCAPNIA

Intracranial hypertension
    Head trauma
    Hemorrhage
    Severe systemic hypertension
    Space-occupying lesions
Cardiovascular instability
Cor pulmonale
β-Blockade
Severe uncorrected metabolic acidosis or hypoxemia

tone and compensatory mechanisms. Permissive hypercapnia may not be advisable or possible to implement safely in the setting of coexisting metabolic acidosis or uncorrected hypoxemia. Especially over the short term, arterial pH may not closely reflect the pH of the intracellular environment. The magnitude of any intracellular acidosis resulting from permissive hypercapnia, however, is almost certain to be less than the profound intracellular pH changes produced by ischemia. Because CO_2 affects cardiac output and influences vascular and bronchomotor tone, it is uncertain if hypercapnia disturbs ventilation-perfusion matching or modulates the extent of lung injury and edema during the course of mechanical ventilatory support. Implementation of permissive hypercapnia often requires deep sedation and/or paralysis, a requirement that may be associated with serious side effects: impaired secretion clearance, fluid retention, and residual muscle weakness.

Recommendations for implementing permissive hypercapnia include utilization of small V_T to minimize transalveolar pressures. P_{aCO_2} is allowed to rise by 10 mm Hg/h until a maximum level of 80 to 100 mm Hg, while maintaining a O_2 saturation greater than 90%. Correction of the respiratory acidosis of permissive hypercapnia may be done with the administration of sodium bicarbonate to maintain the arterial pH greater than 7.15 (9,10).

The efficacy of permissive hypercapnia in the treatment of ARDS has not as yet been examined in a large randomized controlled trial. Several small descriptive, prospective, uncontrolled studies have suggested that permissive hypercapnia is well-tolerated, allows the reduction of peak inspiratory pressure, and does not adversely affect hemodynamics. In addition, these small nonrandomized studies suggested that permissive hypercapnia may provide a mortality benefit for patients with ARDS (11–13).

PERMISSIVE HYPERCAPNIA IN ACUTE RESPIRATORY DISTRESS SYNDROME	
Summary Statement	**Level of Evidence**
Permissive hypercapnia, a ventilatory strategy that deliberately hypoventilates a patient to minimize high transalveolar pressures, may improve mortality.	Nonrandomized, prospective case series

Adjuncts to the Ventilatory Management of Acute Respiratory Distress Syndrome

In recent years, there has been renewed interest in devising ways in which to accomplish effective arterial oxygenation without inflicting further damage on the injured lung. Some of these innovations modify the fundamental nature of ventilatory support (high-frequency ventilation [HFV]), but others provide gas exchange external to the lungs (extracorporeal or intravenacaval gas exchange), alter body position (prone positioning), or administer therapeutic agents designed to improve ventilation-perfusion matching (nitric oxide [NO], aerosolized prostacyclin). One technique modifies the nature of the gas-carrying medium itself (partial liquid ventilation [PLV]). Each of these adjuncts should be considered as a promising technique that is currently just beyond the perimeter of routine clinical practice.

High-Frequency Ventilation

HFV is a mode of ventilation that uses very small V_T and rapid respiratory rates to achieve adequate oxygenation and ventilation. Types of HFV include high-frequency jet ventilation (HFJV), high-frequency oscillation, and high-frequency positive-pressure ventilation. The proposed mechanisms for gas transport during HFV are direct bulk flow, longitudinal dispersion, pendelluft, asymmetric velocity profile, cardiogenic mixing, and molecular diffusion. Direct bulk flow occurs when alveoli in the proximal tracheobronchial tree receive a direct flow of inspired air. Longitudinal dispersion occurs when convective flow is superimposed on diffusion with the creation of turbulence. Pendelluft is defined as gas flow between lung regions in close proximity because of variation in the airway resistance and compliance of these regions. The velocity profile of air moving in the airway is parabolic, with air along the bronchial walls moving slower than air in the center of the airway. During respiratory cycles, the air in the center of the lumen will advance further into the lung. The contracting heart produces physical agitation that can contribute to gas mixing in the lung units near the heart. Molecular diffusion is the mixing of air in the peripheral bronchioles and alveoli (14). HFV has been tried as a ventilatory modality in ALI/ARDS because it uses very small V_T, which minimizes lung injury from overinflation, and the higher respiratory rates allow for the normalization of the $Paco_2$ levels.

A randomized trial of 113 surgical intensive care unit (ICU) patients compared high-frequency percussive ventilation and conventional volume-cycled mechanical ventilation. No statistically significant differences in mortality, surgical ICU days, hospital days, or incidence of barotrauma were seen between the two groups. The investigators concluded that there was no statistical benefit of HFV over conventional mechanical ventilation (15). A prospective randomized trial of 309 patients compared HFJV with conventional volume-cycled mechanical ventilation. Again, there was no significant difference in the physiologic parameters, duration of mechanical support, or mortality between the two groups. The investigators concluded that HFJV did not demonstrate an advantage compared with conventional therapy (16). Two small case series have been published comparing HFV with conventional ventilation. Both studies also concluded that HFV did not demonstrate an advantage over conventional mechanical ventilation (17,18). At this time, HFV remains an experimental mode of ventilation for ALI/ARDS until further prospective, randomized, controlled clinical trials are completed.

HIGH-FREQUENCY VENTILATION IN ACUTE RESPIRATORY DISTRESS SYNDROME	
Summary Statement	**Level of Evidence**
High-frequency ventilation does not improve mortality, intensive care unit length of stay, or number of ventilator-free days in acute respiratory distress syndrome.	Prospective, randomized trials

Extrapulmonary Gas Exchange

Partial substitution for the gas-exchanging function of the lung reduces the requirement for ventilating pressure. Methods for assisting in the process of exchanging respiratory gases include extracorporeal membrane oxygenation (ECMO), extracorporeal CO_2 removal, and intravenacaval gas exchange. ECMO removes CO_2 and adds O_2 to venous blood, and the oxygenated blood is then returned to the patient through either a venous or arterial route. All are costly, highly technical methods best undertaken by an experienced and dedicated team.

In 1974, the National Institutes of Health conducted a randomized controlled trial comparing the additive benefit of ECMO to conventional mechanical ventilation in patients with ARDS. The study was terminated after an interim analysis revealed a mortality rate of 90% in both groups (19). Retrospective reports of ECMO in patients with ARDS have demonstrated survival rates between 45% to 56% (20–28). The Extracorporeal Life Support Organization registry report published data for 483 cases of ECMO for adult respiratory failure, with a survival rate to hospital discharge of 49% (29). There has been one randomized controlled trial of extracorporeal CO_2 removal with tracheal insufflation in patients with ARDS versus conventional ventilation. This trial was terminated because the interim analysis determined that there was a poor chance of demonstrating a survival benefit (30).

Extracorporeal life-support techniques cannot be recommended for the routine management of ALI/ARDS based on the published data.

EXTRAPULMONARY GAS EXCHANGE IN ACUTE RESPIRATORY DISTRESS SYNDROME	
Summary Statement	**Level of Evidence**
Extracorporeal gas exchange in acute respiratory distress syndrome has not been shown to improve mortality.	Randomized, controlled trial

Prone Positioning

Prone positioning has been used as a therapeutic maneuver in ARDS to improve oxygenation. The mechanisms proposed for this effect include an increase in end-expiratory volume, better ventilation-perfusion matching, and regional changes in ventilation because of an alteration in chest-wall mechanics. The literature contains case series and small prospective studies that demonstrate that prone positioning improves oxygenation in 60% to 80% of patients with ARDS. A prospective, multicenter, randomized trial of 304 ALI/ARDS patients compared conventional treatment in the supine position with prone positioning for six or more hours a day for 10 days. The results of this study demonstrated that while placing patients with ARDS in the prone position improved their oxygenation, it did not improve survival (31). One suggested explanation for the lack of a mortality benefit in this study was that the ventilator strategy used large V_T and low PEEP levels. At this time, prone positioning can be recommended as a technique to improve oxygenation in 60% to 80% of patients with ALI/ARDS; however, it has not been shown to improve survival. Further study is necessary to determine whether prone positioning using a lung-protective ventilatory strategy would affect outcomes, determination of the effective time interval for the prone position, and the optimal length of treatment in this manner.

PRONE POSITIONING IN ACUTE RESPIRATORY DISTRESS SYNDROME	
Summary Statement	**Level of Evidence**
Prone positioning can improve oxygenation in ALI/ARDS; however, it has not been shown to improve mortality.	Prospective, multicenter, randomized, controlled trial Case series Small prospective series

ALI, acute lung injury; ARDS, acute respiratory distress syndrome.

Practical Points in Prone Positioning

Although hemodynamic parameters tend to remain unchanged, hypotension, desaturation, and arrhythmias may occur during the process of turning from the supine to the prone position (Table 50.7). These transient problems do not generally persist and can be minimized by using sedation, prior airway suctioning, and 100% O_2 during the maneuver. Continuous arterial pressure monitoring, electrocardiography, and pulse oximetry are also strongly advised. Deep sedation and occasionally paralysis will be required to secure patient compliance. Attention must also be given to preserving the position and patency of intravascular lines and the endotracheal tube during the turning process. Use of a soft (air-cushioned) bed is mandatory for comfort. Pillows must be used to support the hips, pelvis, shoulders, and head. Patients with tracheostomies present a particular challenge. The compliance of the respiratory system generally changes little

TABLE 50.7. PRACTICAL POINTS FOR PRONE POSITIONING IN ACUTE RESPIRATORY DISTRESS SYNDROME

Soft bed
Secure endotracheal tube and all lines before transition
Sedate and preoxygenate before turning
Monitor carefully during transitions
Support shoulders and hips
Adjust PEEP and tidal volume after positioning
Protect eyes and facial areas
Exercise special caution if bronchopleural fistula present
Alternate prone and supine positions one to three times daily

PEEP, positive end-expiratory pressure.

in shifting to the prone position. This is variable; however; V_T should be monitored (and adjusted if necessary) during pressure-controlled ventilation, which is influenced by any position-related changes in chest wall compliance. Furthermore, for the same plateau pressure, peak pressures may change if flow-controlled volume-cycled ventilation is used. For similar reasons, a given level of PEEP may be more or less effective in one position than in another. Although the optimal frequency of supine/prone interconversions is not clear, in current practice, most experienced centers turn patients once or twice daily. Supine repositioning allows certain nursing procedures (washing, line dressing changes, etc.) to be delivered and helps resolve facial edema. It seems reasonable to assign the relative duration of each position in proportion to the gas-exchange response. (For example, equal times would be assigned if only a minor important gas-exchange difference is observed between positions.) Prone repositioning should be reevaluated often in the first 3 to 5 days of illness, after which time it tends to lose its O_2-exchange effectiveness.

Partial Liquid Ventilation

Perfluorochemicals proposed for clinical purposes are environmentally innocuous liquids at room temperature that have a high O_2- and CO_2-carrying capacity, allowing effective gas exchange to take place. Biologically inert and immiscible in both aqueous and lipid media, they cause no known tissue reaction—even during extended use. Perfluorooctyl bromide (Perflubron), a perfluorochemical currently undergoing clinical trials, has a desirably low vapor pressure (it clears itself by evaporating slowly), a high spreading coefficient (it distributes homogeneously), and a low surface tension. Although its viscosity is similar to water, Perflubron has nearly twice the density; airway secretions and alveolar exudates float on it, allowing such debris to migrate centrally for airway suctioning. Infections may occur less commonly in a lung filled with inert nonnutritive liquid hostile to bacterial growth, but this is unproven. Its radiodensity may interfere with conventional imaging (Fig. 50.7). Perflubron has the potential to keep surfactant-deficient alveoli open by two distinct mechanisms: (a) reduction of interfacial surface

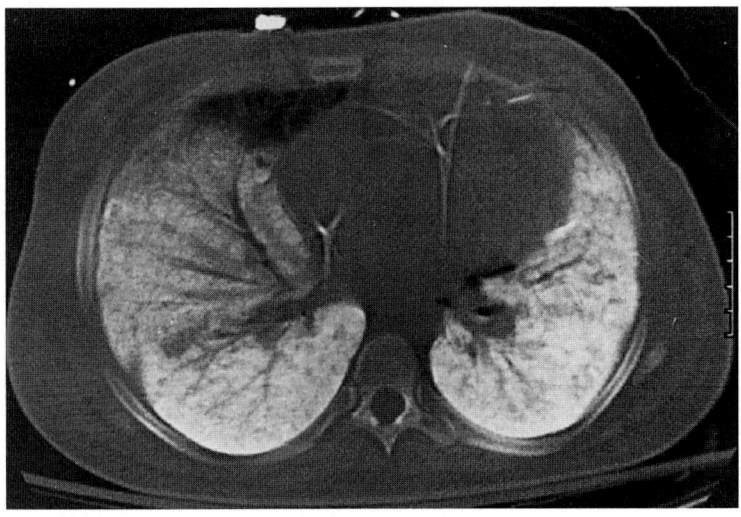

FIGURE 50.7. Computed tomographic scan of a patient with acute respiratory distress syndrome receiving partial liquid ventilation with Perflubron. (From Marini JJ. Evolving concepts in the ventilatory management of acute respiratory distress syndrome. *Clin Chest Med* 1996;17:555–575, with permission.)

tension and (b) physical distention by noncompressible fluid (liquid PEEP). The former property may be especially important in the infant respiratory distress syndrome, whereas alveolar splinting may assume primacy in ARDS.

Sustained PLV preserves the key benefits of liquid breathing while allowing gas ventilation to proceed with standard mechanical ventilators and connecting circuitry. The lung is filled to functional residual capacity with perfluorocarbon, but VT ventilation with gas is performed with conventional mechanical ventilation. The liquid preferentially distends the dependent alveoli most in need of expansion during the initial phase of ARDS, providing the vertically graded PEEP-like effect required by the underlying pathoanatomy. Simultaneously, blood flow diverts toward nondependent regions, which receive a disproportionate share of the gaseous VT. Reduced venous admixture, therefore, has at least two explanations—effective O_2 exchange directly across alveolar units reopened by liquid, and redirection of pulmonary arterial blood toward the better-ventilated nondependent regions, which improves ventilation-perfusion matching and reduces intrapulmonary shunt.

The first report of PLV in adults with ARDS was on 10 patients who were treated with extracorporeal life support and PLV. The instillation of perfluorochemical was safe, and there was improvement in lung compliance and physiologic shunt; however, the lack of a control group does not allow efficacy conclusions to be made (32). A prospective, noncontrolled, phase I/II trial of PLV in nine adults with ARDS showed improvement in gas exchange, reduced FIO_2, and increased mean venous oxygenation at 48 hours. There was no significant improvement in lung compliance, and mortality was 50% (33). PLV for the treatment of ARDS was evaluated for safety and efficacy in a prospective, multicenter, controlled, randomized, exploratory clinical trial. Ninety patients with ALI/ARDS for no more than 24 hours were randomized to either PLV or conventional mechanical ventilation for a maximum of 5 days. There was a significant

reduction in progression to ARDS in the PLV group, but there were no significant differences in the number of days free from the ventilator at 28 days or in mortality (34). A subgroup analysis suggested that there was a trend toward an increase in the number of ventilator-free days for patients with ALI/ARDS who were age 55 years or less. Based on the current clinical evidence, PLV cannot be recommended as standard therapy for ALI/ARDS.

PARTIAL LIQUID VENTILATION IN ACUTE RESPIRATORY DISTRESS SYNDROME

Summary Statement	Level of Evidence
Partial liquid ventilation in ALI/ARDS has been shown to be safe; however, it has not been shown to improve mortality	Uncontrolled case series Small prospective noncontrolled trial Prospective, multicenter, randomized, controlled trial

ALI, acute lung injury; ARDS, acute respiratory distress syndrome.

Tracheal Gas Insufflation

Tracheal gas insufflation (TGI) is an alternative adjunct to mechanical ventilation that allows ventilation with low VT while enhancing the clearance of CO_2.

This minimally invasive approach reduces the effective series (anatomic) dead space by bypassing the airway proximal to the carina during inspiration, by washing out the PCO_2 of this same region during expiration, or both (Fig. 50.8). During TGI-aided ventilation, fresh gas delivery occurs either throughout the respiratory cycle (continuous catheter flow) or only during a segment of it (phasic catheter flow). In either mode, the crucial variable appears to be the volume of fresh gas injected per breath during expiration. During expiration, low-to-moderate continuous flows of fresh gas introduced near the carina dilute the proximal anatomic dead space (dead space flushing). At high catheter flow rates,

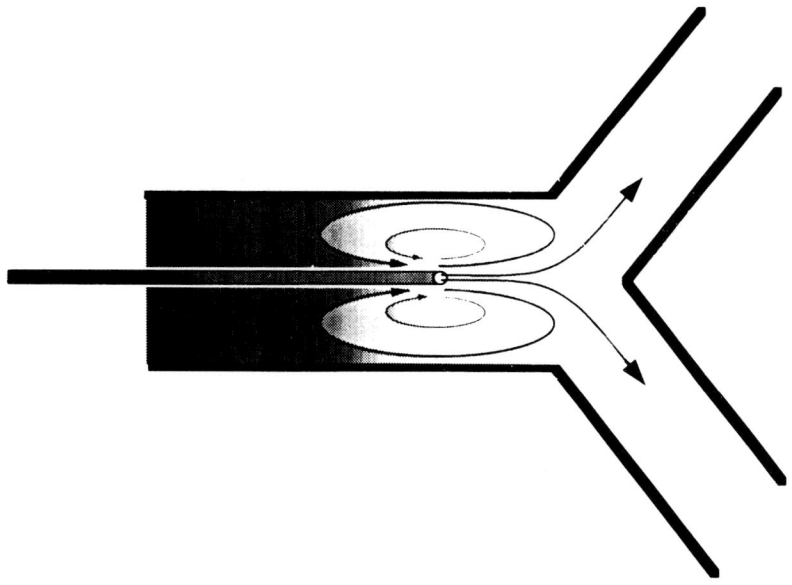

FIGURE 50.8. Tracheal gas insufflation. Carbon dioxide (CO_2)–laden gas that fills the central airways at end-expiration is recycled to the alveolus with the subsequent inspiration. Expiratory flushing of CO_2 from the central airway by fresh gas helps improve CO_2 elimination and reduces dead space. The effectiveness of tracheal gas insufflation is reduced when a high alveolar dead space lowers the end-expiratory tracheal CO_2.

turbulence generated at the catheter tip can also enhance gas mixing in regions beyond its orifice, thereby contributing to CO_2 elimination. Expiratory insufflation appears to be the safest and most effective modality of implementing TGI, avoiding problems with overpressuring the airway, allowing manipulation of the inspiratory time fraction without influencing inspired V_T, and minimizing the volumes of fresh gas that must be injected to achieve a given level of CO_2 elimination.

Because much lower concentrations of CO_2 are delivered to the central airway, TGI loses its effectiveness when there is a large amount of alveolar (as opposed to anatomic and apparatus) dead space. Acute respiratory distress syndrome, emphysema, and pneumonia are typical examples of such diseases. Conversely, permissive hypercapnia boosts the CO_2 concentration, improving the utility of TGI.

Used improperly, TGI has the clear potential to cause mucosal damage, secretion retention, and interference with catheter suctioning. These effects should be mitigated by adequate humidification, using selective expiratory TGI, and the injection of fresh gas via channels imbedded within the walls of the endotracheal tube itself. Injection of catheter gas retrograde to the exhalation stream tends to increase expiratory resistance and generate auto-PEEP; continuous gas injection allows the TGI injector to act as a constant-flow generator during inspiration, when the valves of the machine are closed, risking overdistention. Auto-PEEP and barotrauma are distinct possibilities when high gas flow rates are used—whatever the injection mode (selective expiratory or continuous).

The efficacy of TGI in the treatment of ARDS has not been evaluated by a large randomized controlled trial. A retrospective review of 68 trauma patients with ARDS treated with permissive hypercapnia demonstrated that nine pa-

tients also received continuous TGI. In these nine patients, there was a significant improvement in pH, $Paco_2$, V_T, and minute ventilation. The investigators concluded that continuous TGI is a useful adjunct in permissive hypercapnia, which allows a reduction in the V_T and maintenance of an acceptable pH (35). There have been several small studies evaluating the efficacy of TGI in adults with ARDS that demonstrated significant reductions in $Paco_2$ (36–38). TGI during volume control ventilation and pressure control ventilation was compared in a study of 12 patients with ARDS, and the study demonstrated equivalent results during both modes of ventilation (39).

TGI may be a useful adjunct to pressure-targeted lung protective ventilatory support in ARDS. Larger randomized controlled trials need to be completed to demonstrate survival benefit.

TRACHEAL GAS INSUFFLATION IN ACUTE RESPIRATORY DISTRESS SYNDROME	
Summary Statement	**Level of Evidence**
Tracheal gas insufflation in ALI/ARDS has been shown to be safe; however, it has not been shown to improve mortality.	Uncontrolled case series Retrospective review

ALI, acute lung injury; ARDS, acute respiratory distress syndrome.

Inhaled Nitric Oxide and Prostacyclin

Pulmonary vascular resistance is elevated in ARDS. This may be caused by an imbalance in the vasoconstriction and vasodilatory controls of the pulmonary endothelium secondary to the lung injury of ARDS. NO is a key biologic mediator of smooth muscle relaxation. In the normal lung, endothelial-derived NO stimulates guanylate cyclase to produce cyclic guanosine monophosphate, which helps to maintain a low vasomotor tone. When inhaled, NO has the therapeutic potential to dilate the pulmonary vasculature in well-ventilated regions, tending to reduce pulmonary hypertension and improve the matching of ventilation and perfusion in an unevenly damaged lung. Inhaled NO is active only locally, as it is quenched immediately on exposure to Hgb. Because inhaled NO cannot influence the vasculature of collapsed lung units, the effectiveness of NO often depends on the provision of sufficient PEEP to fully recruit the lung and maintain alveolar patency. Extremely low concentrations of NO achieve nearly full effect; biologic activity is often detectable at concentrations as low as 2 ppm, and beneficial effects on gas exchange are fully saturated at 5 to 20 ppm in most patients. Somewhat higher concentrations of NO may be needed to maximize its pulmonary vasodilating effects. The physiological effects of NO in ARDS are highly variable—sometimes dramatic, but often quite modest. Although the onset and offset of the effects of NO are extremely rapid, gradual accommodation to its beneficial vasodilatory effects can result in rebound vasoconstriction when it is abruptly terminated. High concentrations of NO and minute quantities of its associated oxides (NO_2^{-1} and NO_3^{-2}) are histotoxic and must be avoided.

Clinical trials completed thus far have not shown inhaled NO to significantly improve outcome in ARDS. A multicenter, double-blind, randomized trial of NO versus placebo in 177 ARDS patients showed an acute increase in Pao_2 in 60% of patients receiving inhaled NO versus 24% in the placebo group. The improvement in the oxygenation was seen during the first 4 days but was not persistent after this time. There were no significant differences between the groups in overall mortality, the number of days not on mechanical ventilation, or number of days necessary to meet oxygenation requirement for extubation (40). A European multicenter study of 260 medical and surgical patients with ARDS found the 30-day mortality for the NO-treated patients to be 45%, with 38% for the control patients (41). A French phase III study of inhaled NO also found no significant mortality benefit (42). A randomized study at one center of 40 patients with ARDS compared inhaled NO with conventional ventilation. Inhaled NO increased the Pao_2/Fio_2 ratio during the first 24 hours, but after this time, the two groups had a similar improvement in oxygenation (43).

Inhaled NO cannot be recommended as a standard therapy for ARDS. It may have a role in the treatment of refractory hypoxemia with symptomatic pulmonary hypertension.

Prostacyclin is synthesized in endothelial cells from arachidonic acid and acts as a vasodilator by increasing smooth muscle cAMP. Inhaled prostacyclin may increase perfusion to well-ventilated areas of the lung. To date, there have been no large prospective randomized trials assessing the efficacy of inhaled prostacyclin in ARDS.

Prostaglandin E_1 (PGE_1) activates adenylate cyclase, increases intracellular cAMP, inhibits platelet aggregation, and

is a pulmonary vasodilator. An early prospective, randomized, phase II study comparing liposomal PGE_1 with placebo showed improvement in Pao_2/Fio_2 ratio and in lung compliance (44). A large randomized, prospective, multicenter, double-blind, placebo-controlled, phase III clinical trial evaluated the safety and efficacy of an intravenous liposomal dispersion of PGE_1 in the treatment of 350 patients with ARDS. Treatment with liposomal PGE_1 accelerated improvement in oxygenation indices, but it did not decrease the duration of mechanical ventilation or improve mortality at day 28 (45). PGE_1 is not recommended for treatment of ARDS based on the data from this large prospective randomized trial.

INHALATIONAL THERAPIES FOR ACUTE RESPIRATORY DISTRESS SYNDROME	
Summary Statement	**Level of Evidence**
1. Inhaled nitric oxide may acutely improve oxygenation in acute respiratory distress syndrome, but it does not improve mortality or length of time on ventilation.	Multicenter, randomized, double-blind, controlled trial Multicenter trial Phase III study One-center randomized trial
2. Inhaled prostaglandin E_1 does not improve mortality or number of days on mechanical ventilation.	Large, multicenter randomized, double-blind, placebo-controlled, phase III trial Prospective, randomized, phase II trial

Pharmacological Treatment Options in Acute Lung Injury/Acute Respiratory Distress Syndrome

Corticosteroids

The routine use of corticosteroids for the treatment of early ARDS is not justified. Several trials have been conducted in which steroids were given to patients at risk for or with established ARDS. One study of 81 patients at risk for ARDS who were given steroids were more likely to develop infectious complications and progress to ARDS than was the control group (46). Another study showed that steroids used early had no benefit on the frequency of occurrence of ARDS in patients with septic shock (47). A third trial of 99 patients with ARDS also demonstrated no mortality benefit when treated with a 24-hour course of high-dose corticosteroids (48). Adverse changes in immunity, mental status, metabolism, and protein wastage tend to outweigh any potential therapeutic benefit of steroids in the first week of the course. Steroids should be provided for treatment of steroid responsive conditions such as adrenal insufficiency, vasculitis, allergic reactions, bronchiolitis obliterans with organizing pneumonia, pulmonary hemorrhage syndromes, and *Pneumocystis carinii* pneumonia.

There may be a role for corticosteroids in the treatment of the fibroproliferative phase of ARDS. It has been suggested that steroids affect the fibroproliferative response in the later stage of ARDS by altering macrophage and fibroblast function. The steroids inhibit proliferation of macrophages, and the production of the inflammatory mediators tumor necrosis factor-α and interleukin-1 by macrophages. Additionally, there is an acceleration of procollagen mRNA degradation, as well as inhibition of fibroblast replication and fibronectin production (49).

Several small uncontrolled series using steroids in late ARDS have suggested there may be a survival benefit (49–53). There is one randomized, double-blind, placebo-controlled trial of steroids for late ARDS. Twenty-four patients with ARDS who did not improve after 7 days were randomized at a 1:2 ratio to either placebo or methylprednisolone. The dosing for methylprednisolone was 2 mg/kg load followed by 2 mg/(kg · d) for 2 weeks, then a weekly tapering dosing schedule of 1, 0.5, and 0.125 mg/(kg · d). The results of this study showed that methylprednisolone improved the lung injury score, PaO_2/FIO_2 ratio; decreased the multiple organ dysfunction score; and improved ICU and hospital mortality (53). The National Institutes of Health ARDS Network Late Steroid Rescue Study is a randomized double-blinded trial comparing corticosteroids to placebo in severe late-phase ARDS and will provide further data regarding the role of steroids in ARDS.

THE ROLE OF CORTICOSTEROIDS IN ACUTE RESPIRATORY DISTRESS SYNDROME

Summary Statement	Level of Evidence
1. The use of corticosteroids in the early-phase of ARDS does not prevent progressive lung injury and does not improve mortality.	Multicenter, randomized trials Prospective, randomized, double-blind study Prospective, randomized, double-blind, placebo-controlled trial
2. Patients with ARDS who fail to improve after 7 days may have an improvement in mortality when treated with steroids during this fibroproliferative phase.	Small uncontrolled series Randomized, double-blinded, placebo-controlled trial

ARDS, acute respiratory distress syndrome.

Ketoconazole

The pathological findings in ALI/ARDS include the migration of inflammatory cells into the interstitium and alveolar spaces with activation of proteases and reactive O_2 species. Release of neutrophil chemoattractants and vasoactive mediators contribute to the lung injury and pulmonary hypertension seen in ARDS. Ketoconazole is an antifungal imidazole that has anti-inflammatory properties. It inhibits 5-lipoxygenase, which decreases leukotriene B_4, a key neutrophil chemoattractant. Thromboxane A_2 aggregates platelets and neutrophils and is a pulmonary vasoconstric-

tor. Ketoconazole inhibits synthesis of thromboxane A_2 by inhibiting thromboxane synthase.

Two small trials of ketoconazole for patients at risk for ARDS suggested that it may be effective in reducing the risk in critically ill patients (54,55). Based on these early data, the ARDS Network conducted a multicenter, randomized, double-blind, placebo-controlled trial of 234 patients with ARDS to test the efficacy of ketoconazole in reducing mortality and morbidity. The results showed that ketoconazole was safe and bioavailable but did not improve lung function or reduce mortality (56). On the basis of this large trial, ketoconazole is not recommended for use in ARDS.

KETOCONAZOLE THERAPY FOR ACUTE RESPIRATORY DISTRESS SYNDROME

Summary Statement	Level of Evidence
Ketoconazole does not improve mortality in acute respiratory distress syndrome.	Multicenter, randomized, double-blinded, placebo-controlled trial

---

Exogenous Surfactant

Surfactant functions to decrease the alveolar surface tension and prevent atelectasis. It also suppresses inflammation and inhibits superoxide production by neutrophils (57). Surfactant abnormalities that have been described in ARDS include alterations in surfactant composition and function. Ineffective surfactant activity may cause worsening of lung compliance in ARDS because of alveolar collapse. Trials have been conducted examining the administration of exogenous surfactant in patients with ARDS.

A multicenter, randomized, double-blind, placebo-controlled trial of 51 patients with ARDS showed that nebulized surfactant was well tolerated, but did not significantly improve oxygenation (58). Another small pilot study instilled surfactant bronchoscopically in 10 patients with ARDS and found improvement in oxygenation (59). A randomized, placebo-controlled, open-label study of endotracheal instillation of bovine surfactant in 59 ARDS patients showed a trend of improved mortality in the treated group (60). A large prospective multicenter, randomized, double-blind, place-controlled trial of 725 ARDS patients showed that aerosolized surfactant caused no significant improvement in 30-day mortality, duration of mechanical ventilation, number of days in the ICU, or oxygenation (61). An open-label, uncontrolled phase Ib trial of 12 patients with ARDS received one of three dosing regimens of dilute surfactant by bronchopulmonary segmental lavage. All of the patients tolerated the procedure, and there was improvement in FIO_2 and PEEP requirements 96 hours after the initiation of treatment (62).

Based on the current literature, exogenous surfactant is not recommended for the routine treatment of ARDS.

EXOGENOUS SURFACTANT IN ACUTE RESPIRATORY DISTRESS SYNDROME

Summary Statement	Level of Evidence
1. Nebulized exogenous surfactant does not improve oxygenation or mortality in acute respiratory distress syndrome.	Multicenter, randomized, double-blinded, placebo-controlled trials
2. Endotracheal instillation of bovine surfactant showed a nonsignificant trend toward improved mortality.	Randomized, placebo-controlled, open-label study
3. Bronchoscopically segmental lavage with surfactant is safe and may improve oxygenation acutely.	Uncontrolled, open-label, phase Ib study

Lisofylline

Lisofylline is a derivative of pentoxifylline that is a phosphodiesterase inhibitor. Lisofylline is effective in decreasing the inflammatory response. A randomized placebo-controlled trial of lisofylline for the treatment of ALI/ARDS was conducted by the ARDS Network to determine whether morbidity and mortality could be reduced. This study was stopped early because the interim analysis did not demonstrate a trend toward improvement (63). Lisofylline is not recommended for the treatment of ALI/ARDS.

LISOFYLLINE FOR ACUTE RESPIRATORY DISTRESS SYNDROME

Summary Statement	Level of Evidence
Lisofylline does not improve mortality in ALI/ARDS.	Multicenter, randomized, placebo-controlled trial

ALI, acute lung injury; ARDS, acute respiratory distress syndrome.

In conclusion, there are no effective treatment modalities available at this time that alter the course of disease in ALI/ARDS. There is evidence to show that a ventilation strategy using a low V_T (6 mL/kg) while maintaining a plateau pressure less than 30 cm H_2O will reduce mortality and increase the number of ventilator-free days in patients with ALI/ARDS.

REFERENCES

1. Bernard GR, Artigas A, Brigham K, et al. Report of the American-European conference on ARDS: definitions, mechanisms, relevant outcomes and clinical trial coordination. The consensus committee. *Intensive Care Med* 1994;20:225.
2. Sachdeva RC, Guntupalli KK. Acute respiratory distress syndrome. *Crit Care Clin* 1997;13:503.
3. Brochard L. Respiratory pressure-volume curves. In Tobin MJ, ed. *Principles and practice of intensive care monitoring,* Vol. 2. Columbus, OH: McGraw-Hill, 1998:597.
4. Maggiore SM, Johnson B, Richard JC, et al. Alveolar derecruitment at decremental positive end expiratory pressure levels in acute lung injury. *Am J Respir Crit Care Med* 2001;164:795.
5. Brower RG, Glemmer T, Lanken P, et al. Effects of recruitment maneuvers in acute lung injury patients ventilated with lower tidal volume and higher positive end-expiratory pressures. *Am J Respir Crit Care Med* 2001:163A(abst).
6. Ventilation with lower tidal volumes as compared with traditional tidal volumes for acute lung injury and the acute respiratory distress syndrome: the Acute Respiratory Distress Syndrome Network. *N Engl J Med* 2000;342:1301.
7. Estaban A, Alia I, Gordo R, et al. Prospective randomized trial comparing pressure-controlled ventilation and volume-controlled ventilation in ARDS. *Chest* 2000;117:1690.
8. Wang SH, Wie TS. The outcome of pressure-controlled inverse ratio on patients with severe ARDS in surgical intensive care unit. *Am J Surg* 2002;182:151.
9. Feihl F, Perret C. Permissive hypercapnia: how permissive should we be? *Am J Respir Crit Care Med* 1994;150[6 pt 1]:1722.
10. Bidani A, Tzouanakis AE, Cardenas VJ et al. Permissive hypercapnia in acute respiratory failure. *JAMA* 1994;272:957.
11. Hickling KG, Henderson SJ, Jackson R. Low mortality associated with low volume pressure limited ventilation with permissive hypercapnia in severe adult respiratory distress syndrome. *Intensive Care Med* 1990;16:372.
12. Hickling KG, Walsh J, Henderson S, et al. Low mortality rate in adult respiratory distress syndrome using low-volume, pressure-limited ventilation with permissive hypercapnia: a prospective study. *Crit Care Med* 1994;22:1568.
13. McIntyre RC, Haenel JB, Moore FA, et al. Cardiopulmonary effects of permissive hypercapnia in the management of adult respiratory distress syndrome. *J Trauma* 1994;37:433.
14. Krisnan JA, Brower RG. High-frequency ventilation for acute lung injury and ARDS. *Chest* 2000;118:795.
15. Hurst JM, Branson RD, Davis K, et al. Comparison of conventional mechanical ventilation and high-frequency ventilation: a prospective randomized trial in patients with respiratory failure. *Ann Surg* 1990;211:486.
16. Carlon GC, Howland WS, Ray C, et al. High frequency jet ventilation: a prospective randomized evaluation. *Chest* 1983;84:551.
17. Schuster DP, Lain M, Snyder JV. Comparison of high frequency jet ventilation to conventional ventilation during acute respiratory failure in humans. *Crit Care Med* 1982;10:625.
18. Holzapfel L, Robert D, Perrin F, et al. Comparison of high frequency jet ventilation to conventional ventilation in adults with respiratory distress syndrome. *Intensive Care Med* 1987;13:100.
19. Zapol WM, Snider MT, Hill JD, et al. Extracorporeal membrane oxygenation in severe acute respiratory failure. A randomized prospective study. *JAMA* 1979;242:2193.
20. Kolla S, Lee WA, Hirschl RB, et al. Extracorporeal life support for cardiovascular support in adults. *ASAIO J* 1996;42:M809.
21. Anderson HL, Steimle C, Shapiro M, et al. Extracorporeal life support for adult cardiorespiratory failure. *Surgery* 1993;114:161.
22. Brunet F, Belghith M, Mira JP, et al. Extracorporeal carbon dioxide removal and low-frequency positive-pressure ventilation. Improvement in arterial oxygenation with reduction of risk of pulmonary barotrauma in patients with adult respiratory distress syndrome. *Chest* 1993;104:889.
23. Kolla S, Awad SS, Rish PB, et al. Extracorporeal life support for 100 adult patients with severe respiratory failure. *Ann Surg* 1997;226:544.
24. Egan TM, Duffin J, Glynn MG, et al. Ten-year experience with extracorporeal membrane oxygenation for severe respiratory failure. *Chest* 1988;194:681.
25. Peek GJ, Moore HM, Moore N, et al. Extracorporeal membrane oxygenation for adult respiratory failure. *Chest* 1997;112:759.
26. Pranikoff T, Hirschl RB, Steimle CN, et al. Efficacy of extracorporeal life support in the setting of adult cardiorespiratory failure. *ASAIO J* 1994;40:M339.
27. Lewandowski K, Rossaint R, Pappert D, et al. High survival rate

in 122 ARDS patients managed according to a clinical algorithm including extracorporeal membrane oxygenation. *Intens Care Med* 1997;23:819.

28. Bartlett RH, Roloff DW, Custer JR, et al. Extracorporeal life support: the University of Michigan experience. *JAMA* 2000;283: 904.

29. Extracorporeal Life Support Organization. *Extracorporeal Life Support Organization registry of the extracorporeal life support organization.* Ann Arbor, MI: Extracorporeal Life Support Organization, 1999.

30. Morris AH, Wallace CJ, Menlove RL, et al. Randomized clinical trial of pressure-controlled inverse ratio ventilation and extracorporeal CO_2 removal for adult respiratory distress syndrome. *Am J Respir Crit Care Med* 1994;149:295.

31. Gattinoni L, Tognoni G, Pesenti A, et al. Effect of prone positioning on the survival of patients with acute respiratory failure. *N Engl J Med* 2001;345:568.

32. Hirschl RB, Pranikoff T, Wise C, et al. Initial experience with partial liquid ventilation in adult patients with the acute respiratory distress syndrome. *JAMA* 1996;275:383.

33. Hirschl RB, Conrad S, Kaiser R, et al. Partial liquid ventilation in adult patients with ARDS: a multicenter phase I-II trial: adult PLV study group. *Ann Surg* 1998;228:692.

34. Hirschl RB, Croce M, Gore D, et al. Prospective, randomized, controlled pilot study of partial liquid ventilation in adult acute respiratory distress syndrome. *Am J Respir Crit Care Med* 2002;165; 781.

35. Barnett CC, Moore FA, Moore EE, et al. Tracheal gas insufflation is a useful adjunct in permissive hypercapnia management of ARDS. *Am J Surg* 1996;172:518.

36. Ravenscraft SA, Burke WC, Nahum A, et al. Tracheal gas insufflation augments CO_2 clearance during mechanical ventilation. *Am Rev Respir Dis* 1993;148:345.

37. Nakos G, Zakinthinos S, Kotanidoce A, et al. Tracheal gas insufflation reduces the tidal volume while $Paco_2$ is maintained constant. *Intensive Care Med* 1994;20:407.

38. Kalfon P, Rao GS, Gallart L, et al. Permissive hypercapnia with and without expiratory washout in patients with severe acute respiratory distress syndrome. *Anesthesia* 1997;87:6.

39. Kuo PH, Wu HD, Yu CJ, et al. Efficacy of tracheal gas insufflation in ARDS with permissive hypercapnia. *Am J Respir Crit Care Med* 1996;154:612.

40. Dellinger RP, Zimmerman JL, Tayer RW, et al. Effects of inhaled nitric oxide in patients with acute respiratory distress syndrome: results of a randomized phase II trial: Inhaled Nitric Oxide in ARDS Study Group. *Crit Care Med* 1998;26:15.

41. Lundin S, Mang H, Smithies M, et al. Inhalation of nitric oxide in acute lung injury: preliminary results of a European multicenter study. *Intensive Care Med* 1997;23:52.

42. Groupe d'Etude sur la NO inhale au couers de l'ARDS. GdEsl-Niacd: inhaled NO in ARDS: presentation of a double blind randomized multicenter study. *Am J Respir Crit Care Med* 1996; 153:A590.

43. Michael JR, Barton RG, Saffle JR, et al. Inhaled nitric oxide versus conventional therapy: effect on oxygenation in ARDS. *Am J Respir Crit Care Med* 1998;157:1372.

44. Holcroft JW, Vasser MJ, Weber CJ. Prostaglandin E_1 and survival in patients with adult respiratory distress *Ann Surg* 1986;203:371.

45. Abraham E, Baughman R, Fletcher E, et al. Liposomal prostaglandin E_1 (TLCG-53) in acute respiratory distress syndrome: a controlled, randomized, double-blind, multicenter clinical trial. *Crit Care Med* 1999;27:1478.

46. Weigelt JA, Norcross JF, Borman KR, et al. Early steroid therapy for respiratory failure. *Arch Surg* 1985;120:536.

47. Luce JM, Montgomery AB, Marks JD, et al. Ineffectiveness of high dose methylprednisolone in preventing parenchymal lung injury and improving mortality in patients with septic shock. *Am Rev Respir Dis* 1988;138:62.

48. Bernard GR, Luce JM, Sprung CL, et al. High-dose corticosteroids in patients with adult respiratory distress syndrome. *N Engl J Med* 1987;317:1565.

49. Meduri GU, Belenchia JM, Estes RJ, et al. Fibroproliferative phase of ARDS: clinical findings and effects of corticosteroids. *Chest* 1991;100:943.

50. Hooper RG, Kearl RA. Established adult respiratory distress syndrome successfully treated with corticosteroids. *South Med J* 1996;89:359.

51. Meduri GU, Chinn AJ, Leeper KV, et al. Corticosteroid rescue treatment of progressive fibroproliferation in late ARDS: patterns of response and predictors of outcome. *Chest* 1994;105:1516.

52. Biffle WL, Moore FA, Moore EE, et al. Are corticosteroids salvage therapy for refractory acute respiratory distress syndrome? *Am J Surg* 1995;170:591.

53. Meduri GU, Headley AS, Golden E, et al. Effect of prolonged methylprednisolone therapy in unresolving acute respiratory distress syndrome: a randomized controlled trial. *JAMA* 1998;280:159.

54. Slotman GJ, Burchard KW, D'Arezzo, et al. Ketoconazole prevents acute respiratory failure in critically ill surgical patients. *J Trauma* 1988;28:648.

55. Yu M, Tomasa G. A double-blind, prospective, randomized trial of ketoconazole, a thromboxane synthetase inhibitor, in the prophylaxis of the adult respiratory distress syndrome. *Crit Care Med* 1993;21:1635.

56. Ketoconazole for early treatment of acute lung injury and acute respiratory distress syndrome: a randomized controlled trial. *JAMA* 2000;283:1995.

57. McIntrye RC, Pulido EF, Bensared DD, et al. Thirty years of clinical trials in acute respiratory distress syndrome. *Crit Care Med* 2000;28:3314.

58. Weg, JG, Balk RA, Tharratt RS, et al. Safety and potential efficacy of an aerosolized surfactant in human sepsis-induced adult respiratory distress syndrome. *JAMA* 1994;272:1433.

59. Walmath D, Gunther A, Ghofrani HA, et al. Bronchoscopic surfactant administration in patients with severe adult respiratory distress syndrome and sepsis. *Am J Respir Crit Care Med* 1996;154:57.

60. Gregory TJ, Steinberg KP, Spragg R, et al. Bovine surfactant therapy for patients with acute respiratory distress syndrome. *Am J Respir Crit Care Med* 1997;155:1309.

61. Anzueto A, Baughman RO, Guntupalli KK, et al. Aerosolized surfactant in adults with sepsis-induced acute respiratory distress syndrome: Exosurf Acute Respiratory Distress Syndrome Sepsis Study Group. *N Engl J Med* 1996;334:1417.

62. Wiswell TE, Smith RM, Katz LB, et al. Bronchopulmonary segmental lavage with Surfaxin (KL4-Surfactant) for acute respiratory distress syndrome. *Am J Respir Crit Care Med* 1999;160:1188.

63. Randomized, placebo-controlled trial of lisofylline for early treatment of acute lung injury and acute respiratory distress syndrome. *Crit Care Med* 2002;30:246.

Mechanical Ventilatory Support

51

Neil R. MacIntyre

Mechanical ventilation is the process of using devices to either totally or partially provide oxygen (O_2) and carbon dioxide (CO_2) transport between the environment and the pulmonary capillary bed. The desired effect of mechanical ventilation is maintaining appropriate levels of arterial partial pressure of oxygen (PaO_2) and carbon dioxide ($PaCO_2$) while also unloading the ventilatory muscles. Although negative pressure chambers or wraps and extracorporeal circuits might achieve the same effect, this chapter will focus on the use of positive airway pressure to effect mechanical ventilatory support.

The use of positive pressure mechanical ventilation is widespread. In the United States, estimates range from 1 to 3 million patients annually requiring mechanical ventilatory support outside the operating room (1). This support is supplied by an installed base of approximately 50,000 positive pressure ventilators that traditionally have been used in intensive care unit settings. There are currently clear trends toward expanding this venue to subacute facilities, long-term care facilities, and the home. As the aged population expands and as more aggressive surgical and immunosuppressive therapies are developed, the need for mechanical ventilation is likely to expand in all of these locations (1).

POSITIVE PRESSURE MECHANICAL VENTILATOR DESIGN FEATURES

Gas Delivery Systems

Positive Pressure Breath Controller

Most modern ventilators use piston/bellows systems or controllers of high-pressure sources to drive gas flow (2,3). Tidal

N. R. MacIntyre: Duke University Medical Center, Durham, North Carolina.

breaths are generated by this gas flow and can be either controlled entirely by the ventilator or interactive with patient efforts. Generally, pneumatic, electronic, or microprocessor systems enable various breath types to be available. Breaths are described according to what initiates the breath (trigger variable), what controls gas delivery during the breath (target or limit variable), and what terminates the breath (cycle variable) (4,5). Trigger variables may be either patient effort (detected by the ventilator as a pressure or flow change; see section "Effort (Demand) Sensors") or a set machine timer. Target or limit variables are generally either a set flow or a set inspiratory pressure. Cycle variables are generally a set volume, a set inspiratory time, or a flow rate. Figure 51.1 uses this classification scheme to describe the five most common breath types available on the current generation of mechanical ventilators.

Mode Controller

The availability and delivery logic of different breath types define the mode of mechanical ventilatory support (2,4,5). The mode controller is an electronic-, pneumatic-, or microprocessor-based system that is designed to provide the proper combination of breaths according to set algorithms and feedback data (conditional variables) (Table 51.1). Newer designs can incorporate advanced monitoring and feedback functions into these controllers to allow for continuous adjustments in mode algorithms as patient conditions change (6).

Subsystems of Mechanical Ventilators

Effort (Demand) Sensors

Current ventilators allow for a number of patient-ventilator interactions (7). Examples include patient-triggered breaths (ventilator initiates flow in response to patient demand) and

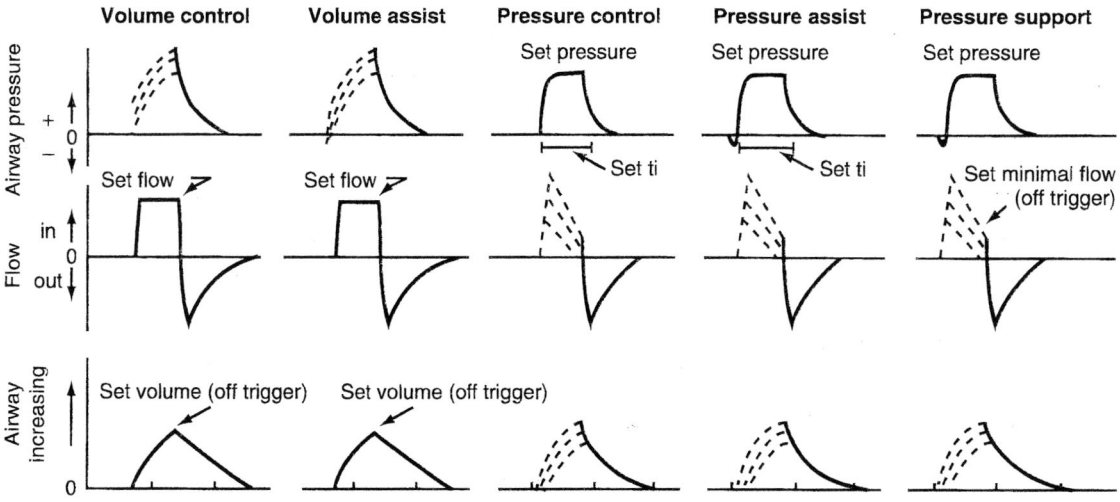

FIGURE 51.1. Airway pressure, flow, and volume tracings over time, depicting the five basic breaths available on most modern mechanical ventilators. Breaths are classified by their trigger, target/limit, and cycle variables. (From MacIntyre NR. Mechanical ventilation. In: Murray J, Nadel JA, eds. *Respiratory diseases*. Philadelphia: WB Saunders, 2000, with permission.)

pressure-targeted/limited breaths (ventilator adjusts flow in response to patient demand) (see section "Patient-Ventilator Interactions"). Patient effort sensors allow the ventilator to properly deliver these interactive breaths. These sensors are usually either pressure or flow transducers in the ventilatory circuitry and are characterized by their sensitivity (how much of a circuit pressure or flow change must be generated to

initiate a ventilator response) and their responsiveness (the delay in providing this response) (8).

Gas Blenders

Blenders mix air and O_2 to produce a delivered fraction of inspired oxygen (FIO_2) ranging from 0.21 to 1.0. On newer systems, blenders are also available to deliver other gases such as Heliox, nitric oxide, and anesthetic agents.

Humidifiers

With the upper airway bypassed by tracheal intubation, sufficient heat and moisture must be added to the inspired gas mixtures to avert mucosal desiccation. Active humidifiers use external water sources and electrical power to adjust blended gas mixtures to near body conditions (tracheal temperature of $>35°C$, water content of >40 mg/L) (9). Passive humidifiers use simple heat/moisture exchange devices in the ventilator circuit to reutilize heat and moisture trapped from expired gas. These disposable units can usually supply adequate heat and moisture (i.e., $>30°C–33°C$ and $>28–32$ mg/L H_2O) for many patients, particularly those receiving mechanical ventilation for only short periods of time (9).

Expiratory Pressure Generator

Positive airway pressure can be sustained throughout expiration (positive end-expiratory pressure [PEEP]) to help maintain alveolar patency and improve ventilation/perfusion ($\dot{V}/\dot{Q}$) matching (see section "Physiologic Effects of Positive Pressure Mechanical Ventilation"). PEEP is usually applied by regulating pressure in the expiratory valve of the ventilator system, but a continuous flow of source gas during the expiratory phase can provide a similar effect. Note that some expiratory valves, even when fully open, have measurable resistance, which may result in some inadvertent PEEP (10). As discussed in more detail below, PEEP may also be produced if expiratory time is inadequate for the lung to return to its

TABLE 51.1. BREATH TYPES AVAILABLE ON COMMON MODES OF MECHANICAL VENTILATION

Modes	Breath Types Available						
	VC	**VA**	**PC**	**PA**	**PS**	**PR**	**SP**
Volume assist control	X[a,b]	X					
Pressure assist control			X[a,b,c]	X[c]			
Volume SIMV	X	X			X[a]		X
Pressure SIMV			X	X	X[a]		X
APRV (BiPAP)						X[b]	X
PSV				X[d]			

In addition to the five basic breaths of Figure 51.1, this table also includes the pressure relief breath (PR, a pressure-targeted breath that allows spontaneous breathing during the inflation phase) and spontaneous unassisted/unsupported breath (SP).
[a] Rate of control breaths can be automatically adjusted according to minute ventilation criteria and called such things as apnea ventilation, and minimum minute ventilation. Rate can also be turned to 0 to pure assist mode of support.
[b] When inspiratory times of these breaths are extended beyond expiratory time, the term inverse ratio ventilation is often used.
[c] Inspiratory pressure can be automatically adjusted according to tidal volume or minute ventilation criteria on some machines (pressure-regulated volume control).
[d] Inspiratory pressure can be automatically adjusted according to tidal volume or minute ventilation criteria on some machines (volume support, pressure augmentation, volume-assured pressure support).
VC, volume controlled; VA, volume assisted; PC, pressure controlled; PA, pressure assisted; PS, pressure supported; APRV, airway pressure release ventilation; BiPAP, bilevel positive airway pressure; PSV, pressure-supported ventilation.

rest volume or if significant flow limitation exists (intrinsic PEEP; sometimes referred to as auto-PEEP, occult PEEP, or air trapping) (11).

Gas Delivery Circuit

This usually consists of flexible tubing that often has pressure or flow sensors and an exhalation valve included. It is important to remember that this tubing has measurable compliance (4 mL/cm H_2O is a representative figure), and significant amounts of delivered gas may serve to distend only this circuitry rather than the patient's lungs under conditions of high airway pressures.

Patient-Ventilator Circuit Interface

Positive pressure ventilation is generally supplied through a tube inserted into the airway via an endotracheal or nasotracheal tube or tracheostomy. These tubes generally have air-filled balloons to provide a proper seal in the airway. An alternative to the tracheal tube is a mask system. Both full face and nasal masks have been used with a variety of ventilatory support systems and modes (12–14). Mask leak, however, can be significant, and thus, support modes using masks must be tested to ensure they can provide adequate volumes and proper inspiratory timing. To this end, special nasal mask ventilators with pressure-targeted and either time-cycled or leak-compensated flow-cycled capabilities have been developed (14).

Aerosol Generators

Therapeutic aerosols (e.g., bronchodilators, steroids, antibiotics) can be delivered through the ventilator circuitry (15). This can be accomplished by either in-line nebulizers or by special chambers designed for metered-dose inhalers. Lung deposition is generally less than in a nonintubated patient because the endotracheal tube serves as a significant barrier to aerosol delivery. Higher dosing is thus advisable.

Monitors and Graphic Displays

Although electronic- and microprocessor-based systems have considerable internal monitoring of electronic and pneumatic function, the three variables generally displayed for clinical use are circuit pressures, flows, and volumes (16). Alarms can be used on all of these monitors (5,17). Most modern positive pressure ventilators also have O_2 sensors in the circuitry to ensure that the desired FIO_2 is being delivered. In addition, some ventilators may also have analyzers for exhaled CO_2 and inhaled therapeutic gases such as nitric oxide or Heliox.

PHYSIOLOGIC EFFECTS OF POSITIVE PRESSURE MECHANICAL VENTILATION

Ventilation and Respiratory System Mechanics

Equation of Motion

Mechanical ventilation produces lung inflation when pressure and flow are applied at the airway opening. The applied pressure interacts with respiratory system compliance (both lung and chest wall components), airway resistance, and, to a lesser extent, respiratory system inertance and lung tissue resistance to effect gas flow (18,19). Because pulmonary inertance and tissue resistance are relatively small, they can be ignored, and the interactions of pressure, flow, and volume with respiratory system mechanics can be expressed by the simplified equation of motion:

$$\text{Driving pressure} = [(\text{flow} \times \text{resistance}) + (\text{volume/system compliance})]$$

In the mechanically ventilated patient, this relationship is expressed as follows:

$$\Delta P_{aw} = [(\dot{V} \times R) + (V_T/CRS)]$$

where ΔP_{aw} is the change in pressure above baseline at the airway opening; $\dot{V}$ is the flow into the patients lungs; R is the resistance of circuit, artificial airway, and native airways; V_T is the tidal volume; and CRS is the respiratory system compliance.

By performing an inspiratory hold at end inspiration (zero flow conditions, $\dot{V} = 0$), the components of ΔP_{aw} required for flow and for respiratory system distention can be separated. Specifically, when $\dot{V} = 0$ at end inspiration, ΔP_{aw} is referred to as the plateau pressure and reflects the static respiratory system compliance ($CRS = V_T/\Delta P_{aw_{plateau}}$). Adding ΔP_{aw} to the baseline pressure yields the total respiratory system distending pressure at end inspiration ($\Delta P_{aw_{plateau}} + \text{baseline pressure} = P_{aw_{plateau}}$). The difference in ΔP_{aw} between flow and no-flow (the peak to plateau difference) equals the inspiratory airway resistance ($R = [\Delta P_{aw_{peak}} - \Delta P_{aw_{plateau}}]/\dot{V}$).

Separating chest wall and lung compliance (CCW and CL, respectively) during a passive machine-controlled positive pressure breath requires an esophageal pressure measurement (P_{es}) to approximate pleural pressure. With this measurement, the inspiratory change in P_{es} (ΔP_{es}) can be used in the following calculations: $CCW = V_T/\Delta P_{es}$ and $CL = V_T/(\Delta P_{aw} - \Delta P_{es})$. In clinical practice, because CCW usually is quite high and ΔP_{es} is thus quite low, $\Delta P_{aw_{plateau}}$ and $P_{aw_{plateau}}$ are often taken as approximations of lung distending pressure. However, in situations in which CCW is reduced (in obesity, anasarca, ascites, and the presence of surgical dressings), the stiff chest wall can have significant effect on $\Delta P_{aw_{plateau}}$ and $P_{aw_{plateau}}$ and must therefore be considered when using these measurements to assess lung stretch.

Pressure-Targeted versus Flow/Volume-Targeted Breaths

There are two basic approaches to delivering positive pressure breaths: pressure targeting and flow/volume targeting (2,4) (Fig. 51.1, Table 51.1). With pressure targeting (breaths 3–5 in Fig. 51.1), an inspiratory pressure target is set such that flow and volume are dependent variables that vary with lung

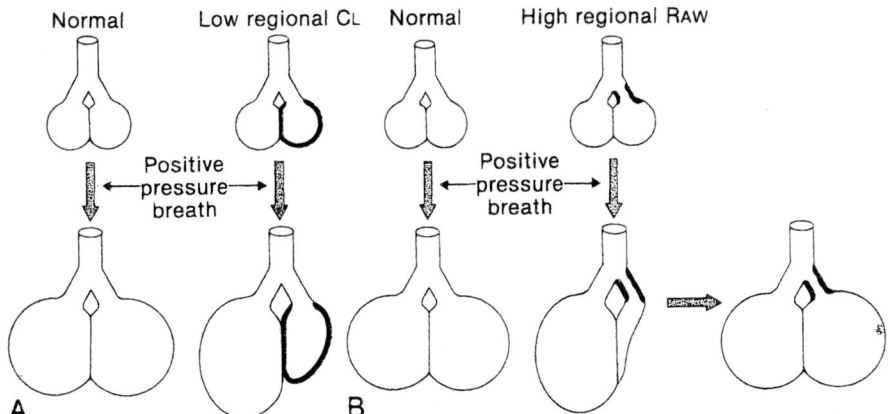

FIGURE 51.2. Schematic effects of the distribution of ventilation in two unit lung models with homogeneous mechanical properties, with abnormal compliance distribution **(A)**, and abnormal resistance distribution **(B)**. Note that in situations with inhomogeneities of lung mechanics, positive pressure breaths are preferentially distributed to healthier regions of the lung and can produce regional overdistention—even when a normal-sized global tidal volume is delivered. (From MacIntyre NR. Mechanical ventilatory support. In: Dantzker D, MacIntyre NR, Bakow E, eds. *Comprehensive respiratory care.* Philadelphia: WB Saunders, 1995, with permission.)

mechanics and patient effort. With flow/volume targeting (breaths 1 and 2 in Fig. 51.1), inspiratory flow and cycling volume are set so that airway pressure is the dependent variable. Changes in compliance or resistance will cause a change of V_T (but not P_{aw}) with the pressure-targeted breath. In contrast, similar changes in compliance or resistance will change P_{aw} (but not flow or volume) with a flow/volume-targeted breath.

Intrinsic Positive End-Expiratory Pressure and the Ventilatory Pattern

Intrinsic PEEP is PEEP that develops within the alveoli because of either inadequate expiratory time or collapsed airways during expiration (or both). Intrinsic PEEP depends on three factors: minute ventilation, expiratory time fraction, and respiratory system expiratory time constant (the product of resistance and compliance) (20). As minute ventilation increases, expiratory time fraction decreases, the time constant lengthens (higher R or CRS values), and the potential to develop intrinsic PEEP increases (20).

Intrinsic PEEP will have different effects on pressure-targeted versus flow/volume-targeted ventilation. In flow/volume-targeted ventilation, the constant delivered volume and ΔP_{aw} in the setting of a rising intrinsic PEEP will increase both the $P_{aw_{peak}}$ and the end-inspiratory $P_{aw_{plateau}}$. In contrast, in pressure-targeted ventilation, the set P_{aw} limit coupled with a rising intrinsic PEEP level will decrease ΔP_{aw} and the delivered V_T (and minute ventilation).

In patients on controlled ventilation, intrinsic PEEP can be assessed in two ways. First, when an inadequate expiratory time is producing intrinsic PEEP, analysis of the flow graphic will show that expiratory flow has not returned to zero before the next breath is given. Second, intrinsic PEEP in alveolar units distal to patent airways can be quantified during a prolonged expiratory hold maneuver that permits equilibration of the intrinsic PEEP throughout the ventilator circuitry (11).

Distribution of Ventilation

A positive pressure tidal breath is distributed among all alveolar units (21,22). Factors affecting the distribution include regional resistances, compliances, functional residual capacities, and the delivered flow pattern (including inspiratory pause). In general, positive pressure breaths will tend to distribute more to units with high compliance and low resistance and away from obstructed or stiff units (Fig. 51.2). This creates the potential for regional overdistention of healthier lung units, even in the face of normal-sized V_T (see section "Lung Stretch Injury and Ventilator-Induced Lung Injury").

Flow pattern may also affect the distribution of ventilation. Specifically, slow and constant flows will tend to distribute more evenly in partially obstructed units and result in a relatively lower end inflation pressure (although consequent shorter expiratory times may worsen air trapping) (21). In contrast, initial rapid flows followed by subsequent decelerating flows (typically seen in pressure-targeted breaths) pressurize lung units quickly and thus produce the highest mean inspiratory alveolar pressure for a given end inflation pressure (23). Finally, inspiratory pauses can also allow pendelluft action to fill slowly filling alveolar units (Fig. 51.2).

It should be noted that a more uniform ventilation distribution does not necessarily result in improved $\dot{V}/\dot{Q}$ matching; the opposite may actually occur in a lung with perfusion inhomogeneities. Because of all these considerations, predicting which flow pattern will optimize $\dot{V}/\dot{Q}$ matching is difficult and is often an empirical trial and error exercise.

Alveolar Recruitment and Gas Exchange

Infiltrative lung disease produces severe $\dot{V}/\dot{Q}$ mismatching through alveolar flooding and collapse (24). In many (but not all) of these disease processes, collapsed alveoli can be recruited during a positive pressure ventilatory cycle (25–29). Three specific techniques that optimize recruitment include the application of PEEP, the use of recruitment maneuvers (RMs), and the prolongation of the inspiratory time.

Positive End-Expiratory Pressure

PEEP is defined as an elevation of transpulmonary pressure at the end of expiration (25,26). As noted above, PEEP can be produced by either expiratory circuit valves (applied PEEP) or as a consequence of ventilator settings interacting with respiratory system mechanics (intrinsic PEEP). Note that expiratory muscle contraction at end expiration can also raise intrathoracic pressures, but this should not be considered PEEP because the mechanism is not that of a transpulmonary pressure increase.

Alveoli prevented from de-recruiting by PEEP provide several potential benefits. First, recruited alveoli improve $\dot{V}/\dot{Q}$ matching and gas exchange (25,26). Second, as discussed in section "Lung Stretch and Ventilator-Induced Lung Injury," alveoli that remain patent throughout the ventilatory cycle are not exposed to the risk of injury from the shear stress of repeated opening and closing (30–32). Third, PEEP prevents surfactant breakdown in collapsing alveoli and thus improves lung compliance (33). PEEP, however, can also be detrimental. Because the tidal breath is delivered on top of PEEP, end-inspiratory pressures are higher than they would be if PEEP were not applied. This must be considered if the lung is at risk for stretch injury. Moreover, because alveolar injury is often quite heterogeneous, appropriate PEEP in one region may be suboptimal in another region and yet excessive in another (27–29). Optimizing PEEP thus involves striking a balance between recruiting potentially recruitable alveoli in diseased regions without overdistending already recruited alveoli in healthier regions. Another potential detrimental effect of PEEP is that it also raises mean intrathoracic pressure, which can reduce cardiac filling in susceptible patients (34).

Recruitment Maneuvers

RMs are based on the concept that alveolar recruitment occurs throughout a positive pressure inflation—all the way to total lung capacity (35). In practice, RMs are performed by using sustained inflations (e.g., 30–40 cm H_2O) for up to 2 minutes (36,37). An alternative approach is to use frequent sigh breaths that take the lung briefly to near total lung capacity on a frequent basis (38). It must be pointed out that RMs only provide initial alveolar recruitment—the sustainability of recruitment almost certainly depends on appropriately setting the level of PEEP to prevent subsequent derecruitment.

Inspiratory Time Manipulations

A positive pressure breath consists of a flow magnitude and profile that, as noted above, can affect ventilation distribution (and thus $\dot{V}/\dot{Q}$). Inspiratory time (and the relationship of inspiratory to expiratory time) are of particular importance.

Prolonging inspiratory time, generally by adding a pause, is often used in conjunction with a rapid decelerating flow (i.e., pressure-targeted) profile and has several physiologic effects. First, the longer inflation period may recruit more slowly recruitable alveoli (39). Second, increased gas mixing time may improve $\dot{V}/\dot{Q}$ matching in infiltrative lung disease (23,40). Third, intrinsic PEEP may develop and be associated with similar effects to those of applied PEEP, as already noted. Indeed, much of the improvement in gas exchange associated with long inspiratory time strategies may be merely a PEEP phenomenon (41). It should be noted, however, that the distribution of intrinsic PEEP (most pronounced in lung units with long time constants) may be different from that of applied PEEP, and thus, $\dot{V}/\dot{Q}$ effects may also be different. Fourth, because long inspiratory times significantly increase total intrathoracic pressures, cardiac output may be adversely affected. Finally, inspiratory/expiratory ratios that exceed 1:1 (so-called inverse ratio ventilation [IRV]) are uncomfortable, and patient sedation/paralysis is often required unless a relief mechanism allows spontaneous breathing during the inflation period (see section "Airway Pressure Release Ventilation") (41–43).

Lung Stretch and Ventilator-Induced Lung Injury

The lung can be injured when it is excessively stretched by positive pressure ventilation. The most well recognized injury is that of alveolar rupture presenting as extra-alveolar air in the mediastinum (pneumomediastinum), pericardium (pneumopericardium), subcutaneous tissue (subcutaneous emphysema), pleura (pneumothorax), and vasculature (air emboli) (44). The risk for extra-alveolar air increases as a function of the magnitude and duration of alveolar overdistention. Thus, interactions of respiratory system mechanics and mechanical ventilation strategies (high regional V_T and PEEP, both applied and intrinsic) that produce regions of excessive alveolar stretch (transpulmonary distending pressures >40 cm H_2O) for prolonged periods create alveolar units at risk for rupture (44).

In experimental animals, parenchymal lung injury (ventilator-induced lung injury [VILI]) can be produced by mechanical ventilation strategies that stretch the lungs beyond the normal maximum (transpulmonary distending pressures of 30–35 cm H_2O). Pathologically, the injury manifests as diffuse alveolar damage but not necessarily as rupture (30–32,45,46), and is associated with cytokine release (47,48) and bacterial translocation (49). VILI appears to be potentiated by a shear-stress phenomenon that occurs when injured alveoli are repetitively opened and collapsed during the ventilatory cycle (30–32,50). Very rapid initial gas flow into the lung may be an additional contributing factor (51).

VILI may occur clinically when low-resistance/high-compliance units receive a disproportionately high regional V_T in the setting of high alveolar distending pressures

(Fig. 51.2). Concern about overdistention injury is the rationale for using lung-protective ventilator strategies that accept less than normal values for pH and partial pressure of O_2 (Po_2) in exchange for lower (and safer) distending pressures (see section "Management Strategies").

Mechanical Loads

Mechanical load describes the mechanical aspects of ventilation with a single number, expressed as either a pressure-time product (PTP) or work (W) (18,19). Because mechanical loads correlate with ventilatory muscle O_2 demands (52–54), the concept of load is useful in considering inspiratory muscle energy requirements during spontaneous or interactive partial ventilatory support. Moreover, when referenced to a muscle strength and/or endurance measure, load tolerance is a useful guide to set levels of partial ventilatory support or to predict the spontaneous breathing capabilities (54).

The PTP expresses load as the integral of pressure over time (PTP = ∫Pdt). Work expresses load as the integral of pressure over volume (W = ∫PdV). Compliance, resistance, and the size of the breath all contribute to the magnitude of the load per breath. During spontaneous breaths, integrating P_{es} over time or volume (referenced to the passive inflation pressure) describes the load borne by the inspiratory muscles to inflate the lungs. During a controlled breath, integrating P_{aw} over time or volume describes the ventilator load necessary to inflate the entire respiratory system (lungs and chest wall), and integrating P_{es} over time or volume describes the load imposed by the chest wall. During interactive, partially supported breaths in which load is shared between patient and ventilator, the sum contributions of patient and ventilator PTP or work is the same as that found during a controlled or spontaneous breath of the same volume and flow profile (55).

Under heavy impedance loading conditions (stiff lung), duration of pressure (PTP) correlates better with muscle energetics and fatigue potential than does volume moved with pressure (work) (52,53). Indeed, during ventilation requiring high pressures, multiplying PTP by the inspiratory time fraction and referencing this to the maximal pressure that the inspiratory muscles can generate results in the pressure-time index. Muscle fatigue can be expected if the pressure-time index exceeds 0.15 (55,56). This concern with high pressure loads in patients receiving partial ventilatory support is one of the rationales for providing ventilator pressure assistance with every spontaneous effort (pressure-assisted or supported breaths), as opposed to alternating fully supported breaths with unsupported breaths (intermittent mandatory ventilation) (57).

Patient-Ventilator Interactions

Mechanical ventilation modes that permit spontaneous ventilatory activity are termed interactive modes, in that patients can influence various aspects of ventilator functions. Interactions range from simple triggering of mechanical breaths

to more complex processes that affect delivered flow patterns and breath timing. Interactive modes allow for muscle exercise, which, when done at nonfatiguing or physiologic levels, may prevent muscle atrophy and facilitate fatigue recovery (57,58). In addition, permitting spontaneous patient ventilatory activity and using comfortable interactive modes may reduce the need for the sedation and/or neuromuscular blockers that are often required to prevent patients from "fighting" machine-controlled ventilation (59,60).

Interactive modes can be either synchronous or dyssynchronous with patient efforts. Synchronous interactions imply that the ventilator is sensitive to the initiation, modulation, and termination of ventilatory effort by the patient (59). Synchrony may occur during any of the three phases of interactive breath delivery: breath triggering, ventilator flow delivery, and breath cycling.

Ventilator Breath Triggering

A spontaneous patient effort (either an airway pressure drop or airway flow change; see section "Effect (Demand) Sensors") must be sensed by an interactive mechanical ventilator in order to trigger a mechanical response (8). Even with modern sensors, however, there is unavoidable dyssynchrony in the triggering process (61). First, a certain level of insensitivity must be built into the sensor to avoid artifacts triggering the ventilator (i.e., auto cycling). Second, even when the patient effort has been sensed, demand valve systems have a certain inherent delay (≥ 100 milliseconds) before they physically open and achieve target flow into the airway (system responsiveness). Both of these factors can result in significant isometric-like pressure loads on the ventilatory muscles during the triggering process (61). In addition, in the setting of air trapping and PEEP (intrinsic PEEP), the elevated alveolar pressure at end expiration can serve as a significant triggering threshold load on the ventilatory muscles (Fig. 51.3). Under these conditions, judicious use of applied PEEP can equilibrate expiratory pressure throughout the lungs and ventilator circuit to reduce this triggering load (62,63).

Ventilator-Delivered Flow Pattern

During an interactive breath, ventilatory muscles are contracting (64,65), and the ventilator flow delivery should be adequate to meet one of three goals:

1. Fully unload the contracting ventilatory muscles in patients with severely overloaded and fatigued muscles
2. Partially unload the contracting ventilatory muscles in patients recovering from muscle fatigue
3. Have no loading effects on contracting ventilatory muscle in patients during spontaneous breathing trials (continuous positive airway pressure [CPAP]).

Synchronous flow interactions can be defined accordingly.

In general, flow synchrony is best assessed by analyzing the airway pressure graphic over time. With assisted/supported breaths designed to near totally unload the ventilatory

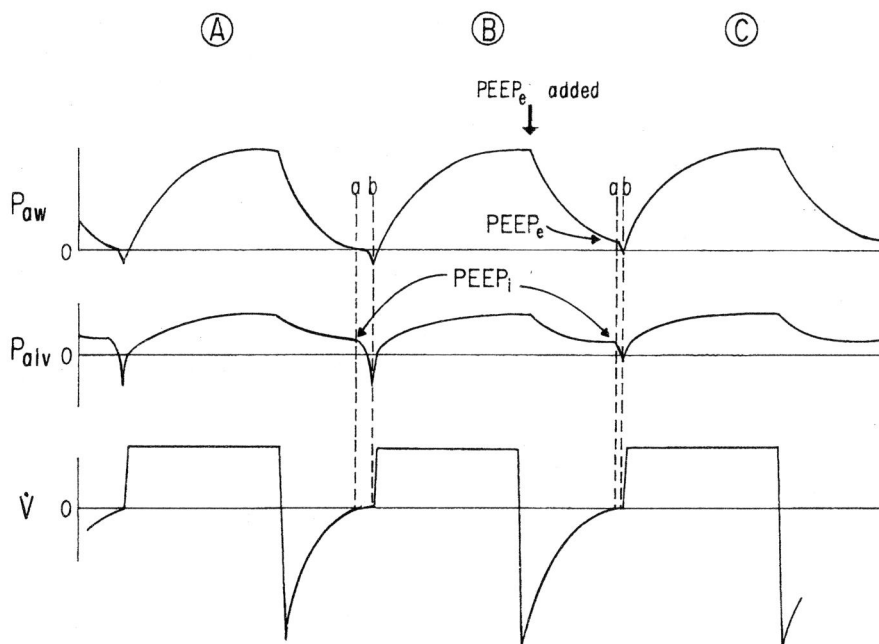

FIGURE 51.3. Schematic tracings of airway pressure (P_{aw}), alveolar pressure (P_{alv}) and flow ($\dot{V}$) during patient-triggered breaths in the setting of dynamic airway collapse and consequent intrinsic positive end-expiratory pressure (PEEP). In breath A, intrinsic PEEP is evident in the P_{alv} tracing at end expiration. Note that this intrinsic PEEP must be overcome so the P_{aw} can be lowered to trigger the assisted breath (point a to b). In breaths B and C, a small amount of applied PEEP (less than intrinsic PEEP) has been added. This serves to partially equilibrate expiratory pressures in the lung and ventilator circuitry, thus reducing the P_{alv} drop that must occur to lower P_{aw}. The inspiratory threshold load imposed by intrinsic PEEP is consequently reduced. (From MacIntyre NR. Intrinsic positive end expiratory pressure. *Prob Respir Care* 1991;4:49, with permission.)

muscles, the assisted/supported airway pressure graphic should mimic the airway pressure graphic of a controlled breath with the same flow and V_T. With assisted/supported breath designed to share loads between the ventilator and the patient, the airway pressure graphic should maintain a convex upward shape, indicating that flow is proportional to demand. Finally, in the setting of providing only CPAP, the airway pressure graphic should be flat. Dyssynchrony (and imposed loading) is said to exist when the airway pressure graphic is literally "sucked downward" below these target patterns.

Breath Cycling

Cycling dyssynchrony can occur in one of two ways. First, if the breath lasts beyond the patient's effort, an inadequate expiratory time may develop (along with air trapping), and/or patient expiratory efforts may be required to terminate the breath (66). Second, if the breath terminates before the patient effort is finished, the patient may be left demanding additional flow without any being delivered. Significant imposed loading and/or double breath triggering may result.

Positive Pressure Ventilation and Cardiac Function

In addition to affecting ventilation and ventilation distribution, intrathoracic pressure applications from positive pressure ventilation can also affect cardiovascular function (34,67,68). In general, as mean intrathoracic pressure is increased, right ventricular filling is decreased and cardiac output/pulmonary perfusion consequently decreases. This is the rationale for using volume repletion to maintain cardiac output in the setting of high intrathoracic pressure. The effect of reduced cardiac filling on cardiac output may be partially

counteracted by improved left ventricular function owing to reduced left ventricular afterload caused by the increased intrathoracic pressure (69). Intrathoracic pressures can also influence the distribution of perfusion by altering the relationship of alveolar pressure to perfusion pressure as modeled by the three-zone lung model of West (70). The supine human lung is generally in a zone 3 (distention) state. As intra-alveolar pressures rise, however, zone 2 and zone 1 conditions are created with high $\dot{V}/\dot{Q}$ units. Indeed, increases in dead space (zone 1 lung) can be a consequence of ventilatory strategies using high ventilatory pressures (IRV).

Positive pressure mechanical ventilation can affect other aspects of cardiovascular function. Specifically, dyspnea, anxiety, and discomfort from inadequate ventilatory support can lead to stress-related catechol release with subsequent increases in myocardial O_2 demands and risk of dysrhythmias (71). In addition, coronary blood O_2 delivery can be compromised by inadequate gas exchange due to injured lung in conjunction with a low mixed venous PO_2 due to high O_2 consumption demands by the ventilatory muscles.

NON–PRESSURE-RELATED COMPLICATIONS OF MECHANICAL VENTILATION

Oxygen Toxicity

O_2 concentrations approaching 100% are known to cause oxidant injuries in airways and lung parenchyma (72). Much of the data supporting the concept of oxidant-induced lung injury, however, have come from studies using animals that often have quite different tolerances to O_2 than that of humans. It is thus not clear what the safe O_2 concentration or duration of exposure is in sick humans. Most consensus groups have argued that exposure to F_{IO_2} levels less than 0.4 are safe for prolonged periods of time and that exposure to F_{IO_2} levels greater than 0.80 should be avoided.

Patient-Ventilator Interface Complications

The patient-ventilator interface includes the ventilator circuitry and the artificial airway. The most important complications associated with this apparatus are ventilator disconnections, including artificial airway dislodgment. This has been reported to occur in up to 8% to 13% of ventilated patients (73) and, if not corrected, can be fatal. Because circuit pressure and flow can still occur with the ventilator not properly connected, as would occur in an esophageally intubated patient or in a partially occluded circuit, it is critical that carefully set, redundant (pressure *and* flow) alarms are present (5). Other complications of the patient-ventilator interface include obstructions from secretions, circuit leaks, airway injury from inadequate heat/humidity, tracheal injury from the artificial airway, and loss of delivered V_T in an overly compliant circuit.

Pulmonary Infectious Complications

Mechanically ventilated patients are at increased risk for pulmonary infections (74–76). First, the natural glottic closure protective mechanism is compromised by an endotracheal tube, which permits continuous seepage of oropharyngeal material into the airways. Second, the endotracheal tube itself impairs the cough reflex and serves as an additional potential portal for pathogens to enter the lungs. This is particularly important if the circuit is contaminated. Third, airway and parenchymal injury from the underlying disease, as well as from management complications noted above, makes the intubated lung more prone to infections. Fourth, the intensive care unit environment with its heavy antibiotic use and presence of very sick patients in close proximity increases the risk for a variety of infections.

Preventing ventilator-associated pneumonia is critical as length of stay in the intensive care unit and associated mortality are both adversely influenced by its development (74–76). Hand-washing and carefully chosen antibiotic regimens can have important beneficial effects. Management strategies that avoid breaking the integrity of the ventilator circuit (changing the circuit only when visibly contaminated) also appear to be helpful (77). Finally, continuous drainage of subglottic secretions may be a simple way of reducing lung contamination with oropharyngeal material (78).

APPLYING MECHANICAL VENTILATORY SUPPORT

Mechanical Ventilatory Support Involves Tradeoffs

To provide adequate support yet minimize VILI, mechanical ventilation goals must involve tradeoffs. Specifically, the need for potentially injurious pressures, volumes, and supplemental O_2 must be carefully weighed against the benefits of gas exchange support. To this end, a re-thinking of gas exchange goals has occurred over the past decade so that pH goals as low as 7.15 to 7.20 and P_{O_2} goals as low as 55 mm Hg are now often considered acceptable if the lung can be protected from VILI (25).

Ventilator settings should be selected to provide at least this level of gas exchange support while at the same time meeting two mechanical goals:

1. Provision of enough PEEP to recruit the recruitable alveoli
2. Avoidance of a PEEP-V_T combination that unnecessarily overdistends lung regions at end inspiration.

These goals embody the concept of a lung-protective mechanical ventilatory strategy, and these principles guide current recommendations for ventilator management (25, 79–81).

Considerations in Choosing Ventilator Settings for Different Forms of Respiratory Failure

Parenchymal Lung Injury

Parenchymal lung injury encompasses disease processes that involve the air spaces and the interstitium of the lung. In general, parenchymal injury produces stiff lungs and reduced lung volumes (24). Functional residual capacity is thus reduced, and the compliance curve is shifted to the right. It is important to realize, however, that in all but the most diffuse diseases, there are often marked regional differences in the degree of inflammation present and thus the degree of mechanical abnormalities that exist. This heterogeneity can have significant impact on the effects of a particular mechanical ventilation strategy. This is because delivered gases will preferentially go to the regions with the highest compliance and lowest resistance, the more normal regions, rather than to sicker regions (Fig. 51.2). A normal-sized V_T may thus be distributed preferentially to healthier regions of the lung and results in a much higher regional V_T and an increased potential for regional overdistention injury.

Parenchymal injury can also affect the airways, especially the bronchioles and alveolar ducts (24). Narrowed and collapsible small airways can contribute to reduced regional ventilation to distally injured lung units. This can lead to regions of air trapping and may be a factor in subsequent cyst formation.

As mentioned, gas exchange abnormalities in parenchymal lung injury are a consequence of alveolar flooding and/or collapse coupled with a misdistribution of ventilation, which results in $\dot{V}/\dot{Q}$ mismatching and shunts. Because dead space ($\dot{V}/\dot{Q} = \infty$) is not a major manifestation of parenchymal lung disease unless there is very severe or end-stage injury, hypoxemia tends to be more of a problem than is CO_2 clearance.

Frequency-V_T (f-V_T) ventilator settings required in parenchymal lung injury should be based on limiting end inspiratory stretch. The importance of this strategy in improving outcome has been demonstrated in several recent clinical trials (79,80) but has been most convincingly shown in the National Institutes of Health (NIH)–sponsored Acute Respiratory Distress Syndrome (ARDS) Network Trial. This trial showed a 10% absolute reduction in mortality with ventilator strategy using a V_T of 6 mL/kg compared with the traditional 12 mL/kg strategy (81). Thus, the current consensus is that the initial V_T setting should be 6 mL/kg ideal body weight. Moreover, strong consideration should be given to further reducing this setting if the end-inspiratory plateau pressure ($P_{aw_{plateau}}$), adjusted for any effects of excessive chest wall stiffness, exceeds 30 cm H_2O. Increases in V_T settings may be considered if there is marked patient discomfort or suboptimal gas exchange provided that the subsequent $P_{aw_{plateau}}$ values do not exceed 30 cm H_2O. Respiratory rate settings are then adjusted to control pH. Unlike obstructive diseases, the potential for air trapping under conditions of parenchymal lung injury is low if the breathing frequency is below 35 breaths/min and may not develop even at frequencies exceeding 50 breaths/min.

The acute phase of severe parenchymal lung injury is generally managed using the assist control mode of ventilation (ACV). This mode assures that the ventilator is providing virtually all of the work of breathing. Choosing pressure-targeted versus flow/volume-targeted ventilation for total support depends on the clinical situation. As noted above, flow/volume-targeted ventilation (volume ACV) guarantees a certain V_T. This, in turn, gives the clinician control over minute ventilation and CO_2 clearance. Under these conditions, however, airway and alveolar pressures are dependent variables and will change in conjunction with changes in lung mechanics or patient effort. Sudden worsening of compliance or resistance will cause abrupt increases in airway and alveolar pressures and result in diversion of the set V_T to healthier regions, causing regional overdistention. Pressure-targeted ventilation, on the other hand, does not guarantee volume but rather controls airway pressure. Volume becomes the dependent variable and will change as lung mechanics or patient effort change. Sudden worsening of compliance or resistance with pressure-targeted ventilation results in a loss of volume and reduced CO_2 clearance, but will avoid regional overdistention. Pressure-targeted ventilation also has a variable decelerating flow waveform, which may improve gas mixing (23) and may interact with patient effort in a more synchronous fashion (82).

The choice of pressure- versus volume-targeted breaths depends on which feature is required for the clinical goal. Specifically, if CO_2 clearance is of primary concern and patient comfort and lung stretch are less of an issue; then volume-targeted ventilation is preferable. On the other hand, if overdistention risk is high and/or patient synchrony is more of an issue than the CO_2 clearance, as is the case in severe ARDS, then pressure-targeted ventilation is preferable.

Setting the inspiratory time and the inspiratory time/expiratory time ratio in cases of parenchymal injury involves several considerations. The normal inspiratory/expiratory ratio is roughly 1:2 to 1:4 and results in the most patient comfort. It is thus a rational initial setting. Assessment of the flow graphic should be done to ensure that an adequate expiratory time is present to avoid air trapping.

Inspiratory prolongation above the normal physiologic range (IRV) can be used as an alternative to increasing PEEP to improve $\dot{V}/\dot{Q}$ matching in severe respiratory failure (40–43). The mechanisms involved include longer mixing times, recruitment of slowly filling alveoli, and development of intrinsic PEEP. A variation on IRV is airway pressure release ventilation (APRV; also known as biphasic ventilation, bilevel ventilation, and bilevel positive airway pressure) (83,84). APRV incorporates the ability to spontaneously breathe during the long inflation period of a pressure-controlled breath—a feature that may enhance recruitment and comfort. APRV is discussed in more detail below (see section "Airway Pressure Release Ventilation").

Generally, IRV strategies are reserved for patients with parenchymal lung injury in whom the $P_{aw_{plateau}}$ has exceeded 30 cm H_2O, and in whom potentially toxic concentrations of FiO_2 are being used without meeting arterial O_2 saturation or O_2 delivery goals. It must be emphasized, however, that although IRV strategies have physiologic appeal, good outcome studies supporting their use do not exist.

There are both mechanical and gas exchange approaches to setting the PEEP/FiO_2 combination in order to support oxygenation. Mechanical approaches use either a static pressure/volume plot to set the PEEP/V_T combination between the upper and lower inflection points of a static pressure/volume plot (85) or else use step increases in PEEP to determine the PEEP level that gives the best compliance (86). With either of these approaches, an RM (sustained inflation to the upper inflection point) may be used to recruit the maximal number of recruitable alveoli before setting the PEEP (36,37). FiO_2 adjustments are then set as low as clinically acceptable. Gas exchange criteria used to guide PEEP application generally involve following algorithms designed to provide adequate values of PaO_2 while minimizing FiO_2. An example would be the NIH ARDS Network PEEP/FiO_2 algorithm in Table 51.2 (81). Note that constructing a PEEP/FiO_2 algorithm is usually an empirical exercise in balancing arterial O_2 saturation with FiO_2 and depends on the clinician's perception of the relative toxicities of high thoracic pressures, high FiO_2, and low arterial O_2 saturation.

Obstructive Airway Disease

Respiratory failure from airflow obstruction is a direct consequence of increases in airway resistance. Airway narrowing and increased resistance lead to two important mechanical changes. First, the increased pressures required for airflow may overload ventilatory muscles, producing a ventilatory

TABLE 51.2. THE POSITIVE END-EXPIRATORY PRESSURE/FRACTION OF INSPIRED OXYGEN

F_{IO_2}	0.30	0.40	0.40	0.50	0.50	0.60	0.70	0.70	0.70	0.80	0.90	0.90	0.90	1.0	1.0	1.0	1.0
PEEP	5	5	8	8	10	10	10	12	14	14	14	16	18	18	20	22	24

Table used during The National Institutes of Health Acute Respiratory Distress Syndrome Network study. The clinical target is a partial pressure of oxygen of 55–80 mm Hg or oxygen saturation of 88%–95%. If the patient is below these target values, move up the row to the right. If the patient is above these targets, move down the row to the left. (From NIH ARDS Network. Ventilation with lower tidal volumes as compared with traditional tidal volumes for acute lung injury and the acute respiratory distress syndromes. *New Engl J Med* 2000;342:1301–1308, with permission.)
F_{IO_2}, fraction of inspired oxygen; PEEP, positive end-expiratory pressure.

pump failure with spontaneous minute ventilation inadequate for CO_2 elimination. Second, the narrowed airways create regions of lung that cannot properly empty and return to their normal resting volume; intrinsic PEEP is a consequence of this mechanism (20). Overly inflated lung regions act as dead space and put inspiratory muscles at a substantial mechanical disadvantage, which further worsens muscle function. Overly inflated lung regions may also compress more healthy regions of the lung, impairing $\dot{V}/\dot{Q}$ matching. Regions of air trapping and intrinsic PEEP also function as a threshold load to trigger mechanical breaths (11,63).

The gas exchange abnormalities in worsening airflow obstruction are several. Although there may be transient initial hyperventilation owing to dyspnea, worsening respiratory failure in obstructed individuals is generally associated with a falling minute ventilation, as respiratory muscles fatigue in the face of large increases in airway resistance (hypercapnic respiratory failure). Then regional lung compression and regional hypoventilation produces $\dot{V}/\dot{Q}$ mismatch that results in progressive hypoxemia. Alveolar inflammation and flooding, however, is not a characteristic feature of respiratory failure owing to pure airflow obstruction, and thus, shunts are less of an issue than they are in parenchymal lung injury. In some patients, overdistended regions of the lung coupled with underlying emphysema result in a reduction in the capillary bed and increasing dead space. This wasted ventilation further compromises the ability of the inspiratory muscles to support adequate ventilation. Emphysematous areas in the lung also have reduced recoil properties that can worsen air trapping. Hypoxemic pulmonary vasoconstriction coupled with chronic pulmonary vascular changes in some airway diseases overload the right ventricle, further decreasing blood flow to the lung and worsening dead space ventilation.

Setting the f/V_T pattern in obstructive diseases involves many considerations that are similar to those above. V_T should be sufficiently low (6 mL/kg ideal body weight) to assure that $P_{aw_{plateau}}$ values are less than 30 cm H_2O (81). In obstructive diseases, however, clinicians should be aware that high peak airway pressures, even in the presence of acceptable values for $P_{aw_{plateau}}$, may transiently overdistend regions of the lung because of a pendelluft effect (Fig. 51.2). As with parenchymal lung injury, V_T reductions should be considered to meet $P_{aw_{plateau}}$ goals. Again, V_T increases can be considered for comfort or gas exchange provided that $P_{aw_{plateau}}$ values do not exceed 30 cm H_2O. The set rate is used to control pH. Unlike parenchymal disease, however, elevated

airway resistance and low recoil pressures greatly increase the potential for air trapping. This phenomenon limits the range of breath rates available.

As with parenchymal injury, substantial muscle unloading is generally required in the initial management of patients with airflow obstruction and thus ACV is often indicated. Both pressure-targeted (pressure ACV) and flow/volume-targeted (volume ACV) modes are effective in this regard. Pressure ACV offers very high initial flows that vary with patient effort. This can help keep the inspiratory time short (and thus expiratory time long) and, if patient triggering is occurring, may synchronize with patient efforts more easily than do set flows (82). Pressure limited breaths also impose an absolute pressure limit on the airway. As in the management of parenchymal lung injury, the choice of pressure- versus volume-targeted breaths generally involves determining the most important management goal. Specifically, if CO_2 clearance is felt to be more important than is overdistention protection or synchrony, volume ACV should be the initial choice. In contrast, if overdistention protection or synchrony are deemed more important than is CO_2 clearance, pressure ACV should be the choice.

The inspiratory/expiratory time ratio in obstructive lung disease is generally set as low as possible to minimize the development of air trapping. For this reason, approaches using IRV strategies are almost always contraindicated.

Because alveolar recruitment is less of an issue in obstructive lung injury compared with parenchymal lung injury, the PEEP-F_{IO_2} steps in Table 51.2 should probably be shifted to emphasize the F_{IO_2} for oxygenation support. Extrinsic PEEP becomes important in the obstructed patient when intrinsic PEEP produces an inspiratory threshold load on the patient attempting to trigger a breath. Under these conditions, judicious application of circuit PEEP (at levels up to 75%–85% of intrinsic PEEP) can balance expiratory pressure throughout the ventilator circuitry to reduce this triggering load and facilitate the triggering process (62,63) (Fig. 51.3).

In severe airflow obstruction, the use of low-density helium gas can help facilitate ventilator settings. Helium is available as 80:20, 70:30, or 60:40 helium/O_2 breathing gas mixtures and can both reduce patient inspiratory work and facilitate lung emptying (recall that driving pressure decreases and/or flow increases through a tube as gas density decreases) (87). Ventilator flow sensors may need to be calibrated to account for the change in gas density when using a helium/O_2 gas mixture.

Neuromuscular Respiratory Failure

The risk of VILI is generally reduced in a ventilated patient with neuromuscular failure because lung mechanics are often near normal, and regional overdistention is thus less likely to occur. More generous VT may be used to improve comfort, maintain recruitment, and prevent atelectasis in these individuals. Maximal distending pressures should still be monitored and should be kept as low as possible consistent with the goals noted above. $P_{aw_{plateau}}$ should always be kept below 30 cm H_2O.

Mode selection in neuromuscular disease patients is often determined by patient comfort. As in other patients, the rapid initial flow and the subsequent variable flow provided by pressure targeted modes is often more synchronous with patient efforts. This consideration must be weighed against the reliability of patient effort to consistently maintain a minute ventilation using pressure-targeted breaths. Volume targeting thus offers an advantage in patients with fluctuating ventilatory drives who may be prone to periods of hypoventilation or atelectasis. Low levels of PEEP help prevent derecruitment (atelectasis) in these patients who are often supine and incapable of secretion clearance or spontaneous sigh breaths.

Recovering Respiratory Failure: Weaning and Discontinuation Process

As respiratory failure stabilizes and begins to reverse, clinical attention shifts to the ventilator withdrawal process. Unfortunately, a number of large clinical trials have clearly demonstrated that current assessment/management strategies are not optimal, and considerable undue delay in ventilator withdrawal is the consequence. Increased length of stay, costs, exposure to pressure, and infection result. Attempts to increase withdrawal aggressiveness, however, must be balanced against the risk of premature withdrawal with consequent airway loss, aspiration, and ventilatory muscle fatigue.

A recent evidence-based task force (88) has recommended a two-step process. A ventilated patient may be considered a candidate for ventilator withdrawal if:

1. The lung injury is stable and/or resolving.
2. Gas exchange is adequate with low PEEP/F_{IO_2} requirements.
3. Hemodynamics are stable without a need for pressors.
4. There is the capability to initiate spontaneous breaths.

When these conditions are met, a spontaneous breathing trial (using T-piece, CPAP, or 5 cm H_2O pressure support) should be performed for 30 to 120 minutes. During this time, the ventilatory pattern, gas exchange, hemodynamics, and patient comfort should be assessed. Patients passing this trial should be considered for ventilator withdrawal.

In patients failing the spontaneous breathing trial, a stable and comfortable level of support should be provided (88). Complete muscle immobility (controlled ventilation) should be avoided, as atrophy and delayed fatigue recovery are theoretical risks. Frequent (q2–12h) ventilatory support reductions should be avoided, as they do not speed up the withdrawal process and only serve to consume resources and expose the patients to fatigue risks.

Partial ventilatory support modes may be used to provide patient comfort. By definition, these modes provide some, but not all, of the work of breathing. Ideally, these modes should provide adequate muscle unloading by providing breaths that are initiated promptly in accordance with patient demand. Accordingly, sensitive and responsive triggering systems should be used. Once the breath is initiated, a flow pattern that is synchronous with the patient's ventilatory demands should be provided.

RECENT INNOVATIONS IN MECHANICAL VENTILATORY SUPPORT

Innovative Strategies for Lung Protection

There are two recently introduced approaches to managing acute respiratory failure. APRV is a variation of pressure-controlled IRV (83,84), and pressure-regulated volume control (PRVC) places pressure-targeting features on the volume-assisted control mode (6).

Airway Pressure Release Ventilation

APRV is a time-cycled, pressure-targeted form of ventilatory support (83). It differs from conventional pressure control in that a pressure release mechanism allows spontaneous breathing to occur during both the inflation and deflation phases. Generally, APRV is used in a strategy of long inspiratory time ventilation and has sometimes been termed CPAP with release or upside-down intermittent mechanical ventilation. The purported advantages of this approach are as follows:

1. The long inflation phase recruits more slowly filling alveoli and raises mean airway pressure without increasing applied PEEP (although intrinsic PEEP can develop with short deflation periods). In this sense, it is similar in concept to older forms of IRV.
2. Additional spontaneous efforts during inflation may enhance both recruitment and cardiac filling compared with other controlled forms of support.
3. The availability of spontaneous breaths may make APRV more tolerable to patients than is pressure- or volume-controlled IRV.

Although IRV strategies are usually reserved for very severe forms of respiratory failure in which airway pressures and F_{IO_2} levels are approaching potentially injurious levels, the comfort and recruitment potential associated with APRV may prompt consideration of its use in less severe forms of lung injury.

Good gas exchange, often with lower maximal airway pressures than in control ventilation, has been demonstrated with APRV in several small observational clinical trials (83). However, the end-inspiratory lung distention in APRV may not be necessarily less than that provided during other forms of support (and, indeed, it could be substantially higher) because spontaneous V_T may occur while the lung is fully inflated by the APRV set pressure. Outcomes have not been routinely assessed in most of these trials, although the most recent reported benefits with APRV compared with a pressure control mode strategy (84). However, this observation is open to criticism because of small patient numbers, the control patients were "sicker" with more extensive ARDS, and different patient management strategies were used (routine paralysis was given for 3 days to the control group). More importantly, the control group was *not* ventilated using settings consistent with the current standard of care—the ARDS Network trial.

Pressure-Regulated Volume Control

Pressure-targeted, time-cycled ventilation uses V_T as a feedback control for continuously adjusting the pressure limit (6). The clinician is required to set a V_T target, and the ventilator will then automatically set the inspiratory pressure within a set range to achieve these goals. The ventilator will set off an alarm if the V_T and maximum pressure limit settings are incompatible.

Conceptually, this technique combines the enhanced gas mixing and patient ventilator synchrony effects of a pressure-targeted breath with a volume guarantee. Moreover, PRVC automatically reduces applied inspiratory pressure as respiratory system mechanics improve. However, it is important to realize that providing a volume guarantee negates the absolute pressure-limiting feature of a set pressure control level. Worsening respiratory system mechanics may drive applied pressures up. Another potential problem with PRVC is that during assisted breaths, if demand increases requiring a larger V_T, the pressure level will diminish. This reduction may not be beneficial depending on the cause of the respiratory failure.

True randomized controlled trials with PRVC using the ARDS Network protocol (81) as the gold standard do not exist. At the present time, PRVC use is based primarily on the physiologic concepts and theoretical advantages noted above.

Tracheal Gas Insufflation (TGI)

TGI utilizes a catheter placed at the distal end of the endotracheal tube to provide fresh gas to flush the endotracheal tube free of CO_2 during exhalation (89). The concept is that the next delivered breath will be free of endotracheal tube CO_2 and thus will have an effectively reduced dead space. This approach has particular appeal during lung-protective ventilatory strategies in which the $Paco_2$ is rising. A number of studies have shown that the TGI concept accomplishes

this physiologic goal of reduced dead space, but PEEP may increase (89).

TGI catheters can deliver fresh gas continuously or just during exhalation. The former approach is easier to implement, but the latter approach reduces the potential for excessive end-inspiratory overinflation. TGI catheters can also be designed to deliver gas directly into the lung or in a retrograde fashion back up the endotracheal tube. The former enhances gas mixing, but the latter reduces inadvertent PEEP buildup. At the present time, it is unclear how to best deliver TGI or whether TGI can significantly affect outcome. Clearly, however, TGI systems need to have safeguards to protect the lung from inadvertent overdistention (89).

High-Frequency Ventilation

High-frequency ventilation (HFV) uses very high breathing frequencies (120–300 breaths/min in the adult) coupled with very small V_T (often less than anatomic dead space) to provide gas exchange (90). Gas transport under these seemingly unphysiologic conditions involve such mechanisms as Taylor dispersion, coaxial flows, and augmented diffusion (91).

HFV can be supplied by either jets or oscillators. Jets inject high-frequency pulses of gas into the airways. Oscillators literally vibrate a fresh bias flow of gas delivered at the tip of the endotracheal tube (92).

The putative advantages to HFV are twofold. First, the high gas flow provides for considerable intrinsic PEEP and thus alveolar recruitment. This is particularly effective after RMs. Second, the very small tidal pressure swings keep the lung well below overdistention thresholds. Because of these features, HFV has sometimes been considered the ultimate lung-protection strategy (92,93).

Clinical experience with HFV has been most extensive in the neonatal and pediatric literature (90,94). Studies have suggested that HFV improves outcome in neonates at risk for overdistention injury (94). Experience with these devices in adults is much less; only recently have HFV devices been available to adequately support gas exchange in this population (95).

Automated Weaning Strategies

Over the years, a number of attempts have been made to automate the weaning process (6). An example is minimum minute ventilation, which adjusted the intermittent mandatory breath rate according to the level of spontaneous ventilation. The concept underlying these attempts was that significant clinician time could be saved, and appropriate ventilatory support reductions could be achieved based on simple ventilator measurements done in a timely fashion.

Volume support (VS) is the latest of these strategies to be used (6). VS is a dual control breath-to-breath pressure support mode that uses V_T as a feedback control for continuously adjusting the pressure support level. All breaths are patient triggered, pressure limited, and flow cycled, but the target V$_T$ is selected. Depending on the specific algorithm used, automatic adjustments in inspiratory pressure are made by the ventilator within a clinician prescribed range.

Proponents claim that this approach could automatically wean a patient by reducing pressure support as patient effort increases and respiratory system mechanics improve. Conversely, pressure support would increase if patient effort diminished or respiratory system mechanics worsened. Similarly, it has also been suggested that VS might be a useful way to maintain a more constant level of partial support in patients with fluctuating levels of effort related to drugs or neurological conditions. All of these effects have been demonstrated in small studies focused on patients with rapidly recovering respiratory failure (6,96).

Unfortunately, the simplicity of VS may produce problems. For instance, if the clinician set volume is excessive for patient demand, a recovering patient may not attempt to take over the work of breathing for that volume, and thus, support reduction and weaning may not progress. In addition, if the pressure level increases in an attempt to maintain an inappropriately high set V$_T$ in the patient with airflow obstruction, intrinsic PEEP may result. On the other hand, a patient may receive inadequate support if the clinician-set V$_T$ is not adequate for patient demand. Under these conditions, a patient will perform excessive work to maintain V$_T$, all the while the inspiratory pressure is being reduced because it exceeds the clinician setting.

Although no outcome studies have been performed using VS, there are specific clinical situations in which there may be some utility (fluctuating patient demand, rapidly recovering patient). However, clinicians need to be aware of the behavior of VS under a variety of circumstances to properly use this mode.

Optimizing Synchrony during Interactive Breaths

Interactive breaths are commonly used during mechanical ventilatory support to improve comfort and to allow sedation levels to be reduced, especially during the recovery phase of respiratory failure. Interactive breaths need to be synchronous with patient efforts during all three phases of breath delivery: trigger, flow delivery, and cycle. To this end, a number of recent innovations have been introduced.

It must be realized that although all of these innovations have conceptual appeal and have been shown to perform as designed in both bench testing and small clinical observational trials, patient outcomes—including sedation needs, ventilator days, or patient comfort assessments—have not been performed.

Automatic Tube Compensation

In this interactive mode, the endotracheal tube provides a measurable resistance to flow during both inspiration and expiration. During the inspiratory phase, this means that pressure buildup in the airways lags behind the pressure buildup in the ventilator circuitry. Thus, the square wave of pressure in the circuitry provided by a pressure-targeted breath is damped to a slower linear pressure rise in the airways. This may create significant initial flow dyssynchrony in patients with vigorous inspiratory efforts. During expiration, a similar gradient between airway pressures and set circuit PEEP can develop.

One way to address this is to target ventilator pressures to a measured tracheal pressure beyond the endotracheal tube. Unfortunately, the reliability of intra-airway pressure sensors over prolonged periods is not good. Another approach is to mathematically account for endotracheal tube resistance in the ventilator flow delivery pattern (96,97). This tends to create a decelerating pattern of delivered inspiratory airway pressure and an initial expiratory airway pressure below the set PEEP. A more square wave pattern of inspiratory and expiratory tracheal pressures is the result.

Applying automatic tube compensation is relatively straightforward. Endotracheal tube characteristics must be entered into the ventilator. Thereafter, the ventilator automatically provides the appropriate circuit pressure profile during both inspiration and expiration to create the desired square wave pattern in the trachea. Although outcome studies using automatic tube compensation have not been performed, the conceptual appeal makes it a consideration in virtually all patients receiving assisted/supported pressure-targeted breaths and especially those with vigorous inspiratory efforts.

Pressure-Targeted Inspiratory Pressure Slope Adjusters

The original design for pressure-targeted breath ventilators (pressure support and pressure assist-control) used a programmed flow-delivery algorithm that attempted to reach the target inspiratory pressure quickly, without causing a discomforting overshoot. Newer ventilators, however, have the capacity to adjust the pressure rate of rise (slope adjusters); clinical studies have suggested that such an adjustment significantly enhances flow synchrony in many patients (98). Specifically, these studies found that a rapid rate of rise of flow was often necessary to match vigorous flow demands, whereas a much slower rate of rise was often preferable in patients with less vigorous demands.

There are several approaches to setting the slope adjuster. The most direct way is to use the airway pressure graphic and adjust the slope to create a smooth square wave appearance in the airway pressure profile. Studies have also shown that an optimal slope setting correlates with the greatest V$_T$ for a given pressure setting (98). Patient comfort should always be considered in determining optimal slope settings.

Pressure Support Cycle Adjusters

Cycle dyssynchrony has recently been recognized as a problem occurring with the flow cycling mechanism of pressure support. In older ventilators, the set flow criteria was usually manufacturer determined (e.g., 25%–35% of peak flow). Although this was effective in most patients, the flow limit could sometimes terminate breaths too early in patients with high inspiratory demands, and it could sometimes terminate breaths too late, typically in patients with obstructive airway disease. In this latter situation, air trapping could also be made worse because of the resulting shorter expiratory time.

There are several approaches to improving cycle synchrony with pressure support. One is to switch from pressure support to a pressure assist breath (patient-triggered, pressure-targeted, time-cycled breath, usually available on most machines providing pressure ACV if the set rate is turned low or off). This breath provides direct clinician control of inspiratory time and, thus, cycling. Another strategy is to adjust the pressure slope setting (see section "Pressure-Targeted Inspiratory Pressure Slope Adjusters") described above on pressure support breaths. A very rapid peak initial flow will have a correspondingly high flow cycle variable (and thus a short inspiratory time); a very slow peak initial flow will have a correspondingly low flow cycle variable (and thus a long inspiratory time).

A newer, more direct approach, however, is to actually allow adjustments of the pressure support cycle flow criteria to assure appropriate synchrony of the cycle with the end of patient effort. As with other adjustments of interactive breaths, airway pressure graphics and assessments of patient comfort should guide adjustments. Proper breath synchrony is characterized by a comfortable patient and no evidence on the airway pressure graphic of expiratory effort during inspiration (delayed cycle) or continued inspiratory effort after cycling (premature cycling). Although no outcome studies have been performed using these cycle adjusters, their physiological appeal, ease of use, and apparent safety should make them a consideration in virtually every patient receiving pressure support.

Proportional Assist Ventilation

Proportional assist ventilation (PAV) is a novel approach to assisted ventilation that uses a set gain on patient-generated flow and volume (99). It thus does not apply a set pressure, flow, or volume. Instead, it boosts the sensed patient effort according to a clinician-set proportion. The greater the patient effort, the greater the delivered pressure, flow, and volume. This contrasts with volume assist, in which flow and volume are not affected by effort, and in fact, applied pressure may be pulled down by effort. PAV also contrasts with pressure assist/support, in which flow and volume are affected by effort but pressure is not.

PAV has been compared with other forms of assisted ventilation and has been found to be comparable in terms of muscle unloading and patient comfort (100). Commercial devices are not currently available, but it appears that both invasive and noninvasive (mask ventilator) versions will be available shortly. Whether PAV improves clinical outcomes remains to be determined.

CONCLUSIONS

Mechanical ventilatory support is a critical component of the management of patients with respiratory failure. It must always be remembered that this technology is supportive and not therapeutic. Mechanical ventilation cannot cure lung injury. Indeed, the best we can hope for is that it will buy time by supporting gas exchange without harming the lungs.

There are exciting innovations on the horizon that will require proper clinical assessment. Assessment will be particularly important for innovations that are associated with significant risks and/or costs. Only with properly conducted clinical trials using such relevant outcomes as mortality, ventilator-free days, barotrauma, and costs will we be able to properly assess the array of new approaches to this vital life-support technology.

REFERENCES

1. MacIntyre, NR. Mechanical ventilation: the next 50 years. *Respir Care* 1998;43:490–493.
2. Mushin M, Rendell-Baker W, Thompson PW, et al. *Automatic ventilation of the lungs.* Oxford: Blackwell Science, 1980:62–160.
3. American Society for Testing and Materials. *Standards specifications for ventilators intended for use in critical care.* Philadelphia: American Society for Testing and Materials, 1991:1123–1155.
4. Chatburn RL. Classification for mechanical ventilators. *Respir Care* 1992;37:1009–1025.
5. Essentials of mechanical ventilators. American Association for Respiratory Care Consensus Group. *Respir Care* 1992;37:1000–1008.
6. Branson RD, MacIntyre NR. Dual control modes of mechanical ventilation. *Respir Care* 1996;41:294–305.
7. MacIntyre, NR. Patient ventilator interactions: dyssynchrony and imposed loads. In: Marini J, Slutsky A, eds. *Physiologic basis of ventilatory support.* New York: Marcel Dekker Inc, 1997.
8. Sassoon Catherine SH. Mechanical ventilator design and unction: the trigger variable. *Respir Care* 1992;37:1056–1069.
9. Branson RD, Peterson BD, Carson KD, eds. Humidification: current therapy and controversy. *Respir Care Clin N Am* 1998;4:189–341.
10. Pinsky MR, Hrehocik D, Culpepper JA, et al. Flow resistance of expiratory positive pressure systems. *Chest* 1988;94:788–791.
11. Pepe PE, Marini JJ. Occult positive end-expiratory pressure in mechanically ventilated patients with airflow obstruction. *Am Rev Respir Dis* 1982;126:166–170.
12. Mehta S, Hill NS. Non-invasive ventilation in acute respiratory failure. *Respir Care Clin N Am* 1996;2:267–292.
13. Non-invasive positive pressure ventilation. American Association for Respiratory Care Consensus Group. *Respir Care* 1997;42:364–369.
14. Drinkwine J, Kacmarck R. Non-invasive positive pressure ventilation: equipment and techniques. *Respir Care Clin N Am* 1996;2:183–194.
15. Hess D. Aerosol therapy. *Respir Care Clin N Am* 1995;1:235–263.

16. Marini JJ. What derived variables should be monitored during mechanical ventilation? *Respir Care* 1992;37:1097–1107.

17. MacIntyre NR, Day S. Essentials for ventilator-alarm systems. *Respir Care* 1992;37:1108–1112.

18. Truwit JD, Marini JJ. Evaluation of thoracic mechanics in the ventilated patient, part I: primary measurements. *J Crit Care* 1988;3:133–150.

19. Truwit JD, Marini JJ. Evaluation of thoracic mechanics in the ventilated patient, part II: applied mechanics. *J Crit Care* 1988;3:192–213.

20. Marini JJ, Crooke PS. A general mathematical model for respiratory dynamics relevant to the clinical setting. *Am Rev Respir Dis* 1993;147:14–24.

21. Macklen PT. Relationship between lung mechanics and ventilation distribution. *Physiology* 1973;16:580–588.

22. Mili-Emili J, Henderson JAN, Dolovich MB, et al. Regional distribution of inhaled gas in the lung. *J Appl Physiol* 1966;21:749–759.

23. Abraham E, Yoshihara G. Cardiorespiratory effects of pressure controlled ventilation in severe respiratory failure. *Chest* 1990;98:1445–1449.

24. Pratt PC. Pathology of the adult respiratory distress syndrome. In: Thurlbeck WM, Ael MR, eds. *The Lung: structure, function and disease.* Baltimore: Williams & Wilkins, 1978:43–57.

25. Slutsky AS. Mechanical ventilation. American College of Chest Physicians' Consensus Conference. *Chest* 1993;104:1833–1859.

26. Kacmarek RM, Pierson DJ, eds. AARC conference on positive end expiratory pressure. *Respir Care* 1988;33:419–527.

27. Gattinoni L, Pesenti A, Baglioni S, et al. Inflammatory pulmonary edema and PEEP: correlation between imaging and physiologic studies. *J Thorac Imaging* 1988;3:59–64.

28. Gattinoni L, Pelosi P, Crotti S, et al. Effects of positive end expiratory pressure on regional distribution of tidal volume and recruitment in adult respiratory distress syndrome. *Am J Respir Crit Care Med* 1995;151:1807–1814.

29. Gattinoni L, Pelosi P, Suter P, et al. ARDS caused by pulmonary and extra pulmonary disease: different syndromes? *Am J Respir Crit Care Med* 1998;158:3–11.

30. Webb HJH, Tierney DF. Experimental pulmonary edema due to intermittent positive pressure ventilation with high inflation pressures: protection by positive end-expiratory pressure. *Am Rev Respir Dis* 1974;110:556–526.

31. Dreyfus D, Soler P, Bassett G, et al. High inflation pressure pulmonary edema. *Am Rev Respir Dis* 1988;137:1159–1164.

32. Muscedere JG, Mullen JB, Gan K, et al. Tidal ventilation at low airway pressures can augment lung injury. *Am J Respir Crit Care Med* 1994;149:1327–1334.

33. Wyszogrodski I, Kyei-Aboagye K, Taaeusch WH Jr, et al. Surfactant inactivation by hyperventilation: conservation by end-expiratory pressure. *J Appl Physiol* 1975;38:461–466.

34. Pinsky MR, Guimond JG. The effects of positive end-expiratory pressure on heart-lung interactions. *J Crit Care* 1991;6:1–15.

35. Crotti S, Mascheroni D, Caironi P, et al. Recruitment and derecruitment during acute respiratory failure. *Am J Respir Crit Care Med* 2001;164:131–140.

36. Rimensberger PC, Prisine G, Mullen BM, et al. Lung recruitment during small tidal volume ventilation allows minimal positive end expiratory pressure without augmenting lung injury. *Crit Care Med* 1999;27:1940–1945.

37. Chumello D, Pristine G, Slutsky AS. Mechanical ventilation affects local and systemic cytokines in an animal model of acute respiratory distress syndrome. *Am J Respir Crit Care Med* 1999;160:109–116.

38. Pelosi P, Cadringher P, Bottino N, et al. Sigh in acute respiratory distress syndrome. *Am J Respir Crit Care Med* 1999;159:872–880.

39. MacIntyre NR. Respiratory system mechanics. In: MacIntyre NR, Branson RD, ed. *Mechanical ventilation.* Philadelphia: WB Saunders, 2001.

40. Armstrong, BW, MacIntyre NR. Pressure controlled inverse ratio ventilation that avoids air trapping in ARDS. *Crit Care Med* 1995;23:279–285.

41. Cole AGH, Weller SF, Sykes MD. Inverse ratio ventilation compared with PEEP in adult respiratory failure. *Intensive Care Med* 1984;10:227–232.

42. Tharratt RS, Allen RP, Albertson TE. Pressure controlled inverse ratio ventilation in severe adult respiratory failure. *Chest* 1988;94:755–762.

43. Shanholtz C, Brower R. Should inverse ratio ventilation be used in ARDS? *Am J Respir Crit Care Med* 1994;149:1354–1358.

44. Samuelson WN, Fulerson WJ. Barotrauma in mechanical ventilation. *Problems in respiratory care.* Philadelphia: Lippincott–Raven Publishers 1991;4:52–67.

45. Kolobow T, Morentti MP, Fumagalli R, et al. Severe impairment in lung function induced by high peak airway pressure during mechanical ventilation. *Am Rev Respir Dis* 1987;135:312–315.

46. Dreyfuss D, Savmon G. Ventilator induced lung injury: lessons from experimental studies. *Am J Respir Crit Care Med* 1998; 157:294–323.

47. Trembly L, Valenza F, Ribiero SP, et al. Injurious ventilatory strategies increase cytokines and c-fos M-RNA expression in an isolated rat lung model. *J Clin Invest* 1997;99:944–952.

48. Ranieri VM, Suter PM, Totorella C, et al. Effect of mechanical ventilation on inflammatory mediators in patients with acute respiratory distress syndrome. *JAMA* 1999;282:54–61.

49. Nahum A, Hoyt J, Schmitz L, Moody J, et al. Effect of mechanical ventilation strategy on dissemination of intratracheally instilled *Escherichia coli* in dogs. *Crit Care Med* 1997;25:1733–1743.

50. Benito S, Lemaire F. Pulmonary pressure-volume relationship in acute respiratory distress syndrome in adults: role of positive and expiratory pressure. *J Crit Care* 1990;5:27–34.

51. Rich BR, Reickert CA, Sawada S, et al. Effect of rate and inspiratory flow on ventilator induced lung injury. *J Trauma* 2000; 49:903–911.

52. MacIntyre NR, Leatherman, NE. Mechanical loads on the ventilatory muscles. *Am Rev Respir Dis* 1989;144:968–973.

53. McGregor M, Bechlake MR. The relationship of oxygen cost of breathing to mechanical work and respiratory force. *J Clin Invest* 1961;40:971–980.

54. Bellemare F, Grassino A. Effect of pressure and timing of contraction on human diaphragm fatigue. *J Appl Physiol* 1982;53:1190–1195.

55. Banner MJ, Kirby RR, MacIntyre NR. Patient and ventilator work of breathing and ventilatory muscle loads at different levels of pressure support ventilation. *Chest* 1991;100:531–533.

56. Marini JJ. Exertion during ventilator support: how much and how important? *Respir Care* 1986;31:385–387.

57. MacIntyre NR. Weaning from mechanical ventilatory support: volume-assisting intermittent breaths versus pressure-assisting ever breath. *Respir Care* 1988;33:121–125.

58. Anzueto A, Peters JI, Tobin MJ, et al. Effects of prolonged controlled mechanical ventilation on diaphragmatic function in healthy adult baboons. *Crit Care Med* 1997;25:1187–1190.

59. MacIntyre NR. Patient-ventilator interactions. In: Grenvik A, ed. *Textbook of critical care medicine,* 4th ed. Philadelphia: WB Saunders, 1999.

60. Hansen-Flaschen J, Brazinsky S, Bassles C, et al. Use of sedating drugs and neuromuscular blockade in patients requiring mechanical ventilation for respiratory failure. *JAMA* 1991;266:2870–2875.

61. Sassoon CSH, Giron AE, Ely E, et al. Inspiratory work of breathing on flow-by and demand-flow continuous positive airway pressure. *Crit Care Med* 1989;17:1108–1114.

62. Petrof BJ, Legare M, Goldberg P, et al. Continuous positive airway pressure reduces work of breathing and dyspnea during weaning from mechanical ventilation in severe chronic obstructive pulmonary disease. *Am Rev Respir Dis* 1990;141:281–289.

63. MacIntyre NR, Cheng KC, McConnell R. Applied PEEP during pressure support threshold reduces the inspiratory load of intrinsic PEEP. *Chest* 1997;111:188–193.

64. Flick GR, Belamy PE, Simmons DH. Diaphragmatic contraction during assisted mechanical ventilation. *Chest* 1989;96:130–135.

65. Marini JJ, Smith TC, Lamb VJ. External work output and force generation during synchronized intermittent mechanical ventilation. *Am Rev Respir Dis* 1988;138:1169–1179.

66. Jubran A, Van de Graaf WB, Tobin MJ. Variability of patient ventilator interactions with pressure support ventilation in patients with chronic obstructive pulmonary disease. *Am J Respir Crit Care Med* 1995;152:129–136.

67. Marini JJ, Culver BH, Butler J. Mechanical effect of lung inflation with positive pressure on cardiac function. *Am Rev Respir Dis* 1979;124:382–386.

68. Scharf SM, Caldini P, Ingram RH Jr. Cardiovascular effects of increasing airway pressure in dogs. *Am J Physiol* 1977;232:1135–1143.

69. Pinsky MR, Summer WR, Wise RA, et al. Augmentation of cardiac function by elevation of intrathoracic pressure. *J Appl Physiol* 1983;54:450–455.

70. Hughes JM, Glazier JB, Maloney JE, et al. Effect of lung volume on the distribution of pulmonary blood flow in man. *Respir Physiol* 1968;4:58–72.

71. Lemaire F, Teboul JL, Cinotti L, et al. Acute left ventricular dysfunction during unsuccessful weaning from mechanical ventilation. *Anesthesiology* 1988;69:171–179.

72. Jenkinson SG. Oxygen toxicity. *New Horizons* 1993;1:504–511.

73. Betbese AJ, Perez M, Bak E, et al. A prospective study of unplanned endotracheal extubation in ICU patients. *Crit Care Med* 1998;26:1180–1186.

74. Craven DE, Kunches LM, Kilinsky V, et al. Risk factors for pneumonia and fatality in patients receiving continuous mechanical ventilation. *Am Rev Respir Dis* 1986;133:792–796.

75. Langer M, Mosconi P, Cigada M, et al. Long-term respiratory support and risk of pneumonia in critically ill patients. *Am Rev Respir Dis* 1989;140:302–305.

76. Fagon J, Chastre J, Domart Y, et al. Nosocomial pneumonia in patients receiving continuous mechanical ventilation. *Am Rev Respir Dis* 1989;139:877–884.

77. Kollef MH, Shapiro SD, Fraser VG, et al. Mechanical ventilation with or without seven day circuit change. *Ann Intern Med* 1995;123:168–174.

78. Mahjul P, Auboyer C, Jospe R, et al. Prevention of nosocomial pneumonia in intubated patients: respective role of mechanical subglottic secretion drainage and stress ulcer prophylaxis. *Intensive Care Med* 1992;18:20–25.

79. Hickling KG, Walsh J, Henderson S, et al. Low mortality rate in adult respiratory distress syndrome using low-volume, pressure-limited ventilation with permissive hypercapnia: a prospective study. *Crit Care Med* 1994;22:1568–1578.

80. Amato MB, Barbas CSV, Medievos DM, et al. Effect of a protective ventilation strategy on mortality in ARDS. *New Engl J Med* 1998;338:347–354.

81. NIH ARDS Network. Ventilation with lower tidal volumes as compared with traditional tidal volumes for acute lung injury and the acute respiratory distress syndrome. *New Engl J Med* 2000;342:1301–1308.

82. MacIntyre NR, McConnell R, Cheng KC, et al. Pressure limited breaths improve flow dyssynchrony during assisted ventilation. *Crit Care Med* 1997;25:167–171.

83. Stock MC, Downs JB, Frolicher DA. Airway pressure release ventilation. *Crit Care Med* 1987;15:462–466.

84. Putensen C, Zech S, Wrigge H, et al. Long term effects of spontaneous breathing during ventilatory support in patients with ALI. *Am J Respir Crit Care Med* 2001;164:43-49.

85. Putensen C, Bain M, Hormann C. Selecting ventilator settings according to the variables derived from the quasi static pressure volume relationship in patients with acute lung injury. *Anesth Analg* 1993;77:436–447.

86. Suter PM, Fairley HB, Isenberg MD. Optimum end expiratory pressure in patients with acute pulmonary failure. *N Engl J Med* 1975;292:284–289.

87. McConnell RR. Adjuncts to mechanical ventilation. In: MacIntyre NR, Branson RD, eds. *Mechanical ventilation.* Philadelphia: WB Saunders, 2001.

88. MacIntyre NR, Cook DJ, Ely EW Jr, et al. Evidence-based guidelines for weaning and discontinuing ventilatory support: a collective task force facilitated by the American College of Chest Physicians; the American Association for Respiratory Care; and the American College of Critical Care Medicine. *Chest* 2001;120 [6 Suppl]:375S–395S.

89. Hess, DR, MacIntyre NR. Tracheal gas insufflation: overcoming obstacles to clinical implementation. *Respir Care* 2001;46:198–199.

90. Froese AB, Bryan C. High frequency ventilation. *Am Rev Respir Dis* 1987;135:1363–1374.

91. Chang HK. Mechanisms of gas transport during high frequency ventilation. *J Appl Physiol* 1984;56:553–563.

92. MacIntyre NR. High frequency ventilation. In: Tobin M, ed. *Mechanical ventilation: principles and practice.* New York: McGraw-Hill, 1994.

93. Froese AB. High frequency oscillatory ventilation for ARDS: let's get it right this time. *Crit Care Med* 1997;25:906–908.

94. Keszler M, Donn SM, Bucciarelli RL, et al. Multicenter controlled trial comparing HFJV and conventional mechanical ventilation in newborns with PIE. *J Pediatr* 1991;119:85–93.

95. Mehta S, Lapinsky SE, Hallett DC, et al. Prospective trial of high frequency oscillation in adults with acute respiratory distress syndrome. *Crit Care Med* 2001;29:1360–1369.

96. MacIntyre NR. Invasive mechanical ventilation in adults: conference summary. *Respir Care* 2002;47:508–518.

97. Fabry B, Zappe D, Guttman J. Breathing pattern and additional work of breathing in spontaneously breathing patients with different ventilatory demand during inspiratory pressure support and automatic tube compensation. *Intensive Care Med* 1997;23:545–552.

98. Ho L, MacIntyre NR. Effects of initial flow rate and breath termination criteria on pressure support ventilation. *Chest* 1991;99:134–138.

99. Younes M. Proportional assist ventilation, a new approach to ventilatory support. *Am Rev Respir Dis* 1992;145:114–120.

100. Grasso S, Ranieri VM. Proportional assist ventilation. *Respir Care Clin N Am* 2001;7:465–473.

Weaning from Ventilatory Support

52

Scott K. Epstein

Invasive mechanical ventilation has beneficial effects on the pathophysiology of acute respiratory failure by increasing delivered fraction of inspired oxygen (FIO_2), re-expanding atelectatic lung, and providing adequate alveolar ventilation. However, invasive mechanical ventilation is also associated with significant risks and complications, including sinusitis, airway injury, thromboembolism, and gastrointestinal bleeding (1). The risk for the most serious complication, ventilator-associated pneumonia, increases with the duration of intubation and appears to contribute to excess mortality (2,3). Therefore, as soon as significant clinical improvement occurs, efforts shift toward rapidly removing the patient from the ventilator.

The process of freeing a patient from mechanical ventilation has been referred to as weaning, but more recently, it has been termed liberation or discontinuation (4,5). The process begins with readiness testing, the recognition that respiratory failure has resolved (partially or completely), respiratory muscle function has been restored, and the patient is ready to undertake trials of spontaneous breathing (SBTs). Although the process will likely be instituted by a physician, increasing evidence indicates that its implementation can be performed by respiratory care practitioners and intensive care unit (ICU) nurses.

Approximately 75% of patients satisfying weaning readiness criteria tolerate an initial SBT, conducted either without ventilator assistance or on low levels of support. These individuals may be safely extubated (6–10) (Fig. 52.1). The remaining minority of patients are initially intolerant of spontaneous breathing and require a gradual process (progressive withdrawal) in which there is a step-by-step shifting of the work of breathing from machine to patient. For these patients, the weaning process can consume 40% of the total time spent on the mechanical ventilator (60% for chronic obstructive pulmonary disease [COPD]) (11,12). Facilitating liberation from the ventilator will depend on identifying and correcting reversible causes for weaning failure. In either case, once spontaneous breathing is tolerated, the clinician must address the separate question of whether the artificial airway (endotracheal tube) is still required or may be removed (Fig. 52.2).

ASSESSMENT OF READINESS

Recently, a set of guidelines for weaning and discontinuing ventilatory support based on a comprehensive evidence-based literature review conducted by the McMaster University Evidence-Based Practice Center has been published (13). In all cases, rapid liberation from mechanical ventilation must be balanced against the risks of premature SBTs. Animal investigations and observational studies in humans suggest that respiratory muscle fatigue may develop during unsuccessful weaning, possibly predisposing to structural respiratory muscle injury and ultimate prolongation of mechanical ventilation (14–21). Weaning failure may also precipitate cardiac dysfunction or be psychologically disturbing to the patient.

An assessment of readiness may commence within hours of the initiation of mechanical ventilation in patients intubated for rapidly reversible processes (e.g., cardiogenic pulmonary edema, some drug overdoses). For other causes of acute respiratory failure, full ventilatory support and respiratory muscle rest should be maintained for 24 to 48 hours before evaluating the patient for a SBT. Subjective assessment alone appears to be insufficient to identify patients appropriate for SBTs (22,23). Subjective criteria to assess

S. K. Epstein: Medical Intensive Care Unit, Pulmonary, Critical Care and Sleep Divisions, New England Medical Center, and Tufts University School of Medicine, Boston, Massachusetts.

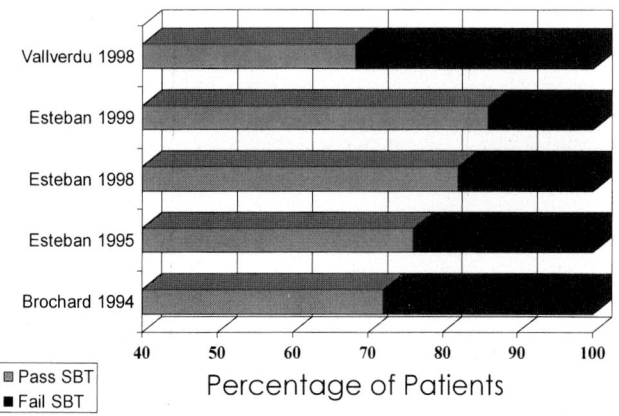

FIGURE 52.1. Percentage of patients passing or failing a trial of spontaneous breathing (SBT) after satisfying readiness criteria.

TABLE 52.1. CRITERIA USED TO DETERMINE READINESS FOR TRIALS OF SPONTANEOUS BREATHING

Required criteria (used by all investigators)
1. $Pao_2/Fio_2 \geq 150^*$ or $Sao_2 \geq 90\%$ on $Fio_2 \leq 40\%$ and PEEP ≤ 5 cm H_2O
2. Hemodynamic stability (no or low-dose vasopressor medications, e.g., dopamine ≤ 5 mcg/[kg · min]) and no active cardiac ischemia

Additional criteria (optional criteria, used by some investigators)
1. Weaning parameters: respiratory rate ≤ 35 breaths/min, spontaneous tidal volume >5 mL/kg, negative inspiratory force <-20 to -25 cm H_2O, f/V_T <105 breaths/(L · min)
2. Hemoglobin ≥ 8–10 mg/DL
3. Core temperature $\leq 38°$–$38.5°$
4. Normal electrolytes
5. Mental status awake and alert or easily arousable

---

*A threshold of $Pao_2/Fio_2 \geq 120$ may be appropriate for patients with chronic hypoxemia. Some patients require higher levels of PEEP (5–8 cm H_2O) to avoid atelectasis during mechanical ventilation.
Pao_2, arterial blood partial pressure of oxygen; Fio_2, fraction of inspired oxygen; Sao_2, arterial oxygen saturation; PEEP, positive end-expiratory pressure; f/V_T, frequency/tidal volume ratio.

patient readiness for spontaneous breathing should be supplemented (6,24), or may be replaced (25,26), by objective assessments that serve as surrogate markers of recovery (Table 52.1). These objective assessments should serve as guidelines rather than rigid criteria because one large randomized controlled trial demonstrated that 30% of patients *never* satisfying objective readiness criteria were still ultimately weaned from mechanical ventilation (27). Another prospective study showed that depressed neurological status (assessed by Glasgow coma scale) in brain-injured patients was not associated with an inability to successfully wean (86). Lastly, a retrospective analysis of a large randomized trial observed that patients managed with a restrictive blood transfusion strategy (goal hemoglobin of 7–9 mg/dL) had the same duration of mechanical ventilation and probability of successful weaning as patients transfused liberally to achieve a hemoglobin greater than 10 mg/d (28). Thus, weaning trials

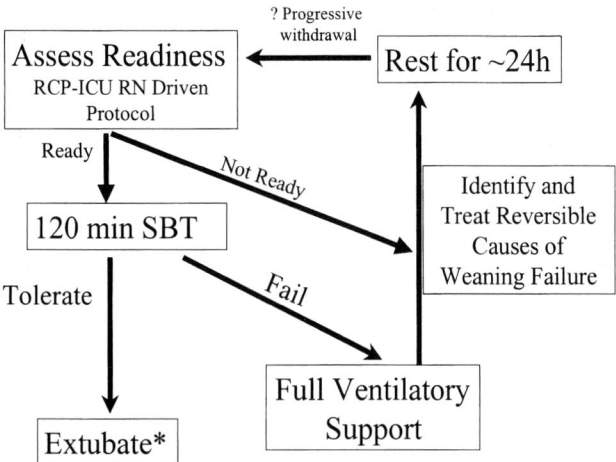

FIGURE 52.2. Overview of the process of weaning a patient from mechanical ventilation. *Extubation is performed if the patient has no evidence of upper airway obstruction, is without excessive airway secretions, and has an adequate cough. RCP, respiratory care practitioner; ICU-RN, intensive care unit nurse; SBT, spontaneous breathing trial. (Adapted from Epstein SK. Weaning from mechanical ventilation. *Respir Care* 2002;47:454–466, with permission.)

should be undertaken even if objective readiness criteria are not completely satisfied.

Various objective physiologic criteria *(weaning predictors)* and their role in assessing readiness have been extensively reevaluated. Important design problems in previous observational studies of weaning predictors have been identified (13,28,29): Weaning predictors were frequently used a priori to determine which patients underwent weaning; measurement techniques and timing differed among studies and were subject to large coefficients of variations; physicians determining weaning tolerance were not adequately blinded to the prediction variables; and there often were absent objective weaning tolerance criteria. These factors inflated the purported accuracy of weaning predictors.

Ideally, decisions regarding weaning based on clear weaning predictors would accelerate liberation from mechanical ventilation while avoiding the adverse consequences of failed weaning trials. Numerous weaning predictors have been investigated over the past three decades (Table 52.2). A comprehensive evidence-based medicine review concluded that relatively few of these predictors were useful in leading to clinically significant changes in the probability of weaning success or failure (13,29). Only five predictors (negative inspiratory force; maximal inspiratory pressure; minute ventilation; airway occlusion pressure/maximal inspiratory pressure; compliance, respiratory rate, oxygenation, pressure [CROP index]) obtained during ventilatory support had possible value in predicting weaning outcome (13). Of these, only the latter two had likelihood ratios suggesting clinical utility, but the small number of patients studied precludes recommending their universal application. The likelihood ratio (LR) is the odds that a given test result will be present (or absent) with a given condition compared with when the condition is absent. When LR >1, the probability of weaning success increases. When

TABLE 52.2. TESTS USED TO PREDICT WEANING OUTCOME (WEANING PREDICTORS)

Measurements of oxygenation and gas exchange
  Pao_2/Fio_2
  Pao_2/Pao_2
  Dead space, V_D/V_T
Simple measurements of respiratory load and muscular capacity
  Negative inspiratory force
  Respiratory system compliance
  Respiratory system resistance
  Minute ventilation
  Respiratory frequency
  Tidal volume
  Maximal voluntary ventilation
  Vital capacity
Measurements integrating multiple factors
  f/V_T
  CROP index (compliance, respiratory rate, oxygenation, pressure)
Complex measurements requiring special equipment
  Airway occlusion pressure
  $P_{0.1}$/maximal inspiratory pressure
  Work of breathing
  Oxygen cost of breathing
  Gastric intramucosal pH

Pao_2, arterial blood partial pressure of oxygen; Fio_2, fraction of inspired oxygen; Pao_2, alveolar partial pressure of oxygen; V_D/V_T, dead space volume/tidal volume; f/V_T, frequency/tidal volume ratio.

LR <1, the probability of weaning success decreases. Three other parameters (respiratory frequency, tidal volume, frequency/tidal volume ratio [f/V_T]), measured during 1 to 3 minutes of unassisted breathing, were more accurate, but even these tests were associated with only small to moderate changes in the probability of predicting weaning success or failure. A preliminary report of a randomized controlled trial of 304 patients indicated that application of a weaning

ASSESSMENT OF READINESS: USING CLINICAL FACTORS AND WEANING PREDICTORS

Summary Statement	Level of Evidence
Assessment of readiness for trials of spontaneous breathing should be based primarily on adequate oxygenation and hemodynamic stability.	Multiple large, randomized, and observational studies
The majority (~70%) of patients satisfying readiness criteria will tolerate their first spontaneous trial and do not require a slow progressive withdrawal from ventilatory support.	Multiple large, randomized, and observational studies
Under most circumstances, weaning predictors are minimally helpful in deciding whether or not to initiate spontaneous breathing trials or reduce the level of ventilatory support. If a weaning predictor is to be used, the frequency/tidal volume ratio appears to be the most accurate.	Comprehensive evidence-based literature review and metaanalysis

predictor (f/V_T) to determine the daily readiness for SBTs tended to impede the process of liberation (30). Although all weaning predictors studied to date have limited positive predictive value, we believe that they may aid decision making in situations in which the risks associated with weaning failure are prohibitively high. In addition, they may help identify reversible causes of weaning intolerance. It is important to note that SBTs appear to be very well tolerated, as only a single patient experienced a clinically detectable weaning complication in a study of more than 1,000 patients (31). This supports the concept that objectively based weaning predictors should not routinely be used to deny a weaning trial.

FORMAL READINESS TESTING

Ventilated patients should undergo formal weaning readiness testing by breathing spontaneously on low levels of pressure support (pressure-support ventilation [PSV] <7 cm H_2O) (7), continuous positive airway pressure (32), or unassisted through a T-piece (7). A SBT is generally mandatory because nearly 40% of patients directly extubated after satisfying readiness criteria alone require reintubation (33).

The optimal form of the SBT has been debated. Proponents of the T-piece method argue that it best approximates the postextubation work of breathing (34–37). In contrast, other experts prefer low levels of pressure support to counterbalance the resistive workload imposed by a narrow endotracheal tube (38). The pressure support level required to offset this imposed load varies widely (3–14 cm H_2O) and cannot be accurately determined noninvasively. Therefore, in any individual patient, a given level of pressure support may either overcompensate or undercompensate for the imposed work (39). Randomized trials comparing pressure support to T-piece, and continuous positive airway pressure to T-piece have shown the techniques to be roughly equivalent in weaning and extubation success (7,32,40). There are, however, practical advantages to performing a SBT through the ventilator: No additional equipment is required; ventilator alarm and monitoring systems can be used to promptly identify the patient who is intolerant of weaning; and, if needed, ventilatory support can be simply and rapidly reestablished. Further, in a randomized trial of 484 patients, the SBT failure rate was higher for the T-piece compared with the pressure support technique (22% versus 14%), suggesting that imposed work causes weaning failure in some patients (7).

The ability to spontaneously breathe for 120 minutes generally indicates that ventilatory support is no longer required (6–8,10,24). The minimal duration of the initial SBT is still unknown. One study found no difference in the weaning success rate in patients randomized to either 30 or 120 minutes of T-piece breathing (8). Of note, these investigators examined only the first attempt at spontaneous breathing. The ideal duration for subsequent SBTs or for trials performed with partial support modes also remains unknown,

TABLE 52.3. CRITERIA INDICATING THAT A PATIENT IS TOLERATING A TRIAL OF SPONTANEOUS BREATHING

Objective criteria
1. $Sao_2 \geq 0.90$ or $Pao_2 \geq 60$ mm Hg on $Fio_2 \leq 0.40–0.50$ or $Pao_2/Fio_2 > 150$
2. Increase in $Paco_2 \leq 10$ mm Hg or decrease in pH ≤ 0.10
3. Respiratory rate ≤ 35 breaths/min
4. Heart rate ≤ 140 bpm or an increase $\leq 20\%$ of baseline
5. Systolic blood pressure ≥ 90 mm Hg or ≤ 160 mm Hg or change of $<20\%$ from baseline

Subjective criteria
1. Absence of signs of increased work of breathing, including thoracoabdominal paradox or excessive use of accessory respiratory muscles
2. Absence of other signs of distress such as diaphoresis or agitation

Sao_2, arterial oxygen saturation; Pao_2, arterial blood partial pressure of oxygen; Fio_2, fraction of inspired oxygen; $Paco_2$, arterial blood partial pressure of carbon dioxide.

but it may be longer than 120 minutes. As an example, a study of 75 COPD patients, ventilated for at least 15 days, found a *median* time to trial failure of 120 minutes (41).

Careful patient assessment while he or she undergoes a SBT is critically important and should be based on both objective and subjective criteria (Table 52.3). Although there are generally accepted criteria, optimal thresholds have not been identified. Nonspecific criteria include tachypnea and tachycardia; these may occur because of psychological distress rather than from true physiologic weaning intolerance. Specific criteria include oximetry, partial pressure of oxygen and carbon dioxide levels, and the absence of clinical signs indicative of increased work of breathing. Criteria may be insufficiently sensitive in detecting incipient respiratory failure. For example, some patients with postextubation respiratory failure had either electromyographic evidence of diaphragmatic fatigue (42) or a chaotic pattern of breathing (43) during a successful pre-extubation SBT.

READINESS TESTING

Summary Statement	Level of Evidence
Readiness testing is best performed with a 120-min spontaneous breathing trial conducted on T-piece or on low levels of CPAP or pressure support. (In some circumstances, a 30-min T-piece trial is adequate.) Tolerance for the trial signals readiness for liberation from mechanical ventilation.	Multiple randomized trials
Tolerance for the spontaneous breathing trial is assessed by monitoring vital signs, oximetry, gas exchange, and absence of clinical signs indicative of increased work of breathing.	Multiple large prospective trials

CPAP, continuous positive airway pressure.

CAUSES OF WEANING FAILURE

As many as one third of patients fail the initial SBT and require a more prolonged weaning process. When failure occurs, a thorough search for the underlying cause with the goal of identifying, and ultimately treating, reversible factors should be undertaken (Fig. 52.3). Hypoxemia is an unusual cause of weaning failure because adequate oxygenation (e.g., arterial partial pressure of oxygen/$Fio_2 > 150$) is a prerequisite for initiating a SBT. When hypoxemia develops during weaning, it likely is secondary to another underlying mechanism for failure.

Depressed central respiratory drive occasionally contributes to weaning intolerance, although more commonly it leads to a delay in the initiation of weaning (44,45). Typically, patients with weaning failure display evidence of an elevated respiratory drive (46–48). Tobin and colleagues reported an elevated mean inspiratory flow (a measure of respiratory drive) at the termination of a failed T-piece trial (48). Similarly, the airway occlusion pressure ($P_{0.1}$), another measure of respiratory drive, is often elevated in patients failing weaning to levels observed in individuals with acute respiratory failure (46). This heightened respiratory drive is likely owing to a mismatch between reduced respiratory muscle capacity and the increased load placed on the system; this load-capacity imbalance may be the most common cause for weaning failure. An excessive load can also be imposed by the endotracheal tube, heat and moisture exchange devices, or the ventilator tubing and valves (49–51). More commonly, factors intrinsic to the patient are responsible. Jubran and Tobin, studying 31 COPD patients at the onset of a SBT, observed higher perceived loads (increased resistance, elastance, and intrinsic positive end-expiratory pressure [PEEP]) in those who failed the trial and also noted that the loads progressively increased to trial termination (17). Rapid shallow breathing was also observed, a response that can worsen dynamic hyperinflation and increase work related to intrinsic PEEP. An investigation of 30 acute respiratory failure patients (using each patient as his or her own control) found markedly elevated inspiratory loads (increased intrinsic PEEP, resistance, tension-time index) and reduced respiratory muscle capacity ($P_I max$) in those who failed weaning (19).

Decreased respiratory muscle strength is frequently observed in patients unable to wean. A number of mechanisms have been identified or postulated, including phrenic nerve injury after cardiac surgery (52), reduced diaphragmatic pressure generation resulting from dynamic hyperinflation, muscle remodeling resulting from inactivity (53), muscle atrophy in cases in which neuromuscular blocking agents have been used (54), neuropathy resulting from critical illness (55), and metabolic abnormalities (e.g., hypothyroidism) or malnutrition. Cohen and colleagues suggested that respiratory muscle fatigue was an important manifestation of weaning failure (16). They observed tachypnea, thoracoabdominal paradox, and an increase in the high/low frequency ratio measured

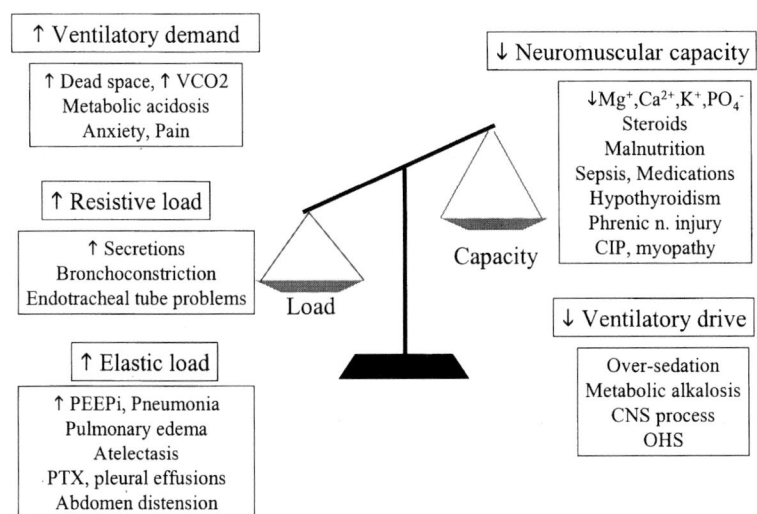

FIGURE 52.3. Weaning failure is usually secondary to an imbalance between the load placed on the respiratory system and the respiratory neuromuscular capacity. Vco_2, carbon dioxide production; PEEPi, intrinsic positive end-expiratory pressure; PTX, pneumothorax; Mg^+, magnesium; Ca^{++}, calcium; K^+, potassium; PO_4^-, phosphorus; CIP, critical illness polyneuropathy; CNS, central nervous system; OHS, obesity hypoventilation syndrome.

by diaphragmatic electromyography in a cohort of patients intolerant of weaning. Subsequently, Tobin and colleagues found that rapid shallow breathing and thoracoabdominal paradox appeared immediately but did not worsen during failed weaning, suggesting that failure was owing to increased loading conditions rather than to a manifestation of muscle fatigue (56). This hypothesis was confirmed when it was demonstrated that normals subjected to a load can develop thoracoabdominal paradox in the absence of fatigue (57). In contrast, Jubran and Tobin and Vassilakopoulos and colleagues found a tension-time index exceeding the 0.15 threshold at which respiratory muscle fatigue occurs during failed weaning trials (17,19). They may have overestimated the tension–time index because the $P_I$max may have been falsely low secondary to poor patient effort. By using the twitch occlusion technique, with magnetic stimulation of the phrenic nerve, Laghi and colleagues found that respiratory muscle fatigue occurred infrequently during a well-monitored SBT (18). Thus, the importance of respiratory muscle fatigue as a cause of weaning failure is questionable.

Weaning intolerance can also occur because of myocardial dysfunction (59–62). Lemaire and colleagues observed that the transition from positive pressure ventilation to spontaneous breathing (e.g., negative intrathoracic pressure) in patients with COPD and cardiac disease, resulted in marked increases in transmural pulmonary artery occlusion pressure and clinical pulmonary edema (61). Large negative swings in intrathoracic pressure increase both left ventricular preload and afterload. A decrease in left ventricular ejection fraction has been observed in COPD patients undergoing T-pieced trials, an effect that can be partially offset by the use of pressure support (62). Cardiac ischemia can occur during weaning trials, as demonstrated in studies using nuclear techniques (63). By using continuous electrocardiography, ischemia was noted in 6% of medical and cardiac patients

during SBTs (59). Cardiac ischemia can result from intrathoracic pressure changes (affecting cardiac loading conditions), diversion of coronary blood flow to the working respiratory muscles, or the adverse effects of increased catecholamine release on myocardial oxygen consumption.

Psychological factors can limit weaning. Criteria generally used to indicate weaning intolerance (e.g., agitation, diaphoresis, tachycardia, and tachypnea) can also be manifestations of anxiety or psychological distress. Small uncontrolled studies have found that biofeedback, relaxation techniques, hypnosis, or therapy for depression (using methylphenidate) contributed to successful weaning (64–67). In a randomized controlled trial of 40 patients, relaxation biofeedback using frontalis and respiratory muscle electromyography reduced the duration of mechanical ventilation (68). Delirium is present in the majority of ventilated patients, and its presence is correlated with prolonged duration of intubation (69). Randomized controlled trials evaluating agents aimed at reversing delirium should be available in the near future.

CAUSES OF WEANING FAILURE

Summary Statement	Level of Evidence
Weaning intolerance most often results from an imbalance between respiratory muscle capacity and respiratory load, cardiac dysfunction, or psychological causes.	Multiple prospective, observational, and physiologic studies
Patients failing spontaneous breathing trials or those intolerant of reductions in ventilatory support should undergo extensive evaluation to identify reversible causes.	Experimental evidence, based on some prospective studies and expert opinion

TABLE 52.4. EXAMPLE OF TREATMENTS AIMED AT REVERSING THE CAUSES OF WEANING FAILURE

Cause	Examples of Treatment	Comment
Increased ventilatory demand	Reduce CO_2 production by suppressing fever and avoiding overfeeding; reduce dead space by treating hypovolemia; treat sepsis; give $NaHCO_3$ for severe metabolic acidosis	Presence suggested by $V_E > 15$ L/min
Increased resistive load	Administer bronchodilators or steroids; antibiotics for respiratory tract infection; airway suctioning for secretions; place larger endotracheal tube	Presence suggested by measured airway resistance $>15–20$ cm $H_2O/(L \cdot s)$
Increased elastic load	Diuretics for increased lung water; drainage of pleural fluid and air; decompression of abdomen with NG tube, paracentesis; bronchodilators to reduce PEEPi; treat pneumonia	Presence suggested by clinical examination, chest radiograph, and respiratory system compliance $<50–70$ mL/cm H_2O
Decreased neuromuscular capacity	Correct electrolyte abnormalities; minimize use of NMBAs; provide adequate nutrition; treat sepsis and hypothyroidism	Presence suggested by poor maximal inspiratory pressure (>-20 to -30 cm H_2O)
Decreased ventilatory drive	Use a sedation algorithm to avoid oversedation; correct metabolic alkalosis with diamox	Presence suggested by unexplained hypercapnia, respiratory frequency <12 breaths/min.

*An imbalance between respiratory load and neuromuscular capacity is also suggested by an elevated respiratory frequency/tidal volume ratio (>100 breaths/[L $\cdot$ min]) or increased airway occlusion pressure ($P_{0.1} >4–6$ cm H_2O).
CO_2, carbon dioxide; $NaHCO_3$, sodium bicarbonate; V_E, minute ventilation; NG, nasogastric; PEEPi, intrinsic positive end-expiratory pressure; NMBAs, neuromuscular blocking agents.

MODES OF PROGRESSIVE WITHDRAWAL

Once the factors limiting weaning are corrected, further efforts to liberate the patient from ventilation are indicated (Table 52.4). Before deciding on the weaning approach, the clinician must decide how long to rest the patient before initiating further attempts at liberation. Laghi and colleagues found that volunteers subjected to a fatiguing inspiratory load required 24 or more hours to fully recover diaphragmatic strength (18). Yet, these same investigators noted that respiratory muscle fatigue is relatively uncommon in patients failing a SBT (58). Indeed, a large randomized controlled study found no difference in outcome between patients undergoing multiple daily SBTs and those undergoing a single daily trial (with 24 hours of rest before the next attempt) (24).

The clinician must next decide whether to perform another SBT or whether to institute a gradual reduction in ventilatory support. The latter approach, termed progressive withdrawal, theoretically slowly shifts work from the ventilator to the patient until tolerance to minimal support signals readiness for liberation. This process, which can be performed using any of several techniques, is designed to avoid respiratory muscle fatigue. Whether this process reconditions (or trains) the respiratory muscles or merely allows more time for further recovery (e.g., reduction in the respiratory load) remains uncertain.

Two large multicenter randomized trials directly compared different progressive withdrawal techniques in patients who satisfied readiness criteria but failed to tolerate a 2-hour SBT (6,24) (Table 52.5). Brochard and colleagues found that pressure support reduced the duration of weaning when compared with that for T-piece *and* synchronized inter-

mittent mandatory ventilation (SIMV) groups (5.7 versus 9.3 days) and was more likely to be associated with weaning success (6). In contrast, Esteban and colleagues also included a strategy of daily SBTs (T-piece) with maintenance on full ventilatory support during intervening periods (24). The T-piece (either once daily or multiple daily trials) technique shortened the median duration of mechanical ventilation when compared with progressive withdrawal with pressure support or SIMV (3 versus 4 versus 5 days) (24). Much has been made of the conflicting results of these studies. Though differences in patient populations and study design may explain the contrasting results, the institution of a daily SBT is likely to have accelerated the process of weaning. An additional major contribution of these studies was the demonstration that SIMV alone slows the weaning process. Similarly, physiologic investigations demonstrate that the degree of respiratory muscle rest achieved with SIMV is *not* proportional to the level of ventilatory support (70,71). For example, during lower levels of SIMV, respiratory muscle contraction was similar during both intervening (unsupported) and mandatory (supported) breaths, indicating that the neuromuscular apparatus poorly adapts to changing loads (70). By adding PSV to the unsupported breaths during SIMV, reductions in work are achieved for the intervening *and* mandatory breaths (72). Indeed, a very small randomized trial of 19 patients with COPD found that patients weaned by SIMV/PSV were liberated more quickly than were patients weaned by SIMV alone (73). To date, no studies are available that examine the utility of combining progressive withdrawal with daily SBTs.

A number of new modes are available on modern ICU ventilators, including volume support, volume-assured pressure support, adaptive support ventilation, and automatic

TABLE 52.5. COMPARISON OF TWO LARGE RANDOMIZED CONTROLLED TRIALS THAT EXAMINED THE BEST APPROACH TO PROGRESSIVE WITHDRAWAL

	Brochard	Esteban
Number of patients screened	456	546
Number randomized	109	130
Duration of mechanical ventilation before randomization	14 d	9 d
Strategies tested	PSV SIMV T-piece (once daily)	PSV SIMV T-piece (once daily) T-piece (multiple daily)
Protocol	PSV: ↓ by 2–4 cm H_2O, twice a day SIMV: ↓ by 2–4 breaths/min, twice a day T-piece: progressively increase to 2 h	PSV: ↓ by 2–4 cm H_2O, twice a day SIMV: ↓ by 2–4 breaths/min, twice a day T-piece (once): as tolerated up to 2 h T-piece (multiple): T-piece or CPAP 5 cm H_2O as tolerated multiple times per day (up to 2 h per trial)
Criteria for success	PSV: 8 cm H_2O for 24 h SIMV: 4 breaths/min for 24 h T-piece: 2 h (1–3 times/24 h)	PSV: 5 cm H_2O for 2 h SIMV: 5 breaths/min for 2 h T-piece: 2 h (once)
Outcome assessed	21 d	14 d
Results	1. PSV decreased percentage of patients with weaning failure (23% versus T-piece 43%, SIMV 42%) 2. Shorter mean duration of weaning with PSV (5.7 d) compared with pooled T-piece and SIMV patients (9.3 d)	1. Weaning failure: once daily T-piece (29%), multiple daily T-piece (18%), PSV (38%), SIMV (31%) 2. Shorter median duration of weaning with T-piece, once (3 d) and T-piece, multiple (3 d) compared with PSV (4 d) and SIMV (5 d)

PSV, pressure-supported ventilation; SIMV, synchronized intermittent mandatory ventilation; CPAP, continuous positive airway pressure.
From Epstein SK. Weaning from mechanical ventilation. *Respir Care* 2002;47:454–466, with permission.

tube compensation. To date, there is no randomized controlled data indicating that these dual control or closed-loop forms of ventilation facilitate the process of weaning compared with the techniques discussed above (74).

There is overwhelming evidence that noninvasive ventilation (NIV) can effectively treat acute respiratory failure complicating COPD (75,76). A number of uncontrolled trials indicate that NIV could be used to facilitate weaning in this population. Nava and colleagues studied 50 intubated COPD patients with acute on chronic hypercapnic respiratory failure (mean arterial partial pressure of carbon dioxide ~90 mm Hg). Patients failing a T-piece trial were randomized to standard pressure support weaning or immediate extubation to noninvasive PSV using a full face mask and a standard ICU ventilator (77). The noninvasive strategy resulted in statistically significant reductions in the duration of mechanical ventilation, length of ICU stay, and 60-day survival. An additional investigation of 53 patients with acute on chronic respiratory failure (approximately one half with COPD) found that NIV led to reduced duration of invasive mechanical ventilation, although other outcomes were equivalent (78). The benefits of NIV include a reduction in the rate of ventilator-associated pneumonias, lower sedation requirements, and better recognition of the readiness for extubation, particularly when psychological factors or the imposed work of breathing are contributing to weaning failure. Larger studies that include patients with other forms of respiratory failure are required before this technique can be generally recommended.

MODES OF PROGRESSIVE WITHDRAWAL

Summary Statement	Level of Evidence
To facilitate weaning, daily spontaneous breathing trials are preferred to slow reductions in ventilatory support. Multiple daily spontaneous breathing trials are permissible as long as there is no evidence of respiratory muscle fatigue. If respiratory muscle fatigue is suspected, patients should rest for 24 hours on full ventilatory support, before another attempt at weaning is made.	Physiologic studies and a large randomized trial
Progressive withdrawal of ventilatory support can be carried out using T-piece, pressure support, or a combination of pressure support and SIMV.	Two large and one small randomized trials
SIMV alone should not be used for weaning.	Two large randomized controlled trials and physiologic studies
Noninvasive ventilation can be used to facilitate weaning in select patients with acute or chronic respiratory failure from COPD.	Two randomized and several uncontrolled trials

SIMV, synchronized intermittent mandatory ventilation; COPD; chronic obstructive pulmonary disease.

Randomized controlled trials have failed to convincingly demonstrate substantial benefits of high-fat/low-calorie enteral nutrition or exogenous growth hormone on weaning outcome (79). A post-hoc analysis of a large randomized trial showed no benefit of a liberal blood transfusion strategy designed to keep the hemoglobin greater than 10 g/dL on duration of mechanical ventilation or likelihood of weaning success (80).

EXTUBATION

When a patient has tolerated a SBT, the clinician must then decide whether the endotracheal tube is still required. Between 2% and 25% of such patients ultimately require reintubation (extubation failure) within 24 to 72 hours of extubation, with the majority of studies reporting rates of 10% to 15% (81). The risk for extubation failure is highest in medical and general surgical ICUs, especially in patients older than 70 years, and for those receiving continuous intravenous sedation (81). Investigators have demonstrated that patients reintubated (after planned extubation) have an increased hospital mortality, have prolonged ICU and hospital stays, and more frequently need long-term acute care (7,8,10,82–85). On the other hand, unnecessary delays in extubation also prolong ICU stays, heighten the risk for developing ventilator-associated pneumonia, and increase hospital mortality (86).

As both extubation delay and extubation failure are associated with adverse outcomes, strategies have been developed to more accurately predict the postextubation course. It must be remembered that passing a properly conducted and monitored SBT has an 85% positive predictive value for successful extubation. In general, the weaning predictors listed in Table 52.2 either have been insufficiently studied or are not satisfactorily accurate in predicting extubation outcome. One explanation is that unlike weaning failure, extubation failure is often caused by excessive respiratory secretions or by obstruction of, or an inability to, protect the upper airway. The risk for postextubation upper airway obstruction increases with traumatic intubation, prolonged duration of intubation, and female sex (81). Upper airway patency can be assessed by detection of an audible air leak when the endotracheal tube balloon is deflated (cuff leak test) (87). The air leak can be quantified by measuring the difference between the inspired and expired tidal volume during assist control ventilation; cuff leak volumes of less than 110 mL (88) or less than 10% of the delivered tidal volume (89) identify patients at elevated risk for postextubation stridor (positive quantitative cuff leak test). Successful extubation is still possible with a positive cuff leak test (90), and postextubation stridor can often be effectively managed without reintubation. In addition, false-positive tests can result from secretions adhering to the outside of the endotracheal tube or when an undetected increase in inspired volume (machine tidal volume plus spontaneous gas inspired around the tube)

contributes to an elevated exhaled tidal volume. Nevertheless, it is recommended that an expert in airway management be immediately available when extubating the patient with a positive cuff leak test. It should be noted that randomized trials have not demonstrated that corticosteroids reduce the rate of postextubation stridor (91).

The effectiveness of cough and the capacity to protect the airway and adequately expel secretions have been quantitatively assessed by measuring maximal expiratory pressure (10) and peak expiratory flow rates (92) in neurologic and neuromuscular patients, respectively. Two components of a six-part semiquantitative airway care score (strong spontaneous cough and infrequent need for airway suctioning), assessed at the time that ventilatory support was no longer required, were predictive of eventual extubation success in brain-injured patients (86). Khamiees and colleagues found that moderate or large volumes of secretions increased the risk for extubation failure sevenfold, weak cough increased the risk for extubation failure fivefold, and the combination of weak cough and moderate or large amounts of secretions was associated with the greatest risk for reintubation (93). This study confirmed previous observations that patients requiring airway suctioning more often than every 2 hours have an increased risk of extubation failure. Adequate neurologic function may be necessary for adequate airway protection after extubation (94). However, abnormal neurologic function alone is not predictive of weaning failure; one study reported that brain-injured patients with reduced Glasgow coma scale scores were not at higher risk for extubation failure (86).

Clinicians often confront patients with unexpected respiratory distress after extubation. Initial efforts are aimed at identifying and reversing the specific cause for extubation failure. Possible therapeutic interventions include using racemic epinephrine or a helium-oxygen mixture (Heliox) for upper airway obstruction; airway suctioning and assisted cough for abundant respiratory secretions; bronchodilators for bronchospasm; and nitrates, diuretics, and afterload reduction for cardiac failure. When these strategies fail, it is imperative to rapidly reestablish ventilatory support. Indeed, rapid reinstitution of invasive ventilatory support (within 12 hours of extubation) is associated with lower mortality (9,82,84). The apparent value of early intervention and the effectiveness of noninvasive positive pressure ventilation (NPPV) in acute respiratory failure has led to the study of NPPV to treat extubation failure. A number of observational studies indicate that NPPV is effective in preventing reintubation in two thirds of patients with extubation failure. In contrast, randomized controlled trials showed that routine use of NPPV in all extubated patients (95) or its application in heterogeneous populations with overt extubation failure (96) did not decrease the need for reintubation or improve survival. On the other hand, a case control investigation observed that NPPV effectively reduced the need for reintubation in COPD patients with early signs and symptoms of postextubation hypercapnic respiratory failure (97). One study randomized 52 patients at high risk for extubation failure (hypercapnia, ventilation >3days, one previous failed weaning attempt, abundant secretions, abnormal upper airway) and demonstrated that NIV (administered for at least 6 h/d) reduced the reintubation rate, ICU mortality, and hospital length of stay when compared with standard care (98).

EXTUBATION	
Summary Statement	**Level of Evidence**
Once a patient has passed a trial of spontaneous breathing, extubation should be carried out if there is adequate cough, minimal secretions, and no evidence of upper airway obstruction.	Large prospective observational studies
Upper airway obstruction should be ruled out in high-risk patients by using either the qualitative or quantitative cuff leak test.	Multiple large observational studies
The amount of secretions should be assessed by measuring the frequency of airway suctioning.	Two prospective studies
A low Glasgow coma scale does not preclude extubation especially when the above criteria are favorable.	Two prospective studies
Noninvasive ventilation can be used in patients with chronic obstructive pulmonary disease (and select others) and early signs of extubation failure. It should not be used routinely after extubation or with overt postextubation respiratory failure when intubation is immediately needed.	Three randomized trials and multiple case controlled or observational studies

APPLICATION OF WEANING PROTOCOLS TO FACILITATE LIBERATION FROM MECHANICAL VENTILATION

Both uncontrolled studies and randomized trials demonstrate improved outcome with an organized approach to weaning from mechanical ventilation (e.g., using a protocol) implemented by physicians or by respiratory care practitioners and ICU nurses. Daily screening protocols can be used to determine readiness for spontaneous breathing, to determine the pace of weaning by using methods of progressive withdrawal, or to direct a search for treatable causes of weaning failure. Of these three applications, the literature indicates that the first is more important than the second; the third strategy has yet to be evaluated in a well-designed trial.

Ely and colleagues randomized 300 mechanically ventilated medical patients to either standard care or an intervention strategy that coupled a daily screen to assess readiness for SBTs (25). Control patients were screened, but further interventions were not made. Those patients who fulfilled the daily screening criteria received a 2-hour SBT (continuous positive airway pressure or T-piece). If patients tolerated the trial, the managing clinicians were queried about

extubation. This strategy resulted in significant reductions in weaning time (1 versus 3 days), duration of mechanical ventilation (4.5 versus 6 days), overall complication rate (20% versus 41%), and ICU costs; no differences were noted in ICU or hospital length of stay, hospital costs, or mortality. Two subsequent randomized controlled trials conducted in medical and surgical ICUs found that a respiratory care practitioner/ICU nurse–directed protocol also shortened the duration of mechanical ventilation compared with that for physician-directed weaning (26, 99). Despite these successes, significant barriers exist to large-scale implementation of weaning protocols. The process is dependent on support from physician leadership and an on-going educational effort directed at all members of the ICU team (31). Though a protocol may serve as the default approach to weaning, flexibility and clinical judgment must be exercised, as too rigid an approach may unnecessarily delay weaning and extubation. Protocols must be adapted to the local ICU environment and should be modified for application to unique patient populations. For example, application of the daily screen/SBT strategy did not improve outcome in a cohort of neurosurgical patients (94).

Randomized trials have demonstrated that protocols directed at minimizing the use of sedative infusions can shorten the weaning process. For example, strategies designed to avoid oversedation by limiting the use of continuous infusions either through sedation assessment scoring (100) or by daily cessation of sedative infusions (44), reduced both the duration of mechanical ventilation and the duration of ICU stay. Additional factors are important, as studies show reduced duration of mechanical ventilation when nurse/patient ratios improve (101) and when a bedside weaning board and flow sheet is used to enhance communication between critical care practitioners (102).

APPLICATION OF WEANING PROTOCOLS TO FACILITATE LIBERATION FROM MECHANICAL VENTILATION	
Summary Statement	**Level of Evidence**
A protocol, driven by respiratory care practitioners and intensive care unit nurses, should be used to assess daily readiness (and monitor) for spontaneous breathing trials and to direct the weaning process.	Multiple large randomized trials
Protocols to decrease the use of continuous intravenous sedation reduce the duration of weaning.	Two large randomized trials

TRACHEOTOMY

The proper timing and indications for tracheotomy remain unclear (103). Surgical and percutaneous dilatational tracheotomy can now be performed at the bedside with a low risk of perioperative complications. The long-term airway risks associated with this procedure are likely similar to those associated with prolonged translaryngeal intubation (103). At present there are no large, well-conducted prospective trials confirming many of the alleged benefits of tracheotomy: increased patient comfort, improved oral care, easier airway suctioning, enhanced patient mobility, and better oral communication. It is thought that tracheotomy reduces the need for sedative medications, a factor that often limits weaning, though this remains to be proven. Robust data is lacking to support the contention that early tracheotomy decreases the probability of acquiring ventilator-associated pneumonia. Prospective randomized trials, conducted primarily in trauma patients, do not convincingly demonstrate favorable effects of performing early (within 3–7 days of intubation) tracheotomy (103). These investigations are further limited by design problems, including quasi-randomization schemes, absence of blinding, and lack of a standard weaning protocol. One physiologic study demonstrated reduced work of breathing through a tracheotomy tube compared with that observed with an endotracheal tube (104). A reduction in the load on the respiratory system might assist weaning from the ventilator in patients with marginal respiratory muscle reserve. For patients incapable of effective secretion clearance or unable to adequately protect the airway, tracheotomy may be necessary, even though mechanical ventilation is no longer required. Tracheotomy ostensibly provides a more secure artificial airway and therefore facilitates transfer of otherwise stable patients from the acute care ICU setting to a long-term care facility or respiratory weaning unit.

ferred to a chronic ventilator or long-term acute care unit, where approximately half (range, 25%–82%) will ultimately be liberated from the ventilator (105). As in the acute ICU setting, standard weaning predictors perform poorly in foretelling outcome for patients with prolonged mechanical ventilation (105). Efforts to wean these patients should commence as early as possible after transfer, as approximately 30% of patients with prolonged mechanical ventilation will tolerate their initial SBT (41). For the remaining patients, an imbalance between respiratory load and neuromuscular capacity often is the basis of ventilator dependence (106). Therefore, continued efforts to identify, and reverse, factors that either increase work of breathing or contribute to respiratory muscle weakness should be undertaken. In addition, although not yet formally studied, general physical reconditioning and proper nutrition may foster eventual liberation from the ventilator.

The only randomized controlled trial evaluating prolonged mechanical ventilation found no difference between pressure support weaning and tracheotomy collar trials of increasing duration in 52 COPD patients (41). This study did support the use of a weaning protocol, as the overall weaning success rate was higher than in historic controls. Indeed, in a prospective observational investigation, a 19-step therapist-implemented, patient-specific weaning protocol decreased the duration of mechanical ventilation by 12 days when compared with that for historic controls (107). Despite these efforts, some patients remain permanently ventilator-dependent, defined as a failure to wean for a minimum of 3 months.

TRACHEOTOMY

Summary Statement	Level of Evidence
Tracheotomy should be considered in stable patients ventilated for 10–14 d, who are likely to require more prolonged mechanical ventilation.	Observational studies, randomized trials, and expert opinion
Tracheotomy should be considered in patients requiring increased sedation in order to tolerate the endotracheal tube, those with persistent inability to protect the airway, or when small reductions in airway resistance may facilitate liberation from ventilator (e.g., when marginal respiratory reserve is present).	Observational and physiologic studies and expert opinion

WEANING PATIENTS WITH PROLONGED MECHANICAL VENTILATION

Summary Statement	Level of Evidence
Stable patients with prolonged mechanical ventilation can be successfully treated in special nonacute care intensive care unit settings. Approximately 50% of such patients will be successfully weaned from mechanical ventilation.	Multiple large prospective, retrospective, observational studies
Weaning protocols can decrease the duration of mechanical ventilation in patients with prolonged mechanical ventilation.	Two prospective, case controlled studies

WEANING PATIENTS WITH PROLONGED MECHANICAL VENTILATION

Approximately 10% to 20% of patients with acute respiratory failure will require prolonged ventilatory support, defined as greater than 21 days of mechanical ventilation. Increasingly this cohort of patients, once stable, will be trans-

REFERENCES

1. Pingleton SK. Complications of acute respiratory failure. *Am Rev Respir Dis* 1988;137:1463–1493.
2. Heyland DK, Cook DJ, Griffith L, et al. The attributable morbidity and mortality of ventilator-associated pneumonia in the critically ill patient. *Am J Respir Crit Care Med* 1999;159:1249–1256.

3. Fagon JY, Chastre J, Domart Y, et al. Nosocomial pneumonia in patients receiving continuous mechanical ventilation: prospective analysis of 52 episodes with use of a protected specimen brush and quantitative culture techniques. *Am Rev Respir Dis* 1989;139: 877–884.

4. Hall JB, Wood LDH. Liberation of the patient from mechanical ventilation. *JAMA* 1987;257:1621–1628.

5. Manthous CA, Schmidt GA, Hall JB. Liberation from mechanical ventilation: a decade of progress. *Chest* 1998;114:886–901.

6. Brochard L, Rauss A, Benito S, et al. Comparison of three methods of gradual withdrawal from ventilatory support during weaning from mechanical ventilation. *Am J Respir Crit Care Med* 1994;150:896–903.

7. Esteban A, Alia I, Gordo F, et al. Extubation outcome after spontaneous breathing trials with t-tube or pressure support ventilation. *Am J Respir Crit Care Med* 1997;156:459–465.

8. Esteban A, Alia I, Tobin M, et al. Effect of spontaneous breathing trial duration on outcome of attempts to discontinue mechanical ventilation. *Am J Respir Crit Care Med* 1999;159:512–518.

9. Esteban A, Anzueto A, Alia I, et al. Mortality of patients receiving mechanical ventilation. *Am J Respir Crit Care Med* 1999;159: A47.

10. Vallverdu I, Calaf N, Subirana M, et al. Clinical characteristics, respiratory functional parameters, and outcome of 2-hour t-piece trial in patients weaning from mechanical ventilation. *Am J Respir Crit Care Med* 1998;158:1855–1862.

11. Nevins M, Epstein S. Predictors of outcome for patients with COPD requiring invasive mechanical ventilation. *Chest* 2001; 119:1840–1849.

12. Esteban A, Alia I, Ibanez J, et al. Modes of mechanical ventilation and weaning: a national survey of Spanish hospitals. The Spanish Lung Failure Collaborative Group. *Chest* 1994;106:1188–1193.

13. MacIntyre N, Cook D, Ely E, et al. Evidence-based guidelines for weaning and discontinuing ventilatory support: a collective task force facilitated by the American College of Chest Physicians, the American Association for Respiratory Care, and the American College of Critical Care Medicine. *Chest* 2001;120:375S–396S.

14. Brochard L, Harf A, Lorino H, et al. Inspiratory pressure support prevents diaphragmatic fatigue during weaning from mechanical ventilation. *Am Rev Respir Dis* 1989;139:513–521.

15. Capdevila X, Perrigault PF, Ramonatxo M, et al. Changes in breathing pattern and respiratory muscle performance parameters during difficult weaning. *Crit Care Med* 1998;26:79–87.

16. Cohen CA, Zagelbaum G, Gross D, et al. Clinical manifestations of inspiratory muscle fatigue. *Am J Med* 1982;73:308–316.

17. Jubran A, Tobin MJ. Pathophysiologic basis of acute respiratory distress in patients who fail a trial of weaning from mechanical ventilation. *Am J Respir Crit Care Med* 1997;155:906–915.

18. Laghi F, D'Alfonso N, Tobin MJ. Pattern of recovery from diaphragmatic fatigue over 24 hours. *J Appl Physiol* 1995;79:539–546.

19. Vassilakopoulos T, Zakynthinos S, Roussos C. The tension-time index and the frequency/tidal volume ratio are the major pathophysiologic determinants of weaning failure and success. *Am J Respir Crit Care Med* 1998;158:378–385.

20. Tobin MJ, Laghi F, Jubran A. Respiratory muscle dysfunction in mechanically-ventilated patients. *Mol Cell Biochem* 1998;179: 87–98.

21. Vassilakopoulos T, Sakynthinos S, Roussos C. Respiratory muscles and weaning failure. *Eur Respir J* 1996;9:2383–2400.

22. Stroetz RW, Hubmayr RD. Tidal volume maintenance during weaning with pressure support. *Am J Respir Crit Care Med* 1995; 152:1034–1040.

23. Afessa B, Hogans L, Murphy R. Predicting 3-day and 7-day outcomes of weaning from mechanical ventilation. *Chest* 1999; 116:456–461.

24. Esteban A, Frutos F, Tobin MJ, et al. A comparison of four methods of weaning patients from mechanical ventilation. *N Engl J Med* 1995;332:345–350.

25. Ely EW, Baker AM, Dunagan DP, et al. Effect on the duration of mechanical ventilation of identifying patients capable of breathing spontaneously. *N Engl J Med* 1996;335:1864–1869.

26. Kollef MH, Shapiro SD, Silver P, et al. A randomized, controlled trial of protocol-directed versus physician-directed weaning from mechanical ventilation. *Crit Care Med* 1997;25:567–574.

27. Ely EW, Baker AM, Evans GW, Haponik EF. The prognostic significance of passing a daily screen of weaning parameters. *Intensive Care Med* 1999;25:581–587.

28. Epstein SK. Weaning parameters. *Respir Care Clin N Am* 2000; 6:253–301.

29. Meade M, Guyatt G, Cook D, et al. Predicting success in weaning from mechanical ventilation. *Chest* 2001;120:400S–424S.

30. Tanios M, Nevins M, Hendra K, et al. The use of weaning parameters prolongs mechanical ventilation time. *Chest* 2001; 129:190S–191S.

31. Ely E, Bennett P, Bowton D, et al. Large scale implementation of a respiratory therapist-driven protocol for ventilator weaning. *Am J Respir Crit Care Med* 1999;159:439–446.

32. Jones D, Byrne P, Morgan C, et al. Positive end-expiratory pressure vs T-piece extubation after mechanical ventilation. *Chest* 1991;100:1655–1659.

33. Zeggwagh AA, Abouqal R, Madani N, et al. Weaning from mechanical ventilation: a model for extubation. *Intensive Care Med* 1999;25:1077–1083.

34. Straus C, Louis B, Isabey D, et al. Contribution of the endotracheal tube and the upper airway to breathing workload. *Am J Respir Crit Care Med* 1998;157:23–30.

35. Ishaaya AM, Nathan SD, Belman MJ. Work of breathing after extubation. *Chest* 1995;107:204–209.

36. Nathan SD, Ishaaya AM, Koerner SK, et al. Prediction of minimal pressure support during weaning from mechanical ventilation. *Chest* 1993;103:1215–1219.

37. Mehta S, Nelson DL, Klinger JR, et al. Prediction of postextubation work of breathing. *Crit Care Med* 2000;28:1341–1346.

38. Wright PE, Marini JJ, Bernard GR. In vitro versus in vivo comparison of endotracheal tube airflow resistance. *Am Rev Respir Dis* 1989;140:10–16.

39. Brochard L, Rua F, Lorino H, et al. Inspiratory pressure support compensates for the additional work of breathing caused by the endotracheal tube. *Anesthesiology* 1991;75:739–745.

40. Farias JA, Retta A, Alia I, et al. A comparison of two methods to perform a breathing trial before extubation in pediatric intensive care patients. *Intensive Care Med* 2001;27:1649–1654.

41. Vitacca M, Vianello A, Colombo D, et al. Comparison of two methods for weaning patients with chronic obstructive pulmonary disease requiring mechanical ventilation for more than 15 days. *Am J Respir Crit Care Med* 2001;164:225–230.

42. Murciano D, Boczkowski J, Lecocguic Y, et al. Tracheal occlusion pressure: a simple index to monitor respiratory muscle fatigue during acute respiratory failure in patients with chronic obstructive pulmonary disease. *Ann Intern Med* 1988;108:800–805.

43. El-Khatib M, Jamaleddine G, Soubra R, et al. Pattern of spontaneous breathing: potential marker for weaning outcome. Spontaneous breathing pattern and weaning from mechanical ventilation. *Intensive Care Med* 2001;27:52–58.

44. Kress JP, Pohlman AS, O'Connor MF, et al. Daily interruption of

sedative infusions in critically ill patients undergoing mechanical ventilation. *N Engl J Med* 2000;342:1471–1477.

45. Kollef MH, Levy NT, Ahrens TS, et al. The use of continuous i.v. sedation is associated with prolongation of mechanical ventilation. *Chest* 1998;114:541–548.

46. Del Rosario N, Sassoon CS, Chetty KG, et al. Breathing pattern during acute respiratory failure and recovery. *Eur Respir J* 1997;10:2560–2565.

47. Sassoon CSH, Te TT, Mahutte CK, et al. Airway occlusion pressure; an important indicator for successful weaning in patients with chronic obstructive pulmonary disease. *Am Rev Respir Dis* 1987;135:107–113.

48. Tobin MJ, Perez W, Guenther SM, et al. The pattern of breathing during successful and unsuccessful trials of weaning from mechanical ventilation. *Am Rev Respir Dis* 1986;134:1111–1118.

49. Le Bourdelles G, Mier L, Fiquet B, et al. Comparison of the effects of heat and moisture exchangers and heated humidifiers on ventilation and gas exchange during weaning trials from mechanical ventilation. *Chest* 1996;110:1294–1298.

50. DeHaven CB, Kirton OC, Morgan JP, et al. Breathing measurement reduces false negative classification of tachypneic preextubation trial failures. *Crit Care Med* 1996;24:976–980.

51. Kirton OC, DeHaven CB, Morgan JP, et al. Elevated imposed work of breathing masquerading as ventilator weaning intolerance. *Chest* 1995;108:1021–1025.

52. Diehl JL, Lofaso F, Deleuze P, et al. Clinically relevant diaphragmatic dysfunction after cardiac operations. *J Thorac Cardiovasc Surg* 1994;107:487–498.

53. Le Bourdelles G, Viires N, Boczkowski J, et al. Effects of mechanical ventilation on diaphragmatic contractile properties in rats. *Am J Respir Crit Care Med* 1994;149:1539–1544.

54. Anzueto A, Peters JI, Tobin MJ, et al. Effects of prolonged controlled mechanical ventilation on diaphragmatic function in healthy adult baboons. *Crit Care Med* 1997;25:1187–1190.

55. Maher J, Rutledge F, Remtulla H, et al. Neuromuscular disorders associated with failure to wean from the ventilator. *Intensive Care Med* 1995;21:737–743.

56. Tobin MJ, Guenther SM, Perez W, et al. Konno-mead analysis of ribcage-abdominal motion during successful and unsuccessful trials of weaning from mechanical ventilation. *Am Rev Respir Dis* 1987;135:1320–1328.

57. Tobin MJ, Perez W, Guenther SM, et al. Does rib cage-abdominal paradox signify respiratory muscle fatigue? *J Appl Physiol* 1987;63:851–860.

58. Laghi F, Jubran A, Parthasarathy S, et al. Can patients who fail a weaning trial develop diaphragmatic fatigue? *Am J Respir Crit Care Med* 2000;161:A790.

59. Chatila W, Ani S, Guaglianone D, et al. Cardiac ischemia during weaning from mechanical ventilation. *Chest* 1996;109:1577–1583.

60. Jubran A, Mathru M, Dries D, et al. Continuous recordings of mixed venous oxygen saturation during weaning from mechanical ventilation and the ramifications thereof. *Am J Respir Care Med* 1998;158:1763–1769.

61. Lemaire F, Teboul J-L, Cinotti L, et al. Acute left ventricular dysfunction during unsuccessful weaning from mechanical ventilation. *Anesthesiology* 1988;69:171–179.

62. Richard C, Teboul JL, Archambaud F, et al. Left ventricular function during weaning of patients with chronic obstructive pulmonary disease. *Intensive Care Med* 1994;20:181–186.

63. Hurford WE, Lynch KE, Strauss HW, et al. Myocardial perfusion as assessed by thallium 201 scintigraphy during the discontinuation of mechanical ventilation in ventilator-dependent patients. *Anesthesiology* 1991;74:1007–1016.

64. Acosta F. Biofeedback and progressive relaxation in weaning the anxious patient from the ventilator: a brief report. *Heart Lung* 1988;17:299–301.

65. LaRicchia PJ, Katz RH, Peters JW, et al. Biofeedback and hypnosis in weaning from mechanical ventilators. *Chest* 1985;87:267–269.

66. Johnson CJ, Auger WR, Fedullo PF, et al. Methylphenidate in the hard to wean patient. *J Psychosom Res* 1995;39:63–68.

67. Rothenhausler HB, Ehrentraut S, von Degenfeld G, et al. Treatment of depression with methylphenidate in patients difficult to wean from mechanical ventilation in the intensive care unit. *J Clin Psychiatry* 2000;61:750–755.

68. Holliday JE, Hyers TM. The reduction of weaning time from mechanical ventilation using tidal volume and relaxation biofeedback. *Am Rev Respir Dis* 1990;141:1214–1220.

69. Ely EW, Margolin R, Francis J, et al. Evaluation of delirium in critically ill patients: validation of the confusion assessment method for the intensive care unit (CAM-ICU). *Crit Care Med* 2001;29:1370–1379.

70. Imsand C, Feihl F, Perret C, et al. Regulation of inspiratory neuromuscular output during synchronized intermittent mechanical ventilation. *Anesthesiology* 1994;80:13–22.

71. Marini JJ, Rodriguez RM, Lamb V. The inspiratory workload of patient-initiated mechanical ventilation. *Am Rev Respir Dis* 1986;134:902–909.

72. Leung P, Jubran A, Tobin MJ. Comparison of assisted ventilator modes on triggering, patient effort, and dyspnea. *Am J Respir Crit Care Med* 1997;155:1940–1948.

73. Jounieaux V, Duran A, Levi-Valensi P. Synchronized intermittent mandatory ventilation with and without pressure support ventilation in weaning patients with COPD from mechanical ventilation. *Chest* 1994;105:1204–1210.

74. Hess D, Branson RD. Ventilators and weaning modes. *Respir Care Clin N Am* 2000;6:407–435.

75. Brochard L, Mancebo J, Wysocki M, et al. Noninvasive ventilation for acute exacerbations of chronic obstructive pulmonary disease. *N Engl J Med* 1995;333:817–822.

76. Kramer N, Meyer TJ, Meharg J, et al. Randomized, prospective trial of noninvasive positive pressure ventilation in acute respiratory failure. *Am J Respir Crit Care Med* 1995;151:1799–1806.

77. Nava S, Ambrosino N, Clini E. Noninvasive mechanical ventilation in the weaning of patients with respiratory failure due to chronic obstructive pulmonary disease: a randomized, controlled trial. *Ann Intern Med* 1998;128:721–728.

78. Girault C, Daudenthun I, Chevron V, et al. Noninvasive ventilation as a systematic extubation and weaning technique in acute-on-chronic respiratory failure: a prospective, randomized controlled study. *Am J Respir Crit Care Med* 1999;160:86–92.

79. Cook D, Meade M, Guyatt G, et al. Trials of miscellaneous interventions to wean from mechanical ventilation. *Chest* 2001; 120:438S–444S.

80. Hebert PC, Blajchman MA, Cook DJ, et al. Do blood transfusions improve outcomes related to mechanical ventilation? *Chest* 2001;119:1850–1857.

81. Epstein SK. Endotracheal extubation. *Respir Care Clin N Am* 2000;6:321–360.

82. Epstein SK, Ciubotaru RL. Independent effects of etiology of failure and time to reintubation on outcome for patients failing extubation. *Am J Respir Crit Care Med* 1998;158:489–493.

83. Epstein SK, Ciubotaru RL, Wong JB. Effect of failed extubation on the outcome of mechanical ventilation. *Chest* 1997;112:186–192.

84. Demling RH, Read T, Lind LJ, et al. Incidence and morbidity of extubation failure in surgical intensive care patients. *Crit Care Med* 1988;16:573–577.

85. Torres A, Gatell JM, Aznar E, et al. Re-intubation increases the

risk of nosocomial pneumonia in patients needing mechanical ventilation. *Am J Respir Crit Care Med* 1995;152:137–141.

86. Coplin WM, Pierson DJ, Cooley KD, et al. Implications of extubation delay in brain-injured patients meeting standard weaning criteria. *Am J Respir Crit Care Med* 2000;161:1530–1536.

87. Fisher MM, Raper RF. The "cuff leak" test for extubation. *Anaesthesia* 1992;47:10–12.

88. Miller R, Cole R. Association between reduced cuff leak volume and postextubation stridor. *Chest* 1996;110:1035–1040.

89. Sandhu RS, Pasquale MD, Miller K, et al. Measurement of endotracheal tube cuff leak to predict postextubation stridor and need for reintubation. *J Am Coll Surg* 2000;190:682–687.

90. Engoren M, Buderer N, Zacharias A, et al. Variables predicting reintubation after cardiac surgical procedures. *Ann Thorac Surg* 1999;67:661–665.

91. Meade MO, Guyatt GH, Cook DJ, et al. Trials of corticosteroids to prevent postextubation airway complications. *Chest* 2001;120:464S–468S.

92. Bach J, Saporito L. Criteria for extubation and tracheostomy tube removal for patients with ventilatory failure. *Chest* 1996;110:1566–1571.

93. Khamiees M, Raju P, DeGirolamo A, et al. Predictors of extubation outcome in patients who have successfully completed a spontaneous breathing trial. *Chest* 2001;120:1262–1270.

94. Namen AM, Ely EW, Tatter SB, et al. Predictors of successful extubation in neurosurgical patients. *Am J Respir Crit Care Med* 2001;163:658–664.

95. Jiang J, Kao S, Wang S. Effect of early application of biphasic positive airway pressure on the outcome of extubation in ventilatory weaning. *Respirology* 1999;4:161–165.

96. Keenan SP, Powers C, Block G, et al. Noninvasive ventilation (NPPV) for post-extubation respiratory distress: a randomized controlled trial. *Amer J Respir Crit Care Med* 2000;161:A263.

97. Hilbert G, Gruson D, Portel L, et al. Noninvasive pressure support ventilation in COPD patients with postextubation hypercapnic respiratory insufficiency. *Eur Respir J* 1998;11:1349–1353.

98. Carlucci A, Gregoretti C, Squadrone V, et al. Preventive use of non-invasive mechanical ventilation (NIMV) to avoid post-extubation respiratory failure: a randomized controlled trial. *Eur Respir J* 2001;in press.

99. Marelich GP, Murin S, Battistella F, et al. Protocol weaning of mechanical ventilation in medical and surgical patients by respiratory care practitioners and nurses: effect on weaning time and incidence of ventilator-associated pneumonia. *Chest* 2000;118:459–467.

100. Brook AD, Ahrens TS, Schaiff R, et al. Effect of a nursing-implemented sedation protocol on the duration of mechanical ventilation. *Crit Care Med* 1999;27:2609–2615.

101. Thorens JB, Kaelin RM, Jolliet P, et al. Influence of the quality of nursing on the duration of weaning from mechanical ventilation in patients with chronic obstructive pulmonary disease. *Crit Care Med* 1995;23:1807–1815.

102. Henneman E, Dracup K, Ganz T, et al. Effect of a collaborative weaning plan on patient outcome in the critical care setting. *Crit Care Med* 2001;29:297–303.

103. Heffner JE. The role of tracheotomy in weaning. *Chest* 2001;120:477S–481S.

104. Diehl JL, El Atrous S, Touchard D, et al. Changes in the work of breathing induced by tracheotomy in ventilator-dependent patients. *Am J Respir Crit Care Med* 1999;159:383–388.

105. Nevins ML, Epstein SK. Weaning from prolonged mechanical ventilation. *Clin Chest Med* 2001;22:13–33.

106. Purro A, Appendini L, De Gaetano A, et al. Physiologic determinants of ventilator dependence in long-term mechanically ventilated patients. *Am J Respir Crit Care Med* 2000;161:1115–1123.

107. Scheinhorn DJ, Chao DC, Stearn-Hassenpflug M, et al. Outcomes in post-ICU mechanical ventilation: a therapist-implemented weaning protocol. *Chest* 2001;119:236–242.

Chronic Respiratory Failure and Noninvasive Ventilation

53

Nicholas S. Hill

The term *chronic respiratory failure* refers to a persistent inability to maintain normal gas exchange. Usually, the term indicates ventilatory failure and applies when blood gases show a chronic respiratory acidosis in the absence of symptoms of an acute deterioration. The term *chronic respiratory insufficiency* is sometimes used interchangeably and denotes compromised respiratory function but not necessarily abnormal gas exchange. Chronic respiratory failure arises from dysfunction of any component or combination of components of the respiratory system. Therapy is contingent on the identification of the dysfunctional component(s). Before ventilatory support is instituted, reversible factors should be sought. In the past, if the cause of respiratory failure could not be quickly identified and reversed, invasive ventilation through a tracheostomy was often deemed necessary. In recent years, however, noninvasive ventilation has become the preferred means of ventilatory support. This chapter considers the various mechanisms that lead to chronic respiratory failure, its presenting manifestations, and current diagnostic and therapeutic approaches. In addition, newer evidence relating to the use of noninvasive ventilation in the acute setting is considered. The various modes of noninvasive ventilation are then presented, with a discussion of the selection of appropriate patients, practical applications, and possible complications. Noninvasive positive-pressure ventilation (NPPV) is the major point of focus.

PATHOPHYSIOLOGY OF CHRONIC RESPIRATORY FAILURE

The normal function of the respiratory system depends on the integrity of each of its components. Chronic respiratory

N. S. Hill: Department of Medicine, Pulmonary, Critical Care, and Sleep Division, Tufts-New England Medical Center, and Department of Internal Medicine, Tufts University School of Medicine, Boston, Massachusetts.

insufficiency arises from a compromise of any one component or combination of components (Table 53.1). Respiratory failure occurs when the compromised system is unable to meet the demand for ventilatory work, because of a limited ability of the system to generate ventilatory work, an excessive demand for ventilatory work, or both. Thus, any pathologic process that interferes with the origination or transmission of the signal to breathe from the respiratory center, through central and peripheral neurons, to the myoneural junction, or with the ability of the respiratory muscles to respond to the signal, may reduce ventilatory function sufficiently to cause respiratory failure. Braun and colleagues (1) observed that carbon dioxide (CO_2) retention is likely when the maximal inspiratory force (P_Imax) is less than 30% of the predicted value. In addition, processes that increase the work of breathing, such as airway obstruction, pulmonary fibrosis, and chest wall deformity, shift the supply-demand balance toward respiratory failure, particularly if respiratory muscle function is compromised. In the case of chest wall deformity, the onset of respiratory failure correlates with an angle of scoliosis exceeding 120 degrees (2).

If respiratory dysfunction develops gradually, the respiratory system may compensate by permitting CO_2 to accumulate in the body. In essence, chronic respiratory failure represents a compromise in which the efficiency of CO_2 excretion is improved (i.e., more CO_2 can be excreted with each breath) at the expense of an increase in both alveolar and arterial P_{CO_2} and a decrease in arterial P_{O_2}. The tendency to make this compromise is partly determined by the sensitivity of the ventilatory control center to CO_2. Evidence for this derives from studies of patients with chronic obstructive pulmonary disease (COPD) who chronically retain CO_2. Close relatives of these patients have less ventilatory sensitivity to CO_2 and hypoxia than relatives of patients with equally severe COPD who are not CO_2 retainers (3). Thus, even though patients with severe COPD and CO_2 retention

TABLE 53.1. CAUSES OF CHRONIC RESPIRATORY FAILURE

Impaired ventilatory control
 Functional
  Obesity-hypoventilation syndrome
  Myxedema
  Drugs (narcotics, sedatives)
  Metabolic abnormalities (hypokalemia, hypophosphatemia,
   hyopmagnesmia, metabolic alkalosis)
 Structural
  Brainstem infarction or neoplasm
 Idiopathic
  Primary alveolar hypoventilation

Neuromuscular disorders
 Myopathies
  Muscular dystrophy
 Neuropathies
  Bilateral diaphragm paralysis
  Poliomyelitis
  Amyotrophic lateral sclerosis
  Cervical spinal cord injury
  Guillain-Barré syndrome
 Disorders of neuromuscular junction
  Myasthenia gravis

Chest wall abnormalities
 Kyphoscoliosis
 Thoracoplasty

Airway obstruction
 Upper airway
  Tracheal stenosis
  Obstructive sleep apnea
  Laryngeal or nasal polyps
  Tonsillar hypertrophy
 Lower airway
  Chronic obstructive pulmonary disease
  Cystic fibrosis

Reduced lung compliance
 Interstitial lung disease
 Surgical resection

**Conditions that may contribute in mixed disorders,
 malnutrition, deconditioning, others**

Source: Adapted from Strumpf DA, Millman RP, Hill NS. The management of
chronic hypoventilation. *Chest* 1990;98:474–480, with permission.

usually have an elevated respiratory drive in comparison with normal persons, a relatively low inherited sensitivity of the respiratory center to CO_2 may contribute to CO_2 retention.

Other factors thought to contribute to chronic respiratory failure include respiratory muscle weakness or fatigue. Defined as an acute reduction in muscle contractility during exhausting work, respiratory muscle fatigue contributes to acute respiratory failure and occurs during exercise in persons with severe COPD. However, the contribution of respiratory muscle fatigue to chronic respiratory failure has not been clearly defined. The concept of central fatigue has been advanced as a mechanism contributing to the development of chronic CO_2 retention (4). This concept proposes that the respiratory center fatigues before actual respiratory

muscle fatigue develops, permitting the gradual accumulation of CO_2. In this way, the overloaded respiratory system prevents or at least postpones the onset of muscle fatigue that would likely presage an acute deterioration.

Other attributes of patients in whom respiratory failure develops include a rapid, shallow breathing pattern. Patients with severe COPD and CO_2 retention breathe more rapidly on average (23 vs. 20 breaths per minute) and may have more ventilation-perfusion mismatching and higher dead space ratios than those without CO_2 retention (5). In addition, during sleep, the respiratory drive is blunted, and the muscle tone of structures in the upper airway is reduced. A magnification of these effects in patients with respiratory insufficiency leads to sleep-disordered breathing and contributes to CO_2 retention. Thus, although patients with chronic respiratory failure have identifiable primary functional disturbances, they also undergo secondary central adaptations that cause alterations in the breathing pattern and breathing disturbances during sleep that are targets for therapeutic interventions.

CAUSES OF CHRONIC RESPIRATORY FAILURE

The most common cause of chronic respiratory failure in the United States is COPD. To gain insight into rates of occurrence of the causes of chronic respiratory failure, Strumpf and colleagues (6) recorded the diagnoses of patients seen at an outpatient chest clinic in a teaching hospital during a 6-month period. As shown in Table 53.2, these authors confirmed that COPD is responsible for chronic CO_2

TABLE 53.2. CAUSES OF CHRONIC HYPOVENTILATION IN AN OUTPATIENT CHEST CLINIC

Cause	No.	Percentage of Total (%)
Chronic obstructive pulmonary disease	46	58
Sleep apnea	6	8
Chest wall deformity		
Thoracoplasty	4	5
Kyphoscoliosis	4	5
Muscular dystrophy	4	5
Interstitial lung disease	3	4
Lung resection for cancer	2	3
Congestive heart failure	1	1
Multifactorial	9	11
	79	100

Note: Data were collected from all patients seen in the outpatient chest clinic at Rhode Island Hospital, a 719-bed general hospital, between January 1, 1989, and July 15, 1989, with a Paco₂ above 45 mm Hg. Patients experiencing an acute exacerbation were excluded. The multifactorial category includes patients with two or more of the causes listed as well as one patient who had chronic obstructive pulmonary disease and laryngeal carcinoma with recurrent aspiration.
Source: From Strumpf DA, Millman RP, Hill NS. The management of chronic hypoventilation. *Chest* 1990;98:474–480, with permission.

retention in the majority of cases. The next most common single cause was the obstructive sleep apnea (OSA) syndrome, which should be considered in any patient with unexplained chronic hypoventilation. Sleep apnea also commonly contributes to chronic hypoventilation in patients with severe COPD or kyphoscoliosis. Restrictive chest wall disease was also a common cause of chronic hypoventilation in this series, but restrictive lung disease was a relatively unusual cause. Chronic respiratory failure secondary to interstitial lung disease was relatively uncommon. CO_2 retention in these patients is usually transient, occurring late in the course as a preterminal event.

The second largest overall etiologic category of chronic CO_2 retention in the series of Strumpf and colleagues was multifactorial, which underscores the fact that a variety of factors often contribute to chronic hypoventilation. As noted in the preceding section, chronic respiratory failure should not be seen as the consequence of a single abnormality of the respiratory system but rather as the interplay of different factors at a number of levels. Chronic CO_2 retention may develop in a patient with severe COPD whose respiratory center is insensitive to CO_2 and who experiences an increased number of apneic episodes during sleep. Another patient with equally severe COPD who is highly sensitive to CO_2 and sleeps normally may not retain CO_2. Multiple factors may also contribute to chronic respiratory failure in patients with the obesity-hypoventilation syndrome. These patients have an increased mechanical load related to their adiposity, may also have a relatively low central sensitivity to CO_2, and often have other contributing factors, such as congestive heart failure. OSA should be excluded in these patients. The multifactorial etiology of chronic respiratory failure should always be considered when patients are being evaluated so that therapeutic results can be maximized (6).

CLINICAL MANIFESTATIONS OF CHRONIC RESPIRATORY FAILURE

Patients with chronic respiratory failure secondary to severe lung disease usually have prominent respiratory symptoms. These prompt a pulmonary evaluation that reveals the hallmark arterial blood gas finding of compensated hypercarbia. However, patients with chronic respiratory failure secondary to neuromuscular disease, central ventilatory defects, or mixed disturbances commonly have few or no respiratory symptoms. Their earliest symptoms are related to the nocturnal exaggeration of CO_2 retention that disrupts normal sleep patterns and causes fretful sleep, nightmares, enuresis, and morning headaches. During the day, fatigue, hypersomnolence, and mood disorders are common, often leading to the misdiagnosis of depression. The physician must be alert to the insidious manner in which chronic hypoventilation may present in these patients so that blood gases are measured and the condition is not missed.

Although the signs of chronic respiratory failure are nonspecific, the physical examination is nevertheless very important for detecting predisposing illnesses. Severe obstructive or restrictive lung diseases should be detectable on physical examination. Morbid obesity, retrognathia, tonsillar hypertrophy, and macroglossia point to the OSA syndrome. An examination of the thoracic cage for scoliosis and a neurologic examination seeking muscle weakness suggestive of a neuromuscular syndrome or cerebrovascular disease are important components of the evaluation. A bedside evaluation of respiratory muscle function should seek evidence of accessory muscle use by inspection or palpation, or evidence of bilateral diaphragmatic paralysis. This is best achieved by having the patient lie supine and observing paradoxical motion of the abdomen during inspiration.

LABORATORY EVALUATION

All patients with symptoms and signs suggestive of chronic hypoventilation should undergo an evaluation beginning with blood gas measurement via arterial puncture (Table 53.3). Noninvasive methods such as pulse oximetry or end-tidal CO_2 monitoring are not sufficiently sensitive to exclude the diagnosis (7), but they may be helpful for following trends. The evaluation should also include a complete blood cell count to exclude polycythemia, thyroid function tests, and serum chemistry studies.

The pulmonary function should be evaluated with spirometry and measurement of the lung volumes and maximal inspiratory and expiratory pressures. These studies identify patients with severe obstructive or restrictive lung diseases in addition to those with muscle weakness. If bilateral diaphragmatic paralysis is suspected, the vital capacity (VC)

TABLE 53.3. DIAGNOSTIC STUDIES FOR PATIENTS WITH CHRONIC RESPIRATORY FAILURE

Routine
  History and physical examination
  Arterial blood gases
  Laboratory studies
    Complete blood cell count
    Serum electrolytes
    Thyroid function tests
    Magnesium, phosphate
  Pulmonary function tests
    Spirometry
    Lung volumes
    Bronchodilator responses
    Maximal inspiratory and expiratory pressures
    Supine and upright vital capacity

For selected patients
  Nocturnal polysomnography
  Transdiaphragmatic pressure measurements

Source: From Strumpf DA, Millman RP, Hill NS. The management of chronic hypoventilation. *Chest* 1990;98:474–480, with permission.

should be measured in the supine and upright positions. If the diaphragm is paralyzed, the supine VC is more than 40% below that measured in the upright position (8). Pulmonary function tests also help to identify patients likely to have additional factors besides lung disease contributing to their chronic hypoventilation. If the forced expiratory volume in 1 second (FEV_1) is more than 1.2 L in a patient with chronic respiratory failure, lung disease is probably not the sole cause of the failure, and other contributing factors should be sought.

Because of the frequency of sleep-disordered breathing in patients with chronic respiratory failure, polysomnography has a central role in their evaluation. Ideally, polysomnography should consist of an overnight sleep study with monitoring of the electroencephalogram, electromyogram, electrooculogram, air flow at the mouth and nose, chest wall motion, and oximetry. The noninvasive monitoring of CO_2 levels by end-tidal or transcutaneous techniques has not proved reliable, so if accurate measurements of the Pco_2 are desired, arterial blood gas sampling via an indwelling catheter is necessary. Afternoon nap studies or overnight monitoring of oximetry are useful if they yield positive results, but a negative study should not be used to exclude sleep apnea (9). Polysomnography is indicated for any patient with chronic respiratory failure and symptoms suggesting OSA, such as snoring or excessive daytime sleepiness, or with an FEV_1 value of more than 1.2 L, even in the absence of suggestive symptoms.

In addition to the evaluation described, other studies may occasionally be useful. Measurement of the transdiaphragmatic pressures with gastric and esophageal balloons is useful to confirm the diagnosis of bilateral diaphragmatic paralysis. Assessment of CO_2 or hypoxic ventilatory responsiveness is primarily a research technique. It is of little value clinically because results are almost invariably abnormal as a consequence of pulmonary dysfunction or blunting of the respiratory drive secondary to chronic CO_2 retention.

THERAPY OF CHRONIC RESPIRATORY FAILURE

Reversal of Contributing Factors

The first priority in the therapy of patients with chronic respiratory failure is to treat any reversible factors that have been identified during the evaluation. The reversal of airway obstruction with bronchodilators or steroids, treatment of congestive heart failure with diuretics, and correction of metabolic alkalosis may be the only interventions necessary to normalize ventilation. Hypothyroidism, hypophosphatemia, and hypomagnesemia are less often encountered, but correction may mitigate the hypoventilation. Drugs such as benzodiazepines or narcotics may contribute to chronic CO_2 retention in patients with compromised pulmonary function or depressed respiratory drive, and their discontinuation may alleviate the hypercapnia.

Pharmacologic Management

Progestational agents stimulate ventilation during pregnancy and can be used to enhance ventilatory drive in normal subjects who are not pregnant. They may reduce hypercarbia in patients with central hypoventilation or the obesity-hypoventilation syndrome (10). Medroxyprogesterone in oral doses of up to 50 mg three times daily is usually well tolerated, but adverse side effects may include acne, ageusia, and sexual dysfunction. Unfortunately, results with progestational agents in the therapy of uncomplicated OSA have been disappointing (11).

Other pharmacologic agents have been used to enhance respiratory drive in patients with chronic respiratory failure, but their efficacy is limited, and none are widely used for this indication. Aminophylline is an acute respiratory stimulant, and when given intravenously to patients with COPD and chronic CO_2 retention, it may acutely reduce hypercarbia (12). However, long-term studies in patients with COPD and chronic hypercarbia have not shown a consistent reversal of chronic respiratory failure with theophyllines. Almitrine bismesylate, a peripheral chemoreceptor agonist, has been used to enhance oxygenation in patients with COPD during both sleep and wakefulness. However, the effect of the drug appears to be related more to an improvement in ventilation-perfusion relationships than to increased respiratory drive, and the role of almitrine in the treatment of chronic respiratory failure remains questionable (13). Doxapram hydrochloride is another agent that has been shown to stimulate ventilation acutely in patients with exacerbations of COPD (14). Unfortunately, adverse side effects, including muscle spasm, agitation, and seizures, occur frequently, the drug is available only in the intravenous form, and its use is not recommended for more than 2 hours consecutively. Thus, it has no role in the therapy of chronic respiratory failure.

Continuous Positive Airway Pressure

Nasal continuous positive airway pressure (CPAP) has become the therapy of choice for symptomatic OSA and can be effective in reversing chronic respiratory failure secondary to OSA (15). Its mechanism of action is to serve as a splint for the upper airway, preventing collapse and permitting unimpeded spontaneous ventilation. Although it does not provide ventilatory assistance per se, CPAP can reduce the work of breathing by raising the functional residual capacity and allowing breathing on a more favorable portion of the respiratory system compliance curve. It also counterbalances intrinsic positive end-expiratory pressure (PEEP) in patients with severe COPD. Accordingly, CPAP has been used to treat respiratory failure in patients who stand to benefit from these mechanisms, such as those with congestive heart failure or acute exacerbations of COPD (16,17). Nasal CPAP may also be beneficial when used nocturnally in patients who have other primary causes of respiratory failure but in whom sleep-disordered breathing appears to be contributory. One acceptable approach is to initiate CPAP in such patients if the respiratory failure is not severe and then proceed to noninvasive ventilation (see next section) if the response to CPAP is inadequate.

Noninvasive Ventilation

Noninvasive ventilation is ventilatory assistance administered without an invasive artificial airway. It has become the ventilatory therapy of choice for patients with many forms of chronic respiratory failure. Although noninvasive ventilators have been available for the past 150 years and were the mainstay of mechanical ventilatory assistance during the polio epidemics that occurred during the first half of the 20th century, invasive positive-pressure ventilators became the preferred means of acute mechanical ventilatory support during the 1960s. Noninvasive ventilators, mainly of the negative-pressure type, continued to be used for chronic respiratory failure until the early 1960s, but invasive positive-pressure ventilation also became more widely used for this indication because of its perceived effectiveness and reliability. With the introduction of nasal ventilation during the mid-1980s, however, NPPV has undergone a resurgence. This mode of administration can provide mechanical ventilatory assistance to selected patients with greater convenience, comfort, safety, and less cost than invasive ventilation. The following sections describe the various techniques and equipment available for noninvasive ventilation and consider the appropriate indications in both chronic and acute forms of respiratory failure and the evidence for efficacy. In addition, general guidelines for the application of NPPV, monitoring, and avoidance of complications are discussed.

Invasive mechanical ventilation has proved effective and reliable, but the placement of an endotracheal airway carries the risk for complications. These have been described in detail and include traumatic complications, such as vocal cord paralysis or tracheal laceration, complications related to the violation of the airway defense system, and discomfort-related complications, including pain and interference with communication and swallowing (18). Similar complications are associated with acute translaryngeal intubations and chronic tracheostomies. Furthermore, airway invasion interferes with normal airway clearance mechanisms such as cough and is a source of continual irritation, increasing the production of mucus and necessitating intermittent suctioning. Special skills are required to care for artificial airways; hence, personnel needs are increased and add to the total cost of care. Thus, noninvasive ventilation has the potential for enhancing patient satisfaction and reducing the cost of care (19). However, it must be emphasized that the techniques are not interchangeable and that candidates for

noninvasive ventilation must be selected carefully according to established guidelines.

EVIDENCE FOR THE EFFICACY OF NONINVASIVE POSITIVE-PRESSURE VENTILATION IN THE TREATMENT OF CHRONIC RESPIRATORY FAILURE	
Summary Statement	**Level of Evidence**
Restrictive thoracic disease: NPPV relieves symptoms and improves gas exchange, sleep quality, quality of life, and survival.	Case series, temporary withdrawal trials; no randomized prospective trials have been performed for ethical reasons.
Central hypoventilation, obstructive sleep apnea: NPPV relieves symptoms and improves gas exchange, sleep quality.	Small case series.
COPD: NPPV relieves symptoms and improves gas exchange, health status; effects on survival, sleep quality, functional status unclear.	Evidence has been conflicting. A number of randomized trials have found little or no benefit, particularly in patients with little or no CO_2 retention.

COPD, chronic obstructive pulmonary disease; NPPV, noninvasive positive-pressure ventilation.

Noninvasive Positive-Pressure Ventilation in Restrictive Thoracic Disease

The restrictive thoracic disorders include those that increase chest wall stiffness (i.e., chest wall deformities) and those that weaken the respiratory muscles. Noninvasive ventilatory approaches have long been used to support patients with such conditions, beginning with negative-pressure ventilation in the form of the iron lung used during the polio epidemics of the past century (20). Some centers first used mouthpiece positive-pressure ventilation some 50 years ago. However, NPPV was not widely used to treat patients with restrictive thoracic disease until the late 1980s, following the demonstration that nocturnal nasal ventilation consistently relieves symptoms and improves gas exchange in patients with chronic respiratory failure caused by restrictive thoracic disease (21,22). Despite the fact that no prospective randomized trial has demonstrated the efficacy of NPPV to treat patients with restrictive thoracic disease, it is now widely accepted as the ventilatory mode of first choice. This view is based on the consistently favorable findings of uncontrolled and nonrandomized clinical trials, in addition to clinical experience. In the following sections, we consider the evidence supporting the efficacy of NPPV for patients with restrictive thoracic disease in regard to a variety of clinical findings.

Symptoms

Virtually every study has reported the alleviation of symptoms such as morning headache and daytime hypersomnolence, even after the first few nights of NPPV therapy (23).

This symptomatic benefit reinforces compliance with therapy and may be sustained for many years, depending on the natural history of the underlying disease.

Gas Exchange

Improvements in gas exchange are also often apparent soon after the initiation of ventilatory assistance. Arterial blood gases can usually be normalized during nocturnal ventilation in patients with restrictive disease, at least those with neuromuscular disease and no lung disease per se. By preventing the worsening of hypoventilation that occurs during sleep in patients with advanced neuromuscular disease, NPPV reverses the blunting of central chemoreceptor sensitivity that is thought to predispose to the gradual development of hypercapnic respiratory failure (24,25). This resetting of respiratory center sensitivity to CO_2 develops over days or weeks, with a gradual reduction in the daytime $Paco_2$. Once a plateau is reached, the daytime $Paco_2$ tends to remain stable for long periods of time, depending on the natural history of the underlying disorder.

Initially, in patients with neuromuscular disease, this improvement in gas exchange is usually sufficient that they can be completely free of supplemental oxygen (O_2) or ventilation during the day. The blood gas values remain remarkably steady during the day between sessions of nocturnal ventilation (26). However, normalization of the $Paco_2$, even during assisted ventilation, may be difficult to achieve in patients with thoracic vertebral deformities because of the severity of the mechanical ventilatory defect. Once achieved, though, the improvement persists indefinitely because of the relative stability of the underlying defect (27). In patients with progressive neuromuscular disease, additional hours of ventilation during the day may become necessary to maintain stable gas exchange as their condition deteriorates. Eventually, round-the-clock ventilatory assistance may be necessary to maintain stable gas exchange.

Some investigators recommend attempting to normalize the daytime $Paco_2$ by adjusting ventilator pressures and prolonging ventilator use, but others advocate accepting a level above normal (up to 50–60 mm Hg) so long as symptoms of hypoventilation and signs of cor pulmonale are controlled (28). The latter strategy allows patients to maintain a steady level of gas exchange at a lower minute volume than would be necessary to normalize the $Paco_2$.

Sleep

The quality of sleep improves with NPPV therapy, as determined by total duration of sleep, efficiency of sleep, and percentage of rapid eye movement (REM) sleep. This response may not be immediate because patients usually require some time (days to weeks) to adapt successfully (24). Symptoms of daytime fatigue, hypersomnolence, and inability to concentrate usually recede as the quality of sleep improves. Conversely, NPPV may disrupt sleep when leakage of air at the mouth during nasal ventilation causes arousals (29). Therefore, although the quality of sleep improves in comparison with baseline when patients respond favorably to NPPV, sleep does not necessarily normalize, and some impairment of sleep quality usually persists.

Pulmonary Function

Although it had been thought that intermittent resting of the respiratory muscles in patients with chronic respiratory failure would translate into improved pulmonary function (30), reported changes in pulmonary function and respiratory muscle force after NPPV have been inconsistent (26). Uncontrolled studies have reported increases in VC and maximal inspiratory and expiratory pressures after periods of NPPV but have not excluded the possibility that improvements in gas exchange alone were responsible for the improved pulmonary function (31). Some studies have reported improvements in more subtle indices of respiratory muscle function, such as the maximum sustained breathing capacity (32). Finally, others have reported stability of gas exchange despite steadily declining pulmonary function (in progressive muscular dystrophies) (27), demonstrating that the benefits of NPPV do not depend on improvements in pulmonary function.

Survival

Without therapy, the life expectancy of patients with restrictive lung disease and chronic respiratory failure is reduced, the extent of the reduction depending on the underlying condition and the severity of CO_2 retention (33). Patients with Duchenne muscular dystrophy die of respiratory failure at an average age of 20 years (33). Fifty percent of patients with amyotrophic lateral sclerosis (ALS) die within 3 years after their illness has been diagnosed, and only 10% are alive at 10 years (34). Patients with kyphoscoliosis in whom chronic hypoventilation develops, complicated by cor pulmonale, have a death rate of 50% within the first year and 80% after 2 years (35). Long-term O_2 therapy alone may improve the prognosis in some patients with chronic respiratory failure (36,37), but as has previously been emphasized, it should be avoided in hypercapnic patients with neuromuscular disease because it may increase the retention of CO_2 and shorten survival (38).

NPPV undoubtedly prolongs survival in patients with restrictive thoracic disorders. By way of comparison, patients with chest wall deformities treated with tracheostomy positive-pressure ventilation had remarkably high survival rates (39). French and English outcome studies showed similar results in a larger population of patients who had restrictive disease treated with NPPV (27,40). These studies indicate that either invasive or noninvasive ventilation results in better survival than O_2 therapy alone (33). Although no controlled trial has directly compared NPPV with tracheostomy positive-pressure ventilation in regard to survival outcome in patients with neuromuscular disease, evidence indicates that both extend life, sometimes for decades after the onset of CO_2 retention.

Nonrandomized trials have evaluated the survival benefit of NPPV. In the study of Vianello and colleagues (41), all five patients with Duchenne muscular dystrophy treated with NPPV survived for the next 2 years, whereas four of the five who declined NPPV died. In the English long-term follow-up study (40), almost 100% of patients with postpolio syndrome (an almost nonprogressive disease) were still using NPPV after 5 years. For patients with various other neuromuscular diseases, the probability of continuing NPPV at 5 years was 81%. The results were not quite as favorable in the French study, which showed only a 47% chance of continuing NPPV beyond 5 years for patients with Duchenne muscular dystrophy. Most patients who discontinued NPPV were switched to tracheostomy ventilation and were still alive after 5 years. Patients with Duchenne muscular dystrophy who continued NPPV experienced progressive ventilatory restriction and eventually required ventilation for 24 hours a day. With the exception of patients at certain specialty centers experienced in administering round-the-clock NPPV (28), patients at most centers decide to switch to tracheostomy ventilation rather than use continuous noninvasive ventilation.

Survival has also been examined in ALS, one of the most challenging of the restrictive disorders because of its rapid progression and tendency to involve the bulbar region. In a retrospective analysis, Gay and colleagues (42) reported success in seven of nine patients with ALS who were part of a larger series of patients using nasal ventilation. In these seven patients, gas exchange improved and symptoms abated, and one patient remained stable after 26 months. However, three of the seven died within 6 months, and most of the survivors had been ventilated for only one year or less. In a nonrandomized prospective trial, Pinto and colleagues (43) used nasal bilevel positive airway pressure (BiPAP) in 10 patients with ALS and an average VC of 48% of the predicted value. The control group had an average VC of 64% of the predicted value and underwent regular medical treatment without ventilation. During the follow-up period, all the controls died within 8 months, whereas the group using BiPAP had a 55% survival at 24 months. In the study of Aboussouan and colleagues (44), nasal NPPV was tolerated in 18 (46%) of 39 patients with respiratory insufficiency secondary to ALS. The risk for death was reduced by a factor of 3.1 if the patient could tolerate NPPV. The risk for death was also reduced in patients with bulbar involvement who could tolerate NPPV, although swallowing dysfunction is ordinarily considered a relative contraindication to the use of noninvasive ventilation. Bulbar involvement halved the likelihood of being able to tolerate the device, however.

These studies demonstrate that NPPV almost certainly extends survival in patients with restrictive thoracic disorders. Survival is much better for those who have relatively static conditions, such as severe chest wall deformity or poliomyelitis, and much worse for those who have rapidly progressive neuromuscular conditions, such as Duchenne muscular dystrophy or ALS. No randomized controlled trials have been performed to prove that NPPV extends survival in these patients, nor is it likely that such a trial will ever be performed. The efficacy of NPPV in restrictive thoracic disorders seems so clear that most investigators would consider it unethical to perform such a randomized trial.

Quality of Life

The effect of NPPV on the quality of life of patients with chronic respiratory failure has been evaluated with health status questionnaires (45,46). Patients with restrictive disorders who use NPPV consistently report relief of symptoms, including cessation of morning headaches, and a better quality of sleep. In a survey by Simonds (47), 73% of the patients were less tired and 44% less breathless, and 48% reported a decreased frequency of respiratory infections. The majority of patients were able to return to work at home, and some returned to professional work. Patients were less frequently hospitalized during the year after they had begun NPPV than in the year before, with the number of hospital days decreasing from 34 to 5 days for patients with scoliosis and from 31 to 9 days for patients with lung restriction secondary to sequelae of tuberculosis ($P < .05$ for both). Compliance with therapy was also very good despite the need to adapt to the mask and ventilator; 7% of the patients with scoliosis, 1% of those with sequelae of tuberculosis, and no patients with Duchenne muscular dystrophy discontinued ventilation during the course of the study. Mean NPPV use was 7.88 h/d for 43 monitored patients, as determined by a clock hidden in the ventilator. The improved quality of life served to reinforce compliance.

Effects of Temporary Withdrawal of Noninvasive Positive-Pressure Ventilation

To determine the efficacy of NPPV, several groups temporarily withdrew NPPV from patients with restrictive thoracic disorders previously stabilized by NPPV (24,48,49). They hypothesized that if NPPV was effective, then its withdrawal would lead to a decline in clinical status. To protect patient safety, NPPV was to be resumed before any serious functional deterioration occurred. Enrolled patients had presented with symptoms and arterial blood gases compatible with chronic respiratory failure and had responded favorably to NPPV.

In all the studies, the condition of patients deteriorated during the period of withdrawal. The earliest and most dramatic change was the reappearance of nocturnal hypoventilation, especially during REM sleep. The quality of sleep also deteriorated as determined by a reduction in total sleep time and duration of REM sleep (48). Symptoms of fatigue, morning headache, and daytime hypersomnolence recurred soon thereafter. Interestingly, measures of pulmonary function did not change significantly during the period of withdrawal (24). Resumption of NPPV relieved the symptoms of nocturnal hypoventilation, and sleep quality was restored.

In these studies, patients served as their own controls, and the results clearly show that NPPV effectively controls nocturnal hypoventilation and symptoms in patients with chronic respiratory failure secondary to restrictive thoracic disease. For safety reasons, the studies were too short to demonstrate that NPPV improves daytime gas exchange and survival, but based on the evidence from earlier uncontrolled studies, it is highly likely that such benefits accrue when these patients use NPPV. NPPV has become the ventilatory mode of first choice in managing patients with chronic respiratory failure caused by restrictive thoracic disorders.

Central Hypoventilation and Obstructive Sleep Apnea

The earliest case reports describing the use of nasal ventilation for chronic respiratory failure were in young children with central hypoventilation (49,50), whose gas exchange abnormalities and symptoms resolved after the initiation of therapy. Little additional information is available, and no controlled studies have been published. Consensus groups have agreed that central hypoventilation is an appropriate indication for NPPV therapy (51). Patients with central hypoventilation usually come to clinical attention because of symptoms of chronic hypoventilation (hypersomnolence and morning headaches) and an arterial blood gas determination revealing chronic CO_2 retention. They almost invariably respond favorably to the prompt initiation of NPPV.

For OSA, nasal CPAP is considered the therapy of first choice. However, some patients with severe OSA present with frank respiratory failure or do not respond to CPAP, and NPPV may be necessary to improve daytime gas exchange and relieve symptoms (52). These patients are often morbidly obese, and BiPAP-type devices may not provide adequate ventilation because of the high airway pressures necessary. Because they can generate high inspiratory pressures, portable volume-limited ventilators are suitable alternatives for these patents. Bilevel ventilation has been touted in patients with OSA as a way to reduce discomfort and improve compliance by virtue of the reduction in positive pressure during expiration (53). However, Reeves-Hoche and colleagues (54) were unable to demonstrate improved compliance rates in patients with OSA treated with bilevel ventilation rather than just CPAP. Hence, the use of NPPV for obstructive apnea is most appropriate for patients with persistent hypoventilation despite adequate CPAP therapy to eliminate the obstructive component.

Chronic Obstructive Pulmonary Disease

Investigators have long thought that noninvasive ventilation would be helpful in patients with chronic respiratory failure caused by severe COPD. The earliest studies used negative-pressure ventilation to rest intermittently the respiratory muscles of patients with severe COPD. It was thought that rest would improve respiratory muscle function and reverse gas exchange abnormalities, thereby improving overall function and promoting a sense of well-being. In 1984, Braun and Marino (55) showed that intermittent daytime sessions with the jacket negative-pressure ventilator improved the daytime gas exchange and inspiratory and expiratory muscle strength of patients with severe COPD. However, this study was uncontrolled, so that other possible causes of the beneficial effect could not be excluded. Later, controlled studies showed similar benefits, but they were very short (<7 d) (56–58). Longer-term controlled studies failed to demonstrate favorable effects of intermittent negative-pressure ventilation in patients with severe COPD. Shapiro and colleagues (59) randomized 184 patients to receive 3 months of wrap or sham ventilation for 4 to 5 hours daily and found no improvements in gas exchange, muscle function, or exercise capacity. Their results mirrored those of Zibrak and colleagues (60), who also found that patients tolerated the ventilators poorly, used them for less time daily than was recommended, and had trouble sleeping while they were in use.

These disappointing results with negative-pressure ventilation prompted investigators to try NPPV for patients with COPD, with the additional hypothesis that NPPV would improve their sleep quality. Findings here have also been conflicting. In a 3-month crossover trial of 19 patients with severe COPD, seven of whom completed the trial, Strumpf and colleagues (61) noted improved neuropsychologic function but could not document any improvements in nocturnal or daytime gas exchange, sleep quality, pulmonary function, exercise tolerance, or symptoms. In contrast, Meecham-Jones and colleagues (62) used a similar design to study 18 patients with severe COPD, 14 of whom completed the trial, and found that NPPV improved nocturnal and daytime gas exchange and total sleep time and relieved symptoms.

These conflicting results may be partially explained by substantial differences in the baseline characteristics of the patients in the two studies. The patients in the study of Meecham-Jones and colleagues had more severe hypercarbia ($Paco_2$, 57 vs. 47 mm Hg) and more nocturnal episodes of O_2 desaturation despite less severe airway obstruction (FEV_1, 0.81 vs. 0.54 L) than the patients in the study of Strumpf and colleagues. These data suggest that patients with more severe daytime CO_2 retention and more nocturnal episodes of O_2 desaturation (blue bloaters) may be a particular subgroup more likely to benefit from NPPV.

Other controlled trials of NPPV in hypercapnic patients with COPD have failed to confirm the hypothesis that NPPV improves their sleep. Gay and colleagues (42) randomized 13 patients with an average initial $Paco_2$ of 51 mm Hg to receive nasal NPPV or sham ventilation in a 3-month trial. Of seven patients who received NPPV, only four completed the trial, and only one had a substantial reduction in daytime $Paco_2$. Subsequently, Lin (63) randomized 12 patients with severe hypercapnic COPD (average $Paco_2$, 51 mm Hg) to sequential 2-week trials of no O_2 or ventilatory assistance (negative control), O_2 supplementation alone, nasal BiPAP alone, or the combination of O_2 and nasal ventilation. No improvements in pulmonary function, exercise capacity, or oxygenation could be attributed to NPPV, and the total sleep time was significantly reduced during periods of NPPV use. More recently, Casanova and colleagues (64) performed a randomized year-long trial in 44 patients with severe COPD and found no improvement in gas exchange, although the patients improved on one test of neuropsychologic function. However, these latter negative studies have been criticized for using relatively low inspiratory pressures (average inspiratory pressure, 10–12 cm H_2O) that may have provided insufficient ventilatory assistance, and the study of Casanova and colleagues did not assess sleep quality or health status. Furthermore, the studies of Lin and of Gay and colleagues included small numbers of patients, and in the case of Lin, inadequate time intervals did not allow successful adaptation to the ventilator.

In summary, the data regarding the effects of NPPV on sleep quality, health status, gas exchange, functional capacity, and survival in patients with severe stable COPD are conflicting. Some uncontrolled trials (65) and preliminary reports of larger randomized trials (66) suggest that NPPV may reduce the need for hospitalization in these patients, with possible reductions in health care costs. Clearly, larger

controlled trials are required to establish the efficacy or lack thereof of NPPV for patients with COPD and chronic respiratory failure. The favorable studies do suggest that patients with substantial CO_2 retention (i.e., >50 mm Hg) are the ones most likely to benefit. Based on this observation, current Medicare guidelines require that to be reimbursed for long-term use of NPPV, patients with COPD must be hypercapnic ($Paco_2 \geq 52$ mm Hg) and have evidence of sleep-related hypoventilation (sustained O_2 saturation $\leq 88\%$ for longer than 5 minutes) (Table 53.4).

THERAPY OF ACUTE RESPIRATORY FAILURE

In recent years, considerable attention has focused on the use of NPPV in acute settings, and evidence from randomized controlled trials is accumulating to support its application for a number of indications. Although a detailed discussion of these trials is beyond the scope of this chapter and may be found elsewhere (67), the following sections summarize the evidence and provide current indications.

Chronic Obstructive Pulmonary Disease

Patients with exacerbations of severe COPD are at risk for the development of respiratory muscle fatigue and failure, and they require intubation. Noninvasive ventilation, by assuming part of the workload of breathing, can help avert muscle fatigue and the need for intubation, serving as a crutch while medical therapy is given time to act. A number of randomized controlled trials have now demonstrated that NPPV is quite effective at achieving this goal, drastically reducing the need for intubation. Most notably, Brochard and colleagues (68) randomized 85 patients to receive NPPV or conventional therapy in a multicenter European trial. The need for intubation was reduced from 74% in controls to 26% in NPPV-treated patients, and NPPV was associated with significant reductions in hospital length of stay (35 vs. 23 days) and mortality rates (30% vs. 9%) ($P < .05$ in both). More recently, Plant and colleagues (69) performed a similar trial at 14 hospitals in England, where nurses with minimal experience in NPPV were responsible for implementation. In this trial, 236 patients were randomized to conventional therapy or NPPV and were treated on a general respiratory ward. The NPPV-treated group showed a significant reduction in the rates of intubation (15% vs. 27%) and mortality (10% vs. 20%), although the benefit was confined to patients with a pH above 7.29. These studies and others have convincingly demonstrated the efficacy of NPPV in improving the outcome of selected patients with exacerbations of COPD and is now considered the ventilatory mode of first choice in managing these patients. Guidelines for the selection of patients are discussed later (see section "Selection Guidelines for Noninvasive Ventilation").

TABLE 53.4. GUIDELINES FOR THE SELECTION OF PATIENTS WITH CHRONIC RESPIRATORY FAILURE FOR NONINVASIVE VENTILATION

Chronic stable or slowly progressive respiratory failure
  1. Significant CO_2 retention ($Paco_2$ >50 mm Hg)
  2. Mild CO_2 retention with symptoms
     a. Morning headache
     b. Daytime hypersomnolence
  3. Nocturnal hypoventilation or oxygen desaturation[a]

Inappropriate candidates excluded
  1. Upper airway function adequate
  2. No excessive airway secretions
  3. Reversible underlying disorders (hypothyroidism, congestive heart failure, others adequately treated)

Appropriate condition
  1. Slowly progressive neuromuscular disorder
  2. Chest wall deformity
  3. Obstructive sleep apnea unresponsive to continuous positive airway pressure
  4. Control of hypoventilation
  5. Obstructive lung disease with[a]
     a. Significant CO_2 retention
     b. Nocturnal episodes of desaturation

[a] Tentative indication.
Source: From Hill NS. *Noninvasive mechanical ventilation in pulmonary and critical care medicine,* update 4. Chicago: Mosby–Year Book, 1997, with permission.

Other Obstructive Lung Diseases

Case series have reported rapid improvements in gas exchange in asthmatic patients treated with NPPV (70), although no randomized studies have documented efficacy. In one randomized trial, too few patients were enrolled to achieve adequate statistical power, partly because of the reluctance of clinicians to enroll patients in a study that might randomize them to a control group (71). As in the case of asthma, controlled trials of patients with cystic fibrosis are lacking, but case series suggest that NPPV can stabilize gas exchange during acute exacerbations of cystic fibrosis (72). Although obstruction of the upper airway has been considered a contraindication to NPPV by some authors, NPPV can be used to stabilize patients with reversible obstruction of the upper airway, such as sometimes occurs when patients are extubated following a bout of acute respiratory failure. Because of the lack of controlled trials, selection criteria for these applications have not been defined, but a trial of NPPV may be warranted so long as standard selection criteria are observed (see section "Selection Guidelines for Noninvasive Ventilation") and the patient is properly monitored.

OBSTRUCTIVE LUNG DISEASES

Summary Statement	Level of Evidence
COPD: NPPV reduces the need for intubation, morbidity, mortality, and hospital lengths of stay in COPD exacerbations.	Multiple randomized trials
Other obstructive diseases: NPPV may improve gas exchange in hypercapnic patients with asthma and cystic fibrosis.	Small case series

COPD, chronic obstructive pulmonary disease; NPPV, noninvasive positive-pressure ventilation.

Hypoxemic Respiratory Failure

Hypoxemic respiratory failure is defined as acute respiratory distress with severe hypoxemia (Pao_2/Fio_2 [fraction of inspired O_2] < 200), tachypnea (>35/min), and a non-COPD diagnosis. Common causes of hypoxemic respiratory failure include acute pulmonary edema, pneumonia, acute respiratory distress syndrome (ARDS), and trauma (73). The use of NPPV for this subcategory has yielded conflicting results. An early randomized trial by Wysocki and colleagues (74) showed no overall benefit of NPPV, but a post hoc analysis revealed that hypoxemic patients with a $Paco_2$ above 45 mm Hg had lower rates of intubation and mortality if treated with NPPV rather than conventional therapy. Subsequently, Antonelli and colleagues (73) randomized 64 patients with hypoxemic respiratory failure to NPPV or immediate intubation. Both groups had equivalent improvements in oxygenation during the first hour, and only 10 of the 32 patients in the NPPV group required intubation. The rate of

sepsis was significantly lower, and strong trends were noted for a shortened ICU stay and reduced mortality in the NPPV group. These results suggest that NPPV can be beneficial in patients with hypoxemic respiratory failure, but the diagnostic category is so broad that it is difficult to apply the study findings to individual patients. For this reason, many studies have focused on individual diagnoses within this general category.

HYPOXEMIC RESPIRATORY FAILURE

Summary Statement	Level of Evidence
Acute pulmonary edema: CPAP and NPPV have both been shown to relieve dyspnea, improve gas exchange, and avoid intubation. One randomized trial has raised the question of increased rates of myocardial infarction with NPPV.	Multiple randomized controlled trials
Pneumonia: NPPV lowers the need for intubation, hospital length of stay, and 2-month mortality in patients with COPD and pneumonia. NPPV reduces the intubation rate, ICU length of stay, and mortality in immunocompromised patients with acute respiratory failure.	Several randomized controlled trials
ARDS and trauma-related respiratory failure: NPPV may have a role in averting intubation in some patients.	Individual case series; no convincing evidence of efficacy

ARDS, acute respiratory distress syndrome; COPD, chronic obstructive pulmonary disease; CPAP, continuous positive airway pressure; ICU, intensive care unit; NPPV, noninvasive positive-pressure ventilation.

Acute Pulmonary Edema

CPAP has been used to treat acute pulmonary edema for more than 60 years (75). In four randomized controlled trials performed during the late 1980s and early 1990s in patients with acute pulmonary edema, CPAP (10 cm H_2O) improved oxygenation and relieved respiratory distress more rapidly and was associated with a lower intubation rate in comparison with O_2 therapy alone (76–79). Masip and colleagues (80) randomized 40 patients with acute pulmonary edema to an NPPV arm (inspiratory pressure of 15 cm H_2O and expiratory pressure of 5 cm H_2O) or a standard O_2 therapy arm. NPPV more rapidly improved oxygenation and drastically reduced the need for intubation (from 33% to 5%), but it did not shorten hospital stay or reduce the mortality rate.

In the only controlled comparison of BiPAP and CPAP, Mehta and colleagues (81) evaluated whether NPPV (i.e., the addition of pressure support to end-expiratory pressure) was more effective than CPAP in relieving dyspnea and improving gas exchange. After 27 patients had been randomized to receive BiPAP ventilation (inspiratory pressure of 15 cm H_2O and expiratory pressure of 5 cm H_2O) or CPAP (10 cm H_2O), the study was stopped prematurely because of an increased rate of myocardial infarction in the BiPAP group (71% vs. 31%). This difference may have been caused by inadequate randomization because more patients in the CPAP group than in the NPPV group presented with chest pain. Pang and colleagues (82) performed a metaanalysis of NPPV modes in the therapy of acute pulmonary edema and concluded that the strongest evidence supported the use of CPAP as the modality of first choice. However, recent controlled trials suggest that NPPV is at least as effective, although the effects on myocardial perfusion raised by the data of Mehta and colleagues require further investigation.

Pneumonia

Earlier studies of the use of NPPV for acute respiratory failure identified pneumonia as a risk factor for NPPV failure (83). More recently, Confalonieri and colleagues (84) randomized 56 patients with severe community-acquired pneumonia to NPPV or conventional therapy. NPPV lowered the intubation rate to 21%, versus 50% in controls ($P = .03$), and shortened the ICU stay to 1.8 days, versus 6 days in controls ($P = .04$). In addition, the mortality rate was significantly lower in the patients with COPD and pneumonia treated with NPPV than in the controls 2 months after discharge. Jolliet and colleagues (85) performed a prospective trial in 24 patients with severe community-acquired pneumonia, specifically excluding patients with underlying COPD. Although 22 of the 24 patients showed an initial improvement in gas exchange and respiratory rate, 66% of them still eventually required intubation, a disturbingly high rate. Thus, the role of NPPV in patients with severe community-acquired pneumonia remains undefined; patients with underlying COPD may benefit, but those without underlying COPD should not be treated with this modality as first-line therapy.

Immunocompromised Patients

Immunocompromised patients in whom respiratory failure from pneumonia or other causes develops are a subgroup for whom NPPV should be considered. This includes patients with severe neutropenia after bone marrow or solid organ transplantation or induction chemotherapy, in addition to patients with AIDS. Antonelli and colleagues (86) randomized 40 patients in whom respiratory failure developed after solid organ transplantation to NPPV or conventional therapy. The NPPV group required significantly fewer intubations (20% vs. 70%), and the rates of ICU mortality, severe sepsis, septic shock, and mortality were lower. However, overall hospital mortality was not significantly reduced in the NPPV group, partly because the study was underpowered.

In a more recent study in which 52 patients, most with hematologic malignancies, were randomized to NPPV or conventional O_2 therapy, the intubation rate was reduced from 76% in the controls to 46% in the NPPV-treated patients, with a concomitant reduction in hospital mortality from 80% to 50% ($P = .02$) (87). These studies demonstrate that even though the mortality rate remains high when immunocompromised patients are managed noninvasively,

it is less than that of intubated patients. The major reason for the reduction in mortality is the avoidance of ventilator-associated pneumonia and septic complications. In one case control series, the rate of ventilator-associated pneumonia was fourfold greater in intubated patients than in physiologically matched patients treated noninvasively. Based on these findings, NPPV should be considered the ventilator mode of first choice for immunocompromised patients unless contraindicated.

Acute Respiratory Distress Syndrome

No controlled trials have examined the use of NPPV in patients with ARDS. One uncontrolled series examined 12 episodes of ARDS in 10 patients and found that NPPV averted intubation in half of the cases (88). Despite this suggestion that NPPV may be of some use in managing ARDS, it should not be considered routine therapy for ARDS. NPPV should be reserved for patients who are hemodynamically stable and do not require high levels of PEEP or sophisticated ventilator modes.

Trauma

Beltrane and colleagues (89) examined outcomes of NPPV therapy in 46 trauma patients with respiratory insufficiency and found rapid improvements in gas exchange and a 72% success rate in avoiding intubation, although the patients with burns did poorly. These findings suggest that NPPV may have a role in treating trauma patients, but controlled trials are needed.

OTHER CATEGORIES OF RESPIRATORY FAILURE

Postoperative Patients

Until recently, the only studies supporting the use of NPPV in postoperative patients were uncontrolled or specifically directed, examining only oxygenation (90) or pulmonary function (91). In 2001, Auriant and colleagues (92) reported that rates of intubation and mortality in patients in whom acute respiratory failure developed after lung resection were diminished if they were treated with NPPV. Therefore, evidence is mounting to support the use of NPPV in this subcategory of patients.

Do-Not-Intubate Patients

Another group of patients with respiratory failure commonly treated with NPPV are those who have declined intubation. Some would argue that there is little to lose in treating such patients with NPPV. However, indiscriminate use of NPPV may waste resources and subject terminally ill patients to the discomfort of a mask in their final moments. Nonetheless, studies of such patients indicate that the overall success rate, defined as survival to hospital discharge, approaches 60%, especially in patients with COPD or congestive heart failure (93). On the other hand, those with underlying malignancies or pneumonia fare less well (94). Therefore, it is reasonable to offer NPPV to do-not-intubate patients so long as they are informed that it is being used as a form of life support and its application is not deemed futile.

Facilitation of Weaning and Extubation

NPPV may also be used to facilitate extubation; it improves outcomes by permitting earlier removal of the endotracheal tube. Udwadia and colleagues (95) were the first group to test this application; they reported that patients who could not be weaned from invasive mechanical ventilation were extubated and weaned rapidly from mechanical ventilation after a brief period of support with NPPV. Most of these patients had a tracheostomy, so that the transition to NPPV was safer because invasive ventilation could easily be resumed if a patient could not tolerate NPPV. The first randomized trial of the use of NPPV as a bridge to extubation was reported by Nava and colleagues (96), who subjected patients with COPD and acute respiratory failure to a T-piece trial after 48 hours of invasive mechanical ventilation. Those who failed were promptly extubated and treated with NPPV, or they were left intubated and weaned with a gradual reduction in pressure support. Patients randomized to NPPV had a higher overall weaning rate (88% vs. 68%), a shorter duration of mechanical ventilation (10.2 vs. 16.6 days), a briefer stay in the ICU (15.1 vs. 24 days), and a better rate of 60-day survival (92% vs. 72%) (NPPV-treated patients vs. controls, $P < 0.05$ for all). In addition, no NPPV-treated patients had nosocomial pneumonia, in comparison with seven of the controls.

In a similar trial, Girault and colleagues (97) randomized 33 patients with acute on chronic respiratory failure, mainly secondary to COPD, to immediate extubation and NPPV or to continued intubation after failure of a 2-hour T-piece trial. The duration of endotracheal intubation was shorter in the NPPV group (4.6 vs. 7.7 days, $P = .004$); however, the total duration of mechanical ventilation was longer in the NPPV group. Furthermore, the weaning and mortality rates and the lengths of ICU and hospital stay were similar, although a trend toward fewer complications was noted in the NPPV group.

These studies support the use of NPPV to expedite extubation in selected patients with COPD, although the study of Girault and colleagues is less compelling than that of Nava and colleagues, indicating that rather than improving outcomes, early extubation shortens the duration of invasive ventilation without worsening outcomes. However, further studies are needed to confirm these promising results, determine whether non-COPD patients may benefit, and define patient selection criteria better. If this approach is used, patients should be selected cautiously, with attention paid

to their ability to cooperate with care and clear secretions. The technique should be avoided in patients who are difficult to intubate or who have a diminished cough reflex or cardiovascular instability. The ethical and medicolegal ramifications of early extubation to NPPV should also be considered.

Another application of NPPV in the weaning process is to avoid reintubation in extubation failures. Epstein and colleagues (98) reported that morbidity and mortality rates are much higher in such patients than in those who are extubated successfully. No randomized controlled trials have yet examined this application of NPPV, but Hilbert and colleagues (99) found that 30 COPD patients with hypercapnic respiratory insufficiency after extubation who were treated with NPPV required reintubation less often (20% vs. 67%) and had a shorter ICU stay than historically matched controls. Jiang and colleagues (100) randomized consecutively extubated patients to receive NPPV or conventional therapy. They found a trend toward a higher reintubation rate in the NPPV group, suggesting that use of this approach for all extubated patients, most of whom are likely to do well without any ventilatory assistance at all, is fruitless.

These findings support the use of NPPV to treat extubation failures, and it is being used routinely for this application at some centers. During the period after extubation, patients with COPD exacerbations, acute pulmonary edema, and possibly increased resistance in the upper airway secondary to glottic swelling appear to be good candidates for NPPV. However, it is important that controlled trials be performed to confirm that NPPV can improve outcomes in this subpopulation of patients with acute respiratory failure, particularly in regard to planned versus unplanned extubations.

OTHER CATEGORIES OF RESPIRATORY FAILURE	
Summary Statement	**Level of Evidence**
Postoperative respiratory failure: NPPV improves oxygenation, preserves pulmonary function, averts intubation, and lowers mortality in certain patient subgroups.	Randomized controlled trials.
Do-not-intubate patients: NPPV use is associated with survival rates to hospital discharge of up to 60%, depending on the diagnosis (patients with CHF and COPD fare the best).	Retrospective and prospective trials. Randomized controlled trials pose ethical dilemmas in this patient subpopulation.
Facilitation of weaning: NPPV can improve weaning rates and lower mortality if used to achieve early extubation in selected COPD patients. NPPV can also avert extubation failure. Caution is advised when NPPV is used to achieve early extubation.	Randomized and historically controlled trials.

CHF, congestive heart failure; COPD, chronic obstructive pulmonary disease; NPPV, noninvasive positive-pressure ventilation.

SELECTION GUIDELINES FOR NONINVASIVE VENTILATION

Restrictive Thoracic Disease

The characteristics that permit the selection of appropriate candidates for noninvasive ventilation are listed in Table 53.5. Patients should have symptoms attributable to hypoventilation and associated poor sleep quality, such as morning headache, daytime hypersomnolence, and energy loss. Unless motivated by the desire for symptomatic relief, patients have difficulty in complying with noninvasive ventilation. In addition, patients with abnormalities of gas exchange, including daytime CO_2 retention and nocturnal hypoventilation as evidenced by sustained O_2 desaturation during sleep, are good candidates. Current Medicare reimbursement guidelines for NPPV in patients with restrictive thoracic disease also allow NPPV to be initiated in patients with a forced vital capacity (FVC) that is less than 50% of the predicted value. However, unless these patients have symptoms or disturbances of gas exchange, they comply poorly with NPPV. Table 53.5 also lists situations in which invasive mechanical ventilation may be preferable. Because NPPV is an open system and provides no direct access to the airway, invasive mechanical ventilation is preferred when maximal prolongation of

TABLE 53.5. FAVORABLE AND UNFAVORABLE CHARACTERISTICS OF PATIENTS WITH RESTRICTIVE THORACIC DISEASE WHO ARE CANDIDATES FOR NONINVASIVE POSITIVE-PRESSURE VENTILATION

Favorable
    Symptomatic (daytime hypersomnolence, morning headaches)
    Hypercapnic ($Paco_2 \geq 45$ mm Hg)
    Nocturnal hypoventilation (O_2 saturation $\leq 88\%$ for ≥ 5 consecutive
        minutes)
    Good upper airway function
    Intact cough
    Medically stable otherwise
    Motivated
    Capable of understanding and managing own illness
    Adequate financial resources
    Adequate family and social support
Unfavorable
    Absence of above
    Excessive secretions
    Depression or agitation
Invasive ventilation preferred
    Good candidate for long-term mechanical ventilation except
        Inadequate upper airway function
        Vocal cord paralysis or other upper airway obstruction
        High level of dependence on assisted ventilation (>20 h/d)[a]
        Failure of noninvasive positive-pressure ventilation to support
          ventilation
        Failure to tolerate noninvasive ventilation

[a]Optional; some centers manage patients with noninvasive positive-pressure ventilation who require continuous ventilatory support.

survival in the face of severe upper airway dysfunction is desired.

The specific diagnosis is also an important consideration when the decision to institute NPPV is being made. Patients with stable or slowly progressive neuromuscular disease or chest wall deformities are the best candidates, provided that the mechanisms of airway protection are intact. Patients with more rapidly progressive syndromes that impair function in the upper airway, such as ALS, respond less well to NPPV than patients with slowly progressive disorders. However, NPPV may be worth trying, even in patients with bulbar involvement, because survival is prolonged if they can adapt to NPPV (44). On the other hand, patients with very rapidly progressive neuromuscular processes, such as Guillain-Barré syndrome, are usually poor candidates because of the almost universal occurrence of upper airway dysfunction and retention of secretions.

Severe Stable Chronic Obstructive Pulmonary Disease

Because the evidence for efficacy has been conflicting, the guidelines for the institution of NPPV in patients with severe stable COPD are controversial. Consensus groups have agreed that substantial CO_2 retention ($Paco_2 > 50$–55 mm Hg) should be a criterion (51). Medicare guidelines also require a demonstration of sustained nocturnal O_2 desaturation while the patient is breathing the prescribed Fio_2 (O_2 saturation $\leq 88\%$ for 5 minutes or longer) and no evidence of OSA (Table 53.6). For qualified patients, a 2-month period of ventilator use without a backup is required, which reduces the reimbursement rates for home care equipment companies. This requirement, along with the additional requirement that sustained O_2 desaturation be demonstrated, has greatly reduced the frequency of NPPV use in patients with COPD.

Central Hypoventilation and Obstructive Sleep Apnea

Noninvasive negative-pressure ventilation has long been used in patients with central hypoventilation who have symptoms

TABLE 53.6. GUIDELINES FOR THE USE OF NONINVASIVE POSITIVE-PRESSURE VENTILATION IN SEVERE STABLE CHRONIC OBSTRUCTIVE PULMONARY DISEASE

Symptomatic despite optimal therapy
Hypercapnic ($Paco_2 \geq 52$ mm Hg)[a]
Evidence of nocturnal hypoventilation (O_2 saturation $\leq 88\%$ for ≥ 5
    consecutive minutes during the use of usual Fio_2)[a]
No clinical evidence of obstructive sleep apnea (if yes, requires sleep study)
Requisite 2-month trial of ventilatory assistance with an assist device
    without a backup rate[a]

[a]Medicare requirement.
Fio_2, fraction of inspired oxygen.

TABLE 53.7. HEALTH CARE FINANCING AGENCY GUIDELINES FOR THE USE OF NONINVASIVE POSITIVE-PRESSURE VENTILATION IN CENTRAL SLEEP APNEA

1. Central sleep apnea demonstrated on a facility-based polysomnogram *and*
2. Obstructive sleep apnea excluded as a major contributor of hypoventilation *or*
3. If obstructive sleep apnea a major contributor, continuous positive airway pressure has been tried and failed *and*
4. O_2 saturation <88% for >5 consecutive minutes at 2 L of O_2 per minute or usual FIO_2 *and*
5. Significant improvement of sleep-associated hypoventilation documented after use of noninvasive positive-pressure ventilation (2 months).

FIO_2, fraction of inspired oxygen.

and CO_2 retention (101). However, these devices can induce OSA (102), and they are now rarely used to provide ventilatory assistance. A polysomnogram is necessary in patients with suspected central hypoventilation to establish the diagnosis and exclude OSA. Presently, patients with confirmed OSA should be started on CPAP; they should be switched to NPPV if they fail to improve. Medicare guidelines (Table 53.7) require that patients with OSA fail CPAP before NPPV can be initiated.

CHRONIC RESPIRATORY FAILURE

Summary Statement	Level of Evidence
Restrictive thoracic disease: NPPV should be used for symptomatic hypoventilation (daytime or nocturnal) in patients without contraindications.	Selection criteria for case series and consensus conferences
COPD: NPPV may benefit hypercapnic patients, particularly those whose hypoventilation intensifies nocturnally.	Single controlled trial and consensus opinion
Central hypoventilation/obstructive sleep apnea: NPPV is indicated in symptomatic, hypoventilating (daytime or nocturnal) patients. Patients with obstructive sleep apnea should have failed CPAP.	Consensus opinion

COPD, chronic obstructive pulmonary disease; CPAP, continuous positive airway pressure; NPPV, noninvasive positive-pressure ventilation.

Acute Respiratory Failure

Consensus groups have reported guidelines for the use of NPPV in acute respiratory failure (103). These include clinical and gas exchange criteria based on the entry criteria used in randomized controlled trials (Table 53.8). First, the criteria aim to exclude patients who are mildly ill and do not require ventilatory assistance while identifying those who may require intubation so that NPPV can be initiated early. Second, the criteria exclude patients who can be more safely

TABLE 53.8. SELECTION GUIDELINES FOR PATIENTS WITH ACUTE RESPIRATORY FAILURE TO RECEIVE NONINVASIVE POSITIVE-PRESSURE VENTILATION

Favorable diagnosis (reversible within days) and with good supportive evidence
    COPD
    Acute cardiogenic pulmonary edema
    Immunocompromised

Reversible, but evidence less clear
    Asthma, cystic fibrosis
    Pneumonia without COPD or immunocompromised

Not advisable unless mild; supporting evidence scanty
    ARDS
    Upper airway obstruction

Need for ventilatory assistance established
    Clinical signs and symptoms
        Moderate to severe respiratory distress
        Tachypnea (>24/min for COPD or cystic fibrosis, >30/min for other diagnoses)
        Abdominal paradox, or excessive accessory muscle use
    Gas exchange abnormalities
        Acute on chronic hypercapnia ($Paco_2$ >45 mm Hg with pH <7.35) or Pao_2/FIO_2 <200

No contraindications to noninvasive positive-pressure ventilation
    Respiratory arrest
    Medically unstable (unstable ischemia, arrhythmias, unstable hemodynamic status, uncontrolled upper gastrointestinal bleed)
    Excessive secretions
    Inadequate cough
    Agitated or uncooperative
    Unable to fit mask
    Recent upper airway or upper gastrointestinal surgery

ARDS, acute respiratory distress syndrome; COPD, chronic obstructive pulmonary disease; FIO_2, fraction of inspired oxygen.

managed with invasive mechanical ventilation, such as those in respiratory arrest; in such cases, there is no time to initiate NPPV.

The diagnosis should always be considered when candidates with acute respiratory failure are selected for NPPV. Patients with conditions that can be reversed within days, such as acute pulmonary edema and exacerbations of COPD, are excellent candidates, whereas those with conditions characterized by excessive secretions (e.g., severe pneumonia) or prolonged bouts of respiratory failure (e.g., ARDS) are poor candidates. Also, the specific criteria should be tailored to the diagnosis. For example, patients with severe COPD benefit from ventilatory assistance when their respiratory rate exceeds approximately 25/min, whereas those with acute pulmonary edema may not be candidates until their respiratory rate exceeds 30/min. In addition, the evidence to support the use of NPPV in a number of applications, such as acute asthma and cystic fibrosis, is scanty, so the selection criteria for these patients are empiric. Although a lack of evidence of efficacy is not the same as a lack of efficacy, practitioners should exercise caution when applying NPPV in patients with these diagnoses.

ACUTE RESPIRATORY FAILURE

Summary Statement	Level of Evidence
Acute hypercapnic respiratory failure: A trial of NPPV is indicated before invasive ventilation if evidence of increased symptoms of respiratory distress and acute deterioration in gas exchange in a patient without contraindications.	Consensus opinion
Acute cardiogenic pulmonary edema: CPAP or NPPV is indicated if moderate to severe respiratory distress, tachypnea (>30/min), and hypoxemia without contraindications. Unclear evidence that NPPV is superior to CPAP; question of increased rates of myocardial infarction with NPPV.	Consensus opinion
Other acute hypoxemic respiratory failure: Selection criteria similar to those for acute cardiogenic pulmonary edema, but NPPV preferred; CPAP not shown to be effective.	Consensus opinion and randomized trial of CPAP

CPAP, continuous positive airway pressure; NPPV, noninvasive positive-pressure ventilation.

TECHNIQUES AND EQUIPMENT FOR NONINVASIVE VENTILATION

Although various noninvasive techniques, such as negative-pressure or abdominal displacement ventilation have been used extensively in the past, NPPV has become the preferred technique. Accordingly, the focus here will be on NPPV, and the reader is referred elsewhere for a discussion of alternative noninvasive ventilators (81,104). Whether used in the acute or chronic setting, NPPV requires a positive pressure ventilator connected via tubing to an interface that delivers positive air pressure to the nose or mouth or both.

Interfaces

Nasal Masks

Nasal masks are the most commonly used interfaces for patients with chronic respiratory failure because they are relatively comfortable and permit normal speech, swallowing, and expectoration. Many different nasal masks are available commercially, largely because of the demand for such devices in the treatment of OSA. The standard nasal mask is a triangular clear plastic device that fits over the nose; a soft cuff is used to form an air seal (Fig. 53.1). These masks exert pressure over the bridge of the nose to achieve an adequate air seal, causing skin redness and irritation and occasionally ulceration. Modifications are available that minimize these complications, such as forehead spacers, gel seals, and very thin silicone seals that minimize the pressure necessary to maintain an adequate air seal. Nasal pillows (Fig. 53.2) can be useful when standard masks cause nasal bridge irritation

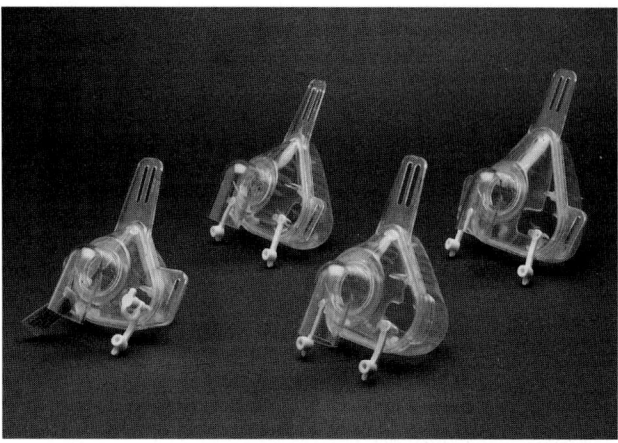

FIGURE 53.1. Example of standard nasal mask commonly used to administer nasal continuous positive airway pressure or noninvasive ventilation.

or ulceration; these are soft cones that are inserted into the nares and do not come in contact with the nasal bridge. Some patients prefer minimasks that are attached just to the tip of the nose, minimizing contact with the face and reducing claustrophobic reactions. Custom-molded masks were used more often in the past, but they are expensive and time-consuming to construct and are rarely used today.

Oronasal (Full Face) Masks

Oronasal masks cover both the nose and mouth and so can prevent air leakage through the mouth, a ubiquitous problem with nasal masks (105). However, they interfere with speech,

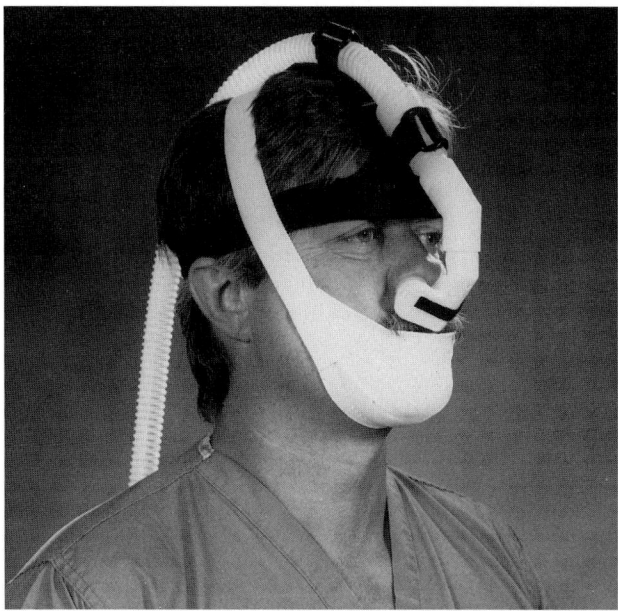

FIGURE 53.2. Example of nasal pillows. These are silicone cones, inserted into each nostril, through which positive pressure is administered to the nose. They are an alternative to the standard nasal mask when pressure over the nasal bridge or claustrophobia poses a problem.

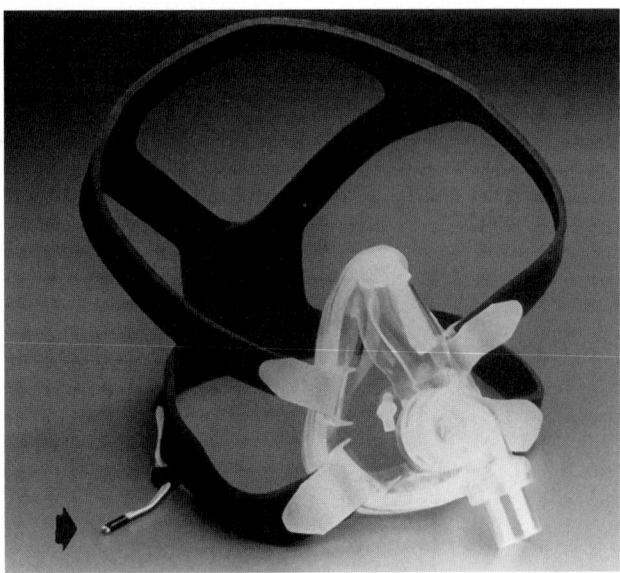

FIGURE 53.3. Example of an oronasal (or full face) mask. This covers both the nose and mouth and may be helpful when air leakage through the mouth interferes with the effectiveness of nasal masks.

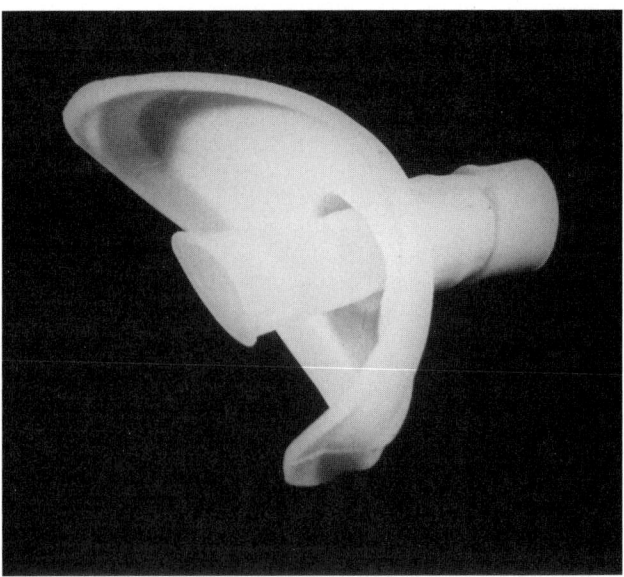

FIGURE 53.4. A mouthpiece inserted through a soft plastic lip seal is strapped in place. The mouthpiece delivers pressurized air to the mouth, and the lip seal reduces air leakage.

eating, and expectoration more than nasal masks and are more apt to cause claustrophobic reactions. Oronasal masks designed specifically for NPPV include valves to minimize rebreathing in the event of ventilator failure and rapid-release straps that permit quick removal if the patient vomits. In addition, recently introduced masks have very soft silicone seals (Mirage, ResMed, San Diego, California; and Image 3, Respironics, Murrysville, Pennsylvania) that greatly increase patient acceptability and long-term compliance (Fig. 53.3).

In a crossover trial of 26 patients with various forms of chronic respiratory failure, Navalesi and colleagues (106) found that oronasal masks were more effective at lowering the $Paco_2$ than nasal masks but that nasal masks were more comfortable. In a randomized trial of patients with acute respiratory failure, Kwok and colleagues (107) found that the oronasal mask was better tolerated than the nasal mask, largely because of its ability to control mouth leaks. Therefore, one approach is to use an oronasal mask initially in the acute setting and then switch to a nasal mask if the patient continues to require NPPV beyond the first few days. Patients beginning NPPV for chronic respiratory failure usually start with a nasal mask, although oronasal masks may be preferable in patients with bulbar muscle weakness, in whom air leakage through the mouth is a problem.

Oral Interfaces

Commercially available oral interfaces use a mouthpiece inserted into a lip seal (Puritan-Bennett, Carlsbad, California) that is strapped tautly to minimize air leakage (Fig. 53.4). This device is difficult to tolerate because it interferes with speech and swallowing. Mouthpieces that are custom-fitted

by an orthodontist may not require a strap for adequate sealing and can be easily expectorated if necessary, even by patients with severe neuromuscular disease. Bach and colleagues (28) reported success in using these devices to administer NPPV to a large number of patients with neuromuscular disease, some with little or no measurable VC. During the daytime, patients received ventilatory assistance via a mouthpiece held by a gooseneck attached to their wheelchairs.

Ventilators

Volume-limited or pressure-limited portable positive-pressure ventilators have been used to deliver NPPV. The choice of ventilator depends largely on practitioner preference and patient needs. For example, sophisticated alarm systems are unnecessary for patients requiring only nocturnal ventilatory assistance, and they can actually be counterproductive because they may needlessly interrupt sleep. In devices intended for long-term use in the home, simplicity and portability are important features.

Volume-Limited Ventilators

Portable volume-limited ventilators commonly used to administer NPPV to patients with chronic respiratory failure include the PLV 100 and 102 (Respironics) and the LP-10 (Puritan-Bennett). The ventilators are usually set in the assist/control mode to allow spontaneous patient triggering, and the backup rate is usually set slightly below the spontaneous breathing rate. The only important difference relative to invasive ventilation is that the tidal volume is usually set at 10 to 15 mL/kg to compensate for air leakage. Currently available volume-limited ventilators have more alarm- and pressure-generating capabilities than most portable pressure-limited ventilators, and they may be better suited for patients who require continuous ventilation, and for those who are obese or have a severe chest wall deformity and require high inflation pressures. In patients with advanced neuromuscular disease and severe impairment of the cough muscles, volume-limited ventilators can be used to stack breaths (i.e., the patient retains the volumes of several consecutive breaths) so that greater before-cough volumes can be achieved to augment cough flow.

Pressure-Limited Ventilators

Portable ventilators that deliver pressure support ventilation ("bilevel" ventilators) are now increasingly used to deliver NPPV in both acute and chronic settings (Fig. 53.5). These deliver a preset inspiratory positive airway pressure (IPAP) that can be combined with positive end-expiratory pressure (PEEP), or expiratory positive airway pressure (EPAP). The difference between IPAP and EPAP is the level of inspiratory assistance, or pressure support. These ventilators have

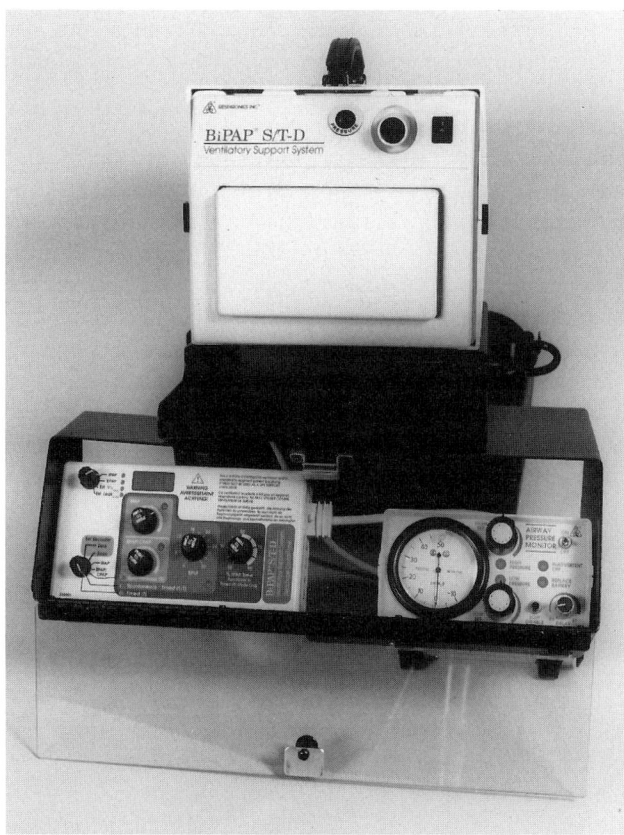

FIGURE 53.5. Example of portable pressure-limited (or "bilevel") ventilators commonly used to deliver noninvasive ventilation. The machines cycle between higher inspiratory and lower expiratory pressures, determined by patient or timed triggers. The difference between the inspiratory and the expiratory pressure determines the amount of inspiratory assistance or pressure support.

sensitive inspiratory triggering and expiratory cycling mechanisms and are well tolerated by most patients. Portable devices that deliver pressure support ventilation (BiPAP Synchrony, Respironics; Knightstar 320, Puritan-Bennett; VPAP, ResMed) are used for long-term applications. These devices are lighter (2–5 kg) and more compact (<1 ft^3) than critical care ventilators, offering greater portability at lower cost.

Most bilevel devices offer not only a spontaneously triggered (S) mode but also time-cycled (T) and combined (S/T) modes. The bilevel devices, by virtue of their portability, compactness, and low cost, have proved ideal for home use in patients with chronic respiratory failure who require only nocturnal ventilatory assistance. In addition, unlike volume-limited ventilators, they are able to adjust inspiratory airflow to compensate for air leaks, thereby potentially providing better support of gas exchange during leaking (107a). However, these devices have limited IPAP capabilities (up to 20–35 cm H_2O, depending on the ventilator), and most lack sophisticated alarm or battery backup systems. Therefore, they are not recommended for patients requiring high inflation pressures, or for those who depend on continuous mechanical ventilation or receive invasive ventilation, unless appropriate alarm and monitoring capabilities have been added.

Although they were initially designed for outpatients with OSA who could not tolerate CPAP, bilevel devices have also been used successfully in the acute setting. Older devices had limited alarm and monitoring capabilities and lacked oxygen blenders, so they were not suitable for patients with significant hypoxemia. In addition, the older devices had problems synchronizing with expiration when air leaks were present (108). Newer bilevel devices have been designed specifically for use in the acute setting; these have graphic screens for monitoring, oxygen blenders, and the capability of limiting inspiratory time for better synchrony (BiPAP Vision, Respironics).

Because bilevel devices use a single tube with a passive exhalation valve, rebreathing may occur if exhaled CO_2 is retained in the exhalation valve. Ferguson and Gilmartin (109) noted substantial rebreathing that interfered with the ability of BiPAP to augment alveolar ventilation, particularly with use of the whisper-swivel valve (Respironics) at low EPAP settings. Using sufficient expiratory pressure (>4 cm H_2O) to ensure adequate bias flow minimizes this problem (109). Rebreathing CO_2 is probably not a significant concern for patients receiving nocturnal nasal ventilation because the leakage of exhaled air via several routes (including the mouth) is substantial (110).

Hybrid Ventilators

In recent years, microprocessor-controlled ventilators have been introduced that offer both pressure- and volume-limited modes in addition to sophisticated monitoring and alarm systems. These ventilators are also highly portable; an example is the LTV (Pulmonetics, Carlsbad, California), which is approximately the size of a laptop computer. Hybrid ventilators can be equipped with oxygen blenders and have backup batteries, so they are suitable for either invasive or noninvasive ventilation. In addition to the LTV, other ventilators in this category include the Achieva (Puritan-Bennett) and Legacy (Viasys, Yorba Linda, California). These ventilators are particularly suitable for the delivery of NPPV in the inpatient setting because they can provide both NPPV and invasive ventilation. Because of their cost, they are not sensible choices for outpatients requiring only intermittent ventilatory assistance.

Other Types of Noninvasive Ventilatory Assistance

Diaphragm pacing and glossopharyngeal breathing are ventilatory methods used in selected patients to enhance independence. In diaphragm pacing, a radiofrequency transmitter and antenna signal a surgically implanted internal receiver and electrode to stimulate the phrenic nerve (111). The use of diaphragm pacing is usually limited to patients who have an intact diaphragm and phrenic nerve, although advances in neurosurgery have permitted the implantation of a spinal nerve into the diaphragm (112). Candidates for diaphragm pacing include patients with central hypoventilation or quadriplegia secondary to a high spinal cord lesion. Diaphragm pacing has a number of limitations, including high cost, the potential to fail abruptly despite a lack of built-in alarms, and a tendency to obstruct the upper airway by the same mechanism as negative-pressure ventilators, so that tracheostomy placement is required in up to 90% of users. In addition, no controlled studies have demonstrated long-term efficacy. Nevertheless, diaphragm pacers are very easy to use once installed and highly portable, and they provide freedom from positive-pressure ventilators. Thus, some patients with high spinal cord lesions may still prefer diaphragm pacing over other types of ventilatory assistance. Its chief applications at the present time are in patients with high spinal cord lesions and in children who have difficulty adapting to noninvasive forms of ventilation (113).

In glossopharyngeal or "frog" breathing, intermittent motions of the tongue and pharyngeal muscles are used to force air into the trachea (114). When gulping, the patient lowers and then raises the tongue against the palate like a piston to inject air into the trachea. With practice, each 0.5-second gulp injects roughly 50 to 150 mL of air. The patient closes the glottis between gulps to prevent escape of air and rapidly repeats the gulping until a tidal volume of approximately 500 or 600 mL is achieved. The air is then exhaled, and the maneuver is repeated eight to 10 times per minute so that a normal minute volume can be achieved. The technique can be used to provide freedom from mechanical ventilation for periods of up to several hours, even in patients with severely weakened lower respiratory muscles. It can also be used to augment individual breaths in patients with low tidal volumes, or to achieve inhaled volumes of 2 to 2.5 L to assist in coughing. However, use of this technique is limited to patients who have intact musculature in the upper airway and more or less normal lungs and chest walls, and who are capable of learning the technique. Good candidates include patients with high spinal cord injuries or post-polio syndrome and appropriate patients with other neuromuscular diseases.

Assisting Cough

Patients with chronic respiratory failure secondary to neuromuscular disease usually have an impaired cough mechanism. During episodes of respiratory infection, this predisposes to retention of secretions, plugging of mucus, and associated complications of hypoxemia, respiratory muscle fatigue, and hypoventilation. Should the situation deteriorate sufficiently, acute respiratory failure can develop, with the need for endotracheal intubation. Respiratory arrest and even death may ensue. Therefore, efforts should be made to avoid secretion retention in these patients.

Techniques to assist cough have been described in detail elsewhere (115). In brief, these consist of manual and mechanical approaches to improve cough efficacy. In manually assisted cough (or quad coughing), an abdominal thrust is used to enhance expiratory airflow. The palms of the assistant's hands are placed just below the costal margins of a reclining patient, and a firm thrust is applied to the upper airway in time with the patient's cough. A twofold or threefold increase in cough flow can be achieved with this technique (116). In addition to stacking breaths with the use of a volume-limited ventilator (see section "Volume-Limited Ventilators"), mechanical techniques for assisting cough include the cough inexsufflator (Cough Assist, J. H. Emerson, Cambridge, Massachusetts). This applies a positive pressure breath of 30 to 40 cm H_2O via a mask or endotracheal tube to inflate the lungs fully, followed by an abrupt switch to an equal negative pressure to simulate airflow during a cough.

Bach and Saporito (117) have shown that the ability of a patient with weakened cough muscles to survive without an artificial airway is correlated with peak cough flow; a value of more than 160 L/s serves as a threshold above which success is very likely. If cough flows exceeding this threshold can be achieved with cough-assistive techniques, then, in the experience of Bach and Saporito (117), the patient can be managed without an artificial airway. Bach and colleagues (118) have described an approach to ventilatory support in patients with neuromuscular disease and chronic respiratory failure in which exclusively noninvasive techniques are used to assist ventilation in addition to cough. In this approach, O_2 saturation is recorded by pulse oximetry. If the O_2 saturation falls below 90%, the patient receives air insufflation from an AMBU bag and cough assistance as previously described until the O_2 saturation is brought back to normal levels. This can be repeated as often as necessary during respiratory infections. Use of this approach was associated with a marked reduction in the need for intubation and even hospitalization. Although the approach has not been tested by a randomized controlled trial, there can be little question about the importance of implementing measures to enhance cough efficacy in patients with severe cough impairment.

Additional measures to assist cough have been developed, including percussion techniques, external chest wall oscillators, and chest physiotherapy and drainage. Detailed descriptions of these approaches are beyond the scope of this text and can be found elsewhere (115).

PRACTICAL APPLICATION

Initiation

In the acute setting, the successful initiation of NPPV requires that the patient adapt rapidly. A comfortable interface must be fitted and strapped in place with minimal air leaks. Letting the patient hold the interface while mechanical ventilation is begun may impart a sense of control and enhance tolerance. Ventilator pressures must then be set optimally. To enhance patient acceptance, the author recommends starting with low pressures (e.g., inspiratory pressure of 8 cm H_2O and expiratory pressure of 4 cm H_2O) and rapidly increasing the pressure as tolerated to alleviate respiratory distress. Alternatively, the inspiratory pressure can be set higher (15–20 cm H_2O) for rapid relief of respiratory distress and then adjusted downward as needed for tolerance. The expiratory pressure can be increased to counterbalance auto-PEEP or improve oxygenation. The selection of optimal pressures requires bedside titration so that mask discomfort and respiratory distress can be minimized. This requires time and patience on the part of practitioners, who must coach patients to adapt.

Unlike patients with acute respiratory failure, who urgently require ventilatory assistance, most patients with chronic respiratory failure can begin NPPV gradually, so that the chances for success are optimized. After an appropriate patient has been identified, a ventilator is selected for the initial trial. Nasal masks should be considered the interfaces of first choice because of their greater comfort in comparison with oronasal masks (107). On the other hand, oronasal masks may be advantageous in patients who have excessive air leaking through the mouth.

The author advises performing the initial trial during the daytime in a relaxed setting on an outpatient basis. To establish continuity, the home respiratory therapist who will follow the patient is asked to bring the necessary equipment to the physician's office or the patient's hospital room. Experienced practitioners then optimize the fit and adjust the initial settings, explaining each step to minimize patient anxiety. When nasal masks are fitted, the smallest standard mask that adequately covers the nose usually works best. Straps are tightened with the least tension necessary to avoid excessive air leakage. Some air leakage is acceptable because the strap tension necessary to eliminate leaking entirely may induce pressure sores, and the ventilator can be adjusted to compensate for leaks. Adjustment of pressures is similar to that in the acute setting, except that the upward adjustment takes place over weeks instead of hours as the patient adapts. If necessary, supplemental O_2 can be connected to ports in the mask or tubing, with the liter flow titrated to maintain the desired O_2 saturation. Patient comfort should be a higher priority initially than improvement in gas exchange or tidal volume, which can be attained later as pressures are increased during the adaptation phase.

The optimal time for the initiation of NPPV in chronic respiratory failure has not been established. Some investigators have hypothesized that early initiation, before the onset of symptoms or daytime hypoventilation, may slow the progression of respiratory dysfunction in patients with neuromuscular disease. Raphael and colleagues (119) tested this hypothesis in patients with Duchenne muscular dystrophy by randomizing asymptomatic patients to receive nasal NPPV or standard therapy. Contrary to their hypothesis, disease progression was not delayed in NPPV-treated patients. In fact, the trial had to be stopped prematurely because of excess mortality in the NPPV group. Shortcomings of the study included failure to document compliance with the device and an excess of patients with severe cardiac dysfunction in the NPPV group, raising doubts about the significance of the mortality findings. However, the study results suggest that early initiation may not be beneficial.

Adaptation and Monitoring

In the acute setting, close attention should be paid to the patient's comfort and tolerance, vital signs, intensity of accessory muscle use, and synchronization with the ventilator. Gas exchange should be monitored with continuous pulse oximetry and occasional blood gas measurement. Inspiratory pressure is increased as tolerated to reduce the $Paco_2$. Numerous studies have shown that improvements in the respiratory rate and blood gas levels within the first 2 hours after initiation presage a favorable outcome.

In the chronic setting, the patient is encouraged to begin with daytime use for a few hours and then institute nocturnal use after a few days. Gradually, the hours of use are extended throughout the night. Comparing the process to that of mastering a musical instrument may be helpful. During this period, frequent visits from an experienced home respiratory therapist help to ensure proper use of the device and allow the adjustments in mask sizes and types, straps, and pressure settings that are often necessary.

Patients should be seen every few weeks by a physician during the initial adaptation period. Once adaptation has been successful, patients can visit the physician less often, as infrequently as twice or thrice yearly. At the time of office follow-up, the symptoms and physical signs should be assessed to detect evidence of nocturnal hypoventilation or cor pulmonale. Spirometry is indicated to assess loss of pulmonary function, particularly in patients with progressive neuromuscular syndromes. Daytime arterial blood gases or pulse oximetry and end-tidal PCO_2 should be obtained at the time of physician visits or when symptoms worsen. Although no consensus has been reached regarding the ideal target level for the daytime $PaCO_2$ in patients receiving noninvasive ventilation, values ranging from approximately 40 to 55 mm Hg are usually associated with good control of symptoms.

Nocturnal monitoring is also useful after adaptation to noninvasive ventilation to ensure the adequacy of oxygenation and ventilation. Nocturnal oximetry at home is helpful in screening, but it cannot be used to diagnose specific problems should episodes of desaturation occur. Thus, home monitoring of chest wall motion, mask pressure, and airflow in addition to oximetry, such as is possible with portable multichannel recorders, is useful to detect evidence of persistent episodes of apnea or excessive air leaking. However, full polysomnography is necessary if information on sleep quality, arousals, or stage is desired. Monitoring of the nocturnal PCO_2 is desirable, but neither transcutaneous nor end-tidal monitoring systems have proved sufficiently reliable to be of much value in characterizing problems (7), other than in a research setting. One practical approach is to establish the adequacy of overnight gas exchange initially with oximetry or portable multichannel monitoring in the home, and then repeat studies as dictated by changes in the symptoms or daytime gas exchange. More sophisticated polysomnographic monitoring can be used when the portable monitor is insufficient to characterize problems.

COMMONLY ENCOUNTERED PROBLEMS AND POSSIBLE SOLUTIONS

Noninvasive ventilation is safe and well tolerated in most properly selected patients. With NPPV, the most commonly encountered problems are interface related (Table 53.9). Patients often report mask discomfort that can be alleviated by minimizing strap tension or trying different mask sizes or types. Excessive air pressure leading to sinus or ear pain is another common problem and can usually be alleviated by lowering the pressure temporarily and then gradually raising it again as tolerance improves. Air leaks toward the eyes can cause conjunctivitis, which is relieved by refitting. Patients may also experience dryness or congestion of the nose or mouth. For dryness, nasal saline solution or efforts to reduce air leaking may help. Flow-by humidifiers may also be helpful, particularly in dry climates, but mask pressure should be verified when these are added to pressure-limited ventilators. For nasal congestion, inhaled steroids or decongestants or oral antihistamine-decongestant combinations may be used.

TABLE 53.9. ADVERSE EFFECTS AND COMPLICATIONS OF NONINVASIVE POSITIVE-PRESSURE VENTILATION

Adverse Effect	Therapeutic Action
Mask-related	
Discomfort	Check fit, adjust straps
Nasal bridge redness or ulceration	Use artificial skin, minimize strap tension
Skin rashes	Skin barrier lotion, topical steroids
Claustrophobic reactions	Try nasal mask, judicious sedation
Airflow- or pressure-related	
Sinus or ear pain	Lower inspiratory pressure if intolerable
Eye irritation	Check for mask leaks, readjust straps
Gastric insufflation	Avoid excessive pressures, simethicone
Pneumothorax	Rare, avoid high inflation pressure (keep <20 cm H_2O)
Complications	
Air leaking	Virtually universal; proper mask fit, head strap tension
Aspiration pneumonia	Exclude patients at risk for aspirating
Failure to tolerate	Reassure, coach breathing pattern, judicious sedation
Failure to ventilate	Use sufficient pressures, optimize patient-ventilator synchrony, minimize leaks

Other commonly encountered problems include erythema and pain or ulceration on the bridge of the nose related to nasal mask pressure. Minimizing strap tension, using artificial skin, or switching to alternative masks such as nasal pillows minimizes this problem. Gastric insufflation is also common but is usually tolerable and can be minimized by avoiding excessive inflation pressure and using simethicone.

Air leaking through the mouth (with nasal masks), through the nose (with mouthpieces), or around the mask (with all interfaces) is inevitable during NPPV. Pressure-limited devices compensate for air leaks by maintaining or increasing inspiratory airflow during leaking. To reduce air leakage through the mouth, patients are coached to keep the mouth shut or use chin straps or oronasal masks. Air leakage occurs during most of sleep in many patients, but fortunately, gas exchange is usually maintained. Leakage may still contribute to arousals and poor sleep quality, however, and ventilatory assistance may occasionally be compromised (30). In this case, options include trials of alternative interfaces or ventilators or, if these fail, tracheostomy. Major complications of noninvasive ventilation, such as aspiration or pneumothorax, are unusual if patient selection guidelines are observed.

Failure of gas exchange to improve may be related to inadequate inflation pressure, excessive leaking, or inability of the patient to synchronize with the ventilator, sometimes because of excessive anxiety. The latter may respond to the judicious use of sedation. Patients with chronic respiratory failure may be unable to tolerate the device and use it for a sufficient number of nocturnal hours. However, if the patient is using the device for most of the night, failure to improve may be related to inadequate inspiratory pressure or tidal volume or to a low backup rate. Further adjustments in the settings and follow-up monitoring are indicated. When daytime gas exchange deteriorates after prior stabilization, the patient's underlying neuromuscular or respiratory disorder may have progressed and often responds to increases in inspiratory pressure, tidal volume, or ventilator rate. If gas exchange fails to respond to repeated adjustments or the patient fails to tolerate NPPV, trials with alternative noninvasive ventilators may be successful. For patients who cannot tolerate NPPV and have persistent symptomatic hypoventilation despite prolonged trials of various noninvasive ventilators, tracheostomy placement may be necessary if they want aggressive ventilatory support.

SUMMARY AND CONCLUSIONS

Chronic respiratory failure is most often caused by mechanical problems of the respiratory system, particularly chronic airway obstruction, neuromuscular weakness, and chest wall deformity. Secondary disturbances may also contribute to CO_2 retention, including insensitivity of the respiratory center to CO_2, hypothyroidism, and sleep-disordered breathing. These secondary contributing factors should be sought in formulating an effective therapy. The first therapeutic intervention should be to reverse the contributing factors. If OSA is found, then nasal CPAP should be tried initially unless CO_2 retention is severe. Nasal ventilation is the preferred choice for chronic hypoventilators who do not have obstructive apnea or who fail CPAP. Oronasal masks are used when excessive mouth leakage occurs during the use of nasal masks. Evidence from uncontrolled and temporary withdrawal studies strongly supports NPPV as the ventilatory mode of first choice for patients with respiratory failure secondary to slowly progressive neuromuscular diseases, chest wall deformities, or central hypoventilation disorders, but the use of noninvasive ventilation in patients with severe COPD remains controversial.

NPPV is also considered the ventilatory mode of first choice for patients with certain types of acute respiratory failure, including exacerbations of COPD and respiratory failure associated with immunocompromise. Patients with acute cardiogenic pulmonary edema also respond well to NPPV, although the strongest evidence supports the use of CPAP alone as the technique of first choice in these cases. Patients with many other forms of acute respiratory failure may respond well to NPPV, including acute asthma, postoperative respiratory failure, failure following extubation, and respiratory failure when intubation has been declined, but they must be selected carefully.

The successful initiation of noninvasive ventilation requires a skilled and attentive staff that is experienced in the selection of patients, masks, and ventilators. They must monitor patients closely and be prepared to make adjustments to optimize patient tolerance of the device. Complications of noninvasive ventilation can be minimized if patients are selected according to established guidelines and are appropriately monitored. Most complications of NPPV are interface-related, such as discomfort caused by air or mask pressure. Because NPPV is an open-circuit system, air leaks may compromise efficacy and interfere with sleep quality. Major complications of NPPV, such as pneumothorax, aspiration pneumonia, and respiratory arrest, are unusual if patients are properly selected and managed, but failure rates still hover in the range of 20% to 40% in most acute care settings, largely related to patient intolerance or progression of the underlying process.

The role of noninvasive ventilation in respiratory care continues to evolve. Some indications are well established, such as chronic respiratory failure secondary to neuromuscular disease and acute respiratory failure secondary to COPD exacerbations, whereas other indications, such as severe stable COPD, await further documentation. Controlled studies aimed at establishing the optimal applications of noninvasive ventilation and technologic advances in ventilators and interfaces should lead to a wider use of NPPV as the indications are expanded and better defined.

REFERENCES

1. Braun NMT, Arora NS, Rochester DF. Respiratory muscle and pulmonary function in polymyositis and other proximal myopathies. *Thorax* 1983;38:616–623.
2. Bergofsky EH. Respiratory failure in disorders of the thoracic cage. *Am Rev Respir Dis* 1979;119:643–669.
3. Mountain R, Zwillich C, Weil J. Hypoventilation in obstructive lung disease. The role of familial factors. *N Engl J Med* 1978;298:521–525.
4. Roussos CH. Respiratory muscle fatigue in the hypercapnic patient. *Bull Eur Physiopathol Respir* 1979;15:117–123.
5. Tobin MJ, Chadha TS, Jenouri TJ, et al. Breathing patterns: 2. Diseased subjects. *Chest* 1983;84:286–294.
6. Strumpf DA, Millman RP, Hill NS. The management of chronic hypoventilation. *Chest* 1990;98:474–480.
7. Sanders MH, Kern NB, Costantino JP, et al. Accuracy of end-tidal and transcutaneous P_{CO_2} monitoring during sleep. *Chest* 1994;106:472–483.
8. Mier A, Brophy C, Moxham J, et al. Assessment of diaphragmatic weakness. *Am Rev Respir Dis* 1988;137:877–883.
9. Meyer TJ, Eveloff SE, Kline LR, et al. One negative polysomnogram does not exclude obstructive sleep apnea. *Chest* 1993;103:756–609.
10. Strohl KP, Hensley MJ, Saunders NA, et al. Progesterone administration and progressive sleep apneas. *JAMA* 1981;245:1230–1232.
11. Rajogopal KR, Abbrecht PH, Jabbari B. Effects of medroxyprogesterone acetate in obstructive sleep apnea. *Chest* 1986;90:815–821.

12. Lakshminarayan S, Sahn SA, Weil JV. Effect of aminophylline on ventilatory responses in normal man. *Am Rev Respir Dis* 1978;117:33–39.

13. Melot C, Naeije R, Rothschild T, et al. Improvement in ventilation-perfusion matching by almitrine in COPD. *Chest* 1983;83:528–533.

14. Burki NK. Ventilatory effects of doxapram in conscious human subjects. *Chest* 1984;85:600–604.

15. Sullivan CE, Issa FG, Berthon-Jones M, et al. Reversal of obstructive sleep apnea by continuous positive airway pressure applied through the nares. *Lancet* 1981;1:862–865.

16. Rasanen J, Heikkila J, Downs J, et al. Continuous positive airway pressure by face mask in acute cardiogenic pulmonary edema. *Am J Cardiol* 1985;55:296–300.

17. Montserrat JM, Martos JA, Alarcon A, et al. Effect of negative pressure ventilation on arterial blood gas pressures and inspiratory muscle strength during an exacerbation of chronic obstructive lung disease. *Thorax* 1991;46:6–8.

18. Pingleton SK. Complications of acute respiratory failure. *Am Rev Respir Dis* 1988;137:1463–1493.

19. Bach JR, Intintola P, Alba AS, et al. The ventilator-assisted individual cost analysis of institutionalization versus rehabilitation and in-home management. *Chest* 1992;101:26–30.

20. Wilson JL. Acute anterior poliomyelitis. *N Engl J Med* 1932;206:887–893.

21. Kerby GR, Mayer LS, Pingleton SK. Nocturnal positive pressure ventilation via nasal mask. *Am Rev Respir Dis* 1987;135:738–740.

22. Bach JR, Alba A, Mosher, et al. Intermittent positive pressure ventilation via nasal access in the management of respiratory insufficiency. *Chest* 1987;94:168–170.

23. Leger P, Jennequin J, Gerard M, et al. Home positive pressure ventilation via nasal mask for patients with neuromuscular weakness or restrictive lung or chest wall deformities. *Respir Care* 1989;34:73–77.

24. Hill NS, Eveloff SE, Carlisle CC, et al. Efficacy of nocturnal nasal ventilation in patients with restrictive thoracic disease. *Am Rev Respir Dis* 1992;101:516–521.

25. Piper AJ, Sullivan CE. Sleep-disordered breathing in neuromuscular disease. In: Saunders NA, Sullivan CE, eds. *Sleep and breathing,* 2nd ed. New York: Marcel Dekker Inc, 1994:761–786.

26. Mohr CH, Hill NS. Long-term follow-up of nocturnal ventilatory assistance in patients with respiratory failure due to Duchenne-type muscular dystrophy. *Chest* 1990;97:91–96.

27. Leger P, Bedicam JM, Cornette A, et al. Nasal intermittent positive pressure. Long-term follow-up in patients with severe chronic respiratory insufficiency. *Chest* 1994;105:100–105.

28. Bach JR, Alba AS, Saporito LR. Intermittent positive pressure ventilation via the mouth as an alternative to tracheostomy for 257 ventilator users. *Chest* 1993;103:174–182.

29. Meyer TJ, Pressman MR, Benditt J, et al. Air leaking through the mouth during nocturnal nasal ventilation: effect on sleep quality. *Sleep* 1997;20:561–569.

30. Hill NS, Braman S. Noninvasive ventilation for neuromuscular disease. In: Cherniack NS, Homma I, Altose M, eds. *Rehabilitation of the patient with respiratory disease.* New York: McGraw-Hill, 1998.

31. Juan G, Calverley P, Talamo C, et al. Effect of carbon dioxide on diaphragmatic function in human beings. *N Engl J Med* 1984;310:874–879.

32. Goldstein RS, De Rosie JA, Avendano MA, et al. Influence of noninvasive positive pressure ventilation on inspiratory muscles *Chest* 1991;99:408–415.

33. Rideau Y, Jankowski LW, Grellet IJ. Respiratory function in the muscular dystrophies. *Muscle Nerve* 1981;4:155–164.

34. Rowland LP. Amyotrophic lateral sclerosis. *Curr Opin Neurol* 1994;7:310–315.

35. Freyschuss V, Nilsonne U, Lundgren KD. Idiopathic scoliosis in old age. I. Respiratory function. *Acta Med Scand* 1968;184:365–372.

36. Ström K, Pehrsson K, Boe J, et al. Survival of patients with severe thoracic spine deformities receiving domiciliary oxygen therapy. *Chest* 1992;102:164–168.

37. Robert D, Leger P, Gerard M, et al. Utilisation de l'oxygénothérapie de longue durée en dehors des bronchopneumopathies chroniques obstructives. *Agressologie* 1988;29:525–528.

38. Gay PC, Edmonds LC. Severe hypercapnia after low-flow oxygen therapy in patients with neuromuscular disease and diaphragmatic dysfunction. *Mayo Clin Proc* 1995;70:327–330.

39. Robert D, Gerard M, Leger P, et al. La ventilation méchanique à domicile définitive par trachéostomie de l'insuffisance respiratoire chronique. *Rev Fr Mal Respir* 1983;11:923–936.

40. Simonds AK, Elliott MW. Outcome of domiciliary nasal intermittent positive pressure ventilation in restrictive and obstructive disorders. *Thorax* 1995;50:604–609.

41. Vianello A, Bevilacqua M, Salvador V, et al. Long-term nasal intermittent positive pressure ventilation in advanced Duchenne's muscular dystrophy. *Chest* 1994;105:445–448.

42. Gay PC, Patel AM, Viggiano RW, et al. Nocturnal nasal ventilation for treatment of patients with hypercapnic respiratory failure. *Mayo Clinic Proc* 1991;66:695–703.

43. Pinto AC, Evangelista T, Carvalho M, et al. Respiratory assistance with a noninvasive ventilator (BiPAP in MND/ALS patients): survival rates in controlled trial. *J Neurol Sci* 1995;129:19–26.

44. Aboussouan LS, Khan SU, Meeker DP, et al. Effect of noninvasive positive pressure ventilation on survival in amyotrophic lateral sclerosis. *Ann Intern Med* 1997;127:450–453.

45. Simonds AK, Muntoni F, Heather S, et al. Impact of nasal ventilation on survival in hypercapnic Duchenne muscular dystrophy. *Thorax* 1998;53:949–952.

46. Bach JR, Campagnolo DI, Hoeman S. Life satisfaction of individuals with Duchenne muscular dystrophy using long-term mechanical ventilatory support. *Am J Phys Med Rehabil* 1991;70:129–135.

47. Simonds AK. Negative pressure ventilation in acute hypercapnic chronic obstructive pulmonary disease. *Thorax* 1996;51:1069–1070.

48. Jimenez JFM, De Cos Escuin JS, Vicente CD, et al. Nasal intermittent positive pressure ventilation. Analysis of its withdrawal. *Chest* 1995;107:382–388.

49. Ellis ER, McCauley VB, Mellis C, et al. Treatment of alveolar hypoventilation in a six-year-old girl with intermittent positive pressure ventilation through a nose mask. *Am Rev Respir Dis* 1987;136:188–191.

50. DiMarco AF, Connors AF, Altose MD. Management of chronic alveolar hypoventilation with nasal positive pressure breathing. *Chest* 1987;92:952–954.

51. Consensus Conference. Clinical indications for noninvasive positive pressure ventilation in chronic respiratory failure due to restrictive lung disease, COPD, and nocturnal hypoventilation—a consensus conference report. *Chest* 1999;116:521–534.

52. Piper AJ, Sullivan CE. Effects of short-term NIPPV in the treatment of patients with severe obstructive sleep apnea and hypercapnia. *Chest* 1994;105:434–444.

53. Sanders MH, Kern NB. Obstructive sleep apnea treated by independently adjusted inspiratory and expiratory positive airway pressure via nasal mask. *Chest* 1990;98:317–324.

54. Reeves-Hoche MK, Hudgel DW, Meck R, et al. Continuous versus bilevel positive airway pressure for obstructive sleep apnea. *Am J Respir Crit Care Med* 1995;151:443–449.

55. Braun NM, Marino WD. Effect of daily intermittent rest of respiratory muscles in patients with severe chronic airflow limitation (CAL). *Chest* 1984;85:59S–60S.

56. Cropp A, Dimarco AF. Effects of intermittent negative pressure ventilation on respiratory muscle function in patients with severe chronic obstructive pulmonary disease. *Am Rev Respir Dis* 1987;135:1056–1061.

57. Scano G, Gigliotti F, Duranti R, et al. Changes in ventilatory muscle function with negative pressure ventilation in patients with severe COPD. *Chest* 1990;97:322–327.

58. Ambrosino N, Montagna T, Nava S, et al. Short-term effect of intermittent negative pressure ventilation in COPD patients with respiratory failure. *Eur Respir J* 1990;3:502–508.

59. Shapiro SH, Ernst P, Gray-Donald K, et al. Effect of negative pressure ventilation in severe chronic obstructive pulmonary disease. *Lancet* 1992;340:1425–1429.

60. Zibrak JD, Hill NS, Federman ED, et al. Evaluation of intermittent long-term negative pressure ventilation in patients with severe chronic obstructive pulmonary disease. *Am Rev Respir Dis* 1988;138:1515–1518.

61. Strumpf DA, Carlisle CC, Millman RP, et al. An evaluation of the Respironics BiPAP bi-level CPAP device for delivery of assisted ventilation. *Respir Care* 1990;35:415–422.

62. Meecham-Jones DJ, Paul EA, Jones PW. Nasal pressure support ventilation plus oxygen compared with oxygen therapy alone in hypercapnic COPD. *Am J Respir Crit Care Med* 1995;152:538–544.

63. Lin CC. Comparison between nocturnal nasal positive pressure ventilation combined with oxygen therapy and oxygen monotherapy in patients with severe COPD. *Am J Respir Crit Care Med* 1996;154:353–358.

64. Casanova C, Celli BR, Tost L, et al. Long-term controlled trial of nocturnal nasal positive pressure ventilation with severe COPD. *Chest* 2000;118:1582–1590.

65. Jones SE, Packham S. Hebden M, et al. Domiciliary nocturnal intermittent positive pressure ventilation in patients with respiratory failure due to severe COPD: long-term follow-up and effect on survival. *Thorax* 1998;53:495–498.

66. Muir JF, De la Salmoniere P, Cuvelier A, et al. Home NIPPV + oxygen versus long-term oxygen therapy alone in severe hypercapnic COPD patients: a European multicenter study. *Am J Respir Crit Care Med* 2000;A262.

67. Mehta S, Hill NS. Noninvasive ventilation—state of the art. *Am J Respir Crit Care Med* 2001;163(2):540–577.

68. Brochard L, Mancebo J, Wysocki M, et al. Noninvasive ventilation for acute exacerbations of chronic obstructive pulmonary disease. *N Engl J Med* 1995;333:817–822.

69. Plant PK, Owen JL, Elliott MW. Early use of noninvasive ventilation for acute exacerbations of chronic obstructive pulmonary disease on general respiratory wards: a multicenter randomized controlled trial. *Lancet* 2000;355:1931–1935.

70. Meduri GU, Cook TR, Turner RE, et al. Noninvasive positive pressure ventilation in status asthmaticus. *Chest* 1996;110:767–774.

71. Holley MT, Morrissey TK, Seaberg DC, et al. Ethical dilemmas in a randomized trial of asthma treatment: can bayesian statistical analysis explain the results? *Academic Emerg Med* 2001;72:1128–1135.

72. Hodson ME, Madden BP, Steven MH, et al. Noninvasive mechanical ventilation for cystic fibrosis patients—a potential bridge to transplantation. *Eur Respir J* 1991;4:524–527.

73. Antonelli M, Conti G, Rocco M, et al. A comparison of non-invasive positive-pressure ventilation and conventional mechanical ventilation in patients with acute respiratory failure. *N Engl J Med* 1998;339:429–435.

74. Wysocki M, Tric L, Wolff MA, et al. Noninvasive pressure support ventilation in patients with acute respiratory failure. A randomized comparison with conventional therapy. *Chest* 1995;107:761–768.

75. Barach AL, Martin J, Eckman M. Positive pressure respiration and its application to the treatment of acute pulmonary edema. *Ann Intern Med* 1938;12:754–795.

76. Rasanen J, Heikkila J, Downs J, et al. Continuous positive airway pressure by face mask in acute cardiogenic pulmonary edema. *Am J Cardiol* 1985;55:296–300.

77. Lin M, Chiang H. The efficacy of early continuous positive airway pressure therapy in patients with acute cardiogenic pulmonary edema. *J Formos Med Assoc* 1991;90:736–743.

78. Bersten AD, Holt AW, Vedig AE, et al. Treatment of severe cardiogenic pulmonary edema with continuous positive airway pressure delivered by face mask. *N Engl J Med* 1991;325:1825–1830.

79. Lin M, Yang Y, Chiany H, et al. Reappraisal of continuous positive airway pressure therapy in acute cardiogenic pulmonary edema: short-term results and long-term follow-up. *Chest* 1995;107:1379–1386.

80. Masip J, Betbese AJ, Paez J, et al. Noninvasive pressure support ventilation versus conventional oxygen therapy in acute cardiogenic pulmonary oedema: a randomized study. *Lancet* 2000;356:2126–2132.

81. Mehta S, Jay GD, Woolard RH, et al. Randomized prospective trial of bilevel versus continuous positive airway pressure in acute pulmonary edema. *Crit Care Med* 1997;25:620–628.

82. Pang D, Keenan SP, Cook DJ, et al. The effect of positive pressure airway support on mortality and the need for intubation in cardiogenic pulmonary edema. *Chest* 1998;114:1185–1192.

83. Ambrosino N, Foglio K, Rubini F, et al. Noninvasive mechanical ventilation in acute respiratory failure due to chronic obstructive pulmonary disease: correlates for success. *Thorax* 1995;50:755–757.

84. Confalonieri M, Potena A, Carbone G, et al. Acute respiratory failure in patients with severe community-acquired pneumonia. *Am J Respir Crit Care Med* 1999;160:1585–1591.

85. Jolliet P, Abajo B, Pasquina P, et al. Noninvasive pressure support ventilation in severe community-acquired pneumonia. *Intensive Care Med* 2001;27:812–821.

86. Antonelli M, Conti G, Bufi M, et al. Noninvasive ventilation for treatment of acute respiratory failure in patients undergoing solid organ transplantation. *JAMA* 2000;283:235–241.

87. Hilbert G, Gruson D, Vargas F, et al. Noninvasive ventilation in immunosuppressed patients with pulmonary infiltrates and acute respiratory failure. *N Engl J Med* 2001;344:481–487.

88. Rocker GM, Mackensie M-G, Williams B, et al. Noninvasive positive pressure ventilation. Successful outcome in patients with acute lung injury/ARDS. *Chest* 1999;115:173–177.

89. Beltrane F, Lucangelo U, Gregori D, et al. Noninvasive positive pressure ventilation in trauma patients with acute respiratory failure. *Monaldi Arch Chest Dis* 1999;54:109–114.

90. Aguilo R, Togores B, Pons S, et al. Noninvasive ventilator support after lung resectional surgery. *Chest* 1997;112:117–121.

91. Joris JL, Sottiaux TM, Chiche JD, et al. Effect of bi-level positive airway pressure (BiPAP) nasal ventilation on the postoperative pulmonary restrictive syndrome in obese patients undergoing gastroplasty. *Chest* 1997;111:665–670.

92. Auriant I, Jallot A, Herve P, et al. Noninvasive ventilation reduces mortality in acute respiratory failure following lung resection. *Am J Respir Crit Care Med* 2001;164:1231–1235.

93. Meduri GU, Fox RC, Abou-Shala N, et al. Noninvasive mechanical ventilation via face mask in patients with acute respiratory failure who refused endotracheal intubation. *Crit Care Med* 1994;22:1584–1590.

94. Nelson DL, Short K, Vespia J, et al. A prospective review of the outcomes of patients with "do-not-intubate" orders who receive noninvasive ventilation. *Crit Care Med* 2000;28:A34.

95. Udwadia ZF, Santis GK, Stevan MH, et al. Nasal ventilation to facilitate weaning in patients with chronic respiratory insufficiency. *Thorax* 1992;47:715–718.

96. Nava S, Ambrosino N, Clini E, et al. Noninvasive mechanical ventilation in the weaning of patients with respiratory failure due to chronic obstructive pulmonary disease: a randomized study. *Ann Intern Med* 1998;128:721–728.

97. Girault C, Daudenthun I, Chevron V, et al. Noninvasive ventilation as a systematic extubation and weaning technique in acute-on-chronic respiratory failure. *Am J Respir Crit Care Med* 1999;160:86–92.

98. Epstein SK, Ciabotaru RL, Wong JB. Effect of failed extubation on outcome of mechanical ventilation. *Am J Respir Crit Care Med* 1997;112:186–192.

99. Hilbert G, Gruson D, Portel L, et al. Noninvasive pressure support ventilation in COPD patients with post-extubation hypercapnic respiratory insufficiency. *Eur Respir J* 1998;11:1349–1353.

100. Jiang J-S, Kao S-J, Wang S-N. Effect of early application of biphasic positive airway pressure on the outcome of extubation in ventilator weaning. *Respirology* 1999;4:161–165.

101. Barlow PB, Bartlett D, Hauri P, et al. Idiopathic hypoventilation syndrome: importance of preventing nocturnal hypoxemia and hypercapnia. *Am Rev Respir Dis* 1980;121:141–145.

102. Hill NS, Redline S, Carskadon MA, et al. Sleep-disordered breathing in patients with Duchenne muscular dystrophy using negative pressure ventilators. *Chest* 1992;102:1656–1662.

103. Bach JR, Brougher P, Hess DR, et al. Consensus statement: noninvasive positive pressure ventilation. *Respir Care* 1997;42:365–369.

104. Hill NS. Clinical applications of body ventilators. *Chest* 1986;90:897–905.

105. Hill NS. Complications of noninvasive positive pressure ventilation. *Respir Care* 1997;42:432–442.

106. Navalesi P, Fanfulla F, Frigerio P, et al. Physiologic evaluation of noninvasive mechanical ventilation delivered by three types of masks in patients with chronic hypercapnic respiratory failure. *Crit Care Med* 2000;28:1785–1790.

107. Kwok H, McCormack J, Cece R, et al. Controlled trial of oronasal versus nasal mask ventilation in the treatment of acute respiratory failure. *Crit Care Med* 2003;31:468–473.

107a. Mehta S, McCool FD, Hill NS. Leak compensation in positive pressure ventilators. *Eur Respir J* 2000;15:A407.

108. Calderini E, Confalonieri M, Puccio PG, et al. Patient-ventilator asynchrony during noninvasive ventilation: the role of expiratory trigger. *Intensive Care Med* 1999;25:662–667.

109. Ferguson GT, Gilmartin M. CO$_2$ rebreathing during BiPAP ventilatory assistance. *Am J Respir Crit Care Med* 1995;151:1126–1135.

110. Hill NS, Carlisle C, Kramer N. Effect of an exhalation valve on long-term nasal ventilation using the BiPAP™ device. *Chest* 2002;122(1):84–91.

111. Glenn WWL, Broullette RT, Dentz B, et al. Fundamental considerations in pacing of the diaphragm for chronic ventilatory insufficiency: a multicenter study. *PACE* 1988;11:2121–2127.

112. Krieger AJ, Gropper MR, Adler RJ. Electrophrenic respiration after intercostal to phrenic nerve anastomosis in a patient with anterior spinal artery syndrome: technical case report. *Neurosurgery* 1994;35:760–764.

113. Moxham J, Shneerson JM. Diaphragmatic pacing. *Am Rev Respir Dis* 1993;148:533–536.

114. Dail CW, Affeldt JR, Collier CR. Clinical aspects of glossopharyngeal breathing. *JAMA* 1953;158:445–449.

115. Bach JR. Update and perspectives on noninvasive respiratory muscle aids: part 2—the expiratory muscle aids. *Chest* 1994;105:1538–1544.

116. Bach JR. Mechanical insufflation-exsufflation: comparison of peak expiratory flows with manually assisted and unassisted coughing techniques. *Chest* 1993;104:1553–1564.

117. Bach JR, Saporito LR. Criteria for extubation and tracheostomy tube removal for patients with ventilatory failure: a different approach to weaning. *Chest* 1996;110:1566–1571.

118. Bach JR, Ishikawa Y, Kim H. Prevention of pulmonary morbidity for patients with Duchenne muscular dystrophy. *Chest* 1997;112:1024–1028.

119. Raphael JC, Chevret S, Chastang C, et al. French multicenter trial of prophylactic nasal ventilation in Duchenne muscular dystrophy. *Lancet* 1994;343:1600–1604.

54 Lung Transplantation

Tim Higenbottam

There is much to celebrate in the development of clinical lung transplant surgery over the past 20 years. It has not only provided a treatment for lung failure but also indirectly has added much to our knowledge of the underlying end-stage lung diseases that cause lung failure. The first reports of success were of heart-lung transplantation for pulmonary hypertension in 1982 (1). In the intervening years, we have learned how to manage many of the "new" diseases of the transplanted lung and so improve survival and quality of life of the recipient. Also, scientific work on the explanted tissue has expanded our knowledge of those diseases that lead to lung failure (2,3). In turn, this knowledge has led to a rapid introduction of effective treatments for some diseases such as primary pulmonary hypertension (PPH) (4–6). The success of these new medical treatments for PPH has reduced need for transplant surgery and may ultimately lead to a cure.

The benefit of transplant surgery derives from the replacement of diseased organs with normal ones, capable of restoring enhanced function to the recipient. However, the cost of transplantation is the risk of developing alternative illnesses that can lead to further lung failure. These illnesses include the discrete causes of pulmonary failure that occur at various times after surgery, such as primary graft failure, acute pulmonary rejection, reimplantation response, pulmonary infections, and airway complications. Although there is overlap in their clinical presentation, each illness is associated with a standardized pathway of investigation and has effective treatments. There still, however, remains a considerable challenge to the long-term success of lung transplant surgery. The obstacle to long-term success is the development of bronchiolitis obliterans syndrome (BOS), which afflicts 50% of lung transplant recipients by 5 years (7). BOS contributes signif-

icantly to the long-term morbidity and mortality rates after adult lung transplant surgery.

Lung transplant surgery requires the premature death of the donor, with the exception of living-related lobar donation. Transplant physicians therefore are obliged to make the most effective use of this precious gift. Two important decisions are required. The first concerns the selection of the individual patient. The second concerns the choice of the most suitable disease to transplant so as to achieve the greatest success from the surgery. Twenty years of experience has provided the necessary information for patient selection criteria and for the diseases suitable for this form of surgery (8). Society also has to make choices in terms of how it spends medical insurance monies or national taxes. Again, detailed analysis of the cost benefits of lung transplant surgery in terms of extension of survival and improvement of quality of life provide guidance on the suitability of this surgical treatment (9).

In the foreseeable future, human donation of organs for transplant surgery is not likely to provide sufficient numbers to treat all suitable patients with terminal lung failure. As only a selected few will benefit, the quest has been to find alternative sources of organs for transplant surgery. Approaches include transgenically modified animals to provide xenografts (10) or development of organs from stem-cell science. Although these notions are still far from realization, they offer a sight of the future potential of lung transplant surgery as a generally applicable, rather than a highly selected, treatment for lung failure.

THE HISTORY OF LUNG TRANSPLANTATION

The advance in immunosuppressive therapy that occurred with the established use of cyclosporine in renal and heart

T. Higenbottam: Division of Clinical Science, The Medical School, University of Sheffield, Sheffield, United Kingdom.

transplant surgery contributed significantly to the successful reintroduction of lung transplantation in the early 1980s. Concern about the frequent development of airway complications that occurred with the earlier immunosuppressive treatments such as azathioprine and corticosteroids had led to abandonment of lung transplant surgery in the 1970s. The first large series of successful heart-lung transplants was reported in 1982, for individuals with PPH (1).

After the successful introduction of heart-lung transplantation, single lung transplant surgery was soon developed, initially for interstitial lung disease (ILD) (11). Major work on surgical techniques was then undertaken to achieve an optimal method to transplant two lungs (12), resulting in the sequential bilateral lung transplant operation. This became the treatment of choice for cystic fibrosis and end-stage chronic obstructive pulmonary disease (COPD) (20).

Combined heart-lung transplant surgery has declined markedly over the past decade, in part as a result of poorer long-term results compared with single lung and bilateral lung transplants, and because donors were needed for an increasing number of cardiac transplants. Heart-lung transplants are now performed only for specific conditions such as congenital heart disease and associated pulmonary hypertension, in which the cardiac abnormality cannot be surgically corrected (13).

LUNG TRANSPLANTS: VOLUME, INDICATIONS, AND SURVIVAL

Since 1994, the yearly rate of lung transplants worldwide has remained constant at around 1,300 to 1,500, roughly split evenly between single and bilateral lung transplants.

The leading indications for lung transplant surgery are COPD, idiopathic pulmonary fibrosis (IPF), cystic fibrosis, emphysema from α_1-antitrypsin deficiency, and PPH (Table 54.1). There have been significant changes over the past 10 years, with a decline in transplants for PPH from

13% in 1990 to 4% in 2000, because of improvements in primary medical treatments for the condition. In contrast, transplants for all forms of COPD and emphysema have risen from 21% to 42% over the same period (7). Individuals with COPD and IPF are usually offered single lung transplants, whereas those with cystic fibrosis and COPD may be offered bilateral lung transplants.

Survival after lung transplantation has improved over the past two decades. Bilateral lung transplants have a half-life of 4.9 years and a conditional half-life (postoperative and perioperative survival time, which is a measure of the effect of the transplant) of 7.9 years compared with a single-lung transplant half-life of 3.7 years and a conditional half-life of 5.9 years. There are differences in the outcome from surgery depending on the disease for which the transplant is performed that may be described by differing perioperative survival. Sarcoidosis, PPH, and IPF have the poorer postsurgical survival figures (7). Such factors influence the size of the differences between the estimated half-lives and the conditional half-lives.

HEART-LUNG TRANSPLANTS: VOLUME, INDICATIONS, AND SURVIVAL

Since 1988, there has been a continuous decline in the annual number of heart-lung transplants. In 2000, the number was only 105, having been almost 250 in 1988.

Over 20% of all heart-lung transplants are performed in patients who are less than 18 years of age. PPH and congenital heart disease with associated pulmonary hypertension are the most frequent indications, followed by cystic fibrosis. As with lung transplantation, effective medical therapies for PPH have led to a decline in the annual rate of heart-lung transplants, from 35% of all operations in 1982–1990 to 20% in 1996–2000. The beneficiary has been the congenital heart group of patients, particularly Eisenmenger syndrome in which the cardiac abnormality could not be surgically

TABLE 54.1. THE COMMON LUNG DISEASES THAT ARE OFFERED LUNG TRANSPLANTS

Diagnosis	Single Lung Transplant (n = 4,663)		Bilateral Lung Transplant (n = 4,118)		Total (n = 8,781)	
Chronic obstructive pulmonary disease/emphysema	2,536	54%	926	22%	3,462	40%
Idiopathic pulmonary fibrosis	1,110	23%	376	9%	1,486	17%
Cystic fibrosis	52	1%	1,360	33%	1,412	16%
α_1-Antitrypsin deficiency emphysema	408	9%	407	10%	815	9%
Primary pulmonary hypertension	61	1%	340	8%	401	5%
Sarcoidosis	126	3%	106	3%	232	3%
Bronchiectasis	14	0.3%	176	4%	190	2%
Congenital heart disease	8	0.2%	95	2%	103	1%
Lymphangiomyomatosis	42	1%	53	1%	95	1%
Connective tissue disease	21	0.4%	18	0.4%	38	0.4%
Cancer	7	0.2%	28	0.7%	35	0.4%

From Hertz MI, Taylor DO, Trulock EP, et al. The Registrary of the International Society for Heart and Lung Transplantation: ninteenth official report—2002. *J Heart Lung Transplant* 2002;21:950–970, with permission.

corrected (13). The percentage of all heart-lung transplants performed for congenital heart disease has risen to 41% in 2000.

Survival from heart-lung transplantation is poorer than survival for lung transplants alone. The half-life is only 2.8 years, largely as a result of poorer perioperative survival as the conditional half-life is 8.2 years.

SELECTION CRITERIA FOR LUNG AND HEART-LUNG TRANSPLANTS

There are optimal ages for lung transplant surgery: For heart-lung transplants, the upper age limit is 55 years; for single lung transplant, the upper age limit is 65 years; and for bilateral lung transplant, the upper age limit is set at 60 years. Patients evaluated for lung transplantation should have received maximal optimal medical treatment for their chronic lung disease and be deemed to be facing a premature fatal outcome as a result of failure of medical therapy to arrest the progress of the disease (8). Concurrent nonpulmonary illness should be adequately treated and preventative care instituted for common illnesses, such as vaccination for influenza and pneumococcal pneumonia. Medical conditions that impact the results of lung transplantation may be considered as relative (Table 54.2) or absolute contraindications to surgery (Table 54.3).

An individual assessment should be performed for every patient, and careful counseling regarding risks and benefits is required. Most centers admit the potential recipient for a period of time to allow the multidisciplinary specialist transplant team members to undertake the detailed evaluation.

Donors and recipient are matched according to ABO blood group. Cytomegalovirus (CMV)-positive donors are usually matched to positive recipients.

TABLE 54.2. RELATIVE CONTRAINDICATIONS

- *Symptomatic* and *asymptomatic osteoporosis* require treatment before transplantation of the lungs. The diagnosis requires full investigation and appropriate objective measures of improvement, as with bone densitometry.
- *Severe musculoskeletal disease of the thorax* is a relative contraindication, and *progressive neuromuscular disease* is an absolute contraindication.
- *Current corticosteroid therapy* is not a contraindication, but the dose should be reduced to ≤20 mg/d.
- *Obesity* or *cachexia* are contraindications; weight needs to be from 70%–130% of ideal body weight.
- *Freedom from substance abuse* for 6 mo is needed, and this includes nicotine, alcohol, and narcotics.
- *Psychosocial problems* must be resolved before surgery.
- *Requirement for invasive ventilation* is a relative contraindication, but this is not applied to patients on noninvasive ventilatory support.
- *Colonization with fungi and mycobacteria* are not absolute contraindications, but special care needs to be observed where single lung transplantation is considered.

TABLE 54.3. ABSOLUTE CONTRAINDICATIONS

- *Major dysfunction of another organ*, such as liver or renal failure, precludes lung transplantation unless combined multiorgan transplant is considered.
- *Infection with HIV.*
- *Infection with hepatitis B (antigen positivity) and hepatitis C with liver disease.*

SELECTION CRITERIA FOR INDIVIDUAL END-STAGE LUNG DISEASES

Lung Transplantation for PPH

"Replacement of pulmonary hypertensive lungs with healthy engrafted ones, that offers the patient a normal pulmonary vascular resistance" is the goal of transplantation for PPH (12,18,20,25,27,58). The natural history of untreated (14) and treated PPH (15) has been known for some time. For the untreated patient, measurements of functional disability (New York Heart Association class, hemodynamic measurements) allow accurate prediction of survival (Table 54.4). More recently, measurements that are predictive of a poor prognosis for patients on "effective" treatments have been described (16,17). Thus, it is now possible to recognize those patients who are failing to respond to medical therapy; this is the population of individuals for whom lung transplantation should be reserved (Table 54.5).

COPD and Emphysema (Including α_1-Antitrypsin Deficiency)

Patients with COPD/emphysema considered for transplant must be optimally medically treated, and asthma must be excluded. The selection is made according to the severity of their disease such that a forced expired volume in 1 second

TABLE 54.4. HOW TO ASSESS PROGNOSIS IN PRIMARY PULMONARY HYPERTENSION AND MONITOR PROGRESS ON TREATMENT

1. Clinical measures
   Modified New York Heart Association functional classes III and IV
Class I and II	5 y mean survival
Class III	2.5 y mean survival
Class IV	0.5 y mean survival

   Falling exercise capacity
   Syncope
   Hemoptysis
   Signs of right ventricular failure
2. Hemodynamic measures
   Pulmonary arterial oxygen saturation <63%
>63%	55% survival at 3 y
<63%	17% survival at 3 y

   Cardiac index <2.1 L/(min · m^2)
<2.1	17 mo median survival

   Right atrial pressure >10 mm Hg
<10 mm Hg	4 y mean survival
>20 mm Hg	1 mo mean survival

   Lack of pulmonary vasodilator response to acute challenge

TABLE 54.5. INDICATIONS FOR LUNG TRANSPLANTATION

- The patient with primary pulmonary hypertension on optimal medical therapy for whom the New York Heart Association functional class is IV and 6-min walk distance is <300 m.
- The patients in whom both a 3-month trial of oral bosentan and a 3-month trial of IV prostacyclin have failed to stabilize or improve functional class, 6-min walking distance, and hemodynamics
- Those patients, who have received bosentan and prostacyclin for 3 mo and have developed pericardial effusions, elevated B-type natriuretic peptide, and arterial oxygen desaturation (>20%) during exercise testing

(FEV_1) less than 25% of predicted without reversibility, and/or an arterial partial pressure of carbon dioxide ($PaCO_2$) of greater than 55 mm Hg (7.3 kPa), and/or elevated pulmonary artery pressure must be present. Preference is shown to those patients with elevated $PaCO_2$ who require long-term oxygen therapy.

Idiopathic Pulmonary Fibrosis

The problem with IPF is that the disease is rapidly progressive and responds poorly to corticosteroids. Most patients are elderly and have concurrent illness.

It is good practice to refer patients to a transplant center once the diagnosis is made, at least for evaluation and subsequent follow-up. Patients with rapidly increasing dyspnea, a vital capacity measurement less than 60% predicted, and a diffusion coefficient for carbon monoxide of less than 60% have a particularly poor prognosis and should be given special consideration.

Cystic Fibrosis

Patients with cystic fibrosis are chosen on the basis of poor lung function, e.g., an FEV_1 less than 30% predicted and a resting $PaCO_2$ greater than 6.5 kPa (50 mm Hg) and an arterial partial pressure of oxygen (PaO_2) less than 7.3 kPa (55 mm Hg). Young female patients with rapidly declining values of FEV_1 are also given special consideration, as they have a poor prognosis. Patients with multiresistant strains of bacteria are not precluded from transplant surgery.

Congenital Heart Disease with Associated Pulmonary Hypertension

Patients are chosen on the basis of New York Heart Association functional class, particularly when the functional class has recently decreased. Special consideration is given to class III and IV patients.

Surgical Techniques Used in Lung and Heart-Lung Transplant Surgery

Twenty years of experience of the efficacy of the different types of lung transplant techniques (13,18–22) and the

additional demands for cardiac donation have empirically led to current practices. An additional important factor is the local experience and skill of the transplant center. The main types of surgery offered for each major indication (7) are listed below:

- COPD/emphysema—most receive single and a smaller number receive bilateral lung transplants
- IPF—mainly receive single lung transplants
- Cystic fibrosis—mainly bilateral lung transplants
- PPH—mainly receive bilateral lung transplants, whereas a significant minority receive heart and lung transplants
- Congenital heart disease—bilateral lung and heart and lung transplants according to the ability to correct the cardiac abnormality.

Heart-Lung Transplantation

The lungs and heart of the recipient are removed en bloc, and the donor trachea is anastomosed to that of the recipient just above the carina (1,22). The integrity of the anastomosis is maintained as a result of extensive collateral arterial blood supply to the lower trachea from the coronary arteries.

The additional advantage of heart-lung transplantation includes the simultaneous engraftment of a heart, allowing immediate restoration of normal cardiac output, which may be an important factor in patients with severe pulmonary hypertension who have long experienced poor cardiac output. The operation requires cardiopulmonary bypass, which sets an age limit of 65 years on the potential recipient.

The major disadvantage of this surgery is that the heart can be involved in chronic rejection, resulting in coronary vascular occlusion (23). Another disadvantage is the limitation of the number of recipients who could potentially benefit from the donor's organs. Alternative use of the organs could theoretically provide two lung disease recipients with single lungs and a heart recipient with a heart. One way around this problem is the "domino" operation in which the recipient's (for the lung transplant) heart is donated to a second cardiac recipient. The long-term results of the domino heart procedure are better than conventional cardiac donation (24).

Internationally, the results of heart-lung transplantation are poorer than the results for other forms of lung transplantation, mainly as a result of worse perioperative survival (7). The half-life of heart and lung transplants is 2.8 years, but the conditional half-life (after excluding the perioperative deaths) is exceptionally good, at 8.2 years. Most patients attain their predicted normal values for FEV_1, vital capacity, and total lung capacity (TLC) within 3 months of the surgery. The elevated pulmonary vascular resistance of PPH is restored to normal, and the disease does not recur in the transplanted lung (25). However, exercise tolerance is not as good as predicted, probably as a result of the denervated heart being unable to increase cardiac output in response to exercise in a normal fashion (26).

At 5 years after transplant, more than 40% of patients are at either full-time or part-time work. Considering the severity of the incapacity associated with either PPH or Eisenmenger syndrome, these long-term results are impressive.

Single Lung Transplantation

Single lung transplantation was first used to treat ILD (20), but quickly gained an indication in the treatment of end-stage emphysema (27). The procedure is performed through a standard lateral thoracotomy incision and does not require cardiopulmonary bypass. An end-to-end bronchial anastomosis is wrapped with omentum tunneled up through the diaphragm. The pulmonary artery is directly reanastomosed, and a cuff of the donor's left atrium (containing the pulmonary veins) is connected to the recipient's left atrium.

Its advantages are that two lung recipients and one cardiac recipient can be potentially treated from one donor. For COPD/emphysema, single lung transplantation also offers a greater chance of a transplant simply because of greater organ availability. As cardiopulmonary bypass is needed only for a minority of the patients, single lung transplants can be offered to those older than 65 years. Indeed, it appears that survival after a single lung transplant is better than is survival after a bilateral lung transplant for patients older than 60 years (28). Survival after single lung transplant for IPF is less good than for other indications, the same is true for PPH and sarcoidosis.

As one native lung remains, the improvement of lung function is less impressive than with double or heart-lung transplants. The hemodynamic improvement is remarkably good, and there is a report of reversal of pulmonary hypertension in the remaining native lung after single lung transplantation in a patient with PPH (29).

If obliterative bronchiolitis (OB) develops in the single lung transplant in an individual with IPF or PPH, a major gas exchange abnormality will ensue. This is because the remaining recipient lung receives little perfusion while the transplanted lung with severe airflow obstruction receives little ventilation (20). It is this issue that has led to the enthusiasm for sequential bilateral lung transplantation.

Sequential Bilateral Lung Transplantation

This operation is performed as two sequential single lung transplants. Donor lungs are transected at the level of the distal trachea and are removed en bloc with the main pulmonary artery and a large left atrial cuff. Because of the high incidence of tracheal anastomotic complications, as well as bleeding complications and poor exposure to the posterior mediastinum, sequential bilateral lung transplantation is performed.

The recipient incision has now been changed from a median sternotomy to an anterior thoracosternotomy (the "clam shell" incision). Donor lungs are implanted as two single lungs with separate vascular and bronchial anastomoses.

This procedure generally eliminates the need for cardiopulmonary bypass. For PPH patients who require bilateral lung transplants, cardiopulmonary bypass is still needed (12,20).

Bilateral lung transplantation offers the best survival outcome for patients under the age of 60 years with emphysema/COPD (28). It is the procedure of choice for cystic fibrosis, because removal of both infected lungs prevents the spread of bacteria from native to engrafted lung, such as occurs in single lung transplants (20).

Bilateral lung transplantation is also the favored technique for PPH because single transplants for this condition are associated with a higher postoperative incidence of reimplantation lung edema. Interestingly, although left ventricular dysfunction is unusual in pulmonary hypertension patients, there is a high incidence of post-transplant left ventricular failure in PPH patients after either single lung or sequential bilateral lung transplantation (30). To some extent, this can be predicted by careful review of a preoperative echocardiogram, in which a relationship between right and left ventricular dysfunction may be found in individuals with severe PPH (31,32). It is also usual practice to perform coronary angiography on all PPH patients above the age of 50 years and on patients when there might be a risk of ischemic heart disease.

Retention of a normally innervated heart, normal lung function, and better exercise capacity of sequential bilateral lung transplantation than with heart-lung or single lung are the principle reasons for preferring this technique. After 5 years, about 35% of patients are at either full-time or part-time work.

Living-Donor Bilateral Lobar Transplants

This technique has been primarily used in children with cystic fibrosis because of the small donor pool. Donations from living relatives have been proposed as life-saving, with minimal risk to an otherwise healthy donor, and the technique is usually performed to provide bilateral implants using bilateral lower lobes (33). It appears that the frequency of acute rejection is less than that for cadaveric transplants (34). Furthermore, there is some evidence of a lower incidence of BOS in these patients than for cadaveric transplant recipients (35). Potential recipients and their relatives are carefully selected with ethical considerations a prime concern (36).

DONOR SELECTION

The procurement of acceptable lungs for transplantation is more difficult than is procurement for other solid organs. Brain death commonly contributes to injury to the lung from hemodynamic instability, noncardiogenic pulmonary edema, or aspiration. This accounts for the limitation of suitable donor organs for lung transplantation.

Ideal donor characteristics include an insignificant smoking history, there being poorer survival among recipients of lungs from smokers (7). ABO compatibility with the recipient is sought. The arterial oxygen tension should be sufficient (Pao$_2$ >300 mm Hg on 100% inspired oxygen with 5 mm Hg of positive end-expiratory pressure [PEEP]). There should be a clear chest radiograph, and absence of purulent secretions at bronchoscopy.

Size matching between the recipient and donor is made from the chest radiograph by using vertical (apex to diaphragm at mid-clavicular line) and horizontal (level of dome of diaphragm) measurements. "Oversizing" of the donor lung(s) is better tolerated in single lung transplantation than in sequential bilateral lung transplants.

The increased demand for donor lungs, together with increased experience, has led to the use of donor lungs previously judged unsuitable. Minimal pulmonary infiltrates, borderline oxygenation, or secretions that can be easily cleared by bronchoscopy may not contraindicate donation. Such cases need to be individualized. Donor lungs are transported cold and inflated. At the present time, cold ischemic times of up to 6 hours appear to be well tolerated.

There is considerable empirical and experimental evidence that pretreatment of the donor with prostacyclin or prostaglandin E$_2$ improves the post-transplant function of the pulmonary graft. Equivalent evidence also exists for the postoperative use of inhaled nitric oxide (37). The present use of these agents is governed by accessibility and cost.

DONOR SELECTION CRITERIA	
Summary Statement	**Level of Evidence**
Non-smoking	Consensus opinions
Preremoval Pao$_2$ >300 mm Hg on 100% inspired oxygen with 5 mm Hg of PEEP; clear chest x-ray and absence of purulent secretions at bronchoscopy	Consensus opinions
Reasonable size matching to recipient	Case-controlled studies
Pretreatment with prostacyclin for vasodilatation	Case-controlled studies

Pao$_2$, partial pressure of oxygen, arterial; PEEP, positive end-expiratory pressure.

POSTOPERATIVE CARE

The complications resulting from the surgery are the principle cause of delayed postoperative recovery after a lung transplant patient. A further risk factor is preexisting end-stage pulmonary disease and the need for cardiopulmonary bypass. Patients without pulmonary hypertension undergoing single lung transplantation tend to require minimal hemodynamic and ventilatory support. They experience the minimal intensive care unit length of stay and have an early discharge from the hospital within 7 to 10 days.

A multidisciplinary team manages the patients after transfer from the operating room to the surgical intensive care unit. This team includes the following staff: the transplant surgeons, the critical care nursing staff, the transplant coordinators, the transplant pulmonologist, physical and respiratory therapists, and nutritionists. Infectious disease specialists are also involved. Routine early postoperative care includes careful monitoring of vital signs, accurate documentation of intake and output, daily chest radiographs, and laboratory analysis, including cyclosporine or tacrolimus levels. The serum creatinine must be monitored particularly closely because keeping the patient relatively intravascularly volume depleted, together with the use of nephrotoxic immunosuppressive agents and antibiotics, may have adverse effects on renal function.

Patients always have a pulmonary artery catheter and arterial line in place on arrival from the operating room. A postoperative perfusion scan is performed to detect pulmonary artery anastomotic abnormalities and thrombosis. Venous thromboembolism and gastrointestinal prophylaxis and adequate pain management are crucial. Placement of an epidural catheter for analgesia is frequently beneficial and facilitates early postoperative ambulation and physical therapy.

Nutrition should be addressed early, particularly in patients with cystic fibrosis. Enteral tube feeding should be initiated early if a patient is unable to be fed orally within a few days. If postoperative ileus prevents this, then total parenteral nutrition should be administered.

Hemodynamic Management

Optimal hemodynamic management is essential after lung or heart-lung transplantation. Because the lymphatic drainage of the lung has been interrupted during transplantation, and because of capillary damage from ischaemia and preservation injury of the transplanted lung(s), there is susceptibility to pulmonary edema formation. Early rejection or infection may also contribute to edema formation. The reimplantation response may result in severe noncardiogenic pulmonary edema and requires aggressive diuresis, cautious use of positive end-expiratory pressure, and, in the single lung transplantation patient, positioning the affected lung up. Independent lung ventilation has been used when pulmonary edema is severe and the lungs have markedly differing compliances.

Patients with pulmonary hypertension undergoing single lung transplantation present particular difficulties, and cardiopulmonary bypass is usually required. These individuals often develop reperfusion edema from the tremendous diversion of blood flow to the new lung. This may result in extreme hemodynamic instability. Discontinuing chronic continuous prostacyclin therapy may produce an acute increase in right ventricular afterload. When sequential bilateral lung transplantation is performed in patients with pulmonary hypertension, hemodynamic management is less difficult.

Mechanical Ventilation

Management of the ventilator after transplantation depends on the underlying disease, the operative procedure, and the stability of the patient. In COPD patients undergoing single lung transplant, minimal or no positive end-expired pressure and lower tidal volumes are used to minimize overdistention of the more compliant native lung. This phenomenon can result in lung herniation with mediastinal shift. Occasionally, replacing the usual single-lumen endotracheal tube with a double-lumen endotracheal tube to permit separate lung ventilation, or even performing volume reduction surgery on the native lung may be helpful. In single lung transplant recipients with underlying pulmonary fibrosis, low tidal volumes and flow rates may help to avoid barotrauma in the stiff native lung.

Bronchoscopy

Examination of the airways is performed in the operating room and again before extubation to evaluate the anastomoses. In patients requiring prolonged mechanical ventilation after transplantation, frequent bronchoscopy may be required to clear secretions and to obtain microbiologic specimens. Impairment of the cough reflex may suggest the need for bronchoscopy as often as daily in some patients during the intensive care unit stay. Aggressive physical therapy is crucial after transplantation. Incentive spirometry, chest physical therapy, frequent turning, and early ambulation are emphasized.

Infection Prophylaxis

Protocols for infection prophylaxis are routinely utilized for bacterial, CMV, *Pneumocystis carinii*, and *Toxoplasma gondii* infections. Certain patients may benefit from fungal prophylaxis as well. Patients with cystic fibrosis should undergo periodic preoperative sputum culture analysis to allow appropriate postoperative antibiotic administration. Synergy studies are often useful in determining appropriate antibiotic combinations. Because CMV is such a frequent pathogen after transplantation, most programs use prolonged prophylaxis, particularly in CMV-seronegative recipients receiving CMV-positive lung grafts. Such prophylaxis will delay but not necessarily prevent the development of CMV infection (see below).

Immunosuppressive Treatment

At the time of surgery about 43% of lung transplant patients (7) receive induction immunosuppressive therapy. This is comprised of either polyclonal antilymphocyte/antithymocyte globulin or an interleukin-2 receptor antagonist. Azathioprine is initiated preoperatively at a dose of 2 mg/kg and is adjusted downward for a white blood cell count

TABLE 54.6. THE CURRENT MAINTENANCE IMMUNOSUPPRESSIVE TREATMENTS USED IN LUNG TRANSPLANTS

- Cyclosporine and mycophenolate mofetil
- Cyclosporine and azathioprine
- Tacrolimus and mycophenolate mofetil
- Tacrolimus and mucophenolate mofetil

Most patients remain on daily prednisolone (at 5 years only 5% patients are steroid free).

of 5,000 or less. Methylprednisolone is administered intravenously at 500 mg before reperfusion of the transplanted lung, followed by 125 mg every 12 hours for 48 hours. It is then switched to oral prednisone in a dose of 20 mg/d, which is then tapered to 10 mg/d over the next 6 months. Mycophenolate mofetil is now replacing azathioprine (38,39).

The principal maintenance immunosuppressive treatments for lung transplants are cyclosporine (20) or the similarly acting calcineurin inhibitor, tacrolimus, a macrolide antibiotic (40,41). These are used in combination with a cell cycle inhibitor, either azathioprine or mycophenolate mofetil, and oral corticosteroids. There is emerging evidence that the tacrolimus/mycophenolate combination is superior to cyclosporine combinations (42). Few patients are free of corticosteroids at 5 years. These combinations are used in over 80% of lung transplant patients (Table 54.6).

Adverse effects of these immunosuppressive agents include nephrotoxicity, hypertension, hypertrichosis, gastrointestinal disturbances, neurotoxicity, gingival hypertrophy, hyperglycemia, and hyperkalemia. Tacrolimus bears no chemical resemblance to cyclosporine but exhibits similar activity. It is also metabolized by cytochrome P_{450} 3A, and as with cyclosporine, certain drug interactions can be expected.

COMPLICATIONS

Summary Statement	Level of Evidence
Hemodynamic measurements are required to minimize accumulation of intravascular and extravascular lung water. A posterior-anterior catheter is necessary for this purpose.	Consensus opinion
Infection prophylaxis will decrease infections with bacteria and cytomegalovirus under certain conditions.	Case-controlled studies
Complications from immunosuppressive use are common and can involve many systems. New immunosuppressive regimens are being tested.	Case-controlled studies
Renal function abnormalities are common owing to multiple factors. The serum creatinine must be frequently monitored.	Consensus opinion

Nonsteroidal anti-inflammatory drugs should be avoided in patients on either agent in view of nephrotoxicity. The principal adverse effects include nephrotoxicity, neurotoxicity (including headache, insomnia, and tremor), gastrointestinal disturbances, hyperglycemia, hyperkalemia, and hair loss. Anaphylaxis has been reported with both tacrolimus and cyclosporine.

Renal function must be carefully monitored, as both cyclosporine and tacrolimus injure the kidneys. Lung transplant patients experience a greater degree of renal failure than do other forms of transplants (43).

MANAGEMENT OF COMPLICATIONS

There are many complications that follow lung transplant, reflecting the intensity of the surgical intervention and the use of high levels of immunosuppressive therapies. The complications differ according to the length of time after surgery (Table 54.7).

A major contribution to the success of lung transplantation was the development of techniques in medical management that allowed early diagnosis of complications, such as rejection and infection (44). Infections and acute rejection are frequent early events after surgery. There are well-established protocols for the investigation and monitoring of the patient during the early phase after transplant. The daily record of the FEV_1 using a hand-held spirometer and transbronchial biopsy (TBB) of the lung are the mainstays of long-term medical surveillance (44–46). The characteristic finding of acute lung rejection on TBB is a lymphocytic perivascular infiltrate. With pulmonary pneumonias, there are intra-alveolar exudates that can show specific features of opportunistic infection. For example, foamy macrophages with pneumocystosis are seen, whereas in CMV, large epithelial cell inclusions are seen.

A decrease in the FEV_1 is an indication for a bronchoscopy, as the chest radiograph is too insensitive to detect these complications. At present, a TBB is the most sensitive and specific test that discriminates between acute rejection and pulmonary infection. Early institution of augmented immunosuppressive therapy—intravenous methylprednisolone, 500 mg/d for 3 days followed by oral prednisolone 20 mg/d for 20 days—can restore the FEV_1 to normal in cases of acute rejection. Alternatively, specific antimicrobial therapy will control infection. This simple method of monitoring patients greatly improves the survival chances of lung transplant patients.

Airway anastomosis complications and acute graft failure are the two other common early causes of death and morbidity. These are the result of surgical problems in the main, or failures in correct donor selection.

Special Problems Associated with Infections

There are two problem infections that afflict lung transplant patients in which there is still uncertainty in management.

The first is CMV infection that causes illness in 60% of lung transplant recipients. The normal host defense against CMV is the innate immune system (47). High-dose corticosteroids used to treat acute rejection and concurrent use of antibiotics to treat bacterial infections can lead to recrudescence of CMV infection in seropositive individuals. However, the greatest risk is to patients who are naive to CMV at the time of transplant surgery who receive donor organs from a seropositive donor. CMV pneumonia is the invariable result (47). CMV infection can also be obtained from blood products. These observations have led to a policy of matching CMV-negative recipients to CMV-negative donors and blood products (48).

Prophylactic treatment of at-risk individuals with ganciclovir must be used but carries high risks of toxic drug responses and drug resistance. Large increases in costs are a particular consequence of postoperative CMV infection. One approach that may have merit is to attempt early detection of CMV infection by measuring increases in viral

TABLE 54.7. THE MOST COMMON CAUSES OF DEATH AFTER LUNG TRANSPLANT

	0–30 d	31 d–1 y	>1–3 y	>3–5 y	5+ y
Coronary artery disease	1.2%	0.8%	1.2%	1.5%	1.3%
Cardiac	9.3%	3.6%	2.1%	3.1%	2.3%
Malignancy	0%	2.0%	4.1%	7.9%	9.0%
Lymphoma	0.1%	3.3%	2.4%	1.7%	4.0%
Cytomegalovirus	0.5%	4.1%	1.7%	0.6%	0.7%
Acute rejection	5.9%	1.8%	2.1%	0.8%	0.7%
Infection, non-cytomegalovirus	24.6%	39.3%	24.9%	18.8%	16.3%
Bronchiolitis	0.7%	6.1%	30.0%	33.0%	34.2%
Primary graft failure	16.4%	6.1%	5.8%	4.0%	4.7%
Other graft Failure	14.7%	11.4%	10.2%	13.8%	8.3%
Technical	8.8%	3.1%	0.9%	0.2%	0.3%
Other	17.7%	18.5%	14.7%	14.6%	18.3%

From Hertz MI, Taylor DO, Trulock EP, et al. The Registry of the International Society for Heart and Lung Transplantation: ninteenth official report—2002. *J Heart Lung Transplant* 2002;21:950–970, with permission.

TABLE 54.8. THE OLD AND NEWLY PROPOSED CLASSIFICATION OF THE BRONCHIOLITIS OBLITERANS SYNDROME

	Original Classification		Current Proposition
BOS 0	FEV_1 ≥80% of baseline	BOS 0	FEV_1 >90% of baseline and $FEF_{25\%-75\%}$ >75% of baseline
		BOS 0-p	FEV_1 81%–90% of baseline and/or $FEF_{25\%-75\%}$ ≤75% of baseline
BOS 1	FEV_1 66%–80% of baseline	BOS 1	FEV_1 66%–80% of baseline
BOS 2	FEV_1 51%–65% of baseline	BOS 2	FEV_1 51%–65% of baseline
BOS 3	FEV_1 ≤50% of baseline	BOS 3	FEV_1 ≤50% of baseline

BOS, bronchiolitis obliterans syndrome; FEV_1, forced expiratory volume in 1s; $FEF_{25\%-75\%}$, forced expiratory flow during the middle half of the forced vital capacity.

load by using a hybrid captive assay and to treat only these individuals (48).

The second unresolved problem of infection is the development of post-transplant proliferative disease (PTLD). This is the result of Epstein-Barr viral infection. Epstein-Barr–seronegative individuals at the time of the lung transplant are 20-fold more likely to develop PTLD. Of those that seroconvert after transplant, 30% to 50% will develop PTLD. This illness carries a 90% mortality rate despite chemotherapy and reductions in immunosuppressive therapy. One new approach is to offer prophylactic treatment to the seronegative recipients by using acyclovir, valacyclovir, or ganciclovir, which appears to block the development of PTLD. (49).

Long-Term Complications of Lung Transplantation

Lung transplant recipients are especially prone to develop cancer. This includes not only basal cell skin cancer but also fatal illnesses such lung cancer and cancer of the bowel and kidney.

However, the main long-term complication of lung transplantation is the development of OB. This complication is the principle cause of death or serious disability in long-term survivors (23,43,44). The development of OB is characterized by an irreversible progressive loss in FEV_1 (23,46).

The function of the lung graft will decline over time, depending on the control of rejection with immunosuppressive treatments (5,20,23,43,44,50). The development of OB is associated with a much faster decline. There are a number of factors that are strongly correlated with the development of OB. These include the frequency of acute rejection, particularly in the first 3 months after transplant. Also, the finding on TBB of a lymphocytic bronchitis or bronchiolitis is strongly associated with the subsequent development of OB. The occurrence of CMV infection or other significant pneumonias does not seem so clearly associated with the development of OB (47,51).

To enhance the diagnosis of OB and in view of the inability of TBB to provide a specific histological diagnosis,

the FEV_1 was proposed as a surrogate measure of its development. The so-called BOS has therefore been based on the development of an irreversible decrease in FEV_1, and the syndrome was classified according to the degree of FEV_1 reduction (Table 54.8). Practical concerns about this system centered on the delayed recognition of BOS as a result of insensitivity of the FEV_1, and as a result, a new classification has been proposed based on flow-volume loop analysis (53) (Table 54.8). The mid-maximal expiratory flow rate (flow rate between 25%–75% of the vital capacity) is the new proxy measurement. The new step of BOS 0-p was introduced based on decrements of mid-maximal expiratory flow rate, which will hopefully allow earlier detection and initiation of therapy for BOS.

However, this new classification of BOS has been questioned (52,53). The serious dilemma is whether or not BOS is a single entity or exists as several forms (52). There is good

MANAGEMENT OF COMPLICATIONS

Summary Statement	Level of Evidence
Transbronchoscopic lung biopsy should be performed to distinguish between infection and acute rejection in the early postoperative period. Infections may be caused by the usual nosocomial pathogens by unusual organisms. Antibiotic use should be specific.	Case-controlled studies
Cytomegalovirus pneumonitis is a major complicating infection in the early postoperative period and should be treated with ganciclovir.	Consensus opinion
Post-transplant proliferative disease is caused by Epstein-Barr viral infection and requires acyclovir therapy.	Case-controlled studies
The bronchiolitis obliterans syndrome is the major long-term complication of lung transplantation. There may be several forms of this condition, and at present, there is no verified test for early detection. It should be managed by manipulation of immunosuppressive therapy.	Case-controlled studies

evidence that two patterns of the syndrome are seen. In one, there is a step-change reduction of FEV_1, often seen in the first 6 months after transplant. Survival when this occurs is poor, in comparison to the second pattern in which the FEV_1 slowly declines at a rate of about 3.7% per annum. This latter form has a better survival (52). It is possible that the two forms represent separate pathophysiologies. Each may require quite distinct therapies.

Earlier recognition of the onset of BOS might allow for the timely introduction of more effective immunosuppressive treatment regimes. For example, the switch from cyclosporine- to tacrolimus-based regimes may halt the refractory acute loss of the FEV_1 (54). Alternatives include rapamycin, which is not a calcineurin inhibitor and may well also influence the development of the fibrotic lesion of OB.

THE HEALTH GAINS OF LUNG TRANSPLANTATION

Lung transplants are expensive procedures and are associated with a continued cost of care that involves not only the immunosuppressive treatments but also the monitoring of lung function and diagnostic procedures. These costs vary considerably across nations and depend on insurance and specific reimbursement models particular to each society.

Early work to estimate the health gain and the cost of lung transplant identified the basic costs and the disparity between the patients who experience many complications compared with those who have few complications (55). A more detailed study of lung transplants in Holland took the community costs into account (56). Measurements of costs per life year gained and of improved quality of life have shown that there is a significant gain by the patient.

What has proved harder to demonstrate is that lung transplant surgery extends life (57). As this treatment has not been subjected to a randomized controlled trial, this aspect is not yet definitively proven. A study of one cohort selected for transplant surgery monitored patients that either received transplant surgery or were wait-listed. Survival benefit was demonstrated in all diseases but in Eisenmenger syndrome, in which the patients awaiting surgery survived longer than did their transplant counterparts (58). Transplanted patients had better survival than did wait-listed individuals for cystic fibrosis, COPD, IPF, PPH, and bronchiectasis. Interestingly, in this cohort, COPD patients survived equally well after heart-lung transplants as from sequential bilateral lung transplants.

SPECIAL ISSUES OF PEDIATRIC LUNG TRANSPLANTATION

Although not a widespread treatment for lung failure in children, experience with pediatric lung transplantation has been

growing apace over the past 20 years. The success rate is improving.

Currently, children have poorer survival figures after lung transplantation than do adults (59). This was argued to be the result of higher incidence rates of pulmonary infections and the greater difficulty in the diagnosis and treatment of acute lung rejection in children (60). Despite these earlier concerns, the survival figures for lung-transplanted children have improved; the half-life figures are 3.5 years for children at age 1 year, 3.5 years for children between 1 and 10 years, and 3.2 years for children between 11 and 17 years (61). For heart-lung-transplanted children, a figure of 2.6 years for half-life has been observed.

Children are managed with the same mixture of calcineurin and cell cycle inhibitors. Although annual global heart-lung transplant numbers for children have fallen to just 20 a year, lung transplant numbers have been sustained between 60 and 80 per year through the 1990s. As in adults, there are fewer patients with PPH receiving lung transplants, but the numbers of patients with cystic fibrosis are increasing. Cystic fibrosis accounts for 67% of the transplants in children over 10 years of age.

OB is the most common cause of death, accounting for 60% of all deaths after 3 to 6 years. Of interest, however, is the finding that children of under 1 year have a much lower incidence of OB (61). It has been argued that immaturity might be associated with greater tolerance of the transplant.

THE FUTURE OF LUNG TRANSPLANTATION

The main limit to transplant surgery is the availability of suitable donor organs. This is likely to remain the limit into the foreseeable future. Presently, human organ transplant surgery is the only means of returning function to a failed organ.

There are a number of emerging therapies that may offer alternatives to human organ transplantation. One area involves the use of stem cells to repair the damaged organ; a discussion of this therapy is outside the compass of this chapter. Another area involves the use of animal organs (xenotransplantation), which would provide an inexhaustible supply of organs for transplant surgery.

Xenotransplants

There are recommendations for lung xenotransplantation (porcine) (62). Its main limitations involve rejection and the risks of xenozoonosis. The latter risk is real, as there is evidence of transmission of porcine endogenous retrovirus from animal to human cells (63). This fear led to the moratorium by the U.S. Food and Drug Administration on xenotransplants in 1997. The severe vascular disease that occurs is owing to circulating xenoreactive antibodies that trigger adverse reactions in the endothelial cells (64).

The activation of complement is facilitated by two receptors expressed on human endothelial cells, the decay accelerating factor, the membrane cofactor protein, and CD59. Use of transgenic pig lungs expressing the human decay accelerating factor and membrane cofactor protein overcome this reaction (65). Also use of the knock-out pig lung that does not express the enzyme α-1,3-galactosyl transferase that adds the α-1,3-galactosyl to the surface of porcine cells also lessens this immediate vasculopathy (66). However, in addition to the problems arising from humorally mediated immunity there remains those related to T cell–mediated rejection (67).

Further obstacles remain for pulmonary xenotransplantation. The porcine lung has a different anatomy than that of the human lung. Also, porcine macrophages release powerful vasoconstrictors, resulting in marked elevation in recipient pulmonary vascular resistance (64).

It is likely to take some time to overcome these obstacles. However, the need to find donor organs provides a powerful incentive to find solutions.

CONCLUSION

The past two decades have witnessed rapid advances in lung transplantation. Early problems have been resolved, and many transplant complications can now be medically managed. The challenge now is to find ways of extending the transplant opportunity to larger numbers of patients.

REFERENCES

1. Reitz BA, Wallwork JL, Hunt SA, et al. Heart-lung transplantation: successful therapy for patients with pulmonary vascular disease. *N Engl J Med* 1982;306:557–564.
2. Tuder RM, Cool CD, Geraci MW, et al. Prostacyclin synthase expression is decreased in lungs from patients with severe pulmonary hypertension. *Am J Respir Crit Care Med* 1999;159:1925–1932.
3. Morrell MW, Yang X, Upton PD, et al. Altered growth responses of pulmonary artery smooth muscle cells from patients with primary pulmonary hypertension to transforming growth factor-β and bone morphogenetic protein. *Circulation* 2001;104:790–795.
4. Olschewski H, Simmoneau G, Galie N, et al. Inhaled Iloprost for severe pulmonary hypertension. *N Engl J Med* 2002;347:322–329.
5. Paramothayan NS, Lasserton TJ, Wells AU, et al. Prostacyclin for pulmonary hypertension. *Cochrane Database Syst Rev* 2002: CD002994.
6. Rubin LJ, Badesch DB, Barst RJ, et al. Bosentan therapy for pulmonary arterial hypertension. *N Engl J Med* 2002;346:896–903.
7. Hertz MI, Taylor DO, Trulock EP, et al. The Registry of the International Society for Heart and Lung Transplantation: nineteenth official report—2002. *J Heart Lung Transplant* 2002;21: 950–970.
8. Maurer JR, Frost AE, Estenne M, et al. International guidelines for the selection of lung transplant candidates. *Am J Respir Crit Care Med* 1998;158:335–339.
9. De Meester J, Smits JM, Persijn GG, et al. Lung transplant waiting list: differential outcome of type of end-stage lung disease, one year after registration. *J Heart Lung Transplant* 1999;18:563–571.
10. Cooper D. Xenografting: how great is the need? *Xenotransplantation* 1993:25–28.
11. Unilateral lung transplantation for pulmonary fibrosis. Toronto Lung Transplant Group. *N Engl J Med* 1986;314:1140–1145.
12. Bando K, Armitage JM, Paradis IL, et al. Indications for and results of single, bilateral, and heart-lung transplantation for pulmonary hypertension. *J Thorac Cardiovasc Surg* 1994;108:1056–1065.
13. Waddell TK, Bennet L, Kennedy R, et al. Heart-lung or lung transplantation for Eisenmengers' syndrome. *J Heart Lung Transplant* 2002;21:731–737.
14. D'Alonzo GE, Barst RJ, Ayres SM, et al. Survival in patients with primary pulmonary hypertension: results from a national prospective registry. *Ann Intern Med* 1991;115:343–349.
15. Higenbottam T, Butt AY, McMahon A, et al. Long term intravenous prostaglandin (epoprostenol or iloprost) for treatment of severe pulmonary hypertension. *Heart* 1998;80:151–155.
16. Sitbon O, Humbert M, Nunez H, et al. Long-term intra-venous epoprostenol infusion in primary pulmonary hypertension prognostic factors and survival. *J Am Coll Cardiol* 2002;40:780–788.
17. Mclaughlin VV, Shillington A, Rich S. Survival in primary pulmonary hypertension the impact of epoprostenol therapy. *Circulation* 2002;106:1477–1482.
18. Bando K, Keenan RJ, Paradis IL, et al. Impact of pulmonary hypertension on outcome after single-lung transplantation. *Ann Thorac Surg* 1994;58:1336–1342.
19. Bando K, Paradis IL, Keenan RJ, et al. Comparison of outcomes after single and bilateral lung transplantation for obstructive lung disease. *J Heart Lung Transplant* 1995;14:692–698.
20. Meyers BF, Lynch J, Trulock EP, et al. Lung transplantation: a decade of experience. *Ann Surg* 1999;230:362–370; discussion 370–371.
21. Pasque MK, Cooper JD, Kaiser LR, et al. Improved technique for bilateral lung transplantation: rationale and initial clinical experience. *Ann Thorac Surg* 1990;49:785–791.
22. Whyte RI, Robbins RC, Altinger J, et al. Heart-lung transplantation for primary pulmonary hypertension. *Ann Thorac Surg* 1999;67:937–941; discussion 941–942.
23. Scott JP, Higenbottam TW, Clelland C, et al. The natural-history of obliterative bronchiolitis and occlusive vascular-disease of patients following heart-lung transplantation. *Transplant Proc* 1989;21:2592–2593.
24. Anyanwu AC, Banner NR, Radley-Smith R, et al. Long-term results of cardiac transplantation from live donors: the Domino Heart Transplant. *J Heart Lung Transplant* 2002;21:971–975.
25. Dawkins KD, Jamieson SW, Hunt SA, et al. Long-term results, hemodynamics, and complications after combined heart and lung transplantation. *Circulation* 1985;71:919–926.
26. Otulana BA, Higenbottam TW, Scott JP, et al. A possible role for mixed venous-blood changes in the hyperventilation of exercise in heart-lung transplant recipients. *Chest* 1990;97[Suppl 3]:S88–S89.
27. Pasque MK, Kaiser LR, Dresler CM, et al. Single lung transplantation for pulmonary hypertension: technical aspects and immediate hemodynamic results. *J Thorac Cardiovasc Surg* 1992;103:475–481; discussion 481–482.
28. Meyer DM, Bennet LE, Novich RJ, et al. Single vs bilateral sequential lung transplantation for end-stage emphysema: influence of recipient age on survival and secondary end-points. *J Heart Lung Transplant* 2001;20:935–941.
29. Levy NT, Liapis H, Eisenberg PR, et al. Pathologic regression of primary pulmonary hypertension in left native lung following right single-lung transplantation. *J Heart Lung Transplant* 2001;20:381–384.

30. Birsan T, Kranz A, Mares P, et al. Transient left ventricular failure following bilateral lung transplantation for pulmonary hypertension. *J Heart Lung Transplant* 1999;18:304–309.

31. Schenk P, Globits S, Koller J, et al. Accuracy of echocardiographic right ventricular parameters in patients with different end-stage lung diseases prior to lung transplantation. *J Heart Lung Transplant* 2000;19:145–154.

32. Vizza CD, Lynch JP, Ochoa LL, et al. Right and left ventricular dysfunction in patients with severe pulmonary disease. *Chest* 1998;113:576–583.

33. Cohen RG, Starnes VA. Living donor lung transplantation. *World J Surg* 2001;25:244–250.

34. Starnes VA, Woo MS, MacLaughlin EF, et al. Comparison of the outcomes between living donor and cadaveric lung transplantation in children. *Ann Thorac Surg* 1999;68:2279–2283.

35. Woo MS, MacLaughlin EF, Horn MV, et al. Bronchiolitis obliterans is not the primary cause of death in pediatric living donor lobar transplants. *J Heart Lung Transplant* 2001;20:491–496.

36. Abecassis M, Adams M, Adams P, et al. Consensus statement on the live organ donor. *JAMA* 2000;284:2919–2926.

37. Bhabra MS, Hopkinson DN, Show TE, et al. Relative importance of prostaglandin/cyclic adenosine monophosphate and nitric oxide/cyclic guanosine monophosphate pathways in lung preservation *Ann Thoracic Surg* 1996;62:1494–1499.

38. Williams R. Randomised trial comparing tacrolimus (FK506) and cyclosporin in prevention of liver allograft rejection. European FK506 Multicentre Liver Study Group. *Lancet* 1994;344:423–428.

39. Pichlmayr R. Placebo-controlled study of mycophenolate mofetil combined with cyclosporin and corticosteroids for prevention of acute rejection. European Mycophenolate Mofetil Cooperative Study Group. *Lancet* 1995;345:1321–1325.

40. van den Berg JW, Postma DS, Keoter GH, et al. New immunosuppressive drugs and lung transplantation: last or least? *Thorax* 1999;54:550–553.

41. Keenan RJ, Konishi H, Kawai A, et al. Clinical trial of tacrolimus versus cyclosporine in lung transplantation. *Ann Thorac Surg* 1995;60:580–584.

42. Treede H, Klepetko W, Riechespurner H, et al Tacrolimus versus cyclosporine after lung transplantation: a randomised controlled two centre trial comparing two different immunosuppressive protocols. *J Heart Lung Transplant* 2001;20:511–517.

43. Broekroelofs J, Stegeman CA, Navis GJ, et al. Creatinine-based estimation of rate of long term renal function loss in lung transplant recipients: which method is preferable? *J Heart Lung Transplant* 2000;19:256–262.

44. Higenbottam T, Stewart S, Penketh A, et al. Transbronchial lung biopsy for the diagnosis of rejection in heart-lung transplant patients. *Transplantation* 1988;46:532–539.

45. Tamm M, Sharples LD, Higenbottam TW, et al. Bronchiolitis obliterans syndrome in heart-lung transplantation: surveillance biopsies. *Am J Respir Crit Care Med* 1997;155:1705–1710.

46. Valentine V, Taylor DE, Dhillon GS, et al. Success of lung transplantation without surveillance bronchoscopy. *J Heart Lung Transplant* 2002;21:319–326.

47. Zamora MR. Controversies in lung transplantation: management of cytomegalovirus infections. *J Heart Lung Transplant* 2002;21:841–849.

48. Bhorade SM, Sandesara C, Garrity ER, et al. Quantification of cytomegalovirus viral load by the hybrid capture assay allows for early detection of CMV disease in lung transplants recipient. *J Heart Lung Transplant* 2001;20:928–934.

49. Malouf MA, Chhajed PN, Hopkins P, et al. Anti-viral prophylaxis reduces the incidence of lymphoproliferative disease in lung transplant recipients. *J Heart Lung Transplant* 2002;21:547–554.

50. Estenne M, Maurer JR, Boehler A, et al. Bronchiolitis obliterans syndrome 2001: an update of the diagnostic criteria. *J Heart Lung Transplant* 2002;21:297–310.

51. Sharples LD, McNeil K, Stewart S, et al. Risk factors for bronchiolitis obliterans: a systematic review of recent publications. *J Heart Lung Transplant* 2002;21:271–281.

52. Jackson CH, Sharples SL, McNeil K, et al. Acute and chronic onset of bronchiolitis obliterans syndrome (BOS): are they different? *J Heart Lung Transplant* 2002;21:658–666.

53. McGiffin DC Classification of bronchiolitis obliterans syndrome: taxonomic realism or skepticism. *J Heart Lung Transplant* 2002;21:941–944.

54. Vitulo P, Oggionni T, Cascina A, et al. Efficacy of tacrolimus rescue therapy in refractory acute rejection after lung transplantation. *J Heart Lung Transplant* 2002;21:435–439.

55. Ramsey SD, Patrick DL, Albert RK, et al. The cost-effectiveness of lung transplantation: a pilot study. University of Washington Medical Center Lung Transplant Study Group. *Chest* 1995;108:1594–1601.

56. TenVergert EM, Essink-Bot ML, Geertsma A, et al. The effect of lung transplantation on health-related quality of life: a longitudinal study. *Chest* 1998;113:358–364.

57. Hosenpud JD, Bennett LE, Keck BM, et al. The Registry of the International Society for Heart and Lung Transplantation: fifteenth official report—1998. *J Heart Lung Transplant* 1998;17:656–668.

58. Charman SC, Sharples LD, McNeil KD, et al. Assessment of survival benefit after lung transplantation. *J Heart Lung Transplant* 2002;21:226–232.

59. Ro PS, Spray TL, Bridges ND. Outcome of infants listed for lung or heart/lung transplantation. *J Heart Lung Transplant* 1999;18:1232–1237.

60. Armitage JM, Kurland G, Michaels M, et al, Critical issues in pediatric lung transplantation. *J Thoracic Cardiovasc Surg* 1995;109:60–66.

61. Boucek MM, Edwards LB, Keck BM, et al. The Registray if the ISHLT: fifth official pediatric report 2001–2002. *J Heart Lung Transplant* 2002;21:827–840.

62. Platt J, Disesa V, Gail D, et al. Recommendations of the NHLB Institute Heart and Lung on xenotransplantation. *Circulation* 2002;106:1043–1047.

63. Butler D. Last hope to stop and think on the risks of xenotransplantation. *Nature* 1998;391:320–324.

64. Hammerman MR. Xenotransplantation of developing kidneys. *Am J Physiol* 2002;283:F601–F606.

65. White DJG. hDAF transgenic pig organs: are they concordant for human transplantation. *Xenotransplantation* 1996:50–55.

66. Butler D. Xenotransplant expert expresses caution over knock out piglets. *Nature* 2002;415:103–104.

67. Dorling A. Clinical xenotransplantation: pigs might fly? *Am J Transplant* 2002;2:695–700.

55 ▷ Immunodeficiency Diseases

Udaya B. S. Prakash · Talmadge E. King, Jr.

Immunodeficiency diseases are encountered in different forms, often in association with other diseases. Disorders of immunodeficiency, whether total or partial, can be congenital or acquired. These disease states are the consequences of impaired function in one or more components of the immune system, including B and T lymphocytes, phagocytes, and the complement system. Immunodeficiency can develop as a sequel of malignancy, long-term corticosteroid therapy, cytotoxic chemotherapy, or an alteration in the ratio of T helper to T suppressor lymphocytes, as occurs in AIDS. Protein-calorie malnutrition adversely affects virtually all immunocompetent cells. It results in an impaired function of phagocytes and decreases both the quantity and quality of lymphocytes. Protein-calorie malnutrition is generally considered the most frequent cause of immunodepression. Additionally, local mechanical factors can predispose immunocompromised patients to special problems, including diseases of the airways, defects in mucociliary clearance, deficiency of secretory immunoglobulin A (IgA), absence of surfactant as a consequence of acute lung injury, and preexisting pulmonary structural damage, such as bullous lesions, bronchiectasis, ancient cavities, and a fibrotic process.

Because the clinical features of the immunodeficiency states are not highly specific and vary from one entity to another, a definitive diagnosis is often delayed. Normally, immunodeficiency syndromes are recognized when a predisposition to unusual or recurrent infections develops in an individual. Most of these infections occur in the respiratory system and are the most frequent cause of morbidity and mortality.

U. B. S. Prakash: Pulmonary and Critical Care Medicine, Mayo Medical School and Mayo Medical Center, Rochester, Minnesota.

T. E. King, Jr.: Department of Medicine, University of California, San Francisco; and Medical Services, San Francisco General Hospital, San Francisco, California.

This chapter addresses the etiologic and diagnostic evaluation of immunocompromised patients and patients with selective immunodeficiency syndromes. The pulmonary complications of infection (including HIV infection) are discussed in Chapter 18, and the pulmonary complications of organ and bone marrow transplantation are discussed in Chapter 56.

PULMONARY DISEASE IN THE IMMUNOCOMPROMISED PATIENT

The term *immunocompromised patient* or *compromised host* generally denotes a person with impaired defense mechanisms, and therefore a greater susceptibility to infection. The most common types of impaired defense mechanisms are reductions in the numbers of granulocytes, B lymphocytes, and T lymphocytes. However, pulmonary abnormalities in immunocompromised patients do not always represent an infectious process (1). The number of immunocompromised hosts is increasing because of the use of more effective and powerful chemotherapeutic agents in the treatment of malignancy and because the number of transplant procedures performed is increasing. As a consequence of these advances in care, opportunities for relapse of the underlying disease and for the development of pulmonary reactions secondary to treatment are more frequent. Consequently, it is becoming increasingly difficult to pinpoint the cause of a pulmonary abnormality in an immunocompromised host (2–4). Fortunately, new molecular diagnostic techniques, more effective prophylactic treatments, and a reduced toxicity of conditioning regimens appear to be contributing to a better prognosis in some of these patients (2,4).

In almost all immunocompromised patients, the first indicator of a respiratory complication is a chest roentgenogram with abnormal findings. Most immunocompromised patients who have diffuse pulmonary opacities on chest imaging studies exhibit similar clinical features: fever, nonproductive cough, dyspnea, anemia, normal or low leukocyte count, decreased platelet count, and hypoxemia to a varying degree. Many of these features may be a manifestation of the underlying primary disease and do not represent a new process.

The mortality rate associated with pulmonary complications in immunocompromised patients is exceedingly high, reaching 85% in some series (3). It is generally agreed that severe pulmonary involvement is an ominous prognostic factor (2,3). Furthermore, Rano and colleagues (3) have shown

that a delay in diagnosing the cause of pulmonary opacities in this setting (>5 days) increases the risk for death more than threefold. In the face of a rapidly deteriorating immunocompromised patient with progressive chest roentgenographic abnormalities, the clinician must quickly consider a myriad of diagnoses (see Fig. 18.1). Unfortunately, the chest roentgenogram rarely aids in making a definitive diagnosis. Simplifying the possibilities by grouping the differential diagnoses is extremely helpful in planning the appropriate diagnostic procedures and administering optimal therapy to an immunocompromised patient (Table 55.1). The etiologic factors contributing to pulmonary abnormalities in

TABLE 55.1. DIFFERENTIAL DIAGNOSIS OF PULMONARY COMPLICATIONS IN THE IMMUNOCOMPROMISED PATIENT

Extension of basic disease process into lungs	*Patterns of pulmonary injury and common causes*
Lymphomas, Hodgkin and non-Hodgkin	**Alveolar hemorrhage**
Leukemias	Leukemia
Plasma cell neoplasms	Bone marrow or organ transplantation
Carcinomatosis, primary and metastatic	Graft versus host disease
Connective tissue diseases	Chemotherapy
Vasculitides	
Kaposi sarcoma	**Nonspecific interstitial pneumonitis**
	Viral infections
Opportunistic infections	Graft versus host disease
	AIDS
Viruses	Bone marrow or organ transplantation
Herpes simplex virus	Drug-induced pulmonary disease
Varicella-zoster virus	
Cytomegalovirus	**Bronchiolitis obliterans**
	Viral infections
Bacteria	Graft versus host disease
Gram-positive bacteria	AIDS
Gram-negative bacteria	Bone marrow or organ transplantation
Anaerobes	Drug-induced pulmonary disease
Mycobacteria	**Pulmonary edema**
M. tuberculosis	Organ transplant recipients
M. avium-intracellulare	Drug-induced pulmonary disease
M. kansasii	
	Lymphocytic interstitial pneumonitis
Fungi	Viral infections
Aspergillus species	AIDS
Candida species	Graft versus host disease
Zygomycetes (Mucorales) species	Agammaglobulinemia
Cryptococcus neoformans	
Histoplasma capsulatum	*New pulmonary process unrelated to*
Blastomyces dermatitidis	*immunodeficiency*
Coccidioides immitis	Pulmonary embolism
Trichosporon species	Aspiration pneumonia
Nocardia asteroides	Community-acquired pneumonia
	Nosocomial pneumonia
Protozoa	Congestive cardiac failure
Pneumocystis carinii	Renal failure
Toxoplasma gondii	Malignant disease
Cryptosporidium species	
	Combination of two or more of the preceding
Parasites	
Strongyloides stercoralis	
Drug-induced pulmonary disease	
Pulmonary cytotoxic drugs	
Oxygen toxicity	
Radiation pneumonitis and fibrosis	
Transfusion-related acute lung injury	

TABLE 55.2. FACTORS PREDISPOSING THE HOST TO OPPORTUNISTIC PULMONARY INFECTION

Basic disease process (see Table 55.1)

Congenital and acquired immunodeficiency states

Altered physical barriers
Indwelling catheters
Nebulizers and ventilators
Local mechanical disruption by tumor and the like
Ciliary dysfunction
Bronchospastic disease
Intubation or tracheostomy

Altered indigenous microbial flora
Systemic illnesses (diabetes mellitus, alcoholism, others)
Surgery
Malnutrition
Aspiration
Hospitalization
Broad-spectrum antibiotic therapy
Change in virulence of microbial flora
Intubation or tracheostomy

Leukopenia
Basic disease process
Decreased migration
Defective phagocytosis
Decreased bactericidal activity
Cytotoxic drug therapy
Protein-calorie malnutrition

Impaired lymphocyte-mediated immunity
Corticosteroid therapy
Cytotoxic drug therapy
Radiation
Transplantation
AIDS
Protein-calorie malnutrition

Underlying pulmonary pathology
Obstructive pulmonary disease
Bronchiectasis
Ancient cavitary disease
Secretory immunoglobulin A deficiency
Surfactant deficiency

---

compromised hosts are outlined in Tables 55.1 and 55.2. Some of the broad categories of diagnostic possibilities listed in Table 55.1 are briefly described in the section "Differential Diagnosis of Lung Disease in the Immunocompromised Patient"; drug-induced pulmonary disease is discussed in Chapter 33.

Diagnostic Approach to Pulmonary Processes in the Compromised Host

Because many of the respiratory problems encountered in this setting are associated with a rapidly downhill clinical course, it is imperative that a diagnostic consideration of an abnormal pulmonary process include the following steps: (a) recognition of the patient as an immunocompromised host, (b) recognition that the patient is at increased risk for infec-

tion, (c) definition of the derangement of the host defense mechanism, (d) categorization of the chest roentgenographic and computed tomographic abnormalities, (e) assessment of the degree of urgency with regard to the various diagnostic procedures, and (f) determination and performance of the most productive diagnostic procedure. This step-by-step approach is most likely to help in designing the optimal therapy for this group of patients (5) (see Chapter 18).

A detailed history and complete physical examination provide important clues to the diagnosis. Routine laboratory procedures, such as blood cell counts, cultures of blood and urine, and other analyses, supply further information when used appropriately. The choice of a particular diagnostic approach depends on the expertise available in one's own institution, the sensitivity of the procedure for the diagnosis of likely processes in the differential diagnoses, the severity of the patient's illness, and the rate at which the illness is progressing (Table 55.3). When routine blood tests, cultures of material from extrapulmonary sources, and biopsies fail to yield a specific answer, the sequence of diagnostic procedures should be that shown in Figure 55.1.

Imaging Procedures

Chest roentgenograms are essential for characterizing abnormalities and narrowing the spectrum of possible diagnoses. However, it should be stressed that the classic roentgenographic features of isolated disease entities may not be apparent in an immunocompromised host because of the effects of various factors in the lung, including opportunistic infections, cytotoxic changes, and radiation pneumonitis (6). Furthermore, because most of these patients are very sick and debilitated, obtaining roentgenograms of optimal quality can be difficult. Lateral decubitus films may help to confirm the presence of free pleural effusions. In a study of chest roentgenograms from 149 consecutive immunocompromised patients with acute pulmonary complications (25 HIV-infected and 125 in non–HIV-infected patients), the most common complication in the patients with AIDS was *Pneumocystis carinii* pneumonia (PCP), and the most common complications in the non-AIDS patients were invasive aspergillosis, drug reaction, and PCP. The radiologists made the correct first-choice diagnosis in 90% of the patients with AIDS and in 34% of the patients without AIDS. In the non-AIDS patients with invasive pulmonary aspergillosis, drug reaction, and PCP, the correct first-choice diagnosis was made in 38%, 26%, and 43% of the readings, respectively.

High-resolution computed tomography of the chest (HRCT) is invaluable in the diagnosis of pulmonary processes in immunocompromised patients. Several studies have documented the usefulness of HRCT in detecting bronchiectasis in patients with immunodeficiency syndromes. The diagnosis of organizing pneumonia may be suggested by HRCT images. CT imaging is helpful in providing both bronchoscopist and surgeon with a road map to the most abnormal

TABLE 55.3. PRACTICAL DIAGNOSTIC APPROACH TO LUNG INVOLVEMENT IN THE IMMUNOCOMPROMISED HOST BASED ON RATE OF PROGRESSION OF LUNG DISEASE, PRESENCE OF FEVER, AND RADIOGRAPHIC PATTERN

Reference Clinical Situation	Underlying Disease	Diagnostic Investigations
■ Slow progression of the disease ■ Absence of fever (or mild fever) ■ Diffuse opacities on chest x-ray films	■ Pulmonary edema ■ Pulmonary localization of the underlying disease ■ Toxic treatment-induced pneumonitis	■ Echocardiography ■ CT ■ Bronchoscopy with BAL and lung biopsy
■ Rapid progression of the condition ■ Fever ■ Diffuse opacities on chest x-ray films	■ Hypersensitivity drug-induced pneumonitis (e.g., methotrexate) ■ Pulmonary localization of the underlying disease ■ Absence of new extrapulmonary symptoms consider *Pneumocystis carinii* ■ Presence of new extrapulmonary symptoms consider another opportunistic infection (e.g., cytomegalovirus infection, cryptococcosis, toxoplasmosis, tuberculosis)	■ Induced sputum ■ Emergency bronchoscopy with BAL and lung biopsy
■ Adult respiratory distress syndrome associated with bacterial pneumonia or sepsis	■ *Streptococcus pneumoniae* ■ *Haemophilus influenzae* ■ *Legionella* species	■ Blood cultures ■ Bronchoscopy with protected bronchial brushing and BAL
■ Rapid to moderate progression of the condition ■ Fever ■ Pulmonary nodules or round opacities on chest x-ray films evolving toward dissemination or cavitation	■ Fungal pneumonia ■ Legionellosis ■ Tuberculosis ■ Pulmonary infarction ■ Vasculitis	■ CT ■ Bronchoscopy with BAL and lung biopsy ■ Percutaneous aspiration or biopsy may be required
■ Focal pulmonary infiltrates that do not respond to antibiotics	■ Opportunistic agents such as *Mycobacteria* species, *Nocardia* species, or *Rhodococcus equi,* organizing pneumonia or tumor	■ CT ■ Bronchoscopy with BAL and lung biopsy ■ Surgical lung biopsy

BAL, bronchoalveolar lavage; CT, computed tomography.
Source: Adapted from Mayaud C, Cadranel J. A persistent challenge: the diagnosis of respiratory disease in the non-AIDS immunocompromised host. *Thorax* 2000;55: 511–517, with permission.

anatomic area to plan procedures such as bronchoscopy and open lung biopsy (7).

When the battery of routine tests fails to provide clues to the cause of the pulmonary process, a direct examination of specimens from the respiratory tract is indicated. This can be accomplished by one or more of the following: (a) study of easily obtained secretions and fluid (sputum, gastric washings, and pleural fluid), (b) percutaneous (transthoracic) needle aspiration and needle biopsy of pleura and lung, (c) diagnostic bronchoalveolar lavage (BAL), (d) bronchoscopic brushing and aspiration or bronchoscopic lung biopsy, and (e) thoracoscopic or thoracotomy biopsy of pleura and lung. To reiterate, the degree of diagnostic urgency and the appropriateness of a given procedure should be weighed against the potential effect of delay on the subsequent outcome. The procedures listed are associated with varying yields and complication rates, which are briefly summarized in the next sections.

Examination of Respiratory Secretions and Fluids

Sputum cultures are usually of limited value in diagnosing bacterial infections in the immunosuppressed host. How-

ever, induced sputum is valuable in the detection of *P. carinii* infection. An overwhelming growth of saprophytic fungi in the oropharyngeal regions of these patients hinders the isolation of true pathogenic bacteria and fungi. Examination of the sputum is also useful in diagnosing mycobacterial infections and bronchogenic carcinoma.

Gastric washings are helpful in diagnosing tuberculosis and certain fungal infections.

Pleural fluid culture is very useful in diagnosing bacterial infections and malignancies. Minor pneumothoraces occur in fewer than 5% of thoracentesis specimens and in fewer than 10% of pleural biopsy specimens.

Transtracheal and transthoracic needle aspirations are rarely indicated in patients with diffuse lung disease. Peripherally localized nodular lesions and lung masses are better approached by CT-guided transthoracic needle aspirations.

Fiberoptic Bronchoscopy

Flexible bronchoscopy has become the procedure of choice for diagnosing opportunistic pulmonary infections in patients with AIDS and other conditions associated with

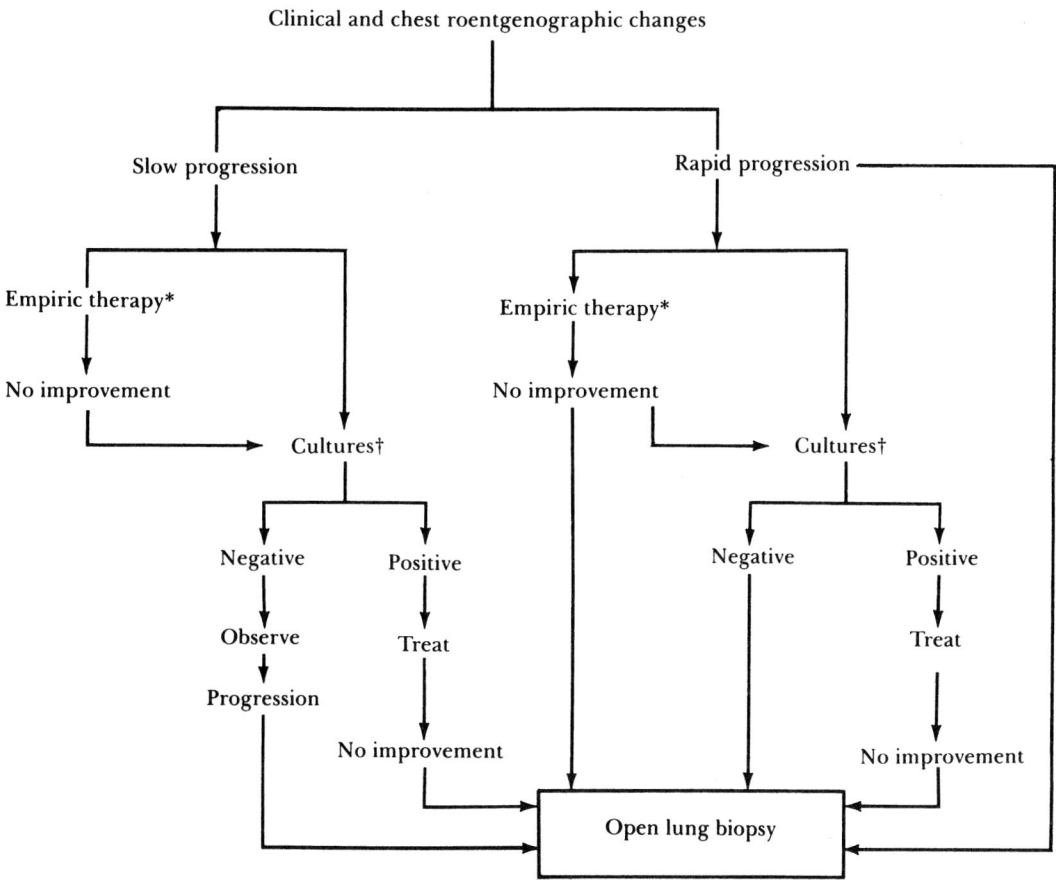

FIGURE 55.1. Diagnostic approach to the immunocompromised patient with abnormal findings on the chest roentgenogram. *Empiric therapy should be individualized and may include antiviral, antibacterial, and antifungal drugs in addition to trimethoprim/sulfamethoxazole against *Pneumocystis carinii*. Other possible components of empiric therapy are the administration of systemic corticosteroids, discontinuation of cytotoxic drugs, and treatment of pulmonary edema. +Cultures should be individualized depending on the clinical situation and chest roentgenographic abnormalities but may be performed on the following: blood, other easily obtained body fluids and secretions, bone marrow, bronchoalveolar lavage fluid, and transbronchial lung biopsy specimens.

immunocompromise (8,9). It is probably the safest of the invasive pulmonary diagnostic procedures. With supplemental oxygenation and appropriate preparation, the procedure can be performed in severely hypoxemic patients. Furthermore, bronchoscopy and BAL can be performed in patients with severe thrombocytopenia, other coagulation disorders, or renal failure; the risk for hemorrhage is minimal (2). Major complications occur in fewer than 1% of patients.

Both diagnostic BAL and bronchoscopic lung biopsy should be considered if diffuse lung infiltrates are present (9). BAL alone, however, is adequate in the diagnosis of infections caused by *P. carinii*, bacteria, viruses, and mycobacteria (10). Mayaud and Cadranel (2) suggest that BAL can be particularly useful in the assessment of patients with (a) extensive pneumonia despite recommended empiric therapy, even after the addition of vancomycin and amphotericin B; (b) nonresolving pneumonia, even after the recovery of neutrophils; and (d) an additional immune defect other than neutropenia, or unusual clinical data.

Lung biopsy is necessary to document tissue invasion by fungi. Bronchoscopic lung biopsy, when used with BAL, increases the diagnostic yield in patients with PCP, mycobacteriosis, and lymphangitic carcinomatosis (8). Bronchoscopic lung biopsy is much more important in the diagnosis of infections caused by organisms other than *P. carinii*. A staged approach is an option for patients in whom PCP is a major diagnostic consideration but whose sputa are negative for *P. carinii*. Only a diagnostic BAL is performed initially; bronchoscopic lung biopsy is added to the initial BAL if other diagnostic possibilities are considered likely; and if the initial BAL is nondiagnostic despite a strong clinical suspicion of *P. carinii* infection, bronchoscopic lung biopsy is performed. Bilateral BAL has been shown to increase the diagnostic yield significantly in patients with opportunistic pulmonary infections. Cytomegalovirus can frequently be detected by examination and culture of the diagnostic BAL fluid. Recovery of *Mycobacterium avium* complex is highest with culture of both washings and BAL fluid. BAL in patients with leukemia and pulmonary infiltrates is not helpful in diagnosing invasive aspergillosis unless a lung biopsy is also performed.

Patients in whom the basic disease process extends into the lungs may require lung biopsy, although BAL provides a high diagnostic yield (>75%) in patients with lymphangitic pulmonary metastasis (8). Bronchoscopic lung biopsy is routinely used by many in the follow-up of patients who have undergone lung or heart-lung transplantation because obliterative bronchiolitis, a common complication in this group of patients, responds to treatment with augmented immunosuppression when detected early by surveillance bronchoscopic lung biopsy.

Lung Biopsy

Thoracoscopy, which allows biopsy of pleura or lung under direct vision, is an excellent way to obtain material for culture and histologic analysis (11). Open lung biopsy is a more invasive pulmonary diagnostic procedure that yields the diagnosis in up to 95% of patients (12,13). As the use of BAL and thoracoscopy has increased, the number of open lung biopsies performed has decreased.

DIAGNOSIS OF LUNG DISEASE IN IMMUNOCOMPROMISED HOSTS

Summary Statement	Level of Evidence
Delays in the diagnosis of lung disease in seriously ill patients have an adverse effect on mortality, particularly as they affects the adequacy of initial therapy.	Observational studies and expert opinion
Chest radiography alone is of limited accuracy for the diagnosis of acute lung disease in the immunocompromised host.	Observational studies and expert opinion
The early use of computed tomography of the chest to investigate unexplained fever in the immunocompromised host expedites the diagnosis of pulmonary processes.	Observational studies and expert opinion
Fiberoptic bronchoscopy with bronchoalveolar lavage or transbronchial lung biopsy allows the diagnosis of many conditions that otherwise would be missed.	Observational studies and expert opinion

DIFFERENTIAL DIAGNOSIS OF LUNG DISEASE IN THE IMMUNOCOMPROMISED PATIENT

The differential diagnosis of an immunocompromised patient with abnormal findings on the chest roentgenogram may include one or more of the following entities: (a) extension of the basic disease process, (b) opportunistic infection, (c) drug-induced lung disease, (d) alveolar hemorrhage, (e) nonspecific interstitial pneumonitis, (f) lymphocytic interstitial pneumonitis, (g) B-cell neoplasia and other cancers

associated with chronic immunosuppression, (h) a new pulmonary problem unrelated to the other conditions. A combination of two or more of the possibilities listed is relatively common. Of these, the first four can cause acute or life-threatening respiratory distress, whereas the others can be subclinical and cause subacute or slowly progressive chronic illness.

Pulmonary Extension of Basic Disease Process

The basic disease processes listed in Table 55.1 are often associated with various degrees of suppression of the immune defense mechanisms. In the present context, patients with such disorders may be considered immunocompromised hosts. Clinicians who encounter pulmonary problems in such patients must ascertain whether the pulmonary manifestations represent an extension of the basic disease into the lungs or other complications. Intrathoracic spread of primary pulmonary and extrapulmonary malignancies is the most common form of pulmonary extension of the basic disease process. Lymphangitic metastases from pulmonary and nonpulmonary malignancies should be included in the differential diagnosis of lung opacities on chest imaging studies in this group of patients.

Hematologic malignancies, especially leukemias and lymphomas, also can cause chest roentgenographic abnormalities (Fig. 55.2). Leukemias as a group are associated with mediastinal and hilar lymphadenopathy in 50% of cases at autopsy and with pulmonary parenchymal involvement in 25%. Occasionally, patients may present with acute respiratory distress resulting from extensive leukemic infiltrates in the lungs. Hodgkin lymphoma causes roentgenographically detectable mediastinal lymphadenopathy in 50% of patients and pulmonary parenchymal lesions in 30%. Non-Hodgkin lymphoma causes mediastinal lymphadenopathy in 35% of cases. A primary pulmonary lymphoma may present as alveolar opacities or as a homogeneous mass. In such cases,

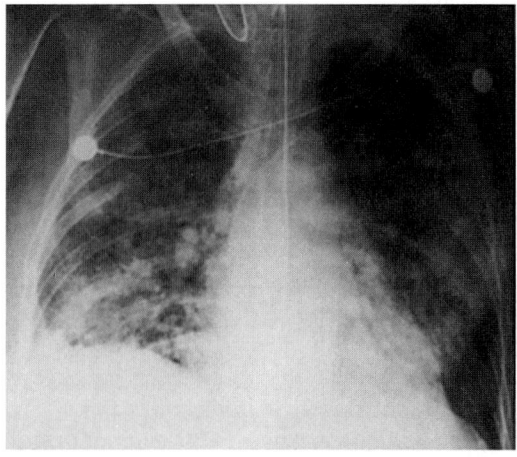

FIGURE 55.2. Pulmonary extension of non-Hodgkin lymphoma refractory to chemotherapy. Diffuse alveolar opacities are seen in both lungs.

elaborate diagnostic investigations may be necessary to rule out an extrapulmonary focus of the lymphoma. Lung involvement is more common in untreated lymphoproliferative diseases than in myeloproliferative diseases. Opportunistic infections are the most common cause of morbidity and mortality in these patients. However, opportunistic infections of the lungs are very uncommon in patients with hematologic malignancies who have no history of chemotherapy, radiation therapy, bone marrow transplantation, or malnutrition.

Connective tissue diseases and the vasculitides are often associated with pulmonary manifestations. Untreated rheumatologic entities, such as rheumatoid arthritis, systemic lupus erythematosus, progressive systemic sclerosis or scleroderma, polymyositis/dermatomyositis, Sjögren syndrome, mixed connective tissue disease, Wegener granulomatosis, temporal arteritis, and Churg-Strauss vasculitis, are well-known causes of pulmonary complications. The pulmonary manifestations of these disorders are discussed at length in Chapters 26 and 30. As in patients with malignancies, pulmonary opportunistic infections are uncommon in these patients unless they have received prolonged immunosuppressive therapy for their disease. Because most patients with symptomatic rheumatologic and vasculitic disorders are treated with immunosuppressive therapy, they become prime targets for opportunistic infections, drug-induced lung disease, and other pulmonary complications.

Opportunistic Pulmonary Infections

Overwhelming pneumonias remain an important cause of morbidity and mortality in immunocompromised patients. Many of these infections progress rapidly and are fatal. An immunocompromised patient is prone to the development of pulmonary infections caused by viruses, bacteria, mycobacteria, fungi, protozoa, and parasites (see Chapter 18).

Patterns of Pulmonary Injury and Common Causes

Alveolar Hemorrhage

Pulmonary alveolar hemorrhage is an important cause of respiratory symptoms and respiratory distress syndrome in immunocompromised patients (14) (see Chapter 31), and it accounts for 11% to 64% of pneumonic infiltrates in this group. However, alveolar hemorrhage is rarely the sole cause of pulmonary infiltrates, with fewer than 5% of patients exhibiting pulmonary hemorrhage as the only respiratory manifestation. Even when it is clinically considered an isolated phenomenon in immunocompromised patients, it is important to exclude occult invasive aspergillosis infection; close to 50% of patients with severe pulmonary hemorrhage may have documented aspergillosis. The association between thrombocytopenia and *Aspergillus* infection

and pulmonary hemorrhage is significant. Alveolar hemorrhage is also associated with other complications, such as mucormycosis, pulmonary veno-occlusive disease, graft versus host disease, mitomycin therapy, and other processes. Alveolar hemorrhage is seen frequently in recipients of heart transplants. In one study, 75% of BAL samples deemed positive for alveolar hemorrhage were in recipients of heart transplants. In another study, alveolar hemorrhage was detected in 21% of 141 consecutive recipients of autologous bone marrow transplants. Alveolar hemorrhage is significantly associated with thrombocytopenia (platelet count <50,000/mm^3), other coagulopathies, renal failure (serum creatinine = 2.5 mg/dL), a history of heavy smoking (>10 pack-years), leukopenia, thoracic radiation, and chemotherapy.

The difficulty of establishing the diagnosis of alveolar hemorrhage can be ascribed to the following factors: highly nonspecific clinical and roentgenographic features, absence of hemoptysis in most patients, and lack of specificity of the imaging procedures, including chest roentgenography, HRCT, and radionuclide scans. The diffusing capacity of the lung for carbon monoxide, when measured serially, has been reported to increase during alveolar bleeding as a result of an increased uptake of carbon monoxide by red blood cells in the alveoli. The need to perform this test serially renders it impractical in sick patients. Furthermore, its reliability in the diagnosis of alveolar hemorrhage has not been established.

Although thoracoscopy and open lung biopsy can document the diagnosis, these are high-risk procedures in immunocompromised patients. BAL has been used to diagnose alveolar hemorrhage in immunocompromised patients. The mere presence of hemosiderin-laden macrophages in the BAL effluent without quantification is not diagnostic. Therefore, estimation of the number of hemosiderin-laden macrophages is used to diagnose this complication. In a study of 240 BAL fluid samples in 194 immunocompromised hosts, a proportion of siderophages of at least 20% was considered to be diagnostic of alveolar hemorrhage (14). By this definition, alveolar hemorrhage was present in 87 (36%) of the samples; a proportion of siderophages of 20% to 65% was correlated with moderate hemorrhage (Golde score between 20 and 100), and a proportion higher than 67% was correlated with severe hemorrhage (Golde score >100). Even when a diagnosis of alveolar hemorrhage is established, it is essential to exclude the coexistence of the basic disease process and infections in the lungs.

Obstructive Airways Disease

Progressive airways disease leading to life-threatening respiratory distress is one of the most serious pulmonary complications encountered in immunocompromised patients. Obstructive airways disease can take the form of bronchospastic disease, lymphocytic bronchitis, or bronchiolitis obliterans.

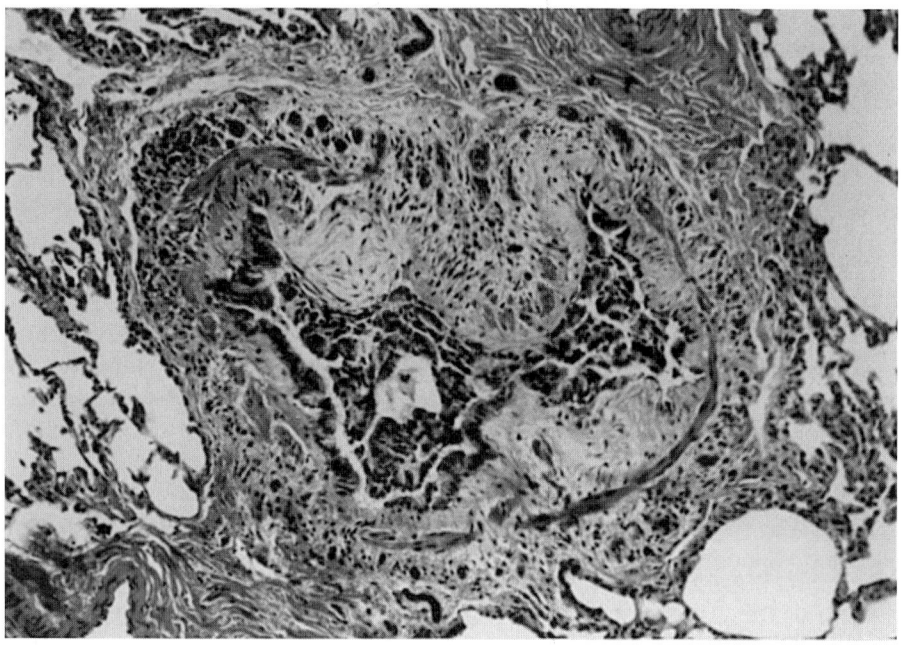

FIGURE 55.3. Bronchiolitis obliterans–associated progressive obstruction of airflow following bone marrow transplantation. Note fibrous thickening of the submucosa and distortion of the muscularis, with resultant compromise of the bronchiolar lumen.

A lymphocyte-mediated pathologic process is most likely responsible for these complications.

Obstructive airways disease secondary to immunocompromise is almost exclusively limited to recipients of organ transplants (Fig. 55.3). Patients with graft versus host disease are at risk for the development of this complication. Bronchiolitis obliterans secondary to rheumatoid arthritis and other collagen diseases is not considered here. However, it is important to recognize that in a patient with rheumatoid arthritis or another collagen disorder who is being treated with specific nonsteroidal antiinflammatory agents (e.g., penicillamine, gold preparations), the development of features of obstructive airways disease may be caused by the drugs themselves.

Nonspecific Interstitial Pneumonitis

The histopathologic findings in the lung tissue of immunocompromised patients with a diffuse pulmonary process may not fit any specific pattern and are therefore described as *nonspecific*. The nonspecificity of a biopsy-based diagnosis is helpful in excluding other causes of an interstitial process (Fig. 55.4). For example, in a study of 70 immunosuppressed patients with diffuse lung disease who underwent open lung biopsy, even though the procedure was diagnostically accurate in 97%, 45% of the diagnoses were nonspecific (fibrosis); no significant difference in mortality was found between the patients with a specific diagnosis and those without, or between the patients whose biopsy diagnosis resulted in an alteration of therapy and those whose biopsy diagnosis did not. In contrast, another study noted a recovery rate of only 25% in patients without a specific diagnosis following lung biopsy, whereas in patients in whom a treat-

able problem had been diagnosed, the overall recovery rate was 70%.

High-dose whole-body irradiation is commonly included in the conditioning regimens that precede bone marrow transplantation in patients with hematologic malignancies. Interstitial pneumonitis is a major complication after bone marrow transplantation, and nearly one fourth of all patients with bone marrow transplants die of this complication. In approximately half of these patients, an infectious agent, particularly cytomegalovirus, is involved. Additional factors, such as remission-induction chemotherapy, cyclophosphamide, methotrexate, cyclosporine, and graft versus host disease, combine to cause interstitial lung disease in these patients.

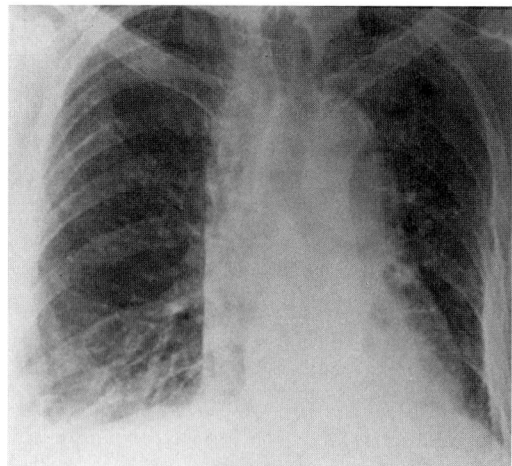

FIGURE 55.4. Nonspecific interstitial pneumonitis in an immunocompromised patient in whom dyspnea and cough developed after thoracic radiation and multiple courses of chemotherapy for Hodgkin lymphoma. Open lung biopsy revealed nonspecific inflammation and fibrosis.

Lymphocytic Interstitial Pneumonitis

The differential diagnosis of lymphocytic interstitial pneumonitis is discussed in Chapter 24. In immunocompromised patients, the causes of lymphocytic interstitial pneumonitis include HIV infection (see Chapter 18), other viral infections, graft versus host disease, and agammaglobulinemia. Because many of the diseases associated with lymphocytic interstitial pneumonitis are forms of lymphoma, immunocompromised patients with lymphocytic interstitial pneumonitis should be closely observed to detect possible lymphoproliferative disease.

Pulmonary "Immune" Neoplasia

The frequency of non-Hodgkin lymphomas is increased in immunocompromised patients as a result of iatrogenic immunosuppressive therapy. Such lymphomas are more common in organ transplant recipients than in other immunocompromised patients. Lymphomas may be oligoclonal or polyclonal in origin (Fig. 55.5), and they may be related to the use of cyclosporine. In contrast, the non-Hodgkin lymphomas seen in patients with AIDS are Burkitt-like lymphomas, B-cell lymphomas, or B-cell immunoblastic sarcomas, with or without plasmacytoid features. They tend to be extranodal.

As a result of successful treatment with radiation, chemotherapy, or both, patients with lymphoma are living longer. The long-term follow-up of these patients has revealed an increased incidence of lung carcinoma. The relative risk for the development of new malignancies in patients treated for Hodgkin or non-Hodgkin lymphoma is two to three times that in the normal population. Previous radiation therapy also may increase the risk for the development of pulmonary nonlymphomatous malignancies.

Small cell carcinoma is the predominant histologic type of lung cancer in both smokers and nonsmokers treated with irradiation. However, patients with Hodgkin lymphoma who receive supradiaphragmatic irradiation or combined-modality therapy may be at increased risk for the development of non–small cell carcinoma of the lung. In a study of such patients, the risk ratio for the development of lung cancer among patients with Hodgkin lymphoma was 5.6 times that expected in the general population. The median ages of patients in whom Hodgkin lymphoma and lung carcinoma were diagnosed were 39 and 45 years, respectively. The interval between the diagnosis of Hodgkin lymphoma and metachronous lung cancer averaged 7 years but appeared to vary inversely with age at diagnosis, a finding that underscores the need for long-term close observation.

Pulmonary Problems Unrelated to Immunodeficiency

Immunocompromised patients are more susceptible to the disease processes that affect nonimmunocompromised subjects. Abnormal findings on a chest roentgenogram in an immunocompromised patient may represent cardiac or noncardiac pulmonary edema, pulmonary embolism, a community-acquired pulmonary infection, aspiration pneumonitis, or delayed effects of thoracic irradiation. More than one third of immunocompromised patients have a combination of two or more of these complications.

IMMUNODEFICIENCY SYNDROMES

X-Linked Agammaglobulinemia

Also known as *Bruton infantile agammaglobulinemia,* X-linked agammaglobulinemia is a disorder of B-lymphocyte maturation. X-linked agammaglobulinemia is caused by a defect in a signal transduction molecule called *Bruton tyrosine kinase* (15). This kinase is expressed in B cells at all stages of development, and also in myeloid and erythroid cells. As a result of the defect, the synthesis and secretion of immunoglobulins and antibodies are deficient or absent, and recurrent infections develop. T-lymphocyte function remains intact, and the number of T cells is usually increased. A diagnosis of X-linked agammaglobulinemia is considered if the serum levels of IgG, IgA, and IgM are significantly below the 95% confidence limits of those for appropriate age- and sex-matched controls. The total immunoglobulin level in patients with X-linked agammaglobulinemia usually is less than 100 mg/dL. Most patients with classic X-linked agammaglobulinemia have fewer than 1% to 2% CD19+ lymphocytes (16). In the context of a positive family

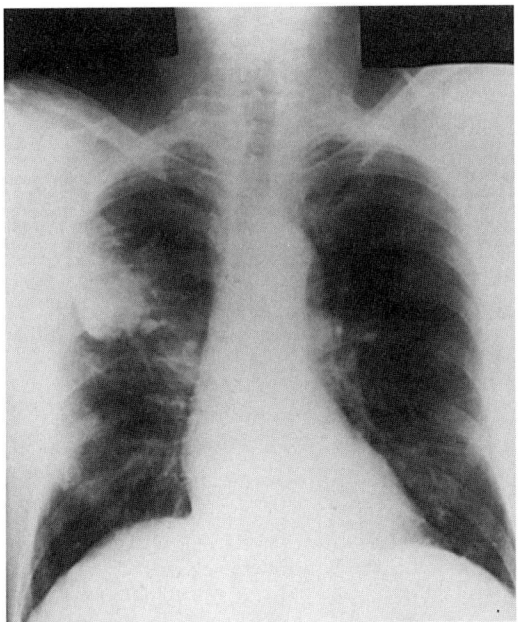

FIGURE 55.5. B-cell lymphoma developing in the right upper lobe of a patient on long-term immunosuppressive therapy after renal transplantation.

history of the disease or when it is possible to establish that the mother is a carrier, low numbers of CD19$^+$ lymphocytes can be diagnostic. However, intermediate B-cell values may make it impossible to distinguish between X-linked agammaglobulinemia, common variable immunodeficiency, and transient hypogammaglobulinemia of infancy (16).

Clinically, recurrent sinopulmonary infections, otitis, meningitis, and skin lesions (eczema) are encountered in infant boys between 4 and 6 months of age (17). In some cases, mild X-linked agammaglobulinemia has been diagnosed in patients as old as 51 years (18). Allergic rhinitis and asthma occur in these patients at a higher rate than in the normal population. Undue susceptibility to bacterial infections is seen, usually after the first year of life. An important clue to the diagnosis is a unique susceptibility to infection with encapsulated pyogenic organisms, including *Streptococcus pneumoniae, Streptococcus pyogenes, Haemophilus influenzae, Pseudomonas aeruginosa,* and staphylococci. This phenomenon probably reflects a requirement for specific opsonization of these bacteria before efficient phagocytic cell ingestion is possible. Recurrent purulent sinusitis, bronchitis, and pneumonia, if untreated, may develop into progressive bronchiectasis and secondary respiratory failure. Adults with the disease are especially prone to *Mycoplasma* infection of the respiratory tract. PCP, although rare in agammaglobulinemia, has been described in congenital cases (19). No evidence of increased susceptibility to viral infections of the respiratory system has been found, but the patients are prone to viral infections of the central nervous system (20). Restrictive lung disease and lymphocytic interstitial pneumonitis are the other long-term pulmonary complications.

In a multicenter study of 96 patients with X-linked agammaglobulinemia (53 familial and 43 nonfamilial cases), pulmonary infections were observed in 65%: pneumonitis in 56%, bronchitis in 9%, and bronchiolitis in 5%. Bacterial cultures of sputum were available from 33 patients with chronic or recurrent pneumonia; isolated bacterial species included *H. influenzae* in 82%, *Staphylococcus aureus* in 27%, and *S. pneumoniae* in 21%. Chronic pulmonary disease was the most frequent long-term complication, occurring in 46% of all patients. The prevalence of lung disease was age-related, present in 13% of those younger than 10 years and 76% of those older than 20 years.

High-dose intravenous immunoglobulin therapy has been shown to prevent recurrent infections (21). In a clinical evaluation of 10 patients with X-linked agammaglobulinemia followed for a mean of 12.5 years, pneumonias developed infrequently in most of the patients treated with intramuscular gamma globulin and long-term oral antibiotics (22).

Common Variable Immunodeficiency

Common variable immunodeficiency, also known as *acquired agammaglobulinemia,* is among the most frequently

encountered primary immunodeficiency disorders (23). A genetic basis is hypothesized for this disorder because it occurs more commonly in first-degree relatives of patients with selective IgA deficiency (24). However, no molecular genetic defects have yet been identified in any patient with common variable immunodeficiency (16). A primary defect in B-cell maturation is the problem. Most patients with this disorder have a normal number of immunoglobulin-bearing B cells in their blood and lymphoid tissue but lack mature plasma cells. A reduced ratio of CD4$^+$ to CD8$^+$ T cells is common, and approximately 60% of patients have depressed T-cell function, with reduced proliferation and reduced production of some cytokines (e.g., interleukins-2, -4, and -5, and interferon-γ) (16,25,26). The serum level of IgG is low or absent, and the IgA and IgM levels are variably diminished; thus, antibody production is diminished. However, a tendency to autoantibody formation has been noted. The role of immunologic defense mechanisms in the development of acute recurrent or chronic sinusitis is obviously important, but the incidence of such immune problems is unknown. Common variable immunodeficiency has been known to be associated with thymoma, hemolytic anemia, gastric atrophy, achlorhydria, follicular lymphoid hyperplasia, celiac disease-like syndrome, and several other disorders (27).

Common variable immunodeficiency occurs in both sexes. A bimodal distribution of incidence by age has been noted, with the major peak between 25 to 45 years and a significant second peak between 5 and 15 years, although the onset may be at any age (16,27,28). The diagnosis may be delayed considerably (23). Pulmonary disease is more frequent and more severe than in patients with X-linked agammaglobulinemia. Sinopulmonary infections begin in the second or third decade (23). Chronic complications include bronchitis, cystic bronchiectasis, patchy pulmonary fibrosis, and interstitial pneumonitis (20,29). Infections caused by encapsulated bacteria are more common. Bronchiectasis and obstructive airways disease occur in up to 40% of patients. Roentgenographic features may include atelectasis, bronchiectasis (Fig. 55.6), and homogeneous and heterogeneous segmental opacities. Patients with late-onset agammaglobulinemia and recurrent pulmonary infections occasionally present with pulmonary hypertrophic osteoarthropathy. In a review of patients in whom pneumonia or empyema developed secondary to infection with *Moraxella catarrhalis,* nearly one third were found to have immunoglobulin abnormalities. Organizing pneumonitis and allergic bronchopulmonary aspergillosis also are described in common variable immunodeficiency (30). Common variable immunodeficiency should be suspected in patients with sarcoidosis who have recurrent infections and hypogammaglobulinemia (31). The mechanism of the apparent relation between these disorders is not known, and it is possible that they are distinct entities with some clinical similarities (16).

A clinical evaluation of 12 patients with common variable immunodeficiency followed for a mean of 10.5 years revealed

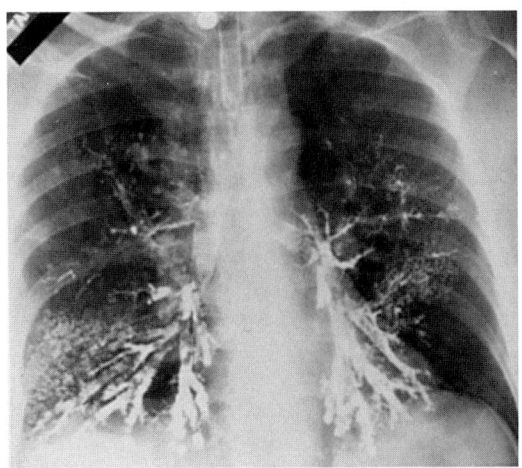

FIGURE 55.6. Bronchography demonstrating bronchiectasis of both lower lobes in a patient with acquired agammaglobulinemia.

few cases of pneumonia among those treated with intramuscular gamma globulin and long-term oral antibiotics (22). The survival rate 20 years after the diagnosis of common variable immunodeficiency was 64% for men and 67% for women, versus the expected 92% survival for men and 94% for women in the general population (32). Factors associated with increased mortality included low levels of serum IgG, poor T-cell responses to phytohemagglutinin, and in particular, a low percentage of peripheral B cells (32).

Selective Immunoglobulin Deficiencies

Selective deficiencies of one or more, but not all, immunoglobulin subclasses are called *dysgammaglobulinemias*. Patients with these disorders usually have normal total serum concentrations of IgG. Thus, it is important to measure the levels of the IgG subclasses in patients suspected of having a selective immunoglobulin deficiency. It is also important to recognize that most patients with a selective deficiency of an IgG subclass are asymptomatic, and the routine administration of intravenous immunoglobulin therapy is not justified unless they are known to have clinical features of the disorder (33).

Immunoglobulin A Deficiency

Immunoglobulin A deficiency (<10 mg/dL) is the most frequent immunoglobulin deficiency (i.e., isolated or in combination with deficiency of another immunoglobulin subclass). The estimated incidence of selective IgA deficiency ranges from 1 in 333 to 1 in 1,000, with most cases occurring sporadically, although some persons inherit the deficiency as an autosomal-dominant or autosomal-recessive trait.

A deficiency of IgA in combination with deficiencies of IgG2 and IgG4 increases the risk for recurrent respiratory infections (34). Bronchitis and bronchiectasis are associated with increased numbers of IgA-producing cells in the bronchi because cells containing IgA1 predominate in the major bronchi and the number of cells containing IgA2 is higher in the bronchi than in nonmucosal lymphoid tissues. In a study of 29 patients with IgA deficiency and recurrent upper and lower respiratory infections, the levels of IgG2 and IgG3 were decreased in 21% of the patients, and low levels of IgG2 and IgG3 were significantly related to abnormal lung function. These findings suggest a causal relationship between low levels of IgG subclasses and reduced lung function and that patients with combined IgA and IgG subclass deficiencies may benefit from immunoglobulin prophylaxis. Like common variable immunodeficiency, selective IgA deficiency is frequently associated with rheumatologic and collagen disorders, including rheumatoid arthritis, systemic lupus erythematosus, dermatomyositis, ankylosing spondylitis, thyroiditis, diabetes mellitus, hepatitis, and a significant number of other disorders. Several medications may also cause an IgA deficiency that resolves once the medication is removed: D-penicillamine, sulfasalazine, aurothioglucose, fenclofenac, gold, captopril, zonisamide, phenytoin, valproic acid, and thyroxine (16,34).

The respiratory complications are usually mild and include atopic asthma, repeated respiratory infections, bronchiectasis, sinusitis, and otitis media. Pulmonary hemosiderosis has been described in some patients. In a prospective study of 43 children, the development of asthma was much more likely in those without any measurable IgA and elevated levels of IgE. Variable deficiencies of IgG and IgA in children have been associated with lymphoid interstitial pneumonitis. The factors responsible for the B-lymphocyte dysfunction and lymphoid infiltrations in the pulmonary parenchyma are unknown.

The treatment of IgA deficiency generally focuses on the prophylaxis and management of infection. Intravenous immunoglobulin is not usually effective in the treatment of selective IgA deficiency. It may be helpful in those patients with associated IgG subclass deficiency (16).

Selective Immunoglobulin G Subclass Deficiencies

Recurrent bacterial infections of the lungs and upper respiratory tract are common in these patients. Selective IgG subclass deficiencies (IgG1, IgG2, IgG3, and IgG4) predispose patients to recurrent infections of the ears, upper respiratory tract, and lungs. Encapsulated bacteria such as *S. pneumoniae* and *H. influenzae* are responsible. Deficiencies of IgG, especially subclasses IgG2 and IgG4 (often in combination with a deficiency of IgA) or IgG4 alone, correlate well with upper respiratory tract infections and chronic bronchial inflammation that contributes to bronchiectasis. Asthma has been noted in some patients with this disorder. A deficiency of IgG3 and a poor response to pneumococcal antigen 7 were demonstrated in more than 50% of 61 children with refractory sinusitis. Isolated IgG4 deficiency appears to be associated with impaired respiratory tract defenses and may occur in the absence of an easily defined antibody deficiency. Acquired hypogammaglobulinemia rarely is associated with obstructive lung disease, and the pathogenesis of the lung disease may be related to an associated increase in the elastase load and a reduction in protease inhibitor function.

Functional Deficiency of Immunoglobulin G

A functional deficiency of IgG may come to light in patients who present with recurrent pulmonary infections, but such patients may have normal serum levels of IgG. Furthermore, combined deficiencies of IgG2 subclass and IgG- and IgM-specific antibodies may be present in persons with normal serum immunoglobulin concentrations. For instance, the IgG2 subclass includes an important group of antibodies against common bacteria such as *S. pneumoniae* and *H. influenzae,* and recurrent sinopulmonary infections may develop in patients with this isolated deficiency even though they have normal total serum levels of IgG. Patients with community-acquired pneumonia of bacterial or unknown cause generally demonstrate decreased serum concentrations of IgG2 at the time of admission, after recovery, and 9 months later. In patients with recurrent lung infections and bronchiectasis who have normal serum concentrations of immunoglobulins, it is important to evaluate both IgG subclasses and antibody production because immunoglobulin replacement has been shown to be beneficial in these patients. Other functional deficiencies of IgG include the absence of an IgG antibody response to polysaccharide antigens and antibody deficiency secondary to IgG degradation, as occurs in cystic fibrosis. IgG subclass deficiencies, particularly deficiencies of IgG1, appear to be related to long-term, low-dose corticosteroid therapy in patients with obstructive lung disease. In patients who have been immunized with pneumococcal vaccine, the increases in serum IgG subclass concentrations and antipneumococcal antibodies do not differ from those in control subjects.

Familial Deficiency of Serum Immunoglobulin E

Familial deficiency of serum IgE, presumably an autosomal-dominant trait with variable penetrance, in association with sinopulmonary infections has been described. The examination of sera from 23 family members, of whom 14 were symptomatic, revealed very low levels (<5 IU/mL) of serum IgE in 12 members of the symptomatic group.

Selective Immunoglobulin M Deficiency

Selective IgM deficiency (<10 mg/dL) is a rare disorder. Described respiratory complications include otitis, bronchiectasis, and lung infections caused by streptococci, mycobacteria,

and other organisms. No specific therapy is available other than appropriate antimicrobial treatment of the bacterial infections.

Hyperimmunoglobulinemia E

Hyperimmunoglobulinemia E, also known as *Job syndrome* or *Buckley syndrome,* is a rare disorder characterized by phagocyte dysfunction, high serum levels of IgE (often >4,000 IU/mL) and IgD, poor antibody- and cell-mediated responses to new antigens, blood and sputum eosinophilia, and normal concentrations of IgG, IgA, and IgM (35). The lymphocytes of patients with hyper-IgE syndrome show an impaired response to interleukin-12 that results in a decreased production of interferon-γ, which may be of key importance in the pathogenesis of the immune abnormalities of hyper-IgE syndrome (36). Persons of both sexes are affected; an autosomal-dominant form of inheritance has been suggested. More than 100 cases of this disorder have been described, mostly in young children. Severe and recurrent staphylococcal abscesses involving skin, lungs, and joints begin in infancy (37–40).

Clinically, the syndrome may include eczematoid dermatitis, dysmorphic syndrome with retarded growth, coarse facies, prognathism, osteogenesis imperfecta, and axial osteoporosis (38,41). Respiratory complications include sinusitis; pneumonia; bronchiectasis caused by *S. aureus, S. pneumoniae,* Gram-negative bacilli, *Candida albicans,* and *Aspergillus* species; pneumatoceles; and chronic dermatitis. Asthma has been reported in approximately 10% of patients (42). The frequency of pneumatoceles is remarkably high, and surgical therapy is often necessary (Fig. 55.7). The primary chest

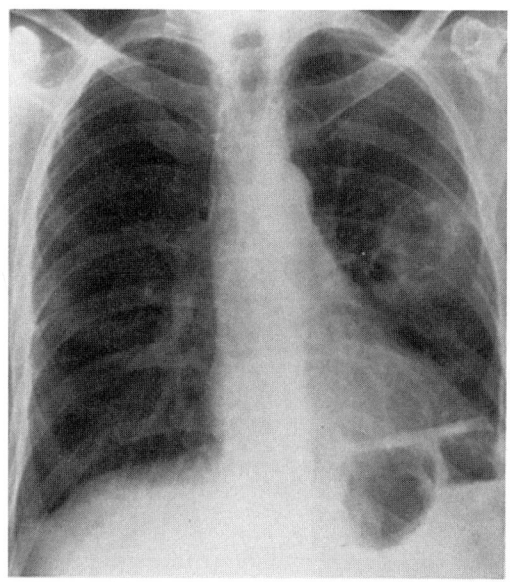

FIGURE 55.7. Hyperimmunoglobulinemia E (Job) syndrome with left lung abscess caused by *S. aureus.* Pneumatoceles, a common complication in this syndrome, can be seen in early stages.

roentgenologic abnormalities include recurrent lung infiltrative process and pneumatoceles (43,44). Pneumothorax may occur occasionally.

Hyperimmunoglobulinemia M

Hyperimmunoglobulinemia M with hypogammaglobulinemia is an uncommon syndrome that has been described as both an X-linked and an autosomal-recessive disease. Patients with this disorder become symptomatic during the first or second year of life. Occasional sporadic cases occur in later life. The results of tests of cellular immunity are normal, but abnormalities in immunoglobulin production are believed to be the consequence of the dysfunctional regulation of B cells by defective T cells (45). Patients with this syndrome usually have elevated levels of IgM and IgD but very low levels of IgA and IgG. They are susceptible to pyogenic infections, including otitis media, sinusitis, and pneumonia. Because they lack the ability to produce IgG antibodies, therapy includes the monthly administration of immunoglobulin.

DiGeorge Syndrome

Congenital thymic aplasia, or DiGeorge syndrome, is characterized by thymic aplasia or hypoplasia resulting from dysmorphogenesis of the third and fourth pharyngeal pouches during embryogenesis (46,47). Associated abnormalities include failed development of the parathyroid glands, neonatal hypocalcemia and tetany, and cardiac defects, including tetralogy of Fallot, right-sided aortic arch, and truncus arteriosus. The facies abnormalities consist of hypertelorism, micrognathia, a short philtrum, and low-set, posteriorly rotated ears with small pinnae. Approximately 80% to 90% of patients with DiGeorge syndrome have microdeletions involving one copy of chromosome 22q11 (48). The immunologic defect is the result of T lymphopenia. The lymphocyte counts are normal, but all the lymphocytes are B cells. The serum immunoglobulin concentrations are usually normal, but the IgG and IgA antibody responses are frequently impaired.

The pulmonary complications described include both viral and bacterial infections and interstitial pneumonitis. Other pulmonary abnormalities reported include hypoplastic lungs with an abnormal anatomic location and hypoplastic pulmonary artery.

Wiskott-Aldrich Syndrome

The Wiskott-Aldrich syndrome is a rare X-linked immunologic disorder characterized by the clinical triad of eczema, profound thrombocytopenia with purpura, and recurrent infections (49). A deficiency of IgM, elevated levels of IgA and IgG, and very high levels of IgE are seen frequently. A defective gene has been identified that encodes a protein designated *Wiskott-Aldrich syndrome–associated protein* (50,51). The function of this protein is unknown, but it appears to act in part to modulate both lymphocyte activation and cytoskeletal rearrangements (50,51).

Respiratory complications in the form of otitis media followed by pneumonia are common. In younger patients, encapsulated organisms more often cause the bacterial infections. Patients are also susceptible to herpes simplex, varicella, and infection with cytomegalovirus and *P. carinii*. Gram-positive and Gram-negative bacterial infections are common. Pulmonary vasculitis with features typical of lymphomatoid granulomatosis has been described. Survival beyond the teens is uncommon. Fatal malignant neoplasms develop in nearly 12% of patients, and more than 80% of these lesions are leukemias and lymphoreticular tumors. However, infections and bleeding (bloody diarrhea) are the major causes of mortality (16). As many as 40% of patients with Wiskott-Aldrich syndrome may have an autoimmune or inflammatory disease such as anemia and neutropenia, various forms of vasculitis, glomerulonephritis, and inflammatory bowel disease (16). The intravenous administration of gamma globulin, antibiotic prophylaxis, and the replacement of blood components have been shown to reduce the morbidity and mortality associated with Wiskott-Aldrich syndrome (16).

Idiopathic CD4$^+$ T Lymphocytopenia

A report of four patients with opportunistic infections and no major risk factors for HIV infection described the phenomenon of idiopathic CD4$^+$ T lymphocytopenia (52). All four patients had severe, persistent CD4$^+$ T lymphocytopenia (range, 12–293 cells per cubic millimeter); the CD4$^+$ cell count progressively declined in only one. All four patients had significantly reduced numbers of circulating CD8$^+$ T cells, natural killer cells, or B cells (or all three). All presented with severe opportunistic infections, including PCP, cryptococcal meningitis (two patients, one with concurrent pulmonary tuberculosis), and histoplasmosis-induced brain abscess. During up to 68 months of observation, none of the four patients showed evidence of infection with HIV.

Ataxia-Telangiectasia

Transmitted as an autosomal-recessive disease, hereditary ataxia-telangiectasia is characterized by progressive cerebellar ataxia that is followed by the development of choreoathetoid movements and, several years later, ocular and cutaneous telangiectasia. Dysfunctional T helper cells may account for the underlying diminished activity of B cells. A lack of both serum and secretory fractions of IgA is

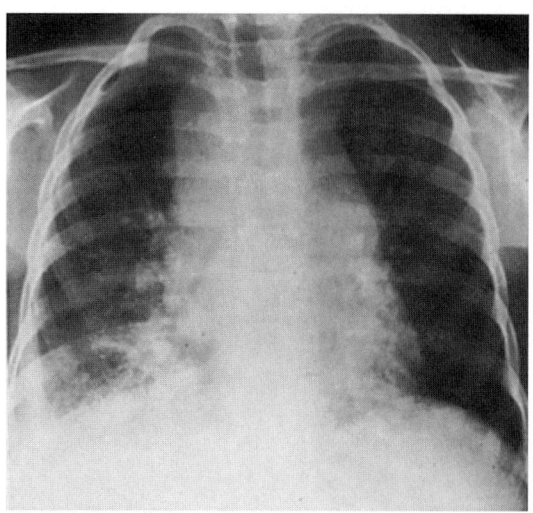

FIGURE 55.8. Bilateral lower lobe infiltrates in a child with ataxia-telangiectasia. This patient had recurrent pulmonary infections caused by *Haemophilus influenzae.*

noted in more than 80% of patients, and serum IgA is absent in approximately 50%. Deficiency of IgG2 is common. Isolated deficiency of IgG4 with normal total levels of IgG and levels of other IgG subclasses occurs. Ataxia-telangiectasia is associated with defective DNA repair mechanisms (16). The estimated incidence of ataxia-telangiectasia is 1 in 20,000 to 1 in 100,000 live births (16,53).

Chronic sinopulmonary infections caused by bacteria develop in 80% of patients. These may lead to severe bronchiectasis. This complication has been observed in both children and adults. Repeated infections of the sinuses and lungs by viral agents and bacteria are common (Fig. 55.8). Chest roentgenograms demonstrate a prominent, symmetric, thicket-like pattern in the lungs. One study of 160 patients with ataxia-telangiectasia reported recurrent sinopulmonary infections in 66% and low levels or an absence of serum IgA in 51%.

The development of lymphoma and acute lymphocytic leukemia is markedly increased in patients with ataxia-telangiectasia, and more than 10% succumb to malignancy (54). No therapies significantly alter the course of the disease (55). Diagnostic tests involving x-rays and ionizing radiation should be kept to a minimum to reduce the risk for somatic mutations and subsequent malignancy (55).

Nezelof Syndrome

Nezelof syndrome consists of thymic dysplasia with normal immunoglobulins. It is an inherited disorder characterized by lymphopenia, diminished lymphoid tissue, abnormal architecture of the thymus, and normal or elevated immunoglobulin levels. Flawed functioning of interleukin-2 has been observed in several patients. Deficient T-cell function is the main abnormality, although Nezelof syndrome is sometimes discussed in conjunction with the severe combined immunodeficiency syndrome. Although Nezelof syndrome is usually a disease of children, several adult cases have been described. Recurrent respiratory infections secondary to bronchiectasis and sinusitis are common (56). Fatal bronchiolitis caused by cytomegalovirus has been described in a child (57).

Hyposplenism

Splenic function is decreased or absent in congenital aplasia, hyposplenism secondary to hemolytic states, malignancy involving the spleen, and chronic sickle cell disease, and after splenectomy. The phagocytosis of encapsulated bacteria depends on normal splenic function. Hyposplenism results in a loss of protection against encapsulated organisms such as *S. pneumoniae* and *H. influenzae.* The administration of pneumococcal vaccine and the prompt treatment of infections are important.

REFERENCES

1. Crawford SW. Noninfectious lung disease in the immunocompromised host. *Respiration* 1999;66:385–395.
2. Mayaud C, Cadranel J. A persistent challenge: the diagnosis of respiratory disease in the non- AIDS immunocompromised host. *Thorax* 2000;55:511–517.
3. Rano A, Agusti C, Benito N, et al. Prognostic factors of non-HIV immunocompromised patients with pulmonary infiltrates. *Chest* 2002;122:253–261.
4. Rano A, Agusti C, Jimenez P, et al. Pulmonary infiltrates in non-HIV immunocompromised patients: a diagnostic approach using noninvasive and bronchoscopic procedures. *Thorax* 2001;56:379–387.
5. Dichter JR, Levine SJ, Shelhamer JH. Approach to the immunocompromised host with pulmonary symptoms. *Hematol Oncol Clin North Am* 1993;7:887–912.
6. Logan PM, Primack SL, Staples C, et al. Acute lung disease in the immunocompromised host. Diagnostic accuracy of the chest radiograph. *Chest* 1995;108:1283–1287.
7. Janzen DL, Adler BD, Padley SP, et al. Diagnostic success of bronchoscopic biopsy in immunocompromised patients with acute pulmonary disease: predictive value of disease distribution as shown on CT. *AJR Am J Roentgenol* 1993;160:21–24.
8. Cazzadori A, Di Perri G, Todeschini G, et al. Transbronchial biopsy in the diagnosis of pulmonary infiltrates in immunocompromised patients. *Chest* 1995;107:101–106.
9. Gruson D, Hilbert G, Valentino R, et al. Utility of fiberoptic bronchoscopy in neutropenic patients admitted to the intensive care unit with pulmonary infiltrates. *Crit Care Med* 2000;28:2224–2230.
10. Cordonnier C, Escudier E, Verra F, et al. Bronchoalveolar lavage during neutropenic episodes: diagnostic yield and cellular pattern. *Eur Respir J* 1994;7:114–120.
11. Feins RH. The role of thoracoscopy in the AIDS/immunocompromised patient. *Ann Thorac Surg* 1993;56:649–650.

12. Toledo-Pereyra LH, DeMeester TR, Kinealey A, et al. The benefits of open lung biopsy in patients with previous nondiagnostic transbronchial lung biopsy. A guide to appropriate therapy. *Chest* 1980;77:647–650.

13. White DA, Wong PW, Downey R. The utility of open lung biopsy in patients with hematologic malignancies. *Am J Respir Crit Care Med* 2000;161:723–729.

14. De Lassence A, Fleury-Feith J, Escudier E, et al. Alveolar hemorrhage. Diagnostic criteria and results in 194 immunocompromised hosts. *Am J Respir Crit Care Med* 1995;151:157–163.

15. Vetrie D, Vorechovsky I, Sideras P, et al. The gene involved in X-linked agammaglobulinaemia is a member of the src family of protein-tyrosine kinases. *Nature* 1993;361:226–233.

16. Bonilla FA. Primary humoral immune deficiencies. In: Rose BD, ed. UpToDate. Wellesley, MA: UpToDate, 2002.

17. Plebani A, Soresina A, Rondelli R, et al. Clinical, immunological, and molecular analysis in a large cohort of patients with X-linked agammaglobulinemia: an Italian multicenter study. *Clin Immunol* 2002;104:221.

18. Kornfeld SJ, Haire RN, Strong SJ, et al. A novel mutation (Cys145→Stop) in Bruton's tyrosine kinase is associated with newly diagnosed X-linked agammaglobulinemia in a 51-year-old male. *Mol Med* 1996;2:619–623.

19. Alibrahim A, Lepore M, Lierl M, et al. *Pneumocystis carinii* pneumonia in an infant with X-linked agammaglobulinemia. *J Allergy Clin Immunol* 1998;101:552–553.

20. Kainulainen L, Nikoskelainen J, Vuorinen T, et al. Viruses and bacteria in bronchial samples from patients with primary hypogammaglobulinemia. *Am J Respir Crit Care Med* 1999;159:1199–1204.

21. Skull S, Kemp A. Treatment of hypogammaglobulinaemia with intravenous immunoglobulin, 1973–93. *Arch Dis Child* 1996;74:527–530.

22. Sweinberg SK, Wodell RA, Grodofsky MP, et al. Retrospective analysis of the incidence of pulmonary disease in hypogammaglobulinemia. *J Allergy Clin Immunol* 1991;88:96–104.

23. Kainulainen L, Nikoskelainen J, Ruuskanen O. Diagnostic findings in 95 Finnish patients with common variable immunodeficiency. *J Clin Immunol* 2001;21:145–149.

24. Schaffer FM, Palermos J, Zhu ZB, et al. Individuals with IgA deficiency and common variable immunodeficiency share polymorphisms of major histocompatibility complex class III genes. *Proc Natl Acad Sci U S A* 1989;86:8015–8019.

25. Sneller MC, Strober W. Abnormalities in the expression of T-cell activation genes in patients with common variable immunodeficiency. *Trans Assoc Am Physicians* 1990;103:163–173.

26. Jaffe JS, Eisenstein E, Sneller MC, et al. T-cell abnormalities in common variable immunodeficiency. *Pediatr Res* 1993;33:S24–S27; discussion S27–S28.

27. Hausser C, Virelizier JL, Buriot D, et al. Common variable hypogammaglobulinemia in children. Clinical and immunologic observations in 30 patients. *Am J Dis Child* 1983;137:833–837.

28. Cunningham-Rundles C. Clinical and immunologic analyses of 103 patients with common variable immunodeficiency. *J Clin Immunol* 1989;9:22–33.

29. Kainulainen L, Varpula M, Liippo K, et al. Pulmonary abnormalities in patients with primary hypogammaglobulinemia. *J Allergy Clin Immunol* 1999;104:1031–1036.

30. Kaufman J, Komorowski R. Bronchiolitis obliterans organizing pneumonia in common variable immunodeficiency syndrome. *Chest* 1991;100:552–553.

31. Fasano MB, Sullivan KE, Sarpong SB, et al. Sarcoidosis and common variable immunodeficiency. Report of 8 cases and review of the literature. *Medicine (Baltimore)* 1996;75:251–261.

32. Cunningham-Rundles C, Bodian C. Common variable immunodeficiency: clinical and immunological features of 248 patients. *Clin Immunol* 1999;92:34–48.

33. Buckley RH. Immunoglobulin G subclass deficiency: fact or fancy? *Curr Allergy Asthma Rep* 2002;2:356–360.

34. Hostoffer R. IgA deficiency. In: Rose BD, ed. *UpToDate*. Wellesley, MA: UpToDate, 2002.

35. Buckley RH, Wray BB, Belmaker EZ. Extreme hyperimmunoglobulinemia E and undue susceptibility to infection. *Pediatrics* 1972;49:59–70.

36. Borges WG, Augustine NH, Hill HR. Defective interleukin-12/interferon-gamma pathway in patients with hyperimmunoglobulinemia E syndrome. *J Pediatr* 2000;136:176–180.

37. Hill HR, Estensen RD, Hogan NA, et al. Severe staphylococcal disease associated with allergic manifestations, hyperimmunoglobulinemia E, and defective neutrophil chemotaxis. *J Lab Clin Med* 1976;88:796–806.

38. Schopfer K, Baerlocher K, Price P, et al. Staphylococcal IgE antibodies, hyperimmunoglobulinemia E, and *Staphylococcus aureus* infections. *N Engl J Med* 1979;300:835–838.

39. Hill HR. The syndrome of hyperimmunoglobulinemia E and recurrent infections. *Am J Dis Child* 1982;136:767–771.

40. Lavoie A, Rottem M, Grodofsky MP, et al. Anti-*Staphylococcus aureus* IgE antibodies for the diagnosis of hyperimmunoglobulinemia E-recurrent infection syndrome in infancy. *Am J Dis Child* 1989;143:1038–1041.

41. Kirchner SG, Sivit CJ, Wright PF. Hyperimmunoglobulinemia E syndrome: association with osteoporosis and recurrent fractures. *Radiology* 1985;156:362.

42. Tsukagoshi H, Nagashima M, Horie T, et al. Kimura's disease associated with bronchial asthma presenting with eosinophilia and hyperimmunoglobulinemia E which were attenuated by suplatast tosilate (IPD-1151T). *Intern Med* 1998;37:1064–1067.

43. Merten DF, Buckley RH, Pratt PC, et al. Hyperimmunoglobulinemia E syndrome: radiographic observations. *Radiology* 1979;132:71–78.

44. Fitch SJ, Magill HL, Herrod HG, et al. Hyperimmunoglobulinemia E syndrome: pulmonary imaging considerations. *Pediatr Radiol* 1986;16:285–288.

45. Oliva A, Quinti I, Scala E, et al. Immunodeficiency with hyperimmunoglobulinemia M in two female patients is not associated with abnormalities of CD40 or CD40 ligand expression. *J Allergy Clin Immunol* 1995;96:403–410.

46. Muller W, Peter HH, Wilken M, et al. The DiGeorge syndrome. I. Clinical evaluation and course of partial and complete forms of the syndrome. *Eur J Pediatr* 1988;147:496–502.

47. Muller W, Peter HH, Kallfelz HC, et al. The DiGeorge sequence. II. Immunologic findings in partial and complete forms of the disorder. *Eur J Pediatr* 1989;149:96–103.

48. Schinke M, Izumo S. Deconstructing DiGeorge syndrome. *Nat Genet* 2001;27:238–240.

49. Sullivan KE, Mullen CA, Blaese RM, et al. A multiinstitutional survey of the Wiskott-Aldrich syndrome. *J Pediatr* 1994;125:876–885.

50. Derry JM, Ochs HD, Francke U. Isolation of a novel gene mutated in Wiskott-Aldrich syndrome. *Cell* 1994;79(5):following 922.

51. Zhu Q, Zhang M, Blaese RM, et al. The Wiskott-Aldrich syndrome and X-linked congenital thrombocytopenia are caused by mutations of the same gene. *Blood* 1995;86:3797–3804.

52. Duncan RA, Von Reyn CF, Alliegro GM, et al. Idiopathic CD4⁺ T-lymphocytopenia—four patients with opportunistic infections and no evidence of HIV infection. *N Engl J Med* 1993;328:393–398.

53. Swift M, Morrell D, Cromartie E, et al. The incidence and gene

frequency of ataxia-telangiectasia in the United States. *Am J Hum Genet* 1986;39:573–583.

54. Morrell D, Cromartie E, Swift M. Mortality and cancer incidence in 263 patients with ataxia-telangiectasia. *J Natl Cancer Inst* 1986;77:89–92.

55. Opal P, Bonilla FA. Ataxia-telangiectasia. In: Rose BD, ed. *UpToDate*. Wellesley, MA: UpToDate, 2002.

56. Novis BH, Gilinsky NH, Wright JP, et al. Plasma cell infiltration of the small intestine, recurrent pulmonary infections, and cellular immunodeficiency (Nezelof's syndrome). *Am J Gastroenterol* 1985;80:891–895.

57. Tanner DD, Buckley PJ, Hong R, et al. Fatal cytomegalovirus bronchiolitis in a patient with Nezelof's syndrome. *Pediatrics* 1980;65:98–102.

Pulmonary Complications in Organ and Bone Marrow Transplant Recipients

56

Vivek N. Ahya · Robert M. Kotloff

Solid organ and bone marrow transplantation emerged in the 1960s as novel therapeutic approaches to many diseases. Propelled by advances in basic immunobiology and clinical medicine, these procedures are now widely applied to treat vital organ dysfunction in addition to various malignant, hematologic, and genetic diseases. Although these procedures offer extended survival to many patients with otherwise lethal conditions, significant complications are common. Pulmonary complications, both infectious and noninfectious, are among the most commonly encountered and contribute significantly to morbidity and mortality. Because the pulmonary complications of solid organ transplantation are somewhat distinct in nature and presentation from those of bone marrow transplantation, each of these topics is discussed separately in this chapter. The section on solid organ transplantation focuses on the experience with the three most frequently performed and long-standing procedures—heart, kidney, and liver transplantation; lung transplantation is discussed in detail in Chapter 54.

SOLID ORGAN TRANSPLANTATION

Infectious Pulmonary Complications

Although the incidence of infectious complications after solid organ transplantation has declined as a result of the introduction of more effective preventive and treatment strategies and more refined immunosuppressive regimens, infection remains the most common life-threatening complication. The lungs are particularly vulnerable and are the leading site of infection in heart transplant recipients (1) and the second most common site (after the abdomen) in liver transplant recipients (2). The incidence of pulmonary infec-

tion is lowest in kidney transplant recipients, reflecting both the less strenuous surgical procedure required to implant the allograft and the decreased level of immunosuppression required to maintain it.

The spectrum of microorganisms responsible for post-transplant infections is similar among the recipients of the various solid organ transplants and is discussed in detail in the next sections. The sequence in which the organisms appear during the post-transplant course is fairly characteristic (Fig. 56.1). In the widely published time line first proposed by Rubin (3), the post-transplant period is divided into three stages: the first month, the second through sixth months, and beyond the sixth month after transplantation. During the first month, the patient is affected primarily by the infectious risks of surgery and intensive care, and less so by the initiation of immunosuppressive agents. Nosocomial bacterial infections predominate, and the pathogenic organisms are similar to those found in the general surgical population. Aspergillosis, which is particularly common early after liver transplantation, is the one exception (4). The second stage extends from the second through sixth months, a period of maximal sustained immunosuppression, and is characterized by the emergence of opportunistic pathogens. Beyond 6 months, allograft function in most patients is sufficiently stable to permit a reduction in the level of immunosuppression. Infections in this group are caused largely by common community-acquired pathogens. Opportunistic infections occur less frequently but continue to plague the subset of patients requiring augmentation of immunosuppression to treat chronic rejection or recurrent episodes of acute rejection.

Bacterial Pneumonia

Bacterial pneumonia may be either nosocomial or community-acquired. The time of onset, responsible pathogens, and outcomes are distinct for the two modes of infection.

V. N. Ahya and **R. M. Kotloff:** Pulmonary, Allergy, and Critical Care Division, University of Pennsylvania Medical Center, Philadelphia, Pennsylvania.

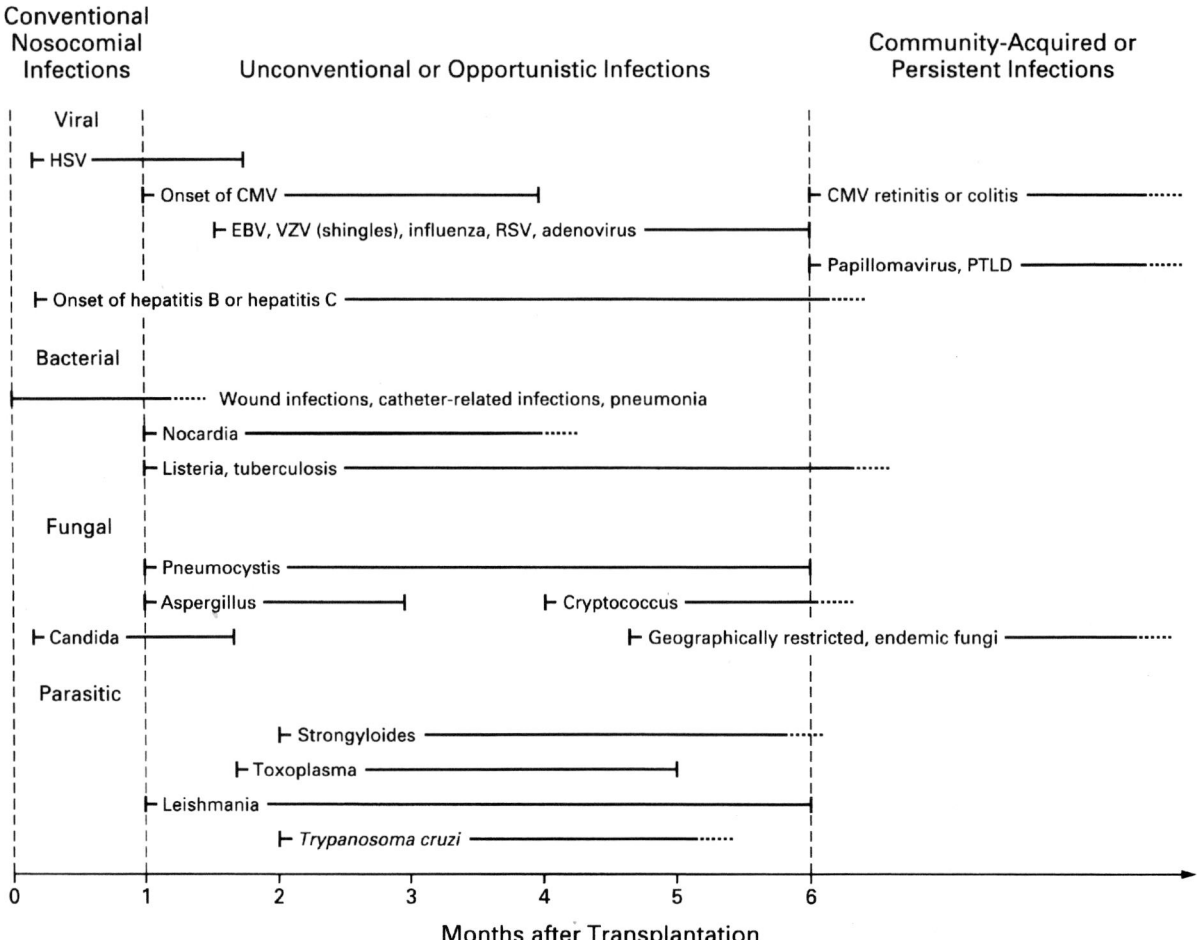

FIGURE 56.1. Time line of infectious complications (pulmonary and nonpulmonary) after solid organ transplantation. (From Fishman JA, Rubin RH. Infection in organ transplant recipients. *N Engl J Med* 1998;338:1741–1751, with permission.)

Nosocomial pneumonia develops almost exclusively in the first month after transplantation. Gram-negative pathogens predominate, but *Staphylococcus aureus* and, in some centers, *Legionella* species are also encountered (1,5–7). Heart and liver transplant recipients are at particular risk for nosocomial pneumonia after having undergone extensive thoracic and abdominal surgery. The need for prolonged postoperative mechanical ventilation has been identified as a major risk factor for nosocomial pneumonia in these groups (6). Although the incidence of nosocomial pneumonia has declined to less than 10% in contemporary series of liver and heart transplantation, mortality remains in the range of 26% to 50% (1,4–6). Community-acquired pneumonia, on the other hand, occurs later in the post-transplant period. *Haemophilus influenzae*, *Streptococcus pneumoniae*, and *Legionella* species are the most commonly identified organisms (1,4,6). In contrast to the poor response to therapy of patients with nosocomial infections, the response to therapy in these cases is generally excellent, with low reported mortality rates in the range of 0 to 33% (1,4,5).

In the early era of solid organ transplantation, *Nocardia* species were relatively common respiratory pathogens, encountered in up to 4% of renal and liver transplant recipients and up to 13% of heart transplant recipients (8,9). The incidence has since declined significantly to 0.2% to 1.3% in contemporary series (1). This change has been attributed to the introduction of cyclosporine-based immunosuppressive regimens permitting the use of reduced doses of corticosteroids, and more recently to the widespread use of sulfonamides for *Pneumocystis carinii* pneumonia (PCP) prophylaxis (1,7). Nonetheless, clinicians must remain particularly vigilant for *Nocardia* infection in patients in whom trimethoprim/sulfamethoxazole has either not been administered because of allergy or has been discontinued after the first year. Infection caused by this aerobic, Gram-positive filamentous rod is most common beyond the first month after transplantation. Patients may be asymptomatic or present subacutely with fever, nonproductive cough, pleuritic chest pain, dyspnea, hemoptysis, and weight loss. Dissemination of *Nocardia* to brain, skin, and soft tissue occurs in up to one third of infected patients. Chest roentgenography and computed tomography (CT) typically demonstrate one or several nodules that may be cavitary (10,11). Sulfonamides are the treatment of choice; minocycline, amikacin, imipenem, and ceftriaxone are alternative agents for patients who are allergic to sulfa drugs. Treatment for at least 3 months is recommended for pulmonary infection, and for up to 12 months for disseminated disease.

Tuberculosis

Tuberculosis (TB) has been reported in approximately 0.5% to 2% of solid organ transplant recipients in the United States and Europe (12–14), but in up to 15% of recipients in endemic regions, such as India (15). Although TB is a relatively uncommon post-transplant infection in developed countries, the annual rate of infection is 30- to 100-fold higher in transplant recipients than in the general population (12–14).

Reactivation of latent infection is postulated to be the prevailing mechanism for the development of active TB following transplantation. Nonetheless, in one series, only 12% of 207 patients with active infection after transplantation had evidence of prior infection on chest radiographs before transplantation, and an additional 5% had a known history of TB (12). Studies of the predictive value of the pre-transplantation purified protein derivative (PPD) status of recipients in whom active TB subsequently developed have been hampered by the lack of routine testing of patients in many transplant programs. In one report of 98 such patients for whom pre-transplant PPD data were available, the PPD status was positive in only 22% (12). In addition to reactivation of latent infection, nosocomial outbreaks and transmission from infected kidney and liver allografts have been documented in rare instances.

A review of the collective published experience with TB in solid organ transplant recipients, encompassing 511 cases through 1997, provided important insight into the clinical presentation of this infection (12). The onset of infection was at a median of 9 months following transplantation, and in nearly two thirds of the cases, infection developed within the first year. In 51% of the patients, TB was restricted to the lungs, whereas 16% had focal extrapulmonary infection and 33% had disseminated disease. When both patients with pulmonary TB and those with lung involvement as part of disseminated disease were counted, the overall rate of lung involvement was 71%. Fever was the most common presenting symptom, occurring in more than 90% of patients with disseminated disease but only 66% of those with pulmonary TB. Chest radiographic abnormalities included focal opacities in 40%, a miliary pattern in 22%, pleural effusions in 13%, diffuse interstitial opacities in 5%, and cavitary lung disease in only 4%.

The treatment of active TB in organ transplant recipients involves the use of combination therapy according to the standard guidelines for the general population. However, the administration of this regimen to transplant recipients can be problematic. The risk for isoniazid-induced hepatotoxicity is markedly enhanced in liver transplant recipients, so that this agent must be discontinued in 41% to 83% of patients (12,16). Other recipient populations tolerate isoniazid better, however, with reported hepatotoxicity rates of 2.5% for kidney transplant recipients and 10% for heart transplant recipients (12). The administration of rifampin, a potent inducer of the hepatic P-450 microsomal enzyme system, dramatically increases the clearance of cyclosporine and tacrolimus, thereby lowering the blood levels of these drugs and enhancing the risk for rejection. The concurrent use of rifampin mandates frequent monitoring of immunosuppressive drug levels and appropriate adjustments in dosing (often on the order of threefold to fivefold increases) to maintain therapeutic levels. Because of difficulties in maintaining therapeutic drug levels, some authors advocate avoiding rifampin in favor of alternative treatment regimens.

Even in contemporary series, mortality among transplant recipients with TB remains in the range of 25% to 40% (12,17). This high rate reflects not only the direct consequences of the infection but also the effects of enhanced rejection and graft loss in treated but suboptimally immunosuppressed patients, and the adverse effects of comorbid conditions that may have contributed to development of TB. In patients who complete a full course of treatment, the response is highly favorable, and mortality rates are low (17).

Given the significant morbidity and mortality associated with active TB in the transplant population, PPD testing and preemptive treatment of latent infection, evidenced by a PPD reaction of 5 mm or larger, is now recommended by the American Thoracic Society and the Centers for Disease Control and Prevention (18). Because waiting times for transplantation frequently exceed 1 year, therapy instituted at the time of listing can often be completed before transplantation. In this way, interactions with immunosuppressive drugs that may enhance the risks for hepatotoxicity and allograft rejection can be avoided.

Cytomegalovirus Infection

Cytomegalovirus (CMV) is the viral pathogen most commonly encountered in all solid organ recipient populations and contributes significantly to post-transplant morbidity. Infection can develop after transfer of the virus with the allograft or after reactivation of latent virus remotely acquired by the recipient. Seronegative recipients who acquire organs from seropositive donors are at greatest risk for the development of infection, and these primary infections tend to be the most severe. The use of antilymphocyte antibody therapy for immunosuppression also enhances the likelihood and severity of infection in susceptible recipients.

CMV infection typically emerges 1 to 3 months after transplantation, although the onset may be delayed in patients receiving prophylaxis. Infection is often subclinical, manifested as asymptomatic viremia or shedding of virus in the respiratory tract or urine. Clinical disease can assume a number of forms, including a mononucleosis-like syndrome with fever and malaise, and organ-specific involvement of the lungs, gastrointestinal tract, liver, and central nervous system. In addition to the direct effects of tissue invasion in causing symptoms and dysfunction of involved organs, CMV infection has been postulated to have a more global immunosuppressive effect, possibly accounting for the frequent emergence of other opportunistic infections in its wake. More insidiously, CMV infection has also been linked to the subsequent development of chronic allograft dysfunction in heart and liver transplant recipients.

Historically, CMV pneumonia developed in 4% to 24% of liver transplant recipients and up to 16% of heart transplant recipients (1,4). Contemporary series in the era of ganciclovir prophylaxis document CMV pneumonia in only 6.5% of liver transplant recipients and 0 to 2.5% of heart transplant recipients (1,4,5). A prodrome of fever, malaise, and myalgias frequently precedes the onset of pneumonia, which is heralded by nonproductive cough and dyspnea. Associated laboratory findings of leukopenia, thrombocytopenia, or elevated liver transaminases provide important clues to the presence of CMV. Radiographically, CMV pneumonia is most commonly associated with bilateral interstitial opacities, but nodular opacities and alveolar consolidation may also be seen.

The demonstration of characteristic inclusion bodies on lung biopsy or cytologic specimens of bronchoalveolar lavage (BAL) fluid unequivocally establishes the diagnosis of CMV pneumonia. In contrast, the detection of virus in BAL fluid by rapid culture technique is nondiagnostic (and possibly misleading) because shedding of virus into the respiratory tract can occur in the absence of tissue invasion. Although lacking specificity, the rapid culture is extremely sensitive; a negative lavage culture makes CMV pneumonia unlikely. A positive result of a CMV antigenemia assay in peripheral blood confirms active CMV infection and provides circumstantial support for a diagnosis of CMV pneumonia in the appropriate clinical setting.

The efficacy of ganciclovir in the treatment of CMV disease in various solid organ transplant populations has been documented repeatedly in uncontrolled clinical series, and ganciclovir has become the standard of care (19). In renal transplant recipients, for example, ganciclovir reduced the overall mortality associated with CMV pneumonia from 50% to 20%, and mortality in the subset requiring mechanical ventilation from more than 90% to 60% (20). Standard treatment consists of a 2- to 3-week course of intravenous ganciclovir at a dosage of 5 mg/kg twice daily, adjusted for renal insufficiency. Some experts advocate the addition of CMV hyperimmune globulin in the treatment of severe disease, but evidence supporting this practice is scant (21). Although treatment is effective, relapse rates of up to 60% in patients with primary infection and 20% in previously

exposed recipients have been reported (22). The administration of a 3-month course of oral ganciclovir following definitive intravenous therapy modestly reduces the risk for relapse (23).

In an attempt to minimize the adverse effects of CMV infection on the post-transplant course, emphasis has shifted to preventive strategies. Numerous prospective randomized trials, summarized in several reviews and one metaanalysis, have documented the efficacy of antiviral prophylaxis in diminishing the risk for post-transplant CMV infection (24–26). Although approaches vary among centers, most administer ganciclovir either intravenously or orally for 3 months. Universal prophylaxis of all seronegative recipients with a seropositive donor is recommended because their risk for CMV infection is high (22,27). In contrast, the risk for infection is significantly lower in seropositive recipients (independently of donor status), so that universal prophylaxis is inefficient and unnecessarily costly. In this population, "preemptive" strategies targeting antiviral therapy exclusively to patients demonstrating asymptomatic viremia are being developed (22,28).

Aspergillosis

Although a number of opportunistic and endemic fungi have been reported to cause pulmonary infections in solid organ transplant recipients, *Aspergillus* species are by far the most frequent and lethal fungal pathogens encountered. The incidence of invasive aspergillosis varies among the recipients of solid organs, with reported rates of 2.5% to 6.2% for heart transplant, 1.7% to 4% for liver transplant, and 0.7% for kidney transplant recipients (1,4,5,29). Infection typically appears within the first month in liver transplant recipients, and patients with poor hepatic or renal function appear to be most vulnerable (29). In contrast, invasive aspergillosis tends to appear 1 to 6 months after transplantation in kidney and heart recipients (29).

Virtually all patients with aspergillosis have pulmonary involvement. Dissemination to distant sites occurs in up to one third of heart recipients and one half of liver recipients but is distinctly uncommon in kidney recipients (29). The brain is most frequently involved in disseminated infection, although virtually any organ can be affected. Symptoms of invasive aspergillosis are nonspecific and include fever, cough, pleuritic chest pain, and hemoptysis. Radiographically, pulmonary aspergillosis may appear as single or multiple nodular opacities, cavities, or alveolar consolidation. In several published series of lung nodules in heart and liver recipients, aspergillosis was the cause most frequently identified (10,11,30). The "halo" sign and "air crescent" sign, characteristic high-resolution CT features of pulmonary aspergillosis in neutropenic patients, are uncommonly seen in solid organ transplant recipients (10).

The diagnosis of *Aspergillus* infection can be problematic. *Aspergillus* is cultured from sputum in only 8% to 34% and from BAL fluid in 45% to 62% of patients with invasive disease (29). Conversely, the false-positive rate associated with the recovery of *Aspergillus* organisms from respiratory tract cultures approaches 50% in solid organ transplant recipients (31). Transthoracic needle aspiration can provide a diagnosis in some cases; thoracoscopic wedge biopsy is reserved for cases that elude diagnosis with less invasive techniques.

Amphotericin B is considered the treatment of choice for invasive aspergillosis. A dose of 1.0 to 1.5 mg/kg daily is recommended, with treatment continued to a total dose of 1 to 1.5 g. Liposomal amphotericin preparations offer the advantage of decreased nephrotoxicity, an important feature for a drug used concurrently with nephrotoxic calcineurin inhibitors (cyclosporine, tacrolimus). A survival advantage in patients treated with liposomal amphotericin in comparison with historical controls treated with conventional preparations has been suggested in a large retrospective case series, but no prospective randomized trials have been conducted to corroborate this observation (29). Itraconazole has also been used in the treatment of invasive aspergillosis, with reported response rates in solid organ transplant recipients as high as 60% (29). Advantages of this agent include the availability of an oral preparation for less ill, nonhospitalized patients and the absence of nephrotoxicity. The capsule formulation is poorly absorbed, with absorption highly dependent on an acidic gastric milieu; treatment failure may thus ensue if optimal serum concentrations are not achieved. An oral suspension is now available that is more reliably absorbed. Itraconazole is a potent inhibitor of the P-450 enzyme system and can lead to dangerously high blood levels of cyclosporine or tacrolimus if appropriate adjustments in the dosing of these agents are not made. In the absence of a prospective randomized comparison of amphotericin with itraconazole, most clinicians remain reluctant to use itraconazole as first-line therapy, although some advocate its use in stable patients after an initial favorable response to amphotericin (29).

Despite the availability of these agents, *Aspergillus* remains the most lethal of all the pulmonary pathogens. Mortality in published series is in the range of 75% to 90% (7,29). In one large series from Stanford, mortality was 40% for patients with infection restricted to the lungs but 100% for those with dissemination to the brain (7). In light of these poor outcomes, some investigators have performed surgical resection as an adjunct to medical therapy in patients with localized pulmonary disease (32).

Pneumocystis carinii *Pneumonia*

Once a common opportunistic infection among solid organ recipients, PCP can be effectively prevented with the administration of low-dose trimethoprim/sulfamethoxazole prophylaxis. In a survey of 1,299 solid organ transplant recipients from the Cleveland Clinic, only 25 cases of PCP were identified, all in patients who had not received prophylaxis (33). Similarly, a series from Stanford documented

43 cases among 620 consecutive heart transplant recipients; all cases occurred in patients who did not take or could not tolerate prophylaxis (7). In light of these observations, it is essential that a clinician evaluating a patient with fever and diffuse pulmonary infiltrates determine whether the patient is receiving effective PCP prophylaxis because this information will dictate the level of suspicion for *Pneumocystis* infection. Vigilance for *Pneumocystis* infection should be greatest during the second to sixth months after transplantation, the period of peak occurrence. Many programs now discontinue prophylaxis after the first year because the incidence declines significantly beyond this point (33). Notably, however, 32% of cases in the Cleveland Clinic series and 23% of cases in the Stanford series occurred beyond the first year and as late as the sixteenth year after transplantation (7,33). Likely because of the need for augmented immunosuppression, patients with refractory acute rejection or chronic rejection appear to be at increased risk for the late development of PCP, and the continuation or resumption of PCP prophylaxis may be warranted under these circumstances (33).

Noninfectious Pulmonary Complications

Perioperative Complications

Liver transplantation entails extensive upper abdominal surgery in a population of patients considered by conventional standards to be poor surgical candidates because of malnutrition, debility, and critical illness. It is therefore not surprising that pulmonary complications are frequent in the perioperative period. In a survey of 546 liver transplant recipients, Glanemann and colleagues (34) found that 11% of them required mechanical ventilatory support beyond 24 hours. Risk factors for the need for prolonged ventilatory support included acute liver failure before transplantation, severe postoperative graft dysfunction, and repeated transplantation. Extubation was eventually achieved in all patients, but 36% of those who had been ventilated for longer than 24 hours and 12% of those ventilated for less than 24 hours required reintubation. The most common indications for reintubation were pneumonia, encephalopathy, and surgical bleeding (35). The need for reintubation was associated with significantly poorer survival.

Acute respiratory distress syndrome is a highly lethal but relatively uncommon cause of postoperative respiratory failure after liver transplantation. The reported incidence ranges from 4.5% to 15.7%, with a mortality rate approximating 80% (36). Sepsis is the most common risk factor reported, but other potential risk factors include massive blood transfusions, transfusion-related acute lung injury, aspiration, and the use of OKT3 antilymphocyte therapy.

Most liver transplant recipients have perioperative pleural effusions (37). The effusions are transudative and either right-sided or bilateral, never exclusively left-sided. Disruption of the diaphragmatic lymphatics during hepatectomy has been postulated to be the principal mechanism of fluid accumulation (37). The effusions may enlarge during the first postoperative week but typically resolve by the third week. The need for drainage because of respiratory compromise has been reported in up to 11% of patients (37). Effusions that continue to enlarge beyond the first week and isolated left-sided effusions should be sampled to rule out other causes.

Right-sided diaphragmatic dysfunction is an underappreciated complication of liver transplantation that is presumed to result from crush injury to the right phrenic nerve by the suprahepatic vena caval clamp placed during surgery (38). McAlister and colleagues (38) performed phrenic nerve conduction studies and diaphragmatic ultrasonography in a prospective series of 48 liver recipients. They found evidence of delayed or absent right-sided phrenic nerve conduction in 79% of them, whereas left phrenic nerve conduction was normal in all cases. In 38% of the patients, associated right diaphragmatic paralysis was documented by ultrasonography. Phrenic nerve injury did not lead to a longer period of mechanical ventilatory support or hospital stay. In a subset of patients followed with serial testing, abnormalities of phrenic nerve conduction and diaphragmatic excursion resolved by 9 months after surgery.

Heart transplant recipients are subject to the same perioperative complications encountered in the general cardiac surgical population. These include atelectasis, pulmonary edema, and pleural effusions. Diaphragmatic dysfunction was documented in 12% of heart transplant recipients in one small series and was predominantly right-sided (39).

Kidney transplantation is carried out with relatively few perioperative pulmonary complications, reflecting the use of a lower abdominal incision and the comparatively good health of the recipients (20,40). The vast majority of patients undergo extubation in the operating room. The most common noninfectious pulmonary complication is pulmonary edema secondary to impaired salt and water excretion in the setting of early allograft dysfunction or rejection. The incidence of thromboembolic events appears to be increased, possibly related in part to surgical manipulation of the pelvic veins (20).

Neoplastic Disorders

Post-transplantation lymphoproliferative disorder encompasses a group of abnormal B-cell proliferative responses ranging from benign polyclonal hyperplasia to malignant lymphomas. In almost all cases, post-transplantation lymphoproliferative disorder is caused by Epstein-Barr virus–mediated B-cell proliferation that proceeds in uncontained fashion in a host lacking the necessary cellular immune response. Recipients of kidney and liver transplants are at relatively low risk for this complication, with reported incidences of approximately 1% and 2.2%, respectively (41). In con-

trast, the cited incidence among heart transplant recipients is in the range of 3.5% to 7% (41). Intrathoracic involvement is particularly common in heart transplant recipients but may also be seen in the recipients of other solid organs. The radiographic appearance is that of solitary or multiple pulmonary nodules, occasionally accompanied by mediastinal adenopathy. Pleural effusions have been reported but are rare. Initial treatment centers on reducing the degree of immunosuppression to permit a partial restoration of host cellular immunity. Tsai and colleagues (42) reported that such a strategy led to regression of tumor in 63% of solid organ recipients. For patients who fail to achieve a complete remission and for those with widespread disease, standard chemotherapy and, more recently, immunotherapy with anti-CD20 antibodies (rituximab) have been used successfully (43).

Other malignancies occasionally present in the lungs after transplantation. Bronchogenic carcinoma has been reported in 1.6% to 4.1% of heart transplant recipients (44). It is unclear whether the numbers represent an increased risk for this cancer or simply reflect the expected occurrence rate in a population comprising a significant number of smokers. Among liver recipients with a pre-transplantation history of hepatocellular carcinoma, the lung is the most common site of recurrence (10). Recurrence is usually within 2 years after transplantation and appears radiographically as a single or multiple lung nodules. An elevated α-fetoprotein level provides an important clue to the possibility of recurrent disease (10).

Metastatic Pulmonary Calcification

The deposition of calcium in lung parenchyma and other organs was first described as a complication of chronic renal failure. Subsequently, cases were documented after kidney transplantation; in only some of these did the complication coincide with a period of graft failure (45–48). Pulmonary calcification has also been described in liver transplant recipients, with a reported incidence in two series of 5.2% and 47% (49,50). Renal failure was a common but not invariable feature in these patients. Munoz and colleagues (50) detected elevated serum levels of parathyroid hormone in all seven liver transplant recipients in their series, including two patients without renal insufficiency. Patients in whom metastatic calcification developed had received significantly more blood products and elemental calcium than those without this complication, but no difference was noted in serum levels of calcium, phosphate, or vitamin D. The authors speculated that hyperparathyroidism secondary to transient hypocalcemia induced by citrate-containing blood products and, in some patients, to renal insufficiency contributed to the deposition of calcium in soft tissue.

Metastatic pulmonary calcification is most often clinically silent but rarely may lead to restrictive lung disease or fulminant respiratory failure (45,47,48). The major import of this disorder lies in its ability to mimic more ominous processes, such as infection or malignancy, radiographically. Single or multiple nodular opacities or areas of alveolar consolidation are seen on plain chest radiographs, but calcification of these lesions may not be apparent. The demonstration of high-attenuation (>100 Hounsfield units) parenchymal opacities by CT or of increased uptake of tracer in the lung by technetium scan is helpful in establishing a diagnosis. In instances of diagnostic uncertainty, transbronchial or surgical lung biopsy may be necessary. No established treatment for pulmonary calcification is available, but given the overall favorable prognosis, this is rarely a consideration.

Drug-Induced Lung Disease

Sirolimus (rapamycin) is a potent immunosuppressive agent that has been introduced into clinical practice. A major advantage of the drug is that it is not nephrotoxic, so that it is an attractive alternative to cyclosporine and tacrolimus. To date, sirolimus has been most widely used in the renal transplant population, but clinical studies are under way in other transplant populations. Since its release, eight cases of associated interstitial pneumonitis have been described in detail in a series from France (51), and an additional 34 cases have been reported to the U.S. Food and Drug Administration (52). In the French series, seven patients presented with symptoms of dry cough, progressive dyspnea, fatigue, and weakness; four of them were febrile, and one had hemoptysis. One patient was asymptomatic. Radiographic studies demonstrated bilateral interstitial infiltrates in all eight patients and concurrent areas of alveolar consolidation in two. Bronchoalveolar lavage studies revealed a lymphocytic alveolitis in seven patients, alveolar hemorrhage in one, and a combination of the two features in one. Transbronchial lung biopsy specimens obtained in two patients demonstrated features of bronchiolitis obliterans–organizing pneumonia, interstitial lymphocytic infiltrates, and nonnecrotizing granulomas without identification of infectious organisms. The histologic pattern was deemed to be consistent with hypersensitivity pneumonitis. Notably, clinical symptoms resolved within 2 weeks and radiographic abnormalities within 2 to 4 months in all patients after sirolimus had been discontinued (seven patients) or the dose reduced (one patient). Although this series provides compelling evidence for sirolimus-induced interstitial pneumonitis, it must be noted that blood levels of the drug were maintained in an unusually high range that would no longer be considered standard.

Hepatopulmonary Syndrome and Portopulmonary Hypertension

Hepatopulmonary syndrome and portopulmonary hypertension are two unusual pulmonary complications of advanced liver disease. The onset of these disorders precedes liver transplantation, and they are not immediately or invariably corrected after liver transplantation, so that they can contribute significantly to post-transplant morbidity and mortality.

Hepatopulmonary syndrome is defined as the triad of liver disease, arterial hypoxemia, and abnormal intrapulmonary vascular dilatation. The vast majority of cases are characterized by diffuse dilatation of the pulmonary microvasculature at the precapillary and capillary level; rarely, discrete arteriovenous communications are present. The presence of intrapulmonary vascular abnormalities is documented by the systemic uptake of technetium-labeled macroaggregated albumin on standard radionuclide perfusion imaging or by the delayed appearance of bubbles in the left atrium on contrast echocardiography. Diffuse microvascular dilatation is postulated to cause hypoxemia by increasing the distance through which oxygen must diffuse and creating a central stream of inadequately oxygenated red cells. Unlike a true shunt, this process can be partially corrected with the administration of 100% oxygen, which serves to increase the pressure gradient favoring the transfer of oxygen from the alveolus to the bloodstream. An unusual feature of hepatopulmonary syndrome is the tendency for oxygenation to worsen in the erect as opposed to the supine position (orthodeoxia), presumably a consequence of the basilar predominance of the vascular abnormalities.

Once considered an absolute contraindication to liver transplantation, demonstration of the resolution of hepatopulmonary syndrome after transplantation has led to the reversal of this stance. Nonetheless, the response to transplantation is neither universal nor necessarily immediate. In a review of 81 patients with hepatopulmonary syndrome undergoing liver transplantation, Krowka and colleagues (53) documented a reduction or normalization of hypoxemia in 82%. Refractory hypoxemia contributed significantly to the observed 16% perioperative mortality, and 21% of the survivors required prolonged mechanical ventilatory support. In published series, the time to resolution of hypoxemia has ranged from several days to more than 30 months (53–55). Late recurrence of hepatopulmonary syndrome coincident with deteriorating allograft function has been reported (56).

Attempts to identify factors predictive of the post-transplantation outcome in patients with hepatopulmonary syndrome have been limited by the scant and retrospective nature of the available data. In the review of Krowka and colleagues (53), a pre-transplantation Po_2 of 50 mm Hg or less in room air was associated with a perioperative mortality rate of 30%, whereas mortality was only 4% when the Po_2 was in excess of 50 mm Hg (53). In contrast, Lange and Stoller (55) were unable to discern any relationship between pre-transplantation blood gases and outcome. Two studies have suggested an association between the magnitude of extrapulmonary radionuclide uptake on perfusion scan and mortality (54,57).

The postoperative care of patients with persistent hypoxemia secondary to hepatopulmonary syndrome consists of the administration of supplemental oxygen pending resolution of the disorder. Based on the positional nature of hypoxemia, mentioned previously, one group reported improved oxygenation in a patient with use of the Trendelenburg position (58). Perhaps most promising, Schenk and colleagues (59) described significant improvements in oxygenation and shunt fraction for up to 10 hours after the administration of a single dose of methylene blue to seven patients with advanced cirrhosis and hepatopulmonary syndrome. This study serves both to implicate a central role for nitric oxide in this disorder (methylene blue is a potent inhibitor of nitric oxide–induced vasodilatation) and potentially to identify a therapeutic approach. However, a greater appreciation of the potential toxicity of the repeated administration of methylene blue is required before routine use of this agent can be recommended.

Portopulmonary hypertension is the development of pulmonary hypertension in patients with advanced liver disease and portal hypertension. The diagnosis rests on the demonstration of a mean pulmonary artery pressure exceeding 25 mm Hg and a normal pulmonary capillary wedge pressure. Some authors also include the criterion of a pulmonary vascular resistance exceeding 120 dynes/s/cm^{-5} to distinguish this syndrome from the more benign and common finding of elevated pulmonary pressures caused solely by increased cardiac output. Histologically, the abnormalities in the pulmonary vascular bed are identical to those seen in primary pulmonary hypertension: medial hypertrophy, intimal fibrosis, and plexiform lesions. Although a mechanistic link has yet to be defined, the observation that the prevalence of pulmonary hypertension in patients with liver disease exceeds that in the general population suggests a connection. Portopulmonary hypertension is encountered in 1% to 2% of patients with chronic liver disease and in up to 12.5% of patients referred for evaluation for liver transplantation (60).

Although mild to moderate pulmonary hypertension does not appear to affect liver transplantation adversely, severe pulmonary hypertension is associated with excessive mortality after transplantation (61,62). In a retrospective review of 43 patients with portopulmonary hypertension who had undergone liver transplantation, Krowka and colleagues (62) documented a mortality rate of 100% for the patients with a mean pulmonary artery pressure of 50 mm Hg or higher and a rate of 50% for those with a mean pressure of 35 to 50 mm Hg in conjunction with a pulmonary vascular resistance exceeding 250 dynes/s/cm^{-5}. In contrast, no deaths occurred in patients with a mean pressure below 35 mm Hg or in those with a pressure of 35 to 50 mm Hg and a pulmonary vascular resistance of less than 250 dynes/s/cm^{-5}. Most deaths occurred in the immediate postoperative period. However, four patients successfully discharged died of progressive right-sided heart failure 5 to 30 months after

surgery (62). Although the experience with severe portopulmonary hypertension has generally been poor, improvement in pulmonary hemodynamics after transplantation has been reported rarely (60,63).

The demonstration that intravenous prostacyclin (epoprostenol) significantly improves pulmonary hemodynamics in patients with portopulmonary hypertension has provided a strategy for optimizing the condition of some patients who would otherwise not be considered for transplantation (64). Several case reports have documented successful transplantation in patients with severe portopulmonary hypertension who responded favorably to the preoperative initiation of prostacyclin (65,66). Additionally, this therapy has been successfully used in the post-transplantation treatment of progressive or recurrent pulmonary hypertension (63,67).

BONE MARROW TRANSPLANTATION

Bone marrow and peripheral blood stem cell transplantation has emerged as an important treatment option for patients with a wide spectrum of nonmalignant and malignant hematologic disorders, genetic disorders, and solid tumors. Transplantation involves the infusion of hematopoietic stem cells to seed and repopulate the ablated bone marrow and reconstitute the immune system. Stem cells can be obtained directly from the bone marrow or, alternatively, from the peripheral circulation or fetal cord blood. The transplantation procedure is further defined by the donor. In allogeneic bone marrow transplantation, stem cells are infused from a donor to a distinct recipient, whereas in autologous transplantation, the patient's own previously harvested stem cells are infused after the administration of high-dose myeloablative chemotherapy.

Despite important advances in the management of complications after transplantation, significant morbidity and mortality are still associated with both autologous and allogeneic bone marrow transplantation. Pulmonary complications are quite common and have been reported to occur in up to 60% of patients (68). Pulmonary complications can be infectious or noninfectious and tend to develop in a rather characteristic sequence (Fig. 56.2). Infectious complications are more common in patients who have undergone allogeneic transplantation because immunosuppressive agents must be administered after transplantation to prevent or mitigate graft versus host disease (GVHD). In addition, GVHD in itself causes an immunodeficient state by affecting mucosal surfaces, organs of the reticuloendothelial system, and bone marrow (69). Recipients of both allogeneic and autologous bone marrow transplants are at risk for acquiring severe infections during the period before engraftment, which is characterized by protracted neutropenia. With both types of transplants, the effective recovery of cellular and humoral immune function may take up to a year, and subtle immunologic abnormalities may persist for many years

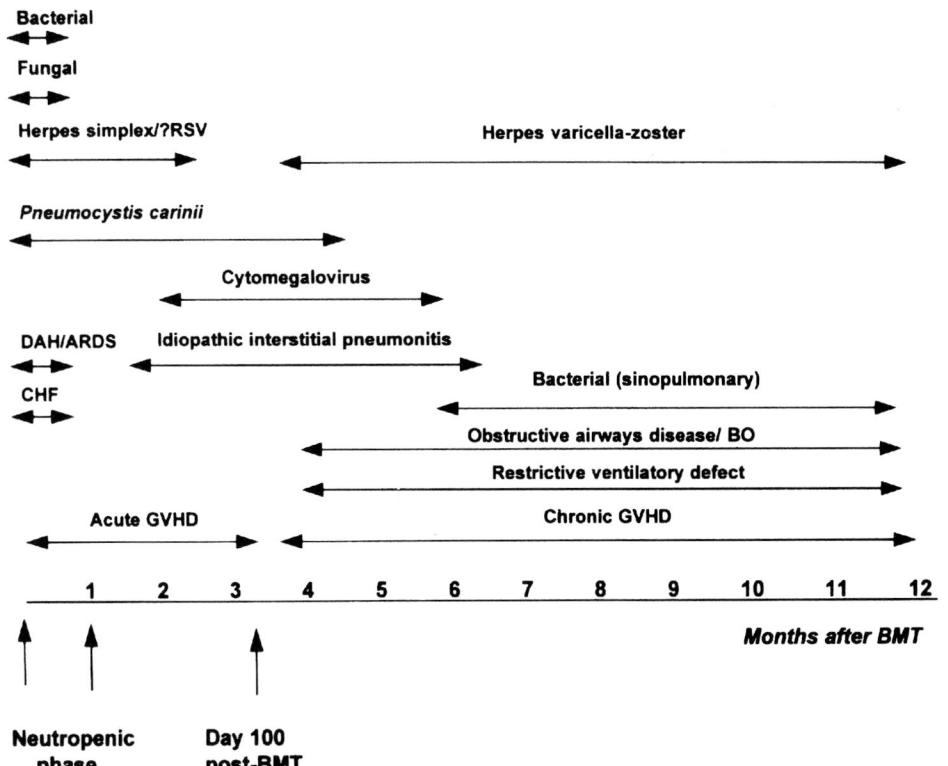

FIGURE 56.2. Time line of pulmonary complications occurring after bone marrow transplantation. *ARDS*, acute respiratory distress syndrome; *BO*, bronchiolitis obliterans; *CHF*, congestive heart failure; *DAH*, diffuse alveolar hemorrhage; *GVHD*, graft versus host disease. (From Soubani AO, Miller KB, Hassoun PM. Pulmonary complications of bone marrow transplantation. *Chest* 1996;109:1066–1077, with permission.)

(70,71). The increased incidence of noninfectious complications after bone marrow transplantation has been blamed largely on pre-transplant conditioning regimens that include numerous chemotherapeutic agents toxic to the lung, often in concert with radiation therapy. In recipients of allogeneic transplants, GVHD may also contribute to injury to the lung parenchyma and small airways.

Infectious Pulmonary Complications

Because of the predictable course of immunosuppression and bone marrow recovery, the risks for the development of infectious complications can be described based on three periods of time: the pre-engraftment (0–30 days), early post-engraftment (30–100 days), and late post-engraftment (beyond 100 days) periods. Variations in the rate of immune system reconstitution and the intensity of administered immunosuppression, however, can shift the boundaries of each period. During the pre-engraftment period, severe neutropenia, mucositis, and the presence of indwelling catheters significantly increase chances for the development of a life-threatening bacterial or fungal infection. The early post-engraftment period is characterized by impaired humoral and cell-mediated immunity, especially in allogeneic recipients receiving immunosuppressive regimens. During this period, allogeneic recipients are particularly susceptible to serious infections with viral and other opportunistic pathogens. By 100 days after transplantation, cytotoxic and

phagocytic function have usually recovered sufficiently to reduce but not eliminate the risk for infection. For those allogeneic transplant recipients in whom significant chronic GVHD develops, the risk for serious infection extends into the late post-engraftment period.

Fiberoptic bronchoscopy is commonly used to evaluate patients with suspected pneumonia. Although multiple studies examining the diagnostic utility of bronchoscopy in bone marrow transplant recipients have been published, a lack of standardized techniques and diagnostic criteria complicates attempts to compare studies. Moreover, the absence of a "gold standard" (e.g., surgical lung biopsy) with which to compare the results of bronchoscopy further limits interpretation, particularly with respect to the recovery of bacterial organisms that may simply represent colonization or contamination from the upper airway. In several series, the diagnostic yield of bronchoscopy varied between 31% and 46% (72–75). Results of bronchoscopy led to changes in therapy (either addition or discontinuation of medications) in 24% to 40% of patients. Notably, survival after the identification of a potential pathogen by bronchoscopy was not better than survival after nondiagnostic procedures (73–75).

Bacterial Infections

Bacterial pneumonia may occur at any time after transplantation but is particularly prevalent during the pre-engraftment period of profound neutropenia. A review of 255 consecutive patients who had undergone allogeneic or autologous bone marrow transplantation revealed a 15% incidence of bacterial pneumonia, with almost half of the cases developing within the first 100 days (76). Gram-negative pathogens, especially *Pseudomonas aeruginosa* and *Klebsiella pneumoniae,* predominated in the first 100 days, whereas Gram-positive organisms such as *Streptococcus pneumoniae* caused most of the late infections. Bacterial pneumonia was fatal in 22% of cases. In another series that included 725 consecutive bone marrow transplant recipients, bacterial pneumonia occurred in only 1.8% (77). The lower incidence most likely reflects the strict diagnostic criteria used by the authors, who required a positive BAL culture in conjunction with isolation of the same organism in blood cultures or with a transbronchial lung biopsy specimen showing acute inflammation. *P. aeruginosa* was the pathogen most frequently identified. Notably, the rates of bacterial pneumonia were similar in recipients of autologous and allogeneic transplants.

Bacterial pneumonia is often heralded by fever, but respiratory symptoms and signs may be absent in the neutropenic host. Presumably because of the paucity of neutrophils, chest radiographic abnormalities may also be subtle or absent. In one series, high-resolution CT revealed evidence of pneumonia in more than 50% of febrile neutropenic patients with normal findings on chest radiographs (78).

Broad-spectrum antibiotics (with anti-*Pseudomonas* activity) should be initiated expeditiously in all suspected cases of bacterial pneumonia. Because of the high risk for infection and the likelihood of rapid progression, empiric antibiotic therapy should also be administered to febrile neutropenic patients, even if a site of infection has not been identified. Because of insufficient data, no consensus has been reached regarding the routine use of prophylactic antibiotics in afebrile, asymptomatic neutropenic patients during the pre-engraftment period (79). Intravenous immunoglobulin may reduce the risk for bacterial infections in the subset of allogeneic transplant recipients with severe hypogammaglobulinemia during the first 100 days after transplantation (79).

Mycobacterial Infections

Mycobacterial infections are uncommon after bone marrow transplantation. In a review of 2,224 bone marrow transplant recipients from the University of Minnesota, the prevalence of mycobacterial disease was 0.6% in the allogeneic recipients and 0.26% in the autologous recipients (80). Of 11 patients identified, only two were infected with *Mycobacterium tuberculosis;* two were infected with *Mycobacterium avium-intracellulare,* and the remaining seven had rapid growers. All treated patients responded completely to antimycobacterial medications. A survey of 8,013 bone marrow transplant recipients from Spain documented an overall prevalence of TB of only 0.25% (81). In the autologous recipients, the rate of

infection was equivalent to that in the general population. In contrast, the risk for TB in the allogeneic recipients was increased approximately threefold, and the mortality rate was 25%. In this series, most infections appeared late (median, 324 days after transplant) and involved the lungs in the majority of cases. Surprisingly, rates of infection also appear to be low in areas of endemicity. In a series of 217 patients who had undergone allogeneic bone marrow transplantation in India, TB developed in only three (82).

Published guidelines recommend the administration of isoniazid to tuberculin-positive transplant recipients (18). Given the low incidence of TB in bone marrow transplant recipients, an alternative approach is to reserve such therapy for tuberculin-positive patients with additional risk factors, such as residence in an area of endemicity or a requirement for augmented immunosuppression (3). This strategy mandates that "low-risk" patients not treated for latent infection be followed with serial chest radiographs.

Aspergillosis

Invasive pulmonary aspergillosis is one of the most devastating complications of bone marrow transplantation, affecting recipients of both autologous and allogeneic transplants and representing the leading cause of infectious deaths in the latter group (83). *Aspergillus* species are ubiquitous, and the organisms have a large sporulating capacity. Humans inhale the organisms continuously, but they usually do not cause invasive disease in immunocompetent hosts. Neutropenia and corticosteroid administration interfere with normal immune defenses against the organisms, permitting germination, proliferation, and eventual tissue invasion within the lung parenchyma. Recipients of both allogeneic and autologous transplants are at increased risk for invasive aspergillosis during the pre-engraftment neutropenic period. Recipients of allogeneic marrow transplants undergo a second period of vulnerability during the early postengraftment phase, coincident with the onset of GVHD and the attendant need to augment immunosuppression.

Of the *Aspergillus* species, *A. fumigatus* accounts for most cases of infection in the bone marrow transplant population. Infection is usually confined to the lungs, but sinusitis and disseminated disease also occur with some frequency. Clinically, invasive pulmonary aspergillosis presents with fever, cough, and dyspnea. Symptoms of pleuritic chest pain and hemoptysis are important, albeit nonspecific, clues to the presence of invasive aspergillosis, reflecting the tendency of the organism to invade blood vessels and cause pulmonary infarction. Massive and sometimes fatal hemoptysis has been reported in up to 15% of patients, typically at the time of neutrophil recovery (84). Characteristic chest radiographic findings include single or multiple nodules, wedge-shaped pleura-based opacities, and in the later stages of infection, an "air crescent" sign (Fig. 56.3A). CT is considered more

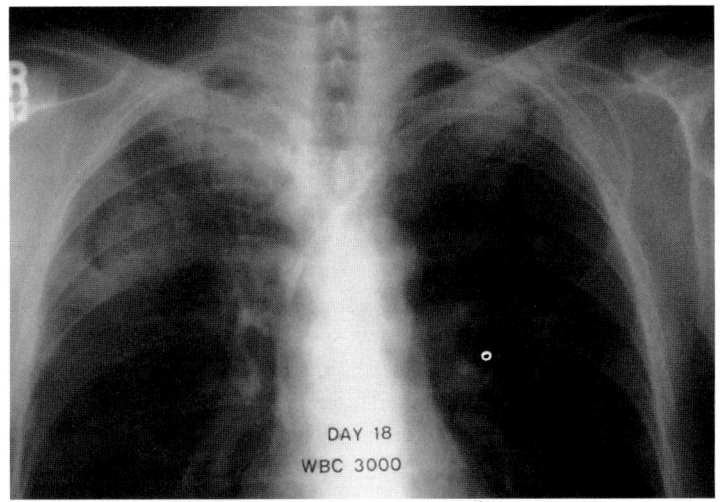

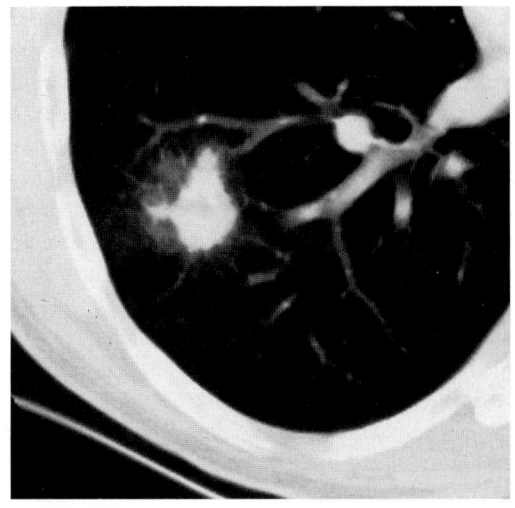

A   B

FIGURE 56.3. Characteristic radiographic features of invasive pulmonary aspergillosis. **A:** Chest radiograph demonstrating an "air crescent" sign (a sequestrum of necrotic lung tissue that has separated from the surrounding parenchyma). **B:** Chest computed tomographic scan demonstrating a "halo" sign (a rim of ground-glass attenuation, representing hemorrhage or edema, surrounding a central nodule).

sensitive in detecting abnormalities and appears to reveal changes at an earlier stage of infection. In addition to the air crescent sign, a highly characteristic CT finding is the "halo" sign, a rim of low attenuation representing edema or hemorrhage surrounding a pulmonary nodule (Fig. 56.3B). In a study by Caillot and colleagues (85), the halo sign was present in more than 90% of neutropenic patients with invasive pulmonary aspergillosis when CT was performed at the onset of fever (85).

Establishing a definitive diagnosis of invasive pulmonary aspergillosis remains difficult, and up to 30% of cases are unrecognized before death (86). The recovery of *Aspergillus* species from respiratory tract cultures is highly suggestive of invasive infection in bone marrow transplant recipients, with a positive predictive value of 82% (31). Unfortunately, respiratory tract cultures, including those obtained by BAL, have a sensitivity of only 35% (87). Cultures appear to be more sensitive if chest CT demonstrates a pattern of bronchopneumonia rather than isolated pulmonary nodules (88). The limitations of available noninvasive diagnostic techniques have prompted the development of new diagnostic tools. One is the enzyme-linked immunosorbent assay (ELISA), which detects galactomannan, a cell wall constituent of *Aspergillus* that is released during invasive disease. In a prospective study, this test had a sensitivity of 89.7% and a specificity of 98.1% (89). Furthermore, a positive test result was obtained before the development of new radiographic findings in 68% of cases and preceded the definitive diagnosis of invasive aspergillosis by a median of 17 days. It is hoped that after the findings of this study have been corroborated, the use of this test in combination with chest CT will facilitate earlier diagnosis and intervention.

Treatment for invasive aspergillosis should be initiated as soon as the diagnosis is suspected, especially in neutropenic patients, because delay adversely affects outcome (86). Intravenous amphotericin B at a dosage of 1 to 1.5 mg/kg daily is considered to be the standard treatment, but the response is suboptimal. In one study, even bone marrow recipients who survived long enough to receive at least 2 weeks of intravenous amphotericin B demonstrated a response rate of only 33% (90). Newer lipid formulations are less nephrotoxic, a particular advantage in the treatment of allogeneic recipients receiving calcineurin inhibitors. However, the efficacy of these preparations in comparison with standard therapy has not been rigorously established.

The use of itraconazole in treating invasive aspergillosis is supported by studies of immunocompromised persons without transplants, but trials in bone marrow transplant recipients are notably lacking. In the absence of such trials, itraconazole is not viewed as first-line therapy, but some experts have suggested a role for itraconazole in completing a course of treatment once infection has been controlled with amphotericin (83). A concern about oral itraconazole is its poor bioavailability; blood levels must be monitored to ensure adequate dosing. A new triazole, voriconazole, has been shown to be more effective and less toxic than amphotericin B in a large randomized trial of invasive aspergillosis in immunocompromised patients, many of them recipients of bone marrow transplants (91). Caspofungin, the first of a new class of antifungal agents to be released, has been approved for salvage therapy of invasive aspergillosis. Exactly how these two new agents will fit into the antifungal armamentarium remains to be established with additional studies.

The surgical resection of localized disease has been proposed as an adjunct to antifungal therapy and as a means of preventing massive hemoptysis. A review of seven small retrospective studies of neutropenic patients (most of whom were not bone marrow transplant recipients) documented an average perioperative mortality rate of 17% and successful eradication of the fungus in more than 90% of the survivors (87). Other than as an emergency treatment for massive hemoptysis, the role of surgery in the management of invasive aspergillosis has not been established.

Effective prophylaxis to prevent *Aspergillus* infection in recipients of bone marrow transplants remains an elusive goal. Low-dose intravenous amphotericin B, aerosolized amphotericin, and itraconazole have all been used in prophylactic strategies, but none has consistently been shown to decrease the incidence of invasive aspergillosis. Measures to minimize environmental exposure to *Aspergillus* spores, including the use of high-efficiency particulate air (HEPA) filters and laminar airflow in patients' rooms and avoidance of areas of hospital construction or renovation, are currently emphasized (79).

Pneumocystis carinii *Pneumonia*

Impaired cell-mediated immunity, chiefly as a consequence of the administration of immunosuppressive agents, increases the risk for the development of PCP after allogeneic transplantation. Without prophylaxis, this infection has been reported to occur in up to 16% of bone marrow transplant recipients, with a median time to onset of 2 months (92). Prophylactic therapy with oral trimethoprim/sulfamethoxazole has reduced the incidence of PCP to a negligible level (93). Inhaled pentamidine and dapsone are alternative prophylactic agents for patients unable to tolerate trimethoprim/sulfamethoxazole, although dapsone was associated with a breakthrough infection rate of 7% in one series of bone marrow transplant recipients (93,94). Many bone marrow transplantation programs discontinue prophylaxis beyond the first 6 to 12 months. However, cases of PCP subsequent to the discontinuation of prophylaxis have been reported, largely confined in one series to patients receiving corticosteroid therapy for chronic GVHD (95).

Patients with PCP typically present with dyspnea, cough, chest tightness, and fever. The onset and course of PCP are generally more fulminant in transplant recipients than in patients with AIDS. Chest radiographs usually reveal bilateral interstitial and alveolar opacities, although isolated nodules, lobar consolidation, and even normal findings have been reported (96).

The diagnostic yield of BAL has been reported to approach 90%; transbronchial or surgical lung biopsy is required in those with nondiagnostic lavage cytology (96).

High-dose trimethoprim/sulfamethoxazole for at least 14 to 21 days remains the treatment of choice. Allergic or intolerant patients can be treated with intravenous pentamidine. The benefit of administering corticosteroids as an adjunct to antimicrobial therapy, which is of proven efficacy in AIDS-related PCP, is uncertain in bone marrow transplant recipients.

Viral Infections

Advancements in the detection, prevention, and treatment of CMV infection have lessened the adverse effects of this virus in bone marrow transplant recipients, but it remains a cause of considerable morbidity and mortality. CMV infection is seen predominantly after allogeneic transplantation, and patients who are seropositive before transplantation are at greatest risk, with a reported incidence of CMV disease in the pre-prophylaxis era of 20% to 35% (97). In contrast to seronegative recipients of solid organ transplants, seronegative recipients of bone marrow transplants who are "CMV-mismatched" (i.e., who receive marrow from a seropositive donor) are at lower risk than seropositive recipients for post-transplantation CMV disease. The risk for CMV disease following autologous bone marrow transplantation is extremely low, with published series documenting an incidence of CMV pneumonia in particular of only 1% to 6% (97). Among the subset of recipients of autologous transplants who receive CD34$^+$-enriched stem cell transplants, however, the incidence of CMV disease is considerably enhanced, possibly because this process results in the infusion of a lower number of T cells and delayed immunologic reconstitution (97).

Before the widespread implementation of antiviral prophylactic measures, the peak incidence of CMV disease was between engraftment and day 100. Prophylaxis appears to have shifted the onset of disease to later in the post-transplantation course. In a series from the Fred Hutchinson Cancer Research Center, the incidence of CMV disease within the first 100 days among seropositive recipients of allogeneic transplants declined from 35% in 1987 to 6% in 1994. During this same period, the incidence of disease beyond the first 100 days increased from 4% to 15% (97). Risk factors for late-onset disease include chronic GVHD, low CD4$^+$ cell counts, and CMV infection before day 100 (79).

Although CMV disease can affect multiple organs, the lung is one of the sites most frequently affected after bone marrow transplantation. CMV pneumonia is particularly virulent in this group of patients, and it is postulated that the pathogenesis involves a combination of infection and an exaggerated host response to the presence of virus. CMV pneumonia typically presents with a nonproductive cough, fever, and hypoxemia, and progression to respiratory failure is rapid in some cases. The chest radiograph most often demonstrates diffuse interstitial opacities, but alveolar consolidation and diffuse nodular opacities have also been reported. The chest CT findings are nonspecific; ground-glass opacities are most commonly seen. The diagnosis of CMV pneumonia requires evidence of virus in the respiratory tract in association with compatible clinical and radiographic features. Although the diagnosis is most securely established by the demonstration of viral inclusion bodies, bronchoscopically derived biopsy and cytology specimens are often inadequate for this purpose. In the proper setting, the detection of virus in BAL fluid by rapid culture technique is considered diagnostic and is likely the most common means by which CMV pneumonia is now diagnosed at most centers. However, the results of rapid culture must be interpreted with caution because viral shedding into the respiratory tract is possible even in the absence of invasive disease.

In early series, CMV pneumonia after bone marrow transplantation was almost invariably lethal. Despite the documented antiviral effects of ganciclovir, its use as a single agent in the treatment of CMV pneumonia did not improve outcomes. In the 1988 study by Reed and colleagues (98), the combination of ganciclovir and CMV immunoglobulin resulted in a survival rate of 52%, compared with a 15% survival rate among historical controls receiving antiviral therapy alone. This approach has become the standard of care despite the fact that no randomized clinical trials have been performed to confirm the observations. Foscarnet, in combination with immunoglobulin, is reserved for patients unable to tolerate ganciclovir and those infected with ganciclovir-resistant strains, but support for this regimen is anecdotal.

In light of the high mortality rate, even with treatment, emphasis has shifted to preventing CMV pneumonia. Two strategies have evolved: universal prophylaxis at the time of engraftment for all patients potentially at risk (seropositive patients and seronegative patients with seropositive donors) and preemptive treatment of patients with subclinical viremia identified by CMV antigen assays or polymerase chain reaction (97). Both approaches have been shown to reduce the risk for early CMV disease, but universal prophylaxis is complicated by a high rate of neutropenia. In a randomized double-blinded study comparing the two strategies, the universal administration of ganciclovir prophylaxis from engraftment to day 100 was associated with a lower incidence of CMV disease within the first 100 days (99). However, this was offset by an increased incidence of late disease, such that no difference in disease frequency was seen at 180 days. Survival was identical in both treatment arms. At the present time, both strategies have been endorsed in published practice guidelines (79).

Emerging immunologic interventions may further reduce the incidence of CMV pneumonia in the future. Walter and colleagues (100) reported that donor-derived CMV-specific cytotoxic T lymphocytes could be expanded *in vitro* and safely infused into recipients, resulting in the effective reconstitution of cellular immunity against CMV. The development of a CMV vaccine is also under active investigation, with the possible strategy of immunizing the donor before transplantation to bolster CMV-specific immunity.

Other respiratory viruses, including respiratory syncytial virus, influenza virus, parainfluenza virus, and ade-

novirus, have been reported to cause pneumonia in bone marrow transplant recipients. Unfortunately, the response of these pathogens to available antiviral agents has been disappointing.

Noninfectious Pulmonary Complications

Diffuse Alveolar Hemorrhage

The frequent occurrence of diffuse alveolar hemorrhage following bone marrow transplantation was first brought to light by Robbins and colleagues (101), who in a retrospective review of 141 consecutive autologous transplant recipients at the University of Nebraska identified 29 patients (21%) with this complication (see Chapter 31). Most cases occurred early after transplantation, with a median time to onset of 12 days after transplantation. Patients presented with dyspnea, nonproductive cough, fever, and diffuse pulmonary infiltrates, but hemoptysis was notably absent in all patients. Although thrombocytopenia was common, the platelet counts were not lower than those of patients without alveolar hemorrhage, and aggressive platelet transfusion did not improve the respiratory status. Since the publication of this initial series, others have reported incidence rates varying from 12% to 35% after autologous bone marrow transplantation (102,103) and 7% to 23% after allogeneic procedures (102,104).

The University of Nebraska group has suggested that in the context of a compatible clinical and radiographic presentation, the recovery from at least three lobes of BAL fluid that becomes progressively bloodier with successive instillations should be considered diagnostic of diffuse alveolar hemorrhage (101). However, data from a small postmortem study of allogeneic bone marrow transplant recipients call this claim into question. Agusti and colleagues (104) reported that four of eight patients with autopsy-proven diffuse alveolar hemorrhage had nonbloody BAL fluid. Conversely, 7 of 13 patients without histologic evidence of diffuse alveolar hemorrhage had bloody lavage fluid.

The pathogenesis of diffuse alveolar hemorrhage in bone marrow transplant recipients remains obscure. Postmortem investigations have shown that most patients with diffuse alveolar hemorrhage have evidence of diffuse alveolar damage, often with an associated infection (101,104). Furthermore, most cases have been noted to occur at the time of engraftment and neutrophil recovery (101). Taken together, these observations suggest that diffuse alveolar hemorrhage may be a manifestation of underlying acute lung injury, possibly induced by conditioning chemotherapy or radiation therapy and exacerbated by infection and neutrophil influx into the lung. Age older than 40 years, total-body irradiation, transplantation for solid tumors, high fevers, severe mucositis, and renal insufficiency all have been identified as risk factors for diffuse alveolar hemorrhage, but these factors shed little light on the pathogenesis (101).

With supportive therapy alone, mortality rates of 80% to 100% have been reported in patients with diffuse alveolar hemorrhage (101–103). The administration of high doses of parenteral corticosteroids (500–1,000 mg of methylprednisolone per day for 3 to 4 days) has been associated with improved survival in several small retrospective series (102,103,105). In the largest of these series, the in-hospital mortality of 35 patients who received high-dose methylprednisolone was 67%, whereas it was more than 90% for groups receiving low-dose steroids or supportive care alone (102).

Engraftment Syndrome

A capillary leak syndrome has been described that is temporally associated with hematopoietic recovery following bone marrow transplantation. The release of proinflammatory cytokines during engraftment has been hypothesized as the cause of this "engraftment syndrome" (106). Clinically, fever, hypoalbuminemia, weight gain, skin rash, and bilateral pulmonary opacities develop. Progression to respiratory failure has been described (107). Care is supportive, and full recovery has been documented, even in patients who required mechanical ventilation (107). The use of granulocyte colony-stimulating factor may increase the incidence and severity of the engraftment syndrome, and discontinuation of this agent is recommended when engraftment syndrome develops (106,107).

Idiopathic Pneumonia Syndrome

Pneumonitis is a common complication after bone marrow transplantation; in approximately one third of cases, no infectious cause is identified. The term *idiopathic pneumonia syndrome* has been coined to describe these episodes of noninfectious diffuse pneumonia (108). A National Institutes of Health workshop panel of experts recommended the following diagnostic criteria for this syndrome: (a) widespread alveolar injury, evidenced by multilobar infiltrates on chest radiographs, symptoms and signs of pneumonia, impaired oxygenation, and restrictive pulmonary function abnormalities; and (b) absence of active lower respiratory tract infection, demonstrated by negative results of BAL fluid studies (108). Applying these criteria in a retrospective review of 1,165 consecutive patients at the Fred Hutchinson Cancer Research Center, Kantrow and colleagues (109) found that the incidence of idiopathic pneumonia syndrome in the first 120 days was 7.6% following allogeneic bone marrow transplantation and 5.7% following autologous procedures. Histopathologic analysis of open lung biopsy specimens from patients with idiopathic pneumonia syndrome revealed two main patterns: interstitial pneumonitis and diffuse alveolar damage (108) (Fig. 56.4). In the later stages of this disorder, pulmonary fibrosis may predominate (110,111).

The pathogenesis of idiopathic pneumonia syndrome is not well characterized. Older age of the recipient, immunosuppression with methotrexate, total-body irradiation before transplantation, malignancy other than leukemia, and high-grade GVHD have been variably identified as risk factors for the development of idiopathic pneumonia syndrome following allogeneic bone marrow transplantation (109). One study suggested that elevated plasma levels of transforming growth factor-β correlated with the development of idiopathic pneumonia syndrome after autologous bone marrow transplantation (110). The similar incidence rates following allogeneic and autologous bone marrow transplantation

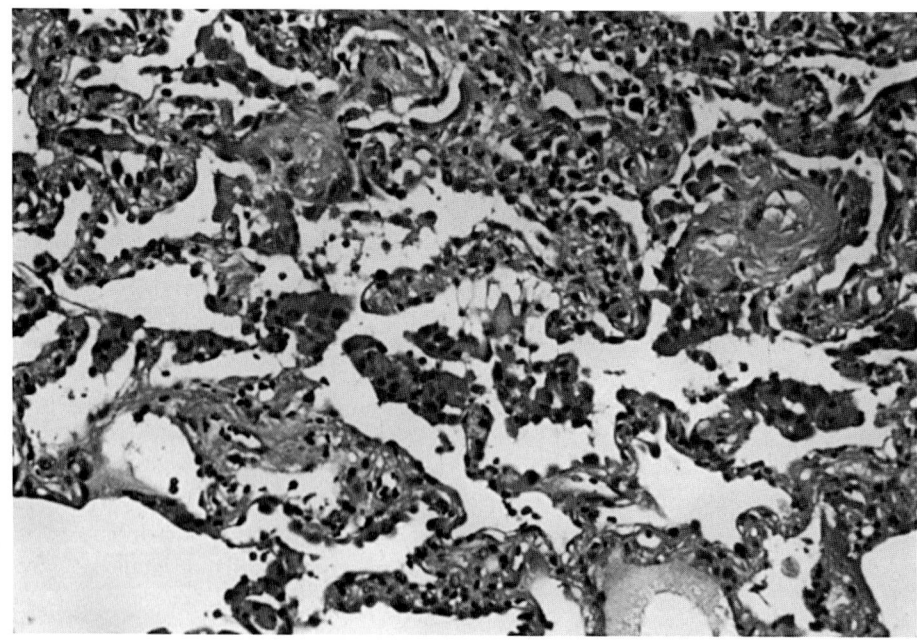

FIGURE 56.4. Idiopathic pneumonia syndrome in a bone marrow transplant recipient shows the pattern of diffuse alveolar damage: mild thickening and inflammatory infiltration of the alveolar septa; proliferation of type II pneumocytes; and edema fluid, exudate, and macrophages in the alveolar air spaces.

suggest that treatment-related toxicities (i.e., chemotherapy and radiation) rather than immunologic mechanisms are principally involved. Animal studies support the view that factors related to the conditioning regimen work in concert with factors related to the transplantation procedure. For example, idiopathic pneumonia syndrome can be induced in a murine model by a combination of pre-transplantation radiation conditioning and allogeneic bone marrow transplantation, but is not seen in mice subjected to either process alone (112). Additional factors that may contribute to lung injury include occult infection, sepsis and the systemic inflammatory response syndrome, and GVHD.

Patients with idiopathic pneumonia syndrome present with dyspnea, fever, nonproductive cough, increasing oxygen requirements, and diffuse radiographic infiltrates. In the Fred Hutchinson Cancer Research Center study, the median time to onset was 21 days after transplantation, although others have reported a longer median time to onset of between 42 and 49 days (108,109). The course is typically rapid, with up to two thirds of patients progressing within several days to respiratory failure and requiring mechanical ventilation. In-hospital mortality in the Fred Hutchinson Cancer Research Center series was 74%. Treatment for idiopathic pneumonia syndrome has been disappointing. The administration of high doses of corticosteroids does not appear to be beneficial (109).

Delayed Pulmonary Toxicity Syndrome

The term *delayed pulmonary toxicity syndrome* has been proposed to describe a form of mild to moderate pulmonary injury observed after high-dose chemotherapy and autologous bone marrow transplantation for breast cancer (113,114). In contrast to idiopathic pneumonia syndrome, this syndrome presents later, is generally responsive to corticosteroid therapy, and carries a better prognosis. In a study by Wilczynski and colleagues (114) of 45 consecutive women who received high-dose chemotherapy with cyclophosphamide, cisplatin, and bischloroethyl-nitrosourea (BCNU) followed by autologous bone marrow transplantation, symptomatic pulmonary toxicity developed in 26 patients (58%) at a mean of 10 weeks after transplantation.

Clinical symptoms include dyspnea on exertion, nonproductive cough, and fever. Pulmonary function testing reveals a marked reduction in the diffusing capacity in association with a mild to moderate restrictive pattern. Ground-glass opacities are the most common radiographic abnormalities demonstrated on CT images, but abnormalities may be absent or delayed in up to one third of patients (114).

The response to corticosteroids is generally favorable. In the study of Wilczynski and colleagues (114), all 26 symptomatic patients and three asymptomatic patients with severely impaired lung function were treated with corticosteroids. Treatment was associated with a mean improvement

in the diffusing capacity of 17%. In addition, none of the patients in this study died of pulmonary toxicity.

It has been postulated that the delayed pulmonary toxicity syndrome represents a form of chemotherapy-induced lung injury. In support of this claim, lung pathology specimens in 10 patients with the syndrome exhibited features consistent with drug toxicity, including alveolar septal thickening, interstitial fibrosis, and type II pneumocyte hyperplasia (113). Moreover, in a study that randomized patients to high-dose or standard chemotherapy before autologous bone marrow transplantation, the incidence of delayed pulmonary toxicity syndrome was 72% in the high-dose group and only 4% in the group receiving standard therapy (115). Two of the chemotherapeutic agents used in the conditioning regimen administered to patients with this syndrome, BCNU and cyclophosphamide, have been associated with lung toxicity. Although the high-dose chemotherapy regimens associated with delayed pulmonary toxicity syndrome included doses of BCNU below the threshold that typically causes pulmonary toxicity, it is possible that the risk for toxicity is enhanced by synergy with concurrently administered cyclophosphamide.

Pulmonary Veno-occlusive Disease

Pulmonary veno-occlusive disease, a form of postcapillary pulmonary hypertension, has been reported as a rare complication of bone marrow transplantation (116). This process is characterized by intimal proliferation and fibrosis of the pulmonary venules and small veins, which lead to progressive vascular obstruction and increased pulmonary arterial and capillary pressures. Patients typically present several months after transplantation with progressive dyspnea on exertion and fatigue. Chest pain, cough, and hemoptysis occur less frequently. Findings on the physical examination include auscultatory crackles and signs of pulmonary hypertension. Chest radiographs may reveal septal (Kerley B) lines, reflective of chronic pulmonary capillary hypertension and the resultant extravasation of edema fluid into the interstitium. CT of the chest reveals interlobular septal thickening, ground-glass opacities, and pleural effusions (117). The triad of pulmonary arterial hypertension, radiographic signs of pulmonary edema, and a normal pulmonary artery occlusion pressure strongly suggest the diagnosis, but all three features may not be present concurrently in all patients. Surgical lung biopsy is required to make a definitive diagnosis.

Because pulmonary veno-occlusive disease has been reported in patients without transplants who have received radiation and chemotherapy and in patients with viral infections, it has been hypothesized that it occurs after bone marrow transplantation as the result of an infectious or toxic injury to the endothelium. BCNU, mitomycin C, and bleomycin have most commonly been associated with this process (118).

Unlike other forms of pulmonary arterial hypertension, pulmonary veno-occlusive disease cannot be treated safely with vasodilators. In this regard, arterial vasodilatation in the setting of fixed pulmonary venous resistance can markedly increase the transcapillary hydrostatic pressure and lead to pulmonary edema. The administration of high doses of corticosteroids has been reported anecdotally to be beneficial (119).

Bronchiolitis Obliterans

Bronchiolitis obliterans is a late complication, occurring beyond the third month, and is seen almost exclusively after allogeneic bone marrow transplantation. Although the cause is unclear, the strong association with chronic GVHD suggests that immune injury to the bronchioles plays an important role (120). Certain conditioning regimens may further increase the risk. For example, a prospective study of 167 patients randomized to receive busulfan or conditioning with total-body irradiation revealed a significantly greater incidence of airflow obstruction in the busulfan group (26%) than in the radiation group (5%) (121).

Presenting symptoms include nonproductive cough, dyspnea, and wheezing. Spirometry reveals airflow obstruction, and chest radiographs typically show normal findings or only hyperinflation. High-resolution CT of the chest may demonstrate evidence of air trapping on expiratory views. Disease progression is variable; some patients experience a rapid decline in lung function, whereas others have a more protracted course (122). Because corticosteroid therapy is typically ineffective in the treatment of bronchiolitis obliterans, alternative treatment strategies have been attempted. These include augmentation of immunosuppression with cyclosporine, azathioprine, or antithymocyte globulin, and the use of immunomodulatory treatments such as photopheresis or thalidomide. Although clinical improvement in response to some of these modalities has been reported anecdotally (123,124), more rigorous clinical trials are necessary before specific treatment regimens can be recommended. Lung transplantation is an option for selected patients with severe bronchiolitis obliterans and no other significant comorbid conditions who are deemed to be cured of the underlying condition for which bone marrow transplantation was performed (125).

Respiratory Failure

Respiratory failure after bone marrow transplantation is a relatively frequent and rather ominous complication. In a review of more than 1,400 consecutive patients who underwent bone marrow transplantation at the Fred Hutchinson Cancer Research Center between 1986 and 1990, Crawford and Petersen (126) documented a need for mechanical ventilation in 23%. Older age, active malignancy at the time of transplantation, and an HLA-nonidentical allogeneic trans-

plant were identified as independent risk factors for respiratory failure. Importantly, only 4% of patients in this series who required ventilation survived to discharge. In a follow-up study encompassing an expanded cohort from the same center, no patients who required mechanical ventilation and had lung injury and either hepatic and renal insufficiency or hemodynamic instability survived (127). The experiences documented in these and other early studies (128–130) have generated a rather pessimistic view of the outcome of respiratory failure and a plea for a limited application of intensive life support in this group of patients (127,131). However, these experiences focused largely on recipients of allogeneic bone marrow transplants, and the findings may not be applicable to other groups of patients. In this regard, among recipients of autologous bone marrow transplants, the incidence of respiratory failure was reported to be only 11%, and

THERAPY FOR INFECTIOUS PULMONARY COMPLICATIONS IN TRANSPLANT RECIPIENTS	
Summary Statement	**Level of Evidence**
Broad-spectrum antibiotics (with anti-*Pseudomonas* activity) should be initiated expeditiously in all suspected cases of bacterial pneumonia.	Observational studies, expert opinion
PPD testing and preemptive treatment of latent tuberculosis infection are recommended.	Observational studies, consensus panel guidelines
Ganciclovir treatment reduces the mortality of CMV pneumonia.	Observational studies
Prophylaxis with ganciclovir reduces the risk for or delays the onset of CMV infection. Universal prophylaxis of donor-seropositive/recipient-seronegative patients is recommended.	Randomized trials, observational studies, consensus panel guidelines
Preemptive therapy with ganciclovir guided by CMV antigenemia may be as effective and less expensive than universal prophylaxis.	Randomized trials, observational studies, consensus panel guidelines
Amphotericin B is currently the treatment of choice for invasive aspergillosis.	Nonrandomized trials, observational studies and expert opinion
Voriconazole may be associated with a better response rate, improved survival, and fewer adverse effects than amphotericin B in the treatment of invasive aspergillosis.	Randomized trial
Environmental control measures (high-efficiency particulate air filters and laminar airflow in patients' rooms) should be taken to minimize environmental exposure to *Aspergillus* spores.	Expert opinion
Trimethoprim/sulfamethoxazole prophylaxis prevents *Pneumocystis carinii* pneumonia.	Nonrandomized trials, observational studies

CMV, cytomegalovirus; PPD, purified protein derivative.

reported survival rates following respiratory failure ranged from 18% to 27% (132,133). Similarly, a prospective study showed that among intubated patients, the survival rate was far better in those who had received a peripheral stem cell transplant than in those who had received a conventional bone marrow transplant (19% vs. 4%) (134).

ACKNOWLEDGMENT

This work was supported in part by the Craig and Elaine Dobbin Pulmonary Research Fund of the University of Pennsylvania Medical Center.

REFERENCES

1. Cisneros JM, Munoz P, Torre-Cisneros J, et al. Pneumonia after heart transplantation: a multi-institutional study. Spanish Transplantation Infection Study Group. *Clin Infect Dis* 1998;27:324–331.
2. Kusne S, Dummer JS, Singh N, et al. Infections after liver transplantation. An analysis of 101 consecutive cases. *Medicine (Baltimore)* 1988;67:132–143.
3. Fishman JA, Rubin RH. Infection in organ-transplant recipients. *N Engl J Med* 1998;338:1741–1751.
4. Singh N, Gayowski T, Wagener M, et al. Pulmonary infections in liver transplant recipients receiving tacrolimus. Changing pattern of microbial etiologies. *Transplantation* 1996;61:396–401.
5. Lenner R, Padilla ML, Teirstein AS, et al. Pulmonary complications in cardiac transplant recipients. *Chest* 2001;120:508–513.
6. Torres A, Ewig S, Insausti J, et al. Etiology and microbial patterns of pulmonary infiltrates in patients with orthotopic liver transplantation. *Chest* 2000;117:494–502.
7. Montoya JG, Giraldo LF, Efron B, et al. Infectious complications among 620 consecutive heart transplant patients at Stanford University Medical Center. *Clin Infect Dis* 2001;33:629–640.
8. Wilson JP, Turner HR, Kirchner KA, et al. Nocardial infections in renal transplant recipients. *Medicine (Baltimore)* 1989;68:38–57.
9. Chapman SW, Wilson JP. Nocardiosis in transplant recipients. *Semin Respir Infect* 1990;5:74–79.
10. Paterson DL, Singh N, Gayowski T, et al. Pulmonary nodules in liver transplant recipients. *Medicine (Baltimore)* 1998;77:50–58.
11. Munoz P, Palomo J, Guembe P, et al. Lung nodular lesions in heart transplant recipients. *J Heart Lung Transplant* 2000;19:660–667.
12. Singh N, Paterson DL. *Mycobacterium tuberculosis* infection in solid-organ transplant recipients: impact and implications for management. *Clin Infect Dis* 1998;27:1266–1277.
13. Meyers BR, Halpern M, Sheiner P, et al. Tuberculosis in liver transplant patients. *Transplantation* 1994;58:301–306.
14. Korner MM, Hirata N, Tenderich G, et al. Tuberculosis in heart transplant recipients. *Chest* 1997;111:365–369.
15. John GT, Shankar V, Abraham AM, et al. Risk factors for post-transplant tuberculosis. *Kidney Int* 2001;60:1148–1153.
16. Meyers BR, Papanicolaou GA, Sheiner P, et al. Tuberculosis in orthotopic liver transplant patients: increased toxicity of recommended agents: cure of disseminated infection with nonconventional regimens. *Transplantation* 2000;69:64–69.
17. Aguado JM, Herrero JA, Gavalda J, et al. Clinical presentation and outcome of tuberculosis in kidney, liver, and heart transplant recipients in Spain. Spanish Transplantation Infection Study Group, GESITRA. *Transplantation* 1997;63:1278–1286.
18. Prevention ATS/CDC. Targeted tuberculin testing and treatment of latent tuberculosis infection. *Am J Respir Crit Care Med* 2000;161:S221–S247.
19. Harbison MA, De Girolami PC, Jenkins RL, et al. Ganciclovir therapy of severe cytomegalovirus infections in solid-organ transplant recipients. *Transplantation* 1988;46:82–88.
20. Ettinger NA, Trulock EP. Pulmonary considerations of organ transplantation. Part I. *Am Rev Respir Dis* 1991;143:1386–1405.
21. D'Alessandro AM, Pirsch JD, Stratta RJ, et al. Successful treatment of severe cytomegalovirus infections with ganciclovir and CMV hyperimmune globulin in liver transplant recipients. *Transplant Proc* 1989;21:3560–3561.
22. Rubin RH. Prevention and treatment of cytomegalovirus disease in heart transplant patients. *J Heart Lung Transplant* 2000;19:731–735.
23. Turgeon N, Fishman JA, Doran M, et al. Prevention of recurrent cytomegalovirus disease in renal and liver transplant recipients: effect of oral ganciclovir. *Transpl Infect Dis* 2000;2:2–10.
24. Griffiths PD. The treatment of cytomegalovirus infection. *J Antimicrob Chemother* 2002;49:243–253.
25. Sia IG, Patel R. New strategies for the prevention and therapy of cytomegalovirus infection and disease in solid-organ transplant recipients. *Clin Microbiol Rev* 2000;13:83–121.
26. Couchoud C, Cucherat M, Haugh M, et al. Cytomegalovirus prophylaxis with antiviral agents in solid organ transplantation: a meta-analysis. *Transplantation* 1998;65:641–647.
27. Singh N. Preemptive therapy versus universal prophylaxis with ganciclovir for cytomegalovirus in solid organ transplant recipients. *Clin Infect Dis* 2001;32:742–751.
28. Van der Bij W, Speich R. Management of cytomegalovirus infection and disease after solid organ transplantation. *Clin Infect Dis* 2001;33[Suppl 1]:S33–S37.
29. Paterson DL, Singh N. Invasive aspergillosis in transplant recipients. *Medicine (Baltimore)* 1999;78:123–138.
30. Haramati LB, Schulman LL, Austin JH. Lung nodules and masses after cardiac transplantation. *Radiology* 1993;188:491–497.
31. Horvath JA, Dummer S. The use of respiratory-tract cultures in the diagnosis of invasive pulmonary aspergillosis. *Am J Med* 1996;100:171–178.
32. Robinson LA, Reed EC, Galbraith TA, et al. Pulmonary resection for invasive *Aspergillus* infections in immunocompromised patients. *J Thorac Cardiovasc Surg* 1995;109:1182–1196; discussion 1196–1197.
33. Gordon SM, LaRosa SP, Kalmadi S, et al. Should prophylaxis for *Pneumocystis carinii* pneumonia in solid organ transplant recipients ever be discontinued? *Clin Infect Dis* 1999;28:240–246.
34. Glanemann M, Langrehr J, Kaisers U, et al. Postoperative tracheal extubation after orthotopic liver transplantation. *Acta Anaesthesiol Scand* 2001;45:333–339.
35. Glanemann M, Kaisers U, Langrehr JM, et al. Incidence and indications for reintubation during postoperative care following orthotopic liver transplantation. *J Clin Anesth* 2001;13:377–382.
36. O'Brien JD, Ettinger NA. Pulmonary complications of liver transplantation. *Clin Chest Med* 1996;17:99–114.
37. Judson MA, Sahn SA. The pleural space and organ transplantation. *Am J Respir Crit Care Med* 1996;153:1153–1165.
38. McAlister VC, Grant DR, Roy A, et al. Right phrenic nerve injury in orthotopic liver transplantation. *Transplantation* 1993;55:826–830.

39. Dorffner R, Eibenberger K, Youssefzadeh S, et al. Diaphragmatic dysfunction after heart or lung transplantation. *J Heart Lung Transplant* 1997;16:566–569.

40. Heino A, Orko R, Rosenberg PH. Anaesthesiological complications in renal transplantation: a retrospective study of 500 transplantations. *Acta Anaesthesiol Scand* 1986;30:574–580.

41. Preiksaitis JK, Cockfield SM. Epstein-Barr virus and lymphoproliferative disorders after transplantation. In: Raleigh A, Bowden RA, Ljungman P, et al., eds. *Transplant infections.* Philadelphia: Lippincott–Raven Publishers, 1998:245–263.

42. Tsai DE, Hardy CL, Tomaszewski JE, et al. Reduction in immunosuppression as initial therapy for post-transplant lymphoproliferative disorder: analysis of prognostic variables and long-term follow-up of 42 adult patients. *Transplantation* 2001;71:1076–1088.

43. Oertel SH, Anagnostopoulos I, Bechstein WO, et al. Treatment of post-transplant lymphoproliferative disorder with the anti-CD20 monoclonal antibody rituximab alone in an adult after liver transplantation: a new drug in the therapy of patients with post-transplant lymphoproliferative disorder after solid organ transplantation? *Transplantation* 2000;69:430–432.

44. Dorent R, Mohammadi S, Tezenas S, et al. Lung cancer in heart transplant patients: a 16-year survey. *Transplant Proc* 2000;32:2752–2754.

45. Justrabo E, Genin R, Rifle G. Pulmonary metastatic calcification with respiratory insufficiency in patients on maintenance haemodialysis. *Thorax* 1979;34:384–388.

46. Ullmer E, Borer H, Sandoz P, et al. Diffuse pulmonary nodular infiltrates in a renal transplant recipient. Metastatic pulmonary calcification. *Chest* 2001;120:1394–1398.

47. Kuhlman JE, Ren H, Hutchins GM, et al. Fulminant pulmonary calcification complicating renal transplantation: CT demonstration. *Radiology* 1989;173:459–460.

48. Giacobetti R, Feldman SA, Ivanovich P, et al. Sudden fatal pulmonary calcification following renal transplantation. *Nephron* 1977;19:295–300.

49. Libson E, Wechsler RJ, Steiner RM. Pulmonary calcinosis following orthotopic liver transplantation. *J Thorac Imaging* 1993;8:305–308.

50. Munoz SJ, Nagelberg SB, Green PJ, et al. Ectopic soft tissue calcium deposition following liver transplantation. *Hepatology* 1988;8:476–483.

51. Morelon E, Stern M, Israel-Biet D, et al. Characteristics of sirolimus-associated interstitial pneumonitis in renal transplant patients. *Transplantation* 2001;72:787–790.

52. Singer SJ, Tiernan R, Sullivan EJ. Interstitial pneumonitis associated with sirolimus therapy in renal-transplant recipients. *N Engl J Med* 2000;343:1815–1816.

53. Krowka MJ, Porayko MK, Plevak DJ, et al. Hepatopulmonary syndrome with progressive hypoxemia as an indication for liver transplantation: case reports and literature review. *Mayo Clin Proc* 1997;72:44–53.

54. Egawa H, Kasahara M, Inomata Y, et al. Long-term outcome of living related liver transplantation for patients with intrapulmonary shunting and strategy for complications. *Transplantation* 1999;67:712–717.

55. Lange PA, Stoller JK. The hepatopulmonary syndrome: effect of liver transplantation. *Clin Chest Med* 1996;17:115–123.

56. Krowka M, Wiseman GA, Steers JL, et al. Late recurrence and rapid evolution of severe hepatopulmonary syndrome after liver transplantation. *Liver Transpl* 1999;5:451–453.

57. Krowka MJ, Wiseman GA, Burnett OL, et al. Hepatopulmonary syndrome: a prospective study of relationships between severity of liver disease, PaO(2) response to 100% oxygen, and brain uptake after (99m)Tc MAA lung scanning. *Chest* 2000;118:615–624.

58. Meyers C, Low L, Kaufman L, et al. Trendelenburg positioning and continuous lateral rotation improve oxygenation in hepatopulmonary syndrome after liver transplantation. *Liver Transpl Surg* 1998;4:510–512.

59. Schenk P, Madl C, Rezaie-Majd S, et al. Methylene blue improves the hepatopulmonary syndrome. *Ann Intern Med* 2000;133:701–706.

60. Kuo PC, Plotkin JS, Gaine S, et al. Portopulmonary hypertension and the liver transplant candidate. *Transplantation* 1999;67:1087–1093.

61. Ramsay MA, Simpson BR, Nguyen AT, et al. Severe pulmonary hypertension in liver transplant candidates. *Liver Transpl Surg* 1997;3:494–500.

62. Krowka MJ, Plevak DJ, Findlay JY, et al. Pulmonary hemodynamics and perioperative cardiopulmonary-related mortality in patients with portopulmonary hypertension undergoing liver transplantation. *Liver Transpl* 2000;6:443–450.

63. Kett DH, Acosta RC, Campos MA, et al. Recurrent portopulmonary hypertension after liver transplantation: management with epoprostenol and resolution after retransplantation. *Liver Transpl* 2001;7:645–648.

64. Krowka MJ, Frantz RP, McGoon MD, et al. Improvement in pulmonary hemodynamics during intravenous epoprostenol (prostacyclin): a study of 15 patients with moderate to severe portopulmonary hypertension. *Hepatology* 1999;30:641–648.

65. Tan HP, Markowitz JS, Montgomery RA, et al. Liver transplantation in patients with severe portopulmonary hypertension treated with preoperative chronic intravenous epoprostenol. *Liver Transpl* 2001;7:745–749.

66. Ramsay MA, Spikes C, East CA, et al. The perioperative management of portopulmonary hypertension with nitric oxide and epoprostenol. *Anesthesiology* 1999;90:299–301.

67. Rafanan AL, Maurer J, Mehta AC, et al. Progressive portopulmonary hypertension after liver transplantation treated with epoprostenol. *Chest* 2000;118:1497–1500.

68. Soubani AO, Miller KB, Hassoun PM. Pulmonary complications of bone marrow transplantation. *Chest* 1996;109:1066–1077.

69. Wick MR, Moore SB, Gastineau DA, et al. Immunologic, clinical, and pathologic aspects of human graft-versus-host disease. *Mayo Clin Proc* 1983;58:603–612.

70. Lum LG. The kinetics of immune reconstitution after human marrow transplantation. *Blood* 1987;69:369–380.

71. Storek J, Joseph A, Espino G, et al. Immunity of patients surviving 20 to 30 years after allogeneic or syngeneic bone marrow transplantation. *Blood* 2001;98:3505–3512.

72. Huaringa AJ, Leyva FJ, Signes-Costa J, et al. Bronchoalveolar lavage in the diagnosis of pulmonary complications of bone marrow transplant patients. *Bone Marrow Transplant* 2000;25:975–979.

73. White P, Bonacum JT, Miller CB. Utility of fiberoptic bronchoscopy in bone marrow transplant patients. *Bone Marrow Transplant* 1997;20:681–687.

74. Dunagan DP, Baker AM, Hurd DD, et al. Bronchoscopic evaluation of pulmonary infiltrates following bone marrow transplantation. *Chest* 1997;111:135–141.

75. Feinstein MB, Mokhtari M, Ferreiro R, et al. Fiberoptic bronchoscopy in allogeneic bone marrow transplantation: findings in the era of serum cytomegalovirus antigen surveillance. *Chest* 2001;120:1094–1100.

76. Lossos IS, Breuer R, Or R, et al. Bacterial pneumonia in recipients of bone marrow transplantation. A five-year prospective study. *Transplantation* 1995;60:672–678.

77. Leung AN, Gosselin MV, Napper CH, et al. Pulmonary infections after bone marrow transplantation: clinical and radiographic findings. *Radiology* 1999;210:699–710.

78. Heussel CP, Kauczor HU, Heussel G, et al. Early detection of pneumonia in febrile neutropenic patients: use of thin-section CT. *AJR Am J Roentgenol* 1997;169:1347–1353.

79. Sullivan KM, Dykewicz CA, Longworth DL, et al. Preventing opportunistic infections after hematopoietic stem cell transplantation: the Centers for Disease Control and Prevention, Infectious Diseases Society of America, and American Society for Blood and Marrow Transplantation practice guidelines and beyond. *Hematology (Am Soc Hematol Educ Program)* 2001;392–421.

80. Roy V, Weisdorf D. Mycobacterial infections following bone marrow transplantation: a 20-year retrospective review. *Bone Marrow Transplant* 1997;19:467–470.

81. De la Camara R, Martino R, Granados E, et al. Tuberculosis after hematopoietic stem cell transplantation: incidence, clinical characteristics and outcome. Spanish Group on Infectious Complications in Hematopoietic Transplantation. *Bone Marrow Transplant* 2000;26:291–298.

82. George B, Mathews V, Srivastava V, et al. Tuberculosis among allogeneic bone marrow transplant recipients in India. *Bone Marrow Transplant* 2001;27:973–975.

83. Bowden RA. Fungal infections after marrow transplantation. In: Raleigh A, Bowden RA, Ljungman P, et al., eds. *Transplant infections*. Philadelphia: Lippincott–Raven Publishers, 1998:325–338.

84. Albelda SM, Talbot GH, Gerson SL, et al. Pulmonary cavitation and massive hemoptysis in invasive pulmonary aspergillosis. Influence of bone marrow recovery in patients with acute leukemia. *Am Rev Respir Dis* 1985;131:115–120.

85. Caillot D, Casasnovas O, Bernard A, et al. Improved management of invasive pulmonary aspergillosis in neutropenic patients using early thoracic computed tomographic scan and surgery. *J Clin Oncol* 1997;15:139–147.

86. Denning DW. Early diagnosis of invasive aspergillosis. *Lancet* 2000;355:423–424.

87. Reichenberger F, Habicht J, Kaim A, et al. Lung resection for invasive pulmonary aspergillosis in neutropenic patients with hematologic diseases. *Am Rev Respir Dis* 1998;158:885–890.

88. Brown MJ, Worthy SA, Flint JD, et al. Invasive aspergillosis in the immunocompromised host: utility of computed tomography and bronchoalveolar lavage. *Clin Radiol* 1998;53:255–257.

89. Maertens J, Verhaegen J, Lagrou K, et al. Screening for circulating galactomannan as a noninvasive diagnostic tool for invasive aspergillosis in prolonged neutropenic patients and stem cell transplantation recipients: a prospective validation. *Blood* 2001;97:1604–1610.

90. Denning DW. Therapeutic outcome in invasive aspergillosis. *Clin Infect Dis* 1996;23:608–615.

91. Herbrecht R, Denning DW, Patterson TF, et al. Voriconazole versus amphotericin B for primary therapy of invasive aspergillosis. *N Engl J Med* 2002;347:408–415.

92. Meyers JD, Pifer LL, Sale GE, et al. The value of *Pneumocystis carinii* antibody and antigen detection for diagnosis of *Pneumocystis carinii* pneumonia after marrow transplantation. *Am Rev Respir Dis* 1979;120:1283–1287.

93. Souza JP, Boeckh M, Gooley TA, et al. High rates of *Pneumocystis carinii* pneumonia in allogeneic blood and marrow transplant recipients receiving dapsone prophylaxis. *Clin Infect Dis* 1999;29:1467–1471.

94. Link H, Vohringer HF, Wingen F, et al. Pentamidine aerosol for prophylaxis of *Pneumocystis carinii* pneumonia after BMT. *Bone Marrow Transplant* 1993;11:403–406.

95. Lyytikainen O, Ruutu T, Volin L, et al. Late-onset *Pneumocystis carinii* pneumonia following allogeneic bone marrow transplantation. *Bone Marrow Transplant* 1996;17:1057–1059.

96. Tuan IZ, Dennison D, Weisdorf DJ. *Pneumocystis carinii* pneumonitis following bone marrow transplantation. *Bone Marrow Transplant* 1992;10:267–272.

97. Boeckh M. Current antiviral strategies for controlling cytomegalovirus in hematopoietic stem cell transplant recipients: prevention and therapy. *Transpl Infect Dis* 1999;1:165–178.

98. Reed EC, Bowden RA, Dandliker PS, et al. Treatment of cytomegalovirus pneumonia with ganciclovir and intravenous cytomegalovirus immunoglobulin in patients with bone marrow transplants. *Ann Intern Med* 1988;109:783–788.

99. Boeckh M, Gooley TA, Myerson D, et al. Cytomegalovirus pp65 antigenemia-guided early treatment with ganciclovir versus ganciclovir at engraftment after allogeneic marrow transplantation: a randomized double-blind study. *Blood* 1996;88:4063–4071.

100. Walter EA, Greenberg PD, Gilbert MJ, et al. Reconstitution of cellular immunity against cytomegalovirus in recipients of allogeneic bone marrow by transfer of T-cell clones from the donor. *N Engl J Med* 1995;333:1038–1044.

101. Robbins RA, Linder J, Stahl MG, et al. Diffuse alveolar hemorrhage in autologous bone marrow transplant recipients. *Am J Med* 1989;87:511–518.

102. Metcalf JP, Rennard SI, Reed EC, et al. Corticosteroids as adjunctive therapy for diffuse alveolar hemorrhage associated with bone marrow transplantation. University of Nebraska Medical Center Bone Marrow Transplant Group. *Am J Med* 1994;96:327–334.

103. Chao NJ, Duncan SR, Long GD, et al. Corticosteroid therapy for diffuse alveolar hemorrhage in autologous bone marrow transplant recipients. *Ann Intern Med* 1991;114:145–146.

104. Agusti C, Ramirez J, Picado C, et al. Diffuse alveolar hemorrhage in allogeneic bone marrow transplantation. A postmortem study. *Am J Respir Crit Care Med* 1995;151:1006–1010.

105. Raptis A, Mavroudis D, Suffredini A, et al. High-dose corticosteroid therapy for diffuse alveolar hemorrhage in allogeneic bone marrow stem cell transplant recipients. *Bone Marrow Transplant* 1999;24:879–883.

106. Lee CK, Gingrich RD, Hohl RJ, et al. Engraftment syndrome in autologous bone marrow and peripheral stem cell transplantation. *Bone Marrow Transplant* 1995;16:175–182.

107. Marin D, Berrade J, Ferra C, et al. Engraftment syndrome and survival after respiratory failure post-bone marrow transplantation. *Intensive Care Med* 1998;24:732–735.

108. Clark JG, Hansen JA, Hertz MI, et al. NHLBI workshop summary. Idiopathic pneumonia syndrome after bone marrow transplantation. *Am Rev Respir Dis* 1993;147:1601–1606.

109. Kantrow SP, Hackman RC, Boeckh M, et al. Idiopathic pneumonia syndrome: changing spectrum of lung injury after marrow transplantation. *Transplantation* 1997;63:1079–1086.

110. Anscher MS, Peters WP, Reisenbichler H, et al. Transforming growth factor-beta as a predictor of liver and lung fibrosis after autologous bone marrow transplantation for advanced breast cancer. *N Engl J Med* 1993;328:1592–1598.

111. Shankar G, Cohen DA. Idiopathic pneumonia syndrome after bone marrow transplantation: the role of pre-transplant radiation conditioning and local cytokine dysregulation in promoting lung inflammation and fibrosis. *Int J Exp Pathol* 2001;82:101–113.

112. Shankar G, Scott Bryson J, Darrell Jennings C, et al. Idiopathic pneumonia syndrome after allogeneic bone marrow transplantation in mice. Role of pretransplant radiation conditioning. *Am J Respir Cell Mol Biol* 1999;20:1116–1124.

113. Todd NW, Peters WP, Ost AH, et al. Pulmonary drug toxicity in patients with primary breast cancer treated with high-dose combination chemotherapy and autologous bone marrow transplantation. *Am Rev Respir Dis* 1993;147:1264–1270.

114. Wilczynski SW, Erasmus JJ, Petros WP, et al. Delayed pulmonary toxicity syndrome following high-dose chemotherapy and bone

marrow transplantation for breast cancer. *Am J Respir Crit Care Med* 1998;157:565–573.

115. Bhalla KS, Wilczynski SW, Abushamaa AM, et al. Pulmonary toxicity of induction chemotherapy prior to standard or high-dose chemotherapy with autologous hematopoietic support. *Am J Respir Crit Care Med* 2000;161:17–25.

116. Williams LM, Fussell S, Veith RW, et al. Pulmonary veno-occlusive disease in an adult following bone marrow transplantation. Case report and review of the literature. *Chest* 1996;109:1388–1391.

117. Mandel J, Mark EJ, Hales CA. Pulmonary veno-occlusive disease. *Am J Respir Crit Care Med* 2000;162:1964–1973.

118. Doll DC, Yarbro JW. Vascular toxicity associated with antineoplastic agents. *Semin Oncol* 1992;19:580–596.

119. Hackman RC, Madtes DK, Petersen FB, et al. Pulmonary veno-occlusive disease following bone marrow transplantation. *Transplantation* 1989;47:989–992.

120. Holland HK, Wingard JR, Beschorner WE, et al. Bronchiolitis obliterans in bone marrow transplantation and its relationship to chronic graft-v-host disease and low serum IgG. *Blood* 1988;72:621–627.

121. Ringden O, Remberger M, Ruutu T, et al. Increased risk of chronic graft-versus-host disease, obstructive bronchiolitis, and alopecia with busulfan versus total body irradiation: long-term results of a randomized trial in allogeneic marrow recipients with leukemia. Nordic Bone Marrow Transplantation Group. *Blood* 1999;93:2196–2201.

122. Clark JG, Crawford SW, Madtes DK, et al. Obstructive lung disease after allogeneic marrow transplantation. Clinical presentation and course. *Ann Intern Med* 1989;111:368–376.

123. Forsyth CJ, Cremer PD, Torzillo P, et al. Thalidomide-responsive chronic pulmonary GVHD. *Bone Marrow Transplant* 1996;17:291–293.

124. Smith EP, Sniecinski I, Dagis AC, et al. Extracorporeal photochemotherapy for treatment of drug-resistant graft-vs.-host disease. *Biol Blood Marrow Transplant* 1998;4:27–37.

125. Rabitsch W, Deviatko E, Keil F, et al. Successful lung transplantation for bronchiolitis obliterans after allogeneic marrow transplantation. *Transplantation* 2001;71:1341–1343.

126. Crawford SW, Petersen FB. Long-term survival from respiratory failure after marrow transplantation for malignancy. *Am Rev Respir Dis* 1992;145:510–514.

127. Rubenfeld GD, Crawford SW. Withdrawing life support from mechanically ventilated recipients of bone marrow transplants: a case for evidence-based guidelines. *Ann Intern Med* 1996;125:625–633.

128. Afessa B, Tefferi A, Hoagland HC, et al. Outcome of recipients of bone marrow transplants who require intensive-care unit support. *Mayo Clin Proc* 1992;67:117–122.

129. Paz HL, Crilley P, Weinar M, et al. Outcome of patients requiring medical ICU admission following bone marrow transplantation. *Chest* 1993;104:527–531.

130. Faber-Langendoen K, Caplan AL, McGlave PB. Survival of adult bone marrow transplant patients receiving mechanical ventilation: a case for restricted use. *Bone Marrow Transplant* 1993;12:501–507.

131. Schuster DP. Everything that should be done—not everything that can be done. *Am Rev Respir Dis* 1992;145:508–509.

132. Shorr AF, Moores LK, Edenfield WJ, et al. Mechanical ventilation in hematopoietic stem cell transplantation: can we effectively predict outcomes? *Chest* 1999;116:1012–1018.

133. Huaringa AJ, Leyva FJ, Giralt SA, et al. Outcome of bone marrow transplantation patients requiring mechanical ventilation. *Crit Care Med* 2000;28:1014–1017.

134. Price KJ, Thall PF, Kish SK, et al. Prognostic indicators for blood and marrow transplant patients admitted to an intensive care unit. *Am J Respir Crit Care Med* 1998;158:876–884.

57   Hematologic Diseases

Udaya B. S. Prakash · Talmadge E. King, Jr.

The erythropoietic system plays a major role in tissue oxygenation because the erythrocytes are the primary carriers of oxygen in the form of oxyhemoglobin. Therefore, anemia, polycythemia, abnormal hemoglobins, and significant changes in blood volume frequently cause alterations in various respiratory functions. Additionally, myeloproliferative, lymphoproliferative, and plasmacytic disorders and other hematologic malignancies frequently affect the pulmonary system. Pulmonary complications are the most common cause of mortality in patients with hematologic malignancies. Respiratory manifestations in these disorders may be caused by pulmonary extension of the basic disease process, cytotoxic drug-induced pulmonary pathology, opportunistic infections, or a combination of these factors. This chapter discusses the various thoracic manifestations of hematologic diseases. The pulmonary complications of bone marrow transplantation are discussed in Chapter 56.

HEMOGLOBINOPATHIES

A *hemoglobinopathy* is an abnormality of hemoglobin synthesis manifested by the production of globin with a structural abnormality (1). More than 90% of these abnormalities result from the replacement of a single amino acid. The clinically significant hemoglobinopathies, as far as the pulmonary system is concerned, include the sickle syndromes, hemoglobinopathies in which oxygen affinity is high (familial erythrocytosis), hemoglobinopathies in which oxygen affinity is low (familial cyanosis), M hemoglobinopathies

U. B. S. Prakash: Pulmonary and Critical Care Medicine, Mayo Medical School and Mayo Medical Center, Rochester, Minnesota.

T. E. King, Jr.: Department of Medicine, University of California, San Francisco; and Medical Services, San Francisco General Hospital, San Francisco, California.

(familial cyanosis), and methemoglobinemia and sulfhemoglobinemia. Although cyanosis as a result of these disorders is rarely encountered in clinical practice, the possibility of abnormal hemoglobin should be considered in the differential diagnosis of a cyanotic patient (Table 57.1).

Hemoglobinopathies with High Oxygen Affinity

More than 120 variants of human hemoglobin are known to exhibit an increased affinity for oxygen. By definition, these hemoglobins demonstrate a shift to the left of the whole-blood oxygen dissociation curve. The hemoglobinopathies associated with high oxygen affinity result from amino acid substitutions at sites crucial to hemoglobin function. These disorders are manifested in the heterozygous state and follow an autosomal-codominant pattern of inheritance. A partial list of abnormal hemoglobins with an increased affinity for oxygen includes Chesapeake, J-Capetown, Malmo, Yakima, Kempsey, Ypsilanti, Hiroshe, Brigham, Rainier, Bethesda, Hiroshima, Little Rock, Olympia, Tarrant, Sureness, Helsinki, Creteil, Hotel Dieu, Radcliffe, Alberta, British Columbia, Heathrow, San Diego, Syracuse, York, and Cowtown.

Many of these hemoglobinopathies are manifested by secondary erythrocytosis (increased red cell mass). Most patients are asymptomatic, and the diagnosis is considered when unexplained erythrocytosis is detected. Patients who have hemoglobin variants with a marked increase in oxygen affinity may demonstrate cyanosis or a slate blue color. Because of the defective hemoglobin function, the arterial blood is partially unsaturated despite a normal oxygen tension; as a result, levels of deoxyhemoglobin in the blood are elevated—hence the cyanosis. However, the cyanosis is a cosmetic problem, and no specific therapy is warranted. Several individuals with high-affinity variants have had persistent leukocytosis, and

TABLE 57.1. DIFFERENTIAL DIAGNOSIS OF CYANOSIS

Inadequate oxygenation of hemoglobin (common)
  Pulmonary diseases
  Cardiac and noncardiac right-to-left shunt
  Vascular collapse (shock)
  Low-oxygen-affinity hemoglobin variant

Methemoglobinemia (uncommon)
  Hereditary (congenital)
    Cytochrome b_5 reductase deficiency
    M hemoglobinopathies

Acquired (toxic)
  Nitrites and nitrates: amyl nitrite, nitroglycerin, nitroprusside, silver nitrate, sodium nitrite
  Other drugs: acetanilid, benzocaine, lidocaine, phenazopyridine, phenacetin, procaine, sulfonamides
  Industrial and environmental toxins: aniline dyes, chlorate, others

Sulfhemoglobinemia (uncommon)
  Congenital (?)
  Acquired: acetaminophen, acetanilid, arylamines, phenacetin, sulfur, toxins, others

Pseudocyanosis
  Argyria
  Hemochromatosis
  Chloroma

an occasional subject has exhibited splenomegaly. Pulmonary fibrosis has been described in several members of a family with hemoglobin Malmo, but the occurrence appears to be coincidental. A low ambient Po_2, as in unpressurized airplanes and at high altitudes, does not pose a risk because high-affinity hemoglobins are avid for oxygen (1).

Hemoglobinopathies with Low Oxygen Affinity

More than a dozen variants of hemoglobin with a low oxygen affinity have been described. A partial list includes Kansas, Beth Israel, St. Mande, Titusville, Connecticut, Bologna, Rothschild, Mobile, Hope, J-Cairo, Raleigh, Vancouver, Presbyterian, and Yoshizuka. Many affected family members have slightly diminished hemoglobin levels. The shift to the right of the oxyhemoglobin dissociation curve reduces the erythropoietin-mediated stimulus to erythropoiesis. The skin and mucous membranes of persons who have a hemoglobin variant with a low ligand affinity may be slate gray in color (1). In heterozygotes with hemoglobin Kansas, cyanosis results from increased levels of deoxyhemoglobin. Individuals with hemoglobin Kansas demonstrate a marked decrease in whole-blood oxygen affinity. Despite the diminished oxygen content of the arterial blood, the shift to the right of the oxyhemoglobin dissociation curve allows adequate oxygen release. A limited tolerance to strenuous muscular exercise, which depends on a greatly increased oxygen unloading, may develop in subjects with hemoglobin Kansas.

In addition to hemoglobin Kansas, hemoglobin variants Beth Israel and St. Mande can be associated with cyanosis.

Both have amino acid substitutions at the same site as hemoglobin Kansas (i.e., a substitution of threonine for asparagine at 102). Familial pulmonary hypertension has been described in association with abnormal hemoglobin with a low oxygen affinity. Persons who have low-affinity hemoglobins usually do not require treatment because oxygen delivery to the tissues is adequate (1). Establishing a correct diagnosis prevents these patients from undergoing unnecessary diagnostic or therapeutic interventions.

M Hemoglobinopathies

The M hemoglobins are the main group of hemoglobins that cause cyanosis. Hemoglobins M-Boston, M-Iwate, M-Saskatoon, M-Hyde Park, and M-Milwaukee exhibit abnormal absorbance spectra secondary to oxidation of the heme iron in the affected subunit. The M hemoglobinopathies behave like autosomal-codominant mutations. In heterozygotes, they cause methemoglobinemia, which results in chronic cyanosis. The Bohr effect is markedly decreased or absent in the α-chain variants, but normal or only slightly decreased in variants of the β chain. Thus, hemoglobins Iwate and Boston, both with α-chain alterations, show a decreased oxygen affinity and a decreased Bohr effect; hemoglobins Hyde Park and Saskatoon, which exemplify β-chain mutations, have essentially a normal oxygen affinity and a normal Bohr effect.

The predominant characteristic of the hemoglobin M disorders is cyanosis from early childhood. Subjects with α-chain variants (M-Boston and M-Iwate) are cyanotic at birth, whereas those with β-chain variants (M-Saskatoon, M-Hyde Park, M-Milwaukee) do not exhibit cyanosis until approximately 5 to 6 months of age, when fetal hemoglobin is replaced by adult hemoglobin. Hemoglobin Freiburg, resulting from a β-chain mutation, is associated with mild cyanosis, whereas hemoglobin Seattle is not associated with cyanosis but does show decreased oxygen affinity. Despite their cyanosis, patients with these hemoglobinopathies show no evidence of cardiac disease or clubbing. Exertional dyspnea is not a feature.

Methemoglobinemia and Sulfhemoglobinemia

Methemoglobinemia results when more than 1% of hemoglobin is oxidized to the ferric form (2). When hemoglobin is oxidized to methemoglobin, the heme iron becomes Fe^{3+} and is incapable of binding oxygen. The methemoglobin content of normal red cells is less than 1%. When the methemoglobin level exceeds 1.5 g/dL (10% of total hemoglobin), cyanosis becomes clinically obvious. Both hereditary (congenital) and acquired forms of methemoglobinemia exist.

Congenital methemoglobinemia results from either hereditary deficiency of the enzyme cytochrome b_5 reductase (methemoglobin reductase) or the presence of one of the M hemoglobins. The major clinical feature is cyanosis without cardiopulmonary problems.

Acquired methemoglobinemia (also known as *toxic methemoglobinemia*) develops when drugs or toxins oxidize hemoglobin directly in the circulation or facilitate its oxidation by molecular oxygen (3) (Table 57.1). Toxic methemoglobinemia may be acute or chronic. In the latter, prolonged administration of the offending agent leads to an increased steady-state concentration of methemoglobin that results in asymptomatic cyanosis. Blood gas analysis usually reveals a normal arterial oxygen tension with a disproportionately low arterial oxygen saturation and increased levels of methemoglobin. Acute methemoglobinemia, especially when the level of methemoglobin exceeds half the total level of hemoglobin, may present a serious medical emergency. When the methemoglobin level exceeds 35%, headaches, weakness, and dyspnea develop. The severity of methemoglobinemia depends on the dose of the causative agent and the susceptibility of the exposed individual. Levels in excess of 80% are incompatible with life. Severe toxic methemoglobinemia should be treated with intravenous methylene blue (2 mg/kg). Methylene blue should not be administered to persons with glucose-6-phosphate dehydrogenase deficiency (e.g., African Americans, people of Mediterranean descent, people from Southeast Asia) (4).

Sulfhemoglobinemia is the presence in peripheral blood of hemoglobin derivatives that are poorly characterized chemically. Occasionally, cyanosis develops in subjects exposed to oxidant compounds that cannot be explained by simple hemoglobin oxidation. Because of high absorbance in the red region of the visible spectrum, sulfhemoglobinemia causes more cyanosis than an equivalent percentage of methemoglobinemia. Congenital and acquired forms of sulfhemoglobinemia have been described. A number of pharmacologic and other agents (Table 57.1) also cause sulfhemoglobinemia and cyanosis.

Sickle Cell Anemia

Sickle cell disease is caused primarily by hemoglobins SS, SC, or Sb thalassemia (5,6). Sickle cell anemia is a chronic, hereditary hemolytic disease resulting from the clinical expression of homozygosity for hemoglobin S. Affected persons are predominantly blacks who have inherited the mutant gene from both parents.

Pulmonary complications are common in patients with sickle cell anemia (hemoglobin SS), less so in patients with hemoglobin SC, and are important causes of morbidity and mortality (7). Pulmonary complications include pneumonia, infarction secondary to in situ thrombosis, embolic phenomena (fat embolism associated with bone marrow infarction), and the acute chest syndrome (7). Sickle cell disease and sarcoidosis are two disorders commonly affecting blacks. Studies have shown the prevalence rates of hemoglobinopathies in patients with sarcoidosis to be 18% to 20%.

Pneumonia

Patients with sickle cell disease are predisposed to the development of pneumonia by impairments in host defenses, including loss of antibody protection (in the setting of autosplenectomy), altered phagocytic function, and defective opsonization (7). Also, local factors, such as previous or concomitant pulmonary damage from vaso-occlusion, probably play a role. Although most acute pulmonary infections were once thought to be caused by pneumococci, subsequent studies (particularly those in adults) have revealed an increasing frequency of infection with *Haemophilus influenzae* (7). Pneumonia, especially in children and probably in all age groups, is the lung disease most commonly encountered in sickle cell anemia; its incidence is 20 times greater in these patients than in the normal population. In children with sickle cell disease, the incidence of pneumonia increases significantly after the age of 8 months. Pneumonia in children is usually caused by *Streptococcus pneumoniae*, whereas in adults, *Staphylococcus aureus* and *Haemophilus* species predominate. Atypical organisms, including *Mycoplasma pneumoniae* and *Chlamydia pneumoniae*, have also been described, particularly in children (7).

Most cases of suspected pneumonia in adults are caused by pulmonary embolism, and the differentiation of infectious pneumonia from acute chest syndrome or pulmonary embolism is difficult. One study of 166 patients with sickle cell anemia reported that 45% were hospitalized because of acute bacterial pneumonia, and half of this group had positive bacterial cultures. However, in another study, of 18 patients with acute chest syndrome, respiratory secretions were obtained by bronchoscopy, and the authors concluded that bacterial pneumonia is uncommon in this group of patients (8). A lower incidence of bacterial pneumonia may result from the use of penicillin prophylaxis and pneumococcal immunization to prevent *S. pneumoniae* infection (9). Multilobar involvement is common, with the upper and middle lobes affected more often than the lower lobes. The administration of pneumococcal vaccine is mandatory in patients with sickle cell anemia.

Fungal infections are uncommon in patients with sickle cell anemia, but occasional cases of cryptococcal infection have been described. Although some have reported a higher incidence of tuberculosis, others have not been able to substantiate this finding.

Acute Chest Syndrome

The acute chest syndrome (also called *sickle chest syndrome, chest crisis, pulmonary sickle crisis,* and *pulmonary infarction*) is seen in up to 35% of patients hospitalized with sickle cell disease; it is associated with significant morbidity and is the leading cause of death in patients with sickle cell disease (10,11). The syndrome is a common manifestation of sickling-induced vaso-occlusive crises. The differentiation of infectious pneumonia from acute chest syndrome is difficult.

A working definition of the acute chest syndrome is the presence of the following signs and symptoms in a patient with sickle cell disease: a new pulmonary infiltrate involving at least one complete lung segment (not atelectasis), chest pain, temperature above 38.5°C, tachypnea, wheezing, and cough (7,12,13).

The acute chest syndrome is characterized by fever, chest pain, and pulmonary infiltrates. A sudden onset of pleuritic chest pains, cough without hemoptysis, fever, and leukocytosis are common. Hypoxemia ($PaO_2 < 50$ mm Hg) is present in up to 40% of patients (14). Dense bilateral consolidations in the lower lung are commonly seen on the chest radiograph. A retrospective analysis of 100 hospitalized children with sickle cell anemia revealed lower lobe pulmonary infiltrates in 86%, upper lobe infiltrates in 25%, and middle lobe infiltrates in 22%; pleural effusions were observed in 38%. Sickle cell crisis may be precipitated by an asthmatic attack.

In a 30-center cooperative study of 671 episodes of acute chest syndrome in 538 patients with sickle cell disease, the causes were identified as follows: unknown cause (46%); pulmonary infarction (16%); fat embolism with or without infection (9%); *Chlamydia pneumoniae* infection (7%); *Mycoplasma pneumoniae* infection (7%); virus infection (e.g., respiratory syncytial virus, parvovirus, rhinovirus) (6%); mixed infection (4%); other pathogens (1%) (12).

Incentive spirometry has been shown to prevent the pulmonary complications of the acute chest syndrome. In a prospective randomized trial of 29 patients (8–21 years of age) with sickle cell diseases who had 38 episodes of acute chest or back pain above the diaphragm and were hospitalized, the incidence of thoracic bone infarction was 40% (15 of 38 hospitalizations). Pulmonary complications in the form of atelectasis or infiltrates developed during only 1 of 19 hospitalizations of patients assigned to the spirometry group, in comparison with 8 of 19 hospitalizations of patients assigned to the nonspirometry group (15).

Fat Embolism

Bone marrow fat embolism in the pulmonary vasculature is a common complication of sickle cell disease and is responsible for many severe cases of acute chest syndrome (16). To diagnose fat embolism, one study evaluated the fatty macrophages recovered by bronchoalveolar lavage (BAL) in 20 consecutive patients with acute chest syndrome; a cutoff of more than 5% of alveolar macrophages containing fat droplets was used (based on a control group) to establish a diagnosis of fat embolism (17). Bronchoalveolar lavage yielded more than 5% fatty macrophages (median, 47%; range, 10%–100%) in 12 episodes of acute chest syndrome, and in 11 cases, fat embolism was associated with proven or probable bone marrow infarction. Overall, the diagnostic yield of BAL for fat embolism was 60%.

Secretory phospholipase A_2 as an important mediator of acute lung injury in the fat embolism syndrome has been used diagnostically; phospholipase A_2 activity appears to correlate with the acute chest syndrome.

Pulmonary pathologic features include vascular occlusion, capillary stasis, thrombus formation, infarction, alveolar wall necrosis, and emboli of necrotic bone marrow. These complications are more common in women, particularly during late pregnancy or shortly after delivery.

In Situ Thrombosis

Patients with hemoglobin SC disease may be at risk for in situ thrombosis of the pulmonary vessels (18,19). The roentgenographic appearance of these lesions is no different from that of thromboemboli. A postmortem study of 36 older patients with sickle cell disease identified thromboemboli in most. However, pulmonary infarction is a much less frequent complication among younger patients. Anticoagulant therapy does not help. Although circulatory stasis may develop in situ, vascular occlusion by marrow emboli is probably a more common cause of pulmonary infarction and has been discovered at autopsy in 13% of patients with sickle cell disease. In patients with sickle cell anemia, pulmonary hemosiderosis may result from repeated blood transfusions.

Pulmonary Edema

Pulmonary edema is another complication of sickle cell crisis (20). Vigorous hypotonic fluid replacement and parenteral analgesic therapy, commonly administered to patients with sickle cell crisis, may contribute to its development. Autopsy findings in patients who died of pulmonary edema are consistent with a diffuse pulmonary vaso-occlusive disease.

Chronic Pulmonary Disease

Sickle cell chronic lung disease is characterized clinically by the development of pulmonary hypertension and cor pulmonale in association with restrictive lung disease (21). Sickle cell chronic lung disease may begin to develop as early as the second decade of life. Pulmonary dysfunction progresses rapidly, and death occurs within 7 years after the diagnosis (7,21). Significant risk factors for sickle cell chronic lung disease include recurrent episodes of acute chest syndrome, painful crises, and aseptic bone necrosis (7,21). Exchange transfusions to maintain a hemoglobin S level of 20%, supplemented with nocturnal or continuous oxygen, have been used to manage this complication (7,21).

Abnormal Pulmonary Physiology

A decreased diffusing capacity of the lung for carbon monoxide has been demonstrated in sickle cell anemia and has been attributed to a loss of membrane area as a result of obstruction of the pulmonary vessels (22). Other physiologic studies have shown a decreased vital capacity, normal maximal breathing capacity, arterial oxygen desaturation, and a widened alveolar-arterial difference in oxygen tension in most patients with the disease (23). Both venoarterial shunting and abnormal ventilation-perfusion relationships play a major role in this finding. Arterial oxygen desaturation predisposes to *in vivo* sickling and its consequences. The heterozygous state of sickle cell trait (hemoglobin AS) may lead to abnormal pulmonary function, as a result of sickling, at high altitudes. The sickling phenomenon can result in pulmonary thromboembolism, which in turn aggravates sickling and worsens hypoxia. Short episodes of hypoxia at high altitudes do not acutely or cumulatively alter the diffusing capacity or spirometric values of healthy persons with sickle cell trait. Upper airway obstruction during sleep secondary to adenoid and tonsillar enlargement has been found in up to one third of children with sickle cell disease (7,24).

TREATMENT OF ACUTE CHEST SYNDROME IN PATIENTS WITH SICKLE CELL DISEASE

Summary Statement	Level of Evidence
Antibiotic regimens that include coverage for community-acquired and atypical organisms should be used, such as a second-generation cephalosporin with or without erythromycin.	Observational studies
Supplemental oxygen, to maintain a PaO_2 of 70 to 100 mm Hg, should be used to prevent further intravascular sickling.	Observational studies
Hydration aimed at the maintenance of a euvolemic state should be a treatment goal.	Observational studies
Empiric anticoagulant therapy is not recommended because of the potential risk for intracranial and renal bleeding (7).	Observational studies
Incentive spirometry (used to prevent atelectasis after rib or sternal infarction) appears to be effective in preventing pulmonary complications (atelectasis and infiltrates) (15).	Randomized controlled trial
Transfusion of leukocyte-depleted red cells that are negative for sickle cells and matched with respect to C, E, and Kell antigens improves oxygenation and decreases the incidence of new red cell antibody formation (7).	Observational studies
Exchange transfusion is recommended in the setting of progressive infiltrates and hypoxemia refractory to conventional therapy. Reduction of the hemoglobin S level to below 30% can lead to marked improvement in most cases (7,25,26).	Observational studies
Inhaled nitric oxide (NO), by reducing the adhesion of sickle erythrocytes to the pulmonary endothelium, may be effective in patients with severe acute chest syndrome (7,27–29).	Observational studies
Hydroxyurea decreases the number of painful crises and episodes of acute chest syndrome (7,30).	Randomized clinical trial

β-Thalassemia Major

Thalassemia major is characterized by an unbalanced synthesis of globin chain that results in ineffective hematopoiesis. Severe hemolytic anemia and ineffective erythropoiesis from infancy are the main characteristics of this disorder, and the ability of the blood to increase its oxygen-carrying capacity during physical stress is limited (31). Patients succumb at a young age to congestive cardiac failure. Patients with thalassemia major subjected to repeated transfusions exhibit a high cardiac output during exercise, regardless of their hemoglobin concentration; the mechanism for this phenomenon is unknown.

Most patients with β-thalassemia have mild abnormalities of pulmonary function, including restrictive and small-airway obstructive defects, hyperinflation, decreased maximal oxygen uptake, and abnormal anaerobic thresholds (32–35). In a cardiopulmonary evaluation of 35 patients with homozygous β-thalassemia, hypoxemia was noted in 85%, reduced lung volumes in 51%, reduced flow rates in 63%, and a diminished diffusing capacity for carbon monoxide in 50% (36). Pulmonary hypertension was present in 75%, and right ventricular dysfunction was more prevalent than left ventricular dysfunction. The possible causes of these complications include left ventricular failure, deposition of iron in the pulmonary vessels, and a hypercoagulable state with thrombotic obstruction of the pulmonary arteries. Transfusion-induced decreases in the forced vital capacity and PaO_2 in the absence of pulmonary edema have been observed, but the mechanism is unclear (37).

HEMORRHAGIC DISEASES

Pulmonary complications such as pulmonary embolism and alveolar hemorrhage can result from an underlying disorder of coagulation. Both hypercoagulable and hypocoagulable states may be associated with these complications. The presence of a hemorrhagic disorder predisposes to pulmonary bleeding, and the risk for bleeding is increased if the patient has a preexisting pulmonary lesion, such as a tumor, bulla (Fig. 57.1), cyst, cavity, or bronchiectasis.

Hemophilia

Hemophilia A (factor VIII deficiency) and hemophilia B (factor IX deficiency) are X-linked recessive diseases (38). The combined incidence of hemophilia A and hemophilia B is 1 in 5,000 live male births (38). The most serious complication is the development of AIDS in persons previously administered factor VIII contaminated with HIV. This risk has significantly diminished as a result of stringent improvements in blood banking. Pulmonary manifestations are unusual in hemophilia but have included spontaneous pneumothorax, hemomediastinum, tracheal obstruction by

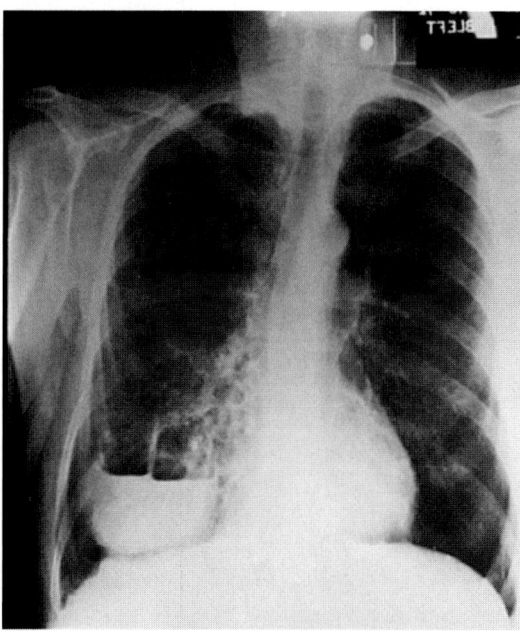

FIGURE 57.1. Hemorrhage into a bullous lesion in the right lower lobe in a patient with a tendency to excessive bleeding secondary to coumarin therapy.

a hematoma, and pleural hematomas (39). In a review of chest roentgenograms, abnormalities were recorded in 26 of 33 adult hemophiliacs; scarring, fibrosis, and pleural thickening were seen in 12 cases; and abnormalities of pulmonary vessels were seen in the remaining 14, of whom four had evidence of hyperinflation (40). Several cases of primary pulmonary hypertension have been described in patients receiving factor VIII infusions (41).

Disseminated Intravascular Coagulation

Pulmonary hemorrhage occurs in patients with disseminated intravascular coagulation and other coagulopathies (42). The incidence of pulmonary hemorrhage is estimated to be approximately 14% in disseminated intravascular coagulation. Often, the hemorrhage is subclinical, with no or very little hemoptysis and patchy, nondescript lung infiltrates. Massive bleeding is uncommon. The pulmonary hemorrhage syndrome shares features with the adult respiratory distress syndrome, such as hyaline membrane formation and pulmonary hypoperfusion. Thrombocytopenia has been shown to lead to the development of pulmonary hematoma, hemothorax, and fatal pulmonary hemorrhage.

Pulmonary infarction has been described in several patients with disseminated intravascular coagulation (43). Thromboembolism and hemorrhage are the main pathologic findings in the lungs of patients dying with disseminated intravascular coagulation. In a postmortem comparative study of 87 patients whose illnesses had been complicated by disseminated intravascular coagulation and 64 control patients, thromboembolism was observed in 51 (59%), infarction in six, hemorrhage in 14, microscopic fibrin thrombosis in 43

(49%), and microthromboembolism in 45 (52%) of the patients with disseminated intravascular coagulation (44). The frequency of pulmonary infarction increased in proportion to the frequency of thromboembolism. In the control group, macroscopic thromboembolism was identified in 20 cases (31%).

MYELOPROLIFERATIVE DISORDERS

Leukemia

Pulmonary involvement in leukemia occurs more often than is usually suspected (45). The reported mortality rate associated with pulmonary complications in leukemia is approximately 60% to 65%. The respiratory complications depend on the type of leukemia, the nature and course of the treatment, and the presence or absence of significant neutropenia (46). Many of the complications, particularly infections, are secondary to the immunocompromised status of leukemic patients, which is caused either by the leukemic state itself or by treatment.

Infectious pneumonia is a frequent and often fatal complication and is responsible for up to 75% of deaths in patients with acute leukemia. In a series of 68 leukemic patients with pulmonary infiltrates, 82% of the focal and 35% of the diffuse infiltrates had an infectious cause. Gram-negative organisms are the most common cause of pneumonia. Fungal pneumonia occurs in up to 30% of patients. *Pneumocystis carinii* pneumonia occurs less often in adults than in children with acute leukemia (47). In a review of 53 cases of *P. carinii* pneumonia, including four in children, leukemia was the underlying hematologic disorder in 28% (48). In another study, 52 episodes of pneumonia were recorded in 68 leukemic patients; Gram-negative bacilli caused most of the pneumonias, with a 25% incidence of fungal pneumonia. The overall mortality was 65%. In childhood leukemia, viruses are more important as respiratory pathogens and are major causes of morbidity.

Granulocytopenia, hypogammaglobulinemia, and lymphocytic bronchitis in graft versus host disease may follow bone marrow transplantation and predispose patients to infectious complications (see Chapter 56). Granulocytopenia in leukemic patients poses a significant risk for invasive aspergillosis and acute respiratory distress syndrome; invasive pulmonary aspergillosis is a life-threatening complication (49,50). The risk for the development of invasive aspergillosis is directly proportional to the duration of granulocytopenia (49). The rate of bone marrow recovery markedly influences the clinical and roentgenographic course of the disease. In patients with acute leukemia, granulocytopenia persisting longer than 3 weeks is the major risk factor for the development of this life-threatening infection. In a study of such patients, granulocyte recovery, with counts exceeding 500/mm^3, was followed by cavitary pulmonary aspergillosis in 73%. Fungal infections develop in nearly one third of the patients with malignancies who receive empiric antibiotic therapy during episodes of granulocytopenia (49). Massive hemoptysis may occur in some patients. The prognosis has been uniformly poor, with mortality rates exceeding 70% in some series. A study reported that aspergillosis can be diagnosed early in leukemic patients on chemotherapy by computed tomography (CT), which reveals a characteristic progression from multiple fluffy masses to cavitation or air crescent formation.

Zygomycosis (mucormycosis) of the lung is another serious fungal infection in severely neutropenic patients. However, it also occurs in patients without neutropenia and in patients who have undergone bone marrow transplantation long after hospital discharge. In a 17-year series of 1,500 consecutive patients with bone marrow transplants, mucormycosis developed in 13 (0.9%)—10 with allogeneic and three with autologous transplants. Seven patients were neutropenic (51). Six infections developed within 90 days after transplantation, and six occurred at or within several days of autopsy. The sites of infection were the lung and brain in four patients, the sinonasal region in three, the lung in two, and the lung and kidney in one. Two patients had disseminated infection. Death from mucormycosis occurred in 10 (77%) of the 13 patients.

Hypogammaglobulinemia, related to inherent abnormalities of B-lymphocyte function and T-cell imbalances, is present in approximately 50% of patients with chronic lymphocytic leukemia. Infections, particularly with encapsulated microorganisms, are a frequent cause of morbidity and mortality.

Hairy cell leukemia is an unusual hematologic malignancy that may be associated with splenomegaly, pancytopenia, and circulating mononuclear cells with prominent cytoplasmic projections (52). Infections are secondary to granulocytopenia and defects in cell-mediated immunity. Bacterial, fungal, and mycobacterial infections develop frequently. Disseminated infections caused by *Mycobacterium kansasii* and *Mycobacterium avium* complex occur in patients with hairy cell leukemia.

Autopsy studies have revealed that noninfectious intrathoracic involvement by leukemia is a common late development. Mediastinal and hilar adenopathy is seen in 50% of cases, and the pulmonary parenchyma is affected in approximately 25%. Acute myelogenous leukemias cause pulmonary parenchymal leukemic infiltrates more commonly than the chronic forms, but among the chronic group, lymphocytic leukemia is more likely than the granulocytic type to invade the pulmonary parenchyma (Figs. 57.2 and 57.3). The usual roentgenographic abnormality within the pulmonary parenchyma is a diffuse bilateral reticulonodular infiltration resembling that of lymphangitic metastasis (Fig. 57.4). This is not uncommon in the terminal stages of leukemia. However, several cases of acute leukemia presenting with diffuse pulmonary infiltrates and respiratory failure have been described. As previously noted, the presence of diffuse lung infiltrates in a patient who is granulocytopenic should warn of the possibility of invasive aspergillosis (Fig. 57.5). Rapidly progressive pulmonary infiltration has been noted as a major clinical problem in chronic myelogenous leukemia. The leukemic infiltrates may be parenchymal (focal or diffuse), pleural, peribronchial, or endobronchial. In the Richter transformation, chronic lymphocytic leukemia may convert from a low-grade histologic pattern to high-grade non-Hodgkin lymphoma and cause hilar or mediastinal lymphadenopathy. Pleural effusion, usually unilateral, is seen in up to 25% of cases.

Pulmonary alveolar hemorrhage is often found at autopsy in leukemic patients. In a necropsy study of 50 patients with acute leukemia, pulmonary hemorrhage was recorded in 54% and leukemic pulmonary infiltrates in 64%. Pulmonary hemorrhage is usually associated with thrombocytopenia

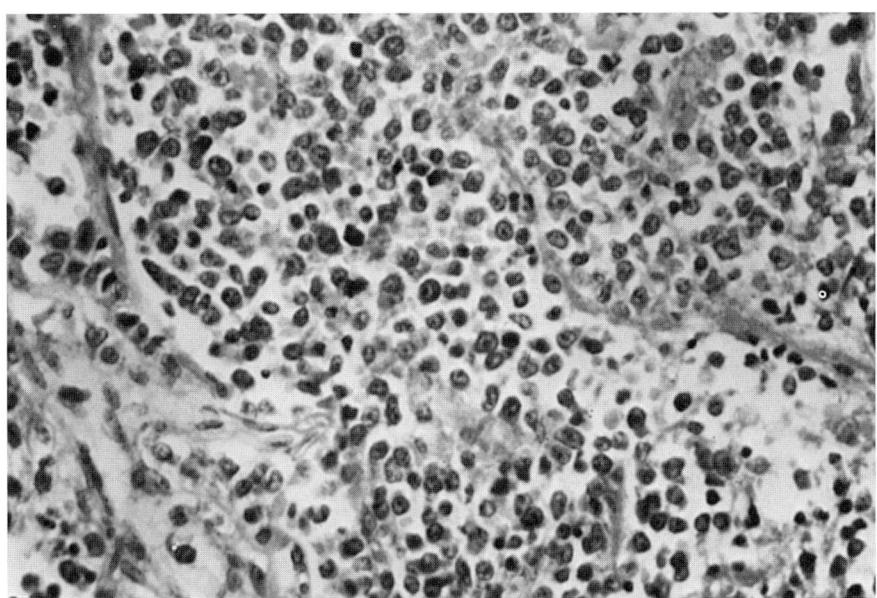

FIGURE 57.2. Pulmonary infiltration by acute granulocytic leukemia.

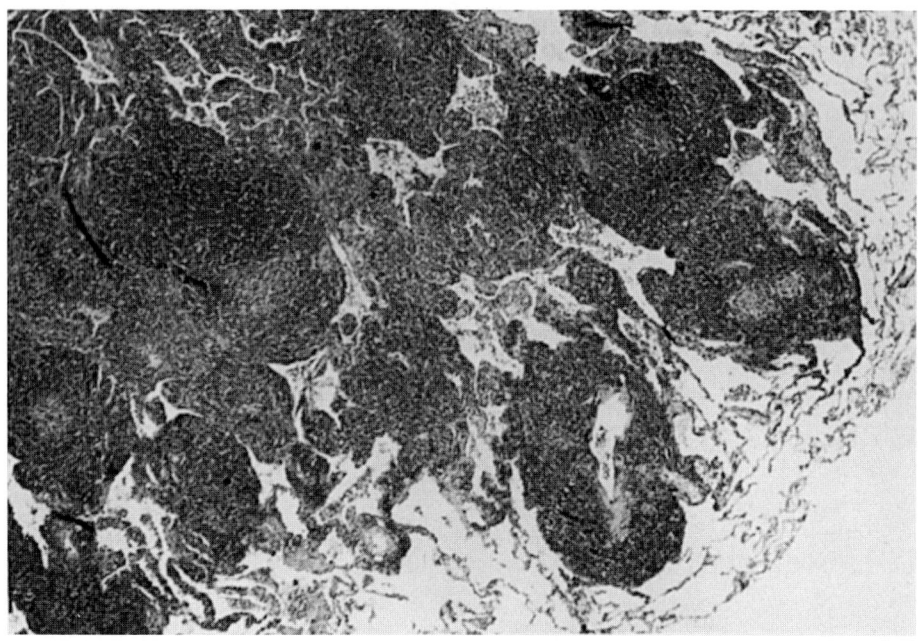

FIGURE 57.3. Pulmonary involvement by chronic lymphocytic leukemia. A dense infiltrate of small lymphocytes can be seen around vessels and in alveolar septa.

and may be extensive. Another predisposing factor is invasive pulmonary aspergillosis. Most patients with pulmonary alveolar hemorrhage do not have hemoptysis.

The term *hyperleukocytosis* denotes peripheral white blood cell counts in excess of 50,000/mm³ (53). This condition has the potential to cause pulmonary leukostasis, which is a serious and frequently fatal complication. Pulmonary leukostasis usually occurs in patients with acute granulocytic leukemias. A clinicopathologic study of 16 leukemic patients with circulating leukocytes counts below 50,000/mm³ and pulmonary

leukostasis concluded that hyperleukocytosis per se cannot be the cause of pulmonary leukostasis but that other factors, such as circulating blasts and the affinity of neoplastic cells for the pulmonary endothelium, may be related to the development of acute respiratory distress (54). Leukemic cell lysis pneumopathy, which develops as a result of pulmonary vascular occlusion by destroyed leukemic cells within 48 hours after the initiation of chemotherapy, may cause respiratory failure. Acute respiratory failure in patients with hematologic disorders is a life-threatening condition. Irrespective of the cause of acute respiratory failure in this group

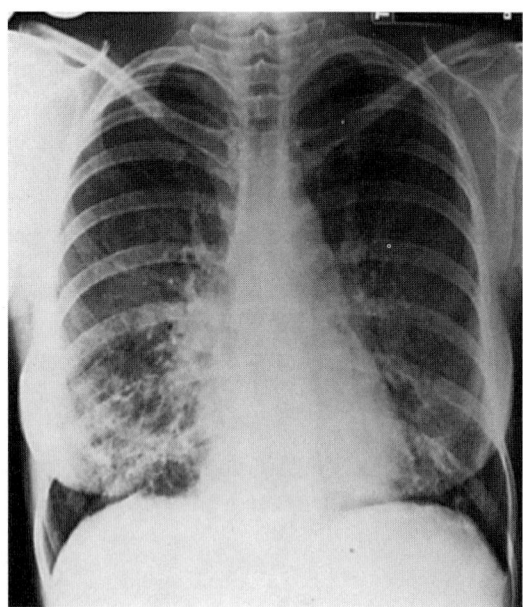

FIGURE 57.4. Leukemic infiltrates in the lower lobes of both lungs in a patient with acute monomyelocytic leukemia.

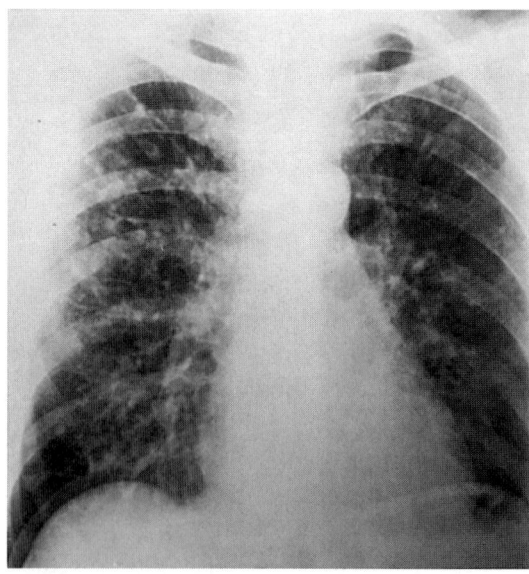

FIGURE 57.5. Diffuse nodular-reticular opacities in a severely granulocytopenic patient on chemotherapy for acute monomyelocytic leukemia.

of patients, the outcome is dismal, with a mortality rate of 80%.

Granulocyte colony-stimulating factor, by augmenting leukocyte production, the pulmonary sequestration of white blood cells, and the margination and production of toxic oxygen radicals, may exacerbate underlying subclinical pulmonary toxic effects of bleomycin. In a series of 12 patients with aggressive non-Hodgkin lymphoma who received chemotherapy that included bleomycin in combination with recombinant human granulocyte colony-stimulating factor, three of four patients in whom a rapidly progressive pneumonic illness developed died; no infection was detected. The lung abnormalities were characterized by diffuse infiltrates and hypoxemia (55). Caution should be exercised when granulocyte-stimulating factors are included in bleomycin-containing regimens.

All-*trans* retinoic acid induces complete remission in most cases of acute promyelocytic leukemia. Its use, however, is associated with potentially fatal pulmonary toxicity in approximately 25% of patients in the setting of a rapidly rising peripheral leukocyte count (56). A prospective multicenter study has shown the efficacy of oral corticosteroid in preventing pulmonary toxicity from retinoic acid.

In patients with leukemia, lung biopsy may suggest areas of pulmonary alveolar phospholipoproteinosis. This is secondary to the monocytopenia of leukemia. Alveolar macrophages are derived from monocytes, and the deficiency of monocytes in leukemia results in an inability of the limited number of alveolar macrophages to ingest intraalveolar phospholipids. In addition, opportunistic infections and cytotoxic drugs may affect the alveolar clearance of phospholipids and cause patchy areas of secondary pulmonary alveolar phospholipoproteinosis. However, this finding is clinically insignificant, and chest roentgenograms may or may not show patchy areas of alveolar infiltrates.

In pseudohypoxemia, or spurious hypoxemia ("leukocyte larceny"), the oxygen tension and saturation in arterial blood are low without clinical evidence of tissue hypoxia. This phenomenon occurs in patients with extreme degrees of leukocytosis. During the *in vitro* transportation of an arterial blood sample from the patient to the laboratory, the large numbers of leukocytes in the syringe consume significant amounts of oxygen, so that the measurement indicates a low PaO_2. Pseudohypoxemia is also seen in patients with severe thrombocytosis.

Polycythemia

Defined as a sustained excess of red blood cell volume, polycythemia occurs in either a primary or a secondary form (57,58). Secondary polycythemia is a compensatory mechanism seen in various chronic hypoxemic states. The pulmonary manifestations in patients with such diseases are those of the underlying disease.

Primary polycythemia, or polycythemia rubra vera, is a chronic disease of unknown cause characterized by hyperplasia of all the cellular elements of the bone marrow, the nucleated red blood cells being more prominently involved. The chest roentgenographic abnormalities consist of accentuated vascular markings and minor infiltrates, and occasionally nodular lesions in the mid lung zones. Thrombosis, stasis, or infarction in the pulmonary veins is believed to cause discrete lesions. Other abnormal roentgenographic findings include enlargement of the hilar vessels and passive pulmonary congestion. The symptoms are those of pulmonary insufficiency resulting from pulmonary edema. Acute airway obstruction caused by spontaneous retropharyngeal bleeding and hematoma formation has been described in a patient with polycythemia rubra vera.

A normal arterial oxygen saturation ($SaO_2 > 92\%$) is regarded as one of the features that differentiate polycythemia vera from the secondary (hypoxemic) form because almost all patients with primary polycythemia have a normal arterial oxygen saturation. However, mild degrees of desaturation may occur in otherwise well-documented polycythemia vera in the absence of cardiopulmonary problems. The pathogenesis of this desaturation is not apparent.

Pulmonary function studies have shown that the vital capacity, airway resistance, and alveolar ventilation are usually normal in patients with polycythemia vera. The diffusing capacity of the lung for carbon monoxide may be slightly increased. This, however, is an inconsistent finding. The pulmonary capillary blood volume and the size of the pulmonary vascular bed may be reduced in some patients, resulting in ventilation-perfusion abnormalities.

LYMPHOPROLIFERATIVE DISORDERS

Hodgkin Disease

Intrathoracic involvement in Hodgkin disease is common, occurring in up to 40% of patients, especially in those with advanced stage IIIB or IV disease. Pulmonary involvement may be seen in more than 50% of cases of Hodgkin lymphoma at autopsy. Intrathoracic involvement is twice as common in Hodgkin as in non-Hodgkin lymphoma (59–62).

Primary pulmonary Hodgkin disease is a distinct entity and denotes involvement of the lung without hilar adenopathy or disseminated disease (63,64). Fewer than 100 cases of pulmonary Hodgkin disease have been reported. This form of Hodgkin lymphoma is more common in women, typically involves upper lung fields, and may appear as a solitary mass or a multinodular process with or without cavitation. Thoracic CT is now recommended for all new patients for its greater accuracy in the detection of parenchymal abnormalities, pericardial involvement, chest wall involvement, and retrocardiac nodes, especially in patients with mediastinal Hodgkin disease (65,66); it can eliminate false-positive findings (66,67). Almost any type of chest roentgenographic

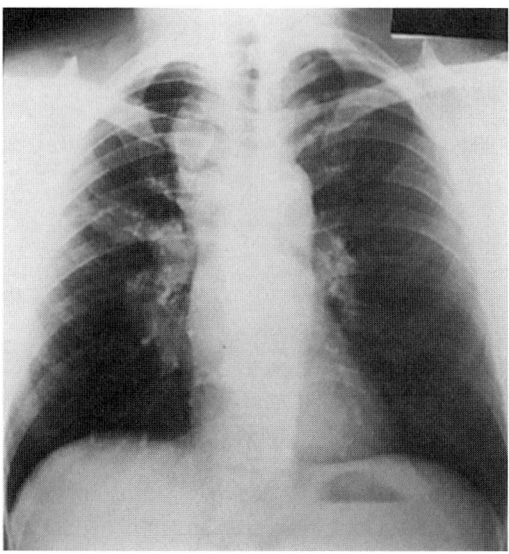

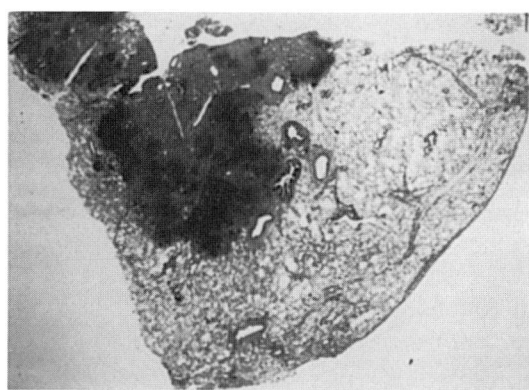

FIGURE 57.8. Hodgkin lymphoma presenting as a localized nodular lesion. The histologic pattern was nodular sclerosing Hodgkin lymphoma. Some of the darker nodules of lymphoid tissue appear to be surrounded by a paler fibrous tissue, indicative of a nodular sclerosing pattern.

FIGURE 57.6. Bilateral hilar and right paratracheal lymphadenopathy caused by Hodgkin lymphoma.

abnormality can be seen in patients with thoracic manifestations of Hodgkin disease. However, the most common abnormality is enlargement of the mediastinal lymph nodes, noted in 50% of cases. Bilateral lymph node enlargement is common, particularly when the paratracheal nodes are involved (Fig. 57.6). The retrosternal nodes, posterior mediastinal nodes, and diaphragmatic group of parietal lymph nodes may also be enlarged. Intrapulmonary lymph node involvement may not be visible on the chest roentgenogram (Fig. 57.7).

Pulmonary parenchymal involvement is seen in up to 30% of patients (Figs. 57.8–57.10), especially those with the nodular sclerosing type of Hodgkin disease, and is usually accompanied by mediastinal lymphadenopathy. In a study of 112 patients with advanced Hodgkin disease, more than 25% were found to have parenchymal disease without lymphadenopathy. The parenchymal features include direct invasion of the lung from regional lymph nodes (characterized by linear, feathery densities), massive homogeneous infil-

trates with lymphadenopathy, nodular infiltrates, and generalized dissemination resembling miliary tuberculosis. Pulmonary parenchymal involvement is ordinarily caused by direct extension from mediastinal nodes along the lymphatics of bronchovascular sheaths. Cavities may develop in the parenchymal masses; usually, these are multiple and located in the lower lobes. Cavitation of pulmonary nodules is rare in Hodgkin disease and has been noted in approximately 55 cases.

Endobronchial involvement occurs in nearly 5% of patients with Hodgkin lymphoma. Lobar or segmental atelectasis, cough, and hemoptysis may result. Bronchial mucosal involvement with non-Hodgkin lymphoma may become severe enough to cause airflow obstruction. Extrinsic compression of the trachea and main bronchi by large mediastinal Hodgkin lymphomas can lead to airway obstruction and respiratory failure. Patients may experience varying degrees of dyspnea in the supine position.

Several cases of the development of acute airway obstruction and respiratory failure during general anesthesia have been described. During general anesthesia, the extrinsic airway compression is exacerbated by diminished lung volumes secondary to reduced inspiratory muscle tone, relaxation of bronchial smooth muscle tone and resultant compressibility of the airway, reduction in the expiratory flow rate, and severely diminished movement of the diaphragm. Pulmonary function tests performed in 43 patients with Hodgkin disease before mantle irradiation (total dose, 36–42 Gy) and at 3, 6, 9, 12, and 15 or more months thereafter revealed only small variations in the functional indices. More than 5 years after therapy, respiratory symptoms and reductions in lung function develop in nearly one third of otherwise healthy survivors of Hodgkin disease (68). Women are at significant risk for pulmonary complications following therapy for Hodgkin disease (68).

Pleural effusion occurs in 30% of patients and is usually associated with other intrathoracic lesions. The main factor

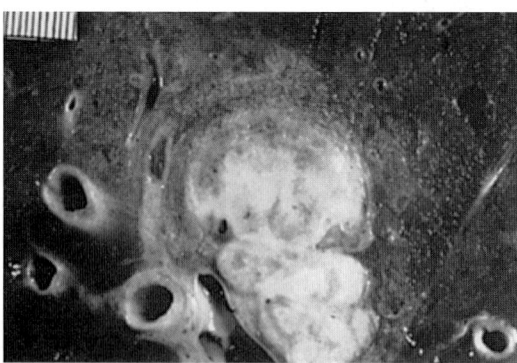

FIGURE 57.7. Involvement of an intrapulmonary peribronchial lymph node by Hodgkin lymphoma, found at autopsy.

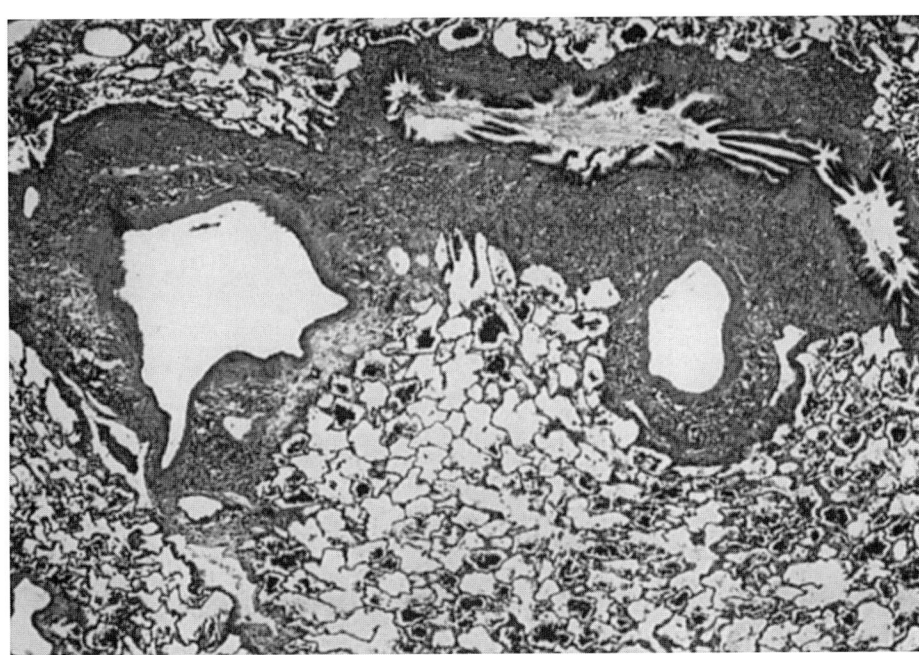

FIGURE 57.9. Hodgkin lymphoma in the lung as part of disseminated disease at presentation. The lung infiltrates were caused by a cellular proliferation around vessels and airways with the cytologic features of Hodgkin lymphoma.

responsible for the collection of pleural fluid is obstruction of the lymphatics by enlarged hilar lymph nodes. The pleural fluid is commonly an exudate, serous, and chylous in one third. Chylothorax is the accumulation of chyle in the pleural space secondary to disruption of the thoracic duct or a major lymphatic tributary. Intrathoracic malignancy is the most common cause of chylothorax, and lymphoproliferative disorders are responsible 75% of the time (69). In a study of 38 patients with chylous effusions, the effusions were caused by lymphomas in 20 of them. Diagnostic thoracentesis and needle biopsy of the pleura may aid in determining whether the pleural space or pleura is involved with

Hodgkin or non-Hodgkin lymphoma. However, the clinical correlation is extremely important in interpreting cytologic preparations. In one report, pleural biopsy was helpful in diagnosing non-Hodgkin lymphoma in 9 of 10 patients. In contrast, a large series demonstrated that the finding of lymphocytic pleuritis on a biopsy specimen or lymphocytosis in pleural fluid was nondiagnostic and that a clinical correlation was essential to confirm the diagnosis. Massive pleural effusions have occurred as a late complication of radiation therapy for Hodgkin lymphoma, probably as a consequence of impaired lymphatic drainage secondary to mediastinal fibrosis induced by radiation.

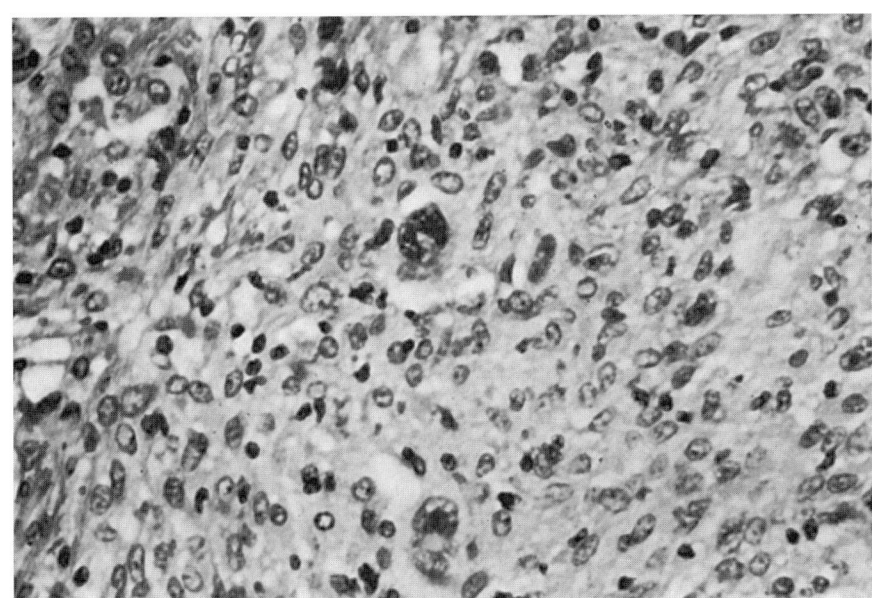

FIGURE 57.10. Hodgkin lymphoma replacing normal lung parenchyma. A Reed-Sternberg cell is at the center.

Spontaneous pneumothorax is an unusual complication of Hodgkin disease (70,71). One study noted 17 episodes of pneumothorax in eight patients, seven with Hodgkin lymphoma and one with non-Hodgkin lymphoma. The observed incidence of pneumothorax among 1,977 patients with lymphoma was 10-fold higher than expected; this finding included a significantly higher incidence in patients younger than 30 years in comparison with those older than 30 years, and a higher incidence in patients with Hodgkin lymphoma than in those with non-Hodgkin lymphoma. The study suggested a strong relationship between radiation and pneumothorax. Pneumothorax associated with lymphoma is more complex and difficult to manage. Other unusual manifestations include involvement of the thoracic cage and diaphragmatic paralysis.

Non-Hodgkin Lymphoma

The most common intrathoracic manifestation of non-Hodgkin lymphoma is mediastinal lymph node enlargement, which is seen in nearly 35% of patients. Primary pulmonary lymphoma ordinarily presents as an alveolar infiltrate or a homogeneous mass. Bronchial obstruction or endobronchial involvement occurs, but less frequently than in Hodgkin lymphoma.

When the lung is involved by non-Hodgkin lymphoma, the typical roentgenographic pattern is one of solitary or multiple nodules 3 mm to several centimeters in diameter that are more frequent in the lower lobes. Other manifestations are similar to those of Hodgkin disease. Endobronchial recurrence of non-Hodgkin lymphoma can be seen in patients who are unresponsive to therapy. Diagnostic BAL provides specimens for lymphocyte subtyping and the classification of lymphoma.

Pleural effusions are common in non-Hodgkin lymphoma. An indolent lymphoma may cause a chylous pleural effusion. Of 26 pleural effusions associated with non-Hodgkin lymphomas, 20 were exudative and five were chylous. The results of cytologic examination were positive in 86% of the exudative effusions, whereas 61% of pleural biopsy specimens were positive for the disease. In a study of 19 patients with pleural effusion caused by non-Hodgkin lymphoma, pleural tissue disclosed lymphoma in 17 patients, supporting the contention that pleural effusion in patients with non-Hodgkin lymphoma is usually secondary to pleural lymphoma rather than to obstruction of the mediastinal lymphatics. Systemic chemotherapy results in resolution of pleural effusion in approximately half of the patients; the prognosis is poor for those with a refractory effusion.

Patients treated for Hodgkin or non-Hodgkin lymphoma should be observed for the appearance of other hematologic and solid neoplasms because they accrue a relative risk two to three times that of the normal population for the development of newer malignancies. Patients with Hodgkin disease who receive supradiaphragmatic irradiation or com-

bined modality therapy may be at higher risk for the development of non–small cell lung cancer (72,73). In a study of such patients, the risk ratio for the development of lung cancer among patients with Hodgkin disease was 5.6 times that expected in the general population. The median age at the diagnosis of Hodgkin disease was 39 years, and at the diagnosis of lung cancer, it was 45 years. The interval between the diagnosis of Hodgkin disease and that of metachronous lung cancer averaged 7 years but appeared to vary inversely with age.

Primary Lymphoma of the Lung

Primary lymphomas of the lung are rare, comprising fewer than 1% of all primary pulmonary malignancies. They usually are well-differentiated B-cell tumors of the immunoglobulin M (IgM) type, although a few cases of IgG and IgA types have been described. Of 62 cases of primary lymphoma of the lung, 58 were B-cell type and two T-cell type; two other cases could not be classified. The largest group (43 cases) were low-grade B-cell lymphomas of bronchus-associated lymphoid tissue (BALT). The histologic features were similar to those of low-grade B-cell lymphoma of mucosa-associated lymphoid tissue (MALT) of the stomach. BALT hyperplasia can vary from multifocal proliferations that arise in and remain in the airway walls (follicular hyperplasia of BALT) to solitary masses or nodules (nodular lymphoid hyperplasia of BALT, or pseudolymphoma) to multifocal or diffuse lymphoid hyperplasia of BALT (lymphoid interstitial pneumonitis).

The definitive diagnosis of primary pulmonary lymphoma rests on the typical histopathologic and immunochemical staining pattern. The peak occurrence of low-grade lymphomas is in the sixth decade of life, whereas high-grade lymphomas occur most often in the seventh decade. A slight male predominance has been noted. Nearly 75% of patients with low-grade B-cell lymphoma of BALT have solitary or multiple sharply defined lung nodules. The prognosis is favorable in those without systemic symptoms.

Most primary extranodal lymphomas (not to be confused with primary lymphoma of lung) originate in MALT, and the term *maltoma* has been applied to them. Maltomas appear to carry a good prognosis. In a study of 161 cases of non-Hodgkin lymphoma and pseudolymphoma of the lung, lymphomas were noted in 32%—plasmacytoid lymphocytic lymphomas in 22% and small cleaved follicular center cell lymphomas in 12%. The remainder were follicular center cell lymphomas and B-immunoblastic sarcomas. Most of the patients were elderly and asymptomatic, and in most cases, a solitary nodule or infiltrate was seen on the chest roentgenogram. Hilar lymphadenopathy was also observed.

Mycosis Fungoides and Sézary Syndrome

The cutaneous T-cell lymphomas encompass a spectrum of diseases, including mycosis fungoides and Sézary syndrome, characterized by the malignant proliferation of pheno-typically mature T lymphocytes with a propensity to infiltrate the skin (74). Microscopic infiltration of the lung parenchyma occurs in 43% to 56% of cases. Lung biopsy and sometimes the sputum cytology show distinctive large and small mononuclear cells with indented cerebriform and hyperchromatic nuclei. Lymphadenopathy precedes visceral involvement. Pulmonary manifestations may include diffuse basilar infiltrates, nodular densities, perihilar densities, pneumonic processes, consolidative lesions, and pleural effusions (75,76). Hemoptysis and hypoxemia are described. Rapid pulmonary dissemination can occur in Sézary syndrome.

Lymphomatoid Granulomatosis (Angiocentric T-cell Lymphoma)

Lymphomatoid granulomatosis is also known as *angiocentric T-cell lymphoma, polymorphic reticulosis, midline malignant reticulosis, midline granuloma,* and *Stewart granuloma.* Even though clinically and roentgenologically lymphomatoid granulomatosis mimics Wegener granulomatosis and is frequently discussed in the context of the vasculitides, lymphomatoid granulomatosis is a lymphoproliferative disorder, not a primary vasculitis (see Chapter 30). Similarities have been noted in the histologic patterns of lymphomatoid granulomatosis and Epstein-Barr virus (EBV)–associated lymphoproliferative disease involving the lung (77). EBV has also been identified by polymerase chain reaction in most cases of pulmonary lymphomatoid granulomatosis. It appears that some cases of lymphomatoid granulomatosis represent B-cell lymphoma associated with EBV infection, whereas others (perhaps those limited to head and neck region) are of T-cell origin and are probably unrelated to EBV infection (78,79).

However, because of the similarity between lymphomatoid granulomatosis and nasal angiocentric lymphoma, the term *angiocentric immunoproliferative lesion* has been proposed for both entities.

Morphologically, lymphomatoid granulomatosis is a destructive angiocentric process characterized by prominent vascular infiltrates and necrosis of medium and small blood vessels with granuloma formation (Fig. 57.11). The histologic features often range from benign-appearing lymphocytic interstitial pneumonitis to overtly malignant lymphoma in the same patient. Progression to non-Hodgkin T-cell lymphoma occurs in more than 50% of patients.

The disease usually presents during middle age, and the prevalence is slightly higher in men. The presenting symptoms are nonspecific and include fever, malaise, and weight loss. Lymphomatoid granulomatosis can affect any organ system, but it is found most frequently in the central nervous system, skin, kidney, and lymphatic system. The central nervous system is involved in nearly one fourth of patients. Ataxia, hemiparesis, blindness, and dizziness are the presenting symptoms. In almost half of patients with lymphomatoid granulomatosis, skin lesions in the form of erythematous, macular, or plaquelike lesions develop on the extremities. Laboratory tests are not helpful in the diagnosis. The diagnosis of lymphomatoid granulomatosis requires a biopsy examination of affected tissue, usually lesions of the lung, skin, or head and neck.

Pulmonary Disease

The lungs are involved in virtually all patients with lymphomatoid granulomatosis. Along with the systemic symptoms, cough and dyspnea are prominent respiratory

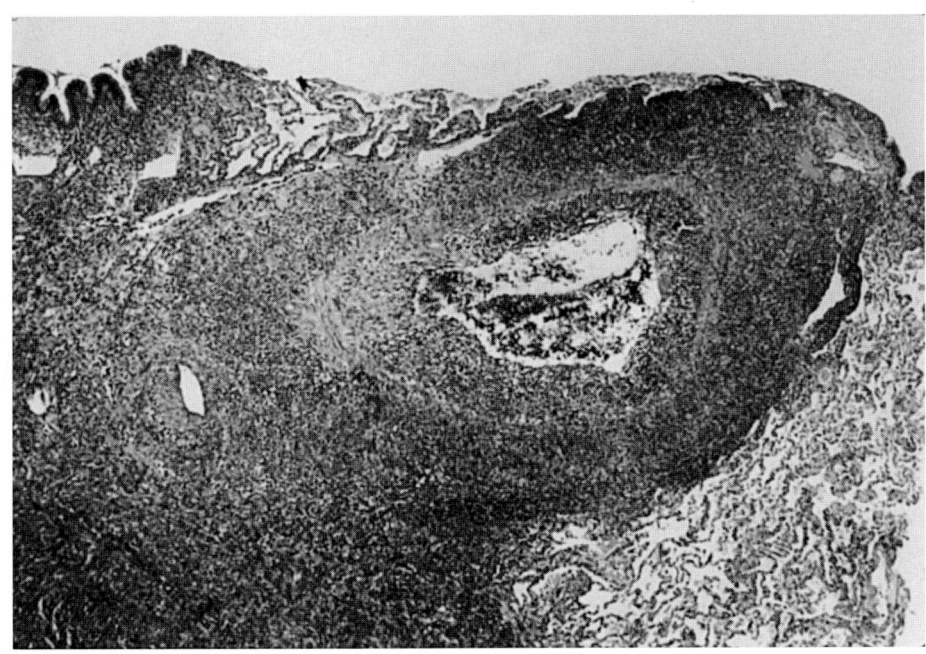

FIGURE 57.11. Lymphomatoid granulomatosis showing angiocentric infiltration by dense lymphoid infiltrates. Cytologically, this case had features of a diffuse large cell lymphoma.

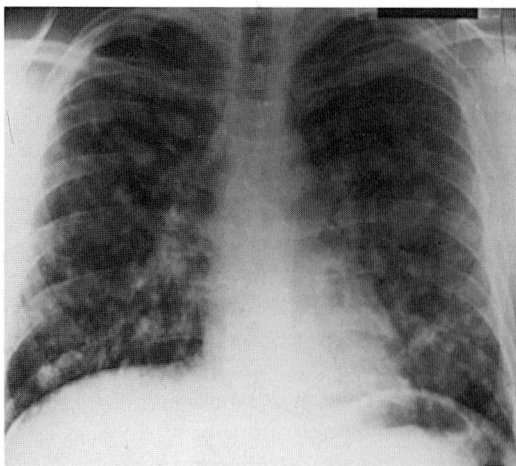

FIGURE 57.12. Bilateral multiple nodular lesions in lymphomatoid granulomatosis.

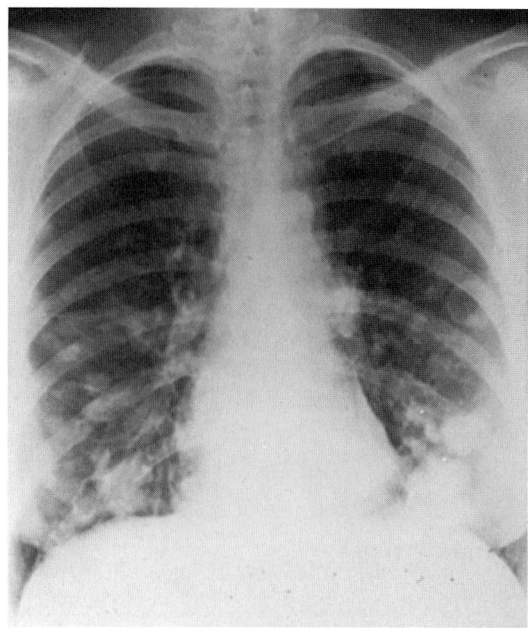

FIGURE 57.13. Bilateral multiple nodules of varying sizes in lymphomatoid granulomatosis. Several nodules are cavitated.

symptoms. If areas of the head and neck are involved, patients may present with symptoms similar to those of Wegener granulomatosis. Hemoptysis is more likely in those with cavitated lung lesions. Chest roentgenograms most frequently disclose nodular infiltrates. Nodular densities may cavitate and are more common in the lower lung zones. In one series, multiple nodules with poorly defined borders were observed in 88% of patients, with cavitation in 25%. Occasionally, alveolar infiltrates are noted. Pleural effusions occur in 25% of patients. One review of 173 patients collected from two separate series noted the following chest roentgenologic abnormalities: multiple bilateral nodules in 80% of patients, cavitation of nodules in 30%, air bronchograms in 35%, pleural effusion in 33%, atelectasis in 30%, pneumonitis or masslike lesions in 30%, and pneumothorax in 5% (Figs. 57.12 and 57.13).

The presence of hilar or mediastinal lymphadenopathy usually signifies lymphomatous transformation. Unilateral or bilateral large pulmonary masses measuring more than 10 cm in diameter often signal the presence of lymphoma.

Airway involvement is unusual but can be extensive. Pathologic findings described include bronchiolitis obliterans, bronchial ulceration, and destruction and occlusion of bronchioles by masses of inflammatory cells and fibrous tissue.

Treatment and Prognosis

No definitive therapy is available for lymphomatoid granulomatosis. In most patients, a therapeutic approach similar to that for highly malignant lymphoma must be considered. Adequate clinical staging and multiple biopsies for a correct assessment of the degree of malignancy are necessary before therapy with multiple drugs can be started. Multiple chemotherapeutic agents with a corticosteroid may be required for patients with highly malignant features. Preliminary reports indicate that interferon-α2b is effective (80).

Localized lesions in the head and neck may respond to radiation. Progressive respiratory involvement, usually with lymphoma and related complications, is the most frequent cause of death. Fever, leukopenia, cutaneous anergy, and hepatomegaly are considered poor prognostic indicators.

Pseudolymphoma

Lymphoid tumors that do not fulfill the criteria for malignant lesions have been called *pseudolymphomas,* although many pseudolymphomas have been reclassified as indolent, well-differentiated lymphocytic and lymphoplasmacytic lymphomas on the basis of immunologic proof of clonality (81). In a study of 161 cases of primary non-Hodgkin lymphoma of the lung, pseudolymphoma was observed in 14%. Pseudolymphoma of the lung is characterized pathologically by a mixed cellular infiltrate (mostly mature lymphocytes), germinal centers, and regional lymph nodes free of lymphoma. Nonetheless, it often is difficult to distinguish between pulmonary pseudolymphoma, lymphoma, and other lymphoid neoplasms and infiltrates by simple histologic examination. Pulmonary manifestations consist of well-delineated nodules, segmental parenchymal consolidation, or diffuse interstitial infiltration. Localized lesions are best treated by resection, whereas patients with diffuse lesions may require immunosuppressive therapy.

Angioimmunoblastic Lymphadenopathy

Angioimmunoblastic lymphadenopathy mimics lymphoma. In this disorder, the lymph node architecture is diffusely obliterated by a proliferation of small vessels and immunoblasts. Both an autoimmune mechanism and a T-cell defect leading to polyclonal B-cell activation may be responsible. The disease is systemic, and the histopathologic features appear benign, although progression to lymphoma can occur. Angioimmunoblastic lymphadenopathy usually presents as generalized lymphadenopathy with hepatosplenomegaly and constitutional symptoms and mimics Hodgkin disease. Differentiating features include polyclonal gammopathy, autoimmune hemolytic anemia, and a predilection for men older than 50 years. The chest roentgenographic features are similar to those of Hodgkin disease—namely, hilar lymphadenopathy, interstitial infiltrates, and pleural effusion (82). Obstruction of the superior vena cava has been described.

Castleman Disease

Originally reported as mediastinal lymph node hyperplasia resembling thymoma, Castleman disease is also described by other terms, including *angiofollicular lymph node hyperplasia, giant lymph node hyperplasia, lymph node hamartoma, benign giant lymphoma,* and *multifollicular lymph node hyperplasia.* The two histologic types of Castleman disease are the hyaline-vascular type (proliferation of hyalinized blood vessels) and the plasma cell type (abundance of plasma cells) (83). The former accounts for 90% of cases and is usually asymptomatic, whereas the latter is associated with systemic manifestations. The disease shows no predilection for any age or race or for either sex. It develops in the thoracic cage in up to 70% of cases. The most common clinical manifestation is a well-defined and lobulated enlargement of the anterior mediastinal lymph nodes adjacent to the thymus and tracheobronchial tree. The symptoms result from compression of the tracheobronchial tree by enlarged lymph nodes and may include cough, dyspnea, and hemoptysis. Intrapulmonary lesions, nodules, and pleural effusion are uncommon (84). CT shows vascular lesions that are well rounded and lobulated. Surgical resection is curative if the disease is limited to resectable lymph nodes.

Cases of paraneoplastic pemphigus with pulmonary involvement have been reported. These have most often been associated with Castleman tumor (85–95). Pulmonary involvement occurs in about 30% of patients with paraneoplastic pemphigus (96). The disease process can directly affect the tracheobronchial tree because the pathogenic autoantibodies against plakin proteins are known to be associated with or induce injury to the epithelium in large and small airways (96). This causes constrictive bronchiolitis that results in severe lung impairment, respiratory failure, and death.

Lymphocytic Interstitial Pneumonitis

Lymphocytic interstitial pneumonitis is characterized by pulmonary parenchymal infiltrates that consist predominantly of small lymphocytes and variable numbers of plasma cells and transformed lymphocytes. Lymphomas develop in many patients with lymphocytic interstitial pneumonitis. Indeed, all cases of lymphocytic interstitial pneumonitis are thought to represent low-grade lymphomas. It is not clear whether the lymphocytic infiltrative lung diseases are premalignant, initially neoplastic, or caused by a hypersensitivity reaction with subsequent development of neoplasia. They comprise a poorly defined group that includes lymphocytic interstitial pneumonitis, immunoblastic lymphadenopathy, plasma cell interstitial pneumonitis, lymphomatoid granulomatosis, and benign lymphocytic angiitis and granulomatosis. The diseases associated with lymphocytic interstitial pneumonitis are listed in Table 57.2. Many of them have similar histologic features, but involvement of the central nervous system, skin, kidneys, and lymph nodes beyond the thorax varies, and the course may be slow or rapidly fatal.

The occurrence of lymphocytic interstitial pneumonitis in patients with AIDS is well recognized. It also occurs frequently in the children of mothers who are at high risk for the development of AIDS.

Low-grade lymphoid malignancies respond well to therapy. The treatments, however, may lead to acute, subacute, or chronic pulmonary complications. A literature analysis of 2,269 patients with low-grade lymphoid malignancies who received more than 7,547 cycles of fludarabine noted the development of opportunistic infections in 3% of the patients; 97% of these were in patients who had been pretreated with alkylating regimens or corticosteroids, and 45 (2%) were of respiratory origin and associated with a 56% mortality rate (97).

TABLE 57.2. DIFFERENTIAL DIAGNOSIS OF LYMPHOCYTIC INTERSTITIAL PNEUMONITIS

Hodgkin lymphoma
Non-Hodgkin lymphoma
Lymphomatoid granulomatosis
Chronic lymphocytic leukemia
Waldenström macroglobulinemia
Angioimmunoblastic lymphadenopathy
Sézary syndrome
Pseudolymphoma
Sjögren syndrome
AIDS
Children of mothers at high risk for AIDS
Graft versus host disease
Congenital agammaglobulinemia
Chronic active hepatitis
Primary biliary cirrhosis
Crohn regional enteritis
Nontropical sprue
Myasthenia gravis
Autoimmune hemolytic anemia
Systemic lupus erythematosus
Chronic thyroiditis
Idiopathic

PLASMA CELL DISORDERS

Amyloidosis

Amyloidosis is a plasma cell disorder of unknown cause that is characterized pathologically by the extracellular deposition of acellular fibrils derived from the light chain of a monoclonal immunoglobulin. In primary amyloidosis, 35% to 70% of cases show roentgenographic evidence of amyloid deposition in the lung, whereas in secondary amyloidosis, pulmonary involvement is rare (98). Pulmonary amyloidosis may be classified as shown in Table 57.3 (see Chapter 32). Diffuse tracheobronchial submucosal plaques result in a generalized narrowing of the tracheobronchial tree that causes progressive stridor, dyspnea, cough, atelectasis, and hemoptysis (Fig. 57.14). The lower respiratory tract is often involved in systemic primary amyloidosis, and occasionally, disease is restricted to the lungs. Chest roentgenograms may exhibit nodular changes or diffuse opacities. Amyloid nodules in the pulmonary parenchyma are peripheral and grow slowly; they may be solitary (amyloidoma) or multiple (Fig. 57.15), and they cavitate in one third of patients. Calcification of the nodule can occur. The diffuse alveolar septal form of pulmonary parenchymal amyloidosis is usually associated with systemic amyloidosis and carries the worst prognosis of all types of pulmonary amyloidosis (Fig. 57.16). Lung biopsy shows diffuse deposition of amyloid in the interstitium and alveolar walls (Fig. 57.17).

Waldenström Macroglobulinemia

Waldenström macroglobulinemia is an uncommon disorder characterized by monoclonal IgM gammopathy, anemia, and lymphocytic or plasmacytic infiltration of the bone marrow. Pleuropulmonary involvement is relatively common (99–102). Of 20 patients, five exhibited abnormalities—asymmetric nodular lesions in four and pleural effusion in one; biopsy specimens showed infiltration of the lungs by lymphocytes and plasmacytes in four, and roentgenograms

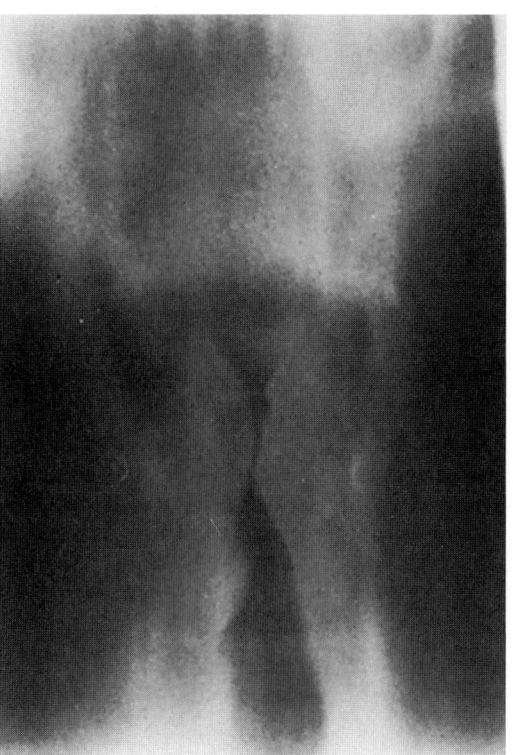

FIGURE 57.14. Tracheal tomogram demonstrates amyloidosis involving the subglottic and upper trachea.

demonstrated resolution of the abnormalities. Characteristically, the chest roentgenogram shows a diffuse reticulonodular pattern and, occasionally, local homogeneous consolidation (Fig. 57.18). Pleural effusion is present in nearly 50% of the patients. Chylothorax is rare.

In a 1980 literature review of the pulmonary complications of Waldenström macroglobulinemia documented by biopsy of the pleura or lung (or both) in 44 patients (26 men, ages 33–84 years; median age, 64 years), mass lesions were noted in 50%, infiltrates in 70%, and pleural effusions in 43%. Mediastinal lymphadenopathy was associated

TABLE 57.3. PULMONARY AMYLOIDOSIS

Type	Pulmonary Symptoms
Macroglossia	Sleep apnea
Laryngeal and subglottic (localized, stenotic)	Stridor, dyspnea
Diffuse tracheobronchial (submucosal plaques)	Stridor, dyspnea, hemoptysis
Localized tracheobronchial (masslike lesions)	Stridor, dyspnea, hemoptysis
Diffuse nodular (parenchymal)	Mild symptoms, bronchiectasis, cavitation in 30%
Solitary nodular (parenchymal, amyloidoma)	Rare, minimal symptoms, incidental finding
Diffuse parenchymal (septal or interstitial)	Progressive dyspnea, hemoptysis
Mediastinal and hilar lymphadenopathy[a]	Seen in 5% of all amyloidoses
Secondary[b]	Incidental (biopsy or autopsy finding, asymptomatic)
Senile	Incidental (autopsy or biopsy finding, asymptomatic)
Malignancy-associated[c]	Incidental

[a] Sometimes associated with multiple myeloma.
[b] Associated with tuberculosis, syphilis, bronchiectasis, and hypergammaglobulinemia.
[c] Pulmonary malignancy, carcinoid, and amyloid associated with medullary thyroid carcinoma.

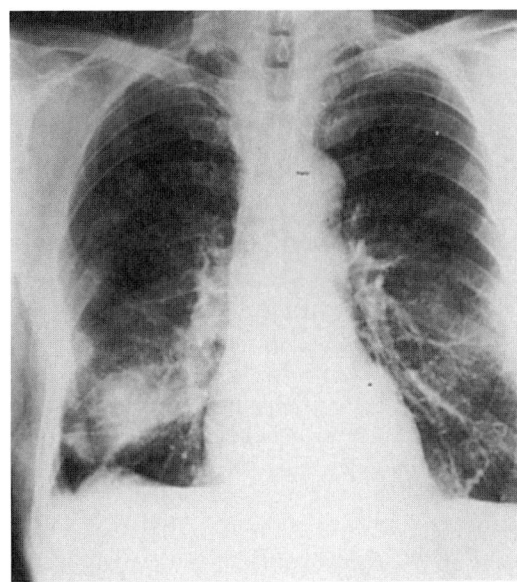

FIGURE 57.15. Localized amyloidosis (amyloidoma) of the right lower lobe treated by surgical resection.

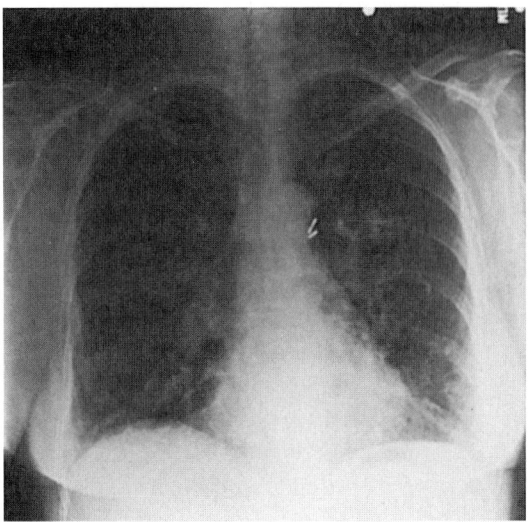

FIGURE 57.16. Diffuse parenchymal amyloidosis showing basal interstitial opacities.

with pulmonary disease in 25%. Two or more of these manifestations were noted in 55% of the patients. Dyspnea (54%), nonproductive cough (33%), and chest pain (7%) were the main pulmonary symptoms, and 15% of the patients were asymptomatic. Many had pulmonary manifestations at the time of the initial disease presentation. Respiratory involvement appeared 2 to 67 months after the diagnosis of Waldenström macroglobulinemia in two thirds. Bronchoalveolar lavage studies in a patient with diffuse pulmonary involvement with Waldenström macroglobulinemia showed abnormal plasma cells (10%–47%) and lymphocytes (60%) and myeloma protein (102).

The pulmonary manifestations respond to alkylating agents, corticosteroids, and radiation and do not appear to affect the prognosis adversely. In one study, 19 of the 31 patients responded to chlorambucil given alone or with corticosteroids.

Multiple Myeloma

A malignant neoplasm of plasma cells, multiple myeloma is manifested primarily by widespread skeletal destruction and is frequently associated with anemia, hypercalcemia, and renal dysfunction. Pulmonary manifestations are rare (103). The chest roentgenographic appearance of a plasmacytoma is typically that of a homogeneous mass associated with an

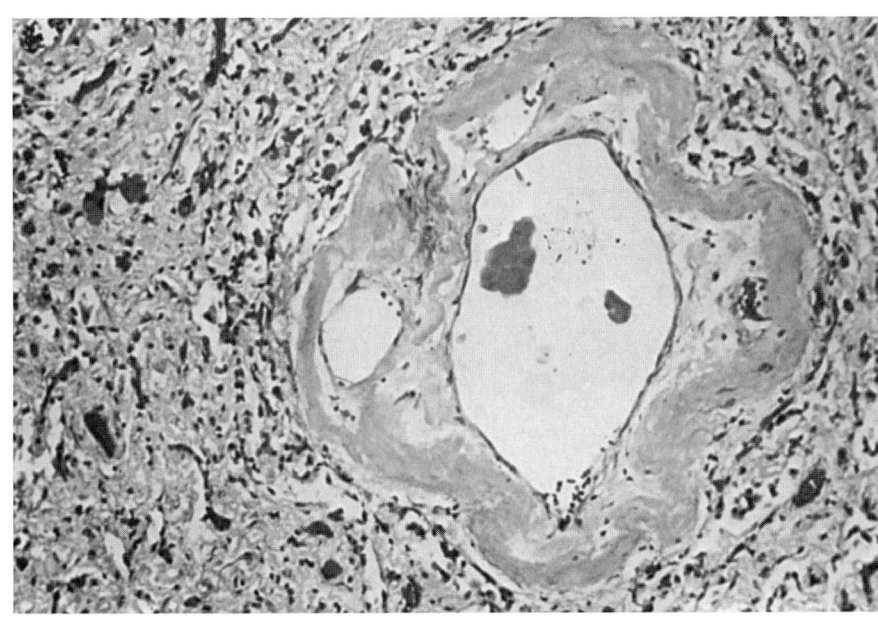

FIGURE 57.17. Amyloid deposits surrounding pulmonary blood vessels in primary amyloidosis.

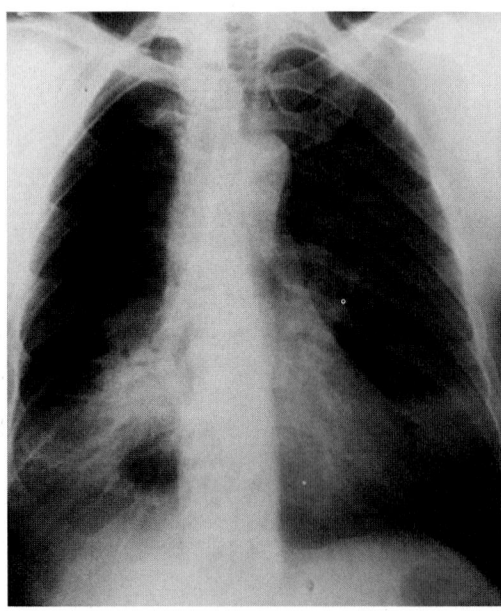

FIGURE 57.18. Bilateral opacities of the lower lung associated with a large right pleural effusion in Waldenström macroglobulinemia.

osteolytic rib lesion; the mass usually protrudes into the thoracic cage (Fig. 57.19). Pulmonary parenchymal involvement by the abnormal plasma cells is unusual. Diffuse pulmonary infiltration by neoplastic plasma cells occasionally causes interstitial changes on the chest roentgenogram.

Solitary plasmacytoma of the upper respiratory tract or pulmonary parenchyma may occur. Primary tracheal plasmacytoma, when present, appears as a solitary mass or multiple masses of homogeneous density. Unusual manifestations

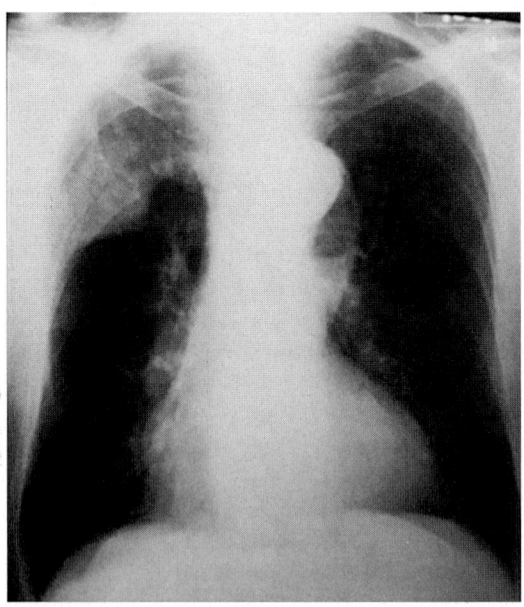

FIGURE 57.19. Multiple myeloma involving the right upper ribs, with protrusion of the bony tumor into the chest cavity.

include nonosseous pleural lesions, pleural effusions, chylothorax, and pulmonary parenchymal calcification. Alveolar hemorrhage has been described as a presenting feature of myeloma. Metastatic pulmonary calcification that resolved with therapy has been described in a patient with multiple myeloma.

POEMS Syndrome

POEMS (polyneuropathy, organomegaly, endocrinopathy, monoclonal gammopathy, and skin changes) syndrome, also known as *Crow-Fukase syndrome,* is a rare variant of plasma cell dyscrasia with multisystemic manifestations. Multiple lung tumorlets have been described. Markedly elevated levels of vascular endothelial growth factor have been observed in this syndrome and perhaps were responsible for the acute arterial obliteration described in several patients. Pulmonary hypertension has been described in this syndrome.

EFFECTS OF TRANSFUSION ON THE LUNG

The use of blood and blood products, even under the best circumstances, carries considerable risk for the recipient. Immediate pulmonary reactions include dyspnea, bronchospasm, and pulmonary edema. It should be emphasized that pulmonary edema following blood transfusion need not be the result of overloading the circulation. In addition to the blood and blood products, patients receive crystalloid solutions and other drugs via the intravenous route. Transfusion-related acute lung injury and the postperfusion syndrome are discussed here.

Transfusion-Related Acute Lung Injury

Transfusion-related acute lung injury (TRALI) is a form of noncardiogenic pulmonary edema (104). The passive transfusion of granulocyte or lymphocyte antibodies, or both, in donor sera is the most common setting for this unusual reaction (105,106). The antibodies in the donor serum may activate granulocytes and complement. Therapeutic or prophylactic granulocyte transfusion has been associated with the development of cytomegalovirus pneumonia. Granulocyte transfusion in combination with amphotericin B or in the setting of endotoxemia has been associated with acute respiratory failure (107).

The incidence of TRALI may be underestimated. One review of 36 cases occurring during a 2-year period indicated an incidence of 0.02% per unit and 0.16% per patient transfused. The clinical features are dramatic. The development of acute respiratory distress within 4 hours after the transfusion (in most cases, after 2 hours) is the sine qua non of this syndrome. Other features include the acute onset of chills, fever, tachycardia, nonproductive cough, and blood eosinophilia. Roentgenograms show patchy opacities in the perihilar and

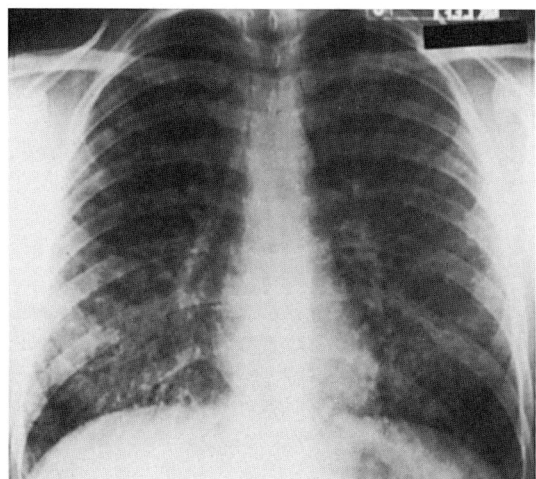

FIGURE 57.20. Diffuse bilateral soft nodular opacities resulting from transfusion-related acute lung injury.

lower lung regions (Fig. 57.20). Although recovery is rapid and complete in 81% of cases, some form of respiratory support may be required in more than two thirds of the patients. Pulmonary infiltrates and hypoxemia have persisted for 7 days in 17% of patients. Granulocyte antibodies in the serum of at least 1 unit of donor blood were demonstrated in 89% of cases, whereas lymphocytotoxic antibodies were present in 72%. Autopsy in a patient with TRALI showed evidence of massive pulmonary edema and granulocyte aggregation within the pulmonary microvasculature and extravasation into alveoli (108). Electron microscopy revealed capillary endothelial damage and activated granulocytes in contact with the alveolar basement membranes (108). These findings provide direct support for the proposed model of the pathogenesis of TRALI.

Postperfusion Syndrome

Pulmonary complications following prolonged cardiopulmonary bypass have been termed *postperfusion syndrome, pump lung, perfusion lung,* and *postperfusion atelectasis.* The cause remains unknown, although immunologic mechanisms have been suggested. After a prolonged period of cardiopulmonary bypass, progressive pulmonary insufficiency develops that is manifested by cyanosis, hypoxemia, increased work of breathing as a result of severely diminished compliance, and widening of the alveolar-arterial oxygen tension gradient. Chest roentgenograms reveal patchy, diffuse alveolar infiltrates that resemble pulmonary edema. Pathologic changes are similar to those seen in the respiratory distress syndrome—namely, diffuse alveolar damage.

Factors that contribute to the postperfusion lung syndrome include hypoxia, interruption of blood supply to the pulmonary tissues (especially the alveolar cells), loss of surfactant, interaction of homologous blood with a pump gas exchanger, and an underlying pulmonary disease process.

Prevention of the postperfusion syndrome is important because treatment is not promising. Corticosteroids given early may help, but the results are similar to those seen in respiratory distress syndrome of other causes.

HISTIOCYTIC RETICULOCYTOSIS

The group of diseases collectively known as *histiocytic reticulocytosis* or *histiocytic reticuloendotheliosis* includes Langerhans cell histiocytosis, Letterer-Siwe disease (acute disseminated histiocytosis X), Hand-Schuller-Christian disease (chronic disseminated histiocytosis X), and localized histiocytosis X (eosinophilic granuloma).

Langerhans Cell Histiocytosis

Langerhans cell histiocytosis is also known as *pulmonary eosinophilic granuloma* or *primary pulmonary histiocytosis X.* This granulomatous disease of unknown cause is characterized by an abnormal proliferation of histiocytes and an unpredictable natural history, although the course is usually slowly progressive (Figs. 57.21 and 57.22). The association between pulmonary Langerhans cell histiocytosis and tobacco smoking is striking; a history of tobacco smoking has been noted in more than 95% of patients with the disorder. Most are 20 to 40 years old, and the male-to-female ratio is approximately 1, although most series have shown a slight male predominance. The main discussion of the pulmonary form of Langerhans cell histiocytosis appears in Chapter 32.

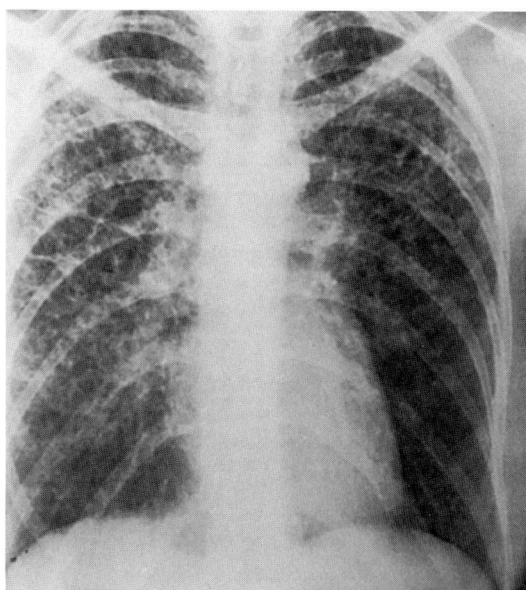

FIGURE 57.21. Pulmonary Langerhans cell histiocytosis with a diffuse reticular and nodular pattern and honeycombing. The distribution of opacities in the upper lung is noteworthy.

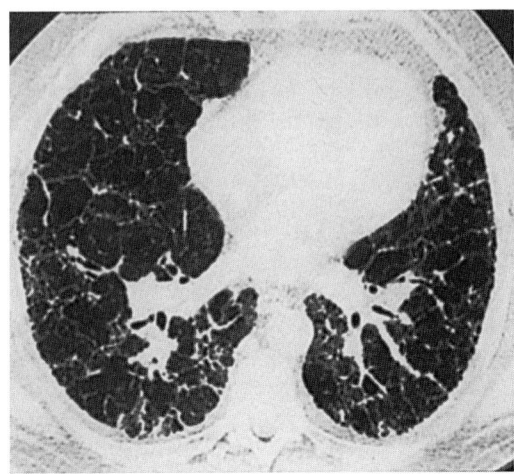

FIGURE 57.22. High-resolution computed tomogram of a lung in an advanced stage of pulmonary Langerhans cell histiocytosis shows extensive cystic changes.

Letterer-Siwe Disease

Letterer-Siwe disease is almost always limited to infants and children and manifests before the age of 2 years. It is characterized by extensive systemic dissemination and a fulminating, fatal course. However, Letterer-Siwe disease has been reported in 26 adult patients, with involvement of the lungs in half of them. If symptoms appear after the age of 2 years, the 10-year survival rate is 85%; when symptoms develop earlier, the 10-year survival is 40%.

Hand-Schuller-Christian Disease

Patients with Hand-Schuller-Christian disease may exhibit one or all of the classic three signs: exophthalmos, diabetes insipidus, and osteolytic lesions of the skull. The characteristic triad, however, is observed in only 10% of children with multifocal Langerhans cell histiocytosis. Hand-Schuller-Christian disease usually becomes apparent during later childhood or adolescence and progresses slowly, so that most patients reach adulthood. It has been suggested that the Hand-Schuller-Christian triad is nonspecific and that the term *multifocal eosinophilic granuloma* should be used to describe the abnormalities in various organs.

MISCELLANEOUS HEMATOLOGIC DISORDERS

Chronic anemia, in addition to its effects on cardiovascular hemodynamics, is known to cause a reduction in the diffusing capacity of the lung for carbon monoxide. The diffusing capacity decreases approximately 7% for each 1-g decrease in hemoglobin per 100 mL. Before the diffusing capacity for carbon monoxide can be used to evaluate lung function, a correction for significant anemia should be made. Ane-

mic patients demonstrate a higher extraction of oxygen from blood, presumably as a result of increased work by the heart.

Paroxysmal nocturnal hemoglobinuria is a hematopoietic stem cell disorder characterized by an increased sensitivity of blood cells to complement-mediated lysis. Thrombosis of the pulmonary vasculature and pulmonary hypertension have been described.

Autoimmune hemolytic anemia has been shown to be associated with pulmonary fibrosis in two patients, and a possible relationship between autoimmune hemolysis and fibrosing alveolitis has been suggested. Primary pulmonary hypertension has been described in association with microangiopathic hemolytic anemia and thrombocytopenia.

Bare lymphocyte syndrome is characterized by an absence of cell surface HLA-A, HLA-B, and sometimes HLA-C antigens and is a form of immunodeficiency in infants. An adult form of this syndrome, complicated by chronic sinusitis and bronchiectasis, has been described.

Hematopoiesis (extramedullary) in the thoracic cage may present as a mediastinal process (109). A case of hematopoiesis occurring in the bronchus has been described. Acute and rapidly fatal respiratory failure resulting from pulmonary interstitial extramedullary hematopoiesis associated with myelofibrosis has been described (110). A ^{99m}Tc-sulfur colloid bone marrow scan may show diffuse replacement of the pulmonary interstitium with bone marrow, and bronchoscopic lung biopsy has revealed interstitial involvement with increased numbers of megakaryocytes and other panhematopoietic staining elements.

Thoracic splenosis may present as a nodular or masslike density in the thoracic cage or lung parenchyma (111). Previous abdominal injuries, in which splenic trauma was followed by the migration of splenic fragments into the chest cage, are usually responsible for this finding. The spleen is absent, usually because of splenectomy, and the peripheral blood smear may be indicative of splenectomy.

Hereditary stomatocytosis is a rare familial disorder of erythrocytes. Nine cases have been described with documented thrombotic complications after splenectomy (112). Three patients became severely ill with pulmonary hypertension.

PULMONARY DIAGNOSTIC PROCEDURES

The diagnostic approach to immunocompromised patients with pulmonary manifestations is discussed in detail in Chapter 55. Chest roentgenography and CT are invaluable in assessing the pulmonary complications of hematologic diseases (113). Pulmonary Langerhans cell histiocytosis and bronchiolitis obliterans–organizing pneumonia are associated with specific findings on high-resolution CT of the chest. CT is frequently helpful in staging Hodgkin and non-Hodgkin lymphomas. Bronchoscopic needle aspiration of the subcarinal, hilar, and paratracheal lymph nodes is facilitated by CT identification of the lymph nodes.

In patients with hematologic diseases in whom lung infiltrates develop, bronchoscopic examination is very useful to identify infectious organisms. In a prospective study of 90 patients with hematologic malignancies (57 acute leukemia, 6 Hodgkin disease, 15 non-Hodgkin lymphoma, 12 other), fever (temperature > 38.4°C), and newly developed lung infiltrates, bronchoscopy was used to obtain culture specimens (114). The results revealed that the most frequent causes of pneumonia were Gram-negative bacteria (n = 38) and fungi (n = 34); the sensitivity of bronchoscopy in diagnosing infectious episodes was 66%, but only 4 of 13 noninfectious lung infiltrates could be identified. Bronchoscopy was most effective in the diagnosis of *P. carinii* and herpesvirus pneumonia, whereas its sensitivity and specificity in detecting fungal and bacterial pneumonia were low. Empiric antibiotic therapy was confirmed by the evaluation of bronchoscopic samples in 25 of 90 cases, and treatment was changed in 34 of 90 cases. Early identification of causative pathogens had a significant effect on survival.

Bronchoscopy and diagnostic BAL are safe in patients with severe thrombocytopenia, other coagulopathies, and alveolar hemorrhage (115). Unless a bronchoscopic lung biopsy is planned, the reversal of a bleeding diathesis with a transfusion of platelets, fresh-frozen plasma, and vitamin K is usually unnecessary when BAL is performed. With appropriate preparation and the administration of supplemental oxygen, these procedures can be performed even in patients with significant hypoxemia.

REFERENCES

1. Nagel RL. Genetic disorders of hemoglobin oxygen affinity. In: Rose BD, ed. *UpToDate.* Wellesley, MA: UpToDate, 2002.
2. Prchal JT. Diagnosis and treatment of methemoglobinemia. In: Rose BD, ed. *UpToDate.* Wellesley, MA: UpToDate, 2002.
3. Dinneen SF, Mohr DN, Fairbanks VF. Methemoglobinemia from topically applied anesthetic spray. *Mayo Clin Proc* 1994;69:886–888.
4. Rosen PJ, Johnson C, McGehee WG, et al. Failure of methylene blue treatment in toxic methemoglobinemia. Association with glucose-6-phosphate dehydrogenase deficiency. *Ann Intern Med* 1971;75:83–86.
5. Lane PA. Sickle cell disease. *Pediatr Clin North Am* 1996;43:639–664.
6. Bunn HF. Pathogenesis and treatment of sickle cell disease. *N Engl J Med* 1997;337:762–769.
7. Hammerman SI, Farber HW. Pulmonary complications of sickle cell disease. In: Rose BD, ed. *UpToDate.* Wellesley, MA: UpToDate, 2002.
8. Kirkpatrick MB, Haynes J Jr, Bass JB Jr. Results of bronchoscopically obtained lower airway cultures from adult sickle cell disease patients with the acute chest syndrome. *Am J Med* 1991;90:206–210.
9. Poncz M, Kane E, Gill FM. Acute chest syndrome in sickle cell disease: etiology and clinical correlates. *J Pediatr* 1985;107:861–866.
10. Aquino SL, Gamsu G, Fahy JV, et al. Chronic pulmonary disorders in sickle cell disease: findings at thin-section CT. *Radiology* 1994;193:807–811.
11. Emre U, Miller ST, Rao SP, et al. Alveolar-arterial oxygen gradient in acute chest syndrome of sickle cell disease. *J Pediatr* 1995;123:272–275.
12. Vichinsky EP, Neumayr LD, Earles AN, et al. Causes and outcomes of the acute chest syndrome in sickle cell disease. National Acute Chest Syndrome Study Group. *N Engl J Med* 2000;342:1855–1865.
13. Platt OS. The acute chest syndrome of sickle cell disease. *N Engl J Med* 2000;342:1904–1907.
14. Comber JT, Lopez BL. Evaluation of pulse oximetry in sickle cell anemia patients presenting to the emergency department in acute vasoocclusive crisis. *Am J Emerg Med* 1996;14:16–18.
15. Bellet PS, Kalinyak KA, Shukla R, et al. Incentive spirometry to prevent acute pulmonary complications in sickle cell diseases. *N Engl J Med* 1995;333:699–703.
16. Vichinsky E, Williams R, Das M, et al. Pulmonary fat embolism: a distinct cause of severe acute chest syndrome in sickle cell anemia. *Blood* 1994;83:3107–3112.
17. Godeau B, Schaeffer A, Bachir D, et al. Bronchoalveolar lavage in adult sickle cell patients with acute chest syndrome: value for diagnostic assessment of fat embolism. *Am J Respir Crit Care Med* 1996;153:1691–1696.
18. Haupt HM, Moore GW, Bauer TW, et al. The lung in sickle cell disease. *Chest* 1982;81:332–337.
19. Oppenheimer EH, Esterly JR. Pulmonary changes in sickle cell disease. *Am Rev Respir Dis* 1971;103:858–859.
20. Haynes J Jr, Allison RC. Pulmonary edema. Complication in the management of sickle cell pain crisis. *Am J Med* 1986;80:833–840.
21. Powars D, Weidman JA, Odom-Maryon T, et al. Sickle cell chronic lung disease: prior morbidity and the risk of pulmonary failure. *Medicine (Baltimore)* 1988;67:66–76.
22. Miller GJ, Serjeant GR, Saunders MJ, et al. Interpretation of lung function tests in the sickle-cell haemoglobinopathies. *Thorax* 1978;33:85–88.
23. Santoli F, Zerah F, Vasile N, et al. Pulmonary function in sickle cell disease with or without acute chest syndrome. *Eur Respir J* 1998;12:1124–1129.
24. Samuels MP, Stebbens VA, Davies SC, et al. Sleep-related upper airway obstruction and hypoxaemia in sickle cell disease. *Arch Dis Child* 1992;67:925–929.
25. Mallouh AA, Asha M. Beneficial effect of blood transfusion in children with sickle cell chest syndrome. *Am J Dis Child* 1988;142:178–182.
26. Emre U, Miller ST, Gutierez M, et al. Effect of transfusion in acute chest syndrome of sickle cell disease. *J Pediatr* 1995;127:901–904.
27. Atz AM, Wessel DL. Inhaled nitric oxide in sickle cell disease with acute chest syndrome. *Anesthesiology* 1997;87:988–990.
28. Sullivan KJ, Goodwin SR, Evangelist J, et al. Nitric oxide successfully used to treat acute chest syndrome of sickle cell disease in a young adolescent. *Crit Care Med* 1999;27:2563–2568.
29. Gladwin MT, Schechter AN, Shelhamer JH, et al. The acute chest syndrome in sickle cell disease. Possible role of nitric oxide in its pathophysiology and treatment. *Am J Respir Crit Care Med* 1999;159:1368–1376.
30. Charache S, Terrin ML, Moore RD, et al. Effect of hydroxyurea on the frequency of painful crises in sickle cell anemia. Investigators of the Multicenter Study of Hydroxyurea in Sickle Cell Anemia. *N Engl J Med* 1995;332:1317–1322.
31. Villa MP, Rotili PL, Santamaria F, et al. Physical performance in patients with thalassemia before and after transfusion. *Pediatr Pulmonol* 1996;21:367–372.
32. Youngchaiyud P, Suthamsmai T, Fucharoen S, et al. Lung function tests in splenectomized beta-thalassemia/Hb E patients. *Birth Defects Orig Artic Ser* 1987;23:361–370.

33. Santamaria F, Villa MP, Ronchetti R. Pulmonary function abnormalities in thalassemia major. *Am J Respir Crit Care Med* 1995;151:919.

34. Piatti G, Allegra L, Ambrosetti U, et al. Beta-thalassemia and pulmonary function. *Haematologica* 1999;84:804–808.

35. Benz EJ Jr. Clinical manifestations of the thalassemias. In: Rose BD, ed. *UpToDate*. Wellesley, MA: UpToDate, 2002.

36. Grisaru D, Rachmilewitz EA, Mosseri M, et al. Cardiopulmonary assessment in beta-thalassemia major. *Chest* 1990;98:1138–1142.

37. Factor JM, Pottipati SR, Rappoport I, et al. Pulmonary function abnormalities in thalassemia major and the role of iron overload. *Am J Respir Crit Care Med* 1994;149:1570–1574.

38. Hoots WK, Shapiro AD. Clinical manifestations and diagnosis of hemophilia. In: Rose BD, ed. *UpToDate*. Wellesley, MA: UpToDate, 2002.

39. Bogdan CJ, Strauss M, Ratnoff OD. Airway obstruction in hemophilia (factor VIII deficiency): a 28-year institutional review. *Laryngoscope* 1994;104:789–794.

40. Putman CE, Gamsu G, Zinn D, et al. Radiographic chest abnormalities in adult hemophilia. *Radiology* 1976;118:41–43.

41. Schulman S, Johnsson H, Blomqvist S. Pulmonary hypertension in hemophilia. *Ann Intern Med* 1988;109:759–760.

42. Robboy SJ, Minna JD, Colman RW, et al. Pulmonary hemorrhage syndrome as a manifestation of disseminated intravascular coagulation: analysis of ten cases. *Chest* 1973;63:718–721.

43. Thomson FJ, Benbow EW, McMahon RF, et al. Pulmonary infarction, myocardial infarction, and acute disseminated intravascular coagulation. *J Clin Pathol* 1991;44:1034–1036.

44. Katsumura Y, Ohtsubo K. Incidence of pulmonary thromboembolism, infarction and hemorrhage in disseminated intravascular coagulation: a necroscopic analysis. *Thorax* 1995;50:160–164.

45. Tamura K, Yokota T, Mashita R, et al. Pulmonary manifestations in adult T-cell leukemia at the time of diagnosis. *Respiration* 1993;60:115–119.

46. Cordonnier C, Escudier E, Verra F, et al. Bronchoalveolar lavage during neutropenic episodes: diagnostic yield and cellular pattern. *Eur Respir J* 1994;7:114–120.

47. Poulsen A, Demeny AK, Bang Plum C, et al. *Pneumocystis carinii* pneumonia during maintenance treatment of childhood acute lymphoblastic leukemia. *Med Pediatr Oncol* 2001;37:20–23.

48. Peters SG, Prakash UB. *Pneumocystis carinii* pneumonia. Review of 53 cases. *Am J Med* 1987;82:73–78.

49. Maschmeyer G, Link H, Hiddemann W, et al. Pulmonary infiltrations in febrile patients with neutropenia. Risk factors and outcome under empirical antimicrobial therapy in a randomized multicenter study. *Cancer* 1994;73:2296–2304.

50. Behre GF, Schwartz S, Lenz K, et al. Aerosol amphotericin B inhalations for prevention of invasive pulmonary aspergillosis in neutropenic cancer patients. *Ann Hematol* 1995;71:287–291.

51. Morrison VA, McGlave PB. Mucormycosis in the BMT population. *Bone Marrow Transplant* 1993;11:383–388.

52. Tallman MS. Clinical features and diagnosis of hairy cell leukemia. In: Rose BD, ed. *UpToDate*. Wellesley, MA: UpToDate, 2002.

53. Gartrell K, Rosenstrauch W. Hypoxaemia in patients with hyperleukocytosis: true or spurious, and clinical implications. *Leukemia Res* 1993;17:915–919.

54. Soares FA, Landell GA, Cardoso MC. Pulmonary leukostasis without hyperleukocytosis: a clinicopathologic study of 16 cases. *Am J Hematol* 1992;40:28–32.

55. Lei KI, Leung WT, Johnson PJ. Serious pulmonary complications in patients receiving recombinant granulocyte colony-stimulating factor during BACOP chemotherapy for aggressive non-Hodgkin's lymphoma. *Br J Cancer* 1994;70:1009–1013.

56. Wiley JS, Firkin FC. Reduction of pulmonary toxicity by prednisolone prophylaxis during all-*trans* retinoic acid treatment of acute promyelocytic leukemia. Australian Leukaemia Study Group. *Leukemia* 1995;9:774–778.

57. Tefferi A, Solberg LA, Silverstein MN. A clinical update in polycythemia vera and essential thrombocythemia. *Am J Med* 2000;109:141–149.

58. Berlin NI. Polycythemia vera: diagnosis and treatment 2002. *Expert Rev Anticancer Ther* 2002;2:330–336.

59. Bragg DG, Chor PJ, Murray KA, et al. Lymphoproliferative disorders of the lung: histopathology, clinical manifestations, and imaging features. *AJR Am J Roentgenol* 1994;163:273–281.

60. Koss MN. Pulmonary lymphoid disorders. *Semin Diagn Pathol* 1995;12:158–171.

61. Lund MB, Kongerud J, Nome O, et al. Lung function impairment in long-term survivors of Hodgkin's disease. *Ann Oncol* 1995;6:495–501.

62. Berkman N, Breuer R, Kramer MR, et al. Pulmonary involvement in lymphoma. *Leukemia Lymphoma* 1996;20:229–237.

63. Radin AI. Primary pulmonary Hodgkin's disease. *Cancer* 1990;65:550–563.

64. Chetty R, Slavin JL, O'Leary JJ, et al. Primary Hodgkin's disease of the lung. *Pathology* 1995;27:111–114.

65. Gallagher CJ, White FE, Tucker AK, et al. The role of computed tomography in the detection of intrathoracic lymphoma. *Br J Cancer* 1984;49:621–629.

66. Diehl LF, Hopper KD, Giguere J, et al. The pattern of intrathoracic Hodgkin's disease assessed by computed tomography. *J Clin Oncol* 1991;9:438–443.

67. Mauch PM. Initial evaluation and diagnosis of Hodgkin's disease. In: Rose BD, ed. *UpToDate*. Wellesley, MA: UpToDate, 2002.

68. Lund MB, Kongerud J, Boe J, et al. Cardiopulmonary sequelae after treatment for Hodgkin's disease: increased risk in females? *Ann Oncol* 1996;7:257–264.

69. Heffner JE. Diagnosis and management of chylothorax and chyliform effusions. In: Rose BD, ed. *UpToDate*. Wellesley, MA: UpToDate, 2002.

70. Plowman PN, Stableforth DE, Citron KM. Spontaneous pneumothorax in Hodgkin's disease. *Br J Dis Chest* 1980;74:411–414.

71. Pezner RD, Horak DA, Sayegh HO, et al. Spontaneous pneumothorax in patients irradiated for Hodgkin's disease and other malignant lymphomas. *Int J Radiat Oncol Biol Phys* 1990;18:193–198.

72. Travis LB, Gospodarowicz M, Curtis RE, et al. Lung cancer following chemotherapy and radiotherapy for Hodgkin's disease. *J Natl Cancer Inst* 2002;94:182–192.

73. Laurie SA, Kris MG, Portlock CS, et al. The clinical course of non–small cell lung carcinoma in survivors of Hodgkin disease. *Cancer* 2002;95:119–126.

74. Hoppe RT, Kim YH. Clinical features, diagnosis, and staging of mycosis fungoides and Sézary syndrome. In: Rose BD, ed. *UpToDate*. Wellesley, MA: UpToDate, 2002.

75. Wolfe JD, Trevor ED, Kjeldsberg CR. Pulmonary manifestations of mycosis fungoides. *Cancer* 1980;46:2648–2653.

76. Ueda T, Hosoki N, Isobe K, et al. Diffuse pulmonary involvement by mycosis fungoides: high-resolution computed tomography and pathologic findings. *J Thorac Imaging* 2002;17:157–159.

77. Hogg JC, Hegele RG. Adenovirus and Epstein-Barr virus in lung disease. *Semin Respir Infect* 1995;10:244–253.

78. Guinee D Jr, Jaffe E, Kingma D, et al. Pulmonary lymphomatoid granulomatosis. Evidence for a proliferation of Epstein-Barr virus–infected B lymphocytes with a prominent T-cell component and vasculitis. *Am J Surg Pathol* 1994;18:753–764.

79. Myers JL, Kurtin PJ, Katzenstein AL, et al. Lymphomatoid

granulomatosis. Evidence of immunophenotypic diversity and relationship to Epstein-Barr virus infection. *Am J Surg Pathol* 1995;19:1300–1312.

80. Wilson WH, Kingma DW, Raffeld M, et al. Association of lymphomatoid granulomatosis with Epstein-Barr viral infection of B lymphocytes and response to interferon-alpha 2b. *Blood* 1996;87:4531–4537.

81. Reich NE, McCormack LJ, Van Ordstrand HS. Pseudolymphoma of the lung. *Chest* 1974;65:424–427.

82. Tishler M, Solomon A, Greif J, et al. Pulmonary changes in angioimmunoblastic lymphadenopathy as demonstrated by computerized tomography. *Comput Radiol* 1985;9:159–162.

83. Shahidi H, Myers JL, Kvale PA. Castleman's disease. *Mayo Clin Proc* 1995;70:969–977.

84. Jones D, Weinberg DS, Pinkus GS, et al. Cytologic diagnosis of primary serous lymphoma. *Am J Clin Pathol* 1996;106:359–364.

85. Fullerton SH, Woodley DT, Smoller BR, et al. Paraneoplastic pemphigus with autoantibody deposition in bronchial epithelium after autologous bone marrow transplantation. *JAMA* 1992;267:1500–1502.

86. Saito K, Morita M, Enomoto K. Bronchiolitis obliterans with pemphigus vulgaris and Castleman's disease of hyaline-vascular type: an autopsy case analyzed by computer-aided 3-D reconstruction of the airway lesions. *Hum Pathol* 1997;28:1310–1312.

87. Kim SC, Chang SN, Lee IJ, et al. Localized mucosal involvement and severe pulmonary involvement in a young patient with paraneoplastic pemphigus associated with Castleman's tumour. *Br J Dermatol* 1998;138:667–671.

88. Chorzelski T, Hashimoto T, Maciejewska B, et al. Paraneoplastic pemphigus associated with Castleman tumor, myasthenia gravis and bronchiolitis obliterans. *J Am Acad Dermatol* 1999;41:393–400.

89. Hasegawa Y, Shimokata K, Ichiyama S, et al. Constrictive bronchiolitis obliterans and paraneoplastic pemphigus. *Eur Respir J* 1999;13:934–937.

90. Wolff H, Kunte C, Messer G, et al. Paraneoplastic pemphigus with fatal pulmonary involvement in a woman with a mesenteric Castleman tumour. *Br J Dermatol* 1999;140:313–316.

91. Takahashi M, Shimatsu Y, Kazama T, et al. Paraneoplastic pemphigus associated with bronchiolitis obliterans. *Chest* 2000;117:603–607.

92. Van der Waal RI, Pas HH, Nousari HC, et al. Paraneoplastic pemphigus caused by an epithelioid leiomyosarcoma and associated with fatal respiratory failure. *Oral Oncol* 2000;36:390–393.

93. Chin AC, Stich D, White FV, et al. Paraneoplastic pemphigus and bronchiolitis obliterans associated with a mediastinal mass: A rare case of Castleman's disease with respiratory failure requiring lung transplantation. *J Pediatr Surg* 2001;36:E22.

94. Cordel N, Ringeisen F, Antoine M, et al. Paraneoplastic pemphigus with constrictive bronchiolitis obliterans. *Dermatology* 2001;202:145.

95. Fujimoto W, Kaneiro A, Kuwamoto-Hara K, et al. Paraneoplastic pemphigus associated with Castleman's disease and asymptomatic bronchiolitis obliterans. *Eur J Dermatol* 2002;12:355–359.

96. Nousari HC, Deterding R, Wojtczack H, et al. The mechanism of respiratory involvement in paraneoplastic pemphigus. *N Engl J Med* 1999;340:1406–1410.

97. Byrd JC, Hargis JB, Kester KE, et al. Opportunistic pulmonary infections with fludarabine in previously treated patients with low-grade lymphoid malignancies: a role for *Pneumocystis carinii* pneumonia prophylaxis. *Am J Hematol* 1995;49:135–142.

98. Urban BA, Fishman EK, Goldman SM, et al. CT evaluation of amyloidosis: spectrum of disease. *Radiographics* 1993;13:1295–1308.

99. Winterbauer RH, Riggins RC, Griesman FA, et al. Pleuropulmonary manifestations of Waldenström's macroglobulinemia. *Chest* 1974;66:368–375.

100. King TE, Schwarz MI, Mathew M. Waldenström's macroglobulinemia. Report of a case with pulmonary involvement and recurrent pneumococcal sepsis after pneumococcal vaccination. *J Natl Med Assoc* 1984;76:184–189.

101. Kobayashi H, Ii K, Hizawa K, et al. Two cases of pulmonary Waldenström's macroglobulinemia. *Chest* 1985;88:297–299.

102. Filuk RB, Warren PW. Bronchoalveolar lavage in Waldenström's macroglobulinaemia with pulmonary infiltrates. *Thorax* 1986;41:409–410.

103. Rodriguez JN, Pereira A, Martinez JC, et al. Pleural effusion in multiple myeloma. *Chest* 1994;105:622–624.

104. Carilli AD, Ramanamurty MV, Chang YS, et al. Noncardiogenic pulmonary edema following blood transfusion. *Chest* 1978;74:310–312.

105. Butt W, Shann F, Duncan A. Deterioration in lung function after neutrophil transfusion. *J Pediatr* 1986;109:393–394.

106. Leger R, Palm S, Wulf H, et al. Transfusion-related lung injury with leukopenic reaction caused by fresh frozen plasma containing anti-NB1. *Anesthesiology* 1999;91:1529–1532.

107. Dutcher JP, Kendall J, Norris D, et al. Granulocyte transfusion therapy and amphotericin B: adverse reactions? *Am J Hematol* 1989;31:102–108.

108. Dry SM, Bechard KM, Milford EL, et al. The pathology of transfusion-related acute lung injury. *Am J Clin Pathol* 1999;112:216–221.

109. Asakura S, Colby TV. Agnogenic myeloid metaplasia with extramedullary hematopoiesis and fibrosis in the lung. Report of two cases. *Chest* 1994;105:1866–1868.

110. Yusem RD, Kollef MH. Acute respiratory failure due to extramedullary hematopoiesis. *Chest* 1995;108:1170–1172.

111. Roucos S, Tabet G, Jebara VA, et al. Thoracic splenosis. Case report and literature review. *J Thorac Cardiovasc Surg* 1990;99:361–363.

112. Stewart GW, Amess JA, Eber SW, et al. Thrombo-embolic disease after splenectomy for hereditary stomatocytosis. *Br J Haematol* 1996;93:303–310.

113. Lee WA, Hruban RH, Kuhlman JE, et al. High-resolution computed tomography of inflation-fixed lungs: pathologic-radiologic correlation of pulmonary lesions in patients with leukemia, lymphoma, or other hematopoietic proliferative disorders. *Clin Imaging* 1992;16:15–24.

114. Von Eiff M, Zuhlsdorf M, Roos N, et al. Pulmonary infiltrates in patients with haematologic malignancies: clinical usefulness of noninvasive bronchoscopic procedures. *Eur J Haematol* 1995;54:157–162.

115. Weiss SM, Hert RC, Gianola FJ, et al. Complications of fiberoptic bronchoscopy in thrombocytopenic patients. *Chest* 1993;104:1025–1028.

58 Renal Diseases

Udaya B. S. Prakash · Talmadge E. King, Jr.

The respiratory and renal systems together maintain normal acid-base equilibrium. Failure of one system promptly elicits a compensatory response from the other. This close relationship is maintained not only in health but also in certain pathologic states. For example, in Goodpasture syndrome, the alterations that develop in the alveolar basement membrane mirror the immunologic process that affects the glomerular basement membrane. Similar relationships exist for most of the disorders classified under the umbrella of pulmonary-renal syndromes. Many of the serious respiratory complications of kidney diseases described in the past are now uncommon because renal disorders are diagnosed and treated early. However, the successful treatment of renal failure by hemodialysis, peritoneal dialysis, and renal transplantation has led to several "new" complications related to the methods themselves. Elucidation of the basis for the pulmonary pathology in chronic hemodialysis has led to an understanding of some of the factors responsible for certain types of acute respiratory distress syndrome. Pulmonary complications after renal transplantation are well recognized. This chapter addresses the pleuropulmonary manifestations of kidney diseases (Tables 58.1 and 58.2) and renal transplantation (see Chapter 56). The pulmonary alveolar hemorrhage syndromes, a common feature in most of the pulmonary-renal syndromes, are described in Chapter 31.

RENAL FAILURE

Pulmonary Edema

Pulmonary changes may be associated with either acute or chronic renal failure. Pulmonary edema is the most se-

rious complication of renal failure. The roentgenographic manifestations—variously referred to as *uremic lung, uremic pneumonia,* and *butterfly shadows* or *bat wing shadows*—are manifestations of pulmonary edema. Similar features can occur in patients with left ventricular failure or noncardiogenic edema of various causes.

In chronic renal failure, pulmonary edema may develop without uremia, in part as a consequence of sodium retention and increased blood volume. The pathogenesis of pulmonary edema in renal failure is unknown. Fluid overload, left ventricular failure, and increased capillary permeability secondary to uremia are among the likely etiologic factors. Studies have shown an increased endothelial permeability to sodium and water and an increased alveolar permeability to ^{99m}Tc-labeled compounds before and during hemodialysis (1). The protein content of edematous fluid sampled by endotracheal aspiration is elevated, suggesting an increased vascular permeability to plasma proteins in renal failure. However, some studies have found no evidence of increased pulmonary endothelial permeability to the plasma protein transferrin in patients with pulmonary edema caused by renal failure (2).

Renal artery stenosis (usually bilateral) may be a specific and treatable predisposing factor to the abrupt onset of pulmonary edema ("flash" edema), which rapidly resolves in azotemic hypertensive patients (3–9). The exact pathophysiology is unknown, but the illness rarely occurs during waking hours, and it has been hypothesized it is a response to nocturnal hypotension in hypertensive patients in whom the nocturnal decrease in blood pressure is maintained (8). Relief of the stenosis by angioplasty or surgical intervention prevents the recurrence of flash pulmonary edema (3,5,6).

The morphologic features of acute pulmonary edema caused by renal failure include septal swelling and edema, proteinaceous fluid in the alveoli, and in some cases hyaline membrane formation. The lung in chronic pulmonary

U. B. S. Prakash: Pulmonary and Critical Care Medicine, Mayo Medical School and Mayo Medical Center, Rochester, Minnesota.

T. E. King, Jr.: Department of Medicine, University of California, San Francisco; and Medical Services, San Francisco General Hospital, San Francisco, California.

TABLE 58.1. PULMONARY COMPLICATIONS IN RENAL DISEASES

Pulmonary Manifestation	Renal Etiology
Hypoxemia	Hemodialysis
	Pulmonary edema
	Pleural effusion
	Pulmonary infections
	Pulmonary calcification
	Pulmonary-renal syndromes (Table 58.2)
Pulmonary edema	Renal failure (acute and chronic)
	Acute glomerulonephritis
	Nephrotic syndrome
	Hemodialysis
	Renal transplantation
"Flash" pulmonary edema	Renal artery stenosis
Pleural effusion	Renal failure (acute and chronic)
	Nephrotic syndrome
	Acute glomerulonephritis
	Hemodialysis
	Peritoneal dialysis
	Ureteral obstruction
	Hydronephrosis
	Perinephric abscess
	Pulmonary embolism
	Pulmonary-renal syndromes
	Renal transplantation
Pleuritis	Uremia
	Hemodialysis
Pulmonary calcification	Hemodialysis
	Transplantation
	Chronic renal failure
Sleep apnea	Chronic renal failure
	Hemodialysis
	Peritoneal dialysis
Infections	Hemodialysis
	Transplantation
	Renal failure
Lymphoma, lung cancer	Renal transplantation
Pulmonary-renal syndromes (Table 58.2)	

TABLE 58.2. PULMONARY-RENAL SYNDROMES

Goodpasture syndrome
Churg-Strauss vasculitis
Wegener granulomatosis
Polyarteritis nodosa
Microscopic polyangiitis
Systemic lupus erythematosus
Lymphomatoid granulomatosis
Henoch-Schönlein purpura
Hemolytic uremic syndrome
Scleroderma
Rheumatoid arthritis
Mixed connective tissue disease
Drug-induced vasculitis
Granulomatous (giant cell) arteritis
Hypocomplementemic urticarial vasculitis
Idiopathic rapidly progressive glomerulonephritis
Essential mixed cryoglobulinemia

but the severity of the changes increases with the degree of azotemia and acidosis. In acute glomerulonephritis, children may die so rapidly of pulmonary edema that the diagnosis is made only postmortem.

Lung function studies in patients with severe renal failure reveal significant decreases in the diffusing capacity of the lung for carbon monoxide (D_{LCO}), presumably as a consequence of pulmonary edema (10). An improvement in midexpiratory flow and a reduction in air trapping after hemodialysis have been described, and it has been suggested that these changes are attributable to the alleviation of peribronchial edema. The degree of restrictive lung dysfunction depends on the chronicity and severity of the renal failure. Muscle weakness, myopathy, and reduced aerobic muscle function are common in chronic renal failure and contribute to pulmonary dysfunction. Furthermore, diaphragmatic weakness caused by phrenic neuropathy is a

edema associated with renal failure shows round hyaline structures in the alveolar septa; these are well circumscribed and coated by a single layer of flat endothelial cells and organized casts of alveoli, alveolar ducts, and bronchioles, many revealing marked cellularity. Repeated episodes of uremic pulmonary edema may result in the development of interstitial fibrosis and the deposition of hemosiderin in the alveoli.

Pulmonary edema (Fig. 58.1) does not occur consistently in uremic patients; its development is unpredictable and cannot be correlated with the degree of azotemia. However, the clearing of chest roentgenographic abnormalities is usually paralleled by a reduction in total body fluid. Even when physical signs in the lungs are scant in comparison with the roentgenographic evidence of pulmonary edema caused by renal failure, the correction of fluid imbalance results in the rapid relief of respiratory symptoms. The chest roentgenogram typically exhibits bilaterally symmetric densities extending laterally from the hilum, with clear apices and peripheral zones (Figs. 58.1 and 58.2). The reason for the central concentration of the abnormal shadows is unclear,

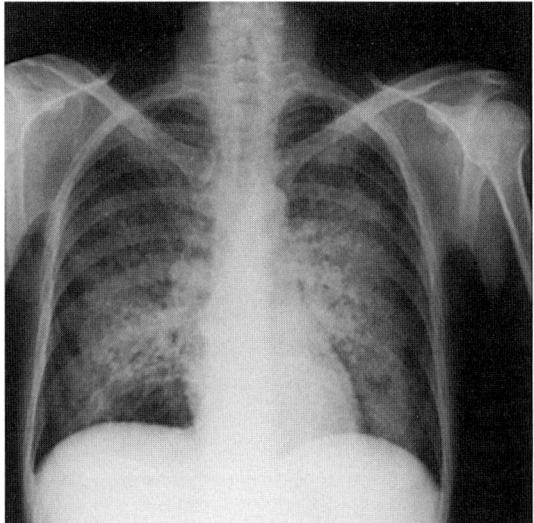

FIGURE 58.1. Typical bat wing (outer one third of lungs) or butterfly (inner two thirds of lungs) appearance in uremic pulmonary edema. Note sparing of both costophrenic angles.

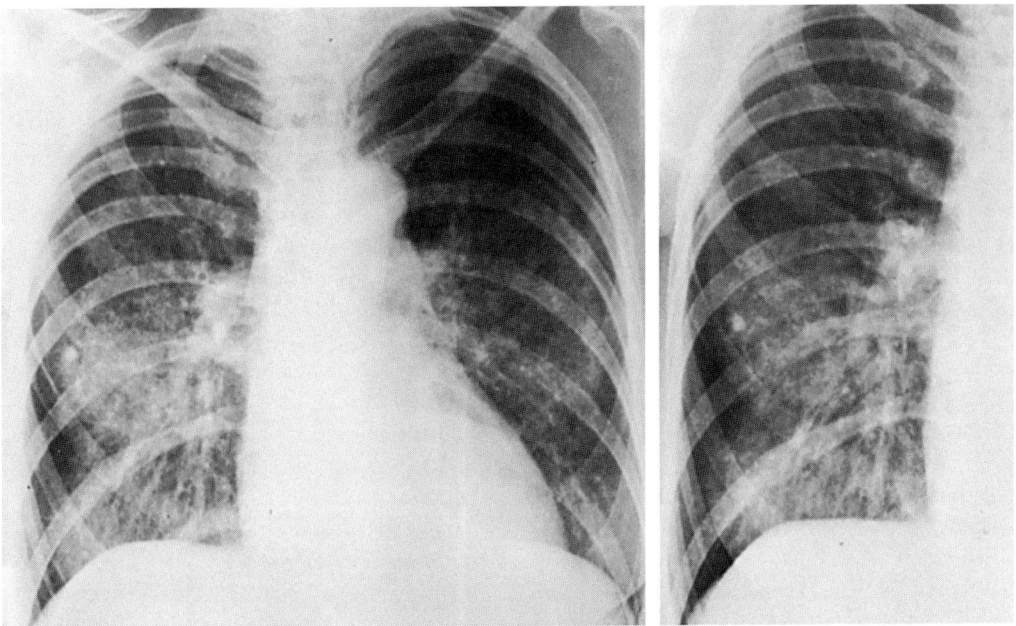

FIGURE 58.2. Bilateral but asymmetric pulmonary edema in acute renal failure (*left*). Close-up shows clear demarcation of normal and abnormal lung.

frequent complication of uremia and contributes to the restrictive pulmonary dysfunction. Pulmonary function tests performed at least 12 hours after hemodialysis in one group of patients revealed a significantly reduced DLCO, even after correction for anemia; there appeared to be no correlation between anemia and the degree of reduction in the DLCO.

Pleural Effusion

Pleural effusion is a common complication of renal diseases (Table 58.1). Hemodialysis, peritoneal dialysis, and renal transplantation are frequently associated with pleural effusion. Although hemodialysis can be associated with pleural effusion, the pleural effusion also resolves after hemodialysis (Fig. 58.3). Pleural effusion occurs in nearly half of children in whom acute glomerulonephritis develops. The effusions are probably secondary to hypervolemia and raised capillary hydrostatic pressures, and they are usually transudative. Many of these patients also exhibit edema and cardiomegaly.

Nephrotic syndrome is one of the common causes of pleural effusion (11). The main factor leading to pleural transudation is diminution of the plasma oncotic pressure, which

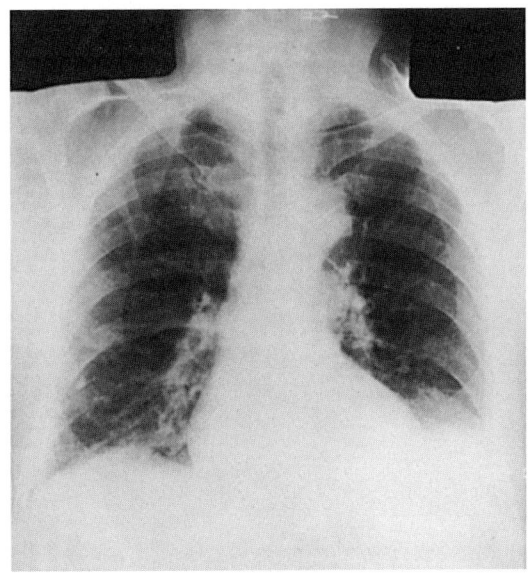
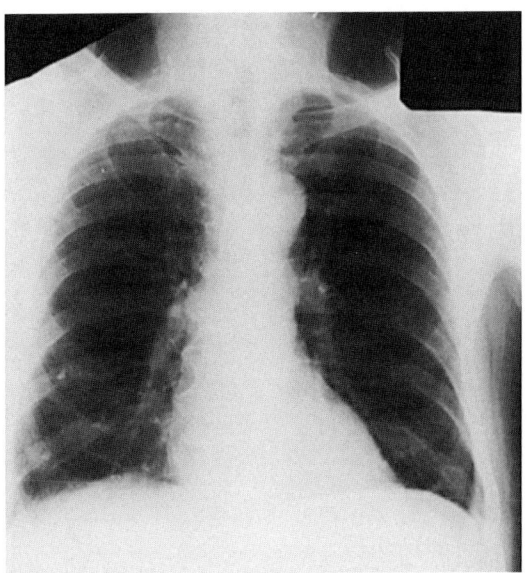

A   B

FIGURE 58.3. Pulmonary edema and pleural effusion before (**A**) and after (**B**) hemodialysis for renal failure.

facilitates the transport of protein-poor fluid into the pleural space. The pleural fluid is usually a transudate with a low protein content. Pleural and pericardial effusions are seen in 20% to 25% of patients with nephrotic syndrome. Usually bilateral and sometimes massive, the pleural effusions may cause significant respiratory distress. A peculiar feature of pleural effusions in patients with uremic syndrome is that they tend to remain subpulmonic in location. A reason for this is that the pleuritis associated with uremia is reported to cause areas of adhesion to form between the parietal diaphragmatic pleura and the visceral pleura; these prevent the fluid from pushing the lung upward. Roentgenologically, subpulmonic effusions do not obliterate the costophrenic angle (Fig. 58.4). The chest roentgenogram may show only an elevated hemidiaphragm on the side of the pleural effusion. A lateral decubitus chest roentgenogram is often necessary to demonstrate free layering of the fluid (Fig. 58.4). Occasionally, pleural effusions are complicated by infection; fibrosing uremic pleuritis complicated by empyema has been described. Medical or surgical pleurodesis may be required in patients with recurrent or symptomatic effusions.

Fibrinous pleuritis is an uncommon but distinct entity and possibly a specific manifestation of uremia, although episodes of fibrinous pleuritis have been noted in patients on long-term hemodialysis. Clinical features consist of recurrent episodes of pleuritic chest pain, dyspnea, and low-grade fever. Pleural friction rubs are commonly heard on auscultation. In many patients, the fluid is an exudate containing high levels of protein and lactate dehydrogenase.

Pleural effusions occasionally develop in patients undergoing long-term hemodialysis. The fluid usually is serosanguineous as a result of heparinization for the dialysis procedure. Correction of the fluid balance by continued hemodialysis and an improvement in renal function result in a gradual clearing of the effusion. Rare case reports have appeared of hemorrhagic effusion that resulted in fibrinous pleuritis and pulmonary restriction with a requirement for pulmonary decortication.

Ureteral obstruction secondary to calculi, ureteral valves, malignancy, or a gravid uterus may result in the extravasation of urine into the pleural space, with formation of a urinothorax or urinoma. Occasionally, retroperitoneal extravasation of urine as a result of hydronephrosis may lead to the development of intrapleural urinomas and mediastinal widening. Urologic procedures, such as the placement of ureteral stents, may cause pleural effusion. Pleural effusions resulting from inflammation of the adjacent pleura may complicate perinephric abscess. These rarely become infected. The pleural fluid in uninfected urinothorax is a transudate with a pH below 7.30 and a creatinine concentration higher than that of the serum.

The possibility that a pleural effusion is caused by pulmonary embolism must be considered because renal vein thrombosis is a known complication of nephrotic syndrome. One study observed pulmonary embolism in 8 (22%) of 36 adult patients with nephrotic syndrome.

The hemolytic uremic syndrome may involve the respiratory system, and pleuritis and pericarditis associated with this syndrome have been described.

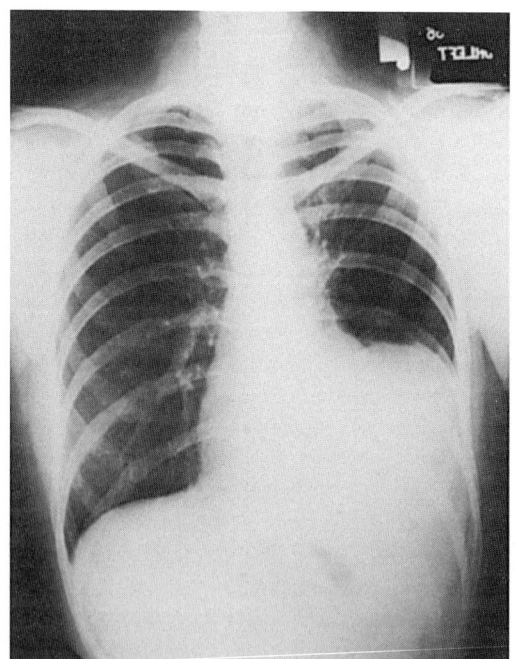
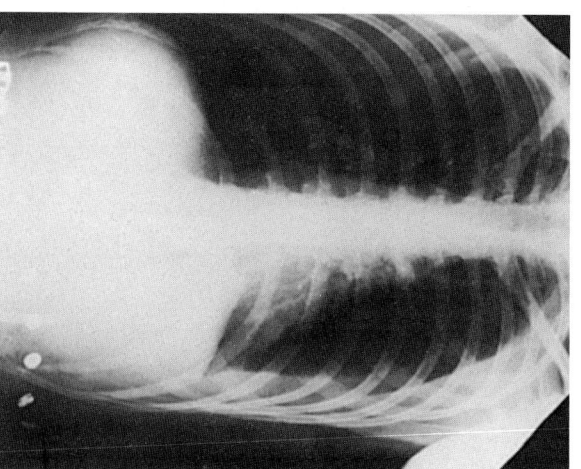

FIGURE 58.4. Subpulmonic left pleural effusion in chronic renal failure demonstrates (**A**) maintenance of sharp costophrenic angle on the left and (**B**) free layering of the pleural effusion in the lateral decubitus position.

Although chylous ascites is known to be associated with nephrotic syndrome, chylous pleural effusion is rare. Edema of the intestines with resultant lacteal leakage or malabsorption may be responsible. Chylous pleural effusion has been described in a patient with nephrotic syndrome.

Pulmonary Calcification

The calcification of soft tissues can be metastatic (i.e., deposition of calcium salts in previously normal tissue) or dystrophic (i.e., deposition at anatomic sites altered by pathologic processes) (12). Pulmonary ossification indicates the formation of bone tissue with or without marrow elements (12). The lung is the primary target of metastatic calcification in patients with chronic renal failure and in those on long-term hemodialysis.

Although the pathogenesis of pulmonary calcification is not fully understood, several pathophysiologic states predispose to pulmonary calcification: hypercalcemia, a local alkaline environment, and previous lung injury (12). Some investigators have suggested that the disorder occurs when the product of calcium and phosphate ions exceeds the solubility constant in the blood (product of plasma calcium and phosphate >75 mg/dL). Others have concluded that the product of calcium and phosphorus is more relevant to the *in vivo* situation.

Crystallographic, spectroscopic, and chemical studies have demonstrated two distinct types of calcium phosphate in the tissues of patients with chronic renal failure. Calcifications in the lungs are microcrystals of magnesium, whitlockite, or an immediate precursor, the formation of which is promoted by the presence of magnesium. Preferential calcification in the upper lung zones may be a consequence of the higher ventilation-perfusion ratio in the apical regions of the lung relative to the basal regions, which results in a lower alveolar carbon dioxide tension and a higher tissue pH (blood pH is approximately 7.51 at the apex, compared with 7.39 at the base) (13). The resultant relative alkalinity may favor the precipitation of calcium phosphate.

Chronic renal failure is complicated by the development of secondary hyperparathyroidism and hypercalcemia. The incidence of pulmonary calcification is greater in hypercalcemic patients with hyperparathyroidism secondary to renal failure. Although pulmonary calcification is considered to be a common occurrence in chronic renal disease, the deposits are usually sparse and identifiable only on histologic examination of the lungs (Fig. 58.5). On the other hand, the pulmonary calcification associated with long-term hemodialysis is clinically more apparent (see section "Hemodialysis: Pulmonary Calcification").

The clinical manifestations of the pulmonary calcification associated with chronic renal failure are nonspecific. Even when pulmonary calcification cannot be demonstrated with certainty, the possibility should be considered in any case of renal failure if the pulmonary opacities remain persistent. High-resolution computed tomography (CT) and ^{99m}Tc-methylene diphosphate (^{99m}Tc-MDP) bone scintigraphy are more sensitive and specific than chest roentgenography in the detection of pulmonary calcification (12).

Chest roentgenograms show areas of calcification that are either localized or diffuse. In most cases, they are identical to the roentgenographic opacities caused by pneumonia or pulmonary edema, but sometimes, definite punctate calcifications are seen (14) (Fig. 58.6). The upper lung zones are more commonly affected.

Several patterns of pulmonary parenchymal calcification may be seen with high-resolution CT: (a) multiple calcified or apparently uncalcified nodules distributed diffusely or more localized in certain regions (Fig. 58.7); (b) diffuse or patchy areas of ground-glass opacification or a poorly defined patchy infiltrate; (c) relatively dense area(s) of consolidation that mimic a lobar community-acquired pneumonia; (d) calcification of the tracheobronchial walls and chest wall blood vessels; and (e) a "ring" pattern of nodular calcification (12,13,15–17). A study of metastatic pulmonary calcification in seven patients (chronic renal failure in four, T-cell leukemia in one, multiple endocrine neoplasia type I syndrome in one, and idiopathic hypercalcemia in one) noted

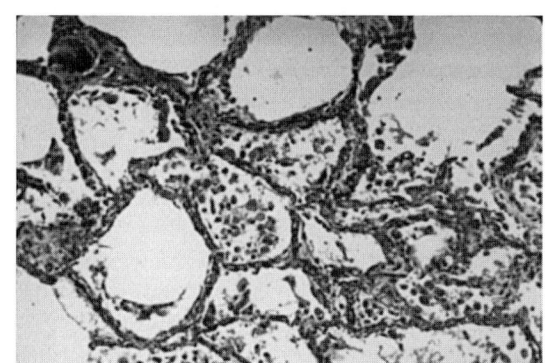
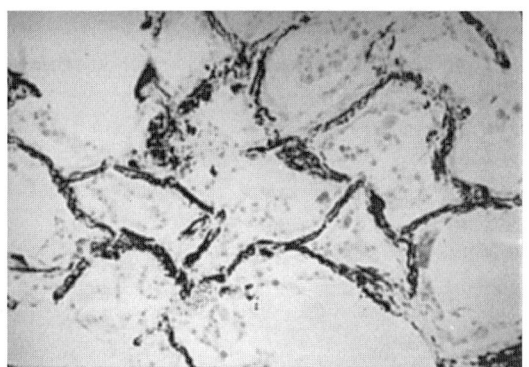

A   B

FIGURE 58.5. Metastatic calcification associated with chronic renal failure or long-term hemodialysis. **A:** Calcium is seen as deposits of dark and platelike material diffusely in the alveolar walls. **B:** Von Kossa stain for calcium shows diffuse black staining of calcium in the alveolar walls.

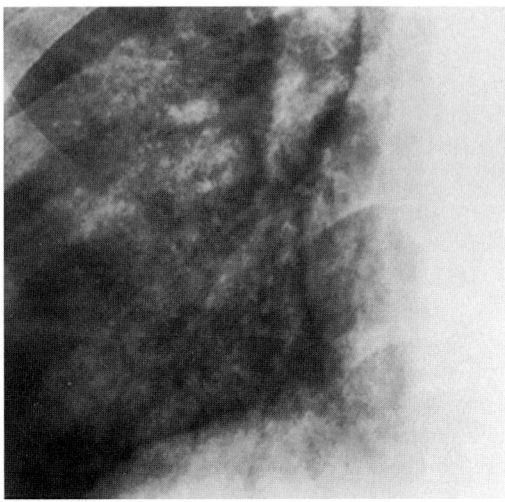

FIGURE 58.6. Diffuse punctate calcification of pulmonary parenchyma in the right lower lung zone in poorly treated chronic renal failure.

the following features on CT scans of the chest: The nodules were predominant in the upper lung zone in three cases, diffuse in three cases, and predominant in the lower lung zone in one case; calcification of the nodules was evident on the CT scans of four of the seven cases; and calcification of vessels in the chest wall was evident on the scans of six of the seven cases (18).

Pulmonary function tests may demonstrate a restrictive defect. Lung scanning with a bone-seeking radionuclide (^{99m}Tc-diphosphonate) has been used to establish an early diagnosis of pulmonary calcification (Fig. 58.8), especially in high-risk patients (12). An unusual form of focal, nodular

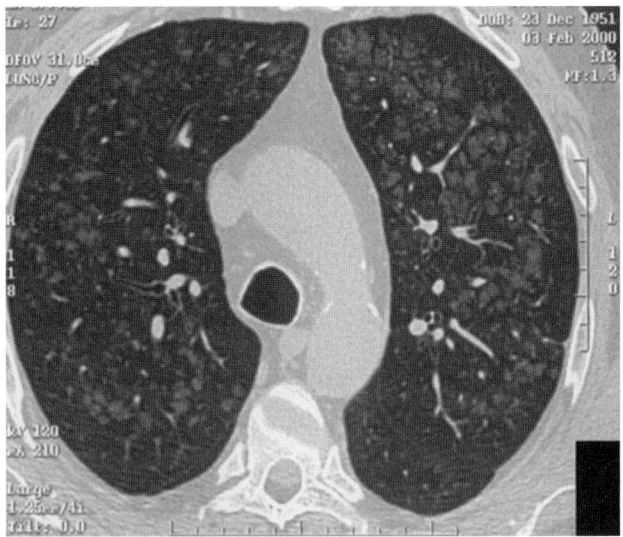

FIGURE 58.7. High-resolution computed tomographic scan of the chest shows diffuse, fluffy, and confluent dense alveolar infiltration. (From Ullmer E, Borer H, Sandoz P, et al. Diffuse pulmonary nodular infiltrates in a renal transplant recipient. Metastatic pulmonary calcification. *Chest* 2001;120:1394–1398, with permission.)

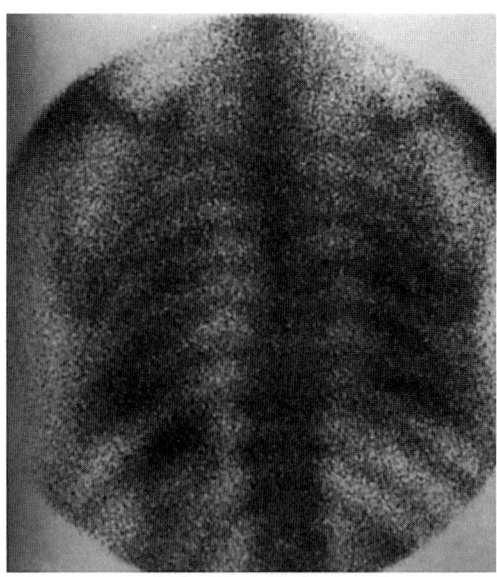

FIGURE 58.8. A posterior view of a ^{99m}Tc scan of the lungs of a patient with pulmonary calcification shows a marked uptake of radionuclide in both lungs and in the stomach (seen below the left lung).

pulmonary calcification has been reported in a patient with renal failure resulting from polycystic kidney disease.

HEMODIALYSIS

Hypoxemia

Hemodialysis-induced hypoxemia has been studied extensively (19–21). In more than 85% of patients, a reduction in the PaO_2 of between 5 and 35 mm Hg below baseline is observed as soon as the procedure is begun. This phenomenon persists for up to 60 minutes after the dialysis has been terminated. The PaO_2, however, seldom drops to below 70 mm Hg. Several mechanisms are responsible for this phenomenon (22–30). Pulmonary arterial microembolization from certain types of dialyzer membranes has been implicated in some studies (31,32). Dialysis membranes also can activate the complement cascade, and complement- and leukocyte-mediated leukostasis can cause hemodialysis-induced hypoxemia. Cuprophane membrane activates the complement cascade to a greater degree than polyacrylonitrile or cellulose membranes (31,33). Larger falls in the PaO_2 have been associated with cuprophane dialysis membrane than with other types of membranes. The interaction of the dialysate and dialysis membrane activates the alternate complement pathway by generating C3a and C5a within minutes after initiation of the dialysis procedure. The deposition of the complement fragments on the dialysis membrane induces an aggregation of platelets and leukocytes on the membrane, from which they migrate to the pulmonary circulation to cause microembolization and hypoxemia. The hypoxemia occurs at the same time as the leukocyte sequestration in the pulmonary vasculature. Histologic analyses of lung tissue from animals undergoing hemodialysis have revealed severe pulmonary vessel leukostasis and interstitial edema. This pathologic process was prevented by prior inactivation of complement and was reproduced by infusions of plasma in which complement was activated by zymosan. Leukostasis or the sequestration of leukocytes within the pulmonary vessels is common in patients undergoing dialysis; leukopenia and impaired pulmonary function are also noted. The leukostasis-induced hypoxemia contributes minimally (<10%) to the development of hemodialysis-induced hypoxemia.

The main cause of hemodialysis-induced hypoxemia appears to be dialysis-induced hypoventilation. Alveolar hypoventilation (compensatory hypoventilation) results from the substantial loss of carbon dioxide across the dialyzer membrane in addition to a decrease in metabolic carbon dioxide production. The consumption of carbon dioxide during the oxidative metabolism of acetate has also been suggested as a mechanism for hypoventilation and hypoxemia. Some studies have indicated that hypoxemia and the reduction in carbon dioxide production are most pronounced during acetate dialysis and minimal during bicarbonate dialysis. Others have opined that whether acetate or bicarbonate is used in the dialysate does not appear to make a difference in dialysis-induced hypoxemia.

Hypoxemia may also result from a decrease in minute ventilation without hypercapnia. It is hypothesized that the decrease in minute ventilation is unrelated to alterations in traditional chemoreceptor output, which depends on changes in arterial oxygen tension. Some have suggested that hypoventilation, localized ventilation-perfusion abnormalities related to changes in the pulmonary vascular volume during dialysis, and increases in arterial pH contribute variably to dialysis-induced hypoxemia.

Is hemodialysis-induced hypoxemia of any clinical significance? The preceding discussion should be considered in the context of when the hypoxemia is detected. Almost all studies of this topic have been performed during hemodialysis. Most patients undergoing hemodialysis are relatively immobile during the procedure because they must remain connected with the dialysis machine. They rarely exert themselves sufficiently—physically, that is—to increase the work of breathing. Therefore, the subjective experience or clinical detection of new or acute dyspnea is unusual during hemodialysis. A clinical caveat is that arterial blood gas analysis should be avoided during active hemodialysis unless respiratory symptoms and signs develop during the procedure. In patients with preexisting hypoxemia resulting from such conditions as chronic obstructive pulmonary disease, the use of cellulose or polyacrylonitrile filters and a bicarbonate bath is likely to minimize hemodialysis-induced hypoxemia.

A decreased D_{LCO} has been noted in both acetate-treated and bicarbonate-treated groups (34). Leukocyte sequestration in the pulmonary capillary network is perhaps one of the reasons for this phenomenon. In a study of 25 uremic pa-tients, hemodialysis-induced reduction in the D_{LCO} in most of them resulted from a reduction in the pulmonary capillary volume brought on by hemodialysis. Another study recorded a significant fall in the peak respiratory flow during the first 30 minutes of dialysis in 30% of patients. The improvements in the flow rates (forced expiratory flow in midcycle [FEF_{25-75}]) after hemodialysis suggested that peribronchial edema, which was present before the hemodialysis, was responsible for the dysfunction of small airways. Pulmonary dysfunction and eosinophilia have been noted in patients undergoing cuprophane dialysis.

Erythropoietin is effective in the treatment of anemia associated with chronic renal failure. Despite a higher hemoglobin concentration and better quality of life after treatment with erythropoietin, however, the peak oxygen uptake is not improved (35,36). In a study of eight patients with chronic renal failure undergoing regular hemodialysis, testing before and after the administration of erythropoietin suggested that this discrepancy results from two factors: First, the increase in hemoglobin induced by erythropoietin therapy is accompanied by a significant reduction in the peak blood flow to exercising muscle, which limits the gain in oxygen transport; and second, even after hemoglobin has been restored, oxygen conductance from the muscle capillaries to the mitochondria remains considerably below normal (35).

Pulmonary Calcification

The limited clinical occurrence and significance of metastatic pulmonary calcification in patients with chronic renal failure has been discussed (see section "Renal Failure: Pulmonary Calcification"). On the other hand, metastatic calcification of the lungs is more common in patients on long-term hemodialysis and may cause clinically significant disease, including respiratory failure (12). Pulmonary calcification occurs more often in patients on long-term hemodialysis than in patients on long-term peritoneal dialysis. Chan and colleagues (12) reported that four conditions lead to metastatic calcification in patients undergoing hemodialysis: (a) Acidosis causes calcium and phosphate to leach from bone; (b) an increased secretion of parathyroid hormone in response to a negative calcium balance, a consequence of failure of the kidneys to convert 25-vitamin D to 1,25-vitamin D, increases the release of calcium and phosphate from bone; (c) intermittent alkalosis, which often accompanies bicarbonate hemodialysis, predisposes to the precipitation of calcium salts in soft tissue; and (d) decreased glomerular filtration of phosphate may contribute to an elevated serum product of calcium and phosphate.

Biochemical analysis of the pulmonary parenchyma of patients with pulmonary calcification has shown that magnesium whitlockite [$(CaMg)_3(PO_4)_2$] is the main constituent. Ultrastructural studies of the lung parenchyma have shown linear or finely granular localization of the calcification along the alveolar septa. The extent of metastatic pulmonary calcification usually reflects the duration of hemodialysis (Figs. 58.6–58.8). Many of the patients in whom pulmonary calcification develops have been undergoing hemodialysis for more than 6 to 8 years. In a prospective study of 31 patients, of whom 15 died, postmortem studies revealed metastatic pulmonary calcification in nine (37). Such calcification also occurs in patients with hyperphosphatemia who are treated with a dialysate high in calcium.

Chest roentgenograms may not reveal obvious abnormalities in patients with pulmonary calcification, which may be indicated by hazy, punctate, or speckled areas of density in the upper and mid lung zones. A pattern of persistent lung opacities despite adequate hemodialysis and normalization of the fluid balance should suggest the possibility of metastatic pulmonary calcification. The findings on high-resolution CT and bone scanning have been described (see section "Renal Failure: Pulmonary Calcification"). Two factors are related to the development of pulmonary calcification in this setting: prolonged dialysis and high serum levels of aluminum.

A literature review in 1979 noted that 7 of 13 patients with pulmonary calcification died of respiratory failure (38).

Sleep Apnea

Hemodialysis is reported to increase the risk for sleep apnea (39–41). Snoring, restless sleep, frequent awakening, morning headaches, daytime sleepiness, and even personality and mood changes are all considered typical symptoms of this syndrome (42). In uremic patients who have at least one of these symptoms, the frequency of sleep apnea is 73% (43). This association does not appear to be altered acutely by conventional hemodialysis treatment and is similar in patients with end-stage renal disease on long-term peritoneal dialysis and those on hemodialysis (40).

Autonomic neuropathy is encountered in some patients with chronic renal failure and may contribute to sleep-disordered breathing. Progressive dialysis encephalopathy and spells of sudden respiratory arrest, in close association with the episodic electroencephalographic abnormalities characteristic of the syndrome, have been reported. Nocturnal hypoxemia secondary to sleep apnea appears to be a cardiovascular risk factor in renal failure (42).

Hemodialysis-Induced Asthma

Episodes of asthma have occurred during hemodialysis, and some believe that bronchial reactivity is more pronounced in this group of patients (44,45). Hemodialysis-induced asthma has been attributed to bronchospasm caused by acetate in the dialysate. Replacing the acetate in the dialysate with bicarbonate has solved this unusual problem. Others have inferred that hemodialysis does not commonly lead to bronchial hyperactivity (44). In a study of six patients without asthma who underwent histamine challenge testing before and after hemodialysis, no change in reactivity was observed, suggesting that hemodialysis does not often cause bronchial hyperreactivity in patients who do not have asthma.

Asthmatic patients who take theophylline as a bronchodilator and are also undergoing hemodialysis require special care. A shortened half-life of theophylline, from 5.7 to 1.6 hours, during hemodialysis has been described. However, the clearance of theophylline during hemodialysis varies substantially and may depend on the dialysis system, rate of blood flow, and dialyzer used.

Pulmonary Embolism

Occlusion of hemodialysis fistulae is a relatively common complication that requires therapy with thrombolysis or thrombectomy. Pulmonary embolism is a potential consequence (46). In a study of 31 patients with 43 acutely thrombosed hemodialysis fistulae, perfusion lung scan abnormalities consistent with the diagnosis of pulmonary embolism were noted in 59% of 22 patients studied (46). However, clinical signs or symptoms were absent in most of the patients.

Renal vein thrombosis is a known complication of nephrotic syndrome (47,48). Therefore, the risk for pulmonary embolism is increased. Pulmonary embolism was detected in 8 (22%) of 36 adults with nephrotic syndrome.

Pulmonary emboli (tumor emboli) from a malignant renal tumor develop when the tumor extends into the renal vein, from which the cancer cells exfoliate and travel to the pulmonary arterial bed. In a patient with renal cell carcinoma, the onset of rapidly progressive dyspnea and the appearance of diffuse interstitial pulmonary infiltrates with Kerley B lines on chest roentgenograms should suggest the possibility of tumor emboli. An acute to subacute onset of secondary pulmonary hypertension can result from tumor emboli.

Postmortem studies of dialysis patients have shown a high incidence of pulmonary atherosclerosis, indicating chronically elevated pulmonary arterial pressure. However, clinical pulmonary hypertension is uncommon in patients with chronic renal failure or in those on long-term dialysis.

Pulmonary Infection

The risk for infection with *Legionella* species is increased in patients on long-term hemodialysis. In some cases, infection of the dialysis fistula by *Legionella* species has been suspected. Patients undergoing hemodialysis and renal transplant recipients are at increased risk for the development of pneumonia caused by *Legionella pneumophila*. Infection of the hemodialysis fistula with *Legionella* organisms can cause *Legionella* pneumonia.

The risk for tuberculosis (TB) is increased in patients with renal failure (49–51). A report from the United Kingdom estimated the risk to be nearly 70 times higher in non-Europeans with chronic renal failure than in the native population. The incidence of TB is also higher in patients on maintenance dialysis. Active TB develops in 3.7% to 6.0% of patients followed longitudinally while on dialysis, an infection rate 12 to 15 times higher than normal. One study of 25 patients on dialysis detected TB in 28%; the majority were women, and extrapulmonary TB was common.

Isoniazid therapy in patients who have TB and also have renal failure or are dialysis-dependent may be complicated by an enhanced risk for isoniazid-induced neurotoxicity (52). The increased susceptibility of dialysis-dependent patients to isoniazid neurotoxicity results mainly from the abnormal metabolism of pyridoxine, which is associated with low serum levels of the active metabolite, pyridoxal phosphate. The rapid clearance of pyridoxal phosphate during hemodialysis results in a pronounced deficiency of this active metabolite. To prevent neurotoxicity, a 100-mg dose of pyridoxine daily is recommended for hemodialysis patients who require therapy with isoniazid.

PERITONEAL DIALYSIS

Diaphragmatic Dysfunction

Many of the pulmonary complications of peritoneal dialysis are similar to those of hemodialysis. However, several complications are peculiar to this group of patients (53–55). Long-term ambulatory peritoneal dialysis essentially causes iatrogenic ascites and its various effects on pulmonary function. Acutely, dialysate volumes of 2 to 3 L cause a mild reduction in vital capacity and total lung capacity. Filling the peritoneal cavity with dialysate induces, in both a supine and an upright position, a significant reduction in the maximal inspiratory pressure and diminished lung volumes. The diaphragmatic dysfunction observed during peritoneal dialysis is most likely a consequence of physical alterations resulting from infusion of the dialysate into the peritoneal cavity. The acute changes usually resolve within 2 weeks after initiation of the procedure as the diaphragmatic and abdominal mechanics adapt. A study of patients on continuous ambulatory peritoneal dialysis for more than 6 weeks indicated that the diaphragm may be capable of an adaptive rightward shift in the force-length relationship when continuously lengthened by continuous ambulatory peritoneal dialysis (53).

Extrapulmonary restrictive ventilatory defects may develop in patients on long-term peritoneal dialysis. The D_{LCO} appears to diminish in patients on continuous ambulatory peritoneal dialysis. A study of 26 patients with chronic renal failure undergoing continuous ambulatory peritoneal dialysis assessed the effects of renal disease on respiratory muscle function (P_{Imax} and P_{Emax}) before dialysis, 4 hours after the administration of 2 L of dialysate into the peritoneal cavity, and just after the next drainage; the authors concluded that respiratory muscle strength is preserved in most patients with chronic renal failure treated by continuous ambulatory peritoneal dialysis (55,56). However, lung volumes and respiratory muscle function, not strength, were decreased during dialysis.

The overall effect of long-term peritoneal dialysis on pulmonary function is minimal, even in patients with mild lung disease of other causes. On the other hand, the peritoneal instillation of large amounts of dialysate fluid in patients with severe chronic obstructive pulmonary disease may aggravate respiratory distress. The common occurrence of phrenic neuropathy in chronic renal failure may exacerbate respiratory distress in patients with severe obstructive lung disease who undergo peritoneal dialysis.

Pleural Effusion

Pleural effusion develops in some patients who undergo peritoneal dialysis. A review of the literature noted 33 cases of pleural effusion associated with peritoneal dialysis. Interestingly, 28 of these cases were in women. The effusion was detected within 48 hours after acute peritoneal dialysis. All cases were unilateral, and all but one were right-sided. The mechanism of fluid accumulation is similar to that in ascites. The instillation of large volumes of fluid intraperitoneally further stretches the diaphragmatic defects, so that dialysate can enter the pleural cavity. The pleural fluid can accumulate acutely and rapidly, within hours after the initiation of peritoneal dialysis, and cause respiratory distress. The effusions tend to recur when peritoneal dialysis is resumed. Massive hydrothorax during continuous ambulatory peritoneal dialysis is a rare complication that may appear at any time during treatment (54). A case has been reported in which peritoneopleural scintigraphy showed a rapid accumulation of the diagnostic agents over the right hemithorax, leading the investigators to suspect that a macroscopic diaphragmatic defect was responsible for the respiratory complication (54).

Sleep Apnea

Disordered sleep is more frequent in patients undergoing long-term peritoneal dialysis or hemodialysis than in the normal population. In a prospective study of 11 patients on long-term peritoneal dialysis, six had obstructive sleep apnea; the amount of dialysate drained in the morning correlated negatively with the minimum arterial oxygen saturation during the night. The association between dialysis and sleep apnea has been discussed (see section "Hemodialysis: Sleep Apnea").

Acid-Base Disturbances

The severe shifts in systemic pH that occur in patients undergoing peritoneal dialysis are usually acidemic and result from an inadequate ability of the kidneys to excrete acid and regenerate bicarbonate. Hypercapnia and acute respiratory acidosis have resulted from an increased carbohydrate load in association with peritoneal dialysis; lipogenesis following a carbohydrate load in patients with renal failure is associated with a respiratory quotient of 8.0, reflecting the much greater production of carbon dioxide per unit of oxygen consumed.

RENAL TRANSPLANTATION

Pulmonary problems in recipients of solid organ transplants are a consequence of the transplant rejection process and immunosuppressive therapy (57). The reader is referred to Chapter 56 for a more detailed discussion of the respiratory complications of organ transplantation. Important pulmonary complications in renal transplant recipients include infection, pulmonary calcification, malignancy, and pulmonary thromboembolism.

Infection

Pulmonary infections are common in renal transplant recipients and are, as a group, the major cause of death. Unusual bacteria or fungi, possibly favored by the suppression of immune mechanisms with drugs and corticosteroids, may cause these infections. The incidence of cytomegalovirus (CMV) infection in patients with cadaveric renal transplants is reported to be as high as 43% to 92%. Although many patients with renal transplants remain asymptomatic during CMV infection, pulmonary dysfunction occurs frequently. One report demonstrated a decreased DLco in virtually every patient with CMV infection. An interesting finding was activation of the complement system (C3d and C3a) in many of these patients, suggesting a causal relationship between complement activation and reduction in the DLco. Earlier studies questioned whether CMV played any role in the development of pneumonia in patients with renal transplants, but other reports indicate that CMV pneumonia has become a leading cause of death in this group of patients.

Studies of pneumonia in patients with renal transplants disclosed single-organism involvement by type 3 *Streptococcus pneumoniae, Staphylococcus aureus, Pseudomonas aeruginosa,* and *Escherichia coli.* Nosocomial pneumonia caused by *L. pneumophila* has been described in renal transplant recipients. Systemic fungal infections associated with pulmonary involvement, particularly candidiasis and aspergillosis, are also common after renal transplantation.

Pneumocystis carinii infection carries a high mortality in renal transplant recipients (58). This complication appears to be more common in older patients and is unrelated to immunosuppressive therapy. A study compared 28 renal transplant recipients who had *P. carinii* pneumonia (PCP) with a control group of 27 renal transplant recipients who did not have any episodes of PCP. The mean age was higher in the former group (50 vs. 38 years) (58). No differences were observed in basic immunosuppressive and rejection treatments or in antibiotic consumption, number of hospitalization days, and incidence of infection caused by CMV.

A study of seven renal transplant recipients in whom PCP developed noted a mean duration of 150 days before diagnosis of the infection; six had at least one episode of acute graft rejection, and CMV pneumonia was diagnosed in six of the patients (59). Overall mortality was 43%.

Prophylactic therapy to prevent PCP usually consists of the long-term oral administration of trimethoprim/sulfamethoxazole. However, up to 20% of patients eventually cannot tolerate this drug combination. A retrospective review of 17 kidney transplant recipients, all of whom were unable to take trimethoprim/sulfamethoxazole, reported that when aerosolized pentamidine was used for prophylaxis against *P. carinii* infection, it was well tolerated and also highly effective (60).

The increased rate of TB in patients with chronic renal failure and in those on long-term hemodialysis has been described (see section "Hemodialysis: Pulmonary Infection"). Renal transplant recipients also are at increased risk for TB, which occurs in this setting as an opportunistic infection. The infection is more frequent in areas where TB is highly prevalent. In a series of 400 transplant patients in a developed country, TB occurred in only five. A South African study of 857 renal transplant recipients noted 21 cases of confirmed or presumed *Mycobacterium tuberculosis* infection; the median time from transplantation to the diagnosis of TB was 14 months (61). The chest roentgenographic findings included consolidation, a miliary pattern, pleural effusion, tuberculoma, cavitation, and hilar lymphadenopathy; the rate of disseminated disease was lower in this study than that reported elsewhere. Several cases of pulmonary infection caused by *Mycobacterium xenopi* have been reported. Simple gastric aspiration is reported to be adequate in the diagnosis of pulmonary TB in renal allograft recipients. In a study of more than 200 renal allograft recipients suspected to have TB, gastric aspirates were more helpful than bronchoalveolar lavage (BAL) in the identification of acid-fast bacilli; positivity for acid-fast bacilli was significantly greater in the patients with chest roentgenographic abnormalities than in those with normal findings on chest roentgenography (62).

The early diagnosis of pulmonary infections in renal transplant recipients is important so that optimal therapy can be instituted promptly. BAL is an important diagnostic procedure in renal transplant recipients in whom respiratory symptoms or chest roentgenographic abnormalities develop. In a study of 70 renal transplant recipients, of whom 48 underwent 58 BAL procedures, 39 etiologic organisms were identified in 32 patients; six patients had more than one infection, and the results of BAL were negative in 22 patients (63). Overall, the results of BAL altered therapy in more than 70% of cases (63).

Pulmonary Calcification

Pulmonary calcification, at times fatal, can develop in renal transplant recipients (see previous discussions of pulmonary calcification in sections "Renal Failure" and "Hemodialysis"). In one patient, extensive pulmonary calcification developed 6 days after renal transplantation, and the patient died of respiratory failure on day 7. Pulmonary calcification and respiratory failure developed in 4 of 17 pediatric patients within 3 to 5 days after renal transplantation. Common clinical features included poor allograft function with persistent uremia requiring dialysis and evidence of moderate to severe hyperparathyroidism. Three patients had a markedly elevated product of calcium and phosphorus, to peak values of 122 to 147 mg/dL. This increase was noted at the time of onset of respiratory failure. All patients died of respiratory failure 5 to 58 days after transplantation.

Malignancy

Long-term immunosuppressive therapy in patients with renal transplants increases the risk for the development of B-cell lymphoma and carcinoma of the lung. Non-Hodgkin lymphoma has been observed in up to 2.5% of renal transplant recipients. Although rare, pulmonary involvement with Kaposi sarcoma has been described in recipients of renal transplants (64).

Parenchymal Lung Disease

Abnormalities of pulmonary function, particularly a reduced D$_{LCO}$, appear to persist after renal transplantation (65). Subclinical pulmonary edema before transplantation is presumed to progress to interstitial fibrosis (44,66). Another plausible hypothesis is that "low-grade pulmonary microvascular injury" in combination with a long-term decrease in pulmonary perfusion is responsible for diffusion abnormalities after kidney transplantation (65).

Pulmonary Thromboembolism

The incidence of pulmonary thromboembolism is increased in renal transplant recipients. Pulmonary embolism was the most frequent complication among 227 renal transplant recipients, observed in 60% of those with a noninfectious pulmonary process.

MISCELLANEOUS RENAL DISEASES

A *hemorrhagic diathesis* associated with renal failure is the result of azotemia-induced platelet dysfunction. The platelet count is normal, but the bleeding time is abnormally elevated. A hemorrhagic diathesis is a relative contraindication to invasive pulmonary diagnostic procedures. When the serum creatinine level exceeds 3.0 mg/dL or the serum urea level exceeds 45 mg/dL, bronchoscopic lung biopsy carries a risk for bleeding of approximately 40%.

Nephrobronchial fistula is a rare sequela of perinephric abscess and other inflammatory renal diseases (67). The successful treatment by nephrectomy of nephrolithiasis and pyelonephritis complicated by obstruction and associated with pyonephrosis, perinephric abscess, and nephrobronchial fistula has been reported. Inflammatory renal disease may involve the perirenal space and spread to contiguous abdominal organs and the adjacent pleural space.

Pulmonary alveolar microlithiasis is an uncommon disease of unknown cause characterized by the deposition of tiny calcispherites in the alveolar spaces (68). Although this disorder is not related to nephrolithiasis, a case of pulmonary alveolar microlithiasis with pleural calcification and nephrolithiasis has been reported.

Renal cell carcinoma is one the tumors with frequent endobronchial metastases (69). Clinically, patients may present with segmental or lobar atelectasis, cough, hemoptysis, and expectoration of endobronchial tumor tissue. Pulmonary parenchymal metastases, usually the result of hematogenous spread of the tumor, may present as rounded nodules ("cannonball" lesions). Some experts recommend that multiple bilateral pulmonary metastatic nodules be resected. One study has reported that in selected patients with renal cell carcinoma and pulmonary metastasis who do not respond to nonsurgical therapy, surgical resection of residual metastatic disease may prolong life. The detection of such lesions may require CT of the chest. However, in a study of 120 patients with renal cell carcinoma who underwent chest roentgenography and CT, follow-up at 24 months showed no significant effect of disagreement between the two imaging methods on therapeutic decisions or ultimate outcome (70). The study also indicated that in patients with a relatively small (T1) tumor, plain chest roentgenography suffices to stage the lung metastasis; indications for CT of chest include a solitary nodule on the chest roentgenogram before salvage resection of the metastasis, respiratory symptoms suggestive of endobronchial metastasis, and extensive regional disease.

Aerosolization therapy with interleukin-2 (IL-2) has been reported to be effective in controlling the progression of pulmonary metastases of renal cell carcinoma (69,71–73). In a study of 15 patients with pulmonary metastases of renal carcinoma treated with high-dose long-term inhalation of IL-2 (90% of the IL-2 dose), none of the pulmonary metastases progressed during treatment; one complete response, eight partial responses, and six cases of stabilization of disease in the lungs were achieved (71).

Renal metastases of primary lung cancer are much less common than pulmonary metastases of renal cancer; however, several cases of primary lung cancer with metastases to the kidneys and acute renal failure have been described (74). The renal changes included extensive bilateral parenchymal infiltration and replacement accompanied by tissue destruction, widespread vascular invasion and thrombosis resulting in ischemia, histologic evidence of foci of distal intratubular obstruction and pyelonephritis, and lymphatic metastases. Common findings in all six reported cases included bilaterally enlarged kidneys and progressive oliguria or anuria despite correction of the pre-renal or post-renal conditions.

Angiomyolipoma of the kidneys is common in patients with pulmonary lymphangioleiomyomatosis (75,76). In one study, 8 (47%) of 17 consecutive patients with pulmonary lymphangioleiomyomatosis had renal angiomyolipomas that were found at surgery or during CT of the abdomen (75). Therefore, patients with pulmonary lymphangioleiomyomatosis should undergo either ultrasonography or CT of the kidneys. Furthermore, serial follow-up by ultrasonography or CT is recommended to identify and monitor patients with renal lesions larger than 4 cm because such lesions present an increased risk for hemorrhage.

Rounded atelectasis, also known as *folded-lung syndrome* or *atelectatic pseudotumor,* has been described in patients with end-stage renal disease (77). It is usually caused by chronic pleural effusion or pleural disease. Uremic pleurisy or recurrent small pleural effusions associated with chronic renal disease may lead to rounded atelectasis.

Interstitial lung disease has been reported in patients with renal tubular acidosis (78–80). The mechanism of this association is unclear. Two siblings with a progressive unrelenting syndrome of bilateral *fibrosing pleuritis* in association with Fanconi syndrome (renal tubular acidosis) have been described (81). The parents of the siblings were second cousins. The condition resulted in the development of severe respiratory failure in both patients and ultimately the death of the older sibling at the age of 21 years (81).

Hypoxemia and hemoptysis with life-threatening consequences have occurred after *lithotripsy* as a result of shock wave–induced pulmonary contusion (82). Acute respiratory distress has been described in a patient undergoing *nephrolithotripsy* (83). The absorption of a large volume of irrigating fluid during the procedure was responsible for this complication.

Hemothorax has occurred as a complication of percutaneous renal biopsy.

REFERENCES

1. Kao CH, Hsu YH, Wang SJ. Evaluation of alveolar permeability and lung ventilation in patients with chronic renal failure using Tc-99m DTPA radioaerosol inhalation lung scintigraphy. *Lung* 1996;174:153–158.
2. Bell D, Nicoll J, Jackson M, et al. Altered lung vascular permeability during intermittent haemodialysis. *Nephrol Dial Transplant* 1988;3:426–431.
3. Pickering TG, Herman L, Devereux RB, et al. Recurrent pulmonary oedema in hypertension due to bilateral renal artery stenosis: treatment by angioplasty or surgical revascularisation. *Lancet* 1988;2:551–552.
4. Harker CP, Steed M, Althaus SJ, et al. Flash pulmonary edema: an acute and unusual complication of renal angioplasty. *J Vasc Interv Radiol* 1995;6:130–132.
5. Weatherford DA, Freeman MB, Regester RF, et al. Surgical management of flash pulmonary edema secondary to renovascular hypertension. *Am J Surg* 1997;174:160–163.
6. Planken, II, Rietveld AP. Rapid onset pulmonary edema (flash edema) in renal artery stenosis. *Neth J Med* 1998;52:116–119.
7. Bloch MJ, Trost DW, Pickering TG, et al. Prevention of recurrent pulmonary edema in patients with bilateral renovascular disease through renal artery stent placement. *Am J Hypertens* 1999;12:1–7.
8. Mansoor S, Shah A, Scoble JE. "Flash pulmonary oedema"—a diagnosis for both the cardiologist and the nephrologist? *Nephrol Dial Transplant* 2001;16:1311–1313.
9. Basaria S, Fred HL. Images in cardiovascular medicine. Flash pulmonary edema heralding renal artery stenosis. *Circulation* 2002;105:899.
10. Kalender B, Erk M, Pekpak MA, et al. The effect of renal transplantation on pulmonary function. *Nephron* 2002;90:72–77.
11. Jenkins PG, Shelp WD. Recurrent pleural transudate in the nephrotic syndrome. A new approach to treatment. *JAMA* 1974; 230:587–588.
12. Chan ED, Morales DV, Welsh CH, et al. Calcium deposition with or without bone formation in the lung. *Am J Respir Crit Care Med* 2002;165:1654–1669.
13. Greenberg S, Suster B. Metastatic pulmonary calcification: appearance on high resolution CT. *J Comput Assist Tomogr* 1994;18:497–499.
14. Neff M, Yalcin S, Gupta S, et al. Extensive metastatic calcification of the lung in an azotemic patient. *Am J Med* 1974;56:103–109.
15. Johkoh T, Ikezoe J, Nagareda T, et al. Metastatic pulmonary calcification: early detection by high-resolution CT. *J Comput Assist Tomogr* 1993;17:471–473.
16. Ullmer E, Borer H, Sandoz P, et al. Diffuse pulmonary nodular infiltrates in a renal transplant recipient. Metastatic pulmonary calcification. *Chest* 2001;120:1394–1398.
17. Lingam RK, Teh J, Sharma A, et al. Case report. Metastatic pulmonary calcification in renal failure: a new HRCT pattern. *Br J Radiol* 2002;75:74–77.
18. Hartman TE, Muller NL, Primack SL, et al. Metastatic pulmonary calcification in patients with hypercalcemia: findings on chest radiographs and CT scans. *AJR Am J Roentgenol* 1994;162:799–802.
19. Davidson WD, Dolan MJ, Whipp BJ, et al. Pathogenesis of dialysis-induced hypoxemia. *Artif Organs* 1982;6:406–409.
20. De Broe ME, De Backer WA. Pathophysiology of hemodialysis-associated hypoxemia. *Adv Nephrol Necker Hosp* 1989;18:297–315.
21. Kishimoto T, Tanaka H, Maekawa M, et al. Dialysis-induced hypoxaemia. *Nephrol Dial Transplant* 1993;8:25–29.
22. Raja R, Kramer M, Rosenbaum JL, et al. Prevention of dialysis-induced hypoxemia with bicarbonate dialysate—role of acetate in etiology. *Proc Clin Dial Transplant Forum* 1980;10:7–11.
23. Nissenson AR. Prevention of dialysis-induced hypoxemia by bicarbonate dialysis. *Trans Am Soc Artif Intern Organs* 1980;26:339–342.
24. Schwarz HP, Luger A, Graf H, et al. Fibronectin and dialysis-induced hypoxemia. *Int J Artif Organs* 1983;6:98.
25. Schwarz HP, Graf H, Luger A, et al. Dialysis hypoxemia: the role of fibronectin and its pathophysiological implication. *Contrib Nephrol* 1984;37:107–110.
26. Vaziri ND, Wilson A, Mukai D, et al. Dialysis hypoxemia. Role of dialyzer membrane and dialysate delivery system. *Am J Med* 1984;77:828–833.
27. Igarashi H, Kioi S, Gejyo F, et al. Physiologic approach to dialysis-induced hypoxemia. Effects of dialyzer material and dialysate composition. *Nephron* 1985;41:62–69.
28. Francos GC, Besarab A, Burke JF Jr, et al. Dialysis-induced hypoxemia: membrane-dependent and membrane-independent causes. *Am J Kidney Dis* 1985;5:191–198.
29. Fontana L, Perricone R, De Carolis C, et al. Dialysis leukopenia and hypoxemia in a patient without measurable complement activity. *Ric Clin Lab* 1985;15:331–336.

30. Wiegmann TB, MacDougall ML, Diederich DA. Dialysis leukopenia, hypoxemia, and anaphylatoxin formation: effect of membrane, bath, and citrate anticoagulation. *Am J Kidney Dis* 1988;11:418–424.

31. Kolb G, Schonemann H, Fischer W, et al. Hemodialysis with cuprophane membranes leads to alteration of granulocyte oxidative metabolism and leukocyte sequestration in the lung. *Adv Exp Med Biol* 1988;240:377–84.

32. Kolb G, Hoffken H, Muller T, et al. Kinetics of pulmonary leukocyte sequestration in man during hemodialysis with different membrane types. *Int J Artif Organs* 1990;13:729–736.

33. Moinard J, Guenard H. Membrane diffusion of the lungs in patients with chronic renal failure. *Eur Respir J* 1993;6:225–230.

34. Herrero JA, Alvarez-Sala JL, Coronel F, et al. Pulmonary diffusing capacity in chronic dialysis patients. *Respir Med* 2002;96:487–492.

35. Marrades RM, Roca J, Campistol JM, et al. Effects of erythropoietin on muscle O_2 transport during exercise in patients with chronic renal failure. *J Clin Invest* 1996;97:2092–2100.

36. Miro O, Marrades RM, Roca J, et al. Skeletal muscle mitochondrial function is preserved in young patients with chronic renal failure. *Am J Kidney Dis* 2002;39:1025–1031.

37. Conger JD, Hammond WS, Alfrey AC, et al. Pulmonary calcification in chronic dialysis patients. Clinical and pathologic studies. *Ann Intern Med* 1975;83:330–336.

38. Justrabo E, Genin R, Rifle G. Pulmonary metastatic calcification with respiratory insufficiency in patients on maintenance haemodialysis. *Thorax* 1979;34:384–388.

39. Mendelson WB, Wadhwa NK, Greenberg HE, et al. Effects of hemodialysis on sleep apnea syndrome in end-stage renal disease. *Clin Nephrol* 1990;33:247–251.

40. Wadhwa NK, Mendelson WB. A comparison of sleep-disordered respiration in ESRD patients receiving hemodialysis and peritoneal dialysis. *Adv Perit Dial* 1992;8:195–198.

41. Wadhwa NK, Seliger M, Greenberg HE, et al. Sleep-related respiratory disorders in end-stage renal disease patients on peritoneal dialysis. *Perit Dial Int* 1992;12:51–56.

42. Zoccali C, Mallamaci F, Tripepi G. Nocturnal hypoxemia predicts incident cardiovascular complications in dialysis patients. *J Am Soc Nephrol* 2002;13:729–733.

43. Kimmel PL, Miller G, Mendelson WB. Sleep apnea syndrome in chronic renal disease. *Am J Med* 1989;86:308–314.

44. Ferrer A, Roca J, Rodriguez-Roisin R, et al. Bronchial reactivity in patients with chronic renal failure undergoing haemodialysis. *Eur Respir J* 1990;3:387–391.

45. Walshaw MJ, Lim R, Ahmad R, et al. Bronchial reactivity in patients undergoing long-term haemodialysis for chronic renal failure. *Blood Purif* 1991;9:70–73.

46. Swan TL, Smyth SH, Ruffenach SJ, et al. Pulmonary embolism following hemodialysis access thrombolysis/thrombectomy. *J Vasc Interv Radiol* 1995;6:683–686.

47. O'Brien AA, O'Donnell JP, Keogh JA. Renal vein thrombosis with recurrent pulmonary emboli in the nephrotic syndrome: use of the Greenfield filter. *Postgrad Med J* 1986;62:223–225.

48. Llach F. Hypercoagulability, renal vein thrombosis, and other thrombotic complications of nephrotic syndrome. *Kidney Int* 1985;28:429–439.

49. Andrew OT, Schoenfeld PY, Hopewell PC, et al. Tuberculosis in patients with end-stage renal disease. *Am J Med* 1980;68:59–65.

50. Iclal I, Bilge BF, Fusun K, et al. Pleuropulmonary tuberculosis in patients with end-stage renal disease: findings on chest radiographs. *Transplant Proc* 1999;31:1719–1720.

51. Quantrill SJ, Woodhead MA, Bell CE, et al. Side-effects of antituberculosis drug treatment in patients with chronic renal failure. *Eur Respir J* 2002;20:440–443.

52. Siskind MS, Thienemann D, Kirlin L. Isoniazid-induced neurotoxicity in chronic dialysis patients: report of three cases and a review of the literature. *Nephron* 1993;64:303–306.

53. Prezant DJ, Aldrich TK, Karpel JP, et al. Adaptations in the diaphragm's *in vitro* force-length relationship in patients on continuous ambulatory peritoneal dialysis. *Am Rev Respir Dis* 1990;141:1342–1349.

54. Lepage S, Bisson G, Verreault J, et al. Massive hydrothorax complicating peritoneal dialysis. Isotopic investigation (peritoneopleural scintigraphy). *Clin Nucl Med* 1993;18:498–501.

55. Siafakas NM, Argyrakopoulos T, Andreopoulos K, et al. Respiratory muscle strength during continuous ambulatory peritoneal dialysis (CAPD). *Eur Respir J* 1995;8:109–113.

56. Bark H, Heimer D, Chaimovitz C, et al. Effect of chronic renal failure on respiratory muscle strength. *Respiration* 1988;54:153–161.

57. Edelstein CL, Jacobs JC, Moosa MR. Pulmonary complications in 110 consecutive renal transplant recipients. *S Afr Med J* 1995;85:160–163.

58. Branten AJ, Beckers PJ, Tiggeler RG, et al. *Pneumocystis carinii* pneumonia in renal transplant recipients. *Nephrol Dial Transplant* 1995;10:1194–1197.

59. Hennequin C, Page B, Roux P, et al. Outbreak of *Pneumocystis carinii* pneumonia in a renal transplant unit. *Eur J Clin Microbiol Infect Dis* 1995;14:122–126.

60. Saukkonen K, Garland R, Koziel H. Aerosolized pentamidine as alternative primary prophylaxis against *Pneumocystis carinii* pneumonia in adult hepatic and renal transplant recipients. *Chest* 1996;109:1250–1255.

61. Hall CM, Willcox PA, Swanepoel CR, et al. Mycobacterial infection in renal transplant recipients. *Chest* 1994;106:435–439.

62. John GT, Juneja R, Mukundan U, et al. Gastric aspiration for diagnosis of pulmonary tuberculosis in adult renal allograft recipients. *Transplantation* 1996;61:972–973.

63. Sternberg RI, Baughman RP, Dohn MN, et al. Utility of bronchoalveolar lavage in assessing pneumonia in immunosuppressed renal transplant recipients. *Am J Med* 1993;95:358–364.

64. Krayem AB, Wali SO, Samman YS. The diagnostic challenge and management of pulmonary Kaposi's sarcoma in renal transplant recipients. *Saudi Med J* 2001;22:1061–1064.

65. Ewert R, Opitz C, Wensel R, et al. Abnormalities of pulmonary diffusion capacity in long-term survivors after kidney transplantation. *Chest* 2002;122:639–644.

66. Bush A, Gabriel R. Pulmonary function in chronic renal failure: effects of dialysis and transplantation. *Thorax* 1991;46:424–428.

67. O'Brien JD, Ettinger NA. Nephrobronchial fistula and lung abscess resulting from nephrolithiasis and pyelonephritis. *Chest* 1995;108:1166–1168.

68. Richardson J, Slovis B, Miller G, et al. Development of pulmonary alveolar microlithiasis in a renal transplant recipient. *Transplantation* 1995;59:1056–1057.

69. Heinzer H, Huland E, Huland H. Systemic chemotherapy and chemoimmunotherapy for metastatic renal cell cancer. *World J Urol* 2001;19:111–119.

70. Lim DJ, Carter MF. Computerized tomography in the preoperative staging for pulmonary metastases in patients with renal cell carcinoma. *J Urol* 1993;150:1112–1114.

71. Huland E, Heinzer H, Huland H. Inhaled interleukin-2 in combination with low-dose systemic interleukin-2 and interferon-alpha in patients with pulmonary metastatic renal cell carcinoma: effectiveness and toxicity of mainly local treatment. *J Cancer Res Clin Oncol* 1994;120:221–228.

72. Huland E, Heinzer H, Mir TS, et al. Inhaled interleukin-2 therapy in pulmonary metastatic renal cell carcinoma: six years of experience. *Cancer J Sci Am* 1997;3[Suppl 1]:S98–S105.

73. Huland E, Heinzer H, Huland H. Treatment of pulmonary metastatic renal cell carcinoma in 116 patients using inhaled interleukin-2 (IL-2). *Anticancer Res* 1999;19:2679–2683.

74. Manning EC, Belenko MI, Frauenhoffer EE, et al. Acute renal failure secondary to solid tumor renal metastases: case report and review of the literature. *Am J Kidney Dis* 1996;27:284–291.

75. Bernstein SM, Newell JD, Adamczyk D, et al. How common are renal angiomyolipomas in patients with pulmonary lymphangioleiomyomatosis? *Am J Respir Crit Care Med* 1995;152:2138–2143.

76. Smolarek TA, Wessner LL, McCormack FX, et al. Evidence that lymphangiomyomatosis is caused by TSC2 mutations: chromosome 16p13 loss of heterozygosity in angiomyolipomas and lymph nodes from women with lymphangiomyomatosis. *Am J Hum Genet* 1998;62:810–815.

77. Yao L, Killam DA. Rounded atelectasis associated with end-stage renal disease. *Chest* 1989;96:441–443.

78. Zalin AM, Weeple J, Gumpel M. Fibrosing alveolitis and renal tubular acidosis. *Br Med J* 1970;4:804.

79. Mason AM, McIllmurray MB, Golding PL, et al. Fibrosing alveolitis associated with renal tubular acidosis. *Br Med J* 1970;4:596–599.

80. Helman CA, Keeton GR, Benatar SR. Lymphoid interstitial pneumonia with associated chronic active hepatitis and renal tubular acidosis. *Am Rev Respir Dis* 1977;115:161–164.

81. Hayes JP, Wiggins J, Ward K, et al. Familial cryptogenic fibrosing pleuritis with Fanconi's syndrome (renal tubular acidosis). A new syndrome. *Chest* 1995;107:576–578.

82. Malhotra V, Rosen RJ, Slepian RL. Life-threatening hypoxemia after lithotripsy in an adult due to shock wave–induced pulmonary contusion. *Anesthesiology* 1991;75:529–531.

83. Rudy DC, Woodside JR, Borden TA, et al. Adult respiratory distress syndrome complicating percutaneous nephrolithotripsy. *Urology* 1984;23:376–377.

59 Gastrointestinal Diseases

Udaya B. S. Prakash · Talmadge E. King, Jr.

The common embryologic origin of the upper gastrointestinal tract and tracheobronchial tree is responsible for their anatomic proximity throughout life. The pathologic importance of this close relationship is illustrated by the fact that some diseases of the esophagus affect the tracheobronchial tree, and vice versa. Furthermore, the intimate relationship between the tracheobronchial tree and esophagus is evident in several congenital and developmental disorders, including tracheoesophageal fistula, abnormalities of the laryngotracheoesophageal cleft, and incomplete development of the trachea and esophagus. Among the acquired diseases, the aspiration of gastric contents as a result of gastroesophageal reflux into the respiratory system is an excellent example of the close relationship between the airways and esophagus. Malignant neoplasms originating in the esophagus frequently invade or compress the tracheobronchial tree and cause respiratory embarrassment. Furthermore, evidence suggests the existence of local neuronal esophagolaryngotracheal reflexes in humans. Pulmonary involvement in hepatic and pancreatic diseases is well known. Respiratory manifestations in other gastrointestinal diseases, however, are less frequent and hence not very familiar to all. This chapter considers the pulmonary manifestations of the common as well as the uncommon gastrointestinal diseases. A discussion of the effects of alcohol on lung function and disease is also included.

ESOPHAGEAL DISORDERS

Fistulae

Tracheoesophageal and bronchoesophageal fistulae may be congenital or acquired. Congenital fistulae are more of-

U. B. S. Prakash: Pulmonary and Critical Care Medicine, Mayo Medical School and Mayo Medical Center, Rochester, Minnesota.

T. E. King, Jr.: Department of Medicine, University of California, San Francisco; and Medical Services, San Francisco General Hospital, San Francisco, California.

ten tracheal than bronchial. In 90% of congenital cases, a proximal esophagus ends blindly, and a connection is usually found between the distal esophagus and the trachea (Fig. 59.1). In the remaining 10% of cases, an H-type fistula is seen. This latter congenital anomaly may remain undetected until adulthood, especially if the communication is small enough that large amounts of solids or liquids are not aspirated through the fistulous tract. The aspiration of small amounts of esophageal contents through the anomalous communication may lead to chronic cough, asthma-like symptoms, and recurrent respiratory infections. A fistula at a more distant site, such as an esophagobronchial fistula, can lead to recurrent infections and ultimately bronchiectasis. Occasionally, surgical resection of a chronically infected bronchiectatic segment of lung may disclose the presence of a previously undiagnosed fistula between the esophagus and the airway.

Approximately 60% of fistulae in adults are tracheoesophageal fistulae acquired as a result of malignancy in the trachea, esophagus, or mediastinum. The remainder are a consequence of infections or mediastinal granulomas secondary to histoplasmosis, broncholithiasis, silicotic lymph nodes, chemical corrosives, or trauma. Esophageal instrumentation (iatrogenic) is an important cause of tracheoesophageal fistula and acute mediastinitis. Esophagoscopy and dilation procedures, inadvertent intubation of the esophagus during endotracheal intubation, rigid bronchoscopic procedures, and endoluminal laser therapy of tracheoesophageal lesions also may lead to the development of fistulae. Radiation necrosis of malignancies involving the tracheoesophageal interphase is a relatively common cause of tracheoesophageal fistulae. Esophagopleural fistulae form (with a frequency of 0.5%) after pneumonectomy for the management of bronchogenic carcinoma (1). They develop when recurrent tumor erodes the esophagus and are more common after right-sided procedures. Mortality approaches 65% in this setting. An uncommon cause of acquired

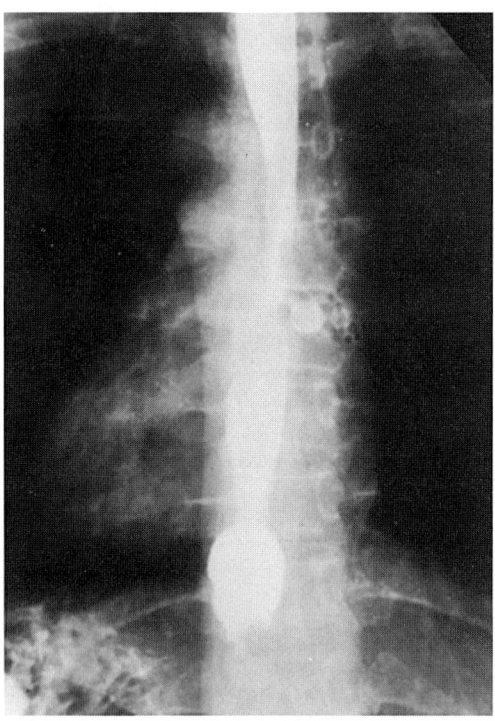

FIGURE 59.1. Situs inversus and congenital fistula between the esophagus and proximal left main bronchus presenting in adulthood as asthma and cough induced by the ingestion of liquids.

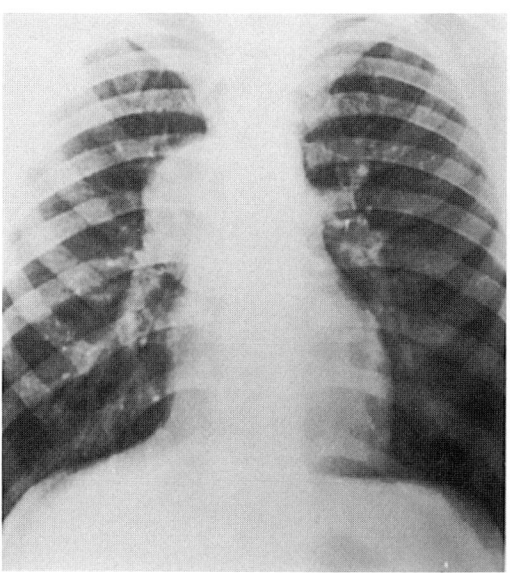

FIGURE 59.2. A large gastroenteric cyst presenting as a posterior mediastinal mass that was asymptomatic and discovered during a routine examination.

tracheoesophageal fistula is Crohn disease, which affects the esophagus in 0.3% of cases. Esophagography in patients with Crohn disease of the esophagus demonstrates stricture in 38% and ulceration in 32%; tracheoesophageal fistula is observed in 6% of patients.

The symptoms depend on the location and size of a fistula, but characteristically, coughing develops when liquids are swallowed. Hemoptysis, recurrent pulmonary infections, wheezing, and bronchiectasis also are commonly encountered. A wrong diagnosis of chronic bronchitis or asthma is not uncommon. The diagnosis is documented by demonstrating in the fistulous tract contrast material introduced through the esophagus. Esophagoscopy and bronchoscopy also are valuable in assessing the location and size of a fistula and in obtaining a biopsy specimen from its edges to exclude malignancy. Furthermore, bronchoscopy and esophagoscopy are important in inserting a tracheobronchial or esophageal prosthesis (stent) to treat a fistula (2,3).

The possibility of satisfactory surgical correction depends on the cause and location of a fistula. Benign fistulous communications are amenable to surgical therapy. In patients with malignant fistulae, repeated aspiration and pneumonia lead to rapid deterioration and death. The prognosis is dismal, and curative resections and surgical bypass have been associated with 25% to 60% mortality (4). The insertion of endoprostheses (stents) by endoscopic

methods carries a perioperative mortality of 15% in these patients.

Gastroenteric Cysts

Gastroenteric cysts develop from the foregut and represent a failure of the originally solid esophagus to become a hollow tube. The cysts occur in the paraspinal region of the posterior mediastinum and are usually round or oval and homogeneous in density (Fig. 59.2). Most of these cysts are detected incidentally when chest roentgenograms are obtained. The typical roentgenologic presentation is in the form of a mediastinal mass (5). Computed tomography (CT) helps in the diagnosis. It is uncommon for these cysts to enlarge greatly. Although the overwhelming majority of patients with gastroenteric cysts are asymptomatic, surgical resection is routine in most cases.

Zenker Diverticulum

A pharyngoesophageal diverticulum of Zenker may be large enough to be identified wrongly as a superior mediastinal mass on chest roentgenograms (6). Symptoms include dysphagia, chronic cough caused by aspiration, and recurrent aspiration pneumonia (Fig. 59.3).

Achalasia

Achalasia (a Greek term meaning "does not relax") is an uncommon disorder with an annual incidence of approximately 1 case per 100,000 (7). An enlarged esophagus (esophagomegaly, megaesophagus) secondary to achalasia can encroach on the upper airway and obstruct airflow

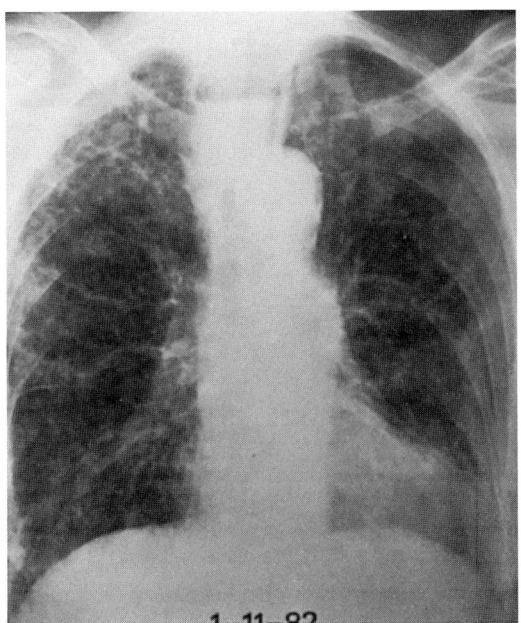

FIGURE 59.3. Acute respiratory failure caused by aspiration from a large pharyngoesophageal diverticulum. Note the air-fluid level in the upper esophagus, just above the aortic arch.

during the expiratory phase. It is not unusual for an enlarged esophagus in achalasia to appear as mediastinal widening or density on routine chest roentgenograms (Fig. 59.4). Aspiration pneumonia is a serious complication of achalasia and may lead to acute respiratory distress syndrome (ARDS). Esophagobronchial fistula has been described in a patient with chronic achalasia. Patients with achalasia are also at substantially increased risk for the development of esophageal cancer, which is typically of the squamous cell type (8).

Mycobacterial infections caused by rapidly growing mycobacteria (*M. fortuitum, M. chelonae,* and others) occur more frequently in patients with achalasia and other esophageal disorders. This complication is more likely if lipoid pneumonia develops as a result of recurrent aspiration. Therapy of both the esophageal disease and mycobacterial infection may be necessary for patients in whom progressive respiratory problems develop.

Chagas Disease

Chagas disease, or American trypanosomiasis, is an infection caused by *Trypanosoma cruzi*. An acute, often asymptomatic illness is followed by a prolonged latent period and chronic cardiac and gastrointestinal sequelae (9). In patients with predominantly esophageal involvement (chagasic megaesophagus), the pleuropulmonary problems include pleural effusion in 36%, pulmonary embolism in 22%, pneumonia in 35%, and aspiration pneumonia in a small percentage. All these complications are more common in patients with chagasic megaesophagus and cardiomyopathy than in those without esophageal involvement.

Esophageal Perforation

Most esophageal perforations are iatrogenic, and fewer than 15% represent spontaneous rupture. Esophagoscopy, especially in the removal of foreign bodies, is the most common cause of iatrogenic perforation (10) (Fig. 59.5). Other causes of esophageal perforation are the insertion of esophageal tubes, external trauma, carcinomas of the esophagus, Mallory-Weiss tear, Boerhaave syndrome, mediastinal malignancy, radiation necrosis of the esophagus, foreign

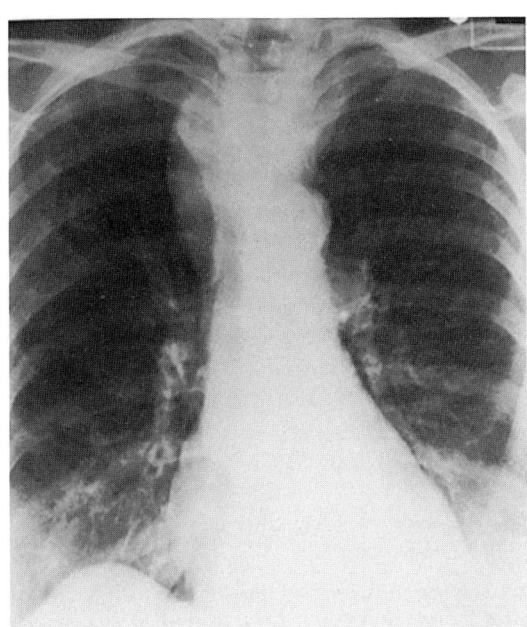

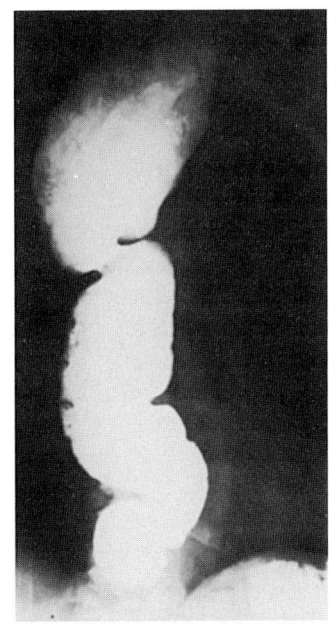

FIGURE 59.4. Achalasia presenting as a superoposterior mediastinal mass. Posteroanterior chest roentgenogram (**A**) and barium contrast study (**B**) demonstrate the megaesophagus.

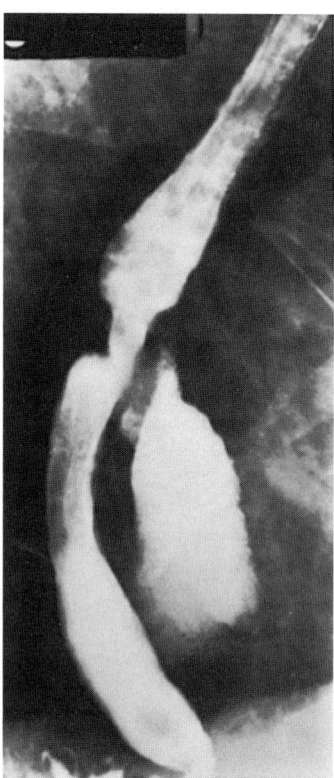

FIGURE 59.5. Instrumental perforation of anterior mid esophagus demonstrated by extravasation of Gastrografin into the mediastinum.

bodies, caustic ingestion, pill esophagitis, Barrett ulcer, and infectious ulcers in patients with AIDS (11).

Acute mediastinitis is the most serious complication of esophageal perforation (11). A pleural effusion develops in approximately 60% of patients with an esophageal perforation, and nearly 25% have a pneumothorax. The pleural effusion is usually left-sided, and analysis reveals a high protein content, high amylase level, low pH, and the presence of squamous epithelial cells and occasionally food particles. The amylase is derived from salivary juices leaking into the pleural space. The extremely low pH results from increased leukocytic and mesothelial metabolism, and also localized acidosis. The diagnosis of esophageal perforation is made by the clinical findings of chest pain, severe back pain, dysphagia, acute fever, and subcutaneous emphysema, and by documentation of the tear with Gastrografin contrast studies of the esophagus. Boerhaave syndrome and Mallory-Weiss tear of the esophagus can lead to acute mediastinitis. Endoscopy has no role in the diagnosis of spontaneous esophageal perforation. Both the endoscope and insufflation of air can extend the perforation and introduce air into the mediastinum (11,12).

Sclerotherapy of Esophageal Varices

Sclerotherapy is one of the therapeutic methods applied to control esophageal variceal hemorrhage (13). Either sodium morrhuate or ethanolamine oleate is used as the sclerosant,

which is injected into the varices under direct vision via the esophagoscope. Within 6 hours after the injection, mediastinal widening develops in some patients, presumably as a consequence of chemical mediastinitis. The overall incidence rates of intrathoracic complications are as follows: pleural effusion, 0 to 50%; mediastinitis, 63%; atelectasis, 16%; bronchitis, 8%; pneumonia, 0 to 5%; esophagopleural fistula, 1% to 2% (14). Other complications, such as esophagobronchial fistula, empyema, ARDS, pulmonary infarction, and late expectoration of sclerosant, are described but rare. Acute pulmonary edema leading to respiratory distress syndrome within 8 to 36 hours after sclerotherapy has been described. A study of 223 patients who underwent 390 esophageal variceal sclerotherapy procedures with either ethanolamine oleate or tetradecyl sulfate evaluated the pulmonary complications and reported the following: retrocardiac or mediastinal widening in 35%, pleural effusion in 27%, atelectasis in 12%, and pulmonary infiltrates in 9% of procedures (15). Respiratory insufficiency was noted after 14 sclerotherapy procedures. Most thoracic manifestations after variceal sclerotherapy are likely caused by a local inflammatory response to the sclerosant.

The injection of sodium morrhuate in sheep causes marked but transient pulmonary hypertension and an increased flow of relatively protein-poor lymph. The constituent unsaturated fatty acids may be responsible for the pathogenesis of pulmonary edema. The edema associated with sodium morrhuate may be another example of hydrostatic (low level of protein in lymph) pulmonary edema caused by the abrupt development of pulmonary hypertension without an increase in pulmonary capillary wedge pressure. The use of a Sengstaken tube immediately after sclerotherapy may increase the risk for pulmonary complications. On the other hand, acute respiratory failure resulting from sclerotherapy has resolved after aspiration of air via a Sengstaken tube.

The reductions in arterial partial pressure of oxygen (Pao_2) and vital capacity observed soon after sclerotherapy have been attributed to pulmonary embolization of the sclerosant, even though a significant occurrence of pulmonary embolism has not been described (16).

Pleural effusion after endoscopic variceal sclerotherapy is reported in 50% of patients (17). The incidence of pleural effusion is related to the amount of sclerosant injected. The effusions are usually small and are bilateral in a third, right-sided in a third, and left-sided in a third. They are usually exudative and transient. The pleural effusions are secondary to mediastinal pleuritis caused by the sclerosant. Chylothorax has also developed after sclerotherapy (18).

GASTROINTESTINAL ENDOSCOPY

Infection can be transmitted during gastrointestinal endoscopy if the instruments are contaminated. Organisms include *Salmonella* species, *Pseudomonas aeruginosa*, *Mycobacterium* species, and *Helicobacter pylori* (19,20). Pulmonary aspiration is a fairly common complication during emergency upper gastrointestinal endoscopy. New pulmonary infiltrates developed in 6 (20%) of 30 patients who underwent upper gastrointestinal endoscopy for the diagnosis and treatment of acute bleeding after the procedure, and all but one exhibited fever, leukocytosis, and oxygen desaturation below 90% (21).

Percutaneous Endoscopic Gastrostomy

Percutaneous endoscopic gastrostomy has become the preferred method of providing enteral nutritional support (22). Pneumonia is a known sequel of this procedure and is reported to occur with an incidence of 10% at 30 days and 56% at 11 months. One study used 24-hour monitoring to demonstrate an increased prevalence of gastroesophageal reflux in patients in whom pneumonia developed after the placement of a percutaneous endoscopic gastrostomy (23).

GASTROESOPHAGEAL REFLUX

Gastroesophageal reflux is an extremely common phenomenon, occurring on a daily basis in 10% and intermittently in 50% of healthy persons (24). Gastroesophageal reflux disease (GERD) is a syndrome that manifests as heartburn and the sequelae of esophagitis, ulceration, stricture, and Barrett epithelium (25). Gastroesophageal reflux and GERD are now known to be important in the pathogenesis of certain lung diseases, particularly laryngospasm, chronic cough, and asthma (24). Strong evidence suggests that both reflux-induced asthma and otolaryngologic complications, including subglottic stenosis, laryngitis, pharyngitis, and cancer, can occur without esophagitis. Mechanical reflux of gastric acid into the tracheobronchial tree is another mechanism responsible for the pulmonary complications. In a study of patients with chronic persistent cough or asthma suspected to be caused by reflux, distal and proximal pH monitoring was used to identify those with reflux-induced pulmonary problems. The study concluded that the abnormal reflux of 17% of the patients whose pulmonary symptoms responded to antireflux therapy would not have been recognized if proximal pH monitoring had not been performed; good to excellent relief of pulmonary symptoms was achieved with antireflux therapy in 71% of patients who had reflux (26). The esophageal pH is of diagnostic significance if intermittent symptoms can be shown to be associated consistently with a decrease in the intraesophageal pH to below 4.0 during testing.

Vagally mediated local neuronal esophagolaryngotracheal reflexes are now known to have an important role in the development of many of the respiratory complications of GERD. Normal vagal reflexes in the respiratory tract include cough, laryngeal closure, forced inspiration, respiratory suppression, bronchoconstriction, and mucus secretion. Abnormal reflexes consist of laryngospasm, prolonged apnea, bronchospasm, and singultus (hiccup). The question remains of whether gastroesophageal reflux is primary or secondary to the pulmonary disease. It is common knowledge that continuous coughing causes retching and vomiting. However, in a study of 12 patients with chronic obstructive pulmonary disease (COPD), esophageal manometry, 24-hour pH monitoring, esophageal acid clearance, and pulmonary function testing were performed to determine that these patients did not have a bronchoconstrictive reflex to distal esophageal acidification and that their esophageal function was normal.

Reflux Laryngitis

The association of gastroesophageal reflux with chronic hoarseness and posterior laryngitis has been referred to as *reflux laryngitis* or *Cherry-Donner syndrome* (24). During 24-hour esophageal pH monitoring, as many as 75% of patients with chronic hoarseness exhibit an abnormal amount of gastroesophageal reflux (27). In a group of 33 patients referred for hoarseness, gastroesophageal reflux was found in almost 80%. Abnormal laryngeal reflexes can be elicited by acidic (pH < 4.5) solutions. GERD also contributes to the development of chronic throat clearing, cough, sore throat, contact ulcer and granuloma, globus pharyngeus, cervical dysphagia, subglottic stenosis, and cricoarytenoid arthritis.

Cough

Controlled studies have shown that chronic persistent cough that remains unexplained after a diagnostic evaluation is associated with increased episodes of otherwise asymptomatic gastroesophageal reflux (28–30). In 4% to 21% of cases, chronic cough is estimated to be secondary to gastroesophageal reflux. Reflux should be considered an etiologic possibility in subjects with chronic persistent cough that remains unexplained after a standard diagnostic assessment. The adjusted odds ratio for the presence of gastroesophageal reflux in adults with unexplained chronic cough has been estimated to be 4.4; indeed, cough may be the sole presenting manifestation of gastroesophageal reflux. Prolonged exposure of the esophageal mucosa to gastric acid may cause cough by stimulating esophagolaryngotracheal reflexes. It has been suggested that a self-perpetuating mechanism may exist in persons with gastroesophageal reflux whereby acid reflux causes cough via a local neuronal esophageal-tracheobronchial reflex, and the cough in turn amplifies the reflux by increasing transdiaphragmatic pressure or by inducing transient relaxation of the lower esophageal sphincter. Impaired clearance of esophageal acid has been documented by 24-hour ambulatory monitoring of the esophageal pH in patients with chronic cough. Postnasal drip also may irritate the receptors located in the pharynx and larynx and contribute to cough; this phenomenon should be excluded in patients who have nocturnal cough and gastroesophageal reflux. Cough caused by tobacco smoke may be aggravated by lowered esophageal sphincter tone induced by the tobacco smoke.

Asthma

The association of asthma with GERD is well documented (31). It has been estimated that as many as 45% to 65% of adults with asthma have gastroesophageal reflux. Both animal and clinical data suggest that gastroesophageal reflux serves as a trigger of bronchospasm, potentiates the bronchomotor response to other triggers, or both. Patients with reflux-associated asthma may manifest symptoms of gastroesophageal reflux, either classic or atypical, but approximately 25% to 30% have clinically silent reflux (32). A questionnaire-based survey of 109 asthmatic patients recorded heartburn in 77%, regurgitation in 55%, and swallowing difficulties in 24%; at least one antireflux medication was required by 37% of them, and none of the asthma medications was associated with an increased likelihood of symptomatic gastroesophageal reflux (33). It is, however, important to recognize that gastroesophageal reflux may develop in asthmatic patients who take theophylline because the drug is known to decrease lower esophageal sphincter tone and predispose to reflux. In addition, theophylline increases gastric acid secretion.

Evidence suggests that microaspiration does not play a significant role in esophageal acid-induced bronchoconstriction (31). The mechanism of bronchospasm in the setting of gastroesophageal reflux is unclear. Although reflux of acid into the airways is well known to produce bronchospasm, asthma does not develop in all persons with gastroesophageal reflux. Asthma and gastroesophageal reflux are more common during sleep, but studies have shown that gastroesophageal reflux does not aggravate nocturnal asthma. It has even been questioned whether asthma causes esophageal reflux because the treatment of asthmatic patients with esophageal reflux diminishes the symptoms of reflux. Nonetheless, in comparison with bronchitic patients who have gastroesophageal reflux, asthmatic patients have more episodes and a shorter duration of gastroesophageal reflux.

One study provided the results of a long-term experience (average follow-up, 7.9 years) with a group of 44 asthmatic patients who had gastroesophageal reflux and underwent Nissan fundoplication; the gastroesophageal reflux cleared in 42 (95%) of them, asthma was markedly relieved or cured in 18 (41%), and the reflux was relieved in 29 (66%) (34). A significant association was found between cure of asthma after fundoplication and the presence of nocturnal attacks, nocturnal tracheitis, intrinsic tracheitis, intrinsic asthma, or a clear history of reflux symptoms preceding the onset of asthmatic symptoms. A clinically useful finding was that the positive response to a trial of medical treatment helped identify the patients who would be cured.

An opposite view of the role of gastroesophageal reflux in asthmatic patients was presented in a report of 90 nonasthmatic patients with adult-onset wheezing. A 90% prevalence of gastroesophageal reflux was noted during a study in which the patients were assigned randomly to receive cimetidine or placebo for 6 months. Those assigned to cimetidine or surgical therapy of gastroesophageal reflux improved significantly. The intake of pulmonary medicine for wheezing decreased significantly. Others have reported that antireflux treatment only minimally improves asthma control in patients with a history of gastroesophageal reflux (35). Unfortunately, no acceptable diagnostic method is available to confirm the presence of gastroesophageal reflux-induced asthma, and controversy about this issue is likely to continue.

No scientific evidence has demonstrated that the treatment of gastroesophageal reflux relieves asthma (31,36). However, subgroups of patients with asthma were identified who might benefit from reflux therapy, but responses were difficult to predict (31,36). Although the otolaryngologic manifestations usually respond to antisecretory medications, reflux-induced asthma responds convincingly only to antireflux surgery (37). A number of studies have documented excellent long-term results after surgical treatment for reflux-induced asthma (38). However, such therapy should be reserved for cases of severe asthma poorly controlled by medications and complicated by severe reflux that leads to ulcerative esophagitis (37).

Aspiration Pneumonia

Aspiration pneumonitis caused by gastroesophageal reflux is a serious acute medical problem and may lead to ARDS. The risk for the development of significant aspiration pneumonia increases when the volume of the gastric contents aspirated exceeds 50 mL and the pH of the aspirate is below 2.5. Although the initial pathologic features are directly related to the damaging effects of gastric acid, aspiration pneumonia is frequently complicated by bacterial pneumonitis. Community-acquired aspiration pneumonia is extremely uncommon except in alcoholics, persons with poor dental hygiene, and debilitated persons. Nosocomial aspiration pneumonia is more likely to be complicated by bacterial pneumonitis. Debility and prolonged supine posture predispose to this complication. Studies in which gastric contents were labeled with ^{99m}Tc-sulfur colloid and endobronchial secretions were subsequently measured in patients on mechanical ventilation have shown that a supine position, particularly when maintained for a prolonged period, is a potential risk factor for the aspiration of gastric contents. The same microorganisms were isolated from stomach, pharynx, and endobronchial samples in 32% of studies performed while patients were semirecumbent and in 68% of studies performed while patients were supine.

Alkalinization of the gastric contents also can predispose to bacterial pneumonia, and gastric colonization by microorganisms is related to the degree of gastric alkalinization. A gastric pH exceeding 4.0 appears to be the most important factor favoring gastric colonization. Hospitalized patients, particularly those on mechanical ventilation, are systematically given antacids or histamine H$_2$ blockers, or both, to prevent the development of stress ulcers. Several studies have shown that the use of these drugs in critically ill patients is associated with a greater incidence of both nosocomial pneumonia and gastric and pharyngeal colonization. These studies also reported that the prophylactic use of a cytoprotective agent such as sucralfate does not alter the gastric pH and thus prevents microbial colonization (see section "Gastric pH and Nosocomial Pneumonia") (39). Others have shown that treatment with cimetidine is an independent risk factor for the development of pneumonia in mechanically ventilated patients. Elevating the head of the bed to 45 degrees is reported to reduce the risk for aspiration pneumonia significantly (40,41).

Pulmonary complications may eventually develop in many subjects who remain asymptomatic despite frequent aspiration. Typical examples of insidious aspiration-induced lung disease include mild basal pulmonary fibrosis and patchy infiltrates. The ingestion of oil-based compounds as a laxative or for other reasons may result in lipoid pneumonia (Fig. 59.6).

Gastric pH and Nosocomial Pneumonia

The clinical practice of neutralizing gastric acid to prevent aspiration pneumonia and nosocomial pneumonia in ventilator- and non–ventilator-dependent patients has been controversial (42). A gastric pH above 4.0 is crucial for the overgrowth of gastric Gram-negative but not Gram-positive bacteria. Intragastric Gram-negative bacteria fre-

quently grow in critically ill patients who receive ulcer prophylaxis with drugs to suppress or neutralize gastric acidity. Gastric colonization with Gram-negative bacteria also occurs in almost all patients receiving enteral feeding. Aspiration of these organisms is an important mechanism in the development of nosocomial pneumonia. In a study of 242 mechanically ventilated trauma patients, pneumonia occurred more frequently in the patients with Gram-negative retrograde colonization from the stomach to the trachea, even though this phenomenon accounted for only 13% of all cases of pneumonia. An endotracheal tube does not afford complete protection from the aspiration of gastric bacteria. In a review of 269 articles including 63 randomized trials of stress ulcer prophylaxis, histamine H$_2$ receptor antagonists decreased the incidence of overt gastrointestinal bleeding, but a trend was noted toward an increased risk for pneumonia in the patients given histamine H$_2$ receptor antagonists in comparison with those given no prophylaxis (43). Sucralfate, however, was associated with a lower incidence of nosocomial pneumonia in comparison with antacids and histamine H$_2$ receptor antagonists. In a study of 242 patients who were randomized to sucralfate, antacid, or ranitidine, no statistically significant difference in pneumonia rates among the treatment groups was found during the first 4 days of therapy, although sucralfate appeared to decrease the incidence of nosocomial pneumonia after this period (44).

Other Complications of Gastroesophageal Reflux Disease

Several other complications of gastroesophageal reflux have been described. These include singultus (hiccup), bronchitis,

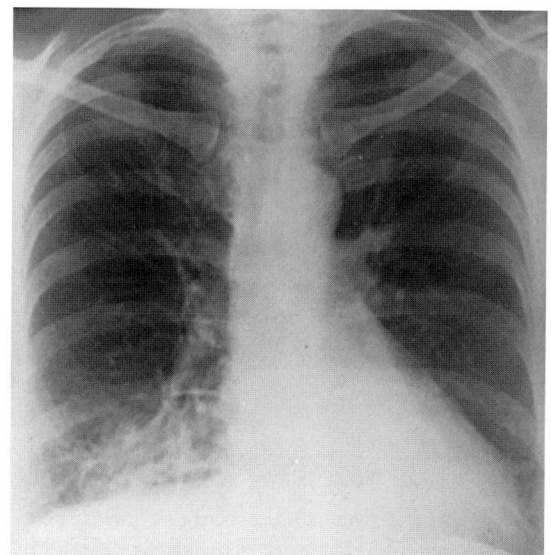
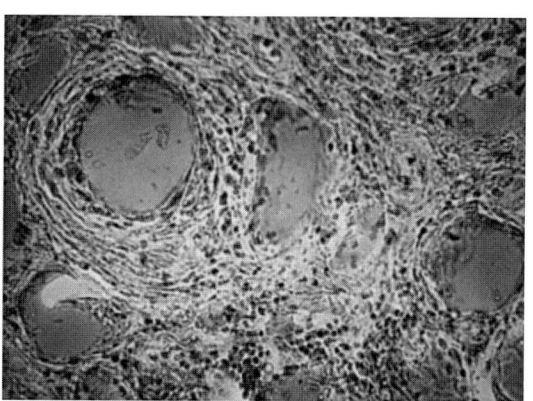

FIGURE 59.6. A: Chronic ingestion of mineral oil for laxative purposes resulting in the formation of an ill-defined mass in the right lower lobe. **B:** Resected portion of the abnormal lung revealed typical findings of lipoid pneumonia.

bronchiectasis, atelectasis, hemoptysis, pulmonary fibrosis, apnea, and seizures related to hypoxia. Many adults with obstructive sleep apnea have gastroesophageal reflux. This may be related to lower intrathoracic pressure caused by obstructive sleep apnea and an increased number of arousals and repetitive body movements during sleep. The treatment of obstructive sleep apnea with nasal continuous positive airway pressure has been shown to decrease thoracic gastroesophageal reflux in these patients. It has been shown that the esophagus and central nervous system of asymptomatic volunteers maintain an awareness of the presence and volume of intraesophageal acid, and the response time of the central nervous system is inversely related to acid volume. Larger volumes of acid in the esophagus are reported to serve as an afferent warning signal to the central nervous system to produce a rapid arousal from sleep along with a shortened interval to the first swallow.

GASTRIC DISORDERS

Hiatal Hernia

In esophageal hiatal hernia, chest roentgenograms often show the herniated portion of the stomach directly behind the heart, suggesting the possibility of a posterior mediastinal mass lesion (45). The presence of an air-fluid level and a barium contrast study usually confirm the diagnosis. Symptoms originating from a hiatal hernia may resemble those of cardiopulmonary disease; however, careful attention to the clinical history often helps in making the distinction. Occasionally, a large hiatal hernia may compromise pulmonary function by occupying a large area of the chest cavity (Fig. 59.7).

One of the most serious respiratory complications of hiatal hernia is aspiration pneumonia secondary to gastroesophageal reflux, as discussed previously (see section "Aspiration Pneumonia") (45). Roentgenologic and endoscopic investigations have reported that from 50% to 94% of patients with GERD have a hiatal hernia (45,46). A study of 34 patients with endoscopically documented hiatal hernia recorded that, in comparison with normal volunteers, those with a hiatal hernia had substantially higher reflux scores and lower pressures in the lower esophageal sphincter.

Hernia through the Foramina of Bochdalek and Morgagni

Hernia through the foramen of Bochdalek results from incomplete fusion of the posterolateral part of the diaphragm. Herniation is seen more frequently in children, and the abnormality is usually located on the left. Chest roentgenograms reveal a space-occupying mass lesion. Large herniations cause dyspnea, chest discomfort, and occasionally respiratory failure. These hernias sometimes mimic pleural effusion, with the lateral chest roentgenogram disclosing free layering. Postmortem studies in infants with congenital diaphragmatic hernia have shown that the lungs are immature, especially the ipsilateral lung. Additionally, intra-alveolar hemorrhage is reported to be a common complication of congenital diaphragmatic hernia. Hernia through the foramen of Morgagni tends to be located on the right and anteriorly. The liver may herniate, although herniation of intestinal segments is more likely (Fig. 59.8).

Peptic Ulcer Disease

Peptic ulcer disease has been found in 10% to 35% of study groups with chronic obstructive lung disease, in contrast with 3% in control groups. The increased incidence of ulcer disease has been explained, at least partly, by gastric

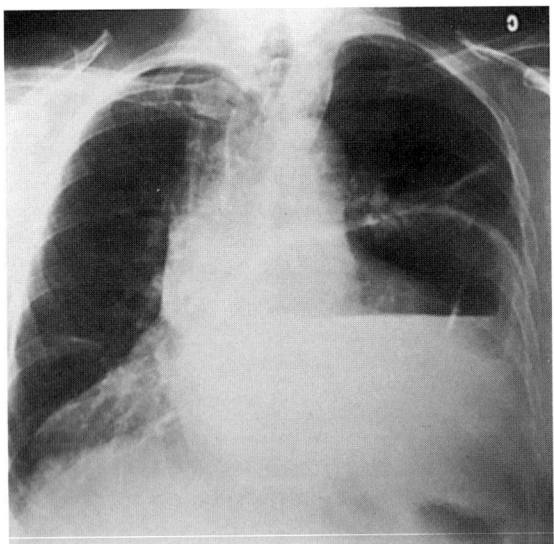
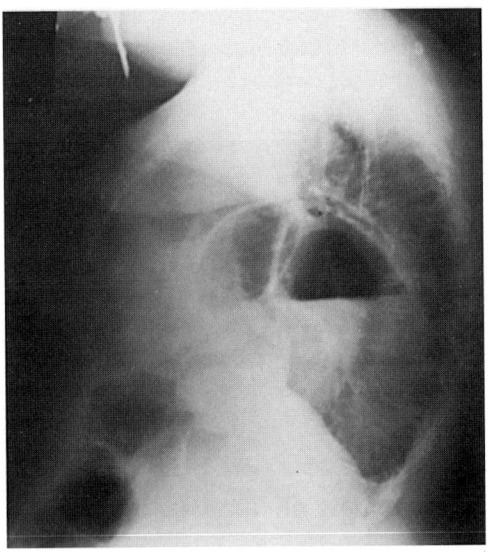

FIGURE 59.7. A large hiatal hernia occupying most of the chest cavity. **A:** Anterior view. **B:** Left lateral view.

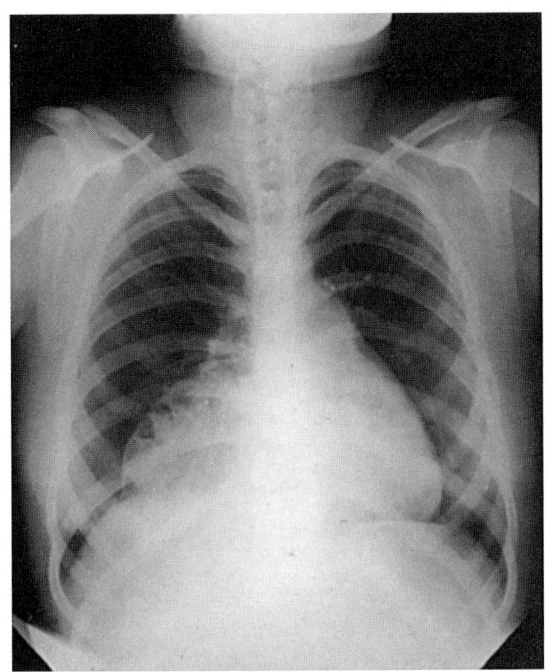
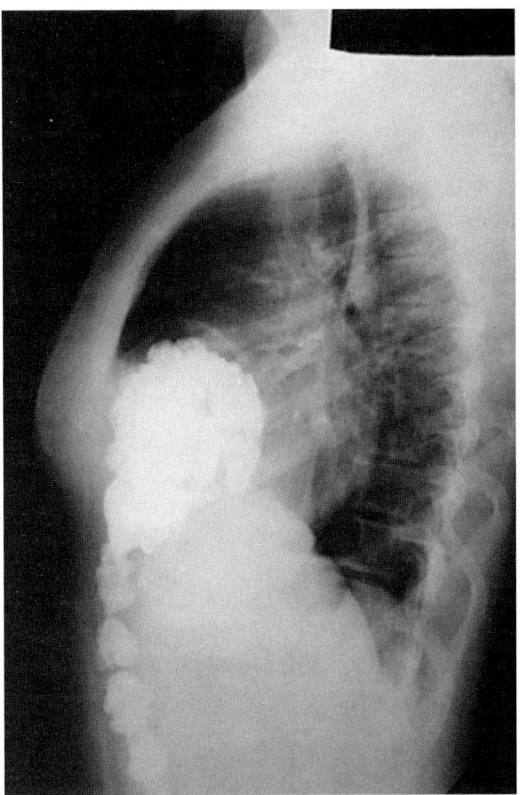

FIGURE 59.8. A: Foramen of Morgagni hernia presenting as an air-filled mass adjacent to the right border of the heart. **B:** A left lateral chest roentgenogram shows that much of the small intestine (containing barium contrast) has herniated through the foramen of Morgagni.

hypersecretion secondary to increased arterial carbon dioxide tension and decreased arterial oxygen tension. This theory applies only to patients in whom persistent hypercarbia develops as a result of their lung disease. The peptic ulcers associated with chronic obstructive lung disease are more commonly duodenal than gastric. Often, the peptic ulcer disease is not accompanied by pain and is recognized only after gastrointestinal hemorrhage occurs. Perforation of a gastric ulcer occasionally may result in pleural effusion. Because many patients who have obstructive lung disease are treated with corticosteroid preparations, the symptoms related to ulcer disease may be masked.

Acute upper gastrointestinal bleeding in patients with COPD is reported to be associated with a higher mortality than upper gastrointestinal bleeding in patients without COPD. In a case control study at a university teaching hospital, the mortality of patients with COPD and ulcer bleeding was 32%, whereas the mortality for those with bleeding but without COPD was 10% (odds ratio, 4.3); the increased mortality was correlated with the severity of COPD (47).

Effect of Gastrectomy on Tuberculosis

Gastrectomy has an adverse effect on preexisting, active pulmonary tuberculosis (TB), and elective surgery is best post-

poned until a reasonable period of antituberculous therapy has been completed. An increased incidence of pulmonary TB after subtotal or total gastrectomy and jejunal or ileal bypass has been noted. The incidence of TB after gastrectomy is estimated at 1% to 5%. The prevalence of prior gastrectomy in patients with TB has ranged from 1.7% to 20%, the higher incidence being more common in elderly patients. A poor response to treatment and an increased rate of reactivation have been noted in patients who have undergone gastrectomy and in whom infection with *Mycobacterium avium* complex later develops. The relationship between gastrectomy and the development of TB several years later is uncertain. A plausible explanation for the increased incidence of TB in this group of patients is the decreased absorption of antituberculous drugs as a result of the gastrectomy. Pharmacokinetic studies have documented this phenomenon in anecdotal cases. All this notwithstanding, fear of TB should not be a factor in a decision for elective gastrectomy.

Total gastrectomy may predispose to the aspiration of esophageal reflux contents. A study concluded that this was the most important risk factor for recurrent pulmonary complications in patients who had undergone total gastrectomy. Among 186 patients who had undergone total gastrectomy, 16 had recurrent respiratory tract inflammation, and 45 had sporadic respiratory tract inflammation (48). The former group frequently had symptoms related to esophageal reflux and the swallowing provocation test.

Gastrobronchial Fistula

Gastrobronchial fistula is extremely rare (49,50). A review in 1985 found only 13 cases (49). The most common cause of this type of fistula is erosion of a subphrenic abscess through the diaphragm with formation of a lung abscess (51). Traumatic rupture of the diaphragm, especially from penetrating injury, is the next most common cause. Perforated ulcer in an incarcerated hiatal hernia and necrosis of gastric tumors and areas of previous esophageal or gastric surgery are the other causes.

INTESTINAL DISEASES

Inflammatory Bowel Disease

Both chronic ulcerative colitis and Crohn disease (regional enteritis) are well-known for their various extraintestinal manifestations (52–54). Pulmonary involvement is an uncommon extraintestinal manifestation of these inflammatory bowel diseases (54,55) (Table 59.1). Pulmonary abnormalities in ulcerative colitis and Crohn disease may present years after the onset of bowel disease and can affect any part of the lungs (53). The pathogenesis of pulmonary disease in inflammatory bowel disease is not known. A common systemic mechanism affecting both the bronchial and colonic epithelium may be responsible. It has also been speculated that similarities in the mucosal immune system of the lung and intestine are responsible for the bronchial hyperreactivity of some patients with active inflammatory bowel disease. A variety of respiratory problems, including pulmonary vasculitis, apical fibrosis, chronic suppurative bronchitis, and bronchiectasis, have been reported (Fig. 59.9). However, in a series of 1,400 patients with inflammatory bowel disease evaluated retrospectively, only three were found to have unexplained bronchopulmonary disease. In a separate review of clinical data for 1,400 patients with inflammatory bowel disease whose diagnoses were recorded in a computerized registry between 1930 and 1970, only six cases of pulmonary disease were unexplained. However, publications in the 1980s and 1990s have reported higher prevalence rates of respiratory problems in patients with inflammatory bowel disease. For instance, abnormalities of pulmonary function have been reported in 36% to 68% of patients with Crohn disease.

A report on the data in an ongoing registry that included 33 patients with pulmonary complications of ulcerative colitis and Crohn disease, of whom 23 were not on any therapy, noted that in 28 of the 33, lung involvement followed the onset of intestinal disease (8 of the 28 had undergone colectomy); in the others, the pulmonary features preceded the intestinal disease (56). Airway manifestations included subglottic stenosis, chronic bronchitis, severe chro-

TABLE 59.1. PULMONARY ABNORMALITIES ASSOCIATED WITH INTESTINAL DISEASES

Intestinal Disease	Pulmonary Abnormality
Inflammatory bowel diseases[a]	Apical pulmonary fibrosis
	Bronchiectasis
	Bronchiolitis
	Bullous lung disease
	Chronic bronchitis
	Desquamative interstitial pneumonitis
	Increased incidence of asthma
	Lymphocytic alveolitis
	Pleural effusion
	Pulmonary edema
	Tracheoesophageal fistula
	Airflow obstruction
	Decreased D$_{LCO}$
	Sulfasalazine- and mesalamine-induced lung disease
Whipple disease	Cough
	Pleuritic chest pain
	Pleural effusion
	Hilar lymphadenopathy
	Pulmonary parenchymal infiltrates
	Restrictive pulmonary dysfunction
	Tracheobronchial nodules
Nontropical sprue (celiac disease)	Interstitial pneumonitis and fibrosis
	Hypersensitivity pneumonitis
	Chronic cough
	Increased incidence of asthma
	Peribronchial fibrosis
	Pulmonary hemosiderosis
Intestinal parasitic diseases	Asthma
	Pulmonary infiltrates with eosinophilia
	Pulmonary parasitic infiltrates
Intestinal lymphangiectasia	Pleural effusion (chylous)

[a]Includes chronic ulcerative colitis and Crohn disease.
D$_{LCO}$, diffusing capacity of the lung for carbon monoxide.

nic bronchial suppuration, bronchiectasis, and chronic bronchiolitis. Bronchoscopy in these patients revealed exuberant inflammatory tissue and mucosal ulcerations and a narrowed tracheal or bronchial lumen. Histologically, dense aggregates of inflammatory cells were noted. Interstitial lung disease consisted mainly of bronchiolitis obliterans–organizing pneumonia, pulmonary infiltrates, and eosinophilia. Neutrophilic necrotic parenchymal nodules were also noted. Corticosteroid therapy was more effective in resolving parenchymal disease than in resolving airway disease.

In another study, of 10 nonsmokers with chronic ulcerative colitis, four had exertional dyspnea, four had abnormalities on their chest roentgenograms, and three had obstructive changes on pulmonary function testing (57). The bronchial biopsy specimens of four patients showed basal cell hyperplasia, submucosal inflammation, and thickening of the basement membrane, similar to the pathologic changes in the colonic mucosa (57). In a study of 18 patients with Crohn disease and no pulmonary symptoms, bronchoalveolar lavage (BAL) revealed lymphocytic alveolitis in 61%, with lymphocyte counts ranging from 18% to 79%. No

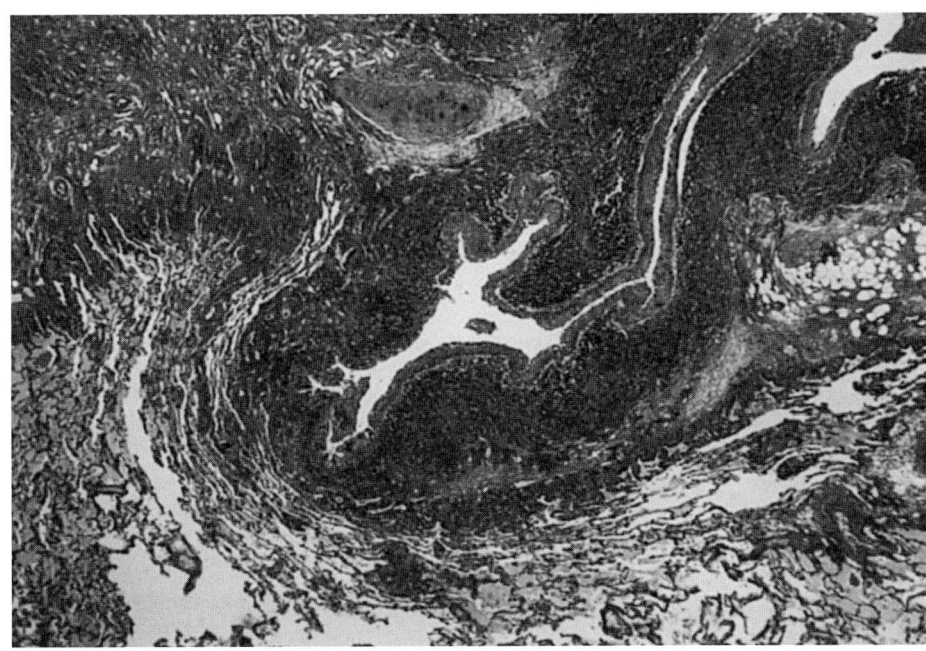

FIGURE 59.9. Chronic bronchiectasis that was symptomatically steroid-responsive in this patient with ulcerative colitis. A dense infiltrate of chronic inflammatory cells involves a small bronchus.

correlation was apparent between the lymphocyte count in the lavage effluent and the pulmonary dysfunction observed in 11 patients. These studies suggest that most patients with Crohn disease have a latent pulmonary involvement mediated by lymphocytes. In one study, 71% of patients with Crohn disease demonstrated increased superoxide production, but the significance of this in the pathogenesis of lung disease is unclear.

Airways Disease

In one study, pulmonary function was assessed in patients with ulcerative colitis or Crohn disease and compared with that in a healthy population, and no statistically significant differences were found between the three groups (58). However, in a prospective study of 58 patients with Crohn disease and 44 patients with chronic ulcerative colitis, the incidence of respiratory abnormalities was high in both groups. Pulmonary function test values were abnormal in 50% of the patients, with diminished flow rates (<50% of the predicted forced expiratory volume in the first second [FEV_1]) in 31% and a decreased diffusing capacity (<75% of the predicted value) in 26%. An abnormally low diffusing capacity was the only abnormality in 16 patients (eight with Crohn disease) (58). Interstitial processes were noted on the chest roentgenograms of four patients with Crohn disease and two with colitis. High-resolution CT changes of bronchiectasis, mosaic perfusion, and air trapping, suggestive of obliterative bronchiolitis, and a pattern of centrilobular nodules and branching linear opacities ("tree in bud" appearance), suggestive of either cellular bronchiolitis or bronchiolectasis with mucoid secretions, have been identified in patients with inflammatory bowel disease (53).

A study disclosed that the prevalence of hay fever and asthma was relatively high in 242 patients with chronic ulcerative colitis and slightly higher in 45 patients with Crohn disease. A report of 29 patients with Crohn disease noted that the lungs are relatively unaffected by Crohn disease. Bronchiolitis with organizing pneumonitis, sclerosing peribronchiolitis, and diffuse panbronchiolitis are the other abnormalities described in ulcerative colitis.

Ulcerative tracheobronchitis, with intense plasma cell infiltration of the tracheal mucosa and submucosa and the destruction of mucous glands, occurred 4 and 8 years after total colectomy in patients with ulcerative colitis (59). Bronchoscopy in Crohn disease has revealed small, diffuse, whitish granulations and erythematous mucosa, and biopsy of the bronchial mucosa has shown ulcerative bronchitis and noncaseous tuberculoid granulomas.

Pulmonary Parenchymal Disease

Pulmonary function testing in a study of 36 outpatients with inflammatory bowel disease revealed a significantly reduced diffusing capacity of the lung for carbon monoxide (D_{LCO}) in comparison with matched controls ($P < .01$). The reason for this reduction was not clear, although it was considered unlikely to be caused by sulfasalazine (salazosulfapyridine). A further study of the lung function of 10 patients with Crohn disease during and after an attack of the disease revealed that the pulmonary volumes and D_{LCO} were not impaired, but that the functional residual capacity was greater during the attack than during remission; it was also greater than in normal subjects. Disease activity, functional residual capacity, and finger clubbing decreased concomitantly during remission. As previously noted (see section "Airways Disease"), some patients have exhibited a low diffusing capacity as the only abnormality.

Although the association of apical fibrosis and ankylosing spondylitis is widely recognized, only one case has been reported in which fibrosis was associated with both spondylitis and ulcerative colitis. Dense basal pulmonary infiltrates responsive to steroid therapy have been reported in two patients; lung biopsy in one revealed changes similar to those in idiopathic pulmonary fibrosis, and the second had nondiagnostic findings. Pulmonary bullous lesions also are described in chronic ulcerative colitis. Hypoproteinemia is common in Crohn disease. A case has been described of a 29-year-old man who presented with recurrent pulmonary edema and hypoalbuminemia. Crohn disease was diagnosed only after several episodes of pulmonary edema.

In an investigation of pulmonary abnormalities in 26 children with acute or quiescent Crohn disease, the chest radiographic findings were normal in all subjects (60). Even though no significant differences were found between acute and quiescent Crohn disease in regard to pulmonary volumes and expiratory flows, the D$_{LCO}$ was significantly decreased during the active phase of the disease in comparison with remission (53% $\pm$ 15% vs. 81% $\pm$ 19% of the predicted value). An 11-year-old child who presented with terminal ileitis associated with pulmonary lesions showing periodic progression has been described; the initial thoracic disorder developed 2 years before roentgenographic evidence of the ileitis, and the second episode coincided with the diagnosis of the ileal lesion. The pulmonary lesions progressed simultaneously with the clinical signs of digestive tract disturbances, which eventually stabilized.

A pathogenetic relationship between sarcoidosis and Crohn disease has been suggested because noncaseating granulomas and BAL fluid lymphocytosis (with an elevated ratio of CD4$^+$ to CD8$^+$ cells) are seen in both disorders (61,62). In patients with inflammatory bowel disease, biopsy of the affected segment of intestine may show granulomatous changes. Noncaseous and nonconfluent granulomas are found in 30% of patients with Crohn disease. A report described three patients with classic chronic ulcerative colitis in whom histologically proven type III sarcoidosis developed during the course of their disease (63). A case of acute segmental inflammation of the terminal ileum in a female patient who presented with signs and symptoms of acute appendicitis has been reported. The patient had associated bilateral pulmonary TB. The role of *Mycobacterium tuberculosis* in the development of segmental ileal disease is well known, but the relationship between TB and inflammatory bowel disease is not clear. The incidence of TB is increased in persons who have undergone a jejunal or ileal bypass.

Other Pulmonary Complications

Pleuropericarditis may complicate ulcerative colitis and Crohn disease. A review of the literature revealed approximately a dozen patients with ulcerative colitis and Crohn disease in whom pleural effusions developed; these were bilateral in a third and left-sided in the rest. Many were associated with pericardial effusion. The pleuropericardial complications of inflammatory bowel disease may run an independent course and may be present when bowel disease is inactive.

Aspiration pneumonia has resulted from esophageal involvement in inflammatory bowel disease. Crohn disease is complicated by esophageal stricture in 38% of cases and by ulcerations in 32%. The most common presenting symptom in Crohn disease of the esophagus is dysphagia, seen in more than two thirds of patients. Cough and repeated bouts of pneumonia occur in a small number of patients.

Enteropulmonary fistula may present as recurrent localized pneumonia. A case of one such fistula originating in the colon of a patient with Crohn disease has been described. Esophagotracheal fistula has been described in 6% of patients. Histologic studies of these areas have shown submucosal fibrosis, lymphocytic infiltration, noncaseous granulomas, and hypertrophy of muscle.

Antineutrophil cytoplasmic antibodies (ANCAs) have been reported in up to 87% of patients with primary sclerosing cholangitis with or without ulcerative colitis and in 68% of patients with only ulcerative colitis. A snowdrift-like perinuclear (p-ANCA) pattern has been described in up to 84% of patients with a high level of disease activity in ulcerative colitis. The cytoplasmic ANCA (c-ANCA) seen in active Wegener granulomatosis and the p-ANCA with myeloperoxidase specificity seen in microscopic polyangiitis are distinctly uncommon in patients with ulcerative colitis. Nevertheless, c-ANCA positivity with histologic features and chest roentgenographic features typical of Wegener granulomatosis has been described in a patient with ulcerative colitis who was treated with sulfasalazine (64). All these features resolved after the withdrawal of sulfasalazine.

Sulfasalazine, used in the treatment of inflammatory bowel disease, is known to cause pulmonary infiltrates and dyspnea (64). Eosinophilia in the peripheral blood is a frequent finding, and chest radiographs often show peripheral infiltrates typical of chronic eosinophilic pneumonia (54). A patient with ulcerative colitis receiving sulfasalazine therapy in whom interstitial pneumonitis and bronchiolitis developed has been described (65). Open lung biopsy in a patient with chronic ulcerative colitis showed severe interstitial fibrosis and bronchiectasis. The pulmonary fibrosis progressed despite the withdrawal of sulfasalazine therapy and a total colectomy. Progressive respiratory distress resulting from desquamative interstitial pneumonitis developed in a child with chronic ulcerative colitis and hepatic cirrhosis despite the withdrawal of sulfasalazine and the initiation of systemic corticosteroid therapy.

Mesalamine, one of the 5-aminosalicylate drugs used to treat inflammatory bowel disease, has been implicated in causing a lung injury characterized by bilateral pulmonary infiltrates, peripheral eosinophilia, and histologic findings consistent with acute pneumonitis (66). Nongranulomatous interstitial diffuse lung disease associated with an inflammatory lymphoid infiltration and mild interstitial collagen fibrosis has been reported in a patient treated with mesalamine for Crohn disease. Bilateral interstitial infiltrates and abnormalities of gas exchange were described in a patient in whom the pulmonary complication developed insidiously after 2 years of treatment with mesalamine.

Tobacco smoking and nicotine gum chewing are reported to have a beneficial effect on the symptoms of patients with ulcerative colitis (67). Current smokers have a 40% lower risk for the development of ulcerative colitis than nonsmokers; however, the disease is approximately 1.7 times more likely to develop in former smokers than in those who have never smoked (68,69). In contrast, several studies have demonstrated a strong association between Crohn disease and smoking. The biologic basis for these unusual associations remains unknown (70).

TREATMENT OF LUNG INVOLVEMENT IN INFLAMMATORY BOWEL DISEASE

Summary Statement	Level of Evidence
Drug-induced disease (sulfasalazine or 5-aminosalicylic acid) and superimposed bacterial infection must be ruled out before therapy is instituted in this setting (54). In the presence of pulmonary infiltrates with eosinophilia, it is reasonable to assume that drug-induced disease is present and discontinue the drug (54).	Expert opinion
Inhaled corticosteroid therapy, often in relatively high doses (e.g., 1,500–2,000 μg of beclomethasone per day), is frequently effective in the various forms of airway inflammation (54).	Observational studies, expert opinion
The pulmonary parenchymal complications of inflammatory bowel disease require oral corticosteroid therapy (54).	Observational studies, expert opinion
Nonsteroidal antiinflammatory therapy is the initial treatment for serositis (e.g., pleural effusions).	Observational studies, expert opinion

Nontropical Sprue

An association of nontropical sprue (celiac disease) and diffuse pulmonary disease has been reported in several cases (71,72). Although each of these disorders may be associated with abnormal immunologic phenomena, the pathogenesis remains unclear. However, studies of patients with this combination of diseases have identified avian protein precipitins in the sera. The influence of extrinsic factors appears to be prominent in cases of pulmonary fibrosis; farmer's lung precipitins (*Micropolyspora faeni*) have been noted in patients with the combination of nontropical sprue and pulmonary fibrosis (73). It has been suggested that both non-tropical sprue and extrinsic allergic alveolitis may be caused by a common immunologic mechanism because extrinsic allergic alveolitis and nontropical sprue are both associated with HLA-D3, and an association between nontropical sprue and hypersensitivity pneumonitis has been reported in Europe (74). However, a study of 18 North American patients with nontropical sprue failed to corroborate such as association (75). Nonetheless, a higher proportion of patients with celiac disease than of control subjects had a history of asthma or chronic cough, and the patients with nontropical sprue showed objective evidence of obstructive lung disease.

Interstitial lung disease has been diagnosed by lung function studies and chest roentgenograms (76–78). A case was reported of a 62-year-old woman with celiac sprue in whom lymphocytic interstitial pneumonia developed followed by abdominal lymphoma (79). The patient presented with dyspnea, cough, weight loss, and bilateral basilar pulmonary infiltrates. Systemic corticosteroids induced an improvement that lasted 1 year. Whereas lymphocytic lymphoma is a well-known complication of sprue, lymphocytic interstitial pneumonitis is not. Postmortem examination of the respiratory system of a patient with nontropical sprue revealed partial fibrous obliteration of small airways and dilation of larger airways (72).

Pulmonary hemosiderosis has been described in several patients with celiac disease (80). A study of seven patients with idiopathic pulmonary hemosiderosis revealed nontropical sprue in three and limited airflow and a decreased D$_{\text{LCO}}$ in five. Clinical documentation that treatment of celiac disease can lead to a remission of idiopathic pulmonary hemosiderosis is worth noting (80). In the cases reported in the literature, both diseases abated in 6 of 10 patients on a gluten-free diet, although histopathologic improvement of the intestinal lesion occurred in only two. Antibodies to reticulin are found in 78% of patients with celiac disease, and antibodies to gliadin in 95%. It has been suggested that if the serology is positive for either reticulin or gliadin in a patient with idiopathic pulmonary hemosiderosis, a gluten-free diet should be considered as part of the therapy.

Whipple Disease

Whipple disease is now recognized as a chronic multisystem granulomatous disorder that affects primarily middle-aged white men (81). Whipple disease typically involves the small intestine and causes malabsorption. Extraintestinal manifestations such as arthritis and fever are common and often develop before the onset of gastrointestinal symptoms. Involvement of the central nervous system can occur and lead to permanent sequelae. Weight loss, hyperpigmentation, and lymphadenopathy are frequent findings. A review of the literature demonstrates a high prevalence of cardiac manifestations, including constrictive pericarditis, valvular deformity, myocarditis, coronary arteritis, and congestive heart failure. The definitive diagnosis is made by biopsy of the small intestinal mucosa, which reveals infiltration of the lamina propria with periodic acid-Schiff (PAS)–positive macrophages. Electron microscopy reveals rod-shaped bacillary bodies that perhaps represent *Tropheryma whippelii*. Therapy with trimethoprim/sulfamethoxazole for 12 months usually results in clinical remission with an excellent prognosis. Several pulmonary complications have been described in patients with Whipple disease.

Pleuropulmonary complications include pleuritic pain, pleural effusion, dyspnea, cough, lung infiltrates, and restrictive lung dysfunction (82). Respiratory involvement without other symptoms, such as arthralgias and fever, has occurred. Cough is noted in nearly half of these cases. Although intestinal and joint manifestations are attributed to intracellular infection, the pulmonary manifestations may be the result of an inflammatory reaction to locally deposited immune complexes containing bacterial antigens. Whipple disease is known to simulate pulmonary sarcoidosis (81). Noncaseous granulomas were found in the peripheral lymph nodes, pleura, and lung parenchyma of one patient in whom chest roentgenographic features of sarcoidosis developed. The pleuropulmonary disease resolved with appropriate treatment of the Whipple disease.

Endobronchial lesions and large pulmonary nodules have been described in Whipple disease. In a 31-year-old man, Whipple disease presented with rapidly enlarging pulmonary nodules (83). A bronchoscopic examination showed several raised yellow endobronchial lesions, mainly at the subcarinae of the lobar bronchi. Biopsy specimens contained multiple foamy macrophages that were PAS-positive and diastase-resistant without granulomas or giant cells. Interestingly, this patient had no gastrointestinal features. Whipple disease presenting as pleuropericarditis in a 48-year-old woman exhibited peribronchiolar and perivascular histiocytic infiltrates in a patchy distribution with characteristic cytoplasmic bacilliform inclusions in the cells.

Other Malabsorption Syndromes

Protein-losing enteropathy may predispose patients to the development of pleural effusions, both transudative and chylous. Primary intestinal lymphangiectasia is a rare condition of uncertain cause characterized by dilated lymphatics in the small bowel and often complicated by anomalous lymphatics elsewhere, typically in the limbs. Protein-losing enteropathy secondary to intestinal lymphangiectasia has been reported to cause chylothorax.

The combination of yellow nails, lymphedema, and pleural effusions is known as the *yellow nail syndrome* (84). Lymphedema can occur as a distinct entity or as a result of lymphatic obstruction or loss of chyle through various mechanisms. More than 20% of patients with primary lymphedema have a protein-losing enteropathy resulting from lymphangiectasia of the small bowel. With significant loss of protein, hypoproteinemia and hypogammaglobulinemia

develop. Persistent pleural effusions and recurrent pulmonary infections may ensue in this setting.

HEPATIC DISEASES

Diseases of the liver cause or are associated with multiple pulmonary problems (Table 59.2). Arterial hypoxemia in conjunction with hemoglobin desaturation, clubbing,

TABLE 59.2. INTRATHORACIC ABNORMALITIES IN HEPATIC DISEASES

Hepatic Disorder	Intrathoracic Complication
Cirrhosis[a]	Intrapulmonary shunting
	Pleural shunting (pleural spider nevi)
	Portopulmonary shunting
	Pleural effusion (without ascites)
	Defective hypoxic vasoconstriction
	Ventilation-perfusion mismatch
	Diffusion abnormalities
	Pulmonary hypertension
	Rightward shift of oxyhemoglobin dissociation curve
Ascites	Diaphragmatic elevation
	Pleural effusion
	Empyema
	Decreased lung volumes
Hepatitis[b]	Pleuritis or pleural effusion
	Interstitial pneumonitis
Primary biliary cirrhosis	Lymphocytic alveolitis (subclinical)
	Lymphocytic interstitial pneumonitis
	Interstitial pneumonitis (nonspecific)
	Desquamative interstitial pneumonitis
	Interstitial noncaseous granulomas
	Airways obstruction (with Sjögren syndrome)
	Restrictive disease (thoracic deformity)
Primary sclerosing cholangitis	Bronchiectasis
	Recurrent bronchitis
Hepatic abscess	Pleurisy or pleural effusion
	Empyema
	Lung abscess
Hepatic amebiasis	Pleurisy or pleural effusion
	Amebic empyema
	Hepatobronchial fistula
Hepatic hydatid disease	Pleurisy or pleural effusion
Hepatic or biliary surgery	Diaphragmatic elevation
	Pleurisy or pleural effusion
	Pulmonary bile embolism
Hepatic malignancy	Pleural effusion
	Pulmonary nodules
	Diffuse lymphangitic infiltration
Liver transplantation	Pleural effusion
	Opportunistic infections
	Atelectasis of right lower lobe
	Diaphragmatic paralysis and dysfunction
	Pulmonary calcification
α_1-Antitrypsin deficiency	Panlobular emphysema
	Bullous lung disease
	Intrapulmonary shunting

[a] Alcoholic, cryptogenic, and postnecrotic cirrhosis.
[b] Viral, drug-induced, and chronic active hepatitis.

pleural effusions secondary to ascites, hyperventilation, and platypnea-orthodeoxia are encountered in 15% to 45% of patients with cirrhosis. The pathologic mechanisms involved in these complications are varied. Pulmonary intravascular macrophages (phagocytes) are mainly responsible for the uptake of circulating particles by lung cells (85). Pulmonary intravascular phagocytosis has been detected in animal models of chronic biliary cirrhosis and in humans with liver diseases. In certain disease states (e.g., biliary cirrhosis), pulmonary phagocytes may develop in the pulmonary capillaries, placing the lungs at risk for pathogen localization and subsequent inflammation leading to respiratory distress.

Hepatic Hydrothorax

Hepatic hydrothorax is a pleural effusion in a patient with cirrhosis and no evidence of underlying cardiopulmonary disease (86). Pleural effusion, usually right-sided and occasionally massive and symptomatic, may occur in cirrhosis or peritonitis. A pleural effusion is found in 6% of patients who have hepatic cirrhosis associated with ascites. The fluid is usually a transudate, and its chemical characteristics are similar to those of ascitic fluid. There are three possible mechanisms for the development of pleural effusion in hepatic cirrhosis: hypoproteinemia, azygos hypertension, and transfer of peritoneal fluid to the pleural cavity through congenital defects in the diaphragm. The intraperitoneal injection of radioactive ^{99m}Tc-sulfur colloid has demonstrated the one-way transdiaphragmatic flow of fluid from the peritoneal to the pleural space, and thoracotomy has made it possible to identify the diaphragmatic defects. In patients with massive pleural effusion secondary to ascites, drainage of the pleural fluid for therapeutic purposes is usually futile because so long as the peritoneal cavity contains fluid, the pleural fluid reaccumulates. Treatment should be aimed at controlling the ascites. Pleural effusions also are seen in viral hepatitis. In a prospective Italian study of hepatitis, some fluid was found in the pleural space of 70% of 156 patients.

Ascites, if large in volume, can interfere with normal pulmonary function by preventing normal diaphragmatic excursion. Ascites and abnormal distention restrict full inflation of the lungs and thus reduce lung volume. This effect of ascites on the pulmonary system is mediated by the hydrostatic pressure exerted from within the peritoneal cavity on the diaphragm. However, the effect varies among patients and appears to depend on the intra-abdominal hydrostatic pressure (thought of as a pressure in excess of the height of the anterior abdominal wall).

Large-volume paracentesis is a safe, rapid, and effective treatment of ascites and usually relieves the respiratory symptoms caused by tense ascites (87). One study investigated the effect of large-volume (5 L) paracentesis on parameters of pulmonary function in eight hemodynamically stable patients with cirrhosis and tense ascites and no known lung disease or abnormalities on chest roentgenograms (88). The

baseline lung volumes, diffusing capacity, and Pao$_2$ were reduced, but the flow rates were normal. Following paracentesis, the lung volumes increased significantly; the diffusing capacity and arterial oxygenation did not change significantly.

Hepatopulmonary Syndrome

Hepatopulmonary syndrome is arterial hypoxemia in a patient with cirrhosis (89–91). Arterial hypoxemia is present in 30% to 50% of patients with hepatic cirrhosis. It may also occur in other chronic liver diseases, such as chronic active hepatitis and nonspecific hepatitis. The pathophysiologic mechanisms include a low level of pulmonary vascular tone characterized by a poor or absent hypoxic pressor response, which results in marked dilation of the pulmonary vasculature. Both the liver and the endothelial cells may play a critical role in the regulation of pulmonary vascular tone in these patients. The abnormal pulmonary vascular tone causes ventilation-perfusion mismatch and mild to moderate hypoxemia (92). As the hepatic damage progresses, the intrapulmonary venoarterial shunt becomes more severe, seriously limiting oxygen diffusion and leading finally to severe respiratory failure. The development of abnormal anatomic communications between the pulmonary arteries and veins with bypass of the capillary-alveolar interphase also contributes to the hypoxemia (91). Other mechanisms may be at play in causing hypoxemia in association with liver cirrhosis. Injection of radioactive krypton into the spleen has revealed definite portopulmonary anastomoses. In some instances, venous blood in the portal system may reach the left side of the heart through anastomotic channels with pulmonary veins. Intrapulmonary shunts can reach considerable proportions (20%–70%) of the cardiac output. Blood gas analysis discloses moderate hypoxemia and respiratory alkalosis.

Orthodeoxia is hypoxemia that develops when a subject is in an erect position and is relieved when the subject assumes a recumbent position (93). Orthodeoxia in patients with hepatic cirrhosis results from the effect of the gravitational forces that increase the blood flow through intrapulmonary venoarterial shunts. When orthodeoxia is severe, patients experience increasing dyspnea while standing (platypnea). Although hypoxemia is common and multifactorial, severe hypoxia is unusual (90). In a large series of cirrhotic patients, 7% had a Pao$_2$ of less than 60 mm Hg while breathing room air.

Chest roentgenograms in hepatopulmonary syndrome normally display bilateral basilar nodular or reticulonodular opacities. Conventional CT reveals that these nodules portray dilated lung vessels. Imaging with technetium 99m-labeled macroaggregated albumin scanning (^{99m}Tc-MAA) perfusion can be utilized to confirm intrapulmonary arteriovenous shunting. High-resolution CT is valuable in eliminating pulmonary fibrosis as the cause of these opacities. Contrast-enhanced echocardiography appears to be the most sensitive diagnostic test for detecting intrapulmonary vascular dilations.

Therapy of hepatopulmonary syndrome with almitrine bimesylate (a somatostatin analogue), indomethacin, and plasmapheresis has been disappointing. Large pulmonary arteriovenous shunts documented by pulmonary angiography have been treated with embolotherapy, with abatement of the hypoxemia (94).

Diffuse Pulmonary Disease

Diffuse interstitial lung disease, occasionally granulomatous, has been observed in patients with primary biliary cirrhosis. Primary biliary cirrhosis is a granulomatous liver disease characterized by chronic intrahepatic cholestasis. The cause is unknown, and it is associated with non–organ-specific antibodies to mitochondria in more than 95% of patients. The frequency and nature of the pleuropulmonary manifestations in primary biliary cirrhosis are poorly documented (95). Many cases of lung involvement in primary biliary cirrhosis have been characterized by granuloma formation in the lung parenchyma and mononuclear cell alveolitis mimicking pulmonary sarcoidosis. One study in which BAL was used showed an increase in the number of alveolar CD4$^+$ lymphocytes (22% vs. 12% in alcoholic cirrhosis) and activated alveolar macrophages in 50% of patients. These data suggest that subclinical alveolar inflammation, involving T lymphocytes and activated alveolar macrophages and mimicking sarcoid alveolitis, is present in a high proportion of patients with primary biliary cirrhosis. Pulmonary nodules simulating pulmonary carcinomatosis and later documented to be lymphocytic interstitial pneumonitis were described in a 51-year-old woman. These changes were unrelated to the activity of the primary biliary cirrhosis and resolved spontaneously. Because sicca complex is often associated with primary biliary cirrhosis, part of the respiratory dysfunction noted in primary biliary cirrhosis may be related to sicca complex rather than to the liver disease.

A prospective study of hepatic and pulmonary function in 47 patients (nonsmokers) with primary biliary cirrhosis found a significant relationship between the histologic stage of the primary biliary cirrhosis and the steady-state diffusing capacity, and between the Mayo risk score for disease severity and the steady-state diffusing capacity (96). Progressive deterioration of the steady-state diffusing capacity was associated with increasing severity of the primary biliary cirrhosis. No relationship was found between pulmonary involvement and the presence of Sjögren syndrome. No significant relationship was observed between expiratory airflow and the severity of primary biliary cirrhosis.

In a prospective study of 170 patients with various types of chronic hepatic disease, mottled pulmonary parenchymal infiltrates were noted in 6%. A decreased D$_{LCO}$ was observed in 20%. Clubbing of the nails appeared to be more frequent in those with liver disease and abnormalities on chest roentgenograms. Pulmonary edema as a result of passive congestion can be seen in patients with liver disease. The incidence of low-pressure pulmonary edema and ARDS appears to be high in patients with fulminant hepatic failure.

Portopulmonary Hypertension

Portopulmonary hypertension is pulmonary hypertension in a patient with portal hypertension (97). The association of hepatic cirrhosis and pulmonary hypertension was first observed more than three decades ago. In a study of 2,459 patients with biopsy-proven cirrhosis and 1,241 patients with cirrhosis diagnosed at autopsy, the incidence rates of idiopathic hypertensive pulmonary vascular disease were 0.6% and 0.73%, respectively, in contrast to 0.13% ($P < .001$) in all autopsies (98). The data from this study suggest an association between cirrhosis and the development of pulmonary hypertension. Whereas the prevalence of cirrhosis alone was highest in the fifth decade of life, the average age of the cirrhotic patients with pulmonary hypertension was 35 years, and they tended to be women. Patients with portopulmonary hypertension present with fatigue, dyspnea, peripheral edema, chest pain, and syncope (99).

The mechanisms responsible for the development of pulmonary hypertension in hepatic cirrhosis are unknown. Recurrent embolization from the portal to the pulmonary circulation, primary vasoconstriction, in situ thrombosis of pulmonary vessels, increased pulmonary vascular resistance caused by vasoactive peptides released as a result of portal hypertension, dietary alterations, and recurrent pulmonary emboli have all been implicated.

Although most cases of pulmonary hypertension have been reported in patients with cirrhosis, hepatic parenchymal disease or failure is not necessary for it to develop. The strongest association appears to be with portal hypertension, and portal hypertension nearly always precedes the diagnosis of pulmonary vascular disease by several years. The histologic features, including plexogenic arteriopathy, are similar to those seen in primary pulmonary hypertension (100). Autopsy studies reveal a high incidence of intravascular thrombosis in association with plexiform lesions (101).

Hepatitis C Virus Infection

Hepatitis C virus (HCV) infection has been suggested as a cause of idiopathic pulmonary fibrosis, based on a Japanese study in which a high prevalence of anti-HCV antibodies was detected. A British study, however, failed to confirm these results (102). In a subsequent study, a 13% prevalence of HCV infection and viral replication was recorded in Italian patients with idiopathic pulmonary fibrosis; the prevalence of anti-HCV antibodies did not differ from that in patients with other lung diseases (103).

In a comparison of lymphocyte subsets in BAL fluid from 13 patients (10 men) with active chronic HCV infection and 13 healthy volunteers, no difference in total cell counts was found between the two groups (104). However, the numbers of lymphocytes and eosinophils were increased in the lavage fluid of the patients with chronic hepatitis C, which led the authors to consider that HCV infection might trigger alveolitis.

Recombinant interferon-α is used to treat HCV infection. Many reports have appeared of diffuse interstitial lung infiltration in patients with chronic HCV infection, and acute respiratory failure in some, after therapy with recombinant interferon-α (105). Increased numbers of lymphocytes, especially CD8$^+$ cells, have been found in BAL fluid, and bronchiolitis obliterans–organizing pneumonia has been detected in lung specimens. In the vast majority of patients, the pulmonary manifestations and chest roentgenographic abnormalities disappeared after interferon therapy was discontinued and corticosteroid therapy was given.

Liver Transplantation

Pulmonary infections occur in 25% of transplant recipients (106). The organisms responsible for pulmonary infections include Gram-negative bacteria, cytomegalovirus (CMV), *Candida* species, *Aspergillus* species, and *Pneumocystis carinii*. Interstitial pneumonia caused by herpes simplex virus 1 (HSV-1) is a severe complication of orthotopic liver transplantation. The combination of acyclovir, mechanical ventilation, and a reduction in the level of immunosuppression has proved to be an effective treatment for HSV-1 pneumonia after orthotopic liver transplantation.

CMV pneumonia is relatively common in orthotopic liver transplant recipients and is associated with a high mortality rate. In a prospective analysis of 141 orthotopic liver transplant recipients, CMV pneumonia developed in 13 (9%) during the first year after transplantation, and the mortality rate in these patients was 85% at 1 year, in comparison with 17% in the patients without CMV pneumonia (107). Overall, a 67% mortality rate was attributed to CMV pneumonia within the first year after liver transplantation.

Noninfectious complications following orthotopic liver transplant are caused by prolonged general anesthesia, extensive upper abdominal surgery, and the massive administration of blood products and colloids. Noninfectious complications include atelectasis, pleural effusion, ARDS, and pulmonary calcification. Although air embolism is common during liver transplantation, the clinical sequelae are few.

Diaphragmatic paralysis after orthotopic liver transplantation may contribute to postoperative pulmonary problems. A crush injury to the right phrenic nerve during transplantation is most likely the cause of right hemidiaphragmatic dysfunction. A prospective study of 48 adult liver transplant recipients assessed by ultrasonography, preoperative and postoperative pulmonary function tests, and transcutaneous phrenic nerve conduction studies recorded right phrenic nerve injury in 79% and hemidiaphragm paralysis in 38%; conduction along the right phrenic nerve was absent in 53% and reduced in 26% (108). Left phrenic nerve conduction and left hemidiaphragm excursion were unaffected. The abnormal findings, however, did not significantly influence the length of time on the ventilator or the hospital stay. Complete recovery of phrenic nerve conduction and diaphragmatic function took as long as 9 months in some patients.

Metastatic pulmonary calcification (calcinosis) has been described after orthotopic liver transplantation. In a series of 91 patients who underwent orthotopic liver transplantation, the chest roentgenograms of 77 patients were reviewed, and pulmonary calcification was observed in 4 (5%) of the 77 (109). Pulmonary calcinosis is a form of dystrophic calcification. Pulmonary calcification, at times fatal, has been described in renal transplant recipients. Many of the renal transplant recipients had a markedly elevated product of calcium and phosphorus, to peak values of 122 to 147 mg/dL. In the four liver transplant recipients, significantly higher levels of serum phosphate and calcium were recorded postoperatively, and these patients had received more intraoperative platelets and other blood products containing exogenous calcium than the other patients. Nonspecific and persistent pulmonary opacities should suggest the possibility of pulmonary calcification. High-resolution CT or lung scanning with a bone-seeking radionuclide (^{99m}Tc-diphosphonate) can be used to establish an early diagnosis of pulmonary calcification.

Miscellaneous Hepatic Disorders

Pulmonary embolism caused by a bile embolus is a rare, occasionally fatal complication of biliary trauma. Communications between the biliary tract and hepatic veins after biliary surgery have been shown to result in the formation of bile emboli in small pulmonary arteries. Among the nine cases reported in the literature up to 1983, five had malignancies encroaching on the biliary tree, and the rest had been subjected to biliary trauma.

Deficiency of α_1-antitrypsin predisposes to the development of pulmonary emphysema, liver cirrhosis, and hepatocellular carcinoma (110). Liver disease or impaired liver function is not a clinically relevant problem in most adults with pulmonary emphysema caused by α_1-antitrypsin deficiency; severe lung and liver disease rarely coexist in the same subject. A review of 19 adult patients with α_1-antitrypsin deficiency and chronic liver disease showed a late onset of symptomatic hepatic abnormalities; 13 patients were 60 years old or older when liver disease was discovered. Low serum levels of α_1-antitrypsin are more likely to be associated with cirrhosis of the liver in children than in adults; significant liver dysfunction develops in approximately 10% of children with PiZZ α_1-antitrypsin deficiency. Chronic liver disease in patients with α_1-antitrypsin deficiency is associated with a high prevalence of hepatic infection by viruses. It has been suggested that the viral infection of the liver, rather than the α_1-antitrypsin deficiency alone, is the cause of liver disease in such patients.

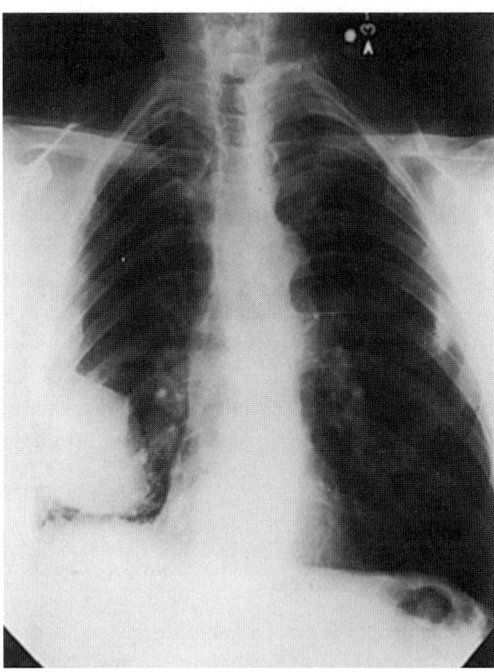

FIGURE 59.10. Right-sided pleuropulmonary involvement by an amebic abscess.

Hepatic amebiasis causes pleuropulmonary complications in 7% to 20% of patients with amebic liver abscesses and in 2% to 3% of those with invasive disease (111). The intrathoracic manifestations include sympathetic effusion over the infradiaphragmatic area of inflammation, rupture of the amebic abscess and amebic empyema, and rupture directly into the bronchial tree with formation of a hepatobronchial fistula (Fig. 59.10).

Pulmonary injury from drugs such as penicillamine, azathioprine, sulfasalazine, and mesalamine may occur in patients to whom they are administered to treat various gastrointestinal diseases.

Alcohol and the Lung

Chronic alcohol consumption increases the risk for pulmonary TB, chronic bronchitis, aspiration pneumonitis, lung abscess, and pulmonary complications of alcoholic cirrhosis and alcoholic cardiomyopathy. The reported effects of alcohol on the respiratory system include diminished ciliary motion, decreased migration of alveolar macrophages, interference with surfactant production, and increased prevalence of oropharyngeal Gram-negative bacilli.

Three large epidemiologic studies in the 1980s critically analyzed the effect of alcohol on respiratory function and concluded that alcohol had little, if any, effect on pulmonary function. The pulmonary functional abnormalities noted in earlier studies were apparently related to smoking, a common habit among subjects who consume alcohol. Furthermore, a study of 27 alcoholic subjects in the United Kingdom concluded that the high prevalence of respiratory disease in alcoholics was largely attributable to their smoking habits

and that evidence of a specific toxic effect of ethanol on the lungs could not be found. A population-based study, however, of more than 8,750 persons, each of whom had consumed 350 g of alcohol per week or more, evaluated the effect of alcohol consumption on pulmonary function during a period of 5 years and reported that alcohol consumption significantly accelerated the loss of FEV_1 and forced vital capacity; these changes were comparable with the effects of smoking 15 g of tobacco daily. Other reports have noted that a short-term cessation of alcohol intake has no effect on parameters of pulmonary function in alcoholics who smoke cigarettes.

Impaired glottic and cough reflexes and the excessive sedation induced by the ingestion of alcohol may play a role in causing community-acquired pneumonia. A case control study concluded that a high level of alcohol intake is the main risk factor for the development of community-acquired pneumonia in middle-aged people (112). In comparison with nonalcoholic patients, alcoholic patients with pneumonia had more severe clinical symptoms and required intravenous therapy and hospitalization for a longer time; multilobar involvement and pleural effusions were more frequent, and their lung infiltrates resolved more slowly. Pneumonia may also result from the gastroesophageal reflux induced by alcohol ingestion. The effect of a moderate amount of alcohol (120 mL of Scotch whiskey, with 40% alcohol) on nocturnal esophageal reflux was studied in healthy volunteers. Monitoring of the esophageal pH of the subjects during ambulation and in a supine posture revealed prolonged episodes of reflux while in the supine position in 41% of those given alcohol, whereas none of the control subjects had reflux. This study also noted a significant exposure of the distal esophagus to acid and an impaired clearance of acid from the esophagus in the supine position after the intake of only moderate amounts of alcohol.

Klebsiella pneumoniae pneumonia with bacteremia is common and associated with a very high mortality in alcoholic subjects. In a study of 28 alcoholic patients (all men) with community-acquired pneumonia who were admitted to a referral medical center, all but a few were heavy smokers; bacteremic *K. pneumoniae* pneumonia was diagnosed in 11 patients, all of whom required management and ventilatory support in the intensive care unit (113). Chest roentgenograms showed pleural effusion and spread of pneumonia in nearly 50% of the patients. Acute renal failure and disseminated intravascular coagulation developed in six patients. Even though the overall mortality was 64%, all patients with *K. pneumoniae* died.

ARDS is reported to occur more frequently in patients with a history of alcohol abuse. A prospective cohort study of 351 medical and surgical intensive care unit patients with one of seven at-risk diagnoses for the development of ARDS noted that the incidence of ARDS was significantly higher in patients with a history of alcohol abuse than in those without such a history (43% vs. 22%) (114). Among patients with sepsis, ARDS developed in 52% of those with a prior history of alcohol abuse but in only 20% of those without such a history. In the subset of patients in whom ARDS developed, the in-hospital mortality rate was 65% for those with a prior history of alcohol abuse. This mortality rate was significantly higher than the mortality rate of the patients without a history of alcohol abuse. It has been shown that chronic alcohol abuse alters antioxidant glutathione homeostasis in the human lung, and this may be a mechanism by which chronic alcohol abuse predisposes susceptible patients to ARDS (115).

Alcoholism is closely associated with TB, the prevalence of alcoholism being 49% in patients with newly diagnosed tuberculous disease. Among 970 subjects in New York City with alcohol and drug addiction, the prevalence of TB was 0.91%, which was 28 times the age-matched rate for the population in the city; screening of only those with a positive tuberculin test result and cough substantially increased the yield of active TB to 7.2%, or 225 times the rate for the city. In view of the rising incidence of TB in the 1990s, screening for TB in the alcoholic population is highly recommended.

A review of 23 patients with primary pulmonary sporotrichosis, presumably acquired by inhalation, revealed that this form of the disease affects middle-aged men with a history of alcoholism or chronic lung disease. Clinically and roentgenographically, the disease mimics chronic cavitary TB and histoplasmosis.

One study reported that a low to moderate rate of alcohol consumption in older persons is associated with a decreased risk for deep venous thrombosis and pulmonary embolism.

The term *alcohol asthma* is defined as chest tightness and wheezing after the ingestion of alcohol; this phenomenon has been described in a small number of persons of Asian and Native American extraction.

A deficiency of immunoglobulin G subclass has been reported in 70% of patients with alcoholic liver disease, and the deficiency was reported to be closely correlated with the number and type of bacterial respiratory infections.

PANCREATIC DISEASES

Pleural Effusion

Pleural effusion occurs in 4% to 17% of patients with acute pancreatitis. Roentgenographic abnormalities include a free or loculated pleural effusion, elevation of a hemidiaphragm, and basilar atelectasis. The effusions are predominantly left-sided. Characteristically, the fluid is an exudate, contains an elevated level of amylase, and is hemorrhagic in 30% of patients. Massive pleural effusions can occur in association with asymptomatic pancreatic disease.

Pleuropancreatic fistula may cause chronic massive pleural effusions. Chronic massive pancreatic pleural effusion may also develop weeks, months, or years after an episode of acute pancreatitis, and most of these patients have no history of pancreatitis. Patients may present with dyspnea, cough, and chest pain. The amylase content of the pleural fluid is always markedly elevated. Chronic massive pancreatic pleural effusion is caused by posterior disruption of the pancreatic duct into the retroperitoneal space, with tracking of secretions from the pancreas along the esophagus or aorta upward into the mediastinum. The fluid occasionally collects in the mediastinum and forms a mediastinal pseudocyst. Pericardial effusion and tamponade have been described. Very high levels of amylase in pleural fluid may also be seen in pleural effusion secondary to esophageal perforation, in this situation as a consequence of leakage of salivary amylase.

Acute Respiratory Distress Syndrome

ARDS is the most serious complication of pancreatitis and is reported to occur in 20% to 50% of patients (116). A prospective study to assess the incidence of pulmonary infiltrates in acute pancreatitis observed this complication in 26% of patients, but not all patients had ARDS (117). Pancreatitis-induced ARDS is usually attributed to the release of active enzymes and vasoactive substances from the pancreas. The mechanism of injury is unknown, but it is believed to be related to defective surfactant production. Lecithin is a main constituent of the pulmonary surfactant dipalmitoyl lecithin. The surfactant is split by a lecithinase, which is increased in acute pancreatitis. An experimental study suggests that pancreatic elastase plays a major role, by direct deleterious action on the pulmonary vasculature, in the development of pulmonary vascular injury after acute pancreatitis. In another experimental model, in which pancreatitis was induced by the injection of trypsin and sodium taurocholate into the pancreas, pulmonary injury was prevented by pretreatment of the animals with aprotinin (Trasylol), an antiprotease drug with activity against trypsin and elastase.

Drainage of the thoracic duct has been used to remove pancreatic enzymes and vasoactive substances before they reach the systemic circulation and cause ARDS (118). This method was used to collect the lymphatic effluent of six patients with severe acute pancreatitis; moderate lymph-to-plasma gradients were noted for interleukin-6, lipase, and trypsin, and similar levels in plasma and lymph were recorded for other substances. These results suggest that cytokines in addition to pancreatic enzymes may contribute to the development of the lung injury and that the lymphatics are potential vectors of these mediators.

Octreotide, a synthetic analogue of somatostatin, effectively palliates the vomiting associated with intra-abdominal malignancies by reducing the volume of secretions. The intravenous administration of octreotide in patients with severe necrotizing pancreatitis significantly reduces the frequency of ARDS, circulatory shock, and mortality (119).

Acute hemorrhagic pancreatitis is frequently associated with acute respiratory failure and pulmonary edema, which is generally believed to be caused by increased alveolar membrane permeability. Hypoalbuminemia in pancreatitis may aggravate the tendency to the development of pulmonary edema.

Pancreatic pseudocysts have been complicated by large intrathoracic collections of fluid. Most, but not all, chronic or persistent pleural effusions are associated with, and caused by, a fistulous tract between the pseudocyst and the pleural space. CT is helpful in detecting the fistulous communication. A subdiaphragmatic collection of fluid is common and may play a role in the formation of a pleural effusion; ultrasonography or CT is necessary to exclude such fluid collections. Other pulmonary complications of chronic pancreatitis include bilateral basilar atelectasis, diaphragmatic elevation caused by a pleural effusion or atelectasis, and pleural calcification. Mediastinal fat necrosis is another reported complication.

GASTROINTESTINAL MALIGNANCIES

Esophageal Cancer

Gastrointestinal malignancies play a major role in respiratory diseases, particularly esophageal cancer. Metastatic pulmonary involvement by esophageal cancer occurs in 20% of patients (120). However, an overwhelming majority of the metastases are the result of direct spread to the tracheobronchial tree as a consequence of the anatomic proximity of the esophagus to the airways. For this reason, some routinely perform bronchoscopy before surgical resection of the esophageal cancer. An important clinical caveat is that positive cytology in the bronchoscopic secretions of patients with esophageal carcinoma does not necessarily indicate airway involvement by cancer. Rather, the abnormal cytology is often the result of the aspiration of cancer cells from the esophagus into the airways.

The respiratory manifestations vary depending on the type of esophageal lesion and degree of pulmonary involvement. An obstructing esophageal lesion can cause the retention of food proximally, which in turn can lead to cough and aspiration pneumonia. Direct extension of the cancer into the airways can result in the formation of an esophagotracheobronchial fistula. This too can cause aspiration pneumonia, in addition to hemoptysis. Extrinsic compression of the tracheobronchial tree may cause respiratory difficulty. Lastly, surgical resection of an esophageal cancer may lead to respiratory complications.

A retrospective study of 309 resections for esophageal cancer (Ivor-Lewis resection for middle thoracic lesions in 182 cases and Akiyama resection for upper thoracic lesions in 127 cases) recorded an overall mortality of 9% and a morbidity of 37% (121). The mortality was four times higher, and the morbidity twice higher, after the Akiyama procedure than after the Ivor-Lewis procedure. Respiratory complications accounted for 64% of the postoperative deaths. The Akiyama procedure was associated with more respiratory complications, especially isolated bronchopneumonia and necrosis of the trachea or the right or left main bronchus. Respiratory complications accounted for 53% of the cases

of postoperative morbidity, mainly recurrent nerve paralysis with false passages and stasis in the transplant. Another mechanism for the formation of an esophageal-airway fistula is necrosis of the esophageal tissue after surgery or high-dose radiation therapy for cancer (122).

Colon Cancer

Metastatic involvement of the lungs occurred in 2,659 (11.7%) of 22,715 patients who underwent colectomy for carcinoma in the U.S. Veterans Administration hospital system (123). Of the patients who had pulmonary metastases, 514 had no prior or other metastatic sites. Of 974 patients who underwent surgery for colorectal cancer during a 20-year period in Japan, pulmonary metastasis developed in 35 (3.6%). Solitary or multiple lung nodules occur more frequently than other forms of pulmonary metastasis. Thus, colorectal carcinoma should always be considered when new or undiagnosed pulmonary nodules are encountered. Obviously, a documented history of previous malignancy of the colon and rectum increases the possibility of pulmonary metastasis. Even though the therapeutic approach to nodular lung metastasis from colon cancer has varied, the surgical resection of pulmonary metastases of colorectal cancer in selected patients may improve the prognosis. Significantly enhanced survival can be expected in patients with only intrapulmonary metastasis documented before thoracotomy.

Several large studies of patients who underwent resection of pulmonary metastases of colorectal cancer recorded survivals of 20% to 41% at 5 years and 20% to 30% at 10 years (124). In the Veterans Administration study previously cited, resections of pulmonary metastases were performed in 76 (2.9%) of the patients; the projected 5-year survival rate was 36%, the mean survival was 8 months, and the 30-day mortality rate was 3%. Of the 974 patients who underwent surgery for colorectal cancer during a 20-year period in Japan, the survival rate was 53% at both 3 and 5 years after resection of pulmonary metastasis.

Predictors of longer survival include total resection of metastatic lung disease, fewer than two pulmonary metastases, and a normal serum level of carcinoembryonic antigen (CEA) before thoracotomy (125). In one study, the estimated 5-year survival rate of patients with a normal serum level of CEA before thoracotomy was 60%, whereas it was 4% in patients with an elevated serum level of CEA (>5 ng/mL). Sex, age, site of the primary tumor (colon or rectum), disease-free interval, size of the metastases, and previous resection of hepatic metastases do not appear to be statistically significant prognostic factors.

Liver and Pancreatic Cancer

The pulmonary metastases of liver cancer may appear as small nodular lesions or, more likely, as interstitial infiltrations. Hepatocellular carcinoma is treated by hepatic artery chemoembolization therapy. One of the therapeutic agents contains iodized oil. In a retrospective study of 336 patients with hepatocellular carcinoma who underwent transcatheter oily chemoembolization of the hepatic artery, 14 of them were administered more than 20 mL of iodized oil (126). In six of these, pulmonary symptoms, including cough, hemoptysis, and dyspnea, developed 2 to 5 days after chemoembolization therapy. The chest roentgenograms demonstrated diffuse bilateral pulmonary parenchymal infiltrates; the PaO_2 on ambient air ranged from 39 to 60 mm Hg. All respiratory features resolved in 10 to 28 days, and five patients survived; one patient died 10 days after the procedure as a result of progression of a pulmonary infiltrate and respiratory arrest.

In consecutive autopsies of 154 patients with exocrine pancreatic cancer, 13 (8%) were found to have pulmonary metastases without hepatic metastasis.

OTHER GASTROINTESTINAL DISEASES AND CONDITIONS

Subphrenic Abscess

Subphrenic abscess is a common complication of intra-abdominal problems such as rupture or perforation of a viscus and of intra-abdominal surgery. Both sides are involved equally often, as are the anterior and posterior subphrenic spaces. Roentgenographically, evidence of a subphrenic abscess appears within the lung and in the pleural and subphrenic spaces. The costophrenic angle is blunted in nearly 90% of patients. Retroperitoneal abscess also can cause pleural effusion.

Abdominal Surgery

Changes in respiratory function after abdominal surgery have been well documented. Intraoperative testing of lung function has shown reductions in both vital capacity and residual capacity. Microatelectasis, seen commonly in the postoperative state, is believed to be a major cause of persistent hypoxemia. Several mechanisms have been hypothesized: diminished production of surfactant secondary to the inhalation of oxygen at high concentrations or altered ventilatory patterns; alveolar collapse resulting from the complete resorption of alveolar gas after the inhalation of 100% oxygen; and peripheral airways obstruction secondary to bronchoconstriction in response to hypocapnia.

Postoperative pulmonary complications of upper abdominal surgery are common. Laparoscopic procedures are less likely to cause respiratory complications. In a case control study of laparoscopic cholecystectomy (37 patients) and open cholecystectomy (58 patients), the incidence of postoperative pulmonary complications was 2.7% after the laparoscopic and 17.2% after the open procedure (127). Increased intra-abdominal pressure during laparoscopic cholecystectomy causes a significant but fully reversible decrease in dynamic compliance. Prospective evaluation of preoperative and postoperative spirometry, arterial blood gases, and chest roentgenograms in patients undergoing laparoscopic cholecystectomy has shown that the physiologic derangements are sufficiently small that all but the most severely impaired patients with pulmonary disease should be able to tolerate this operation.

Pleural effusions frequently develop after abdominal procedures. The amount of fluid that accumulates, however, is small. In one study, pleural fluid could be detected in 49% of 200 patients 48 to 72 hours after surgery. The incidence was higher after upper abdominal surgery and in patients with atelectasis on the side on which the operation was performed. Thoracentesis revealed that the fluid was an exudate in 16 of 20 patients. Almost all the effusions resolved spontaneously.

Miscellaneous Disorders

Pulmonary embolism can be triggered by the act of defecation in patients with deep vein thrombosis. One retrospective chart review estimated that defecation-induced pulmonary embolism occurred in 6.8% of all patients with the discharge diagnosis of pulmonary embolism, and of the nine patients with this combination, six died. It has been hypothesized that increased intra-abdominal pressure (from the Valsalva maneuver) during defecation, followed by a sudden decrease in pressure (vacuum effect), dislodges clots from deep veins.

Ventral hernia and other abnormalities of the abdominal wall may interfere with normal pulmonary function. Large defects such as ventral hernia may cause respiratory embarrassment and therefore require surgical correction, especially in patients with chronic obstructive lung disease.

Pneumatosis coli is a rare condition characterized by multiple gas-filled cysts within the bowel wall (128). A review of 25 patients (mean age, 59 years; 15 women and 10 men) treated during a period of 30 years observed an association with chronic lung disease in 20%. Oxygen therapy relieves the symptoms (128). Hyperbaric oxygen therapy has also been successful in treating patients with pneumatosis coli and may help to avoid the pulmonary and central nervous system toxicity associated with the prolonged use of oxygen at high flow rates (128).

Strongyloides stercoralis infestation is postulated to be associated with asthma. However, a study found no statistically significant difference in the prevalence of asthma between patients with *S. stercoralis* infestation and those without parasitic infection.

REFERENCES

1. Kopec SE, Irwin RI. Sequelae and complications of pneumonectomy. In: Rose BD, ed. *UpToDate.* Wellesley, MA: UpToDate, 2002.
2. Saxon RR, Barton RE, Katon RM, et al. Treatment of malignant

esophagorespiratory fistulas with silicone-covered metallic Z stents. *J Vasc Intervent Radiol* 1995;6:237–242.

3. Saltzman JR. Endoscopic palliation of esophageal cancer. In: Rose BD, ed. *UpToDate*. Wellesley, MA: *UpToDate*, 2002.

4. Talamonti MS. Management of locally advanced unresectable esophageal cancer. In: Rose BD, ed. *UpToDate*. Wellesley, MA: UpToDate, 2002.

5. Thurer RL. Evaluation of mediastinal masses. In: Rose BD, ed. *UpToDate*. Wellesley, MA: UpToDate, 2002.

6. Mulder CJJ. Zenker's diverticulum. In: Rose BD, ed. *UpToDate*. Wellesley, MA: UpToDate, 2002.

7. Howard PJ, Maher L, Pryde A, et al. Five-year prospective study of the incidence, clinical features, and diagnosis of achalasia in Edinburgh. *Gut* 1992;33:1011–1015.

8. Sandler RS, Nyren O, Ekbom A, et al. The risk of esophageal cancer in patients with achalasia. A population-based study. *JAMA* 1995;274:1359–1362.

9. Marin-Neto JA. Pathology and pathogenesis of Chagas' disease. In: Rose BD, ed. *UpToDate*. Wellesley, MA: UpToDate, 2002.

10. Pasricha PJ, Fleischer DE, Kalloo AN. Endoscopic perforations of the upper digestive tract: a review of their pathogenesis, prevention, and management. *Gastroenterology* 1994;106:787–802.

11. Triadafilopoulos G. Boerhaave's syndrome: effort rupture of the esophagus. In: Rose BD, ed. *UpToDate*. Wellesley, MA: UpToDate, 2002.

12. Gubbins GP, Nensey YM, Schubert TT, et al. Barogenic perforation of the esophagus distal to a stricture after endoscopy. *J Clin Gastroenterol* 1990;12:310–312.

13. Sanyal AJ. Prevention of recurrent variceal hemorrhage in patients with cirrhosis. In: Rose BD, ed. *UpToDate*. Wellesley, MA: UpToDate, 2002.

14. Ikezoe J, Morimoto S, Akira M, et al. Computed tomography following endoscopic sclerotherapy of esophageal varices. *Acta Radiol* 1987;28:415–420.

15. Zeller FA, Cannan CR, Prakash UB. Thoracic manifestations after esophageal variceal sclerotherapy. *Mayo Clin Proc* 1991;66:727–732.

16. Samuels T, Lovett MC, Campbell IT, et al. Respiratory function after injection sclerotherapy of oesophageal varices. *Gut* 1994;35:1459–1463.

17. Parikh SS, Amarapurkar DN, Dhawan PS, et al. Development of pleural effusion after sclerotherapy with absolute alcohol. *Gastrointest Endosc* 1993;39:404–405.

18. Nygaard SD, Berger HA, Fick RB. Chylothorax as a complication of oesophageal sclerotherapy. *Thorax* 1992;47:134–135.

19. Spach DH, Silverstein FE, Stamm WE. Transmission of infection by gastrointestinal endoscopy and bronchoscopy. *Ann Intern Med* 1993;118:117–128.

20. Wu MS, Wang JT, Yang JC, et al. Effective reduction of *Helicobacter pylori* infection after upper gastrointestinal endoscopy by mechanical washing of the endoscope. *Hepatogastroenterology* 1996;43:1660–1664.

21. Lipper B, Simon D, Cerrone F. Pulmonary aspiration during emergency endoscopy in patients with upper gastrointestinal hemorrhage. *Crit Care Med* 1991;19:330–333.

22. DeLegge MH. Prevention and management of complications from percutaneous endoscopic gastrostomy. In: Rose BD, ed. *UpToDate*. Wellesley, MA: UpToDate, 2002.

23. Short TP, Patel NR, Thomas E. Prevalence of gastroesophageal reflux in patients who develop pneumonia following percutaneous endoscopic gastrostomy: a 24-hour pH monitoring study. *Dysphagia* 1996;11:87–89.

24. Spiess AE, Kahrilas PJ. Complications of gastroesophageal reflux. In: Rose BD, ed. *UpToDate*. Wellesley, MA: UpToDate, 2002.

25. Kahrilas PJ. Gastroesophageal reflux disease. *JAMA* 1996;276:983–988.

26. Schnatz PF, Castell JA, Castell DO. Pulmonary symptoms associated with gastroesophageal reflux: use of ambulatory pH monitoring to diagnose and to direct therapy. *Am J Gastroenterol* 1996;91:1715–1718.

27. Kambic V, Radsel Z. Acid posterior laryngitis. Aetiology, histology, diagnosis and treatment. *J Laryngol Otol* 1984;98:1237–1240.

28. Irwin RS, Zawacki JK, Curley FJ, et al. Chronic cough as the sole presenting manifestation of gastroesophageal reflux. *Am Rev Respir Dis* 1989;140:1294–1300.

29. Irwin RS, Curley FJ, French CL. Chronic cough. The spectrum and frequency of causes, key components of the diagnostic evaluation, and outcome of specific therapy. *Am Rev Respir Dis* 1990;141:640–647.

30. Irwin RS, French CL, Curley FJ, et al. Chronic cough due to gastroesophageal reflux. Clinical, diagnostic, and pathogenetic aspects. *Chest* 1993;104:1511–1517.

31. Harding SM. Gastroesophageal reflux and asthma. In: Rose BD, ed. *UpToDate*. Wellesley, MA: UpToDate, 2002.

32. Simpson WG. Gastroesophageal reflux disease and asthma. Diagnosis and management. *Arch Intern Med* 1995;155:798–803.

33. Field SK, Underwood M, Brant R, et al. Prevalence of gastroesophageal reflux symptoms in asthma. *Chest* 1996;109:316–322.

34. Spivak H, Smith CD, Phichith A, et al. Asthma and gastroesophageal reflux: fundoplication decreases need for systemic corticosteroids. *J Gastrointest Surg* 1999;3:477–482.

35. Harding SM, Richter JE, Guzzo MR, et al. Asthma and gastroesophageal reflux: acid-suppressive therapy improves asthma outcome. *Am J Med* 1996;100:395–405.

36. Coughlan JL, Gibson PG, Henry RL. Medical treatment for reflux oesophagitis does not consistently improve asthma control: a systematic review. *Thorax* 2001;56:198–204.

37. Schwaitzberg SD. Surgical management of gastroesophageal reflux. In: Rose BD, ed. *UpToDate*. Wellesley, MA: UpToDate, 2002.

38. Ekstrom T, Johansson KE. Effects of anti-reflux surgery on chronic cough and asthma in patients with gastro-oesophageal reflux disease. *Respir Med* 2000;94:1166–1170.

39. Tryba M, Cook DJ. Gastric alkalinization, pneumonia, and systemic infections: the controversy. *Scand J Gastroenterol* 1995;210[Suppl]:53–59.

40. Torres A, Serra-Batlles J, Ros E, et al. Pulmonary aspiration of gastric contents in patients receiving mechanical ventilation: the effect of body position. *Ann Intern Med* 1992;116:540–543.

41. Drakulovic MB, Torres A, Bauer TT, et al. Supine body position as a risk factor for nosocomial pneumonia in mechanically ventilated patients: a randomised trial. *Lancet* 1999;354:1851–1858.

42. Galil K, Zaleznik DF. Nosocomial pneumonia. In: Rose BD, ed. *UpToDate*. Wellesley, MA: UpToDate, 2002.

43. Cook DJ, Reeve BK, Guyatt GH, et al. Stress ulcer prophylaxis in critically ill patients. Resolving discordant meta-analyses. *JAMA* 1996;275:308–314.

44. Prod'hom G, Leuenberger P, Koerfer J, et al. Nosocomial pneumonia in mechanically ventilated patients receiving antacid, ranitidine, or sucralfate as prophylaxis for stress ulcer. A randomized controlled trial. *Ann Intern Med* 1994;120:653–662.

45. Spiess AE, Kahrilas PJ. Hiatus hernia. In: Rose BD, ed. *UpToDate*. Wellesley, MA: UpToDate, 2002.

46. Wright RA, Hurwitz AL. Relationship of hiatal hernia to endoscopically proved reflux esophagitis. *Dig Dis Sci* 1979;24:311–313.

47. Cappell MS, Nadler SC. Increased mortality of acute upper gastrointestinal bleeding in patients with chronic obstructive pulmonary disease. A case controlled, multiyear study of 53 consecutive patients. *Dig Dis Sci* 1995;40:256–262.

48. Marumo K, Homma S, Fukuchi Y. Postgastrectomy aspiration pneumonia. *Chest* 1995;107:453–456.

49. Moeller DD, Carpenter PR. Gastrobronchial fistula: case report and review of the English literature. *Am J Gastroenterol* 1985;80:538–541.

50. Richardson AJ, Tait N, O'Rourke IO. Gastrobronchial fistula owing to non-malignant causes. *Br J Surg* 1992;79:331–332.

51. Angelillo VA, O'Donohue WJ Jr, Campbell JC, et al. Gastrobronchial fistula secondary to a subphrenic abscess. *Chest* 1983;84:85–86.

52. Levine JB, Lukawski-Trubish D. Extraintestinal considerations in inflammatory bowel disease. *Gastroenterol Clin North Am* 1995;24:633–646.

53. Mahadeva R, Walsh G, Flower CD, et al. Clinical and radiological characteristics of lung disease in inflammatory bowel disease. *Eur Respir J* 2000;15:41–48.

54. Weinberger SE, Peppercorn MA. Pulmonary complications of inflammatory bowel disease. In: Rose BD, ed. *UpToDate.* Wellesley, MA: UpToDate, 2002.

55. Garg K, Lynch DA, Newell JD. Inflammatory airways disease in ulcerative colitis: CT and high-resolution CT features. *J Thorac Imaging* 1993;8:159–163.

56. Camus P, Piard F, Ashcroft T, et al. The lung in inflammatory bowel disease. *Medicine* 1993;72:151–183.

57. Higenbottam T, Cochrane GM, Clark TJ, et al. Bronchial disease in ulcerative colitis. *Thorax* 1980;35:581–585.

58. Tzanakis N, Bouros D, Samiou M, et al. Lung function in patients with inflammatory bowel disease. *Respir Med* 1998;92:516–522.

59. Vasishta S, Wood JB, McGinty F. Ulcerative tracheobronchitis years after colectomy for ulcerative colitis. *Chest* 1994;106:1279–1281.

60. Munck A, Murciano D, Pariente R, et al. Latent pulmonary function abnormalities in children with Crohn's disease. *Eur Respir J* 1995;8:377–380.

61. Smiejan JM, Cosnes J, Chollet-Martin S, et al. Sarcoid-like lymphocytosis of the lower respiratory tract in patients with active Crohn's disease. *Ann Intern Med* 1986;104:17–21.

62. Bewig B, Manske I, Bottcher H, et al. Crohn's disease mimicking sarcoidosis in bronchoalveolar lavage. *Respiration* 1999;66:467–469.

63. Theodoropoulos G, Archimandritis A, Davaris P, et al. Ulcerative colitis and sarcoidosis: a curious association—report of a case. *Dis Colon Rectum* 1981;24:308–310.

64. Salerno SM, Ormseth EJ, Roth BJ, et al. Sulfasalazine pulmonary toxicity in ulcerative colitis mimicking clinical features of Wegener's granulomatosis. *Chest* 1996;110:556–559.

65. Hamadeh MA, Atkinson J, Smith LJ. Sulfasalazine-induced pulmonary disease. *Chest* 1992;101:1033–1037.

66. Bitton A, Peppercorn MA, Hanrahan JP, et al. Mesalamine-induced lung toxicity. *Am J Gastroenterol* 1996;91:1039–1040.

67. Pullan RD, Rhodes J, Ganesh S, et al. Transdermal nicotine for active ulcerative colitis. *N Engl J Med* 1994;330:811–815.

68. Boyko EJ, Koepsell TD, Perera DR, et al. Risk of ulcerative colitis among former and current cigarette smokers. *N Engl J Med* 1987;316:707–710.

69. Peppercorn MA. Definition of and risk factors for inflammatory bowel disease. In: Rose BD, ed. *UpToDate.* Wellesley, MA: UpToDate, 2002.

70. Silverstein MD, Lashner BA, Hanauer SB, et al. Cigarette smoking in Crohn's disease. *Am J Gastroenterol* 1989;84:31–33.

71. Coeliac lung disease. (Editorial.) *Lancet* 1978;1:917–918.

72. Edwards C, Williams A, Asquith P. Bronchopulmonary disease in coeliac patients. *J Clin Pathol* 1985;38:361–367.

73. Faux JA, Hendrick DJ, Anand BS. Precipitins to different avian serum antigens in bird fancier's lung and coeliac disease. *Clin Allergy* 1978;8:101–108.

74. Muers MF, Faux JA, Ting A, et al. HLA-A, B, C and HLA-DR antigens in extrinsic allergic alveolitis (budgerigar fancier's lung disease). *Clin Allergy* 1982;12:47–53.

75. Tarlo SM, Broder I, Prokipchuk EJ, et al. Association between celiac disease and lung disease. *Chest* 1981;80:715–718.

76. Karlish AJ. Coeliac disease and diffuse lung disease. *Lancet* 1971;1:1077.

77. Morris JS, Read AE, Jones B, et al. Coeliac disease and lung disease. *Lancet* 1971;1:754.

78. Brightling CE, Symon FA, Birring SS, et al. A case of cough, lymphocytic bronchoalveolitis and coeliac disease with improvement following a gluten-free diet. *Thorax* 2002;57:91–92.

79. Neil GA, Lukie BE, Cockcroft DW, et al. Lymphocytic interstitial pneumonia and abdominal lymphoma complicating celiac sprue. *J Clin Gastroenterol* 1986;8:282–285.

80. Wright PH, Buxton-Thomas M, Keeling PW, et al. Adult idiopathic pulmonary haemosiderosis: a comparison of lung function changes and the distribution of pulmonary disease in patients with and without coeliac disease. *Br J Dis Chest* 1983;77:282–292.

81. Sharma OP. Unusual systemic disorders associated with interstitial lung disease. *Curr Opin Pulm Med* 2001;7:291–294.

82. Symmons DP, Shepherd AN, Boardman PL, et al. Pulmonary manifestations of Whipple's disease. *Q J Med* 1985;56:497–504.

83. Kelly CA, Egan M, Rawlinson J. Whipple's disease presenting with lung involvement. *Thorax* 1996;51:343–344.

84. Beer DJ, Pereira W Jr, Snider GL. Pleural effusion associated with primary lymphedema: a perspective on the yellow nail syndrome. *Am Rev Respir Dis* 1978;117:595–599.

85. Warner AE. Pulmonary intravascular macrophages. Role in acute lung injury. *Clin Chest Med* 1996;17:125–135.

86. Lazaridis KN, Frank JW, Krowka MJ, et al. Hepatic hydrothorax: pathogenesis, diagnosis, and management. *Am J Med* 1999;107:262–267.

87. Chao Y, Wang SS, Lee SD, et al. Effect of large-volume paracentesis on pulmonary function in patients with cirrhosis and tense ascites. *J Hepatol* 1994;20:101–105.

88. Berkowitz KA, Butensky MS, Smith RL. Pulmonary function changes after large-volume paracentesis. *Am J Gastroenterol* 1993;88:905–907.

89. Agusti AG, Roca J, Rodriguez-Roisin R. Mechanisms of gas exchange impairment in patients with liver cirrhosis. *Clin Chest Med* 1996;17:49–66.

90. Vachiery F, Moreau R, Hadengue A, et al. Hypoxemia in patients with cirrhosis: relationship with liver failure and hemodynamic alterations. *J Hepatol* 1997;27:492–495.

91. Lange PA, Stoller JK. Hepatopulmonary syndrome. In: Rose BD, ed. *UpToDate.* Wellesley, MA: UpToDate, 2002.

92. King PD, Rumbaut R, Sanchez C. Pulmonary manifestations of chronic liver disease. *Dig Dis* 1996;14:73–82.

93. Seward JB, Hayes DL, Smith HC, et al. Platypnea-orthodeoxia: clinical profile, diagnostic workup, management, and report of seven cases. *Mayo Clin Proc* 1984;59:221–231.

94. Poterucha JJ, Krowka MJ, Dickson ER, et al. Failure of hepatopulmonary syndrome to resolve after liver transplantation

and successful treatment with embolotherapy. *Hepatology* 1995;21:96–100.

95. Costa C, Sambataro A, Baldi S, et al. Primary biliary cirrhosis: lung involvement. *Liver* 1995;15:196–201.

96. Krowka MJ, Grambsch PM, Edell ES, et al. Primary biliary cirrhosis: relation between hepatic function and pulmonary function in patients who never smoked. *Hepatology* 1991;13:1095–1100.

97. Hadengue A, Benhayoun MK, Lebrec D, et al. Pulmonary hypertension complicating portal hypertension: prevalence and relation to splanchnic hemodynamics. *Gastroenterology* 1991;100:520–528.

98. McDonnell PJ, Toye PA, Hutchins GM. Primary pulmonary hypertension and cirrhosis: are they related? *Am Rev Respir Dis* 1983;127:437–441.

99. Robalino BD, Moodie DS. Association between primary pulmonary hypertension and portal hypertension: analysis of its pathophysiology and clinical, laboratory and hemodynamic manifestations. *J Am Coll Cardiol* 1991;17:492–498.

100. Schraufnagel DE, Kay JM. Structural and pathologic changes in the lung vasculature in chronic liver disease. *Clin Chest Med* 1996;17:1–15.

101. Edwards BS, Weir EK, Edwards WD, et al. Coexistent pulmonary and portal hypertension: morphologic and clinical features. *J Am Coll Cardiol* 1987;10:1233–1238.

102. Irving WL, Day S, Johnston IDA. Idiopathic pulmonary fibrosis and hepatitis C virus infection. *Am Rev Respir Dis* 1993;148:1683–1684.

103. Meliconi R, Andreone P, Fasano L, et al. Incidence of hepatitis C virus infection in Italian patients with idiopathic pulmonary fibrosis. *Thorax* 1996;51:315–317.

104. Kubo K, Yamaguchi S, Fujimoto K, et al. Bronchoalveolar lavage fluid findings in patients with chronic hepatitis C virus infection. *Thorax* 1996;51:312–314.

105. Chin K, Tabata C, Sataka N, et al. Pneumonitis associated with natural and recombinant interferon alfa therapy for chronic hepatitis C. *Chest* 1994;105:939–941.

106. O'Brien JD, Ettinger NA. Pulmonary complications of liver transplantation. *Clin Chest Med* 1996;17:99–114.

107. Falagas ME, Snydman DR, George MJ, et al. Incidence and predictors of cytomegalovirus pneumonia in orthotopic liver transplant recipients. *Transplantation* 1996;61:1716–1720.

108. McAlister VC, Grant DR, Roy A, et al. Right phrenic nerve injury in orthotopic liver transplantation. *Transplantation* 1993;55:826–830.

109. Libson E, Wechsler RJ, Steiner RM. Pulmonary calcinosis following orthotopic liver transplantation. *J Thorac Imaging* 1993;8:305–308.

110. Stoller JK. Extrapulmonary manifestations of alpha-1-antitrypsin deficiency. In: Rose BD, ed. *UpToDate.* Wellesley, MA: UpToDate, 2002.

111. Weller PF. Pulmonary manifestations of amebiasis. In: Rose BD, ed. *UpToDate.* Wellesley, MA: UpToDate, 2002.

112. Fernandez-Sola J, Junque A, Estruch R, et al. High alcohol intake as a risk and prognostic factor for community-acquired pneumonia. *Arch Intern Med* 1995;155:1649–1654.

113. Jong GM, Hsiue TR, Chen CR, et al. Rapidly fatal outcome of bacteremic *Klebsiella pneumoniae* pneumonia in alcoholics. *Chest* 1995;107:214–217.

114. Moss M, Bucher B, Moore FA, et al. The role of chronic alcohol abuse in the development of acute respiratory distress syndrome in adults. *JAMA* 1996;275:50–54.

115. Moss M, Guidot DM, Wong-Lambertina M, et al. The effects of chronic alcohol abuse on pulmonary glutathione homeostasis. *Am J Respir Crit Care Med* 2000;161:414–419.

116. Banerjee AK, Haggie SJ, Jones RB, et al. Respiratory failure in acute pancreatitis. *Postgrad Med J* 1995;71:327–330.

117. Lankisch PG, Droge M, Becher R. Pulmonary infiltrations. Sign of severe acute pancreatitis. *Int J Pancreatol* 1996;19:113–115.

118. Montravers P, Chollet-Martin S, Marmuse JP, et al. Lymphatic release of cytokines during acute lung injury complicating severe pancreatitis. *Am J Respir Crit Care Med* 1995;152:1527–1533.

119. Fiedler F, Jauernig G, Keim V, et al. Octreotide treatment in patients with necrotizing pancreatitis and pulmonary failure. *Intensive Care Med* 1996;22:909–915.

120. Quint LE, Hepburn LM, Francis IR, et al. Incidence and distribution of distant metastases from newly diagnosed esophageal carcinoma. *Cancer* 1995;76:1120–1125.

121. Dumont P, Wihlm JM, Hentz JG, et al. Respiratory complications after surgical treatment of esophageal cancer. A study of 309 patients according to the type of resection. *Eur J Cardiothorac Surg* 1995;9:539–543.

122. Muto M, Ohtsu A, Miyamoto S, et al. Concurrent chemoradiotherapy for esophageal carcinoma patients with malignant fistulae. *Cancer* 1999;86:1406–1413.

123. Wade TP, Virgo KS, Li MJ, et al. Outcomes after detection of metastatic carcinoma of the colon and rectum in a national hospital system. *J Am Coll Surg* 1996;182:353–361.

124. Okumura S, Kondo H, Tsuboi M, et al. Pulmonary resection for metastatic colorectal cancer: experiences with 159 patients. *J Thorac Cardiovasc Surg* 1996;112:867–874.

125. Van Halteren HK, Van Geel AN, Hart AA, et al. Pulmonary resection for metastases of colorectal origin. *Chest* 1995;107:1526–1531.

126. Chung JW, Park JH, Im JG, et al. Pulmonary oil embolism after transcatheter oily chemoembolization of hepatocellular carcinoma. *Radiology* 1993;187:689–693.

127. Hall JC, Tarala RA, Hall JL. A case-control study of postoperative pulmonary complications after laparoscopic and open cholecystectomy. *J Laparoendosc Surg* 1996;6:87–92.

128. Goldberg E, LaMont JT. Pneumatosis intestinalis. In: Rose BD, ed. *UpToDate.* Wellesley, MA: UpToDate, 2002.

Endocrine and Metabolic Diseases

60

Udaya B. S. Prakash · Talmadge E. King, Jr.

It is not commonly recognized in clinical practice that the respiratory system can be involved in many endocrine and metabolic diseases. The lung, under certain conditions, may secrete or release various humoral substances that can cause specific endocrine syndromes or otherwise influence the functions of many organ systems. Ectopic endocrine syndromes, which most often develop with pulmonary malignancies, are the best-known and most dramatic.

In addition to the well-known respiratory compensatory mechanisms that occur in metabolic acidosis and alkalosis, the pulmonary system may become involved in both common and uncommon metabolic disorders. This chapter deals with the pulmonary problems resulting from or associated with various endocrine and metabolic diseases. The pulmonary effects of the reproductive organs are discussed in Chapter 64.

ENDOCRINE DISORDERS

Acromegaly

Cardiopulmonary complications are responsible for significant mortality in acromegalic patients.

Pneumomegaly

The lungs are involved in the general visceromegaly of acromegaly, and if an excess of growth hormone is present in adult life, the lungs are capable of additional growth. The total lung capacity in acromegaly is significantly greater than the predicted value measured by body plethysmography. In one study, large lungs, defined as those with a vital capacity of more than 120% of the predicted normal value, were noted in 34% of 35 patients with acromegaly (1). Studies of pulmonary function in 10 male patients with acromegaly and one male pituitary giant revealed a tremendous increase in all lung volumes. No evidence was found of airflow obstruction or air trapping; lung compliance was increased, but lung elastic recoil was normal. Despite the large lung volumes, the diffusing capacity of the lung for carbon monoxide (D_{LCO}) was normal. However, others have reported a D_{LCO} of more than 120% of the predicted normal value in 22% of patients with acromegaly. Furthermore, physiologic studies in acromegalic patients indicate that lung growth is achieved by an increase in alveolar number rather than by an increase in size (2). Reports disagree regarding whether abnormal lung growth occurs in women with acromegaly.

In children with hypopituitarism, the mechanical properties of the lung are consistent with height-related rather than age-related variations (2).

Airways Obstruction

Extrathoracic airway narrowing has been noted in acromegalic patients. Even though the pulmonary function test values are normal in most, reduced airflow as a result of upper airway involvement has been noted in 50% of patients. Pulmonary function testing and roentgenographic assessment of the larynx and trachea in a group of 26 acromegalic patients demonstrated upper airway obstruction in 23%, whereas laryngeal tomography revealed marked narrowing of the true and false vocal cords in 54%.

The airway obstruction in acromegaly is believed to be related to osseous and soft tissue changes surrounding the upper airway, which cause narrowing and subsequent collapse during sleep. Macroglossia and hypertrophy of the hypopharyngeal tissues, regressive after surgical therapy, have

---

U. B. S. Prakash: Pulmonary and Critical Care Medicine, Mayo Medical School and Mayo Medical Center, Rochester, Minnesota.

T. E. King, Jr.: Department of Medicine, University of California, San Francisco; and Medical Services, San Francisco General Hospital, San Francisco, California.

also been noted. Flexible bronchoscopy in acromegalic patients has revealed collapsible upper airways at the level of the soft palate, whereas at the base of the tongue, little, if any, dynamic narrowing occurs. The clinical importance of these observations is that attention to the laryngeal anatomy is important in acromegalic patients scheduled for tracheal intubation and anesthesia. Thickening of the laryngeal mucosa has caused stridor and progressive dyspnea in acromegalic patients.

Sleep Apnea

Obstructive sleep apnea is a recognized complication in acromegaly (3). In one series of 11 patients, five had obstructive sleep apnea. Contributing factors include the large tongue and thickened tissues in the upper airways of acromegalic patients. The reduced ratio of airway space to tissue mass increases the resistance to airflow. As previously noted, obstruction of the airways by an enlarged tongue further exaggerates airway narrowing. However, bronchoscopic examination in some patients with sleep apnea and acromegaly has shown that during inspiration, the soft tissue of the posterior and lateral hypopharynx invaginates into the lateral vestibule before any posterior movement of the tongue occurs; thus, enlargement of the tongue does not appear to be a primary factor in causing sleep apnea.

Central sleep apnea occurs more frequently in patients with acromegaly (4,5). In a study of 53 patients with acromegaly, central sleep apnea was the predominant type of apnea in 33% of patients (4). Biochemical evidence of increased disease activity was associated with the presence of central apnea rather than with the degree of sleep apnea. Another study of 21 patients with sleep apnea and acromegaly suggested that central sleep apnea in acromegaly may result from a defective respiratory drive caused by the elevated level of growth hormone. The resolution of sleep apnea after treatment of acromegaly indicates that it may indeed resolve after a normal level of growth hormone has been restored. The hypercapnic ventilatory response remains normal and unaffected by the level of growth hormone.

The results of a case control study of 11 patients with treated acromegaly who underwent nocturnal sleep studies, cephalometry, and endocrinologic studies revealed abnormal nocturnal breathing in 10 of them (6). The predominant abnormality of breathing was periodic breathing with symmetrically waxing and waning respiratory effort without a major component of body movement. Treated acromegaly was the most powerful predictor of breathing abnormalities independently of the other significant predictors, which were age and body mass index.

Results of clinical investigations suggest that the pituitary tumors of acromegalic patients with sleep apnea should be treated to reduce the level of growth hormone before surgery to enlarge or bypass the upper airway is considered. In a report of seven patients with both sleep apnea and acromegaly,

four were treated by transsphenoidal hypophysectomy alone, with resolution of the sleep apnea syndrome (7). One patient underwent hypophysectomy followed by postoperative radiation therapy, which relieved his apnea, and surgery was unsuccessful in three patients.

Octreotide, a somatostatin analogue, has been shown to lower the indices of severe sleep apnea in patients with sleep apnea caused by acromegaly (8).

Thyroid Disorders

Goiter

Respiratory symptoms can be caused by both extrathoracic and intrathoracic goiters (Table 60.1). An intrathoracic goiter may be defined as any thyroid enlargement in which the

TABLE 60.1. PULMONARY COMPLICATIONS IN THYROID DISEASES

Goiter
  Cough
  Mediastinal mass
  Tracheal obstruction
  Superior vena cava syndrome
  Recurrent laryngeal nerve paralysis
  Chylothorax
Hyperthyroidism
  Thyrotoxic dyspnea
    Thyrotoxic myopathy
    Increased work of breathing
    Increased oxygen consumption
    Decreased compliance
  Exacerbation of asthma
    Thyrotoxic dyspnea
    ?Diminished cyclic adenosine monophosphate
    ?Diminished adrenergic responsiveness
    ?Decreased catecholamines
    ?Increased metabolism of bronchodilators
  Anterior mediastinal mass
    Benigh thymic hyperplasia
  Aspiration pneumonia in thyrotoxic bulbar paralysis
Hypothyroidism
  Depressed respiratory center
    Decreased response to hypercapnia
    Decreased hypoxic drive
    Central sleep apnea
  Hypoventilation
    Myxedema coma
    Central hypoventilation
    Muscle weakness
  Decreased bronchospasm in asthma
  Pleural effusion
  Pulmonary edema (in myxedema heart)
  Leftward shift of oxyhemoglobin dissociation curve
  Myxedematous pulmonary infiltrates
  Aspiration pneumonia (in myxedema coma)
Riedel thyroiditis
  Cough
  Tracheal obstruction
  Massive upper lobe pulmonary fibrosis

greater portion of the mass is inferior to the thoracic inlet. Although a goiter extends into the thorax in only 1% to 3% of patients who undergo thyroidectomy, thyroid masses comprise a considerable percentage of anterior mediastinal tumors (9). In most of these, a retrosternal mass is directly connected to a palpable thyroid gland in the neck. The masses are usually nodular colloid goiters, and thyrotoxicosis occurs in some cases. Malignant changes are extremely uncommon, even though a rare case of tracheal invasion by a papillary carcinoma in an intrathoracic goiter has been reported. An intrathoracic location of a goiter is not in itself associated with a predisposition to malignant change. Up to 80% of the intrathoracic goiters arise from the isthmus or lower pole and extend into the anterior mediastinum in front of the trachea. The rest arise from the posterior aspect of the thyroid gland and extend into the posterior mediastinum, behind the trachea and almost always on the right.

Among patients with a total of 2,908 goiters who underwent surgery during a 17-year period, 22 had severe or acute dyspnea, and four required immediate tracheal intubation. Chronic dyspnea without cyanosis was noted in 36 patients. In a study of 91 patients who underwent thyroidectomy, 29 had a markedly enlarged thyroid, 13 were unilateral (mean weight, 122 g), and 16 were bilateral (mean weight, 160 g) (10). Of the 25 patients with symptoms of airway compression, 18 exhibited tracheal narrowing or displacement, 19 had substernal extension, and one had superior vena cava syndrome. Histologic analysis revealed nodular goiter in 11 patients, adenoma in five, carcinoma in three, Graves disease in five, and toxic multinodular goiter in five (11).

Most patients with intrathoracic goiters are women, and many have a history of thyroid surgery. From 50% to 96% of such patients have symptoms. The most common manifestations of an intrathoracic goiter are dyspnea, stridor, dysphagia, hoarseness, coughing, wheezing, and a cervical mass. A small percentage of intrathoracic goiters cause stridor and respiratory embarrassment. In a study of 273 patients with benign goiters, 33% had signs of tracheal compression, mostly caused by colloid goiters. Another study of 132 patients used flow-volume loops to evaluate the upper airways and reported upper airway obstruction in 31% of those with a goiter. The incidence of tracheoesophageal compression was higher (67%) in the patients with thyroiditis. Acute or subacute tracheal obstruction necessitated tracheostomy in 3% of these. Severe expiratory flow obstruction requiring surgical removal of a goiter has been described. Acute life-threatening tracheal obstruction has been noted in patients with an intrathoracic goiter. Histologic studies have shown that the acute problem is very likely related to the presence of multiple foci of hemorrhage in the goiter.

Goiters may present with obstruction of the superior vena cava. Among 32 patients with superior vena cava syndrome, four had thyroid goiters. Recurrent laryngeal nerve paralysis is uncommon in patients with benign goiters, having

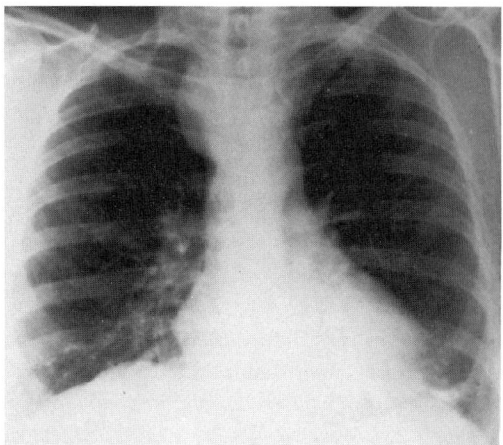

FIGURE 60.1. Intrathoracic extension of thyroid goiter.

been associated with fewer than 1% of 3,279 goiters. A retrosternal goiter can compress the thoracic duct and brachiocephalic vessels and cause chylothorax. Intrathoracic goiter with hyperthyroidism, tracheal compression, superior vena cava syndrome, and Horner syndrome has been described.

In the evaluation of chronic cough, thyroid disease is usually ignored as a cause. The close proximity of the thyroid gland to the laryngotracheal structures is occasionally responsible for distressing chronic cough. The cough usually disappears after the goiter has been removed. Thyroiditis also may present with chronic cough.

Chest roentgenograms reveal a sharply defined, lobulated or smooth mass of homogeneous density displacing the trachea posteriorly and laterally if the goiter is located in the anterior mediastinum (Fig. 60.1). Calcification is very common (Fig. 60.2). Most intrathoracic goiters cause no symptoms and are discovered incidentally on a routine chest roentgenogram. A small percentage of patients have symptoms: inspiratory and expiratory stridor, hoarseness, and rarely respiratory distress. The results of radioisotope studies (^{131}I thyroid scans) are diagnostic when positive, but these goiters are rarely, if ever, functioning. To evaluate the

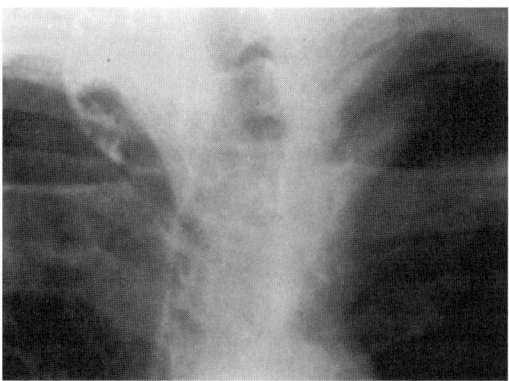

FIGURE 60.2. Close-up view of upper middle chest demonstrating calcification within an intrathoracic goiter.

degree of tracheal obstruction caused by a thyroid goiter or mass, flow-volume loops may be superior to conventional roentgenologic methods. Cine computed tomography (CT) and bronchoscopy provide dynamic assessment of the airway during all phases of respiration.

In a retrospective study of patients with 2,908 goiters who underwent surgery during a 17-year period, it was noted that a long-standing goiter did not preclude the possibility of compressive respiratory distress. Therefore, preventive removal of all large or substernal goiters should be considered. Thyroidectomy is the treatment of choice in patients with thyroid enlargement complicated by compression or displacement of the trachea. In patients who cannot undergo surgery, a bronchoscopically inserted tracheal prosthesis (stent) may provide airway patency.

Hyperthyroidism

Dyspnea at rest (thyrotoxic dyspnea) is a common symptom in patients with thyrotoxicosis. Proximal myopathy appears to play a major role because weakness of the skeletal muscles has been reported in as many as 82% of thyrotoxic patients, and electromyographic evidence of myopathy is found in 93%. Significant decreases in both inspiratory and expiratory maximal pressures have been demonstrated (12). The vital capacity and compliance also may be reduced; however, the D$_{LCO}$ is normal. The respiratory muscle strength is inversely proportional to the degree of thyroid dysfunction, and the thyrotoxic myopathy is reversible with medical treatment (13). Thyrotoxic patients have a higher rate of ventilation than normal subjects during exercise (14). The increased ventilation is secondary to enhanced central drive, which is correlated with the level of circulating thyroid hormone, and the abnormal drive can be normalized by β-blockade. These findings suggest that the inappropriately increased ventilatory drive may be the result of enhanced adrenergic stimulation (15).

Dyspnea in thyrotoxic patients is also caused by decreased compliance, increased dead space ventilation, and increased work of breathing. These are further aggravated by the greater oxygen requirement of the hypermetabolic body tissues. A study of 12 patients during hyperthyroid and euthyroid states indicated that exercise intolerance in hyperthyroidism, despite an elevated resting cardiac output, is the result of diminished work efficiency of the skeletal muscles (16).

Hyperthyroidism occasionally causes benign thymic hyperplasia. In most instances, the thymic enlargement is minimal and remains unnoticed. On rare occasions, thymic hyperplasia may present as an anterior mediastinal mass. An enlarged thymus associated with hyperthyroidism may occasionally cause dyspnea as a consequence of extrinsic compression of the trachea, but the thymic hyperplasia is usually detected by CT performed for other reasons. Thymic hyperplasia regresses promptly after hyperthyroidism has been treated. Bulbar palsy is a known complication of thyrotoxi-

cosis; aspiration pneumonia and respiratory failure have been described in this setting.

Hypothyroidism

Hypothyroidism is associated with several respiratory problems because of a combination of factors, including hypoactivity of the respiratory center, disturbances of neuronal and neuromuscular transmission (hypothyroid neuropathy), respiratory muscle weakness, and changes in the pulmonary alveolar capillary membranes (17).

Hypoventilation

Alveolar hypoventilation occurs in myxedema, and nearly 10% of patients with myxedema have a diminished hypoxic drive. The minute ventilation and oxygen and carbon dioxide tension in arterial blood are normal in patients with myxedema. However, their response to breathing higher concentrations of carbon dioxide is decreased. The hypoventilation is related to a depressed hypoxic ventilatory drive. The abnormal hypoventilatory response resolves with thyroid replacement therapy. A less-known mechanism is the myopathy that occurs in 30% to 40% of all hypothyroid patients. Dysfunction of the diaphragm, in addition to weakness of other inspiratory and expiratory muscles, also develops in these patients (18,19). Indeed, hypothyroidism can present as dyspnea secondary to phrenic neuropathy, which is reversible with therapy for hypothyroidism. Diminished muscle strength, indicated by diminished maximal voluntary ventilation, has been observed in patients with hypothyroidism (19). Rapid resolution of hypercapnia after thyroid replacement despite persistent muscle weakness in some patients suggests that the thyroid hormone deficiency is hierarchically more important than the myopathy. It has also been documented that the significantly diminished maximal inspiratory and expiratory strength returns to normal after thyroid replacement therapy. Prolonged hypothyroidism with the gradual onset of respiratory failure and predominant hypercapnia has been described. Myxedema coma usually occurs in elderly, obese women; hypoventilation appears to be responsible for the coma in a third of patients.

Sleep Apnea

Obstructive sleep apnea and oxygen desaturation are important complications of hypothyroidism (20). However, in a study of 65 patients with documented obstructive sleep apnea, only two (3%) had hypothyroidism, and, among 20 patients with hypothyroidism, two had moderate to severe obstructive sleep apnea (21). All the hypothyroid patients in this study were snorers. Whereas obstructive sleep apnea without hypothyroidism is more common in men, obstructive sleep apnea associated with hypothyroidism is more common in women. Obstructive sleep apnea in hypothyroidism is caused by macroglossia and narrowing of the upper airways secondary to the submucosal deposition of mucopolysaccharides and extravasation of protein.

Central sleep apnea results from abnormalities in ventilatory control (5). Episodes of sleep apnea are more frequent in hypothyroid patients who are obese than in those who are not obese. The impaired respiratory drive is corrected by thyroid hormone replacement therapy. Thyroxine replacement decreases the frequency of apnea, even without a change in body weight. Increases in the loaded respiratory effort and ventilation during thyroxine therapy have been demonstrated. The restoration of a euthyroid status usually results in the complete resolution of obstructive sleep apnea.

Pleural Effusion

Myxedema is an uncommon cause of pleural effusion, and the incidence of this complication in hypothyroidism is unknown. A review of the literature in 1983 revealed 13 cases, of which 11 were in women whose mean age was 52 years. The pleural effusions were frequently associated with ascites. Congestive heart failure was also noted in many patients. Usually, myxedematous patients with pleural effusion have a concomitant pericardial effusion. The pleural effusion associated with pericardial effusion is a transudate (Fig. 60.3). A report in 1990 reviewed the records of 60 patients with hypothyroidism and noted a pleural effusion in 15 (25%), but the effusions in most cases were caused by other diseases or hypothyroidism-related nonpulmonary complications. When the 15 patients in this study were combined with another group of 13, for a total of 28 patients who had a pleural effusion associated with hypothyroidism, it was found that only 5 (18%) of the 28 had a pleural effusion that could be ascribed to hypothyroidism; the protein levels in the pleural fluid of four patients varied from 1.1 to 3.2 g/dL (22). Usually, effusions are evident only on roentgenographic examination, and they are rarely sufficiently large to cause symptoms. The observation that the pleural effusions disappear after myxedema has been treated supports an etiologic relationship. Increased pulmonary or pleural capillary permeability may play a role in the collection of fluid in the pleural space.

Other Complications

A decrease in the vital capacity in the absence of heart failure has also been noted in myxedema. Hypothyroidism is a good example of a leftward shift of the oxyhemoglobin dissociation curve; hence, the tissue supply of oxygen is worse than indicated by hypoxemia alone. Soft, patchy, nodular infiltrates (myxedematous lesions) have been reported in myxedema. Roentgenographic clearing of these infiltrates has been reported after replacement therapy with thyroid hormone. The pathogenesis of these lesions is unknown, but studies have shown that atelectasis related to decreased surfactant develops in thyroidectomized rats, and thyroxine therapy stimulates surfactant synthesis. Thyroxine is reported to promote maturation in fetal rabbit lungs.

The coexistence of autoimmune hypothyroidism with pulmonary hemosiderosis has been described in a patient. Pulmonary hemosiderosis has also been described in four patients with thyrotoxicosis.

Asthma and the Thyroid Gland

The relationship between thyroid function and bronchial asthma has very interesting clinical implications. However, the coexistence of asthma and thyroid disease has been reported only sporadically. In a retrospective cohort mortality study of 3,696 women treated for thyrotoxicosis, asthma was the underlying cause of death in seven patients, in comparison with 2.6 expected deaths in the normal population. Another retrospective study of 1,107 patients found only 12 with coexistent hypothyroidism and asthma. Treatment of hypothyroidism in three of these patients was associated with worsening of their asthma. A similar experience was described after the administration of triiodothyronine for hypothyroidism. In contrast, some patients with coexistent intractable asthma and hyperthyroidism experienced prompt and striking relief of their asthma after they were treated for hyperthyroidism. In one study, however, thyrotoxicosis that was induced by administering triiodothyronine (T_3) to subjects with mild asthma had no effect on lung function, airway responsiveness, or exercise capacity (23). A proposed mechanism for the worsening of asthma in hyperthyroidism is increased airways reactivity. Reduced β-adrenergic responsiveness and the down-regulation of β-receptors in asthma may contribute to the worsening of bronchospasm. However, a positive response to the treatment of hyperthyroidism in patients with asthma is not uniformly achieved.

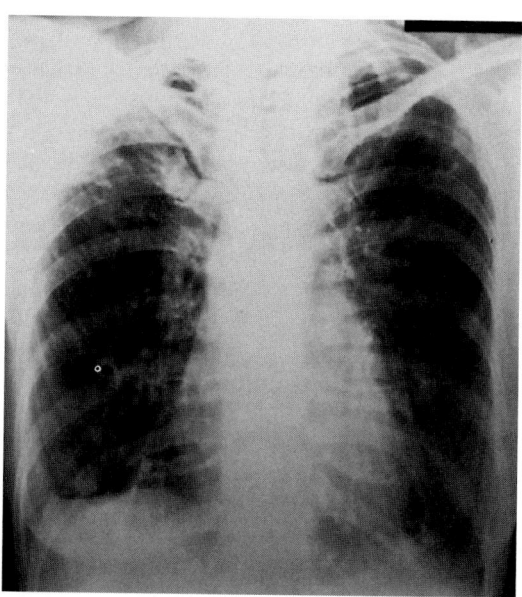

FIGURE 60.3. Right-sided pleural effusion and pulmonary edema in a patient with severe myxedema. These resolved with thyroid replacement therapy.

An entirely opposite airway response is seen in hyperthyroid patients without asthma. There appears to be an inverse relationship between the level of thyroid function and β-adrenergic receptor responsiveness. Acute hypothyroidism has been reported to increase nonspecific bronchial reactivity in subjects without asthma (24). However, a report of 11 hyperthyroid patients without asthma concluded that hyperthyroidism actually reduced the severity of carbachol-induced changes in airways reactivity as measured by airway specific conductance (sG_{aw}).

It should be recognized that patients with hyperthyroidism may not benefit from bronchodilator therapy. This is because bronchodilators accelerate the metabolic rate. The administration of β-adrenergic blockers such as propranolol to treat thyrotoxicosis may exacerbate asthma. An asthmatic patient in whom hyperthyroidism develops should be closely monitored for worsening asthma. Similarly, even slow and cautious restoration of the euthyroid state in hypothyroid patients may exacerbate asthma.

Iodide-induced thyrotoxicosis occasionally develops after the long-term administration of iodine or iodide-containing compounds to patients with preexisting thyroid disorders, particularly goiter. Interestingly, a saturated solution of potassium iodide (SSKI) was used in the past as an expectorant in asthmatic patients. In some cases, this caused hyperthyroidism, which in turn aggravated the asthma. Iodinated glycerol (Organidin), a mucolytic agent used to treat chronic obstructive pulmonary disease, has been reported to induce thyrotoxicosis (25).

Riedel Thyroiditis

Riedel thyroiditis is a rare disease characterized by extensive dense fibrosis of the thyroid gland, often extending into the strap muscles and adjacent structures in the neck. The condition is rare; 20 cases were discovered among 42,000 patients seen at a tertiary center. Respiratory symptoms result from tracheal compression. A massive fibrotic process has been described in the upper lobes of both lungs. Severe upper airway obstruction has been described in a patient with Hashimoto thyroiditis. Lymphocytic interstitial pneumonitis has been described in four patients with autoimmune thyroiditis. An association of idiopathic pulmonary hemosiderosis and autoimmune thyroiditis has been noted.

Thyroid Cancer

Pulmonary involvement in thyroid carcinoma may be related to direct or contiguous spread, with intraluminal extension into the airway, extrinsic compression of the trachea, or the development of metastatic nodules in the lungs (26). The latter can be solitary or multiple. Tracheal obstruction can be life-threatening and requires immediate, bronchoscopically guided stent therapy or tracheostomy. Paralysis of the recurrent laryngeal nerve increases the risk for aspiration pneumonia.

Pulmonary metastases are not uncommon in children and young adults with differentiated thyroid cancer. Metastases in the lungs may be overlooked unless nearly total thyroidectomy is followed by total-body radioiodine scanning in these patients (27). In a study of 209 patients younger than 25 years who were treated for thyroid cancer, 19 (9%) had pulmonary metastases at presentation, and all 19 had regional lymphadenopathy at the time of diagnosis (28). This study observed that lung metastases almost always concentrate radioiodine diffusely and that chest roentgenographic findings may be normal in almost half of patients. Nevertheless, it is important to note that radioiodine uptake in the lung can also represent an unrelated pulmonary disease, uptake by the breasts, or external contamination.

Parathyroid Disorders

Parathyroid tumors rarely present as anterior mediastinal masses. They are usually small and encapsulated growths in the upper mediastinum. They may become large enough to widen the mediastinum, usually unilaterally. Mediastinal parathyroid tissue is identified in approximately 11% of patients who undergo surgical exploration and resection as therapy for primary hyperparathyroidism. In a study of 573 patients who underwent surgical exploration to treat hypercalcemia, the number of mediastinal parathyroid glands was 68, of which 55 (81%) were enlarged and 13 were of normal size (29). The preoperative serum levels of calcium are generally higher in patients with mediastinal parathyroid tissue than in those with hyperactive parathyroid glands in the neck. Among patients who are suspected to have primary hyperparathyroidism, approximately 60% of the mediastinal glands are found on first exploration of the neck; in the rest (35%), more than one surgical exploratory procedure is usually required to detect and resect the parathyroid tissue.

Ectopic parathyroid glands in the thoracic cavity have been detected with great accuracy by means of sestamibi scintigraphy, whereas single photon emission CT (SPECT) has been helpful in distinguishing adenomas in the aortopulmonary recess from those in the anterior mediastinum, a more frequent location. Both CT and magnetic resonance imaging also can make this distinction.

Because most of these tumors are functioning, patients present with clinical hyperparathyroidism, which, along with hypercalcemic crisis, has been reported to cause pulmonary edema. This, however, is uncommon. The hypercalcemic state is also associated with metastatic calcification or calcinosis (or calciphylaxis) of the visceral organs. In the lungs, calcium deposits are found in the bronchi, alveoli, and venous channels. A review of more than 7,000 autopsies disclosed 13 cases of metastatic pulmonary calcification; chronic renal disease and parathyroid abnormalities accounted for seven of them, and the remainder were associated with malignancies. Roentgenograms in patients with metastatic pulmonary calcification reveal calcification of the bronchi and an amorphous, diffuse, finely dispersed calcification of the lungs radiating from the hilar regions. Although primary hyperparathyroidism, malignancies, and chronic renal failure are the more common causes of the hypercalcemic state, metastatic lung calcification is also seen in recipients of renal and liver transplants and in patients with hypervitaminosis D, sarcoidosis, or milk alkali syndrome. It may also develop after the intravenous infusion of calcium.

In a study of 49 patients with persistent primary hyperparathyroidism caused by mediastinal parathyroid adenoma, angiographic ablation performed by injecting large doses of contrast material into the feeding artery was successful in the long-term control of persistent primary hyperparathyroidism in 17 (63%) of 27 patients; the unsuccessful cases were treated by surgical resection via median sternotomy (30).

Parathyroid carcinoma is associated with nodular metastases in the lungs. After resection of the pulmonary metastases of six patients with such lesions, the serum calcium level returned to normal after each thoracotomy in three patients, who were alive and well 3, 8, and 12 years after the first thoracotomy; however, the hypercalcemia persisted in the other three patients (31).

Adrenal Disorders and Corticosteroids

Cushing syndrome and *long-term corticosteroid therapy* can result in an abnormal accumulation of fat in the upper mediastinum (mediastinal lipomatosis) and both pleuropericardial angles. Roentgenograms reveal a smooth, symmetric widening of the upper mediastinum (Fig. 60.4A) extending from the thoracic inlet to both hilar areas. CT (Fig. 60.4B) is diagnostic because it can demonstrate the lipid density in the mediastinum.

Cushing syndrome can be the initial clinical presentation in patients with bronchial carcinoid tumors (32). In a study of 15 consecutive patients with Cushing syndrome, all of whom were subsequently found to have bronchial carcinoid tumors, biochemical studies showed a marked elevation of circulating corticotropin (mean serum value, 156 ± 58 pmol/L; normal, 4–22 pmol/L), hypokalemia in six patients, and a glucocorticoid response to either high-dose dexamethasone or metyrapone in six of 13 patients. The carcinoid tumors were frequently radiographically occult, with 10 of 15 patients initially having normal chest roentgenographic findings. CT was successful in locating the lesions. Surgery resulted in complete remission in 10 patients and partial remission in two; three patients continued to have symptomatic glucocorticoid excess caused by metastatic disease.

Long-term corticosteroid therapy suppresses some of the immune defense mechanisms of the body and predisposes the patient to a number of unusual and opportunistic infections. Tuberculosis (TB) is more frequent in patients receiving long-term corticosteroid therapy. *Pneumocystis carinii* pneumonia is a serious complication in patients taking significant doses of corticosteroid therapy for long periods. Endogenous Cushing syndrome has been complicated by cryptococcosis. This syndrome, secondary to a hormonally active thymic carcinoid, has been noted to be associated with *P. carinii* infection. Patients with endogenous Cushing syndrome in whom pulmonary infiltrates develop should be carefully evaluated to exclude the possibility of opportunistic infection.

Aerosolized corticosteroid therapy in asthmatic patients, particularly in megadoses, has been of concern in regard to an increased risk for oropharyngeal candidiasis and also

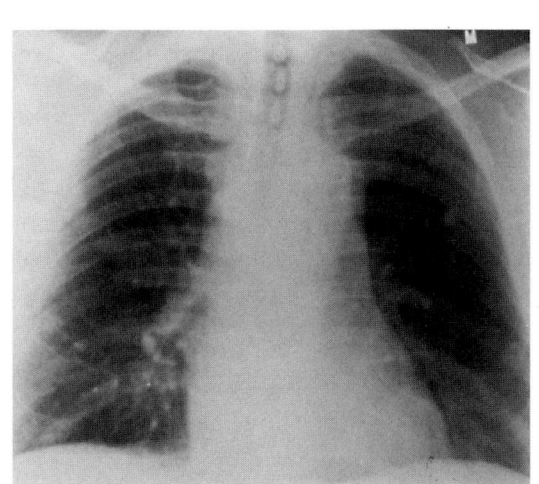

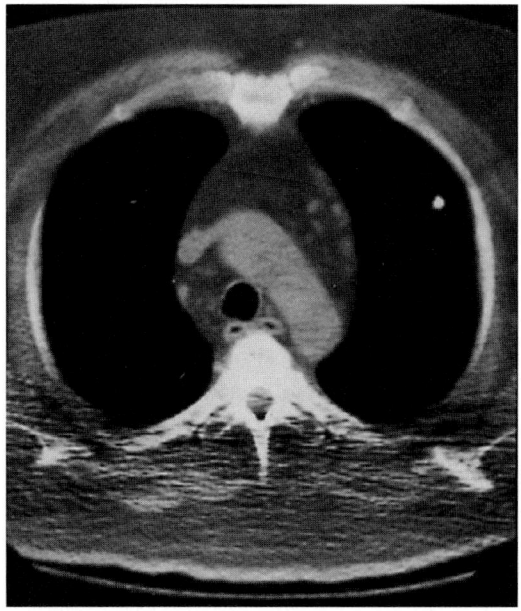

A

B

FIGURE 60.4. A: Cushing syndrome with mediastinal widening. **B:** Computed tomography in mediastinal lipomatosis reveals typical lipid density in the anterior mediastinum.

suppression of adrenal function. In one report, prolonged administration of 200 μg of inhaled budesonide daily to young children with severe asthma did not impair growth or pituitary-adrenal function.

Pheochromocytoma in association with a catecholamine-induced cardiomyopathy has led to the development of recurrent bilateral and unilateral pulmonary edema; special radionuclide studies indicated that excessive amounts of catecholamines influenced both the heart and lungs. Acute respiratory distress syndrome has been observed in a patient with pheochromocytoma. A surge of catecholamines from a pheochromocytoma may induce pulmonary edema; the mechanism is similar to that in neurogenic pulmonary edema. Hemoptysis during paroxysms of hypertension caused by a pheochromocytoma that was cured by surgical resection of the tumor has been reported.

Paragangliomas (chemodectomas) are tumors of the extra-adrenal paraganglion system. The most common paragangliomas are carotid body chemodectomas, glomus jugulare tumors, and globus tympanicum. Paraganglioma of the mediastinum is an indolent and slowly growing tumor. A review of the world literature noted 79 cases of mediastinal paraganglioma (33). The tumors were locally invasive, with a high local recurrence rate (56%) and a true metastatic capacity in 27%; the overall survival was 62%, with a mean survival time of 98 ± 12 months. In a retrospective study of 16 patients (10 men and 6 women with a mean age of 43 years) with mediastinal paraganglioma, 13 tumors were located in the posterior mediastinum and three in the anterior mediastinum. Some, however, have reported that these neoplasms are usually located in the anterior mediastinum (Fig. 60.5). In the thorax, they are generally found above the aortic arch near the subclavian arteries. A preponderance of cases in women, an average age at the time of diagnosis of 49 years, and an average tumor size of 7.5 cm were reported in a review of 40 patients. Nearly 50% of the patients are asymptomatic; the reported symptoms include hoarseness,

cough, dysphagia, and chest pain. Distant metastases were noted in 23% of the 40 cases reported in 1979. Surgical resection is recommended.

Carney triad is a syndrome of pulmonary chondroma, multicentric gastric epithelioid leiomyosarcoma, and extra-adrenal paraganglioma (34). It has been described in more than 35 patients since 1977. Several clinically significant features of this unusual syndrome include the following: multicentricity of both the paragangliomas and the epithelioid leiomyosarcomas, an often indolent progression of metastatic leiomyosarcoma, and a potential for late recurrence. It is important to distinguish intra-adrenal from peri-adrenal catecholamine-producing tumors (paragangliomas). The majority of the patients have been girls with an average age of 16.5 years. The most common clinical features are hematemesis and anemia as a result of the gastric lesion. Hypertension is the next most common finding. Multiple pulmonary tumors (two thirds are uncalcified) and mediastinal widening are seen on the chest roentgenograms (Fig. 60.6). None of the reported patients had symptoms caused by the pulmonary lesions. If a new catecholamine-producing tumor is suspected, urine biochemical assays and CT of the chest and abdomen are the first-choice localization procedures.

The uncommon concurrence of duodenal epithelioid stromal sarcoma, pulmonary chondromatous hamartoma, and pancreatic islet cell tumor in a patient has been described as a variant or analogue of Carney triad. Gastric leiomyosarcoma and extra-adrenal paraganglioma have been described in a 7-year-old child.

Adrenal carcinoma is rare. A review of the records of 24 patients with adrenal cortical carcinoma and pulmonary metastases during a 14-year period revealed that 10 patients underwent pulmonary resection (35). The 5-year survival of seven patients in the surgical group was significantly longer than that of the patients with unresected tumors, none of whom survived more than 3 years (median survival, 11 months).

METABOLIC DISORDERS

Diabetes Mellitus

Diabetes mellitus is a common disease that is often complicated by the involvement of "target" organs, such as the eyes, kidneys, and peripheral nervous system. Based on the pathophysiologic abnormalities observed in various studies, the lung has also been considered a "target" organ (36). The pulmonary pathologic changes, such as thickened alveolar epithelial and pulmonary capillary basal laminae, are considered to be secondary to pulmonary microangiopathy, akin to the diabetic vasculopathy encountered in the retinal, renal, and systemic vasculature. Pulmonary complications may manifest clinically in different ways (37). The reported complications of diabetes mellitus are listed in Table 60.2.

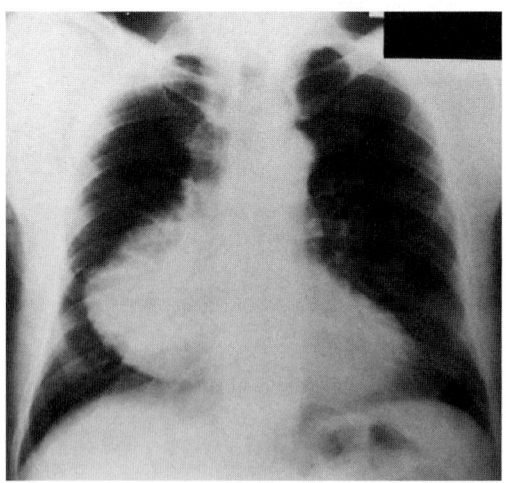

FIGURE 60.5. Paraganglioma located in the lower anterior mediastinum.

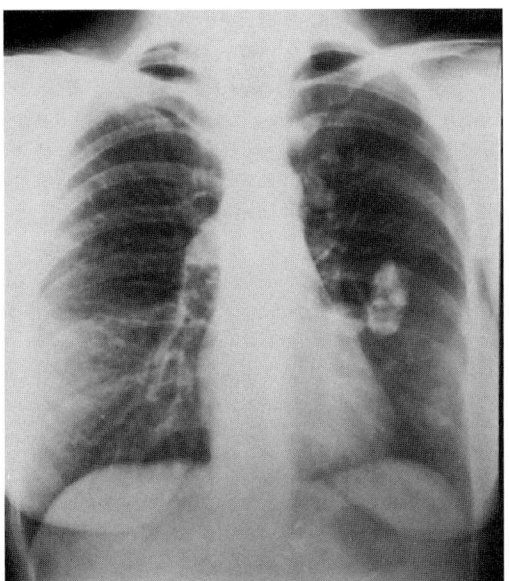
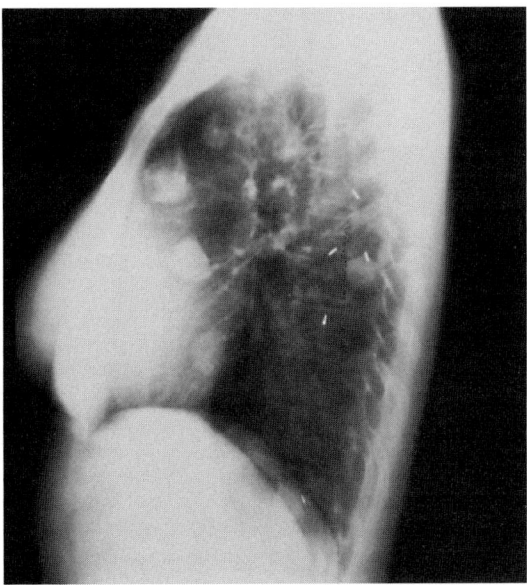

FIGURE 60.6. Multiple pulmonary chondromas in the triad of multicentric gastric epithelioid leiomyosarcoma, functioning extra-adrenal paraganglioma, and pulmonary chondroma.

Pulmonary Infections

Diabetes mellitus is often identified as an independent risk factor for the development of lower respiratory tract infections. The rates of carriage of aerobic Gram-negative rods in pharyngeal secretions have been found to be higher in diabetics and alcoholics. Bacterial pneumonias are by far the most common type of respiratory infection. The causative agents include Gram-negative organisms (*Escherichia coli, Klebsiella pneumoniae*) and Gram-positive bacteria (*Staphylococcus aureus*). Infections caused by *Streptococcus pneumoniae, Legionella,* and influenza virus may be associated with increased morbidity and mortality. The frequency of nonbacterial lung infections (mycobacteria and *Mucor*) is also increased.

TABLE 60.2. PULMONARY COMPLICATIONS IN DIABETES MELLITUS

Reduced elastic lung recoil
Reduced diffusing capacity for carbon monoxide
Viral and bacterial infections
Tuberculosis
Mucormycosis
Pneumomediastinum
Pneumothorax
Acute pleuritic pain (in ketoacidosis)
Pulmonary fibrosis
Pulmonary edema (in ketoacidosis)
Mucous plugging of major airways (in ketoacidosis)
Central hypoventilation (in autonomic neuropathy)
Sleep apnea (with autonomic neuropathy)
Aspiration pneumonia (in diabetic gastroparesis)
Pulmonary xanthogranulomatosis
Respiratory alkalosis (in ketoacidosis)
Increased endogenous production of carbon dioxide

Diabetics are particularly prone to the development of TB, frequently to an advanced stage (38). Among 106 patients with both diseases, diabetes appeared first in 48 and TB first in 40; the two were diagnosed simultaneously in 18. The increased incidence of TB in patients with diabetes mellitus is paralleled by the increased incidence of diabetes in those with TB. Tuberculous infection of lungs in diabetics may present with infiltrates in any lobe (Fig. 60.7) rather than the classic posterior-apical segments of the upper lobes (39). In a study of 20 patients with both pulmonary TB and diabetes mellitus, lower lobe involvement was noted in 10%.

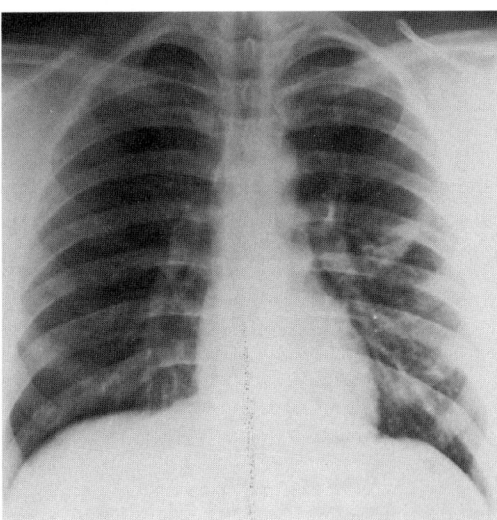

FIGURE 60.7. Localized lesion secondary to *Mycobacterium tuberculosis* infection in a young patient with type I diabetes mellitus. The pulmonary lesion is located in the superior segment of the left lower lobe.

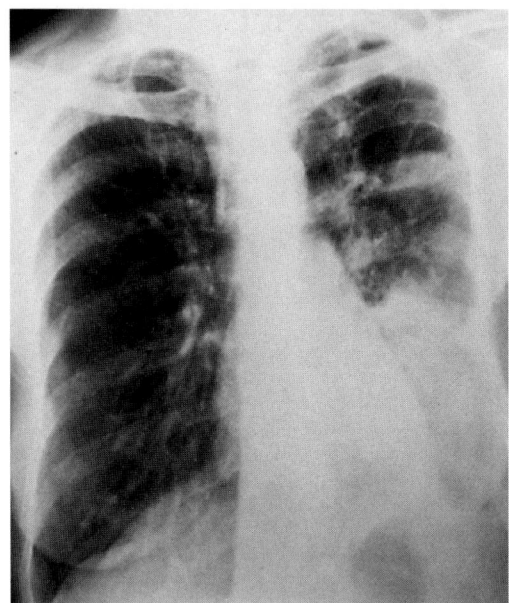

FIGURE 60.8. Pneumonia of the left lower lobe secondary to infection with *Mucor* species in a patient with poorly controlled diabetes mellitus.

Diabetics have also been found to be more susceptible to mucormycosis, particularly patients with poorly controlled diabetes mellitus and multiple complications (Fig. 60.8). In a literature review of 255 patients with pulmonary mucormycosis, diabetes mellitus was noted in 32%. Other associated medical conditions included leukemia or lymphoma, chronic renal failure, a history of organ transplantation, and a known solid tumor. The overall mortality was 80%; the most common causes of death were fungal sepsis (42%), respiratory insufficiency (27%), and hemoptysis (13%).

A striking tendency to the development of lesions in major airways has been noted in diabetics with pulmonary mucormycosis. Because of the propensity of *Mucor* species to invade vascular structures, pulmonary infarction or massive hemoptysis can occur. The diagnostic features of involvement of the major airways include hoarseness, gross hemoptysis, and mediastinal widening on chest roentgenograms. Sudden, massive hemoptysis is a common fatal complication of endobronchial mucormycosis. Pulmonary zygomycosis causes a spectrum of roentgenographic findings: normal patterns, lung abscess, subacute or chronic pneumonia that often evolves into a lung abscess, and rapidly progressive fatal pneumonia.

Pulmonary Dysfunction

Pulmonary dysfunction in diabetics is reported to be related to the severity of diabetes mellitus. A study of 284 diabetics reported that on average, the forced vital capacity and forced expiratory volume in 1 second (FEV_1) were reduced by 334 and 239 mL, respectively, in insulin-treated diabetics and by 184 and 117 mL, respectively, in diabet-

ics treated with oral hypoglycemic agents. An earlier study of 31,691 patients with diabetes mellitus noted pulmonary emphysema in 4.2%, asthma in 0.9%, and pulmonary fibrosis in 0.8%. Although the incidence of asthma and emphysema among diabetics was the same as in the total hospital population, the incidence of fibrosis was reported to be moderately elevated. Parameters of pulmonary function in 36 patients with insulin-dependent diabetes mellitus were compared with those of 40 nondiabetic controls, and the inspiratory vital capacity in the former group was found to be significantly reduced (40). The authors concluded that this abnormality may have been caused partly by a reduced capacity of the inspiratory muscles.

Significant abnormalities of lung function have included reduced lung volumes in young (younger than 25 years of age) insulin-dependent diabetic subjects, reduced pulmonary elastic recoil in both young and adult (older than 25 years of age) diabetic subjects, and impaired diffusion caused by a reduced volume of pulmonary capillary blood in the adult group (41,42). Nonenzymatic glycosylation-induced alteration of lung connective tissue is reported to be the most likely pathogenetic mechanism underlying mechanical pulmonary dysfunction in diabetic subjects, and the most tenable explanation for impaired diffusion is pulmonary microangiopathy. Diminished total lung capacity in insulin-dependent diabetics has been ascribed to limited expansion of the ribs. The clearance of inhaled ^{99m}Tc-diethyltriaminepentaacetic acid (DTPA) aerosol from the lungs has been used to show that the development of decreased epithelial permeability in diabetic patients, particularly those with other complications of diabetes, leads to pulmonary dysfunction (43). Other studies, however, have shown that insulin-dependent diabetes mellitus does not affect pulmonary function.

Physiologic studies of juvenile diabetics have shown that their elastic lung recoil is significantly less than that of normal persons, and their total lung capacity is also diminished. It is postulated that the disordered lung mechanics are a manifestation of elastin and collagen abnormalities. In a comparison of 40 adult insulin-dependent diabetics, all lifelong nonsmokers without evidence of lung disease, with a matched group of healthy controls, detailed pulmonary function tests demonstrated mild abnormalities of lung elastic recoil and D$_{LCO}$ in the diabetics, in addition to a reduction in pulmonary capillary blood volume (42). The degree of lung dysfunction was related directly to the duration of insulin-dependent diabetes mellitus.

Histopathologic studies of rats with streptozotocin-induced diabetes have shown ultrastructural alterations in the granular pneumocytes of the alveolar septum, nonciliated bronchiolar epithelial (Clara) cells, and collagen and elastin in the alveolar wall. Postmortem studies of diabetics have also documented thickening of the epithelial and capillary basal laminae of alveoli, centrilobular emphysema, and diabetic microangiopathy in the capillaries of the alveolar septa and the alveolar and pleural arterioles (44).

The threshold for the cough response to nebulized citric acid is higher in diabetics with autonomic neuropathy, which suggests that vagal innervation of the bronchial tree is damaged in this condition. Additional evidence of damaged vagal innervation is the observation that bronchoconstriction in response to cold air and methacholine is impaired in patients with diabetic autonomic neuropathy. Further studies in patients with diabetic autonomic neuropathy have demonstrated a reduction in parasympathetic bronchomotor tone that results in an increased basal airway caliber. Even though diaphragmatic dysfunction is reported to be common in type I diabetes, the impairment in diaphragmatic function is not caused by phrenic neuropathy (45).

Physiologic studies in patients with insulin-dependent diabetes (type I) have shown that the endogenous opioid system does not respond to the stress caused by breathing against fatiguing inspiratory resistive loads (46). Furthermore, whereas breathing against resistive loads caused a further increase in the plasma β-endorphin concentration in the control group, absolutely no increase was noted in the diabetic patients.

What are the clinical implications of these observations? Clinical experience suggests that pulmonary parenchymal defects and pulmonary dysfunction are insufficient to cause significant respiratory embarrassment in the vast majority of patients with insulin-dependent diabetes mellitus. Despite the overwhelming information published in the medical literature on the subject, as is evident from this discussion, clinically significant lung disease based solely on pulmonary dysfunction induced by diabetes mellitus is seldom encountered in clinical practice. Despite the extensive studies of pulmonary dysfunction in patients with diabetes mellitus, routine pulmonary function testing is not indicated in the absence of pulmonary symptoms or a history of smoking.

Pulmonary Edema

Pulmonary edema has been associated with diabetic ketoacidosis. It has been suggested that altered pulmonary capillary permeability is the cause of the extravascular leakage of fluids. Patients with diabetic ketoacidosis are usually administered large quantities of intravenous crystalloids within a short period. These solutions elevate the hydrostatic pressure and diminish the oncotic pressure, thereby facilitating the development of pulmonary edema. Pulmonary vascular diabetic angiopathy may predispose some diabetics to pulmonary edema. Additionally, endogenous fluid shifts resulting from severe hyperglycemia may contribute to pulmonary edema. Recurrent episodes of acute alveolar and interstitial pulmonary edema have been noted on chest roentgenograms in anephric diabetics during periods of severe hyperglycemia. Clinical and chest roentgenographic resolution occurs immediately after insulin therapy and the restoration of normoglycemia.

Disordered Sleep

Sleep-related abnormalities of breathing are more frequent in diabetic patients with autonomic neuropathy. The ventilatory and heart rate responses to hypoxia are impaired in diabetics, whereas the ventilatory response to hypercapnia is well preserved. Although a diminished hypercapnic ventilatory response to progesterone therapy has been described in a patient with diabetic autonomic neuropathy, detailed studies of the effect of this neuropathy on the respiratory system have shown no difference between the ventilatory responses to hypoxemia and hypercapnia of patients with autonomic neuropathy and the responses of those without autonomic neuropathy. Diabetic microangiopathy of muscles, resulting in a myopathic process, muscle weakness, and central hypoventilation, may cause hypercapnia and respiratory failure. Another explanation for the diminished ventilatory response to hypoxia is that the medullary depression of ventilation by hypoxia is greater in diabetic patients than in control subjects. Others have reported normal breathing patterns in diabetics with severe autonomic neuropathy. A relationship has been shown between neuropathy and sleep-related abnormalities of breathing in patients with insulin-dependent (type I) diabetes.

Other Complications

The oxygen tension in arterial blood is usually high in patients with diabetic ketoacidosis as a consequence of hyperventilation secondary to acidosis and an increased glucose load. Additionally, the production of endogenous carbon dioxide in metabolic acidosis causes a higher respiratory quotient and thus a higher-than-expected increase in the oxygen tension in arterial blood. Rarely, hypokalemic hypoventilation may complicate severe diabetic ketoacidosis.

Pleural effusion is reported to occur more commonly in diabetic patients, particularly those with left ventricular failure. In a study of 40 patients with similar degrees of left ventricular dysfunction, pleural effusions were more common in the diabetic patients, and four of five diabetic patients who had persistent pleural effusions had no evidence of either cardiomegaly or congestive cardiac failure (47). Although several mechanisms were postulated to be responsible, the exact mechanism remains unclear.

Pneumomediastinum has been reported in several cases of diabetic ketoacidosis. The cause remains obscure, although ketoacidosis is believed to change the pressure gradient within the lungs as a consequence of hyperpnea induced by the acidosis, severe vomiting, or a combination of both. The prognosis is excellent, and the pneumomediastinum regresses promptly after the ketoacidosis has been corrected.

Mucous plugging of major airways has been described as a specific complication of diabetic ketoacidosis. Lethargy, altered vagal tone, and autonomic neuropathy have been proposed as contributing factors responsible for occult mucous plugging. Reduced airway vagal tone and diminished responsiveness to cold have been documented in nonsmoking, nonasthmatic diabetic patients with autonomic neuropathy.

Aspiration pneumonia secondary to recurrent vomiting in unsuspected gastroparesis has been observed in diabetic patients. This is important during anesthetic procedures.

Xanthogranulomatosis has been demonstrated in the perivascular spaces of the lungs in 6% of diabetic patients (vs. 2% in nondiabetics), but the effect of this abnormality on pulmonary function is unknown.

Acute pulmonary edema was observed in patients in whom hypoglycemic coma was induced as therapy (insulin shock therapy) for schizophrenia in the 1930s. In one series of seven patients treated with insulin shock, acute pulmonary edema was the second most frequent cause of death (after irreversible coma). Most of the patients were otherwise healthy and younger than 35 years. Animal studies support the hypothesis that the pulmonary edema seen in hypoglycemic coma has neurogenic causes.

Pulmonary maturation in the fetus has been linked to the level of maternal glucose control in diabetic pregnancies (48). Amniocentesis performed in pregnant diabetic women has shown that adequate glucose control may lower the risk for fetal pulmonary immaturity to the same level as in nondiabetic pregnancies.

Obesity

Pulmonary Dysfunction

Obesity, even when mild, has been reported to impair lung function significantly. The most persistent abnormalities of pulmonary function in obesity are a decreased expiratory reserve volume and a decreased functional residual capacity. In a comparison of 144 men with mild obesity (mean weight, 81.1 ± 9.0 kg) and 28 subjects of normal weight, the functional residual capacity, expiratory reserve volume, and arterial oxygen tension were decreased in 63% of the obese subjects. Spirometric evaluation of parameters of lung function in morbidly obese patients before weight loss has shown no significant abnormalities and no significant improvement in lung functions after considerable weight loss. Several studies have reported decreases in the forced expiratory flow in midcycle (FEF_{25-75}) and mild decreases in arterial oxygen tension. A study of 63 obese men without overt obstructive lung disease detected a subgroup with normal flow rates but significantly diminished maximum voluntary ventilation (49). These findings have been interpreted to indicate disease of the small airways.

Several studies in obese subjects have shown decreases in the tidal volume, vital capacity, and functional residual capacity but a normal diffusing capacity. Another study has shown an increase in the DLco in patients with weight-to-height ratios exceeding 0.6. It is postulated that the increase in the DLco is caused by the increase in pulmonary blood volume that accompanies the elevated cardiac output noted in obesity. These findings suggest that the diminished DLco in morbidly obese subjects indicates intrinsic pulmonary pathology. Abnormal ventilation-perfusion ratios have been demonstrated in the bases of the lungs of obese patients with hypoxemia and low or normal carbon dioxide tension in arterial blood.

The alterations in respiratory function that develop in obesity may result from a combination of mechanical impedance to breathing exerted by thoracic and abdominal fat and ventilation-perfusion mismatch. Increased work of breathing and decreased efficiency of the respiratory system are also seen. Studies suggest greater diaphragmatic efficiency in the upright than in the supine position in most obese subjects, a reversal of the normal response. Diaphragmatic overstretching may be an important mechanism in the development of hypoventilation in the morbidly obese. The overall incidence of postoperative pulmonary complications in a large group of obese patients undergoing abdominal surgery (ileojejunal bypass) was 25%.

Hypoventilation

The hypoventilation seen in obese patients with both hypoxemia and hypercapnia may result from one or more of the following proposed mechanisms: an increase in fat deposits around the chest wall with a resultant increase in the work of breathing, an extremely low ventilation-perfusion ratio at the lung bases resulting from a lower expiratory reserve volume, obstruction of the upper airways, and a disturbance in the respiratory center itself that makes it insensitive to carbon dioxide. Considerable weight loss may reverse the symptoms in many cases. However, in some instances, a low arterial oxygen tension may persist, whereas in others, the number of episodes of sleep-disordered breathing and nocturnal desaturation has been significantly reduced, lending support to the concept that obesity is the cause and not an effect of the sleep apnea syndrome in these patients.

A detailed discussion of sleep-disordered breathing in obese subjects can be found in Chapter 69.

Malnutrition

Clinically significant malnutrition is a common complication of long-term mechanical ventilation and of severe emphysematous obstructive lung disease. These forms of malnutrition, like the malnutrition resulting from starvation, affect the respiratory system. Prolonged starvation significantly alters the structure and function of the lungs. Morphometric and ultrastructural changes similar to those observed in elastase-induced emphysema have been noted in hamsters subjected to starvation. The pulmonary defense mechanisms, like those of other organ systems, depend on an optimal nutritional status. A diminished respiratory clearance of microbial organisms, a decrease in the number of pulmonary alveolar macrophages, and marked decreases in the levels of secretory immunoglobulin A and other immunoglobulins (as a result of hypoproteinemia) may predispose these patients to infection with various organisms. Furthermore, the ventilatory drive is reduced in malnourished subjects as a consequence of the effects of nutritional depletion on both the central nervous system and the respiratory muscles. The diaphragmatic muscle mass is also reduced in malnourished subjects.

The effects of starvation and renutrition on pulmonary function have been studied in patients with anorexia nervosa. In a study of 15 patients with anorexia nervosa, results of spirometry, lung volumes, arterial blood gases, and diaphragmatic function were recorded at admission and at days 7, 30, and 45 (50). The mean body weight at admission was 37 ± 4.7 kg (63% of ideal body weight) and increased significantly to 43 ± 4.6 kg by day 45. The vital capacity and FEV_1 increased significantly by day 30; the lung volumes were unchanged. The most significant change was in diaphragmatic contractility, which was severely depressed initially but increased significantly with nutritional support by day 30. These results support earlier assertions that diaphragmatic function is markedly impaired in severely malnourished patients, even in the absence of lung disease, and that renutrition partially reverses the weakness.

Rachitic lung demonstrates roentgenographic abnormalities as lobar or segmental atelectasis, compression atelectasis, and interstitial pneumonitis (51). These changes are attributed to hypoventilation in a distorted, small chest along with chronic and recurrent pulmonary infections. Hypoventilatory failure has been described in these patients. In a large group of children with vitamin A deficiency, the incidence of respiratory disease was twice that in normal children, and the risk for respiratory disease was more closely associated with vitamin A status than with general nutritional status.

Gaucher Disease

Gaucher disease is an autosomal-recessive error of lipoprotein metabolism caused by a deficiency of glucocerebrosidase, the enzyme that catalyzes glucocerebroside metabolism. It occurs predominantly in Jewish women in a neurologic, a visceral, and an osseous form. As glucocerebroside accumulates in cells of the reticuloendothelial system, they are transformed into Gaucher cells, which accumulate both in the reticuloendothelial system and in the lungs and other organs. Whereas pulmonary involvement and symptoms are common in the infantile form of Gaucher disease, they are distinctly uncommon in the adult form (type I disease) (52).

The pulmonary manifestations consist of an interstitial infiltration of Gaucher cells in the peribronchial, perivascular, and septal regions (53). Pulmonary hypertension has resulted from pulmonary capillary plugging by Gaucher cells. Roentgenograms of the lung show a diffuse reticulonodular or miliary pattern. Microscopic examination reveals an impressive consolidation of lung parenchyma by Gaucher cells (54). Elevated serum levels of angiotensin-converting enzyme have been noted in this disease.

Of 95 patients with type I Gaucher disease studied in Israel, 68% had abnormalities of pulmonary function; the total lung capacity was reduced in 22%, the ratio of residual volume to total lung capacity was elevated in 18%, and the FEV_1 was reduced in one third of the patients (55). The functional residual capacity and transfer coefficient for carbon monoxide (K_{CO}) were reduced in 45% and 42% of the patients, respectively. The incidence of reduced expiratory flow was higher in male than in female subjects. Even though chest roentgenographic abnormalities were found in 17% of the patients, only 4% had significant symptoms. No association was found between abnormal pulmonary function and genotype or age.

In a patient with pulmonary involvement in type I Gaucher disease, high-resolution CT demonstrated thickening of the interlobular septa and between four and six small nodules within secondary lobules, each probably corresponding to an acinus (56). An interstitial disease pattern or a combination of interstitial and alveolar disease with a mosaic pattern may be seen on high-resolution CT scans (57,58).

Intrathoracic extramedullary hematopoiesis in the form of a thoracic paravertebral mass has been described in an asymptomatic woman with type I Gaucher disease.

Replacement therapy with glucocerebrosidase has improved the pulmonary status.

Niemann-Pick Disease

Niemann-Pick disease is characterized by an absolute or relative deficiency of the enzyme sphingomyelinase. Severe nodular pulmonary disease leading to cor pulmonale has been noted. An association of widespread pulmonary nodules, linear strands, and honeycombing has been reported. Large, multivacuolated foam cells (sea blue histiocytes) can be found in the pulmonary alveoli.

Angiokeratoma Corporis Diffusum (Fabry Disease)

Fabry disease, an X-linked sphingolipid storage disorder caused by a lack of α-galactosidase, is reported to be associated with multiple angiomas of the tracheobronchial tree and bullous emphysema leading to hyperinflation of the lungs. Recurrent pulmonary infections and hemoptysis may indicate respiratory involvement. Bronchial inclusion bodies and alveoli filled with ceramide hexosidase have been observed in patients with obstructive lung disease secondary to Fabry disease. The deposition of ceramide hexosidase in the bronchial tree may contribute to intrinsic airways disease and functional airways obstruction.

Mucopolysaccharidosis

Lung involvement occurs in several mucopolysaccharidoses. The deposition of mucopolysaccharides in the tracheal wall resulted in tracheal narrowing and airways compromise in 9 of 56 patients with various mucopolysaccharidoses. Pulmonary complications in 21 patients with mucopolysaccharidosis or mucolipidosis included the following: (a) upper airway narrowing by hypertrophic tongue, tonsils, adenoids, and mucous membranes; (b) lower airway narrowing as a result of glycosaminoglycan deposition within the tracheobronchial mucosa; and (c) thoracic dimensions decreased by scoliosis and thoracic hyperkyphosis (59). The pulmonary consequences include an increased risk for respiratory tract infections, airway compromise during or after anesthesia or sedation, dyspnea on exertion, obstructive lung disease, obstructive sleep apnea, and cor pulmonale.

Hunter syndrome is one of a group of heritable metabolic disorders in which decreased activity of one or more of the lysosomal enzymes responsible for mucopolysaccharide catabolism results in the excessive deposition of mucopolysaccharides in the skeletal and soft tissues. Airway obstruction is a frequent problem. Progressive obstruction sequentially involving the upper, mid, and lower airway, characterized by the gradual deformation and collapse of the trachea (tracheobronchomalacia), has been described. Autopsy analyses have demonstrated anteroposterior flattening of the trachea and bronchi and submucosal thickening leading to the structural alterations peculiar to this disease. Sleep apnea syndrome, atelectasis, recurrent pneumonia, and difficult endotracheal intubation are known to be associated with this rare disorder.

Hurler syndrome is a rare mucopolysaccharide storage disease that becomes clinically apparent during early childhood as deposits of mucopolysaccharide form in the skeletal and soft tissues. The progressive deposition of mucopolysaccharide in the oropharynx and tracheal connective tissues leads to airway obstruction if untreated. Tonsillectomy, adenoidectomy, and tracheostomy have been performed to relieve symptoms of upper airway obstruction. Carbon dioxide laser excision of tracheal lesions is an alternative method for the management of airway obstruction.

Hurler-Scheie syndrome is a genetic compound of two mucopolysaccharidoses, the Hurler and Scheie syndromes. The genetic error of metabolism responsible for this syndrome causes intermediate systemic effects. Because of a lack of the enzyme α-L-iduronidase, glycosaminoglycans are deposited in the tissues, causing multiple systemic effects and airway lesions.

Morquio syndrome (mucopolysaccharidosis type IVA) is a rare inherited connective tissue disorder characterized by a distinct form of skeletal dystrophy (spondyloepiphyseal dysplasia), restrictive pulmonary disease, and normal intelligence. Tetraplegia secondary to the subluxation of C1 over C2 as a consequence of marked odontoid dysplasia or hypoplasia is common in these patients. Pulmonary function studies have noted the restrictive nature of the ventilatory defects. Collapse of the upper airways during head flexion may be an important cause of pulmonary disability in Morquio disease.

Krabbe leukodystrophy leading to rapidly progressive respiratory failure in an 8-week-old boy has been described. Ultrastructural examination of the lungs revealed numerous intra-alveolar macrophages.

Sleep apnea is common in patients with mucopolysaccharidoses. In the past, all reported cases of sleep apnea in these patients were treated with tonsillectomy/adenoidectomy or tracheostomy. Some patients have been successfully treated with nasal continuous positive airway pressure and supplemental oxygen. Bone marrow transplantation has resulted in effective metabolic correction and the relief of obstructive apnea in Hurler syndrome.

Lipoid Proteinosis

A rare hereditary disorder of the autosomal-recessive type, lipoid proteinosis is characterized by the deposition of an amorphous eosinophilic glycoprotein in multiple organs. The pulmonary abnormality consists of an infiltration of the anomalous glycoprotein into capillary walls. Roentgenograms reveal a diffuse reticulonodular pattern throughout both lungs.

Bronchoalveolar lavage in patients with pulmonary involvement in the lipid storage disorders shows lipid-containing foamy cells and both periodic acid-Schiff– and Scharlach red stain–positive vacuoles in the cytoplasm of alveolar macrophages. These abnormal cells are the same cells found in bone marrow biopsy specimens.

Lysinuric Protein Intolerance

Lysinuric protein intolerance is an autosomal-recessive disorder caused by the defective transport of cationic amino acids. Pulmonary disease is a potentially fatal complication. In a study of nine patients with lysinuric protein intolerance, a 10-year-old patient died of severe respiratory insufficiency caused by alveolar proteinosis (60). The remaining patients were asymptomatic at the time of the study, although high-resolution CT revealed acinar nodules, interlobular or intralobular thickening of the interstitial septa, and subpleural cysts in five of them. No abnormalities of pulmonary function were evident. Radionuclide studies showed an uneven distribution of perfusion and ventilation and confirmed the presence of segmental or diffuse pulmonary functional defects.

Acute Intermittent Porphyria

Acute intermittent porphyria results from an inborn error of metabolism. Occasionally, this entity may present as acute respiratory insufficiency or with neurologic, psychiatric, or gastrointestinal manifestations. In patients with respiratory involvement, the mortality may be high. The pulmonary features are usually similar to those of Guillain-Barré syndrome, in which the disease process involves the respiratory muscles and causes alveolar hypoventilation. Acute intermittent porphyria should be considered in the differential diagnosis of respiratory failure.

Carcinoid Syndrome

Carcinoid tumors of the bronchus and lung are discussed fully elsewhere. The following is a review of the pulmonary manifestations of the carcinoid syndrome, the classic form of which is caused by a hormonally active carcinoid tumor located most frequently in the terminal ileum. The tumor arises from the Kulchitsky (argentaffin) cells, which contain neurosecretory granules filled with serotonin (5-hydroxytryptamine). This hormone is responsible for most of the clinical features, which include episodic flushing, purplish cyanosis, diarrhea, bronchospasm, and valvular disease of the right side of the heart.

Of 3,718 cases of abdominal carcinoid tumor, 3.7% had symptomatic endocrine activity. In a Mayo Clinic series, the carcinoid syndrome was associated with 7% of gastrointestinal carcinoids and 2% of bronchial carcinoids (61).

The pulmonary manifestations of the syndrome may include hyperventilation and wheezing. Most frequently, however, patients do not have symptoms referable to the chest, and evidence of bronchoconstriction is found only during attacks of flushing. The most prominent cardiac symptoms are caused by stenosis of the pulmonic and tricuspid valves, and these lesions can lead to intractable failure of the right side of the heart. Elevated urinary levels of 5-hydroxyindoleacetic acid are helpful in establishing the diagnosis.

Other Metabolic Disorders

Volume contraction is a common clinical problem, and its effects on pulmonary function have been studied. During hypohydration induced by the administration of diuretics to normal volunteers, lung volumes increased significantly. In addition, the peak expiratory flow rate, FEV_1, maximal voluntary ventilation, and flow rates at low lung volumes also increased, but returned to normal on rehydration (62). The DLCO was unchanged. The mechanism is probably related to loss of water in the airway walls or peribronchial space. The clinical significance of these findings is unclear.

Hypokalemia is a commonly encountered clinical problem. Respiratory muscle weakness may result from severe hypokalemia. Periodic hypokalemic paralysis has been associated with hypoventilation. Severe diarrhea, dehydration, and marked hypokalemia in a child were followed by fatal respiratory failure as a result of respiratory muscle paralysis.

Hypophosphatemic states are known to cause muscle weakness followed by respiratory failure. A decrease in the level of phosphate in the body diminishes the level of adenosine triphosphate and results in muscle weakness. Phosphate replacement therapy in such cases dramatically improves muscle function and reverses respiratory failure. Chronic hypophosphatemia causes a decrease in 2,3-diphosphoglycerate, which increases the affinity of oxygen for hemoglobin and so decreases the delivery of oxygen to tissues.

Hypomagnesemia may contribute to respiratory muscle weakness. Next to potassium, magnesium is the most abundant intracellular cation in the human body. It is required as a cofactor by many enzymes and is a cofactor in all transphosphorylation reactions. The incidence of hypomagnesemia varies from 30% in alcoholics to 2% in normal individuals. In patients with respiratory muscle weakness, hypomagnesemia should be sought as an etiologic factor because magnesium replacement therapy has been shown to improve all indices of muscle power measured after treatment.

Hypermagnesemia as a result of the excessive ingestion of antacids, bowel obstruction, or renal failure may be followed by respiratory depression and coma. These features can be reversed by lowering the magnesium level.

Metabolic alkalosis is a common acid-base disorder in hospitalized patients. Compensatory hypoventilation may lead to atelectasis, deterioration of the ventilation-perfusion relationship, and an increased alveolar-arterial difference in oxygen tension. The resultant hypoxia can be corrected significantly by reversing the alkalosis with hydrochloric acid.

High carbohydrate loads have led to acute respiratory failure. This is a potential problem in patients on total parenteral nutrition. Because the infused glucose is used as the primary source of energy, carbon dioxide production and the respiratory quotient are substantially increased. Respiratory failure is more likely to occur in patients with limited pulmonary reserve.

Total parenteral nutrition is associated with increased carbon dioxide production in patients on ventilation, whose inability to match carbon dioxide excretion with the carbon dioxide load leads to an increase in arterial carbon dioxide tension. This risk can be minimized by increasing the minute ventilation before total parenteral nutrition is begun.

Hyperlipidemia is reported to cause falsely low DLCO measurements as a result of interference with a hemoglobin-combining coefficient. This is of no clinical significance in healthy subjects.

Glycogen storage diseases predispose patients to bacterial infections. Staphylococcal infections may cause lung abscesses and pneumatoceles (Fig. 60.9).

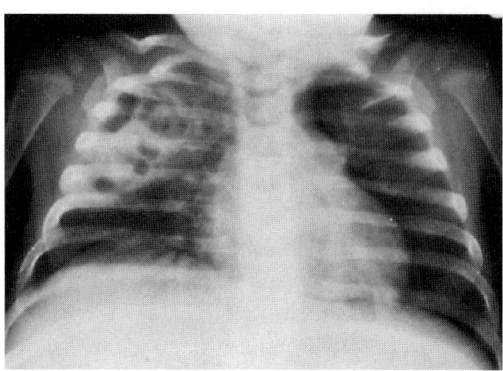

FIGURE 60.9. Glycogen storage disease in an infant complicated by *Staphylococcus aureus*–induced abscesses in the right upper lobe.

Gouty tophi of the larynx and vocal cords have been described, with accompanying stridor, hoarseness, and signs of extensive gouty disease.

REFERENCES

1. Trotman-Dickenson B, Weetman AP, Hughes J. Upper airflow obstruction and pulmonary function in acromegaly: relationship to disease activity. *Q J Med* 1991;79:527–538.
2. Donnelly PM, Grunstein RR, Peat JK, et al. Large lungs and growth hormone: an increased alveolar number? *Eur Respir J* 1995;8:938–947.
3. Rosenow F, Reuter S, Deuss U, et al. Sleep apnoea in treated acromegaly: relative frequency and predisposing factors. *Clin Endocrinol (Oxf)* 1996;45:563–569.
4. Grunstein RR, Ho KY, Sullivan CE. Sleep apnea in acromegaly. *Ann Intern Med* 1991;115:527–532.
5. Grunstein RR, Ho KY, Berthon-Jones M, et al. Central sleep apnea is associated with increased ventilatory response to carbon dioxide and hypersecretion of growth hormone in patients with acromegaly. *Am J Respir Crit Care Med* 1994;150:496–502.
6. Pelttari L, Polo O, Rauhala E, et al. Nocturnal breathing abnormalities in acromegaly after adenomectomy. *Clin Endocrinol (Oxf)* 1995;43:175–182.
7. Mickelson SA, Rosenthal LD, Rock JP, et al. Obstructive sleep apnea syndrome and acromegaly. *Otolaryngol Head Neck Surg* 1994;111:25–30.
8. Grunstein RR, Ho KK, Sullivan CE. Effect of octreotide, a somatostatin analog, on sleep apnea in patients with acromegaly. *Ann Intern Med* 1994;121:478–483.
9. Madjar S, Weissberg D. Retrosternal goiter. *Chest* 1995;108:78–82.
10. McHenry CR, Piotrowski JJ. Thyroidectomy in patients with marked thyroid enlargement: airway management, morbidity, and outcome. *Am Surg* 1994;60:586–591.
11. Melliere D, Saada F, Etienne G, et al. Goiter with severe respiratory compromise: evaluation and treatment. *Surgery* 1988;103:367–373.
12. McElvaney GN, Wilcox PG, Fairbarn MS, et al. Respiratory muscle weakness and dyspnea in thyrotoxic patients. *Am Rev Respir Dis* 1990;141:1221–1227.
13. Siafakas NM, Milona I, Salesiotou V, et al. Respiratory muscle strength in hyperthyroidism before and after treatment. *Am Rev Respir Dis* 1992;146:1025–1029.
14. Kahaly G, Hellermann J, Mohr-Kahaly S, et al. Impaired cardiopulmonary exercise capacity in patients with hyperthyroidism. *Chest* 1996;109:57–61.
15. Small D, Gibbons W, Levy RD, et al. Exertional dyspnea and ventilation in hyperthyroidism. *Chest* 1992;101:1268–1273.
16. Kimura H, Kawagoe Y, Kaneko N, et al. Low efficiency of oxygen utilization during exercise in hyperthyroidism. *Chest* 1996;110:1264–1270.
17. Wilson WR, Bedell GN. The pulmonary abnormalities in myxedema. *J Clin Invest* 1960;39:42.
18. Martinez FJ, Bermudez-Gomez M, Celli BR. Hypothyroidism. A reversible cause of diaphragmatic dysfunction. *Chest* 1989;96:1059–1063.
19. Siafakas NM, Salesiotou V, Filaditaki V, et al. Respiratory muscle strength in hypothyroidism. *Chest* 1992;102:189–194.
20. Rajagopal KR, Abbrecht PH, Derderian SS, et al. Obstructive sleep apnea in hypothyroidism. *Ann Intern Med* 1984;101:491–494.
21. Lin CC, Tsan KW, Chen PJ. The relationship between sleep apnea syndrome and hypothyroidism. *Chest* 1992;102:1663–1667.
22. Gottehrer A, Roa J, Stanford GG, et al. Hypothyroidism and pleural effusions. *Chest* 1990;98:1130–1132.
23. Hollingsworth HM, Pratter MR, Dubois JM, et al. Acute hypothyroidism has no effect on pulmonary vascular resistance. Effect of triiodothyronine-induced thyrotoxicosis on airway hyperresponsiveness. *J Appl Physiol* 1991;71:438–444.
24. Wieshammer S, Keck FS, Schauffelen AC, et al. Effects of hypothyroidism on bronchial reactivity in nonasthmatic subjects. *Thorax* 1990;45:947–950.
25. Becker CB, Gordon JM. Iodinated glycerol and thyroid dysfunction. Four cases and a review of the literature. *Chest* 1993;103:188–192.
26. Samaan NA, Schultz PN, Haynie TP, et al. Pulmonary metastasis of differentiated thyroid carcinoma: treatment results in 101 patients. *J Clin Endocrinol Metab* 1985;60:376–380.
27. Casara D, Rubello D, Saladini G, et al. Different features of pulmonary metastases in differentiated thyroid cancer: natural history and multivariate statistical analysis of prognostic variables. *J Nucl Med* 1993;34:1626–1631.
28. Vassilopoulou-Sellin R, Klein MJ, Smith TH, et al. Pulmonary metastases in children and young adults with differentiated thyroid cancer. *Cancer* 1993;71:1348–1352.
29. Conn JM, Goncalves MA, Mansour KA, et al. The mediastinal parathyroid. *Am Surg* 1991;57:62–66.
30. Doherty GM, Doppman JL, Miller DL, et al. Results of a multidisciplinary strategy for management of mediastinal parathyroid adenoma as a cause of persistent primary hyperparathyroidism. *Ann Surg* 1992;215:101–106.
31. Obara T, Okamoto T, Ito Y, et al. Surgical and medical management of patients with pulmonary metastasis from parathyroid carcinoma. *Surgery* 1993;114:1040–1048.
32. Arioglu E, Doppman J, Gomes M, et al. Cushing's syndrome caused by corticotropin secretion by pulmonary tumorlets. *N Engl J Med* 1998;339:883–886.
33. Lamy AL, Fradet GJ, Luoma A, et al. Anterior and middle mediastinum paraganglioma: complete resection is the treatment of choice. *Ann Thorac Surg* 1994;57:249–252.
34. Margulies KB, Sheps SG. Carney's triad: guidelines for management. *Mayo Clin Proc* 1988;63:496–502.
35. Kwauk S, Burt M. Pulmonary metastases from adrenal cortical carcinoma: results of resection. *J Surg Oncol* 1993;53:243–246.
36. Sandler M. Is the lung a "target organ" in diabetes mellitus? *Arch Intern Med* 1990;150:1385–1388.
37. Hansen LA, Prakash UBS, Colby TV. Pulmonary complications in diabetes mellitus. *Mayo Clin Proc* 1989;64:791–799.

38. Kim SJ, Hong YP, Lew WJ, et al. Incidence of pulmonary tuberculosis among diabetics. *Tuber Lung Dis* 1995;76:529–533.

39. Morris JT, Seaworth BJ, McAllister CK. Pulmonary tuberculosis in diabetics. *Chest* 1992;102:539–541.

40. Wanke T, Formanek D, Auinger M, et al. Inspiratory muscle performance and pulmonary function changes in insulin-dependent diabetes mellitus. *Am Rev Respir Dis* 1991;143:97–100.

41. Cooper BG, Taylor R, Alberti KG, et al. Lung function in patients with diabetes mellitus. *Respir Med* 1990;84:235–239.

42. Sandler M, Bunn AE, Stewart RI. Cross-section study of pulmonary function in patients with insulin-dependent diabetes mellitus. *Am Rev Respir Dis* 1987;135:223–229.

43. Caner B, Ugur O, Bayraktar M, et al. Impaired lung epithelial permeability in diabetics detected by technetium-99m-DTPA aerosol scintigraphy. *J Nucl Med* 1994;35:204–206.

44. Farina J, Furio V, Fernandez-Acenero MJ, et al. Nodular fibrosis of the lung in diabetes mellitus. *Virchows Arch* 1995;427:61–63.

45. Wanke T, Paternostro-Sluga T, Grisold W, et al. Phrenic nerve function in type I diabetic patients with diaphragm weakness and peripheral neuropathy. *Respiration* 1992;59:233–237.

46. Wanke T, Lahrmann H, Auinger M, et al. Endogenous opioid system during inspiratory loading in patients with type I diabetes. *Am Rev Respir Dis* 1993;148:1335–1340.

47. Chertow BS, Kadzielawa R, Burger AJ. Benign pleural effusions in long-standing diabetes mellitus. *Chest* 1991;99:1108–1111.

48. Piper JM, Langer O. Does maternal diabetes delay fetal pulmonary maturity? *Am J Obstet Gynecol* 1993;168:783–786.

49. Sahebjami H, Gartside PS. Pulmonary function in obese subjects with a normal FEV_1/FVC ratio. *Chest* 1996;110:1425–1429.

50. Murciano D, Rigaud D, Pingleton S, et al. Diaphragmatic function in severely malnourished patients with anorexia nervosa. Effects of renutrition. *Am J Respir Crit Care Med* 1994;150:1569–1574.

51. Khajavi A, Amirhakimi GH. The rachitic lung. Pulmonary findings in 30 infants and children with malnutritional rickets. *Clin Pediatr (Phila)* 1977;16:36–38.

52. Zimran A, Kay A, Gelbart T, et al. Gaucher disease. Clinical, laboratory, radiologic, and genetic features of 53 patients. *Medicine* 1992;71:337–353.

53. Mistry P, Sirrs S, Chan A, et al. Pulmonary hypertension in type 1 Gaucher's disease: genetic and epigenetic determinants of phenotype and response to therapy. *Mol Genet Metab* 2002;77:91.

54. Ross DJ, Spira S, Buchbinder NA. Gaucher cells in pulmonary capillary blood in association with pulmonary hypertension. *N Engl J Med* 1997;336:379–381.

55. Kerem E, Elstein D, Abrahamov A, et al. Pulmonary function abnormalities in type I Gaucher disease. *Eur Respir J* 1996;9:340–345.

56. Tunaci A, Berkmen YM, Gokmen E. Pulmonary Gaucher's disease: high-resolution computed tomographic features. *Pediatr Radiol* 1995;25:237–238.

57. Aydin K, Karabulut N, Demirkazik F, et al. Pulmonary involvement in adult Gaucher's disease: high-resolution CT appearance. *Br J Radiol* 1997;70:93–95.

58. Yassa NA, Wilcox AG. High-resolution CT pulmonary findings in adults with Gaucher's disease. *Clin Imaging* 1998;22:339–342.

59. Semenza GL, Pyeritz RE. Respiratory complications of mucopolysaccharide storage disorders. *Medicine* 1988;67:209–219.

60. Santamaria F, Parenti G, Guidi G, et al. Early detection of lung involvement in lysinuric protein intolerance: role of high-resolution computed tomography and radioisotopic methods. *Am J Respir Crit Care Med* 1996;153:731–735.

61. Galanis E, Kvols LK, Rubin J. Carcinoid syndrome. *J Clin Oncol* 1998;16:796–798.

62. Javaheri S, Bosken CH, Lim SP, et al. Effects of hypohydration on lung functions in humans. *Am Rev Respir Dis* 1987;135:597–599.

61 Neurologic Diseases

Udaya B. S. Prakash · Talmadge E. King, Jr.

The central and peripheral nervous systems play significant roles in the normal functioning of the respiratory system. The central component of the respiratory system resides mainly in the respiratory centers located in the medulla oblongata. Internuncial pathways connect these centers with higher brain centers, which also play a role in the normal breathing mechanism. The peripheral nervous system is responsible for normal functioning of the respiratory musculature. Depending on the type and extent of injury to either the central or peripheral nervous system, the respiratory system may exhibit various abnormalities. In this chapter, the pulmonary manifestations of disease processes at various levels of the nervous system are discussed.

NEUROGENIC BREATHING DISORDERS

The most common respiratory feature noted in intracranial disorders is a change in the breathing pattern (1). Elevation of intracranial pressure is the main pathologic event responsible for the breathing abnormalities. When damage is limited to one hemisphere, breathing is often normal. In contrast, acute bilateral hemispheric injury commonly elicits abnormal pattern of breathing. Abnormal breathing patterns have been related to prognosis after brain damage. Abnormal breathing is equally common in each of three large groups of patients: those with head injury, intracranial tumor, or subarachnoid hemorrhage. Depending on the anatomic location of brain injury, patients may demonstrate hypoventilation, hyperventilation, or both at different times during their illness. In one

U. B. S. Prakash: Pulmonary and Critical Care Medicine, Mayo Medical School and Mayo Medical Center, Rochester, Minnesota.
T. E. King, Jr.: Department of Medicine, University of California, San Francisco; and Medical Services, San Francisco General Hospital, San Francisco, California.

report of 100 consecutive patients with severe head injuries who arrived at a major trauma center, hypoxia was noted in 30% and hypercapnia in 4% (1a). Abnormalities in the rate and depth of respiration occur in approximately 40% of cases of cerebral hemorrhage. Extensive lesions—such as massive cerebral hemorrhage, major cerebral embolism, and those caused by severe head trauma—are accompanied by a higher incidence of abnormalities in breathing pattern.

Several types of breathing abnormalities, including periodic breathing, irregular breathing, and tachypnea, have been described in patients with central nervous system trauma, tumor, or cerebrovascular accidents. In one report of 227 patients with these types of abnormalities, 60% demonstrated some type of abnormal breathing (2). All patients with medullary lesions demonstrated respiratory abnormalities, whereas pontine lesions were associated with respiratory abnormalities in 60% to 70% of patients. Poor prognosis was associated with respiration exceeding 25 breaths/min and an arterial carbon dioxide tension ($Paco_2$) of less than 30 mm Hg (see section "Neurogenic Hyperventilation").

Cheyne-Stokes Breathing

Cheyne-Stokes breathing is characterized by regularly alternating phases of hyperventilation and apnea and usually persists for long periods. It occurs in approximately 25% of cases of cerebral embolism and nearly 10% of cases of cerebral infarction (3). This respiratory dysrhythmia is also seen in other clinical conditions, including lactic acidosis, diabetic ketoacidosis, and uremic coma. Instability of the ventilatory control system is the main cause of Cheyne-Stokes breathing. Another possible cause is abnormal sensitivity of respiratory neurons to carbon dioxide, resulting in hyperventilation that is unduly prolonged by impairment of forebrain ventilatory inhibition. Patients with Cheyne-Stokes respiration exhibit a progressively increased tidal volume during the hyperpneic phase, with subsequent decreases without change in respiratory rate.

Patients with Cheyne-Stokes breathing in whom respiratory alkalosis develops have a higher mortality. Cardiac and pulmonary monitoring in 44 patients admitted within 48 hours of onset of stroke disclosed that the presence of intermittent Cheyne-Stokes breathing or tachypnea, seen in 88%, was associated with increased mortality. In one study reporting on 11 patients with a Paco$_2$ of less than 35 mm Hg and a pH of more than 7.46, only one patient survived. There is an increase in mortality associated with Cheyne-Stokes respiration in patients with congestive heart failure (4). Hypoxemia is frequently present owing to concomitant heart and lung disease (1).

Periodic Breathing

Periodic breathing is a variant of Cheyne-Stokes respiration. Periodic breathing is characterized by regular recurrent cycles of changing tidal volumes in which the lowest tidal volume is less than half the maximal tidal volume in that cycle (1). It is the most frequent abnormal respiratory pattern directly related to stroke, and may be more common among patients with subarachnoid hemorrhage (1).

Ataxic Breathing

Ataxic breathing, sometimes known as *chaotic breathing*, comprises periodic hypoventilation, slow regular breathing, Biot respiration, apneusis-like inspiratory pauses, and inspiratory gasps. Ataxic breathing is caused by dysfunction of the dorsal respiratory neurons in the medulla that control the rhythmicity of breathing (1). Ataxic breathing is seen in lower pontine and medullary disorders, morphine poisoning, hypercapnic stupor, infarctions of the brainstem, meningitis, and tumors of the central nervous system (5).

Biot respiration is another term that was used in the past to describe some abnormal breathing patterns. The terms *ataxic breathing* and *Biot breathing* are often used synonymously. The breathing pattern consists of irregular cycles of uniformly deep or shallow breaths separated by apnea. Biot breathing can be seen in patients with lower pontine and medullary disorders, meningitis, lesions in the posterior fossa, morphine poisoning, and hypercapnic stupor.

Apneustic breathing refers to prolonged inspiratory "cramps" with cessation of breathing in the inspiratory phase. It is a rare clinical entity. Dissociation of cerebral pathways is believed to cause this. A report on five patients with achondroplasia, all of whom demonstrated apneustic breathing, speculated that compression of the lower medullary respiratory centers and afferent pathways in the spinal cord was responsible for the breathing abnormality. Apneustic breathing can be seen in patients with lower pontine and medullary disorders, brainstem infarction, hypercapnic stupor, menin-

gitis, and hypoglycemia. The pattern is rarely observed because patients usually have severe bulbar dysfunction and require mechanical ventilation (1,2). Weaning from mechanical ventilation is often difficult, and long-term ventilation via tracheostomy is often necessary (1). A classic example of apneustic breathing has been described in a patient with Dandy-Walker syndrome, in which hydrocephalus associated with a cystic fourth ventricle, hypoplasia or agenesis of the cerebellar vermis, and atresia of the foramina of Luschka and Magendie are noted. Although the breathing pattern may revert to normal after a shunt procedure, respiratory failure is the major complication leading to death in infants with this syndrome.

Cluster breathing is characterized by clusters of normal breaths separated by irregular pauses. Cluster breathing is seen in patients with high medullary or low pontine lesions.

In *respiratory inhibitory apraxia,* the patient is unable to stop breathing voluntarily. However, voluntary spontaneous respiration is unaffected. This abnormal breathing pattern is often associated with other forms of apraxia or motor impersistence. Respiratory inhibitory apraxia has been described in association with lesions in the internal capsule and areas supplied by the middle cerebral artery.

Gasping is an abnormal breathing pattern characterized by an attenuated inspiratory period followed by a disproportionately long period of expiration. Respiratory failure almost invariably follows the development of this breathing pattern (1). Gasping is more commonly seen in medullary strokes but overall has poor localizing value (1).

Neurogenic Hyperventilation

A rare phenomenon, neurogenic hyperventilation is characterized by very regular rapid breathing (24 to 38 breath/min, a rate three to six times greater than normal) for hours or days at a time (6). The diagnosis of central hyperventilation is based on the presence of normal arterial partial pressure of oxygen (Pao$_2$; 80 mm Hg) and a volume of breathing that is increased out of proportion and beyond body needs. Lesions in the region of the midbrain and upper pontine tegmentum—as seen in brainstem infarctions, acute encephalitis, hypoglycemia, severe sustained anoxia, trauma, and carbon monoxide poisoning—may cause central neurogenic hyperventilation. The mortality is very high when central neurogenic hyperventilation or Cheyne-Stokes breathing is associated with respiratory alkalosis (7).

The mechanism of respiratory alkalosis in central neurogenic hyperventilation is unclear. Lessened sensitivity of peripheral chemoreceptors to hypoxia may allow the Pao$_2$ to fall to 45 mm Hg, at which point central hypoxic drive produces hyperventilation and respiratory alkalosis. The presence of hyperventilation itself has been used as a diagnostic aid in patients with partial complex seizures. In a study of a large number of patients with partial complex seizures, hyperventilation maneuvers evoked abnormal electroencephalographic discharges and clinical seizures in 11%. Central neurogenic hyperventilation has never been induced experimentally, and it is rare even in patients with severe neurologic problems.

Neurogenic Hypoventilation

Hypoventilation is defined as elevation in $Paco_2$ of 45 mm Hg. Neurogenic hypoventilation can be either central or peripheral in origin (8). The direct depressant effects of overdoses of narcotic medication are a well-known cause of centrally induced hypoventilation. Cerebral trauma, vascular accidents, and infections also may result in alveolar hypoventilation. Neurogenic hypoventilation, as result of microinfarctions of basal ganglia, has been described in patients with familial hemiplegic migraine. Patients with severe cerebrovascular disease show a reduced steady-state ventilatory response to hypercapnia. The mechanism for this phenomenon is unknown.

Ondine's curse or "true" central alveolar hypoventilation (i.e., hypoventilation without any neurologic, cardiopulmonary, or metabolic disorder) is extremely rare, with only a few cases having been reported. If, however, disorders such as syringomyelia, Parkinson disease, schizophrenia, and mental retardation are included, approximately 50 cases of central alveolar hypoventilation have been described. Clinical features in these patients included cyanosis in all, polycythemia in one third, somnolence in one third, and headache in 25%. Frequent findings noted among these patients have included pulmonary hypertension and congestive cardiac failure. Bilateral phrenic nerve pacing has been tried with varying success. Pharmacologic agents, including medroxyprogesterone acetate and nocturnal administration of oxygen, have been used to stimulate respiration in patients with central hypoventilation.

Neurogenic Pulmonary Edema

The clinical occurrence of neurogenic pulmonary edema is uncommon (9–11). In a report of 2,100 patients with serious head injuries and 132 with serious cervical spinal cord or spinal column injuries, there were only two clear examples of neurogenic pulmonary edema. In contrast, an autopsy study of 100 soldiers dying of combat wounds in Vietnam revealed pulmonary edema and alveolar hemorrhage in 89%, most commonly in those who died within 1 week of injury (12,13). Respiratory disease was discovered frequently, whether or not thoracic injury was present. Furthermore, pulmonary edema is a common postmortem finding in patients with bulbar poliomyelitis, hydrocephalus, tumors of the central nervous system, intracerebral hematomas, intraventricular and subarachnoid hemorrhages, and especially trauma to the central nervous system (14).

Sustained acute elevation of intracranial pressure is probably the most important factor in the pathogenesis of neurogenic pulmonary edema. Elevation of intracranial pressure stimulates hypothalamic centers, resulting in massive α-adrenergic sympathetic discharge. Damage to the hypothalamus probably initiates the response just discussed; indeed, the postchiasmatic area has been referred to as the *edematogenic center*. These events result in severe vasoconstriction of the systemic and pulmonary vessels. Additionally, increases in microvascular pressure attributed to changes in the distribution of lung perfusion are believed to play a major pathogenic role in pulmonary edema (Fig. 61.1). These hemodynamic events occur within seconds after injury to the central nervous system. The stiffening of the left ventricle further contributes to the development of pulmonary edema. Pulmonary edema develops during these hemodynamic alterations and persists after the vascular pressures return to normal. The persistence of edema is a consequence of pulmonary capillary endothelial damage caused by the abrupt changes in pressure and volume within the pulmonary vasculature. Protein also leaks into the alveoli.

Head trauma is one of the most common causes of severe but nonfatal neurogenic pulmonary edema. Analysis of a large autopsy database and head-injured patient database showed the incidence of neurogenic pulmonary edema in patients with isolated head injury dying at the scene to be 32%; in patients with isolated head injury dying within 96 hours, the incidence was 50% (15). The implication of these findings is that neurogenic pulmonary edema begins very early after head injury. In a retrospective, clinical, and pathologic analysis of 78 cases of fatal subarachnoid hemorrhage, a pathologic diagnosis of pulmonary edema was made in 71%, and 31% of this group had a clinical diagnosis of pulmonary edema (16). Neurogenic pulmonary edema after subarachnoid hemorrhage carries a poor prognosis, and postmortem studies indicate the presence of pulmonary edema in 33% to 71% of patients with fatal subarachnoid hemorrhage.

Severe cerebral hypoxia of any cause can lead to neurogenic pulmonary edema. The overall frequency of postictal edema is low; the literature yields approximately 100 cases. Postictal pulmonary edema has recurred in the same patient. It shows a predilection for young epileptic patients. It may develop immediately after an epileptic seizure or several hours later. Electric shock therapy for seizure disorder has resulted in fatal pulmonary edema. Guillain-Barré syndrome, old poliomyelitis, and meningitis have caused neurogenic pulmonary edema. In a report of the pathologic findings in 200 cases of fatal meningococcal meningitis, pulmonary edema was noted in 60%. Neurogenic pulmonary edema has followed trigeminal blockade.

The clinical features of neurogenic pulmonary edema include the obvious evidence of damage to the central nervous system; progressive respiratory distress, tachycardia, hypertensive and bilateral crackles are found on chest examination (1). The chest radiograph reveals bilateral opacities that tend to be more interstitial than alveolar (Fig. 61.2), and the

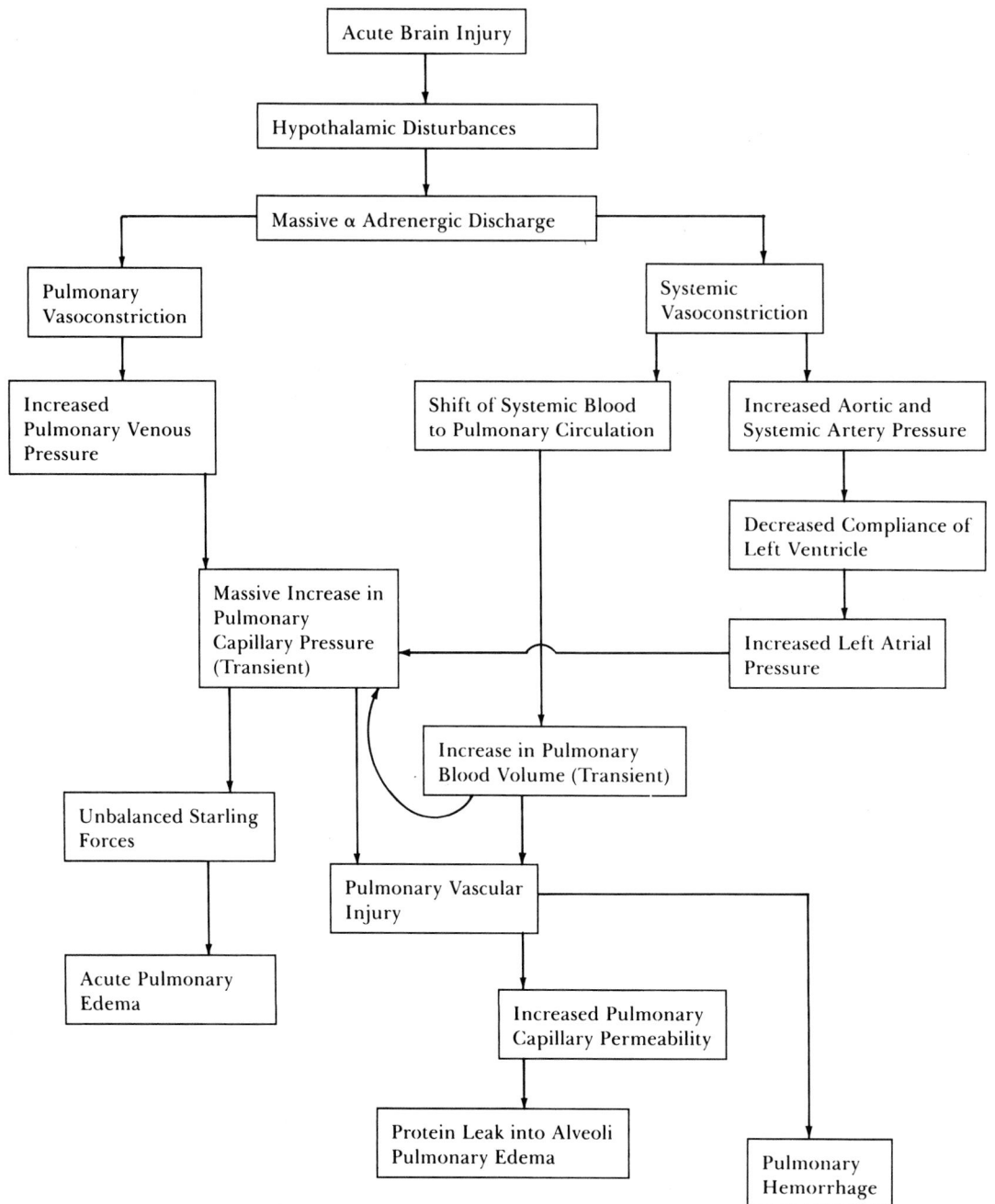

FIGURE 61.1. Mechanism of neurogenic pulmonary edema. (From Theodore J, Robin ED. Speculations on neurogenic pulmonary edema [NPE]. *Am Rev Respir Dis* 1976;113:405–411, with permission.)

cardiac silhouette may appear normal or enlarged. Unlike aspiration pneumonia in this setting, neurogenic pulmonary edema develops abruptly and progresses quickly after the onset of the neurological insult (1). Delayed onset of edema is unusual, but it has been observed in a number of cases. The diagnosis requires a high index of suspicion when pulmonary congestion develops in patients with head trauma (especially with elevated intracranial pressure), seizures or status epilepticus, or subarachnoid hemorrhage (1). Treatment of neurogenic pulmonary edema is largely supportive and directed

mainly toward treatment of the underlying neurologic condition (1,11,17).

ABNORMAL STATES OF CONSCIOUSNESS

Unconsciousness and Coma

Unconsciousness and coma predispose to the development of aspiration pneumonitis, nosocomial pneumonia, hypoventilatory respiratory failure, and pulmonary

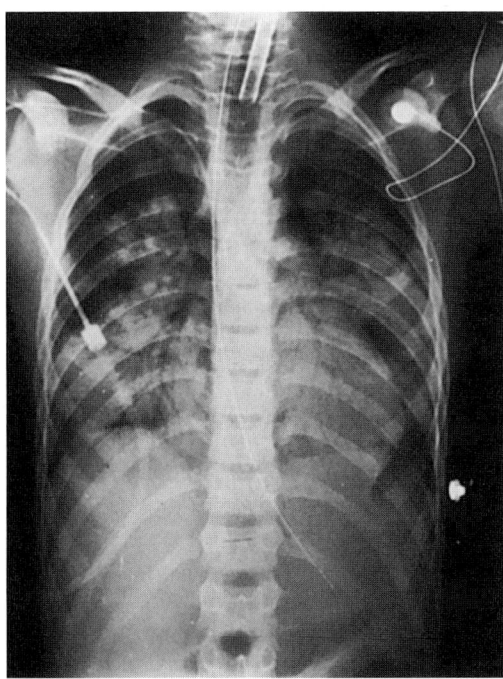

FIGURE 61.2. Neurogenic pulmonary edema. Bilateral alveolar infiltrates with air bronchograms are noted.

thromboembolism. Neurogenic pulmonary edema also is seen in these patients. Abnormal breathing patterns are common, especially at the lowest level of consciousness. However, no significant association has been found between a particular abnormal pattern and level of consciousness. The unconscious patient breathes more rapidly and regularly than does a conscious patient. Increasing regularity of respiration correlates well with deepening coma and accurately reflects ultimate outcome, even when other clinical signs remain unchanged.

Aspiration pneumonia and nosocomial pneumonia resulting from infection with Gram-positive, Gram-negative, and anaerobic organisms are the major causes of morbidity and mortality in this group of patients. Approximately 50% of patients who are unconscious or comatose aspirate. Aspiration is significantly associated with reduced pharyngeal sensation, dysphagia, and stroke severity (18). Aspiration is common in the early period after acute stroke. Therefore, each patient admitted with acute stroke should be carefully tested for disordered pharyngeal sensation. Even though aspiration is a transient phenomenon in most cases of acute stroke, it is associated with a high incidence of lower respiratory tract infection. In a prospective study of 60 consecutive patients with acute stroke, videofluoroscopy detected aspiration in 42% of patients within 72 hours of stroke onset, and aspiration had resolved in all but three patients after 3 months (19). Aspiration was closely related to the presence of dysphagia, which itself resolved within 2 weeks in all but the persistent aspirators (20). Lower respiratory tract infection was more common in aspirators than in nonaspi-

rators. In an analysis of 125 patients with closed head injury, development of early pneumonia was noted in 48% (21). Patients in whom early pneumonia developed were found to have a lower score on the Glasgow coma scale (5). In a study of 441 patients with recent stroke, videofluoroscopic barium swallow detected aspiration of thin liquids in 84 patients (19%), and aspiration pneumonia developed in 12% of this group (22). A prospective, longitudinal, cohort study of 114 consecutive inpatients admitted for stroke rehabilitation estimated that the relative risk for development of pneumonia was 6.95 times greater for those patients who aspirated compared with those who did not, 5.57 times greater for those who aspirated silently compared with those who coughed during aspiration or who did not aspirate, and 8.36 times greater for those who aspirated more than 10% on one or more barium test swallows compared with those who aspirated less than 10% or did not aspirate (23). In a study of 38 patients with bilateral stroke, the investigators observed that abnormal gag reflex and impaired voluntary cough accurately predicted radiographically verified aspiration. By using this prediction model, patients can be grouped into three risk strata: low risk of (cough and gag normal), moderate risk (one of two behaviors abnormal), and high risk of (cough and gag abnormal) (24).

Head Trauma

Neurogenic pulmonary edema and other complications also can result from closed head injury. The pulmonary complications depend on the degree of trauma, level of consciousness, and involvement of other organs. Among 47 consecutive patients with severe craniocerebral trauma who underwent computed tomography of the head and prospective limited computed tomography examination of the thorax, nine patients had pneumothorax (bilateral in one) (25). Thirty-one areas of pulmonary parenchymal contusions were seen in 19 subjects, and rupture of thoracic aorta and right diaphragmatic rupture each in one patient. The limited computed tomography examination of the chest supplied additional information (compared with chest roentgenography) in 30% of patients (25).

Closed head injury commonly requires endotracheal intubation and mechanical ventilation. A study of 109 initially comatose patients with isolated closed head injuries who were ventilated for 24 hours or more showed that closed head injury is associated with a high incidence of pneumonia, and pneumonia occurs earlier in patients with closed head injury than in other patient groups. Pneumonia usually does not occur after the first week of hospitalization in this group of patients.

Barbiturates are commonly administered to patients with cerebral edema. A prospective study in mechanically ventilated patients with brain edema discovered that the rate of nosocomial pneumonia was significantly higher in patients receiving barbiturates than in the control group, with those receiving higher doses being at greater risk for development of pneumonia. Colonization of the respiratory tract was observed in all barbiturate-treated patients and in 70% of the control group.

Epilepsy

Short periods of apnea almost always occur in *petit mal* seizures. Prolonged apnea also has been noted. Apneic periods have been observed in partial epilepsy, especially the temporal lobe type. However, respiratory changes only rarely appear to be the principal and important components of the seizure. Several cases of respiratory failure as a seizure phenomenon have been reported. The sudden death of epileptic patients, unexplained by autopsy, is reported to be relatively frequent. Such deaths have been attributed to acute functional disturbances in cardiorespiratory centers as a result of seizure discharges. It is theorized that acute respiratory failure develops from the propagation of seizure discharges that lead to brainstem dysfunction.

Laryngospasm has been noted as a presenting symptom in patients with temporal lobe seizures. Severe hypoxia and acidosis after local anesthetic-induced convulsions have been reported; the convulsions were induced by topical application of bupivacaine. Neurogenic pulmonary edema also occurs after epileptic seizures. Prolonged spasm of the respiratory muscles leading to ventilatory problems has been reported in patients with status epilepticus.

Phenytoin, used in the therapy of epilepsy, has been noted to predispose to immune deficiency (immunoglobulin A) and frequent symptoms of respiratory disease. Phenytoin also is reported to cause mild lymphadenopathy.

Exaggerated vagal response has been described in 58 children in whom reflex anoxic seizures secondary to provoked cardiac inhibition (also known as *white breath-holding attacks*) were diagnosed (26). The seizures were diagnosed initially as epileptic in nature; however, it appears that these seizures resulted from vagally mediated reflex cardiac arrest.

SPINAL CORD DISORDERS

Approximately 200,000 people living in the United States have suffered spinal cord injury (27). Damage to the cervical spinal cord can interfere with both afferent and efferent spinal pathways concerned with respiratory function (27). Transection or other severe injury to the cervical spinal cord at a high level causes weakness of the respiratory muscles and may result in ventilatory failure. Transection of the cord below the level of the fifth cervical vertebra results in intercostal muscle paralysis. In such an instance, although the accessory neck muscles of respiration are affected, diaphragmatic function is preserved, and so hypoventilation is rare. However, the work done by the diaphragm (work of breathing) is

significantly exaggerated, and therefore, most patients with transection of the spinal cord experience dyspnea. Spinal cord injury causes restrictive ventilatory changes, with reductions in vital capacity (VC), functional residual capacity, and expiratory reserve volume. Vital capacity often is used as an indicator of overall pulmonary function in these patients (28).

The term *hemiplegia* denotes loss of neuromuscular function on one side of the body, usually owing to a cerebrovascular accident on the contralateral side. The functional classification of spinal cord injuries includes *pentaplegia, quadriplegia (tetraplegia),* and *paraplegia.* In quadriplegia, the C4 through C8 levels are involved, with motor and sensory loss in the arms and legs. In respiratory quadriplegia, the spinal cord is involved at the second through third cervical vertebral levels, and findings include motor and sensory loss of the arms, legs, and diaphragm. Pentaplegia results when the lesion is located in the brainstem to the first cervical vertebral level, with resultant motor and sensory loss of the neck, arms, legs, and diaphragm. In paraplegia, sensory and motor loss is noted in the legs as a result of involvement of the spinal cord between the levels of the first thoracic and first sacral vertebrae.

Quadriplegia (Tetraplegia)

In quadriplegic patients, the VC is approximately two thirds of normal, and the maximal breathing capacity is half of normal. A mean decrease in VC to 42% of the predicted value has been reported. The impaired ventilatory function in quadriplegic patients is caused by the elimination of supraspinal control of respiratory muscles innervated by spinal segments below the level of the lesion. The spastic paralysis results in decreased compliance of the chest wall and reduction of both inspiratory and expiratory reserve volumes. The decrease in VC is also caused by altered body posture. Duration of quadriplegia does not seem to alter the response to pulmonary function testing (29). In the early stages of quadriplegia, the intensity of the compensatory respiratory function of the sternomastoid muscle varies, and its development to full strength as an auxiliary force in the act of breathing may require some time and the use of systematic exercises. Indeed, the role of another accessory muscle, the pectoralis major, is such that its causes dynamic airway compression during expiratory efforts in a substantial proportion of tetraplegic subjects (30).

The most conspicuous feature of the respiratory mechanics of the supine quadriplegic patient is the paradoxical inward movement of the rib cage during inspiration. This results in functional deformity of the chest wall and increased work of breathing. In the sitting posture, the paradoxical inward motion disappears in the lower rib cage, whereas it is decreased but still present in the upper rib cage. The disappearance of paradoxical motion of the upper rib cage with time in quadriplegics has been attributed to the development of spasticity of the intercostal muscles, with better support of the rib cage preventing it from drawing in during inspiration.

The work done by the diaphragm in quadriplegic patients is estimated to be nine times greater than that in normal individuals. This increased work of breathing is associated with dyspnea, which is minimized by a decrease in the respiratory rate to an inadequate level, which is the basis for the chronic alveolar hypoventilation seen in such cases. Tracheostomy in these patients has been associated with a higher mortality. Radiofrequency electrophrenic respiratory pacing has been used to support quadriplegic patients in whom hypoventilation develops. Milder degrees of hypoventilation may respond to noninvasive ventilatory therapies, such as continuous positive airway pressure (CPAP) (31). Mechanical ventilatory assistance is required in many.

Abnormal airway reactivity has also been reported in the spinal cord injury population (32–35). A study evaluating the airway responsiveness to methacholine in subjects with spinal cord injury reported that smokers and former smokers with quadriplegia are hyper-responsive to methacholine and that the response is comparable with that found in persons who have never smoked. The airway hyper-responsiveness in these subjects is thought to represent loss of sympathetic innervation of the lung, leaving bronchoconstrictor cholinergic activity intact and unopposed (33).

Bronchorrhea (mucous secretion >100 mL/d) or bronchial mucous hypersecretion is reported to occur in 20% of quadriplegic patients, with the quantity of mucus produced occasionally exceeding 1.0 L/d. The sudden onset of and spontaneous recovery from quadriplegic bronchorrhea is probably a consequence of disturbed neuronal control of bronchial mucous gland secretions and the initial disappearance and later reappearance of peripheral sympathetic nervous system tone.

Most deaths that follow acute quadriplegia are caused by pulmonary complications. Respiratory problems include hypoventilation, recurrent infections resulting from aspiration and ineffective cough, neurogenic pulmonary edema in the acute quadriplegic state, and an increased incidence of thromboembolic phenomena. In a prospective study of 22 consecutive patients with quadriplegia, a high mortality was noted during the first months; a 15% to 40% mortality was seen in the first year. Most deaths were related to respiratory failure. A retrospective analysis of 22 quadriplegic patients showed a 41% mortality within 5 years after quadriplegia. With time, respiratory function improved in the survivors, especially diaphragmatic function.

Hemiplegia

In hemiplegia, spastic paralysis or weakness of the affected side of the body may affect the diaphragm and intercostal muscles. However, respiratory complications ordinarily are not regarded as a complication of hemiplegia, even though ipsilateral diaphragmatic dysfunction occurs frequently. The left diaphragm is more commonly involved in left hemiplegia than is the right hemidiaphragm in right hemiplegia. Forced VC (FVC) and forced expiratory volume may be decreased to 60% of normal. Ventilatory failure becomes imminent when the VC is reduced to 25% or less of the predicted normal value. Spirometry has shown reduction of FVC and forced expiratory volume in 1 second (FEV_1) to approximately 60% and 70%, respectively, of the predicted values. Also, a mild restrictive pulmonary dysfunction occurs in patients with hemiplegia. The lack of significant clinical symptoms is attributed to the physical inactivity.

Paraplegia

Paraplegia usually is accompanied by a slight ventilatory restriction. Lung function tests have shown both VC and maximal voluntary ventilation (MVV) in the ranges of 60% to 100% of predicted normal values. One study reported a VC diminished to 60% in patients with high thoracic transections and to 78% in patients with low thoracic lesions.

DIAPHRAGMATIC PARALYSIS

The diaphragm is the most important muscle of respiration, and therefore, diaphragmatic paralysis can cause significant respiratory abnormalities (36). The paralysis can be unilateral or bilateral, and transient or permanent. It may result from interruption of the nerve supply, from muscular atrophy, or transiently from diaphragmatic pleurisy. Acute unilateral diaphragmatic paralysis usually results from interruption of the phrenic nerve by bronchogenic carcinoma or another tumor in the mediastinum, whereas chronic unilateral paralysis usually is idiopathic. Unilateral or bilateral paralysis can be caused by motor neuron disease, paralytic poliomyelitis, high cervical cord injuries, infectious polyneuritis of Guillain-Barré, or peripheral neuritis associated with measles, tetanus, typhoid, or diphtheria. Diaphragmatic involvement is often a late manifestation of generalized neuromuscular disease. Diaphragmatic weakness has also been noted in patients with Charcot-Marie-Tooth disease. Diaphragmatic paralysis has been associated with Erb palsy, which is a well-circumscribed complication of birth trauma to the shoulder and neck; with thoracotomy; and as a complication of central venous alimentation.

Unilateral phrenic nerve paralysis occurs in 2% to 10% of patients who undergo cardiac procedures, most frequently with Blalock-Taussig shunts (37). Hypothermic cardioplegia, induced by placing ice around the heart before open heart surgery, is complicated by transient unilateral phrenic nerve palsy ("frost-bitten" phrenic nerve) that lasts for 6 to 8 weeks. In recipients of orthotopic liver transplants, crush injury to the right phrenic nerve during transplantation is most likely the cause of right hemidiaphragmatic dysfunction. A prospective study of 48 adult recipients of liver transplants recorded right phrenic nerve injury and hemidiaphragmatic paralysis in 79% and 38% of patients, respectively (38). Complete recovery of phrenic nerve conduction and diaphragmatic function took as long as 9 months in some patients.

The etiology of diaphragmatic paralysis remains undetermined in more than two thirds of cases. The majority of patients studied in clinical investigations were asymptomatic and remained so on follow-up examination. Approximately 25% of them regained diaphragmatic function after a period of several months to 3 years. In another study, of 247 patients with diaphragmatic paralysis, a cause was found in 42.5% of the cases, whereas no reason for the paralysis could be identified in the remaining 57.5% (142 patients) (39). Among this group, left-sided paralysis was seen in 58%, right-sided involvement in 41%, and bilateral involvement in 1% (39). Intrathoracic malignant lesions were subsequently diagnosed in 3.5%, and progressive neurogenic atrophy was seen in one patient. During a 1-year period, two cases of bilateral diaphragmatic paralysis were found among 360 prospectively studied patients who underwent hypothermic cardioplegia; both patients had insulin-dependent diabetes mellitus (40). Phrenic nerve isolation and protection from hypothermia during surgery resulted in no case of phrenic paralysis in a group of 76 control patients, compared with an 18% incidence in 76 patients whose phrenic nerves were exposed to cold (41).

Parsonage-Turner syndrome, also referred to as *paralytic brachial neuritis, neuralgic amyotrophy,* or *brachial plexus neuropathy,* is characterized by sudden onset of pain in shoulder, chest, or upper arm followed by paresis of the shoulder girdle or upper arm. Although rare, both unilateral and bilateral diaphragmatic paralysis has been described in this syndrome (42). The diseases associated with diaphragmatic paralysis are listed in Table 61.1.

Unilateral Diaphragmatic Paralysis

A diagnosis of unilateral diaphragmatic paralysis often is difficult to establish with certainty. Study of the motion of the abdominal wall and rib cage in the supine position with magnetometry has failed to show paradoxical movements of the abdomen in unilateral paralysis. This is in contrast to the findings in bilateral diaphragmatic paralysis, in which the anterior abdominal wall moves inward paradoxically with inspiration. Measurement of transdiaphragmatic pressure using two balloon catheters has shown that at rest and expiration, when the diaphragm is relaxed, the transdiaphragmatic pressure is zero. During maximal inspiration, the change in pressure exceeds 25 cm H_2O in normal individuals, whereas in patients with weakness of the diaphragm, this pressure is 6 cm H_2O.

TABLE 61.1. CAUSES OF DIAPHRAGMATIC PARALYSIS

Cerebral hemispheric stroke
Spinal cord disorders
Trauma to the cervical spinal cord
Syringomyelia
Poliomyelitis
Motor neuron diseases
Peripheral neuropathies
Trauma to the phrenic nerve (surgery, radiation, tumor)
Phrenic nerve compression by tumor
Landry-Guillain-Barré syndrome
Brachial plexus neuritis
Nutritional or alcoholic neuropathy
Lead neuropathy
Postinfectious neuropathies
Diphtheria
Tetanus
Typhoid
Measles
Myasthenia gravis
Muscular disorders
Myotonic dystrophies
Duchenne muscular dystrophy
Metabolic myopathies
Polymyositis
Idiopathic

Symptoms of unilateral phrenic paralysis are orthopnea and difficulty in inspiration. Significant arterial oxygen desaturation can occur in the supine position but is unusual. Carbon dioxide retention also is unusual. Roentgenographic findings include elevation of the diaphragm; diminished, absent, or paradoxical movements on inspiration; mediastinal shift on inspiration; and paradoxical movements of the diaphragm under conditions of augmented load, such as sniffing. Paradoxical motion of the affected diaphragm during a "sniff test" under fluoroscopic guidance is a widely accepted test to establish the diagnosis (43) (Fig. 61.3). It should be noted, however, that nearly 6% of normal people may demonstrate paradoxic movement of either hemidiaphragm. If paradoxical excursion during sniffing exceeds 2 cm and involves the whole leaf of the diaphragm as seen on the oblique view, it probably is pathologic, provided that the abdominal muscles are relaxed during the test. Measurement of transdiaphragmatic pressure or diaphragmatic electromyography are more reliable for the diagnosis. The diagnostic evaluation of respiratory muscle weakness primarily involves the assessment of diaphragmatic function. An algorithmic approach is depicted in Figure 61.4 (44).

Pulmonary function studies in patients with unilateral diaphragmatic paralysis have shown total lung capacity (TLC) to be decreased by 37%, and VC and MVV to be decreased by 20%. The effects of posture on lung volume, airway closure, and gas exchange studied in eight patients with hemidiaphragmatic paralysis showed the mean VC in the sitting

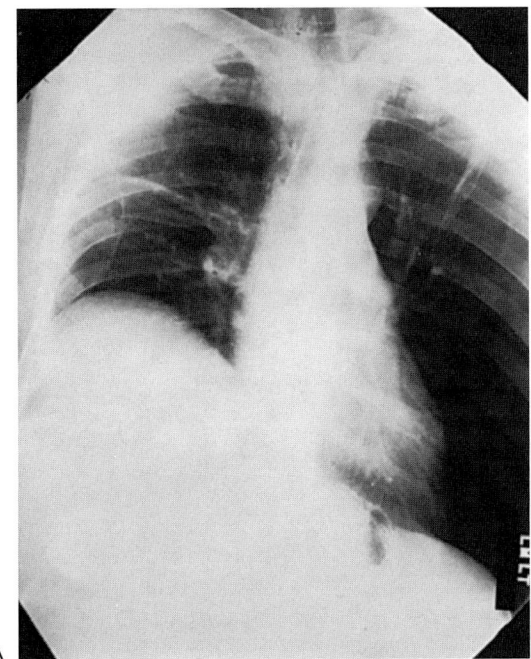 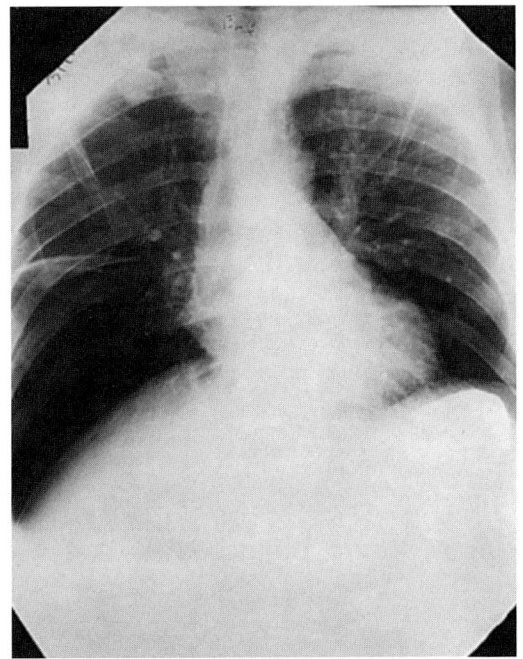

A   B

FIGURE 61.3. Diaphragmatic motion in diaphragmatic paralysis. **(A)** Paradoxical upward motion of the paralyzed right diaphragm during sudden inspiratory breathing. **(B)** Paradoxical downward motion during expiration.

position to be 81% of the predicted normal value; in the supine posture, it decreased by a further 19% in right-sided paralysis but by only 10% in left-sided paralysis. Diffusing capacity for carbon monoxide (D_{LCO}) was normal in all cases. Overall pulmonary function in the sitting position in 17 subjects with hemidiaphragmatic paralysis revealed VC, MVV, and FEV_1 to be reduced by an average of approximately 25%. Studies of regional lung function in the same body position have shown a considerable decrease in perfusion (19%), ventilation (20%), and lung volume (7%) in the diseased side compared with reference values obtained in healthy volunteers.

Ipsilateral diaphragmatic dysfunction occurs frequently in hemiplegia. As stated previously, the left hemidiaphragm is more commonly involved in left hemiplegia than is the right hemidiaphragm in right hemiplegia. FVC and FEV_1 may be decreased to 60% of normal values in these patients. Ventilatory failure becomes imminent when the VC is reduced to 25% or less of the predicted normal value. Determination of maximal inspiratory and expiratory pressures is helpful in assessing respiratory muscle strength. Serial measurements aid in recognizing respiratory muscle fatigue or recovery of muscle strength. Unilateral diaphragmatic paralysis is associated with an abnormal pattern of use of the respiratory muscles during quiet breathing, characterized by the use of intercostal and accessory inspiratory muscles or compensatory use of abdominal expiratory muscles. A detailed physiologic study in one patient with right hemidiaphragmatic paralysis has suggested that to compensate for paralysis of a hemidi-

aphragm, a new pattern of inspiratory muscle recruitment develops, involving more rapid contraction of the remaining inspiratory muscles.

Bilateral Diaphragmatic Paralysis

Bilateral diaphragmatic paralysis is not as common as unilateral paralysis. Acute bilateral paralysis can be life-threatening. Bilateral paralysis or severe weakness of the diaphragm alone does not lead to respiratory failure unless weakness of other respiratory muscles is present. The most striking clinical feature is severe orthopnea in the absence of heart and lung disease (45). The VC is reduced to 50% of the predicted normal value in upright posture, with further decrease in the supine position accompanied by orthopnea (46). Lung compliance is reduced, especially in the supine posture, perhaps because of atelectasis. Although the $Paco_2$ is usually normal in the erect position, in some cases an elevated $Paco_2$ in the supine position and during sleep has been observed. Bilateral diaphragmatic paralysis leads to chronic respiratory failure, with worsening of hypoxemia and hypercapnia during sleep.

An increased alveolar-arterial oxygen tension difference ($Pao_2 - Pao_2$) and further mismatch of ventilation-perfusion relationships occur when the supine posture is assumed. A retrospective review of 118 consecutive adult patients with a diagnosis of neuromuscular disease and diaphragmatic dysfunction found that the mean $Paco_2$ increased 28.2 $\pm$ 23.3 torr after low-flow oxygen treatment (47). The investigators concluded that in patients with

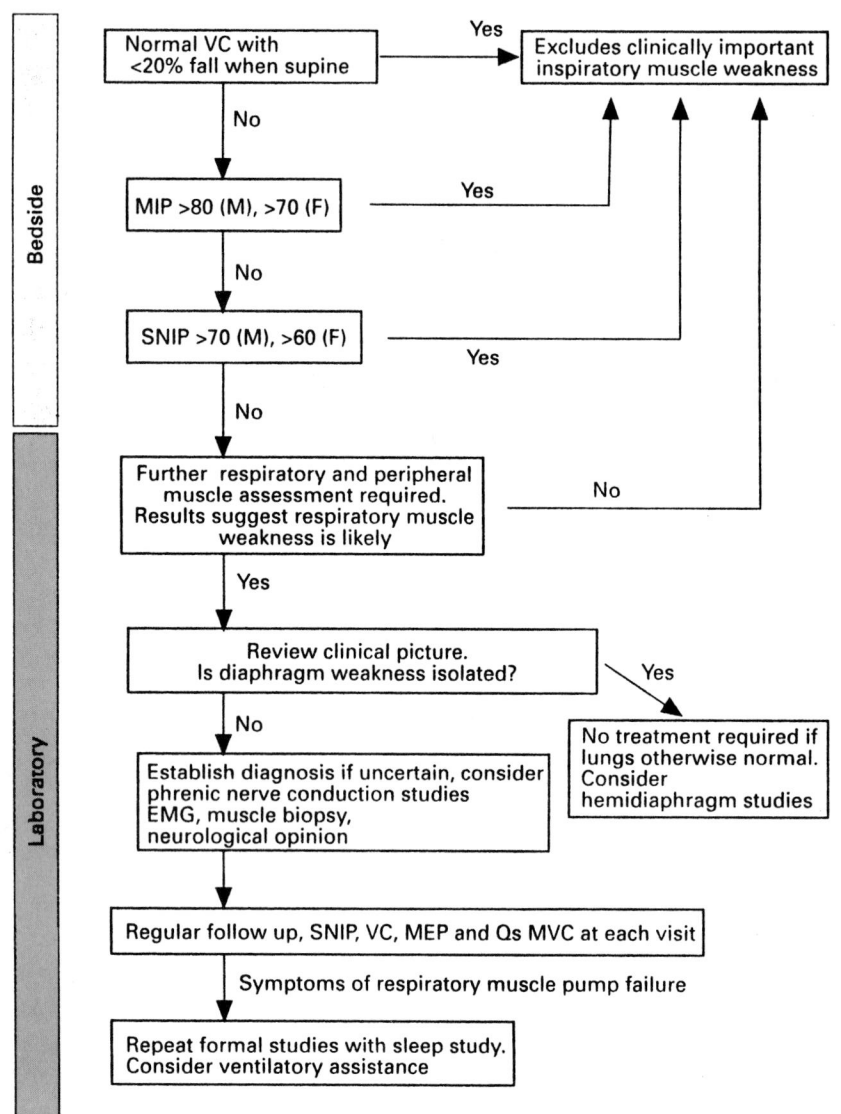

FIGURE 61.4. Algorithm for approach to assessment of respiratory muscles. An incremental approach is used for most patients. For the remainder, comprehensive specialized tests are indicated. *VC,* vital capacity; *MIP,* maximal inspiratory pressure; *MEP,* maximal expiratory pressure; *SNIP,* sniff nasal inspiratory pressure; *Qs,* quadriceps; *MVC,* maximal voluntary contraction force. (From Polkey MI, Green M, Moxham J. Measurement of respiratory muscle strength. *Thorax* 1995;50:1131–1135, with permission.)

neuromuscular disease and diaphragmatic dysfunction, even low-flow supplemental oxygen should be administered with caution. Inspiratory muscle training can improve force and endurance in patients with neuromuscular weakness (48).

Radiofrequency electrophrenic pacing has been used successfully in some patients. Nocturnal ventilatory support, nasal CPAP, and chest cuirass have been used as therapies. The increased incidence of respiratory infection may be caused by chronic atelectasis and impaired mucociliary clearance.

MYONEURAL AND MUSCULAR DISORDERS

Among these disorders are various neuromyopathies, demyelinating diseases, motor neuron diseases, and dystrophic muscle disorders. Although the etiology, pathogenesis, and nonrespiratory manifestations vary greatly in these diverse diseases, the main pulmonary problem relates to respiratory muscle weakness and chronic hypoventilation (49). In fact, respiratory failure may be the presenting symptom in many of these diseases (Table 61.2), and in their later stages, respiratory failure is common and frequently the cause of death (50).

Myasthenia Gravis

Several pulmonary complications occur in myasthenia gravis (51,52). They can be categorized as complications of the disease itself and respiratory complications associated with therapy (53) (Table 61.3). The respiratory muscles are involved in approximately 10% of patients with myasthenia

TABLE 61.2. MYOPATHIC DISEASES ASSOCIATED WITH RESPIRATORY DYSFUNCTION

Inherited muscular disorders
  Muscular dystrophy
  Duchenne muscular dystrophy
  Myotonic dystrophy
  Facioscapulohumeral muscular dystrophy
  Limb girdle dystrophy
  Oculopharyngeal dystrophy
  Congenital myopathies
  Nemaline (rod) myopathy
  Centronuclear myopathy
  Metabolic myopathies
  Acid maltase deficiency
  Mitochondrial myopathies
  Periodic paralysis

Acquired myopathies
  Inflammatory myopathies (polymyositis and dermatomyositis)
  Systemic lupus erythematosus
  Endocrine myopathies
  Hyperthyroidism
  Hypothyroidism
  Hyperadrenocorticism and corticosteroid therapy
  Acute steroid myopathy
  Electrolyte disorders
  Rhabdomyolysis

From Lynn DJ, Woda RP, Mendell JR. Respiratory dysfunction in muscular dystrophy and other myopathies. *Clin Chest Med* 1994;15:661–674, with permission.

TABLE 61.3. EFFECTS OF MYASTHENIA GRAVIS ON THE RESPIRATORY SYSTEM

Reduced global respiratory muscle strengh (reduced PImax and PEmax)
Reduced vital capacity as a result of
■ inspiratory muscle weakness, resulting in a reduction in inspiratory capacity
■ expiratory muscle weakness, resulting in a reduction in expiratory reserve volume
Fall in vital capacity of >25% in supine position with severe diaphragmatic weakness
Increased residual volume in some patients
Decreased FRC
Decreased transpulmonary pressure at FRC
Decreased maximal transdiaphragmatic pressure
Rapid shallow breathing
Blunted ventilatory response to hypercapnia

Acute changes after anticholinesterase therapy
  Improved global respiratory muscle function (increased PImax and PEmax)
  Increased FRC because of greater respiratory muscle tone
  Increased static compliance
  Increased maximal transdiaphragmatic pressure
  Minimal change in lung volumes
  Improved ventilatory response to hypercapnia

PImax, maximal inspiratory pressure; PEmax, maximal expiratory pressure; FRC, functional residual capacity.
From Zulueta JJ, Fanburg BL. Respiratory dysfunction in myasthenia gravis. *Clin Chest Med* 1994;15:683–691, with permission.

gravis; the resultant respiratory failure may require prolonged ventilatory assistance. The risk for respiratory insufficiency is increased by surgery, infectious diseases, and the administration of corticosteroids or antimicrobial drugs. Untreated myasthenic patients show decreases in VC, TLC, dynamic lung volumes, and functional residual capacity (FRC), as well as in maximal inspiratory and expiratory forces (54). Patients with myasthenia gravis may have severe respiratory muscle involvement, even when peripheral muscle weakness is mild. Repetitive surface electrode stimulation of the phrenic nerves is a useful and noninvasive method for identifying patients with myasthenia gravis in whom weakness of the diaphragm is suspected.

The patient with myasthenia gravis undergoing thymectomy presents special problems during and after anesthesia. In a study of 24 myasthenic patients who underwent thymectomy, assessment of four factors—duration of myasthenia, presence or absence of respiratory disease, pyridostigmine dosage, and VC—made it possible to predict in which patients postoperative mechanical ventilation would be needed and in which patients extubation could readily be performed. In addition, bulbar symptomatology and a prior history of respiratory failure should be considered in identifying patients who will need mechanical ventilation. Previous reports advocated tracheostomy in all instances to deal with complications in postoperative myasthenic patients. Others recommend that tracheostomy be performed if bulbar weakness is present, if the patient has a history of respiratory and myasthenic crises, or if the VC is 2 L. One study reported that repeated measurements of VC and blood gas parameters do not help to identify those in whom respiratory failure eventually develops (55). The anesthetic management of patients with myasthenia gravis is complicated by their increased sensitivity to nondepolarizing myoneural blocking drugs and resistance to depolarizing neuromuscular blocking drugs. Consequently, it is common practice to leave the endotracheal tube in place for 24 to 48 hours after surgery, and usually the patient's response to doses of anticholinesterase drugs is used as a guide to the progress of myasthenia after surgery. The major problems in myasthenic patients undergoing general anesthesia involve maintenance of adequate ventilation and provision of adequate relaxation and clearance of secretions.

Studies of the effect of administration of an anticholinesterase agent (pyridostigmine) on lung mechanics in eight patients with myasthenia gravis demonstrated impaired respiratory muscle function; the average VC increased by 14% after therapy. Pyridostigmine did not seem to modify specific airway conductance or the relationship between static lung recoil pressure and maximal expiratory flow. It did, however, markedly increase the peak expiratory flow and maximal inspiratory flow. This study suggested that the changes observed in patients were related solely to the increase in respiratory muscle force, and the major effect of the drug was an increase in the ability to inflate the lungs. Further studies using edrophonium chloride (Tensilon) have shown that this drug reduces the VC and the maximal inspiratory flows. Hence, the use of edrophonium chloride may be limited in patients with myasthenic crisis, especially those with obstructive lung disease. The increased airway resistance signals the limits of drug quantity that can be administered, especially in myasthenic patients who also have obstructive lung disease.

Plasmapheresis, immunosuppressive therapy, and thymectomy may prove effective in improving the respiratory function of some patients with myasthenia gravis (56). In a study of 22 patients who required prolonged mechanical ventilation because of respiratory failure secondary to myasthenia gravis, the most frequent cause of respiratory failure was surgery, and the most common type of procedure was thymectomy. All but one of the patients were weaned from the ventilator after 1 to 32 days of respiratory support.

Myasthenic Syndrome

Also known as *Eaton-Lambert syndrome,* myasthenic syndrome is a disorder of neuromuscular transmission in which the presence of immunoglobulin G antibodies to presynaptic calcium channels causes them to be down-regulated, thereby reducing the calcium-dependent, nerve impulse–evoked release of acetylcholine. Nearly 70% of patients with this syndrome have an underlying small-cell carcinoma of the lung (57). In approximately half of all cases of myasthenic syndrome, a tumor is not detectable. The syndrome is characterized by proximal muscle weakness, tendency to fatigue, and progressive respiratory failure.

Myotonic and Progressive Muscular Dystrophy

Myotonic dystrophy and progressive muscular dystrophy can lead to insidious, chronic respiratory failure (50). This complication develops in approximately 10% of patients with myotonic dystrophy. Myotonic patients demonstrate decreased minute ventilation, hypoxemia, hypercapnia, and pulmonary hypertension, whereas patients with nonmyotonic dystrophy exhibit a greater decrease in VC and maximal breathing capacity. FVC and MVV were decreased to 67% of predicted values and peak expiratory flow rate was reduced to 72% in 14 men with pseudohypertrophic muscular dystrophy. Pulmonary involvement in the form of respiratory muscle weakness is frequently observed in patients with limb girdle muscular dystrophy and occurs early in the disease (58). Children with nonmyotonic muscular dystrophy of the Duchenne type normally have well-preserved diaphragmatic function, but they commonly die of respiratory failure or pulmonary infection. In a nonrandomized, prospective, descriptive study of 11 patients with spinal muscular atrophy type II and 14 patients with Duchenne muscular dystrophy, the investigators observed that the seven

patients who needed mechanical ventilation were those with Duchenne muscular dystrophy who had the greatest disability and the smallest values for FVC (FVC, 30%) (59). Also, marked abnormalities in the thoracoabdominal pattern of breathing were noted in patients with spinal muscular atrophy (60). Blunted respiratory drive is occasionally seen in congenital myopathies. Chronic alveolar hypoventilation has been reported in all major forms of muscular dystrophy. Studies of lung mechanics in patients with severe respiratory muscle weakness have shown that both maximal transpulmonary pressure and static expiratory compliance are low (61). The low compliance results from either microatelectasis or a generalized alteration of alveolar elastic properties (61).

Patients with muscular dystrophies face the same problems as those with other neuromyopathic diseases—i.e., aspiration pneumonia, hypoventilation, and, in patients with dystrophic myocardial involvement, cardiomyopathy and pulmonary edema (62). The VC improves following vigorous respiratory therapy, including breathing exercises and intermittent positive-pressure therapy. A study of seven patients with mild myotonic dystrophy showed a consistently decreased hypoxic ventilatory response with a varying hypercapnic response. The high incidence of respiratory failure in such patients is most likely related to the decreased hypoxic ventilatory response, which occurs because of an underlying neurogenic deficit.

Daytime hypersomnolence is frequently reported by patients with myotonic dystrophy, and they often exhibit hypoxia during sleep (63). Obese patients with myotonic dystrophy are particularly at risk for the development of sleep apnea. These patients may demonstrate central apnea, an obstructive type of apnea, or a combination of the two (64). Detailed sleep studies in six young male patients with mild myotonic dystrophy and excessive daytime sleepiness showed evidence of sleep apnea syndrome, with high apnea indices in all. Other studies have shown no relation between hypoxic and hypercapnic ventilatory responses during wakefulness and sleep apnea indices. Both hypoxemia and hypercapnia worsen considerably during rapid-eye-movement (REM) sleep. Pulmonary and systemic arterial pressures are increased during sleep in these patients.

Ventilatory aids and mechanical respiratory assistance have been used in a domiciliary setting to support the respiratory function of such patients (65). They can have a meaningful life even though they require continuous mechanical ventilatory assistance. Spinal stabilization is one of the therapies available for patients with Duchenne muscular dystrophy. A retrospective study of 17 boys with Duchenne muscular dystrophy who underwent spinal stabilization found that the procedure did not alter the decline in pulmonary function or survival (66). On the other hand, a study of 16 patients with spinal muscular atrophy who underwent surgical spinal stabilization demonstrated not only a reversal in the decline in lung function seen preoperatively but also a significant improvement at final follow-up.

Friedreich Ataxia

Friedreich ataxia is characterized by cardiac myopathy with decreased ventricular compliance, varying degrees of hypertrophy, and, less frequently, obstruction to ventricular outflow (67). Cardiopulmonary dysfunction is a primary cause of death in patients in whom the disease develops at a young age (average, 28 years). Progression of the neuromuscular disease leads to total respiratory failure. Three mechanisms contribute to the eventually fatal outcome: (a) severe scoliosis, common in these patients, leads to respiratory failure; (b) neuromuscular dysfunction decreases the efficiency of the respiratory muscles; and (c) pulmonary edema occurs secondary to cardiomyopathy. Pulmonary function shows decreases in TLC and VC with elevation of the residual volume (RV) and FRC (68). Scoliosis itself may cause most of the respiratory difficulty in patients with Friedreich ataxia.

A follow-up and a study repeated 3 years later in a group of 15 patients with classic Friedreich ataxia showed striking decreases in RV and FRC (69). These changes could not be attributed entirely to the progression of scoliosis, as RV has been shown to be independent of the degree of scoliosis. Hence, it was concluded that the deterioration of cardiopulmonary function was multifactorial and that neuromyopathy appeared to be the main contributing factor to the deterioration in cardiopulmonary function, which is exacerbated by scoliosis and cardiomyopathy of varying degrees of severity.

Another unusual feature in these patients is the low incidence of pulmonary infections.

Steinert Myotonic Dystrophy

Steinert myotonic dystrophy is a genetically transmitted (autosomal-dominant) neuromuscular disease in which premature death is caused by cardiopulmonary complications. Both acute and chronic respiratory failure develop. Acute respiratory insufficiency is first diagnosed by the failure to generate the first postnatal breath, leading to a requirement for ventilatory support in the neonatal period. In adults with Steinert dystrophy, acute respiratory disease can be precipitated during recovery from general anesthesia. Chronic respiratory complications include pneumonia, weakness of the respiratory muscles and hypoventilation, increased work of breathing, and altered central control of respiration (70). Both the blunted chemical drive of breathing and the respiratory muscle weakness have been cited in the pathophysiology of premature death in these patients. Studies have shown that the sensitivity of chemoreceptors in the respiratory centers is well preserved; however, the output to breathing is modulated by the impaired ventilatory mechanics, which causes tachypnea even in the absence of restricted lung volume.

Demyelinating Diseases

Multiple sclerosis, a relatively common demyelinating disease in Western countries, may lead to several types of respiratory complications (71) (Table 61.4). The pulmonary

TABLE 61.4. PATTERNS OF RESPIRATORY INVOLVEMENT IN MULTIPLE SCLEROSIS

Abnormality	Anatomic Localization	Clinical Findings at Bedside
Paralysis of voluntary respiration	Bilateral corticospinal tracts, brainstem, or upper cervical cord	Inability to voluntarily increase tidal volume or hold breath; automatic respirations intact
Paralysis of automatic respiration	Dorsomedial medulla, nucleus ambiguus, and medial lemnisci	Apnea during drowsiness; normal voluntary control of respiration while awake
Diaphragmatic paralysis (unilateral or bilateral)	Upper cervical cord (C1–C4 level)	■ Paradoxical movements of chest wall and abdomen; use of accessory muscles ■ Orthopnea
Apneustic breathing	Lower brainstem	Inspiratory apneusis; voluntary control between episodes
Paroxysmal hyperventilation	Lower brainstem	Apneic pauses after hyperventilation with or without bulbar "tonic spasms"
Obstructive sleep apnea	Tegmentum of medulla	Snoring, sleep apnea with or without hiccups
Neurogenic pulmonary edema	Medulla in region of nucleus tractus solitarii and floor of fourth ventricle	Pulmonary edema without signs of heart failure

From Carter JL, Noseworthy JH. Ventilatory dysfunction in multiple sclerosis. *Clin Chest Med* 1994;15:693–703, with permission.

complications, however, tend to be mild in the majority of patients (72). In a report of the natural history of multiple sclerosis in 840 patients, it was noted that involvement of the vital centers of the central nervous system was rare and confined to patients with acute disease who died within a few months of onset. This series included three deaths caused by respiratory failure, one of which occurred within 3 months of onset.

Pulmonary function was studied in patients with clinically definite multiple sclerosis with a range of motor impairment. FVC, MVV, and maximal expiratory pressure were normal in the ambulatory patients but reduced in bedridden patients and wheelchair-bound patients with upper extremity involvement (73). In a report of four cases of respiratory failure associated with multiple sclerosis, the presence of lesions in high segmental sensory levels was emphasized (74). In these patients, respiratory failure was secondary to demyelinating lesions involving the bulbar area (especially the region of the respiratory center) and pyramidal tracts bilaterally and possibly the anterior horns. Severe involvement of the spinal cord by the demyelinating process may be complicated by respiratory failure. Hyperventilation, decreased response to carbon dioxide, irregular breathing, and sleep-induced apnea have been noted. Three cases of spontaneous pneumothorax were noted among 141 patients identified as incidence cases of spontaneous pneumothorax in an epidemiologic study (75). This occurrence was reported to be unlikely on the basis of chance alone. A statistically low incidence (less than expected) of pulmonary embolism has been noted (76). A study of 40 patients with multiple sclerosis concluded that descriptive clinical indices and clinical assessment were superior to spirometry as predictors of clinical illness; however, determination of MVV uncovered subtle respiratory muscle weakness (77).

Other Neuropathies

Charcot-Marie-Tooth disease encompasses a collection of chronic degenerative neuropathic conditions and includes cases of hereditary motor and sensory neuropathies (78). The major clinical feature is slowly progressive weakness, predominantly of the distal lower limbs. Diaphragmatic dysfunction has been described in several patients with this disease. Neuropathic changes characteristic of the disease have been observed in phrenic nerves.

Other Myopathies

Metabolic Myopathies

Acid maltase deficiency, also called *Pompe disease,* is a type II glycogen storage disease known to cause respiratory failure (79). The deficiency of the enzyme acid maltase leads to engorgement of cellular vacuoles with glycogen excess. Acid maltase deficiency can present with respiratory failure. Prox-

imal myopathy and weakness, as well as diaphragmatic dysfunction, occurs; isolated diaphragmatic paralysis also has been noted. Acid maltase deficiency classically affects infants and children, with a few sporadic cases appearing in adults.

Respiratory involvement, including ventilatory failure and diaphragmatic paralysis, has been described in various types of myopathies, including centronuclear myopathies (congenital myotubular myopathy), progressive congenital myopathy with type I fiber atrophy, Isaac syndrome (myokymia, generalized muscular stiffness, and decreased tendon reflexes), and Kearns-Sayre syndrome (also known as *oculocraniosomatic neuromuscular disease,* characterized by a combination of all or some of the following: ptosis, external ophthalmoplegia, retinal degeneration, axial muscle weakness, deafness, ataxia, pyramidal tract abnormalities, small stature, mental retardation, endocrine abnormalities, and cardiac conduction defects). Mitochondrial myopathy leading to chronic respiratory failure with the need for mechanical ventilation has been described.

The porphyrias (acute intermittent porphyria, porphyria variegata, and hereditary coproporphyria) are disorders of porphyrin metabolism. Each of these may be associated with ascending paralysis and respiratory failure. The neuropathy in these diseases probably is caused by the toxic effect of the accumulated porphyrin precursors aminolevulinic acid and porphobilinogen.

Muscular weakness and respiratory failure have been noted in rhabdomyolysis (myoglobinuria), hypophosphatemia, hypokalemia, polymyositis-dermatomyositis, and familial periodic paralysis.

Toxic Myopathies

Organic phosphate poisoning is a common occurrence in certain regions of the world where these compounds are used as agricultural insecticides. Accidental or suicidal ingestion can lead to serious respiratory problems as a result of muscarinic and nicotinic effects (80). Organic phosphates cause muscle paralysis by inhibiting acetylcholinesterase. The pulmonary features include rhinorrhea, excessive bronchial secretions, pulmonary edema, laryngospasm, bronchospasm, respiratory muscle paralysis, and paralysis of the respiratory centers. In a report of 107 subjects in Taiwan exposed to organic phosphate or carbonate, respiratory failure developed in 40%, and 51% died. The use of pralidoxime did not reduce the incidence of respiratory failure. Importantly, aggressive treatment within the first 96 hours resulted in prevention of respiratory failure.

Botulism is a disorder of the neuromuscular junctions caused by the binding of neurotoxins elaborated by the bacterium *Clostridium botulinum* (81). Botulism characteristically causes multiple cranial motor neuropathies. Clinical findings include blurred vision, paralysis of pupillary muscles, ileus, dry mouth, and descending paralysis involving extraocular and bulbar muscles, with frequent progression to respiratory muscle weakness. Muscle weakness of the upper airways may result in dysphonia and nasal regurgitation. In a study of six patients with botulism, weakness of the ventilatory muscles was noted early in the course of poisoning in all patients, but recovery was the rule, although it took several months (82). Long-term follow-up in 13 patients revealed that residual symptoms, including dyspnea and fatigue, were common at 2 years after intoxication, even though lung function had returned to normal in all (83).

Summary of Respiratory Problems in Myoneural and Muscular Disorders

The main respiratory complications in neuropathies and dystrophic muscular diseases include hypoventilation with progressive respiratory failure, restrictive pulmonary dysfunction, aspiration pneumonia, recurrent infection, and cardiopulmonary problems in patients with cardiomyopathy-associated muscular dystrophies. Pulmonary embolism also occurs with greater frequency. Depending on the severity of the underlying disease, patients may have symptoms of anxiety, lethargy, headaches, dyspnea, and occasionally a sensation of suffocation. Severe hypoventilation leads to confusion, coma, cyanosis, severe hypoxemia, hypercapnia, and death. In patients with severe, protracted, respiratory muscle weakness, marked alterations develop in the static mechanical properties of the lungs. Alveolar collapse produces low pulmonary compliance. Spirometric evaluation of lung function and assessment of respiratory muscle function by measurement of inspiratory and expiratory pressures aid in gauging the severity of respiratory involvement. A step-by-step approach to the evaluation and diagnosis of respiratory muscle weakness is important in the management of these patients (Fig. 61.4).

DISEASES OF PERIPHERAL NERVES AND ANTERIOR HORN CELLS

Poliomyelitis

Poliomyelitis is a typical example of an anterior horn cell disease that can lead to respiratory failure. Respiratory involvement from poliomyelitis may go undetected. Indeed, many patients remain in a state of chronic hypoventilation. Pulmonary function studies in patients who have recovered from poliomyelitis but who have residual muscle weakness have demonstrated that the majority experience exertional dyspnea and recurrent respiratory tract infections (84). Late onset of respiratory failure and polycythemia have been described in a significant number of patients with previous poliomyelitis (85). Respiratory failure is more common in poliomyelitis patients who have kyphoscoliosis and diaphragmatic paralysis. In a study of 55 patients with previous poliomyelitis, VC was reduced to approximately 20% to 40% of the predicted normal values and TLC was correspondingly reduced

in the majority of patients, but RV was within normal limits. The PaO_2 is usually normal despite severe reduction in VC. However, 60% of patients with a VC that is <50% of the predicted value have exhibited a PaO_2 of less than 80 mm Hg. Hypercapnia is seen at some stage in 35% of patients. The decreased VC is a consequence of diminished compliance of the chest wall and lung parenchyma.

In patients with previous poliomyelitis and severe respiratory failure, long-term ventilatory assistance is required. Four years after the epidemic of poliomyelitis in Copenhagen in 1952, in which 264 patients underwent tracheostomy and 232 were treated with positive-pressure ventilation, 24 of 138 survivors were considered to be chronically respirator-dependent. Nine of these died during the next 17 years. Among the 24 chronically respirator-dependent patients, 13 were alive in 1975 and were receiving constant ventilatory assistance.

Guillain-Barré Syndrome

Guillain-Barré syndrome (acute polyneuritis) is the most common cause of acute paralysis and neuromuscular ventilatory failure (86). Guillain-Barré syndrome is probably the most common neuromuscular cause of acute respiratory failure. It is a demyelinating disease of motor neurons, and it is manifested clinically as symmetric ascending paralysis and a lack of cellular response in the cerebrospinal fluid despite an increase in protein concentration. A typical patient is younger than 26 years or between 45 and 60 years of age. Seasonal clustering (late summer and autumn) is a feature. However, atypical clinical features may make Guillain-Barré syndrome difficult to diagnose, and therefore, a process of exclusion is necessary. Respiratory complications develop in nearly half the patients. The diaphragmatic and intercostal muscular paralysis produce progressive alveolar hypoventilation. The patient frequently is not disturbed by this weakness because of its gradual onset and slow progression. Indeed, significant respiratory muscle insufficiency can be present without being detected clinically. Paralysis of the ninth and tenth cranial nerves may lead to dysphagia, laryngeal paralysis, and aspiration. Neurogenic pulmonary edema has occurred in patients with Guillain-Barré syndrome.

The clinical course of Guillain-Barré syndrome is variable, but complete recovery can be expected in most cases. Systemic corticosteroids have been used as treatment, but because of the extremely variable course of the disease, it is difficult to evaluate their role. Treatment with plasma exchange and immune globulins has decreased the duration of mechanical ventilation by half (86). Respiratory failure requires mechanical ventilatory support in 10% to 30% of patients (86). In a series of 79 patients with acute Guillain-Barré syndrome, 27% required admittance to the respiratory intensive care unit for 14 to 105 days, and nasotracheal intubation followed by tracheostomy and mechanical ventilation were required in 18% (87). The mortality was 4%.

Repeated measurements of VC have been used as predictive parameters of the need for mechanical ventilation and weaning success. Up to 10% of patients remain seriously disabled, and approximately 5% die as a result of complications (86). Most deaths are caused by cardiopulmonary complications.

Amyotrophic Lateral Sclerosis

Amyotrophic lateral sclerosis is the most common motor neuron disease in the United States. Destruction of the anterior horn cells in the spinal cord leads to atrophy and muscle weakness. The loss of anterior horn cells is most marked in the cervical, lumbosacral, and lower thoracic spinal segments. Most patients with amyotrophic lateral sclerosis exhibit progressive neurologic deterioration without remission, with an average life expectancy of 4 years after the onset of symptoms.

Respiratory muscle involvement can be detected in most patients before respiratory symptoms begin, and respiratory failure occurs as the initial manifestation in some (88). However, patients who have respiratory symptoms, decreased FVC, and an abnormal $Pao_2/Paco_2$ ratio are more likely to exhibit increased phrenic nerve latencies or absent response than are patients with amyotrophic lateral sclerosis who have no respiratory problems (89). Irreversible hypoventilation leading to fatal respiratory failure is common in the later stages of the disease. Hypopnea during sleep as the presenting symptom has been described. Sleep and breathing were assessed in 18 patients with amyotrophic lateral sclerosis involving the bulbar muscles involvement and 10 controls (90). The patients had more arousals per hour, more stage 1 sleep, a shorter total sleep time, and mild sleep-disordered breathing with a greater apnea-hypopnea index than did the control subjects. Eight patients had sleep-disordered breathing consisting of periods of hypoventilation, predominantly during REM sleep. No obstructive sleep apnea was observed.

Among 218 patients with amyotrophic lateral sclerosis, indications of abnormal lung function were detected in 94%. Decreased MVV and FVC were the significant findings. Severe diminution of maximal inspiratory and expiratory pressures, as well as MVV, is observed in most, and the majority of patients have low lung volumes and unaltered RV volume and FRC. Some studies have found that TLC is well preserved even in an advanced stage of the disease, provided that diaphragmatic function is not grossly compromised. Obstructive pulmonary disease, although clinically not well recognized, has been noted in up to 19% of patients. Repetitive aspiration caused by bulbar incoordination perhaps is responsible.

The second major problem is aspiration pneumonia, as 25% of patients with amyotrophic lateral sclerosis have bulbar paralysis, which aggravates the problem of aspiration (Fig. 61.5). Respiratory insufficiency in patients with amy-

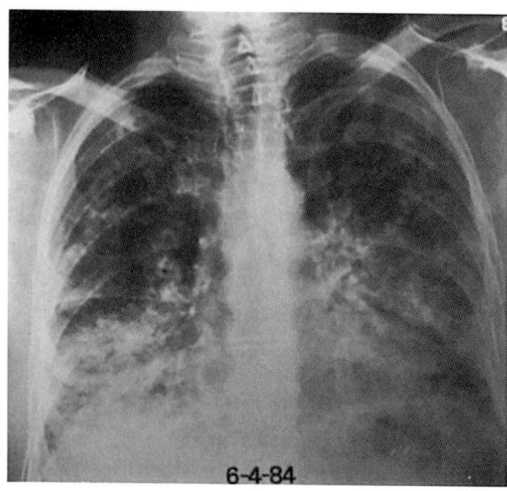

FIGURE 61.5. Recurrent episodes of aspiration pneumonia secondary to bulbar involvement in amyotrophic lateral sclerosis.

otrophic lateral sclerosis also may be a consequence of unilateral or bilateral diaphragmatic paralysis.

The prognosis in the motor neuron diseases depends on the rapidity with which the underlying disorder progresses and the degree of respiratory muscle involvement. Aggressive long-term ventilatory assistance and tracheostomy usually are not recommended because of the relentless progression of the disease (91). Selected patients, those who demonstrate slow progression of disease, are occasionally treated by using CPAP or tracheostomy with ventilator assistance. In one study of 18 patients with amyotrophic lateral sclerosis, significantly prolonged survival was demonstrated in subjects who elected to receive noninvasive mechanical ventilation: 80 days for patients who had therapy versus 19 days for patients who did not (88). Prevention of aspiration pneumonia and nonaggressive palliative therapy are the prudent goals.

DYSKINETIC DISORDERS

Extrapyramidal diseases, such as parkinsonian syndrome, may produce severe, prolonged spasm of the respiratory musculature and consequent respiratory insufficiency. Respiratory abnormalities described in extrapyramidal diseases are now believed to involve the nigrostriatal dopaminergic system. In addition, these patients have episodes of respiratory spasms or tics associated with grunting, snorting, or puffing. It is postulated that the respiratory dyskinesias are related to destruction of mesencephalic and pontine respiratory centers governing the lower bulbar regions.

Parkinson Disease

Parkinson disease is a common dyskinetic disorder, and although pulmonary involvement is frequent and considered to be the common cause of death, it rarely is recognized clinically. Pneumonia and pulmonary embolism are the two most frequent causes of overall mortality in Parkinson disease (92). Parkinson disease is associated with pathologic changes in the reticular formation of the brainstem, and hence, the afferent or efferent pathways involved in the control of respiration may be affected. More than 85% of patients have impaired ventilatory function, which is related to the severity of disease rather than to underlying lung disease. Patients with more severe disease tend to exhibit more pronounced pulmonary dysfunction. In a detailed study of 63 patients with Parkinson disease, a restrictive ventilatory defect was noted in 54 patients, all of whom had an FEV_1/FVC ratio that was more than 80% of predicted (93).

The more common pulmonary function abnormality, however, is the obstructive type. It is been postulated that the obstructive lung disease in Parkinson disease may be related to increased parasympathetic tone and infection. It is more likely that the airway abnormalities reflect involvement of the upper airway musculature.

Upper airway obstruction is relatively common in patients with Parkinson disease. Among 31 patients with Parkinson disease who underwent detailed pulmonary function testing, evidence of obstructive pulmonary function was identified in one third; lung function did not improve after therapy with levodopa (94). However, significant abatement of symptoms of Parkinson disease was noted, and hence, it was concluded that the obstructive pulmonary disease did not result from the Parkinson disease. In contrast, 10 patients in another study exhibited a significant improvement in MVV after therapy with levodopa, but no correlation was found between clinical and pulmonary functional improvement.

An abnormal flow-volume loop contour is a frequent finding in patients with Parkinson disease (Fig. 61.6). A study of the maximal inspiratory and expiratory flow-volume curves in 63 patients with different stages of Parkinson disease, of whom 59 were undergoing treatment, showed that 31 patients (49%) had abnormal flow-volume curves. Physiologic evidence of upper airway obstruction was observed in three cases. The clinical aspects and duration of disease did not influence the pattern of the curve.

Erratic breathing, also known as *chaotic breathing,* is common. The ventilatory defect is caused by rigidity and weakness of the respiratory muscles, which abate with treatment.

Levodopa is commonly used to treat Parkinson disease. In patients with neuroleptic-induced tardive dyskinesia or levodopa-induced dyskinesia, acute dyspnea and chest pain may develop secondary to severe involuntary muscle incoordination. Bromocriptine has been used in the treatment of Parkinson disease (95). In a review of 123 patients treated with bromocriptine, six had pleurisy accompanied by effusion, pleural thickening, and pulmonary infiltrates. The daily dose of bromocriptine ranged from 20 to 90 mg, and the duration of treatment ranged from 6 to 27 months. Three of the patients were also taking levodopa with benserazide, from

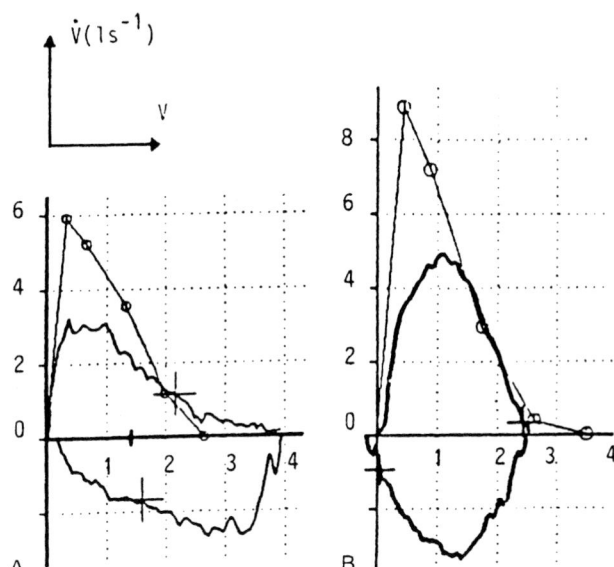

FIGURE 61.6. Flow-volume loops described in patients with Parkinson disease. **(A)** Loop exhibits "saw-toothing" of both inspiratory and expiratory limbs, believed to result from rapid changes in laryngeal and supraglottic diameter. **(B)** Loop exhibits a delay in achieving peak flow and a decrease in peak flow. (From Bogaard JM, Hovestadt A, Meerwaldt J, et al. Maximal expiratory and inspiratory flow-volume curves in Parkinson's disease. *Am Rev Respir Dis* 1989;139:610, with permission.)

400 to 800 mg/d. The pleuropulmonary complications are believed to have been caused by bromocriptine rather than by levodopa. Similar complications have been noted in a patient receiving cabergoline. Bromocriptine-induced myocardial infarction and secondary pulmonary edema should be considered in any patient using this drug, because bromocriptine is reported to cause coronary vasospasm and myocardial infarction; 24 such cases have been identified in the literature.

Respiratory Dyskinesia

The term *respiratory dyskinesia* has been used to describe extrapyramidal dysfunction with dyspnea that is not related to Parkinson disease (96). It may mimic chronic psychogenic hyperventilation syndrome, and so it has been called *pseudopsychogenic hyperventilation.* Respiratory dyskinesia is probably related to destruction of mesencephalic and pontine respiratory centers governing the lower bulbar regions. When these areas of the brainstem are affected by pathologic process, irregular respiratory movements result. In both respiratory dyskinesia and chronic hyperventilation syndrome, abnormal respiratory movements worsen with stress and disappear with sleep.

In patients with respiratory dyskinesia, speech is interrupted by involuntary sounds or grunts, snorting, and puffing; respiration is awkward; and the patient appears distressed and anxious even when pain or dyspnea is absent (97). In a report of four patients with severe involuntary respiratory dyskinesia, respiratory findings included irregular respiratory rate, shortness of breath, and discomfort in the chest. Three of these patients had neuroleptic-induced tardive dyskinesia (98), and one had levodopa-induced dyskinesia. Many of these initially were believed to have cardiopulmonary disorders. Dopaminergic manipulation was successful in correcting the subjective discomfort and respiratory abnormalities in all these patients. Reserpine was used in three patients, and the dose of levodopa was lowered in another (99).

Tardive Dyskinesia

Tardive dyskinesia is a syndrome of involuntary movement characterized by facial involvement and temporal association with ingestion of neuroleptic drugs (100). Respiratory dyskinesia may well be a part of tardive dyskinesia syndrome (101). Patients with subjective tardive dyskinesia should undergo an assessment of respiratory function. Stiff-man syndrome is reported to be associated with progressive respiratory failure.

Respiratory tardive dyskinesia (clinical evidence of irregular respiration) was observed in 2% of a large group of continuously hospitalized patients with tardive dyskinesia and psychiatric illness. The prevalence of respiratory irregularities was significantly greater in patients with an organic mental disorder (11%) than in those without. None had respiratory symptoms.

CEREBELLAR DISORDERS

Arnold-Chiari Malformation

Arnold-Chiari malformation is a congenital anomaly characterized by caudal displacement of the inferior cerebellar vermis, kinking of the medulla oblongata, a small posterior fossa, a low tentorium cerebelli, and displacement of the fourth ventricle into the spinal canal (102). Coexistence of spina bifida, hydrocephalus, and other anomalies of the neural axis is common. The most common respiratory problem is the dramatic onset of laryngeal stridor, which appears precipitously and is closely correlated with increased intracranial pressure. Three vagally mediated mechanisms have been postulated: brainstem disease, compression of the vagus nerves at the level of the foramen magnum, and traction of the vagus nerves by caudal displacement of the brainstem. Respiratory obstruction and apnea with bilateral abductor vocal cord paralysis also has been described (103,104). Depressed ventilatory response to carbon dioxide has been observed. However, physiologic studies have shown that patients with uncomplicated Arnold-Chiari malformation have normal respiratory function.

Respiratory abnormalities, such as respiratory distress, apnea, vocal cord paralysis, and inability to swallow, are known complications of Arnold-Chiari malformation. Hemorrhages in the medulla oblongata in addition to compression

or traction of the vagus and other lower cranial nerves may cause these symptoms. Respiratory problems result from impaired function of the 9th, 10th, and 12th cranial nerves. In a study of 14 children who had Arnold-Chiari malformation, vascular lesions resulting in hemorrhage, hemorrhagic necrosis, or bland infarctions in the tegmentum of the medulla oblongata were found in 12 children with clinical abnormalities of respiratory function and dysfunction of the lower cranial nerves. Surgical decompression of the posterior fossa has been shown to relieve respiratory symptoms in some cases. Respiratory problems frequently cause death or markedly shorten the life expectancy of affected children.

Joubert Syndrome

Joubert syndrome, caused by agenesis of the cerebellar vermis, is characterized by abnormal eye movements, ataxia, retardation, and episodic hyperpnea. An abnormal respiratory pattern—i.e., persistent tachypnea from birth—is the clinical hallmark of Joubert syndrome and may be detectable in utero, thus permitting prenatal diagnosis. Peak respiratory rates in excess of 200 breaths/min during wakefulness and of 150 breaths/min with tachypneic episodes lasting up to 150 seconds have been described. Apneic episodes in non-REM sleep lasting 10 to 20 seconds, with a maximal duration of 45 seconds, have been observed.

PERIPHERAL CHEMORECEPTORS

Carotid Body Resection

Respiratory hypoxic drive is controlled primarily by peripheral chemoreceptors situated in the carotid bodies. Although the carotid bodies initiate the hyperpneic response to hypoxia, they have no part in ventilatory control in normal persons at sea level, either at rest or after exercise. Therapeutic carotid body resection has been advocated for bronchial asthma, but beneficial effects have not been proved. Bilateral carotid endarterectomy may abolish compensatory hyperventilation and cause hypoxemia. Furthermore, bilateral carotid body resection may preclude compensatory ventilation when hypoxemia develops. However, it has been reported that in patients who underwent bilateral carotid body resection for asthma, the ventilatory response to increased $Paco_2$ was reduced, but hypoventilation did not occur. A patient with cough syncope has been described who was found to have carotid sinus hypersensitivity and mixed cardioinhibitory and vasodepressor responses. The cough syncope improved after denervation of the more hypersensitive carotid sinus.

Sympathectomy

Dorsal sympathectomy is performed for a wide spectrum of vascular diseases. Most patients have some shortness of breath during the first days after the operation. Pulmonary function tests in a group of 15 patients before and 1 to 3 months after upper dorsal sympathectomy showed significant decreases in all lung volumes and maximal expiratory flows. The reasons for these include a loss of diaphragmatic tone as a result of the surgical procedure, surgical transection of the scalenus anticus muscle leading to impairment of maximal inspiration and decreases in TLC and VC, and pulmonary constriction caused by sympathetic denervation.

DISORDERS OF THE AUTONOMIC NERVOUS SYSTEM

Familial Dysautonomia (Riley-Day Syndrome)

The term *dysautonomia* denotes autonomic dysfunction. Both acquired and familial dysautonomia can lead to respiratory problems. Central and obstructive sleep apnea both occur in patients with dysautonomia. Familial dysautonomia is a mendelian recessive disease associated with a relative unresponsiveness to hypoxia and hypercapnia, believed to result from a defect in the carotid body. Breath-holding attacks have been seen in 66% of 210 children with familial dysautonomia, and fleeting episodes of hyperventilation followed by profound hypoxia have been observed. Hyperventilation followed by hypoxia, attributed to incoordinated central depression consequent to reduced cerebral blood flow, has been reported in these patients. Familial dysautonomia in 13 patients was associated with abnormal sleep patterns (decreased amounts of REM sleep and increased REM latencies) in all patients; the average number of apneic spells was 73 per night.

Acquired Dysautonomia

Dysautonomia is acquired as a result of diabetic autonomic neuropathy, amyloidosis, Shy-Drager syndrome, Arnold-Chiari malformation, botulism, generalized neuropathy, neoplasms, Parkinson disease, bilateral cervical cordotomy, and bulbar poliomyelitis. A 6-year-old girl in whom sleep-induced hypoventilation and apnea with diffuse dysautonomic changes developed died 2 years later during sleep; detailed pathologic analysis revealed a ganglioneuroma originating in the sympathetic ganglia. This type of acquired progressive dysautonomia is rare. Dysautonomia can be associated with respiratory failure resulting from inability of the chemoreceptors to respond to hypoxia.

Aspiration pneumonia is a significant complication in patients with diabetic autonomic neuropathy. Studies of gastric volume and pH have shown solid, undigested food particles to be present more often in the gastric contents of diabetic patients with autonomic neuropathy than in diabetic patients without autonomic neuropathy (105).

MISCELLANEOUS NEUROLOGIC DISORDERS

Alzheimer Disease

Pulmonary complications are being recognized more frequently in patients with progressive or advanced Alzheimer disease. A prospective study of 25 patients with moderate or severe Alzheimer disease used videofluoroscopy to assess the incidence of oropharyngeal swallowing abnormalities (106). Six patients (28.6%) exhibited aspiration, and only four patients showed unequivocally normal performance. Swallowing abnormalities were associated significantly with duration of dementia, eating dependency, and abnormal oral praxis. A trend toward a higher incidence of aspiration in patients with more severe dementia was noted.

Cerebral Palsy

Patients with cerebral palsy are predisposed to respiratory infection because respiratory neuromotor control is affected. In one study of dynamic and static lung volumes in children with cerebral palsy, total capacity was significantly reduced, averaging 85% of the predicted normal values; a 50% decrease in VC was noted in subjects with dyskinesia, and a 67% decrease in patients with spasticity. The features of lung disease in these children were similar to those of chronic obstructive pulmonary disease. Breathing exercises in a study of 10 children with spastic cerebral palsy showed a mean increase in VC to 30% of pretest values, and this increase in VC nearly matched the normal predicted levels.

Migraine

Severe hyperventilation occasionally encountered in patients with migraine has led to diagnostic difficulties. In the reported cases, hyperventilation occurred at the peak of the migraine, making the attack seem worse to the patient. It is speculated that in these cases the migraine was exacerbated by the vasoconstrictor effect of hyperventilation. The term *pulmonary migraine* was suggested to describe a localized atelectasis of the lung associated with migraine headaches in a 14-year-old girl. Neuropathologic findings included deep areas of microinfarction in the basal ganglia and a remarkable sparing of brainstem nuclei associated with respiratory function.

Dystonia

Dystonia is a rare disorder characterized by involuntary sustained muscle contractions that frequently cause twisting and repetitive movements or abnormal postures. The disorder can be primary or secondary and may affect any muscle.

A combination of upper airway and diaphragmatic dysfunction has been described in these patients. The results of a study of 26 patients with dystonia indicated that dyspnea in dystonia appeared to be caused by excessive and/or desynchronized contractions of the upper airways and/or diaphragm, with usually normal gas exchange (107).

Reye Syndrome

Reye syndrome is characterized by encephalopathy and fatty accumulation in visceral organs, especially in children. Excessive lipolysis and mobilization of fat occur in this disorder, which has been shown to be associated with hypoxemia, hypocapnia, and tachypnea, as well as interstitial pneumonitis, thickening of the alveolar walls, and the presence of intraalveolar foamy histiocytes.

Krabbe Globoid Cell Leukodystrophy

Krabbe globoid cell leukodystrophy is a hereditary degenerative brain disease caused by lack of the enzyme galactosylceramide galactosidase. The disease is characterized by the progressive development of retardation, failure to thrive, seizures, spasticity, and blindness, culminating in death by the age of 2 to 3 years. Symptoms begin at 4 to 8 months of age. In an 8-week-old boy who presented with rapidly progressive respiratory failure and died shortly thereafter, lung biopsy revealed numerous intra-alveolar and a few interstitial macrophages containing intracellular structures that stained positively with periodic acid-Schiff (108).

Pulmonary Effects of Electroconvulsive Therapy

Electroconvulsive therapy is used in the treatment of major depressive disorders, schizophrenia, mania, and other conditions. Aspiration may occur, especially in elderly patients (109). Neurogenic pulmonary edema after electroconvulsive therapy has been observed in these patients (110).

Pulmonary Effects of Ventriculoatrial Shunt

Ventriculoatrial and ventriculoperitoneal shunts are placed to treat high-pressure hydrocephalus. The catheter tips occasionally become blocked or infected. Recurrent discharge of the proteinaceous debris from the catheter tip into the pulmonary circulation can produce recurrent embolic phenomena and secondary pulmonary hypertension. The onset of pulmonary hypertension in these patients is insidious and invariably leads to right ventricular failure. Empyema has been described as a complication of ventriculoperitoneal shunt.

Pulmonary Embolism in Neurologic Diseases

Pulmonary embolism is a common occurrence in patients with neurologic disorders and in those who undergo neu-

rosurgery (111). A major etiologic factor is venous thromboembolism, especially in the lower extremities, as a result of stasis caused by significant immobilization. The risk for venous thromboembolism and pulmonary embolism is higher in patients with head trauma, stroke, spinal cord injury, brain tumor, and subarachnoid hemorrhage and in patients who have undergone neurosurgical operations (112). In one study, spinal cord injury accounted for 31% of all pulmonary embolisms in the total trauma population of 2,525 patients (113). Subacute or chronic neurologic disorders also are associated with a higher risk for pulmonary embolism. For instance, a review of the results of 60 complete autopsies performed in patients with parkinsonian syndrome revealed that pulmonary embolism was second only to pneumonia as the most common cause of overall mortality.

Anticoagulant therapy in patients with intracranial diseases is fraught with the risk of causing or aggravating hemorrhage in the brain or other areas within the cranium. Excessive anticoagulation has resulted in fatal intracerebral hemorrhage in patients with brain tumors. The risk for pulmonary embolism, however, exceeds the risk for severe or fatal bleeding from prophylactic or therapeutic anticoagulation. Studies have noted that prophylactic insertion of a filter in the inferior vena cava is effective in preventing pulmonary emboli in these patients.

REFERENCES

1. Chalela JA, Kasner SE. Cardiac and respiratory complications of stroke. In: Rose BD, ed. *UpToDate*. Wellesley, MA: UpToDate, 2002.
1a. Miller JD, Sweet RC, Narayan R, et al. Early insults to the injured brain. *JAMA* 1978;240:439–442.
2. Lee MC, Klassen AC, Resch JA. Respiratory pattern disturbances in ischemic cerebral vascular disease. *Stroke* 1974;5:612–616.
3. Lee MC, Klassen AC, Heaney LM, et al. Respiratory rate and pattern disturbances in acute brain stem infarction. *Stroke* 1976;7:382–385.
4. Hanly PJ, Zuberi-Khokhar NS. Increased mortality associated with Cheyne-Stokes respiration in patients with congestive heart failure. *Am J Respir Crit Care Med* 1996;153:272–276.
5. North JB, Jennett S. Abnormal breathing patterns associated with acute brain damage. *Arch Neurol* 1974;31:338–344.
6. Rodriguez M, Baele PL, Marsh HM, et al. Central neurogenic hyperventilation in an awake patient with brainstem astrocytoma. *Ann Neurol* 1982;11:625–628.
7. Rout MW, Lane DJ, Wollner L. Prognosis in acute cerebrovascular accidents in relation to respiratory pattern and blood gas tensions. *Br Med J* 1971;3:7–9.
8. Gozal D, Marcus CL, Shoseyov D, et al. Peripheral chemoreceptor function in children with the congenital central hypoventilation syndrome. *J Appl Physiol* 1993;74:379–387.
9. Colice GL, Matthay MA, Bass E, et al. Neurogenic pulmonary edema. *Am Rev Respir Dis* 1984;130:941–948.
10. Simon RP. Neurogenic pulmonary edema. *Neurol Clin* 1993;11:309–323.

11. Drislane FW, Mandel J. Neurogenic pulmonary edema. In: Rose BD, ed. *UpToDate*. Wellesley, MA: UpToDate, 2002.

12. Simmons RL, Martin AM Jr, Heisterkamp CA 3rd, et al. Respiratory insufficiency in combat casualties, II: pulmonary edema following head injury. *Ann Surg* 1969;170:39–44.

13. Simmons RL, Heisterkamp CA 3rd, Collins JA, et al. Acute pulmonary edema in battle casualties. *J Trauma* 1969;9:760–775.

14. Mayer SA, Fink ME, Homma S, et al. Cardiac injury associated with neurogenic pulmonary edema following subarachnoid hemorrhage. *Neurology* 1994;44:815–820.

15. Rogers FB, Shackford SR, Trevisani GT, et al. Neurogenic pulmonary edema in fatal and nonfatal head injuries. *J Trauma* 1995;39:860–866.

16. Weir BK. Pulmonary edema following fatal aneurysm rupture. *J Neurosurg* 1978;49:502–507.

17. Hemmer M. Ventilatory support for pulmonary failure of the head trauma patient. *Bull Eur Physiopathol Respir* 1985;21:287–293.

18. Johnson ER, McKenzie SW, Sievers A. Aspiration pneumonia in stroke. *Arch Phys Med Rehabil* 1993;74:973–976.

19. Kidd D, Lawson J, Nesbitt R, et al. Aspiration in acute stroke: a clinical study with videofluoroscopy. *Q J Med* 1993;86:825–829.

20. Kidd D, Lawson J, Nesbitt R, et al. The natural history and clinical consequences of aspiration in acute stroke. *QJM* 1995;88:409–413.

21. Woratyla SP, Morgan AS, Mackay L, et al. Factors associated with early onset pneumonia in the severely brain-injured patient. *Conn Med* 1995;59:643–647.

22. Teasell RW, McRae M, Marchuk Y, et al. Pneumonia associated with aspiration following stroke. *Arch Phys Med Rehabil* 1996;77:707–709.

23. Holas MA, DePippo KL, Reding MJ. Aspiration and relative risk of medical complications following stroke. *Arch Neurol* 1994;51:1051–1053.

24. Horner J, Brazer SR, Massey EW. Aspiration in bilateral stroke patients: a validation study. *Neurology* 1993;43:430–433.

25. Karaaslan T, Meuli R, Androux R, et al. Traumatic chest lesions in patients with severe head trauma: a comparative study with computed tomography and conventional chest roentgenograms. *J Trauma* 1995;39:1081–1086.

26. Stephenson JB. Reflex anoxic seizures ("white breath-holding"): nonepileptic vagal attacks. *Arch Dis Child* 1978;53:193–200.

27. Lieberman SL, Brown R. Pulmonary physiologic changes following spinal cord injury. In: Rose BD, ed. *UpToDate*. Wellesley, MA: UpToDate, 2002.

28. Roth EJ, Nussbaum SB, Berkowitz M, et al. Pulmonary function testing in spinal cord injury: correlation with vital capacity. *Paraplegia* 1995;33:454–457.

29. Anke A, Aksnes AK, Stanghelle JK, et al. Lung volumes in tetraplegic patients according to cervical spinal cord injury level. *Scand J Rehabil Med* 1993;25:73–77.

30. Estenne M, Van Muylem A, Gorini M, et al. Evidence of dynamic airway compression during cough in tetraplegic patients. *Am J Respir Crit Care Med* 1994;150:1081–1085.

31. Harvey LA, Ellis ER. The effect of continuous positive airway pressures on lung volumes in tetraplegic patients. *Paraplegia* 1996;34:54–58.

32. Spungen AM, Dicpinigaitis PV, Almenoff PL, et al. Pulmonary obstruction in individuals with cervical spinal cord lesions unmasked by bronchodilator administration. *Paraplegia* 1993;31:404–407.

33. Dicpinigaitis PV, Spungen AM, Bauman WA, et al. Bronchial hyperresponsiveness after cervical spinal cord injury. *Chest* 1994;105:1073–1076.

34. Almenoff PL, Alexander LR, Spungen AM, et al. Bronchodilatory effects of ipratropium bromide in patients with tetraplegia. *Paraplegia* 1995;33:274–277.

35. Grimm DR, Chandy D, Almenoff PL, et al. Airway hyperreactivity in subjects with tetraplegia is associated with reduced baseline airway caliber. *Chest* 2000;118:1397–1404.

36. Celli BR. Causes and diagnosis of bilateral and unilateral diaphragmatic paralysis. In: Rose BD, ed. *UpToDate*. Wellesley, MA: UpToDate, 2002.

37. DeVita MA, Robinson LR, Rehder J, et al. Incidence and natural history of phrenic neuropathy occurring during open heart surgery. *Chest* 1993;103:850–856.

38. McAlister VC, Grant DR, Roy A, et al. Right phrenic nerve injury in orthotopic liver transplantation. *Transplantation* 1993;55:826–830.

39. Piehler JM, Pairolero PC, Gracey DR, et al. Unexplained diaphragmatic paralysis: a harbinger of malignant disease? *J Thorac Cardiovasc Surg* 1982;84:861–864.

40. Mazzoni M, Solinas C, Sisillo E, et al. Intraoperative phrenic nerve monitoring in cardiac surgery. *Chest* 1996;109:1455–1460.

41. Laub GW, Muralidharan S, Chen C, et al. Phrenic nerve injury: a prospective study. *Chest* 1991;100:376–379.

42. Mulvey DA, Aquilina RJ, Elliott MW, et al. Diaphragmatic dysfunction in neuralgic amyotrophy: an electrophysiologic evaluation of 16 patients presenting with dyspnea. *Am Rev Respir Dis* 1993;147:66–71.

43. Alexander C. Diaphragm movements and the diagnosis of diaphragmatic paralysis. *Clin Radiol* 1966;17:79–83.

44. Polkey MI, Green M, Moxham J. Measurement of respiratory muscle strength. *Thorax* 1995;50:1131–1135.

45. Sandham JD, Shaw DT, Guenter CA. Acute supine respiratory failure due to bilateral diaphragmatic paralysis. *Chest* 1977;72:96–98.

46. Mier-Jedrzejowicz A, Brophy C, Moxham J, et al. Assessment of diaphragm weakness. *Am Rev Respir Dis* 1988;137:877–883.

47. Gay PC, Edmonds LC. Severe hypercapnia after low-flow oxygen therapy in patients with neuromuscular disease and diaphragmatic dysfunction. *Mayo Clin Proc* 1995;70:327–330.

48. McCool FD, Tzelepis GE. Inspiratory muscle training in the patient with neuromuscular disease. *Phys Ther* 1995;75:1006–1014.

49. Garcia-Pachon E, Marti J, Mayos M, et al. Clinical significance of upper airway dysfunction in motor neurone disease. *Thorax* 1994;49:896–900.

50. Lynn DJ, Woda RP, Mendell JR. Respiratory dysfunction in muscular dystrophy and other myopathies. *Clin Chest Med* 1994;15:661–674.

51. Drachman DB. Myasthenia gravis. *N Engl J Med* 1994;330:1797–1810.

52. DeLisser HM. Respiratory considerations in myasthenia gravis. In: Rose BD, ed. *UpToDate*. Wellesley, MA: UpToDate, 2002.

53. Zulueta JJ, Fanburg BL. Respiratory dysfunction in myasthenia gravis. *Clin Chest Med* 1994;15:683–691.

54. Garcia Rio F, Prados C, Diez Tejedor E, et al. Breathing pattern and central ventilatory drive in mild and moderate generalised myasthenia gravis. *Thorax* 1994;49:703–706.

55. Rieder P, Louis M, Jolliet P, et al. The repeated measurement of vital capacity is a poor predictor of the need for mechanical ventilation in myasthenia gravis. *Intensive Care Med* 1995;21:663–668.

56. Walter Allan W. Treatment of myasthenia gravis. In: Rose BD, ed. *UpToDate*. Wellesley, MA: UpToDate, 2002.

57. Chartrand-Lefebvre C, Howarth N, Grenier P, et al. Association of small cell lung cancer and the anti-Hu paraneoplastic syndrome: radiographic and CT findings. *AJR Am J Roentgenol* 1998;170:1513–1517.

58. Stubgen JP, Ras GJ, Schultz CM, et al. Lung and respiratory muscle function in limb girdle muscular dystrophy. *Thorax* 1994;49:61–65.

59. Lyager S, Steffensen B, Juhl B. Indicators of need for mechanical ventilation in Duchenne muscular dystrophy and spinal muscular atrophy. *Chest* 1995;108:779–785.

60. Perez A, Mulot R, Vardon G, et al. Thoracoabdominal pattern of breathing in neuromuscular disorders. *Chest* 1996;110:454–461.

61. Estenne M, Gevenois PA, Kinnear W, et al. Lung volume restriction in patients with chronic respiratory muscle weakness: the role of microatelectasis. *Thorax* 1993;48:698–701.

62. Darras BT. Duchenne and Becker muscular dystrophies. In: Rose BD, ed. *UpToDate*. Wellesley, MA: UpToDate, 2002.

63. Finnimore AJ, Jackson RV, Morton A, et al. Sleep hypoxia in myotonic dystrophy and its correlation with awake respiratory function. *Thorax* 1994;49:66–70.

64. Khan Y, Heckmatt JZ. Obstructive apnoeas in Duchenne muscular dystrophy. *Thorax* 1994;49:157–161.

65. Fukunaga H, Okubo R, Moritoyo T, et al. Long-term follow-up of patients with Duchenne muscular dystrophy receiving ventilatory support. *Muscle Nerve* 1993;16:554–558.

66. Kennedy JD, Staples AJ, Brook PD, et al. Effect of spinal surgery on lung function in Duchenne muscular dystrophy. *Thorax* 1995;50:1173–1178.

67. Durr A, Cossee M, Agid Y, et al. Clinical and genetic abnormalities in patients with Friedreich's ataxia. *N Engl J Med* 1996;335:1169–1175.

68. Bureau MA, Ngassam P, Lemieux B, et al. Pulmonary function studies in Friedreich's ataxia. *Can J Neurol Sci* 1976;3:343–347.

69. Cote M, Bureau M, Leger C, et al. Evolution of cardiopulmonary involvement in Friedreich's ataxia. *Can J Neurol Sci* 1979;6:151–157.

70. Pradella M, Sunseri M, Ferriere G. Effects of body position on sleep related disordered breathing in a patient with Steinert's disease. *Arq Neuropsiquiatr* 1993;51:529–531.

71. Carter JL, Noseworthy JH. Ventilatory dysfunction in multiple sclerosis. *Clin Chest Med* 1994;15:693–703.

72. Buyse B, Demedts M, Meekers J, et al. Respiratory dysfunction in multiple sclerosis: a prospective analysis of 60 patients. *Eur Respir J* 1997;10:139–145.

73. Smeltzer SC, Utell MJ, Rudick RA, et al. Pulmonary function and dysfunction in multiple sclerosis. *Arch Neurol* 1988;45:1245–1249.

74. Yamamoto T, Imai T, Yamasaki M. Acute ventilatory failure in multiple sclerosis. *J Neurol Sci* 1989;89:313–324.

75. Melton LJ 3rd, Bartleson JD. Spontaneous pneumothorax and multiple sclerosis. *Ann Neurol* 1980;7:492.

76. Kaufman J, Khatri BO, Riendl P. Are patients with multiple sclerosis protected from thrombophlebitis and pulmonary embolism? *Chest* 1988;94:998–1001.

77. Smeltzer SC, Skurnick JH, Troiano R, et al. Respiratory function in multiple sclerosis. Utility of clinical assessment of respiratory muscle function. *Chest* 1992;101:479–484.

78. Cruse RP. Hereditary primary motor sensory neuropathies, including Charcot-Marie-Tooth disease. In: Rose BD, ed. *UpToDate*. Wellesley, MA: UpToDate, 2002.

79. Darras BT. Metabolic myopathies: Nonlysosomal and lysosomal glycogenoses. In: Rose BD, ed. *UpToDate*. Wellesley, MA: UpToDate, 2002.

80. Zwiener RJ, Ginsburg CM. Organophosphate and carbamate poisoning in infants and children. *Pediatrics* 1988;81:121–126.

81. Pegram PS, Stone SM. Botulism. In: Rose BD, ed. *UpToDate*. Wellesley, MA: UpToDate, 2002.

82. Wilcox PG, Morrison NJ, Pardy RL. Recovery of the ventilatory and upper airway muscles and exercise performance after type A botulism. *Chest* 1990;98:620–626.

83. Wilcox P, Andolfatto G, Fairbarn MS, et al. Long-term follow-up of symptoms, pulmonary function, respiratory muscle strength, and exercise performance after botulism. *Am Rev Respir Dis* 1989;139:157–163.

84. Midgren B. Lung function and clinical outcome in postpolio patients: a prospective cohort study during 11 years. *Eur Respir J* 1997;10:146–149.

85. Stanghelle JK, Festvag L, Aksnes AK. Pulmonary function and symptom-limited exercise stress testing in subjects with late sequelae of poliomyelitis. *Scand J Rehabil Med* 1993;25:125–129.

86. Teitelbaum JS, Borel CO. Respiratory dysfunction in Guillain-Barré syndrome. *Clin Chest Med* 1994;15:705–714.

87. Gracey DR, McMichan JC, Divertie MB, et al. Respiratory failure in Guillain-Barré syndrome: a 6-year experience. *Mayo Clin Proc* 1982;57:742–746.

88. Sherman MS, Paz HL. Review of respiratory care of the patient with amyotrophic lateral sclerosis. *Respiration* 1994;61:61–67.

89. Evangelista T, Carvalho M, Pinto A, et al. Phrenic nerve conduction in amyotrophic lateral sclerosis. *J Neurol Sci* 1995;129[Suppl]:35–37.

90. Ferguson KA, Strong MJ, Ahmad D, et al. Sleep-disordered breathing in amyotrophic lateral sclerosis. *Chest* 1996;110:664–669.

91. Kaplan LM, Hollander D. Respiratory dysfunction in amyotrophic lateral sclerosis. *Clin Chest Med* 1994;15:675–681.

92. Mosewich RK, Rajput AH, Shuaib A, et al. Pulmonary embolism: an under-recognized yet frequent cause of death in parkinsonism. *Mov Disord* 1994;9:350–352.

93. Izquierdo-Alonso JL, Jimenez-Jimenez FJ, Cabrera-Valdivia F, et al. Airway dysfunction in patients with Parkinson's disease. *Lung* 1994;172:47–55.

94. Langer H, Woolf CR. Changes in pulmonary function in Parkinson's syndrome after treatment with L-DOPA. *Am Rev Respir Dis* 1971;104:440–442.

95. Todman DH, Oliver WA, Edwards RL. Pleuropulmonary fibrosis due to bromocriptine treatment for Parkinson's disease. *Clin Exp Neurol* 1990;27:79–82.

96. Hayashi T, Nishikawa T, Koga I, et al. Prevalence of and risk factors for respiratory dyskinesia. *Clin Neuropharmacol* 1996;19:390–398.

97. Yassa R, Lal S. Respiratory irregularity and tardive dyskinesia: a prevalence study. *Acta Psychiatr Scand* 1986;73:506–510.

98. Kruk J, Sachdev P, Singh S. Neuroleptic-induced respiratory dyskinesia. *J Neuropsychiatry Clin Neurosci* 1995;7:223–239.

99. Ivanovich M, Glantz R, Bone RC, et al. Respiratory dyskinesia presenting as acute respiratory distress. *Chest* 1993;103:314–316.

100. Wilcox PG, Bassett A, Jones B, et al. Respiratory dysrhythmias in patients with tardive dyskinesia. *Chest* 1994;105:203–207.

101. Rich MW, Radwany SM. Respiratory dyskinesia: an underrecognized phenomenon. *Chest* 1994;105:1826–1832.

102. Omer S, al-Kawi MZ, Bohlega S, et al. Respiratory arrest: a complication of Arnold-Chiari malformation in adults. *Eur Neurol* 1996;36:36–38.

103. Doherty MJ, Spence DP, Young C, et al. Obstructive sleep apnoea with Arnold-Chiari malformation. *Thorax* 1995; 50:690–691.

104. Choi SS, Tran LP, Zalzal GH. Airway abnormalities in patients with Arnold-Chiari malformation. *Otolaryngol Head Neck Surg* 1999;121:720–724.

105. Ishihara H, Singh H, Giesecke AH. Relationship between diabetic autonomic neuropathy and gastric contents. *Anesth Analg* 1994;78:943–947.

106. Horner J, Alberts MJ, Dawson DV, et al. Swallowing in Alzheimer's disease. *Alzheimer Dis Assoc Disord* 1994;8:177–189.

107. Braun N, Abd A, Baer J, et al. Dyspnea in dystonia: a functional evaluation. *Chest* 1995;107:1309–1316.

108. Clarke JT, Ozere RL, Krause VW. Early infantile variant of Krabbe globoid cell leucodystrophy with lung involvement. *Arch Dis Child* 1981;56:640–642.

109. Zibrak JD, Jensen WA, Bloomingdale K. Aspiration pneumonitis following electroconvulsive therapy in patients with gastroparesis. *Biol Psychiatry* 1988;24:812–814.

110. Tsutsumi N, Tohdoh Y, Kawana S, et al. A case of pulmonary edema after electroconvulsive therapy under propofol anesthesia. *Masui* 2001;50:525–527.

111. Hamilton MG, Hull RD, Pineo GF. Venous thromboembolism in neurosurgery and neurology patients: a review. *Neurosurgery* 1994;34:280–296.

112. Quevedo JF, Buckner JC, Schmidt JL, et al. Thromboembolism in patients with high-grade glioma. *Mayo Clin Proc* 1994;69:329–332.

113. Wilson JT, Rogers FB, Wald SL, et al. Prophylactic vena cava filter insertion in patients with traumatic spinal cord injury: preliminary results. *Neurosurgery* 1994;35:234–239.

114. Theodore J, Robin ED. Speculations on neurogenic pulmonary edema (NPE). *Am Rev Respir Dis* 1976;113:405–411.

62 Skeletal Diseases

Udaya B. S. Prakash · Talmadge E. King, Jr.

The skeletal thorax is as much a part of the respiratory system as are the lungs, and hence, it plays a major role in normal pulmonary function. Instability of the chest wall can lead to respiratory failure, as exemplified by ventilatory failure in patients with flail chest (1). Congenital and acquired defects and diseases of the thoracic cage may interfere with normal respiratory mechanics. Occasionally, diseases of the extrathoracic skeleton may be associated with lung problems. An excellent example of this is the pulmonary parenchymal process that occurs in patients with ankylosing spondylitis. In this chapter, some common and uncommon skeletal diseases in which the respiratory system is involved are discussed. Certain disease entities, such as Marfan syndrome, that are not primary skeletal diseases are nonetheless covered here, because skeletal abnormalities are clinically evident in such patients. The major spinal deformities are scoliosis, kyphosis, pectus excavatum, pectus carinatum, and straight-back syndrome. Discussions of respiratory complications in ankylosing spondylitis and several other skeletal disorders are also included.

KYPHOSCOLIOSIS

Scoliosis is deformity of the spine characterized by marked lateral curvature, kyphosis is the abnormally accentuated posterior curvature of the spine, and kyphoscoliosis is the combination of the two, which results in a lateral bending and rotation of the vertebral column. Pulmonary problems occur in both scoliosis and kyphoscoliosis (2) (Fig. 62.1).

U. B. S. Prakash: Pulmonary and Critical Care Medicine, Mayo Medical School and Mayo Medical Center, Rochester, Minnesota.

T. E. King, Jr.: Department of Medicine, University of California, San Francisco; and Medical Services, San Francisco General Hospital, San Francisco, California.

Scoliosis is by far the most common spinal deformity. An incidence of four of 1,000 population was found by a roentgenographic survey. Scoliosis is classified etiologically into five varieties: idiopathic, congenital, neuropathic (poliomyelitis, cerebral palsy, and syringomyelia), myopathic (muscular dystrophy, amyotonia, and Friedreich ataxia), and traumatic. Scoliosis also is seen in mesenchymal disorders and in association with neurofibromatosis. In practice, 80% of cases of scoliosis are idiopathic (1). Among infants, the male-to-female ratio is 6:4, but among cases that begin in adolescence—the largest group—the ratio is 1:9; overall, it is 2:8. Infantile scoliosis is reported usually to involve a curvature toward the left, whereas scoliosis in adolescent girls is usually toward the right. A familial basis for idiopathic scoliosis exists. Among first-, second-, and third-degree relatives of children with idiopathic scoliosis, abnormal spinal curvature occurs 20 times as often as in a comparable group of the general population. In congenital scoliosis of early onset, there is failure of alveolar multiplication, whereas in idiopathic scoliosis, the alveoli do not enlarge normally.

Idiopathic scoliosis in adolescent girls usually involves seven to 10 vertebrae. The curvature or angulation of a scoliotic spine is best measured by the Cobb method (Fig. 62.2). Pulmonary symptoms are not seen until the curvature exceeds 70 degrees. Adolescent idiopathic thoracic curves of 60 to 80 degrees have been observed to increase by an average of 30 degrees during a period of 25 years after completion of growth. The Cobb angle has been traditionally used in the clinical assessment and correlation of spinal deformity and pulmonary function tests. However, a study of 70 adolescents (mean age, 13.8 years) with idiopathic right thoracic scoliosis found that the mean values for the Cobb angle, vertebral rotational flexibility, kyphosis, and rib-vertebral angle asymmetry (in radiographs of standing and supine bending positions) differed significantly between patients with more than 80% of predicted vital capacity (VC) and those

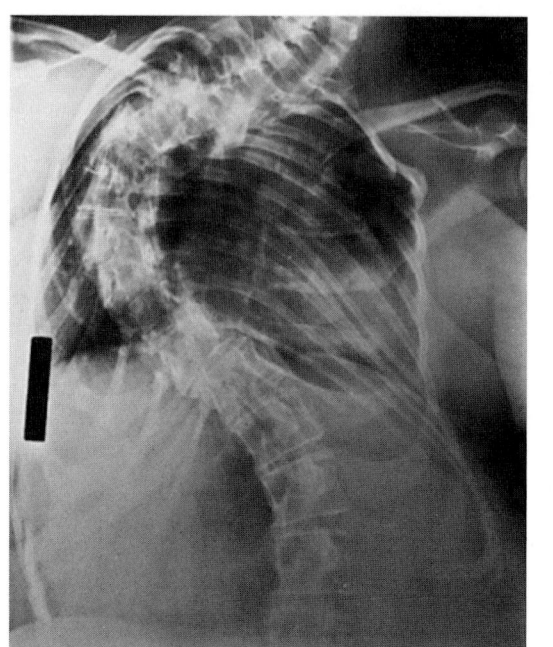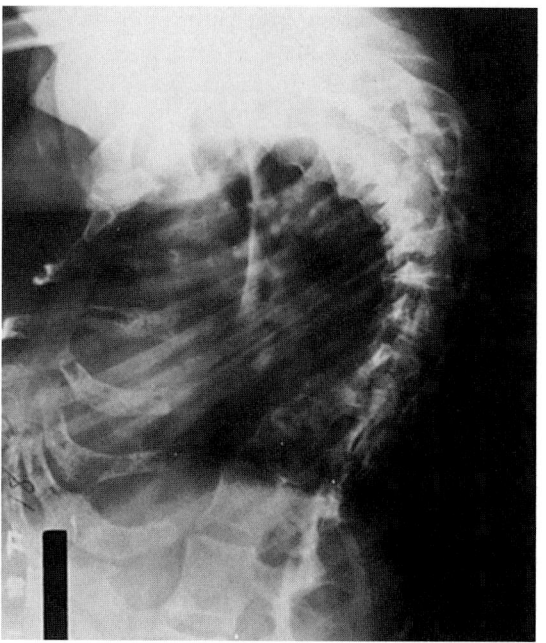

FIGURE 62.1. Severe thoracic kyphoscoliosis. **(A)** Posteroanterior view. **(B)** Left lateral view.

whose VC was 60% of predicted values (3). Roentgenologic features indicative of better pulmonary function included rotational flexibility exceeding 55%, rib-vertebral angle asymmetry (standing) of less than 25 degrees, and kyphosis of 15 degrees. The two parameters of deformity, vertebral rotational flexibility and rib-vertebral angle asymmetry, provided a better prediction of respiratory function than does the commonly used Cobb angle.

The scoliotic angle is an important predictor of respiratory failure. In a long-term study of 24 patients with unfused scoliosis, pulmonary function tests were performed 20 years apart, and respiratory failure occurred only in patients who had a VC of 45% of the predicted value during the initial testing and an angle of 110 degrees; the initial VC was the strongest predictor of the development of respiratory failure, followed by scoliotic angle. In a study of 29 patients with adolescent idiopathic thoracic scoliosis of 60 degrees, maximal inspiratory pressure was found to be reduced, but maximal expiratory pressure was normal. The low maximal inspiratory pressure was attributed to the mechanical disadvantage resulting from the chest deformity.

Abnormalities of Pulmonary Function

The most common abnormality of pulmonary function is a reduction in static lung volumes, including VC and total lung capacity (TLC). An inverse relationship exists between the angle of scoliotic curvature and the values (as a percentage of predicted values) for VC, TLC, functional residual capacity, residual volume, and static compliance of the total respiratory system. The ventilatory function may be impaired even in mild forms of scoliosis. The force developed by the respiratory muscles is a more important determinant of ventilatory defect than is the degree of spinal curvature. The decreased lung compliance is most pronounced in scoliotic patients with muscle weakness. In kyphoscoliosis, prediction of lung volume from body height results in significant

FIGURE 62.2. The Cobb angle is determined by lines drawn perpendicularly to the tangents from the end plates of the most tilted superior and inferior vertebrae.

underestimation, but arm span serves satisfactorily for this purpose. A method has evolved by which the theoretic height of these patients is predicted from the angle of scoliosis, length of spine, and actual height.

Even though restrictive lung dysfunction is typical in patients with severe scoliosis, obstructive airway disease and positive bronchodilator response are present. Extensive pulmonary function testing in 44 children (36 girls, 8 boys) between the ages of 10 and 18 years with idiopathic scoliosis before surgical correction showed significant restrictive defect in 41% of subjects, whereas air flow obstruction was noted in 7% of subjects (4). However, the ratio of total gas volume (by plethysmography) to functional residual capacity (by helium dilution) demonstrated moderate or severe gas trapping in 20 subjects (46%). Bronchodilator administration resulted in significant improvement in airway mechanics. Other studies of pulmonary function studies in children with idiopathic scoliosis have shown diminished VC, 1-second forced expiratory volume (FEV_1), gas transfer, and maximal static expiratory airways pressure, but no significant diminution in TLC or maximal inspiratory pressure.

The characteristic deformity seen in scoliosis causes one hemithorax to become smaller than the other (5). This inherent mechanical inefficiency of ventilation is the major factor in causing respiratory embarrassment. However, the impairment of exercise performance found in adults with moderate scoliosis cannot be attributed to any important ventilatory limitation, abnormality in lung volume, or impaired chemoreceptor sensitivity (5,6). Kesten and coworkers suggest that the reduced maximum oxygen consumption (Vo_2max) likely arises from deconditioning and lack of regular aerobic exercise (5). Patients with moderate to severe kyphoscoliosis have significant oxygen desaturation during exercise and should thus routinely be tested by oximetry during exercise for assessment of ambulatory oxygen therapy. Although hypoxemia often is present and has been attributed to alveolar hypoventilation resulting from small tidal volumes, arterial carbon dioxide partial pressure ($Paco_2$) usually is normal. In advanced cases, however, increased $Paco_2$ is common and signifies the onset of serious respiratory insufficiency. Increased ratios of physiologic dead space to tidal volume (Vd/Vt) and elevated alveolar-arterial oxygen tension gradients ($Pao_2 - Pao_2$) have been demonstrated. Studies employing ^{133}Xe have shown that the gas exchange abnormality in idiopathic scoliosis is primarily a consequence of ventilation-perfusion maldistribution resulting from deformity of the ribs (7–9). The proportion of ventilation, oxygen consumption, and volume on the side of convexity is less than on the side of concavity. However, a study with radionuclide methods did not find consistent differences in perfusion between the convex and concave sides of the curvature. Although adolescents with mild asymptomatic scoliosis (thoracic curvature of 35 degrees) demonstrate little or no impairment of lung volumes at rest, abnormal ventilatory patterns develop during exercise, hypoxia, or hypercapnia.

Clinical Features

Symptoms and signs of respiratory failure usually do not appear until the fourth or fifth decade. Cardiorespiratory failure is likely to occur when the VC is 40% of the predicted normal value. Patients in whom cor pulmonale develops exhibit severely diminished TLC. A retrospective survey of approximately 800 scoliotic subjects attending a chest clinic during a 25-year period revealed that cardiorespiratory failure attributable to scoliosis was the cause of death in 11 patients; in 10 of these, the scoliotic curve had first been observed at 5 years of age, whereas the onset was during early adolescence (11 years) in only one (10).

The term *Quasimodo syndrome* is used to describe severe kyphoscoliosis with abnormal sleep patterns. Sleep apnea and hypopnea occur more frequently in patients with kyphoscoliosis. Derangements in breathing pattern and arterial oxygen saturation apparently are unrelated to the degree of thoracic deformity, pulmonary function, $Paco_2$, or chemical drives to breathe. Hypoventilation occurs in patients with kyphoscoliosis during sleep, particularly rapid-eye-movement (REM) sleep. Hypoventilation secondary to reduced chest wall movements is the main mechanism responsible for hypoxemia and hypercapnia during sleep. Pure obstructive sleep apnea caused by spinal deformity alone is uncommon.

An interesting observation has been the significant association between scoliosis and pulmonary infection with *Mycobacterium avium* complex. In an evaluation of 67 patients with pulmonary disease caused by *M. avium* complex, 52% of patients were discovered to have scoliosis (11). This skeletal abnormality was significantly more common among all patients with *M. avium* complex infection than among patients with *M. tuberculosis* infection or the general population. This increased risk for infection among scoliotic subjects is most likely related to structural bronchopulmonary abnormalities rather than to immunologic or other well-known risk factors.

Atelectasis of a lobe as a result of scoliosis-related bronchial stenosis has been described. Clinically, significant bronchiectasis is a late complication in patients with severe kyphoscoliosis. Subclinical lung damage by this mechanism may predispose to secondary infections observed in some patients.

Treatment of Kyphoscoliosis

Significant improvements in pulmonary function test results is unlikely in the majority of patients who undergo corrective surgery. The aim of all therapies in this group of patients is to halt progression of the spinal deformity and thereby prevent further progression of pulmonary dysfunction. In a study of 14 adults who underwent anterior spinal surgery for correction of scoliosis, a follow-up evaluation 32 months later revealed a decrease in mean forced VC of 0.21 L despite improvement in the Cobb angle of 31% (12). The inference from this study is that in adults with reasonable lung function, the decrease in forced VC is small and clinically insignificant. Another study noted that whereas pulmonary function test values normalize in adolescent patients by 2 years after thoracoplasty, long-term pulmonary function in adults remains diminished (13). In advanced cases with hypercapnic respiratory failure, the treatment is mainly aimed at assisted ventilation to improve oxygenation and treat hypercapnia (14). It has been recommended that children with congenital scoliosis caused by multiple anomalies undergo surgery at an early age, before deformity becomes too severe (15).

Milwaukee brace or spinal fusion and reduction of the deformity by the posterior placement of Harrington distraction strut bars have been the standard approaches to therapy of kyphoscoliosis. Many studies have shown no appreciable difference in lung function between patients with the Milwaukee brace and those with surgical correction. In severe respiratory failure resulting from kyphoscoliosis, cuirass respirators have been used with varying success. In a meta-analysis of five studies comprising a total of 173 patients, the Harrington rod therapy resulted in an increase in mean VC ranging from 2% to 11% of predicted VC (16).

Nighttime ventilatory support using continuous positive airway pressure is helpful in many patients with respiratory failure caused by secondary scoliosis (17,18). A comparison study of 13 clinically stable patients with kyphoscoliosis treated by nocturnal positive-pressure ventilation via a nasal mask and of 13 patients with kyphoscoliosis and acute respiratory insufficiency treated by nocturnal ventilation via tracheostomy concluded that both treatments are effective in the long-term management of respiratory failure in these patients (19). It appears that if nocturnal positive-pressure ventilation via a nasal mask is initiated earlier in patients with chronic respiratory failure, the need to use an invasive technique, such as tracheostomy, is delayed.

Acute respiratory failure in adults with severe thoracic spinal deformity is associated with a higher mortality, but successful management of acute respiratory failure is possible in the majority of patients. Pulmonary function deteriorates at a slower rate after acute respiratory failure in these patients, who tend to be middle-aged, than in patients in whom acute respiratory failure develops as a result of chronic obstructive respiratory disease.

Postoperative Respiratory Complications

Postoperative respiratory complications after spinal fusion are common in patients with nonidiopathic scoliosis who are 20 years of age or older, undergo anterior spinal fusion, are mentally retarded, and have relative arterial hypoxemia or obstructive pulmonary dysfunction. In a report of 32 pediatric patients (18 boys and 14 girls; mean age, 13 years) with severe restrictive lung disease (mean VC, 31% of predicted normal), 54 reconstructive spinal surgical procedures were followed by pulmonary complications in six patients (19%) (20). The complications included pneumonia, reintubation, pneumothorax, respiratory arrest, or the need for tracheostomy, with three patients requiring tracheostomy. Patients in whom thoracotomy or a thoracoabdominal approach was used had a significantly higher number of pulmonary complications. Lung function measurements in anesthetized young patients undergoing spinal correction have shown immediate and short-term deterioration of respiratory mechanics. However, in one study that assessed the effects of spinal fusion on pulmonary function test values in a homogeneous population of 42 women with idiopathic scoliosis by measuring lung function before surgery and a minimum of 3 years (mean, 7.7 years) after surgery, the only significant preoperative abnormality found was VC reduced to 81% of predicted. A scoliotic angle exceeding 50 degrees was associated with a significantly lower VC. Postoperative evaluations showed that VC increased significantly, by 12%.

KYPHOSCOLIOSIS	
Summary Statement	**Level of Evidence**
Surgery is of questionable benefit and carries a significant complication rate established in adults with kyphoscoliosis; both surgery and brace treatment improve lung function in scoliotic adolescents.	Observational studies, expert opinion
Pulmonary rehabilitation and supplemental oxygen as needed are useful therapies in established kyphoscoliosis in adults.	Observational studies, expert opinion
Adults with kyphoscoliosis benefit from intermittent nocturnal or longer-term use of noninvasive positive pressure ventilation.	Observational studies, expert opinion

PECTUS DEFORMITIES

Pectus Excavatum

The congenital deformity pectus excavatum (also called *funnel chest*) is characterized by a depressed sternum (usually above the xiphisternal junction) and symmetric or asymmetric prominence of the ribs on either side. The origin of pectus excavatum is unknown, but it is believed to be caused by excessive diaphragmatic traction on the lower sternum or a more lateral displacement of the heart into the left hemithorax. A report of 10 cases of pectus excavatum noted pulmonary sequestration and other pulmonary abnormalities in nine patients and suggested a connection between pulmonary sequestration and the development of this deformity. However, when the common occurrence of pectus excavatum in clinical practice is considered, this incidence seems unusually high. Pectus excavatum usually occurs sporadically, although a dominant pattern of inheritance has been described. It may be associated with Marfan syndrome and other connective tissue diseases. The majority of patients are asymptomatic, but some experience exertional dyspnea, precordial pain, palpitation, and a sensation of dizziness. Pulmonary function is usually normal, but with very severe deformity, the VC, TLC, and maximal breathing capacity may be decreased.

Chest roentgenograms may reveal displacement of the heart to the left. The right parasternal soft tissues of the anterior chest wall give rise to the appearance of right middle lobe disease on posteroanterior roentgenograms (Fig. 62.3A). Sternal depression is best appreciated on lateral views (Fig. 62.3B). Paradoxical increase in cardiac size on inspiration has been described. Chuang and Wan showed that in children with pectus excavatum, a pectus index based on the central section taken through the deepest part of the deformity as measured on computed tomography scans provided useful information regarding the approach to conservative or surgical management (21).

In the study mentioned earlier, 27% of 67 patients with *M. avium* complex infection were found to have pectus excavatum deformity (11). By comparison, only 5% with *M. tuberculosis* infection had this skeletal abnormality. The prevalence of pectus excavatum among women with *M. avium* complex infection was significantly different from that among either the general population or patients infected with *M. tuberculosis,* whereas the prevalence of *M. avium* infection in male patients with pectus excavatum was significantly different from that in the general population but not from that in patients infected with *M. tuberculosis.* Possible mechanisms for this putative association include bronchopulmonary structural abnormalities secondary to pectus excavatum, impaired mucociliary function, im-

paired pulmonary lymphatic drainage, and altered alveolar macrophage function. It is unlikely that the skeletal abnormalities occurred as a result of mycobacterial infection, because there were no indications of chronic or past tuberculous infections.

An earlier study reported an apparent increase in infections of the lower respiratory tract among a series of U.S. Air Force recruits with pectus excavatum. Three cases of congenital bronchial atresia with pectus excavatum are reported (22,23); the investigators indicate that costosternal retraction during the efforts to overcome the airway obstruction may have played a part in causing pectus excavatum.

In patients with significant pectus excavatum, pulmonary function tests usually show restrictive phenomena. The restrictive lung dysfunction does not appear to be related to age, severity of the deformity at physical examination, or pulmonary symptoms (24). In a study of 152 patients who underwent surgery for pectus excavatum at a mean age of 15 years, lung function was reevaluated after 8 years, and it was noted that the restrictive pulmonary dysfunction worsened despite a reduction in the symptoms of most patients and despite a significant increase in anteroposterior diameter of the chest (25).

Pectus Carinatum

Pectus carinatum is a congenital or acquired deformity of the chest cage characterized by protrusion of the sternum. It is a relatively rare chest deformity with an occurrence rate of 1 to 2 per 1,000 population. Type I pectus carinatum, or "pigeon breast," is caused by an overgrowth of rib cartilages, resulting in forward buckling of the sternum. Pectus carinatum type II, or "pouter pigeon breast"

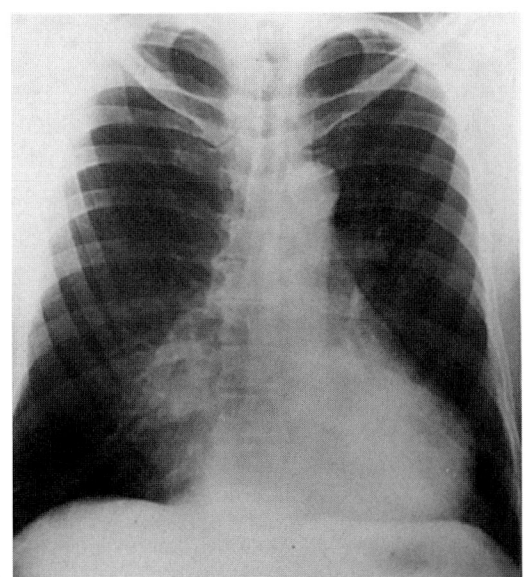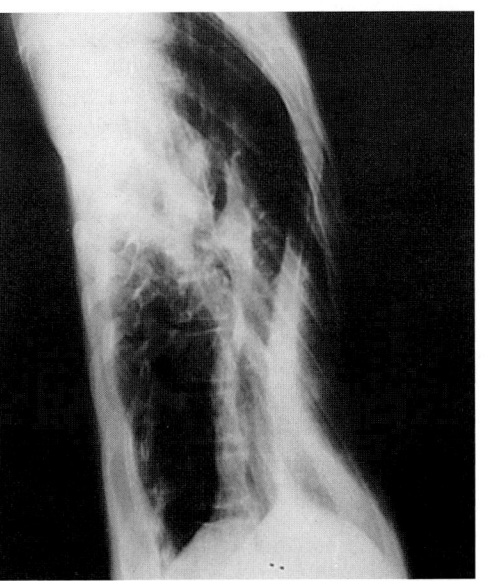

FIGURE 62.3. Pectus excavatum. **(A)** Right border of the heart is obliterated, and an infiltrate is apparent in the right middle lobe. The ribs on the right appear crowded. **(B)** Right lateral view shows sternal depression.

(Currarino-Silverman syndrome), is characterized by premature fusion of the manubriosternal joint and sternal segments, resulting in high carinate chest deformity. Both types of pectus carinatum deformities are frequently associated with congenital heart disease (26). The common cardiac anomalies in type I deformity are congenital atrial or ventricular septal defects. Conversely, nearly 50% of patients with those forms of heart disease have pectus carinatum. Some have reported that chronic and prolonged asthmatic attacks produce this deformity. Most patients with pectus carinatum are asymptomatic, but it has been suggested that they are subject to recurrent respiratory infections.

Pectus Deformatum

Pectus deformatum is the term used to describe an axially rotated sternum with an S-shaped frontal or sagittal plane. Among 80 patients with various abnormalities of the thoracic cage, pectus deformatum was noted in 13 (16%), and the incidence was identical to that of pectus carinatum. Pulmonary function abnormalities are usually mild, somewhat similar to those in pectus excavatum and pectus carinatum.

Surgical Correction of Pectus Deformities

Pectus deformities are surgically corrected for cosmetic reasons, for alleviating cardiopulmonary dysfunctions, and for preventing progressive postural deformities (27–30). In a study of 88 patients who underwent surgical correction of any of the pectus deformities just discussed, the operation appeared to have a favorable effect on chest roentgenologic indices but resulted in undercorrection in pectus excavatum and overcorrection in pectus carinatum (31). Furthermore, the study revealed that patients with preoperative lung function values that were 75% of predicted values experienced a functional improvement after corrective surgery. Interestingly, the pulmonary dysfunction worsened if lung function values were 75% of predicted. Another pulmonary function study of 138 patients before and after surgical correction of pectus excavatum reported that although the corrective procedures produced an excellent cosmetic result, there was no beneficial effect on pulmonary function. Among 227 children with pectus excavatum and 25 with pectus carinatum (195 boys and 57 girls) who underwent repair of pectus deformities, preoperative exercise limitation was reported by 51%, and frequent respiratory infections or asthma were reported by 32% (32). Surgical repair through a transverse incision, with subperiosteal resection of the lower four or five costal cartilages from sternum to costochondral junction bilaterally, resulted in improvements in exercise tolerance, endurance, respiratory symptoms, and cosmetic appearance in 98% of patients. The investigators of this study recommend operation at an early age with routine use of substernal support (32). Although technically more difficult than in children, pectus deformities may be repaired in adults with low

morbidity, short hospital stay, and very good physiologic and cosmetic results (33).

ANKYLOSING SPONDYLITIS

Ankylosing spondylitis, also known by other names, including *rheumatoid spondylitis* and *Marie-Strümpell disease,* is a chronic disorder characterized by progressive inflammation of the spine and adjacent soft tissues. The sacroiliac, hip, and shoulder joints are commonly affected. The disease affects men (male-to-female ratio, 10:1) 16 to 40 years of age but begins most often in the third decade. The cause is unknown. Ankylosing spondylitis may be inherited by a single autosomal-dominant factor, with a 70% penetrance in men and a 10% penetrance in women. A high association exists between ankylosing spondylitis and the histocompatibility antigen HLA-B27. Extraskeletal manifestations are numerous and include incompetence of the aortic valve, varying degrees of heart block, acute anterior uveitis, fever, anemia, fatigue, and weight loss.

The most widespread involvement of the respiratory system occurs when ankylosing spondylitis causes chest wall pain, diminished chest wall movement, and a dorsal stoop (34). Although pulmonary involvement has been reported in 2% to 70% of these patients in the clinical setting, only a small percentage (5%) demonstrate clinically discernible pulmonary problems. In a review of 2,080 patients with ankylosing spondylitis, pleuropulmonary manifestations were noted in only 28 (1.3%). The most common chest roentgenologic finding was fibrobullous apical lesions, in 26 patients. Other pleuropulmonary features included aspergilloma in five patients and pleural effusion with nonspecific pleuritis in three patients. A peculiar type of fibrotic process in the upper lobes characterized by nodular and linear lesions has been observed in 14% to 30% of patients. The process initially appears as linear strands in the upper lobes, beginning medially and radiating laterally. When the spine resembles bamboo, these linear strands give rise to a "telephone pole" appearance. Occasionally, the linear strands are replaced by small nodules that show cavitation or appear cystic (Fig. 62.4). Computed tomography may reveal bullous changes, mycetomas, parenchymal fibrosis, and pleural thickening. The cystic spaces and cavities occasionally become infected by *Aspergillus* species, *M. avium* complex, *M. kansasii,* or *M. scrofulaceum.*

Diffuse interstitial pneumonitis and fibrosis are uncommon (35,36). Bronchoalveolar lavage and bronchial biopsies in patients with ankylosing spondylitis have failed to indicate subclinical alveolitis (37). Bilateral pleural effusion has been described in a patient with quiescent ankylosing spondylitis. A case of tracheobronchomegaly is reported in association with ankylosing spondylitis.

Upper airway involvement in the form of cricoarytenoid ankylosis occurs in some patients. Respiratory failure

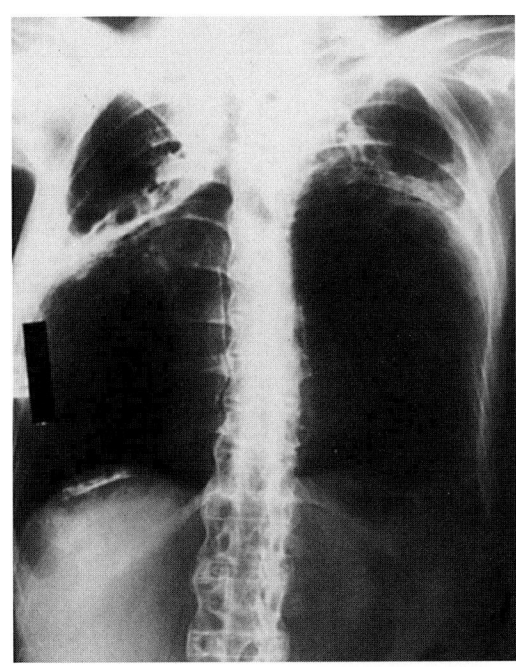

FIGURE 62.4. Ankylosing spondylitis demonstrates "bamboo spine," bilateral apical fibrous cavitary process, and right diaphragmatic calcification.

resulting from cricoarytenoid ankylosis has necessitated therapeutic tracheostomy in four patients (38). Calcification and ossification of cartilaginous structures may occur in the large airways. Obstruction by ossified arytenoid cartilage has been treated by endoscopic arytenoidectomy. Carcinoma of the upper lobes of lungs is another unusual long-term complication. Pathologic analysis of lung tissue in ankylosing spondylitis has demonstrated nonspecific fibrosis with lymphocytic infiltrates, dilated bronchi, and thin-walled bullae and cavities. Diaphragmatic calcification is seen in a small number of patients.

Ankylosing spondylitis alters lung function by modifying the mechanical properties of the thoracic cage. The ankylosis of the costovertebral joints rarely produces symptoms, even though pulmonary function test values are abnormal in these patients. Pulmonary function tests reveal diminished TLC, VC, and diffusing capacity for carbon monoxide (D_{LCO}) (39). Increases in residual volume and functional residual capacity are the other findings, although in some studies the functional residual capacity was decreased. Lung function studies in 16 patients with ankylosing spondylitis recorded a mean TLC of 83% of predicted and normal total respiratory resistance. Ventilation studies using ^{133}Xe have shown decreases in ventilation and gas volumes in the upper lobes; however, one study concluded that the upper zones of the lungs are not underventilated in patients with ankylosing spondylitis except in the presence of radiographically visible fibrosis. In a study of 32 patients with ankylosing spondylitis, pulmonary function test findings were compared with those of a control population. The patients had no lung symptoms,

and their chest roentgenographic findings were normal. The main findings were reduced lung volumes, a raised closing volume–to-VC ratio, and decreased airways conductance. The lung volume reduction correlated with disease duration, thoracic mobility, and degree of acute phase reaction. The stiff spondylitic thorax probably was the main contribution to the impairment of lung function in these patients, but the findings in this study also suggested involvement of the small airways. Despite abnormal pulmonary function test findings, the majority of patients with ankylosing spondylitis are able to perform normal physical activities (40). The exercise capacity in patients with ankylosing spondylitis is not influenced by the limitation of chest wall movements, probably owing to the maintenance of moderate physical activity along with an active life style (41). Although diaphragmatic calcification occurs in some patients with ankylosing spondylitis, diaphragmatic function is unimpaired and compensates well for the minor restrictive changes found in tests of respiratory function.

In a report of the coexistence of seronegative spondyloarthropathy and sarcoidosis in 12 patients, the investigators observed that the pelvic and spinal manifestations of sarcoidosis can mimic those of spondyloarthropathy. The coexistence of sarcoidosis and spondyloarthropathy is probably caused by chance, as there are no shared predisposing genetic factors and the number of reported cases is small.

Treatment is by mobilizing physiotherapy coupled with a home exercise program to encourage mobility and improve cardiovascular fitness. The role of medication is to ease symptoms and, hence, enable exercise. No treatments exist that can prevent the development of fibrobullous disease or halt its progression, although this may happen spontaneously. Treatment of established aspergillosis, especially when aspergillomas have formed, is unsatisfactory and carries substantial risks for morbidity and death.

CERVICAL HYPEROSTOSIS

Cervical hyperostosis of the spine is anatomically manifested by bony outgrowths arising from the anterior aspects of the vertebral bodies and extending over the disk spaces. Also known as *diffuse idiopathic skeletal hyperostosis (DISH)*, the condition was observed in 12% of 215 routine autopsies. The abnormality is most common in men; the average age is 66 years. The pharyngeal masses formed by the bony outgrowths can be extensive and may occasionally be visualized or palpated at the time of physical examination. These hyperostotic spurs are known to cause dysphagia, foreign-body sensation, aspiration, respiratory distress, and dysphonia. Dysphagia occurs in 17% to 28% of patients with this disorder (42).

Bilateral vocal cord paralysis with airways obstruction has been described in patients with DISH (43). The pathogenesis is infection superimposed on ulceration of the cricoid produced by laryngeal movement over a large sharp osteophyte. Severe acute airway obstruction caused by a cervical osteophyte pressing on the posterior trachea is described in a 68-year-old man; tracheostomy followed by resection of the osteophyte was therapeutically successful. Dysphagia and aspiration are the results of mechanical compression (44–46). Nonsteroidal anti-inflammatory drugs and antireflux precautions should be suggested for patients who have dysphagia. Surgical removal of the hyperostotic process is required in severe cases (47).

Cervical spondylosis can be associated with pressure symptoms in the neck area. Dyspnea and paresis of the left hemidiaphragm, relieved by laminectomy, are described.

OSTEOPOROSIS

Compression fractures of multiple thoracic vertebral bodies as a result of osteoporosis produce an anatomic anomaly akin to kyphosis. With severe compression fracture, a gentle (nonacute angle) thoracic gibbus or hyperkyphosis develops in some patients. Furthermore, a markedly shortened thoracic vertebral column leads to reduced lung volumes. A study of the effect of thoracic kyphosis on respiratory mechanics in 15 women with kyphosis resulting from spinal osteoporosis showed the VC, inspiratory capacity, TLC, and lateral expansion of the thorax to be lower in the osteoporotic group (48). These mechanical factors and the pain secondary to compression fracture have the potential to cause respiratory dysfunction. The pulmonary effects of significant osteoporosis are similar to those observed in scoliosis. Seventy-four women referred for evaluation of osteoporosis were subjected to pulmonary function testing, and those with thoracic wedge compression fractures secondary to osteoporosis had a significantly lower predicted forced VC than did those without fractures. The degree of hyperkyphosis as measured by the Cobb angle had an appreciable effect on this parameter. The study estimated that a decrease of approximately 9% in the predicted forced VC might be expected for each thoracic vertebral fracture.

STERNOTOMY

Median sternotomy is a common surgical procedure used in the vast majority of cardiac surgeries, particularly coronary artery bypasses and valve replacement procedures. A restrictive ventilatory defect follows median sternotomy. VC, FEV_1, and functional residual capacity may decline to as little as 40% of preoperative values 1 to 3 days after coronary artery bypass grafting. These changes are more pronounced after the use of internal mammary artery bypass than after saphenous vein grafting. This is reported to be related to disruption of the internal mammary artery–derived vascular supply of the phrenic nerves. The diminished lung function begins to reverse by the end of the first postoperative week, and recovery is almost total at 3 weeks. The causes of lung dysfunction include pain, atelectasis, pulmonary edema, pulmonary embolism, hemothorax, diaphragmatic paralysis ("frost-bitten" phrenic nerve), pleurotomy, and chest wall instability. A study of rib cage mechanics in 16 men before and 1 week and 3 months after median sternotomy for coronary artery grafting revealed that reduced and uncoordinated rib cage expansion contributed to the restrictive ventilatory defect. Pre-existing cardiopulmonary disease influences the reduction in lung volumes. Obviously, resection of pulmonary parenchyma will result in permanent loss of lung function contributed by the resected segment or lobe.

MARFAN SYNDROME

A heritable generalized disorder of connective tissue, Marfan syndrome is manifested clinically by abnormalities of the skeletal system (excessive length of long bones), eyes (ectopia lentis), and cardiovascular system (aneurysm of the thoracic aorta, septal and valvular cardiac anomalies). Pulmonary abnormalities are observed in approximately 10% of patients with Marfan syndrome and include generalized honeycombing of the lungs, spontaneous pneumothorax, and bronchiectasis (Fig. 62.5). Of these, spontaneous pneumothorax is the most common and is seen in nearly 5% of adolescents and adults. Spontaneous pneumothorax and bullae are causally related to Marfan syndrome. Necropsy studies of four infants with this syndrome and pulmonary emphysema showed that the elastic fibers in alveolar ducts and sacs were irregularly thickened, wavy, fragmented, and clumped

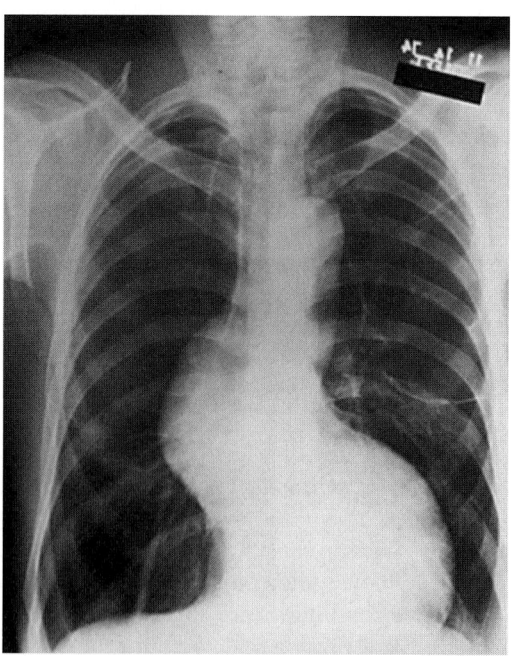

FIGURE 62.5. Marfan syndrome with hyperinflation, bullous changes, dilated tortuous aorta, and "tall" lungs.

(49). Diffuse honeycombing of the lungs and spontaneous pneumothorax were reported as the presenting features of Marfan syndrome in a boy (50). In two cases, bilateral bullous disease with spontaneous pneumothorax was reported (51). Fibrosis of the upper lobes also is reported in Marfan syndrome. A report described three members of a family—a father and two sons, all afflicted with Marfan syndrome—who had multiple bilateral episodes of pneumothorax that required repeated drainage procedures (52).

Structural abnormalities of the right middle lobe have been described. Ciliary dyskinesia also has been observed in a patient with Marfan syndrome. Additionally, deformities of the thoracic cage resulting from abnormalities of the vertebral column, ribs, and sternum are common in this syndrome and may occur in any combination and degree of severity. Both scoliosis and pectus excavatum occur and may cause pulmonary dysfunction. Tracheal weakness, presumably resulting from structural deficiency of the cartilages, has been reported in a patient.

A review of published reports disclosed nearly 50 patients with bullous lesions, lung cysts, or emphysema, 22 of whom were younger than 20 years and two thirds of whom were male (53). In the same review of an additional 100 patients with Marfan syndrome, 11 had spontaneous pneumothorax, with recurrence in 10 patients and bilateral appearance in six patients, pneumonia or recurrent respiratory infections in eight patients, and bronchiectasis in two patients (53). Chest roentgenograms revealed emphysematous bullae in five patients, fibrosis of the upper lobes in four patients, and aspergilloma in two patients. Another review of 249 patients older than 12 years reported the frequency of pneumothorax to be 4.4%, with recurrent or bilateral pneumothorax in 3% (54). This review suggested that definitive surgical therapy should be considered at the first occurrence of pneumothorax because of the high rate of recurrence after treatment with a chest tube (54).

Pulmonary dysfunction occurs in the absence of thoracic cage abnormality. An important aspect of interpreting the pulmonary function test results is the recognition that the values are based on age, sex, and standing height. The unusually long length of the legs in patients with Marfan syndrome contributes disproportionately to these calculations. Studies of pulmonary function in patients with Marfan syndrome have revealed diminished TLC and VC and mildly lowered flow rates at low lung volumes, with decreased diffusing capacity and elastic lung recoil, but only minimal abnormalities of pulmonary function have been noted in some cases. A study involving 79 patients with Marfan syndrome concluded that persons with this syndrome who have, at most, mild thoracic deformity do not have significant abnormalities of static pulmonary function, and thus, the connective tissue defects in the lungs seem to have minimal clinical impact beyond the risk for pneumothorax (55). However, tests of dynamic lung function were not performed in this group of subjects. In a report of 11 children with Marfan syndrome, airway reactivity as measured by methacholine challenge was noted in all children, even though only one patient had a diagnosis of asthma. An unusual case of Marfan syndrome with hypercoagulability complicated by multiple pulmonary emboli has been described.

The prevalence of obstructive sleep apnea is higher in patients with Marfan syndrome. Sleep apnea in these patients is not related to obesity. Indeed, patients with Marfan syndrome usually are tall and thin rather than obese. Excessive collapsibility of the upper airway resulting from connective tissue defect has been postulated as one of the reasons (56). A more likely mechanism is related to the characteristically constricted maxilla and the high-arched palate. Measurement of nasal airway resistance by posterior manometry in patients with Marfan syndrome has shown high resistance (57). The indices of maxillary constriction as determined by measurement of nasal airway resistance have been shown to correlate with the severity of sleep apnea.

ACHONDROPLASIA

Achondroplasia is the most common skeletal dysplasia resulting in short-limbed dwarfism. The disorder results from abnormal endochondral bone formation. Pulmonary complications are common in achondroplastic infants and children younger than 2 years (58). Factors that influence respiratory manifestations include associated deformities of the chest wall and involvement of respiratory centers at the level of the brainstem and upper cervical cord. The thoracic skeletal abnormalities include reduced chest cage measurements, pectus excavatum, accentuated thoracic kyphosis, or thoracic lordosis. Detailed physiologic abnormalities in 12 healthy subjects with achondroplasia showed that the reduction in VC was out of proportion to what would be expected if these subjects had limbs of normal size; the other pulmonary function parameters were normal (59). In a study of 58 female and 44 male achondroplastic subjects between 7 and 60 years of age, the values for VC were 68% and 72% of predicted normal values for normally proportioned men and women, respectively.

Upper airway involvement, nasal obstruction, hypoxemia, and obstructive sleep apnea are more common in younger achondroplastic subjects (60). The most important breathing disorder during sleep in children with achondroplasia is upper airway obstruction. The short cranial base and midfacial hypoplasia increase the risk for upper airway obstruction during sleep. Sleep apnea and death caused by acute or chronic compression of the lower brainstem or cervical spinal cord have been noted in infants with achondroplasia. One study found no relationship between apnea type and foramen magnum stenosis. Obstructive sleep apnea is reported to occur more often in older subjects with achondroplasia. Resolution of sleep apnea by tracheostomy in achondroplastic dwarfs has resulted in normalization of growth hormone release and normal growth. Apneustic breathing is a rare pattern of neurogenic breathing characteristic of some patients with achondroplasia. In a report of five patients with achondroplasia, all of whom demonstrated apneustic breathing, the investigators speculated that compression of the lower medullary respiratory centers and afferent pathways in the spinal cord were responsible for the abnormal breathing pattern (61).

RIGID SPINE SYNDROME

In rigid spine syndrome, a rigid spine is associated with a myopathy predominantly affecting proximal limb muscles. Histologic analysis of skeletal muscles, including the diaphragm, may show the presence of autophagic vacuoles in muscle fibers. Although this syndrome is more common in children, respiratory failure secondary to respiratory muscle weakness has been described in adults. The cause of respiratory failure is extreme flattening of the chest and fixation of the thorax as a result of contracture of costovertebral joints. In almost all reported cases of rigid spine syndrome, the patients have died of respiratory failure. Respiratory muscle involvement is a significant feature of rigid spine syndrome, resulting in hypercapnic ventilatory failure in some patients. Investigation of thoracic abnormalities and respiratory muscle function in nine patients with rigid spine syndrome showed a severe restrictive chest wall defect and limited mobility of the spine. Most importantly, significant respiratory muscle weakness was present in all patients. Respiratory muscle strength and endurance were 60% of control values (62). Even though six of the patients were emaciated and one patient was underweight, no relationship was seen between body mass index and respiratory muscle strength (62). Patients with hypoventilation demonstrated more pronounced respiratory muscle dysfunction.

Nocturnal ventilatory assistance has been employed to assist patients with severe hypoventilation and respiratory failure.

CRANIOFACIAL DEFORMITIES

Several types of craniofacial deformities have been described. These structural aberrations frequently are associated with upper airway problems. Severe sleep apnea, sometimes necessitating tracheostomy, is a recognized complication of various craniofacial structural abnormalities. Different grades of respiratory distress resulting from obstructive sleep apnea have been described in adults with craniofacial dysostosis, achondroplasia, metatropic dwarfism, Hallermann-Streiff syndrome, and Treacher Collins syndrome. Sleep apnea is a well-recognized aspect of micrognathia and Pierre Robin syndrome (bird-face syndrome). Tracheostomy is recommended in pediatric cases of craniofacial abnormalities with sleep apnea before reconstructive surgery is undertaken.

Pierre Robin syndrome is characterized by mandibular hypoplasia (micrognathia) and glossoptosis, often associated with a cleft palate. Upper respiratory obstruction is commonly present in this disorder (63). The tongue is posteriorly displaced (glossoptosis) as a consequence of micrognathia and anterior insertion of the tongue to the mandible. Severe airway obstruction may persist for months but may improve with time.

Because of micrognathia, patients with Treacher Collins syndrome are at greater risk for development of obstructive sleep apnea. Surgical correction of the micrognathia may relieve sleep apnea.

GORHAM DISEASE

Gorham disease, or Gorham-Stout disease (disappearing or vanishing bone disease), is characterized by massive osteolysis (64). It generally appears in the second and third decades of life, with an equal sex distribution. A report in 1994 recorded that 146 cases of Gorham syndrome were documented in the literature (65). Although any skeletal bone can be affected, the commonly involved bones are the innominate bones, thorax, and spine. Clinically, patients present with dull aching and weakness in an affected extremity. Pain is usually caused by pathologic fractures, which are a prominent feature of this disease. Histologically, lymphangiomatous tissue is observed in the affected skeletal structures. The predominant feature is the lymphatic dysplasia in skeletal structures and in the thorax.

Pleuropulmonary manifestations include pleural effusion and development of lymphangiomatous tissue in the mediastinum (66). Massive pleural effusions, sometimes chylous, with high mortality have been described. Of the 146 cases of Gorham syndrome documented in the literature, chylothorax was diagnosed in 26 (17%) of patients (65). Pneumothorax may be associated with chylothorax and may be seen in conjunction with chylous pleural effusion. Pulmonary lymphangiectasia, described in patients with some of these skeletal abnormalities, may be responsible for the chylous pleural effusion. Reports of successful treatment of chylothorax by high-dose radiotherapy and bleomycin have been published.

ADULT STILL DISEASE

Adult Still disease is characterized by high fever, arthritis, evanescent rash, serositis, lymphadenopathy, splenomegaly, leukocytosis, and absence of rheumatoid factor and antinuclear antibodies. Pleuropulmonary complications, such as pleuritis and pneumonitis, occur frequently. The incidence of pleuropulmonary complications is reported to be approximately 30%, but estimates of up to 60% are recorded. The most common symptom is pleurisy with or without effusion. Persistent or severe pulmonary parenchymal infiltrates

are uncommon. Diffuse interstitial lung disease has been described in a patient with adult-onset Still disease (67). Fatal adult respiratory distress syndrome complicated by opportunistic pulmonary infections has been described in a 65-year-old woman.

OSTEOGENIC SARCOMA AND OTHER SKELETAL NEOPLASMS

Pulmonary metastatic disease is a relatively common complication of osteogenic sarcoma and other soft tissue sarcomas, including Ewing sarcoma of bone, rhabdomyosarcoma, and synovial sarcoma. The pulmonary lesions almost always present as lung nodules, either solitary nodules or multiple bilateral nodules. Pulmonary metastases may appear with the primary tumor or follow it by several months to years after therapy of the primary tumor. The median doubling time for pulmonary metastatic nodules secondary to bone or soft tissue sarcomas is estimated to be 35 days (estimated 95% range, 3.9 to 352 days) (68). Follow-up chest roentgenography should be considered in the majority of these patients. Periodic computed tomography of the chest is more accurate in detecting smaller nodules than is the plain chest roentgenogram. One of the unusual features of metastatic osteogenic sarcoma is calcification of the metastatic lung lesion.

Spontaneous regression of pulmonary metastatic osteosarcoma is extremely rare, even after curative therapy of the primary tumor. Therefore, pulmonary metastasectomy with or without adjuvant therapy is the accepted therapy. Up to 50% of patients with osteogenic sarcoma in whom pulmonary metastases develop can be satisfactorily treated with continued effective chemotherapy and pulmonary metastasectomies, as long as good local control is achieved in the primary tumor (69,70). The presence of bilateral, extensive, or recurrent disease is not a contraindication to thoracotomy, because aggressive resection of multiple nodules and improved chemotherapy appear to prolong survival of these patients in comparison with survival rates of historical control subjects. In patients presenting with simultaneous primary tumor and pulmonary metastatic disease, the cure rate is potentially as high as it is in those patients who present with primary tumor alone. Because the majority of patients are young and otherwise healthy, thoracotomy with resection of lung nodules—sometimes repeated and bilateral—is associated with low morbidity and mortality. Patients who undergo resection of pulmonary metastatic osteogenic sarcoma generally have a better prognosis than do those with other soft-tissue tumors. The long-term pulmonary toxicity of multiagent chemotherapy, including bleomycin and cyclophosphamide, in osteosarcoma survivors include significant declines in all mean values for TLC, FEV_1, and Dlco in the first year. However, this was not associated with significant long-term abnormalities of pulmonary function (71).

In a report of 152 patients (median age, 19 years; range, 5 to 33 years) who underwent 258 thoracic explorations for resection of metastatic Ewing sarcoma (28), rhabdomyosarcoma (6), soft tissue sarcoma other than rhabdomyosarcoma (42), and osteosarcoma (76), the thoracic procedures consisted of 218 wedge resections, 19 anatomic resections, 14 wedge and anatomic resections, four wedge and chest wall resections, and three wedge resections/other procedures. Complete resection was achieved in 121 patients (80%) (72). The median survival from initial thoracotomy was 2.2 years. Unfavorable prognostic factors included three or more positive nodules, histology other than osteosarcoma, and incomplete resection. Predictors of shorter survival included the following: two or more metastatic lung nodules, left-sided thoracic location of metastatic lesion(s), age 14 years or older at diagnosis, or histology that depicted rhabdomyosarcoma. In a study of 36 patients with pulmonary metastatic osteogenic sarcoma, the 5-year survival rate after pulmonary metastasectomy was 23% (73).

In a study of 12 patients with Ewing sarcoma of bone who relapsed with pulmonary metastases alone and were treated with surgical resection of the metastatic lesions but no additional radiotherapy or chemotherapy, five were continuously free of disease at follow-up, ranging between 3 and 14 years (mean, 9 years) (74). The remaining seven patients died with uncontrolled disease 12 to 39 months (mean, 22 months) after thoracotomy. These results seem to indicate that an aggressive surgical approach should be considered for a selected group of patients with Ewing sarcoma who relapse with only lung metastases.

Extraskeletal osteosarcomas are rare malignancies that account for about 1% of all soft tissue sarcomas. One study of 40 patients (mean age, 51 years; male-to-female ratio, 1.9:1) with extraskeletal osteosarcoma found pulmonary metastases in 81% (75). The primary tumors originated in the lower limbs in 68% of cases and presented in 90% of patients as an enlarging soft tissue mass; nine patients had a history of trauma. Morphologically, all were high-grade osteosarcomas. Distant metastases occurred, usually within 3 years, in 65%, but lung involvement was noted in 81%. The overall 5-year survival rate was 37%.

Benign giant-cell tumor of bone demonstrates the unusual ability to metastasize to the lungs. It is estimated that 9% of such tumors may metastasize to the lungs. Approximately 50 such cases have been reported. In a report of six patients with pulmonary metastasis of giant-cell tumor, one patient exhibited spontaneous regression and another died of pulmonary complications (76).

MISCELLANEOUS TOPICS

The increased risk for deep vein thrombophlebitis and pulmonary embolism in patients who undergo orthopedic procedures—particularly arthroplasty of the hip, knee, and other joints—is discussed elsewhere, as is the topic of fat embolism after fractures of bone and orthopedic procedures. Orthopedic procedures such as intramedullary femoral nailing and arthroplasty in which chemical adhesive cement (methyl methacrylate) is used have been followed by pulmonary complications.

Femoral nailing after reaming has been shown to be associated with higher risk for development of adult respiratory distress syndrome in comparison with unreamed femoral nailing (77). The risk for respiratory complications is even higher in those with "borderline pulmonary status."

REFERENCES

1. Baron RM, Schwartzstein RM. Diseases of the chest wall. In: Rose BD, ed. *UpToDate*. Wellesley, MA: UpToDate, 2002.
2. Kearon C, Viviani GR, Kirkley A, et al. Factors determining pulmonary function in adolescent idiopathic thoracic scoliosis. *Am Rev Respir Dis* 1993;148:288–294.
3. Upadhyay SS, Mullaji AB, Luk KD, et al. Evaluation of deformities and pulmonary function in adolescent idiopathic right thoracic scoliosis. *Eur Spine J* 1995;4:274–279.
4. Boyer J, Amin N, Taddonio R, et al. Evidence of airway obstruction in children with idiopathic scoliosis. *Chest* 1996;109:1532–1535.
5. Kesten S, Garfinkel SK, Wright T, et al. Impaired exercise capacity in adults with moderate scoliosis. *Chest* 1991;99:663–666.
6. Shneerson JM. The cardiorespiratory response to exercise in thoracic scoliosis. *Thorax* 1978;33:457–463.
7. Bjure J, Grimby G, Kasalicky J, et al. Respiratory impairment and airway closure in patients with untreated idiopathic scoliosis. *Thorax* 1970;25:451–456.
8. Bake B, Bjure J, Kasalichy J, et al. Regional pulmonary ventilation and perfusion distribution in patients with untreated idiopathic scoliosis. *Thorax* 1972;27:703–712.
9. Littler WA, Brown IK, Roaf R. Regional lung function in scoliosis. *Thorax* 1972;27:420–428.
10. Branthwaite MA. Cardiorespiratory consequences of unfused idiopathic scoliosis. *Br J Dis Chest* 1986;80:360–369.
11. Iseman MD, Buschman DL, Ackerson LM. Pectus excavatum and scoliosis: thoracic anomalies associated with pulmonary disease caused by *Mycobacterium avium* complex. *Am Rev Respir Dis* 1991;144:914–916.
12. Wong CA, Cole AA, Watson L, et al. Pulmonary function before and after anterior spinal surgery in adult idiopathic scoliosis. *Thorax* 1996;51:534–536.
13. Lenke LG, Bridwell KH, Blanke K, et al. Analysis of pulmonary function and chest cage dimension changes after thoracoplasty in idiopathic scoliosis. *Spine* 1995;20:1343–1350.
14. Jones DJ, Paul EA, Bell JH, et al. Ambulatory oxygen therapy in stable kyphoscoliosis. *Eur Respir J* 1995;8:819–823.
15. Day GA, Upadhyay SS, Ho EK, et al. Pulmonary functions in congenital scoliosis. *Spine* 1994;19:1027–1031.
16. Kinnear WJ, Johnston ID. Does Harrington instrumentation improve pulmonary function in adolescents with idiopathic scoliosis?: a meta-analysis. *Spine* 1993;18:1556–1559.
17. Ellis ER, Grunstein RR, Chan S, et al. Noninvasive ventilatory support during sleep improves respiratory failure in kyphoscoliosis. *Chest* 1988;94:811–815.
18. Finlay G, Concannon D, McDonnell TJ. Treatment of respiratory failure due to kyphoscoliosis with nasal intermittent positive pressure ventilation (NIPPV). *Ir J Med Sci* 1995;164:28–30.
19. Zaccaria S, Ioli F, Lusuardi M, et al. Long-term nocturnal mechanical ventilation in patients with kyphoscoliosis. *Monaldi Arch Chest Dis* 1995;50:433–437.
20. Rawlins BA, Winter RB, Lonstein JE, et al. Reconstructive spine surgery in pediatric patients with major loss in vital capacity. *J Pediatr Orthop* 1996;16:284–292.
21. Chuang JH, Wan YL. Evaluation of pectus excavatum with repeated CT scans. *Pediatr Radiol* 1995;25:654–656.
22. Scholl RJ 3rd, Neumann DP, Yamase HT. Case report: bronchial atresia associated with pectus excavatum. *Conn Med* 1997;61:263–267.
23. van Klaveren RJ, Morshuis WJ, Lacquet LK, et al. Congenital bronchial atresia with regional emphysema associated with pectus excavatum. *Thorax* 1992;47:1082–1083.
24. Quigley PM, Haller JA Jr, Jelus KL, et al. Cardiorespiratory function before and after corrective surgery in pectus excavatum. *J Pediatr* 1996;128:638–643.
25. Morshuis W, Folgering H, Barentsz J, et al. Pulmonary function before surgery for pectus excavatum and at long-term follow-up. *Chest* 1994;105:1646–1052.
26. Chidambaram B, Mehta AV. Currarino-Silverman syndrome (pectus carinatum type 2 deformity) and mitral valve disease. *Chest* 1992;102:780–782.
27. Goertzen M, Baltzer A, Schulitz KP. Long-term results after operation for funnel chest. *Arch Orthop Trauma Surg* 1993;112:289–291.
28. Prevot J. Treatment of sternocostal wall malformations of the child: a series of 210 surgical corrections since 1975. *Eur J Pediatr Surg* 1994;4:131–136.
29. Haller JA Jr, Colombani PM, Humphries CT, et al. Chest wall constriction after too extensive and too early operations for pectus excavatum. *Ann Thorac Surg* 1996;61:1618–1624;discussion 1625.
30. Lancaster L, McIlhenny J, Rodgers B, et al. Radiographic findings after pectus excavatum repair. *Pediatr Radiol* 1995;25:452–454.
31. Derveaux L, Clarysse I, Ivanoff I, et al. Preoperative and postoperative abnormalities in chest x-ray indices and in lung function in pectus deformities. *Chest* 1989;95:850–856.
32. Fonkalsrud EW, Salman T, Guo W, et al. Repair of pectus deformities with sternal support. *J Thorac Cardiovasc Surg* 1994;107:37–42.
33. Fonkalsrud EW, DeUgarte D, Choi E. Repair of pectus excavatum and carinatum deformities in 116 adults. *Ann Surg* 2002;236:304–312.
34. Haslock I. Ankylosing spondylitis. *Baillieres Clin Rheumatol* 1993;7:99–115.
35. Turner JF, Enzenauer RJ. Bronchiolitis obliterans and organizing pneumonia associated with ankylosing spondylitis. *Arthritis Rheum* 1994;37:1557–1559.
36. Ferdoutsis M, Bouros D, Meletis G, et al. Diffuse interstitial lung disease as an early manifestation of ankylosing spondylitis. *Respiration* 1995;62:286–289.
37. Wendling D, Dalphin JC, Toson B, et al. Bronchoalveolar lavage in ankylosing spondylitis. *Ann Rheum Dis* 1990;49:325–326.
38. Miller FR, Wanamaker JR, Hicks DM, et al. Cricoarytenoid arthritis and ankylosing spondylitis. *Arch Otolaryngol Head Neck Surg* 1994;120:214–216.
39. Vanderschueren D, Decramer M, Van den Daele P, et al. Pulmonary function and maximal transrespiratory pressures in ankylosing spondylitis. *Ann Rheum Dis* 1989;48:632–635.
40. Fisher LR, Cawley MI, Holgate ST. Relation between chest expansion, pulmonary function, and exercise tolerance in patients with ankylosing spondylitis. *Ann Rheum Dis* 1990;49:921–925.

41. Seckin U, Bolukbasi N, Gursel G, et al. Relationship between pulmonary function and exercise tolerance in patients with ankylosing spondylitis. *Clin Exp Rheumatol* 2000;18:503–506.

42. Suzuki K, Ishida Y, Ohmori K. Long term follow-up of diffuse idiopathic skeletal hyperostosis in the cervical spine: analysis of progression of ossification. *Neuroradiology* 1991;33:427–431.

43. Hassard AD. Cervical ankylosing hyperostosis and airway obstruction. *Laryngoscope* 1984;94:966–968.

44. Joseph MG, Matheson JM, Blum PW. Hyperostosis of anterior cervical vertebrae: a rare cause of dysphagia. *Med J Aust* 1988;149:442–443.

45. Warnick C, Sherman MS, Lesser RW. Aspiration pneumonia due to diffuse cervical hyperostosis. *Chest* 1990;98:763–764.

46. Mader R. Clinical manifestations of diffuse idiopathic skeletal hyperostosis of the cervical spine. *Semin Arthritis Rheum* 2002;32:130–135.

47. Krause P, Castro WH. Cervical hyperostosis: a rare cause of dysphagia: case description and bibliographical survey. *Eur Spine J* 1994;3:56–58.

48. Culham EG, Jimenez HA, King CE. Thoracic kyphosis, rib mobility, and lung volumes in normal women and women with osteoporosis. *Spine* 1994;19:1250–1255.

49. Dominguez R, Weisgrau RA, Santamaria M. Pulmonary hyperinflation and emphysema in infants with the Marfan syndrome. *Pediatr Radiol* 1987;17:365–369.

50. Lipton RA, Greenwald RA, Seriff NS. Pneumothorax and bilateral honeycombed lung in Marfan syndrome: report of a case and review of the pulmonary abnormalities in this disorder. *Am Rev Respir Dis* 1971;104:924–928.

51. Turner JA, Stanley NN. Fragile lung in the Marfan syndrome. *Thorax* 1976;31:771–775.

52. Yellin A, Shiner RJ, Lieberman Y. Familial multiple bilateral pneumothorax associated with Marfan syndrome. *Chest* 1991;100:577–578.

53. Wood JR, Bellamy D, Child AH, et al. Pulmonary disease in patients with Marfan syndrome. *Thorax* 1984;39:780–784.

54. Hall JR, Pyeritz RE, Dudgeon DL, et al. Pneumothorax in the Marfan syndrome: prevalence and therapy. *Ann Thorac Surg* 1984;37:500–504.

55. Streeten EA, Murphy EA, Pyeritz RE. Pulmonary function in the Marfan syndrome. *Chest* 1987;91:408–412.

56. Cistulli PA, Sullivan CE. Sleep apnea in Marfan's syndrome. Increased upper airway collapsibility during sleep. *Chest* 1995;108:631–635.

57. Cistulli PA, Richards GN, Palmisano RG, et al. Influence of maxillary constriction on nasal resistance and sleep apnea severity in patients with Marfan's syndrome. *Chest* 1996;110:1184–1188.

58. Tasker RC, Dundas I, Laverty A, et al. Distinct patterns of respiratory difficulty in young children with achondroplasia: a clinical, sleep, and lung function study. *Arch Dis Child* 1998;79:99–108.

59. Stokes DC, Wohl ME, Wise RA, et al. The lungs and airways in achondroplasia. Do little people have little lungs? *Chest* 1990;98:145–152.

60. Zucconi M, Weber G, Castronovo V, et al. Sleep and upper airway obstruction in children with achondroplasia. *J Pediatr* 1996;129:743–749.

61. Mador MJ, Tobin MJ. Apneustic breathing: a characteristic feature of brainstem compression in achondroplasia? *Chest* 1990;97:877–883.

62. Ras GJ, van Staden M, Schultz C, et al. Respiratory manifestations of rigid spine syndrome. *Am J Respir Crit Care Med* 1994;150:540–546.

63. Wilson AC, Moore DJ, Moore MH, et al. Late presentation of upper airway obstruction in Pierre Robin sequence. *Arch Dis Child* 2000;83:435–438.

64. Green HD, Mollica AJ, Karuza AS. Gorham's disease: a literature review and case reports. *J Foot Ankle Surg* 1995;34:435–441.

65. Tie ML, Poland GA, Rosenow EC 3rd. Chylothorax in Gorham's syndrome: a common complication of a rare disease. *Chest* 1994;105:208–213.

66. Tie ML, Poland GA, Rosenow EC 3rd. Pleural effusion: a complication of Gorham's disease. *Pediatr Radiol* 1994;24:542.

67. Van Hoeyweghen RJ, De Clerck LS, Van Offel JF, et al. Interstitial lung disease and adult-onset Still's disease. *Clin Rheumatol* 1993;12:418–421.

68. Blomqvist C, Wiklund T, Tarkkanen M, et al. Measurement of growth rate of lung metastases in 21 patients with bone or soft-tissue sarcoma. *Br J Cancer* 1993;68:414–417.

69. Heij HA, Vos A, de Kraker J, et al. Prognostic factors in surgery for pulmonary metastases in children. *Surgery* 1994;115:687–693.

70. Rosen G, Holmes EC, Forscher CA, et al. The role of thoracic surgery in the management of metastatic osteogenic sarcoma. *Chest Surg Clin N Am* 1994;4:75–83.

71. Kharasch VS, Lipsitz S, Santis W, et al. Long-term pulmonary toxicity of multiagent chemotherapy including bleomycin and cyclophosphamide in osteosarcoma survivors. *Med Pediatr Oncol* 1996;27:85–91.

72. Temeck BK, Wexler LH, Steinberg SM, et al. Metastasectomy for sarcomatous pediatric histologies: results and prognostic factors. *Ann Thorac Surg* 1995;59:1385–1389.

73. Ward WG, Mikaelian K, Dorey F, et al. Pulmonary metastases of stage IIB extremity osteosarcoma and subsequent pulmonary metastases. *J Clin Oncol* 1994;12:1849–1858.

74. Bacci G, Briccoli A, Picci P, et al. Metachronous pulmonary metastases resection in patients with Ewing's sarcoma initially treated with adjuvant or neoadjuvant chemotherapy. *Eur J Cancer* 1995;31A:999–1001.

75. Lee JS, Fetsch JF, Wasdhal DA, et al. A review of 40 patients with extraskeletal osteosarcoma. *Cancer* 1995;76:2253–2259.

76. Kay RM, Eckardt JJ, Seeger LL, et al. Pulmonary metastasis of benign giant cell tumor of bone. Six histologically confirmed cases, including one of spontaneous regression. *Clin Orthop* 1994:219–230.

77. Pape HC, Regel G, Dwenger A, et al. Influences of different methods of intramedullary femoral nailing on lung function in patients with multiple trauma. *J Trauma* 1993;35:709–716.

63 Dermatologic Diseases

Udaya B. S. Prakash · Talmadge E. King, Jr.

Dermatologic manifestations of diseases that originate in other organs are commonly encountered in clinical practice. Frequently, the dermatologic sign is the initial signal of an internal illness. The best example of this is the presentation of paraneoplastic manifestations in the form of clubbing, dermatomyositis, acanthosis nigricans, bullous pemphigoid, and other external clinical features that point toward the possibility of an underlying malignancy (1). Among the malignant disorders, respiratory neoplasms are well known to cause paraneoplastic syndromes listed above. Many vasculitic syndromes and collagenoses also produce significant cutaneous lesions. These disorders are discussed in Chapters 28 and 32. Nonmalignant disorders such as pulmonary infections and pulmonary sarcoidosis may demonstrate dermal response in the form of erythema nodosum or erythema multiforme. This chapter addresses several of these entities and the respiratory manifestations of primary dermatologic diseases. However, many of these disorders cannot be classified as primary dermatoses, although their clinical presentations with cutaneous lesions warrant their inclusion here. Because of the lack of connection among most of the diseases included here, which makes an appropriate classification difficult, the diseases are discussed in alphabetic order.

ACANTHOSIS NIGRICANS AND OTHER PARANEOPLASTIC DERMATOSES

Acanthosis (*acantho,* thorn) nigricans (black) is an uncommon cutaneous disorder characterized by hyperpigmentation and epidermal hypertrophy (Fig. 63.1). The majority

U. B. S. Prakash: Pulmonary and Critical Care Medicine, Mayo Medical School and Mayo Medical Center, Rochester, Minnesota.

T. E. King, Jr.: Department of Medicine, University of California, San Francisco; and Medical Services, San Francisco General Hospital, San Francisco, California.

of cases of acanthosis nigricans are benign and associated with obesity. Insulin resistance is a common finding in all nonmalignancy-associated cases of acanthosis nigricans, e.g., diabetes mellitus, Cushing syndrome, and hypothyroidism (2–4). The paraneoplastic category of acanthosis nigricans is associated, in 90% of cases, with gastric adenocarcinoma and other intra-abdominal malignancies (5). Skin changes and an underlying neoplasm appear together in 60% of cases, whereas the cutaneous changes appear before clinical evidence of carcinoma in 20% of patients. Acanthosis nigricans may be the presenting clinical feature of lung cancer, with adenocarcinoma of the lung being the most common type of pulmonary malignancy associated with this skin disorder. Acanthosis nigricans has also been observed in a patient with bronchoalveolar cell carcinoma (6). The prognosis in patients with acanthosis and associated cancer is dismal. Progressive skin changes signify a higher mortality.

Tripe palms (paraneoplastic acrokeratosis), sometimes called Bazex syndrome, are characterized clinically by rugose, thickened, velvety palms with pronounced dermatoglyphic ridges and sulci. Tenderness around the fingernails also has been observed in this entity. Histologic examination reveals an undulant epidermis with hyperkeratosis, acanthosis, and papillomatosis. Over two thirds of the patients with tripe palms exhibit associated acanthosis nigricans. More than 90% of patients with tripe palms have an associated cancer, most commonly involving the lung or the stomach (7). Among the 77 patients with tripe palms, the most common underlying neoplasm was lung cancer (in 53%), whereas patients with both tripe palms and acanthosis nigricans had gastric cancer (in 35% of cases) or lung cancer (11% of cases) (8). Importantly, in more than 40% of patients, tripe palms were the presenting feature of a previously undiagnosed malignancy. Therefore, any patient with tripe palms must have a complete cancer workup, especially for lung and stomach cancer.

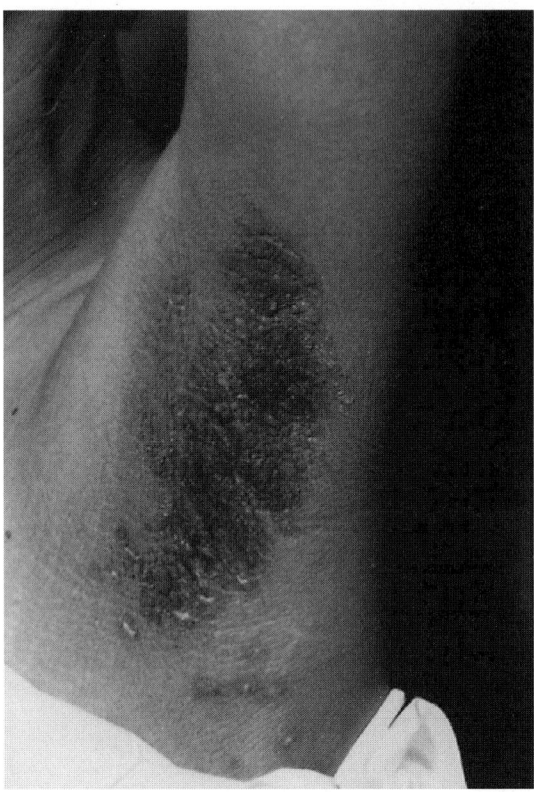

FIGURE 63.1. Acanthosis nigricans involving left axilla in a patient with adenocarcinoma of the lung. Marked hyperpigmentation and epidermal hypertrophy are the pathologic features.

Bowen disease is a chronic dermatosis characterized by the development of in situ epidermoid carcinoma of the skin (9). This disease has been linked to arsenic exposure in some cases; arsenic is a known carcinogen (10). The arsenic content of American tobacco was quite high until the early 1960s. This may explain some of the cases of lung cancer associated with Bowen disease described in the past.

Paraneoplastic pemphigus is a syndrome in which patients have a severe mucocutaneous eruption with clinical features similar to those of both erythema multiforme major (Stevens-Johnson syndrome) and pemphigus vulgaris, in association with non-Hodgkin lymphomas and other malignant neoplasms (11,12). Paraneoplastic pemphigus is an autoimmune disease characterized by the production of autoantibodies mainly directed against proteins of the plakin family (11). A patient has been described in whom non-Hodgkin lymphoma, in apparent complete remission after autologous bone marrow transplantation, developed bullous pemphigoid-like reaction and respiratory disease (13). Deposits of immunoglobulin (Ig) G were observed within the epithelium of the bronchial mucosa.

Tylosis or hyperkeratosis palmaris et plantaris, *epidermolysis bullosa, porphyria cutanea tarda,* and *acquired hypertrichosis lanuginosa* are among the other paraneoplastic cutaneous dermatoses associated with bronchogenic carcinoma. Many of these dermatoses precede the onset of the malignancy (1,14).

ACUTE FEBRILE NEUTROPHILIC DERMATOSIS

Acute febrile neutrophilic dermatitis (Sweet syndrome) is an uncommon, recurrent, often dramatic cutaneous disease manifested by fever; painful erythematous plaque-forming inflammatory papules on the face, neck, and limbs; arthralgias; and leukocytosis (15). Most cases are associated with a viral upper respiratory infection. There is a striking female predominance (4:1) (16). Approximately 10% of patients have associated malignancies, particularly hematologic neoplasms (17).

Pulmonary involvement has been described in several cases. Chest roentgenograms have revealed patchy pulmonary parenchymal infiltrates. Histologic features in lung biopsies have included diffuse interstitial edema, neutrophilic interstitial and alveolar exudates, bronchiolitis obliterans with organizing pneumonitis, recent hemorrhages, and hyperplasia of type I and II cells. Pulmonary pathologic findings in one patient consisted of marked intraalveolar neutrophilic infiltrates similar to skin biopsy findings, chronic interstitial pneumonitis, and minimal fibrosis; resolution was reported after corticosteroid therapy (18). A report on a 54-year-old woman with myelodysplasia described severe dyspnea and pulmonary infiltrates associated with recurrent episodes of Sweet syndrome (19). Lung and skin biopsies revealed a sterile infiltration of the interstitial tissues by mature neutrophils. Although corticosteroid therapy resulted in rapid clinical improvement, recurrent episodes became increasingly resistant to therapy, and she ultimately died from respiratory failure. Rare cases of primary lung cancer have been described in association with Sweet syndrome (20).

ANHIDROTIC ECTODERMAL DYSPLASIA

Anhidrotic ectodermal dysplasia is a hereditary, usually X-linked disorder characterized by insufficient sweating, sparse hair, and scanty teeth (21). Predisposition to severe bronchitis has been observed (22). Common upper respiratory infections occur often in these patients and have been ascribed to scanty mucus and deficient cilia. Absence of mucous glands in the tracheobronchial tree and increased incidence of asthma are the other respiratory features described in this disorder.

ATAXIA-TELANGIECTASIA

Also known as Louis-Bar syndrome, ataxia-telangiectasia is characterized by a progressive cerebellar ataxia, oculocutaneous telangiectasia, and recurrent sinopulmonary infections (23). This disorder is associated with deficiency of IgA and IgE and the development of lymphoreticular malignancies (24). In addition, granulocytopenia, noted in many of these patients, is a factor in frequent infections. Repeated sinopulmonary infections are noted in three fourths of patients with ataxia-telangiectasia, usually starting at approximately 4 to 6 years of age. Infection in nonrespiratory organs is uncommon. Severe neurologic impairment, bronchiectasis, and pulmonary fibrosis are usually progressive, leading to death by the time of adolescence (23). Roentgenologically, abnormalities are similar to those in cystic fibrosis, and both diseases manifest as chronic paranasal sinusitis. Upper airway dysfunction, identified by abnormal maximum inspiratory and expiratory flow-volume loops, has been described in patients with olivopontocerebellar atrophy.

BLUE RUBBER BLEB NEVUS SYNDROME

Less than 150 cases of the blue rubber bleb nevus syndrome (Bean syndrome), which is characterized by the presence of rubbery blue hemangiomas of the skin and gastrointestinal tract associated with gastrointestinal hemorrhage, have been reported in the literature (25). The rubbery angiomas of skin are variable in size, are compressible, and refill on release of pressure. Hemangiomas may occur in other organs, including the pleura. Those of the gastrointestinal tract cause profuse hemorrhage, whereas hemothorax has resulted from pleural hemangiomas. Hemothorax and hemopericardium are described in a patient with this syndrome (26). Histologic examination of pleural specimens has shown features similar to those in the skin.

CHEST WALL LESIONS

Confusion arises when chest roentgenograms reveal unusual abnormalities caused by lesions located in the chest wall. Initially diagnosed as pulmonary parenchymal lesions, many of these undergo extensive diagnostic testing. Good physical examination with a posteroanterior stereo chest roentgenogram and a lateral view will exclude an intrathoracic lesion. Unusual density, significant calcification, and association with skin lesions in areas other than the thoracic cage assist in excluding an intrathoracic lesion (Figs. 63.2 and 63.3).

CHRONIC MUCOCUTANEOUS CANDIDIASIS

Mucocutaneous candidiasis is an uncommon disorder associated with certain immunologic defects (27). Deficiency of the IgG_2/IgG_4 subclass and absence of antibodies against pneumococcal and *Hemophilus* polysaccharide occur in patients with this disorder (28). Detailed studies of a pediatric patient with mucocutaneous candidiasis and recurrent pulmonary infections revealed a severe defect in cell-mediated immunity, but humoral immune responses were normal. The disease may be complicated by candidiasis involving the

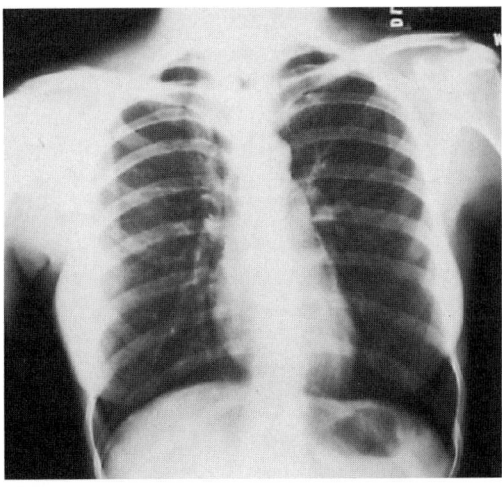

FIGURE 63.2. Thick braid of hair masquerading as a superior mediastinal mass in the right paratracheal region.

larynx, trachea, bronchi, and esophagus. Symptoms consist of hoarseness, hemoptysis, and dysphagia. Bacterial pneumonia, bronchopneumonic infiltrates, and bronchiectasis are some of the pulmonary manifestations described.

COGAN SYNDROME

Cogan syndrome is a disease of unknown origin characterized by audio-vestibular symptoms, nonsyphilitic interstitial keratitis, and systemic manifestations that include fever, anemia, elevated sedimentation rate, leukocytosis, and thrombocytosis (29). Complications include deafness, blindness, vasculitis, aortic insufficiency, and death. Variable

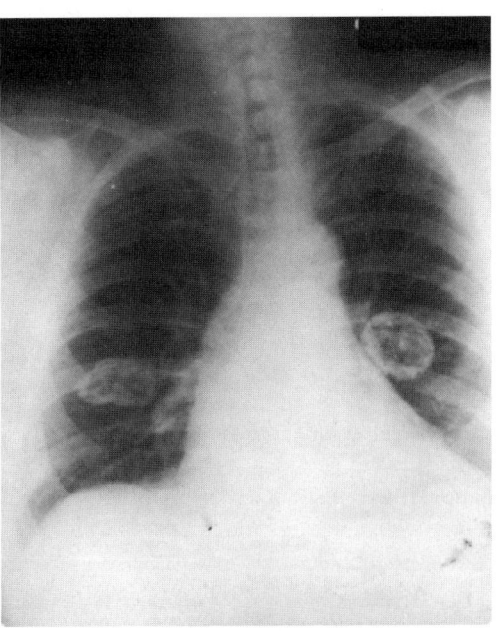

FIGURE 63.3. Calcified skin lesions appearing as intrapulmonary lesions on a single posteroanterior view.

cardiovascular involvement leading to aortic insufficiency or orificial stenosis of coronary or aortic arch vessels is a common complication (29,30).

Respiratory involvement is present in approximately 20% of patients and includes mild, sometimes transient, chest roentgenologic abnormalities and pleuropericarditis. An upper respiratory tract infection precedes onset of the syndrome in approximately 40% of patients. A review of 78 patients noted transient pulmonary infiltrates and pleuritis in 9% and 5%, respectively (31). Recurrent lung infiltrates have been described.

CUTIS LAXA

Cutis laxa (generalized elastolysis) is a rare systemic disorder of connective tissue in which the elastic fibers become fragmented, disorganized, and fewer in number (32). A congenital (X-linked recessive) and an acquired variety have been described. The acquired cases manifest in midlife, and their origin, genetic or otherwise, is unknown. The dermatologic abnormalities in cutis laxa seem to result mainly from a developmental defect of the elastic network in the papillary dermis. Both the congenital and acquired varieties exhibit identical clinical, physiological, and pathologic abnormalities. Cutaneous pathologic findings are characterized by the disappearance of elastic fibers of the skin (Fig. 63.4). The skin changes lead to an appearance of early senility. Because the disease affects connective tissues all over the body,

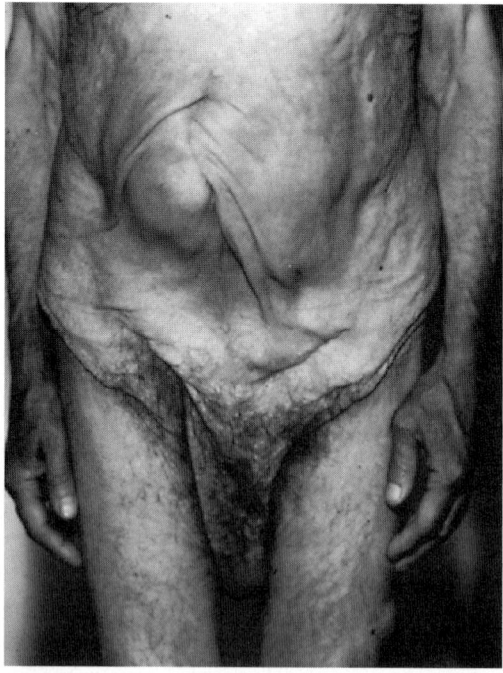

FIGURE 63.4. Cutis laxa (generalized elastolysis) shows loss of skin elasticity over lower trunk and external genitalia. This patient also had severe emphysema.

the clinical manifestations can be varied. Cutis laxa (loose skin), emphysema, aortic aneurysms, diverticula of bowel, and hernias are some of the complications. This disorder is distinct from Marfan syndrome, Ehlers-Danlos syndrome, and pseudoxanthoma elasticum.

The respiratory system ranks second only to the skin as the most commonly affected organ. The most frequent and serious pulmonary problem associated with cutis laxa is panlobular emphysema (32). Markedly elevated activity of an elastase-like serum enzyme, observed in some patients with cutis laxa, may predispose to the development of emphysema. Severe and rapidly progressive emphysema leads to early cor pulmonale, which is the most common cause of death among patients with the congenital variety. Emphysema also occurs in nearly 5% of patients with acquired cutis laxa. Other respiratory complications include pneumothorax, pulmonary fibrosis, pulmonary artery stenosis, eventration of the diaphragm, recurrent pulmonary infections, bronchiectasis, tracheobronchomegaly, and aneurysms of the thoracic aorta.

EHLERS-DANLOS SYNDROME

Ehlers-Danlos syndrome is a group of inherited disorders in which connective tissue diseases result from disorganization of collagen fibers (33). Deficiency of type III collagen may be responsible for the respiratory complications. Ultrastructural and biochemical analysis of the lung tissue have revealed a marked decrease in type III collagen and the production of less type III procollagen relative to type I procollagen by fibroblasts cultured from the abnormal lung. Electron microscopic examination of the lung tissue has shown dilated endoplasmic reticulum of the fibroblasts with normal collagen. Of the nine subtypes of Ehlers-Danlos syndrome, which generally are too difficult to distinguish from one another, only types I and IV are reported to be associated with a substantial risk of arterial rupture. Specifically, type IV, which is also known as the vascular or ecchymotic type, is associated with many serious complications. The disorder is clinically characterized by abnormal skin flaccidity, hyperextensibility of the joints, bleeding tendencies, atrophic scars, easy skin bruising, and pseudotumors.

Pulmonary involvement in Ehlers-Danlos syndrome results from weakness of the collagen in the lung tissue. Respiratory complications recorded include pneumothorax and bullous lung disease (33,34). Severe panacinar emphysema of lungs has been observed, and transient pulmonary cysts have been reported with this syndrome. Bronchiectasis resulting from weakened bronchial walls also has been reported. A dilated trachea, similar to that in Mounier-Kuhn syndrome, was noted in a patient with this disorder. Weakness of the pulmonary arterial wall may result in rupture and hemoptysis. Massive recurrent hemoptysis over a 6-year period followed by fatal lung hemorrhage has been described in a 27-year-old man. Pulmonary artery regurgitation and pulmonary valvular stenosis are described as well (35). An 18-year-old patient with Ehlers-Danlos syndrome, type IV, who developed recurrent large, thick-walled, lung cavitary lesions, probably a manifestation of focal lung rupture, has been described (36). A patient with Ehlers-Danlos syndrome that presented acutely with clinical and roentgenologic features suggestive of aortic dissection was found to have mediastinal hematoma with no evidence of aortic dissection and was treated conservatively with no complications (37).

EOSINOPHILIC FASCIITIS

The syndrome of eosinophilic fasciitis consists of symmetric thickening of the deep fascia between muscle and subcutis of the arms, legs, and torso. Skin biopsy reveals a normal epidermis and an inflammatory infiltrate in the deep fascia. More than 200 cases of this unusual syndrome have been reported. Visceral involvement is generally mild or absent. Clinically, the affected skin is thickened and indurated.

Pulmonary or pleural involvement are unusual features of eosinophilic fasciitis (38). When the skin around the thoracic cage becomes involved, the work of breathing is increased by the constricting effect of the thickened noncompliant skin ("hidebound chest") (39). Physical examination may reveal marked induration of the thoracic integument with a severely limited chest wall excursion. This extrapulmonary thoracic restriction has led to progressive respiratory limitation, documented by pulmonary function tests. Pulmonary parenchymal disease is not a feature, even though the diffusing capacity of carbon monoxide (DLCO) in some patients with this disorder has been found to be reduced to a very low level.

EPIDERMOLYSIS BULLOSA DYSTROPHICA

Epidermolysis bullosa represents a group of rare hereditary bullous disorders marked by blister formation after relatively minor trauma. Three types of the disease occur, depending on the site of disruption within the skin: simplex (above the basement membrane), dystrophic (below the basement membrane), and junctional (at the lamina lucida). Epidermolysis bullosa dystrophica generally presents in newborns and is characterized by noninflammatory bullous lesions that may affect the tracheobronchial mucosa and cause respiratory distress (40). Postmortem analysis of the airways in a 29-month-old boy who died from laryngeal obstruction secondary to this disorder showed intense mucosal inflammation and swelling of the seromucinous glands in the supraglottic airway (41). Localized subglottic edema and the formation of an inflammatory membrane in the trachea have led to chronic subglottic stridor. Even minimal trauma is reported to result in stricture formation. In one series of five children, three required tracheostomies acutely, and one died of airway obstruction (42). The laryngeal cysts are distinct from the cutaneous bullae or bullous pemphigoid.

ERYTHEMA MULTIFORME

Erythema multiforme, Stevens-Johnson syndrome, and toxic epidermal necrolysis are three disorders that have similar clinical features (43). There is controversy as to whether all three of these disorders exist along a single spectrum. Erythema multiforme is a systemic disorder characterized by generalized eruptions of red or violaceous macules that are similar to urticaria, papules, vesicles, or bullae; involvement of various internal organs; and fever (44). The most characteristic skin lesion is known as a target or bull's eye. A more severe form is generally described as Stevens-Johnson syndrome, in which mucocutaneous ulcerations are seen. The histopathology of Stevens-Johnson syndrome and toxic epidermal necrolysis are similar and distinct from that of erythema multiforme (43).

Although the association of erythema multiforme with respiratory infection caused by *Mycoplasma pneumoniae* is well known, the most common association of this disorder is with bacterial pneumonias caused by streptococci, *Pseudomonas* species, pneumococci, *Legionella* species, and *Hemophilus influenzae* (45,46). Erythema multiforme is also seen in association with histoplasmosis and blastomycosis. Noninfectious causes of erythema multiforme include penicillin, antipyretics, barbiturates, and sulfonamides. A literature review of 70 cases of *Mycoplasma* pneumoniae infections associated with the Stevens-Johnson syndrome recorded that none of the cases exhibited erythema multiforme (47). Most patients had prodromal symptoms of an upper respiratory tract infection before the onset of the eruption and an underlying pneumonia. These findings led the investigators to conclude that *M. pneumoniae* is the most common infectious agent associated with the Stevens-Johnson syndrome and that the infection is not associated with erythema multiforme.

Respiratory complications include bronchopneumonic infiltrates, massive pneumonic consolidations, miliary lesions, hilar lymphadenopathy, and, uncommonly, pleural effusions. Clinically, the pulmonary manifestations are indicated by laryngotracheobronchitis, cough, hemoptysis, dyspnea, and cyanosis. In a 46-year-old woman with active systemic lupus erythematosus, severe Stevens-Johnson syndrome developed 8 hours after intravenous urography with the nonionic contrast medium iopamidol. The illness included erythema multiforme, intrahepatic cholestasis, pulmonary infiltrates, and acute renal failure, which led to her death. Rapidly progressive and fatal bronchiolitis obliterans was observed in a middle-aged woman. Stevens-Johnson syndrome with supraglottic laryngeal obstruction has been described.

The diagnosis and management of erythema multiforme and Stevens-Johnson syndrome are complex and controversial. Systemic corticosteroids have been used successfully in many instances.

ERYTHEMA NODOSUM

Erythema nodosum is a self-limited cutaneous disorder characterized by inflammatory nodules in the dermis and subcutaneous tissues, commonly along the extensor aspects of the legs. This form of panniculitis is clinically characterized by pain in the anterior tibial area, followed by development of tender pink nodules on the shins. The lesions normally resolve spontaneously over a period of several weeks. The appearance is so characteristic that biopsy is seldom required. Erythema nodosum is most likely a hypersensitivity reaction to a broad variety of disorders, especially drug reactions and infection by viruses, bacteria, and fungi. The cause of erythema nodosum remains unknown in approximately half the patients.

Sarcoidosis is one of the common diseases associated with erythema nodosum (48). Erythema nodosum has been observed in 13% of two large series of patients with sarcoidosis. Erythema nodosum can be the presenting manifestation of sarcoidosis. The presence of erythema nodosum in patients with sarcoidosis is associated with a good prognosis, and an acute onset of sarcoidosis with erythema nodosum signifies a good prognosis and spontaneous resolution. Erythema nodosum in conjunction with non-Hodgkin lymphoma that presents as a solitary pulmonary nodule has also been described.

Histoplasmosis and coccidioidomycosis are common causes of erythema nodosum in the United States. Pulmonary blastomycosis associated also with erythema nodosum has been described (49). Tuberculosis, although an uncommon cause of erythema nodosum in most developed countries, should always be looked for and excluded, especially in endemic areas. Among 305 children with postprimary tuberculosis, erythema nodosum was observed in 37 (12%). As in sarcoidosis, erythema nodosum in association with these infections denotes a good prognosis because such a combination confirms the development of antibodies or hypersensitivity to the pathogenic antigens. Erythema nodosum was observed in 28% of 88 cases of tularemia in northern Finland, and pulmonary tularemia was present in 27% of the patients (50). Erythema nodosum was seen more often in patients with pulmonary tularemia than in other forms of the disease.

FAMILIAL MEDITERRANEAN FEVER

Familial Mediterranean fever, also known as periodic disease, is an autosomal-recessive inherited disorder characterized by recurrent episodes of fever accompanied by inflammation of the peritoneum, pleura, synovial membranes (recurrent polyserositis), and skin. The disorder predominantly affects persons of Mediterranean origin (Sephardic Jews, Armenians, and Arabs) and is rare in other groups. The familial Mediterranean fever gene, named MEFV, is located on the short arm of chromosome 16 (51,52).

The most serious complication of the disease is amyloidosis, which is the cause of death in a substantial proportion of adult patients (53). Abdominal pain, which occurs in more than 95% of patients, is an important aspect of the disease. Acute arthritis occurs in 17% to 75% of patients.

Pulmonary manifestations commonly occur in the form of pleuritic chest pain in 35% to 85% of patients (54,55). Recurrent pleuritic chest pains are common and may be associated with small pleural effusions. Right-sided effusions are reported to be more common. Pulmonary hypertension and pulmonary amyloidosis have been described in familial Mediterranean fever.

Asthma is reported to occur less commonly in patients with familial Mediterranean fever, but this remains unproven (54,55). A study of 148 parents of patients with familial Mediterranean fever and of 148 ethnically matched control persons demonstrated an apparently reduced prevalence of asthma in the heterozygotes compared with those of the control subjects (three versus six) (56). The investigators of this study concluded that their data were in agreement with previous studies that demonstrated decreased asthma prevalence in patients with familial Mediterranean fever.

HEREDITARY HEMORRHAGIC TELANGIECTASIA

Hereditary hemorrhagic telangiectasia (Osler-Weber-Rendu disease) is an autosomal-dominant inherited disorder characterized by telangiectasia of the skin and mucous membranes and by intermittent bleeding from arteriovenous malformations and fistulas. The prevalence of simultaneous hereditary hemorrhagic telangiectasia and pulmonary arteriovenous malformation during a 10-year period in one Scandinavian county of more than 429,207 inhabitants was 2.6 per 100,000 (57). Investigators from the Mayo Clinic documented 194 cases of pulmonary arteriovenous malformation over a total of 45 years, for an annual incidence at that center of 4.3 cases/y (58–60). The male–female ratio was 1:2. Telangiectasias of the skin and oral, nasal, and conjunctival mucosa manifest in the second and third decades of life. They appear bright red, punctate, or linear, and they blanch under pressure. Gastrointestinal bleeding occurs in approximately 15% of patients.

Hereditary hemorrhagic telangiectasia is the most common cause of pulmonary arteriovenous fistula. In a study of seven families that participated in screening for pulmonary arteriovenous malformations and hereditary hemorrhagic telangiectasia, 36 (80%) of the 45 screened family members were found to have hereditary hemorrhagic telangiectasia, and 13 (36%) of the 36 family members with hereditary hemorrhagic telangiectasia were proven to have pulmonary arteriovenous malformations by pulmonary angiography (61). A report on 53 patients with pulmonary arteriovenous malformations observed that 42 (79%) patients had associated hereditary hemorrhagic telangiectasia.

The rate of occurrence of pulmonary arteriovenous fistulas is determined by the mutations in endoglin. In a genetic study, members of families with the mutation in endoglin (the locus has been designated ORW1) exhibited a 29% prevalence of pulmonary arteriovenous malformations compared with a prevalence rate of 3% in families in which ORW1 was excluded (62). A genetically determined location for a second ORW locus with linkage to chromosome 12 has been identified in patients with significantly reduced incidence of pulmonary involvement (63).

Pulmonary arteriovenous malformation is a rare cause of cyanosis in the newborn (64). Among the nine previously reported neonatal cases, typical signs at presentation included cyanosis, murmur, and congestive cardiac failure. Chest roentgenographs commonly exhibited cardiomegaly, oligemia, and focal pulmonary density. The majority of pulmonary fistulas are detected in the third and fourth decades of life. The pulmonary fistulas usually occur in the lower lobes of lungs and are multiple in nearly 35% of patients. Typically, chest roentgenograms show the pulmonary arteriovenous fistulas as oval or round homogeneous nodular lesions that measure from a few millimeters to several centimeters in diameter. These fistulas tend to evolve and continue to enlarge over long periods, sometimes as long as 24 years. A standard chest roentgenogram may show a nodular shadow but can easily obscure small afferent and efferent vessels attached to the fistula (Fig. 63.5). The risk of relying solely on the standard chest roentgenogram becomes apparent when a transthoracic needle aspiration is performed, with resultant serious hemorrhage. Simple tomography generally discloses an artery entering the fistula and a vein leaving it (Fig. 63.6). Pulmonary angiography confirms the diagnosis in virtually all cases and is required before embolotherapy or surgical resection of a fistula is undertaken (Fig. 63.7). Cases of spontaneous pneumothorax and hemothorax secondary to intrapleural rupture of an arteriovenous fistula have been observed. Endobronchial mucosal or submucosal telangiectasias are distinctly uncommon. They may come to light when bronchoscopy is performed to investigate hemoptysis. Telangiectasia of the nasal mucosa occurs more frequently than does endobronchial fistula and leads to recurrent bouts of epistaxis.

Dyspnea and hemoptysis are the two common symptoms. The severity of dyspnea depends on the degree of right-to-left shunting. Although dyspnea is present in nearly 60% of patients, hemoptysis (occurring in 10%–20%) is the most common presenting symptom. This can be brisk but usually is not life-threatening. In a study of 143 patients

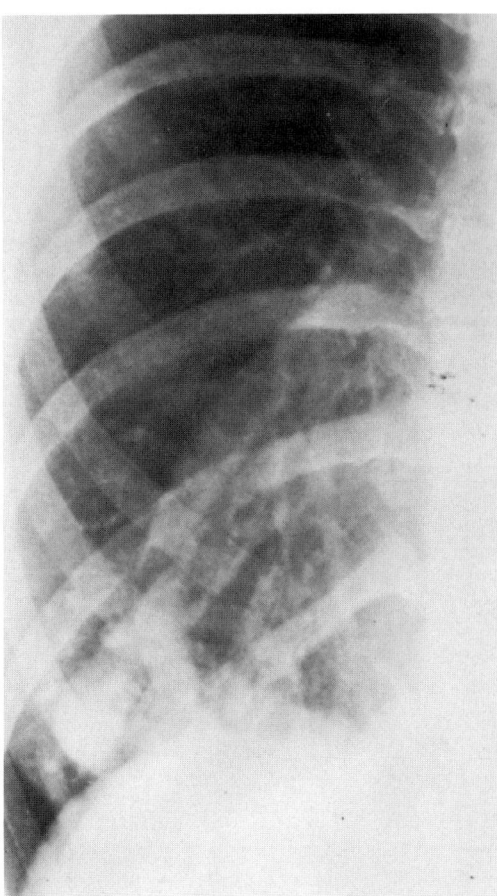

FIGURE 63.5. Pulmonary arteriovenous malformation in right lower lobe of a patient with hereditary hemorrhagic telangiectasia reveals afferent and efferent vessels attached to the fistula.

with pulmonary arteriovenous malformations associated with hereditary hemorrhagic telangiectasia, 11 (8%) patients (seven women and four men) had a history of either massive hemoptysis or hemothorax; one patient died because of the pulmonary hemorrhage (65). Among the seven women, three had pulmonary hemorrhage during pregnancy. The increased risk of bleeding from the arteriovenous malformations during pregnancy has been reported in several cases.

Among the 93 patients with pulmonary arteriovenous fistulas seen at the Mayo Clinic, 15 patients (16%) were asymptomatic (60). Notable clinical findings included epistaxis in 46 (49%), hemoptysis in 14 (15%), cyanosis in 27 (29%), clubbing in 18 (19%), dyspnea in 53 (57%), and pulmonary bruits/murmurs in 32 (34%) (60). Pulmonary artery catheterization generally reveals diminished arterial oxygen tension and saturation but normal pulmonary artery pressure. Echocardiography is a less invasive method for detecting extracardiac right-to-left shunts. After venous injection of indocyanine green dye or agitated saline, the characteristic contrast flow pattern consists of a markedly delayed appearance of echoes in the left ventricle. However, this type

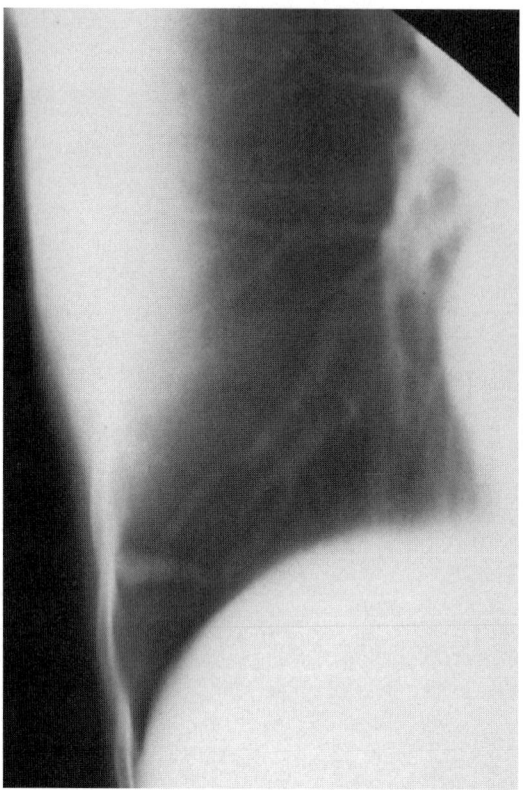

FIGURE 63.6. Localized tomography sometimes is necessary to identify pulmonary arteriovenous malformation, especially when the fistula is small.

of assessment does not calculate the degree of shunt. Administering 100% oxygen and obtaining blood samples for measurements of gas tensions allow calculation of the physiological shunt.

Paradoxic embolism is a common and serious complication of pulmonary arteriovenous fistulas; the occurrence of

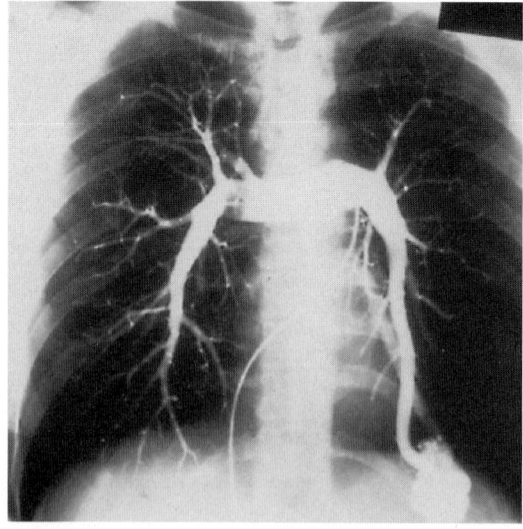

FIGURE 63.7. Pulmonary angiogram in hereditary hemorrhagic telangiectasia shows a large arteriovenous malformation in the left lower lobe.

this complication has been noted at presentation in more than one third of patients. A report on 53 patients with pulmonary arteriovenous malformations indicated that 19 (36%) patients had neurologic problems compatible with paradoxic embolization (66). Among 67 patients with pulmonary arteriovenous malformations associated with hereditary hemorrhagic telangiectasia, strokes and transient ischemic attacks were recorded in 37% (67). Another report observed that four of five patients with asymptomatic small- or moderate-sized pulmonary arteriovenous malformations presented with stroke caused by paradoxic embolism. A review of the English-language literature in 1990 disclosed 52 cases of neurologic complications, but not all were caused by paradoxic emboli originating in pulmonary arteriovenous fistulas. Indeed, among a series of more than 200 reported patients with hereditary hemorrhagic telangiectasia and associated neurologic sequelae, 61% developed neurologic lesions secondary to pulmonary arteriovenous fistula, whereas 36% of the patients with neurologic manifestations exhibited vascular malformations of the brain and spinal cord.

Various neurologic manifestations are reported in up to 30% of patients. Brain abscess, estimated to occur in approximately 1% of patients, can be the presenting feature of hereditary hemorrhagic telangiectasia. Mental obtundation, headache, visual disturbances, hemiplegia, and seizures are the most common presenting features of paradoxic embolism to the neurologic system (68). Leukocytosis and fever are not prominent features, and blood cultures are generally sterile. However, in patients with brain abscesses, anaerobic and microaerophilic streptococci are the most common pathogens isolated. In a series of 31 patients with hereditary hemorrhagic telangiectasia and neurologic involvement, 13 patients died, and patients without abscess drainage or with delayed diagnosis had a higher mortality.

Unusual complications described in patients with hereditary hemorrhagic telangiectasia include high-output congestive cardiac failure, portosystemic encephalopathy (from hepatic arteriovenous malformations), and disseminated intravascular coagulation. In a report on 47 patients with documented hereditary hemorrhagic telangiectasia, disseminated intravascular coagulation was observed in 51%.

The treatment of choice is pulmonary artery embolotherapy (therapeutic embolization) using coils and other intravascular devices (66). The aim of such treatments is to reduce right-to-left shunts. As new fistulas evolve in the same patient, or recanalization occurs in the embolized fistulas over a period of time, repeated embolizations may be necessary (Figs. 63.8 and 63.9). A publication on embolotherapy in 67 patients with pulmonary arteriovenous malformations associated with hereditary hemorrhagic telangiectasia reported that the physiological improvements remained stable for 5 years after embolotherapy, complications were minimal, and surgery was not required in any patient. In another report on 11 patients with pulmonary arteriovenous malformations, lung function tests before

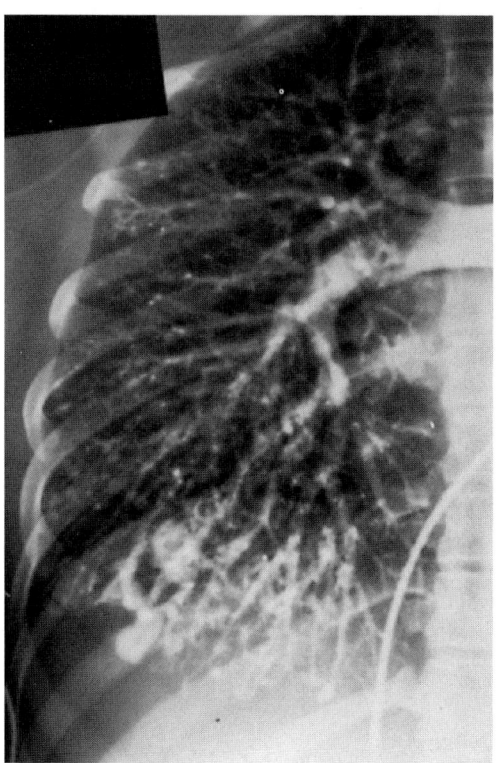

FIGURE 63.8. Multiple arteriovenous malformations in the right lower lobe. This patient had multiple bilateral arteriovenous malformations.

embolotherapy disclosed normal vital capacity and FEV_1/FVC ratios, reduced $DLCO$ (mean, 71% of predicted; range, 36%–123%), a resting supine arterial oxygen saturation of 86% (range, 67%–95%), mean shunt fraction of 33% (range, 15%–47%), and well-preserved exercise capacity (69). Six months after therapy, the mean shunt fraction decreased

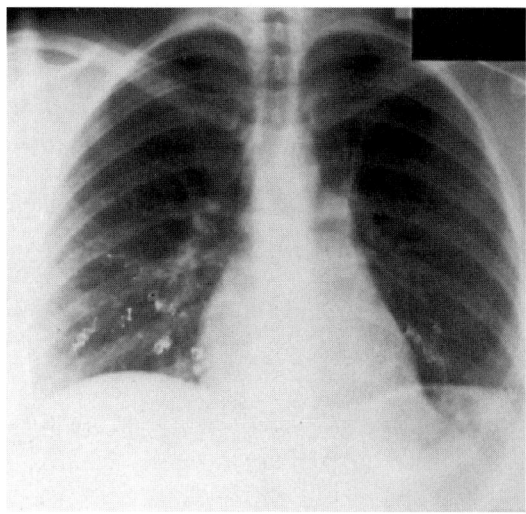

FIGURE 63.9. Chest roentgenogram of the patient shown in Figure 63.8 after multiple steel-coil embolizations. This patient has required several embolizations for recurrent arteriovenous malformations.

from 33% to 19%, and resting arterial oxygen saturation increased from 86% to 92%. A consistent improvement in $DLCO$ was also seen. There were no long-term complications after embolotherapy. In another report, 32 patients with 92 pulmonary arteriovenous malformations (with feeding arteries >3 mm) were treated by coil embolization and followed up for a mean period of 25 months, and the mean shunt fraction decreased from 16.6% to 7.4%; treatment was incomplete in two patients, one of whom was subsequently treated surgically (70). Others also have documented the immediate improvement in respiratory symptoms, exercise capacity, and gas exchange at rest and during exercise as a result of the embolization-induced reduction in right-to-left shunt. Even though hypoxia induced by right-to-left shunt does not respond to oxygen therapy, many patients subjectively feel better with supplemental oxygen.

Complications of coli embolization therapy have been noted in 10% of procedures (71). They have included potentially serious problems such as systemic coil embolization, cerebrovascular accident, and myocardial puncture.

Large arteriovenous fistulas (diameter of efferent vessel >10 mm) may require surgical resection. The life expectancy of patients with hereditary hemorrhagic telangiectasia is not reduced provided treatable complications are diagnosed and treated promptly.

HYPERHIDROSIS

Hyperhidrosis, or abnormally excessive production of sweat, can signify an underlying malignancy (72). Idiopathic hyperhidrosis (seen in approximately 1% of the population) is a benign increase in eccrine sweating without pathologic cause (73). Unilateral hyperhidrosis of the chest cage has been described in patients with lung cancer. In most reported cases, hyperhidrosis has been limited to the same side as the tumor. It is speculated that direct irritation of nerves may excite the autonomic efferent fibers. The presence of hyperhidrosis indicates a poor prognosis. Resection of a cervical rib may abolish the hyperhidrosis.

ANHIDROSIS

Anhidrosis or abnormally diminished production of sweat can be encountered as part of the paraneoplastic syndrome. An example of this is the anhidrosis seen in Horner syndrome, in which the other features include ipsilateral miosis and ptosis. These changes and anhidrosis occur on the same side as the pulmonary neoplasm.

MALIGNANT ATROPHIC PAPULOSIS

Malignant atrophic papulosis (Degos disease) is a rare multisystemic disorder characterized by typical skin and gastrointestinal symptoms. The distinctive skin lesions begin as rose-colored dome-shaped papules, which subsequently develop an umbilicated atrophic porcelain-white center (74). Approximately 150 cases have been reported worldwide (74). The male-to-female ratio is 3:1. The age of reported cases ranges from 7 to 70 years, although it most commonly presents in the third and fourth decades (74). Many patients demonstrate a rapidly fatal course. The presenting clinical feature is the appearance of crops of asymptomatic oval skin lesions that range from 2 to 8 mm in diameter. A review of 60 reported cases of Degos disease found that 17 included intrathoracic abnormalities, most of which were found incidentally at postmortem (75). The most common intrathoracic findings were pleuritis and pericarditis. Bilateral hemorrhagic pleural effusions, pleural plaques, pulmonary infarcts, and pulmonary abscesses also were noted.

MASTOCYTOSIS

Systemic mastocytosis, or mast cell disease, is an uncommon disorder characterized by urticaria pigmentosa, hepatosplenomegaly, osteosclerotic bone lesions, diarrhea, nausea, vomiting, and flushing. There are four forms of systemic mastocytosis distinguished by clinical presentation, degree and type of extracutaneous organ involvement, and associated hematologic syndromes or malignancies (76). Respiratory manifestations include interstitial lung disease and extensive peribronchial and alveolar infiltration with mast cells. There are several reports of systemic mastocytosis associated with mediastinal germ cell tumors.

NEUROFIBROMATOSIS

Neurofibromatosis (von Recklinghausen disease) is a common disease of variably expressive autosomal-dominant inheritance characterized by café-au-lait spots, freckling, and neurofibromas of skin and internal organs. The neurofibromatosis type 1 gene has been mapped to chromosome 17q11.2 and cloned (77). Its incidence is one per 3,000; approximately half the cases occur sporadically (78). Cutaneous lesions are the result of the maldevelopment of neural crest cells. The number of dermal neurofibromas varies from individual to individual. Large plexiform neurofibromas develop along peripheral nerves and involve deeper tissues. Extracutaneous (visceral) involvement may not be apparent during life unless such lesions produce symptoms.

Respiratory involvement occurs in 10% to 15% of patients with neurofibromatosis. Although neurofibromatosis is a congenital disorder, the lung involvement does not become evident until adulthood. Up to 20% of patients older than 35 years develop diffuse interstitial fibrosis (79). Diminished perfusion and ventilation to apices of the lungs has been documented by radionuclide studies in a patient with

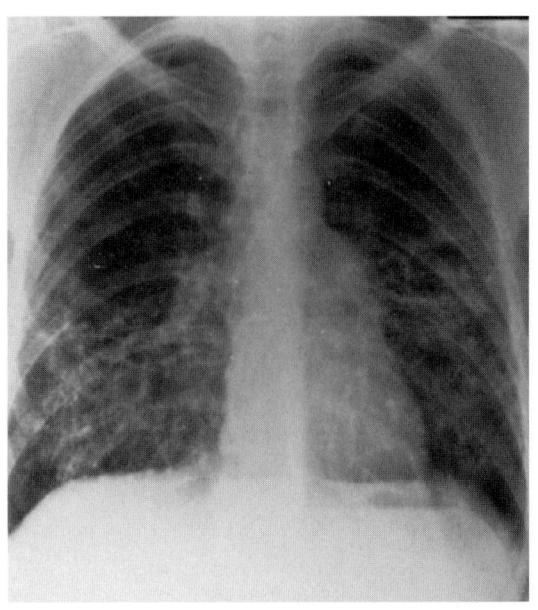

FIGURE 63.10. Neurofibromatosis with pulmonary manifestations showing bullous changes in the upper lung zone and honeycomb changes in the lower lungs.

cutaneous neurofibromatosis. Bullous lung disease may occur alone or in combination with diffuse pulmonary fibrosis. Pulmonary fibrosis usually is seen in the basal areas of the lungs, whereas the bullous lesions occur predominantly in the apical areas (Fig. 63.10). Cystic lung disease resembling honeycomb lung also has been described.

The pulmonary parenchymal disease is attributed to a mesenchymal defect resulting in primary deposition of collagen. The histologic features mimic those of idiopathic pulmonary fibrosis. Ultrastructural studies have shown fragmentation of collagen fibers in the lung. The clinical manifestations are mild, usually consisting only of exertional dyspnea, but a restrictive pattern of pulmonary function and diminished diffusing capacity often are observed.

Intrathoracic neurofibromas and meningoceles may be associated with a dermal form of neurofibromatosis, but these usually remain undetected because they rarely are symptomatic (Fig. 63.11). An earlier review of the literature reported 27 cases of intrathoracic meningoceles with neurofibromatosis. Since then, more than a dozen such associations have been reported. When these lesions are situated in the posterior mediastinum, as they commonly are, they may represent so-called dumbbell tumors with intraspinal extension (80). Magnetic resonance imaging of the involved spinal area is helpful in assessing the anatomic extent of such tumors.

Neurofibromatosis can involve the mediastinum. A 44-year-old woman with a dumbbell-shaped mediastinal mass developed a large pleural effusion, respiratory failure, and fatal hemoptysis (81). Autopsy revealed systemic neurofibromatosis involving the mediastinum and pleura. Mediastinal and pleural hemorrhage probably occurred as a result of

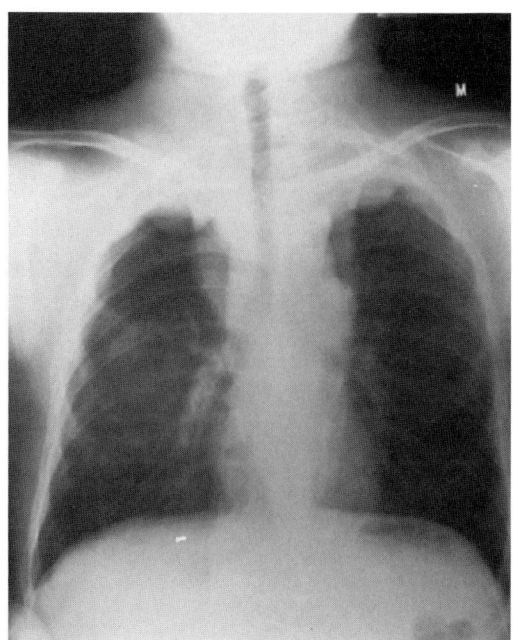

FIGURE 63.11. Neurofibromatosis with intrathoracic neurofibromas.

an eroded thoracic artery. Primary pulmonary parenchymal neurofibromas are rare. Benign neurogenous tumors arising in the trachea are also uncommon. Laryngeal involvement in neurofibromatosis is rare, and the predominant pulmonary features include dyspnea, stridor, loss or change of voice, and dysphagia (82). A report described a patient with neurofibromatosis who presented with dyspnea caused by endotracheal neurofibroma (83). Hoarseness may result from recurrent laryngeal nerve involvement.

Primary or secondary malignancy in the lung has been overlooked in two patients with generalized neurofibromatosis because of roentgenographic confusion caused by overlying cutaneous lesions (see section "Chest Wall Lesions"). Neurofibromatosis is associated with an increased incidence of malignancy, ranging from malignant tumors of the central nervous system to Wilms tumor, rhabdomyosarcoma, leukemia, and pheochromocytoma. In 5% of patients, the neurofibromas in neurofibromatosis undergo transformation to malignant degeneration and commonly metastasize to the lungs. Scar cancer of the lung has been reported as a complication of the chronic pulmonary process in neurofibromatosis.

NONSUPPURATIVE PANNICULITIS

Sometimes referred to as *Weber-Christian disease,* nonsuppurative panniculitis is characterized by cutaneous nodular fat necrosis of the panniculus adiposum (84,85). Tender, erythematous, subcutaneous nodules appear over the extremities and trunk.

A review in 1976 reported pulmonary involvement in only five cases (86). Pulmonary manifestations include pulmonary fat emboli and infarcts, lipogranulomatous pneumonitis with nodules measuring 0.8 to 3 cm in diameter, and fluffy roentgenographic densities bilaterally. Recurrent pneumonia and pleural effusion also occur (87). Interestingly, α_1-antitrypsin deficiency has been found in some patients with acute panniculitis (88–91). There is no report of emphysematous lung disease occurring as a result of this. A recent case report described recurrent panniculitis in a man with asthma who was receiving treatment with leukotriene-modifying agents (92).

OCULOCUTANEOUS ALBINISM

Sometimes called *pulmonary ceroidosis* or the *Hermansky-Pudlak syndrome,* oculocutaneous albinism is an autosomal-recessive disorder characterized by oculocutaneous tyrosinase-positive albinism, platelet pool disease with moderate bleeding tendency, and lysosomal accumulation of ceroid-lipofuscin, an amorphous lipid-protein complex in the reticuloendothelial system. A review of the literature in 1989 recorded more than 200 cases of the Hermansky-Pudlak syndrome, the most striking feature of which is the presence of clinically recognizable oculocutaneous albinism. However, the most frequent clinical complication is hemorrhage, and epistaxis is the most common hemorrhagic manifestation.

Respiratory involvement is a recognized complication in oculocutaneous albinism (93). Ceroid-lipofuscin, which accumulates in a variety of cells, including alveolar macrophages, may cause pulmonary fibrosis (93). The primary disease affects men and women equally, but the incidence of lung disease is twice as high in women as in men. The pulmonary disease is similar to idiopathic pulmonary fibrosis and usually begins in the third or fourth decade of life (94). Bronchoalveolar lavage in asymptomatic patients has shown that the concentration of platelet-derived growth factor–related peptides is six times greater in patients with Hermansky-Pudlak syndrome than in normal subjects (95). These peptides are important in the initiation of alveolar remodeling in the fibrotic lung disorders and are perhaps involved in the pathogenesis of lung disease in this syndrome.

Clinically, constant nonproductive cough and progressive dyspnea are the chief symptoms. Dyspnea can develop suddenly over several weeks or gradually over years, and the respiratory disease can progress to end-stage fibrosis and death. High-resolution computed tomography (CT) was more sensitive than was chest radiography in evaluating the extent of pulmonary disease in patients with Hermansky-Pudlak syndrome (93). Common chest radiographic findings included reticular or nodular interstitial pattern, perihilar fibrosis, and pleural thickening. High-resolution CT showed septal thickening, ground-glass opacities, and peribronchovascular thickening (93). The pulmonary pathology in oculocutaneous albinism is compatible with oxidant injury as it parallels pathologic alterations seen with pulmonary oxygen toxicity. Bronchoalveolar lavage may show alveolar macrophages containing typical ceroid-like material. Brown-pigmented histiocytes have been demonstrated in the alveolar spaces. Increased levels of immunoglobulins, numbers of IgG- and IgA-secreting cells, and normal percentages of helper and suppressor T cells are observed. The pulmonary fibrosis is an irreversible and progressive process. No specific therapy is available for the lung disease.

Pulmonary ceroidosis occurs in many of the approximately 30 disorders in which systemic or localized deposition of ceroid occurs. Sea-blue histiocytosis syndrome is an example of ceroidosis, and lung involvement is present in 11% of these patients. Idiopathic pulmonary ceroidosis may represent pulmonary alveolar deposition of ceroid-like material in the absence of clinical or biochemical data characteristic of any specific ceroid storage disease. Interestingly, deposition of ceroid-like pigment in the pulmonary alveolar macrophages has been reported in eight patients with carcinoma of the stomach.

PEMPHIGOID

The association of bullous pemphigoid with lung cancer was discussed earlier. Cicatricial pemphigoid, however, is a non-paraneoplastic chronic vesiculobullous disease of the mucosal epithelium that primarily involves the oral cavity and the eyes (96). This chronic mucosal blistering disorder exhibits a predilection for subsequent scar formation. Airway obstruction and laryngeal stenosis, several of which required tracheostomy, have been described in patients with cicatricial pemphigoid. An unusual case of a 20-year-old woman who died of respiratory failure and was noted to have cicatricial pemphigoid of the bronchi is reported (97). A case of a 22-year-old man with cicatricial pemphigoid in whom severe stenosis of the left mainstem bronchus developed 2 years after onset of the disease is described; therapy by sleeve resection and end-to-end anastomosis was successful. Pulmonary hemorrhage associated with bullous pemphigoid of the lung has been described. Stenosis of the nasopharynx or larynx has resulted in obstructive sleep apnea.

PSEUDOXANTHOMA ELASTICUM

Pseudoxanthoma elasticum is a rare disorder characterized by fragmentation and calcification of elastic fibers in skin, blood vessels, and retina. Both autosomal-dominant and -recessive forms have been described. Adenosine triphosphate–binding cassette subfamily C member 6 gene has been demonstrated to be responsible for pseudoxanthoma elasticum, and 43 mutations have been identified to date (98). One patient with pseudoxanthoma elasticum has been reported in whom the lung biopsy showed widespread deposition of calcium in the walls of some arteries, arterioles, and venules, with swollen, short, irregularly clumped elastic fibers and irregularity of the elastic laminae (99).

PYODERMA GANGRENOSUM

Pyoderma gangrenosum is a painful, chronic, destructive, and ulcerating skin disease of unknown origin. The occurrence of this disorder in intestinal diseases is well known. In a report on 86 patients with this disease, inflammatory bowel disease was present in 36% (100). Asthma or chronic obstructive pulmonary disease was noted in 5%. Pulmonary abscess has been described in a patient with pyoderma gangrenosum, but the relationship between pyoderma gangrenosum and pulmonary disease remains unclear (101). Pyoderma gangrenosum of the skin and trachea has been described in a 9-month-old boy.

TUBEROUS SCLEROSIS

Tuberous sclerosis (Bourneville disease) is an autosomal-dominant disease of mesodermal development characterized clinically by epilepsy and mental retardation and pathologically by congenital tumors and malformations of the brain, skin, and viscera. (see Chapter 32). The classic clinical triad in tuberous sclerosis consists of adenoma sebaceum, mental retardation, and seizures. Skin lesions, in addition to adenoma sebaceum or dermal angiofibroma, include ash leaf spots (a hypopigmented skin lesion, the earliest to appear in tuberous sclerosis), shagreen patches (hamartomas of connective tissue seen in 50% of patients and located over the lumbosacral area), and periungual fibromas (benign pink fibrous neoplasms adjacent to the nails and seen in 15%–20% of patients). Poliosis, or hypopigmentation of the scalp hair or eyelashes, also is seen. Extracutaneous manifestations include seizure disorder, electroencephalographic abnormalities, or both in 80% to 90% of patients; mental retardation of wide-ranging severity; a hamartomatous lesion of the central nervous system; retinal phakomas; angiomyolipomas of the kidney; renal and bone cysts; and cardiac rhabdomyomas.

Some consider tuberous sclerosis and pulmonary lymphangioleiomyomatosis to be the same clinical entity because of the many striking similarities in clinical, roentgenologic, and pathologic features. However, the presence of hormonal (estrogen, progesterone) receptors in lymphangioleiomyomatosis may distinguish it from tuberous sclerosis, although not all patients with lymphangioleiomyomatosis exhibit these receptors. Chylous effusion is more common in lymphangioleiomyomatosis, whereas angiomyolipomas are much more common in tuberous sclerosis. The difficulty of separating these two entities as distinct diseases is further enhanced by the observation that several patients reported in the literature with the diagnosis of tuberous sclerosis have responded favorably to hormonal therapy that is used to treat pulmonary lymphangioleiomyomatosis. Furthermore, the clinical features are not overt in many patients; indeed, a study of nine patients with pulmonary tuberous sclerosis noted that there was an average delay of 8 years before the correct diagnosis was made. Details on pulmonary lymphangioleiomyomatosis are included in Chapter 32.

Morphologic analysis of the lungs affected by tuberous sclerosis reveals multiple cysts measuring a few millimeters in diameter. The walls of the cysts are formed of hypertrophied smooth muscle cells. The compression of the bronchioles caused by the hypertrophied smooth muscles leads to obstruction, air trapping, bulla formation, and pneumothorax. The compression of the pulmonary venules results in venous congestion and hemoptysis, whereas the compression of the pulmonary arterioles may lead to pulmonary hypertension. The same mechanism, when it involves the lymphatic channels, causes chylothorax. Ultrastructural morphologic analysis of the lung in tuberous sclerosis has shown findings identical to those in lymphangioleiomyomatosis. Cystic disease of the lung with focal adenomatoid proliferation is among the least common pathologic features of tuberous sclerosis.

Pulmonary function tests demonstrate obstructive pulmonary dysfunction despite the nodular interstitial appearance of lungs on the chest roentgenograms. Obstruction to airflow is caused by the compression of the smaller airways by the smooth muscles that undergo hyperplasia. This mechanism also contributes to the increased lung volumes and thoracic hyperinflation. Air space lesions, however, are reported to be more important than is muscular proliferation in bringing about these physiological abnormalities.

Respiratory disease is seen in less than 2% of patients with tuberous sclerosis (102). Often, there is a delay in the diagnosis of pulmonary disease, and many patients are treated for asthma or emphysema. A review of the literature in 1971 noted that there were only 31 reported cases of pulmonary tuberous sclerosis (103). Pulmonary tuberous sclerosis usually involves other organs. Indeed, in the largest series of nine patients with pulmonary tuberous sclerosis reported in 1995, seizure was the most common presenting feature (104). The pulmonary disease tends to develop in adult life and occurs much more commonly among women of childbearing age (18–34 years) who do not have mental retardation and epileptic seizures. Lung disease has been observed in a mother and daughter from a family with tuberous sclerosis for four generations. Only two male patients with pulmonary tuberous sclerosis are described; neither had pathologic documentation of lung disease. The disease may be rapidly fatal after the onset of respiratory symptoms. Exertional dyspnea is the most common respiratory symptom and may progress to the point of disability. Hemoptysis occurs in up to 25% of patients. The diffuse pulmonary interstitial process may progress to honeycombing and cyst formation, spontaneous pneumothorax, and cor pulmonale (Fig. 63.12). An earlier review of the literature revealed 19 cases of spontaneous

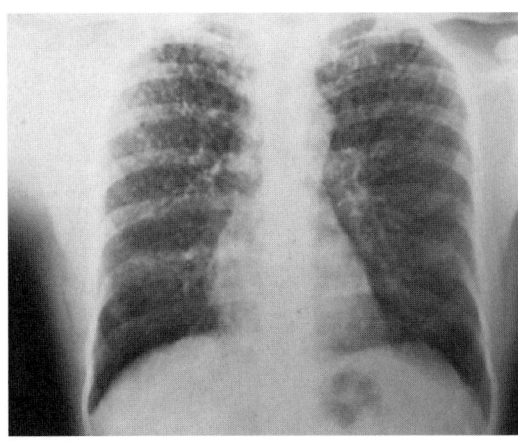

FIGURE 63.12. Tuberous sclerosis with extensive reticulonodular infiltrates with some sparing of lower lung zones.

pneumothorax secondary to tuberous sclerosis, with eight patients dying of this complication. Chylous pleural effusion secondary to lymphatic obstruction from mediastinal lymphadenopathy can occur. Significant pulmonary hypertension also has been reported.

Chest roentgenograms in tuberous sclerosis may show diffuse interstitial infiltrates in later stages of the disease. In the early stages, reticular or reticulonodular changes are found. Bullous changes and hyperinflation of lungs are also common. Spontaneous pneumothorax is common. Pleural effusion may be secondary to pneumothorax or to chylous effusion. In up to 25% of patients, normal chest roentgenograms may contribute to missed diagnoses. In such cases, a high-resolution CT scan of the lung is helpful. High-resolution CT scans of lungs in tuberous sclerosis have shown thin-walled cysts less than 20 mm in diameter scattered randomly in all parts of the lungs, with normal-appearing lung tissue between cysts. The CT findings are identical in tuberous sclerosis and pulmonary lymphangioleiomyomatosis (Fig. 63.13). The CT findings correlate better with Dlco than do chest roentgenograms.

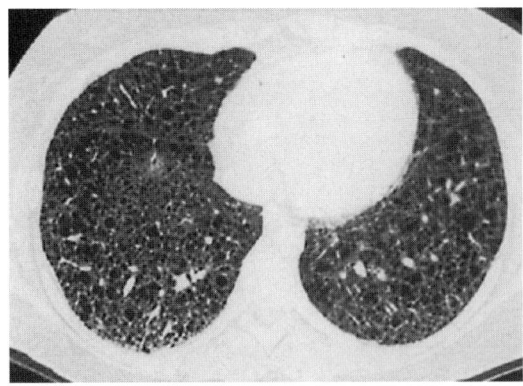

FIGURE 63.13. Tuberous sclerosis of lung evaluated by high-resolution computed tomography, showing typically diffuse fine honeycombing.

YELLOW NAIL SYNDROME

The term yellow nail syndrome was first used in 1964 to describe yellow discoloration of the fingernails in association with lymphedema in 13 patients (Fig. 63.14). Further experience with more than 150 patients portrayed in the literature has demonstrated the association of yellow nails with pleural effusion and bronchiectasis (105). Lymphedema of the breasts has been described in many patients with the yellow nail syndrome. The origin of yellow nail syndrome is unknown, although a few cases seemed to follow episodes of pneumonia. The mechanism of nail discoloration is undefined, and the nail changes are not present in all patients. Histopathologic changes in the nail matrix and bed demonstrate dense, fibrous tissue replacing subungual stroma with numerous ectatic, endothelium-lined vessels that mimic pleural alterations in this syndrome. Based on these findings, it is hypothesized that primary stromal sclerosis may lead to lymphatic obstruction and lymphedema.

Among 97 patients with yellow nail syndrome, most developed the disease in early middle age; the male-to-female ratio was 1:1.6 (106). Yellow nail syndrome has been described in an 8-year-old. Although more than half the patients develop nail changes, the majority do not notice the nail discoloration because its onset is subtle. Nails of both hands and feet are affected, becoming thickened, excessively curved along both axes, very slow growing, and of yellowish-gray hue. Cuticle and lunula are usually absent, and onycholysis generally is evident. Nail discoloration may precede or follow pleural effusion and lymphedema. Lymphangiography of the lower extremities has shown hypoplasia or aplasia of the lymphatics, similar to that occurring in primary lymphedema.

The recurrent pleural effusions are most likely the result of lymphatic hypoplasia. Measurements of the rate of pleural fluid turnover have indicated that accumulation of pleural fluid in yellow nail syndrome results from defective lymphatic drainage rather than excess production. Histologic examination of the pleura shows thickening with fibrosis,

chronic inflammatory infiltration, and dilation of lymphatic capillaries in the visceral pleura. The pathologic process affects not only the lymphatic system but also the pleural capillaries. Ectasia of lymphatic capillaries has been documented by electron microscopy. Pleural effusion may precede the onset of nail changes by several years. The fluid may be an exudate or a transudate. In some patients, the pleural fluid glucose level may be reduced. Pleural effusions range from small, unilateral, and asymptomatic to large, bilateral, recurrent, and debilitating. The pulmonary symptoms depend on the size of the pleural effusion and the severity of associated bronchiectasis. Empyema thoracis has been reported as a complication of the yellow nail syndrome.

Bronchiectasis of lower lobes is now included in the definition of yellow nail syndrome. Bronchiectasis limited to upper lung zones has been noted in a patient, but the mechanism responsible for its development is unknown. Many patients develop sinus infections. Among 17 patients with yellow nail syndrome, 14 (83%) suffered severe rhinosinusitis that predated nail changes in four, coincided with yellow nails in six, and occurred later in the remaining patients (107). In general, patients responded poorly to conventional medical and surgical treatment, with the exception of endoscopic sinus surgery.

Even though several cases have been described in association with carcinomas of breast, lung, and larynx, there is no clear indication that yellow nail syndrome is a paraneoplastic process. Nevertheless, the nail changes have resolved with successful treatment of the malignancy. There has been one report of a case of yellow nail syndrome after penicillamine therapy that resolved after discontinuation of the drug. A report of eight patients with proved diagnoses of AIDS and *Pneumocystis carinii* pneumonia described yellow discoloration of the distal portions of the nails in four patients, with some showing ridging, loss or decrease in size of lunulae, and opaqueness. Yellow nail syndrome has been described in association with rheumatoid arthritis in three patients and in two mentally retarded siblings.

Nonpulmonary complications of yellow nail syndrome include keratosis obturans involving the external ear and excess cerumen, chylous ascites, hypoalbuminemia, chyluria, intestinal lymphangiectasia, pericardial effusion, giant-cell interstitial infiltrates, lymphedema of the eyelids, nephrotic syndrome, and Raynaud phenomenon.

Large, recurrent, or debilitating pleural effusions require repeated thoracentesis, pleuroperitoneal shunting, medical or surgical pleurodesis, or pleurectomy. Chylous effusions are more difficult to cure, although successful therapy has been achieved with dietary restriction of fat and supplements of medium-chain triglycerides. Treatment of pulmonary disease (bronchiectasis and sinus infections) also may resolve the nail changes. There are reports of resolution of the nail changes after topical vitamin E solution. There also are reports of spontaneous resolution of nail discoloration without change in the patient's respiratory status.

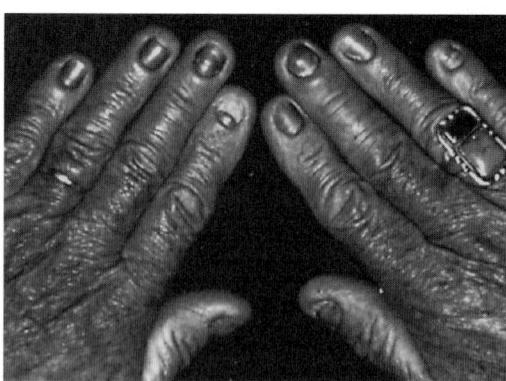

FIGURE 63.14. Yellow nail syndrome with characteristic yellow discoloration of nails.

URTICARIAL VASCULITIS

Urticarial vasculitis is a systemic disorder characterized by urticarial wheals or papules similar to those in the usual urticaria, with itching and arthralgias in 60% of cases, arthritis in 28%, abdominal pain in 25%, and glomerulonephritis in 5%. Angioedema, fever, uveitis, episcleritis, and seizures also may occur. Urticarial vasculitis with or without hypocomplementemia occurs in systemic lupus erythematosus. The erythrocyte sedimentation rate is elevated in 66% of patients, and hypocomplementemia is seen in 38%. The hypocomplementemic form of urticarial vasculitis has been associated with pulmonary complications (108).

Vasculitis of the pulmonary vasculature is not characteristic of this disease. However, obstructive pulmonary disease occurs in many of these patients. Airways disease results from a combination of smoking and an immunologic process that has yet not been identified. Up to 62% of patients with hypocomplementemic urticarial vasculitis develop chronic obstructive pulmonary disease, with tobacco smoking contributing to rapid progression of the disease. A publication reported that among 17 patients with hypocomplementemic vasculitis, 11 had dyspnea, and all dyspneic patients had moderate to severe airflow obstruction, which progressed in all 11 and subsequently improved in only one (108). Six of the 11 patients died of respiratory failure, one underwent lung transplantation, and three of the remaining four had moderately severe to life-threatening respiratory insufficiency. Treatment did not appear to alter the progression of obstructive lung disease. In contrast, renal insufficiency in two patients improved with treatment. Another report on 16 patients with hypocomplementemic urticarial vasculitis reported severe obstructive airways disease in eight of 10 smokers studied, one of which died of lung disease (109). Severe obstructive pulmonary disease developed in three patients at a young age after smoking cigarettes for a relatively low number of pack-years. A review of 72 cases of biopsy-proven urticarial vasculitis revealed that 32% had hypocomplementemia and 21% had obstructive lung disease (110). Case reports of bilateral pleural effusion and pulmonary capillaritis characterized by repeated episodes of diffuse alveolar hemorrhage and of progressive irreversible airway dysfunction have been published (111,112).

LEUKOCYTOCLASTIC VASCULITIS

Leukocytoclastic vasculitis is characterized by necrotizing vasculitis and fibrinoid necrosis of the vessel walls, with leukocytoclasis of the inflammatory cells in the wall of the vessel. Leukocytoclastic vasculitis may occur in association with inflammatory, autoimmune, and malignant disease. It commonly presents as palpable purpura.

Several respiratory complications have been described (113). Patchy pneumonitis secondary to biopsy-proven leukocytoclastic vasculitis of the pulmonary veins, manifested by hemoptysis and pleuritic chest pains, has been described in a patient who also exhibited obstructive airways disease.

MIXED CRYOGLOBULINEMIA

Mixed cryoglobulinemia is manifested by recurrent purpura, arthralgias, systemic involvement, and, frequently, elevated cryoglobulin and rheumatoid factor. Biopsy of vascular structures reveals findings similar to those in leukocytoclastic vasculitis. The most serious complication is glomerulonephritis caused by deposition of immune complexes. Lung function tests in 19 patients (17 of whom were women, with a mean age of 49.6 years) showed diminished DLco and maximal expiratory flow at 50% of forced vital capacity, total lung capacity, and functional residual capacity (114). Respiratory complications described include bronchiectasis, pulmonary fibrosis, pulmonary insufficiency, and Sjögren syndrome-like illness with lung involvement (115). Severe pulmonary hemorrhage also has been described in cryoglobulinemia (116).

Bronchoalveolar lavage and pulmonary function tests in 16 nonsmoking women with mixed cryoglobulinemia associated with hepatitis C virus, free of clinical pulmonary symptoms, and with normal chest roentgenograms showed a subclinical T-lymphocytic alveolitis without evidence of deterioration in lung function (117). No correlations between bronchoalveolar lavage results and pulmonary function tests were found; a 5-year follow-up of five patients did not demonstrate deterioration in lung function. Several reports have been published on the occurrence of diffuse pulmonary vasculitis with alveolar hemorrhage and bronchiolitis obliterans organizing pneumonia in association with essential mixed cryoglobulinemia (118).

EOSINOPHILIA-MYALGIA SYNDROME

The eosinophilia-myalgia syndrome is a multisystem inflammatory disease with characteristic features of myalgia and eosinophilia. This syndrome occurred in epidemic proportions in the United States during 1989, affecting more than 1,500 persons and causing approximately 30 deaths. Cases of the eosinophilia-myalgia syndrome have been reported from Canada, Europe, and other countries.

Epidemiologic studies have demonstrated that the eosinophilia-myalgia syndrome is the result of ingestion of L-tryptophan, used by lay people as a remedy for insomnia, depression, premenstrual syndrome, and other health disorders. Several contaminants—3(phenylamine)alanine, 1,1′-ethylidenebis(tryptophan), and 3-anilino-L-alanine—involved in the manufacturing of L-tryptophan have been implicated as the causative agents of both the

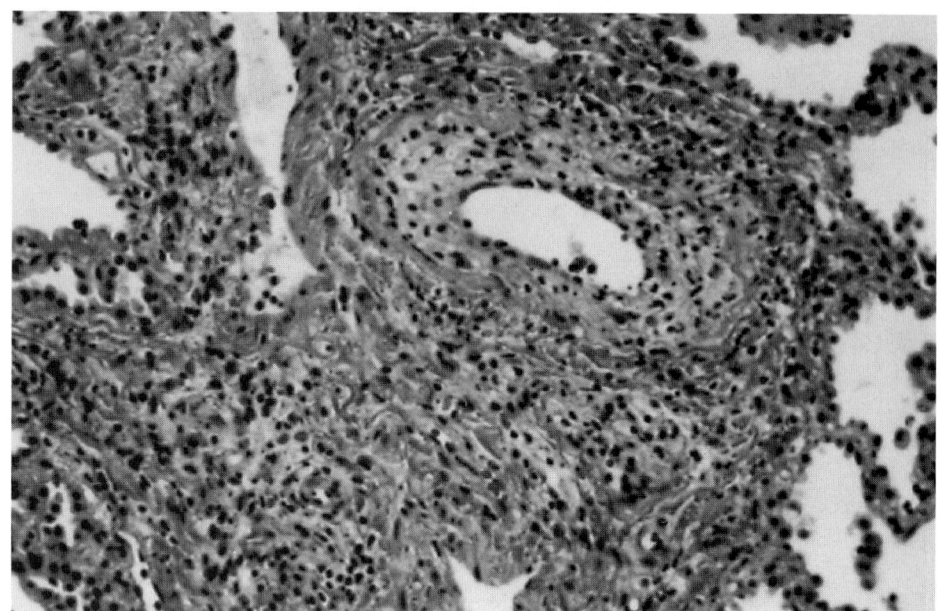

FIGURE 63.15. Pulmonary involvement in L-tryptophan–induced eosinophilia-myalgia syndrome. A mixed inflammatory infiltrate involves a septal vein. There is marked intimal proliferation and infiltration by cells that include relatively numerous eosinophils.

eosinophilia-myalgia syndrome and the Spanish toxic oil syndrome (119,120).

The clinical manifestations resemble those of the Spanish toxic oil syndrome, caused by ingestion of adulterated rapeseed oil. Symptoms and signs include myalgias, fatigue, muscle weakness, arthralgias, edema of the extremities, skin rash, oral and vaginal ulcers, scleroderma-like changes, fasciitis, ascending neuropathy, and profound eosinophilia.

Respiratory complications were observed in approximately 60% of patients with the eosinophilia-myalgia syndrome (121,122). Pulmonary manifestations included parenchymal lung infiltrates associated with severe respiratory distress and progressive hypoxemia, pleural effusion, diffuse bilateral reticulonodular infiltrates, and pulmonary hypertension. In a study of five cases of pathologically proven eosinophilia-myalgia syndrome, all patients were women ranging in age from 34 to 65 years, and all presented with pulmonary symptoms that began after 1 to 9 months of L-tryptophan therapy (123). Four patients exhibited peripheral eosinophilia and bilateral interstitial infiltrates (one had a normal chest roentgenogram). Lung specimens revealed vasculitis and perivasculitis associated with eosinophilia and mild interstitial pneumonitis. Clinical or morphologic evidence of pulmonary hypertension was noted in three, and one patient had follicular bronchiolitis. Whereas four patients responded promptly to discontinuation of L-tryptophan ingestion and systemic corticosteroids, one patient showed only minimal symptomatic improvement.

Other histologic changes described in the lungs of patients with the eosinophilia-myalgia syndrome have included alveolar exudate made up of eosinophils and histiocytes, changes characteristic of hypersensitivity pneumonitis, interstitial and perivascular infiltrates, and fibrointimal hyperplasia of small pulmonary vessels (Fig. 63.15) (124).

REFERENCES

1. Selkin BA, Reynolds RV, Selkin G. Cutaneous manifestations of internal malignancy. In: Rose BD, ed. *UpToDate*. Wellesley, MA: UpToDate, 2002.
2. Rogers DL. Acanthosis nigricans. *Semin Dermatol* 1991;10:160–163.
3. Mellor-Pita S, Yebra-Bango M, Alfaro-Martinez J, et al. Acanthosis nigricans: a new manifestation of insulin resistance in patients receiving treatment with protease inhibitors. *Clin Infect Dis* 2002;34:716–717.
4. Torley D, Munro CS. Genes, growth factors and acanthosis nigricans. *Br J Dermatol* 2002;147:1096–1101.
5. Rigel DS, Jacobs MI. Malignant acanthosis nigricans: a review. *J Dermatol Surg Oncol* 1980;6:923–927.
6. Menzies DG, Choo-Kang J, Buxton PK, et al. Acanthosis nigricans associated with alveolar cell carcinoma. *Thorax* 1988;43:414–415.
7. Bolognia JL. Bazex syndrome: acrokeratosis paraneoplastica. *Semin Dermatol* 1995;14:84–89.
8. Cohen PR, Grossman ME, Almeida L, et al. Tripe palms and malignancy. *J Clin Oncol* 1989;7:669–678.
9. Col M, Col C, Soran A, et al. Arsenic-related Bowen's disease, palmar keratosis, and skin cancer. *Environ Health Perspect* 1999;107:687–689.
10. Heddle R, Bryant GD. Small cell lung carcinoma and Bowen's disease 40 years after arsenic ingestion. *Chest* 1983;84:776–777.
11. Joly P, Richard C, Gilbert D, et al. Sensitivity and specificity of clinical, histologic, and immunologic features in the diagnosis of paraneoplastic pemphigus. *J Am Acad Dermatol* 2000;43:619–626.

12. Goldstein BG, Goldstein AO. Pemphigus and bullous pemphigoid. In: Rose BD, ed. *UpToDate.* Wellesley, MA: UpToDate, 2002.
13. Fullerton SH, Woodley DT, Smoller BR, et al. Paraneoplastic pemphigus with autoantibody deposition in bronchial epithelium after autologous bone marrow transplantation. *JAMA* 1992;267:1500–1502.
14. Cuzick J, Harris R, Mortimer PS. Palmar keratoses and cancers of the bladder and lung. *Lancet* 1984;1:530–533.
15. Sweet RD. An acute febrile neutrophilic dermatoses. *Br J Dermatol* 1964;76:349.
16. Moschella SL. Neutrophilic dermatoses. In: Rose BD, ed. *UpToDate.* Wellesley, MA: UpToDate, 2002.
17. Cohen PR, Talpaz M, Kurzrock R. Malignancy-associated Sweet's syndrome: review of the world literature. *J Clin Oncol* 1988;6:1887–1897.
18. Fett DL, Gibson LE, Su WPD. Sweet's syndrome: systemic signs and symptoms and associated disorders. *Mayo Clin Proc* 1995;70:234–240.
19. Takimoto CH, Warnock M, Golden JA. Sweet's syndrome with lung involvement. *Am Rev Respir Dis* 1991;143:177–179.
20. Nielsen I, Donati D, Strumia R, et al. Sweet's syndrome and malignancy: report of the first case associated with adenocarcinoma of the lung. *Lung Cancer* 1993;10:95–99.
21. Wisniewski SA, Kobielak A, Trzeciak WH, et al. Recent advances in understanding of the molecular basis of anhidrotic ectodermal dysplasia: discovery of a ligand, ectodysplasin A and its two receptors. *J Appl Genet* 2002;43:97–107.
22. Beahrs JO, Lillington GA, Rosan RC, et al. Anhidrotic ectodermal dysplasia: predisposition to bronchial disease. *Ann Intern Med* 1971;74:92–96.
23. Opal P, Bonilla FA, Lederman HM. Ataxia-telangiectasia. In: Rose BD, ed. *UpToDate.* Wellesley, MA: UpToDate, 2002.
24. Waldmann TA, Broder S, Goldman CK, et al. Disorders of B cells and helper T cells in the pathogenesis of the immunoglobulin deficiency of patients with ataxia telangiectasia. *J Clin Invest* 1983;71:282–295.
25. Rodrigues D, Bourroul ML, Ferrer AP, et al. Blue rubber bleb nevus syndrome. *Rev Hosp Clin Fac Med Sao Paulo* 2000;55:29–34.
26. Langleben D, Wolkove N, Srolovitz H, et al. Hemothorax and hemopericardium in a patient with Bean's blue rubber bleb nevus syndrome. *Chest* 1989;95:1352–1353.
27. Lilic D. New perspectives on the immunology of chronic mucocutaneous candidiasis. *Curr Opin Infect Dis* 2002;15:143–147.
28. Bragger C, Seger RA, Aeppli R, et al. IgG$_2$/IgG$_4$ subclass deficiency in a patient with chronic mucocutaneous candidiasis and bronchiectases. *Eur J Pediatr* 1989;149:168–169.
29. St Clair EW, McCallum R. Cogan's syndrome. In: Rose BD, ed. *UpToDate.* Wellesley, MA: UpToDate, 2002.
30. Gaubitz M, Lubben B, Seidel M, et al. Cogan's syndrome: organ-specific autoimmune disease or systemic vasculitis? A report of two cases and review of the literature. *Clin Exp Rheumatol* 2001;19:463–469.
31. Vollertson RS, McDonald T, Younge BR, et al. Cogan's syndrome: 18 cases and a review of the literature. *Mayo Clin Proc* 1986;61:344–361.
32. Corbett E, Glaisyer H, Chan C, et al. Congenital cutis laxa with a dominant inheritance and early onset emphysema. *Thorax* 1994;49:836–837.
33. Clark JG, Kuhn C 3rd, Uitto J. Lung collagen in type IV Ehlers-Danlos syndrome: ultrastructural and biochemical studies. *Am Rev Respir Dis* 1980;122:971–978.
34. Ayres JG, Pope FM, Reidy JF, et al. Abnormalities of the lungs and thoracic cage in the Ehlers-Danlos syndrome. *Thorax* 1985;40:300–305.
35. Yost BA, Vogelsang JP, Lie JT. Fatal hemoptysis in Ehlers-Danlos syndrome: old malady with a new curse. *Chest* 1995;5:1465–1467.
36. Herman TE, McAlister WH. Cavitary pulmonary lesions in type IV Ehlers-Danlos syndrome. *Pediatr Radiol* 1994;24:263–265.
37. Eng J, Oommen PK, Nair UR. Mediastinal haematoma in Ehlers-Danlos syndrome. *Int J Cardiol* 1991;31:247–249.
38. Killen JW, Swift GL, White RJ. Eosinophilic fasciitis with pulmonary and pleural involvement. *Postgrad Med J* 2000;76:36–37.
39. Chalker RB, Dickey BF, Rosenthal NC, et al. Extrapulmonary thoracic restriction (hidebound chest) complicating eosinophilic fasciitis. *Chest* 1991;100:1453–1455.
40. Gonzalez C, Roth R. Laryngotracheal involvement in epidermolysis bullosa. *Int J Pediatr Otorhinolaryngol* 1989;17:305–311.
41. Davies H, Atherton DJ. Acute laryngeal obstruction in junctional epidermolysis bullosa. *Pediatr Dermatol* 1987;4:98–101.
42. Lyos AT, Levy ML, Malpica A, et al. Laryngeal involvement in epidermolysis bullosa. *Ann Otol Rhinol Laryngol* 1994;103:542–546.
43. Nirken M. Stevens-Johnson syndrome and toxic epidermal necrolysis in adults. In: Rose BD, ed. *UpToDate.* Wellesley, MA: UpToDate, 2002.
44. Bastuji-Garin S, Rzany B, Stern RS, et al. Clinical classification of cases of toxic epidermal necrolysis, Stevens-Johnson syndrome, and erythema multiforme. *Arch Dermatol* 1993;129:92–96.
45. Villiger RM, von Vigier RO, Ramelli GP, et al. Precipitants in 42 cases of erythema multiforme. *Eur J Pediatr* 1999;158:929–932.
46. Leaute-Labreze C, Lamireau T, Chawki D, et al. Diagnosis, classification, and management of erythema multiforme and Stevens-Johnson syndrome. *Arch Dis Child* 2000;83:347–352.
47. Tay YK, Huff JC, Weston WL. Mycoplasma pneumoniae infection is associated with Stevens-Johnson syndrome, not erythema multiforme (von Hebra). *J Am Acad Dermatol* 1996;35:757–760.
48. Pietinalho A, Ohmichi M, Hiraga Y, et al. The mode of presentation of sarcoidosis in Finland and Hokkaido, Japan: a comparative analysis of 571 Finnish and 686 Japanese patients. *Sarcoidosis Vasc Diffuse Lung Dis* 1996;13:159–166.
49. Miller DD, Davies SF, Sarosi GA. Erythema nodosum and blastomycosis. *Arch Intern Med* 1982;142:1839.
50. Syrjala H, Karvonen J, Salminen A. Skin manifestations of tularemia: a study of 88 cases in northern Finland during 16 years (1967–1983). *Acta Dermatol Venereol (Stockholm)* 1984;64:513–516.
51. Ancient missense mutations in a new member of the RoRet gene family are likely to cause familial Mediterranean fever: the International FMF Consortium. *Cell* 1997;90:797–807.
52. A candidate gene for familial Mediterranean fever.: the French FMF Consortium. *Nat Genet* 1997;17:25–31.
53. Pras M. Amyloidosis of familial Mediterranean fever and the MEFV gene. *Amyloid* 2000;7:289–293.
54. Livneh A, Langevitz P, Pras M. Pulmonary associations in familial Mediterranean fever. *Curr Opin Pulm Med* 1999;5:326–331.
55. Lidar M, Pras M, Langevitz P, Livneh A. Thoracic and lung involvement in familial Mediterranean fever (FMF). *Clin Chest Med* 2002;23:505–511.
56. Brenner-Ullman A, Melzer-Ofir H, Daniels M, et al. Possible protection against asthma in heterozygotes for familial Mediterranean fever. *Am J Med Genet* 1994;53:172–175.
57. Vase P, Holm M, Arendrup H. Pulmonary arteriovenous

fistulas in hereditary hemorrhagic telangiectasia. *Acta Med Scand* 1985;218:105–109.

58. Dines DE, Arms RA, Bernatz PE, et al. Pulmonary arteriovenous fistulas. *Mayo Clin Proc* 1974;49:460–465.

59. Dines DE, Seward JB, Bernatz PE. Pulmonary arteriovenous fistulas. *Mayo Clin Proc* 1983;58:176–181.

60. Swanson KL, Prakash UB, Stanson AW. Pulmonary arteriovenous fistulas: Mayo Clinic experience, 1982–1997. *Mayo Clin Proc* 1999;74:671–680.

61. Haitjema T, Disch F, Overtoom TT, et al. Screening family members of patients with hereditary hemorrhagic telangiectasia. *Am J Med* 1995;99:519–524.

62. Berg JN, Guttmacher AE, Marchuk DA, et al. Clinical heterogeneity in hereditary haemorrhagic telangiectasia: are pulmonary arteriovenous malformations more common in families linked to endoglin? *J Med Genet* 1996;33:256–257.

63. Johnson DW, Berg JN, Gallione CJ, et al. A second locus for hereditary hemorrhagic telangiectasia maps to chromosome 12. *Genome Res* 1995;5:21–28.

64. Allen SW, Whitfield JM, Clarke DR, et al. Pulmonary arteriovenous malformation in the newborn: a familial case. *Pediatr Cardiol* 1993;14:58–61.

65. Ference BA, Shannon TM, White RI Jr, et al. Life-threatening pulmonary hemorrhage with pulmonary arteriovenous malformations and hereditary hemorrhagic telangiectasia. *Chest* 1994;106:1387–1390.

66. Dutton JA, Jackson JE, Hughes JM, et al. Pulmonary arteriovenous malformations: results of treatment with coil embolization in 53 patients. *AJR Am J Roentgenol* 1995;65:1119–1125.

67. White RI Jr, Lynch-Nyhan A, Terry P, et al. Pulmonary arteriovenous malformations: techniques and long-term outcome of embolotherapy. *Radiology* 1988;169:663–669.

68. Press OW, Ramsey PG. Central nervous system infections associated with hereditary hemorrhagic telangiectasia. *Am J Med* 1984;77:86–92.

69. Chilvers ER, Whyte MK, Jackson JE, et al. Effect of percutaneous transcatheter embolization on pulmonary function, right-to-left shunt, and arterial oxygenation in patients with pulmonary arteriovenous malformations. *Am Rev Respir Dis* 1990;142:420–425.

70. Haitjema TJ, Overtoom TT, Westermann CJ, et al. Embolisation of pulmonary arteriovenous malformations: results and follow up in 32 patients. *Thorax* 1995;50:719–723.

71. Haitjema TJ, ten-Berg JM, Overtoom TT, et al. Unusual complications after embolization of a pulmonary arteriovenous malformation. *Chest* 1996;109:1401–1404.

72. Smetana GW. Approach to the patient with night sweats. In: Rose BD, ed. *UpToDate.* Wellesley, MA: UpToDate, 2002.

73. Leung AK, Chan PY, Choi MC. Hyperhidrosis. *Int J Dermatol* 1999;38:561–567.

74. Chave TA, Varma S, Patel GK, et al. Malignant atrophic papulosis (Degos' disease): clinicopathological correlations. *J Eur Acad Dermatol Venereol* 2001;15:43–45.

75. Pierce RN, Smith GJW. Intrathoracic manifestations of Degos' disease (malignant atrophic papulosis). *Chest* 1978;73:79–84.

76. Bingham CO 3rd, Castells MC. Mastocytosis. In: Rose BD, ed. *UpToDate.* Wellesley, MA: UpToDate, 2002.

77. Feldkamp MM, Gutmann DH, Guha A. Neurofibromatosis type 1: piecing the puzzle together. *Can J Neurol Sci* 1998;25:181–191.

78. North K. Neurofibromatosis type 1: review of the first 200 patients in an Australian clinic. *J Child Neurol* 1993;8:395–402.

79. Burkhalter JL, Morano JU, McCay MB. Diffuse interstitial lung disease in neurofibromatosis. *South Med J* 1986;79:944–946.

80. Bourgouin PM, Shepard JO, Moore EH, et al. Plexiform neu-

rofibromatosis of the mediastinum: CT appearance. *AJR Am J Roentgenol* 1988;151:461–463.

81. Baydur A, Cabula OS, Krishnareddy N, et al. Fatal intrathoracic hemorrhage in a patient with von Recklinghausen's disease. *Respiration* 1995;62:104–106.

82. Masip MJ, Esteban E, Alberto C, et al. Laryngeal involvement in pediatric neurofibromatosis: a case report and review of the literature. *Pediatr Radiol* 1996;26:488–492.

83. el Oakley R, Grotte GJ. Progressive tracheal and superior vena caval compression caused by benign neurofibromatosis. *Thorax* 1994;49:380–381.

84. Panush RS, Yonker RA, Dlesk A, et al. Weber-Christian disease: analysis of 15 cases and review of the literature. *Medicine (Baltimore)* 1985;64:181–191.

85. Requena L, Yus ES. Panniculitis, part I: mostly septal panniculitis. *J Am Acad Dermatol* 2001;45:163–183.

86. Federman Q, Abrams RM, Lee T. Pulmonary radiographic findings in a case of febrile, relapsing, nonsuppurative panniculitis (Weber-Christian disease). *Mt Sinai J Med* 1976;43:174–179.

87. Kumagai-Kurata N, Kunitoh H, Nagamine-Nishizawa M, et al. Idiopathic lobular panniculitis with specific pleural involvement. *Eur Respir J* 1995;8:1613–1615.

88. Breit SM, Clark P, Robinson JP, et al. Familial occurrence of α_1-antitrypsin deficiency and Weber-Christian disease. *Arch Dermatol* 1983;119:198–202.

89. Pottage JC Jr, Trenholme GM, Aronson IK, et al. Panniculitis associated with histoplasmosis and α_1-antitrypsin deficiency. *Am J Med* 1983;75:150–153.

90. Bleumink E, Klokke HA. Protease-inhibitor deficiencies in a patient with Weber-Christian panniculitis. *Arch Dermatol* 1984;120:936–940.

91. Bleumink E, Klokke AH. Relationship between Weber-Christian panniculitis and the ZZ phenotype of α_1-antitrypsin. *Arch Dermatol Res* 1985;277:328–329.

92. Dellaripa PF, Wechsler ME, Roth ME, et al. Recurrent panniculitis in a man with asthma receiving treatment with leukotriene-modifying agents. *Mayo Clin Proc* 2000;75:643–645.

93. Avila NA, Brantly M, Premkumar A, et al. Hermansky-Pudlak syndrome: radiography and CT of the chest compared with pulmonary function tests and genetic studies. *AJR Am J Roentgenol* 2002;179:887–892.

94. Garay SM, Gardella JE, Fazzini EP, et al. Hermansky-Pudlak syndrome: pulmonary manifestations of a ceroid storage disease. *Am J Med* 1979;66:737–747.

95. Harmon KR, Witkop CJ, White JG, et al. Pathogenesis of pulmonary fibrosis: platelet-derived growth factor precedes structural alterations in the Hermansky-Pudlak syndrome. *J Lab Clin Med* 1994;123:617–627.

96. Hanson RD, Olsen KD, Rogers RS II. Upper aerodigestive tract manifestations of cicatricial pemphigoid. *Ann Otol Rhinol Laryngol* 1988;97:493–499.

97. de Carvalho CR, Amato MB, Da Silva LM, et al. Obstructive respiratory failure in cicatricial pemphigoid. *Thorax* 1989;44:601–602.

98. Ohtani T, Furukawa F. Pseudoxanthoma elasticum. *J Dermatol* 2002;29:615–620.

99. Jackson A, Loh CL. Pulmonary calcification and elastic tissue damage in pseudoxanthoma elasticum. *Histopathology* 1980;4:607–611.

100. Powell FC, Schroeter AL, Su WPD, et al. Pyoderma gangrenosum: a review of 86 patients. *Q J Med* 1985;55:173–186.

101. Vignon-Pennamen MD, Zelinsky-Gurung A, Janssen F, et al. Pyoderma gangrenosum with pulmonary involvement. *Arch Dermatol* 1989;125:1239–1242.

102. Shepherd CW, Gomez MR, Lie JT, et al. Causes of death in

patients with tuberous sclerosis. *Mayo Clin Proc* 1991;66:792–796.

103. Dwyer JM, Hickie JB, Garvan J. Pulmonary tuberous sclerosis: report of three patients and a review of the literature. *Q J Med* 1971;40:115–125.
104. Castro M, Shepherd CW, Gomez MR, et al. Pulmonary tuberous sclerosis. *Chest* 1995;107:189–195.
105. Hiller E, Rosenow EC 3rd, Olsen AM. Pulmonary manifestations of the yellow nail syndrome. *Chest* 1972;61:452–458.
106. Nordkild P, Kromann-Andersen H, Struve-Christensen E. Yellow nail syndrome–the triad of yellow nails, lymphedema, and pleural effusion: a review of the literature and a case report. *Acta Med Scand* 1986;219:221–227.
107. Varney VA, Cumberworth V, Sudderick R, et al. Rhinitis, sinusitis and the yellow nail syndrome: a review of symptoms and response to treatment in 17 patients. *Clin Otolaryngol* 1994;19: 237–240.
108. Wisnieski JJ, Baer AN, Christensen J, et al. Hypocomplementemic urticarial vasculitis syndrome. Clinical and serologic findings in 18 patients. *Medicine (Baltimore)* 1995;74:24–41.
109. Schwartz HR, McDuffie FC, Black LF, et al. Hypocomplementemic urticarial vasculitis: association with chronic obstructive pulmonary disease. *Mayo Clin Proc* 1982;57:231–238.
110. Mehregan DR, Hall MJ, Gibson LE. Urticarial vasculitis: a histopathologic and clinical review of 72 cases. *J Am Acad Dermatol* 1992;26:441–448.
111. Falk DK. Pulmonary disease in idiopathic urticarial vasculitis. *J Am Acad Dermatol* 1984;11:346–352.
112. Paira SO. Bilateral pleural effusion in a patient with urticarial vasculitis. *Clin Rheumatol* 1994;13:504–506.
113. Odeh M, Misselevich I, Oliven A. Squamous cell carcinoma of the lung presenting with cutaneous leukocytoclastic vasculitis: a case report. *Angiology* 2001;52:641–644.
114. Viegi G, Fornai E, Ferri C, et al. Lung function in essential mixed cryoglobulinemia: a short-term follow- up. *Clin Rheumatol* 1989;8:331–338.
115. Bombardieri S, Paoletti P, DiMunno O, et al. Lung involvement in essential mixed cryoglobulinemia. *Am J Med* 1979;66:748–756.
116. Gomez-Tello V, Onoro-Canaveral JJ, de la Casa Monje RM, et al. Diffuse recidivans alveolar hemorrhage in a patient with hepatitis C virus-related mixed cryoglobulinemia. *Intensive Care Med* 1999;25:319–322.
117. Manganelli P, Salaffi F, Subiaco S, et al. Bronchoalveolar lavage in mixed cryoglobulinaemia associated with hepatitis C virus. *Br J Rheumatol* 1996;35:978–982.
118. Zackrison LH, Katz P. Bronchiolitis obliterans organizing pneumonia associated with essential mixed cryoglobulinemia. *Arthritis Rheum* 1993;36:1627–1630.
119. Silver RM. Eosinophilia-myalgia syndrome, toxic-oil syndrome, and diffuse fasciitis with eosinophilia. *Curr Opin Rheumatol* 1992;4:851–856.
120. Philen RM, Posada M. Toxic oil syndrome and eosinophilia-myalgia syndrome: May 8–10, 1991, World Health Organization meeting report. *Semin Arthritis Rheum* 1993;23:104–124.
121. Catton CK, Elmer JC, Whitehouse AC, et al. Pulmonary involvement in the eosinophilia-myalgia syndrome. *Chest* 1991;99:327–329.
122. Campagna AC, Blanc PD, Criswell LA, et al. Pulmonary manifestations of the eosinophilia-myalgia syndrome associated with tryptophan ingestion. *Chest* 1992;101:1274–1281.
123. Tazelaar HD, Myers JL, Drage CW, et al. Pulmonary disease associated with L-tryptophan induced eosinophilic myalgia syndrome: clinical and pathologic features. *Chest* 1990;97:1032–1036.
124. Herrick MK, Chang Y, Horoupian DS, et al. L-tryptophan and the eosinophilia-myalgia syndrome: pathologic findings in eight patients. *Hum Pathol* 1991;22:12–21.

Obstetrics, Gynecology, and Reproductive Organs

64

Udaya B. S. Prakash · Talmadge E. King, Jr.

The respiratory system is affected by the normal anatomic and physiologic alterations that take place throughout pregnancy, parturition, and early postpartum. A healthy pregnant woman experiences minimal or tolerably mild respiratory symptoms. A pre-existing pulmonary problem, however, can be exacerbated by pregnancy. On the other hand, the normal course of the pregnancy can be adversely affected by pre-existing respiratory disorders to the point of threatening the pregnancy itself. In pregnancy, the clinical course of primary pulmonary diseases such as asthma, sarcoidosis, and certain infectious processes may vary from that in the nonpregnant patient. Likewise, the treatment of pulmonary disease in the pregnant patient may differ because some of the drugs normally used may interfere with pregnancy or cross the placental barrier and adversely affect the fetus. Pathologic processes can also involve the pulmonary system in pregnancy, such as amniotic fluid embolism and trophoblastic pulmonary emboli that can occur after removal of a benign hydatidiform mole. The various pulmonary complications described in pregnancy and the postpartum are listed in Table 64.1 (1). In this chapter, the physiologic changes noted in normal pregnancy, lung involvement by obstetric and gynecologic pathology, and the pulmonary manifestations in the disorders of the reproductive organs are included (2).

PREGNANCY

Effect of Pregnancy on Respiration

Pregnancy alters lung function, and breathlessness is a common complaint in pregnant patients. These changes result

U. B. S. Prakash: Pulmonary and Critical Care Medicine, Mayo Medical School and Mayo Medical Center, Rochester, Minnesota.

T. E. King, Jr.: Department of Medicine, University of California, San Francisco; and Medical Services, San Francisco General Hospital, San Francisco, California.

from alterations in breathing pattern, changes in rib cage displacement, increased laxity of abdominal musculature, and mismatch in ventilation and perfusion (3). Resting ventilation and, to a lesser extent, oxygen consumption are increased at rest and during exercise in pregnancy (as well as during labor). Hyperventilation is a common feature of pregnancy, but the overall pH remains relatively intact because of increased renal excretion of bicarbonate. Severe hyperventilation, however, during labor has resulted in tetany. Changes in concentrations of progesterone, a known stimulant of respiration and respiratory drive, play a role in producing the ventilatory changes in pregnancy.

The total lung capacity remains relatively unchanged because the inspiratory capacity and the inspiratory reserve volume increase; in addition, the transverse diameter of the lower chest wall expands and diaphragmatic motion is maintained (3,4). Late pregnancy is commonly associated with a decrease in expiratory reserve volume, a mild decrease in functional residual capacity, and a slightly reduced total lung capacity. Airway closure is too insignificant to cause clinical problems.

Arterial oxygen partial pressure (Pa_{O_2}) is elevated because of the hyperventilation (ranging from 106–108 mm Hg in the first trimester to 101–104 mm Hg in the third trimester) (5). However, an abnormally high alveolar-arterial oxygen tension difference near term, possibly because of small-airway closure, partially offsets the high Pa_{O_2}. Diffusing capacity during early pregnancy is unchanged or slightly increased over nonpregnant values in the same patient and then diminishes to a plateau during the latter half of pregnancy. The arterial partial pressure of carbon dioxide (Pa_{CO_2}) falls to a plateau of 27 to 32 mm Hg during pregnancy (5). This respiratory alkalosis is followed by compensatory renal excretion of bicarbonate, so that the resultant arterial pH is normal to slightly alkalotic (usually between 7.40–7.45) (5,6).

TABLE 64.1. PULMONARY COMPLICATIONS IN PREGNANCY

Pulmonary Complications	Obstetric Causes
Dyspnea of pregnancy	Mechanical
	Hormonal (biochemical)
	Hemodynamic changes
	Pulmonary disease (see below)
Pneumothorax and pneumomediastinum	Valsalva maneuver (second stage of labor)
Pulmonary edema	Aspiration
	Eclampsia
	Tocolytic therapy
	Pulmonary embolism
	Amniotic fluid embolism
	Disseminated intravascular coagulation
	Trophoblastic embolism
	Transfusion reactions
	Sepsis (septic abortion)
Pleural effusion	Postpartum
	Eclampsia
	Pulmonary edema (see above)
	Pulmonary embolism
	Amniotic fluid embolism
	Metastatic choriocarcinoma
Pulmonary embolism	Thromboembolism
	Amniotic fluid embolism
	Septic embolism (septic abortion)
Pulmonary hypertension	Unknown
	Recurrent pulmonary embolism
	Trophoblastic emboli

Sarcoidosis, rhinitis, asthma, coccidioidomycosis, tuberculosis, and cystic fibrosis, although not complications owing to pregnancy, may be present in conjunction with, and thereby affect, pregnancy, and vice versa.

By the 12th week of pregnancy, more than 20% of women experience dyspnea at rest, whereas nearly two thirds are dyspneic on exertion. The incidence of dyspnea increases from 15% in the first trimester to 50% by the 19th week and 75% by the 31st week of gestation. Upward displacement of the diaphragm by the enlarging uterus results in slightly diminished lung volumes in the second half of pregnancy. However, diaphragmatic excursion during respiration is not impaired (5). Diaphragmatic fatigue after prolonged contractions, particularly before and during labor, may contribute to dyspnea.

Smoking and Pregnancy

There are many documented adverse outcomes associated with cigarette smoking during pregnancy including spontaneous pregnancy loss, placental abruption, preterm premature rupture of membranes, placenta previa, preterm labor and delivery, stillbirth, and low birth weight (7). Cigarette smoking during pregnancy increases the risk of postnatal morbidities including neonatal death (death within 28 days of birth), sudden infant death syndrome, respiratory infections, reactive airway disease, otitis media, bronchiolitis, short stature, lower reading and spelling scores, shorter atten-

tion spans, hyperactivity, and decreased school performance (7–10).

Studies in children have demonstrated a clear association between passive exposure to maternal smoking and frequency of acute respiratory illness and chronic pulmonary conditions such as wheezing or asthma. Infants of mothers who smoke during pregnancy have reduced respiratory function and are more likely to develop wheezing. In a study in which healthy infants born to women who smoked during pregnancy were compared with infants born to women who did not smoke during pregnancy, maternal smoking was associated with significant reductions in forced expiratory flow in their young offspring. Maternal smoking during pregnancy may impair in utero airway development or alter lung elastic properties, and these effects may be important factors predisposing infants to the occurrence of wheezing illness later in childhood. In another study, respiratory-function data from 461 infants showed that in utero smoke exposure, a family history of asthma, and maternal hypertension during pregnancy were associated with reduced respiratory function after birth (11). This led the investigators to speculate that these factors adversely affect lung development in utero. A study of the relationship between maternal smoking during pregnancy and lung function in 493 white and 383 black schoolchildren 9 to 11 years of age in three areas of Philadelphia observed that maternal smoking during pregnancy was associated with significant deficits in the midexpiratory phase of the forced expiratory flow and forced expiratory volume in 1 second/forced vital capacity (FEV_1/FVC), and the observed deficits were larger for black children than for white children, and they were larger for boys than for girls (12). Suburban white schoolchildren whose mothers smoked during pregnancy had significantly reduced lung function.

A reduction in the number of cigarettes smoked during pregnancy has not produced consistent improvement in perinatal outcomes (7,13). Therefore, smoking cessation is the goal of treatment in pregnant women. Given the known risks of continued smoking during pregnancy, a reasonable approach is to offer pharmacotherapy (e.g., nicotine replacement or sustained release bupropion) to pregnant women who are at high risk for continued smoking: heavy smokers (>10 cigarettes/d), those smoking later in pregnancy, and those who have attempted to stop previously (7,10). Pregnancy provides a unique opportunity for medical intervention that can lead to significant reductions in the number of women smoking during pregnancy. Unfortunately, only about half of obstetricians routinely advise and provide follow-up for smoking cessation; furthermore, less than one third of obstetricians discuss actual strategies for cessation (7,14,15).

Asthma

Asthma is encountered in pregnancy with an estimated frequency of 0.4% to 1.3% and is reported to complicate

PREGNANCY AND SMOKING

Summary Statement	Level of Evidence
Because of the serious risks of smoking to the pregnant smoker and the fetus, pregnant smokers should, whenever possible, be offered extended or augmented psychosocial interventions that exceed minimal advice to quit (7, 16).	Randomized controlled trials
Although abstinence early in pregnancy will produce the greatest benefits to the fetus and mother, quitting at any point in pregnancy can yield benefits. Thus, clinicians should offer effective smoking cessation interventions to pregnant smokers at the first prenatal visit, as well as throughout the course of pregnancy (7, 16).	Observational studies, expert opinion
Use of adjunct pharmacotherapy substantially increases quit rates when compared with placebo (7, 16).	Randomized controlled trials
Pharmacotherapy has not been recommended for all women during pregnancy but is primarily targeted for women who are unlikely to quit owing to concern over the potential for adverse fetal effects (7, 16).	Observational studies expert opinion

gestation in approximately 1% of pregnant women. Publications have reported both an improvement and worsening of asthma during pregnancy in approximately 5% to 46% of women (5,17,18). A study of 31 asthmatic women reported that mild to moderately severe asthmatics exhibit an improvement in asthma in the last trimester, but more than one-third of these may have a postpartum deterioration. In contrast, a prospective study of 198 pregnancies among 181 asthmatics reported that asthma caused no emergencies during labor, and there was no difference between asthmatic and control subjects with regard to length of gestation, birth weight, incidence of perinatal deaths, low Apgar scores, neonatal respiratory difficulties, hyperbilirubinemia, or malformations. However, the study observed that severe asthma or systemic corticosteroid treatment (or both) during pregnancy increased the incidence of preeclampsia in the mother and hypoglycemia in the infant. Another significant finding was that among the asthmatic women, 28% of births were by cesarean section, compared with 17% in the control group.

Two cross-sectional community studies indicated that asthmatic mothers were more likely to have a preterm delivery than were nonasthmatic mothers and that asthmatic mothers did not have an increased risk of delivering small growth-retarded babies (19). Maternal asthma, paternal asthma, and premature birth, in that order, increased the risk of later childhood respiratory morbidity. Another study analyzed the hormonal factors and clinical and physiologic parameters during the preconception period (in 20 asthmatic women) and after conception and delivery (in 16 of 20 women), and noted that both airway responsiveness and asthma severity showed statistically and clinically significant improvements during pregnancy and returned toward preconception levels postpartum (20). A significant association between pregnancy-induced hypertension and asthma during pregnancy has been observed (21). It also appears that there is a significant upward trend in the incidence of asthma during pregnancy in women without, with moderate, and with severe pregnancy-induced hypertension. The reasons for this relationship are not obvious.

The improvement in asthma during pregnancy may be induced by progesterone and other hormone-induced reduction in the contractility of airway smooth muscle, increased free serum cortisol, and the prolonged duration of action of the steroid. The latter explanations are supported by the observation that other inflammatory conditions, such as rheumatoid arthritis, also improve during pregnancy. The effect of mechanical factors responsible for dyspnea in nonasthmatic pregnant patients, discussed above, is also important in the deterioration of asthma during pregnancy. Bronchial responsiveness improves in most patients during pregnancy (20).

Management of asthma during pregnancy is similar to that in the nonpregnant patient (22,23). A study of 504 pregnant asthmatic subjects who were prospectively monitored and treated showed that patients with inadequate inhaled anti-inflammatory treatment during pregnancy run a higher risk of suffering an acute attack of asthma than those adequately treated with an anti-inflammatory agent (24). The investigators concluded that if the acute attack of asthma is relatively mild, and promptly treated, it does not have a serious effect on the pregnancy, delivery, or the health of the newborn infant. In a prospective study of 181 asthmatic women with 198 pregnancies, 40% of the patients were managed during pregnancy with the same antiasthmatic medications as before pregnancy, 18% required less medication and 42% needed more. Theophylline therapy at term did not influence labor or delivery. During the second and third trimesters until term, moderate doses of theophylline are safe. However, the safety of theophylline treatment during the first trimester with regard to teratogenicity remains to be determined. β-Agonists are also safe, but an increased risk of fetal malformation has been mentioned with the use of epinephrine. Catecholamines inhibit uterine contractions. Corticosteroids may cause fetal adrenal insufficiency, but this risk is believed to be negligible. Hypoglycemia in the infant is a complication of maternal corticosteroid therapy, and therefore, plasma glucose must be carefully monitored in the newborn. Status asthmaticus unresponsive to medical therapy during pregnancy may necessitate termination of the pregnancy. Respiratory distress can complicate pregnancy in women with severe obstructive pulmonary disease. Endotracheal intubation and mechanical ventilation in the postpartum period may be required. Bronchiectasis, if mild, does not seem to pose special problems for the pregnant patient. The National Institute of Health has indicated that undertreatment of pregnant asthmatic women, partially because of unfounded fears of adverse pharmacologic effects on the developing fetus, remains the major problem in the management of asthma during pregnancy in the United States (25).

PREGNANCY AND ASTHMA	
Summary Statement	**Level of Evidence**
Prepregnancy severity of asthma does not reliably predict the course of asthma during pregnancy (5, 26).	Observational studies
There is a relatively small but significant increase in the complications of pregnancy in asthmatic women. However, neither the effect of pregnancy on asthma nor the effect of asthma on pregnancy should be considered a contraindication to pregnancy for the asthmatic patient (27).	Observational studies, case control studies, and expert opinion
Exacerbations of asthma in the majority of women will respond to the usual treatment of bronchial asthma.	Observational studies, expert opinion
Combined oral contraceptive pill or gonadotrophin-releasing hormone analogs may be effective in patients who do not respond to usual therapy.	Observational studies, expert opinion

Sleep Apnea

Even though several cases of obstructive sleep apnea in pregnancy are reported, the prevalence of sleep apnea in pregnancy is unknown. The effects of pregnancy on the severity of pre-existent sleep apnea also are unknown. More important is the effect of obstructive sleep apnea–induced hypoxemia on fetal maturation. Chronic hypoxemia induced in an animal model has caused fetal polycythemia, but the heart rate and respiratory movements were not greatly affected. Intrauterine growth retardation in maternal obstructive sleep apnea has been reported and may be present even if external cardiotocography shows normal fetal heart rate reactivity to fetal movements, despite apneic episodes and periods of desaturation in the pregnant woman. Early recognition and treatment of obstructive sleep apnea in pregnancy might prevent problems with fetal development. Nasal continuous positive airway pressure treatment and other nonhormonal therapies pose no threat to the development of the fetus, but careful monitoring of fetal status and maternal cardiopulmonary condition is imperative.

Barotrauma

Spontaneous pneumothorax and pneumomediastinum may appear during pregnancy, but these are more likely to occur during the second stage of labor (28). Repeated Valsalva maneuvers are the most frequent cause of these problems. Pneumomediastinum is a rare complication of pregnancy, and symptoms usually are not noted until after delivery.

Pulmonary Hypertension

The incidence of primary pulmonary hypertension in pregnancy is higher than that in nonpregnant young women. A review of 602 cases of primary pulmonary hypertension from 51 medical centers recorded that 4.5% of the cases were associated with pregnancy. Another analysis of 73 women with primary pulmonary hypertension showed that 8% of the cases were related to pregnancy (29). A rigorous screening of these patients (all of whom were referred for heart-lung transplantation) to detect an underlying etiology for the pulmonary hypertension failed to disclose evidence of thromboembolic disease. Recurrent noncardiogenic pulmonary edema has been described in patients with pregnancy-induced hypertension. The reason for the increased incidence of primary pulmonary hypertension in pregnancy remains unknown.

Pulmonary Edema

Obstetric causes of pulmonary edema include aspiration pneumonia, sepsis, transfusion reactions, allergic reactions, disseminated intravascular coagulation, amniotic fluid embolism, toxemia of pregnancy, tocolytic therapy, and eclampsia, the latter being the most common cause of pulmonary edema in pregnancy. In a report on 32 obstetric patients who required admission to a critical care unit, preeclampsia was the most common reason (22%). Eclampsia remains the leading cause of maternal mortality in developing countries. A study of 126 patients with eclampsia showed acute respiratory insufficiency in 24% and a mortality of 6%. Morphologic changes in the lungs include intravascular coagulation, fibrin deposition, and intra-alveolar hemorrhage. Focal areas of bronchopneumonia also may occur. Hemodynamic studies have shown reductions in colloid osmotic pressure, pulmonary capillary leak, and left ventricular failure (30). Left ventricular dysfunction is common enough that echocardiography has been recommended to evaluate all pregnant women who develop pulmonary edema (31). Decreased venous tone and venous resistance have been suggested as the reasons for iatrogenic pulmonary edema. Surgical procedures, pyelonephritis, and other infections during pregnancy pose an increased risk for the development of pulmonary edema and acute respiratory distress syndrome. Bromocriptine therapy to suppress lactation can also cause postpartum pulmonary edema in cocaine-addicted mothers through effects on central dopamine receptors (32).

Tocolytic therapy, used to arrest uterine contractions, is associated with the development of pulmonary edema in up to 4.5% of pregnant women who are thus treated. Women with twin gestations are more likely to develop this complication, and the syndrome can occur within 12 hours postpartum. The mechanisms responsible for tocolytic therapy–induced pulmonary edema likely include a combination of volume overload, decreased colloid oncotic pressure, and increased hydrostatic pressure.

A review of tocolytic therapy–induced pulmonary edema from 1966–1988 revealed 58 cases (33). Terbutaline, a β-adrenergic agonist was the most commonly used tocolytic agent, in 41% of patients, followed by isoxsuprine in 33%, ritodrine in 17%, and salbutamol in 10%. The mean duration of tocolytic therapy was 54 hours. Symptoms included dyspnea (76%), chest pain (24%), and cough (17%), and these occurred before delivery in 70% of cases. The mean Pao_2 was 50 mm Hg. Chest roentgenograms showed bilateral alveolar opacities and a normal-sized heart. The response to diuresis was usually rapid, with full recovery over a period of 24 hours, but there were two deaths.

Pleural Effusion

Pleural effusions occur with toxemia of pregnancy, preeclampsia, pulmonary edema, pulmonary embolism, choriocarcinoma, and amniotic fluid embolism (34). Small pleural effusions are common in the postpartum period in normal pregnancy. In a retrospective study of 112 pregnant women who underwent normal delivery, pleural effusion was noted in 46%, whereas a prospective study of 30 normal pregnancies revealed pleural effusion in 67% (35). These effusions were noted within 24 hours of delivery, and all were asymptomatic and small. The factors that promote pleural effusion include increased blood volume and decreased colloid osmotic pressure normally seen in pregnancy, as well as the impaired lymphatic drainage secondary to elevated systemic venous pressure from Valsalva maneuvers during the second stage of labor. Pleural effusion as an uncommon complication of ureteral obstruction by the gravid uterus has been described in a patient. Several cases of transudative pleural effusion in connection with severe preeclampsia are reported.

Pulmonary Embolism

Thrombophlebitis and pulmonary embolism are important complications of pregnancy. Pulmonary embolism is second only to abortion as a cause of maternal death. In pooled data from the Center for Disease Control's National Pregnancy Mortality Surveillance System from 1987–1990, pulmonary embolism was the most common cause of pregnancy-related death when the fetus was undelivered and accounted for 20% of all pregnancy-related deaths, second only to postpartum hemorrhage (36,37). It occurs with higher frequency during the postpartum period, especially after a difficult labor and an abnormal postpartum hemorrhage. An earlier review of several series observed the incidence of deep vein thrombosis (DVT) to be 0.29 per 100 deliveries. Among the 32,337 pregnancies reviewed at the Mayo Clinic, superficial phlebitis

was seen in 12 per 1,000 patients, and deep phlebitis was seen in two per 1,000 pregnancies. The prepartum and postpartum incidences of thrombophlebitis were one in 1,902 patients and one in 622 patients, respectively. More than 75% of phlebitic episodes occurred during the first month after delivery, especially within the first 3 days postpartum. Calf veins were involved in 50%. Pulmonary embolism was noted to have an incidence of 0.4 per 1,000 persons (13 of 32,337 pregnancies), and 10 of these occurred during the first postpartum month. The incidence of pulmonary embolism is increased also during the first trimester.

Pregnancy and the postpartum period may be marked by venous stasis, endothelial injury, and a hypercoagulable state (37–39). There is a strikingly consistent finding of a greater incidence of DVT in the left versus the right leg in pregnant women (37,40). This distribution has been attributed to increased venous stasis in the left leg related to compression of the left iliac vein by the right iliac artery as it issues from the aorta, coupled with compression of the inferior vena cava by the gravid uterus itself (37,40–42). Pregnancy is a hypercoagulable state associated with a progressive increase in several coagulation factors, such as factors I, II, VII, VIII, IX, and X, along with a decrease in protein S (37). The factor V Leiden mutation that leads to activated protein C resistance is an important risk factor for thrombophlebitis and pulmonary embolism during pregnancy (especially the first trimester), after pregnancy, or during oral contraceptive use (43,44). A study of 50 women who had DVT and/or pulmonary embolism identified 10 women with activated protein C resistance caused by factor V Leiden mutation (45). First-trimester DVT and/or pulmonary embolism developed in six of the 10 women with the mutation compared with three of 40 women without the mutation. Another coagulopathy that plays a significant role in pregnancy-associated thrombophlebitis and pulmonary embolism is the presence of antiphospholipid antibody syndrome (46,47). Also known as lupus anticoagulant syndrome or anticardiolipin antibody syndrome, the antiphospholipid antibody syndrome is characterized by the presence of antiphospholipid antibodies in serum. Obstetric complications attributed to this syndrome include recurrent (three or more) miscarriages, fetal death in utero, intrauterine growth restriction, preterm delivery, early or severe eclampsia, and abruptio placentae (46,47).

The diagnosis of venous thromboembolism during pregnancy can be complicated by physiologic changes associated with pregnancy and by reluctance of parents and physicians to expose the fetus to even small amounts of ionizing radiation (37). Coumarin drugs, unlike heparin, cross the placenta and may cause fetal hemorrhage and congenital malformations, with a perinatal mortality of 18%. Treatment of antepartum thrombophlebitis or pulmonary embolism should start with intravenous heparin, followed by coumarin after the first trimester (48). Coumarin should be replaced by intravenous heparin at the 37th week of gestation. All anticoagulants are withheld from the time of labor to 6 hours after delivery. Then heparin and coumarin should be resumed as in conventional patients. The availability of low-molecular-weight heparin for prophylactic use in patients with high or known risk for development of thromboembolic diseases has been shown to be effective. The use of prophylactic low-molecular-weight heparin therapy during part of their pregnancy in 24 women carrying 27 pregnancies with known risk of venopulmonary thromboembolic diseases showed that none of the treated women developed clinical signs of thromboembolic diseases during pregnancy or 6 weeks postpartum (49). All the babies were born healthy, and none of the women had any side effects owing to the treatment.

PREGNANCY AND VENOUS THROMBOEMBOLISM

Summary Statement	Level of Evidence
Documented venous thromboembolism requires treatment for the duration of pregnancy with either unfractionated or low-molecular-weight heparin (37).	Observational studies, expert opinion
Prophylaxis of venous thromboembolism should be undertaken in women with a prior history of idiopathic venous thromboembolism and/or a documented hypercoagulable state (37).	Observational studies, expert opinion
All patients should avoid the supine position in favor of the left lateral decubitus position in late pregnancy (37).	Observational studies, expert opinion
Graduated elastic compression stockings may be useful (37, 50).	Observational studies, expert opinion

Amniotic Fluid Embolism

Amniotic fluid embolism is an uncommon complication of parturition (51). In the United States, the incidence is in the range of one in 20,000 to 30,000 deliveries (51–53). Amniotic fluid embolism carries an exceedingly high mortality, with a fatal outcome in 86% of cases (54). Nearly 10% of maternal deaths in the 1960s were attributed to this complication. As the frequency of other causes of mortality in pregnancy has diminished, the percentage of deaths owing to amniotic fluid embolism has risen, and it is reported to be second only to pulmonary thromboembolism.

The average age at occurrence of amniotic fluid embolism is 32 years, and the risk factors include multiparity, very strong (tetanic) uterine contractions during labor, a large fetus, a dead fetus, and large quantities of particulate matter, including meconium. In one study of 40 cases of amniotic fluid embolism, the occurrence of abruptio placentae and placenta previa was noted in 45%. Rupture of the cervix (in 54%–60% of cases), amniocentesis, and legal abortions also have caused amniotic fluid embolism.

Originally, the pathogenesis was attributed to an anaphylactoid reaction, but there has been no proof of this. The pathogenesis probably comprises a combination of three fac-

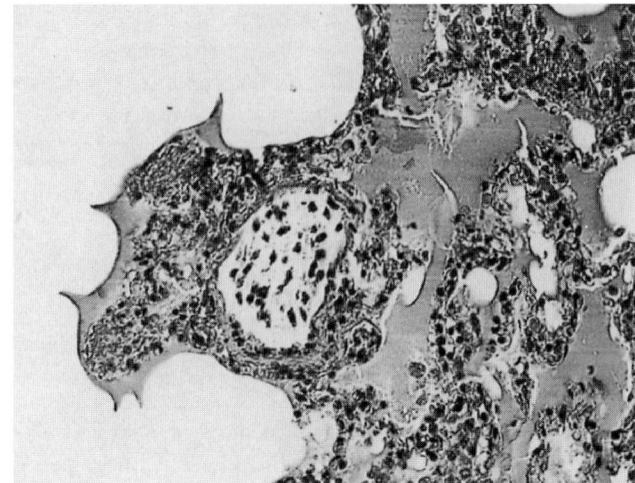

FIGURE 64.1. Amniotic fluid embolism. Pulmonary arteriole occluded by fetal cells, vernix, and mucin.

tors: pulmonary microvascular obstruction with subsequent systemic hypotension, pulmonary hypertension with acute cor pulmonale, and ventilation-perfusion inequality (54). Detailed studies have shown that left ventricular failure is the only consistent abnormality. Pathologic examination of the lungs show overwhelming obstruction of the pulmonary arteries are by amniotic fluid contents—i.e., mucin, fetal squamous cells, vernix fat globules, meconium, and lanugo hairs (Fig. 64.1). Mucin is usually present, and the cellular elements are seen 80% of the time, with special stains and immunoperoxidase.

Clinically, the patient develops chills, shivering, cough, cyanosis, convulsions, and profound shock during labor or immediately postpartum (55). The survivors usually develop disseminated intravascular coagulopathy, resulting in excessive uterine hemorrhage. The diagnosis is made on a clinical basis presumptively and definitively at postmortem. The diagnosis also can be made by identifying mucin and squamous cells in a blood smear taken from a central venous line such as a pulmonary artery catheter. Treatment is supportive, as the use of corticosteroids and anticoagulants has not changed the course of the disease.

Tuberculosis

The annual incidence of tuberculosis among pregnant women has varied depending on the period during which the data were collected (56). The rate of tuberculosis among American women of childbearing age (15–45 years) declined from 3.8 per 100,000 in 1977 to 2.35 per 100,000 in 1987, then increased to 2.5 per 100,000 in 1989 among Hispanic white women.

Pregnancy neither predisposes to the development or progression of tuberculosis nor alters the clinical presentation of the disease (57,58). Because prenatal care is often the only contact that many high-risk women have with the health care system, screening for tuberculosis is recommended during pregnancy (59). A study of 1,565 pregnancies during which tuberculosis was active showed no evidence of a negative consequence of pregnancy on tuberculosis during gestation, although most of the relapses developed in the postpartum period. A corollary to this is that tuberculosis neither affects nor complicates the course of pregnancy or the type of delivery (60). However, mother-to-fetus or -newborn transmission of tuberculosis is an important clinical consideration in the management of the pregnant tuberculous patient. The modes of spread of *tubercle bacilli* from mother to fetus or newborn include hematogenous or lymphogenous spread, transmission through placenta, and tuberculous endometritis during pregnancy. A detailed review of the topic concluded that despite the potential for transmission in utero, the newborn is at greater risk of acquiring tuberculosis postpartum than congenitally, particularly if born to a mother whose sputum contains *tubercle bacilli* and whose condition remains undiagnosed and untreated.

The presentation of tuberculosis in pregnant women is similar to that in nonpregnant women, but diagnosis may be delayed by the nonspecific nature of early symptoms and the frequency of malaise and fatigue in pregnancy (61–63). The most common site of tuberculosis in pregnant women is pulmonary (61). The most common symptom and signs include cough, weight loss, fever, malaise or fatigue, and hemoptysis (61). Although up to 20% of pregnant women with pulmonary tuberculosis are asymptomatic, all have abnormal chest radiographs (61). Extrapulmonary disease is becoming more prevalent, and the increase is more pronounced among young women and immigrants from countries with a high prevalence of tuberculosis. (64) Radiation hazard from repeated chest roentgenography should be minimized in pregnant women. In those suspected of having tuberculosis, a chest roentgenogram should be obtained after the 12th week of gestation with proper shielding of the abdomen, and it should be performed only when a positive result of a tuberculin skin test requires exclusion of active pulmonary tuberculosis. However, it may be necessary sooner if the patient has symptoms that are highly suggestive of pulmonary tuberculosis. Tuberculin skin testing is not contraindicated in pregnancy, as it does not affect pregnancy or the fetus. The tuberculin response in pregnancy is no different from that in nonpregnant woman. Induced sputum and gastric washings on a repeated basis are valuable.

Active pulmonary tuberculosis diagnosed during pregnancy should be treated promptly, the initial drug combination being isoniazid (300 mg/d) and rifampin (600 mg/d) for at least 9 months (65). Ethambutol may be used if the clinical situation warrants addition of the third or alternate drug. Because of their potential to cause fetal toxicity, pyrazinamide, streptomycin, and other aminoglycosides should be avoided. Active disease detected at the time of delivery should be treated. During the postpartum period, antituberculous drugs are continued until the prescribed treatment period

is completed. Antituberculous therapy is not a contraindication to breast-feeding. Other precautions—i.e., the isolation precautions, study of contacts, and preventive therapy for the infant and close contacts—are similar to the approach in nonpregnant tuberculous patients. Tuberculosis is not an indication for routine therapeutic interruption of pregnancy.

Gestational Trophoblastic Disease

Gestational trophoblastic disease defines a heterogeneous group of interrelated lesions that represent an aberrant fertilization event (66). These diseases occur after any gestational experience (e.g., abortion, ectopic, or term pregnancy). The pathogenesis is unique because the maternal tumor arises from fetal, not maternal, tissue (66).

Molar Pregnancy

Thoracic complications can occur after removal of a benign hydatidiform mole. The incidence of trophoblastic pulmonary emboli varies between 2% and 11%. Clinically, a wide spectrum of pulmonary findings occurs, including the development of pulmonary hypertension and pulmonary edema. Among 128 women who underwent evacuation of hydatidiform mole, 9.4% developed acute severe respiratory distress, and trophoblastic embolism was identified in seven patients. The incidence of respiratory complications increased from zero at less than 16 weeks' gestation to 27% when the uterus had developed beyond 16 weeks. In a review of 60 patients with benign trophoblastic disease, five developed pulmonary complications, with two progressing into acute respiratory distress syndrome from pulmonary edema. Possible etiologies for the respiratory manifestations include trophoblastic emboli, hypervolemia, and intravascular coagulation. Chest roentgenograms may reveal rounded lesions.

Choriocarcinoma

Choriocarcinoma is a form of gestational trophoblastic disease that commonly metastasizes to lung, vagina, uterus, and brain because of the propensity of trophoblastic tissue to disseminate hematogenously. Choriocarcinoma is most often preceded by molar pregnancy. It is a fetal neoplasm that invades maternal tissue and it occurs in one in 20,000 pregnancies. The diagnosis can be confirmed by the finding of high plasma human chorionic β-gonadotropin levels in a nonpregnant patient. Pulmonary metastases occur frequently in patients with gestational choriocarcinoma. The interval between pregnancy and pulmonary metastases varies from 1 to 60 months. Pulmonary metastases have been reported in 68% of patients with choriocarcinoma. The pulmonary lesions may be multiple, discrete, calcified, and associated with pleural effusion. Hemoptysis is seen in patients with chest roentgenographic abnormalities. In a series of 179 patients, 36 presented with pulmonary symptoms, and all but one had abnormal chest roentgenograms. Among 131 patients with gestational trophoblastic tumor, 57% had pulmonary metastases detected on plain chest roentgenography (67). Computed tomography scans of the chest may reveal lesions not seen on plain chest roentgenography. Pulmonary involvement was commonly extensive, with 43% having more than 10 pulmonary metastases and 60% having a pulmonary lesion more than 5 cm in diameter (67). Eleven percent developed early respiratory failure, requiring mechanical ventilation within 1 month of presentation. Other pulmonary features included greater than 50% lung opacification in 25 patients, mediastinal involvement in 25 patients, and pleural effusion in 36 patients.

Most patients with pulmonary metastasis from choriocarcinoma achieve remission with chemotherapy alone. The major aspect of management of patients with high-risk, metastatic, gestational trophoblastic tumors includes polychemotherapy. Therapeutic regimen using etoposide, high-dose methotrexate, actinomycin D, cyclophosphamide, and vincristine is reported to result in complete response rates of 80% to 94% and survival rates of 82% to 100%. The factors that determine poor response to treatment are metastases to sites other than the lung and vagina, more than eight metastases, previous failed chemotherapy and a World Health Organization score greater than eight. Tumor emboli and hemothorax also can occur. Gestational choriocarcinoma has presented as an endobronchial lesion. The indications for surgical resection of lung metastasis are limited, but in appropriately selected patients, resection of a lesion resistant to chemotherapy can be curative (68).

Miscellaneous Obstetric Disorders

Sarcoidosis

Sarcoidosis does not seem to have any adverse effects on the course of pregnancy (69). Pregnancy, on the other hand, is reported to lead to improvement of sarcoidosis in some patients. In patients whose chest roentgenograms demonstrate disease resolution before pregnancy, a normal chest roentgenogram is likely to persist through the prenatal period and gestation. Patients with active sarcoidosis usually experience partial or complete resolution of chest roentgenographic abnormalities during pregnancy, although many in this group will experience exacerbation of sarcoid within 3 to 6 months after delivery (70,71). Those with a fibrotic process secondary to sarcoidosis are likely to show no changes in their chest roentgenograms. One possible explanation for the frequent ameliorating effect of pregnancy on sarcoidosis is the increased serum levels of corticosteroids.

Rhinitis

Rhinitis occurs frequently during pregnancy, and although many causes (e.g., altered vagal function, and hormonal imbalance) have been proposed, the rhinitis of pregnancy may not be a distinct entity.

Varicella

Varicella pneumonia seems to occur more commonly in pregnant women. The incidence of varicella is estimated to be one to five cases per 10,000 pregnancies (72). A review of the literature in 1980 noted that approximately 10% of all reported cases of varicella pneumonia were in pregnant women, and the maternal mortality rate was approximately 45%. A study in 1996 of 28 pregnant women with varicella infection observed the incidence of pneumonia to be 3.6% and reported that pregnant women are not at increased risk of developing varicella pneumonia (73). Furthermore, all pregnant patients recovered uneventfully, and no congenital anomalies or perinatal complications were noted in the infants of the 26 mothers who were followed up. A case control study of 18 pregnant women with varicella pneumonia and 72 pregnant controls with varicella but no pneumonia found that smoking and the occurrence of 100 skin lesions or more were risk factors for the development of pneumonia (74). Importantly, varicella pneumonia in pregnancy is a medical emergency (75). The mortality rate in untreated pregnant women is in excess of 40% (76). Prompt supportive care and acyclovir are the mainstays of therapy (74,77).

Coccidioidomycosis

Coccidioidomycosis shows a propensity to disseminate during pregnancy (78,79). One report on 50 pregnant women observed a 50% rate dissemination. The risk of dissemination was higher in those who contracted the infection during pregnancy, particularly in the second and third trimesters. Amphotericin B, the drug of choice in disseminated coccidioidomycosis, has no detrimental effects on pregnancy and poses minimal risk to the fetus.

Cystic Fibrosis

Cystic fibrosis poses special problems in pregnancy (80). As women with cystic fibrosis are living longer, pregnancy is becoming increasingly common in this group of women. The incidence of female infertility may be as high as 20% (81). It is caused by both secondary amenorrhea (induced primarily by malnutrition) and the production of abnormally tenacious cervical mucus (82). Premature labor and delivery remain a significant risk for pregnant women with cystic fibrosis, contributing to a high rate of perinatal death. Maternal illness and death result from deteriorating pulmonary function. In a study of 11 pregnancies among eight women with cystic fibrosis, the maternal condition deteriorated during and after pregnancy and did not return to the pregravidic state. Prepregnancy FEV_1 appears to be the most useful predictor of important outcome measures in pregnancies in women with cystic fibrosis. A retrospective study of 22 pregnancies in 20 patients with cystic fibrosis noted that 18 pregnancies were completed producing healthy noncystic fibrosis infants (12 female) (83). Even though there was a 13% decrease in FEV_1 and 11% decrease in FVC during pregnancy, these values returned to normal after labor.

Connective Tissue Diseases

Systemic Lupus Erythematosus

Systemic lupus erythematosus (SLE) may be exacerbated during pregnancy. Several cases of lupus pneumonitis developing during the postpartum period have been described. A prospective study of 80 pregnant women with SLE demonstrated that worsening of SLE is uncommon in pregnancy, and prophylactic prednisone therapy is unnecessary (84). Prematurity and fetal death is the greatest hazards in patients with SLE (85,86).

Progressive Systemic Sclerosis

In progressive systemic sclerosis, significant renal involvement is a major contraindication to pregnancy because of the very poor fetal prognosis and the risk of maternal death owing to a lethal progression of renal failure (87–89). Women with early, rapidly progressive, diffuse skin thickening should avoid becoming pregnant because, intrinsically, they are at higher risk of developing renal crisis (90). A case control study showed that women with scleroderma had twice the rate of spontaneous abortion and three times the rate of fertility problems (no successful pregnancy by the age of 35) compared with rates for control women (91).

Wegener Granulomatosis

Wegener granulomatosis is reported to relapse during pregnancy. A review noted that there were 15 pregnancies recorded in 10 women with Wegener granulomatosis (92). Among these, the diagnosis of Wegener granulomatosis was documented during pregnancy in four cases and during the postpartum period in three cases. Eight pregnancies occurred in women with known Wegener granulomatosis, and the disease relapsed during five pregnancies. Two cases ended with maternal death.

Pulmonary Arteriovenous Malformations

Pulmonary arteriovenous malformations associated with hereditary hemorrhagic telangiectasia (Osler-Rendu-Weber syndrome) pose several additional pulmonary problems. Pregnant women with this syndrome face the risk of deterioration of pulmonary shunt, pulmonary hemorrhage, and stroke (93,94). There are several reports of the arteriovenous fistulas enlarging during pregnancy, rupturing into the lungs or pleura, causing serious complications such as massive hemothorax, and increasing hypoxia. Transcatheter

embolotherapy of maternal pulmonary arteriovenous malformations performed by an experienced radiologist appears to be safe and effective after 16 weeks of gestational age (94).

Diaphragmatic Rupture

Diaphragmatic rupture leading to respiratory failure is another rare but potentially lethal complication of pregnancy (95,96).

Appendicitis during Pregnancy

A case control study of 49 patients with appendicitis during pregnancy noted pulmonary edema or lung opacities in seven patients and adult respiratory distress syndrome in two patients (97). By multivariate analysis, the following factors were estimated to predict 99% of the pulmonary complications: a fluid overload of 4 L, respiratory rate of 24 breaths/min, maximum temperature of 100.4°F, and tocolytic usage.

GYNECOLOGIC DISORDERS

Several gynecologic diseases produce pulmonary complications. Some of these represent a peculiar association of pulmonary and gynecologic disorders rather than complications. Table 64.2 lists the pulmonary complications of the gynecologic diseases.

Thoracic Endometriosis

Endometriosis is defined as the presence of endometrial glands in stroma outside the confines of the uterine cavity and musculature (98). A literature review in 1996 of 110 cases of thoracic endometriosis observed the following clinical features: pneumothorax in 73%, hemothorax in 14%, hemoptysis in 7%, and lung nodules in 6% (99). The

TABLE 64.2. PULMONARY COMPLICATIONS IN GYNECOLOGIC DISEASES

Pulmonary Complication	Gynecologic Etiology
Pneumothorax, pneumo-mediastinum (catamenial)	Pleural endometriosis
	Air entry via genital tract into pleural space
Hemoptysis	Endobronchial endometriosis
Pulmonary nodules or atelectasis	Endobronchial endometriosis
	Benign metastasizing leiomyoma
	Pulmonary lymphangioleiomyomatosis
Pleural effusion	Ovarian neoplasm (Meigs-Salmon syndrome)
	Pulmonary lymphangioleiomyomatosis
	Uterine fibroids
	Pleural endometriosis
Premenstrual exacerbation of asthma	Hormonal imbalance (?)

right hemithorax was involved in more than 90% of all manifestations except for nodules. Hemothorax was more often associated with presence of pleural and pelvic endometriosis compared with other manifestations. Spontaneous pneumothorax has also been described in a patient with carcinoma of the cervix.

Pulmonary Endometriosis

Pulmonary endometriosis is rare (100). The endometrial tissue in the lung is presumed to originate from hematogenous spread or celomic metaplasia. Pleural endometriosis is believed to spread from pelvic or peritoneal deposits. Another possibility is the hematogenous metastasis of viable endometrial tissue after uterine surgery or cesarean section. This argument is supported by the finding that pulmonary endometriosis is almost always detected in the lower lung, which receives a higher blood supply. Pathologic analysis of pleuropulmonary tissue in patients with thoracic endometriosis shows changes typical of endometriosis.

Pulmonary parenchymal endometriosis appears most often in women in their fourth or fifth decade (mean age, 39 years) and is associated with pelvic endometriosis in only 10% of cases, catamenial hemoptysis in 82% of cases, and catamenial pain and dyspnea in 18% of cases. A literature review in 1996 of 110 cases of thoracic endometriosis observed the lung nodules in 6% (99). Endobronchial endometriosis has been reported to cause catamenial hemoptysis and airway obstruction with segmental atelectasis. Other symptoms include chest pain, dyspnea, or pleural effusion. Asymptomatic pulmonary density is another manifestation. Chest roentgenograms have revealed solitary pulmonary nodules in parenchymal endometriosis.

Catamenial Pneumothorax

Catamenial pneumothorax is a syndrome of spontaneous recurrent pneumothorax occurring within 48 to 73 hours of the onset of menses (101). Pleural disease is associated more frequently with pelvic endometriosis. Until pneumothorax recurs, it is impossible to determine clinical coincidence from the specific syndrome of catamenial pneumothorax. Catamenial pneumothorax is the most common thoracic complication of endometriosis. A review in 1990 noted that there were approximately 100 cases in the literature (102). Among 196 cases of spontaneous pneumothoraces in women younger than 50 years, 5.6% were catamenial. Usually seen in women between the ages of 30 and 35 years, catamenial pneumothorax is almost always (90%–95%) right-sided and small. The majority of patients present with chest pain or mild dyspnea; however, the syndrome can be asymptomatic. Chest computed tomography scan findings of pulmonary and pleural nodules have been noted, but the scan may be negative unless it is obtained during menses (103).

Pneumothorax is believed by some to be caused by pleural endometriosis (Fig. 64.2). However, clinical and pathologic

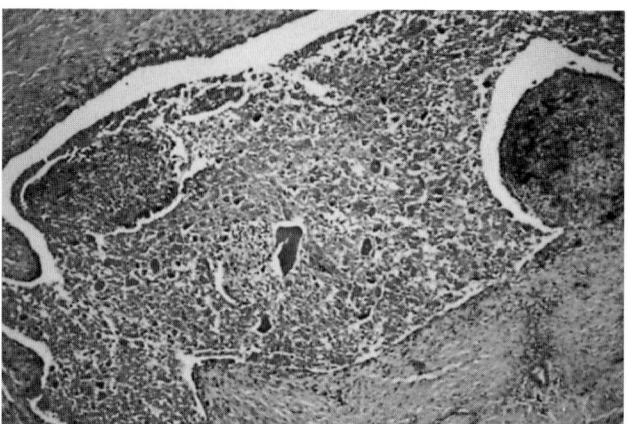

FIGURE 64.2. Pleural endometriosis causing pneumothorax.

evidence of pelvic endometriosis is demonstrated in only 22% to 37% of cases. Pleural or diaphragmatic endometrial implants have been visualized at thoracotomy in 23% to 35% of patients. Air originating in the genital tract is believed to make its way through defects in the diaphragm. Examination at the time of thoracotomy for treatment of catamenial pneumothorax has revealed defects in the diaphragm, and closure of these defects has resulted in the absence of recurrent pneumothorax. However, such diaphragmatic defects or fenestrations have been found in only 19% to 33% of the cases explored. The diaphragmatic defects have been observed with thoracoscopy using a bronchoscope.

Ovulation-suppressing agents such as danazol sometimes are helpful in preventing recurrent pneumothorax. A case of catamenial pneumomediastinum that responded to danazol has been described.

Premenstrual Asthma

Premenstrual worsening of asthma (premenstrual asthma) has been reported in several publications (104). Severe asthmatics are reported to be more prone to premenstrual deterioration of asthma. In a study involving 126 consecutive women age 14 to 46 years who attended an outpatient asthma clinic, a detailed questionnaire and twice-daily peak expiratory flow (PEF) measurements revealed premenstrual deterioration of asthma in 40% (105). The falls in peak flow were modest and of a degree that would not be expected to result in increased dyspnea. No correlations were found between premenstrual exacerbation of asthma and symptoms of premenstrual tension, consumption of aspirin, use of the contraceptive pill, cycle length, or behavior of asthma during pregnancy. Even mild asthmatics who were previously unaware of premenstrual asthma have been shown to observe a premenstrual deterioration of asthmatic symptoms and PEF rate without showing any significant changes in spirometry or airway reactivity.

The mechanism of premenstrual exacerbation of asthma is unclear. Progesterone level reaches a peak approximately 7 days before menstruation and rapidly decreases almost to

zero at the onset of the period. It is known that progesterone is a smooth-muscle relaxant in the gastrointestinal
tract, genitourinary system, and vascular tree, and the decrease in progesterone concentration in the late luteal phase
might be associated with the withdrawal of a relaxant effect on bronchial smooth muscle. There are earlier reports
on treatment of ovarian asthma by irradiation of the ovaries
and progesterone preparations. Progesterone is a well-known
respiratory stimulant and is known to cause hyperventilation, which may heighten the sensation of breathlessness.
However, the peak serum concentrations of progesterone
are reached several days before symptomatic deterioration of
asthma, and therefore, progesterone-induced hyperventilation is an unlikely explanation for premenstrual exacerbation
of asthma. Analysis of clinical data from 182 nonpregnant
women with asthma, ages 13 years to menopause, showed a
fourfold variation in asthma presentations during the perimenstrual interval, indicating that the monthly variations in
serum estradiol levels may influence the severity of asthma
in women (106). A role for long-acting bronchodilators and
leukotriene-modifying agents in controlling perimenstrual
asthma exacerbations has been suggested (107,108).

Estrogen Replacement Therapy

Estrogen replacement therapy may play a role in the pathophysiology of asthma. Long-term use and/or high doses of
postmenopausal hormone therapy may increase subsequent
risk of asthma. A prospective study of a cohort of premenopausal and postmenopausal women 34 to 68 years of
age during 582,135 person-years of follow-up documented
726 new cases of asthma (109). Postmenopausal women who
were never users of replacement hormones had a significantly
lower age-adjusted risk of asthma than that of premenopausal
women. Those who had 10 or more years of replacement
hormones had twice the age-adjusted risk of asthma compared with that of women who never used postmenopausal
hormones.

Ozone exposure during the follicular phase of the menstrual cycle is reported to elicit enhanced airway response and
lead to airway inflammation. One study noted although the
socioeconomic status appeared to affect FEV$_1$ responsiveness
to ozone, with the middle socioeconomic group being the
most responsive, the phase of menstrual cycle did not have
an impact on individual responsiveness to ozone (110).

Effect of Menses on Respiration

Menses also affect normal respiration in nonasthmatic
women. The respiratory-stimulating effect of progesterone
was mentioned above. The level of progesterone varies during the menstrual cycle in adult women. In a study of 30
healthy women, respiratory muscle function, measured by
maximal static inspiratory and expiratory pressures, was assessed during the midfollicular and midluteal phases of the
menstrual cycle; the results showed that inspiratory muscle

endurance was 26% higher in the midluteal phase than in the
midfollicular phase, whereas the respiratory muscle strength
and pulmonary function were unchanged (111). Other studies have shown that resting ventilation, ventilatory response
to hypoxia or hypercapnia, and resistance to genioglossal
activity are elevated during the luteal phase. These findings
imply that the high inspiratory muscle endurance in the midluteal phase may be related, at least in part, to high plasma
progesterone levels. A study of variations in carbon monoxide diffusing capacity (D$_{LCO}$) during the menstrual cycle in
14 healthy women (eight were using oral contraceptives),
with a mean age of 29 years, observed the D$_{LCO}$ to vary significantly during the menstrual cycle, with the highest values
occurring before menses and the lowest values occurring on
the third day of menses, with a mean difference between
them of 9% (112).

Metastasizing Benign Leiomyoma

Metastasizing benign leiomyoma is an oddity in pulmonary
diseases and an oxymoron. Uterine fibroleiomyomas (also
called well-differentiated leiomyosarcoma) are known to be
associated with multiple pulmonary fibroleiomyomas. Although slow-growing, these are believed to be pulmonary
metastases, hence the term metastasizing benign leiomyoma
(113). A review of 23 reported cases revealed the following:
The age span among patients studied was 30 to 74 years
(mean, 47 years), three fourths had uterine leiomyomas, and
all but two were white (114). Most cases were discovered
during routine chest roentgenographic examination. The lesions were nodular, bilateral in 15 patients, recurrent in three
patients, and increased in size in seven patients. Roentgenographically, these nodular densities may range from 0.5 to 4.5
cm in diameter (Figs. 64.3 and 64.4) and, occasionally, pleural effusion is also seen. Nodules may grow in premenopausal
women and remain stationary in postmenopausal women.

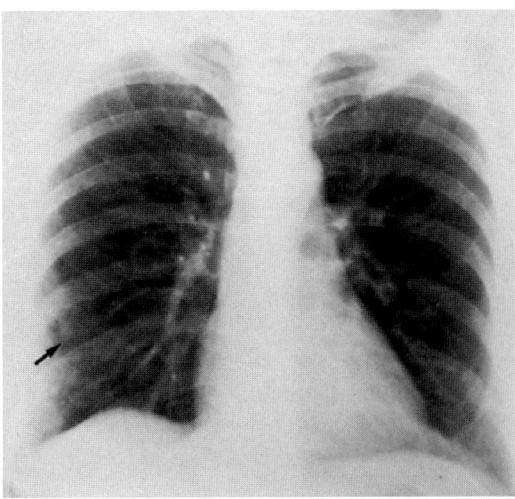

FIGURE 64.3. Benign metastasizing leiomyoma in the lungs. *Arrows* point
to small nodules in the lungs.

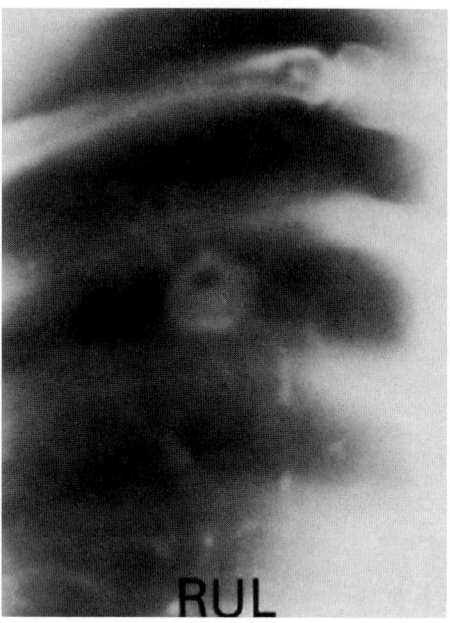

FIGURE 64.4. Benign metastasizing leiomyoma in right upper lobe (RUL); cavitation as a result of secondary infection is demonstrated.

REPRODUCTIVE ORGANS

Diseases of the reproductive organs are occasionally associated with pulmonary problems. The main entities included in this discussion are Meigs-Salmon syndrome, Klinefelter syndrome, Turner syndrome, and Young syndrome. Lymphangioleiomyomatosis is a rare disorder that affects women of childbearing age and is discussed in Chapter 32. Pleuropulmonary metastases are common in patients with malignancies of the reproductive organs.

Meigs-Salmon Syndrome

Meigs-Salmon syndrome, also known as Meigs-Salmon-Cass syndrome, is characterized by the coexistence of ovarian fibroma or other solid ovarian tumors, ascites, and pleural effusion. Pleural effusion occurs in 3% of patients with ovarian neoplasms that measure more than 6 cm in diameter. A variant of this syndrome is described in which the clinical features were highly suggestive of Meigs-Salmon syndrome, but the ovary showed degenerative changes without tumor. The pleural effusions in this syndrome are more common on the right, are transudative chemically, and may become voluminous. The transportation of fluid from the peritoneum to the pleural space is via the diaphragmatic lymphatics. Massive edema of the ovary without neoplastic changes has been reported to cause hydrothorax and ascites. Very large ovarian tumors are capable of producing respiratory failure by upward push on the diaphragm. The effusions and ascites usually disappear with removal of the ovarian tumor.

Uterine Cancer

Endometrial cancer is the most common female genital cancer, and approximately 90% of the cases are diagnosed while they are still confined to the uterus (115,116). Among 1,665 patients with uterine cancer, 100 patients (6%) who had pulmonary metastases showed the following clinical features: median age of 65.5 years, 59 adenocarcinomas, 21 sarcomas, and 14 adenosquamous carcinomas (116). Lung metastases were found at the time of diagnosis of the primary tumor in 22 patients. Of all patients with lung metastases, 75% did not survive 1 year; however, 6% survived more than 5 years after diagnosis of metastatic disease.

Uterine Fibroids

Uterine fibroids have been responsible for the occurrence of pleural effusion in several cases. These patients were between the ages of 30 and 45 years and presented with abdominal distention and mass. There were no menstrual abnormalities. The pleural effusions were right-sided in 75% and hemorrhagic in one patient. Both transudates and exudates have been described. The pathogenesis of the pleural effusion in these patients and in Meigs-Salmon syndrome is unknown, although there exists the possibility of active exudation of fluid by the tumors or inflamed peritoneum and lymphatic or venous obstruction.

Klinefelter Syndrome

Klinefelter syndrome is the most common example of male hypogonadism in phenotypic men, characterized by the presence of two or more X chromosomes, the most common karyotype being XXY. It is morphologically manifested by varying degrees of seminiferous tubular failure and decreased Leydig cell function. Clinical features include small and firm testes, infertility, decreased testosterone level, gynecomastia, and, frequently, eunuchoid features and mild mental retardation. Respiratory disease is known to be more prevalent in these patients than in the population at large. Pulmonary manifestations described have included asthmatic bronchitis, recurrent pulmonary infections, bronchiectasis, pectus excavatum, kyphoscoliosis, pulmonary cysts, respiratory infections, and emphysema. Restrictive lung dysfunction is attributed to chest wall abnormalities, even though pulmonary restriction has been demonstrated in the absence of parenchymal or musculoskeletal abnormalities. A detailed physiologic study of 13 patients with Klinefelter syndrome reported that none exhibited chest wall restriction, but four patients demonstrated significantly reduced lung compliance. The investigators concluded that the likely cause of pulmonary restriction, noted in eight patients (62%), was a decrease in the compliance of the lung matrix, probably related to the absence of testosterone.

Turner Syndrome

Turner syndrome is a disorder of sex differentiation. Its clinical features include an XO sex chromosome constitution, dwarfism, sexual infantilism, webbing of the neck, and cubitus valgus. Thoracic manifestations consist of square and shield-like chest, pleural effusions, coarctation of the aorta, and rib notching.

Young Syndrome

Young syndrome, or obstructive azoospermia, denotes primary infertility in men who have normal spermatozoa in the epididymides but none in the ejaculate (117). This entity differs from the well-known links between infertility and lung diseases noted in ciliary dysmotility syndromes and cystic fibrosis (118). Unlike the immotile cilia syndrome, Young syndrome has no demonstrable ultrastructural ciliary disorders, and unlike cystic fibrosis, normal sweat and pancreatic functions are present. Indeed, electron microscopy of nasal cilia in 12 patients with Young syndrome has confirmed normal ciliary ultrastructure. Young syndrome is estimated to have a prevalence rate comparable to that of Klinefelter syndrome and higher than that of either cystic fibrosis or the immotile cilia syndrome.

The underlying abnormality in Young syndrome is unknown, although it is presumed to be a mucous defect. Mucociliary clearance, as determined by nasal ciliary beat frequency, is shown to be abnormal in Young syndrome. It is not clear whether this is the cause or effect of sinusitis. The relative disorientation of distal ciliary axoneme in patients with Young syndrome may be owing to a structural defect but is more likely a consequence of abnormal mucus. However, use of mucoregulatory agents in these patients has not been helpful.

Mercury intoxication has been proposed as an etiologic factor in the development of Young syndrome. Calomel (mercurous chloride) was removed from teething powders and worm medication in the United Kingdom in 1955. An interesting study of 274 men with obstructive azoospermia undergoing epididymovasostomy observed that the incidence of Young syndrome fell significantly from 114 of 227 men born up to 1955 to eight of 47 men born since then (119). This decline in incidence of Young syndrome in those born after 1955 was similar to that observed with pink disease (mercury intoxication).

More than half the patients in the original series had severe chest disease in childhood. In a study of 34 infertile men with obstructive azoospermia and normal controls, the following abnormalities were noted in those with Young syndrome: grossly abnormal sinus roentgenograms (59%), sinusitis (56%), repeated otitis media (32%), chronic bronchitis (35%), abnormal chest roentgenograms (53%), and bronchiectasis (29%) (120) (Fig. 64.5). Airflow obstruction was observed in 15 patients. Although this controlled

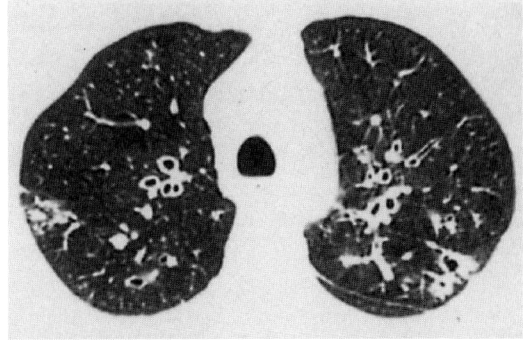

FIGURE 64.5. Young syndrome with bronchiectasis documented by high-resolution computed tomography showing bilateral bronchiectasis.

study confirmed that a significant excess of sinopulmonary disease exists in this group, the reason for the relationship between obstructive azoospermia and lung disease remains undefined.

Pregnancies, with paternity documented by genotyping, have occurred in several couples (117). Thus, improved microsurgical and medical therapy might restore fertility.

Sexual Activity and the Lung

The coital act is physically strenuous, even in healthy humans. The presence of chronic respiratory disease affects this function in many patients in the form of functional impotence or lack of libido. Although a considerable number of patients with respiratory diseases are concerned about their inability to have normal sexual intercourse, very few mention this aspect of their health to their physicians. Part of the reason is the patients' embarrassment in bringing up this seemingly medically irrelevant topic, and part is owing to physicians' failure to inquire about it. Several medications, particularly β-blocking agents, cause impotence. However, none of the drugs used in chronic obstructive pulmonary disease or other common lung diseases is known to affect sexual function. Medroxyprogesterone used in some patients with central sleep apnea may result in impotence after long-term therapy. In hypoxemic patients, supplemental oxygen therapy during sexual intercourse may be helpful.

Coital Hemoptysis

Coital hemoptysis has been described in a patient with coronary artery disease. Despite recurrent episodes of hemoptysis that necessitated several visits to his physician, the patient did not provide the history of sexual activity in relation to hemoptysis. Increased cardiovascular demands and left ventricular dysfunction brought on by sexual activity were concluded to be physiologic reasons for the hemoptysis. Postcoital catamenial pneumothorax not associated with endometriosis has also been reported.

Postcoital Asthma

Postcoital asthma and rhinitis (honeymoon rhinitis) brought on by sexual activity have been described in several patients (121,122). A study of three men and one woman with postcoital asthma or rhinitis observed clinically significant attacks of asthma or rhinorrhea during and immediately after sexual intercourse; indeed, one man required several visits to the emergency department and hospitalization on one occasion. All had a previous history of asthma, and anxiety was noted to be a predominant feature in the patients and their sexual partners. Sexual excitement, rather than exercise, may have caused asthma in one of the patients who developed asthmatic symptoms before sexual intercourse. Allergy to human seminal plasma in female subjects has also been reported to cause postcoital asthma.

Reflux Dyspareunia

Reflux dyspareunia denotes heartburn occurring during sexual intercourse. In a prospective study of 100 women with known gastroesophageal reflux, 77% suffered from reflux symptoms (severe in six, moderate in 22, and mild in 49) during sexual intercourse (123). The supine position and increased intra-abdominal pressure may account for the reflux symptoms during sexual intercourse. Although the number of women with hiatal hernia was not mentioned, the presence of gastroesophageal reflux during coitus is as important as other factors in causing reflux dyspareunia. No mention has been made in the literature on reflux dyspareunia-related aspiration.

REFERENCES

1. Lapinsky SE, Kruczynski K, Slutsky AS. Critical care in the pregnant patient. *Am J Respir Crit Care Med* 1995;152:427–455.
2. Rizk NW, Kalassian KG, Gilligan T, et al. Obstetric complications in pulmonary and critical care medicine. *Chest* 1996;110:791–809.
3. Tenholder MF, South-Paul JE. Dyspnea in pregnancy. *Chest* 1989;96:381–388.
4. Noble PW, Lavee AE, Jacobs MM. Respiratory diseases in pregnancy. *Obstet Gynecol Clin North Am* 1988;15:391–428.
5. Weinberger SE. Dyspnea during pregnancy. In: Rose BD, ed. *UpToDate*. Wellesley, MA: UpToDate, 2002.
6. Lim VS, Katz AI, Lindheimer MD. Acid-base regulation in pregnancy. *Am J Physiol* 1976;231:1764–1769.
7. Rodriguez-Thompson D. Smoking and pregnancy. In: Rose BD, ed. *UpToDate*. Wellesley, MA: UpToDate, 2002.
8. Alm B, Milerad J, Wennergren G, et al. A case-control study of smoking and sudden infant death syndrome in the Scandinavian countries, 1992–1995: the Nordic Epidemiological SIDS Study. *Arch Dis Child* 1998;78:329–334.
9. Brown HL, Hopf SK. Clinical perspectives on smoking during pregnancy. *Female Patient* 1998;23:59.
10. American College of Obstetricians and Gynecologists. Smoking and women's health. Washington, DC: American College of Obstetricians and Gynecologists, 1997; Educational Bulletin No. 240.
11. Stick SM, Burton PR, Gurrin L, et al. Effects of maternal smoking during pregnancy and a family history of asthma on respiratory function in newborn infants. *Lancet* 1996;348:1060–1064.
12. Cunningham J, Dockery D, Gold DR, et al. Racial differences in the association between maternal smoking during pregnancy and lung function in children. *Am J Respir Crit Care Med* 1995;152:565–569.
13. Dolan-Mullen P, Ramirez G, Groff JY. A meta-analysis of randomized trials of prenatal smoking cessation interventions. *Am J Obstet Gynecol* 1994;171:1328–1334.
14. Orleans CT, Barker DC, Kaufman NJ, et al. Helping pregnant smokers quit: meeting the challenge in the next decade. *Tob Control* 2000;9:III-6–III-11.
15. Orleans CT, Johnson RW, Barker DC, et al. Helping pregnant smokers quit: meeting the challenge in the next decade. *West J Med* 2001;174:276–281.
16. U.S. Department of Health and Human Services. Women and smoking: a report of the surgeon general. Rockville, MD: U.S. Department of Health and Human Services, Public Health Service, Office of the Surgeon General, 2001.
17. Schatz M, Harden K, Forsythe A, et al. The course of asthma during pregnancy, post partum, and with successive pregnancies: a prospective analysis. *J Allergy Clin Immunol* 1988;81:509–517.
18. Nelson-Piercy C. Asthma in pregnancy. *Thorax* 2001;56:325–328.
19. Kelly YJ, Brabin BJ, Milligan P, et al. Maternal asthma, premature birth, and the risk of respiratory morbidity in schoolchildren in Merseyside. *Thorax* 1995;50:525–530.
20. Juniper EF, Daniel EE, Roberts RS, et al. Improvement in airway responsiveness and asthma severity during pregnancy: a prospective study. *Am Rev Respir Dis* 1989;140:924–931.
21. Lehrer S, Stone J, Lapinski R, et al. Association between pregnancy-induced hypertension and asthma during pregnancy. *Am J Obstet Gynecol* 1993;168:1463–1466.
22. Schatz M. The efficacy and safety of asthma medications during pregnancy. *Semin Perinatol* 2001;25:145–152.
23. Weinberger SE. Asthma medications during pregnancy. In: Rose BD, ed. *UpToDate*. Wellesley, MA: UpToDate, 2002.
24. Stenius-Aarniala BS, Hedman J, Teramo KA. Acute asthma during pregnancy. *Thorax* 1996;51:411–414.
25. Clark SL. Asthma in pregnancy. National Asthma Education Program Working Group on Asthma and Pregnancy. National Institutes of Health, National Heart, Lung and Blood Institute. *Obstet Gynecol* 1993;82:1036–1040.
26. Schatz M, Hoffman C. Interrelationships between asthma and pregnancy: clinical and mechanistic considerations. *Clin Rev Allergy* 1987;5:301–315.
27. Weinberger SE. Pregnancy in patients with asthma. In: Rose BD, ed. *UpToDate*. Wellesley, MA: UpToDate, 2002.
28. VanWinter JT, Nichols FC III, Pairolero PC, et al. Management of spontaneous pneumothorax during pregnancy: case report and review of the literature. *Mayo Clin Proc* 1996;71:249–252.
29. Dawkins KD, Burke CM, Billingham ME, et al. Primary pulmonary hypertension and pregnancy. *Chest* 1986;89:383–388.
30. Desai DK, Moodley J, Naidoo DP, et al. Cardiac abnormalities in pulmonary oedema associated with hypertensive crises in pregnancy. *Br J Obstetr Gynaecol* 1996;103:523–528.
31. Mabie WC, Hackman BB, Sibai BM. Pulmonary edema associated with pregnancy: echocardiographic insights and implications for treatment. *Obstet Gynecol* 1993;81:227–234.
32. Bakht F, R., Kirshon B, Baker T, et al. Postpartum cardiovascular

complications after bromocriptine and cocaine use. *Am J Obstet Gynecol* 1990;162:1065–1066.

33. Pisani RJ, Rosenow EC III. Pulmonary edema associated with tocolytic therapy. *Ann Intern Med* 1989;110:714–718.

34. Heffner JE, Sahn SA. Pleural disease in pregnancy. *Clin Chest Med* 1992;13:667–678.

35. Hughson WG, Friedman PJ, Feigin DS, et al. Postpartum pleural effusion: a common radiologic finding. *Ann Intern Med* 1982;97:856–858.

36. Rochat RW, Koonin LM, Atrash HK, et al. Maternal mortality in the United States: report from the Maternal Mortality Collaborative. *Obstet Gynecol* 1988;72:91–97.

37. Schwartz DR, Malhotra A, Weinberger SE. Venous thromboembolism in pregnancy. In: Rose BD, ed. *UpToDate.* Wellesley, MA: UpToDate, 2002.

38. Toglia MR, Weg JG. Venous thromboembolism during pregnancy. *N Engl J Med* 1996;335:108–114.

39. Greer IA. Thrombosis in pregnancy: maternal and fetal issues. *Lancet* 1999;353:1258–1265.

40. Ginsberg JS, Brill-Edwards P, Burrows RF, et al. Venous thrombosis during pregnancy: leg and trimester of presentation. *Thromb Haemost* 1992;67:519–520.

41. Cockett F, Thomas M, Negus D. Iliac vein compression: its relation to iliofemoral thrombosis and the post-thrombotic syndrome. *Br Med J* 1967;2:14.

42. Hull RD, Raskob GE, Carter CJ. Serial impedance plethysmography in pregnant patients with clinically suspected deep-vein thrombosis: clinical validity of negative findings. *Ann Intern Med* 1990;112:663–667.

43. Grandone E, Margaglione M, Colaizzo D, et al. Genetic susceptibility to pregnancy-related venous thromboembolism: roles of factor V Leiden, prothrombin G20210A, and methylenetetrahydrofolate reductase C677T mutations. *Am J Obstet Gynecol* 1998;179:1324–1328.

44. Gerhardt A, Scharf RE, Beckmann MW, et al. Prothrombin and factor V mutations in women with a history of thrombosis during pregnancy and the puerperium. *N Engl J Med* 2000;342:374–380.

45. Hirsch DR, Mikkola KM, Marks PW, et al. Pulmonary embolism and deep venous thrombosis during pregnancy or oral contraceptive use: prevalence of factor V Leiden. *Am Heart J* 1996;131:1145–1148.

46. Branch DW, Silver RM, Blackwell JL, et al. Outcome of treated pregnancies in women with antiphospholipid syndrome: an update of the Utah experience. *Obstet Gynecol* 1992;80:614–620.

47. Silver RM, Draper ML, Scott JR, et al. Clinical consequences of antiphospholipid antibodies: an historic cohort study. *Obstet Gynecol* 1994;83:372–377.

48. Sanson BJ, Lensing AW, Prins MH, et al. Safety of low-molecular-weight heparin in pregnancy: a systematic review. *Thromb Haemost* 1999;81:668–672.

49. Rasmussen C, Wadt J, Jacobsen B. Thromboembolic prophylaxis with low molecular weight heparin during pregnancy. *Int J Gynaecol Obstet* 1994;47:121–125.

50. Norgren L, Austrell C, Nilsson L. The effect of graduated elastic compression stockings on femoral blood flow velocity during late pregnancy. *Vasa* 1995;24:282–285.

51. Killam A. Amniotic fluid embolism. *Clin Obstet Gynecol* 1985;28:32–36.

52. Sperry K. Amniotic fluid embolism: to understand an enigma. *JAMA* 1986;255:2183–2186.

53. Gilbert WM, Danielsen B. Amniotic fluid embolism: decreased mortality in a population-based study. *Obstet Gynecol* 1999;93:973–977.

54. Masson RG. Amniotic fluid embolism. *Clin Chest Med* 1992;13:657–665.

55. Morgan M. Amniotic fluid embolism. *Anaesthesia* 1979;34:20–32.

56. Ormerod P. Tuberculosis in pregnancy and the puerperium. *Thorax* 2001;56:494–499.

57. Carter EJ, Mates S. Tuberculosis during pregnancy: the Rhode Island experience, 1987–1991. *Chest* 1994;106:1466–1470.

58. Espinal MA, Reingold AL, Lavandera M. Effect of pregnancy on the risk of developing active tuberculosis. *J Infect Dis* 1996;173:488–491.

59. American College of Obstetricians and Gynecologists. Pulmonary disease in pregnancy. Washington, DC: American College of Obstetricians and Gynecologists, 1996; Technical Bulletin No. 224.

60. Robinson CA, Rose NC. Tuberculosis: current implications and management in obstetrics. *Obstet Gynecol Survey* 1996;51:115–124.

61. Good JT Jr., Iseman MD, Davidson PT, et al. Tuberculosis in association with pregnancy. *Am J Obstet Gynecol* 1981;140:492–498.

62. Hamadeh MA, Glassroth J. Tuberculosis and pregnancy. *Chest* 1992;101:1114–1120.

63. Doveren RF, Block R. Tuberculosis and pregnancy: a provincial study (1990–1996). *Neth J Med* 1998;52:100–106.

64. Jana N, Vasishta K, Saha SC, et al. Obstetrical outcomes among women with extrapulmonary tuberculosis. *N Engl J Med* 1999;341:645–649.

65. Bothamley G. Drug treatment for tuberculosis during pregnancy: safety considerations. *Drug Safety* 2001;24:553–565.

66. Ainbinder S, Berek JS. Epidemiology and pathology of gestational trophoblastic disease. In: Rose BD, ed. *UpToDate.* Wellesley, MA: UpToDate, 2002.

67. Bakri YN, Berkowitz RS, Khan J, et al. Pulmonary metastases of gestational trophoblastic tumor. Risk factors for early respiratory failure. *J Reprod Med* 1994;39:175–178.

68. Jones WB, Romain K, Erlandson RA, et al. Thoracotomy in the management of gestational choriocarcinoma: a clinicopathologic study. *Cancer* 1993;72:2175–2181.

69. Agha FP, Vade A, Amendola MA, et al. Effects of pregnancy on sarcoidosis. *Surg Gynecol Obstet* 1982;155:817–822.

70. Haynes deRegt R. Sarcoidosis and pregnancy. *Obstet Gynecol* 1987;70:369–372.

71. Selroos O. Sarcoidosis and pregnancy: a review with results of a retrospective survey. *J Intern Med* 1990;227:221–224.

72. Stagno S, Whitley RJ. Herpesvirus infections of pregnancy, part II: herpes simplex virus and varicella-zoster virus infections. *N Engl J Med* 1985;313:1327–1330.

73. Baren JM, Henneman PL, Lewis RJ. Primary varicella in adults: pneumonia, pregnancy, and hospital admission. *Ann Emerg Med* 1996;28:165–169.

74. Harger JH, Ernest JM, Thurnau GR, et al. Risk factors and outcome of varicella-zoster virus pneumonia in pregnant women. *J Infect Dis* 2002;185:422–427.

75. Riley LE. Varicella-zoster virus infection in pregnancy. In: Rose BD, ed. *UpToDate.* Wellesley, MA: UpToDate, 2002.

76. Haake DA, Zakowski PC, Haake DL, et al. Early treatment with acyclovir for varicella pneumonia in otherwise healthy adults: retrospective controlled study and review. *Rev Infect Dis* 1990;12:788–798.

77. Smego RA Jr, Asperilla MO. Use of acyclovir for varicella pneumonia during pregnancy. *Obstet Gynecol* 1991;78:1112–1116.

78. Peterson CM, Schuppert K, Kelly PC, et al. Coccidioidomycosis and pregnancy. *Obstet Gynecol Surv* 1993;48:149–156.

79. Wack EE, Ampel NM, Galgiani JN, et al. Coccidioidomycosis during pregnancy. An analysis of ten cases among 47,120 pregnancies. *Chest* 1988;94:376–379.

80. Kent NE, Farquharson DF. Cystic fibrosis in pregnancy. *Can Med Assoc J* 1993;149:809–813.

81. Katkin JP. Clinical manifestations and diagnosis of cystic fibrosis. In: Rose BD, ed. *UpToDate.* Wellesley, MA: UpToDate, 2002.

82. Gilljam M, Antoniou M, Shin J, et al. Pregnancy in cystic fibrosis: fetal and maternal outcome. *Chest* 2000;118:85–91.

83. Edenborough FP, Stableforth DE, Webb AK, et al. Outcome of pregnancy in women with cystic fibrosis. *Thorax* 1995;50:170–174.

84. Lockshin MD. Pregnancy does not cause systemic lupus erythematosus to worsen. *Arthritis Rheum* 1989;32:665–670.

85. Kaufman RL, Kitridou RC. Pregnancy in mixed connective tissue disease: comparison with systemic lupus erythematosus. *J Rheumatol* 1982;9:549–555.

86. Lockshin MD, Qamar T, Druzin ML. Hazards of lupus pregnancy. *J Rheumatol* 1987;13:214–217.

87. Smith CA, Pinals RS. Progressive systemic sclerosis and postpartum renal failure complicated by peripheral gangrene. *J Rheumatol* 1982;9:455–458.

88. Challan BP, Nisand I, Dellenbach P, et al. Scleroderma and pregnancy: new case and review of the literature. *Ann Med Interne (Paris)* 1984;135:435–439.

89. Maymon R, Fejgin M. Scleroderma in pregnancy. *Obstet Gynecol Surv* 1989;44:530–534.

90. Steen VD, Conte C, Day N, et al. Pregnancy in women with systemic sclerosis. *Arthritis Rheum* 1989;32:151–157.

91. Silman AJ, Black C. Increased incidence of spontaneous abortion and infertility in women with scleroderma before disease onset: a controlled study. *Ann Rheum Dis* 1988;47:441–444.

92. Pauzner R, Mayan H, Hershko E, et al. Exacerbation of Wegener's granulomatosis during pregnancy: report of a case with tracheal stenosis and literature review. *J Rheumatol* 1994;21:1153–1156.

93. Shovlin CL, Winstock AR, Peters AM, et al. Medical complications of pregnancy in hereditary haemorrhagic telangiectasia. *QJM* 1995;88:879–887.

94. Gibson PG, Robinson BW, McLennan G, et al. The role of bronchoalveolar lavage in the assessment of diffuse lung diseases. *Aust N Z J Med* 1989;19:281–291.

95. Hill R, Heller MB. Diaphragmatic rupture complicating labor. *Ann Emerg Med* 1996;27:522–524.

96. Flick RP, Bofill JA, King JC. Pregnancy complicated by traumatic diaphragmatic rupture. A case report. *J Reprod Med* 1999;44:127–130.

97. de Veciana M, Towers CV, Major CA, et al. Pulmonary injury associated with appendicitis in pregnancy: who is at risk? *Am J Obstet Gynecol* 1994;171:1008–1013.

98. Sahn SA. Thoracic endometriosis. In: Rose BD, ed. *UpToDate.* Wellesley, MA: UpToDate, 2002.

99. Joseph J, Sahn SA. Thoracic endometriosis syndrome: new observations from an analysis of 110 cases. *Am J Med* 1996;100:164–170.

100. Yu Z, Fleischman JK, Rahman HM, et al. Catamenial hemoptysis and pulmonary endometriosis: a case report. *Mt Sinai J Med* 2002;69:261–263.

101. Choong CK, Smith MD, Haydock DA. Recurrent spontaneous pneumothorax associated with menstrual cycle: report of three cases of catamenial pneumothorax. *ANZ J Surg* 2002;2:678–679.

102. Carter EJ, Ettensohn DB. Catamenial pneumothorax. *Chest* 1990;98:713–716.

103. Kalapura T, Okadigwe C, Fuchs Y, et al. Spiral computerized tomography and video thoracoscopy in catamenial pneumothorax. *Am J Med Sci* 2000;319:186–188.

104. Pauli BD, Reid RL, Munt PW, et al. Influence of the menstrual cycle on airway function in asthmatic and normal subjects. *Am Rev Respir Dis* 1989;140:358–362.

105. Gibbs CJ, Coutts II, Lock R, et al. Premenstrual exacerbation of asthma. *Thorax* 1984;39:833–836.

106. Skobeloff EM, Spivey WH, Silverman R, et al. The effect of the menstrual cycle on asthma presentations in the emergency department. *Arch Intern Med* 1996;156:1837–1840.

107. Nakasato H, Ohrui T, Sekizawa K, et al. Prevention of severe premenstrual asthma attacks by leukotriene receptor antagonist. *J Allergy Clin Immunol* 1999;104:585–588.

108. Magadle R, Berar-Yanay N, Weiner P. Long-acting bronchodilators in premenstrual exacerbation of asthma. *Respir Med* 2001;95:740–743.

109. Troisi RJ, Speizer FE, Willett WC, et al. Menopause, postmenopausal estrogen preparations, and the risk of adult-onset asthma: a prospective cohort study. *Am J Respir Crit Care Med* 1995;152:1183–1188.

110. Seal E Jr, McDonnell WF, House DE. Effects of age, socioeconomic status, and menstrual cycle on pulmonary response to ozone. *Arch Environ Health* 1996;51:132–137.

111. Chen HI, Tang YR. Effects of the menstrual cycle on respiratory muscle function. *Am Rev Respir Dis* 1989;140:1359–1362.

112. Sansores RH, Abboud RT, Kennell C, et al. The effect of menstruation on the pulmonary carbon monoxide diffusing capacity. *Am J Respir Crit Care Med* 1995;152:381–384.

113. Drevelengas A, Kalaitzoglou I, Sichletidis L. Benign pulmonary leiomyomatosis with cyst formation and breast metastasis: case report and literature review. *Eur J Radiol* 1995;19:121–123.

114. Horstmann JP, Pietra GG, Harman JA, et al. Spontaneous regression of pulmonary leiomyomas during pregnancy. *Cancer* 1977;39:314–321.

115. Bouros D, Papadakis K, Siafakas N, et al. Patterns of pulmonary metastasis from uterine cancer. *Oncology* 1996;53:360–363.

116. Bouros D, Papadakis K, Siafakas N, et al. Natural history of patients with pulmonary metastases from uterine cancer. *Cancer* 1996;78:441–447.

117. Handelsman DJ, Conway AJ, Boylan LM, et al. Young's syndrome: obstructive azoospermia and chronic sinopulmonary infections. *N Engl J Med* 1984;310:3–9.

118. Friedman KJ, Teichtahl H, De Kretser DM, et al. Screening Young syndrome patients for CFTR mutations. *Am J Respir Crit Care Med* 1995;152:1353–1357.

119. Hendry WF, A'Hern RP, Cole PJ. Was Young's syndrome caused by exposure to mercury in childhood? *BMJ* 1993;307:1579–1582.

120. Neville E, Brewis R, Yeates WK, et al. Respiratory tract disease and obstructive azoospermia. *Thorax* 1983;38:929–933.

121. Picado C. Postcoital severe exacerbation of asthma requiring mechanical ventilation. *Eur J Respir Dis* 1987;71:52–53.

122. Shah A, Sircar M. Postcoital asthma and rhinitis. *Chest* 1991;100:1039–1041.

123. Kirk AJ. Reflux dyspareunia. *Thorax* 1986;41:215–216.

65 Genetics of Lung Disease

David G. Morris · Esteban González Burchard

HISTORICAL PERSPECTIVE

The hereditary basis of disease has fascinated physicians, scientists, and the general public for centuries. However, our understanding of genetics was limited until important milestones increased our understanding of the hereditary basis of disease. Discoveries by Gregor Mendel in 1865 of the basis of genetic heredity, extensive theoretic work by population geneticists, and advances in molecular genetics spurred by the discovery of DNA, and the description of its basic structure by Watson and Crick in 1953 have dramatically advanced our understanding of hereditary factors and the genetic blueprint.

Gregor Mendel introduced the concept of discrete heritable factors and described specific properties that explained observations of physical traits observed in pea plants. Mendel's idea of discrete units of inheritance was novel and controversial because the predominant school of thought during his time was that each offspring represented a blending of parental characteristics. Mendel also proposed that inheritance units were transmitted independently and with equal frequency from parent to offspring. This proposition went on to become Mendel's first law, which is otherwise known as the law of segregation. Mendel's second law, independent assortment, is that these heritable factors would be transmitted to offspring independently from one another. The debate between the school of thought that believed in the blending-type theory and those that believed in discrete heritable units was not resolved until 1918 when Ronald

D. G. Morris: Pulmonary and Critical Care Medicine, Yale University; and Pulmonary and Critical Care Medicine, Yale–New Haven Hospital, New Haven, Connecticut.

E. González Burchard: Pulmonary and Critical Care Medicine, University of California, San Francisco; and San Francisco General Hospital, San Francisco, California.

Fisher published his seminal paper describing polygenic inheritance.

James Watson and Francis Crick identified the double-helical structure of the DNA molecule, and their work helped to bring about the spectacular advances in molecular genetics in the past five decades. Although we still have much to learn, the Human Genome Project, which was initiated to thoroughly map and characterize the human genome, has sparked a revolution in health care and biomedical sciences by accelerating the pace of novel discoveries. The mapping of the genome will open new horizons and may have a significant impact on the elucidation of all diseases that have a genetic basis.

This chapter will outline the general approach to genetic analysis that is applicable to any trait or disease of interest. Thereafter, it will focus on three well-known genetic lung diseases: cystic fibrosis (CF), α_1-antitrypsin (AAT) deficiency, and ciliary dysmotility syndrome. It will then close with a discussion of the genetics of asthma as an example of applying genetic principles to understanding diseases with complex inheritance patterns.

GENETIC APPROACHES TO LUNG DISEASE

Establishing a Genetic Basis

Before embarking on the long journey of gene discovery, one must define the trait (phenotype) or clinical parameter under investigation. Clinical definitions must be consistent, discriminatory, accurate, and consistently applied. The clinical definition of the trait should differentiate the exact phenotype of interest from subphenotypes or syndromes that overlap with the trait of interest. However, the clinical definition should also be sensitive enough to include the full range of affected individuals.

Once the phenotype is clearly defined, evidence for a genetic basis of the trait must be established. Family studies, twin studies, and adoption studies may all be helpful in evaluating the evidence for a genetic basis of a trait. A disease is said to segregate in families if the incidence or prevalence of the disease or trait among relatives of affected individuals (probands) is higher than the disease incidence or prevalence in relatives of healthy controls (1). However, additional investigations are needed in order to declare that a disease has a genetic basis because there are several nongenetic reasons (confounders) that may explain why a trait may segregate in families, which include environmental, cultural, and socioeconomic factors or an ascertainment bias. Adoption studies are also an important methodology that allows investigators to differentiate between genetic versus environmental contributions to a trait.

The relative risk of disease among relatives of affected individuals (often referred to as λ) is often used to quantify the risk associated with shared ancestry with an affected individual. λ_R is defined as the ratio of risk to relatives (e.g., siblings, parents, offspring) versus the general population risk. Many studies assess risk as the risk to siblings of probands, also known as λ_S. A higher value of λ is generally thought to indicate a stronger genetic effect, with a λ_S above 2.0 indicative of a significant genetic component. For example, λ_S for CF is approximately 500, and for Huntington disease, it is 5,000. The λ_S is approximately 20 to 30 for multiple sclerosis, 15 for insulin-dependent diabetes, and 2 to 4 for asthma. However, direct comparisons of λ are not always an optimal way to compare the genetic contribution of one disease relative to another because the λ value depends on and is inversely proportional to the prevalence of disease.

As mentioned, a valuable resource for determining genetic contributions to a phenotype is twin studies. Twin studies provide a simple manner in which to differentiate genetic from environmental influences. Monozygotic twins share 100% of their genes, whereas dizygotic twins share 50% of their genes on average. One can take advantage of the difference in monozygotic and dizygotic twins by assessing the concordance rate of disease among twins to determine the relative environmental contributions compared with genetic contributions. Concordance rate is defined as the probability that the second twin will be affected given that the first twin is affected. If there is evidence that the concordance rates of the phenotype of interest are higher among monozygotic twins compared with dizygotic twins, then one can assume that there is a genetic contribution to the phenotype under study. Furthermore, twin studies allow the calculation of heritability, defined as the proportion of variation in a trait attributable to genetic causes.

These data provide evidence as to both the strength of the genetic contribution to the trait and to the underlying model. There are two broad categories of genetic models: single gene disorders and complex or multifactorial disorders. Single gene disorders such as CF are owing to a single or major gene and are often referred to as mendelian disorders because the inheritance pattern follows that predicted by mendelian law. Complex disorders such as asthma and hypertension are thought to be owing to multiple genes interacting with environmental factors. Furthermore, the contribution of any one gene in complex disorders may vary. It is estimated that more than 7,000 diseases are inherited in a mendelian fashion, and more than 1,000 genes associated with these disorders have been mapped to a chromosomal region (2). However, relatively few genes for common diseases have been mapped.

Identifying Disease Susceptibility Genes

There are two major strategies that have been used to identify genes related to disease: linkage analysis and association studies. The suspected mode of inheritance and strength of the genetic contribution will influence the design of any study to identify the putative gene or genes responsible to the disease in question. For example, if a single gene with a strong genetic contribution is suspected, a linkage analysis using large extended families may be most effective. This approach may not work as well for complex diseases in which there are multiple genes contributing to the phenotype, each with a potentially modest and undetectable effect.

Linkage Analysis

The broad aim of linkage analysis is to establish genetic landmarks that tend to be inherited along with the trait of interest and are therefore linked and located in a nearby chromosomal region. Modern linkage methods are nonparametric (i.e., not model-based) and typically involve allele-sharing methods (most commonly, affected sibling pairs). Polymorphic genetic markers that are spaced equidistant throughout the genome—much like mile markers—are used as landmarks to localize the locus of the trait of interest on a map of the human genome. Linkage analysis relies on the cosegregation of two or more loci (genes, markers, and traits) in families to determine whether alleles are physically close to each other on a strand of DNA. Loci that are quite removed from one another, such as loci on separate chromosomes, segregate independently according to Mendel's law. Linked loci, on the other hand, tend to segregate more often than would be expected by chance. This implies a close proximity of one to the other. For example, if a genetic marker and trait segregate together, also known as being linked, then one can conclude that the causative gene for the trait under study and genetic marker are in close physical proximity to each other. This allows investigators to narrow down the entire genome to more manageable genetic regions, or linked regions, that likely contain the gene or genes associated with their trait of interest. Fine mapping of these genetic regions with genetic markers spaced at even smaller intervals can further narrow this to a region encompassing a few genes. An advantage of linkage analysis is that novel chromosomal regions associated with a particular trait can be identified. Furthermore, one does not need to know the exact pathogenesis of the trait in order to identify linked genetic regions. These linked chromosomal regions may be located near or may contain disease-causing genes. A major disadvantage of this approach, however, is the requirement for a large number of families that include multiple affected individuals (e.g., two or more affected siblings). This is particularly true for complex diseases such as asthma, because there are likely to be multiple genetic risk factors, each with only modest effects (3,4). In such cases, the large sample size required to demonstrate linkage can limit the ability to detect a region in which disease susceptibility loci do actually exist.

Association Studies

Association studies examine the relationship between a particular genetic variant of an allele and a disease. Candidate genes are those genes that have biologic plausibility as candidates for causing or contributing to the pathogenesis of the disease or a phenotype of interest. The detection of an allele that is more frequent in persons with the disease than among those without the disease allows the inference that the particular allele may be causally associated with the disease or that the allele is in linkage disequilibrium with another disease-causing gene at a nearby locus. Linkage disequilibrium occurs when two alleles from separate loci occur together more (or less) often than would be expected by chance. Alleles at closely linked loci are often found to be in linkage disequilibrium. If one of these alleles is associated with a particular disease, then other nearby alleles may also be associated with that disease; however, it may be difficult to determine which allele is actually the disease-causing allele. Association studies are potentially a very powerful strategy for identifying genes of modest effect in complex diseases such as asthma, hypertension, and diabetes (3). The simplest form of association study is the case control, in which markers are genotyped in a sample of cases, and unrelated matched controls are then tested for allele frequency differences. Another approach, called the transmission disequilibrium test (TDT), compares the transmission of alleles from parents to affected offspring or probands (5). The TDT involves determining whether a particular allele is transmitted from parents to an affected offspring more often than expected by chance based on mendelian inheritance. The TDT only requires families with one affected offspring; however, it can be applied to families with multiple affected offspring.

Proving the Gene as the Cause of the Disease

After a gene has been identified as being linked or associated with the trait of interest, the next step is to determine whether there are variants in a gene that are associated with or may predispose individuals to disease. By comparing the DNA sequence of a gene in affected and unaffected individuals, one can easily identify genetic variants of candidate genes. Once these genetic variants are identified, the next step is determining whether these variants result in functional change of the biologic behavior of the gene. Functional changes can be assessed in many ways, including studies of modified gene expression, altered protein structure, cell-based assays of protein function, or genetically manipulated animal models.

Genetically manipulated animal models typically have as their goal the recapitulation of human disease in a mouse and often involve the generation of either a transgenic mouse, in the case of a dominant disease-causing gene, or a knockout mouse, in the case of a recessive phenotype. In a transgenic mouse, the putative disease-causing gene is artificially introduced and is expressed in a restricted manner under the control of tissue-specific and/or drug-inducible promoters. In a knockout mouse, the putative disease-causing gene is inactivated either in all cells or in a selected subset of cells within particular tissues. Such models have been used extensively in the study of pulmonary fibrosis, asthma, and emphysema (6–13). Recently, efforts have turned toward identifying disease-causing genes by introducing random or near-random mutations using chemicals or insertion-prone sequences of DNA coupled to a gene-inactivating cassette into the germ-lines of mice and analyzing the offspring for abnormalities (so-called phenodeviants). Once heritable phenotypes are identified, investigators use the conventional genetic approaches of selective breeding, linkage analysis, and repeated phenotyping to eventually identify the causative mutation. Both approaches to genetic manipulation are complementary and will undoubtedly lead to a rapid acceleration of knowledge concerning the genetic determinants of lung disease in the coming years.

GENETIC LUNG DISEASES

Cystic Fibrosis

Overview

Cystic fibrosis (CF) is the most common lethal genetic disease in white populations. Although it was long categorized as a pediatric disease, with a median age at diagnosis of 6 months (14), CF is increasingly becoming a disease of adults as a result of improved early diagnosis and treatment. In fact, within the past 10 years, the median survival of patients with CF has risen from approximately 29 to 32 years (14). Nevertheless, despite dramatic improvements in survival, CF remains a lethal disease, with over 90% of affected individuals dying of pulmonary complications. The identification of the CF transmembrane conductance regulator (CFTR)—a kinase-regulated ion channel that mediates chloride ion permeability in both secretory and absorptive epithelium—as the gene responsible for this disease represents one of the most dramatic achievements of classical and molecular human genetics.

Clinical Manifestations

The diagnosis of CF is typically considered in patients with recurrent lower respiratory tract infections or unexplained parenchymal lung disease, pancreatic insufficiency, and azoospermia. CF is characterized by the clinical triad of excessive concentrations of sodium and chloride in sweat, chronic obstructive pulmonary disease (COPD), and exocrine pancreatic insufficiency. The severity of these manifestations varies among affected patients and depends, at least to some extent, on the particular combination of mutant alleles (or genes). Despite identification of the CF mutation more than a decade ago, the precise pathogenesis of increased susceptibility to pulmonary bacterial infection, particularly with *Staphylococcus* and *Pseudomonas* species, remains unresolved. Currently, it is thought that increased bacterial susceptibility may be owing to abnormalities in innate mucosal defense related to impaired function of salt-sensitive defensins, and to abnormalities in ciliary function owing to dehydrated mucous (15,16).

Genetics

CF has a classic autosomal-recessive mendelian inheritance pattern and affects approximately one in 2,500 to 3,500 newborns in North America. CF results from a mutation in the *CFTR* gene located on the long arm of chromosome 7 (7q31.3).

The identification of the *CFTR* gene is one of the great accomplishments of a genetic approach known as positional cloning. By using linkage analysis of large kindreds of affected families, geneticists mapped the position of the CF gene to a guanosine and cytosine–rich region (GpC island) on chromosome 7. Subsequent sequencing of this region in DNA derived from normal and affected individuals identified a previously unknown gene, expressed in appropriate tissues, with a 3-bp deletion corresponding to the deleted phenylalanine at amino acid 508 of the epithelial chloride channel (ΔF508). Subsequent screening of DNA from CF patients revealed a high prevalence of this mutation (17). About two thirds of all CF chromosomes examined to date carry this mutation. Several hundred other less common mutations have been documented in this same gene, some of which are associated with relatively mild clinical disease. Transfer of a normal copy of the *CFTR* gene into pancreatic and airway cells derived from CF patients restored normal cAMP-dependent chloride permeability, hence proving that the mutant protein was responsible for the genetic defect (see review by Davis et al. [17]).

Approximately one in 25 to 35 clinically normal whites in North America carries a single copy of the ΔF508 mutation in the *CFTR* gene. Such a high prevalence of a disease-associated allele is surprising, and various theories have been proposed to explain a potential survival advantage. A biologically plausible hypothesis is that heterozygotes may be protected against the effects of chloride-secreting diarrhea, especially infantile or epidemic diarrhea such as cholera, which are mediated in part by CFTR overstimulation (18).

The *CFTR* gene product is a glycosylated 1,480-amino-acid protein. It consists of 12 transmembrane domains separated in the middle by two nucleotide-binding regions and a single regulatory domain. The majority of the protein is cytoplasmic and is within the cell membrane, with only a small portion located in the extracellular space. It is a member of the ATP-binding cassette membrane transporter superfamily of proteins, which includes the multidrug-resistance protein, the sulfonylurea receptor, and the transporter for antigen presentation, among others (18). CFTR functions as a chloride-selective ion channel located on either the apical or basal membrane of secretory or absorptive epithelium in the airways, sweat glands, or digestive tract. The function of CFTR is regulated by phosphorylation of the protein and is ATP dependent. Different mutations lead to different abnormalities of the *CFTR* gene product. These abnormalities are generally broken down into five different classes (I–V) based on whether they result in an absence of synthesis (class I), defective intracellular protein processing (class II), abnormal regulation (class III), altered conductance (class IV), or reduced synthesis (class V). CF is discussed in detail in Chapter 13.

α_1-Antitrypsin Deficiency

Overview

AAT (α_1-antiprotease, α_1-protease inhibitor [PI]) is a member of the serine PI family of proteins (serpins) and the major PI in human plasma. The vast majority of AAT is synthesized by hepatocytes, but mononuclear cells, polymorphonuclear leukocytes, intestinal epithelium, and the kidney parenchyma make small amounts. AAT is an acute phase reactant, and concentrations in plasma may vary by as much as fourfold in response to acute infection or inflammation. Despite its name, the primary role of AAT appears to be to neutralize elastase derived from neutrophils. It does this by tightly binding to elastase and then undergoing a dramatic refolding, much like a mousetrap, to form a stable AAT-elastase complex that immediately neutralizes elastinolytic activity and opens the elastase molecule for catabolism (19). Any mutation that reduces the ability of AAT either to tightly bind neutrophil elastase or refold reduces its anti-elastinolytic activity (20).

AAT deficiency is an autosomal-codominant disorder in which both alleles are expressed and affect the clinical phenotype. It was identified shortly after the development of protein electrophoresis for clinical use and is characterized by a loss of the α_1 globulin band in serum, which normally contains albumin and the globulins $\alpha_{1,2}$, $\beta_{1,2}$, and γ. The α_1 globulin band contains the vast majority of trypsin-inhibitory biochemical activity in serum so the syndrome was named AAT deficiency. The history and early phenotyping and genetic studies are nicely outlined in studies by Erikkson (21,22). Abnormalities in gene transcription, translation, or intracellular processing of the AAT protein cause AAT deficiency. The resulting mutant proteins are characterized by their abnormal electrophoretic mobility, decreased serum levels, or malfunction. Deficiency of AAT activity or amount results in excessive proteolytic breakdown of lung tissue owing to decreased inhibition of the endogenous proteolytic enzyme elastin. This then results in the development of characteristic early onset pulmonary emphysema. Intracellular accumulation of insoluble aggregates of a particular form of the AAT protein (ZZ) in hepatocytes can lead to liver disease, primarily in the pediatric population.

Genetics

AAT deficiency results from inheritance of two abnormal alleles on chromosomal segment 14q32.1–32.3 in the AAT gene locus (23–26). The gene, designated *SERPINA1*, is 12.2 kb in length and is composed of seven exons (27–29) that code for a 1,584-bp messenger RNA. It is situated in a cluster of genes that code for related proteins of the serpin superfamily, which includes cortisol-binding globulin, α_1-antichymotrypsin, AAT itself, and the protein C inhibitor. All of these proteins have substantial amino acid and structural homologies. Translation of AAT mRNA results in a 418-amino-acid protein with a 24-amino-acid leader signal peptide that directs the protein to the rough endoplasmic reticulum. Here, the signal peptide is cleaved, and glycosylation of the protein takes place. The glycosylated protein is then transported to the Golgi, where further processing occurs. After this, the fully folded 52-kDa globular glycoprotein is secreted into the serum (30). Defects at any stage of this processing can result in clinically significant deficiencies in functional protein.

Molecular Epidemiology, Incidence, and Prevalence

Population-based studies show a frequency of AAT deficiency of one in 3,500 live births in the United States and therefore predict a prevalence of 100,000 severely deficient Americans (31). Current estimates of the number of patients diagnosed with AAT deficiency, however, suggest that fewer than 10% of affected individuals have been detected (31). The presumed reasons for this are both under-recognition of this disorder in individuals with premature emphysema and lack of clinical consequences in many individuals despite severe deficiency.

DNA sequencing has revealed the presence of at least 75 AAT allelic variations of the *SERPINA1* gene, and about 100 phenotypic PI variants of AAT may be detected by the isoelectric focusing technique and determination of circulating levels of the protein. PI classification is based on electrophoretic mobility of the AAT protein isoforms and is denoted as Pi followed by the allele forms. The allelic forms are named for their electrophoretic mobility by using isoelectric focusing and are designated by the letters A (isoelectric at pH around 4.0) through Z (isoelectric at pH around 5.0). The M allele (with its several subtypes) is the most common allele, migrates in middle-zone of the electropherogram, and is associated with normal levels of elastase inhibitory activity (32). Each allele is associated with a characteristic serum level of protein, and the final serum level of protein depends on the particular combination of alleles. Therefore, these multiple allelic PI forms can be divided into four functional classes based on serum level and function: (a) normal, (b) deficient (associated with serum AAT levels of less than 35% of normal), (c) null (no detectable AAT in serum), or (d) dysfunctional (normal levels of malfunctioning isoforms) (32).

The most common mutant allele of AAT is the S form, with an allelic frequency in whites in the United States of 2% to 4% (32) and in Europe of 7% (33). Individuals homozygous for this Glu^{264} to Val mutation have a 40% reduction in their serum AAT levels and typically do not manifest any clinical symptoms (20). Interestingly, this allele is more common in southern Europe (33).

The majority (95%) of individuals with severe AAT deficiency are homozygous with a PI type of ZZ. The allelic frequency of the Z form in whites in the United States is 1% to 2% (32) and approximately 3% in Europe (33). Population genetic studies suggest that this mutation arose in an individual who lived in northern Europe approximately 6,000 years ago (34). This allele is not found in pure Asian or African populations. The remaining 5% of AAT-deficient persons exhibit a wide range of other variants (30,32,35).

About one in 25 individuals of northern European ancestry carry the Z allele of AAT. Individuals homozygous for this particular mutation, in which Lys is substituted for Glu at position 342 (Glu342Lys) results in improper intracellular protein folding. PiZZ individuals synthesize normal amounts of the protein in the liver but secrete only 15% into the blood. The remaining 85% remains in the hepatocyte and is either degraded or accumulates as large intracellular inclusions (36).

Other variants may be associated with substantially reduced levels of functional protein, substantially reduced or normal levels of nonfunctional AAT, or with undetectable levels of the protein (null mutation). Homozygous individuals with null alleles (PiQ_0Q_0) have either zero or less than 1% of the normal amount of AAT. The frequency of this mutation is estimated to be about 1.7×10^{-4}, which is approximately one-hundredth of the frequency of the PiZZ genotype. Most null mutations (e.g., $PiQ_{0GraniteFalls}$, $PiQ_{0Bellingham}$) are the result of premature stop codon mutations. Eleven forms of null mutation have been reported.

Other mutants are associated with abnormalities in mRNA splicing or stability or abnormal retention in the rough endoplasmic reticulum or Golgi with subsequent degradation. For continually updated information of identified alleles and a comprehensive review of the genetic aspects of this disorder, the reader is referred to Online Mendelian Inheritance in Man, maintained by the National Center for Biotechnology Information and Johns Hopkins University, at *http://www.ncbi.nlm.nih.gov/entrez/dispomim.cgi?id = 107400.*

Clinical Manifestations

The clinical manifestations of AAT deficiency involve primarily the lung, although some young patients have hepatic or dermatologic involvement. The most common syndrome associated with AAT deficiency is emphysema, which is typically panacinar and basilar in location. Clinical findings are similar to those of patients with other forms of emphysema-associated COPD (see Chapter 12). Hepatic disease is the second most frequent clinical manifestation of AAT deficiency and usually presents in the postnatal period as cholestatic jaundice. Only patients with the PiZZ variant develop hepatic disease, which is caused by intracellular accumulation of aggregates of AAT protein in the hepatocytes. Although liver disease in most AAT-deficient children is mild, with only 10% having clinically significant disease, AAT-deficient children with severe hepatic disease may require liver transplantation. In general, the risk for liver disease among adults with AAT deficiency is low; however, it may increase in those who survive beyond 50 years (37). Finally, panniculitis, characterized by inflammatory and necrotizing lesions of the skin, is the least common manifestation of AAT deficiency. It occurs in individuals with a variety of phenotypes, including PiZZ, PiMZ, PiSS, and PiMS.

Pathophysiology and Risk Factors for Lung Disease

The panacinar emphysema in AAT-deficient individuals is produced by excessive breakdown of lung elastin (elastinolysis), which occurs by several mechanisms. Generally, AAT-deficient individuals have a relative deficiency of anti-elastase activity in lung tissue at all times. In addition, smoking causes a large influx of elastase-producing neutrophils and macrophages into the lung, thus increasing the total elastase burden. Furthermore, oxidant components of cigarette smoke also inactivate AAT that is present in lung by oxidizing a crucial methionine (position 358) at the center of the active site of the molecule and thereby potentiate the effects of neutrophil- and macrophage-derived elastase (38).

Understandably, then, chronic tobacco smoke exposure is the most important associated risk factor for the development of COPD in AAT-deficient individuals. Less is known about the deleterious effects of environmental air pollution on the development or severity of lung disease in individuals with AAT deficiency, although it is likely that breathing ozone, sulfur dioxide, oxides of nitrogen, and other such pollutants will increase the rate of worsening of lung disease occurring in the AAT-deficient setting. Respiratory infections in early childhood may also be a risk factor for the early development of emphysema in individuals with severe AAT deficiency. Chronic bronchitis with repeated acute bacterial exacerbations by the usual offending organisms in AAT-deficient adults also seems to be a risk factor. Finally, other unidentified genetic modifiers may be additional risk factors because the risk of an AAT-deficient individual developing COPD is increased if a parent has emphysema, bronchitis, or asthma.

Diagnosis

When a diagnosis of AAT deficiency has been established by low serum levels, the PI phenotype should be determined. Direct determination of the genotype may be required in the case of unusual clinical phenotypes.

Screening

The overwhelming majority of patients with emphysema are not AAT deficient, so that screening for this condition is both costly and not generally effective. About 3% of this population will have AAT levels below the normal range. Screening of siblings of known AAT-deficient individuals is useful because the positive yield will be 25%. These individuals can be counseled to stop smoking and can be evaluated for therapy.

Historically, screening for AAT deficiency has been performed in three ways. The first is general screening of adults, usually done in the blood donor population. This has been useful for estimating the prevalence of undiagnosed AAT deficiency in the community, but it is not cost-effective because of its low yield (39). Directed screening of adults who have a higher-than-average risk of having AAT deficiency is useful. Such screening has been offered by the AAT Deficiency Detection Center in Salt Lake City since 1991 to individuals who have a family history of AAT deficiency and have chronic bronchitis, emphysema, or asthma. Last, several neonatal screening programs have provided knowledge about the prevalence of the disease and eventually will provide information about the natural history of the disease in children and adults.

Therapy

Treatment of AAT deficiency may be divided into measures directed at the primary defect (low levels of AAT) and those directed at the secondary effects of the disease (i.e., emphysema, bronchitis, bronchiectasis). The latter measures are similar to those in other patients with COPD. Smoking cessation should play a prominent role in any therapy program for AAT deficiency, as smoking is the most important single risk factor for development of lung disease in AAT-deficient individuals. Cessation of smoking should be confirmed prior to undertaking augmentation therapy.

Intravenous α_1-Antitrypsin Augmentation

A serum AAT level exceeding 80 mg/dL (11 μM; normal, 200–53 μM) is thought to protect against the development of emphysema. Recent observational data from the National Heart, Lung, and Blood Institute (NHLBI) α_1-Antitrypsin Deficiency Registry have shown enhanced survival (risk ratio, 0.64; $P < .05$) in patients receiving intravenous augmentation therapy, and a decreased rate of decline of forced expiratory volume at 1 second (FEV_1) in patients with American Thoracic Society (ATS) stage II COPD (FEV_1, 35%–49% of predicted) (40). Similar results have been found in other registry-based studies (41). Repeated weekly infusions of partially purified, plasma-derived AAT at a dose of 60 mg/kg body weight result in a mean nadir AAT level of 20 μM in 21 patients whose pretreatment level was 5 μM. Antibodies were not produced in response to the AAT, and the infusion was shown to result in increases in serum and bronchoalveolar lavage fluid antineutrophil elastase activity, suggesting that the infused AAT was active in the lung and might afford some protection against continued elastinolysis, alveolar wall destruction, and progression of emphysema. The half-life of the infused AAT was between 4 and 5 days (42). AAT may also be administered as monthly infusions. In patients given AAT at a dose of 250 mg/kg once every 28 days for 1 year, serum AAT levels of 11–13 μM were maintained for 20 days. Even at 28 days, the bronchoalveolar lavage AAT levels and antineutrophil-elastase capacities were above threshold, suggesting that alveoli were protected over the whole cycle (43).

Recombinant AAT is a 45,000-kDa nonglycosylated protein produced by yeast. This protein does not contain the terminal methionine or the three carbohydrate chains of the native molecule. Recombinant AAT has a half-life of hours because of rapid renal clearance, and its clinical use is not appropriate.

Randomized prospective trials to evaluate whether augmentation therapy prevents worsening of emphysema and prolongs life have not yet been undertaken because of the long time frame of such a study, difficulties in the reliable quantitation of emphysema, the large numbers of patients needed to treat, and the expense. Recent estimates, based on data from the NHLBI α_1-Antitrypsin Deficiency Registry, suggest that 147 patients per treatment arm would be needed for such a trial to detect a significant difference in the rate of FEV_1 decline over 4 years, and 342 patients per treatment arm would be required to detect a 40% decline in mortality over 5 years (44). Investigators are focusing on developing other reliable surrogate markers of disease progression, such as quantitative high-resolution chest computed tomography scanning to measure changes in lung density, in the hopes of providing improved statistical power with fewer patients (45).

Although therapy is expensive (31), side effects of AAT are few and include headache, myalgias, arthralgias, and low back pain. Some patients with pulmonary hypertension related to their disease develop worsening dyspnea during or shortly after the infusion. This may be secondary to the protein load and water retention. All patients slated to receive AAT should be vaccinated against hepatitis B, although no cases have been reported. Acute allergic or anaphylactic reactions have been few. Rare patients with severe AAT deficiency may also be immunoglobulin (Ig) A deficient; because they may receive some IgA with the AAT infusion, acute anaphylactic reactions have been noted in these individuals.

Patient selection for intravenous AAT augmentation therapy is somewhat controversial. The ATS has published guidelines for therapy, but they are not universally accepted, given the uncertainty of therapeutic efficacy and the cost involved (46). In general, only patients with clearly deficient AAT levels (PiZZ, PiQ$_0$-PiQ$_0$, PiZ-PiQ$_0$, PiS-PiQ$_0$, and a few PiSZ) should be treated. The age at which therapy should begin is unclear; although a priori reasoning would suggest initiation of therapy at a young age, there are no data on which to base judgment on this issue. The ATS recommends that patients who continue to smoke not be treated, as they are unlikely to benefit from the treatment.

Aerosol delivery of AAT is currently under investigation. This could potentially offer effective enhancement of AAT levels in the airway surface liquid while using much less protein (and thus be more cost-effective).

Lung Transplantation

More than 4,300 patients, about 30% with COPD, have undergone lung transplantation worldwide. Approximately 12% of these transplants were performed for emphysema caused by AAT deficiency. Although the 6-year actuarial survival for all lung transplantation recipients is approximately 40%, patients with emphysema have a 4-year survival rate of 54%, the best survival among all groups. Recipients who are AAT deficient have an actuarial survival of 45% at 5 years. Most lung transplantation survivors have reported functional improvement. Because of the shortage of suitable lung donors, most patients now receive single lung transplantation.

Liver Transplantation

Liver transplantation is associated with normal circulating levels of AAT and, presumably, with a normal pulmonary prognosis. Liver transplantation is not a viable form of therapy for isolated lung disease but is an option in those few (mostly pediatric) patients with end-stage liver disease.

Lung Volume Reduction Surgery

Lung volume reduction is a surgical technique that attempts to reduce hyperinflation and improve lung function by removing multiple emphysematous areas of lung identified by computed tomography. Physiological function has been shown to improve in selected individuals through partial restoration of the normal domed shape of the diaphragm and its mechanical advantage. In addition, elastic recoil of the lung may increase after reduction pneumoplasty, thereby increasing compliance and improving function.

Patients with end-stage emphysema—i.e., those with generalized severe disease associated with pulmonary hypertension (mean pulmonary artery pressure >35 mm Hg), severe hypercapnia (arterial partial pressure of carbon dioxide >55 mm Hg), low FEV_1 (<20% of predicted), and barrel chests—are not good candidates for resection. In a recent study of 1,033 patients, high mortality rates (16% compared with zero among medically treated patients) were seen in patients with an FEV_1 <20% of predicted and either a diffusing capacity for carbon monoxide of less than 20% or predicted or diffuse emphysema. Ninety percent of the deaths were from respiratory causes (47). Functional improvement with increased FEV_1 is variable, although many patients report lessened dyspnea and an increase in exercise tolerance. Long-term benefits more than 1 year after surgery have not yet been reported.

Gene Therapy

Although AAT deficiency may be treated with weekly infusions of AAT, this treatment is expensive and inconvenient. Investigations are currently ongoing regarding transfection of the complete α_1-antiprotease cDNA to the respiratory tract of deficient individuals. Expression of the protein in the airway and alveolar space would theoretically provide levels of AAT sufficient to prevent reductions in pulmonary function.

Similar to what has been used for genetic therapy of CF, nonviral vectors and modified nonreplicating retroviruses and adenoviruses have been used to deliver AAT cDNA to the lung or other tissues. Retroviral delivery systems are effective in placing the AAT cDNA into cells, and AAT protein has been produced by cells that do not normally synthesize the protein. However, serum therapeutic levels have not been achieved.

Unlike retroviruses, adenoviruses function in the cytoplasm of the cell. They have also been shown to be effective in transfecting respiratory epithelium of rats with human AAT cDNA and in producing AAT protein that can be detected in cells and bronchoalveolar lavage fluid. Administration of the modified vector must be repeated on a periodic basis because the transfection is not stable. This form of therapy is undergoing active investigation at this time; clinical application of this approach may be limited by the recipient's immune response to the viral vector.

Plasmids containing AAT cDNA and a cytomegalovirus promoter contained within cationic liposomes have been given to rabbits by the aerosol or intravenous route. Respiratory tract epithelial cells take up the liposomes and express and release AAT protein into bronchoalveolar lavage fluid.

Other Therapies

Novel therapies for pulmonary emphysema, such as retinoic acid therapy, are currently under investigation. Studies in rats have shown that all-*trans*-retinoic acid reversed protease-mediated emphysema and studies in patients are ongoing (48,49). Other novel approaches, including use of chemical chaperones to improve export of misfolded proteins have been effective in animal models of disease (50).

Prognosis

The natural history of lung dysfunction in AAT deficiency is one of progressive decline, and severe AAT deficiency generally shortens life. Only about 16% of ZZ homozygotes survive to age 60 compared with 85% of normal age-matched individuals. Although lung function is relatively normal during the first two decades of life, it declines thereafter at a variable rate that ranges from about 40 to 300 mL of FEV_1 lost per year. Death among homozygotes is usually from respiratory failure, although some deaths may be ascribed to complications of hepatic disease.

α_1-Antitrypsin Deficiency Registries

The natural history and the efficacy of intravenous augmentation therapy with human AAT in patients with severe AAT deficiency and pulmonary emphysema is currently being studied in three large multicenter registries, including a U.S. NHLBI registry, a Danish–Dutch registry (European Randomized Placebo-Controlled Trial of α_1-PI Replacement Therapy), and a German registry (the Wissenschaftliche Arbeitsgemeinschaft zur Therapie von Lungenerkrankungen, WATL, or the Multicenter Trial of α_1-PI Augmentation Therapy in Patients with α_1-PI Deficiency). The α_1 National Association (A1NA) is the main source of information for AAT-deficient patients regarding new developments and support groups. Free screenings, an informational CD-ROM for patients and health professionals (AlphaMedia), and information about patient infusion services (AlphaNet) are available. The α_1 *News* is produced by the association, as is an information hotline and website (*AlphaLine*, 1-800-4ALPHA1; www.alpha1.org).

Primary Ciliary Dyskinesia (Immotile Cilia Syndrome, Kartagener Syndrome)

The clinical triad of situs inversus, bronchiectasis, and pansinusitis was recognized as a distinct entity in 1936 by Kartagener, who also noted the occurrence of the triad in siblings. Kartagener syndrome remained a clinical oddity until Afzelius and colleagues reported that sperm from these patients were immotile and that their ciliary ultrastructure was abnormal. Subsequently, the generalized nature of the ciliary abnormality was recognized. Several kindreds have since been reported to have a variety of ultrastructural abnormalities and a common clinical picture of chronic sinus and bronchial disease, with or without situs inversus. Because many patients with similar clinical syndromes have abnormal cilia with disordered but not absent movement, the preferred term today is *primary ciliary dyskinesia* (PCD) rather than *immotile cilia syndrome.*

Incidence and Prevalence

Situs inversus occurs with an incidence of one in 8,000 to 24,000 live births, and of these, only 12% to 25% have the complete triad of Kartagener syndrome. It is not clear whether situs inversus occurs with a 50% (i.e., random) incidence in all patients with immotile cilia. However, with a few assumptions, it may be estimated that the incidence of PCD may be as high as one in 20,000 live births.

Genetics

The familial pattern of Kartagener syndrome is consistent with an autosomal-recessive mode of inheritance. The syndrome has been documented in siblings of both sexes but has rarely been seen in two consecutive generations. Other variants of PCD have been observed in siblings. At least one family has been reported with an X-linked inheritance pattern. From the estimated incidence figures above, it may be calculated that approximately one in 70 persons is heterozygous for one form or another of the disorder.

Pathophysiology

Mucociliary function depends on a number of factors, including the number, orientation, and beat frequency of cilia and the dimensions and viscoelastic properties of the mucus and the aqueous periciliary fluid layers. Virtually any structural abnormality of cilia that results in an abnormal ciliary beat can result in clinical abnormalities. The ultrastructure of cilia is quite constant, with two central microtubules surrounded by nine outer microtubule doublets. The microtubules are composed of tubulin, a protein with no intrinsic contractile activity. Radial spokes extend from the central doublet to the outer tubules, and nexin links help maintain the structure. Other structures projecting from the outer doublets (dynein arms) have ATPase activity. Motion of the cilia is thought to occur by interaction of the dynein arms with adjacent microtubules via a sliding mechanism similar to that of muscle contraction.

Electron microscopy of cilia from sperm tails and from nasal and bronchial epithelium of patients with Kartagener syndrome reveals the partial or complete absence of dynein arms. Other kindreds with absent radial spokes or with other ultrastructural patterns have also been reported. Familial clusters of patients with ciliary aplasia have also been reported; these patients have similar clinical manifestations to those with classical PCD.

Not all patients with chronic sinopulmonary disease have immotile cilia, yet many of these patients do demonstrate abnormal ciliary ultrastructure. Chronic infection or inflammation may itself produce abnormalities. Clinical and ultrastructural data must be interpreted with caution, and it is difficult to assign a genetic basis to a particular patient's problem unless the ultrastructure is classic (i.e., absence of dynein arms) or there is familial clustering. It also should be pointed out that fixation and staining techniques may have a great impact on the ultrastructure visualized, and artifacts are common.

It has been postulated that ciliary beat is necessary for the normal embryonic rotation of the primitive foregut and that the situs inversus commonly associated with immotile cilia results from an essentially random rotation. Although this hypothesis is unproven, it is clear that siblings of patients with Kartagener syndrome often have pansinusitis and bronchiectasis without situs inversus. Many other patients with immotile cilia who do not have situs inversus have been reported. In 65 patients with Polynesian bronchiectatic disease, there were none with situs inversus. These patients have been reported to have deficient dynein arms on their ciliary microtubules, but the relationship between the two syndromes remains unclear.

Patients with PCD develop bronchial disease much more slowly than do those with CF and do not usually have the extensive mucous hypersecretion and airway plugging so characteristic of CF. Also, in striking contrast to CF, they do not have a high frequency of infection with *Pseudomonas aeruginosa.* The very existence of the clinical syndrome emphasizes the physiological importance of cilia in the respiratory tract, but it is clear that other factors are of importance in the pathogenesis of severe bronchopulmonary disease.

Clinical Manifestations

The clinical manifestations of PCD may begin early in life, or they may not become apparent until the second or third decades. In infants and children, cough and recurrent otitis media may be the primary signs. Patients are often suspected of having CF, but sweat testing will exclude this possibility. The usual signs and symptoms of sinusitis, bronchitis, and bronchiectasis are present in most patients; cough and sputum production, recurrent fevers, hemoptysis, digital clubbing, and eventually cyanosis may be present. Recurrent otitis media and conductive hearing loss are common. Although sperm counts may be normal, most men are infertile. Nevertheless, some patients with well-documented PCD have fathered children.

Diagnosis

The diagnosis of PCD may be suspected on the basis of the clinical picture, and it must be emphasized that situs inversus is not a necessary finding. A simple screening test may be performed by microscopic examination of scrapings of nasal epithelium (obtained from the middle to posterior third of the nose and placed into tissue culture medium). If adequate specimens are obtained, and the patient does not have an acute infection, the absence of ciliary beat on repeated testing is presumptive evidence of immotile cilia. In adult men, sperm also may be examined. It is important to obtain sheets of ciliated epithelium rather than isolated cells for examination and to compare the ciliary motility of the specimen with that of control material. Most isolated cells will not be viable, and their cilia will not beat. Confirmation of the diagnosis depends on the demonstration of characteristic ciliary ultrastructural abnormalities. No other laboratory findings are diagnostic. Specimens for ultrastructural study may be obtained from the nose or a bronchus.

Patients may have defective mucociliary transport for reasons other than immotile cilia, and the demonstration of normal ciliary beat or normal ciliary ultrastructure does not mean that mucociliary function is normal.

Pathology

PCD affects all ciliated epithelia, including those of the middle ear, eustachian tube, nose, paranasal sinuses, tracheobronchial tree, and perhaps other locations. However, there is no distinctive histologic picture, and these patients cannot be distinguished from those with other forms of bronchiectasis or sinusitis on the basis of light microscopy. Electron microscopy reveals characteristic ultrastructural abnormalities, including disorientation of the ciliary basal bodies. The classic finding is absence of inner or outer dynein arms (or both), but microtubular transposition, absence of radial spokes, and other abnormalities have been reported as well.

Treatment

There is no specific treatment that will alter ciliary function in patients with PCD. The bronchopulmonary disease is treated by chest physiotherapy, antibiotics, and bronchodilators as needed. Sinusitis should be treated with antibiotics and surgical drainage if necessary. Attention to the management of upper respiratory tract infections and otitis media should help reduce the complications of conductive hearing loss. When bronchiectasis is localized and severe, excision of involved areas of the lung may be indicated if medical management is insufficient.

The ultimate therapy for PCD is correction of the genetic defect. Techniques being developed for gene transfer therapy of other diseases such as CF will have direct and immediate application to PCD once the defective gene has been identified. The Human Genome Project can be expected to result in the identification of the gene or genes involved in PCD, so it is not unreasonable to anticipate successful gene transfer therapy in the foreseeable future.

Prognosis

The complete spectrum of PCD is not yet defined. What is clear is that the involvement and severity are quite variable. The classical patient develops severe bronchiectasis in the third to fourth decade and may succumb to pulmonary complications. Patients can reach advanced age, and many live a comparatively normal life. The majority of patients appear to develop bronchitis in childhood and to demonstrate findings of airway obstruction after two to three decades. Infections may be most severe in childhood and adolescence, with a partial clinical remission in adult life. Effective gene therapy would be expected to substantially improve prognosis.

OTHER FORMS OF AIRWAYS DISEASE WITH POSSIBLE GENETIC BASES

Genetics of Complex Diseases

Complex diseases are those diseases, including asthma, in which there is no clearly defined inheritance pattern and in which there appears to be gene-environment and/or gene-gene interactions. In addition to gene-environment interactions, asthma appears to be under the influence of multiple genes, and there appear to be gene-gene interactions (51). The exact contribution of each gene is unclear. For example, it is unknown if there are a few major genes and several minor genes or if there are several genes, each with a modest effect on the development of asthma. Another possibility, often ignored, is that there are a large number of genes that can contribute to the development of asthma in the population, but major effects on a small subset of genes explain the disease in each affected individual. This possibility would be especially difficult to detect with any of the commonly used statistical approaches to population genetics.

Asthma

Defining the Genetic Component

To date, no genes have been demonstrated to be unequivocally associated with asthma. Nevertheless, family studies suggest that asthma has a genetic basis. Clinical studies have demonstrated an increased prevalence of asthma among first-degree relatives of asthmatic subjects (20%–25%), compared with the general population prevalence of 4% (52–54), and greater concordance rates among monozygotic than dizygotic twins (50% versus 33%, respectively) (53,55,56). The exact mechanisms that underlie this familial aggregation are unknown. However, what is known is that asthma does not follow a simple mendelian pattern of inheritance, which qualifies asthma as a complex disease. Despite the inconsistencies, there are several genomic regions that are consistently identified in linkage analyses of asthma; however, it must be said that there have been an equal number of studies that did not replicate these results. These areas include chromosomal regions 5q31–33 (57–59), 11q (60, 61), and 12q (62–65).

Genetic Variation

Naturally occurring genetic variants, sequence variants, and polymorphisms are all referred to as alleles of genes and are an important source of genetic diversity. These variants may come in the form of single nucleotide polymorphisms (SNPs), repeats, insertions, or deletions. SNPs account for over 90% of all human DNA polymorphism (66). Although these alleles may or may not be associated with disease, identifying them provides data on genetic diversity and also provides useful markers for gene mapping and, possibly, for predicting disease susceptibility. Genetic variants in key regulatory regions (i.e., promoter regions) or in the gene itself may alter the normal biologic behavior of the gene. When these variants alter the function of the gene, they are often referred to as mutations. Many sequence variants in asthma candidate genes have been studied using association-based investigations and have been found to be associated with asthma or asthma subphenotypes, including IgE levels, bronchial hyperresponsiveness, and skin test reactivity. However, as with linkage analysis results, many of the results from association studies have been inconsistent. For example, sequence variants in the interleukin-4 gene (67) have been related to elevated levels of plasma IgE; this locus has been associated with the diagnosis of asthma in some studies (68,69) but not in others (70). SNPs located within the promoter or other key regulatory regions of these genes may alter biologic function of gene regulation and thus be important in the pathogenesis of asthma and other allergic disease phenotypes. In addition to SNPs, it has become evident that patterns of genetic variants, haplotypes, within a given gene or across a genetic region may also be associated with disease (71). Haplotypes among the $\beta_2 AR$ gene have been demonstrated to have a pharmacogenetic effect or influence the response to bronchodilators among subjects with asthma (72).

In addition to candidate genes located in the chromosomal region 5q23–31, there are other areas that have been linked to asthma including but not limited to 2q, 11q, and 12q, which may also contain potentially important candidate genes. Linkage results varied by the ethnicity and race, possibly suggesting that the genetic regulation of asthma may differ between racial groups (57,62).

CONCLUSIONS AND FUTURE DIRECTIONS

The study of the genetic basis of lung diseases offers great promise. Despite several recent advances in our understanding of human genetics, we are still at the edge of a new horizon, which promises to be filled with many challenges and the potential for great benefit to human kind. Equally possible is the potential for great harm if this technology is abused. Beyond the science, we as a medical community, society, and citizens must take great efforts to ensure that the fruits of the Human Genome Project will benefit all members of our society and not just those who can afford these benefits. Furthermore, we must take measures to prevent the abuse of our newfound understanding of potential benefits and risks associated with knowing an individual's genetic background.

REFERENCES

1. Risch N. Linkage strategies for genetically complex traits, II: the power of affected relative pairs. *Am J Hum Genet* 1990;46:229–241.
2. McKusick VA. *Mendelian inheritance of man.* Baltimore: Johns Hopkins University Press, 1994.
3. Risch N, Merikangas K. The future of genetic studies of complex human diseases. *Science* 1996;273:1516–1517.
4. Schork NJ, Cardon, LR, Xu X. The future of genetic epidemiology. *Trends Genet* 1998;14:266–272.
5. Spielman RS, McGinnis RE, Ewens WJ. Transmission test for linkage disequilibrium: the insulin gene region and insulin-dependent diabetes mellitus (IDDM). *Am J Hum Genet* 1993;52:506–516.
6. Elias JA, Geba GP, Tang W, et al. Transgenic modeling of cytokines in the investigation of pulmonary disease. *Chest* 1996;109:69S–73S.
7. Hautamaki RD, Kobayashi DK, Senior RM, et al. Requirement for macrophage elastase for cigarette smoke-induced emphysema in mice. *Science* 1997;277:2002–2004.
8. Munger JS, Huang X, Kawakatsu H, et al. The integrin α v β 6 binds and activates latent TGF β_1: a mechanism for regulating pulmonary inflammation and fibrosis. *Cell* 1999:96:319–328.
9. Kaminski N, Allard JD, Pittet JF, et al. Global analysis of gene expression in pulmonary fibrosis reveals distinct programs regulating lung inflammation and fibrosis. *Proc Natl Acad Sci U S A* 2000;97:1778–1783.
10. Zheng T, Zhu Z, Wang Z, et al. Inducible targeting of IL-13 to the adult lung causes matrix metalloproteinase- and cathepsin-dependent emphysema. *J Clin Invest* 2000;106:1081–1093.
11. Wang Z, Zheng T, Zhu Z, et al. Interferon gamma induction of pulmonary emphysema in the adult murine lung. *J Exp Med* 2000;192:1587–1600.
12. Elias JA. Airway remodeling in asthma. Unanswered questions. *Am J Respir Crit Care Med* 2000;161:S168–S171.
13. Zuo F, Kaminski N, Eugui E, et al. Gene expression analysis reveals matrilysin as a key regulator of pulmonary fibrosis in mice and humans. *Proc Natl Acad Sci U S A* 2002;99:6292–6297.
14. Cystic Fibrosis Foundation. *Patient registry: 2000 annual data report.* Bethesda, MD: Cystic Fibrosis Foundation, 2001.
15. Bals R, Weiner DJ, Wilson JM. The innate immune system in cystic fibrosis lung disease. *J Clin Invest* 1999;103:303–307.
16. Knowles MR, Boucher RC. Mucus clearance as a primary innate defense mechanism for mammalian airways. *J Clin Invest* 2002;109:571–577.
17. Davis PB, Drumm M, Konstan MW. Cystic fibrosis. *Am J Respir Crit Care Med* 1996;154:1229–1256.
18. Akabas MH. Cystic fibrosis transmembrane conductance regulator: structure and function of an epithelial chloride channel. *J Biol Chem* 2000;275:3729–3732.

19. Huntington JA, Read RJ, Carrell RW. Structure of a serpin-protease complex shows inhibition by deformation. *Nature* 2000;407:923–926.

20. Carrell RW, Lomas DA. α_1-Antitrypsin deficiency: a model for conformational diseases. *N Engl J Med* 2002;346:45–53.

21. Eriksson S. α_1-Antitrypsin deficiency: lessons learned from the bedside to the gene and back again: historic perspectives. *Chest* 1989;95:181–189.

22. Eriksson S. A 30-year perspective on α_1-antitrypsin deficiency. *Chest* 1996;110:237S–242S.

23. Cox DW, Markovic VD, Teshima IE. Genes for immunoglobulin heavy chains and for α_1-antitrypsin are localized to specific regions of chromosome 14q. *Nature* 1982;297:428–430.

24. Turleau C, de Grouchy J, Chavin-Colin F, et al. Two patients with interstitial del (14q), one with features of Holt-Oram syndrome: exclusion mapping of PI (α_1-antitrypsin). *Ann Genet* 1984;27:237–240.

25. Schroeder WT, Miller MF, Woo SL, et al. Chromosomal localization of the human α_1-antitrypsin gene (PI) to 14q31-32. *Am J Hum Genet* 1985;37:868–872.

26. Rabin M, Watson M, Kidd V, et al. Regional location of α_1-antichymotrypsin and α_1-antitrypsin genes on human chromosome 14. *Somat Cell Mol Genet* 1986;12:209–214.

27. Lai EC, Kao FT, Law ML, et al. Assignment of the α_1-antitrypsin gene and a sequence-related gene to human chromosome 14 by molecular hybridization. *Am J Hum Genet* 1983;35:385–392.

28. Long GL, Chandra T, Woo SL, et al. Complete sequence of the cDNA for human α_1-antitrypsin and the gene for the S variant. *Biochemistry* 1984;23:4828–4837.

29. Yamamoto Y, Sawa R, Okamoto N, et al. Deletion 14q(q24.3 to q32.1) syndrome: significance of peculiar facial appearance in its diagnosis, and deletion mapping of Pi(α_1- antitrypsin). *Hum Genet* 1986;74:190–192.

30. Brantly M, Nukiwa T, Crystal RG. Molecular basis of α_1-antitrypsin deficiency. *Am J Med* 1988;84:13–31.

31. Mullins CD, Huang X, Merchant S, et al. The direct medical costs of α_1-antitrypsin deficiency. *Chest* 2001;119:745–752.

32. Crystal RG, Brantly ML, Hubbard RC, et al. The α_1-antitrypsin gene and its mutations: clinical consequences and strategies for therapy. *Chest* 1989;95:196–208.

33. Carrell RW, Jeppsson JO, Laurell CB, et al. Structure and variation of human α_1-antitrypsin. *Nature* 1982;298:329–334.

34. Cox DW, Woo SL, Mansfield T. DNA restriction fragments associated with α_1-antitrypsin indicate a single origin for deficiency allele PI Z. *Nature* 1985;316:79–81.

35. Crystal RG. α_1-antitrypsin deficiency, emphysema, and liver disease: genetic basis and strategies for therapy. *J Clin Invest* 1990;85:1343–1352.

36. Lomas DA, Evans DL, Finch JT, et al. The mechanism of Z α_1-antitrypsin accumulation in the liver. *Nature* 1992;357:605–607.

37. Cox DW, Smyth S. Risk for liver disease in adults with α_1-antitrypsin deficiency. *Am J Med* 1983;74:221–227.

38. Hubbard RC, Ogushi F, Fells GA, et al. Oxidants spontaneously released by alveolar macrophages of cigarette smokers can inactivate the active site of α_1-antitrypsin, rendering it ineffective as an inhibitor of neutrophil elastase. *J Clin Invest* 1987;80:1289–1295.

39. Silverman EK, Miletich JP, Pierce JA, et al. α_1-Antitrypsin deficiency: high prevalence in the St. Louis area determined by direct population screening. *Am Rev Respir Dis* 1989;140:961–966.

40. Survival and FEV1 decline in individuals with severe deficiency of α_1-antitrypsin. The α_1-Antitrypsin Deficiency Registry Study Group. *Am J Respir Crit Care Med* 1998;158:49–59.

41. Seersholm N, Wencker M, Banik N, et al. Does α_1-antitrypsin augmentation therapy slow the annual decline in FEV_1 in patients with severe hereditary α_1-antitrypsin deficiency? Wissenschaftliche Arbeitsgemeinschaft zur Therapie von Lungenerkrankungen (WATL) α_1-AT study group. *Eur Respir J* 1997; 10:2260–2263.

42. Wewers MD, Casolaro MA, Sellers SE, et al. Replacement therapy for α_1-antitrypsin deficiency associated with emphysema. *N Engl J Med* 1987;316:1055–1062.

43. Hubbard RC, Sellers S, Czerski D, et al. Biochemical efficacy and safety of monthly augmentation therapy for α_1-antitrypsin deficiency. *JAMA* 1988;260:1259–1264.

44. Schluchter MD, Stoller JK, Barker AF, et al. Feasibility of a clinical trial of augmentation therapy for α_1- antitrypsin deficiency. The α_1-Antitrypsin Deficiency Registry Study Group. *Am J Respir Crit Care Med* 2000;161:796–801.

45. Dirksen A, Dijkman JH, Madsen F, et al. A randomized clinical trial of α_1-antitrypsin augmentation therapy. *Am J Respir Crit Care Med* 1999;160:1468–1472.

46. Guidelines for the approach to the patient with severe hereditary α_1-antitrypsin deficiency. American Thoracic Society. *Am Rev Respir Dis* 1989;140:1494–1497.

47. Patients at high risk of death after lung-volume-reduction surgery. *N Engl J Med* 2001;345:1075–1083.

48. Massaro GD, Massaro D. Retinoic acid treatment abrogates elastase-induced pulmonary emphysema in rats. *Nat Med* 1997;3:675–677.

49. Mao JT, Goldin JG, Dermand J, et al. A pilot study of all-trans-retinoic acid for the treatment of human emphysema. *Am J Respir Crit Care Med* 2002;165:718–723.

50. Burrows JA, Willis LK, Perlmutter DH. Chemical chaperones mediate increased secretion of mutant α_1-antitrypsin (α_1-AT) Z: a potential pharmacological strategy for prevention of liver injury and emphysema in α_1-AT deficiency. *Proc Natl Acad Sci U S A* 2000;97:1796–1801.

51. Howard TD, Koppelman GH, Xu J, et al. Gene-gene interaction in asthma: IL4RA and IL13 in a Dutch population with asthma. *Am J Hum Genet* 2002;70:230–236.

52. Sibbald B, Turner-Warwick M. Factors influencing the prevalence of asthma among first degree relatives of extrinsic and intrinsic asthmatics. *Thorax* 1979;34:332–337.

53. Hopp RJ, Bewtra AK, Watt GD, et al. Genetic analysis of allergic disease in twins. *J Allergy Clin Immunol* 1984;73:265–270.

54. Sandford A, Weir T, Pare P. The genetics of asthma. *Am J Respir Crit Care Med* 1996;153:1749–1765.

55. Duffy DL. A population-based study of bronchial asthma in adult twin pairs. *Chest* 1992;102:654.

56. Duffy DL, Mitchell CA, Martin NG. Genetic and environmental risk factors for asthma: a cotwin-control study. *Am J Respir Crit Care Med* 1998;157:840–845.

57. A genome-wide search for asthma susceptibility loci in ethnically diverse populations. The Collaborative Study on the Genetics of Asthma (CSGA). *Nat Genet* 1997;15:389–392.

58. Noguchi E, Shibasaki M, Arinami T, et al. Evidence for linkage between asthma/atopy in childhood and chromosome 5q31-q33 in a Japanese population. *Am J Respir Crit Care Med* 1997;156:1390–1393.

59. O'Donnell CJ, Lindpaintner K, Larson MG, et al. Evidence for association and genetic linkage of the angiotensin-converting enzyme locus with hypertension and blood pressure in men but not women in the Framingham Heart Study. *Circulation* 1998;97:1766–1772.

60. Cookson WO, Young RP, Sandford AJ, et al. Maternal inheritance of atopic IgE responsiveness on chromosome 11q. *Lancet* 1992;340:381–384.

61. Cookson WO. 11q and high-affinity IgE receptor in asthma

and allergy. *Clin Exp Allergy* 1995;25[Suppl 2]:71–73; discussion 95–96.

62. Barnes KC, Neely JD, Duffy DL, et al. Linkage of asthma and total serum IgE concentration to markers on chromosome 12q: evidence from Afro-Caribbean and Caucasian populations. *Genomics* 1996;37:41–50.

63. Nickel R, Wahn U, Hizawa N, et al. Evidence for linkage of chromosome 12q15-q24.1 markers to high total serum IgE concentrations in children of the German Multicenter Allergy Study. *Genomics* 1997;46:159–162.

64. Ober C, Cox NJ, Abney M, et al. Genome-wide search for asthma susceptibility loci in a founder population. The Collaborative Study on the Genetics of Asthma. *Hum Mol Genet* 1998;7:1393–1398.

65. Wilkinson J, Grimley S, Collins A, et al. Linkage of asthma to markers on chromosome 12 in a sample of 240 families using quantitative phenotype scores. *Genomics* 1998;53:251–259.

66. Collins FS, Brooks LD, Chakravarti A. A DNA polymorphism discovery resource for research on human genetic variation. *Genome Res* 1998;8:1229–1231.

67. Rosenwasser LJ, Klemm DJ, Dresback JK, et al. Promoter polymorphisms in the chromosome 5 gene cluster in asthma and atopy. *Clin Exp Allergy* 1995;25:[Suppl 2]:74–78; discussion 95–96.

68. Kawashima T, Noguchi E, Arinami T, et al. Linkage and association of an interleukin 4 gene polymorphism with atopic dermatitis in Japanese families. *J Med Genet* 1998;35:502–504.

69. Noguchi E, Shibasaki M, Arinami T, et al. Association of asthma and the interleukin-4 promoter gene in Japanese. *Clin Exp Allergy* 1998;28:449–453.

70. Walley A J, Cookson WO. Investigation of an interleukin-4 promoter polymorphism for associations with asthma and atopy. *J Med Genet* 1996;33:689–692.

71. Martin ER, Monks SA, Warren LL, et al. A test for linkage and association in general pedigrees: the pedigree disequilibrium test. *Am J Hum Genet* 2000;67:146–154.

72. Drysdale CM, McGraw DW, Stack CB, et al. Complex promoter and coding region β_2-adrenergic receptor haplotypes alter receptor expression and predict in vivo responsiveness. *Proc Natl Acad Sci U S A* 2000;97:10483–10488.

Developmental Anomalies of the Respiratory Tract Manifesting in the Adult

66

Linda S. Snyder · Fernando D. Martinez

The frequency of congenital pulmonary anomalies ranges from 7.5% to 18.7% of all congenital malformations (1). Most cases are diagnosed and treated in the newborn period, infancy, or early childhood. However, some patients with congenital lung malformations that were once fatal early in life now survive into adulthood. Pulmonologists need to be aware of congenital lung anomalies that may first become manifest in the adult, either with symptoms or as an incidental radiographic finding. Therefore, it is necessary for pulmonologists to be knowledgeable regarding developmental anomalies of the respiratory tract and their long-term outcomes.

This chapter will focus on specific developmental anomalies of the respiratory tract, and when data are available, long-term outcome and presentation in adulthood will be addressed. The anomalies have been divided into seven anatomic groups: (a) larynx and trachea, (b) bronchi, (c) cystic structures, (d) pulmonary vasculature, (e) diaphragm, (f) chest wall, and (g) pleural fissures.

OVERVIEW OF THE DEVELOPMENT OF THE HUMAN RESPIRATORY TRACT

A simplified review of normal development of the human respiratory tract is necessary to conceptualize congenital lung malformations. Intrauterine fetal lung development can be divided into five stages, based on the description by Boyden (2):

1. In the *embryonic stage,* the lung begins to form with bud-

ding of epithelium from the ventral floor of the foregut at 21 to 24 days of gestation. The first outgrowth of the entodermal tube forms the larynx and trachea. The bronchial buds form and branch to become the right and left bronchi and the main bronchi of the five lobes of the lung. At 7 weeks of gestation, third-order bronchi are present and continue to develop into 18 bronchopulmonary segments.

2. In the *glandular stage* (5–16 weeks), ongoing bronchial branching occurs, as does pulmonary vasculature development. Mesenchyme around the lung bud contains a vascular network from the foregut, which is important for vessel formation. By the end of 16 weeks of gestation, formation of all airways through the terminal bronchioles is complete.

3. The *canalicular stage* (16–24 weeks) includes respiratory bronchiole formation and vascularization. It is a critical phase of development, as capillaries now start to penetrate the lining of the tubules and are in close contact with the epithelium of the developing airway. The close association of airways and blood vessels begins early in development. Vascular growth proceeds rapidly, and the capillaries thin the lining of the respiratory bronchioles. Early gas exchange units form during this phase.

4. The *saccular stage* (24–35 weeks) includes further airway growth and the formation of acini. The two types of epithelial lining cells are seen, and surfactant is produced.

5. The *alveolar stage* (35 weeks–2 years) is when the lungs are getting ready for gas exchange, and alveoli continue to develop and increase 10-fold between birth and 2 years of age. The number of alveoli reaches adult levels by 8 years of age. Airway growth continues after birth as well, with increases in diameter and length.

L. S. Snyder and F. D. Martinez: Arizona Respiratory Center, University of Arizona; and Arizona Health Sciences Center, Tucson, Arizona.

DEVELOPMENTAL ANOMALIES OF THE LARYNX AND TRACHEA

Laryngomalacia

Laryngomalacia is the most common congenital anomaly in the upper airway—it is also called congenital stridor. It accounts for 60% of laryngeal problems in infants (3). It is a delay in development of the supporting structures of the larynx and leads to flaccidity of the epiglottis and upper airway. This results in collapsibility of the larynx in inspiration and stridor. The stridor may be present at birth or develop within the first 6 weeks of age. Some patients will present at a few months of age when the stridor becomes noticeable after an upper respiratory tract infection. The stridor is usually more prominent during respiratory infections, crying, and feeding.

The history and physical examination are very important for diagnosis; however, the gold standard is direct laryngoscopy. It should be noted that laryngomalacia often coexists with other laryngeal anomalies such as esophageal atresia (EA) and tracheoesophageal atresia. Most cases are mild and self-limited, with symptoms usually resolving by 2 years of age. Rare cases of significant airway obstruction and obstructive apneas have been described.

The long-term outlook for patients with laryngomalacia is very good, with little evidence of significant sequelae in adulthood. One follow-up study of patients with laryngomalacia into late childhood found a small number with persistent obstructive findings on flow volume loops (4).

Laryngotracheoesophageal Cleft

Laryngeal cleft anomalies are rare congenital defects of the posterior laryngotracheal wall that are associated with significant morbidity and mortality in the neonatal period. It is an abnormal communication between the esophagus and the larynx and the trachea, usually leading to aspiration. These defects are typically present from birth and manifest with clinical features that include difficulty with swallowing secretions, respiratory distress (especially with feedings), and aspiration pneumonia. It is often associated with other laryngotracheal malformations such as EA or tracheoesophageal fistula (TEF).

There is a spectrum in clinical severity that depends on the length of involvement of the laryngotracheal airway. Mild defects may not require surgical correction. Timing of surgery for severe defects depends on the clinical condition of the child at the time of diagnosis. Overall survival for infants who undergo aggressive surgery is nearly 70%; however, survival is significantly less for those patients with complicated defects or associated anomalies. It is possible for the diagnosis of a laryngotracheal cleft to be delayed until adulthood because mild cases may be asymptomatic or have minimal symptomatology. Therefore, rarely will patients present with laryngotracheal clefts in adult life. Two case reports document posterior laryngeal clefts presenting in adults 19 and 50 years of age and emphasize the importance of maintaining suspicion of the diagnosis into adulthood in the proper clinical setting (5,6).

Tracheomalacia and Vascular Compression Syndromes

Tracheomalacia is the result of congenital absence or deficiency of the tracheal cartilage, which leads to collapse of the trachea during the respiratory cycle. Tracheomalacia can be owing to intrinsic weakness of the tracheal cartilage or to extrinsic compression by a mass or vascular structure. Primary tracheomalacia is rare and has been associated with Down syndrome and certain congenital heart defects.

The Williams-Campbell syndrome is a rare familial form of tracheobronchomalacia characterized by a deficiency of cartilage in the bronchi, leading to airway collapse and bronchiectasis. Although the syndrome was originally described in children, there have been reports in adults. The clinical course of Williams-Campbell syndrome is variable, and long-term follow-up is limited. However, there are reports of survival into adulthood with chronic pulmonary symptoms and progression to respiratory failure (7).

More frequently, tracheomalacia occurs as a localized abnormality secondary to extrinsic compression from a vascular structure or cyst. The clinical presentation of airway compression by vascular structures ranges from patients with minimal symptoms or incidental radiographic findings to severe airway compromise that requires intervention. A review of vascular tracheobronchial compression syndromes in 22 patients (ages, 8 days–46 years) documents the type of anomalies leading to tracheal compression, such as double aortic arch, right aortic arch plus left ligamentum arteriosum, and left pulmonary artery sling syndrome (8).

Vascular rings are congenital abnormalities of the aortic arch that lead to complete or partial encirclement of the trachea or esophagus. In most cases, vascular rings present in infancy or early childhood with respiratory symptoms, wheezing, stridor, or infections. Occasionally, asymptomatic adults with vascular rings will develop symptoms of tracheal obstruction or tracheomalacia owing to enlargement of the vascular structures with aging (9).

A review of vascular rings in 25 adult patients (ages, 18–57 years) found the most common vascular anomaly was double aortic arch (46%), followed by right aortic arch with aberrant left subclavian artery and ligamentum arteriosum (30%) and by right aortic arch and left ligamentum arteriosum (19%) (10). The most frequent symptoms involved the respiratory tract and occurred in 42% of adult patients. Clinical symptoms included dyspnea on exertion, stridor, bronchitis, and recurrent pneumonia. Dysphagia occurred in 33% of patients. Vascular rings in adults are not usually associated with congenital cardiac abnormalities. Magnetic resonance imaging (MRI) and computed tomography (CT) imaging are excellent radiographic modalities to define these anomalies.

In this review, 59% of patients underwent surgery, and follow-up was available in 11 of 14 patients who had surgery and nine who did not. The majority of patients were clinically improved after surgery, but some had persistent problems, including tracheomalacia.

Tracheobronchomegaly

Congenital tracheobronchomegaly, or Mounier-Kuhn syndrome, is a rare disorder characterized by marked dilation of the trachea and main bronchi. It is associated with tracheal wall weakening and mucosal herniations between the cartilaginous rings, leading to diverticulosis, retained secretions, and recurrent lower respiratory tract infections (11).

Clinicians may see a spectrum of clinical findings that range from minimal disease with good lung function to progressive disease, leading to respiratory failure. Symptoms are nonspecific and indistinguishable from chronic bronchitis or bronchiectasis and include chronic sputum production, cough, recurrent pulmonary infections, dyspnea, and occasional hemoptysis. Many patients remain asymptomatic until adulthood, and the diagnosis is made in most patients after 30 years of age.

Marked dilation of the trachea may be obvious on chest roentgenogram. The diagnosis is easily confirmed by CT scans of the chest (12). Treatment is focused on secretion clearance, postural drainage, and antibiotic therapy. It is recommended that patients with this disease who require mechanical ventilation have an uncuffed endotracheal tube.

Secondary tracheobronchomegaly has been described in association with Ehlers-Danlos syndrome, Marfan syndrome, ankylosing spondylitis, and cutis laxa (11,13).

Tracheoesophageal Fistula

TEF and other congenital anomalies of the esophagus and trachea occur in about one in 3,000 live births (1). There are a number of anatomic types; the most common is EA with TEF (85% of cases); other types include isolated EA (5%–10% of cases) and TEF without EA (or H-type fistula) (<5% of cases). This group of anomalies is an important cause of respiratory distress in the newborn period. Approximately 50% of infants with TEF have associated anomalies of the skeletal, cardiac, or gastrointestinal systems. Management is surgical, and postoperative complications are relatively common. It should be noted that variable degrees of tracheomalacia persist beyond the time of surgical closure of the TEF in the majority of patients. This may lead to chronic respiratory symptoms of cough, bronchitis, and pneumo-

nia later in life. However, the overall prognosis for children born with the EA/TEF group of anomalies is about 70% (14). Pulmonary function testing in patients with repaired TEF usually shows mild restrictive impairment. In addition, many patients continue to have esophageal motility problems, leading to dysphagia and gastroesophageal reflux in adulthood (14).

Congenital TEF without EA, also known as H-type fistula, can go undetected for years or decades and may not manifest until adulthood (15). Clinical symptoms include recurrent respiratory infections, coughing, and choking during eating. The nonspecific nature of the symptoms, together with difficulty in identifying the fistula, leads to a delayed diagnosis. This type of fistula can masquerade in adulthood as idiopathic chronic lung disease. A review of nine adults noted the duration of symptoms in many patients was greater than 15 years (16). The diagnosis was made by esophagram in the majority of patients, with two patients diagnosed by bronchoscopy or at surgery. Treatment is surgical ligation, with fewer postoperative complications than for other forms of TEF. In this review, all patients did well after surgical repair.

Tracheal Stenosis

Congenital tracheal stenosis is a rare disorder that usually presents in infancy and causes severe respiratory distress. Three types have been described, including generalized tracheal hypoplasia (30% of cases), funnel-like stenosis tapering down to the carina (20% of cases), and short-segment stenosis (50% of cases) (3). Congenital complete tracheal rings is another condition that leads to tracheal stenosis. In this anomaly, the tracheal rings are fused posteriorly with no membranous tracheal wall. Various forms of congenital tracheal stenosis have been associated with other anomalies, including congenital heart defects, TEF, skeletal abnormalities, and left pulmonary artery sling syndrome (1).

Most cases of congenital tracheal stenosis present in infancy and have a high mortality rate. Less severe short-segment stenosis of the trachea may cause mild symptoms and resolve with time or be surgically repaired. Patients with tracheal stenosis usually present with stridor, wheezing, cyanosis, cough, or tachypnea. A definitive diagnosis of tracheal stenosis is made by radiographic studies (CT or MRI) and endoscopy. Radiographic studies are important in evaluating the extent of stenosis, determining the size of the airway, ruling out extrinsic compression syndromes, and diagnosing concomitant anomalies.

Management of congenital tracheal stenosis is difficult. Tracheal surgical techniques are complex, have high morbidity and mortality rates, and should be performed at institutions with expertise in this area (3).

Adult presentation of congenital tracheal stenosis is very rare. A recent case report documented the first adult patient

(21 years of age) with complete tracheal rings causing congenital long-segment tracheal stenosis, which masqueraded as asthma (17).

DEVELOPMENTAL ANOMALIES OF THE BRONCHI

Abnormal Bronchial Branching

Isolated lobar or segmental bronchial abnormalities are recognized and usually cause minimal symptoms and, therefore, are not usually detected until adulthood. The most common anomalies are tracheal bronchus and abnormal segmental bronchial branching, including double right upper lobe bronchus and accessory cardiac bronchus.

Tracheal bronchus always occurs on the right side, usually arising from the mid intrathoracic trachea and supplying a segment of the right upper lobe. A radiographic review of congenital bronchial abnormalities noted a variety of bronchial anomalies originating from the trachea or main bronchus to the upper lobe (18). Out of 35 cases of tracheal bronchi, only eight originated from the trachea and 24 originated from the bronchi. This may be associated with stenosis or malacia, as well as poor drainage leading to recurrent infections, atelectasis, or bronchiectasis later in life. The diagnosis is usually made at bronchoscopy, although CT imaging can detect this anomaly as well. Knowledge of congenital bronchial abnormalities is important for airway procedures such as bronchoscopy, surgery, brachytherapy, and intubation.

Bronchial Atresia

A blind-ending lobar or segmental bronchus and hyperinflation of the obstructed lung characterizes congenital bronchial atresia. Ventilation of the segment is thought to occur through the pores of Kohn and results in gas trapping. When detected in adults, it is usually an incidental radiographic finding, and most patients are asymptomatic. On chest radiograph, a rounded perihilar mass with distal hyperinflation is seen. Chest CT is used to confirm the diagnosis and typically shows mucous plugging in a branching pattern with associated segmental hyperinflation (19). A review of 86 cases of congenital bronchial atresia noted the majority of patients presented in early adulthood (20). Although most patients are asymptomatic, a small number will present with recurrent pulmonary infections.

Bronchoesophageal Fistula

Congenital bronchoesophageal fistula (BEF) without EA is a rare anomaly but can present in adulthood. A review of 13 adult patients notes that the most common site of communication is the mid esophagus and right lower lobe (21). Clinical symptoms are nonspecific and include chronic cough, cough with ingestion of liquids, and recurrent pulmonary infections. The diagnosis is often delayed because of the nonspecific nature of these symptoms. In this report, barium esophagram was useful in making the diagnosis of bronchoesophageal fistula. Surgical intervention or fistulectomy is relatively straightforward, and only rarely is pulmonary resection needed secondary to severe bronchiectasis (21,22).

CYSTIC ANOMALIES OF THE LUNGS AND MEDIASTINUM

The major forms of congenital cystic lesions of the lungs discussed in this section are bronchogenic cysts (BCs), cystic adenomatoid malformation (CAM), congenital lobar emphysema (CLE), and sequestration.

Bronchogenic Cysts

BCs are congenital anomalies of the tracheobronchial tree with a clinical presentation that ranges from respiratory distress at birth to an asymptomatic radiographic finding in adulthood. BCs form when a developing bronchus is disrupted at a particular stage and a piece of bronchial tissue separates to form the cyst. On histological examination, cysts are lined by ciliated columnar epithelium and surrounded by muscle and fibrous tissue. The cyst is usually single and may be large.

Clinical findings are variable, depending on the location of the cyst. BCs are located in five areas in the thorax: (a) carinal region (51%), (b) right peritracheal region (19%), (c) periesophageal (14%), (d) hilar (9%), and (e) others such as pericardial, retrosternal, or paravertebral (7%) (23). Compression of the trachea leads to symptoms of stridor and respiratory distress. Compression of smaller bronchi can cause cough, wheeze, atelectasis, chest pain, or recurrent respiratory infections. The cyst can also become infected, leading to enlargement and worsening of compression symptoms. Many patients have no symptoms, and the cyst is found incidentally on a chest radiograph. BCs appear radiographically as a cystic lesion, located near the hilum and often displacing the adjacent bronchus, leading to postobstructive hyperlucency (Fig. 66.1). Chest CT is an excellent imaging modality to localize and define the anatomy of the cystic lesion. CT of BCs typically shows sharply marginated mediastinal masses of soft tissue or water attenuation. MRI can be useful for elucidating the cystic nature of the minority of lesions that appear solid on CT examination. Surgical resection is generally recommended in patients with suspected BCs who are operable candidates, even if they are asymptomatic, to confirm the diagnosis and avoid potential complications (24–26).

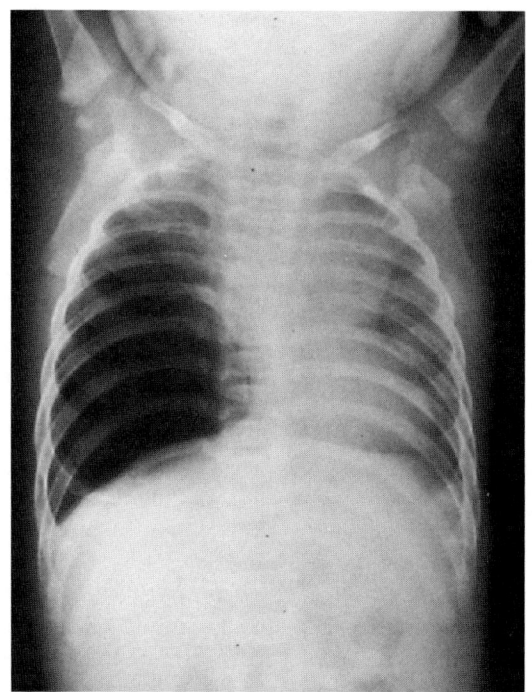

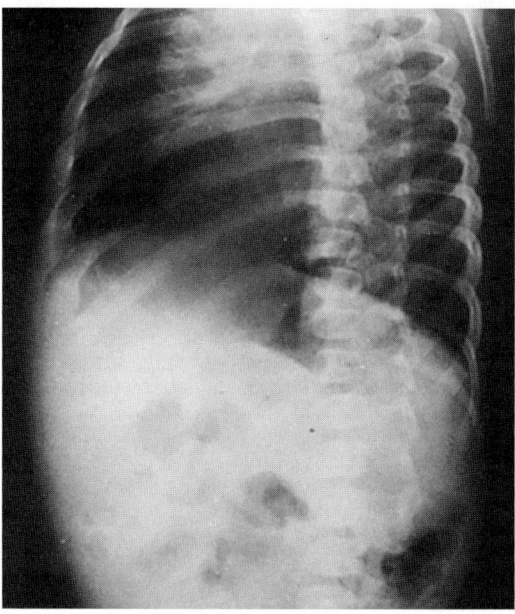

FIGURE 66.1. Bronchogenic cyst. Hyperaeration with definable boundary within a lobe.

BRONCHOGENIC CYSTS	
Summary Statement	**Level of Evidence**
More than 50% of patients are diagnosed after 15 years of age, and 37%–80% of patients are asymptomatic.	Observational studies, expert opinion
Symptomatic patients may have chest pain, dysphagia, cough, or hemoptysis.	Observational studies, expert opinion
Adults with bronchogenic cysts may develop symptoms over time, which can be serious (respiratory distress secondary to compression and infection).	Observational studies, expert opinion
Surgery is the treatment of choice and carries an excellent prognosis.	Observational studies, expert opinion

Cystic Adenomatoid Malformation

CAM is a rare anomaly characterized by solid, cystic, or mixed parenchymal masses that communicate with the normal bronchial tree. It may involve part of a lobe, more than one lobe, or an entire lung (Fig. 66.2). Three types of adenomatoid malformations have been described: type I (macroscopic) is characterized by large cysts 3 to 10 cm in diameter, type II (microscopic) is characterized by numerous cysts between 0.5 and 3 cm in diameter, and type III (solid) has many small cysts less than 0.5 cm in diameter. CAM usually presents in the newborn period with symptoms of severe respiratory distress. The malformation can cause mediastinal shift to the opposite side with compression atelectasis. CAM may have features that overlap with those of other congenital lung lesions, such as sequestration or bronchial atresia. Occasionally, it is difficult to distinguish CAM from congenital diaphragmatic hernia (DH) or CLE in an infant with severe respiratory distress.

CAM has rarely been described in older children and adults, in whom it is localized to one area of the lung (27,28). The older children can present with nonresolving pulmonary infiltrates, failure to thrive, or pneumothorax. The rare adult cases have been discovered as an incidental finding on a chest radiograph or in patients with symptoms such as recurrent pneumonia and pyopneumothorax (29). Malignancies complicating CAM, such as bronchioloalveolar cancer and rhabdomyosarcoma, are rare but have been reported in both adults and children (30,31).

Congenital Lobar Emphysema

CLE is massive overinflation of one or more lobes of the lung and usually occurs in neonates. In approximately 50% of patients, it occurs within the first month of life. The overexpanded lung, usually an upper or middle lobe, compresses the remaining lung parenchyma and leads to severe respiratory distress (Fig. 66.3). The defect is owing to partial obstruction of the lobar bronchus with air trapping. The partial obstruction may be caused by defective or absent cartilage in the affected bronchus. Concomitant congenital heart anomalies are frequently seen in these patients. The majority of patients require early surgical intervention, particularly newborns with severe pulmonary compromise.

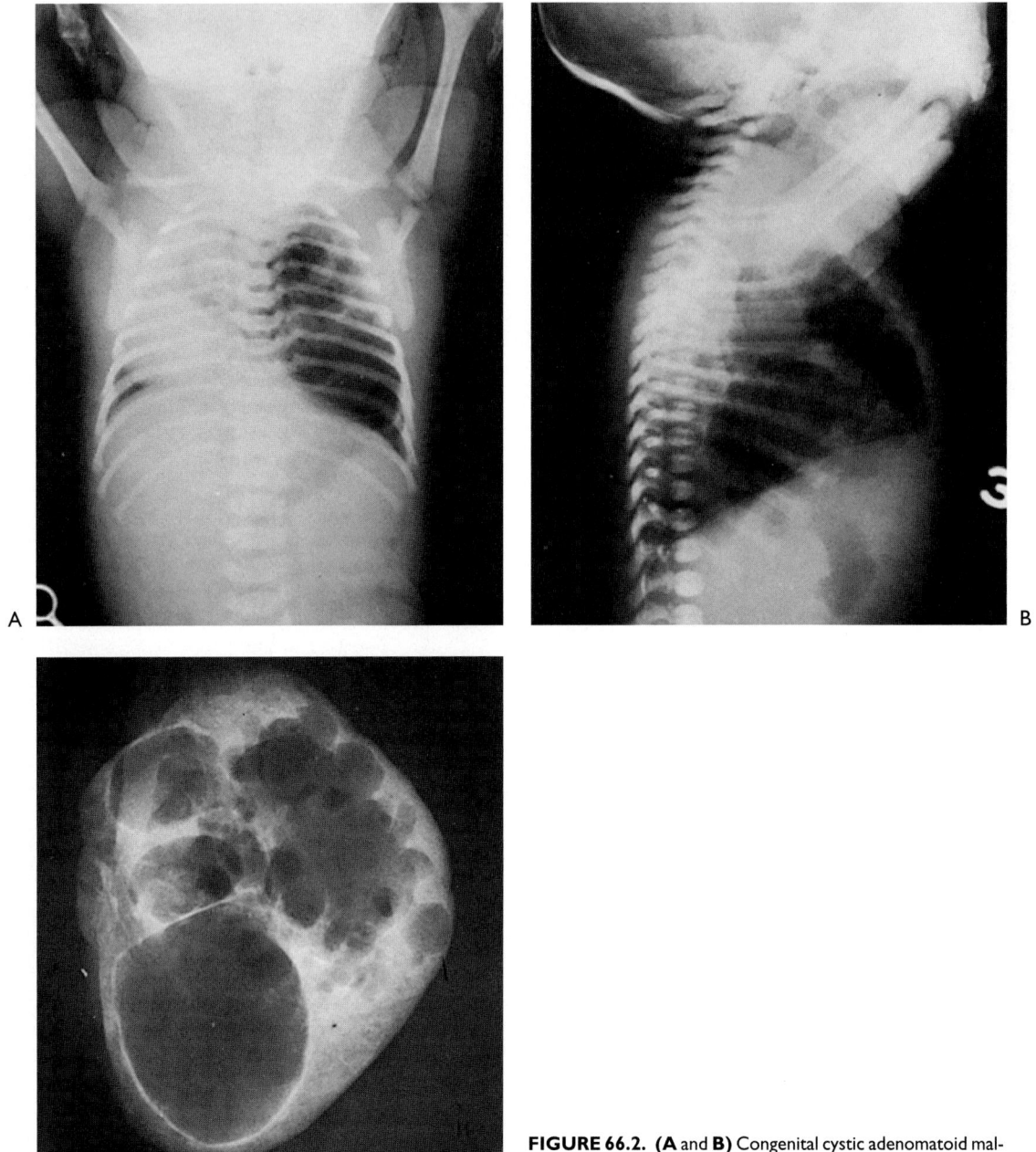

FIGURE 66.2. (A and **B)** Congenital cystic adenomatoid malformation of the lung. **(C)** A roentgenogram of the surgically resected specimen.

There are a few case reports of CLE discovered in adulthood. Generally, symptoms are not severe, or the abnormality is incidentally found on a chest radiograph (32).

Sequestration

A pulmonary sequestration can be defined as a disconnected or abnormally communicating bronchopulmonary mass or cyst with a normal or anomalous arterial supply or venous drainage (1). Two anatomic types are described: the more common intrapulmonary form lying within the normal visceral pleura (intralobar), and the rare extrapulmonary form lying outside the visceral pleura, enclosed in its own pleural sac (extralobar).

Intrapulmonary sequestrations form more than 85% of sequestrations, and 60% of these are found in the posterior basal segment of the left lower lobe. Bronchial communication is usually absent or abnormal. The aberrant systemic arterial blood supply usually arises from the lower thoracic or upper abdominal aorta and is typically large. A small percentage of cases receive blood supply from the other sources such as the subclavian, intercostal, bronchial, celiac, or internal

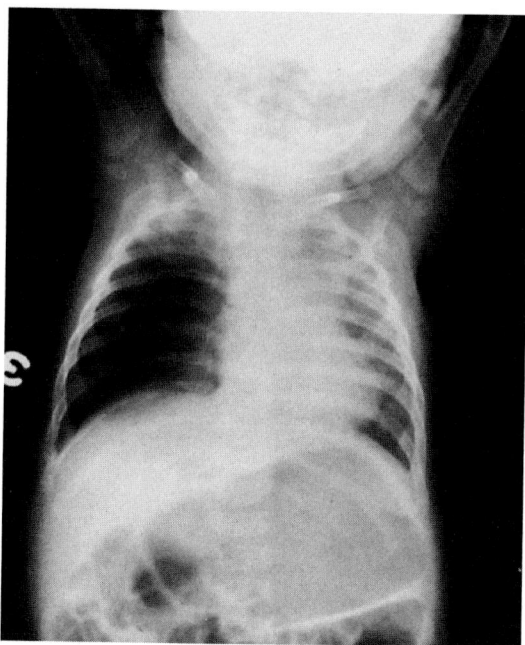

FIGURE 66.3. Congenital lobar emphysema with hyperexpansion of the right middle lobe. The compressed lower lobe is visible as a triangular shadow in the cardiophrenic angle.

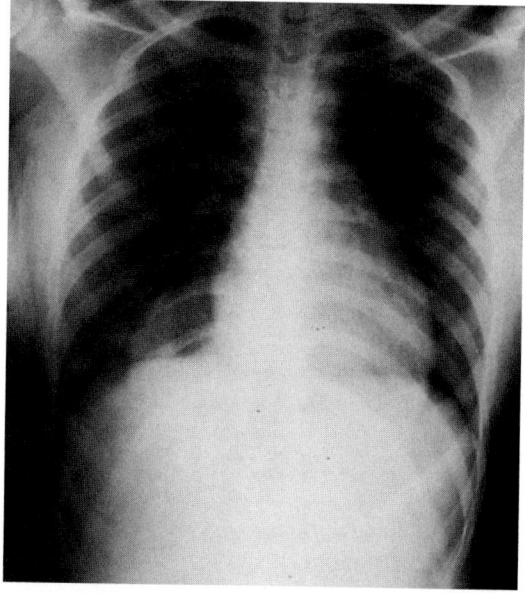

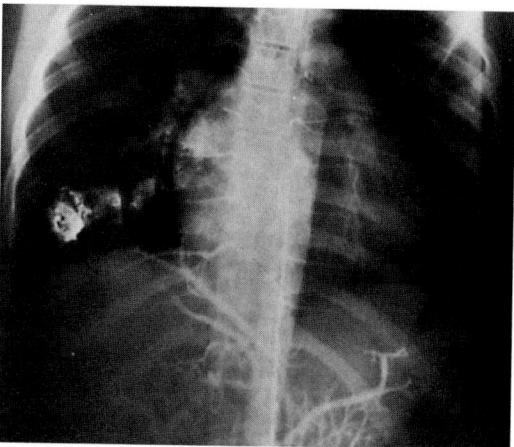

FIGURE 66.4. Intralobar sequestration in the right lower lobe. Retrograde arteriogram shows that the blood supply is from the aorta below the level of the diaphragm. Opaque material remains from the previous bronchogram.

mammary arteries. The venous drainage is typically normal to the left atrium, but may be anomalous to the right atrium or vena cava.

Intrapulmonary sequestration affects males and females equally and usually presents with symptoms of cough and fever in early adulthood. More than 50% of patients are older than 20 years of age at presentation (33, 34). The symptoms of intrapulmonary sequestration are related to pulmonary infections and include cough, sputum production, recurrent pulmonary infections, fever, and hemoptysis. Left ventricular enlargement and heart failure from left-to-right shunt may also develop. A small number of patients (15%) may be asymptomatic when the lesion is incidentally discovered on a chest radiograph (33). Intrapulmonary sequestration is infrequently associated with other congenital anomalies (12%).

A chest radiograph of a patient with intrapulmonary sequestration usually shows a homogenous opacity or cystic lesion with air-fluid levels in the lung base. Traditionally, aortography is used in the diagnosis of pulmonary sequestrations with excellent definition of the anomalous arterial supply and venous drainage (Fig. 66.4). CT and MRI are also useful studies and can show the parenchymal changes and the aberrant vessels supplying the sequestration (35). Preoperative diagnosis and assessment of sequestration is crucial because much of the morbidity and mortality of surgical resection is related to unexpected vascular complications.

The less common extrapulmonary sequestration frequently presents in the neonate and early childhood and affects male patients more frequently (80% of cases). Approx-

imately 90% of extrapulmonary sequestrations occur on the left side, often between the left lower lobe and diaphragm. The aberrant artery usually arises within the thorax, most commonly from the thoracic aorta, and is usually small in caliber. Venous drainage is often anomalous to the right atrium, vena cava, or azygous system. Extrapulmonary sequestration is often associated with other congenital anomalies (58%), including DH, skeletal deformities, cardiac malformations, and renal anomalies. Clinical symptoms are usually minor, and this anomaly is usually diagnosed during an evaluation of an associated malformation. Surgical resection may be necessary in symptomatic patients, and prognosis is related to the presence of other anomalies (33). In addition, the presentation of sequestrations can overlap with that of other lung lesions such as CAM, BCs, and scimitar syndrome (36). A recent review comparing pediatric and adult patients with sequestrations noted significantly more pulmonary infections in patients with intrapulmonary sequestrations (37). In addition, adult patients had more respiratory infections and required lobectomy more often than did pediatric patients.

DEVELOPMENTAL ANOMALIES OF THE PULMONARY VASCULATURE

Scimitar Syndrome

The scimitar syndrome is a rare malformation defined as partial anomalous pulmonary venous return of the right pulmonary veins to the inferior vena cava. Hypoplasia of the right lung is an integral part of the syndrome. Other features include anomalies of the right pulmonary arterial tree, dextrocardia and other cardiac defects, and bronchial abnormalities. The arterial supply to the right lung is variable and can arise from the pulmonary, bronchial, or systemic arterial system. In more than 50% of cases, the aberrant systemic artery arises below the diaphragm. A scimitar-shaped shadow of an anomalous pulmonary vein along the right heart border, which can be seen on chest radiograph in about 40% of cases, is how the name was derived (1) (Fig. 66.5).

The chest radiograph may suggest the diagnosis with the scimitar shadow; however, CT scan, angiogram, and cardiac catheterization may be necessary for diagnosis and definition of the anatomic relationships.

Clinically, patients can present with a spectrum of symptoms that range from severe to mild. In the severe form,

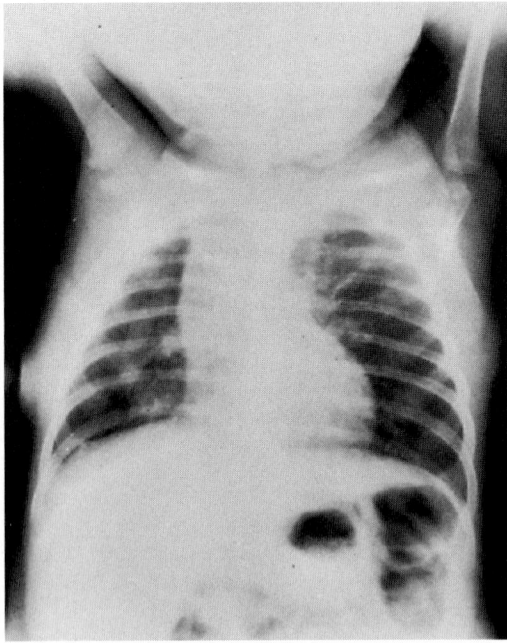

FIGURE 66.5. Scimitar syndrome in a child. The pulmonary vein on the right runs parallel to the right atrium to its connection with the inferior vena cava below the diaphragm.

patients present in the neonatal period with congestive heart failure, pulmonary hypertension, left-to-right shunt, and respiratory failure. A review of 32 cases of surgical repair of this syndrome noted surgery seldom results in normal blood flow to the right lung but does repair the left-to-right shunt (38). Postoperative pulmonary venous obstruction was common, especially in infants. Patients with milder forms of scimitar syndrome can be asymptomatic or have minor symptoms of cough and recurrent pulmonary infections. Older children and adults are more likely to present in this fashion. In a review of 122 cases of "adult" scimitar syndrome, 43 patients were 12 years or older at the time of diagnosis, and the eldest was 73 years of age (39). The typical chest radiograph finding of the scimitar-shaped anomalous pulmonary venous drainage was overlooked in more than half the cases. The pulmonary artery pressure was normal in 94 of 122 patients and slightly elevated in 28 patients. The prognosis of adults with scimitar syndrome without pulmonary hypertension is very good, and conservative management is usually adequate. In this review, 85 patients were monitored without surgical intervention and were asymptomatic. Surgery was done in 37 cases, and postoperative respiratory problems were common. The syndrome can show familial clustering, with an affected father and daughter described in one family and with sisters described in another (40).

Pulmonary Arteriovenous Malformation

A pulmonary arteriovenous malformation is an abnormal communication between the pulmonary arterial and venous system, which results in intrapulmonary right to left shunting. They are usually congenital, and in approximately 70% of cases are associated with hereditary hemorrhagic telangiectasia (HHT) (41). Conversely, approximately 15% to 25% of patients with HHT have pulmonary arteriovenous malformation. Pulmonary arteriovenous malformations occur more frequently in female patients than in male patients. Approximately 10% of cases of pulmonary arteriovenous malformation are identified in infancy or childhood. Although the pulmonary arteriovenous malformation in HHT should be present at birth, it usually does not become clinically manifest until the third or fourth decade of adult life.

The three most common symptoms are epistaxis, dyspnea, and hemoptysis. Epistaxis is an early symptom, and nearly 90% of patients develop it by 45 years of age (41). Dyspnea is the most common pulmonary complaint and is seen in patients with large or multiple pulmonary arteriovenous malformations. Some patients have platypnea (shortness of breath in upright position, relieved on reclining). Hemoptysis can be a presenting complaint, and may be massive. The presence of symptoms correlates with the size of the pulmonary arteriovenous malformation, and the incidence is higher in patients with multiple malformations. Usually, a pulmonary arteriovenous malformation less than 2 cm in diameter does not cause symptoms.

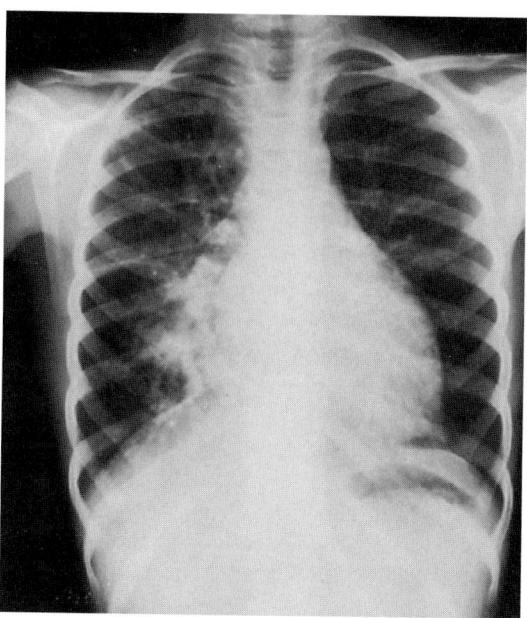

FIGURE 66.6. An irregular density in the right lower lobe of a patient with arterial hypoxemia, a continuous murmur, dyspnea, and palpitations.

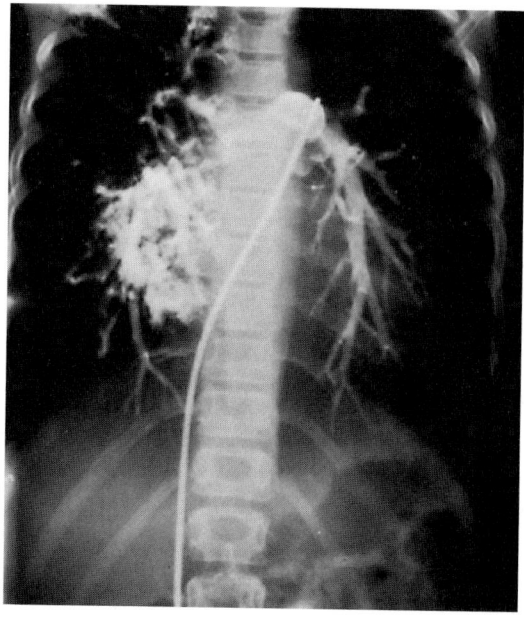

FIGURE 66.7. Angiographic demonstration of a single pulmonary arteriovenous fistula in the patient shown in Figure 66.6.

Physical signs of pulmonary arteriovenous malformation include superficial telangiectasias of the face, mouth, and lips that is attributable to HHT. In a seven-consecutive-case series from 1962–1993, digital clubbing and cyanosis were seen in 39% and 34% of patients, respectively. Murmurs over the site of the pulmonary arteriovenous malformation (most audible during inspiration) were heard in 46% of patients (41).

Chest radiographs are abnormal in nearly 98% of patients with pulmonary arteriovenous malformation and show a round mass of uniform density with smooth borders usually located in the lower lobes (Fig. 66.6). Single lesions are seen in two thirds of cases. Pulmonary arteriovenous malformation can be difficult to see on chest radiograph if there is parenchymal hemorrhage or atelectasis. Patients with microvascular telangiectasia may have a normal chest radiograph, with only a vague increase in pulmonary vascular markings at the bases. The findings on chest radiograph may be subtle, and further evaluation may be necessary with a contrast-enhanced CT or angiography if clinically indicated (Fig. 66.7). Whether CT imaging will replace standard pulmonary angiography in the diagnosis of pulmonary arteriovenous malformation is not known, and additional comparative studies are needed. However, CT imaging is a very useful technique for follow-up of patients with proven pulmonary arteriovenous malformation and for diagnosis in patients who cannot tolerate angiography (41).

Many complications occur in patients with pulmonary arteriovenous malformation. Neurological problems are seen in about 30% of patients and include stroke, transient ischemic attack, brain abscess, and headache. Although serious neurological problems are typically seen in symptomatic patients, there are reports of asymptomatic patients presenting with strokes or brain abscesses. Less common, but potentially life-threatening, complications include hemothorax and hemoptysis. Hemothorax can be secondary to rupture of a subpleural pulmonary arteriovenous malformation, and hemoptysis may be owing to either a ruptured pulmonary arteriovenous malformation or endobronchial telangiectasias. Hematologic abnormalities such as polycythemia (25%) and anemia (17%) are seen in some patients. Of note, the pulmonary artery pressure is normal or low in nearly all patients with pulmonary arteriovenous malformation.

The natural history of patients with untreated pulmonary arteriovenous malformation results in considerable morbidity and mortality. Pulmonary arteriovenous malformations may remain stable in size over time, but 25% will slowly enlarge. The data from three studies of consecutive patients with untreated pulmonary arteriovenous malformation showed the incidence of stroke was 11.4%, incidence of brain abscess was 6.8%, and total morbidity and mortality was 23% (41).

Treatment options for pulmonary arteriovenous malformation include embolization therapy and surgical resection. Embolization therapy consists of occluding the feeding artery to the malformation. Overall, results with this therapy are quite good, with recent series documenting successful occlusion rates of 95%. Complications of embolization are infrequent and self-limited. Pleuritic chest pain can be seen in about 13% of patients, usually within the first 2 days after embolization. Long-term follow-up of patients treated with embolization therapy is variable. Some patients can develop pulmonary hypertension after embolization owing to a reduction in the low-resistance vascular communications. In one study of follow-up CT scans more than 1 year after embolization, 96% of pulmonary arteriovenous malformations were either not visible or reduced in size. Some experts recommend CT scans every 3 to 5 years after embolization to assess the size of malformations. Surgical resection of pulmonary arteriovenous malformation can also be performed with few complications and minimal mortality. However, there are a few reports of acute right heart failure within hours of pulmonary arteriovenous malformation resection, presumably owing to the removal of the low-resistance pulmonary arteriovenous malformation.

In summary, treatment of pulmonary arteriovenous malformation with embolization therapy is associated with minimal morbidity. Treatment is recommended for all symptomatic patients with pulmonary arteriovenous malformations and patients with pulmonary arteriovenous malformations larger than 2 cm in diameter (41). Embolization therapy is preferable in many patients, especially those with multiple pulmonary arteriovenous malformations. The management of asymptomatic patients with pulmonary arteriovenous malformations less than 2 cm in diameter is not clear, but some experts recommend that if the feeding vessel is greater than 3 mm, embolization therapy should be considered.

Other Congenital Pulmonary Vascular Anomalies

Unilateral pulmonary artery agenesis is a rare congenital anomaly that usually presents in infancy or childhood. In many cases, it is associated with other cardiovascular abnormalities, such as right aortic arch, septal defects, tetralogy of Fallot, and patent ductus arteriosus. This anomaly is usually surgically treated in the patient's first year of life. However, there are reports of patients being diagnosed in adulthood. A recent review documented the clinical presentation of this anomaly in six adults (42). Five of these six patients had symptoms of recurrent mild pulmonary infections since childhood. On physical examination, decreased breath sounds on the involved side and slight ipsilateral deviation of the trachea were noted. All patients had radiographic abnormalities, including a smaller-than-normal hyperlucent lung. Ventilation-perfusion lung scans showed absence of perfusion to one lung and no air trapping during the washout phase. These characteristic findings help to differentiate this abnormality from Swyer-James syndrome. MRI was felt to be a useful noninvasive imaging technique in this group of patients with unilateral pulmonary artery agenesis.

Congenital unilateral pulmonary vein atresia usually presents in infancy or childhood with recurrent pneumonia or hemoptysis in association with congenital heart defects and pulmonary hypertension. Presentation in adulthood is rare but does occur. A recent report of three adults (ages, 25–43 years) revealed presenting symptoms of significant hemoptysis in two and recurrent pneumonia and

progressive dyspnea in the third (43). The findings on chest radiograph may mimic lung cancer or fibrosing mediastinitis. However, a chest CT can suggest the diagnosis and shows a small hemithorax with ipsilateral shift, a diminutive ipsilateral pulmonary artery, and absence of ipsilateral pulmonary vein drainage into the left atrium. Two patients underwent pneumonectomy, and one underwent percutaneous coil embolization of the systemic arterial collateral vessels.

DEVELOPMENTAL ANOMALIES OF THE DIAPHRAGM

Diaphragmatic Hernia

DHs are common congenital anomalies, representing approximately 8% of major congenital lesions (1). The defect originates from the incomplete development of the septum transversum that normally separates the pleural and peritoneal cavities between 3 and 9 weeks of fetal life. In more than one third of cases, other severe congenital anomalies are present, including cardiac defects, neural tube defects, skeletal anomalies, and sequestration. DHs occur at three main sites: foramen of Bochdalek (>85%), anterior foramen of Morgagni (1%–5%), and esophageal hiatus (1%–5%) (1).

The most common type of congenital DH is Bochdalek, and it is found on the left side in 80% to 90% of cases (Fig. 66.8). However, the most significant associated problem is pulmonary hypoplasia, which is secondary to the abdominal contents in the chest and restriction of normal lung. Of the 60% of patients without other major anomalies, the prognosis is related to the degree of pulmonary hypoplasia. Timing of herniation, as well as the amount of abdominal contents in the thoracic cavity, affects the degree of pulmonary hypoplasia. A large hernia early in fetal life would lead to severe lung hypoplasia and higher mortality than if the hernia occurs later in fetal life when the more developed lung would have a chance for recovery after surgical repair.

Most cases of congenital DH present in the first days of life with severe tachypnea and cyanosis. Treatment is surgical repair with the patient stabilized with ventilatory and cardiovascular support if needed. Aggressive postoperative treatment, including extracorporeal membrane oxygenation, has led to improved survival. Mortality is approximately 30% when surgery is required within the first 24 hours and is 70% in untreated cases (1).

Children who survive the repair have been reported to do well into adulthood (44). Long-term follow-up of survivors of surgery for congenital DH is available. A study of 60 long-term survivors (mean age at follow-up, 30 years) revealed obstructive ventilatory impairment in 15%, restrictive impairment in 12%, and a mixed picture in 25% of patients (45). The diffusion capacity of carbon monoxide was normal in all patients in which it was measured. Chest asymmetry and scoliosis were also noted to be common among adults

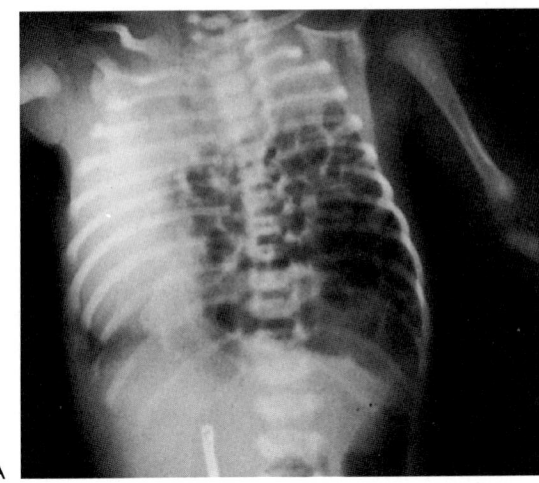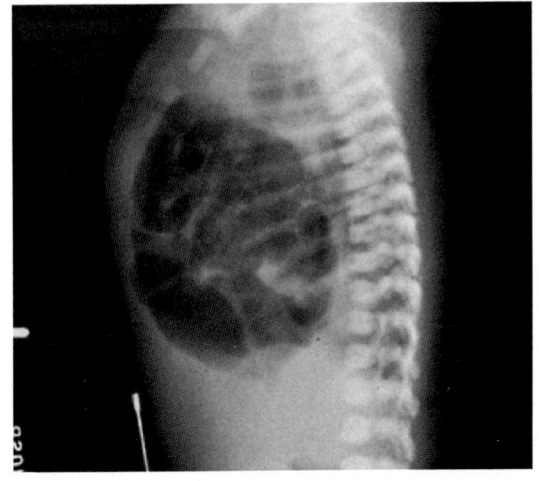

A

B

FIGURE 66.8. Congenital diaphragmatic hernia. There is herniation of small intestine, large intestine, and stomach (or parts thereof) into the left hemithorax. Note the air in the descending colon.

with repaired congenital DH. In general, the ventilatory impairment and thoracic deformity is mild; surveillance of these patients into adulthood is appropriate (45,46).

There are a small number of cases in which presentation of a congenital DH is delayed until adulthood. When this occurs, presenting symptoms are usually related to the gastrointestinal tract (vomiting, abdominal pain, diarrhea, and abdominal distention), and the ipsilateral lung is minimally hypoplastic (47). Chest radiographs may show elevation of the hemidiaphragm or a pleural effusion. Additional radiographic studies are usually needed and include CT scans of the chest and abdomen or MRI. In addition, incidental Bochdalek hernias are seen in adults. A radiologic review of this entity documented an incidence of 0.17%, with a mean age of 67 years. None of the patients were symptomatic (48).

A Morgagni hernia is the rarest congenital DH. The average age at diagnosis is 50 years. The size of the hernia is usually limited because the defect is small. The danger is bowel strangulation, and surgery is indicated even in asymptomatic patients because of this risk. It can present in adulthood as an incidental radiographic finding or as symptoms of abdominal pain, obstruction, or chest tightness (49).

DEVELOPMENTAL ANOMALIES OF THE CHEST WALL

Pectus Deformities

Pectus deformities are common congenital anomalies of the anterior chest wall and occur in more than one of every 1,000 live births (1) (see Chapter 62). The basic defect appears to be abnormal development of diaphragmatic tendons. Pectus excavatum is more frequent than is carinatum, and males are affected more often than females.

The physiologic and functional consequences of pectus deformities are controversial. A recent review of surgical

repair of pectus deformities in 25 adults (mean age, 31 years) noted all patients were symptomatic with loss of stamina and exercise capacity (50). However, many reviews note a high incidence of symptoms in patients seeking surgical correction. Studies of pulmonary function tests in patients with pectus deformities show mild-to-moderate restrictive abnormalities. Some patients with pectus excavatum have displacement of the heart into the left chest with compression of the right ventricle. The data regarding the significance of cardiac compression and its potential improvement after surgery are inconsistent and difficult to interpret. There appears to be limited evidence for an increase in cardiac performance after repair in some patients. Many patients do not require surgical intervention. The operation in adults is more difficult than that in children, although long-term results have been similar (50).

DEVELOPMENT ANOMALIES OF THE PLEURAL FISSURES

Anomalous Fissures

Anomalous fissures are a common congenital abnormality involving the lung. They are rarely associated with symptoms; however, their recognition is important for accurate radiologic interpretation and knowledge for surgical procedures such as lobectomy. The most common supernumerary fissure anomaly is trilobation of the left lung, occurring in 8% of routine chest radiographs. Accessory fissures are responsible for the formation of accessory lobes, including dorsal lobe, cardiac lobe, anterior basal lobe, and a true lingular lobe.

The azygous lobe is a portion of the right upper lobe. It is separated from the rest of the lobe by the azygous vein. The azygous vein remains embedded in the right lung and forms an accessory fissure that is seen in approximately 1% of routine chest radiographs.

REFERENCES

1. Clements BS. Malformation of the lungs and airways. In: Taussig LM, Landau LI, eds. *Pediatric respiratory medicine*. St. Louis: Mosby, 1999:1106–1136.
2. Boyden EA. Development of the human lung. In: Brennermann, ed. *Practice of pediatrics*, Vol. 4. Hagerstown, MD: Harper & Row, 1972:Chapter 64.
3. Wiatrak BJ. Congenital anomalies of the larynx and trachea. *Otolaryngol Clin N Am* 2000;33:91–111.
4. Smith GC, Cooper DM. Laryngomalacia and inspiratory obstruction in later childhood. *Arch Dis Child* 1981;56:345–349.
5. Lancaster JL, Hanafi Z, Jackson SR. Adult presentation of a tracheoesophageal fistula with co-existing laryngeal cleft. *J Laryngol Otol* 1999;113:469–472.
6. Thornton M, Rowley H, Conlon BJ, et al. Type I laryngeal cleft: late presentation. *J Laryngol Otol* 2001;115:821–822.
7. Palmer SM Jr, Layish DT, Kussin PS, et al. Lung transplantation for Williams-Campbell syndrome. *Chest* 1998;113:534–537.
8. Sebening C, Jakob H, Tochtermann U, et al. Vascular tracheobronchial compression syndromes: experience in surgical treatment and literature review. *Thorac Cardiovasc Surg* 2000;48:164–174.
9. Van Son JAM, Julsrud PR, Hagler DJ, et al. Surgical treatment of vascular rings: the Mayo Clinic experience. *Mayo Clin Proc* 1993;68:1056–1063.
10. Grathwohl KW, Afifi AY, Dillard TA, et al. Vascular rings of the thoracic aorta in adults. *Am Surg* 1999;65:1077–1083.
11. Lazzarini-de-Oliveira LC, Costa de Barros Franco CA, Gomes de Salles CL, et al. A 38-year-old man with tracheomegaly, tracheal diverticulosis, and bronchiectasis. *Chest* 2001;120:1018–1020.
12. Woodring JH, Howard RS 2nd, Rehm SR. Congenital tracheobronchomegaly (Mounier-Kuhn syndrome): a report of 10 cases and review of the literature. *J Thorac Imaging* 1991;6:1–10.
13. Schwartz M, Rossoff L. Tracheobronchomegaly. *Chest* 1994;106:1589–1590.
14. Zach MS, Eber E. Adult outcome of congenital lower respiratory tract malformations. *Thorax* 2001;56:65–72.
15. Stephens RW, Lingeman RE, Lawson LJ. Congenital tracheoesophageal fistulas in adults. *Ann Otol Rhin Laryn* 1976;85:613–617.
16. Azoulay D, Regnard JF, Magdeleinat P, et al. Congenital respiratory-esophageal fistula in the adult: report of nine cases and review of the literature. *J Thorac Cardiovasc Surg* 1992;104:381–384.
17. Nagappan R, Parkin G, Wright CA, et al. Adult long-segment tracheal stenosis attributable to complete tracheal rings masquerading as asthma. *Crit Care Med* 2002;30:238–240.
18. Ghaye B, Szapiro D, Fanchamps JM, et al. Congenital bronchial abnormalities revisited. *Radiographics* 2001;21:105–119.
19. Rappaport DC, Herman SJ, Weisbrod GL. Congenital bronchopulmonary diseases in adults: CT findings. *AJR Am J Roentgenol* 1994;162:1295–1299.
20. Jederlinic PJ, Sicilian LS, Baigelman W, et al. Congenital bronchial atresia: a report of four cases and a review of the literature *Medicine (Baltimore)* 1986;66:73–83.
21. Kim JH, Park KH, Sung SW, et al. Congenital bronchoesophageal fistulas in adult patients. *Ann Thorac Surg* 1995;60:151–155.
22. Deb S, Ali MB, Fonseca P. Congenital bronchoesophageal fistula in an adult. *Chest* 1998;114:1784–1786.
23. Majer HC. Bronchogenic cysts of mediastinum. *Ann Surg* 1948;122:476.
24. Patel SR, Meeker DP, Biscotti CV, et al. Presentation and management of bronchogenic cysts in the adult. *Chest* 1994;106:79–85.
25. Cioffi U, Bonavina L, DeSimone M, et al. Presentation and surgical management of bronchogenic and esophageal duplication cysts in adults. *Chest* 1998;113:1492–1496.
26. Ribet ME, Copin MC, Gosselin BH. Bronchogenic cysts of the lung. *Ann Thorac Surg* 1996;61:1636–1640.
27. Plit ML, Blott JA, Lakis N, et al. Clinical, radiographic and lung function features of diffuse congenital cystic adenomatoid malformation of the lung in an adult. *Eur Respir J* 1997;10:1680–1682.
28. Hulnick DH, Naidich DP, McCauley DI, et al. Late presentation of congenital cystic adenomatoid malformation of the lung. *Radiology* 1984;151:569–573.
29. DiGiorgio A, Al Mansour M, Cardini CL, et al. Congenital cystic adenomatoid malformation of the lung presenting as pyopneumothorax in an 18-year-old woman. *J Thorac Cardiovasc Surg* 2001;122:1034–1036.
30. Granata C, Gambini C, Balducci T, et al. Bronchioloalveolar carcinoma arising in congenital cystic adenomatoid malformation in a child: a case report and review on malignancies originating in congenital cystic adenomatoid malformation. *Pediatr Pulmonol* 1998;25:62–66.
31. Ozcan C, Celik A, Ural Z, et al. Primary pulmonary rhabdomyosarcoma arising within cystic adenomatoid malformation: a case report and review of the literature. *J Pediatr Surg* 2001;36:1062–1065.
32. Critchley PS, Forrester-Wood CP, Ridley PD. Adult congenital lobar emphysema in pregnancy. *Thorax* 1995;50:909–910.
33. Savic B, Birtel FJ, Tholen W, et al. Lung sequestration: report of seven cases and review of 540 published cases. *Thorax* 1979;34:96–101.
34. Satinder P, Singh, SP, Nath H. A 53-year-old man with hemoptysis. *Chest* 2001;120:298–301.
35. Ikezoe J, Murayama S, Godwin JD, et al. Bronchopulmonary sequestration: CT assessment. *Radiology* 1990;176:375–379.
36. Bratu I, Flageole H, Chen MF, et al. The multiple facets of pulmonary sequestration. *J Pediatr Surg* 2001;36:784–790.
37. Van Raemdonck D, De Boeck K, Devlieger H, et al. Pulmonary sequestration: a comparison between pediatric and adult patients. *Eur J Cardiothorac Surg* 2001;19:388–395.
38. Najm HK, Williams WG, Coles JG, et al. Scimitar syndrome: twenty years' experience and results of repair. *J Thorac Cardiovasc Surg* 1996;112:1161–1168.
39. Dupuis C, Charaf LA, Breviere GM, et al. The "adult" form of the scimitar syndrome. *Am J Cardiol* 1992;70:502–507.
40. Ashida K, Itoh A, Naruko T, et al. Familial scimitar syndrome: three-dimensional visualization of anomalous pulmonary vein in young sisters. *Circulation* 2001;103:E126–E127.
41. Gossage JR, Kanj G. Pulmonary arteriovenous malformations: a state of the art review. *Am J Respir Crit Care Med* 1998;158:643–661.
42. Bouros D, Pare P, Panagou P, et al. The varied manifestation of pulmonary artery agenesis in adulthood. *Chest* 1995;108:670–676.
43. Heyneman LE, Nolan RL, Harrison JK, et al. Congenital unilateral pulmonary vein atresia: radiologic findings in three adult patients. *AJR Am J Roentgenol* 2001;177:681–685.
44. Falconer AR, Brown RA, Helms P, et al. Pulmonary sequelae in survivors of congenital diaphragmatic hernia. *Thorax* 1990;45:126–129.

45. Vanamo K, Rintala R, Sovijarvi A, et al. Long-term pulmonary sequelae in survivors of congenital diaphragmatic defects. *J Pediatr Surg* 1996;31:1096–1099.

46. Vanamo K, Peltonen J, Rintala R, et al. Chest wall and spinal deformities in adults with congenital diaphragmatic defects. *J Pediatr Surg* 1996;31:851–854.

47. Bujanda L, Larrucea I, Ramos F, et al. Bochdalek's hernia in adults. *J Clin Gastroenterol* 2001;32:155–157.

48. Mullins ME, Stein J, Saini SS, et al. Prevalence of incidental Bochdalek's hernia in a large adult population. *AJR Am J Roentgenol* 2001;177:363–366.

49. Lev-Chelouche D, Ravid A, Michowitz M, et al. Morgagni hernia: unique presentations in elderly patients. *J Clin Gastroenterol* 1999;28:81–82.

50. Fonkalsrud EW, Bustorff-Silva J. Repair of pectus excavatum and carinatum in adults. *Am J Surg* 1999;177:121–124.

Pathophysiology and Diagnosis of Pleural Diseases

67

Veena B. Antony

The pleura is a membrane that covers a closed space in the chest cavity. It covers the entire surface of the lung, including fissures and the inner surface of the thoracic cage, diaphragm, and mediastinum. The visceral pleura and the parietal pleura are joined together at the hilum. The two pleural cavities, the right and the left, are separated from each other by the mediastinum and the pericardial cavity (1,2). During respiration, because of the movement of the lungs, the visceral and parietal pleura move against each other. The dome of the pleura extends above the first rib for 2 to 3 cm along the medial one third of the clavicle behind the sternal cleidomastoid muscles (2). The surface of the pleura is a smooth glistening membrane on the visceral surface, through which the lung can be easily visualized. The pleura varies in thickness in different areas of the chest cavity and is, however, usually made up of five separate layers: (a) a single layer of mesothelial cells, (b) a thin submesothelial connective tissue layer including a basal lamina, (c) a thin superficial elastic layer, (d) a loose connective tissue layer, and (e) a deep fibroelastic layer (3–5). The pleural mesothelial cell comprises the surface of the pleura and ranges from 16.4 ± 68 to 41.9 ± 9.5 μm in diameter and from less than 1 to 4 μm in thickness (6,7). Pleural mesothelial cells are covered with microvilli on electron microscopic examination of the mesothelial cell (6,8,9). A number of pinocytic vesicles are present in the mesothelial cell. The cytoplasm is full of organelles such as mitochondria, both rough and smooth endoplasmic reticulum, and dense bodies. Golgi apparatus and phagocytic vacuoles are also visible. Mesothelial cells are metabolically active cells that produce multiple cytokines and chemokines (10). They are joined together by intercellular junctional structures and demonstrate the presence of focal adhesions, adherens

junctions, and tight junctions. During homeostasis, the junctional proteins play a quiescent role, allowing for movement and overlap between the mesothelial cells. During the process of inflammation, the junctional protein responses are specific and vary with the inflammatory stimulus (11). For example, mycobacteria causes down-regulation of β-catenin, an adherens junction protein. The surface of the mesothelial cell is covered by glycoproteins and hyaluronic acid (12). Hyaluronic acid is a large-molecular-weight protein that allows for smooth movement between the two surfaces of the pleura. The volume of pleural fluid in healthy humans ranges from 0.2 to 1 mL and forms a thin layer between the two surfaces (13). It contains a small amount of protein, about 1 to 2 g/100 mL, and a small number of cells that are mostly mononuclear cells. These range between 1,400 to 4,500 cells/mL of pleural fluid (5,13,14). During homeostasis, the pleural fluid is maintained at a constant volume, with tightly regulated restrictions on transport of other proteins and cells into the pleural space. The pleural cavity communicates with the lymphatics of the chest wall through stomas, membrana cribriformis, and lacunae and lymphatic channels (15–18). The pleura has well-described mechanisms that help repair its surface after denudation after injury (19).

FORMATION OF PLEURAL LIQUID

Stomas in the parietal pleura, which connect to lymphatic channels, permit normal physiological movement of fluid from the pleural space into the lymphatics under homeostasis. Indeed, most of the liquid outflow into the pleural space is provided by lymphatic drainage (20). Normal pleural fluid is formed by filtration from systemic pleural microvessels. Though both parietal and visceral pleural microvessels contribute to the formation of normal pleural fluid, the

V. B. Antony: Department of Medicine, Indiana University School of Medicine; and Veterans Affairs Medical Center, Indianapolis, Indiana.

majority of the fluid is formed via leakage of the parietal pleural microvessels. Pleural lymphatics originate in stomas on the parietal pleural surface and are present in the form of a network beneath the mesothelial monolayer. During homeostasis, fluid and protein is clear through the lymphatics. In patients with congestive heart failure, the pulmonary capillary wedge pressure correlates best with the presence of pleural effusions (21,22). In volume-overloaded sheep, protein concentration in pleural fluid increased and was similar to that found in the lung interstitial liquid after volume overload. In pulmonary edema owing to lung microvascular injury, there is leakage of the pleural fluid across the visceral pleura. Movement of fluid and proteins from the lung into the pleural space requires a pressure gradient from the lung interstitium to the pleural space, and this has been demonstrated by Bhattacharya and colleagues (23). Abnormal fluid accumulation in the pleural space has many postulated mechanisms and may occur with changes in pleural membrane permeability such as that seen in inflammation. There may be changes in microvascular oncotic pressure such as that seen in patients with hypoalbuminemia, a decrease in pleural pressure such as in atelectasis, and an increase in hydrostatic pressure as seen in congestive heart failure. The rate of fluid entry and the capacity of the pleura for clearance control the formation and accumulation of pleural fluid.

DIAGNOSTIC APPROACHES TO PLEURAL EFFUSIONS

Chest Radiography

The chest radiograph remains a vital and standard imaging technique for assessment of pleural disease. A pleural effusion that causes minimal blunting of the costophrenic angle in a standard upright posterior-anterior chest radiograph is caused by the presence of at least 300 mL of pleural liquid (24). Decubitus films are important to determine if the fluid is free flowing or loculated. Bilateral decubiti film allows the underlying lung to be viewed. If the fluid margin is greater than 10 mm in diameter from the chest wall to the outside margin of the lung, the fluid is usually amenable to thoracentesis. Changes in the contour of the diaphragm may signify subpulmonic effusions. Decubitus film will allow for definition of their presence. Occasionally, pleural fluid can be found in the minor fissure, the so-called pseudotumor (25). Chest x-ray films should be evaluated for mediastinal shift either toward or away from the pleural effusion. The presence of a pleural effusion should move the mediastinum to the contralateral side. When the mediastinum is shifted toward the ipsilateral side, it may imply atelectasis of the underlying lung secondary to possible bronchial obstruction by a tumor mass, fixation of the mediastinum by fibrosis, malignant invasion, or the encasing of the lung in a malignant peel in diseases such as mesothelioma (26). Pleural effusions with a

parenchymal abnormality are more likely to be exudates and involve the pleura in inflammation. Pleural effusions in the absence of pulmonary parenchymal abnormalities are seen with heart failure, primary tuberculosis (TB), and abdominal inflammatory disease such as pancreatitis, hepatitis, liver abscess, viral pleurisy, or pulmonary embolism.

Ultrasound, Computed Tomography, and Magnetic Resonance Imaging in Pleural Disease

Ultrasound is used for localizing pleural masses or pleural fluid loculations and for guiding thoracentesis or pleural biopsy. Computed tomography (CT) is particularly helpful in differentiating pulmonary parenchymal abnormalities from pleural abnormalities (27). Loculated effusions will have a lenticular configuration with smooth margins and displace adjacent parenchyma (25,28). This atypical appearance is helpful in differentiating pleural from parenchymal lesions. The edge of lung abscess as it touches the chest wall usually forms in an acute angle, whereas that of an empyema is usually obtuse (29). The split pleura sign is particularly useful in differentiating empyemas from lung abscesses. Thoracostomy tube placement in empyema can be placed under CT or ultrasound guidance. Image-guided thoracostomy tube placement combined with fibrinolytic agents can obviate surgical decortication in some cases of empyema. Pleural metastasis produces diffuse pleural thickening with lobular masses, as does malignant mesothelioma. The CT of the chest can be particularly helpful in assessing the extent and staging of malignant mesothelioma (30). Magnetic resonance imaging (MRI) is advantageous because of its ability to image the thorax directly in multiple planes, but its role in evaluation of the pleura is somewhat limited. However, MRI may be helpful in evaluating the extent of chest wall involvement by tumor (31). Pleural deoxyglucose positron emission tomography (PET scanning) has been reported to be helpful in evaluating the extent of malignant involvement of the pleura (32). Ultrasound is a readily available technique that allows for bedside imaging of the pleural space. Ultrasound can be useful in determining the presence, size, and location of pleural fluid collections (33–35), particularly in a complicated parapneumonic effusion in which there may be multiple loculation. Ultrasound allows for the visualization of septae within the effusion, which appear as thin echogenic bands within the fluid, which suggests that the fluid is an exudate. Ultrasound can also identify pleural masses in patients who have malignant pleural effusions. Directed thoracentesis into anechoic or hypoechoic collections under visual guidance allows for fewer complications in patients in whom thoracentesis is seen as essential. Ultrasound is often used to evaluate pleural involvement in patients who cannot be moved to the radiology department. Also, ultrasound-guided thoracentesis is useful in a small effusion or in a ventilated patient. Ultrasound-guided thoracentesis or chest tube insertion may be helpful in a multiloculated effusion. The technique may also be used for evaluation for pleural masses in patients with malignant disease, TB, and calcified or noncalcified plaques (36–39). Finally, for evaluation of pneumothorax, ultrasound may provide additional information than that obtained via a chest radiography (40,41).

USE OF ULTRASOUND IMAGING FOR PLEURAL DISEASE

Summary Statement	Level of Evidence
Ultrasound should be used for aspirating small effusions or in ventilated patients.	Expert opinion
Use ultrasound for chest tube insertion or aspiration of loculated effusions.	Expert opinion
Ultrasound may aid evaluation of pleural mass.	Nonrandomized trials
Ultrasound aids in detection of pneumothorax.	Nonrandomized trials

Thoracentesis

A diagnostic thoracentesis should be performed in any individual with a unilateral or bilateral free-flowing effusion and a normal heart size. Patients who have heart failure can reasonably be observed; however, unusual features such as a fever or an elevated white count justify thoracentesis (42). A volume of 50 mL is usually sufficient for diagnostic evaluation. Evaluation of pleural fluid that is removed by thoracentesis will often lead to a diagnosis. In about 75% of cases, relevant information is obtained after thoracentesis. There are relative contraindications of thoracentesis, which include a bleeding diathesis, anticoagulation, and small pleural effusions that may be difficult to tap without the guide of ultrasound sonography. Complications associated with thoracentesis include pneumothorax in up to 10%; only 2% of cases require tube thoracostomy placement. Pneumothorax is rare when experienced operators perform thoracentesis and/or ultrasound guidance is involved in localizing the pleural fluid (43). Chest pain is common and occurs in about 30% of patients. Cough; hypoxemia; vasovagal reactions; bleeding secondary to intercostal artery laceration; hemothorax; infections; subdiaphragmatic needle placement with hepatic, splenic, or renal laceration; and reexpansion pulmonary edema after large volume thoracentesis (>1,500 mL) have been noted. If pleural fluid is withdrawn rapidly and the pleural pressure falls below −20 cm of water, reexpansion pulmonary edema is more commonly reported. A chest radiograph after thoracentesis is not indicated in an asymptomatic patient; however, if the pleural fluid obscured the underlying parenchyma, a chest radiograph after the thoracentesis may reveal underlying lung pathology (44).

The appearance of the pleural fluid on thoracentesis may offer visual clues to the etiology of the effusion. Pleural fluid

TABLE 67.1. CHARACTERISTICS OF PLEURAL FLUID

Characteristic	Probable Cause
Bloody	Trauma, malignancy
White	Chylothorax, empyema
Black	Aspergillosis, amebic liver abscess
Brown	Draining into pleural space
Yellow-green	Rheumatoid pleurisy
Viscous	Malignant mesothelioma (resulting from high levels of hyaluronic acid)
Ammonia odor	Urinothorax
Food particles	Esophageal rupture

may be bloody in patients with trauma, in malignancy, or in patients with pulmonary infarction. It is white to light yellow with chylothorax and empyema; it may be black or brown with aspergillosis and amebic liver abscesses, which drain into the pleural space. Pleural effusions in patients with rheumatoid pleurisy have been described to be yellow to green in nature (45). Malignant mesothelioma pleural fluid has been described as viscous. The appearance of food particles and other particulates in the pleural fluid can signify esophageal rupture (Table 67.1).

Pleural fluid is classically differentiated into either a transudate or an exudate. Separating pleural fluid into exudates or transudates does not provide a diagnosis, but allows one to provide a probability evaluation on the likely nature of the pleural fluid (46). The classic criteria defining an exudate were established by Light in 1972 (47). An effusion is an exudate if it meets one of the criteria, which include (a) an absolute pleural fluid serum lactate dehydrogenase (LDH) concentration of greater than 200 IU/L, (b) pleural fluid LDH divided by LDH ratio greater than 0.6, and (c) pleural fluid protein divided by serum protein ratio greater than 0.5. The sensitivity and specificity of these criteria for defining an exudate are high (97.9% sensitivity and 74.3% specificity). Since then, several other diagnostic tests have been suggested that also have a high sensitivity, such as pleural fluid LDH and pleural fluid cholesterol, with a sensitivity of 97.5% and a specificity of 71.9% (48). If a serum sample is not obtained at the time of thoracentesis, pleural fluid LDH or cholesterol allows a physician to still define pleural fluid as an exudate without affecting diagnostic accuracy (Table 67.2). It should be recognized that differentiating a transudate from an exudate provides a probability statement as to the likely nature of a pleural effusion, but it is not diagnostic for a particular effusion. Pleural fluid results of LDH and cholesterol, without serum levels, clearly have both cost-saving and convenience benefits, with equivalent diagnostic sensitivity and specificity to Light's criteria. A metaanalysis of existing studies, including Light's criteria, suggests that Light's criteria provide excellent discriminative properties but that the pleural fluid cutoff point should be set at greater than 45% of the upper limit of normal for LDH values (49). These are identified as the modified Light's

TABLE 67.2. LIGHT'S CRITERIA FOR EXUDATE

Fluid/serum protein ratio >0.5
Fluid/serum LDH ratio >0.6
Absolute LDH greater than two-thirds upper limit of normal

Modified Light's criteria
    Fluid/serum protein ratio >0.5
    Fluid/serum LDH ratio >0.6

Abbreviated Light's criteria
    Fluid/serum protein ratio >0.5

Other criteria
    Fluid/LDH >0.45, upper limit of normal
    Fluid/cholesterol >45 mg/dL
    Fluid protein >2.9 mg/dL

LDH, lactate dehydrogenase.

TABLE 67.3. DISEASES ASSOCIATED WITH A LOW PLEURAL FLUID pH AND LOW GLUCOSE

Diagnosis	Usual pH	Usual Glucose
Empyema	5.50–7.29 (~100%)	<40 mg/dL
Esophageal rupture	6.00 (~100% by 48 h)	<60 mg/dL
Rheumatoid pleurisy	7.00 (80%)	0–30 mg/dL
Malignancy	6.95–7.29 (33%)	30–59 mg/dL
Tuberculous pleurisy	7.00–7.29 (20%)	30–59 mg/dL
Lupus pleuritis	7.00–7.29 (20%)	30–59 mg/dL

criteria. In fact, pleural fluid LDH can be removed entirely from Light's criteria, which would then be defined as the abbreviated Light's criteria, without affecting any diagnostic accuracy.

Pleural fluid tests usually obtained should include those to define an exudate protein, LDH, cholesterol plus glucose, pH, and total cell count with a differential cell count. Additional studies should be performed based on clinical suspicion and include Gram stain and culture, fungal culture, potassium hydroxide preparation, acid-fast bacilli serum culture, and cytology. Other tests that may be ordered include rheumatoid factor, antinuclear antibody, adenosine deaminase (ADA), amylase, triglyceride levels, and complement levels.

A serosanguinous pleural effusion, or frankly bloody pleural effusion, is seen in a limited number of disease entities. Importantly, traumatic effusions secondary to trauma caused during the process of thoracentesis should be differentiated from truly bloody pleural effusions. Typically, during a traumatic thoracentesis, the second or the third vial of pleural fluid obtained will be less sanguinous than is the first vial. Fresh traumatic effusions will also clot, whereas effusions owing to other causes in which the blood in the pleural fluid has undergone fibrinolysis will not clot. A red blood cell count of greater than 100,000 mL is associated with trauma, malignancy, pulmonary infarction, asbestos-induced pleural effusions, and postcardiac injury syndrome (Dressler syndrome). Importantly, if malignant cells are present in the pleural fluid, a diagnosis of pleural involvement with malignancy can be made (50). Evaluation of the total pleural fluid cell count is valuable and may offer clues for the diagnosis of a variety of diseases. The white blood cell differential count is often less than $1,000/\mu L$, with mononuclear cells predominating in transudative effusions, whereas exudative effusions such as TB or malignancy will have a white cell count of 5,000 to 10,000 μ/L (51). In parapneumonic effusions, both uncomplicated and complicated, the white cell count can rise dramatically to greater than 10,000 cells/μL. Malignant pleural effusions are usually predominant in mononuclear cells,

whereas acute processes such as inflammation secondary to bacterial infections are usually predominant in neutrophils. Eosinophils are seen in the pleural fluid in diseases such as parasitic infections, fungal infections, and drug-induced effusions, as well as asbestos effusions and Churg-Strauss vasculitis. Eosinophilia of greater than 10% often implies the presence of blood or air in the pleural space (52,53). Eosinophils have been found to be elevated in patients with hemothorax, pulmonary embolism, or infarction, as well as patients who have had several prior thoracenteses. Mesothelial cells are usually not present in patients with TB pleurisy. Pleural fluid glucose is usually equivalent to the serum value. Pleural fluid glucose correlates with pleural fluid pH. A pleural fluid glucose of less than 60 mg/dL is associated with diseases such as rheumatoid effusions, parapneumonic effusions, malignant effusions, TB, and esophageal rupture (54) (Table 67.3). Significantly depressed pleural fluid glucose (0–30 mg/dL) is seen in rheumatoid effusions and in empyema. The mechanism of a low glucose in the pleural fluid has been suggested to be owing to decreased transport of glucose into the pleural fluid in diseases such as rheumatoid arthritis in which the pleura may be covered in the fibrotic peel or increased consumption by cells in the pleural space, such as bacteria or white blood cells in empyema. A low pleural fluid pH is defined as less than 7.3. It is seen in the same set of diseases in which a low glucose is noted, i.e., esophageal rupture, empyema, malignancy, rheumatoid effusions (55,56), lupus pleuritis, and systemic acidosis. In parapneumonic effusions, a decreasing pH is an excellent marker for complications that may require thoracostomy tube placement. Approximately one third of patients with malignant effusions will have a low pH. Although malignant pleural effusions with a low pH and a low glucose concentration have been shown by some to have worse survival and poorer response to pleurodesis than those with normal pH and glucose, other investigations have not found an association among pleural fluid, pH, survival, or success of pleurodesis (57). Pleural fluid pH in malignant pleural effusions should be used in conjunction with clinical evaluation of the patient's general health and performance status in making decisions related to therapy such as pleurodesis. Cytology in malignant pleural effusions will yield a diagnosis in 62% to 90% of cases. Diagnosis of mesothelioma is usually at the lower end of this yield, and often a tissue biopsy is required to make a definitive diagnosis of this particular tumor. Pleural fluid amylase may be elevated in malignancy and in esophageal rupture.

Elevated triglycerides (>110 mg/dL) are seen in chylous effusions (58). A chylothorax is formed when there is a leakage of chyle from the thoracic duct and usually has a pleural fluid triglyceride concentration of greater than 110 mg/dL. Pseudochylous effusion can occur with other diseases, typically those associated with a long-standing trapped lung from either rheumatoid pleurisy, TB pleurisy, or the results of therapy for TB with pneumothorax. The diagnosis of a true chylous effusion can be established by identifying cholesterol crystals on a smear of the pleural fluid or the presence of a high triglyceride content (59). ADA (levels of greater than 50 IU/L) is seen in TB, effusions secondary to lymphoma, and parapneumonic effusions (60). Because elevation of ADA is nonspecific, it is helpful only in narrowing the differential diagnosis.

CLOSED PLEURAL BIOPSIES

Closed pleural biopsies are performed via a percutaneous approach and are often used in the evaluation of a lymphocyte predominant pleural effusion that is exudative and remains undiagnosed after thoracentesis. The diagnostic yield in cytology negative malignant pleural effusions can range between 40% and 75% (61–65). In TB, pleural effusions, granulomas, or acid-fast bacilli stain may be positive 50% to 80%, and mycobacterial cultures may be positive in up to 75% (66–69). The relatively low yield of blind pleural biopsies is owing to several factors that may be relevant to the stage of the disease when pleural biopsy is done, the absence of visualization of the area being sampled, and operator inexperience. Contraindications include a bleeding diathesis, anticoagulation, local chest wall infection, tenuous respiratory status, and the absence of pleural fluid. The risks are similar to thoracentesis, but with an increased incidence of pneumothorax.

MEDICAL THORACOSCOPY

Medical thoracoscopy allows full exploration of the thoracic cavity by using an endoscopic telescope of high optical quality. A rigid thoracoscope with a cold light source is used, which allows high-quality visual exploration of both the pleural surfaces and the lung and facilitates multiple and large biopsies of the pleura under direct visualization (70). Medical thoracoscopy performed by pulmonologists uses local anesthesia and conscious sedation and has a diagnostic yield of greater than 90% (71). The sensitivity for malignant disease approaches 95% (72,73). Medical thoracoscopy is primarily a diagnostic procedure. Indications include evaluation of exudative effusions for unknown cause, staging of malignant mesothelioma and cancers, and treatment of malignant and other recurrent effusions with talc pleurodesis. The sensitivity of medical thoracoscopy for diagnosis of malignancy is 97% when combined with pleural fluid cytology and closed pleural biopsy (71). Medical thoracoscopy may also be useful in staging patients with lung cancer and diffuse mesothelioma. It may allow a physician to avoid an exploratory thoracotomy. Pleural metastasis commonly involves the visceral and parietal pleura and the diaphragmatic surfaces of the pleura (74). These are usually positioned in the lower half of the thorax; thus, access to the sites of malignant deposits is usually difficult if blind pleural biopsy is the only procedure used. These are, however, readily visualized by thoracoscopy. The contraindications to the procedure include a trapped lung, coagulopathy, hypoxemia, and cardiac disease. Complications may include postoperative fever, air leak, hypoxemia, and bleeding. Fewer than 10% of effusions remain undiagnosed after thoracoscopy.

Fiberoptic and rigid bronchoscopy procedures have minimal yield in the diagnosis of patients with pleural disease; however, if an endobronchial lesion is suspected in a patient with hemoptysis or atelectasis, a bronchoscopy may be performed for evaluation of the airways (75,76).

SURGICAL PROCEDURES

Video-assisted thoracic surgery or open thoracotomy will require general anesthesia and single lung ventilation. A surgeon will usually undertake a more extensive procedure than medical thoracoscopy and may combine therapy with a diagnostic biopsy (75).

TRANSUDATIVE EFFUSIONS

Congestive Heart Failure

Congestive heart failure is the most common cause of pleural effusions and occurs in up to 70% of patients with congestive heart failure at some point during the course of their disease (76). The effusions are typically bilateral, whereas some of them (up to 20%) may be right-sided; a few left-sided effusions have also been noticed (up to 9%) (77–79). Pleural effusions specifically indicate left ventricular dysfunctions secondary to congestive heart failure. Patients with isolated right ventricular abnormalities, with or without pulmonary hypertension, do not usually present with pleural effusions. The pulmonary capillary wedge pressure in patients with congestive heart failure is elevated. Patients with congestive heart failure and pleural effusions will often present with dyspnea on exertion and other evidence of congestive heart failure, which may include pedal edema, jugular venous distention, and an S_3 gallop. Long-standing pleural effusions secondary to congestive heart failure, particularly after the use of diuretics, can result in an increase in pleural fluid protein and/or LDH, leading to confusion in the diagnosis of the effusion. Pleural fluid cholesterol is resistant to changes secondary to diuresis and can be useful in differentiating the pleural effusion. In a well-diagnosed patient with congestive heart failure, the presence of a pleural effusion does not necessitate thoracentesis unless the patient presents with fever or elevated white count, which should prompt the clinician to evaluate the patient for underlying infections, pulmonary embolism, etc.

Transudative Effusions from Other Causes

Transudative pleural effusions may also be found in patients with cirrhosis, in which it can occur in up to 6% of patients who also have ascites (80). These pleural effusions are often right-sided, occurring in up to 67% of patients on the right, whereas left-sided and bilateral effusions are seen much less commonly, in up to 16% to 17%. The mechanism for fluid accumulation is the flow across diaphragmatic defects into the pleural space. Some other causes of transudative effusions are nephrotic syndrome, myxedema, pulmonary embolism, superior venacaval obstruction, and peritoneal dialysis. A small percentage of patients being treated with continuous ambulatory peritoneal dialysis develop pleural effusions (81). The mechanisms for the development of the effusion are similar to hepatic hydrothorax. The cause of the low plasma oncotic pressure because of a low albumin contributes to the development of pleural effusions in patients with nephrotic syndrome; about 20% of these patients will present with pleural effusions. Myxedema is associated with pleural effusions in 25% to 50% of patients and can be transudative or exudative in nature.

EXUDATIVE PLEURAL EFFUSIONS

Parapneumonic Effusions and Empyema

Infections in the pleural space are a diverse group of heterogenous expression of the underlying pleural infection. Parapneumonic effusions occur in patients with bacterial pneumonia, and during the earliest presentation, they may present with less than 10 mm layering of fluid on a decubitus radiograph. At the opposite end of the spectrum is empyema in which the pleural space is filled with frank pus, the presence of organisms with multiple loculations in the pleural space (82). Infectious pleural effusions secondary to bacterial pneumonia can be separated into uncomplicated and complicated effusions. Uncomplicated parapneumonic effusions are defined as those that do not require drainage and will respond to antibiotic therapy alone for the underlying pneumonia. At the other extreme, complicated parapneumonic effusions are defined as those that will not respond to antibiotic therapy and will require drainage to prevent the formation of a frank empyema. It is extremely important to remember that pleural space infections are a continuum, from the uncomplicated free-flowing fluid to the development of a frank empyema (82). The transition to the more severe forms of pleural infection can occur extremely rapidly, in some cases within a 24-hour period. Characteristically, uncomplicated parapneumonic effusions will have a pH of greater than 7.30, a glucose of greater than 60 mg/dL, and an LDH of less than 1,000 IU/L.

During the process of pleural inflammation incited by the presence of infectious organisms and cytokines, several factors come into play. The interaction of the mesothelium with bacteria and LPS causes a rapid evolution of changes in both vascular and pleural permeability. This injury of the alveolar epithelium, the microscopic capillary endothelium, and the pleural mesothelium allows the exudative stage of parapneumonic effusions to ensue. A neutrophil predominance, an elevated protein, and a normal pH and glucose characterize the fluid at this stage. This process may progress to the fibrinopurulent stage, which is characterized by a further influx of neutrophils and protein with the accumulation in the pleural space of cellular debris and clotting factors. The decline in fluid pH and glucose is thought to be caused by a net increase in cellular glycolysis from bacterial and cellular metabolism. The fluid turns into a coagulum, which provides a fibrin network for fibroblast proliferation. The final stage is characterized by organization. During this stage, multiple fibrinous strands on which cells such as fibroblasts grow link the two surfaces of the pleura. These fibroblasts lay down collagen and other matrix proteins that eventually become a fibrotic peel that surrounds the lung. The most common etiology of infections in the pleural space is secondary to an underlying bacterial pneumonia, which accounts for 70% of reported empyemas. However, pleural space infection can be associated with trauma, can occur as a result of a penetrating or blunt thoracic injury, and can result from iatrogenic pleural space compromise after procedures such as thoracentesis and open or endoscopic surgical procedures. Underlying systemic immune deficiencies can also promote pleural infections.

Bacterial infections of the lung and the pleural space have emerged as a frequent cause of pulmonary infections in HIV-infected individuals. Compared with immunocompetent individuals, HIV-infected individuals have more bacteremia and more frequent development of parapneumonic effusions or empyema. In a series of 983 patients with parapneumonic effusions from Spain, 9% of patients had concomitant HIV infection (83). Twenty-one percent of the HIV-infected individuals developed parapneumonic effusions compared with 13% of non–HIV-infected individuals.

Alcohol abuse may also, in part, contribute to the development of infections in the pleural space. Alcoholism was found in 10% of patients in one series (84). The predisposing factors in the patient's clinical history may give a clue to the underlying microbial cause of pleural space infections. If the patient has an underlying pneumonia, the organisms most frequently isolated from pleural fluid are *Streptococcus pneumoniae*, *Staphylococcus aureus*, and

TABLE 67.4. UNDERLYING FACTORS AND PROBABLE ORGANISMS IN PLEURAL SPACE INFECTIONS

Predisposing Factors	Organisms Most Frequently Isolated from Infected Pleural Fluid
Pneumonia	*Streptococcus pneumoniae, Staphylococcus aureus, Haemophilus influenzae**
Aspiration pneumonia or lung abscess	Mixed oropharyngeal anaerobes, *S. aureus*, enteric Gram-negative bacilli, viridans streptococci
Thoractomy	*S. aureus*, anaerobes, enteric Gram-negative bacilli
Esophageal rupture or perforation	Mixed oropharyngeal organisms
Contiguous intra-abdominal infection	Mixed enteric Gram-negative bacilli and anaerobes
Chest trauma	Enteric Gram-negative bacilli, *S. aureus*
HIV	Same as pneumonia, tuberculosis, fungal

*Invasive *H. influenzae* infections have largely disappeared in countries where immunization with *H. influenzae* type b conjugate vaccine has been introduced.

Haemophilus influenzae (85) (Table 67.4). If aspiration pneumonia or lung abscess is the underlying cause, mixed oropharyngeal anaerobes, *S. aureus,* or Gram-negative bacilli may be involved (86). If the infection is after thoracotomy, *S. aureus,* anaerobes, and Gram-negative bacilli should be considered. After esophageal rupture or perforation, mixed oropharyngeal organisms are the most common cause of infections. When there is a contiguous intra-abdominal infection, mixed enteric Gram-negative bacilli and anaerobes are the leading causes of pleural space contamination. For evaluation of bacterial pleural space infections, a sample of the pleural fluid should be collected under sterile conditions and immediately processed by the laboratory. Bacteremia has been detected in 15% to 54% of pleural space infections. A Gram stain may provide vital diagnostic information before initiation of therapy. The sensitivity of microscopy in Gram stain in pleural infections has been reported to be 55% to 63% (87,88). Pleural fluid should be cultured in an aerobic media.

TUBERCULOUS PLEURAL EFFUSIONS

Tuberculous pleural effusions are a common presentation of clinical TB and may be the initial presentation of TB in up to 30% of patients in sub-Saharan Africa and up to 5% of cases in the United States (89). TB effusions represent a delayed hypersensitivity reaction in the pleural space, which leads to increased permeability of the underlying capillaries and pleural membranes (90). Typically, the rate of culture negative pleural fluid is high. Lymphocytic pleural effusions can be produced in sensitized animals with killed mycobacteria, and pleural effusions can be produced in nonsensitized animals after introduction of T cells from immunized animals. The pleural fluid is usually a serosanguinous exudate

with a total protein concentration of greater than 4 gm/dL and an LDH greater than 500 IU/L. The pleural fluid is typically predominant in lymphocytes, with a total cell count of less than 5,000 cells/mL (66,91,92). Occasionally if the effusion is acute, a neutrophil predominance will be noted. Pleural fluid pH is low, is in only 20% of patients, and ranges between 7.0 and 7.3. Mesothelial cells and eosinophils are notable by their absence (52). TB empyema is a distinct and separate entity from the more common TB pleural effusions and can occur when there is progression of the primary TB pleural effusion leading to a trapped lung, an extension of infection from thoracic lymph nodes, and hematogenous spread; or it can occur after therapeutic pneumothorax therapy, which may also lead to a trapped lung. In these patients, there is a low-grade inflammatory process that can continue for several years. It may lead to the development of empyema necessitatis.

MALIGNANT PLEURAL EFFUSIONS

Pleural effusions occur commonly in patients with underlying malignancy. In these patients, a pleural effusion, when found, does not necessarily imply the presence of malignant cells in the pleural space (93). Effusions in patients with malignancy may also be secondary to multiple other causes that are unrelated to direct tumor involvement of the pleura. The mechanisms for these effusions include atelectasis secondary to bronchial obstruction, postobstructive pneumonia, hypoalbuminemia associated with malnutrition, pulmonary emboli, and complications from radiation therapy or chemotherapy. True malignant pleural effusions occur when the visceral or the parietal pleura is the site for seeding of malignant metastases. Malignant pleural effusions are the second most common cause of exudative pleural effusions, and imply a poor prognosis with limited survival (94,95). The most common cause of malignant pleural effusions is lung cancer, followed by breast cancer, lymphoma, and then other malignancies (96,97). The annual incidence of malignant pleural effusions in the United States is estimated to be greater than 150,000 cases (98,99). Pleural metastases arise from tumor contiguous to the visceral pleural surface with secondary seeding to the parietal pleura in patients with lung cancer. Other possible mechanisms include tumor emboli, direct tumor invasion, hematogenous spread to the pleura, and lymphatic involvement (96). Malignant cells that are metastatic to the pleural surface initiate local inflammatory changes that cause an increase in pleural permeability. The pleural fluid in patients with true malignant pleural effusions is usually a mononuclear predominant exudate with 50% of them being grossly hemorrhagic (100). One third of pleural effusions have a pH of less than 7.3, and this is often associated with a glucose level of less than 60 mg/dL.

A recent analysis of data by Heffner and colleagues (57), encompassing more than 400 patients, found that pleural fluid pH was an independent predictor of survival; however, only 55% of patients identified by pleural fluid pH of less than or equal to 7.28 died within 3 months. The investigators concluded that pleural fluid pH was insufficiently predictive for selecting patients for pleurodesis based on survival data. Thus, the pleural fluid pH should be used only in conjunction with the patient's performance status and primary tumor type in decisions for therapy.

At the time of diagnosis, pleural effusions are rare in patients with Hodgkin disease but are not infrequent in non-Hodgkin lymphoma. They may be the only radiologic manifestations of the disease in these patients, and lymphomatous invasion of the pleura is a common finding in non-Hodgkin lymphoma. However, in patients with untreated Hodgkin disease, up to 30% of patients will eventually develop pleural effusions (101).

Malignant mesothelioma and asbestos exposure, especially to crocidolite fiber, is a risk factor for the development of malignant mesothelioma. The clinical course of the disease is relentless, and survival of the patient is usually between 6 and 18 months (102).

Distant metastasis is rare in the early stages of the disease, but may be present in patients presenting at end stage of the disease. The patient may often present with pleural effusions, shortness of breath, or a dry hacking cough. Pleural effusions will typically have a low pH, and the diagnosis of mesothelioma is challenging because pleural fluid cytology, which is positive in about 25% of cases, may be difficult to distinguish from adenocarcinoma. Pleural biopsies are diagnostic. In about one fifth of cases, medical thoracoscopy and thoracotomy may be required, leading to diagnosis in up to 90% of patients. The pleural fluid hyaluronic acid level is a nonspecific finding and does not add to the diagnosis of the disease. Specific immunohistochemistry and electron microscopy may be essential to aid in the differentiation of the disease. Patients with breast cancer have the longest survival time of metastatic pleural disease. Pleural effusion may be the initial sign in up to 43% of patients with metastatic breast cancer (103), and up to 11% of patients will develop a malignant pleural effusion during the course of their disease. Fentiman and colleagues found that in 1,999 patients with breast cancers, 50% of effusions were ipsilateral, 40% were contralateral, and 10% were bilateral to the site of the breast tumor (104).

PLEURAL EFFUSIONS WITH PULMONARY EMBOLISM AND INFARCTION

A small pleural effusion with a peripheral wedge-shaped infiltrate can raise the suspicion of pulmonary embolism in a patient with underlying cause. Pleural effusions occur in 50% of patients with pulmonary emboli. In patients with pulmonary infarction, about 30% of the effusions are grossly bloody and exudates. Pulmonary emboli may cause atelectasis of the lung, in which case the pleural fluid will be a transudate (105,106). Chest x-ray typically shows a small pleural effusion. The effusion is usually unilateral and has a volume of less than one third of the hemithorax. The presence of an infiltrate is seen in approximately 50% of patients with pulmonary embolism and effusion. The pleural fluid is grossly bloody in two thirds of patients; however, the number of red blood cells exceeds 100,000 mL in less than 20% of patients. The leukocyte count ranges from less than 100 cells/mL to greater than 50,000 cells/mL with pulmonary infarction.

COLLAGEN VASCULAR DISEASE

Rheumatoid pleural effusions are a common intrathoracic manifestation and are seen in 5% of patients. The patient with active disease typically is male. In patients with pleural effusions, interstitial disease is seen in 30% of patients, whereas cutaneous nodules are seen in 80% of patients. The pleural fluid is characteristically a neutrophil- or monocyte-predominant exudate with a low pH and an elevated LDH, which may be greater than 1,000 U/L. Pleural fluid rheumatoid factor may be tested and is often greater than 1:320, which will indicate active pleural disease. In systemic lupus erythematosus, some 15% to 45% of patients will have pleural effusions. These effusions are more common in women and are symptomatic with cough, fever, chest pain, and dyspnea. The effusion here too is typically an exudate with neutrophil or monocyte predominance, of a low pH and an elevated LDH, usually less than 500 IU/L. The pleural fluid antinuclear antibody titer is greater than 1:160 (107). Patients may also have drug-induced lupus. There has been a definite association of chlorpromazine, hydralazine, isoniazid, phenantoin, procainamide, and quinidine implicated in the production of drug-induced lupus. Criteria for the diagnosis of drug-induced lupus are not definitive; however, the appearance of lupuslike symptoms, the presence of an antinuclear antibody, the resolution of symptoms, and immunological abnormalities after discontinuation of the drug suggest evidence of drug-induced lupus. Patients with procainamide-induced lupus and pleural effusions usually have antibodies to denature DNA and nucleohistone but have little or no antibody to native DNA. The renal function in patients with drug-induced lupus remains normal. The incidence of lupus syndrome with hydralazine is more common in women and is dose dependent.

PNEUMOTHORAX

Pneumothorax is defined as the presence of air in the pleural space. Typically, the patient will present with the acute onset of dyspnea. They may have tachycardia, decreased breath sounds, and decreased tactile fremitus. A pleural friction rub may also be heard. The Hamman sign is a crunching sound synchronous with the heartbeat, which suggests mediastinal emphysema. A tension pneumothorax may cause acute deterioration and implies the continuous leak of air into the pleural space, leading to mediastinal shift and hemodynamic compromise. Pneumothoraces can either occur from primary causes without evidence of underlying lung disease, or be secondary to the presence of underlying parenchymal abnormalities. The pathogenesis is typically described as the rupture of a subpleural bleb, allowing air to enter into the pleural space and elevating the pleural pressure, which causes the lung to collapse (108).

On chest x-ray, the visceral parietal pleura can be seen separated from the parietal pleura by air. Typically, an end expiratory radiograph will increase the density of the lung while reducing its volume, thus demonstrating the difference between the density of the lung parenchyma and the pleural gas (109). The size of a pneumothorax can be estimated by the following formula: percent pneumothorax $= 100 - $ (diameter of lung)^3/(diameter of hemithorax)^3.

In primary spontaneous pneumothorax, the patients are typically slender young men who may have a history of smoking. The annual incidence is 40 per 100,000 (110,111). Patients may also have marfanoid features. The pathogenesis is the increase in the height of the patient with rapid change in the chest cavitary size without concurrent increase in lung size. This leads to stretching of the underlying lung parenchyma and apical bullous formation. Some 40% of patients with a first pneumothorax will develop a recurrent pneumothorax within 5 years.

In secondary pneumothorax, the patient has underlying lung disease with formation of bullae or blebs under the visceral pleural surface. A wide variety of disorders may cause secondary pneumothorax (Table 67.5). Pneumothoraces recur in about 45% of patients with increasing risk for subsequent recurrences. Catamenial pneumothorax occurs in patients who have subpleural and diaphragmatic endometriosis (112). The rupture of these endometrial nodules, at the time of menstruation, can cause development of pneumothoraces.

Pneumothorax secondary to barotrauma occurs in up to 3% to 15% of patients receiving mechanical ventilation. Barotrauma and pneumothoraces secondary to high positive end-expiratory pressure and elevated peak airway pressures will develop in mechanically ventilated patients. Patients with underlying lung pathology such as acute respiratory distress syndrome, necrotizing pneumonia, chronic obstructive pulmonary disease, and asthma will have a higher incidence of the disease. Diagnosis can be made acutely because of the sudden rise in peak airway pressure with a narrow peak-plateau pressure gradient, signifying an acute decrease in system compliance. These pneumothoraces may often be tension pneumothoraces. Barotrauma is more common with controlled mechanical ventilation than with synchronous intermittent mandatory ventilation.

TABLE 67.5. CAUSES OF SECONDARY PNEUMOTHORAX

Chronic obstructive pulmonary disease	Pulmonary infarction
Pertussis	Eosinophilic granuloma
Pulmonary alveolar proteinosis	Sarcoidosis
Rheumatoid lung	Lymphangiomyomatosis
Tuberculosis	Asthma
Ehlers-Danlos syndrome	Tuberous sclerosis
Interstitial pneumonitis	Necrotizing pneumonia
Scleroderma	Cystic fibrosis
Pulmonary fibrosis	Lung cancer
Marfan syndrome	Thoracic irradiation

REFERENCES

1. Hayek v. The parietal pleura (pleura parietalis) and the visceral pleura (pleura pulmonalis). In: *The human lung*. New York: Hafner Publishing, 1960:34.
2. Wang NS. Anatomy of the pleura. *Clin Chest Med* 1998;19:229–240.
3. Mariassay AT, Wheeldon EB. The pleura: a combined light microscopic, scanning, and transmission electron microscopic study in the sheep, I. Normal pleura. *Exp Lung Res* 1983;4:293–314.
4. Michailova KN. The serous membranes in the cat: electron microscopic observations. *Anat Anz* 1996;178:413–424.
5. Miserocchi G, Agostoni E. Contents of the pleural space. *J Appl Physiol* 1971;30:208–213.
6. Albertine KH, Wiener-Kronish JP, et al. Structure, blood supply, and lymphatic vessels of the sheep's visceral pleura. *Am J Anat* 1982;165:277–294.
7. Wang NS. The regional difference of pleural mesothelial cells in rabbits. *Am Rev Respir Dis* 1974;110:623–633.
8. Andrews PM, Porter KR. The ultrastructural morphology and possible functional significance of mesothelial microvilli. *Anat Rec* 1973;177:409–426.
9. Legrand M, Pariente R, Andre J. Ultrastructure de la pleure parietale humaine. *Press Med* 1971:2514.
10. Antony VB, Mohammed KA. Pathophysiology of pleural space infections. *Semin Respir Infect* 1999;14:9–17.
11. Mohammed KA, Nasreen N, Hardwick J, et al. Bacterial induction of pleural mesothelial monolayer barrier dysfunction. *Am J Physiol* 2001;281:L119–L125.
12. Wang NS. Mesothelial cells in situ. In: Chretien J, Bignon J, Hirsch A, eds. *The pleura in health and disease*. New York: Marcel Dekker Inc, 1985:23.
13. Yamada S. Ueber die serose Flüssigkeit in der Pleurahöhle der gesunden Menschen. *Z Ges Exp Med* 1933;90:342.
14. Sahn SA, Willcox ML, Good JT Jr, et al. Characteristics of normal rabbit pleural fluid: physiologic and biochemical implications. *Lung* 1979;156:63–69.
15. Wang NS. The preformed stomas connecting the pleural cavity and the lymphatics in the parietal pleura. *Am Rev Respir Dis* 1975;111:12–20.
16. Wheeldon EB, Mariassy AT, McSporran KD. The pleura: a combined light microscopic and scanning and transmission electron microscopic study in the sheep, II. Response to injury. *Exp Lung Res* 1983;5:125–140.
17. Courtice F, Morris B. The effect of diaphragmatic movement on the absorption of protein and of red blood cells from the pleural cavity. *Aust J Exp Biol Med Sci* 1953;31:227.
18. Miserocchi G, Venturoli D, Negrini D, et al. Model of pleural fluid turnover. *J Appl Physiol* 1993;75:1798–1806.
19. Nasreen N, Mohammed KA, Galffy G, et al. MCP-1 in pleural injury: CCR2 mediates haptotaxis of pleural mesothelial cells. *Am J Physiol* 2000;278:L591–L598.
20. Negrini D, Pistolesi M, Miniati M, et al. Regional protein

absorption rates from the pleural cavity in dogs. *J Appl Physiol* 1985;58:2062–2067.

21. Weiner-Kronish J, Broaddus V, Goldstein R, et al. Pulmonary hypertension and right atrial hypertension in the absence of left heart failure are not associated with pleural effusion. *Am Rev Respir Dis* 1986;133:A130.

22. Broaddus V, Weiner-Kronish J, Jerome E, et al. Pleural effusions in volume overload pulmonary edema. *Physiologist* 1986;29:104.

23. Bhattacharya J, Gropper MA, Staub NC. Interstitial fluid pressure gradient measured by micropuncture in excised dog lung. *J Appl Physiol* 1984;56:271–277.

24. Levin DL, Klein JS. Imaging techniques for pleural space infections. *Semin Respir Infect* 1999;14:31–38.

25. Müller NL. Imaging of the pleura. *Radiology* 1993;186:297–309.

26. Sahn SA. State of the art: the pleura. *Am Rev Respir Dis* 1988;138:184–234.

27. McLoud TC. CT and MR in pleural disease. *Clin Chest Med* 1998;19:261–276.

28. McLoud TC, Flower CD. Imaging the pleura: sonography, CT, and MR imaging. *AJR Am J Roentgenol* 1991;156:1145–1153.

29. Schabel SI. Radiological techniques in pleural disease. *Semin Respir Med* 1987;9:13–21.

30. Mossman BT, Gee JB. Asbestos-related diseases. *N Engl J Med* 1989;320:1721–1730.

31. Rusch VW, Godwin JD, Shuman WP. The role of computed tomography scanning in the initial assessment and the follow-up of malignant pleural mesothelioma. *J Thorac Cardiovasc Surg* 1988;96:171–177.

32. Al-Sugair A, Coleman RE. Applications of PET in lung cancer. *Semin Nucl Med* 1998;28:303–319.

33. Yang PC, Luh KT, Chang DB, et al. Value of sonography in determining the nature of pleural effusion: analysis of 320 cases. *AJR Am J Roentgenol* 1992;159:29–33.

34. Hirsch JH, Rogers JV, Mack LA. Real-time sonography of pleural opacities. *AJR Am J Roentgenol* 1981;136:297–301.

35. Conces DJ. Pleural imaging. *Semin Respir Crit Care Med* 1995;16:279–287.

36. Martinez O, Serrano B, Romero R. Real-time ultrasound evaluation of tuberculous pleural effusions. *J Clin Ultrasound* 1989;17:407–410.

37. Akhan O, Demirkazik FB, Ozmen MN, et al. Tuberculous pleural effusions: ultrasonic diagnosis. *J Clin Ultrasound* 1992;20:461–465.

38. Bradley MJ, Metreweli C. Ultrasound in the diagnosis of the juxta-pleural lesion. *Br J Radiol* 1991;64:330–333.

39. Morgan RA, Pickworth FE, Dubbins PA, et al. The ultrasound appearance of asbestos-related pleural plaques. *Clin Radiol* 1991;44:413–416.

40. Dulchavsky SA, Schwarz KL, Kirkpatrick AW, et al. Prospective evaluation of thoracic ultrasound in the detection of pneumothorax. *J Trauma* 2001;50:201–205.

41. Maury E, Guglielminotti J, Alzieu M, et al. Ultrasonic examination: an alternative to chest radiography after central venous catheter insertion? *Am J Respir Crit Care Med* 2001;164:403–405.

42. Sahn SA. The diagnostic value of pleural fluid analysis. *Semin Respir Crit Care Med* 1995;16:269–278.

43. Grogan D, Irwin R, Channick R, et al. Complications associated with thoracentesis: a prospective, randomized study comparing three different methods. *Arch Intern Med* 1990;150:873–877.

44. Capizzi S, Prakash UB. Chest roentgenography after outpatient thoracentesis. *Mayo Clin Proc* 1998;73:948–950.

45. Lillington GA, Carr DT, Mayne JG. Rheumatoid pleurisy with effusion. *Arch Intern Med* 1971;128:764–768.

46. Heffner JE. Evaluating diagnostic tests in the pleural space: dif-

ferentiating transudates from exudates as a model. *Clin Chest Med* 1998;19:277–293.

47. Light RW, MacGregor MI, Luchsinger PC, et al. Pleural effusions: the diagnostic separation of transudates and exudates. *Ann Intern Med* 1972;77:507–513.

48. Hamm H, Brohan U, Bohmer R, et al. Cholesterol in pleural effusions: a diagnostic aid. *Chest* 1987;92:296–302.

49. Heffner JE, Brown LK, Barbieri CA. Diagnostic value of tests that discriminate between exudative and transudative pleural effusions. Primary Study Investigators. *Chest* 1997;111:970–980.

50. Light RW, Erozan YS, Ball WC Jr. Cells in pleural fluid: their value in differential diagnosis. *Arch Intern Med* 1973;132:854–860.

51. Light RW. *Pleural diseases,* 4th ed. Philadelphia: Lippincott Williams & Wilkins, 2001.

52. Adelman M, Albelda SM, Gottlieb J, et al. Diagnostic utility of pleural fluid eosinophilia. *Am J Med* 1984;77:915–920.

53. Spriggs AI, Boddington MM. *The cytology of effusions,* 2nd ed. New York: Grune and Stratton, 1968.

54. Sahn SA. The pleura in health and disease. In: Hirsch A, ed. *Pathogenesis and clinical features of diseases associated with a low pleural fluid glucose.* New York: Marcel Dekker, 1985:267–285.

55. Good JT Jr, Antony VB, Reller LB, et al. The pathogenesis of the low pleural fluid pH in esophageal rupture. *Am Rev Respir Dis* 1983;127:702–704.

56. Sahn SA, Reller LB, Taryle DA, A et al. The contribution of leukocytes and bacteria to the low pH of empyema fluid. *Am Rev Respir Dis* 1983;128:811–815.

57. Heffner JE, Nietert PJ, Barbieri C. Pleural fluid pH as a predictor of pleurodesis failure: analysis of primary data. *Chest* 2000;117:87–95.

58. Staats BA, Ellefson RD, Budahn LL, et al. The lipoprotein profile of chylous and nonchylous pleural effusions. *Mayo Clin Proc* 1980;55:700–704.

59. Coe J, Aikawa J. Cholesterol pleural effusion. *Arch Intern Med* 1961;108:763–774.

60. Fontan BJ, Verea HH, Garcia-Buela JP, et al. Diagnostic value of simultaneous determination of pleural adenosine deaminase and pleural lysozyme/serum lysozyme ratio in pleural effusion. *Chest* 1988;93:303–307.

61. Rodriguez-Panadero F, Lopez Mejias J. Low glucose and pH levels in malignant pleural effusions. Diagnostic significance and prognostic value in respect to pleurodesis. *Am Rev Respir Dis* 1989;139:663–667.

62. Starr RL, Sherman ME. The value of multiple preparations in the diagnosis of malignant pleural effusions: a cost-benefit analysis. *Acta Cytol* 1991;35:533–537.

63. Loddenkemper R, Grosser H, Gabler A, et al. Prospective evaluation of biopsy methods in the diagnosis of malignant pleural effusions: intra-patient comparison between pleural fluid cytology, blind needle biopsy and thoracoscopy. *Am Rev Respir Dis* 1983;127[Suppl 4]:114.

64. Poe RH, Israel RH, Utell MJ, et al. Sensitivity, specificity, and predictive values of closed pleural biopsy. *Arch Intern Med* 1984;144:325–328.

65. Escudero BC, Garcia CM, Cuesta CB, et al. Cytological and bacteriologic analysis of fluid and pleural biopsy specimens with Cope's needle. *Arch Intern Med* 1990;150:1190–1194.

66. Berger HW, Mejia E. Tuberculous pleurisy. *Chest* 1973;63:88–92.

67. Scharer L, McClement JH. Isolation of tubercle bacilli from needle biopsy specimens of parietal pleura. *Am Rev Respir Dis* 1968;97:466–468.

68. Levine H, Metzger W, Lacera D, et al. Diagnosis of tuberculous pleurisy by culture of pleural biopsy specimen. *Arch Intern Med* 1970;126:269–271.

69. Scerbo J, Keltz H, Stone DJ. A prospective study of closed pleural biopsies. *JAMA* 1971;218:377–380.

70. Boutin C, Astoul P. Diagnostic thoracoscopy. *Clin Chest Med* 1998;19:295–309.

71. Loddenkemper R. Thoracoscopy: state of the art. *Eur Respir J* 1998;11:213–221.

72. Menzies R, Charbonneau M. Thoracoscopy for the diagnosis of pleural disease. *Ann Intern Med* 1991;114:271–276.

73. Canto A, Blasco E, Casillas M, et al. Thoracoscopy in the diagnosis of pleural effusion. *Thorax* 1977;32:550–554.

74. Boutin C, Viallat JR, Aelony Y. *Practical thoracoscopy.* New York: Springer-Verlag New York, 1991.

75. Kelly P, Fallouh M, O'Brien A, et al. Fibreoptic bronchoscopy in the management of lone pleural effusion: a negative study. *Eur Respir J* 1990;3:397–398.

76. Poe RH, Levy PC, Israel RH, et al. Use of fiberoptic bronchoscopy in the diagnosis of bronchogenic carcinoma: a study in patients with idiopathic pleural effusions. *Chest* 1994;105:1663–1667.

77. Peterman TA, Brothers SK. Pleural effusions in congestive heart failure and in pericardial disease. *N Engl J Med* 1983;309:313.

78. Weiss JM, Spodick DH. Laterality of pleural effusions in chronic congestive heart failure. *Am J Cardiol* 1984;53:951.

79. Race GA, Schiefley CH, Edwards JE. Hydrothorax in congestive heart failure. *Am J Med* 1957;22:83–89.

80. Lieberman FL, Hidemura R, Peters RL, et al. Pathogenesis and treatment of hydrothorax complicating cirrhosis with ascites. *Ann Intern Med* 1966;64:341–351.

81. Nomoto Y, Suga T, Nakajima K, et al. Acute hydrothorax in continuous ambulatory peritoneal dialysis: a collaborative study of 161 centers. *Am J Nephrol* 1989;9:363–367.

82. Strange C, Sahn SA. The definitions and epidemiology of pleural space infection. *Semin Respir Infect* 1999;14:3–8.

83. Gil Suay V, Cordero PJ, Martinez E, et al. Parapneumonic effusions secondary to community-acquired bacterial pneumonia in human immunodeficiency virus-infected patients. *Eur Respir J* 1995;8:1934–1939.

84. Jerng JS, Hsueh PR, Teng LJ, et al. Empyema thoracis and lung abscess caused by viridans streptococci. *Am J Respir Crit Care Med* 1997;156:1508–1514.

85. Fine NL, Smith LR, Sheedy PF. Frequency of pleural effusions in mycoplasma and viral pneumonias. *N Engl J Med* 1970;283:790–793.

86. Kelly JW, Morris MJ. Empyema thoracis: medical aspects of evaluation and treatment. *South Med J* 1994;87:1103–1110.

87. Maziah W, Choo KE, Ray JG, et al. Empyema thoracis in hospitalized children in Kelantan, Malaysia. *J Trop Pediatr* 1995;41:185–188.

88. Alfageme I, Munoz F, Pena N, et al. Empyema of the thorax in adults. Etiology, microbiologic findings, and management. *Chest* 1993;103:839–843.

89. Mlika-Cabanne N, Brauner M, Mugusi F, et al. Radiographic abnormalities in tuberculosis and risk of coexisting human immunodeficiency virus infection: results from Dar-es-Salaam, Tanzania, and scoring system. *Am J Respir Crit Care Med* 1995;152:786–793.

90. Leibowitz S, Kennedy L, Lessof MH. The tuberculin reaction in the pleural cavity and its suppression by antilymphocyte serum. *Br J Exp Pathol* 1973;54:152–162.

91. Seibert AF, Haynes J Jr, Middleton R, et al. Tuberculous pleural effusion: 20-year experience. *Chest* 1991;99:883–886.

92. Epstein DM, Kline LR, Albelda SM, et al. Tuberculous pleural effusions. *Chest* 1987;91:106–109.

93. Sahn SA. Pleural diseases related to metastatic malignancies. *Eur Respir J* 1997;10:1907–1913.

94. Marel M, Zrustova M, Stasny B, et al. The incidence of pleural effusion in a well-defined region: epidemiologic study in central Bohemia. *Chest* 1993;104:1486–1489.

95. Valdes L, Alvarez D, Valle JM, et al. The etiology of pleural effusions in an area with high incidence of tuberculosis. *Chest* 1996;109:158–162.

96. Chernow B, Sahn SA. Carcinomatous involvement of the pleura: an analysis of 96 patients. *Am J Med* 1977;63:695–702.

97. Johnston WW. The malignant pleural effusion: a review of cytopathologic diagnoses of 584 specimens from 472 consecutive patients. *Cancer* 1985;56:905–909.

98. Cohen S, Hossain SA. Primary carcinoma of the lung: a review of 417 histologically proved cases. *Dis Chest* 1966;49:67–74.

99. Parker SL, Tong T, Bolden S, et al. Cancer statistics, 1997. *CA Cancer J Clin* 1997;47:5–27.

100. Benard F, Sterman D, Smith RJ, et al. Metabolic imaging of malignant pleural mesothelioma with fluorodeoxyglucose positron emission tomography. *Chest* 1998;114:713–722.

101. Wong RM, Grace WJ. Pleural effusions, ascites, pericardial effusions, and edema in Hodgkin's disease. *Am J Med* 1963;146:678.

102. Johansson L, Linden CJ. Aspects of histopathologic subtype as a prognostic factor in 85 pleural mesotheliomas. *Chest* 1996;109:109–114.

103. Weichselbaum R, Marck A, Hellman S. Pathogenesis of pleural effusion in carcinoma of the breast. *Int J Radiat Oncol Biol Phys* 1977;2:963–965.

104. Fentiman IS, Rubens RD, Hayward JL. Control of pleural effusions in patients with breast cancer: a randomized trial. *Cancer* 1983;52:737–739.

105. Bynum J, Wilson J III. Radiographic features of pleural effusions in pulmonary embolism. *Am Rev Respir Dis* 1978;117:829–834.

106. Bynum J, Wilson J III. Characteristics of pleural effusions associated with pulmonary embolism. *Arch Intern Med* 1976;136:159–162.

107. Good JT Jr, King TE, Antony VB, et al. Lupus pleuritis. Clinical features and pleural fluid characteristics with special reference to pleural fluid antinuclear antibodies. *Chest* 1983;84:714–718.

108. Warner BW, Bailey WW, Shipley RT. Value of computed tomography of the lung in the management of primary spontaneous pneumothorax. *Am J Surg* 1991;162:39–42.

109. Lesur O, Delorme N, Fromaget JM, et al. Computed tomography in the etiologic assessment of idiopathic spontaneous pneumothorax. *Chest* 1990;98:341–347.

110. Lange P, Mortensen J, Groth S. Lung function 22 to 35 years after treatment of idiopathic spontaneous pneumothorax with talc poudrage or simple drainage. *Thorax* 1988;43:559–561.

111. Anderson B, Nielsen JB. Recurrence risk in spontaneous pneumothorax. *Acta Chir Scand* 1965;356:160–165.

112. Lippert HL, Lund O, Blegvad S, et al. Independent risk factors for cumulative recurrence rate after first spontaneous pneumothorax. *Eur Respir J* 1991;4:324–331.

Management of Pleural Diseases

68

Steven A. Sahn · John E. Heffner

Pleural effusions, pleural inflammation, and pneumothorax can be the consequence of disease localized to the chest or a manifestation of systemic disease. Pleural effusions are the most common form of pleural disease; pleurisy without effusion and pneumothorax are seen less frequently. Chest physicians are asked not only to diagnose the cause of a newly formed pleural effusion but also to manage recurrent malignant and nonmalignant effusions, complicated parapneumonic effusions, and pneumothoraces. A substantial percentage of pulmonary consultations are directly related to pleural disease, or else a pleural effusion is an important feature of the illness. This is not surprising because disease in virtually any organ can manifest as a pleural effusion, and pneumothorax can be a manifestation of many parenchymal and airway diseases. The two most frequent consultations for pleural disease are for the management of malignant effusions and parapneumonic effusions. Other less common but nonetheless therapeutically challenging pleural problems are chylothorax, hepatic hydrothorax, and trapped lung.

In this chapter, after reviewing pleural fluid analysis with a bayesian approach to diagnosis, we focus on the management of common pleural diseases, such as pleurodesis for malignant and nonmalignant pleural effusions, drainage of the pleural space for complicated parapneumonic effusions and empyema, and pneumothorax. We also address the medical and surgical approaches to chylothorax, the treatment of patients with hepatic hydrothorax, the diagnosis and treatment of trapped lung, and the management of hemothorax. Lastly, the role of corticosteroid treatment in pleural disease is discussed.

S. A. Sahn: Department of Medicine, Medical University of South Carolina; Division of Pulmonary and Critical Care Medicine, Medical University Hospital, Charleston, South Carolina.

J. E. Heffner: Department of Medicine, Medical University of South Carolina; and Division of Pulmonary and Critical Care Medicine, Medical University Hospital, Charleston, South Carolina.

DISCRIMINATING BETWEEN EXUDATIVE AND TRANSUDATIVE EFFUSIONS

When the history, physical examination, and routine laboratory assessment do not establish the cause of a pleural effusion, patients undergo thoracentesis for pleural fluid analysis to categorize the effusion as either an exudate or a transudate. The presence of a transudative effusion narrows the differential diagnosis to conditions that are usually apparent from the history, physical examination findings, and routine laboratory studies (Table 68.1). In contrast, exudative effusions present a broad differential diagnosis of predominantly inflammatory and neoplastic disorders that necessitate further diagnostic testing (Table 68.2). It is therefore important to discriminate accurately between exudative and transudative pleural effusions.

Light and colleagues proposed a diagnostic rule for categorizing a pleural effusion as an exudate (1). According to this rule, an effusion is exudative if any one of the following three criteria is fulfilled: (a) The pleural fluid lactate dehydrogenase (LDH) level is more than two thirds of the laboratory's upper limits of normal for the serum value, (b) the pleural fluid-to-serum LDH ratio is higher than 0.6, or (c) the pleural fluid-to-serum protein ratio is higher than 0.5. The use of a three-test combination with an "or" rule maximizes the diagnostic sensitivity of these criteria for detecting exudative pleural effusions but lowers their specificity (2). A high level of sensitivity is desirable, however, in screening for conditions, such as exudative effusions, that have important clinical implications.

Since the initial report of the criteria of Light and colleagues, multiple studies have examined other tests of pleural fluid and rules for testing and compared the results with those obtained with the Light criteria. Alternative tests include the pleural fluid-to-serum albumin ratio, pleural fluid cholesterol level, pleural fluid-to-serum cholesterol ratio, and

TABLE 68.1. CAUSES OF TRANSUDATIVE PLEURAL EFFUSIONS

Diagnosis	Comment
Congestive heart failure	Acute diuresis can increase pleural fluid protein and lactate dehydrogenase concentrations
Cirrhosis	Rare without clinical ascites
Nephrotic syndrome	Typically small and bilateral; unilateral, larger effusion may be caused by pulmonary embolism
Peritoneal dialysis	Large right effusion develops within 48 hours after start of dialysis
Hypoalbuminemia	Edematous fluid rarely isolated to pleural space; small, bilateral effusions
Urinothorax	Unilateral effusion caused by ipsilateral obstructive uropathy
Atelectasis	Small effusion caused by increased intrapleural negative pressure; common in patients in intensive care
Constrictive pericarditis	Bilateral effusions with normal heart size
Trapped lung	Unilateral effusion caused by imbalance in hydrostatic pressures resulting from a remote inflammatory process
Superior vena cava obstruction	Caused by acute systemic venous hypertension or acute obstruction of lymphatics
Dural-pleural fistula	Cerebrospinal fluid in pleural space

pleural fluid-to-serum bilirubin ratio. Some reports have suggested that several of the alternative pleural fluid tests are preferable to the Light criteria on the basis of a higher rate of diagnostic accuracy or a lower cost of testing. In contrast, other observers opine that the Light criteria are already sufficiently accurate and that further attempts to identify better testing strategies are not warranted.

To address this controversy, a metaanalysis used primary, patient-level data to examine the relative diagnostic accuracy of several pleural fluid tests in comparison with the Light criteria (2). The analysis included data from 1,448 patients and summarized the cutoff points (decision thresholds) in the various primary reports (Table 68.3). The study determined that the diagnostic accuracy was statistically similar for all the diagnostic tests and combinations of tests examined, in comparison with the Light criteria, except for the pleural fluid-to-serum bilirubin ratio. Consequently, clinicians can select among several tests to evaluate pleural effusions, depending on the clinical circumstances. For instance, the Light criteria require that the serum LDH and protein levels be determined from blood samples drawn near the time of thoracentesis. Several of the alternative pleural fluid test strategies, such as the combination of pleural fluid protein and pleural fluid cholesterol, do not require the results of serum tests.

The high sensitivity and lower specificity of the three-test combination used in the Light criteria often classify incorrectly patients with transudative pleural effusions secondary

TABLE 68.2. CAUSES OF EXUDATIVE PLEURAL EFFUSIONS

Infectious	Malignancy	Immunologic disease
Bacterial pneumonia	Carcinoma	Lupus pleuritis
Tuberculous pleurisy	Lymphoma	Rheumatoid pleurisy
Fungal disease	Mesothelioma	Mixed connective tissue disease
Atypical pneumonias	Leukemia	Churg-Strauss syndrome
Nocardia, Actinomyces infection	Chylothorax	Wegener granulomatosis
Subphrenic abscess	**Other inflammatory causes**	Postcardiac injury syndrome
Hepatic abscess	Pancreatitis	Familial Mediterranean fever
Splenic abscess	BAPE	**Endocrine dysfunction**
Hepatitis	Pulmonary infarction	Hypothyroidism
Spontaneous esophageal rupture	Radiation therapy	Ovarian hyperstimulation syndrome
Parasites	Uremic pleurisy	**Lymphatic abnormalities**
Iatrogenic	Sarcoidosis	Malignancy
Drug-induced	Hemothorax	Yellow nail syndrome
Esophageal perforation	ARDS	Lymphangioleiomyomatosis (chylothorax)
Esophageal sclerotherapy	**Increased negative intrapleural pressure**	Lymphangiectasis
Central venous catheter misplacement/migration	Atelectasis	**Movement of fluid from abdomen to pleural space**
Enteral feeding tube in pleural space	Trapped lung (with malignancy)	Acute pancreatitis
	Cholesterol effusion	Pancreatic pseudocyst
		Meigs syndrome
		Carcinoma
		Chylous ascites
		Urinothorax

ARDS, acute respiratory distress syndrome; BAPE, benign asbestos pleural effusion.

TABLE 68.3. CUTOFF POINTS REPORTED IN THE LITERATURE FOR VARIOUS PLEURAL FLUID TESTS

Test	Reported Cutoff Points
Pleural fluid protein	>3 g/dL (326)
Ratio of pleural fluid to serum protein	>0.5 (1)
Pleural fluid LDH	>0.66 (327) and 0.82 (328) of upper limits of normal for serum LDH
Ratio of pleural fluid to serum LDH	>0.6 (1)
Pleural fluid cholesterol	>45 mg/dL
	>54 mg/dL
	>55 mg dL
	>60 mg/dL
Ratio of pleural fluid to serum cholesterol	>0.3
Albumin gradient	≤1.2 g/dL
Ratio of pleural fluid to serum bilirubin	>0.6

LDH, lactate dehydrogenase.

to congestive heart failure who have been treated with diuretics (3). Diuretics cause pleural fluid to be resorbed at a faster rate than the proteins and LDH within the fluid. Consequently, the protein and LDH become more concentrated in the pleural space after diuresis, causing one or more of the Light criteria to move slightly into the exudative range and suggesting the presence of a "borderline" exudate. Chakko and colleagues (3) define such borderline pleural effusions in patients with heart failure who undergo diuresis as pseudoexudates.

Pseudoexudates, however, actually represent false-positive test results, which always occur when tests with continuous numeric results are used to categorize patients as being "with" or "without" disease. The case of a patient with a borderline test result near a cutoff point presents a higher degree of uncertainty to a clinician than a patient with an extremely abnormal result. Rather than coining new diagnostic categories, such as pseudoexudates, clinicians can use a bayesian

approach to pleural fluid analysis to evaluate borderline test results that do not fit the clinical circumstances. This approach estimates the likelihood that a patient has an exudative effusion rather than placing the patient in an exudative or transudative category.

A bayesian approach combines the physician's estimate of the pretest probability that an effusion is an exudate with the results of pleural fluid analysis to generate a post-test probability. The pretest probability is a percentage estimate but can be converted to a pretest odds by the following formula: pretest odds = pretest probability/(1 − pretest probability). The pretest odds is multiplied by a likelihood ratio, which is derived from the pleural fluid test result, to calculate the post-test odds. The post-test odds is converted to a post-test probability by the following formula: post-test odds/(post-test odds + 1). The post-test probability quantifies the possibility that the pleural effusion is an exudate in light of the clinician's knowledge of the pleural fluid test result.

Likelihood ratios are defined by the likelihood of a given test result in patients with a target disorder (i.e., exudative effusion) in comparison with the likelihood of the same result in patients without the target condition (i.e., transudative effusion) (4). Test result values above or below 1 indicate that the test result is either more or less likely to occur in patients with an exudative effusion. Unfortunately, likelihood ratios are not available for most diagnostic studies in clinical medicine. Likelihood ratios for discriminating between exudative and transudative effusions, however, have been reported (4) (Tables 68.4 and 68.5).

The value of a bayesian approach in pleural fluid analysis can be demonstrated by examining the use of likelihood ratios for patients with congestive heart failure who have undergone diuretic therapy. In this example, a clinician may consider an exudative effusion unlikely (e.g., a 10% probability) before testing in the evaluation of a patient with known congestive heart failure and a pleural effusion that has diminished but failed to resolve with diuretic therapy. If

TABLE 68.4. LIKELIHOOD RATIOS FOR PLEURAL FLUID PROTEIN AND PLEURAL FLUID-TO-SERUM PROTEIN RATIOS

P-PF Test Results (g/dL)	Exudates (n)	Transudates (n)	LR	P-R Test Results	Exudates (n)	Transudates (n)	LR
>5.0	265	2	47.25	>0.70	475	1	168.65
4.6–5.0	184	2	32.80	0.66–0.70	150	1	53.26
4.1–4.5	138	3	16.40	0.61–0.65	117	6	6.92
3.6–4.0	120	18	2.38	0.56–0.60	102	12	3.02
3.1–3.5	66	23	1.02	0.51–0.55	70	14	1.78
2.6–3.0	51	35	0.52	0.46–0.50	47	34	0.49
2.1–2.5	21	42	0.18	0.41–0.45	27	34	0.28
1.6–2.0	18	88	0.07	0.36–0.40	13	37	0.12
≤1.5	12	99	0.04	0.31–0.35	8	44	0.06
				≤0.30	19	182	0.04

P-PF, pleural fluid protein; P-R, pleural fluid-to-serum protein ratio; LR, likelihood ratio.

TABLE 68.5. LIKELIHOOD RATIOS FOR PLEURAL FLUID LACTATE DEHYDROGENASE AND PLEURAL FLUID-TO-SERUM LACTATE DEHYDROGENASE RATIOS

LDH-PF Test Results[a]	Exudates (n)	Transudates (n)	LR	LDH-R Test Results	Exudates (n)	Transudates (n)	LR
>1.00	626	5	44.33	>1.10	657	6	38.92
0.91–1.00	57	2	10.09	1.01–1.10	47	1	16.71
0.81–0.90	43	7	2.17	0.91–1.00	50	3	5.92
0.71–0.80	61	6	3.60	0.81–0.90	56	10	1.99
0.61–0.70	78	13	2.12	0.71–0.80	64	17	1.34
0.51–0.60	56	31	0.64	0.61–0.70	50	18	0.99
0.41–0.50	59	49	0.43	0.51–0.60	34	26	0.46
0.31–0.40	54	73	0.26	0.41–0.50	27	54	0.18
0.21–0.30	18	97	0.07	0.31–0.40	21	94	0.08
≤0.20	10	93	0.04	≤0.30	18	135	0.05

[a]LDH-PF is shown as a fraction of the upper limit of the serum value for the primary laboratory.
LDH-PF, pleural fluid lactate dehydrogenase; LDH-R, pleural fluid-to-serum lactate dehydrogenase ratio; LR, likelihood ratio.

the patient then undergoes thoracentesis and has a pleural fluid-to-serum LDH ratio of 0.75, an exudate (or pseudoexudate) is diagnosed by the Light criteria. With the use of likelihood ratios, however, the pretest probability of 10% is converted to a pretest odds of 0.11. The pretest odds is multiplied by the likelihood ratio for an LDH ratio of 0.75 (i.e., 1.34 from Table 68.4), which results in a post-test odds of 0.15. This post-test odds is converted to a post-test probability of 13%. The LDH ratio of 0.75, therefore, only marginally increases the clinician's estimate of the probability that the patient has an exudative effusion (13%), so the effusion is still more likely to be a transudate.

Alternatively, if the pretest probability is 50%, the post-test probability with the same laboratory results becomes 57%, and an exudative effusion becomes more likely. A pretest probability of 50% with a more extreme pleural fluid-to-serum LDH ratio of 1.15, however, generates a high degree of clinical confidence that the patient has an exudative effusion because the likelihood ratio is 16.71 (Table 68.5) and the post-test probability is 94%.

Pocket tools are available for converting pretest probabilities to post-test probabilities so that calculations are unnecessary (5). Also, if clinicians use sequential test combinations to determine the post-test probability of a pleural effusion, the post-test probability calculated from one pleural fluid test can be used as the pretest probability for a second pleural fluid test. When the Light criteria are used in a sequential manner, however, only two of the three criteria must be fulfilled. Because the test results for the pleural fluid LDH and the pleural fluid-to-serum LDH ratio both contain the value for pleural fluid LDH, the results of these two tests are highly correlated (Pearson coefficient of correlation = 0.84) (2). Combining two tests that are highly correlated in a diagnostic strategy does not enhance diagnostic performance. Consequently, it has been recommended that "abbreviated" Light criteria be used, which include the pleural fluid-to-serum protein ratio and either the pleural fluid LDH or pleural fluid-to-serum LDH ratio (2). The operating char-

acteristics of these two-test strategies are similar to those of the full three-test strategy.

Summary: Discriminating between Exudative and Transudative Effusions

Several diagnostic strategies are available for discriminating between exudative and transudative pleural effusions. Because the presence of an exudative effusion has important clinical implications, the diagnostic approaches for identifying patients with pleural fluid exudates should have excellent sensitivity. Therefore, most clinicians use combinations of two or three tests to maximize sensitivity, but these decrease specificity. Among the available tests, the Light criteria are diagnostically adequate. However, the abbreviated Light criteria should be used because the pleural fluid LDH and the pleural fluid-to-serum LDH are highly correlated, and both need not be included in the diagnostic model. If serum test results are not available, test combinations that rely only on pleural fluid test results can be used with a diagnostic accuracy similar to that of the Light criteria. A bayesian approach, in which likelihood ratios are applied to pretest estimates of the probability of an exudative effusion, improves diagnostic accuracy.

PARAPNEUMONIC EFFUSIONS

Parapneumonic effusions develop during the clinical course of 20% to 60% of patients hospitalized with pneumonia (6). In 5% to 10% of these cases, the course is complicated, and drainage is required to treat or prevent a frank empyema. An established empyema is associated with a high rate of morbidity and an overall mortality of 5% to 20% in general patient populations (7,8) and of 70% in elderly patients with comorbid conditions.

Parapneumonic effusions develop when a pulmonary infection involves the pleura and alters the permeability characteristics of the pleural membrane. Central to fluid formation is the activation of mesothelial cells and the release of neutrophils. Protein-rich exudative fluid enters the pleural space with an influx of inflammatory cells (9). In patients who recover with antibiotic therapy, the pleural fluid is resorbed through the subpleural parietal lymphatics. Patients with a pleural infection that evolves to a frank empyema have been described to progress through three pathophysiologic stages: exudative, fibrinopurulent, and organizing (10).

The exudative stage is the earliest phase of empyema formation. In this stage, the pleural fluid is nonviscous and freely flowing; the permeability of the pleural membranes is increased, but the membranes remain pliable and minimally inflamed. Patients are likely to respond to antibiotics if treated early. The early fibrinopurulent stage of empyema formation is characterized by increasing viscosity of the pleural fluid and thickening of the pleural membranes that predispose to the formation of intrapleural loculations. Patients may respond to antibiotic therapy alone but often require a pleural fluid drainage procedure as they progress to the late fibrinopurulent stage, which is characterized by one or more loculations. In the organized stage of a parapneumonic effusion, surgical drainage of an established empyema is required to manage a thick pleural peel and highly viscous pleural fluid. In a patient with an organized empyema, the development of trapped lungs interferes with lung reexpansion during management with chest tube insertion alone.

Detection

The expert consensus recommendations are that every patient hospitalized for pneumonia undergo an imaging examination to detect a parapneumonic effusion and determine whether drainage is required. No prospective randomized studies have been performed to show that mortality and morbidity are reduced by early detection and drainage. Existing observational studies, however, support a prompt diagnostic and therapeutic approach, having demonstrated that mortality is increased and hospitalization prolonged in hospitalized patients managed with delayed thoracentesis and drainage (6,8,11).

The initial two-view chest radiograph should be examined to determine the presence of clear diaphragmatic margins. Moderate to large effusions warrant thoracentesis guided by physical examination. Smaller collections of free-flowing fluid, subpulmonic effusions, and loculated effusions should be sampled by ultrasound-guided thoracentesis (12).

The sensitivity of standard chest radiographs in detecting parapneumonic effusions is low (~65%–70%). The detection threshold of standard radiographs is between 200 and 500 mL of pleural fluid (13). Subtle signs of subpulmonic effusions include an absence of lung markings in the posterior sulcus on lateral views or flattening of the medial diaphragmatic surfaces. Supine radiographs may demonstrate only a subtle increase in the radiopacity of a hemithorax secondary to the posterior layering of fluid.

Among the other imaging studies commonly used to determine whether a patient has a parapneumonic effusion, chest ultrasonography is exceptionally sensitive, being able to detect pleural effusions as small as 5 mL. Ultrasonography is often used to guide thoracentesis in patients with small or loculated parapneumonic effusions. Although ultrasonographically guided thoracentesis is adequate for most patients, chest computed tomography (CT) allows the image-guided sampling of central pleural fluid loculations adjacent to the mediastinum. Chest ultrasonography, however, is more sensitive than chest CT for detecting septa within fluid loculi. An advantage of CT is its ability to demonstrate contrast enhancement of inflamed pleural surfaces, thereby discriminating between lung abscesses adjacent to the pleura and empyemas (14). Magnetic resonance imaging plays a less important role in the management of parapneumonic effusions; it is used predominantly in patients who cannot undergo contrast CT studies because of allergy to iodinated contrast.

Sampling a parapneumonic effusion by thoracentesis makes it possible to identify an etiologic pathogen in cases of pneumonia, establish the need for pleural fluid drainage, and drain the pleural space if the fluid is freely flowing and not loculated. The microbiologic yield of thoracentesis is better if it is performed before antibiotics are administered, but the administration of antibiotics to treat pneumonia should not be delayed until thoracentesis is performed because such delay increases mortality.

A variety of tests may be ordered to evaluate a parapneumonic effusion. A positive Gram stain or culture can assist in identifying patients who require pleural drainage. Unfortunately, the Gram stain is positive in only 55% to 65% of patients with an empyema (15). To increase the diagnostic yield of the Gram stain, samples should be centrifuged before staining. Staining specimens with acridine orange makes it possible to detect bacteria killed by the initial antibiotic therapy (16). The demonstration of pleural pus indicates the presence of an empyema and the need for surgical drainage. A high concentration of salivary amylase or the detection of food particles during the cytologic examination of pleural fluid establishes the presence of a ruptured esophagus (17).

Samples of pleural fluid obtained by thoracentesis must be transported immediately to the microbiology laboratory in appropriate containers. The diagnostic accuracy is increased when anaerobic transport containers are used rather than liquid blood culture bottles. Gram staining or quantitative cultures cannot be performed on samples transported in liquid blood culture bottles. The use of liquid media also increases the probability that contaminating organisms will grow in culture. It is important to keep samples at room temperature before they are plated on solid culture media, so that colony counts can be determined.

LABORATORY TESTS THAT ASSIST IN THE EVALUATION OF PARAPNEUMONIC EFFUSIONS

Evaluation: Findings and Interpretations	Evidence
Cell count and differential: Leukocyte count of little diagnostic value; predominance of neutrophils establishes acute infection. Differential provides no diagnostic value.	Nonrandomized studies; expert opinion
Glucose, pH, lactate dehydrogenase: Adjunctive value to determine need for drainage.	Randomized controlled studies
pH < 7.00 suggests presence of a ruptured esophagus.	Observational studies; expert opinion
Amylase: Elevated concentrations of salivary amylase establish the presence of a ruptured esophagus.	Expert opinion
Aerobic/anaerobic cultures: Positive cultures establish etiologic pathogen and need for drainage.	Observational studies; expert opinion
Gram stain: Establishes need for drainage. Identifies pathogen morphology.	Observational studies; expert opinion
Special studies in selected patients: Mycobacterial stains and cultures, fungal stains and cultures, special stains and culture techniques for *Nocardia* species.	Expert opinion
Cytology: Establishes presence of unusual pathogens. Cytology also diagnoses underlying malignancy and detects food particles in patients with a ruptured esophagus.	Expert opinion

Antibiotic Therapy

The initial antibiotic therapy of a patient with a parapneumonic effusion is guided by the general recommendations for the antibiotic management of patients with community-acquired pneumonia (18). Various antibiotics penetrate the pleural membranes to varying degrees (19), but no clinical trials have demonstrated the superiority of any particular regimen in patients with a parapneumonic effusion. A positive Gram stain or culture of pleural fluid, however, allows antibiotic therapy to be targeted. Patients with an established empyema should be managed with antibiotics other than aminoglycosides. Although no outcome data are available, in vitro studies have shown that aminoglycosides are inactivated in purulent fluid with a low pH (20).

Determination of the Need for Drainage

The decision to drain the pleural space depends on the ability of the clinician to predict at the initiation of therapy the prob-

ability that the effusion will resolve with antibiotics alone. No prospective trials have identified independent variables that can predict the clinical course of a patient with a parapneumonic effusion with a high degree of certainty. Experts agree, however, that when multiple loculations, a trapped lung, or frank intrapleural pus is present and the result of Gram stain or culture of the pleural fluid is positive, drainage is warranted. Unfortunately, none of these clinical factors may be noted in many patients who nevertheless require drainage. In up to 35% of patients with an established empyema, the results of microbiologic examination are negative (15).

Other clinical factors should be considered in determining the need for drainage. Drainage of the pleural fluid should be considered for patients with leukocytosis and fever that persist several days after the initiation of antibiotic therapy if other causes of ongoing sepsis cannot be identified. In patients with comorbid conditions such as severe anemia and hypoalbuminemia or risk factors for aspiration (alcoholism, chronic swallowing difficulties) at the initial presentation, the presence of anaerobic pathogens in the pleural space is likely, and drainage is warranted (15,21).

Observational studies have suggested that if certain configurations of the pleural fluid are apparent on imaging studies, drainage is warranted. Multiple loculations increase the likelihood that drainage will be needed (22), although single loculi are sometimes present in patients with preexisting pleural symphysis who may respond to antibiotic therapy alone (22). An air-fluid level within the pleural space indicates a bronchopleural fistula and the need for pleural fluid drainage (15).

In one observational study, only 24% of patients with a parapneumonic effusion occupying more than 40% of the hemithorax responded to antibiotic therapy alone without pleural drainage (21). Chest ultrasonographic evidence that a loculus contains a complex structure of internal septa or fibrin strands with necrotic debris increases the probability that drainage will be necessary (21,23). These findings, however, are not absolute indications for drainage. Thickened pleural membranes (>5 mm) suggest a trapped lung, and consideration of drainage is warranted (24). CT may demonstrate thickened extrapleural subcostal tissues with increased attenuation of extrapleural fat, associated with an empyema (25,26).

The decision to drain the pleural space also depends on the virulence of the underlying pathogen causing the pneumonia. Pleural infections with *Streptococcus pyogenes* (27), *Staphylococcus aureus* (28), anaerobic pathogens (29), or *Klebsiella pneumoniae* (30) are more likely to progress to loculated, complicated parapneumonic effusions than are infections with *Streptococcus pneumoniae* (6).

Pleural fluid cell counts are of limited value in determining the need for drainage. Leukocyte counts and cell differentials do not assist in the decision. Evidence of squamous cells on cytologic examination of the pleural fluid suggests a ruptured esophagus and the need for drainage (17), but in nearly all these patients, other signs are present that suggest that the course will be complicated.

It has been suggested that the pH of the pleural fluid and the levels of glucose and LDH can assist in the decision to drain a parapneumonic effusion. These are parameters of the severity of pleural inflammation. In parapneumonic effusions with a high load of bacteria and activated neutrophils, the pH and glucose level are low because these cells metabolize glucose to carbon dioxide and lactate (31–34). The lysis of intrapleural inflammatory cells during progressive infection increases the content of LDH in pleural fluid (31–34).

Multiple studies have examined the value of the pleural fluid pH and glucose and LDH levels in identifying parapneumonic effusions that require drainage, and these tests were evaluated in a metaanalysis of discrete patient-level data from the primary studies (35). The metaanalysis determined that the pleural fluid pH is of greater diagnostic value (n = 197; area under the receiver operating curve [AUC], 0.89; 95% confidence interval [CI], 0.86–0.92) than the pleural fluid glucose (n = 105; AUC, 0.71; 95% CI, 0.65–0.77) or LDH (n = 91; AUC, 0.71; 95% CI, 0.63–0.79). These observations suggest that the pleural fluid pH should be used in preference to the glucose and LDH levels. The glucose or LDH level can be used if the pleural fluid pH is not available.

The metaanalysis suggested that if the pleural fluid pH was to be used to determine the need for pleural fluid drainage, a bayesian approach could assist in decision making. It recommended draining fluid with a pH below 7.30 in patients at high risk for progression to an empyema. High-risk patients were those who had other features associated with a need to drain (large effusions, loculations), features associated with a poor outcome (advanced age, comorbid conditions), or infections with virulent pathogens. A pH cutoff below 7.20 was recommended for low-risk patients. The test performance indices of pleural fluid pH, LDH, and glucose, along with the cutoff points for high- and low-risk patients, are shown in Table 68.6.

Several precautions must be taken when biochemical indices are used in pleural fluid analysis. Pleural fluid samples for a pH determination must be transported on ice or processed promptly, like blood samples for arterial blood gas measurement. Also, the primary studies on which the metaanalysis of the pleural fluid pH and glucose and LDH level determinations was based contained multiple design flaws (35). Consequently, the pleural fluid pH and glucose and LDH levels should play an adjunctive role in determining the need for drainage.

A consensus statement from the American College of Chest Physicians recommended that a staging system be used to determine the need to drain a parapneumonic effusion (36) (Table 68.7). The statement emphasized the general principle, however, that the decision to drain a parapneumonic effusion should be individualized, with clinicians erring on the side of early drainage to avoid the increased

TABLE 68.6. TEST PERFORMANCE INDICES FOR PLEURAL FLUID pH, GLUCOSE, AND LACTATE DEHYDROGENASE IN THE DECISION TO DRAIN A PARAPNEUMONIC EFFUSION

	Nonpurulent Complicated		
	pH	Glucose	LDH
AUC	0.81 ± 0.05	0.71 ± 0.06	0.71 ± 0.08
Cutoff point			
Patient A[a]	7.21	78 mg/dL	800
Patient B[b]	7.30	100 mg/dL	620
Sensitivity			
Patient A	0.62	0.52	0.65
Patient B	0.73	0.76	0.71
Specificity			
Patient A	0.93	0.86	0.78
Patient B	0.79	0.66	0.68
+ Predictive value			
Patient A	0.50	0.29	0.25
Patient B	0.54	0.43	0.43
− Predictive value			
Patient A	0.96	0.94	0.95
Patient B	0.90	0.89	0.88
Likelihood ratio			
Patient A	8.9	3.7	3.0
Patient B	3.5	2.2	2.2

[a] Low-risk patient.
[b] High-risk patient. See text for explanation.
AUC, area under the curve; LDH, lactate dehydrogenase.

morbidity and mortality associated with the delayed management of complicated parapneumonic effusions.

DETERMINING NEED FOR DRAINING PARAPNEUMONIC EFFUSIONS

Summary Statement	Evidence
Drain if:	
Frank pus, trapped lung, positive fluid Gram stain/culture, persistent fever/leukocytosis (other causes excluded).	Expert opinion
Multiple loculations, intrapleural air-fluid level, large (i.e., >40% hemithorax) effusion.	Observational study
Consider if:	
Pleural membranes thickened (0.5 mm), complex loculum, virulent organism.	Expert opinion
Low pleural fluid pH more predictive than glucose or lactate dehydrogenase.	Observational study

Approaches to Draining the Pleural Space

No randomized controlled trials guide clinicians in determining the ideal method for draining parapneumonic effusions. The goals of drainage are clear, however. Once the decision to drain has been made, a method should be selected that promptly and completely removes the pleural fluid and allows the lung to reexpand against the chest wall.

TABLE 68.7. STAGING SYSTEM FOR EMPYEMA PROPOSED BY THE AMERICAN COLLEGE OF CHEST PHYSICIANS CONSENSUS CONFERENCE

Pleural Space Anatomy		Pleural Fluid Bacteriology		Pleural Fluid Chemistry	Category	Risk for Poor Outcome	Drainage
A0 Minimal, free-flowing effusion (<10 mm on lateral decubitus)	*and*	**BX** Culture and Gram stain results unknown	*and*	**CX** pH unknown	1	Very low	No
A1 Small to moderate free-flowing effusion (>10 mm and <1/2 hemithorax)	*and*	**B0** Negative culture and Gram stain	*and*	**C0** pH ≥ 7.20	2	Low	No
A2 Large, free-flowing effusion (>1/2 hemithorax), loculated effusion, or effusion with thickened parietal pleura	*or*	**B1** Positive culture or Gram stain	*or*	**C1** pH <7.20	3	Moderate	Yes
		B2 Pus			4	High	Yes

A0, A1, A2 denote the three pleural space anatomic categories; BX, B0, B1, B2 denote the four pleural fluid bacteriologic categories; CX, C0, C1 denote the three pleural fluid chemical categories.
Source: From Colice GL, Curtis A, Deslauriers J, et al. Medical and surgical treatment of parapneumonic effusions: an evidence-based guideline. *Chest* 2000;118:1158–1171, with permission.

Among the available drainage techniques, therapeutic thoracentesis effectively drains parapneumonic effusions in the exudative stage of empyema development. Suitable candidates should have freely flowing fluid without any loculations. Some clinicians repeat the thoracentesis if the first procedure successfully drained the pleural space but fluid has reaccumulated. Other clinicians perform a pleural lavage with saline solution and antibiotics during the thoracentesis (37). If the initial thoracentesis is not definitive, however, patients may experience a prolonged hospital course if managed with serial thoracenteses. No evidence indicates that therapeutic thoracentesis decreases the morbidity of patients in the exudative stage or prevents progression to empyema.

The insertion of intercostal chest tubes is a traditional method for draining parapneumonic effusions. Unfortunately, the success rates of standard 22F to 34F chest tubes in managing parapneumonic effusions range between 5% and 78%, with a mortality of 5% (38,39). Standard chest tubes are most effective in managing exudative or early fibrino-purulent parapneumonic effusions that are nonviscous and freely flowing. Inserting chest tubes away from intrapleural fluid loculations is a common cause of chest tube failure (40). Some patients with sepsis may require chest tube drainage as stabilizing care while being prepared for a more definitive drainage procedure (41). Patients treated with chest tubes should undergo imaging studies after insertion to determine the adequacy of drainage. If a standard chest radiograph does not clearly show that the parapneumonic effusion is completely drained, chest ultrasonography or chest CT is indicated. Chest tubes that have adequately drained the pleural space may be removed when the pleural drainage decreases to 50 to 100 mL/d. Major complications of standard chest tubes

are tube misplacement outside the pleural space, lung perforation, and transdiaphragmatic or intra-abdominal placement with visceral damage (42).

The placement of percutaneous chest catheters under imaging guidance with a trocar or Seldinger technique has been extensively evaluated in observational studies of the management of parapneumonic effusions (40,43). CT with fluoroscopy as an imaging modality combines the advantages of cross-sectional imaging with the real-time visualization of guidewires and catheters (44). Small catheters (8F–16F) can effectively drain nonviscous fluid collections. Larger-bore catheters (28F) are required for draining viscous or bloody parapneumonic effusions. Percutaneous catheters rarely drain organized empyemas successfully, although some patients with organized empyemas who are poor surgical candidates may benefit from percutaneous drainage until their condition stabilizes and they can undergo more definitive drainage (40,41).

With imaging techniques, catheters can be placed percutaneously to drain fluid collections in the apex and paramediastinal regions of the chest that cannot be drained by standard chest tubes. We place percutaneous catheters to create a water seal with or without suction and monitor them closely to maintain patency with periodic instillations of saline solution.

Parapneumonic effusions that fail to drain after chest tube or catheter placement may respond to the intrapleural instillation of fibrinolytic agents. Streptokinase, urokinase, and recombinant tissue plasminogen activator (45) can lyse fibrin adhesions and thin viscous intrapleural fluid (46) to promote drainage. Four controlled studies have evaluated the efficacy of fibrinolytic therapy in the management of parapneumonic effusions (47–50). Two of these studies used a placebo control design (48,50). The study of Chin and Lim (47) was nonrandomized and used natural history controls. The intrapleural instillation of streptokinase in 23 patients with complicated parapneumonic effusions or empyemas was associated with a greater volume of chest tube drainage than simple chest tube drainage in the 29 control patients but no decrease in time to defervescence, duration of hospital stay, need for surgical intervention, or mortality. Wait and colleagues (49) compared video-assisted thoracoscopic surgery (VATS) (n = 11) versus chest tube drainage with the intrapleural instillation of streptokinase (n = 9). The VATS group had a higher success rate (10 of 11 [91%] vs. 4 of 9 [44%], $P < .05$), a shorter duration of chest tube placement (5.8 ± 1.1 vs. 9.8 ± 1.3 days, $P = .03$), and a lower total number of hospital days (8.7 ± 0.9 vs. 12.8 ± 1.1 days, $P = .009$). Davies and colleagues (48) compared the instillation of streptokinase with saline solution control and noted an accelerated resolution of radiographic pleural abnormalities but no decrease in hospital stay. Bouros and colleagues (50) reported in a double-blinded study comparing intrapleural urokinase with saline solution placebo that streptokinase was associated with a higher rate of chest tube drainage success (13 of 15 [87%] vs. 4 of 16 [25%]; relative risk for failure, 0.27; 95% CI, 0.09–0.76), a decreased need for surgical drainage (2% vs. 38%), and a shorter hospitalization (mean, 13 days vs. 18 days).

A Cochrane Review of fibrinolytic therapy for patients with parapneumonic effusions, however, concluded that insufficient data are available to support the efficacy of fibrinolytic therapy in managing parapneumonic effusions (51). Faulty study design, small numbers of patients, and inconsistent findings across reports limit existing studies. In contrast, the American College of Chest Physicians consensus statement on empyema management recommends fibrinolytic therapy for all patients with parapneumonic effusions undergoing catheter drainage (36).

We take a middle course and recommend a course of intrapleural fibrinolysis for patients with loculated or poorly draining parapneumonic effusions. Patients with a parapneumonic effusion in the exudative or early fibrinopurulent stage are most likely to respond. If the effusion does not respond after a short 1- to 2-day trial of fibrinolysis (two to six instillations), good surgical candidates are referred for definitive surgical drainage.

Intrapleural fibrinolytic therapy appears safe in that systemic fibrinolysis has not been observed (52–54). However, associations of intrapleural fibrinolysis with dissection of the thoracic aorta (55), ventricular fibrillation (56), hemorrhage (57,58), and hypoxic respiratory failure (59) have been reported. We recommend avoiding fibrinolytic therapy in the setting of bronchopleural fistulae.

Patients in the late fibrinopurulent stage or with an organized empyema usually require primary surgical drainage. A thick pleural peel and viscous pleural fluid prevent effective catheter drainage, and these patients experience prolonged

hospital stays. Surgical drainage is also indicated for patients who fail catheter drainage with or without a trial of intrapleural fibrinolysis. Surgical interventions are directed toward rapidly establishing effective pleural drainage and allowing full lung reexpansion (11,60).

Patients in the early fibrinopurulent stage of empyema formation can be adequately managed with VATS. In up to 10% to 20% of patients who undergo VATS, an intraoperative conversion to a full thoracotomy is required to allow sufficient drainage of the pleural space (61–66). Some surgeons use VATS to manage patients with an organized empyema (usually < 4 weeks), although they recognize that conversion to an open procedure is frequently needed (62).

Muscle-sparing limited thoracotomy continues to play a role in the management of patients with parapneumonic effusions. No prospective randomized studies have compared the outcomes of limited thoracotomy with those of VATS. One series argues that VATS is superior because it results in a better cosmesis and fewer surgical sequelae (67).

Patients in the late fibrinopurulent or organized stage of empyema formation with congealed pleural fluid and dense loculations require open thoracotomy for debridement, decortication, and drainage to allow the lung to reexpand (68–71). As many as 90% of properly selected patients recover fully after an open thoracotomy (38,63).

Patients with chronic empyemas and extensive pleural peels and patients with bronchopleural fistulae require long-term open drainage. Several reports have reviewed the indications for and outcomes of long-term open drainage (72,73).

EVALUATION OF PARAPNEUMONIC EFFUSIONS	
Recommendation	**Evidence**
Urgently evaluate all hospitalized patients with pneumonia for parapneumonic effusion.	Observational studies
Parapneumonic effusions should be staged to determine likely response to antibiotics and need for drainage.	Nonrandomized studies
Delay in effective drainage of infected pleural fluid increases morbidity and mortality.	Nonrandomized and observational studies

MALIGNANT PLEURAL EFFUSIONS

The estimated incidence of malignant pleural effusion in the United States is 150,000 cases per year (74). The diagnosis of malignant involvement of the pleura by fluid cytologic examination, percutaneous pleural biopsy, or thoracoscopy or thoracotomy biopsy signals incurability and a poor prognosis. The median survival of patients after a malignant effusion has been diagnosed is 4 months, with survival rates of 80% at 1 month, 64% at 3 months, 31% at 6 months, and only

13% at 1 year (75). Patients with gastrointestinal, lung, or ovarian cancers have a worse prognosis than those with breast cancer or lymphoma (75).

The primary goal of management in these cases is relief of dyspnea. The decision to palliate should be made after a careful consideration of all aspects of the patient's clinical status, not just a single factor.

Pathogenesis

Pleural seeding and independent tumor growth depend on the occurrence of a sequence of events (76,77). After a malignant cell separates from the primary tumor site, it must attach to and migrate through a blood vessel wall, then be transported in the blood to the visceral pleural surface. Autocrine growth factors and angiogenesis are necessary for the local growth and spread of tumor cells.

Pleural effusions develop in progressive pleural metastasis as a consequence of increased vascular permeability and new vessel growth, caused by angiogenic factors such as vascular endothelial growth factor (VEGF) (78), and of lymphatic obstruction at any point from the stoma of the parietal pleura to the mediastinal lymph nodes (79,80).

In a series of 191 patients who died with malignancy, autopsy revealed pleural metastasis in 55 (29%; 95% CI, 23%–36%) and pleural effusion in 30 (16%; CI, 16%–22%) (81). Whether the primary tumor is a lung cancer or a malignancy of extrapulmonic origin, the visceral pleura is virtually always involved as a consequence of neoplastic invasion of the pulmonary vasculature (80,81). The parietal pleura subsequently becomes involved when malignant cells spread from the visceral pleura along preformed or tumor-induced adhesions or attach to the parietal pleura after exfoliation into the pleural space.

Causes

In most large series of malignant pleural effusions, lung cancer most frequently involves the pleura, causing about 40% of malignant pleural effusions (82). Breast cancer is the second most common malignancy to metastasize to the pleura, accounting for 25% of cases. Cancer of virtually every organ has been reported to involve the pleura, with ovarian and gastric cancer each causing about 5% of malignant pleural effusions. Lymphoma accounts for about 10% of malignant pleural effusions in most series, and approximately 7% to 10% of patients have an unknown primary at the time a malignant pleural effusion is diagnosed.

Dyspnea

The most common and distressing symptom in patients with a malignant pleural effusion is dyspnea (79). Breathlessness initially occurs only during exertion, but as the disease progresses, it manifests at rest. The degree of breathlessness generally parallels the size of the pleural effusion, but premorbid lung disease or the development of tumor infiltration, lymphangitic carcinomatosis, or tumor emboli can cause dyspnea without an increase in the size of the pleural effusion. The pathogenesis of dyspnea in large pleural effusions is probably multifactorial: decreased compliance of the chest wall (83), a contralateral shift of the mediastinum, inversion of the diaphragm, and decreased ipsilateral lung volume modulated by neurogenic reflexes from the lungs and chest wall.

Management

Palliative therapy should be considered for all patients with a malignant pleural effusion. The patient's degree of breathlessness and expected survival are two of the most important factors influencing a decision to institute palliative therapy. Other factors that should be considered include the patient's performance status (84), type of primary tumor (75), and pleural fluid pH (75,85). Several options are available to the clinician for palliating symptoms. The management strategies include therapeutic thoracentesis, chemical pleurodesis through a small-bore catheter or standard chest tube, talc poudrage or pleural abrasion at thoracoscopy, placement of an indwelling catheter, pleuroperitoneal shunting, and parietal pleurectomy. The aforementioned local treatments should be considered if the patient is not a candidate for or has failed treatment with chemotherapy or radiation therapy.

Chemotherapy and Radiation Therapy

A limited number of malignant pleural effusions are likely to be controlled by chemotherapy alone. Malignant effusions that may be responsive to chemotherapy include those associated with small cell lung cancer (86), breast carcinoma (87), and lymphoma. Other effusions that may be responsive include those associated with prostate and ovarian cancer, germ cell tumors, and thyroid cancer. Lymphomatous chylothorax may be treated successfully with radiation therapy (88).

Local Treatment

Local treatment should focus on relieving dyspnea, avoiding or minimizing hospitalization, limiting costs, and preventing complications.

Therapeutic Thoracentesis

All patients with a symptomatic pleural effusion should undergo a therapeutic thoracentesis to determine whether dyspnea is relieved and assess the rate and degree of recurrence. If a therapeutic thoracentesis does not relieve breathlessness, the clinician should consider several possibilities, including trapped lung, lymphangitic carcinomatosis, microscopic tumor embolism, venous thromboembolism, and atelectasis. Thoracentesis may also fail to relieve dyspnea as a consequence of a complication of the procedure, such as a hemothorax or pneumothorax. Hemothorax should be suspected if the pleural effusion has enlarged on a chest radiograph obtained after the procedure. Pneumothorax, which can be diagnosed on the chest radiograph by visualizing a visceral pleural line, is typically accompanied by chest pain. If the effusion enlarges after thoracentesis, thoracentesis should be repeated immediately to evaluate the patient for hemothorax.

Patients with far-advanced disease, a poor performance status, and an expected survival of less than 3 months should be treated with therapeutic thoracentesis when they become breathless (74). Therapeutic thoracentesis can be performed in the ambulatory setting to avoid the cost and inconvenience of hospitalization. The volume of fluid that can be safely aspirated at therapeutic thoracentesis is unknown. However, if the patient has a large pleural effusion with a contralateral mediastinal shift, it is highly unlikely that the thoracentesis will cause a large decrease in pleural pressure; therefore, unilateral pulmonary edema should not develop. However, it is best to monitor the pleural liquid pressure when a large volume of pleural fluid is withdrawn. We currently monitor pleural pressures as fluid is withdrawn from the pleural space by attaching the catheter to a transducer and signal conditioner; this arrangement provides continuous pleural space manometry. Because continuous pleural space manometry is not available to most clinicians, it is advisable to stop the fluid withdrawal after 1 L has been removed and observe the patient for symptoms of increased dyspnea, chest discomfort, or cough before the procedure is resumed.

Caution should be exercised when pleural fluid is withdrawn from a patient who does not have a contralateral mediastinal shift or has an ipsilateral mediastinal shift on the chest radiograph because these findings suggest trapped lung or endobronchial obstruction. In patients with either of these two conditions, withdrawal of fluid will cause a marked decrease in pleural pressure, thereby increasing the transpulmonary pressure gradient and the likelihood of unilateral pulmonary edema.

Trapped Lung

In far-advanced malignancy of the pleural space, a large tumor burden can encase the lung and prevent expansion to the chest wall, creating an increased negative pleural pressure and a transient space in vacuo. This mechanism increases the parietal pleural interstitial–pleural space pressure gradient, promoting the movement of interstitial fluid into the pleural space to reach a new steady-state volume for the formation and removal of pleural fluid (89). Fluid reaccumulates rapidly within a few days to the pre-thoracentesis volume. Trapped lung is likely if any of the following are noted in the absence of endobronchial obstruction: (a) failure of the lung to expand completely on the chest radiograph after most of the fluid has been removed; (b) an initial negative pleu-

ral pressure, usually below 5 cm H_2O; and (c) an increased pleural space elastance (large change of ≥ 25 cm H_2O in the pleural pressure after 1 L of fluid withdrawal) (90–93). Thoracentesis in patients with a trapped lung greatly increases the likelihood of unilateral pulmonary edema and should be attempted with caution. However, dyspnea can be relieved if a portion of the pleural fluid volume represents the malignant process, in addition to the hydrostatic pressure gradient caused by the trapped lung; this clinical situation explains the success of pleuroperitoneal shunting in patients with trapped lung who have failed chemical pleurodesis (89). A clue that failure to relieve dyspnea with thoracentesis is caused by a trapped lung is that the effusion is a transudate resulting from a hydrostatic pressure gradient; the effusion associated with a trapped lung and concomitant malignant involvement of the pleura is typically exudative and less likely to lead to pulmonary edema, and dyspnea is relieved to some degree after thoracentesis (89).

Short-Term Chest Tube Drainage

Five case series comprising a total of 126 patients treated with chest tube drainage alone have been reported during the past 30 years (94–98). The success of pleurodesis with short-term (3–12 days) standard chest tube drainage alone ranges from 0 to 77%, the average being 60%. In three of the studies, chest tube drainage alone was compared with radioactive phosphorus, talc, and mitoxantrone. The success rate of tube drainage alone was 60% (95% CI, 50%–70%), and with a pleurodesis agent, it was 79% (95% CI, 69%–86%) (96–98). This success rate is lower than that achieved with the agents currently used for chemical pleurodesis. If a chest tube is placed, a chemical agent should be instilled in patients with complete lung expansion because relief of dyspnea is more likely to be sustained.

Chemical Pleurodesis

Several chemical agents have consistently produced pleurodesis and prevented the symptomatic recurrence of malignant effusion. However, assessments of efficacy have been hampered by small case series; the use of different techniques, criteria of success, and follow-up times; and limited direct comparisons between agents. In a review of the English literature from 1966 through 1992 on the use of pleurodesis in malignant pleural effusion, complete success was achieved in 752 (64%; 95% CI, 62%–67%) of 1,168 patients (no recurrence of pleural fluid by radiologic or clinical assessment) (99). Talc was the most successful agent, with 153 complete responses in 165 (93%; 95% CI, 88%–96%) patients. *Corynebacterium parvum* (no longer available) was successful in 76%, doxycycline in 72% (95% CI, 69%–75%), and bleomycin in 54%. The complete response rate with agents that produce fibrosis (talc, tetracyclines, *C. parvum*, and others) was 72% (95% CI, 69%–75%), whereas it was only 44% (95% CI, 39%–49%) with antineoplastic agents (bleomycin, interferon-β, cisplatin/cytarabine, doxorubicin, mitomycin, fluorouracil, and etoposide) (99). In a review of the literature on pleurodesis from 1958 to 1992, the rate of complete or partial success (no requirement for repeated thoracentesis) with talc poudrage was 91% (95% CI, 88%–93%), and it was similar with slurry, at 91% (95% CI, 86%–94%) (100). In a series of 57 patients randomized to talc slurry through a chest tube or talc poudrage with thoracoscopy, the success rates of the two methods did not differ when 5 g of talc was used (101). In a completed but not yet published randomized trial of talc slurry versus talc poudrage for malignant effusion in more than 200 patients, the two methods were equally effective in achieving pleurodesis, although the success rate was purportedly lower than the previously reported 90%.

Technique. Several controversial issues concerning the methodology of pleurodesis remain; these are related to chest tube size, dwell time, patient rotation, timing of the instillation of the chemical agent, and chest tube removal. In 12 case series with a total of 245 patients in which small-bore (7F–16F) catheters were used for chemical pleurodesis, the overall success rate was 78%, comparable with that achieved by using standard chest tubes (102–113). Talc produced complete or partial success in 87% (95% CI, 76%–94%) of 55 patients. Doxycycline had a success rate of 80%, bleomycin of 75%, and tetracycline of 75%. Based on these small case series, it appears that small-bore catheters are as effective as standard chest tubes and are associated with less patient morbidity.

It has been shown that tetracycline labeled with a radioactive substance disperses immediately and completely throughout the pleural space when instilled through a chest tube (114). A randomized study comparing tetracycline pleurodesis in patients whose position was rotated with those who remained supine showed no difference in success, suggesting that it is not necessary to rotate patients when a soluble agent such as tetracycline is used (115). We think that when talc is used as a slurry, the patient should be rotated during a 1-hour period, placed both in the lateral decubitus position, with the head of the bed at 60 degrees, and in the Trendelenburg and supine positions, because the slurry may not disperse as completely as a soluble agent.

Experimental data have shown that mesothelial cells are injured within minutes after contact with a chemical agent (116). Because mesothelial cell injury initiates the inflammatory response that leads to pleural fibrosis, a dwell time of only 1 hour is probably sufficient, and the two pleural surfaces should be juxtaposed as soon as possible to promote pleurodesis.

In the current methodology, based on consensus opinion, pleurodesis agent is instilled through the chest tube when the lung is fully expanded on the chest radiograph and fluid drainage is less than 150 mL/24 h. It is also dogma that the chest tube should not be removed until drainage is less than 100 to150 mL/24 h after instillation of the pleurodesis agent. Twenty-five patients with malignant pleural effusions were randomized to the standard procedure (15 patients) or "short-term" chest tube drainage (10 patients) (117). In the standard group, doxycycline was instilled when complete lung expansion was noted on the chest radiograph and the volume of fluid drainage was less than 100 mL/24 h. The chest tube was removed when the volume of fluid drainage was less than 100 mL/24 h after tetracycline had been administered. In the short-term group, tetracycline was instilled as soon as the chest radiograph showed complete lung expansion, regardless of the volume of drainage; the chest tube was removed the day after tetracycline instillation. The pleurodesis success rate was 80% in both groups, but the duration of chest tube drainage was significantly shorter in the short-term group (median, 2 days; range, 2–9 days) than in the group undergoing the standard procedure (median, 7 days; range, 3–19 days; $P < .01$). This small randomized study suggests that as soon as the lung is fully expanded, the pleurodesis agent should be instilled regardless of the volume of chest tube drainage, and that the chest tube can be removed as early as 24 hours after instillation regardless of the chest tube drainage. Short-term chest tube drainage can substantially shorten the hospital stay or can be performed in an ambulatory care setting; in either case, costs are minimized.

Although some suggest that intrapleural lidocaine is helpful in diminishing or abolishing chest pain, we believe that the effect is inconsistent. In our experience, small doses of intravenous morphine and midazolam provide excellent pain control and cause an amnestic response during pleurodesis. The drugs should be given 5 to 10 minutes before the chemical agent is instilled.

Adverse Effects. The most common adverse effects of the chemical pleurodesis agents are chest pain and fever. The retrospective incidence rates are variable and range from 7% to 43% for chest pain and from 10% to 59% for fever (99). Fever tends to develop within the first 12 hours after talc instillation and generally resolves by 48 hours (100). Knowledge of this febrile response to pleural inflammation should prevent the immediate initiation of a diagnostic evaluation for fever unless the clinical presentation suggests another cause. Surveillance for up to 40 years has documented neither mesothelioma (117–119) nor lung cancer (117) after the use of asbestos-free talc. In addition, no clinically important short-term (120,121) or long-term (118) physiologic restriction has been reported after talc pleurodesis.

Acute Respiratory Failure Associated with Talc Pleurodesis. Talc has been used since 1958 and has an excellent record of success and safety. However, several cases of acute respiratory failure associated with talc pleurodesis have been reported. For this reason, we reviewed the English language literature from 1958 through 2001 in an attempt to determine the incidence and causes of acute respiratory failure after talc pleurodesis with either poudrage or slurry. The total number of reported talc poudrage and slurry pleurodesis procedures was 4,252 in case series that included a few to more than 350 patients. We noted 43 episodes of acute respiratory failure (1.0%; 95% CI, 0.8%–1.3%). Acute respiratory failure developed in 41 (1.3%; 95% CI, 1.0%–1.8%) of 3,064 patients with malignant effusion, in 2 (0.2%) of 1,009 patients with pneumothorax, and in none of 178 patients with nonmalignant pleural effusion (100,101,122–135). Based on a retrospective review of these series, it was our opinion that only 18 (0.4%) of the episodes of acute respiratory failure were probably related to talc, although other circumstances may have placed these patients at increased risk for respiratory failure. Nine of the 18 patients were treated with talc slurry and nine with poudrage, with an average dose of 5.5 g and a range of 2 to 10 g (122,124,125,127,128,132–134). Of the 18 patients, 16 (89%; 95% CI, 67%–97%) required mechanical ventilation, and 9 (50%; 95% CI, 29%–71%) of them died. One of the 18 had undergone simultaneous bilateral pleurodesis and two pleural abrasion, and biopsy samples had been taken at multiple sites from one. Of the other 25 of the 43 cases, nine most likely were not primarily talc-related; other factors were present (e.g., excessive narcotic use, very severe chronic obstructive pulmonary disease, widespread cancer, severe contralateral pneumonia, widespread lymphoma involving the lung and mediastinum) (122), and four had "very limited lung function" (128). In the remaining 16 patients, no information was provided that could be used to assess causality.

The literature suggests that patients with malignancy are at greatest risk for acute respiratory failure after talc pleurodesis and that those with nonmalignant effusions or pneumothorax are essentially not at risk. It is likely that the minimal pulmonary reserve of severely debilitated patients with end-stage malignancy markedly increases the risk for acute respiratory failure. We suspect most of the patients in whom acute respiratory failure develops are probably not appropriate candidates for pleurodesis (see section "Recommendations for Chemical Pleurodesis").

Possible causes of acute respiratory failure after talc pleurodesis include systemic inflammatory response syndrome leading to acute respiratory distress syndrome, reexpansion pulmonary edema, excessive premedication, severe comorbidity, diffuse malignancy involving the lung, a terminal state, sepsis resulting from the use of unsterile talc or a poor chest tube technique, and excessive doses of talc (high-dose or simultaneous bilateral pleurodesis). If the talc is culpable, it may be because of a small particle size ($< 30 \mu$m) (136) or the presence of endotoxin (137). Simultaneous bilateral chemical pleurodesis should never be performed with any agent. Furthermore, we believe that pleural abrasion should not be performed before talc pleurodesis because it may allow talc to move more rapidly into the lung and systemic circulation.

Recommendations for Chemical Pleurodesis. Factors that should be considered before chemical pleurodesis is undertaken include response of the patient to therapeutic thoracentesis, general health and performance status (84) of the patient, pleural space anatomy on the chest radiograph or chest CT scan, pleural space elastance (89–93), primary malignancy (75,79), and pleural fluid pH (85,138–140). Absolute contraindications to pleurodesis include failure of therapeutic thoracentesis to relieve dyspnea, extensive trapped lung, and occlusion of a main bronchus. Relative contraindications include a terminal state, widespread metastatic disease, poor performance status, active air leak, low pleural fluid pH, severe underlying lung disease, prior extensive pleural abrasion or pleural biopsy sampling, and partially trapped lung.

Although the pleural fluid pH is directly correlated with survival and the response to chemical pleurodesis, it should not be used alone to decide whether pleurodesis should be offered to the patient. The pleural fluid pH should be used as adjunctive information and considered together with other factors.

Options for Patients with Failed Pleurodesis or Trapped Lung

Long-term Indwelling Catheterization

Two studies of long-term indwelling pleural catheterization (15.5F catheters) have shown that it is a safe and effective means of relieving dyspnea and as effective as chest tube drainage with doxycycline or talc (141,142). It would appear, however, that catheterization does not offer a significant advantage over chemical pleurodesis because the patient is burdened with the chest tube for an extended period. Catheterization may have a role in patients who have failed chemical pleurodesis, whose effusion is not caused solely by a trapped lung, or who are not candidates for parietal pleurectomy.

Pleuroperitoneal Shunting

Pleuroperitoneal shunting has been performed in patients who have failed chemical pleurodesis, chemotherapy, and radiation therapy, or who have a trapped lung or malignant chylothorax. Petrou and colleagues (125) reported a 10-year experience of patients referred for surgical palliation of malignant pleural effusion. Of 180 patients, 134 (74%) had undergone previous treatment; 117 patients demonstrated full lung expansion at surgery and underwent talc pleurodesis, and the remaining 63 patients had a trapped lung and received a pleuroperitoneal shunt. Palliation was obtained in 98% of the patients. The major complication was shunt occlusion, which developed in 14% of the patients. Occlusion was managed by shunt replacement, revision, removal, or open drainage. No intraoperative deaths occurred. It appears that pleuroperitoneal shunting can provide effective palliation in patients who have failed chemical pleurodesis and in whom trapped lung is not the sole cause of the effusion, malignancy also being responsible for the accumulation of pleural fluid. Shunting may also be an effective means of recirculating chyle in patients with chylothorax.

Parietal Pleurectomy

Parietal pleurectomy offers a definitive treatment for patients with recurrent malignant effusions, but it carries a high rate of morbidity and some mortality and is not justified in patients with a poor prognosis. In two studies of 130 patients who underwent thoracotomy and parietal pleurectomy for malignant pleural effusion, good palliation was obtained, but the postoperative mortality rate was 10% (143,144). In a small study of 19 patients in whom VATS was performed, the postoperative mortality was zero (145). Because it is associated with significant morbidity and mortality, parietal pleurectomy should be reserved for patients who are severely symptomatic and have failed chemical pleurodesis or who

---

LOCAL THERAPEUTIC OPTIONS FOR PATIENTS WITH RECURRENT SYMPTOMATIC MALIGNANT PLEURAL EFFUSIONS

Procedure: Comments	Evidence
Therapeutic thoracentesis: For acute relief of dyspnea, as primary treatment of end-stage disease in patients with poor performance status.	Expert opinion
Short-term (3–12 d) chest tube drainage: 60% success; range, 0–77%.	Observational studies
Chemical pleurodesis with chest tube (small-bore or standard): Success varies with agent, technique, and patient selection.	
Talc slurry: >90% success, inexpensive, associated with respiratory failure (<1%).	Randomized and nonrandomized studies
Doxycycline: Expensive, 60%–70% success, can be very painful.	Randomized and nonrandomized studies
Bleomycin: Less successful than talc and doxycycline, expensive.	Nonrandomized and observational studies
Talc poudrage: >90% success, expense of thoracoscopy, associated with respiratory failure (<1%).	Randomized and nonrandomized studies
Chronic indwelling catheter (2–3 mo): Option with failed pleurodesis and trapped lung.	Expert opinion
Pleuroperitoneal shunt: Can provide palliation with failed pleurodesis and trapped lung.	Expert opinion
Parietal pleurectomy: Effective; high rate of morbidity and some mortality; for failed pleurodesis, trapped lung, or at diagnostic surgery; should not be offered to patients with poor performance status and expected survival <6 mo.	Expert opinion

---

have a trapped lung in addition to a malignant effusion; it can also be performed when a malignant effusion is found during thoracotomy to resect an intrathoracic tumor. The procedure should not be offered to patients with a poor performance status and an expected survival of less than 6 months.

Recommendations for the Management of Malignant Pleural Effusion

The least invasive, morbid, and costly therapy should be recommended to patients with a malignant pleural effusion and a limited anticipated survival. The most important goal is to improve quality of life, mainly by relieving breathlessness. It is important to minimize hospitalization and patient discomfort and to avoid multiple procedures and increased costs. Patients must be selected for palliation and a specific procedure chosen after a careful consideration of the various factors discussed in the preceding sections. Unfortunately, clinicians cannot at present rely on the results of randomized controlled trials in making these important therapeutic decisions. Prospective studies are needed to evaluate the course of small, asymptomatic malignant effusions, assess the potential role of intrapleural immunomodulators, compare ambulatory and hospital-based management, and study of the issue of talc-associated respiratory failure.

PLEURODESIS IN NONMALIGNANT PLEURAL EFFUSION

The term *pleurodesis* is derived from the Greek words *pleura* ("rib") and *desis* ("binding together"). A successful pleurodesis creates fibrous adhesions between the visceral and parietal pleurae and obliterates the pleural space. Pleurodesis can be accomplished medically or surgically. Surgical pleurodesis can be performed at thoracotomy or thoracoscopy with gauze abrasion, parietal pleurectomy, or talc poudrage. Medical pleurodesis is achieved by instilling a chemical agent through a chest tube that should have a small bore (8F–16F). Although the major indication for pleurodesis is to manage recurrent, symptomatic malignant pleural effusion and recurrent pneumothorax, pleurodesis has also been used successfully to manage symptomatic nonmalignant effusions associated with chylothorax, yellow nail syndrome, hepatic chylothorax, congestive heart failure, and other conditions.

Pathogenesis

For pleurodesis to be successful, several events must occur: (a) widespread mesothelial injury; (b) recruitment of inflammatory cells, neutrophils, and mononuclear phagocytes to the pleural space; (c) recruitment and proliferation of fibroblasts in the pleural space; (d) activation of the pleural coagulation cascade; and (e) inhibition of pleural fibrinolytic activity (146). The process of pleurodesis begins with substantial injury to the mesothelial cells, which triggers a biologic cascade. The production and release of inflammatory and profibrotic mediators are essential for pleurodesis to occur after mesothelial injury (147–150). The importance of widespread exposure of the mesothelium to the inciting inflammatory agent is supported by the clinical observation that when extensive tumor covers the mesothelium, reflected by a low pleural pH and glucose level, pleurodesis is less likely to be successful (85,138). In addition to the mesothelial cells, neutrophils and mononuclear phagocytes recruited to the pleural space most likely play a role in pleural fibrosis (147,148). For example, pleural fibrosis does not develop without active fibroblast recruitment and proliferation. It has been shown that mesothelial cells produce fibroblastic growth factor when stimulated by either tetracycline or talc (149,150). Fibroblasts migrate into the pleural space from their location in the submesothelial connective tissue unimpeded by the mesothelial barrier, which has been injured or disrupted by the chemical agent or the induced inflammatory mediators. Fibroblasts must be able to attach to a matrix and proliferate therein (151). Pleural space injury promotes procoagulant activity (152–154) and decreases fibrinolysis (153–155), thereby generating a fibrin matrix. A poor response to talc pleurodesis in humans has been associated with increased pleural fibrinolysis (156). Why some pleurodesis agents are more effective than others is unknown. However, a common pathway from pleural injury to fibrosis appears to start with mesothelial cell injury and involve activation of the coagulation cascade in conjunction with diminished fibrinolysis and finally fibroblast migration and proliferation in the fibrin matrix.

Pleurodesis

In comparison with reports of the use of pleurodesis to manage malignant pleural effusions and pneumothorax, the data on the use of pleurodesis to manage symptomatic nonmalignant effusions are scarce. In a review of the English language literature from 1966 through 1991, only 24 patients were found to have undergone chemical pleurodesis for 25 nonmalignant pleural effusions (hepatic hydrothorax, congestive heart failure, nephrotic syndrome, continuous ambulatory peritoneal dialysis, chylothorax, lupus pleuritis, and yellow nail syndrome) (130). Pleurodesis was reported to be effective in preventing recurrence in 20 (80%; 95% CI, 61%–91%) of the 25 effusions. Tetracycline was used in 12 of the pleurodesis procedures, talc in six, and quinacrine, fibrin glue, nitrogen mustard, and silver nitrate in the remainder. Recurrence was noted in one patient with hepatic hydrothorax, one with congestive heart failure, one with lupus pleuritis, and two on continuous ambulatory peritoneal dialysis.

In that same year, a group from Brazil reported on the use of talc poudrage in 22 patients with nonmalignant or undiagnosed pleural effusions (157). Six of the patients had hepatic hydrothorax, two had lupus pleuritis, five had chylothorax, and nine had an idiopathic effusion. Recurrence was noted in 2 (9.1%; 95% CI, 2.5%–27.8%) of the 22 patients. Others have reported 100% success in small case series with the use of talc poudrage and talc slurry (158,159).

In a report from Israel by Glazer and colleagues (129), 16 patients (six with congestive heart failure, six with hepatic hydrothorax, one with yellow nail syndrome, one with lupus pleuritis, one with chylothorax, three with an unknown cause) were treated with 2 to 3 g of talc slurry by either standard chest tube or small-bore catheter. The authors reported complete success in 12 patients, partial success (some reaccumulation of fluid not requiring repeat thoracentesis) in three, and failure in one. The same authors reviewed the English language literature on pleurodesis for nonmalignant pleural effusions and found an additional 114 pleurodesis procedures that had been reported (129). Of the 130 patients undergoing pleurodesis, 92 were treated with talc poudrage or slurry and 38 with other chemical agents. The success rate in those treated with talc was 97% (95% CI, 91%–99%), and in those treated with other agents, it was 61% (95% CI, 45%–74%). Talc was virtually 100% successful in the patients with chylothorax, congestive heart failure, yellow nail syndrome, lupus pleuritis, or an idiopathic effusion, and more than 80% successful in 28 patients with hepatic hydrothorax. The same group from Brazil reported their 15-year experience in using thorascopic talc poudrage to treat 108 patients with nonmalignant pleural effusions (128). Some of these patients had previously been reported by Glazer and colleagues (129) in their literature review. Of the 108 patients, 51 had an idiopathic effusion, 24 had hepatic hydrothorax, 18 had chylothorax, and 12 had lupus pleuritis. During the follow-up period of 1 to 84 months, recurrence developed in 7 (7%; 95% CI, 3%–13%) of the 108 patients, and they underwent a second successful thorascopic procedure. Three patients who appeared to have trapped lung did not respond to talc poudrage. Therefore, pleurodesis was effective in 105 (97%; 95% CI, 92%–99%) of the 108 patients. Adverse effects were prolonged drainage in 5%, fever in 4%, reexpansion pulmonary edema in 4%, and empyema in 2%. Acute respiratory failure did not develop in any of the 178 patients reported in the literature who underwent chemical pleurodesis (the majority of whom received talc) for nonmalignant pleural effusion.

Conclusions for Pleurodesis in Nonmalignant Pleural Effusion

It appears that the success rate of chemical pleurodesis is higher in the management of nonmalignant effusion than in the management of malignant effusion. One might expect this higher success rate in patients with a normal pleura because no tumor covers the pleural surface, preventing mesothelial cell injury and the migration of fibroblasts into the pleural space. The failure of pleurodesis in nonmalignant effusion may be caused by pleural fibrosis (lupus pleuritis or rheumatoid pleurisy), trapped lung (rheumatoid pleurisy), or the rapid reaccumulation of pleural fluid (hepatic hydrothorax and chylothorax).

CHYLOTHORAX

Chylothorax, a relatively uncommon cause of pleural effusion, is often a perplexing therapeutic problem. Approximately half of the reported cases of chylothorax are secondary to malignancy, the most common tumor being non-Hodgkin lymphoma (160–162). Trauma sustained during surgery (especially in the vicinity of the aortic arch or involving the esophagus) or invasive diagnostic and therapeutic procedures and penetrating and blunt injuries account for approximately 25% of cases of chylothorax (160,161,163). A number of cases are caused by infection or are idiopathic (many secondary to minor trauma) (160,161,163). Neonatal chylothorax accounts for approximately 15% of cases (163); the remainder are caused by a miscellaneous group of diseases that include lymphangioleiomyomatosis (164), Noonan syndrome (165), and other conditions associated with lymphangiectasia (166).

Pathogenesis

A chylothorax develops when chyle accumulates in the pleural cavity secondary to rupture of the thoracic duct or impairment of thoracic lymphatic flow. Chyle can enter the pleural space via leakage from the thoracic duct or its tributaries or extravasation from the pleural lymphatics, and chylous ascitic fluid can move into the pleural space through diaphragmatic defects that open when the peritoneal pressure is increased.

Although the lymphatic anatomy varies substantially, the thoracic duct most often originates in the cisterna chyli and traverses the diaphragm at the aortic hiatus (163). As it approaches the fifth thoracic vertebra, it crosses from right to left and moves cephalad behind the arch of the aorta. After advancing a short distance into the neck, the thoracic duct empties into the left subclavian vein near its junction with the left jugular vein. The anatomic course of the thoracic duct explains why right-sided chylothorax develops after injury below the level of T5 and a left chylothorax after injury above this level.

Chyle is classically described as a whitish fluid, but in many instances, chyle may appear bloody, turbid, serosanguinous, or serous (160). An accumulation of chyle can be confused with an empyema or a cholesterol pleural effusion. Therefore, the diagnosis of chylothorax requires a high index of suspicion based on the clinical presentation.

Chyle is an alkaline, bacteriostatic fluid with a variable total protein concentration and fat content. The protein concentration of chyle can range from transudative to exudative and has been reported as between 2 and 6 g/dL (163). The variability in the protein and fat content is related to the timing and fat content of meals (167). Most (usually 80%–100%) of the nucleated cells in chyle are lymphocytes (168). The flow of chyle varies from 15 to 100 mL/h, the former rate noted during fasting and the latter after meals. Therefore, in persons consuming a high-fat diet, the flow of chyle can be up to 2.5 L in a 24-hour period (169). The loss of large volumes of chyle from the body through tube drainage can lead to immunologic and nutritional deficiencies because chyle contains a large number of T lymphocytes and fat-soluble vitamins.

Diagnosis

If the pleural fluid triglyceride concentration is above 110 mg/dL, the diagnosis of chylothorax is virtually certain (160). If the pleural fluid triglyceride concentration is below 50 mg/dL, a chylothorax is highly unlikely (160). With values between 50 and 110 mg/dL, pleural fluid lipoprotein electrophoresis should be performed to determine whether the pleural fluid contains chylomicrons; if chylomicrons are present, the diagnosis is confirmed (160,170). The cholesterol concentration or the ratio of cholesterol to triglyceride is not helpful in diagnosing a chylothorax. The triglyceride concentration of a chylothorax tends to reflect the patient's nutritional status; triglyceride concentrations above 1,000 mg/dL are usual in idiopathic cases, whereas very low triglyceride concentrations tend to occur in the postoperative state; patients with lymphoma tend to have intermediate triglyceride concentrations (160).

Management

Because chylothorax is a relatively uncommon cause of pleural effusion and has numerous causes, the optimal treatment is controversial. When the underlying cause has been determined, specific treatment, such as radiation of the mediastinum to control lymphomatous chylothorax, may be effective. In most cases, management must be individualized. The primary goal of management is to relieve breathlessness by removing pleural fluid; another goal is to prevent recurrence yet minimize the morbidity associated with removing protein, vitamins, and lymphocytes from the body. Factors that must be considered in planning treatment include the volume of chyle in the pleural space, degree of dyspnea, chronicity of the chylothorax, underlying cardiopulmonary physiology, and nutritional status. For example, if a patient has a small chylothorax and is asymptomatic, observation would be more appropriate than prolonged chest tube drainage, which increases the risk for malnutrition and immunodeficiency. Because chyle is bacteriostatic and nonfibrogenic, its presence in the thorax will not cause a spontaneous empyema or trapped lung (Table 68.8).

TABLE 68.8. MANAGEMENT OF CHYLOTHORAX

Option	Comments
Observation	Small, stable effusion; asymptomatic
Treat specific disease	Malignancy, infections
Repeated therapeutic thoracentesis	Rarely successful, complications
Tube thoracostomy	Monitor cycle output, nutrition, lymphocyte count
Bowel rest and total parenteral nutrition	Effective in traumatic chylothorax
Thoracoscopic talc pleurodesis	Successful in lymphoma with failed chemotherapy and radiation
Somatostatin or octreotide	Success in case reports
Thoracic duct embolization	Some success in postoperative and trauma-related chylothorax
Thoracic duct ligation/closure of fistula	Thoracoscopy or thoracotomy

Conservative Management

Conservative management in a symptomatic patient entails chest tube drainage, which is usually followed by complete lung expansion because chyle does not cause pleural adhesions. However, the underlying disease process or previous thoracentesis procedures may prevent complete lung expansion. It is necessary to monitor the daily output of chyle, nutritional parameters, protein concentration, lymphocyte counts, and electrolytes. The role of chyle reinfusion is controversial because it is associated with adverse events, such as anaphylaxis. Success with medium-chain triglyceride diets has been variable (171), and most clinicians prefer total parenteral nutrition and complete bowel rest to reduce chyle flow. The latter regimen appears to be effective in cases of traumatic chylothorax because these effusions tend to resolve spontaneously in 10 to 14 days (172,173). Oral intake can be resumed when the lung has reexpanded, the amount of pleural fluid is minimal, and the volume of fluid drained through the chest tube is small. Once the patient has ingested a normal diet without recurrence of the effusion, the chest tube can be removed.

Somatostatin or its analogue octreotide, which inhibits the secretion of digestive fluids and so decreases the flow of chyle in the thoracic duct, has been used successfully in selected cases of chylothorax refractory to chest tube drainage and total parenteral nutrition (174). Percutaneous transabdominal embolization of the thoracic duct and cisterna chyli has been reported to be successful in postoperative chylothorax (175). Cope (175), in a prospective study of 11 consecutive patients, 10 with postoperative trauma-related chylothorax and one with lymphangioleiomyomatosis, reported that the thoracic duct was successfully catheterized in five patients and embolized in four. The effusions of two patients resolved, and no morbidity was associated with the procedure.

Surgical Management

The mortality associated with traumatic chylothorax decreased about 40% after Lampson (176) reported transpleural ligation of the thoracic duct about a half century ago. Several surgical options can be used individually or in combination. These include closure of the thoracic duct fistula, thoracic duct ligation, mass ligation of the thoracic duct and adjacent tissue, suture of the mediastinal pleural leak, pleurodesis, pleurectomy, pleuroperitoneal shunt, and lymphovenous anastomosis (161,166,169). The surgical approach (thoracotomy or thoracoscopy) is dictated by the surgeon's expertise. Identifying the site of leakage, suturing the defect, and using Teflon pledgets to compress the leakage site allow the major portion of the thoracic duct to remain patent. In cases of bilateral chylothorax, the thoracic duct is usually ligated supradiaphragmatically on the right, whereas in cases of unilateral chylothorax, the ligation is accomplished ipsilaterally by either thoracotomy or thoracoscopy. After duct ligation, parietal pleurectomy or mechanical abrasion is usually performed if the site of the leak is not identified. Anastomosis of the thoracic duct and azygos vein does not appear to be effective.

Currently, VATS or medical thoracoscopy appears to be the method of choice for evaluating and managing chylothorax (177,178). Talc poudrage, clipping of the thoracic duct or pleural defect, the application of fibrin glue, selective lymphatic clipping, and pleuroperitoneal shunting have all been used with VATS.

No controlled trials have validated a 2-week period of conservative management for chylothorax. Although the rate of chyle formation, operative intervention, age of the patient, and survival may be correlated (179), each patient's management must be individualized. Patients with traumatic chylothorax whose condition does not improve with conservative management probably should undergo surgery early. Factors that indicate a need for early thoracic duct ligation include a loss of more than 1,500 mL of chyle per day for 5 days, no reduction in chyle flow within 2 weeks, the development of nutritional complications, and a reaccumulation of chyle despite tube drainage (179). Following esophagectomy, patients had a better outcome and a shorter hospital stay with early surgical intervention (180,181). The chyle output may be the best indicator of treatment for chylothorax following esophagectomy; if the output of chyle is less than 10 mL/kg on day 5, medical treatment is usually successful (182). In children who have undergone cardiothoracic surgery and in whom chylothorax develops, conservative management with a medium-chain triglyceride diet or total parenteral nutrition is usually successful (173).

Pleurodesis

Talc poudrage, talc slurry, and other sclerosing agents have been used successfully to treat chylothorax (132,157,178,

183,184). As in other types of nonmalignant effusion, pleurodesis is usually successful if the rate of chyle flow is not excessive and the two pleural surfaces can be brought into close approximation during the inflammatory process.

Pleuroperitoneal Shunting

A pleuroperitoneal shunt should be considered when surgery is not an option and nonoperative management is ineffective. The shunt relieves breathlessness and recirculates the chyle so that malnutrition and immunodeficiency do not develop. Pleuroperitoneal shunting has been shown to be effective in idiopathic postoperative chylothorax (185) and in malignancy (186). In properly selected patients, the shunt is safe and effective. Shunt occlusion (incidence of 10%) is the most common complication, and the shunt can be revised or replaced (186). This procedure cannot be performed in the setting of chylous ascites.

Conclusions for the Management of Chylothorax

No approach to the patient with chylothorax is standard. The method of treatment must be individualized, and the decision should be based on the underlying cause of the chylothorax and the general health and symptoms of the patient. Asymptomatic patients should be observed without chest tube drainage. For symptomatic patients, initial therapy should be directed at the underlying disease if possible. The literature suggests that certain patients should undergo early surgical intervention rather than 2 weeks of conservative therapy, including those with a persistently large output of chyle or with post-esophagectomy chylothorax. Early surgical management prevents nutritional and immunologic compromise and prolonged hospitalization and reduces costs. The initial surgical approach should be thoracoscopic direct closure of the thoracic duct leak or supradiaphragmatic ligation of the thoracic duct. If the site of the leak cannot be identified, parietal pleurectomy or chemical pleurodesis should be performed. No randomized controlled studies have compared surgical with conservative management of chylothorax. For debilitated patients with advanced malignancies, intermittent thoracentesis or chest tube pleurodesis may be the best approach. Those with nonsurgical traumatic chylothorax are best managed with chest tube drainage, bowel rest, and total parenteral nutrition; spontaneous resolution usually occurs within 10 to14 days.

PNEUMOTHORAX

Pneumothorax is the collection of air within the pleural space. Pneumothorax is classified on the basis of the underlying cause (Table 68.9). The estimated annual incidence of primary spontaneous pneumothorax is between 7.4 and 18 cases per 100,000 population in men and between 1.2 and 6 cases per 100,000 population in women (187,188). Pneumothorax occurs most typically in tall, thin men younger than 30 years of age (189). Smoking increases the risk for primary spontaneous pneumothorax by a factor of 20. Risk correlates with the number of cigarettes smoked (188).

Secondary spontaneous pneumothorax complicates the course of patients with a wide variety of underlying lung diseases (Table 68.10). The annual incidence is approximately 6.3 cases per 100,000 population in men and 2.0 cases per 100,000 population in women (187). The peak occurrence is during the seventh decade of life, which parallels the peak

TABLE 68.9. CLASSIFICATION OF PNEUMOTHORAX

Spontaneous (without antecednet trauma or other cause)
Primary: no clinical lung disease
Secondary: a complication of clinically manifested lung disease

Traumatic
Penetrating chest injury
Blunt chest injury

Iatrogenic (associated with diagnostic and therapeutic procedures)
Transthoracic needle aspiration
Subclavian vein catheter placement
Thoracentesis
Barotrauma

Source: From Sahn SA, Heffner JE. Spontaneous pneumothorax. *N Engl J Med* 2000;342:868–874, with permission.

TABLE 68.10. CAUSES OF SECONDARY SPONTANEOUS PNEUMOTHORAX

Diseases of the airways
Chronic obstructive pulmonary disease (chronic bronchitis and emphysema)
Cystic fibrosis
Acute asthma

Parenchymal lung infection
Pneumocystis carinii pneumonia
Necrotizing infections (anaerobes, Gram-negative bacteria, *Staphylococcus aureus*, *Nocardia* species, *Mycobacterium tuberculosis*, fungi)

Malignancy
Lung cancer
Sarcoma
Metastases

Interstitial lung disease
Langerhans cell granulomatosis
Sarcoidosis
Connective tissue disease
Tuberous sclerosis
Idiopathic pulmonary fibrosis

Others
Thoracic endometriosis (catamenial)
Lymphangioleiomyomatosis
Marfan syndrome
Ehlers-Danlos syndrome

Source: From Sahn SA, Heffner JE. Spontaneous pneumothorax. *N Engl J Med* 2000;342:868–874, with permission.

occurrence of chronic lung disease in the general population (189). Traumatic and iatrogenic pneumothorax occurs as a complication of conditions that cause penetrating injuries to the chest wall or airways or marked increases in airway pressure that rupture lung tissue.

Although primary spontaneous pneumothorax is defined by the absence of clinically apparent lung disease, subpleural bullae are noted in 56% to 100% of patients with primary spontaneous pneumothorax on chest CT scans or thoracic surgery (190–195). Studies comparing patients with a history of primary spontaneous pneumothorax (n = 20) and age-matched controls (n = 20) found a higher incidence of emphysematous lesions on the CT scans of patients with pneumothorax (16 vs. 0) (195). However, the relationship between the bullae and pneumothorax is unclear. Some experts suggest that rupture of the bullae allows air to track through lung tissue planes and enter the mediastinum, from which it ruptures into the pleural space (196,197). Other investigators have not observed a relationship between CT evidence of bullae and recurrence of pneumothorax (193). The causes of bullae in patients with primary spontaneous pneumothorax are also unknown. It has been suggested that inflammation in the small airways induced by smoking leads to tissue injury and airway obstruction that increases distal airway pressures through one-way ball-valve mechanisms (196).

Secondary spontaneous pneumothorax results from mechanical defects in the lung architecture associated with a predisposition to alveolar rupture; coughing and increased respiratory rates with dynamic hyperinflation further increase the risk. Chronic obstructive pulmonary disease and lung infection with *Pneumocystis carinii* in patients with HIV infection are the two most common causes of secondary spontaneous pneumothorax. The incidence of pneumothorax increases with the severity of measured airway obstruction, and patients with a forced vital capacity less than 40% of the predicted value are at greatest risk (198). A spontaneous pneumothorax develops in up to 6% of patients with HIV infection (199). Langerhans cell granulomatosis and lymphangioleiomyomatosis warrant special mention because a pneumothorax develops in 25% of patients with Langerhans cell granulomatosis and in 80% of patients with lymphangioleiomyomatosis at some time during their clinical course (164,200). Catamenial pneumothorax occurs in women of childbearing age with a history of endometriosis (201).

Patients with a primary spontaneous pneumothorax usually present with ipsilateral pleuritic chest pain and varying degrees of dyspnea (202). Because their underlying lung function is normal, the dyspnea is usually mild to moderate, even in patients with a large pneumothorax. A tension pneumothorax, which is a rare event in this setting, is associated with more severe symptoms. The symptoms usually resolve within 24 hours, even if the pneumothorax persists. Tachycardia and tachypnea are the most common physi-

cal findings. The chest examination results may be normal in patients with a small pneumothorax (<20% of the volume of the hemithorax). Large pneumothoraces are associated with an increased percussion note, diminished fremitus, and decreased or absent breath sounds. The arterial blood gases may demonstrate varying degrees of hypoxia and acute hypocapnia.

The onset of a secondary spontaneous pneumothorax manifests as chest pain. Even in the case of a small pneumothorax, severe dyspnea develops as a result of the underlying pulmonary compromise (203–205). Other evidence of cardiopulmonary compromise may appear, such as severe hypoxemia (mean Pao_2, 60 mm Hg), hypotension, cyanosis, labored breathing, altered mental status, and hypercapnia (204–206). The manifestations of the pneumothorax may be obscured by those of the underlying lung disease.

Primary spontaneous pneumothorax is readily diagnosed by the characteristic acute onset of chest pain and dyspnea and the radiographic features of pneumothorax. The chest radiograph demonstrates pleural air and a 1-mm-thick white line that represents the visceral pleura displaced from the chest wall. Although not recommended in routine practice (207), a chest radiograph obtained during expiration can help to detect an apical pneumothorax.

A secondary spontaneous pneumothorax may be more difficult to diagnose because the respiratory symptoms are sometimes falsely ascribed to the underlying lung disease. The chest radiograph of a patient with interstitial lung disease usually provides clear evidence of a pneumothorax because the rim of air in the pleural space contrasts with the increased density of the diseased lung. A secondary spontaneous pneumothorax may be more difficult to diagnose from the chest radiograph of a patient with chronic obstructive pulmonary disease because the density of the hyperlucent, emphysematous lungs is similar to that of pleural air. Moreover, subpleural giant bullae may simulate pneumothorax in these patients. Chest CT can assist in the differentiation between giant bullae and pneumothorax (208).

The goals of therapy in spontaneous pneumothorax focus on reexpanding the collapsed lung and preventing recurrence. Primary spontaneous pneumothorax recurs in 30% (range, 16%–52%) of patients (198,209,210). Patients with a second primary spontaneous pneumothorax are at even greater risk for the development of a third pneumothorax. The risk for recurrence of a secondary spontaneous pneumothorax is 39% to 47% (198,210,211), and each recurrence presents a potentially life-threatening event.

Multiple approaches are used to treat pneumothorax. Unfortunately, few results of prospective randomized trials are available to guide treatment recommendations, and design flaws mar the studies that exist. The American College of Chest Physicians recognized the absence of level I data when it published a consensus report on the management of spontaneous pneumothorax (212). Consensus was attained through an explicit Delphi process that allowed readers to note the degree of consensus among experts for each treatment recommendation.

Patients with a small (<15%) primary spontaneous pneumothorax usually require only observation because symptoms are minimal. Supplemental oxygen accelerates the rate at which a pneumothorax resolves by increasing the gradient for nitrogen resorption from the pleural space into the bloodstream. An otherwise healthy, young patient with a small pneumothorax may be managed without hospitalization after 6 hours of observation in an emergency department to determine that the pneumothorax is stable or decreasing in size. Larger primary spontaneous pneumothoraces or expanding pneumothoraces may be treated with insertion of a small-bore (7F–14F) intercostal catheter (213–216) or by simple aspiration. Simple aspiration entails the temporary placement of a needle or narrow-caliber catheter connected to a syringe into the pleural space to withdraw air. Simple aspiration may be successful in 70% of patients, although the need to aspirate more than 2.5 L of air predicts failure of this approach (217). Patients can be observed for several hours and discharged to home if a follow-up chest radiograph demonstrates lung reexpansion.

Patients who fail simple aspiration can be treated with a small-bore catheter attached to a Heimlich valve (215,218), which allows ambulation, or to a water seal device (214,215). The application of suction to a water seal device does not clearly improve outcome (219). We reserve suction for patients with large air leaks and for those whose lungs fail to reexpand under water seal drainage. When a small catheter is used to manage a primary spontaneous pneumothorax, close monitoring is required to ensure tube patency (215). Catheter drainage is successful in 91% of patients with a first-time spontaneous pneumothorax (220). The success rate decreases to 52% in patients with a first recurrence and to 15% for patients with a second recurrence (220).

For patients with a secondary spontaneous pneumothorax, 20F to 28F chest tubes are needed to manage ongoing air leaks and to ensure early lung reexpansion and prompt resolution of the respiratory symptoms. These patients require hospitalization and close monitoring because of the risk for cardiopulmonary decompensation (221).

The air leaks of most patients with a primary spontaneous pneumothorax resolve within the first several days after the initiation of chest tube drainage; 75% to 100% resolve by day 7 to 15 of hospitalization (222,223). The air leaks of only 60% to 79% of patients with a secondary spontaneous pneumothorax resolve by day 15 (222,223). In most patients with a primary spontaneous pneumothorax, therefore, a persistent air leak will resolve without a surgical procedure. The recurrence rate of 30% in patients with a first-time pneumothorax, however, justifies consideration of a pleurodesis procedure after 7 days of hospitalization. Patients may elect to wait 14 days for the air leak to resolve or proceed to pleurodesis earlier to speed recovery and prevent a recurrence (196). We recommend a pleurodesis procedure for all suitable surgical candidates with a secondary pneumotho-

rax because of the potential lethality of a recurrence. Other physicians may elect to wait 14 days before recommending surgery (222).

In patients with a primary or secondary spontaneous pneumothorax, pleurodesis can be performed by instilling a sclerosing agent, such as talc, through a chest tube or by thoracoscopy or a limited thoracotomy (128,131,212,224–229). The American College of Chest Physicians expert consensus panel favors thoracoscopy with resection of bullae and insufflation of talc for pleurodesis (212). No randomized controlled trials have demonstrated the superiority of thoracoscopy over a limited, muscle-sparing thoracotomy. Most experts, however, do not recommend chemical pleurodesis through a chest tube (212).

Conclusions for the Management of Pneumothorax

The management of pneumothorax differs for patients with and without clinically apparent underlying lung disease. Patients with a small (<15%) primary spontaneous pneumothorax do well with observation but benefit from simple aspiration or small-bore catheter drainage to speed recovery from larger pneumothoraces. A pleurodesis procedure to prevent further recurrence is indicated after the first recurrence of a primary spontaneous pneumothorax. Because patients with underlying lung disease tolerate pneumothorax poorly, secondary spontaneous pneumothorax requires catheter drainage. Most clinicians recommend a pleurodesis procedure for the majority of patients with a first episode of secondary spontaneous pneumothorax.

TRAPPED LUNG

Trapped lung is one of the few causes of a persistent benign pleural effusion. This condition develops when the lung is covered by fibrous tissue that prevents it from expanding to the chest wall, so that a persistent fluid-filled space is left (230). Trapped lung is an uncommon consequence of fibrinous or granulomatous pleuritis, in which a fibrous membrane covers the visceral pleura while the lung is removed from the chest wall. Trapped lung may be considered a form of abnormal healing of the pleural space, with the formation of scar tissue on the visceral pleura while the lung is partially collapsed. The diagnosis of trapped lung implies a chronic, constant-volume effusion and a mechanical cause for the persistent fluid-filled pleural space. The protein and LDH concentrations of the pleural fluid in trapped lung are low, consistent with a transudate (89).

It is important to define the difference between a trapped lung and a lung that is "entrapped" by an active inflammatory process. For example, a number of conditions prevent the lung from expanding, such as malignancy involving the visceral pleura or the fibrous peel of an empyema. These conditions are distinguished from trapped lung by the presence of an active pleural process that may be progressive or that may resolve spontaneously or with specific therapy. The mechanism of pleural fluid accumulation in an active inflammatory process or malignant condition is associated with lung entrapment and differs from the mechanism in trapped lung. In patients with a trapped lung, no other explanation can be found for the mechanical restriction of lung expansion or the persistence of a pleural effusion. In contrast, in patients with intense inflammation, as in empyema, other pathophysiologic mechanisms, in addition to the trapped lung, are causing the production of pleural fluid. Therefore, lung entrapment, as in malignancy, can cause a pleural effusion by two mechanisms: (a) a hydrostatic mechanism secondary to the inability of the lung to expand to the chest wall, and (b) a capillary leak or lymphatic obstruction resulting from the malignancy. A trapped lung, however, is caused solely by a failure of lung expansion that results in a hydrostatic imbalance, and no other mechanism of pleural fluid formation is involved. Therefore, a trapped lung produces a transudate and an entrapped lung an exudate.

Causes

A trapped lung develops secondary to pleural inflammation or hemothorax. A pleural effusion must be chronic so that mature fibrous tissue can form on the visceral pleural surface while the pleural spaces remain separated. Conditions associated with the development of a trapped lung include cardiac surgery, infection, inflammation, and malignancy (231–235) (Table 68.11). Because so many cardiac surgical procedures are performed today, especially procedures in which internal mammary artery vascularization is used for coronary bypass grafting, cardiac surgery is now one of the most common causes of trapped lung.

Inadequate management of any of the conditions mentioned in the preceding paragraph, whether therapy of the underlying condition, drainage of the pleural space, or both, should be considered causative in the development of a trapped lung. Some patients present with a trapped lung resulting from a condition for which they never sought medical attention.

Pathophysiology

The generation and removal of pleural fluid in trapped lung take place under normal pleural space conditions, with intact

TABLE 68.11. CAUSES OF TRAPPED LUNG

After cardiac surgery
Complicated parapneumonic effusion/empyema
Postcardiac injury syndrome
Uremic pleuritis
Rheumatoid pleurisy
Tuberculous pleurisy
Malignancy
Pneumothorax therapy for tuberculosis

hydrostatic and oncotic pressure gradients. In trapped lung, the factors promoting the generation and removal of pleural fluid are in equilibrium (236). The loss of lung volume causes a decrease in the pleural pressure and a decrease in the thoracic volume on the affected side. Moderate decreases in lung volume, such as occur in lobar atelectasis or interstitial lung disease or after lobectomy, do not usually cause a pleural effusion; the fact that trapped lung, associated with no greater volume loss, results in a pleural effusion requires explanation. After lobectomy, the remaining lung expands, the diaphragm may be displaced upward, and the pleural space assumes its usual width, with the remaining lung assuming the shape of the thoracic cavity. In trapped lung, the fibroelastic membrane usually involves only the dependent portion of the lung, although the entire lung may be involved. The affected lung is prevented from expanding by the fibrous membrane, and it is also prevented from conforming to the shape of the thoracic cavity. The unaffected lung expands normally during breathing and therefore occupies any void left by the lung that is trapped. For the effusion of a partially trapped lung to persist, the shape of the trapped lung must differ sufficiently from that of the opposing parietal pleural surface, and the unaffected lung must be mechanically prevented from expanding into that space. Otherwise, the space would be obliterated during the reestablishment of negative pleural pressures after resolution of the inflammatory process. Conditions in the pleural effusion of the trapped lung are closer to the conditions along the lobar margins, with wider separation of the pleural surfaces, a steeper pressure gradient, and more negative pressures (237,238).

It has been shown that the mean pleural liquid pressure in patients with trapped lung is initially negative and rapidly and substantially decreases after fluid removal. However, the initial pleural pressures in trapped lung overlap considerably, not only with those in effusions secondary to malignancy but also with those in transudates and exudates not associated with entrapment, in which pressures are occasionally negative; therefore, the specificity of initial pleural pressure measurements is limited for diagnostic purposes (90–92). The pleural space elastance (change in the pleural pressure with the removal of fluid) is consistently higher in trapped lung than in either transudative or exudative effusions unless malignancy or endobronchial obstruction is present. The occasional finding of a negative initial pleural pressure and increased elastance in malignancy is not surprising, given the potential for concomitant lung entrapment (90–93). A negative initial pleural pressure and an elastance of greater than or equal to 25 cm H_2O after 1 L of fluid is removed, in the absence of malignancy or endobronchial obstruction, supports the diagnosis of trapped lung.

Clinical Presentation

Most patients with trapped lung present with a chronic, asymptomatic unilateral pleural effusion. Usually, a history of pleurisy or a remote history of an infection or inflammatory process known to involve the pleural space can be elicited. The thickened visceral pleura of a completely collapsed lung may be seen on the chest CT scan. In an asymptomatic patient, a trapped lung presents a diagnostic dilemma rather than a condition requiring treatment. However, some patients with trapped lung experience varying degrees of dyspnea and exhibit restrictive physiology on pulmonary function testing, and they should be considered for treatment.

Diagnosis

The sole cause of persistent pleural fluid in trapped lung should be hydrostatic imbalance. The detection of malignancy, active infection, intense inflammation, a fibrinous exudate, or blood in the pleural space implies the presence of other causes of fluid accumulation. Thoracentesis with pleural fluid analysis, including cytology, is the first diagnostic step. A sterile, lymphocyte-predominant (usually > 80%) effusion with a low concentration of protein and LDH and without malignant cells is characteristic, but not diagnostic, of trapped lung. The initial pleural liquid pressure is typically negative, usually below 5 cm H_2O, and the pressure drops precipitously during fluid withdrawal (90–92). An initial positive pleural liquid pressure makes the diagnosis unlikely. The fluid volume usually returns to that measured before thoracentesis within 48 to 72 hours after thoracentesis. The patient generally does not experience significant relief after therapeutic thoracentesis. Complete expansion of the lung following thoracentesis is inconsistent with the diagnosis of trapped lung. If the diagnosis is not established and the lung has not expanded after therapeutic thoracentesis, chest CT should be performed to exclude severe parenchymal disease, and fiberoptic bronchoscopy should be considered to exclude endobronchial obstruction. At thoracoscopy, a thin, resilient membrane is seen covering the lung and preventing reexpansion. On histologic examination, mature fibrosis is evident, with few inflammatory cells. If chronicity and stability over time have been demonstrated, trapped lung can be diagnosed with reasonable confidence. These patients often have a history of a persistent pleural effusion for months to years. Complete resolution of the effusion after decortication confirms the diagnosis.

Therapy

A trapped lung can be prevented by appropriate management of the pleural space during the acute inflammatory process. For example, in the setting of a complicated parapneumonic effusion or empyema, appropriate antimicrobial therapy and drainage of the pleural space will usually prevent a fibrous peel from developing over the visceral pleural surface. Effusions following cardiac surgery or secondary to tuberculous pleurisy tend to resolve spontaneously or with drug therapy before visceral pleural fibrosis develops (239). The key point

to remember about trapped lung is that it results in a chronic benign effusion. When a specific active pleural process has been excluded and nothing other than a mechanical cause of the persistent pleural effusion has been found, a decision can be reached regarding therapy. An asymptomatic patient with a partially trapped lung does not appear to be at risk for a secondary infection or other complications and therefore will not benefit from decortication. For a symptomatic patient, the likelihood of symptomatic relief following decortication and the feasibility of surgery should be assessed. If the trapped lung is severely diseased, reexpansion following decortication is unlikely, and therefore surgery should not be expected to result in symptomatic relief. The underlying lung is best assessed with chest CT. When surgery is contemplated, the general health of the patient and the mechanics of the surgery itself must be carefully considered. Ideally, the elastic membrane that covers the visceral pleura can be easily separated from the pleura without creating extensive air leaks. However, at times, the resection plane is lacking, and the likelihood of complications is increased in this setting. CT may be helpful by showing the extension of fibrous tissue from the pleura into the lung parenchyma. In properly selected candidates, decortication can be achieved successfully years after the acute pleural injury has resolved.

Conclusions for Trapped Lung

Trapped lung should be included in the differential diagnosis of a stable, persistent effusion. The diagnosis requires that an active pleural process be excluded. Trapped lung is characterized by failure of the lung to expand after thoracostomy or thoracentesis, an initial negative pleural pressure, and a high degree of pleural space elastance. The fibrous membrane covering the visceral pleura can be demonstrated by CT after replacement of the pleural fluid with air. Asymptomatic patients with trapped lung do not require therapy. Decortication should be considered for patients with dyspnea on exertion and restrictive physiology. Full expansion of the lung and resolution of the pleural effusion after decortication confirm the diagnosis.

HEPATIC HYDROTHORAX

Hepatic hydrothorax results from the transdiaphragmatic migration of ascitic fluid into the pleural space through acquired defects that open when the peritoneal pressure is increased (240). The patient must have documented cirrhosis of the liver without primary pulmonary or cardiac disease. The reported prevalence is 4% to 6%, and in patients with advanced liver disease, it may reach 12% (241,242). Although most patients with hepatic hydrothorax have alcoholic cirrhosis, hepatic hydrothorax can develop in end-stage liver disease of any cause (241).

Pathophysiology

After ascitic fluid forms as a consequence of portal hypertension and hypoalbuminemia, it may move across the diaphragm from the peritoneal to the pleural space. The ascitic fluid may reach the pleural space by convection across the two mesothelial layers. However, the only mechanism for the rapid movement of fluid across the diaphragm that has been demonstrated is through acquired defects in the diaphragm (243). No evidence has been found of the existence of direct lymphatic channels connecting the peritoneal and pleural spaces across the diaphragm. When radioactive contrast is instilled into the peritoneal cavity, the dye enters lymphatics that drain into the mediastinum, but not the pleural space.

The defects are probably the result of thinning and separation of the collagenous fibers of the diaphragm (244). Diaphragmatic defects 1 mm in diameter are more common on the right and tend to develop in the tendinous portion of the diaphragm (245,246). As the peritoneal pressure increases, blebs develop on the mesothelium covering the defects and eventually rupture, forming one-way valves that promote the movement of fluid into the pleural space. A hepatic hydrothorax develops when fluid accumulates in the pleural space more rapidly than it is removed through the parietal pleural lymphatics. In a report from 1997, 85% of hepatic hydrothoraces were found to occur on the right side, 13% on the left, and 2% bilaterally (247).

Diagnosis

A presumptive diagnosis of hepatic hydrothorax can be made in a patient with known cirrhosis, a right-sided pleural effusion, and no cardiac or renal disease. A thoracentesis showing a serous transudate with fewer than 1,000 nucleated cells, predominantly mononuclear cells, a pH above 7.40, and a glucose concentration similar to that of serum supports the clinical diagnosis. In a comparison of pleural and ascitic fluid, the protein and LDH concentrations are similar but tend to be slightly higher in the pleural fluid (241). The definitive diagnosis can be established by the appearance of radionuclide in the pleural space within a few hours after injection into the peritoneal space.

Management

Patients with hepatic hydrothorax have end-stage liver disease, and their management is problematic and often leads to iatrogenic complications.

Medical Management

The initial management of a patient with hepatic hydrothorax should be sodium restriction and the administration of diuretics, including spironolactone. Approximately one third of patients respond transiently to medical management

(248). Prolonged diuretic therapy may result in volume depletion and, subsequently, renal failure. The successful treatment of hepatic hydrothorax with octreotide, an arteriolar vasoconstrictor with preferential action on the splenic vascular bed, has been reported (249). If sodium restriction and diuretics fail, therapeutic paracentesis and thoracentesis may temporarily relieve dyspnea.

Chest tube drainage is ineffective and can cause serious, life-threatening complications (250). Prolonged drainage can be associated with protein, electrolyte, and volume depletion, renal failure, infection, and leakage around the chest tube site after removal. In general, chemical pleurodesis, especially with talc, is effective in the management of nonmalignant pleural effusions (129,157,241). However, the success rate is lowest in hepatic hydrothorax because the rapid movement of ascitic fluid into the pleural space prevents apposition of the two pleural surfaces, which is necessary for pleurodesis (241). Attempts at chemical pleurodesis usually lead to prolonged tube drainage, a long hospital stay, and increased costs.

Surgical Therapy

De Campos and colleagues (251) reported on 24 patients who underwent 29 procedures with VATS and medical thoracoscopy with talc slurry pleurodesis. Only 13 (45%; 95% CI, 28%–63%) of the 29 procedures were effective. Four recurrences developed in the thoracoscopy group; the patients were re-treated, but only one re-treatment was successful. Of the five patients who received talc slurry, recurrence developed in three, and re-treatment was unsuccessful in two. When the diaphragmatic defect cannot be identified, the patient is usually subjected to a prolonged period of drainage, which increases the risk for complications in someone who is extremely ill. However, if the diaphragmatic defect can be visualized, the defect can be patched or treated with fibrin glue followed by talc poudrage, with better results. Although thoracotomy may allow better visualization of the diaphragm and repair of the defect, it should not be the first option; these patients are poor surgical candidates, and the defect may be microscopic and difficult to detect (251).

Transjugular intrahepatic portosystemic shunting (TIPS) was first reported by Strauss and colleagues in 1994 (244). The shunt, which functions similarly to a side-to-side surgical portacaval shunt, creates a decompressive channel between the hepatic and portal veins. TIPS appears to be the best initial approach for patients with refractory hepatic hydrothorax who require frequent thoracenteses (252). The benefit of TIPS is a reduction in the rate of production of ascitic fluid and therefore pleural fluid, so that dyspnea is relieved while general anesthesia and major abdominal surgery are avoided; furthermore, the extrahepatic vascular anatomy is not altered in potential transplant candidates. The success of TIPS is operator-dependent, and when performed by an experienced operator, it is a safe and effective temporizing measure for carefully selected patients with hepatic hydrothorax (253,254).

TIPS is associated with 10% morbidity and 2% mortality; shunt malfunction and hepatic encephalopathy are the two most significant chronic complications (255). Some investigators believe that TIPS should be used to manage hepatic hydrothorax only in patients who are awaiting transplantation (256). There do not appear to be any reliable predictors for a good response to TIPS.

Conclusions for the Management of Hepatic Hydrothorax

No treatment for refractory hepatic hydrothorax appears to be universally effective. VATS to repair an observed diaphragmatic defect with talc poudrage is effective and should be considered for patients who fail medical management. TIPS relieves dyspnea by reducing the production of ascitic fluid and is safe and effective when performed by a skilled operator. Both TIPS and VATS should be considered temporizing measures because the survival of these patients remains poor. The procedures should be considered a bridge to liver transplantation.

HEMOTHORAX

A *hemothorax* is arbitrarily defined as sufficient bleeding into the pleural space to raise the pleural fluid hematocrit to 50% of the peripheral blood hematocrit. A bloody pleural effusion in which the pleural fluid hematocrit is less than 50% of the peripheral blood hematocrit but in which the erythrocyte count is above 100,000/μL is a *hemorrhagic pleural effusion*. A pleural effusion in which the erythrocyte count is below 100,000/μL and the fluid appears pink or red is a *sanguinous pleural effusion*.

Causes

Cases of hemothorax are categorized according to whether they are of traumatic, iatrogenic, or nontraumatic (spontaneous) origin (Table 68.12). Blood enters the pleural space from injured blood vessels in the chest wall, diaphragm, mediastinum, or lung. Prompt drainage is the primary therapy for hemothorax because large volumes of retained blood rapidly form intrapleural loculations and create a risk for empyema and fibrothorax.

Traumatic hemothorax is the result of penetrating or blunt chest trauma. Nearly 50% of patients have an associated pneumothorax, and diaphragmatic injuries are common (257). Initial chest radiographs may fail to demonstrate a pleural effusion. Patients who have sustained significant chest trauma, therefore, require an initial chest radiograph and a second study 24 hours later if a pleural effusion is not initially apparent, or sooner if the peripheral blood hematocrit decreases. The early use of chest CT in patients with chest

TABLE 68.12. CATEGORIZATION AND ETIOLOGY OF HEMOTHORAX

Traumatic
  Penetrating chest trauma
  Blunt chest trauma

Iatrogenic
  Central line insertion
  Esophagoscopy
  Invasive chest wall procedures
  Systemic anticoagulation
  Intrapleural thrombolysis therapy

Nontraumatic (spontaneous)
  Vascular amyloid
  Pulmonary arteriovenous malformation
  Extramedullary hematopoiesis
  Spontaneous rupture of the thoracic aorta
  Ruptured pulmonary infarction
  Endometriosis
  Congenital cystic adenomatoid malformation
  Chronic myeloid leukemia
  Mediastinal tumors
  Ehlers-Danlos syndrome
  Neurofibromatosis
  Aortic pseudocoarctation
  Ruptured internal mammary artery
  Ectopic pregnancy
  Hemodialysis
  Ruptured mediastinal bronchial artery aneurysm
  Costal exostosis
  Pneumothorax
  Pleural metastases
  Idiopathic
  Lymphangiohemangioma
  Chest wall sarcomas
  Lung cancer
  Mycotic aneurysms
  Sarcoidosis
  Lupus
  Idiopathic thrombotic thrombocytopenia

trauma has made it possible to diagnose traumatic hemothorax earlier (257).

Management

Tube thoracostomy with a large-bore chest tube to drain pleural blood is the mainstay of therapy. Chest tubes are used to remove blood, monitor bleeding, and reexpand the lung to promote tamponade of sites of bleeding on the visceral pleura. Patients with traumatic hemothorax complicated by cardiac tamponade, injury to major intrathoracic vessels, sucking chest wounds, major air leaks from bronchopleural fistulae, or ongoing bleeding require thoracotomy or VATS. Thoracoscopy can successfully treat traumatic hemothorax if performed during the first several days, before extensive pleural adhesions form (258). Thoracotomy is reserved for patients with massive hemothorax. Patients with retained blood in the pleural space despite chest tube drainage do not require surgical drainage if the hemothorax occupies less than 30% of the hemithorax (259). Small- to medium-sized hemothoraces resolve without causing pleural restriction. Some patients with retained intrapleural blood have been successfully treated with the intrapleural instillation of fibrinolytic agents (260). Pleural effusions commonly develop after a chest tube placed to manage a hemothorax has been removed (261). These nonspecific exudates should be evaluated by thoracentesis to exclude pleural infection. Hemothorax progresses to fibrothorax in only 1% of cases, most often in patients with hemopneumothorax and empyema. In most instances, pleural thickening that develops after hemothorax has been treated resolves spontaneously within 3 to 6 months.

Iatrogenic hemothoraces occur most often after an intrathoracic artery or vein has been perforated during placement of a central venous catheter. Hemothorax can also develop as a complication of invasive diagnostic procedures, such as thoracentesis, transbronchial biopsy, percutaneous lung biopsy, and pleural biopsy. Hemothorax is a rare complication in patients receiving anticoagulant therapy with heparin (262) or warfarin (263), and in patients undergoing intrapleural fibrinolytic therapy (55). Iatrogenic hemothorax is managed by chest tube drainage; thoracoscopy or thoracotomy is considered for patients with ongoing hemorrhage. Anticoagulation is reversed in patients with hemothorax secondary to anticoagulant therapy.

Nontraumatic or spontaneous hemothorax affects patients with a variety of acquired and congenital conditions (262). Patients may be managed initially with chest tube placement and observation; surgical intervention is undertaken for those with ongoing hemorrhage.

Conclusions for Hemothorax

Hemothorax has multiple traumatic iatrogenic, and spontaneous causes. Confirmation of a pleural fluid hematocrit that is 50% of the peripheral blood hematocrit establishes the clinical diagnosis. Patients with hemothorax require placement of a chest tube to monitor intrapleural bleeding and remove pleural blood, which increases the risk for the development of empyema and pleural fibrosis with pulmonary restriction.

CORTICOSTEROID TREATMENT OF PLEURAL DISEASE

Several pleural diseases have been reported to respond to corticosteroid therapy. The data are derived primarily from case reports or small case series. Small randomized controlled studies have been reported only in tuberculous pleurisy (Table 68.13).

Rheumatoid Pleurisy

Pleural involvement is the most common thoracic manifestation of rheumatoid arthritis, with an incidence of 5% (264,265); however, autopsy series show a 40% to 70% incidence of pleuritis (266). The clinicopathologic difference suggests either that patients are asymptomatic or that antiinflammatory medications mask pleural symptoms. The prototypic patient with rheumatoid pleurisy is a man older than 45 years of age with subcutaneous nodules (264,265). Although a pleural effusion may develop at any time during the course of rheumatoid arthritis, the onset is most often within 5 years after the appearance of articular manifestations, although in approximately 20% of patients, the effusion develops before or simultaneously with the disease (265).

Rheumatoid effusions are typically unilateral and small-to medium-sized, but they can be large or massive. Effusions can be transient, chronic, or relapsing (265,267). It is uncommon for an effusion to resolve in less than 1 month, the time to resolution being most typically 3 to

TABLE 68.13. CORTICOSTEROID THERAPY IN PLEURAL DISEASE

Disease	Response	Evidence	Recommendations
Rheumatoid pleurisy	Variable	Case reports	Early systemic or intrapleural trial
Lupus pleuritis	Resolution of symptoms and effusion in 1–2 wk	Small case series	Prednisone 60–80 mg qd and taper when inflammation resolves
Postcardiac injury syndrome	Resolution of symptoms and effusion in 1–2 wk	Case reports	Prednisone 40–60 mg qd with taper over 2–4 wk if symptoms persist after nonsteroidal antiinflammatory drugs
Sarcoidosis	Resolution of symptoms and effusion by 2 wk	Case reports	Prednisone 20–40 mg qd and taper over 2–4 wk for symptomatic patients
Tuberculous pleurisy	May reduce resolution time and symptoms; no effect on residual pleural thickening	Three randomized clinical trials with different methodologies	Routine use of steroids not recommended; prednisone 20–40 mg qd with antituberculosis medications if acute severe symptoms

4 months (264,265,268). Approximately half of patients have a protracted course that lasts from 7 months to 5 years (264,265,268); occasionally, patients' progression to severe pleural thickening and trapped lung necessitates decortication (235,264).

No controlled studies have evaluated the effectiveness of corticosteroids or nonsteroidal antiinflammatory drugs in the management of rheumatoid pleural effusions. Both systemic and intrapleural corticosteroids have been used with variable results (264,265,269–274). The degree of inflammation in the pleural space and joints does not determine the response to therapy. In the 50% of patients with a protracted course, effective therapy may prevent the development of trapped lung. Because it is not possible to predict which patients will have a protracted course by clinical variables, a reasonable strategy is to institute either systemic or intrapleural corticosteroids early in the disease process. If the patient appears to respond clinically, then therapy should be continued for several weeks before being stopped. If the effusion does not resolve or recurs, therapeutic thoracentesis and intrapleural steroids should be considered.

Lupus Pleuritis

Pleural inflammation is a common feature of systemic lupus erythematosus and is virtually always associated with chest pain with or without a pleural effusion (275–277). The incidence of pleural effusion is 45% to 55% during the course of the disease (276,277). Pleural effusions are more common in women and are usually a later manifestation of the disease, but they may be the presenting feature in 5% of patients (276,278,279). The effusions are usually small- to medium-sized and bilateral, although unilateral and massive effusions have been reported (275,278).

In contrast to the pleural effusions of rheumatoid pleurisy, those of lupus pleuritis resolve rapidly with corticosteroid therapy. Hunder and colleagues (272) reported that the pleural effusions of five of six patients resolved quickly with corticosteroid therapy; the effusion of the sixth patient resolved gradually after 6 months of therapy. Winslow and colleagues (278) reported that the effusions of 11 patients treated with corticosteroids resolved in less than 2 weeks, whereas only 10 of 16 effusions cleared at 2 weeks without corticosteroid therapy. Others have reported that effusions resolved in 7 days to 6 weeks with the daily administration of 20 to 30 mg of prednisone (280–282).

Based on small case series and clinical experience, patients with lupus pleuritis should be treated with 60 to 80 mg of prednisone and the dose rapidly tapered once the acute inflammation has resolved. Massive effusions refractory to steroid therapy have been reported rarely. Responses have been reported after the addition of a second immunosuppressive drug, such as cyclophosphamide or azathioprine. Alternative treatments for refractory cases have also included intravenous immunoglobulins (283), chemical pleurodesis with tetracycline (284) and talc (157), and pleurectomy (285).

Postcardiac Injury Syndrome

Postcardiac injury syndrome occurs days, weeks, or months after an array of myocardial or pericardial injuries (286). It has been reported after cardiac surgery (286–289), myocardial infarction (290,291), blunt chest trauma (292,293), pacemaker implantation (294,295), and angioplasty (296,297). This immunologic syndrome is manifested by pericarditis, fever, leukocytosis, an increased erythrocyte sedimentation rate, and pulmonary infiltrates and pleural effusions (286). The incidence is highest after cardiac surgery (range, 17%–31%) (288,289,295,298), with pleural effusions occurring in 47% (95% CI, 31%–63%) (299) to 68% (95% CI, 52%–81%) (289) of those with the syndrome. The reported incidence of postcardiac injury syndrome after myocardial infarction is 1% to 7% (290,291,300), with effusions occurring in 40% (95% CI, 26%–55%) (300) to 68% (95% CI, 52%–81%) (289) of patients.

The pleural effusions resolve during a variable period, depending on the response to antiinflammatory drugs. The effusions of patients who have had a myocardial infarction are reported to resolve within 1 to 5 weeks with nonsteroidal antiinflammatory drugs or prednisone (290,300). Although spontaneous resolution after cardiac surgery usually occurs by 2 months, the effusions of some patients resolve within 3 weeks with antiinflammatory drugs (289). Although salicylates and other nonsteroidal antiinflammatory drugs are usually effective in these patients, some require corticosteroid therapy for the treatment of more severe forms of postcardiac injury syndrome. The response is usually rapid, and tapering of the prednisone is typically successful within a 2- to 4-week period.

Sarcoidosis

Pleural involvement is an uncommon manifestation of sarcoidosis, with the incidence of pleural effusions ranging from 0 to 7.5% (301–304). Patients in whom a pleural effusion develops usually have extensive parenchymal disease and extrathoracic manifestations (301–304). The chest radiograph typically shows a unilateral, small- to medium-sized effusion, but bilateral and massive effusions have been reported (301,303–306). Pleural sarcoidosis is diagnosed in the proper clinical setting after tuberculosis and fungal disease have been excluded.

Sarcoid pleural effusions may resolve spontaneously, or corticosteroids may be required. The time to spontaneous resolution is variable, but most effusions resolve within 1 to 3 months (302,303,307,308). Resolution after 2 weeks with steroid therapy (305,309) and after as long as 6 months with or without steroids (302,309) has been reported.

The management of sarcoid pleural effusions should be individualized based on the clinical presentation. A small effusion in an asymptomatic patient usually resolves spontaneously. If a patient is symptomatic or the effusion is recurrent, corticosteroid therapy should be administered to relieve symptoms and enhance resolution of the effusion. Incomplete resolution of a sarcoid pleural effusion with progression to chronic pleural thickening has been reported (304).

Tuberculous Pleural Effusions

The incidence of tuberculous pleural effusions varies from 4.0% (95% CI, 3.7%–4.0%) of all cases of tuberculosis in the United States (310) to 23% (95 CI, 20%–26%) in Spain (311). The chest radiograph typically shows a small-to medium-sized unilateral effusion, although massive effusions have been reported in 14% to 29% of patients with primary disease (312–315). Bilateral effusions occur in approximately 10% of cases and are more commonly seen in patients who are HIV-positive (313,315,316).

Tuberculous effusions resolve spontaneously in 8 to 16 weeks. When the effusions were left untreated, pulmonary or extrapulmonary tuberculosis developed in 19 (65%) of 141 of patients within 5 years (312). Therapy with isoniazid and rifampin for 6 months was effective in patients who were not HIV-infected, with a relapse rate of zero after a mean follow-up of 3 years (317,318); the radiographs showed complete resolution by 6 months, but no data were provided on the resolution rate of the pleural effusions. With a 9-month course of isoniazid and rifampin, pleural effusions resolved within 6 weeks, although pleural thickening sometimes persisted (319).

The currently recommended treatment for tuberculous pleural effusions is isoniazid, rifampin, and pyrazinamide for 2 months, followed by isoniazid and rifampin for the next 4 months (320). In 75% of cases, the effusions resolve after 6 months of therapy, with a relapse rate of zero at 20 months (321). During the initial weeks of therapy, the effusions may enlarge in a small minority of patients; however, this does not imply treatment failure (322).

Corticosteroids have been advocated as adjunctive therapy to hasten the resolution of symptoms and the resorption of pleural fluid and to prevent pleural thickening. Three randomized, double-blinded, placebo-controlled trials have been reported, but they had important methodologic differences. Lee and colleagues (323) treated patients with isoniazid, rifampin, and ethambutol for the initial 3 months and with isoniazid and rifampin for the subsequent 6 to 9 months; one group received prednisolone (0.75 mg/kg per day) and the other placebo. Diagnostic thoracentesis was performed on the first day of hospitalization. The pleural effusion in the 21 patients who received corticosteroids resolved after a mean of 55 days, whereas the mean time to resolution in the 19 patients who did not receive corticosteroids was 123 days ($P < .01$). The authors did not observe a significant

difference between the groups with respect to residual pleural thickening. Galarza and colleagues (324) treated patients with isoniazid and rifampin for 6 months and either prednisone (1 mg/kg per day) or placebo. The pleural effusions of all patients were drained by thoracentesis to equal amounts of approximately one third of the hemithorax. The resorption rates at 1 month were 93% (95% CI, 83%–97%) in the corticosteroid group and 89% (95% CI, 78%–94%) in the placebo group ($P = .01$); however, the difference between groups disappeared thereafter. No difference was found between the groups with respect to residual pleural thickening. Wyser and colleagues (325) treated patients with isoniazid, rifampin, and pyrazinamide for 6 months and then 34 patients with prednisone (0.75 mg/kg per day) and 36 patients with placebo. The effusions of all patients were completely drained via thoracoscopy. No differences in symptoms, rates of recurrence of the effusion after drainage, or residual pleural thickening were observed between the groups.

Based on the current data, the routine use of corticosteroids is not recommended; they should be used only if patients have acute, severe symptoms, such as fever, chest pain, and dyspnea. A reasonable strategy is to perform a diagnostic and therapeutic thoracentesis, especially in patients with large pleural effusions, with an attempt made to evacuate as much fluid as possible, and to initiate antituberculous chemotherapy.

Conclusions for the Corticosteroid Treatment of Pleural Disease

Patients with lupus pleuritis, who virtually all have symptoms, should be treated with corticosteroids; this therapy typically results in a rapid resolution of symptoms and effusions. In most patients with sarcoid pleural effusions, the effusions are small and asymptomatic and do not require therapy; however, when patients have dyspnea and chest pain, the response to corticosteroids is significant and rapid. Patients with acute rheumatoid pleural effusions should probably be given a trial of corticosteroid therapy, with tapering of the dose during several weeks if the response is good. If patients with postcardiac injury syndrome do not respond to nonsteroidal antiinflammatory drugs, corticosteroids should be instituted and tapered during 2 to 4 weeks. Patients with tuberculous pleurisy should be treated with corticosteroids only if they have acute, severe symptoms and only under the umbrella of antituberculous chemotherapy.

REFERENCES

1. Light RW, MacGregor I, Luchsinger PC, et al. Pleural effusion: the diagnostic separation of transudates and exudates. *Ann Intern Med* 1972;77:507–513.
2. Heffner JE, Brown LK, Barbieri C. Diagnostic value of tests that discriminate between exudative and transudative pleural effusions. *Chest* 1997;111:970–980.

3. Chakko SC, Caldwell SH, Sforza PP. Treatment of congestive heart failure. Its effect on pleural fluid chemistry. *Chest* 1989;95: 798–802.

4. Heffner JE, Sahn SA, Brown LK. Multilevel likelihood ratios for identifying exudative pleural effusions. *Chest* 2002;121(6): 1916–1920.

5. Sackett DL, Haynes RB, Tugwell P. *Clinical epidemiology, a basic science for clinical medicine,* 2nd ed. Boston: Little, Brown and Company, 1991.

6. Taryle DA, Potts DE, Sahn SA. The incidence of clinical correlates of parapneumonic effusion in pneumococcal pneumonia. *Chest* 1978;74:170–173.

7. Smith JA, Mullerworth MH, Westlake GW, et al. Empyema thoracis: 14-year experience in a teaching center. *Ann Thorac Surg* 1991;51:39–42.

8. Forty J, Yeatman M, Wells FC. Empyema thoracis: a review of a 4 1/2 year experience of cases requiring surgical treatment. *Respir Med* 1990;84:147–153.

9. Antony VB, Godbey SW, Holm KA, et al. Mesothelial cell derived epithelial neutrophil activating protein-78 (ENA-78): a major neutrophil chemokine in parapneumonic effusions. *Am J Respir Crit Care Med* 1996;153:A44.

10. Andrews NC, Parker EF, Shaw RR, et al. Management of nontuberculous empyema. *Am Rev Respir Dis* 1962;85:935–936.

11. Ashbaugh DG. Empyema thoracis. Factors influencing morbidity and mortality. *Chest* 1991;99:1162–1165.

12. Rasmussen OS, Boris P. Ultrasound-guided puncture of pleural fluid collections and superficial thoracic masses. *Eur J Radiol* 1989;9:91–92.

13. Müller NL. Imaging of the pleura. *Radiology* 1993;186:297–309.

14. Stark DD, Federle MP, Goodman PC, et al. Differentiating lung abscess and empyema: radiography and computed tomography. *AJR Am J Roentgenol* 1983;141:163–167.

15. Alfageme I, Munoz F, Pena N, et al. Empyema of the thorax in adults. Etiology, microbiologic findings, and management. *Chest* 1993;103:839–843.

16. Bryant RE, Salmon CJ. Pleural empyema. *Clin Infect Dis* 1996; 22:747–762.

17. Drury M, Anderson W, Heffner JE. Diagnostic value of pleural fluid cytology in occult Boerhaave's syndrome. *Chest* 1992; 102:976–978.

18. Niederman MS, Mandell LA, Anzueto A, et al. Guidelines for the management of adults with community-acquired pneumonia. Diagnosis, assessment of severity, antimicrobial therapy, and prevention. *Am J Respir Crit Care Med* 2001;163:1730–1754.

19. Teixeira LR, Vargas FS, Carmo AO, et al. Effectiveness of sodium hydroxide as a pleural sclerosing agent in rabbits: influence of concomitant intrapleural lidocaine. *Lung* 1996;174:325–332.

20. Thys JP, Vanderhoeft P, Herchuelz A, et al. Penetration of aminoglycosides in uninfected pleural exudates and in pleural empyemas. *Chest* 1988;93:530–532.

21. Ferguson AD, Prescott RJ, Selkon JB, et al. The clinical course and management of thoracic empyema. *QJM* 1996;89:285–289.

22. Himmelman RB, Callen PW. The prognostic value of loculations in parapneumonic pleural effusions. *Chest* 1986;90:852–856.

23. Chen KY, Liaw YS, Wang HC, et al. Sonographic septation: a useful prognostic indicator of acute thoracic empyema. *J Ultrasound Med* 2000;19:837–843.

24. Aquino SL, Webb WR, Gushiken BJ. Pleural exudates and transudates: diagnosis with contrast-enhanced CT. *Radiology* 1994;192:803–808.

25. Takasugi JE, Godwin DJ, Teefey SA. The extrapleural fat in empyema: CT appearance. *Br J Radiol* 1991;64:580–583.

26. Waite RJ, Carbonneau RJ, Balikian JP, et al. Parietal pleural changes in empyema: appearance at CT. *Radiology* 1990;175: 145–150.

27. Braman SS, Donat WE. Explosive pleuritis: manifestation of group A beta-hemolytic streptococcal infection. *Am J Med* 1986; 81:723–726.

28. Watanakunakorn C. Staphylococcal aureus pneumonia. *Scand J Infect Dis* 1987;19:624–627.

29. Bartlett JG, Finegold SM. Anaerobic infections of the lung and pleural space. *Am Rev Respir Dis* 1974;110:56–77.

30. Torres A, Serra-Batlles J, et al. Severe community-acquired pneumonia: epidemiology and prognostic factors. *Am Rev Respir Dis* 1991;144:312–318.

31. Taryle D, Good JT Jr, Sahn SA. Metabolic activity of pleural fluid: possible role in production of pleural fluid acidosis. *J Lab Clin Med* 1979;93:1041–1046.

32. Good JT Jr, Taryle DA, Maulitz RM, et al. The diagnostic value of pleural fluid pH. *Chest* 1980;78:55–59.

33. Sahn SA, Reller LB, Taryle DA, et al. The contribution of leukocytes and bacteria to the low pH of empyema fluid. *Am Rev Respir Dis* 1983;128:811–815.

34. Sahn SA, Taryle DA, Good JT Jr. Time course and pathogenesis of pleural fluid acidosis and low pleural fluid glucose. *Am Rev Respir Dis* 1979;120:355–361.

35. Heffner JE, Brown LK, Barbieri C, et al. Pleural fluid chemical analysis in parapneumonic effusions. A meta-analysis. *Am J Respir Crit Care Med* 1995;151:1700–1708.

36. Colice GL, Curtis A, Deslauriers J, et al. Medical and surgical treatment of parapneumonic effusions: an evidence-based guideline. *Chest* 2000;118:1158–1171.

37. Storm HKR, Krasnik M, Bang K, et al. Treatment of pleural empyema secondary to pneumonia: thoracocentesis regimen versus tube drainage. *Thorax* 1992;47:821–824.

38. Pothula V, Krellenstein DJ. Early aggressive surgical management of parapneumonic empyemas. *Chest* 1994;105:832–836.

39. Varkey B, Rose HD, Kutty CP, et al. Empyema thoracis during a ten-year period. Analysis of 72 cases and comparison to a previous study (1952–1967). *Arch Intern Med* 1981;141:1771–1776.

40. VanSonnenberg E, Nakamoto SK, Mueller PR, et al. CT-and ultrasound-guided catheter drainage of empyemas after chest-tube failure. *Radiology* 1984;151:349–353.

41. Mathiesen DJ. A surgeon's view of interventional radiology in general thoracic surgery patients. *Semin Intervent Radiol* 1991;8:85–87.

42. Milliken JS, Moore EE, Steiner E, et al. Complications of tube thoracostomy for acute trauma. *Am J Surg* 1980;140:738–741.

43. Klein JS, Schultz S, Heffner JE. Interventional radiology of the chest: image-guided percutaneous drainage of pleural effusions, lung abscess, and pneumothorax [see Comments]. *AJR Am J Roentgenol* 1995;164:581–588.

44. White CS, Meyer CA, Templeton PA. CT fluoroscopy for thoracic interventional procedures. *Radiol Clin North Am* 2000;38:303–322.

45. Moulton JS. Image-guided management of complicated pleural fluid collections. *Radiol Clin North Am* 2000;38:345–374.

46. Simpson G, Roomes D, Heron M. Effects of streptokinase and deoxyribonuclease on viscosity of human surgical and empyema pus. *Chest* 2000;117:1728–1733.

47. Chin NK, Lim TK. Controlled trial of intrapleural streptokinase in the treatment of pleural empyema and complicated parapneumonic effusions. *Chest* 1997;111:275–279.

48. Davies RJO, Traill ZC, Gleeson FV. Randomized, controlled trial of intrapleural streptokinase in community-acquired pleural infection. *Thorax* 1997;52:416–421.

49. Wait MA, Sharma S, Hohn J, et al. A randomised trial of empyema therapy. *Chest* 1997;111:1548–1551.

50. Bouros D, Schiza S, Patsourakis G, et al. Intrapleural streptokinase versus urokinase in the treatment of complicated parapneumonic effusions: a prospective, double-blind study. *Am J Respir Crit Care Med* 1997;155:291–295.

51. Cameron R. Intra-pleural fibrinolytic therapy vs. conservative management in the treatment of parapneumonic effusions and empyema. *Cochrane Data Base Syst Rev* 2000;3:CD002312.

52. Davies CW, Lok S, Davies RJ. The systemic fibrinolytic activity of intrapleural streptokinase. *Am J Respir Crit Care Med* 1998;157:328–330.

53. Fraedrich G, Hofmann D, Effenhauser P, et al. Instillation of fibrinolytic enzymes in the treatment of pleural empyema. *Thorac Cardiovasc Surg* 1982;30:36–38.

54. Berglin E, Ekroth R, Teger-Nilsson A-C, et al. Intrapleural instillation of streptokinase: effects on systemic fibrinolysis. *Thorac Cardiovasc Surg* 1981;29:124–126.

55. Srivastava P, Godden DJ, Kerr KM, et al. Fatal haemorrhage from aortic dissection following instillation of intrapleural streptokinase. *Scott Med J* 2000;45:86–87.

56. Alfageme I, Vazquez R. Ventricular fibrillation after intrapleural UK. *Intensive Care Med* 1997;23:352.

57. Godley PJ, Bell RC. Major hemorrhage following administration of intrapleural streptokinase. *Chest* 1984;86:486–487.

58. Temes RT, Follis F, Kessler RM, et al. Intrapleural fibrinolytics in the management of empyema thoracis. *Chest* 1996;110:102–106.

59. Frye MD, Jarratt M, Sahn SA. Acute hypoxemic respiratory failure following intrapleural thrombolytic therapy for hemothorax. *Chest* 1994;105:1595–1596.

60. Ali I, Unruh H. Management of empyema thoracis. *Ann Thorac Surg* 1990;50:355–359.

61. Cunniffe MG, Maguire D, McAnena OJ, et al. Video-assisted thoracoscopic surgery in the management of loculated empyema. *Surg Endosc* 2000;14:175–178.

62. Lackner RP, Hughes R, Anderson LA, et al. Video-assisted evacuation of empyema is the preferred procedure for the management of pleural space infections. *Am J Surg* 2000;179:27–30.

63. Mackinlay TAA, Lyons GA, Chimondeguy DJ, et al. VATS debridement versus thoracotomy in the treatment of loculated postpneumonia empyema. *Ann Thorac Surg* 1996;61:1626–1630.

64. Landreneau RJ, Keenan RJ, Hazelrigg SR, et al. Thoracoscopy for empyema and hemothorax [see Comments]. *Chest* 1996;109:18–24.

65. Karmey-Jones R, Sorenson V, Horst M, et al. Rigid thoracoscopic debridement and continuous pleural irrigation in the management of empyema. *Chest* 1997;111:272–274.

66. Lawrence DR, Ohri SK, Moxon RE, et al. Thoracoscopic debridement of empyema thoracis. *Ann Thorac Surg* 1997;64:1448–1450.

67. Angelillo-Mackinlay T, Lyons GA, Piedras MB, et al. Surgical treatment of postpneumonic empyema. *World J Surg* 1999;23:1110–1113.

68. Muskett A, Burton NA, Karwande SV, et al. Management of refractory empyema with early decortication. *Am J Surg* 1988;156:529–532.

69. Spagnuolo PJ, Paune VD. Clostridial pleuropulmonary infection. *Chest* 1980;78:622–625.

70. Fishman NH, Ellertson DG. Early pleural decortication for thoracic empyema in immunosuppressed patients. *J Thorac Cardiovasc Surg* 1981;74:537–541.

71. Mayo P. Early thoracotomy and decortication for nontuberculous empyema in adults with and without underlying disease: a twenty-five year review. *Am Surg* 1985;51:230–236.

72. Miller JI, Jr. The history of surgery of empyema, thoracoplasty, Eloesser flap, and muscle flap transposition. *Chest Surg Clin N Am* 2000;10:45–53.

73. Shapiro MP, Gale ME, Daly BDT. Eloesser window thoracostomy for treatment of empyema: radiographic appearance. *AJR Am J Roentgenol* 1988;150:549–552.

74. Statement of the American Thoracic Society. Management of malignant pleural effusions. *Am J Respir Crit Care Med* 2000;162:1987–2001.

75. Heffner JE, Nietert PJ, Barbieri C. Pleural fluid pH as a predictor of survival for patients with malignant pleural effusions. *Chest* 2000;117:79–86.

76. Jiang W. *In vitro* models of cancer invasion and metastasis: recent developments. *Eur J Surg Oncol* 1994;20:493–499.

77. Zetter B. Adhesion molecules in tumor metastasis. *Semin Cancer Biol* 1993;4:219–229.

78. Verheul HMW, Hoekman K, Jorna AS, et al. Targeting vascular endothelial growth factor blockade: ascites and pleural effusion formation. *Oncology* 2000;5:45–50.

79. Chernow B, Sahn SA. Carcinomatous involvement of the pleura: an analysis of 96 patients. *Am J Med* 1977;63:695–702.

80. Meyer PC. Metastatic carcinoma of the pleura. *Thorax* 1966;21:437–443.

81. Rodriguez-Panadero F, Borderas-Naranjo F, Lopez-Mejias J. Pleural metastatic tumours and effusions. Frequency and pathogenic mechanisms in a post-mortem series. *Eur J Respir Dis* 1989;2:366–369.

82. Sahn SA. Malignant pleural effusions. In: Fishman AP, Elias JA, Fishman JA, et al., eds. *Pulmonary diseases and disorders*, 3rd ed. New York: McGraw-Hill, 1998:1429–1438.

83. Estenne M, Yernault JC, Detroyer A. Mechanism of relief of dyspnea after thoracentesis in patients with large pleural effusions. *Am J Med* 1983;74:813–819.

84. Burrows CM, Mathews C, Colt HG. Predicting survival in patients with recurrent symptomatic malignant pleural effusions. An assessment of the prognostic values of physiologic, morphologic, and quality-of-life measures of extensive disease. *Chest* 2000;117:73–78.

85. Sahn SA, Good JT Jr. Pleural fluid pH in malignant effusions. Diagnostic, prognostic, and therapeutic implications. *Ann Intern Med* 1988;108:345–349.

86. Livingston RB, McCracken JD, Trauth CJ, et al. Isolated pleural effusion in small-cell lung carcinoma: favorable prognosis. *Chest* 1982;81:208–210.

87. Fentiman IS, Rubens RD, Hayward JL. Control of pleural effusions in patients with breast cancer. *Cancer* 1983;52:737–739.

88. Xaubet A, Diumenjo MC, Marin A, et al. Characteristics and prognostic value of pleural effusions in non-Hodgkin's lymphomas. *Eur J Respir Dis* 1985;66:135–140.

89. Doelken P, Sahn SA. Trapped lung. *Semin Respir Crit Care Med* 2001;22:631–635.

90. Light RW, Jenkinson SG, Minh V, et al. Observations on pleural pressures as fluid is withdrawn during thoracentesis. *Am Rev Respir Dis* 1980;121:799–804.

91. Light RW, Stansbury DW, Brown SE. The relationship between pleural pressures and changes in pulmonary function after therapy to thoracentesis. *Am Rev Respir Dis* 1986;133:658–661.

92. Villena V, Lopez-Encuentra A, Pozo F, et al. Management of pleural pressures during therapeutic thoracentesis. *Am J Respir Crit Care Med* 2001;162:1534–1538.

93. Lan RS, Lo SK, Chuang ML, et al. Elastance of the pleural space: a predictor for the outcome of pleurodesis in patients with malignant pleural effusion. *Ann Intern Med* 1997;126:768–774.

94. Lambert CJ, Shah HH, Urschel HC, et al. The treatment of

malignant pleural effusions by closed trocar tube drainage. *Ann Thorac Surg* 1967;3:1–5.

95. Anderson CB, Philpott GW, Ferguson TB. The treatment of malignant pleural effusions. *Cancer* 1974;33:916–922.

96. Izbicki R, Weyhing BT III, Baker L, et al. Pleural effusion in cancer patients. A prospective randomized study of pleural drainage with the addition of radioactive phosphorus to the pleural space vs. pleural drainage alone. *Cancer* 1975;36:1511–1518.

97. Sorensen PG, Svendsen TL, Enk B. Treatment of malignant pleural effusion with drainage, with and without instillation of talc. *Eur J Respir Dis* 1984;65:131–135.

98. Groth G, Gatzemeier U, Haussingen K, et al. Intrapleural palliative treatment of malignant pleural effusions with mitoxantrone versus placebo (pleural tube alone). *Ann Oncol* 1991;2:213–215.

99. Walker-Renard PB, Vaughan LM, Sahn SA. Chemical pleurodesis for malignant pleural effusions. *Ann Intern Med* 1994;120:56–64.

100. Kennedy L, Sahn SA. Talc pleurodesis for the treatment of pneumothorax and pleural effusion [see Comments]. *Chest* 1994;106:1215–1222.

101. Yim AP, Chan AT, Lee TW, et al. Thoracoscopic talc insufflation versus talc slurry for symptomatic malignant pleural effusion [see Comments]. *Ann Thorac Surg* 1996;62:1655–1658.

102. Walsh FW, Alberts M, Solomon DA, et al. Malignant pleural effusions: pleurodesis using small-bore catheter. *South Med J* 1989;82:963–972.

103. Parker LA, Charnock GC, Delany DJ. Small-bore catheter drainage and sclerotherapy for malignant effusions. *Cancer* 1989;64:1218–1221.

104. Morrison MC, Mueller PR, Lee MJ, et al. Sclerotherapy of malignant pleural effusion through sonographically placed small-bore catheters. *AJR Am J Roentgenol* 1992;158:41–43.

105. Goff BA, Mueller PR, Muntz HG, et al. Small chest-tube drainage followed by bleomycin sclerosis from malignant pleural effusions. *Obstet Gynecol* 1993;81:993–996.

106. Seaton KG, Patz EFJ, Goodman PC. Palliative treatment of malignant pleural effusions: value of small-bore catheter thoracostomy and doxycycline sclerotherapy. *AJR Am J Roentgenol* 1995;164:589–591.

107. Patz EF, Jr, McAdams HP, Goodman PC, et al. Ambulatory sclerotherapy for malignant pleural effusions. *Radiology* 1996;199:133–135.

108. Hsu WH, Chiang CD, Chen CY, et al. Ultrasound-guided small-bore Elecath tube insertion for the rapid sclerotherapy of malignant pleural effusion. *Jpn J Clin Oncol* 1998;28:187–191.

109. Patz EF, Jr, McAdams HP, Erasmus JJ, et al. Sclerotherapy for malignant pleural effusions. A prospective randomized trial of bleomycin versus doxycycline with small-bore catheter drainage. *Chest* 1998;113:1305–1311.

110. Thompson RL, Yau JC, Donnelly RF, et al. Pleurodesis with iodized talc for malignant effusions using pigtail catheters. *Ann Pharmacother* 1998;32:739–742.

111. Marom EM, Patz EF Jr, Erasmus JJ, et al. Malignant pleural effusions. Treatment with small-bore-catheter thoracostomy and talc pleurodesis. *Radiology* 1992;210:277–281.

112. Bloom AI, Wilson MW, Kerlan RK Jr, et al. Talc pleurodesis through small-bore percutaneous tubes. *Cardiovasc Intervent Radiol* 1999;22:433–438.

113. Saffran L, Ost DE, Fein AM, et al. Outpatient pleurodesis of malignant pleural effusions using a small-bore pigtail catheter. *Chest* 2000;118:417–421.

114. Lorch DG, Gordon L, Wooten S, et al. Effect of patient positioning on the distribution of tetracycline in the pleural space during pleurodesis. *Chest* 1988;93:527–529.

115. Dryzer SR, Allen ML, Strange C, et al. A comparison of rotation and nonrotation in tetracycline pleurodesis. *Chest* 1993;104:1763–1766.

116. Heuvel van den MM, Smit HJ, Barbierato SB, et al. Talc-induced inflammation in the pleural cavity. *Eur Respir J* 1988;12:1419–1423.

117. Chappell AG, Johnson A, Charles WJ, et al. A survey of the long-term effects of talc and kaolin pleurodesis. *Br J Dis Chest* 1979;73:285–288.

118. Lange P, Mortensen J, Groth S. Lung function 22 to 25 years after the treatment of idiopathic spontaneous pneumothorax with talc poudrage or simple drainage. *Thorax* 1988;43:559–561.

119. Viskum K, Lange P, Mortensen J. Long-term sequelae after talc pleurodesis for spontaneous pneumothorax. *Pneumologie* 1989;43:105–106.

120. Paul JS, Geattie EJ, Blades B. Lung function studies in the poudrage treatment of recurrent spontaneous pneumothorax. *J Thorac Surg* 1951;22:52–61.

121. Knowles JH, Storey CF. Effects of pleural talc poudrage on pulmonary function. *J Thorac Surg* 1957;340:250–256.

122. Kennedy L, Rusch VW, Strange C, et al. Pleurodesis using talc slurry. *Chest* 1994;106:342–346.

123. Viallat JR, Rey F, Astoul P, et al. Thoracoscopic talc poudrage pleurodesis for malignant effusions. A review of 360 cases [see Comments]. *Chest* 1996;110:1387–1393.

124. De Campos JRM, Werebe EC, Vargas FS, et al. Respiratory failure due to insufflated talc. *Lancet* 1997;349:251–252.

125. Petrou M, Kaplan D, Goldstraw P. Management of recurrent malignant pleural effusions. The complementary role of talc pleurodesis and pleuroperitoneal shunting. *Cancer* 1995;75:801–805.

126. Weissberg D, Ben-Zeev I. Talc pleurodesis: experience with 360 patients. *J Thorac Cardiovasc Surg* 1993;106:689–695.

127. Rehse DH, Aye RW, Florence MG. Respiratory failure following talc pleurodesis. *Am J Surg* 1999;177:437–440.

128. De Campos JR, Vargas FS, De Campos Werebe E, et al. Thoracoscopy talc poudrage: a 15-year experience. *Chest* 2001;119:801–806.

129. Glazer M, Berkman N, Lafair JS, et al. Successful talc slurry pleurodesis in patients with nonmalignant pleural effusion. *Chest* 2000;117:1404–1409.

130. Sudduth CD, Sahn SA. Pleurodesis for nonmalignant pleural effusions: recommendations. *Chest* 1992;102:1855–1860.

131. Cardillo G, Facciolo F, Giunti R, et al. Video thoracoscopic treatment of primary spontaneous pneumothorax: a 6-year experience. *Ann Thorac Surg* 2000;69:357–361.

132. Mares DC, Mathur PN. Medical thoracoscopic talc pleurodesis for chylothorax due to lymphoma. *Chest* 1998;114:731–735.

133. Rinaldo JE, Owens GR, Rodgers RM. Adult respiratory distress syndrome following the intrapleural instillation of talc. *J Thorac Cardiovasc Surg* 1983;85:523–526.

134. Bouchama A, Chastre J, Gaudiched A, et al. Acute pneumonitis with bilateral pleural effusion after talc pleurodesis. *Chest* 1984;86:795–797.

135. Lineau C, Le Coz A, Quinquenel ML, et al. Acute respiratory insufficiency after pleural talcage of pneumothorax. Apropos of a case. *Rev Pneumol Clin* 1993;49:153–155.

136. Ferrer J, Villarino MA, Tura JM, et al. Comparison of size and composition of nine different talcs. Its relevance for pleurodesis. *Am J Respir Crit Care Med* 1998;157:A66.

137. Shaffer JP, Allen JN, Prior RB. Detection of endotoxin in talc preparations used for pleurodesis. *Chest* 2000;118:130S.

138. Rodriguez-Panadero F, Lopez Mejias J. Low glucose and pH levels in malignant pleural effusions. Diagnostic significance and

prognostic value in respect to pleurodesis. *Am Rev Respir Dis* 1989;139:663–667.

139. Sanchez-Armengol A, Rodriguez-Panadero F. Survival and talc pleurodesis in metastatic pleural carcinoma, revisited. *Chest* 1993;104:1482–1485.

140. Heffner JE, Nietert PJ, Barbieri C. Pleural fluid pH as a predictor of pleurodesis failure. *Chest* 2000;117:87–95.

141. Putnam JB Jr, Light RW, Rodrigues RM, et al. A randomized comparison of indwelling pleural catheter and doxycycline pleurodesis in the management of malignant pleural effusion. *Cancer* 1999;86:1992–1999.

142. Putnam JB Jr, Walsh GL, Swisher SG, et al. Outpatient management of malignant pleural effusion by a chronic indwelling pleural catheter. *Ann Thorac Surg* 2000;69:369–375.

143. Martini N, Bains M, Beattie EJ Jr. Indications for pleurectomy in malignant effusions. *Cancer* 1975;35:734–738.

144. Fry WA, Khandekar JD. Parietal pleurectomy for malignant pleural effusion. *Ann Thorac Oncol* 1995;2:160–164.

145. Waller DA, Morritt GN, Forty J. Video-assisted thoracoscopic pleurectomy in the management of malignant pleural effusion. *Chest* 1995;107:1454–1456.

146. Rodriguez-Panadero F, Antony VB. Pleurodesis: state of the art. *Eur Respir J* 1997;10:1648–1654.

147. Antony VB, Godbey SW, Kunkel SL, et al. Recruitment of inflammatory cells to the pleural space. Chemotactic cytokines, IL-8, and monocyte chemotactic peptide-1 in human pleural fluids. *J Immunol* 1993;151:7216–7223.

148. Antony VB, Hott JW, Kunkel SL, et al. Pleural mesothelial cell expression of C-C (monocyte chemotactic peptide) and C-X-C (interleukin-8) chemokines. *Am J Respir Crit Care Med* 1995;12:581–588.

149. Antony VB, Rothfuss KJ, Godbey SW, et al. Mechanism of tetracycline hydrochloride–induced pleurodesis: tetracycline hydrochloride–stimulated mesothelial cells produced a growth factor–like activity for fibroblasts. *Am Rev Respir Dis* 1992;146:1009–1013.

150. Godbey SW, Holm KA, Yu L, et al. Role of mesothelial cell in pleural fibrosis following successful talc poudrage: identification of basic fibroblast growth factor (FGF-2) in pleural fluids. *Am J Respir Crit Care Med* 1995;151:A353.

151. Dryzer SR, Joseph J, Baumann M, et al. Early inflammatory response of minocycline and tetracycline on the rabbit pleura. *Chest* 1993;104:1585–1588.

152. Agrenius V, Chmielewska J, Widström O, et al. Increased coagulation activity of the pleura after tube drainage and quinacrine instillation in malignant pleural effusion. *Eur Respir J* 1991;4:1135–1139.

153. Good JT Jr, Taryle DA, Hyers TM, et al. Clotting and fibrinolytic activity of pleural fluid in a model of pleural adhesions. *Am Rev Respir Dis* 1978;118:903–908.

154. Strange C, Baumann MA, Sahn SA, et al. Effects of intrapleural heparin or urokinase on the extent of tetracycline-induced pleural disease. *Am J Respir Crit Care Med* 1995;151:508–515.

155. Agrenius V, Chmielewska J, Widstrom O, et al. Pleural fibrinolytic activity is decreased in inflammation as demonstrated in the quinacrine pleurodesis treatment of malignant pleural effusion. *Am Rev Respir Dis* 1989;140:1381–1385.

156. Rodriguez-Panadero F, Segado A, Martin Juan J, et al. Failure of talc pleurodesis is associated with increased pleural fibrinolysis. *Am J Respir Crit Care Med* 1995;151:785–790.

157. Vargas FS, Milanez JR, Filomeno LT, et al. Intrapleural talc for the prevention of recurrence in benign or undiagnosed pleural effusions. *Chest* 1994;106:1771–1775.

158. Aelony Y, King R, Boutin C. Thoracoscopic talc poudrage pleu-

rodesis for chronic recurrent pleural effusions. *Ann Intern Med* 1991;115:778–782.

159. Webb WR, Ozmen V, Moulder PV, et al. Iodized talc pleurodesis for the treatment of pleural effusions. *J Thorac Cardiovasc Surg* 1992;103:881–885.

160. Staats BA, Ellefson RD, Budahn LL, et al. The lipoprotein profile of chylous and nonchylous pleural effusions. *Mayo Clin Proc* 1980;55:700–704.

161. Valentine VG, Raffin TA. The management of chylothorax. *Chest* 1992;102:586–591.

162. Ryu JH, Havermann TM. Pulmonary lymphoma: primary and secondary disease. *Semin Respir Crit Care Med* 1997;18:341–352.

163. Johnstone DW, Feins RH. Chylothorax. *Chest Surg Clin N Am* 1994;4:617–628.

164. Taylor JR, Ryu J, Colby TV, et al. Lymphangioleiomyomatosis. Clinical course in 32 patients. *N Engl J Med* 1990;323:1254–1260.

165. Smith S, Schulman A, Weir EK, et al. Lymphatic abnormalities in Noonan syndrome. *S Afr Med J* 1979;56:271–274.

166. Faul JL, Bery GJ, Colby TV, et al. Thoracic lymphangiomas, lymphangiectasis, lymphangiomatosis, and lymphatic dysplasia syndrome. *Am J Respir Crit Care Med* 2000;161:1037–1046.

167. Staats BA. Lipid metabolism. In: Chretien J, Bignon J, Hirsch A, eds. *Pleura in health and disease*. New York: Marcel Dekker Inc, 1985:287–307.

168. Yoffey JM, Cortice FC. *Lymphatics, lymph, and lymphoid tissue*. Cambridge: Harvard University Press, 1956.

169. Miller JI, Jr. Diagnosis and management of chylothorax: techniques of mediastinal surgery. *Chest Surg Clin N Am* 1996;6:139–148.

170. Serif NS, Cohen ML, Samuel P, et al. Chylothorax: diagnosis by lipoprotein electrophoresis of serum and pleural fluid. *Thorax* 1977;32:98–100.

171. Jensen GL, Mascili EA, Meyer LP, et al. Dietary modification of chyle composition in chylothorax. *Gastroenterology* 1989;97:761–765.

172. Marts BC, Naunheim KS, Fiore AC, et al. Conservative versus surgical management of chylothorax. *Am J Surg* 1992;164:532–534.

173. Beghetti M, Lascala G, Belli D, et al. Etiology and management of pediatric chylothorax. *J Pediatr* 2000;136:653–658.

174. Demos NJ, Kozel J, Scerbos JE. Somatostatin in the treatment of chylothorax. *Chest* 2001;119:964–966.

175. Cope C. Diagnosis and treatment of postoperative chyle leakage via percutaneous transabdominal catheterization of the cisterna chyli: a preliminary study. *J Vasc Intervent Radiol* 1998;9:727–734.

176. Lampson RS. Traumatic chylothorax: a review of the literature and report of a case treated by mediastinal ligation of the thoracic duct. *J Thorac Surg* 1948;17:778–791.

177. Mason PF, Ragoowansi RH, Thorpe JAC. Post-thoracotomy chylothorax: a cure in the abdomen? *Eur J Cardiothorac Surg* 1997;11:567–570.

178. Graham DD, McGahren ED, Tribble CG, et al. Use of video-assisted thoracic surgery in the treatment of chylothorax. *Ann Thorac Surg* 1994;57:1507–1512.

179. Selle JG, Snyder WH, Schreiber JT. Chylothorax: indications for surgery. *Ann Surg* 1973;177:245–249.

180. Cerfolio RJ, Allen MS, Deschamps C, et al. Postoperative chylothorax. *J Thorac Cardiovasc Surg* 1996;112:1361–1366.

181. Merigliano S, Molena D, Ruol A, et al. Chylothorax complicating esophagectomy for cancer: a plea for early thoracic duct ligation. *J Thorac Cardiovasc Surg* 2000;119:453–457.

182. Dugue L, Sauvanet A, Farges O, et al. Output of chyle as an

indicator of treatment for chylothorax complicating oesophagectomy. *Br J Surg* 1998;85:1147–1149.

183. Robinson CLN. The management of chylothorax. *Ann Thorac Surg* 1985;39:90–95.

184. Browse NL, Allen DR, Wilson NM. Management of chylothorax. *Br J Surg* 1997;84:1711–1716.

185. Murphy MC, Newman VM, Rodgers BM. Pleuroperitoneal shunts in the management of persistent chylothorax. *Ann Thorac Surg* 1989;48:195–200.

186. Little A, Kadowaki M, Ferguson M, et al. Pleuroperitoneal shunting: alternative therapy for pleural effusions. *Ann Surg* 1988;208:443–450.

187. Melton LJ 3rd, Hepper NG, Offord KP. Incidence of spontaneous pneumothorax in Olmsted County, Minnesota: 1950 to 1974. *Am Rev Respir Dis* 1979;120:1379–1382.

188. Bense L, Eklund G, Wiman LG. Smoking and the increased risk of contracting spontaneous pneumothorax. *Chest* 1987;92:1009–1012.

189. Primrose WR. Spontaneous pneumothorax: a retrospective review of aetiology, pathogenesis and management. *Scott Med J* 1984;29:15–20.

190. Nkere UU, Griffin SC, Fountain SW. Pleural abrasion: a new method of pleurodesis. *Thorax* 1991;46:596–598.

191. Hazelrigg SR, Landreneau RJ, Mack M, et al. Thoracoscopic stapled resection for spontaneous pneumothorax. *J Thorac Cardiovasc Surg* 1993;105:389–392.

192. Inderbitzi RG, Leiser A, Furrer M, et al. Three years' experience in video-assisted thoracic surgery (VATS) for spontaneous pneumothorax. *J Thorac Cardiovasc Surg* 1994;107:1410–1415.

193. Smit HJ, Wienk MA, Schreurs AJ, et al. Do bullae indicate a predisposition to recurrent pneumothorax? *Br J Radiol* 2000;73:356–359.

194. Mitlehner W, Friedrich M, Dissmann W. Value of computed tomography in the detection of bullae and blebs in patients with primary spontaneous pneumothorax. *Respiration* 1992;59:221–227.

195. Lesur O, Delorme N, Fromaget JM, et al. Computed tomography in the etiologic assessment of idiopathic spontaneous pneumothorax. *Chest* 1990;98:341–347.

196. Sahn SA, Heffner JE. Spontaneous pneumothorax. *N Engl J Med* 2000;342:868–874.

197. Ohata M, Suzuki H. Pathogenesis of spontaneous pneumothorax. With special reference to the ultrastructure of emphysematous bullae. *Chest* 1980;77:771–776.

198. Light RW, O'Hara VS, Moritz TE, et al. Intrapleural tetracycline for the prevention of recurrent spontaneous pneumothorax. *JAMA* 1990;264:2224–2230.

199. Brynes TA, Brevig JK, Yeoh CB. Pneumothorax in patients with acquired immunodeficiency syndrome. *J Thorac Cardiovasc Surg* 1989;98:546–550.

200. Lewis JG. Eosinophilic granuloma and its variants with special reference to lung involvement: a report of 12 patients. *QJM* 1964;33:337–359.

201. Joseph J, Sahn SA. Thoracic endometriosis syndrome: new observations from an analysis of 110 cases. *Am J Med* 1996;100:164–170.

202. Seremetis MG. The management of spontaneous pneumothorax. *Chest* 1970;57:65–68.

203. Tanaka F, Itoh M, Esaki H, et al. Secondary spontaneous pneumothorax. *Ann Thorac Surg* 1993;55:372–376.

204. Dines DE, Clagett OT, Payne WS. Spontaneous pneumothorax in emphysema. *Mayo Clin Proc* 1970;45:481–487.

205. Shields TW, Oilschlager GA. Spontaneous pneumothorax in patients 40 years of age and older. *Ann Thorac Surg* 1966;2:377–383.

206. George RB, Herbert SJ, Shames JM, et al. Pneumothorax complicating pulmonary emphysema. *JAMA* 1975;234:389–393.

207. Bradley M, Williams C, Walshaw MJ. The value of routine expiratory chest films in the diagnosis of pneumothorax. *Ann Emerg Med* 1991;8:115–116.

208. Bourgouin P, Cousineau G, Lemire P, et al. Computed tomography used to exclude pneumothorax in bullous lung disease. *J Can Assoc Radiol* 1985;36:341–342.

209. Schramel FM, Postmus PE, Vanderschueren RG. Current aspects of spontaneous pneumothorax [see Comments]. *Eur Respir J* 1997;10:1372–1379.

210. Lippert HL, Lund O, Blegvad S, et al. Independent risk factors for cumulative recurrence rate after first spontaneous pneumothorax. *Eur Respir J* 1991;4:324–331.

211. Videm V, Pillgram-Larsen J, Ellingsen O, et al. Spontaneous pneumothorax in chronic obstructive pulmonary disease: complications, treatment and recurrences. *Eur J Respir Dis* 1987;71:365–371.

212. Baumann MH, Strange C, Heffner JE, et al. Management of spontaneous pneumothorax: an American College of Chest Physicians Delphi consensus statement. *Chest* 2001;119:590–602.

213. Martin T, Fontana G, Olak J, et al. Use of pleural catheter for the management of simple pneumothorax. *Chest* 1996;110:1169–1172.

214. Minami H, Saka H, Senda K, et al. Small-caliber catheter drainage for spontaneous pneumothorax. *Am J Med Sci* 1992;304:345–347.

215. Conces DJ, Tarver RD, Gray WC, et al. Treatment of pneumothoraces utilizing small-caliber chest tubes. *Chest* 1988;94:55–57.

216. Casola G, VanSonnenberg E, Keightley A, et al. Pneumothorax: radiologic treatment with small catheters. *Radiology* 1988;166:89–91.

217. Soulsby T. British Thoracic Society guidelines for the management of spontaneous pneumothorax: do we comply with them and do they work? *J Accid Emerg Med* 1998;15:317–321.

218. Ponn RB, Silverman HJ, Federico JA. Outpatient chest tube management. *Ann Thorac Surg* 1997;64:1437–1440.

219. So SY, Yu DY. Catheter drainage of spontaneous pneumothorax: suction or no suction, early or late removal? *Thorax* 1982;37:46–48.

220. Jain SK, Al-Kattan KM, Hamdy MG. Spontaneous pneumothorax: determinants of surgical intervention. *J Cardiovasc Surg (Torino)* 1998;39:107–111.

221. Chee CB, Abisheganaden J, Yeo JK, et al. Persistent air-leak in spontaneous pneumothorax—clinical course and outcome. *Respir Med* 1998;92:757–761.

222. Schoenenberger RA, Haefeli WE, Weiss P, et al. Timing of invasive procedures in therapy for primary and secondary spontaneous pneumothorax. *Arch Surg* 1991;126:764–766.

223. Weissberg D, Refaely Y. Pneumothorax: experience with 1,199 patients. *Chest* 2000;117:1279–1285.

224. Yim AP, Ng CS. Thoracoscopy in the management of pneumothorax. *Curr Opin Pulm Med* 2001;7:210–214.

225. Noppen M. Management of primary spontaneous pneumothorax: does cause matter? *Monaldi Arch Chest Dis* 2001;56:344–348.

226. Lang-Lazdunski L, De Kerangal X, Pons F, et al. Primary spontaneous pneumothorax: one-stage treatment by bilateral videothoracoscopy. *Ann Thorac Surg* 2000;70:412–417.

227. Baumann MH. Treatment of spontaneous pneumothorax. *Curr Opin Pulm Med* 2000;6:275–280.

228. Ayed AK, Al-Din HJ. The results of thoracoscopic surgery for primary spontaneous pneumothorax. *Chest* 2000;118:235–238.

229. Heffner JE, McDonald J, Barbieri C, et al. Management of parapneumonic effusions. An analysis of physician practice patterns. *Arch Surg* 1995;130:433–438.

230. Stead WW, Eichenholz A, Stauss H-K. Operative and pathologic findings in twenty-four patients with the syndrome of idiopathic pleurisy with effusion, presumably tuberculosis. *Am Rev Tuberc Pulm Dis* 1955;71:473–502.

231. Farber JE, Lincoln NS. The unexpandable lung. *Am Rev Tuberc* 1939;47:704–709.

232. Young D, Simon J, Pomerantz M. Current indications for and status of decortication for "trapped lung." *Ann Thorac Surg* 1972;14:631–634.

233. Kollef MH, Peller T, Knodel A, et al. Delayed pleuropulmonary complications following coronary artery revascularization with the internal mammary artery. *Chest* 1988;94:68–71.

234. Berger HW, Rammohan G, Neff MS, et al. Uremic pleural effusion. A study in 14 patients on chronic dialysis. *Ann Intern Med* 1975;82:362–364.

235. Brunk JR, Drash EC, Swineford O. Rheumatoid pleuritis successfully treated with decortication: report of a case and review of the literature. *Am J Med Sci* 1966;251:545–551.

236. Black LF. The pleural space and pleural fluid. *Mayo Clin Proc* 1972;47:493–506.

237. Lai-Fook SJ. Mechanics of the pleural space: fundamental concepts. *Lung* 1987;165:249–267.

238. Boggs DS, Kinasewitz GT. Pathophysiology of the pleural space. *Am J Med Sci* 1995;309:53–59.

239. Cohen M, Sahn SA. Resolution of pleural effusions. *Chest* 2001;119:1547–1562.

240. Zenda T, Miyamoto S, Murata S, et al. Detection of diaphragmatic defect as the cause of severe hepatic hydrothorax with magnetic resonance imaging. *Am J Gastroenterol* 1998;93:2288–2289.

241. Alberts WM, Salem AJ, Solomon DA, et al. Hepatic hydrothorax: cause and management. *Arch Intern Med* 1991;151:2383–2388.

242. Gordon FD, Anastopoulos HT, Crenshaw W, et al. The successful treatment of symptomatic, refractory hepatic hydrothorax with transjugular intrahepatic portosystemic shunt. *Hepatology* 1997;25:1366–1369.

243. Lieberman FL, Hidemura R, Peters RL, et al. Pathogenesis and treatment of hydrothorax complicating cirrhosis with ascites. *Ann Intern Med* 1966;64:341–351.

244. Strauss RM, Martin LG, Kaufman SL, et al. Transjugular intrahepatic portal systemic shunt for the management of symptomatic cirrhotic hydrothorax. *Am J Gastroenterol* 1994;94:1520–1522.

245. Giacobbe A, Facciorusso D, Barbano F, et al. Hepatic hydrothorax: diagnosis and management. *Clin Nucl Med* 1996;21:56–60.

246. Kirschner PA. Porous diaphragm syndromes. *Chest Surg Clin N Am* 1998;8:449–472.

247. Strauss RM, Boyer TD. Hepatic hydrothorax. *Semin Liver Dis* 1997;17:227–232.

248. Haitjema T, Maat CEM. Pleural effusion without ascites in a patient with cirrhosis. *Neth J Med* 1994;44:207–209.

249. Dumortier J, Lepetre J, Scalone O, et al. Successful treatment of hepatic hydrothorax with octreotide. *Eur J Gastroenterol Hepatol* 2000;12:817–820.

250. Runyon BA, Greenblatt M, Ming RHC. Hepatic hydrothorax is a relative contraindication to chest tube insertion. *Am J Gastroenterol* 1986;81:566–567.

251. De Campos JRM, Filho LOA, De Campos Werebe E, et al. Hepatic hydrothorax. *Semin Respir Crit Care Med* 2001;22:665–673.

252. Degawa M, Hamasaki K, Yano K, et al. Refractory hepatic hydrothorax treated with transjugular intrahepatic portosystemic shunt. *J Gastroenterol* 1999;34:123–131.

253. Rossle M, Siegerstetter V, Huber M, et al. The first decade of the transjugular intrahepatic portosystemic shunt (TIPS): state of the art. *Liver* 1998;18:73–89.

254. Jeffries MA, Kazanjian S, Wilson M, et al. Transjugular intrahepatic portosystemic shunts in liver transplantation in patients with refractory hepatic hydrothorax. *Liver Transpl Surg* 1998;4:416–423.

255. Freedman AM, Sanyal AJ, Tisnado J, et al. Complications of transjugular intrahepatic portosystemic shunt: a comprehensive review. *Radiographics* 1993;13:1185–1210.

256. Ong JP, Sands M, Younossi ZM. Transjugular hepatic portosystemic shunts TIPS: a decade later. *J Clin Gastroenterol* 2000;30:14–28.

257. Guerrero-Lopez F, Vazquez-Mata G, Alcazar-Romero PP, et al. Evaluation of the utility of computed tomography in the initial assessment of the critical care patient with chest trauma. *Crit Care Med* 2000;28:1370–1375.

258. Ambrogi MC, Lucchi M, Dini P, et al. Videothoracoscopy for the evaluation and treatment of hemothorax. *J Cardiovasc Surg (Torino)* 2002;43:109–112.

259. Coselli JS, Mattox KL, Beall AC, Jr. Reevaluation of early evacuation of clotted hemothorax. *Am J Surg* 1984;148:786–790.

260. Aye RW, Froese DP, Hill LD. Use of purified streptokinase in empyema and hemothorax. *Am J Surg* 1991;161:560–562.

261. Wilson JM, Boren CH Jr, Peterson SR, et al. Traumatic hemothorax: is decortication necessary? *J Thorac Cardiovasc Surg* 1979;77:489–495.

262. Martinez FJ, Villanueva AG, Pickering R, et al. Spontaneous hemothorax. Report of 6 cases and review of the literature. *Medicine (Baltimore)* 1992;71:354–368.

263. Kollef MH, Gronski TJ. Hemothorax and an abdominal hematoma after treatment of ischemic cardiomyopathy with warfarin. *Heart Lung* 1994;23:125–127.

264. Horler AR, Thompson M. The pleural and pulmonary complications of rheumatoid arthritis. *Ann Intern Med* 1959;50:1179–1203.

265. Walker WC, Wright V. Rheumatoid pleuritis. *Ann Rheum Dis* 1967;26:467–474.

266. Baggenstoss AH, Rosenberg EF. Visceral lesions associated with chronic infectious rheumatoid arthritis. *Arch Pathol* 1943;35:503–516.

267. Jones JS. An account of pleural effusions, pulmonary nodules and cavities attributable to rheumatoid disease. *Br J Dis Chest* 1978;72:39–56.

268. Carr DT, Mayne JG. Pleurisy with effusion in rheumatoid arthritis, with reference to the low concentration of glucose in pleural fluid. *Am Rev Respir Dis* 1962;85:345–350.

269. Campbell GD, Ferrington E. Rheumatoid pleuritis with effusion. *Dis Chest* 1968;53:521–527.

270. Jurik AG, Grudal H. Pleurisy in rheumatoid arthritis. *Scand J Rheumatol* 1983;12:75–80.

271. Faurschou P, Francis D, Faarup P. Thoracoscopic, histologic, and clinical findings in nine cases of rheumatoid pleural effusion. *Thorax* 1985;40:371–375.

272. Hunder GG, McDufie FC, Heppern GG. Pleural fluid complement in systemic lupus erythematosus in rheumatoid arthritis. *Ann Intern Med* 1972;76:357–362.

273. Russell ML, Gladman DD, Mintz S. Rheumatoid pleural effusion: lack of response to intrapleural corticosteroids. *J Rheumatol* 1986;13:412–415.

274. Chapman PT, O'Donnell JL, Moller PW. Rheumatoid pleural

effusion: response to intrapleural corticosteroids. *J Rheumatol* 1992;19:478–480.

275. Good JT Jr, King TE, Antony VB, et al. Lupus pleuritis. Clinical features and pleural fluid characteristics with special reference to pleural fluid antinuclear antibodies. *Chest* 1983;84:714–718.

276. Harvey AM. Systemic lupus erythematosus: a review of the literature and clinical analysis of 138 patients. *Medicine* 1954;33:291–437.

277. Dubois EL. *Lupus erythematosus: a review of the current status of discoid and systemic lupus erythematosus and their variance,* 2nd ed. New York: McGraw-Hill, 1974.

278. Winslow WA, Ploss LN, Loitman B. Pleuritis in systemic lupus erythematosus: its importance as an early manifestation in diagnosis. *Ann Intern Med* 1958;49:70–88.

279. Alacon-Segovia D, Alarcon DG. Pleuro-pulmonary manifestations of systemic lupus erythematosus in the U.S. *Dis Chest* 1961;39:7–17.

280. Bouros D, Panagou P, Papandreou L, et al. Massive bilateral pleural effusion as the first presentation of systemic lupus erythematosus. *Respiration* 1992;59:173–175.

281. Wang D, Chang D, Kuo S, et al. Systemic lupus erythematosus presenting as pleural effusion: report of a case. *J Formos Med Assoc* 1995;94:746–749.

282. Goel MK, Banavaliker JN, Bhalotra B. An uncommon presentation of systemic lupus erythematosus. *Indian J Chest Dis Allied Sci* 1996;38:119–122.

283. Ben-Chetrit E, Putterman C, Naparstek Y. Lupus refractory pleural effusion: transient response to intravenous immunoglobulins. *J Rheumatol* 1991;18:1635–1637.

284. McKnight KM, Adair NE, Agudelo CA. Successful use of tetracycline pleurodesis to treat massive pleural effusion secondary to systemic erythematosus. *Arthritis Rheum* 1991;34:1483–1484.

285. Bell R, Lawrence S. Chronic pleurisy in systemic lupus erythematosus treated with pleurectomy. *Br J Dis Chest* 1979;73:314–316.

286. Stelzner TJ, King TE, Antony VB, et al. The pleuropulmonary manifestations of the postcardiac injury syndrome. *Chest* 1983;84:383–387.

287. Ito T, Engle MA, Goldberg HP. Postpericardiotomy syndrome after surgery for nonrheumatic heart disease. *Circulation* 1958;17:549–556.

288. Engle MA, Zabriskie JB, Senterfit LB, et al. Postpericardiotomy syndrome: a new look at an old condition. *Mod Concepts Cardiovasc Dis* 1975;44:59–64.

289. Kiminsky ME, Rodan BA, Osborne DR, et al. Postpericardiotomy syndrome. *Am J Roentgenol* 1982;138:503–508.

290. Dressler W. The post-myocardial-infarction syndrome. *Arch Intern Med* 1959;103:28–42.

291. Liem KL, Ten Veen JH, Lie KI, et al. Incidence and significance of heart-muscle antibodies in patients with acute myocardial infarction and unstable angina. *Acta Med Scand* 1979;206:473–475.

292. Tabatznik B, Isaacs JP. Postpericardiotomy syndrome after traumatic hemopericardium. *Am J Cardiol* 1961;7:83–96.

293. Weigand L, Zwillich CW. The post-cardiac injury syndrome following blunt chest trauma. *J Trauma* 1993;34:445–447.

294. Hargreaves M, Bashir Y. Postcardiotomy syndrome after transvenous pacemaker insertion. *Eur Heart J* 1994;15:1005–1007.

295. Miller GL, Coccio EB, Sharma SC. Postpericardiotomy syndrome and cardiac tamponade after transvenous pacemaker placement. *Clin Cardiol* 1996;19:255–256.

296. Escaned J, Ahmad RA, Shiu MF. Pleural effusion after coronary perforation during balloon angioplasty: an unusual presentation

of the postpericardiotomy syndrome. *Eur Heart J* 1992;13:716–717.

297. Velander M, Grip L, Mogensen L. The post-cardiac injury syndrome after percutaneous transluminal coronary angioplasty. *Clin Cardiol* 1993;16:353–354.

298. Soloff LA, Zatuchni J, Janton OH, et al. Reactivation of rheumatic fever after mitral commissurotomy. *Circulation* 1953;8:481–493.

299. Nishimura RA, Fuster V, Burgert S, et al. Clinical features in long-term natural history of the postpericardiotomy syndrome. *Int J Cardiol* 1983;4:443–450.

300. Toole JC, Silverman ME. Pericarditis of acute myocardial infarction. *Chest* 1975;67:647–653.

301. Chusid EL, Siltzbach LE. Sarcoidosis of the pleura. *Ann Intern Med* 1974;81:190–194.

302. Sharma OP, Gordonson J. Pleural effusion in sarcoidosis: a report of six cases. *Thorax* 1975;30:95–101.

303. Beekman JF, Simmert SM, Chun BK, et al. Spectrum of pleural involvement in sarcoidosis. *Arch Intern Med* 1976;136:323–330.

304. Wilen SB, Rabinowitz JG, Ulreich S, et al. Pleural involvement in sarcoidosis. *Am J Med* 1974;57:200–209.

305. Johnson NM, Martin NDT, McNicol MW. Sarcoidosis presenting with pleurisy and bilateral pleural effusions. *Postgrad Med J* 1980;56:266–267.

306. Claiborne RA, Kerby G. Pleural sarcoidosis with massive pleural effusion in lung entrapment. *Kans Med* 1990;91:103–105.

307. Nicholls AJ, Friend JAR, Legge JS. Sarcoid pleural effusions: three cases and review of the literature. *Thorax* 1980;35:277–281.

308. Serloos O. Exudative pleurisy and sarcoidosis. *Br J Dis Chest* 1996;60:191–196.

309. De Vuyst P, De Troyer A, Yernault JC. Bloody pleural effusion in a patient with sarcoidosis. *Chest* 1979;76:607–609.

310. Reider HL, Snider DE Jr, Cauthen GM. Extrapulmonary tuberculosis in the United States. *Am Rev Respir Dis* 1990;141:437–451.

311. Vidal R, De Garcia J, Ruiz J, et al. Estudio contralata des 637 patientes: tuberculosis: diagnostico y resultatos terapeuticos con esquemas de nine y six meses. *Med Clin (Barc)* 1986;87:368–370.

312. Roper WH, Waring JJ. Primary serofibrinous pleural effusion in military personnel. *Am Rev Tuberc* 1955;71:616–635.

313. Sibley JC. A study of 200 cases of tuberculous pleurisy with effusion. *Am Rev Tuberc* 1950;62:314–323.

314. Chan CHS, Arnold M, Chan CY, et al. Clinical and pathological features of tuberculous pleural effusion and its long-term consequences. *Respiration* 1991;58:171–175.

315. Epstein DM, Cline LR, Albelda SM, et al. Tuberculous pleural effusions. *Chest* 1987;91:106–109.

316. Richter C, Perenboom R, Mtoni I, et al. Clinical features of HIV-seropositive and HIV-seronegative patients with tuberculous pleural effusions in Dar es Salaam, Tanzania. *Chest* 1994;106:1471–1476.

317. Dutt AK, Moers D, Stead WW. Tuberculous pleural effusion: six-month therapy with isoniazid and rifampin. *Am Rev Respir Dis* 1992;145:1429–1432.

318. Canete C, Galarza I, Granados A, et al. Tuberculous pleural effusion: experience with six months of treatment with isoniazid and rifampicin. *Thorax* 1994;49:1160–1161.

319. Matthay RA, Neff TA, Iseman MD. Tuberculous pleural effusions developing during chemotherapy for pulmonary tuberculosis. *Am Rev Respir Dis* 1974;109:469–472.

320. Bass JB, Farer LS, Hopewell P, C., et al. Treatment of tuberculosis and tuberculous infection in adults and children. *Am J Respir Crit Care Med* 1994;149:1359–1374.

321. Ormerod LP, McCarthy OR, Rudd RM, et al. Short-course chemotherapy for tuberculous pleural effusion in

culture-negative pulmonary tuberculosis. *Tuberc Lung Dis* 1995;
76:25–27.

322. Al-Majed S. Study of paradoxical response to chemotherapy in tuberculous pleural effusion. *Respir Med* 1996;90:211–214.

323. Lee C, Wang W, Lan R, et al. Corticosteroids in the treatment of tuberculous pleurisy: a double-blind, placebo-controlled, randomized study. *Chest* 1988;94:1256–1259.

324. Galarza I, Canete C, Granados A, et al. A randomised trial of corticosteroids in the treatment of tuberculous pleurisy. *Thorax* 1995;50:1305–1307.

325. Wyser C, Walz LG, Smedema JP, et al. Corticosteroids in the treatment of tuberculous pleurisy: a double-blind, placebo-controlled, randomized study. *Chest* 1996;110:333–338.

326. Leuallen EC, Carr DT. Pleural effusion, a statistical study of 436 patients. *N Engl J Med* 1955;1955:79–83.

327. Light RW. *Pleural diseases,* 3rd ed. Baltimore: Williams & Wilkins, 1995:38–39.

328. Joseph J, Badrinath P, Basran G, et al. Is the pleural fluid transudate or exudate? A revisit of the diagnostic criteria. *Thorax* 2001;56:867–870.

Pathophysiology of Sleep-Disordered Breathing

69

Safwan Badr · Kingman P. Strohl

Sleep-disordered breathing (SDB) involves a collection of medical disorders characterized by intermittent disruptions in breathing and gas exchange during sleep. According to cross-sectional studies, SDB is common, and a conservative estimate is that 2% of people in the community could be candidates for treatment on the basis of the sequelae of SDB, i.e., excessive daytime sleepiness, cardiac co-morbidity, and cognitive dysfunction (1). In addition, there are epidemiological data to suggest that snoring (partial upper airway obstruction during sleep) is associated with risks for common diseases such as systemic hypertension, myocardial infarction, and diabetes (2–5). Finally, a positive association between SDB and motor vehicle accidents exists, and treatment of SDB reduces this risk to that found in the general population (6–8). Clearly, SDB has an important medical and social impact on the community.

The purpose here is to describe elements in the physiology of sleep and breathing and factors relevant to clinical management of SDB (see Chapter 70). The focus will be on those factors that are particularly relevant to the goals of treatment, whether it be restoring respiratory rhythm or upper airway patency, and modifiable preclinical risk.

DEFINITIONS

Diagnosis of SDB depends on observations of respiratory rate and depth during sleep (9, 10). Three patterns of apnea, i.e., cessation of breathing, can be observed during sleep. These are schematically shown in Figure 69.1. A central apnea

S. Badr: Pulmonary, Critical Care, and Sleep Medicine, Department of Internal Medicine, Wayne State University School of Medicine; and Section of Pulmonary and Critical Care, Harper Hospital, Detroit, Michigan.

K. P. Strohl: Department of Medicine, Case Western Reserve University; and Center for Sleep Disorders Research, Louis Stokes DVA Medical Center, Cleveland, Ohio.

occurs when both airflow and respiratory efforts are absent. Other terms used in the early literature that are equivalent to central apnea are diaphragmatic or arrhythmic apnea (Table 69.1). These terms imply a cessation of respiratory effort at a brainstem level. During obstructive apnea, respiratory efforts persist although airflow is absent at the nose and mouth. Other terms previously used for obstructive apnea are upper airway or peripheral apnea. Obstructive and central apneas are related clinically and pathophysiologically. Many adult patients exhibit apnea in which both central and obstructive patterns occur, which is termed mixed apnea. In a single apneic episode, there may be a period in which no efforts occur, followed by the appearance of respiratory efforts, also without airflow. In addition, in the same night, patients may have central, mixed, and obstructive apneas.

Hypopneas, or hypoventilation, during sleep may arise by mechanisms similar to those producing apnea. Hypoventilation (hypopnea) leads to increased carbon dioxide (CO_2) and decreased oxygen (O_2) levels in arterial blood and to arousals from sleep; as do apneas, hypopneas may result from reduction in respiratory efforts or partial upper airway obstruction. Snoring is a form of partial airway obstruction and is called obstructive hypopnea. Snoring is a common report, but those patients who snore may present with symptomatic features of sleep apnea syndrome even if complete cessation of airflow (apnea) never occurs during sleep. Moreover, such patients may exhibit abnormal sleep and cardiorespiratory changes as well.

There are certain summary measures (Table 69.1) used to describe respiratory disturbances during sleep (9). The *apnea-hypopnea index* is the total number of apneas and hypopneas during sleep divided by the hours of sleep time. Values of the apnea-hypopnea index can be computed for the different stages of sleep. Another term used is the *respiratory disturbance index,* which is equivalent to the apnea-hypopnea index. The term *desaturation index,* also called O_2

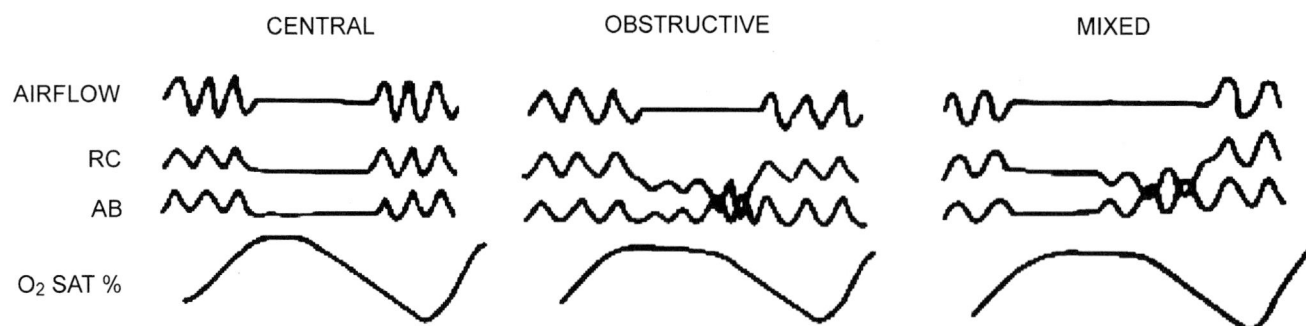

FIGURE 69.1. Shown are examples of the three patterns of apnea found during sleep. An apnea is defined as a cessation of airflow for at least 10 seconds. In a central apnea, there appears no ribcage of abdominal movements during the period of apnea. In an obstructive event, movements of the rib cage (RC) and abdomen (AB) occur with each occluded inspiratory event. In this example as the abdomen moves out the rib cage moves in ("paradoxical movement") with obstructions; both move out with unoccluded breaths. In a mixed apnea, there is a combination of central and obstructive events. For each apnea, there often occurs a decrease in oxygen saturation greater than 4%. The rate of decrease and the depth of hypoxemia resulting from an apnea depend mainly on the baseline oxygen saturation and the length of the apnea.

desaturation index, refers to the number of times per hour that O_2 saturation falls by more than 3% to 4%, and may be reported as an independent measure of cardiorespiratory instability. If measured, there are also summary measures for snoring; the *snoring index* is the percentage of time spent snoring during sleep.

If sleep is directly measured, an *arousal index* is computed as the number of transient awakenings per hour, as defined by a change in state from sleep to waking that is longer than 2 seconds but less than 3 minutes (11). This number is used to estimate individual exposure to central nervous system arousals from sleep, and is distinguished from nocturnal awakenings by the length of the bout of wakefulness. Arousals may occur in the context of other causes such as leg jerks, and spontaneous brief awakenings from both external and internal stimuli are also included in this metric. The number of arousals per hour of sleep may not be equivalent to the apnea-hypopnea index or respiratory disturbance index because many (approximately 20%) apneas or hypop-

neas are not accompanied by arousals and/or other causes for arousals are present.

Distribution plots of values of O_2 saturation over time estimate the extent of exposure to hypoxemia during sleep. One way to understand this data is called the *O_2 saturation profile,* in which values of O_2 saturation over time are presented in the frequency domain (12). Values reported include estimations of the lowest O_2 saturation, as well as more relevant features of the time spent below an O_2 saturation of 90%, 85%, 80%, etc. In addition, recordings can be examined in the time domain to estimate the degree to which O_2 saturation exhibits periodic behavior.

Hypoventilation is clinically not directly measured, as it is uncomfortable and potentially risky to routinely measure arterial blood gases. Surrogate markers for partial pressure of CO_2 ($Paco_2$) include end-tidal values of CO_2 or transcutaneous estimates of CO_2. The former can be unreliable as it depends on adequate sampling of alveolar gases, and the latter provides trends rather than precise numbers. Neither is used routinely during polysomnography in adults.

TABLE 69.1. TERMS USED TO DESCRIBE SLEEP DISORDERED BREATHING

Apnea Index	Number of Apneas Per Hour of Sleep
Apnea hypopnea index	Number of apneas and/or hypopneas per hour of sleep
Respiratory disturbance index	Equivalent to apnea hypopnea index
Snoring index	Amount of time of sleep (%) during which snoring is recorded
Desaturation index	The number of "dips" in oxygen saturation >3 or >4% per hour of sleep
Lowest oxygen saturation	Lowest oxygen saturation recorded during sleep
Values for oxygenation in a frequency domain	Time spent (%) below an oxygen saturation of 90%, 50%, 10%

THE PHYSIOLOGY OF SLEEP AND BREATHING

Sleep is a behavioral state characterized by inactivity and reduced responsiveness to external stimuli. Neurophysiologic monitoring results in a classification (in humans) into two distinct broad states termed non–rapid eye movement (NREM) sleep and rapid eye movement (REM) sleep. States are distinguished by recording electroencephalogram (EEG), electrooculogram, and electromyogram of the chin muscles (13). The combination of these measures and the cardiopulmonary monitoring of airflow, respiratory effort, O_2 saturation, and heart rate, along with identification of body position, comprise polysomnography (14).

By polysomnography, NREM sleep is further classified into four stages, which correlate with the difficulty in producing an arousal. Stage I is light sleep, slightly beyond drowsiness, whereas stage IV represents deep sleep. The EEG shows decreased frequency and increased amplitude as sleep progresses from stage I to stage IV. REM sleep is the stage when most dreaming occurs, and there occurs presynaptic inhibition of antigravity muscles. There is, however, activation of the cortex, the EEG being fast mixed frequencies with low amplitude (resembling awake EEG). Thus, REM sleep is described as paradoxical sleep: active central nervous system and paralysis of skeletal muscle. REM sleep occurs in cycles every 90 to 110 minutes, and the longer bouts of REM sleep occur more toward the end a nocturnal sleep period.

Ventilatory behavior refers to the elements of tidal volume and frequency that contribute to minute ventilation (15). Phases of inspiration and expiration are thought of as having a neural and mechanical element (16). Ventilatory rate and rhythm are organized at a neural level by interactions between groups of neurons located in the medulla: a dorsal group located in the vicinity of the nucleus tractus solitarius and a ventral group consisting of neurons in the nucleus retroambigualis and paraambigualis, the nucleus retrofacialis, and the nucleus ambigualis (17). Efferent activity of the nerves that supply upper airway muscles is adjusted by nucleus ambigualis activity, and activity to the chest-wall muscles by dorsal medullary nuclei. The activity of these medullary groups of respiratory neurons can be altered by descending pathways from pontine and suprapontine areas and can be affected by the sleep/wake cycle, in particular the waxing and waning of the median raphe, or reticular activating system.

The medulla helps coordinate the activation of the chest wall and upper airway muscle groups in both time and amplitude (18). The electric activity of upper airway muscles precedes the onset of activation of the diaphragm and is entrained to the respiratory rhythm (19). Phasic amplitude increases and decreases in the activity of many upper airway muscles are altered by the same chemical stimuli (CO_2 and hypoxia) that affect diaphragm and intercostal muscle activity. Uncoupling or mismatches in upper airway and chest wall muscle activation can occur as a result of local reflexes and of changes in medullary outflow. The effects of such mismatch on ventilation will depend in part on the mechanical properties of the lungs/chest wall or the upper airway.

Elements of respiratory control relevant to understanding ventilatory behavior in SDB are schematically presented in Figure 69.2. Breathing rate and depth are the result of a feedback control system in which the brainstem (controller) organizes neuromuscular output to the respiratory muscles of the upper airway and chest wall. Muscle action generates tidal volume through the mechanical actions of the chest wall and lungs (the controlled system). Sensors monitor the success/failure of controlled system outputs of ventilation and gas exchange; these are the peripheral (carotid body) and

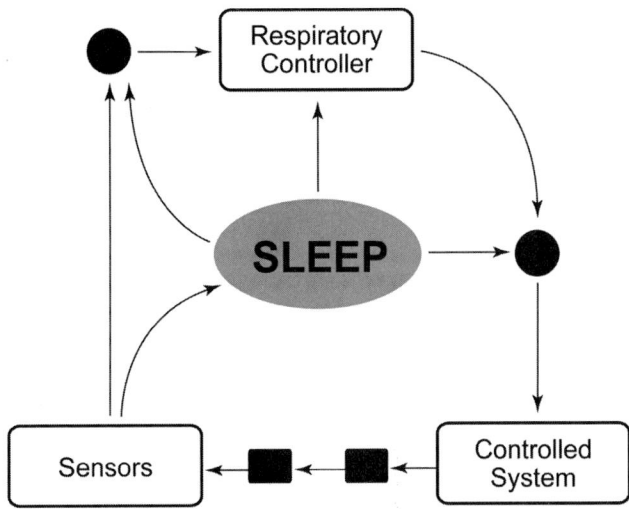

FIGURE 69.2. This schematic representation of the respiratory control system includes the respiratory controller (the brain regions generating neuromuscular drive), the controlled system (upper airway, lung, and chest wall), and the sensors located at the carotid body and ventral medulla. The controlled system alters arterial pH, carbon dioxide, and oxygen. Sleep and other states of consciousness alter the brain and affect neural outflow. There is also evidence that the chemosensors affect sleep-wake behavior. This scheme of respiratory feedback control is a basic concept for understanding how sleep affects ventilation and gas exchange.

central (medullary) chemoreceptors, and mechanoreceptors distributed along the upper and lower airways, joints, lungs, and skeletal muscles.

There are putative set points for this system based on a need for homeostatic control of pH and O_2 delivery. These set points are altered in sleep at various points in this system. One example of the operation of a set point is the apneic threshold, also defined as that level of arterial (or central) CO_2 below which there is no threshold for activation of inspiration. Certainly, brain centers other than the medulla and pons contribute to breathing rate and depth and can override to a certain extent brainstem mechanisms for breathing. However, during sleep these "higher" centers appear to have less influence on and be actively inhibiting respiration, unless engaged in an arousal response from sleep, something that can happen not only with respiratory abnormalities but also with a variety of external stimuli and intrinsic mechanisms.

Changes in Ventilatory Behavior with Sleep

Sleep is accompanied by a reduction in movements and a passive appearance of a sleeping subject. There is a reduction in metabolic rate and, therefore, a reduced need to breathe. In addition, there is a loss of a wakefulness stimulus. Thus, breathing during sleep becomes generally more responsive to chemoreceptor and mechanoreceptor stimuli, and less responsive to higher centers. Consequences of sleep onset include reduced tidal volume, changes in lung mechanics, reduced activity of upper airway dilators, and reduced upper airway caliber of loss of load compensation (20).

Sleep alters postural muscle tone and autonomic outflow, resulting in alterations in chest-wall, lung, and upper airway mechanics. Furthermore, in NREM sleep, the ratio of rib cage to abdominal displacement is greater than that during wakefulness, whereas in REM sleep, it is less (9). These changes in movement may affect the distribution of ventilation in the lungs, increasing ventilation-perfusion mismatching, and so contribute to hypoxia, necessitating changes in respiratory output and possibly initiating an unstable breathing pattern.

Upper Airway Caliber and Compliance

Reduced motor output during sleep is associated with reduced tidal volume, alveolar hypoventilation, and elevated $Paco_2$. Upper airway dilating muscle activity is reduced during NREM sleep, especially in those muscles with tonic ac-

tivity (independent of the phase of respiration), such as the tensor palatini muscle, which is reduced at sleep onset (21). Upper airway caliber is reduced during sleep, likely owing to decreased upper airway dilating muscle activity (22,23). The mechanical corollary of reduced caliber is increased upper airway resistance (24,25). In addition, pharyngeal compliance increases during NREM sleep relative to wakefulness (22,26), so that the normal negative pressures produced by the chest wall muscles during inspiration tend to further stress the patency of the upper airway. The degree of upper airway rigidity can depend on the bony and cartilaginous structures supporting the airway, on the soft tissue features of the upper airway, and on the level of activity in upper airway muscles. If upper airway caliber or compliance is compromised, inspiratory flow limitation develops secondary to negative intrathoracic pressure, manifesting by a plateau in flow despite continued development of negative pressure (25). Figure 69.3 is an example of the changes in pressure-flow relationships between wakefulness and sleep,

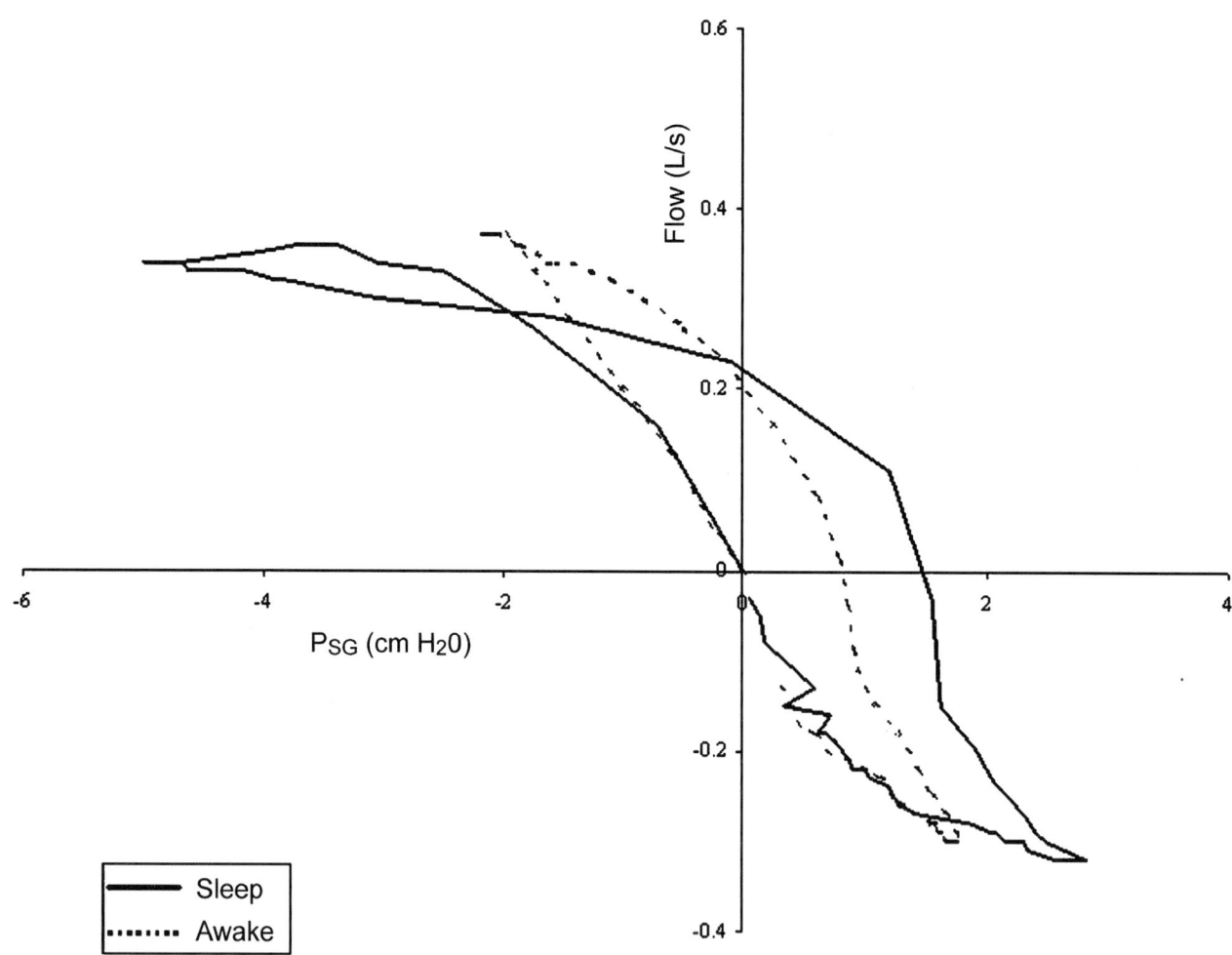

FIGURE 69.3. The axes represent flow (vertical) and trans-upper airway pressure (horizontal). Shown are the pressure-flow relationships for two breaths representative of quiet wakefulness and slow wave sleep in the supine position. The higher pressures for any given flow during inspiration **(top left quadrant)** and expiration **(bottom right quadrant)** indicate that flow resistance increases during sleep. The flattening of inspiratory flow (increasing subglottic pressure with no increase in flow) is by definition flow limitation and is seen in healthy subjects during sleep.

and shows an increased upper airway resistance and flow limitation during sleep in a normal subject.

In REM sleep, despite muscle atonia, pharyngeal compliance is not increased (22,26). In fact, the retropalatal airway is less compliant during REM sleep relative to NREM (22). This finding indicates the significance of nonneuromuscular factors in maintaining upper airway patency during sleep. REM sleep is a special case because peripheral atonia is accompanied by augmented inspiratory medullary neuronal activity and because the REM sleep EEG shares many features of the awake EEG.

Load Compensation

The ability of the ventilatory control system to compensate for changes in resistance is essential for the preservation of alveolar ventilation. Breathing through a resistor during wakefulness (loading) leads to increased ventilatory effort to maintain ventilation and $Paco_2$. During sleep, in contrast, immediate and subsequent compensation to added loads is compromised. Therefore, resistive loading results in decreased tidal volume and minute ventilation and, hence, alveolar hypoventilation. The ensuing elevation of arterial $Paco_2$ restores ventilation toward normal levels (27). This inability to perceive and immediately respond to loads allows for sleep to continue undisturbed. For instance, the main

consequence of sleep is an increase in $Paco_2$ of 4 to 5 mm Hg. Such elevations in $Paco_2$ result in mild acidosis in both healthy individuals and in those with cardiopulmonary disorders but without SDB.

A consequence of an upstream resistor is the imposition of an internal load. A substantial increase in resistance may cause fluttering of the soft palate owing to turbulent flow (28). This fluttering is responsible for the acoustic phenomenon known as snoring. Like those experiencing experimentally applied loads, spontaneous snorers demonstrate inspiratory flow limitation by flow plateaus during inspiration; they do not arouse from sleep despite continuous generation of subatmospheric intraluminal pressure, as shown in Figure 69.4. If increased resistance and inspiratory flow limitation are prolonged, the increased work of breathing and/or hypoventilation leads to frequent arousals from sleep and to ensuing excessive daytime sleepiness. This occurrence of partial upper airway obstruction with arousals in association with increasing respiratory effort, accompanied by daytime symptoms, comprises the pathophysiology of what is referred to as upper airway resistance syndrome (29).

The Hypocapnic-Apneic Threshold

Loss of wakefulness renders ventilation during NREM sleep critically dependent on chemoreceptor stimuli (arterial

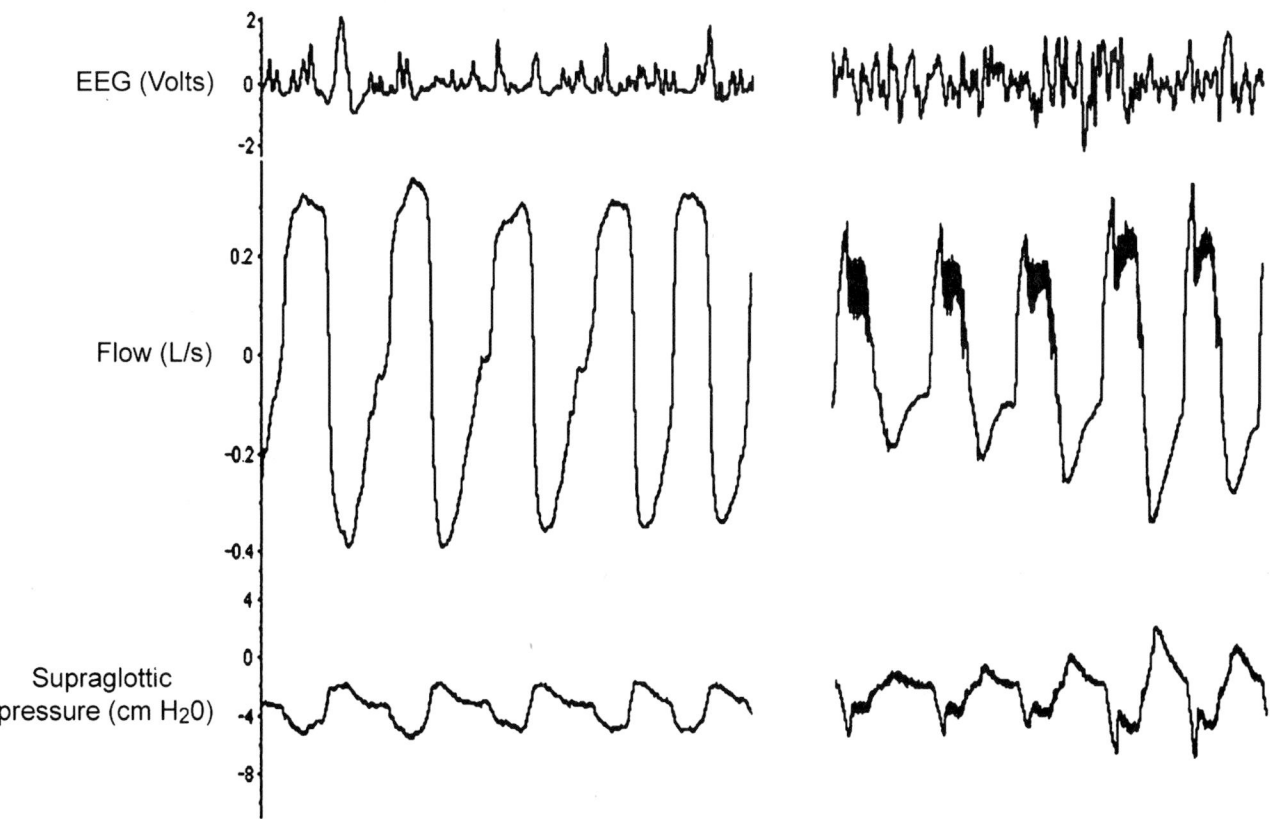

FIGURE 69.4. Several cycles of breathing during electroencephalogram defined wakefulness and sleep are shown for wakefulness **(left)** and quiet sleep **(right)** in a healthy subject. Flow limitation (See Fig. 69.5) is present during inspiration with flow fluctuations indicative of snoring.

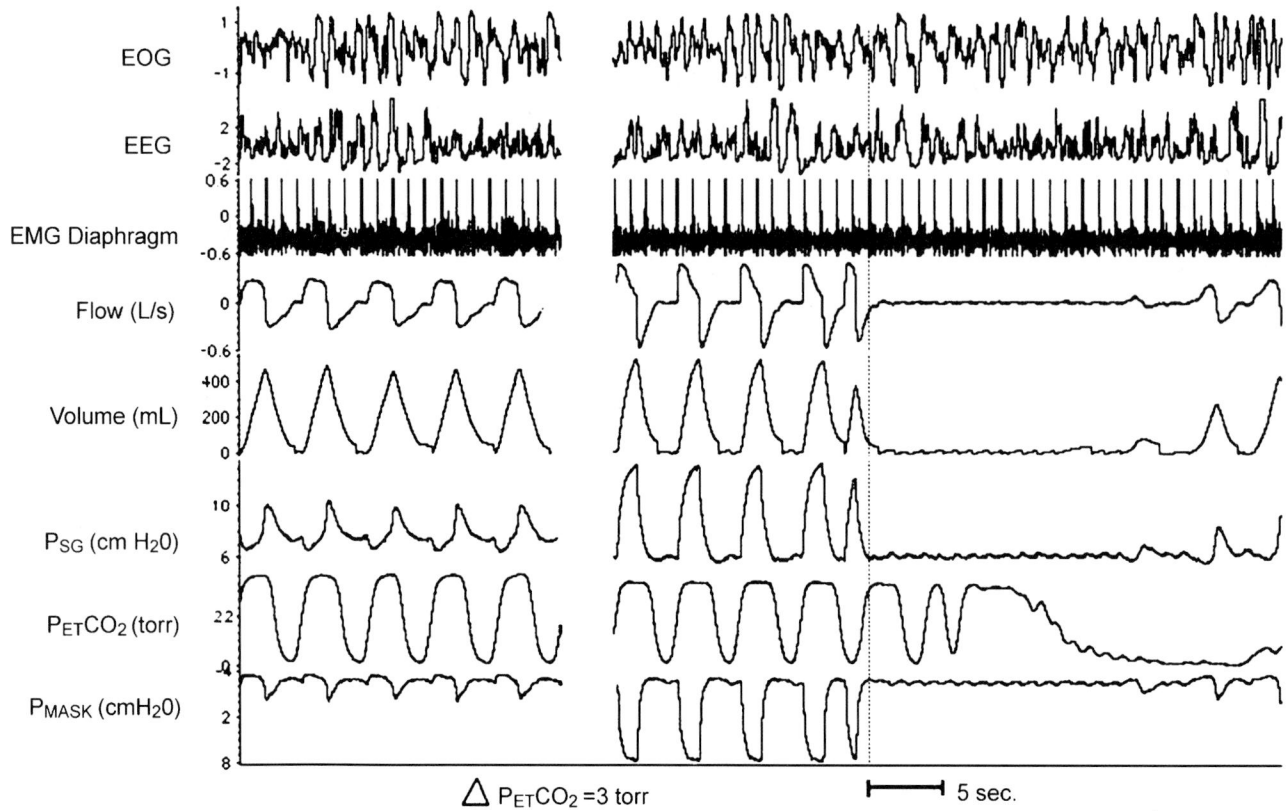

EOG

EEG

EMG Diaphragm

Flow (L/s)

Volume (mL)

P$_{SG}$ (cm H$_2$O)

P$_{ET}$CO$_2$ (torr)

P$_{MASK}$ (cmH$_2$O)

$\triangle$ P$_{ET}$CO$_2$ =3 torr   5 sec.

FIGURE 69.5. This is a study of the effect of passive mechanical ventilation on breathing pattern. The subject is breathing through a nasal continuous positive airway pressure mask during sleep **(left)** and then is placed on mechanical ventilation through the mask **(right)** along with supplemental carbon dioxide to maintain a stable end-tidal value of approximately 3 torr below that during sleep. When mechanical ventilation is stopped, there occurs a central apnea for 10 seconds, demonstrating the effect of the hypocapnic threshold. This is not as apparent during wakefulness.

partial pressure of O$_2$ and Paco$_2$). Reduced Paco$_2$ is a powerful inhibitory factor of ventilation. Therefore, central apnea develops when Paco$_2$ is reduced below a highly reproducible hypocapnic-apneic threshold, unmasked by NREM sleep (30) (Fig. 69.5). Hypocapnia is probably the most important inhibitory factor during NREM sleep. This threshold level of Paco$_2$ is decreased by hypoxia, possibly by excitation caused by miscellaneous nonchemical stimuli. One major cause for SDB is breathing instability produced by this threshold effect and by arousals, hypoxia, and other factors that alter this threshold over time. Periodic breathing is discussed in more depth in the section "Pathogenesis of Central Sleep Apneas/Hypopneas."

Cardiovascular Effects of Sleep

Ventilatory behavior during sleep acts in concert with the cardiovascular system to deliver O$_2$ to peripheral tissue and excrete CO$_2$. The cardiovascular system is not a passive bystander either during the transition from wakefulness to sleep, or in the change in gas exchange that accompanies sleep or that may interrupt sleep. Normally, with NREM sleep

there is a rather sudden withdrawal of sympathetic tone, both humoral and neural, and an increase in parasympathetic tone. As a result, there occurs a reduction in heart rate, blood pressure, cardiac output, and autonomic activity (31). There is decreased cardiac workload and O$_2$ demand, and the ability to provoke arrhythmia is reduced, both experimentally and observationally.

With spontaneous arousals, however, there occurs an abrupt increase in sympathetic drive, manifested by increases in sympathetic nerve activity, blood pressure and heart rate, and parasympathetic withdrawal. In contrast, full awakening, rather than transient arousals from sleep, is accompanied by a modest increase in sympathetic outflow without much evidence for parasympathetic withdrawal (32,33).

In REM sleep, cardiovascular and breathing systems are less dependent on metabolic drive. Sympathetic activation increases to levels seen during wakefulness but are often episodic, leading to transient changes in heart rate, blood pressure, and breathing. Thus, sympathetic outflow is uncoupled from the presynaptic inhibition that is characteristic of skeletal muscle control during this state (31).

In general, however, sleep is cardioprotective for the cardiovascular system in a healthy subject. SDB disrupts cardiovascular regulation during sleep because of repetitive arousals, hypoxemia, intrathoracic pressure changes, and preload and afterload effects (34).

COMMUNITY EXPRESSION OF SLEEP-DISORDERED BREATHING

Subjects without clinical problems may exhibit obstructive or central apneas at sleep onset or during periods of REM sleep (35). Apneic episodes are usually less than 15 seconds in duration and are not repetitive. Occasionally, longer periods of apnea lasting 30 seconds or more are seen in normal subjects, particularly during REM sleep (36). These episodes may not be accompanied by arousal or sleep-state changes.

In healthy young subjects, some studies have shown that more boys than girls have frequent apneas during sleep, but others report little sex difference in the occurrence of apneas. After the sixth decade, however, respiratory disturbances during sleep seem to increase in number and occur with equal frequency in men and women (37). Patients with a clinically important sleep apnea may be distinguished from normal by the existence of repetitive apneas greater than 10 seconds in duration during stages I and II and REM sleep and by improvement in daytime symptoms and general performance with treatment of SDB.

In U.S. communities, 9% to 12% of women and 27% to 35% of men may have an apnea-hypopnea index greater than five, a number often quoted as a threshold value for normality; however, many people with an apnea-hypopnea index greater than five have no symptoms or apparent illness (1) (see Chapter 70). If the definition of illness is the presence of daytime sleepiness or cardiovascular complications such as hypertension, the estimates are that 2% to 4% of those in the community have symptomatic SDB. These studies also suggest that these subjects have higher accident rates and substantial disability.

Snoring is believed to be a predisposing feature in the development of disease (38,39). Snoring increases with age, so that approximately 45% of men and 30% of women age 65 years are said to snore. Hypertension is two to three times (3) and diabetes is 1.5 times more likely among persons who snore, even after age and obesity are taken into account (5,40).

SDB has been shown to exhibit familial clustering, and if snoring is considered as a variant of SDB, the familial incidence of snoring and sleep apnea is quite striking. There is some evidence from cephalometric measurements that the arrangement of the jaw to the head and neck is inherited (41,42). Conceivably, individuals with a certain structural framework would be predisposed to snoring and/or apneas. It is also known that there are familial traits in hypercapnic and hypoxic sensitivity; these could relate to the tendency to breathe periodically during sleep. It is not known if there is a familial trait involving the respiratory coordination of

muscles of the chest wall and upper airway. In addition, obesity and alcoholism (factors associated with SDB) can be family traits and, to the extent that these factors are causally related to apneas, are bases for familial clustering of sleep apnea.

There is increasing evidence that sleep apnea has a genetic component (43). Symptoms relating to apnea are present with two to six times greater frequency in family members of affected patients than in a control population. Sleep apneic activity itself is present more often in first-degree relatives of patients than in age-, sex-, and socioeconomic-matched control families. These family studies also suggest that the frequency of sleep apnea is underestimated in the community and that the symptomatic sequelae of multiple apneas are quite variable. The experience in directly measuring for genetic factors in SDB is limited. Taking a candidate gene approach, there was observed an increased prevalence (twofold) in a polymorphism for apolipoprotein E, which is also associated with cardiovascular disease and Alzheimer disease (44). This has not been confirmed in other studies (45,46), perhaps because the observation may occur as a function of age or of the ascertained population. From human studies of families with one (or more) affected members (the Cleveland Family Study), there is statistical evidence for an oligogenic transmission explaining some 27% of the variation in apnea-hypopnea index expression in the community (47). In whites, analysis of an age-adjusted (log-transformed) apnea-hypopnea index suggests recessive mendelian inheritance with separate distributions for each sex, accounting for 21% to 27% of the variance, with an additional 8% to 9% of the variation owing to other familial factors, either environmental or polygenic. Similarly, transmission patterns in the African-American sample were consistent with mendelian inheritance, accounting for 25% of the total variation with an additional 8% due to other familial effects. Consideration of body mass index (BMI) in the analytic model showed different results according to each race. Adjustment for BMI in whites significantly reduced the major gene effect; however, in African Americans, there remained an effect accounting for 19% of the total variation with an additional 8% of the variance owing to other familial effects. These results provide support for an underlying genetic basis for obstructive sleep apnea independent of the contribution of BMI to the disease in African Americans. The analyses in whites suggested that a major gene for obstructive sleep apnea might be closely related to genes for or effects of obesity.

A role for genetic transmission of ventilatory behavior (respiratory frequency, tidal volume, and minute ventilation) is directly supported by reports of nearly absent respiratory depression in response to brief hypoxia in nitric oxide synthase-3 mutant mice (48) and an altered breathing pattern in knock-out nitric oxide synthase-1 mice (49,50). Other studies of knock-out mouse models report loss of ventilatory function in regard to hypoxic response attributed to endothelin-converting enzyme-1, to endothelin-1, to dopamine, to the neutral endopeptidase, and to HIF; on the other hand, knock-out animals for other supposedly critical factors for hypoxic or hypercapnic responses show no effect on ventilation (neither nicotinamide adenine dinucleotide phosphate nor endothelin-3) (15). Development of CO_2 responses results from action involving the mammalian achaetescute homologous gene (Mash-1) system (51), but this is a developmental pathway and less likely to operate in an independent fashion in adult responses. More complex models that are still based on single mutant genes include the effects of leptin in the ob/ob mutant B6 mouse (52). This is an example of a modifier gene effect, as the basic structure of resting breathing is unaffected, but the functions of CO_2 responses are modified by leptin, even in the absence of obesity. Thus, a candidate gene/protein approach has shown proof-of-principle for providing insight into functions of individual genes possibly relevant in SDB. It is likely that sleep apnea is not just the result of a single mutation or protein action.

Pathogenesis of Central Sleep Apneas/Hypopneas

Illness from central events is associated with recurring episodes of apnea/hypopnea during sleep (Fig. 69.6). To summarize this section, the instability of breathing with central apnea/hypopneas reflects a brainstem interplay between the hypocapnic threshold and the tendency for short-term potentiation of ventilation. The latter determines the occurrence of stable breathing during sleep; however, the duration of hyperventilation may determine whether medullary P_{CO_2} is reduced sufficiently for the development of central apnea. There is however a contribution to both the appearance and recurrence of apneas by the upper airway and upper airway reflex action on the medullary controller. Certain risk factors (age, gender, and sleep) and clinical conditions such as stroke and congestive heart failure (CHF) are associated with the occurrence of central apneas and can be thought of as contributing factors.

Hypocapnia

Hypocapnia is the most ubiquitous and consistent inhibitory (more aptly described as disfacilitatory) influence during NREM sleep, resulting in central apnea if Pa_{CO_2} is lowered below a hypocapnic-apneic threshold by steady-state passive or active hyperventilation. However, the state of vigilance influences stability of respiration as hyperpnea during wakefulness is not followed by apnea, even in the face of substantial hypocapnia and alkalosis. The duration of hyperpnea during sleep is also a determinant of central apnea. Central apnea occurrs infrequently after passive hyperventilation for 1 minute (53), possibly owing to insufficient inhibitory influences. Likewise, transient-induced cortical arousals cause

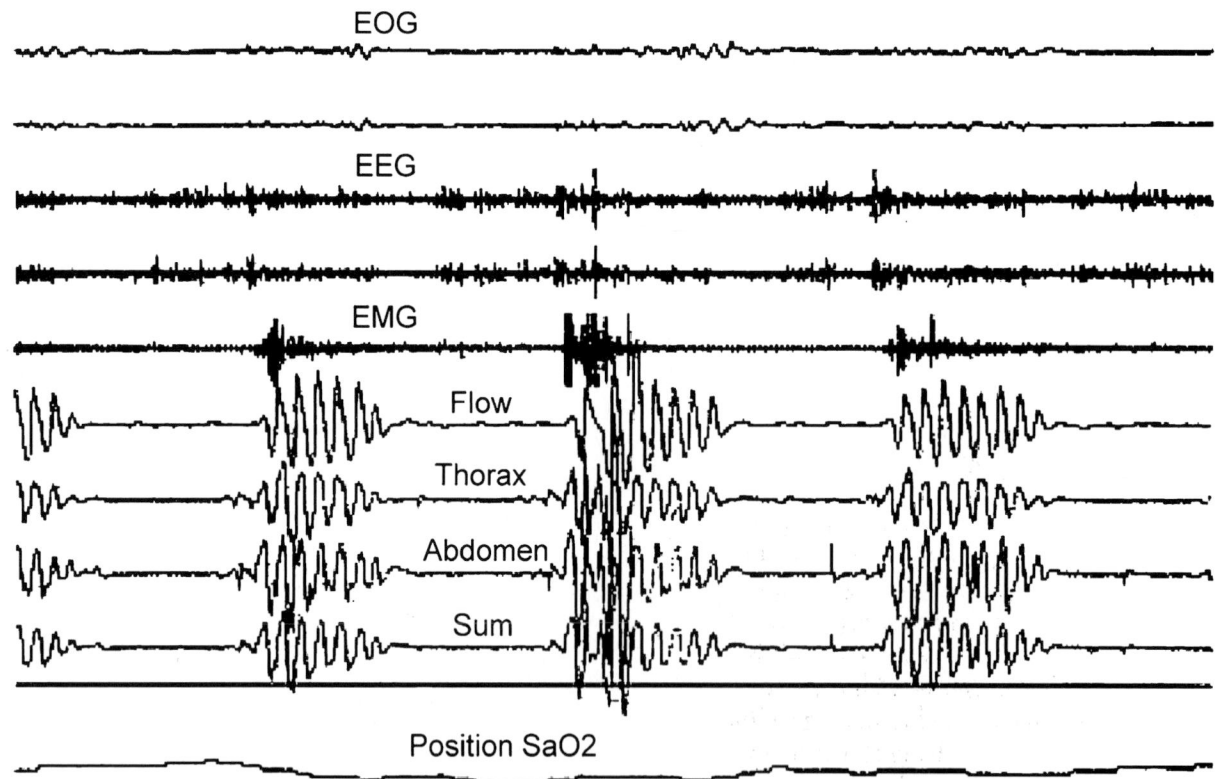

FIGURE 69.6. These are a series of central apneas during sleep. Each episode of absent flow is accompanied by a cessation of thoracoabdominal efforts.

brief hyperpnea but no apnea or hypopnea in the recovery period (54).

The inhibitory effects of hypocapnia during sleep are offset by neural mechanisms stabilizing ventilation. The most widely studied mechanism, short-term potentiation, occurs after transient stimuli (55); the decay of short-term potentiation (also called after-discharge) has a time domain of minutes. Short-term potentiation is activated by brief isocapnic hypoxia in humans during NREM sleep, resulting in brief, but gradually diminishing, hyperpnea upon removal of the hypoxic stimulus and lasting for several breaths. Thus, short-term potentiation preserves ventilatory motor output in the face of transient hypocapnia. As an example, central apnea rarely occurs after termination of brief hypoxia, despite hypocapnia at or below the apneic threshold (56). Similarly, although hypocapnia occurs during transient arousals from sleep, the occurrence of central apnea is probably minimized by the activation of short-term potentiation.

Short-term potentiation may be abolished by prolonged hypoxia, which may explain the development of periodic breathing after a period (20–25 minutes) of hypoxia, as well as the occurrence of central apnea on termination of prolonged hypoxic exposure (55).

Upper Airway Effects

Central apnea during sleep may also occur without preceding hyperventilation. Laryngeal stimulation and negative pressure–induced deformation in sleeping dogs precipitate central apnea. There is indirect evidence suggesting that negative pressure or deformation of the upper airway may contribute to the development of central apnea in humans. For example, central apnea occurs more frequently in the supine position and may be reversed with nasal continuous positive airway pressure (CPAP). Some investigators speculate that upper airway obstruction or prolapse of the epiglottis may reflexly abolish central neural ventilatory output and cause central apnea in some patients (57–62). The presence and relevance of such reflexes to the treatment of central apnea in sleeping humans remains speculative at the present time.

The Nature of Repetitive Apneas

The occurrence of a central (or for that matter any apnea) apnea appears to set in motion several consequences that conspire to promote further breathing instability (63). First, the inertia of the ventilatory control system prevents resumption of rhythmic breathing after apnea until arterial CO_2 levels increase by 4 to 6 mm Hg above eupnea (64,65). Second, central apnea is associated with narrowing or occlusion of the pharyngeal airway (66). This narrowing of the upper airway may explain the overlap between central and obstructive apnea (i.e., mixed apnea) and the successful use of nasal CPAP in some patients with central sleep apnea. Thus, resumption of ventilation in a central apnea requires opening of

a narrowed or occluded airway, overcoming tissue adhesion forces, and overcoming craniofacial gravitational forces (67). Third, a combination of hypoxia, hypercapnia, and transient arousal results in ventilatory overshoot, subsequent hypocapnia, and further apnea/hypopnea.

As discussed above, short-term potentiation of ventilation, or ventilatory after-discharge, can be evoked by brief hypoxia exposure, and it promotes ventilatory stability and protects against dysrhythmic breathing, as represented by repetitive apnea and Cheyne-Stokes respiration. Conversely, an absence of short-term potentiation would promote periodic breathing (PB). Such proposals are supported by studies on patients with obstructive sleep apnea hypopnea syndrome (68) or CHF patients with Cheyne-Stokes respiration (69), in whom the impairment of short-term potentiation appears in the context of the breathing disorders during sleep. Dysrhythmic breathing is common to Cheyne-Stokes respiration, obstructive sleep apnea hypopnea syndrome, and the appearance of dysrhythmic breathing at altitude (55,70). Indeed, central and obstructive apneas may occur in the same patient over one night, indicating that dysrhythmic breathing is a fundamental event in sleep apnea syndrome (71).

Hypoxia, imposed through either inhalation of low O_2 mixtures or ascent to altitude is well known to induce dysrhythmic breathing in animals and humans. Sleep, increased time delay, and decreased damping of the system are all known to promote respiratory instability through loop gain (71). Mathematical models and studies on humans have focused on statistical correlations between the incidence of dysrhythmic breathing and hypoxic sensitivities (72). Posthypoxic dysrhythmic breathing during sleep occurs more frequently in individuals, including those with Cheyne-Stokes respiration, with higher peripheral chemosensitivity (73,74).

Alternative explanations for repetitive apneas during sleep are (a) that oscillations in those with repetitive apneas reflect those with the same amplitude as in normal individuals, but excitatory stimuli contribute to a larger extent to total respiratory drive of patients with sleep apnea (72), and (b) recurrent apneas result from an intrinsic property in the feedback control of breathing in regard to either stability or instability in ventilation over time (75). A system could be intrinsically designed in such a way as to produce a spontaneous oscillatory phenomenon that in turn would promote central apneas (76). Theoretically at least, if, in response to the cyclic changes in drive, the mechanical outputs of chest wall muscles and upper airway muscles are not identical either in phase or in amplitude, there could be an occurrence of obstructive events in the context of central apneas (67).

Modifiers of the Expression of Central Apnea

Age

Central sleep apnea occurs more frequently in older adults (Table 69.2). The pathophysiology of central apnea in older

TABLE 69.2. RISK FACTORS FOR SLEEP DISORDERED BREATHING

Increasing age	CSA, OSA
Male gender predominance	CSA, OSA
Family history of apnea or snoring	OSA
Head form (craniofacial morphology)	OSA
Fitness	OSA
BMI	CSA (lower BMI); OSA (higher BMI)
Alcohol exposure	OSA
Smoking exposure	OSA
Sleep restriction	OSA
Presence of cardiovascular disease	CSA, OSA

CSA, central sleep apnea and Cheyne-Stokes respiration; OSA, obstructive sleep apnea; BMI; body mass index.

adults is explained by sleep-state instability leading to breathing instability. Interestingly, it is unclear whether central sleep apnea in older adults is pathologic. In other words, it is not known whether adverse health consequences result from this condition.

Gender

SDB is more common in men relative to women. However, it is unclear whether the manifestations of SDB are similar in both genders. Specifically, susceptibility to periodic breathing has not been studied systematically. However, published case series clearly show strong male predominance. In patients with CHF and Cheyne-Stokes respiration, male gender is a risk factor for the development of central sleep apnea. Similarly, periodic breathing occurs after prolonged hypoxic exposure during sleep; however, all participants in these studies were men, raising the possibility that dysrhythmic breathing could not be induced in women. The pathophysiologic explanation is that women have a lower hypocapnic-apneic threshold during NREM sleep (77). In other words, more pronounced hyperventilation and lower $Paco_2$ is required in women to develop central sleep apnea. This effect does not seem to be caused by progesterone but is likely caused by male sex hormones. The central susceptibility to develop hypocapnic central apnea may play a major role.

Sleep State

Sleep onset is a particularly vulnerable period for the development of transient breathing instability and central apnea as sleep state oscillates between wakefulness and light sleep (78). It may be that the level of $Paco_2$ is at or below the hypocapnic level required to maintain rhythmic breathing during sleep (i.e., the apneic threshold), resulting in central apnea; recovery from apnea is associated with transient wakefulness and hyperventilation. The subsequent hypocapnia elicits apnea once sleep is resumed. Thus, sleep state and breathing continue to oscillate until sleep is consolidated,

a higher $Paco_2$ set point is established, and $Paco_2$ is maintained above this level. Central apnea at sleep onset is perhaps a normal phenomenon that should be distinguished from repetitive sleep fragmentation secondary to central apnea, which may result in clinical symptoms.

In contrast to sleep onset, central sleep apnea occurs less commonly in REM sleep relative to NREM sleep, as breathing during REM sleep may be uncoupled to the presence of hypocapnia (8). However, apparent central apnea secondary to transient hypoventilation may occur during phasic REM sleep in patients with neuromuscular disease, owing to REM-induced loss of intercostal and accessory muscle activity. This may be manifested as central hypopnea, but the events may be interpreted as central apnea in patients with severe diaphragm dysfunction given the pronounced reduction in tidal volume. Thus, central apnea during REM sleep may be owing to decreased respiratory muscle activity rather than to posthyperventilation hypocapnia and, hence, is more relevant to hypercapnic rather than to nonhypercapnic central apnea.

Cerebrovascular Disease

Sleep apnea is more common in stroke patients than in age-, weight-, and BMI-matched controls (79). Parra and colleagues investigated the time course for sleep apnea after transient ischemia attack or cerebrovascular accident (80). They found that sleep apnea is very common after a stroke; 70% of patients have an apnea-hypopnea index above 10 events/h of sleep. Sleep apnea was predominantly central in 40% of patients of sleep apnea after a cerebrovascular accident. Interestingly, there was no difference in the prevalence of stroke between patients with hemispheric or brainstem involvement. The prevalence of sleep apnea decreased to 61% during the stable phase, so did the prevalence of predominantly central apnea, decreasing to 29% of the patients with an AHI above 10/h. Although central sleep apnea may be a result of cerebrovascular disease; the natural history and consequences of central apnea in this group of patients remain uncertain. Based on the available data on the acute consequences of sleep apnea on blood pressure and sympathetic motor output, it seems prudent to attempt to identify and treat sleep apnea in the poststroke period (81).

Congestive Heart Failure

It is estimated that 50% of patients with CHF (even compensated) have clinically significant central sleep apnea (82). Apnea occurs at the nadir of ventilatory drive during cycles of Cheyne-Stokes respiration. Although mechanism(s) of central apnea in patients with CHF are yet to be deciphered, apnea is induced by hyperventilation, which is common even during wakefulness in patients with CHF. In addition, resting Pco_2 is precariously close to the apneic threshold in patients with CHF and central sleep apnea owing to increased hypercapnic chemoresponsiveness during wakefulness relative to healthy and to CHF patients without central apnea. The perpetuation of central apnea is often ascribed to prolongation of circulation time; this explanation has been difficult to prove. In fact, a study in animals has demonstrated that the development of central apnea requires a several-fold increase in circulation time (83), which is more than the observed prolongation in CHF. In addition, circulation time is prolonged in patients with CHF regardless of the presence of Cheyne-Stokes respiration (84). Conversely, prolonged circulation time correlates with the cycle length (the sum of apneic and hyperpneic periods) both in mathematical models (85) and in patients with CHF and central sleep apnea (84).

Metabolic Disorders

Patients with hypothyroidism and renal failure have an unexpectedly high prevalence of both central and obstructive sleep apnea (86,87). Similarly, patients with acromegaly have a high rate of central and obstructive apnea, which correlates with higher biochemical markers of disease activity and higher chemoresponsiveness.(88–90). Other disorders associated with sleep apnea include hypothyroidism and hypercorticism (91,92).

The Pathogenesis of Obstructive Sleep Apnea/Hypopnea

The fundamental feature of obstructive apneas and hypopneas (including snoring) is instability of the upper airway in regard to its function as a channel for air to and from the lungs. Illness occurs in the context of repetitive events (Fig. 69.7). The upper airway in wakefulness has many functions other than breathing, and it is proposed that the existence of these functions and the requirements in human evolution for successful vocal communication resulted in an airway more vulnerable to collapse during sleep (67). Factors that affect upper airway function during sleep are identified in Figure 69.8, and are in the next section.

Anatomic Considerations

Many people with clinically significant SDB and obstructive sleep apnea in particular have normal upper airway functions during wakefulness and on physical examination. The

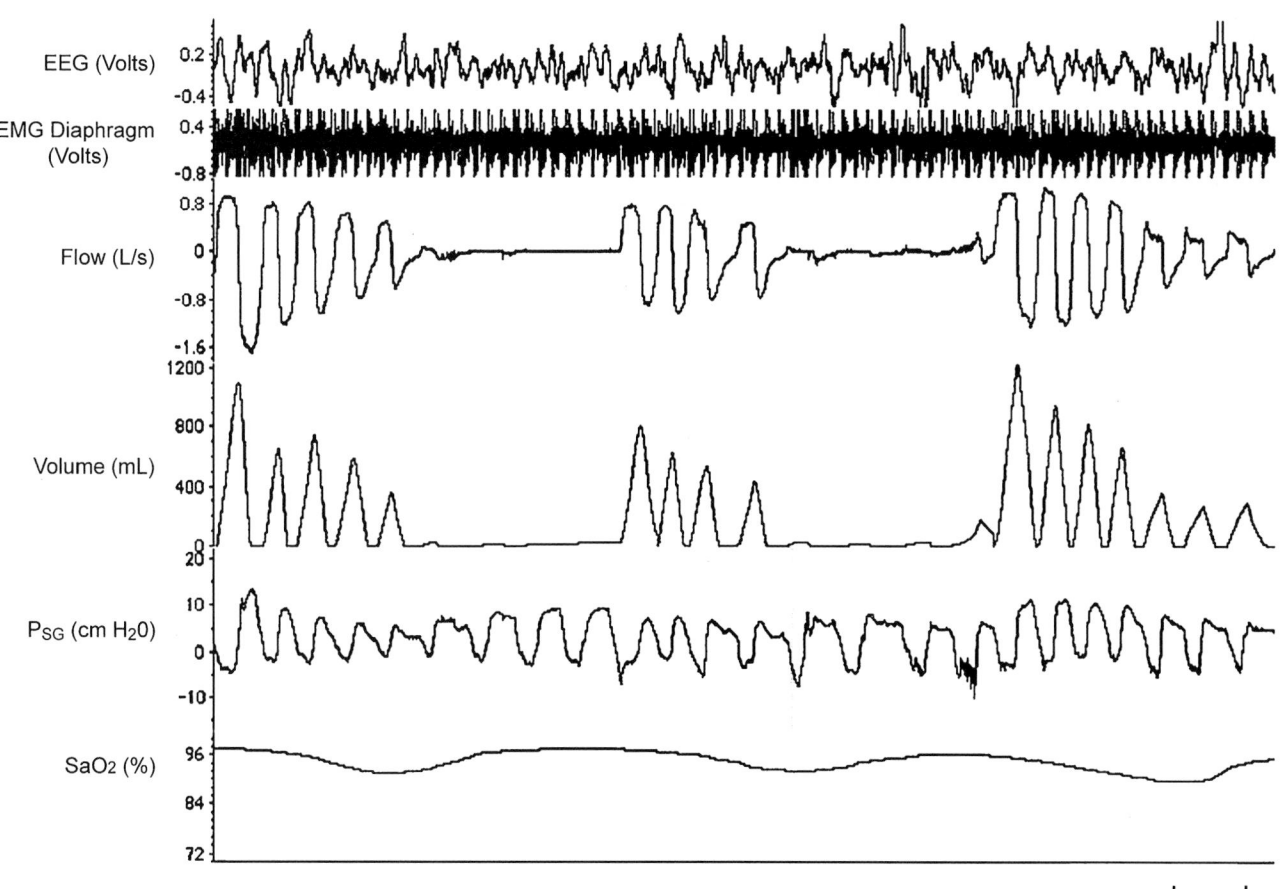

FIGURE 69.7. These are a series of obstruction apneas during sleep. Each episode of absent flow is accompanied by continued thoracoabdominal efforts.

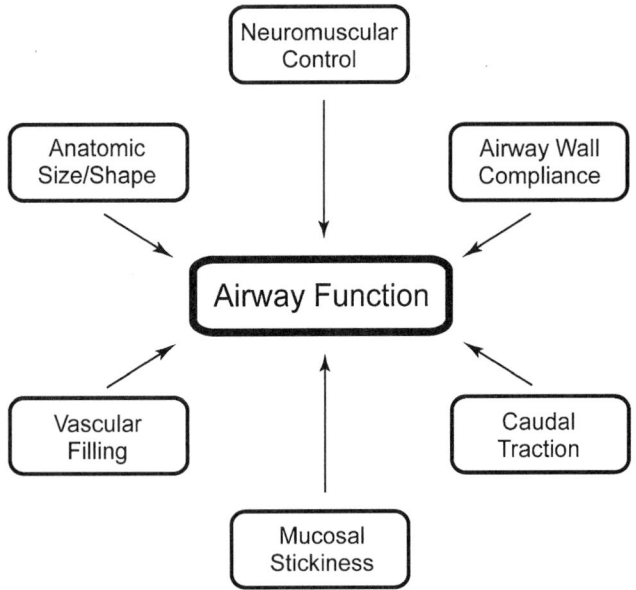

FIGURE 69.8. This schematic identifies the elements that impact on upper airway function during sleep. The upper airway regions of most interest are the posterior nasopharynx and the oropharynx.

presence of an anatomic abnormality is not sufficient or necessary to produce overt disease. Nevertheless, there is evidence that the pharyngeal airway is smaller during wakefulness in patients with obstructive sleep apnea relative to that of normal people (93). In addition, the pharyngeal airway in patients with obstructive sleep apnea syndrome has an anterior/posterior configuration unlike the horizontal configuration in normal subjects (93). The implications of the observed lateral narrowing to the treatment of upper airway obstruction during sleep are not determined.

The upper airway, being an extrathoracic structure, is exposed to pressures generated in the act of taking a breath in a manner different from that of the intrathoracic airway. When breathing out, there occurs a potential dilating pressure and a constricting pressure. A collapsing transmural pressure can be generated either by a negative intraluminal pressure or by a collapsing surrounding pressure. The role of negative intraluminal pressure in the pathogenesis of upper airway obstruction is widely presumed (67). Accordingly, a subatmospheric intraluminal pressure generated by the thoracic pump muscles causes upper airway obstruction by "sucking" the hypotonic upper airway. However, there are no data showing that subatmospheric intraluminal pressure causes upper airway obstruction in sleeping human beings. In addition, pharyngeal obstruction does not require negative pressure. By using fiberoptic nasopharyngoscopy, Badr and colleagues found complete upper airway collapse during central apnea in patients with clinically significant sleep apnea (66). The occurrence of upper airway obstruction in the absence of negative intraluminal pressure is consistent with the hypothesis that the intrinsic properties of the upper airway will permit collapse to occur or to not occur. Sim-

ilarly, Isono and colleagues (94) compared the mechanics of the pharynx in anesthetized paralyzed healthy controls and patients with obstructive steep apnea. The pharynx was patent at atmospheric intraluminal pressure in the controls and required negative intraluminal pressure for closure. In contrast, patients with obstructive sleep apnea had positive closing pressure; i.e., the pharynx was closed at atmospheric intraluminal pressure. Thus, the surrounding extraluminal pressure is an important contributor to the collapsing transmural pressure during sleep (67).

The compliance of the pharyngeal wall is an important modulator of the effect of collapsing transmural pressure; a stiff tube is more likely than a compliant tube to remain open, even in the face of a collapsing transmural pressure (67). The intrinsic stiffness of the pharyngeal wall is owing to neuromuscular and nonneuromuscular factors. However, studies regarding the effect of upper airway muscle activity on pharyngeal compliance are inconclusive. For example, patients with obstructive sleep apnea demonstrate increased pharyngeal compliance and increased activity of the genioglossus muscle during wakefulness (21) and sleep (19), perhaps as a compensation for anatomically reduced caliber. Other studies have shown dissociation between compliance and reported muscle activity. Rowley and colleagues using nasopharyngoscopy showed that pharyngeal compliance at the retroglossal level is not increased during REM sleep relative to NREM sleep (i.e., stiffness is unaltered), despite the known inhibition of phasic upper airway dilator (22,23). This finding clearly speaks for a major role for nonneuromuscular factors as determinants of pharyngeal compliance.

Another factor acting on upper airway mechanical properties is the anatomic connection to the thoracic cage and the mediastinum. Increased lung volume during inspiration is associated with increased upper airway caliber in awake human beings, likely because of thoracic inspiratory activity providing caudal traction on the upper airway independent of upper airway dilating muscle activity (95). Caudal traction may transmit subatmospheric pressure through the trachea and ventrolateral cervical structures to the soft tissues surrounding the upper airway, increasing transmural pressure and, hence, dilating the pharyngeal airway. This mechanism has been shown in sleeping subjects by reduced upper airway resistance and increased retropalatal airway size when end-expiratory lung volume was increased by passive inflation (96). Caudal traction may either dilate or stiffen the pharyngeal airway. It is likely that patients with obstructive sleep apnea are more dependent on the effects of increased lung volume because dilatation and/or stiffening may be more prominent in a highly compliant upper airway.

The wall of the pharynx is comprised not only of slowly varying structures, such as muscles and cartilage, but also of rapidly changing structures such as muscles and the vasculature. Vasoconstriction and vasodilatation have been shown to cause a decrease and increase in upper airway resistance, respectively (97). The effect of changes in vascular blood volume in the neck on upper airway patency in sleeping human beings remains unknown.

Once upper airway closure occurs, surface mucosal forces ("stickiness") may impede subsequent upper airway opening and promote further narrowing/occlusion; mucosal lining forces may be particularly important in patients with obstructive sleep apnea caused by mucosal inflammation from repeated trauma (98,99). Data about sleeping human beings are limited. A recent study on sleeping people showed that pharyngeal mucosal surface tension is associated with decreased apnea/hypopnea index (100). The relative contribution of reducing mucosal surface tension to the treatment of sleep apnea is yet to be determined.

Thus, the pathogenesis of pharyngeal obstruction during sleep can be different in different patients or can occur as a result of a combination of factors. However, common features can be assembled in plausible proposed mechanisms involving alterations in the neuromuscular control of upper airway muscle, the resting size of the channels for airflow through the upper airway, and the stiffness (or lack thereof) of the airway wall. The underlying defect is a pharynx susceptible to narrowing and collapse. The change in respiratory drive with sleep onset leads to reduced ventilatory motor output to upper airway dilators and is the critical trigger setting in motion a cascade of events that lead to pharyngeal obstruction during sleep (101). In fact, upper airway obstruction often occurs during experimentally induced periodic breathing at the nadir of ventilatory motor output (102). The presence of a central breathing instability has been demonstrated when periodic breathing persists after tracheostomy in patients with obstructive sleep apnea (103). Accordingly, central ventilatory control instability may be a key mechanism of upper airway obstruction (103).

The reduction in ventilatory drive leads to reduced pharyngeal stiffness via reduction of neural output to upper airway dilating muscles. The ensuing pharyngeal narrowing occurs because of the collapsing transmural pressure caused by collapsing intraluminal and extraluminal forces.

A narrowing of the pharyngeal airway leads to increased velocity of flow and, subsequently, to a further reduction in intraluminal pressure (the Bernoulli principle) and further pharyngeal narrowing. Eventually, complete pharyngeal obstruction occurs. Mucosal adhesive forces and gravity lead to prolongation of apnea, asphyxia, and arousal from sleep. The ensuing ventilatory overshoot leads to hyperpnea, hypocapnia, and subsequent reduction of ventilatory motor output as sleep is resumed (63).

The aforementioned sequence does not explain how the cycle is initiated. In patients with severe sleep apnea, removal of the wakefulness stimulus to breathe per se may be an adequate reduction of ventilatory motor output to cause upper airway obstruction. Sleep-state instability at sleep onset may be the trigger in others. It is clear, however, that nasal CPAP can eliminate obstructive apneas during sleep in adult patients with sleep apnea syndrome. Nasal CPAP acts as a pneumatic splint, preventing airway collapse in association with a reduction in upper airway muscle activity (9). So a key component in the pathogenesis of obstructive apneas and snoring is the mechanical instability of the upper airway.

In conclusion, upper airway occlusion is a result of an interaction between multiple anatomic and physiological abnormalities; the common features are the development of a collapsing transmural pressure and a small compliant pharynx. Although subatmospheric intraluminal pressure contributes to the generation of a collapsing transmural pressure, it is unlikely to be the sole mechanism of upper airway obstruction during sleep.

Modifiers of Disease Expression

Arousals and Sleep Loss

Restless sleep and observed apneas are sensitive and specific indications of the recurrent apneas. Sleep complaints include either excessive daytime sleepiness or insomnia. Both are related to the number and type of nocturnal arousals. It is said that patients with insomnia generally have fewer, shorter, primarily central apneas with little hypoxemia, whereas patients with excessive daytime sleepiness have more, longer, primarily mixed obstructive apneas with greater hypoxemia.

Snoring

It is proposed that snoring in early life leads to the insidious development of hypersomnolence and cardiovascular disease in patients with obstructive sleep apnea. In support of these suggestions are the findings that a history of heavy snoring is reported in more than 70% of adult patients with obstructive sleep apnea syndrome (104–106). Patients and family members often report minor symptoms of hypersomnolence occurring 10 to 20 years before diagnosis. Most clinical reports have emphasized the recognition of sleep apnea syndrome in the middle-aged man, and little is known about the natural history of these disorders in women, the elderly, or children (106). However, it is likely that in all groups, symptoms will increase abruptly with the appearance of increased hypoxemia and cardiopulmonary complications.

People with simple snoring generally are not sleepy, although they are perhaps more susceptible to behavioral influences and morbidity from alcohol or sedatives than are individuals who do not snore at all. This group would comprise one half of the male population and one third of the female population. Respiratory disturbance indices are usually low, and a positional component to snoring and apnea may be present. Aspects of the association between snoring and other common diseases and the distinction between heavy snoring and mild snoring have been reviewed in the section "Community Expression of Sleep-Disordered Breathing." The major epidemiologic associations with hypertension, cardiovascular disease, myocardial infarction, and stroke possibly include these individuals, as well as those with mild or moderate disease severity.

Hypoventilation

It is clear that in the case of the excessively sleepy individual with cor pulmonale, CO_2 retention, and polycythemia, elimination of apneas during sleep by tracheostomy or by nasal CPAP is desirable, leads to clinical remission, and, as indicated by retrospective studies, reduces mortality. The same studies suggest that elimination of apneas in those with moderate disease can reduce mortality; perhaps more importantly, therapy will improve symptoms of sleepiness to the extent that there may be less morbidity from complications such as automobile or industrial accidents.

Obesity

Several factors could predispose the obese patient to apneas during sleep (107). Hypoxemia occurs in the supine posture as a result of decreased functional residual capacity. Patients with obesity can show a decreased ability to respond with increased respiratory muscle output to added loading of the respiratory system. Another factor could be narrowing of the upper airway. Yet, the fact is that many obese people do not have sleep apnea or a history of snoring; it also cannot be shown that sleep apneas cause obesity. Thus, the association between obesity and sleep apnea is indirect.

Gender

The gender difference in the susceptibility to develop hypocapnic central apnea may influence the development of obstructive sleep apnea. As mentioned above, the occurrence of central apnea (rather than hypopnea) may set in motion several events that conspire to perpetuate periodic breathing after central apnea. Thus, periodic breathing is perpetuated (apnea begets apnea), with pharyngeal occlusion occurring at the nadir of ventilatory drive. Accordingly, the occurrence of a hypopnea rather than apnea in women may mitigate the subsequent overshoot and prevent the development of sustained periodic breathing.

Although there are known gender differences in upper airway structure (108) and the soft tissue volume surrounding the upper airway (109), the upper airway cross-sectional area is similar in the supine position (93). Similarly, upper airway resistance is similar between both genders during wakefulness (110). Nevertheless, studies in humans have yielded conflicting results regarding upper airway resistance during sleep in men and women; higher upper airway resistance during sleep in males has been reported in some (111) but not all studies (23,112). Inconsistency of findings also extends to upper airway function. For example, the genioglossus electromyogram activity is higher in women compared with men during wakefulness (113). Similarly, Pillar and colleagues have shown that women are less susceptible

to loading-related hypoventilation during NREM sleep, a finding consistent with a gender difference in collapsibility (114). In contrast, Rowley and colleagues demonstrated no difference in the critical closing pressure between men and women (23). The aforementioned discussion suggests that gender differences in the prevalence of obstructive sleep apnea cannot be attributed to differences in upper airway structure or function alone.

Cardiovascular Associations with Obstructive Apnea

Bradyarrhythmias during sleep are found in patients with obstructive sleep apnea (115). During obstructive apneas, the depressive effects of the carotid body on heart rate predominate, whereas quickening of heart rate occurs when ventilation occurs. Patients with sleep apnea who exhibit bradycardia during sleep may have normal findings on His bundle studies and have otherwise normal cardiac function during wakefulness, indicating the functional nature of the events. Other cardiac arrhythmias include ventricular ectopy and escape rhythms, but in addition, reflexes elicited by forceful respiratory efforts against a closed airway and the resulting swings in pleural pressure have significant effects on circulatory function. Arrhythmias in patients with sleep apnea often disappear when the apneas are relieved (9).

Pulmonary hypertension (PH) can be a feature in the presentation of patients with clinically significant sleep apnea; if looked for in a systematic fashion, only 20% to 40% of patients without significant cardiopulmonary diseases have PH (116). Such patients tend to be slightly older and heavier than those without pulmonary artery pressures greater than 20 cm H_2O. It is unclear at this time whether such elevations in pulmonary artery pressures reflect cumulative effects of hypoxia or arousals or perhaps indicate that there is a subpopulation that is intrinsically more susceptible to developing this complication. In those with mild elevations in pressure, there can be a reduction below 20 cm H_2O within 6 months (117,118), but other studies emphasize that the time course of recovery can be 18 months or longer.

Hypoventilation occurs in 10% to 20% of patients with sleep apnea and is believed to be associated with alterations in the chemoresponsiveness to hypoxia or CO_2 (9,119). The current literature suggests that as in the presentation for pulmonary hypertension, this hypoventilation does not require morbid obesity or age. In one study, patients with normal weight and lung function showed an improvement in chemoresponsiveness and reduction in $Paco_2$ to within normal limits within 6 weeks of initiation of treatment with CPAP or bilevel ventilation for obstructive sleep apnea.

Stroke is associated with obstructive sleep apnea (120–122). One potential mechanism relates to the rapid and severe fluctuations in cardiac output and blood pressure that occur during apneas and that are transmitted to the brain vasculature. Such nightly effects combined with other effects of hypoxia on vascular regulation may provide a substrate for the development of stroke or the propagation of apneas over time through alterations in central neural systems (123).

PATHOPHYSIOLOGY OF SLEEP-DISORDERED BREATHING	
Summary Statement	**Level of Evidence**
The fundamental event in the production of an apnea is a reduction in neuromuscular drive.	Case collections and physiologic studies from a number of laboratories, with convincing data
Some abnormality in the upper airway promotes the appearance of obstructive apneas.	Paired case-control physiologic studies
Compliance of the upper airway is an important structural component.	Paired case-control physiologic studies
Size of the airway is not as fundamental as a structural component as is compliance.	Paired case-control physiologic studies of children, women, and men
Obesity precedes the onset of clinical disease in obstructive sleep apnea.	A handful of longitudinal studies
Periodic breathing is a fundamental event in the propagation of all apneas over time.	Case collections and physiologic reports from different laboratories, with convincing theory
Sleep is a vulnerable state for patients with respiratory disease.	Case collections and physiologic studies from a number of laboratories, with convincing theory

NATURAL HISTORY OF SLEEP APNEA

Death and sleep apnea are associated, but the nature of the association and extent of causality have not been satisfactorily explained. Early reports of patients with the pickwickian syndrome noted high in-hospital mortality from cardiorespiratory failure, pulmonary embolus, and renal failure. Death has been reported to result from sedative drug use, particularly preoperative medications. However, it is the impression of some that automobile accidents related to excessive daytime sleepiness may have a greater impact on morbidity and mortality than do cardiovascular complications or other nonaccidental sudden death.

Taking a broader view, sleep quantity and quality are associated epidemiologically with early mortality, hypertension, and all-cause cardiovascular risk (124–126). Self-reported snoring appears important in this association, probably as a marker for respiratory disorders of sleep, including obstructive sleep apnea. How one asks the question about snoring is important because snoring is usually recognized by the "snoree" rather than the "snorer." However, studies have suggested that snoring reports by the patient and bedpartner are similar (127), so that subjective estimates are probably sufficient to avoid egregious misclassification in population studies.

Several reports now suggest a relationship between responses "occasional snoring" and "regular snoring" to a subsequent diagnosis of diabetes. From the analysis, snoring could be a novel independent risk associated with the risk of developing diabetes. There are potential pathways between snoring and diabetes and, in particular, the notion that sleep apnea produces a "neuroexcitatory state" through sympathetic activation by repetitive apneas and hypoxemia. There is reasonable support for this position. There is, however, emerging literature showing that sleep itself is important in glucose and insulin regulation. Sleep restriction in healthy subjects results in higher fasting glucose levels and decreased insulin sensitivity, markers often found in subjects at risk for diabetes (5). Common to sleep apnea, sleep restriction, and fragmentation could be the activation of the hypothalamic-pituitary stress axis, resulting in higher circulating cortisol (128,129). Alternatively, short sleep and interrupted sleep flatten growth hormone surges known to be associated with uninterrupted slow wave sleep, which may disrupt energy balance and satiety (130). Snoring could be a marker for other characteristics. Snoring subjects are more likely to have allergies and nasal obstruction during the day and possibly are less fit than are nonsnorers. As sleep interruption in snorers results in daytime fatigue, snorers may drink more coffees or cola drinks, which have a more noticeable alerting effect in sleepy than in nonsleepy persons. Snoring and sleep apnea are linked to alcohol consumption, which in turn is linked to insulin resistance.

The occurrence of sleep apnea with the features of syndrome X hypertension, obesity, diabetes, and hyperlipidemia has prompted a call to change the syndrome to syndrome Z (131). This cluster of diseases and disorders may occur through a common set of neuroendocrine factors and/or genetic predispositions. The strength of both the physiologic plausibility of sleep problems relating to insulin resistance and the epidemiologic associations of snoring to cardiovascular risk factors offers a rationale to begin to explore the pathogenesis of obstructive sleep apnea and its associations with obesity, race, and cardiovascular disease, as well as the occurrence of central apneas and its associations with aging, cardiovascular disease, and stroke.

It may be that prevention of progression of disease related to sleep apnea may be nestled within those risk factors that are proposed to modify cardiovascular risk, i.e., obesity, alcohol, lack of exercise, and hypertension.

VARIANT PRESENTATIONS OF SLEEP-DISORDERED BREATHING

Upper Airway Disease

Patients with disease of the nose, larynx, and pharynx will present with two major classes of sleep problems: sleep apnea and aspiration. Aspiration of secretions may occur because of excessive production of mucus, as exemplified by chronic allergic rhinitis, or because of inadequate neuromuscular tone, as in bilateral recurrent laryngeal nerve paralysis. In both instances, there occur frequent arousals from sleep associated with cough and/or a choking sensation. In sleep and, in particular, in REM sleep, the cough response is less than that during wakefulness. As a result, greater amounts of secretions are tolerated before a cough ensues. After awakening, this larger amount of material may precipitate paroxysmal cough. It is important to recognize that in these cases, the disturbed sleep and what might sound like apnea result from problems with secretions or aspiration. Treatment with hypnotic medications may be particularly harmful because greater amounts of secretions may be tolerated before arousal from sleep, increasing the likelihood of aspiration injury to the lungs. In the patient with allergic rhinitis, nasal decongestants given before bedtime may be helpful. In the patient with neuromuscular impairment, elevation of the bed may diminish the tendency to aspirate pharyngeal contents.

Chronic Obstructive Pulmonary Disease

Patients with chronic obstructive pulmonary disease (COPD) may present with a variety of sleep problems. Nocturnal cough can be related to bronchitis. Insomnia may be the consequence of therapy with drugs such as aminophylline. Hypoxemia during sleep may occur as a consequence of mechanical impairment of the airways already present during wakefulness but exacerbated by the normal changes in gas exchange during sleep. There seems to be an association between the occurrence of hypoxemia only during sleep and the development of cor pulmonale in the patient with moderately severe COPD. Recognition of these individuals occurs when it is noticed that features of hypoxemia and hypercapnia are not associated with a severe mechanical defect on pulmonary function testing. Certainly other diagnostic entities such as recurrent pulmonary emboli or chest wall muscle weakness also should be explored. Hypoventilation will occur during sleep not only because of sleep apnea but also because of changes in ventilation-perfusion matching and a decrease in respiratory drive, especially during REM sleep. If the problem is sleep apnea, there is usually historical evidence for snoring and restless sleep, and the patient should be treated appropriately (see Chapter 70). If apneas are not the problem, treatment with supplemental O_2 only during sleep may be indicated.

Asthma

The most common sleep problem associated with asthma is cough. Cough and arousals from sleep with cough may be the presenting complaints of the patient with asthma and increased airway reactivity. Cough may result from changes

in airway smooth-muscle tone during sleep and of bronchoconstriction during REM sleep. There is some indication that gastroesophageal reflux may precipitate bronchoconstriction; however, patients with reflux are usually symptomatic during wakefulness as well as sleep. Cough occurring in the patient with uncomplicated asthma may indicate inadequate therapeutic effect of medication throughout the night or exacerbation of airway disease.

A related clinical problem is that of morning dipping, which refers to the fall in lung function that occurs in the early morning hours. Morning dipping has been reported in severe asthmatic attacks and has been held somewhat responsible for deaths from asthma. Morning dipping represents an extreme form of diurnal variation in lung function present in most patients with airway reactivity. Reports describing morning dipping emphasize that lung function measured some hours later during the day may be normal, whereas values during the night may show moderately severe airway obstruction. Symptoms suggestive of morning dipping are an indication that additional treatment is needed. If nocturnal symptoms are persistently bothersome, instruction of the patient in the use of a peak-flow measurement device and in the frequent recording of values of peak flow at night may be helpful in identifying changes in lung function throughout the day and in monitoring the effectiveness of medications over the course of a night's sleep.

Neuromuscular Disorders

Respiratory disturbances caused by obstructive apneas during sleep may occur because the underlying disease process affects upper airway muscles such as the genioglossus. Inadequate respiratory activation of upper airway muscles makes the upper airway vulnerable to collapse during inspiratory efforts by the muscles of the chest wall. Indeed, respiratory failure in the patient with neuromuscular disease may be related to upper airway muscle disease and may not have as dire prognostic consequences as does primary involvement of chest wall muscles such as the diaphragm.

Disturbances of sleep and respiration during sleep may be the first indication of involvement of the respiratory system in the patient with neuromuscular disease. Occasionally, sleep fragmentation and the effects of sleep deprivation dominate the clinical presentation of the patient with neuromuscular disease. After treatment for SDB, the clinical manifestations of the primary neuromuscular disorder may not appear so severe.

Kyphoscoliosis

Severe kyphoscoliosis is associated with restrictive lung disease and cor pulmonale; however, recently it has been shown that treatment of hypocapnic respiratory failure by tracheostomy with or without positive-pressure ventilator support during sleep can reverse cor pulmonale and improve the appearance of the chest roentgenogram.

Interstitial Lung Disease

Restrictive lung disease also can be associated with respiratory disturbances during sleep because of cough or hypoxemia. Patients also may have a concomitant sleep apnea. Sleep hypoxemia may be a factor in the development of pulmonary hypertension. Treatment of sleep hypoxemia is directed at apneas, or if apneas are not present, a trial of O_2 therapy may be indicated.

A restrictive defect on pulmonary function testing and interstitial fibrosis on the chest roentgenogram can reflect a history of chronic aspiration. There are ongoing investigations on aspiration during sleep and its acute and chronic effect on lung function. During sleep, the tone of the gastroesophageal junction relaxes, allowing stomach contents to regurgitate to the level of the pharynx. In patients in whom such a phenomenon is suspected, it may be useful to measure pH levels in the pharynx and esophagus during sleep in order to document gastroesophageal reflux during sleep as a potential cause for aspiration pneumonitis.

REFERENCES

1. Boehlecke BA. Epidemiology and pathogenesis of sleep-disordered breathing. *Curr Opin Pulm Med* 2000;6:471–478.
2. Nieto FJ, Young TB, Lind BK, et al. Association of sleep-disordered breathing, sleep apnea, and hypertension in a large community-based study. Sleep Heart Health Study. *JAMA* 2000;283:1829–1836.
3. Peppard PE, Young T, Palta M, et al. Prospective study of the association between sleep-disordered breathing and hypertension. *N Engl J Med* 2000;342:1378–1384.
4. Peppard PE, Young T, Palta M, et al. Longitudinal study of moderate weight change and sleep-disordered breathing. *JAMA* 2000;284:3015–3021.
5. Elmasry A, Lindberg E, Berne C, et al. Sleep-disordered breathing and glucose metabolism in hypertensive men: a population-based study. *J Intern Med* 2001;249:153–161.
6. Horstmann S, Hess CW, Bassetti C, et al. Sleepiness-related accidents in sleep apnea patients. *Sleep* 2000;23:383–389.
7. George CF. Reduction in motor vehicle collisions following treatment of sleep apnoea with nasal CPAP. *Thorax* 2001;56:508–512.
8. Cassel W, Ploch T, Becker C, et al. Risk of traffic accidents in patients with sleep-disordered breathing: reduction with nasal CPAP. *Eur Respir J* 1996;9:2606–2611.
9. Strohl KP, Cherniack NS, Gothe B. Physiologic basis of therapy for sleep apnea. *Am Rev Respir Dis* 1986;134:791–802.
10. American A. Indications and standards for cardiopulmonary sleep studies. American Thoracic Society Consensus Report. *Am Rev Respir Dis* 1989;139:559–568.
11. Systematic review of the literature regarding the diagnosis of sleep apnea. *Evid Rep Technol Assess (Summ)* 1999:i–viii, 1–154.
12. Slutsky AS, Strohl KP. Quantification of oxygen saturation during episodic hypoxemia. *Am Rev Respir Dis* 1980;121:893–895.
13. EEG arousals: scoring rules and examples. A preliminary report from the Sleep Disorders Atlas Task Force of the American Sleep Disorders Association. *Sleep* 1992;15:173–184.
14. Chesson AL Jr, Ferber RA, Fry JM, et al. The indications for polysomnography and related procedures. *Sleep* 1997;20:423–487.
15. Han F, Strohl KP. Inheritance of ventilatory behavior in rodent models. *Respir Physiol* 2000;121:247–256.
16. Richter DW, Spyer KM. Studying rhythmogenesis of breathing: comparison of in vivo and in vitro models. *Trends Neurosci* 2001;24:464–472.
17. Ramirez JM, Richter DW. The neuronal mechanisms of respiratory rhythm generation. *Curr Opin Neurobiol* 1996;6:817–825.
18. van Lunteren E, Strohl KP. The muscles of the upper airway. *Clin Chest Med* 1986;7:171–188.
19. Suratt PM, McTier RF, Wilhoit SC. Upper airway muscle activation is augmented in patients with obstructive sleep apnea compared with that in normal subjects. *Am Rev Respir Dis* 1988;137:889–894.
20. Dempsey JA, Skatrud JB. Apnea following mechanical ventilation may be caused by nonchemical neuromechanical influences. *Am J Respir Crit Care Med* 2001;163:1297–1298.
21. Mezzanotte WS, Tangel DJ, White DP. Influence of sleep onset on upper-airway muscle activity in apnea patients versus normal controls. *Am J Respir Crit Care Med* 1996;153(6 pt 1):1880–1887.
22. Rowley JA, Zahn BR, Babcock MA, et al. The effect of rapid eye movement (REM) sleep on upper airway mechanics in normal human subjects. *J Physiol* 1998;510(pt 3):963–976.
23. Rowley JA, Zhou X, Vergine I, et al. Influence of gender on upper airway mechanics: upper airway resistance and P_{crit}. *J Appl Physiol* 2001;91:2248–2254.
24. Hudgel DW, Martin RJ, Johnson B, et al. Mechanics of the respiratory system and breathing pattern during sleep in normal humans. *J Appl Physiol* 1984;56:133–137.
25. Henke KG, Dempsey JA, Badr MS, et al. Effect of sleep-induced increases in upper airway resistance on respiratory muscle activity. *J Appl Physiol* 1991;70:158–168.
26. Rowley JA, Sanders CS, Zahn BR, et al. Effect of REM sleep on retroglossal cross-sectional area and compliance in normal subjects. *J Appl Physiol* 2001;91:239–248.
27. Henke KG, Badr MS, Skatrud JB, et al. Load compensation and respiratory muscle function during sleep. *J Appl Physiol* 1992;72:1221–1234.
28. Badr MS, Kawak A, Skatrud JB, et al. Effect of induced hypocapnic hypopnea on upper airway patency in humans during NREM sleep. *Respir Physiol* 1997;110:33–45.
29. Guilleminault C, Quo SD. Sleep-disordered breathing. A view at the beginning of the new Millennium. *Dent Clin North Am* 2001;45:643–56.
30. Dempsey JS, Skatrud JB. A sleep-induced apneic threshold and its consequences. *Am Rev Respir Dis* 1986;133:1163–1170.
31. Somers VK, Dyken ME, Mark AL, et al. Sympathetic-nerve activity during sleep in normal subjects. *N Engl J Med* 1993;328:303–307.
32. Ringler J, Basner RC, Shannon R, et al. Hypoxemia alone does not explain blood pressure elevations after obstructive apneas. *J Appl Physiol* 1990;69:2143–2148.
33. Launois SH, Averill N, Abraham JH, et al. Cardiovascular responses to nonrespiratory and respiratory arousals in a porcine model. *J Appl Physiol* 2001;90:114–120.
34. Phillips BG, Somers VK. Neural and humoral mechanisms mediating cardiovascular responses to obstructive sleep apnea. *Respir Physiol* 2000;119:181–187.

35. Young T, Palta M, Dempsey J, et al. The occurrence of sleep-disordered breathing among middle-aged adults. *N Engl J Med* 1993;328:1230–1235.

36. Block AJ, Boysen PG, Wynne JW, et al. Sleep apnea, hypopnea, and oxygen desaturation in normal subjects. *N Engl J Med* 1979;300:513–517.

37. Redline S, Strohl KP. Recognition and consequences of obstructive sleep apnea hypopnea syndrome. *Clin Chest Med* 1998;19:1–19.

38. Partinen M. Epidemiology of obstructive sleep apnea syndrome. *Curr Opin Pulm Med* 1995;1:482–7.

39. Dalmasso F, Prota R. Snoring: analysis, measurement, clinical implications and applications. *Eur Respir J* 1996;9:146–59.

40. Al-Delaimy WK, Manson JE, Willett WC, et al. Snoring as a risk factor for type II diabetes mellitus: a prospective study. *Am J Epidemiol* 2002;155:387–93.

41. Guilleminault C, Partinen M, Hollman K, et al. Familial aggregates in obstructive sleep apnea syndrome. *Chest* 1995;107:1545–1551.

42. Kulnis R, Nelson S, Strohl K, et al. Cephalometric assessment of snoring and nonsnoring children. *Chest* 2000;118:596–603.

43. Redline S, Tosteson T, Tishler PV, et al. Studies in the genetics of obstructive sleep apnea. Familial aggregation of symptoms associated with sleep-related breathing disturbances. *Am Rev Respir Dis* 1992;145(2 pt 1):440–4.

44. Kadotani H, Kadotani T, Young T, et al. Association between apolipoprotein E ε4 and sleep-disordered breathing in adults. *JAMA* 2001;285:2888–2890.

45. Foley DJ, Masaki K, White L, Redline S. Relationship between apolipoprotein E ε4 and sleep-disordered breathing at different ages. *JAMA* 2001;286:1447–1448.

46. Saarelainen S, Lehtimaki T, Kallonen E, et al. No relation between apolipoprotein E alleles and obstructive sleep apnea. *Clin Genet* 1998;53:147–148.

47. Buxbaum S. Segregation analysis of the respiratory disturbance index: evidence supporting oligogenic transmission. *Genetic Epidemiol (in press).*

48. Kline DD, Yang T, Huang PL, et al. Altered respiratory responses to hypoxia in mutant mice deficient in neuronal nitric oxide synthase. *J Physiol* 1998;511:273–287.

49. Kline DD, Prabhakar NR. Peripheral chemosensitivity in mutant mice deficient in nitric oxide synthase. *Adv Exp Med Biol* 2000;475:571–579.

50. Kline DD, Yang T, Premkumar DR, et al. Blunted respiratory responses to hypoxia in mutant mice deficient in nitric oxide synthase-3. *J Appl Physiol* 2000;88:1496–1508.

51. Dauger S, Guimiot F, Renolleau S, et al. MASH-1/RET pathway involvement in development of brain stem control of respiratory frequency in newborn mice. *Physiol Genomics* 2001;7:149–157.

52. O'Donnell CP, Tankersley CG, Polotsky VP, et al. Leptin, obesity, and respiratory function. *Respir Physiol* 2000;119:163–170.

53. Badr MS, Kawak A. Post-hyperventilation hypopnea in humans during NREM sleep. *Respir Physiol* 1996;103:137–145.

54. Badr MS, Morgan BJ, Finn L, et al. Ventilatory response to induced auditory arousals during NREM sleep. *Sleep* 1997;20:707–714.

55. Dempsey JA, Smith CA, Harms CA, et al. Sleep-induced breathing instability. *Sleep* 1996;19:236–247.

56. Badr MS, Skatrud JB, Dempsey JA. Determinants of poststimulus potentiation in humans during NREM sleep. *J Appl Physiol* 1992;73:1958–1971.

57. White DP, Edwards JK, Shea SA. Local reflex mechanisms: influence on basal genioglossal muscle activation in normal subjects. *Sleep* 1998;21:719–728.

58. Tomori Z, Benacka R, Donic V, et al. Contribution of upper airway reflexes to apnoea reversal, arousal, and resuscitation. *Monaldi Arch Chest Dis* 2000;55:398–403.

59. Widdicombe J. Upper airway reflexes. *Curr Opin Pulm Med* 1998;4:376–382.

60. Malhotra A, Fogel RB, Edwards JK, et al. Local mechanisms drive genioglossus activation in obstructive sleep apnea. *Am J Respir Crit Care Med* 2000;161:1746–1749.

61. Huang L, Williams JE. Neuromechanical interaction in human snoring and upper airway obstruction. *J Appl Physiol* 1999;86:1759–1763.

62. Eastwood PR, Curran AK, Smith CA, et al. Effect of upper airway negative pressure on inspiratory drive during sleep. *J Appl Physiol* 1998;84:1063–1075.

63. Cherniack NS. Apnea and periodic breathing during sleep. *N Engl J Med* 1999;341:985–987.

64. Leevers AM, Simon PM, Xi L, et al. Apnoea following normocapnic mechanical ventilation in awake mammals: a demonstration of control system inertia. *J Physiol* 1993;472:749–768.

65. Leevers AM, Simon PM, Dempsey JA. Apnea after normocapnic mechanical ventilation during NREM sleep. *J Appl Physiol* 1994;77:2079–2085.

66. Badr MS, Toiber F, Skatrud JB, et al. Pharyngeal narrowing/occlusion during central sleep apnea. *J Appl Physiol* 1995;78:1806–1815.

67. Olson LE, Fouke JM, Hoekje PL, et al. A biomechanical view of the upper airway. 1988;359–389.

68. Georgopoulus D, Giannouli E, Tsara V, et al. Respiratory short-term poststimulus potentiation (after-discharge) in patients with obstructive sleep apnea. *Am Rev Respir Dis* 1992;146(5 pt 1):1250–1255.

69. Ahmed M, Serrette C, Kryger MH, et al. Ventilatory instability in patients with congestive heart failure and nocturnal Cheyne-Stokes breathing. *Sleep* 1994;17:527–534.

70. White DP, Gleeson K, Pickett CK, et al. Altitude acclimatization: influence on periodic breathing and chemoresponsiveness during sleep. *J Appl Physiol* 1987;63:401–412.

71. Younes M. Apnea following mechanical ventilation may not be caused by neuromechanical influences. *Am J Respir Crit Care Med* 2001;163:1298–1301.

72. Khoo MC, Anholm JD, Ko SW, et al. Dynamics of periodic breathing and arousal during sleep at extreme altitude. *Respir Physiol* 1996;103:33–43.

73. Khoo MC. Determinants of ventilatory instability and variability. *Respir Physiol* 2000;122:167–182.

74. Javaheri S. Treatment of central sleep apnea in heart failure. *Sleep* 2000;23[Suppl 4]:S224–S227.

75. Gottschalk A, Khoo MC, Pack AI. Multiple modes of periodic breathing during sleep. *Adv Exp Med Biol* 1995;393:105–110.

76. Han F, Subramanian S, Price ER, et al. Periodic breathing in the mouse. *J Appl Physiol* 2002;92:1133–1140.

77. Zhou XS, Shahabuddin S, Zahn BR, et al. Effect of gender on the development of hypocapnic apnea/hypopnea during NREM sleep. *J Appl Physiol* 2000;89:192–199.

78. Pack AI, Cola MF, Goldszmidt A, et al. Correlation between oscillations in ventilation and frequency content of the electroencephalogram. *J Appl Physiol* 1992;72:985–992.

79. Bassetti C, Aldrich MS. Sleep apnea in acute cerebrovascular diseases: final report on 128 patients. *Sleep* 1999;22(2):217–23.

80. Parra O, Arboix A, Bechich S, et al. Time course of sleep-related breathing disorders in first-ever stroke or transient ischemic attack. *Am J Respir Crit Care Med* 2000;161:375–80.

81. Parra O, Arboix A, Bechich S, et al. Time course of sleep-related breathing disorders in first-ever stroke or transient ischemic attack. *Am J Respir Crit Care Med* 2000;161:375–80.

82. Javaheri S, Parker TJ, Wexler L, et al. Occult sleep-disordered breathing in stable congestive heart failure. *Ann Intern Med* 1995;122:487–492.

83. Guyton A, Crowell J, Moore J. Basic oscillating mechanism of Cheyne-Stokes breathing. *Am J Physiol* 1979;187:18522.

84. Moskowitz MA, Fisher JN, Simpser MD, et al. Periodic apnea, exercise hypoventilation, and hypothalamic dysfunction. *Ann Intern Med* 1976;84:171–173.

85. Khoo MC, Kronauer RE, Strohl KP, et al. Factors inducing periodic breathing in humans: a general model. *J Appl Physiol* 1982;53:644–659.

86. Zoccali C, Mallamaci F, Tripepi G. Sleep apnea in renal patients. *J Am Soc Nephrol* 2001;12:2854–2859.

87. Zoccali C. Sleep apnoea and nocturnal hypoxaemia in dialysis patients: mere risk- indicators or causal factors for cardiovascular disease? *Nephrol Dial Transplant* 2000;15:1919–1921.

88. Grunstein RR, Ho KY, Berthon-Jones M, et al. Central sleep apnea is associated with increased ventilatory response to carbon dioxide and hypersecretion of growth hormone in patients with acromegaly. *Am J Respir Crit Care Med* 1994;150:496–502.

89. Grunstein RR, Ho KY, Sullivan CE. Sleep apnea in acromegaly. *Ann Intern Med* 1991;115:527–532.

90. Hochban W, Ehlenz K, Conradt R, et al. Obstructive sleep apnoea in acromegaly: the role of craniofacial changes. *Eur Respir J* 1999;14:196–202.

91. Rosenow F, McCarthy V, Caruso AC. Sleep apnoea in endocrine diseases. *J Sleep Res* 1998;7:3–11.

92. Clark RW, Schmidt HS, Malarkey WB. Disordered growth hormone and prolactin secretion in primary disorders of sleep. *Neurology* 1979;29:855–861.

93. Schwab RJ, Gupta KB, Gefter WB, et al. Upper airway and soft tissue anatomy in normal subjects and patients with sleep-disordered breathing: significance of the lateral pharyngeal walls. *Am J Respir Crit Care Med* 1995;152(5 pt 1):1673–1689.

94. Isono S, Feroah TR, Hajduk EA, et al. Interaction of cross-sectional area, driving pressure, and airflow of passive velopharynx. *J Appl Physiol* 1997;83:851–859.

95. van de Graaf WB. thoracic influence on the upper airway. *J Appl Physiol* 1988;65:2124–2133.

96. Begle RL, Badr MS, Skatrud JB, et al. Effect of lung inflation on pulmonary resistance during NREM sleep. *Am Rev Respir Dis* 1990;141(4 pt 1):854–860.

97. Wasicko MJ, Hutt DA, Parisi RA, et al. The role of vascular tone in the control of upper airway collapsibility. *Am Rev Respir Dis* 1990;141:1569–1577.

98. Olson LG, Strohl KP. Airway secretions influence upper airway patency in the rabbit. *Am Rev Respir Dis* 1988;137:1379–1381.

99. Olson LG, Strohl KP. Non-muscular factors in upper airway patency in the rabbit. *Respir Physiol* 1988;71:147–155.

100. Jokic R, Kilmaszewski A, Mink J. Surface tension forces in sleep apnea: the role of soft-tissue lubricant. *Am J Respir Crit Care Med* 1998;157:1522–1525.

101. Morrell MJ, Arabi Y, Zahn B, et al. Progressive retropalatal narrowing preceding obstructive apnea. *Am J Respir Crit Care Med* 1998;158:1974–1981.

102. Onal E, Burrows DL, Hart RH, et al. Induction of periodic breathing during sleep causes upper airway obstruction in humans. *J Appl Physiol* 1986;61:1438–1443.

103. Onal E, Lopata M. Periodic breathing and the pathogenesis of occlusive sleep apneas. *Am Rev Respir Dis* 1982;126:676–680.

104. Lindberg E. Snoring and sleep apnea: a study of evolution and consequences in a male population. Minireview based on a doctoral thesis. *Ups J Med Sci* 1998;103:155–202.

105. Ohayon MM, Guilleminault C, Priest RG, et al. Snoring and breathing pauses during sleep: telephone interview survey of a United Kingdom population sample. *BMJ* 1997;314:860–863.

106. Strohl KP, Redline S. Recognition of obstructive sleep apnea. *Am J Respir Crit Care Med* 1996;154(2 pt 1):279–289.

107. Bloom JW, Kaltenborn WT, Quan SF. Risk factors in a general population for snoring. Importance of cigarette smoking and obesity. *Chest* 1988;93:678–683.

108. Brooks LJ, Strohl KP. Size and mechanical properties of the pharynx in healthy men and women. *Am Rev Respir Dis* 1992;146:1394–1397.

109. Whittle AT, Marshall I, Mortimore IL, et al. Neck soft tissue and fat distribution: comparison between normal men and women by magnetic resonance imaging. *Thorax* 1999;54:323–328.

110. White DP, Lombard RM, Cadiex RG, et al. Pharyngeal resistance in normal humans: Influence of gender, age and obesity. *J Appl Physiol* 1985;58:365–371.

111. Trinder J, Kay A, Kleiman J, et al. Gender differences in airway resistance during sleep. *J Appl Physiol* 1997;83:1986–1997.

112. Thurnheer R, Wraith PK, Douglas NJ. Influence of age and gender on upper airway resistance in NREM and REM sleep. *J Appl Physiol* 2001;90:981–988.

113. Popovic RM, White DP. Influence of gender on waking genioglossal electromyogram and upper airway resistance. *Am J Respir Crit Care Med* 1995;152:725–731.

114. Pillar G, Malhotra A, Fogel RF, et al. Airway mechanics and ventilation in response to response to resistive loading during sleep: influence of gender. *Am J Respir Crit Care Med* 2000;162:1627–1632.

115. Bauer T, Ewig S, Schafer H, et al. Heart rate variability in patients with sleep-related breathing disorders. *Cardiology* 1996;87:492–496.

116. Apprill M, Weitzenblum E, Krieger J, et al. Frequency and mechanism of daytime pulmonary hypertension in patients with obstructive sleep apnoea syndrome. *Cor Vasa* 1991;33:42–49.

117. Sajkov D, Wang T, Saunders NA, et al. Continuous positive airway pressure treatment improves pulmonary hemodynamics in patients with obstructive sleep apnea. *Am J Respir Crit Care Med* 2002;165:152–158.

118. Alchanatis M, Tourkohoriti G, Kakouros S, et al. Daytime pulmonary hypertension in patients with obstructive sleep apnea: the effect of continuous positive airway pressure on pulmonary hemodynamics. *Respiration* 2001;68:566–572.

119. Han F, Chen E, Wei H, et al. Treatment effects on carbon dioxide retention in patients with obstructive sleep apnea-hypopnea syndrome. *Chest* 2001;119:1814–1819.

120. Lawrence E, Dundas R, Higgens S, et al. The natural history and associations of sleep disordered breathing in first ever stroke. *Int J Clin Pract* 2001;55:584–588.

121. Leung RS, Bradley TD. Sleep apnea and cardiovascular disease. *Am J Respir Crit Care Med* 2001;164:2147–2165.

122. Lanfranchi P, Somers VA. Obstructive sleep apnea and vascular disease. *Respir Res* 2001;2:315–319.

123. Netzer N, Werner P, Jochums I, et al. Blood flow of the middle cerebral artery with sleep-disordered breathing: correlation with obstructive hypopneas. *Stroke* 1998;29:87–93.

124. Bliwise DL, King AC, Harris RB. Habitual sleep durations and health in a 50–65 year old population. *J Clin Epidemiol* 1994;47:35–41.

125. Nieto FJ, Young TB, Lind BK, et al. Association of sleep-disordered breathing, sleep apnea, and hypertension in a large community-based study. Sleep Heart Health Study. *JAMA* 2000;283:1829–1836.

126. Vgontzas AN, Kales A. Sleep and its disorders. *Annu Rev Med* 1999;50:387–400.

127. Kump K, Whalen C, Tishler PV, et al. Assessment of the validity and utility of a sleep-symptom questionnaire. *Am J Respir Crit Care Med* 1994;150:735–741.

128. Brooks B, Cistulli PA, Borkman M, et al. Obstructive sleep apnea in obese noninsulin-dependent diabetic patients: effect of continuous positive airway pressure treatment on insulin responsiveness. *J Clin Endocrinol Metab* 1994;79:1681–1685.

129. Brooks D, Horner RL, Kimoff RJ, et al. Effect of obstructive sleep apnea versus sleep fragmentation on responses to airway occlusion. *Am J Respir Crit Care Med* 1997;155:1609–1617.

130. Strohl KP. Diabetes and sleep apnea. *Sleep* 1996;19[10 Suppl]: S225–S228.

131. Wilcox I, McNamara SG, Collins FL, et al. "Syndrome Z": the interaction of sleep apnoea, vascular risk factors and heart disease. *Thorax* 1998;53[Suppl 3]:S25–S28.

Diagnosis and Treatment of Respiratory Disorders of Sleep

70

Michael L. Stanchina · Atul Malhotra · David P. White

OBSTRUCTIVE SLEEP APNEA-HYPOPNEA SYNDROME

Definition of the Syndrome

The current definition of obstructive sleep apnea syndrome (OSA) is based on the consensus conference statement ("Chicago criteria") of an American Academy of Sleep Medicine task force convened in 1999. OSA is characterized by recurrent episodes of partial or complete upper airway obstruction during sleep. These episodes are manifested as a reduction (hypopnea) or cessation (apnea) of airflow with ongoing respiratory effort and are associated with repeated disruptions of sleep. Overnight monitoring should demonstrate five or more events of obstructed breathing per hour of sleep. These events may include any combination of obstructive hypopneas/apneas or arousals related to respiratory effort. Obstructive hypopneas must last 10 seconds or longer and can be defined as either a clear decrease ($>50\%$) from baseline in the amplitude of a valid measure of breathing during sleep or a lesser decrease in amplitude ($<50\%$) from baseline associated with either arousal or oxygen desaturation ($>3\%$). Obstructive apneas are characterized by a complete absence of airflow. Recurrent arousals from sleep, combined with hypoxemia and hypercapnia (Fig. 70.1), are the physiologic mechanisms believed to cause the daytime symptoms, such as excessive somnolence, that are characteristic of this disorder (1). Thus, in addition to the polysomnographic criteria for OSA, the patient must exhibit excessive daytime somnolence that is not explained by other factors or at least two of the following: choking/gasping during sleep, recur-

rent awakenings from sleep, unrefreshing sleep, and daytime fatigue or impaired concentration. The severity of OSA is often characterized according to the symptoms, frequency of breathing events recorded during overnight polysomnography, and degree of oxygen desaturation (Table 70.1).

Risk Factors for Obstructive Sleep Apnea

Substantial work has been completed identifying the genetic, environmental, and physiologic risk factors associated with OSA (see Chapter 69).

Collectively, genetic studies suggest a strong familial component in OSA. The factors explaining this aggregation are likely combinations of genetic influences on the size of the upper airway (anatomy), pharyngeal mechanics and activation of upper airway dilator muscles, stability of ventilatory control, and as yet unidentified physiologic mechanisms (see Chapter 69).

Obesity

The strongest risk factor for the development of OSA is obesity; several cross-sectional studies have identified the body mass index (BMI) and waist-to-hip ratio as independent risk factors for the development of apnea. The strongest incidence data for an association of apnea and obesity come from the Wisconsin Sleep Cohort, in which Peppard and colleagues (2) demonstrated that a 10% increase in weight predicted a sixfold increase in the odds for the development of sleep-disordered breathing. Their model also predicted a 32% higher apnea-hypopnea index in obese persons than in their nonobese counterparts. In addition, a 10% decrease in weight during an 11-year follow-up led to a significant reduction in the apnea-hypopnea index, suggesting that weight loss does improve outcome in this disorder.

OSA is common in morbidly obese patients, although obesity-related hypoventilation syndromes are also

M. L. Stanchina: Department of Medicine, Brown Medical School; and Sleep Disorders Center, Rhode Island Hospital, Providence, Rhode Island.

A. Malhotra, and **D. P. White:** Sleep Medicine and Pulmonary/Critical Care Divisions, Brigham and Women's Hospital; and Department of Medicine, Harvard Medical School, Boston, Massachusetts.

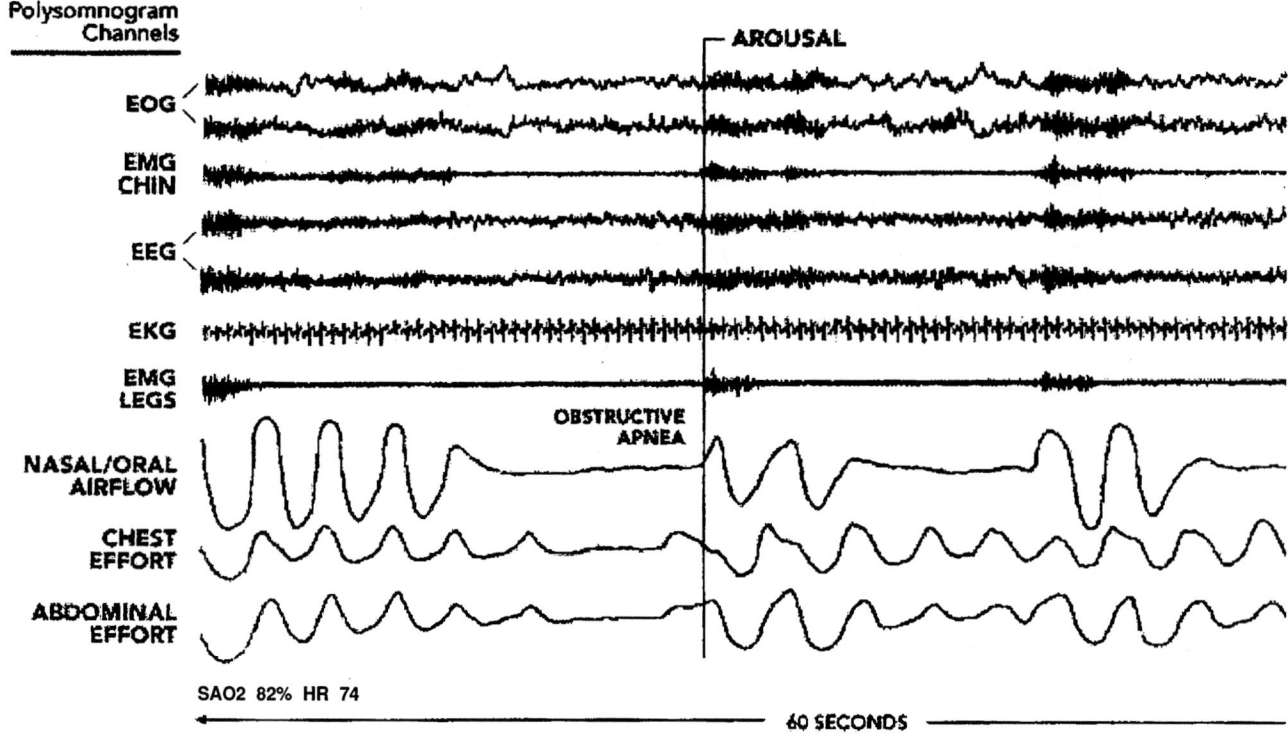

FIGURE 70.1. Polysomnogram showing the different signals recorded during a typical night. This example reveals obstructive apneas, noted by the absence of flow and ongoing abdominal and rib cage effort that is terminated by an electroencephalographic arousal.

frequently encountered in these subjects. Resta (3) estimated that 50% of morbidly obese patients (BMI >40) have an apnea-hypopnea index of at least 10 events per hour of sleep. Severe OSA, defined as more than 30 events of obstructed breathing per hour, was seen in 25% of this cohort. In addition, several studies have demonstrated a good correlation between the degree of obesity (BMI or upper body obesity) and the severity of OSA. However, many obese patients do not experience sleep-disordered breathing (see Chapter 69). Thus, despite evidence that obesity is a major risk factor,

TABLE 70.1. DISEASE SEVERITY AND SYMPTOMS OF OBSTRUCTIVE SLEEP APNEA

Severity	Respiratory Events per Hour	Symptoms of Sleepiness
Mild	5–15	Sleepiness during activity requiring little attention (reading, watching television)
Moderate	15–30	Sleepiness during activity requiring some attention (attending meetings, concerts)
Severe	>30	Sleepiness during activity requiring active attention (driving, conversation)

Source: Summarized from the report of the American Academy of Sleep Medicine Task Force. Sleep-related breathing disorders in adults: recommendations for syndrome definition and measurement techniques in clinical research. *Sleep* 1999;22:667–689, with permission.

the causal link between obesity and OSA remains poorly defined.

Aging

The prevalence of OSA increases with age. OSA affects approximately 4% of male Americans and 2% of female Americans (4). However, at each level of apnea severity, the prevalence of OSA is higher in older subjects (see Chapter 69 for a discussion of the potential mechanisms of age-related differences in prevalence).

The importance of OSA as a cause of morbidity and mortality in the elderly has been questioned. Lavie and colleagues (5) reported a decreased relative risk for dying of OSA (0.33) in elderly persons (older than 70 years of age) in comparison with the risk for death in a younger population with OSA. However, Ancoli-Israel and colleagues (6) observed an increased mortality in nursing home residents and elderly, institutionalized patients with Alzheimer disease and concomitant OSA (6). It remains unclear whether treatment of this population with continuous positive airway pressure (CPAP) substantially improves cognitive outcomes or decreases mortality.

Gender

Despite consistent evidence that sleep apnea is more common in men than in women, the explanation for these gender-related differences in the prevalence of OSA remains unclear (see Chapter 69). However, regardless of the mechanism, men and postmenopausal women should be considered at higher risk for the development of sleep apnea.

Exogenous Influences

Other variables, such as alcohol and nicotine intake, are modifiable clinical risk factors that influence the prevalence of sleep-disordered breathing. Large doses of ethanol were shown to increase the frequency of apnea and the duration and severity of oxygen desaturation (7,8). An increase in the apnea-hypopnea index was also observed when ethanol was given in smaller doses to normal subjects without sleep disordered breathing (9–11). Nicotine has been associated with an increased risk for sleep-disordered breathing. As part of the Wisconsin Sleep Cohort questionnaire, subjects were asked about their smoking habits. Heavy current smoking (>40 cigarettes per day) put subjects at the greatest risk for sleep-disordered breathing (odds ratio of 40.47 in comparison with nonsmokers). However, former smoking was not found to be a substantial risk factor for snoring or sleep-disordered breathing after control for confounders (12). Based on these studies, physicians should encourage smoking cessation and avoidance of ethanol during the evening hours.

Clinical Predictors of the Severity of Apnea

History and Physical Examination Findings

In assessing the clinical probability of sleep apnea, the physician should be aware of relevant symptoms and airway examination findings that are associated with an increased likelihood of sleep-disordered breathing. Since the description by Guilleminault and colleagues (13), sleep apnea has been associated with snoring, witnessed apneas, choking, restless sleep, morning headaches, excessive daytime somnolence, and occasionally impotence.

Tools for the subjective assessment of sleepiness, such as the Epworth Sleepiness Scale (14) and the Stanford Sleepiness Scale (15), were developed as psychometric aids for quantifying subjective symptoms of sleepiness or alertness. The Epworth Scale, which is the most commonly used instrument, rates sleepiness behaviorally and has been validated clinically. People are asked to rate their ability to fall asleep in settings that are typically conducive to sleep (i.e., in a car, in church, while talking to someone, while watching television). Overall, the Epworth Scale is helpful in subjectively quantifying how sleepy a person feels during a 30-day period. However, it does not accurately predict objective sleepiness as measured by the multiple sleep latency test, nor does it accurately predict the severity of sleep apnea.

Many clinical prediction rules have been developed to assess the probability of OSA based on combinations of the risk factors and clinical variables previously noted (see section "Risk Factors for Obstructive Sleep Apnea") (16–21). In a study of 594 persons, the patients with OSA had more sub-

jective complaints of snoring, nocturnal choking, excessive daytime sleepiness, and impotence than the controls without apnea (19). However, these subjective findings do not correlate well with the severity of sleep-disordered breathing as assessed by overnight polysomnography. Entering both subjective complaints and objective measures such as the BMI, age, and blood pressure into regression models explains more of the variance (46%, $P < .05$) in the apnea-hypopnea index than any single factor, suggesting that the clinical impression alone is not sufficient to predict the severity of apnea reliably. In a study from Oxford of 1,001 patients, the apnea-hypopnea index correlated best with neck size, BMI, age, and ethanol consumption in a regression model (17). A report by Flemons and colleagues (22) included both clinician a priori predictions of OSA and the clinical variables previously described to develop a clinical scoring system for sleep apnea. They reported that a large neck circumference, hypertension, habitual snoring, and bed partner reports of gasping and choking were the most significant predictors of severe apnea-hypopnea ($R^2 = 0.34$). Notably missing from the predictors of severe apnea-hypopnea were daytime sleepiness and cognitive deficits, such as an inability to concentrate, neither of which was found to correlate well with severe sleep-disordered breathing.

Anatomic Assessment

A number of anatomic risk factors are important in the development of sleep-disordered breathing; some of these can be assessed by physical examination, whereas others require either cephalometric techniques (i.e., lateral x-ray films) or magnetic resonance imaging (Fig. 70.2).

A crowded pharynx with a low-lying uvula and soft palate is a frequent finding in patients with OSA. Macroglossia and retrognathism are also common. Occasionally, large tonsils are noted. In one report, large tonsils and lateral narrowing of the pharyngeal airway were the most important physical findings that predicted sleep-disordered breathing (23). A neck circumference larger than 17 in (43.7 cm) in a male patient also increases the odds of OSA substantially (22,24), probably as a consequence of increased amounts of neck fat and large lateral pharyngeal fat pads. The analysis of cephalometric radiographs has been used by several groups to identify subjects at risk for OSA and to predict successful upper airway surgery (25–27). Cephalometry is widely available, easily performed, and a less expensive way to study the upper airway than computed tomography or magnetic resonance imaging. However, specific, standardized radiographic equipment and techniques and interpretive skills are required. Collectively, these data suggest that a diagnosis of OSA should be considered in a patient who on cephalometry has enlarged tonsils, a large tongue, a narrow crowded airway, or retrognathism (defined by specific soft tissue and bony structures). Cephalometric x-rays may thus confirm the findings but are generally not helpful as a screening tool for OSA.

RISK FACTORS FOR OBSTRUCTIVE SLEEP APNEA

Summary Statement	Level of Evidence
Obesity is the strongest risk factor for OSA, and evaluation should be considered for obese patients with hypertension or daytime sleepiness. In addition, most patients treated for obesity experience a reduction in the severity of OSA.	Population-based prospective cohort data
The prevalence of OSA substantially increases with age, and the diagnosis should be considered in older patients with symptoms of sleepiness or neurocognitive dysfunction.	Population-based prospective cohort, cross-sectional epidemiologic cohort
OSA has a strong familial component. The pathogenesis likely involves multiple genetic influences.	Case control series
Men and postmenopausal women are at greater risk for the development of OSA than premenopausal women.	Case control series and paired physiologic studies
Ethanol and nicotine may promote upper airway collapse.	Population-based prospective cohort studies and paired physiologic studies
Patients with OSA typically have a crowded airway, with thickening of the lateral pharyngeal walls noted on CT scans.	Case control studies
Common reported complaints in patients with OSA include snoring, witnessed apneas, choking, restless sleep, excessive daytime sleepiness (not universal), and a neck size >17 in (43.7 cm) in men.	Case series, large cross-sectional database entry.

CT, computed tomography; OSA, obstructive sleep apnea.

Diagnosis of Obstructive Sleep Apnea

Overnight Polysomnography

The current gold standard for the diagnosis of OSA is full overnight polysomnography (28,29). This is typically a monitored test (i.e., performed in a laboratory), although home-based polysomnography is also now available. During the standard study, multiple physiologic channels are recorded: the electroencephalogram (EEG), electrooculogram (EOG), chin electromyogram (EMG) (sleep staging), respiration (nasal pressure or thermistor), abdominal/chest wall motion, body position, anterior tibialis EMG, electrocardiogram (ECG), arterial oxygen saturation (Sao_2), and often snoring. Previous reports of diurnal nap studies (with full instrumentation) found substantial variability in the reported sleep architecture and severity of sleep-disordered breathing. Thus, these studies have been largely abandoned in the diagnosis of OSA.

Recording Sleep

Sleep is typically monitored with four EEG leads positioned on the scalp according to the international 10–20 system, with the leads named by position. Eye movements (EOG) are recorded at each lateral canthus, and submental leads are used to measure the chin EMG (30). These signals differentiate between wakefulness, non–rapid eye movement (NREM) sleep (stages 1–4), and REM sleep. Sleep is staged according to the rules of Rechtshaffen and Kales (31).

Recording Respiratory Signals

Both respiratory effort and measures of inspiratory flow are necessary to distinguish obstructive from central apneic events. Obstructive events are recognized by decrements in or an absence of inspiratory flow during continued respiratory effort, whereas an absence of flow and effort characterizes central events. The definitions of disordered breathing events have been discussed (see section "Definition of the Syndrome").

Airflow

Currently, the tools most commonly used to quantify airflow are thermistors (or thermocouples) and nasal pressure transducers. Thermistors measure temperature change as a surrogate for flow and are generally accurate in detecting a cessation of airflow. However, this signal is minimally quantitative and thus less helpful in identifying hypopneas (32). Measurements of nasal pressure have become standard in many laboratories for quantifying flow; the drop in pressure across the nares is measured with a standard nasal cannula connected to a sensitive pressure transducer (33,34). In a study by Hosselet and colleagues (33), flattening of the cannula flow-time waveform was a more quantitative measure of flow limitation than the thermistor reading and correlated well with the degree of inspiratory airway resistance. As can be seen in Figure 70.3, a greater flattening of the flow-time contour indicates a greater limitation of inspiratory flow.

Thus, the sensitivity to small decrements in airflow is substantially increased with the use of nasal cannulae and pressure transducers, and nasal pressure is an excellent parameter of airflow. In one study, 25% of hypopneas identified by nasal pressure were missed with thermistors (33). In addition, this technology has been helpful in identifying patients with respiratory effort–related arousals, characterized by progressively more negative esophageal pressure lasting for 10 seconds and terminated by an arousal from sleep. Ayappa and colleagues (35) reported strong agreement between esophageal manometry and nasal pressure, indicating that nasal pressure measurement is a comparable noninvasive means of detecting fluctuations in pleural pressure in patients with increased upper airway resistance.

Respiratory Effort

In clinical sleep laboratories, strain gauge technology, with either piezoelectric crystals or respiratory inductance

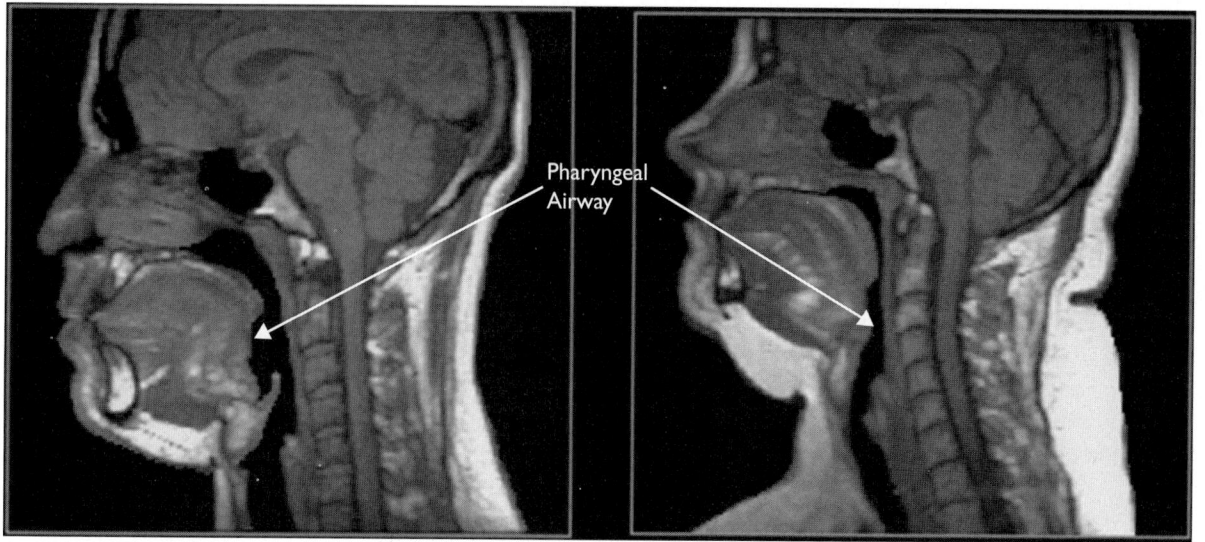

FIGURE 70.2. Comparison of the upper airway size of a normal subject with that of a patient with obstructive sleep apnea. (From Schwab RJ. Radiographic imaging in the diagnostic evaluation of sleep apnea. *UpToDate* 2002 [*www.uptodate.com*], with permission.)

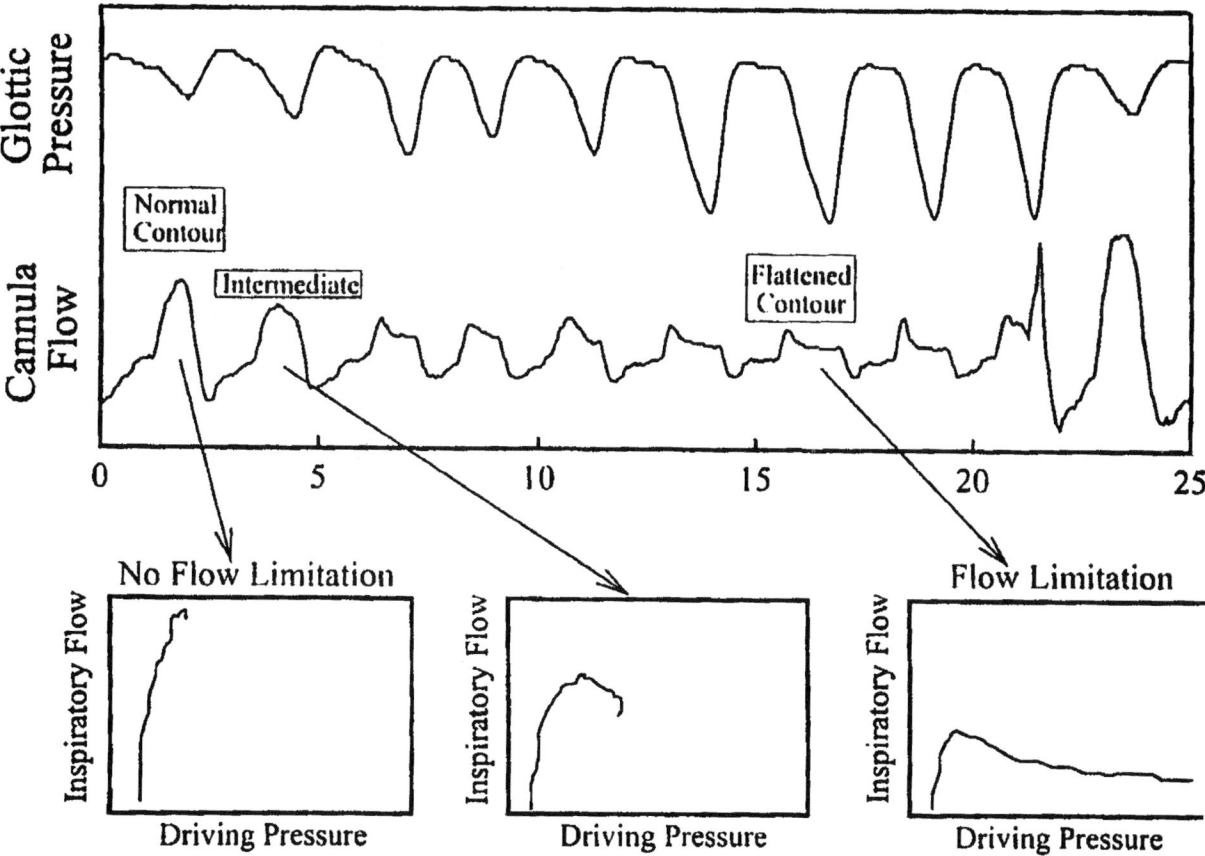

FIGURE 70.3. **Top graph:** Pressure-flow relationships of a single respiratory event. The x-axis shows time in seconds. Breaths with normal, intermediate, and flattened contours are labeled. **Bottom graph:** Pressure-flow relationships for the three breaths noted in the upper graph. The breath with a flattened flow-time contour shows a nonlinear flow-pressure relationship, characteristic of flow limitation. (From Hosselet J, Norman RG, Ayappa I, et al.. Detection of flow limitation with a nasal cannula/pressure transducer system. *Am J Respir Crit Care Med* 1998;157:1461–1467, with permission.)

plethysmography, is generally used to assess chest/abdominal wall movement as a measure of ventilatory effort. These signals often reveal a pattern of abdominal/chest wall paradox during obstructive apneas and an absence of effort during central apneas (36). Esophageal manometry has been used in both clinical and research settings, and the esophageal pressure is a relatively direct parameter of the pleural pressure. It is still considered essential by some to diagnose upper airway resistance syndrome, a disorder characterized by increasing respiratory effort followed by arousal from sleep, notably in the absence of quantifiable apneas or hypopneas. However, most investigators now believe these events to be subtle hypopneas that can be detected by nasal pressure measurement, obviating the need for esophageal pressure measurement in routine polysomnography.

Oximetry

Oximetry has been used alone, during cardiorespiratory home studies, and routinely during overnight polysomnography to measure the arterial oxygen saturation. Series and colleagues assessed oximetry alone in 240 patients, simply quantifying the number of fluctuations in the Sao_2 per hour. They found the sensitivity of oximetry to be high but the specificity relatively low in the diagnosis of OSA (20,37). Algorithms that empirically quantify the number and severity of dips in the Sao_2 increase the specificity of this test but reduce its sensitivity (38). Thus, based on the currently available evidence, including guidelines previously published by the American Sleep Disorders Association (39), oximetry alone cannot be recommended for either screening or diagnosis in OSA. However, it should certainly be used with more complete respiratory monitoring.

Split-Night Studies

Although full-night polysomnography has been used for years, split-night studies are now probably the approach most often used. A split-night study typically includes 2 to 3 hours of diagnostic monitoring followed by CPAP titration if a threshold frequency of apnea-hypopnea is exceeded (40). With this approach, effective positive-pressure determinations are possible in 60% to 80% of patients (40–43). The major limitation of split-night studies is that less time is available for CPAP titration. However, this is not generally a problem, and no convincing data have shown that acceptance of CPAP by patients is diminished following split-night as opposed to full-night studies.

Home Monitoring

Portable devices have been used to diagnose sleep-disordered breathing and titrate CPAP in the home; studies can be carried out with the patient attended or unattended. The number of recorded signals is highly variable, depending on the device (44), so that it is difficult to make general state-

ments about the suitability of the devices (45). However, the Sleep Heart Health Study, a large multicenter trial investigating the cardiovascular complications of sleep-disordered breathing, used in-home polysomnography with great success. In this study of more than 6,000 participants, 94.7% of the studies acquired from patients unattended in the home were adequate for evaluation (46). Despite the appeal of home studies, no cost analysis has demonstrated that they are less expensive than in-laboratory studies. In addition, Fry and colleagues (45) found that most patients preferred the laboratory-based study to home evaluation. Thus, diagnosing OSA in the home remains controversial.

DIAGNOSIS OF OBSTRUCTIVE SLEEP APNEA	
Summary Statement	**Evidence**
Overnight polysomnography is the current gold standard for the diagnosis of OSA and should be considered for any patient in whom this disorder is suspected.	Consensus conference opinion, multiple comparative trials
Split-night polysomnograms allow adequate time for both diagnosis and proper CPAP pressure prescription.	Prospective case control studies
Home-based studies provide data comparable with those of in-lab studies. However, devices vary substantially, so that general conclusions are difficult to make. Oximetry alone cannot be recommended as a screening tool for OSA.	Cross-sectional studies and case control/correlation trials
Nasal pressure changes detected during inspiration and expiration reflect changes in airflow more accurately than thermistors.	Correlational studies

CPAP, continuous positive airway pressure; OSA, obstructive sleep apnea.

Consequences of Obstructive Sleep Apnea

As previously noted (see section "Clinical Predictors of the Severity of Apnea: History and Physical Examination Findings"), recurrent apneas-hypopneas may disrupt sleep and lead to excessive daytime sleepiness in patients with OSA. In addition, arousals from sleep with concomitant hypoxia and hypercapnia may lead to neurocognitive and cardiovascular sequelae; these are described in more detail in the next sections.

Neurocognitive Deficits

The cognitive deficits reported in patients with OSA may be characterized as deficits in attention/psychomotor function (driving performance, trail-making tests), memory/learning, and executive/frontal lobe function (verbal fluency, mazes) (47). Several studies have reported cognitive deficits in all these domains that worsen as sleep-disordered breathing becomes more severe (48–51). Kim and colleagues (52) studied 841 patients in a cross-sectional design protocol and reported a relationship between attention/concentration deficits and worsening OSA. This relationship was linear, suggesting that subtle cognitive deficits may be found in patients with mild OSA (≥5 events per hour). Trials of treatment with CPAP have reported substantial improvements in cognitive outcomes and sleepiness scores in patients with OSA who experience daytime somnolence (53,54) (see section "Treatment of Obstructive Sleep Apnea").

Automobile Accidents

Several studies have shown that automobile accidents are more common in patients with untreated OSA, whose risk for accidents is increased 2 to 6.3 times (55–57). CPAP effectively reduces this risk in most patients with OSA, indicating the increased risk is secondary to OSA (see section "Treatment of Obstructive Sleep Apnea").

Health-Related Quality Of Life

In a large-scale epidemiologic study of patients with OSA, Finn and colleagues (58) reported lower quality-of-life scores on the Short Form 36 (SF-36), a general health-screening questionnaire. They observed an inverse relationship between health-related quality-of-life scores and sleep-disordered breathing events that was independent of age, BMI, and cardiovascular disease in 737 patients from the Wisconsin Sleep Cohort. Flemons and colleagues (59,60) developed a questionnaire for patients with OSA and noted a substantial improvement in many disease-specific measurements after treatment with CPAP (see section "Treatment of Obstructive Sleep Apnea").

Cardiovascular Complications

Rigorous, large, population-based studies have yielded convincing evidence linking cardiovascular disease to sleep apnea. The association of four major cardiovascular outcomes—hypertension, stroke, coronary artery disease and congestive heart failure—with OSA is discussed in the next sections.

Hypertension

Cross-sectional data from the Sleep Heart Health Study, a cohort of 6,132 subjects, indicated an increased risk for hypertension in patients with moderate-severe OSA (>30 events per hour) (odds ratio [OR], 1.37; confidence interval [CI], 1.03–1.83) (61). More convincing results were reported in a prospective study of 893 patients from the Wisconsin Sleep Cohort. The investigators observed a significant linear increase in daytime blood pressure as the apnea-hypopnea index increased (OR, 2.89 for an apnea-hypopnea index >15) (62). These results corroborate the findings of Brooks and colleagues (63), who noted a sustained increase in systolic

NEUROCOGNITIVE COMPLICATIONS OF OBSTRUCTIVE SLEEP APNEA	
Summary Statement	**Level of Evidence**
Attention/concentration deficits are common in OSA patients with reported daytime hypersomnolence and are linearly related to the apnea-hypopnea index. CPAP reduces sleepiness and cognitive dysfunction in this hypersomnolent group. However, patients with no reported daytime hypersomnolence may have a lesser degree of cognitive dysfunction that is not substantially reduced by CPAP.	Randomized placebo-controlled trials, epidemiologic cross-sectional cohort trials
Automobile accidents are more common in OSA patients than controls despite control for age, weight, and ethanol intake. CPAP reduces crash rates. Thus, OSA patients should be counseled about driving and the risk for automobile accidents and should be offered therapy when clinically indicated.	Epidemiologic cohorts, interventional trials
HRQL is decreased in persons with untreated OSA. Several studies have shown improvements in HRQL scores after treatment with CPAP.	Randomized placebo-controlled trials, epidemiologic cross-sectional cohort trials

CPAP, continuous positive airway pressure; HRQL, health-related quality of life; OSA, obstructive sleep apnea.

blood pressure of 15.7 ± 4.3 mm Hg in a group of dogs exposed to repeated airway occlusion during the night for a period of 1 to 3 months (Fig. 70.4).

Several randomized trials and a number of uncontrolled observational studies have also reported that treating OSA with CPAP decreases daytime blood pressure (64–66). Thus, despite considerable prior controversy (67), these studies provide evidence that OSA contributes to sustained daytime hypertension and suggest that treatment with CPAP leads to improvement.

Stroke

Sleep-disordered breathing is quite common after stroke and is reported to occur in from 43% to 91% of such patients (68–72). In most of the studies, the cerebrovascular event preceded the documentation of OSA, so that a cause-and-effect relationship was not clear. However, OSA was associated with worse functional outcomes and higher mortality rates in stroke victims (68,73). The best data linking stroke and OSA were reported by the Sleep Heart Health Study investigators. Shahar and colleagues (74) reported an increased risk for stroke in patients with OSA (OR, 1.6). Future studies of treatment are necessary to determine whether the risk for stroke can be reduced with CPAP therapy, thereby supporting a relationship between OSA and cerebrovascular disease.

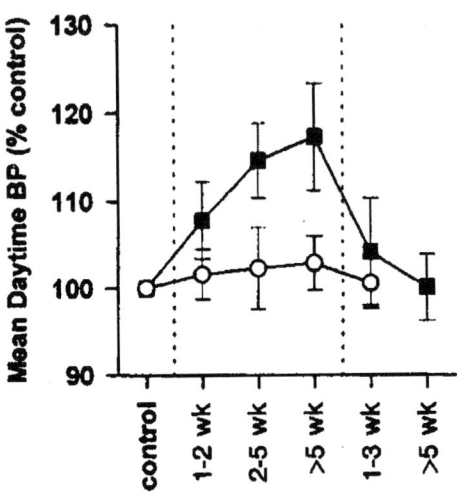

FIGURE 70.4. Mean daytime arterial blood pressure in four dogs during obstructive sleep apnea (*filled squares*) and sleep fragmentation (*open circles*). (From Brooks D, Horner RL, Kozar LF, et al. Obstructive sleep apnea as a cause of systemic hypertension. *J Clin Invest* 1997;99:106–109, with permission.)

Coronary Artery Disease

Cross-sectional data from the Sleep Heart Health Study indicate that OSA is an independent risk factor for coronary artery disease. Shahar and colleagues (74) observed an odds ratio of 1.27 (CI, 0.99–1.62) for coronary artery disease in patients with an apnea-hypopnea index of 11 or more events per hour (74). The clinical significance of this finding is unclear. However, several smaller studies have suggested that the prevalence of OSA is high among patients with coronary artery disease (75,76), and that mortality rates are higher in these patients. Peker and colleagues (77) studied 16 patients with known coronary artery disease and OSA. During the 3-year follow-up, 37.5% of the patients with OSA died, in comparison with 9.3% of the non-OSA patients matched for severity of cardiovascular disease. A Cox model identified the respiratory disturbance index as an independent predictor of cardiovascular mortality. An increased incidence of myocardial infarction has also been associated with OSA. Hung and colleagues (78) identified a 23.3 times greater odds for the development of an acute myocardial infarction in patients with OSA. Mooe and colleagues (79) similarly observed an increased risk (OR, 4.1) for the development of coronary artery disease in women with an apnea-hypopnea index of more than 5 events per hour. Thus, these studies suggest an important relationship between OSA and coronary artery disease. However, further studies are needed to determine whether treatment of OSA (CPAP) prevents the development of coronary artery disease or reduces the number of secondary cases once coronary artery disease is established.

Congestive Heart Failure

The prevalence of OSA in patients with congestive heart failure ranges from 11% to 37% (80,81). Shahar and colleagues (74), in cross-sectional data from the Sleep Heart Health Study, also reported increased odds for the development of congestive heart failure (OR, 2.38) in patients with an apnea-hypopnea index of 11 or higher. This was the largest association in the Sleep Heart Health Study for any OSA-related cardiovascular complication. Thus, although the evidence linking OSA and congestive heart failure appears strong, further intervention trials are necessary to see whether CPAP treatment effectively improves cardiac function. Improvement in these variables has been observed in patients with congestive heart failure and Cheyne-Stokes respiration (Fig. 70.5).

CARDIOVASCULAR COMPLICATIONS OF OBSTRUCTIVE SLEEP APNEA	
Summary Statement	**Level of Evidence**
OSA is associated with an increased risk for the development of hypertension, stroke, CHF, and coronary artery disease. The data are strongest for hypertension.	Hypertension, stroke, CHF, and coronary artery disease: prospective case control or cross-sectional prevalence studies

CHF, congestive heart failure; OSA, obstructive sleep apnea.

Treatment of Obstructive Sleep Apnea

As previously discussed (see section "Consequences of Obstructive Sleep Apnea"), compelling evidence suggests that recurrent obstructive apnea-hypopnea leads to daytime sleepiness, impaired cognitive performance, impaired driving skills, and hypertension. Current data also suggest that OSA may be associated with a higher incidence of stroke, myocardial infarction, and congestive heart failure (61,71,74,82–85). Treatment to eliminate events of obstructed breathing substantially relieves daytime somnolence and improves cognitive performance. CPAP remains the mainstay of therapy based on the results of several randomized controlled trials. Other forms of therapy include bilevel or auto-titration positive-pressure devices, upper airway surgery, oral appliances, and positional therapy. Each of these modalities has a potential therapeutic role and is discussed in more detail in the next sections.

Continuous Positive Airway Pressure

CPAP has been used to treat obstructive sleep apnea since 1981 and has virtually supplanted tracheostomy (86) (Fig. 70.6).

Positive airway pressure prevents collapse of the upper airway during sleep by increasing the transmural pressure across the upper airway, thereby acting as a pneumatic splint. The raised intraluminal pressure during CPAP overcomes both the collapsing forces generated during inspiration (negative pressure) and the tissue forces generated in the relaxed

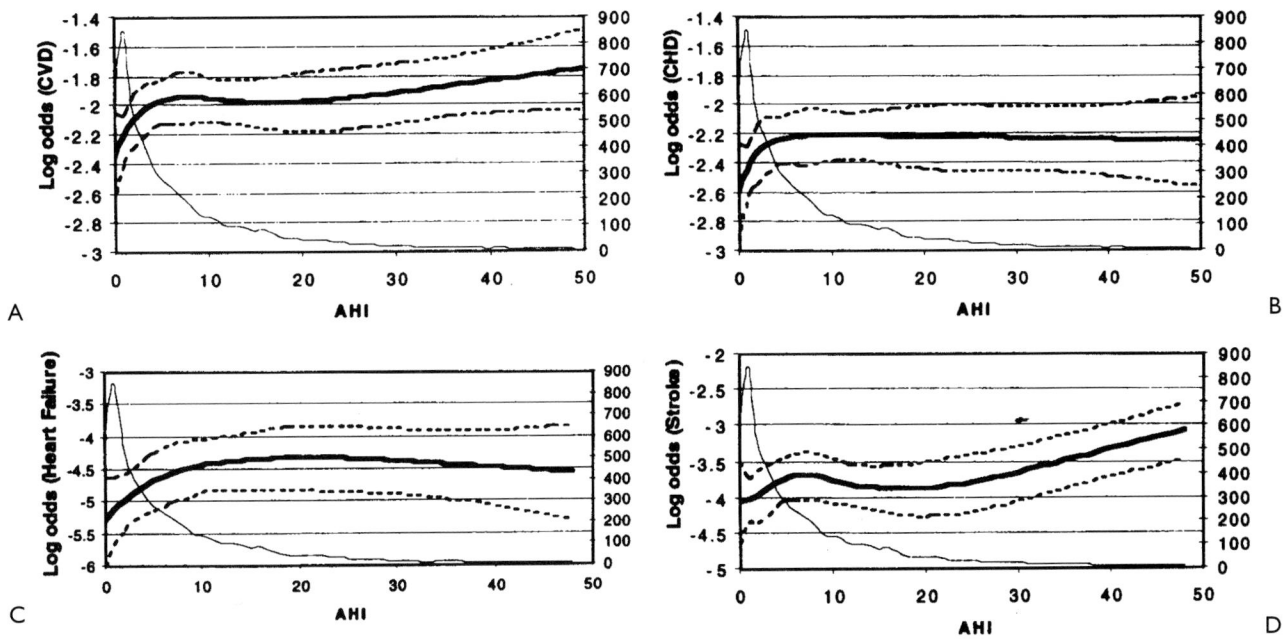

FIGURE 70.5. Regression of the log odds of cardiovascular disease (*CVD*) (**A**), coronary heart disease (*CHD*) (**B**), heart failure (**C**), and stroke (**D**) on the apnea-hypopnea index (*AHI*). *Solid thick line*, predicted odds; *dashed lines*, 95% confidence intervals; *solid thin line*, number of participants at various values of the apnea-hypopnea index (*right axis*, frequency distribution). (From Shahar E, Whitney CW, Redline S, et al. Sleep-disordered breathing and cardiovascular disease: cross-sectional results of the Sleep Heart Health Study. *Am J Respir Crit Care Med* 2001;163:19–25, with permission.)

pharynx during sleep (87). In addition, CPAP increases the functional residual capacity and thus may promote upper airway patency through mechanisms independent of upper airway muscle splinting (88,89). Multiple observational trials and several randomized trials have reported that CPAP

effectively reduces sleep-disordered breathing events, pathologic sleepiness, and the cognitive dysfunction characteristic of this disorder. Early trials by Issa and Sullivan (90) compared CPAP with conventional therapy, which included weight loss, maintenance of nasal patency, and avoidance

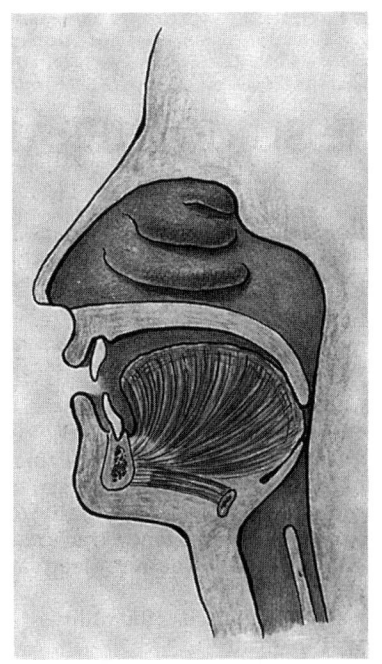

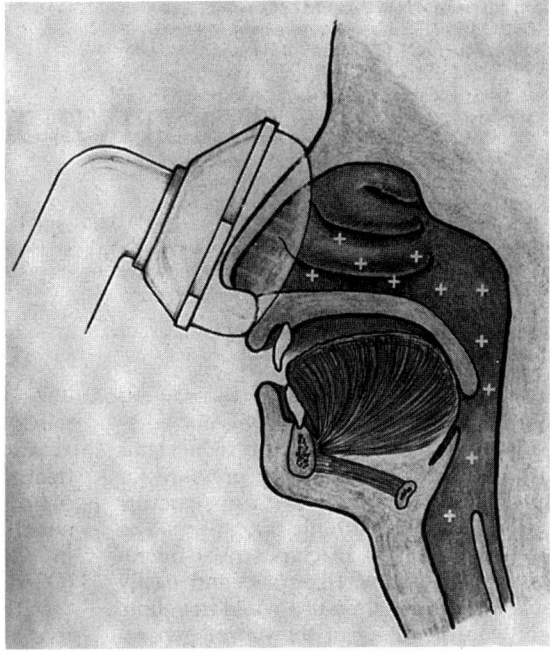

FIGURE 70.6. Nasal continuous positive airway pressure acting as a pneumatic splint in the upper airway. (From Strollo PJ, Sanders MH, Atwood CW. Positive pressure therapy. *Clin Chest Med* 1998;19:55–68, with permission.)

of alcohol. Positive pressure delivered by a nasal mask at approximately 10 cm H_2O prevented recurrent collapse of the upper airway, decreased sleep fragmentation, improved sleep quality, and often led to rebounds in slow-wave and REM sleep. After a longer period of treatment with CPAP (1–3 months), the quality-of-life scores of patients with moderate-severe OSA (>30 events of obstructed breathing per hour of sleep) improved substantially (91–93).

Findley and colleagues (94) demonstrated a reduction in crash rates after treatment with CPAP (0.07 vs. 0 crashes per driver per year, $P < .02$). They estimated that CPAP treatment in 36 hypersomnolent patients with OSA prevented five crashes during 2 years. In a larger study, George (95) suggested that CPAP treatment prevented 75 motor vehicle crashes in 210 patients during 3 years. Thus, therapy for OSA (CPAP) effectively reduces automobile accidents in patients with OSA and should be recommended.

Randomized Trials with Oral Placebo

The randomized trials investigating CPAP have used either a pill or sham CPAP as placebo. Four randomized trials comparing oral (pill) placebo with nasal CPAP (66,76–78) showed substantial improvements in cognitive function and a reduction in sleepiness in both subjective and objective assessments. However, the patients who derived the greatest benefit had subjectively reported sleepiness before enrollment and had had more severe OSA. A pill placebo–controlled study by Faccenda and colleagues (66) showed a decrease in diastolic blood pressure after treatment with CPAP in a group of normotensive patients with moderate OSA. This study supports the findings of animal studies, several intervention trials in humans, and large cross-sectional epidemiologic cohorts investigating the cardiovascular sequelae of OSA (61–63,96,97).

Despite these results and those of many similar but smaller uncontrolled case series, CPAP therapy for OSA was questioned in a controversial systematic review of the literature in 1997 from the United Kingdom. Wright and colleagues (67) stated that without adequate placebo-controlled trials, good evidence was not available to support the use of nasal CPAP in the treatment of OSA. Since that report, several randomized placebo-controlled trials in which sham CPAP was used have been conducted.

Randomized Trials with Sham Placebo

Jenkinson and colleagues (98) compared therapeutic with sham CPAP in a trial with a randomized prospective parallel design. Extra holes were placed in the mask of their sham CPAP device so that leakage was sufficient to prevent the airway pressure from rising above 1 cm H_2O yet rebreathing of carbon dioxide was prevented. Subsequently, Montserrat and colleagues (99) used this approach (sham CPAP) in a trial with a crossover design of patients with moderate-severe apnea. They found substantial and significantly greater improvements in Epworth Scale scores, measured vigilance, and

productivity scores after 6 weeks of treatment in comparison with placebo. Henke and colleagues (100) noted similar improvements in psychologic test scores after 2 weeks of CPAP in comparison with a sham device. However, a randomized controlled study in which sham CPAP placebo was used to address the effectiveness of CPAP in patients with moderate-severe OSA but no subjective sleepiness (Epworth Scale score <10) reported no significant changes in measured daytime sleepiness, quality-of-life scores, cognitive performance, or blood pressure after 6 weeks of therapy (101).

Collectively, these data end the debate regarding the effectiveness of CPAP in persons with moderate-severe OSA and pathologic sleepiness. CPAP therapy clearly relieves sleep-disordered breathing and daytime hypersomnolence, and in patients with concomitant dips in oxygen saturation, it lowers daytime blood pressure. In addition, driving performance, cognitive function, and self-reported functional outcome scores are substantially better in patients treated with CPAP than in those receiving placebo (pill or sham CPAP). These data confirm the previous recommendations for the use of CPAP to treat OSA published by the American Thoracic Society and the American College of Chest Physicians (102,103). However, improvement in neurocognitive function is less predictable in patients without pathologic sleepiness (101).

Role of Continuous Positive Airway Pressure in Mild Obstructive Sleep Apnea

The correlation between the apnea-hypopnea index and the sequelae of OSA is poor, so that the cutoff apnea-hypopnea index at which treatment should be initiated is controversial. Three additional studies investigated CPAP therapy in patients with mild OSA, defined as an apnea-hypopnea index of 5 to 15 events per hour, who reported daytime somnolence (104–106). These studies collectively demonstrated improvements in subjective sleepiness scores and cognitive tasks, such as driving simulation. Redline and colleagues (106) found that the treatment responses were not related to the degree of baseline sleepiness or sleep-disordered breathing, suggesting that patients with milder OSA should be treated with CPAP. However, Engleman and colleagues (104) found that only 14 of 34 patients preferred CPAP to a placebo pill, thus highlighting the potential lack of acceptability of CPAP to patients with mild OSA. Therefore, questions remain regarding the effectiveness of CPAP in patients with milder disease and those without pathologic sleepiness, regardless of the severity of their apnea. Given the cardiovascular complications potentially associated with OSA, previously described (see section "Cardiovascular Complications"), treatment with CPAP should at least be considered for patients with moderate-severe apnea, regardless of symptoms. However, the current consensus conference recommendation to treat moderate to severe OSA (>30 events per hour of sleep) regardless of subjective sleepiness cannot be fully supported by the available data (103).

Continuous Positive Airway Pressure Interfaces

The nasal mask has become the most popular interface for modern CPAP devices (Fig. 70.6). However, full-face masks are still used on occasion. Mask technology has exploded during the past decade, such that nearly everyone can be fitted with a comfortable interface. The nasal masks are designed to cover the nares or be inserted into the nostrils (nasal pillows) while various types of headgear hold the mask in place. Device-related problems such as nasal congestion, oral drying, skin breakdown at pressure points of the mask, and rarely conjunctivitis have all been attributed to the interface. Thus, nasal problems may affect compliance.

CONTINUOUS POSITIVE AIRWAY PRESSURE TREATMENT

Summary Statement	Level of Evidence
CPAP therapy is very effective at reducing obstructed respiratory events, relieving symptoms of daytime hypersomnolence, and improving cognitive function and health-related quality of life.	Randomized placebo-controlled prospective trials
CPAP therapy reduces daytime blood pressure in subjects with symptoms of sleepiness and oxygen desaturation and disordered breathing events.	Randomized intervention trials
CPAP therapy may not be as effective at reducing blood pressure or changing symptom scores in patients with moderate-severe OSA and minimal subjective sleepiness.	Single interventional trial

CPAP, continuous positive airway pressure; OSA, obstructive sleep apnea.

Compliance with Continuous Positive Airway Pressure

Although CPAP can prevent pharyngeal collapse in virtually all patients who wear a device, poor patient adherence to treatment may limit its overall effectiveness. Discomfort from the facial mask, excessive air pressure, and nasal symptoms often limit the time patients are willing to use this therapy. Compliance with CPAP varies depending on the study and style of reporting but has ranged from 3.9 to 7 hours a night. Disparity between reported use and actual CPAP meter readings remains common. Kribbs and colleagues (107) noted that the reported use of CPAP was 6 hours a night, whereas objective meter readings indicated use for only 5.0 ± 0.46 hours a night. McArdle and colleagues (108) studied 1,103 patients prospectively, with follow-up to 4 years, and found that 84% of patients who initiated therapy with CPAP used their device regularly (at least 2 hours a night) at 12 months. This number reached a plateau at 4 years, with 68% of patients remaining on therapy. The primary determinants of CPAP compliance in their multivariate model were an apnea-hypopnea index of more than 15, daytime sleepiness (Epworth Scale score >10), and evidence of CPAP use for longer than 2 hours a night at 3 months after the start of therapy. Similarly, Pepin and colleagues (109) found that CPAP compliance at 3 months was nearly 80%. Finally, Weaver and colleagues (110) showed that early and frequent use of CPAP, by day 4, predicted better longer-term compliance with the device. Methods aimed at improving compliance with CPAP include (a) a pressure ramp, (b) heated humidification if substantial nasal drying occurs, (c) chin straps or full face masks for mouth leaks, (d) nasal steroids or humidity to treat nasal congestion, and (e) bilevel pressure or auto-titration devices when difficulty with exhalation is a problem.

Ramp Feature. Most modern CPAP devices have a ramp feature that increases the airway pressure over 10 to 45 minutes to increase comfort. Ideally, the patient with OSA will fall asleep before the highest airway pressure delivered is reached. No studies have investigated whether compliance is improved with this feature; however, it is commonly used and can be abused. A study by Pressman and colleagues (111) identified a patient who repeatedly used his remotely controlled ramp feature, so that despite good compliance, pressures remained suboptimal for most of the night.

Heated Humidification, Face Masks, and Nasal Steroids. Nasal obstruction, whether resulting from CPAP or some other malady, is quite common and may compromise the efficacy of the device. An increase in nasal resistance potentially decreases the pharyngeal pressure and may reduce effectiveness, compliance, or both (112). Heated humidification systems may lower nasal resistance, alleviate congestion, and reduce dryness in the airway. Massie and colleagues (113) noted a better quality of sleep and increased objective use of CPAP (5.52 ± 2.1 vs. 4.93 ± 2.2 hours a night) with heated humidification. Nasal steroids are also administered frequently to reduce the nasal congestion induced by CPAP or allergic rhinitis. McNicholas and colleagues (114) reported that nasal resistance and the apnea-hypopnea index were increased in a group of patients during the peak ragweed season in comparison with a control period 6 to 8 weeks later ($P < .05$). Although this was not an interventional trial, the results support the concept that treatment should be considered for patients with OSA and nasal obstruction and that nasal steroids may improve compliance with CPAP. Full-face masks are occasionally used successfully in patients bothered by substantial air leakage from the mouth that cannot be relieved with a chin strap. However, Mortimore and colleagues (115) found that objective compliance and overall comfort were greater with a nasal mask than with a full-face mask.

Bilevel versus Fixed Airway Pressure. Fixed airway pressure devices are engineered to maintain a constant airway pressure throughout the respiratory cycle. However, patients occasionally have difficulty exhaling against fixed airway pressure. Bilevel positive airway pressure to treat OSA was introduced in the late 1980s in an attempt to improve compliance, based on the premise that partitioning the inspiratory and expiratory pressures would allow a lower expiratory pressure yet maintain airway patency. Sanders and colleagues (116) observed that obstructed respiratory events could be eliminated at expiratory pressures lower than those of conventional nasal CPAP therapy. However, a subsequent study by Reeves-Hoche and colleagues (117) of 83 OSA patients randomized to either CPAP or bilevel pressure showed no significant difference in objective machine use (5.0 ± 0.19 vs. 4.9 ± 0.23 hours a night), although more complete dropouts were noted in the CPAP than in the bilevel group. Thus, although lower expiratory pressures can be delivered with bilevel pressure devices, no convincing evidence indicates that compliance is affected.

Auto-titration Devices. "Intelligent" CPAP devices have been designed to vary the pressures applied to the upper airway according to the pressure required to maintain patency (118–121). The technology was developed to provide the lowest adequate pressure through the night. These devices can also be used to titrate CPAP levels in the home or laboratory once the diagnosis of OSA has been established. Several studies have reported that auto-titration devices maintain lower mean airway pressures in comparison with conventional CPAP devices. Sharma and colleagues (119) studied 20 patients (mean apnea-hypopnea index, 50.8 ± 28.8) and reported a mean pressure of 10.1 ± 3.8 cm H_2O in the auto-titration group versus 12.3 ± 3.9 cm H_2O in the group using fixed-level CPAP (118). Similar reductions were reported in a study by Behbehani and colleagues (8.4 ± 3.3 vs. 11.5 ± 3.1 cm H_2O) (122). Conceivably, auto-titration may improve compliance with positive airway pressure, although this has not been a consistent observation. However, the devices do abolish apneas-hypopneas as effectively as conventional CPAP. Ficker and colleagues (120) observed equivalent reductions in the apnea-hypopnea index with auto-titration and conventional CPAP (post-treatment apnea-hypopnea indices of 4.2 and 3.6 events per hour). Auto-titration devices have also been used to predict future fixed-level CPAP needs. Lloberes and colleagues (123) found auto-titration of CPAP to be as effective as standard titration in determining the optimal positive pressure. However, the variation in pressure in many patients was more than 2 cm H_2O with the auto-titration device in comparison with conventional CPAP titration in REM sleep. Thus, the role of auto-titration CPAP devices, both as therapy for OSA and as a means to determine the fixed CPAP requirement, remains controversial.

Oral Positive Airway Pressure. A device has been developed to deliver positive airway pressure through the mouth with a dental appliance interface. This device is intended to reduce the airway pressures required to prevent pharyn-geal collapse during sleep and allow oral ventilation in patients with nasal disease. However, no trials comparing efficacy or side effects in comparison with conventional CPAP have been published, so that it is impossible to make any conclusions.

COMPLIANCE WITH CONTINUOUS POSITIVE AIRWAY PRESSURE THERAPY

Summary Statement	Level of Evidence
Heated humidification devices improve CPAP compliance and reduce symptoms of nasal obstruction.	Comparative intervention trials and expert opinion
Bilevel pressure has not been shown to improve compliance with CPAP therapy substantially; however, bilevel pressure is able to eliminate apneas with a lower expiratory pressure.	Comparative intervention trials
Auto-titrating devices eliminate apneas similarly to CPAP devices; however, their use at home as pressure-titrating devices requires further study.	Comparative intervention trials

CPAP, continuous positive airway pressure.

Oral Appliances

The American Academy of Sleep Medicine practice guidelines for the use of oral appliances recommended them as a treatment for snoring or mild OSA. In addition, a trial of oral appliance therapy was suggested for patients with severe OSA who could not tolerate CPAP (124). Since that time, randomized placebo-controlled trials have further justified their use. These devices are mouth guards that simply advance the mandible or hold the tongue forward, favorably affecting airway size and relieving apnea. Lowe and colleagues (125) observed substantial increases in airway size with these devices in place. A study in which computed tomography was used reported similar results, with a mean increase of 2.83 cm² in the size of the pharyngeal airway noted during wakefulness with an appliance in place (126).

Currently, more than 55 devices are available, but only three have undergone rigorously controlled or randomized trials. The most popular oral appliances are adjustable, allowing for progressive mandibular advancement over time (Fig. 70.7).

Lowe reported better comfort and tolerance with progressively advanced devices than with devices that had a single setting (127). Ferguson and colleagues (128), in a small randomized crossover study of a group of patients with mild OSA, found that 85% of them preferred oral appliances to CPAP despite greater reductions in the apnea-hypopnea index with CPAP. Although many patients with OSA accept these devices, side effects are common. In a study of 22 patients, Fritsch and colleagues (129) reported mucosal

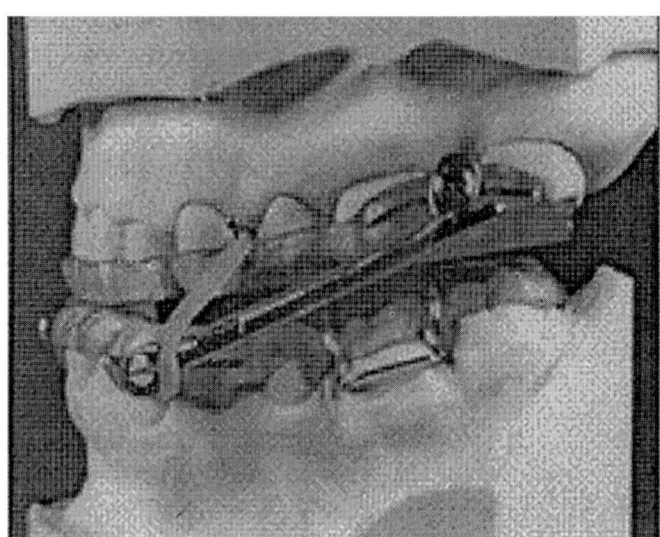
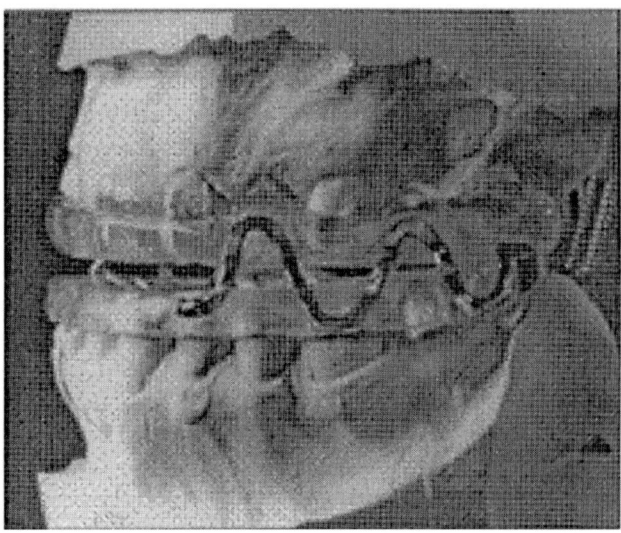

A   B

FIGURE 70.7. Two examples of oral appliances for the treatment of obstructive sleep apnea: OSA-Herbst (**A**) and OSA-Monoblock (**B**). (From Bloch KE, Iseli A, Zhang J, et al. A randomized, controlled crossover trial of two oral appliances for sleep apnea treatment. *Am J Respir Crit Care Med* 2000;162:246–251, with permission.)

dryness in 86%, tooth discomfort in 59%, and hypersalivation in 55% as the most common side effects of two commercially available oral appliances. However, no patient withdrew from the trial or had to discontinue the treatment. Furthermore, the devices effectively reduced both the apnea-hypopnea index (27.6 ± 3.5 vs. 6.3 ± 1.4 events per hour) and the arousal index. Similarly, Bloch and colleagues (130) compared two oral appliances in a group of 24 patients who could not tolerate CPAP and found substantial reductions in both the apnea-hypopnea index and subjective sleepiness (Epworth Scale score) (Fig. 70.8).

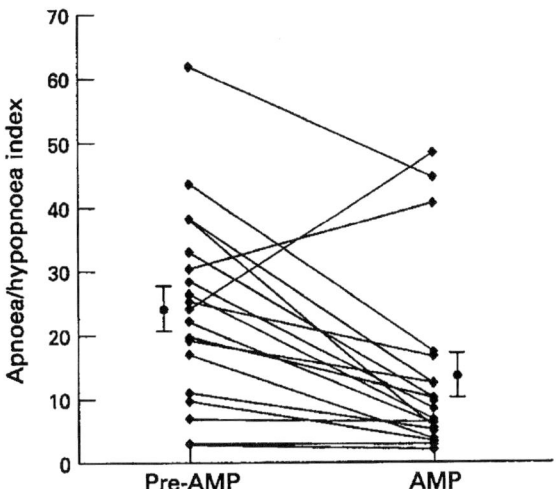

FIGURE 70.8. Apnea-hypopnea index before and after placement of an anterior mandibular positioner. The apnea-hypopnea index was significantly reduced by the positioner ($P < .005$). (From Ferguson KA, Ono T, Lowe AA, et al. A short-term controlled trial of an adjustable oral appliance for the treatment of mild to moderate OSA. *Thorax* 1997;52:362–368, with permission.)

In a randomized trial in which a lower dental plate was used as a control, Mehta and colleagues (131) showed substantial reductions in the apnea-hypopnea index, with 35% of patients experiencing a complete response, defined as an apnea-hypopnea index of fewer than 5 events per hour. Multiple regression analysis identified four independent predictors of a complete response to therapy: (a) neck circumference, (b) baseline apnea-hypopnea index, (c) size of the retropalatal air space on cephalometry, and (d) degree of jaw protrusion on cephalometric films. However, despite the inclusion of the apnea-hypopnea index in this regression model, more severe OSA was not associated with an increase in oral appliance treatment failures. Liu and colleagues (132) provided further support for these predictors, observing that young persons and those with narrower airways had the best response to oral appliances.

Objective compliance with oral appliances is more difficult to measure than objective compliance with CPAP. Lowe and colleagues (133) reported the use of a temperature-sensitive monitor embedded in the oral appliance that made it possible to determine compliance. The mean duration of use was 6.8 hours a night, which reduced the apnea-hypopnea index (32.6 ± 2.1 vs. 12.1 ± 1.7 events per hour of sleep).

Collectively, these data provide strong evidence that oral appliances effectively reduce the apnea-hypopnea index, relieving daytime sleepiness, and are useful alternatives for patients who cannot tolerate CPAP. Major disadvantages are few; however, the therapy may not be effective in patients with severe OSA. Minor side effects, such as increased salivation, mouth and tooth discomfort, and tooth movement, are rarely prohibitive. As previously noted, the American Academy of Sleep Medicine recommends oral appliances for patients with moderate-severe OSA who cannot tolerate CPAP therapy and for patients with mild disease. In addition, Millman and colleagues (134) suggested that oral appliances are useful for reducing the apnea-hypopnea index after failed uvulopalatopharyngoplasty (UPPP) (see section "Uvulopalatopharyngoplasty"). However, further trials are needed to define the appropriate groups better and to determine what patient characteristics suggest the greatest benefit.

ORAL APPLIANCE THERAPY	
Summary Statement	**Level of Evidence**
Oral appliance therapy is effective at reducing the apnea-hypopnea index, arousal index, symptoms of daytime sleepiness, and nadir oxygen saturation in patients with mild-moderate OSA. Patients with moderate OSA and those with severe OSA who are intolerant of CPAP should be considered for oral appliance therapy.	Randomized placebo-controlled trial comparing placebo (mouth guard) with oral appliance
Oral appliances are preferred to CPAP therapy; however, the apnea-hypopnea index is reduced further with CPAP.	Randomized crossover trial

CPAP, continuous positive airway pressure; OSA, obstructive sleep apnea.

Surgical Therapy

Nasal CPAP remains the first-line treatment for OSA. However, a major drawback of CPAP therapy is that the device must be used every night for life, which limits compliance (109). Thus, upper airway surgery may be considered for patients in whom other noninvasive treatments for OSA have been unsuccessful or rejected on a long-term basis. Surgical therapy is often approached in a staged manner. However, five procedures are addressed individually in the next sections, with the order reflecting increasing invasiveness.

Radiofrequency Volumetric Tissue Reduction of the Palate

Radiofrequency energy has been used for several years to reduce the size of the palate in patients with sleep-disordered breathing (135). Frequencies of 465 kHz are delivered directly to the tissue of the soft palate, tongue, or nares with custom-fabricated needle electrodes. This procedure induces swelling in the local tissues and ultimately shrinkage after repeated applications. It can be performed in an outpatient setting with minimal sedation, and the patients do not often report substantial discomfort. Troell and colleagues (136) reported that only 9% of a radiofrequency group but 100% of a laser-assisted uvulopalatoplasty (LAUP) group required postoperative narcotic medicine for pain. Despite the fa-

vorable side effect profile, radiofrequency ablation appears most useful for simple snoring, not sleep apnea. Powell and colleagues (135) noted a reduction in upper airway resistance (characterized by less-negative esophageal balloon deflections) in 22 patients with either mild OSA, increased upper airway resistance, or primary snoring. However, the apnea-hypopnea index did not substantially change in this cohort. In a prospective nonrandomized study by Brown and colleagues (137), the apnea-hypopnea index decreased modestly (from 31.2 ± 5.1 to 23.5 ± 4.2 events per hour, $P < .05$), with none of the patients demonstrating a reduction in daytime sleepiness or an improvement in sleep architecture. Lastly, Woodson and colleagues (138) compared CPAP therapy with radiofrequency palatal tissue reduction in patients with OSA. They reported modest improvements in the apnea-hypopnea index (from 40.5 to 32.8 events per hour) after radiofrequency and similar daytime sleepiness scores for the two groups. Thus, one study suggests that radiofrequency palatal ablation may be a viable alternative to CPAP in patients with mild OSA. However, this was a small, nonrandomized trial. Before radiofrequency palatal ablation can be fully accepted as therapy for mild apnea, further large-scale trials are required.

Collectively, these studies suggest that radiofrequency palatal ablation is minimally effective at treating anything more than very mild OSA. However, it is moderately effective in reducing or eliminating snoring, although the durability of this effect is questionable.

Laser-Assisted Uvulopalatoplasty

LAUP is a surgical procedure in which a carbon dioxide laser is used to vaporize the uvula and portions of the soft palate. In comparison with UPPP (see next section), this procedure removes less palatal tissue, spares tonsillar tissue, and is generally performed as an outpatient procedure during one to several visits. To date, randomized placebo-controlled studies of the effectiveness of LAUP in OSA are lacking. The results of early studies in which LAUP was used to treat snoring were encouraging. Kamami and colleagues (139) reported the elimination of virtually all snoring in 77.4% of their cohort. However, longer-term follow-up studies reported a reduction in snoring in only 62.2% of patients beyond 2 years (140). These results are comparable with those of UPPP for snoring (141).

The data for LAUP in treating OSA and reducing the apnea-hypopnea index are less compelling. Ryan and Lowe (142) reported a reduction in the apnea-hypopnea index to below 10 in only 27% of their cohort despite improvements in airway size (anteroposteriorly but not laterally) and quality-of-life measures. However, the postoperative decrements in the sleepiness scores did not correlate with decrements in the apnea-hypopnea index, suggesting that the surgery may not have been responsible for the observed symptomatic improvements. In addition, patients with mild

OSA (mean apnea hypopnea index, 19 ± 13 events per hour) showed an increase in the apnea-hypopnea index postoperatively (142). Small improvements in the apnea-hypopnea index have been reported by Seeman and colleagues (143) and in several other small cohorts (144–147). Seeman and colleagues (143) reported modest reductions in the apnea-hypopnea index in 60% of their patients, with the greatest improvements seen in the patients with the most severe disease (apnea-hypopnea index >30 events per hour). Thus, LAUP does not appear to be particularly effective in the treatment of sleep apnea.

The pain that patients experience after LAUP is considerable and actually comparable with that experienced after UPPP. However, the latter procedure requires an inpatient hospital stay. In addition to pain, the most common side effects include choking at meals, dry throat, persistent globus sensation in the throat, and nasal congestion (136).

Based on the available literature, practice parameters for the use of LAUP were published by the Standards of Practice Committee of the American Academy of Sleep Medicine in 2001 (148). The report concluded that insufficient evidence is available to recommend LAUP for the treatment of OSA. The decision, based on all available data, cited a paucity of large studies and only small reductions in the apnea-hypopnea index, with an occasional increase in the apnea-hypopnea index. In addition, data are lacking on the long-term efficacy of the procedure and predictive strategies to determine responders to this surgery (148).

Uvulopalatopharyngoplasty

UPPP, introduced in 1981 by Fujita and colleagues (149), remains a common form of therapy for OSA. Patients with clinically important OSA in whom medical treatment has failed or who are unwilling to comply with medical therapy are considered candidates for this surgical intervention. The improvement is attributed to enlargement of the velopharynx because the procedure removes the uvula, tonsillar pillars, and a portion of the soft palate (150). In addition, reductions in pharyngeal collapsibility, measured by the critical closing pressure of the airway (Pcrit), have been reported after successful UPPP (151).

Despite early excitement about this procedure, the postoperative outcomes are highly variable, with approximately half of the patients undergoing UPPP showing at least a 50% reduction in the apnea-hypopnea index (152). In a meta-analysis of 37 studies, Sher and colleagues (153) reported a favorable response to UPPP in 40.7% of patients; a favorable outcome was defined as an apnea-hypopnea index of fewer than 20 events per hour and at least a 50% reduction in the apnea-hypopnea index.

Identifying the collapsing segment of the upper airway has been helpful in determining which patients are more likely to have a favorable outcome after UPPP. UPPP is most effective when collapse occurs in the palatal region but is ineffective in preventing collapse in either the retroglossal space or the oropharynx. Launois and colleagues (154) reported greater reductions in the apnea-hypopnea index and arousal index when the nasopharynx (defined as the region extending from the nasal septum to the free margin of the soft palate) was the primary site of obstruction. In a follow-up study, Isono and colleagues (155) determined the static pressure and area characteristics of the upper airway in 13 anesthetized, paralyzed patients undergoing UPPP. They noted that patients with less collapse in the pharyngeal segment behind the tongue had a better outcome after UPPP. Unfortunately, such measurements are cumbersome and require specialized equipment and so are impractical for clinical assessment. In addition, efforts to determine the site of airway collapse with nasopharyngoscopy during Müller maneuvers were not able to discriminate adequately between surgical responders (defined as patients with at least a 50% reduction in the apnea-hypopnea index) and nonresponders (156).

Cephalometric examinations have been used with variable success to predict outcomes after UPPP. Absence of a retrognathic jaw and a short distance between the mandibular plane and hyoid bone predicted a successful UPPP (157).

Long-term outcomes after UPPP vary depending on the time to follow-up. Boot and colleagues (158) reported long-term follow-up in 50 patients after UPPP at 6, 21, and 46 months. Surgical success was defined as an apnea-hypopnea index of fewer than 10 events per hour. At 6 months (first assessment), 60% of patients had a successful outcome, whereas at 21 months, only 38% were still responders. The patients whose apnea-hypopnea index increased with time also had an increase in their BMI of 2.2 ± 1.5 kg/m². After weight loss and abstinence from alcohol, the success rate for this group increased to 50% at 46 months (158). Thus, long-term (to 46 months) outcomes after UPPP are not substantially different from the early results, after control for confounders such as weight gain and alcohol consumption.

Mandibular Osteotomy with Genioglossus Advancement

Hypopharyngeal obstruction is common in OSA and may be relieved surgically by a limited osteotomy of the mandible with advancement of the hyoid-genioglossus complex (Fig. 70.9).

This surgery was first described by Powell and colleagues as part of the Stanford stepped approach to surgical intervention for OSA. It is sometimes combined with a hyoid suspension procedure. The operation theoretically increases airway size and prevents posterior displacement of the tongue during sleep. The efficacy of the procedure is limited by the extent of anterior displacement of the tongue that is possible and depends on the thickness of the mandible. Riley and colleagues (159) determined that the apnea-hypopnea index of only 37.5% of patients with hypopharyngeal collapse

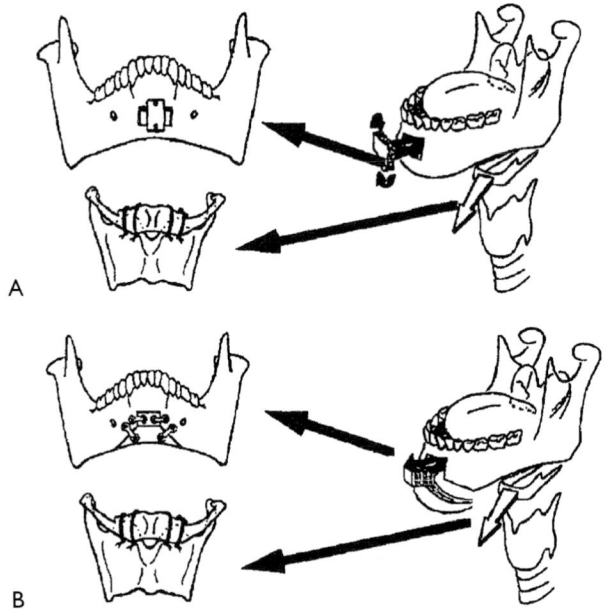

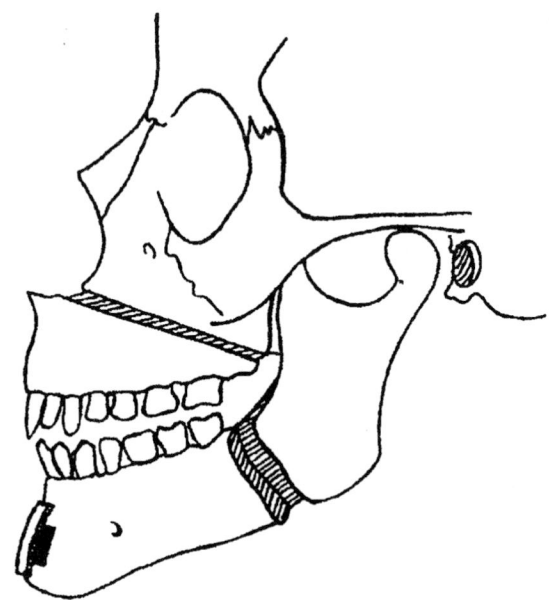

FIGURE 70.9. Genioglossus advancement, hyoid myotomy, and hypothyroidopexy. **A:** The genioglossus advancement procedure is usually performed via an inferior rectangular sagittal osteotomy of the mandible (*upper arrow*, A). **B:** Alternatively, the osteotomy can be started at the inferior border of the mandible and followed under visual control by trapezoidal osteotomy for advancement of the genioglossus muscle (*upper arrow*, B). Late modifications to either procedure involve stabilization of the hyoid bone inferiorly by attachment to the superior border of the thyroid cartilage (*lower arrow*, A and B). (From Bettega G, Pepin JL, Deschaux C, et al. Obstructive sleep apnea syndrome: 51 consecutive patients treated by maxillofacial surgery. *Am J Respir Crit Care Med* 2000;162:641–649.)

FIGURE 70.10. Maxillomandibular advancement osteotomy procedure. Bilateral sagittal split osteotomy and maxillary advancement by Le Fort I osteotomy. (From Bettega G, Pepin JL, Deschaux C, et al. Obstructive sleep apnea syndrome: 51 consecutive patients treated by maxillofacial surgery. *Am J Respir Crit Care Med* 2000;162:641–649, with permission.)

improved substantially after osteotomy and genioglossus advancement alone. The addition of hyoid myotomy and suspension improved response rates to 65.3%. However, UPPP was also performed in all these cases. Other groups have reported more limited success with this procedure. Bettega and colleagues (160) presented the results in 51 consecutive patients treated with a stepped surgical approach in which step 1 consisted of a mandibular osteotomy with genioglossus advancement (with or without hyoid myotomy and UPPP). Overall, the apnea-hypopnea index of only 22.7% of their patients was reduced to fewer than 15 events per hour. These inconsistencies have also been observed in smaller studies of the osteotomy procedure, with success rates ranging from 17% to 78% (161,162). Nearly half of the Bettega cohort eventually underwent more definitive surgery, the maxillomandibular advancement osteotomy (Fig. 70.10). To date, no studies have identified clinical factors that predict the surgical outcome.

Maxillomandibular Advancement Osteotomy

Refractory hypopharyngeal obstruction that is not amenable to medical therapy (CPAP) or that has failed to improve after less invasive upper airway surgical procedures may be corrected with a maxillomandibular advancement procedure.

Typically, this invasive procedure is reserved for failures of prior surgical therapy because the sleep-disordered breathing of a substantial number of patients is eliminated or significantly reduced by lesser procedures. Maxillomandibular advancement osteotomy consists of a maxillary osteotomy with rigid plate fixation and bilateral sagittal split mandibular osteotomies (Fig. 70.10). The result is advancement of both the maxilla and mandible by at least 10 mm to allow more room for the tongue and pharyngeal airway (163).

This procedure often cures OSA in selected patients; some centers report success rates of more than 90% when maxillomandibular advancement osteotomy is performed after genioglossus advancement (164). Riley and Powell (163) reported substantial improvements in the apnea-hypopnea index after maxillomandibular advancement osteotomy (72.0 ± 25.8 vs. 8.8 ± 6.1 events per hour), with reductions in the nadir oxygen saturation. However, reported success rates from both Riley and Powell (163) and Waite and colleagues (165) are approximately 78% for maxillomandibular advancement osteotomy alone (without previous genioglossus advancement). Bettega and colleagues (160) reported reductions in the apnea-hypopnea index from 59 ± 29 to 11 ± 9 events per hour, with a favorable outcome in 75% of patients (apnea-hypopnea index <10 events per hour and a 50% reduction in obstructed breathing events). As with genioglossus advancement, no clear preoperative clinical predictors of success are available for these procedures.

SURGICAL THERAPY

Summary Statement	Level of Evidence
Radiofrequency volumetric reduction of the palate is not an effective therapy for OSA. However, as a treatment for primary snoring, it may be successful in some patients.	Nonrandomized cohort, case series
Laser-assisted uvulopalatoplasty is not effective as a treatment for OSA; however, it may be helpful in treating primary snoring.	Nonrandomized concurrent case series and expert opinion/position papers
UPPP is effective in approximately 40%–50% of patients in reducing the apnea-hypopnea index to <20 events per hour and by 50%. This therapy is more effective when obstruction occurs in the velopharynx. UPPP is less effective than CPAP.	Comparative trials observing moderate efficacy in treating OSA; small randomized study comparing UPPP with oral appliances for treatment
Mandibular osteotomy with genioglossus advancement and hyoid myotomy with suspension is variably effective (22%–78%) in reducing the apnea-hypopnea index to <10 events per hour.	Small cohort studies and case series
Maxillomandibular advancement lowers the apnea-hypopnea index and reduces oxygen desaturation in approximately 75% of patients. This therapy should be used for people who have failed other surgical interventions for OSA, unless they have facial deformities preventing less invasive surgical procedures.	Nonrandomized concurrent prospective cohort studies

CPAP, continuous positive airway pressure; OSA, obstructive sleep apnea; UPPP, uvulopalatopharyngoplasty.

Positional Therapy

Obstructive apneas that occur primarily when patients are in a supine position are often amenable to positional therapy, in which patients try not to sleep on their back. This can be accomplished in some cases by placing an uncomfortable object, such as a ball or backpack, in the midthoracic region posteriorly, effectively eliminating or substantially reducing the amount of time spent in a supine position. Cartwright and colleagues (166) studied 60 men with an apnea-hypopnea index above 12.5 that was clearly positional. The apnea-hypopnea index was reduced to below 5 in more than 50% of the patients when they avoided sleeping in a supine position. Jokic and colleagues (167) studied positional OSA in a smaller cohort, randomizing the patients to CPAP or positional therapy. They reported a lower mean apnea-hypopnea index in the CPAP group (difference of 6.1 events per hour). However, the sleepiness

scores and cognitive outcome studies of the two groups did not differ significantly. Thus, despite small differences in the apnea-hypopnea index, positional therapy may be an adequate therapeutic alternative for patients with mild positional OSA.

Pharmacologic Therapy

The pharmacologic treatment of sleep-disordered breathing is appealing because CPAP is often difficult to tolerate, and many patients are unwilling to undergo potentially complicated upper airway surgery. However, no currently available pharmacologic agents effectively treat OSA. Several classes of drugs are promising and may ultimately prove useful.

Medroxyprogesterone

Medroxyprogesterone is a steroid moiety that increases the hypercapnic ventilatory response during wakefulness (168). It has been reported to increase minute ventilation in some patients with chronic obstructive lung disease and obesity hypoventilation syndrome. However, two randomized, double-blinded, placebo-controlled trials reported no significant reduction in apnea severity (169,170) after this drug was administered, especially in patients with normocapnia. Patients with resting hypercapnia (obesity hypoventilation) do seem to derive some benefit; however, they likely represent a different subgroup from the patients with standard sleep apnea.

Acetazolamide

Acetazolamide is a carbonic anhydrase inhibitor that increases central respiratory drive and lowers the carbon dioxide apneic threshold, thus preventing the development of central apneas. White and colleagues (171) treated six men who had central sleep apnea (CSA) with acetazolamide four times per day. They observed a decrease in central apneas (from 54 to 12 events per hour), a decrease in arterial P_{CO_2} and pH, and relief of daytime symptoms. However, one randomized and two small subsequent nonrandomized interventional trials showed no substantial benefit of acetazolamide in the treatment of OSA (172–174). In addition, the apnea-hypopnea index of some patients increased during therapy. Finally, Whyte and colleagues (175) reported modest reductions in the apnea-hypopnea index with acetazolamide but no symptomatic improvement. These data suggest that acetazolamide is not effective therapy for OSA, although it may have a role in CSA.

Protriptyline

Protriptyline is a nonsedating tricyclic antidepressant that was fortuitously found to reduce the apnea-hypopnea index during treatment for narcolepsy (176). Subsequent studies of protriptyline showed that the primary benefit of this agent is to reduce REM sleep and thus the frequency of apneas, which tend to occur in REM rather than in NREM sleep.

One randomized placebo-controlled trial (crossover design with acetazolamide) observed no significant reduction in apneas, oxygen desaturation, or symptom scores (175). Other studies have shown improvements in the apnea-hypopnea index, but the effects are generally minor and related to REM-associated events (177–180). Collectively, these studies suggest that protriptyline reduces the apnea-hypopnea index in patients with primarily REM-related events. Side effects of the tricyclic agents also limit their general acceptance. Therefore, they are not often used to treat sleep apnea.

Serotonin Reuptake Inhibitors, Trazodone, and L-Tryptophan

Importantly, serotoninergic neurons modulate activation of the genioglossus muscle, the major upper airway dilator muscle, through the serotonin (5-HT) receptors 2A, 2C, 6, and 7 (181). Both Kubin and colleagues (182) and Douse and colleagues (183) observed increased activity in the hypoglossal nerve (or genioglossus muscle) after the direct application of serotoninergic agonists to the hypoglossal motor nucleus in cats. During sleep, a substantial decrease in the activity of serotoninergic neurons projecting to the hypoglossal motor nucleus may contribute to upper airway collapse in patients with OSA. Therefore, serotonin reuptake inhibitors might be expected to increase the activity of the genioglossus muscle and thus relieve sleep-disordered breathing. Berry and colleagues (184) observed an increase in the peak activity of the genioglossus muscle (29.8% vs. 24.4%, $P < .05$) in eight subjects given a single 40-mg dose of paroxetine before bedtime. However, the apnea-hypopnea index did not substantially differ after therapy. Kraiczi and colleagues (185) performed a double-blinded, randomized, placebo-controlled trial to test the effect of 20 mg of paroxetine per day for 6 weeks and found a 35% reduction in the NREM apnea-hypopnea index; however, no effect was seen in REM-related apneas. In addition, no significant improvement in cognitive function was reported. Collectively, serotonin reuptake inhibitors have only a modest effect on the apnea-hypopnea index and thus are not currently recommended for the treatment of OSA.

Another approach taken to activate the serotoninergic system has been to administer a serotonin precursor (L-tryptophan) and a 5-HT$_2$ receptor agonist (trazodone). Veasey and colleagues (181) administered L-trytophan and trazodone to English bulldogs (OSA model) and observed substantial reductions in the apnea-hypopnea index, sleep fragmentation, and sleep-related suppression of upper airway dilator muscle activation. Although these data provide interesting insights into the pathophysiology of sleep-disordered breathing, trazodone and L-tryptophan have not been studied in humans.

Cholinergic Agonists

Nicotine has been shown to be a potent activator of the genioglossus in animals and may act through either local or central cholinergic mechanisms. Gothe and colleagues (186) observed modest reductions in the apnea-hypopnea index after nicotine gum was given to a group of patients with OSA. However, Davila and colleagues (187) reported no significant changes in the apnea-hypopnea index after the application of a nicotine patch. Slamowitz and colleagues (188) studied normal subjects before and after transmucosal nicotine patches were attached to an upper molar and observed no significant changes in genioglossus activation. Thus, based on the available data, nicotine cannot be recommended for the treatment of OSA.

Modafinil

Modafinil is a novel wakefulness-promoting agent that has primarily been used to treat the excessive daytime sleepiness associated with narcolepsy. Two randomized, placebo-controlled trials have investigated its use in the treatment of daytime sleepiness in OSA. Kingshott and colleagues (189) studied 30 hypersomnolent patients with OSA who had Epworth Scale scores of 11 or higher and sleep onset latencies of

PHARMACOLOGIC THERAPY	
Summary Statement	**Level of Evidence**
Medroxyprogesterone is not effective therapy for OSA in patients with normocapnia. The evidence for its effectiveness in the treatment of hypercapnic patients is mixed, and thus it cannot be recommended.	Comparative intervention trials
Acetazolamide therapy is not effective treatment for OSA. It may reduce the carbon dioxide apneic threshold and thus relieve central sleep apnea.	Comparative trials and one randomized trial
Protriptyline may modestly reduce the apnea-hypopnea index but should be used with caution given the anticholinergic side effects associated with tricyclic antidepressant medications. It is therefore not recommended.	Comparative and small randomized trials
Serotonin agonists (or SSRIs) do not substantially affect the apnea-hypopnea index or the neurocognitive defects associated with the disorder. Thus, these agents are not recommended for the treatment of OSA.	Mostly comparative trials with one randomized placebo-controlled trial
Cholinergic agonists (nicotine) may modestly reduce the apnea-hypopnea index in patients with OSA; however, they cannot be routinely recommended for the treatment of OSA.	Conflicting nonrandomized comparative trials
Modafinil may reduce residual daytime sleepiness after CPAP therapy for OSA.	Conflicting randomized controlled trials

CPAP, continuous positive airway pressure; OSA, obstructive sleep apnea; SSRI, selective serotonin reuptake inhibitor.

10 minutes or less. The patients were treated with modafinil or placebo and concomitant CPAP for 2 weeks. No changes in subjective assessments of sleepiness or scores on the Multiple Sleep Latency Test were observed. However, a significant increase in alertness, measured by the Maintenance of Wakefulness Test, was reported (18.3 vs. 16.6 minutes, $P < .02$), although a small portion of this treatment effect may have been attributable to worsening CPAP compliance in the treatment group (6.3 vs. 6.5 hours per night, $P < .03$). In a study by Pack and colleagues (190), the treatment of hypersomnolent patients (mean baseline Epworth Scale score, 14; Multiple Sleep Latency Test, 7.5 minutes) with modafinil for 4 weeks led to improvements in subjective assessments of daytime sleepiness and improved scores on the Multiple Sleep Latency Test.

Further studies are needed to determine specific patient characteristics that predict a response to modafinil in the treatment of residual daytime sleepiness and the most effective dose.

CENTRAL SLEEP APNEA AND CHEYNE-STOKES RESPIRATION WITH CONGESTIVE HEART FAILURE

CSA is defined as a cessation of ventilation without concomitant respiratory effort. It is a manifestation of breathing instability that occurs in a variety of clinical conditions and is classified as hypercapnic or nonhypercapnic depending on the daytime $P\text{co}_2$. Patients with predominantly CSA comprise fewer than 10% of apneic patients in most sleep laboratory populations, with studies suggesting a prevalence of only 4% (191–193).

Hypercapnic Central Sleep Apnea

This relatively rare form of CSA is characterized by daytime hypercapnia and nocturnal episodes of CSA. Adults with obesity hypoventilation syndrome (pickwickian syndrome) hypoventilate during the daytime, and the hypoventilation worsens during sleep (194). Their chemoresponsiveness to carbon dioxide is significantly blunted, so that the daytime $P\text{co}_2$ is elevated (195). The sequelae of chronic alveolar hypoventilation, including cor pulmonale, polycythemia, and peripheral edema, are common in these patients (195). They also commonly experience daytime hypersomnolence and disrupted sleep, both secondary to nocturnal arousals associated with CSA. However, obstructive apneas also occur in this population and likely contribute to their daytime symptoms. Other diseases can be responsible for inducing hypercapnic CSA, including Shy-Drager syndromes, familial dysautonomia, brainstem strokes, encephalitis, neuromuscular disease, and diabetes. The abnormal control of breathing in some of these disorders is associated with diffuse abnormalities of the brain-

stem or autonomic nervous system that are quite rare (196). Thus, therapy for hypercapnic CSA is focused on improving alveolar ventilation by administering nocturnal ventilation. Noninvasive ventilatory support via a nasal mask is effective (197) and has largely supplanted tracheostomy, diaphragmatic pacing, and negative-pressure ventilators (iron lung or cuirass).

Nonhypercapnic Central Sleep Apnea

Transient instability of the ventilatory control system, rather than a defect of ventilatory control, is the hallmark of nonhypercapnic CSA. This form of CSA is typically associated with an increased hypercapnic ventilatory sensitivity that leads to hyperventilation and recurrent apneas during sleep. Although metabolic disorders such as acromegaly can be associated with this form of CSA (198), the two most common forms of nonhypercapnic CSA are Cheyne-Stokes respiration and idiopathic CSA, which are discussed in the next sections.

Idiopathic Central Apnea

Idiopathic CSA is a disorder characterized by recurrent central apneas/hypopneas and an unstable sleep state for which no cause can be readily identified. Nonetheless, these patients typically have an increased ventilatory response to carbon dioxide and thus are prone to hyperventilation and recurrent apneas during both wakefulness and sleep. They typically have a low resting $P\text{co}_2$ while awake (35.1 vs. 38.8 mm Hg) and during sleep (37.8 vs. 42.7 mm Hg) (199). Thus, at the onset of sleep, patients with idiopathic CSA have a $P\text{co}_2$ that is typically below the apneic threshold and are prone to the development of central apneas. They may experience daytime hypersomnolence but more often experience insomnia, restless sleep, frequent awakenings, and occasionally shortness of breath. Successful treatment has been reported with acetazolamide, supplemental oxygen, and CPAP. White and colleagues (171) found that acetazolamide, a carbonic anhydrase inhibitor, substantially reduced central apneas in six patients treated for 1 to 2 weeks. Martin and colleagues (200) observed that oxygen therapy reduced the frequency of apnea in eight patients, and in a similar study, McNicholas and colleagues (201) reported reductions in central apneas after the administration of oxygen that were sustained after 5 months of therapy. Both Issa and Sullivan (202) and Hoffstein and Slutsky (203) have shown CPAP therapy to be effective in some patients with CSA.

Cheyne-Stokes Respiration

Cheyne-Stokes respiration with CSA is characterized by central apneas/hypopneas alternating with ventilatory periods that have a waxing-waning pattern of tidal volume (204). This pattern of breathing occurs in 30% to 40% of patients with congestive heart failure; however, Cheyne-Stokes respiration with CSA is also seen in a variety of neurologic conditions, including cerebrovascular disease and dementia (205). The exact mechanism leading to Cheyne-Stokes respiration with CSA in these neurologic conditions is not known. However, combinations of hypocapnia, hypoxia, increased chemosensitivity, and a delayed circulatory time contribute to the pathophysiology of Cheyne-Stokes respiration with CSA seen in congestive heart failure (204).

Patients who have congestive heart failure and Cheyne-Stokes respiration with CSA have a higher mortality rate and a greater need for cardiac transplantation (206–208). CPAP therapy in patients with stable chronic congestive heart failure and Cheyne-Stokes respiration with CSA has been shown to reduce Cheyne-Stokes respiration with CSA, left ventricular afterload, plasma catecholamines, and sympathetic nervous system activity, and to improve left ventricular ejection fraction and quality of life (204) (Fig. 70.11). In a pilot study of 66 patients with congestive heart failure and Cheyne-Stokes respiration with CSA performed by Sin and colleagues (208), those patients who were randomized to treatment with CPAP and complied with therapy up to 6 hours per night had a significantly higher rate of transplantation-free survival (25% vs. 56%).

Supplemental oxygen has also been shown to reduce the severity of Cheyne-Stokes respiration with CSA and to decrease urinary catecholamine levels. Andreas and colleagues (209) demonstrated improvements in exercise capacity after treatment with oxygen for 4 weeks. Theophylline has been used to treat patients with congestive heart failure and CSA. Javaheri and colleagues (210) reported reductions in the severity of CSA (6 vs. 26 apneas per hour, $P < .001$) after 5 days of oral theophylline therapy (210). Pesek and colleagues (205) reported the successful use of intravenous theophylline to reduce the severity of Cheyne-Stokes respiration with CSA in a patient who suffered a nearly fatal cardiorespiratory arrest during dialysis. However, despite the reported effectiveness of theophylline, some caution should be exercised when it is used to treat Cheyne-Stokes respiration with CSA. Proarrhythmic effects during the long-term use of theophylline are not uncommon (211), and sustained benefits are unproven. Thus, the data support CPAP as the

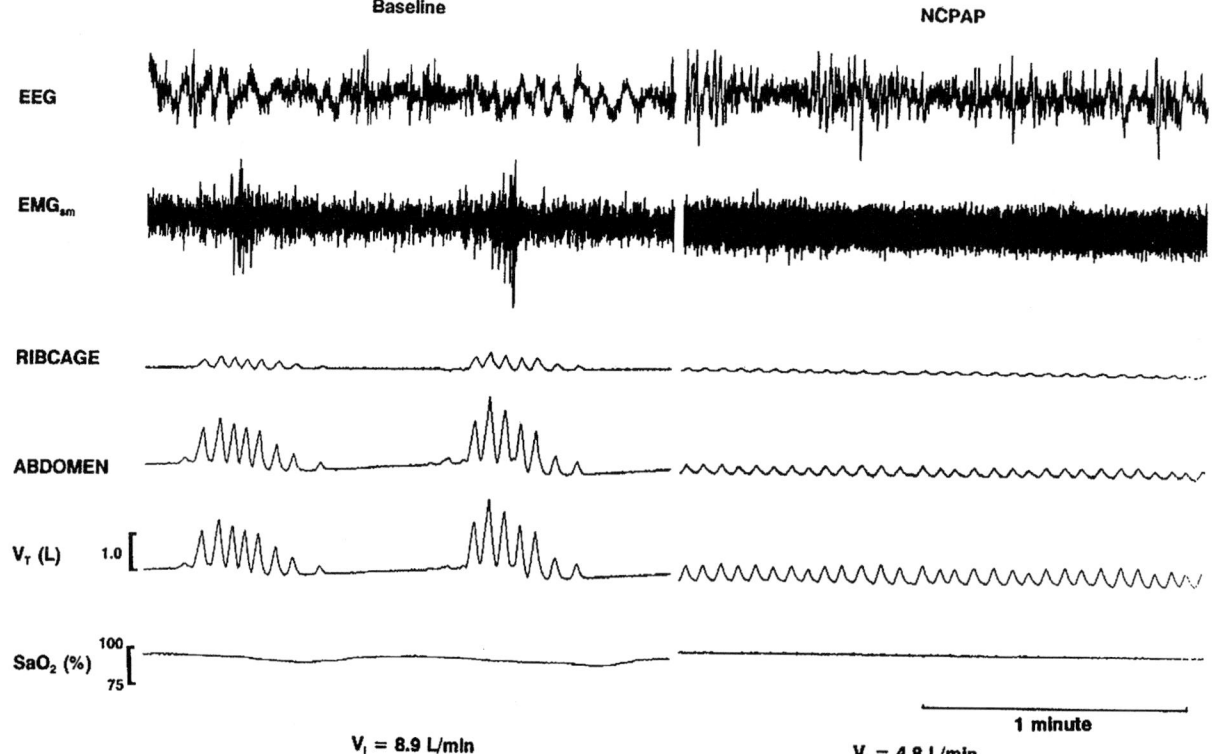

FIGURE 70.11. Two polysomnographic recordings from the same patient at baseline and 1 month after nasal continuous positive airway pressure therapy. The baseline shows typical Cheyne-Stokes respiration with central sleep apnea, in which a pattern of hyperpnea alternates with central apneas accompanied by mild dips in the Sao₂. Note the arousals from sleep, indicated by a change on the electroencephalogram and electromyogram at the peak of ventilation. After nasal continuous positive airway pressure therapy, no further breathing events or arousals are evident. EMG_{sm}, submental electromyogram; *EEG*, electroencephalogram; V_T, tidal volume. (From Naughton MT, Benard DC, Rutherford R, et al. Effect of continuous positive airway pressure on central sleep apnea and nocturnal Pco₂ in CHF. *Am J Respir Crit Care Med* 1994;150:1598–1604, with permission.)

most effective therapy for Cheyne-Stokes respiration with congestive heart failure.

CENTRAL SLEEP APNEA AND CHEYNE-STOKES RESPIRATION WITH CONGESTIVE HEART FAILURE

Summary Statement	Level of Evidence
CHF with secondary CSR portends a worse prognosis than CHF without CSR, and so CSR should be treated if present. CPAP has been shown to reduce CSR, improve the LVEF, and reduce catecholamine levels, and it may improve transplant-free survival.	Randomized trials; multiple observational treatment trials
Theophylline and supplemental oxygen have also been used to treat CSR. Despite reductions in CSR events, no effect on cardiac function and no long-term effects have been reported. In addition, theophylline may cause arrhythmias. Thus, further study is necessary before theophylline or oxygen therapy can be recommended in preference to CPAP.	Several observational treatment trials
Nonhypercapnic idiopathic CSA without CSR may be relieved by supplemental oxygen therapy or treatment with acetazolamide.	Randomized interventional trials
Treatment for hypercapnic CSA, a disorder of the ventilatory control system, should be aimed at improving alveolar ventilation. Noninvasive ventilation or tracheostomy and mechanical ventilation should lower the P_{CO_2} and relieve cor pulmonale and symptoms of daytime hypersomnolence.	Nonrandomized intervention trials

CHF, congestive heart failure; CPAP, continuous positive airway pressure; CSA, central sleep apnea; CSR, Cheyne-Stokes respiration; LVEF, left ventricular ejection fraction.

REFERENCES

1. American Academy of Sleep Medicine Task Force. Sleep-related breathing disorders in adults: recommendations for syndrome definition and measurement techniques in clinical research. *Sleep* 1999;22:667–689.
2. Peppard P, Young T, Palta M, et al. Longitudinal study of moderate weight change and sleep-disordered breathing. *JAMA* 2000;284:3015–3021.
3. Resta O. Sleep-related breathing disorders, loud snoring and excessive daytime sleepiness in obese subjects. *Int J Obes* 2001;25:669–675.
4. Young T, Palta M, Dempsey J, et al. The occurrence of sleep-disordered breathing among middle-aged adults. *N Engl J Med* 1993;32:1230–1235.
5. Lavie P, Herer P, Peled R, et al. Mortality in sleep apnea patients: a multivariate analysis of risk factors [see Comments]. *Sleep* 1995;18:149–157.
6. Ancoli-Israel S, Klauber MR, Kripke DF, et al. Sleep apnea in female patients in a nursing home. Increased risk of mortality. *Chest* 1989;96:1054–1058.
7. Issa FG, Sullivan CE. Alcohol, snoring and sleep apnea. *J Neurol Neurosurg Psychiatry* 1982;45:353–359.
8. Tassan VC, Block AJ, Boysen PG, et al. Alcohol increases sleep apnea and oxygen desaturation in asymptomatic men. *Am J Med* 1981;71:240–245.
9. Robinson RW, White DP, Zwillich CW. Moderate alcohol ingestion increases upper airway resistance in normal subjects. *Am Rev Respir Dis* 1985;132:1238–1241.
10. Krol RC, et al. Selective reduction of genioglossal muscle activity by alcohol in normal human subjects. *Am Rev Respir Dis* 1984;129:247–250.
11. Berry RB, Desa MM, Light RW. Effect of ethanol on the efficacy of nasal continuous positive airway pressure as a treatment for obstructive sleep apnea. *Chest* 1991;99:339–343.
12. Wetter DW, Young TB, Bidwell TR, et al. Smoking as a risk factor for sleep-disordered breathing. *Arch Intern Med* 1994;154:2219–2224.
13. Guilleminault C, Eldridge FL, Tilkian A, et al. Sleep apnea syndrome due to upper airway obstruction: a review of 25 cases. *Arch Intern Med* 1977;137:296–300.
14. Johns MW. A new method for measuring daytime sleepiness: the Epworth Sleepiness Scale. *Sleep* 1991;14:540–545.
15. Hoddes E, Zarcone VP, Smythe H. Quantification of sleepiness: a new approach. *Psychophysiology* 1973;10:431–436.
16. Kapuniai LE, Andrew DJ, Crowell DH, et al. Identifying sleep apnea from self-reports. *Sleep* 1988;11:430–436.
17. Stradling JR, Crosby JH. Predictors and prevalence of obstructive sleep apnoea and snoring in 1001 middle-aged men. *Thorax* 1991;46:85–90.
18. Scharf SM, Garshick E, Brown R, et al. Screening for subclinical sleep-disordered breathing. *Sleep* 1990;13:344–353.
19. Hoffstein V, Szalai JP. Predictive value of clinical features in diagnosing obstructive sleep apnea. *Sleep* 1993;16:118–122.
20. Crocker BD, Olson LG, Saunders NA, et al. Estimation of the probability of disturbed breathing during sleep before a sleep study. *Am Rev Respir Dis* 1990;142:14–18.
21. Viner S, Szalai JP, Hoffstein V. Are history and physical examination a good screening test for sleep apnea? *Ann Intern Med* 1991;115:356–359.
22. Flemons WW, Whitelaw WA, Brant R, et al. Likelihood ratios for a sleep apnea clinical prediction rule. *Am J Respir Crit Care Med* 1994;150(5 Pt 1):1279–1285.
23. Schellenberg JB, Maislin G, Schwab RJ. Physical findings and the risk for obstructive sleep apnea. The importance of oropharyngeal structures. *Am J Respir Crit Care Med* 2000;162(2 Pt 1):740–748.
24. Katz I, Stradling J, Slutsky AS, et al. Do patients with obstructive sleep apnea have thick necks? [see Comments]. *Am Rev Respir Dis* 1990;141(5 Pt 1):1228–1231.
25. Woodson BT, Conley SF, Dohse A, et al. Posterior cephalometric radiographic analysis in obstructive sleep apnea. *Ann Otol Rhinol Laryngol* 1997;106:310–313.
26. Woodson BT, Conley SF. Prediction of uvulopalatopharyngoplasty response using cephalometric radiographs. *Am J Otolaryngol* 1997;18:179–184.
27. Ryan CF, Dickson RI, Lowe AA, et al. Upper airway measurements predict response to uvulopalatopharyngoplasty in obstructive sleep apnea. *Laryngoscope* 1990;100:248–253.

28. American Thoracic Society/American Sleep Disorders Association. Statement on health outcomes research in sleep apnea. *Am J Respir Crit Care Med* 1998;157:335–341.

29. American Thoracic Society. Indications and standards for cardiopulmonary sleep studies. *Am Rev Respir Dis* 1989;139:559.

30. Polysomnography Task Force, American Sleep Disorders Association Standards of Practice Committee. Practice parameters for the indications for polysomnography and related procedures. *Sleep* 1997;20:406–422.

31. Rechtschaffen A, Kales A. *A manual of standardized terminology, techniques and scoring system for sleep stages of human subjects.* NIH Publication No. 204, 1968.

32. Norman RG, Ahmed MM, Walsleben JA, et al. Detection of respiratory events during NPSG: nasal cannula/pressure. *Sleep* 1997;20:1175–1184.

33. Hosselet JJ, Norman RG, Ayappa I, et al. Detection of flow limitation with a nasal cannula/pressure transducer system. *Am J Respir Crit Care Med* 1998;157(5 Pt 1):1461–1467.

34. Montserrat JM, Farre R, Ballester E, et al. Evaluation of nasal prongs for estimating nasal flow. *Am J Respir Crit Care Med* 1997;155:211–215.

35. Ayappa I, Norman RG, Krieger AC, et al. Non-invasive detection of respiratory effort-related arousals (REras) by a nasal cannula/pressure transducer system. *Sleep* 2000;23:763–771.

36. Staats BA, Bonekat HW, Harris CD, et al. Chest wall motion in sleep apnea. *Am Rev Respir Dis* 1984;130:59–63.

37. Gyulay S, Olson LG, Hensley MJ, et al. A comparison of clinical assessment and home oximetry in the diagnosis of obstructive sleep apnea. *Am Rev Respir Dis* 1993;147:50–53.

38. Slutsky AS, Strohl K. Quantification of oxygen saturation during episodic hypoxemia. *Am Rev Respir Dis* 1980;121:893–895.

39. Standards of Practice Committee of the American Sleep Disorders Association. Practice parameters for the use of portable recording in the assessment of obstructive sleep apnea [see Comments]. *Sleep* 1994;17:372–377.

40. Sanders MH, Black J, Costantino JP, et al. Diagnosis of sleep-disordered breathing by half-night polysomnography. *Am Rev Respir Dis* 1991;144:1256–1261.

41. Sanders MH, Kern NB, Costantino JP, et al. Adequacy of prescribing positive airway pressure therapy by mask for sleep apnea on the basis of a partial-night trial. *Am Rev Respir Dis* 1993;147:1169–1174.

42. Sanders MH, Kern NB, Costantino JP, et al. Prescription of positive airway pressure for sleep apnea on the basis of a partial-night trial. *Sleep* 1993;16[8 Suppl]:S106–S107.

43. Iber C, O'Brien C, Schulter J, et al. Single night studies in obstructive sleep apnea. *Sleep* 1991;14:381–382.

44. White DP. Complex home monitoring [Review]. *Sleep* 1996;19[10 Suppl]:S248–S250.

45. Fry JM, Diphillipo MA, Curran K, et al. Full polysomnography in the home. *Sleep* 1998;21:635–642.

46. Kapur VK, Rapoport DM, Sanders MH, et al. Rates of sensor loss in unattended home polysomnography: the influence of age, gender, obesity and sleep-disordered breathing. *Sleep* 2000;23:682–688.

47. Engleman HM RK, SE Martin, NJ Douglas. Cognitive function in the sleep apnea/hypopnea syndrome. *Sleep* 2000;23:S102–S107.

48. Redline S, Strauss ME, Adams N, et al. Neuropsychological function in mild sleep-disordered breathing. *Sleep* 1997;20:160–167.

49. Bedard MA, Montplaisir J, Richer F, et al. Obstructive sleep apnea syndrome: pathogenesis of neuropsychological deficits. *J Clin Exp Neuropsychol* 1991;13:950–964.

50. Naegele B, Thouvard V, Pepin JL, et al. Deficits of cognitive executive functions in patients with sleep apnea syndrome. *Sleep* 1995;18:43–52.

51. Greenberg GD, Watson RK, Deptula D. Neuropsychological dysfunction in sleep apnea. *Sleep* 1987;10:254–262.

52. Kim HC, Young T, Matthews CG, et al. Sleep-disordered breathing and neuropsychological deficits. A population-based study. *Am J Respir Crit Care Med* 1997;156:1813–1819.

53. Engleman HM, Martin SE, Deary IJ, et al. Effect of CPAP therapy on daytime function in patients with mild sleep apnoea/hypopnoea syndrome [see Comments]. *Thorax* 1997;52:114–119.

54. Engleman HM, Martin SE, Kingshott RN, et al. Randomised placebo-controlled trial of daytime function after continuous positive airway pressure (CPAP) therapy for the sleep apnoea/hypopnoea syndrome [see Comments]. *Thorax* 1998;53:341–345.

55. Strohl K, Bonnie R, Findley L. Sleep apnea, sleepiness and driving risk. *Am J Respir Crit Care Med* 1994;150:1463–1473.

56. Barbe, Pericas J, Munoz A, et al. Automobile accidents in patients with sleep apnea syndrome. *Am J Respir Crit Care Med* 1998;158:18–22.

57. Teran-Santos J, Jimenez-Gomez A, Cordero-Guevara, J. The association between sleep apnea and the risk of traffic accidents. Cooperative Group Burgos-Santander. *N Engl J Med* 1999;340:847–851.

58. Finn L, Young T, Palta M, et al. Sleep-disordered breathing and self-reported general health status in the Wisconsin sleep cohort. *Sleep* 1998;21:701–706.

59. Flemons W. Measuring health-related quality of life in sleep apnea. *Sleep* 2000;23:S109–S114.

60. Flemons WW, Reimer MA. Development of a disease-specific health-related quality of life. *Am J Respir Crit Care Med* 1998;158:494–503.

61. Nieto F, Young TB, Lind BK, et al. Association of sleep-disordered breathing, sleep apnea, and hypertension in a large community-based study. Sleep Heart Health Study. *JAMA* 2000;283:1829–1836.

62. Peppard P, Young T, Palta M, et al. Prospective study of the association between sleep-disordered breathing and hypertension. *N Engl J Med* 2000;342:1378–1384.

63. Brooks D, Horner RL, Kozar LF, et al. Obstructive sleep apnea as a cause of systemic hypertension. Evidence from a canine model [see Comments]. *J Clin Invest* 1997;99:106–109.

64. Somers VK, Dyken ME, Clary MP, et al. Sympathetic neural mechanisms in obstructive sleep apnea. *J Clin Invest* 1995;96:1897–1904.

65. Dimsdale JE, Profant J. Effect of continuous positive airway pressure on blood pressure: a placebo trial. *Hypertension* 2000;35:144–147.

66. Faccenda J, Boon NA, Mackay TW, et al. CPAP effects on blood pressure in the sleep apnea/hypopnoea syndrome during a randomized controlled trial. *Am J Respir Crit Care Med* 2001;163:344–348.

67. Wright J, Johns R, Watt I, et al. Health effects of obstructive sleep apnoea and the effectiveness of CPAP. *BMJ* 1997;314:851–860.

68. Good DC, Henkle JQ, Gelber D, et al. Sleep-disordered breathing and poor functional outcome after stroke. *Stroke* 1996;27:252–259.

69. Dyken ME, Somers VK, Yamada T, et al. Investigating the relationship between stroke and obstructive sleep apnea. *Stroke* 1996;27:401–407.

70. Bassetti C, Aldrich MS, Chervin RD, et al. Sleep apnea in patients with transient ischemic attack and stroke: a prospective study of 59 patients. *Neurology* 1996;47:1167–1173.

71. Wessendorf TT, Wang Y. Schriber A, et al. Fibrinogen levels and obstructive sleep apnea in ischemic stroke. *Am J Respir Crit Care Med* 2000;162:2039–2042.

72. Parra O, Arboix A, Bechich S, et al. Time course of sleep-related breathing disorders in first-ever stroke or transient ischemic attack. *Am J Respir Crit Care Med* 2000;161:375–380.

73. Spriggs DA, French JM, Murdy JM, et al. Snoring increases the risk of stroke and adversely affects prognosis. *QJM* 1992;83:555–562.

74. Shahar E, Whitney CW, Redline S, et al. Sleep-disordered breathing and cardiovascular disease: cross-sectional results of the Sleep Heart Health Study. *Am J Respir Crit Care Med* 2001;163:19–25.

75. De Olazabal JR, Miller MJ, Cook WR, et al. Disordered breathing and hypoxia during sleep in coronary artery disease. *Chest* 1982;82:548–552.

76. Koehler U, Schafer H. Is obstructive sleep apnea (OSA) a risk factor for myocardial infarction and cardiac arrhythmias in patients with coronary heart disease (CHD)? *Sleep* 1996;19:283–286.

77. Peker Y, Hedner Y, Kraiczi H, et al. Respiratory disturbance index: an independent predictor of mortality in coronary artery disease. *Am J Respir Crit Care Med* 2000;162:81–86.

78. Hung J, Whitford EG, Parsons RW, et al. Association of sleep apnoea with myocardial infarction in men [see Comments]. *Lancet* 1990;336:261–264.

79. Mooe T, Rabben T, Wiklund U, et al. Sleep-disordered breathing in women: occurrence and association with coronary artery disease [see Comments]. *Am J Med* 1996;101:251–256.

80. Javaheri S, Parker TJ, Liming JD, et al. Sleep apnea in 81 ambulatory male patients with stable heart failure. *Circulation* 1998;97:2154–2159.

81. Sin D, Fitzgerald F, Parker J. Risk factors for central and obstructive sleep apnea in 450 men and women with congestive heart failure. *Am J Respir Crit Care Med* 1999;160:1101–1106.

82. Engleman HM, Douglas NJ. Cognitive effects and daytime sleepiness. *Sleep* 1993;16[8 Suppl]:S79.

83. Findley LJ, Weiss JW, Jabour ER. Drivers with untreated sleep apnea. A cause of death and serious injury. *Arch Intern Med* 1991;151:1451–1452.

84. Findley LJ, Fabrizio MJ, Knight H, et al. Driving simulator performance in patients with sleep apnea. *Am Rev Respir Dis* 1989;140:529–530.

85. Lavie P, Here P, Hoffstein V. Obstructive sleep apnea syndrome as a risk factor for hypertension. *Br Med J* 2000;320:479–482.

86. Sullivan CE, Issa FG, Berthon-Jones M, et al. Reversal of obstructive sleep apnoea by continuous positive airway pressure applied through the nares. *Lancet* 1981;1:862–865.

87. Remmers JE, DeGroot WJ, Sauerland EK, et al. Pathogenesis of upper airway occlusion during sleep. *J Appl Physiol* 1978;44:931–938.

88. Hoffstein V, Zamel N, Phillipson EA. Lung volume dependence of pharyngeal cross-sectional area in patients with obstructive sleep apnea. *Am Rev Respir Dis* 1984;130:175–178.

89. Van de Graaff WB. Thoracic influence on upper airway patency. *J Appl Physiol* 1988;65:2124–2131.

90. Issa FG, Sullivan CE. The immediate effects of nasal continuous positive airway pressure treatment on sleep pattern in patients with obstructive sleep apnea syndrome. *Electroencephalogr Clin Neurophysiol* 1986;63:10–17.

91. Ballester E, Badia JR, Hernandez L, et al. Evidence of the effectiveness of continuous positive airway pressure in the treatment of sleep apnea/hypopnea syndrome. *Am J Respir Crit Care Med* 1999;159:495–501.

92. Meslier N, Lebrun T, Grillier-Lanoir V, et al. A French survey of 3,225 patients treated with CPAP for obstructive sleep apnea: benefits, tolerance, compliance and quality of life. *Eur Respir J* 1998;12:185–192.

93. Bennett LS, Barbour C, Langford B, et al. Health status in obstructive sleep apnea. *Am J Respir Crit Care Med* 1999;159:1884–1890.

94. Findley L, Smith C, Hooper J, et al. Treatment with nasal CPAP decreases automobile accidents in patients with sleep apnea. *Am J Respir Crit Care Med* 2000;161:857–859.

95. George CF. Reduction in motor vehicle collisions following treatment of sleep apnoea with nasal CPAP. *Thorax* 2001;56:508–512.

96. Davies RJ, Crosby J, Prothero A, et al. Ambulatory blood pressure and left ventricular hypertrophy in subjects with untreated obstructive sleep apnoea and snoring, compared with matched control subjects, and their response to treatment. *Clin Sci (Colch)* 1994;86:417–424.

97. Akashiba T, Minemura H, Yamamoto H, et al. Nasal continuous positive airway pressure changes blood pressure "non-dippers" to "dippers" in patients with obstructive sleep apnea. *Sleep* 1999;22:849–853.

98. Jenkinson C, Davies RJ, Mullins R, et al. Comparison of therapeutic and subtherapeutic nasal continuous positive airway pressure for obstructive sleep apnoea: a randomised prospective parallel trial. *Lancet* 1999;353:2100–2105.

99. Montserrat J, et al. Effectiveness of CPAP treatment in daytime function in sleep apnea syndrome. A randomized controlled study with an optimized placebo. *Am J Respir Crit Care Med* 2001;164:608–613.

100. Henke KG, Grady JJ, Kuna ST. Effect of nasal continuous positive airway pressure on neuropsychological function in sleep apnea-hypopnea syndrome. *Am J Respir Crit Care Med* 2001;163:911–917.

101. Barbe F, Mayoralas LR, Duran J, et al. Treatment with continuous positive airway pressure is not effective in patients with sleep apnea but no daytime sleepiness. A randomized, controlled trial. *Ann Intern Med* 2001;134:1065–1067.

102. American Thoracic Society. Indications and standards for the use of nasal continuous positive airway pressure (CPAP) in sleep apnea syndromes. Official statement adopted March 1944 [published erratum appears in *Am J Respir Crit Care Med* 1995 Feb;151(2 Pt 1):578]. *Am J Respir Crit Care Med* 1994;150 (6 Pt 1):1738–1745.

103. Loube D, Gay PC, Strohl KP, et al. Indications for positive airway pressure treatment of adult obstructive sleep apnea patients: a consensus statement. *Chest* 1999;115:863–866.

104. Engleman HM, Kingshott RN, Wraith PK, et al. Randomized placebo-controlled crossover trial of continuous positive airway pressure for mild sleep apnea/hypopnea syndrome. *Am J Respir Crit Care Med* 1999;159:461–467.

105. Montaserio C, Vidal S, Duran J. Effectiveness of continuous positive airway pressure in mild sleep apnea-hypopnea syndrome. *Am J Respir Crit Care Med* 2001;164:939–943.

106. Redline S, Adams N, Strauss ME, et al. Improvement of mild sleep-disordered breathing with CPAP compared with conservative therapy. *Am J Respir Crit Care Med* 1998;157(3 Pt 1):858–865.

107. Kribbs NB, Pack AI, Kline LR, et al. Objective measurement of patterns of nasal CPAP use by patients with obstructive sleep apnea [see Comments]. *Am Rev Respir Dis* 1993;147(4):887–895.

108. McArdle N, Devereux G, Heidarnejad H, et al. Long-term use of CPAP therapy for sleep apnea/hypopnea syndrome. *Am J Respir Crit Care Med* 1999;159(4 Pt 1):1108–1114.

109. Pepin J, Krieger J, Rodenstein D, et al. Effective compliance during the first three months of continuous positive airway pressure. *Am J Respir Crit Care Med* 1999;160:1124–1129.

110. Weaver TE, Kribbs NB, Pack AI, et al. Night-to-night variability in CPAP use over the first three months of treatment. *Sleep* 1997;20:278–283.

111. Pressman MR, Peterson DD, Meyer TJ, et al. Ramp abuse. A novel form of patient noncompliance to the administration of nasal continuous positive airway pressure for the treatment of obstructive sleep apnea. *Am J Respir Crit Care Med* 1995;151:1632–1634.

112. Lafond C, Series F. Influence of nasal obstruction on auto-CPAP behavior during sleep in apnea/hypopnea syndrome. *Thorax* 1998;53:780–783.

113. Massie CA, Hart RW, Peralez K, et al. Effects of humidification on nasal symptoms and compliance in sleep apnea patients using continuous positive airway pressure. *Chest* 1999;116:403–408.

114. McNicholas WT, Tarlo S, Cole P, et al. Obstructive apneas during sleep in patients with seasonal allergic rhinitis. *Am Rev Respir Dis* 1982;126:625–628.

115. Mortimore IL, Whittle AT, Douglas NJ. Comparison of nose and face mask CPAP therapy for sleep apnoea. *Thorax* 1998;53:290–292.

116. Sanders MH, Kern N. Obstructive sleep apnea treated by independently adjusted inspiratory and expiratory positive airway pressure via nasal mask. *Chest* 1990;98:317–324.

117. Reeves-Hoche MK, Hudgel DW, Meck R, et al. Continuous versus bilevel positive airway pressure for obstructive sleep apnea. *Am J Respir Crit Care Med* 1995;151(2 Pt 1):443–449.

118. Scharf MB, Brannen DE, McDannold MD, et al. Computerized adjustable versus fixed NCPAP treatment of obstructive sleep apnea. *Sleep* 1996;19:491–496.

119. Sharma S, Wali S, Pouliot Z, et al. Treatment of obstructive sleep apnea with a self-titrating continuous positive airway pressure (CPAP) system. *Sleep* 1996;19:497–501.

120. Ficker JH, Wiest GH, Lehnert G, et al. Evaluation of an auto-CPAP device for the treatment of obstructive sleep apnea. *Thorax* 1998;53:643–648.

121. Hudgel DW, Fung C. A long-term randomized cross-over comparison of auto-titrating and standard nasal continuous airway pressure. *Sleep* 2000;23:645–648.

122. Behbehani K, Yen F, Lucas E, et al. A sleep laboratory evaluation of an automatic positive airway pressure system for the treatment of obstructive sleep apnea. *Sleep* 1998;21:485–491.

123. Lloberes P, Ballester E, Montserrat JM, et al. Comparison of manual and automatic CPAP titration in patients with sleep apnea/hypopnea syndrome. *Am J Respir Crit Care Med* 1996;154 (6 Pt 1):1755–1758.

124. American Sleep Disorders Association. Practice parameters for the treatment of snoring and obstructive apnea with oral appliances: a review. *Sleep* 1995;18:511–513.

125. Lowe A, Fleetham J, Ryan F, et al. Effects of a mandibular repositioning appliance used in the treatment of obstructive sleep apnea on tongue muscle activity. *Prog Clin Biol Res* 1990;345:395–404; discussion 405.

126. Gale DJ, Sawyer RH, Woodcock A, et al. Do oral appliances enlarge the airway with obstructive sleep apnea? A prospective computerized tomographic study. *Eur J Orthod* 2000;22:159–168.

127. Lowe A. The tongue and the airway. *Otolaryngol Clin North Am* 1990;23:677–698.

128. Ferguson KA, Ono T, Lowe AA, et al. A randomized crossover study of an oral appliance vs nasal-continuous positive airway pressure in the treatment of mild-moderate obstructive sleep apnea [see Comments]. *Chest* 1996;109:1269–1275.

129. Fritsch KM, Iseli A, Russi EW, et al. Side effects of mandibular advancement devices for sleep apnea treatment. *Am J Respir Crit Care Med* 2001;164:813–818.

130. Bloch KE, Iseli A, Zhang J, et al. A randomized, controlled crossover trial of two oral appliances for sleep apnea treatment. *Am J Respir Crit Care Med* 2000;162:246–251.

131. Mehta A, Qian J, Petocz P, et al. A randomized, controlled study of a mandibular advancement splint for obstructive sleep apnea. *Am J Respir Crit Care Med* 2001;163:1457–1461.

132. Liu Y, Lowe AA, Fleetham JA, et al. Cephalometric and physiologic predictors of the efficacy of an adjustable oral appliance for treating obstructive sleep apnea. *Am J Orthod Dentofacial Orthop* 2001;120:639–647.

133. Lowe AA, Sjoholm TT, Ryan CF, et al. Treatment, airway and compliance effects of a titratable oral appliance. *Sleep* 2000;15[23 Suppl 4]:S172–S178.

134. Millman RP, Rosenberg CL, Carlisle CC, et al. The efficacy of oral appliances in the treatment of persistent sleep apnea after uvulopalatopharyngoplasty. *Chest* 1998;113:992–996.

135. Powell NB, Riley RW, Troell RJ, et al. Radiofrequency volumetric tissue reduction of the palate in subjects. *Chest* 1998;113:1163–1174.

136. Troell RJ, Powell NB, Riley RW, et al. Comparison of postoperative pain between laser-assisted uvulopalatoplasty, uvulopalatopharyngoplasty and radiofrequency volumetric tissue reduction of the palate. *Otolaryngol Head Neck Surg* 2000;122:402–409.

137. Brown DJ, Kerr P, Kryger M. Radiofrequency tissue reduction of the palate in patients with moderate sleep-disordered breathing. *J Otolaryngol* 2001;30:193–198.

138. Woodson BT, Nelson L, Mickelson S, et al. A multi-institutional study of radiofrequency volumetric tissue reduction for OSAS. *Otolaryngol Head Neck Surg* 2001;125:303–311.

139. Kamami Y. Laser CO_2 for snoring. Preliminary results. *Acta Otorhinolaryngol Belg* 1990;44:451–456.

140. Mickelson SA, Ahuja A. Short-term objective and long-term subjective results of laser-assisted uvulopalatoplasty for obstructive sleep apnea. *Laryngoscope* 1999;109:362–367.

141. Finkelstein Y, Shapiro-Feinberg M, Stein G, et al. Uvulopalatopharyngoplasty vs. laser-assisted uvulopalatoplasty. Anatomical considerations [see Comments]. *Arch Otolaryngol Head Neck Surg* 1997;123:265–276.

142. Ryan CF, Lowe LL. Unpredictable results of laser-assisted uvulopalatoplasty in the treatment of obstructive sleep apnea. *Thorax* 2000;55:399–404.

143. Seeman RP, DiToppa JC, Holm MA, et al. Does laser-assisted uvulopalatoplasty work? An objective analysis using pre- and postoperative polysomnographic studies. *J Otolaryngol* 2001;30:212–215.

144. Walker RP, Grigg-Damberger MM, Gopalsami C, et al. Laser-assisted uvulopalatoplasty for snoring and obstructive sleep apnea: results in 170 patients. *Laryngoscope* 1995;105(9 Pt 1):938–943.

145. Walker RP, Grigg-Damberger MM, Gopalsami C. Uvulopalatopharyngoplasty versus laser-assisted uvulopalatoplasty for the treatment of obstructive sleep apnea. *Laryngoscope* 1997;107:76–82.

146. Utley DS, Shin EJ, Clerk AA, et al. A cost-effective and rational surgical approach to patients with snoring, upper airway resistance syndrome, or obstructive sleep apnea syndrome. *Laryngoscope* 1997;107:726–734.

147. Walker RP, Garrity T, Gopalsami C. Early polysomnographic findings and long-term subjective results in sleep apnea patients treated with laser-assisted uvulopalatoplasty. *Laryngoscope* 1999;109:1438–1441.

148. Littner M. Practice parameters for the use of laser-assisted uvulopalatoplasty. *Sleep* 2001;24:603–619.

149. Fujita S, Conway W, Zorick F, et al. Surgical correction of anatomic abnormalities in obstructive sleep apnea syndrome: uvulopalatopharyngoplasty. *Otolaryngol Head Neck Surg* 1981;89:923–934.

150. Katsantonis GP, Schweitzer PK, Branham GH, et al. Management of obstructive sleep apnea: comparison of various treatment modalities. *Laryngoscope* 1988;98:304–309.

151. Schwartz AR, et al. Effect of uvulopalatopharyngoplasty on upper airway collapsibility in obstructive sleep apnea. *Am Rev Respir Dis* 1992;145:527–532.

152. Shepard JWJ, Olsen KD. Uvulopalatopharyngoplasty for the treatment of obstructive sleep apnea. *Mayo Clin Proc* 1990;65:1260–1267.

153. Sher AE, Schechtman KB, Piccirillo JF. The efficacy of surgical modifications of the upper airway in adults with obstructive sleep apnea syndrome. *Sleep* 1996;19:156–177.

154. Launois SH, Feroah TR, Campbell WN, et al. Site of pharyngeal narrowing predicts outcome of surgery for obstructive sleep apnea [see Comments]. *Am Rev Respir Dis* 1993;147:182–189.

155. Isono S, Shimada A, Tanaka A, et al. Efficacy of endoscopic static pressure/area assessment of the passive pharynx in predicting uvulopalatopharyngoplasty outcomes. *Laryngoscope* 1999;109:769–774.

156. Doghramji K, Jabourian ZH, Pilla M, et al. Predictors of outcome for uvulopalatopharyngoplasty. *Laryngoscope* 1995;105 (3 Pt 1):311–314.

157. Millman RP, Carlisle CC, Rosenberg C, et al. Simple predictors of uvulopalatopharyngoplasty outcome in the treatment of obstructive sleep apnea. *Chest* 2000;118:1025–1030.

158. Boot H, Van Wegen R, Poublon RM, et al. Long-term results of UPPP for obstructive sleep apnea syndrome. *Laryngoscope* 2000;110:469–475.

159. Riley RW, Powell NB, Guilleminault C. Obstructive sleep apnea and the hyoid: a revised surgical procedure. *Otolaryngol Head Neck Surg* 1994;111:717–721.

160. Bettega G, Pepin JL, Deschaux C, et al. Obstructive sleep apnea syndrome: 51 consecutive patients treated by maxillofacial surgery. *Am J Respir Crit Care Med* 2000;162:641–649.

161. Johnson NT, Chinn J. Uvulopalatopharyngoplasty and inferior sagittal mandibular osteotomy with genioglossus advancement for treatment of obstructive sleep apnea. *Chest* 1994;105:278–283.

162. Bittencourt LR, Palombini P, Morgado S, et al. Clinical and PSG findings in surgically treated patients with OSA. *Am J Respir Crit Care Med* 1997;155:A667.

163. Riley RW, Powell NB. Maxillofacial surgery and obstructive sleep apnea syndrome. *Otolaryngol Clin North Am* 1990;23:809–826.

164. Hochban W, Conradt R, Brandenburg U, et al. Surgical maxillofacial treatment of obstructive sleep apnea. *Plast Reconstr Surg* 1997;99:619–626; discussion 627–628.

165. Waite PD, Wooten V, Lachner J, et al. Maxillomandibular advancement surgery in 23 patients with obstructive sleep apnea syndrome. *J Oral Maxillofac Surg* 1989;47:1256–1261; discussion 1262.

166. Cartwright RD, Diaz F, Lloyd S. The effects of sleep posture and sleep stage on apnea frequency. *Sleep* 1991;14:351–353.

167. Jokic R, Klimaszewski A, Crossley M, et al. Positional treatment vs continuous positive airway pressure in patients with positional obstructive sleep apnea syndrome. *Chest* 1999;115:771–781.

168. Zwillich CW, Natalino MR, Sutton FD, et al. Effects of progesterone on chemosensitivity in normal men. *J Lab Clin Med* 1978;92:262–269.

169. Cook WR, Benich JJ, Wooten SA. Indices of the severity of the obstructive sleep apnea syndrome do not change during medroxyprogesterone acetate therapy. *Chest* 1989;96:262–266.

170. Block AJ, Wynne JW, Boysen PG, et al. Menopause, medroxyprogesterone and breathing during sleep. *Am J Med* 1981;70:506–510.

171. White DP, Zwillich CW, Pickett CK, et al. Central sleep apnea. Improvement with acetazolamide therapy. *Arch Intern Med* 1982;142:1816–1819.

172. Tojima H, Kunitomo F, Kimura H, et al. Effects of acetazolamide in patients with the sleep apnoea syndrome. *Thorax* 1988;43:113–119.

173. Sharp JT, Druz WS, Diamond E. Effect of metabolic acidosis upon sleep apnea. *Chest* 1985;87:619–624.

174. DeBacker WA, Verbraecken J, Willemen M, et al. Central sleep apnea decreases after prolonged treatment with acetazolamide. *Am J Respir Crit Care Med* 1995;151:87–91.

175. Whyte KF, Gould GA, Airlie MA, et al. Role of protriptyline and acetazolamide in the sleep apnea/hypopnea syndrome. *Sleep* 1988;11:463–472.

176. Hudgel DW, et al. Pharmacologic treatment of sleep-disordered breathing. *Am J Respir Crit Care Med* 1998;158:691–699.

177. Hanzel DA, Proia NG, Hudgel DW. Response of obstructive sleep apnea to fluoxetine and protriptyline. *Chest* 1991;100:416–421.

178. Smith PL, Haponik EF, Allen RP, et al. The effects of protriptyline in sleep-disordered breathing. *Am Rev Respir Dis* 1983;127:8–13.

179. Clark RW, Schmidt HS, Schaal SF, et al. Sleep apnea: treatment with protriptyline. *Neurology* 1979;29(9 Pt 1):1287–1292.

180. Conway WA, Zorick F, Piccione P, et al. Protriptyline in the treatment of sleep apnoea. *Thorax* 1982;37:49–53.

181. Veasey SC, Fenik P, Panckeri K, et al. The effects of trazodone with l-tryptophan on sleep-disordered breathing in the English bulldog. *Am J Respir Crit Care Med* 1999;160(5 Pt 1):1659–1667.

182. Kubin L, Tojima H, Davies RO, et al. Serotonergic excitatory drive to hypoglossal motoneuron in the decerebrate cat. *Neurosci Lett* 1992;139:243–248.

183. Douse MA, et al. Serotoninergic effects on hypoglossal neural activity and reflex responses. *Brain Res* 1996;726:213–222.

184. Berry RB, Yamaura EM, Gill K, et al. Acute effects of paroxetine on genioglossus activity in obstructive sleep apnea. *Sleep* 1999;22:1087–1092.

185. Kraiczi H, Hedner J, Dahlof P, et al. Effect of serotonin uptake inhibition on breathing during sleep and daytime symptoms in obstructive sleep apnea. *Sleep* 1999;22:61–67.

186. Gothe B, Strohl KP, Levin S, et al. Nicotine: a different approach to the treatment of obstructive sleep apnea. *Chest* 1985;87:11–17.

187. Davila DG, Hurt RD, Offord KP, et al. Acute effects of transdermal nicotine on sleep architecture, snoring, and sleep-disordered breathing in nonsmokers. *Am J Respir Crit Care Med* 1994;150:469–474.

188. Slamowitz DA, Shea SA, Edwards JK, et al. Serotoninergic and cholinergic influences on pharyngeal muscles. *Sleep* 1998;21:418.C(abst).

189. Kingshott RN, Vennelle M, Coleman EL, et al. Randomized, double-blind, placebo-controlled crossover trial of modafinil in the treatment of residual excessive daytime sleepiness in the sleep apnea/hypopnea syndrome. *Am J Respir Crit Care Med* 2001;163:918–923.

190. Pack AI, Black JE, Schwartz JRL, et al. Modafinil as adjunct therapy for daytime sleepiness in obstructive sleep apnea. *Am J Respir Crit Care Med* 2001;164:1675–1681.

191. Guilleminault C. Diagnosis, pathogenesis, and treatment of the

sleep apnea syndromes. *Ergeb Inn Med Kinderheilkd* 1984;52:1–57.

192. Roehrs T, Conway W, Wittig R, et al. Sleep-wake complaints in patients with sleep-related respiratory disturbances. *Am Rev Respir Dis* 1985;132:520–523.

193. DeBacker WA, Verbraecken J, Willemen M, et al. Central apnea index decreases after prolonged treatment with acetazolamide. *Am J Respir Crit Care Med* 1995;151:87–91.

194. Zwillich CW, Sutton FD, Pierson DJ, et al. Decreased hypoxic ventilatory drive in the obesity-hypoventilation syndrome. *Am J Med* 1975;59:343–348.

195. Bradley TD, McNicholas WT, Rutherford R, et al. Clinical and physiologic heterogeneity of the central sleep apnea syndrome. *Am Rev Respir Dis* 1986;134:217–221.

196. Wuyam B, Pepin J, Tremel F, et al. Pathophysiology of central sleep apnea syndrome. *Sleep* 2000;23:S213–S215.

197. Guilleminault C, Stoohs R, Schneider H, et al. Central alveolar hypoventilation and sleep. Treatment by intermittent positive-pressure ventilation through nasal mask in an adult. *Chest* 1989;96:1210–1212.

198. Grunstein RR, Ho KY, Berthon-Jones M, et al. Central sleep apnea is associated with increased ventilatory response to carbon dioxide and hypersecretion of growth hormone in patients with acromegaly. *Am J Respir Crit Care Med* 1994;150:496–502.

199. Xie A, Rutherford R, Rankin F, et al. Hypocapnia and increased ventilatory responsiveness in patients with idiopathic central sleep apnea. *Am J Respir Crit Care Med* 1995;152(6 Pt 1):1950–1955.

200. Martin RJ, Sanders MH, Gray BA, et al. Acute and long-term ventilatory effects of hyperoxia in the adult sleep apnea syndrome. *Am Rev Respir Dis* 1982;125:175–180.

201. McNicholas WT, Carter JL, Rutherford R, et al. Beneficial effect of oxygen in primary alveolar hypoventilation with central sleep apnea. *Am Rev Respir Dis* 1982;125:773–775.

202. Issa FG, Sullivan CE. Reversal of central sleep apnea using nasal CPAP. *Chest* 1986;90:165–171.

203. Hoffstein V, Slutsky AS. Central sleep apnea reversed by continuous positive airway pressure. *Am Rev Respir Dis* 1987;135:1210–1212.

204. Leung RST, Bradley TD. Sleep apnea and cardiovascular disease. *Am J Respir Crit Care Med* 2001;164:2147–2165.

205. Pesek CA, Cooley R, Narkiewicz K, et al. Theophylline therapy for near-fatal Cheyne-Stokes respiration. A case report. *Ann Intern Med* 1999;130:427–430.

206. Hanley PJ, Zuberi-Khokhar NS. Increased mortality associated with Cheyne-Stokes respiration in patients with congestive heart failure. *Am J Respir Crit Care Med* 1996;153:272–276.

207. Lanfranchi PA, Braghiroli A, Bosimini E, et al. Prognostic value of nocturnal Cheyne-Stokes respiration in chronic heart failure. *Circulation* 1999;99:1435–1440.

208. Sin D, Logan A, Fitzgerald F, et al. Effects of continuous positive airway pressure on cardiovascular outcomes in heart failure patients with and without Cheyne-Stokes respiration. *Circulation* 2000;102:61–66.

209. Andreas S, Clemens C, Sandholzer H, et al. Improvement of exercise capacity with treatment of Cheyne-Stokes respiration in patients with congestive heart failure. *J Am Coll Cardiol* 1996;27:1486–1490.

210. Javaheri S, Parker TJ, Wexler L, et al. Effect of theophylline on sleep-disordered breathing in heart failure. *N Engl J Med* 1996;335:562–567.

211. Sessler CN, Cohen MD. Cardiac arrhythmias during theophylline toxicity. A prospective continuous electrocardiographic study. *Chest* 1990;98(3):672–678.

SUBJECT INDEX

Note: Page numbers followed by *f* indicate figures; those followed by *t* indicate tables.

A

Abdominal surgery, postoperative
  complications, 1233
ABIH (American Board of Industrial
  Hygiene), 938
ABMAs. *See* Antibasement membrane
  antibodies (ABMAs)
Abscesses
  acute, 410
  causes, 409
  chronic, 410
  classification, 409–410
  clinical features, 410–411
  complication, 412, 412*t*
  definition, 409
  differential diagnosis, 410
  epidemiology, 409
  fiberoptic bronchoscopy, 410
  microbiology, 409, 410*t*
  pathogenesis, 409
  secondary, 409
  subphrenic, 1233
  treatment, 411–412
Acanthosis nigricans, 929, 1293–1294
ACCP (American College of Chest
  Physicians), 289–290
ACE. *See* Angiotensin-converting enzyme
  (ACE)
Acetazolamide, for obstructive sleep apnea,
  1441
Acetylcysteine, nebulized, for chronic
  obstructive pulmonary disease,
  234
ACGIH (American Conference of
  Governmental Industrial
  Hygienists), 938
ACGIH TLVs (American Conference of
  Governmental Industrial
  Hygienists Threshold Limit
  Levels), 945–946
Achalasia, esophagomegaly secondary to,
  1214–1215, 1215*f*
Achondroplasia, 1287–1288
Acid anhydrides, 984
Acid-fast bacillus stains, 381–382, 382*t*
Acinetobacter, 426
Acquired immune deficiency syndrome
  (AIDS). *See also*
    Immunodeficiency diseases
  Aspergillus, 326–328
  bacteria, 323–325

Blastomyces dermatitidis, 332
Candida, 328
Coccidioides immitis, 332
Cryptococcus, 330–331
definition, 319
diagnostic procedures, 321–323
empiric therapy, 323
epidemiology, 319
Histoplasma capsulatum, 331–332
Mucormycosis, 328
mycobacteria, 325–326
Paracoccidioides brasiliensis, 332
Pneumocystis carinii infection in, 319,
  320, 321, 328–330
protozoa, 332
pulmonary disorders associated with, 319
viruses, 332–335
Acromegaly
  airway obstruction, 1237–1238
  cardiopulmonary complications, 1238
  lung volume, 1237
  sleep apnea, 1238
Actinic cell carcinoma, 874
Actinomyces israelii, 368
Actinomycosis, 368
Acute chest syndrome, 1177–1178
Acute interstitial pneumonia (AIP),
  476–477, 499
  clinical findings of, 476–477
  histopathologic findings of, 477
  treatment of, 477
Acute respiratory distress syndrome (ARDS)
  as complication of pancreatic disease,
    1231–1232
  noninvasive positive pressure ventilation,
    1113
Adenocarcinoma
  classification of, 806–808, 808*f*
  histopathology of, 793–794, 793*t*
  pathology of, 806–808, 808*f*
Adenoid cystic carcinoma, 874
Adenomatoid malformation, cystic, 1347,
  1348*f*
Adenosine triphosphate (ATP), 226
Adenovirus, 334
Adrenal disorders, 1243–1244, 1243*f,* 1244*f*
B-Adrenergic receptor agonists, asthma
  treatment
  albuterol, 185*t,* 189, 189*t*
  bitolterol, 185*t,* 189, 189*t*
  fenoterol, 185*t,* 189, 189*t*

formoterol, 185*t,* 189, 189*t*
leukotriene modifiers, 190–191
metaproterenol, 185*t,* 189, 189*t*
pirbuterol, 185*t,* 189, 189*t*
salmeterol, 185*t,* 189, 189*t*
terbutaline, 185*t,* 189, 189*t*
theophylline, 189–190
Adrenocorticotropin, 915, 916*f,* 917
Adult Still's disease, 1288–1289
Aerosols
  characteristics of, 133
  definition, 133
  deposition in lung, 137–138, 138*f*
  devices for generating, 138–141
    dry-powder inhalers, 139, 140*f,* 141
    metered-dose inhalers, 138–139, 139*f*
    nebulizers, 141, 141*t*
  during mechanical ventilation, 142–143
  for medication delivery, 143
    systemic bioavailability, 143
  particle size in, 136
  research applications, 143
Agammaglobulinemia, X-linked, 1147–1148
Age-related effects
  in obstructive sleep apnea, 1426
  postoperative risk, 116
β_2-Agonists, for chronic obstructive
  pulmonary disease, 232
AIDS. *See* Acquired immune deficiency
  syndrome (AIDS)
AIHA (American Industrial Hygiene
  Association), 938
Air crescent sign, 22, 23*f*
Airways. *See also specific disease*
  in acromegaly, 1237–1238
  in asthma, 159–160, 168
  in bronchiectasis, 257–258
  in chronic obstructive pulmonary disease,
    208
  in chronic respiratory failure, 1106–1107
  chronic respiratory failure and,
    1106–1107
  cystic fibrosis and, 249–250
  in immunodeficiency diseases,
    1145–1146, 1146*f*
  inflammatory bowel disease and, 1223
  nitric oxide and, 166–167
  in obstructive sleep apnea, 1408–1409,
    1408*f,* 1432–1434, 1433*f*
  pressure release ventilation, 1083–1084
  sarcoidosis and, 546–547, 547*f*